The Lippincott Manual of Nursing Practice

Lillian Sholtis Brunner
R.N., M.S.N., Sc.D., Litt.D., F.A.A.N.

Doris Smith Suddarth
R.N., B.S.N.E., M.S.N.

Vice Chairman (Education and Research):
Board of Trustees; Consultant in Nursing,
Presbyterian–University of Pennsylvania Medical
Center, Philadelphia, Pennsylvania

Member, Board of Overseers,
School of Nursing, University of Pennsylvania,
Philadelphia, Pennsylvania

Formerly Assistant Professor of Nursing,
Yale University School of Nursing,
New Haven, Connecticut

Formerly Consultant in Health Occupations,
Job Corps Health Office, U.S. Department of Labor

Formerly Coordinator of the Curriculum,
The Alexandria Hospital School of Nursing,
Alexandria, Virginia

Dorothy Brooten, R.N., PhD., F.A.A.N.
(Part II: Maternity Nursing)
Chair, Health Care of Women and the Childbearing
Family Section,
School of Nursing, University of Pennsylvania,
Philadelphia, Pennsylvania

Anne Schwalenstocker Klijanowicz, R.N., M.S.
(Part III: Pediatric Nursing)
Assistant Professor and Clinician II (Pediatrics),
University of Rochester School of Nursing,
Rochester, New York

Donnajeanne Bigos Lavoie, R.N., M.S.N.
(Part III: Pediatric Nursing)
Assistant Professor, College of Nursing, Department
of Maternal and Child Health, Howard University,
Washington, DC; and
Neonatology Nurse Consultant;
formerly Neonatology Nurse Consultant, Children's
al National Medical Center,
ton, DC

The Lippincott

Joyce E Anderson

Manual of Nursing Practice

Fourth Edition

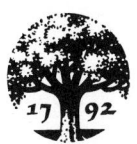

J. B. Lippincott Company   Philadelphia

London   Mexico City   New York   St. Louis   São Paulo   Sydney

Sponsoring Editor: Diana Intenzo
Manuscript Editor: Helen Ewan
Indexer: Deana Fowler
Production Supervisor: Kathleen P. Dunn
Production Assistant: Carol A. Florence
Compositor: TAPSCO, Inc.
Printer/Binder: R. R. Donnelley & Sons Company

Fourth Edition

6 5 4 3

Library of Congress Cataloging-in-Publication Data

Brunner, Lillian Sholtis.
    The Lippincott manual of nursing practice.

    Includes bibliographies and index.
    1. Nursing—Handbooks, manuals, etc.   I. Suddarth,
Doris Smith.   II. Title. [DNLM: 1. Nursing Care—
handbooks. WY 39 B895L]
RT51.B78   1986   610.73   85-19876
ISBN 0-397-54499-5

The authors and publisher have exerted every effort to ensure
that drug selection and dosage set forth in this text are in
accord with current recommendations and practice at the time
of publication. However, in view of ongoing research, changes
in government regulations, and the constant flow of
information relating to drug therapy and drug reactions, the
reader is urged to check the package insert for each drug for
any change in indications and dosage and for added warnings
and precautions. This is particularly important when the
recommended agent is a new or infrequently employed drug.
It is assumed that treatment is given under the supervision of a
physician.

Contributors

Brenda G. Bare, R.N., M.S.N.
Acting Director, The Alexandria Hospital School of
Nursing, Alexandria, Virginia
Chapter 1: The Nursing Process
Chapter 2: Health Education and the Nursing Process
*Chapter 3: Data Collection and Record Keeping: Patient
    History and Problem Oriented Records*

Elizabeth W. Bayley, R.N., M.S.
Director: Burn, Emergency and Trauma Nursing,
Widener University School of Nursing, Chester,
Pennsylvania
Chapter 13, Part 2: Burns

Susan M. Foster, R.N., M.S.
Educational Coordinator, Critical Care, The Alexandria
Hospital, Alexandria, Virginia
Chapter 9: Cardiovascular Disorders

David Goodman, M.D., Ph.D.
Director, Division of Pathology and Laboratory
Medicine, Hospital of the University of Pennsylvania,
Philadelphia, Pennsylvania
Appendix I: Diagnostic Studies and Their Meaning

Marilyn Hravnak, R.N., M.S.N., C.C.R.N., C.R.T.T.
Clinical Instructor, Surgical Intensive Care Unit,
Presbyterian–University Hospital of Pittsburgh,
Pittsburgh, Pennsylvania
Chapter 7, Part 3: Respiratory Function and Therapy

Donna D. Ignatavicius, R.N., M.S.
Instructor, University of Maryland School of Nursing,
Baltimore, Maryland
Chapter 14: Connective Tissue Disorders
Chapter 15: Allergy Problems

Leslie H. Kirilloff, R.N., Ph.D.
Associate Professor, Pulmonary Nursing Specialty,
University of Pittsburgh, Pittsburgh, Pennsylvania
Chapter 7, Part 3: Respiratory Function and Therapy

Debra A. Kramer, R.N., M.S.N.
Urology Clinical Nurse Specialist, The Children's
Hospital, Philadelphia, Pennsylvania
Chapter 28: Pediatric History Taking
Chapter 29: Pediatric Physical Examination

Dorothy B. Liddel, R.N., M.S.N.
Curriculum Coordinator, The Alexandria Hospital
School of Nursing, Alexandria, Virginia
Chapter 19: Musculoskeletal Conditions

Rita Nemchik, R.N., M.S.
Director, Center for Continuing Education, University of
Pennsylvania School of Nursing, Philadelphia,
Pennsylvania
Chapter 16, Part 5: Diabetes Mellitus

Janet N. Pavel, R.N.
Supervisory Nurse, Clinical Center Blood Bank, National
Institutes of Health, Bethesda, Maryland
Chapter 8, Part 2: Transfusion Therapy

Gerry Stossel Pratsch, R.N., M.P.H.
Education Coordinator, Emergency Medical Services,
Children's Hospital National Medical Center,
Washington, DC
*Chapter 46: Trauma, Prehospital Management of the
    Injured Child*

Suzanne C. O'Connell Smeltzer, R.N., Ed.D.
Assistant Professor, Adult Health and Illness Section,
University of Pennsylvania School of Nursing,
Philadelphia, Pennsylvania; and
Robert Wood Johnson Clinical Nursing Scholar,
University of Rochester School of Nursing, Rochester,
New York
*Chapter 10, Part 3: Conditions of the Hepatic and
    Biliary System*
*Chapter 16, Part 1: Disorders of the Thyroid Gland
            Part 2: Disorders of the Parathyroid Glands
            Part 3: Disorders of the Adrenal Glands*

Loretta Spittle, R.N., M.S., C.C.R.N.
Clinical Specialist, Cardiovascular Nursing,
The Alexandria Hospital, Alexandria, Virginia
*Chapter 9, Part 2: Fundamentals of
    Electrocardiography*

Contents

Part I   Medical–Surgical Nursing

List of Guidelines

Maternity Nursing

Pediatric Nursing

Health Education/Patient Education

Page numbers followed by *f* indicate illustrations; *t* following a page number indicates tabular material.

Entries followed by the designation *pediatric* deal with pediatric considerations and include parental teaching.

Letters in parentheses that follow page numbers refer to specific outline subheadings containing material on patient or parental teaching. Example: 1430 (B, D)

Preface

The winds of change are dramatically affecting the kind and quality of health care being delivered. This is apparently a result of a number of concurrent happenings. The prime initiator has been governmental cutbacks introduced in 1984 with diagnostic-related groupings. Cost constraints have reduced hospital patient days and have extended the need for acute-care service into the community.

Another dramatic change has been the more widespread use of diagnostic and treatment aids that are markedly less invasive, less traumatic, and more accurate. Examples are imaging techniques (CT, PET, and MRI), fiberoptics, and lasers.

In addition, an ever-increasing awareness of health promotion, physical fitness, and the concept of self-care continues, while the numbers of persons living longer are increasing this more illness-vulnerable older age-group.

The purpose of *The Lippincott Manual of Nursing Practice* is to help nurses keep abreast of these changes and to enhance clinical judgment, nursing practice, and high-level health care. The authors have sought to set forth nursing concepts and strategies commensurate with research findings, technological advances, different treatment modalities, and new knowledge and understanding from the behavioral, biological, and physical sciences.

The nursing process is incorporated widely throughout this volume. Nursing assessment, diagnosis, mutual goal-setting, planning and implementing nursing interventions, patient education, and evaluation are highlighted to present an organized approach. Not every problem could be addressed with this detail because of space limitations. The nurse practitioner is encouraged to focus on the individual patient's strengths and what can be done, while using the principles set forth to understand and manage complex care options.

The sections on health education have been extended to help the patient make informed decisions, minimize health-thwarting behaviors, and effect positive changes toward optimum health.

We thank those who have shared their knowledge and clinical expertise and express our admiration of and respect for our nursing colleagues who translate these principles into high-quality professional practice. Although perfection is elusive, the essence of nursing continues to be concern for and improvement of the human condition.

Lillian Sholtis Brunner
and Doris Smith Suddarth

Acknowledgments

Randy Caine, R.N., M.S., C.C.R.N.
Assistant Professor, California State University, Long Beach, Department of Nursing, Long Beach, California

Josephine M. Cantone, R.N., B.S.N.
Acting Director, School of Nursing, Presbyterian School of Nursing, Philadelphia, Pennsylvania

Carol Case, R.N., M.Ed.
Chief, Public Inquiry, National Cancer Institute, Bethesda, Maryland

Cynthia Chrystal, R.N., C.R.N.I., M.S.
Clinical Director IV Therapy, Grant Hospital, Chicago, Illinois; and Chairperson, Standards Committee, National Intravenous Therapy Association (NITA)

Jane B. Dengler, M.Ed., M.S.N., R.N.
Associate Director, Nursing Service, Bryn Mawr Hospital, Bryn Mawr, Pennsylvania

Margaret P. Cunningham Duprey, R.N., M.S.N.
Instructor, Psychiatric Nursing, Bryn Mawr Hospital School of Nursing, Bryn Mawr, Pennsylvania

Mervyn L. Elgart, M.D.
Professor and Chairman, Department of Dermatology, George Washington University School of Medicine, Washington, DC

Anne B. Fletcher, M.D.
Associate Professor of Child Health and Development, George Washington University School of Medicine; and Associate Director of Neonatology, Children's Hospital National Medical Center, Washington, DC

Mary Lou Frain, R.N., B.S.
Assistant Director, Nursing Service, Presbyterian–University of Pennsylvania Medical Center, Philadelphia, Pennsylvania

Marilyn B. Hartsell, R.N., M.S.N.
Clinical Specialist, Home Disabled Respiratory Children (formerly Coordinator for Infant Apnea Program), Children's Hospital National Medical Center, Washington, DC

Bertha Y. Hawk, R.N., B.S.N.
Instructor, Psychiatric Nursing, Bryn Mawr Hospital School of Nursing, Bryn Mawr, Pennsylvania

Joan Holihan, R.N., M.S.N.
Director, Burn Unit Nursing Service, Children's Hospital National Medical Center, Washington, DC

Karen E. Javie, R.N., B.S.N.
Assistant Director, Nursing Service, Presbyterian–University of Pennsylvania Medical Center, Philadelphia, Pennsylvania

Brian J. Kelly, M.D.
Neurology Resident, Associate Professor of Medicine, Uniformed Services University of the Health Sciences, National Naval Medical Center, Bethesda, Maryland

Susan F. Leitman, M.D.
Acting Chief, Blood Services Section, Clinical Center Blood Bank, National Institutes of Health, Bethesda, Maryland

Etta J. Liberi, R.N., B.S.N., M.S.
Director, School of Practical Nursing, Presbyterian–University of Pennsylvania Medical Center, Philadelphia, Pennsylvania

Catherine D. McMahon, R.N., C.C.R.N.
Director of Pediatric Intensive Care Nursing Services, Children's Hospital National Medical Center, Washington, DC

Mary Ann Morgan, R.N., B.S.N., M.S.N.
Formerly Director, School of Nursing, Presbyterian–University of Pennsylvania Medical Center, Philadelphia, Pennsylvania

Donald M. Poretz, M.D.
Chief of Infectious Diseases, The Fairfax Hospital, Falls Church, Virginia

Mary S. Rieser, R.N., M.S.
Director of Staff Development, Division of Nursing, Hospital of the University of Pennsylvania, Philadelphia, Pennsylvania

Eileen F. Riviello, R.N., B.S.N., M.S.N.
Acting Assistant Director, Presbyterian School of Nursing, Philadelphia, Pennsylvania

Mary Evan Robinson, Ph.D.
Pediatric Psychologist, Private Practice; formerly of Children's Hospital National Medical Center, Washington, DC

Gary J. Starecheski, R.Ph., B.Sc.
Assistant Director of Pharmacy and Hospice Pharmacist, The Bryn Mawr Hospital, Bryn Mawr, Pennsylvania

Harry Wollman, M.D.
Robert Dunning Dripps Professor, Chairman,
Department of Anesthesia, Professor of Pharmacology,
University of Pennsylvania, Philadelphia, Pennsylvania

Research/Library

Kathy Ahrens, M.S., Director, Medical/Nursing Library
Presbyterian–University of Pennsylvania Medical Center,
Philadelphia, Pennsylvania

James Caine, Deputy Chief
Reference Services Division, National Library of
Medicine, Bethesda, Maryland

Ann Campisi, Library Technician
Medical/Nursing Library, Presbyterian–University of
Pennsylvania Medical Center, Philadelphia, Pennsylvania

Shirley W. Chilson, for research assistance

Leslie D. Gundry, Chief Medical Librarian
Joseph N. Pew, Jr., Medical Library, The Bryn Mawr
Hospital and School of Nursing, Bryn Mawr,
Pennsylvania

Alexander G. Kulchar, Medical Librarian
Clothier Nursing Library, The Bryn Mawr Hospital and
School of Nursing, Bryn Mawr, Pennsylvania

Alice Makov, Reference User Education
Scott Memorial Library, The Thomas Jefferson
University, Philadelphia, Pennsylvania

Reference Librarians and Reference Technicians
National Library of Medicine, Bethesda, Maryland

Barbara H. Suddarth, for research assistance

Gladys L. Taylor and Staff, Head Monograph Processing
Group Circulation and Control Section
National Library of Medicine, Bethesda, Maryland

Jacqueline van de Kamp, Technical Information
Specialist
National Library of Medicine, Bethesda, Maryland

We acknowledge the following persons with special
appreciation:

Diana Intenzo, our Executive Editor, for her editorial
insight, discrimination, judgment, and support.

Tracy Baldwin for her unique frame of art reference and
June Melloni who translated ideas into illustrations with
grace and artistic expertise.

Helen Ewan for the quiet, efficient manner in which she
checks reams of manuscript and her organized
dedication to maintaining a strict schedule.

Mary Murphy, for her unending source of support and
sustenance as well as her kindness and courtesy.

Barton H. Lippincott and **John Connolly** for their interest
and many kindnesses.

David T. Miller. The authors wish to pay special tribute
to David because he conceived the idea for *The
Lippincott Manual of Nursing Practice* and has provided
continuing encouragement and support.

Of course, our deepest tributes and most sincere
appreciations are reserved for those who mean the most
to us, our husbands, Mat and Hilton.

Medical-Surgical Nursing

The Nursing Process

The *nursing process* is a systematic, decision-making process that involves assessment (data collection), planning, and implementation and uses evaluation and subsequent modifications as feedback mechanisms that promote the ultimate resolution of the patient's nursing problems. The process as a whole is cyclic, the steps being interrelated, interdependent, and recurrent.

Steps of the Nursing Process

1. *Assessing*—systematic assessment of the patient's actual and potential health needs for the purpose of establishing nursing diagnoses. (Analysis of data is included as part of the assessment. For those who wish to emphasize its importance, analysis may be identified as a separate step of the nursing process.)
2. *Planning*—development of a plan of care designed to meet the patient's actual and potential health needs.
3. *Implementing*—implementation of the plan of care or supervision of others who implement the plan.
4. *Appraisal*—evaluation of the patient's response to the nursing interventions and the extent to which the goals have been achieved.

Assessing

Assessment begins with the nurse's first encounter with the patient. It involves the systematic collection of data about the patient's nursing needs and the use of this data to formulate nursing diagnoses. Pre-hospital admission assessment is often conducted by nurses in physicians' offices, clinics, and outpatient departments. This assessment includes a nursing history and an appraisal of the patient's readiness for hospitalization or outpatient services. Any special instructions and preparation that the patient needs are given at this time.

A. The Nursing History (see details, p. 13)

1. Is carried out for the purpose of determining the patient's state of wellness or illness and is best accomplished as part of a planned interview.
2. Provides the nurse with the opportunity to collect data and also to convey interest, support, and understanding to the patient and to establish a relationship of mutual trust and respect.

B. The Physical Examination (see details, p. 18)

1. To determine the patient's physical alterations and limitations.
2. To determine the patient's assets, which may serve to offset his limitations.

C. Other Sources of Assessment Data

1. Patient's family and/or significant others
2. Members of the health team
3. Patient's health record

D. Nursing Diagnoses

Those actual or potential health problems that are amenable to resolution by means of nursing actions.

1. Organize, analyze, synthesize, and summarize the collected data.
2. Identify the patient's health problem(s), its particular characteristic(s) and etiology(ies).
3. State nursing diagnoses concisely and precisely.

Planning

See Example of a Nursing Care Plan, page 4.

1. Assign priorities to the nursing diagnoses. Highest priority is given to problems that are the most urgent and critical.
2. Establish goals for nursing interventions.
   a. Specify short-term, intermediate, and long-term goals as established by nurse and patient together.
   b. State goals in realistic and measurable terms.
3. Identify nursing interventions appropriate for goal attainment.
4. Establish expected outcome criteria.
   a. State outcomes in terms of patient behaviors.
   b. Outcomes must be realistic and measurable.
   c. Identify critical time periods for the attainment of outcomes.
5. Formulate the nursing care plan (see sample nursing care plan, p. 4).
   a. Include nursing diagnoses in order of priority, goals, nursing interventions, outcome criteria, and critical time periods.
   b. Write entries precisely, concisely, and systematically.
   c. Keep the plan current and flexible to meet the patient's changing needs.
   d. Involve the patient, his family and/or significant others, nursing team members, other health team members, and community agencies in all aspects of planning.

Implementing

1. Put the nursing care plan into action.
2. Coordinate the activities of the patient, his family and/or significant others, nursing team members, and other health team members.
3. Delegate specific nursing interventions to other members of the nursing team, as appropriate.
   a. Consider the capabilities and limitations of the members of the nursing team.
   b. Supervise the performance of the nursing interventions.
4. Record the patient's responses to the nursing interventions.

Example of a Nursing Care Plan

Mr. John Preston, a 52-year-old businessman, was admitted to the hospital with a diagnosis of angina pectoris. He stated that he had experienced substernal chest pain and weakness in his arms and hands after having lunch with a business associate. The pain had lessened by the time he arrived at the hospital. The nursing history revealed that he had been hospitalized 5 months previously with the same complaints and had been told by his physician to go to the emergency department if the pain ever recurred. He had been placed on a low-fat diet and had stopped smoking. Physical examination revealed that Mr. Preston's vital signs were within normal ranges and that his chest pain had been relieved with nitroglycerin. He stated that he had feared that he was having a "heart attack" until his pain subsided and until he was told that his ECG was normal. He verbalized that he wanted to find out how he could prevent the attacks of pain in the future. The physician's requests upon admission included activity as tolerated, low-cholesterol diet, and nitroglycerin 0.4 mg. ($^1/_{150}$ gr.) sublingually prn.

Nursing Diagnosis: Alteration in comfort—pain related to myocardial ischemia.
Goals—Short-term: Relief of pain.
Long-term: Altered life-style to include measures that decrease myocardial oxygen demands. Adherence to therapeutic regimen.

Nursing Interventions	Outcome Criteria	Critical Time*	Outcome
Continue assessment of cardiac function:			
Monitor blood pressure (BP), pulse (P), respirations (R) q. 4 hr.	BP, P, R remain within normal limits.	24 hr.	BP: stable at 116–122/72–84. P: stable at 68–82. R: stable at 16–20.
Assess frequency of chest pain and precipitating events.	Free of chest pain.	24 hr.	Denies chest pain; able to walk length of hall, eat meals, and visit with family and friends without chest discomfort.
Encourage food and fluid intake that promotes normal nutrition, digestion, and elimination and that does not precipitate chest pain: light, regular meals; foods low in cholesterol; 1500–2000 ml. fluid/day.	Tolerates dietary regimen. Absence of chest pain after meals. Maintains normal bowel elimination. Intake of 1500–2000 ml. fluid/ day.	48 hr.	Denies chest pain after meals; no constipation or diarrhea; fluid intake 1700–2100 ml./ day.
Request consultation with dietitian—for diet teaching.	Identifies foods low in cholesterol and those foods that are to be avoided. Selects well-balanced diet within prescribed restrictions.	48 hr.	Selects and eats a balanced diet consisting of foods low in cholesterol; dietitian reviewed diet restrictions with patient and wife; wife counseled in meal planning.
Encourage alterations in activities and exercise that are necessary to prevent episodes of anginal pain.	Identifies activities and exercises that could precipitate chest pain: those that require sudden bursts of activity and heavy effort. Identifies emotionally stressful situations. Explains the necessity for alternating periods of activity with periods of rest.	3 days	Patient and wife have identified activities and situations that should be avoided; patient and wife have studied their usual daily routine and have made plans to alter the routine to allow for rest periods; teenage son had volunteered to assist with strenuous home-maintenance chores.
Teaching; nitroglycerin regimen.	(See teaching plan, p. 8)		

* These times have not been standardized, but are individualized according to the patient's needs.

a. Record the responses precisely, concisely, and objectively.
b. Recordings should be related to the nursing diagnoses.
c. Include any additional pertinent assessment data.

Evaluating

1. Collect objective data.
2. Compare the patient's behavioral outcomes to the outcome criteria. Determine the extent to which the goals were achieved.
3. Include the patient, his family and/or significant others, nursing team members, and other health team members in the evaluation.
4. Identify alterations that need to be made in the nursing care plan.

Continuation of the Nursing Process

1. Continue all steps of the nursing process: assessing, planning, implementing, and evaluating.
2. Continuous evaluation provides the means for maintaining the viability of the entire nursing process and for demonstrating accountability for the quality of nursing care rendered.

Bibliography

Books

Atkinson LD and Murray ME. Understanding the Nursing Process. New York, Macmillan, 1983

Campbell C. Nursing Diagnosis and Intervention in Nursing Practice. New York, John Wiley & Sons, 1984

Carnevali DL. Diagnostic Reasoning in Nursing. Philadelphia, JB Lippincott, 1984

Carnevali DL. Nursing Care Planning: Diagnosis and Management. Philadelphia, JB Lippincott, 1983

Carpenito LJ. Nursing Diagnosis. Application to Clinical Practice. Philadelphia, JB Lippincott, 1983

Gordon M. Nursing Diagnosis. Process and Application. New York, McGraw-Hill, 1982

Griffith JW and Christensen PJ. Nursing Process. Application of Theories, Frameworks, and Models. St Louis, CV Mosby, 1982

Kim MJ, McFarland GK and McLane AM (eds). Pocket Guide to Nursing Diagnoses. St Louis, CV Mosby, 1984

Kim MJ and Moritz DA. Classification of Nursing Diagnoses. New York, McGraw-Hill, 1982

Marriner A. The Nursing Process. A Scientific Approach to Nursing Care. St Louis, CV Mosby, 1983

Yura H and Walsh MB. Human Needs and the Nursing Process. Norwalk, CT, Appleton-Century-Crofts, 1978

Yura H and Walsh MB. Human Needs 2 and the Nursing Process. Norwalk, CT, Appleton-Century-Crofts, 1982

Yura H and Walsh MB. Human Needs 3 and the Nursing Process. Norwalk, CT, Appleton-Century-Crofts, 1983

Yura H and Walsh MB. The Nursing Process. Norwalk, CT, Appleton-Century-Crofts, 1983

Articles

Barnard KE. Nursing diagnosis: A descriptive method. MCN 1983 May/June; 8(3):223

Bockrath M. Your patient needs two diagnoses—medical and nursing. Nurs Life 1982 Mar/Apr; 2(2):29–32

Bruce JA and Snyder ME. The right and responsibility to diagnose. Am J Nurs 1982 Apr; 82(4):645–646

Case BA and Rooney DS. Patient care planning strategies. Nurs Manage 1982 April; 13(4):23–26

Dossey B and Guzetta CE. Nursing diagnosis. Nursing '81 1981 June; 11(6):34–38

Fadden TC and Seiser GK. Nursing diagnosis. A matter of form. Am J Nurs 1984 April; 84(4):470–472

Fredette SL and Gloriant FS. Nursing diagnosis in cancer chemotherapy. In practice. Am J Nurs 1981 Nov; 81(11): 2021–2022

Fredette SL and Gloriant FS. Nursing diagnosis in cancer chemotherapy. In theory. Am J Nurs 1981 Nov; 81(11): 2013–2020

Gray JW and Aldred H. Care plans in long-term facilities. Am J Nurs 1980 Nov; 80(11):2054–2057

Guzzetta CE and Dossey BM. Nursing diagnosis: Framework, process, and problems. Heart Lung 1983 May; 12(3):281–291

Leslie FM. Nursing diagnosis: Use in long-term care. Am J Nurs 1981 May; 81(5):1012–1014

Lillesand KM and Korff S. Nursing process evaluation: A quality assurance tool. Nurs Adm Q 1983 Spring; 7(3): 9–14

Lunney M. Nursing diagnosis: Refining the system. Am J Nurs 1982 Mar; 82(3):456–459

Moughton M. The patient: A partner in the health care process. Nurs Clin North Am 1982 Sept; 17(3):467–479

Nodhturft VL and MacMullen JA. Standardized nursing care plans. Nurs Manage 1982 Oct; 13(10):33–42

Popkiss SA. Diagnosing your patient's strengths. Nursing '81 1981 July; 11(7):34–37

Health Education and the Nursing Process

Health Education

Health education is an essential component of nursing care and is directed toward promotion, maintenance, and restoration of health, and toward adaptation to the residual effects of illness.

Objective:
To teach people to live life to its healthiest—that is, to strive toward achieving one's maximum health potential.

Principles of Teaching and Learning

1. The teaching–learning process requires the active involvement of both the teacher and the learner.
2. The desired outcome of the teaching–learning process is a change in the learner's behavior.
3. The teacher serves as a facilitator of learning.
4. Learning is facilitated by progressing from the simple to the complex and from the known to the unknown.
5. Learning is facilitated when the learner is aware of his progress toward the learning goals.

Variables that Affect Learning Readiness

A. Physical Readiness

1. Physical distress that absorbs the patient's attention prevents effective learning.
2. Readiness to learn can be promoted by alleviating or at least minimizing as much as possible the patient's physical distress.

B. Emotional Readiness

1. Motivation to learn depends upon
   a. Acceptance of the illness or acceptance of the fact that illness is a threat.
   b. Recognition of the need to learn.
   c. A therapeutic regimen compatible with the patient's life-style or altered life-style.
2. Motivation to learn can be promoted by
   a. Creating a warm, accepting, positive atmosphere.
   b. Encouraging the patient to participate in the establishment of acceptable, realistic, attainable learning goals.
   c. Providing feedback about progress, that is, positive reinforcement when the patient is successful, constructive criticism when he is unsuccessful.

C. Experimental Readiness

1. The patient's previous experiences, especially learning experiences, affect the learning process.
   a. Success in past learning experiences usually serves to motivate future learning.

b. Failure in past learning experiences often causes the learner to be hesitant to make new attempts to learn; this learner must be helped to gain confidence in his ability to learn.
2. Learning is dependent upon attainment of those behaviors that are prerequisites to the specific learning task, for example, knowledge of the basics of normal nutrition is a prerequisite to understanding a special diet.

The Learning Atmosphere

1. The physical environment should be conducive to learning: quiet, uninterrupted, and comfortable.
   Consider the following variables:
   a. temperature
   b. lighting
   c. noise level
   d. traffic
   e. seating facilities and arrangement
2. The time of the teaching–learning session should be scheduled to meet the patient's needs.
   a. Encourage the patient and his family to participate in the scheduling of the teaching–learning session.
   b. Select a time when the patient is most alert, most comfortable, and least fatigued.
   c. Select a time when the patient is not anticipating immediate diagnostic or therapeutic procedures.
   d. Select a time when family members who are to be included in the teaching plan are available.

Teaching Strategies

Learning is facilitated by selecting teaching techniques and methods that are most appropriate to meet the individual patient's needs.

A. Lecture

1. Is most useful in teaching groups of patients who share the same learning needs.
2. Should always be accompanied by discussion, which allows the individual patient to
   a. Express his feelings and concerns.
   b. Ask questions.
   c. Clarify information.

B. Group Discussion

1. Is most useful for patients who relate well in groups.
2. Allows patients to experience security through being a member of a group of patients with similar problems or learning needs.

3. Provides patients with the opportunity to gain support, assistance, and encouragement from group members.

C. Demonstration and Practice

1. Is most useful when skills are to be learned.
2. Ample opportunity must be provided for practice sessions.
3. Equipment should be the same as that which the patient will use after leaving the hospital.

D. Teaching Aids

1. Are useful to supplement the resources of the nurse in helping the patient to learn.
2. Include books, pamphlets, pictures, films, slides, tapes, and models.

3. Must be reviewed prior to presentation to ensure that they are appropriate for meeting the patient's individual learning needs.

E. Reinforcement and Follow-up

1. Allow ample time for the patient to learn and to have his learning reinforced.
2. Follow-up sessions promote the patient's confidence in his ability to retain his newly learned behaviors.
3. Evaluate the patient's progress, which is imperative, and plan additional teaching sessions, as necessary.
4. Follow-up sessions after discharge may be needed to assist the patient in transferring what he has learned in the hospital to his home setting.

The Nursing Process in Patient Teaching

The teaching–learning process is an integral part of the nursing process. With a focus on learning and with regard for the principles, variables, techniques, and strategies of teaching and learning, the steps of the nursing process—assessing, planning, implementing, and evaluating—are used for the purpose of meeting the teaching and learning needs of the patient and his family.

Assessing

1. Assess the patient's learning needs and his physical, emotional, and experiential readiness for health education.
   a. What are his health beliefs and behaviors?
   b. What psychosocial adaptations is he making?
   c. Is he ready to learn?
      (1) Is he able to learn these behaviors?
      (2) What are his expectations?
      (3) What additional information is needed about him?
2. Assess the patient's need for education and preparation related to the self-care activities for which he will be responsible after discharge.
3. Use appropriate assessment guides to facilitate data collection.
   Adapt such guides to the individual responses, problems, and needs of the patient.
4. Formulate nursing diagnoses that relate to the patient's learning needs.
   a. Organize, analyze, synthesize, and summarize the collected data.
   b. Identify the patient's learning need(s), its particular characteristic(s) and etiology(ies).
   c. State nursing diagnoses concisely and precisely.

Planning

1. Assign priority to the nursing diagnoses.
2. Specify the short-term, intermediate, and long-term learning goals established by both the nurse and patient.
3. Identify teaching actions appropriate for goal attainment.
4. Establish expected outcome criteria.
5. Identify critical time periods for the attainment of outcomes.
6. Develop a written teaching plan (see sample teaching plan, p. 8).
   a. Include diagnoses (in order of priority), goals, teaching strategies, outcome criteria, and critical time periods.

   b. Write entries precisely, concisely, and systematically.
   c. Include a topical outline of the information to be presented.
   d. Select appropriate teaching techniques and methods.
   e. Keep the plan current and flexible to meet the patient's changing learning needs.
7. Involve the patient, his family and/or significant others, nursing team members, and other health team members in all aspects of planning.

Implementing

1. Put the teaching plan into action.
2. Know the material to be presented.
3. Provide an atmosphere conducive to learning.
4. Use language the patient can understand.
5. Use appropriate teaching techniques and methods.
6. Use the same equipment that the patient will use after discharge.
7. Encourage the patient and his family to participate actively in learning.
8. Coordinate the activities of the patient, his family and/or significant others, nursing team members, and other health team members.
9. Emphasize the importance of learning to care for self after discharge.
10. Record the patient's responses to the teaching actions.

Evaluating

1. Collect objective data.
   a. Observe the patient.
   b. Ask questions to determine if the patient understands.
   c. Use rating scales, checklists, anecdotal notes, and written tests when appropriate.
2. Compare the patient's behavioral outcomes with the outcome criteria. Determine the extent to which the goals were achieved.
3. Include the patient, his family and/or significant others, nursing team members, and other health team members in the evaluation.
4. Identify alterations that need to be made in the teaching plan.
5. Make referrals to appropriate resource persons or agencies for reinforcement of learning after discharge.
6. Continue all steps of the teaching–learning process: assessing, planning, implementing, and evaluating.

Example of a Teaching Plan (For background information see nursing care plan example, p. 4)

Assessment of Mr. Preston's teaching and learning needs revealed the following: Basic knowledge about the etiology and pathology of angina pectoris • Definitive plans for adherence to the dietary regimen • Definitive plans for alteration of life-style to attempt to prevent episodes of anginal pain • Inadequate knowledge about nitroglycerin therapy regimen.

Nursing Diagnosis: Nonadherence to nitroglycerin therapy regimen related to inadequate knowledge about the regimen.

Goals—Short-term: Describes action, use, and correct administration of nitroglycerin.

Long-term: Adheres to nitroglycerin therapy regimen.

Teaching Interventions	Outcome Criteria	Critical Time*	Outcome
Explain and discuss the action and use of nitroglycerin for treatment and prevention of anginal episodes.	Explains in his own words the action and use of nitroglycerin to treat anginal episodes.	3 days	Stated explanation accurately.
	Identifies activities and exercises prior to which nitroglycerin should be taken for its prophylactic effects.	3 days	Accurately identified activities and exercises.
Explain and discuss the necessity for keeping a record of his use of nitroglycerin and providing the physician with this record.	Explains in his own words the necessity for recording the following data and reporting to his physician: Date and time of drug use Factors that precipitated pain Time required for relief of pain Amount of drug taken	3 days	Stated explanation accurately.
Explain and discuss the need to have nitroglycerin available at all times and the precautions to take to maintain its potency.	Explains in his own words the necessity to carry nitroglycerin with him at all times and the following precautions to take: Keep nitroglycerin in tightly capped, dark-colored glass bottle. Discard the cotton filler/packing. Avoid carrying bottle in contact with body. Discard tablets after 5 months.	3 days	Stated explanation accurately.
Explain and discuss the procedure for use of nitroglycerin.	Explains in his own words the correct procedure for use of nitroglycerin: Place tablet under the tongue at first sign of chest discomfort. Rest in the upright position until all pain subsides. Take an additional tablet in 3 to 5 minutes if pain is not relieved after the second tablet is taken, or if it recurs after a short interval, go to the nearest emergency facility.	3 days	Stated explanation accurately.
	Takes nitroglycerin according to procedure.	After discharge	

Encourage to wear Medic Alert bracelet and carry medication identification on his person.	Wears Medic Alert bracelet. Carries medication identification on his person.	3 days 3 days	Obtained Medic Alert bracelet and wears it at all times. Filled out medication identification card and placed it in a visible place in his wallet.
Explain and discuss the necessity for keeping all physician appointments.	Explains in his own words the importance of keeping all appointments with physician. Keeps all appointments with physician.	3 days After discharge	Stated explanation accurately.

* These times have not been standardized, but are individualized according to the patient's needs.

Bibliography

Books

Rankin SH and Duffy KL. Patient Education: Issues, Principles, and Guidelines. Philadelphia. JB Lippincott, 1983

Redman BK. The Process of Patient Teaching in Nursing. St Louis, CV Mosby, 1984

Articles

Bille DA. Process-oriented patient education. DCCN 1983 Mar/Apr; 2(2): 108–115.

Blackwell B. What do we really know about noncompliance? Consultant 1981 Jan; 21(1):259–266

Burke LE. Learning and retention in the acute care setting. CCQ 1981 Dec; 4(3):67–73

Corkadel L and McGlashan R. A practical approach to patient teaching. J Contin Educ Nurs 1983 Jan/Feb; 14(1):9–15

George G. If patient teaching tries your patience, try this plan. Nursing '82 1982 May; 12(5):50–55

Grosser LR. All nurses can be involved in teaching patient and family. AORN J 1981 Feb; 33(2):217–219

Johnson J. The effects of a patient education course on persons with a chronic illness. Cancer Nurs 1982 April; 5(2):117–123

Lyons C et al. Interactive computerized patient education. Heart Lung 1982 July/Aug; 11(4):340–341

McCauzhrin WC. Patient understanding: The key to quality patient education. QRB 1981 May; 7(5):2–4

McClurg E. Developing an effective patient teaching program. AORN J 1981 Sept; 34(3):474–487

Shaw LM. The patient as an adult learner. AORN J 1981 Feb; 33(2):233–239

Zemble S. Teaching people to manage their health. Nurs Manage 1983 Mar; 14(3):36–38

Data Collection and Record Keeping:
Patient History and Problem Oriented Records

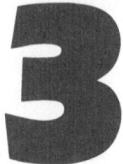

Data Collection

Purpose

1. Data collection is the first step in the process of defining problems.
2. A thorough and accurate assessment of a patient's problems or condition depends on the completeness and accuracy of the data collected.

Types of Data Collected

A. The Patient's History (see details, p. 13)

1. Is elicited in an interview.
2. The history, in final written form, logically presents the *patient's views* of:
   a. His health problems
   b. General health condition
   c. Past medical history
   d. Family health history
   e. A profile of the patient's personal and social life and well-being
3. The patient history will also reveal what the patient knows about his health, what is important in terms of health care, and expectations of the health care being sought.

    This may be supplemented by information from the patient's hospital record, conversations with other care-givers, parents (in the case of children and infants), or consultants.
4. The patient history is always *subjective* information in that it is presented from the point of view of the person reporting to the interviewer rather than directly observed by the interviewer.

B. The Physical Examination (see details, Chap. 4)—is performed by the practitioner for the following purposes:

1. To corroborate the patient's history.
2. To observe any findings not reported in the history.
3. To obtain *objective* information about the individual's health state and/or status of a health problem.

    Objective information is that body of data about a person that can be perceived by another person.

C. Laboratory Data—from test results

It is important to know that laboratory data constitute another source of *objective data* that is important in assessing many health problems and conditions; these must be considered by all nurses engaged in caring for and understanding patients.

Principles of Data Collection

1. All data collection should be well-organized and should follow a format that promotes thoroughness.
2. There is no room for bias in data collection, since the practitioner's mind must be open to clues and cues that might otherwise be missed.
3. Understanding the techniques of interviewing is basic to collecting accurate data in the patient's history and to establishing the basis for a working relationship with the patient.
4. Information gathered must be organized and recorded so that it has meaning for members of the health care team and can guide patient assessment and care.

Recording the Data Gathered

General Guidelines

1. Keep in mind the purpose of recording the information and the audience for whom it is intended. This serves to guide the form and content of the record.
2. Remember that the patient's record is a legal document.

    The record must present the information about the patient as completely, concisely, and accurately as possible, without unnecessary duplication of material.

3. Avoid redundancy.

    Redundancy obscures important information and makes careful reading of the record unnecessarily time-consuming. As a result, the record is not read carefully.

General Principles

1. *When to record*

    As soon as the information is gathered—to minimize omission and distortion of facts.

2. *Organization*

    Information must be organized and recorded systematically. (This applies to complete history, physical examination, or progress notes.)

    a. The history, or subjective information, is recorded first.

    b. Then the physical examination, or objective data, is recorded.

    c. From a systematic recording of the facts must stem a logical assessment of the subjective and objective data.

    d. Therefore, facts must be reported so that their meaning is clear and they tell a connected story.

3. *Detail*

    Describe the data gathered, using the appropriate vocabulary.

4. *Language*

    a. The written record must be succinct, yet understandable to the reader.

    b. Avoid using abbreviations.

5. *Legal considerations*

    a. Since the patient's record is a legal document, facts must be identified and stated precisely and objectively.

    b. Both inaccuracy and interpretation must be avoided.

    c. Assessment or judgment can be made only after facts are obtained and recorded with great care.

    d. The document must be signed and dated.

6. *Ethical considerations*

    a. The patient should be fully informed of all aspects of the data collection process.

    b. The patient's decision to participate in the data collection process should be made freely.

    c. The interview should be conducted in private, and confidentiality must be maintained.

Recording the History

(The general principles listed above apply to recording the history.)

1. The present illness must be recorded chronologically, beginning with the onset of the problem.

Often it is helpful to think of a beginning phrase such as "The patient was well until. . . ." Each paragraph should then describe events in sequence up to the time that the patient is being interviewed.

2. Quantify anything related to measurement.

    For example: "the patient has *frequent* headaches" is less accurate than "the patient has an average of 3 headaches a week . . ."

Recording the Physical Examination

(It is important to follow the above principles.) Other specific guidelines include the following:

1. Describe any abnormality in detail.

2. Carefully describe a normal finding in conditions where one might expect the normal to be abnormal.

    For instance, in the patient with hypertension, it would be important to report the absence of hemorrhages and exudates in the fundoscopic examination report.

3. If there are any laboratory results, they are recorded after the physical examination and before the assessment and plan.

Progress Notes

1. Progress notes are records of the patient's health status from visit to visit, day to day, or shift to shift, as the case may be.

2. They are usually written in relation to a specific problem or condition and report the relevant subjective (history) and objective (physical examination and laboratory results) data that bring the record up to date.

3. Progress notes also include an assessment of the data and a plan dealing with the problem.

    (The Problem Oriented Medical Record format developed by Dr. Lawrence Weed is an extremely useful and instructive guide in organizing and recording the initial data base and the progress notes.)

The Problem Oriented Record (POR)

A *problem oriented record* is a patient's health record organized so that specific problems are defined, numbered, and then referred to by number throughout the record. Problems are identified and numbered after the initial data base is collected.

Components of the POR

These may vary according to the particular setting in which the system is used. However, every system includes the following:

A. Initial Data Base

Consists of:

a. The patient's comprehensive health history

b. A complete physical examination

c. Nursing assessment

d. Patient profiles from other members of the health team

e. Available laboratory and radiologic data

B. Problem List

1. Consists of a numbered list of medical, social, environmental, and psychological problems and past problems derived from the initial data base.

2. Includes active and inactive problems, date of onset, and date of resolution when applicable.

    a. Often this list appears at the very beginning of the record and serves as an index.

    b. A number is never used twice even though new problems arise, some old ones are resolved, or several problems are found to be related to one common problem.

3. It is important to remember that the numbered problem list should serve as an index to the record, so that information can be systematically ordered around a problem and not get lost or be misinterpreted as the volume of the record grows in the course of many visits.

C. Progress Notes

See Sample Progress Note below.
1. Organization of the progress note varies, but the basic format remains the same.
2. The note begins with the problem and its number and then continues as follows:

S = *Subjective* data (history, consultation) concerning the problem and covering the time interval since the last entry.

O = *Objective* data (physical examination, laboratory reports) concerning the problem and covering the same time period.

A = *Assessment* of the S and the O. Includes, as appropriate, statements about probable etiology; course of the problem; the patient's response to therapy and his coping ability; general diagnostic, therapeutic, and health education plans; and a rationale for the entire plan. It should include a statement about the patient's participation in planning and his reaction to the plan.

P = *Plan*—This is a statement *specifying* what is to be done regarding the problem, who is to do it, and when it is to be done. A timetable is provided when possible. The plan stems directly from the rationale in the assessment and may include any or all of the following:

(1) *Diagnostic plan*—states what is to be done to make the data base more complete.
(2) *Therapeutic plan*—indicates projected methods for curing, improving, or palliating the patient's problem.
(3) *Health education plan*—outlines content of health teaching concerning the problem and the diagnostic and/or therapeutic plan.

I = *Intervention*—Includes nursing actions done for or with the patient.

E = *Evaluation*—Patient outcomes are used as the basis for evaluation. The evaluation may appear in the next progress note because more time is needed to observe the patient's response to nursing interventions.

Computer Documentation

Purpose
1. Documentation of nursing care
2. Standardization of assessment and nursing care plans
3. Communication and information transferral
4. Facilitation of clinical and statistical data retrieval

General Guidelines
1. Computers are compatible with the problem oriented record system.
2. Computers do not replace nursing care and the nursing process—they are facilitators of care.
3. Computers facilitate the recording of the nursing care plan, but they do not exclude individualization of the plan.
4. The information processed and displayed by computers is only as reliable and as valuable as the data that have been entered into the computer.

Sample Progress Note

Hypertension

S. The patient has felt well since he was seen 3 months ago. He has had no headaches, no visual or gastrointestinal problems, no chest pain or palpitations, no shortness of breath. His activity is unchanged, he sleeps on one pillow, has no nocturia or ankle swelling. He is taking his medications, knows their names and dosages. Drinks orange juice with fluid pill qd. He is following a diet that has "no added" salt, drinks 5 beers a week; lunchmeat sandwiches for lunch. He thinks he is gaining weight—his "clothes are tighter."

O. P 72 regular
Wt 82.5 kg. (182 pounds)
BP 148/95 right arm lying
    140/100 right arm standing

Respiratory. Chest expands symmetrically; fremitus (perceptible vibration) normal bilaterally; bronchovesicular sounds present, no adventitious (unnatural) sounds.

Cardiovascular: No heaves or thrills; point of maximal impulse (PMI) at 5th intercostal space in midclavicular line; normal sinus rhythm without murmurs, gallops, or extrasystoles; trace of pedal edema.

A. BP is fairly well controlled. Weight is up 2.3 kg. (5 pounds). The patient is taking his medication. However, his diet contains a lot of sodium, even though none is "added." If he can cut out some of the high-salt foods and lose 2.3–4.5 kg. (5–10 pounds), his pressure will no doubt be under better control. He seems motivated to lose some weight, since his clothes are tighter. He needs to know about sodium content of food, and his wife needs instruction too, since she does the shopping. Will continue the same medications and try having the patient lose weight to bring BP under better control. The patient comprehends the consequences of uncontrolled hypertension and the need for sustained weight control and medical follow-up. His wife sounds very supportive. Patient will need routine yearly blood work and cardiogram by next visit.

P. 1. Diet instruction for patient and wife. Patient will call to suggest a convenient time and will set up appointment then.
2. Continue same medications: Aldomet 250 mg. tid, hydrochlorothiazide 50 mg. qd with dietary K^+ supplement.
3. Return visit in 3 months to check BP and weight.
4. Blood work before next visit (Na^+, K^+, CO_2, urea-N, glucose, creatinine).
5. Electrocardiogram before next visit.

I. Patient given the following instructions:
1. Dietitian's name and telephone number to make appointment for diet instruction
2. Prescriptions for medications
3. Appointment for return visit
4. Prescription for blood work and electrocardiogram

The Patient History

General Principles

1. The first step in caring for a patient and in soliciting his active cooperation is to gather a careful and complete history.
   a. In *all* patient concerns and problems, an accurate history is the foundation on which data collection and the process of assessment are based.
   b. The comprehensiveness of the history elicited will depend on the information available in the patient's record.
2. Time spent early in the nurse–patient relationship gathering detailed information about what the patient knows, thinks, and feels about his problems will prevent time-consuming errors and misunderstandings later.
3. Skill in interviewing will affect both the accuracy of information elicited and the quality of the relationship established with the patient.
   This point cannot be overemphasized; the reader is encouraged to consult other sources for detailed discussion of techniques of health interviewing.
4. The purpose of the interview is to encourage an interchange of information between the patient and the nurse.
   a. The patient must feel that his words are understood and that his concerns are being listened to and dealt with sensitively.
   b. Some basic techniques for achieving these ends include the following:
      (1) Provide privacy for the patient in as quiet a place as possible and see that he is comfortable.
      (2) Begin the interview with a courteous greeting and an introduction. Explain who you are and why you are there.
      (3) Be sure that facial expressions, body movements, and tone of voice are pleasant, unhurried, and nonevaluative, and that they convey the attitude of a sensitive listener, so that the patient will feel free to express his thoughts and feelings.
      (4) Avoid reassuring the patient prematurely (before you have adequate information about the problem). This only serves to cut off discussion; the patient may then be unwilling to bring up a problem causing concern.
      (5) At times a patient gives cues or suggests information, but does not tell enough. It may be necessary to probe for more information in order to obtain a thorough history; the patient must realize that this is done for his benefit.
      (6) Guide the interview so that the necessary information is obtained, without cutting off discussion. Controlling the rambling patient is often difficult, but with practice, it can be done skillfully, without jeopardizing the quality of the information gained.

Identifying Information

A. Purposes

1. To eliminate confusion about the patient's identity; to obtain the information required for contacting him if the need arises.
2. To provide an introduction to the patient and some indication of his habits, life-style, and beliefs, which may be explored in greater depth in the personal and social history.
3. To initiate a relationship based on recognition of the importance of the informant's role in sharing in the care of the patient (when this is the case).

B. Types of Information Needed

1. Date and time
2. Patient's name, address, telephone number, race, religion, birthdate, and age
3. Name of referring practitioner
4. Insurance data
5. Name of informant—the patient may be the person giving this history; if not, record the name, address, telephone number, and relationship to the patient of the person giving the history
6. Accuracy and reliability of informant—this is a judgment based on the consistency of responses to questions and on a comparison of information in the history with your own observations in the physical examination

C. Method of Collecting Data

1. Careful interviewing of the patient or his "care person" will provide most of the information.
2. The patient's hospital or clinic record may also be a valuable source.
3. Repeat information when necessary to verify accuracy (e.g., to ensure that there has been no change in address or telephone number).
4. Assume a direct and courteous manner.
5. Explain the reasons why the information is needed—to help put the patient at ease.

Chief Complaint

A. Purposes

1. To allow the patient to describe his own problems and expectations with little or no direction from the interviewer.
2. To identify the overriding problem for which the person is seeking help.
   a. Adults with chronic conditions often have numerous complaints.
   b. If possible, focus on a single problem or concern—the one most important to the patient.
3. To identify the patient's feelings about his symptoms. The patient may show fear, guilt, or defensiveness in this first statement.

B. Types of Information Needed

The patient's primary problem(s) or concern in his own words. A statement describing the duration of the complaint.

C. Method of Collecting Data

1. Ask the patient a direct question, for example, "How may I help you?" or "For what reason have you come to the hospital (clinic, etc.)?"
2. Avoid confusing questions, for example, "What brings you here?" ("The bus.") or "Why are you here?" ("That's what I came to find out.")
3. Ask how long the concern or problem has been present. If necessary, establish the time of onset precisely by offering such clues as "Did you feel this way a month (6 months or 2 years) ago?"

4. Let the patient speak freely without offering your opinion until he has had an opportunity to identify the problem as clearly as possible.
5. Write down what the patient says, using quotation marks to identify his words.

History of Present Illness

A. Purposes

1. To amplify the description of the chief complaint and to clarify its relationship to other symptoms and events.
2. To carefully describe a symptom or problem that may be a clue to future diagnosis.

B. Types of Information Needed

1. A *detailed chronological* picture beginning with the time the patient was last well (or, in the case of a problem with an acute onset, the patient's condition just prior to the onset of the problem) and ending with a description of the patient's current condition.
2. If there is more than one important problem, each is described in a separate, chronologically organized paragraph in the written history of present illness.
3. The outline for reporting the present illness will vary with each case.

C. Method of Collecting Data

1. For each problem investigate the following:
   a. Quality (e.g., sharp, dull, knife-like—referring to pain)
   b. Quantity (e.g., ½ cup sputum)
   c. Location of symptoms, intensity, periodicity (e.g., epigastric area; daily; after meals)
   d. Aggravating and alleviating factors (e.g., medications, prescribed and over-the-counter; rest; diet)
   e. Associated phenomena (e.g., shortness of breath)
2. Date of onset of the problem as accurately as possible, since chronology is of the utmost importance (see Chief Complaint, p. 13).
3. Describe the character of the symptoms and state whether they have changed over time.
4. In the case of acute infections, inquire about possible exposure or an incubation period.
5. When the present illness has been characterized by attacks separated by free intervals, obtain the history of a typical attack.
   Onset, duration, and associated symptoms—pain; fever; chills; relation to any activity, either physical or emotional, or to such factors as diet, medication, etc.
6. In both acute and chronic illnesses, note whether and when the patient stopped working and/or went to bed.
7. Get the patient's subjective appraisal of whether the symptom or problem is getting better or worse.
8. When a particular organ or system is disturbed, ask for a review of that system and related systems so that important negative and positive information may be included in the written history.
   For instance, if a patient complains of chest pain, ask about both the respiratory and cardiac systems, as well as the musculoskeletal history of the chest.
9. Questioning may reveal that other systems must also be reviewed.
10. Ask about previous treatment, including medications, prescribing physician or practitioner, and place where treatment was obtained (name of hospital, clinic, etc.).
11. At the end, review the chronology and specifics with the patient and ask him to affirm or correct the information.
12. Organize the information for recording or presentation.

Past Medical History

A. Purposes

1. To determine any change in the patient's normal patterns of living that may or may not be caused by illness.
2. To identify clues that may aid in diagnosing the present illness.
3. To participate in gathering and recording information that may be helpful in making a diagnosis, even though the nurse may not have the final responsibility for diagnosing the patient's particular problem.

B. Types of Information Needed

1. *General health and strength*—sleeping patterns, appetite, stability of weight, usual activities.
2. *Acute infectious diseases*—measles, mumps, whooping cough, chickenpox, pneumonia, pleurisy, tuberculosis, scarlet fever, acute rheumatic fever, rheumatic heart disease, tonsillitis, hepatitis, polio, sexually transmitted disease, tropical or parasitic diseases, any other acute infectious problem the patient describes.
3. *Immunization*—polio, diphtheria, pertussis, tetanus, influenza, last PPD or other skin test, any abnormal or unusual reactions. Give date when possible.
4. *Operation*—indications, diagnosis, dates, hospital, surgeon, complications.
5. *Previous hospitalizations*—physician, hospital date (year), diagnosis, treatment.
6. *Injuries*—type; resulting disabilities.
7. *Major illnesses* (any prolonged illnesses not requiring hospitalization)—dates, symptoms, course, treatment.
8. *Allergies* (may appear in review of systems)—asthma, hay fever, hives, food allergies, drug reactions, previous treatment with penicillin and any reactions.
9. *Obstetrical history* (may appear in review of systems)
   a. Pregnancies, miscarriages, abortions.
   b. Describe course of pregnancy, labor, and delivery; date, place of delivery.
10. *Psychiatric history* (may appear in review of systems)—treatment by a psychiatrist or psychologist, indications, date, place, medications for "nerves."

C. Method of Collecting Data

1. Begin by explaining the purpose and type of questions you will be asking; for example, "I am now going to ask you some questions about your past health."
2. Explain that these questions are important in order to obtain an accurate picture of all the events that affected or that *did not* affect the patient's health in the past.
3. Use direct questions, for example, "How would you describe your general health?" and then proceed with more specific queries, such as "Has your weight been stable over the past 5 years?"

Family History

A. Purposes

1. To present a picture of the patient's family health, including specifically that of grandparents, parents, brothers, and sisters.

It also involves the health of close relatives, since some diseases show a familial tendency or are hereditary.

2. To describe the health of the patient's spouse and children, since this may give clues about possible communicable disease problems.

It also will be important in determining what sort of condition a family is in and how this affects the patient.

B. Types of Information Needed

1. Age and health status of (or age at and cause of death of) parent, sibling.
2. History, in immediate and close relatives, of heart disease, hypertension, stroke, diabetes, gout, kidney disease or stones, thyroid disease, asthma or other allergies, blood problems, cancer (types), epilepsy, mental illness, arthritis, alcoholism, obesity.
3. Hereditary diseases such as hemophilia or sickle cell disease.
4. Age and health status of spouse and children.

C. Method of Collecting Data

1. Begin with an explanation of what you are asking and why, since the patient may not understand the purpose of your questions. For example:

"I am going to ask now about the health of your immediate family and relatives. It is important to know if there are any conditions which tend to or could occur in your family, or in you as a member of the family."

2. Ask direct questions.
   a. Begin with the patient's siblings.
      "Do you have any brothers and sisters?"
      "How old are they and what is the state of their health?"
   b. List each sibling separately, giving age and state of health.

Review of Systems

A. Purpose

To obtain detailed information about the current state of the patient and any past symptoms, or lack of symptoms, he may have experienced related to a particular body system.

B. Types of Information Needed

Subjective information about what the patient feels or sees with regard to the major systems of the body.

1. *Skin*—rash, itching, change in pigmentation or texture, sweating, hair growth and distribution, condition of nails.
2. *Skeletal*—stiffness of joints, pain, deformity, restriction of motion, swelling, redness, heat. If there are problems, ask the patient to specify any activities of daily life that he finds difficult or impossible to perform.
3. *Head*—headaches, dizziness, syncope, head injuries.
4. *Eyes*—vision, pain, diplopia, photophobia, blind spots, itching, burning, discharge, recent change in appearance or vision, glaucoma, cataracts, glasses/contact lenses worn, date of last refraction, infection.
5. *Ears*—hearing acuity, earache, discharge, tinnitus, vertigo.
6. *Nose*—sense of smell, frequency of colds, obstruction, epistaxis, postnasal discharge, sinus pain or therapy, use of nose drops or sprays (type and frequency).
7. *Teeth*—pain; bleeding, swollen or receding gums; recent abscesses, extractions; dentures; dental hygiene practices.
8. *Mouth and tongue*—soreness of tongue or buccal mucosa, ulcers, swelling.
9. *Throat*—sore throats, tonsillitis, hoarseness, dysphagia.
10. *Neck*—pain, stiffness, swelling, enlarged glands or lymph nodes.
11. *Endocrine*—goiter, thyroid tenderness, tremors, weakness, tolerance to heat and cold, changes in hat or glove size, changes in skin pigmentation, libido, bruisability, muscle cramps, polyuria, polydipsia, polyphagia, hormone therapy.
12. *Respiratory*
    a. Pain in the chest and relationship to respirations.
    b. Dyspnea, wheezing, cough, sputum (character, quantity), hemoptysis.
    c. Night sweats (Does the patient have to change his bedding?).
    d. Last chest x-ray and result; (indicate where obtained).
    e. Exposure to tuberculosis.
13. *Cardiac*
    a. Presence of pain or distress and location (have patient point to location); radiation of pain; precipitating/aggravating causes; alleviating measures; timing and duration.
    b. Palpitations, dyspnea, orthopnea (note number of pillows required for sleeping), edema, cyanosis.
    c. Exercise tolerance (determine in relation to patient's regular activities—how much can he do before stopping to rest?).
    d. Blood pressure (if known); last ECG and results (indicate where obtained).
14. *Hematologic*—anemia (if so, treatment received), tendency to bruise or bleed, thromboses, thrombophlebitis, any known abnormalities of blood cells.
15. *Lymph nodes*—enlargement, tenderness, suppuration, duration and progress of abnormality.
16. *Gastrointestinal*
    a. Appetite and digestion, intolerance to certain classes of foods.
    b. Pain associated with hunger or eating, eructation, regurgitation, heartburn, nausea, vomiting, hematemesis.
    c. Regularity of bowel movement; (describe normal bowel habits and whether they have changed recently or not); diarrhea, flatulence, stools (color—brown, black, clay; tarry, fresh blood, mucus, etc.).
    d. Hemorrhoids, jaundice, dark urine, use of laxatives—type; frequency. (This should be included under past medical history with medications, but may be repeated here.)
    e. History of ulcer, gallstones, polyps, tumors.
    f. Previous x-rays—where, when, results.
17. *Genitourinary*—dysuria, pain, urgency, frequency, hematuria, nocturia, polydipsia, polyuria, oliguria, edema of the face, hesitancy, dribbling, loss in size or force of stream, passage of stones, stress incontinence, hernias.
    a. Males
       (1) Puberty—onset, voice change, erections, emissions
       (2) Libido—satisfaction with sexual relations
    b. Females
       (1) Menses—onset, regularity, duration of flow, dysmenorrhea, last period, intermenstrual bleeding or discharge, dyspareunia

(2) Libido—satisfaction with sexual relations
(3) Pregnancies (see past medical history)
(4) Methods of contraception
(5) Breasts—pain, tenderness, discharge, lumps, mammograms, breast self-examination—techniques and timing with regard to menstrual cycle

18. *Neuromuscular*
   a. Mental status—orientation to time, place, person, and distance. "How far is your home from the hospital?" (Interviewer must be able to verify the answer.)
   b. Memory—distant memory shown by recalling past medical history.
      —recent memory shown by recalling what was eaten for breakfast.
   c. Cognition, or ability of patient to conceptualize (very useful information in determining a health education plan for the patient).
   d. Patient's description of his personality—how he views himself.
   e. Presence of tics, twitching, weakness, paralysis, tremor, wasting of muscles, incoordination, fatigue, sensory loss with respect to pain, temperature, touch, muscle pain, cramps.
   f. Psychiatric history may be entered here.

19. *General constitutional symptoms*—fever, chills, malaise, fatigability, recent loss or gain of weight.

C. Method of Collecting Data

1. Begin by explaining to the patient—"I am going to ask you many questions about your body which will help in understanding your present problem."
2. Ask direct questions about each system, using terms that the patient understands.
3. Whenever the patient complains or suggests a symptom, ask the questions outlined under method of collecting data about the present illness (onset, duration, etc.).
4. Never assume that things are "OK" if the patient fails to mention something.
   a. Ask about every aspect of the function of a particular system and be sure to record the patient's responses.
   b. Often the fact that a body system has been free of any symptoms is as important as any symptoms that have been experienced.
5. If necessary, memorize a list of questions for each system or use a list when interviewing the patient.
   Knowing what to ask about each system is based on knowledge of the function of each body system and of the way that normal function manifests itself.

Personal and Social History

A. Purposes

1. To describe the patient's life situation—may have bearing on the present condition and/or the patient's ability to cope with this problem.
2. To develop a plan of care that "fits" the patient.
   Here the interviewer finds out the many personal and family resources an individual has to aid him in coping with the situation—both long-term and short-term.

3. To have some idea of how the patient patterns his life.
   a. Certain habits and patterns are more easily assimilated and changed, when necessary, than others.
   b. Knowing the patient's patterns is useful in helping to organize hospital routine in ways that will be least disruptive to the patient.
4. To help the patient develop a workable plan of care at home, based on knowledge of home conditions.
5. To determine if the patient's occupation is directly or indirectly related to his condition.
6. To determine if the patient's religious affiliation may affect therapy.

B. Types of Information Needed

1. *Personal status*—birth place, education, armed service affiliation, position in the family, satisfaction with life situations (home and job), personal concerns.
2. *Habits/patterns*
   a. Sleeping, activities/hobbies, nutrition/eating habits (diet for a typical day).
   b. Consumption of alcohol, coffee, tea, drugs (marijuana, over-the-counter medications).
   c. Tobacco (what form; how long).
   d. Sexual habits (can be part of GU history)—relationships, frequency, satisfaction.
3. *Home conditions*
   a. Marital status, nature of family relationships.
   b. Economic conditions—source of income; health insurance, Medicare, Medicaid.
   c. Living arrangements and housing (owning/renting, heating, sewage, pets, etc.).
   d. Involvement with agencies (name, case worker, etc.).
4. *Occupation*
   a. Past and present employment and working conditions, including exposure to stress/tension, noise, pollution.
   b. Working hours.
   c. Job satisfaction.
5. *Religion*—name, whether practicing or not, any stipulations with regard to health practices.

C. Method of Collecting Data

1. Begin by explaining that you are now going to ask questions about the patient's life situation in order to gain a clearer perspective of the patient's condition and of how you might help him.
2. Your manner should be matter-of-fact, yet concerned. If you are uncomfortable asking the questions, most likely the patient will sense that and be uneasy answering them.
3. A sensitive interviewer can ask most of the questions listed above in an initial interview without alienating the patient. For instance, ask "What has been your education?" instead of "How far have you gone in school?"

Ending the History

When you have completed the history, it is often helpful to say: "Is there anything else you would like to tell me?" or "What do you think is the matter with you?" This allows the patient to end the history by saying what is on his mind and what concerns him most.

Bibliography

Books

Brozino JD. Computer Applications for Patient Care. Menlo Park, CA, Addison-Wesley, 1982

Burns KR and Johnson PJ. Health Assessment in Clinical Practice. Englewood Cliffs, NJ, Prentice-Hall, 1980

Grimes J and Iannopollo E. Health Assessment in Nursing Practice. Monterey, CA, Wadsworth Health Sciences Division, 1982

Jones DA, Lepley MK and Baker BA. Health Assessment Across the Life Span. New York, McGraw-Hill, 1984

Malasanos L, Barkauskas V and Moss M. Health Assessment. St Louis, CV Mosby, 1981

Sherman JL and Fields SK. Guide to Patient Evaluation. Garden City, NY, Medical Examination Publishing Co, 1982

Weed L. Medical Records. Medical Education and Patient Care. Cleveland, Case Western Reserve University Press, 1968

Articles

Cook M. Selecting the right computer system. Nurs Manage 1982 Aug; 13(8): 26–28

DeMilliano M. 8 Common charting mistakes to avoid. Nurs Life 1984 May/June; 4(3):30–32

Edmunds L. Computer-assisted nursing care. Am J Nurs 1982 July; 82(7): 1076–1079

Gamberg D, Hushower G and Smith N. Outcome charting. Nurs Manage 1981 Oct; 12(10):36–38

Haggard BA. Coping with anxiety about patient interviews. AORN J 1983 Feb; 37(2):195–198

Happ B. Should computers be used in the nursing care of patients? Nurs Manage 1983 July; 14(7):31–35

Keithley JK and Tasic PW. A unified approach to assessment of the surgical patient. Am J Nurs 1982 April; 82(4): 612–614

Kiley M et al. Computerized nursing information systems (NIS). Nurs Manage 1983 July; 14(7):26–29

Kuehnel C and Rowe B. Patient education and the audit. Superv Nurse 1980 Dec; 11(12):15–19

Lee AA. What computers can do for you. RN 1982 Sept; 45(9):43–44+

Lombard N and Light N. On-line nursing care plans by nursing diagnosis. Comput Healthc 1983 Nov; 4(11):22–23

Mallick MJ. Patient assessment—based on data, not intuition. Nurs Outlook 1981 Oct; 29(10):600–605

Mengel A. Getting the most from patient interviews. Nursing '82 1982 Nov; 12(11):46–49

Milholland DK and Cardona VD. Computers at the bedside. Am J Nurs 1983 Sept; 83(9):1304–1307

Perin GA. Promoting informed consent. Top Clin Nurs 1981 Jan; 2(4):61–65

Randall AM. The nursing system—a computer challenge of the 80's! Comput Hosp 1982 May/June; 3(3): 50–53

Reeves DM and Underly NK. Computerization of nursing. Nurs Manage 1982 Aug; 13(8):50–53

Rich PL. Make the most of your charting time. Nursing '83 1983 Mar; 13(3):34–39

Romano C, McCormick KA and McNeely LD. Nursing documentation: A model for a computerized data base. Adv Nurs Sci 1982 Jan; 4(2):43–56

Sherman LG. Nursing and computers: The present and implications for the future. Va Nurse 1983 Winter; 51(4): 211–216

Viers VM. Introducing nurses to computer world. Nurs Manage 1983 July; 14(7):24–25

Zielstorff RD. Nurses can affect computer systems. J Nurs Adm 1978 Mar; 8(3):49–51

Adult Physical Examination

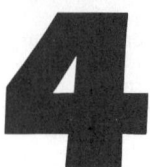

General Principles

1. A complete or partial physical examination is conducted following a careful comprehensive or problem-related history.
2. It is conducted in a quiet, well-lit room with consideration for patient privacy and comfort.

Approach to the Patient

1. When possible, begin with the patient in a sitting position, so that both front and back can be examined.
2. Completely expose the part to be examined but drape the rest of the body appropriately.
3. Conduct the examination systematically from head to foot so as not to miss observing any system or body part.
4. While examining each region, consider the underlying anatomical structures, their function, and possible abnormalities.
5. Since the body is bilaterally symmetrical, for the most part, compare findings on one side with those on the other.
6. Explain all procedures to the patient while the examination is being conducted—to avoid alarming or worrying the patient and to encourage his cooperation.

Techniques of Examination and Assessment

Use the following techniques of examination as appropriate for eliciting findings.

Inspection

1. Begins with first encounter with the patient and is the most important of all the techniques.
2. Is an organized scrutiny of the patient's behavior and body.
3. With knowledge and experience, the examiner can become highly sensitive to visual clues.
4. The examiner begins each phase of the examination by inspecting the particular part with the eyes.

Palpation

1. Involves touching the region or body part just observed and noting what the various structures feel like.
2. With experience comes the ability to distinguish variations of normal from abnormal.
3. Is performed in an organized manner from region to region.

Percussion

1. By setting underlying tissues in motion, percussion helps in determining whether the underlying tissue is air-filled, fluid-filled, or solid.

2. Audible sounds and palpable vibrations are produced, which can be distinguished by the examiner.

There are five basic notes produced by percussion, which can be distinguished by differences in the qualities of sound, pitch, duration, and intensity.

	Relative Intensity	Relative Pitch	Relative Duration	Example Location
Flatness	Soft	High	Short	Thigh
Dullness	Medium	Medium	Medium	Liver
Resonance	Loud	Low	Long	Normal lung
Hyperresonance	Very loud	Lower	Longer	Emphysematous lung
Tympany	Loud	*	*	Gastric air bubble or puffed out cheek

* Distinguished mainly by its musical timbre.
(From Bates B. A Guide to Physical Examination, 2nd. ed. Philadelphia, JB Lippincott, 1983)

3. The technique for percussion may be described as follows:
   a. Hyperextend the middle finger of your left hand, pressing the distal portion and joint firmly against the surface to be percussed.
      (1) Other fingers touching the surface will damp the sound.
      (2) Be consistent in the degree of firmness exerted by the hyperextended finger as you move it from area to area or the sound will vary.
   b. Cock the right hand at the wrist, flex the middle finger upwards, and place the forearm close to the surface to be percussed. The right hand and forearm should be as relaxed as possible.
   c. With a quick, sharp, *relaxed* wrist motion, strike the extended left middle finger with the flexed right middle finger, using the tip of the finger, not the pad. (A very short fingernail is a must!)
      Aim at the end of the extended left middle finger (just behind the nail bed) where the greatest pressure is exerted on the surface to be percussed.
   d. Lift the right middle finger rapidly to avoid damping the vibrations.
   e. The movement is at the wrist, not at the finger, elbow, or shoulder; the examiner should use the lightest touch capable of producing a clear sound.

Auscultation

1. Is a method that uses the stethoscope to augment the sense of hearing.
2. The stethoscope must be constructed well and must fit the user. Earpieces should be comfortable, the length of the tubing should be 25–38 cm. (10–15 inches), and the head should have a diaphragm and a bell.
   a. The bell is used for low-pitched sounds such as certain heart murmurs.
   b. The diaphragm screens out low-pitched sounds and is good for hearing high-frequency sounds such as breath sounds.
   c. Extraneous sounds can be produced by clothing, hair, and movement of the head of the stethoscope.

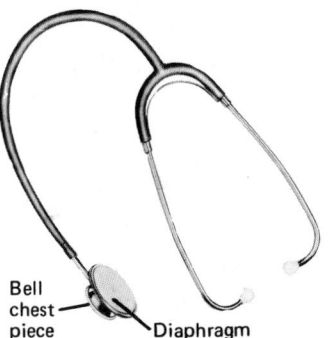

Bell chest piece — Diaphragm

Equipment

Thermometer	Cotton applicator stick
Sphygmomanometer	Stethoscope
Oto-ophthalmoscope	Reflex hammer
Flashlight	Tuning fork
Tongue depressor	Safety pin

Additional items include disposable gloves and lubricant for rectal examination and a speculum for examination of female pelvis.

| Technique | Findings |

Vital Signs

Importance—Many major therapeutic decisions are based on the vital signs; therefore, accuracy is essential.

Temperature

1. Routinely, where accuracy is not crucial, an oral temperature will suffice.
2. A rectal temperature is the most accurate.
3. Unless contraindicated (as in a patient with a severe cardiac arrhythmia), a rectal temperature is often preferred.

Temperature—may vary with the time of day.
Oral: 37°C. (98.6°F.) is considered normal. May vary from 35.8°C. to 37.3°C. (96.4°F. to 99.1°F.).
Rectal: Higher than oral by 0.4°C. to 0.5°C. (0.7°F. to 0.9°F.).

Pulse

1. Palpate the radial pulse and count for at least 30 seconds.
2. If the pulse is irregular, count for a full minute and note the number of irregular beats/minute.
3. Note whether the beat of the pulse against your finger is strong or weak, bounding or thready.

Pulse—Normal adult pulse is 60–80 beats/minute; regular in rhythm. Elasticity of the arterial walls, blood volume, and mechanical action of the heart muscle are some of the factors that affect strength of the pulse wave, which normally is full and strong.

Respiration

1. Count the number of respirations taken in 15 seconds and multiply by 4.
2. Note rhythm and depth of breathing.

Respiration—Normally 16–20 respirations/minute.

Blood Pressure

1. Measure the blood pressure in both arms.
2. Palpate the systolic pressure before using the stethoscope in order to detect an auscultatory gap.*
3. Apply cuff firmly; if too loose, it will give a falsely high reading.
4. Use cuff in appropriate size: a pediatric cuff for children; a leg cuff for obese people (see p. 380, Vascular Disorders).
5. The cuff should be approximately 2.5 cm. (1 inch) above the antecubital fossa.

Normal range
Systolic—95–140 mm. Hg.
Diastolic—60–90 mm. Hg.
A difference of 5–10 mm. Hg between arms is common.
Systolic pressure in lower extremities is usually 10 mm. Hg higher than reading in upper extremities.
Going from a recumbent to a standing position can cause the systolic pressure to fall 10–15 mm. Hg and the diastolic pressure to rise slightly (by 5 mm. Hg).

Height and Weight

Determine the patient's height and weight.

General Appearance

Begin observation on first contact with the patient (in the waiting room or while the patient is in bed); continue throughout the interview systematically—as the first step in the examination of each body part.

---

* Auscultatory gap:
1. The first sound of blood in the artery is usually followed by continuous sound until nothing is audible with the stethoscope.
2. Occasionally the sound is not continuous and there is a gap after the first sound, after which the sound of blood in the vessel is heard again.
3. If one uses only the auscultatory method and pumps the cuff up until the sound is no longer heard, it is possible, when there is a gap in the sound or when the sound is not continuous, to get a falsely low systolic reading.

Technique	Findings

Inspection

Observe for: race, sex, general physical development, nutritional state, mental alertness, evidence of pain, restlessness, body position, clothes, apparent age, hygiene, grooming.

Careful observation of the general state of the individual provides many clues about a person's body image and how he behaves and also some idea of how well or ill he is.

Skin

1. Examination of the skin is correlated with the information obtained in the history and other parts of the physical examination.
2. Examine the skin as you proceed through each body system.

Inspection

Observe for: skin color, pigmentation, lesions (distribution, type, configuration, size), jaundice, cyanosis, scars, superficial vascularity, moisture, edema, color of mucous membranes, hair distribution, nails.

1. "Normal" varies considerably depending on racial or ethnic background, exposure to sun, complexion, pigmentation tendencies (e.g., freckles).

Palpation

Examine skin for temperature, texture, elasticity, turgor.

2. The skin is normally warm, slightly moist, and smooth and returns quickly to its original shape when picked up between two fingers and released. There is a characteristic hair distribution over the body associated with gender and normal physiologic function. Nails are present and smooth and cared for in some way.

Head

Inspection

Observe for: symmetry of face, configuration of skull, hair color and distribution, scalp.

1. Normally, the skull and face are symmetrical, with distribution of hair varying from person to person. (However, determine by history if there has been any change.)

Palpation

Examine: hair texture, masses, swelling or tenderness of scalp, configuration of skull.

2. The scalp should be free of flaking, with no signs of nits (small, white louse eggs), lesions, deformities, or tenderness.

Eyes and Vision

Equipment

Ophthalmoscope

Anatomical Landmarks

Globes	Sclerae
Palpebral fissures	Pupils
Lid margins	Iris
Conjunctivae	

Eye diagram labels: Pupil, Punctum, Sclera covered by bulbar conjunctiva, Lower eyelid, Limbus (corneoscleral juncture), Iris, Upper eyelid

Inspection

1. *Globes*—for protrusion.
2. *Palpebral fissures* (longitudinal openings between the eyelids)—for width and symmetry.

2. *Palpebral fissures*—appear equal in size when the eyes are open.
   Upper lid—covers a small portion of the iris and cornea.
   Lower lid—margin is just below the junction of the cornea and sclera (limbus).
   Ptosis—drooping of eyelids.

3. *Lid margins*—for scaling, secretions, erythema, position of lashes.

3. *Lid margins*—are clear; the lacrimal duct openings (puncta) are evident at the nasal ends of the upper and lower lids.
   Eye lashes—normally are evenly distributed and turn outward.

Technique	Findings

4. *Bulbar and palpebral conjunctivae*—for congestion and color.
  Bulbar conjunctiva—membranous covering of the sclera (contains blood vessels).
  Palpebral conjunctiva—membranous covering of the inside of the upper and lower lids (contains blood vessels).
	4. *Bulbar conjunctiva* (cover of sclera)—consists of transparent, red blood vessels, which may become dilated and produce the characteristic "bloodshot" eye.
	  Palpebral conjunctivae—are pink and clear.
	  Conjunctivitis—inflammation of the conjunctival surfaces.

5. *Sclerae*—for color; *iris* for color.	5. *Sclerae*—should be white and clear.
6. *Pupils*—for size, shape, symmetry, reaction to light and accommodation (ability of the lens to adjust to objects at varying distances).	6. *Pupils*—normally constrict with increasing light and accommodation. Pupils are normally round and can range in size from very small ("pinpoint") to large (occupying the entire space of the iris).

7. *Eye movement*—extraocular movements, nystagmus, convergence.
  (Nystagmus: rapid, lateral, horizontal or rotary movement of the eye.)
  (Convergence: ability of the eye to turn in and focus on a very close object.)
  (See neurologic examination, p. 43.)
	7. *Extraocular movement*—movement of the eyes in conjugate fashion. (Six muscles control the movement of the eye.) Eyes normally move in conjugate fashion, except when converging on an object that is moving closer.
	  Nystagmus—may be seen normally as a result of eye fatigue.
	  Convergence—fails when double vision occurs, usually 10–15 cm. (4–6 inches) from nose.

8. *Gross visual fields*—by confrontation. (See neurologic examination, p. 44.)	8. *Peripheral vision*—is full (medially and laterally, superiorly and inferiorly) in both eyes.

9. *Visual acuity*
  Check with a Snellen chart (with and without glasses).
	9. *Normal vision*—20/20.
	  Myopia—nearsightedness.
	  Hyperopia—farsightedness.

Palpation	
1. Determine strength of upper lids by attempting to open closed lids against resistance.	1. The examiner should not be able to open the lids when the patient is squeezing them shut.
2. Palpate globes through closed lids for tenderness and tension.	2. Globes normally are not tender when palpated.
Fundoscopic Examination (ends eye examination).	
1. *Red retinal reflex*—check the transparency of the anterior and posterior chambers.	1. *Red retinal reflex*—can be spotted by the examiner while standing 30 cm. (12 inches) from the eye. The anterior and posterior chambers should be transparent.
2. *Cornea*—check for transparency.	2. *Cornea*—should be transparent.
3. *Lens*—check for transparency.	3. *Lens*—should be transparent (i.e., retina can be seen).

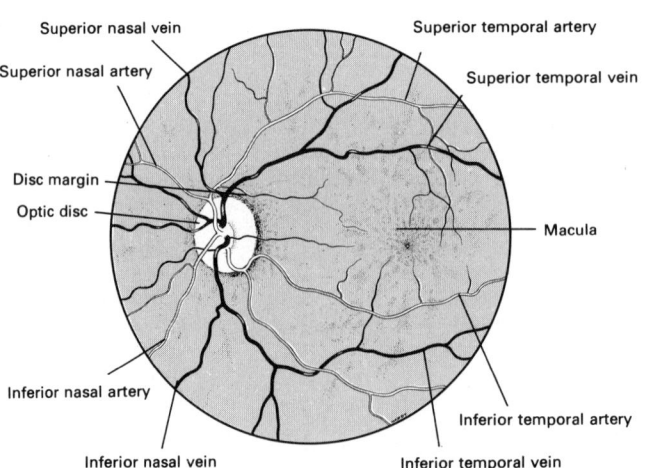

Superior nasal vein
Superior nasal artery
Disc margin
Optic disc
Inferior nasal artery
Inferior nasal vein
Superior temporal artery
Superior temporal vein
Macula
Inferior temporal artery
Inferior temporal vein

<table>
<tr><td>**Technique**</td><td>**Findings**</td></tr>
</table>

Technique	Findings
4. *Retina*—check for color, pigmentation, hemorrhages, and exudates.	4. *Retina*—color varies according to the amount of pigment present. There should be no hemorrhages or exudates.
5. *Optic disc*—check for color, distinction of margins, pigmentation, degree of elevation, cupping.	5. *Optic disc*—is circular and has a yellowish-pink color. Although disc appearance may vary, the margins are normally distinct and regular, with varying amounts of pigment.
6. *Macula*—check for color. (Lies at a distance of 2 optic disc diameters laterally from the optic disc.)	6. *Macula*—since it is free of blood vessels, it is lighter in color than the rest of the retina.
7. *Blood vessels*—check for diameter; arteriovenous (A/V) ratio; origin and course; venous-arterial crossings. (Both arteries and veins are present and move outward from the disc nasally and temporally.)	7. *Retinal arteries and veins*—arteries are approximately $\frac{4}{5}$ the size of the veins and lighter in color. Where arteries and veins cross, there is usually no disturbance in the course of either. Pulsations may occur in the vein near the optic disc.

Use of the Ophthalmoscope

1. Hold the instrument in your right hand and use your right eye to examine the patient's right eye.
   a. Reverse the procedure to examine the patient's left eye.
   b. This approach allows you to get close to the patient without bumping noses.
2. Hold the instrument so that your last 2 fingers are straight, rather than curved around the handle.
   You can place these fingers against the patient's cheek to steady the instrument and to avoid hitting the patient with it.
3. Begin the fundoscopic examination standing about 30 cm. (a foot) from the patient. The room should be darkened.
4. Turn the dial on the head of the ophthalmoscope to +8 or +10 (black numbers).
5. Turn on the ophthalmoscope light and place the eyepiece up to your eye.
   If you wear glasses or contact lenses, it is best to wear them during the examination so that you do not have to accommodate for your vision by turning the dial on the ophthalmoscope.
6. Aim the light at the pupil of the eye. You should see the red reflex immediately.
7. Slowly move in toward the patient, continuing to look through the eyepiece and keeping the light directed at the pupil, beyond which is the fundus.
8. With the index finger of the hand holding the ophthalmoscope, turn the dial toward zero as you move in.
   a. This allows you to focus on the various chambers of the eye.
   b. A way to find the eye and pupil is to put your hand on top of the patient's head and your thumb at the outer corner of the eye. If you lose the fundus, you can return to your thumb and get your bearings by moving medially from the thumb nail.
9. Once your hand is resting on the patient's cheek, continue to turn the dial until you can focus on the retina, and the blood vessels and the optic disc appear sharp.
10. Once you are focused on the optic disc, it is possible to follow the blood vessels out from the disc inferiorly and superiorly, medially and laterally. (See Chapter 15, [Eye] for visual fields, color vision tests, refraction, gonioscopy, tonometry.)

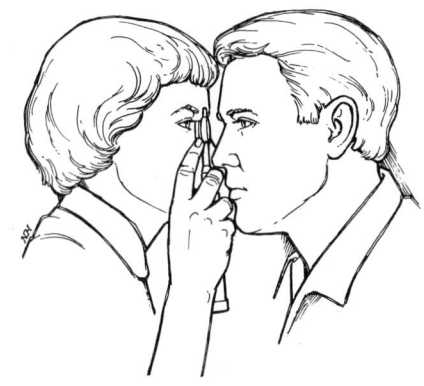

Ears and Hearing

Equipment

Tuning fork, otoscope

To Examine with Otoscope

1. Hold the helix of the ear and gently pull the pinna upward and back toward the occiput to straighten the external canal.
2. Gently insert the lighted otoscope, using an earpiece that is a comfortable size for the patient.
3. Once the otoscope is in place, put your eye up to the eyepiece and examine the external canal.

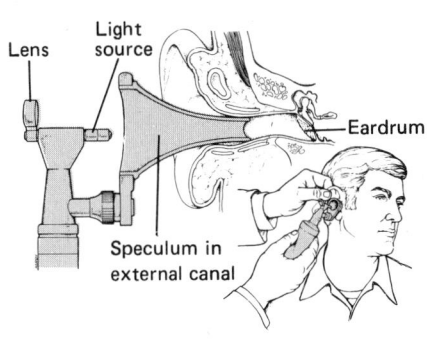

Lens   Light source   Eardrum

Speculum in external canal

Technique

Findings

Examination Techniques

Inspection

1. *Pinna*—examine for size, shape, color, lesions, masses.
2. *External canal*—examine with the otoscope for discharge, impacted cerumen, inflammation, masses, or foreign bodies.
3. *Tympanic membrane*—examine for color, luster, shape, position, transparency, integrity, and scarring.
4. *Landmarks*—note cone of light, umbo, handle and short process of the malleus, pars flaccida, and pars tensa.
    Gently move the otoscope to observe the entire drum. (Cerumen may obscure visualization of the drum.)

Palpation

Pinna—examine for tenderness, consistency of cartilage, swelling.

2. *External canal*—is normally clear with perhaps minimal cerumen.

3. *Tympanic membrane and landmarks.*

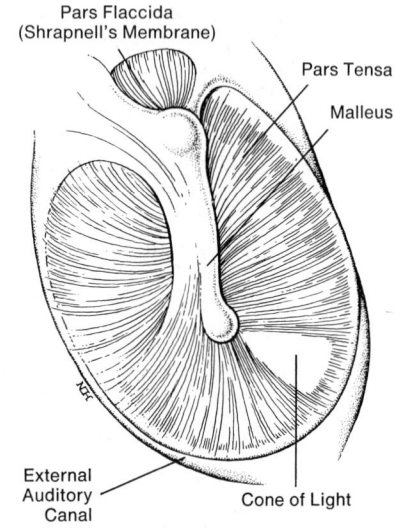

Mechanical Tests

1. Test each ear for gross hearing acuity using whispered word or watch. Cover the ear not being tested.
2. *Weber test*—test for lateralization of vibration. Place tuning fork in the center of the scalp near the forehead (*A*).
    (Also see Chapter 16 [Ear], p. 741).
3. *Rinne Test*—compares air and bone conduction.
    a. Place vibrating tuning fork on the mastoid process behind the ear and have the patient tell you when the vibration stops (*B*).
    b. Then quickly hold the buzzing end of the tuning fork *near* the ear canal and ask if patient can hear it (*C*).
    (See p. 741 for Audiogram.)

1. A person with normal hearing can hear a whispered word from approximately 4.5 meters (15 feet) and a watch from 30 cm. (12 inches). The patient should hear the sound equally well in both ears, that is, there is no lateralization.

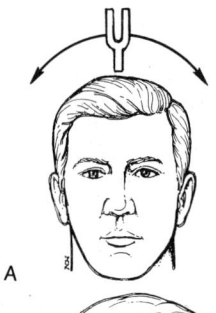

A

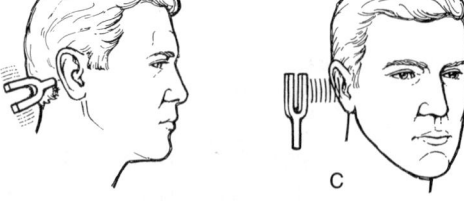

B   C

Normally, sound should be heard after vibration can no longer be felt, that is, air conduction is greater than bone conduction. Lateralization and conduction findings are altered by damage to the 8th cranial nerve and damage to the ossicles in the middle ear.

Technique	Findings

Nose and Sinuses

Equipment

Otoscope, nasal speculum

Techniques of Examination

Inspection

1. Observe for general deformity.
2. With nasal speculum (otoscope, if speculum is unavailable) examine for:
   a. Nasal septum (position and perforation).
   b. Discharge (anteriorly and posteriorly).
   c. Nasal obstruction and airway patency.
   d. Mucous membranes for color.
   e. Turbinates for color and swelling.

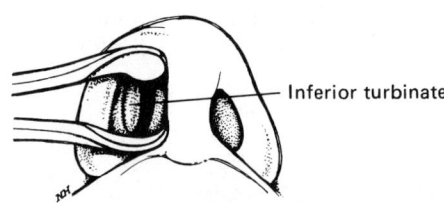

Nasal septum—is normally straight and not perforated.

Discharge—none should be present.

Airways—are patent.

Mucous membranes—are normally pink.

Turbinates—3 bony projections on each lateral wall of the nasal cavity covered with well vascularized, mucus-secreting membranes. They serve to warm the air going into the lungs and may become swollen and pale with colds and allergies.

Palpation

Sinuses (frontal and maxillary)—for tenderness.

Frontal—direct manual pressure upward toward wall of sinus. Avoid pressure on eyes.

Maxillary—with thumbs, direct pressure upward over lower edge of maxillary bones.

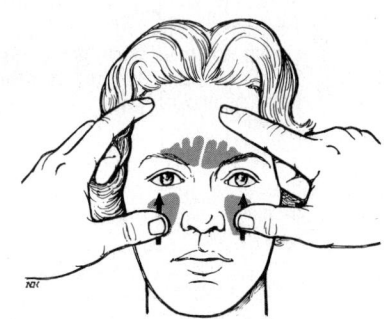

Mouth

Equipment

Flashlight, tongue depressor, gloves, gauze sponges

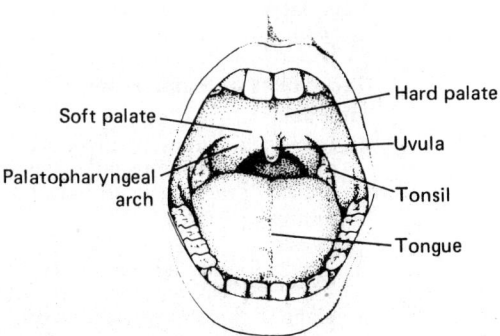

Techniques of Examination

Inspection

1. Observe lips for color, moisture, pigment, masses, ulcerations, fissures.
2. Use tonge depressor and penlight to examine:
   a. *Teeth*—number, arrangement, general condition.
   b. *Gums*—for color, texture, discharge, swelling, or retraction.

Teeth—the adult normally has 32 teeth.

Gums—commonly recede in adults.
　　—bleeding is fairly common and may result from trauma, gingival disease, or systemic problems (less common).

Technique	Findings

c. *Buccal mucosa*—for discoloration, vesicles, ulcers, masses.

d. *Pharynx*—for inflammation, exudate, and masses.

e. *Tongue* (protruded)—for size, color, thickness, lesions, moisture, symmetry, deviations from midline, fasciculations.

Tongue—is normally midline and covered with papillae, which vary in size from the tip of the tongue to the back. (The circumvallate papillae are large and posterior.)

f. *Salivary glands*—for patency.
   Parotid glands

   Sublingual and submaxillary glands.

Parotid glands—open in the buccal pouch at the level of the upper teeth halfway back.
Sublingual and submaxillary glands—open underneath the tongue.

g. *Uvula*—for symmetry when patient says "ah."

h. *Tonsils*—for size, ulceration, exudates, inflammation.

i. *Odor of breath.*

j. *Voice*—for hoarseness.

Lingual tonsils—can often be seen on the posterior portion of the tongue.
Odor of breath—may indicate dental caries.

Palpation

1. Examine oral cavity with gloved hand for masses and ulceration. Palpate beneath tongue and explore laterally the floor of the mouth (*A*).

2. Grasp tongue with gauze sponge to retract; inspect sides and undersurface of tongue and floor of mouth (*B*).

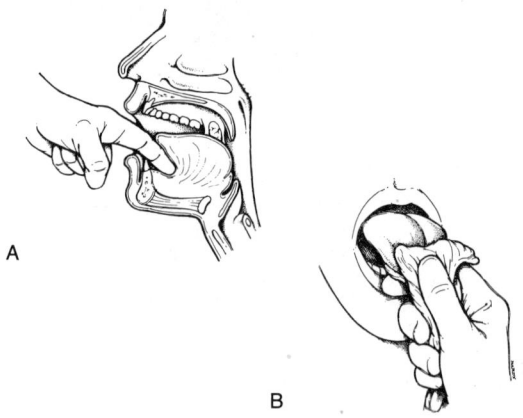

A

B

Neck

Equipment
Stethoscope

Techniques of Examination

Inspection

1. Inspect all areas of the neck anteriorly and posteriorly for muscular symmetry, masses, unusual swelling or pulsations, and range of motion.

1. *Range of motion*—normally, the chin can touch the anterior chest, the head can be extended at least 45 degrees from the vertical position and can be rotated 90 degrees from midline to side.

2. *Thyroid*—Ask the patient to swallow and observe for movement of an enlarged thyroid gland at the suprasternal notch.

2. *Thyroid*—is not usually visible, except in extremely thin persons.

3. *Muscular strength*
   a. *Cervical muscles*—have patient turn his chin forcefully against your hand.
   b. *Trapezius muscles*—exert pressure on the patient's shoulders while he shrugs his shoulders.

3. *Strength*—see Findings, 11th cranial nerve, p. 46.

4. *External jugular veins*—observe with patient sitting and then lying at 30–40 degree angle; patient's neck should not be flexed.

Jugular veins—when the patient is lying with head elevated 30–40 degrees, the jugular veins are approximately at the level of the right atrium, and pulsations that are transmitted from the right atrium can normally be seen with tangential lighting. Veins are not distended when the patient is sitting.

Technique	**Findings**

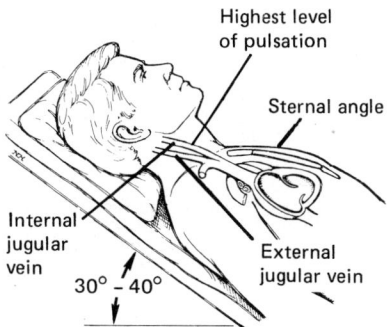

This serves as a fairly constant and therefore reliable landmark, when patient is supine or sitting, for estimating venous pressure, that is, the height in cm. measured from level of distended internal jugular veins to level of sternal angle.

Note the sternal angle, the point on the surface anatomy that is approximately 5–7 cm. (2–2.75 inches) above the right atrium.

Palpation
1. *Cervical nodes and salivary glands.*

Cervical nodes—in the adult, the cervical lymph nodes are not normally palpable unless the patient is very thin, in which case the nodes are felt as small, freely movable masses.

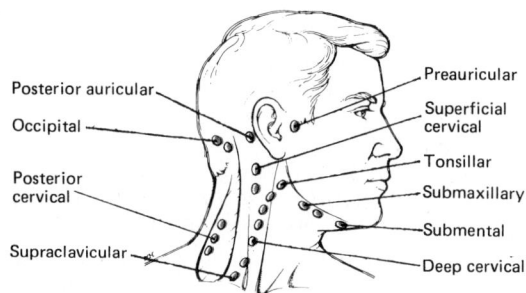

2. *Trachea*—palpate at the sternal notch. Stand behind (or in front of) patient and allow the middle finger of each hand to glide off the head of the clavicle into the sternal notch. Palpate for deviation and tracheal tug.

2. *Trachea*—should be midline.
Landmarks are easy to identify using this procedure.

This is the downward pull synchronous with cardiac pulsation, usually the result of aneurysm of aorta.

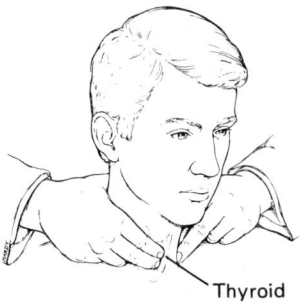

Thyroid

3. *Thyroid*
   a. Stand behind the patient and have him flex his neck to relax the cervical muscles.
   b. Place the fingertips of your left hand behind the left sternocleidomastoid muscle adjacent to the trachea just below larynx.
   c. Palpate the area over the trachea and to the left of the trachea.
   d. Note any enlargement, nodules, masses, consistency.
   e. Reverse the procedure and examine the right lobe of the thyroid.
   f. Since the thyroid gland moves upward upon swallowing, have the patient swallow to facilitate examination.

To discern the outline of the isthmus of the left lobe of the thyroid gland.

If the thyroid is palpable, it is normally smooth, without nodules, masses, or irregularities, or bruits (gushing sound produced by blood moving through a narrow vessel).

Technique Findings

4. *Carotid arteries*
   a. Palpate the carotids 1 side at a time.
   b. The carotids lie anterolaterally in the neck—avoid palpating the carotid sinuses at the level of the thyroid cartilage just below the angle of the jaw, since this may cause slowing of heart rate.
   c. Note symmetry of pulsations, strength, and amplitude.

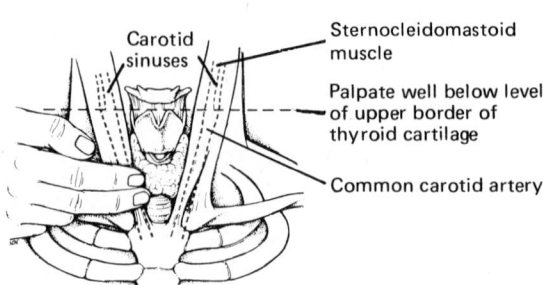

Lymph Nodes

1. It is important at some point in the examination to palpate all areas where lymphadenopathy might appear.
2. Often this is done as each region of the body is examined, for example, the cervical nodes are examined when the neck is examined.
3. However, in the record, the condition of the lymph nodes is described under a separate heading.

Techniques of Examination

Inspection

Note size, shape, mobility, consistency, tenderness, and inflammation.

Palpation

1. *Cervical, supra- and infraclavicular nodes.*

   Cervical nodes and supra- and infraclavicular nodes—are not normally palpable.

2. *Axillary nodes*

   Axillary nodes—are not normally palpable.

   a. Examine while the patient is sitting.
   b. Place the patient's arm at his side and insert the examining fingers to the apex of the patient's axilla. (Use the fingers of your right hand to examine the left axilla and vice versa.)
   c. Rotate the examining hand, so that the fingers can palpate the anterior and posterior axillary fossae pressing against the chest wall. Press against the humerus bone in the axilla to examine the lateral fossa for nodes. Conclude the axillary examination by moving the fingers from the apex of the axilla downward in the midline along the chest wall.

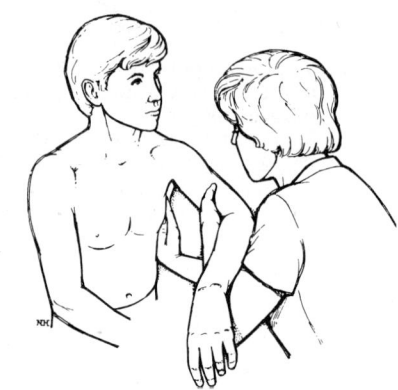

3. *Inguinal nodes*—are located in inguinal canal and are usually examined when the abdomen is examined.

   Inguinal nodes—a few may be felt, but are small, movable, and nontender.

4. *Epitrochlear nodes*—are palpated just above the olecranon process.

   Epitrochlear nodes—not usually palpable.

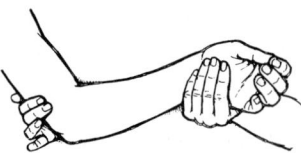

Technique

Findings

Breasts (Male and Female)

Female Breast

Inspection

(With the patient sitting, arms relaxed at sides.)

1. Inspect the areolae and nipples for position, pigmentation, inversion, discharge, crusting, and masses.

   Extra, or supernumerary, nipples may occur normally, most commonly in the anterior axillary region or just below the normal breasts.
2. Examine the breast tissue for size, shape, color, symmetry, surface, contour, skin characteristics, and level of breasts. Note any retraction or dimpling of the skin.
3. Ask the patient to elevate her hands over her head; repeat the observation.

4. Have patient press her hands to her hips; repeat the observation.

Palpation

(This is best done with the patient recumbent.)

1. The patient with pendulous breasts should be given a pillow to place under the ipsilateral scapula of the breast being palpated so that the tissue is distributed more evenly over the chest wall.
2. The arm on the side of the breast being palpated should be raised above the patient's head.
3. Palpate one breast at a time, beginning with the "asymptomatic" breast if the patient complains of symptoms.
4. To palpate, use the palmar aspects of the fingers in a rotating motion, compressing the breast tissue against the chest wall. (This is done quadrant by quadrant until the entire breast has been palpated—including the "tail" of the breast tissue which extends into the axillary region in the upper outer quadrant of the breast.)
5. Note skin texture, moisture, temperature, or masses.

6. Gently squeeze the nipple and note any expressible discharge.

7. Repeat examination on the opposite breast and compare findings.

Male Breast

Examination of the male breast can be brief and should never be omitted.

1. Observe the nipple and areola for ulceration, nodules, swelling, or discharge.
2. Palpate the areola for nodules and tenderness.

1. The *nipples* should be at the same level and protrude slightly.
   An *inverted nipple* (one that turns inward), if present since puberty, may be normal.
   A *supernumerary nipple* usually consists of a nipple and a small areola and may be mistaken for a mole.
2. *Breast size*—In the female it is not uncommon to find a difference in the size of the 2 breasts. Normal asymmetry has usually been present since puberty and is not a recent phenomenon.
3. If there is a mass attached to the pectoral muscles, contracting the muscles will cause retraction of the breast tissue.

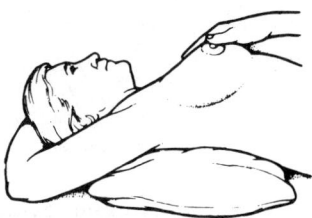

3. This allows the examiner to palpate the "normal" breast first and then compare the "symptomatic" breast to it.
4. *Breast texture*—varies according to the amount of subcutaneous tissue present.
   a. In young females, tissue is fairly soft and homogeneous; in postmenopausal women, tissue may feel nodular or stringy.
   b. Consistency also varies with menstrual cycle, being more nodular and edematous just prior to menstruation.*
5. *Masses*—If a mass is palpated, its location, size, shape, consistency, mobility, and associated tenderness are reported.
6. *Discharge*—In the normal nonpregnant or nonlactating female, there is no nipple discharge.

1. There should be no discharge.

---

 * In teaching women about breast self-examination, explain that the best time for performing the examination is a week after the menstrual period, when the breasts are least engorged and tender.

Technique   **Findings**

Thorax and Lungs

General Information

1. Methodical inspection of the thorax requires reference to established "landmarks" in order to locate specific structures and to report significant findings.
2. The same structural landmarks are used in examining both the lung and the heart.
3. It is important to visualize the underlying structures and organs when examining the thorax.

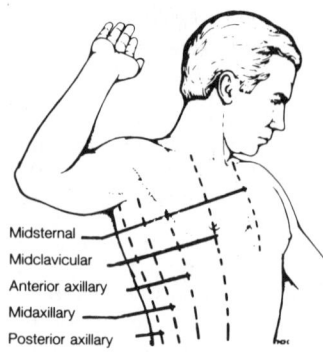

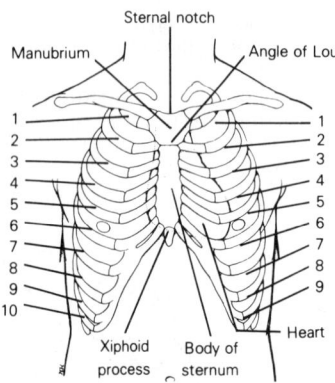

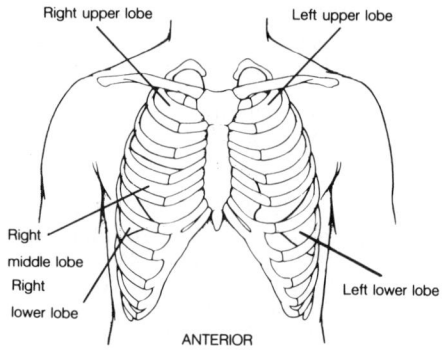

ANTERIOR

Techniques of Examination

Posterior Thorax and Lungs

Begin the examination with the patient seated; examine posterior chest and lungs.

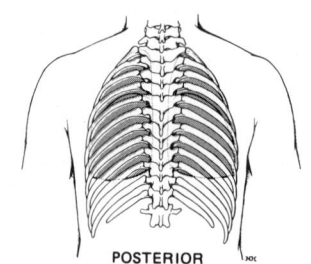

POSTERIOR

Inspection

1. Inspect the spine for mobility and any structural deformity.
2. Observe the symmetry of the posterior chest and the posture and mobility of the thorax upon respiration. (Note any bulges or retractions of the costal interspaces upon respiration or any impairment of respiratory movement.)
3. Note the anteroposterior diameter in relation to the lateral diameter of the chest.

2. The thorax is normally symmetrical; it moves easily and without impairment upon respiration. There are no bulges or retractions of the intercostal spaces.

3. The anteroposterior (AP) diameter of the thorax in relation to the lateral diameter is approximately 1:2.

Palpation

1. Palpate the posterior chest with the patient sitting; identify areas of tenderness, masses, inflammation.
2. Palpate the ribs and costal margins for symmetry, mobility, and tenderness and the spine for tenderness and vertebral position.
3. To assess respiratory excursion—place the thumbs at the level of the 10th vertebra; with hands held parallel to the 10th ribs as they grasp the lateral rib cage, ask the patient to

2. On palpation there should be no tenderness; chest movement should be symmetrical and without lag or impairment.

Technique	Findings

inhale deeply. Observe the movement of the thumbs while feeling the range, and observe the symmetry of the hands.

4. To elicit vocal and tactile *fremitus* (palpable vibrations transmitted through the broncho-pulmonary system upon speaking).
    a. Ask the patient to say "99"; palpate and compare symmetrical areas of the lungs with the ball of one hand.
    b. Note any areas of increased or decreased fremitus.
    c. If fremitus is faint, ask the patient to speak louder and in a deeper voice.

4. Posteriorly, fremitus is generally equal throughout the lung fields.
    It may be increased near the large bronchi.
    It may be decreased or absent anteriorly and posteriorly when vocal loudness is decreased, when posture is not erect, or when excessive tissue or underlying structures are present.
    One must distinguish the various normal causes of increased or decreased fremitus from the pathologic causes.

Percussion

As with palpation, the posterior chest is percussed with the patient sitting.

1. Percuss symmetrical areas, comparing sides.
2. Begin across the top of each shoulder and proceed down between the scapulae and then under the scapulae, both medially and laterally in the axillary lines.
3. Note and localize any abnormal percussion sound.
4. For diaphragmatic excursion, percuss by placing the pleximeter (stationary) finger parallel to the approximate level of the diaphragm below the right scapula.
    a. Ask the patient to inhale deeply and hold his breath; percuss downward to the point of dullness. Mark this point.
    b. Let the patient breathe normally and then ask him to exhale deeply; percuss upward from the mark to the point of resonance.

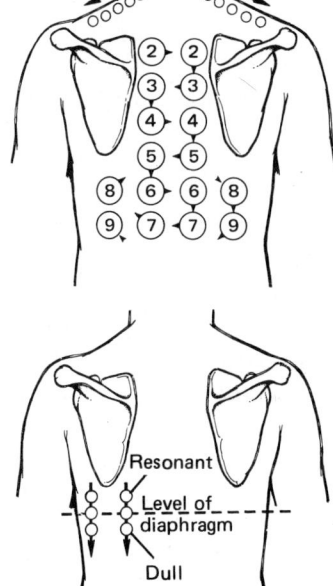

    c. Mark this point and measure between the 2 marks—normally 5–6 cm. (2–2.3 inches).
    d. Repeat this procedure medially and laterally on the right and left sides of the chest.
    The lower border of the lungs on normal respiration is approximately at the level of the 10th thoracic spinous process.

Percussion normally reveals resonance over symmetrical areas of the lung.
Percussion sound may be altered by poor posture and/or presence of excessive tissue.

Auscultation

Aids in assessing air flow through the lungs, the presence of fluid or mucus, and the condition of the surrounding pleural space and lungs.

1. Have patient sit erect.*
2. With a stethoscope, listen to the lungs as the patient breathes somewhat more deeply than normally with mouth open. (Let the patient pause, as needed, to avoid hyperventilation.)
3. Place the stethoscope in the same areas on the chest wall as those percussed, and listen

Breath Sounds

On auscultation, breath sounds vary according to proximity of the large bronchi.
    a. They are louder and coarser near the large bronchi and over the anterior.
    b. They are softer and much finer (vesicular) at the periphery over the alveolae.

Breath sounds also vary in duration with inspiration and expiration.

Sounds may normally decrease in obese individuals.

---

* Note: if patient is unable to sit with or without assistance for examination of the posterior chest and lungs, position the patient first on one side and then on the other as you examine the lung fields.

<table>
<tr><td>**Technique**</td><td>**Findings**</td></tr>
</table>

to a complete inspiration and expiration in each area.

4. Compare symmetrical areas methodically from the apex to the lung bases.

5. It should be possible to distinguish 3 types of normal breath sounds as indicated in the following table.

Pathology will alter the normal bronchial, bronchovesicular, and vesicular breath sounds. (Abnormal breath sounds or adventitious sounds are to be noted and localized.)

Breath Sounds	Duration of Inspiration and Expiration	Pitch of Expiration	Intensity of Expiration	Sample Location
Vesicular	Insp. > Exp.	Low	Soft	Most of lungs
Broncho-vesicular	Insp. = Exp.	Medium	Medium	Near the main stem bronchi, *i.e.,* below the clavicles and between the scapulae, especially on the right
Bronchial or tubular	Exp. > Insp.	High	Usually loud	Over the trachea

(From Bates BL. A Guide to Physical Examination, 2nd ed. Philadelphia, JB Lippincott, 1983)

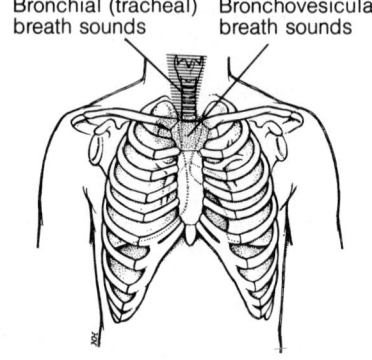
Bronchial (tracheal) breath sounds   Bronchovesicular breath sounds

Anterior Thorax and Lungs

(The patient should be recumbent with arms at sides and slightly abducted.)

Inspection

1. Inspect the chest for any structural deformity.
2. Note the width of the costal angle.

3. Observe rate and rhythm of breathing, any bulging or retraction of intercostal spaces on respiration, use of accessory muscles of respiration (sternocleidomastoid and trapezius on inspiration and abdominal muscles on expiration).

4. Note any asymmetry of chest wall movement on respiration.

Palpation

(Serves the same purposes in examining the anterior chest as in the posterior chest.)

1. To assess diaphragmatic excursion, place hands along the costal margins and note symmetry and degree of expansion as the patient inhales deeply.

2. Palpate for fremitus with the ball of the hand anteriorly and laterally.
   (Underlying structures, e.g., heart, liver, etc., may damp, or decrease, fremitus.)

3. Compare symmetrical areas.

4. If necessary, displace the female breast gently if necessary.

2. The angle at the tip of the sternum is determined by the right and left rib margins at the xiphoid process. Normally, the angle is less than 90 degrees.

3. The thorax is normally symmetrical and moves easily without impairment on respiration. There are no bulges or retractions of the intercostal spaces.

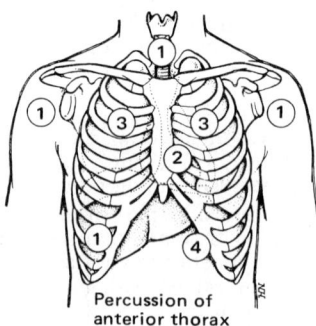
Percussion of anterior thorax

① Flat   ③ Resonant

② Dull   ④ Tympanic

Technique	Findings

Percussion

1. With patient's arms resting comfortably at his sides, examiner percusses the anterior and lateral chest.

   Begin just below the clavicles and percuss downward from one interspace to the next, comparing the sound from the interspace on one side with that of the contralateral interspace.

2. Displace the female breast, so that breast tissue does not damp the vibration. Continue downward, noting the intercostal space where hepatic dullness is percussed on the right and cardiac dullness on the left.

3. Note effect of underlying structures.

2. A tympanic sound is produced over the gastric air bubble on the left somewhat lower than the point of liver dullness on the right.

3. Percussion over heart will produce a dull sound. The upper border of the liver will be percussed on the right side, producing a dull note.

Auscultation

Listen to the chest anteriorly and laterally for the distribution of resonance and any abnormal or adventitious sounds.

Heart

General Approach

1. The examiner must visualize the position of the heart under the sternum and the ribs and know certain landmarks for identification of specific structures and significant findings.

2. It is also important to identify those "areas" on the chest wall that will yield the most information initially about the function of the heart and its valves.

   a. In locating the intercostal spaces, begin by identifying the angle of Louis, which is felt as a slight ridge approximately 2.5 cm. (1 inch) below the sternal notch, where the manubrium and the body of the sternum are joined.

   b. The 2nd ribs extend to the right and left of this angle.

   c. Once the 2nd rib is located, palpate downward and obliquely away from the sternum to identify the remaining ribs and intercostal spaces.

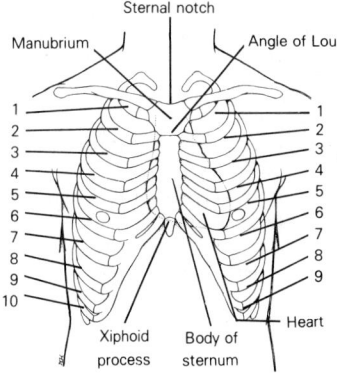

Inspection

1. Inspect the precordium for any bulging, heaving, or thrusting.

2. Look for the apical impulse approximately in the 5th or 6th intercostal space at or just medial to the midclavicular line.

3. Note any other pulsations. Tangential lighting is most helpful in detecting pulsations.

1. Normally there are no bulges.

2. An apical impulse may or may not be observable.

3. There should be no other pulsations.

Palpation

1. Use the ball of the hand to detect vibrations, or "thrills," which may be caused by murmurs. (Use the fingertips and/or palmar surface to detect pulsations.)

2. Proceed methodically through the examination so that no area is omitted. Palpate for thrills and pulsations in each area (aortic, pulmonic, tricuspid, mitral).

1. There should be no thrills or other pulsations. (Thrills are vibrations [caused by turbulence of blood moving through valves] that are transmitted through the skin—feels similar to a purring cat.)

Technique	**Findings**

a. Begin in the aortic area (2nd right intercostal space, close to the sternum) and proceed downward to the apex of the heart. (The mitral area is considered the apex of the heart.)

b. In the tricuspid area, use the palm of the hand to detect any heaving or thrusting of the precordium (tricuspid area—5th intercostal space next to the sternum).

Ordinarily, no heaving of the ventricle is felt, except, possibly, in the pregnant female.

c. In the mitral area (5th intercostal space, at or just medial to the midclavicular line) palpate for the apical beat; identify the point of maximal impulse (PMI) and note its size and force.

The apical pulse should be felt approximately in the 5th intercostal space, at or just medial to the midclavicular line. In the young, thin person, it is a sharp, quick impulse no larger than the intercostal space. In the older person, the impulse may be less sharp and quick.

Percussion

1. Outline the border of the heart or area of cardiac dullness.
   a. The left border generally does not extend beyond 4, 7, and 10 cm. left of the midsternal line in the 4th, 5th, and 6th intercostal spaces, respectively.
   b. The right border usually lies under the sternum.
2. Percuss outward from the sternum with the stationary finger parallel to the intercostal space until dullness is no longer heard. Measure the distance from the midsternal line in centimeters.

Auscultation

1. Place the stethoscope in the pulmonic or aortic area.
2. Begin by identifying the 1st (S_1) and 2nd (S_2) heart sounds.
   a. S_1 is caused by the closing of the tricuspid and mitral valves.
   b. S_2 results from the closing of the aortic and pulmonary valves.
   The 2 sounds are separated by a short systolic interval; each pair of sounds is separated from the next pair by a longer diastolic interval. Normally, 2 sounds are heard—"lub," "dub."
   a. In the aortic and pulmonic areas, S_2 is usually louder than S_1. In this way, each of the paired sounds can be distinguished from the other.
   b. In the tricuspid area, S_1 and S_2 are of almost equal intensity, and in the mitral area, S_1 is often slightly louder than S_2.

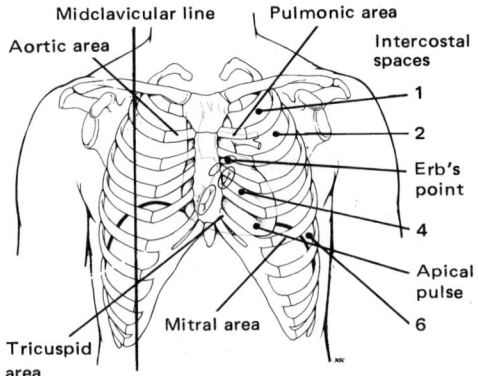

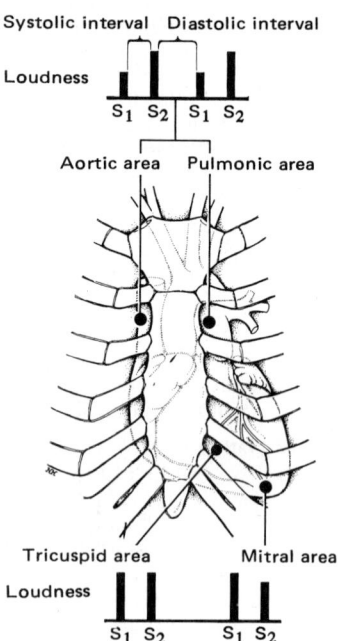

Technique	Findings
3. Once the heart sounds are identified, count the rate and note the rhythm as discussed under vital signs. If there is an irregularity, try to determine if there is any pattern to the irregularity in relation to the intervals, heart sounds, or respirations.	Normally, the heart sounds are regular, with a rate of 60–80 beats/minute (in the adult). In the athlete or jogger, the resting pulse may be between 40 and 60 beats/minute.
4. Once rate and rhythm are determined, listen in each of the 4 areas and at Erb's point (3rd left interspace, close to the sternum) systematically, first with the diaphragm (detects higher pitched sounds) and then with the bell (detects lower pitched sounds).	
a. In each area, listen to S_1 and then to S_2 for intensity and splitting.	a. Occasionally, there may be a splitting of S_2 in the pulmonary area. This is normal. Splitting of S_2 (2 contiguous sounds are heard instead of 1) is best heard at the end of inspiration, when right ventricular stroke volume is sufficiently increased to delay closure of the pulmonic valve *slightly* behind closure of the aortic valve.
b. Listen to the intervals 1 at a time and note any extra sounds or murmurs.	b. There are usually no extra sounds.

Peripheral Circulation

Jugular Veins

Evaluation of jugular venous distention is most useful in patients with suspected compromise of cardiac function.

Inspection

1. Inspect neck for internal jugular venous pulsations.	1. Jugular venous pulsations can be distinguished from carotid pulsations by the following chart:

Internal Jugular Pulsations	Carotid Pulsations
Rarely palpable	Palpable
Soft, undulating quality, usually with 2 or 3 outward components (a, c, and v waves)	A more vigorous thrust with a single outward component
Pulsation eliminated by light pressure on the vein just above the sternal end of the clavicle	Pulsation not eliminated
Level of pulsation usually descends with inspiration	Pulsation not affected by inspiration
Pulsations vary with position	Pulsations are unchanged by position

(From Bates B. A Guide to Physical Examination, 2nd ed. Philadelphia, JB Lippincott, 1983)

2. Identify the highest point at which the pulsations can be seen and measure the vertical line between the point and the sternal angle. With the head raised to 45 degrees, the internal jugular venous pulsations should not be visible above 3 cm. (1.18 inch).

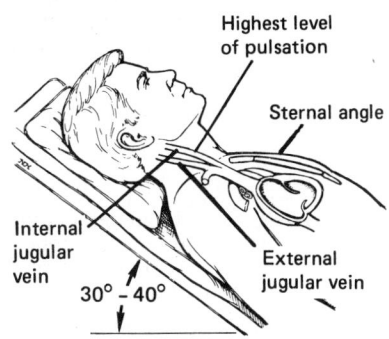

Highest level of pulsation
Sternal angle
Internal jugular vein
External jugular vein
30° – 40°

Technique	Findings

Extremities

Inspection

1. Observe skin over extremities for color, pallor, rubor, hair distribution.
2. Inspect for any superficial vessels.

1. Extremities should be symmetrically even in color, warmth, and moisture, without swelling. Swelling of feet may occur after prolonged standing or sitting, but will disappear readily when extremity is elevated.

Palpation

1. Note temperature of skin over extremities, comparing one side to the other.
2. Palpate pulses (radial, femoral, posterior tibial, dorsalis pedis), comparing symmetry from side to side.

2. There should be no arterial bruits.

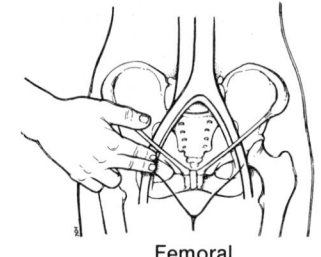

Radial and ulnar   Femoral

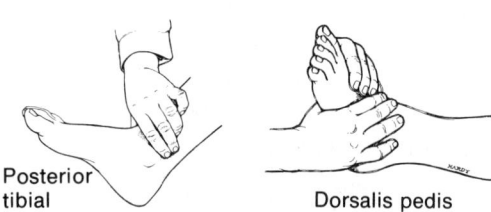

Posterior tibial   Dorsalis pedis

3. Palpate skin over the tibia for edema by pressing skin between thumb and index finger for 30 seconds to 1 minute.
   Then run pads of fingers over the area pressed and note indentation.
   If indentation is noted, repeat procedure, moving up the extremity, and note the point at which no more swelling is present.

3. Edema is usually graded from trace to 3+ or 4+ pitting (note scale used when recording data). Trace is a slight indentation that disappears in a short time. Grade 3+ or 4+, depending on the scale, is *deep* pitting that does not disappear readily. At best, these are subjective measurements, which are tried and confirmed through practice and comparison of findings with associates.

Abdomen

General Approach

1. Be sure the patient has an empty bladder.
2. The patient should be lying comfortably with arms at the side. Often, bending the knees slightly will help to relax the abdominal muscles and make palpation easier.
3. Expose the abdomen fully. Make sure your hands and the stethoscope diaphragm are warm.
4. Be methodical in visualizing the underlying organs as you inspect, auscultate, percuss, and palpate each quadrant or region of the abdomen.

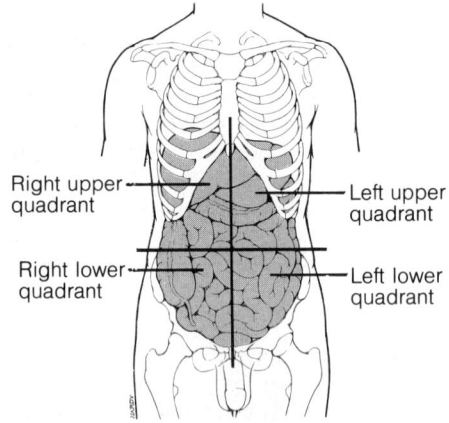

Right upper quadrant   Left upper quadrant

Right lower quadrant   Left lower quadrant

Inspection

1. Observe the general contour of the abdomen (flat, protuberant, scaphoid, or concave; local bulges). Also note symmetry, visible peristalsis, aortic pulsations.
2. Check the umbilicus for contour or hernia and the skin for rashes, striae, and scars.

The abdomen may or may not have any scars and should be flat or slightly rounded in the nonobese person.

Technique	Findings

Auscultation

1. This is done before percussion and palpation, since the latter may alter the character of bowel sounds.
2. Note the frequency and character of bowel sounds (pitch, duration).
3. Listen over the aorta and renal arteries (either side of the umbilicus) for bruits.

2. Anywhere from 5–35 bowel sounds/minute. May have familiar sound of "growling."
3. There should be no bruits or rubs.

Percussion

1. Percussion provides a general orientation to the abdomen.
2. Proceed methodically from quadrant to quadrant, noting tympany and dullness.
3. In right upper quadrant (RUQ) in the midclavicular line, percuss the borders of the liver.
   a. Begin at a point of tympany in the midclavicular line of the right lower quadrant (RLQ) and percuss upward to the point of dullness (the lower liver border); mark the point.
   b. Percuss downward from the point of lung resonance above the RUQ to the point of dullness (the upper border of the liver); mark the point.
   c. Measure in centimeters the distance between the 2 marks in the midclavicular line (the liver span).
   d. Tympany of the gastric air bubble can be percussed in the left upper quadrant (LUQ) over the anterior lower border of the rib cage.

2. Tympany should predominate.

3. Percussion of the liver should help guide subsequent palpation. The liver border in the midclavicular line should normally range from 6–12 cm. (2.3–4.6 inches).

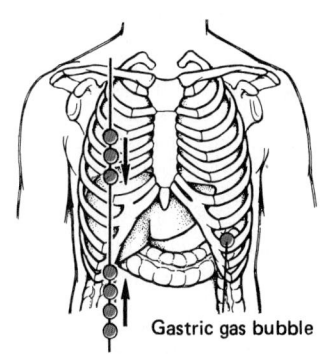

Gastric gas bubble

Midclavicular line

Kidney

1. Next palpate for the left and right kidneys.
2. Place the left hand under the patient's back between the rib cage and the iliac crest.
3. Support the patient while you palpate the abdomen with the right palmar surface of the fingers facing the left side of the body.
4. Palpate by bringing the left and right hands together as much as possible slightly below the level of the umbilicus on right and left.

4. The kidney is usually felt only in persons with very relaxed abdominal muscles (the very young, the aged, multiparous women). The right kidney is slightly lower than the left. The kidney is felt as a solid, firm, smooth elastic mass.

5. If the kidney is felt, describe its size and shape, and any tenderness.
6. Costal vertebral angle (CVA) tenderness is palpated with the patient sitting—usually during the examination of the posterior chest. Locate the CVA in the flank region and strike firmly with the ulnar surface of your hand. Note any tenderness over the area.

6. There should be no CVA tenderness.

Aorta

1. Next, palpate for the aorta with the thumb and index finger.

The aorta is soft and pulsatile.

Technique	Findings

2. Press deeply in the epigastric region (roughly in the midline) and feel with the fingers for pulsations, as well as for the contour of the aorta.

Other Findings

1. Palpation of the RLQ may reveal the part of the bowel called the cecum.
2. The sigmoid colon may be palpated in the LLQ.
3. The inguinal and femoral areas should be palpated bilaterally for lymph nodes.

1. The cecum will be soft.
2. The sigmoid colon is rope-like and vertical and, if filled with feces, may be quite firm.
3. Often small inguinal nodes are present; they are nontender, freely movable, and firm.

Male Genitalia and Hernias

This part of the examination, especially for hernias, is best done with the patient standing. (A *hernia* is the protrusion of a portion of the intestine through an abnormal opening.)

1. Drape the patient's chest and abdomen.
2. Expose the groin and genitalia.

Inspection

1. Inspect the pubic hair distribution and the skin of the penis.
2. Retract or have the patient retract the foreskin, if present.
3. Observe the glans penis and the urethral meatus. Note any ulcers, masses, or scars.
4. Note the location of the urethral meatus and any discharge.

5. Observe the skin of the scrotum for ulcers, masses, redness, or swelling. Note size, contour, and symmetry. Lift the scrotum to inspect the posterior surface.
6. Inspect the inguinal areas and groin for bulges (without and with the patient bearing down—as though having a bowel movement).

2. The foreskin of the penis, if present, should be easily retractable.
3. The skin of the glans penis is smooth, without ulceration.
4. The urethral meatus normally is located ventrally on the end of the penis. Normally, there is no discharge from the urethra.
5. The scrotum descends approximately 4 cm. (1.5 inches) in the adult; the left side is often larger than the right side.

Palpation

Use gloves if there are any inflammatory lesions present.

1. Palpate any lesions, nodules, or masses, noting tenderness, contour, size, and induration. Palpate the shaft of the penis for any induration (firmness in relation to surrounding tissues).
2. Palpate each testis and epididymis separately between the thumb and first 2 fingers, noting size, shape, consistency, and undue tenderness (pressure on the testis normally produces pain).
3. Also palpate the spermatic cord, including the vas deferens within the cord, from the testis to the inguinal ring. Note any nodules or tenderness.
4. Palpate for inguinal hernias, using the left hand to examine the patient's left side and the right hand to examine the patient's right side.
   a. Insert the right index finger laterally, in-

2. The testes are usually rubbery and of equal size. The epididymis is located posterolaterally on each testis and is most easily palpable on the superior portion of the testis.

4. Normally, there is no palpable herniating mass in the inguinal area.

Technique	Findings

vaginating the scrotal sac to the external inguinal ring.

b. If the external ring is large enough, insert the finger along the inguinal canal toward the internal ring and ask the patient to strain down, noting any mass that touches the finger.

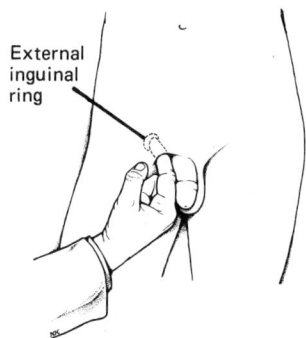

External inguinal ring

5. Also palpate the anterior thigh for a herniating mass in the femoral canal. Ask patient to strain down. (Femoral canal—not palpable, but is a potential opening in the anterior thigh, medial to the femoral artery below the inguinal ligament.)

5. Ordinarily, there is no palpable mass in the femoral area.

Female Genitalia

Equipment

Disposable gloves, lubricant, speculum of appropriate size, excellent direct lighting, cervical scraper, glass slide, fluid for fixing Papanicolaou smear, cotton tip applicator

General Approach

1. The patient's bladder should be empty.
2. The patient should lie in the lithotomy position with her buttocks extending slightly over the end of the examining table.
3. Her thighs are flexed and abducted; her feet are in the stirrups.
4. Her arms are at her side or crossed over her chest.
5. If a male is performing the examination, a female attendant must be present.
6. The examination will be most successful if the patient is relaxed. This can best be accomplished by draping the patient well so that the drape extends over the knees.
7. Explain each step of the procedure and avoid any quick, unexpected movements.
8. Be sure that your hands and the speculum are warm.

Inspection and Palpation

(These are performed almost simultaneously through the course of the examination.)

1. Begin with inspection of the pubic hair distribution.

1. Normally, the pubic hair is distributed in an inverted triangle over the symphysis pubis.

2. Inspect the labia majora, the mons pubis, and the perineum (tissue between the anus and the vaginal opening).

2. In the virgin, the labia majora are full and rounded. They become thinner in older and multiparous women.

3. With gloved hand, separate the labia majora and inspect the clitoris, urethral meatus, and vaginal opening. Note skin color, ulcerations, nodules, discharge, or swelling.

3. The labia minora and the prepuce around the clitoris are pinkish.

4. Note the area of the Skene's and Bartholin's glands. If there is any history of swelling of the latter, palpate the glands by placing the index finger in the vagina at the posterior end of the opening and the thumb outside the posterior portion of the vagina. Palpate between the finger and thumb for nodules, tenderness, or swelling. Repeat on each side of the posterior vaginal opening.

4. The hymen, or membranous fold that may partially occlude the vaginal opening, may or may not be present.

<table>
<tr><td align="center">**Technique**</td><td align="center">**Findings**</td></tr>
</table>

Speculum Examination

1. Have the appropriate size speculum available and lubricated with warm water. (Other lubricants may interfere with cytologic studies.)

2. Begin by inserting the first 2 fingers of the gloved hand into the vagina; locate the cervix, noting the angle of the fingers and the distance from the vaginal opening to the cervix.

3. Proceed by removing the 2 fingers to the edge of the vaginal opening. Press the 2 fingers downward against the perineum. Take the speculum in your other hand and, with the blades closed and held obliquely, guide the speculum past the 2 gloved fingers while exerting pressure downward. (This avoids putting painful pressure on the anterior urethral structures.) Avoid pinching the vagina with the speculum.

4. Once the speculum is inserted, remove the gloved fingers from the introitus (vaginal opening) and return the speculum blades to a horizontal position, maintaining pressure posteriorly.

5. Next, open the speculum blades and, with direct light, visualize the cervix. Maneuver the speculum, so that the cervix comes into full view.
(The cervix lies within the *fornix,* or posterior portion of the vagina, dividing the fornix into the anterior, posterior, right, and left fornices.)

6. Inspect the cervix and its opening (os), noting position, color, and shape of the os, ulceration, nodules, bleeding, and discharge. (For Papanicolaou smear, see page 564).

7. As you slowly pull the speculum out of the vagina, inspect the vaginal mucosa for color, inflammation, ulcers, masses, or discharge.

8. Close the blades before reaching the introitus, and remove the speculum without pinching the vaginal wall. (Also see Guidelines in Chap. 12, p. 564).

2. Normally, the uterus is positioned forward with the cervix at almost a right angle to the vagina.

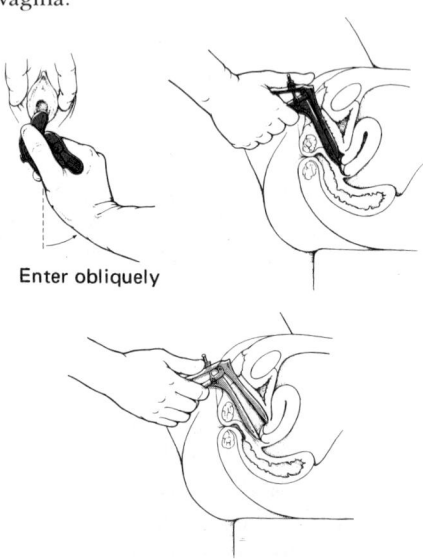

Enter obliquely

6. The cervix of the nonpregnant woman is pink and smooth.

7. A small amount of clear lubricating mucus is normal in the vagina. Normally, there is no bleeding from the nonmenstruating female.

Palpation (Bimanual Examination)

1. Lubricate the index and middle fingers of the gloved hand and insert them into the vagina, noting nodules, masses, or irregularities anteriorly and posteriorly.

2. Locate the cervix and fornices and note tenderness, shape, size, consistency, regularity, and mobility of the cervix.

3. Place the gloved finger in the posterior fornix and the ungloved hand on the abdomen approximately midway between the umbilicus and the symphysis pubis.

4. Press the 2 hands toward one another and palpate the uterus, noting its size, shape, regularity, consistency, mobility and tenderness, and any masses.

5. Next, place the gloved fingers in the right lateral fornix and the ungloved hand in the right lower quadrant. Palpate the ovaries, if possible, noting shapes, sizes, consistency,

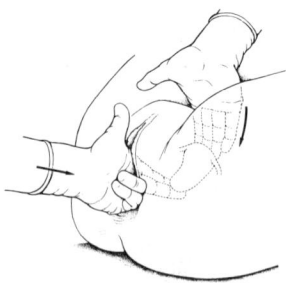

The cervix of the nonpregnant woman is smooth, firm, and slightly movable. It is nontender. The uterus is firm, smooth, and nontender.

5. The ovaries vary in size considerably, but average about $3.5 \times 2 \times 1.5$ cm. ($1.4 \times 0.8 \times 0.6$ inches). The uterine (fallopian) tubes are generally not palpable.

Technique	**Findings**

regularity, mobility, pain (the ovary is usually tender), or masses. Repeat the procedure on the left side.

6. Next, withdraw the gloved hand, leaving the index finger in the vagina and placing the middle finger in the rectum. Repeat the procedure of the bimanual examination.

6. Explain what you are doing, since this is uncomfortable for the patient and may produce the sensation of wanting to defecate.

7. If possible, press the uterus downward toward the rectal finger, so that as much of the posterior surface of the uterus as possible can be examined.

8. Proceed with the rectal examination (see below).

9. Upon completing the examination, wipe genitalia and perineum with a tissue or offer the patient one so that she may do it herself.

Rectum

Equipment
Glove, lubricant

Techniques of Examination
Male

General Approach
1. If the patient is ambulatory, have him stand and bend over the edge of the table.
2. It is also possible to examine the anus and rectum with the patient lying on his left side, knees drawn up and buttocks close to the edge of the table. (This is generally an uncomfortable position, and the patient should be told that he may feel as though he wants to move his bowels.)
3. The patient should be draped so that only his buttocks are exposed.

Inspection
Spread the buttocks and inspect the anus, perianal region, and sacral region for inflammation, nodules, scars, lesions, ulcerations, or rashes. Ask the patient to bear down; note any bulges.

In males and females, the perianal and sacrococcygeal areas are dry, with varying amounts of hair covering them. In the sacrococcygeal region, it is not uncommon to find a small opening or sinus surrounded by a tuft of hair. This is a *pilonidal cyst;* it should be nontender and noninflamed.

Palpation
1. Palpate any abnormal area noted on inspection.
2. Lubricate the index finger of the gloved hand. Rest the finger over the anus as the patient bears down and, as the sphincter relaxes, insert finger slowly into the rectum.

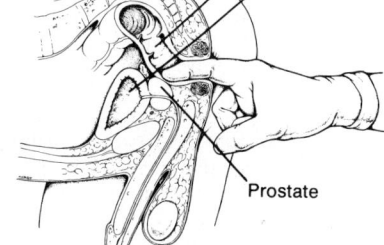

3. Note sphincter tone, any nodules or masses, or tenderness.

3. The anal canal is approximately 2.5 cm. (1 inch) long; it is bordered by the external and internal anal sphincters, which are normally firm and smooth.

4. Insert the finger further and palpate the walls of the rectum laterally and posteriorly while rotating your index finger. Note irregularities, masses, nodules, tenderness.

4. The wall of the rectum in males and females is smooth and moist.

5. Anteriorly, palpate the 2 lateral lobes of the prostate gland and its median sulcus for irregularities, nodules, swelling, or tenderness.

5. The male prostate gland is approximately 2.5 cm. (1 inch) long, smooth, regular, nonmovable, nontender, and rubbery.

<table>
<tr><td align="center">**Technique**</td><td align="center">**Findings**</td></tr>
</table>

Technique	Findings
6. If possible, palpate the superior portion of the lateral lobe, where the seminal vesicles are located. Note induration, swelling, or tenderness.	6. The seminal vesicles are generally not palpable unless swollen.
7. Just above the prostate anteriorly, the rectum lies adjacent to the peritoneal cavity. If possible, palpate this region for peritoneal masses and tenderness.	
8. Continue to insert the finger as far as possible and have the patient bear down so that more of the bowel can be palpated.	
9. Gently withdraw your finger. Any fecal material on the glove should be tested for occult blood (see p. 414).	9. There is normally no occult blood in the stools.

Female

General Approach

1. The examination is usually performed following the pelvic examination with the patient still in the lithotomy position.
2. If only the rectal examination is done, the patient may be positioned laterally, as for examination of the male.
   The lateral position permits better visualization of the sacral region.

Technique	Findings
1. The technique is basically the same for the female as for the male.	
2. Anteriorly, the cervix, and perhaps a retroverted uterus, may be felt.	2. Anteriorly, the cervix is round and smooth.

Musculoskeletal System

General Approach

1. Examine the muscles and joints, keeping in mind the structure and functions of each.
2. This discussion will center on the technique for examining the patient who is asymptomatic and, therefore, will not present in detail the techniques for inspecting and palpating joints that are symptomatic or deformed.
3. It is important to ask in the history and to note in the examination whether the patient has difficulty performing activities of daily living:
   a. Bathing
   b. Dressing (buttoning, using zippers, tying shoelaces)
   c. Combing hair
   d. Brushing teeth
   e. Walking up and down stairs
   f. Bending
   g. Sitting
   h. Grasping and holding items without dropping them
   i. Standing from a sitting position, unaided
4. Once the above facts have been ascertained, the examination proceeds. Observe and palpate joints and muscles for symmetry and then examine each joint individually as indicated.
5. The examination is performed with the joints both at rest and in motion—moving through a full range of motion; joints and supporting muscles and tissues are noted.

Inspection

Technique	Findings
1. Inspect the upper and lower extremities for size, symmetry, any deformity, and muscle mass.	For the purpose of this text, it is sufficient to say that in the course of the history and examination, the examiner should not find any compromise or restriction of the patient's activities of daily living or any other normal activities. If any activity is restricted because of muscular or skeletal problems, the reader is referred to a more detailed book on physical examination.
2. Inspect the joints for range of motion (in degrees), enlargement, redness.	
3. Note gait and posture; observe the spine for range of motion, lateral curvature, or any abnormal curvature.	
4. Observe the patient for signs of pain during the examination.	

Technique	Findings

Palpation

1. Palpate the joints of the upper and lower extremities and the neck for tenderness, swelling, temperature, and range of motion.
2. Hold the palm of the hand over the joint as it moves, or move the joint through the fullest range of motion and note any crepitation (crackling feeling within the joint).
3. Palpate the muscles for size, tone, strength, and tenderness.
4. Palpate the spine for bony deformities and crepitation. Gently hit the spine with the ulnar surface of your fist from the cervical to the lumbar region and note any pain or tenderness.

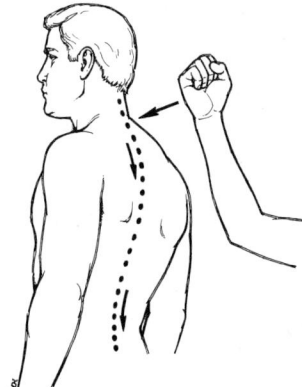

Neurologic System

Equipment

Safety pin, cotton, tuning fork, reflex hammer, flashlight, tongue blade

General Information

1. The examination described in this section is a screening neurologic examination.
   a. It is performed on individuals without specific neurologic complaints.
   b. There is a more detailed examination for patients with specific signs and symptoms.
   c. The student is referred to another text for the content and technique of a detailed neurologic examination.
2. The examination is performed with the patient in either the sitting or supine position.
3. Much of the neurologic examination can be performed as different regions of the body are being examined. This facilitates the flow of the entire examination.
   Example: The cranial nerves can be examined at the same time as the head and neck.
   A mental status evaluation can be done while the history is elicited and while the entire physical examination is performed.

Components of the Neurologic Examination

There are 6 components of the neurologic examination:
1. Mental status (cerebral function)
2. Cranial nerve function
3. Cerebellar function
4. Motor function
5. Sensory function
6. Deep tendon reflexes (DTRs)

The screening neurologic examination involves testing all of these components at least superficially. Learning these components in order will help in organizing the examination and in avoiding the omission of any part.

Basic Principles

1. Symmetry of function and findings on both sides of the body is important to note.
   Always compare one side of the body with the other side (e.g., compare degree of motor strength of the right biceps with that of the left biceps).
2. Integrating the neurologic examination into the examination of the various body regions is advisable, although the results of the neurologic findings should be recorded together as an entity.

Carrying Out the Examination

Mental Status

Components of the mental status examination include the following:
—State of consciousness (alert, somnolent, stuporous, comatose)
—Memory (short-term, long-term, intermediate)

In a screening examination, mental status is evaluated by observing the patient's affect during the history and the content of what he or she says.

Technique	Findings
—Cognition (calculations, current events) —Affect (mood) —Ideational content (hallucinations)	
1. While recording the history ask the patient for identifying information (how to spell his name, where he lives), and ask what the date is. This tests orientation.	1. Normally the individual is alert, knows who he is and where he lives, and can tell you the date.
2. The patient's ability to remember is also evaluated as the history is taken—by asking for his past medical history (long-term memory) and dietary habits: "What did you eat for breakfast?" (intermediate memory).	2. The patient remembers recent and past events consistently, and willingly admits forgetting something. Elderly people often have much better long-term memory than recent memory.
3. Cognition and ideational content are evaluated throughout the history by what the patient says and by his articulateness, consistency, and reliability in reporting events.	
4. Affect or mood is evaluated by observing the patient's verbal and nonverbal behavior in response to questions asked, to sudden noises, to interruptions—for example, does the patient laugh or smile when talking about normally sad events; is he easily startled by unexpected noises?	4. Mood should be appropriate to the content of the conversation.

Cranial Nerve Function

First (Olfactory) Nerve

(Is not usually tested unless the patient complains of a disturbance in sense of smell.)

1. The airway must be patent.
2. Occlude 1 nostril; ask the patient to close his eyes and then present various subtances to smell (e.g., coffee, tobacco). Occlude the other nostril and repeat.
3. Use substances that do not have a lingering effect.

Second (Optic) Nerve

(Includes tests of visual acuity and of gross visual fields and examination of the optic disc with a fundoscope.)

Visual acuity:

Is tested with the use of a Snellen chart (patient uses glasses if required).

1. Have the patient cover 1 eye at a time and read the smallest print possible on the chart from a distance of 6 meters (20 feet).	1. Normal vision and corrected vision should be 20/20.

Visual fields:

1. Measure by having patient cover his right eye with his right hand. (You cover your left eye with your left hand.)	
2. Stand approximately 60 cm. (2 feet) from the patient and have him fix his gaze on your nose.	
3. Bring 2 wagging fingers in from the periphery (in a plane equidistant from the patient and you) in all quadrants of the visual field and ask the patient to tell you when he sees your wagging fingers.	3. Assuming your visual fields are grossly normal, the patient and you should see the wagging fingers approximately simultaneously. (The patient's peripheral vision should approximate the examiner's, assuming that it is normal.)

Optic disc:

Is visualized as part of the fundoscopic examination (see p. 22).

Technique   **Findings**

Third (Oculomotor), **Fourth** (Trochlear),
and Sixth (Abducens) **Nerves**

(Are tested together.) These nerves control the
movements of the extraocular muscles of the
eye—the superior and inferior oblique and the
medial and lateral rectus muscles.
  The oculomotor nerve also controls pupillary
constriction.

1. Hold your index finger approximately 30 cm.
   (1 foot) from the patient's nose. Ask the
   patient to hold his head steady.
2. Ask the patient to follow your finger with his
   eyes.
3. Move your finger to the right as far as the
   patient's eye moves. Before bringing your
   finger back to the center, move it up and then
   down, so that the patient glances up and
   peripherally and then down and peripherally.
4. Repeat the test, moving your finger to the
   left.

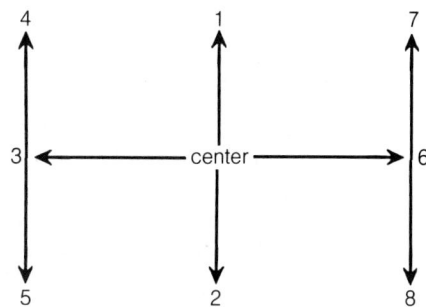

Fifth (Trigeminal) **Nerve**

(Has motor component that controls muscles of
mastication and a sensory component that controls sensations of the face.)

Motor:

1. Have the patient bite down on a tongue
   depressor with one side of his mouth while
   you try to pull the blade out.
2. Repeat the test on the other side of the mouth
   and compare muscle strength of the 2 sides.

Muscle strength in the face should be present
and should be symmetrical.

Sensory:
(Sensation to light touch.)

1. Have the patient close his eyes.
2. Touch first one side of the patient's face and
   then the other (forehead, cheek, and chin),
   asking the patient if the sensation is present
   and feels the same on both sides.
3. Sensation to pain (pinprick) is tested similarly.

Sensation should be present and symmetrical.
Always demonstrate to the patient how and with
what you are testing sensation—to avoid startling
the patient and to encourage cooperation.

Seventh (Facial) **Nerve**

(Motor function is tested by observing facial
expression and symmetry of facial movement.)
  Ask the patient to frown, close his eyes, and
  smile.

The facial muscles should look symmetrical when
the patient frowns, closes his eyes, and smiles.
Notice particularly the symmetry of the nasolabial
folds.

Eighth (Acoustic) **Nerve**

(Has 2 branches.)
  Cochlear (mediates hearing). See ear exami-
  nation, p. 23.
  Vestibular (helps control equilibrium).

Romberg test: Have the patient stand erect with
his eyes closed and feet close together.

Slight swaying may occur, but the patient should
not fall. (Stand close to the patient, so that you
can assist if he begins to fall.)

Ninth (Glossopharyngeal) **and Tenth** (Vagus) **Nerves**

(Are tested together, since both have a motor
portion innervating the pharynx.)

1. Ninth: Test the presence of the gag reflex.
2. Tenth: Ask the patient to say "ah" and observe
   the movement of the uvula and palate for
   deviation and asymmetry.

The gag reflex should be present, and there
should be no difficulty in swallowing.
The palate and uvula should move symmetrically
without deviation.

Technique

Findings

Eleventh *(Spinal Accessory)* **Nerve**
(Mediates the sternocleidomastoid and upper portion of the trapezius muscles.)
1. Ask the patient to turn his head to the side against resistance while your fingers apply pressure to the jaw.
2. Palpate the sternocleidomastoid muscle on the opposite side.

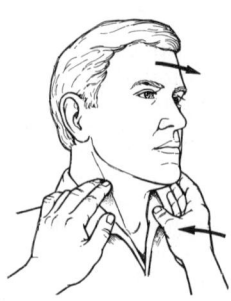

3. Then have the patient shrug his shoulders while you place your hands on his shoulders and apply slight pressure.

Neck and shoulder muscle strength should be symmetrical.

Twelfth *(Hypoglossal)* **Nerve**
(Innervates muscles of the tongue.)
Test by noting articulation and by having the patient stick out his tongue, noting any deviation or asymmetry.

The tongue should be symmetrical and should not deviate.

Cerebellar Function

(Purpose: to screen for coordination.)
1. Observe posture and gait.
2. Ask the patient to walk forward (and then backward) in a straight line.
3. To test for muscle coordination in the lower extremities, have the patient run his right heel down his left shin and vice versa.
4. To test coordination in upper extremities, have the patient close his eyes and touch his nose with his index finger (starting position: arms outstretched) first left, then right, in rapid succession.

The patient should be able to perform all the tests described with smooth, even movement and without losing balance.

The normal person can do this with rapid, smooth movements without undershooting or overshooting the target.

Motor Function

(Tested in conjunction with the skeletal system, since any bony deformity will affect motor function.)
Evaluate muscle mass, tone, strength, and any abnormal movements (tics, fasciculations, twitching).
Muscle mass: Note symmetry between sides of the body and distribution distally and proximally.
Tone: Test by noting the resistance the muscle offers to movement upon passive motion.

Muscle mass: Is usually considered in relation to sex and body build and to use of various muscle groups.
Tone: Generally there is slight resistance to passive movement of muscles as opposed to flaccidity (no resistance) or rigidity (increased muscle tone).
Strength: Will vary from person to person.

Strength:
Lower extremity—have the patient do deep knee bends; walk on his toes and then his heels; hop on 1 foot and then the other.
Upper extremity—have the patient squeeze your fingers with both hands; compare sides of the body.
Also, apply resistance (1) to the patient's outstretched arms and (2) when the patient flexes the wrist and elbow; compare sides.

Technique	Findings

Unusual muscle movements: If present, are noted both when muscle is at rest and when it is moving.

Normally, tremors, tics, or fasciculations are not present either at rest or with movement.

Sensory Function

(Should test sensitivity to light touch [cotton], pain [pinprick], vibration [tuning fork], and position.) Compare both sides of body.

Light touch:
Ask the patient to close his eyes. Brush his skin with a piece of cotton (on back of hands, forearms, upper arms, dorsal portion of foot laterally and medially; and along the tibia and thigh laterally and medially). Ask the patient to indicate when he feels the cotton and to compare the sensation bilaterally.

Pain: Use a safety pin; touch the skin as lightly as possible to elicit a sharp sensation.

Vibration sense: Test by placing a vibrating tuning fork on a bony prominence (wrist, medial and lateral malleoli). Ask the patient to tell you when he no longer feels vibration. Stop the vibration with your hand.

The patient should normally feel no vibration within a very short time.

Position sense:
1. Have the patient close his eyes.
2. Move the patient's digit (finger, great toe) up or down and ask the patient to say in what direction his finger or toe is pointing.
3. Place your thumb and index finger on either side of the digit being moved, so that the patient will not sense any pressure from your finger in the direction in which you are moving the digit.

Normally the patient can tell you without hesitation in what direction his digit is pointing.

Deep Tendon Reflexes

1. Have the patient relax; provide support for the extremity being tested.
2. Compare reflex amplitude of the same tendons on either side of the body.

Amplitude of the reflex may vary for different tendons.

Upper Extremities

Biceps:
1. Place your right thumb on the patient's right biceps tendon (located in the antecubital fossa).
2. Rest the patient's forearm on your left hand and strike your thumb with the pointed end of the hammer head. (Hold the hammer loosely, so that it pivots in your hand when it is moved with a wrist action.)

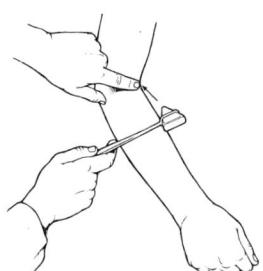

3. Strike your thumb with the least amount of pressure needed to elicit the reflex.

The forearm may move, and your thumb should feel the tendon jerk.

Triceps tendon:
1. Hold the patient's arm abducted and bent at the elbow.

Technique	**Findings**

2. Posteriorly, about 2.5 cm. (1 inch) above the olecranon process, strike the tendon directly, using the pointed end of the hammer.

The forearm should move slightly.

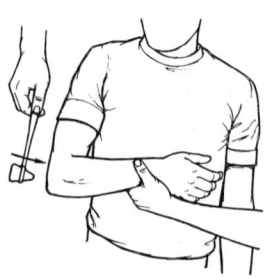

Brachioradialis tendon:

1. Strike the forearm with the hammer about 2.5 cm. (1 inch) above the wrist over the radius.
2. Be sure the forearm is supported and relaxed.

The thumb may be observed moving downward.

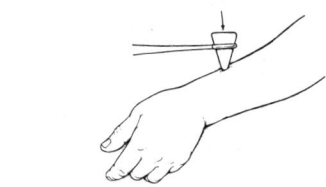

Lower Extremities

Quadriceps reflex:

1. Have the patient sitting with his legs hanging over the edge of the table or lying down while you support the legs at the knee (slightly bent).
2. Strike the tendon just below the patella.
3. If reflexes are difficult to elicit, have the patient interlace the fingers of both hands and then have him try to pull his hands apart. While he is thus distracted, inhibition of the quadriceps reflex is diminished, and the reflex can be elicited more easily. If such a distraction is used to elicit the reflex, record this fact with the physical findings.

Achilles reflex:

1. Support the foot in dorsiflexed position.
2. Tap the Achilles tendon with the hammer head.

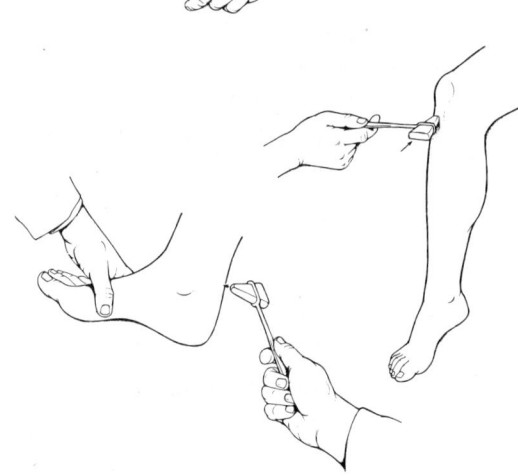

The foot should move downward into your hand.

Nutritional Assessment

Purposes

1. To determine the nutritional status of the patient, which may directly or indirectly affect his state of health.
2. To note that different populations in different geographic areas suffer from different illnesses and that these factors, along with mobility of populations, are affecting disease patterns.
3. To recognize that nutritional patterns may have lifelong effects (e.g., victims of famine in early childhood can have permanent alterations in physical size and behavior).
4. To appreciate the profound effect (catabolism) on the body from surgery, trauma, and severe infections when there is little intake of nutrients.
5. To relate the value of clinical nutrition to the whole biophysiologic and psychological make-up of the individual.
6. To refer potential nutritional problems to the nutritionist or metabolic specialist.

Types of Information Needed

Specific information about the patient's nutritional pattern and the correlation of this information with pertinent physical findings and laboratory determinations are necessary. Age and health status should already be known.

1. *Appetite*—How is it described by the patient (good, fair, poor, too good)?
2. *Weight*—Has it been stable? How has it changed?
3. *Diet*—Describe the type: regular, special. If not regular, why not? (E.g., teeth a problem, sensitive mouth?)
4. *Usual mealtimes*—How many meals a day? When? Which are heavy meals?
5. *Food preferences*—Size of servings; any imbalance such as craving for salt; prefers beef to other meats; dislikes seafood; prefers desserts but not fruit.
6. *Food dislikes*—What and why? Culture related?
7. *Usual eating places*—Home, snack shops, restaurants.
8. *Ability to eat*—Describe inabilities—dental problems; ill-fitting dentures; difficulties with chewing, swallowing.
9. *Elimination* (micturition and defecation)—Nature, frequency, problems.
10. *Exercise and physical activity*—How extensive or deficient?
11. *Psychosocial–cultural factors*—Review any having a bearing on proper nutrition.
12. *Medications*—May be obtained from nursing or medical history.
13. *Laboratory determinations*

Blood: hemoglobin	Urine: protein
hematocrit	glucose
protein	acetone
albumin	
cholesterol	

14. *Specific physical examination information*
    Height
    Weight   Desired or preferred weight
    Body type: Small   Medium   Large
15. *Anthropometric measurement**
    a. Mid-upper arm circumference (MUAC)
       (1) Locate midpoint between the acromial process of the scapula (bony protrusion on posterior of the upper shoulder) and the olecranon process of the elbow (bony point of the elbow).
       (2) Place a tape measure around the upper arm at the previously marked midpoint, tighten it snugly (do not pinch), and note the measurement in centimeters.
    b. Triceps/subscapular skin fold (TSF)
       This is an objective estimate of subcutaneous fat reserves.
       With the patient standing with left arm hanging by his side, grasp a vertical pinch of skin and subcutaneous fat about 1 cm. above the midpoint mark. Place an adipometer (caliper) over the skin fold using the left hand while the right hand maintains its grasp of the skin fold. Three readings are taken and averaged.
    c. Arm muscle circumference (AMC)
       This is determined using the above calculations in centimeters as follows:

$$AMC = MUAC - (3.14 \times TSF)$$

Method of Obtaining Data

1. Eating and food usually are topics that can be talked about easily. The items listed above under "Types of Information Needed" are readily adapted to a conversational-type interview.
2. As in all history taking, ensure the privacy of the patient. The use of the caliper in obtaining anthropometric measurements can serve as a conversation piece.
3. Be alert for questions that this assessment may stimulate in the patient.
4. After obtaining information, summarize your findings and determine the nutritional diagnosis and nutritional plan of care.

---

* Courtesy of Ross Laboratories, Columbus, OH.

Bibliography

Books

Bates B. A Guide to Physical Examination, 2nd ed. Philadelphia, JB Lippincott, 1983

Bouchier LAD and Morris JS. Clinical Skills: A System in Clinical Examination. Philadelphia, WB Saunders, 1982

Brown MS. Student Manual of Physical Examination, 2nd ed. Philadelphia, JB Lippincott, 1983

Burnside JW. Physical Diagnosis, 16th ed. Baltimore, Williams & Wilkins, 1981

DeGowin EL and DeGowin RL. Bedside Diagnostic Examination, 4th ed. New York, Macmillan, 1981

Delp MH and Manning RT. Major's Physical Diagnosis, 9th ed. Philadelphia, WB Saunders, 1981

Frantz A. The Well Adult (RN Nursing Assessment Series). Oradell, NJ, Medical Economic Books, 1982

Grimes J and Iannopollo E. Health Assessment in Nursing Practice, Monterey, CA, Wadsworth Health Sciences Division, 1982

Hillman RS et al. Clinical Skills: Interviewing, History Taking and Physical Diagnosis. New York, McGraw-Hill, 1981

Jones DA. Lepley MK and Baker BA. Health Assessment Across the Life Span. New York, McGraw-Hill, 1984

Judge RD, Zuidema GD and Fitzgerald FT. Clinical Diagnosis, 4th ed. Boston, Little, Brown & Co, 1982

Malasanos L et al. Health Assessment. St Louis, CV Mosby, 1981

Nurse's Reference Library: Assessment. Springhouse PA, Intermed Communication, 1982

Perloff JK. Physical Examination of the Heart and Circulation. Philadelphia, WB Saunders, 1982

Prior JA, Silberstein JS and Stang JM. Physical Diagnosis, 6th ed. St Louis, CV Mosby, 1981

Rudy EB and Gray VR. Handbook of Health Assessment. Bowie, MD, Robert J Brady, 1981

Sana JM and Judge RD. Physical Assessment Skills for Nursing Practice, 2nd ed. Boston, Little, Brown & Co, 1982

Seedor MM. The Physical Assessment, 2nd ed. New York, Teachers College Press, 1981

Sherman JL Jr and Fields SK. Guide to Patient Evaluation. Garden City, NY, Medical Examination Publishing Co, 1982

Swartz MH (ed). An Introduction to Physical Diagnosis. New York, Raven Press, 1981

Articles

Blackers HM et al. Evaluating sensory and motor systems. Pat Care 1983 Sept 30; 17(17):121–164

Brewer LM. The periodic health examination. Postgrad Med 1983 Nov; 74(5):125–129

Brown MS. Test your knowledge of nursing assessment. Nursing '83 1983 Oct; 13(10):81–86

Farrell J. The human side of assessment. Nursing '80 1980 Apr; 10(4):74–75

Hayden GF. Olfactory diagnosis in medicine. Postgrad Med 1980 Apr; 67(4):110–118

Hudson MF. Safeguard your elderly patient's health through accurate physical assessment. Nursing '83 1983 Nov; 13(11):58–64

King RD. A systematic plan for assessing the head and face. RN 1982 Jan; 45(1):55–58

Machenzie TB. The initial patient interview. Postgrad Med 1983 Oct; 74(4):259–265

Partridge SA. Cardiac auscultation. DCCN 1982 May–June; 1(3):152–164

Performing percussion. Nursing '83 1983 Feb; 13(2):63–64

Prager D. Evaluating the mouth and the hypopharynx during the routine physical examination. CA 1980 Nov/Dec; 30(6):322–323

Refining the chest examination. Pat Care 1982 Sept 30; 16(16):15–20

Rubin BA. Black skin. RN 1979 Mar; 42(3):31–35

Saul L. Heart sounds and common murmurs. Am J Nurs 1983 Dec; 83(12):1679–1689

Rehabilitation Concepts

5

Rehabilitation Nursing

Rehabilitation involves an active, dynamic program and learning process aimed at enabling an ill or disabled person to achieve the highest level of physical, mental, social, emotional, educational, and vocational self-sufficiency of which he is capable.

Goal of Rehabilitation

To enable an ill or disabled person to function optimally by the use of an individualized approach.

Rehabilitation Team

Rehabilitation is a creative process; it calls for a team of health care professionals working together and contributing their specialized services for a common goal for one person. In group sessions the team members evaluate the patient's progress and make necessary program changes.

1. *Patient*—key member of the health care team; he participates in goal-setting, learning, and working on his individual rehabilitation program so that he eventually can control his own life.
2. *Rehabilitation nurse*—responsible for developing a plan of patient care directed toward defined patient goals and for coordinating the actions of other team members toward these goals. Included in the rehabilitation nurse's responsibilities are the following:
   a. Prevention of complications.
   b. Restoration and maintenance of optimal physical and psychosocial health.
   c. Application of the nursing care plan, with interventions in skin care, positioning, transfer techniques, bladder and bowel management, nutrition, psychosocial support, and patient education.
3. *Physician*—makes the medical diagnosis, so that therapy can be directed toward realistic goals, designs the patient program, and directs the team.
4. *Physiatrist*—a physician who is a specialist in physical medicine and rehabilitation.

a. Tests the patient's physical functioning.
b. Determines the potential functional goal.
c. Supervises the rehabilitation program.

5. *Physical therapist*—strengthens weak muscles and prevents deformity; teaches and supervises the patient during his prescribed exercise program, teaches new ways of locomotion, transportation, and daily activities; uses physical agents and materials as aids to restoration of bodily function after illness and injury.
6. *Psychologist*—helps patient in exploring and expressing feelings about himself; assesses the patient's motivation, values, and attitude toward his disability; provides consultation about behavioral interventions that will facilitate the patient's mainstreaming back into society; helps ease the stress of staff members involved in patient care; works with the family to help them cope with problems that have arisen as a result of the patient's disability.
7. *Occupational therapist*—develops skills that can be transferred to home and work situations; devises practical projects for the patient to pursue that will develop his active participation in purposeful living and lead to the mastery of self and environment.
8. *Social worker*—investigates patient's background and socioeconomic status and assists the patient and family as the patient adjusts to home and social environments.
9. *Vocational counselor*—tests the patient to determine his interests and aptitudes, so that vocational training can be instituted.
10. *Rehabilitation engineer*—uses science and technology in designing and constructing devices that help severely and multiply handicapped persons to function despite their disabilities.
11. *Sex counselor*—is trained to diagnose and treat sexual dysfunctions of disabled persons. This role may also be assumed by a prepared health professional (social worker, nurse, psychologist).

51

Causes of Disability

Primary disability—the result of a pathologic process (congenital disorders, disease, injury).
Secondary disability—the result of either inactivity or contraindicated and injurious activity.
Disuse syndrome—disabilities due to inactivity.

Disuse Phenomena

Condition	Cause	Prevention
1. Muscle atrophy (diminution in muscle strength and size)	Lack of exercise	Exercise
2. Joint contracture (limited range of motion)	Lack of joint motion	Passive range of motion: splinting: proper positioning
3. Metabolic disturbances		
Osteoporosis	Lack of weight-bearing ability Postmenopausal problem Demineralization of bone Immobilization	Tilt table and stand-up exercises Mobilization
Urinary tract stones	Dehydration/urine concentration	High fluid intake No excess vitamins or minerals Prompt treatment of urinary infections: minimal use of catheter
4. Circulatory disturbances		
Orthostatic hypotension	Recumbent position	Tilt table and stand-up exercises
Venous thrombosis	Slowing of venous return Lack of motion in lower extremities	Change of position; exercise; elastic stockings
Hypostatic pneumonia	Poor position/prolonged rest in one position	Change of position Prone position to drain bronchial tree: exercise and deep breathing
Pressure sores	Pressure Immobility	Frequent change of position
5. Sphincter disturbances		
Urinary incontinence	Lack of opportunity	Urinal or bedpan instead of indwelling catheter Increased sensory input
Bowel incontinence/constipation	Improper diet Lack of activity Lack of opportunity	Regular bowel routine Adequate fluids; diet
6. Psychological deterioration	Inactivity Isolation Separation from accustomed environment Institutional routine	Maximum activity Active participation in goal-setting and planning own care Participation in decision making Increase sensory input; build self-esteem with meaningful activity

Psychological Reactions to a Disability

Disability has a tremendous impact on the patient's body image (physical appearance, bodily sensations, beliefs and emotions about the body). A patient with a disability has normal needs, which must sometimes be met in different ways. The mode of the patient's interpersonal relations will be altered by the changes he makes concerning his body image.

Assessment

Stages of Psychological Reaction

A. **Period of Confusion, Disorganization, and Denial**

1. Is in a state of conflict; has to cope with problems of forced dependence, with loss of self-esteem, and

with feeling that personal and family integrity are threatened.
2. Uses mechanisms of denial as a psychological defense against accepting information that is overwhelming. (Denial has a survival value.)
   a. Receives and processes only limited amounts of information; may have restricted problem-solving abilities.
   b. May have false hopes of a speedy and complete recovery.
   c. Likely to be self-centered and child-like.
   d. May attempt to remain "normal" and nondisabled.
   e. Denial is the mechanism used by those who have placed great value on strength and attractive appearance.

B. Period of Depression and/or Anxiety and Grief; a Period of Situational Reaction

1. Emotionally acknowledges losses.
2. Appears to mourn for his lost function or missing body part.
3. May have body-image distortions.
4. May be depressed because of sensory deprivation and restricted environmental stimulation.
5. Limited mobility and sensory stimulation may produce behavioral disruptions.

C. Period of Adaptation and Adjustment

1. Redirects energies toward coping with physical functioning, etc.
2. Revises his body image and modifies his former picture of himself; has a reorientation of values.
3. Accepts a degree of dependency.
4. Accepts limitations imposed by the disability.
5. Begins to develop realistic goals for the future.

Patient Problems/Nursing Diagnoses

Depression and grief related to losses
Ineffective individual coping related to effects of disability

Planning and Implementation
Nursing Interventions

1. Provide atmosphere of acceptance.
   a. Develop a trusting relationship.
   b. Use open-ended questions to elicit and clarify information.
   c. Allow open expression of feelings; assist the patient to identify sources of hostility/anger.
   d. Avoid displaying value judgments regarding the patient's feelings.
   e. Give emotional support to help patient work through shock, anger, and grief.
   f. Clarify and validate reality.
2. Determine the patient's remaining resources for maintaining an effective life-style.
   a. Find out about previous interests, values, and goals.
   b. Assist the patient in identifying positive coping patterns used in the past that can be used in present.
   c. Work with the patient, emphasizing his assets, while, at the same time, listening, encouraging, and sharing his problems and triumphs.
   d. Help the patient to think of substitutions and attaining goals of "being" (new joys, attitudes, perspectives, opportunities for fulfillment).
   e. Help the patient to think about and resume previously rewarding activities.
   f. Encourage the patient to assume increasing responsibility for his rehabilitation program.
   g. Reassure the patient that the support of other caring professionals/family/friends is available.

Evaluation

1. Works through grieving process.
   a. Uses thought-stopping techniques when grief seems intolerable.
   b. Expresses anger and frustration.
   c. Reveals less emotional lability (i.e., less frequent periods of crying).
2. Demonstrates beginning ability to cope with situation.
   a. Verbalizes feelings about disability.
   b. Verbalizes alternate methods of dealing with problems.
   c. Begins to structure a daily program.
   d. Accepts suggestions from rehabilitation personnel.
   e. Discusses the future in more optimistic terms.

Sexuality: A Part of the Rehabilitation Program

Sexuality is part of a person's self-concept and involves feelings of self-worth, acceptance, sharing, affection, and intimacy, as well as feelings of masculinity or femininity. It includes physical, psychological, emotional, and social elements and is reflected in everything a person says and does.
   The handicapped person is also a sexual human being.

Assessment

Sexual History

Includes present sexual activity, level of satisfaction, and concerns.

Patient Problem/Nursing Diagnosis

Potential for sexual dysfunction related to disability, problems in self-esteem, effects of treatment, and inability to have sexual intercourse.

Planning and Implementation
Nursing Interventions

1. Be comfortable with your own sexuality; avoid imposing your values on the patient.
2. Establish an atmosphere that is conducive to acceptance and open communication.
3. Let the patient know that sexual rehabilitation is part of the total rehabilitation program.

4. Inform the patient that there is a breadth and depth of sexual expression possible and that he/she is a person of value.
5. Recognize that feelings of warmth, approval, and friendship, as well as sharing and touching, are important.
6. Be aware that patients with long-standing disabilities may need training in communication and assertiveness skills.
7. Inform the patient of the availability of the following services:
   Social-skills training
   Sex education/counseling services (individual, couples, and family)
   Genetic/contraceptive counseling
   Sex therapy
   Reading materials; audiovisual materials
   Group discussion
8. See the bibliography at the end of this chapter. The quarterly journal, *Sexuality and Disability,* is devoted to the sexual implications of disability.

Evaluation

Expected Outcomes

Feels more positive about self.
1. Demonstrates improvement in hygiene and grooming.
2. Discusses alternate methods of sexual pleasure.
3. Expresses satisfaction over changes in social relationships.
4. Plans to join a support group.

Preventing Complications and Deformities

Deformities and complications of illness or injury can often be prevented by *frequent changes of position, proper positioning in bed, exercise, and progressive ambulation.*

Positioning

Purposes for Changing Positions

1. To prevent contractures.
2. To stimulate circulation and to help prevent thrombophlebitis, pressure sores, and edema of the extremities.
3. To promote lung expansion and drainage of respiratory secretions.
4. To relieve pressure on a body area.

Patient Self-Care Activities

After receiving positioning instructions and turning schedules, the patient is encouraged to assume increasing responsibility for his positioning program.

Principles of Body Alignment in Body Positioning

A. **Dorsal or Supine Position**
1. The head is in line with the spine, both laterally and anteroposteriorly.
2. The trunk is positioned so that flexion of the hips is minimized.
3. The arms are flexed at the elbow with the hands resting against the lateral abdomen.
4. The legs are extended in a neutral position with the toes pointed toward the ceiling.
5. The heels are suspended in a space between the mattress and the footboard.
6. Trochanter rolls are placed under the greater trochanters in the hip joint areas.

B. **Side-lying or Lateral Position**
1. The head is in line with the spine.
2. The body is in alignment and is not twisted.
3. The uppermost hip joint is slightly forward and supported by a pillow in a position of slight abduction.
4. A pillow supports the arm, which is flexed at both the elbow and shoulder joints.

C. **Prone Position**
1. The head is turned laterally and is in alignment with the rest of the body.
2. The arms are abducted and externally rotated at the shoulder joint; the elbows are flexed.
3. A small, flat support is placed under the pelvis, extending from the level of the umbilicus to the upper third of the thigh.
4. The lower extremities remain in a neutral position.
5. The toes are suspended over the edge of the mattress.

Therapeutic Exercises

Exercise involves the function of muscles, nerves, bones, and joints, as well as the cardiovascular and respiratory systems. The return of function depends on the strength of the musculature that controls the joint.

Objectives

1. To develop and retrain deficient muscles.
2. To restore as much normal movement as possible to prevent deformity.
3. To stimulate the functions of various organs and body systems.
4. To build strength and endurance.

Accomplishments of Exercise Programs

1. Maintain and build muscle strength.
2. Maintain joint function.
3. Prevent deformity.
4. Retrain for neuromuscular coordination.
5. Stimulate circulation.
6. Build tolerance and endurance.

Types of Exercises

1. Passive
2. Active assistive
3. Active
4. Resistive
5. Isometric or muscle-setting

A. **Passive**—an exercise carried out by the therapist or the nurse without assistance from the patient.

1. Purpose: to retain as much joint range of motion as possible.
   to maintain circulation.

2. Action
   a. Stabilize the proximal joint and support the distal part.
   b. Move the joint smoothly, slowly, and gently through its full range of motion (below).
   c. Avoid producing pain.

B. Active Assistive—an exercise carried out by the patient with the assistance of the therapist or the nurse.

1. Purpose: to encourage normal muscle function.
2. Action
   a. Support the distal part and encourage the patient to take the joint actively through its range of motion.
   b. Give only the amount of assistance necessary to accomplish the action.
   c. Short periods of activity are followed by adequate rest periods.

C. Active—an exercise accomplished by the patient without assistance.

1. Purpose: to increase muscle strength.
2. Action
   a. When possible, active exercise should be done against gravity.
   b. The joint is moved through the full range of motion without assistance.
   c. The patient should not substitute another joint movement for the one intended.
   d. Other active forms of exercise include turning from side to side, turning from back to abdomen, and moving up and down in bed.

D. Resistive—an active exercise carried out by the patient working against resistance produced by either manual or mechanical means.

1. Purpose: to provide resistance in order to increase muscle power.
2. Action
   a. The patient moves the joint through its range of motion while the therapist provides slight resistance at first and then progressively increases resistance.
   b. Sandbags and weights can be used and are supplied at the distal point of the involved joint.
   c. The movements should be done smoothly.

E. Isometric or Muscle-Setting—alternately contracting and relaxing a muscle while keeping the part in a fixed position. This exercise is performed by the patient.

1. Purpose: to maintain strength when a joint is immobilized.
2. Action
   a. The patient contracts or tightens the muscle as much as possible without moving the joint.
   b. He holds for several seconds, then "lets go" and relaxes.
   c. He breathes deeply during the contraction phase.

Range-of-Motion Exercises

Range of motion is the movement of a joint through its full range in all appropriate planes. It may be passive, active, or resistive.

Goals

To prevent limitation of range of motion.
To maintain function and prevent deterioration.
To maintain or increase the maximal motion of a joint.

Underlying Principles

1. Range-of-motion testing is done by the physician to determine the movement that exists at the joint areas. Testing helps set realistic and positive goals.
2. The patient's range of motion is affected by his physical condition, the disease process, and his genetic make-up.
3. Each joint of the body has a normal range of motion (Table 5-1).
4. Joints may lose their normal range of motion, stiffen, and produce a permanent disability; frequently seen in neuromuscular conditions—hemiplegia.
5. Range-of-motion exercises are individually planned, since there is wide variation in the degrees of motion of which patients of varying body builds and age-groups are capable.
6. Range-of-motion exercises should be carried out whenever there is physical inactivity, provided the patient's clinical status allows such activity.

Techniques of Range of Motion

1. Place the patient in a supine position with his arms to the side and the knees extended.
2. Hold the extremity at the joint (e.g., elbow, wrist, or knee) and move the joint smoothly, slowly, and gently through its range. If the joint is painful (as in arthritis) support the extremity in the muscular area.
3. Move each joint through its range of motion about 3 to 5 times, at least once and preferably twice daily—smoothly, rhythmically, slowly.
4. Avoid moving a joint beyond its free range of motion; avoid forcing movement. The motion should be stopped at the point of pain.
5. When painful muscle spasm is present, move the joint slowly to the point of resistance. Then exert gentle, steady pressure until the muscle relaxes.
6. Refer to the figures in Table 5-1 for joint motion.

Definitions

Abduction—movement away from the midline of the body
Adduction—movement toward the midline of the body
Flexion—bending of a joint so that the angle of the joint diminishes
Extension—the return movement from flexion; the joint angle is increased
Inversion—movement that turns the sole of the foot inward
Eversion—movement that turns the sole of the foot outward
Dorsiflexion—flexing or bending the foot toward the leg
Plantar flexion—flexing or bending the foot in the direction of the sole
Pronation—rotating the forearm so that the palm of the hand is down
Supination—rotating the forearm so that the palm of the hand is up

(*Text continues on p. 59*)

Table 5-1 **Range of Motion**

SHOULDER

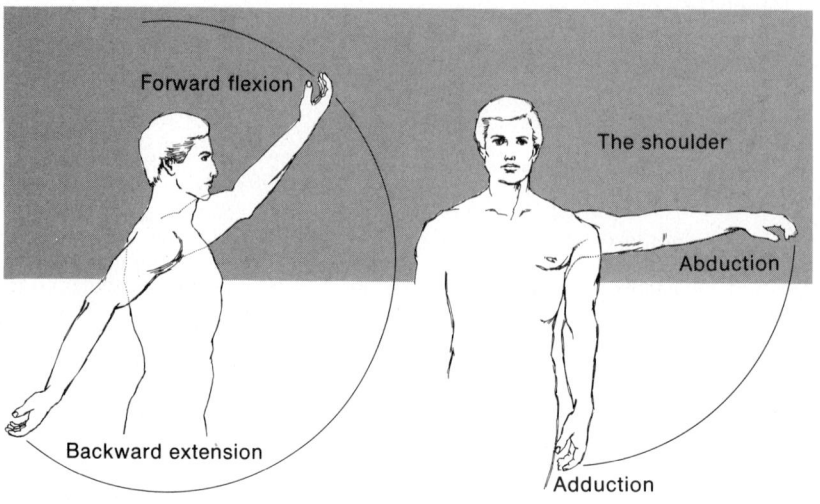

ELBOW

FOREARM

WRIST

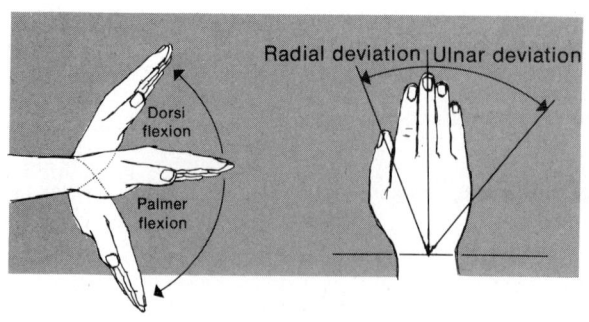

Table 5-1   Range of Motion (continued)

THUMB

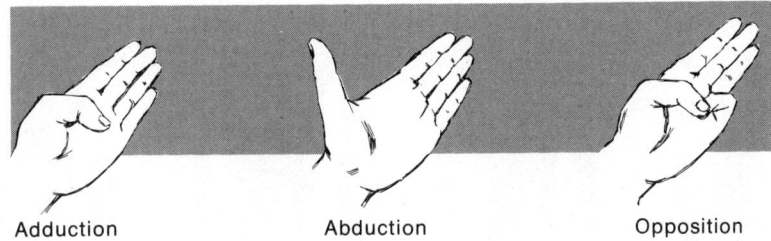

Adduction   Abduction   Opposition

FINGERS

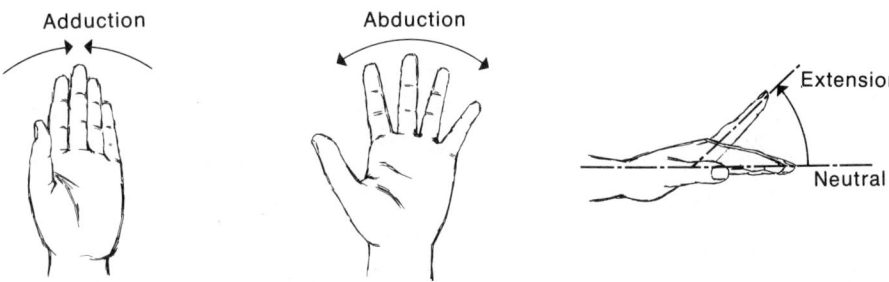

Adduction   Abduction   Extension / Neutral

ANKLE   **FOOT**

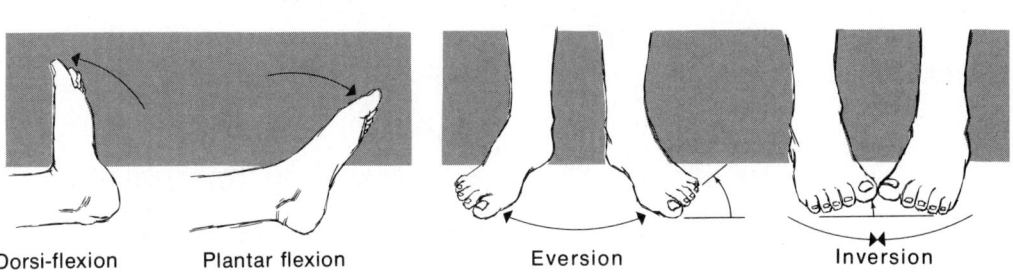

Dorsi-flexion   Plantar flexion   Eversion   Inversion

TOES

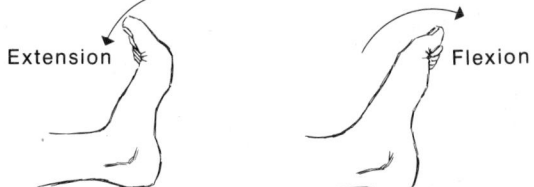

Extension   Flexion   Adduction   Abduction

Table 5-1   Range of Motion (continued)

HIP

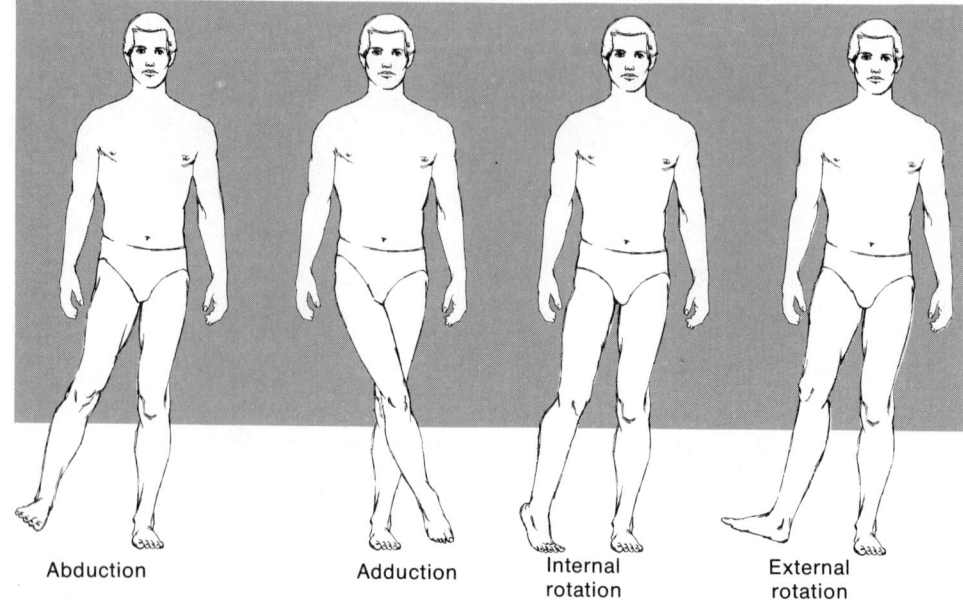

Abduction   Adduction   Internal rotation   External rotation

KNEE

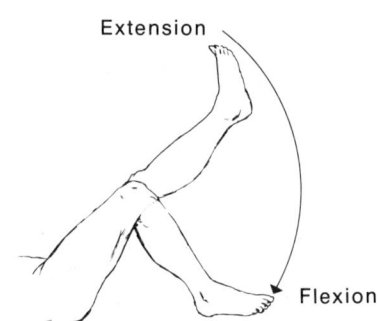

Extension

Flexion

CERVICAL SPINE

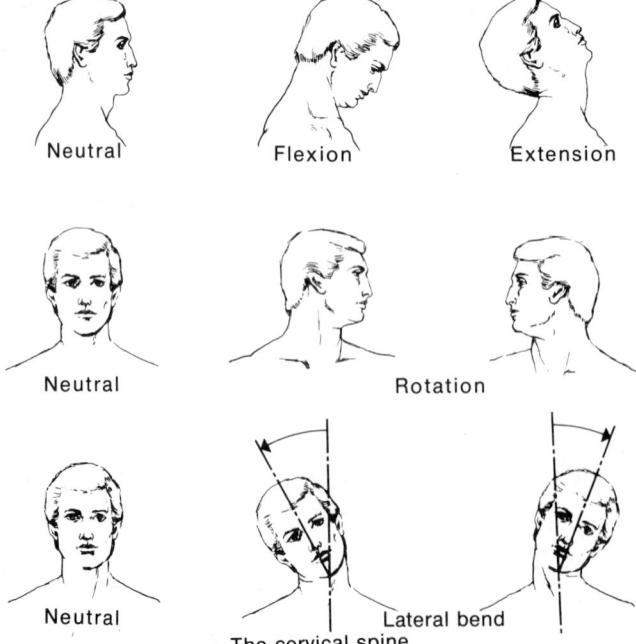

Neutral   Flexion   Extension

Neutral   Rotation

Neutral   Lateral bend

The cervical spine

Rotation—turning or movement of a part around its axis
Internal: turning inward toward the center
External: turning outward, away from the center

Preventing External Rotation of Hip

Patients on prolonged bed rest may develop external rotation deformity of the hip. The hip (being a ball-and-socket joint) has a tendency to rotate outward when the patient lies on his back.

Nursing Management

1. To prevent this deformity, use a trochanter roll extending from the crest of the ilium to the midthigh when the patient is lying on his back. A trochanter roll serves as a mechanical wedge under the projection of the greater trochanter.
2. Use a footboard when the patient is in the dorsal position.
3. To make and position a trochanter roll:
   a. Take both ends of a large Turkish towel and bring them to the center. The towel is now folded in half with the edges at the center.
   b. Turn the towel over so that the ends are facing downward.
   c. Turn the patient on his side with his upper leg flexed.
   d. Place one side of the towel in the midline of the buttock. The towel should extend from the crest of the ilium to the midthigh.
   e. Then place the patient in a dorsal position with his leg extended.
   f. Grasp the remaining side of the towel and roll inward in an underneath fashion until the entire roll is well under the patient's buttocks. The roll should be kept taut and smooth.
   g. For the larger patient, a drawsheet or a bath blanket may be used.

Preventing Footdrop

Footdrop (plantar flexion) is a deformity caused by contraction of both the gastrocnemius and the soleus muscles; it may be produced by loss of flexibility of the Achilles tendon.

Causes

1. Prolonged bed rest and lack of exercise
2. Incorrect positioning in bed
3. Weight of bedding forcing the toes into plantar flexion (ankle bends in the direction of the sole of the foot)

Clinical Problem

If footdrop continues without correction, the patient will walk on his toes without the heel of his foot touching the ground.

Nursing Management

1. Use a footboard or pillows to keep feet at right angles to the legs when the patient is lying on his back.
   a. Position the feet with the entire plantar surface firmly against the footboard.
   b. Maintain the legs in a neutral position. Use a trochanter roll.
2. Encourage the patient to flex and extend (curl and stretch) his feet and toes frequently.
3. Have the patient rotate ankles clockwise and counterclockwise several times each hour.

Preventing Pressure Sores

Pressure sores (decubitus ulcers; bedsores) are localized areas in which necrosis of skin and subcutaneous tissues have been produced by pressure.

Altered Physiology

Pressure $\rightarrow$ compression of small nutrient vessels of skin and underlying tissue $\rightarrow$ tissue anoxia and ischemia $\rightarrow$ necrosis of tissue cells $\rightarrow$ sloughing and ulceration $\rightarrow$ invasion by microorganisms $\rightarrow$ infection $\rightarrow$ sepsis $\rightarrow$ involvement of underlying fascia, muscle, and bone $\rightarrow$ rapidly irreversible condition.

Causes

A. **Pressure**—exerted on skin and subcutaneous tissues by bony prominences and by the object on which the body part rests (mattress, cast, etc.); pressure interferes with the blood supply of the tissues and, if prolonged, will cause tissue death.

B. **Contributing Factors**

1. Immobilization and lack of normal movement—from neurologic, orthopedic, circulatory inadequacies, and other conditions.
2. Friction, moisture (incontinence), and heat—irritate skin, making it less resistant to injury.
3. Shearing force—caused by gravitational forces that pull the patient's body down toward the foot of the bed and by resisting forces created by friction taking place on the skin surface.
   a. Pulls tissues so that tissues and blood vessels are stretched and injured.
   b. Occurs when the patient is pulled up in bed, is allowed to slump in the bed or chair, or moves in bed by digging heels or elbows into the mattress.
4. Sensory and motor deficits
   a. Sensory loss—produces lack of awareness of pain and pressure.
   b. Motor paralysis with associated muscular atrophy—causes lack of movement and reduction in amount of padding between overlying skin and underlying bone.
5. Circulatory deficiencies
6. Poor nutrition (obesity, underweight, protein deficiency; anemia; dehydration)—negative nitrogen, phosphorus, sulfur, and calcium balance will produce wasting of tissue, osteoporosis, and loss of weight.
   a. Anemia—may determine whether hypoxia and necrosis will occur.
   b. Hypoproteinemia
   c. Vitamin deficiencies (particularly ascorbic acid)
   d. Malabsorption syndromes
7. Edema—impairs circulation and interferes with supply of nutrients to the cells.
8. Infection—lowers resistance of skin to breakdown; destroys tissue.
9. Advancing age and debilitation—may cause changes in skin from reduced production of sebum.
10. Equipment—traction, casts, restraints, improper bedding and seats.

Sites (See Fig. 5-1)

A. **Weight-bearing bony prominences covered only by skin and small amounts of subcutaneous fat**—75% of all pressure sores located at such sites.

1. Ischial tuberosities—especially in patients who sit for prolonged periods.

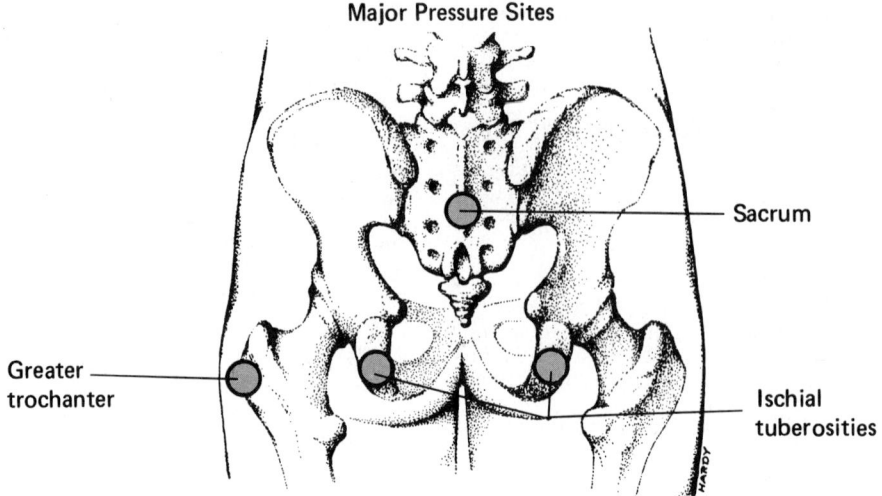

Figure 5-1. Sites of pressure sores.

2. Trochanters
3. Sacrum
B. Other bony prominences—knees, malleoli, heels, and elbows.

Assessment
Clinical Manifestations

1. Redness (a danger sign); redness will blanch on pressure; skin temperature is increased because of vasodilatation.
2. Dusky, cyanotic blue-gray area (fails to blanch on pressure)—shows capillary occlusion and subcutaneous weakening.
3. Vesiculation (blistering)
4. Break in skin, progressing to deep, penetrating necrosis; may involve deeper soft tissues, bursae, muscles, tendons, bone and/or joints.

Nursing Assessment

1. Inspect each pressure area for erythema.
   a. Press on the area; look for blanching; redness that does not disappear when finger pressure is applied indicates impending ulcer formation.
   b. Note how long hyperemia persists following removal of pressure.
2. Inspect for dry skin, moist skin, and breaks in the skin.
3. Palpate for warmth.
   Is the skin temperature increased? Compare with other parts of the body.
4. Palpate the peripheral pulses to evaluate circulatory status.
5. Take the patient's temperature; pressure sores cause fever of unknown origin in the elderly.
6. Check the patient's record for hematocrit, hemoglobin, and serum albumin levels.

Diagnostic Evaluation

Sinography, direct magnification radiography, and computerized tomography—useful in detecting sinus tracts/bony involvement.

Patient Problem/Nursing Diagnosis

Potential impairment of skin integrity related to pressure.

Planning and Implementation
Nursing Interventions

A. Relieving or removing pressure to prevent occurrence of pressure sore

1. Recognize those patients in whom pressure sores are likely to develop. *Pressure sores may appear in a matter of hours.*
2. Relieve pressure by encouraging the patient to keep active.
   a. Set up and adhere to a turning schedule.
   b. Turn the patient hourly or at 2-hour intervals—shifting of weight allows blood to flow back into tissues and helps tissues to recover from pressure.
   c. Position the patient on all four sides (laterally, prone, dorsally) in sequence unless contraindicated.
3. Avoid shearing forces and friction.
   a. Avoid elevating head of bed more than 30 degrees—to reduce shearing forces.
   b. Avoid placing the patient in semi-recumbent positions; discourage activities that increase exposure to shearing forces.
      (1) Use good transfer techniques to reduce friction and consequent loss of epidermis.
      (2) Roll and lift the patient; do not slide or pull body across supporting surface.
      (3) Use turning sheets.
      (4) Employ heel and elbow protectors.
   c. Avoid the use of rubber rings or doughnuts—they merely increase pressure around bony prominences.
   d. Keep the foundation sheet dry and tightly stretched to prevent wrinkles.
4. Position the patient with pillows, pads, etc. to relieve pressure.
5. Use devices to support specific areas of the body; the supporting medium should mold to the patient to ensure uniformly distributed pressure and should allow evaporation of perspiration.
   a. Gel-type flotation pad—reduces pressure, since the gel-like material (similar in consistency to human adipose tissue) ''gives'' with the patient's weight.

b. Fleeces (synthetic; wool)—softness and resilience of padding provides resistance to shear and results in even distribution of pressure; provides freedom from wrinkles and friction, and dissipation and absorption of moisture.

c. Fluid-supported mattresses (waterbeds) and fluid-supported seats—eliminates pressure points; as the body sinks into the fluid, additional surface area becomes available for weight-bearing, thereby further decreasing body weight per unit area.

6. Use of an alternating pressure mattress or alternating pressure chair—alternating inflation and deflation of pad produces constriction of vessels followed by dilation of superficial blood vessels of the skin; pressure on any one part is reduced, and blood supply is increased.

7. Relieve pressure over bony prominences by correct positioning with pillows and bridging techniques.

8. Relieve pressure on bony prominences of patients sitting in wheelchairs for prolonged periods.

a. Have wheelchair cushions fitted and adjusted on an individualized basis, using pressure-measurement techniques as a guide to selection and fitting.

b. Teach the paraplegic patient to raise himself from his wheelchair for a few seconds every 20–30 minutes for intermittent relief of pressure from ischial tuberosities and prevention of ischial pressure sores.

c. Adjust foot rests, etc., so that body weight is distributed evenly over the thighs and buttocks.

d. Have the patient wear shoes when in a wheelchair.

9. Inspect, adjust, and pad casts, braces, splints, and compression bandages.

B. Maintaining skin in a clean and healthy condition

1. Inspect the skin frequently for signs of pressure—especially for redness over bony prominences.

a. Teach the patient to use a mirror for inspecting posterior areas if he is paraplegic or has another neuromuscular disorder.

b. Massage and stroke lightly around bony prominences (only if tissue damage is not present)—promotes venous return, reduces edema, and increases vascular tone.

c. Keep the patient's weight off any reddened area until it has completely cleared.

2. Maintain meticulous skin hygiene.

a. Inspect the skin several times daily, especially if an area is prone to breakdown or if a new activity/circumstance arises that increases the risk of pressure sore formation.

b. Wash the skin with mild soap, rinse, and *blot* dry with a soft towel.

c. Keep local areas dry, clean, and free of body waste material.

d. Lubricate the skin with a bland lotion to keep the skin soft and pliable. Be sure the lotion is rubbed into the skin around the coccyx and buttocks.

e. Avoid placing the patient on a poorly ventilated mattress that is covered with plastic or impermeable material.

3. Employ active and passive exercises—to improve muscular, skin, and vascular tone.

4. Employ bladder and bowel programs in incontinent patient to prevent skin soilage.

5. Ambulate or use a tilt table whenever possible—the degree of mobility is an important criterion for prognosis and treatment.

C. Ensuring optimal nutrition

1. Improve nutritional status and maintain a positive nitrogen balance—pressure sores develop more quickly and are more resistant to treatment in patients suffering from nutritional disorders.

a. High-protein diet—adequate protein reserves are necessary to maintain tissue vitality.

b. Vitamins and protein supplements

c. Iron preparations and transfusions of whole blood—hemoglobin level is a critical factor in the development of pressure sores.

d. Zinc supplements (improve appetite and increase rate of wound healing)

2. Carry out frequent hemoglobin, hematocrit, and blood sugar determinations.

Evaluation
Expected Outcomes

1. Avoids pressure.

a. Shifts weight and changes position every 1–2 hours.

b. Changes from supine to side lying to prone positions.

c. Uses trapeze to raise self from bed at 30-minute intervals while awake.

d. Raises self from seat/wheelchair every 30 minutes.

2. Monitors self for manifestations of skin reddening and change in skin.

a. Uses hand mirror to inspect hard-to-see areas.

b. Palpates susceptible areas for increased skin temperature.

c. Inspects susceptible areas at least twice daily.

3. Maintains intact skin—no redness, breakdown, excoriation.

Treating Pressure Sores

Goals:
Relieve all pressure from the area.
Continue with preventive measures of a more vigorous nature.
Encourage restoration of circulation and cellular function.
Prevent necrosis of deeper structures.

Principles:
Treatment is related to the extent and depth of the wound and any associated infection.

1. Relieve pressure from the area; a pressure sore will not heal when subjected to continuous pressure.

a. Continue preventive measures.

b. Improve general health of the patient to provide optimal healing.

2. Treat the underlying disorder—underlying conditions must be managed to allow the ulcer to heal.

3. Take bacterial cultures (and sensitivity studies) early if infection is present; pressure sores contain bacterial flora.

4. Employ daily mechanical cleansing of the ulcer—clears up sepsis and stimulates regeneration of epithelium.

a. Deep ulcers may need to be irrigated with prescribed sterile solution or cleansed in a whirlpool or Hubbard tank.

b. Debride ulcer—devitalized tissue promotes infection, delays granulation, and impedes healing.
(1) Use sharp dissection (scalpel blade) to remove eschar covering the ulcer.
(2) Cross-hatching of the eschar with the scalpel blade may facilitate penetration of enzymatic debriding agent (collagenase therapy).
(3) Debridement of deep necrotic ulcers is performed in the operating room.
5. Control infection—may be a precipitating cause and may inhibit healing of ulcer; chronic infection contributes to anemia, hypoalbuminemia, and malnutrition.
a. Assess for systemic infection—fever, cellulitis, lymphangitis.
b. Give systemic antimicrobial therapy based on identification of pathogens and antimicrobial sensitivity determinations.
c. Place the patient on drainage and secretion precautions if the decubitus ulcer is infected, minor, or limited, and on contact isolation if the ulcer is draining.
6. Utilize physical modalities of treatment.
a. Expose ulcer to air and sunlight.
b. Employ light stroking around lesion—promotes venous return and reduces edema.
c. Use ultraviolet irradiation—
(1) Clean discharges from surface of ulcer.
(2) Cover normal skin surrounding ulcer during irradiation.
d. Whirlpool treatments—increase circulation and have debriding action.
e. Use oxygen under pressure applied directly on ulcer (hyperbaric oxygen therapy)—directs more oxygen to tissues; hastens metabolic processes and reduces healing time.
7. Utilize topical applications as directed. There is a wide variety of opinion concerning these agents.
a. Skin barriers—Karaya powder, Stomahesive, etc.
b. Antiseptic plastic sprays
c. Aerosol spray containing a corticosteroid and an antibiotic
d. Absorbable gelatin sponges (Gelfoam)—placed at base of ulcer to improve healing and decrease plasma loss from pressure sores.
e. Enzymatic debriding agents (collagenase therapy)—digests necrotic tissue and purulent exudate and is applied using the following procedure:
(1) Remove eschar covering ulcer or crosshatch eschar with scalpel blade to allow enzyme to come in contact with the material to be digested.
(2) Remove loose debris with forceps.
(3) Irrigate with prescribed sterile solution.
(4) Assess wound for inflammation, pus, odor.

(5) Apply enzymatic debriding ointment in thin, even layer over surface of ulcer.
(6) Cover with dry sterile dressing secured with hypoallergenic tape or gauze bandage.
f. Transparent, elastic, self-adhesive film (Op-Site)—purported to seal in body's normal defenses (leukocytes, plasma, fibrin).
g. Dextranomer (Debrisan)—useful when depth of ulcer exceeds 2 mm. or for a moist sloughing wound.
(1) Cleanse ulcer thoroughly with prescribed solution for each treatment and damp-dry.
(2) Apply dextranomer directly onto lesion—contains dry porous beads with hydrophilic (water absorbing) properties; also absorbs debris, allowing granulation tissue to develop.
(3) Cover with a dry porous dressing and secure with a gauze bandage.
h. Absorption (copolymer starch) dressing (Bard Absorption Dressing).
8. Ensure good nutrition—to reverse catabolism, correct anemia and edema, and increase tissue oxygenation and perfusion.
a. High-protein feedings may be employed to correct protein deficiency; loss of serum from a draining ulcer depletes the body stores of protein, specifically albumin.
b. Iron and ascorbic acid (vitamin C) given as directed—vitamin C is necessary for collagen formation. (Wound healing is dependent on collagen.)
c. Zinc supplements—to accelerate healing.
9. Prepare the patient for surgical intervention if ulcer does not respond to conservative measures.
a. Prepare the patient for lying prone before surgery is performed.
b. Assist with diagnostic workup in addition to presurgical management for spasticity and contractures.
c. Surgical procedures:
(1) Incision and drainage—if ulcer is not draining properly, is suppurating, or is not undermined.
(2) Grafting procedures—different types of grafts are used according to size of ulcer.
(3) Closure of defect—removal of ulcer, surrounding scar, underlying bursa, affected bone.
d. Postoperative nursing intervention:
(1) Relieve pressure by proper positioning and elimination of shearing forces for 4–6 weeks.
(2) Allow controlled pressure on site (after 6 weeks) for 10–15 minutes, 2–3 times a day under close nursing surveillance; watch for redness or abrasion.

Supporting the Patient in Daily Self-Care

Activities of Daily Living

Activities of daily living are those self-care activities that must be accomplished each day in order for the patient to care for his own needs and participate in society. They include:

1. Getting in and out of bed (transfers)
2. Personal hygiene and toilet management
3. Dressing
4. Eating
5. Mobility
6. Environmental management

Assessment

Physical examination
Functional neuromuscular examination (sitting, balance, transfers, ADL skills, ambulation)

The Activities of Daily Living (ADL) Sheet

The ADL sheet is an information sheet for those who are caring for the patient. It is a guide to the assessment of the patient's functional capabilities.

Purposes:

to inform each member of the rehabilitation team what activities the patient can carry out.
to serve as an index of progress.

Nurse's Responsibility in Using ADL Sheet
1. Review the ADL sheet each morning to know what the patient is capable of doing and what activities he is learning.
2. Avoid doing for the patient what he can do for himself.

Patient Problems/Nursing Diagnosis

Self-care deficits related to general complex problems of disability, limited mobility and access, and potential for dependency.

Planning and Implementation

Nursing Interventions

1. Define the goal with the patient.
2. Identify the patient's strengths and indications of wellness; point these out to the patient.
3. Determine how much the patient can do (and would like to do) for himself.
4. Study each component motion of the desired activity.
5. Ascertain what methods can be used to accomplish the task.
   Example: There are several ways of putting on a given garment.
6. Determine what the patient can do by watching him perform.
7. Encourage the patient to exercise the muscles used in performing the motions involved in the activity.
8. Select activities that encourage gross functional movements of the upper and lower extremities (e.g., bathing, holding larger objects).
9. Gradually include activities that use finer motions (e.g., buttoning clothes, eating with a spoon).
10. Set appropriate limits to allow the patient to move toward self-care.
11. Allow the patient to achieve mastery.
12. Extend the period of activity as much and as fast as the patient can tolerate.
13. Teach use of adaptive equipment.
14. Have the patient perform and practice the activity in a real-life situation.
15. Encourage the patient to perform every activity up to his maximal capabilities within the framework of his ability.
16. Support the patient by giving justifiable praise, reinforcement, and feedback for effort put forth and for acts accomplished.

Evaluation

Expected Outcomes

Moves toward self-care in activities of daily living (as competently as residual functioning permits); shows progress in specific activities as indicated by ADL sheet.

Assisting the Patient with Ambulation

Guidelines: Using a Tilt Table

A *tilt table* is a board or table that can be tilted gradually from a horizontal to a vertical (upright) position.

Keep patient active to increase skin and vascular tone

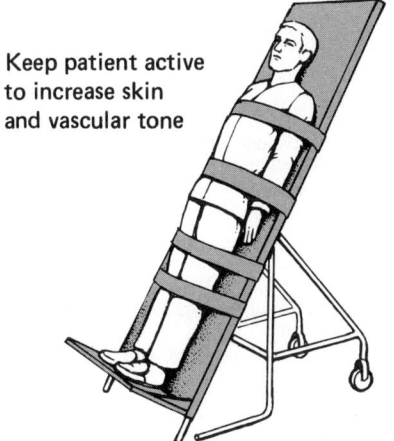

(continued)

Guidelines: Using a Tilt Table (continued)

Purposes
1. To help the patient adjust gradually to varying degrees of the upright posture and ultimately to complete upright position.
2. To help the patient start weight-bearing activities.
3. To increase standing tolerance.
4. To prevent disuse syndrome.
5. To prevent demineralization of bone and development of urinary tract stones.
6. To condition the vascular system.

Clinical Usefulness

Spinal cord injuries
Orthostatic hypotension
Brain damage

Equipment

Tilt table with footboard
Straps
Sphygmomanometer and stethoscope
Abdominal binder, elastic stockings, or venous pressure gradient leotard*

Procedure

Nursing Action	Rationale/Amplification
Preparatory Phase	
1. Apply snug-fitting abdominal binder, elastic compression bandages from toes to groin on both legs or a leotard (waist-high venous pressure gradient support*).	1. Compression of abdomen prevents pooling of blood in splanchnic area and subsequent postural hypotension and inadequate cerebral circulation. Compression of legs restricts the vascular walls of the blood vessels and prevents pooling of blood in the legs, with development of edema.
Performance Phase	
1. Transfer the patient to the tilt table by 3-person carry method. Place the patient in a dorsal position with his feet placed firmly against the footboard. Position the body in correct alignment.	
2. Fasten the straps across the pelvis, knees, chest, and abdomen.	
3. Apply the blood pressure cuff to the arm and take and record the blood pressure while the patient is lying flat.	3. This serves as a baseline recording for future comparisons.
4. Tilt the table 15–30 degrees. Take the blood pressure every 3–5 minutes.	4. Tilting the patient from a supine to an upright position causes a decrease in systolic pressure.
5. Evaluate the patient constantly and assess for a drop in blood pressure. If the patient feels dizzy and the blood pressure drops, return him to a flat position.	
6. Observe for pallor, diaphoresis, tachycardia, and nausea.	6. These are signs and symptoms of insufficient cerebral circulation.
7. Increase the standing tolerance by 5- to 10-degree increments.	7. The angle of tilt will be determined by the patient's tolerance, blood pressure stability, and the desired amount of weight-bearing.
8. Continue the procedure until the patient tolerates the desired tilt (usually between 45–80 degrees).	
9. Avoid allowing the patient to stand for prolonged periods.	9. Prolonged standing may cause pressure ulceration on plantar surfaces of feet.
10. Do not leave patient unattended.	
Follow-up Phase	
1. Place the patient back in bed at the end of the prescribed period or when his condition indicates.	
2. Record degree of tilt, amount of time on tilt table, and reaction of patient.	

* Jobst Venous Pressure Gradient Support

Transfer Activities

A *transfer* is the movement of the patient from one piece of furniture or equipment to another (from bed to chair, bed to commode, bed to wheelchair).

Weight-bearing transfers—carried out by patients who have at least one stable lower extremity (hemiplegics, unilateral lower extremity amputees, patients with hip fractures).

Non–weight-bearing transfers—done by double lower-extremity amputees, or paraplegics who are not wearing braces.

Preparation for Transfers

Goal:
Develop ability to raise and move the body in different positions.

A. Exercises to Strengthen Arm and Shoulder Extensors

1. Have the patient sit upright in bed.
2. Place a book under each hand.
3. Instruct the patient to push down on the book, thus raising his body weight.

B. Technique for Moving the Patient to the Edge of the Bed

1. Move the patient's head and shoulders toward the edge of the bed.
2. Move the patient's feet and legs to the edge of the bed. (The patient is now in a crescent position, giving good range of motion to the lateral trunk muscles.)
3. Place both of your arms well under the patient's hips. (Before the next maneuver, tighten or set the muscles of your back and abdomen.)
4. Straighten your back while moving the patient toward you.

C. Technique for Sitting the Patient on the Edge of the Bed

1. Place one hand under the patient's shoulders.
2. Instruct the patient to push his elbow into the bed while you lift his shoulders with one arm and swing his legs over the edge of the bed with the other. (Gravity pulls the legs downward, which aids in raising the patient's trunk.)

D. Technique for Assisting the Patient to Stand

1. Place the patient's feet well under him.
2. Face the patient and firmly grasp each side of his rib cage.
3. Push your knee against one of the patient's knees.
4. Rock the patient forward as he comes to a standing position. (Your knee is pushed against the patient's knee as he comes to the standing position.)
5. Ensure that the patient's knees are "locked" (full extension) while he is standing. (Locking the patient's knees is a safety measure for those patients who are weak or who have been in bed for a period of time.)
6. Give the patient enough time to balance himself.
7. Pivot the patient, positioning him to sit in the chair.

E. Technique for Transfer by Sliding Board

1. A *sliding board* (or transfer board) is a polished light-weight board that is used to bridge the gap between the bed and the chair (or chair and tub, etc.).
2. When the muscles that the patient uses to lift himself off the bed are not strong enough to overcome the resistance of body weight, use the following maneuver:
   a. Place one side of the sliding board under the patient's buttocks and the other side on the surface of the chair, bed, toilet, etc., to which the transfer is being made.
   b. Instruct the patient to push up with his hands, to shift his buttocks, and to slide across the board to the other surface.

Crutch Walking

Crutches are artificial supports that assist patients who need aid in walking because of disease, injury, or a birth defect.

Preparation for Crutch Walking

Goals:
Develop power in the shoulder girdle and upper extremities that bear the patient's weight in crutch walking.

Strengthen and condition the patient.

A. To Strengthen the Muscles Needed for Ambulation

Instruct the patient as follows:
1. For *quadriceps setting*
   a. Contract the quadriceps muscle while attempting to push the popliteal area against the mattress and raise the heel.
   b. Maintain the muscle contracture for the count of 5.
   c. Relax for the count of 5.
   d. Repeat this exercise 10–15 times hourly.
2. For *gluteal setting*
   a. Contract or pinch the buttocks together for the count of 5.
   b. Relax for the count of 5.
   c. Repeat 10–15 times hourly.

B. To Strengthen the Muscles of the Upper Extremities and Shoulder Girdle

Instruct the patient as follows:
1. Flex and extend arms slowly while holding traction weights; gradually increase poundage of weight and number of repetitions to increase strength and endurance.
2. Do pushups while lying in a prone position.
3. Squeeze rubber ball—increases grasping strength.
4. Raise head and shoulders from bed; stretch hands forward as far as possible.
5. Sit up on bed or chair.
   a. Raise body from chair by pushing hands against chair seat (or mattress).
   b. Raise body out of seat. Hold. Relax.

C. To Measure for Crutches

1. When the patient is lying down (an approximate measurement)
   a. Instruct the patient to wear the shoes he will be using for walking.
   b. Measure from the anterior fold of the axilla to the sole of the foot. Then add 5 cm. (2 inches).
   c. Or subtract 40 cm. (16 inches) from the patient's height.
2. When the patient is standing erect.
   a. Stand the patient against the wall with feet slightly apart and away from the wall.

b. Mark 5 cm. (2 inches) out to the side from the tip of the toe.

c. Measure 15 cm. (6 inches) straight ahead from the first mark. Mark this point.

d. Measure from 5 cm. (2 inches) below the axilla to the second mark. This measurement is the approximate crutch length.

D. Crutch Stance

1. Have the patient wear well-fitting shoes with firm soles.
2. The crutches should be fitted with large rubber suction tips.
3. Have the patient stand by a chair on the unaffected leg to achieve balance.
4. Position the patient against a wall with his head in a neutral position.
5. *Tripod position*—basic crutch stance for balance and support
   a. Crutches rest approximately 20–25 cm. (8–10 inches) in front of and to the side of patient's toes. (Fig. 5-2)
   b. Taller patient requires a wider base, whereas shorter patient needs a narrower base.
6. Teach the patient to support his weight on his hands; weight borne on the axillae can damage the brachial plexus nerves and produce "crutch paralysis."
   a. The hand piece should be adjusted to allow a 30-degree elbow flexion.
   b. There should be a 2-finger-width insertion between the axillary fold and the arm piece.

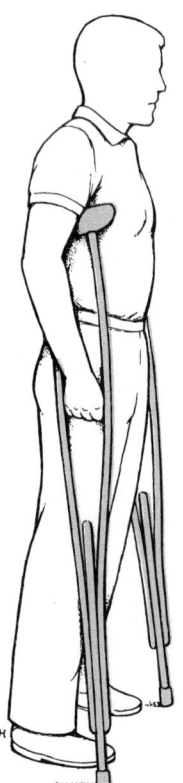

Figure 5-2. The tripod position is the basic crutch stance for balance and support.

c. A foam-rubber pad on the underarm piece will relieve pressure on the upper arm and thoracic cage.

Teaching the Crutch Gait

1. Crutch walking requires balance, coordination, and a high energy cost; these can be acquired with diligent and regular practice.
2. Practice balancing with crutches while leaning against the wall.
3. Practice shifting body weight in different positions, while standing with crutches.
4. The selection of the crutch gait depends on the type and severity of the disability and the patient's physical condition, arm and trunk strength, and/or body balance.
5. Teach the patient at least 2 gaits—a faster gait to be used for making speed, and a slower one to be used in crowded places.
6. Instruct the patient to change from one gait to another—relieves fatigue, since a different combination of muscles is used.
7. Make sure the patient is bearing weight on his hands—if the weight is borne on the axilla, the pressure of the crutch can damage the brachial plexus and produce crutch paralysis.

Crutch Gaits

A. 4-Point Gait (4-point alternate crutch gait)

1. This is a slow but stable gait; the patient's weight is constantly being shifted.
2. 4-point gait can be used only by patients who can move each leg separately and bear a considerable amount of weight on each of them.

Crutch–foot sequence (Fig. 5-3)

1. Right crutch
2. Left foot
3. Left crutch
4. Right foot

B. 2-Point Gait (2-point alternate crutch gait)

1. There is a faster gait but requires more balance, since there are only 2 points of contact with the floor.

Crutch–foot sequence (Fig. 5-4)

1. Right crutch and left foot
2. Left crutch and right foot simultaneously

C. 3-Point Gait

1. This is a fairly rapid gait but requires more strength and balance.
2. The patient's arms must be strong enough to support his entire body weight.

Crutch–foot sequence (Fig. 5-5)

1. Both crutches and the weaker lower extremity are moved forward simultaneously.
2. Then the stronger lower extremity is moved forward, while putting most of the body weight on the extremities.

D. Tripod Crutch Gaits

1. The patient constantly maintains a tripod position.
2. At the start, both crutches are held fairly widespread out front while both feet are held together in the back.
3. These gaits are slow and labored.

Tripod Alternate Crutch Gait

Crutch–foot sequence

1. Right crutch
2. Left crutch
3. Drag body and legs forward

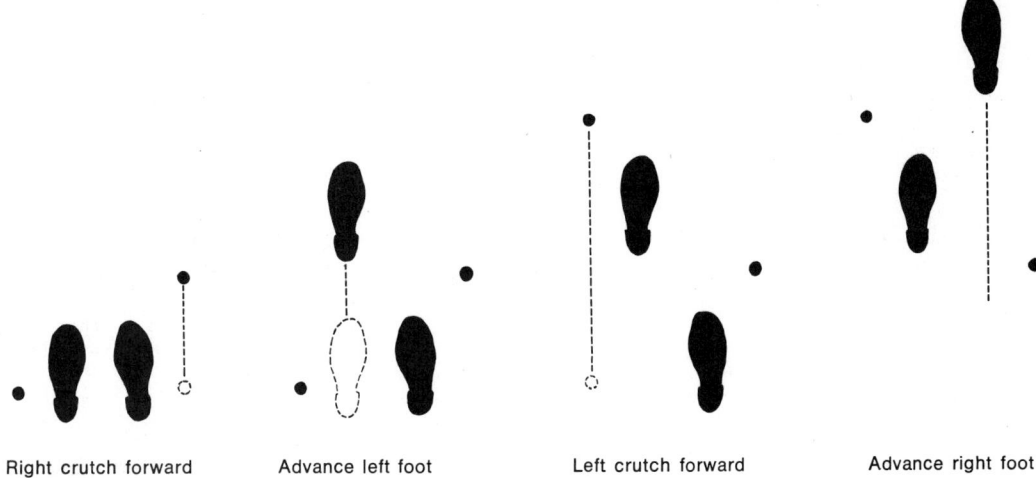

Right crutch forward   Advance left foot   Left crutch forward   Advance right foot

Figure 5-3. Four-point gait.

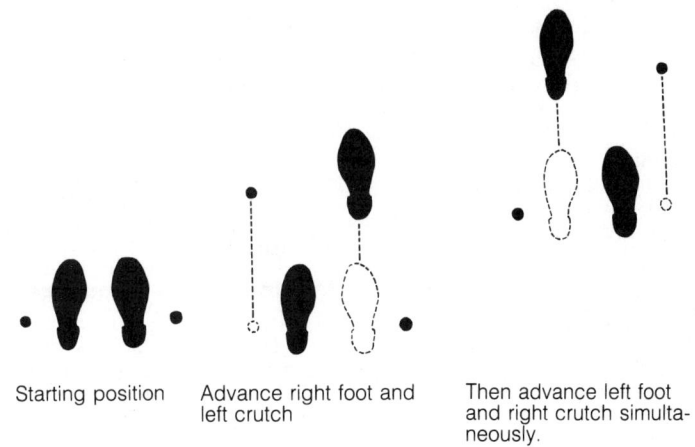

Starting position   Advance right foot and left crutch   Then advance left foot and right crutch simultaneously.

Figure 5-4. Two-point gait.

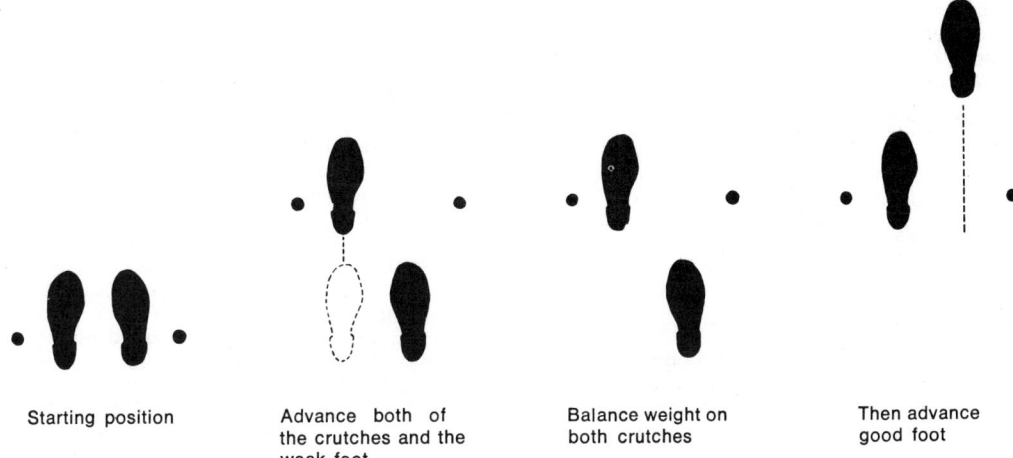

Starting position   Advance both of the crutches and the weak foot   Balance weight on both crutches   Then advance good foot

Figure 5-5. Three-point gait.

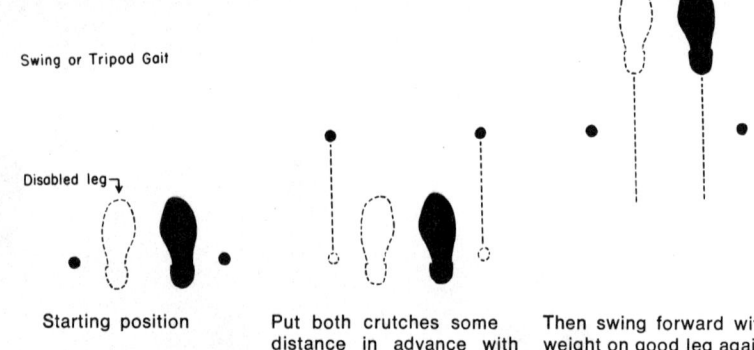

Swing or Tripod Gait

Disabled leg

Starting position

Put both crutches some distance in advance with weight on good leg

Then swing forward with weight on good leg again

Figure 5-6. Tripod simultaneous crutch gait.

Tripod Simultaneous Crutch Gait
Crutch–foot sequence (Fig. 5-6)
    1. Both crutches
    2. Drag body and legs forward

E. Swinging Crutch Gaits

1. In the swinging crutch gaits, both legs are lifted off the ground simultaneously and swung forward while the patient pushes up on the crutches.

Swinging-to Gait
Crutch–foot sequence
    1. Bear weight on good leg.
    2. Advance both crutches forward simultaneously.
    3. While leaning forward, swing the body to a position that is even with the crutches.

Swinging-through Gait
Crutch–foot sequence
    1. Advance both crutches forward.
    2. Lift both legs off ground and swing forward, landing in advance of the crutches.
    3. Bring crutches forward again—rapidly to prevent being caught off balance.

Other Crutch Maneuvering Techniques

A. To Stand Up

1. Move forward to the edge of the chair with the strong leg slightly under the seat.
2. Place both crutches in the hand on the side of the affected extremity.
3. Push down on the hand pieces while raising the body to a standing position.

B. To Sit In a Chair

1. Grasp the crutches at the hand pieces for control and bend forward slightly while assuming a sitting position.

C. To Go Up Stairs

1. Advance the stronger leg first up to the next step.
2. Then advance the crutches and the weaker extremity.

D. To Go Down Stairs

1. Place feet forward as far as possible on the step.
2. Advance crutches to the lower step. The weaker leg is advanced first and then the stronger one—the stronger extremity shares the work of raising and lowering the body weight with the patient's arms.

Note: Strong leg goes up stairs first and down stairs last.

Ambulation with a Cane

Purposes

A cane is used for balance and support:
1. To assist the patient to walk with greater balance and support and less fatigue.
2. To compensate for deficiencies of function normally performed by the neuromuscular skeletal system.
3. To relieve pressure on weight-bearing joints.
4. To provide forces to push or pull the body forward or to restrain the forward motion of the patient while walking.

Underlying Principles

1. An adjustable aluminum cane, fitted with a 3.75 cm. (1½-inch) rubber suction tip to provide traction while walking, gives optimal stability to the patient.
2. To fit for a cane
    a. Have patient flex his elbow at a 30-degree angle and hold the cane 15 cm. (6 inches) lateral to the base of his fifth toe.
    b. Adjust the cane so that the handle is approximately level with the greater trochanter. (Fig. 5-7)

Technique for Walking with a Cane

Instruct the patient as follows:
1. Hold the cane in the hand opposite to the affected extremity (i.e., the cane should be used on the good side).
2. Advance the cane at the same time the affected leg is moved forward.
3. Keep the cane fairly close to the body to prevent leaning.
4. If the patient is unable to use the cane in the opposite hand, the cane may be carried on the same side and advanced when the affected leg is advanced.
5. To go up and down stairs
    a. Step up on *unaffected* extremity.
    b. Then place cane and affected extremity on the step.
    c. Reverse this procedure for descending steps.
    d. The strong leg goes up first and comes down last.

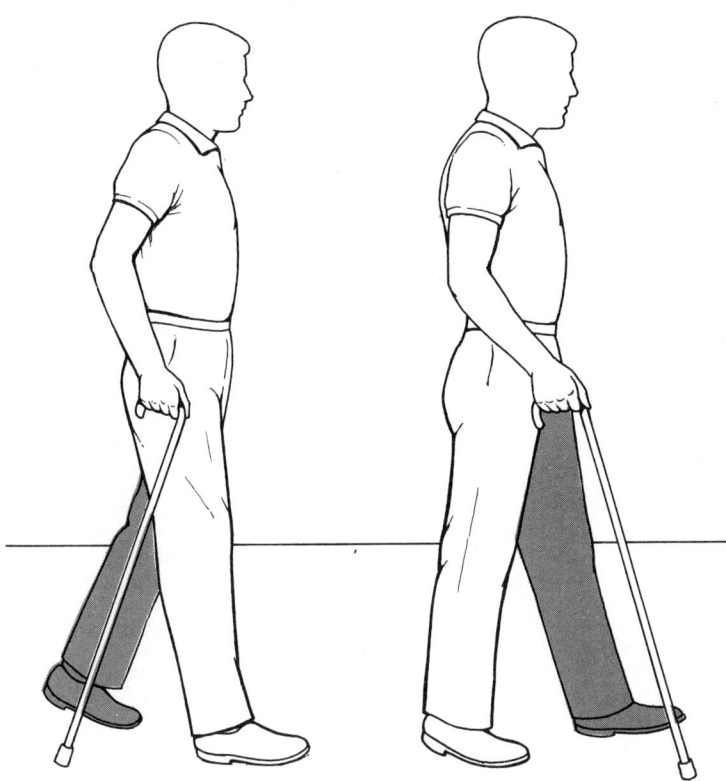

Figure 5-7. Walking with cane.

Prosthetic and Orthotic Devices

A *prosthesis* is an artificial replacement for a missing portion of the body. An *orthosis* is an orthopedic appliance/device used to provide support and alignment, to prevent or correct deformities, and to improve the function of the body (includes braces and splints).

Preprosthetic Nursing Management*

1. Help the patient to develop an attitude of realistic hopefulness and acceptance.
2. *Prevent deformities*—to limit the time between the healing of tissues and the fitting of a prosthesis.
3. Bandage an extremity stump correctly so that proper shrinkage and shaping of the stump occur.

Support and Health Education of the Patient Using Braces

A *brace* is a support that protects weakened muscles, prevents and corrects deformities, aids in controlling involuntary muscle movements, and immobilizes and protects a diseased or injured joint.

The following are the main points to emphasize in teaching the patient to care for his brace:
1. Place the brace on a table or the floor, or prop it

---

* Specific prostheses are described in this volume under the clinical conditions requiring such devices. Information concerning prosthetic and orthopedic appliances may also be obtained from the American Orthotic and Prosthetic Association, 717 Pendleton Street, Alexandria, VA 22314.

against the wall when it is not in use; hanging may cause distortion of its position.
2. Twisting of the brace may occur with use; check alignment frequently. Look down the full length of the brace. The joints should coincide with the body joints.
3. Before putting a brace on, check carefully for worn areas, missing or loose screws, and the condition of straps and buckles.
4. Pressure areas may occur if metal or plastic rubs the skin.
5. Check the skin for reddened areas immediately after removing the brace.
6. Keep the heels and soles of the shoes in good condition.
7. Clean and dry the brace, when necessary, at night.
8. To clean the plastic parts:
   a. Wipe the plastic parts with a damp cloth.
   b. Do not oil plastic surfaces and joints.
   c. Check the plastic parts for stress fractures.
   To clean the metal parts:
   a. Remove rust or corrosion spots with steel wool.
   b. Clean dirt out of metal joints and locks with a pipe cleaner dipped in a solvent.
   c. Clean the metal parts with a solvent.
   d. Apply a light coat of paste wax to the metal parts to prevent rust.
   e. Put oil in metal joints with an eyedropper or toothpick.
9. Have the brace checked periodically; any changes in body size will alter the fit of the brace.

Overcoming Elimination Problems: Bladder and Bowel Training

Urinary Elimination Problems

Assessment
Clinical Manifestations
1. Urine incontinence
2. Dribbling

Nursing Assessment
1. History of onset and precipitation factors
2. Assessment of patient's awareness and ability to concentrate
3. Urologic assessment (see p. 499) to determine type of bladder problem

Patient Problems/Nursing Diagnosis
Alteration in patterns of urinary elimination (incontinence) related to urologic dysfunction.

Planning and Implementation
Nursing Interventions
Bladder training
1. Set up a schedule of definite times for the patient to try to empty his bladder using a toilet or commode.
2. Give the patient a measured amount of fluid to drink at regularly scheduled times.
3. Have the patient wait 30 minutes and then ask him to attempt to void; *regularity is the key to success.*
   a. Position the patient with thighs flexed and feet and back supported; sufficient daily fluid intake (2500 ml.) is essential.
   b. Instruct him to press or massage over bladder area or increase intra-abdominal pressure by *leaning forward*—helps to initiate evacuation of bladder.
   c. Have the patient concentrate on voiding.
   d. Have the patient try to void every 2 hours; interval may be lengthened as control is gained.
      (1) Set alarm clock at 2–3-hour intervals during the daytime.
      (2) Set alarm clock 2 times during night.
      (3) Curtail or limit fluids after 5 p.m.
4. Have the patient keep a voiding calendar—a continuous record of time and amount of fluid ingested and time and amount of each voiding.
5. Encourage the patient to hold his urine until the specified voiding time if possible.
6. Assess for signs of urinary retention; test (catheterize) for residual urine as directed.
7. Encourage the patient to continue self-care and exercise programs; encourage the patient to wear his own clothing.
8. Stress the abilities (not the disabilities) of the patient.
9. Have a positive approach; the patient needs an atmosphere of encouragement and support.

Management of the Incontinent Patient
(Not due to neurogenic bladder impairment)
1. Assist the patient to bathroom at a regularly scheduled time—delay in responding to call for bedpan or urinal or for assistance to toilet is a common cause of incontinence.
2. Encourage the patient to perform self-care activities—boredom and frustration lead to incontinence.

3. Give adequate amounts of fluids.
4. Avoid overt encouragement of incontinence such as the routine use of pads, diapers, and other depersonalizing procedures.
5. Create an environment that keeps sensory monotony to a minimum.
   a. Use orienting aids to discriminate day/night, seasons.
      (1) Have wall clock and calendar to orient patient to time and place.
      (2) Hang wall posters, pictures, etc. for visual stimulus.
   b. Use telephone, radio, and television selectively.
   c. Encourage the patient to make decisions (menu selection, keeping intake/output chart)—improves self-esteem.
   d. Have the patient do meaningful tasks (sort mail, straighten his bureau drawers, etc.).
   e. Use reminders and schedules.
   f. Extend the patient's environment beyond the confines of his room.
   g. Increase the patient's social contacts.
6. Encourage the patient to wear his own clothes—enhances his self-esteem and dignity and is a strong deterrent to regressive behavior.

Evaluation
Expected Outcomes
1. Remains dry and free from odor.
2. Empties bladder at first sensation of pressure.
3. No residual urine.
4. Shows no signs of bacteriuria.
5. Drinks prescribed amount of fluid.
6. Maintains social contacts.

Bowel Elimination Problems

Assessment
Clinical Manifestations
Irregularity, fecal incontinence, diarrhea, fecal impaction.

Nursing Assessment
Bowel history, nutrition history, physical status, and functional ability.

Patient Problems/Nursing Diagnosis
Alteration in bowel elimination (incontinence) related to inactivity, neuromuscular disorder.

Planning and Implementation
Nursing Interventions
Bowel training
1. Secure a bowel history; bowel schedule should be normal and comfortable for the patient.
2. Establish a *specific and definite time* for the bowel movement; *regularity is necessary to establish reflex assistance.*
   a. The exact time period depends on the patient's schedule.
   b. Attempts at evacuation should be made within 15 minutes of this same time daily.
   c. Establish bowel evacuation 20–40 minutes after

a regularly scheduled meal—utilizes the stimulation of peristalsis and the gastrocolic and duodenocolic reflexes.

  d. Stimulate anorectal reflex if necessary.

    (1) Insert a glycerin suppository into the rectum 15–30 minutes before the scheduled bowel time.

    (2) *OR* insert a gloved finger into the rectum and gently dilate the anal sphincter.

      (a) If glycerin suppository is not effective, a suppository of bisacodyl (Dulcolax) may be tried.

      (b) Eventually, the patient may evacuate without any stimulation.

  e. Have the patient use a normal posture for defecation—a toilet seat or commode most nearly approximates the physiologic position for defecation.

    (1) Instruct the patient to bear down and contract the abdominal muscles.

    (2) Have the patient lean forward to increase intra-abdominal pressure by compression against the thighs.

3. Ensure adequate fiber and fluid intake 2–4 liters (2.1–4.2 quarts) daily.

  a. Give 120 ml. (4 oz.) of prune or fig juice at the same time daily (i.e., 30 minutes before breakfast)—helps establish regularity.

  b. Encourage high-fiber diet (vegetables, fruits, salads, bran, cereals)—to prevent hard stools and to stimulate peristalsis.

4. Encourage patient to exercise—good abdominal muscle tone and muscular activity is helpful in bowel training.

Evaluation

Expected Outcomes

Achieves regular bowel functioning

Absence of fecal soiling/incontinence

Family Support

Goal:

The family becomes an integral part of the rehabilitation process.

1. Develop a trusting relationship with the family.
2. Assess the family's attitude toward the patient, his disability, and his return home.
3. Involve the family in the patient's care in order to develop and practice skills that help the patient reach his rehabilitation goals.
4. Teach the family as much about the patient's condition as possible, so that they will not fear his return home. Encourage the family to ask questions.
5. Provide some type of counseling and support system for the family—they need direction and support in coping with personality and intellectual impairment/psychiatric symptoms.
6. Consider day-care programs or respite care arrangements with an extended care facility to give the family relief.
7. Give positive reinforcement; encourage the family to return to their normal activities and interests.
8. Help each family member understand his feelings.

Discharge Planning and Referral for Follow-up Care

Goals:

Improve the future quality of life.

Maintain continuity of care during transfer from the health care facility to another setting (home, extended care facility, or independent living arrangement).

1. Plan for care at home or in another setting as soon after hospital admission as possible.
2. Gather information about the patient's home environment (from patient, family, social worker, community health nurse and other resources).
3. Estimate the patient's functional potential; make plans with this in mind.
4. Plan, with the patient, ways and methods of coping with problems that may arise, and make realistic plans for the future.
5. Encourage the family to be involved with the patient. (See Family Support.)
6. Send referral form to local community health agency so nurse can evaluate the home environment.

  a. Review patient's ADL sheet with community health or visiting nurse—so community nurses will know exactly what activities patient can perform.

  b. Determine what modifications will be necessary in the home (for wheelchair, for self-care activities).

  c. Inquire how the patient expects to be transported for clinic visits, special therapy, etc.

7. Send referral to the State Vocational Rehabilitation Agency if the patient will require additional educational or job training.
8. Assist with transfer of the patient to extended-care facility if he is unable to return to home situation.

  a. Recognize that not all families can be expected to carry on the rehabilitation program that the patient may require.

  b. Send the ADL sheet to the extended-care facility with the patient to help orient staff to the patient's goals and programs.

Bibliography

Books

Abreu BC (ed). Physical Disabilities Manual. New York, Raven Press, 1981

Basmajian JV (ed). Medical Rehabilitation—A Student's Textbook. Baltimore, Williams & Wilkins, 1984

Basmajian JV. Therapeutic Exercise, 4th ed. Baltimore, Williams & Wilkins, 1984

Bell CW et al. Home Care and Rehabilitation in Respiratory Medicine. Philadelphia, JB Lippincott, 1983

Breur JA. Handbook of Assistive Devices for the Handicapped Elderly: New Help for Independent Living Handicapped. New York, Haworth Press, 1982

Burish TG and Bradley LA. Coping with Chronic Disease: Research and Applications. New York, Academic Press, 1983

Caird FI, Kennedy RD and Williams BO. Practical Rehabilitation of the Elderly. Marshfield, MA, Pitman, 1983

Cole TM and Cole SS. "Rehabilitation of Problems of Sexuality in Physical Disability" in Krusen's Handbook of Physical Medicine and Rehabilitation. Kottke FJ, Stillwell GK and Lehmann JF. Philadelphia, WB Saunders, 1982

Cook AM and Webster JG (eds). Therapeutic Medical Devices. Englewood Cliffs, NJ, Prentice-Hall, 1982

Cornett SJ and Watson JE. Cardiac Rehabilitation: An Interdisciplinary Team Approach. New York, John Wiley & Sons, 1984

Davis WM. Aids to Make You Able. New York, Beaufort Books, 1981

Downey JA, Riedel C and Kutscher AH (eds). Bereavement of Physical Disability: Recommitment to Life, Health, and Function. New York, Arno Press, 1982

Eisenberg M, Griggins C and Duval RJ (eds). Disabled People as Second-Class Citizens. New York, Springer, 1982

Fraser BA and Hensinger RN. Managing Physical Handicaps. Baltimore, Paul H Brookes, 1983

Godou AG. Human Sexuality. St Louis, CV Mosby, 1982

Greif E and Matarazzo RG. Behavioral Approaches to Rehabilitation: Coping With Change. New York, Springer, 1982

Hale G. The Source Book for the Disabled. Philadelphia, WB Saunders, 1982

Hollis M. Practical Exercise Therapy, 2nd ed. Boston, Blackwell Scientific Pub, 1981

Horsley JA et al. Preventing Decubitus Ulcers. New York, Grune & Stratton, 1981

Kamenetz HL. Dictionary of Rehabilitation Medicine. New York, Springer, 1983

Kaplan PE and Materson RS. The Practice of Rehabilitation Medicine. Springfield, IL, Charles C Thomas, 1982

Katz AH and Martin K. A Handbook of Services for the Handicapped. Westport, CT, Greenwood Press, 1982

Kohn KH et al. Physical Medicine and Rehabilitation, 4th ed. New Hyde Park, NY, Medical Examination Pub, 1983

Kottke FJ, Stillwell GK and Lehman JF. Krusen's Handbook of Physical Medicine and Rehabilitation, 3rd ed. Philadelphia, WB Saunders, 1982

Kreisler N and Kreisler J. Catalog of Aids for the Disabled. New York, McGraw-Hill, 1982

Krueger DW. Rehabilitation Psychology. Rockville, MD, Aspen Systems Corporation, 1984

Lief HI. Sexual Problems in Medical Practice. Chicago, AMA, 1981

Lindemann JE. Psychological and Behavioral Aspects of Physical Disability: A Manual for Health Practitioners. New York, Plenum Press, 1981

Lion EM. Human Sexuality in Nursing Process. New York, John Wiley & Sons, 1982

Marinelli RP and DellOrto AE. The Psychological and Social Impact of Physical Disability. New York, Springer, 1984

Martin N, Holt NB and Hicks D. Comprehensive Rehabilitation Nursing. New York, McGraw-Hill, 1981

Nickel VL (ed). Orthopedic Rehabilitation. New York, Churchill Livingstone, 1982

Miller JF. Coping with Chronic Illness: Overcoming Powerlessness. Philadelphia, FA Davis, 1983

Minor MA and Minor SD. Patient Care Skills. Reston, Reston Pub Co, 1984

Nichols PJR (ed). Rehabilitation Medicine, 2nd ed. Boston, Butterworths, 1980

Okamoto GA and Phillips TJ. Physical Medicine and Rehabilitation. Philadelphia, WB Saunders, 1984

O'Sullivan SB, Cullen KE and Schmitz TJ. Physical Rehabilitation: Evaluation and Treatment Procedures. Philadelphia, Davis, 1981

Pedretti LW. Occupational Therapy—Practice Skills for Physical Dysfunction. St Louis, CV Mosby, 1981

Pepper NH. Fundamentals of Care of the Aging, Disabled, and Handicapped. Springfield, IL, Charles C Thomas, 1982

Power PW. A Guide to Rehabilitation Assessment. Baltimore, University Park Press, 1983

Power PW and DellOrto AE. Role of the Family in the Rehabilitation of the Physically Disabled. Baltimore: University Park Press, 1980

Providing Early Mobility: Nursing Photobook. Horsham, PA, Intermed Communications, 1980

Rule WR. Lifestyle Counseling for Adjustment to Disability. Rockville, MD, Aspen Systems, 1984

Simpson JEP and Levitt R. Going Home: A Guide for Helping the Patient on Leaving the Hospital. New York, Churchill Livingstone, 1981

Sine RD et al (eds). Basic Rehabilitation Techniques: A Self-Instructional Guide. Rockville, MD, Aspen Systems, 1981

Smith DW. Survival of Illness: Implications for Nursing. New York, Springer, 1981

Spiegel AD and Podair S. Rehabilitating People With Disabilities Into the Mainstream of Society. Park Ridge, NJ, Noyes Medical, 1981

Stolov WC and Clowers MR (eds). Handbook of Severe Disability. Washington, DC, US Government Printing Office, US Department of Education, Rehabilitation Services Administration, 1981

Trombly CA (ed). Occupational Therapy for Physical Dysfunction, 2nd ed. Baltimore, Williams & Wilkins, 1983

Vash CL. The Psychology of Disability. New York, Springer, 1981

Washburn KB. Physical Medicine and Rehabilitation: Essentials of Primary Care, 2nd ed. Garden City, NY, Medical Examination Publishing Co, 1981

Wright RA. Physical Disability: A Psychosocial Approach, 2nd ed. New York, Harper & Row, 1983

Articles

Ahmed MC. Op-site for decubitus care. Am J Nurs 1982 Jan; 82(1):61–64

Arnell I. Treating decubitus ulcers: Two methods that work. Nursing '83 1983 June; 13(6):50–55

Cammer MM. Growth model of self-care for neurologically impaired people. J Neurosurg Nurs 1983 Oct; 15(5):299–305

Cooney TC and Reuler JB. Protecting the elderly patient from pressure sores. Geriatrics 1983 Feb; 38(2):125–134

Daniels SM et al. Sexuality and disability: The need for services. Ann Rev Rehabil 1981; 2:83–112

Donnelly DC. Rehabilitation and the occupational health nurse. Occup Health Nurs 1983 Aug; 31(8):39–41

Drugs that cause sexual dysfunction. Med Lett Drugs Ther 1983 Aug 5; 25(641):73–76

Dudas S. Rehabilitation concepts of nursing. J Enterostomal Ther 1984 Jan–Feb; 11(1):6–15

Eisenberg MG and Jansen MA. Rehabilitation psychology: State of the art. Ann Rev Rehabil 1983; 3:1–31

Fowler E. Once-daily pressure sore dressing speeds healing. RN 1983 Apr; 46(4):56–57

Fowler WM. Viability of physical medicine and rehabilitation in the 1980s. Arch Phys Med Rehabil 1982 Jan; 63(1):1–5

Getz PA and Blossom BM. Preventing contractures: The little "extras" that help so much. RN 1982 Dec; 45(12): 44–48

Goodgold J et al. Using prothetics to gain independence. Patient Care 1983 Jan 15; 17(1):45

Gurevich I. Infected decubiti: The problem of patient placement and care. Top Clin Nurs 1983 July; 5(2): 55–63

Levitt R. Sex and physical disability. J Neurosurg Nurs 1981 June; 13(3):127–128

Loomis J et al. Discharge planning: Planning means fewer hospitalizations for the chronically ill. Nursing '81 1981 May; 11(5):70–75

Natow AB. Nutrition in prevention and treatment of decubitus ulcers. Top Clin Nurs 1983 July; 5(2):39–44

Oliver M. Have crutch will travel. Am J Nurs 1983 Aug; 83(8):1228

Reddy MP. Decubitus ulcers: Principles of prevention and management. Geriatrics 1983 July; 38(7):55–61

Ross T. Nursing process: Activities of living. Nurs Mirror 1983 Feb 9; 156: 28–29

Schuster EA (ed). Symposia on sexuality and nursing practice. Nurs Clin North Am 1982 Sep; 17(3):343–454

Staas WE and LaMantia JG. Decubitus ulcers and rehabilitation medicine. Int J Dermatol 1982 Oct; 21(8):437–444

Zinn WM (ed). Sexuality and disablement. Int Rehabil Med 1981; 3(1):18–42

Care of the Surgical Patient

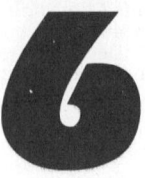

1: Perioperative Nursing

Concept of Perioperative Patient Care

Perioperative role in operating room nursing is a term used to describe the nursing functions in the total surgical experience of the patient: preoperative, intraoperative, and postoperative.

Preoperative phase—from the time the decision is made for surgical intervention to the transference of the patient to the operating room.

Intraoperative phase—from the time the patient is received in the operating room until he is admitted to the recovery room.

Postoperative phase—from the time of admission to the recovery room to the follow-up home/clinic evaluation.

Examples of nursing interventions in the perioperative role are presented in the chart below.

Examples of Nursing Interventions in the Perioperative Role

Preoperative Phase	Intraoperative Phase	Postoperative Phase
Preoperative Assessment Home/clinic 1. initiates initial preoperative assessment	Maintenance of Safety 1. assures that the sponge, needle, and instrument counts are correct	Communication of Intraoperative Information 1. gives patient's name 2. states type of surgery performed

2. plans teaching methods appropriate to patient's needs
3. involves family in interview

Surgical unit
1. completes preoperative assessment
2. coordinates patient teaching with other nursing staff
3. explains phases in perioperative period and expectations
4. develops a plan of care

Surgical suite
1. assesses patient's level of consciousness
2. reviews chart
3. identifies patient
4. verifies surgical site

Planning
1. determines a plan of care

Psychological Support
1. tells patient what is happening
2. determines psychological status
3. gives prior warning of noxious stimuli
4. stands near/touches patient during procedures/induction
5. communicates patient's emotional status to other appropriate members of the health care team

2. positions the patient
   a. functional alignment
   b. exposure of surgical site
   c. maintenance of position throughout procedure
3. applies grounding device to patient
4. provides physical support

Physiological Monitoring
1. calculates effects on patient of excessive fluid loss
2. distinguishes normal from abnormal cardiopulmonary data
3. reports changes in patient's pulse, respirations, temperature, and blood pressure

Psychological Monitoring (Prior to Induction and if Patient Conscious)
1. provides emotional support to patient
2. continues to assess patient's emotional status
3. communicates patient's emotional status to other appropriate members of the health care team

Nursing Management
1. provides physical safety for the patient
2. maintains aseptic, controlled environment
3. effectively manages human resources

3. provides contributing intraoperative factors, ie, drain, catheters
4. states physical limitations
5. states impairments resulting from surgery
6. reports patient's preoperative level of consciousness
7. communicates necessary equipment needs

Postoperative Evaluation
Recovery area
1. determines patient's immediate response to surgical intervention

Surgical unit
1. evaluates effectiveness of nursing care in the OR
2. determines patient's level of satisfaction with care given during perioperative period
3. evaluates products used on patient in the OR
4. determines patient's psychological status
5. assists with discharge planning

Home/clinic
1. seeks patient's perception of surgery in terms of the effects of anesthetic agents. Impact on body image, distortion, immobilization
2. determines family's perceptions of surgery

(Operating room nursing: Perioperative role. AORN J 1978 May; vol. 27; reprinted with permission)

Nursing Process Overview in the Preoperative Period

Preoperative Assessment
Nursing History, Physical Examination, and Diagnostic Determinations

1. Engage the patient in conversation to determine his reaction to and concerns about hospitalization and the forthcoming operation.
2. Take a nursing history and perform a general physical examination (see Chap. 4).
3. Assess nutritional status (weight-loss history, albumin and transferrin levels, total protein, mid-arm muscle circumference, triceps skin fold).
4. Prepare the patient for various diagnostic tests by explaining why and how they are done and how the patient may contribute to the success of the test. Record reactions to tests, as well as the outcome of such tests. (Diagnostic studies are specific for each patient and are presented in detail in each condition discussed in following chapters.)
5. Ascertain risk factors and develop individualized preventive strategies (see p. 79).
6. Determine the patient's level of understanding of his condition; develop a plan for preoperative patient education (see p. 76).

Patient Problems/Nursing Diagnoses

1. Knowledge deficit: inadequate or insufficient information about the operation
2. Fear, worry, and depression related to the diagnosis, to the outcome of surgery, and to risk factors and postoperative pain
3. Disturbance in self-concept (body image and role performance) related to surgery and postoperative care
4. Possible risk factors related to life-style and health status

Planning and Implementation
Nursing Interventions

1. Assist the patient in understanding the physical and psychosocial aspects of the surgical experience
2. Acquaint the patient and his family with the environ-

ment, protocols, and expectations as surgery is anticipated

3. Teach the patient certain procedures that will help in reducing postoperative complications and in increasing comfort and enhancing recovery
4. Prepare the patient physically and psychologically for the anesthetic and operative procedure
5. Collaborate with other members of the health team in coordinating all preoperative preparations

Evaluation
Expected Outcomes

1. Approaches planned surgery with a positive attitude
2. Demonstrates and explains the major postoperative activities he will be required to perform
3. Reduces potential risks to acceptable levels
4. Cooperates during immediate presurgical preparation and tells why he is receiving presurgical medication

Preoperative Patient Education

Preoperative patient education is the giving of information to the patient who is scheduled to have an operation; such instruction may be offered through conversation, discussion, the use of audiovisual aids, demonstrations, and return demonstrations. It is designed to help the patient understand what he is about to experience so that he can participate intelligently and recover more effectively from surgery and anesthesia.

Note: Parts of this program may be initiated before hospitalization.

Patient Education (May include the family or significant others)

A. Obtain data base and plan modus operandi.

1. Determine what the patient already knows and what he wishes to know. This can be accomplished by reading the patient's chart, by interviewing the patient, and by communicating with his physician, family, and other members of the health team.
2. Plan this presentation or series of presentations for this individual patient or a group of patients.
3. Encourage active participation of patients in their care and recovery.
4. Demonstrate essential techniques; provide opportunity for patient practice and return demonstration.
5. Provide time for and encourage patient to ask questions and express his concerns; make every effort to answer all queries truthfully and in basic agreement with the overall therapeutic plan.

B. Constantly assess needs of patient as teaching progresses.

1. Begin at the patient's level of understanding and proceed from there.
2. Correct misinformation—provide opportunity for him to express himself.
3. Provide general information and be alert for patient needs as intercommunication takes place. Assess his ability to absorb, his curiosity or lack of it.
   a. Explain details of preoperative preparation.
   b. Offer general information on his specific surgery. (Physician is the resource person.)
   c. Tell when surgery is scheduled (if known) and how long it will take; explain that afterwards he will go to the recovery room.
   d. Let him know that his family will be kept informed and that they will be told where to wait and when they can see him; note visiting hours.
   e. Explain to him how a procedure or test may *feel* during or after.
   f. Describe the recovery room; what personnel and equipment the patient may expect to see and

hear (specially trained personnel, monitoring equipment, tubing for various functions, and a moderate amount of activity by nurses and physicians).
   g. Explain the importance of his participation in his postoperative recovery. Tell him you will demonstrate to him some of the activities he will be doing postoperatively.
   h. Utilize other resource persons; physicians, therapists, chaplain, interpreters, and so forth.
   i. Document in outline form what has been taught, as well as the patient's reaction and level of understanding.

▶ **NURSING ALERT:** Touch is a useful modality in preoperative teaching of patients that appears to reduce anxiety significantly.

C. Utilize audiovisual aids if available.

1. Videotapes with sound or film strips with narration are effective in giving basic information to a single patient or group of patients.
2. Booklets, brochures and models, if available, are helpful.
3. Demonstrate any equipment that will be specific for the particular patient. Examples:

Drainage equipment   Monitoring equipment
Side rails   Incentive spirometer
Ostomy bag

▶ **NURSING ALERT:** The extent of preoperative patient teaching is determined on an individual basis; determinants are the patient's previous knowledge, his desire to learn and willingness to use this new knowledge, his psychoemotional and physical condition, the amount of time available, and the quality of teaching. Effectiveness is greater when time is provided for patient participation and discussion.

Preoperative Practice of Postoperative Activities

Activities that the patient will practice and do postoperatively include the following:

A. Diaphragmatic Breathing

This is a mode of breathing in which the dome of the diaphragm is flattened during inspiration resulting in enlargement of the upper abdomen as air rushes into the chest. During expiration, abdominal muscles and the diaphragm relax (also see p. 151).

For the patient:

1. Assume bed position similar to that most likely to be used postoperatively (semi-Fowler's).

2. Place both hands over lower rib cage; make a loose fist and rest the flat surface of the fingernails against the chest (to feel chest movement).
3. Exhale gently and fully; ribs will sink downward and inward toward midline.
4. Inhale deeply through mouth and nose; permit abdomen to rise as lungs fill with air.
5. Hold this breath through a count of 5.
6. Exhale and let *all* air out through mouth and nose.
7. Repeat 15 times with a brief rest following each group of five.
8. Practice this twice each day preoperatively.

B. Incentive Spirometry

Preoperatively, the patient uses a spirometer to measure his deep breaths (inspired air) while exerting his maximum effort (see Guidelines, p. 208).

The preoperative measurement becomes the goal to be achieved as soon as possible after the operation.
1. Postoperatively, the patient is encouraged to use the incentive spirometer (available commercially) about 10–12 times an hour. (He does this on his own.)
2. Deep inhalations expand alveoli, which, in turn, prevents atelectasis and other pulmonary complications.
3. There is less pain with inspiratory concentration than with expiratory concentration, such as with coughing and using blow bottles.

C. Coughing

Coughing promotes the removal of chest secretions.
1. Interlace the fingers and place the hands over the proposed incision site; this will act as a splint during coughing and not harm the incision.

2. Lean forward slightly while sitting in bed.
3. Breathe, using the diaphragm as described under diaphragmatic breathing (see above, item A).
4. Inhale fully with the mouth slightly open.
5. Let out 3 or 4 sharp "hacks."
6. Then, with mouth open, take in a deep breath and quickly give 1 or 2 strong coughs.
7. Secretions should be readily cleared from the chest to prevent respiratory complications (pneumonia, obstruction, etc.).

D. Turning

Changing positions from his back to side-lying (and vice versa) stimulates circulation, encourages deeper breathing, and relieves pressure areas.
1. Assist the patient to move onto his side if he is unable to do this himself.
2. Place the uppermost leg in a more flexed position than that of the lower leg and place a pillow comfortably between the legs.
3. Ensure that the patient is turned from one side to his back and onto the other side every 2 hours.

E. Foot and leg exercises

Moving the legs improves circulation and muscle tone.
1. Have the patient lie on his back; instruct him to bend the knee and raise the foot—hold it a few seconds, extend the leg, and lower it to the bed.
2. Repeat above for about 5 times with 1 leg and then with the other. Repeat the set 5 times every 3–5 hours.
3. Then have the patient lie on his side; exercise the legs by pretending to pedal a bicycle.
4. Suggest the following foot exercise: Trace a complete circle with the great toe.

Informed Consent (Operative Permit)

An *informed consent* (operative permit) is a form signed by the patient (and witnessed), granting permission to have the operation performed as described by the patient's physician; this is a medicolegal requirement. The consent form should be written using short words and brief, simple sentences. Such forms should be reviewed by patients and the hospital attorney prior to being adopted as a standard form.

Purposes

1. To ensure that the patient understands the nature of the treatment, including potential complications.
2. To indicate that the patient's decision was made without pressure.
3. To protect the patient against unauthorized procedures.
4. To protect the surgeon and hospital against legal action by a patient who claims that an unauthorized procedure was performed.

Prior to signing an informed consent, the patient should:
1. Be told in clear and simple terms by the surgeon what is to be done (drawings or audiovisual aids may help).
2. Be aware of the risks, possible complications, disfigurement, and removal of parts.
3. Have a general idea of what to expect in the early and late postoperative periods.

4. Have a general idea of the time frame involved from surgery to recovery.
5. Have an opportunity to ask any questions.
6. Sign a separate form for each operation.

Informed Consent and the Adolescent Patient

1. An *emancipated minor* is usually recognized as one who is not subject to parental control or regulation.
   a. Married minor
   b. Those in military service
   c. College student who is under age 18 but living away from home
2. Most states have enacted *minor-treatment statutes.*
   a. This applies to persons 14 to 18 years of age (statutes vary widely).
3. Standards of informed consent are the same for adolescents and adults.
   a. If a patient of any age does not understand all material facts, the consent given will be held legally insufficient; no treatment should be given without parental consent except in an acute emergency.

Circumstances Requiring a Permit

1. Any surgical procedure where scalpel, scissors, suture, hemostats, or electrocoagulation may be used.

2. Entrance into a body cavity—paracentesis, bronchoscopy, cystoscopy.
3. General anesthesia, local infiltration, and regional block (e.g., for reduction of a fracture).

Obtaining Informed Consent

1. *Written* permission is best and is legally acceptable.
2. Signature is obtained with the patient's complete understanding of what is to occur; it is obtained before he receives sedation and is secured without pressure or duress.

3. A witness is desirable—nurse, physician, or other authorized person.
4. In an emergency, permission via telephone or telegram is acceptable.
5. For a minor (or a patient who is unconscious or irresponsible), permission is required from a responsible member of the family—parent or legal guardian.
6. For a married minor, permission from the husband or wife is acceptable.
7. If the patient is unable to write, an ''X'' to indicate his sign is acceptable if there are 2 signed witnesses to his mark.

Types of Surgery and Surgical Incisions

A. Types of Surgery

1. *Optional*
   Surgery is scheduled completely at the preference of the patient (e.g., cosmetic surgery).
2. *Elective*
   The approximate time for surgery is at the convenience of the patient; failure to have surgery is not catastrophic (e.g., superficial cyst).
3. *Required*
   The condition requires surgery within a few weeks (e.g., eye cataract).

4. *Urgent*
   Surgical problem requires attention within 24 to 48 hours (e.g., cancer).
5. *Emergency*
   Requires immediate surgical attention without delay (e.g., intestinal obstruction).
6. Ambulatory (see next section).

B. Regions and Incisions of the Abdomen

See Figure 6-1.

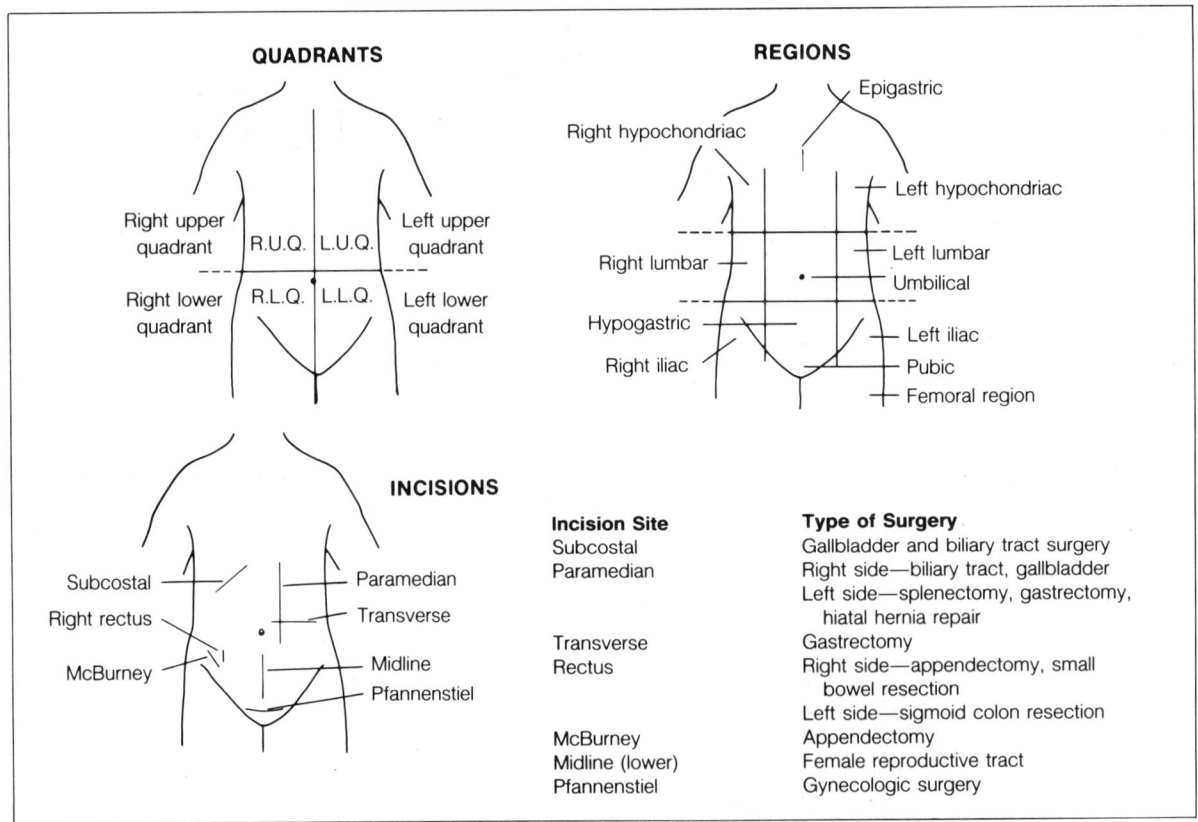

Figure 6-1. Regions and incisions of the abdomen.

Ambulatory (Day) Surgery

Ambulatory surgery (day surgery, in-and-out surgery, outpatient surgery) is not a new idea but is becoming more prevalent. The nurse is in a key role to assess patient status, plan perioperative experience, monitor, instruct, and evaluate the patient.

Advantages

1. Reduced cost to patient, hospital, and insuring and governmental agencies
2. Reduced psychological stress to the patient
3. Less evidence of hospital-acquired infection
4. Less time lost from work by patient; minimal disruption of patient's activities and family life

Disadvantages

1. Less time to assess and evaluate patient
2. Less time to establish rapport between patient and health personnel
3. No opportunity to assess for late postoperative complications (this is in the hands of the patient and lay individuals)

Patient Selection

Criteria for selection include:
1. Surgery of short duration (15–90 minutes)
2. Noninfected conditions
3. Type of operation in which postoperative complications are predictably low
4. Age is usually not a factor, although too risky in a premature infant
5. Patient should be willing and have a positive outlook (someone frightened or unwilling to have the surgery is a poor risk).
6. Types of frequently performed procedures:
    a. Dilatation and curettage
    b. Tubal ligation
    c. Myringotomy
    d. Excision of skin lesions
    e. Oral surgery (T & A)
    f. Cystoscopy
    g. Diagnostic laparoscopy
    h. Vasectomy

Nursing Management

A. Initial Assessment
1. Develop a nursing history for the day surgical patient.
2. Obtain signed informed consent form.
3. Explain what laboratory studies are needed and why.
4. Determine during initial assessment, his physical and psychological status
    Calm or agitated? Overweight? Disabilities or limitations? Clean or dirty? Allergies? Medications being taken? Condition of teeth (dentures, caps, crowns)? Blood pressure problems? Major illnesses? Other surgeries? Seizures? Severe headaches?
5. Begin health education regimen. Instructions to patient:
    a. Notify surgical unit immediately if you get a cold, have a fever, or have any illness before date of surgery.
    b. Arrive at specified time.
    c. No food or fluid since midnight previous to day of surgery.
    d. No make-up or nail polish.
    e. Comfortable, loose clothing; low-heeled shoes.
    f. No valuables or jewelry.
    g. Brush teeth in morning, rinse, but do not swallow liquid.
    h. Have a responsible adult accompany you and drive you home—have person stay with you for 24 hours after surgery.

B. Preoperative Preparation
1. Administer preanesthetic medication; check vital signs.
2. Escort the patient to surgery after he has emptied his bladder.

C. Postoperative Care
1. Check vital signs frequently until stable.
2. Administer oxygen if necessary; check temperature.
3. Change patient's position as he progresses in activity—head of bed elevated, dangling, ambulating with no dizziness or nausea.
4. Ascertain, using the following criteria, that the patient has recovered adequately to be discharged:
    a. Vital signs stable
    b. Stands without dizziness and nausea; begins to walk
    c. Comfortable and free of excessive pain
    d. Able to void
    e. Oriented as to time, place, person
    f. Understands postoperative instructions and takes instruction sheet home

Surgical Risk Factors and Preventive Strategies

A. Obesity
1. Danger
    a. Increases difficulty involved in technical aspects of performing surgery (e.g., sutures are difficult to tie because of fatty secretions); wound dehiscence is greater.
    b. Increases likelihood of infection because of lessened resistance.
    c. Postoperatively, more difficult to turn and ventilate the patient when he is lying on his side. This leads to hypoventilation, pneumonia, and other pulmonary problems.
    d. Increases demands on the heart, leading to cardiovascular embarrassment.
    e. Increases possibility of renal, biliary, hepatic, and endocrine disorders.
2. Therapeutic Approach
    Encourage weight reduction if time permits.

B. Fluid, Electrolyte, and Nutritional Status
1. Danger
    Dehydration and malnutrition have adverse effects in terms of a general anesthetic, the shock of surgery, and postoperative recovery—can disturb fluid and electrolyte balance and lead to shock.

2. Therapeutic Approach
   a. Administer fluids (parenteral) as prescribed.
   b. Keep a detailed input and output record.
   c. Provide high-calorie diet to alleviate malnutrition; supplement with protein and vitamin C—helps repair tissue and serves as a deterrent to infection.
   d. Recommend repair of dental caries and proper mouth hygiene to prevent respiratory tract infection.
   e. Assist with administration (and surveillance) of blood transfusion or protein hydrolysates if there is a protein deficiency.
   f. Assist with hyperalimentation.
   g. Monitor for evidence of electrolyte imbalance (Na^+, K^+, Ca^{++}, etc.).

C. Aging

1. Danger
   a. Recognize that reactions to injury are not as obvious and are slower in appearing.
   b. Be aware that the cumulative effect of medications is greater in the older person than it is in younger people.
   c. Note that medications such as morphine and barbiturates in the usual dosages may cause confusion and disorientation; morphine may cause respiratory depression.
2. Therapeutic Approach
   a. Consider using lesser doses for desired effect.
   b. Anticipate problems from long-standing chronic disorders such as anemia, obesity, diabetes, hypoproteinemia.
   c. Adjust nutritional intake to conform to higher protein and vitamin needs.
   d. When possible, cater to set patterns in older patients (sleeping and eating patterns, use of alcohol and laxatives).

D. Presence of Disease

1. *Cardiovascular*
   a. Increased diligence is required when surgical problem is complicated by a cardiovascular problem.
   b. Avoid overloading the body with fluids (oral, parenteral, blood) because of possible congestive failure and pulmonary edema.
   c. Prevent prolonged immobilization, which results in stasis of circulating fluids.
   d. Encourage change of position but avoid sudden exertion.
   e. Note evidence of hypoxia and initiate therapy.
2. *Diabetes*
   a. Be aware that hypoglycemia due to inadequate carbohydrate intake or insulin overdosage is life-threatening in uncontrolled diabetes.
   b. Recognize the signs and symptoms of ketoaci-

dosis and glucosuria (p. 706), which can threaten an otherwise smooth surgical experience.
   c. Reassure the diabetic patient that when his disease is controlled, the surgical risk may be no greater than it is for the nondiabetic person.
3. *Alcoholism*
   a. Anticipate the additional problem of malnutrition in the presurgical alcoholic patient.
   b. Recognize that the acutely intoxicated person is susceptible to injury and may receive serious injuries without being aware of them.
   c. Be prepared to perform gastric lavage on the intoxicated patient if surgery cannot be postponed; this may lessen the chance of vomiting and aspiration during anesthesia induction.
   d. Note that risk due to surgery is greater for the individual who is a chronic alcoholic.
   e. Anticipate the acute withdrawal syndrome (delirium tremens).
4. *Pulmonary and Upper Respiratory Disease*
   a. Surgery may be contraindicated in the patient who has an upper respiratory infection because an acute upper respiratory infection may be the forerunner of more serious illness, such as pneumonia.
   b. Patients with chronic pulmonary problems such as emphysema, bronchiectasis, etc. should be treated for several days preoperatively with bronchodilators, aerosol medications, and conscientious mouth care, along with a reduction in weight and smoking, and methods to control secretions.
5. *Concurrent or Prior Pharmacotherapy*
   a. Hazards exist when certain medications are given concomitantly with others; therefore, an awareness of prior drug therapy is essential. (Example: interaction of some drugs with anesthetics can lead to arterial hypotension and circulatory collapse.)
   b. Notify anesthesiologist if the patient is taking any of the following drugs:
      (1) Certain antibiotics*—may, when combined with a curariform muscle relaxant, interrupt nerve transmission, causing respiratory paralysis and apnea.
      (2) Antidepressants, particularly monoamine oxidase inhibitors (MAOs), increase hypotensive effects of anesthesia.
      (3) Phenothiazines increase hypotensive action of anesthetics.
      (4) Diuretics, particularly thiazides, cause electrolyte imbalance and respiratory depression during anesthesia.

* Neomycin, streptomycin, dihydrostreptomycin, polymyxin A and B, colistin, viomycin, paromomycin, and kanamycin.

Preoperative Prophylaxis to Prevent Postoperative Venous Thromboembolism*

Low-dose heparin administered to all *hemostatically competent* patients over the age of 40 who are to undergo

* Council on Thrombosis of The American Heart Association. Special Report—Prevention of Venous Thromboembolism in Surgical Patients by Low-Dose Heparin. Circulation 1977 Feb.; Vol. 55, No. 2.

major elective abdominal or thoracic surgical procedures will effect an 80% reduction in postoperative pulmonary emboli.

Significance

This could prevent 4,000–8,000 postoperative deaths annually.

Preoperative Screening

1. Administer no aspirin or other platelet antiaggregating drugs for 5 days prior to an operation.
2. Administer no coumarin therapy at time of operation.
3. Note laboratory results for hematocrit, prothrombin time, partial thromplastin time, and platelet count; these should be within normal ranges prior to operation.

Dose and Duration of Prophylaxis

1. Administer 5,000 USP units of heparin (s.c.) 2 hours before operation.
2. Repeat above dosage every 12 hours until discharge from hospital.

Limitations and Contraindications

1. Of limited value in:
   a. Repair of femoral fracture
   b. Hip and knee joint reconstruction
   c. Open prostatectomy

2. Not recommended for operations:
   a. On the eye
   b. On the brain
   c. With spinal anesthesia
3. *The regimen is ineffective in patients with an active thrombotic process.*
4. This regimen is followed only at the discretion of the physician.

Monitoring of Heparin Therapy

1. Since low-dose heparin does not significantly prolong coagulation time, no laboratory test (whole blood clotting time, partial thromboplastin time, antithrombin III assay) is necessary during therapy.
2. With this regimen, there may be a *slight increase in minor wound hematoma.* Report this immediately.
3. Employ adjunctive measures—early ambulation, leg exercises, and elastic stockings.
4. Avoid positioning of legs that could compromise venous return.

Skin Preparation of Specific Operative Areas

Pharmacophysiologic Emphasis

1. Human skin normally harbors transient and resident bacterial flora, some of which are pathogenic.
2. Skin cannot be sterilized without destroying skin cells.
3. Friction enhances the action of detergent antiseptics.
4. No existing antiseptic produces instant skin disinfection.

5. Unless contraindicated, it may be desirable for the nonemergency patient to bathe with a bacteriostatic soap for several days prior to surgery.
6. Numerous studies indicate that shaving the skin may produce nicks and breaks in the skin, which, in turn, breaks down the skin barrier to infection. However, many surgeons still prefer that the skin be shaved prior to surgery.

Guidelines: Preparing the Patient's Skin for Surgery by Shaving

Goal   To cleanse the skin and reduce the number of organisms on the skin to eliminate as far as possible the transference of such organisms into the incision site.

For Specific Areas

See Figure (pp. 82–83)
For head surgery, obtain specific instructions from the surgeon concerning the extent of shaving.

Equipment

Disposable tray with essentials, or a tray containing
   2 bowls for detergent–germicide
   1 emesis basin
   2 applicator sticks
   6 or 8 (4 × 4-inch) gauze squares
   Razor and blades
   Scissors for cutting long hair, if required

Procedure

Preparatory Phase

1. Explain to the patient the purpose of the activity.
2. Instruct the patient to assume the most comfortable and satisfactory position for the required skin preparation.
3. Cover the patient with a bath blanket, protect bedding, and expose the area to be shaved.

Nursing Action	Rationale/Amplification
Performance Phase	
1. Apply warm detergent–germicide with gauze pledgets and cleanse area using light friction; begin at incision site and, in a circular pattern, work outward from the center.	1. Oils, soil, and organisms are removed from skin surface. Working away from incision site prevents the clean area from becoming recontaminated.

(continued)

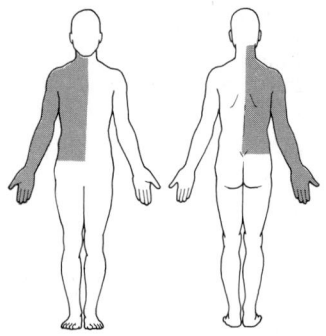

Shoulder prep. Shave fingertips to hairline, midline chest to midline spine on operative side and to iliac crest, including axilla.

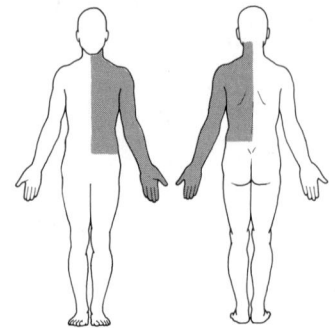

Upper arm prep. Shave fingertips to neckline (hairline), on operative side from midline chest to midline spine on operative side from axilla to iliac crest. Trim and clean fingernails. Use brush on hand and nails.

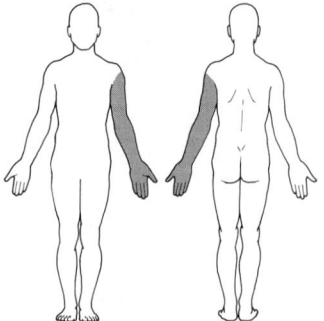

Hand prep. Shave fingertips to shoulder. Trim and clean fingernails. Use brush on hand and nails.

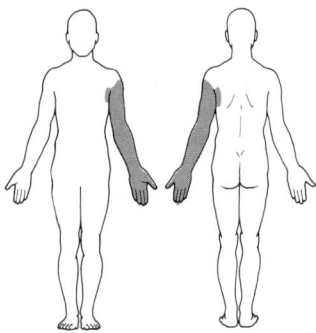

Forearm and elbow prep. Shave from fingernails to shoulder including axilla. Trim and clean fingernails. Use brush on hand and nails.

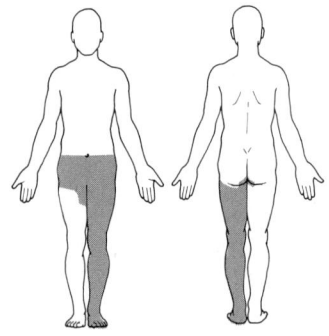

Saphenous vein ligation prep. Shave from umbilicus to toes of affected leg, or both legs. Include pubis and perineal area. Prep entire leg posteriorly.

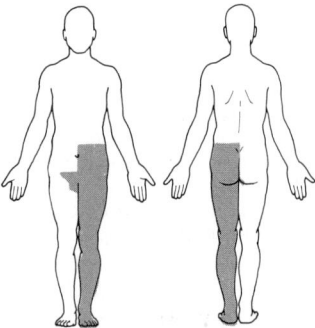

Thigh prep. Shave from toes to 3 inches above the umbilicus, midline front and back. Complete pubic shave. Clean and trim toenails. Use brush on foot and nails.

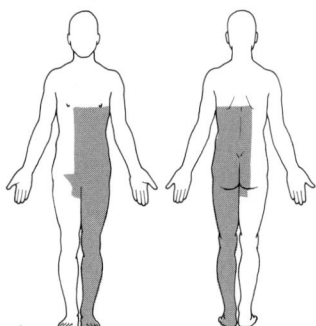

Hip prep. Shave toes to nipple line and at least 3 inches beyond midline back and front. Complete pubic shave. Clean and trim toenails. Use brush on foot and nails. Hip fractures—all preps done in the operating room.

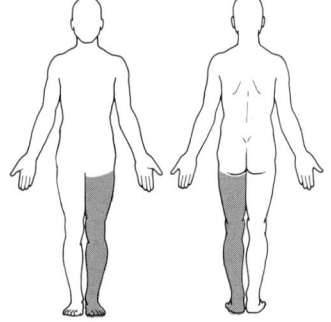

Knee and lower leg prep. Shave entire leg, toes to groin. Clean and trim toenails. Use brush on foot and nails.

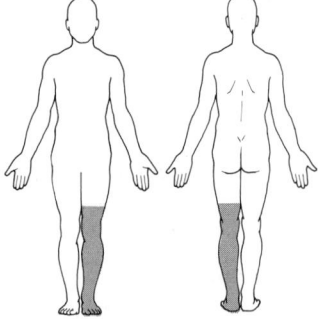

Ankle and foot prep. Shave entire leg, toes to 3 inches above the knee. Clean and trim toenails. Use brush on foot and nails.

(From Committee on Control of Surgical Infections of the Committee on Pre- and Postoperative Care, American College of Surgeons: Manual on Control of Infection in Surgical Patients, Philadelphia, JB Lippincott, 1977).

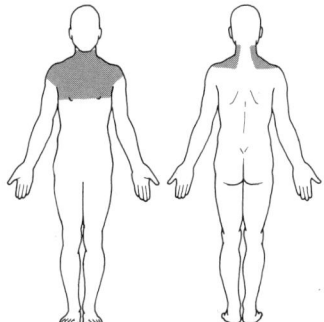

Thyroid prep. Shave from chin line to nipples, including axillary region. Extend to back of neck and upper shoulder as sketched.

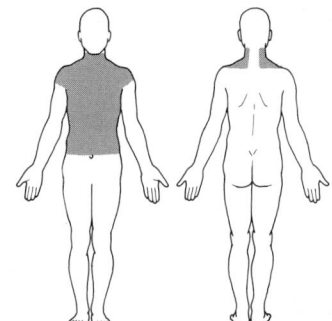

Parathyroid prep (as for sternal splitting). Shave from chin line to umbilicus, shoulder to shoulder in the front. Extend to back of neck and upper shoulder in back as shown. Prep laterally for chest tubes if so prescribed.

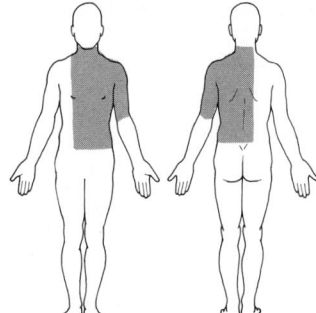

Thoracotomy prep. Shave from chin line to iliac crest, from nipple on unaffected side to at least 2 inches beyond the midline in back. Include axilla and entire arm to elbow.

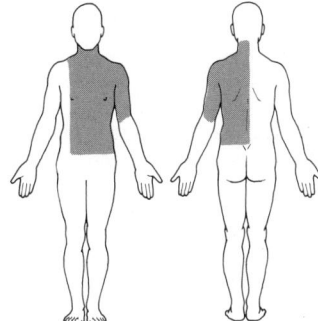

Mastectomy prep. Shave from upper neck to iliac crest, from nipple line on unaffected side to midline of back (affected side). Prep axilla and entire arm to elbow on affected side.

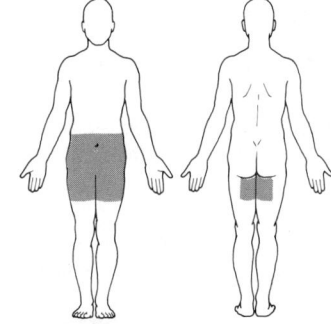

Lower abdominal prep (as for hernia, femoral vein ligation, femoral embolectomy). Shave from 2 inches above the umbilicus to mid-thigh, including the pubic area. Femoral ligation—shave to midline of thigh posteriorly. Hernia and embolectomy—shave to costal margin and down to knee as prescribed.

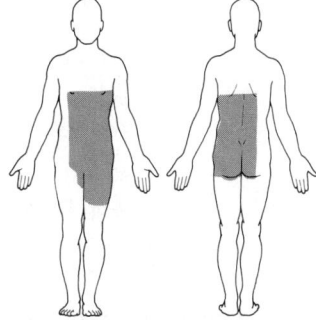

Flank prep (as for renal procedures, adrenalectomy, sympathectomy). Shave from nipple line to pubis and 3 inches beyond the midline in back. Shave pubic area. Shave upper thigh on the affected side.

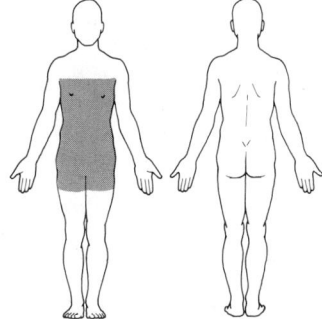

Abdominal prep. Shave from 3 inches above the nipple line to upper thighs, including pubis.

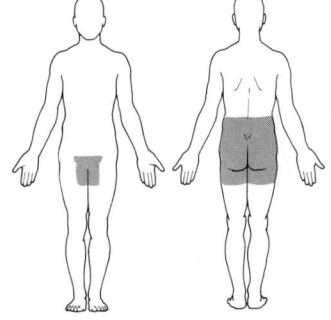

Perineal prep (as for hemorrhoidectomy, fistula-in-ano). Shave pubis, perineum, and perianal area. Shave from the waist in back to at least 3 inches below the groin.

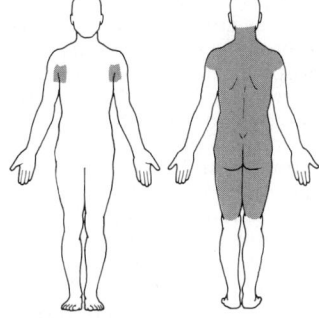

Spine prep. Shave entire back, including shoulders and neck, to hairline and down to knees and to both sides, including axillae.

(continued)

Guidelines: Preparing the Patient's Skin for Surgery by Shaving (continued)

Procedure
(Cont.)

Nursing Action	Rationale/Amplification
2. Cut long hairs with scissors.	2. Much easier and quicker than with a razor.
3. Provide extra attention to areas where there are folds of skin (e.g., axillae, pubic area, umbilicus). Draw loose skin taut. Use cotton-tipped applicators where necessary.	3. Greater numbers of organisms are harbored in folds of skin; removal requires extra effort.
4. If the operative area includes calloused areas or the nails, use a soft-bristled brush.	4. Facilitates cleansing in out-of-the-way areas
5. Soak hairy areas about 4 minutes before shaving.	5. Provides time to permit the keratin of the hair to absorb fluid, which makes the hair softer.
6. Shave with the direction of hair growth—not the opposite direction of hair growth.	6. This leaves a blunt rather than a sharp hair stub, which could penetrate the wall of the hair follicle and inject itself into the skin (risking postoperative pseudofolliculitis).

▶ **NURSING ALERT:** *Pseudofolliculitis barbae* is a papulopustular inflammation of hair follicles in areas that have been shaved so closely that the sharp-pointed tip may inject itself into the side of the hair follicle, carrying bacteria into the skin. It simulates folliculitis barbae, which develops in bearded areas. Note above items 5 and 6 to prevent this condition.

7. Use a disposable or sterilized razor and a sharp, new blade.	7. Avoids risk of infectious hepatitis from contaminated razor.
8. For denuded or sensitive areas, soak gently with detergent and flush thoroughly with saline or sterile water.	8. Prevents additional trauma.
9. Avoid nicking the skin; report any skin abrasions.	9. An opening in the skin increases the hazard of infection.
10. Gently scrub the skin area after the shaving is completed; rinse carefully and blot dry.	10. Prevents irritation and chapping.

Follow-up Phase

1. Remove all equipment and dispose of expendable materials according to local policy.
2. Remind the patient of the necessity for keeping the prepared area clean for surgery; provide for his comfort.

Immediate Presurgical Preparation of the Patient

Physical and Psychological Attention to the Patient

1. Provide patient with a short gown to be worn to the operating room.
2. Remove hairpins; braid long hair; cover hair with a cap.
3. Remove dentures or plates (unless anesthesiologist requests that they be left in to reduce respiratory tract obstruction); inspect mouth for foreign material such as chewing gum.
4. Remove jewelry, identify properly, and place in the hospital safe; if wedding ring cannot be removed, tie with gauze bandage fastened around wrist.
5. Remove contact lenses; have the patient place them in properly marked receptacle (left and right), identify properly, and deposit in the hospital safe.
6. Have the patient void before receiving preoperative medication and immediately before leaving for the operating room; measure amount and note time of voiding; document.
7. Continue to support the patient emotionally and correct any misconceptions he may have.
8. Permit the patient to relax as the medication becomes effective prior to his being called to the operating room; instruct the patient to call for assistance if necessary. Raise side rails.

Preanesthetic Medication

(Prescribed to meet individual needs)

Goals

1. To facilitate the administration of any anesthetic
2. To minimize respiratory tract secretions and changes in heart rate
3. To relax the patient and reduce anxiety

▶ **NURSING ALERT:** Administer preanesthetic medication precisely at the time it is prescribed. If given too early, the maximum potency will have passed before it is needed; if given too late, the action will not have begun before anesthesia is started.

"On Call" Medications

1. Have medication ready and administer as soon as call is received.
2. Proceed with remaining preparation activities.
3. Indicate on the chart or preoperative check list the time when medication was administered.

Transporting Patient to the Operating Room

1. Adhere to the principle of maintaining the comfort and safety of the patient.
2. Accompany operating room attendants to the patient's bedside for introduction and proper identification.
3. Assist in transferring the patient from bed to stretcher (unless bed goes to OR floor).
4. Complete chart and preoperative check list; include

laboratory reports and x-rays as required in the operating room.
5. Recognize importance of coordinating team effort to ensure arrival of the patient in the operating room at the proper time.

The Patient's Family

1. Direct the patient's family to the proper waiting room where magazines, television, and coffee may be available.
2. Inform them that the surgeon will probably come to this room immediately after surgery to inform them of the operation.
3. Acquaint the family with the fact that a long interval of waiting does not mean the patient is in the operating room all the while; anesthesia preparation and induction take time, and after surgery the patient is taken to the recovery room.
4. Tell the family what to expect postoperatively when they see the patient—tubes, monitoring equipment, and blood transfusion, suctioning, and oxygen equipment.

The Nursing Process in the Immediate Postoperative Period

Assessment

Immediate Nursing Assessment

Upon receiving a patient in the recovery room from the anesthesiologist and circulating nurse, the following determinations are made:
1. Appraise the air-exchange status of the patient and note his skin color.
2. Verify the patient's identity, the operative procedure, and the surgeon who performed the procedure.
3. Request a briefing on problems encountered in the operating room and those that may arise in the recovery period.
4. Determine vital signs and establish with the anesthesiologist an agreement as to their meaning.
5. Examine the operative site and check dressings for drainage.
6. Perform safety checks to verify that padded side rails are in place and restraints properly applied for infusions, transfusions, etc.

Patient Problems/Nursing Diagnoses

1. Possible ineffective airway clearance related to effects of general anesthesia
2. Possible fluid volume deficit related to blood loss, food and fluid deprivation, potential vomiting
3. Alteration in sensory perception related to effects of medications and anesthesia
4. Alteration in comfort (pain) related to surgical incision and tissue trauma
5. Impairment of skin integrity related to operative incision
6. Alteration in nutrition related to reduced intake preoperatively and during day of surgery
7. Potential for injury due to sensory deprivation as a result of preanesthetic medications and anesthesia

Planning and Implementation

Nursing Interventions

A. Ensure the Maintenance of a Patent Airway and Adequate Respiratory Function.

1. Place the patient in the lateral position with neck extended (if not contraindicated)—this permits the best possible expansion of the lungs.
2. Allow metal, rubber, or plastic airway to remain in place until the patient begins to waken and is trying to eject the airway.
   a. The airway keeps the passage open and prevents the tongue from falling backward and obstructing the air passages.
   b. Leaving the airway in after the pharyngeal reflex has returned may cause the patient to gag and vomit.

Note: Many seriously ill patients return from the operating room with a tracheal tube in place; this may be left in place for hours or days and requires special management.

3. When the patient is partially awake and the airway is removed, he may show signs of gagging, nausea, or vomiting; place him in the lateral position with the upper arm supported on a pillow.
   a. This will promote chest expansion.
   b. Turn the patient every hour or two to facilitate breathing and ventilation.
4. Aspirate excessive secretions when they are heard in the nasopharynx and oropharynx.
   a. Using a Y-connecting tube with catheter, turn suction machine on, insert catheter into pharynx 15–20 cm. (6–8 inches), then close Y-tube outlet with finger to activate suction; withdraw slowly while rotating catheter.
   b. If secretions are lower in the tracheobronchial tree, intratracheal suctioning may be necessary. (See procedure for tracheal suctioning, p. 153.)
5. Encourage patient to take deep breaths to aerate lungs fully and prevent hypostatic pneumonia; use incentive spirometer to aid in this function (p. 208).
6. Administer humidified oxygen if required.
   a. Heat and moisture are normally lost during exhalation.
   b. Dehydrated patients may require oxygen and humidity because of higher incidence of irritated respiratory passages in these patients.
   c. Secretions can be kept soft to facilitate removal.
7. Employ mechanical ventilation to maintain adequate pulmonary ventilation if required (see p. 227).

B. Assess Status of Circulatory System.

1. Take vital signs (blood pressure, pulse, and respiration) frequently, as clinical condition indicates, until the patient is well stabilized. Then check every 4 hours thereafter.
   a. Know the patient's preoperative blood pressure in order to make significant comparisons.
   b. Report immediately a falling systolic pressure.
   c. Variations in blood pressure and cardiac arrhythmias are reportable.
   d. Respirations over 30 should be reported.
   e. Evaluate pulse pressure to determine status of perfusion.
2. Recognize the variety of factors that may alter circulating blood volume.

a. Reactions to anesthesia and medications
b. Blood loss and organ manipulation during surgery
c. Moving the patient from one position on the operating table to another on the stretcher
3. Monitor temperature hourly to be alert for hyperthermia and to detect hypothermia. A temperature over 37.7°C. (100°F.) or under 36.1°C. (97°F.) is reportable.
4. Be aware of early symptoms of shock or hemorrhage.
   a. Cool extremities, decreased urine output, and narrowing of pulse pressure may be indicative of decreased cardiac output.
   b. Rapid, thready pulse and a falling blood pressure may indicate hemorrhage, leading to a decrease in blood volume.
   c. Initiate oxygen therapy to increase oxygen availability from the circulating blood.
   d. Place the patient in shock position with feet elevated (unless contraindicated).
   e. See page 90 for more detailed consideration of shock.

C. Promote Comfort and Maintain Safety.

1. Provide a therapeutic environment with proper temperature and humidity; remove unnecessary blanket, which might cause loss of body fluid through excessive perspiration; when cold, provide warm blankets.
2. Place side rails in protecting position until the patient is fully awake.
3. Protect the extremity into which intravenous fluids are running so that the needle will not become accidentally dislodged.
4. Turn the patient frequently and maintain good body alignment.
5. Avoid nerve damage and muscle strain by properly supporting and padding pressure areas.
6. Assess pain by observing behavioral and physiologic manifestations.
7. Administer analgesics (low blood pressure may be a result of pain).

D. Continue Constant Surveillance of the Patient Until He Is Completely Out of Anesthesia.

▶ **NURSING ALERT:** This phase of nursing care is geared to *recognizing* the significance of signs and *anticipating* and *preventing* postoperative difficulties.
Carefully monitor the patient coming out of general anesthesia until:
1. Vital signs are stable for at least 30 minutes and are within *his* normal range.
2. He is breathing easily.
3. Reflexes have returned to normal.
4. He is out of anesthesia, responsive, and oriented to time and place.
For the patient who had regional anesthesia, observe carefully until:
1. Sensation has been recovered.
2. Reflexes have returned.
3. Vital signs have stabilized for at least 30 minutes.

1. Be aware of the fact that the patient cannot complain of injury such as the pricking of an open safety pin, or a clamp that is exerting pressure.
2. Examine dressings for unexpected drainage or bleeding.
3. Check dressings for constriction.
4. Observe drainage tubes and catheters for proper connection and patency.
5. Note proper functioning of monitoring and suctioning devices, oxygen therapy equipment, etc.
6. Observe the patient for bladder distention (see Fig. 11-9, p. 514).
7. Inspect skin and tissue surrounding intravenous needles to detect early infiltration.
8. Evaluate periodically the patient's status of orientation—how he responds to being addressed by his name or performs simple movements upon receiving a command.

Patient: Smith, Raymond
Room: B 1083
Date: 3/7/-

POST-ANESTHESIA RECOVERY ROOM
SCORING CARD

Final Score: 10
Physician: Dr. J. Evans
Nurse: Mrs. Peggy Fay, R.N.

Physical Signs → TIME ↓	ACTIVITY Score	Comment	RESPIRATION Score	Comment	CIRCULATION Score	Comment	CONSCIOUSNESS Score	Comment	COLOR Score	Comment	TOTAL SCORE
Admission A.M. 11:15 P.M.	1	Spinal anesth.	1	chest & abdom. pain.	1		1	Semi-conscious	1		5
½ Hour A.M. 11:45 P.M.	1		1		2		1		1	Slight pallor	6
½ Hour A.M. P.M.											
Dismissal A.M. 12:15 P.M.	2		2		2		2	alert verbally responsive	2	color improved	10
FINAL SCORE A.M. P.M.	2		2		2		2		2		10

Figure 6-2. Recovery room scoring card.

Note: Alterations in cerebral function may suggest impaired oxygen delivery to tissues.

9. Determine return of motor control following spinal anesthesia—indicated by how the patient responds to a pinprick or a request to move a part. *See Postanesthesia Recovery Room Scoring Guide* (Fig. 6-2).

E. Recognize Stress Factors That May Affect the Patient in the Recovery Room and Attempt to Minimize These Factors.

1. Know that the ability to hear returns more quickly than other senses as the patient emerges from anesthesia.
2. Avoid saying anything in the patient's presence that may disturb him; he may appear to be sleeping but still consciously hears what is being said.
3. Explain procedures and activities at the patient's level of understanding.
4. Minimize the patient's exposure to emergency treatment of nearby patients by drawing curtains and lowering voice and noise levels.
5. Treat the patient as a person who needs as much attention as the equipment and monitoring devices.
6. Respect his feeling of sensory deprivation and simultaneous bombardment of sensory stimuli; make any necessary adjustments to minimize this problem.
7. Make every effort to demonstrate concern for and understanding of this patient—anticipate his needs and feelings.

8. Tell the patient repeatedly that the surgery is over and that he is in the recovery room.

F. Transfer the Patient from the Recovery Room to his Unit.

1. Relay appropriate information to the unit nurse regarding his condition; point out significant needs (e.g., drainage, fluid therapy, incision and dressing requirements, intake needs, urinary output).
2. Assure the patient of his value as a person and reinforce his positive thoughts of recovering.

Evaluation

Expected Outcomes

(Criteria for leaving recovery unit)

1. Breathes easily with clear lung sounds noted via stethoscopic auscultation.
2. Reaches stable vital signs and achieves adequate circulatory perfusion.
3. Responds well to commands when asked to cough, breathe deeply, or move extremities.
4. Approaches a satisfactory level of awareness and consciousness.
5. Complains minimally of pain that is being controlled with increasingly less potent medications.
6. Maintains acceptable levels of urinary output (at least 30 ml./hr.).
7. Appears to have vomiting well under control, if not absent.

Postanesthesia Recovery Room Scoring Guide*

Many hospitals use a scoring system to determine the patient's general condition and his readiness to be released from the recovery room. As the patient progresses through the recovery period, his physical signs are observed and evaluated by means of an objective scoring guide.

Objective:

To provide the recovery room staff with a guideline to the patient's condition following surgery and anesthesia. This evaluation system is a modification of the Apgar score.

Physical Signs and Criteria for Their Assessment

1. Activity
   Muscle activity is assessed by observing the ability of the patient to move his extremities spontaneously or on command.
   Score: 2—able to move all extremities
   1—able to move 2 extremities
   0—not able to control any extremity
2. Respiration
   Respiratory efficiency evaluated in a form that permits accurate and objective assessment without complicated physical tests.
   Score: 2—able to breathe deeply and cough
   1—limited respiratory effort (dyspnea or splinting)
   0—no spontaneous respiratory effort
3. Circulation
   Use changes in arterial blood pressure from preanesthetic level.
   Score: 2—systolic arterial pressure between plus or minus 20% of preanesthetic level (Riva–Rocci method)
   1—systolic arterial pressure between plus or minus 20% to 50% of preanesthetic level
   0—systolic arterial pressure between plus or minus 50% or more of the preanesthetic level
4. Consciousness
   Determination of the patient's level of consciousness.
   Score: 2—full alertness seen in patient's ability to answer questions and acknowledge his/her location
   1—aroused when called by name
   0—failure to elicit a response upon auditory stimulation
   Physical stimulation should not be considered reliable since even a decerebrated patient might react to it.
5. Color
   This is an objective sign that is easy to recognize.
   Score: 2—normal skin color and appearance
   1—any alteration in skin color: pale, dusky, blotchy, jaundiced, etc.
   0—frank cyanosis

Implications of Score

1. The patient's score is taken at stated intervals, such as every 15 or 30 minutes, and totaled on the official scorecard (Fig. 6.2).
2. Patients with a total score of less than 7 must remain in the recovery room until improved or transferred to an intensive care area.
3. This guide permits a more objective evaluation of the patient's physical condition in the recovery area (Fig. 6-2).

* Margaret Furay Rozman. Introduction to Recovery Room Nursing. Denver, Association of Operating Room Nurses

Postoperative Discomforts

Many patients experience some discomforts postoperatively. These are usually related to the general anesthetic and/or the surgical procedure. The most common discomforts are nausea, vomiting, restlessness, sleeplessness, thirst, constipation, and pain.

Nausea and Vomiting

Incidence

1. Occurs in many postoperative patients.
2. Results from an accumulation of fluid or food in the stomach before peristalsis returns.
3. May occur as a result of abdominal distention, which follows manipulation of abdominal organs.
4. Induced during anesthesia from inadequate ventilation.
5. Likely to occur if the patient believes preoperatively that he will vomit (psychological induction).
6. May be a side effect of narcotics.

Preventive Measures

1. Insert nasogastric tube preoperatively for operations on gastrointestinal tract to prevent abdominal distention, which triggers vomiting.
2. Determine whether patient is sensitive to morphine and meperidine (Demerol), since they may induce vomiting in some patients.
3. Be alert for any significant comment such as, "I just know I will vomit under anesthesia." Report such a comment to the anesthesiologist, who may prescribe an antiemetic drug and also talk to the patient before the operation.

Nursing Interventions

1. Encourage patient to breathe deeply to facilitate elimination of anesthetic.
2. Support the wound during retching and vomiting; turn head to side to avoid aspiration.
3. Discard vomitus and refresh patient—mouthwash for mouth, clean linens for bed, etc.
4. Suspect idiosyncratic response to a drug if vomiting is worse when a medication is given (but diminishes thereafter).
5. Administer antiemetic medication such as prochlorperazine (Compazine).
6. Offer hot tea with lemon or small sips of a carbonated beverage such as ginger ale, if tolerated.
7. Report excessive or prolonged vomiting so that the cause may be investigated.
8. Detect presence of abdominal distention, hiccups, suggesting gastric retention.
9. Suspect the possibility of paralytic ileus.

Restlessness and Sleeplessness

Promoting Factors	Relief Measures
1. Discomfort such as back pain, headache, and thirst	1. Massage the back gently, using an emollient lotion. Administer acetylsalicylic acid as prescribed.
2. Tight dressings or drainage-soaked dressings	2. Change dressings and check for tightness.
3. Urinary retention	3. Utilize nursing measures to initiate voiding (see p. 93).
4. Abdominal distention	4. Ambulation; insert rectal tube to relieve flatus—stimulates peristalsis and propels gas to rectum.
5. Noise and environmental stimuli	5. Keep noise level at a minimum. Limit visitors to those who may promote rest in the patient. For rest periods, provide privacy, darkness, and quiet. Schedule treatments with this in mind.
6. Worry and anxiety	6. Attempt to find cause of concern. Provide time to talk with the patient and permit him to vent his feelings. Seek advice of spiritual counselor or psychologist if necessary. Offer sedatives or hypnotics as required.

Thirst

Causes

1. Inhibition of secretions by preoperative medication with atropine.
2. Fluid lost via perspiration, blood loss, and dehydration due to preoperative fluid restriction.

Nursing Intervention

1. Administer fluids by vein or by mouth if tolerated.
2. Offer sips of hot tea with lemon juice to dissolve mucus.
3. Apply a moistened gauze square over lips occasionally to humidify inspired air.
4. Allow the patient to rinse mouth with mouthwash; lemon juice and glycerin swabbing of the mouth is also refreshing.
5. Obtain hard candies or chewing gum to help in stimulating saliva flow and in keeping the mouth moist.

Constipation

Causes

1. Trauma and irritation to the bowel during surgery.
2. Local inflammation, peritonitis, or abscess.
3. Long-standing bowel problem: This may lead to fecal impaction.

Preventive Measures

1. Early ambulation to aid in promoting peristalsis.
2. Adequate fluid intake to keep stool soft and promote hydration.
3. Proper diet to promote peristalsis and maintain adequate fluid balance.
4. Query patient as to his usual remedy for constipation; try this.

Treatment (Fecal Impaction)

(See also p. 465.)
1. Insert a gloved finger and break up the impaction manually.
2. Administer an oil enema (180–200 ml.) to help soften the mass and facilitate evacuation.

Pain

Pain is a subjective symptom in which the patient exhibits a feeling of distress caused by stimulation of certain nerve endings; usually it indicates that tissue damage is beginning to take place or has taken place as a result of surgery.

Incidence

1. Pain is one of the earliest symptoms that the patient expresses upon return to consciousness.
2. Maximal postoperative pain occurs between 12 and 36 hours after surgery and usually disappears by 48 hours.
3. Anesthetic agents that are soluble are slow to leave the body and therefore control pain for a longer time than agents that are insoluble; the latter produce rapid recovery, but the patient is more restless and complains more of pain.
4. Older persons seem to have a higher tolerance for pain than younger or middle-aged persons.
5. There is no documented proof that one sex tolerates pain better than the other.

Clinical Manifestations

1. Autonomic
   a. Outpouring of epinephrine
   b. Elevation of blood pressure
   c. Increase in heart and pulse rate
   d. Rapid and irregular respiration
   e. Increase in perspiration
2. Skeletal muscle
   Increase in muscle tension or activity
3. Psychological
   a. Increase in irritability
   b. Increase in apprehension
   c. Increase in anxiety
   d. Attention focused on pain
   e. Complaints of pain

Patient's reaction depends upon:
1. Previous experience
2. Anxiety or tension
3. State of health
4. His ability to concentrate away from the problem or be distracted
5. Meaning that pain has for him

Nursing Interventions

1. Employ comfort measures in caring for the patient.
   a. Provide therapeutic environment—proper temperature and humidity, ventilation, visitors.
   b. Increase the patient's bodily comfort by adding a blanket if he is cold, and vice versa.
   c. Massage the patient's back in soothing strokes—move him easily and gently.
   d. Offer diversional activities, soft radio music, or favorite quiet television program.
   e. Provide for fluid needs by giving a cool drink, offering a bedpan.
   f. Investigate possible causes of pain such as bandage or adhesive that is too tight, full bladder, cast that is too snug, or elevated temperature suggestive of inflammation or infection.
2. Initiate measures to reduce the likelihood of pain.
   a. Encourage the patient to turn frequently.
   b. Massage pressure areas; support vulnerable areas—strategic placement of pillow, anchoring a footboard, placing a pillow between legs in the Sims's lateral position.
   c. Determine the patient's need to void and need for relief from intestinal distension.
   d. Loosen constricting dressings.
   e. Keep bedding clean, dry, and free from crumbs.
   f. Maintain the patient in correct physiologic position.
   g. Encourage the patient to verbalize—to ease pain reaction, raise threshold.
   h. Give analgesic drugs as prophylaxis to prevent pain.
3. Relieve localized pain.
   a. Carefully support the painful area and elevate painful extremities.
   b. Apply medications or counterirritants gently; use hot or cold applications as prescribed.
   c. Encourage and assist the patient to follow prescribed exercise program.
4. Recognize the power of suggestion; mention that relief of pain will take place when a "reasonable" method is selected and used.
   a. Combine chosen method of pain relief with verbal assurance that it will help.
   b. Explain why the method chosen will help in relieving pain—positive assurance has been recognized as enhancing the effect of the "reasonable" action.
   c. Indicate to the patient that you understand that he has pain, that you have time to listen and to help him, and that you care.
5. Be selective in administering pain-relieving agents; recognize individual differences.
   a. First determine the patient's respiratory rate and level of activity (arousal); use this information in making subsequent assessments.
   b. Administer tranquilizers to relieve anxiety.
   c. Use narcotic analgesics when postoperative pain justifies such medication.
   d. Patients who have had abdominal or chest surgery are more likely to need narcotics. The exchange of respiratory gases can be reduced by pain that causes reflex chest-muscle contraction.
   e. Potent drugs such as morphine may produce depression of the patient's respiratory center, thereby reducing rate and depth of breathing; also, such drugs tend to constrict bronchiolar smooth muscles and increase tracheal bronchial secretions—leading to atelectasis and pneumonia.
   f. Give narcotic agonist–antagonist (capable of reversing effects of narcotics, but in absence of narcotic, they produce a narcotic-like action) when prescribed.
   g. Provide soporifics for sleep induction.
   h. Administer muscle-relaxant and antispasmodic medications for uncontrolled muscle tension.
   i. Utilize specific medications for specific conditions

such as relief of nausea, relief of undesirable coughing, relief of headache.
j. Administer Narcan to relieve significant respiratory depression when brought about by a narcotic or narcotic agonist–antagonist.

▶ **NURSING ALERT:** "Potentiators" (hydroxyzine, promethazine) appear to sedate the patient, but it has not been proven that they are effective in potentiating the effects of an analgesic.

6. Recognize desired effects and untoward reactions of all medications given.

a. Observe patient for desired effect of medication.
b. Note respiratory rate; compare it with rate noted before medication was given. Assess the difference. A narcotic is more likely to cause respiratory depression.
c. Be alert to toxic manifestations and hypersensitivity reactions.
  (1) Unpleasant psychic reactions (anxiety, hallucinations) may occur in some patients after taking a narcotic agonist–antagonist.
d. Be knowledgeable about drug interactions.
e. Note signs of respiratory embarrassment, adverse vital signs, rashes.

Postoperative Complications

Shock

Shock is a response of the body to a decrease in the circulating volume of blood; tissue perfusion is impaired culminating, eventually, in cellular hypoxia.

Classification

1. *Oligemic* (hematogenic)—shock resulting from loss of plasma or whole blood; this may be external or internal. When 10% of the blood volume is lost, *hypovolemic* shock occurs.
2. *Bacteremic* (septic or toxic shock)—characterized by a change in the capillary endothelium, permitting loss of blood and plasma through capillary walls into surrounding tissues; no actual fluid volume is lost from the body.
3. *Cardiogenic*—observed when there is interference with heart pumping action, as might occur in myocardial infarction, cardiac tamponade, which results in inadequate vascular circulation.
4. *Neurogenic* (vasogenic)—marked vasodilation and reflex inhibition, which results in a sluggish circulating system, depriving vital centers of proper blood supply.
5. *Psychic*—results from extreme pain or deep fear.

Altered Physiology and Clinical Manifestations

1. Loss of effective circulating blood volume—initiates metabolic and physiologic reactions resulting in poor tissue perfusion (see Table 6-1).
2. Hyperventilation, caused by stress, leads to respiratory alkalosis; this is the earliest acid–gas change of shock.
3. Pituitary hormones are released:
  ACTH (adrenocorticotropic)—stimulates the adrenal cortex to secrete glucocorticoids.
  ADH (antidiuretic)—stimulates kidney tubules to absorb more fluid.
  ASH (aldosterone-stimulating)—stimulates potassium excretion by kidney, stimulates sodium chloride retention and water retention.
4. Epinephrine and norepinephrine promote capillary vasoconstriction—increases flow through vital organs but diminishes flow through peripheral tissues. Later, peripheral vasoconstriction produces *pale, cold, clammy skin.*
5. Acidemia causes lung to compensate—increased rate (tachypnea) and volume.
6. Heart rate accelerates; diastole lessens.
  With lessened coronary perfusion during diastole,

Table 6-1 Correlation of Magnitude to Volume Deficit and Clinical Presentation

		Shock	
Approximate Deficit	Decrease in Blood Volume	Degree	Signs
ml.	%		
0–500	0–10	None	None
500–1200	10–25	Mild (compensated)	Slight tachycardia Mild hypotension Mild peripheral vasoconstriction
1200–1800	25–35	Moderate	Thready pulse, 100–120 beats/min. Blood pressure, 90–100 mm. Hg systolic Marked vasoconstriction Diaphoresis Anxiety, restlessness Decreased urinary output
1800–2500	35–50	Severe	Thready pulse, 120 beats/min. Blood pressure, 60 mm. Hg systolic Marked vasoconstriction Marked diaphoresis Obtundation No urinary output

(Wilkins EW Jr [ed]. MGH Textbook of Emergency Medicine, 2nd ed, p. 40. Baltimore, Williams & Wilkins, 1983)

cardiac output falls, resulting in *reduced systolic pressure, lowered pulse pressure,* and generalized vasoconstriction.
7. Weak, thready pulse and subnormal temperature.
8. Lip cyanosis, circumoral pallor; decreased salivary secretions.
9. At first patient appears *nervous* and *apprehensive;* later, *apathy develops* and *sensations are dulled. Muscle weakness* and *fatigue* become apparent.

Effects of Shock

1. *Anoxia*—lack of oxygen in the body
2. *Anoxemia*—decreased amount of oxygen in the blood
3. *Hyperpyrexia*—an excessive fever, about 42.2 to 42.8°C. (108–109°F.), which occurs shortly before death
4. *Oliguria*—decreased kidney secretion and urinary output
5. *Anuria*—absence of urinary secretion
6. Thrombosis with subsequent emboli due to blood stasis

Nursing Interventions

A. Prevention

1. Prepare adequately the mental as well as the physical condition of the patient.
2. Anticipate any complications that may arise during and after surgery.
3. Have blood available if there is any indication that it may be needed.
4. Measure accurately any blood loss.
5. Keep operative trauma to a minimum; minimize postoperative disturbance of the patient.
6. Anticipate progression of symptoms upon earliest manifestation.
7. Monitor vital signs frequently until they are stable.
8. Assess vital sign deviations; evaluate blood pressure in relation to other parameters.
9. Institute therapy immediately following an injury, etc., that is likely to lead to shock.
10. Recognize that blood pressure limits vary with individuals; in some patients 90/60 may be normal, whereas in others it may indicate severe shock.
11. Prevent infection; this will prevent septic shock.

B. Definitive Management

1. KEEP THE AIRWAY PATENT
    a. Use an airway or place an endotracheal tube.
    b. Remove oral and tracheal secretions.
    c. Institute resuscitative measures if necessary.
2. Arrest hemorrhage (not present in septic shock). Ascertain where hemorrhage is occurring; if external, utilize pressure control.
3. Place patient in most physiologically desirable position for shock (Fig. 6-3).
    a. Elevate the head on a pillow.
    b. Keep the trunk horizontal.
    c. Elevate lower extremities about 20 to 30 degrees, keeping knees straight.

▶ **NURSING ALERT:** Do not use Trendelenburg head-low position because (1) after initial increase of blood to the head, a reflex compensatory action takes place causing vasoconstriction and thereby decreasing blood supply to the brain; and (2) viscera tend to fall against the diaphragm, causing increased resistance to breathing and inadequate ventilation.

4. Ensure an adequate venous return.
    a. Insert intravenous catheter for infusion in upper extremities; 2 may be required.
    b. Place a central venous pressure (CVP) catheter in or near the right atrium (see Fig. 9-3 and Guidelines, p. 287).
        (1) Note direction and degree of change from initial reading.
        (2) Utilize route established by CVP catheter for emergency fluid volume and electrolyte replacement.
    c. Start plasma expanders if needed until whole blood is available.
    d. Begin blood transfusion when blood is available.
5. Obtain blood for determinations of pH, PO_2, PCO_2, and hematocrit; correct deviations.
    a. pH—may indicate acidosis resulting from anaerobic metabolism.
    b. PCO_2—assesses function of pulmonary alveolar membrane.
    c. PO_2—determines level of oxygen tension.
    d. Hematocrit—reveals losses due to obstruction or peritonitis.

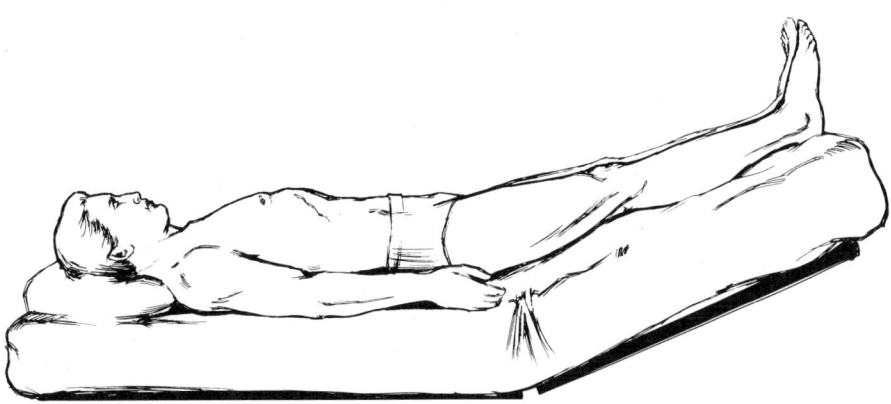

Figure 6-3. Proper positioning of the patient who shows signs of shock. Elevate the lower extremities about 20 degrees, keeping the knees straight, trunk horizontal, and head slightly elevated.

6. Insert a urinary catheter to monitor hourly urinary output.

   Objective is to maintain a 1 ml./kg./hr. urinary volume output to ensure adequate kidney perfusion.

7. Administer antimicrobials in order to offset infection, which can occur due to stagnant hypoxia in wounds and in peripheral tissues.

   Utilize large doses of penicillin, streptomycin, or broad-spectrum chemotherapeutic agents.

8. Support the defense mechanisms of the patient.
   a. Comfort and reassure the patient if he is conscious.
   b. Resort to sedation and analgesia with discriminating judgment.
   c. Keep the patient warm, but do not apply too much external covering, since it will produce unnecessary vasodilation resulting in more fluid loss.

9. Recognize signs of impending cardiac failure—increasing CVP, distended neck veins, pulmonary crackles, etc.

   Initiate prophylactic inotropic drugs.

   Use rapid-acting medications in the very young and very old (dopamine, isoproterenol).

10. If the patient does not respond to fluid loading and inotropic drugs, expect steroids to be prescribed.

11. If response to conventional methods fails, it may be necessary to resort to mechanical assistance, such as use of intra-aortic balloon pump to increase diastolic aortic pressure.

12. Throughout the entire panorama of impending shock, continue flow sheet, recording of vital signs, observations, and interventions.

13. Septic shock is most often due to gram-negative infection: peritonitis, meningitis; it may have a direct toxic effect on the heart resulting in depressed cardiac function.

Hemorrhage

Hemorrhage is copious escape of blood from a blood vessel.

Classification

A. General

1. *Primary*—occurs at the time of operation.
2. *Intermediary*—occurs within the first few hours after surgery.

   Blood pressure returns to normal and causes loosening of poorly tied vessels and flushing out of weak clots from untied vessels.

3. *Secondary*—occurs some time after surgery.
   a. Ligature slips from blood vessel.
   b. Erosion of blood vessel.

B. According to Blood Vessels

1. *Capillary*—slow general oozing from capillaries.
2. *Venous*—bleeding that is dark in color and bubbles out.
3. *Arterial*—bleeding that spurts and is bright red in color.

C. According to Location

1. *Evident or external*—visible bleeding on the surface.
2. *Concealed or internal*—bleeding that cannot be seen.

Clinical Manifestations

1. Apprehension, restlessness, thirst; cold, moist, pale skin.
2. Pulse increases, respirations become rapid and deep ("air hunger"), temperature drops.
3. With progression of hemorrhage
   a. Decrease in cardiac output.
   b. Rapidly decreasing arterial and venous blood pressure as well as hemoglobin.
   c. Circumoral pallor, spots appear before the eyes, ringing in the ears.
   d. Patient grows weaker until death occurs.

Nursing Interventions

1. Treat the patient as described for shock (p. 90).
2. Inspect the wound as a possible site of bleeding.

   If an extremity is bleeding, apply a gauze-pad pressure dressing.

3. Administer blood (typed) or blood substitute until blood is available.

▶ **NURSING ALERT:** In giving fluids by vein, recognize that, in the case of hemorrhage, giving too large a quantity or administering fluids too rapidly may elevate the blood pressure sufficiently to recycle the hemorrhaging process.

Femoral Phlebitis or Deep Thrombophlebitis

Phlebitis often occurs after operations on the lower abdomen or during the course of septic conditions such as ruptured ulcer or peritonitis. (See p. 362, Chap. 9.)

Causes

1. Injury—damage to vein resulting from
   a. Tight straps or leg holders during surgery.
   b. Compression of a blanket roll under the knees.
2. Fluid loss or dehydration leading to concentration of blood.
3. Lowered metabolism and circulatory depression after surgery leading to slowing of blood flow.
4. Combinations of the above.

Clinical Manifestations

1. Left leg appears to be affected more frequently than right.
2. Pain or cramp in the calf, progressing to painful swelling of entire leg.
3. Slight fever, chills, perspiration.
4. Marked tenderness over anteromedial surface of thigh.
5. Intravascular clotting without marked inflammation may develop, leading to phlebothrombosis.

▶ **NURSING ALERT:** A complaint of slight soreness of the calf is never ignored. The danger inherent in femoral thrombosis is that a clot may be dislodged and produce an embolus.

Nursing Interventions

A. Prophylaxis

1. Hydrate the patient adequately postoperatively to prevent blood concentration.
2. Encourage leg exercises and ambulate the patient as soon as permitted by the surgeon. (Exercises are taught preoperatively—see p. 77.)
3. Avoid any restricting devices such as tight straps that can constrict and impair circulation.

4. Prevent the use of bed rolls, knee gatches, even "dangling" over the side of the bed, because there is danger of constricting the vessels under the knee.

B. Active Intervention

1. Initiate anticoagulant therapy either intravenously, intramuscularly, or subcutaneously (see p. 80).
2. Prevent swelling and stagnation of venous blood by wrapping the legs from the toes to the groin with elastic bandage or elastic stockings.
3. Control pain in the extremities by bandaging.

Pulmonary Complications

Preventive Measures

1. Report any evidence of upper respiratory infection to the surgeon.
2. Postoperatively, initiate measures to prevent chilling.
3. Aspirate secretions that might cause respiratory embarrassment.
4. Recognize the predisposing causes of pulmonary complications:
   a. Infections—mouth, nose, throat
   b. Aspiration of vomitus
   c. History of heavy smoking, chronic respiratory disease
   d. Obesity

Complications

1. *Atelectasis*—collapse of pulmonary alveoli caused by a mucous plug closing a bronchus.
2. *Bronchitis*—inflammation of bronchi, causing a cough with considerable mucous secretion.
3. *Bronchopneumonia*—a chest complication with elevated temperature, pulse, and respiratory rate plus a productive cough.
4. *Lobar pneumonia*—onset of a chill followed by a high temperature, pulse and respiration elevation, flushed cheeks, respiratory embarrassment.
5. *Hypostatic pulmonary congestion*—more common in the debilitated or elderly patient, whose weakened heart and vascular system permit stagnation of secretions at base of lungs.
6. *Pleurisy*—knife-like pain in the chest on the affected side, particularly on intake of a deep breath, and elevated temperature, pulse, and respirations.

Nursing Interventions

1. Appraise the patient's progress very carefully on a daily basis for the first postoperative week to detect early signs and symptoms of respiratory difficulties.
   a. Slight temperature, pulse, and respiration elevations
   b. Apprehension and restlessness
   c. Complaints of chest pain, signs of dyspnea or cough
2. Promote full aeration of the lungs.
   a. Turn the patient frequently.
   b. Encourage the patient to take 10 deep breaths hourly.
   c. Utilize a spirometer or any device that encourages the patient to ventilate. Inspiratory exercises are more effective than expiratory (see p. 208).
   d. Assist the patient in coughing in an effort to bring up mucous secretions (Fig. 7-11, p. 180).
   e. Assist the patient to ambulate as early as the physician will allow.

3. Initiate specific measures for particular pulmonary problems.
   a. Provide cool mist or steam (electric vaporizer) for the patient who exhibits signs of bronchitis.
   b. Encourage the patient to take fluids and expectorants if he appears to be developing pneumonia.
   c. Administer antibiotics to patients with pulmonary infections.
   d. Prevent abdominal distention—causes pulmonary and circulatory embarrassment.
   e. Provide analgesics for discomfort.
   f. Note that the patient who has pleurisy with effusion may need chest aspiration; have a thoracentesis tray ready and be prepared to assist.
   g. Be prepared to administer oxygen to assist in aeration of the lungs for oxygenation of blood.

Pulmonary Embolism

An *embolus* is a foreign body in the bloodstream—usually a blood clot that has become dislodged from the original site. When such a clot is carried to the heart, it is forced into the pulmonary artery or one of its branches. (See also p. 168.)

Clinical Manifestations

1. Sharp, stabbing pains in the chest
2. Anxiousness and cyanosis
3. Pupillary dilation, profuse perspiration
4. Rapid and irregular pulse becoming imperceptible—leads rapidly to death
5. Dyspnea

Immediate Treatment

1. Administer oxygen and inhalations with the patient in an upright sitting position.
2. Reassure and quiet the patient.
3. Administer morphine to control panic, as prescribed.

Urinary Difficulties

Retention of Urine

1. *Incidence*—occurs most frequently after operations on the rectum, anus, vagina, or lower abdomen; caused by spasm of bladder sphincter.
2. *Nursing Measures*
   a. Assist patient to sit or even stand up (if permissible), since many patients are unable to void while lying in bed.
   b. Provide the patient with privacy.
   c. Use the psychological aid of running the tap water—frequently the sound or sight of running water relaxes the spasm of the bladder sphincter.
   d. Catheterize only when all other measures are unsuccessful.
      (1) May lead to possible bladder infection.
      (2) Subsequent catheterizations are often required.

▶ **NURSING ALERT:** Recognize that when a patient voids small amounts (30–60 ml. every 15–30 minutes) this may be a sign of overdistended bladder ("overflow of retention").

Urinary Incontinence

1. *Cause*—loss of tone of the bladder sphincter.
2. *Incidence*—occurs as a complication in the aged after surgery or shocking injury.

3. *Recovery*—disappears as patient gains strength and muscle tone.
4. *Management*
   a. Offer a bedpan hourly.
   b. Provide extra padding under patient; use special disposable pants.
   c. Initiate a consistent plan for special care of the skin to avoid skin breakdown.

Intestinal Obstruction

Causes

1. May occur following surgery on lower abdomen and pelvis, especially when there is drainage.
2. A loop of intestines may kink because of inflammatory adhesions.
3. A loop of intestine may become involved in the drainage tract.

Clinical Manifestations

1. Most commonly occurs between the 3rd and 5th postoperative day.
2. Sharp, colicky abdominal pains with pain-free intervals.
3. Pain is localized and should be noted, since it may become more generalized later; location may pinpoint source of difficulty.
4. Peristaltic activity can be assessed by listening to the abdomen with a stethoscope.
5. Pain-free intervals grow shorter as time advances.
6. With completion of obstruction, intestinal contents back up into stomach and cause vomiting.
7. Abdominal distention and perhaps hiccups occur, but no bowel movements, if obstruction is complete; if obstruction is partial or incomplete, diarrhea may occur.
8. Following a simple enema, returns are clear, indicating very small amount of intestinal contents has reached large intestines.
9. If obstruction is not relieved, vomiting continues, distention becomes more pronounced, pulse increases, shock develops, and death occurs.

Management

1. Relieve abdominal distention by passing a nasoenteric suction tube.
2. Administer body-deficient electrolytes per intravenous infusion as prescribed.
3. Consider preparing the patient for surgical intervention if obstruction continues unresolved (see pp. 457–458).

Hiccups (Singultus)

Hiccups are intermittent spasms of the diaphragm causing a sound ("hic") that results from the vibration of closed vocal cords as air rushes suddenly into the lungs.

Cause

Irritation of phrenic nerve between spinal cord and terminal ramifications on undersurface of diaphragm.
   a. *Direct*—distended stomach, peritonitis, abdominal distention, chest pleurisy, tumors pressing on nerves, or surgery performed near the diaphragm
   b. *Indirect*—toxemia, uremia
   c. *Reflex*—exposure to cold, drinking very hot or very cold liquids, intestinal obstruction

Management

1. Remove the cause if possible.
   a. Gastric lavage for gastric distention
   b. Treatment for pleurisy
   c. Removal of drainage tubes causing irritation
2. When removal of cause is not possible, favorite simple remedies may be tried.
   a. Holding breath while taking a large swallow of water.
   b. Applying finger pressure on the eyeballs through closed lids for several minutes.
   c. Inhaling carbon dioxide (breathing in and out of a paper bag).
3. Medications may be prescribed (chlorpromazine, Benzedrine, quinidine, or barbiturates). The degree of success with these drugs varies widely.
4. Introduce a catheter (No. 16 Fr.) into the patient's pharynx about 7–10 cm. (3–4 inches); rotate gently and jiggle back and forth; this action interrupts impulses from vagus nerve, and hiccups stop.
5. For intractable hiccups, an extreme procedure is surgical crush of the phrenic nerve.

Wound Infection

Infection in a wound occurs when there is growth of bacteria; infection may be limited to a single area or may affect a patient systemically.

A. Causative Organisms

1. *Staphylococcus aureus*
2. *Escherichia coli*
3. *Proteus vulgaris*
4. *Pseudomonas aeruginosa*
5. Anaerobic bacteria (e.g., *Bacteroides fragilis*). Anaerobes have become more prominent in wound infections, particularly following bowel surgery; a characteristic odor can be detected. Often this infection is detected only if anaerobic cultures are performed.

B. Clinical Manifestations

1. Redness, excessive swelling, tenderness
2. Red streaks in the skin near the wound
3. Pus or other discharge from the wound
4. Tender lymph nodes in axillary region or groin closest to wound
5. Foul smell from wound
6. Generalized body chills or fever
7. Elevated temperature and pulse

▶ **NURSING ALERT:** A useful rule of thumb is that an elevated temperature occurring within 24 hours suggests a pulmonary infection; within 48 hours suggests a urinary tract infection; after 72 hours suggests a wound infection.

C. Factors Affecting the Extent of an Infection

1. The kind, virulence, and quantity of contaminating microorganisms
2. Presence of foreign bodies or devitalized tissue
3. Location and nature of the wound
4. Amount of dead space or presence of hematoma
5. Immune response of the patient
6. Presence of ischemia leading to wound compression
7. Condition of the patient, such as whether he is elderly, alcoholic, diabetic, malnourished

Preventive Medical and Nursing Interventions

1. Insist on housekeeping cleanliness in the surgical environment.

2. Instruct the patient in how to keep a wound clean; include aseptic technique in the handling of dressings.

A. Preoperative

1. Encourage the patient to achieve an optimal nutritional level.
   If hypoproteinemic with weight loss, provide oral or parenteral alimentation.
2. Reduce preoperative hospitalization to barest minimum to avoid acquiring "hospital infection" (nosocomial infection).
3. When the risk of developing an infection is high (or when infection would have grave consequences) antibiotic therapy is initiated preoperatively.
4. Most clinically effective antibiotics given as prophylaxis are the cephalosporins (spectrum includes gram-positive and gram-negative).
5. Antibiotic bowel preparation for colon surgery may benefit from a combination of oral and possibly perioperative systemic antibiotics.

B. Operative

1. Follow strict asepsis when the wound is made and thereafter until it is completely healed.
2. When a wound has exudate, fibrin, dessicated fat, or nonviable skin, it should not be approximated by primary closure but should be delayed for secondary closure.

C. Postoperative Care of an Infected Wound

1. Surgeon removes one or more stitches, separates wound edges, and examines for infection using a hemostat as a probe.
2. A culture is taken and sent to the bacteriology laboratory.
3. Wound irrigation may be done; have asepto syringe and saline available.
4. A drain (rubber or gauze) may be inserted.
5. Antibiotics are prescribed.
6. Hot wet dressings may be suggested.

Wound Complications

Hemorrhage and Hematoma

A. Manifestations

1. Inspect dressings frequently during the first 24 hours postoperatively.
   a. Note evidence of bright red blood on dressings.
   b. Look for bulging, which may indicate bleeding and clot formation (hematoma) under the skin.
   c. Examine bedding directly underneath incision site for evidence of trickling ooze.
   d. Check drainage bottle for undue amount of red drainage.
2. Check vital signs for evidence of bleeding—elevated pulse, apprehension, air hunger (see p. 92).

B. Management

1. Notify physician.
2. If bleeding continues, it may be necessary for the patient to return to surgery to have bleeding vessel ligated, to remove large hematoma, to resuture wound.

Dehiscence (Rupture, Disruption, Evisceration)

A. Causes

1. The wounds of elderly patients do not heal as readily as those of younger patients.
2. Pulmonary and cardiovascular diseases contribute to wound breakdown, since they impede delivery of nutritional essentials to the wound (circulatory and pulmonary difficulties).
3. Abdominal distention, obesity, infection, poor nutritional status, and systemic diseases (e.g., diabetes).

B. Prophylaxis

1. Apply abdominal binder for heavy or elderly patients or those with weak or pendulous abdominal walls.
2. Encourage proper nutrition with emphasis on adequate amounts of protein and vitamin C.

C. Clinical Manifestations

1. Patient complains that something suddenly gave way in his wound.
2. In an intestinal wound, the edges of the wound may part and the intestines may gradually push out—observe for drainage of peritoneal fluid on dressings (clear or serosanguineous fluid).

D. Management

1. Stay with the patient and have someone notify the surgeon immediately.
2. If intestines are exposed, cover with sterile moist saline dressings.
3. Keep the patient on absolute bed rest.
4. Instruct the patient to bend his knees—relieves tension on abdomen.
5. Assure the patient that his wound will be properly cared for; keep him quiet and relaxed.
6. Prepare the patient for surgery and repair of the wound.

Postoperative Psychological Disturbances

Delirium is a mental aberration that occurs only occasionally in some postoperative patients.

Classification

A. Toxic

1. Incidence—occurs in combination with symptoms of general toxemia (e.g., peritonitis, sepsis).
2. Symptoms—acutely ill, restless patient with elevated temperature and pulse, flushed face, bright and roving eyes—indicates mental confusion.
3. Management
   a. Administer fluids to aid in elimination of toxins.

Note: Not all delirious patients can tolerate fluids. It is also inappropriate to administer fluids if it may lead to cerebral fluid retention and delirium; treatment in this instance is fluid restriction.

   b. Control infection by giving the proper antibiotics.

B. Traumatic

1. *Incidence*—develops following sudden trauma, particularly in the highly nervous person.
2. *Symptoms*—manifests itself by wild excitement, hallucinations, delusions, or melancholic depression.
3. Management
   a. Administer tranquilizing medications; chloral hydrate, paraldehyde.
   b. This state of delirium begins and ends abruptly.

C. Delirium Tremens

1. Incidence—patients who have used alcohol excessively are poor surgical risks and take anesthetic agents poorly.
2. Symptoms—postoperatively, after continued abstinence from alcohol, patient shows signs of delirium tremens.

a. Restless, nervous, easily irritated.

b. Sleeps poorly, disturbed by unreal dreams, momentarily appears to be in a strange place and does not know nursing or medical staff.

c. Later, loses control of mental functions; his mind is filled with haunting hallucinations that torment him constantly.

d. Additional symptoms include sleeplessness, excessive perspiration, and marked tremor of the extremities. Patient eventually becomes stuporous.

3. Medical and Nursing Management

a. Administer sedatives to keep the patient quiet and comfortable; stimulation may be required by older patients with alcoholism.

b. Give glucose intravenously and concentrated vitamins by mouth to control nutritional deficiencies.

c. Recommend that the patient remain in bed; it may be necessary to restrain him so that injuries are minimized. (Bear in mind that restraining should be a last resort, since this often makes such a patient quite rebellious.)

d. Encourage ambulation as soon as the surgical condition permits.

e. See also pages 951–952.

2: The Patient Receiving Infusion Therapy

Goals and Principles

Goals:

1. Maintain or replace body stores of water, electrolytes, vitamins, proteins, calories, and nitrogen in the patient who cannot maintain an adequate intake by mouth.
2. Restore acid–base balance.
3. Replenish blood volume.
4. Provide avenues for the administration of medications.

Physiologic Assimilation of Infusion Solutions

A. Principles

1. Blood cells (erythrocytes, etc.) are surrounded by a semipermeable membrane.
2. *Osmotic pressure* is the pressure demonstrated when a solvent moves through the semipermeable membrane from weaker to stronger concentrations.
3. Osmotic characteristics of different solutions are often determined by the way they affect red blood cells.

B. Types of Fluids

1. *Isotonic*—a solution that has the same osmotic pressure externally as that found across the semipermeable membrane within the cell.
   a. Normal saline 0.9%
   b. Dextrose 5% in water
   c. Lactated Ringer's
   d. Balanced isotonic
2. *Hypotonic*—a solution that has less osmotic pressure than that of blood serum; this causes the cells to expand or swell.
   Sodium chloride 0.45%
3. *Hypertonic*—a solution that has higher osmotic pressure than that of blood serum; this causes the cells to shrink.
   a. Dextrose 5% in saline
   b. Dextrose 10% in saline
   c. Dextrose 10% in water
   d. Dextrose 5% in ½-strength saline
   e. Dextrose 20% in water

C. Composition of Fluids

1. Saline solution—fluids and electrolytes (Na^+, Cl^-)
2. Dextrose—fluid and calories
3. Lactated Ringer's—fluid, electrolytes (Na^+, K^+, Cl^-, Ca^{++}, lactate)
4. Balanced isotonic—fluid, electrolytes, some calories (Na^+, K^+, Mg^{++}, Cl^-, HCO_3^-, gluconate)
5. Whole blood and blood components (see Chap. 8)
6. Plasma expanders: albumin, dextran, plasminate
   To improve circulating blood volume
7. Parenteral hyperalimentation nutrients
8. Administration of a particular medication or combination of medications

Nursing Process Overview

Nursing Assessment

A. Diagnosis and Need for Fluid Therapy

It is important to know the major and minor medical problems of the patient as indicated in the physician's diagnostic evaluation and the nurse's assessment of the patient.

1. Can the patient's illness affect his fluid balance?
2. What medication or treatment is he receiving that can affect fluid components? How?
3. What is the relation of his fluid intake to fluid output?
4. Does he have dietary restrictions?
5. Is he taking adequate fluids by mouth?
6. What is the physician's plan of treatment?

B. Evidence of Fluid Imbalance in the Patient

1. Determine body temperature—febrile conditions suggest loss of body fluids through perspiration.
2. Is he thirsty? Possible dehydration.
3. Observe for dry, warm skin, cracked lips—signs of dehydration.
4. Check skin for elasticity—lightly pull up a pinchfold of skin, release it. Does it rapidly resume its normal position?

In an elderly patient, check for tongue furrows—this may be more significant than skin turgor.

5. Note color and amount of urine—concentrated, scanty urine indicates lack of fluids.
6. Compare present weight with admission weight—it may indicate fluid change.
7. Absence of moisture in axillae or groin may indicate dehydration.

C. Inspection of Prescribed Fluid and Equipment to be Used for the Infusion

1. Observe fluid for discoloration, foreign particles, cloudiness, film—if present, do not use.
2. Fluid in a bag:
   Gently squeeze and observe for leakage.
3. Fluid in a glass bottle:
   a. Hold flask up to light.
   b. Slowly rotate flask in upright position and then on its side; carefully inspect for a flash of light that could indicate a crack.
4. Check IV tubing for discoloration or defects; if noted, secure new equipment.
5. Follow instructions for assembling equipment, using aseptic technique when inserting drip chamber spike into flask; flush equipment with 20–30 ml. of fluid from receptacle before using. (See Guidelines p. 102.)
6. Return defective equipment with a note describing defect to the proper department.

Patient Problems/Nursing Diagnoses

1. Fluid volume deficit related to possible dehydration, shock, hemorrhage, decreased venous filling, use of diuretics, etc.
2. Knowledge deficit; unfamiliarity with intravenous or infusion procedures.
3. Fear related to expected discomfort of procedure.
4. Potential for injury related to IV infiltration.

Planning and Implementation
Nursing Interventions

1. Acquaint the patient with the requirements for intravenous infusion and his need for it.
2. Select a suitable vein for venipuncture to optimize benefits of infusion and minimize discomfort to patient.
3. The use of arm boards are considered when IV devices are placed over or near areas of flexion to prevent injury to vein.
4. Cleanse infusion site to prevent infection.
5. Utilize best method of distending a vein to permit easiest access to a vessel.
6. Consider local anesthesia for the unusually sensitive patient after verifying presence of allergies.
7. Adjust rate of flow of fluids appropriate to needs of patient as prescribed (see pp. 99 and 100).

Evaluation
Expected Outcomes

1. Receives adequate IV therapy as prescribed
2. Shows no untoward side effects of IV therapy
3. Communicates an understanding of the reason for IV therapy
4. Experiences a comfortable and safe intravenous infusion with no signs of infiltration or pain.

Procedural Considerations in IV Therapy

Criteria for Selecting a Vein Suitable for Venipuncture

1. Use distal branches of a large vein rather than the best sites—these are then available for emergencies.

▶ **NURSING ALERT:** Select most distal vein on hand or arm initially for venipuncture or infusion. If, with subsequent venipunctures, this site is difficult to enter, move up higher on the arm. Conversely, if the antecubital fossa area is used first, and if later there is difficulty entering at this site, none of the lower veins can be used.

2. Suitable veins include the following:
   a. Back of the hand—metacarpal vein (Fig. 6-4A). Avoid digital veins.
      (1) The advantage of this site is that it permits arm movement.
      (2) If later a vein problem develops at this site, another vein higher up the arm may be used.
   b. Forearm—basilic or cephalic vein (Fig. 6-4B).
   c. Inner aspect of elbow, antecubital fossa—median basilic and median cephalic for relatively short-term infusion.
      (1) These veins are large and easily accessible.
      (2) Note, however, that this site precludes arm movement.
      (3) Choose site below elbow crease for patient's comfort.

3. In adult patients, veins in lower extremities are used as a last resort.
   a. Thigh—great saphenous and femoral veins
   b. Ankle—great saphenous; foot—venous plexus of dorsum, dorsal venous arch, medial marginal vein
   c. When varicose veins are present, the extremity must be carefully monitored.

▶ **NURSING ALERT:** Veins in lower extremities are avoided because of venous stasis, increased risk of thrombosis, and limitations imposed on ambulating patient.

4. Central veins are used:
   a. When medications are hypertonic or highly irritating requiring rapid, high-volume dilution to prevent systemic reactions and local venous irritation (e.g., protein hydrolysate, hypertonic sodium chloride; (see Table 6-2).
   b. During shock or cardiac arrest; peripheral blood flow is diminished.

Methods of Distending a Vein

1. Apply manual compression above site where cannula is to be inserted.
2. Have the patient periodically clench his fist (if arm is used).
3. Massage area in direction of venous flow.

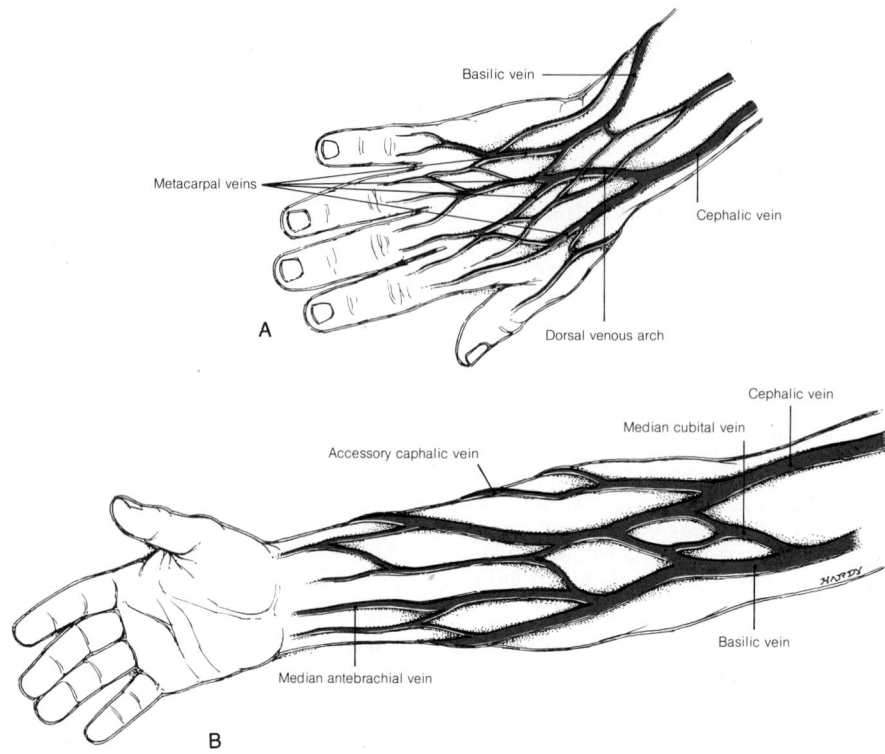

Figure 6-4. (A) Superficial veins, dorsal aspect of hand. (B) Superficial veins, forearm.

4. Apply sphygmomanometer cuff (keep pressure just below systolic pressure).
5. Fasten soft rubber tubing with a hemostat.
6. Tie soft rubber tubing as a slip knot.
7. Lightly tap vein site; this is to be done gently so that the vein is not injured.
8. Allow extremity to be dependent for a few minutes.
9. Apply moist heat by wringing out a Turkish towel and wrapping the part. (Currently controversial—when heat is withdrawn, there may be venous stasis.)
10. Apply external heat to extremity using a thermostatically controlled electric blanket.

Hand-operated hair dryer can be used to direct heat to a possible needle site.

Table 6-2   Factors in the Selection of Peripheral or Central Sites for Intravenous Insertion

Factor	Peripheral Veins		Central Veins	
	Suitable	Unsuitable	Suitable	Unsuitable
Type of drug or solution	Most drugs Isotonic fluids	Irritating drugs or hypertonic fluids, which require maximal dilution	Irritating drugs or hypertonic fluids	Drugs that if injected centrally could cause arrhythmias, shock, or other complications
Duration of therapy	Short-term or intermittent therapy; is less hazardous	Long-term therapy; in which all available veins would be used up	Moderate to long-term continuous therapy	Short-term therapy; the patient is subjected to greater risks
Accessibility of veins	Patients with adequate peripheral veins	Very obese patients; IV drug abusers; conditions that impair peripheral circulation	When peripheral veins inaccessible, especially if intravenous line is needed in an emergency	At times not accessible after repeated use (e.g., pacemaker). May be accessible, but increased risks due to location near lung
Cooperation of patient	Extremity can usually be restrained sufficiently to allow insertion and maintenance of line	Disoriented or agitated adult or child may be more likely to attempt removal of intravenous line located in upper extremity	Central lines, especially subclavian, are less likely to be disrupted once inserted	Patient must lie absolutely still during the insertion to prevent pneumothorax and other complications

(Sager DP and Bomar SK. Intravenous Medications, p. 40. Philadelphia; Lippincott, 1980)

Note: Should the above measures fail, it may be necessary to perform a "cutdown"—this is a surgical procedure exposing the vein for venipuncture; the incision site is treated as a surgical wound.

Stabilizing Extremity with a Padded Armboard

1. This is done if the patient is restless, disoriented, elderly, or a child and if motion could result in infiltration into tissues or phlebitis.
2. Various kinds of armboards are available; an armboard should be padded.

▶ **NURSING ALERT:** If hand and arm are to be immobilized, place in normal functional position. *Contractures may occur if hand is immobilized in flat position.*
For hand: Dorsiflexion of wrist about 20–25 degrees.
Flexion of metacarpophalangeal joint about 45–50 degrees.
Palm slightly cupped with finger flexion increasing from index to little finger.
Thumb should be extended in relaxed position and not flexed under fingers.

3. Prevent compression of nerves or blood vessels; check pulse and ask patient if pressure is too great.

Cleansing Infusion Site

1. If skin is unusually soiled, then use a good surgical soap to cleanse the infusion site thoroughly. Dirt, dead skin, blood, mucus, and oil are to be removed so that action of antiseptic is not hindered.
2. Rinse the area with water or alcohol.
3. Apply an iodine-base antiseptic; 1% or 2% iodine in water or in 70% alcohol is effective. After 30 seconds, tr. of iodine can be washed off with alcohol.
   a. In patients sensitive to iodine, iodophors may be used. Do not wash off an iodophor, since it provides sustained release of free iodine, which may enhance the germicidal action.
   b. If iodine preparations are not available, 70% alcohol is an alternative if it is applied vigorously for 1 minute after the area has been cleansed.
4. Wait until area is dry before inserting needle; this is done to prevent carrying antiseptic solution into the vein.

▶ **NURSING ALERT:** In applying antiseptic, swab the infusion site first; then, covering an ever-widening circular area, move out to the periphery, preparing a 2″–3″ area.

Providing Local Anesthesia for Unusually Sensitive Patients

1. Because of risk of anaphylaxis and increased costs, local anesthetics should be used only for special circumstances.
2. Use 0.1 ml. of 1% lidocaine without epinephrine intradermally over IV site.

Equipment

A. Needle or Catheter

Infusion may be administered through a needle (short-term) or through a catheter (long-term). (See Table 6-3.)

B. Bevel

To facilitate entering a vein with least injury to skin, the bevel should face—

1. Upward—when entering a vein lumen that is larger than the needle.
2. Downward—when entering a small vein with lumen that approaches the size of the needle.

C. Solution Container

1. Soft polyvinyl chloride and semirigid polyolefin containers are more convenient than glass containers.
2. Polyolefin containers are less likely to leak; they do not introduce DEHP (di-2-ethylhexyl phthalate) into IV solution.
3. Polyolefin containers require more storage space.
4. When plastic containers are used, adsorption of added medications may be greater than when glass bottles are used.

Adjusting Rate of Flow of Fluid in Infusion Therapy

The physician prescribes the flow rate. However, the nurse is responsible for regulating and maintaining the proper rate.

A. Patient Determining Factors

1. Surface area of the patient
   The larger the person, the more fluid he requires and the faster he utilizes it.
2. Patient condition
   If patient has cardiovascular or renal problems, the rate should be carefully monitored.
3. Age of patient
   Administer intermittent medication more slowly to the very young or elderly.
4. Tolerance to solutions
   Example: Test protein sensitivity by administering protein hydrolysates slowly.
5. Fluid composition for this particular patient
   When drugs are administered via infusion, the effect desired often depends on speed of administration.
6. Patient movement and activity

B. Factors Affecting Rate of Flow

1. Pressure gradient—the difference between 2 levels in a fluid system
2. Friction—the interaction between fluid molecules and surfaces of inner wall of tubing
3. Diameter and length of tubing; gauge of cannula
4. Height of column of fluid
5. Size of opening through which fluid leaves receptacle
6. Characteristics of fluid
   a. Viscosity
   b. Temperature—refrigerated fluids may cause diminished flow and vessel spasm; bring fluid to room temperature.
7. Vein trauma, clots, plugging of vents, venous spasm, vasoconstriction, etc.
8. Flow-control-clamp derangement
   a. Some clamps may slip and loosen, resulting in a very rapid, or "runaway," infusion.
   b. Plastic tubing may distort, causing "creep" or "cold flow"—the inside diameter of tubing will continue to change long after clamp is tightened or relaxed.
   c. Marked stretching of tubing may cause distortions of tubing and render clamp ineffective (may occur when patient turns over and pulls on a short tubing).
9. If there is any question regarding rate of fluid administration, check with the physician.

Table 6-3   Comparison of Different Types of Intravenous Cannulae

Type of Cannula	Indications for Use	Advantages	Disadvantages
A. Needles			
1. Straight needles	Cooperative adult patients who require very short-term (1–3 days) therapy	Ease of insertion Less likely to cause phlebitis	Rigid, difficult to secure so more prone to infiltration especially in active or agitated patients Less comfortable
2. Winged-needle unit (scalp-vein needle)	Short-term therapy for any patient, especially for infants and children, geriatric and other patients with fragile or rolling veins	Wings enable easy insertion and securing to prevent movement and dislodgement Less likely to cause phlebitis	Needle rigid and short so may infiltrate if patient very active or if needle not securely taped
3. Intermittent winged-needle unit (heparin-lock)	Intermittent administration of drugs such as heparin, antibiotics, frequent blood sampling, or to keep vein open when no fluids are needed	Allows prompt access to the vein without giving fluids Economical; greater comfort and mobility for the patient	Will clot if not flushed with heparinized saline; part of clot can be injected into the patient when the next dose of drug is given
B. Plastic Catheters			
1. Over-the-needle catheter	Active or moderately agitated patients who require a secure venous line for uninterrupted delivery of drugs and/or fluids	Easy to insert More comfortable for the patient Less prone to infiltration than needles	More likely to cause phlebitis, particularly if not changed every 48–72 hours Can kink if inserted near an area of flexion (such as elbow)
2. Over-the-needle catheter with resealable cap	Patients on intermittent drugs without need for fluids, yet who require a secure device	Combines advantages of over-the-needle catheter with those of intermittent winged-needle unit (heparin-lock)	Same as those of other over-the-needle catheters Will clot unless flushed with heparinized saline periodically
3. Through-the-needle catheter	Administration of hypertonic fluids or irritating drugs, which must be given via a central vein to ensure adequate dilution; for monitoring of CVP; emergencies in which life-sustaining drugs and fluids must be given rapidly and accurately	Very secure Available in many sizes and lengths so it can be inserted directly into a central vein or via a peripheral vein	Greater risk of infection and other complications especially when inserted into central vein Insertion requires a high degree of skill; incorrect insertion or guarding of needle can cause severing and embolization of catheter fragment
4. In-lying (cutdown) catheter	Patients in whom percutaneous access to veins is unsuccessful such as those in shock or cardiac arrest, those with sclerosed veins due to IV drug abuse, markedly obese patients	Provides access to superficial or deep veins May be the only means of establishing an intravenous line during emergencies Once inserted is very secure	Must be inserted by a physician Creates a surgical wound so the risk of infection is greater

(Sager DP and Bomar SK. Intravenous Medications, p. 37. Philadelphia, JB Lippincott, 1980)

Table 6-4   Calibrating IV Fluids

Prescription	Regular (15 drops/ml.)		Microdrip (60 drops/ml.)		Macrodrip (10 drops/ml.)	
	Drops/min.	Drops/¼ min.	Drops/min.	Drops/¼ min.	Drops/min.	Drops/¼ min.
40 ml./hr.	10	2¼	40	10	7	2
50 ml./hr.	12	3	50	12½	8	2
60 ml./hr.	15	4	60	15	10	2½
80 ml./hr.	20	5	80	20	13	3
100 ml./hr.	25	6	100	25	16	4
125 ml./hr.	30	7½	125	30	20	5
150 ml./hr.	38	9½	150	38	25	6

24-Hour Fluids	
ml./24 hr	ml./hr.
1000	40
1500	60
2000	80
2500	100
3000	125
3500	145

(Norcross MB. Am J Nurs Nov. 75:2003)

C. Calculation of Flow Rate*

1. Drops per milliliter vary with commercial parenteral sets. (Check directions on set or calculate by timing for 1 minute.) (Also see Table 6-4, Calibrating IV Fluids, p. 100.)
2. Utilize the following formula:

* Metheny NM and Snively WD, Jr. Nurse's Handbook of Fluid Balance, 4th ed. Philadelphia, JB Lippincott, 1983.

$$\text{Drops/min.} = \frac{\text{Total volume infused} \times \text{drops/ml.}}{\text{Total time for infusion in minutes}}$$

Example:
Infuse 1000 ml. of 5% D/W in 2 hours
(Set indicates 10 drops in 1 ml.)

$$\frac{1000 \times 10}{120 \text{ min.}} = 80 \text{ drops/min. (approximately)}$$

Note: Convenient calculators are available from manufacturers of parenteral solutions.

Guidelines: Venipuncture/Phlebotomy

Venipuncture is the puncturing of a vein with a sterile cannula (needle or catheter) attached to a syringe.
Phlebotomy is the aspiration of blood from a vein.

Purpose
1. To obtain blood samples for analysis, cross matching
2. To administer fluids, blood, medications
3. To perform diagnostic tests requiring the administration of IV medications

Equipment

Tourniquet, usually rubber tubing or flat latex rubber, approximately 37.5 cm. (15 in.). (Blood pressure cuff is effective because it can be pumped to the desired 100 mm. Hg.)

Foil-wrapped alcohol or povidone-iodine sponges

Sterile syringe; 10 or 20 ml. depending on amount of blood desired

No. 18 needle—with disposable needles, the likelihood of a burr is practically nonexistent. If there is any question, draw needle through sterile gauze—a burr will pick up threads. A needle with a burr should be discarded.

Procedure

Nursing Action	Rationale/Amplification
Preparatory Phase	
1. Wash hands thoroughly.	
2. Explain procedure to patient.	2. Most patients have had experience with blood drawing.
3. Select site The back of the hand, the back of the arm, or the antecubital vein is used (in order of preference). Vein selection is determined by size, elasticity, and distance below skin. (Clip hair if necessary.) Vein should be distinct, easily observable, and palpable; it should be large enough for a needle to enter.	
4. Ascertain if there is satisfactory distention of the vein.	4. This is done by observation or by palpation.
5. Make decision about whether to use a tourniquet or not.	5. If vein is easily identified (i.e., full or pliable), a tourniquet may not be required.
6. If tourniquet is used, do not apply too tightly—venous flow should be stopped but arterial flow should continue (radial pulse should be palpable).	6. Improperly applied tourniquet may cause blood stasis and may result in blood chemistry alterations. This is why some prefer to apply a blood pressure cuff to 100 mm. Hg.
7. Scrub area with iodine-base antiseptic. Allow to dry.	7. To reduce number of skin microorganisms.
8. If vein is prominent, it is not necessary to request patient to make a fist.	8. Fist-making may increase ammonia concentration in the blood.
Performance Phase	
1. Insert the needle, bevel up, through the skin and at a 45-degree angle.	1. Usually, a single sliding stroke can be used to enter skin and vessel.
2. If vessel rolls, it may be necessary to penetrate the skin first at a 20-degree angle and then apply a second thrust parallel to the skin to enter the vessel.	2. Satisfactory penetration is evidenced by appearance of blood coming back into syringe.
3. Direct needle into vein, this usually means a slight change in direction to avoid going through the other side of the vessel.	3. If tourniquet was used, remove at this time to prevent extravasation of blood.
4. For blood sampling. Draw desired amount of blood into syringe.	4. Blood should flow easily; if suction is required, reposition needle to avoid hemolysis.

(continued)

Guidelines: Venipuncture/Phlebotomy (continued)

Procedure
(Cont.)

Nursing Action	Rationale/Amplification
Follow-up Phase	
1. Place a sterile sponge over vein at site of puncture and withdraw needle.	1. Instruct the patient to hold the cotton ball in place with slight pressure for 2–3 minutes. If oozing continues, apply a strip of adhesive tape over a fresh sterile cotton ball.
2. Slowly inject blood specimen into proper receptacle, label, and see that specimen is delivered to proper laboratory.	2. Record venipuncture and purpose of blood specimen.

Note: For Arterial Puncture, see p. 143, Conditions of the Respiratory Tract.

Guidelines: Administering an Intravenous Infusion Using the Antecubital Fossa

Procedure

Nursing Action	Rationale/Amplification
Preparatory Phase	
1. Place the patient in bed in semi-Fowler's position.	1. This is comfortable for the patient and permits the selected arm to assume a flexed comfortable position.
Inform him of the procedure and its purpose.	To secure his understanding and cooperation.
2. Remove the patient's arm from sleeve of garment.	2. To permit removal of gown or pajama top if necessary while infusion is in progress (without cutting sleeve).
3. Position (but do not tighten) tourniquet under lower end of upper arm (5 cm. [2 inches] above joint).	
4. An arm board may be required after successful cannulation to minimize complications. (see p. 99).	4. To immobilize arm while needle or catheter is in vein; this will prevent dislodging of needle and injury to vein. Padding will prevent constriction of nerves or blood vessels.
5. Connect intravenous material; hang fluid receptacle after checking label for proper solution.	5. Intravenous fluids are considered medications; labeling must be verified.
6. Allow fluid to flow through the system; tighten the clamp; maintain sterility until arm is prepared.	6. To eliminate air bubbles, which could cause air emboli in the circulatory system.
Performance Phase	
1. Tighten tourniquet.	1. To distend veins (for better visualization) by preventing blood flow back to heart.
Ends of tubing should be opposite or away from infusion site.	To prevent contamination of injection area by tubing ends.
2. Request patient to open and close his fist. Palpate and note suitable vein for injection.	2. Contracting muscles of lower arm forces blood into veins, which distends them further.
3. Cleanse skin thoroughly, using an antiseptic swab and apply friction in a circular pattern outward from injection site.	3. To remove skin pathogens and sebum which might otherwise be drawn into the subcutaneous tissue or vein as the needle is advanced.
4. Use thumb to apply tension on tissue and vein about 5 cm. (2 inches) distal to injection site.	4. To aid in anchoring the vein as the needle is introduced.
5. Hold the device at a 30-degree angle alongside the wall of the vein in the direction of and near the intended site of injection; pierce skin.	5. This angle permits greatest ease and accuracy in entering the vein and prevents contamination of device.
6. Decrease angle of needle until it is nearly parallel with the skin and slightly to one side of the vein; apply pressure in same direction as puncture and enter the vein.	
7. If there is a backflow of blood through the needle, the vein has been entered; decrease angle of needle 10 degrees and advance cannula.	7. To prevent the needle from becoming dislodged and puncturing the posterior wall of the vein.
8. Release tourniquet.	8. To permit infusion solution to enter circulatory system.
9. Release clamp on infusion tubing and relax skin tension.	9. To allow flow of solution and to prevent blood from clotting in the needle.
10. Sterile topical ointment may be applied (optional).	10. Inconclusive data on effectiveness of antibiotic on these sites.
11. Secure catheter hub with tape to insure placement. (Fig 6-5).	11. Effective anchoring allows some mobility for the patient and retains safe inflow of solution.
12. Apply gauze or transparent IV dressing.	
13. Regulate flow rate of solution.	13. Proper monitoring of solution will prevent overloading of the circulatory system.

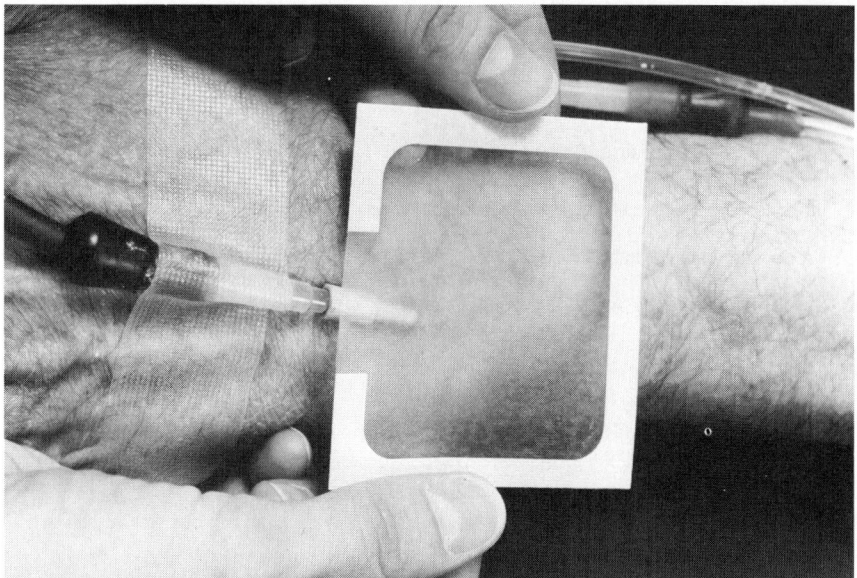

Figure 6-5. Tegaderm® Transparent IV Dressing and Transpore® Surgical Tape combine to provide a neat, secure, and visible peripheral IV site. The Tape's bidirectional tear and good adhesion allow for quick taping to fit any application. (Courtesy of 3M Medical Products Division)

Procedure
(Cont.)

Follow-up Phase
1. Change catheter site q. 48–72 hours; reduces potential for infection (NITA Standards; CDC Guidelines) (If longer than 72 hours, there is risk of infection—extensive documentation required.)
2. Change gauze dressings q. 24–48 hours; allows one to inspect catheter site.
3. Transparent dressing remains in place for duration of catheter—48–72 hours.

Discontinuance of Intravenous Infusion
1. Gently loosen dressing and fixation near injection site.
2. Place a sterile gauze square over cannula where it enters vein; withdraw cannula and exert pressure at site. Examine catheter tip to be sure catheter embolus has not occurred.
3. Remove adhesive marks with solvent.
4. Record (a) Nature of therapy and time given; (b) type of solution and rate of flow; (c) total amount of solution; (d) appearance of catheter tip; (e) patient's reaction and/or presence of IV-related complications.

Guidelines: Intravenous Infusion with Insertion of Plastic Catheter
(Mounted on Metal Needle)

Equipment
Rubber tourniquet
Foil-wrapped alcohol sponges or iodine-base antiseptic
Sterile infusion set containing:
    Gauze squares
    Hollow intravenous needle with catheter (Teflon, Silastic, polyurethane or polyvinyl chloride) attached to rigid hub
      Note: Thorough hand washing is required before handling sterile supplies.

Procedure
As described on page 101, then as follows.

(continued)

Guidelines: Intravenous Infusion with Insertion of Plastic Catheter
(Mounted on Metal Needle) (continued)

Procedure
(Cont.)

<table>
<tr><td align="center">Nursing Action</td><td align="center">Rationale / Amplification</td></tr>
<tr><td>

1. Insert needle into vein; when blood return is present, advance needle and catheter as one unit another ⅛″.
2. Hold onto catheter and pull back on needle to separate needle from catheter hub (about ¼″); advance catheter into vein.
3. Slowly remove needle while holding catheter hub in place.
4. Apply pressure on vein beyond catheter with the small or ring finger (Fig. 6-6).
5. Connect infusion tubing to hub of catheter.
6. Apply sterile antibiotic ointment (optional).
7. Tape catheter securely and apply a sterile dressing.

8. Loop tubing and fasten to arm.

</td><td>

1. To ensure entry of needle and catheter into vein lumen.
2. Pulling back on needle places needle inside catheter which prevents inadvertent puncture of vein and provides stability of catheter for insertion.
3. If catheter is not held in place, it is possible to pull catheter out of vein.
4. This will reduce blood leakage while removing needle and connecting tubing to infusion set.

6. Inconclusive data on effectiveness.
7. To prevent catheter movement, which could irritate vein and lead to phlebitis.
8. To prevent any tension on tubing from affecting or moving catheter in the vein.

</td></tr>
</table>

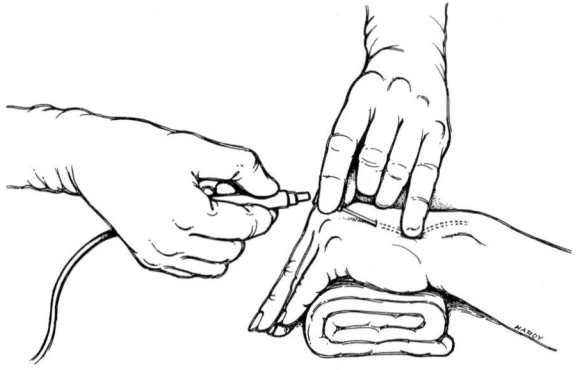

Figure 6-6. Finger palpation of dorsal venous arch.

Follow-up

<table>
<tr><td>

1. Frequent inspection of venipuncture site.
2. Record date of insertion, size and type of catheter.

3. Change gauze dressing every 24–48 hours.
4. Change catheter q. 48–72 hours; change transparent dressing at this time also.
5. Change IV tubing every 24–48 hours.
6. Use 0.22-micron filter unless contraindicated.

</td><td>

1. To ensure proper functioning of infusion.
2. This is done on the patient's chart as well as on adhesive tape near infusion puncture site.
3. Permits one to check catheter site.
4. Increased potential for infection when use of IV site exceeds 72 hours.
5. New IV tubing is used when IV site is established.
6. Decreases risk of IV-related complications.

</td></tr>
</table>

Guidelines: Intravenous Infusion by Insertion of Catheter Through Needle (IntraCatheter)

Equipment

Infusion set containing (sterile):
Rubber tourniquet
Gauze squares
Foil wrapped alcohol sponges or iodine-base antiseptic
Intravenous needle with plastic catheter through needle

Procedure

As described on page 101, then as follows:

Procedure
(Cont.)

Nursing Action	Rationale/Amplification
1. When needle has punctured vein wall, gently thread catheter through needle until desired length of catheter in vein has been achieved.	1. *Catheter damage is prevented by proper needle angle.*
2. Place index finger over vein (with catheter in place) and withdraw needle.	2. To hold catheter in proper position.
3. Apply pressure at puncture site for several seconds.	3. To control bleeding.
4. Slide needle shield to cover bevel of needle.	4. This will prevent cutting of the catheter by the needle.
5. An effective splint for the needle (and its junction with catheter) is made by taping a wooden tongue blade to needle and catheter.	5. This will prevent kinking of catheter and possibility of its breaking at bevel of needle.
6. Apply dressing and tape.	

▶ **NURSING ALERT:** If insertion of catheter through the needle is unsuccessful, remove both catheter and needle *at the same time.* Otherwise, if catheter is pulled through needle, *it may break and slip into the circulatory system.*

Follow-up

1. Frequent inspection of venipuncture site.	1. To detect possible complications.
2. Record date of insertion, size, and type of catheter.	2. This is done on the patient's chart as well as on adhesive tape near puncture site.
3. Change gauze dressing q. 24–48 hours.	3. Permits one to check catheter site.
4. Change catheter q. 48–72 hours; change transparent dressing also.	4. Increased potential for infection when IV site use exceeds 72 hours.
5. Change IV tubing q. 24–48 hours.	5. New IV tubing is used when IV site is established.
6. Use 0.22-micron filter unless contraindicated.	6. Decreases risk of IV-related complications.

Guidelines: Use of Winged Infusion Set (Venipuncture) "Butterfly"

Winged Infusion is the puncturing of a vein with a needle that has a pair of plastic wings attached to a flattened hub (Fig. 6-7).*

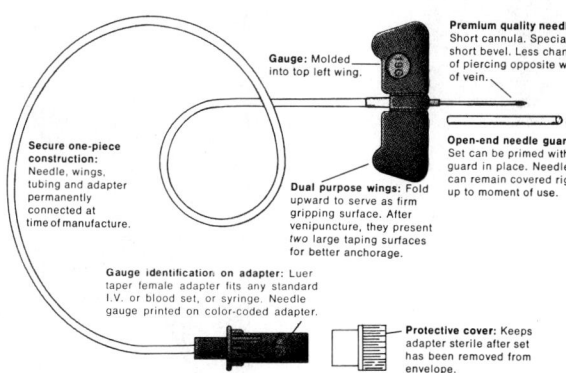

Gauge: Molded into top left wing.

Premium quality needle: Short cannula. Special short bevel. Less chance of piercing opposite wall of vein.

Secure one-piece construction: Needle, wings, tubing and adapter permanently connected at time of manufacture.

Open-end needle guard: Set can be primed with guard in place. Needle can remain covered right up to moment of use.

Dual purpose wings: Fold upward to serve as firm gripping surface. After venipuncture, they present two large taping surfaces for better anchorage.

Gauge identification on adapter: Luer taper female adapter fits any standard I.V. or blood set, or syringe. Needle gauge printed on color-coded adapter.

Protective cover: Keeps adapter sterile after set has been removed from envelope.

Figure 6-7. "Butterfly" winged infusion set.

Advantages

1. Wings can be folded upward for easy manipulation and control of needle during insertion into vein.
2. A short length and small gauge facilitate insertion of cannula.
3. Usually, this type of commercially prepared set has a shorter needle with a short bevel that may lessen possibility of puncturing the opposite vein wall.
4. Following insertion of the needle, the wings are released; they spread flat against the patient's skin and provide 2 anchor surfaces for taping. Absence of hub reduces possibility of pressure irritation.

* Figures courtesy of Abbott Laboratories.

(continued)

Guidelines: Use of Winged Infusion Set (Venipuncture) *"Butterfly"* (continued)

Procedure

As described on p. 101, then as follows.

Nursing Action	**Rationale/Amplification**
1. Position wing set so that bevel of needle is up.	1. This permits proper introduction of needle through skin into vein.
2. Note gauge of needle on left wing.	2. Most sets are marked for easy recognition of needle gauge.
3. Pinch wings firmly together between thumb and index finger.	3. Needle is held firmly and comfortably for insertion.
4. Follow usual procedure, described on p. 101, for inserting needle.	
5. Advance needle cautiously into vein; simultaneously, lift wings up slightly.	5. To avoid piercing opposite vein wall.
6. Release tourniquet and release wings; hold flat against patient's skin and permit fluid to flow temporarily.	6. This will anchor needle in vein and permit checking of flow of fluid.
7. Apply tape parallel to needle on each side. Make a protective loop and fasten to arm with tape.	7. To anchor needle position.
8. Apply dressing over site, and tape.	

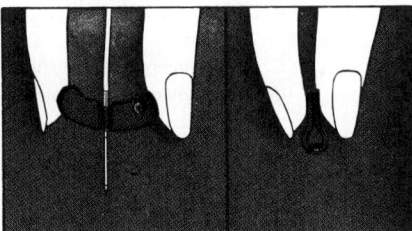
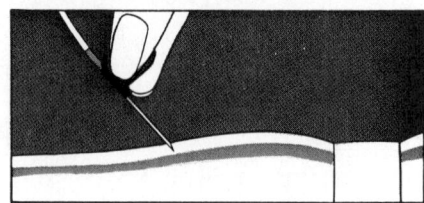
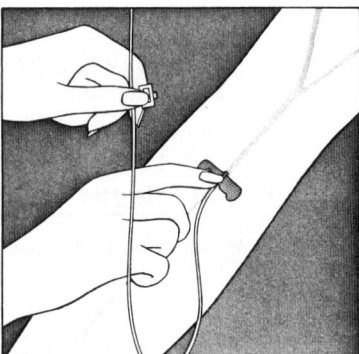
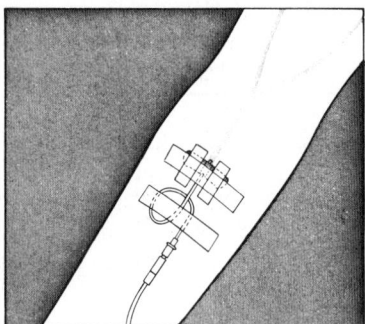

Guidelines: Setting Up An Automatic IV "Piggyback"

"Piggyback" intravenous administration is a means of administering medication via the fluid pathway of an established primary infusion line.

Features and Advantages

1. Drugs may be given on an intermittent basis through a "keep-open" infusion.
2. The secondary bottle contains the medication; this may be single dose or multiple dose.
3. When desired, the primary infusion is clamped off, and the prescribed amount of medication from the secondary bottle is administered; or 2 solutions may run simultaneously depending on tubing design.

Features and Advantages
(Cont.)

4. When a check-valve is present, it performs the following functions:
   a. Permits the primary infusion to flow after the medication has been administered.
   b. Prevents air from entering the system.
   c. Prevents secondary fluid from "running dry."
   d. Permits less mixing of primary fluid with secondary solution.
5. Higher flow rates can be achieved by elevating either of the receptacles.

Equipment

Sterile infusion set (primary)
Sterile infusion set with admixture (secondary)
Sterile gauze squares and iodine-base antiseptic
Tourniquet
Tape

Procedure

Follow procedure of particular manufacturer of "piggyback" infusion set.
In general, most procedures are similar to the following:

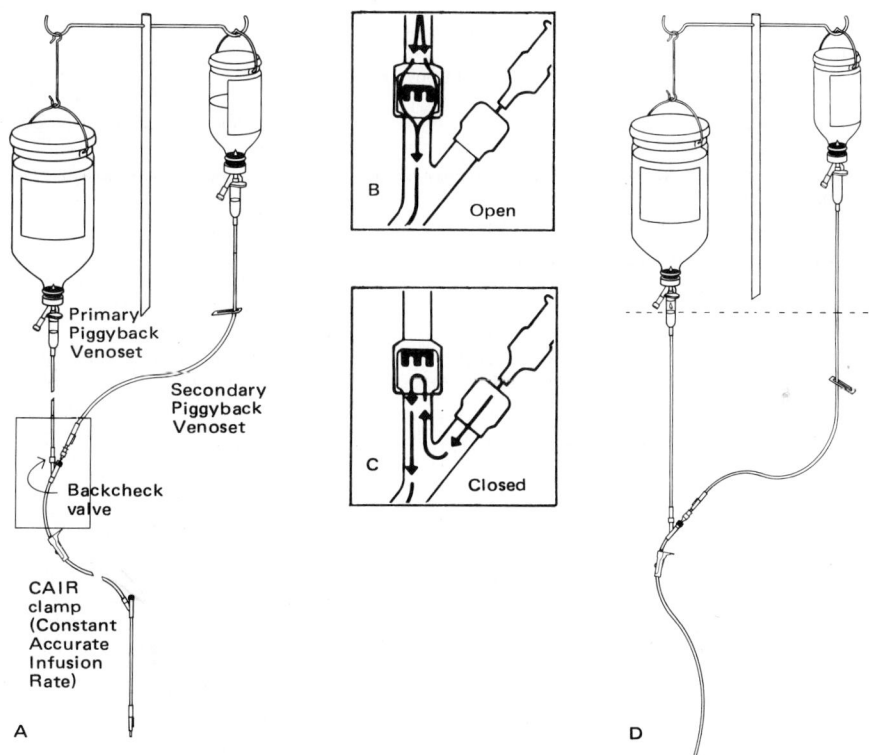

Figure 6-8. *(A) "Piggyback" IV. On left is the primary infusion flask. Note use of extension hook (hanging from IV pole) to suspend primary flask. Backcheck valve is seen more clearly in B and C. Secondary "piggyback" source is seen on the right.*
(B) Open check-valve. Fluid from primary source flows down on either side of movable disc. Fluid from secondary source is closed off with clamp (not visible).
(C) Closed check-valve. Note that fluid source from secondary flask (where pressure is greater because flask source is higher) is forcing movable disc upward, thereby closing off fluid from primary source.
(D) When last of fluid from secondary source reaches the level of the fluid in the primary set drip chamber (as indicated by broken line), hydrostatic pressure between both sets will equalize. This releases check-valve; flow will shift from secondary to primary source. (Adapted from Abbott Laboratories)

(continued)

Guidelines: Setting Up An Automatic IV "Piggyback" (continued)

Procedure
(Cont.)

Nursing Action	Rationale/Amplification
1. Wash hands thoroughly.	1. Minimizes possibility of infection.
2. Set up primary infusion set as described on p. 107, this may have a check-valve (Fig. 6-8A)	2. The primary set should be functioning effectively before the secondary (piggyback) set can be attached.
3. Lower the primary flask on the IV pole; usually, an extension hook accompanies the set.	3. This will permit the check-valve to function (Fig. 6-8A)
4. Prime secondary set; hang it on IV pole. Ideally the system should be maintained as a closed system since each entry increases the risk of infection.	4. This may be a partial-fill bottle or special additive container. Priming allows all air to escape from the system.
5. Use antiseptic swab to carefully cleanse injection site.	5. Usually this is a Y-connection on the primary set.
6. Open clamp on secondary set; inspect the check-valve to ensure that it closes off the flow of solution from the primary source (Fig. 6-8C).	6. Pressure is greater from the secondary source, since it is more elevated; increased pressure forces the disc upward in the check-valve. This closes off the flow from the primary source.
7. When fluid from secondary source reaches level of fluid in primary set drip chamber, hydrostatic pressure between the two sets equalizes (Fig. 6-8D).	7. This releases check-valve (Fig. 6-8B), and flow will then resume automatically from primary source.

Follow-up

1. Follow specific instructions on manufacturer's set for secondary replacement.	
2. Discontinuation of primary source is as for conventional infusion set.	
3. Same as Follow-up on page 105.	3. NITA Standards of Practice; CDC Guidelines.

Intravenous "Push"

IV "Push" refers to the administration of a medication from a syringe and needle directly into an ongoing intravenous infusion. It may also be given directly into a vein or heparin lock. Although called "push," it is administered *slowly,* and the patient is carefully observed throughout the procedure.

Note: IV "push" medication is usually restricted to intensive care units and is administered by specially prepared personnel.

Advantages

1. Avoids incompatibility problems that may occur when several medications are mixed in one bottle.
2. Reduces patient discomfort because there are fewer IM injections and need for venipunctures.
3. Provides for immediate absorption of drugs; the effects are rapid and observable.
4. Permits rapid concentration of a medication in the patient's bloodstream.

Precautions and Recommendations

1. Determine the patient's condition and his ability to accept the drug.
   Perhaps a more dilute medication is indicated.
   Example: Does the patient have heart disease? limited cardiac output? diminished urinary output? pulmonary congestion?
2. Many medications require dilution because of their irritating effect on veins Further dilution of the drug may be obtained by administering the drug simultaneously with the primary IV solution if the 2 are compatible. If 2 solutions are incompatible, the line must be flushed before and after administering the drug with the solution that is compatible with this drug and primary solution.

3. Administer medication *slowly.* The shortest time to spend in emptying a syringe should be 1 minute; the longest could be 6 or 7 minutes. Slow administration provides an opportunity to observe the patient; if untoward effects occur, stop the injection.
4. Check the list of incompatible medications; often, the local hospital pharmacy prepares this list in collaboration with the medical staff based on medications used by the local hospital. Frequent updating is needed because of new drugs and research.
5. Watch for major patient reactions such as anaphylaxis, respiratory distress, tachycardia, bradycardia, seizures. Also note "minor" side effects such as nausea, flushing, vomiting, skin rash, confusion, gastrointestinal distress.
   If a major reaction occurs, or if a minor one is increasing in severity, stop the medication and notify the physician.
6. Be familiar with antidotes for side effects and be prepared to administer them if prescribed:
   Examples: Skin reactions—Benadryl
   Anaphylaxis—Epinephrine
   Vomiting—Tigan
   Diarrhea—Lomotil
   Emergency medications should be available.
7. Cardiopulmonary resuscitative procedures should be familiar to nurses giving IV "push" medications.
8. Vesicants are always given through the side arm of a running IV.

Procedure Methods

1. Directly into the vein (See Guidelines: Venipuncture, p. 101)
2. Into IV tubing ("push")
   a. As with venipuncture, aseptic technique is rigidly observed.

b. The distal port is carefully swabbed with alcohol before it is punctured.

c. Usually, 10 cm. (up to 4 inches) is used for IV "push" medications.

3. Via "piggyback" (see Guidelines: IV "Piggyback," p. 106)

4. Into a "heparin lock" (Butterfly-21 Abbott)
   a. This is similar to the "butterfly" shown in Fig. 6-7.
   b. A winged needle is positioned in a vein; to the winged hub is attached a 9–10 cm. (3½ inch) length of plastic tubing.

c. At the end of this short tubing is a permanently attached latex reseal injection site.

d. This is used to inject medications or withdraw periodic blood samples.

For indwelling needle sets or catheters for intermittent procedures, the system must be flushed at regular intervals with saline or heparinized saline solution (10–100 units) to prevent clotting.

Guidelines: Heparin Lock

Heparin lock is an intermittent infusion reservoir that permits administration of periodic intravenous medications/solutions without continuous fluid administration and aspiration of blood samples for laboratory analysis.

Equipment

#21 gauge intermittent infusion reservoir, cannula or catheter infusion device with Latex port adapter attached
Foil-wrapped alcohol sponges or iodine-base antiseptic
Rubber tourniquet
Antimicrobial ointment
2 × 2-inch gauze squares
½-inch tape
Tuberculin syringe containing prescribed 0.5 ml. heparin solution (100 U./ml.) or other prescribed amount of heparin
One 6-ml. syringe containing normal saline solution with #25 gauge needle.

Procedure

Nursing Action	Rationale / Amplification
1. Explain nature and purpose of heparin lock to patient.	1. His understanding will facilitate proper functioning of the lock.
2. Follow Guidelines: Use of Winged Infusion Set, p. 105, using #21 gauge intermittent infusion reservoir: a. Prepare selected site for infusion reservoir as described on p. 101 in Guidelines: Venipuncture b. Apply tourniquet to the patient's arm.	
3. Cleanse rubber injection port of heparin lock.	3. Firmly rub, using alcohol sponge.
4. Insert #25 gauge needle of syringe containing normal saline solution into injection port.	4. Small-gauge needle will prevent large puncture openings.
5. Flush cannula–reservoir system with flush solution (usual volume is 1–2 ml.).	5. This will release air bubble from reservoir.
6. Perform venipuncture as described on p. 101 (Guidelines: Venipuncture/Phlebotomy).	
7. After confirming the position of the needle in the vein, secure wings with adhesive.	7. Carefully aspirate blood to verify needle position.
8. Inject 2 ml. of normal saline solution.	8. Observe site for evidence of infiltration.
9. Remove saline syringe with needle from injection port.	9. Continue to observe site for evidence of infiltration.
10. Apply antimicrobial ointment to insertion site; cover with 2 × 2-inch gauze square; secure with ½-inch tape.	10. To reduce possibility of infection.
11. Replace with needle and syringe containing heparin-holding solution.	11. Strict asepsis is observed in making this switch.
12. Inject 0.5 ml. heparinized saline solution (or other prescribed dose).	12. Heparinized saline solution will keep the line open for the next injection.
13. Remove needle and syringe from injection port.	

To Administer Medication

1. Prepare the medication to be administered by drawing it into the appropriate syringe.	
2. Draw 2 ml. of normal saline solution into each of 2 syringes.	2. Heparin is incompatible with many antibiotics; saline solution is used before and after administration to prevent mixing of 2 incompatible drugs.
3. Draw heparinized saline solution into a syringe if prescribed.	
4. Explain to the patient what are you about to do.	

(continued)

Guidelines: Heparin Lock (continued)

Procedure
(Cont.)

Nursing Action	Rationale/Amplification
5. Cleanse injection port of the heparin lock with alcohol. Insert normal saline syringe needle into port and aspirate slightly.	5. When positive blood return is not obtained, monitor site carefully to detect infiltration.
6. Inject normal saline solution to flush reservoir of heparinized saline and remove.	6. Note any signs of inflammation or infiltration, also observe the patient for signs of discomfort. If such signs are present, discontinue injection.
7. Insert medication syringe, administer drug, and remove syringe.	7. Maintain stability of system by inserting sterile equipment.
8. Insert saline syringe, and flush reservoir slowly, then remove syringe.	8. Saline solution will clear the reservoir of medication and prepare the way for heparinized saline solution.
9. Inject heparinized saline solution into reservoir if prescribed.	9. The usual heparin is 10–100 units in 1–2 ml.
10. Remove heparin syringe and needle from injection port.	10. Treatment is completed.

Follow-up Phase

1. Maintain patency of heparin lock by flushing it q. 8 hours.	1. If resistance is met, device should not be flushed. Attempt to remove occlusion via aspiration. If unable to restore patency, remove IV device.
2. Record all actions and medications.	
3. Heparin lock should not be left in place longer than 48–72 hours.	3. NITA Standards; CDC Guidelines.
4. IV administration sets for intermittent therapy should be changed q. 24 hours or immediately upon contamination. A new sterile needle should be used for each entry into the intermittent cannula device.	4. Since the tubing is not maintained as a closed system, it is at higher risk for infection.

Discontinuance of Heparin Lock

1. Remove immediately when IV therapy no longer indicated.	1. To minimize infection.

Electronic Flow Rate Regulators

Types

1. *Controller*—An electronic device that is mechanically different than the pump (described next); it regulates by electronically monitoring drop rate* or regulating fluid passage by a magnetically activated metal ball valve.†
   Advantages:
   a. More accurate than nonelectronic regulators.
   b. Has alarms to alert for problems.
   c. Takes care of a wide range of fluid and medication needs of patients.
2. *Infusion pump*—An electronic device that exerts pressure (1) on tubing or (2) on fluid.
   By pumping against pressure gradients, a constant, accurate, and preselected fluid rate and volume can be maintained.
   Types:
   a. Peristaltic—Moves fluid by exerting externally applied forces on tubing.
      (1) Linear   (2) Rotary
   b. Piston–cylinder—Exerts pressure on fluid in a cylinder by pumping action of a piston.
   c. Syringe—A motor-driven device in which plunger is depressed at a constant preset rate to eject medication.

* IVAC 230, IVAC Corporation, LaJolla, CA 92038
† Epic 100, Burton Medical Products, Bethlehem, PA 18018

   d. Volumetric—A device that uses the piston–cylinder principle. Chief advantage is that most models will not pump air (a safeguard against air emboli).

Advantages of Electronic Flow Rate Regulators

1. Ability to infuse large volumes of fluid with accuracy.
2. Usually an alarm warns of problems.
3. Can be used for intra-arterial infusions.

Disadvantages of Electronic Flow Rate Regulators

1. Cost considerations; however, studies (Rapp et al) have demonstrated that not only are these devices cost-effective, but complications (such as infiltration, postinfusion phlebitis, and the necessity for infusion restarts) are reduced significantly.
2. Some require special tubing.
3. Special precautions must be employed if vesicant drugs are used.

Indications for Use of Controlled Infusions

1. Intra-arterial infusions
2. Critical care fluid and medication management
3. Forcing fluids—TPN, enteral alimentation
4. Closed wound irrigation

5. Antacid titration via nasogastric tube
6. Continuous heparin administration
7. Minute doses of medications for systemic use
8. Chemotherapy and oxytocic drugs
9. Regional arterial perfusion
10. Antiarrhythmic drugs; pressor agents
11. Bronchoactive and hypoglycemic agents

Considerations When Selecting Infusion Devices

(Also see Pediatric Techniques, Infusion Pumps p. 1165.)
1. Cost vs. budget
2. Specific needs of institution
3. Inservice facilities
4. Vesicants or irritants

Complications of Intravenous Therapy

Infection

A local reaction due to contamination; this may spread systemically.
1. Causes (Fig. 6-9)
   a. Fluid contamination; this may be due to faulty preparation, crack in flask, puncture in plastic container, fluid additives. No container should hang longer than 24 hours; some solutions expire in less time.
   b. Peripheral IV catheters are changed in 48–72 hours; when catheter is in place for a longer period, there is greater chance of infection.
   c. Failure to "prep" skin rigorously—to remove dead skin, dirt, mucus, etc., before inserting cannula.
   d. Ineffective handwashing technique can result in cross-contamination.
   e. Use of contaminated bar soap, liquid soap, and hand lotion may result in infection.
   f. May be transmitted within the patient from another infected part of his body to the catheter site.
   g. The practice of manipulating the system for administration of medication, tubing changes, dressing changes, etc. may provide the opportunity for introducing contaminants.
2. Preventive nursing
   a. Practice rigid aseptic technique when inserting a cannula; consider the procedure a minor operation.
   b. Thoroughly cleanse the infusion site; follow this with an iodine-base antiseptic.
   c. Avoid the use of aqueous benzalkonium chlorides, since they have been demonstrated to be ineffective against some gram-negative organisms, especially *Pseudomonas.*
   d. Take care to anchor the catheter/cannula firmly in order to prevent excessive movement that might traumatize the cannulated vein and possibly facilitate entry of organisms at infusion site. Use 0.22-micron filter unless contraindicated.
   e. Change solution every 24 hours or more frequently depending on manufacturer's recommendations.
   f. Whenever admixtures are made, they should be done in the pharmacy under a laminar–air flow hood.

Mechanical Failures

Solution flow slowing down or stopping, etc.
1. Causes
   a. Needle may be lying against the side of the vein, cutting off fluid flow. (Patient may have moved his arm.)

b. Level of intravenous receptacle may change rate of flow (gravity):
   (1) Higher—more rapid
   (2) Lower—less rapid
c. Needle may be clogged due to clotting.
d. Regulator of flow rate may be faulty; the clamp with a tapered **V**-shaped groove seems to provide greater dependability than the regular clamp.

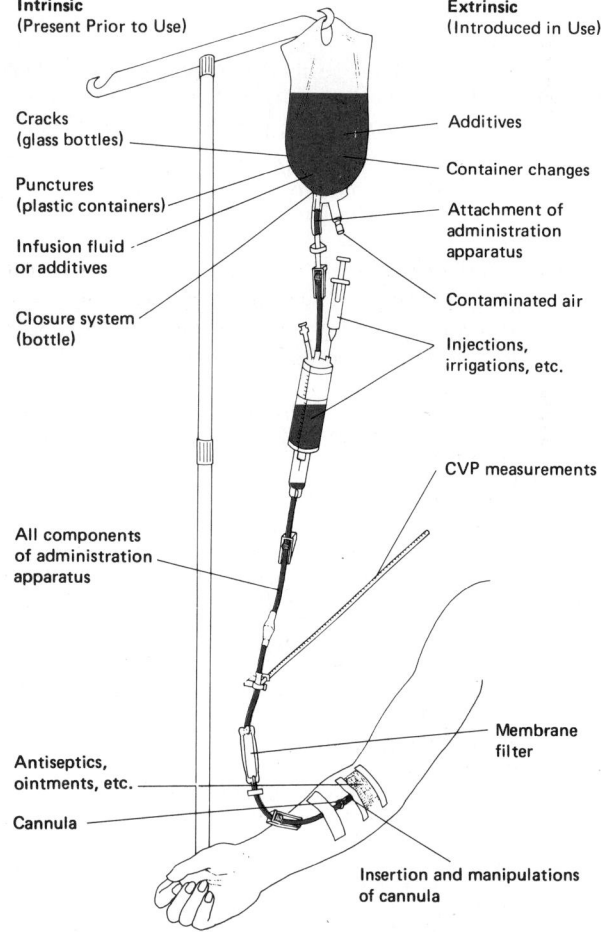

Intrinsic (Present Prior to Use)
Extrinsic (Introduced in Use)

Cracks (glass bottles)
Additives
Punctures (plastic containers)
Container changes
Infusion fluid or additives
Attachment of administration apparatus
Closure system (bottle)
Contaminated air
Injections, irrigations, etc.
CVP measurements
All components of administration apparatus
Antiseptics, ointments, etc.
Membrane filter
Cannula
Insertion and manipulations of cannula

Figure 6-9. Potential mechanisms for contamination of IV infusion systems (Maki DG. Preventing infection in intravenous therapy. Hospital Practice)

2. Nursing assessment and approach
    a. Note whether there is swelling at needle site; if edema is present, it suggests infiltration (see below).
    b. Remove tape and check for kinking of tubing.
    c. Pull back cannula because it may be lying against wall of vein.
    d. Move the patient's arm to a new position.
    e. Elevate or lower needle to prevent occlusion of bevel of needle; if necessary to maintain a slightly different position use a gauze pad or cotton ball as a prop and maintain position by placing a few adhesive straps.
    f. Try pulling the needle or catheter back a short distance, since it may be occluded at a bifurcation.
    g. Check for infiltration; apply tourniquet to stop venous flow; if catheter is in vein, IV flow will also stop.
    h. Never irrigate (override undue resistance) a cannula or needle with syringe since it may force a clot into the circulation.
    i. If none of the preceding steps produces the desired flow, remove needle and restart infusion.

▶ **NURSING ALERT:** Sterile distilled water is never added to an intravenous set-up because it is hypotonic.

Bacteremia

A generalized reaction due to contaminated equipment or solutions (less apparent with disposable equipment).
1. Symptoms (occur about 30 minutes to 1 hour after start of infusion)
    a. Abrupt temperature elevation, chills
    b. Face flushing, sudden pulse rate change
    c. Complaints of backache, headache
    d. Nausea and vomiting
    e. Hypotension—vascular collapse
    f. Cyanosis—vascular collapse
2. Preventive nursing
    a. Solutions never hang more than 24 hrs. or even less as recommended by manufacturer's directives.
    b. Use of 0.22 micron filter decreases risk of IV-related complications.
    c. Cannula site is to be changed every 48–72 hours.
    d. Change IV administration set every 24–48 hours.
3. Nursing treatment
    a. Discontinue infusion and IV cannula.
    b. Check vital signs; reassure patient.
    c. Notify physician.
    d. Save all equipment for further laboratory study.
    e. Record name, lot number, and information—i.e., manufacturer of solution and any medications that have been added.

Nerve Damage

May result from tying the arm too tightly to the splint.
1. Symptoms
    Numbness of fingers or hands
2. Nursing preventive measures
    Place padding around arm where bandage is to be applied.
3. Nursing treatment measures
    a. Massage arm and move shoulder through its range of motion.
    b. Instruct the patient to open and close hand several times each hour.
    c. Physical therapy may be required.

Infiltration

Dislodging of needle will cause fluid to infiltrate tissues.
1. Symptoms at site
    a. Edema, blanching of skin—also check undersurface of arm for puffiness.
    b. Discomfort, depending on nature of solution.
    c. Fluid flows more slowly or stops.
    d. Note temperature of skin; since solution is much cooler than patient, infiltration site will feel cool to touch.
    e. With a vasoconstrictor, such as norepinephrine (Levophed), infiltration can cause serious injury leading to necrosis and sloughing of tissues.
2. Preventive nursing
    a. Fasten needle securely.
    b. Check IV site for complications hourly.
    c. Check IV flow rate at least hourly.
    d. Avoid looping of tubing below bed level.
3. Nursing treatment
    a. Stop infusion and institute immediate treatment if vesicant infiltrated.
    b. Notify intravenous therapist, physician, etc.
    c. Place a sterile 3 × 3-inch gauze pad over needle and vein; withdraw needle and apply firm pressure over venipuncture site for several minutes.
    d. Apply warm compresses to increase fluid absorption if not contraindicated.
    e. Infusion may be restarted elsewhere.

Circulatory Overload

Patient receives an excessive amount of solution (happens more frequently in elderly patients or in infants).
1. Symptoms
    a. Headache, flushed skin, rapid pulse
    b. Venous distention (engorged neck veins)
    c. Increased blood pressure
    d. Increased venous pressure
    e. Coughing, shortness of breath, increased respirations
    f. Syncope, shock
    g. Pulmonary edema leading to dyspnea and cyanosis
2. Preventive nursing
    a. Know whether patient has existing heart condition—more prone to develop acute pulmonary edema.
    b. Monitor solution flow.
    c. Place patient in semi-sitting position during infusion.
    d. Be especially attentive to the elderly or the infant.
3. Nursing treatment
    a. Slow infusion to a "keep-open" rate (available for emergency medication); notify physician.
    b. Raise patient to sitting position—will ease the breathing problem.

Drug Overload

Patient receives an excessive amount of fluid containing drugs.
1. Toxic concentrations of drug are collected in main organs: brain and heart.
2. Symptoms
    a. Dizziness, fainting leading to shock.
    b. Specific symptoms related to the offending drug.
3. Preventive nursing interventions—monitor flow rate carefully.

4. Nursing treatment—related to the nature of the medication.

Superficial Thrombophlebitis

1. Causes
   a. Overuse of a vein, which may cause vasospasm; this may lead to an inflammatory process.
   b. Irritating infusion solution (strong acids or alkalies, hypertonic glucose solutions, and certain drugs such as cytotoxic agents, methacillin, barbiturates).
   c. Clot formation in an inflamed vein.
   d. Anatomic location—veins of the lower extremities (relatively sluggish blood flow) are more vulnerable than cephalad vessels.
   e. Length of time the cannula is in place—the longer the cannulation, the greater the possibility of infection.
   f. Polyvinyl chloride catheters appear to be associated with infection more often than steel needles.
   g. Catheter diameter: large-bore catheters are more often associated with phlebitis than small-bore.
2. Symptoms
   a. Tenderness at first, then pain along course of the vein
   b. Edema and redness at injection site
   c. Arm feels warmer than other arm
3. Preventive nursing interventions
   a. Change intravenous site so that the same vein is used no longer than 72 hours (preferably no longer than 48 hours).
   b. Use large veins for irritating fluids because of higher rate of blood flow, which rapidly dilutes irritant.

   c. Stabilize venipuncture at area of flexion.
   d. Use 0.22-micron filter.
4. Nursing treatment interventions
   a. Apply cold compresses immediately to relieve pain and inflammation.
   b. Later follow with moist warm compresses to stimulate circulation and promote absorption.

Air Embolism

Air manages to get into the circulatory system.

▶ **NURSING ALERT:** Recognize the high possibility of air embolism when a physician pumps in blood (e.g., 500 ml.–1 pint in 10 minutes), since this builds high pressure in blood receptacle.

1. Symptoms
   a. Hypotension, cyanosis, tachycardia
   b. Increased venous pressure, loss of consciousness
2. Nursing preventive interventions
   a. Replace initial bottle before it is completely empty with a fresh, full bottle; check attachment to be certain it is tight.
   b. In "Y" type sets, tightly clamp the nearly empty bottle to prevent air from being sucked into the tubing.
   c. Allow fluid to flow through tubing and needle or catheter to force air out—before starting infusion.
   d. Use 0.22-micron filter.
3. Nursing treatment
   Unless prompt action is taken, the patient may die within minutes.
   a. *Immediately* turn patient on left side in Trendelenburg position—air will rise to feet or right atrium. The trapped air will be slowly absorbed.

3: Care of the Wound

A *wound* is an injury to the tissues of the body causing disruption of the normal tissue pattern; such an injury is caused by physical means.

Classification

According to the manner in which it is made:
   Incised—made by a clean cut with a sharp instrument; e.g., a surgeon's incision with a scalpel.
   Contused—made by a blunt force, which does not break through the skin but causes considerable soft tissue damage (e.g., a rock, when thrown, bruises a person).
   Lacerated—made by an object that tears tissues, producing jagged irregular edges (e.g., blunt knife, jagged wire, glass.
   Puncture—made by a pointed instrument, such as an ice pick, bullet, knife stab, nail.

Surgical Classification

Clean—an aseptically made wound, as in surgery, in which all bleeding vessels have been ligated (tied).
Contaminated—exposed to excessive amounts of bacteria (e.g., unprepared colon surgery, dirty laceration). These wounds are not grossly infected but have been exposed to bacteria (contaminated) and have higher risk of infection.

Infected—a wound that may not be closed may contain devitalized or infected material.
Debridement—the process whereby devitalized or necrotic tissue is cut out and flushed clean with saline solution.

Physiology of Wound Healing (Fig. 6-10)

A. First Intention Healing (Primary Union)

Healing that takes place aseptically with a minimum of tissue damage and tissue reaction; this is the ideal sought by the surgical staff; surgically closed (sutures or surgical tapes).

B. Second Intention Healing (Granulation)

Wounds that are left open to heal spontaneously; not surgically closed. They need not be infected.
1. If infected, pus forms; drainage is accomplished by incision and perhaps insertion of drains.
2. Necrotic material disintegrates and sloughs off.
3. Cavity fills with a red, soft, sensitive tissue, which bleeds easily.
4. Buds, called granulation tissue, enlarge to fill area formerly destroyed and thus form a scar (cicatrix).

C. Third Intention Healing (Secondary Suture)

1. Occurs when a wound breaks down and is resutured or when a wound has been kept open and fills with granulation tissue and then is closed with sutures (2

First Intention

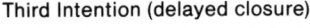

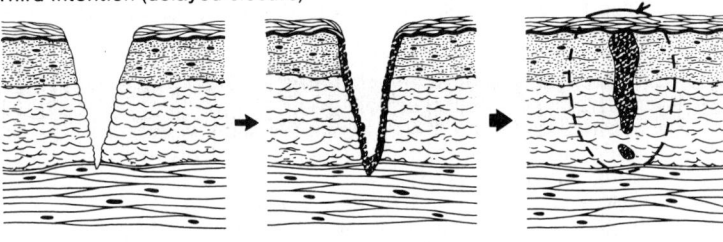

Second Intention (contraction and epithelialization)

Third Intention (delayed closure)

Figure 6-10. Classification of wound healing. *First intention*—A clean incision is made with primary closure; there is minimal scarring. *Second intention* (contraction and epithelialization)—The wound is left open to granulate in with resultant large scab and abnormal dermal–epidermal junction. *Third intention* (delayed closure)—The wound is left open and closed secondarily when there is no evidence of infection. (Hardy JD. Hardy's Textbook of Surgery. Philadelphia, JB Lippincott, 1983, p. 109)

faces of granulation tissue are brought together in apposition).
2. Scar tissue formation is deeper, wider, and more pronounced.

Wound Healing Without Dressings

Preferred by some surgeons; may be desirable for a simple, clean wound.

A. Advantages

1. Permits better observation and early detection of problems.
2. Promotes cleanliness and facilitates bathing.
3. Eliminates conditions necessary for growth of organisms.
   a. Warmth
   b. Moisture
   c. Darkness
4. Avoids adhesive tape reaction.
5. Facilitates patient activity.
6. Is economical.

B. Disadvantages

1. Psychologically, a patient may object to an exposed wound.
2. Wound is more vulnerable to injury.
3. Bedding and clothing may catch on stitches.

The Purpose of Dressings

1. To protect the wound from mechanical injury.
2. To splint or immobilize the wound.
3. To absorb drainage and fluid wastes.
4. To promote homeostasis and minimize accumulation of fluid, as in a pressure dressing.
5. To prevent contamination from bodily discharges.
6. To provide physical and psychological comfort for the patient as well as a physiological environment conducive to wound healing.
7. To debride a wound by combining capillary action and the entwining of necrotic tissue within its mesh.
8. To inhibit or kill organisms by using dressings that contain antiseptic medications.
9. To support a fractured or reconstructed area.
10. To provide information about the nature of the underlying wound.

Transparent Wound Dressings

Synthetic, clear transparent wound dressings are available that are permeable to oxygen and water vapor but impermeable to liquids and bacteria. (Tegaderm®—3M, Bioclusive®—Johnson & Johnson, Op-Site®—Acme United, and others); see Fig. 6-11).

A. Characteristics

1. Most are made of polyurethane film with the opposite side coated with hypoallergenic water-resistant adhesive.
2. Highly elastic and conforms to body contours.
3. Apply unstretched and unwrinkled to dry, clean wound with sufficient margin to avoid leakage of fluids that may accumulate under the dressing.
4. If excessive fluid does not accumulate or infection does not occur, dressing may be left in place until re-epithelialization is complete.

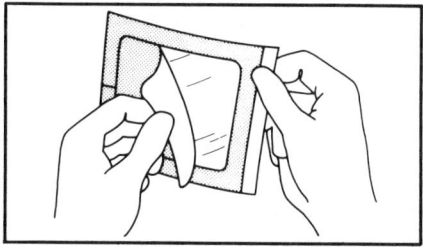

1. Clean and thoroughly dry application area; remove and discard center cut-out window.

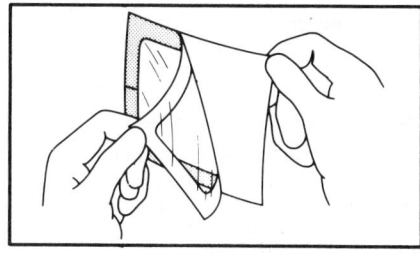

2. Peel paper liner from paper-framed dressing, exposing adhesive surface.

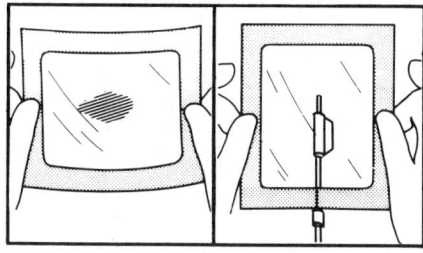

3. Position over wound or IV site. Smooth dressing from center toward edges.

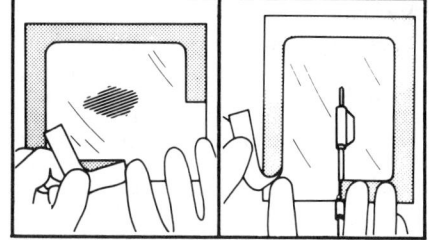

4. Remove paper frame. Smooth dressing edges. Over IV, seal dressing securely around IV tubing or hub.

Figure 6-11. These diagrams show how Tegaderm® Transparent Dressing is applied. *Part 3* indicates the placement of Tegaderm® Transparent IV Dressing. (*Part 4*) Below the dressing, the adaptor and IV tubing are stabilized with Transpore® Surgical Tape to provide a neat, secure, and visible peripheral IV site. (Courtesy of 3M Medical Products Division)

B. Indications

1. Covering arterial and venous catheter sites
2. Pressure and stasis ulcers
3. Peristomal and peri-fistulas
4. Donor sites for skin grafts
5. Surgical wounds
6. Minor burn areas

C. Advantages

1. Decreased pain noted.
2. Wound is visible.
3. Infection can be noted early and treated immediately.
4. Greater freedom of movement.
5. Patient bathing is facilitated.

Nursing Process Overview

Assessment

Factors that Affect Wound Healing

1. What type of surgery did patient have?
2. Where is the wound? How extensive?
   a. Was hemostasis in the operating room effective?
   b. What is nature of vascularity? (e.g., adequate blood supply)
   c. Evidence of edema? Inflammation?
3. How is the wound held together?
   Butterfly tapes, wire sutures, tension sutures, clips?
4. Are there drains in place? What kind? How many? Portable suction?
5. What kinds of dressings are being used?
   a. Are they saturated with exudate?
   b. Is drainage consistent with nature of surgery?
6. How does the patient appear?
   Signs or complaints of wound pain or discomfort? Fever?
7. How old is the patient?
   a. What is his nutritional status?
   b. Has his intake of protein and vitamin C been adequate? (These are needed for wound healing.)
8. Was he given packed cells to maintain adequate levels of red blood cells?
9. What conditions does patient have, and what medications is he taking that could affect wound healing?
   a. Check his medications—steroids, etc.
   b. Note all listed diagnoses—diabetes mellitus, etc.
10. How long has patient been in the hospital preoperatively?
    (Longer preoperative hospitalization increases risk of nosocomial infections.)

11. Does he understand principles of asepsis and importance of not touching sterile parts of dressing and the incision line?

Patient Problems/Nursing Diagnoses

1. Alteration in comfort (pain) related to incision site, drains, nature of surgery, dressing changes, etc.
2. Knowledge deficit: lack of understanding of principles of asepsis and potential for contaminating wound
3. Potential for infection related to incision
4. Fear related to possibility of rupturing skin stitches
5. Potential for injury related to unhealed wound and altered mobility

Planning and Implementation
Nursing Interventions

1. Ensure patient comfort by changing dressings when required.
2. Minimize strain on wound utilizing tape, bandage, and binders, in order to promote proper healing.
3. Maintain asepsis during dressing change and wound cleansing.
4. Discard soiled dressings in proper receptacle for incineration.

5. Monitor incision site for signs of irritation, inflammation.
6. Support the patient's need for mobility by providing adequate support of incision site.
7. Document condition of incision site (drainage, if present, color, smoothness, etc.) when dressings are changed.

Evaluation
Expected Outcomes

1. Relates that incision site is comfortable, looks clean, improves each day
2. Enumerates restrictions on certain physical activities to prevent wound dehiscence
3. Tells why it is important to wash hands when changing dressings
4. Demonstrates how to change his own dressings
5. Indicates the need for proper disposition of soiled dressings to avoid contamination or spread of infection, if wound is still draining
6. Lists conditions that need to be reported: dehiscence, bleeding when wound appeared to have approximated; oozing or drainage after wound appeared to be dry; heat, redness, pain, swelling

Procedural Considerations in Wound Care

Guidelines: Assisting with a Change of Surgical Dressings

Surgical Dressing Technique

The procedure of changing dressings, examining and cleansing the wound, utilizing principles of asepsis.
1. A team works together to change a patient's dressing—nurse with surgeon or nurse with a colleague.
2. The condition of the wound is noted in order to better understand the nature of the patient's surgical recovery.
3. The healing process is facilitated by keeping the wound clean.
4. Stitches or clips are removed after the 5th or 6th day, since wound edges have begun to knit together.

Equipment

Sterile
Gloves—disposable
Pack containing scissors, forceps, grooved director, dressings, cotton tipped swabs, solution cup
Antiseptic solution, sterile saline
Culture tubes
For draining wound: add sterile safety pin, packing, irrigation set

Unsterile
Plastic bag for discarded dressings
Adhesive, proper size
Pads to protect patient's bed
Gown for nurse, if wound is purulent

Procedure

Preparatory Phase
1. Inform the patient that his dressing is to be changed. Explain procedure to him. Have him lie in bed.
2. Avoid changing dressings at mealtime.
3. Ensure his privacy by drawing the curtains or closing the door; expose the dressing site.
4. If the dressings have a foul odor, perhaps they can be changed in a separate treatment area that is adequately ventilated.
5. Prevent undue exposure of the patient; respect his modesty and prevent him from being chilled.
6. Wash your hands thoroughly; this should be done before and after each patient.

Procedure
(Cont.)

Nursing Action	Rationale/Amplification
Removing Adhesive Tape	
1. Remove tape along longitudinal axis, slowly and gently.	1. Removing tape in the same plane is less injurious and less painful.
2. Peel back edges by holding skin taut and pushing away from tape.	2. It is less traumatic to push skin away from tape than to pull tape from skin.
3. Remove tape near a wound by pulling toward the wound.	3. Pulling away from a wound may tear some of the delicate newly formed tissues.
4. Use a suitable solvent, such as baby oil, if the tape does not pull away easily.	4. Oil is safe, works as well as true solvents, and, in addition, lubricates and soothes the sensitive skin beneath.
Removing Old Dressing	
Method A (Using disposable gloves)	
1. Don sterile disposable gloves, remove top dressings carefully, and discard into plastic bag.	1. Dressings are not to be handled by ungloved hands because of the possibility of transmitting pathogenic organisms.
2. Gradually loosen last dressing and observe skin and wound site.	2. If dressings adhere, moisten them with sterile saline and slowly withdraw dressing.
3. Remove and discard disposable gloves into plastic bag.	3. This will go to the incinerator later.
Method B (Using a sterile plastic bag)	
1. After washing hands, open package containing sterile plastic bag.	1. Bag should extend several centimeters (inches) above wrist.
2. Put right hand into sterile bag, being careful not to touch outside of bag (this bag acts as a sterile glove).	2. Bag acts as a glove to protect hand from the dressings.
3. Pick up all soiled dressings as above and hold them in right hand; use left hand to grasp top edge of bag and pull it down over the hand and dressings.	3. This encloses soiled dressings in a plastic container; this bag can be used to receive soiled cotton balls or dressings used to clean wound.

Cleansing the Simple Wound and Obtaining a Wound Culture

Assistant Nurse	Nurse or Surgeon	Rationale
1. Use aseptic technique.		1. To prevent contamination of a clean wound or to prevent further contamination of a ''dirty'' wound. Also to prevent transmission of pathogenic organisms to clean areas.
2. Open sterile package of gloves.	2. Don sterile gloves.	
3. Open package containing sterile syringe and needle.	3. Aspirate generous amount of liquid material into syringe; inject into anaerobic tube.	3. Collect specimen before wound is cleansed to obtain true sample of microorganisms present.
4. If liquid material is not obtainable, use cotton applicator swab.	4. Swab desired area, attempting to get maximum saturation of cotton applicator with tissue fluid.	4. Used when there is insufficient liquid material to aspirate with a syringe.
5. Receive specimen and see that it gets to the laboratory.		
6. Open a sterile pack containing a scissors, forceps, a grooved director, dressings, and solution container.	6. Pick up dressing with forceps and hold it over emesis basin.	
7. Pour antiseptic solution over dressing.	7. Clean wound gently but thoroughly.	
	8. Use forceps to pick up each stitch, cut with scissors, and pull stitch out. Deposit in emesis basin or on a sterile gauze square.	8. After 5th or 6th day; stitches serve no useful purpose. If they remain in place, they can act as wicks carrying pathogenic organisms from the skin.

(continued)

Guidelines: Assisting with a Change of Surgical Dressings (continued)

Procedure
(Cont.)

Assistant Nurse	Nurse or Surgeon	Rationale

Completion of Dressing

Assistant Nurse	Nurse or Surgeon	Rationale
1. Select proper size and type of adhesive for securing dressing; rubber-based or acrylate adhesive.	1. Place minimal dressing over wound.	1. *Rubber-based* (cloth-backed or plastic-backed) dressing is used principally for heavy support and where a high level of adhesion is required. *Acrylate* (nonwoven or fabric backing) usually is used for surgical taping because of hypoallergenic quality.
2. A thin layer of ''Skin Prep'' may be applied.	2. This is sprayed on area before tape is applied.	2. This enhances sticking of tape.
3. Apply minimal amount of taping necessary to keep dressing in place.	3. Remove gloves and complete dressing fixation with adhesive.	
4. Avoid placing adhesive in areas where sweat glands are numerous.		4. Adhesive does not adhere easily; when it is removed, it is more traumatizing.

Follow-up Care

Nursing Action	Rationale/Amplification
1. Make patient comfortable.	
2. Remove emesis basin and dispose of soiled dressings in proper receptacle. Discard disposable items and clean equipment which is to be reused.	2. To prevent transmission of pathogenic organisms.
3. Record nature of procedure and condition of wound, as well as patient reaction.	

Guidelines: Dressing a Draining Wound

Reinforcement of Dressings

Draining wounds may require frequent changes of dressings.

Outer layers may be removed and fresh dressings applied without disturbing wound site.
   a. Saturated dressings cause discomfort to the patient.
   b. Dressing edges may become dry, hard, and scratchy.
   c. Odor may be unpleasant.

Auxiliary Aids to Facilitate Dressing Changes

Montgomery Straps

Strips of adhesive tape, the edges of which have been folded back for a short distance with a small hole cut in the folded portion and threaded with gauze strips or cotton tape. Two opposing strips are brought together and the tapes tied (Fig. 6-12).

Removal of Adherent Dressings

1. To prevent the discomfort of removing dry, sticking dressings, moisten the dressing with sterile saline or hydrogen peroxide using an asepto bulb syringe.
2. Provide an emesis basin to catch excess fluid.

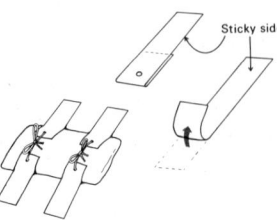
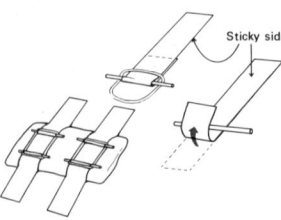

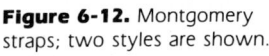
Figure 6-12. Montgomery straps; two styles are shown.

Anchoring and Gradual Withdrawal of Drainage Tubes

1. With each dressing change, the drainage tube is often pulled out of the wound a few centimeters and the excess tube is cut.
2. Hollow hard rubber or polyethylene tubes are used occasionally to drain a cavity. After the tube is anchored with a suture, the tube is taped to the skin.
    a. Cut a 5-cm. (2-inch) length of adhesive tape; trifurcate the tape lengthwise to the middle.
    b. Place right half of tape on skin up to emerging rubber drain; allow 2 end tails to straddle tube and neatly fasten middle tail around drain in a spiral fashion.
    c. Repeat process in opposite direction. Then place 2 cross strips of 5-cm. (2-inch) adhesive tape on either side of drain.

Skin Care

1. Drainage is often irritating to surrounding skin tissues, particularly if it contains gastrointestinal secretions.
2. Apply protective ointment if prescribed (caution—ointments may cause maceration and may prevent drainage).
    a. Petrolatum gauze
    b. Zinc oxide ointment
    c. Stomahesive (by Squibb)
3. Recognize value of portable wound suction in maintaining cleanliness of surrounding tissues (see below).
4. Attach drainage tubing to suction bottle.
    Check tubing frequently for kinking or looping which would restrict flow of drainage.

Guidelines: Using Portable Wound Suction (HemoVac, Porto-Vac)

Portable wound suction is a suction system that gently removes adventitious fluid and debris from a wound by means of a perforated catheter connected to a portable suction apparatus.

Purpose To speed healing of the wound by removing fluids that could retard tissue granulation and by exerting negative pressure, which permits two layers of tissue to adhere and thus eliminates dead space.

Advantages

1. Tubing rarely becomes occluded because it is siliconized and has multiple perforations.
2. Pressure exerted is gentle and even, suction is quiet.
3. Equipment is lightweight, permitting patient to move easily.
4. It is easy to measure amount of wound drainage.

Equipment

1. A long (0.25–0.5 cm.) (⅛–¼ inch) malleable stainless steel introducing needle with a cutting edge on one end and a fine screw thread at the other.
2. A long 0.25-cm. (⅛ inch) calibre, siliconized, noncollapsible, polyethylene catheter with many small perforations in the center.
3. A noncollapsible, siliconized, polyethylene connecting tube. The wound catheter fits snugly into the lumen of this tube.
4. A vacuum source (evacuator) consisting of an unbreakable plastic container with rigid ends and collapsible sides (may be a size to collect 200, 400, or 800 ml. of fluid).
    Box has 1 cuffed hole into which the connecting tube fits snugly and an airhole supplied with a plug. This box may be of accordion-like collapsible plastic, or it may have steel coil springs on the inside to hold the ends of the box apart.
5. A plastic Y-connector, which fits between wound catheters and connecting tube and allows 2 wound tubes to be connected to 1 evacuator if desired.

Method of Inserting Drainage Tube(s)

1. In the operating room, the surgeon places the perforated drainage tubing in the desired wound area.
2. A stab wound is made with the needle, and excess tubing is drawn through the wound (stab wound is preferred because a more tightly sealed porthole is created; if the wound opening is used, drainage may seep through the incision line).
3. Needle is cut off, and tubing is attached via adapter to evacuator tubing (Fig. 6-13).

(continued)

Guidelines: Using Portable Wound Suction (HemoVac, Porto-Vac) (continued)

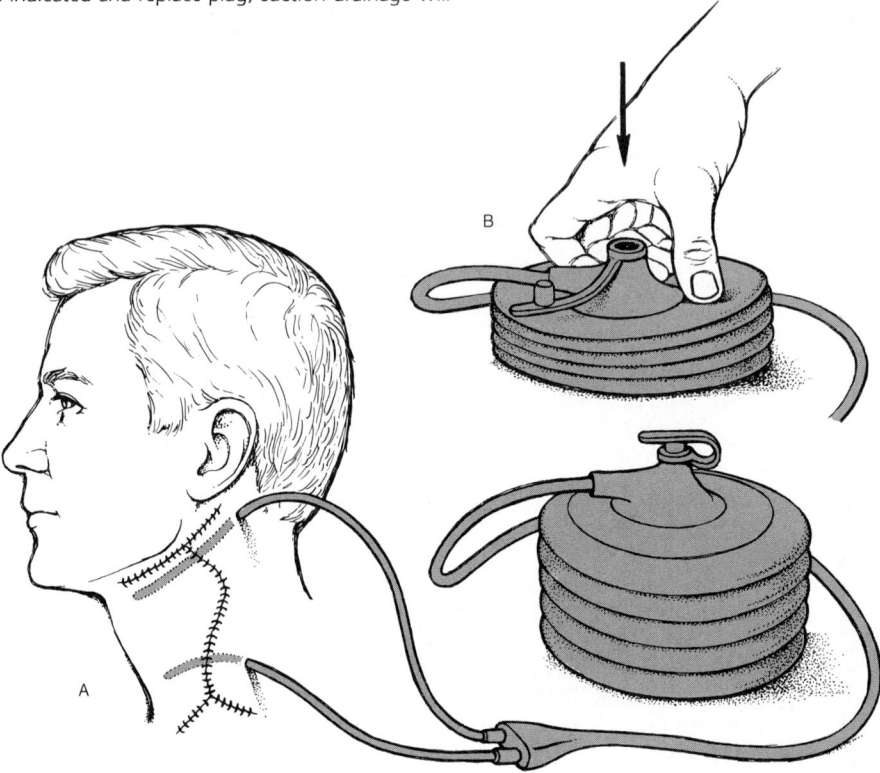

Figure 6-13. (*A*) Two perforated catheters are draining the incisional area following a radical neck dissection. By means of a Y-tube, drainage is drawn into a portable wound-suction receptacle. When full, open top plug of receptacle and empty. (*B*) To reestablish negative pressure, compress receptacle as indicated and replace plug; suction drainage will resume.

Method of Initiating Suction

Nursing Action	Rationale/Amplification
1. Connect tubes to evacuator.	
2. Squeeze ends of box together.	2. This will expel air.
3. Plug air hole.	3. To create a negative pressure.
4. As spring expands, a negative pressure of approximately 45 mm. Hg is produced.	4. Any fluid and blood in tissues is sucked into evacuator. Negative pressure is not great enough to suck the soft tissues into the holes of the catheters.
5. When evacuator is full (200, 400, or 800 ml.—depending on size of evacuator), it is time to empty. A good rule is to empty every 8 hours, or more frequently if necessary.	5. Negative pressure has been fully dissipated.

Emptying Evacuator

1. Carefully remove plug, maintaining its sterility.	
2. Empty contents of evacuator into calibrated container.	2. Measure drainage.
3. Place evacuator on flat surface.	3. To permit adequate compression.
4. Cleanse opening, as well as plug, with an alcohol sponge.	4. To maintain cleanliness of outlet.
5. Compress evacuator completely (Fig. 6-13).	5. To remove air.
6. Replace plug while evacuator is compressed.	6. To reestablish negative pressure (suction).
7. Check system for proper operation.	7. Look for fluid entering receptacle.
8. Secure evacuator to bedding; if patient is ambulatory, fasten evacuator to his clothing.	8. This permits patient to move without disturbing closed suction.
9. Record character and amount of drainage.	

Wound Irrigation Combined with Portable Wound Suction

1. Perforated wound tubes are placed side by side in wound. One is connected to irrigating fluid (or antibiotic solution), the other to portable wound suction.
2. At least 30% of the perforated section of one tube should be positioned parallel to the perforated area of the other.
3. If tubes are to remain for some time, a suture (usually stainless steel wire) is used.
4. Having the drainage tube exit through a stab wound (away from main incision line) makes it convenient to manipulate, inspect, and remove the drainage tube without disturbing the wound dressing.
5. After drip fluid has been stopped, all remaining tubes should have suction applied for at least 48 hours.

Tube Removal

1. At conclusion of use, discard tubing and evacuator by placing in a paper bag and depositing in trash container for incineration.
2. See Guidelines: Assisting with a Change of Surgical Dressings (p. 116).

4: Suturing

Guidelines: Suturing for Simple Wound Closure

Purpose   To close a small wound using nonabsorbable sutures such as black silk or dermal suture.

Equipment

Sterile gloves
Sterile suture set containing:
   Drape with aperture
   Needle holder for curved needles
   Needles: cutting edge—straight and/or curved
   Toothed forceps
   Scissors to cut sutures
   Suture material
   Dressings
Saline solution to cleanse suture line
Antiseptic solution or soap and water to cleanse area surrounding wound

Procedure

Nursing Action	Rationale/Amplification
1. Thoroughly cleanse small wound using detergent–germicidal soap.	1. To remove foreign bodies, debris, crusted blood; to minimize the possibility of contamination.
2. Apply an antiseptic that will be nonirritating to exposed subcutaneous tissues.	2. To reduce microbial contamination.
3. Don sterile gloves and apply drape with opening centered over wound.	3. This will present a sterile field.
4. Usually a straight cutting-edge needle is preferable for suturing skin.	4. Less motion is required with a straight needle; if wound is deeper, a curved needle is more effective.
5. Thread needle with desired suture material. 37.5 cm. (15 inches) is a convenient suture length; when threaded, allow 30 cm. (12 inches) on one side of needle and 7.5 cm. (3 inches) on the other. A curved needle is threaded from inner curve outward. This method helps prevent suture from falling out of needle.	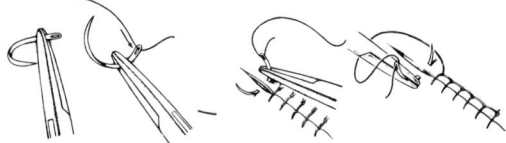
6. Grasp wound edge gently with toothed forceps.	6. This will anchor tissue when needle is forced through.
7. Stitches may be interrupted or continuous. Interrupted stitches are independent of each other; continuous sutures are applied more rapidly, but if there is a break in the suture line, the entire wound is affected. Figure shows straight cutting edge–needle, which is held by gloved fingers (not in needle holder).	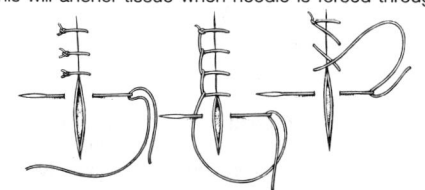
8. Space stitches evenly; tie a square knot (Fig. 6-14). *Tissues need only be approximated.*	8. Do not tie knots with excess tension, since this will traumatize the wound. If tied too tightly, stitches will be even tighter the next day due to edema.

(continued)

Guidelines: Suturing for Simple Wound Closure (continued)

Procedure
(Cont.)

Nursing Action	Rationale/Amplification
9. When cutting sutures, hold scissors almost closed in right hand; hold suture ends taut and at right angle to skin. Glide scissors down along suture, holding scissors parallel to skin.	9. This will provide control when cutting and prevent cutting of skin or tissue. 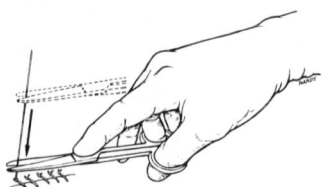
10. Cut stitch, leaving 0.65-cm. (¼-inch) tails extending from knot.	10. To prevent knot from becoming undone; such a cut stitch will be easy to grasp when it is time for stitch removal.
11. Continue with stitches to close wound.	
12. Cleanse suture line with saline dampened gauze; apply dressing and tape.	12. Remove dried blood to lessen irritation to skin.

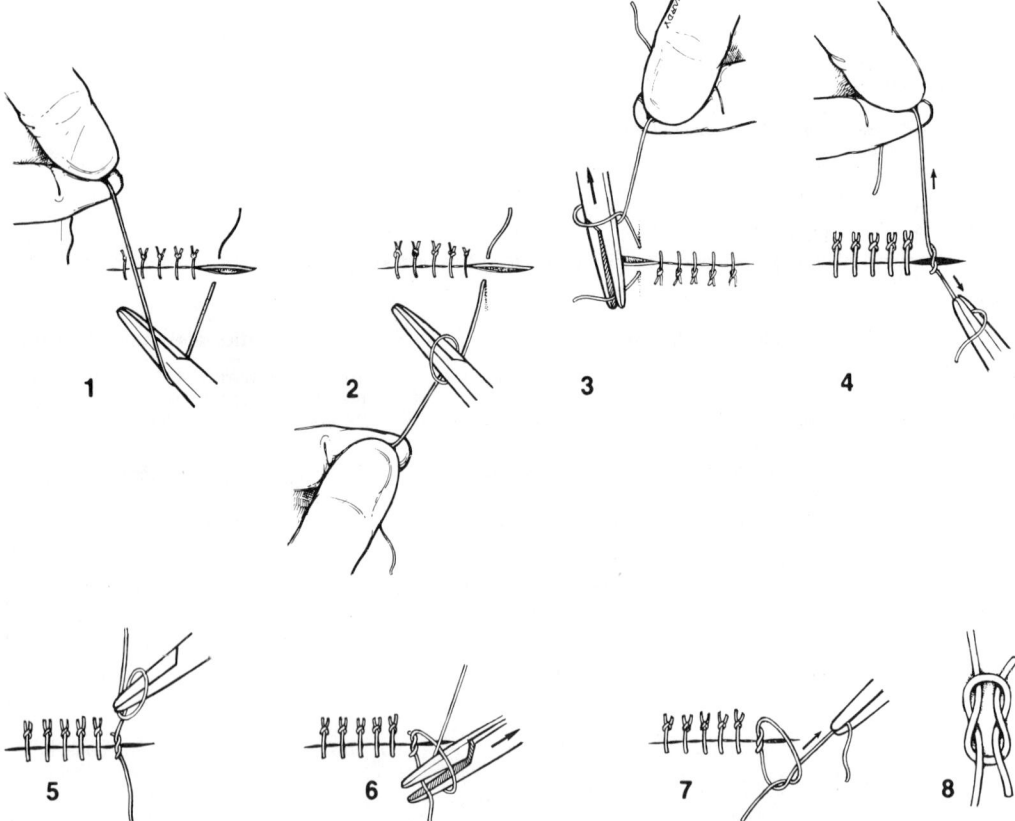

Figure 6-14. (1) After the suture is drawn through both sides of the wound, allow a short end of suture to remain. (2) Remove curved needle from holder and with the long end of the suture make a loop around the needle holder, starting with the holder in front of the suture. (3) Grasp the short end of the suture with the needle holder, which is through the loop. (4) Pull the suture through the loop and carefully tie the first part of the knot, using the needle holder to pull one end. Traction is exerted parallel to the skin, with short end toward you. (5) To complete the square knot, reverse the suture ends so that the short end is away from you. (6) Tie second part of knot. (7) Again tighten by pulling ends parallel to skin. (8) Square knot is completed.

Guidelines: Suture Removal

The timing of stitch removal (of nonabsorbable stitches) depends on the location of the stitch on the body: head and neck, 3–5 days; chest and abdomen, 5–7 days; lower extremities, 7–10 days.

Equipment

Stitch removal tray containing:
Antiseptic pledgets
Smooth forceps
Scissors
Dressings

Procedure

Nursing Action	Rationale/Amplification
1. Cleanse the stitch area carefully and thoroughly, using alcohol sponges.	1. Stitches provide pathways for microorganisms to invade tissues; therefore, skin surface must be rendered as clean as possible.
2. Use hydrogen peroxide if there are dried blood encrustations.	2. In the process of liberating oxygen, peroxide will loosen dried serum.
3. Grasp the knot of the suture with a pair of smooth forceps and gently pull upwards.	3. This will pull stitch away from skin.

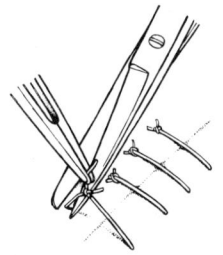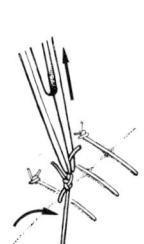

4. Cut the shortened end of the stitch as close to the skin as possible.	4. This will allow the stitch to be pulled free of wound so that only that part of the stitch which is under the skin touches subcutaneous tissues.

▶ **NURSING ALERT:** Note that no segment of the stitch that is on the surface of the skin should be drawn below the skin surface. To permit this would introduce skin-surface contaminants subcutaneously with risk of infection.

5. For continuous suture removal, cut the suture at each skin orifice on one side and remove the suture through the opposite side.	5. The objective here again is to avoid subcutaneous contamination.
6. Pat the wound site with an alcohol sponge. If there is any oozing, apply a small dressing.	6. Any orifice is a potential site for infection.
7. Avoid injury to the tender and newly healed wound.	

Bibliography

Books

Groer MW. Physiology and Pathophysiology of the Body Fluids. St Louis. CV Mosby, 1981
Gruendemann BJ and Meeker MH. Alexander's Care of the Patient in Surgery. St Louis, CV Mosby, 1983
Hunt TK (ed). Wound Healing and Wound Infection: Theory and Surgical Practice. New York, Appleton-Century-Crofts, 1980
Kee JL. Fluids and Electrolytes with Clinical Applications, 3rd ed. St Louis, CV Mosby, 1982
Kneedler J and Dodge GH. Perioperative Nursing Care. St Louis, CV Mosby, 1983

Metheny NM and Snively WD, Jr. Nurses' Handbook of Fluid Balance, Philadelphia, JB Lippincott, 1983
Nursing Photobook. Caring for Surgical Patients. Springhouse, PA, Springhouse, 1982
Nursing Photobook. Controlling Infection. Springhouse, PA, Springhouse, 1982
Perry AG and Potter PA et al (eds). Shock: Comprehensive Nursing Management. St Louis, CV Mosby, 1983
Roderick MA. Infection Control in Critical Care. Rockville, MD, Aspen Systems, 1983
Rosoff AJ. Informed Consent. A Guide for Health Care Providers.

Gaithersburg, MD Aspen Systems Corp., 1981

Perioperative Nursing
Articles
Alexander RM. Fire in the OR! RN 1982 Aug; 45(8):92L–92R
Barness SK and Long CS. Perioperative nursing. AORN J 1984 Mar; 39(4):609–615
Brocklehurt G. Face masks and wedding rings. Lancet 1983; July 16; 2(8342): 157
Hauer JM. Current uses of autotransfusion in surgery. NITA 1983 July–Aug; 6(4):261–264

Hazzard ME. Linking the OR to curriculum goals. AORN J 1980 Nov; 32(5):807–814

Hercules P. OR experience teaches continuity of care. AORN J 1980 Nov; 32(5):799–806

Kaminski S. OR orientation. Today's OR Nurse 1983 July; 5(5):24–29

Larke GA. Perioperative charting; OR nursing on display. AORN J 1980 Feb; 31(2):194–198

Pesetski JD. A practical guide for perioperative practice. AORN J 1980 June; 32(6):1049–1058

Phippen ML. Perioperative nursing. AORN J 1984 Mar; 39(4):601–608

Proposed recommended practices for OR sanitation. AORN J 1981 June; 33(7):1262–1266

Standards of administrative nursing practice: Operating Room. AORN J 1981 Aug; 34(2):268–280

Statements of basic competency for perioperative nurses. AORN J 1982 April; 35(5):882–884

Stein TP and Buzby GP. Protein metabolism in surgical patients. Surg Clin North Am 1981 June; 61(3):519–527

Preoperative Patient Care

Abbott NK, Brala G and Pollock W. The impact of preoperative assessment on intraoperative nurse performance. AORN J 1983 Jan; 37(1):43–58

Brennan PE. Preoperative visits—controlling the stress. Today's OR Nurse 1982 Dec; 4(10):9–13

Cushing M. Informed consent. Am J Nurs 1984 Apr; 84(4):437–440

Brown MS. Test your knowledge of nursing assessment. Part 4. Nursing '83 1983 Dec; 13(12):73–77

Dean KA. Informed consent. Focus on Critical Care 1983 Aug; 19(4):62–63

DeLapp TD. Accidental hypothermia. Am J Nurs 1983 Jan; 83(1):63–67

Fraser I. Removing starch powder from gloves. Br Med J 1982 June 19; 284(6332):1835

Greenwood BS. Presurgery fears. Nursing '82 1982 July; 12(7):34–35

Highfield MF and Cason C. Spiritual needs of patients: Are they recognized? Cancer Nurs 1983 June; 6(3):187–192

How we can overcome barriers to preoperative interviews? (opinions) AORN J 1984 Apr; 33(5):931–942

Kochler JS. Perioperative nursing can be cost effective. AORN J 1980 Dec; 32(6):1068–1076

Mattia MA. Hazards in the hospital environment. The sterilants ethylene oxide and formaldehyde. Am J Nurs 1983 Feb; 83(2):240–243

McClurg E. Developing an effective patient teaching program. AORN J 1981 Sept; 34(3):474–487

Metheny N. Preoperative fluid balance assessment. AORN J 1981 Jan; 33(1):51–56

Parker CB. Endoscopic movies for patient teaching. AORN J 1981 Aug; 34(2):254–259

Perin GA. Promoting informed consent. Topics Clin Nurs 1981 Jan; 2(4):61–65

Phippen ML. Nursing assessment of preoperative anxiety. AORN J 1980 May; 31(6):1019–1026

Preoperative depilation. Lancet 1983 June 11; 1(8337):1311

Preston CA, Ivancevich JM and Matteson MT. Stress and the OR nurse. AORN J 1981 Mar; 33(4):662–671

Rice VH and Johnson JE. Preadmission self-instruction booklets, postadmission exercise performance, and teaching time. Nurs Res 1984 May–June; 33(3):147–151

Silva MC. Ethics, informed consent and the OR nurse. Today's OR Nurse 1982 Mar; 4(1):21–24, 62–63

Stotts N. Nutritional assessment before surgery. AORN J 1982 Feb; 35(2):207–214

Surgical sepsis—a delicate balance. AORN J 1982 March; 35(4):786–790

Intraoperative Nursing Care

Belkin NL. Evaluating surgical gowning, draping fabrics. AORN J 1981 Sept; 34(3):499–511

Can OR garb be stylish and functional? AORN J 1980 Sept; 32(3):423–444

Dineen P and Poncy M. Testing an externally powderless surgical glove. AORN J 1980 Oct; 32(4):633–645

Hurwitz M. Intraoperative ultrasound. AORN J 1983 Dec; 38(6):979–984

McDonald NE. Patient representatives come to the operating room. AORN J 1981 Aug; 34(2):332–340

McNameer C and McLean B. Nerve palsies: The preventable sort. Can Nurse 1980 July–Aug; 76:38–40

Recommended practices. OR attire. AORN J 1984 Mar; 39(4):710–720

Recommended practices. Sponge, sharps, and instrument counts. AORN J 1984 Mar; 39(4):699–706

Recommended practices. Surgical scrubs. AORN J 1984 May; 39(6):1080–1083

Anesthesia

Cleaning and processing anesthesia equipment. AORN J 1984 Jan; 39(1):92–98

Grinde JW, Grina R and Gellatly T. Pain management by epidural analgesia: The challenge for nursing. Heart & Lung 1984 Mar; 13(2):105–110

Manchikanti L, Kraus JW and Edds SP. Cimetidine and related drugs in anesthesia. Anesth Analg 1982 July; 61(7):595–608

Mattia MA. Anesthesia gases and methylmethacrylate. Am J Nurs 1983 Jan; 83(1):73–77

Recommended practices. Monitoring the patient receiving local anesthesia. AORN J 1984 May; 39(6):1080–1083

Reducing the risks from ethylene oxide. Amer J Nurs 1983 Dec; 83(12):1643

Rogers AG. What to expect from the most common analgesics. RN 1983 May; 46(5):44–46

Schwarz T. Prolonged regional analgesia

with morphine—epidurally. RN 1982 May; 45(5):32–35

Seamans DJ. Shortcuts to a more complete postanesthesia room transfer. Nursing '83 1983 Sept; 13(9):47–49

Surgical suite is no place for jewelry, watches, or nail polish. AORN J 1981 June; 33(7):1294–1295

Wetchler BV. Anesthesia for outpatient surgery. AORN J 1981 Aug; 34(2):282–296

Day Surgery

Ambulatory surgery. AORN J 1984 May; 39(6):1036–1040

Becker A. Same day surgery—a psychological approach. Today's OR Nurse 1983 July; 5(5):8–11, 43

Bradley DE and Boswick J. Ambulatory hand surgery. Today's OR Nurse 1983 July; 5(5):14–17, 46

Brandon J and Radoszewski. Ambulatory surgery. AORN J 1984 May; 39(6):1036–1040

Burns LA. Ambulatory surgery growing at a rapid pace. AORN J 1982 Feb; 35(2):260–270

Mauldin BC. Ambulatory surgery. AORN J 1984 Apr; 38(5):770–771

Spielman FJ. Ambulatory surgery. Med Times 1983 Sept; 3(9):62–66

Strategies for ambulatory surgery. AORN J 1984 June; 39(7):1245–1253

Postoperative Nursing Care

Ayres SM et al. Coping with postoperative circulatory collapse. Pat Care 1983 July 15; 17(13):199–254

Ayres SM et al. Rescuing the patient in cardiogenic shock. Pat Care 1983 July 15; 17(13):255–278

Bailey CJ et al. Epidural morphine infusion. AORN J 1984 May; 39(6):997–1008

Banyard SG. New drug-free technique cuts postoperative pain. RN 1982 Apr; 45(7):31–33

Barrows JJ. Shock demands drugs. Nursing '82 1982 Feb; 12(2):34–41

Bobb J. What happens when your patient goes into shock? RN 1984 Mar; 47(3):26–29

Bohen M. Herpetic whitlow. DCCN 1982 May–June; 1(3):172–173

Burns ED. Promoting healing of bone tissue. AORN J 1982 May; 35(6):1186–1191

Cardona VD. Trauma post-operative. RN 1982 Mar; 45(3):23–29

Danielson DA. Drug monitoring of surgical patients. JAMA 1982 Sept 24; 248(12):1482–1485

Darden ML. Blood loss determination. AORN J 1981 June; 33(7):1368–1380

DeCrosta T. MAST—not just for the emergency department anymore. Nurs Life 1983 July/Aug; 3(4):50–55

Defective spore strips cause misleading results. AORN J 1981 Aug; 34(2):245–246

Digregorio GJ and Fruncillo RJ. Antiemetics. Am Fam Physician 1982 July; 26(1):200–202

Drain CB. Managing postoperative

pain—it's a matter of sighs. Nursing '84 Aug; 84(8):52–55

Dufek SR and Finch JS. Radiant heat lamps in the recovery room. Am J Nurs 1983 Apr; 83(4):570

Elwyn DH, Kinney JM and Askonazi J. Energy expenditure in surgical patients. Surg Clin North Am 1981 June; 61(3):545–556

Ennis CE and Andrassy RJ. Nutritional management of the surgical patient. AORN J 1980 June; 31(6):1217–1224

Farr L. Alterations in circadian excretion of urinary variables and physiological indicators of stress following surgery. Nurs Res 1984 May–June; 33(3):140–146

Fernsebner B. A protocol for malignant hyperthermia. AORN J 1980 Apr; 31(8):814–818

Fraulini KE and Gorski DW. Don't let perioperative medications put you in a spin. Nursing '83 1983 Dec; 13(12):26–30

Fraulini KE and Murphy P. R.E.A.C.T. A new system for measuring postanesthesia recovery. Nursing '84 1984 Apr; 14(4):101–102

Friedman FB. PRN analgesics: Controlling the pain or controlling the patient? RN 1983 March; 46(3):67, 70, 72, 74, 76, 78

Fuchs P. Before and after surgery: Stay right on respiratory care. Nursing '83 1983 May; 13(5):47–50

Fuller BF. Hemostasis: A balanced system. AORN J 1981 Aug; 34(2):225–230

Getz PA and Blossom BM. Preventing contractures. RN 1982 Dec; 45(12):45–48

Gever LN. Dopamine. Nursing '83 1983 June; 13(6):30

Gever LN. Naloxone. Nursing '83 1983 May; 13(5):102

Greenburg AG. Operative mortality in general surgery. Am J Surg 1982 July; 144(1):22–28

Heaman DJ and Mattle LF. Adolescent emergence excitement. AORN J 1982 Feb; 35(2):230–242

Higgins PG. Improving estimation of blood loss. DCCN 1983 Mar/Apr; 2(2):120–123

Hudelson E. A 'just in case' guide to postanesthetic recovery for the non-recovery room nurse. RN 1982 Mar; 45(3):51–53

Lamb LS. Think you know septic shock? Nursing '82 1982 Jan; 12(1):34–43

Larson E. Hands: The healers and killers. Top Clin Nurs 1979 July; 1(2):59–65

Martin S. Fat embolism syndrome. DCCN 1983 Nov/Dec; 2(6):158–161

Mathewson M. A Homan's sign is an effective method of diagnosing thrombophlebitis in bedridden patients. Crit Care Nurse 1983 July/Aug; 3–4:64–65

McConnell EA. After surgery. Nursing '83 1983 Feb; 13(2):74–84

Meador B. Cardiogenic shock. RN 1982 July; 45(4):38–42

Merrill S. A teaching plan for positioning. AORN J 1982 Jan; 35(1):63–66

Moss G. Postoperative ileus is an avoidable complication. Surg Gyn Obstet 1979 Jan; 148(1):81–82

Mullen JL. Consequences of malnutrition in the surgical patient. Surg Clin North Am 1981 June; 61(3):465–487

Nicola M and DeChavio D. A transparent polyurethane membrane used as an IV dressing. NITA 1984 Mar–Apr; 7(2):139–142

Petlin A and Carolan JM. Halt hypovolemic shock. RN 1982 May; 45(5):36–42

Redmond C. Student nurses in the recovery room. AORN J 1981 Sept; 34(3):534–538

Robusto N. Advising patients on sex after surgery. AORN J 1980 July; 32(1):55–61

Rosen T and Mills JM. What does this nurse have in common with this patient? (pseudomonas) RN 1982 Jan; 45(1):45, 100

Schneider M. The recovery room as special procedures unit. AORN J 1981 Sept; 34(3):490–498

Siskind J. Handling hemorrhage wisely. Nursing '84 1984 Jan; 14(1):34–41

Stillwell SB. Importance of visiting needs as perceived by family members of patients in the intensive care unit. Heart & Lung 1984 May; 13(3):238–242

Sumner SM and Lewandowski V. Guidelines for using artificial breathing devices. Nursing '83 1983 Oct; 13(10):54–57

Swedberg J, Driggers D and Johnson R. Hemorrhagic shock. Am Fam Physician 1983 July; 28(1):173–177

Taylor AG et al. How effective is TENS for acute pain? Am J Nurs 1983 Aug; 83(8):1171–1174

Voshall B. The effects of preoperative teaching on postoperative pain. Top Clin Nurs 1980 Apr; 2(1):39–43

Warmbrod LLS. Supporting families of critically ill patients. Crit Care Nurse 1983 Sept/Oct; 3(5):49–52

Wells N. The effect of relaxation on postoperative muscle tension and pain. Nurs Res 1982 July/Aug; 31(4):236–238

Williams WW. CDC Guidelines for the prevention and control of nosocomial infections: Guidelines for infection control in hospital personnel. Am J Infect Control 1984 Feb; 12(1):43

Zumer MM. Effects of information on postsurgical coping. Nurs Res 1983 Sept–Oct; 32(5):282–287

Infusions and Fluid Balance
Articles

Acevedo ML. Electronic flow control. NITA 1983 Mar–Apr; 6(2):105–106

Boyle P. Calculating IV flow rates. Nursing '83 1983 July; 13(7):70–71

Brendel V. Current concepts in the care of central line catheters. NITA 1983 July–Aug; 6(4):272–274

Brown EA. Patient emotional response to intravenous therapy. NITA 1982 Nov–Dec; 6(5):374

Caman W (letter) Positioning for air embolism. Nursing '83 1983 Nov; 13(11):66

Carlquist K. Understanding the psychological needs of the patient on IV therapy: A stress reducing approach. NITA 1981 Sept–Oct; 5(1):368–370

Computing IV flow rate. Nursing '81 1981 Jan; 11(1):89–92

Courtemanche JB. Imagery enhance venipuncture. NITA 1984 Jan–Feb; 7(1):36

Crowley M and Baker M. Preparing nurses for Hickman catheter care: A self-learning module. Onc Nurs Forum 1980 Fall; 7(4):17–19

DiGiacinto E. Behavioral management in IV therapy. NITA 1982 July–Aug; 5(4):280–281

Dobson J. IV tube changing—24 or 48 hours? NITA 1981 Sept–Oct; 5(1):349–350

Dolby BA. Caution: Abused veins, handle with care. NITA 1983 Mar–Apr; 6(2):95–96

Engram B. Computing IV flow rates. Nursing '81 1981 Jan; 11(1):89–92

Erickson R. Tube talk; principles of fluid flow in tubes. Nursing '82 1982 July; 12(7):54–62

Faehnrich J. Extravasation. NITA 1984 Jan–Feb; 7(1):49–52

Freeman P and Boyer JK. How to get the most out of Op-site. RN 1982 Jan; 45(1):36–39

Friedman FB. KVO's: How fast is fast enough? RN 1982 Sept; 45(9):69, 73–74

Garner JS. Nosocomial infections: Risks and preventive measures for IV nurses. NITA 1982 July–Aug; 5(4):250–254

Gever LN. Intravenous lipids. Nursing '81 1981 Nov; 11(11):160–161

Gong H, Jr., Finnerty MA and Robinson LE. Nursing techniques in preparing and administering intravenous admixtures. NITA 1982 Mar–Apr; 5(2):132–135

Gorgone PA. Multiple intravenous solutions delivered via the manifold system. NITA 1983 Sept–Oct; 6(5):369–371

Grabbe M. Clinical product evaluation and proposal justification in product selection. NITA 1983 July–Aug; 6(4):268–271

Guarriello DL. Intravenous therapy and the law. NITA 1983 July–Aug; 6(4):278–281

Haessler RM. Transparent IV dressings vs traditional dressings. NITA 1983 May–June; 6(3):169–170

Hill B. Helpful hints on how to read a plastic IV container. Can Nurse 1981 Sept; 77(8):43

Intravenous admixtures. Am J Nurs 1981 Mar; 81(3):574–575

Introduction to CDC's guidelines for

prevention of intravascular infections. NITA 1982 Jan–Feb; 5(1):39–50

IV taping technique. Am J Nurs 1981 Feb; 81(2):349

Jemison-Smith P and Thrupp LD. Phlebitis, infections, and filtration. NITA 1982 Sept–Oct; 5(5):328–335

Johnston-Early A, Cohen MH and White KS. Venipuncture and problem veins. Am J Nurs 1981 Sept; 81(9):1636–1640

Jones BC, Briggs CD and Norton DA. This new type IV dressing can save you time. Nursing '82 1982; 12(12):70–73

Keithley JK and Fraulina KE. What's behind that IV line? Nursing '82 1982 Mar; 12(3):33–42

Koszuta LE. Choosing the right control device for your patient. Nursing '84 1984 Mar; 14(3):55–56

Labry J. Infusion monitoring devices. NITA 1981 Mar–Apr; 5(1):366–367

Lane G and Peirce AG. When persistence pays off. Nursing '82 1982 Jan; 12(1):44–47

Larkin M. Home intravenous care. NITA 1984 Jan–Feb; 7(1):10–11

Levitt DZ. Use of the heparin lock on an outpatient basis. Can Nurs 1981 Apr; 4(2):115–119

MacLaughlin JE. Intravenous containers—variability in measurement. Can Nurs 1981 Sept; 77(8):29–30

Metheny NA. The interstitial (third-space) phenomenon. NITA 1983 July–Aug; 6(4):251–254

Millan DA. Tips for improving your venipuncture techniques. Nursing '83 1983 Aug; 13(8):40–43

Moore RA and Terry BE. Nafcillin necrosis. NITA 1984 Jan–Feb; 7(1):61–62

Nawrocki HR. Administering IV bolus injections. Nursing '81 1981 Nov; 11(11):124–130

Parent B. In-line IV filters. Nursing '81 1981 Aug; 11(8):58–60

Pelletier GM. Responding to a need: Home intravenous therapy. NITA 1982 Nov–Dec; 6(5):383–384

Peterson PJ and Freeman PT. Use of a transparent polyurethane dressing for peripheral intravenous catheter care. NITA 1982 Nov–Dec; 6(5):387–390

Rapp RP et al. Effects of electronic infusion control on the efficacy, complications and cost of IV therapy. Hosp Forum 1979 Nov; 14(11):975–982

Rosenthal KA. Converting micrograms/kilograms/minute to microdrops. DCCN 1982 Nov–Dec; 1(6):326

Santolla A and Weckel C. A new closed system for arterial lines. RN 1983 June; 46(6):49–52

Shinozaki T et al. Bacterial contamination of arterial lines. JAMA 1983 Jan 14; 249(2):223–225

Steel J. Too fast or too slow—the erratic IV. Am J Nurs 1983 June; 83(6):898–901

Stiklorius C. A safe approach to IV antibiotics. RN 1981 Apr; 44(4):37–39

Terry J. Home care utilizing silastic catheters. NITA 1983 Sept–Oct; 6(5):348–350

Treating air emboli. Am J Nurs 1982 Apr; 82(4):554

Weinstein S. Intravenous therapy within the scope of home health services. NITA 1984 Jan–Feb; 7(1):39–41

Williams DN et al. Infusion thrombophlebitis and infiltration associated with intravenous cannulae. NITA 1982 Nov–Dec; 6(5):379–382

Zenowich D. IV flow control. NITA 1984 Jan–Feb; 7(1):21–25

Fluids and Electrolytes

Carveth ML et al. Acid–base assessment with peripheral venous blood. Heart & Lung 1984 Jan; 13(1):48–54

Flomenbaum N. Acid–base disturbances. Emerg Med 1980 Oct 15; 12(17):24–45

Folk-Lighty M. Fluid imbalance. Nursing '84 1984; 14(2):34–41

Gammon SS. Respiratory acidosis. Nursing '82 1982 Aug; 12(8):65

Gever LN. Administering potassium chloride supplements. Nursing '81 1981 Oct; 11(10):32

Glass LB and Jenkins CA. The ups and downs of serum pH. Nursing '83 1983 Sept; 13(9):34–41

Mandell HN. Gases and lytes without anguish. Postgrad Med 1981 Feb; 69(2):67–74

Quinlan M. Would you recognize this dangerous electrolyte imbalance? RN 1983 Mar; 46(3):51–55

Quinlan M. Solving the mysteries of calcium imbalance: An action guide. RN 1982 Nov; 45(11):50–54

Rice V. Magnesium, calcium, and phosphate imbalances; their clinical significance. Crit Care Nurse 1983 May–June; 3(3):90–112

Shamsi S and De Monaco HJ. Use of hydrochloric acid in metabolic alkalosis. NITA 1982 Mar–Apr; 5(2):136–137

When potassium therapy is needed. Pat Care 1982 Sept 30; 16(16):63–94

Wright TR and Murray M. Potassium problems: Which patient is in danger? RN 1982 June; 45(6):56–61

Intravenous Therapy Standards

CDC's Guidelines for prevention of intravascular infections. NITA 1982 Jan–Feb; 5(1):39–50

Chrystal C. Making the NITA standards work for you. NITA 1983 Jan–Feb; 6(1):19–20

Chrystal C. Making the NITA standards work for you. NITA 1983 Mar–Apr; 6(2):87–92

Chrystal C. Making the NITA standards work for you. NITA 1983 May–June; 6(3):188–190

Larkin M. NITA's I.V. Standards/CDC's I.V. guidelines. NITA 1982 Jan–Feb; 5(1):8–11

The National Intravenous Therapy Association, Inc. Outline for Standards. NITA 1982 Jan–Feb; 5(1):19–24

The National Intravenous Therapy Association, Inc. Standards—Recommendations of Practice. NITA 1982 Jan–Feb; 5(1):24–34

The National Intravenous Therapy Association's Intravenous Nursing Standards of Practice. Home I.V. Therapy. NITA 1984 Mar–Apr; 7(2):93

Wound Care—Infection

Articles

Alexander J et al. The influence of hair-removal methods on wound infections. Arch Surg 1983 March; 118:347–352

Allen JR. Wound infection. Today's OR Nurse. 1983 Sept; 6(9):11–17

Altemeier WA. Infection control in the operating room and perioperative areas, pp. 63–71 *in* Roderick MA. Infection Control in Critical Care. Rockville, MD, Aspen Systems, 1983

Baron MC. The skin and wound healing. Top Clin Nurs 1983 July; 5(2):11–22

Bartley J and Chamberlin DA. The barriers to infection. Today's OR Nurse 1983 Sept; 6(9):26–34

Bauman B. Update your technique for changing dressings dry to dry. Nursing '82 1982 Jan; 12(1):64–67

Bauman B. Update your technique for changing dressings wet to dry. Nursing '82 1982 Feb; 12(2):68–71

Bremer C. Promoting health of trauma wounds. AORN J 1982 May; 35(6):1150–1170

Fernandez A and Finley JM. Wound healing. Postgrad Med 1983 Oct; 74(4):311–317

Frogge MH. Promoting wound healing in the irradiated patient. AORN J 1982 May; 35(6):1088–1093

Fry DE and Polk HC Jr. Infection in the surgical patient: Prevention and treatment. Drug Ther 1982 Aug; 82(8):19–28

Gallucci BB and Reheis CE. Infection, nutrition and the compromised patients. Top Clin Nurs 1979 July; 1(2):23–33

Garner JS, Dixon RE and Aber RC. Epidemic infections in surgical patients. AORN J 1981 Oct; 34(4):700–724

Georgiade GS. Wound contamination. Postgrad Med 1983 Mar; 73(3):247–254

Glickman R and DeTorres OH. Antibiotic prescribing. Postgrad Med 1982 July; 72(1):223–230

Groszek DM. Promoting wound healing in the obese patient. AORN J 1982 May; 35(6):1132–1138

Humphreys PT and Barthel CS. Power spray cleaning for those hard-to-clean wounds. Nursing '83 1983 Apr; 13(4):42–43

Jackson MM and Lynch P. Infection control—too much or too little? Am J Nurs 1984 Feb; 84(2):208–211

Keithley JK. Wound healing in malnourished patients. AORN J 1982 May; 35(6):1094–1099

Kottra CJ. Wound healing in the immunosuppressed host. AORN J 1982 May; 35(6):1142–1148

Lutz D, Schimeneck G and Troiani Y. A new use for hollihesive. RN 1983 March; 46(3):47–49

Lyons RJ. Promoting healing of skin flaps and grafts. AORN J 1982 May; 35(6):1174–1183

Narcotic and opioid analgesics. Nursing '83 1983 Oct; 13(10):64–66

Nichols RL. Postoperative wound infection. N Engl J Med 1982 Dec 30; 307(27):1701–1702

Schumann D. The nature of wound healing. AORN J 1982 May; 35(6): 1068–1077

Stotts NA. The most effective method of wound irrigation. Focus on Critical Care 1983 Oct; 10(5):45–48

Taylor DL. Wound healing. Nursing '83 1983 May; 13(5):44–45

Transparent wound dressings. Med Lett 1983 Nov 11; 25(648):103–104

Westaby S. Wound care. Nurs Times 1982 No. 11, July 21; 78:41–44; No. 12. Aug 18; 78:45–48, No. 13. Sept 22; 78:49–52

Wineland MD. Invasive procedures and infection control. Top Clin Nurs 1979 July; 1(2):53–57

Winters B. Promoting wound healing in the diabetic patient. AORN J 1982 May; 35(6):1083–1087

Yordan EL Jr and Bernhard LA. The surgeon's role in wound healing. AORN J 1982 May; 35(6):1078–1082

Conditions of the Respiratory Tract

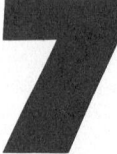

1: Conditions of the Nose and Throat

Problems of the Nose

Rhinitis

Rhinitis is an inflammation of the mucous membrane of the nose.

Clinical Manifestations

1. From allergic reaction, in infection (coryza), or early stages of viral infection

2. Congested and swollen mucous membranes; when persistent → "chronic catarrh"
3. Chronic rhinitis → abnormally large amounts of connective tissue → spurs, polyps, and hypertrophies on nasal septum → atrophy of mucous membrane and cartilage → abundant foul-smelling exudate (ozena)

▶ **NURSING ALERT:** Instruct patient as follows:
1. Do not blow nose too frequently or too hard; doing so may cause infection to spread, sinuses to become infected, and an eardrum to be perforated.
2. Blow through both nostrils at the same time to equalize pressure.

Treatment

1. Fundamental therapy is antihistamine administration (e.g., chlorpheniramine maleate). This may be supplemented with a decongestant, such as pseudo-ephedrine hydrochloride.
2. Also see Allergic Rhinitis, p. 666, Allergy Problems.

Nasal Obstruction

Causes

1. Deflected septum
2. Hypertrophy of turbinate bones
3. Polyps
4. Tumors
5. Common cold
6. Foreign bodies
7. Fractures
8. Allergic rhinitis
9. Adenoid hypertrophy

Related Problems

1. Chronic infection of nose, such as nasopharyngitis
2. Sinusitis, which may include pain in sinus regions
3. Recurrent otitis media

Primary Care Nurse as a Case Finder

School and community nurses particularly will be able to detect children with nasal obstruction; these should be referred to the physician.

Treatment

1. Nasal obstruction should be removed.
2. Measures employed to curb chronic infection:
    a. Nasal allergy corrected
    b. Nasal sinuses drained (may be an operating room procedure)
    c. Nasal polyps clipped
    d. Hypertrophied turbinates shrunk with astringent solutions
    e. Hypertrophied adenoids removed
    f. Submucous resection or nasal septal reconstruction may be performed to remove deflected bone and cartilage (see following on SMR and NSR)

Submucous Resection (SMR) or Nasal Septal Reconstruction (NSR) Fracture of the Nose

Submucous resection of the septum is an operation in which cartilaginous and/or osseous portions of the septum that lie between the flaps of the mucous membrane and perichondrium are removed or straightened—to establish an adequate partition between the right and left nasal cavities in order to provide a clear nasal airway.

Nasal septal reconstruction involves resection or removal of cartilaginous (or bony septum) followed by reconstruction of all parts of the septum that may produce nasal airway obstruction.

Nasal fracture results from direct trauma, for example, a blow inflicted by an object (ball or fist) or an injury sustained in an automobile collision.

Assessment

Clinical Manifestations

1. Observe for nasal obstruction and swelling → impaired breathing or complete obstruction.
2. Determine whether there is nasal displacement → cosmetic deformity.
3. Note bleeding—not only external bleeding, but also any trickling of blood into the oropharynx.
4. In the event of a fracture of the nose, assess general condition of the patient for related injuries to head and face; these may take priority over a nasal injury as far as treatment is concerned.

Patient Problems/Nursing Diagnoses

1. Ineffective airway clearance related to deviated nasal cartilage, osseous or cartilaginous blockage, or edema.
2. Pain related to injury or obstruction.
3. Altered sense of smell related to nasal obstruction.
4. Knowledge deficit of surgical procedure and plan of care.

Planning and Implementation

Nursing Interventions

A. Relief of Nasal Obstruction and Concomitant Problems of Pain, Headache, Bleeding, and Recurrent Rhinitis

1. Control bleeding.
    a. Raise head of bed to promote drainage—to make the patient more comfortable and to lessen edema.
    b. Apply cold compresses as soon as possible.
    c. Place patient in a comfortable position with head somewhat elevated to control bleeding; if in sitting position, the patient might faint during manipulation of nasal fracture.
2. Administer medication for comfort.
    Maintain patient comfort by administering meperidine or morphine as prescribed, inasmuch as there is a fair amount of postoperative discomfort for several hours.
3. With fracture, prepare for reduction.
    The physician will determine whether fracture reduction can be maneuvered without anesthesia; often, pressure can be exerted on the convex side of the nose and the bones and septum manipulated into position.

B. Pre- and Postoperative Care

1. Preoperative
    a. Describe what is to happen; explain that if local anesthesia is used, pain will be minimal; pressure sensation in the nasal area may be felt during surgery.
    b. Indicate that ecchymosis (facial or periorbital) may be present postoperatively but that it will gradually subside.

c. Project that there is a good possibility of nasal packing being in place for 24–36 hours.

2. Postoperative
   a. Promote comfort and prevent complications.
   b. Reassure the patient about the sucking sound that will be experienced upon swallowing; the nasal packing prevents air from moving through the nose and a partial vacuum is created in the throat during swallowing.
   c. Change the gauze pad under the nose as it becomes soaked with blood; this is usually done 2 or 3 times the first day. Each time there should be less blood.
   d. Notify the surgeon if bleeding increases rather than decreases.
   e. Apply cold compresses or ice packs for first 24 hours—to lessen edema and discoloration and to promote comfort.
   f. Instruct the patient not to blow his nose but to blot secretions with tissue.
   g. Administer frequent mouth care, since the patient is forced to breathe through the mouth.
   h. Administer sedative/antibiotics as prescribed to promote comfort.
   i. Report excessive bleeding; return for follow-up visit.

Evaluation
Expected Outcomes

1. Is free of edema and nasal obstruction which permits easier breathing; tests both sides by pressing one nostril with finger
2. Reports no pain or discomfort in nasal area
3. Requires no medications for nasal problem
4. Relates awareness that excessive bleeding is to be reported

---

Specific Infections of the Upper Respiratory Tract

General Considerations
A. Predisposing Conditions

Nasal septum and turbinate pathology, allergy, emotional problems

B. Preventive Health Measures

1. Intended to support body defenses and reduce susceptibility to infection.
2. Patient should set up a conscientious health regimen—adequate exercise, plenty of sleep, nutritious diet, relaxing hobbies.
   a. Avoid chilling, particularly of the feet, since this lowers resistance.
   b. Employ humidifying measures indoors during winter months.
   c. Avoid emotionally upsetting experiences.
   d. Minimize indulgence in alcohol, smoking, drugs.
   e. Avoid inhaling irritating substances such as hair spray or other sprays, dust, chemicals, smoke, etc.

Adenoviral Infections
Types
A. Acute Respiratory Disease (ARD)

Symptoms
    Cold
    Sore throat
    Headache
    Temperature elevation
    Malaise

B. Pharyngoconjunctival Fever

1. Duration—1 to 10 days
2. Symptoms (common in summer in children who swim in pools)
    Fever
    Sore throat
    Cold
    Large and tender cervical lymph nodes
    Headache
    Hoarseness
    Acute conjunctivitis
    Malaise

C. Rhinoviral Infections

Examples: Common cold, croup, and bronchitis, which may lead to bronchopneumonia.

Treatment

1. Symptomatic
2. No specific antimicrobial or chemotherapy

Herpes Simplex Infection

This infection produces common herpes labialis (fever blisters, cold sores, cankers).

Clinical Manifestations

1. Small vesicles, single or in groups, located on lips, tongue, cheeks, or pharynx.
2. Sore ruptures and becomes shallow ulcer covered with gray membrane.
3. Signs associated with other febrile conditions; pneumococcus pneumonia, meningococcal meningitis, malaise.
4. Virus remains latent in cells of lips or nose and is activated by febrile illnesses.

Treatment

1. Chemotherapy and antimicrobials appear to be of no value.
2. Analgesics and perhaps codeine are helpful in relieving pain.
3. Spirits of nitre or Campho-Phenique applied locally is helpful in drying the lesion.

Sinusitis

Sinusitis is an inflammation of the sinuses. (Sinuses are often involved in upper respiratory tract infections.) Recovery is based on the condition that the nasal passage be clear. If passage is obstructed (blocked by deviated septum, polyps, spurs, enlarged turbinates) sinusitis may become chronic.

Acute Sinusitis

Clinical Manifestations

1. Pain
   a. Frontal headache—related to frontal sinusitis
   b. In and about eyes—related to ethmoidal sinusitis
   c. Lateral to nose, upper teeth—related to maxillary sinusitis
   d. Occipital headache—related to sphenoidal sinusitis
2. Nasal congestion and discharge may or may not be present
3. Mild fever; anosmia
4. Acute suppurative infection
   If frontal sinus involved, this can be serious because it may rupture posteriorly and lead to brain abscess.
5. Nasal mucosa may be red and edematous

Medical and Nursing Interventions

1. Bed rest; analgesics for pain; hot compresses to midface and forehead
2. Nonsurgical drainage of sinuses
   a. Instill vasoconstrictor: Neo-Synephrine ¼% spray or drops.
   b. Use penicillin to speed recovery and lessen possibility of complications.
   c. Administer an antihistaminic.

Chronic Sinusitis

Chronic sinusitis is a suppurative inflammation of the sinuses with chronic irreversible change in the mucosa and sinus bony area.

Clinical Manifestations

1. Persistent nasal obstruction; purulent nasal discharge
2. Cough—produced by constant dripping of discharge back into nasopharynx
3. Headache—more noticeable in the morning

Medical and Nursing Interventions

1. Administration of vasoconstricting drugs to promote drainage
   Recognize danger of prolonged use of nasal decongestants. It may lead to *rhinitis medicamentosa,* which is a recurring cycle of: nasal congestion → use of decongestants → relief → leading to nasal congestion → more decongestants, etc.
2. Repair of structural deformities
   a. Polyps excised or cauterized
   b. Deviated septum removed
3. Draining of sinuses
   a. Frontal—incision through eyebrow

b. Maxillary—*Caldwell-Luc operation,* in which the incision is made along the upper gum line above canine teeth under the upper lip. An opening is made into the anterior wall of the sinus to permit stripping out of infected contents. A "window" is created between maxillary sinus and nose.
   (1) Postoperative nursing management is similar to that for a patient who has had a submucous resection (see p. 129).
   (2) Be prepared to support the patient and assist the physician when sinus packing is withdrawn through nose.
      (a) Drape patient, who is in a sitting position in bed.
      (b) Place emesis basin under nasal area.
      (c) Observe for bleeding while instructing patient to keep his eyes closed if he appears squeamish.
   (3) Administer mouth care carefully; limit this to mouth rinses at first; when a toothbrush is used it should be of the soft type. Care is taken not to injure the incision area.
   (4) Apply cold compresses over lip to help in reducing edema.
   (5) Inform patient that swelling and a "black eye" are often in evidence for a week or two; the latter is due to extravasation of blood into soft tissues under the eye.
   (6) Offer liquid diet for the first few days and then progress to soft diet.

Health Education

1. Advise patient that numbness in the operative area may be present for several weeks or months.
2. Instruct patient not to blow his nose for at least 2 weeks after packing has been removed to avoid forcing nasal secretions back into the maxillary sinus.
3. Prevent irritation along incision line for several weeks; upper dentures should not be worn, since they could injure the operative area.

Streptococcal Sore Throat

Clinical Manifestations

1. Rapid onset of sore throat, chills, temperature above 38.3°C. (101°F.), headache, general malaise.
2. Children may have (in addition to the above) acute abdominal pain, nausea, perhaps repeated vomiting.
3. Red pharynx, enlarged tonsils and tonsillar nodes below angle of the mandible, edematous uvula.
4. Mouth breathing, halitosis, annoying tickling cough.
5. Tonsils and pharynx may be covered with an exudate.
6. Throat pain may prevent swallowing.
7. Patient may present with a flushed face and leukocyte count over 12,000.

Diagnostic Evaluation

1. Physical examination—enlarged inflamed tonsils
2. Throat culture (see Guidelines: Obtaining a Throat Culture, p. 132)

Treatment

Goal:
Eliminate infection, reduce fever, and avoid complications

Early intervention with chemotherapeutic agents is important to prevent serious complications such as acute rheumatic fever, acute glomerulonephritis.
1. Initiate penicillin therapy for 24 hours.
2. If culture is positive in 24 hours for group A *hemolytic Streptococci,* continue treatment for 10 days.
3. If culture is negative and if there is no significant clinical improvement in the patient, discontinue penicillin.
4. If culture is negative and patient has improved clinically, continue penicillin for 10 days. (This means penicillin is effective; discontinuing penicillin too soon may cause a return of infection.)
5. If throat culture shows other microbial infection, utilize specific antimicrobial agent.

Note: See also page 316 for role of streptococcal infection in rheumatic heart disease—treatment and nursing management, pages 316–317.

6. If the patient is hypersensitive to penicillin, he may be treated with erythromycin.

Guidelines: Obtaining a Throat Culture

Purpose   To determine the nature of microbial throat infection, secretion or material from the mucous surface of the throat may be transferred to a medium that encourages the growth of microorganisms. This growth is subsequently studied in the laboratory.

Equipment

  Tongue blade
  Sterile cotton or Dacron swab
  Blood agar plate or required culture medium
  Adequate light source

Procedure
(Fig. 7-1)

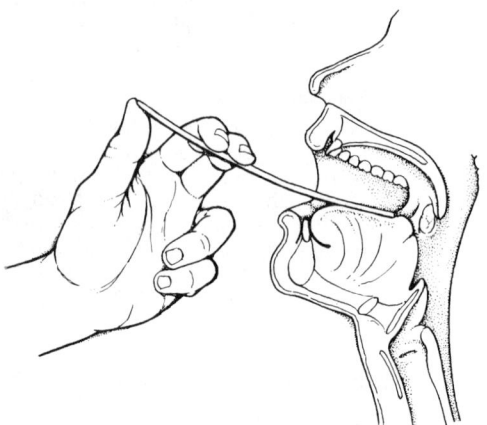

A. Grasp the tongue blade so that the thumb pushes the end upward (as a fulcrum) while the fingers push the middle section downward.

B. Vigorously rub a cotton or dacron swab over each tonsillar area and posterior pharynx.

Labels: Uvula, Vallate papillae, Swab, Palatine tonsil, Fungiform papillae

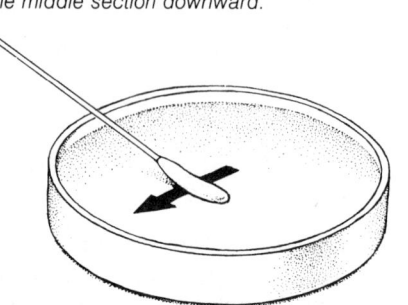

C. Streak the swab on a blood agar plate and place in an incubator for 24 hours. Plate can then be read grossly.

Figure 7-1. Throat culture.

Procedure
(Cont.)

Nursing Action	Rationale/Amplification
1. Inform the patient of the need for a throat culture.	1. When the patient is cooperative, procedure is facilitated and is more acceptable to him.
2. Place the patient in a comfortable sitting or lying position; instruct him to tilt the head backward.	
3. Have patient open his mouth wide; direct maximum lighting toward back of throat.	3. A good light source illuminates back of throat and assists nurse in identifying structures.
4. Depress the tongue as shown in Fig. 7-1A. (Some patients object to the use of a tongue blade; if such a patient can relax his tongue while panting, this may be satisfactory.)	4. This permits access of the swab to the tonsillar area and posterior pharynx. (The tongue blade may stimulate the gag reflex.)
5. Vigorously swab the involved tonsillar area and posterior pharynx with the cotton or Dacron swab (Fig. 7-1B).	5. *Avoid* swabbing the tongue. Use aseptic technique in handling swab.
6. Immediately streak the swab on the plate or follow directions of the laboratory for transport medium (Fig. 7-1C).	6. In some instances, it may be required to submit the swab; in this instance, swab must not be allowed to dry, but should be brought to the laboratory in transporter-handling medium.
7. All specimens are to be labeled—include patient's name and unit, nature and source of specimen, date.	7. This is recorded on label attached to specimen and also on patient's chart.
8. Patient is permitted to resume activity.	

Cancer of the Larynx

Incidence
1. Occurs in men over 50; ratio of men to women is 10:1.
2. Greater predisposition to laryngeal cancer in some families and in people who smoke heavily or use their voices excessively.
3. In North America, about ⅔ of carcinomas of the larynx arise in the glottis, almost ⅓ arise in the supraglottic region, and about 3% in the subglottic region of the larynx.

Clinical Expectations
1. When treated early, the likelihood of cure is great.
2. When limited to the vocal cords (intrinsic), spread is slow because of lessened blood supply.
3. When cancer involves the epiglottis (extrinsic), cancer spreads more rapidly because of abundant supply of blood and lymph and soon involves the lymph nodes of the neck.

Treatment
Goal:
Provide relief of symptoms by various treatment modalities (endoscopic removal of small tumor, radiation, surgery), the extensiveness of which is determined by the nature of the malignancy.

A. Endoscopic Removal of Early Malignancy
1. By means of an endoscope, the earliest cancer, or carcinoma in situ, is removed without an incision.
2. This does not affect the voice, and there are usually no other problems.
3. Close supervision is required (through follow-up visits to the physician).

B. Radiation—treatment is effective in controlling early cancers that are not deeply invasive and are without nodal metastasis.
1. The greater the extent of malignancy, the more likely radiation therapy will be used in conjunction with surgery.
2. Surgeons and radiologists vary as to the role of radiation therapy pre- and postoperatively; the quality of life is a strong consideration.

C. Surgery—varies with extensiveness of invasion.
1. Partial laryngectomy—removal of small lesion on true cord, along with a substantial margin of healthy tissue.
2. Supraglottic laryngectomy—removal of hyoid bone, epiglottis, and false vocal cords; tracheostomy may be done to maintain adequate airway; radical neck dissection may be done.
3. Hemilaryngectomy—removal of one true vocal cord, false cord, one half of thyroid cartilage, arytenoid cartilage.
4. Total laryngectomy—removal of entire larynx (epiglottis, false or true cords, cricoid cartilage, hyoid bone, 2 or 3 tracheal rings are usually removed when there is extrinsic cancer of the larynx [extension beyond the vocal cords]). A radical neck dissection may also be done because of metastasis to cervical lymph nodes.
5. Total laryngectomy with laryngoplasty—voice rehabilitation may be attempted through the *Asai operation.*
   a. A dermal tube is made from the upper end of the trachea into the hypopharynx.
   b. The tracheostomy opening is closed off with a finger.
   c. Then the patient expires air up the dermal tube into the pharyngeal cavity.
   d. The sound produced is transformed into almost normal speech.
6. Palliative therapy—For even more advanced cancer, palliative therapy may be initiated in the form of intra-arterial infusion with chemotherapeutic agents, followed by deep roentgen ray therapy (see p. 918).
7. Variations utilizing implants—specific with surgeon.

Assessment
Clinical Manifestations

1. Hoarseness or voice change is usually the earliest sign: this symptom is apparent because the vocal cords are inhibited from approximating (coming close together) by the diseased tissue.
2. A feeling that there is a lump in the throat, dyspnea, dysphagia.
3. Pain in laryngeal prominence (Adam's apple), enlarged cervical nodes, cough.
4. Persistent sore throat (6 weeks).

Diagnostic Evaluation

1. Laryngoscopy, either indirect (mirror) or direct (using a laryngoscope), can be effective for early diagnosis.
2. Biopsy under local or general anesthesia.
   a. Toluidine blue contrast medium may be used to stain the larynx and pinpoint biopsy site (cancer cells have an affinity for the contrast medium).
3. Other diagnostic modalities are roentgenographic, such as:
   (a) Anesthetizing larynx with cocaine and injecting Lipiodal for roentgenogram visualization
   (b) Tomography
   (c) Barium esophagogram

Patient Problems/Nursing Diagnoses

For patient with total laryngectomy
1. Anxiety related to diagnosis of cancer
2. Impaired verbal communication related to disrupted laryngeal function and inability to speak
3. Disturbance in self-concept related to communication problems and physical impact of laryngectomy
4. Knowledge deficit of treatment modalities and available rehabilitation measures

Planning and Implementation
Nursing Interventions

A. **Psychosocial Preparation of the Patient for a Total Laryngectomy**

1. Collaborate with the physician in preparing the patient; amplify and interpret what the surgeon has already told the patient.
2. Inform him that he will breathe through an opening made in his neck.
3. Apprise him of the fact that his speech will be altered by surgery.
4. Expect reactions of depression, since the above information has a direct effect on his future.
5. Arrange for him to be visited by a laryngectomee (one who has had his larynx removed either totally or partially); such a person is able to transmit hope and encouragement to the patient.
6. Inform him of the services available for speech rehabilitation. Many patients make remarkable adjustments and pursue normal activities.
7. Practice a means of communication that is comfortable for the patient (i.e., sign language, pictures, word cards, pad and pencil).

B. **Preoperative Nursing Management**

1. Maintain good mouth hygiene; suggest that male patient shave beard to allow for easier and safer postoperative care.
2. Teach what patient is to expect postoperatively:

   a. Tracheostomy, suctioning, feeding methods, monitoring devices
   b. Nature of recovery room experience
3. Administer prescribed analgesics and antibiotics.

C. **Postoperative Nursing Management**

1. Laryngectomy management
   The laryngectomy tube is shorter but thicker than the tracheostomy tube. Care is similar to that for a tracheostomized patient (see p. 218).
2. Monitor vital signs and change patient's position to facilitate breathing as he emerges from anesthesia.
3. Maintain patent airway by suctioning secretions as they accumulate.
4. Supply humidification to liquefy thick secretions.
5. Clean tracheostomy cannula as required; have available a sterile tracheostomy set.
6. Watch for evidence of subcutaneous emphysema (occurs occasionally).
7. Reassure the patient that someone is always near to help; keep call bell within his reach.
8. Administer food and fluids for the first 48 hours by nasogastric tube or intravenously because of the possibility of swallowing difficulty if given by mouth.
9. Gradually offer fluid by mouth as tolerated.
10. The patient's diet is supplemented with vitamins and infusions to maintain proper fluid, electrolyte, and nutritional balance.

    Note: Some physicians do not employ a nasogastric tube postoperatively but begin early oral feedings.

11. Usually a laryngectomy tube is worn for a week or 10 days until the stoma heals. Thereafter, observe the stoma area for crusting; crust can be softened and removed with a thin coating of petrolatum, antimicrobial ointment, and perhaps moist gauze over the opening; proper room humidification is helpful.
    a. Aseptic technique is practiced to avoid tracheal and respiratory infection.
    b. If there is danger of incisional contamination, antimicrobial therapy may be prescribed.

D. **Promotion of Self-Care Activities**

1. Explain all procedures to allay any anxieties.
2. Encourage slow, gradual resumption of vocal sounds; have the patient begin with a whisper until healing is complete, and then add more substantial sounds. He will have to occlude his tracheostomy tube to speak.
3. Demonstrate procedure for cleaning stoma and changing tube and draw strings; encourage the patient's questions and participation.
4. Provide communication aids as necessary.
5. Maintain nutritional and fluid levels as required; cater to the patient's personal likes and provide supplemental feedings if necessary.

E. **Rehabilitation, Discharge Planning, and Health Education**

1. Speech rehabilitation
   a. Reassure the patient that speech rehabilitation can be very successful. Laryngeal or esophageal speech or one of the artificial larynxes can be used (Fig. 7-2).
   b. Through the combined efforts of the surgeon, nurse, patient, family, other persons who have had laryngectomies, and a speech therapist, a plan of speech rehabilitation is initiated.

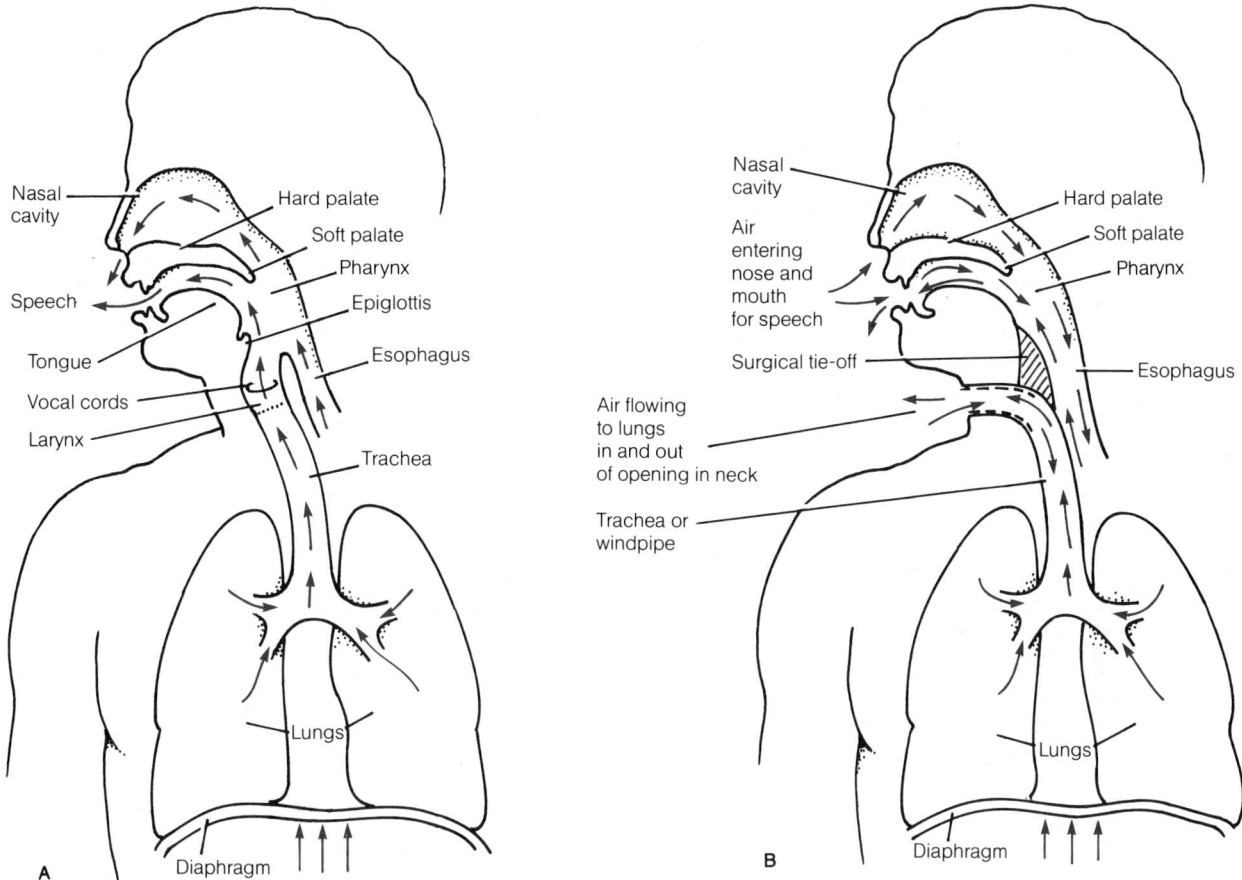

Figure 7-2. *(A)* Normal physiology of respiration and speech—note arrows indicating flow of air. *(B)* This diagram illustrates the effect of a laryngectomy on the physiology of respiration and speech—again note air-flow patterns. *(Adapted from American Cancer Society)*

c. Postlaryngectomy patients utilize the technique of taking in a bolus of air as an energy source and then, by compression of the lips, simulating sounds by "plosive" speech. Esophageal speech is similar, but utilizes a belch to create a speech sound.

d. Various mechanical aids are available; it becomes a matter of selecting the best aid for the particular patient.

e. Tracheo-esophageal puncture (TEP) is a relatively new technique utilizing a prosthetic device (duck-bill).

A fistula is made at the posterior trachea and anterior esophageal wall; a one-way valve is formed through the fistula. The finger is used to close the stoma during speech.

f. Motivation, determination, and relaxation are necessary for the patient to learn a new means of communication. He needs encouragement and support, which the nurse and his family can provide.

g. Affiliation with a group of similar individuals promotes the patient's progress. Addresses of organizations that offer assistance follow:

American Speech–Language–Hearing Association
10801 Rockville Pike
Rockville, Maryland 20852

International Association of Laryngectomees
American Cancer Society
777 Third Avenue
New York, New York 10017

Local groups of "Lost Chord Clubs"
"New Voice Clubs"

2. Stoma cleanliness
Instruct the patient as follows:
a. Wash hands before touching stoma to prevent infection.
b. Wet wash cloth with warm water; wring dry, spread it over the stoma to cleanse tissue.
c. Do not use soap, tissues, or loose cotton, since these substances may get into the airway.
d. Apply petrolatum thinly around exterior of (but not in) stoma. Wipe away excess lubricant.

3. Stoma bib
a. A bib acts as a filter and warms the air about to enter the stoma. A crocheted cover or a cotton

cloth that hangs over the stoma may be used. The bib can be fastened with ties around the neck.

b. For men: Ascot or turtle neck sweaters may be worn. When a regular shirt is worn, the second button from the top can be sewed over the buttonhole as though it were fastened—this leaves a wide opening through which a handkerchief can be inserted when coughing.

For women: A variety of fashionable scarves, jewelry, high-neck dresses, and turtleneck sweaters can be worn.

4. Mouth care
   a. Oral mucosa is not "aired" as before, and the patient's ability to detect mouth odors is lessened; therefore, special mouth care is required.
   b. In addition to normal dental cleaning, a soft toothbrush is used to scrub the tongue and sides of the mouth; a turkish wash cloth is also effective in cleaning.
   c. The mouth can be rinsed with a deodorizing mouthwash.

5. Drugs and medications
   Instruct the patient as follows:
   a. Because many drugs tend to dry the stoma, always check with the physician before taking any medication.
   b. Avoid undiluted alcohol, since it has a tendency to dry the stoma; alcohol is also an irritant.

6. During a "cold"
   a. Use steam inhalation—place a container of steaming water on a stool and sit in front of it with a towel draped around the neck and shoulders to form a hood. A steam inhalator can be used.

7. Complications to avoid
   Instruct the patient as follows:
   a. Fistula—observe suture line daily to note preliminary signs of redness, swelling, and possible secretions. If the temperature rises, this may be indicative of infection.
      (1) Protect skin around stomal orifice, since secretions can cause breakdown of dermal tissues.
      (2) Use a nasogastric tube for feedings; otherwise, whatever is eaten could leak through fistula and delay healing.
      (3) Maintain intake and output records and be alert for signs of dehydration.
   b. Occlusion of opening
      (1) Protect stoma when showering by wearing a protective plastic cover.
      (2) Swimming is not recommended.
      (3) Protect stoma during a haircut and when powdering to prevent dust and hair from entering stoma.
      (4) When shaving, use a dry towel around the neck to prevent hairs from entering stoma.
      (5) In the event of an obstruction to the stoma, see Guidelines: Emergency First Aid for the Laryngectomee, below.

Evaluation

Expected Outcomes

1. Demonstrates an optimistic view of future following perioperative experience
2. Accepts the treatment regimen as a means of controlling cancer spread
3. Participates actively in voice rehabilitation program
4. Follows the convalescent plan; lists the activities involved in maintaining satisfactory recovery

Guidelines: Emergency First Aid for the Laryngectomee

Nature of the Problem

Clogging or obstruction of the neck stoma is a life-threatening problem.

Equipment (if available):

Suction equipment
Sterile disposable catheter
   #14–16 Fr. (adult)
   #8–10 Fr. (child)

Sterile gloves
Sterile saline
Portable mask and bag

Procedure for Total Neck Breather

One who breathes ONLY through the neck opening
1. There is no connection between lungs and nose or mouth.
2. A tracheostomy or laryngectomy tube may or may not be in the neck opening.

▶ **NURSING ALERT:** No air can get through the mouth or nose of a total laryngectomee when stoma is clogged.

Nursing Action	Rationale/Amplification
1. PLACE PATIENT ON HIS BACK, head straight, chin up. Bare the neck down to the sternum.	1. Access to the laryngeal stoma and observation of thoracic movement are facilitated.
2. Position a blanket or any article of clothing under the shoulders.	2. This promotes extension of the neck area permitting access.
3. Make a rapid assessment of the situation:	3.
a. Is victim wearing a tracheostomy or laryngectomy tube?	a. In a laryngectomee, tube removal cannot cause immediate danger.

Procedure for Total Neck Breather
(Cont.)

Nursing Action	Rationale/Amplification
b. Has he been operated on recently? c. Check for tracheal obstruction. Clean stomal opening of mucus and encrusted matter.	b. If so, tracheostomy tube cannot be removed. c. Mucus, etc. may account for obstruction. Use a clean cloth or handkerchief—never tissue.
4. START MOUTH-TO-NECK BREATHING PROMPTLY: Position yourself at side of victim. Place your mouth and lips tightly over neck opening or around the tracheal tube if the person is wearing one.	4. SECONDS COUNT Do not remove the tube.
5. If suction equipment is available, insert a soft rubber tube 7.5–12.5 cm. (3–5 in.) into opening for a few seconds.	5. A partially open airway transporting air to the victim is infinitely better than a clean airway that does not supply air at this crucial time.
6. Blow in a sufficient amount of air to see chest rise.	
7. For the first 5 seconds, repeat every 1–2 seconds; then slow down to a steady pace of every 4–5 seconds (12–20 times per minute).	
8. Continue until spontaneous breathing returns.	

Follow-up Phase

1. When victim recovers, provide oxygen from a portable supply.	
2. If breathing fails again, resume mouth-to-neck breathing.	
3. You can also use mechanical resuscitation with the rubber or plastic inflatable bag and mask combination.	3. Attach baby-sized mask; be sure there is a tight seal against neck opening. Because a tight seal is difficult to maintain and because pressure of the mask on the major blood vessels of the neck may interfere with blood supply to the brain, mouth-to-neck breathing is safer and better.
4. Watch the chest rise	
5. Observe the patient constantly.	

Procedure for Partial Neck Breather

One who breathes MAINLY through the neck opening.
1. A connection between the lungs and the nose and mouth still exists.
2. The larynx may or may not be present.
3. A tracheostomy or laryngectomy tube may or may not be in the neck opening.

▶ **NURSING ALERT:** With mouth-to-neck breathing, FAILURE OF THE CHEST TO RISE is reliable proof that the patient is a partial neck breather. The rescuer may hear or feel air escaping from the victim's nose or mouth, but it is not getting into the lungs.

1. a. Immediately place the palm of your hand (the one nearest to the patient's head) over the lips and mouth. b. Pinch the nose shut between your third and fourth fingers. c. Place your thumb in the soft space under the chin and firmly press upward and backward.	1. This will close the area between the trachea and throat and at the same time raise the base of the tongue against the palate and pharynx.
2. Remove the patient's dentures.	2. To ensure better lip closure and effective underchin thumb closure.
3. Now mouth-to-neck breathing will fill the lungs and the chest will rise.	

2: Conditions of the Chest

Major Manifestations of Bronchopulmonary Disease

Cough and Sputum Production

A. Causes

1. Coughing is a protective mechanism that serves to clear the airways.
2. Cough-producing stimuli may be inflammatory, mechanical, chemical, or thermal.
3. Clinical problems producing cough are infection, inflammation, neoplasms, cardiovascular disorders, trauma, physical agents, and allergic disorders.

4. Violent coughing may cause bronchial obstruction and syncope, and cause further irritation of the bronchi.
5. Thick, mucopurulent sputum, which is difficult to remove, is more apt to cause violent coughing.

B. Nursing Assessment

1. Evaluate the character of the cough.
    a. Throat-clearing cough—postnasal drip.
    b. Dry and hacking—may be due to nervousness, viral infections, bronchogenic carcinoma, early congestive heart failure.
    c. Loud and harsh—irritation in upper airway.
    d. Wheezing—associated with bronchospasm.
    e. Severe or changing in character or with position—may be bronchogenic cancer (cough, chest pain, hemoptysis).
    f. Loose—indicates problems in peripheral bronchi and lung parenchyma.
    g. Painful—may indicate pleural involvement, chest wall disease.
    h. Chronic, productive—sign of bronchopulmonary disease.
2. Note relationship of cough to time, to patient's position, and to environmental exposure.
    a. Recent onset of cough (hours or days) suggests infection.
    b. Cough most noticeable upon awakening—suppurative lung disease; bronchitis.
    c. Coughing paroxysms at night—may indicate bronchial asthma or left-sided heart failure.
    d. Cough that worsens when patient is supine—may be due to postnasal drip from sinusitis, bronchiectasis.
    e. Cough associated with food intake—may be the result of aspiration into tracheobronchial tree.
    f. Cough of recent onset or gradually progressive over a period of weeks or months suggests tuberculosis or bronchogenic carcinoma.
3. Determine the patient's:
    a. Smoking history: Current? Past?
    b. Environmental or occupational exposure to dusts, fumes, or gases?
    c. Allergies, asthma, sinusitis, upper respiratory infection?
4. Observe character, quantity, and color of expectorated material and ability of patient to clear his secretions. Ask if there has been a change in the character or frequency of coughing.
    a. Clear or mucoid—stems from viral infection, chronic bronchitis, postnasal drip.
    b. Thick yellow or green sputum—due to primary or secondary bacterial infections.
    c. Rusty—may indicate bacterial pneumonia (if patient not receiving antibiotics).
    d. Malodorous—due to lung abscess, infection from fusospirochetal or anaerobic organisms.
    e. Frothy pink sputum—indicates acute pulmonary edema.
    f. Note amount of sputum produced daily. A sudden decrease in the quantity of sputum may indicate inspissation (drying and thickening) in tracheobronchial tree and may lead to respiratory insufficiency and failure.
    g. Layering of sputum in sputum cup occurs in lung abscess or bronchiectasis.

C. Nursing Interventions

1. Give cough suppressants, expectorants, and mucolytic agents as prescribed.

2. Make sure the patient is adequately hydrated to liquefy sputum.
3. Assist the patient to cough productively by controlled coughing, postural drainage, and chest percussion.
4. Discourage smoking—interferes with lung defense mechanisms: interferes with ciliary action, increases bronchial secretions, causes inflammation and hyperplasia of mucous glands, reduces production of surfactant, impairs function of alveolar macrophages (scavenger cells).
5. Encourage oral hygiene—odor and taste of sputum depresses appetite.

Dyspnea

(Breathlessness or difficult breathing) May be acute, chronic, progressive, recurrent, or paroxysmal

A. Causes

1. In lung disease, shortness of breath is due to change in lung rigidity or increased airway resistance.
2. Lung disease places strain on the right ventricle—may cause right ventricular failure.

B. Clinical Implications

1. In general, the acute lung diseases produce a more severe grade of dyspnea than do the chronic diseases.
2. Sudden dyspnea in a healthy person may indicate pneumothorax (air in pleural cavity).
3. Sudden dyspnea in ill or postoperative patient may indicate pulmonary embolus; pneumothorax.
4. Orthopnea—characteristic of cardiogenic pulmonary congestion.
5. Expiratory wheeze—arises from obstructive disease in peripheral airways (asthma, chronic bronchitis, emphysema).
6. Noisy respirations—related to localized obstruction of major branches, tumor, foreign body, or narrowing of smaller airways.
7. Inspiratory stridor—indicates partial obstruction at laryngeal or tracheal level.
8. Paroxysmal wheezing unrelated to exertion—may arise from bronchial (allergic) asthma or bronchitis.

C. Nursing Assessment

Ascertain circumstances that cause dyspnea
1. Relation to exertion, position, or environmental exposure.
2. Quantify exertion and specify type producing dyspnea (housework, mowing lawn, walking a set distance).
3. Mode of onset? Sudden? Gradual?
4. Quantify change in dyspnea. (What could patient do a year ago, a month ago that he cannot do now?)
5. Can the patient take a deep breath?
6. At what time of day/night is it obvious?
7. Is there associated cough?
8. Is there expiratory wheeze?
9. Is dyspnea associated with other symptoms?

D. Nursing Interventions

The treatment depends on alleviating the cause.
1. Place the patient on rest with his head elevated.
2. Administer oxygen as prescribed.

Hemoptysis

(Coughing up or expectoration of blood or bloodstained sputum from the respiratory tract)

A. Causes

1. Chronic bronchitis; bronchiectasis
2. Bronchial carcinoma

3. Bronchial or parenchymal infections
4. Cardiovascular conditions (mitral stenosis)

B. Nursing Assessment

1. Question the patient about ingestion of aspirin or aspirin-containing medication within the past 24 hours.
2. Ascertain whether blood is coming from nose or throat, gastrointestinal tract, or lungs.
   a. Nose (*epistaxis*)—usually there is a discharge of blood from nose.
      (1) During severe epistaxis, the patient may swallow or aspirate blood.
      (2) Look for dried blood in nose or nasopharynx.
   b. Gastrointestinal tract (*hematemesis*)
      (1) Usually preceded by nausea and accompanied by retching and vomiting.
      (2) Blood appears dark red in color; may contain food particles.
      (3) Blood is acid in reaction (pH less than 7.0).
   c. Lungs (*hemoptysis*)
      (1) Blood is *coughed* up; patient may have tickling in throat, salty taste, burning or bubbling sensation in chest.
      (2) Usually bright red and frothy; blood-tinged sputum may persist for days.
      (3) Blood is alkaline in reaction (pH greater than 7.0).

C. Nursing Interventions

1. Place the patient on bed rest and give mild sedation as prescribed.
   a. Place on affected side (if known)—to avoid flooding the contralateral lung.
   b. Maintain a calm reassuring approach—fright in a patient promotes hyperventilation.
2. Recognize the patient's fear and apprehension due to this threatening symptom and give him understanding and support.
3. Record quantity, color, and character (mixed with mucus, pure blood).
4. Save all coughed up blood for inspection by physician.
5. Have equipment for emergency bronchoscopy/laryngoscopy in readiness—for removal of blood clots and identification of bleeding site.
6. In event of asphyxia or massive hemoptysis, prepare for balloon catheter insertion and inflation to occlude bleeding site and/or for surgical intervention.

Chest Pain.

A. Causes

1. Parietal pleura has rich supply of sensory nerves coming from intercostal nerves to the diaphragm. These nerve endings may be stimulated by inflammation and stretching of membranes and by respiratory movements—produces a characteristic sharp, knife-like pain.
2. Pleuropulmonary pain—bacterial pneumonia, infarction, spontaneous pneumothorax.

B. Clinical Manifestations and Nursing Assessment

1. Pleural pain is a common manifestation of inflammatory and malignant disease, but also accompanies pneumothorax and pulmonary embolism.
2. Pleural pain (usually well localized, sharp, and stabbing) occurs at end of inspiration.
3. Assess quality, intensity, and radiation of pain.
4. Note factors that precipitate pain.
5. Evaluate whether position of the patient changes character of pain.
6. Determine the effect of inspiration and expiration on the patient's pain.

C. Nursing Interventions

1. Should be directed towards relieving underlying causes.
2. Give prescribed analgesic taking care not to depress respiratory center or productive cough.
3. Assist with regional anesthetic block—procaine is injected along the intercostal nerves that supply the painful area in cases where pain is intractable.

Hoarseness

A. Causes

1. Acute
   When associated with febrile episode, suggests viral laryngotracheobronchitis.
2. Persistent
   May indicate intrinsic neoplasm of vocal cord, bronchogenic cancer, mediastinal lesion.

Constitutional Manifestations of Bronchopulmonary Disease

A. Constitutional Symptoms of Bronchopulmonary Disease

1. Anorexia
2. Fever
3. Weight loss
4. Fatigue, malaise, weakness
5. Sweats
6. Chills

related to duration and severity of disease

B. Constitutional Signs of Bronchopulmonary Disease

1. Cyanosis
2. Clubbing of fingers
3. Wasting

Diagnostic Studies*

Radiography

A. Chest Roentgenogram

1. Normal pulmonary tissue is radiolucent. Thus densities produced by tumors, foreign bodies, etc. can be detected.

2. Shows position of normal structures, displacement, and presence of abnormal shadows.
3. Chest x-rays may reveal extensive pathology in the lungs in the absence of symptoms.

B. Tomography (planigraphy)

1. Provides films of sections of lungs at different levels within the thorax.
2. Useful in demonstrating presence of small, solid lesions, calcification, or cavitation within a lesion.

* For physical examination of lungs and thorax, see page 30.

C. Computed Tomography

An imaging method in which the lungs are scanned in successive layers by a narrow beam x-ray. A computer printout is obtained of the absorption values of the tissues in the plane that is being scanned.

It may be used to define pulmonary nodules, small tumors adjacent to pleural surfaces (which may be invisible on routine roentgenograms), and to demonstrate mediastinal abnormalities and hilar adenopathy.

D. Positron Emission Tomography (PET)

Uses high-energy physics and computer techniques to study lung function; useful for quantitative measurements of regional pulmonary perfusion and for studying ventilation–perfusion relationships.

E. Fluoroscopy

Enables roentgenologist to view heart, lungs, and diaphragm in the dynamic (moving) state.

F. Barium Swallow

Outlines the esophagus and reveals displacement of esophagus and encroachment on its lumen by cardiac, pulmonary, and mediastinal abnormalities.

G. Bronchography

A radiopaque medium is instilled directly into the trachea and bronchi, and the entire bronchial tree or selected areas may be visualized. This is a diagnostic test for any disease that alters the caliber or patency of the bronchial tree or that causes its displacement. It is infrequently used since the advent of fiberoptics.

1. The patient is assessed for allergic reaction to anesthetic agent or contrast media before the test is started.
2. The patient is kept fasting—to avoid aspiration of gastric contents.
3. Preoperative medication may include atropine to decrease secretions and vagally mediated reflex bradycardia and diazepam (Valium) for sedation/tranquilization.
   a. Topical anesthesia is sprayed in the mouth, on tongue and posterior pharynx.
   b. Local anesthetic is injected into the larynx and tracheal tree to prevent gagging and coughing when the tube is passed.
      (1) Extreme caution is indicated in patients with respiratory insufficiency, since these patients may experience temporary problems with ventilation and diffusion.
      (2) Oxygen, antispasmodic agents, and cortisone should be available.
4. *Nursing Responsibilities after Bronchogram*
   a. Withhold fluids and food until patient demonstrates a cough reflex.
   b. Check vital signs as indicated.
   c. Encourage the patient to cough and clear his bronchial tree; postural drainage may be required. A slight elevation of temperature is common following a bronchogram.

H. Angiographic Studies of Pulmonary Vessels

Radiopaque medium is rapidly injected into vasculature of the lungs for radiographic study of pulmonary vessels.

1. It can be performed by
   a. Venous injection into one or both arms (or femoral vein) through a needle or catheter, OR
   b. Introducing a catheter into main pulmonary artery or its branches
2. Films are taken in rapid sequence after injection.

I. Aortography

Opacification studies of either thoracic aorta or abdominal aorta; taken when aneurysm of thoracic aorta is suspected.

Endoscopic Procedures

A. Bronchoscopy

The direct inspection and observation of the larynx, trachea, and bronchi through a flexible or rigid bronchoscope; has both diagnostic and therapeutic uses in pulmonary conditions.

1. *Diagnostic Uses*
   a. To collect secretions for cytologic/bacteriologic studies.
   b. To determine location and extent of a pathologic process and to obtain biopsy for diagnosis.
      (1) *Tissue biopsy*—use of small biopsy forceps to obtain sample of tissue for examination.
      (2) *Brush biopsy*—target bronchus is brushed using a small wire with brush on one end that is introduced through bronchoscope. Material (cells and secretions) can be examined cytologically or cultured to look for pathogenic organisms.
   c. To determine whether a tumor can be resected surgically.
   d. To diagnose bleeding sites (source of hemoptysis).
2. *Therapeutic Uses*
   a. To remove foreign bodies from tracheobronchial tree.
   b. To remove secretions obstructing the tracheobronchial tree when the patient is unable to clear them.
   c. To fulgurate and excise lesions.

B. Flexible Fiberoptic Bronchoscopy

Passage of thin, flexible bronchofiberscope that can be directed into segmental bronchi; by its smaller size, flexibility, and excellent optical system, it allows increased visualization of peripheral airways.

1. May be done transnasally, transorally, or through an endotracheal tube; allows for brush biopsy (see above).
2. Causes very little patient discomfort; better patient acceptance even under local anesthetic.
3. Clinical applications for flexible fiberoptic bronchoscopy: allows diagnostic visualization of airways to segmental bronchi; permits brushing for malignant cells/infecting agents; biopsy of lesions; therapeutic removal of secretions; localization of source of hemoptysis.
   Bronchoalveolar lavage—injection of saline through fiberoptic bronchoscope, which is immediately withdrawn; recovers alveolar cells, secretions, and pathogens by washing them from distal airways.
4. Possible complications: reaction to anesthetic agent, pneumothorax, arrhythmias, bronchospasm.

C. Rigid Bronchoscopy

Hollow metallic tube with light at its end used for removal of foreign bodies, suctioning thick secretions, and investigating source of massive hemoptysis, or for endobronchial surgical procedures (resection of tumors, dilation of strictures, etc.).

1. May be done under local or general anesthesia.
2. Rigid bronchoscope preferred in following instances: small children, endobronchial tumor resection, mas-

sive hemorrhage, foreign body retrieval; otherwise it is being replaced by flexible fiberoptic bronchoscopy.
  3. Nursing interventions
     a. See that an informed consent form has been signed.
     b. Administer medication to reduce secretions and block the vasovagal reflex and relieve anxiety. Give encouragement and nursing support.
     c. Restrict fluid and food for 6 hours before procedure—to reduce risk of aspiration when reflexes are blocked.
     d. Remove dentures, contact lenses, and other prostheses.
     e. After the procedure, wait until the patient demonstrates that he can cough before giving him cracked ice or fluids. A return to his usual diet is resumed in a few hours.
     f. Following bronchoscopy watch patient for
        (1) Cyanosis
        (2) Hypotension
        (3) Tachycardia and arrhythmia
        (4) Hemoptysis
        (5) Dyspnea
        (6) Confusion and lethargy in elderly

D. Mediastinoscopy (See p. 142.)

Radioisotope Diagnostic Procedures

Ventilation and perfusion scintigraphy—Refers to radioisotope imaging of ventilation and blood flow to the lungs. The camera may be interfaced to a computer to record, collate, and refine data.

A. Perfusion Lung Scan

Following injection of a radioactive isotope, scans are made with a scintillation camera.
  1. Measures blood perfusion through the lungs; evaluates lung function on a regional basis.
  2. Useful in perfusion (vascular) abnormalities—pulmonary embolism.

B. Ventilation Scan

  1. Inhalation of radioactive gas (xenon, krypton), which diffuses throughout the lungs.
  2. Useful in detecting ventilation abnormalities (emphysema).

C. Gallium Scan

Radioisotope lung scan used to detect inflammatory conditions of the lungs.

Examination of Sputum

A. Purpose

  1. Sputum is obtained for evaluation of gross appearance, for microscopic examination, for gram staining and culture to identify the predominant organisms, and for cytologic examination.
     a. Direct smear—shows presence of white blood cells and intracellular (pathogenic) bacteria and extracellular (mostly nonpathogenic) bacteria.
     b. Sputum culture—to make diagnosis, to determine drug sensitivity, and to serve as a guide for drug treatment (choice of antibiotic).
     c. Sputum cytology (exfoliative cytology)—used to identify tumor cells.
  2. Patients receiving antibiotics, steroids, and immunosuppressive agents for prolonged periods may have periodic sputum examinations, since these agents may give rise to opportunistic pulmonary infections.

B. Methods of Obtaining Sputum

  1. By deep breathing and coughing
     a. Secure early morning specimen—yields best sample of deep pulmonary material from all lung fields.
     b. Clear nose and throat and rinse mouth—to decrease sputum contamination.
     c. Instruct patient to take several deep breaths, exhale, and perform a series of short coughs.
     d. Cough deeply and expectorate the sputum into a sterile container.
     e. See that specimen is transported to laboratory immediately; allowing it to stand in a warm room will result in overgrowth of organisms, making identification of pathogen difficult; also alters cell morphology.
     f. Give oral hygiene frequently, especially if the patient has foul sputum.
  2. By ultrasonic and/or heated hypertonic saline nebulization
     a. Patient inhales through mouth slowly and deeply for 10–20 minutes.
     b. Increases the moisture content of air going to lower tract; particles will condense on tracheobronchial tree and aid in expectoration.
  3. Tracheal aspiration (see Guidelines, p. 153)
  4. Bronchoscopic removal (p. 140)—provides sputum sampling by aspiration of secretions; brushing through a sterile catheter; bronchoalveolar lavage, and transbronchial biopsy.
  5. Gastric aspiration (rarely necessary since advent of ultrasonic nebulizer).
     a. Nasogastric tube is inserted into the stomach to siphon out swallowed pulmonary secretions.
     b. This test is useful only for culture of tubercle bacilli, but not for direct examination.
  6. Transtracheal aspiration (see Fig. 7-4). See Guidelines, page 145.

Examination of Pleural Fluid and Pleural Biopsy

A. Pleural Fluid

Pleural fluid is continuously produced and reabsorbed, with a thin layer of fluid normally in the pleural space; abnormal accumulation of pleural fluid (effusion) occurs in diseases of the pleura, heart, or lymphatics. The pleural fluid is studied along with other tests to determine underlying cause.
  1. Pleural fluid is obtained by aspiration (thoracentesis, p. 146) or by tube thoracotomy.
  2. Pleural fluid is examined for cell count, differential, specific gravity, cytology, protein, glucose, pH, LDH, and amylase.
     a. Pleural fluid, usually light straw color
     b. Purulent fluid—suggests empyema
     c. Blood-tinged fluid—pulmonary infarction; neoplastic disease
     d. Milky fluid (chylothorax)—invasion of thoracic duct by tumor or inflammatory process; traumatic rupture of thoracic duct
  3. Observe and record total amount of fluid withdrawn, nature of fluid, and its color and viscosity.
  4. Prepare sample of fluid for laboratory evaluation if prescribed.

B. Pleural Biopsy

Accomplished via needle biopsy of pleura or via pleuroscopy (visual exploration of pleural space through a bronchofiberscope inserted into pleural space).

Biopsy Procedures of the Lung

Goal:
Obtain histologic material from lung to aid in diagnosis.

A. Transbronchoscopic Biopsy

Biopsy forceps inserted through bronchoscope and specimen of lung tissue obtained.

B. Transthoracic Needle Aspiration Biopsy
(needle biopsy through thoracic wall)

1. Skin site is cleansed and anesthetized.
2. Small skin incision is made, and a needle is advanced under fluoroscopic control to the desired site.
3. With the needle in the periphery of the lesion, the stylet is removed, the syringe attached, and suction applied while 2 or 3 short needle thrusts are made into mass.
4. Specimen is smeared and fixed on a slide for cytologic examination if neoplasm is suspected. Smears may also be made for bacteria, acid-fast organisms, and fungi.
5. A fluoroscopic survey is done to determine if a pneumothorax has developed that will require chest tube drainage.
6. Postbiopsy care
   a. Observe for possible complications: pneumothorax, hemoptysis, bacterial contamination of the pleural space.
   b. Encourage the patient to remain in bed for several hours with his aspirated lung in a dependent position.

C. Transcatheter Bronchial Brushing

D. Open Lung Biopsy

1. Used in making a diagnosis when other biopsy methods fail.
2. Usually done by a small anterior thoracotomy; does not usually involve a rib resection.
3. Subsequent pneumothorax controlled by chest tube connected to a water-seal drainage system.
4. Complications include hemorrhage, pneumothorax, and local and systemic infection.

Lymph Node Biopsy
(Scalene or Mediastinal Nodes)

Goal:
Detect lymph node spread of pulmonary disease. It is used as a diagnostic and prognostic measure.

1. Mediastinoscopy—endoscopic examination of the mediastinum for evaluation of tumor spread and biopsy of mediastinal nodes.
   a. Incision is usually made in suprasternal notch isthmus.
   b. The edges of incision are spread with forceps; the tissues overlying the trachea are dissected, and a channel is prepared for introduction of the mediastinoscope.
   c. Lymph nodes in the area are biopsied utilizing a small forcep.
   d. Useful in diagnosing and staging bronchogenic cancer to predict if tumor can be resected, and to obtain tissue for diagnosis in other conditions.
2. Mediastinotomy—surgical resection of second anterior costal cartilage for access to anterior mediastinum to evaluate lung lymphatic drainage.
   Procedure most frequently used to evaluate left upper lobe disease processes.
3. Scalene lymph nodes are enmeshed in deep cervical

pad of fat; these nodes drain lungs and mediastinum and may show histologic changes from intrathoracic disease.

Pulmonary Function Studies

Pulmonary function studies (see Ventilatory Function Tests [Table 7-1]) are done to detect and measure abnormalities in respiratory function. Such tests include measurements of lung volumes, ventilatory function, diffusing capacity, gas exchange, lung compliance, airway resistance, and distribution of gases in the lung.

A. Ventilatory Studies (Spirometry)

1. Most commonly used test.
2. Requires water spirometer, electronic spirometer, or wedge spirometer that plots volume against time (*timed vital capacity*).
3. Patient is asked to take as deep a breath as possible and then to exhale into spirometer as completely and as forcefully as possible. Results are compared with normals for patient's age, height, and sex (see Table 7-1).
4. A reduction in the vital capacity *alone* may indicate a restrictive form of lung disease (disease due to increased lung stiffness).
5. A reduction in several parameters usually indicates an obstructive form of lung disease (obstruction to flow due to bronchial obstruction or loss of lung elastic recoil).

B. Lung Volumes

1. Are determined by asking the patient to inhale known concentration of inert gas such as helium or 100% oxygen and measuring concentration of inert gas or nitrogen in exhaled air (dilution method). May also be measured in plethysmograph.
2. Yields thoracic gas volume (total lung capacity, plus any unventilated blebs or bullae).
3. An increased residual volume is found in air-trapping due to obstructive lung disease.
4. A reduction in several parameters usually indicates a restrictive form of lung disease or chest wall abnormality.

C. Diffusing Capacity

1. Measures lung surface effective for the transfer of gas in the lung.
2. Requires the patient to inhale gas containing known low concentration of carbon monoxide.
3. Measures carbon monoxide concentration in exhaled air (difference between inhaled and exhaled concentrations is related directly to uptake of carbon monoxide across alveolar–capillary membrane).
4. Is reduced in parenchymal lung disease, possibly in severe anemia, and in some forms of heart disease.

Arterial Blood Gas Studies

A. Purpose

1. A measurement of partial pressure of oxygen and carbon dioxide in arterial blood, as well as the pH of the blood.
2. The partial pressure of oxygen, together with hemoglobin, is a measurement of the amount of oxygen in the arterial blood.
3. Provide a means of assessing the adequacy of oxygenation and ventilation (i.e., the lungs supplying O_2 to the body and removing CO_2).
4. Help assess the acid–base status of the body—whether acidosis or alkalosis is present and to what degree.

B. Clinical Uses of Arterial Blood Gas Studies

1. Unexplained tachypnea, dyspnea (especially in patients with cardiovascular or pulmonary disease).
2. Unexplained restlessness, anxiety, drowsiness, or confusion in patients at risk for respiratory insufficiency or respiratory failure.
3. Assessment of preoperative pulmonary status.
4. Assessment before and during long-term oxygen therapy and during mechanical ventilator support.
5. Potential or actual impairment in acid–base balance.
6. Assessment of disease progression or reversibility.

C. See Guidelines, below.

Guidelines: Assisting with Arterial Puncture for Blood Gas Analysis

Terminology

Partial pressure—pressure exerted by each type of gas in a mixture of gases.
The following is a list of symbols used in reference to arterial blood gas studies:

P = pressure
PO_2—partial pressure of oxygen
PCO_2—partial pressure of carbon dioxide
P_AO_2—partial pressure of alveolar oxygen
P_ACO_2—partial pressure of alveolar carbon dioxide
PaO_2—partial pressure of arterial oxygen
$PaCO_2$—partial pressure of arterial carbon dioxide
PvO_2—partial pressure of venous oxygen
$PvCO_2$—partial pressure of venous carbon dioxide
P_{50}—oxygen tension at 50% hemoglobin saturation

Equipment

(Disposable kit is available)
2-ml. glass syringe with No. 25 gauge needle
10-ml. glass syringe with No. 20 or 21 gauge needle (adult), or No. 22 or 25 gauge needle (child)
Sodium heparin
Stopper or cap
Procaine
Sterile sponges and skin germicide
Basin containing ice

Assessment

Nursing Action	Rationale/Amplification
1. Record patient's inspired oxygen concentration.	1. Changes in inspired oxygen concentration alter the PaO_2. Degree of hypoxemia cannot be assessed without knowing the inspired oxygen concentration.
2. Take patient's temperature.	2. May be taken into consideration when results are evaluated. Hyperthermia and hypothermia influence oxygen release from hemoglobin at the tissue level.

Planning/Implementation

Preparatory Phase

1. Heparinize the syringe	
a. Withdraw a small amount of heparin into the syringe to wet the plunger and fill dead space in the needle.	a. This action coats the interior of the syringe with heparin to prevent blood from clotting.
b. Hold syringe in an upright position and expel excess heparin and air bubbles.	b. Air in the syringe may affect measurement of PaO_2. Heparin in the syringe may effect measurement of the pH.

Performance Phase (by physician, nurse, or respiratory therapist with special instruction)

1. Palpate the radial or femoral artery.	1. Arterial puncture is performed on areas where a good pulse is palpable.
2. If puncturing the radial artery, perform the Allen test. *In the conscious patient:*	2. The Allen test is a simple method for assessing collateral circulation in the hand. Ensures circulation if radial artery thrombosis occurs.
a. Obliterate the radial and ulnar pulses simultaneously by pressing on both blood vessels at the wrist.	a. Impedes arterial blood flow into the hand.
b. Ask patient to clench and unclench his fist until blanching of the skin occurs.	b. Forces blood from the hand.

(continued)

Guidelines: Assisting with Arterial Puncture for Blood Gas Analysis (continued)

Planning/Implementation
(Cont.)

Nursing Action	Rationale/Amplification
c. Release pressure on ulnar artery (while compressing radial artery). Watch for return of skin color within 15 seconds. *In the unconscious patient:* a. Obliterate the radial and ulnar pulses simultaneously at the wrist. b. Elevate patient's hand above his heart and squeeze or compress his hand until blanching occurs. c. Lower patient's hand while compressing radial artery (release pressure on ulnar artery) and watch for return of skin color.	c. Documents that ulnar artery alone is capable of supplying the hand, since radial artery is still occluded. **Note:** If the ulnar artery does not have sufficient blood flow to supply the entire hand, another artery should be used.
3. Feel along the course of the radial artery and palpate for maximum pulsation with the middle and index fingers. Prepare the skin with germicide. The skin and subcutaneous tissues may be infiltrated with a local anesthetic agent (procaine).	3. The wrist should be stabilized to allow for finer control of the needle.
4. The needle is at a 45–60° angle (Fig. 7-3) and is inserted into the artery. Once the artery is punctured, arterial pressure will push up the hub of the syringe and a pulsating flow of blood will easily fill the syringe.	4. In most patients the artery is located close to the surface of the skin.

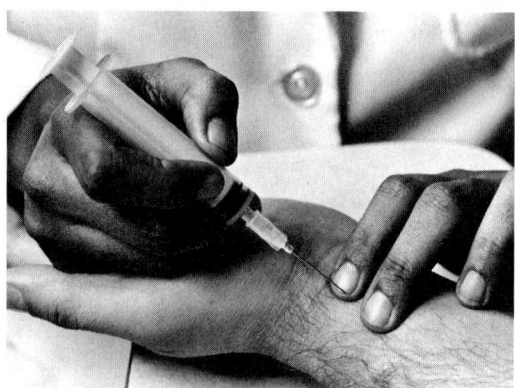

Figure 7-3. Technique of arterial puncture for blood gas analysis.

5. After blood is obtained, withdraw needle and apply firm pressure over the puncture.	5. Significant bleeding can occur because of pressure in the artery.
6. Cap the syringe tightly or plunge it into a rubber stopper.	6. Immediate capping of the needle prevents room air from mixing with the blood specimen.
7. Place the capped syringe in the container of ice.	7. The lower temperature reduces metabolism and minimizes the alteration of the true values of oxygen, carbon dioxide, and pH.
8. *Maintain firm pressure on the puncture site for 5 minutes* (by the clock). If the patient is on anticoagulant medication, apply direct pressure over puncture site for 15 minutes and then apply a firm pressure dressing.	8. Firm pressure on the puncture site prevents further bleeding and hematoma formation.
9. For patients requiring serial monitoring of arterial blood, an arterial catheter (connected to a flush solution of heparinized saline), is inserted into the femoral or radial artery.	9. All connections must be tight to avoid disconnection and rapid blood loss. The arterial line also allows for direct pressure monitoring in the critically ill patient.

Follow-up Phase

1. Send the basin of ice with the syringe containing blood to the laboratory immediately.	1. Blood gas analysis should be done as soon as possible, since tension and pH can change rapidly.
2. Palpate the pulse (distal to the puncture site), inspect the puncture site and assess for cold hand, numbness, tingling or discoloration.	2. Hematoma and arterial thrombosis are complications following this procedure.

Evaluation/Outcome

Nursing Action	Rationale/Amplification
1. Change ventilator settings, inspired oxygen concentration, or type and settings of respiratory therapy equipment if indicated by the results.	1. The PaO_2 results will determine whether to maintain, increase, or decrease the F_IO_2. The $PaCO_2$ and pH results will detect if any changes are needed in tidal volume or rate in patient ventilator.
2. Palpate the pulse (distal to the puncture site), inspect the puncture site and assess for cold hand, numbness, tingling, and discoloration.	2. Hematoma and arterial thrombosis are complications of this procedure.

Table 7-1 Ventilatory Function Tests

Description	Term Used	Symbol	Remarks
The maximum volume of air exhaled from the point of maximum inspiration	Vital capacity	VC	Slow vital capacity may be normal or reduced in COPD* patients.
Vital capacity performed with a maximally forced expiratory effort	Forced vital capacity	FVC	Forced vital capacity is often reduced in COPD owing to air trapping.
Volume of air exhaled in the specified time during the performance of forced vital capacity	Forced expiratory volume (qualified by subscript indicating the time interval in seconds)	FEV_t, usually FEV_1	A valuable clue to the severity of the expiratory airway obstruction.
FEV_t expressed as a percentage of the forced vital capacity	Ratio of timed forced expiratory volume to forced vital capacity	$FEV_t/FVC\%$, usually $FEV_1/FVC\%$	Another way of expressing the presence or absence of airway obstruction.
Mean forced expiratory flow between 200 ml. and 1200 ml. of the FVC	Forced expiratory flow	$FEF_{200-1200}$	Formerly called maximum expiratory flow rate (MEFR). An indicator of large airway obstruction.
Mean forced expiratory flow during the middle half of the FVC	Forced mid-expiratory flow	$FEF_{25\%-75\%}$	Formerly called maximum and mid-expiratory flow rate. Slowed in small airway obstruction.
Mean forced expiratory flow during the terminal portion of the FVC	Forced end-expiratory flow	$FEF_{75\%-85\%}$	Slowed in obstruction of smallest airways.
Volume of air expired in a specified period during repetitive maximal effort	Maximal voluntary ventilation	MVV	Formerly called maximum breathing capacity. An important factor in exercise tolerance.

* Chronic obstructive pulmonary disease
(American Lung Association: Chronic Obstructive Pulmonary Disease, 5th ed. New York, 1981)

Guidelines: Assisting with Transtracheal Aspiration

Transtracheal aspiration involves passing a needle and then a catheter through a percutaneous puncture of the cricothyroid membrane (Fig. 7-4). Transtracheal aspiration bypasses the oropharynx and avoids specimen contamination by mouth flora.

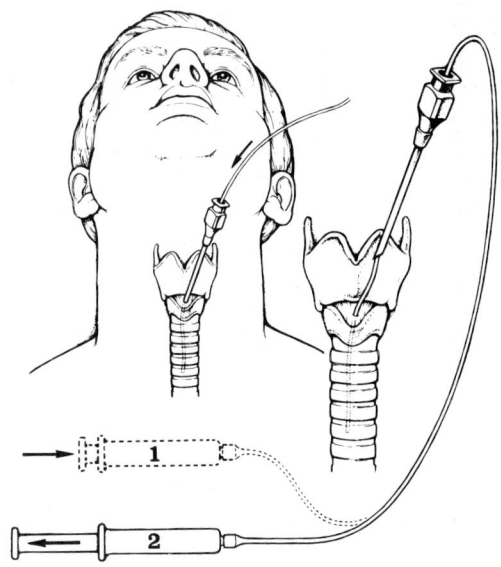

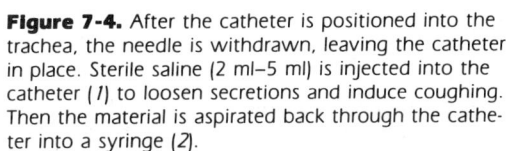

Figure 7-4. After the catheter is positioned into the trachea, the needle is withdrawn, leaving the catheter in place. Sterile saline (2 ml–5 ml) is injected into the catheter (*1*) to loosen secretions and induce coughing. Then the material is aspirated back through the catheter into a syringe (*2*).

Purposes
1. To obtain an uncontaminated sputum specimen for culture and sensitivity studies.
2. To promote coughing in the patient with an absent cough reflex.

(continued)

Guidelines: Assisting with Transtracheal Aspiration (continued)

Equipment

Sterile transtracheal set:
    No. 14, No. 16, and No. 18 gauge needles
    Polyethylene catheter
    Syringe
    Skin germicide
    Local anesthetic
    Sterile gloves

ECG monitoring equipment
Endotracheal tube
Suction apparatus with catheters
Cardiac resuscitation equipment

Procedure

Nursing Action	Rationale / Amplification
Preparatory Phase	
1. Explain the procedure and give reassurance by skilled and empathetic attention to the patient's needs.	1. Inform the patient that the procedure will cause coughing.
2. Administer supplemental oxygen as directed during the procedure if the patient's arterial oxygen tension is below normal while the patient is breathing room air.	2. This prevents worsening of hypoxemia.
3. Extend the patient's neck and place a pillow under his shoulders.	3. This is the optimum position for cricothyroid puncture.
Performance Phase (by the physician)	
The cricothyroid membrane is identified by palpation.	
1. The skin over the cricothyroid area is cleansed and the area infiltrated with local anesthetic.	1. The cricothyroid membrane is less vascular and offers more safety in preventing posterior wall puncture than other areas.
2. A No. 14, 16, or 18 gauge needle is inserted through the cricothyroid membrane into the trachea and a polyethylene catheter is inserted through the needle into the trachea.	2. Caution the patient against swallowing or talking while the needle is introduced through the cricothyroid membrane.
3. The needle is withdrawn leaving the catheter in place.	
4. A small amount of sterile saline (2–5 ml.) is injected into the trachea through the catheter.	4. Saline loosens secretions and initiates a paroxysm of coughing.
5. The secretions and exudates are aspirated back into the syringe as the patient coughs.	
6. Air is removed from the syringe and the syringe is capped or the sample is injected into an anaerobic transfer vial. The specimen is sent to the laboratory immediately.	6. This ensures anaerobic conditions.
7. The catheter is withdrawn and pressure applied over the puncture site.	7. Gentle, firm pressure over the site for about 5 minutes will help prevent subcutaneous or mediastinal emphysema.
Follow-up Care	
1. Instruct the patient to rest quietly for an hour or so.	
2. Observe for the following complications: bleeding, pneumomediastinum, subcutaneous emphysema, cardiac arrhythmias.	2. Assess for hoarseness after the procedure; this may be from a submucosal tracheal hematoma, which can cause suffocation. Inform the patient that minor blood-streaking of sputum almost always occurs following this procedure.

Guidelines: Assisting the Patient Undergoing Thoracentesis

Thoracentesis is the aspiration of fluid or air from the pleural space. It may be a diagnostic or a therapeutic procedure.

Purposes
1. To remove fluid and air from the pleural cavity (for diagnostic and therapeutic purposes).
2. To obtain diagnostic aspiration of pleural fluid.
3. To obtain pleural biopsy.
4. To instill medication into the pleural space.

Equipment

Syringes: 5-, 20-, 50-ml. syringes
Needles: No. 22, No. 26, No. 16 (7.5 cm. long)
Stopcock and tubing
Hemostat
Biopsy needle
Germicide solution
Local anesthetic
Sterile gauze dressings
Sterile towels and drape
Sterile specimen containers
Sterile gloves

Or for ultrasound-directed thoracentesis:
Needle–syringe assembly (needle, extension tubing, syringe)

Procedure

Nursing Action	Rationale/Amplification
Preparatory Phase	
1. Ascertain in advance if chest roentgenograms and/or other tests have been prescribed and completed. These should be available at the bedside.	1. Localization of pleural fluid is accomplished by physical examination, chest roentgenogram, ultrasound localization, or fluoroscopic localization.
2. See if consent form has been explained and signed.	
3. Determine if the patient is allergic to the local anesthetic agent to be used. Give sedation if prescribed.	
4. Inform the patient about the procedure and indicate how he can be helpful. Explain: a. The nature of the procedure. b. The importance of remaining immobile. c. Pressure sensations to be experienced. d. That no discomfort is anticipated after the procedure.	4. An explanation helps orient the patient to the procedure, assists him to mobilize his resources, and gives him an opportunity to ask questions and verbalize anxiety.
5. Make the patient comfortable with adequate supports. If possible place him upright and in one of the following positions (Fig. 7-5): a. Sitting on the edge of the bed with feet supported and head on a padded over-the-bed table. b. Straddling a chair with his arms and head resting on the back of the chair. c. If patient is unable to sit in a chair or side of bed, elevate head of bed 30–45° or place him on unaffected side and elevate head of bed.	5. The upright position ensures that the diaphragm is most dependent and facilitates the removal of fluid that usually localizes at the base of the chest. A comfortable position helps the patient to relax.

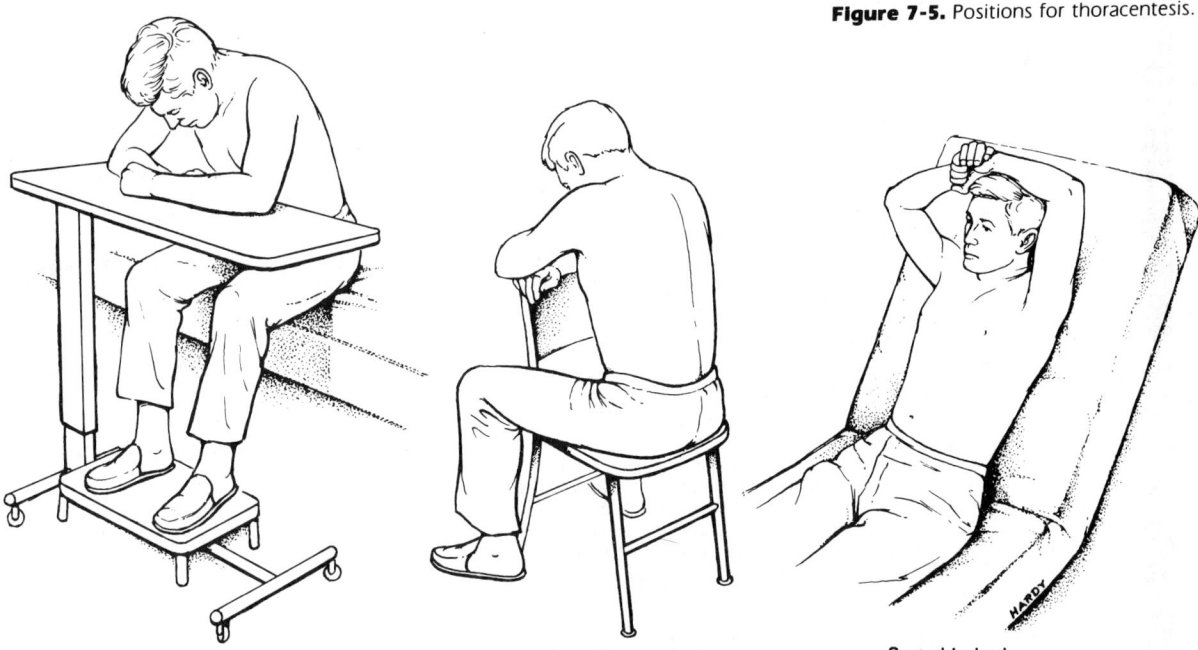

Figure 7-5. Positions for thoracentesis.

Over the bed table   Straddling a chair   Seated in bed

(continued)

Guidelines: Assisting the Patient Undergoing Thoracentesis (continued)

Procedure
(Cont.)

Nursing Action	Rationale/Amplification
6. Support and reassure the patient during the procedure.	6. Sudden and unexpected movement by the patient can cause trauma to the visceral pleura with resultant trauma to the lung.
a. Prepare the patient for sensations of cold from skin germicide and for pressure and sting from infiltration of local anesthetic agent.	
b. Encourage the patient to refrain from coughing.	A local anesthetic inhibits nerve conduction and is used to prevent pain during the procedure.

Performance Phase

1. The site for aspiration is determined from chest x-rays, by percussion, or by fluoroscopic or ultrasound localization. If fluid is in the pleural cavity, the thoracentesis site is determined by study of the chest x-ray and physical findings, with attention to the site of maximal dullness on percussion.

1. If air is in the pleural cavity, the thoracentesis site is usually in the 2nd or 3rd intercostal space in the midclavicular line (Fig. 7-6). Air rises in the thorax because the density of air is much less than the density of liquid.

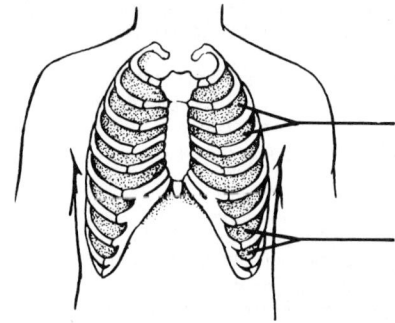

2nd or 3rd interspace for air

Site for aspiration of fluid determined by study of x-ray of chest and physical findings

Figure 7-6. Sites for thoracentesis.

2. The procedure is done under aseptic conditions. After the skin is cleansed, the physician slowly injects a local anesthetic with a small caliber needle into the intercostal space.

2. An intradermal wheal is raised slowly; rapid intradermal injection causes pain. The parietal pleura is very sensitive and should be well infiltrated with anesthetic before the thoracentesis needle is passed through it.

3. The physician advances the thoracentesis needle with the syringe attached. When the pleural space is reached, suction may be applied with the syringe.

a. A 20-ml. or 50-ml. syringe with a 3-way adapter (stopcock) is attached to the needle. (One end of the adapter is attached to the needle and the other to the tubing leading to a receptacle that receives the fluid being aspirated.)

a. When a large quantity of fluid is withdrawn, a 3-way adapter serves to keep air from entering the pleural cavity.

b. If a considerable quantity of fluid is to be removed, the needle is held in place on the chest wall with a small hemostat.

b. The hemostat steadies the needle on the chest wall and prevents too deep a penetration of pleural space. Sudden pleuritic pain or shoulder pain may indicate that the visceral or diaphragmatic pleura are being irritated by the needle point.

c. A pleural biopsy may be performed.

4. After the needle is withdrawn, pressure is applied over the puncture site and a small sterile dressing is fixed in place.

4. This is done to prevent air entry into pleural space.

Follow-up Phase

1. Place the patient on bed rest. A chest x-ray is usually obtained following thoracentesis.

1. Chest x-ray verifies that there is no pneumothorax.

2. Record vital signs every 15 minutes for 1 hour.

3. Record the total amount of fluid withdrawn and the nature of the fluid, its color and viscosity. If prescribed, prepare samples of fluid for laboratory evaluation (usually bacteriology, cell count and differential, determinations of protein, glucose, LDH, specific gravity). A small amount of heparin may be needed for several of the specimen containers, to prevent coagulation. A specimen container with formalin may be needed if a pleural biopsy is to be obtained.

3. The fluid may be clear, serous, bloody, purulent, etc.

4. Evaluate the patient at intervals for increasing respirations, faintness, vertigo, tightness in the chest, uncontrollable cough, blood-tinged frothy mucus, and rapid pulse and signs of hypoxemia.

4. Pneumothorax, tension pneumothorax, hemothorax, subcutaneous emphysema, or pyogenic infection may result from a thoracentesis.

Chest Physical Therapy

Postural Drainage Exercises

Postural drainage is the use of specific positions so that the force of gravity can assist in the removal of bronchial secretions from the affected bronchioles into the bronchi and trachea by means of expectoration (Fig. 7-7).

Underlying Principles

1. The patient is positioned so that the diseased area(s) are in a near vertical position, and gravity is used to assist drainage of the specific segment(s).
2. The positions assumed are determined by the location, severity, and duration of mucus obstruction.

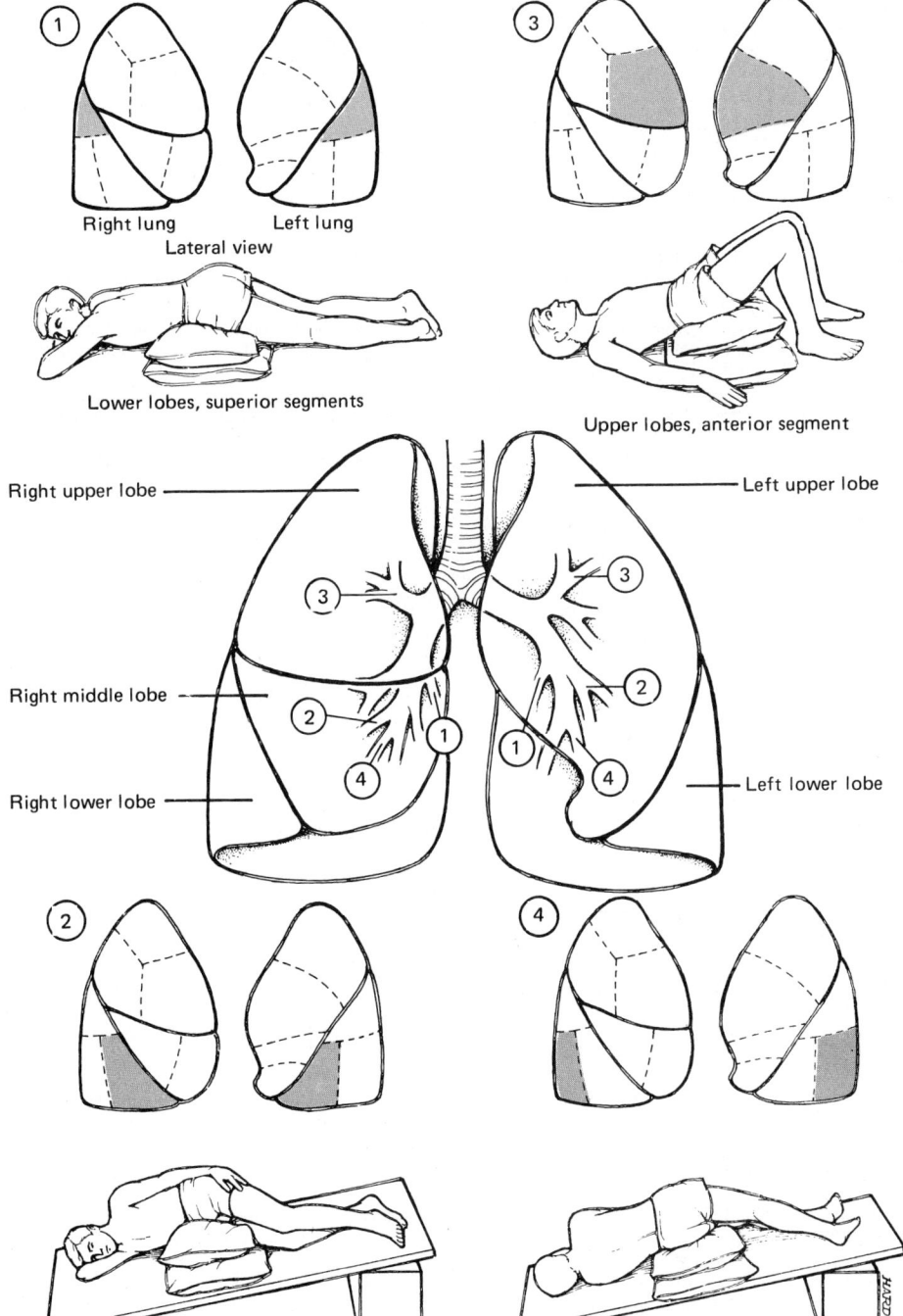

Right lung   Left lung
Lateral view
Lower lobes, superior segments

Upper lobes, anterior segment

Right upper lobe — — Left upper lobe

Right middle lobe —

Right lower lobe —

— Left lower lobe

Lower lobes, anterior basal segment

Lower lobe, lateral basal segment

Figure 7-7. Postural drainage. The patient is positioned to allow the involved segments of the lung to drain by gravity.

3. The exercises are usually performed 2 to 4 times daily, before meals and at bedtime.
4. Discontinue the procedure if tachycardia, palpitations, dyspnea, chest pain, or other symptoms occur—may indicate hypoxemia.

Nursing Management

1. Make the patient comfortable before the procedure starts and as comfortable as possible while he assumes each position.
   a. Bronchodilators, broncholytic agents, water, or saline may be nebulized and inhaled before postural drainage to reduce bronchospasm, decrease thickness of mucus and sputum, and combat edema of the bronchial walls.
   b. Use a folding cot to prop up patient to desired height if his bed is not adjustable; have an emesis basin ready for draining mucus.

2. Use a stethoscope to determine the areas of needed drainage.
3. Upper lobes are generally drained by upright positions; lower and middle lobes are drained by head-down positions.
4. Have patient assume left prone and left oblique positions (simultaneously)—this will give additional drainage to middle lobe and lateral segments of the right lower lobe; assuming the right prone and right oblique position (simultaneously) will give additional drainage to middle lobe and lateral segments of the left lower lobe.
5. Encourage the patient to cough after he has spent the allotted time in each position.
6. Encourage diaphragmatic breathing (p. 151) throughout postural drainage exercises; this helps widen airways so that secretions can be drained.
7. Chest wall percussion may be desirable to loosen and propel sputum in the direction of gravity drainage.

Guidelines: Percussion (Clapping) and Vibration

Percussion and vibration are manual techniques designed to loosen secretions and promote drainage of mucus and secretions from the lungs while the patient is in the position of postural drainage indicated for his specific lung problem. The procedure requires trained personnel.

1. *Percussion*—movement done by striking the chest wall in a rhythmic fashion with cupped hands over the chest segment to be drained. The wrists are alternately flexed and extended so that the chest is cupped or clapped in a painless manner.
2. *Vibration*—technique of applying manual compression and tremor to the chest wall during the exhalation phase of respiration.

Purposes
1. To dislodge mucus adhering to the bronchioles and bronchi.
2. To help mobilize secretions.

Clinical Indications

Lung conditions that cause increased production of secretions:
Bronchiectasis
Empyema
Cystic fibrosis
Chronic bronchitis

Contraindications

1. Lung abscess or tumors
2. Pneumothorax
3. Diseases of the chest wall
4. Lung hemorrhage
5. Painful chest conditions
6. Tuberculosis

▶   **NURSING ALERT:** Postural drainage and chest percussion may result in hypoxia and should only be used if secretions are believed to be present.

Procedure

Nursing Action	Rationale / Amplification
Performance Phase	
1. Instruct the patient to use diaphragmatic breathing (p. 151).	1. Diaphragmatic breathing helps the patient to relax and helps to widen airways.
2. Position the patient in prescribed postural drainage position(s) (p. 149). The spine should be straight to promote rib cage expansion.	2. The patient is positioned according to the area of the lung that is to be drained.
3. Percuss (or clap) with cupped hands over the chest wall for 1 or 2 minutes from: a. The lower ribs to shoulders in the back b. The lower ribs to top of chest in front	3. This action helps to dislodge mucous plugs and mobilize secretions toward the main bronchi and trachea. The air trapped between the operator's hand and chest wall will produce a characteristic hollow sound.
4. Avoid clapping over the spine, liver, kidneys, spleen, breast, scapula, clavicle, or sternum.	4. Percussion over these areas may cause injuries to the spine and internal organs.

Procedure
(Cont.)

Nursing Action	Rationale/Amplification
5. Instruct the patient to inhale slowly and deeply. Vibrate the chest wall as the patient exhales slowly through pursed lips.	5. This sets up a vibration that carries through the chest wall and helps free the mucus.
a. Place one hand on top of the other over affected area or place one hand on each side of the rib cage.	
b. Tense the muscles of the hands and arms while applying moderate pressure and vibrate hands and arms.	b. This maneuver is performed in the direction in which the ribs move upon expiration.
c. Relieve pressure on the thorax as the patient inhales.	
d. Encourage the patient to cough, using his abdominal muscles, after 3 or 4 vibrations.	d. Contracting the abdominal muscles while coughing increases cough effectiveness. Coughing aids in the movement and expulsion of secretions.
6. Allow the patient to rest several minutes.	
7. Listen with a stethoscope for changes in breath sounds.	7. The appearance of moist sounds (crackles) indicates movement of air around mucus in the bronchi.
8. Repeat the percussion and vibration cycle according to the patient's tolerance and his clinical response; usually 15 to 20 minutes.	

Guidelines: Teaching the Patient Breathing Exercises

Breathing exercises are techniques utilized to compensate for respiratory deficits by increasing efficiency of breathing. They are aimed at conserving energy through controlled breathing.

Purposes
1. To relax muscles and relieve anxiety.
2. To eliminate useless uncoordinated patterns of respiratory muscle activity.
3. To slow the respiratory rate.
4. To decrease the work of breathing.

General Instructions
1. Clear the nasal passages before beginning breathing exercises.
2. Always inhale through the nose—permits filtration, humidification, and warming of air.
3. Breathe slowly in a rhythmic and relaxed manner—permits more complete exhalation and emptying of lungs; helps overcome anxiety associated with dyspnea and decreases oxygen requirement.
4. Avoid sudden exertion.
5. Practice breathing exercises in several positions, since air distribution and pulmonary circulation vary according to position of the chest.

Diaphragmatic Breathing

Purposes:
1. To strengthen the diaphragm—the main respiratory muscle
2. To decrease the use of the accessory muscles of respiration

Teaching Procedure	Rationale/Amplification
Instruct the patient as follows:	
1. Place one hand on stomach just below the ribs and the other hand on the middle of the chest.	1. This helps the patient to become aware of the diaphragm and its function in breathing.
2. Breathe in slowly and deeply through the nose, letting the abdomen protrude as far as it will (Fig. 7-8A) The abdomen enlarges during inspiration and decreases in size during expiration.	2. Slow inhalation provides ventilation and hyperinflation of the lungs.
3. Breathe out through pursed lips while contracting (tightening) the abdominal muscles. Press firmly inward and upward on the abdomen while breathing out (Fig. 7-8B).	3. Contracting the abdominal muscles assists the diaphragm in rising to empty the lungs.

(continued)

Guidelines: Teaching the Patient Breathing Exercises (continued)

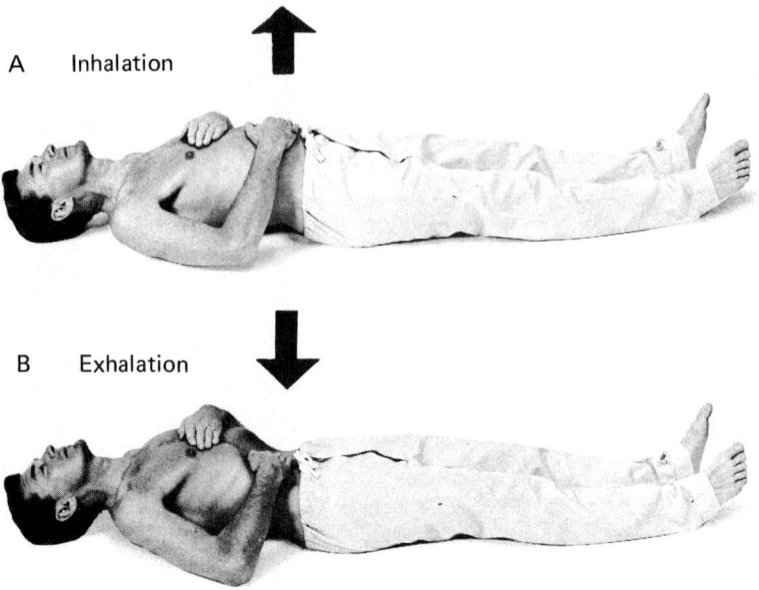

A   Inhalation

B   Exhalation

Figure 7-8. Breathing exercises for inhalation and exhalation. (Living with Asthma, Chronic Bronchitis, and Emphysema. Riker Laboratories, Inc., Northridge, California)

Diaphragmatic Breathing
(Cont.)

Teaching Procedure	Rationale/Amplification
4. The chest should not move; attention is directed at the abdomen, not the chest.	4. Contraction of the abdominal muscles should take place during expiration.
5. Repeat for approximately 1 minute (followed by a rest period of 2 minutes). Work up to 10 minutes, 4 times daily.	
6. Learn to do diaphragmatic breathing while lying, then sitting, and ultimately standing and walking. a. Coordinate diaphragmatic breathing with stair climbing, lifting, etc. b. Carry out activity (lifting) during the prolonged expiration phase.	6. Diaphragmatic breathing helps the patient breathe in a controlled manner during activities that produce dyspnea. If the patient becomes short of breath, have him stop the exercises until his breathing pattern comes under control.

Pursed-lip Breathing

Purposes
1. To slow the respiratory rate
2. To assist in emptying the lungs
3. To combat dyspnea due to exertion

Instruct the patient as follows:

1. Inhale through the nose.	
2. Exhale slowly and evenly against pursed lips while contracting (tightening) the abdominal muscles. Count to 7 while prolonging expiration through pursed lips.	2. Pursing the lips increases intrabronchial pressure (helps maintain the bronchi in an open position) as well as intra-alveolar pressure. The pursed-lip maneuver also prolongs the expiratory phase of breathing, makes it easier to empty the air in the lungs and promotes carbon dioxide elimination.
3. Sit in a chair. Fold the arms across the abdomen. a. Inhale through the nose. b. Bend over and exhale slowly through pursed lips while counting to 7.	b. Leaning forward pushes the abdominal organs upward.
4. While walking: a. Inhale while walking 2 steps. b. Exhale through pursed lips while walking 4 steps.	4. Try any similar combinations according to breathing tolerance of patient.

Other Exercises

Lower Side Rib Breathing

1. Place hands on sides of lower ribs.
2. Inhale deeply and slowly while sides expand moving hands outward.
3. Exhale slowly through pursed lips and feel the hands and ribs move inward.
4. Rest.

Lower Back and Rib Breathing

1. Sit in a chair. Place hands behind back; hold flat against lower ribs.
2. Inhale deeply and slowly while rib cage expands backward; the hands will move outward.
3. Keep hands in place. Blow out slowly; hands will move in.

Segmental Breathing

1. Place hands on sides of lower ribs.
2. Inhale deeply and slowly while concentrating on moving the right hand outward by expanding the right rib cage.
3. Ensure that the right hand moves outward more than the left hand.
4. Keeping hands in place, exhale slowly and feel the right hand and ribs moving in.
5. Repeat, concentrating on expanding left side more than the right side.
6. Rest.

Guidelines: Nasotracheal (NT) Suctioning

Suctioning of the tracheobronchial tree in a patient without an artificial airway is possible by inserting a suction catheter through the nares into the nasal passage, down through the oropharynx, past the glottis and into the trachea (Fig. 7-9).

(a) In addition to direct removal of secretions, nasotracheal suctioning stimulates strong paroxysms of coughing, enabling mobilization of secretions.

(b) Nasotracheal suctioning may be indicated in patients who are mechanically capable of coughing but do not do so because of central nervous system (CNS) depression, in those who have an inadequate cough secondary to "splinting" as a result of pain, or in patients whose cough is ineffective.

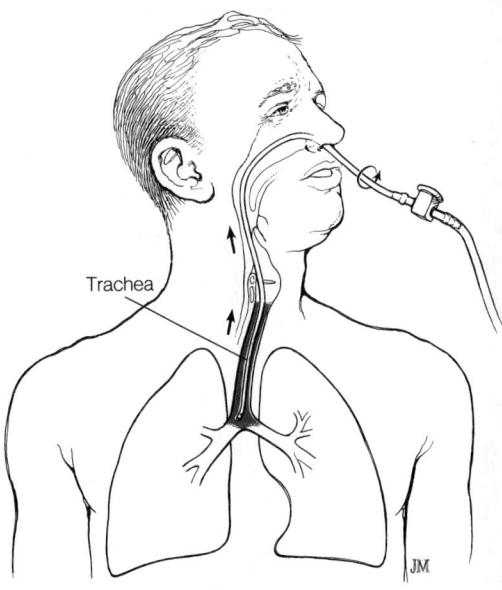

Figure 7-9. Placement of nasotracheal tube.

Contraindications

Bleeding disorder (disseminated intravascular coagulation [DIC], thrombocytopenia, leukemia, etc.)
Laryngeal edema, laryngeal spasm
Esophageal varices
Tracheal surgery
Gastric surgery with high anastomosis
Myocardial infarction (check with physician)

Caution

1. Trauma to the nasal passages may occur. Do not attempt to force the catheter if resistance is met. Trauma to nasal membranes or polyps may occur. If significant bleeding occurs, notify the physician.
2. Repeated suctioning may produce irritation of the nasal passages, resulting in pain and swelling. Insertion of a nasal airway may help to protect the nasal passages from trauma.
3. Repeated NT suctioning may promote laryngeal edema due to irritation and trauma. Stop if suctioning becomes difficult or if the patient develops new upper airway noise or obstruction.

(continued)

Guidelines: Nasotracheal (NT) Suctioning (continued)

Equipment

Assemble the following equipment or obtain a prepackaged kit.
Disposable curved-tipped suction catheter
Sterile towel
Sterile disposable gloves
Sterile water
Anesthetic water soluble lubricant jelly
Suction source at −80 to −120 mm. Hg
Resuscitation bag with face mask—connect 100% O_2 source with flow 10 liters/min.

Nursing Action	Rationale / Amplification
Assessment	
1. Monitor heart rate, respiratory rate, color, ease of respirations. If the patient is on monitor, continue monitoring heart rate or arterial blood pressure. Discontinue the suctioning and apply oxygen if heart rate decreases by 20 beats per minute or increases by 40 beats per minute, if blood pressure decreases, or if cardiac dysrhythmia is noted.	1. Suctioning may cause the occurrence of: a. Hypoxemia—initially resulting in tachycardia and increased blood pressure, and later causing cardiac ectopy, bradycardia, hypotension, and cyanosis. b. Vagal stimulation resulting in bradycardia.
Planning/Implementation	
Preparatory Phase	
1. Ascertain that the suction apparatus is functional. Place suction tubing within easy reach.	1. The procedure must be done aseptically, since the catheter will be entering the trachea below the level of the vocal cords, and introduction of bacteria is contraindicated.
2. Inform and instruct the patient regarding procedure. a. At a certain interval the patient will be requested to cough to open the lung passage so that the catheter will go into the lungs and not into the stomach. He will also be encouraged to try not to swallow, as this will also cause the catheter to enter the stomach. b. The postoperative patient can splint his wound to make the coughing produced by NT suctioning less painful.	2. A thorough explanation will decrease patient anxiety and promote patient cooperation (which is necessary for successful implementation of this procedure).
3. Place the patient in a semi-Fowler's or sitting position if possible.	3. NT suctioning should follow chest physical therapy, postural drainage, and/or ultrasonic nebulization therapy. The patient should not be suctioned after eating or after a tube feeding is given unless absolutely necessary to decrease the possibility of emesis and aspiration.
Performance Phase	
1. Place sterile towel across the patient's chest. Squeeze small amount of sterile anesthetic water soluble lubricant jelly onto the towel.	
2. Open sterile pack containing curved-tipped suction catheter.	
3. Aseptically glove both hands. Designate one hand (usually the dominant one) as "sterile" and the other hand as "contaminated."	3. The "contaminated" hand must also be gloved to ensure that organisms in the sputum do not come in contact with the nurse's hand, possibly resulting in infection of the nurse.
4. Grasp sterile catheter with sterile hand.	
5. Lubricate catheter with the anesthetic jelly and pass the catheter into the nostril and back into the pharynx.	5. If obstruction is met, do not force the catheter—remove it and try the other nostril.
6. Pass the catheter into the trachea. To do this, ask the patient to cough or say "ahh." If he is incapable of either, try to advance the catheter on inspiration. Asking the patient to stick out his tongue, or hold his tongue extended with a gauze sponge may also help to open the airway.	6. These maneuvers may aid in opening the glottis and allowing passage of the catheter into the trachea. To evaluate proper placement, listen at the catheter end for air, or feel for air movement against the cheek. An increase in intensity of breath sounds or more air movement against cheek indicates nearness to the larynx. Gagging or sudden lessening of sound means the catheter is in the hypopharynx. Draw back and advance again. The presence of the catheter in the trachea is indicated by: a. Sudden paroxysms of coughing.

Planning/Implementation
(Cont.)

Nursing Action	Rationale/Amplification
	b. Movement of air through the catheter. c. Vigorous bubbling of air when the distal end of the suction catheter is placed in a cup of sterile water. d. Inability of the patient to speak. If a protracted amount of time is needed to position the catheter in the trachea, stop and oxygenate the patient with his face mask or the resuscitation bag–mask unit at intervals. If three attempts to place the catheter are unsuccessful, request assistance.
7. Specific positioning of catheter for deep bronchial suctioning: a. For left bronchial suctioning, turn the patient's head to the extreme right, chin up. b. For right bronchial suctioning, turn the patient's head to the extreme left, chin up.	7. Turning the patient's head to one side elevates the bronchial passage on the opposite side, making catheter insertion easier. Suctioning of a particular lung segment may be of value in patients with unilateral pneumonia, atelectasis, or collapse. **NOTE:** The value of turning the head as an aid to entering the right or left main stem bronchi is not accepted by all clinicians.
8. Never apply suction until catheter is in the trachea. a. Once correct position is ascertained, apply suction and gently rotate catheter while pulling it slightly upward. Do not remove catheter from the trachea.	a. Because entry into the trachea is often difficult, less change in arterial oxygen may be caused by leaving the catheter in the trachea than by repeated insertion attempts.
9. Disconnect the catheter from the suctioning source after 5–15 seconds. Apply oxygen by placing a face-mask over the patient's nose, mouth, and catheter, and instruct the patient to breathe deeply.	9. Be sure that adequate time is allowed to reoxygenate the patient, since oxygen is removed, as well as secretions, during suctioning.
10. Reconnect suction source. Repeat suction as necessary.	10. No more than 3–4 suction passes should be made per suction episode.
11. During the last suction pass, remove the catheter completely while applying suction and rotating the catheter gently. Apply oxygen when catheter is removed.	11. Never leave the catheter in the trachea after the suction procedure is concluded, since the epiglottis is splinted open and aspiration may occur.

Follow-up Phase

Dispose of disposable equipment.

1. Measure heart rate and blood pressure. Record the patient's tolerance of procedure, type and amount of secretions removed, and complications.	1. Notify physician of any patient intolerance of procedure (changes in vital signs, bleeding, laryngospasm, upper airway noise).

Clinical Conditions

The Pneumonias

Pneumonia is an inflammatory process, involving the terminal airways and alveoli of the lung, because of an infection (bacteria, viruses, *Mycoplasma,* fungi). See Table 7-2, p. 156.

Predisposing Factors and Features

1. Pneumonia may be community-acquired (due to a limited number of organisms, namely *Streptococcus pneumoniae*) or hospital-acquired (nosocomial), due primarily to aerobic gram-negative bacilli and staphylococci.
2. Pathogens producing pneumonia may be carried in the nasopharynx of a healthy person.
3. Pathogens may invade tissues when the host's natural resistance is lowered by severe underlying illness.
4. Colds and upper respiratory tract infections lead to more serious illnesses by allowing bacterial invasion of lower respiratory tract.
5. Immunocompromised patients (those receiving corticosteroids; those with cancer; those being treated with chemotherapy or radiotherapy; those undergoing organ transplantation) have an increased chance of developing overwhelming infection.
6. A wide variety of pulmonary infections may develop in patients receiving immunosuppressive drugs (aerobic and anaerobic gram-negative bacilli, *Staphylococcus, Nocardia,* fungi, *Candida,* viruses [including cytomegalovirus], *Pneumocystis carinii,* reactivation of tuberculosis, and others).
7. Any condition interfering with normal drainage of the lung will predispose the person to pneumonia (*e.g.,* cancer of the lung).
8. Postoperative patients may develop bronchopneumonia, since anesthesia impairs respiratory defenses and decreases diaphragmatic movement.
9. Depression of the central nervous system (from drugs [including alcohol], head injury) predispose the patient to pneumonia.

Table 7-2 Commonly Encountered Pneumonias

Type	Organism Responsible	Manifestations	Clinical Features	Treatment	Complications
Bacterial					
Streptococcal pneumonia	*Streptococcus pneumonia*	May be history of previous respiratory infection Sudden onset, with shaking and chills Rapidly rising fever; tachypnea Cough; with expectoration of rusty or green (purulent) sputum Pleuritic pain aggravated by cough Chest dull to percussion; crackles, bronchial breath sounds Confusion may be only presenting feature in elderly	Herpes simplex lesions often present on face or lips Usually involves one or more lobes	Penicillin G Alternate drug therapy; erythromycin, clindamycin, cephalosporins, other penicillins, trimethoprim-sulfamethoxazole	Shock Pleural effusion Superinfections Pericarditis Bacteremia
Staphylococcal pneumonia	*Staphylococcus aureus*	Often prior history of viral infection, especially influenza Insidious development of cough, with expectoration of yellow, blood-streaked mucus Onset may be sudden if patient is outside hospital Fever, pleuritic chest pain, progressive dyspnea Pulse varies; may be slow in proportion to temperature	Frequently seen in hospital setting; during influenza epidemics; in intravenous drug abuse These infections often lead to necrosis and destruction of lung tissue Treatment must be vigorous and prolonged owing to disease's tendency to destroy the lungs Organism may develop rapid drug resistance Prolonged convalescence usual	Penicillinase-resistant penicillins	Effusion/pneumothorax Lung abscess Empyema Meningitis
Pneumonia due to gram-negative enteric bacilli	*Klebsiella pneumoniae, Pseudomonas aeruginosa, Escherichia coli, Enterobacter,* and other species	Sudden onset with fever, chills, dyspnea Pleuritic chest pain and production of purulent sputum	Usually infection occurs from aspiration of pharyngeal flora into bronchioles Seen in persons with severe illness; among the more common causes of hospital-acquired pneumonia	Usually multiple drug regimens recommended; combinations of a cephalosporin, carbenicillin, ticarcillin or other penicillins with an aminoglycoside	Early necrosis of lung tissue with rapid abscess formation
Legionnaires' disease	*Legionella pneumophila*	Prodromal period of abdominal pain and diarrhea High fever, chills, cough, chest pain, tachypnea	Peak incidence in persons over 50 who are cigarette smokers and have underlying diseases that increase susceptibility to infection; may be hospital-acquired	Erythromycin	Respiratory failure
Hemophilus influenza pneumonia	*H. influenzae*	Abrupt onset of coughing, fever, chills, chest pain	May affect healthy young adults	Depends on patient's previous or current use of antibiotic and on ampicillin-resistance rate in community	High mortality rate in patients with underlying disease (cancer; COPD) Pleural effusion common
Pittsburgh pneumonia agent (PPA)	*Legionella micdadei*	Fever, myalgias, nonproductive cough, dyspnea; pleuritic pain may occur. Patchy alveolar infiltrates on chest x-ray	May be hospital-acquired Generally seen in immuno-compromised patient	Erythromycin; rifampin; trimethoprim-sulfamethoxazole	Involves multiple lobes; bilateral consolidation common High mortality rate; clinical recovery slow
Nonbacterial Pneumonias					
Mycoplasma pneumonia	*Mycoplasma pneumoniae*	Gradual onset; severe headache; irritating, hacking cough producing scanty, mucoid sputum Anorexia; malaise Fever; nasal congestion; sore throat	Occurs most commonly in children and young adults, as well as in older adults in community hospital setting Rise in serum-complement-fixing antibodies to the organism	Erythromycin; tetracycline	Persisting cough, meningoencephalitis, polyneuritis, monoarticular arthritis, pericarditis, myocarditis
Viral pneumonia	Influenza viruses Parainfluenza viruses Respiratory syncytial viruses	Cough Constitutional symptoms may be pronounced (severe headache, an-	In majority of patients influenza begins as an acute coryza; others have bronchitis, pleurisy, etc., while	Treat symptomatically Does not respond to treatment with	Persons with underlying disease have increased risk of complications; primary in-

Table 7-2 Commonly Encountered Pneumonias (continued)

Type	Organism Responsible	Manifestations	Clinical Features	Treatment	Complications
	Rhinoviruses Adenovirus Varicella, rubella, rubeola, herpes simplex, cytomegalovirus, Epstein–Barr virus	orexia, fever, and myalgia)	still others develop gastrointestinal symptoms Risk of developing influenza related to crowding and close contact of groups of individuals	presently available antimicrobials Prophylactic vaccination recommended for high-risk persons (over 65; chronic cardiac or pulmonary disease, diabetes, and other metabolic disorders)	fluenzal pneumonia; secondary bacterial pneumonia
Pneumocystis carinii pneumonia	*Pneumocystis carinii*	Insidious onset Increasing dyspnea and nonproductive cough Tachypnea; progresses rapidly to intercostal retraction, nasal flaring, and cyanosis Lowering of arterial oxygen tension Chest x-ray will reveal diffuse, bilateral interstitial pneumonia	Usually seen in host whose resistance is compromised; seen also in male homosexual population Organism invades lungs of patients who have suppressed immune system (from cancer, AIDS, leukemia) or following immunosuppressive therapy for cancer, organ transplant, or collagen disease Frequently associated with concurrent infection by viruses, (cytomegalovirus) bacteria, and fungi	Pentamidine methanesulfonate Trimethoprim-sulfamethoxazole	Patients are critically ill Prognosis guarded, since it usually is a complication of a severe underlying disorder
Fungal pneumonia	*Aspergillus fumigatus*	Fever, productive cough, chest pain, hemoptysis Chest x-ray reveals broad range of abnormalities from infiltration to consolidation, cavitation, and empyema	Neutropenic individual most susceptible May develop *Aspergillus* as a superinfection	Amphotericin B; ketoconazole	High fatality rate Invades blood vessels and destroys lung tissue by direct invasion and vascular infarction

10. Persons over 50 have a higher fatality rate even with appropriate antimicrobial therapy.

▶ **NURSING ALERT:** Recurring pneumonia often indicates underlying disease (cancer of the lung, multiple myeloma).

Health Maintenance and Preventive Measures

1. Natural resistance should be maintained (adequate nutrition, rest, exercise).
2. Avoid contact with people who have upper respiratory infections.
3. Obliteration of cough reflex and aspiration of secretions should be avoided.
4. Adequate bronchial hygiene should be employed.
5. Immobilized patients should be turned every 2 hours and encouraged to breathe deeply, sigh, and cough.
6. Use every measure to reduce bacterial colonization and superinfection of the hospitalized patient.
7. Highly susceptible persons (elderly and chronically ill) should be immunized against influenza.
8. Pneumococcal vaccine should be given to those at greatest risk—persons over 50 with chronic systemic diseases, COPD, sickle cell anemia, absence of spleen, immunosuppression patients who have had a pneumonectomy.

Assessment
Clinical Manifestations

See Table 7-2, pp. 156–157.

Diagnostic Evaluation

1. Chest auscultation and percussion—listen for dullness to percussion, bronchial breath sounds, crackles.
2. Lateral and posteroanterior chest x-rays—to localize the process and determine presence or absence of fluid.
3. Gram stain, culture, and sensitivity studies of sputum.
4. Blood culture—to recover causative organism; bloodstream invasion (bacteremia) occurs frequently with bacterial pneumonia.
5. Thoracentesis—if pleural effusion is present.
6. Other serologic tests for *Legionella pneumophila*, psittacosis, etc.
7. Counter immunoelectrophoresis (CIE) and immunofluorescence microscopy—for immunologic detection of microbial antigens or their products.

Patient Problems/Nursing Diagnoses

1. Ineffective breathing patterns and cough related to infection of lung.
2. Potential for complications (pain, alteration in tissue perfusion, impaired gas exchange, fluid volume deficit) related to respiratory toxicity and pneumonic disease process.
3. Knowledge deficit of therapeutic and preventive program.

Planning and Implementation
Nursing Interventions

For patient with bacterial pneumonia:

A. Assessment

1. Take a careful history to help establish etiologic diagnosis.
   a. What was the mode of onset?
   b. Number, frequency, and duration of chills
   c. Description of chest pain
   d. Patient taking any recent antimicrobial drugs?
   e. Any family illness?
   f. Alcohol, tobacco, drug abuse?
2. Identify the etiologic agent causing the pneumonia and determine the drug sensitivity.
   a. Obtain freshly expectorated sputum for direct smear (gram stain) and culture.
      (1) Be sure the patient *coughs* up sputum, not saliva.
      (2) Instruct the patient to expectorate into sterile container for culture. The expectorate may become contaminated with colonizing upper respiratory flora.
   b. Utilize percussion (p. 150) with or without IPPB treatment as directed; tenacious sputum may be liquefied by inhaling nebulized aerosol of water or saline solution by mask.
   c. Aspirate trachea with catheter if patient is too ill to raise sputum (see Guidelines, p. 153).
   d. Sputum may also be collected by transtracheal aspiration (p. 145).
3. Give prescribed antimicrobial agent—the therapy of pneumonia depends on laboratory identification of the agent causing the infection and on the drainage of purulent secretions.

B. Clearing the bronchi of collected secretions—retained secretions interfere with gas exchange and may cause slow resolution (subsidence).

1. Encourage high level of fluid intake within limits of patient's cardiac reserve—adequate hydration thins mucus and serves as an effective expectorant; replaces fluid losses due to fever, diaphoresis, dehydration, and dyspnea.
2. Humidify air to loosen secretions and improve ventilation.
3. Encourage the patient to cough; avoid suppressing the cough reflex, especially in patients who sound "bubbly."
4. Employ chest wall percussion (p. 150) and postural drainage (p. 149) to mobilize secretions.
5. Utilize tracheal aspiration in patients with poor cough response.
6. Assist in bronchoscopic removal of inspissated (thickened) mucous plugs if patient is too weak to cough effectively.
7. Auscultate the chest for crackles.
8. Control cough when coughing is nonproductive and paroxysms cause serious hypoxemia; give moderate doses of codeine as prescribed.
9. Avoid hypoxemia, especially in patients with existing heart disease.

C. Careful and continuous observation of the patient until clinical condition improves

1. Remember that fatal complications may develop during the early period of antimicrobial treatment.
2. Monitor temperature, pulse, respiration, and blood pressure at regular intervals to assess the patient's response to therapy.
3. Listen to lungs and heart—heart murmurs or friction rub may indicate acute bacterial endocarditis, pericarditis, or myocarditis.
4. Assess for resistant fever or return of fever from:
   a. Drug allergy—usually skin eruptions appear 7–10 days after the beginning of treatment.
   b. Drug resistance or slow response to therapy.
   c. Inadequate or inappropriate antimicrobial therapy.
   d. Inadequate lung drainage.
   e. Superinfection (infection with a second organism resistant to antibiotics used).
   f. Failure of pneumonia to resolve; raises suspicion of underlying carcinoma of bronchus.
   g. Pneumonia caused by unusual bacteria, fungi, tuberculosis, or *Pneumocystis carinii.*
5. Obtain chest x-rays to follow resolution (subsidence) of pneumonic process.

D. Supportive modalities of treatment

1. Do blood gas analysis to determine oxygen need and patient response to the concentration of oxygen selected.
   An arterial oxygen tension (PaO_2) below 55 mm. Hg indicates hypoxemia.
2. Administer oxygen at concentration to maintain PaO_2 at acceptable level—hypoxemia may be encountered because of abnormal ventilation/perfusion ratios in affected lung segments.
3. Avoid high concentrations of oxygen in patients with chronic obstructive pulmonary disease (chronic bronchitis, emphysema)—*the use of high oxygen concentrations may worsen alveolar ventilation by removing the patient's only remaining ventilatory drive.*
4. Observe the patient for cyanosis, dyspnea, hypoxemia, and confusion.
5. Patients with pneumonia and coexisting chronic ventilatory insufficiency may require mechanical ventilation.
6. Relieve the pleuritic pain.
   a. Avoid suppressing a productive cough.
   b. Avoid narcotics in patient with history of COPD.
   c. Administer moderate doses of analgesics to relieve pleuritic pain.
   d. Treat dry cough and laryngospasm with aerosolized water produced by an ultrasonic nebulizer.
   e. Evaluate the patient's sensorium, before administering sedatives or tranquilizers, to assess for signs and symptoms suggestive of meningitis.

▶ **NURSING ALERT:** Restlessness, confusion, aggressiveness may be due to cerebral hypoxia. In such instances, sedatives are inappropriate.

7. Maintain adequate hydration, since fluid loss is high from fever, dehydration, dyspnea, and diaphoresis.
8. Encourage modified bed rest during febrile period.
9. Treat abdominal distention or ileus, which may be due to swallowing of air during intervals of severe dyspnea.
   a. Pass nasogastric tube for acute gastric distention.
   b. Use a rectal tube and give neostigmine methylsulfate to facilitate intestinal decompression.

E. Prevention of complications

1. Patients should respond to treatment within 24–48 hours. However, be on the alert for complications such as the following:

a. Pleural effusion
b. Sustained hypotension and shock, especially in gram-negative bacterial disease, particularly in the elderly
c. Delayed resolution
d. Superinfection: pericarditis, bacteremia, meningitis
e. Atelectasis—from obstruction of bronchus by accumulated secretions; may occur at any stage of acute pneumonia
f. Delirium—*this is considered a medical emergency*
g. Congestive heart failure, cardiac arrhythmias, pericarditis, myocarditis
h. Peripheral thrombophlebitis, with or without pulmonary emboli
i. Acute respiratory insufficiency

2. Employ special nursing surveillance for patients with the following conditions:
   a. Alcoholism or chronic obstructive pulmonary disease; these persons, as well as elderly patients, may have little or no fever.
   b. Chronic bronchitis; it is difficult to detect subtle changes in condition, since the patient may have seriously compromised pulmonary function.
   c. Epilepsy: pneumonia may result from aspiration following a seizure.
   d. Delirium, which may be caused by hypoxia, meningitis, delirium tremens of alcoholism.
      (1) Prepare for lumbar puncture; meningitis may be lethal.
      (2) Ensure adequate hydration and give mild sedation.
      (3) Give oxygen.
      (4) Delirium must be controlled to prevent exhaustion and cardiac failure.

3. Assess these patients for *unusual behavior,* alterations in mental status, stupor, and congestive heart failure.

Discharge Planning and Health Education

1. Fatigue, weakness, and depression may be prolonged after pneumonia.
2. Encourage chair rest after fever subsides; gradually increase activities to bring energy level back to pre-illness stage.
3. Encourage breathing exercises (p. 151) to clear lungs and promote full expansion and function after the fever subsides.
4. Explain that a chest x-ray is taken 4–6 weeks after discharge; should show cleared lungs.
5. It is wise to stop smoking. Cigarette smoking destroys tracheobronchial cilial action, which is the first line of defense of lungs; also irritates mucosa of bronchi and inhibits function of alveolar scavenger cells (macrophages).
6. Advise the patient to keep up natural resistance with good nutrition, adequate rest—one episode of pneumonia may make the individual susceptible to recurring respiratory infections.
7. Instruct the patient to avoid fatigue, sudden extremes in temperature, and excessive alcohol intake, which lower resistance to pneumonia.
8. Encourage the patient to obtain influenza vaccine at prescribed times. Influenza increases susceptibility to secondary bacterial pneumonia.
9. Encourage the patient to seek medical advice about

receiving pneumococcal vaccine against *Streptococcus pneumoniae,* which is effective against the majority of bacteremic pneumococcal diseases.

Evaluation
Expected Outcomes

1. Demonstrates improved respiratory function—normal blood gases, respiratory rates, breathing patterns
2. Is free of complications—diminished cough and sputum production, improved check x-rays, decline in fever
3. Adheres to therapeutic and preventive program—takes prescribed antimicrobial drug and does breathing exercises; stops smoking and verbalizes preventive measures

Aspiration Pneumonia

Aspiration is the inhalation of oropharyngeal secretions and/or stomach contents into the lungs. It may produce an acute form of pneumonia.

Etiology

Patients at risk and factors associated with risk:
1. Loss of protective airway reflexes—swallowing, laryngeal, cough
   a. Altered state of consciousness (general anesthesia, head injury, stroke, coma, convulsions)
   b. Alcohol; drug overdose
   c. During resuscitation procedures
   d. Seriously ill, debilitated patients
   e. Abnormalities of normal pharnygeal and gag reflexes
2. Nasogastric tube feedings
3. Obstetrical patients—from general anesthesia, lithotomy position, delayed emptying of stomach from enlarged uterus, labor contractions
4. Esophageal disease—hiatal hernia
5. Delayed emptying time of stomach—intestinal obstruction, abdominal distention
6. Prolonged endotracheal intubation/tracheostomy—can depress glottic and laryngeal reflexes from disuse

Prevention

1. Be on guard constantly and monitor patients at risk as described above.
2. Elevate head of bed for debilitated patients, for those receiving tube feedings, and for those with motor diseases of the esophagus.
3. Place patients with impaired reflexes in a lateral position.
4. Be sure that nasogastric tube is patent.
5. Give tube feedings slowly, with patient sitting up in bed. See page 414.
   a. Check position of tube in stomach before feeding.
   b. Check seal of cuff of tracheostomy or endotracheal tube before feeding.
6. Keep the patients in a fasting state before anesthesia (at least 8 hours).
7. Place the comatose patient on his side and elevate the foot of the bed 15–23 cm. (6–9 inches) unless medically contraindicated.

Assessment
Clinical Manifestations

1. Depends on volume and character of aspirated contents

a. Food particles—mechanical blockage of airways and secondary infection
b. Pathogenic bacteria—from oropharyngeal secretions containing bacteria
c. Gastric juice—destructive to alveoli and capillaries; results in outpouring of protein-rich fluids into the interstitial and intra-alveolar spaces—impairs exchange of oxygen and carbon dioxide, producing hypoxemia, respiratory insufficiency and failure
d. Fecal contamination—endotoxins may be absorbed or thick proteinaceous material found in the intestinal contents may obstruct airway, leading to atelectasis and secondary bacterial infection
2. Tachycardia/tachypnea
3. Dyspnea and cough
4. Cyanosis
5. Crackles, rhonchi, wheezing
6. Pink, frothy sputum (may simulate acute pulmonary edema)
7. Fever

▶ **NURSING ALERT:** The morbidity and mortality rate of aspiration pneumonia remains high even with optimum treatment. Prevention is the key to the problem.

Patient Problems/Nursing Diagnoses

1. Ineffective airway clearance and alteration in breathing pattern (dyspnea) related to aspiration of secretions or stomach contents into lungs
2. Impaired gas exchange
3. Potential fluid volume deficit
4. Potential for complications (infection, respiratory or metabolic acidosis)

Planning and Implementation
Nursing Interventions

A. Improvement of Respiratory Function

(The therapy depends on the material aspirated.)
1. Clear the obstructed airway.
   a. If foreign body becomes lodged in the patient's throat, remove object with forceps (see also p. 927).
   b. Place the patient in tilted head-down position on right side (right side more frequently affected if patient has aspirated solid particles).
   c. Suction trachea/endotracheal tube—to remove any particulate matter.
   d. Prepare for laryngoscopy/bronchoscopy if the patient is asphyxiated by solid material.
2. Correct hypoxia by immediate ventilation.
   a. Give oxygen.
   b. Place patient on assisted ventilation—if adequate PO$_2$ cannot be maintained with other means of administering oxygen (see p. 227).
3. Correct hypotension (usually the result of hypovolemia and hypoxia) by fluid volume replacement.

B. Prevention or Resolution of Complications

1. Monitor for fever, purulent sputum and x-ray evidence of pulmonary infiltrate.
2. Give supportive therapy as indicated.
   a. Antimicrobials—if there is evidence of superimposed bacterial infection; pulmonary infection usually occurs 1–2 weeks after initial insult.
   b. Correct acidosis—respiratory acidosis and meta-

bolic acidosis indicate a severe reaction due to aspiration of gastric contents.
   c. Monitor arterial blood gases.
3. Watch for development of later complications; lung abscess, necrotizing pneumonia, empyema.

Evaluation
Expected Outcomes

1. Demonstrates improved respiratory function: normal blood gases, respiratory rate, breathing pattern
2. Shows no signs of complications: no fever or acidosis, no coughing or dypnea, no evidence of pneumonitis on chest x-ray

Pleurisy

Pleurisy is a clinical term to describe *pleuritis,* (inflammation of the pleura).
Fibrinous pleurisy is deposition of a fibrinous exudate on the pleural surface.

Causes
May occur in the course of many pulmonary diseases:
1. Pneumonia (bacterial, viral)
2. Tuberculosis
3. Pulmonary infarction, embolism
4. Pulmonary abscess
5. Upper respiratory tract infection
6. Pulmonary neoplasm

Clinical Manifestations

1. Chest pain—becomes severe, sharp, and knife-like upon inspiration (pleuritic pain).
   a. Pain may become minimal or absent when breath is held.
   b. Pain may be localized or radiate to shoulder or abdomen.
2. Intercostal tenderness.
3. Pleural friction rub—grating or leathery sounds heard in both phases of respiration; heard low in the axilla or over the lung base posteriorly; may be heard only a day or so.
4. Evidence of infection; fever, malaise, increased white cell count.

Diagnostic Evaluation

1. Chest x-ray
2. Sputum examination
3. Examination of pleural fluid obtained by thoracentesis for smear and culture
4. Pleural biopsy (selected patients)

Treatment and Nursing Management

1. Implement treatment for the underlying primary disease (pneumonia, infarction, etc.). Inflammation usually resolves when the primary disease subsides.
2. Relieve the pain.
   a. Give prescribed analgesics.
   b. Splint the rib cage (Fig. 7-11, p. 180) when the patient coughs.
   c. Apply heat or cold—to provide symptomatic relief.
   d. Instruct the patient to lie on affected side occasionally—to splint chest wall.
   e. Assist with procaine intercostal block.
3. Watch for signs of development of pleural effusion (collection of fluid in pleural space): shortness of breath, pain, local decreased excursion of chest wall.

Pleural Effusion

Pleural effusion refers to a collection of fluid in the pleural space. It is rarely a primary disease, but is usually secondary to other diseases.

Etiology

Complication of:
1. Disseminated cancer (particularly lung and breast); lymphoma
2. Infection: tuberculosis, bacterial pneumonia, pulmonary infection
3. Congestive heart failure
4. Cirrhosis
5. Kidney disease
6. Others: sarcoidosis, systemic lupus erythematosus, peritoneal dialysis, etc.

Clinical Manifestations

(Usually caused by underlying disease)
1. Increasing dyspnea
2. Dullness or flatness to percussion (over areas of fluid) with minimal or absent breath sounds

Diagnostic Evaluation

1. Chest x-ray
2. Thoracentesis—biochemical, bacteriologic, and cytologic studies of pleural fluid
3. Physical examination
4. Pleuroscopy (visual exploration of pleural space through a thoracoscope inserted into the pleural space); pleural biopsy

Treatment

1. The treatment depends on the cause.
2. The following modalities of treatment have been advocated for malignant effusions.
   a. Thoracentesis (aspiration) for fluid removal and relief of dyspnea
      In malignant diseases, thoracentesis may provide only transient benefits since effusion may reaccumulate within a few days.
   b. Tube drainage (chest catheter) connected to underwater seal drainage system or suction; instillation of sclerosing agent (tetracycline; cytotoxic agent) into pleural space to obliterate pleural space by formation of adhesions between the visceral and parietal pleurae (*pleurodesis*).
      (1) Chest tube inserted into pleural space to drain the fluid and reexpand the lung.
      (2) Drug is introduced through tube into pleural space; tube is clamped; patient is helped to assume the following positions for 1–5 minutes each to ensure uniform distribution of the drug and maximize drug contact with pleural surfaces: prone, left side down, supine, right side down, knee to chest (if able).
      (3) Tube is unclamped as prescribed.
      (4) Chest drainage continued for 24 hours or longer.
      (5) Resulting pleural irritation, inflammation, and fibrosis causes fusion of the visceral and parietal surfaces when they are brought together by the negative pressure caused by chest suction.
   c. Radiation of the chest wall.
   d. Surgical procedures to control malignant effusions—parietal pleurectomy; pleural abrasion.

Lung Abscess

A *lung abscess* is a localized, pus-containing, necrotic lesion in the lung characterized by cavity formation.

Etiology

1. Aspiration of vomitus or infected material from upper respiratory tract
2. Aspiration of foreign body into lung
3. Bronchial obstruction (usually a tumor causes obstruction to the bronchus, causing distal stasis and infection of secretions, or there is necrosis within the tumor mass)
4. Necrotizing pneumonias
5. Tuberculosis
6. Pulmonary embolism

Clinical Features

1. The right lung is involved more frequently than the left—owing to dependent position of the right bronchus, the less acute angle which the right main bronchus forms within the trachea, and its larger size.
2. In the initial stages, the cavity in the lung may or may not communicate with the bronchus.
3. Eventually the cavity becomes surrounded or encapsulated by a wall of fibrous tissue, except at 1 or 2 points where the necrotic process extends until it reaches the lumen of some bronchus or pleural space and establishes a communication with the respiratory tract, the pleural cavity (bronchopleural fistula), or both.

Assessment
Clinical Manifestations

1. Cough
2. Fever and malaise—from segmental pneumonitis and atelectasis
3. Headache, anemia, weight loss
4. Pleuritic chest pain—from extension of suppurative pneumonitis to pleural surface
5. Production of mucopurulent sputum—often foul-smelling; blood streaking common; may become profuse after abscess ruptures into bronchial tree.

Diagnostic Evaluation

1. History of patient
2. X-ray of chest—for diagnosis and location of lesion
3. Direct bronchoscopic visualization—to exclude possibility of tumor or foreign body; bronchial washings and brush biopsy may be done for cytopathologic study
4. Bronchogram—may be necessary to differentiate between lung abscess and bronchiectasis
5. Leukocytosis in acute stage
6. Sputum culture and sensitivity—to determine causative organism(s) and antimicrobial sensitivity
7. Dullness and bronchial breath sounds—may be heard over diseased segment

Patient Problems/Nursing Diagnoses

1. Alteration in respiratory function (cough, dyspnea, sputum production) related to presence of suppurative lung disease
2. Alteration in comfort (chest pain and headache) related to underlying condition
3. Potential nonadherence to therapeutic regimen related to extended course of treatment
4. Potential for infection and nutritional imbalance

Planning and Implementation
Nursing Interventions

1. Carry out drainage procedures.
   a. Postural drainage (hastens resolution)—positions to be assumed depend on the segmental localization of the abscess (see p. 149).
   b. Percussion, coughing, and breathing exercises.
   c. Prepare patient for therapeutic bronchoscopy—to drain abscess.
2. Give appropriate antimicrobial based on culture and sensitivity studies of organisms—mixed infections are common and may require multiple antibiotics.
3. Measure and record the volume of sputum—to follow the course of healing.
4. Utilize supportive measures during the acute phase of illness.
   a. Support respiratory and cardiac function.
   b. Give a high-protein, high-calorie diet—chronic infections are associated with catabolic state, which requires calories and protein to facilitate healing.
   c. Care for the patient having blood component therapy—anemia may be advanced in the patient with infection.
5. Prepare the patient for serial radiographs—to judge effectiveness of therapy.
6. Prepare for surgical intervention if indicated—done only if the patient fails to respond to adequate medical treatment.
   a. Excision—usually lobectomy (occasionally segmental resection); usually performed when there is a thick-walled abscess with purulent drainage.
   b. Thoracotomy tube drainage—usually done for patients who cannot tolerate major thoracotomy (elderly, patients with alcoholism, and those with low pulmonary functional reserve).
   c. See page 179 for care of the patient having thoracic surgery.

Health Education

1. Teach the patient that an extended course of antimicrobial therapy (4–8 weeks) is usually necessary, depending on demonstration of improved/clear chest film.
2. Encourage the patient to have patience.
3. Encourage the patient to assume responsibility for attaining and maintaining an optimal state of health through a planned program of good nutrition, rest, and exercise.

Evaluation
Expected Outcomes

1. Achieves improved respiratory function: temperature in normal range, less purulent sputum coughed up, improved x-ray
2. Adheres to therapeutic regimen by taking antimicrobials and reporting for follow-up care

Bronchiectasis

Bronchiectasis is a chronic dilatation of the bronchi and bronchioles due to inflammation and destruction of their walls.

Causes

1. Pulmonary infections and obstruction of bronchi
2. Aspiration of foreign bodies, vomitus, or material from upper respiratory tract
3. Extrinsic pressure from tumors, dilated blood vessels, enlarged lymph nodes

Altered Physiology

Impairment of bronchial clearance → increased bronchial secretions → stasis → infection → weakening and further destruction of bronchial walls → increased dilatation → atelectasis → inflammatory scarring → fibrosis of involved areas → respiratory insufficiency → ventilation and perfusion imbalance → hypoxemia.

Health Maintenance and Prevention

1. Treat all respiratory infections promptly.
2. Teach the family to seek medical treatment and ongoing surveillance if child has recurrent respiratory infections; more than half of cases start in childhood.
3. All stuporous or comatose patients should be turned (prone position to lateral)—to drain all bronchial segments.
4. Encourage individual immunization program to prevent pertussis and measles (which can lead to bronchiectasis).

Assessment
Clinical Manifestations

The patient experiences symptoms when he has superimposed infection.
1. Persistent and/or productive cough with mucopurulent sputum
2. Intermittent hemoptysis
3. Recurrent fever and bouts of localized pulmonary infection/pneumonia
4. Crackles (rales) and rhonchi over involved areas
5. Dyspnea (depending on amount of lung tissue involved)
6. Wheezing
7. Clubbing of fingers (long-standing disease)

Diagnostic Evaluation

1. Chest roentgenogram (may reveal areas of atelectasis with widespread dilatation of bronchi)
2. Bronchogram (to map the entire bronchial tree to determine narrowing, dilatation, or obstruction of the bronchi)
3. Bronchoscopy—to rule out obstructive lesion
4. Sputum examination

Patient Problems/Nursing Diagnoses

1. Ineffective airway clearance and breathing patterns related to copious sputum production and irreversible dilation of the bronchial tree
2. Potential for infection
3. Potential for nonadherence to therapeutic regimen related to prolonged course of disease
4. Weight loss, weakness, dyspnea, and cyanosis related to advanced disease

Planning and Implementation
Nursing Interventions

1. Empty the bronchi of their accumulated secretions.
   a. Use postural drainage suitable to segment(s) involved to drain the bronchiectatic areas by gravity, thus reducing degree of infection and amount of secretions (see p. 149).
      (1) Postural drainage should be done for 20 minutes twice daily or more frequently as clinical condition indicates.
      (2) Affected chest area may be percussed or

"cupped" to assist in raising secretions (see p. 150).

b. Encourage copious fluid intake to reduce viscosity of sputum and make expectoration easier.
c. Utilize vaporizer to provide humidification and to keep secretions liquid.
d. Eliminate smoking and dusts, which are bronchial irritants that increase secretions.
e. Give expectorants and bronchodilator drugs when indicated. (See treatment of patient with emphysema, p. 164.)
f. Prepare patient for bronchoscopy when necessary to drain sputum and/or remove foreign body.

2. Implement treatment for the patient during periods of acute infection.
   a. Employ judicious antimicrobial therapy guided by sensitivity studies on organisms cultured from sputum.
   b. Patients with repeated infections may be given short courses of antimicrobials prophylactically during the winter months.

3. Prepare patient for surgical intervention when conservative treatment is inadequate.
   a. Segmental resection to spare as much healthy, functioning lung parenchyma as possible. (See p. 179 for principles of nursing following chest surgery.)
   b. Evaluate for postoperative complications.
      (1) Pneumonia
      (2) Empyema

Health Education

1. Instruct the patient to avoid noxious fumes, dusts, and other pulmonary irritants (cigarette smoking).
2. Teach the patient to monitor sputum. Report to physician/clinic if change in quantity (increase/decrease) or character occurs.
3. Instruct the patient and family about importance of pulmonary drainage.
   a. Teach drainage exercises and chest physical therapy techniques.
   b. Encourage postural drainage before rising in the morning, since sputum accumulates during night.
   c. Engage in physical activity throughout day to help move mucus.
4. Encourage regular dental care.
5. Emphasize the importance of influenza immunization.
6. See page 166 for other health teaching aspects (patient with emphysema).

Evaluation

Expected Outcomes

1. Demonstrates ability to clear airway of secretions
2. Breathes with increased ease
3. Adheres to therapeutic program: takes prescribed medications, carries out pulmonary drainage exercises, has regular check-up

Chronic Obstructive Pulmonary Disease (COPD)

Chronic obstructive pulmonary disease (COPD) is a term that refers to a group of conditions associated with chronic obstruction of airflow entering or leaving the lungs.
COPD includes:
1. Chronic bronchitis
2. Emphysema
3. Asthma (see p. 667)

Altered Physiology

1. Basically, the person with COPD may have:
   a. Excessive secretion of mucus and chronic infection within the airways not due to specific causes (bronchitis)
   b. An increase in size of air spaces distal to the terminal bronchioles, with loss of alveolar walls and elastic recoil of the lungs (emphysema)
   c. Narrowing of the bronchial airways that changes in severity (asthma, see page 667, since the triggering device in asthma is allergic in origin)
   d. There may be an overlap of these conditions.
2. As a result of these conditions, there is a subsequent derangement of airway dynamics (e.g., obstruction to airflow).

Causes of COPD (Emphysema–Bronchitis Complex)

1. Cigarette smoking
2. Air pollution
3. Occupational exposure
4. Allergy
5. Autoimmunity
6. Infection
7. Genetic predisposition
8. Aging

Chronic Bronchitis

Chronic bronchitis is a chronic infection of the lower respiratory tract characterized by excessive mucus secretion, cough, and dyspnea associated with recurring infections of the lower respiratory tract. There is often reduced ability to ventilate the lungs.

Altered Physiology

Infection, irritation, hypersensitivity → local hyperemia → hypertrophy of mucous glands → increase in size and number of mucus-producing elements in bronchi (mucous glands and goblet cells) → inflammation and changes in bronchial and bronchiolar walls.

Health Maintenance and Prevention

1. Avoid respiratory irritants, particularly tobacco smoke; chronic bronchitis is most often a smoker's disease.
2. Persons who are prone to respiratory infections should be immunized against influenza and *Streptococcus pneumoniae*.
3. Acute respiratory infections should be treated.

Clinical Features

1. A wide range of viral, bacterial, and mycoplasmal infections can produce acute exacerbations of bronchitis.
2. Exacerbations of chronic bronchitis are most apt to occur during winter months—patients have bronchospasm due to inhalation of cold air.
3. Secretions must be expelled; otherwise they produce chronic bronchial obstruction, air trapping, hypoxemia, carbon dioxide retention, and localized infection.
4. Chronic bronchitis often progresses to emphysema.
5. Hypoxemia may lead to right ventricular failure (cor pulmonale).

Clinical Manifestations

Usually insidious, developing over a period of years
1. Persistent bouts of cough and sputum production
2. Recurrent acute respiratory infections followed by persistent cough

3. Production of thick, gelatinous sputum (greater amounts produced during superimposed infections)
4. Wheezing and dyspnea as disease progresses

Diagnostic Evaluation

1. Chest roentgenogram—to exclude other diseases of the chest
2. Pulmonary function and arterial blood gas studies

Management

Goals:

Maintain patency of peripheral bronchial tree.
Facilitate removal of bronchial exudates.
Prevent disability.
See below (emphysema) for management, health education, and evaluation.

Pulmonary Emphysema

Pulmonary emphysema is a complex lung disease characterized by destruction of the alveoli, enlargement of distal airspaces, and a breakdown of alveolar walls. There is a slowly progressive deterioration of lung function for many years before the development of illness.

Causes

(See Causes of Chronic Obstructive Pulmonary Disease, p. 163.)

Clinical Manifestations

1. *Dyspnea;* slow in onset and steadily progressive
2. Cough—may be minimal, except with respiratory infection
3. Fatigue, sleep difficulties, irritability, anorexia, weight loss—due to hypoxia, increased respiratory muscular effort, and respiratory acidosis.

Diagnostic Evaluation

1. Clinical assessment of patient
2. History of cough, exertional dyspnea, wheezing, smoking, exposure to dusts, fumes, gases
3. Pulmonary function tests
4. Chest roentgenogram—abnormal only in advanced disease
5. Arterial blood gas analysis (with exercise if possible) to detect hypoxemia
6. Alpha$_1$-antitrypsin assay—useful in identifying person at risk

Complications

1. Respiratory acidosis
2. Cor pulmonale
3. Congestive heart failure
4. Spontaneous pneumothorax
5. Overwhelming respiratory infections
6. Cardiac arrhythmias
7. Profound depression
8. Malnutrition

Patient Problems/Nursing Diagnoses

1. Hypoxemia related to severe chronic obstructive pulmonary disease
2. Faulty breathing patterns related to effects of disease
3. Activity intolerance related to impaired pulmonary function and fatigue
4. Potential for infection related to compromised pulmonary function
5. Alteration in nutrition (less than body requirements) related to shortness of breath at meal times, loss of muscle mass, tenacious sputum, potassium depletion
6. Coping difficulties and emotional lability related to shortness of breath and fatigue
7. Sleep pattern disturbance related to hypoxia
8. Potential for nonadherence to the therapeutic program related to chronic nature of disease

Planning and Implementation

Nursing Interventions

A. **Removal of bronchial secretions to improve pulmonary ventilation and gas exchange**

1. *Eliminate all pulmonary irritants, particularly cigarette smoking.*
   a. Cessation of smoking usually results in decreased pulmonary irritation, sputum production, and cough.
   b. Avoid outside physical activities when air pollutants are high.
   c. Keep bedroom as dust-free as possible.
   d. Consider the use of air filters to remove particles and pollutants from air in areas where this is a problem.
   e. Use a room humidifier during winter months—allows dust particles to settle and makes air less irritating.
2. Control bronchospasm to decrease the work of breathing—many patients with chronic obstructive pulmonary disease have some degree of bronchospasm.
   a. Bronchospasm is detected by auscultation with a stethoscope.
   b. Administer prescribed bronchodilators, which dilate airways by relieving bronchial mucosal edema and smooth muscle contraction.
      (1) See page 188 for table of bronchodilators.
      (2) Drugs may be administered orally, subcutaneously, intravenously, or rectally; or via nebulization (by pressurized aerosols, hand-held nebulizers, pump-driven nebulizers, metered-dose devices, ultrasonic unit, or IPPB).
      (3) Assess patient for unwanted side effects—tremulousness, tachycardia, cardiac arrhythmias, central nervous system stimulation, hypertension.
      (4) Follow inhalation of bronchodilator drug with inhalation of moisture—to thin secretions.
      (5) Avoid excessive use of bronchodilators.
      (6) Auscultate the chest after administration of aerosol bronchodilators to assess improvement of air entry and reduction of adventitious breath sounds.
      (7) Assess if patient has reduction in dyspnea.
3. Keep secretions liquid.
   a. Encourage high level of fluid intake (8–10 glasses; 2–2½ liters daily) within level of cardiac reserve.
   b. Give inhalations of nebulized water to humidify bronchial tree and liquefy sputum.
4. Use postural drainage positions to aid in clearance of secretions, since mucopurulent secretions are responsible for airway obstruction.
   a. Positions that drain lower and middle lobes appear to be most helpful in patients with COPD.
   b. Other patients achieve effective cough and sputum clearance while seated and leaning forward.

    c. Employ percussion of thorax (p. 150) to assist in propulsion of sputum through the bronchi, when necessary.

5. Use controlled coughing.
    a. Inhale slowly and deeply.
    b. Exhale through pursed lips—empties lungs of residual volume.
    c. Cough in short bursts of "huffing" rather than vigorously forcing cough which causes airways to collapse.
    d. Inhale slowly.

6. Prepare patient for bronchoscopic removal of secretions if he is unable to cough and raise his sputum.

7. Prepare patient for endotracheal intubation or tracheostomy if indicated, to permit more effective suctioning of secretions and to provide ventilatory assistance.

▶ **NURSING ALERT:** Patients with acute respiratory failure along with acute ventilatory failure and rapid CO_2 retention will require mechanical ventilation.

B. Control of infection

1. Recognize early manifestations of respiratory infection—increased dyspnea, fatigue; change in color, amount, and character of sputum; nervousness; irritability; low-grade fever.

2. Obtain sputum for smear and culture.

3. Give prescribed antimicrobials (ampicillin; erythromycin; tetracycline) at first sign of respiratory infection to control secondary bacterial infection in the bronchial tree, thus clearing the airways.

4. Periodic sputum cultures for possible superinfection should be done for patients on long-term antibiotic therapy.

5. Advise patient to avoid exposure to persons with respiratory tract infections.

6. Give corticosteroids as prescribed; these drugs have an anti-inflammatory effect, and thus help to relieve airway obstruction.
    a. Short course of corticosteroids may be beneficial to persons who have acute attacks of bronchial obstruction, severe wheezing, or marked eosinophilia in sputum or blood.
    b. Antacids may be prescribed to prevent development of an ulcer.

▶ **NURSING ALERT:** Watch for increased susceptibility to infections, for gastrointestinal discomfort, and for bleeding tendencies.

C. Nutritional considerations

1. Dyspnea, with accompanying air swallowing, cough, and sputum production, combined with intake of medications, contributes to loss of appetite and weight loss. Nutritional depletion may influence rate of decline in lung function.

2. Encourage 6 small meals daily if patient is dyspneic—even a small increase in abdominal contents may press on diaphragm and cause dyspnea.

3. Offer high-protein diet with between-meal snacks to improve caloric intake and counteract weight loss.

4. Avoid foods producing abdominal discomfort.

5. Give supplemental oxygen while patient is eating to relieve dyspnea (when directed).

D. Relief of severe hypoxemia and related symptoms

1. Give low-flow oxygen to selected patients with severe, chronic, obstructive pulmonary disease—to correct hypoxemia in a controlled manner and thereby minimize CO_2 retention.
    a. In patients with COPD, poor exchange of gases may result in chronically elevated CO_2 (which is then a less effective stimulus to respiration). Giving a high concentration of oxygen may remove the hypoxic drive—leading to increased hypoventilation, respiratory decompensation, and the development of a worsening respiratory acidosis.
    b. Low-flow oxygen dosage is individualized and is given after analysis of arterial blood gases.
    c. Graded exercises with low-flow oxygen may be given to increase exercise capacity.

2. Avoid narcotics, sedatives, and tranquilizers. Watch for excessive somnolence, restlessness, aggressiveness, anxiety, or confusion which is frequently caused by acute respiratory insufficiency.

E. Techniques of breathing retraining to strengthen diaphragm and muscles of expiration and to decrease the work of breathing

1. Relaxation exercises—to reduce stress, tension, and anxiety.

2. Teach lower costal, diaphragmatic, and abdominal breathing (p. 151), using a slow and relaxed breathing pattern to reduce respiratory rate and decrease energy cost of breathing.

3. Use pursed-lip breathing (p. 152) at intervals and during periods of dyspnea to control rate and depth of respiration and improve respiratory muscle coordination.

F. Reconditioning of patient and increase in physical activity

1. Employ graded exercise and physical conditioning programs (enhances delivery of oxygen to tissues; allows functioning at a higher level of activity with greater comfort)—walking, stationary bicycle. Portable oxygen system for low-flow oxygen may be used for ambulation in selected patients—useful for patients with hypoxemia with marked disability

2. Encourage patient to carry out regular exercise training program to increase physical endurance and promote sense of well-being and independence.

3. Train patient in energy-saving methods.

G. Psychosocial support

1. Understand that the constant shortness of breath and fatigue makes the patient irritable, apprehensive, anxious, and depressed, with feelings of helplessness/hopelessness.

2. Assess the patient for reactive behaviors (anger, depression, acceptance).

3. Demonstrate a positive and interested approach to the patient.
    a. Be a good listener and show that you care.
    b. Be sensitive to his fears, anxiety, and depression; helps give emotional relief and insight.

4. Strengthen the patient's self-image.

5. Allow the patient to express his feelings and retain (within a controlled degree) the mechanisms of denial and repression.

6. Be aware that sexual dysfunction is common in patients with COPD.

7. Support spouse/family members.

Health Education

1. Give the patient a clear explanation of his disease, what to expect, how to treat and live with it.
   Reinforce by frequent explanations, reading material, demonstrations, and question and answer sessions.
2. Review with the patient the objectives of treatment and nursing management (pp. 164–165).
3. Work with the patient to set goals (i.e., stair climbing, return to work, etc.).

Instruct the patient as follows:

1. Avoid exposure to respiratory irritants—cigarette smoke, pollens, fumes, aerosols, dust, cold.
   a. Stop smoking and avoid smoke-filled rooms.
   b. Avoid sweeping, dusting, and exposure to paint, aerosols, bleaches, and other respiratory irritants.
   c. Keep kitchen ventilated.
   d. Stay out of extremely hot/cold weather to avoid aggravating bronchial obstruction and sputum production.
      (1) Keep a warming mask or scarf over nose and mouth to warm inspired air in cold weather.
      (2) Stay indoors with air conditioning when pollution level is high.
      (3) Try to avoid abrupt environmental changes.
      (4) Shower in warm (not too hot or too cold) water.
   e. Humidify indoor air in winter; maintain 30%–50% humidity for optimal mucociliary function.
2. Prevent and treat respiratory infections.
   a. Avoid exposure to persons with respiratory infections; a respiratory infection makes symptoms worse and can produce further irreversible damage.
   b. Avoid crowds and areas with poor ventilation.
   c. Take influenza immunization (if not allergic) to decrease likelihood of developing infection.
   d. Recognize and report evidence of respiratory infection *promptly* to the physician/clinic—chest pain, changes in character of sputum (amount, color, or consistency), increasing difficulty in raising sputum, increasing cough/wheezing, increasing shortness of breath.
   e. Take prescribed antimicrobial at first sign of infection.
      (1) Have a home supply available.
      (2) Have periodic sputum cultures when receiving long-term antimicrobial therapy.
3. Reduce bronchial secretions.
   a. Maintain an adequate fluid intake (8–10 glasses daily); mark down the amount of liquid consumed daily.
   b. Take bronchodilators only as directed.
   c. Follow postural drainage exercises as prescribed.
      (1) Stay in each position 5–15 minutes.
      (2) Utilize controlled cough after each position.
   d. Take medications prescribed for cough and expectoration.
   e. Avoid drugs that suppress cough and dry secretions (certain cough medicines, antihistamines).
4. Increase pulmonary ventilation.
   a. Use respiratory therapy consistently and faithfully.
      (1) Learn how to assemble and disassemble equipment.
      (2) Do the procedure immediately upon arising in the morning, before retiring, and as prescribed. Use the *exact* amount of medication prescribed.

      (3) Inhale and exhale as evenly as possible during the treatment.
      (4) Try to cough *productively* (with *controlled coughing*) after the treatment.
         (a) Breathe slowly and deeply, using diaphragmatic breathing.
         (b) Hold breath several seconds.
         (c) Cough—2 short, forceful coughs with the mouth open; the first cough loosens mucus, and the second cough moves it.
         (d) Pause and inhale by sniffing quietly. (Inhaling vigorously may initiate unproductive coughing, which is energy consuming.)
         (e) Rest.
      (5) Practice oral hygiene after each treatment.
      (6) Clean respiratory therapy equipment daily to prevent contamination and secondary infection and ensure equipment functioning.
         (a) Allow equipment to dry thoroughly before reassembling.
         (b) Do not re-use medications/solution/water left standing in a humidifier/nebulizer.
5. Do breathing exercises to strengthen muscles of expiration, to strengthen and coordinate muscles of breathing, and to lessen fatigue and to help empty lungs more completely.
   a. Learn the importance of slow and relaxed breathing (controlled breathing).
   b. Practice diaphragmatic breathing and pursed-lip breathing.
   c. Consciously use pursed-lip breathing during episodes of dyspnea and stress.
   d. Maintain muscle tone of the body by regular exercise.
6. Maintain general health at highest attainable level.
   a. Follow good habits of nutrition—patients with COPD may have loss of muscle mass with poor nutritional status, poor appetite, potassium depletion, sodium retention, and dehydration.
   b. Follow high-protein diet with adequate mineral, vitamin, and fluid intake.
   c. Avoid excessive hot or cold fluids/foods that may provoke an irritating cough.
   d. Avoid hard-to-chew foods (causes tiring) and gas-forming foods, which cause distention and restrict diaphragmatic movement.
   e. Eat 5–6 small meals daily—to ease shortness of breath during and after meals.
   f. Have rest periods before and after meals if eating produces shortness of breath.
   g. Do not eat when upset/angry.
   h. Avoid potassium depletion—patients with COPD tend to have low potassium levels; also patient may be taking diuretics.
      (1) Watch for weakness, numbness, tingling of fingers, leg cramps.
      (2) Foods high in potassium include bananas, dried fruits, dates, figs, orange juice, grape juice, milk, peaches, potatoes.
   i. Restrict sodium as directed.
   j. Use community resources (Meals on Wheels) if energy level is low.
7. Avoid activities that produce excessive shortness of breath.
   a. Live within the limitations that emphysema imposes.
   b. Learn to relax and work at a slower pace.

c. Obtain vocational counseling to secure a sedentary job if presently in a demanding manual job.

d. Avoid overfatigue, which is a factor in producing respiratory distress.

e. Adjust activities according to individual fatigue patterns.

f. Use pursed-lip breathing in a slow and relaxed manner during periods of breathlessness and physical exertion.

g. Try to cope with emotional stress as positively as possible—such stress triggers attacks of dyspnea.

h. Study individual life-style and avoid energy-wasting activities.

i. Exercise to improve physical condition.

8. Understand the importance of preserving existing function.

a. Become familiar with the nature of emphysema and reasons for a therapeutic program.

b. Accept the fact that therapy and medical supervision must be continued for a lifetime.

Evaluation
Expected Outcomes

1. Increases activity level: takes bronchodilators/medications as prescribed, demonstrates improved exercise tolerance (walks longer distances; climbs more stairs), identifies time when energy levels are high/low.

2. Avoids and seeks treatment for infection.

3. Improves nutritional status; times meals to coincide with periods of improved breathing; rests before and after meals.

4. Demonstrates some relief of hypoxemia with low-flow oxygen and graded exercises as prescribed.

5. Works to breathe more effectively; performs breathing exercises at scheduled periods.

6. Demonstrates improved emotional outlook; expresses feelings; seeks support group.

7. Adheres to therapeutic program for controlling respiratory environment, preventing infection, reducing bronchial secretions, increasing pulmonary ventilation, practicing breathing exercises, maintaining health, avoiding tiring activities, and continuing with follow-up care.

Pulmonary Heart Disease
(Cor Pulmonale)

Pulmonary heart disease (cor pulmonale) is an alteration in the structure or function of the right ventricle resulting from disease affecting lung structure or function or its vasculature (except when this alteration results from disease of the left side of the heart or from congenital heart disease). Cor pulmonale refers to heart disease caused by lung disease.

Etiology

1. Chronic obstructive pulmonary disease—chronic bronchitis, emphysema most common

2. Conditions that restrict ventilatory function—kyphoscoliosis

3. Pulmonary vascular disease—pulmonary emboli

Pathophysiology

Chronic obstructive pulmonary disease → hypoxia → hypercapnia → acidosis → circulatory complications → pulmonary hypertension → right heart enlargement → right heart failure.

Assessment
Clinical Manifestations

1. Increasing dyspnea and fatigue; progressive dyspnea (orthopnea, paroxysmal nocturnal dyspnea), chronic cough

2. Right heart enlargement demonstrated by:
   a. Physical examination
   b. ECG changes
   c. Chest x-ray—may show change in heart size

3. Peripheral edema

4. Manifestations of carbon dioxide narcosis—headache, confusion, somnolence, coma

Clinical Evaluation

1. Arterial blood gas analysis

2. Pulmonary function tests

Patient Problems/Nursing Diagnoses

1. Ineffective breathing pattern (dyspnea) related to right ventricular hypertrophy and pulmonary hypertension

2. Impaired gas exchange

3. Potential fluid volume excess

4. Activity intolerance

Planning and Implementation
Nursing Interventions

1. Improve ventilation and correct hypoxemia with its consequent pulmonary hypertension.
   a. Use oxygen with mechanical ventilatory aids or continuous low-flow oxygen to reduce pulmonary artery pressure and pulmonary vascular resistance.
   b. Monitor arterial blood gases as a guide in assessing adequacy of alveolar ventilation.
   c. Avoid central nervous system depressants (narcotics, barbiturates, hypnotics)—have depressant action on respiratory centers.
   d. See page 185 for management of respiratory failure.

2. Combat respiratory infection, which commonly precipitates pulmonary heart disease—respiratory infection causes carbon dioxide retention and hypoxemia, resulting in constriction of pulmonary arterioles and subsequent pulmonary hypertension.

3. Implement measures to treat heart failure when it exists.
   a. Reverse the patient's hypoxemia and hypercapnia. (See above treatment first in order to improve cardiac action.)
   b. Limit physical activity.
   c. Restrict sodium intake.
   d. Give diuretics to lower pulmonary artery pressure by reducing total blood volume.
   e. Watch electrolyte levels, especially potassium, as hypokalemia increases risk of arrhythmias.
   f. Give digitalis as prescribed if right ventricular failure is present. Digitalis is given with caution, since digitalis toxicity is a serious problem in management of respiratory failure because of hypoxemia, acidosis, and electrolyte abnormalities.
   g. Employ ECG monitoring when necessary—high incidence of arrhythmias in these patients.
   h. Administer vasodilators and beta-adrenergic drugs as directed.

Health Education

1. Emphasize the importance of stopping cigarette smoking; cigarette smoking is a major cause of pulmonary heart disease.

a. Query the patient about his smoking habits.
b. Inform the patient of risks of smoking and benefits to be gained when smoking is stopped.
2. Teach the patient to recognize and treat infections immediately.
3. Inform the patient of interrelationship between infection, air pollution, and cardiopulmonary disease.
4. Explain to the patient/family that restlessness, depression, and poor sleeping, as well as irritable and angry behavior, may be characteristic; patient should improve with rise in O_2 and fall in CO_2 levels in arterial blood gas values.
5. Explain that if the patient has chronic lung disease it may be necessary to have continuous low-flow oxygen therapy at home.

Evaluation
Expected Outcomes

1. Demonstrates improved respiratory function: decreased hypoxemia, improved breathing patterns, normal blood gas values, etc.
2. Demonstrates increased activity tolerance and less fatigue
3. Follows diet protocol for reducing salt intake

Pulmonary Embolism

Pulmonary embolism refers to the obstruction of one or more pulmonary arteries by a thrombus (or thrombi) originating somewhere in the venous system or in the right side of the heart, which becomes dislodged and is carried to the lungs.

Pulmonary infarction—necrosis of lung tissue that can result from interference with blood supply.

Predisposing Factors

1. Stasis of venous circulation, especially in blood vessels with injury to the endothelial lining—leads to intravascular clotting.
   Immobilization, sitting, prolonged standing contribute to venous stasis of lower extremities.
2. Injury to the vessel wall.
3. Hypercoagulability of the blood.
4. Septic foci related to drug abuse.
5. Most emboli originate in the deep veins of the lower extremities or pelvis, where they become detached and are carried to the lungs.

Health Maintenance and Prevention

1. Assess each patient with a high index of suspicion for pulmonary embolism.
2. Be aware of high-risk patients—immobilization, trauma to pelvis (especially surgical) and lower extremities (especially hip fracture), obesity, history of thromboembolic disease, varicose veins, pregnancy, congestive heart failure, myocardial infarction, malignant disease, postoperative patients, elderly.
3. Prevent stasis of blood in extremities due to dependent position of legs, prolonged sitting, immobility, constricting clothing.
   a. Encourage early mobilization and weight bearing.
   b. Elevate legs 15–20 degrees at intervals—to minimize stasis and increase venous return.
   c. Apply fitted elastic stockings—to increase blood flow to deep leg veins.
   d. Instruct the patient to wiggle toes, move feet, raise and lower legs frequently—to increase venous return.
   e. Do not allow the patient's legs and feet to dangle in a dependent position; have the patient place his feet on a chair when sitting on the edge of the bed (if bed is in a high position). Instruct the patient to avoid crossing the legs.
   f. External pneumatic compression of calves—boots alternately inflate and deflate to pump blood from calf veins; used postoperatively.
4. Avoid hemoconcentration and immobilization of patients confined to bed.
5. Encourage higher levels of fluid intake during periods of immobility.
6. Avoid leaving catheters in veins (parenteral therapy, measurement of central venous pressure) for prolonged periods.
7. Examine the patient's legs carefully, since thrombi frequently originate in deep veins of legs, particularly those of the calf. Assess for swelling of leg, duskiness, pain upon pressure over gastrocnemius muscle, pain upon dorsiflexion of the foot (positive Homan's sign).
8. Use agents for preventing venous thrombi and pulmonary embolism in high-risk patients; the approach depends on the patient's status.
   a. Oral anticoagulants (warfarin sodium)—antithrombotic agent useful in hip surgery.
   b. Low dose heparin—for patients over 40 undergoing major surgery.
   c. Antiplatelet agents (aspirin; dipyridamole).

Assessment
Clinical Manifestations

Underlying considerations
1. The size and location of the embolus determines the physiologic effect. Symptoms therefore vary from none to cardiovascular collapse.
2. The physiologic effects develop from pulmonary artery obstruction and heightened resistance to blood flow through partially obstructed vessels.
3. Small emboli tend to be multiple and recurrent.
4. Chest pain with apprehension and a sense of impending doom; occurs when most of the pulmonary artery is obstructed.
5. Dyspnea, pleuritic pain, cough; tachypnea.
6. Subtle deterioration in patient's condition with no explainable cause.
7. Pallor, cyanosis, tachyarrhythmias, clinical shock.
8. Engorgement of neck veins.
9. Pleural friction rub, accentuated pulmonic second sound, gallop rhythm.

▶ **NURSING ALERT:** Have a high index of suspicion if there is a subtle deterioration in the patient's condition and unexplained cardiovascular and pulmonary findings.

Diagnostic Evaluation

1. Physical findings: clinical signs and symptoms are elusive.
2. Arterial blood gases—systemic arterial hypoxemia is usually found, due to perfusion abnormality of the lung.
3. Radioisotope lung scans—perfusion scan investigates regional blood flow to determine presence of perfusion defects; ventilation scan may be done in patient with large perfusion defects.

4. Pulmonary angiogram (most definitive)—emboli seen as "filling defects."
5. Contrast phlebography or impedance phlebography—for detecting deep vein thrombosis of the legs.

Patient Problems/Nursing Diagnoses

1. Ineffective breathing pattern (dyspnea) related to acute increase in alveolar dead space and possible changes in lung mechanics from embolism
2. Alterations in tissue perfusion related to decreased blood circulation
3. Potential for recurrence
4. Potential for bleeding related to thrombolytic/anticoagulant therapy
5. Anxiety related to inability to breathe.

Planning and Implementation

Nursing Interventions

A. Restoration of pulmonary function

1. Provide respiratory assistance to eliminate hypoxemia.
   a. Oxygen via face mask or nasal catheter.
   b. Monitor vital signs, ECG, and arterial blood gases.
2. Give IV fluids and/or vasopressors to preserve right ventricular filling pressure and increase blood pressure.
3. Treat patient for heart failure when present.
4. Give analgesics and sedatives as directed for pain control and apprehension.

B. Preventing recurrence and extension of thromboembolism

1. Administer heparin (IV)—stops further thrombus formation and extends the clotting time of the blood; it is an anticoagulant and antithrombotic.
   a. IV loading dose usually followed by continuous pump or drip infusion or given intermittently every 4–6 hours.
   b. Dosage adjusted to maintain the activated partial thromboplastin time (PTT) at 1.5 to 2.5 times the pretreatment value (if the value was normal).
   c. Assess patient for untoward bleeding; major bleeding may occur from GI tract, brain, lungs, nose, and GU tract.
   d. Have protamine available to neutralize heparin during episodes of acute bleeding.
2. Give warfarin sodium (Coumadin) as anticoagulant (prevents formation and extension of stasis thrombi in the venous system); may be given simultaneously at the beginning or after 5–6 days of heparin therapy.
   a. Dosage is controlled by monitoring serial tests of prothrombin time; desired prothrombin time is 2 to 2.5 times normal value.
   b. Have phytonadione (Mephyton) available to counteract effects of prothrombin depressant drugs (warfarin sodium)—bleeding is the most important side effect.
   c. Anticoagulants may be contraindicated in certain situations: recent brain, spinal cord, joint, or urinary surgery; certain bleeding tendencies; fracture of pelvis or extremity; recent bleeding from peptic ulceration.
   d. Be aware that many drugs interact with anticoagulants.
3. Give thrombolytic agents (streptokinase; urokinase) as directed—lyse thrombi in deep venous system and emboli in pulmonary circulation, causing more rapid resolution of the thrombi/emboli and restoring pulmonary circulation to normal; improve circulatory and hemodynamic status.
   a. Effective in acute pulmonary embolism and thrombosis in popliteal and proximal deep veins.
   b. Administered intravenously in a loading dose followed by constant infusion.
   c. Limit invasive procedures (CVP line, arterial puncture, IM injections) during infusion to minimize bleeding.
      (1) Perform essential arterial blood gas studies on upper extremities; apply digital compression at puncture site for 30 minutes.
      (2) Apply pressure dressing to previously involved sites.
      (3) Maintain patient on strict bed rest during thrombolytic therapy.
      (4) Take vital signs every 4 hours during infusion.
      (5) Discontinue infusion in the event of uncontrolled bleeding.
   d. Thrombolytic therapy usually followed with heparin and warfarin treatment to prevent additional thrombus formation.
4. Prepare patient for surgical intervention when anticoagulation is contraindicated or has failed, or when the patient has a major embolization.
   a. Inferior vena cava interruption—reduces channel size to prevent passage of emboli and at the same time permits some blood to flow. One of the following may be done:
      (1) Plication with suture or clips.
      (2) Intraluminal obstruction achieved with umbrella filters, balloon catheters, trapping catheters. All methods of venacaval interruption may produce venous insufficiency of lower extremities with subsequent stasis and leg swelling.
   b. Embolectomy by:
      (1) Transvenous pulmonary embolectomy—transvenous suction catheter introduced into affected pulmonary artery to aspirate emboli.
      (2) Surgical removal of embolus from pulmonary artery; performed with cardiopulmonary bypass in patient with massive embolism with shock.

Health Education

1. See Preventive Measures, page 168.
2. Patient may have to continue taking anticoagulant therapy for 6 weeks to 6 months following his initial episode.
3. Female patients who have experienced thromboembolism should be advised against taking oral contraceptives.
4. Instruct the patient to watch for signs of overanticoagulation: bleeding gums, nosebleeds, bruising, hematuria, blood in stools, etc.
5. Patient should avoid taking any medications unless approved by physician, since many drugs interact with anticoagulants.
6. The patient should notify the dentist that he is on an anticoagulant.
7. Avoid inactivity for prolonged periods or sitting with legs crossed.

8. Wear a Medic-Alert bracelet identifying patient as anticoagulant user.
9. Lose weight if applicable; obesity is an important risk factor for women.

Evaluation

Expected Outcomes

1. Shows improved respiratory function: absence of dyspnea, tachypnea, or pleural friction rub; normal breath sounds upon auscultation
2. Demonstrates need to avoid bleeding: applies pressure to puncture site after laboratory tests; verbalizes the need for regular laboratory monitoring during treatment; participates in self-monitoring for bleeding (bruising, blood in urine/stools, etc.); wears identification bracelet
3. Prevents recurrence: takes prescribed anticoagulant to protect against further thromboembolism; avoids sitting for prolonged periods; avoids alcohol and over-the-counter drugs; wears gradient support stockings

Occupational Lung Diseases

Diseases of the lungs can occur in a variety of occupations as a result of exposure to organic or inorganic (mineral) dusts and noxious gases.

Altered Physiology

1. Effects of inhaling noxious particles, gases, or fumes depends on composition of inhaled substance, its antigenic (precipitating an immune response) or irritating properties, the dose inhaled, the length of time inhaled, and the host's response.
2. Exposure to inorganic dusts stimulates pulmonary interstitial fibroblasts, resulting in pulmonary interstitial fibrosis.
3. Noxious fumes may cause acute injury to alveolar wall with increasing capillary permeability and pulmonary edema.
4. Occupational lung diseases usually develop slowly (20–30 years) and are asymptomatic in the early stages.

Prevention and Health Maintenance

Goal:

Reduce exposure of workers to industrial products that may be hazardous to breathing.

1. Preserve, in every way possible, the general health of the worker/miner exposed to occupational dusts.
2. Enclose toxic substances, and reduce their concentration in the air.
   a. Engineering controls to reduce exposure
   b. Monitoring of air samples
3. Ventilate properly to reduce dust content of work atmosphere.
4. Have workers use protective devices (face masks, respirators, hoods, etc.).
5. Monitor workers who are exposed to high concentrations of industrial dusts.
6. Encourage workers to stop smoking.

Pneumoconioses

The *pneumoconioses* refer to a non-neoplastic alteration of the lung resulting from exposure to inorganic dust (e.g., "dusty lung") and the tissue reaction to its presence. The most common pneumoconioses are silicosis, asbestosis, and coal worker's pneumoconiosis.

Silicosis

Silicosis is a chronic pulmonary fibrosis caused by inhalation of silica dust.

A. Etiology and Altered Physiology

1. Exposure to silica dust is encountered in almost any form of mining because the earth's crust is composed of silica and silicates (gold, coal, tin, copper mining); also stone cutting, quarrying, manufacture of abrasives, ceramics, pottery, and foundry work.
2. When silica particles (which have fibrogenic properties) are inhaled, nodular lesions are produced throughout the lungs. These nodules undergo fibrosis, enlarge, and fuse.
3. Dense masses form in the upper portion of the lungs; restrictive and obstructive lung disease results.

B. Clinical Manifestations

1. Chronic productive cough
2. Dyspnea upon effort
3. Susceptibility to lower respiratory tract infections

C. Management

1. There is no specific treatment; the patient is treated symptomatically.
2. Give prophylactic isoniazid (INH) to patients with positive PPD skin tests; silicosis is associated with tuberculosis.
3. *Prevention:* See Prevention and Health Maintenance.

Asbestosis

Asbestosis is a diffuse pulmonary fibrosis caused by inhalation of asbestos dust and particles.

A. Altered Physiology

1. Asbestos fibers are inhaled and enter alveoli, which in time are eventually obliterated by fibrous tissue that surrounds the asbestos particles.
2. Fibrous pleural thickening and pleural plaque formation produce restrictive lung disease, decrease in lung volume, diminished gas transfer, and hypoxemia with subsequent development of cor pulmonale.

B. Etiology

1. Found in workers involved in manufacture, cutting, and demolition of asbestos-containing materials; there are over 4000 known uses of asbestos fiber (asbestos mining and manufacturing, construction, roofing, demolition work, brake linings, floor tiles, paints, plastics, shipyards, insulation).

▶ **NURSING ALERT:** Asbestosis is strongly associated with bronchogenic cancer, also with mesotheliomas of the pleura and peritoneum and probably with neoplasms in other sites.

C. Clinical Manifestations (may develop 20–40 years after exposure)

1. Dyspnea on exertion: severe, progressive, irreversible
2. Cough
3. Crackles heard at lung bases
4. Clubbing of fingers and toes; cor pulmonale

D. Treatment

1. No treatment will affect the progressive fibrosis. Most of the asbestos fibers already in the lungs will remain there.
2. Persuade persons who have been exposed to asbestos fibers to stop smoking. The risk of developing lung cancer for an asbestos worker who smokes is consid-

ered to be 50–100 times greater than that for a nonexposed nonsmoker.

3. Keep worker under cancer surveillance; watch for changing cough, hemoptysis, weight loss, melena, etc.
4. Continuous low-flow oxygen may be prescribed for patients with severe gas transport abnormalities.
5. *Prevention:* See Prevention and Health Maintenance.

Coal Worker's Pneumoconiosis

Coal worker's pneumoconiosis (CWP; "black lung") is a variety of respiratory disease found in coal workers in which there is an accumulation of coal dust in the lungs, causing a tissue reaction in its presence.

A. Altered Physiology

1. Dusts (coal, kaolin, mica, silica) are inhaled and deposited in the alveoli and respiratory bronchioles.
2. There is an increase of macrophages that engulf the particles and transport them to terminal bronchioles.
3. When normal clearance mechanisms no longer can handle the excessive dust load, the respiratory bronchioles and alveoli become clogged with coal dust, dying macrophages, and fibroblasts, which lead to the formation of the coal macule, the primary lesion of CWP.
4. As macules enlarge, there is dilation of the weakening bronchiole with subsequent development of focal or centrilobular emphysema.

B. Clinical Manifestations

1. Progressive dyspnea
2. Cough and sputum production; expectoration of varying amounts of black fluid

C. Management

1. There is no specific treatment; the treatment is symptomatic (e.g., bronchodilator drugs, antibiotics for infection).
2. See also treatment of emphysema, page 164.
3. *Prevention:* See page 170.

Cancer of the Lung
(Bronchogenic Cancer)

Bronchogenic cancer refers to a malignant tumor of the lung arising within the wall or epithelial lining of the bronchus. The lung is also a common site of metastasis from cancer elsewhere in the body via venous circulation or lymphatic spread.

Classification (according to cell type)

1. Epidermoid (squamous cell)—most common
2. Adenocarcinoma
3. Small (oat cell) carcinoma—usually widespread and not as resectable as other types
4. Large cell (undifferentiated) carcinoma

Predisposing Factors

1. Cigarette smoking—amount, frequency, and duration of smoking have positive relationship to cancer of the lung.
2. Occupational exposure to asbestos, arsenic, chromium, nickel, iron, radioactive substances, isopropyl oil, coal tar products, petroleum oil mists alone or in combination with tobacco smoke.

Health Maintenance and Prevention

1. Encourage patients to abstain from cigarette smoking.
   a. Teach by example.
   b. Refer patients to smoking cessation programs within the community.
   c. Continue efforts to discourage young people from starting smoking.
2. Maintain close watch of patients who are smokers—disease is insidious and exists before producing symptoms.

▶ **NURSING ALERT:** Suspect cancer of the lung in patients who belong to a susceptible age-group and who have repeated unresolved respiratory infections.

Assessment
Clinical Manifestations

Usually occur late and are related to size and location of tumor, extent of spread, and involvement of other structures.

1. Cough—especially a new type or changing cough
2. Hemoptysis
3. Wheezing or recent increase in shortness of breath
4. Thoracic discomfort; chest pain; hoarseness
5. Repeated infections of upper respiratory tract
6. Neural or humoral manifestations; hypertrophic pulmonary osteoarthropathy, Cushing's syndrome; hypoglycemia
7. Constitutional symptoms; weight loss, fatigue, anorexia (appear late)
8. Usual sites of metastases: lymph nodes, bone, brain, contralateral lung, and adrenal glands

Diagnostic Evaluation

1. Roentgenogram of chest—including fluoroscopy and tomography; lung cancers may be partly or completely hidden by other structures.
2. Cytologic examination of sputum/chest fluids for malignant cells.
3. Bronchoscopic evaluation (p. 140).
   Fluorescence bronchofiberoscopy—intravenous injection of a hematoporphyrin derivative given 72 hours before bronchoscopy; this is accumulated and retained in malignant tissue and emits a red fluorescence upon excitation by violet light during bronchofiberoscopy.
4. Lymph node biopsy; mediastinoscopy—to establish lymphatic spread; to plan treatment.
5. Lung, brain, and bone scans, if indicated.
6. Computed tomography—sensitive in detecting small pulmonary nodules and metastatic lesions.
7. Pulmonary function tests combined with split-function perfusion scan to determine if patient will have adequate pulmonary reserve to withstand surgical procedure.

Management

1. The treatment depends on the cell type, the stage of disease, and the physiologic status of the patient.
2. Treatment includes surgery (pneumonectomy, lobectomy, sleeve resection [removal of portion of a main bronchus with reestablishment of tracheobronchial continuity]), radiotherapy (p. 912), chemotherapy (p. 905), and immunotherapy (see below), used separately or in combination.

A. Immunotherapy

1. Patients with lung cancer tend to be immunosuppressed; severe immunodeficiency may exist before operation.

2. Immunotherapy may be tried to reverse this immunosuppression; in theory this may lead to tumor rejection.
3. Objective of immunotherapy: to restore or augment the normal mechanisms of host defense against the tumor cells or suppression of tumor cell proliferation.
4. Immunotherapeutic approaches:
   a. BCG (bacille Calmette Guérin), an immune stimulating agent, is injected into pleural space (either into clamped pleural drainage system, via thoracentesis), or via needle injection into peripheral lung tumor through a fiberoptic bronchoscope. Theoretical rationale: Immunostimulating agent is brought into contact with tumor antigens; also allows stimulation of regional lymph nodes draining tumor.
   b. Levamisole—theoretically restores depressed immune responses to normal.
   c. Transfer factors—material extracted from sensitized lymphocytes of lymphocyte donors; injected into patient to stimulate cell-mediated immunity.

Patient Problems/Nursing Diagnoses

1. Cough and dyspnea related to lung tumor, possible obstructive infection, superior vena cava obstruction, invasion of adjacent structures
2. Malnutrition related to hypermetabolic state, taste aversion, anorexia from radiotherapy/chemotherapy
3. Potential for complications
4. Anxiety and depression related to uncertain outcome and possible recurrence of disease

Planning and Implementation
Nursing Interventions

A. Relief of respiratory symptoms

1. Prepare patient physically, emotionally, and intellectually for prescribed therapeutic program.
2. Elevate head of bed to promote gravity drainage and prevent fluid collection in upper body (from superior vena cava syndrome).
3. Teach breathing retraining exercises to increase diaphragmatic excursion with resultant reduction in work of breathing.
4. Give appropriate treatment for productive cough (expectorant; antimicrobial agent) to prevent inspissated secretions and subsequent dyspnea.
5. Support patient undergoing removal of pleural fluid (by thoracentesis or tube thoracostomy) and instillation of sclerosing agent (p. 161) to obliterate pleural space and prevent fluid recurrence.

B. Improvement of nutritional status

1. Emphasize that nutrition is an important part of the treatment of lung cancer.
   a. Eat small amounts of high-calorie and high-protein foods frequently, rather than three daily meals.
   b. Eat major meal in the morning if rapidly becoming satiated and feeling full are problems.
   c. Be sure protein intake is adequate.
      (1) Substitute milk, eggs, chicken, fowl, fish, and oral nutritional supplements if aversion to meat is present.
      (2) Take prescribed vitamin supplement to avoid deficiency states, glossitis, and cheilosis.
2. Give enteral or total parenteral nutrition for malnourished patient who is unable or unwilling to eat.

C. Prevention of complications

1. Monitor for complications:
   a. Superior vena cava syndrome—interference in the return of blood through superior vena cava to the right atrium; manifested by facial and upper extremity edema, dyspnea/orthopnea and cough, dilated venous collateral channels
   b. Hypercalcemia, manifested by polyuria, nocturia, GI symptoms, mental obtundation, profound weakness
   c. Pleural effusion (see p. 161)
   d. Infectious complications, especially upper respiration infections

D. Other Nursing Interventions

1. See Health Education, below, for emotional support of patient.
2. Encourage sufficient hydration to thin secretions and to return calcium levels to normal if hypercalcemia is present.
3. Encourage patient to use muscles (range of motion and other exercises) to avoid complications of inactivity and disuse.
4. Use all known safeguards, including meticulous handwashing techniques, to reduce incidence of nosocomial infections since the patient with lung cancer tends to be immunosuppressed.

Health Education

A. Quality of Life

1. Focus on carrying on as normal a life as possible; an improved quality of life can be maintained.

B. Concerns About Pain

1. Realize that not every ache and pain is due to the results of lung cancer; some patients do not even experience pain.
2. Use aspirin or prescription medication as necessary. Do not be concerned about "addiction."
3. Radiation therapy may be used for pain control if tumor has spread to bone.
4. Report any new or persistent pain; it may be due to some other cause, such as arthritis.

C. Emotional Reactions

1. Shock, disbelief, denial, anger, and depression are all normal reactions to the diagnosis of lung cancer.
2. Try to have the patient express any concerns; share these concerns with health professionals.
3. Encourage the patient to communicate feelings to significant persons in his life.
4. Expect some feelings of anxiety and depression to recur during illness.
5. Encourage the patient to keep busy and remain in the mainstream. Continue with usual activities (work, recreation, sexual) as much as possible.
6. Secure services of a trained counselor if emotional stresses become overwhelming.
7. Talk to social service worker about financial assistance as money problems are a major concern to many.
8. Be aware that the American Cancer Society offers services and support modes to persons with cancer.

Evaluation
Expected Outcomes

1. Achieves relief of cough and dyspnea
2. Maintains nutritional balance; absence of excessive weight loss

3. Absence of preventable complications
4. Copes with emotional distress; communicates feelings about lung cancer

Chest Trauma

Chest trauma is an injury to the chest caused by any form of violence.

1. Chest injuries are potentially life-threatening because of (1) immediate disturbances of cardiorespiratory physiology and hemorrhage; and (2) later developments of infection, damaged lung and thoracic cage.
2. Patients with chest trauma may have injuries to multiple organ systems.
3. The patient should be examined for intra-abdominal injuries, which must be treated aggressively.

Altered Physiology

1. In penetrating injuries, some air escapes into the pleural space. (Negative intrapleural pressure is replaced by atmospheric pressure.)
2. The loss of normal negative pressure within the pleural cavity causes collapse of the lung.

Assessment

Clinical manifestations
1. Dyspnea
2. Asymmetric chest movement
3. Pain with breathing
4. Cyanosis

Emergency Management

Goal:
Restore normal cardiorespiratory function as quickly as possible.

This is accomplished by performing effective resuscitation while simultaneously assessing the patient, restoring chest wall integrity, and reexpanding the lung. The order of priority is determined by the clinical status of the patient.

Nursing Interventions

A. Relief of acute respiratory distress

1. Evaluate the status of the respiratory and circulatory systems.
   a. Examiner's ear is placed close to patient's mouth and nose, allowing him to listen at the airway, watch uncovered chest movements, and monitor pulse—this provides a rough estimate of the adequacy of ventilation.
   b. Assess for signs of obstruction, sternal retraction, stridor, wheezing, and cyanosis.
   c. Check neck for position of trachea, subcutaneous emphysema, and distended neck veins.
2. Establish and maintain an open airway and ventilation.
   a. Aspirate secretions, vomitus, and blood from nose and throat via:
      (1) Tracheal aspiration, if patient is unable to clear the tracheobronchial tree by coughing (p. 153).
      (2) Utilize endotracheal tube if patient is bleeding from nasopharynx or if trachea is injured (short-term use).
      (3) Employ bronchoscopic aspiration if necessary.
      (4) Prepare for tracheostomy if necessary.
         (a) Tracheostomy helps to obtain clear, dry tracheobronchial tree, helps the pa-

tient breathe with less effort, decreases amount of dead air space in the respiratory tree, and helps reduce paradoxical motion.
         (b) The use of a cuffed tracheostomy tube permits a closed system for air exchange when connected to a ventilator.
   b. Stabilize the chest wall.
   c. Free the pleural cavity of blood and air.
   d. Sucking chest wounds should be closed with an emergency dressing. The presence of lung injury and chest tube drainage must also be considered.
3. Control hemorrhage.
4. Treat for shock. (Shock may be due to blood loss, impairment of cardiorespiratory function.)
   a. Use one or more intravenous infusion lines; obtain blood for baseline studies.
   b. Restore blood volume to adequate levels—plasma expanders, electrolyte solutions.
   c. Give infusion rapidly.
   d. Monitor serial central venous pressure readings to prevent hypovolemia and circulatory overload (p. 286).
5. Apply electrodes for ECG monitoring—dysrhythmias are a frequent cause of death in chest trauma victims.
6. Assist with treatment of specific type of injury (see following discussion).
7. Ongoing nursing surveillance includes:
   a. Monitoring of arterial blood pressure, CVP, and respirations
   b. Arterial blood gas measurements—to determine need for mechanical ventilation
   c. Urinary output (hourly)—to evaluate tissue perfusion
   d. Thoracic drainage—to provide information about rate of blood loss, whether or not bleeding has stopped, whether surgical intervention is necessary
   e. ECG monitoring—for early detection and treatment of cardiac dysrhythmias
8. Complicatons of chest injuries: aspiration, atelectasis, pneumonia, mediastinal/subcutaneous emphysema, respiratory failure.

Types of Chest Injuries

A. Hemothorax

Blood in the pleural space as a result of penetrating or blunt chest trauma.

1. Blood in the pleural cavity produces a compression of the lungs and can result in hidden blood loss, causing signs and symptoms of shock.
2. Patient may be asymptomatic; or he may be dyspneic, apprehensive, or in shock.
3. Management
   a. Blood and air are aspirated via needle thoracentesis *or*
   b. An intercostal catheter (thoracotomy tube) is inserted and drainage instituted to accomplish more complete and continuous removal of blood and air—effects reexpansion of lung and permits monitoring of blood loss.
      The chest catheter is sutured in position and connected to a water-seal drainage-bottle.
   c. Record the volume of fluid drained into the collection-bottle hourly for the first several hours to alert for a sudden increase in drainage.
   d. Prepare for immediate blood replacement and thoracotomy if bleeding continues.

B. Pneumothorax

Air in the pleural space occurring spontaneously from injury or disease. In patients with chest trauma, it is usually the result of a laceration to the lung parenchyma, tracheobronchial tree, or esophagus.

The patient's clinical status depends on the rate of air leakage and size of wound.

1. Assessment
   a. Hyperresonance; diminished breath sounds
   b. Reduced mobility of affected half of thorax
2. Spontaneous pneumothorax
   a. May occur in healthy individuals; is usually due to rupture of a subpleural bleb of the lung.
   b. Treatment is generally nonoperative if pneumothorax is not too extensive; needle aspiration or chest tube drainage may be necessary to achieve reexpansion of collapsed lung.
   c. Surgical intervention (thoracotomy) is advised for patients with recurrent spontaneous pneumothorax.
3. Tension pneumothorax—buildup of pressure in the pleural space, resulting in compromise of ventilation; produces a collapse of the lung and decreased ventilation of other lung because of compression, and decreased venous return to the heart.
   a. Clinical picture is one of air hunger, agitation, hypotension, and cyanosis; there is an *acute threat to life.*
   b. Management
      (1) Insert chest tube drain immediately to allow air to escape (chest tube then connected to underwater-seal suction).
      (2) Use thoracentesis for emergency decompression of pleural space until tube thoracostomy can be accomplished.

C. Open pneumothorax (sucking wound of chest)

Implies an opening in the chest wall large enough to allow air to pass freely in and out of thoracic cavity with each attempted respiration; the rush of air through the hole in the chest wall produces a "sucking sound." This represents an acute threat to life.

1. When there is a large open hole in the chest wall, the patient will have a "steal" in ventilation of other lung.
2. A portion of the tidal volume will move back and forth through the hole in the chest wall rather than the trachea as it normally does.
3. Management
   a. Close the chest wound immediately to restore adequate ventilation and respiration.
   b. Instruct the patient to inhale and exhale forcefully against a closed glottis (Valsalva maneuver) as the pressure dressing (petrolatum gauze secured with elastic adhesive) is laid in place. (This maneuver helps to expand collapsed lung.)
   c. Prepare for chest tube insertion and drainage to permit evacuation of fluid/air and produce reexpansion of the lung. Surgical intervention may be necessary.
   d. If condition permits, place patient in semi-sitting position to permit greater ventilatory efficiency.

D. Fracture of Ribs and Sternum (most common chest injury)

▶ **NURSING ALERT:** Rib fractures should be regarded as potentially serious because they may result in underlying lung contusion. Older individuals with preexisting pulmonary disease may develop atelectasis and pneumonia following a rib fracture. If rib fragments are driven inward, there may be lacerations of the pleura, a pneumothorax, hemothorax, or hemopneumothorax.

1. Manifestations
   a. Localized tenderness or crepitus (crackling) over fracture site.
   b. Chest pain referred to the fracture site.
   c. Painful, shallow respirations (due to splinting of involved chest).
2. Management
   a. Give analgesics (usually non-narcotic) to assist in effective coughing and deep-breathing.
   b. Encourage deep-breathing with strong inspiration; give local support to injured area with nurse's hands.
   c. Assist with intercostal nerve block (see below)—to relieve pain so that coughing and deep breathing may be accomplished.
   d. For multiple rib fractures, epidural anesthesia may be used.

E. Flail Chest

Loss of stability of chest wall, with subsequent respiratory impairment. This is usually the result of multiple rib fractures or combined fractures of the sternum and ribs.

1. Pathophysiology
   a. When this occurs, one portion of the chest has lost its bony connection to the rest of the rib cage.
   b. During respiration, the detached part of the chest will be pulled in on inspiration and blown out on expiration (paradoxical movement).
   c. Normal mechanics of breathing impaired to a degree that seriously jeopardizes ventilation.
   d. Generally associated with some degree of lung contusion (see below).
2. Clinical manifestations
   a. Pain, dyspnea, cyanosis
   b. Paradoxical (reverse of normal) movements of involved chest wall
3. Management
   a. Stabilize the flail portion of the chest with the hands; apply a pressure dressing and turn the patient on his injured side, or place 10-pound sandbag at site of flail.
   b. If respiratory failure is present, prepare for immediate endotracheal intubation and ventilation therapy with controlled ventilation or positive-end expiratory pressure (PEEP)—treats underlying pulmonary contusion and serves to stabilize the thoracic cage for healing of fractures, improves alveolar ventilation, and restores thoracic cage stability and intrathoracic volume by decreasing work of breathing, *or*
   c. Thoracic epidural analgesia may be used for some patients to relieve pain and improve ventilation.
   d. See also treatment for lung contusion, which follows.

G. Pulmonary Contusion (lung contusion)

Damage to the lung parenchyma that results in leakage of blood and fluid into the interstitial space of the lung.

1. Clinical manifestations
   a. Tachypnea, tachycardia
   b. Crackles (rales) on auscultation
   c. Pleuritic chest pain

d. Copious secretions

e. Cough—constant, loose, rattling

2. Management (for moderate lung contusion)

   a. Employ endotracheal intubation and ventilatory support; place the patient on ventilator with low concentration of oxygen and positive-end expiratory pressure (PEEP)—to maintain the pressure and keep lungs inflated.

   b. Administer diuretics—to reduce edema.

   c. Correct metabolic acidosis with IV sodium bicarbonate.

   d. Utilize pulmonary artery pressure monitoring.

H. Cardiac Tamponade

Compression of the heart as a result of accumulation of fluid within the pericardial space.

1. Clinical manifestations

   a. Falling blood pressure

   b. Rising venous pressure/distended neck veins/elevated venous pressure

   c. Distant heart sounds

   d. Pulsus paradoxus (systolic blood pressure drops and fluctuates with respiration)

   e. Dyspnea, cyanosis, shock

▶ **NURSING ALERT:** A rapidly developing effusion interferes with ventricular filling and causes impairment of circulation. Thus, there is a reduced cardiac output and poor venous return to the heart. Cardiac collapse can result. In the patient with hypovolemia due to associated injuries, the venous pressure may not rise, thus masking the signs of cardiac tamponade.

2. Management (for penetrating injuries)

   a. Emergency thoracotomy to control bleeding and to repair cardiac injury.

   b. Pericardial aspiration (pericardiocentesis), aspiration or drainage of the pericardium (see p. 289); to transiently improve hemodynamic function enabling transfer to OR.

      (1) Repeated aspirations may be necessary.

Guidelines: Assisting with an Intercostal Nerve Block (Fig. 7-10)

An *intercostal nerve block* is the injection of a local anesthetic into the area surrounding the intercostal nerves to relieve pain temporarily following rib fracture(s), chest wall injury, or thoracotomy.

Purpose   To decrease pain and improve the patient's ability to cough.

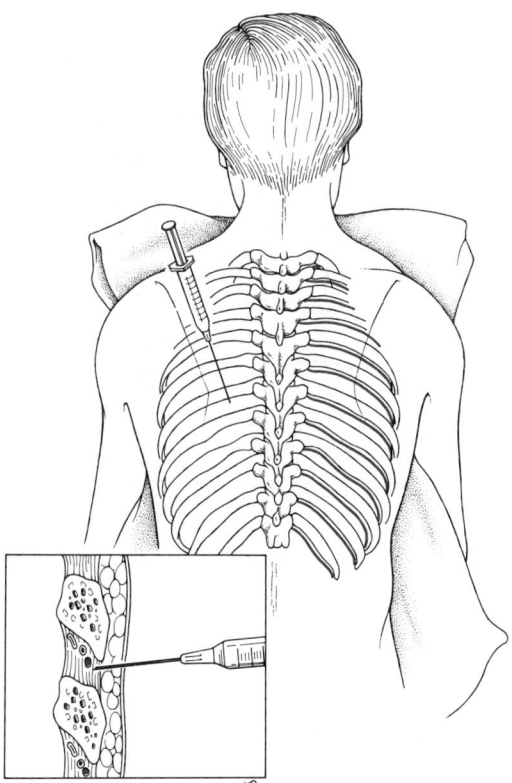

Figure 7-10. Intercostal nerve block.

(continued)

Guidelines: Assisting with an Intercostal Nerve Block (continued)

Equipment

Syringes, 10 ml. Luer–Lok
Needles, No. 22–30 gauge
Anesthetic solution (Xylocaine, bupivacaine, Pontocaine, procaine)
Skin germicide; sterile gloves

Procedure

Nursing Action	Rationale / Amplification
Preparatory Phase	
1. Inform the patient that he will experience the prick of the needle and a slight sensation of pressure.	
2. Position the patient according to the physician's preference:	
a. Have the patient sit up, bend forward, and hug a pillow, OR	a. This posture moves the scapulae forward and out of the way.
b. Place the patient prone with pillow under his chest, OR	b. The prone position helps immobilize the patient.
c. Have the patient lie on his unaffected side with his upper arm hanging over the side of the table.	c. This pulls the scapula out of the way.
3. Ask the patient to identify the site of pain.	3. To determine which intercostal nerves are to be injected.
Performance Phase (by the physician)	
1. After the skin is prepared, the lower margin of the rib is palpated and a small skin wheal is raised, using a 25–30 gauge needle.	1. This is infiltration anesthesia.
2. Usually nerve blocks are done at the posterior angle of the ribs between the posterior axillary line and the spine.	2. The posterior angle is the most prominent and accessible, and an injection at this area produces a block of the entire distal nerve.
3. A fine needle is advanced through the wheal and directed downward so that it slips under the edge of the rib into the upper portion of the interspace.	3. The intercostal nerve runs in a groove along the under-surface of the above rib.
4. The syringe (needle in place) is aspirated.	4. To ensure that the needle has not punctured the lung or that an intercostal vessel has been entered.
5. The local anesthetic (usually 3–5 ml.) is injected into the area.	5. Usually the local anesthetic is injected above and below the painful rib to obtain complete relief of pain, since the sensory fields of intercostal nerves overlap.
Follow-up	
1. Assess for relief of pain and less painful coughing.	1. This is the expected outcome.
2. Obtain a chest x-ray.	2. To ensure that a pneumothorax has not occurred.

Guidelines: Assisting with Tube Thoracostomy (Chest Tube Insertion)

A *tube thoracostomy* is the insertion of one or more flexible tubes into the pleural space to evacuate air, blood, or fluid collections.

Equipment

Tube thoracostomy tray:
  Syringes
  Needles/trocar
  Basins/skin germicide
  Sponges
  Scalpel/sterile drape/gloves
  Two large clamps

Suture material
Local anesthetic
Chest Tube (appropriate size); connector
Chest drainage system—connecting tubes and tubing, collection-bottles or commercial system, vacuum pump (if required)

Sites for Chest Tube Placement

For pneumothorax—2nd interspace along mid-clavicular or anterior axillary line
For pleural effusion or hemothorax—6th–7th lateral interspace in the mid-axillary line

Procedure

Nursing Action	Rationale/Amplification

Preparatory Phase

1. Assess patient for pneumothorax, hemothorax, presence of respiratory distress.

2. Obtain a chest x-ray. Other means of localization of pleural fluid include ultrasound and/or fluoroscopic localization.

    2. To evaluate extent of lung collapse or amount of bleeding in pleural space.

3. Assemble drainage system.

4. Reassure the patient and explain the steps of the procedure. Tell the patient to expect a needle prick and a sensation of slight pressure during infiltration anesthesia.

    4. The patient can cope by remaining immobile and doing relaxed breathing during tube insertion.

5. Position the patient as for an intercostal nerve block.

    5. See page 176.

Performance Phase (by the physician)

Needle or IntraCath Technique

A needle or IntraCath catheter is used for removal of small amounts of air or a minimal air leak from the lung.

1. The skin is prepared and anesthetized using local anesthetic with a short 25-gauge needle. A larger needle is used to infiltrate the subcutaneous tissue, intercostal muscles, and parietal pleura.

    1. The area is anesthetized to make tube insertion and manipulation relatively painless.

2. An exploratory needle is inserted.

    2. To puncture the pleura and determine the presence of air/blood in the pleural cavity.

3. The IntraCath catheter is inserted through the needle into the pleural space. The needle is removed, and the catheter is pushed several centimeters into the pleural space.

4. The catheter is taped to the skin.

    4. To prevent it from being pushed out of the chest during patient movement or lung expansion.

5. The catheter is attached to a connector/tubing and attached to a drainage system (underwater-seal or commercial system).

Trocar Technique for Chest Tube Insertion

A trocar catheter is used for the insertion of a large-bore tube for removal of a modest to large amount of air leak or for the evacuation of serous effusion.

1. A small incision is made over the prepared, anesthetized site. Blunt dissection (with a hemostat) through the muscle planes in the interspace to the parietal pleura is performed.

    1. To admit the diameter of the chest tube.

2. The trocar is directed into the pleural space, the cannula removed, and a chest tube inserted into the pleural space and connected to a drainage system.

    2. There is a trocar catheter available equipped with an indwelling pointed rod for ease of insertion.

Hemostat Technique Using a Large-Bore Chest Tube

A large bore chest tube is used to drain blood or thick effusions from the pleural space.

1. After skin preparation and anesthetic infiltration, an incision is made through the skin and subcutaneous tissue.

    1. The skin incision is usually made one interspace below proposed site of penetration of the intercostal muscles and pleura.

2. A curved hemostat is inserted into the pleural cavity and the tissue is spread with the clamp.

    2. To make a tissue tract for the chest tube.

3. The tract is explored with an examining finger.

    3. Digital examination helps confirm the presence of the tract and penetration of the pleural cavity.

4. The tube is held by the hemostat and directed through the opening up over the rib and into the pleural cavity.

5. The clamp is withdrawn and the chest tube is connected to a chest drainage system.

    5. The chest tube has multiple openings at the proximal end for drainage of air/blood.

6. The tube is sutured in place and covered with a sterile dressing.

Follow-up Care

1. Observe the drainage system for blood/air.
   Observe that there is free fluctuation in the tube upon respiration. (See water-seal drainage, p. 183.)

    1. If a hemothorax is draining through a thoracostomy tube into a bottle containing sterile normal saline, the blood is available for autotransfusion.

2. Secure a follow-up chest x-ray.

    2. To confirm correct chest tube placement and reexpansion of the lung.

3. Look for bleeding, infection, leakage of air and fluid around the tube.

Thoracic Surgery

▶ **NURSING ALERT:** Meticulous attention must be given to the preoperative and postoperative care of patients undergoing thoracic surgery. These operations are wide in scope and represent a major stress on the cardiorespiratory system; patients requiring thoracotomy often have preexisting pulmonary disease with a limited cardiopulmonary reserve.

Preoperative Care

Goals:

Determine if the patient can survive planned procedure.

Ensure optimal condition of the patient for surgery.

A. **Determine the preoperative status of the patient, his physical assets and liabilities.**

1. Assist the patient undergoing diagnostic studies.
   a. History and physical examination
   b. Chest roentgenograms
   c. Pulmonary function studies to ascertain if patient will have adequately functioning lung tissue postoperatively; incidence of postoperative pulmonary complications is closely correlated with preoperative pulmonary disease.
   d. Special diagnostic studies as required; radionuclide lung scanning may show if gas exchange will be affected by procedure.
   e. Baseline studies to ascertain any unsuspected abnormalities and to serve as a baseline reference during the postoperative period.
      (1) ECG—to disclose presence of atherosclerotic heart disease or conduction defect
      (2) Prothrombin time, partial thromboplastin time, platelet count—to confirm integrity of coagulation system
      (3) Blood urea nitrogen, serum creatinine—to obtain a "rough" measurement of renal function
      (4) Blood sugar or glucose tolerance—to detect unrecognized diabetes
      (5) Blood electrolytes, serum protein studies, and blood volume determinations as indicated
      (6) Arterial blood gas studies to determine presence of hypoxemia/hypercapnia
2. Nursing assessment of the patient.
   a. What signs and symptoms are present? (cough, expectoration, wheeze, hemoptysis, chest pain)
   b. What is his smoking history (amount and duration)? How much is he presently smoking?
   c. What is the patient's cardiopulmonary tolerance while bathing, eating, walking, etc.?
   d. What is the "physiologic age" of the patient? (general appearance, mental alertness, behavior, degree of nutrition)
   e. What other medical conditions exist?
   f. What is his breathing pattern?
   g. How much exertion is required to produce dyspnea?
   h. What are his personal preferences and dislikes?

B. **Improve alveolar ventilation and overall respiratory function.**

1. Encourage the patient to stop smoking, since this increases bronchial irritation.

2. Teach an effective coughing technique.
   a. Sit the patient upright with knees flexed and body bending slightly forward.
   b. Splint the incision with your hands; show the patient how to splint the painful area with firm hand pressure or support it with a pillow or folded towel while coughing.
   c. Instruct the patient to take three short breaths, followed by a deep inspiration, inhaling slowly and evenly through the nose.
   d. Instruct him to contract (pull in) his abdominal muscles and cough twice forcefully with his mouth open and tongue out.
   e. Have the patient lie on his side with his hips and knees flexed if he is unable to sit.
   f. "Huffing technique" for the patient with diminished expiratory flow rate or for the patient who refuses to cough:
      (1) Take a deep diaphragmatic breath and exhale forcefully against your hand; exhale in a quick distinct pant, or "huff."
      (2) Practice doing small "huffs" and progress to one strong "huff" while exhaling.
3. Employ all measures to minimize pulmonary secretions.
   a. Measure sputum daily in patients with large volume of secretions to determine if volume of secretion is decreasing.
   b. Encourage patient to cough effectively (see above).
   c. Humidify the air to loosen secretions.
   d. Administer bronchodilators for bronchospasm.
   e. Give antimicrobials for infection.
   f. Encourage deep breathing with the use of incentive spirometer or blow bottles.
   g. Teach diaphragmatic breathing preoperatively (see p. 151).
   h. Set up a schedule of breathing exercises that encourage the use of abdominal muscles.
   i. Carry out postural drainage in patients having increased mucus production (see p. 149).

C. **Evaluate cardiovascular and pulmonary status so that complications may be anticipated and prevented.**

1. Study the results of diagnostic tests to learn of existing deviations from normal.
2. Observe the patient and his reactions to various activities of daily living.
3. Give cardiac drugs to patients with congestive heart failure.
4. Correct anemia, dehydration, and hypoproteinemia—intravenous infusions, tube feedings, blood transfusions as indicated.
5. Give prophylactic anticoagulant (low-dose heparin) as prescribed to reduce perioperative incidence of deep vein thrombosis and pulmonary embolism.

D. **Prepare the patient for the surgical experience by offering reassurance, explanations, and skillful preoperative nursing care.**

1. Orient the patient to events in the postoperative period.
   a. Coughing with chest support and breathing routine

b. Presence of chest tube and drainage-bottles
c. Oxygen therapy; ventilator therapy
d. Measures used to control discomfort
e. Leg exercises and range of motion exercises for affected shoulder
f. Coping measures (breathing, turning, analgesics) for postoperative discomfort

2. Encourage expression of psychologic and safety needs.
3. See that consent form has been explained and signed.

Postoperative Care

Patient Problems/Nursing Diagnoses

1. Ineffective breathing pattern related to altered physiology secondary to opening the pleural cavity and ineffective airway clearance
2. Pain related to chest incision and presence of chest tubes
3. Impaired mobility of affected shoulder and arm related to location of incision and presence of chest tubes
4. Potential for complications

Planning and Implementation
Nursing Interventions

A. Maintenance of effective respiration and gas exchange

1. Maintain an open airway and assure adequate respiratory function.
   a. Look and listen at the patient's open mouth as he breathes for evidences of obstruction, and listen to his chest (auscultation) with a stethoscope.
   b. Monitor for adequacy of pulmonary function:
      (1) Measure PaO_2, $PaCO_2$, and tidal volume.
      (2) Use indwelling arterial line to facilitate drawing arterial blood samples and provide a continuous measurement of systemic arterial pressures.
   c. Most patients have endotracheal tubes in place with ventilatory support until adequate respiratory function and stable cardiovascular status is attained. Ventilatory weaning is started as early as possible.
   d. Aspirate all secretions with suctioning until the patient is able to raise secretions effectively—endotracheal secretions are present in excessive amounts in post-thoracotomy patients because of trauma to the tracheobronchial tree during operation, diminished lung ventilation, and diminished cough reflex.
      Excessive secretions will produce airway obstruction; air in the alveoli distal to the obstruction will become absorbed, and the lung will collapse.

▶ **NURSING ALERT:** Look for changes in color and consistency of aspirated sputum. Colorless, fluid sputum is not unusual; opacification or coloring of sputum may mean dehydration or infection.

2. Maintain continuing nursing surveillance of the patient's hemodynamic status:
   a. Take blood pressure, pulse, and respiration every 15 minutes or more frequently as indicated; extend the time intervals according to the patient's clinical status.
   b. Evaluate *character* of respirations and patient's color—depth of respiration is an important criterion in evaluating whether lungs are being adequately expanded.
   c. Auscultate and percuss chest frequently to determine adequacy of ventilation—detects early respiratory embarrassment.
   d. Monitor heart rate and rhythm via auscultation and ECG, since arrhythmias are more frequently seen after thoracic surgery.
      (1) Arrhythmias can occur anytime and contribute significantly to postoperative mortality rate.
      (2) *Rate of occurrence of arrhythmias increases with patients over 50 and with those undergoing pneumonectomy or esophageal surgery.*
      (3) Begin anti-arrhythmic measures immediately if indicated.
   e. Monitor the central venous pressure for prompt recognition of hypovolemia and for evidence of excessive fluid administration.
   f. Monitor cardiac output and pulmonary artery wedge or left atrial mean pressures.
   g. Elevate the head of the bed 30–40 degrees when patient is oriented and his blood pressure stabilized.

3. Maintain surveillance and careful management of the chest drainage system, which is used to eliminate any residual air or fluid following thoracotomy.*
   a. Chest tube(s) inserted at time of surgery to prevent fluid and air from accumulating in pleural or mediastinal space and to assist in reexpansion of remaining lung tissue.
   b. Check amount and character of drainage immediately postoperatively and at necessary intervals thereafter—drainage should progressively decrease after first 12 hours.
   c. The drainage is usually bloody immediately after surgery but becomes serous in 24 hours or so.
   d. Persistence of bloody drainage indicates bleeding. Prepare for blood replacement and possible reoperation to achieve hemostasis.
   e. See page 183 for summary of the nurse's role in the management of water-seal drainage.

4. Give humidified, warmed oxygen in immediate postoperative period to ensure maximum oxygenation—respirations are still depressed, and residual secretions in the peripheral respiratory passages may partially block gas exchange. Warming and humidification of inspired gases promotes ciliary action and prevents loss of body heat. Monitoring by means of arterial blood gas analysis is the most accurate method of detecting existing or impending hypoxemia.
   a. Assess for respiratory distress and a feeling of tightness in the chest.
   b. Watch for restlessness—often the first sign of hypoxia.

B. Pain relief

1. Provide intelligent pain relief—pain limits chest excursions, thereby decreasing ventilation.
   a. Severity of pain varies with type of incision and with the patient's reaction to and ability to cope

---

* A patient with a pneumonectomy usually does not have water-seal chest drainage, since it is desirable that the pleural space fill with an effusion, which eventually obliterates this space. Some surgeons do use a "modified" water-seal system.

with pain. Usually a posterolateral incision is the most painful.

b. Give narcotics (usually in frequent small doses) for pain relief, to permit patient to breathe more deeply and cough more effectively; place on oral analgesic as soon as possible.

c. Avoid depressing respiratory and vascular systems with too much narcotic; patient should not be so somnolent that he does not cough.

d. Assist patient having intercostal nerve block for pain control.

2. Position in bed correctly.

a. Position patient upright (15–30 degrees) if cardiovascular system is stable to facilitate optimal ventilation; allows diaphragm to descend and lung volume to increase; this also helps residual air to rise in upper portion of pleural space where it can be removed by the chest tube.

b. Patients with limited respiratory reserve may not be able to turn on unoperated side as this may limit ventilation of the operated side.

c. Vary the position from horizontal to semi-erect; remaining in one position tends to promote the retention of secretions in the dependent portion of the lungs.

3. Encourage and promote an effective cough routine (Fig. 7-11); a persistent and ineffective cough exhausts the patient, and retained secretions lead to atelectasis and pneumonia.

a. Sit the patient on side of bed with feet supported on a chair if his condition permits.

b. Support the chest firmly over the operated side and against opposite chest to lessen incisional pain or support the thorax with one hand pressing on the mid-sternum and the other arm around the back if there is a median sternotomy incision.

c. Instruct the patient to take a deep breath (to increase cough pressure), to pull in his abdominal muscles, and to cough vigorously.

d. Assist the patient to cough at least every 1–2 hours during the first 24 hours and when necessary thereafter.

C. Mobility of the affected shoulder

1. Restore normal range of motion and function of shoulder and trunk.
2. Encourage breathing exercises to mobilize thorax (p. 151).
3. Encourage skeletal exercises to promote abduction and mobilization of the shoulder.
4. Ambulate as soon as pulmonary and circulatory systems are compensated.
5. Encourage progressive activities according to diminution of fatigue.

D. Prevention of complications

1. Anticipate and forestall complications.
   a. Hypoxia; watch for restlessness, tachycardia, tachypnea, and elevated blood pressure

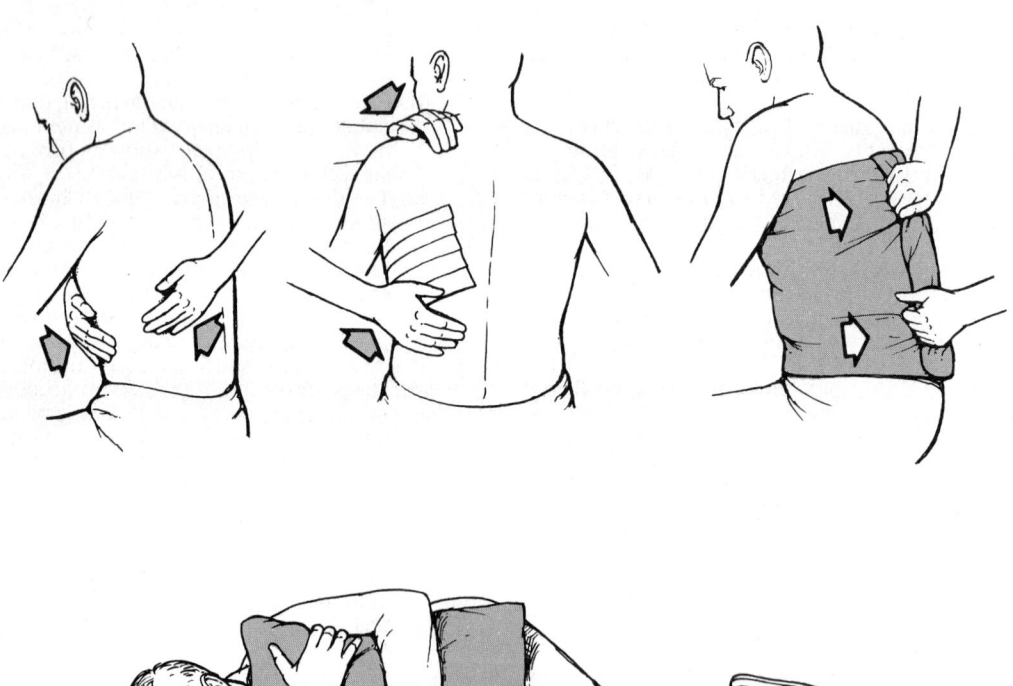

Figure 7-11. Promotion of an effective cough.

b. Postoperative bleeding; watch for restlessness, anxiety, pallor, tachycardia, and hypotension
c. Low cardiac output syndrome
d. Pneumonitis; atelectasis
e. Cardiac arrhythmias, myocardial infarction, pulmonary edema
f. Gastric distension
g. Renal failure

E. Other Nursing Interventions

1. Administer blood and parenteral fluids at a slower rate after thoracic surgery—pulmonary edema due to transfusion/infusion overload is an ever-present threat; following pneumonectomy, the pulmonary vascular system has been greatly reduced.
2. Continue to monitor blood gas and serum electrolyte values.
3. Monitor hourly urine output from indwelling catheter, since urine volume reflects cardiac output and organ perfusion.

Health Education

1. There will be some intercostal pain for a period of time, which can be relieved by local heat and oral analgesia.
2. Weakness and fatigability are common during the first 3 weeks following a thoracotomy.
3. Range-of-motion exercises for the arm and shoulder on the affected side should be carried out several times daily to avoid ankylosis of the shoulder ("frozen shoulder").
4. Carry out deep-breathing exercises for the first few weeks at home.
5. Consciously practice good body alignment, preferably in front of a full-length mirror.
6. The chest muscles may be weaker than normal for 3 to 6 months following surgery. Avoid lifting more than 20 pounds until complete healing has taken place.
7. Alternate walking and other activities with frequent short rest periods. Walk at a moderate pace and gradually extend walking time and distance.
8. Stop any activity immediately that causes undue fatigue, increased shortness of breath, or chest pain.
9. Because all or part of one lung has been removed, stay away from respiratory irritants (smoke, fumes, high level of air pollution).
   a. Avoid anything that may cause spasms of coughing.
   b. Sit in nonsmoking areas in public places.
10. Have an annual influenza injection (pneumonectomy patients).
11. Report for follow-up care by the surgeon or clinic as necessary.

Evaluation
Expected Outcomes

1. Maintains effective respiration: normal respiratory rate and blood gas measurements, absence of wheezes and crackles; able to cough up secretions
2. Achieves pain relief by requesting pain medication and splinting incision with hands when coughing
3. Attains/maintains mobility of affected shoulder: extends arm at hourly intervals; checks posture; consciously tries to use affected arm; ambulates increasing distances
4. Avoids preventable complications: absence of bleeding, hypoxia

Chest Drainage
Pathophysiology

1. The normal breathing mechanism operates on the principle of negative pressure (the pressure in the chest cavity is lower than the pressure of the outside air, causing air to move into the lungs during inspiration).
2. Whenever the chest is opened, from any cause, there is loss of negative pressure, which can result in collapse of the lung. The collection of air, fluid, or other substances in the chest can compromise cardiopulmonary function and even cause collapse of the lung, because these substances take up space.
3. Pathologic substances that collect in the pleural space include: fibrin, or clotted blood, liquids (serous fluids, blood, pus, chyle) and gases (air from the lung, tracheobronchial tree, or esophagus).
4. Surgical incision of the chest wall almost always causes some degree of pneumothorax. Air and fluid collect in the intrapleural space, restricting lung expansion and reducing air exchange.
5. It is necessary to keep the pleural space evacuated postoperatively and to maintain negative pressure within this potential space. Therefore, during or immediately after thoracic surgery, chest tubes are positioned strategically in the pleural space, sutured to the skin, and connected to some type of drainage apparatus to remove the residual air and drainage fluid from the pleural or mediastinal space. This assists in the reexpansion of remaining lung tissue.

Principles of Chest Drainage

1. A chest drainage system must be capable of removing whatever collects in the pleural space so that a normal pleural space and normal cardiopulmonary function may be restored and maintained.
2. There are many types of commercial chest drainage systems in use, most of which use the water-seal principle. The chest catheter is attached to a bottle, using a one-way valve principle. Water acts as a seal and permits air and fluid to drain from the chest, but air cannot reenter the submerged tip of the tube (Fig. 7-12).
3. Chest drainage can be categorized into three types of mechanical systems (Fig. 7-12):

A. The Single-Bottle Water-Seal System

1. The end of the drainage tube from the patient's chest is covered by a layer of water, which permits drainage of air and fluid from the pleural space, but does not allow air to move back into the chest. Functionally, drainage depends on gravity, on the mechanics of respiration, and, if desired, on suction by the addition of *controlled* vacuum.
2. The tube from the patient extends approximately 2.5 cm. (1 inch) below the level of the water in the container. There is a vent for the escape of any air that is drained from the lung. The water level fluctuates as the patient breathes; it goes up when the patient inhales and down when the patient exhales.
3. At the end of the drainage tube, bubbling may or may not be visible. Bubbling can mean either persistent leakage of air from the lung or other tissues or a leak in the system.

B. The Two-Bottle System

1. The two-bottle system consists of the same water-seal chamber, plus a fluid-collection bottle.

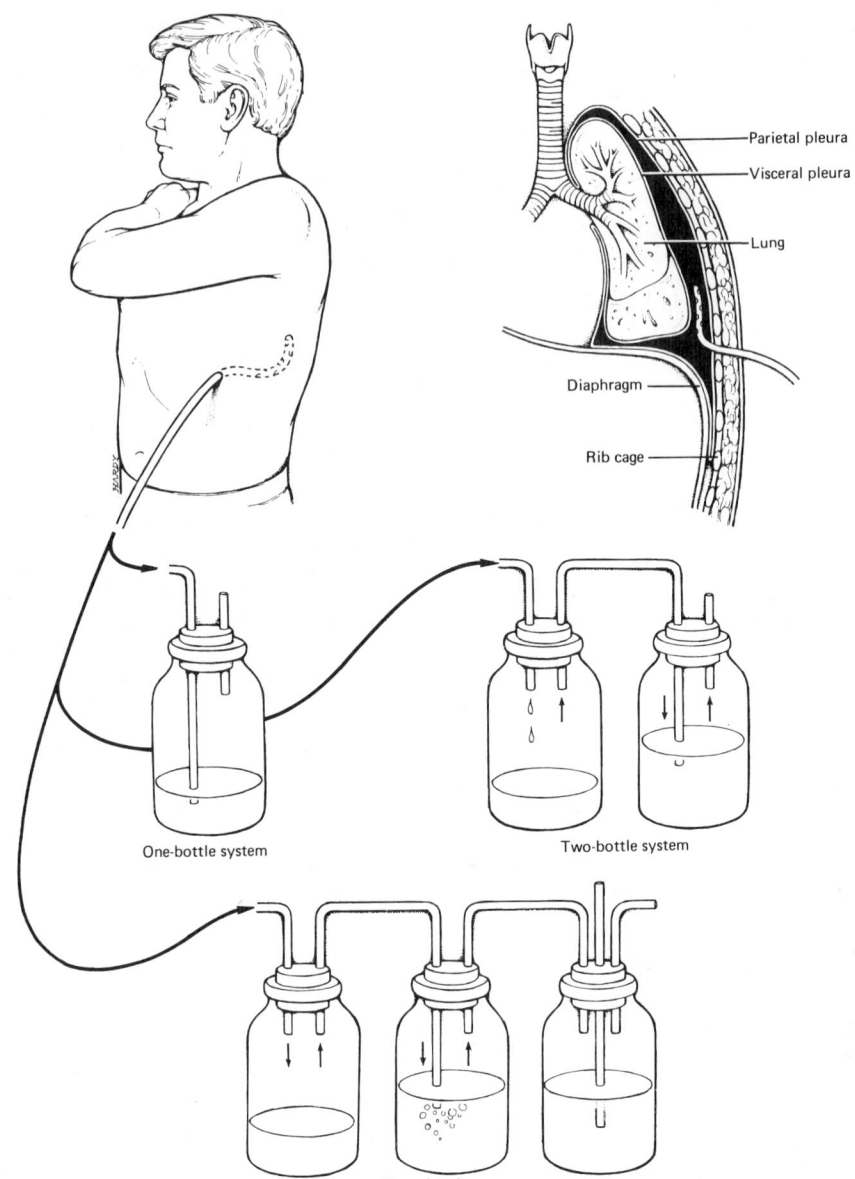

Figure 7-12. One-, two-, and three-bottle chest drainage systems.

2. Drainage is similar to that of a single unit, except that when pleural fluid drains, the underwater-seal system is not affected by the volume of drainage.
3. Effective drainage depends on gravity or on the amount of suction added to the system. When vacuum (suction) is added to the system from a vacuum source, such as wall suction, the connection is made at the vent stem of the underwater-seal bottle.
4. The amount of suction applied to the system is regulated by the wall gauge.

C. The Three-Bottle System

1. The three-bottle system is similar in all respects to the two-bottle system, except for the addition of a third bottle to control the amount of suction applied.
2. The amount of suction is determined by the depth to which the tip of the venting glass tube is submerged in the water.
3. In the three-bottle system (as in the other two systems), drainage depends on gravity or the amount of suction applied. The amount of suction in the three-bottle system is controlled by the manometer bottle. The mechanical suction motor or wall suction creates and maintains a negative pressure throughout the entire closed drainage system.
4. The manometer bottle regulates the amount of vacuum in the system. This bottle contains three tubes: (1) A short tube above the water level comes from the water-seal bottle; (2) another short tube leads to the vacuum or suction motor, or to wall suction; (3) the third tube is a long tube that extends below the water level in the bottle and opens to the atmosphere

outside the bottle. This tube regulates the amount of vacuum in the system, depending on the depth to which the tube is submerged—the usual depth is 20 cm. (7.6 inches).

5. When the vacuum in the system becomes greater than the depth to which the tube is submerged, outside air is sucked into the system. This results in constant bubbling in the manometer bottle, which indicates that the system is functioning properly.

Note: When the motor or the wall vacuum is turned off, the drainage system should be open to the atmosphere so that intrapleural air can escape from the system. This can be done by detaching the tubing from the suction port to provide a vent.

Guidelines: Managing the Patient with Water-Seal Chest Drainage*

An intrapleural drainage tube is used after most intrathoracic procedures. One or more chest catheters are held in the pleural space by suture to the chest wall and are attached to a drainage system.

Purposes
1. To remove solids, liquids and gas from the pleural space or thoracic cavity and the mediastinal space. (Liquids are serous fluid, blood, pus, and occasionally other fluids; gas and air from the lung, tracheobronchial tree, or esophagus.)
2. To bring about reexpansion of the lung and restore normal cardiorespiratory function after surgery, trauma, or medical conditions.

Equipment

Closed chest drainage system
Holder for drainage system (if needed)
Vacuum motor
Sterile connector for emergency use

Procedure

Nursing Action	Rationale/Amplification
1. Attach the drainage tube from the pleural space to the tubing that leads to a long tube with end submerged in sterile normal saline.	1. Water-seal drainage provides for the escape of air and fluid into a drainage bottle. The water acts as a seal and keeps the air from being drawn back into the pleural space.

2. Check the tube connections periodically. Tape if necessary.
  a. The tube should be approximately 2.5 cm. (1 inch) below the water level.
 	
  b. The short tube is left open to the atmosphere.
	2. Tube connections are checked to ensure tight fit and patency of the tubes.
	  a. If the tube is submerged too deep below the water level, a higher intrapleural pressure is required to expel air.
	  b. Venting the short glass tube lets air escape from the bottle.

3. Mark the original fluid level with tape on the outside of the drainage-bottle. Mark hourly/daily increments (date and time) at the drainage level.	3. This marking will show the amount of fluid loss and how fast fluid is collecting in the drainage-bottle. It serves as a basis for blood replacement, if the fluid is blood. Grossly bloody drainage will appear in the bottle in the immediate postoperative period and, if excessive, may necessitate reoperation. Drainage usually declines progressively after the first 24 hours.
4. Make sure that the tubing does not loop or interfere with the movements of the patient.	4. Fluid collecting in the dependent segment of the tubing will decrease the negative pressure applied to the catheter. Kinking, looping, or pressure on the drainage tubing can produce back pressure, thus possibly forcing drainage back into the pleural space or impedes drainage from the pleural space.
5. Encourage the patient to assume a position of comfort. Encourage good body alignment. When the patient is in a lateral position, place a rolled towel under the tubing to protect it from the weight of the patient's body. Encourage the patient to change his position frequently.	5. The patient's position should be changed frequently to promote drainage and his body kept in good alignment to prevent postural deformity and contractures. Proper positioning helps breathing and promotes better air exchange. Pain medication may be indicated to enhance comfort and deep-breathing.
6. Put the arm and shoulder of the affected side through range-of-motion exercises several times daily. Some pain medication may be necessary.	6. Exercise helps to avoid ankylosis of the shoulder and assist in lessening postoperative pain and discomfort.
7. "Milk" the tubing in the direction of the drainage bottle hourly. (Some polyvinyl tubes are too rigid to be "milked.")	7. "Milking" the tubing prevents it from becoming plugged with clots and fibrin. Constant attention to maintaining the patency of the tube will facilitate prompt expansion of the lung and minimize complications.

* There are numerous commercial disposable chest drainage devices available for collecting pleural fluid that use the water-seal principle.

(continued)

Guidelines: Managing the Patient with Water-Seal Chest Drainage (continued)

Procedure
(Cont.)

Nursing Action	Rationale/Amplification
8. Make sure there is fluctuation ("tidaling") of the fluid level in the long glass tube.	8. Fluctuation of the water level in the tube shows that there is effective communication between the pleural space and the drainage bottle, provides a valuable indication of the patency of the drainage system, and is a gauge of intrapleural pressure.
9. Fluctuations of fluid in the tubing will stop when: a. The lung has reexpanded b. The tubing is obstructed by blood clots or fibrin c. A dependent loop develops (see #4) d. Suction motor or wall suction is not operating properly	
10. Watch for leaks of air in the drainage system as indicated by contant bubbling in the water-seal bottle. a. Report excessive bubbling in the water-seal chamber immediately. b. "Milking" of chest tubes in patients with air leaks should be done only if requested by surgeon.	10. Leaking and trapping of air in the pleural space can result in tension pneumothorax.
11. Observe and report immediately signs of rapid, shallow breathing, cyanosis, pressure in the chest, subcutaneous emphysema, or symptoms of hemorrhage.	11. Many clinical conditions may cause these signs and symptoms, including tension pneumothorax, mediastinal shift, hemorrhage, severe incisional pain, pulmonary embolus, and cardiac tamponade. Surgical intervention may be necessary.
12. Encourage the patient to breathe deeply and cough at frequent intervals. If there are signs of incisional pain, adequate pain medication is indicated.	12. Deep breathing and coughing help to raise the intrapleural pressure, which allows emptying of any accumulation in the pleural space and removes secretions from the tracheobronchial tree so that the lung expands and atelectasis is prevented.
13. Stabilize the drainage-bottle on the floor or in a special holder. *Caution visitors and personnel against handling equipment or displacing the drainage-bottle.*	13. If any part of the apparatus is damaged, the closed system of drainage will be destroyed and the patient will be endangered by atmospheric pressure in the pleural space and resultant collapse of the lung. The drainage system must be kept airtight to reestablish negative intrapleural pressure.
14. If the patient has to be transported to another area, place the drainage-bottle below the chest level (as close to the floor as possible) if he is lying on a stretcher. If the tube becomes disconnected, cut off the contaminated tips of the chest tube and tubing, insert a sterile connector in the chest tube and tubing and reattach to the drainage system.	14. The drainage apparatus must be kept at a level lower than the patient's chest to prevent backflow of fluid into the pleural space.
15. When assisting the surgeon in removing the tube: a. Instruct the patient to perform the Valsalva maneuver (forcible exhalation against a closed glottis, holding one's breath) b. The chest tube is clamped and quickly removed c. Simultaneously, a small bandage is applied and made airtight with petrolatum gauze covered by 4 X 4-inch gauze and thoroughly covered and sealed with tape.	15. The chest tube is removed as directed when the lung is reexpanded (usually 24 hours to several days). During removal of the tube, the chief priorities are prevention of entrance of air into the pleural space as the tube is withdrawn and prevention of infection.

3: **Respiratory Function and Therapy**

Respiratory Function

Basic Terminology

1. *Ventilation*—movement of air in and out of the lungs by means of inspiration and expiration.
2. *Tidal volume* (V_T)—total volume of each breath.
   a. Normal: 7–8 ml./kg. of body weight.
   b. Not all of the tidal volume reaches the alveoli to participate in oxygen and carbon dioxide exchange.

   c. Dead space (V_D)
   (1) Portion of inspired air that remains in conducting airways from nose and mouth to bronchioles (not included in gas exchange).
   (2) Normal dead space: 150 ml.
   (3) Diseases that cause alveoli to lose venous blood flow add to dead space (pulmonary embolism, primary pulmonary hypertension, emphysema).

3. *Minute ventilation* ($\dot{V}_E$)—product of the amount of air moved per breath (V_T) and the number of breaths per minute. Consists of (1) alveolar ventilation ($\frac{2}{3}$), and (2) dead space ventilation ($\frac{1}{3}$).
4. *Vital capacity* (V_C)—maximum volume of gas that can be expelled from lungs by forceful effort following a maximal inspiration.
   a. Indicates patient's ability to take a deep breath.
   b. Normal: 70 ml./kg. of body weight.
   c. Reduction in vital capacity is important index of respiratory failure.
5. *Inspiratory force*—maximum negative pressure that the patient can exert against the occluded airway. (Minimum safe level—25 cm. H_2O.)
6. *Diffusion*—transfer of a gas from alveoli to blood. Occurs when tension exerted by gas in alveoli differs from that in the blood.
7. *Alveolar*—arterial gradient or difference (A-aDO_2); a measure of the difference between oxygen tension in the alveolar and arterial blood.
   a. Indicates efficiency of gas transfer; diseases that impair gas exchange increase the A-aDO_2.
   b. Normal: 10 mm. Hg.
   c. Increased in diseases involving the lung paren-

chyma and conducting airways. Extent of increase reflects amount of gas exchange impairment.
8. *Perfusion*—filling of the pulmonary capillaries with venous blood, which has returned to the heart from the general circulation and is pumped via the right ventricle to the lungs.
9. *Shunting*
   a. Normally 2% of the blood that is pumped to the lungs by the right ventricle bypasses the alveoli and does not participate in blood gas exchange.
   b. This blood is returned unoxygenated to the left heart and mixes with arterial blood.
   c. Increase in shunting occurs in atelectasis, pneumonia, pulmonary edema, and adult respiratory distress syndrome (ARDS).

Abbreviations

$PACO_2$—partial pressure of alveolar carbon dioxide
$PaCO_2$—partial pressure of arterial carbon dioxide
PAO_2—partial pressure of alveolar oxygen
PaO_2—partial pressure of arterial oxygen
FiO_2—fractional concentration of oxygen in the inspired air (ambient air 21% or 0.21)
For ventilatory function test symbols see Table 7-1, p. 145.

Respiratory Failure and Insufficiency

Lung Function

The major function of the lung is to supply oxygen and remove carbon dioxide. When gas exchange becomes inadequate, changes occur in the amount of O_2 and CO_2 transported in the arterial blood. Changes in arterial oxygen tension (PaO_2) and arterial carbon dioxide tension ($PaCO_2$) can be determined by analyzing a sample of the patient's arterial blood. The degree of change (mild, moderate, severe), parameters that change (PaO_2, $PaCO_2$, or both), and rapidity of change (acute, chronic) define the type of respiratory failure experienced.

Pathophysiology

The primary defect is impaired gas exchange. Development of respiratory failure can be conceptualized as a continuum, with progression from normal respiratory function → respiratory insufficiency → respiratory failure.

A. Respiratory Insufficiency

An alteration in the function of the respiratory system that produces clinical symptoms—usually includes dyspnea. The term signifies that respiratory function is abnormal but not sufficiently impaired to cause respiratory failure.

B. Respiratory Failure

An alteration in the function of the respiratory system that causes the PaO_2 to fall below 50 mm. Hg or the $PaCO_2$ to rise above 50 mm. Hg. Respiratory failure is determined by analysis of arterial blood drawn while the patient is at rest and breathing room air. Patients may experience three types of respiratory failure:
1. Oxygenation failure
   a. Characterized by a decrease in PaO_2 and a normal or decreased $PaCO_2$.
   b. Primary problem is inability to adequately oxygenate the blood, resulting in hypoxemia.

   c. Hypoxemia occurs because damage to the alveolar–capillary membrane, leakage of fluid into the interstitial space or into the alveoli slows or prevents movement of oxygen from the alveoli to the pulmonary capillary blood. Typically this damage is widespread, resulting in many areas of the lung being poorly ventilated or nonventilated. Consequences are severe ventilation–perfusion imbalance and shunt.
   d. Hypocapnia results from hypoxemia and decreased pulmonary compliance. Fluid within the lungs makes the lung less compliant (stiffer). This change in compliance reflexively stimulates the juxtacapillary receptors (J reflex) to increase ventilation. Ventilation is also increased as a response to hypoxemia. Ultimately, if treatment is unsuccessful, the $PaCO_2$ will increase, and the patient will experience both an increase in $PaCO_2$ and a decrease in PaO_2.
2. Ventilatory failure with normal lungs
   a. Characterized by an increased $PaCO_2$ and a decreased PaO_2 with normal or nearly normal lung function.
   b. Primary problem is insufficient respiratory center stimulation or insufficient chest wall movement, resulting in alveolar hypoventilation.
   c. Hypercapnia occurs because impaired neuromuscular function or chest wall expansion limits the amount of carbon dioxide removed from the lungs. In this type of respiratory failure, the primary problem is not the lungs. The patient's minute ventilation (tidal volume times the number of breaths per minute) is insufficient to allow normal alveolar gas exchange.
   d. Hypoxemia occurs as a consequence of hypercapnia. When the $PaCO_2$ rises, the PaO_2 must

fall unless increased amounts of oxygen are added to the inspired air.

3. Ventilatory failure with intrinsic lung disease
   a. Characterized by an increased $PaCO_2$ and a decreased PaO_2 with preexisting lung disease.
   b. Primary problem is acute exacerbation or chronic progression of previously existing lung disease, resulting in CO_2 retention.
   c. Hypercapnia occurs because damage to the lung parenchyma and/or airway obstruction limit the amount of carbon dioxide removed by the lungs. In this type of respiratory failure, the primary problem is preexisting lung disease—usually chronic bronchitis, emphysema or severe asthma. Respiratory rate and minute ventilation are normal or increased.
   d. Hypoxemia occurs as a consequence of hypercapnia. In addition, damage to the lung parenchyma and/or airway obstruction limit the amount of oxygen that enters the pulmonary capillary blood.

Respiratory failure may develop within minutes or hours, or over months or years. A sudden further deterioration in respiratory function may also occur in patients with long-standing respiratory failure. Several additional terms are used to describe these conditions:

C. Acute Respiratory Failure

1. Characterized by hypoxemia (PaO_2 less than 50 mm. Hg) or hypercapnia ($PaCO_2$ greater than 50 mm. Hg).
2. Occurs rapidly, usually in minutes to hours or days.

D. Chronic Respiratory Failure

1. Characterized by hypoxemia (decreased PaO_2) or hypercapnia (increased $PaCO_2$).
2. Occurs over a period of months to years—allows for activation of compensatory mechanisms.

E. Acute and Chronic Respiratory Failure

1. Characterized by an abrupt increase in the degree of hypoxemia or hypercapnia in patients with preexisting chronic respiratory failure.
2. May occur following acute bronchitis or pneumonia, or without obvious cause.
3. Extent of deterioration is best assessed by comparing the patient's present arterial blood gases with previous arterial blood gases (patient "normals").

▶ **NURSING ALERT:**

1. Arterial blood gases should be obtained whenever the history or physical examination suggests that the patient is at risk for developing respiratory failure. Optimally, these values should be recorded on a flow sheet so that comparisons can be made over time.
2. A slow deterioration in PaO_2 and $PaCO_2$ is better tolerated than a rapid change. For example, a patient with previously normal arterial blood gas values who suddenly develops a PaO_2 of 40 mm. Hg and a $PaCO_2$ of 60 mm. Hg will probably experience severe mental confusion or coma and arrhythmias. In contrast, a patient with chronic respiratory failure who typically has a PaO_2 of 50 mm. Hg and a $PaCO_2$ of 60 mm. Hg may experience only slight cognitive dysfunction and a morning headache. Sudden further deterioration would, however, cause more symptoms.

3. Frequent bedside measurements of respiratory rate, vital capacity, inspiratory force, and minute ventilation are helpful in following the progress of patients with ventilatory failure with normal lungs. Again, these data should be recorded on a flow sheet and values compared over time.

Etiology

Oxygenation failure (primary inability to oxygenate arterial blood)

1. Cardiogenic pulmonary edema (left ventricular failure; mitral stenosis)
2. Adult respiratory distress syndrome or ARDS (shock of any etiology; infectious causes—gram-negative sepsis, viral pneumonia, bacterial pneumonia; trauma—fat emboli, head injury, lung contusion; aspiration—gastric fluid, near drowning; inhaled toxins—oxygen in high concentrations, smoke, corrosive chemicals; hematologic disorders—massive transfusions, post cardiopulmonary bypass; metabolic disorders—pancreatitis, paraquat ingestion, uremia).

Assessment
Clinical Manifestations

1. Hypoxemia—PaO_2 will be low (<50 mm. Hg) on room air, and will increase minimally following administration of oxygen.
2. Hyperventilation—$PaCO_2$ will initially be low (25–35 mm. Hg). May become normal or increase (if treatment is ineffective).
3. Markedly increased A-aDO_2—reflects presence of shunt and severe ventilation–perfusion imbalance.
4. Low or normal pulmonary wedge pressure in ARDS; high wedge pressure in left heart failure.

Patient Problems/Nursing Diagnosis

1. Impaired gas exchange related to interstitial edema and alveolar flooding.
2. Potential alteration in fluid volume (excess or deficit) related to underlying disorder (see above).
3. Potential alteration in cardiac output (decreased) related to left ventricular failure.

Planning and Implementation
Nursing Interventions

1. Give specific treatment for underlying disorder (i.e., antibiotics for sepsis and pneumonia; cardiotonics and diuretics for pulmonary edema due to left ventricular failure).
2. Administer oxygen to maintain PaO_2 of 60 mm. Hg using devices that provide increased oxygen concentrations (aerosol mask, partial rebreathing mask, nonrebreathing mask).
3. If PaO_2 of 60 mm. Hg cannot be achieved with devices described above or if inspired oxygen concentration required is greater than 60% for 24 hours, patient may require intubation and the use of positive end-expiratory pressure (PEEP) with mechanical ventilation or continuous positive airway pressure (CPAP) without mechanical ventilation.
4. Monitor fluid balance by direct measurement of pulmonary capillary wedge pressure to detect presence of hypo/hypervolemia.

Evaluation

Expected Outcomes

1. Demonstrates reversal of symptomatology related to underlying disorder
2. Achieves normal PaO_2 and $PaCO_2$ without use of mechanical ventilation/supplemental oxygen
3. Maintains adequate cardiac output and fluid balance

Ventilatory Failure With Normal Lungs

Etiology

1. Insufficient respiratory center activity (drug intoxication—drug overdose, general anesthesia; vascular disorders—cerebral vascular insufficiency, cerebral tumor; trauma—head injury, increased intracranial pressure)
2. Insufficient chest wall function (neuromuscular disease—Guillain–Barré, myasthenia gravis, poliomyelitis, demyelinating disease, muscular dystrophy; trauma to the chest wall resulting in multiple fractures; spinal cord trauma; kyphoscoliosis)

Assessment

Clinical Manifestations

1. Hypoxemia and hypercapnia
2. Decreased vital capacity, decreased inspiratory force
3. Decreased respiratory rate (insufficient respiratory center activity) *or* increased respiratory rate (insufficient chest wall function)
4. Normal $A\text{-}aDO_2$—reflects lungs' ability to move O_2 and CO_2 normally in the absence of respiratory center/chest wall dysfunction.

Patient Problems/Nursing Diagnoses

1. Impaired gas exchange related to inadequate respiratory center activity or chest wall movement
2. Potential alteration in airway clearance related to inability to cough and breathe deeply
3. Impaired physical mobility related to underlying disorder (see above)

Planning and Implementation

Nursing Interventions

1. Give specific treatment for cause of respiratory failure (i.e., narcotic antagonist for narcotic or narcotic analogue intoxication, pyridostigmine for myasthenia gravis).
2. Initiate measures to prevent atelectasis and promote chest expansion (incentive spirometer, intermittent positive pressure breathing, out of bed, or head of bed elevated 30 degrees).
3. Monitor adequacy of alveolar ventilation by frequent measurement of respiratory rate, vital capacity, and inspiratory force.
4. If respiratory rate is >35/minute, vital capacity < 15 ml./kg. body weight, or inspiratory force is less than −25 cm. H_2O, the patient may require intubation and mechanical ventilation.

Evaluation

Expected Outcomes

1. Demonstrates reversal of symptomatology related to underlying disorder: achieves normal respiratory rate, vital capacity, and inspiratory force

2. Achieves normal PaO_2 and $PaCO_2$
3. Prevents development of atelectasis and secretion retention: coughs and breathes deeply at frequent intervals
4. Regains optimal physical mobility

Ventilatory Failure With Intrinsic Lung Disease

Etiology

1. Chronic obstructive pulmonary disease or COPD (chronic bronchitis, emphysema, cystic fibrosis).
2. Severe asthma.

Assessment

Clinical Manifestations

1. Hypoxemia and hypercapnia that is increased in relation to patient's normal values.
2. Use of accessory muscles (scalene, sternomastoid, and pectoralis) and intercostal retraction—reflects difficulty moving air through passages in bronchospasm or obstructed by secretions.
3. Crackles (rales) or wheezing—indicates fluid in alveoli and airways, bronchospasm.
4. Altered level of consciousness—indicates decreased cerebral perfusion.
5. Moderately increased $A\text{-}aDO_2$.

Patient Problems/Nursing Diagnoses

1. Ineffective airway clearance related to increased or tenacious secretions.
2. Impaired gas exchange related to lung parenchyma damage and/or airway obstruction.
3. Alteration in fluid volume (excess) related to right ventricular failure.

Planning and Implementation

Nursing Interventions

1. Administer oxygen at 24%–38% by Venturi mask, or 1–2 liters per minute by nasal cannula.
2. Begin intravenous fluids to reduce sputum viscosity.
3. Initiate measures to increase alveolar ventilation—bronchodilators to reduce bronchospasm (Table 7-3), corticosteroids to reduce airway inflammation, chest physical therapy to remove mucus, slow respiratory rate with pursed-lip breathing.
4. Give specific treatment for cause of the exacerbation (i.e., antibiotics for respiratory infection).
5. Initiate intubation and mechanical ventilation only if patient is apneic on admission—usually from sedative drugs or excessive oxygen concentration (>28%); patient becomes increasingly lethargic, cannot cough or expectorate secretions, or cannot cooperate with therapy; or pH falls below 7.25 and the P_aCO_2 continues to increase despite use of the above therapy.

Evaluation

Expected Outcomes

1. Demonstrates ability to clear airway of secretions (decrease in volume and tenacity of respiratory secretions)
2. Achieves blood gas values that are within the patient's normal limits
3. Demonstrates normal fluid balance

Table 7-3 **Drugs Commonly Used to Prevent or Reverse Bronchospasm**

Drugs/Administration	Pharmacologic Effects	Indications	Undesired Effects	Nursing Implications
Bronchodilators				
Aminophylline (intravenous injection)	Methyl xanthine compound—relaxes smooth muscle by increasing level of cyclic adenosine monophosphate	Acute exacerbation of asthma or bronchitis	CNS—irritability, restlessness, insomnia CV—palpitations, tachycardia, hypotension GI—nausea, vomiting, diarrhea	Too rapid administration can cause hypotension, extra systoles, muscle tremors. Administer at prescribed rate with an intravenous infusion pump.
Theophylline preparations (oral)	Methyl xanthine compound—relaxes smooth muscle by increasing cyclic adenosine monophosphate	Maintenance therapy for bronchospasm	CNS—irritability, restlessness, insomnia CV—palpitations, tachycardia, hypotension GI—nausea, vomiting, diarrhea	Teach patients to take at equal intervals throughout the day. To decrease GI irritation, take with milk or crackers.
Epinephrine (subcutaneous injection)	Sympathomimetic—acts on alpha (vasoconstrictor), $beta_1$ (cardiac stimulation), and $beta_2$ (bronchial smooth muscle relaxation) receptors	Acute exacerbation of asthma or bronchitis	Tachycardia, arrhythmias, elevation of blood pressure, headache, nausea, vomiting, paradoxical increase in bronchospasm	Use with extreme caution in patients who are elderly or who have heart or thyroid disease; stop treatment and monitor pulse and blood pressure if undesired effects occur.
Isoproterenol (metered-dose inhaler, solution for inhalation)	Sympathomimetic—acts on $beta_1$ and $beta_2$ receptors	Maintenance therapy for bronchospasm	Nervousness, tachycardia, palpitations, headache, nausea, tremors	Use with extreme caution in patients who are elderly or who have heart or thyroid disease; now used infrequently because of development of drugs with selective $beta_2$ activity.
Isoetharine (metered-dose inhaler, solution for inhalation)	Sympathomimetic—claimed to act more selectively on $beta_2$ than on $beta_1$ receptors	Maintenance therapy for bronchospasm	Nervousness, tachycardia, palpitations, headache, nausea, tremors	Although safer than the preceding drug, caution should still be used in patients with heart disease.
Terbutaline (oral, subcutaneous injection)	Sympathomimetic with selective $beta_2$ activity	Acute exacerbation of asthma or bronchitis (subcutaneous preparation) Maintenance therapy for bronchospasm (oral preparation)	Nervousness, tachycardia, headache, nausea (subcutaneous preparation) Hand tremors (subcutaneous and oral preparations)	Caution patients that hand tremors may occur. Tremors decrease with prolonged oral use.
Metaproterenol (oral, metered-dose inhaler, inhalant solution)	Sympathomimetic with selective $beta_2$ activity	Maintenance therapy for bronchospasm	Rare	Observe inhalation by patient to be certain that correct technique is used.
Albuterol (oral, metered-dose inhaler)	Sympathomimetic with highly selective $beta_2$ activity; longest acting aerosol bronchodilator	Maintenance therapy for bronchospasm	Rare	Observe inhalation by patient to be certain that correct technique is used.
Corticosteroids				
Hydrocortisone/prednisone (intravenous injection, oral preparation)	Potent anti-inflammatory activity	Acute exacerbation of asthma or bronchitis (IV preparation) Maintenance therapy (oral preparation)	CNS—depression, euphoria GI—gastric irritation, peptic ulcer Metabolic—hypernatremia, hypokalemia	Should not be abruptly discontinued, since causes supression of adrenal function.
Beclomethasone (metered-dose inhaler)	Synthetic corticosteroid with potent anti-inflammatory activity; effective only by inhalation	Steroid dependent asthma (alternative to use of oral steroids)	Oral candidiasis Systemic side effects associated with oral steroids do not occur	Inhaled as a powder. May precipitate bronchospasm in acute exacerbation. Not used with status asthmaticus or acute asthma episodes.
Miscellaneous				
Cromolyn sodium (solution for inhalation, powder used with special inhaler)	Inhibits release of histamine from mast cells in the respiratory tract, *prevents* bronchospasm Not effective in acute attack; must be used for 2–4 weeks to show effectiveness	Maintenance therapy for asthma	Cough, bronchospasm	Should not be used with status asthmaticus or acute asthma episodes. May be given in combination with bronchodilator if administration causes bronchospasm.

Oxygen Therapy

General Considerations

1. Oxygen is an odorless, tasteless, colorless, transparent gas that is slightly heavier than air.
2. Because oxygen supports combustion, there is always danger of fire when oxygen is being used.

   a. Avoid using oil or grease around oxygen connections.
   b. Eliminate antiseptic tinctures, alcohol, and ether in immediate oxygen environment.
   c. Do not permit any electrical devices (radios,

heating pads, electric razors) in or near an oxygen tent.
  d. Keep the oxygen cylinder (if used) secured in an upright position away from heat.
  e. Post "NO SMOKING" signs on the patient's door and in view of the patient's visitors.
  f. Have a fire extinguisher available.
3. Oxygen can be dispensed from a cylinder, piped-in system, liquid oxygen reservoir, or oxygen concentrator. Oxygen supplied to the patient is controlled by using:
  a. Reduction gauge—reduces pressure to that of the atmosphere.
  b. Flow meter (flow gauge, flow control)—regulates control of oxygen in liters per minute.
4. Oxygen is given to relieve hypoxemia or hypoxia.
  a. *Hypoxemia*—present when the oxygen tension in arterial blood is below normal.
  b. *Hypoxia*—present when there is an insufficient amount of oxygen available in the tissue cells to meet the requirements of an organ or tissue at that moment.

Assessment

1. Suspect need for oxygen when patients predisposed to impaired gas exchange have:
  a. Tachypnea
  b. Tachycardia or arrhythmias (premature ventricular contractions)
  c. A change in level of consciousness (symptoms of decreased cerebral oxygenation are irritability, confusion, lethargy, and coma, if untreated)
2. Early use of oxygen therapy may prevent development of:
  a. Cyanosis—occurs as a late sign ($PaO_2 \leq 45$ mm. Hg)
  b. Labored respirations—indicates severe respiratory distress
  c. Myocardial stress—increase in heart rate and stroke volume (cardiac output) is the primary mechanism for compensation for hypoxemia or hypoxia
3. Measurement of the arterial blood gases is the best method of determining the need for and adequacy of oxygen therapy (p. 143).

Planning and Implementation
Nursing Interventions

1. Select the appropriate form of oxygen therapy after obtaining arterial blood gases and assessing the patient's current oxygenation status and acid–base balance. Choices are:
  a. Low concentration—appropriate for patients prone to retain carbon dioxide (chronic obstructive pulmonary disease, drug overdose). Such patients may be dependent on hypoxemia (hypoxic drive) to maintain respiration. If hypoxemia is suddenly reversed, hypoxic drive may be lost. Respiratory arrest may then occur.
  b. High concentration—appropriate in patients not predisposed to carbon dioxide retention.
2. Monitor response to therapy by arterial blood gas evaluations.
3. Increase or decrease the inspired oxygen concentration (FiO_2), as appropriate, to correct arterial blood gases to patient normals. **NOTE:** Oxygen toxicity should always be of concern in the patient receiving inspired concentrations over 60% for longer than 24 hours.

Evaluation
Expected Outcomes

Responds to oxygen therapy successfully by attaining desired PaO_2 and $PaCO_2$, adequate tissue oxygenation, decreased work of breathing

Oxygen Delivery Systems

1. Oxygen may be administered by nasal cannula, various types of face masks, or a tent. It may also be applied directly to endotracheal or tracheal tube via a mechanical ventilator, T-piece, or hyperinflation bag.
2. The method selected depends on the required concentration of oxygen (low, medium, high), desired variability in delivered oxygen concentration (none, minimal, moderate), and required ventilatory assistance (mechanical ventilator, spontaneous breathing).

Monitoring Oxygen Therapy

▶ **NURSING ALERT:**
Arterial blood gas evaluations are the best means of assessing the effectiveness of oxygen therapy and guiding appropriate changes. Of particular importance is the effect of oxygen therapy on the patient who has chronic obstructive pulmonary disease and who may retain carbon dioxide if given too much oxygen. Frequent blood gas evaluations may be necessary in this type of patient to make sure that respiratory drive is not suppressed.

Guidelines: Administering Oxygen by Nasal Cannula (Fig. 7-13)

Equipment

Oxygen source
Plastic nasal cannula with connecting tubing (disposable)
Humidifier filled with sterile distilled water to indicated level
Flowmeter
"NO SMOKING" signs

Assessment

Nursing Action	Rationale/Amplification
1. Assess the patient's respiratory rate and level of consciousness.	1. Nasal cannula oxygen administration is often used for patients prone to CO_2 retention. Oxygen may depress

(continued)

Guidelines: Administering Oxygen by Nasal Cannula (Fig. 7-13) (continued)

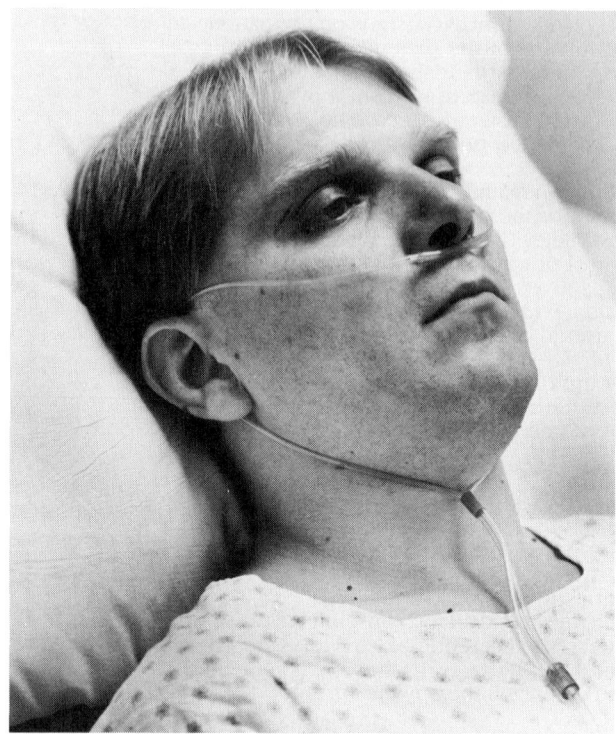

Figure 7-13. Administering oxygen by nasal cannula. Patient's inspiration consists of a mixture of supplemental oxygen supplied via the nasal cannula and room air. Oxygen concentration is variable and depends on patient's tidal volume and ventilatory pattern. (Courtesy of Photography Department, Montefiore Hospital, Pittsburgh, Pennsylvania)

Assessment
(Cont.)

Nursing Action	Rationale/Amplification
	the hypoxic drive of these patients (evidenced by a decreased respiratory rate, altered mental status, and further $PaCO_2$ elevation).
	NOTE: If $PaCO_2$ is decreased or normal, the patient is not experiencing CO_2 retention and can use oxygen without fear of the above consequences.
2. Determine current arterial blood gases if available.	

Planning/Implementation

Preparatory Phase

1. Post "NO SMOKING" signs on the patient's door and in view of patient and visitors.	
2. Show the nasal cannula to the patient and explain the procedure.	
3. Make sure that the humidifier is filled to the appropriate mark.	3. If the humidifier bottle is not sufficiently full, less moisture will be delivered.
4. Attach the connecting tube from the nasal cannula to the humidifier outlet.	

Planning/Implementation
(Cont.)

Nursing Action	Rationale/Amplification
5. Set the flow rate at prescribed liters/minute. Feel to determine if oxygen is flowing through the tips of the cannula.	5. *Approximate* oxygen concentrators delivered by nasal cannula are: 1 liter = 24% 2 liters = 28% 3 liters = 32% 4 liters = 36% 5 liters = 40%

Performance Phase

1. Place the tips of the cannula in the patient's nose.	1. Position the cannula so that the tips do not extend more than 2.5 cm. (1 inch) into the nares.
2. Adjust flow to prescribed rate.	2. **NOTE:** Because a nasal cannula is a low-flow system (patient's tidal volume supplies part of the inspired gas), oxygen concentration will vary, depending on the patient's respiratory rate and tidal volume.

▶ **NURSING ALERT:** Patients who require low, constant concentrations of oxygen and whose breathing pattern varies greatly may need to use a Venturi mask, particularly if they are carbon dioxide retainers.

Follow-up Phase

1. Change cannula, humidifiers, tubing, and other equipment exposed to moisture frequently.	1. Contaminated equipment may cause nosocomial infection in debilitated patients.
2. Assess patient's condition, arterial blood gases, and the functioning of equipment at regular intervals.	2. Depression of hypoxemic drive is most likely to occur within the first hours of oxygen use.

Evaluation/Outcome

1. Record flow rate used, patient response.	1. Note the patient's tolerance of treatment. Notify the physician if intolerance is noted.
2. Determine patient comfort with oxygen use.	2. Flow rates in excess of 4 liters/minute may lead to air swallowing and cause irritation to the nasal and pharyngeal mucosa. If higher concentrations are required, consider an alternate form of therapy.

Guidelines: Administering Oxygen by Venturi Mask (Figs. 7-14 and 7-15)

Underlying Principles

1. To ensure precise control of the oxygen concentration, total gas flow at the patient's face must meet or exceed peak inspiratory flow rate. When mask output does not meet inspiratory flow rate, room air (drawn through mask side holes) mixes with the gas mixture provided by the face mask, lowering the inspired oxygen concentration.
2. The Venturi mask mixes a fixed flow of oxygen with a high but variable flow of air to produce a constant oxygen concentration. Oxygen enters via a jet (restricted opening) at a high velocity. Room air also enters and mixes with oxygen at this site. The higher the velocity (smaller the opening), the more room air is drawn into the mask. Mask output ranges from 84 liters/minute (24%) to 44 liters per minute (40%).
3. Excess gas leaves through openings in the mask, carrying with it the expired carbon dioxide; this virtually eliminates rebreathing of carbon dioxide.

Equipment

Oxygen source
Flowmeter
Venturi mask for correct concentration (24%, 28%, 31%, 35%, 40%) or correct concentration adaptor if interchangeable color-coded adaptors are used
If high humidity desired:
    Compressed air source and flowmeter
    Nebulizer with sterile distilled water
    Large-bore tubing
"NO SMOKING" signs

(continued)

Guidelines: Administering Oxygen by Venturi Mask (Figs. 7-14 and 7-15) (continued)

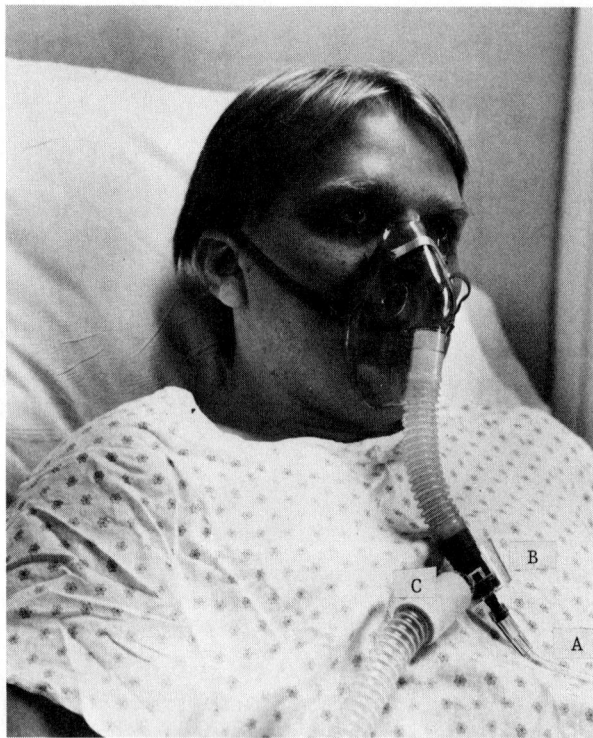

Figure 7-14. Administering oxygen by Venturi mask. Oxygen (A) is diluted to a precise inspired oxygen concentration (24%–40%) by room air as it enters the specially constructed openings (B) of the mask. Additional humidity can be supplied via a humidification port (C), which is connected to a nebulizer and compressed air source. (Courtesy of Photography Department, Montefiore Hospital, Pittsburgh, Pennsylvania)

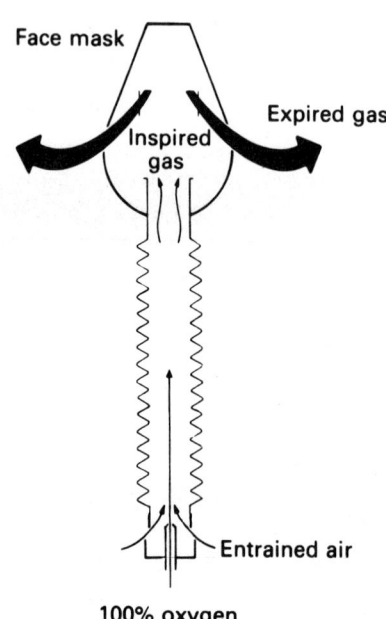

Figure 7-15. Air flow diagram with Venturi mask. Arrows indicate direction of flow. (Burton GC and Hodgkin JE [eds]. Respiratory Care: A Guide to Practice, 2nd ed. Philadelphia, JB Lippincott, 1984, p. 409)

Assessment

Nursing Action	Rationale/Amplification
1. Assess patient's respiratory rate and level of consciousness.	1. Venturi masks are used for patients prone to CO_2 retention. Oxygen may depress the hypoxic drive of these patients (evidenced by a decreased respiratory rate, altered mental status, and further $PaCO_2$ elevation).
2. Determine current arterial blood gases if available.	

Planning/Implementation

Preparatory Phase

1. Post "NO SMOKING" signs on the door of the patient's room and in view of patient and visitors.	
2. Show the Venturi mask to the patient and explain the procedure.	
3. Connect the mask by lightweight tubing to the oxygen source.	
4. Turn on the oxygen flowmeter and adjust to the prescribed rate (usually indicated on the mask). Check to see that oxygen is flowing out the vent holes in the mask.	4. To ensure the correct air/oxygen mix, oxygen must be set at the prescribed flow rate. Prescribed flow rates differ for different oxygen concentrations. Usually this information is printed on the mask or interchangeable color-coded adaptor.

Planning/Implementation
(Cont.)

Nursing Action	Rationale/Amplification

Performance Phase

1. Place Venturi mask over the patient's nose and mouth and under the chin. Adjust elastic strap.
2. Check to make sure holes for air entry are not obstructed by the patient's bedding.
3. If high humidity is used:
   a. Connect the nebulizer to a compressed air source.
   b. Attach large-bore tubing to the nebulizer and connect the tubing to the fitting for high humidity at the base of the Venturi mask.

2. Proper mask function depends on mixing of sufficient amount of air and oxygen.
3. When a Venturi mask is used with high humidity, both an oxygen source and compressed air source are required. The compressed air source provides air for the air/oxygen mix. Excessive oxygen would be inspired if both tubings were connected to an oxygen source.

Follow-up Phase

1. Change the mask, nebulizer, and tubing at frequent intervals.
2. Assess the patient's condition and arterial blood gases, and the functioning of the equipment at regular intervals.

1. Nebulizers, tubing, and masks may become contaminated and cause nosocomial infections.
2. Depression of hypoxic drive is most likely to occur within the first hours of oxygen use.

Evaluation/Outcome

1. Record inspired oxygen concentration, patient response.

2. Determine patient comfort with oxygen use.

1. Note the patient's tolerance of treatment. Notify the physician if intolerance occurs.
2. Venturi masks are best tolerated for relatively short periods of time because of their size and appearance. They also must be removed for eating and drinking. With improvement in patient condition, a nasal cannula may often be substituted.

Guidelines: Administering Oxygen by Simple Face Mask With/Without Aerosol (Fig. 7-16)

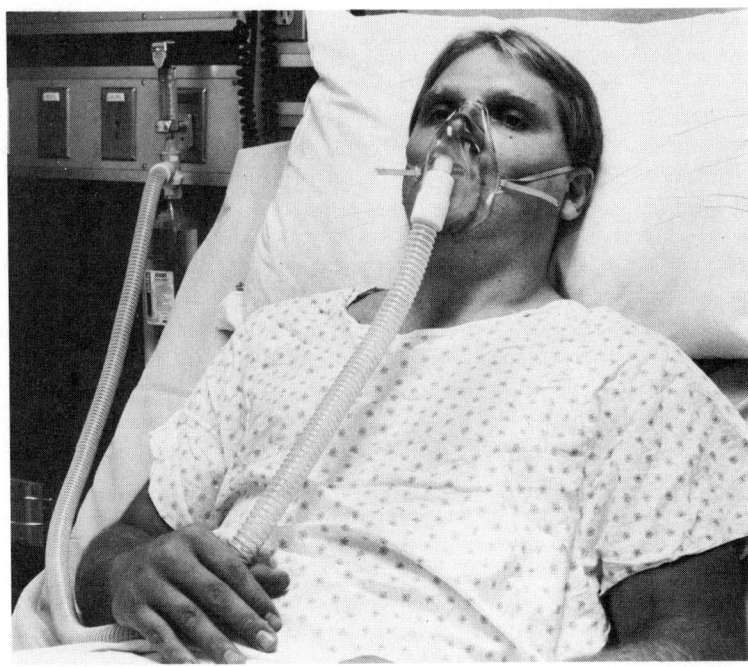

Figure 7-16. Administering oxygen by simple face mask with aerosol. Simple face masks are inexpensive and relatively comfortable and often are used when the patient requires humidification or aerosol therapy with oxygen. (Courtesy of Photography Department, Montefiore Hospital, Pittsburgh, Pennsylvania)

(continued)

Guidelines: Administering Oxygen by Simple Face Mask With/Without Aerosol (continued)

Equipment

Oxygen source
Nebulizer bottle with sterile distilled water, if high humidity is desired
Plastic aerosol mask
Large-bore tubing (high humidity) or small-bore tubing
Flowmeter
"NO SMOKING" signs
For heated aerosol therapy:
    Nebulizer heating element

Assessment

Nursing Action	Rationale/Amplification
1. Assess the patient's respiratory rate, level of consciousness, and arterial blood gases, if available.	1. Because the aerosol face mask is a low-flow system (patient's tidal volume may supply part of inspired gas), oxygen concentration will vary depending on the patient's respiratory rate and rhythm. Oxygen delivery may be inadequate for tachypneic patients (flow does not meet peak inspiratory demand) or excessive for patients with slow respirations.
2. Assess viscosity and volume of sputum produced.	2. Aerosol is given to assist in mobilizing retained secretions.

Planning/Implementation

Preparatory Phase

1. Post "NO SMOKING" signs on patient's door and in view of the patient and visitors.	
2. Show the aerosol mask to the patient and explain the procedure.	
3. Make sure the nebulizer is filled to the appropriate mark.	3. If the nebulizer bottle is not sufficiently full, less moisture will be delivered.
4. Attach the large-bore tubing from the mask to the nebulizer outlet.	
5. Set desired oxygen concentration on nebulizer bottle and plug in the heating element, if used.	5. The inspired oxygen concentration is determined by the nebulizer setting. Usual percentages are 35%–40%.
6. If the patient is tachypneic and a concentration of 50% oxygen or greater is desired, two nebulizers and flowmeters should be yoked together.	6. The aerosol mask is a low-flow system. Yoking two nebulizers together doubles nebulizer flow but does *not* change the inspired oxygen concentration.

Performance Phase

1. Adjust the flow rate until the desired mist is produced (usually 10–12 liters/minute).	1. This ensures that the patient is receiving flow sufficient to meet inspiratory demand and maintains a constant accurate concentration of oxygen.
2. Apply the mask to the patient's face and adjust the straps so that the mask fits securely and there are no leaks.	

Follow-up Phase

1. Change mask, tubing, nebulizer, and other equipment exposed to moisture at frequent intervals.	1. Contaminated equipment may cause nosocomial infection in debilitated patients.
2. Assess the patient's condition and the functioning of equipment at regular intervals.	2. Assess the patient for change in mental status, diaphoresis, changes in blood pressure, and increasing heart and respiratory rates.
3. If the patient's condition changes, assess arterial blood gases.	3. Inadequate flow rates may cause symptoms of hypoxemia and hypoxia.
4. Drain the tubing frequently. If a heating element is used, the tubing will have to be drained more often.	4. The tubing must be kept free of condensate. Condensate allowed to accumulate in the delivery tube will block flow and alter oxygen concentration.
5. If a heating device is used, the temperature must be checked often.	5. Excessive temperatures can cause airway burns; patients with elevated temperatures should be humidified with an unheated device.

Evaluation/Outcome

1. Record inspired oxygen concentration, patient response.	1. Note the patient's tolerance of treatment. Notify the physician if intolerance occurs.
2. Record changes in volume and tenacity of sputum produced.	2. Indicates effectiveness of therapy.

Guidelines: Administering Oxygen by Partial Rebreathing Mask (Figs. 7-17 and 7-18)

A *partial rebreathing mask* has an inflatable bag that stores 100% oxygen. On inspiration, the patient inhales from the mask and bag; on expiration, the bag refills with oxygen. Perforations on both sides of the mask serve as exhalation ports. High concentrations of oxygen are indicated in the acute phase of some diseases (pneumonia, pulmonary edema, pulmonary embolism).

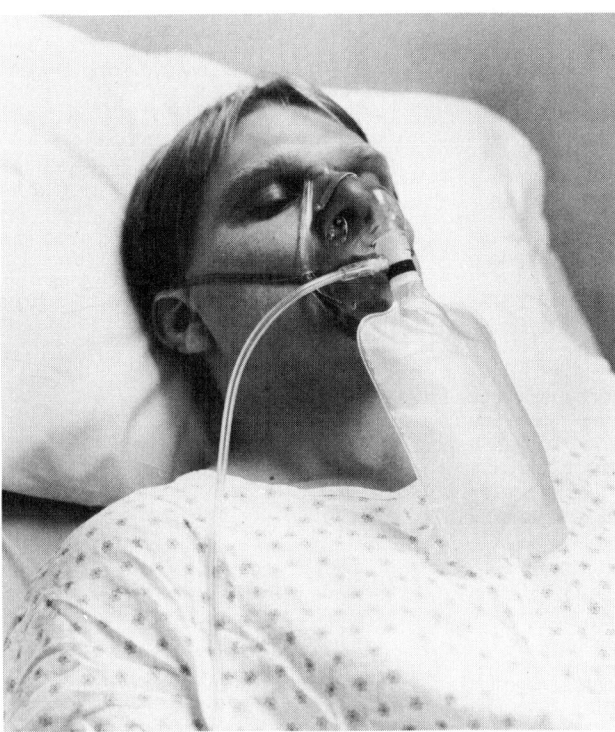

Figure 7-17. Administering oxygen via a partial rebreathing mask. Liter flow is adjusted so that the rebreathing bag does not collapse even with deep inspiration. This prevents expired carbon dioxide from entering the bag. (Courtesy of Photography Department, Montefiore Hospital, Pittsburgh, Pennsylvania)

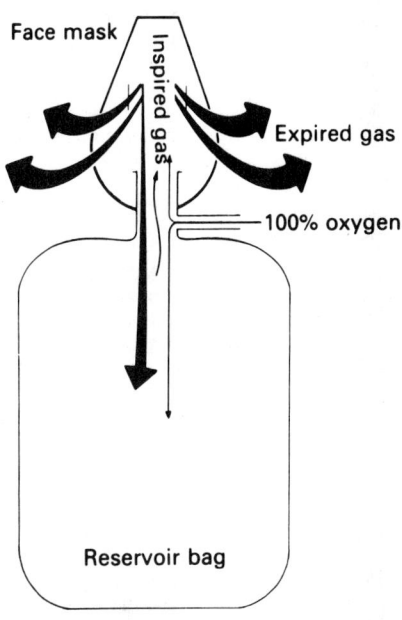

Figure 7-18. Air flow diagram with partial rebreathing mask. Arrows indicate direction of flow. (Burton GC and Hodgkin JE [eds]. Respiratory Care: A Guide to Practice, 2nd ed. Philadelphia, JB Lippincott, 1984, p. 410)

Equipment

Oxygen source
Plastic face mask with reservoir bag and tubing
Humidifier with distilled water
Flowmeter
"NO SMOKING" signs

Assessment

Nursing Action	Rationale/Amplification
1. Assess the patient's respiratory rate and level of consciousness.	1. Provides a baseline for evaluating patient response. Typically used for short-term support of patients who require a high inspired oxygen concentration.
2. Determine current arterial blood gases, if available.	2. Allows objective evaluation of patient response.

Planning/Implementation

Preparatory Phase

1. Post "NO SMOKING" signs on the patient's door and in view of the patient and visitors.

(continued)

Guidelines: Administering Oxygen by Partial Rebreathing Mask (continued)

Planning/Implementation
(Cont.)

Nursing Action	Rationale/Amplification
2. Fill humidifier with sterile distilled water.	2. If the humidifier bottle is not sufficiently full, less moisture will be delivered.
3. Attach tubing to outlet on humidifier.	
4. Attach flowmeter.	
5. Show the mask to the patient and explain the procedure.	
6. Flush the reservoir bag with oxygen to inflate the bag and adjust flowmeter to 6–10 liters/minute.	6. Bag serves as a reservoir, holding oxygen for patient inspiration.

Performance Phase

Nursing Action	Rationale/Amplification
1. Place the mask on the patient's face.	1. Be sure that the mask fits snugly, since there must be an airtight seal between the mask and the patient's face.
2. Adjust liter flow so that the rebreathing bag will not collapse during the inspiratory cycle, even during deep inspiration.	2. With a well-fitting rebreathing bag adjusted so that the patient's inhalation does not deflate the bag, inspired oxygen concentration of 60%–80% can be achieved. Some patients may require flow rates higher than 10 liters/minute to ensure that the bag does not collapse on inspiration.

▶ **NURSING ALERT:** A partial rebreathing mask does not have a one-way valve between the mask and reservoir bag. Exhaled air enters the bag very early (first ⅓ expiration). This is dead space ventilation and contains little CO_2. If the bag is allowed to collapse on inspiration, more exhaled air can enter the reservoir and the patient can inhale high concentrations of CO_2.

Nursing Action	Rationale/Amplification
3. Stay with the patient for a period of time to make him comfortable and observe his reactions.	3. Be sure that oxygen is not escaping from the sides of the mask.

Follow-up Phase

Nursing Action	Rationale/Amplification
1. Remove mask periodically (if the patient's condition permits) to dry the face around the mask. Powder skin and massage face around the mask.	1. These actions reduce moisture accumulation under the mask. Massage of the face stimulates circulation and reduces pressure over the area.
2. Observe the patient for change of condition. Assess equipment for malfunctioning and low water level in humidifier.	2. Assess the patient for change in mental status, diaphoresis, change in blood pressure, and increasing heart and respiratory rates.
3. If the patient's condition changes, assess arterial blood gases.	3. Inadequate oxygen concentration may cause hypoxemia or hypoxia. Rebreathing of CO_2 may cause CO_2 retention.

Evaluation/Outcome

Nursing Action	Rationale/Amplification
1. Record patient response.	1. Note the patient's tolerance of treatment. Notify the physician if intolerance occurs.
2. Determine patient comfort with oxygen use.	2. Moisture accumulation and tight fit of the mask predispose to skin breakdown, generally limiting mask to short-term use.

Guidelines: Administering Oxygen by Nonrebreathing Mask (Fig. 7-19)

A *nonrebreathing mask* has (1) an inflatable bag to store 100% oxygen, (2) a one-way valve between the bag and mask to prevent exhaled air from entering the bag (diverts it into the atmosphere), (3) one-way valves covering one or both exhalation ports to prevent entry of room air on inspiration, and (4) flap or spring-loaded valves to permit entry of room air should the oxygen source fail or patient needs exceed the available oxygen flow. Optimally, all the patient's inspiratory volume will be provided by the mask/reservoir, allowing delivery of nearly 100% oxygen.

Equipment

Oxygen source
Plastic face mask with reservoir bag and tubing
Humidifier with sterile distilled water
Flowmeter
"NO SMOKING" signs

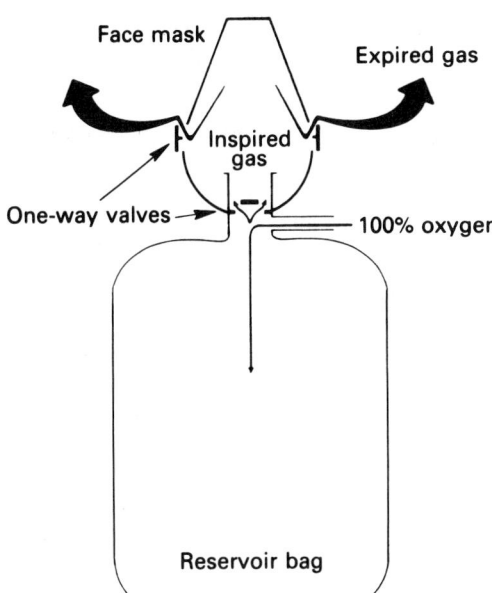

Figure 7-19. Air flow diagram with nonrebreathing mask. Arrows indicate direction of flow. (Burton GC and Hodgkin JE [eds]. Respiratory Care: A Guide to Practice, 2nd ed. Philadelphia, JB Lippincott, 1984, p. 410)

Assessment

Nursing Action	Rationale/Amplification
1. Assess the patient's respiratory rate and level of consciousness.	1. Provides a baseline for evaluating patient response. Method is typically used for short-term support of patients with oxygen failure. Goal is to avoid intubation until treatment of the underlying disorder is effective.
2. Determine current arterial blood gases, if available.	2. Allows objective evaluation of patient response.

Planning/Implementation

Preparatory Phase

1. Post "NO SMOKING" signs on patient's door and in view of patient and visitors.
2. Show the mask to the patient and explain the procedure.
3. Make sure the humidifier is filled to the appropriate mark.

3. If the humidifier bottle is not sufficiently full, less moisture will be delivered.

Performance Phase

1. Place the mask on the patient's face.

1. Be sure that the mask fits snugly, since there must be an airtight seal between the mask and the patient's face.

2. Adjust liter flow so that the reservoir bag will not collapse during the inspiratory cycle, even during deep inspiration.

2. Since the patient is receiving all of his ventilation from the reservoir bag, the flow rate must be sufficient to provide the patient's required ventilation.

▶ **NURSING ALERT:** With a well-fitting mask and bag adjusted so that the patient's inhalation does not deflate the bag, inspired oxygen concentrations of up to 90% can be achieved. If oxygen flow is not sufficient to keep reservoir bag filled, oxygen concentration will be reduced as room air is drawn in through the flap or spring-loaded valves.

3. Stay with the patient for a period of time to make him comfortable and observe his reactions.

3. Be sure that oxygen is not escaping from the sides of the mask.

Follow-up Phase

1. Remove mask periodically (if patient's condition permits) to dry the face around the mask. Powder skin and massage face around the mask.

1. These actions reduce moisture accumulation under the mask. Massage of the face stimulates circulation and reduces pressure over the area.

(continued)

Guidelines: Administering Oxygen by Nonrebreathing Mask(continued)

Planning/Implementation
(Cont.)

Nursing Action	Rationale/Amplification
2. Observe for change of condition. Assess equipment for malfunctioning and low water level in humidifier.	2. Assess the patient for change in mental status, diaphoresis, change in blood pressure, and increasing heart and respiratory rates. Determine that the reservoir bag never completely collapses as the patient's ventilatory pattern varies.
3. If the patient's condition changes, assess arterial blood gases.	3. Inadequate oxygen concentration may cause hypoxemia or hypoxia. Even though this system is designed to provide high oxygen concentrations, such concentrations are inconsistently achieved because of air leaks around the mask or air entry through the flap or spring-loaded safety valves. If patient's condition deteriorates, continuous positive airway pressure (CPAP) by face mask or intubation and mechanical ventilation may be indicated.

Evaluation/Outcome

1. Record patient response.	1. Note the patient's tolerance of treatment. Notify the physician if intolerance occurs.
2. Determine patient comfort with oxygen use.	2. Moisture accumulation and tight fit of the mask predispose to skin breakdown, generally limiting the mask to short-term use.

Guidelines: Administering Oxygen by Face Mask
(Continuous Positive Airway Pressure; CPAP) (Fig. 7-20)

Continuous positive airway pressure (CPAP) provides expiratory and inspiratory positive airway pressure in a manner similar to positive end-expiratory pressure (PEEP) during mechanical ventilation but without endotracheal intubation. The mask has (1) an inflatable cushion and head strap designed to tightly seal the mask against the face, (2) a PEEP valve incorporated into the exhalation port to maintain positive pressure on exhalation, and (3) uses high inspiratory flow rates to maintain positive pressure on inspiration.

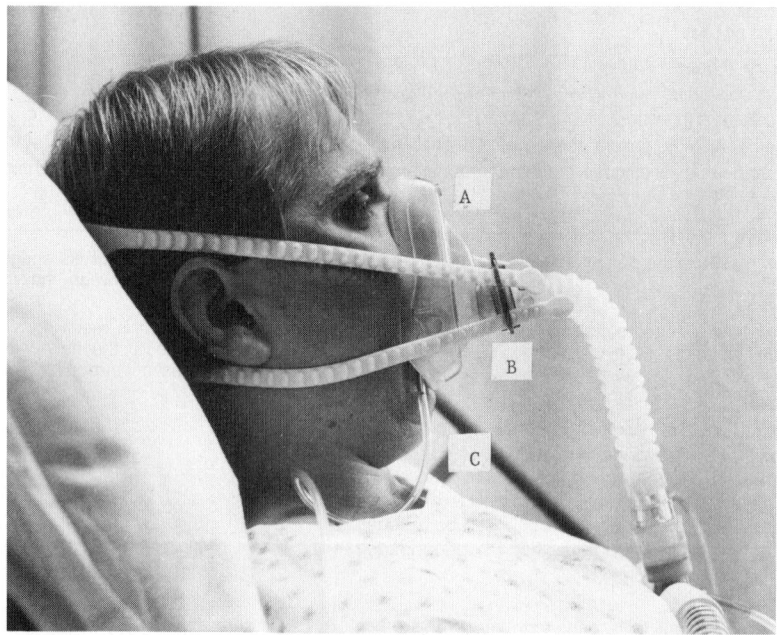

Figure 7-20. Administering oxygen by face mask with continuous positive airway pressure (CPAP). The CPAP mask has a cushion (*A*), head strap (*B*), and positive end-expiratory pressure (PEEP) valve incorporated into the exhalation port (not shown). Nasogastric suction (*C*) diminishes the risk of gastric distention or emesis. (Courtesy of Photography Department, Montefiore Hospital, Pittsburgh, Pennsylvania)

Equipment

Oxygen blender
Flowmeter
CPAP mask
Valve for prescribed PEEP (2.5, 5, 7.5, 10, or 12.5 cm. H_2O)
Nebulizer with sterile distilled water
Large-bore tubing
Nasogastric tube
Sealing pad to accommodate nasogastric tube

Assessment

Nursing Action	Rationale/Amplification
1. Assess the patient's level of consciousness and gag reflex.	1. CPAP by face mask may lead to aspiration in patient not sufficiently alert to swallow oral secretions.
2. Determine current arterial blood gases.	2. Provides a baseline for evaluating response.

▶ **NURSING ALERT:**

1. CPAP is used when patients have not responded to attempts to increase PaO_2 with other types of masks.
2. The patient will require frequent assessment to detect changes in respiratory status, cardiovascular status and level of consciousness.
3. If the patient's level of consciousness decreases or arterial blood gases deteriorate, intubation may be necessary.

Planning/Implementation

Preparatory Phase

1. Post "NO SMOKING" signs on the patient's door and in view of the patient and visitors.	
2. Show the mask to the patient and explain the procedure.	
3. Make sure nebulizer is filled to the appropriate mark.	
4. Insert nasogastric tube.	4. With CPAP, the patient may swallow air, causing gastric distention, emesis, and/or distention of gastric suture line. Prophylactic nasogastric suction diminishes this risk.
5. Attach nasogastric tube adaptor.	5. Use of adaptor may decrease air leak around the mask.

Performance Phase

1. Set desired concentration of oxygen blender and adjust flow rate so that it is sufficient to meet the patient's inspiratory demand.	1. O_2 blenders are devices that mix air and O_2 using a proportioning valve. Concentrations of 21%–100% may be delivered at flows of 2–100 liters per minute, depending on the model. Because the patient will be receiving all of his minute ventilation from this "closed system," it is essential that the flow rate be adequate to meet changes in the patient's breathing pattern.
2. Place the mask on the patient's face, adjust the head strap, and inflate the mask cushion to ensure a tight seal.	2. To maintain CPAP, an airtight seal is required. Head straps and the inflatable cushion help to ensure that difficult areas, such as the nose and chin, are sealed with greater comfort to the patient.
3. Stay with the patient to observe his reaction.	3. If the CPAP level is too high for a particular individual (CPAP is usually not used in levels above 10 cm.), the patient's work of breathing may actually be increased rather than diminished.

Follow-up Phase

1. Assess patient's mental status, respiratory status, cardiovascular status, and fluid balance frequently.	1. Provides objective documentation of patient response. CPAP may increase work of breathing, resulting in patient tiring and inability to maintain ventilation without intubation. CPAP may also decrease venous return (PEEP effect), resulting in decreased cardiac output.
2. Assess patency of nasogastric tube at frequent intervals.	2. May become obstructed, causing gastric distention.
3. Organize care to remove the mask as infrequently as possible.	3. If mask is removed (for coughing, suctioning), CPAP is not maintained and inspired oxygen concentrations drop.
4. Assess patient comfort and functioning of the equipment frequently.	4. Tight fit of the mask may predispose to skin breakdown. System may develop leaks, resulting in air escaping between the patient's face and mask.

(continued)

Guidelines: Administering Oxygen by Face Mask
(Continuous Positive Airway Pressure; CPAP) (continued)

Evaluation/Outcome

Nursing Action	Rationale/Amplification
1. Record patient response. With improvement, oxygen therapy without positive airway pressure can be substituted. With deterioration, intubation and mechanical ventilation may be required.	1. Face mask CPAP is usually continued only for short periods (72 hours) because of patient tiring and the necessity to remove mask for suctioning and coughing. Note the patient's tolerance of treatment. Notify physician if intolerance occurs.
2. Determine patient comfort with oxygen use.	2. Moisture accumulation and tight fit of the mask predispose to skin breakdown.

Guidelines: Administering Oxygen via Endotracheal and Tracheostomy Tubes With a T-Piece (Briggs) Adapter (Fig. 7-21)

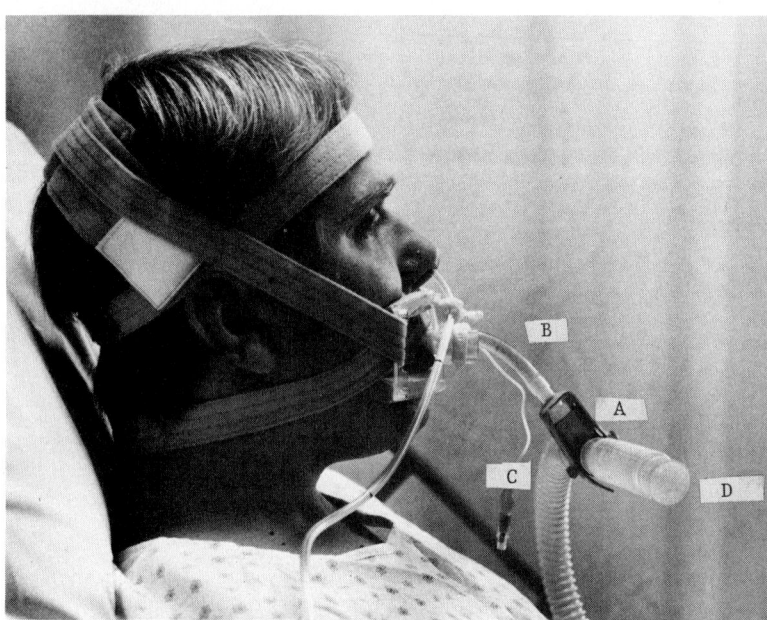

Figure 7-21. Administering oxygen via endotracheal tube with a T-piece adapter. A T-piece adapter (A) is attached to the endotracheal tube (B) and large-bore tubing (C), which serves as a source of oxygen and humidity. On inspiration, aerosol mist should not be withdrawn into the reservoir tubing (D). (Courtesy of Photography Department, Montefiore Hospital, Pittsburgh, Pennsylvania)

Equipment

Oxygen
Oxygen blender
Flowmeter
Nebulizer and sterile distilled water (heating element may be used as described in aerosol masks)
Large-bore tubing
T-piece and reservoir tubing

If oxygen blender is not used and precise O_2 concentrations are required:
    Venturi tube
    Humidity device and large-bore tubing
    Compressed air source (as described in use of Venturi mask)
"NO SMOKING" signs

Assessment

Nursing Action	Rationale/Amplification
1. Assess the patient's respiratory rate, level of consciousness and arterial blood gases, if available.	1. Provides baseline to assess response.
2. Assess viscosity and volume of sputum produced.	2. Aerosol is given to assist in mobilizing retained secretions.

Planning/Implementation

Nursing Action	Rationale/Amplification
Preparatory Phase	
1. Post "NO SMOKING" signs on the patient's door and in view of the patient and visitors.	
2. Show the T-tube or Venturi tube to the patient and explain the procedure.	
3. Make sure the nebulizer is filled to the appropriate mark.	3. If nebulizer is not sufficiently full, less aerosol will be delivered.
4. Attach the large-bore tubing from the T-tube to the nebulizer outlet.	
5. Set desired oxygen concentration of O_2 blender or nebulizer bottle and plug in heating element if used.	5. O_2 blenders are devices that mix air and O_2 using a proportioning valve. Concentrations of 21%–100% may be delivered at flows of 2–100 liters per minute, depending on the model. Used in situation when precise control is required.
Performance Phase	
1. Adjust the flow rate until the desired mist is produced and meets the patient's inspiratory demand.	1. The aerosol mist in the reservoir tubing attached to the T-tube should not be completely withdrawn on patient inspiration. If mist is withdrawn (does not extend from reservoir tubing) on inspiration, room air may be inspired and O_2 concentration decreased.
Follow-up Phase	
1. Change mask, tubing, nebulizer, and other equipment exposed to moisture daily.	1. Contaminated equipment may cause nosocomial infection in debilitated patients.
2. Assess the patient's condition and the functioning of equipment at regular intervals.	2. Assess the patient for change in mental status, diaphoresis, perspiration, changes in blood pressure, and increasing heart and respiratory rates.
3. Drain the tubing frequently. If a heating element is used, the tubing will have to be monitored and drained more often.	3. The tubing must be kept free of condensate. Condensate allowed to accumulate in the delivery tube will block flow and alter oxygen concentration.
4. If a heating device is used, the temperature must be checked often.	4. Excessive temperatures can cause airway burns; patients with elevated temperatures will be better humidified with an unheated device.
5. If the patient appears tachypneic, assess arterial blood gases.	5. Inadequate flow rates may cause hypoxemia or hypoxia.

Evaluation/Outcome

Nursing Action	Rationale/Amplification
1. Record patient response.	1. Note the patient's tolerance of treatment. Notify physician if intolerance occurs.
2. Record changes in volume and tenacity of sputum produced.	2. Indicates effectiveness of therapy.

Guidelines: Administering Oxygen by Tracheostomy Collar

A *tracheostomy collar* fits over the tracheostomy and delivers humidity and oxygen. If the patient does not require precise or high concentrations of oxygen, he is usually more comfortable with a tracheostomy collar than with a T-tube or Venturi tube.

Equipment

Oxygen or compressed air source
Flowmeter
Nebulizer and sterile distilled water (heating element may be used as described in use of aerosol masks)
Large-bore tubing
Tracheostomy collar
"NO SMOKING" signs

Assessment

Nursing Action	Rationale/Amplification
1. Assess the patient's respiratory rate, level of consciousness and arterial blood gases, if available.	1. Provides baseline to assess response.
2. Assess viscosity and volume of sputum produced.	2. Aerosol is given to assist in mobilizing retained secretions.

(continued)

Guidelines: Administering Oxygen by Tracheostomy Collar*(continued)*

Planning/Implementation

Nursing Action	Rationale/Amplification
Preparatory Phase	
1. Post "NO SMOKING" signs on the patient's door and in view of the patient and visitors.	
2. Show the tracheostomy collar to the patient and explain the procedure.	
3. Make sure the nebulizer is filled to the appropriate mark.	3. If nebulizer is not sufficiently full, less aerosol will be delivered.
4. Attach the large-bore tubing to the tracheostomy collar and nebulizer outlet.	
5. Set desired O_2 concentrations of nebulizer bottle and plug in heating element, if used.	
Performance Phase	
1. Adjust the flow rate until the desired mist is produced and meets the patient's inspiratory demand.	1. The aerosol mist in the tracheostomy collar should not be completely withdrawn on patient inspiration. If the mist is withdrawn (does not flow from the tracheostomy collar) on inspiration, room air may be inspired and O_2 concentration and/or humidification decreased.
Follow-up Phase	
1. Change mask, tubing, nebulizer, and other equipment exposed to moisture at frequent intervals.	1. Contaminated equipment may cause nosocomial infection in debilitated patients.

Evaluation/Outcome

1. Record patient response.	1. Note patient's tolerance of treatment. Notify physician if intolerance occurs.
2. Record changes in volume and tenacity of sputum produced.	2. Indicates effectiveness of therapy.

Guidelines: Administering Oxygen by Bag-Mask or Bag-Airway System
(Manual Resuscitation Bag)

A *bag–mask* is used when a patient is not intubated. The need to use a bag–mask usually occurs primarily during a cardiopulmonary arrest episode. Bag–airway systems are used to hyperinflate ventilator patients during suctioning and when they are being transported (Fig. 7-23).

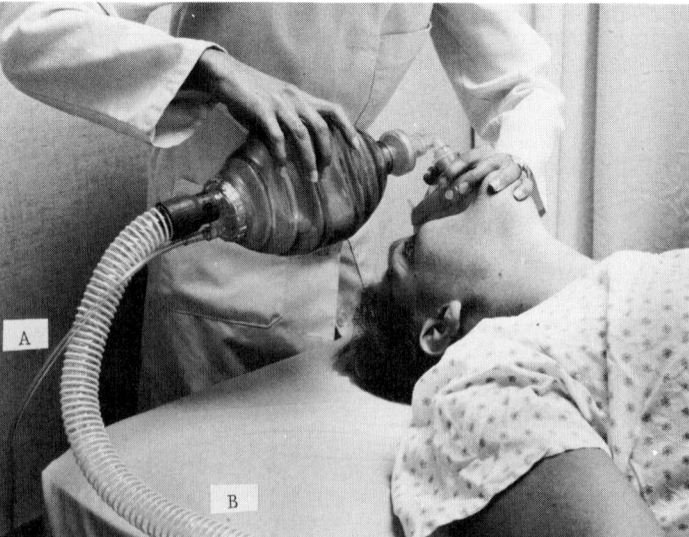

Figure 7-22. Using a resuscitation bag with a mask. The patient's head is positioned to ensure an open airway. The mask is held tightly against the face to prevent an air leak; the bag is connected to an oxygen source (*A*) and supplied with a reservoir tubing (*B*). (Courtesy of Photography Department, Montefiore Hospital, Pittsburgh, Pennsylvania)

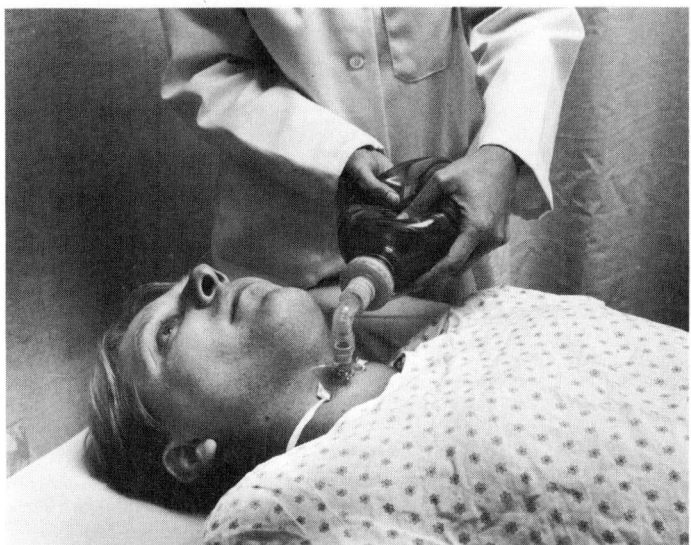

Figure 7-23. Using a resuscitation bag connected to an artificial airway. This method is used to provide supplemental oxygen before, during, and after suctioning, during patient transport or during cardiopulmonary resuscitation. (Courtesy of Photography Department, Montefiore Hospital, Pittsburgh, Pennsylvania)

Equipment

Oxygen source
Resuscitation bag and mask
Reservoir tubing or reservoir bag
O_2 connecting tubing
Nipple adaptor to attach flowmeter to connecting tubing
Flowmeter

Assessment

Nursing Action	Rationale / Amplification
1. In cardiopulmonary arrest, shake victim to validate arrest situation, shout for help, and place ear to patient's nose and mouth to determine presence/absence of respirations. If respirations are absent, give 4 breaths, then palpate carotid pulse.	1. Establishes that cardiopulmonary arrest has occurred. Initiates call for assistance. Gives initial ventilatory support.
2. In suctioning or transport situation, assess patient's heart rate, level of consciousness, and respiratory status.	2. Provides a baseline to estimate patient's tolerance of procedure.

Planning/Implementation

Preparatory Phase

1. Attach connecting tubing from flowmeter and nipple adaptor to resuscitation bag.	1. A humidifier bottle is not used, since the high flow rates of oxygen required would force water into the tubing and clog it.
2. Turn flowmeter to ''flush'' position.	2. A high flow rate or ''flush'' position is necessary to meet the minute ventilation of the patient.
3. Attach reservoir tubing or reservoir bag to resuscitation bag.	3. A high inspired O_2 concentration is required. Without a reservoir, inspired O_2 concentration will be low (.28–.56) because inspired gas will be air/O_2 mix. With a reservoir, manual resuscitation bags can achieve a F_iO_2 of >.96 at a flow rate of 15 liters/minute.
4. In a cardiopulmonary arrest situation, every effort should be made to establish a patent airway.	4. If the patient is not intubated, attach mask to the bag, insert an oral airway, and while tilting back the patient's head, place the mask over the patient's face.

Performance Phase

1. If cardiac massage is being given: a. Breaths will have to be quickly interposed between cardiac compressions. If the patient needs only respiratory assistance, watch for chest expansion and listen with the stethoscope to ensure adequate ventilation.	a. Squeeze resuscitation bag with sufficient force and at the rate necessary to maintain adequate minute ventilation.

(continued)

Guidelines: Administering Oxygen by Bag–Mask or Bag–Airway System
(Manual Resuscitation Bag) (continued)

Planning/Implementation
(Cont.)

Nursing Action	Rationale/Amplification
b. A rate of approximately 14–18 breaths per minute is used unless the patient is being given external cardiac compressions (see p. 925).	b. Continue squeezing bag at appropriate intervals until CPR (cardiopulmonary resuscitation) is no longer required.
2. If hyperinflation is being used with suctioning, ventilate the patient before and after each suctioning pass (*including* after the last suction pass). See Sterile Tracheobronchial Suction Via Tracheostomy or Endotracheal Tube, p. 220).	2. Hyperinflation prior to suctioning helps prevent hypoxemia. Hyperinflation after suctioning replaces O_2 removed during the procedure and helps to prevent atelectasis. The larger tidal volumes may also assist in mobilizing secretions and promote surfactant secretion.
3. If hyperinflation is used in transport, suction patient prior to disconnection for transport; monitor heart and respiratory rates and level of consciousness during procedure.	3. Establishes a patent airway before patient is moved. Provides information for assessing tolerance of transport.

Evaluation/Outcome

1. In cardiopulmonary arrest, verify return of spontaneous pulse and respirations. Initiate further support as needed.	1. Establishes patient's need for definitive therapy (drugs, defibrillation, intensive care).
2. In suctioning or transport, return patient to previous support. Note patient tolerance of procedure.	2. Note heart rate, rate and ease of respirations, arterial blood pressure (if monitored), level of consciousness. Notify physician if intolerance occurs.

Other Respiratory Therapeutic Modalities

Guidelines: Assisting the Patient Undergoing Intermittent Positive Pressure Breathing (IPPB)

The *IPPB unit* is a piece of equipment that delivers air or oxygen under positive pressure (above atmospheric pressure) during inspiration. (Fig. 7-24)

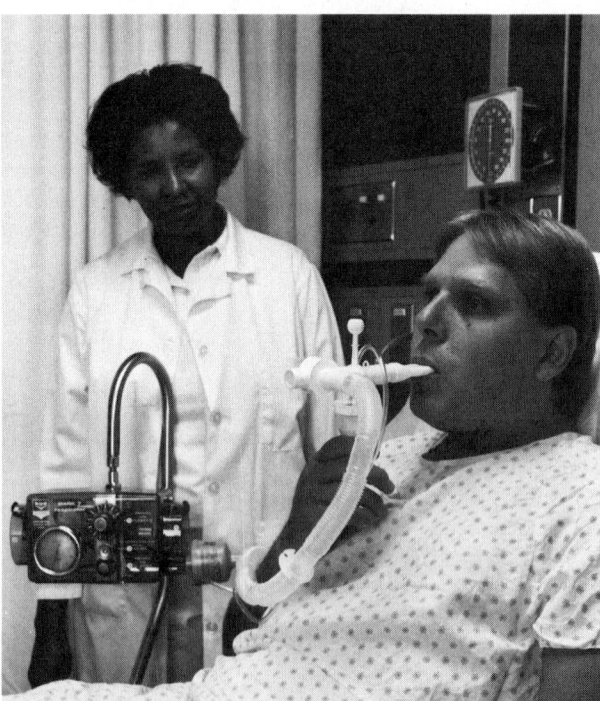

Figure 7-24. Intermittent positive pressure breathing (IPPB) treatment. (Courtesy of Photography Department, Montefiore Hospital, Pittsburgh, Pennsylvania)

Contraindications

Untreated pneumothorax

Mediastinal and subcutaneous emphysema

Tracheoesophageal fistula

Use with caution in patients with gastrointestinal surgery, hemoptysis, bullous disease, cardiovascular insufficiency, active tuberculosis.

Hazards Excessive ventilation

Excessive oxygenation

Decreased venous return

Gastric insufflation

Equipment

According to the type of machine used (each machine may have different controls and settings)

IPPB circuitry

Medication or fluid for aerosolization

"NO SMOKING" signs if oxygen is used as the drive gas

Nursing Action	Rationale/Amplification

Assessment

1. Monitor the heart rate before and after the treatment, especially for patients using bronchodilator drugs.

2. Assess the patient's breath sounds.

1. Bronchodilators may produce tachycardia, precordial distress, palpitations, dizziness, nausea, and excessive perspiration.

2. This will help in evaluating post-treatment changes.

Planning/Intervention

Preparatory Phase

1. Post "NO SMOKING" signs if oxygen is used as the drive gas. Explain the procedure to the patient.
2. Place the patient in a comfortable sitting or semi-Fowler's position.

3. Plug the machine into the pressure source (oxygen or compressed air).
4. Place the prescribed medication or saline solution in the nebulizer.
5. Adjust all controls on tentative settings according to the machine directions or physician request.
   a. Sensitivity—adjusted to −1.5 cm./H_2O to −2 cm./H_2O.

   b. Flow—usually set at 15 cm./H_2O.

   c. Pressure—set at 10–15 cm./H_2O.

6. Check the nebulizer for mist.

1. Proper explanation of the procedure helps to ensure the patient's cooperation.
2. The diaphragmatic excursion and lung compliance is greater in this position, and the upright position helps prevent air swallowing.
3. The machine is driven by pressure. No electricity is needed.
4. An IPPB treatment should not be given with dry gas.

5. Standard or individualized settings may be used for sensitivity, pressure and flow.
   a. Must be adjusted to particular patient. A setting that is not sensitive enough may cause increased work of breathing.
   b. Adjustments may be needed to ensure that the patient's gas flow needs are met or exceeded. Insufficient flow will result in increased work of breathing, patient discomfort, and insufficient ventilation.
   c. The patient's chest should appear to have adequate expansion. Measured tidal volume should be 1½ times the baseline. Test the unit to make sure that the desired pressure is achieved before treating the patient.
6. Adequate fog and particle size is essential for effective distribution of medication and moisture.

Performance Phase

1. Instruct the patient to bite down gently on the mouthpiece and seal the mouthpiece with his lips. Noseclips are sometimes used only if the patient has difficulty breathing through his mouth.

2. Tell the patient to breathe slowly and normally and let the machine do the work.

3. Observe expansion of the patient's chest and measure exhaled tidal volume to ensure adequate ventilation.

1. The mouthpiece (or mask) must provide an airtight seal. This will enable the airway pressure to build and allow the unit to cycle properly. If air escapes through the patient's nose when the mouthpiece is used, the unit will be unable to attain the desired pressure.
2. A slight inspiratory effort will activate the positive pressure phase, and the lungs will be inflated with the flow of gas until the predetermined pressure is reached. Gas flow will then cease, and passive exhalation will occur.
3. Measurement of tidal volume is particularly important in the patient who has a high arterial PCO_2 and needs an adequate tidal volume to lower it.

(continued)

Guidelines: Assisting the Patient Undergoing Intermittent Positive Pressure Breathing
(IPPB) (continued)

Planning/Intervention
(Cont.)

Nursing Action	Rationale/Amplification
a. The machine will exert the regulated pressure on inhalation, helping the patient to breath more deeply.	a. The patient should take 8–10 breaths per minute.
b. Instruct the patient to hold his breath 3–4 seconds at the end of each inspiration.	b. This encourages settling of aerosal particles on bronchiolar mucosa.
4. Remind the patient to exhale completely and slowly through the mouthpiece in a relaxed manner. The patient controls exhalation.	4. This type of breathing encourages good diaphragmatic motion and reduces residual air volume.
5. Monitor the treatment.	5. Ensure that the patient is taking the treatment correctly: a. Make sure the patient has a good seal around the mouthpiece. b. Monitor for hyperventilation. c. Make sure the patient does not cycle the machine prematurely. d. Make sure the patient is not expectorating into the nebulizer.
6. Encourage the patient to continue the treatment until all the medication is given.	6. The treatment should last 10–15 minutes, depending on the clinical problem.

Follow-up Phase

Nursing Action	Rationale/Amplification
1. Disassemble and clean the exhalation unit and nebulizer after each use. Keep this equipment in the patient's room. The equipment is changed every 24 hours.	1. Each patient has his own breathing circuit (exhalation valve, nebulizer and tubing, mouthpiece and mask). Through proper cleaning, sterilization, and storage of equipment, organisms can be prevented from entering the lungs.

Evaluation/Outcome

Nursing Action	Rationale/Amplification
1. Record medication used, patient's respiratory rate and effort, pre- and post-treatment heart rate (especially if bronchodilator is used), pre- and post-treatment breath sounds, and description of secretions expectorated. Also record pressure limit and flow rate. Subjective comments may also be added.	1. Note the patient's tolerance of the treatment. Notify physician if intolerance is noted.

Guidelines: Assisting the Patient Undergoing Nebulizer Therapy Without Positive Pressure
(Sidestream Jet Nebulizer) (Fig. 7-25)

A *nebulizer* is a device that produces a stable aerosol of fluid particles. The nebulizer most commonly used for medication administration to the spontaneously breathing patient is the *sidestream jet nebulizer*. The nebulizer is powered by either oxygen or compressed air.

Contraindications

Inability of patient to cooperate in taking deep breaths
Adverse reactions encountered with medication

Hazards

Swelling of dried, retained secretions
Precipitation of bronchospasm

Equipment

Air compressor or oxygen/air flowmeter
Oxygen nipple adapter
Connection tubing
Nebulizer manifold
Medication or saline solution

Nursing Action	Rationale/Amplification

Assessment

Nursing Action	Rationale/Amplification
1. Monitor the heart rate before and after the treatment for patients using bronchodilator drugs.	1. Bronchodilators may produce tachycardia, precordial distress, palpitation, dizziness, nausea, and excessive perspiration.

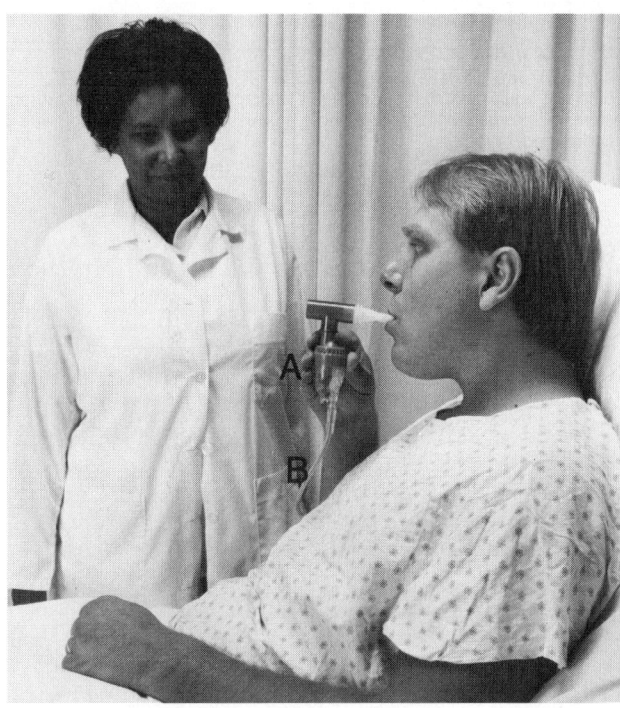

Figure 7-25. A sidestream jet nebulizer. The nebulizer is filled with the prescribed amount of saline or medication (*A*) and attached to compressed air or oxygen source (*B*). (Courtesy of Photography Department, Montefiore Hospital, Pittsburgh, Pennsylvania)

Planning/Implementation

Nursing Action	Rationale/Amplification
Preparatory Phase	
1. Explain the procedure ot the patient. *This therapy depends on patient effort.*	1. Proper explanation of the procedure helps to ensure the patient's cooperation.
2. Place the patient in a comfortable sitting or a semi-Fowler's position.	2. The diaphragmatic excursion and lung compliance is greater in this position. This ensures maximal distribution and deposition of aerosolized particles to basilar areas of the lungs.
3. Connect the nebulizer (containing medication or saline) and connecting tubing to the oxygen flowmeter and set flow at 4–5 liters/minute, or to the air compressor.	3. A fine mist from the device should be visible.
Performance Phase	
1. Instruct the patient to exhale.	
2. Tell the patient to take in a deep breath from the mouthpiece, hold his breath briefly, then exhale.	2. This encourages optimal dispersion of the medication.
3. Nose clips are sometimes used if the patient has difficulty breathing only through his mouth.	
4. Observe expansion of the patient's chest to ascertain that he is taking deep breaths.	4. This will ensure that medication is deposited below the level of the oropharynx.
5. Instruct the patient to breathe slowly and deeply until all the medication is nebulized.	5. Medication usually will be nebulized within 10–15 minutes at a gas flow of 4–5 liters/minute.
6. Upon completion of the treatment, encourage the patient to cough after several deep breaths.	6. The deep lung inflation will allow forceful coughing and facilitate the expectoration of secretions.
Follow-up Phase	
1. Disassemble and clean nebulizer after each use. Keep this equipment in the patient's room. The equipment is changed every 24 hours.	1. Each patient has his own breathing circuit (nebulizer, manifold, tubing, and mouthpiece). Through proper cleaning, sterilization, and storage of equipment, organisms can be prevented from entering the lungs.

Evaluation/Outcome

1. Record medication used, patient's respiratory rate and effort, pre- and post-treatment heart rate, and description of secretions.	1. Note the patient's tolerance of the treatment. Notify physician of any intolerance.

Guidelines: Assisting the Patient Using an Incentive Spirometer (Fig. 7-26)

The *incentive spirometer* is a piece of equipment that encourages performance by the patient of active maximum sustained inspiration. Because this maneuver helps to open closed alveoli, it is used in the prevention and treatment of atelectasis. Patient self-administration is encouraged.

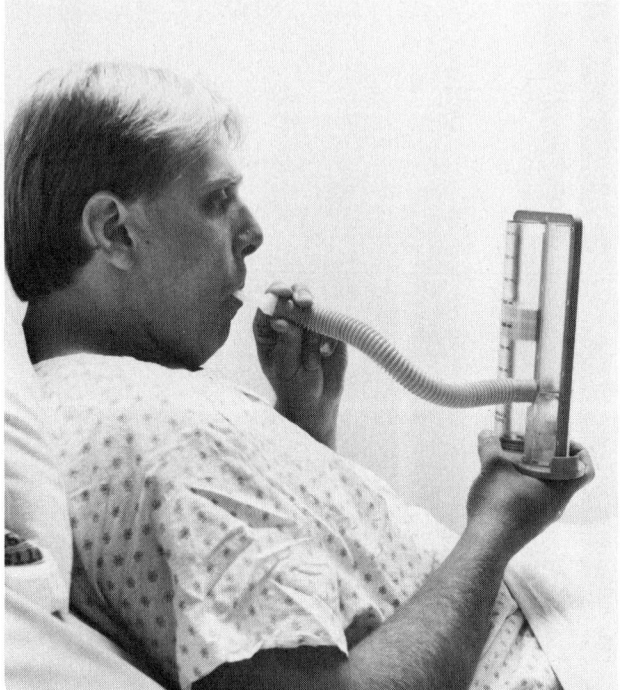

Figure 7-26. An incentive spirometer, designed to encourage sustained maximum inspiration for patients who are predisposed to atelectasis. (Courtesy of Photography Department, Montefiore Hospital, Pittsburgh, Pennsylvania)

Equipment

According to the type of device used

Nursing Action	Rationale/Amplification
Assessment	
1. Measure the patient's normal resting tidal volume and auscultate the chest.	1. The patient's baseline is established.
Planning/Implementation	
Preparatory Phase	
1. Explain the procedure and its purpose to the patient.	1. Optimal results are achieved when the patient is given pretreatment instruction. Preoperative instruction is also beneficial for the surgical patient.
2. Place the patient in a comfortable sitting or semi-Fowler's position.	2. The diaphragmatic excursion is greater in this position; however, if the patient is medically unable to be in this position, the exercise may be done in any position.
3. For the postoperative patient, try as much as possible to avoid discomfort with the treatment administration.	3. Try to coordinate treatment with administration of pain-relief medications. Instruct and assist the patient with splinting of incision.
4. Set the incentive spirometer tidal volume indicator at the desired goal the patient is to reach or exceed (500 ml. is often used to start). The tidal volume is set according to the manufacturer's instructions.	4. The initial tidal volume may be prescribed by the physician, but the purpose of the device is to establish a baseline tidal volume and provide incentive to achieve greater volumes progressively.

Planning/Implementation
(Cont.)

Nursing Action	Rationale / Amplification

Performance Phase

1. Demonstrate the technique to the patient.
2. Instruct the patient to exhale fully.
3. Tell the patient to take in a slow, easy deep breath from the mouthpiece.

4. When the desired goal is reached (lungs fully inflated), ask the patient to continue the inspiratory effort for 3 seconds, even though he may not actually be drawing in more air.
5. Instruct the patient to remove the mouthpiece, relax, and passively exhale. He should take several normal breaths before attempting another one with the incentive spirometer.
6. Continue to monitor the patient's spirometer breaths, periodically increasing the tidal volume as the patient tolerates it.
7. At the conclusion of the treatment, encourage the patient to cough after a deep breath.

3. Noseclips are sometimes used if the patient has difficulty breathing only through his mouth—this will ensure full credit for each breath measured.
4. Sustaining the inspiratory effort helps to open closed alveoli.

5. Usually one incentive breath per minute minimizes patient fatigue. No more than 4–5 maneuvers should be performed per minute to minimize hypocarbia.

7. The deep lung inflation may loosen secretions and enable the patient to expectorate them.

Follow-up Phase

1. Have the patient take the prescribed number of breaths and note the tidal volumes.

1. A total of 10 sustained maximal inspiratory maneuvers per hour during waking hours is a frequent request. A counter on the incentive spirometer indicates the number of breaths the patient has taken.

Outcome/Evaluation

1. Auscultate the chest. Chart any improvement or variation, the volume attained, effectiveness of cough, description of any secretions expectorated.

1. Note the effectiveness and patient tolerance of the treatment.

Guidelines: Assisting the Patient Using an Ultrasonic Nebulizer

Ultrasonic nebulizers employ fluid contained in a chamber, which is rapidly vibrated, causing the fluid to break into small particles. A flow of gas then carries these particles to the patient to be inhaled. This treatment will be administered to the patient at atmospheric pressures, or may be incorporated into an IPPB treatment or mechanical ventilation.

Equipment

Ultrasonic nebulizer and nebulizer cup
Circuitry set-up (according to manufacturer's instructions)
Disposable aerosol mask

Nursing Action	Rationale / Amplification

Assessment

1. Auscultate the chest and monitor vital signs.

1. The patient's baseline is established.

Planning/Implementation

Preparatory Phase

1. Explain the procedure to the patient.
2. Fill the coupling compartment (water reservoir) of the machine with tap water.
3. Place the nebulizer chamber in the coupling compartment and fill with the prescribed fluid.
4. Assemble circuitry according to manufacturer's instruction.
5. Plug in the machine and adjust the setting until the desired amount of mist is obtained.

3. Normal saline is usually used.

(continued)

Guidelines: Assisting the Patient Using an Ultrasonic Nebulizer (continued)

Planning/Implementation
(Cont.)

Nursing Action	Rationale/Amplification
Performance Phase	
1. Place the mask on the patient's face. Instruct the patient to breathe in slowly through his mouth and to exhale the same way.	1. This allows maximal particle deposition.
2. Have the patient continue to breathe in this manner for the prescribed length of the treatment.	2. The procedure usually lasts approximately 15 minutes.
3. Observe the patient for any adverse reaction to the treatment. a. Wheezing (bronchospasm) b. Excessive fluid deposition, causing suffocation	3. The patient may develop wheezing because of the irritating effects of the fluid on the airways, or may not be able to expectorate the delivered fluid and secretions. The fluid may also cause dried retained secretions to swell, resulting in airway narrowing or closure. He may need assistance in draining his secretions by suctioning or postural drainage.
4. Encourage the patient to periodically cough and expectorate any secretions loosened during the treatment.	
Follow-up Phase	
1. Keep this equipment in the patient's room. The equipment should be changed every 24 hours.	1. Ultrasonic nebulizers have a high contamination rate. It is desirable that each patient have his own device in his room.

Outcome/Evaluation

1. Record the medication used, the patient's respiratory rate and effort, and description of secretions expectorated.	1. Note any adverse reactions. Notify physician of any patient intolerance of the treatment.

Artificial Airway Management

An *artificial airway* is a tube that is inserted at the mouth or nose (endotracheal tube) or level of the second or third tracheal ring (tracheostomy) to permit mechanical ventilation and/or facilitate secretion removal. The distal end of the tube is located in the trachea below the vocal cords.

Indications

1. Acute respiratory failure, CNS depression, neuromuscular disease, pulmonary diseases, chest wall injury
2. Upper airway obstruction (tumor, inflammation, foreign body, laryngeal spasm)
3. Anticipated upper airway obstruction from edema or soft tissue swelling due to head and neck trauma, some postoperative head and neck procedures involving the airway, facial or airway burns, decreased level of consciousness
4. Aspiration prophylaxis
5. Fractured cervical vertebrae with spinal cord injury requiring ventilatory assistance

Route of Insertion

A. Endotracheal

May be inserted through the nose or the mouth (Fig. 7-27). A cuff is always located at the distal end of the tube.
1. Orotracheal—insertion of an oral tube is technically easier, since it is done under direct visualization. Disadvantages are increased oral secretions, decreased patient comfort, difficulty with stabilization, and inability of patient to use lip movement as a communication means.
2. Nasotracheal—may be more comfortable to the patient and is easier to stabilize. Disadvantages are that blind insertion is required; possible development of pressure necrosis of the nasal airway, sinusitis, and otitis media.

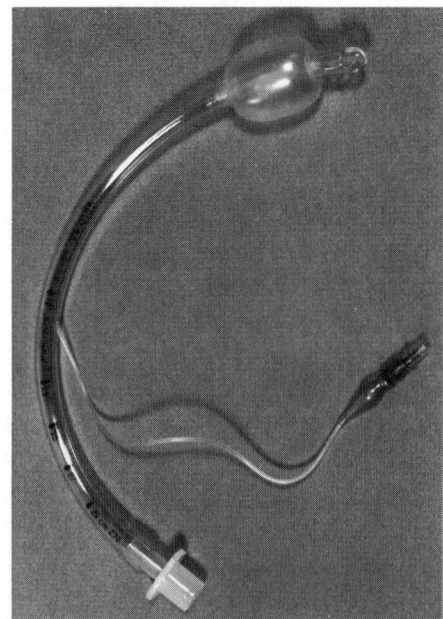

Figure 7-27. Endotracheal tube. (Courtesy of Photography Department, Montefiore Hospital, Pittsburgh, Pennsylvania)

Tube types:
  a. Vary according to length and inner diameter in millimeters. Usual sizes for adults are 6.0, 7.0, 8.0, and 9.0 mm.
  b. Vary according to cuff. Most are high volume, low pressure, with self-sealing inflation valves, or the cuff may be of foam rubber (Fome-Cuff®).

B. Tracheostomy

Inserted into the trachea via an incision created at the level of the 2nd or 3rd cartilage ring; totally bypasses the upper airway. These tubes may or may not be cuffed. Patients with tracheostomies requiring mechanical ventilation are given cuffed tracheostomy tubes. Patients who are awake and alert, are able to protect the airway, and do not require mechanical ventilation may be given a cuffless tracheostomy tube. This same group of patients may be given cuffed "trach" tubes, with the cuff inflated only during feeding (see Nursing Management below). Tube types (Fig. 7-28):
  1. Vary according to composition and cuff type: synthetic Teflon, nylon, polyvinyl chloride, polyethylene, or silastic. May or may not have inner cannula. Usually are cuffed.
     a. Tubes with high-volume, low-pressure cuffs, self-sealing inflation valves. With or without inner cannula.
     b. Pressure-limiting cuffs
     c. Polyurethane foam-filled cuffs
     d. Speaking tracheostomy tube
     e. Fenestrated
     f. Silver (Silver tracheostomy tubes are rarely used.)
  2. May vary according to length and inner diameter in millimeters. Usual sizes for an adult are 6.0, 7.0, 8.0, and 9.0 mm.

Nursing Management

A. Physical Management

  1. Ensure adequate ventilation and oxygenation through the use of mechanical ventilation, continuous positive airway pressure (CPAP) device, Briggs T-piece adapter (or O_2 "trach" mask).
  2. Provide adequate humidity, since the natural humidifying pathway of the oropharynx is bypassed. Clear airway of secretions as needed with suctioning.
  3. Use aseptic technique when entering the artificial airway. The artificial airway bypasses the upper airway, and the lower airways are sterile below the level of the vocal cords.
  4. Frequently assess the patient's need for ventilatory assistance.
  5. Elevate the patient to a semi-Fowler's or sitting position, when possible, since these positions result

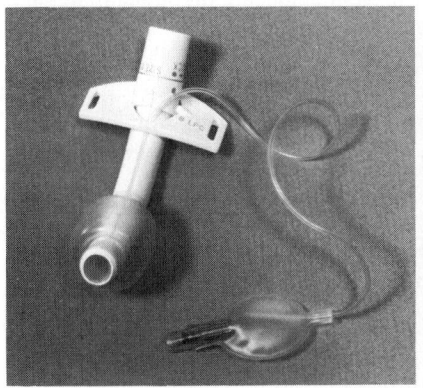

A. Low pressure cuff (Shiley)

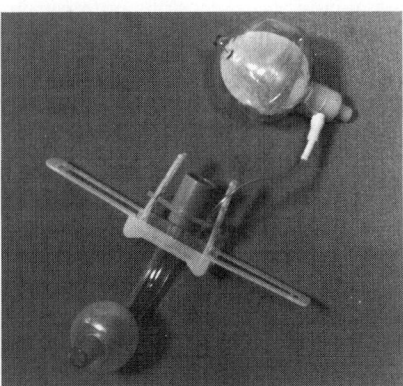

B. Pressure limiting cuff (Lanz)

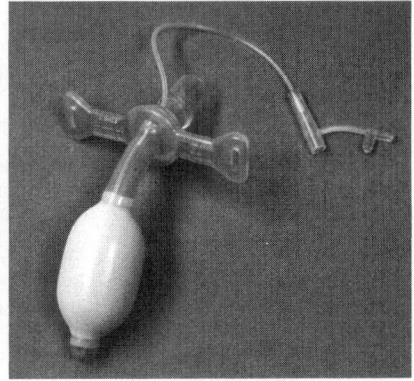

C. Polyurethane foam filled cuff (Fome-Cuf)

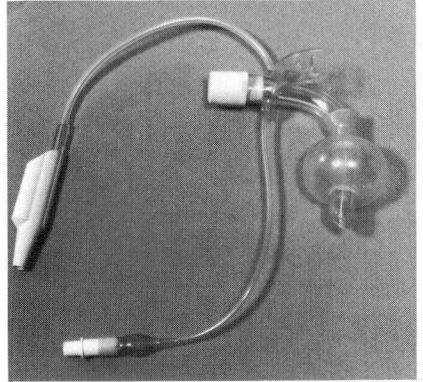

D. Speaking tube (Pitt)

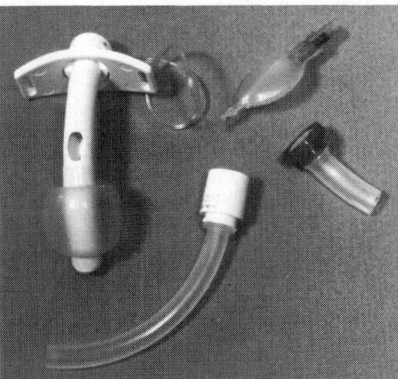

E. Fenestrated tube (Shiley)

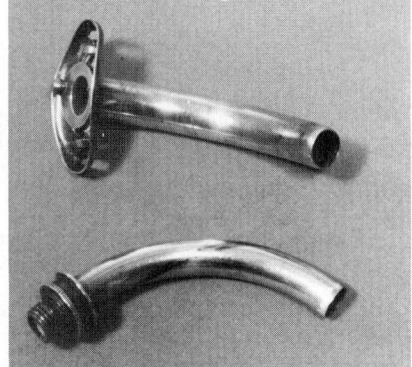

F. Silver tube

Figure 7-28. Types of tracheostomy tubes. (Courtesy of Photography Department, Montefiore Hospital, Pittsburgh, Pennsylvania)

in improved lung compliance. The patient's position, however, should be changed at least every 2 hours to ensure ventilation of all lung segments and prevention of secretion stagnation. Position changes are also necessary to avoid skin breakdown.

6. Nutrition
   a. Endotube—recognize that the tube holds open the epiglottis. Therefore only the inflated cuff prevents the aspiration of oropharyngeal contents into the lungs. *The patient must not receive oral feeding.* Nutrition must take the form of enteral tube feedings, or parenteral hyperalimentation.
   b. Tracheostomy—if the tracheostomy tube is cuffed, the nurse should determine whether the patient is able to eat with the cuff inflated or deflated.

      Note: patients on mechanical ventilation or CPAP must have the cuff inflated at all times. The inflated cuff prevents aspiration of food contents into the lungs, but bulging of the tracheal wall caused by the inflated cuff may push against the esophagus and make swallowing more difficult. Patients who are not on mechanical ventilation and are awake, alert, and able to protect the airway are candidates for eating with the cuff deflated.

      (1) To assess ability to protect the airway:
          (a) Sit the patient upright.
          (b) Feed the patient colored gelatin.
          (c) If color from gelatin can be suctioned from the tracheostomy tube, aspiration is occurring and the cuff must be inflated during feeding and for 1 hour afterward.

7. Be aware of the complications and damage that inflated cuffs may have on the tracheal mucosa. Endotracheal tube cuffs should be inflated continuously and deflated only during intubation, extubation, and tube repositioning. The internal cuff pressure should be checked every 2 hours. Tracheostomy tube cuffs also should be inflated continuously in patients on mechanical ventilation or CPAP. Tracheostomized patients who are breathing spontaneously may have the cuffs inflated continuously (in the patient having suppressed levels of consciousness with an inability to protect airway), deflated continuously, or inflated only for feeding if the patient is at risk for aspiration. (See Cuff Inflation for technique.)

8. External tube site care
   a. Endotracheal tubes—patients with endotracheal tubes have mouth care every shift, or as frequently as needed. Oral secretions tend to stagnate, and risk of oral infection is increased. An oral endotracheal tube may also stimulate an increase in the production of oral secretions. The tube must be secured at all times (see Endotracheal Intubation for technique), and the ventilator, CPAP, or T-piece tubing supported so that traction is not applied to the tube.
   b. Tracheostomy tube—the stoma should be cleaned once a shift or more frequently if needed, and the tracheostomy ties changed once a day (see Tracheostomy Site Care for technique). The ventilator, CPAP, or T-piece tubing must be supported so that traction is not applied to the tracheostomy tube.

9. Have available at all times at the patient's bedside a resuscitation bag, oxygen source, and mask to ventilate the patient in the event of accidental tube removal. Anticipate your course of action in such an event.
   a. Endotracheal tube—know location and assembly of reintubation equipment. Know method of contact of personnel capable of reintubation.
   b. Tracheostomy—have extra tracheostomy tube at bedside. Be aware of reinsertion technique, or know method of contact of personnel capable of reinserting the tube. **Note:** Remember that with tracheostomized patients, as long as the airway is patent (from upper to lower), it is possible to bag/mask ventilate with the resuscitation bag if the stoma is covered. Only patients with complete airway obstruction, an open stoma, or laryngectomy need have mouth to stoma ventilation performed.

Psychological Care of the Patient

1. Recognize that the patient is usually apprehensive, particularly about choking, inability to communicate verbally, being unable to remove secretions, difficulty in breathing, or mechanical failure.
2. Explain the function of the equipment carefully.
3. Inform the patient and his family that he will not be able to speak while the tube is in place (the exception being a tracheostomy tube with a deflated cuff, a fenestrated tube, or a speaking tracheostomy tube). Develop with the patient the best method of communication (e.g., sign language, lip movement, letter boards, paper and pencil, magic slate, or coded messages). Patients with tracheostomy tubes or nasal endotracheal tubes may effectively use orally operated electrolarynx devices. Devise a means for the patient to get the nurse's attention when someone is not immediately available at the bedside, such as call bell, hand-operated bell, rattle, etc.
4. Anticipate some of the patient's questions by discussing "Is it permanent?" "Will it hurt to breathe?" "Will someone be with me?"

Complications

1. Mechanical
   a. Cuff leaks
   b. Cuff herniation
   c. Tube obstruction (biting, kinking, mucus plug, blood clot)
   d. Tube displacement
   e. Inadvertent extubation
   f. Right main stem intubation (endotracheal tube)
2. Laryngeal and tracheal
   a. Sore throat
   b. Hoarse voice
   c. Glottic edema
   d. Ulceration of tracheal mucosa
   e. Vocal cord ulceration, granuloma, or polyps
   f. Vocal cord paralysis
   g. Laryngotracheal web—formation of a web of fibrin and cellular debris initiated by necrotic tissue at the glottic or subglottic level. Most often seen 4–5 days after tracheal extubation.
   h. Postextubation tracheal stenosis
   i. Tracheal dilatation
   j. Formation of tracheal–esophageal fistula
   k. Formation of tracheal–arterial fistula
   l. Inominate artery erosion
   m. See additional complications under specific procedures dealing with artificial airways.

Guidelines: Endotracheal Intubation (Fig. 7-29)

An *endotracheal tube* may be inserted via the nose or the mouth. The indications for use are the same as those for any artificial airway.

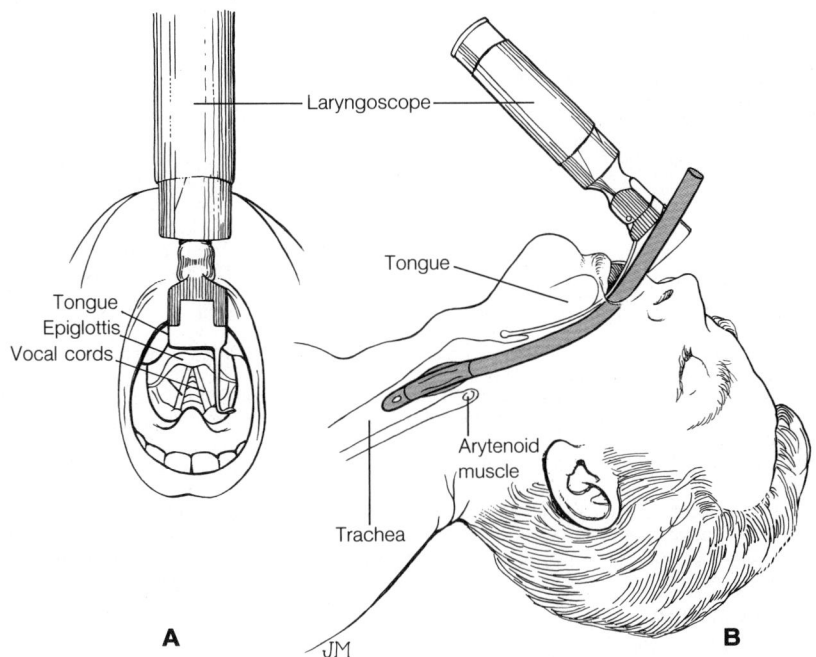

Figure 7-29. Endotracheal intubation. (*A*) The primary glottic landmarks for tracheal intubation as visualized with proper placement of the laryngoscope. (*B*) Positioning the endotube.

Equipment

Laryngoscope with curved or straight blade and working light source (Check batteries and bulb periodically.)
Endotracheal tube with low-pressure cuff and adapter to connect tube to ventilator or resuscitation bag
Stylet to guide the endotracheal tube
Oral airway (assorted sizes) or bite block to keep patient from biting into and occluding the endotracheal tube
Adhesive tape or tube fixation system
Sterile anesthetic lubricant jelly (water-soluble)
Syringe
Suction source
Suction catheter and tonsil suction
Resuscitation bag and mask connected to oxygen source
Anesthetic spray
Sterile towel

Nursing Action	Rationale / Amplification
Assessment	
1. Monitor the patient's heart rate, level of consciousness, and respiratory status.	1. Provides a baseline to estimate patient's tolerance of procedure.
Planning/Implementation	
1. Remove the patient's dental bridgework and plates.	1. May interfere with insertion. Will not be able to remove easily from patient once intubated.
2. Remove headboard of bed (optional).	

(continued)

Guidelines: Endotracheal Intubation (continued)

Planning/Implementation
(Cont.)

Nursing Action	Rationale/Amplification
3. Prepare equipment	
a. Ensure function of resuscitation bag with mask, and suction.	a. Patient may require ventilatory assistance during procedure. Suction should be functional, since gagging and emesis may occur during procedure.
b. Assemble the laryngoscope—make sure the light bulb is tightly attached and functional.	
c. Select an endotracheal tube of the appropriate size (6.0–9.0 mm. for average adult).	
d. Place the endotracheal tube on a sterile towel.	d. Although the tube will pass through the contaminated mouth or nose, the airway below the vocal cords is sterile, and efforts must be made to prevent iatrogenic contamination of the distal end of the tube and cuff. The proximal end of the tube may be handled, since it will reside in the upper airway.
e. Inflate the cuff to make sure it assumes a symmetrical shape and holds volume without leakage. Then deflate maximally.	e. Malfunction of the cuff must be ascertained before tube placement occurs.
f. Lubricate the distal end of the tube liberally with the sterile anesthetic water soluble jelly.	f. Aids in insertion.
g. Insert the stylet into the tube (if oral intubation is planned—nasal intubation does not employ use of the stylet).	g. Stiffens the soft tube, allowing it to be more easily directed into the trachea.
4. Aspirate stomach contents if nasogastric tube is in place.	
5. If time allows, inform the patient of impending inability to talk and discuss alternate means of communication.	5. Discuss alternate means of communication (see Artificial Airway, Psychological Care, Step 3).
6. If the patient is confused, it may be necessary to apply soft wrist restraints.	6. Restraint of the confused patient may be necessary to promote patient safety and maintain sterile technique.

Performance Phase

1. If cervical spine is not injured, for oral intubation place head in a "sniffing" position—flexed at the junction of the neck and thorax and extended at the junction of the spine and skull.	1. Upper airway is open maximally in this position and mouth of the unconscious patient will often open.
2. Spray the back of the patient's throat with an anesthetic spray if time is available.	2. Will decrease gagging.
3. Ventilate and oxygenate the patient with the resuscitation bag and mask before intubation.	3. This decreases the likelihood of cardiac arrhythmias or respiratory distress secondary to hypoxemia.
4. Hold the handle of the laryngoscope in the left hand and hold the patient's mouth open with the right hand by placing crossed fingers on the teeth.	4. Leverage is improved by crossing the thumb and index fingers when opening the patient's mouth (scissor-twist technique).
5. Insert the curved blade of the laryngoscope along the right side of the tongue, push the tongue to the left, and use right thumb and index finger to pull patient's lower lip away from lower teeth.	5. Rolling the lip away from teeth prevents injury by being caught between teeth and blade.
6. Lift laryngoscope forward (toward ceiling) to expose the epiglottis.	6. Do not use teeth as a fulcrum which could lead to dental damage.
7. Lift laryngoscope upward and forward at a 45-degree angle to expose glottis and visualize vocal cords.	7. This stretches the hypoepiglottis ligament, folding the epiglottis upward and exposing the glottis.
8. As the epiglottis is lifted forward (toward ceiling) the vertical opening of the larynx between the vocal cords will come into view (Fig. 7-29A).	8. Do not use wrist. Use shoulder and arm to lift epiglottis.
9. Once vocal cords are visualized, insert tube into the right corner of the mouth and pass the tube—guided by blade, but keeping vocal cords in constant view.	9. Make sure you do not insert tube into esophagus (Fig. 7-29B); the esophageal mucosa is pink and the opening is horizontal rather than vertical.
10. Gently push the tube through the triangular space formed by the vocal cords and back wall of trachea.	10. If the vocal cords are in spasm (closed), wait a few seconds before passing tube.
11. Stop insertion just after the tube cuff has disappeared from view beyond the cords.	11. Advancing tube further may lead to its entry into a mainstem bronchus (usually the right bronchus) causing collapse of the unventilated lung.
12. Withdraw laryngoscope while holding endotracheal tube in place. Disassemble mask from resuscitation bag and ventilate the patient.	
13. Inflate cuff with the minimal amount of air required to occlude the trachea.	13. The amount of air used for cuff inflation depends on the size of the cuff and the diameter of the patient's trachea. Occlusion occurs when no air is felt or heard passing through the patient's nose or mouth.

Planning/Implementation
(Cont.)

Nursing Action	Rationale/Amplification
14. Insert oral airway or bite block if necessary.	14. This keeps patient from biting down on the tube and obstructing the airway.
15. Ascertain expansion of both sides of the chest by observation and auscultation of breath sounds.	15. Observation and auscultation help in determining that tube remains in position and has not slipped into the right main stem bronchus.
16. Mark proximal end of tube with marking pen or tape at the point where the tube reaches the corner of the patient's mouth.	16. This will allow for detection of any later change in tube position.
17. Secure tube to the patient's face with adhesive tape or apply a commercially available endotracheal tube stabilization device. The patient in Fig. 7-21 is wearing such a device.	17. The tube must be fixed securely to ensure that it will not be dislodged. Dislodgement of a tube with an inflated cuff may result in damage to the vocal cords.
18. Obtain chest x-ray to verify tube position.	

Follow-up Phase

Nursing Action	Rationale/Amplification
1. Measure cuff pressure with manometer; adjust pressure (see Cuff Inflation). Make adjustment in tube placement on the basis of the chest x-ray results.	1. The tube may be advanced or removed several centimeters for proper placement on the basis of the chest x-ray results.

Evaluation/Outcome

Nursing Action	Rationale/Amplification
1. Record tube type and size, cuff pressure, and patient tolerance of the procedure. Auscultate breath sounds every one to two hours or if signs and symptoms of respiratory distress occur. Assess arterial blood gases after intubation if requested by the physician.	1. Arterial blood gases may be prescribed to ensure adequacy of ventilation and respiration. Tube displacement outward may result in extubation (cuff above vocal cords). Tube displacement forward may result in tube touching carina (causing paroxysmal coughing) or intubation of a mainstem bronchus (resulting in collapse of the unventilated lung).

Guidelines: Extubation

Extubation consists of removal of the oral or nasal endotracheal tube.
NOTE: Extubation may be performed only if personnel qualified to reintubate are available. The occurrence of laryngospasm or tracheal edema postextubation may require immediate tube replacement.

Equipment

Tonsil suction (surgical suction instrument)
10-ml. syringe
Resuscitation bag and mask with oxygen flow
Aerosol face mask connected to aerosol tubing and nebulizer with oxygen source
Sterile towel
Suction catheter and tonsil suction

Nursing Action	Rationale/Amplification

Assessment

Nursing Action	Rationale/Amplification
1. Monitor heart rate, lung expansion, and breath sounds pre-extubation. Record tidal volume, vital capacity, and inspiratory force.	1. Tidal volume, vital capacity, and negative inspiratory force are measured to assess respiratory muscle function and adequacy of ventilation.
2. Assess the patient for other signs of recovered muscle power. a. Instruct the patient to tightly squeeze the index and middle fingers of your hand. Resistance to removal of your fingers from the patient's grasp must be demonstrated. b. Ask the patient to lift his head from the pillow and hold for 2–3 seconds.	2. Adequate muscle strength is necessary to ensure maintenance of a patent airway.

Planning/Implementation

Preparatory Phase

Nursing Action	Rationale/Amplification
1. Obtain orders for extubation and post extubation oxygen therapy from the physician.	1. Do not attempt extubation until postextubation oxygen therapy is available and functioning at the bedside.

(continued)

Guidelines: Extubation (continued)

Planning/Implementation
(Cont.)

Nursing Action	Rationale/Amplification
2. Explain the procedure to the patient: a. He will have the artificial airway removed. b. He will be suctioned prior to extubation. c. He will be asked to take deep breaths on command. d. He will be asked to cough after extubation.	2. Increases patient cooperation.
3. Prepare necessary equipment for extubation. Have ready for use: tonsil suction, 10-ml. syringe, bag/mask unit, and oxygen via face mask.	
4. Place patient in sitting or semi-Fowler's position (unless contraindicated).	4. Increases lung compliance and decreases work of breathing. Facilitates coughing.

Performance Phase

Nursing Action	Rationale/Amplification
1. Suction endotracheal tube (see Sterile Tracheobronchial Suctioning).	
2. Suction oropharyngeal airway above the endotracheal cuff as thoroughly as possible.	2. Secretions left above the cuff may be aspirated when the cuff is deflated.
3. Loosen tape or endotracheal tube securing device.	
4. Extubate the patient: a. Ask the patient to take as deep a breath as possible (if the patient is not following commands, give a deep breath with the resuscitation bag). b. At peak inspiration, deflate the cuff completely and pull the tube out in the direction of the curve (out and downward).	a. At peak inspiration, the trachea and vocal cords will dilate, allowing atraumatic tube removal.
5. Once the tube is fully removed, ask the patient to cough or exhale forcefully to remove secretions. Then suction the back of the patient's airway with the tonsil suction.	5. Frequently, old blood is seen in the secretions of newly extubated patients. Monitor for the appearance of bright red blood due to trauma occurring during extubation.
6. Evaluate immediately for any signs of airway obstruction, stridor, or difficult breathing. If the patient develops any of the above problems, attempt to ventilate the patient with the resuscitation bag and mask and prepare for reintubation.	6. Immediate complications: a. Laryngospasm may develop causing obstruction of the airway. b. Edema may develop at the cuff site. Signs of narrowing airway lumen are high pitched crowing sounds, decreased air movement, and respiratory distress.
7. Administer oxygen as directed.	

Follow-up Phase

Nursing Action	Rationale/Amplification
1. Observe patient closely postextubation for any signs and symptoms of airway obstruction or respiratory insufficiency.	1. Tracheal or laryngeal edema may develop postextubation (a possibility for up to 24 hours). Signs and symptoms include high-pitched, crowing upper airway sounds and respiratory distress.
2. Observe character of voice.	2. Hoarseness is a common postextubation complaint. Observe for worsening hoarseness or vocal cord paralysis.

Evaluation/Outcome

Nursing Action	Rationale/Amplification
1. Note patient tolerance of procedure, upper and lower airway sounds postextubation, description of secretions.	1. Establishes a baseline to assess improvement/development of complications.

Guidelines: Assisting With Tracheostomy Insertion

Tracheostomy is usually performed when the need for an artificial airway is protracted (usually greater than 14 days). Tracheostomy may also be performed when the surgical interruption of the airway is necessary (i.e., laryngectomy).

Equipment

Tracheostomy tube (sizes 6.0–9.0 mm. for most adults)
Sterile instruments: hemostat, scalpel and blade, forceps, suture material, scissors
Sterile gown and drapes, gloves
Cap and mask
Antiseptic prep solution
Gauze sponges
Shave prep kit
Sedation

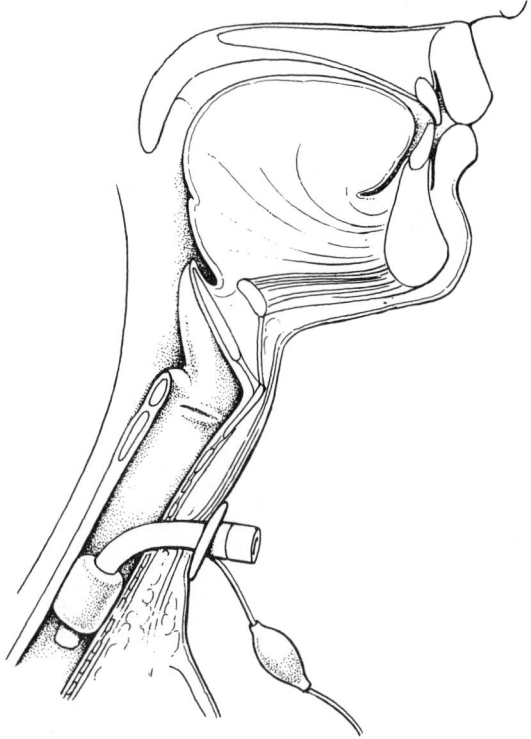

Figure 7-30. Tracheostomy tube placement.

Local anesthetic and syringe
Resuscitation bag and mask with oxygen source
Suction source and catheters
Syringe for cuff inflation
Respiratory support available for post-tracheostomy (mechanical ventilation, tracheal oxygen mask, CPAP, T-piece)

Nursing Action	Rationale / Amplification

Assessment

1. Monitor vital signs (heart rate, respiration, blood pressure, temperature) before insertion.

1. Provides baseline for assessment of progress or complications.

Planning/Implementation

Preparatory Phase

1. Explain the procedure to the patient. Discuss a communication system with the patient.

1. Apprehension about inability to talk is usually a major concern of the tracheostomized patient.

2. Obtain consent for operative procedure.

3. Shave neck region.

3. Hair and beard may harbor harmful microorganisms. If beard is to be removed, inform the patient or family.

4. Assemble equipment. Using aseptic technique, inflate tracheostomy cuff and evaluate for symmetry and volume leakage. Deflate maximally.

4. Ensures that the cuff is functional prior to tube insertion.

5. Position the patient (supine with head extended, with a support under shoulders).
   Apply soft wrist restraints if the patient is confused.

5. This position brings the trachea forward.
   Restraint of the confused patient may be necessary to ensure patient safety and preservation of aseptic technique.

6. Give medication per physician request.

7. Position light source.

8. Assist with antiseptic prep.

9. Assist physician with gowning and gloving.

10. Assist with sterile draping.

(continued)

Guidelines: Assisting With Tracheostomy Insertion (continued)

Planning/Implementation
(Cont.)

Nursing Action	Rationale/Amplification
Performance Phase	
1. The physician performs the procedure with the nurse circulating. He or she or another designated nurse also monitors the patient's vital signs, suctions as necessary, gives medication as prescribed, or administers emergency care.	1. Bradycardia may result from vagal stimulation due to tracheal manipulation, or hypoxemia. Hypoxemia may also cause cardiac irritability.
2. Immediately after the tube is inserted, inflate the cuff. The chest should be auscultated for the presence of bilateral breath sounds.	2. Ensures ventilation of both lungs.
Follow-up Phase	
1. Apply respiratory assistive devices (mechanical ventilation, tracheostomy oxygen mask, CPAP, T-piece adapter).	
2. Check the tracheostomy tube cuff with the pressure manometer.	2. Excessive cuff pressure may cause tracheal damage.
3. "Tie sutures" or "stay sutures" of 00 silk may have been placed through either side of the tracheal cartilage at the incision and brought out through the wound. Each is to be taped to the skin at a 45-degree angle laterally to the sternum.	3. Should the tracheostomy tube become dislodged, the stay sutures may be grasped and used to spread the tracheal cartilage apart, facilitating placement of the new tube.

Evaluation/Outcome

1. Assess vital signs and ventilatory status; note tube size used, physician performing procedure, type, dose and route of medications given.	1. Provides baseline.
2. Obtain chest x-ray.	2. Documents proper tube placement.
3. Assess and chart condition of stoma: a. Bleeding	a. Some bleeding around the stoma site is not uncommon for the first few hours. Monitor and inform the physician of any increase in bleeding. Clean site aseptically when necessary (see Tracheostomy Care). Do not change tracheostomy ties for first 24 hours, since accidental dislodgement of the tube could result when the ties are loose, and tube reinsertion through the as yet unformed stoma may be difficult or impossible to accomplish.
b. Swelling c. Subcutaneous air	c. When positive pressure respiratory assistive devices are used (mechanical ventilation, CPAP) before the wound is healed, air may be forced into the subcutaneous fat layer. This can be seen as enlargement of the neck and facial tissues and felt as crepitus or "crackling" when the skin is depressed. The physician is informed.

4. An extra tube, obturator, and hemostat should be kept at the bedside. In the event of tube dislodgement, reinsertion of a new tube may be necessary. For emergency tube insertion:
   Spread the wound with a hemostat or stay sutures;
   Insert replacement tube (containing the obturator) at an angle;
   Point cannula downward and insert the tube maximally; remove the obturator.
	4. The hemostat will open the airway and allow ventilation in the spontaneously breathing patient. Avoid inserting the tube horizontally, as the tube may be forced against the back wall of the trachea.

Guidelines: Tracheostomy Care (Routine)

Tracheostomy care keeps the area clean and dry, preventing skin irritation and infection. Secretions collected above the tracheostomy tube cuff ooze out of the surgical incision. The resultant wetness promotes irritation of the skin, and the wetness, coupled with the transmission of bacteria via the secretions, sets up a medium for infection to occur.

Equipment

Assemble the following equipment or obtain a prepackaged tracheostomy care kit;

Sterile towel

Sterile gauze sponges (12)

Sterile cotton swabs

Equipment
(Cont.)

Sterile gloves
Hydrogen peroxide
Sterile water
Antiseptic solution and ointment (optional)
Tracheostomy tie tapes

Nursing Action	Rationale/Amplification
Assessment	
1. Assess condition of stoma prior to tracheostomy care (redness, swelling, character of secretions, presence of purulence or bleeding).	1. The presence of skin breakdown or infection must be monitored. Culture of the site may be warranted by appearance of these signs.
Planning/Implementation	
Preparatory Phase	
1. Suction the trachea and pharynx thoroughly prior to tracheostomy care.	1. Removal of secretions prior to tracheostomy care keeps the area clean longer.
2. Explain procedure to the patient.	
3. Wash hands thoroughly.	
4. Assemble equipment:	
a. Place sterile towel on patient's chest under tracheostomy site.	a. Provides sterile field.
b. Open 4 gauze sponges and pour hydrogen peroxide on them.	b. For removing mucus and crust, which promotes bacterial growth.
c. Open 2 gauze sponges and pour antiseptic solution on them.	c. May be applied to fresh stoma or infected stoma—not necessary for clean, healed stoma.
d. Open 2 gauze sponges, keep dry.	
e. Open 2 gauze sponges and pour sterile water on them.	
f. Place tracheostomy tube tapes on field.	
g. Put on sterile gloves.	g. Sterile gloves prevent contamination of the wound by nurse's hands and also protect the nurse's hands from infection.
Performance Phase	
1. Clean the external end of the tracheostomy tube with 2 gauze sponges with hydrogen peroxide; discard sponges.	
2. Clean the stoma area with 2 peroxide-soaked gauze sponges. Make only a single sweep with each gauze sponge before discarding.	2. Hydrogen peroxide may help loosen dry crusted secretions.
3. Loosen and remove any crust with sterile cotton swabs.	
4. Repeat step 2 using the sterile water-soaked gauze sponges.	4. Ensures that all hydrogen peroxide is removed.
5. Repeat two using dry sponges.	5. Ensures dryness of the area—wetness promotes infection and irritation.
6. (Optional) An infected wound may be cleaned with gauze saturated with an antiseptic solution, then dried. A thin layer of antibiotic ointment may be applied to the stoma with a cotton swab.	6. May help clear infection of the wound.
7. Change the tracheostomy tie tapes:	
a. Cut soiled tape while holding tube securely with other hand.	a. Stabilization of the tube helps prevent accidental dislodgement and keeps irritation and coughing due to tube manipulation at a minimum. Two persons may participate in the procedure at this point.
b. Remove old tapes carefully.	
c. Grasp slit end of clean tape and pull it through opening on side of the tracheostomy tube.	
d. Pull other end of tape securely through the slit end of the tape.	
e. Repeat on the other side.	
f. Tie the tapes at the side of the neck in a square knot. Alternate knot from side to side each time tapes are changed.	f. To prevent irritation and rotate pressure site.
g. Tape should be tight enough to keep tube securely in the stoma but loose enough to permit two fingers to fit between the tapes and the neck.	g. Excessive tightness of tapes will compress jugular veins and decrease blood circulation to the skin under the tape, as well as being uncomfortable for the patient.

(continued)

Guidelines: Tracheostomy Care (Routine) (continued)

Planning/Implementation
(Cont.)

Nursing Action	Rationale/Amplification

8. Some clinicians elect to place a gauze pad between the stoma site and the tracheostomy tube to absorb secretions and prevent irritation of the stoma. Other clinicians feel that this is unnecessary (Fig. 7-31). Many clinicians feel that gauze should not be used around the stoma. In their opinion, the dressing keeps the area moist and dark, promoting stomal infection. They believe the stoma should be left open to the air and the surrounding area kept dry. A dressing is used only if secretions are draining onto subclavian or neck IV sites or chest incisions.

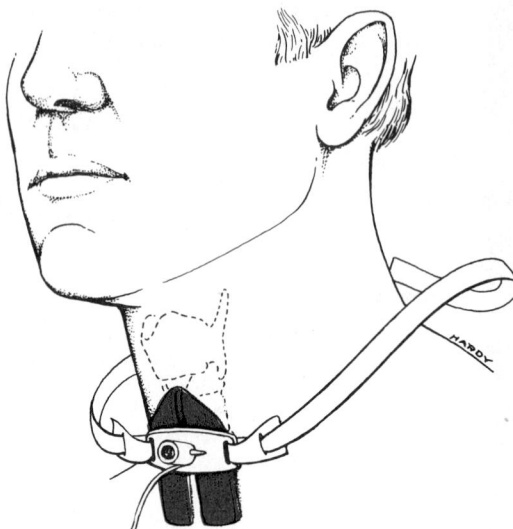

Figure 7-31. Placement of tracheostomy tube tapes and elective gauze pad.

Follow-up Phase

1. Cleaning of the fresh stoma should be performed every 8 hours, or more frequently if indicated by accumulation of secretions. Ties should be changed every 24 hours, or more frequently if soiled or wet.

   1. The area must be kept clean and dry to prevent infection or irritation of tissues.

Evaluation/Outcome

1. Document procedure performance, observations of stoma (irritation, redness, edema, subcutaneous air), and character of secretions (color, purulence).

   1. Provides a baseline. Notify physician of changes in stoma appearance or secretions.

Guidelines: Sterile Tracheobronchial Suction via Tracheostomy or Endotracheal Tube
(Spontaneous or Mechanical Ventilation) (Fig. 7-32)

The patient with an ineffective cough cannot clear his secretions and requires mechanical aspiration (suctioning). It is a sterile procedure. Secretion collection in the artificial airway or tracheobronchial tree may result in narrowing of the airway, respiratory insufficiency, increased work of breathing, and stasis of secretions.

Indications

1. When secretions can be seen or sounds resulting from secretions are heard with or without the use of a stethoscope.
2. Following postural drainage or chest physiotherapy.
3. Following respiratory treatments aimed at liquefying secretions (i.e., ultrasonic nebulization).
4. Following a sudden rise or the "popping off" of the peak airway pressure in mechanically ventilated patients that is not due to kinking of the artificial airway or ventilator tube, patient biting the tube, the patient coughing or struggling against the ventilator, or pneumothorax.

   NOTE: Patients with ineffective cough mechanisms do not require "routine" suctioning. The need for suctioning may be assessed by pulmonary physical examination (especially auscultation) and chest x-ray findings. To aid in assessing for the need for suctioning, the patient may be ventilated with a resuscitation bag to increase ventilation and facilitate auscultation. Bagging may also stimulate the cough reflex, decreasing the need for suctioning.

Equipment

Assemble the following equipment or obtain a prepackaged suctioning kit:

Sterile suction catheters—No. 14 or 16 (adult), No. 8 or 10 (child). The outer diameter of the suction catheter should be no greater than two thirds of the inner diameter of the artificial airway.

Two sterile gloves

Sterile towel

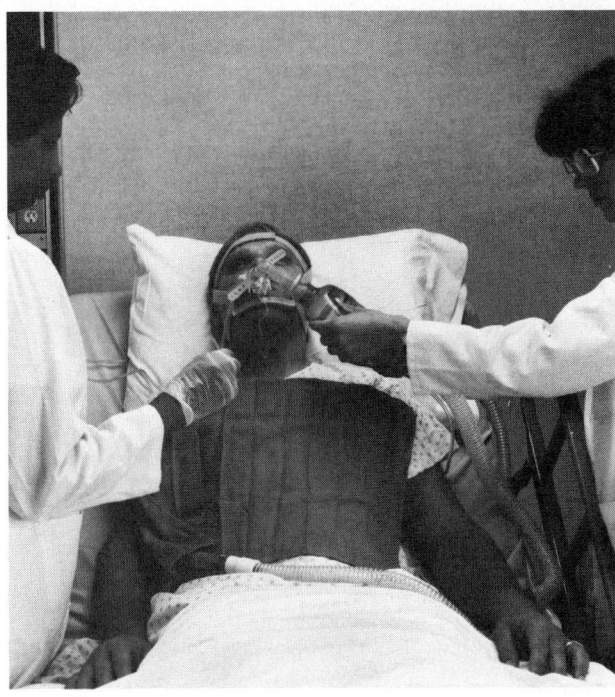

Figure 7-32. Suctioning through an endotracheal or tracheostomy tube. (Courtesy of Photography Department, Montefiore Hospital, Pittsburgh, Pennsylvania)

Equipment
(Cont.)

Suction source set at −80 to −120 mm. Hg

Sterile water

Resuscitation bag with a reservoir connected to 100% oxygen source (If patient is on PEEP or CPAP, add positive end-expiratory pressure (PEEP) valve to exhalation valve on resuscitation bag in an amount equal to that on the ventilator or CPAP device.)

Normal saline solution (in syringe or single-dose packet)

Sterile cup for water

Alcohol swabs

Sterile water-soluble lubricant jelly

Nursing Action	Rationale/Amplification

Assessment

1. Monitor heart rate, color, ease of respiration. If the patient is monitored, continuously monitor heart rate and arterial blood pressure. If arterial blood gases are done routinely, know baseline values. (It is important to establish a baseline, since suctioning should be discontinued and oxygen applied or manual ventilation reinstituted if, during the suction procedure, the heart rate decreases by 20 beats per minute or increases by 40 beats per minute, blood pressure drops, or cardiac dysrhythmia is noted.)

1. Suctioning may cause:
   a. Hypoxemia, initially resulting in tachycardia and increased blood pressure, progressing to cardiac ectopy, bradycardia, hypotension, and cyanosis.
   b. Vagal stimulation, which may result in bradycardia.

Planning/Implementation

Preparatory Phase

1. Instruct the patient how to "splint" surgical incision, as coughing will be induced during the procedure. Explain the importance of performing the suction procedure in an aseptic manner.

2. Assemble equipment. Check function of suction and manual resuscitation bag connected to 100% O₂ source.

3. Wash hands thoroughly.

1. Thorough explanation lessens patient's anxiety and promotes cooperation.

2. Make sure that all equipment is functional before sterile technique is instituted to prevent interruption once the procedure is begun. Use of 100% O₂ will help to prevent hypoxemia.

(continued)

Guidelines: Sterile Tracheobronchial Suction via Tracheostomy or Endotracheal Tube

(Spontaneous or Mechanical Ventilation) (continued)

Planning/Implementation
(Cont.)

Nursing Action	Rationale/Amplification
Performance Phase	
1. Open sterile towel—place in a bib-like fashion on patient's chest. Open alcohol wipes and place on corner of towel. Place small amount of sterile water-soluble jelly on towel.	
2. Open sterile gloves—place on towel.	
3. Open suction catheter package.	
4. If the patient is on mechanical ventilation, test to make sure that disconnection of ventilator attachment may be made with one hand.	
5. Don sterile gloves. Designate one hand as contaminated for disconnecting, bagging, and working the suctioning control. Usually the dominant hand is kept sterile and will be used to thread the suction catheter.	5. The hand designated as sterile must remain uncontaminated so that organisms are not introduced into the lungs. The contaminated hand must also be gloved to prevent sputum from contacting the nurse's hand, possibly resulting in an infection of the nurse.
6. Use the sterile hand to remove carefully the suction catheter from the package, curling the catheter around the gloved fingers.	
7. Connect suction source to the suction fitting of the catheter with the contaminated hand.	
8. Using the contaminated hand, disconnect the patient from the ventilator, CPAP device, or other oxygen source. (Place the ventilator connector on the sterile towel and flip a corner of the towel over the connection to prevent fluid from spraying into the area).	8. Prevents contamination of the connection.
9. Ventilate and oxygenate the patient with the resuscitator bag, compressing firmly and as completely as possible approximately 5–6 times (try to approximate the patient's tidal volume). This procedure is called "bagging" the patient. In the spontaneously breathing patient, coordinate manual ventilations with the patient's own inspiratory effort.	9. Ventilation prior to suctioning helps prevent hypoxemia. When possible, two nurses work as a team to suction. Attempting to ventilate against the patient's own respiratory efforts may result in high airway pressures, predisposing the patient to barotrauma (lung injury due to pressure).
10. Lubricate the tip of the suction catheter. Gently insert suction catheter as far as possible into the artificial airway without applying suction. Most patients will cough when the catheter touches the trachea.	10. Suctioning on insertion would unnecessarily decrease oxygen in the airway.
11. Apply suction and quickly rotate the catheter while it is being withdrawn.	11. Failure to rotate catheter may result in damage to tracheal mucosa. Release suction if a pulling sensation is felt.
12. Limit suction time to 10–15 seconds. Discontinue if heart rate decreases by 20 beats per minute or increases by 40 beats per minute, or if cardiac ectopy is observed.	12. Suctioning removes oxygen as well as secretions and may also cause vagal stimulation.
13. Bag patient between suction passes with approximately 4–5 manual ventilations.	13. The oxygen removed by suctioning must be replenished before suctioning is attempted again.
14. At this point, sterile nonbacteriostatic saline may be instilled into the trachea via the artificial airway if secretions are tenacious.	14. Some clinicians feel that secretion removal may be facilitated with saline instillation. Others feel that saline does not mix with mucus and that suctioning of the saline just instilled is the only effect produced by performing this step.
a. Remove needle from syringe and inject 3–5 ml. nonbacteriostatic saline into the artificial airway during spontaneous inspiration. Alternately, a saline "bullet" or small prepackaged container of saline may be used.	a. Removal of the needle will prevent accidental loss of the needle into the airway. Instillation of the saline during inspiration will prevent the saline from being blown back out of the tube.
b. Bag vigorously and then suction.	b. Bagging stimulates cough and distributes saline to loosen secretions.
15. Rinse catheter between suction passes by inserting tip in cup of sterile water and applying suction.	
16. Continue making suction passes, bagging the patient between passes, until the airways are clear of accumulated secretions. No more than 4 suction passes should be made per suctioning episode.	16. Repeated suctioning of a patient in a short time interval predisposes to hypoxemia, as well as being tiring and traumatic to the patient.
17. Give the patient 6–8 "sigh" breaths with the bag.	17. Sighing is accomplished by depressing the bag slowly and completely with 2 hands to deliver approximately 1½ times the normal tidal volume to the patient, allowing for maximal lung expansion and prevention of atelectasis.

Planning/Implementation
(Cont.)

Nursing Action	Rationale/Amplification
18. Return the patient to the ventilator or apply CPAP or other oxygen-delivery device.	
19. Suction oral secretions from the oropharynx above the artificial airway cuff.	

Follow-up Phase

1. Clean elbow fitting of resuscitation bag with alcohol; wipe before storing.
2. Assess need for further suctioning at least every 2 hours, or more frequently if secretions are copious.

Evaluation/Outcome

1. Note any change in vital signs or patient's intolerance to the procedure. Record amount and consistency of secretions.	1. Evaluate the effectiveness of procedure.

Guidelines: Artificial Airway Cuff Inflation/Deflation (Cuff Pressure Measurement)

The cuffs of endotracheal and tracheostomy tubes must be inflated continuously when the patient is on mechanical ventilation or CPAP. The cuff is then deflated only for tube removal or repositioning. The cuffs of spontaneously breathing tracheostomized patients may require inflation at all times if the patient has a sufficiently depressed level of consciousness, or neuromuscular deficiency that does not permit the patient to protect his airway. The cuffs of spontaneously breathing tracheostomized patients not on mechanical ventilation or CPAP may be deflated:

1. At times when the patient can adequately protect the airway.
2. Between meals, if the patient is at aspiration risk only during feeding. The cuff may be inflated prior to feeding and for 1 hour after feeding.

Complications of Excessive Cuff Pressure

Tracheal swelling	Tracheoarterial fistula
Tracheal ulceration	Tracheal necrosis
Tracheoesophageal fistula	Tracheal malacia

Equipment

Suction catheter
Tonsil suction
Suction source
10-ml. syringe
Pressure manometer (mercury or anaeroid)
Manual resuscitation bag with reservoir, connected to 100% oxygen at 10–15 liters/min.

Nursing Action	Rationale/Amplification
Assessment	
1. Note degree of air leakage around cuff by listening over the cuff area with a stethoscope. Note and report excessive bleeding from tube (or around stoma of tracheostomized patient).	1. Provides a baseline. Air leakage is heard as a crowing sound at peak airway pressure.
Planning/Implementation	
Preparatory Phase	
1. Explain procedure to the patient.	1. Decreases the patient's anxiety and promotes cooperation.
Deflating the Cuff	
1. Suction the trachea, then the oral and nasal pharynx. Then replace the suction catheter with a stent catheter.	1. Removes secretions collected above the cuff, which could be aspirated into the lungs when the cuff is deflated. Do not reenter the trachea with the same catheter used for suctioning the mouth.
2. Deflate the cuff slowly.	2. The small test balloon at the end of the tubing remains inflated as long as the cuff at the distal end of the tube is inflated. A vacuum within the syringe is sensed when no more air can be aspirated.

(continued)

Guidelines: Artificial Airway Cuff Inflation/Deflation (Cuff Pressure Measurement) (continued)

Planning/Implementation
(Cont.)

Nursing Action	Rationale/Amplification
3. (Concomitant with step 2) Have the patient cough, or manually inflate the lungs with the resuscitation bag. Be ready to receive secretions in a tissue, or aspirate with a tonsil suction.	3. Positive pressure in the airways may help force secretions upward and prevent aspiration.

4. Suction through the tracheostomy or endotracheal tube.	4. Secretions that may have been present above the inflated cuff and around the exterior tube have now seeped downward. The coughing reflex may be stimulated, helping to mobilize secretions.
	  a. Continue observation of color, pulse, etc.
	  b. Monitor patient closely for tolerance. Loss of tidal volume or PEEP may promote hypoxemia and hypocarbia. Cuff should not be deflated for more than 30–45 seconds.

5. Provide adequate ventilation while the cuff is deflated.
  a. If the patient does not require assisted ventilation, maintain humidified oxygen as directed.
  b. If the patient requires assisted ventilation, provide manual ventilation via a resuscitation bag. Leave cuff deflated for as long as the tube repositioning requires; then reinflate.	

Inflating a Cuff

Nursing Action	Rationale/Amplification

1. No leak technique:
  a. Attach air-filled syringe to cuff injection port.
  b. Slowly inject air until no air escapes from the patient's lungs around the cuff.
  c. Note amount of air injected to provide the seal.
	1. Air leakage will be heard when the intra-airway pressure is most positive (maximum peak airway pressure). For the spontaneously breathing patient, air leakage will be heard on exhalation. For the patient on positive pressure ventilation, air leakage will be heard at maximum ventilator inspiration.

2. Minimal leak technique (for mechanical ventilation):
  a. Attach air-filled syringe to cuff injection port.
  b. Slowly inject air until no leak is heard at maximum peak airway pressure.
  c. Slowly remove air from cuff until a small air leak is heard at maximum peak airway pressure.
  d. Note amount of air injected.
	c. Adjustment in tidal volume setting may be necessary to compensate for the leak.

3. Inflation using intracuff pressure measurement:
  a. Insert male port of three-way stopcock into cuff injection port. One female port of stopcock holds the air-filled syringe, and one port holds the pressure manometer.
  b. Inject air into cuff until desired intracuff pressure is reached at maximum peak airway pressure.
	b. Anaeroid manometer measures cuff pressure in cm. H_2O; end pressure of 20–25 cm. H_2O is desired. Mercury manometer pressure should be 15–20 mm. Hg. Pressure greater than upper limit may cause compression of tracheal vessels. Pressure less than lower limit may allow aspiration of gastric or oral secretions.

c. Note amount of air needed to achieve the desired intracuff pressure.	
5. Remove the stopcock from the injection port.	5. Most injection ports have self-sealing valves. If not, a cap or closed stopcock may be left in the injection port (clamping of the inflation tubing is discouraged as it may result in cracking or kinking of the line permanently).
6. While the cuff is inflated, assess inflation every 2 hours. The cuff pressure manometer is useful for this.	6. Leakage of air from the cuff or cuff injection port may occur. Assess the inflation status and adjust as needed.

Inability to Maintain a Seal

Nursing Action	Rationale/Amplification

1. Assess the degree of leakage and length of time elapsed since cuff volume was replenished.	1. If a cuff seal reverts to air leakage (or greater leakage if minimal leak technique is used) within 10 minutes, assessment is necessary. Possibilities may be:
	  a. Cuff positioned above the vocal cords (direct visualization necessary for repositioning).
	  b. Incompetence of artificial airway cuff balloon.
	  c. Incompetence of self-sealing valve on injection port.
	  d. Tracheal dilatation (requiring larger size tube).
	  e. Cuff may be ruptured, requiring a new tube.

2. Inflate the cuff to desired level.	
3. Disconnect syringe (and manometer if used).	
4. Assess for leakage.	
5. If leakage recurs, place three-way stopcock between syringe and injection port, inflate cuff, close stopcock. Remove syringe (and manometer if used) leaving closed stopcock in injection port.	5. Closed stopcock left in injection port acts as "plug" if self-sealing valve is incompetent.
6. If air leak persists, tube repositioning or replacement may be necessary. Consult with appropriate personnel.	

Planning/Implementation
(Cont.)

Nursing Action	Rationale/Amplification
Follow-up Phase	
1. Assess cuff inflation status at least every 2 hours.	
Evaluation/Outcome	
1. Note and record amount of air used for adequate seal, intracuff pressure, and inability to achieve seal.	1. Notify physician or personnel qualified to intubate, or change tracheostomy tube if unable to achieve desired seal.

Mechanical Ventilation

The *mechanical ventilator* is a device that functions as a substitute for the bellows action of the thoracic cage and diaphragm. The mechanical ventilator can maintain ventilation automatically for prolonged periods of time. It is indicated when the patient is unable to maintain safe levels of oxygen or carbon dioxide by spontaneous breathing even with the assistance of other oxygen delivery devices.

Types of Ventilators

A. Negative Pressure Ventilators

1. Applies negative pressure around the chest wall. This causes intra-airway pressure to become negative, thus drawing air into the lungs through the patient's nose and mouth.
2. No artificial airway is necessary—patient must be able to control and protect own airway.
3. Indications—may be used for selected patients with respiratory neuromuscular problems, or as adjunct to weaning from positive pressure ventilation.

B. Positive Pressure Ventilators

During mechanical inspiration, air is actively delivered to the patient's lungs under positive pressure. Requires use of a cuffed artificial airway. Exhalation is passive.
1. Pressure limited:
   a. Terminates the inspiratory phase when a preselected airway pressure is achieved.
   b. Volume delivered is dependent on lung compliance (ml. volume/cm. H_2O airway pressure).
   c. Use of volume-based alarms are recommended because any obstruction between the machine and lungs that allows a buildup of pressure in the ventilator circuitry will cause the ventilator to cycle, but the patient will receive no volume.
2. Volume limited:
   a. Terminates the inspiratory phase when a designated volume of the gas is delivered into the ventilator circuit (12–15 ml./kg. body weight—usual starting volumes).
   b. Delivers the predetermined volume regardless of changing lung compliance (although airway pressures will increase as compliance decreases). Airway pressures vary from patient to patient and from breath to breath.
   c. Pressure-limiting valves (fixed or adjustable), which prevent excessive pressure buildup within the patient–ventilator system, are usually incorporated. Without this valve, pressure could increase indefinitely and pulmonary barotrauma could result. Usually equipped with a system that alarms when selected pressure limit is exceeded and vents excess inspired air to the atmosphere.

Modes of Operation

A. Controlled Ventilation (CV)

1. Cycles automatically at rate that is selected by operator.
2. A fixed level of ventilation is provided. Will not cycle or have gas available or circuitry to respond to patient's own inspiratory efforts (may result in increase in work of breathing for patients attempting to breathe spontaneously).
3. Possibly indicated for patients whose respiratory drive is absent.

B. Assist Ventilation (AV)

1. Inspiratory cycle of ventilator activated by detection of decrease in airway pressure caused by the patient's voluntary inspiratory activity.
2. Once inspiration initiated, ventilator will deliver gas flow until desired volume, pressure, or time limit is reached.
3. No minimum level of minute ventilation is provided. Indicated for the patient who is making regular inspiratory efforts but who cannot achieve an adequate tidal volume.

C. Assist/control (A/C)

1. Inspiratory cycle of ventilator activated by detection of the patient's voluntary inspiratory effort.
2. Ventilator additionally cycles at a rate predetermined by the operator. Should the patient stop breathing, or breathe so weakly that the ventilator cannot function as an assistor, this mandatory baseline rate will prevent apnea. A minimum level of minute ventilation is provided.
3. Indicated for patients who are breathing spontaneously but who have the potential to lose their respiratory drive or muscular control of ventilation. In this mode, the patient's work of breathing is greatly reduced.

D. Intermittent Mandatory Ventilation (IMV)

1. Allows patient to breathe spontaneously through ventilator circuitry.
2. Periodically, at preselected rate and volume, cycles to give a "mandated" ventilator breath. A minimum level of ventilation is provided.
3. Gas provided for spontaneous breathing usually flows continuously through the ventilator circuitry.
4. Indications—patients requiring ventilator assistance in whom it may be desirable to do some of the work of breathing.

E. Synchronized Intermittent Mandatory Ventilation (SIMV):

1. Allows patient to breathe spontaneously through the ventilator circuitry.

2. Periodically, at a preselected time, a mandatory breath is delivered. The patient may initiate the mandatory breath with his own inspiratory effort, and the ventilator breath will be synchronized with the patient's efforts, or will be "assisted." If the patient does not provide inspiratory effort, the breath will still be delivered, or be "controlled".
3. Gas provided for spontaneous breathing is usually delivered through a demand regulator which is activated by the patient.
4. Indicated for patients who needs ventilator assistance, but in whom it may be desirable to perform some of the work of breathing.

Special Positive Pressure Ventilation Techniques

A. Positive End-Expiratory Pressure (PEEP)

1. Maneuver by which pressure during mechanical ventilation is maintained above atmospheric at end of exhalation, resulting in an increased functional residual capacity. Airway pressure is therefore positive throughout the entire ventilatory cycle.
2. Purpose—the increase in functional residual capacity (or the amount of air left in the lungs at the end of expiration) is greater than atmospheric pressure:
   a. Increasing the surface area for gas exchange.
   b. Preventing collapse of alveolar units and development of atelectasis.
   c. Decreasing intrapulmonary shunt.
3. Benefits
   a. Since a greater surface area for diffusion is available and shunting is reduced, it is often possible to use a lower fraction of inspired oxygen concentration (F_IO_2) than would otherwise be required to obtain adequate arterial oxygen levels. This reduces the risk of oxygen toxicity.
   b. Positive intra-airway pressure may be helpful in reducing the transudation of fluid from the pulmonary capillaries in situations where capillary pressure is increased (i.e., left heart failure) or when the alveolar–capillary membrane is damaged (i.e., adult respiratory distress syndrome).
   c. Increased lung compliance resulting in decreased work of breathing.
4. Hazards
   a. Since the mean airway pressure is increased by PEEP, venous return is impeded. This may result in a decrease in cardiac output (especially noted in hypovolemic patients).
   b. The increased airway pressure may possibly result in alveolar rupture. The likelihood is greater in patients with noncompliant lungs. This barotrauma may result in pneumothorax, tension pneumothorax, or development of subcutaneous emphysema.
   c. The decreased venous return may cause antidiuretic hormone formation to be stimulated, resulting in decreased urine output.
5. Precautions
   a. Monitor frequently for signs and symptoms of pneumothorax (increased pulmonary artery pressure, increased size of hemithorax, decreased lung movement, hyperresonant percussion note, diminished breath sounds).
   b. Monitor for signs of decreased venous return:
      (1) Decreased arterial blood pressure
      (2) Decreased cardiac output
      (3) Decreased urine output; formation of peripheral edema
   c. Abrupt discontinuance of PEEP is not recommended. The patient should not be without PEEP for longer than 15 seconds. The manual resuscitation bag used for ventilation during suction procedure or patient transport should be equipped with a PEEP device. Some clinicians feel that loss of PEEP for short periods of time is not detrimental in the lower ranges (less than 10 cm. H_2O). An exception might be patients with increased intracranial pressure.
   d. Intrapulmonary blood vessel pressure may increase because of compression of the vessels by increased intra-airway pressure. Therefore, CVP and PA pressures and wedge may be increased. The clinician must bear this in mind when determining the clinical significance of these pressures.

B. Continuous Positive Airway Pressure (CPAP)

1. Also provides for positive airway pressure during all parts of a respiratory cycle but refers to spontaneous ventilation rather than mechanical ventilation.
2. May be delivered through ventilator circuitry when ventilator rate is at "0," or may be delivered through a separate CPAP circuitry that does not require the ventilator.
3. Indicated for patients who are capable of maintaining an adequate tidal volume, but have pathology preventing maintenance of adequate levels of tissue oxygenation.
4. CPAP has the same benefits, hazards, and precautions noted with PEEP. Mean airway pressures may be lower because of lack of mechanical ventilation breaths. This results in less risk of barotrauma and impedence of venous return.

Underlying Principles

1. Variables that control ventilation and oxygenation:
   a. Ventilator rate—adjusted by rate knob. On some ventilators, it is set by adjusting the inspiratory and expiratory times.
   b. Tidal volume—set by tidal volume knob. Measured as inhaled volume.
   c. Fraction inspired oxygen concentration (F_IO_2)—set on ventilator or with an oxygen blender. Measured with an oxygen analyzer.
   d. Ventilator dead space—circuitry common to inhalation and exhalation. Tubing is calibrated.
   e. PEEP—set within the ventilator or with the use of external PEEP devices. Measured at the proximal airway.
2. CO_2 elimination—controlled by tidal volume, rate, and dead space.
3. Oxygen tension—controlled by oxygen concentration and PEEP (also by rate and tidal volume).
4. The duration of inspiration should not exceed exhalation. Rate, tidal volume, gas flow in liters per minute, and inspiratory pause all control inspiratory time. Inverse inspiration—exhalation ratio results in "stacking" of breaths or buildup of pressure within the airway. Barotrauma and decreased cardiac output can result.
5. The inspired gas must be warmed and humidified to prevent thickening of secretions and decrease in body temperature. Sterile distilled water is warmed and humidified via a heated humidifier or nebulizer.

Clinical Indications

1. Mechanical failure of ventilation
   a. Neuromuscular disease
   b. Central nervous system disease
   c. Central nervous system depression (drug intoxication, respiratory depressants, cardiac arrest)
   d. Musculoskeletal disease
   e. Inefficiency of thorax cage in generating pressure gradients necessary for ventilation (chest injury, thoracic malformation)
2. Disorders of pulmonary gas exchange
   a. Acute respiratory failure
   b. Chronic respiratory failure
   c. Left ventricular failure
   d. Pulmonary diseases resulting in diffusion abnormality

   e. Pulmonary diseases resulting in ventilation/perfusion mismatch

Complications

1. Airway obstruction (thickened secretions, mechanical problem with artificial airway or ventilator circuitry)
2. Tracheal damage (see artificial airway)
3. Pulmonary infection
4. Barotrauma (pneumothorax or tension pneumothorax)
5. Cardiac embarrassment
6. Atelectasis
7. GI malfunction (dilatation, bleeding)
8. Renal malfunction
9. Central nervous system malfunction
10. Psychiatric trauma

Guidelines: Managing the Patient Requiring Mechanical Ventilation

Equipment

Artificial airway
Mechanical ventilator
Ventilator circuitry
Humidifier
See manufacturer's directions for specific machine

Nursing Action	Rationale / Amplification
Assessment	
1. Obtain baseline samples for blood gas determinations (pH, PaO_2, $PaCO_2$, HCO_3) and chest x-ray.	1. Baseline measurements serve as a guide in determining progress of therapy.
Planning/Implementation	
Preparatory Phase	
1. Give a brief explanation to the patient.	1. Emphasize that mechanical ventilation is a temporary measure. The patient should be prepared psychologically for weaning at the time the ventilator is first used.
2. Establish the airway by means of a cuffed endotracheal or tracheostomy tube (see Endotracheal Intubation, Tracheostomy, and Cuff Inflation).	2. A closed system between the ventilator and patient's lower airway is necessary for positive pressure ventilation.
3. Prepare the ventilator:	
a. Set up desired circuitry.	
b. Connect oxygen and compressed air source.	
c. Turn on power.	
d. Set tidal volume (usually 12–15 ml./kg. body weight).	d. Adjusted according to $PaCO_2$ and PaO_2.
e. Set oxygen concentration.	e. Adjusted according to PaO_2.
f. Set PEEP.	f. Adjusted according to $PaCO_2$.
g. Set rate at 12–14 breaths per minute (variable).	g. This setting approximates normal respiration. These machines settings are subject to change according to the patient's condition and response, and the ventilator type being used.
h. Adjust flow rate (velocity of gas flow during inspiration). Usually set at 40–60 liters per minute. Is dependent on rate and tidal volume. Set to avoid inverse inspiratory:expiratory (I:E) ratio. Usual I:E ratio is 1:2.	h. The slower the flow, the lower will be the peak airway pressure resulting from set volume delivery. This results in lower intrathoracic pressure and less impedance of venous return. However, a flow that is too low for the rate selected may result in inverse inspiratory: expiratory ratios.
i. Check machine function—measure tidal volume, rate, I:E ratio, analyze oxygen, check all alarms.	i. Ensures safe function.
Performance Phase	
1. Couple the patient's airway to the ventilator.	1. Be sure that all connections are secure. Prevent ventilator tubing from ''pulling'' on artificial airway, possibly resulting in tube dislodgement or tracheal damage.

(continued)

Guidelines: Managing the Patient Requiring Mechanical Ventilation (continued)

Planning/Implementation
(Cont.)

Nursing Action	Rationale/Amplification
2. Assess patient for adequate chest movement and rate. Do not depend on digital rate readout of ventilator. Note peak airway pressure and PEEP. Adjust gas flow if necessary to provide safe I:E ratio.	2. Ensures proper function of equipment.
3. Set airway pressure alarms according to patient's baseline: a. High pressure alarm	a. High airway pressure or "pop off" pressure is set at about 20 cm. H_2O above peak airway pressure. An alarm sounds if airway pressure selected is exceeded. Alarm activation indicates: decreased lung compliance (worsening pulmonary disease, increased pulmonary blood volume, decreased lung volume such as pneumothorax, tension pneumothorax, hemothorax, pleural effusion), increased airways resistance (secretions, coughing, breathing out of phase with the ventilator), loss of patency of airway (mucous plug, blood clot, airway spasm, biting or kinking of tube).
b. Low pressure alarm	b. Low airway pressure alarm set at 5–10 cm. H_2O below peak airway pressure. Alarm activation indicates inability to build up airway pressure because of disconnection or leak, or inability to build up airway pressure because of insufficient gas flow to meet patient's inspiratory needs.
4. Assess frequently for change in respiratory status via arterial blood gas, spontaneous rate, use of accessory muscles, color, and vital signs. Other means of assessing are through the use of exhaled carbon dioxide or continuous mixed venous oxygen saturation.	4. If change is noted, notify appropriate personnel. In emergency condition, disconnect from ventilator and ventilate with manual resuscitation bag.
5. Monitor and trouble-shoot alarm conditions. Ensure appropriate ventilation at all times.	5. Priority is ventilation and oxygenation of the patient. In alarm conditions that cannot be immediately corrected, disconnect the patient from mechanical ventilation and manually ventilate with resuscitation bag.
6. Positioning a. Turn patient from side to side every 2 hours, or more frequently if possible.	a. For patients on long-term ventilation, this may result in sleep deprivation. Evolve a turning schedule best suited to a particular patient's condition.
b. Lateral turns of 120 degrees are desirable; from right semi-prone to left semi-prone. c. Sit the patient upright at regular intervals if possible. d. Position the patient in postural drainage positions as requested.	c. Upright posture increases lung compliance. d. Adequate postural drainage decreases the need for deep tracheobronchial catheter aspiration by preventing retention of secretions in the peripheral areas of the lungs.
e. Carry out passive range of motion exercises of all extremities for patients unable to do so.	
7. Deep breaths a. Augment the patient's spontaneous tidal volume periodically by giving him 6–8 deep breaths with a manual resuscitator bag, or use sigh mechanism available on some ventilators. Provide patient with adequate oxygenation during this maneuver.	a. Periodic sighing with greater than normal tidal volumes (usually 1½ times normal) helps to prevent alveolar collapse, promotes coughing, and reveals the presence of retained secretions.
8. Assess for need of suctioning every 2 hours (see suctioning).	8. Patients with artificial airways on mechanical ventilation are unable to clear secretions on their own. Suctioning may help to clear secretions and stimulate the cough reflex.
9. Assess breath sounds every 2 hours: a. Listen with stethoscope to the chest from bottom to top on both sides. b. Determine whether breath sounds are present or absent, normal or abnormal, and whether a *change* has occurred. c. Observe the patient's diaphragmatic excursions and use of accessory muscles of respiration.	a. Auscultation of the chest is a means of assessing airway patency and ventilatory distribution. It also confirms the proper placement of the endotracheal or tracheostomy tube.
10. Humidification a. Check the water level in the humidification reservoir to ensure that the patient is never ventilated with dry gas. Empty the water that condenses in the delivery and exhalation tubing. Humidifier and nebulizer must be changed every 24 hours.	a. Water condensing in the inspiratory tubing may cause increased resistance to gas flow. This may result in increased peak airway pressures. Water collection in the exhalation line may cause an increase in the PEEP. Warm, moist tubing is a perfect breeding area for bacteria. Emptying the tubing

Planning/Implementation
(Cont.)

Nursing Action	Rationale/Amplification
	prevents introduction of water into the patient's airways. Always wash hands after emptying fluid from ventilator circuitry.
11. Assess airway pressures at frequent intervals.	11. Monitor for changes in compliance, or onset of conditions that may cause airway pressure to increase or decrease (see step 3).
12. Measure delivered tidal volume and analyze oxygen every 4 hours or more frequently if indicated.	
13. Monitor cardiovascular function. Assess for depression. a. Monitor pulse rate and arterial blood pressure; intra-arterial pressure monitoring may be carried out.	a. To accomplish intra-arterial pressure monitoring, a catheter is introduced into an artery, usually the radial or femoral, and the pressure at the catheter tip transmitted to a pressure transducer that converts the pressure wave into an electrical signal that is displayed for continuous visual observation on an oscilloscope and digital readout.
b. Use Swan–Ganz catheter to monitor pulmonary capillary wedge pressure, mixed venous oxygen ($P\bar{v}O_2$), and cardiac output.	b. Intermittent and continuous positive pressure ventilation may increase the pulmonary artery pressures and decrease cardiac output.
14. Monitor for pulmonary infection. a. Aspirate tracheal secretions into a sterile container and send to laboratory for culture and sensitivity testing. This is done immediately after endotracheal intubation and in some instances on an every-other-day basis. b. Daily gram staining of secretions may also be done in some institutions. c. Monitor for systemic signs and symptoms of pulmonary infection (pulmonary physical examination findings, increased heart rate, increased temperature, increased WBC count).	a. This technique allows the earliest detection of infection or change in infecting organisms in the tracheobronchial tree.
15. Evaluate need for sedation or muscle relaxants.	15. Sedatives may be prescribed by the physician to decrease patient anxiety, or to relax the patient so that he is not "competing" with the ventilator. At times, pharmacologically induced paralysis may be necessary in order to permit mechanical ventilation. Paralysis is prescribed by the physician.
16. Report intake and output precisely and attain an accurate daily weight to monitor fluid balance.	16. Positive fluid balance resulting in increase in body weight and interstitial pulmonary edema is a frequent problem in patients requiring mechanical ventilation. Prevention requires early recognition of fluid accumulation. An average adult who is dependent on parenteral nutrition can be expected to lose 0.25 kg. (½ lb.)/day; therefore, constant body weight indicates positive fluid balance.
17. Monitor nutritional status.	17. Patients on mechanical ventilation require inflation of artificial airway cuffs at all times. Patients with tracheostomy tubes may eat, if capable, or may require enteral feeding tubes or parenteral nourishment. Patients with endotracheal tubes are to be NPO (the tube splints the epiglottis open) and must be enterally tube fed or parenterally nourished.
18. Monitor GI function. a. Test all stools and gastric drainage for occult blood. b. Measure abdominal girth daily.	18. Mechanically ventilated patients are at risk for development of stress ulcers. a. About ¼ of patients requiring mechanical ventilation develop GI bleeding. Many of these patients require blood transfusions. b. Abdominal distention occurs frequently with respiratory failure and further hinders respiration by elevation of the diaphragm. Measurement of abdominal girth provides objective assessment of the degree of distention.
19. Provide for care and communication needs of patient with an artificial airway (see Artificial Airway Management, Tracheobronchial Suctioning, Cuff Inflation/Deflation/Pressure Measurement, Tracheostomy Care).	
20. Provide psychological support. a. Assist with communication. b. Orient to environment and function of mechanical ventilation. c. Ensure that the patient has adequate rest and sleep.	20. Mechanical ventilation may result in sleep deprivation and loss of touch with surroundings and reality.

(continued)

Guidelines: Managing the Patient Requiring Mechanical Ventilation (continued)

Planning/Implementation
(Cont.)

Nursing Action	Rationale/Amplification
Follow-up Phase	
1. Change ventilator circuitry every 24 hours; assess ventilator's function every 4 hours or more frequently if problem occurs.	1. Prevents contamination of lower airways.
Evaluation/Outcome	
1. Maintain a flow sheet to record ventilation patterns, arterial blood studies, venous chemical determinations, hemoglobin and hematocrit, status of fluid balance, weight, and assessment of the patient's condition. Notify appropriate personnel of changes in the patient's condition.	1. Establishes means of assessing effectiveness and progress of treatment.

Guidelines: Weaning the Patient From the Mechanical Ventilator

Weaning is the process by which the patient is gradually allowed to assume the responsibility for regulating and performing his own ventilation. Before weaning is instituted, the patient should have acceptable arterial blood gases while on the ventilator, have no evidence of acute pulmonary complication or dead space ventilation, have an intrapulmonary shunt less than 30%, and be hemodynamically stable while on the ventilator.

Equipment

Varies according to technique used
Briggs T-piece (see earlier section)
IMV or SIMV (set up in addition to ventilator or incorporated in ventilator and circuitry)

Nursing Action	Rationale/Amplification
Assessment	
1. For weaning to be successful, the patient must be physiologically capable of maintaining spontaneous respirations. Assessments must ensure that:	1. Provides baseline; ensures that patient is capable of having adequate neuromuscular control to provide adequate ventilation.
a. The underlying disease process is significantly reversed, as evidenced by pulmonary examination, arterial blood gas, chest x-ray.	
b. The patient can mechanically perform ventilation. Should: have vital capacity greater than 10–15 ml./kg; have tidal volume greater than 5 ml./kg.; have spontaneous respiratory rate of less than 25 min.; be without significant tachycardia; not be hypotensive; have optimal hemoglobin for his condition.	
2. Assess for other factors that may cause respiratory insufficiency.	2. Weaning is difficult when these conditions are present.
a. Acid–base abnormality	
b. Caloric depletion	
c. Electrolyte abnormality	
d. Exercise intolerance	
e. Fever	
f. Abnormal fluid balance	
g. Hyperglycemia	
h. Infection	
i. Pain	
j. Protein loss	
k. Sleep deprivation	
l. Decreased level of consciousness	
Planning/Implementation	
Preparatory Phase	
1. Ensure psychological preparation. Explain procedure. Explain that weaning is not always successful on the initial attempt.	1. Explaining procedure to patient will decrease patient anxiety and promote cooperation. The patient should not be discouraged if weaning is unsuccessful on the first attempt.

Planning/Implementation
(Cont.)

Nursing Action	Rationale/Amplification

2. Prepare appropriate equipment.
   a. Briggs adapter (T-tube), or
   b. IMV or SIMV circuitry (frequently incorporated in ventilator circuitry)
3. Position the patient in sitting or semi-Fowler's position.
4. Pick optimal time of day.
5. Perform bronchial hygiene necessary to ensure that the patient is in best condition (postural drainage, chest physical therapy, and suctioning) prior to weaning attempt.

3. Increases lung compliance, decreases work of breathing.
4. The patient should be rested.
5. The patient should be in best pulmonary condition for weaning to be successful.

Performance Phase

T-piece

This system provides oxygen enrichment and humidity to a patient with an endotracheal or tracheostomy tube while allowing completely spontaneous respirations (for set-up and function see oxygen therapy section).

1. Discontinue mechanical ventilation and apply T-piece adapter.
2. Time on T-piece may vary from 5–10 min./hr. to 15–30 min./hr.
3. Monitor the patient for factors indicating need for reinstitution of mechanical ventilation.
   a. Blood pressure increase or decrease greater than 20 mm. Hg systolic or 10 mm. Hg diastolic
   b. Heart rate increase of 20 beats/min or rate greater than 110
   c. Respiratory rate increase greater than 10 breaths per minute or rate greater than 30
   d. Tidal volume less than 250–300 ml. (in adults)
   e. Appearance of new cardiac ectopy, or increase in baseline ectopy
   f. P_aO_2 less than 60, P_aCO_2 greater than 55, or pH less than 7.35 (may accept lower P_aO_2 and pH, and higher P_aCO_2 in patients with COPD)
4. Increase time off ventilator with each weaning attempt as the patient's condition indicates. Evaluate for toleration before moving to the next increment.
5. Institute other techniques helpful in encouraging weaning.
   a. Mental stimulation
   b. Biofeedback
   c. Participation in care
   d. Provision of rewards
   e. Contact with successfully weaned patients.
6. When the patient tolerates 40–60 min. of continuous weaning, weaning increments can increase rapidly.
7. When the patient can maintain spontaneous ventilation throughout day with only periodic IPPB treatments, begin night weaning.

1. Stay with the patient during weaning time to decrease patient anxiety and monitor for tolerance of procedure.

3. Indicates intolerance of weaning procedure.

4. The patient will progress as he becomes mentally and physically able to perform adequate spontaneous ventilation.
5. Provides motivation and positive feedback.

IVM or SIMV Weaning

1. Set ventilator to IMV or SIMV mode.
2. Set rate interval.

3. If the patient is on continuous flow IMV circuitry, observe reservoir bag to be sure that it remains mostly inflated during all phases of ventilation.
4. If gas for the patient's spontaneous breath is delivered via a demand valve regulator, ensure that machine sensitivity is at maximum setting.
5. Evaluate for tolerance of procedure. Monitor for factors indicating need for increase or decrease of mandatory respiratory rate (see step 3 of T-piece adapter section above). In rapid weaning, changes may be made approximately every 20–30 minutes.
6. If intolerance is not indicated, decrease mandatory rate as patient tolerates.

2. This determines the time interval between machine-delivered breaths, during which the patient will breathe on his own.
3. The gas flow rate into the bag must be adequate to prevent the bag from collapsing during inspiration. Flow rates of 6–10 liters per minute are usually adequate.
4. Aids in decreasing work of breathing necessary to open demand valve.

5. Indicates intolerance of weaning procedure.

6. May be done as frequently as every 20–30 minutes with arterial blood gas monitoring, ear or pulmonary artery (PA) oximetry, documentation of successful weaning.

(continued)

Guidelines: Weaning the Patient From the Mechanical Ventilator (continued)

Planning/Implementation
(Cont.)

Nursing Action	Rationale/Amplification
7. Institute other techniques helpful in encouraging weaning (see step 6, T-piece section above).	7. Provides motivation and positive feedback.

Evaluation/Outcome

1. Record at each weaning interval: heart rate, blood pressure, respiratory rate, F_1O_2, arterial blood gas, ear or PA oximetry value, rate (if IMV or SIMV), or length of time off ventilator (if T-piece weaning).	1. Provides record of procedure and assessment of progress.
NOTE: It is not within the scope of this book to establish criteria for the use of one weaning modality as opposed to another.	

Bibliography

Conditions of the Nose and Throat

Books

Ballenger JJ. Diseases of the Nose, Throat, Ear, Head and Neck, 13th ed. Philadelphia, Lea & Febiger, 1984

Boone DR. The Voice and Voice Therapy, 3rd ed. Englewood Cliffs, NJ, Prentice-Hall, 1983

DeWeese D and Saunders WH. Textbook of Otolaryngology, 6th ed. St Louis, CV Mosby, 1982

Farb SN. The Ear, Nose & Throat Book. New York, Appleton-Century-Crofts, 1980

Gluckman JL. Medical Management of Common Problems of the Ear, Nose & Throat. Philadelphia, WB Saunders, 1984

Goode R and Levine P. Common Problems in Otolaryngology. Philadelphia, JB Lippincott, 1984

Karmody CS. Textbook of Otolaryngology. Philadelphia, Lea & Febiger, 1983

Lesavoy MA. Reconstruction of the Head and Neck. Baltimore, Williams & Wilkins, 1980

Paparella MM. 1984 Yearbook of Otolaryngology. Chicago, Year Book Medical Publishers, 1983

Paparella MM and Shumrick DA (eds). Otolaryngology, 2nd ed. Philadelphia, WB Saunders, 1980

Snow JB Jr (ed). Controversy in Otolaryngology. Philadelphia, WB Saunders, 1980

Wilson W and Nadol J. Quick Reference of Ear, Nose, & Throat Disorders. Philadelphia, JB Lippincott, 1982

Articles

Nose

Beekhuis GJ. Silastic alar—columellar prosthesis in conjunction with rhinoplasty. Arch Otolaryngol 1982 Aug; 108(7):429–432

Busse WW. Chronic rhinitis. Postgrad Med 1983 Feb; 73(2):325–335

Crawford LV Jr et al. When your patient has rhinitis. Pat Care 1983 Oct 15; 17(17):186–207

Giordano AM and Gaskins RE. Correct, cautious management of epistaxis. ER Reports 1983 Jan 10; 10(1):1–6

Goode RL. Magnetic intranasal splints. Arch Otolaryngol 1982 May; 108(5): 319

Gordon CB. Practical approach to the loss of smell. Am Fam Physician 1982 Sept; 26(3):191–193

Hayden GF. Olfactory diagnosis in medicine. Postgrad Med 1980 Apr; 67(4):110–118

Ingram NM. Stanching nosebleeds. RN 1982 Sept; 45(9):51–53, 115

Intranasal corticosteroid aerosols— noninfectious rhinitis. Med Lett Drugs Ther 1981 Nov 27; 23(24):101–102

Johnson JT. Epistaxis management. Postgrad Med 1981 Nov; 70(5):231– 235

Kveton JF, Pillsbury HC and Sasaki CT. Nasal obstruction (adenoiditis vs adenoid hypertrophy). Arch Otolaryngol 1982 May; 108(5):315– 318

Lavie P et al. Excessive daytime sleepiness and insomnia (association with deviated nasal septum and nocturnal breathing disorders). Arch Otolaryngol 1982 June; 108(6):373– 377

Malkiewicz J. Examining the nose. RN 1982 Apr; 45(4):55–57

Newman RK and Johnson JT. Nasal airway obstruction. Postgrad Med 1980 Aug; 68(2):184–191

Tag AR. Toxic shock syndrome: Otolaryngologic presentations (nasal and sinus packing). Laryngoscope 1982 Sept 12; 92(9):1070–1072

Thomas JR, Mechlin DC and Templer J. Skin grafts (nose). Arch Otolaryngol 1982 July; 108(7):437–438

Sinuses and Throat

Beamis JF and Shapshay SM. ND-YAG laser therapy for tracheobronchial disorders. Postgrad Med 1984 Feb 15; 75(3):173–180

Cunningham CA and Sergent JB. Contamination of suction apparatus. Focus Crit Care 1983 Aug; 10(4):10– 14

Current care for pharyngitis. Pat Care 1980 Dec 15; 14(21):50–92

Dick EC et al. Common cold: What's known? What's new? Pat Care 1983 Nov 15; 17(19):20–45

Johnson JT, Newman RK and Olson JE. Persistent hoarseness. Postgrad Med 1980 May; 67(5):212–216

Kern EB. Is it really sinusitis? Postgrad Med 1983 Oct; 74(4):156–160

Kern EB. Why and how to drain a sinus. Postgrad Med 1983 July; 74(1):224– 230

Mandell HN. A moratorium on tonsillectomy. Postgrad Med 1983 Sept; 74(3):22–26

Neel HB and McDonald TJ. Chronic sinusitis. Postgrad Med 1981 Mar; 69(3):109–113

Neel HB and McDonald TJ. Tonsillectomy and adenoidectomy. Postgrad Med 1981 Sept; 70(3):107– 112

Rhea JT and Deluca SA. Acute sinusitis. Am Fam Physician 1982 Apr; 25(4): 121–122

Tonsillectomy justified for severe recurrent throat infections. AORN J 1981 Jan; 33(1):97

Head and Neck

Dropkin MJ. Development of a self-care teaching program for postoperative head and neck patients. Cancer Nurs 1981 April; 4(2):103–106

Vikram B and Farr HW. Adjuvant radiation therapy in locally advanced head and neck cancer. CA 1983 May– June; 33(3):134–138

Larynx

Baker BM and Cunningham CA. Vocal rehabilitation of the patient with a laryngectomy. Part I. Pre- and postoperative counseling. Oncol Nurs Forum 1980; 7(4):23–27

Baker BM and Cunningham CA. Vocal

rehabilitation of the patient with a laryngectomy. Part II. Assessment for vocal rehabilitation. Oncol Nurs Forum 1980; 7(4):28–33

Baker BM and Cunningham CA. Vocal rehabilitation of the patient with a laryngectomy. Part III. Specific techniques in laryngectomee vocal rehabilitation. Oncol Nurs Forum 1980; 7(4):33–36

Baker HW. Staging of cancer of the head and neck: Oral cavity, pharynx, larynx, and paranasal sinuses. CA 1983 May–June; 33(3):130–133

Bradenburg JH. Vocal rehabilitation after laryngectomy. Arch Otolaryngol 1980 Nov; 106(11):688–690

Gartside G. Mr. Smith's total laryngectomy. Nurs Times 1980 Oct 23; 76(43):1884–1885

Graber RF. Laryngoscopy. Patient Care 1984 Jan 15; 18(1):207–214

Knapp BA and Panje WR. A voice button for laryngectomees. AORN J 1982 Aug; 36(2):183–192

Lidocaine may prevent post-op laryngospasm. AORN J 1980 Jan; 31(1):76

Markus JF and Konrad HR. The right-angle laryngeal telescope in undergraduate medical education. Arch Otolaryngol 1982 June; 108(6):344–346

McCormick GP et al. Artificial speech devices. Am J Nurs 1982 Jan; 82(1):121–122

More laryngectomy patients speaking due to advances. AORN J 1982 Jan; 35(1):75–78

Pilcher L. Carbon dioxide lasers in laryngeal surgery. AORN J 1981 June; 33(7):1402–1407

Scully PA and Stratton CJ. Argon laser use in papillomas of the larynx. Laryngoscope 1982 Oct; 92(10):1164–1167

Weaver TE. Bronchography, laryngography, and their potential complications. RN 1982 Dec; 45(12):64–65

Weinberg B. Airway resistance of the voice button. Arch Otolaryngol 1982 Aug; 108(8):498–500

Agency

International Association of Laryngectomees, c/o American Cancer Society, 777 Third Ave, New York, NY 10017

Conditions of the Chest
Books

American Hospital Association. Staff Manual for Teaching Patients About Chronic Obstructive Pulmonary Diseases, 1982 ed. Chicago, American Hospital Association, 1982

Baue AE and Glenn WL (eds). Thoracic and Cardiovascular Surgery, 4th ed. Norwalk, CT, Appleton-Century-Crofts, 1982

Brody JS and Snider GL. Current Topics in the Management of Respiratory Disease. New York, Churchill Livingstone, 1981

Burki NK. Pulmonary Diseases. Garden City, NY, Medical Examination Publishing Company, 1982

Burns MD (ed). Pulmonary Care: A Guide for Patient Education. Norwalk, CT, Appleton-Century-Crofts, 1983

Burrows B et al. Respiratory Disorders: A Pathophysiologic Approach, 2nd ed. Chicago, Year Book Medical Publishers, 1983

Davies GM. Office Diagnosis and Management of Chronic Obstructive Pulmonary Disease. Philadelphia, Lea & Febiger, 1981

Drage CW (ed). Respiratory Medicine for Primary Care. New York, Academic Press, 1982

Epstein J and Gaines J. Clinical Respiratory Care of the Adult Patient. Bowie, MD, RJ Brady, 1983

Fishman AP (ed). Assessment of Pulmonary Function: Pulmonary Diseases and Disorders. New York, McGraw-Hill, 1980

Fishman NH. Thoracic Drainage. Chicago, Year Book Medical Publishers, 1983

George RB, Light RW and Matthay RA (eds). Chest Medicine. New York, Churchill Livingstone, 1983

Glauser FL (ed). Signs and Symptoms in Pulmonary Medicine. Philadelphia, JB Lippincott, 1983

Glinz W. Chest Trauma: Diagnosis and Management. New York, Springer-Verlag, 1981

Gracey DR (ed). Pulmonary Disease in the Adult. Chicago, Year Book Medical Publishers, 1981

Greco FA, Oldham RK and Bunn PA Jr (eds). Small Cell Lung Cancer. New York, Grune & Stratton, 1981

Grenville-Mathers R. The Respiratory System, 2nd ed. New York, Churchill Livingstone, 1983

Harper RW. A Guide to Respiratory Care: Physiology and Clinical Applications. Philadelphia, JB Lippincott, 1981

Hinshaw HC and Murray JF. Diseases of the Chest, 4th ed. Philadelphia, WB Saunders, 1980

Humphrey EW and McKeown DL. Manual of Pulmonary Surgery. New York, Springer-Verlag, 1982

James DG and Studdy PR. Color Atlas of Respiratory Diseases. Chicago, Year Book Medical Publishers, 1982

Jay SJ and Stonehill RB (eds). Manual of Pulmonary Procedures. Philadelphia, WB Saunders, 1980

Kaplan JA. Thoracic Anesthesia. New York, Churchill Livingstone, 1982

Kiss GT. Diagnosis and Management of Pulmonary Disease in Primary Practice. Menlo Park, CA, Addison-Wesley, 1982

Kwaan HC and Bowie EJW. Thrombosis. Philadelphia, WB Saunders, 1982

Miller WC. Chronic Obstructive Pulmonary Disease. Garden City, NY, Medical Examination Publishing Co, 1980

Moser KM and Spragg RG (eds). Respiratory Emergencies, 2nd ed. St Louis, CV Mosby, 1982

Newman GE, Effman EL and Putman CE.

Pulmonary Aspiration Complexes in Adults. Chicago, Year Book Medical Publishers, 1982

Orr WC, Altshuler KZ and Stahl ML. Managing Sleep Complications. Chicago, Year Book Medical Publishers, 1982

Paré JAP and Fraser RG. Synopsis of Diseases of the Chest. Philadelphia, WB Saunders, 1983

Parkes WR. Occupational Lung Disorders, 2nd ed. Boston, Butterworths, 1982

Pennington JE (ed). Respiratory Infections: Diagnosis and Management. New York, Raven Press, 1983

Petty TL and Cotton EK. Intensive and Rehabilitative Respiratory Care: A Practical Approach to the Management of Acute and Chronic Respiratory Failure, 3rd ed. Philadelphia, Lea & Febiger, 1982

Poe RH and Israel RH (eds). Problems in Pulmonary Medicine for the Primary Physician. Philadelphia, Lea & Febiger, 1982

Putman CE (ed). Pulmonary Diagnosis: Imaging and Other Techniques. New York, Appleton-Century-Crofts, 1981

Rarey KP and Youtsey JW. Respiratory Patient Care. Englewood Cliffs, NJ, Prentice-Hall, 1981

Sabiston DC Jr and Spencer FC (eds). Gibbon's Surgery of the Chest, Vol I and II, 4th ed. Philadelphia, WB Saunders, 1983

Sahn SA (ed). Pulmonary Emergencies. New York, Churchill Livingstone, 1982

Selawry OS and Hansen HH. Lung Cancer, pp. 1709–1744. In Cancer Medicine by Holland JF and Frei E III, 2nd ed. Philadelphia, Lea & Febiger, 1982

Selecky PA (ed). Pulmonary Disease. New York, John Wiley & Sons, 1982

Sexton DL. Chronic Obstructive Pulmonary Disease: Care of the Child and Adult. St Louis, CV Mosby, 1981

Sharma OP and Balchum OJ (eds). Key Facts in Pulmonary Disease. New York, Churchill Livingstone, 1983

Shields TW. General Thoracic Surgery, 2nd ed. Philadelphia, Lea & Febiger, 1983

Snider GL. Clinical Pulmonary Medicine. Boston, Little, Brown & Co, 1981

Straus MJ (ed). Lung Cancer: Clinical Diagnosis and Treatment, 2nd ed. New York, Grune & Stratton, 1983

Stringer LW. Emergency Treatment of Acute Respiratory Diseases, 3rd ed. Bowie, MD, Robert J Brady, 1983

Traver GA (ed). Respiratory Nursing: The Science and the Art. New York, John Wiley & Sons, 1982

Weiss W. Lung Cancer, pp. 417–435. In Concepts in Cancer Medicine by Kahn SB et al. New York, Grune & Stratton, 1983

White R. Respiratory Infections and Tumors. Lancaster, England, MTP Press, 1981

Williams MH. Essentials of Pulmonary Medicine. Philadelphia, WB Saunders, 1982

Ziment I (ed). Practical Pulmonary

Disease. New York, John Wiley & Sons, 1983

Articles

Assessment/Diagnosis

Davis GS and Kelley J. Invasive techniques for the diagnosis of respiratory infections. Clin Lab Med 1982 June; 2(2):269–283

Estenne M, Yernault J-C and DeTroyer A. Mechanism of relief of dyspnea after thoracentesis in patients with large pleural effusions. Am J Med 1983 May; 74(5):813–819

Fink I et al. CT-guided aspiration biopsy of the thorax. J Comput Assist Tomogr 1982 Oct; 6(5):958–962

Hornsberger HR, Lee TG and Mukuno DH. Rapid inexpensive real-time directed thoracentesis. Radiology 1983 Feb; 146(2):545–546

Matalon TA et al. Noncardiac chest sonography. The state of the art. Chest 1983 Apr; 83(4):675–678

Sanderson DR. Diagnostic techniques. Semin Resp Med 1981 July; 3(1): entire volume

Ward PCJ. Pleural fluid data 1. Postgrad Med 1982 Oct; 72(4):281–287

Ward PCJ. Pleural fluid data 2. Postgrad Med 1982 Nov; 72(5):291–304

Weaver T. Helping your patient through thoracentesis and pleural biopsy. RN 1983 Jan; 46(1):64–65

Weaver TE. Bronchoscopy, laryngography, and their related complications. RN 1982 Dec; 45(12): 64–65

Pneumonia/Lung Abscess

Bradsher RW. Overwhelming pneumonia. Postgrad Med 1983 Aug; 74(2):201–217

Carden DL and Gibb KA. Pneumonia and lung abscess. Emerg Med Clin North Am 1983 Aug; 1(2):345–370

Choosing antibiotic therapy for pneumonia. Am Fam Physician 1983 Nov; 28(5):246–251

Donowitz GR and Mandell GL. Empiric therapy for pneumonia. Rev Infect Dis 1983 Mar–Apr; 5(Suppl 1):S40–S54

Fick RB Jr and Reynolds HY. Changing spectrum of pneumonia—news media creation or clinical reality. Am J Med 1983 Jan; 74(1):1–8

Larson GL, Parrish DA and Itenson PM. Lung defences. The paradox of inflammation. Chest 1983 May; 83 (5 Suppl):1S–5S

McCue JD. Dyspnea and confusion after a febrile illness. Hosp Pract 1983 Apr; 18(4):96–97

Muder RR et al. Nosocomial legionnaires' disease uncovered in a prospective pneumonia study. JAMA 1983 June 17; 249(23):3184–3188

Muder RR, Yu VL and Zuravleff JJ. Pneumonia due to the Pittsburgh pneumonia agent: New clinical perspectives with a review of the literature. Medicine 1983 Mar; 62(2): 120–128

Ort S et al. Pneumococcal pneumonia in hospitalized patients. JAMA 1983 Jan 14; 249(2):214–218

Parker RH. Hemophilus influenzae respiratory infections in adults. 2. Treatment guidelines. Postgrad Med 1983 Mar; 73(3):187–191

Tafuro P and Cunha BA. Prevention of hospital-acquired pneumonias. DCCN 1983 Sept–Oct; 2(5):287–292

Chronic Obstructive Pulmonary Disease

D'Agostino JS. You *can* breathe new life into your COPD patients. Nursing '83 1983 Sept; 13(9):72–77

Dunlap CI and Marchionno P. Help your COPD patient take a better breath—with inhalers. Nursing '83 1983 May; 13(5):42–43

Hager T. Cigarettes pose dual threat in emphysema [news]. JAMA 1983 June 10; 249(22):3007

Kinsman RA et al. Symptoms and experiences in chronic bronchitis and emphysema. Chest 1983 May; 83(5): 755–761

Matthay RA and Berger HJ. Cardiovascular function in cor pulmonale. Clin Chest Med 1983 May; 4(2):269–295

Mennies JH. Smoking: One way to stop. Am J Nurs 1983 Aug; 83(8):1147–1148

Openbrier DR et al. Nutritional status and lung function in patients with emphysema and chronic bronchitis. Chest 1983 Jan; 83(1):17–22

Pierson DJ and Hudson LD. Pneumonia in the elderly: The fatal complication. Geriatrics 1982 Jan; 37(1):40–50.

Polacek L et al. Teaming up to send the end-stage COPD patient home. Nursing '84 1984 Jan; 14(1):65–68, 71

Schuman E and Cohen AB. Effective therapy for chronic bronchitis and emphysema. Geriatrics 1982 Sept; 37(9):71–74, 76

Sjoberg EL. Nursing diagnosis and the COPD patient. Am J Nurs 1983 Feb; 83(2):244–248

Pulmonary Embolism

Barker AF. Clinical and laboratory management of pulmonary embolism. Geriatrics 1983 Apr; 38(4):105–7, 110–111, 115

Bell WR. Pulmonary embolism: Progress and problems. Am J Med 1982 Feb; 72(2):181–183

Bell WR and Simon TL. Current Status of pulmonary thromboembolic disease: Pathophysiology, diagnosis, prevention, and treatment. Am Heart J 1982 Feb; 103(2):239–262

Bomalaski JS et al. Inferior vena cava interruption in the management of pulmonary embolism. Chest 1982 Dec; 82(6):767–774

Brown AK. Diagnosis and treatment of pulmonary embolus. Compr Ther 1983 Mar; 9(3):68–74

Fowler AA and Hyers TM. Thrombolytic therapy. For pulmonary embolism and deep venous thrombosis. Postgrad Med 1982 Apr; 71(4):149–154, 158

Goldhaber SZ et al. Risk factors for pulmonary embolism. The Framingham study. Am J Med 1983 June; 74(6):1023–1028

Gomez GA, Cutter BS and Wheeler HB.

Transvenous interruption of the inferior vena cava. Surgery 1983 May; 93(5):612–619

Greenfield LJ and Jay SJ. Immediate management of massive pulmonary embolism. Chest 1982 Dec; 82(6): 775–778

Hull RD et al. Pulmonary angiography, ventilation lung scanning, and venography for clinically suspected pulmonary embolism with abnormal perfusion lung scan. Ann Intern Med 1983 June; 98(6):891–899

Mattox KL et al. Pulmonary embolectomy for acute massive pulmonary embolism. Ann Surg 1982 June; 195(6):726–731

Peri-operative low-dose heparin. Drug Ther Bull 1982 Jan 22; 20(2):5–7

Russell JC. Prophylaxis of postoperative deep vein thrombosis and pulmonary embolism. Surg Gynecol Obstet 1983 July; 157(1):89–104

Sasahara AA et al. Pulmonary thromboembolism. JAMA 1983 June 3; 249(21):2945–2950

Satiani B. Management of acute deep venous thrombosis. Am Fam Physician 1982 Apr; 25(4):103–109

Stewart JR and Greenfield LJ. Transvenous vena caval filtration and pulmonary embolectomy. Surg Clin North Am 1982 June; 62(3):411–430

Unger KM. Pulmonary embolism. Am Fam Physician 1982 Oct; 26(4):189–198

Walsh PN. Oral anticoagulant therapy. Hosp Pract 1983 Jan; 18(1):101–120

Occupational Lung Diseases

Brooks SM, Lockey JE and Harber P (eds). Occupational lung diseases. Clin Chest Med 1981 Sept; 2(3): entire volume

Brooks SM, Lockey JE and Harber P (eds). Occupational Lung Diseases. Clin Chest Med 1981 May; 2(2):entire volume

Turner-Warwick M. Occupational lung disease: The scope of the problem. Lung Biol Health Dis 1981; 18:1–33

Lung Cancer/Thoracic Surgery

Bodai BI et al. Emergency thoracotomy in the management of trauma. JAMA 1983 Apr 8; 249(14):1891–1896

Carr DT (ed). Cancer of the Lung: Part 1. Semin Resp Med 1982 Jan; 3(3): entire volume

Carr DT. Cancer of the lung: Part 2. Semin Resp Med 1982 July; 4(1): entire volume

Chlebowski RT, Heber D and Block JB. Lung cancer cachexia. Cancer Treat Res 1983; 11:125–142

Conacher ID et al. Epidural analgesia following thoracic surgery. A review of two years' experience. Anaesthesia 1983 June; 38(6):546–551

Fentiman IS, Rubens RD and Hayward JL. Control of pleural effusions in patients with breast cancer. Cancer 1983 Aug 15; 52(4):737–739

Gorty SR. Recovery room care after thoracic surgery. Int Anesthesiol Clin 1983 Spring; 21(1):173–184

James EC et al. Epidural analgesia for post-thoracotomy patients. J Thorac Cardiovasc Surg 1981 Dec; 82(6):898–903

Matthay RA (ed). Symposium on recent advances in lung cancer. Clin Chest Med 1982 May; 3(2):entire volume

Smith AS and Stewart JA. Oncologic emergencies. Am J Nurs 1983 Sept; 83(9):1282–1285

Zaloznik AJ et al. Intrapleural tetracycline in malignant pleural effusions. Cancer 1983 Feb 15; 51(4): 752–755

Trauma

Cogbill TH et al. Rationale for selective application of emergency department thoracotomy in trauma. J Trauma 1983 June; 23(6):453–460

Dittmann M et al. Epidural analgesia or mechanical ventilation for multiple rib fractures? Intensive Care Med 1982 Mar; 8(2):89–92

Heimlich HJ. Heimlich valve for chest drainage. Med Instrum 1983 Jan–Feb; 17(1):29–31

Hoyt KS. Chest trauma: When the patient looks bad, act fast, and when he looks good, act fast. Nursing '83 1983 May; 13(5):34–41

Lewis FR. Thoracic trauma. Surg Clin North Am 1982 Feb; 62(1):97–104

Mattox KL. Thoracic injury requiring surgery. World J Surg 1983 Jan; 7(1): 49–55

Pinilla JC. Acute respiratory failure in severe blunt chest trauma. J Trauma 1982 Mar; 22(3):221–226

Rich W and Reichenberger M. Managing flail chest. Nursing '81 1981 Dec; 11(12):26–31

Respiratory Function and Therapy

Books

Burton GG and Hodgkin JE (eds). Respiratory Care, 2nd ed. Philadelphia, JB Lippincott, 1984

Campbell JW and Frisse M (eds). Manual of Medical Therapeutics, 24th ed. Boston, Little, Brown & Co, 1983

Freitag JJ and Miller LW (eds). Manual of Medical Therapeutics, 23rd ed. Boston, Little, Brown & Co, 1982

Guenter CA and Welch MH. Pulmonary Medicine, 2nd ed. Philadelphia, JB Lippincott, 1982

Johanson BC et al. Standards For Critical Care. St Louis, CV Mosby, 1981

Luce JM, Tyler MC and Pierson DJ. Intensive Respiratory Care. Philadelphia, WB Saunders, 1984

Shapiro BA, Harrison RA and Trout CA. Clinical Application of Respiratory Care, 2nd ed. Chicago, Year Book Medical Publishers, 1979

Spearman CB, Sheldon RL and Egan DF. Egan's Fundamentals of Respiratory Therapy, 4th ed. St Louis, CV Mosby, 1982

Tisi GM. Pulmonary Physiology in Clinical Medicine. Baltimore, Williams & Wilkins, 1980

Wade JF. Comprehensive Respiratory Care: Physiology and Technique, 3rd ed. St Louis, CV Mosby, 1982

Zagelbaum GL and Paré, JAP. Manual of Acute Respiratory Care. Boston, Little, Brown & Co, 1982

Articles

Barnes TA, and Watson ME. Oxygen delivery performance of old and new designs of the Laerdal, Vitalograph and AMBU adult manual resuscitators. Resp Care 1983 Sept; 28(9):1121–1128

Bone RC (ed). Adult respiratory distress syndrome. Clin Chest Med 1982 Jan; 3(1):1–212

Brown SE et al. Prevention of suctioning-related arterial oxygen desaturation: Comparison of off-ventilator and on-ventilator suctioning. Chest 1983 Apr; 83(4):621–627

Celli BR, Rodriguez KS and Snider GL. A controlled trial of intermittent positive pressure breathing, incentive spirometry and deep breathing exercises in preventing postoperative pulmonary complications after abdominal surgery. Am Rev Resp Dis 1984 Jul; 130(1):12–15

Fuchs PL. O_2 Delivery systems. Nursing '80 1980 December; 10(12):34–43

Fuchs PL. Streamlining your suctioning techniques: Nasotracheal suctioning (part I). Nursing '84 1984 May; 14(5): 55–61

Fuchs PL. Streamlining your suctioning techniques: Endotracheal suctioning (part II). Nursing '84 1984 June; 14(6):46–51

Fuchs PL. Streamlining your suctioning techniques: Tracheostomy suctioning (part III). Nursing '84 1984 July; 14(7):39–43

Kirilloff LH and Maszkiewicz RC. Guide to respiratory care in critically ill adults. Am J Nurs 1979 Nov; 79(11): 2005–2012

Petty TL and Fowler AA. Another look at ARDS. Chest 1982 Jul; 82(1):98–103

Powner DJ and Eross B. Oxygen therapy for the adult patient. Postgrad Med 1981 Oct; 70(4):223–232

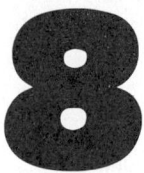

1: Blood Disorders

Cellular Components of Normal Blood

Erythrocytes (Red Blood Cells)
1. Comprise the vast majority of all blood cells; chiefly responsible for the color of blood.
2. Approximately 5 million erythrocytes per cu. mm. of blood.
3. Normal red cell has no nucleus; it is a biconcave disc.
4. Mature red blood cells consist primarily of hemoglobin, which makes up 95% of cell mass.
   a. Presence of a large amount of hemoglobin enables the cell to perform its principal function, the transport of oxygen from the lungs to the tissues.
   b. Iron is present in the heme portion of the molecule and is necessary for oxygen transport.
5. Whole blood normally contains about 14–15 gm. of hemoglobin per 100 ml. of blood.
6. Red blood cells are produced in red bone marrow, which also provides most of the blood's leukocytes and all of its platelets.
7. For normal erythrocyte production, the bone marrow requires iron, vitamin B$_{12}$, folic acid, and other factors.
   If any of these factors is deficient during erythropoiesis (production of erythrocytes), decreased red blood cell production and anemia result.
8. Normal life expectancy of a red cell is between 115 and 130 days—then eliminated by phagocytosis in the reticuloendothelial system, predominantly in spleen and liver.

Leukocytes (White Blood Cells)
1. Normally the total leukocyte count is 5,000 to 10,000 cells per mm.^{3}. Leukocytes can be differentiated from erythrocytes by the presence of a nucleus, their larger size, and different staining properties.
2. Leukocytes are divided into two general categories: granulocytes and mononuclear cells.
   a. *Granulocytes* (produced in marrow) account for 70% of all white cells.
      (1) Called *granulocytes* because of the abundant granules contained in their cytoplasm, or *polymorphonuclear leukocytes,* since their mature nuclei are of a highly irregular, multilobed configuration.
      (2) Granulocytes are divided into 3 subgroups according to their staining properties: eosinophils, basophils, neutrophils.
   b. *Mononuclear leukocytes* (lymphocytes and monocytes) are white blood cells with a single-lobed nucleus and a granule-free cytoplasm. In normal adult blood, lymphocytes account for approximately 30% and monocytes approximately 5% of the total leukocytes.
      (1) Mature lymphocytes are derived from marrow stem cells that undergo further differentiation in the lymph nodes and in the lymphoid tissue of the intestine, spleen, and thymus gland.
      (2) Monocytes are the largest of the blood leukocytes and are produced by the bone marrow.
3. Function of the leukocytes is to protect the body from invasion by foreign cells (e.g., bacteria)—provide protection by phagocytosis, production of antibodies, and rejection of foreign tissue.
   a. The chief function of some granulocytes is

phagocytosis and intracellular kill of ingested organisms; others (eosinophils and basophils) function as reservoirs of potent biological materials such as histamine, serotonin, and heparin. Release of these compounds alters blood supply to the tissues and helps mobilize body defense mechanisms.

   b. Lymphocytes produce substances (interferon, transfer factor, antibodies, etc.) that aid in attacking foreign material; responsible for the immunocompetence of an individual and for the long-term immunologic memory.

4. Reduction in leukocyte number or activity causes a patient to have decreased resistance to infections.

Platelets (Thrombocytes)

1. Are the smallest and most fragile of the formed elements; are small particles (devoid of nuclei) that arise as a result of budding from giant cells, called *megakaryocytes,* in the bone marrow.

2. Number approximately 150,000–450,000 platelets per cu. mm. of blood.

3. Prime function is to control bleeding—important in the formation of clots at sites of injury to blood vessels; maintain the integrity of the vascular endothelium.

   a. Their granules contain adenosine diphosphate (ADP), calcium, serotonin, phospholipids, and other chemical substances.

   b. After tissue injury, circulating platelets stick to the damaged blood vessel walls, release their granules, and form a primary hemostatic plug.

   c. Platelet phospholipid metabolites such as thromboxane A_2 cause vasoconstriction at the site of injury, and ADP promotes platelet aggregation as well as the release of granules from other platelets.

   d. Additional substances released from platelets activate coagulation factors in the blood plasma.

Common Problems of Patients with Blood Disorders

Patient Problems/Nursing Diagnoses	Goals and Interventions	Evaluation
Fatigue and weakness related to effects of disease, anemia, stress of coping with disease and its treatment	*GOAL:* Modification of life-style to cope with fatigue and weakness. Plan nursing care to conserve the patient's strength and emotional energy. Give frequent rest periods. Encourage ambulation activities as tolerated. Encourage conditioning exercises to increase endurance. Avoid disturbing activities, noise, stress, or any activity that ordinarily increases heart rate or cardiac output. Encourage optimal nutrition—high-protein and high-calorie foods and beverages.	Follows a progressive plan of rest, activities, and exercise Paces activities according to energy level

Hemorrhagic tendencies (easy bruising, petechiae, purpura, ecchymoses, menorrhagia, bleeding in mucous membranes of mouth, retina, GI tract) related to thrombocytopenia, abnormalities of platelet function, thrombocytosis, blood vessel and connective tissue disease; depression of bone marrow from toxic effects of chemotherapy.	*GOAL:* Prevention or management of bleeding episodes.
	Use measures to prevent bleeding:
	  Handle skin gently; avoid use of adhesive tape.
	  Use small-gauge needles when administering medication by injection; apply pressure to venipuncture site for 5 minutes with patient's arm extended above the level of his heart.
	  Give required IM injections with thin needles, Z-track technique, and pressure.
	  Rotate extremities for blood pressure measurement.
	  Use electric shaver instead of razor.
	  Avoid rectal instrumentation (thermometer; enemas; suppositories).
	  Avoid use of vaginal tampons.
	  Employ stool softeners to prevent
		Identifies factors/circumstances that cause bleeding
		
		Reports early manifestaitons of bleeding

(continued)

Patient Problems/Nursing Diagnoses	Goals and Interventions	Evaluation
	rupture of blood vessels from straining.	
	Keep the patient at rest during the bleeding episodes.	
	Apply gentle pressure to the bleeding site.	Can recall appropriate interventions to manage bleeding
	Apply cold compresses to the bleeding site when indicated.	
	Avoid disturbing clots.	
	Give a Popsicle to the patient who is bleeding orally—induces vasoconstriction; stop oral hygiene measures, including rinsing, during periods of active bleeding.	
	Measure blood loss; weigh linens, bandages, and note saturation of pads during menses.	
	Test urine, stool, and emesis for occult blood.	
	Monitor hematocrit and hemoglobin levels.	
	Observe for symptoms of internal bleeding.	
	Check supine and standing blood pressure and pulse; if pulse increases or BP goes down, patient is not stable.	
	Have a tracheostomy set available for the patient who is bleeding from the mouth or throat; observe for signs of asphyxiation.	
	Support the patient during transfusion therapy.	
	Educate the patient to:	
	Protect himself from injury.	
	Avoid medications containing aspirin.	
	Blow his nose gently with his mouth open.	
	Avoid the Valsalva maneuver.	
Alteration in oral mucous membranes related to: bacterial flora, presence of infections, cytotoxic action of chemotherapeutic agents on oral mucosal cells, and effects of radiation.	*GOAL:* Decrease in oral discomfort and increase in integrity of oral mucous membranes.	Uses preventive oral care
Bleeding gums	Develop and follow a plan for oral care based on oral assessment.	Notifies health care personnel of early signs and symptoms of oral complications.
Pain/ulcerations	Encourage regular dentist visits—bleeding gums occur when there is gross tartar on the teeth.	Follows oral hygiene regimen before and after eating.
Periodontal infection		
Pain with chewing and swallowing related to mucosal damage	Use mechanical cleansing procedures to remove plaque and debris.	
Xerostomia (dry mouth)	a. Use a soft, multitufted nylon toothbrush.	Requests measures for comfort
Cheilitis; lip cracking	b. Employ careful flossing with short, delicate strokes to avoid damage to the gingiva; discontinue flossing if it causes pain.	
Candidiasis (white curds, plaques, ulcerations)		
Herpes simplex (painful vesicles that rupture and become encrusted)	Offer mouthwash (normal saline solution or Cepacol® diluted with water, 1:5) before and after meals.	

Patient Problems/Nursing Diagnoses	Goals and Interventions	Evaluation
	Moisten lips with water-soluble lubricant (K-Y jelly) every 2–4 hours.	
	For patients with mucositis, pain, periodontal infection, xerostomia:	Uses appropriate interventions if complications arise
	Remove dentures	
	Control moderate to severe pain of mucous membranes with topical anesthetic agents for mucous membranes	
	Give systemic analgesics (acetaminophen; codeine) as directed for severe pain to allow pain relief for sleep and consumption of fluids.	
	Cleanse teeth with moistened gauze wrapped around finger; use Water Pik® on low setting.	
	Employ normal saline for mouth rinse every 2–4 hours; avoid alcohol-containing mouth washes.	
	Employ prophylactic nystatin rinses for candidiasis.	
	Offer a bland diet avoiding temperature extremes.	Makes dietary changes to compensate for oral soreness
	Encourage a high intake (3,000 ml.) of bland, chilled fluids.	Eliminates tart, acidic, and highly seasoned food from diet
	Offer lemon drops, sugarless gum, ice chips, and saliva substitute (Salivart® Synthetic Saliva) to stimulate saliva and as a mouth moisturizer.	Reports signs and symptoms of infection immediately
Dyspnea related to reduction of oxyhemoglobin and possible bleeding into pulmonary system	*GOAL:* Management of symptoms. Elevate the head of the bed. Use pillows to support the patient in the orthopneic position. Administer oxygen when indicated. Prevent unnecessary exertion. Avoid gas-forming foods.	Uses comfort measures to alleviate shortness of breath
Bone and joint pains related to proliferation of neoplastic cells; bleeding	Provide appropriate pain relief on a regular schedule. Relieve pressure of bedding by using a cradle. Administer either hot or cold compresses as prescribed. Provide for joint immobilization when prescribed.	Requests interventions for pain control Attempts to achieve control over pain by following optimal lifestyle management (rest, nutrition, activity, elimination)
Fever related to infection, hematologic malignancy	Assist in determining cause of fever (infection). Administer cool sponges. Give antipyretic (acetaminophen) drugs as prescribed. Encourage liberal fluid intake unless contraindicated. Maintain a cool environmental temperature.	Avoids potential sources of infection Relates early signs and symptoms of infections
Alteration in skin integrity (pruritus or skin eruptions) related to pathophysiologic process of hematologic malignancy, release	Keep the patient's fingernails short. Use soap sparingly. Apply emollient lotions in skin care.	Monitors and protects skin integrity Absence of skin excoriation

(continued)

Patient Problems/Nursing Diagnoses	Goals and Interventions	Evaluation
of proteolytic enzymes by tumor, chemotherapy	Give antihistamines as prescribed. See page 606.	
Fear (of patient and family) related to diagnosis, diagnostic procedures, therapy, and prognosis	*GOAL:* Psychosocial support. Provide emotional support to facilitate the process of coping with the diagnosis and treatment of a hematologic disorder.	Attempts to maintain control; asks questions, makes wishes known
	Explain the nature, the discomforts, and limitations of activity associated with the diagnostic procedures and treatments.	Identifies support person/system
	Offer the service of listening about anxieties, guilt, doubts, finances, etc.	
	Provide an atmosphere of acceptance and understanding.	
	Encourage the patient to verbalize his *feelings*.	Verbalizes feelings and concerns
	Give skilled care; promote relaxation and comfort.	
	Remember the patient's individual preferences.	
	Promote a sense of independence and self-care within the patient's limitations.	
	Teach the patient stress reduction techniques; progressive relaxation, distraction, guided imagery.	Uses diversion and relaxation techniques
	Encourage the family to participate in the patient's care (as desired).	
	Create a comfortable atmosphere for the family's visits with the patient.	

Blood and Bone Marrow Specimens

Blood may be obtained by (1) skin puncture (finger, toe, heel, or ear lobe) or (2) venipuncture.*

A *skin puncture* is performed when only a small amount of blood is needed (for red and white cell counts,

hemoglobin and hematocrit determinations, reticulocyte counts, blood films for differential smear). However, the values for the red blood cells, hematocrit, hemoglobin, and platelets are lower in capillary blood than in venous blood.

A *venipuncture* is a puncture of a vein to obtain blood; used when larger amounts of blood are needed (preferred method).

* The most common hematologic tests are described in the Appendix 1, p. 1509.

Guidelines: Obtaining Blood by Skin Puncture

Equipment

Disposable lancet
Pipette and tubing
Slides
Alcohol sponges and dry sterile sponges

Procedure

Nursing Action	Rationale/Amplification
Performance Phase	
1. Cleanse site (preferably ball of finger) with alcohol and dry with sterile gauze square.	1. If any alcohol remains, it will alter red cell morphology; also, blood will not collect into a compact drop but will run down the patient's finger.
2. Create stasis by pressing on the distal joint of the finger to produce redness at the end of the finger.	
3. Use a sterile disposable lancet, or an automated lancet.	3. This avoids the possibility of the transference of the hepatitis virus.
4. Prick the skin sharply and quickly with the lancet.	4. Pricking the skin sharply and quickly minimizes pain and produces a free-flowing sample.
5. Release pressure on the finger. Wipe off the first drop of blood.	5. Epithelial or endothelial cells may be found in the first drop of blood and render the count inaccurate. Also, platelets will begin to clump immediately in the blood at the puncture site.
6. Allow the blood to flow freely with an adequate puncture.	6. Pressing out the blood dilutes it with tissue fluid.
7. Obtain the blood sample: a. Fill the pipette or microhematocrit tube. b. Make blood slides according to the study required.	b. Gently touch the drop of blood to glass slides or cover slip.
8. Apply pressure over the wound with a dry gauze sponge until bleeding stops.	

Guidelines: Obtaining Blood by Venipuncture

Veins Used

Antecubital area
Wrist
Dorsum (back) of hand
Top of foot

Equipment

70% alcohol and tincture of iodine
Dry sterile sponges
5- and 10-ml. syringe
No. 20 gauge needle(s)

Procedure

Nursing Action	Rationale/Amplification
Performance Phase	
1. Reassure the patient. Explain that relatively little blood will be taken.	1. The patient is reassured when the nurse displays self-assurance and competence in relating to people and when performing technical skills.
2. Instruct the patient to extend his arm; the arm should be held straight at the elbow.	
3. Apply the tourniquet directly above the elbow with just sufficient pressure to prevent venous return.	3. A tourniquet increases venous pressure and makes the vein more prominent and easier to enter.
4. Inspect the area to visualize the vein. Palpate the vein.	4. Select a vein that is visible, palpable, and well fixed to surrounding tissue so that it does not roll away. (Not all veins are visible; some may be deep and can only be palpated.)
5. Cleanse the skin with iodine and alcohol. Dry.	5. Cleansing the skin reduces pathogens.
6. Fix chosen vein with the thumb and draw the skin taut immediately below the site before inserting needle to stabilize the vein.	6. The vein may roll beneath the skin when the needle approaches its outer surface (especially in elderly and extremely thin patients).
7. Hold the syringe between the thumb and last 3 fingers with the bevel up and directly in line with the course of the vein. Insert the needle quickly and smoothly under the skin and into the vein.	

(continued)

Guidelines: Obtaining Blood by Venipuncture (continued)

Procedure
(Cont.)

Nursing Action	Rationale/Amplification
8. Obtain blood sample by *gently* pulling back on the plunger.	8. Use minimal suction to prevent hemolysis of blood and collapse of the vein.
9. Release the tourniquet.	
10. Withdraw the needle slowly.	10. Slow withdrawal of the needle is less painful.
11. Gauze is applied with pressure over the puncture site for 2–4 minutes.	11. Firm pressure over the puncture site prevents leakage of blood into surrounding tissues with subsequent hematoma development. Merely flexing the arm may not prevent a hematoma as the vein can slip to the side of the area where pressure is applied.
12. Make the blood smear from the needle as desired.	
13. Remove the needle from the syringe. As soon as possible after drawing the blood, gently eject the blood sample into a test tube containing an anticoagulant.	13. Slowly transfer the blood into the test tube *without* forming bubbles.
14. Place stopper on the test tube.	
15. Invert the tube gently several times to mix blood with anticoagulant.	15. For some tests, the blood is allowed to coagulate in the test tube.
16. Label specimens correctly and send to laboratory immediately.	16. Specimens should go to the laboratory with a minimum of delay for optimum reliability.
17. Dispose needle and syringe in appropriate containers to avoid possible spread of hepatitis. Clean all spills with alcohol and peroxide or other antiseptic agents according to agency policy.	

Guidelines: Bone Marrow Aspiration and Biopsy

Bone marrow aspiration and/or *biopsy* is done so that specimens of bone marrow and bone can be obtained for establishing a diagnosis.

Purposes
1. To diagnose hematologic disorders—enables the precursors of cells in peripheral blood to be examined and their relative numbers determined; to evaluate for iron content.
2. To follow the course of disease and the patient's response to treatment.
3. To diagnose diseases other than pure hematologic disorders, such as primary and metastatic tumors, infectious diseases, and certain granulomas.
4. To isolate bacteria and other pathogenic agents by culture or animal inoculation.

Complications
1. Bleeding and hematoma in patients with bleeding disorders

Equipment

Bone marrow aspiration tray
   Marrow aspiration needles with stylets
   Towels
   No. 25 and 22 gauge needles
   Two 20-ml. syringes
   Three 5-ml. syringes
Local anesthetic (1% procaine or xylocaine)
Sterile gauze squares
Sterile gloves, drape
Skin antiseptic
Laboratory equipment
   Coverslips
   Microscopic slides
   Test tubes (plain and heparinized)
Scalpel blade and handle

Procedure

Nursing Action	Rationale/Amplification

Preparatory Phase

1. Explain the procedure to the patient. Tell patient when the skin will be marked, antiseptic applied, and the needle puncture performed.

2. Give medication (meperidine) or tranquilizer as requested; usually not necessary for aspiration.

3. Place the patient in prone or supine position.
4. The following sites are most frequently used:
   a. Posterior superior iliac crest
   b. Anterior iliac crest (if patient is very obese)
   c. Sternum

1. An explanation helps the patient to cope with anticipated stress. Tactile sensations (pressure, cold) can be misinterpreted as pain unless the patient is forewarned.

2. Demerol may be used as an analgesic and sedative for apprehension. Anxiety may produce excessive discomfort.

Iliac Crest Aspiration/Biopsy

Performance Phase (by physician)

1. Position the patient on his abdomen (prone) or on his side with top knee flexed.
   a. The posterior iliac crest is located and marked.

   b. The skin area is prepared and draped. The marked area is infiltrated with local anesthetic through the skin and subcutaneous tissue to the periosteum of the bone.
   c. A small incision may be made.

   d. The bone marrow needle, with stylet in place, is introduced through the incision.

   e. The needle is advanced and rotated by using firm and steady pressure. When the needle is felt to enter the outer cortex of the bone marrow cavity, the stylet is removed and the syringe attached. Negative pressure is applied, and a small volume of blood and marrow is aspirated (0.5 ml.).
   f. A biopsy is taken by using a special needle equipped with a sharp cutting edge and a hollow core.

a. The iliac crest provides a large marrow cavity at the posterior superior iliac spine away from nearby abdominal organs.
b. Tell the patient he will experience a needle prick followed by a burning sensation.
   The periosteum is the region of greatest sensitivity.

c. The biopsy needle is large, and a small incision facilitates insertion.
d. The needle is pointed toward the anterior superior iliac spine and brought into contact with the posterior iliac spine.
e. There is usually decreased resistance when the bone marrow cavity is entered.
   The actual aspiration may cause brief pain, and the patient should be forewarned.
   Bone marrow appears rusty-red and normally has a thick, fluid-like consistency.

Sternal Aspiration

Performance Phase (by physician)

1. The skin is prepared and the site infiltrated with procaine or xylocaine.
2. The site selected is usually the midsternal line at the level of the 2nd interspace.
3. A small stab incision may be made before bone marrow needle insertion.
4. The marrow needle with stylet in place is inserted through the cortex of the bone with a slight rotating motion. The physician usually feels a "give" in the marrow needle when the marrow cavity has been penetrated.
5. The stylet is removed and a syringe attached to the hub of the needle. The plunger is withdrawn slowly until marrow appears in the syringe (0.2 ml. of fluid is aspirated).
6. Warn the patient that he will feel a brief episode of sharp pain.
7. The syringe and needle are removed and passed to a technician for preparation of smears.
8. Pressure is applied over the puncture site for a brief period to ensure hemostasis.
9. A small dressing is applied with pressure over the puncture site.
10. Remove dressing after 24 hours and inspect area for inflammation.

2. The sternum is thinner and marrow more plentiful between the sternal interspaces.
3. This technique avoids pushing the skin into the bone marrow.
4. A sternal puncture is considered more dangerous than other sites because of its proximity to vital structures in the mediastinum.

5. The marrow will appear as thick, dark reddish fluid.

6. The pain is caused by suction of the syringe and lasts only a few seconds.
7. Smears of aspirated marrow are made; technique is similar to that of preparing blood smears.
8. If the patient has thrombocytopenia, pressure should be applied for 10–15 minutes.

(continued)

Guidelines: Bone Marrow Aspiration and Biopsy (continued)

Procedure
(Cont.)

Nursing Action	Rationale/Amplification
Follow-up Phase	
1. Give mild analgesic if needed.	1. Most patients have no discomfort after aspiration, but the site of a biopsy may ache for a day or so.
2. Assess the patient for discomfort, continued bleeding, and untoward symptoms.	

Anemia

Anemia is a laboratory definition that implies a low red cell count and a hemoglobin or hematocrit level that is below normal. Physiologically, anemia exists when there is an insufficient amount of hemoglobin to deliver oxygen to the tissues.

Altered Physiology

1. The appearance of anemia may reflect (1) decreased production of red cells, (2) red cell loss, or (3) increased destruction.
2. Marrow failure may occur as a result of nutritional deficiency, toxic exposure, tumor invasion, or unknown causes.
3. Red cells may be lost through hemorrhage or hemolysis (increased destruction).
   a. This problem may be rooted in an intrinsic red-cell defect that is incompatible with normal red-cell survival or is explainable on the basis of some factor extrinsic to the red cell that promotes red-cell destruction.
   b. Red-cell lysis occurs mainly within the phagocytic cells of the reticuloendothelial system, notably within the liver and spleen.
   c. As a by-product of this process, bilirubin, formed by the metabolism of hemoglobin within the phagocyte, enters the bloodstream, and an increase in hemolysis is promptly reflected by an increase in total plasma bilirubin.

Clinical Manifestations

(Most manifestations are attributable to a decrease in the oxygen-carrying capacity of the blood, and are the same regardless of the cause of anemia.)
1. The more rapidly the anemia develops, the more severe its symptoms:
   a. Pallor
   b. Susceptibility to fatigue
   c. Shortness of breath
   d. Headache; disturbed cerebration; dizziness
   e. Development of angina pectoris or congestive heart failure in susceptible individuals
2. Severity of symptoms dependent on:
   a. The speed with which and the degree to which the anemia has developed
   b. Its prior duration (i.e., its chronicity)
   c. The metabolic requirements of the particular patient
   d. Any other disorders currently afflicting the patient, particularly cardiac conditions, etc.
   e. Special complications or concomitant features of the condition producing the anemia

Iron Deficiency Anemia

Iron deficiency anemias are conditions in which the total body iron content is decreased below normal. It is the most common type of anemia in all age-groups and is a major health problem in developing countries.

Etiology

Iron deficiency develops when the body's need for iron exceeds the supply.
1. Chronic blood loss—gastrointestinal (GI) bleeding (secondary to gastritis, peptic ulcer, hemorrhoids, malignancy), excessive menstrual bleeding, multiple pregnancies, hookworm infestation
2. Impaired gastrointestinal absorption of iron—small bowel disease, certain gastric resections
3. Insufficient intake
4. Increased iron requirements—during pregnancy, periods of rapid growth, menstruation (average of 20 mg. of iron lost per menstrual cycle)
5. Excessive ingestion of aspirin (leading to occult GI blood loss)

Iron Balance and Stores

1. Approximately 6 mg. of iron is ingested per 1000 Kcal.; or 16–20 mg./day.
2. The amount of iron ingested is related to the number of calories consumed.
   Normally about 5%–10% of ingested iron is absorbed by the gastrointestinal mucosa, bound to transferrin (main iron-binding protein in plasma), and carried through the bloodstream to the bone marrow. In the marrow, iron is transported to red blood cells and reticuloendothelial cells.
3. Normal adult male has iron stores of 900 mg.; adult female has 300 mg.
4. Adult male loses about 1 mg. iron per day; premenopausal woman loses about 1.5 mg. iron per day.

Management
A. Oral Iron Therapy

1. Allows patient to regenerate hemoglobin. (Hematologic values should return to normal in 4–8 weeks.) Therapy is continued approximately 6 months following normalization of blood values to restore hemoglobin and iron stores. It is continued longer in patients with continued blood loss.
2. Choice of iron depends on (1) patient tolerance, (2) gastrointestinal absorption, (3) dosage according to estimate of hemoglobin deficiency.

3. Oral iron preparations
   a. Ferrous sulfate (preferred and least expensive)
   b. Ferrous gluconate

B. Parenteral Iron Therapy

1. Parenteral iron therapy is given only (1) when the patient is unable to tolerate iron preparations orally, (2) when the patient has severe gastrointestinal disorders, (3) when there is continuing negative iron balance while patient is taking maximum oral dose tolerated, or (4) when there is nonadherence by patient.

▶ **NURSING ALERT:** Extravasation of iron medication results in painful local induration. An anaphylactic reaction may occur following either intramuscular or intravenous injection of iron dextran.

2. Parenteral iron preparations
   a. Iron dextran (Imferon)
   b. Iron sorbitex (Jectofer)—may cause patient's urine to turn black on standing, since about 50% of iron is excreted in the urine within 24 hours.

Assessment
Clinical Manifestations

Reduction in hemoglobin concentration decreases the capacity of the blood to transport and deliver oxygen to the tissues.
1. Easy fatigability
2. Headache, dizziness, tinnitus
3. Palpitations and dyspnea on exertion
4. Pallor of skin and mucous membranes
5. Smooth, sore tongue associated with a burning sensation
6. Cheilosis (lesions at corners of mouth)
7. Pica (craving to eat unusual substances)
8. Koilonychia (spoon-shaped fingernails)

Laboratory Evaluation

Measurements of hemoglobin, hematocrit, red cell indices, serum iron level, total iron binding capacity, serum ferritin (occasionally bone marrow iron stain), examination of peripheral blood smear.

Note: It is important to recognize and correct the underlying cause.
1. Question the patient concerning hematemesis, melena, epistaxis, hematuria, menometrorrhagia, multiple diagnostic procedures.
2. Send urine and stool specimens to laboratory for occult blood examination.
3. Prepare patient for sigmoidoscopy, colonoscopy, barium enema, upper gastrointestinal studies.

Patient Problems/Nursing Diagnoses

1. Fatigue related to anemia
2. Discomfort (headache, etc.) related to anemia
3. Activity intolerance related to reduced energy
4. Inadequate nutritional intake related to dyspepsia
5. Ineffective individual coping related to altered lifestyle resulting from activity limitations
6. Diarrhea or constipation related to iron ingestion

Planning and Implementation
Nursing Interventions

A. Oral Iron Therapy

1. Iron preparations are absorbed at all levels of the gastrointestinal tract below the stomach; maximal absorption occurs in the duodenum and upper jejunum.
2. Iron is usually given between meals, on an empty stomach, with a 4-hour interval between doses—to prevent reduced absorption by presence of food.
   a. Iron may be started with smaller doses and increased slowly over 7–10 days to minimize side effects.
   b. If side effects (epigastric distress, nausea, constipation, diarrhea) occur, iron may be taken with meals (which drastically reduces absorption) and then shifted to a between-meal schedule for maximum absorption.
3. Educate patient to anticipate a certain amount of dyspepsia from time to time.
4. Iron salts alter the color of the stools; tell the patient to expect color changes (dark green to black).
5. Ferrous sulfate is apt to deposit on the teeth and the gums; advise patient to use frequent oral hygiene measures.
6. The dosage of iron may be gradually increased over a few days, from 1 tablet daily up to 3 tablets daily.
7. Iron administration should be continued approximately 6 months after hemoglobin levels return to normal—to replenish iron stores.

B. Parenteral Iron Therapy

1. Technique of parenteral iron administration:
   a. Discard needle that is used to draw medication into syringe; use a fresh needle for injection—to avoid tracking medication through subcutaneous tissue.
   b. Allow a small amount of air in syringe.
   c. Use a needle 5 cm. (2 inches) long—medication is injected deep into upper outer quadrant of buttock.
   d. Retract the skin over the muscle *laterally* before inserting needle (Z-track)—to prevent leakage along injection tract and staining of skin.
   e. Inject solution slowly followed by air in syringe. Wait a few seconds before withdrawing needle.

Health Education

1. Emphasize that the patient should take the iron faithfully.
   See oral iron therapy, steps 1–7, above.
2. Encourage the selection of a well-balanced diet. Adolescent girls should receive nutritional counseling—fad diets may limit amount of absorbable iron ingested.
3. Keep iron medications out of reach of small children—iron tablets are dangerous when ingested by small children.

Evaluation
Expected Outcomes

1. Demonstrates a return to normal hemoglobin levels
2. Adheres to medication schedule
3. Increases daily activities

Megaloblastic Anemias

1. A *megaloblast* is a nucleated red cell with delayed and abnormal nuclear maturation.
2. The most common megaloblastic anemias are caused by B_{12} deficiency (pernicious anemia) and/or folic acid deficiency.
3. Anemias due to deficiencies of vitamins B_{12} and folic

acid show identical bone marrow and peripheral blood changes. This is because both vitamins are essential for normal DNA synthesis.

Pernicious Anemia

Pernicious anemia is caused by lack of intrinsic factor, which normally is produced by gastric mucosal parietal cells. (B_{12} deficiency is also seen in diseases of the small intestine—i.e., malabsorption, blind loop syndrome, following gastrectomy.)

Altered Physiology

1. Pernicious anemia is produced by a defect in the gastric mucosa; the stomach wall becomes atrophic and fails to secrete intrinsic factor.
2. This substance ordinarily binds dietary vitamin B_{12} and travels with it to the ileum, where the vitamin is absorbed. Without intrinsic factor, orally administered B_{12} cannot be absorbed.
3. Therefore, after the body's store of B_{12} is used up, the patient begins to show signs of the anemia.
4. Vitamin B_{12} is necessary for normal DNA synthesis in maturing red cells.

Clinical Manifestations

1. Symptoms due to anemia
   a. Pallor
   b. Dyspnea, tachycardia, easy fatigability
   c. Angina pectoris, arrhythmias, congestive heart failure
   d. Edema of legs
2. Symptoms due to physiologic changes in gastrointestinal tract
   a. Sore mouth with smooth, red, "beefy" tongue
   b. Loss of appetite
   c. Indigestion and epigastric discomfort
   d. Recurring diarrhea or constipation
   e. Weight loss
3. Symptoms due to neurologic changes (neuropathy occurs in high percentage of untreated patients)
   a. Tingling and numbness or burning pain (paresthesia) involving hands and feet
   b. Loss of position sense, leading to disturbances of gait
   c. Disturbances of bladder and bowel function
   d. Psychiatric symptoms—from cerebral dysfunction

Diagnostic Evaluation

1. Blood smear—reveals marked variation in size and shape of cells and a variable number of unusually large cells containing a normal concentration of hemoglobin.
2. Tests for serum and red cell folate levels and serum vitamin B_{12} level.
3. Gastric analysis—the gastric juice lacks free hydrochloric acid (achlorhydria).
4. *Schilling Test*—a test for vitamin B_{12} absorption.
   Purpose:
   To prove that the patient cannot absorb oral vitamin B_{12} unless intrinsic factor is added.
   a. The patient is given a small dose of radioactive B_{12} in water to drink followed by a nonradioactive intramuscular dose.
   b. When the oral vitamin is absorbed, it will be excreted in the urine; the IM dose helps to flush it into the urine.
   c. A 24-hour urine specimen is collected and measured for radioactivity. All urine must be collected. Patients with renal disease may require longer periods of collection.
   d. If very little has been excreted, the test is repeated several days later (the "second stage") with a capsule of oral intrinsic factor added to the oral vitamin B_{12}.
   e. If the patient has pernicious anemia, this time much more radioactivity will be found in the 24-hour urine specimen.

Management

A. Management During Acute Stage

1. Hydroxocobalamin or cyanocobalamin (vitamin B_{12} IM) as directed (daily for 7 days, weekly for 10 weeks, and then monthly for rest of life; many protocols for administration of B_{12} are in use).
   a. Parenteral vitamin therapy is necessary, since most of these patients are unable to absorb the vitamin by mouth.
   b. Reticulocytes begin to increase on 4th day after therapy is started; normal hemoglobin values are obtained in approximately 6 weeks.
   c. Patient begins to improve in general well-being and mental status in a few days.
   d. Recent neurologic changes will usually be reversed.
2. Give transfusion of packed cells (rarely necessary); *administer very slowly.*
   a. Transfusions are given only to patients whose anemia is life-threatening (symptoms of hypoxia to heart or brain).
   b. Place the patient in a sitting position in bed.
      Too rapid administration of transfusion to a patient with anemia may produce acute pulmonary or cerebral edema. These patients are particularly susceptible to volume overload because they have an expanded plasma volume.
3. Support the patient with neurologic involvement (see p. 540 for management of patient with neurogenic bladder).

Health Education

1. Impress upon the patient that vitamin B_{12} must be continued for his lifetime.
   a. Maintenance dose schedule—vitamin B_{12} IM every 4 weeks.
   b. Teach patient and family or have community health nurse give maintenance therapy.
   c. Untreated pernicious anemia is fatal.
2. Instruct the patient to report for follow-up examinations every 6 months—for hematocrit and physical examination.
   a. Patient may develop hematologic or neurologic relapse if therapy is inadequate.
   b. Patients with pernicious anemia have a higher incidence of gastric cancer and thyroid problems; therefore, periodic stool examinations for occult blood and gastric cytology, along with thyroid function tests, should be made.
3. Following total gastrectomy (and occasionally subtotal gastrectomy), patient should receive maintenance dose of vitamin B_{12} as often as indicated—removal of gastric fundus deprives the patient of all intrinsic factor; may take as long as 10 years for clinical symptoms to appear, because of the small amount of

daily vitamin B_{12} required and the large body stores available for use.

Folic Acid Deficiency

Folic acid is necessary for normal red blood cell production. Folate depletion results in progressive anemia.

Causes

1. Inadequate dietary intake
   a. Common in alcoholics
   b. Elderly individuals who live on "tea and toast"
   c. Patients on hyperalimentation or chronic hemodialysis
2. Impaired absorption—most absorption of folic acid takes place in upper jejunum
3. Increased requirements—chronic hemolytic anemias; pregnancy, etc.
4. Impaired utilization—from folic acid antagonists (methotrexate)

Clinical Manifestations

Symptoms of anemia—fatigue, weakness, pallor
Sore tongue, cracked lips

Diagnostic Evaluation

Assay of serum folate

Management

1. Give oral folic acid replacement as prescribed.
2. Inform the patient that a proper diet will prevent most instances of folate deficiency: green vegetables (asparagus, broccoli, spinach); yeast, liver, organ meats, some fresh fruits.

Aplastic Anemia

Anemia from bone marrow aplasia (failure) is characterized by deficiency in all the cellular elements of the blood.

Aplastic anemia is a stem cell disorder characterized by bone marrow failure with pancytopenia (deficiency in all cellular elements of the blood).

Causes

1. Idiopathic (50% of all cases)
2. Chemical toxins
3. Idiosyncratic response to drugs
4. Virus, especially hepatitis
5. Congenital (Fanconi's anemia)

Note: Secondary bone marrow aplasia is a predictable marrow suppression induced by antineoplastic agents and radiation therapy or bone marrow transplantation.

Clinical Course

1. The clinical course is variable, and the overall mortality rate is high; patients with severe pancytopenia with totally aplastic marrow have a poor prognosis.
2. Patients with aplastic anemia are at serious risk of infection, hemorrhage, and other complications of chronic anemia.

Treatment

1. Search for cause/prevention of toxic exposure
2. Bone marrow transplant (treatment of choice for patients with severe aplastic anemia who have matched donors)
3. Androgens (oxymetholone or testosterone enanthate)—controversial
4. Immunosuppressive treatment (splenectomy; cyclophosphamide)
5. Immunologic therapy (antithymocyte globulin [ATG])

Assessment
Clinical Manifestations

1. Abnormal bleeding—resulting from thrombocytopenia
   a. Bleeding from gums, nose, gastrointestinal and genitourinary tracts
   c. Purpura; petechiae; ecchymoses
2. Anemia—resulting from depression of hemoglobin; symptoms pronounced because of rapidity of blood cell change
   a. Pallor; weakness
   b. Exertional dyspnea, palpitations
3. Infections with high fever—resulting from granulocytopenia
   a. Pharyngitis and oropharyngeal mucositis
   b. Sepsis via gastrointestinal tract or genitourinary tract

Diagnostic Evaluation

1. Peripheral blood smear shows pancytopenia.
2. Bone marrow aspiration and biopsy—bone marrow is hypoplastic or aplastic; reduction of its cellular elements occurs, and there is an almost complete absence of hemopoietic activity.

Patient Problems/Nursing Diagnoses

1. Ineffective coping related to anxiety about achieving a remission
2. Potential for infection related to lack of circulating granulocytes
3. Potential for hemorrhage related to thrombocytopenia

Planning and Implementation
Nursing Interventions

A. Recovery of Adequate Bone Marrow Function

1. Attempt to identify and eliminate the underlying toxic agent(s)—gives marrow opportunity to recover before being damaged too severely. However, permanent damage often occurs.
   a. Question the patient regarding all agents (drugs, chemicals) to which he has been exposed.
   b. Instruct the patient to discontinue all unnecessary medications and eliminate exposure to toxins.
2. Support the patient undergoing bone marrow transplantation (see p. 273) (replacement of affected bone marrow with marrow from healthy donor—preferably matched sibling).
   a. Bone marrow transplantation should be carried out *early,* since subsequent blood and platelet transfusions can cause irreversible sensitization of patient and result in graft rejection.
   b. This modality of treatment is performed at specialized transplant centers.
   c. Drawbacks in bone marrow transplantation include immunologic problems (graft-versus-host disease) and marrow graft rejection.
3. Give agents (androgenic steroids) to attempt to stimulate marrow regeneration and bring about a remission; may be indicated in a few patients.

B. Prevention of Infection

1. Maintain continuing surveillance for evidence of infection—infection is major cause of death.
   a. Organisms not usually pathogenic may become so, particularly those of the *Pseudomonas, Proteus,* and *Klebsiella* species.
   b. Sources of infection in these patients are endogenous bacteria from gastrointestinal and upper respiratory tracts, particularly in those patients hospitalized for prolonged periods.
2. Attempt to reduce potential endogenous pathogens in the hospitalized patient.

▶ **NURSING ALERT:** Place the patient in a protected environment (private room) with handwashing precautions strictly enforced.

   a. Pay scrupulous attention to skin infections. Regard any small break in the skin as hazardous.
      (1) Use antibacterial agent (povidone-iodine solution) in bathwater—to diminish resident body flora.
      (2) Encourage the use of an electric rather than plain razor.
   b. Examine axillae and groin areas—apt to harbor pathogens and develop pustules.
   c. Monitor temperature—fever implies bacterial, fungal, or viral infection.
3. Give antibiotics at first sign of infection.
   a. Oral antifungal agent is frequently administered to eradicate colonization of GI tract with yeast; absence of bacteria may encourage fungal overgrowth.
   b. Broad-spectrum antibiotics usually given IV.
   c. Granulocyte transfusions may be given to the neutropenic patient with infection who fails to respond to antibacterial or antifungal therapy.

C. Supportive Treatment When Bone Marrow Transplantation Is Not Feasible

1. Give blood components—to supply red cells, platelets, and granulocytes when bone marrow has ceased to produce them.
   a. Keep veins open—patient may require frequent transfusions for long periods; monitor IV sites carefully.
   b. Give packed red cell transfusions carefully—to maintain hemoglobin level compatible with patient's activities and to relieve symptoms of dyspnea, palpitation, and weakness.
   c. Give platelet transfusions from histocompatible donors when necessary—to arrest bleeding in the patient hemorrhaging from thrombocytopenia. (Hemorrhagic complications occur with platelet counts below 20,000/cu. mm.)
   d. Keep patient who receives multiple transfusions over a period of time under careful nursing surveillance—these patients may develop transfusion complications.
      (1) Eventually, patient may develop antibodies to minor red cell antigens and to platelet antigens so that transfusions no longer raise the counts sufficiently.
      (2) Multiple transfusions decrease chance for successful bone marrow transplantation.
2. Make the patient comfortable during febrile episodes.
   a. Acetaminophen (avoid aspirin, which interferes with platelet aggregation).
   b. Cooling blankets; tepid sponges; cool packs to axilla, groin.
3. Support the patient who is bleeding (in skin, nose, GI tract, genitourinary tract, lungs, optic fundi, brain).
   a. See page 237.
   b. Exercise care with IM injections—use thin needle, Z-track technique and pressure.
   c. Menses may be suppressed (androgens or contraceptive agents).
   d. Maintain effective oral hygiene.
4. Prepare patient for splenectomy if indicated—the spleen sequesters and accelerates the removal of red cells, white cells, and platelets; splenectomy may cause slight elevation of hemoglobin levels and decrease the transfusion requirements.

Discharge Planning and Health Education

Instruct the patient as follows:
1. Be aware of drugs that may damage the bone marrow.
2. When taking drugs that can produce blood dyscrasias (chloramphenicol, phenylbutazone, sulfonamides), have regular blood counts; however, aplastic anemia may develop after drug has been discontinued.
3. Prevent minor infections. Any abrasion or wound of mucous membranes or skin is a potential site of infection.
4. Report any infection, no matter how trivial.
5. Report any fever >37.8°C. (100°F.).

Evaluation
Expected Outcomes

1. Achieves remission of disease
2. Avoids infection
3. Manages bleeding episodes
4. Copes with uncertain outcome; talks about this to mental health professionals

---

Polycythemia Vera

Polycythemia vera (primary polycythemia) is a myeloproliferative disorder with hyperplasia of bone marrow resulting in increased numbers of circulating erythrocytes, granulocytes, and platelets. The underlying defect is unknown. It is a multiple organ system disease.

Altered Physiology

1. Increased blood volume because of increase in red cell mass
2. Increased supply of precursor cells

3. Hyperplasia of all bone marrow elements
4. Striking increase in total blood volume; gradually increasing blood viscosity
5. Decreased marrow iron
6. Enlargement of spleen

Clinical Course

1. Insidious and gradual onset—probably measured in years.
2. More frequent in males; most common during middle and later years of life.
3. Peptic ulcers are common in these patients; cerebral, gastrointestinal, and nasal hemorrhages may occur at any time during the course of the disease.
4. Acute leukemia may be a terminal complication of polycythemia vera; myelofibrosis (replacement of marrow with fibrotic tissue) may also occur.

Clinical Manifestations

(Clinical manifestations are referable to increased blood volume and viscosity from erythrocytosis [increased red cells].)
1. Plethoric appearance (reddish-purple hue of skin and mucosa)
2. Pruritus (worsens after bathing/showering)
3. Painful fingers and toes—from arterial and venous insufficiency
4. Bleeding tendency
5. Headache, dizziness, impaired mental ability, vertigo, visual abnormalities (scotomata; double or blurred vision)—from disturbed cerebral circulation
6. Splenomegaly, producing abdominal discomfort
7. Hepatomegaly
8. Hypertension
9. Hyperuricemia—from increased formation and destruction of erythrocytes and leukocytes and increased metabolism of nucleic acids
10. Weakness and easy fatigability

Diagnostic Evaluation

1. Increased red cell mass (measured by isotopic technique).
2. Thrombocytosis; often abnormal platelet aggregation
3. Leukocytosis (in majority of patients)
4. Elevated granulocyte alkaline phosphatase activity
5. Increased serum B_{12}
6. Normal PO_2 (used to differentiate primary from secondary polycythemia)

Management

(Optimal therapy is controversial.)
1. Phlebotomy (withdrawal of blood) to reduce red cell mass; frequency of phlebotomy determined by hematocrit

2. Myelosuppressive therapy
3. Allopurinol—to control hyperuricemia

Nursing Management

A. Symptomatic Relief of Discomfort

1. Assist with phlebotomy (venesection) to decrease blood volume and to reduce viscosity of blood by removal of the excessive numbers of red blood cells.
    a. 250–500 ml. of blood removed every other day until hematocrit reaches desired level.
    b. Repeated phlebotomies may be performed to lower hemoglobin, hematocrit, and red cell mass to normal ranges.
    c. Elderly persons with compromised cardiovascular systems are phlebotomized with caution!
2. Myelosuppressive therapy—radioactive phosphorus (^{32}P) either orally or intravenously—acts on hyperplastic bone marrow to suppress panmyelosis.
3. Administer allopurinol when necessary—to control hyperuricemia.
4. Support patient troubled with pruritus.
    a. May subside with myelosuppressive therapy.
    b. Antihistamine drugs such as cyproheptadine may give relief.

B. Prevention of Complications

1. Evaluate (and treat) complications—the clinical course of polycythemia is determined by the development of complications.
    a. Thromboembolic complications—due to hyperviscosity which leads to reduced blood flow and subsequent infarction.
        Includes deep vein thrombophlebitis, myocardial and cerebral infarction, and thrombotic occlusion of the splenic, hepatic, portal, and mesenteric veins.
    b. Hemorrhagic tendency—bleeding occurs spontaneously from increasing blood volume and capillary and venous distention. Platelets may also be qualitatively abnormal.
    c. Gout—from overproduction of uric acid (secondary to nucleoprotein turnover of marrow cells).
    d. Congestive failure—from increased blood volume and hypertension.
    e. Acute leukemia—may be a terminal complication.
2. Keep the patient ambulatory, since the likelihood of thrombosis increases when the patient is at bed rest.

Health Education

1. Report at prescribed intervals for follow-up blood (hematocrit) studies.
2. Avoid taking *hot* baths/showers—worsens pruritus.

The Leukemias

The *leukemias* are neoplastic disorders of the blood-forming tissues (spleen, lymphatic system, and bone marrow). The common features of the leukemias are an unregulated proliferation of white cells in the bone marrow with replacement of normal marrow elements. There may also be proliferation in the liver, spleen, and lymph nodes, and invasion of nonhematologic organs such as the meninges, gastrointestinal tract, kidney, and skin.

Classification

Classified according to:
1. The cell type involved (lymphocytic, granulocytic, or monocytic)

2. The maturity of malignant cells
    a. Acute (immature cells)
    b. Chronic (differentiated cells)

Predisposing Factors

Etiology unknown—several factors are associated with increase in incidence:
1. Exposure to radiation
2. Chemical agents—benzene
3. Infectious agents—viruses (currently being investigated)
4. Genetic abnormalities—increased risk of leukemia in patients with Down's syndrome (see p. 1474)
5. Chemotherapeutic agents — particularly alkylating agents
6. Myeloproliferative disorders — polycythemia vera, myelofibrosis (fibrosis of bone marrow)
7. Genetic influence—some families with incidence of leukemia

Acute Leukemia*

Acute leukemia is a rapidly progressive disease involving primitive cells (blasts) that proliferate at an uncontrolled rate. It may involve lymphocytic, granulocytic (myelocytic), or monocytic cell types. The clinical course of the acute leukemias is similar for all types.

Assessment

Clinical Manifestations

1. Easy fatigability and generalized malaise; pallor—secondary to anemia
2. Bleeding of gums, epistaxis, petechiae, prolonged bleeding following a surgical procedure—from thrombocytopenia (lowered platelet count)
3. Fever or infection—secondary to granulocytopenia
4. Enlarged lymph nodes and spleen; abdominal discomfort—from organ infiltration
5. Bone pain, arthralgia—from rapidly expanding marrow in bone
6. Tachycardia, weight loss, dyspnea on exertion, intolerance to heat—from increased metabolism
7. Leukemic infiltration of the skin—tendency for leukemic cells to infiltrate other organs and tissues
8. Cerebral hemorrhage, cranial nerve paralysis, increased intracranial pressure—from neurologic complications (leukemic cells frequently invade the central nervous system)
9. Pain—from infarction, particularly the spleen

▶ **NURSING ALERT:** Undiagnosed patients may appear in the emergency department for treatment of acute infections. Suspect leukemia.

Diagnostic Evaluation

1. Blood evaluation—total peripheral white count varies widely (1,000–100,000/cu. ml.)
2. Bone marrow examination—characteristically large percentage of bone marrow's nucleated cells are immature leukocyte forms called "blasts"
3. Lymph node biopsy
4. Chest x-ray—to detect mediastinal node and lung involvement
5. Skeletal x-ray—to detect skeletal lesions

* For discussion of acute leukemia in children, see page 1457.

Patient Problems/Nursing Diagnoses

1. Fatigue, nausea, constipation, discomfort, related to chemotherapy
2. Ineffective individual coping related to toxicity encountered during chemotherapy
3. Potential development of infection related to granulocytopenia and mucosal damage
4. Bleeding tendencies related to thrombocytopenia from leukemia and chemotherapy
5. Pain related to proliferation of leukemia cells and enlargement of abdominal organs
6. Fear related to the prognosis of the disease

Management

1. The therapy for leukemia causes severe bone marrow suppression. Failure to improve is usually due to complications—infection and hemorrhage.
2. Initial treatment in a specially equipped medical facility that treats patients with leukemia with a multidisciplinary team approach gives the best promise for prolonged remission.

A. Chemotherapy

1. The drugs are classified on the basis of their effects on cell chemistry. (See p. 908 for complete list of drugs used in cancer chemotherapy.)
2. Goal of chemotherapy—to induce remission (disappearance of all abnormal cell forms in the bone marrow and peripheral blood).

B. Underlying Principles of Chemotherapy

1. Chemotherapy inhibits growth of leukemic cells by destroying or inactivating nucleic acids or by interfering with their synthesis; causes bone marrow depression and depresses the patient's immunologic defense mechanism.
2. Drugs are usually given in combination (exert different biological effects) at high dose levels to produce greater leukemic cell damage.
3. The treatment regimen is designed to affect cells in different phases of the mitotic cycle.
4. Commonly, there is intensive treatment with multiple agents at the beginning of therapy (induction) to induce a remission, followed by long-term continuation (maintenance) therapy. No one regimen produces successful responses in all patients.
5. The drugs used to treat leukemia produce major toxicity to the hematopoietic system, resulting in prolonged periods of pancytopenia.
6. The nursing management of the patient with acute leukemia includes constant assessment of the patient for effects of drug toxicity.

C. Drugs Used for Acute Lymphocytic Leukemia

1. Combinations of vincristine, prednisone, daunorubicin, and L-asparaginase are used during the induction phase. Maintenance therapy employs combinations of 6-mercaptopurine, methotrexate, vincristine, and prednisone.

D. Drugs Used for Acute Nonlymphocytic Leukemias*

1. Combinations of daunorubicin, cystosine arabinoside, and 6-thioguanine are used for induction therapy. Unlike the situation with acute lymphocytic leukemia,

* Acute nonlymphocytic leukemias include acute myelocytic, myelomonocytic, monocytic, progranulocytic and erythroleukemia.

in nonlymphocytic leukemia, maintenance therapy is not helpful in prolonging remission.

2. Patients should be given allopurinol, increased amounts of fluids, and urinary alkalinization for hyperuricemia, which occurs as a result of drug-induced cell breakdown.

E. Bone Marrow Transplantation (see p. 273, marrow transplantation)

1. High-dose chemotherapy and total body irradiation given first to destroy all residual leukemic cells.
2. The patient is then given intravenous infusion of allogeneic bone marrow.
3. The patient requires excellent supportive nursing care during the 3 weeks following bone marrow transplantation, since he is unable to make WBCs, RBCs, or platelets: he is transfusion-dependent and susceptible to overwhelming opportunistic infection.

F. Vascular Access

Hickman catheter may be implanted intravenously to facilitate vascular access for chemotherapy, multiple blood sampling and antibiotic administration.

G. Cranial Irradiation—followed by intrathecal methotrexate (given by lumbar puncture into the subdural space) to destroy meningeal foci of leukemic cells. This is most commonly performed as part of induction therapy for lymphocytic leukemia.

Planning and Implementation
Nursing Interventions

A. Administration of Chemotherapy

1. Obtain baseline information before chemotherapy is started.
   a. Know the patient's "normal" TPR and BP.
   b. Follow the WBC, differential count, hemoglobin measurements, platelet counts—to be aware of the drug's effect on the body.
   c. Follow blood chemistry studies, electrolytes, urea nitrogen, creatinine, liver enzymes, bilirubin.
   d. Weigh the patient daily.
   e. Assist with bone marrow aspirations as directed (see p. 242).
2. Watch for toxic manifestations during chemotherapy.
   a. Modifications of the patient's chemotherapy regimen are based on laboratory and physical examinations before each course of treatment.
   b. Monitor intravenous infusion of drugs (see p. 905)—may cause local irritation in the veins; the patient may complain of burning sensations during infusions of methotrexate and prednisone.
      (1) Adjust infusion flow to a slower rate.
      (2) Change position of extremity to prevent muscle cramping.
      (3) The patient may complain of nausea, vomiting, and burning sensation along the gastrointestinal tract during or immediately after drug infusion.
      (4) Certain agents such as daunorubicin, mitomycin, and vincristine are "sclerosing" agents and cause extensive tissue damage and necrosis if infiltrated into subcutaneous spaces. These drugs should be given only by a physician or a specially trained oncology nurse.
   c. Watch for mouth ulcers—frequently occur when the patient is taking methotrexate. Offer medicated mouth rinses frequently to relieve oral discomfort.
   d. Expect the patient to experience loss of hair during antileukemic treatment—alopecia occurs in high percentage of patients receiving daunorubicin. Encourage the patient to experiment with wigs, hair pieces, head scarves.
   e. Check deep tendon reflexes. Assess patient for footdrop, weakening hand grasp, ptosis of eyelids—vincristine may cause neuropathy.
   f. Assess for constipation and abdominal pain—vincristine may produce adynamic ileus.
   g. Watch for personality changes, fluid retention, hypertension, gastric ulcers, and diabetes mellitus—occur with prednisone therapy.
   h. Watch for other drug side effects—diarrhea, maculopapular rash, stomatitis, phlebitis, bone marrow depression, evidences of cardiac toxicity (tachycardia, arrhythmias, tachypnea, dyspnea).
   i. Take ECG readings as prescribed—cardiac toxicity is associated with certain chemotherapeutic agents.
   j. See page 905 for nursing management of the patient undergoing chemotherapy.
3. Encourage patient to endure discomfort associated with the treatment.

B. Prevention of Infection

1. Prevent and treat infection, which is the major morbidity and mortality factor associated with leukemia.
2. Monitor for *temperature elevation,* flushed appearance, chills, tachycardia, appearance of white patches in mouth, redness, swelling, heat or pain of eyes, ears, throat, skin, joints, abdomen, rectal and perineal areas; cough; changes in character and/or color of sputum, stool; skin rash.

   Remember that the usual manifestations of infection are altered in patients with leukemia. Prednisone may blunt the normal febrile response to infection.
3. Monitor the concentration of circulating granulocytes. Concentrations under $500/\mu l$ make the patient at serious risk of infection.
4. *Avoid mucosal and epithelial damage.*
   a. Avoid venipuncture, subcutaneous, and intramuscular injections unless absolutely necessary.
      (1) Wash hands.
      (2) Provide daily IV site care.
      (3) Change cannula according to protocol of hospital.
   b. Avoid urinary catheterization if possible. See page 505 for nursing interventions for patient requiring catheterization.
   c. Avoid the use of vaginal tampons; use sanitary napkins.
   d. Avoid constipation by use of stool softeners, etc.—mucosal damage may develop by force of bowel movements pushing bacteria into damaged cells.
   e. Avoid rectal thermometers—perianal cellulitis and perirectal abscess are common complications.
5. Prevent infectious complications by control of environmental contamination.
   a. Use careful handwashing techniques before and after every patient contact.
   b. Instruct patient to make sure that each individual

washes his hands before coming into contact with him (e.g., handwash in his presence).

c. Use intensive environmental cleaning procedures; double-bucket mopping; daily disinfecting of sink, toilet, horizontal surfaces in room, etc.

d. Use ice that falls out of machine into container (without coming into hand contact), since ice is a source of contamination.

e. Consider a laminar air flow room (a unidirectional air flow "barrier" that establishes an air environment in which the infection-prone patient is free from contact with exogenous microorganisms) for the patient with greatly reduced granulocyte count.

6. Employ meticulous personal hygiene measures.

a. Inspect all body sites that are at high risk for infection daily: orifices; perianal area; axilla and groin; IV sites; wounds.

b. Bathe the patient daily.

c. Wash perineum from front to back following defecation (males and females); women should wash after urination.

d. Establish and maintain oral hygiene regimen.

7. Treat infection promptly as directed.

a. Obtain cultures (for both aerobes and anaerobes) of blood, urine, sputum, spinal fluid.

b. Obtain serial chest x-ray.

c. Broad-spectrum antimicrobials are usually given until organism is identified; oral nonabsorbable antibiotic regimens may be given to prevent enteric colonization and systemic infection.

d. Watch for development of fungal infection (especially *Candida* and *Aspergillus*)—from indwelling catheters, immunosuppressive effects of chemotherapy, bacterial suppression by antimicrobials, and decreased resistance of patient.

e. Granulocyte transfusions may be of benefit.

C. Prevention or Management of Bleeding Episodes

1. Assess the patient for signs of bleeding:

a. Monitor platelet count daily; major cause of hemorrhage is thrombocytopenia (decrease in platelets).

b. Minor bleeding—petechiae, ecchymoses, conjunctival hemorrhage, epistaxis, bleeding gums; guaiac-positive emesis and stools; heme-positive urine, bleeding at puncture sites, vaginal spotting.

c. Serious bleeding—headache; change in responsiveness; blurred vision; hemoptysis; hematemesis; melena; hypotension with tachycardia; dizziness.

d. Check the mouth and nose for bleeding; monitor urine, feces and emesis for occult bleeding.

e. Monitor pad count/amount of saturation during menses.

2. Support the patient receiving blood component therapy; transfusion requirements depend on the type of leukemia, stage of the disease, and the intensity of chemotherapy (see Transfusion Therapy, p. 263).

3. Teach the patient to remain at rest during active bleeding episodes—helps to lower pulse rate and blood pressure and promotes clot formation.

4. Control bleeding—keep injections to a minimum; take blood samples and give analgesics through Hickman catheter.

5. Nose and mouth bleeding

a. Apply firm pressure to bridge of nose.

b. Avoid tilting the head back (blood draining down throat will be swallowed; resultant nausea and emesis will exacerbate bleeding).

c. Apply ice compresses to bridge of nose.

d. Apply vasoconstricting agents as directed.

6. Gastrointestinal bleeding—see page 419.

7. Intracranial bleeding

a. See page 763 for assessment.

b. Avoid the Valsalva maneuver or activity that increases intracranial pressure.

D. Relief of Pain and Discomfort

1. Control the pain and discomfort.

a. Use milder analgesics when possible; change to a stronger narcotic as the patient's condition requires.

b. Give tranquilizers as directed to enhance the effects of narcotics.

c. Give antiemetic medication before meals—to help assuage the patient's nausea; sedatives may also be helpful.

2. Maintain oral intake between 3 and 4 liters daily—to prevent precipitation of uric acid crystals in the urine.

3. Control fever—employ cool sponges, increased fluid intake, antipyretic drugs.

4. Give frequent and special mouth care—to remove dried blood, combat odor, and soothe oral ulcerations.

a. Reduce the number of commensal organisms in mouth by:

(1) Prophylactic dental visits for regular removal of plaque and mucus.

(2) Regular toothbrushing (with small automatic toothbrush) except in presence of gross gingival hypertrophy with associated pain and bleeding; use Water Pic® on low setting.

(3) Use of mouthwashes (with sodium perborate, hydrogen peroxide, sodium bicarbonate)—effervescent action helps remove detritus and inspissated mucus from teeth, dentures, and ulcers.

(4) Use of analgesic mouthwash for patients with painful gingival problems.

b. Watch for development of candidiasis and infective processes of the mouth—from corticosteroids and some antibiotics.

E. Promotion of Coping Mechanisms to Deal with Physiologic and Emotional Distress

1. Assist the patient to understand that the range of feelings about leukemia is normal—may help patient gain control.

a. The patient may react with shock and anger when disease is first recognized; anger may be directed at health-care personnel.

b. Anger is a defense mechanism; patient realizes that death is inevitable; anger is also a defense against anxiety.

c. Develop ability to accept and deal with this anger—important for establishing a therapeutic patient-nurse relationship.

d. Allow patient and family to ventilate their emotions.

e. Patient may use mechanism of denial—denial may need to be supported or worked through.

2. Use support group (American Cancer Society) to help diffuse anger and dependency and to provide support and education.

Health Education

1. Avoid possible sources of infection—crowds, unnecessary hospital visits, etc.
    a. Employ good, frequent handwashing practices.
    b. Report any sign of infection to physician/clinic promptly.
    c. Report any exposure to varicella, measles, hepatitis, etc.
2. Pay careful attention to nutrition—undernourished person does not tolerate antileukemic drugs as well as well-nourished individual.
3. Follow instructions on proper Hickman catheter care, including daily heparin-flushes.
4. Monitor weight to be certain a significant amount of weight is not lost.
5. See your dentist—oral disease is frequently present; request dentist to contact your physician before initiating dental examination.
6. Avoid rectal mucosal trauma by preventing constipation; use stool softeners, increase fluid intake, high-fiber foods; wash perineum with soap and water after each elimination.
7. Shower/bathe daily, paying attention to axillae, skin folds, groin, and perineum. Use an electric shaver.
8. Use a deodorant rather than an antiperspirant (antiperspirant blocks sweat glands and may cause infection).
9. Practice oral hygiene after each meal.
10. Watch for signs of bleeding—avoid use of sharp objects, straining at stool, forceful nose blowing, products containing aspirin.
11. Use birth control pills as directed to prevent breakthrough bleeding.
12. Remember that leukemia is a treatable disease, and that advances in treatment are continually being made; most side effects of antileukemic drugs are short-term and treatable.

Evaluation

Expected Outcomes

1. Copes with chemotherapy; reports for treatments
2. Remains free of infection and infectious complications
3. Shows no evidence of bleeding; manages bleeding episodes when present
4. Achieves relief of pain/discomfort
5. Copes with distress; adjusts to new body image (hair loss, skin discoloration, indwelling Hickman catheter); uses support groups; verbalizes feelings and concerns

Chronic Lymphocytic Leukemia

Chronic lymphocytic leukemia (CLL) is a type of leukemia characterized by a marked increase in mature lymphocytes in the circulation and in the lymphoid organs of the body.

Clinical Manifestations

1. Insidious onset affecting older populations (mean age greater than 60 years); the disease may run a protracted, relatively asymptomatic course over a number of years.
2. Symptoms and signs are related to infiltration of lymph nodes, bone marrow, liver, and spleen with lymphocytes.
    a. Gradual appearance of generalized lymph node enlargement—cervical region, axillae, groin; splenomegaly (may be painful)
    b. Anemia, thrombocytopenia—may be due to bone marrow infiltration, to immune destruction, or to hypersplenism
    c. Weight loss, fever, enhanced susceptibility to infection

Laboratory Evaluation

1. White blood cells may be in excess of 100,000/cu. mm. of blood; small, mature lymphocytes may comprise 90%–99% of cells.
2. Decrease in erythrocyte, granulocyte, and platelet counts are common.

Management

A. **Asymptomatic Patient with Chronic Lymphocytic Leukemia**

1. May not require treatment for a period of years.
2. Support the patient with optimal nutrition, rest, exercise, recreation, and mental activity.

B. **Symptomatic Patient** (with Massive Adenopathy, Severe Anemia, Thrombocytopenia, Skin Involvement, Recurring Infections)

1. Chemotherapy—brings symptomatic relief; decreases size of lymph nodes and spleen.
    a. Single-agent therapy—chlorambucil (Leukeran)
    b. Combination drug therapy (3- or 4-drug regimen) may be given to patients with poorly differentiated lymphocytes who are unresponsive to a single chemotherapeutic agent—reduces white blood cell count; improves constitutional symptoms
2. Radiation therapy
    a. To obtain cosmetic control of local disease
    b. To reduce size and relieve symptoms of splenomegaly
3. Corticosteroids (prednisone)—are lymphocytic and helpful in controlling autoimmune complications.
4. Transfusion therapy—red cells and/or platelet concentrates as indicated by symptoms and counts.
5. Splenectomy — occasionally done for refractory thrombocytopenia.
6. See page 905 for nursing support of patient receiving chemotherapy and page 251 for other aspects of management of a patient with leukemia.

Chronic Granulocytic Leukemia

Chronic granulocytic (myelocytic, myelogenous) leukemia is a chronic condition characterized by an increased proliferation of myeloid elements, including granulocytes, monocytes, platelets, and occasionally red cells. It is often associated with great enlargement of the spleen and liver. The condition may also occur in an acute or accelerated form.

Clinical Features

1. Appears most often between ages 35 and 50, and 60 and 70.
2. Gradual, insidious onset; the disease runs a progressive course over several years.
3. The Philadelphia chromosome is present in cells of bone marrow origin in over 90% of patients.

Clinical Manifestations

1. Pallor, palpitations, dyspnea—from anemia
2. Dragging sensation or enlargement of left side of abdomen—from splenic enlargement
3. Hematologic features: elevated platelet count, elevated granulocyte count; blood smear shows predominance of granulocytes at all stages of maturation
4. Weakness, loss of weight, loss of appetite—from increased metabolic rate due to high granulocyte turnover and anorexia from splenomegaly
5. Tenderness and pain in long bones (particularly tibia, ribs, lower part of sternum)—due to invasion by abnormal marrow
6. Thrombocytosis—manifested clinically as thromboembolic or hemorrhagic phenomena

Laboratory Evaluation

1. Elevated leukocyte count
2. Low leukocyte alkaline phosphatase
3. Demonstration of Philadelphia chromosome in bone marrow cells

Treatment

1. Chemotherapy—treatment with cytotoxic drugs usually will reduce size of spleen, restore leukocyte count to normal, and alleviate symptoms.
   a. Busulfan (Myleran)—will induce a complete or partial remission in majority of patients.
      (1) Following initial treatment, the patient may be placed on long-term, low-dose maintenance therapy. This is known as the chronic phase of the disease. Second-line drugs or more aggressive multi-drug combinations may be used if disease enters an accelerated phase.
      (2) Hydroxyurea—is often given to control myeloproliferative acceleration when the patient becomes relatively resistant to busulfan and other effective therapy.
      (3) Eventually, the patient will no longer respond; the acute exacerbation phase is termed myeloblastic or "blast" crisis, which is refractory to treatment and is a terminal phase. The patient is then treated as for acute leukemia (see p. 250).
         (a) Patient experiences fever and bone pain; spleen enlarges and becomes painful.
         (b) Lymphadenopathy and osteolytic lesions in bone may respond to local irradiation.
2. Bone marrow transplantation may be attempted during the chronic or early accelerated phase if suitable donor can be found.
3. Leukapheresis (removal of white blood cells from whole blood; red blood cells transfused back into patient) may be used for the patient who needs white blood cell count reduced rapidly.
4. See page 905 for nursing support of the patient receiving chemotherapy.
5. See page 251 for other aspects of management of a patient with leukemia.

Malignant Lymphomas

The *lymphomas* are a group of neoplastic diseases of the lymphoreticular system and include Hodgkin's disease and the non-Hodgkin's lymphomas.

1. Lymphomas are classified both according to the predominant malignant cell type—as lymphocytic lymphomas, histiocytic lymphomas, or Hodgkin's disease—as well as by degree of malignant cell differentiation—well-differentiated, poorly differentiated, or undifferentiated.
2. These tumors usually start in lymph nodes, but can involve any lymphoid tissue in the spleen, gastrointestinal tract (tonsils, walls of stomach), liver, or bone marrow.
3. They may spread to all these areas and to extralymphatic tissues (lungs, kidneys, skin).
4. The etiology of these diseases is unknown.

Hodgkin's Disease

Hodgkin's disease is a malignant disease of unknown etiology that originates in the lymphoid system and involves predominantly the lymph nodes. It may occur in nearly any lymphoid tissue: spleen, bone marrow, liver.

Altered Physiology

1. The malignant cell of Hodgkin's disease is the "Reed–Sternberg" cell, which is a gigantic, atypical tumor cell, morphologically unique and of uncertain lineage.
2. The different histopathologic types of Hodgkin's disease are associated with varying prognoses.
3. Hodgkin's disease shows a highly predictable pattern of spread—usually via the lymphatic channels from one chain of lymph nodes to another, often to the spleen, and ultimately to extralymphatic sites.
4. Hodgkin's disease may also have a hematogenous mode of spread as extra nodal sites involved include the gastrointestinal tract, bone marrow, skin, upper air passages, and other organs.

Clinical Manifestations

1. Painless enlargement of lymph nodes (usually on one side of neck)
2. Slight to high fever; chills, night sweats, weight loss
3. Pruritus (itching), (either local or generalized)
4. Progressive anemia
5. Enlargement of lymph nodes in other regions of the body
6. Enlargement of mediastinal and retroperitoneal lymph nodes producing pressure symptoms
   a. Dyspnea from pressure against the trachea
   b. Dysphagia from pressure against the esophagus
   c. Laryngeal paralysis due to pressure against the recurrent laryngeal nerve
   d. Brachial, lumbar, or sacral neuralgias due to pressure on the nerve
   e. Edema of the extremities due to pressure on the veins
   f. Enlargement of spleen and liver

7. Effusions into the pleura or peritoneum
8. Obstructive jaundice—from pressure on the bile duct

Diagnostic Evaluation

The extent of the disease is determined before treatment.
1. Biopsy of lymph node(s) to identify characteristic histologic features
2. Complete blood count
3. Chest x-ray and tomography—to detect mediastinal, hilar, or intrapulmonary disease
4. Computed tomography—to determine precise location of nodal involvement; used in treatment planning and follow-up
5. Bone marrow biopsy
6. Liver function tests and scan
7. Lymphangiogram
   a. Reveals size of lymph nodes
   b. Detects abdominal lymph node involvement, which may not be seen on tomography
8. Surgical staging (laparotomy with splenectomy, liver biopsy, multiple lymph node biopsies)—to identify disease in the spleen and lymph nodes below the diaphragm and to guide decisions regarding therapy

Patient Problems/Nursing Diagnoses

1. Discomfort related to lymph node enlargement, fever, and itching
2. Potential for fever
3. Alteration in breathing patterns related to tracheal pressure
4. Alteration in nutrition related to dysphagia
5. Potential nonadherence to treatment program related to side effects and length of therapy

Management

A. Depends on Stage, Symptoms, and Cell Type

Radiotherapy and combination chemotherapy are the two primary therapeutic modalities.

1. Radiotherapy (delivery of a lethal dose of ionizing radiation to tumor cells) is the first choice of treatment in early Hodgkin's disease; potentially curable by radiotherapy. An important factor in treatment is the radiation dose administered.
2. Hodgkin's disease may be eradicated from any site that has received 4,000–4,400 rads within the space of 4 weeks. Megavoltage radiation techniques permit the delivery of such a dose to one or more entire lymph node chains.
3. Areas of the body in which the lymph node chains are located can tolerate doses of this magnitude without serious damage.
   a. Males may wish to consider sperm banking before beginning therapy, since sterility is a complication. Females may wish to undergo oophoropexy (surgical placement of ovaries outside the radiation field).
   b. Vital structures such as the heart, lungs, liver, kidney, and bone marrow are protected by lead shields.
4. Radiotherapy usually given daily over a period of weeks.
5. Complications of intensive radiotherapy
   a. Radiation pneumonitis and fibrosis; pericarditis; nephritis, myelitis, prolonged myelosuppression; hypothyroidism, and sterility.
   b. Acute reactions to irradiation—dryness of mouth; loss of taste; dysphagia; nausea and vomiting; apathy and lassitude; skin redness, dry peeling

in treatment fields; loss of hair at back of neck and under areas treated; reduction of white blood cells.

B. Treatment of Patients with Localized or Systemic Disease Plus Constitutional Symptoms

1. Combination chemotherapy—many chemotherapy strategies in current use. The response rate varies.
   a. Nitrogen mustard, vincristine, procarbazine, and prednisone (MOPP).
      Many programs modify the MOPP combination with deletion of an agent, substitution of one or more drugs with agents from the same class or new agents effective for Hodgkin's disease.
   b. Adriamycin, bleomycin, vinblastine, decarbazine (ABVD).
2. Three or four drugs may be given in intermittent or cyclical courses with periods off therapy to allow recovery of normal tissues.
   a. Toxic effects of these drugs often overlap, especially bone marrow depression.
   b. Late complications: cardiotoxicity, lung fibrosis, infertility, second neoplasms, avascular necrosis of bone.
3. Combination chemotherapy in addition to extended field radiation may be used.

Planning and Implementation
Nursing Interventions

1. Help the patient cope with unpleasant side effects of radiation.
   a. Esophagitis—bland soft foods at mild temperatures, aspirin gum (use moderately), anesthetic lozenges, pain medication before eating if patient unable to eat.
   b. Loss of taste—serve palatable meals.
   c. Anorexia—encourage patient to make the effort to eat.
   d. Nausea and vomiting—antiemetics given to cover peak time of nausea.
   e. Diarrhea—antidiarrheal medication.
   f. Skin reaction (sunburned/tanned appearance of treatment area)—avoid rubbing, heat, cold, application of lotions.
   g. Lethargy—rest/sleep to keep energy level up; diversional activities to prevent boredom.
   h. Tingling with numbness in hands, toes; weakness in knees, hands—use a cane for stability.
2. Support the patient having toxic effects from chemotherapy.
   a. Encourage the patient by saying that the therapy will end in "a period of time"—serves as an incentive for the patient to continue with therapy. Emphasize high likelihood of cure.
   b. Give stool softeners to control constipation that accompanies chemotherapy, or place on a bowel-conditioning program (see p. 70). Offer high fiber foods (bran) to maintain intestinal tone.
   c. Anticipate that patients on chemotherapy will develop leukopenia, thrombocytopenia, and anemia.
   d. See page 905 for nursing management of patient undergoing chemotherapy.
3. Prepare the patient for surgical staging (laparotomy). Surgery may also be used to alleviate complications caused by pressure or obstruction due to tumor masses.

▶ **NURSING ALERT:** There is an apparent increase in second malignancies (primarily leukemia) of patients who are long-term survivors of Hodgkin's disease, especially in those who have received combination chemotherapy as well as radiation therapy.

Health Education

The control of the disease requires continuing observation by the patient.
1. Report fever or any sign of infection (skin redness, tenderness, lesions, cough) immediately, since the disease and its treatment make one susceptible to infection.

    Herpes zoster occurs frequently; may become generalized in immunosuppressed patients.
2. Use humidifier/throat lozenges for dry throat and to control desire to cough.
3. Express feelings and anxieties; seek supportive persons and groups.
    a. Depression and fear are normal reactions to diagnosis, treatment, and stress of uncertain outcome.
    b. Expect to feel fatigued up to a year after therapy.
    c. Remain active and employed (if possible); seek to enjoy the present.
4. Expect some degree of hair loss if taking vincristine or nitrogen mustard; almost always reversible after therapy is completed.
5. Avoid taking alcohol, narcotics, antihistamines, tranquilizers, or sympathomimetic agents when taking procarbazine.
6. Report for follow-up.

Evaluation
Expected Outcomes
1. Is free of symptoms
2. Adheres to therapeutic program
3. Achieves a cure/remission

Non-Hodgkin's Lymphomas

Non-Hodgkin's lymphomas are a group of lymphoid malignancies in which the most frequent presenting manifestations are enlarged lymph nodes and splenomegaly. Dissemination to other organs (liver, gastrointestinal system, CNS, lungs) is common. Marrow damage, manifested by anemia and thrombocytopenia, and immune dysfunction, with heightened susceptibility to bacterial and mycotic infections, are also evident in these patients.

Clinical Manifestations
1. Prominent generalized lymphadenopathy
2. Fatigue—attributable primarily to anemia from impaired erythropoiesis and, rarely, hemolysis
3. Malaise, anorexia, weight loss
4. Fever and sweating
5. Abdominal distention—due to enlargement of spleen
6. Respiratory symptoms—from lymphoma involving the mediastinum, pulmonary parenchyma, pleura
7. Gastrointestinal symptoms (abdominal pain, intestinal obstruction, diarrhea)—from extranodal involvement

Diagnostic Evaluation
1. Biopsy of lymph node
2. Blood tests; bone marrow aspirate and biopsy.
3. Liver and renal function tests
4. Computed tomography of the abdomen, if indicated
5. Laparotomy—for staging

Treatment and Nursing Interventions
1. The treatment approach depends on the stage of the disease and histopathologic classification. Many of these patients have disseminated disease at the time of diagnosis.
    a. Surgery—for staging laparotomy and for diagnosis of suspicious lesions.
    b. Radiation therapy (may be curative in localized disease) (see p. 912).
    c. Chemotherapy—for the patient with widespread disease. Multi-agent approach using cyclophosphamide, vincristine, doxorubicin, bleomycin, and prednisone as standard first-line agents. Methotrexate, cytarabine hydrochloride, and procarbazine also effective.
2. Be constantly vigilant for complications.
    a. Infection—by bacteria, viruses, fungi; due to deficiencies of cellular immunity.
    b. Anemia—from bone marrow invasion, hemorrhage, chemotherapy, hypersplenism, hemolysis.
    c. Spinal cord compression—from lymphomatous meningitis.
    d. Hyperuricemia.
3. See also discussion of the care of patients with Hodgkin's disease (see above).

Mycosis Fungoides
(Cutaneous T-cell Lymphoma)

Mycosis fungoides is a T-cell lymphoma that often begins in the skin and frequently involves the lymph nodes and internal organs.

The term "mycosis fungoides" describes the mushroom-like appearance of the skin tumors. The late stage of the disease closely resembles malignant lymphoma.

Assessment
Clinical Manifestations
1. Generalized severe itching—may last for several years
2. Erythematous, urticarial, eczematous, or psoriasis-like lesions—there are exacerbations and remissions of these eruptions
3. Ulcerating crusting and necrotic tumors of the skin—lesions become indurated and more fungoidal until they are mushroom-like growths (scarlet or purplish in color), varying in size from 1–5 cm.; the body may be covered with these lesions
4. Once the disease involves extracutaneous sites (nodes, liver, spleen), there is usually a progressively downward course

Diagnostic Evaluation
1. Biopsy of skin lesion—gives distinctive diagnostic pattern of mycosis fungoides
2. Biopsies of lymph nodes, bone marrow, liver
3. Liver scan

Patient Problem/Nursing Diagnosis
1. Alteration in comfort (generalized itching, burning in affected areas of skin, pain) related to lymphomatous skin lesions
2. Ineffective coping related to body image problems and general discomforts of the disease

Management
(Selection of treatment is based on clinical staging.)
1. Topical (local) therapy used for cutaneous manifestations.

a. Nitrogen mustard used as topical therapy—effective in certain stages of the disease—allergic dermatitis may develop as a response to mustard.

b. Other agents used include topical corticosteroids (under plastic occlusive dressings).

2. Radiation therapy (electron beam therapy, ultraviolet light, photochemotherapy with Psoralen, and Long-wave ultraviolet light [PUVA]).

3. Systemic chemotherapy—used when visceral involvement is suspected, when skin tolerance limits further radiation therapy, or other methods fail to control the disease.

a. A combination of topical therapy, radiotherapy, and systemic therapy may be used.

b. Antimetabolites, cytotoxic antibiotics, alkylating agents and corticosteroids may be used.

Planning and Implementation
Nursing Interventions

A. Relief of Discomfort

1. Support the patient who has painful open weeping lesions.

a. See care of burn patient, page 634.

b. Line pajamas and bed linens with Telfa®—to absorb drainage and prevent bedding from adhering to skin.

c. Give analgesics for discomfort.

d. Handle the patient with care.

(1) Give the patient time to move slowly.

(2) Use 2 health care personnel to lift and turn the patient.

(3) Use distraction techniques when nursing care causes pain.

(4) Watch for development of contractures and pressure sores.

e. Keep up nutritional status, since the patient loses protein and fluid from body surface.

2. Assist the patient to cope with foul odor from bacterial growth in lesions.

a. Wash hands before and after patient contact to reduce bacterial spread.

b. Continue with excellent skin care to keep bacterial levels low.

c. Use whirlpool therapy to aid in skin cleansing and debridement.

d. Apply prescribed topical cream—as prophylaxis against infection and to promote comfort by excluding air from exposed nerve endings.

3. Monitor for evidences of infection, which is the major cause of death.

4. See page 255 for discussion of the nursing management of the patient with Hodgkin's disease and page 622 for management of exfoliative dermatitis.

Health Education

1. Emphasize the importance of personal hygiene and skin care.

a. Daily bathing with a mild superfatted soap and medicated bath oil.

b. Application of prescribed creams/ointments.

2. Discuss modifications that may need to be made in life-style (role changes, sexual relations); psychotherapy may be helpful, especially for patient in terminal phase of illness.

3. Avoid using perfumes and after-shave lotion.

4. Wear nonrestrictive cotton clothing.

5. Report to the physician any flare-up in skin condition, fever, signs and symptoms of systemic illness; hospitalization is usually necessary.

Evaluation
Expected Outcomes

1. Gains some relief from pain and discomfort

2. Demonstrates coping ability in relation to body image

Multiple Myeloma

Multiple myeloma (plasma cell myeloma; plasmacytoma; myelomatosis) is a malignant disease of the plasma cell that infiltrates bone and soft tissues. The cause is not known. It is a disease of older people and is not classified as a lymphoma.

Altered Physiology

1. The malignant cell is the plasma cell; a widespread proliferation of immature plasma cells takes place in the bone marrow throughout the skeleton.

2. The bones most commonly affected are the vertebrae, skull, ribs, sternum, pelvis, upper ends of humerus. In later stages, the liver, spleen, and kidneys may become involved.

3. Plasma cells are derived from B-lymphocytes and normally produce physiologic levels of immunoglobulins. Malignant plasma cells produce abnormal amounts of an immunoglobulin or parts of an immunoglobulin protein (Bence Jones protein) that can usually be detected in the serum and in urine by immunoelectrophoresis.

4. There is a constant threat of hypercalcemia and hyperuricemia because of osteoclast activation by the myeloma cells, leading to bone resorption and skeletal destruction.

5. Increased loss of bone substance leads to collapse of vertebral bodies and pathologic or spontaneous fractures in areas of cortical thinning.

Assessment
Clinical Manifestations

1. Constant severe bone pain, especially on movement.

a. Low back pain—the most characteristic symptom

b. Lytic skeletal lesions—producing swelling, tenderness, pain, and *pathologic fractures*

2. Anemia—due to malignancy and/or replacement of marrow with myeloma cells. May be associated with thrombocytopenia and granulocytopenia—causes increased susceptibility to infection and abnormal bleeding.

3. Marked weight loss.

4. Symptoms of renal failure—may be due to precipitation of the immunoglobulin in the tubules or to pyelonephritis, hypercalciuria, increased uric acid, infiltration of the kidney with plasma cells (myeloma kidney), renal vein thrombosis.

5. Nausea, vomiting, constipation, lethargy (late stage)—these are symptoms of marked hypercalcemia.

Diagnostic Evaluation

1. Bone marrow aspiration and biopsy—should show increased numbers of plasma cells.
2. Malignant plasma cells produce abnormal globulins, which appear in serum electrophoresis as a monoclonal paraprotein "spike"—fragments of these globulins are excreted in urine as Bence Jones proteins.
3. Numerous osteolytic bone lesions may appear on x-ray; generalized demineralization of skeleton (osteoporosis) is also common.
4. Radioactive technetium bone scans—involved areas show increased uptake of technetium.

Patient Problems/Nursing Diagnoses

1. Bone pain related to bone erosion and possible pathologic fractures
2. Potential for complications related to plasma cell proliferation
3. Fatigue related to anemia
4. Weight loss related to disease process
5. Potential for injury related to frailty of bones
6. Coping difficulties related to change in life-style and body image

Management

1. Chemotherapy—to suppress plasma cell growth. Melphalan or cyclophosphamide given as single agents or combined with prednisone and other agents in a variety of schedules.
2. Radiation therapy—very helpful in palliating bone pain associated with lytic lesions and pathologic fractures.
3. Treatment of concomitant anemia related to tumor burden of myeloma cells.
   a. Packed red cell transfusions for patients with severe anemia.
   b. Chemotherapy may be administered to decrease degree of marrow infiltration; may improve anemia.

Planning and Implementation
Nursing Interventions

A. Relief of Bone Pain

1. Keep the patient ambulatory and avoid immobilization unless lesions in spine (extradural plasmacytomas) produce danger of cord compression; ambulation prevents further bone resorption and hypercalcemia.
   a. Allow the patient to set own pace.
   b. Use walker and assistive devices to keep the patient active.
   c. Determine methods to conserve energy; note these on patient's care plan.
2. Control pain.
   a. Avoid excessive lifting and straining. Handle the patient with smooth, unhurried movements.
   b. Try to *prevent* pain.
      (1) Administer pain-relieving medication at a scheduled time around the clock until pain control is attained.
      (2) Oral narcotic mixture—methadone or morphine, cocaine, alcohol with an antiemetic and flavorings (or other combinations) can be used to lower sensory dimension of pain and diminish fear.

(3) Assess the effectiveness of pain intervention in order to decrease dosage or change medication until pain relief is achieved without sedation.
(4) Radiation therapy to focal lesions, splinting, back brace, relaxation techniques—are other measures used for pain.

B. Prevention and Management of Complications

1. Assess the patient for signs and symptoms of renal insufficiency—abnormal proteins may exert a nephrotoxic effect at tubular level; or renal failure may develop from pyelonephritis; hypercalcemia (from bony destruction and immobilization), amyloidosis, hyperuricemia, myeloma kidney.
   a. Encourage liberal fluid intake and keep urine flow rate high—to prevent protein precipitation and to minimize hypercalciuria.
   b. Give allopurinol as prescribed—to control hyperuricemia.
   c. Watch for symptoms of hemorrhagic cystitis in patient taking cyclophosphamide; maintain on liberal fluid intake.
   d. Avoid dehydration—can precipitate acute renal failure; IV fluids may be necessary.
   e. Give prednisone as prescribed by physician—may be used in management of hypercalcemia. Weigh patient daily to monitor fluid retention.

▶ **NURSING ALERT:** Patients with multiple myeloma should *not* have their fluid intake restricted prior to diagnostic tests, since dehydrating procedures can precipitate acute renal failure.

   f. Monitor renal status through blood studies and urinalysis.
   g. Dialysis may be required in severely hypercalcemic patients with advanced renal insufficiency.
2. Watch for recurrent infections—from decrease in normal circulating antibodies because of proliferation of abnormal plasma cells, which produce ineffective globulins; chemotherapy and radiotherapy cause marrow depression; steroids increase susceptibility to opportunistic infection.
   a. Monitor temperature—patients on steroids may not have overt symptoms of infection. Assess for apathy, lethargy, and tachycardia.
   b. Assess for symptoms of urinary tract and respiratory tract infections.
   c. Secure cultures from skin lesions, blood, sputum, and urine as indicated.

Health Education and Emotional Support

1. Instruct the patient about proper body mechanics and avoiding heavy lifting.
2. Make the patient aware of potentially nephrotoxic factors such as *dehydration* or drugs.
3. Instruct the patient to wear a back brace as prescribed and to use muscle strengthening exercises to maintain performance status.
4. Report the presence of fever, bone pain, bleeding, or neurologic complications; report for regular follow-up.
5. Support the patient emotionally and demonstrate continuing interest.
   a. Reinforce the patient's understanding of treatment and its possible side effects.

b. Take a positive approach emphasizing the benefits of therapy.
c. Emphasize the patient's strengths.
   (1) Share and work through the patient's anxieties.
   (2) Explore precisely what the patient fears.
   (3) Allow the patient to talk about his problems. Give *specific* help (for pain, breathlessness, depression, etc.).
   (4) Anticipate the patient's anxieties after leaving the hospital.
6. Use diet supplement during periods of anorexia.

Evaluation
Expected Outcomes

1. Reports relief of disabling bone pain; increases activities
2. Demonstrates minimal/no complications; shows reduction of tumor cell mass by laboratory evaluation; achieves reversal of symptoms
3. Demonstrates improved results of blood studies—hemoglobin, platelet count, white blood cell count
4. Increases weight and has good appetite
5. Becomes more alert and is able to cope with life changes

Bleeding Disorders

Bleeding disorders may be classified as congenital or acquired and single or multifactorial.

Nursing History

1. Is there a history of abnormal or excessive bleeding? Following previous surgery? Dental extraction? Tonsillectomy? Family history of bleeding tendencies?
2. What medications is the patient taking? (Many drugs impair platelet function.) Taking aspirin? (More than 250 preparations contain aspirin.)
3. Has there been occupational exposure to toxic agents? Ionizing radiation?

Clinical Manifestations

1. Mucocutaneous bleeding—petechiae or ecchymosis on skin, nosebleeding, gum oozing while brushing teeth, hemorrhagic bullae in oral mucosa, gastrointestinal bleeding, lower urinary tract bleeding
2. Bleeding into soft tissue, joints, viscera
3. Palpable liver and spleen (hepatomegaly and splenomegaly)
4. Bleeding in central nervous system

Laboratory Evaluation

1. Falling hemoglobin/hematocrit levels
2. Thrombocytopenia
3. Prolonged prothrombin time (PT)
4. Prolonged partial thromboplastin time (PTT)
5. Prolonged bleeding time

Nursing Interventions

1. Maintain integrity of skin.
   a. Use electric razor for shaving.
   b. Avoid intramuscular injections when possible.
   c. Handle the skin gently; try to avoid use of adhesive tape.
   d. Avoid the use of tourniquets.
   e. Rotate extremities for blood pressure measurement.
2. Promote integrity of mucous membranes.
   a. Lubricate lips.
   b. Cleanse mouth carefully (see Common Problems of Patients with Blood Disorders, p. 237).
   c. Encourage soft, bland, and nonirritating foods.
3. Monitor integrity of gastrointestinal tract.
   a. Avoid constipation by enhancing hydration and motility.
   b. Administer stool softeners to prevent rupture of blood vessels from straining.
   c. Avoid rectal instrumentation (rectal thermometers; enemas).
4. Measure blood loss.
   a. Weigh linens, bandages.
   b. Monitor the pad count/amount of saturation during menses.
   c. Measure drainage.
5. Evaluate hemoglobin and hematocrit levels.
6. Conserve the patient's strength during and after bleeding episodes.
7. See page 252 for other nursing interventions.

Vascular Purpuras

The term *purpura* refers to extravasation (escape) of blood into the skin and mucous membranes. Purpuric lesions may occur spontaneously as an isolated phenomenon or as an accompaniment of obvious disease.

Types of Purpura

1. *Petechiae*—small pinpoint hemorrhages under the skin.
2. *Ecchymoses*—escape of blood into tissues; producing a large bruise.
3. Petechiae and ecchymoses may occur as the result of vascular rupture, permitting the leakage of blood into the subcutaneous tissue of the mucous membranes.
4. *Symptomatic or secondary purpura*—certain types of bloodstream infections (e.g., meningococcemia and infective endocarditis) exhibit this phenomenon because of damage to the vascular walls by the infectious agent or by immune complexes.
5. Severe arterial hypertension—may cause the patient to bruise easily; Valsalva maneuver may cause petechiae.
6. *Anaphylactoid purpura*—generally regarded as an allergic disorder in which there are various skin lesions (purpuric and otherwise) and episodes of arthritis, abdominal pain, hematuria, gastrointestinal hemorrhages, and fever.
   a. Attacks last several weeks and recur for years.
   b. Steroid therapy is often effective.
7. *Familial hemorrhagic telangiectasia*—a hereditary

disorder manifested by an abnormal tendency to bleed and bruise.
   a. Precise nature of defect is obscure.
   b. Condition does not respond to any proved method of treatment.
8. *Toxic purpura*—a condition observed after exposure to certain drugs and poisons.
9. *Vitamin C deficiency*—a vascular purpura.
10. Senile purpura.
11. Rheumatic and collagen–vascular diseases—associated with *palpable purpura* caused by deposition of immune complexes in blood vessels of the skin.
12. Steroid purpura—associated with loss of capillary integrity.

Thrombocytopenia

Thrombocytopenia is a decrease in the circulating platelet count, which may result in bleeding or hemorrhage.

Altered Physiology and Causes

1. Decreased platelet production (infiltrative diseases of bone marrow, leukemia, myelosuppressive therapy, other tumors, myelofibrosis, radiation therapy, drug effect, aplastic anemia, etc.).
2. Increased platelet destruction (infection, immune thrombocytopenic purpura, disseminated intravascular coagulation, drug-induced, etc.).
3. Abnormal distribution or sequestration—hypersplenism.
4. Loss of platelets from body (extracorporeal circulation, dilution due to blood loss and multiple blood transfusions).

Clinical Manifestations

When the platelet count drops below 20,000/mm.^{3}:
1. Petechiae occur spontaneously.
2. Ecchymoses occur at sites of minor trauma (venipuncture, bruises).
3. Hematomas occur at sites of more significant trauma (surgical wounds).
4. Bleeding from mucosal surfaces, nose, GI, and genitourinary (GU) tracts, respiratory tract, and central nervous system may occur.
5. Menorrhagia is common.
6. Excessive bleeding after dental extractions is seen.

Treatment and Nursing Management

1. Treat the underlying disease (e.g., treat the leukemia, discontinue offending drugs, etc.).
2. Assist with administration of platelet transfusions if platelet production is impaired; if excessive destruction of platelets is the problem, transfused platelets will also be destroyed and will not raise the count. Steroids are helpful in autoimmune thrombocytopenia.
3. Hormonal control of menstrual periods is usually carried out.
4. Teach the patient to avoid any maneuver that increases intracranial pressure when platelet count is <20,000/mm.^{3}.
5. See Bleeding Disorders, page 259.

Immune Thrombocytopenic Purpura

Immune thrombocytopenic purpura is a group of bleeding disorders due to immune destruction of platelets. Antiplatelet antibodies are produced for unknown reasons, so that the platelet life span is markedly shortened. Antibody-coated platelets are removed from the circulation by reticuloendothelial cells of the spleen and liver.

Clinical Manifestations

1. History of easy bruising
2. Bleeding—mild to severe (thrombocytopenia not usually accompanied by bleeding unless the platelet count falls below 20,000/mm.^{3}).
   a. Skin lesions—small red hemorrhages; do not blanch on pressure
   b. Purpuric lesions may occur in vital organ (brain)
   c. Bleeding may occur from nose, mouth, genitourinary tract

Laboratory Manifestations

1. Platelets may be absent or only slightly decreased in number; abnormalities may be seen in platelet size or morphologic appearance.
2. Increased levels of immunoglobulins (IgG) or complement components on the platelet surface.
3. Bone marrow examination—bone marrow megakaryocytes are increased in number.

Treatment

Management depends on severity of clinical situation.
1. Immunosuppression by corticosteroids (prednisone). Therapeutic response usually seen in days to weeks; dose is then reduced, and the process of tapering prednisone is started.
2. Splenectomy (see p. 262). Is necessary in up to two thirds of patients with immune thrombocytopenic purpura.
3. Immunosuppression by cytotoxic drugs (azathioprine; cyclophosphamide; vincristine)—reserved for those patients not responding to steroids and splenectomy.

Nursing Management

1. Give corticosteroids (prednisone) for acute bleeding as directed—causes a decrease in the production of antibody and a decrease in the clearance of antibody-coated platelets by the spleen, and also reduces capillary fragility.
2. Prepare the patient for a splenectomy if patient fails to respond to steroids—spleen is the primary organ of platelet clearance.
3. Support the patient receiving platelet transfusions (see p. 265)—given to patients with life-threatening hemorrhage.
4. Keep the patient at bed rest during periods of active bleeding.
5. See also page 237.

Health Education

Instruct the patient as follows:
1. Employ self-monitoring for infectious complications if you are on long-term steroid therapy.
2. Avoid aspirin or aspirin-containing products.
3. Avoid potential sources of accidents; protect yourself from injury.

Bleeding Disorders Due to Coagulation Defects

Disseminated Intravascular Coagulation (DIC)

Disseminated intravascular coagulation is an acquired hemorrhagic syndrome in which there is widespread clotting in small vessels of the body, leading to consumption of the clotting factors and platelets so that bleeding and thrombosis are occurring simultaneously. It is seen as a complication of a variety of disorders.

Clinical Features

1. Seen in a variety of diseases.
   a. Overwhelming infections; bacterial and viral sepsis
   b. Obstetrical complications
   c. Disseminated malignancies
   d. Massive tissue injuries (burns and trauma)
   e. Vascular and circulatory collapse; shock
   f. Anaphylaxis
   g. Hemolytic transfusion reactions
2. Hemorrhagic tendency is the consequence of the acute activation of the clotting mechanism of the blood—results in intravascular consumption of the plasma clotting factors.
3. Clotting factors are consumed more quickly than they can be replenished by the liver.

Assessment

Clinical Manifestations

1. Bleeding or a tendency to bleed—from occult internal bleeding to profuse hemorrhaging from all orifices
2. Acrocyanosis (cold, mottled fingers and toes)
3. Dyspnea, hemoptysis, crackles—from involvement of pulmonary circulation due to microcirculatory obstruction
4. Signs and symptoms of acute renal failure—from fibrin deposition in small vessels of kidneys

Diagnostic Evaluation

1. Platelet count
2. Clotting tests (prothrombin time; activated partial thromboplastin time, fibrin split products)
3. Fibrinogen level

Management

1. Removal and treatment of precipitating cause
2. Antibiotics to treat overwhelming infection
3. Supportive measures (fluid replacement, oxygenation, maintenance of blood pressure and urine output)—to restore circulating blood volume and deliver oxygen to ischemic tissues
4. Replacement therapy for serious hemorrhagic manifestations (transfusions of red cells, platelet concentrates, and, if indicated by very low fibrinogen level, cryoprecipitate)

Patient Problems/Nursing Diagnoses

1. Bleeding related to inability to form a stable clot
2. Alteration in tissue and organ perfusion related to microthrombi of fibrin and/or platelets obstructing microcirculation/organ function
3. Altered breathing patterns related to microcirculatory obstruction of pulmonary circulation
4. Alteration in urinary elimination related to underlying disease

Planning and Implementation
Nursing Interventions

A. **Relief of Bleeding Episodes and Related Complications**

1. Remove the underlying condition responsible for DIC.
   a. Correct any condition that exaggerates coagulopathy (shock, acidosis, sepsis).
   b. Give antisepsis treatment for coagulation changes produced by bacteremia.
2. Administer blood component replacement (platelet concentrates, fresh frozen plasma or cryoprecipitate) See page 271 for nursing interventions to prevent complications, recognize adverse factors and treatment of untoward reactions.
3. Take every measure to prevent and control hemorrhage.
   a. Give medications orally or through intravenous lines when possible; avoid IM injections.
   b. Document all attempts at venipuncture.
      (1) Use small-gauge needles.
      (2) Use infusion control equipment to ensure constant, accurate flow rates.
      (3) Avoid excessive skin handling and tape removal.
      (4) Apply pressure to IV and IM sites.
   c. Check and mark skin for progression of subcutaneous bleeding.
   d. Check stools, urine, and emesis for occult blood.
   e. Monitor vital signs.
   f. Measure blood loss; weigh bandages and linen.
   g. Stay calm during episodes of bleeding; help the patient control fear.

B. **Establishment of Adequate Tissue and Organ Perfusion**

1. Carry out ongoing nursing assessment for occult bleeding and thromboembolic occlusion from formation of thrombi in multiple body sites.
   a. Look for bleeding from suture line, and oozing of blood from IV sites.
   b. Assess color of skin and mucosa, petechiae, cold mottled hands and feet, gingival bleeding, nosebleeding, bleeding/jaundice of conjunctivae and sclerae, hemoptysis.
   c. Monitor for vascular occlusion, which produces circulatory obstruction and organ hypoperfusion.
      (1) Kidneys—monitor for urine volume and hematuria.
      (2) Skin—petechiae, purpura, ecchymoses—reflect bleeding into skin.
      (3) Lungs (interstitial hemorrhage)—monitor for

dyspnea, respiratory distress, hemoptysis, cyanosis; auscultate for crackles.
(4) CNS (cerebral thromboemboli/dysfunction)—assess level of responsiveness, orientation, sensory and motor dysfunction, convulsions, and coma.
2. Ask about bone and joint pain; changes in vision (retinal hemorrhage).
3. Evaluate cardiopulmonary function; assess for tachypnea, orthopnea, tachycardia, palpitations, orthostatic hypotension—reflect inadequacy of tissue oxygenation and/or fall in blood volume.
4. Examine for abdominal tenderness.
5. Monitor for falling platelet count, and prolonged prothrombin time and partial thromboplastin time.

Evaluation

Expected Outcomes

1. Absence of bleeding
2. Demonstrates tissue and organ perfusion
3. Absence of dyspnea
4. Maintains adequate urine output

Hemophilia

Hemophilia is a hereditary coagulation disorder (see p. 1285).

Von Willebrand's Disease

Von Willebrand's disease is a common bleeding disorder with either autosomal dominant or recessive inheritance, which is due to an abnormality of the factor VIII complex. There are several genetic variants.

Clinical Manifestations

1. Epistaxis; gingival oozing; easy bruising
2. Gastrointestinal bleeding
3. Menorrhagia
4. Prolonged bleeding from cuts
5. Postoperative bleeding

Laboratory Evaluation

1. Prolonged bleeding time
2. Immunologic tests of subcomponents of the factor VIII macromolecular complex

Management

1. Infusions of cryoprecipitate—correct the defects of Von Willebrand's disease. May be repeated every 12 hours until bleeding stops or postoperative period stabilizes.
2. See page 237 for nursing management of the patient who is bleeding.

Acquired Defects in Coagulation

Acquired defects in coagulation may be associated with many conditions, including:
1. Anticoagulant administration
   a. Coumarin-like drugs
   b. Heparin
2. Diseases of the liver
3. Disseminated intravascular coagulation
4. Uremia
5. Massive transfusions (dilutional clotting factor deficiency)
6. Certain antibiotics—inhibit coagulation factors

Splenectomy

Splenectomy is surgical removal of the spleen.

Indications for Splenectomy

1. Bleeding from trauma/rupture of the spleen
   a. History of injury
   b. Persistent abdominal pain
   c. Abdominal rigidity, rebound tenderness, shock
2. Staging procedure for lymphomas
3. Primary hematologic problems
   a. Hypersplenism (sequestration and premature destruction of red and white blood cells and of platelets by an enlarged spleen)
   b. Autoimmune hemolytic anemia, immune thrombocytopenia and/or immune neutropenia. Spleen is the major clearance site for antibody and/or complement-coated blood cells.

Underlying Consideration

New approaches are being tried following trauma to conserve splenic tissue, since the spleen has a vital role in host defense.

A. Preoperative Care

1. Carry out studies of coagulation status of patient.
   a. Have units of platelets available (may be transfused during operation to assist in hemostasis); surgeon usually waits until splenic vascular pedicle is cross-clamped before giving platelet concentrates.
   b. Administer vitamin K for abnormalities of prothrombin time.
   c. Prepare for transfusion of packed red cells if patient has significant anemia.
2. Assist with preoperative pulmonary physical therapy—to reduce incidence of pulmonary complications; patient may be debilitated from hematologic disease, from immunosuppressants, etc.
3. Preoperative preparation for patient with rupture of spleen
   a. Administer whole blood if rupture of spleen has occurred.
   b. Evacuate stomach with nasogastric tube—to prevent aspiration.
   c. Check the patient for pneumothorax/hemothorax—thoracotomy tube may be in place before anesthesia is started.

B. Postoperative Care

1. See page 440 for general aspects of nursing management following abdominal surgery.
2. Watch for the development of complications—related to location (anatomic) of spleen, the reason for its removal, and sequelae of splenectomy.
   a. Bleeding

(1) Measure abdominal girth for persistent or recurring hemorrhage.

(2) Prepare for surgical reexploration after ensuring coagulation defects have been corrected with transfusions of platelets (for thrombocytopenia) or fresh frozen plasma (for abnormal clotting factors).

b. Respiratory complications
Atelectasis of left lower lobe with pneumonia; pleural effusion—operations on left upper quadrant predispose to hypoventilation and limited diaphragmatic movement.

(1) Employ aggressive chest physiotherapy and incentive spirometry.

(2) Encourage early and progressive mobilization.

c. Infection
Assess for persistent fever—may indicate subphrenic abscess/hematoma

▶ **NURSING ALERT:** Adult asplenic patients are at above normal risk of developing overwhelming sepsis years after splenectomy.

Assess for persistent fever—may indicate subphrenic abscess/hematoma.

d. Thrombocytosis (elevation of platelets above normal) may follow a few days after elective splenectomy; platelet count usually increases progressively during first 2 weeks; this postoperative physiologic thrombocytosis may be conducive to thromboembolic complications.

(1) Monitor daily platelet count to detect postsplenectomy thrombocytosis.

e. Postsplenectomy fever (not always the result of infection).

Discharge Planning/Health Education

1. Emphasize that febrile illness should be reported immediately. An antimicrobial agent is usually given at the first sign of infection and may be taken on a long-term basis in some circumstances.
2. Encourage immunization with polyvalent pneumococcal vaccine several weeks prior to splenectomy if possible—an individual undergoing splenectomy is at risk for pneumococcal infections and sepsis.
3. Inform the patient that there is a relatively high incidence of viral illness in asplenic individuals.

2: Transfusion Therapy

Basic Immunohematology

Antigens, Antibodies, and Crossmatching

A. **Antigens**—complex proteins on the red cell surface. Antigens may stimulate the formation of antibodies.

1. Antigens are inherited from parents.
   a. Positive—antigens present
   b. Negative—antigens absent
2. If an antigen is present on the red cell, the immune system recognizes it as "self" and does not normally produce antibody.

B. **Antibodies**—proteins circulating in the plasma, produced in response to an antigen that the individual is lacking.

1. The most potent red cell antigens are in the ABO system (see Table 8-1 and Fig. 8-1); they are so potent that antibody production is stimulated soon after birth by antigenically similar substances in the

Table 8-1   ABO and Rh Systems and Their Significance in Transfusion Therapy

Recipient Blood Group	Incidence	Description	Antibody	Antibody Development	Compatible Donor Blood	Compatible Donor Plasma
A	42%	A antigen on red cell membranes	anti-B	Naturally occurring at age 3 months	A whole blood and red cells; O red cells	A plasma; AB plasma
B	10%	B antigen on red cell membranes	anti-A	Naturally occurring at age 3 months	B whole blood and red cells; O red cells	B plasma; AB plasma
AB	3%	A and B antigens on red cell membranes	None	Body sees both A and B antigens as "self"	AB whole blood and red cells; A red cells; B red cells; O red cells	AB plasma
O	45%	Neither A or B antigen on red cell membranes	anti-A and anti-B	Naturally occurring at age 3 months	O whole blood and red cells	O plasma; AB plasma; A plasma; B plasma
Rh positive	85%	D (Rh) antigen on red cell membranes	None	Body sees D antigen as "self"	Rh positive or Rh negative cellular products	Rh positive or Rh negative plasma
Rh negative	15%	No D (Rh) antigen present on red cells	anti-D	May occur after exposure to D antigen (transfusion or pregnancy)	Rh negative cellular products (whole blood, red cells, granulocytes, platelets)	Rh positive or negative plasma (red cell free)

See Figure 8-1.

Blood Group	Red Cell Antigen	Antibody Stimulated
A	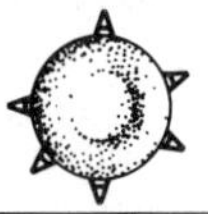	B B B B B B
B	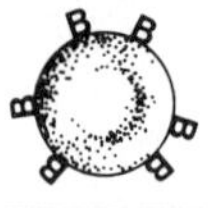	A A A A A A
AB	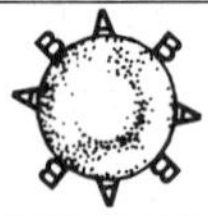	None
O	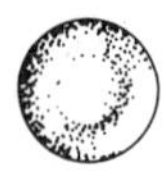	A B A B A B A B A B
Rh Positive	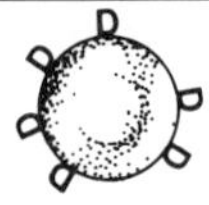	None
Rh Negative	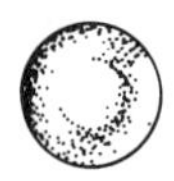	D D D D D D

Figure 8-1. Red cell antigen activity by blood groups.

environment. Example: Individuals lacking A antigen—blood groups B and O—make anti-A by age 3 months (naturally occurring).

2. The Rh system is the second most potent (see Table 8-1), but those lacking Rh antigens (Rh negative) are stimulated to produce antibody only after exposure to Rh positive red cells (transfusion or pregnancy). Such stimulated antibodies are called *alloantibodies* or atypical antibodies.

C. **Crossmatching** (compatibility testing)— accomplished by incubating a sample of the patient's plasma with the donor's red cells to detect signs of incompatibility, which are:

Agglutination—clumping of cells
   and
Hemolysis—destruction of red cells
Both are seen as the result of the interaction of antigen and antibody.

1. A compatible crossmatch between donor and recipient is necessary before a transfusion is given.

▶ **NURSING ALERT:** Compatibility testing is the best available method of providing a safe transfusion, but it does not guarantee that a reaction will not occur.

2. Blood products that require crossmatch/compatibility testing prior to transfusion are those containing a significant number of red cells, such as whole blood, red blood cells, and granulocytes.
3. A routine crossmatch requires 1–2 hours. In an emergency, an abbreviated crossmatch can be performed, or ABO compatible uncrossmatched blood can be transfused with minimal risk.

Whole Blood and Blood Components

Whole Blood

A unit of blood (drawn from a donor) consists of 450 ml. of blood collected into 60–70 ml. preservative/anticoagulant.

1. Blood collected into a sealed container can be stored for 21 to 35 days (depending on type of preservative/anticoagulant).
2. Whole blood stored more than 24 hours does not contain functional platelets or practical amounts of coagulation factors V and VIII.

A. **Indications**

1. Acute massive blood loss when oxygen-carrying properties of red cells, as well as volume expansion of plasma, is required.
2. The loss of up to one-third of the total blood volume (1,000–1,200 ml.) can usually be managed with crystalloid and/or colloid solutions.

B. **Nursing Interventions**

1. Transfuse through a standard blood infusion set with a 170-micron blood filter. If the patient is receiving massive transfusions, a microaggregate filter may be used (see p. 268).
2. The indications for giving whole blood (severe bleeding) usually necessitate the rapid infusion of blood; observe closely for adverse reactions.

3. For rapid infusion, a special pressure cuff may be placed around the unit of blood. Pressure should not exceed 300 mm. of mercury.

Note: Infusion devices—A variety of volumetric infusion pumps are available that deliver fluid at rates as low as 1 ml./hour. While some are tested and approved for blood, others may induce red cell hemolysis attributable to excessive pressure. The manufacturer should be consulted prior to use of infusion devices.

Blood Components

1. Approximately 10%–20% of the blood collected is transfused as whole blood, while the remaining 80%–90% is separated into components.
2. Components provide optimal therapeutic benefit while reducing the risk of circulatory overload.
3. Advanced technology—provides methods of separating red blood cells, platelets, plasma, and plasma derivatives from one unit, thereby supporting multiple patients from a single donation.

Packed Red Cells

Red cells (packed red cells)—are erythrocytes separated from a unit of whole blood prepared by removing up to 80% of the plasma by centrifugation or sedimentation.

1. Red cells provide a concentrated form of hemoglobin.

2. If plasma is removed without breaking the seal of the original container (through pre-attached satellite bag), red cells can be stored for 21 to 49 days, depending on the type of preservative/anticoagulant used. If the seal is broken, storage time is reduced to 24 hours due to possible bacterial contamination.

A. **Indications**—to restore or maintain oxygen-carrying capacity with a minimal expansion of blood volume.

B. **Nursing Interventions**

1. Use a No. 19 gauge needle (or larger). Red cells are viscous, making it difficult to achieve an adequate flow rate. If the patient's condition permits, normal saline (0.9%) may be added to the cells.
2. A Y-type blood infusion set (Fig. 8-2) allows the addition of saline.
   a. Close all clamps on blood infusion set. Insert couplers into saline and red cells.
   b. Open clamp to saline and flush tubing to needle adaptor. Close clamp to recipient.
   c. Lower the red cell container and open clamp to red cell container.
   d. Allow desired amount of saline to enter red cells.

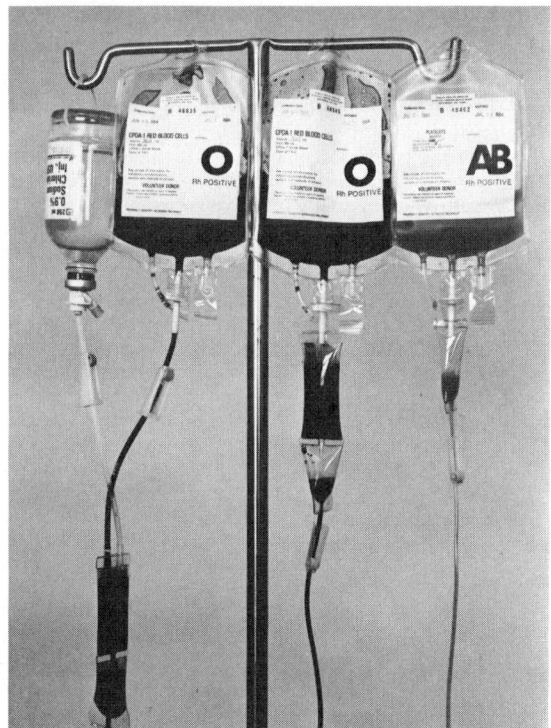

Figure 8-2. *Standard blood administration sets with 170-micron filters include:*
1. *Y-type blood infusion set—recommended for viscous products requiring predilution. Convenient for maintaining saline drip pretransfusion and in the event of a reaction (Left).*
2. *Straight blood infusion set—can be used for all products, excluding granulocytes and platelets (Middle).*
3. *Component infusion set—for use with platelets and granulocytes; made without rubber connections (Right).*

▶ **NURSING ALERT:** Solutions other than *0.9% saline* can cause red cell agglutination and/or hemolysis and must not be used as an IV flush or diluent. Medications are never added to blood products.

3. Infuse red cells over 2–3 hours. If the patient's condition or size prohibits the infusion of the entire unit within 4 hours, notify the physician. It may be necessary to divide the unit into small volumes, allowing the remaining portions to be properly refrigerated until requested.

Platelet Concentrates

Platelet concentrates are large numbers of platelets in a minimum amount of plasma. They also contain some lymphocytes and red blood cells, the amount varying with preparation techniques.

A. **Random Donor Platelets**—platelets prepared by centrifugation of a unit of whole blood. Approximately 60% of the available platelets are removed resulting in a minimum of 5.5×10^{10} platelets per unit.

1. *Indications*—to stop or prevent bleeding in patients with thrombocytopenia (patients receiving chemotherapy, etc.).
2. *Nursing Considerations*
   a. Each unit is suspended in 50–70 ml. of plasma. The usual dose for a thrombocytopenic, bleeding adult is 6–10 units.
   b. The units may be pooled prior to release from the blood bank or issued in separate bags.
   c. If the seal is unbroken, platelets are stored at room temperature with continuous agitation for 3–5 days (varies according to type of container). If the container is entered, platelets must be transfused within 4 hours.

B. **Single Donor Platelets**—6–8 units of platelets collected from a single donor by apheresis. Platelets and a small amount of plasma are removed from the donor; red blood cells and the remaining plasma are returned to the donor. The volume of plasma varies from 200–500 ml., and platelets can be stored 1–5 days.

1. *Indications*
   a. Platelets from a single donor reduce the risk of donor-related transmissible disease (see p. 273) and antigen sensitivity.
   b. It is also the most efficient means of obtaining HLA matched platelets.

C. **HLA Matched Platelets**—platelets that are histocompatible with the recipient's HLA type. HLA (histocompatibility antigens/human leukocyte antigens) are present on all human cells except red cells and are critical factors in tissue transplantation.

1. *Indications*—for platelet transfusion to patients who do not respond to unmatched platelets due to the development of HLA antibodies.
   a. HLA matching is complicated and expensive. There are hundreds of combinations of antigens determining HLA type.
   b. A family member is the most likely identical match.

D. **Nursing Interventions for Platelet Transfusions**

1. Verify plasma compatibility (see p. 263) prior to transfusion, particularly if the volume exceeds 100 ml. or if the recipient is an infant or child. Platelets

contain few red cells and therefore do not require ABO crossmatching, but transfusing large volumes of incompatible plasma can cause a positive direct Coombs and red cell destruction.

2. Infuse through a *component* administration set with a standard 170-micron filter.

▶ **NURSING ALERT:** DO NOT use a microaggregate filter or administration set with rubber connections. Platelets will aggregate and adhere to the filter and rubber.

3. Infuse as rapidly as the patient's condition permits (not to exceed 4 hours). Most reactions are related to foreign protein (allergic) or white cell sensitivity (febrile).

Granulocyte Concentrates

Granulocyte concentrates are large numbers of granulocytes (1.0×10^{10}) and some lymphocytes, platelets, and red cells prepared by centrifugation leukapheresis of a single donor.

A. Indications—only patients with severe granulocytopenia (less than 500/mm.^{3}) or rare patients with nonfunctional granulocytes should receive granulocytes. Other indications include:

1. Documented bacterial infection (granulocytes are not usually effective against viral or fungal infections)
2. Fever or progressive local infection unresponsive to appropriate 24–48 hours of antibiotic therapy
3. Reasonable chance for bone marrow recovery
4. Neonatal sepsis

B. Nursing Interventions

1. *Transfuse immediately* following notification by blood bank that unit of granulocytes is available. Granulocytes remain functional for only hours after collection. Viability is best preserved by storage at room temperature; granulocyte concentrates are not refrigerated.
2. Check ABO compatibility before transfusion. Granulocyte preparations are heavily contaminated with red blood cells and do require crossmatching.
3. Transfuse through a standard blood administration set with 170-micron filter.

▶ **NURSING ALERT:** DO NOT use a microaggregate filter (see Fig. 8-4). Granulocytes will be removed by the filter.

4. Infuse slowly (2 ml./minute) for the first 30 minutes. Transfuse total volume over 1½ to 2½ hours.
5. Observe the patient closely during transfusion, since reactions due to hypersensitivity are frequent. The patient may require medication (antihistamine; analgesic) to reduce the incidence and severity of reactions.
Allergic reactions range from mild symptoms (hives, urticaria) to anaphylaxis. Severe episodes of fever and chills are occasionally seen.

Plasma

Plasma is the liquid portion of blood after removal of cellular components (red cells, platelets, leukocytes). Plasma is composed of approximately 91% water, 7% protein, and 2% carbohydrates and lipids. The method of preparation determines the use and effectiveness of plasma.

Note: Plasma carries a risk of hepatitis equal to that of whole blood. If only volume expansion is required, albumin, plasma protein fraction, or crystalloid solutions are safe products.

A. Fresh Frozen Plasma (FFP)—prepared from whole blood by separating and freezing the plasma within 6 hours of collection. FFP contains clotting factors V and VIII (the labile factors) as well as factors I, II, VII, IX, X, XI, XII, and XIII. One milliliter of FFP contains 1 unit of coagulation factor activity.
Indications:

1. FFP is transfused for coagulation factor deficiencies related to liver disease, DIC, and dilutional coagulopathy resulting from massive blood replacement.
2. It may also be indicated for congenital coagulation deficiencies (i.e., hemophilia A or B) but commercially prepared concentrates are more commonly used when available.

B. Single Donor Plasma—plasma that has been removed from a unit of whole blood up to 5 days after the expiration date of the unit. It can be stored frozen up to 5 years. It contains all the stable coagulation factors but reduced levels of factors V and VIII.
Indications—Single-donor plasma can be used in the treatment of deficiencies of stable coagulation factors. It is the preferred product for reversal of Coumadin-induced anticoagulation.

C. Nursing Interventions for Plasma Transfusion

1. Verify ABO compatibility. Plasma contains no red cells and does not require crossmatching, but the plasma must be compatible with the recipient's red cells (see Compatibility chart). Rh negative patients may safely receive Rh positive plasma.
2. Observe color and appearance. Notify Blood Bank prior to beginning transfusion if any of the following abnormalities are noted:
   a. Cloudiness—normal plasma is a clear, yellow color but a green color may be a harmless manifestation of the use of oral contraceptives.
   b. Fibrin strands or clots—indicates improper thawing.
3. Transfuse through 170-micron filter over 1–2 hours.
4. The most common complications are related to circulatory overload and allergic reactions to foreign proteins.

Plasma Derivatives

Plasma derivatives are specific proteins removed from plasma for administration in concentrated form. Examples of plasma derivatives are cryoprecipitate, coagulation factors VIII and IX, albumin, and gamma globulin.
Indications—Plasma derivatives provide large quantities of a specific protein while limiting the plasma volume.

A. Cryoprecipitate—a product rich in factor VIII, factor VIII: vWF (von Willebrand's factor), fibrinogen, factor XIII, and fibronectin. It is prepared by thawing one unit of fresh frozen plasma at 4°C. and removing all but 10–15 ml. of plasma and the cold-insoluble globulins. The product is refrozen and used for up to 1 year.

1. *Indications*—cryoprecipitate is used in the treatment of:

a. Hemophilia A (factor VIII: C deficiency)
b. Von Willebrand's disease (factor VIII: vWF deficiency)
c. Disseminated intravascular coagulation
d. Uremic bleeding
2. Nursing interventions for cryoprecipitate transfusion:
a. Store cryoprecipitate after thawing at room temperature and transfuse within 4 hours. Cryoprecipitate contains a negligible number of red cells making crossmatching unnecessary, but if the total plasma volume exceeds 100 ml., it is advisable to transfuse ABO-compatible cryoprecipitate. Rh-negative patients may safely receive cryoprecipitate from Rh-positive donors.
b. Be aware that cryoprecipitate may be pooled into a single container or provided in individual units. Rinse bags thoroughly with saline to remove all cryoprecipitate.
c. Transfuse through component recipient set with 170-micron filter over 30–60 minutes.
d. Know that the most common reaction is related to foreign protein substances (allergic).

B. Factor VIII Concentrate (antihemophiliac factor, AHF)—a concentrated form of factor VIII prepared by pooling, fractionating, and lyophilizing (freeze-drying) large volumes of human plasma. This product is stable at refrigerated temperature for long periods but once reconstituted should be given within 3 hours.
1. Indications
a. Used in treatment of moderate to severe congenital factor VIII deficiency (hemophilia A).
b. To lower the risk of hepatitis transmission, a heat-treated product has recently been licensed for use. The cost per unit is considerably greater.
2. Nursing intervention
a. Reconstitute with sterile diluent provided.
b. Administer IV push through a filtered needle or drip through a component administration set.

Note: Many patients receive home treatment and administer their own concentrate.

c. Observe for side effects, which include malaise, fever, nausea, and chills. Hives are common.

C. Factor IX Concentrate (prothrombin complex)—a concentrated form of factor IX prepared by pooling, fractionating and lyophilizing large volumes of human plasma. Stable at refrigerated temperatures for long periods but once reconstituted should be given within 3 hours.
1. Indications
a. Used primarily for treatment of patients with factor IX deficiency (hemophilia B, or Christmas disease). Also contains factors II, VII, and X.
b. This product carries a high risk of transmissible disease (i.e., hepatitis) because preparation requires plasma pooling from many paid donors and is not processed to destroy infectious agents.
2. Nursing interventions
a. Reconstitute with sterile diluent provided. Administer intravenously, through a filter.
b. Observe for side effects—malaise, fever, nausea, chills, and hives. Disseminated intravascular coagulation has been reported, but is rare.

D. Albumin and Plasma Protein Fraction (PPF)—protein solutions prepared from plasma by fractionation. These products are heat-treated to inactivate the hepatitis virus. Albumin is composed of 96% albumin and 4% globulins, while PPF is a cruder fraction, containing 83% albumin and 17% globulin.
1. Indications—colloid solutions are used primarily in the treatment of hypovolemia or shock. Less commonly, these products have been used for major burns, plasma exchange, hemolytic disease of the newborn, and liver failure.
2. Nursing intervention for albumin and PPF
a. Transfuse intravenously through tubing provided by the manufacturer or a standard IV infusion set. These products do not require crossmatching or filtering.
b. Infuse at the rate indicated by the physician. Dose and rate will vary according to the clinical situation.
c. Be alert for signs of circulatory overload (see p. 272). Other side effects include nausea, chills, fever, headache, and hypotension. Because of reports of hypotension, PPF is contraindicated for use intra-arterially or during cardiopulmonary bypass.

E. Immune Serum Globulin (ISG)—proteins precipitated from pools of human plasma, which provide specific or nonspecific passive immunity. Processing inactivates the hepatitis virus.
1. *Specific Immune Globulins* are prepared by processing plasma from donors with high levels of antibody to such agents as hepatitis B (hepatitis B immune globulin, HBIG), tetanus, and herpes zoster (varicella zoster immune globulin, VZIG). Rh immune globulin (an example of specific immune globulin) is prepared from donors with high titers of Rh antibody (anti-D).
a. Indications
(1) Administered to Rh-negative individuals exposed to Rh-positive red cells through transfusion or pregnancy to prevent the formation of Rh antibody.
(2) Rh immune globulin has significantly reduced the incidence of hemolytic disease of the newborn.
b. *Nursing intervention*
(1) Administer by deep IM injection. Intramuscular injections can be *painful* and cause local irritation.
(2) Rare side effects include nausea, vomiting, hypotension, syncope, tachycardia, and arrhythmias.
2. *Nonspecific immune serum globulin* is prepared by fractionating human plasma from random normal donors. It provides nonspecific immunity to individuals with immunodeficiency syndromes such as hypogammaglobulinemia and agammaglobulinemia.
a. *Nursing interventions*
(1) Administer by deep IM injection. An IV preparation is available that is recommended for patients who require an immediate increase in intravascular immunoglobulin levels, who have small muscle mass, or those with bleeding tendencies for whom IM injections are contraindicated.
(2) IV preparations must be given via a separate line. Drug and solution compatibility has not been evaluated.

▶ **NURSING ALERT:** Only the preparation specifically prepared for IV use may be given IV.

      (3) Side effects are rare but include back pain, nausea, and flushing.

Special Blood/Component Products

Special blood products are sometimes necessary to alleviate or prevent transfusion complications. The products listed below require additional preparation.

A. Washed Red Cells—red cells that have been depleted of leukocytes and plasma by the addition and removal of normal saline. The shelf life after washing is 24 hours.

1. Indications
   a. To reduce the risk of febrile reactions by removing 70% of the leukocytes.
   b. To remove plasma when there is incompatibility with the recipient's red cells.
2. Nursing interventions (same as for red cells)

B. Deglycerolized Red Cells—red blood cells that have been frozen within 6 days of collection and thawed prior to transfusion. The cryoprotective agent (glycerol) added to red cells prior to freezing is hypertonic and must be removed before infusion. The "deglycerolization" process removes virtually all leukocytes, plasma, and anticoagulant. Frozen red cells can be stored for 3 years. Deglycerolization requires 1–2 additional hours of preparation time and reduces the shelf life to 24 hours.

1. Indications
   a. For storage of rare blood types for autologous, or homologous transfusion.
   b. To stockpile blood when donations are plentiful for use during blood shortages.
   c. For transfusion of IgA deficient recipient having IgA antibody.
   d. To reduce the risks of transfusing incompatible plasma and anticoagulant to neonates.
   e. To reduce the risk of febrile, nonhemolytic reactions related to white cell sensitivity when other methods fail.
2. Nursing interventions (same as for red cells)

C. Irradiated Blood Products—blood products that have been exposed to a radioactive substance. Radiation alters the ability of donor lymphocytes to engraft and divide.

1. The amount of radiation exposure varies, but as little as 1,500 rads is usually effective. The process requires minutes and does not alter the shelf life of the product.
2. The product carries *no* radiation risk.
3. Indications
   a. Prevention of graft-versus-host disease in immunosuppressed patients receiving blood products containing viable white blood cells (whole blood, red cells, platelets, granulocytes).
   b. Used most often for recipients of bone marrow transplants.

D. Prewarmed Blood Products—those that are warmed to 37°C. prior to infusion. Blood warmers are of two types: (1) a coil of plastic tubing placed in a monitored waterbath and (2) electrically heated plates warming the blood as it passes through a plastic bag (Fig. 8-3).

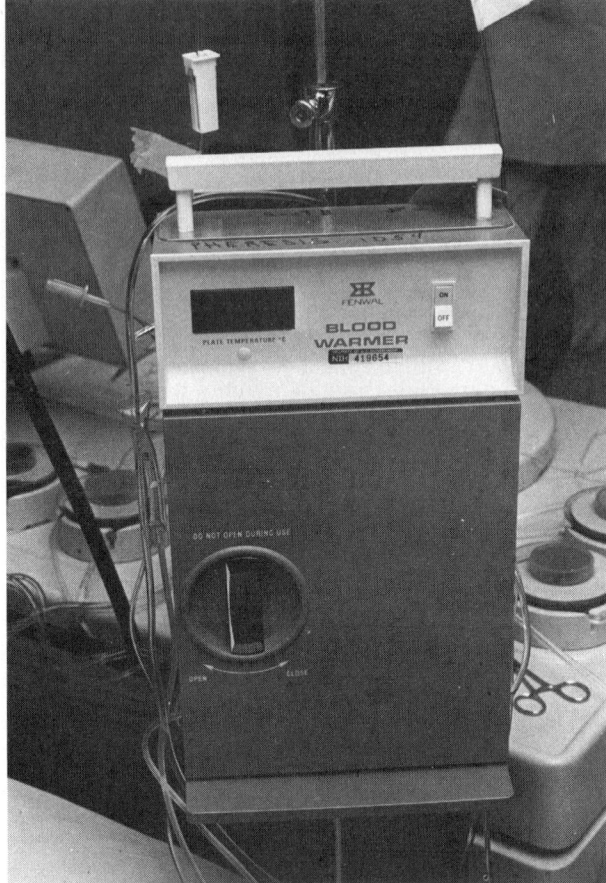

Figure 8-3. Blood Warmer, passing the blood through a plastic bag placed between electrically heated warming plates. This model (Fenwal Corp.) provides a digital reading of the temperature and has both audio and visual alarms.

▶ **NURSING ALERT:** These devices require frequent temperature monitoring by the nurse. Red cells exposed to temperatures greater than 40°C. can hemolyze and cause serious harm to the recipient.

1. Indications:
   a. For patients receiving rapid, massive transfusions. The transfusion of cold blood at rates greater than 100 ml./minute has been associated with arrhythmias and cardiac arrest.
   b. For exchange transfusion in infants.
   c. For patients with cold agglutinin disease.

E. Microaggregate Filtered Blood—the infusion of whole blood or red cells through a filter with a 20- or 40-micron pore size. Several such filters are commercially available (Fig. 8-4). The most common types are "in-line" filters, inserted by the nurse/transfusionist at the time of blood infusion.

1. Indications
   a. To remove aggregated leukocytes and platelets accumulated during blood storage. These aggregates have been noted in the lungs following

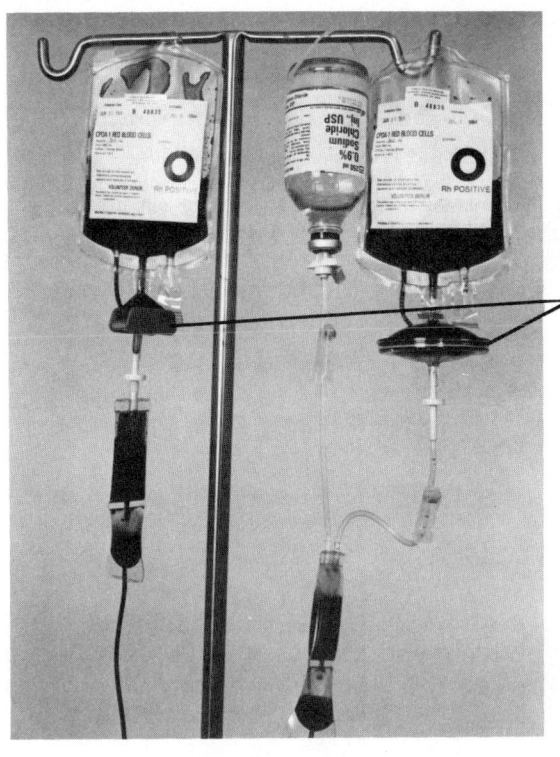

Microaggregate filters

Figure 8-4. Two types of microaggregate filters are:
1. 40-micron screen type filter (Pall Biomedical Products; *Left*).
2. 20-micron depth type filter (Fenwal Corp.; *Right*).

massive transfusion (replacement of one or more total blood volumes over 24 hours).
b. To remove leukocytes and reduce the risk of febrile, nonhemolytic transfusion reactions.

▶ **NURSING ALERT:** Microaggregate filters should not be used for the transfusion of platelets or granulocytes.

2. Nursing interventions (see manufacturer's directives)

Guidelines: Administering Blood/Blood Components

Purpose
1. To restore circulating blood volume.
2. To stop bleeding due to platelet deficiencies or defects and coagulation factor deficiencies.
3. To increase oxygen-carrying capacity of the blood.
4. To combat infection due to decreased or defective white cells or antibodies.

Equipment

Blood or component administration set (see Fig. 8-2)
Blood/blood component as prescribed
Needles (No. 19 gauge or larger)
Normal saline
Iodine-containing skin antiseptic
Tourniquet

Procedure

Nursing Action	Rationale/Amplification
Preparatory Phase	
1. Inform the patient of the procedure, blood product to be given, approximate length of time, and desired outcome of transfusion.	1. Instruct the patient to report unusual symptoms immediately.

(continued)

Guidelines: Administering Blood/Blood Components (continued)

Procedure
(Cont.)

Nursing Action	Rationale/Amplification
2. Obtain and record baseline vital signs.	2. Useful for later comparison.
3. Prepare infusion site. Select a large vein that allows patient some degree of mobility. Start the prescribed intravenous infusion.	3. Antecubital veins are not recommended for lengthy infusions. Prolonged restriction of arm movement is uncomfortable and inconvenient for the patient.

▶ **NURSING ALERT:** Crystalloid solutions other than 0.9% saline and all medications are incompatible with blood products. They may cause agglutination and/or hemolysis.

4. Obtain blood product from blood bank. Inspect for abnormal color, cloudiness, clots, and excess air. Read instructions on the product label regarding storage and infusion. Check expiration date.	4. Platelets are normally cloudy.

▶ **NURSING ALERT:** If the transfusion cannot begin immediately, return product to blood bank. Blood out of the refrigerator more than 30 minutes (above 10°C. [50°F.]) cannot be reissued. *Never* store blood in unauthorized areas such as the nursing unit refrigerator.

5. *Verify patient identification.*
  a. Ask the patient to state his full name. If the patient is unable to state his name, verify his identity with an individual who is familiar with the patient.
  b. Compare name and hospital ID number on the patient's wrist band to that on blood compatibility tag (Fig. 8-5).
	5. This is the single most important function of the nurse. Meticulous attention to detail is essential to avoid giving the wrong blood to the wrong patient, perhaps causing a fatal reaction.

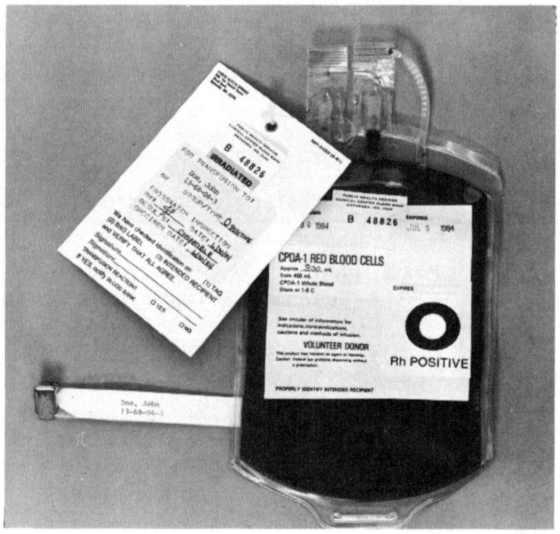

Figure 8-5. To properly identify intended recipient compare:
1. Name as stated by the recipient to name on identification bracelet (*a*).
2. Name and patient identification number on ID bracelet (*a*) to those on bag tag (*b*).
3. Blood donor number on bag tab (*c*) to donor number on bag label (*d*).
4. Blood group and Rh type on bag tag (*e*) and bag label (*f*). Verify compatibility (*g*).
5. Expiration date to current date (*h*).
6. Read all instructions on bag label thoroughly (*i*).

c. Verify product compatibility.	c. This is done by comparing group and type on blood compatibility tag, bag label, and patient's chart.

▶ **NURSING ALERT:** Any discrepancy must be investigated before beginning the transfusion. It is recommended that two qualified individuals verify patient identification and product compatibility.

Performance Phase

1. Start infusion slowly at 2 ml./minute. Remain at bedside for 15–30 minutes. If there are no signs of adverse reaction or circulatory overloading, the infusion rate may be increased.	1. The rate of infusion depends on the patient's condition and the product transfused. Signs or symptoms of an acute untoward reaction are usually manifested during infusion of the initial 50–100 ml. of blood.

Procedure
(Cont.)

Nursing Action	Rationale / Amplification
2. Observe the patient closely and check vital signs at least hourly until 1 hour post-transfusion. Report signs and symptoms of adverse reaction to physician immediately.	2. Acute reactions may occur at any time during the transfusion.
3. Record the following information on the patient's chart:	3. Facts relating to the transfusion should be charted exactly.
a. Product and volume transfused b. Product identification number	b. It must be possible to trace each transfusion product to the original blood donor.

c. Time transfusion started and ended
   d. Names of individuals verifying patient ID; name of person starting and ending transfusion;
   e. Patient's immediate response—for example, "no apparent reaction"	

Adverse Effects of Blood Transfusion

General Reactions

1. Based on the fact that every patient who receives blood is subject to the possible development of complications of transfusion therapy, the patient's major problems include:
   a. Acute reactions (allergic, febrile [nonhemolytic])
   b. Septic reactions
   c. Circulatory overload
   d. Hemolytic reactions
   e. Delayed reactions
2. See Table 8-2 for causes, clinical manifestations, management, and prevention.

Overview of Acute Reactions

1. Because many reactions exhibit similar clinical manifestations, every symptom should be considered potentially serious and the transfusion discontinued until the cause is determined.
2. When a reaction is suspected, blood bags with tubing from all products transfused within 4 hours should be returned to the blood bank for reevaluation.
   a. A postreaction blood sample from the patient is tested to reverify blood group and type and determine the presence of free hemoglobin in the plasma.
   b. A direct Coombs test is performed to detect antibody on the red cells.
   c. A urine sample is tested for hemoglobinuria.
   d. If the only symptoms are those resulting from a mild allergic reaction (urticaria), extensive evaluation is not required. In the event of a severe reaction, more tests may be necessary.

Table 8-2   Adverse Effects of Blood Transfusion

Acute Reaction	Cause	Clinical Manifestations	Management	Prevention
Allergic	Sensitivity to plasma protein or donor antibody, which reacts with recipient antigen	1. Flushing 2. Itching, rash 3. Urticaria, hives 4. Asthmatic wheezing 5. Laryngeal edema 6. Anaphylaxis	1. Stop transfusion immediately. Keep vein open (KVO) with normal saline. 2. Give antihistamine as directed (diphenhydramine). 3. Observe for anaphylaxis—prepare epinephrine if respiratory distress is severe. 4. If hives are the only clinical manifestation, the transfusion can sometimes continue at a slower rate.	Prior to transfusion, ask patient about past reactions. If patient has history of anaphylaxis, alert physician, have emergency drugs available, and remain at bedside for the first 30 minutes.
Febrile, non-hemolytic	Hypersensitivity to donor white cells, platelets, or plasma proteins	1. Sudden chills and fever 2. Headache 3. Flushing 4. Anxiety	1. Stop transfusion immediately and KVO with normal saline. Notify physician and blood bank. 2. Send blood samples and blood bags to blood bank. Collect urine sample for testing. 3. Check temperature ½ hour after chill and as indicated thereafter. 4. Give antipyretics as prescribed—treat symptomatically.	Give antipyretic (acetaminophen or aspirin) before transfusion as directed. Leukocyte-poor blood products may be recommended for future transfusions.

(continued)

Table 8-2   Adverse Effects of Blood Transfusion (continued)

Acute Reaction	Cause	Clinical Manifestations	Management	Prevention
Septic reactions	Transfusion of blood or components contaminated with bacteria	1. Rapid onset of chills 2. High fever 3. Vomiting; diarrhea 4. Marked hypotension	1. Stop transfusion immediately and KVO with normal saline. Notify physician and blood bank. 2. Obtain cultures of patient's blood and return blood bags with administration set to blood bank for culture. 3. Treat septicemia as directed—antibiotics, IV fluids, vasopressors, steroids.	Do not permit blood to stand at room temperature longer than necessary. Warm temperatures promote bacterial growth. Inspect blood for gas bubbles, clotting, or abnormal color before transfusion. Complete infusions within 4 hours. Change administration set after 4 hours of use.
Circulatory overload	Fluid administered at a rate or volume greater than the circulatory system can accommodate. Increased blood in pulmonary vessels and decreased lung compliance.	1. Rise in venous pressure 2. Distended neck veins 3. Dyspnea 4. Cough 5. Crackles at base of lungs	1. Stop transfusion and KVO with normal saline. Notify physician. 2. Place patient upright with feet in dependent position. 3. Administer prescribed diuretics, oxygen, morphine, and aminophylline.	Concentrated blood products should be given whenever possible. Transfuse at a rate within the circulatory reserve of the patient. Monitor CVP of patient with heart disease.
Hemolytic reaction	Infusion of incompatible blood products: 1. Antibodies in recipient's plasma attach to transfused red cells, hemolyzing the cells either in circulation or in the reticuloendothelial system. 2. Antibodies in donor plasma attach to recipient red cells, causing hemolysis (may result from infusion of incompatible plasma—less severe than incompatible red cells).	1. Chills; fever 2. Low back pain 3. Feeling of head fullness; flushing 4. Oppressive feeling 5. Tachycardia, tachypnea 6. Hypotension, vascular collapse 7. Hemoglobinuria, hemoglobinemia 8. Bleeding 9. Acute renal failure 10. Death	1. Stop transfusion immediately—keep vein open with 0.9% saline. 2. Notify physician and blood bank. 3. Treat shock, if present. 4. Draw testing samples, collect urine sample. 5. Maintain BP with IV colloid solutions. Give diuretics as prescribed to maintain urine flow, glomerular filtration, and renal blood flow. 6. Insert indwelling catheter to monitor hourly urine output. Patient may require dialysis if renal failure occurs.	Meticulously verify patient identification—from sample collection to product infusion. Begin infusion slowly and observe closely for 30 minutes—consequences are in proportion to the amount of incompatible blood transfused.

Delayed Reactions

1. Transfusion complications can occur days to months posttransfusion. Symptoms exhibited within this time frame should be investigated thoroughly to rule out a delayed transfusion reaction.

2. Examples of delayed reaction include:
   a. Delayed hemolytic reaction
   b. Iron overload (hemosiderosis)
   c. Graft-versus-host disease
   d. Infectious diseases
      (1) Hepatitis B

Table 8-3   Delayed Reactions to Transfusion Therapy

Delayed Reaction	Cause	Clinical Manifestations	Management	Prevention
Delayed hemolytic reaction	The destruction of transfused red cells by antibody not detectable during crossmatch but formed rapidly after transfusion. Rapid production may occur because of antigen exposure during previous transfusions or pregnancy.	1. Fever 2. Mild jaundice 3. Decreased hematocrit	Generally, no acute treatment is required, but hemolysis may be severe enough to cause shock and renal failure. If this occurs, manage as outlined under acute hemolytic reactions.	The crossmatch blood sample should be drawn within 48 hours of blood transfusion. Antibody formation may occur within 90 days of transfusion and/or delivery.
Iron overload (hemosiderosis)	Deposition of iron in the heart, endocrine organs, liver, spleen, skin, and other major organs as a result of multiple, long-term transfusions (aplastic anemia, thalassemia).	1. Diabetes 2. Decreased thyroid function 3. Arrhythmias 4. Congestive heart failure and other symptoms related to major organ failure	1. Treat symptomatically. 2. Deferoxamine (Desferal), which chelates and removes accumulated iron through the kidneys, may be administered IV, IM, or subcutaneously.	Transfusion of young red cells (neocytes) to extend periods between transfusion is currently under study. Collection techniques result in low neocyte yields, usually limiting use to pediatric patients.

Table 8-3 Delayed Reactions to Transfusion Therapy (continued)

Delayed Reaction	Cause	Clinical Manifestations	Management	Prevention
Graft-versus-host disease	Engraftment of lymphocytes in the bone marrow of immunosuppressed patients setting up an immune response of the graft against the host.	(See p. 274)	(See p. 274)	Transfuse with irradiated blood products.
Infectious disease 1. Hepatitis B	Virus transmitted from recipient via infected blood products.	1. Elevated liver enzymes (SGPT and SGOT) 2. Anorexia, malaise 3. Nausea and vomiting 4. Fever 5. Dark urine 6. Jaundice	Usually resolves spontaneously within 4–6 weeks. Can result in permanent liver damage. Treat symptomatically.	1. Screen blood donors, temporarily rejecting those who may have had contact with the virus. Those with a history of hepatitis are permanently deferred. 2. Pretest all blood products (radioimmunoassay).
2. NonA, nonB hepatitis	Agent has not been identified. Accounts for 90% of all posttransfusion hepatitis.	Similar to serum B hepatitis, but symptoms are usually less severe. Chronic liver disease and cirrhosis may develop.	Symptoms usually mild and require no treatment.	No screening test available. Careful donor screening only available method of disease control.
3. Epstein–Barr virus, cytomegalovirus, malaria, toxoplasmosis	Transmitted through infected blood products.			Question prospective blood donors regarding colds, flu, foreign travel.
4. Acquired immunodeficiency syndrome	Probably transmitted by a retrovirus (HTLV—III). In rare cases, transmission has been associated with transfusion of blood products.	1. Night sweats 2. Unexplained weight loss 3. Lymphadenopathy 4. Pneumocystis pneumonia 5. Kaposi's sarcoma 6. Diarrhea	Treat symptomatically. Frequently, no treatment is effective (see p. 886).	HTLV-III antibody test (detects antibodies in virus). Individuals in high-risk groups should be discouraged from donation: 1. Sexually active homosexual or bisexual males with multiple partners 2. Recent Haitian entrants 3. Present or past IV drug abusers 4. Those with symptoms suggestive of AIDS
5. Syphilis	Spirochetemia caused by *Treponema pallidum*. Incubation 4–18 weeks	1. Presence of chancre 2. Regional lymphadenopathy 3. Generalized rash	Penicillin therapy	Test blood prior to transfusion (rapid plasma reagin—RPR). Organism will not remain viable in blood stored 24–48 hours at 4°C.

(2) NonA nonB hepatitis

(3) Epstein–Barr virus, cytomegalovirus, malaria, toxoplasmosis

(4) AIDS (acquired immunodeficiency syndrome)

(5) Syphilis

3. See Table 8-3 for causes, clinical manifestations, management, and prevention of these delayed reactions.

▶ **NURSING ALERT:** Careful handwashing with solutions containing iodine are recommended after handling blood products. Gloves should be worn when handling body fluids of patients having known infectious agents. Clean blood spills thoroughly with a 1:10 solution of sodium hypochlorite (bleach). Health workers routinely exposed to patients with hepatitis B may elect to receive hepatitis B vaccine, which stimulates the production of antibody to the hepatitis B virus.

Bone Marrow Transplantation

Bone marrow transplantation is the aspiration of nucleated cells (polymorphonuclear leukocytes, monocytes, and lymphocytes) from the bone marrow of a donor for peripheral reinfusion to a recipient who needs reconstitution of hematologic and immunologic function.

The infused donor marrow migrates to the recipient marrow spaces, where engraftment occurs. The donor cells proliferate in the marrow, releasing functional cells into the peripheral circulation.

Indications for Bone Marrow Transplantation

1. When the patient's disease is refractory to conventional therapy

2. The following diseases have been successfully treated with bone marrow transplantation:
   a. Leukemia, lymphoma, neuroblastoma
   b. Aplastic anemia; Fanconi's anemia
   c. Thalassemia

Donor Selection

Successful transplant usually depends on the availability of a compatible donor. Compatibility testing includes:

1. ABO testing—ABO compatible donors are preferred. If donor is ABO incompatible, recipient alloantibody titers must be reduced through methods such as plasma exchange.
2. Human leukocyte antigen typing (HLA)—One set of HLA genes (one haplotype) is inherited from each parent, making four possible combinations and a 25% chance of a match between siblings.
3. Mixed lymphocyte culture (MLC)—establishes donor/recipient HLA-D compatibility.

Types of Bone Marrow Transplants

1. Autologous—cryopreservation of patient's own marrow during a remission of neoplastic disease for reinfusion as autograft in the event of relapse.
2. Syngeneic—donor and recipient are identical twins.

3. Allogeneic HLA matched—transplant between HLA identical sibling or nonsibling.
4. Allogeneic HLA mismatched—transplantation of nonhistocompatible marrow. Successful only if T-lymphocytes are removed from donor marrow.

Marrow Collection

1. Both the marrow donor and recipient must be well-informed prior to treatment.
2. The donor spends 1–3 days in the hospital for a complete workup to ensure donor suitability. To avoid anemia, many donors give their own blood months or weeks prior to donation to be stored and returned during bone marrow aspiration. The risks of disease transmission are therefore eliminated.
3. In the operating room, a general anesthetic is given and 400–800 ml. of marrow is aspirated from multiple sites in the iliac crest or sternum.
4. A large pressure dressing is applied to the sites and should remain intact for several hours. No long-term adverse effects have been documented following bone marrow donation.
5. The marrow is filtered, and if storage is to exceed a few days, it is usually placed in a cryoprotective substance, placed in a freezing container, and frozen until immediately prior to transfusion.

Table 8-4 Complications of Bone Marrow Transplantation

Complication	Clinical Manifestations	Treatment/Nursing Interventions	Prevention
Infection	Fever, chills, hypotension, flushing, localized inflammation, cough, white patches in mouth, urinary frequency or burning	Broad-spectrum antibiotics until organism is identified, then more specific antibiotic Antifungal agents for persistent fevers Tepid sponge baths, hypothermia blankets, and acetaminophen may relieve symptoms.	"Sterilize" the alimentary tract with nonabsorbable antibiotics prior to the initiation of chemotherapy and/or radiation. Provide a pathogen-free environment (laminar flow room), if available. Otherwise, reverse isolation should be maintained until the peripheral polymorphonuclear count is >500/mm³. In spite of precautions, infection is a major cause of death.
Bleeding	Petechiae, ecchymoses, epistaxis, bleeding gums, hematuria, guaiac-positive stools, uncontrolled menses, headache, and neurologic changes	Prophylactic platelet transfusions if peripheral platelet count less than 20,000/mm³. Actively bleeding patients should be transfused if <50,000/mm³. Provera is administered to control menses.	Avoid invasive procedures such as IM injections. Use Toothettes® to administer mouth care, rather than toothbrush. Instruct patient to avoid blowing the nose or straining with stools.
Stomatitis	Ulcerations, white plaques, red swollen gums, reduced salivation	Meticulous mouth care every 2–4 hours—including saline rinse and gentle swabbing. Antifungal rinses (nystatin) may be prescribed. Local and even IV analgesics may be required.	Stomatitis is usually an unpreventable side effect of both radiation and chemotherapy.
Venocclusive disease (VOD)	Hepatomegaly, elevated bilirubin, heart failure, encephalopathy	Treat symptomatically	No measures prevent the occurrence of this complication in 25% of bone marrow transplant (BMT) patients; fatal in 40% of those patients.
Graft-versus-host disease (GVHD)	Acute—faint, red maculopapular rash 7–14 days posttransplant Chronic—firm, inelastic skin, ulcerations, and/or contractures Mucosal degeneration leading to guaiac-positive diarrhea, nausea, vomiting, ascites, and malnutrition Hepatosplenomegaly	Apply creams and ointments to relieve itching and skin discomfort. Administer IV fluids and hyperalimentation. Parenteral analgesics may be required to relieve pain. ATG—anti-thymocyte globulin may be administered to reduce donor lymphocytes. Observe closely during administration. ATG is made from horse serum and can cause an anaphylactic response.	Select histocompatible donor. Irradiate all blood products prior to infusion. Administer chemotherapy agents and steroids to inhibit immune response. In spite of preventive measures, GVHD occurs in 30%–70% of BMT patients—fatal in 20%–40% of those affected.

Recipient Preparation

1. To inhibit the natural immune response to a foreign substance, the recipient marrow must be ablated.
   a. Marrow ablation is accomplished by the administration of high-dose cytotoxic drugs, sometimes in combination with total body irradiation.
   b. After the chemotherapeutic drugs have left the circulatory system (usually within 2–3 days), the donor marrow is infused.
2. Bone marrow is similar in appearance to red blood cells and identical precautions must be used to ensure accurate recipient identification.
3. Begin the infusion slowly, periodically comparing temperature, pulse, and BP with baseline vital signs. Bone marrow infusion can provoke the same adverse reactions as blood transfusion, chills, fever, and rash being most common.
4. Exactly how the marrow migrates to the marrow spaces is not known, but signs of engraftment—the appearance of erythrocytes, leukocytes, and thrombocytes—should begin within a few weeks.
5. Complete marrow recovery may require 6–8 weeks.

Posttransfusion Observation

1. During total marrow aplasia, the patient requires intensive nursing care.
2. The nurse must observe the patient for the complications outlined in Table 8-4.
   a. Infection
   b. Bleeding
   c. Stomatitis
   d. Venocclusive disease (VOD)
   e. Graft-versus-host disease (GVHD)
3. The patient must be prepared to deal with prolonged confinement, discomfort, and possibly sterility, disfigurement, and death.
4. Be an empathetic resource to the patient and family.

Bibliography

Blood Disorders

Books

Colman RW et al. Hemostasis and Thrombosis. Philadelphia, JB Lippincott, 1982

Everson LK. Hematologic Diseases. New Hyde Park, NY, Medical Examination Publisher, 1983

Gunz FW and Henderson ES. Leukemia, 4th ed. New York, Grune & Stratton, 1983

Hocking WG. Practical Hematology. New York, John Wiley & Sons, 1983

Lindenbaum J (ed). Nutrition in Hematology. New York, Churchill Livingstone, 1983

Newcom SR and Kadin ME. Hematologic Malignancies in the Adult. Menlo Park, CA, Addison-Wesley, 1982

Richards JDM, Linch DC and Goldstone AH. A Synopsis of Haematology. Boston, Wright, 1983

Spivak JL. Fundamentals of Clinical Hematology, 2nd ed. New York, Harper & Row, 1984

Sun NCJ. Hematology. Philadelphia, WB Saunders, 1983

Yasko JM. Guidelines for Cancer Care: Symptom Management. Reston, VA, Reston, 1983

Articles

Anemias

Alavi JB. Aplastic anemia associated with intravenous chloramphenicol. Am J Hematol 1983; 15(4):375–379

Camitta BM, Storb R and Thomas ED. Aplastic anemia (first of two parts): Pathogenesis, diagnosis, treatment, and prognosis. N Engl J Med 1982 Mar 18; 308(11):645–652

Camitta BM, Storb R and Thomas ED. Aplastic anemia (second of two parts): Pathogenesis, diagnosis, treatment, and prognosis. N Engl J Med 1982 Mar 25; 306(12):712–718

Charlton RW and Bothwell TH. Definition, prevalence and prevention of iron deficiency. Clin Haematol 1982 June; 11(2):309–325

Cook JD and Reusser ME. Iron fortification: An update. Am J Clin Nutr 1983 Oct; 38(4):648–659

Dinsmore R and O'Reilly RJ. Bone marrow transplantation: Current status. Pathobiol Annu 1982; 12:213–231

Evans DL, Edelsohn GA and Golden RN. Organic psychosis without anemia or spinal cord symptoms in patients with vitamin B12 deficiency. Am J Psychiatry 1983 Feb; 140(2):218–221

Fairbanks VF, Wahner HW and Phyliky RL. Tests for pernicious anemia: The "Schilling test." Mayo Clin Proc 1983 Aug; 58(8):541–544

Hutchison MM. Aplastic anemia. Care of the bone-marrow-failure patient. Nurs Clin North Am 1983 Sept; 18(3):543–551

Levine AS (ed). Proceedings of the conference on aplastic anemia: A stem cell disease. US Department of Health and Human Services, Washington, DC, NIH Pub, 81-1008; June 1981

Maxfield DL and Boyd WC. Pernicious anemia: A review, an update, and an illustrative case. J Am Osteopath Assoc 1983 Oct; 83(2):133–142

Ramsay NKC et al. Total lymphoid irradiation and cyclophosphamide conditioning prior to bone marrow transplantation for patients with severe aplastic anemia. Blood 1983 Sept; 62(3):622–626

Rappeport JM and Nathan DG. Acquired aplastic anemias: Pathophysiology and treatment. Adv Intern Med 1982; 27:547–590

Spruce W, McMillan R and Beutler E. Bone marrow transplantation for the treatment of severe aplastic anaemia. Clin Haematol 1983 Feb; 12(1):285–310

Polycythemia/Agranulocytosis

Adamson JW. The polycythemias: Diagnosis and treatment. Hosp Pract 1983 Dec; 18(12):49–57

dePauw BE et al. Randomized study of ceftazidime versus gentamicin plus cefotaxime for infections in severe granulocytopenic patients. J Antimicrob Chemother 1983 July; 12(Suppl):93–99

Heit WFW. Hematologic effects of antipyretic analgesics. Drug-induced agranulocytosis. Am J Med 1983 Nov 14; 75(5A):65–69

Klastersky J. Management of infection in granulocytopenic patients. J Antimicrob Chemother 1983 Aug; 12(2):102–104

Leukemia

Campbell JB, Preston R and Smith KY. The leukemias. Nurs Clin North Am 1983 Sept; 18(3):523–541

Cork A. Chromosomal abnormalities in leukemia. Am J Med Technol 1983 Oct; 49(10):703–714

Dwyer JE and Held DM. Home management of the adult patient with leukemia. Nurs Clin North Am 1982 Dec; 17(4):665–675

Frenkel EP and Graham MS. Clinical forms of chronic lymphocytic leukemia. Postgrad Med 1984 Mar; 75(4):101–110

Goldman JM and Baughan A. Application of bone marrow transplantation in chronic granulocytic leukemia. Clin Haematol 1983 Oct; 12(3):739–753

Green BG, Adler SS and Knospe WH. Bone marrow transplantation in leukemia. Postgrad Med 1983 Aug; 74(2):123–140

Kelly JO. Standards of clinical nursing practice for leukemia: Neutropenia and thrombocytopenia. Cancer Nurs 1983 Dec; 6(6):487–494

Martin JK Jr et al. Hickman catheter implantation in the treatment of acute leukemia. Arch Surg 1983 Oct; 118(10):1224–1226

Peterson D and Sonis S (eds). Oral complications of cancer

chemotherapy. Devel Oncology 1983; 12:entire volume

Sondel PM. Bone marrow transplantation as immunotherapy. Wis Med J 1983 Oct; 82(10):17–19

Storb R and Santos GW. Application of bone marrow transplantation in leukaemia and aplastic anaemia. Clin Haematol 1983 Oct; 12(3):721–737

Talpaz M et al. Human leukocyte interferon to control thrombocytosis in chronic myelogenous leukemia. Ann Intern Med 1983 Dec; 99(6):789–792

Wessler RM. Care of the hospitalized adult patient with leukemia. Nurs Clin North Am 1982 Dec; 17(4):649–663

Lymphomas

Bonadonna G. Chemotherapy strategies to improve the control of Hodgkin's disease. Cancer Res 1982 Nov; 42(11):4309–4320

Bonadonna G and Santoro A. Evolution in the treatment strategy of Hodgkin's disease. Adv Cancer Res 1982; 36:257–293

Canellos GP, Come SE and Skarin AT. Chemotherapy in the treatment of Hodgkin's disease. Semin Hematol 1983 Jan; 20(1):1–24

Cotter GW et al. Palliative radiation treatment of cutaneous mycosis fungoides—A dose response. Int J Radiat Oncol Biol Phys 1983 Oct; 9(10):1477–1480

DeVita VT Jr et al. The cure of Hodgkin's disease with drugs. Adv Intern Med 1983; 28:277–302

Drug selection in the treatment of Hodgkin's disease. Hematol Oncology 1983 Jan–Mar; 1(1):3–12

Durie BGM and Salmon SE. The current status and future prospects of treatment for multiple myeloma. Clin Hematol 1982 Feb; 11(1):181–210.

Eddy JL, Selgas-Cordes R and Curran M. Cutaneous T-cell lymphoma. Am J Nurs 1984 Feb; 84(2):202–206

Eddy J, Cordes RS and Curran M. Sam was dying—We had to help him live again. Nursing '81 1981 Aug; 11(8):42–45

Ganeval D et al. Kidney involvement in multiple myeloma and related disorders. Contrib Nephrol 1982; 33:210–222

Hagan SJ. Bring help and hope to the patient with Hodgkin's disease. Nursing '83 1983 Aug; 13(8):58–63

Haserick JR, Richardson JH and Grant DJ. Remission of lesions in mycosis fungoides following topical application of nitrogen mustard. Cleve Clin Q 1983 Summer; 50(2):91–95

Hays K and Rafferty DC. Care of the patient with malignant lymphoma. Nurs Clin North Am 1982 Dec; 17(4):677–695

Price NM, Hoppe RT and Deneau DG. Ointment-based mechlorethamine treatment for mycosis fungoides. Cancer 1983 Dec 15; 52(12):2214–2219

Rotstein H. The management of minimal extent mycosis fungoides. Int J Dermatol 1983 Nov; 22(9):515–517

Rowan RM. Multiple myeloma: Some recent developments. Clin Lab Haematol 1982; 4(3):211–230

Vonderheid EC and Van Scott EJ. Commentary and update: Topical chemotherapy with mechlorethamine for mycosis fungoides. Cleve Clin Q 1983 Summer; 50(2):97–100

Yasko JM. Care of the patient receiving radiation therapy. Nurs Clin North Am 1982 Dec; 17(4):631–648

Bleeding Disorders

Aster RH. Immune thrombocytopenias. Hosp Pract 1983 Nov; 18(11):187–190, 194–195, 198–199

Burns TR and Saleem A. Idiopathic thrombocytopenic purpura. Am J Med 1983 Dec; 75(6):1001–1007

Caplin M. Disseminated intravascular coagulation: A multisystem problem. Dimens Crit Care Nurs 1984 Mar–Apr; 3(2):76–83

Feinstein DI. Diagnosis and management of disseminated intravascular coagulation: The role of heparin therapy. Blood 1982 Aug; 60(2):284–287

Hewitt PE and Davies SC. The current state of DIC. Intensive Care Med 1983; 9(5):249–252

Kelton JG and Gibbons S. Autoimmune platelet destruction: Idiopathic thrombocytopenic purpura. Semin Thrombo Hemost 1982 Apr; 8(2):83–104

Kigan R and Laros RK. Immune thrombocytopenia. Clin Obstet Gynecol 1983 Sept; 26(3):537–546

Kirchner CW and Reheis CE. Two serious complications of neoplasia: Sepsis and disseminated intravascular coagulation. Nurs Clin North Am 1982 Dec; 17(4):595–606

Rosse WT. Treatment of chronic immune thrombocytopenia. Clin Haematol 1983 Feb; 12(1):267–284

Sherman LA. DIC in massive transfusion. Prog Clin Biol Res 1982; 108:171–189

Walter J. Care of the patient receiving antineoplastic drugs. Nurs Clin North Am 1982 Dec; 17(4):607–629

Weinstein SM. Disseminated intravascular coagulation. NITA 1982 May–June; 5(3):169–172.

Zimmerman TS and Ruggeri ZM. Von Willebrand's disease. Clin Haematol 1983 Feb; 12(1):175–200

Splenectomy/Polycythemia

Ellison EC and Fabri PJ. Complications of splenectomy. Etiology, prevention, and management. Surg Clin North Am 1983 Dec; 63(6):1313–1330

Forward AD. Splenectomy for hematologic disease. Can J Surg 1983 Nov; 26(5):441–442

Karpatkin S. The spleen and thrombocytopenia. Clin Haematol 1983 June; 12(2):591–604

Merl SA et al. Splenectomy for thrombocytopenia in chronic lymphocytic leukemia. Am J Hematol 1983 Nov; 15(3):253–259

Mitchell A and Morris PJ. Surgery of the spleen. Clin Haematol 1984 June; 12(2):565–590

Sekikawa T and Shatney CH. Septic sequelae after splenectomy for trauma in adults. Am J Surg 1983 May; 145(5):667–673

Transfusion Therapy

Books

Chisari F, Alter H and Dienstag J. Advances in Hepatitis Research, pp 281–292. New York, Masson, 1984

Mollison PL. Blood Transfusion in Clinical Medicine, 7th ed. Boston, Blackwell Scientific Publications, 1983

Rutnam RC and Miller WV. Transfusion Therapy Principles and Procedures. Rockville, MD, Aspen Systems Corp, 1982

Snyder EL. Blood Transfusion Therapy. Arlington, American Association of Blood Banks, 1983

Widman FK. Technical Manual of the American Association of Blood Banks, 8th ed. Washington, JB Lippincott, 1981

Articles

Berkman SA. The spectrum of transfusion reactions. Hosp Pract 1984 June; 19(6):205–219

Bourn R. The blood transfusion nurse. Nurs. Mirror 1983 Jun 1; 156(22):50

Clough JD and Paganini EP. Therapeutic plasmapheresis. Postgrad Med 1984 May 15; 75(7):77–84

Cowart VS. Blood substitutes: Two ways to get there. JAMA 1983 Jan 14; 249(2):159–164

Masoorli ST and Piercy S. A step-by-step guide to trouble free transfusions. RN 1984 May; 47(5):34–42

Nuscher R et al. Bone marrow transplantation. Am J Nurs 1984 June; 84(6):764–772

Parker N and Cohen T. Acute graft-versus-host disease in allogeneic marrow transplantation. Nurs Clin North Am 1983 Sept; 18(3):569–577

Pauley SY. Administrative aspects of transfusion. NITA 1983 Mar–Apr; 6(2):117–121

Querin JJ and Stahl LD. 12 simple sensible steps for successful blood transfusions. Nursing '83 1983 Nov; 13(11):34–43

Sadler C. Banking on blood. Nurs Mirror 1983 Apr 13; 156(15):18–22

Salinger J. If your patient gets a bone marrow transplant. RN 1984 May; 47(5):62–68

Schmidt PJ. Transfusion mortality. AORN J 1981 Dec; 34(6):1114–1122

Weir JA. Blood components and transfusion reactions. NITA 1982 Sept–Oct; 5(5):320–323

Woods ME and Mazza I. Blood and component therapy. Nurs Clin North Am 1980 Sept; 15(3):629–646

Agencies

American Association of Blood Banks
1828 L Street, NW
Washington, DC 20036

Leukemia Society of America
800 Second Avenue
New York, NY 10017

US Department of Health and Human Services
National Heart, Lung and Blood Institute
Blood Diseases and Resources Division
National Institutes of Health
Bethesda, MD 20205

Cardiovascular Disorders

9

1: Cardiac Disorders

Manifestations of Heart Disease

The patient's symptoms of heart disease depend on:
1. Nature of cardiopathy
2. Resultant physiological disturbances of the circulation

Dyspnea

Dyspnea is undue breathlessness, an awareness of discomfort associated with breathing.

A. General Features
1. Dyspnea of cardiac origin—failure of left ventricle characterized by increased left atrial, pulmonary venous and capillary pressures; as left atrial pressure rises, the lungs become congested resulting in dyspnea.
2. The threshold (tolerance) for dyspnea varies with the individual.

B. Types of Cardiac Dyspnea
1. *Exertional dyspnea*—breathlessness upon moderate exertion, which is relieved by rest.
2. *Orthopnea*—shortness of breath when lying down, which is relieved by promptly sitting upright.
3. *Paroxysmal nocturnal dyspnea*—sudden dyspnea at night while lying down.
4. *Cheyne–Stokes respiration*—periodic breathing characterized by gradual increase in depth of respiration, followed by a decrease in respiration resulting in apnea; periods of hyperpnea alternating with periods of apnea.
   a. Cheyne–Stokes respiration is usually considered a serious sign.
   b. Associated with left ventricular failure (severe), cerebral vascular disease.

C. Nursing Assessment of Dyspnea

1. What precipitates or relieves the dyspnea?
2. What position does the patient assume?
3. What is the skin color? Pallor? Cyanosis?

Chest Pain

A. Cardiac Causes of Chest Pain

1. Ischemia caused by an increase in demand for coronary blood flow and oxygen delivery, which exceeds available blood supply; due to coronary artery disease (angina pectoris, myocardial infarction).
2. Excruciating pain radiating to back and flanks—from acute dissecting aneurysm of the aorta.
3. Sharp precordial pain (over heart area) radiating to left shoulder and upper back, aggravated by respirations—indicates acute pericarditis.

B. Assessment of Patient with Chest Pain

1. Where is pain located? Does it radiate? To neck? Face? Back? Abdominal area?
2. What is the character of the pain—dull, sharp, boring, crushing?
3. Are there associated symptoms and signs? Diaphoresis? Light-headedness? Nausea? Shortness of breath?
4. What are the time and mode of onset?
5. How long does the episode last?
6. What factors precipitate pain (breathing, coughing, swallowing, rapid walking, emotional stress, exposure to cold)?
7. What factors alleviate pain (rest, change in position, nitroglycerin)?

Palpitation

Palpitation is a rapid, forceful, or irregular heartbeat felt by the patient.

A. General Features

1. The patient complains of pounding, jumping, stopping sensations in his chest.
2. May be associated with heart disease—enlargement of heart, disturbances of rhythm.
3. Other causes—anxiety, fever, anemia, thyroid disturbances, and reactions to certain drugs.

B. Nursing Assessment

1. Notify physician and take ECG during episodes of palpitation—for later interpretation.
2. Compare apical and a peripheral pulse.
3. Note concomitant symptoms—dizziness, chest pain, dyspnea.
4. Take blood pressure to check for hemodynamic changes.

Edema

Edema is an abnormal accumulation of serous fluid in the connective tissues.

A. General Features

1. Cardiac causes of edema—congestive heart failure
2. Other causes of edema—sodium retention, liver disease, renal disease, hypoproteinemia, venous or lymphatic obstruction

B. Types

1. Ascites—excessive fluid in peritoneal cavity
2. Pleural effusion—excessive fluid in the pleural cavity
3. Anasarca—gross generalized edema

C. Nursing Implications

1. In heart conditions the location of edema is influenced by gravity. Fluid collects in the lower parts of the body (dependent edema).
   a. Evaluate for edema of ankles and feet in the ambulatory patient.
   b. Evaluate for edema of sacral area and posterior thighs in patients confined to bed.
2. Avoid undue pressure on edematous areas. Edematous patients are prone to develop pressure sores.

Fatigue

1. Fatigue associated with heart disease is produced by low cardiac output.
2. As heart disease advances, fatigue is precipitated by less and less effort.

Dizziness and Syncope

May be caused by fall in cardiac output with resulting cerebral ischemia: may be secondary to arrhythmias, atrioventricular block, carotid-sinus sensitivity, and cerebrovascular obstructive disease.

Skin Color and Temperature

Examine for change in skin color: pallor, flushing, cyanosis, jaundice. *Cyanosis* is a bluish discoloration of the skin and mucous membranes.

A. Types of Cyanosis

1. Central cyanosis—low oxygen saturation of arterial blood
2. Peripheral cyanosis—reduction of oxyhemoglobin in capillaries from restricted circulation (low output or vasoconstriction)

B. Cardiac Causes of Cyanosis

1. Congenital heart disease—due to mixing of arterial stream with venous blood
2. Congestive heart failure and pulmonary edema—due to hypoxia resulting from low cardiac output and poor oxygenation of blood by lungs

C. Nursing Assessment

1. Look at lobes of ears, fingernail beds, and palms.
2. Look in mouth—less color variation in mucous membranes.
3. Palpate for sweaty, cold, clammy, warm, or dry skin.
4. Evaluate for jaundice—may indicate congestive heart failure associated with severe liver congestion.

Hemoptysis

Hemoptysis is the coughing up of blood.

1. Small quantities of dark, clotted blood may indicate mitral stenosis, but more commonly associated with pulmonary embolism and pulmonary infarction.
2. Mixture of blood and pus—indicates pulmonary suppuration.
3. Pink, frothy sputum—indicates acute pulmonary edema.
4. Blood-streaked sputum—indicates acute pulmonary congestion.
5. Frank hemoptysis—due to lung pathology.

Abdominal Pain or Discomfort

1. Epigastric (upper abdominal) pain—due to myocardial infarction, distention of liver capsule from congestive heart failure.
2. Severe abdominal pain—may be due to dissection of the abdominal aorta or rupture of an aortic abdominal aneurysm.
3. Intermittent abdominal pain (related to food intake) may indicate circulatory insufficiency of mesenteric arteries or noncardiac pain.

Other Manifestations of Heart Disease

1. Distention of neck veins—may be produced by pressure on liver (hepatojugular reflux), congestive heart failure, pericardial compression due to effusion, or constrictive pericarditis.
2. Digital clubbing (clubbing of fingers)—due to cyanotic congenital heart disease, bacterial endocarditis, certain forms of lung pathology; may also be familial.
3. Jaundice—congestive heart failure associated with severe liver congestion.

Diagnostic Evaluation for Heart Disease

Physical Assessment

A. Arterial Pulse

1. Examine the pulses bilaterally; peripheral pulses should be equal.
   a. Note amplitude (fullness), which depends on pulse pressure (difference between systolic and diastolic pressures); this gives an estimate of stroke volume.
      (1) Small volume pulse may be from low stroke volume and peripheral vasoconstriction (myocardial infarction, shock, constrictive pericarditis, vasoconstrictive drugs).
      (2) Large volume pulse produced by large stroke volume (aortic regurgitation, pregnancy, thyrotoxicosis, bradycardia, patent ductus arteriosus).
   b. Palpate carotid artery—reveals character of pulse in the proximal aorta and provides indication of any abnormality causing disease of left ventricle.

B. Blood Pressure

1. Take on both arms; subsequently blood pressure is taken on right arm.
2. Measure blood pressure with patient supine and standing.
3. Document site of blood pressure measurement and position of patient. (See also page 380 for further discussion of technique.)

C. Respiration

Note rate, depth, and respiratory pattern.

D. Jugular Venous Pulse

1. Venous pulsation can be more easily seen than felt.
2. Identification of venous pulse permits assessment of height of venous pressure.
3. See page 35 for technique.

E. Heart Auscultation

1. Heart auscultation requires knowledge, experience, and a "listening ear" tuned to hear each event of the cardiac cycle.
2. Heart auscultation should be systematic, and the stethoscope should "inch" from one area to another.
3. Four main areas of auscultation: aortic area, pulmonary area, mitral area, and the tricuspid area.
4. Listen for rate and regularity of rhythm.
   a. Determine if an irregularity is related to respiratory movements.
   b. Evaluate the sequence in which an irregularity occurs.

5. During auscultation, the examiner assesses the venous pulse, feels the pulsation of the right carotid artery and the radial artery, feels precordial movement, and listens to the heart.
6. See Chapter 4 for a more complete discussion of heart examination and examination of abdomen and extremities.

Cardiographic Studies

A. Electrocardiogram—a visual representation of the electrical activity of the heart as reflected by changes in electrical potential at the skin surface.

1. ECG is obtained by placing leads on various body parts and recording the electrical impulse as a tracing on a strip of paper or on the screen of an oscilloscope.
2. Clinical usefulness—evaluation of conditions that interfere with normal electrophysiological function—disturbances of rhythm, disorders of cardiac muscle, enlargement of chambers of heart, presence of myocardial infarction, electrolyte disturbances.
3. See page 334 for a more detailed account.

B. Echocardiography (Ultrasound Cardiography)—a record of high-frequency sound vibrations that have been sent into the heart through the chest wall. The cardiac structures return the echoes derived from the ultrasound. The motions of the echoes are traced on an oscilloscope and recorded on film.

1. The patient is placed in supine position, and the transducer is placed on his chest.
2. Transducer is applied (left sternal border) with ultrasonic gel to maintain airless contact between skin and transducer.
3. ECG is recorded simultaneously to time the events within cardiac cycle. (Two-dimensional echocardiography now in use.)
4. *Clinical usefulness*
   a. Demonstration of valvular and other structural deformities
   b. Detection of pericardial effusion
   c. Evaluation of prosthetic valve function
   d. Diagnosis of cardiac tumors; asymmetric thickening of interventricular septum
   e. Diagnosis of cardiomegaly (heart enlargement)

C. Ambulatory Electrocardiographic Monitoring—continuous recording of an ECG to monitor the heartbeat while the patient goes about his daily routine.

1. Patient wears miniaturized tape-recording device us-

ing a single- or double-lead system attached to belt or worn on a shoulder strap.

2. Patient keeps a diary—records his activities and any symptoms that are noted; useful when symptoms are provoked by specific activities (jogging, stress); used for assessing patients who suffer from transient dizziness, syncope, or near syncope; detecting arrhythmias; assessing response to therapy; and evaluating patients after myocardial infarction.

D. Exercise Stress Testing—exercise testing on a treadmill or a bicycle-like device carried out to identify ischemic heart disease, to evaluate patients with chest pain, to assess results of therapy, and to aid in developing individual physical fitness programs.

1. Obtain informed consent—patient advised of purpose and risks of test.
2. ECG electrodes applied to patient and tracings made before, during, and after exercise testing.
3. Patient is exercised by increasing walking speed and the incline of the treadmill or by increasing the load against which he pedals.
4. Instruct patient to avoid smoking, eating, and drinking for 4 hours prior to test and to rest and avoid stimulants or extreme temperature changes after the test.

E. Phonocardiography—graphic recording of the heart sounds and pulse waves and their relation to time.

1. Helps to identify, to accurately time, and to differentiate various sounds and murmurs.
2. Provides a permanent record for future comparison.

F. Vectorcardiography—presents a three-dimensional view of the electrical forces of the heart.

1. Amplifies understanding of the ECG.
2. Gives more specific information in certain situations than the standard electrocardiogram.

G. Myocardial Imaging (Radionuclide imaging)

With the use of radionuclides and scintillation cameras, radionuclide angiograms can be utilized to assess left ventricular performance.

1. *"Hot spot" or positive imaging*
   a. Technetium-99m stannous pyrophosphate is a radionuclide most commonly utilized. Necrosed or ischemic myocardium takes up the phosphate and produces a "hot spot" indicative of a positive scan.
   b. Scans become positive within 12–36 hours and are usually negative after 7 days.
   c. Utilized when diagnosis of myocardial infarction (MI) is unclear. Not employed in routine workup for diagnostic evaluation of MI.
2. *"Cold spot" imaging*
   a. Thallium-201 most common isotope utilized. Thallium-201 concentrates in myocardial cells relative to blood flow. Areas of low concentration are termed "cold spots."
   b. Differentiation between old and new infarctions cannot be determined with this method and no distinction can be made between areas of infarction and ischemia.
   c. A normal thallium scan is likely to rule out the diagnosis of myocardial infarction. Usually not

employed in routine workup for diagnostic evaluation of MI.

3. *Radionuclide ventriculogram*
   a. A noninvasive method for accurate assessment of ventricular hemodynamics, and regional wall motion.
   b. Provides measurements of right and left ventricular ejection fraction, distinguishes regional from global ventricular wall motion, and allows for subjective analysis of cardiac anatomy to detect intracardiac shunts, and valvular or congenital abnormalities.
   c. A radiopharmaceutical (usually Technetium-99m) is injected rapidly through a central venous catheter, Swan–Ganz catheter, or antecubital vein.
   d. Indices of ventricular performance are measured from the initial transit of the radiotracer through the heart.

Roentgenologic Studies

A. Chest X-Ray—shows heart size, contour, and position; reveals cardiac and pericardial calcifications and demonstrates physiologic alterations in pulmonary circulation.

B. Fluoroscopy—provides visual observation of the heart on a luminescent x-ray screen.

1. Shows heart and vascular pulsations; useful in the assessment of unusual cardiac contours and especially calcifications.
2. Useful in placement and positioning of intravenous electrodes and for guiding the catheter in cardiac catheterization.

C. Angiocardiography—injection of contrast medium into the vascular system (to outline the heart and blood vessels) accompanied by *cineangiograms* (rapidly changing films or movies on an intensified fluoroscopic screen), which record the passage of contrast media through the vascular tree.

Useful for providing information regarding coronary anatomy, structural abnormalities (occlusions, defects, fistulae) or abnormal heart valve function.

1. *Selective angiocardiography*—contrast medium is injected through a catheter directly into one of the heart chambers, coronary arteries, or greater vessels, and the angiocardiogram is recorded by means of a rapid film changer or motion picture camera.
2. *Aortography*—a form of angiography that outlines the lumen of the aorta and major arteries arising from it.
3. *Coronary arteriography* (most common form of selective angiocardiography)—a radiopaque catheter is introduced into the right brachial artery via open arteriotomy (or femoral artery via percutaneous puncture), passed into the ascending aorta, and manipulated into appropriate coronary artery under fluoroscopic control.
   a. Used as an evaluation tool before coronary artery surgery or myocardial revascularization and after surgery to evaluate graft patency.
   b. Used to study suspected congenital anomalies of the coronary arteries.
4. *Nursing implications in angiocardiography*
   a. Before angiogram
      Keep the patient in a fasting state prior to

examination—to minimize danger of pulmonary aspiration should emesis occur.

b. After angiogram
   (1) Record vital signs every 15 minutes (or more often as patient's condition indicates) until vital signs are stable.
   (2) Check for bleeding at puncture or cutdown site.
   (3) Check distal extremity for normal color and intact pulses.
   (4) The patient may complain of mild headache and/or discomfort in the groin or other site, depending on route by which contrast medium was administered.
   (5) Check for bed rest and special fluid directives from physician.

Cardiac Catheterization

Cardiac catheterization is a diagnostic procedure in which a catheter(s) is (are) introduced into the heart and blood vessels to (1) measure oxygen concentration, saturation, tension, and pressure in the various heart chambers; (2) detect shunts; (3) provide blood samples for analysis; and (4) determine cardiac output and pulmonary blood flow. Cardiac catheterization is also done to assess heart status before heart surgery.

Angiography is usually combined with heart catheterization for coronary artery visualization. During the procedure, the patient is monitored electrocardiographically by means of an oscilloscope.

A. Right-Heart Catheterization—a radiopaque catheter is passed from an antecubital or femoral vein into the right atrium, right ventricle, and pulmonary vasculature under direct visualization with a fluoroscope.

1. Right atrium and right ventricle pressures measured; blood samples taken for hematocrit and oxygen saturation.
2. After entering the right atrium, the catheter is then passed through the tricuspid valve, and similar tests are performed on blood within the right ventricle.
3. Finally the catheter is passed through the pulmonic valve and as far as possible beyond that point; capillary samples are obtained and "capillary pressures" (wedge pressure) are recorded.
4. Complications—cardiac arrhythmias, venous spasm, thrombophlebitis, infection of cutdown site, cardiac perforation, and cardiac tamponade.

B. Left-Heart Catheterization—usually done by retrograde catheterization of the left ventricle or by transseptal catheterization of the left atrium.

1. Retrograde approach—catheter inserted under direct vision into right brachial artery and advanced under fluoroscopic control into the ascending aorta and into the left ventricle; or, catheter may be introduced percutaneously by puncture of femoral artery.
2. Transseptal approach—catheter is passed from the right femoral vein (percutaneously or by saphenous vein cutdown) into right atrium. A long needle is passed up through the catheter and is used to puncture the septum separating the right and left atria; needle is withdrawn and the catheter advanced under fluoroscopic control into left ventricle. Patient is monitored by ECG during both retrograde and transseptal techniques.

a. Gives hemodynamic data—permits flow and pressure measurements of left heart.
b. Most often performed to evaluate the function of the left ventricular muscle and mitral and aortic valves, or the patency of coronary arteries.
c. Used to evaluate patients before and after cardiac surgery.
d. Complications of left heart catheterization and implications for nursing assessment are
   (1) Arrhythmias (ventricular fibrillation), syncope, vasospasm
   (2) Pericardial tamponade, myocardial infarction, pulmonary edema
   (3) Allergic reaction to contrast medium
   (4) Perforation of great vessels of heart; systemic embolization (stroke, MI)
   (5) Loss of pulse distal to arteriotomy and possible ischemia of lower arm and hand.

C. Nursing Management in Heart Catheterization

1. Preceding heart catheterization
   a. Know which approach is to be used in order to anticipate possible complications.
   b. Withhold food and fluid 6 hours before procedure—to prevent vomiting and aspiration.
   c. Ascertain history of previous allergies.
   d. Mark distal pulses—for easy reference after catheterization.
   e. Explain to the patient that he will be lying on an examining table for a prolonged period and that he may experience certain sensations:
      (1) Occasional thudding sensations in the chest—from extrasystoles, particularly when the catheter is manipulated in ventricular chambers.
      (2) Strong desire to cough—may occur during contrast medium injection into right heart during angiography.
      (3) Transient feeling of heat, particularly in the head—from injection of contrast medium.
   f. Remove dentures; give prescribed medication.
2. Following heart catheterization
   a. Record the blood pressure and apical pulse every 15 minutes (or more frequently) until vital signs are stable after the procedure—to discern arrhythmias.
   b. Check peripheral pulses in affected extremity (dorsalis pedis, posterior tibial pulse in the lower extremity, and radial pulse in upper extremity); evaluate extremity temperature, color, and complaints of pain, numbness, or tingling sensation—to determine signs of arterial insufficiency.
   c. Watch puncture (cutdown) sites for hematoma formation. Question patient about increase in pain/tenderness at site.
   d. Assess for complaints of chest pain and report occurrence immediately—myocardial infarction may occur and is a serious complication of cardiac catheterization.
   e. If protocol requires, see that the patient remains in bed with little movement of the involved extremity until the following morning.

Blood Studies

1. CBC
2. Blood electrolytes (potassium, sodium, chloride, car-

bon dioxide)—for patients treated with digitalis or diuretics

3. Blood urea nitrogen and creatinine—to evaluate cardiac output
4. Sedimentation rate, C-reactive protein and antistreptolysin O titer—to rule out inflammatory heart disease
5. Blood culture—to exclude bacterial endocarditis

Enzyme and Isoenzyme Tests

A. Rationale of Tests—the release of enzymes from cells into body fluids and into the circulation provides an indication of tissue damage and of changes taking place within the cells.

B. Underlying Concepts

1. Heart muscle is rich in enzymes that promote different biochemical reactions.
2. When myocardial tissue is damaged (myocardial infarction) certain cardiac enzymes are released into the bloodstream and result in elevated peripheral blood enzyme levels:

Creatine kinase (CK)
Glutamic oxaloacetic transaminase (GOT)
Lactic dehydrogenase (LDH)

3. However, these enzymes may be widely distributed in tissues and elevated in conditions not associated with myocardial infarction (i.e., damage to skeletal muscles, liver, brain, kidneys, and other organs).

C. Isoenzymes—forms of protein species that promote the same biochemical action as enzymes but differ chemically, physically, and/or immunologically.

1. Isoenzymes can be identified by laboratory methods to reveal the specific tissue that is damaged; creatine kinase can be separated into 3 isoenzymes, known as MM, MB, and BB.
2. An elevation of serum CK-MB activity signifies that an adverse effect on myocardial cells has taken place; thus, it is the most specific and sensitive enzymatic criterion of myocardial injury now available. CK-MB greater than 5 IU is significant.

Hemodynamic Monitoring

Hemodynamic monitoring is the assessment of the patient's circulatory status; it includes measurements of heart rate, intra-arterial pressure, pulmonary artery and pulmonary capillary wedge pressures (see below), central venous pressure (p. 286), cardiac output (p. 289), and blood volume.

Guidelines: Measuring Pulmonary Artery Pressure by Flow-Directed Balloon-Tipped Catheter (Swan–Ganz Catheter)

The *Swan–Ganz catheter* is a flow-directed, balloon-tipped, 4-lumen catheter (2- or 3-lumen also available), allowing for ease of right heart catheterization at the bedside and permitting continuous monitoring of right and left ventricular function, pulmonary artery pressures, cardiac output, and arterial venous oxygen difference.
The catheter is 110-cm. long, marked at increments of 10 cm., and is available in diameters of No. 5 and 7 French (Fig. 9-1).

Purposes*

1. To obtain precise hemodynamic data concerning pressures in the right atrium, right ventricle, pulmonary artery, and distal branches of the pulmonary artery (pulmonary capillary wedge pressure). The latter reflects the level of the pressure in the left atrium (or filling pressure in the left ventricle), thus, pressures on the left side of the heart are inferred from pressure measurements obtained on the right side of the circulation.
2. To evaluate the patient and permit rational selection of therapy when critical changes in cardiac dynamics occur.
3. To evaluate the patient's response to implemented therapy.
4. To obtain cardiac output through thermodilution.
5. To obtain mixed venous blood samplings from pulmonary artery.

Underlying Considerations

1. Left atrial pressure is closely related to left ventricular end-diastolic pressure (LVEDP) (filling pressure of the left ventricle) and is therefore an indicator of left ventricular function.
2. Pulmonary artery pressures are important in evaluating patients with cardiogenic shock, severe left ventricular failure with pulmonary edema, mitral regurgitation, and/or ventricular-septal rupture, etc.

Equipment

Swan–Ganz catheter set	Heparin
ECG, monitor and display unit	Antiarrhythmic drugs
Defibrillator	Local anesthetic
Pressure transducer; transducer holder	Skin antiseptic
Cutdown tray	Elastoplast tape
Syringes: tuberculin; 2.5-ml. syringe	Sterile drape/gloves
Sterile saline solution	

* With the placement of 2 or more fine wires into the catheter, additional functions such as intra-atrial electrocardiography, as well as atrial and ventricular pacing, may be achieved.

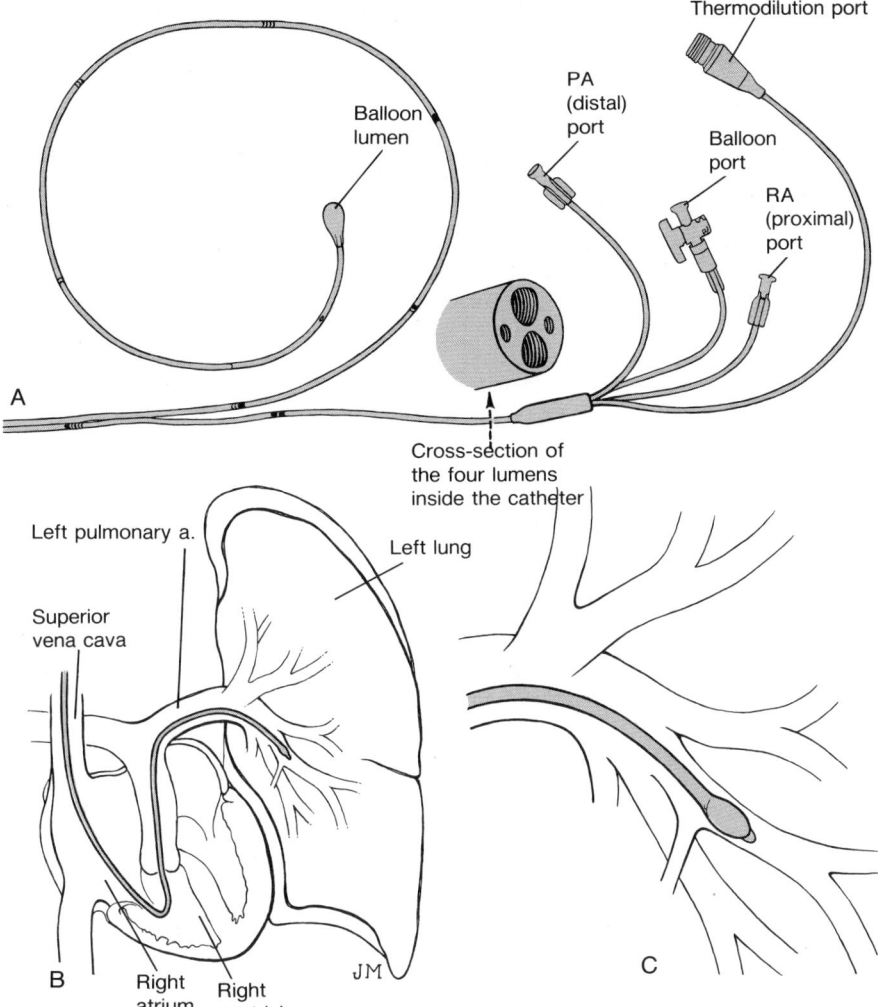

Figure 9-1. (*A*) Swan–Ganz catheter.
(*B*) Location of the Swan–Ganz catheter within the heart. The catheter enters the right atrium via the superior vena cava. The balloon is then inflated, allowing the catheter to follow the blood flow through the tricuspid valve, through the right ventricle, through the pulmonic valve, and into the main pulmonary artery. Wave form and pressure readings are noted during insertion to identify location of the catheter within the heart. The balloon is deflated once the catheter is in the pulmonary artery and properly secured.
(*C*) Pulmonary capillary wedge pressure (PCWP). The catheter floats into a distal branch of the pulmonary artery when the balloon is inflated, and becomes "wedged." The wedged catheter occludes blood flow from behind, and the tip of the lumen records pressures in front of the catheter. The balloon is then deflated, allowing the catheter to float back into the main pulmonary artery.

Procedure (Fig. 9-1)

Nursing Action	Rationale/Amplification
Preparatory Phase (by nurses)	
1. Explain procedure to the patient and family/significant other.	1. Tell the patient he may feel the catheter moving through his vein, and this is normal.
2. Check vital signs and apply ECG electrodes.	
3. Place patient in a position of comfort; this is the baseline position.	3. Note the angle of elevation if patient cannot lie flat as subsequent pressure readings are taken from this baseline position to ensure consistency.

(continued)

Guidelines: Measuring Pulmonary Artery Pressure by Flow-Directed Balloon-Tipped Catheter (Swan-Ganz Catheter) (continued)

Procedure
(Cont.)

Nursing Action	Rationale/Amplification

4. Set up equipment according to manufacturer's directives:
  a. The pulmonary artery catheter requires a transducer; recording, amplifying, and flush systems (Fig. 9-1).
 	
  b. Flush system according to manufacturer's directions.
 	
5. Lower transducer to level of patient's right atrium (phlebostatic level) (Fig. 9-2).
	4. a. Monitoring systems may vary greatly. The complexity of equipment requires an understanding of the equipment in use. A constant microdrip is maintained except when reading pressures.
	  b. Flushing of the catheter system ensures patency and eliminates air bubbles.
	
	5. Pressure is monitored through a fluid-filled column. Any difference between the level of the right atrium where the catheter tip lies and the transducer will result in incorrect pressure readings.

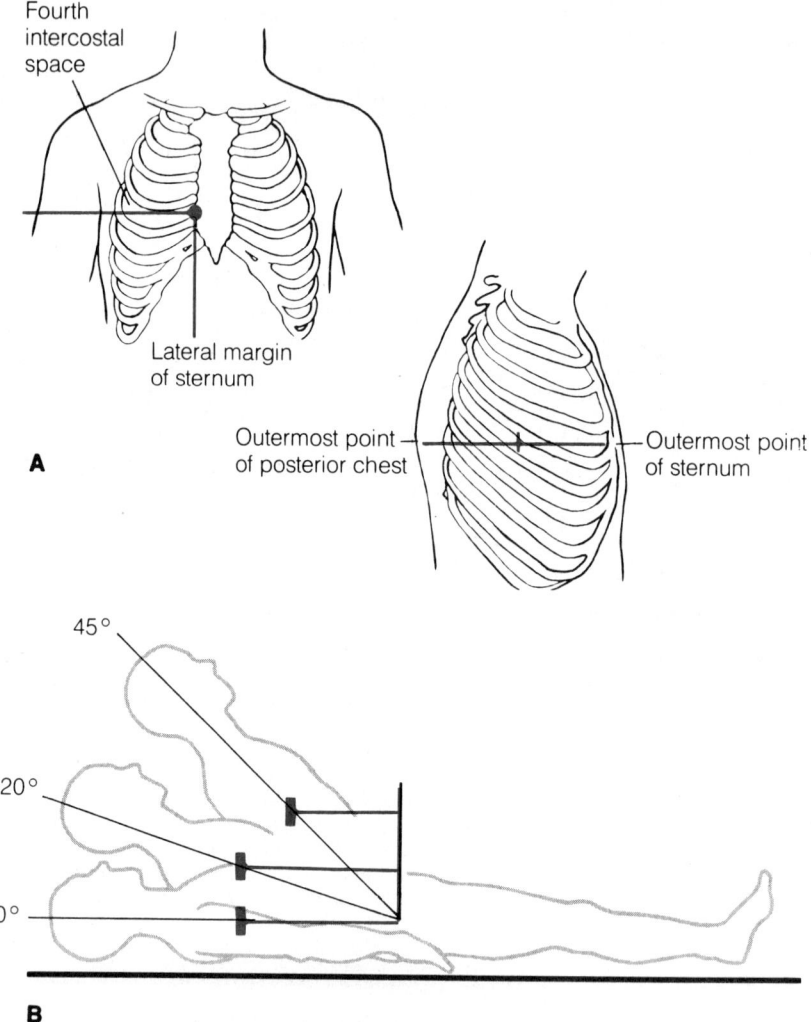

Figure 9-2. The phlebostatic axis and the phlebostatic level. (A) The phlebostatic axis is the crossing of two reference lines: (1) a line from the fourth intercostal space at the point where it joins the sternum, drawn out to the side of the body beneath the axilla; (2) a line midpoint between the anterior and posterior surfaces of the chest. (B) The phlebostatic level is a horizontal line through the phlebostatic axis. The transducer or the zero mark on the manometer must be level with this axis for accurate measurements. As the patient moves from the flat to erect positions, he moves his chest and therefore the reference level; the phlebostatic level stays horizontal through the same reference point. (After Shinn J et al: Heart Lung 8[2]:324, 1979)

Procedure
(Cont.)

Nursing Action	Rationale/Amplification
6. Calibrate pressure equipment.	6. A known quantity of pressure is applied to the transducer (usually by mercury manometer) to ensure accurate monitoring of pressure readings.
7. Shave and prepare skin over insertion site.	7. The catheter is inserted percutaneously at the bedside under sterile conditions.

Performance Phase (by the physician)

1. Physician dons sterile gown and gloves, and places sterile drapes over patient.	1. Sterile field is established to prevent chance of infection.
2. The balloon is inflated with air and then deflated, or it is inflated with air under sterile water or saline to test for leakage (bubbles).	2. To ensure that the balloon is intact.
3. The Swan–Ganz catheter is inserted through the internal jugular, subclavian, or any easily accessible vein by either percutaneous puncture or venotomy.	3. The internal jugular vein establishes a short route into the central venous system.
4. The catheter is advanced to the superior vena cava. Oscillations of the pressure waveforms will indicate when the tip of the catheter is within the thoracic cavity. The patient may be asked to cough.	4. Catheter placement may be determined by characteristic wave forms and changes. Coughing will produce deflections in the pressure tracing when the catheter tip is in the thorax.
5. When the catheter is in the superior vena cava, it is inflated with air and advanced gently.	5. The amount of air to be used is indicated on the catheter.
6. The inflated balloon at the tip of the catheter will be guided by the flowing stream of blood through the right atrium and tricuspid valve into the right ventricle. From this position, it finds its way into the main pulmonary artery carried by blood flow. The catheter tip pressures are recorded continuously by specific pressure wave forms as the catheter advances through the various chambers of the heart.	6. Watch ECG monitor for signs of ventricular irritability as catheter enters the right ventricle. Report any signs of arrhythmia to the physician.
7. The flowing blood will continue to direct the catheter more distally into the pulmonary tree. When the catheter reaches a pulmonary vessel that is approximately the same size or slightly smaller in diameter than the inflated balloon, it cannot be advanced any further. This is the wedge position, called pulmonary capillary wedge pressure (PCWP) or pulmonary artery wedge pressure (PAWP).	7. With the catheter in the wedge position, the balloon blocks the flow of blood from the right side of the heart toward the lungs and the resulting capillary wedge pressure is equal to the mean left atrial pressure.
8. The pressure is recorded with the balloon wedged in the pulmonary vascular bed. Normal PCWP is 8–12 mm. Hg. Optimal LV function appears to be at a wedge between 14–18 mm. Hg.	8. Wedge pressure reading provides information about the level of pulmonary congestion and is closely related to left atrial pressure and to left ventricular end-diastolic pressure (in the absence of mitral valve disease). This is a valuable parameter of cardiac function. Filling pressures less than 8–10 mm. Hg in an acutely injured heart are often associated with reduction in cardiac output, hypotension, and tachycardia.
9. The balloon is deflated, causing the catheter to retract spontaneously into a larger pulmonary artery. This gives a continuous pulmonary artery systolic, diastolic, and mean pressure.	9. The normal systolic pulmonary pressure ranges are 15–25 mm. Hg, and the diastolic pulmonary pressure ranges are 8–12 mm. Hg. The normal mean pulmonary artery pressure (average pressure in pulmonary artery throughout the entire cardiac cycle) ranges from 10–20 mm. Hg.
10. The catheter is sutured in place.	10. An antibactericidal ointment may be placed around the site and covered with a sterile dressing.
11. The patency of the catheter is maintained with a low-flow continuous irrigation.	11. A chest x-ray to confirm catheter position and to provide a baseline for future reference is obtained after Swan–Ganz insertion. A constant microdrip is maintained.

To obtain a wedge pressure reading

1. Note amount of air to be injected into balloon, usually 1 ml.	
2. Inflate the balloon slowly until the contour of the pulmonary arterial pressure changes to that of pulmonary wedge pressure. As soon as a wedge pattern is observed, no more air is introduced. Do not introduce more air into balloon than specified.	2. The transducer converts the pressure wave into an electronic wave that is displayed on a screen. Pulmonary capillary wedge pressure is only measured intermittently. Do not allow catheter to remain in the wedge position when patient is unattended or when not directly making the measurement.

(continued)

Guidelines: Measuring Pulmonary Artery Pressure by Flow-Directed Balloon-Tipped Catheter (Swan-Ganz Catheter) (continued)

Procedure
(Cont.)

Nursing Action	Rationale/Amplification
3. Deflate the balloon as soon as the pressure reading is obtained.	3. Segmental lung infarction may occur if the catheter balloon is left inflated for long periods.
4. Record PCWP reading and amount of air needed to obtain wedge reading. Document recorded waveform by placing a strip of the waveform in patient's chart showing wedge tracing reverting to pulmonary artery waveform.	4. Overinflation of balloon may cause a "superwedge" waveform, and data obtained will be inaccurate. Overinflation of balloon may cause balloon to loose elastic properties and rupture. The strip provides documentation that catheter was not left in wedge position.

Follow-up Phase

1. Inspect the insertion site daily. Look for signs of infection, swelling, and bleeding. Culture the site every 48 hours.	1. A foreign body (catheter) in the vascular system increases the risk of sepsis.
2. Record date and time of dressing change and IV tubing change.	
3. Assess the extremity for color, temperature, capillary filling, and sensation.	3. Ischemia (with possible loss of digits) may occur from inadequate arterial flow.
4. Assess contour of waveform frequently and compare with previous documented waveforms.	4. Catheter may move forward and become lodged in wedge position or drift back into right ventricle. Turn patient to left side and ask him to cough (may dislodge catheter from wedge position). If not dislodged, notify physician.
5. Assess for complications: pulmonary embolism, arrhythmias, heart block, damage to tricuspid valve, intracardiac knotting of catheter, thrombophlebitis, infection, balloon rupture, rupture of pulmonary artery.	5. Blood coming back into syringe indicates balloon rupture. Notify physician immediately.

Postinsertion Phase (Physician)

The catheter is removed without excessive force or traction; pressure dressing is applied over the site.	The site should be checked periodically for bleeding.

Guidelines: Central Venous Pressure

Central venous pressure (CVP) is the pressure within the right atrium or in the great veins within the thorax.

Central venous pressure monitoring serves as a guide for assessment of right-sided cardiac function.

Central venous pressure monitoring serves as a guide for assessment of left-sided cardiac function only in the absence of cardiorespiratory disease.

Purposes
1. To serve as a guide for fluid replacement in seriously ill patients.
2. To estimate blood volume deficits.
3. To determine pressures in the right atrium and central veins.
4. To evaluate for circulatory failure (in context with total clinical picture of patient).

Vein Sites for Catheter Placement

The most commonly used sites are:
Subclavian
Internal or external jugular
Median basilic

Equipment

Venous pressure tray
Cutdown tray
Infusion solution and infusion set
3- or 4-way stopcock (a pressure transducer may be used)
IV pole attached to bed; arm board; adhesive tape
ECG monitor
Carpenter's level (for establishing zero point)

Procedure

Nursing Action	Rationale/Amplification
Preparatory Phase	
1. Assemble equipment according to manufacturer's directions.	
2. Explain that the procedure is similar to an IV and that the patient may move in bed as desired after the passage of the CVP catheter.	
3. Place the patient in a position of comfort. This is the baseline position used for subsequent readings.	3. Serial CVP readings should be made with the patient in the same position. Inaccuracies in CVP readings can be produced by changes in position, coughing, or straining during the reading.
4. Attach manometer to the IV pole. The zero point of the manometer should be on a level with the patient's right atrium. Mark the midaxillary line on the patient with an indelible pencil.	4. The right atrium is at the midaxillary line, which is about ⅓ of the distance from the anterior to the posterior chest wall (Fig. 9-3). The midaxillary line is an external reference point for the zero level of the manometer (which coincides with the level of the right atrium).

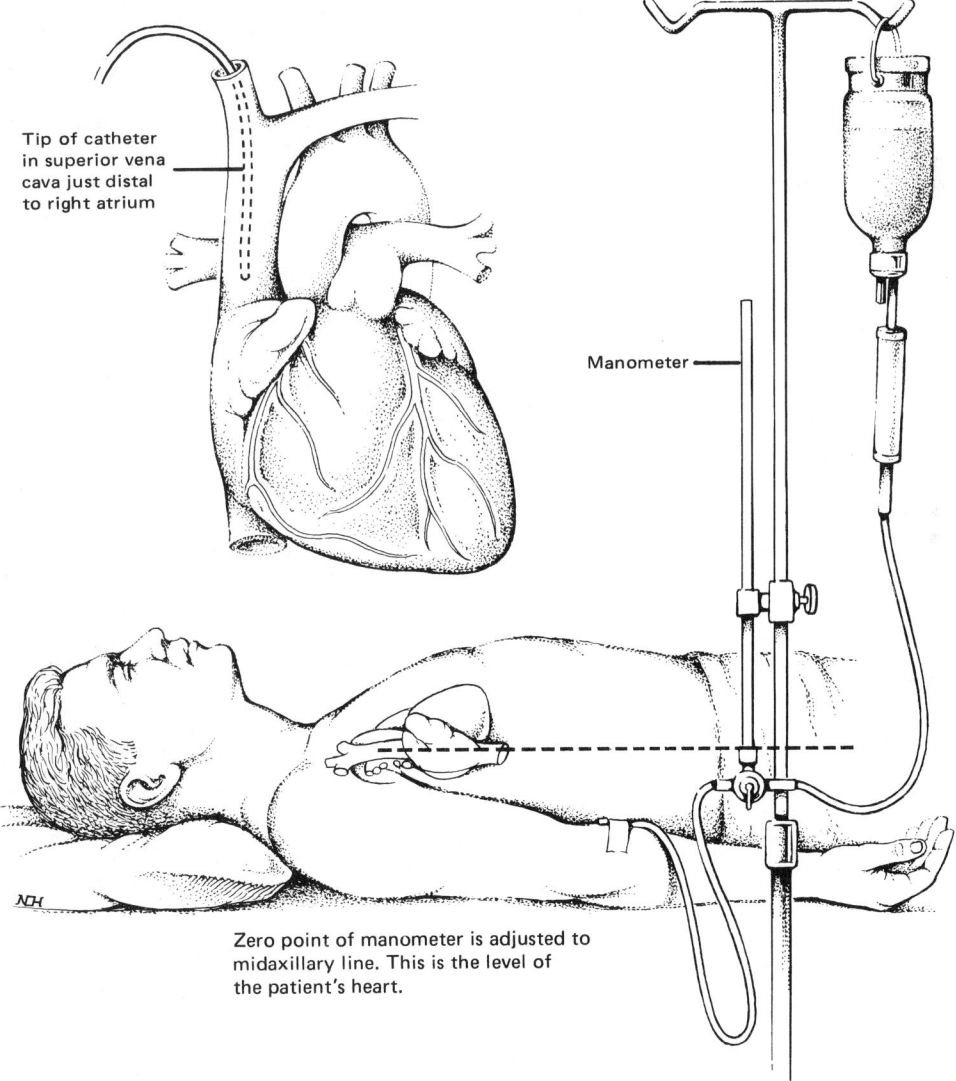

Tip of catheter in superior vena cava just distal to right atrium

Manometer

Zero point of manometer is adjusted to midaxillary line. This is the level of the patient's heart.

Figure 9-3. Central venous pressure.

(continued)

Guidelines: Central Venous Pressure (continued)

Procedure
(Cont.)

Nursing Action	Rationale/Amplification
5. The CVP catheter is connected to a 3-way stopcock that communicates to an open IV (e.g., saline and heparin) and to a manometer (the measuring device).	5. Or, the CVP catheter may be connected to a transducer and an electrical monitor with either digital or calibrated CVP wave readout.
6. Start the IV flow and fill the manometer 10 cm. above anticipated reading (or until the level of 20 cm. H_2O is reached). Turn the stopcock and fill the tubing with fluid.	
7. The CVP site is surgically cleansed. The physician introduces the CVP catheter percutaneously or by direct venous cutdown and threaded through an antecubital, subclavian, or internal or external jugular vein into the superior vena cava just before it enters the right atrium.	7. If the catheter is inserted through the subclavian or internal jugular vein, place patient in a head-down position to increase venous filling and reduce risk of air embolism. The correct catheter placement can be confirmed by fluoroscopy or chest x-ray.
8. When the catheter enters the thorax, an inspiratory fall and expiratory rise in venous pressure are observed.	8. The fluid level fluctuates with respiration. It rises sharply with coughing, straining.
9. The patient may be monitored by ECG during catheter insertion.	9. When the tip of the catheter contacts the wall of the right atrium (or right ventricle) it may produce aberrant impulses and disturb cardiac rhythm.
10. The catheter may be sutured and taped in place. A sterile dressing is applied.	10. Label dressing with time and date of catheter insertion.
11. The infusion is adjusted to flow into the patient's vein by a slow continuous drip.	11. The infusion may cause a significant increase in venous pressure if permitted to flow too rapidly.

To Measure the CVP

1. Place the patient in the identified position and confirm the zero point. (See step 3 under Preparatory Phase.) Intravascular pressures are measured to the atmospheric pressure at the middle of the right atrium; this is the zero point or external reference point.	1. The zero point or baseline for the manometer should be on a level with the patient's right atrium. The middle of the right atrium is the midaxillary line in the 4th intercostal space.
2. Position the zero point of the manometer at the level of the right atrium.	2. All personnel taking the CVP measurement use the same zero point.
3. Turn the stopcock so that the IV solution flows into the manometer, filling to about the 20–25-cm. level. Then turn stopcock so that solution in manometer flows into patient.	
4. Observe the fall in the height of the column of fluid in manometer. Record the level at which the solution stabilizes or stops moving downward. This is the central venous pressure. Record CVP and the position of the patient.	4. The column of fluid will fall until it meets an equal pressure (i.e., the patient's central venous pressure). The CVP reading is reflected by the height of a column of fluid in the manometer when there is open communication between the catheter and the manometer. The fluid in the manometer will fluctuate slightly with the patient's respirations. This confirms that the CVP line is not obstructed by clotted blood.
5. The CVP may range from 5–12 cm. H_2O. (Absolute numerical values have not been agreed upon.)	5. The change in CVP is a more useful indication of adequacy of venous blood volume and alterations of cardiovascular function. CVP is a dynamic measurement. The normal values may change from patient to patient. The management of the patient is not based on one reading but on repeated serial readings in correlation with patient's clinical status.
6. Assess the patient's clinical condition. Frequent changes in measurements (interpreted within the context of the clinical situation) will serve as a guide to detect whether the heart can handle its fluid load and whether hypovolemia or hypervolemia is present.	6. CVP is interpreted by considering the patient's entire clinical picture; hourly urine output, heart rate, blood pressure, cardiac output measurements. a. A CVP near zero indicates that the patient is hypovolemic (verified if rapid IV infusion causes patient to improve). b. A CVP above 15–20 cm. H_2O may be due to either hypervolemia or poor cardiac contractility.
7. Turn the stopcock again to allow IV solution to flow from solution bottle into the patient's veins.	7. When readings are not being made, flow is from a very slow microdrip to the catheter, bypassing the manometer.

Follow-up Phase

1. Observe for complications. a. From catheter insertion: pneumothorax; hemothorax; hematoma; cardiac tamponade. b. Secondary to presence of indwelling venous catheter: air embolism, catheter embolization; colonization of organisms.	1. The incidence of complications rises rapidly the longer the CVP catheter is left in place. The patient's complaint of a new or different pain should be assessed and acted upon.

Procedure
(Cont.)

Nursing Action	Rationale/Amplification

2. Carry out ongoing nursing surveillance of the insertion site and maintain aseptic technique.
   a. Inspect entry site twice daily for signs of local inflammation/phlebitis. Remove immediately if there are any signs of infection.
   b. Change dressings as prescribed.
   c. Label to show date/time of change.
   d. Send the catheter tip for bacteriologic culture when it is removed.	

▶ **NURSING ALERT:** A CVP line is a potential source of septicemia.

Cardiac Output

Cardiac output is the amount (volume) of blood ejected by one ventricle in 1 minute.

Clinical Assessment of Cardiac Output

A low cardiac output may be detected by:
1. Cyanosis or duskiness of buccal mucosa, nailbeds, and ear lobes
2. Cool, moist skin
3. Low urine output
4. Falling blood pressure

Underlying Concepts

1. Cardiac output depends on cardiac function, tone of the blood vessels, and blood volume.
2. Cardiac output is expressed in liters per minute and is equal to the stroke volume × heart rate (SV × HR).
   a. SV = amount of blood ejected from ventricle per beat
   b. HR = number of cardiac contractions
   c. Normal cardiac output = 5 to 6 liters/minute
3. Cardiac output is usually expressed as the cardiac index (CI).
   a. CI = indicator for peripheral perfusion of organs
   b. CI = CO divided by body surface area; the body surface area is determined by standard charts
   c. Normal CI = 2.7–4.3 $l/min/m^2$ indicates normal peripheral perfusion
4. Cardiac output is measured by a variety of techniques. In the clinical setting, it is usually measured by the thermodilution technique used in conjunction with a flow-directed balloon catheter (Swan–Ganz catheter, p. 282).

Method

1. The Swan–Ganz catheter is positioned in its final position in a branch of the pulmonary artery; it has a thermistor (external heat-sensing device) situated 4 cm. from the tip of the catheter, which measures the temperature of the blood that flows by it.
2. Sterile dextrose or saline solution at 0°C. is injected through 1 lumen of the catheter. The solution mixes with the blood in the right side of the heart and flows to the pulmonary artery where blood temperature is detected by the thermistor.
3. A small computer converts the temperature changes into a direct reading of cardiac output.

Special Therapeutic Modalities

Guidelines: Assisting the Patient Undergoing Pericardiocentesis (Pericardial Aspiration)

Pericardiocentesis is the puncturing of the pericardial sac in order to aspirate fluid and thereby relieve cardiac tamponade (Fig. 9-4).

Acute cardiac tamponade is life-threatening, and emergency needle pericardiocentesis is indicated. Stable tamponade, which presents no immediate threat to life, may indicate techniques to determine etiologic diagnosis to be performed: xiphoid pericardiostomy; pericardial window; visceral pericardiectomy.

Cardiac tamponade is compression of the heart by blood, effusion, or a foreign body in the pericardial sac, which impairs normal heart action.

1. Acute—a rapid increase of fluid into pericardial space (as little as 200 ml.) causes a marked rise in intrapericardial pressure. Emergency intervention is required to prevent severe circulatory compromise.
2. Stable—slow accumulation of fluid into pericardial sac over weeks or months, causing pericardium to stretch and accommodate up to 2 liters of fluid without severe increases in intrapericardial pressure.

Clinical Manifestations of Cardiac Tamponade

1. Rising venous pressure
2. Falling arterial blood pressure
3. Small, quiet heart, muffled heart sounds (evidenced by fluoroscopy and chest auscultation)

(continued)

Guidelines: Assisting the Patient Undergoing Pericardiocentesis (Pericardial Aspiration) (continued)

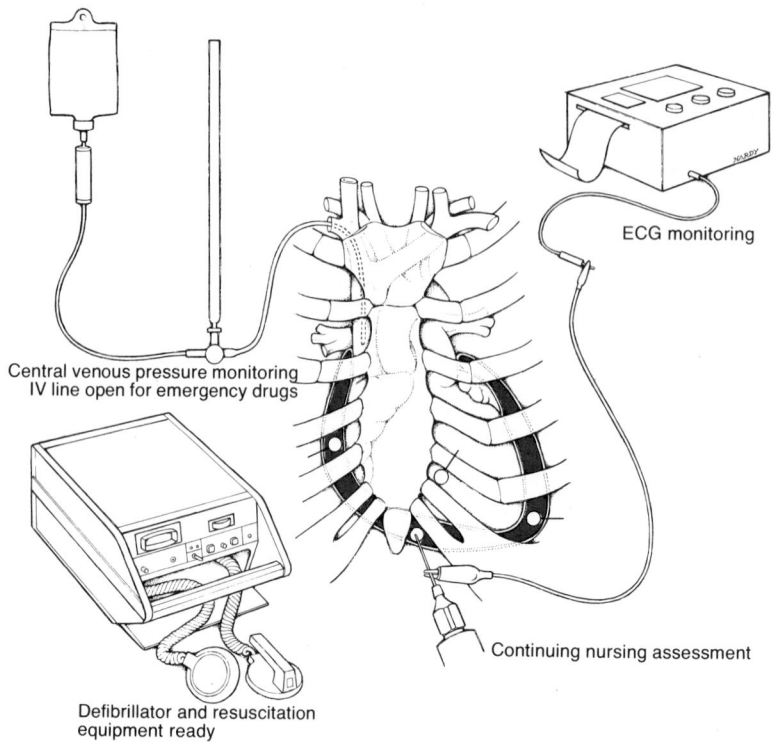

Figure 9-4. *Nursing support of the patient undergoing pericardiocentesis. (Small circles indicate sites for pericardial aspiration.)*

4. Narrowing pulse pressure (difference between systolic and diastolic pressures)
5. Paradoxical pulse (abnormal degree of decline in systolic arterial blood pressure during inspiration). Assessment for paradoxical pulse (pulsus paradoxus) with cuff sphygmomanometry.
   a. Place the patient in recumbent position.
   b. Inflate cuff above the patient's palpated systolic pressure and the disappearance of Korotkoff sounds.
   c. Adjust the patient's position to enable reading of manometer and observation of patient's respiratory pattern.
   d. Slowly deflate cuff (2 mm. Hg per second) and listen for first Korotkoff sound at expiration; then observe the number of mm. the manometer falls while Korotkoff sounds cease on inspiration but are heard on expiration.
6. Decrease cuff until Korotkoff sounds are heard throughout respiratory cycle.
7. Record blood pressure and paradoxical pulse.
8. Palpation
   a. A decrease in amplitude during inspiration can be palpated at radial, femoral, or carotid arteries.
   b. Provides a gross assessment of paradoxical pulse and can be confirmed by cuff method. (Usually palpable if paradox is 15 mm. Hg.)
9. Distention of neck veins and inspiratory rise in venous pressure (Kussmaul's sign)
10. Apprehension; dyspnea
11. Tachypnea; pallor or cyanosis
12. Characteristic posture—sitting upright and leaning forward
13. Clinical shock

Purpose
1. To remove fluid from the pericardial sac caused by:
   a. Pericarditis
   b. Effusion from malignant neoplasm or lymphoma
   c. Trauma
      (1) Accidental—blunt or penetrating wounds
      (2) Iatrogenic—cardiac surgery; cardiopulmonary resuscitation; perforation of heart by catheter or transvenous pacemaker
   d. Infection

Purpose
(Cont.)

   2. To obtain fluid for diagnosis
   3. To instill certain therapeutic drugs

Equipment

Pericardiocentesis tray
Intracath set
Skin antiseptic
1%–2% procaine
Sterile gloves
ECG for monitoring purposes
Sterile ground wire—to be connected between pericardial needle and V lead of ECG (use alligator clip type connectors)
Equipment for cardiopulmonary resuscitation

Sites for Pericardiocentesis

1. Subxiphoid—needle inserted in the angle between left costal margin and xiphoid
2. Near cardiac apex, 2 cm. (0.8 inch) inside left border of cardiac dullness
3. To the left of the 5th or 6th interspace at the sternal margin
4. Right side of 4th intercostal space just inside border of dullness

Procedure (Fig. 9-4)

Nursing Action	Rationale/Amplification
Preparatory Phase	
1. Medicate the patient as prescribed.	
2. Start a slow intravenous drip of saline or glucose.	2. This preserves a route for intravenous therapy in the event of an emergency.
3. Place the patient in a comfortable position with the head of the bed or treatment table raised to a 60-degree angle.	3. This position makes it easier to insert needle into pericardial sac.
4. Apply the limb leads of the ECG to the patient.	4. The patient is monitored during the procedure by ECG.
5. Have defibrillator available for immediate use.	5. In case the procedure has severe adverse effect.
6. Have pacemaker available.	
7. Open the tray, using aseptic technique.	
Performance Phase (by physician)	
1. The site is prepared with skin antiseptic; the area is draped with sterile towels and injected with procaine solution.	
2. The pericardial aspiration needle is attached to a 50-ml. syringe by a 3-way stopcock. The V lead (precordial lead wire) of the ECG is attached to the hub of the aspirating needle by a sterile wire and alligator clips or clamp.	2. There is danger of laceration of myocardium/coronary artery and of cardiac arrhythmias.
3. The needle is advanced slowly until fluid is obtained.	3. Fluid is generally aspirated at a depth of 2.5–4 cm. (1 to 1½ inches).
4. When the pericardial sac has been entered, a hemostat is clamped to the needle at the chest wall just where it penetrates the skin. Pericardial fluid is aspirated slowly.	4. This prevents movement of the needle and further penetration while fluid is being removed.
5. Monitor the patient's ECG, blood pressure, and venous pressure constantly.	5. a. The ST segment rises if the point of the needle contacts the ventricle; there may be ventricular ectopic beats. b. The PR segment is elevated when the needle touches the atrium. c. Large, erratic QRS complexes indicate penetration of the myocardium.
6. If a large amount of fluid is present, a polyethylene catheter may be inserted through a needle (an intracath) and left in the pericardial sac; it is then attached to a drainage bottle.	6. An indwelling catheter left in the pericardial space permits further slow drainage of fluid and prevents recurrence of cardiac tamponade.
7. Watch for presence of bloody fluid. If blood accumulates rapidly, an immediate thoracotomy and cardiorrhaphy (suturing of heart muscle) may be indicated.	7. Bloody pericardial fluid may be due to trauma. Bloody pericardial effusion fluid does not clot readily, whereas blood obtained from inadvertent puncture of one of the heart chambers *does* clot.

(continued)

Guidelines: Assisting the Patient Undergoing Pericardiocentesis (Pericardial Aspiration) (continued)

Procedure
(Cont.)

Nursing Action	Rationale/Amplification
Follow-up Phase	
1. Place patient in intensive care unit or cardiac care unit.	1. Following pericardiocentesis, careful monitoring of blood pressure, venous pressure, and heart sounds will be necessary to indicate possible recurrence of tamponade. A repeated aspiration is then necessary.
2. Watch for rising venous pressure and falling arterial pressure.	2. In the presence of these signs, the patient is probably experiencing cardiac tamponade.
3. Auscultate the area over the heart.	3. Listen for decrease in intensity of heart sounds indicating recurring cardiac tamponade.

4. Prepare for surgical drainage of pericardium if:
  a. Pericardial fluid repeatedly accumulates, or
  b. The aspiration is unsuccessful, or
  c. Complications develop	

5. Assess for complications:
  Inadvertent puncture of heart chamber
  Arrhythmias
  Puncture of lung, stomach, or liver
  Laceration of coronary artery or myocardium	

Cardiopulmonary Resuscitation for Cardiac Arrest

See Chapter 23, Emergency Nursing, p. 925.

Guidelines: Direct Current Defibrillation for Ventricular Fibrillation

Defibrillation (or countershock) is the passing of an electrical shock of short duration through the heart to terminate ventricular fibrillation or ventricular tachycardia without pulse.

A *defibrillator* is an instrument that delivers an electric shock to the heart to convert ventricular fibrillation to normal sinus rhythm. (Defibrillators are also used to convert other abnormal and rapid cardiac rhythms.)

Purpose   To terminate ventricular fibrillation or ventricular tachycardia without pulse.

Equipment

DC defibrillator with paddles
Interface material (saline-soaked gauze pads, electrode gels and pastes, disposable conductive gel pads)
Resuscitative equipment

Procedure

Nursing Action	Rationale/Amplification
Performance Phase (by nurse)	
1. *Monitored patient*—if ventricular fibrillation recognized within 2 minutes, give precordial thump, assess rhythm and carotid pulse, and expose anterior chest. *Unmonitored patient*—expose anterior chest.	
2. *Unmonitored patient*—START CARDIOPULMONARY RESUSCITATION IMMEDIATELY. *Monitored patient*—if within 2 minutes of detection of ventricular fibrillation, defibrillate before initiating cardiopulmonary resuscitation. Beyond 2 minutes, START RESUSCITATION EFFORTS IMMEDIATELY.	2. This procedure should be carried out immediately after ventricular fibrillation is detected to minimize cerebral and circulatory deterioration. Cardiopulmonary resuscitation is essential before and after defibrillation to ensure blood supply to the cerebral and coronary arteries.
3. Apply interface material (gel, paste, saline pads) to the paddles. The electrode paddles should be in firm contact with the patient's skin.	3. The interface material helps provide better contact and prevents skin burns. Do not allow any paste on the skin between the electrodes. If the paste areas touch, the current may short circuit (severely burning the patient) and may not penetrate the heart.
4. Disconnect the oxygen.	4. Prevents danger of fire or explosion.

Procedure
(Cont.)

Nursing Action

5. A second person should turn on the defibrillator to the prescribed setting. The American Heart Association* recommends that initial defibrillation should be 200–300 watt seconds of *delivered* energy. A second attempt at same level should be given if first attempt unsuccessful. A third attempt with an increase of energy level to 360 watt seconds should be attempted only after assessment of arterial blood gases for presence of hypoxia and acidosis.

6. Apply one electrode just to the right of the upper sternum below the clavicle and the other electrode just to the left of the cardiac apex or left nipple (Fig. 9-5). About 20–25 lb. of pressure is applied to paddles to ensure good contact with the patient's skin.

Rationale / Amplification

5. The shock is measured in joules or watt seconds (the dose is based on estimated body weight). The ideal energy dose for defibrillation remains controversial.

6. The paddles are placed so that the electrical discharge flows through as much myocardial mass as possible. If anteroposterior paddles are used, the anterior paddle is held with pressure on the middle sternum while the patient lies on the posterior paddle under the left infrascapular region. In this method the countershock more directly traverses the heart.

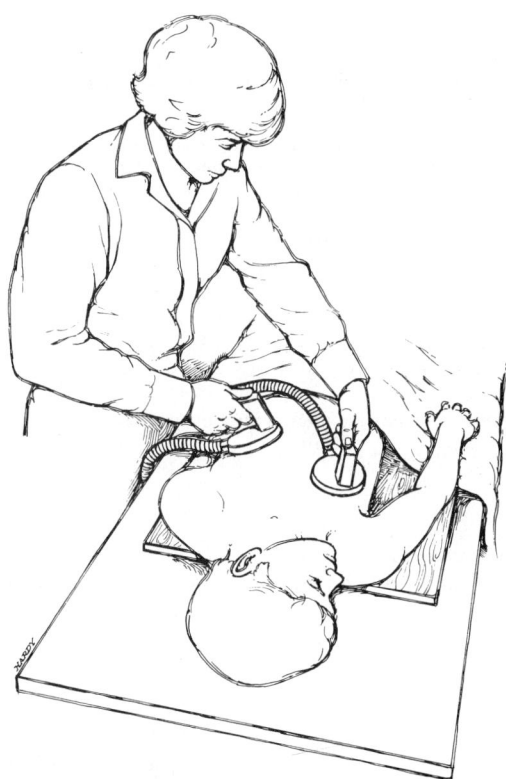

Figure 9-5. Paddle placement in ventricular defibrillation.

7. Grasp the paddles only by the insulated handles.
8. GIVE THE COMMAND FOR PERSONNEL TO STAND CLEAR OF THE PATIENT AND THE BED. Look quickly to make sure all are away from the patient and bed.
9. Push the discharge buttons in both paddles simultaneously.
10. Remove the paddles from the patient *immediately* after the shock is administered (unless monitoring leads are in the paddles).

8. If a person touches the bed, he may act as a ground for the current and receive a shock, especially if there are electrolyte solutions on the floor.

* McIntyre KM and Lewis AJ (eds). The Textbook of Cardiac Life Support, p. 92. Dallas, American Heart Association, 1983.

(continued)

Guidelines: Direct Current Defibrillation for Ventricular Fibrillation (continued)

Procedure
(Cont.)

Nursing Action	Rationale/Amplification
11. Resume cardiopulmonary resuscitation efforts until stable rhythm, spontaneous respirations, pulse, and blood pressure return.	11. After discharge of the countershock, CPR efforts should be resumed, total delay should be no more than 5 seconds in order to oxygenate the patient and restore circulation.
12. Look at the ECG monitor to determine the specific therapy for the resultant electrical mechanism. Further high energy countershocks may be necessary.	

Follow-up Phase

Nursing Action	Rationale/Amplification
1. After the patient is defibrillated and rhythm is restored, lidocaine is usually given to prevent recurrent episodes, and sodium bicarbonate administered to treat metabolic acidosis.	1. Any resultant arrhythmia may require appropriate drug intervention. Metabolic acidosis is due to accumulation of acidic products in blood because of cessation of respiration.
2. Continue with intensive monitoring/care.	

Guidelines: Application of Rotating Tourniquets or Automatic Inflating Cuffs

Rotating tourniquets refers to a technique whereby tourniquets are systematically rotated on the extremities to remove a volume of blood from the central circulation in order to decrease venous return and right ventricular output; this technique aids in decongesting the lungs.

Purpose To decrease circulating blood volume temporarily in the extremities in order to reduce venous return to the heart.

Underlying Principles

1. Three of the 4 extremities are compressed while 1 extremity is usually free at all times.
2. No single extremity should be compressed continuously for more than 45 minutes.
3. Tourniquets may have to be rotated at 5-minute intervals on the elderly patient to prevent gangrene and other complications.
4. These principles are important, since they can reduce the risks of phlebothrombosis and fatal pulmonary embolism.

Equipment

Equipment for extremity compression
   4 Sphygmomanometer cuffs, or
   4 Tourniquets, 61 cm. (2 feet) long with outside diameter 0.8–3.8 cm. ($^5/_{16}$ to 1½ inches), or
   Equipment designed to inflate and deflate blood pressure cuffs automatically (Danzer apparatus)
Small towels
Watch—to note time interval
Work sheet

Procedure

Nursing Action	Rationale/Amplification
Performance Phase (Fig. 9-6)	
1. Explain to the patient (if his condition permits) the purpose of the compression and that the skin of the extremities may become discolored.	1. To relieve anxiety.
2. Take the blood pressure.	2. Initial blood pressure reading serves as a baseline for future comparison.
3. Assess peripheral pulses and mark peripheral pulses with water-soluble ink pen.	3. Facilitates checking of pulses during treatment.
4. a. Apply the 4 blood pressure cuffs (or Danzer apparatus if available) several inches below shoulders and groin. Inflate 3 cuffs to a pressure 10 mm. Hg below diastolic blood pressure.	4. a. Venous flow must be occluded, but arterial flow must not be impeded. Peripheral pulses distal to cuff will be palpable if appropriate pressure is selected.
b. Apply tourniquets as high as possible on 3 extremities. Place tourniquets over gown or small towel in a definite rotation pattern.	b. Tourniquet should be placed in such a way that the arterial pulse can be palpated. One extremity should be free of a tourniquet during each time interval.

Procedure
(Cont.)

▶ **NURSING ALERT:** Do not apply tourniquets or cuffs to ischemic or infected extremities or extremities with intravenous lines.

Nursing Action	Rationale/Amplification
5. Release 1 tourniquet every 15 minutes. Then apply a tourniquet to the previously free extremity.	5. The venous outflow in any 1 extremity will be occluded for 45 minutes and unoccluded for 15 minutes. The time interval may be shorter if the patient's condition indicates.
6. Rotate cuff inflation systematically, OR Rotate tourniquets in definitive clockwise pattern.	6. Ensures pressure released on appropriate extremity at proper time.
7. Monitor blood pressure every 15–30 minutes after tourniquets/cuffs have been applied.	7. Application of tourniquets/cuffs may precipitate hypotension in some patients.
8. Measure urinary output at frequent intervals. (Usually an indwelling catheter is used.)	8. Watch for sudden reduction in plasma volume with hypotension and oliguria after administration of rapid-acting diuretics (ethacrynic acid, furosemide).
9. Observe for complication of shock or arterial emboli.	9. Contact physician if shock occurs or if there is suspicion of arterial emboli. If extremity becomes tender, loses pulse, or is cool to touch, remove cuffs/tourniquets according to designated protocol (see step 10).
10. At the completion of the rotation, remove 1 tourniquet/ cuff at a time according to the specified time interval (usually 15 minutes).	10. Releasing the tourniquets 1 at a time prevents a sudden increase in circulatory blood volume and thus prevents circulatory overload.
11. Examine each extremity after tourniquet removal for color, warmth, and the presence of a palpable pulse.	

Follow-up Phase

1. Record starting time of procedure, rotation intervals, clinical response, medications given, and the time tourniquets were discontinued.

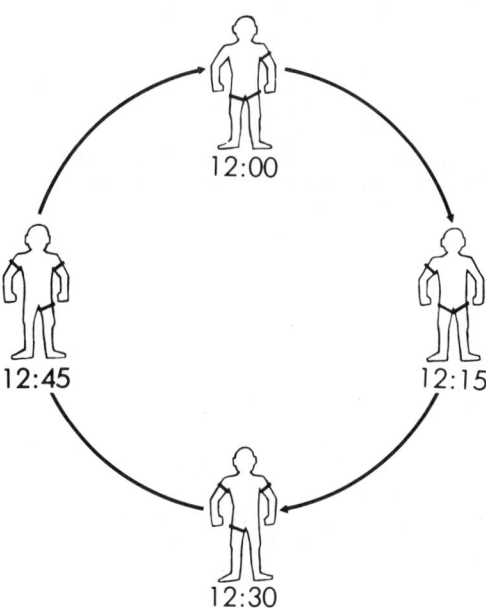

Figure 9-6. One method of rotating tourniquets. This illustration shows a clockwise pattern.

Cardiac Arrhythmias

Arrhythmia is a clinical disorder of the heart beat; it may include a disturbance of rate, rhythm (sequence), or both. Arrhythmias are derangements of heart function and not of heart structure.

Etiology

1. Arrhythmias due to organic heart disease
   a. Inflammatory heart disease

b. Degenerative heart disease (atherosclerosis)
c. Congenital heart disease
d. Hypertensive heart disease
2. Arrhythmias due to disturbances of other organ systems
   a. Disease of central nervous system—from sympathetic and vagal stimulation
   b. Pulmonary disease
   c. Endocrine disorders (hyper- and hypothyroidism, hypoglycemia, diabetic ketoacidosis)
   d. Gastrointestinal disorders (fluid and electrolyte imbalance)
   e. Renal disorders (renal failure)
3. Arrhythmias from other causes
   a. Drugs (digitalis intoxication, quinidine, procainamide)
   b. Infection
   c. Disturbances of electrolyte balance
   d. Anemia
   e. Following cardiac surgery

Classification of Arrhythmias Based on Disturbed Physiology

1. Disturbance of impulse formation—heartbeat activated for one or more beats by a pacemaker other than the SA node.
2. Disturbances of conduction—due to delayed transmission of impulses, to failure of some impulses to be conducted, or to a block of impulses at the affected site.
3. Combined disorders—combination of abnormally rapid impulse formation and decreased ability to conduct the impulses.

Clinical Manifestations

(Depends on ventricular rate, condition of heart, and the patient's psychological reaction.)
1. Symptoms and signs of rapid arrhythmias
   a. Palpitation
   b. Dizziness and fainting
   c. Throbbing in head and neck
   d. Shortness of breath
   e. Precordial discomfort and pain
   f. Anxiety
2. Symptoms and signs of slow heart action (bradyarrhythmia)
   a. Shortness of breath
   b. Fatigue on exertion
   c. Dizziness and fainting—may indicate syncopal attacks, leading to convulsive seizures

Clinical Effects

1. Some arrhythmias are relatively harmless, while others are harbingers of cardiac arrest.
2. Cardiac arrhythmias impair pumping action of the heart and reduce cardiac output, which has the effect of lowering the blood pressure and decreasing blood perfusion of the brain, heart, kidneys, gastrointestinal tract, muscles, and skin.
3. Cardiac arrhythmias often produce attacks of transient cerebral ischemia, which may result in stroke from reduction in cerebral blood flow.
4. Arrhythmias can precipitate congestive heart failure or angina pectoris in certain patients.
5. Bradyarrhythmias (rate below 60) predispose to electrical instability of the heart and decreased cardiac output.
6. A marked degree of disability may accompany an arrhythmia.

Management

1. Evaluate the patient's general appearance: pallor, cyanosis, sweating—may indicate peripheral arteriolar constriction.
2. How does the patient describe his symptoms?
3. What is the duration and frequency of the arrhythmia?
4. Observe carotid pulsation: Rapid and vigorous? Irregular with varying amplitude?
5. Listen to the heartbeat with a stethoscope.
   a. Listen for rate, presence of irregularity, increase in intensity of first heart sound.
      (1) 30 beats or lower—complete AV block, partial AV block, or sinus bradycardia
      (2) 40–60 beats per minute—varying degrees of AV block, sinus bradycardia
      (3) 60–110 beats per minute—sinus arrhythmia, premature beats, AV heart block, atrial fibrillation, atrial flutter, atrial tachycardia with block
      (4) 140–180 beats per minute—atrial tachycardia, atrial flutter, junctional or ventricular tachycardia
   b. If possible, have an electrocardiogram taken during an episode of arrhythmia.
   c. Take the blood pressure and pulse—distal pulses give clue to heart's ability to perfuse the periphery.
6. Take respiratory rate: note depth and effort.
7. Evaluate for:
   a. Mental confusion with arrhythmia—indicates cerebral ischemia.
   b. Presence of signs and symptoms of congestive heart failure—may indicate arrhythmia causing serious effect.
   c. Chest pains with arrhythmia—due to myocardial ischemia.
   d. Weakness.
8. Use ambulatory cardiac monitoring for persons with suspected arrhythmias (patients with dizzy spells, palpitations, chest pain) and to evaluate antiarrhythmic therapy.
   a. One lead sensor is taped to the patient's chest and connected to portable recording equipment. Recorder is started.
   b. The patient goes about his daily routine while keeping a diary of times and activities during which he feels his symptoms.
   c. After 8–30 hours, the tape is put through a scanner for oscilloscope reading (computer scanning now available).
9. Offer calm explanations and convey optimism—patients with arrhythmias are likely to be anxious, and anxiety tends to aggravate symptoms; fear and anxiety can outweigh all other factors.
10. The treatment of arrhythmias includes pharmocologic, electrical (pacing; cardioversion), and surgical (excision of the "foci," etc.) therapy. See page 338 for a complete discussion of the most common arrhythmias, their ECG interpretations and treatment.

Health Education

Involve family in the teaching as follows:
1. Take prescribed medication on schedule.
2. Stop smoking.
3. Modification of the diet may be indicated; in general, avoid caffeine (coffee, cola, cocoa, chocolate, tea) and pain medications that contain caffeine or stimulants.

4. Notify physician if unusual symptoms or unexpected intolerance to exercise, emotional states, or cold occurs.

Cardiac Pacing

A *cardiac pacemaker* is an electronic device that delivers direct stimulation to the heart, causing electrical depolarization and cardiac contraction. The pacemaker initiates and maintains the heart rate when the natural pacemakers of the heart are unable to do so.

Cardiac pacing is accomplished through stimulation of either the atrium, the ventricle, or both.

Pacemaker functions are described by an international code developed in 1974 and revised in 1980 by the International Society Commission for Heart Disease Resources (ICHD) (see Table 9-1).

Cardiac pacing can be internal or external.
1. Internal—electrical stimulation of endocardium or epicardium.
2. External—external electrical stimulation through electrodes applied to chest wall. Requires large amount of electrical current to cause significant muscle contraction. Rarely used because of complications of pain and skin burns.

Pacemaker Design

Pacemakers consist of two component parts:
1. *Pulse generator,* which contains the circuitry and batteries that generate the electrical signal; the battery cells are usually lithium cell units with a projected life of 8–12 years, or less frequently, mercury–zinc batteries with a projected life of 2–5 years and isotopic (nuclear) batteries with a projected life of 20 years.
   Pulse generators may be external or implanted (internal).
2. *Pacemaker electrodes,* which transmit the pacemaker impulses to the heart. The stimuli from the pacemaker travel through a flexible catheter electrode (lead) that is threaded through a vein into the right ventricle (endocardial approach), or introduced by direct penetration of the chest wall (requires thoracotomy or upper abdominal surgical approach—epicardial approach).
   a. Pacemaker electrode may be unipolar or bipolar: *unipolar* catheter has one electrode in contact

with heart; *bipolar* has two electrodes in contact with heart. Bipolar may be converted to unipolar. Unipolar catheters sense intrinsic cardiac signals better and produce a larger pacer spike on an ECG recording.

Clinical Indications

1. Symptomatic bradyarrhythmias
   a. Sinoatrial bradyarrhythmias
   b. Sinoatrial arrest
   c. Sick sinus syndrome
2. Heart Block
   a. Mobitz I—second-degree AV block (Wenckebach phenomenon); rate variable, usually 60–100 beats per minute
   b. Mobitz II—second-degree AV block; rate usually 30–55 per minute
   c. Complete heart block
3. Prophylaxis
   a. Following acute MI; arrhythmia and conduction defects
   b. Before or following cardiac surgery
   c. During coronary arteriography
   d. Before permanent pacing
4. Tachyarrhythmias; to break rapid rhythm disturbances
   a. Supraventricular
   b. Ventricular

Pacing Modes

1. *Demand* (synchronous, noncompetitive) atrial/ventricular
   Most commonly used; has the advantage of working only when the heart rate goes below a certain level. Therefore, it does not compete with the heart's basic rhythm. If the patient's heart rate falls below a predetermined escape interval (programmed into pulse generator), an electrical stimulus is delivered to the heart.
2. Fixed rate (asynchronous, competitive) atrial/ventricular
   This unit delivers an electrical stimulus at a preset constant rate that is independent of the patient's own rhythm. However, it can compete with the patient's own rhythm. Used infrequently, usually in patients with complete and unvarying heart block. Does not allow atrial contribution to cardiac output.
3. Synchronous atrial/ventricular
   A demand form of pacing, which is able to increase heart rate to accompany the physiologic demands of the body. An atrial electrode senses the patient's atrial depolarization, waits for a preset interval (simulated PR interval), and triggers firing of ventricular pacer. If rapid atrial rhythm occurs, the ventricular pacemaker stimulates the ventricle at a fixed rate independent of atrial activity.
4. Bifocal atrioventricular sequential
   Mode of choice for pacing patients with borderline cardiac function and selected dysrhythmias. Offers stimulation of both atria and ventricles.
   a. Continuous sequential A-V pacing—delivers continuous stimuli to atria and ventricles in sequence (fixed rate). The pacemaker is unable to sense patient's intrinsic rhythm.
   b. QRS inhibited sequence A-V pacing—simulates normal cardiac function through stimulation of atria and ventricles sequentially at a preset fixed interval. The pacemaker is able to detect the patient's intrinsic ventricular depolarization and will shut off both atrial and ventricular pacing stimuli.

Table 9-1 International Pacemaker Classification—Three-letter Identification Code

1st Letter	2nd Letter	3rd Letter
Chamber Paced	Chamber Sensed	Mode of Response
V—Ventricle	I—Inhibited	
A—Atrium	T—Triggered	
D—Double Chamber	O—Not Applicable	

First letter—The paced chamber is identified by V for ventricle, A for atrium, or D for double—both atrium and ventricle.

Second letter—The sensed chamber of either is again V for ventricle, A for atrium.

Third letter—The mode of response, if any, is either:
 I for inhibited, a pacemaker whose output is blocked by a sensed signal, or
 T for triggered, a unit whose output is discharged by a sensed signal.
 O indicates a specific comment is not applicable.

(Parsonnet V, Furman S, and Smyth NPD: Implantable cardiac pacemakers status report and resource guideline. Circulation 1974 Oct; 50(4):A21. Used by permission of the American Heart Association, Inc.)

5. New developments
Programmable pacemaker allows noninvasive adjustment (programming) of implanted pacemaker.

Temporary and Emergency Pacemaker Systems

Temporary pacing of the heart is usually an emergency procedure that permits observation of the effects of pacing on heart function so that an optimal pacing rate can be selected before a permanent pacer is implanted. Temporary pacing may be done for hours, days, or weeks; it is continued until the patient improves or a permanent pacemaker is implanted.

A. Approaches

Accomplished by either an endocardial (transvenous) approach or a transthoracic approach to the myocardium.

1. The transvenous electrode is passed under fluoroscopic guidance through a peripheral vein (subclavian, femoral, jugular, brachial, etc.), and the catheter

(electrode) is positioned in the apex of the right ventricle.

2. The pacing wire protrudes from the incision or percutaneous site and is connected to an external pulse generator attached to the patient or fastened to the bed linens. The catheter is anchored in place to allow motion of the extremity (Fig. 9-7). The external pacemaker is powered by standard batteries that require proper maintenance.

Permanent Pacemakers

A. Approaches

1. Transvenous (endocardial)—electrodes (unipolar or bipolar) are threaded through cephalic or external jugular vein and into the right ventricle. The peripheral end of the electrode is connected to the pulse generator, which is implanted underneath the skin below the right or left pectoral region (Fig. 9-8*A*).
   a. Performed under local anesthesia
   b. Thoracotomy unnecessary
   c. Majority of pacemakers inserted transvenously
2. Transthoracic (epicardial)—anterior chest is opened,

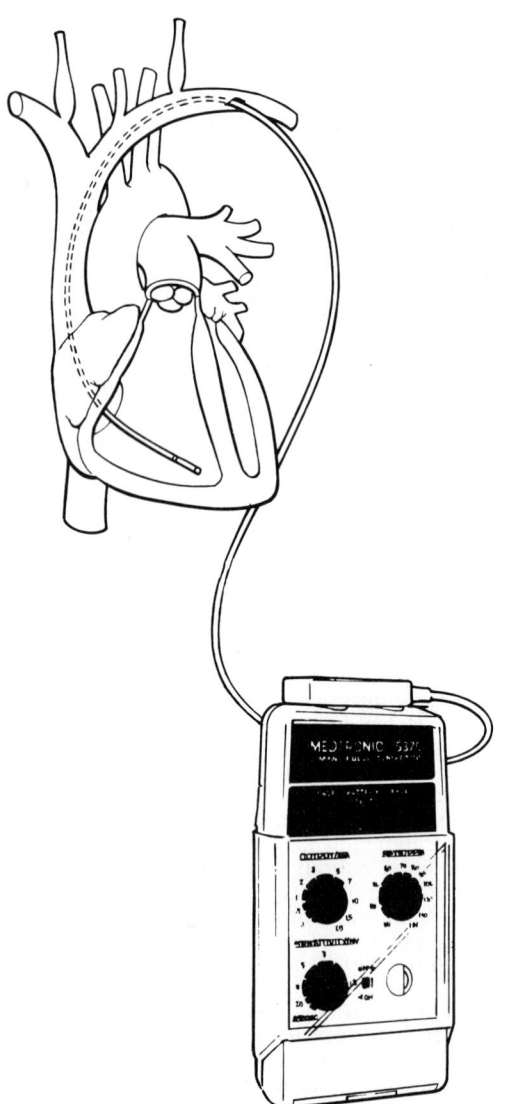
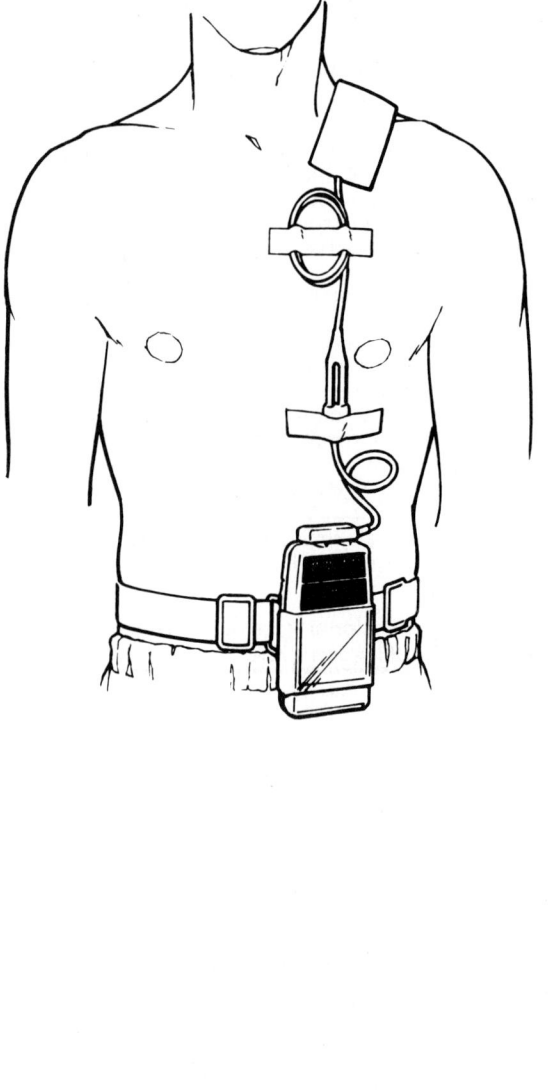

Figure 9-7. Temporary external pacemaker. (Courtesy of MEDTRONIC, Inc.)

and electrodes are sutured to the surface of the right or left ventricle or atrium, then threaded subcutaneously to the abdominal wall either above or below the waist (Fig. 9-8*B*).

    a. Offers electrode stability

    b. Greater selection of pacing modes

    c. Method of choice for children to allow for vertical chest growth

Patient Problems/Nursing Diagnoses

1. Potential for injury related to pacemaker malfunction and from the presence of the pacemaker within the body.
2. Potential for infection related to foreign body implantation.
3. Anxiety related to pacemaker insertion and hospitalization.
4. Fear of death related to pacemaker failure.
5. Body image disturbances (potential) related to pacemaker implant.
6. Powerlessness related to independence–dependence conflict.

Planning and Implementation
Nursing Interventions

A. Maintaining optimal cardiac rhythm

1. Observe for complications of pacemaker malfunction—failure in one or more components of the pacing system; battery exhaustion; wire (electrode) fractures; failure to capture and/or sense properly.

    a. Monitor ECG following implantation (high risk if electrode is displaced soon after insertion).

    b. Take pulse regularly for one full minute to assess rate and rhythm.

    c. Assess for dizziness, light-headedness, chest pain, shortness of breath (may indicate pacer malfunction).

    d. Place ECG strip in the patient's chart every 4 hours.

2. Record the following information after insertion of pacemaker:

    a. Note the data about the model, date of insertion, location of pulse generator, stimulation threshold, and pacer rate on the patient's record. Report and record changes in these parameters.

    b. Place a card at the head of the bed indicating that the patient has a pacemaker.

3. Assist the patient in and out of bed when ambulatory—a fall can dislodge an electrode. (There is a high incidence of associated disease in elderly patients; the mean age of these patients is 70 years—have associated arteriosclerotic heart disease and heart failure, hypertension, and diabetes.)

4. Observe for complications related to presence of pacemaker in body: Arrhythmias—ventricular ectopic activity—from irritation of the ventricular wall by the electrode. Pacemakers can create baffling arrhythmias. Complications from electrode malposition, or perforation; high ventricular threshold may cause abrupt loss of pacing.

    a. Maintain intravenous infusion to have an accessible vein in the event of an arrhythmia.

    b. Make sure all equipment is grounded with 3-pronged plugs inserted into a proper outlet—improperly grounded equipment can generate currents capable of producing ventricular fibrillation.

        A clinical engineer, electrician, or other qualified person should make certain that the patient is in an electrically safe environment.

    c. Avoid using electrocautery, electrocoagulating equipment, and electric razors—external interference may suppress output of temporary pacemaker. Check to see that no metal parts are

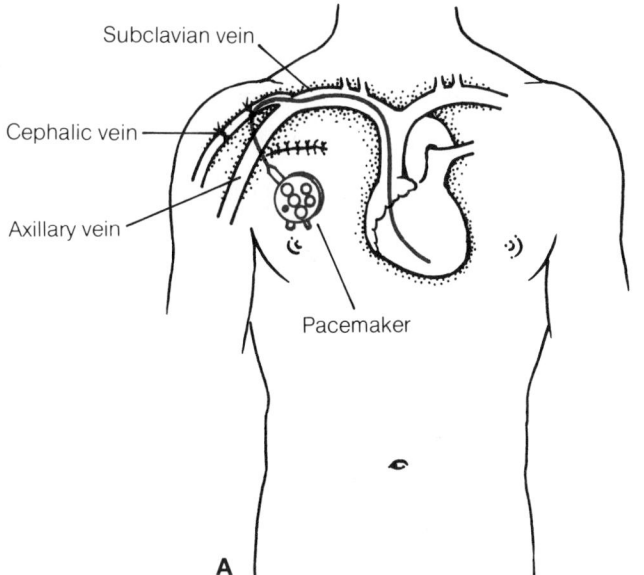

Subclavian vein

Cephalic vein

Axillary vein

Pacemaker

A

Transvenous installation of a permanent pacemaker.

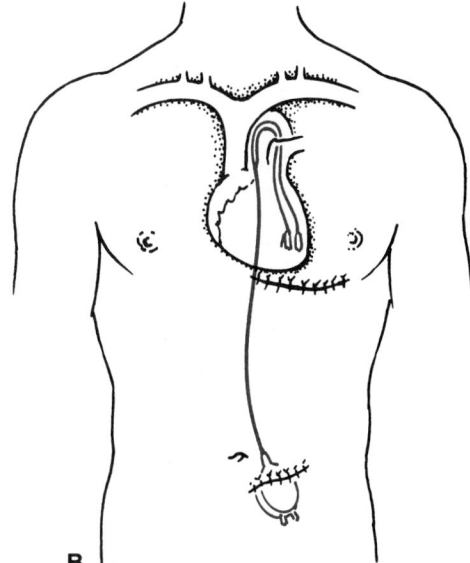

B

Transthoracic installation of a permanent pacemaker.

Figure 9-8. *(A) The catheter is unipolar and is threaded to the apical area of the right ventricle via a major vein. (B) The catheter is bipolar and is passed through an opening in the chest wall and is sutured to the external surface of the left ventricle.*

exposed and electrode insulation is intact—to prevent accidental ventricular fibrillation from stray electrical currents.

  d. Monitor blood pressure and hemodynamic status.
  e. Question the patient about symptoms experienced.
  f. Observe for hiccups—may be caused by chest/diaphragmatic stimulation.
  g. Implement passive range of motion to side of pacemaker implant to avoid pain and stiffness of muscles and joints.

B. Avoidance of infection

1. Observe wound for infection—local infection (sepsis or hematoma formation)—occurs at the site of venous cutdown or subcutaneous pacemaker placement.
  a. Inspect the incision site under the pressure dressings for bleeding and hematoma—hematoma appears to be a contributing factor to wound infection.
  b. Observe the vein through which the pacing catheter has been placed for evidences of phlebitis.
2. Utilize sterile technique for dressing changes.
3. Take temperature regularly (note elevations—38.5°C. [100.5°F.]).
4. Observe for signs/symptoms of bacteremia (see Endocarditis, Clinical Manifestations).

C. Reduction in anxiety

1. Assess anxiety level of patient preoperatively and postoperatively: *mild*—increased alertness; *moderate*—decreased ability to communicate; *severe*—drastic decrease in ability to communicate; and *panic*—inability to communicate, distortion of reality. Learning cannot take place in severe or panic level of anxiety.
2. Offer careful explanations regarding anticipated procedures and treatments and answer the patient's questions with concise explanations. Repeat as necessary. Information is geared to level of patient. (Patients have difficulty processing input—do not overload.)
  a. Preoperatively—reinforce explanation of procedure to the patient and family. Explain that the patient will be awake (for transvenous pacing), will lie on a hard table 20–30 minutes, but discomfort will be minimal.
  b. Postoperatively—explain to the patient the nature and purpose of monitoring equipment (ECG). Monitoring will be continuous for several days, but the patient will be able to walk around in room and use bedside commode while being monitored.
    Explain to the patient that analgesics will be administered for pain at implantation site.
3. Explore with patient (preoperatively and postoperatively) those factors that evoke feelings of anxiety. Converse with the patient frequently and convey willingness to listen.
4. Encourage the patient to utilize coping mechanisms to overcome anxieties—talking, crying, walking.
5. Offer measures to ensure patient comfort—prescribed analgesics, backrubs.
6. Discuss with the patient the plan of care, allowing the patient to make decisions where appropriate.
7. Encourage family members to offer support and un-

derstanding to the patient through a willingness to listen to the patient's concerns.

D. Perceptions as to cause of fears

1. Encourage patient verbalization regarding pacemaker implantation—"What thoughts are you having about receiving and living with a pacemaker?"
2. Listen and encourage the patient's attempt to discuss fears.
3. Assess for unwarranted fears expressed by the patient (commonly, pacemaker failure) and provide explanations to alleviate fear. Explain to the patient life expectancy of batteries and the measures taken to check for failure (see Health Education, below).
4. Talk to family members about their fears and offer explanations to help allay the fears (avoids the transmission of unwarranted fears to the patient).

E. Maintaining a positive body image

1. Assess for verbal and nonverbal cues (inability to look at insertion site) indicative of nonacceptance of pacemaker.
2. Encourage the patient to express concerns regarding self-image and pacer implant.
3. Reassure the patient that sexual activity and modes of dressing will not be altered by pacemaker implantation.
4. Offer the patient the opportunity to talk to others who have had a pacemaker implantation.
5. Encourage spouse of patient or significant other to discuss concerns of self-image with the patient.

F. Resumption of previous roles and activities prior to pacemaker implantation with minimal limitations

1. Explore with the patient his feelings toward limitations secondary to illness.
  a. Discuss with the patient current life-style prior to need for pacemaker.
  b. Discuss with the patient areas of independence and dependence in his life.
  c. Discuss with the patient the importance of learning how to live with a pacemaker.
  d. Encourage family members to offer support and express to the patient their willingness to help.
2. Encourage the patient's readiness to learn.
  a. Assess the patient's readiness to learn about his pacemaker.
  b. Offer literature to the patient to review as desired (suggestion: American Heart Association Publication, "Living With a Pacemaker").
3. Encourage the patient to accept responsibility for care.
  a. Review plan of care with the patient.
  b. Encourage the patient to make decisions regarding a daily schedule of self-care activities.
  c. Engage the patient in goal-setting—establish with the patient priorities of care, time frames to accomplish goals up until discharge.
4. See Health Education, below.

Health Education

A. General Principles

1. Patient teaching should be individualized, provide for active participation by patient, and if possible, include at least one significant other of patient.

2. To evaluate the patient's retention of material, the patient should be asked to repeat in his own words the concepts discussed and return a demonstration of the skills presented.

B. Anatomy and Physiology of the Heart—utilize diagrams to identify heart structure, conduction system, and area where pacemaker is inserted.

C. Introduction to Pacemaker

1. Give the patient the manufacturer's instructions (for his particular pacemaker) and help him to become familiar with his pacemaker.
2. If available, give the patient a pacemaker to hold and identify unique features of patient's pacemaker.
3. Reassure the patient so that he will develop confidence in his pacemaker and new life-style.
   a. Physical activity does not usually have to be curtailed because of an implanted pacemaker.
   b. Sexual activity may be resumed when desired.
   c. Caution the patient not to manipulate pulse generator by twisting or retracting electrode catheter ("twiddler's syndrome").

D. Pacemaker Failure

1. Teach the patient to check his own pulse rate daily for 1 full minute at rest to be certain that preset rate remains constant.
2. Teach the patient to evaluate daily pulse rate by comparing it with a normal pulse range.
   a. To identify normal pulse range, tell the patient to record pulse rate every day for 1 month after returning to normal living pattern.
   b. Tell the patient to use the 1-month record of pulse to evaluate his daily pulse rates.
3. Teach the patient to:
   a. Report *immediately* any sudden slowing of pulse greater than 4–5 beats per minute, or any increase in pulse rate.
   b. Report signs and symptom of dizziness, fainting, palpitation, prolonged hiccups, and chest pain to physician immediately—indicative of pacemaker failure.
   c. Take pulse while these feelings are being experienced.
4. Encourage the patient to wear identification bracelet and carry pacemaker identification card that lists his pacemaker type, rate, physician's name, and the hospital where the pacemaker was inserted.

E. Electromagnetic Interference

1. Advise the patient that improvements in pacemaker design have reduced problems of electromagnetic interference (EMI). Give general instructions to the patient unless specific instructions are included with pacemaker.
   a. Sources of electromagnetic interference that still affect a number of pulse generators include high-energy radar, television and radio transmitters, industrial arc welders, certain electrocautery machines used in hospitals, airport screening devices (metal triggers alarm), antitheft devices found in jewelry and department stores, microwave oven.
   b. Teach the patient that if dizziness occurs, he should move 5–10 feet away from source (3 feet from microwave) and check pulse. Pulse should return to normal. Patient should explain to appropriate individual that he has a pacemaker.
   c. Advise the patient to sit in the back of airplanes away from the kitchens (microwaves present).
   d. Advise the patient to inform his dentist that he has a pacemaker.

F. Care of Pacemaker Site

1. Advise patient to wear loose-fitting clothing around the area of pacemaker implantation until healing has taken place.
2. Watch for signs and symptoms of infection around generator and leads—fever, heat, pain, skin breakdown at implant site.
3. Advise patient to keep incision clean and dry. Avoid showers until healing has taken place (tub bath may be taken).

G. Follow-up

1. See that the patient has a copy of his ECG tracing (according to agency policy)—for future comparisons. Encourage patient to have regular pacemaker checkup (preferably at a pacemaker clinic) for monitoring function and integrity of his pacemaker.
2. Transtelephonic evaluation of implanted cardiac pacemakers for battery and electrode failure is available.
3. Review medications with the patient prior to discharge.
4. Inform the patient that the pulse generator will have to be surgically removed for a variety of reasons (battery failure) and replaced; improved power sources and circuitry make reoperation less frequent.
   a. Relatively simple procedure performed under local anesthesia.
   b. Incision made; old generator disconnected from electrode catheter.
   c. New generator connected and placed in existing subcutaneous pocket; incision closed.
   d. Prophylactic antibiotics usually administered.
   e. Patient discharged from hospital 1–3 days postoperatively.

Evaluation
Expected Outcomes

1. Maintains an optimal cardiac output; does not demonstrate signs and symptoms of pacemaker malfunction
2. Remains free of infection—exhibits no signs/symptoms of septicemia or phlebitis; temperature normal; incision free of redness
3. Achieves a reduction in anxiety—identifies sources of anxiety and communicates ability to cope with anxiety
4. Recognizes factors causing fears—identifies fears related to pacemaker implant, utilizes family members for support, communicates ability to cope with fears
5. Resumes previous roles and activities (prior to pacemaker insertion)—demonstrates independence with daily self-care activities, verbalizes need for assistance when appropriate
6. Maintains a positive body image—expresses feelings of well-being

Atherosclerotic Heart Disease

Angina Pectoris

Angina pectoris is a clinical syndrome characterized by paroxysms of pain or oppression in the anterior chest caused by insufficient coronary blood flow and/or inadequate oxygen supply to the myocardial muscle.

Altered Physiology

Atherosclerosis of major vessels → critical obstruction with diminution of coronary blood flow → decreased myocardial oxygen delivery in response to myocardial oxygen demand → anginal pain.

Etiology

1. Usually due to atherosclerotic heart disease—is almost invariably associated with a significant obstruction of a major coronary artery.
2. May be from severe aortic stenosis or insufficiency, aortitis, hyperthyroidism, anemia, tachycardia.

Clinical Manifestations

Pain—(caused by myocardial ischemia).
1. *Location*—behind middle or upper third of sternum (retrosternal) felt deep in chest. The patient may make a fist over site of pain.
2. *Radiation*—usually radiates to neck, jaw, shoulders, and upper extremities (on left side more often than on right).
   a. Frequently may be localized.
   b. The patient often experiences tightness, choking, or a strangling sensation.
3. *Character*—constrictive, oppressive, strangling, vise-like, insistent.
   a. May be mild to severe.
   b. May produce numbness or weakness in arms, wrist, hands.
   c. Accompanied by severe apprehension and feeling of impending death.
4. *Duration*—attack usually lasts less than 3 minutes. Attacks occurring when the patient is at rest—persist 5–15 minutes.

▶ **NURSING ALERT:** Suspect an evolving acute myocardial infarction if anginal pain lasts more than 20–30 minutes.

5. *Factors precipitating anginal pain*
   a. Exertion
   b. Exposure to cold
   c. Eating a heavy meal
   d. Emotion and excitement

Diagnostic Evaluation

1. Evaluation of clinical manifestations (pain)
2. Nitroglycerin test—positive response (relief of pain) to nitroglycerin
3. ECG and stress testing—ST and T wave changes indicative of myocardial ischemia

Treatment

The objective of treatment is to reduce the work load of the heart, thereby decreasing myocardial oxygen demands, to relieve pain, and to prevent myocardial infarction.

Drug therapy combined with life-style modification and/or surgical intervention (coronary artery bypass graft surgery) are employed for the treatment of symptoms.

Pharmacotherapy

A. Nitroglycerin

(Mainstay of treatment)
1. Purpose—to reduce myocardial oxygen consumption
2. Effects—decreases ischemia and relieves anginal pain
3. Mechanism of action (not clearly established)
   a. Nitroglycerin has an effect on peripheral circulation—by increasing the capacity of the venous bed, it causes venous pooling of blood throughout the body.
   b. As a result, less blood is returned to the heart, and there is a reduction in ventricular volume, stroke volume, and cardiac output.
   c. Nitrates also relax the systemic arteriolar bed and thus may cause a fall in blood pressure.
   d. Nitrates also increase coronary blood flow and oxygen supply dilation of coronary collaterals.
4. Nitroglycerin should be taken *before* pain develops. The patient regulates the drug usage, taking the smallest dose that relieves pain.
5. Nitroglycerin is usually given sublingually (under tongue) or in buccal pouch while the patient is seated (see Health Education, p. 304).
   a. Pain relief usually begins within 3 minutes.
   b. Caution the patient not to take more than 2–3 sublingual nitroglycerin tablets over a 15-minute period.
6. Side effects—headaches, transient dizziness, weakness, syncope (may be caused by cerebral ischemia from postural hypotension); some side effects may subside with continued therapy.

B. Nitroglycerin Ointment

Appears to protect against anginal pain and promote its relief. Useful for patients experiencing nocturnal angina or whose angina occurs frequently.
1. Ointment is measured with a calibrated strip of paper that comes with the product and is smoothed onto the skin in a thin uniform layer; can be applied on any convenient skin surface, since it is topically absorbed.
2. May be covered with plastic wrap—protects clothing and enhances absorption.
3. Appears to have beneficial effects persisting up to 4–6 hours.

C. Transdermal Nitroglycerin

Impregnated on an adhesive circular bandage and applied topically to skin to provide 24-hour constant drug absorption through the skin into the systemic circulation.
1. The circular discs are applied daily to skin that is free of hair and in an area not subject to excessive movement. The site of application should be changed slightly each time to avoid undue skin irritation.

D. Beta-adrenergic Blocking Drugs

To decrease myocardial oxygen need.
1. Propranolol—reduces oxygen consumption by blocking sympathetic impulses to the heart. This produces

a reduction in heart rate, systemic blood pressure, and myocardial contractility, which is associated with a decrease in myocardial oxygen consumption. This allows the patient to work or exercise while requiring less myocardial oxygen delivery.

2. Given daily in divided doses at equally spaced intervals; dosage titrated to the patient's symptoms.
3. Side effects—fatigue, hypotension, severe bradycardia, mental depression, bronchospasm in susceptible individual; may precipitate congestive heart failure.
4. Take blood pressure and heart rate with the patient in upright position 2 hours after administration to assess for postural hypotension.
5. Do not give if pulse rate drops below 50 beats per minute.
6. Propranolol also used in conjunction with sublingual isosorbide dinitrate for antianginal and antiischemia prophylaxis.
7. Exercise ECG testing may be used to determine when optimal therapy has been achieved.

E. Calcium Channel Blockers (Calcium Antagonists)

1. Purpose—to reduce myocardial oxygen demand and decrease net myocardial oxygen consumption.
2. Effect—alter the electrochemical function of myocardial cells by blocking the influx of calcium. This causes a reduction in the mechanical activity of the cells, since the myocardial cells are unable to respond vigorously to the electrical stimulation of the pacemaker cells.
3. Mechanism of action
   a. *Coronary arterial dilation*—calcium channel blockers decrease smooth muscle tone in the coronary arteries, causing a decrease in coronary vascular resistance and a resultant increase in coronary blood flow. Coronary collateral circulation is also increased.
   b. *Negative inotropic effect*—calcium channel blockers (verapamil and diltiazem only) exert a dose-dependent negative inotropic effect, resulting in a decrease in myocardial contractility and a lowering of myocardial oxygen consumption. A low dose produces a negative inotropic effect. High doses produce substantial peripheral dilation, resulting in a reflex positive inotropic effect. The net myocardial oxygen consumption, however, remains decreased.
   c. *Peripheral arterial dilation*—calcium channel blockers cause widespread vasodilatation with a resultant decrease in systemic vascular resistance.
   d. *Automaticity*—calcium channel blockers (verapamil and diltiazem only) reduce the rate of sinus node discharge and inhibit conduction through the AV node.
4. Calcium channel blockers are used alone, in combination with either nitrates or beta-adrenergic blocking agents, or in combination with nitrates and beta-adrenergic blocking agents. Calcium channel blockers used after therapy with nitrates or beta-adrenergic blocking agents have been ineffective or only partially effective in relieving angina. Calcium channel blockers are usually added when angina occurs at rest or there is evidence of coronary spasm.
   a. *Verapamil*—side effects include dizziness, headache, constipation, hypotension, AV conduction disturbances; may increase serum concentration of digoxin.

▶ **NURSING ALERT:** Caution should be observed when combining verapamil with beta-adrenergic blocking agents, since the potency of the drugs is enhanced.

   b. *Nifedipine*—side effects include dizziness, headache, constipation, nausea, fatigue, and hypotension; may increase serum digoxin levels.
   c. *Diltiazem*—side effects include dizziness, headaches, fatigue, nausea, constipation, and rash; may produce AV conduction disturbances (to a lesser degree than verapamil).

Assessment

A. Assess and record all facets of the patient's activities that precede or precipitate attacks of anginal pain.

1. When do attacks tend to occur? Following a meal? After engaging in certain activities? After physical activities in general? After visits of family/others?
2. Where is the pain located?
3. How does the patient describe the pain?
4. Was the onset of pain sudden? Gradual?
5. How long did it last—seconds? minutes? hours?
6. Was the pain steady and unwavering in quality?
7. Is the discomfort accompanied by other symptoms? Sweating? Light-headedness? Nausea? Palpitations? Shortness of breath?
8. How many minutes after taking nitroglycerin did the pain last?
9. What was the mode of abatement?

B. Try to take an ECG during episodes of pain— ECG may show transient ST segment shifts or T wave changes that revert to normal when pain is relieved.

Patient Problems/Nursing Diagnoses

1. Chest pain related to myocardial ischemia.
2. Anxiety related to fear of impending death and uncertainty of etiology and prognosis.
3. Activity intolerance related to loss of balance between myocardial oxygen supply and demand.

Planning and Implementation
Nursing Interventions

A. Relief of pain and avoidance of complications

1. Administer medication as prescribed. (For details see Pharmacotherapy, pp. 302–303)
2. Assess effect of drug therapy, especially upon initiation of therapy or an increase in dosage.
   a. Take frequent orthostatic vital signs to evaluate the hemodynamic effects of the drugs.
   b. Notify physician if diastolic pressure falls below 60 mm. Hg.
   c. Monitor ECG for conduction disturbances in patients receiving diltiazem or verapamil.
   d. Observe for side effects of medications and be alert to possible hazard of drug interactions.
   e. Review manufacturer's instructions before administering agents, noting mechanism of action, dosage, and side effects (agents are still being studied, and dosage, side effects may change).
3. Assess for development of unstable angina (progressive increase in frequency, intensity, and duration of anginal attacks); these patients are at high risk for

myocardial infarction and sudden death; may be admitted to CCU.

    a. Assessment of acute anginal attack

      (1) How long did it take for the nitroglycerin to relieve discomfort?

      (2) Was the relief partial or complete?

      (3) Take blood pressure every 3 minutes (1–2 minutes after drug administration) to evaluate adequacy of drug effect (should be a moderate decline in systolic pressure).

      (4) Assess for dizziness and faintness after drug administration; check blood pressure and heart rate with the patient in upright position.

    b. If anginal pain undergoes a change in pattern, intensifying, lasting longer, or becoming more easily provoked, suspect an acute myocardial infarction.

4. Watch for development of congestive heart failure and arrhythmias.

5. Correct other problems in order to decrease oxygen demands of myocardium—hypertension, hyperthyroidism, aortic stenosis, anemia.

6. Prepare for surgical intervention (coronary artery bypass surgery) to bring a new blood supply to ischemic myocardium when symptoms cannot be controlled (see p. 329).

B. Decrease in anxiety

1. Explain to the patient and family reasons for hospitalization, diagnostic tests, and therapies administered.

2. Encourage the patient to verbalize fears and concerns regarding illness through frequent conversations—conveys to the patient a willingness to listen.

3. Answer the patient's questions with concise explanations.

4. Continually assess the patient's and family's level of anxiety and utilization of appropriate coping mechanisms.

5. Explain to the patient the importance of anxiety reduction to assist in control of angina. (Anxiety and fear put an increased stress on the heart, requiring the heart to use more oxygen. The result may be an imbalance of myocardial oxygen supply and demand, causing pain.)

6. Administer drugs to relieve patient anxiety.
Sedatives and tranquilizers—may be used to prevent attacks precipitated by aggravation, excitement, or tension.

7. Support the patient having coronary arteriography to determine if surgical intervention is advisable.

C. Modification of activity level

Activity considerations

1. Help the patient to participate in self-assessment to determine the provoking factors/events that precipitate the onset of angina—including physical activity, emotional pressures, worries, family, financial problems.

2. Reduce activity to below the point at which anginal pain occurs.

3. Nitroglycerin should be used prophylactically to avoid pain known to occur with certain activities (stair climbing, sexual intercourse, exposure to cold).

4. See Health Education, below.

Health Education

Instruct the patient as follows:

1. Chest discomfort or pain may be provoked by any activity that puts too much load on the heart and increases heart rate and blood pressure.

2. Use moderation in all activities to prevent an episode of anginal pain.

    a. Participate in a normal daily program of activities that do not produce chest discomfort, shortness of breath, and undue fatigue.

    b. Avoid activities known to cause anginal pain—sudden exertion, walking against the wind, extremes of temperature, high altitude, emotionally stressful situations; may accelerate heart rate, raise blood pressure, and increase cardiac work.

    c. Refrain from engaging in physical activity for 2 hours after meals. Rest after each meal if possible.

    d. Do not undertake activities requiring heavy effort (carrying heavy objects).

    e. Try to avoid cold weather if possible; dress warmly and walk more slowly. Wear scarf over nose and mouth when in cold air.

    f. Reduce weight, if necessary, to reduce cardiac load.

    g. Avoid overeating.

      (1) Avoid excessive caffeine intake (coffee, cola drinks) that can increase the heart rate and produce angina.

      (2) Do not use "diet pills," nasal decongestants, or any over-the-counter medications that can increase the heart rate or stimulate high blood pressure.

      (3) Avoid the use of alcohol or drink alcohol only in moderation (alcohol can increase hypotensive side effects of drugs).

3. Use prescribed nitroglycerin effectively.

    a. Carry nitroglycerin at all times.

      (1) Nitroglycerin is volatile and is inactivated by heat, moisture, air, light, and time.

      (2) Keep nitroglycerin in original dark glass container, tightly closed—to prevent absorption of drug by other pills or pillbox.

      (3) Do not carry nitroglycerin in a plastic or metal pillbox or mixed with other pills.

      (4) Renew supply every 5–6 months.

      (5) Nitroglycerin should cause a slight burning or stinging sensation under the tongue when it is potent.

    b. Place nitroglycerin under tongue at first sign of chest discomfort.

      (1) Stop all effort/activity; sit, and take nitroglycerin tablet—relief should be obtained in a few minutes.

      (2) Do not swallow saliva until tablet is dissolved.

      (3) Bite the tablet between front teeth and slip under tongue to dissolve if quick action is desired.

      (4) Repeat dosage in a few minutes for total of 3 tablets if relief is not obtained.

      (5) Keep a record of number of tablets taken—to evaluate any change in anginal pattern.

      (6) Take nitroglycerin prophylactically to avoid pain known to occur with certain activities.

4. If taking a beta blocker, do not interrupt therapy without first consulting the physician—abrupt withdrawal can produce exacerbation of angina, myocardial infarction.

5. Go to nearest health care facility if pain persists more than 20 minutes or becomes more intense or widespread. (Do not drive yourself.)

6. If dizziness or faintness occurs, lower head between legs and breathe deeply to enhance recovery from symptoms.

7. Mild headaches are common. If severe headaches

occur (lasting longer than 15 minutes) consult physician. Dosage may have to be reduced.

8. Provide information to the patient regarding vocational rehabilitation if a less stressful job is needed.
9. Inform the patient of available cardiac rehabilitation programs.
10. Inform the patient of available methods of learning stress management: biofeedback, Transcendental Meditation, etc.
11. Encourage the patient to obtain a medication information card and carry card at all times. Cards may be obtained from Medical Alert Foundation, Turlock, California 95380.

Evaluation

Expected Outcomes

1. Maintains balance between myocardial oxygen supply and demand; absence of chest pain, takes appropriate measures to relieve pain, calls nurse, takes nitroglycerin, and stops activity.
2. Experiences no complications; normal sinus rhythm, chest pain duration less than 5 minutes, chest pain relieved with nitroglycerin.
3. Achieves a decrease in anxiety; verbalizes lessening anxiety, verbalizes ability to cope.
4. Adheres to modified activity level; avoids activities that precipitate angina attacks.

Guidelines: Percutaneous Transluminal Coronary Angioplasty (PTCA)

Percutaneous transluminal coronary angioplasty (PTCA) is a technique utilized for the treatment of coronary artery disease (CAD) unresponsive to medical therapy. A balloon-tipped catheter is introduced through a guidewire into a coronary vessel with a proximal, accessible, noncalcified atheromatous lesion. The balloon of the catheter is then inflated, causing disruption of the intima and changes in the atheroma. The result is an increase in the diameter of the lumen of the coronary vessel (as judged by angiographic criteria) and improvement of blood flow below the lesion. Balloon inflation/deflation may be repeated until satisfactory results are achieved (Fig. 9-9).

Contraindications

1. Patients with left main coronary artery disease are generally not good candidates for this procedure.
2. Patients with multi-vessel disease (role of procedure remains unclear).

Complications

Coronary occlusion occurs in approximately 5% of patients. Necessitates immediate coronary artery bypass graft surgery to avert myocardial infarction. A cardiac surgical team must be on standby during all PTCA procedures.

Procedure

Nursing Actions	Rationale / Amplification
Preparatory Phase	
1. Assess the patient's level of understanding of PTCA procedure.	1. Cardiologist will initially explain procedure to the patient.
a. Ask the patient to describe in own words the procedure and the events that will occur before, during, and after the procedure.	a. Teaching is geared to the patient's comprehension level to minimize stress.
2. Reinforce all information about the procedure and accompanying events. Instruct the patient as follows:	2. Preparation for procedure minimizes anxiety and enhances recovery.
a. Procedure will be performed in cardiac catheterization laboratory and is approximately 2 hours in length (see Heart Catheterization, p. 281).	a. Procedure similar to coronary arteriography. All tactile and auditory stimuli should be explained to the patient.
b. Discuss diagnostic tests to be done prior to procedure.	b. Chest x-ray, ECG, blood tests: coagulation, complete blood count, electrolytes; urinalysis, myocardial imaging
c. The location of coronary vessels and a description of the patient's lesion.	c. Use diagrams of heart if possible.
d. Local anesthesia will be given at catheter insertion site.	d. Promotes patient comfort.
e. The patient will be alert throughout procedure and will be asked to cough.	e. Coughing enhances catheter placement.
f. A temporary pacemaker will be inserted.	f. Used for emergency pacing if necessary.
g. Medication (heparin, nitroglycerin) will be given.	g. Heparin prevents clot formation. Nitroglycerin reduces incidence of coronary spasm.
h. Stress importance of reporting chest pain to nurse or physician prior to, during, or after procedure.	h. Indicates myocardial ischemia, which could precipitate complications.
i. Food and fluid will be restricted the night and morning before procedure.	i. Reduces incidence of stomach upset during procedure.
j. Bed rest will be maintained for 6 to 12 hours after procedure, with head of bed elevated no more than 30 degrees, and immobilization of affected extremity.	j. Activity may cause bleeding and prolong healing of vessel lining.
k. Patient may eat after procedure.	k. IV line will remain in place for 6 hours.
l. Vital signs will be observed frequently.	l. Necessary for detection of complications.

(continued)

Guidelines: Percutaneous Transluminal Coronary Angioplasty (PTCA) (continued)

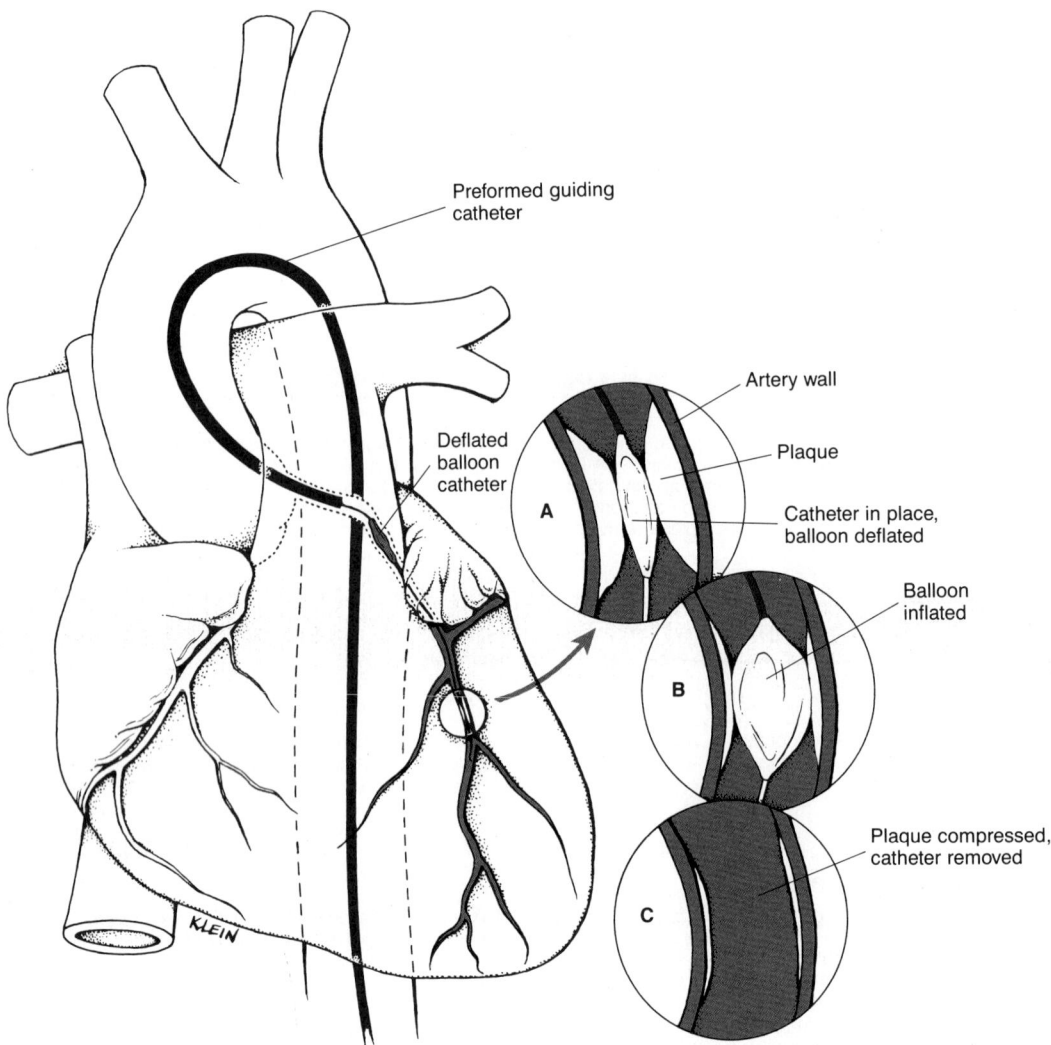

Figure 9-9. Percutaneous transluminal coronary angioplasty. (*A*) The balloon-tipped catheter is passed into the affected coronary artery. (*B*) The balloon is then rapidly inflated and deflated with controlled pressure. (*C*) The balloon disrupts the intima and causes changes in the atheroma, resulting in an increase in the diameter of the lumen of the vessel and improvement of blood flow. (Redrawn after Purcell JA and Giffin PA: Percutaneous transluminal coronary angioplasty. Am J Nurs 81[9]:1620–1626, Sept 1981)

Procedure
(Cont.)

Nursing Action	Rationale / Amplification
m. Indwelling urethral catheter will remain for 6 hours after procedure.	m. Diuresis caused by contrast medium used during procedure may cause intense thirst.
n. Discharge will be the following day.	
3. Prepare the patient for complications of procedure. (Prior to procedure, patient must be a suitable candidate for heart surgery and have consented to heart surgery as alternative treatment.)	3. Coronary artery occlusion, coronary artery rupture, or acute coronary artery spasm may necessitate cardiopulmonary bypass graft surgery.
a. Provide preoperative teaching to the patient and family regarding heart surgery (see Heart Surgery, p. 328).	

Procedure
(Cont.)

Nursing Action	Rationale / Amplification
4. Record the patient's vital signs prior to going to catheterization laboratory. a. Assess peripheral pulses and color and temperature of extremities.	4. Provides baseline data for comparison after procedure.

Post Procedure Phase

Nursing Action	Rationale / Amplification
1. Check vital signs every 15 minutes for 1 hour, then every half hour for 2 hours, and finally every hour for 4 hours.	1. Allows for frequent assessment of possible complications—bleeding, bradycardia, hypotension.
2. Place sandbag over insertion site.	2. Prevents bleeding.

3. Check peripheral pulse of affected extremity and insertion site after each vital sign check.
   a. Look for presence of hematoma and mark hematoma to note change in size.
   b. Check bed linen for blood under patient.
   c. Mark peripheral pulse of affected extremity with water-soluble ink.
   d. Observe color and temperature of affected extremity.
	3. Because intraprocedure heparinization is not reversed, there is increased chance of bleeding after procedure.
	   a. Notify physician if hematoma continues to enlarge or if bleeding is not controlled after pressure is applied at site with fingers.
	   c. Facilitates pulse checks.
	   d. Notify physician if extremities become cool and pale, and pulses become significantly diminished or absent.

4. Record intake and output and monitor serum electrolytes.	4. Contrast medium used during procedure causes diuresis and potassium depletion.

Follow-up Phase

Nursing Action	Rationale / Amplification

1. Instruct the patient as follows:
   a. Modification of cardiac risk factors as means of controlling progression of coronary artery disease.
 	
   b. Name of medications, action, dosage, and side effects.
 	
   c. Dates and importance of follow-up tests—exercise ECG, thallium-201 perfusion imaging.
   d. Symptoms for which patient should seek medical attention—side effects of medications, chest pain, or weight increases greater than 5 pounds.
	a. PTCA is palliative treatment for coronary artery disease, not a cure.
	   Refer patient to outpatient cardiac rehabilitation program.
	   b. Common medications prevent clot formation (aspirin, Anturane, Persantine); increase blood flow to heart (Isordil); or slow heart rate/decrease chest pain (Inderal).
	   c. Stenosis can recur within 6 months. Second angioplasty usually successful for more than 1 year.
	   d. Chest pain unrelieved with nitroglycerin and persisting longer than 15 minutes after rest is significant.

Myocardial Infarction (MI)

Myocardial infarction refers to the process by which myocardial tissue is destroyed in regions of the heart that are deprived of their blood supply because of a reduced coronary blood flow.

Causes

1. Critical narrowing of a coronary artery—due to atherosclerosis, spasm, or complete occlusion of artery from emboli or thrombus.
2. Decreased coronary blood flow—causes a profound imbalance between myocardial oxygen supply and demand.

Assessment
Clinical Manifestations

1. Chest pain—steady, constrictive pain (central portion of chest and epigastrium) not relieved by rest or nitrates; pain may radiate widely; may produce arrhythmias, hypotension, shock, cardiac failure
2. Profuse perspiration; moist, clammy skin with pallor
3. Drop in blood pressure
4. Dyspnea, weakness, and fainting

5. Nausea and vomiting
6. Anxiety and restlessness
7. Tachycardia or bradycardia

▶ **NURSING ALERT:** Many patients do not have symptoms; these are the "silent myocardial infarctions." Nevertheless there is still resultant damage to the myocardium.

8. Atypical symptoms—extreme fatigue, epigastric or abdominal distress, shortness of breath.

Diagnostic Evaluation

1. Clinical history and findings from physical examination.
2. ECG changes (within 2–12 hours, but may take as long as 72–96 hours). See page 338 for ECG interpretation of MI.
3. Elevation of serum isoenzymes (see CPK-MB test).
4. Radionuclide imaging—see page 280; allows recognition of areas of decreased perfusion as "cold spots," which are seen in areas of ischemia and infarction.

Treatment

The objective of treatment is to promote adequate circulatory function with healing of the myocardium, to limit size of infarct, and to prevent death.

Patient Problems/Nursing Diagnoses

1. Alteration in cardiac output related to mechanical factors (preload, afterload, contractility).
2. Pain related to myocardial ischemia.
3. Anxiety related to fear of death, complex environment, and uncertainty of etiology and prognosis.
4. Activity intolerance related to imbalance between myocardial oxygen supply and demand.
5. Altered pattern of elimination; constipation related to restricted activity level.
6. Potential for depression related to threats to self-esteem and disturbances in sleep–rest patterns.

Planning and Implementation

Nursing Interventions

A. Maintaining hemodynamic stability

1. Admit to cardiac care unit for constant monitoring.
   a. Lift patient from stretcher to bed; place in position of comfort.
   b. Start an intravenous infusion running slowly—to keep vein open for administration of IV medications in event of an arrhythmia.
2. Attach ECG monitoring electrodes to monitor the heart rhythm and to confirm clinical impression of MI.
3. Utilize hemodynamic monitoring for critically ill patient (see Swan–Ganz, p. 282).
4. Continually assess peripheral perfusion (blood supply to organs and tissues).
   a. Measure and record vital signs every 1–2 hours to determine presence of impending cardiogenic shock and other complications.
      (1) Note on record, method of taking blood pressure (palpation/auscultation).
      (2) Evaluate both apical and radial pulse rates. Note strength of femoral pulse.
   b. Count respirations—tachypnea may indicate congestive heart failure, pulmonary embolism.
   c. Monitor body temperature—gives some indication of tissue perfusion.
   d. Assess skin temperature and color.
   e. Auscultate for breath sounds, crackles.
   f. Auscultate the heart for gallop, friction rub, murmurs.
   g. Assess neck veins for distention—elevation of venous pressure may indicate failure of heart to pump effectively.
   h. Assess for changes in mental status (apathy, confusion, restlessness)—from inadequate cerebral perfusion.
   i. Evaluate urine output (30 ml./hour)—decrease in urine volume reflects a decrease in renal blood flow.
5. Be alert for indications of complications.
   a. *Cardiogenic shock*
      (1) Falling arterial blood pressure.
      (2) Reduced urinary volume (30 ml./hour or less).
      (3) Cool, moist skin; may be peripheral cyanosis—due to systemic vasoconstriction caused by reduction in cardiac output.
      (4) Restlessness, apathy, lessening of responsiveness—from systemic vasoconstriction.
      (5) See page 310 for management of cardiogenic shock. A patient with cardiogenic shock should, ideally, be transferred to cardiac center with hemodynamic monitoring capabilities.
   b. *Congestive heart failure*—myocardial infarction reduces ability of left ventricle to eject blood, diminishes cardiac output, produces an elevation of left ventricular end pressure with ensuing pulmonary vascular complications.
      (1) Assess for tachycardia and gallop rhythm, dyspnea, orthopnea, edema, hepatomegaly.
      (2) Watch for development of pulmonary edema (see p. 327)—represents extreme left ventricular failure. Assess for extreme dyspnea, frothy, blood-stained mucus, tachycardia, distended neck veins, and diffuse crackles.
      (3) See page 324 and page 327 for treatment of congestive heart failure and acute pulmonary edema.
   c. *Other complications*
      (1) Papillary muscle rupture, ventricular septal rupture, ventricular aneurysm.
      (2) Postmyocardial infarction syndrome (Dressler's syndrome)—a recurrent febrile illness with pericarditis, pleuritis, and pneumonitis.
      (3) Cerebral and peripheral emboli; pulmonary emboli.
   d. *Prepare for surgical intervention if indicated*—insertion of intra-aortic counterpulsation device, coronary artery bypass, repair of ventricular septal defect, mitral valve replacement. (See nursing management of patient undergoing heart surgery, p. 328.)
6. Monitor dietary intake.
   a. Diet is prescribed according to status of circulatory condition.
   b. Full liquids for 24 hours (per physician request) to reduce increase in cardiac output needed for digestion. Diet progresses depending on the patient's lipid analysis, body weight, etc.
   c. Avoid large meals, which increase demand for splanchnic blood flow and increase cardiac workload.

B. Avoidance of life-threatening arrhythmias

1. *Arrhythmias*—occur frequently in first few days after infarction. The reduction in myocardial oxygenation produces myocardial ischemia. Ischemic muscle is electrically unstable and produces arrhythmias. Risk of ventricular fibrillation and death is greatest in first few hours following MI.
   a. Assess, prevent, and treat conditions that may initiate an arrhythmia—congestive heart failure, pulmonary embolus, inadequate pulmonary ventilation, electrolyte disturbances, underoxygenation of blood.
   b. Draw arterial blood for blood gas analysis.
   c. Watch for ventricular fibrillation, ventricular tachycardia, AV block, asystole.
   d. See page 296 for management of arrhythmias.
2. Be vigilant for occurrence of any type of premature ventricular beats—may presage ventricular tachycardia and ventricular fibrillation. (See p. 339 for discussion of arrhythmias.)
   a. Correct arrhythmia immediately—may unfavorably alter the balance between oxygen supply and demand at the periphery of the infarct.
   b. Lidocaine may be given prophylactically—to protect patient against ventricular fibrillation.

c. Other antiarrhythmic drugs include procainamide, quinidine, propranolol, atropine, etc.—selected by classification.

d. Prepare patient for prophylactic pacing (p. 297), if indicated.

3. Administer oxygen by nasal cannula (p. 189) if prescribed by physician, and encourage patient to take deep breaths—may decrease incidence of arrhythmias by allowing the myocardium to be less ischemic and thus less irritable; may reduce size of infarct.

C. Establishing balance between myocardial oxygen supply and demand

1. Offer psychological support and reassurance to patient to decrease anxiety.

2. Give analgesic, morphine, or meperidine—decreases sympathetic activity and reduces myocardial oxygen consumption with subsequent decreases in heart rate, blood pressure, and muscle tension.

3. Give in small IV doses repeated every 15–20 minutes until relief is obtained (if vital signs are within safe parameters).

▶ **NURSING ALERT:** Assess for persistent or recurring pain, which suggests an extension or threatened extension of infarct; urgent and aggressive intervention is required. Notify physician immediately.

4. Monitor blood pressure, pulse, and respiratory rate before administering narcotics—narcotics depress arterial pressure and may contribute to development of shock and arrhythmias. Do not leave patient in a sitting position.

5. Assess for complications of narcotic administration, such as respiratory impairment (especially in patients with chronic obstructive pulmonary disease) and hypotension.

6. Avoid intramuscular injections of analgesic agents, since they may cause falsely elevated serum CK values, resulting in an incorrect diagnosis of myocardial infarction.

D. Decreasing anxiety

1. Assess levels of anxiety and coping mechanisms of patient and his family.

2. Relieve the patient's pain and anxiety—anxiety and fear increase the heart rate (which puts heart under more stress), raise the blood pressure, and cause the adrenal glands to release epinephrine, which may produce an arrhythmia.

3. Administer antianxiety agents—anxiety is associated with increased sympathetic drive.

4. Discuss with patient CCU environment and what can be anticipated in the coming days, to allay anxiety and help him mobilize his resources for coping.

5. Explain all procedures to the patient and invite questions.

6. If severe anxiety is present, try to maintain consistency of care, with one or two nurses assisting patient regularly.

7. Before discharge from coronary care unit, prepare the patient for non-intensive care environment through discussions with family and patient, focusing on the decreased need to monitor patient continually.

E. Adjustment in activity level

1. Promote bed rest with increased mobilization.
   a. Place the patient at rest—to lower heart rate and blood pressure and oxygen demands of heart and to maintain cardiac work at its lowest level.

The following is an example of an activity schedule:
   (1) Day 1—bed rest with commode; requires less cardiovascular work than bedpan.
   (2) Day 2—sitting on side of bed 3 times daily for 5 minutes.
   (3) Day 3—out of bed to chair, as tolerated, for 5–15 minutes (usually 3 times daily is sufficient).
   (4) Day 4—lengthen time allotted for chair rest.
   (5) Day 5—ambulation in room as tolerated and beginning walks to corridor.

2. Assist with implementation of self-care activities on a gradual basis.
   a. Initially, patient may feed self.
   b. Complete bed bath on day one.
   c. Assist with bed bath on day two to day five.
   d. After discharge from coronary care unit, a warm shower may be taken with chair in shower, or assistance.

3. Instruct patient to avoid any sudden effort.

4. Offer patient diversional activities, such as light reading and listening to the radio.

5. Apply antiembolism stockings.

F. Establishing normal elimination pattern

1. Administer stool softeners as directed.

2. Offer diet with bulk and fiber.

3. Limit foods known to produce excess gas.

4. Allow use of bedside commode rather than bedpan.

G. Developing adaptive coping abilities

1. Assess the patient's stage of grieving.

2. Give intelligent reassurance and assist the patient in establishing a positive attitude toward his illness.
   a. Most persons use the mechanism of denial during initial stages of MI.
   b. Depression is commonly encountered on about the 3rd day in CCU, although it may not surface until the patient returns home.
      (1) Depression following MI is normal; the patient is grieving over his losses—health, confidence, independence.
      (2) The patient may feel pressure from having to alter his life-style (i.e., eating, drinking, smoking).

3. Assess for maladaptive coping patterns—inappropriate denial, withdrawal, changes in usual communicative patterns, destructive behavior. Ask the patient what he is thinking about and feeling; try to draw out specific concerns.

4. Involve family in support and education.

5. Allow the patient to have control over plan of care as much as possible; include the patient in decision-making when appropriate.

6. Compliment the patient on activities he is able to do; avoid false reassurance.

7. Discuss with the patient usual sleep patterns—onset of sleep, usual waking time, number of hours of rest needed daily.

8. Manipulate environment to provide and maintain the patient's normal sleep patterns.

Health Education

Goals:

Restore patient to his optimal physiologic, psychological, social, and work level.

Aid in restoring confidence and self-esteem.

Prevent progression of underlying disease (atherosclerosis).

1. Inform the patient about what has happened to his

heart and explain that myocardial healing starts early but is not complete for 6–8 weeks.

2. A myocardial infarction may require some modification of life-style.

3. Exercise tolerance testing will be done after myocardial healing to determine optimal level of activity and to plan rehabilitation program.

4. A program of exercise training will be prescribed at this time to improve cardiovascular functional capacity.

5. Physical limitations are usually only temporary. The following guidelines usually apply until the patient is reevaluated after complete myocardial healing:
   a. Expect to feel weak and tired for a period of time; depression is not uncommon.
   b. Walk daily, gradually increasing the distance and time.
   c. Avoid doing anything that tenses the muscles (isometric exercises, weight lifting, straining, lifting heavy objects, pushing/pulling heavy loads)—may place strain on coronary reserve.
   d. Rest after meals and before doing any exercise.
   e. Space activities throughout the day to alternate rest and work.
      (1) Stop as soon as fatigued.
      (2) Avoid tenseness and rushing.
   f. Avoid working with arms above shoulder level.
   g. Shorten work hours when first returning to work.

6. Advise the patient to eat 3–4 meals daily (each containing about the same amount of food).
   a. Avoid large meals.
   b. Avoid hurrying while eating.
   c. Limit caffeine intake (coffee and cola) and cigarette smoking.
   d. Maintain prescribed diet (modifications in calories, fats, and sodium).

7. Extremes in temperature and walking against the wind should be avoided.
   a. Stop immediately for shortness of breath.
   b. Sit down and take nitroglycerin for chest pain.

8. Sexual relations may be resumed upon advice of physician, usually after exercise tolerance is assessed.
   a. If patient can walk briskly or climb two flights of stairs, he can usually resume sexual activity with familiar partner; resumption of sexual activity parallels resumption of usual activities.
   b. Sexual activity should be avoided after eating a heavy meal, after drinking alcohol, or when tired.

9. Instruct the patient to notify the physician when the following symptoms appear:
   a. Chest pressure or pain not relieved in 15 minutes by nitroglycerin or rest
   b. Shortness of breath
   c. Unusual fatigue
   d. Swelling of feet and ankles
   e. Fainting, dizziness
   f. Very slow or rapid heart beat

10. Explain pharmacologic regimen.

Evaluation
Expected Outcomes

1. Maintains hemodynamic stability; exhibits no signs/symptoms of heart failure—diaphoresis, hypotension, change in mental status, cool, clammy skin

2. Experiences no life-threatening arrhythmias; heart rate 60–100 beats per minute; rhythm—normal sinus rhythm

3. Maintains balance between myocardial oxygen supply and demand; experiences no chest pain; calls nurse if experiences pain

4. Experiences a decrease in anxiety; exhibits calm speech pattern, relaxed facial expression, verbalizes feelings about death

5. Adheres to limited activity prescription; engages in activities according to CCU protocol

6. Maintains normal elimination pattern; soft, formed stool per normal pattern for patient

7. Copes adaptively to illness; communicates self-confidence in future life-style; requests information regarding illness, environment, and routines; participates in self-care activities

Cardiogenic Shock

Cardiogenic shock (power failure), the end stage of left ventricular dysfunction, occurs when the left ventricle is extensively damaged by myocardial infarction. The heart muscle loses its contractile power, and there is marked reduction in cardiac output with decreased perfusion (lack of blood and oxygen) to vital organs (heart, brain, and kidneys). The degree of pump dysfunction is related to the extent of damage to the heart muscle.

Cardiogenic shock now accounts for the majority of hospital deaths from myocardial infarction and has a high mortality rate.

Assessment
Clinical Manifestations

1. Low systolic pressure (90 mm. Hg or 30 mm. Hg less than previous levels)

2. Oliguria—urine output less than 30 ml./hour—from impaired renal circulation

3. Cold, clammy skin, weak pulse, cyanosis—from circulatory insufficiency

4. Mental lethargy, confusion—from poor cerebral perfusion

Diagnostic Evaluation

1. Physical examination—signs/symptoms of decrease in cerebral, renal, and peripheral perfusion, pulmonary congestion, and hypotension.

2. Medical history—reduction in cardiac output unrelated to hypovolemia, significant arrhythmias, depressive drug therapy, arterial hypoxia, or acute pain.

3. Diagnosis of MI—ECG, medical history, physical examination.

Treatment

1. The management of cardiogenic shock is directed at decreasing pulmonary congestion, improving cardiac output, and decreasing systemic congestion while preserving the borderline areas of the myocardium and limiting infarct size.

2. Measures to decrease pulmonary congestion focus on reduction of venous return or reduction of circulating blood volume. Cardiac output is improved through therapy that decreases cardiac workload and stimulates cardiac contractility while maintaining balance of myocardial oxygen supply and demand. Systemic congestion is treated by decreasing circulating blood volume.

Patient Problems/Nursing Diagnoses

1. Impaired cardiac output related to massive ischemic damage to the left ventricle.

2. Impaired gas exchange related to pulmonary congestion.
3. Alteration in mental status related to impaired cerebral blood flow.
4. Impaired tissue perfusion related to decreased peripheral blood flow.

Planning and Implementation
Nursing Interventions

A. Improvement in cardiac output

1. Start hemodynamic monitoring at the *first* indication of deterioration of the patient's condition—hemodynamic monitoring is necessary for continuing patient evaluation and serves as a guideline for therapy. Measure left ventricular pressure—oxygen demands of ischemic myocardium are determined by left ventricular pressure and heart rate, myocardial contractility, size, shape, and wall thickness of left ventricle.
    a. Measurement of left ventricular end-diastolic pressure is estimated by the pulmonary arterial wedge pressure as measured by the Swan–Ganz catheter.
        (1) Values are elevated in patients with left ventricular failure, mitral valve disease, pulmonary hypertension.
        (2) See page 282 for technique.
    b. Pulmonary capillary wedge pressure (PCWP) provides an accurate estimate of left ventricular filling pressure only in the absence of mitral valve disease.
        (1) Used also as a guide for infusion therapy; pulmonary congestion is indicated by PCWP greater than 18 mm. Hg; the increase signifies that the left side of the heart is in failure.
        (2) See page 285 for technique.
    c. Evaluate cardiac output—pulmonary artery catheters are also used to evaluate cardiac output by thermodilution technique.
2. Measure intra-arterial pressure by direct arterial cannulization—more accurate measurement of blood pressure.
3. Administer continuous oxygen at percentages needed to combat hypoxemia.
4. Correct hypovolemia.
    a. Administer IV fluids until left ventricular pressure increases to 18–20 mm. Hg (the value associated with highest cardiac output).
    b. Watch for development of pulmonary edema, which may occur abruptly.
5. Give appropriate drug therapy if the patient is still in shock—to lessen ischemia and limit size of infarct and decrease the work of the heart.
    a. *Vasodilator therapy*—vasodilator drugs dilate capacitance vessels (veins and venules) and/or resistance vessels (arterioles), reducing impedance to left ventricular outflow and venous return to the heart; decreases myocardial oxygen consumption; improves perfusion to organs. Vasodilators in current use include sodium nitroprusside, phentolamine, and nitroglycerin.
    b. *Inotropic agents*—used to increase cardiac output by direct effect on myocardium. Include digitalis, dopamine, and dobutamine.
    c. *Diuretics*—may reduce tissue edema at site of infarct and improve myocardial perfusion and oxygenation.
6. Measure urine volume via indwelling catheter every ½–1 hour—urine flow reflects renal blood flow and the status of central circulation.
7. Relieve psychological stress and anxiety—explain all procedures to the patient, allow family members to visit, administer sedation per physician request (anxiety may cause an increase in myocardial oxygen demand).
8. Be alert for significant arrhythmia.
9. Auscultate for extra heart sounds and murmurs every 2–4 hours—report abnormalities to physician.
    a. Utilize counterpulsation to decrease ventricular work of the patient with severe shock. (See description of method, which follows.)
    b. Prepare the patient for surgical intervention to correct defects that are interfering with pump function and to reperfuse the heart (see Patient Undergoing Heart Surgery, p. 328).

B. Decrease in pulmonary congestion

1. Assess for signs/symptoms of acute pulmonary congestion.
    a. Auscultate lung fields every 2–4 hours and evaluate for crackles and wheezes.
    b. Note and record respiratory rate of patient, evidence of dyspnea, cough, hemoptysis, orthopnea.
2. Monitor arterial blood gases to assess for hypoxia and metabolic acidosis.
3. Place the patient in semi-Fowler's or Fowler's position (decreases venous return).
4. Administer drug therapy as directed.
    a. Morphine sulfate—aids in decreasing venous return.
    b. Aminophylline—reduces bronchospasm caused by severe congestion; also can act as peripheral vasodilator.
    c. Vasodilators—dilate venous and arterial beds to varying degrees, causing a decrease in venous return and systemic vascular resistance (nitroprusside, nitroglycerin).
    d. Diuretics—decrease circulating blood volume and may have an effect on decreasing venous return.
5. Be alert for complications of drug therapy (aminophylline may cause nausea, vomiting, tachyarrhythmias).
6. Monitor the patient closely during administration of mechanical ventilation (positive end-expiratory pressure [PEEP] may be implemented to aid in decreasing venous return and to improve arterial oxygenation) and plasmapheresis (decreases blood volume by removing blood from circulation).

C. Improvement in level of consciousness

1. Assess for mental status changes every 2 hours utilizing a systematic approach (i.e., Glasgow Coma Scale).
2. Report changes to physician immediately.

D. Adequate tissue perfusion

1. Assess for tissue symptoms indicative of heart failure progressing to shock (see Clinical Manifestations, #3).
2. Report symptoms to physician immediately.

Evaluation
Expected Outcomes

1. Demonstrates improved cardiac output—CO greater than 2.5 liter/minute, CI (cardiac index) greater than 2.2 liter/minute/m², PCWP less than 18 mm. Hg, urine output greater than 30 ml./hour
2. Exhibits a decrease in pulmonary congestion—spon-

taneous respirations in range of 14–18, breath sounds clear on auscultation, blood gas values (arterial) within normal limits for patient

3. Demonstrates improved level of conciousness—alert (follows commands), absence of confusion, pupils equal and reactive to light
4. Exhibits adequate tissue perfusion—skin warm and dry, nailbeds and lips with normal coloring

Counterpulsation
(Mechanical Cardiac Assistance)

Counterpulsation (diastolic augmentation) is a method of assisting the failing heart and circulation by mechanical support that may be accomplished by (1) intra-aortic balloon pump or (2) external counterpulsation pressure. Counterpulsation with an intra-aortic balloon pump (IABP) during the acute phase of myocardial infarction eases the workload of a damaged heart and if started before irre-versible change takes place, may limit infarct size by increasing coronary blood flow.

A. Intra-aortic Balloon Pump—introduction of a balloon catheter via the femoral artery or via a percutaneous route into the descending thoracic aorta; it is inflated and deflated in sequence with the cardiac cycle and acts as an auxiliary pump assisting forward blood flow (Fig. 9-10). This provides an augmentation of diastole, which results in an increase in coronary blood flow and cardiac output, and it reduces left ventricular end pressure (by causing a more complete emptying of the left ventricle). This decreases the resistance in the arterial tree against which the heart must pump and reduces myocardial oxygen requirements.

1. Using synchronization with the patient's ECG, the balloon is inflated at the onset of diastole ("diastolic augmentation"); this results in increased diastolic pressure, which increases coronary blood flow and myocardial nutrition.
2. The balloon is deflated at the onset of cardiac systole

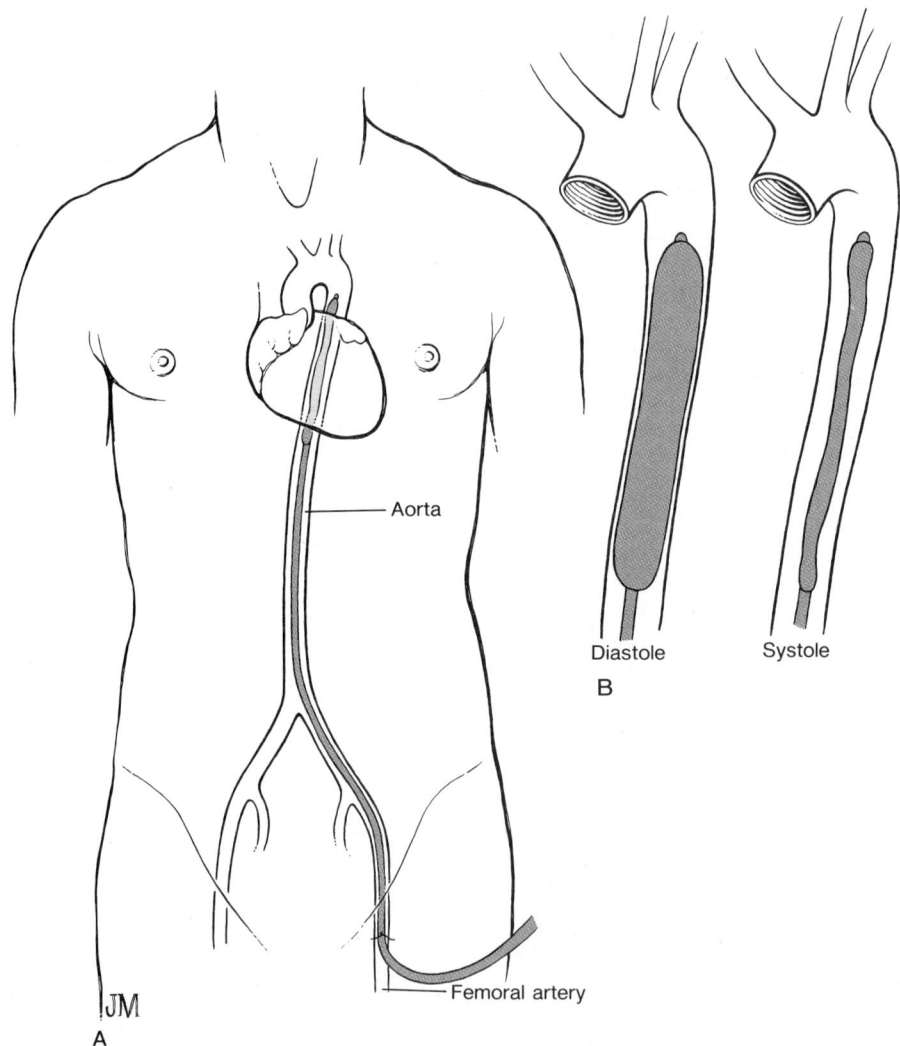

Aorta

Diastole

Systole

B

Femoral artery

A

Figure 9-10. Counterpulsation. (*A*) Introduction of the intra-aortic bal-loon catheter via the femoral artery. (*B*) The intra-aortic balloon pump augments diastole, resulting in in-creased perfusion of the coronary ar-teries and myocardium and a de-crease in the left ventricular work load.

to lower the aortic blood pressure so that the work of the left ventricle is reduced (reduction in left ventricular impedance and afterload).

3. A bedside console provides gas for balloon inflation and controls the inflation/deflation cycle to accommodate variations in the patient's heart rate.

It is timed by the ECG and triggered by the arterial pulse wave.

4. *Clinical Uses*
   a. Treatment of cardiogenic shock following myocardial infarction
   b. Low cardiac output states—following open heart surgery; life-threatening arrhythmias
   c. High cardiac output states—sepsis, hemorrhage
   d. Myocardial ischemia unresponsive to medical therapy and external counterpulsation pressure.

B. **External Counterpulsation Pressure** (ECP)—a noninvasive method of assisting the circulation; it is designed to boost the heart temporarily during a period of pump failure. It helps maintain adequate perfusion of vital organs and tissues until the heart is able to resume its function.

1. The counterpulsation device is positioned around the lower extremities from thighs to ankles; the legs are encased in 2 rigid troughs, and the system is closed to make an airtight seal.

2. A pump is positioned between the patient's ankles.

3. Water is pumped through the system during diastole in response to an electronic signal triggered by the ECG; squeezing the legs during diastole forces a column of arterial blood back to the heart, which provides diastolic augmentation and improves coronary arterial filling pressure.

4. The pressure is released (application of negative pressure) during cardiac systole, which lowers the systolic pressure (and thus the peak left ventricular pressure).

5. In cardiogenic shock, ECP increases the coronary blood flow by raising diastolic pressure, which may improve cardiac function; compression of the legs also increases venous return to the heart and thus increases cardiac output. Left ventricular work is thus reduced.

6. *Clinical Uses*
   a. Chest pain associated with MI unrelieved by medical therapy
   b. Mild to moderate heart failure

7. See Myocardial Infarction, page 307 and Cardiogenic Shock, page 310.

Patient Problems/Nursing Diagnoses
(Patient receiving IABP therapy)

1. Fear related to invasive therapy, environment, and death.
2. Impaired cardiac output related to refractory left ventricular failure.
3. Potential for injury related to thrombus formation, thrombocytopenia and infection.
4. Immobility related to IABP therapy.
5. Sleep pattern disturbance related to ICU environment.

Planning and Implementation
Nursing Interventions

A. **Reduction of fear**

1. Explain procedure to the patient and invite questions.
2. Allow the patient to verbalize fears regarding illness and therapy.

3. Offer reassurance and comfort measures.
4. Explain therapy to family and encourage them to visit and discuss fears with the patient.
5. Obtain consent form from patient or authorized family member prior to procedure.

B. **Establishing hemodynamic stability**

1. Assist physician and patient during insertion of IABP catheter.
2. Monitor hemodynamic parameters with Swan–Ganz catheter and intra-arterial line (see Hemodynamic Monitoring, p. 282).
   a. Record CVP, PCWP, PAP, CO, HR, BP.
   b. Record date, time, and the patient's tolerance of procedure.
3. Start IABP immediately after insertion according to physician's request.
   a. Note timing of inflation and deflation of balloon every hour and adjust as necessary.
   b. Record vital signs every 15–30 minutes for 4–9 hours and then hourly.
   c. Record gas utilized for pumping (CO_2 or helium).
   d. Review manufacturer's manual for IABP equipment in use.
4. Monitor and record urine output from indwelling catheter every hour.
5. Record daily intake and output.
6. Treat arrhythmias as directed by physician.
7. Auscultate lung fields every 2 hours.
8. Auscultate for extra heart sounds and murmurs as necessary.
9. Report any chest pain experienced by patient.
10. Record effectiveness of therapy.
11. See Cardiogenic Shock, page 310.

C. **Avoiding complications**

1. Check peripheral pulses with Doppler every hour (especially left brachial, radial, and popliteal arteries).
2. Assess color and temperature of extremities every hour. Notify physician if extremities are dusky or cold.
3. Monitor rectal temperature every 2–4 hours and report temperature greater than 38.5°C. (100.5°F.).
4. Obtain blood, sputum, and urine cultures per physician request.
5. Utilize sterile technique for all dressing changes.
6. Assess for redness, swelling, warmth, and IV sites.
7. Incorporate good handwashing techniques during care.
8. Administer prescribed anticoagulation therapy.
9. Evaluate prothrombin times daily.

D. **Normal skin integrity and joint motion**

1. Implement passive range of motion exercises with exception of extremity with IABP catheter.
2. Turn patient from side to side as a unit every 2 hours (patients are usually debilitated and prone to pressure sores).
3. Keep head of bed elevated 15–30 degrees or flat (catheter may migrate upward and obstruct left subclavian artery).

E. **Minimum sleep deprivation**

1. Manipulate environment to allow patient uninterrupted rest periods.
2. Monitor for signs/symptoms of ICU psychosis (hallucinations, disorientation).
3. Orient the patient to time and place as appropriate.
4. Keep the patient informed of progress of therapy.

Evaluation

Expected Outcomes

1. Maintains hemodynamic stability: CI (cardiac index) greater than 2.4 liter/min/m², urine output greater than 30 ml./hour, no chest pain
2. Recognizes factors causing fear—verbalizes ability to cope with fears
3. Free of preventable complications—peripheral pulses present, skin warm and color normal, temperature within normal limits
4. Maintains normal skin integrity and joint motion—absence of skin breakdown, able to perform active ROM of extremities
5. Experiences minimum sleep deprivation—sleeps 5 hours daily without interruption

Endocardial Disease

Diseases Affecting the Endocardium

1. Infective endocarditis (see below)
2. Rheumatic endocarditis (complication of acute rheumatic fever, p. 316)
3. Chronic valvular heart disease (p. 320)

Altered Physiology

1. When an area of the endocardium becomes inflamed, a fibrin clot (vegetation) may form that in time becomes converted into a mass of scar tissue.
2. The scarred endocardium becomes thickened, stiffened, contracted, and deformed.
3. A fringe of vegetations along the free margins of the valve flaps represents the basic lesion of endocarditis and is the forerunner of chronic valvular heart disease.

Infective Endocarditis

Infective endocarditis (IE) (bacterial endocarditis) is an infection of the valves and inner lining of the heart caused by direct invasion of bacteria or other organisms; leading to deformity of the valve leaflets.

Prosthetic valve endocarditis—infection of previously inserted mechanical or biological heart valve.

Etiology

1. Bacteria
   a. *Streptococcus viridans*—bacteremia occurs after dental work or upper respiratory infection.
   b. *Staphylococcus aureus*—bacteremia occurs after cardiac surgery or parenteral drug abuse.
   c. *Enterococci* (penicillin-resistant group D streptococci)—bacteremia usually occurs in elderly (over 60) with genitourinary tract infection.
2. Fungi (*Candida albicans, Aspergillus*)
3. Rickettsiae

Characteristics

1. Infective endocarditis may develop on a heart valve already injured by other disease (rheumatic fever, congenital defects), on abnormally vascularized valves, normal heart valves.
2. Infective endocarditis may be acute or subacute, depending on the microorganisms involved. Acute IE manifests rapidly with danger of intractable heart failure. Subacute IE manifests a prolonged chronic course with a lesser chance of complications.
3. Infective endocarditis may follow cardiac surgery, especially when prosthetic heart valves are used. (Foreign bodies, such as prosthetic valves, dialysis shunts, and pacemakers, predispose to infection.)
4. The vegetations on the affected endocardial surface may travel to various organs and tissues and cause emboli—spleen, kidney, coronary arteries, central nervous system, and lungs.

5. High incidence among narcotic addicts, in whom the disease mainly affects normal valves, usually the tricuspid.
6. Hospitalized patients with indwelling catheters, those on prolonged intravenous therapy or prolonged antibiotic therapy, and those on immunosuppressive drugs or steroids may develop fungal endocarditis.
7. Relapse due to metastatic infection is possible, usually within the first 2 months after completion of antibiotic regimen.

Assessment

Clinical Manifestations

Severity of manifestations depends on invading microorganism.

A. General Manifestations

1. Fever, chills, sweats (fever may be absent in elderly or in patients with uremia)
2. Anorexia, weight loss, weakness
3. Cough; back and joint pain (especially in elderly over 60)
4. Splenomegaly

B. Skin and Nail Manifestations

1. Petechiae—conjunctiva, mucous membranes
2. Splinter hemorrhages in nail beds
3. Osler's nodes—painful red nodes on pads of fingers and toes; usually late sign of infection and found with a subacute infection
4. Janeway lesions—light pink macules on palms or soles, nontender, may change to light tan within several days, fade in 1–2 weeks. Usually an early sign of endocardial infection

C. Heart Manifestations

1. New pathologic or changing murmur—no murmur with other signs/symptoms may indicate right heart infection
2. Tachycardia—related to decreased cardiac output

D. Central Nervous System Manifestations

1. Localized headaches
2. Transient cerebral ischemia
3. Altered mental status, aphasia
4. Hemiplegia
5. Cortical sensory loss

E. Pulmonary Manifestations

1. Usually occur with right-sided heart involvement
2. Pneumonitis, pleuritis, pulmonary edema, pulmonary infiltrates

F. Embolic Phenomena

1. Lung—hemoptysis, chest pain, shortness of breath
2. Kidney—hematuria

3. Spleen—pain in upper left quadrant of abdomen radiating to left shoulder
4. Heart—myocardial infarction
5. Brain—sudden blindness, paralysis, brain abscess, meningitis
6. Blood vessels—mycotic aneurysms
7. Abdomen—melena, acute pain

Diagnostic Evaluation

Varied clinical manifestations and similarities to other diseases make early diagnosis of IE difficult.
1. Blood cultures—at least two positive serial blood cultures isolating bacteria or fungi
2. Medical history—elicitation of a history of symptoms of disease
3. Physical examination—especially cardiac auscultation and funduscopic
4. Elevated sedimentation rate, tests indicative of anemia, mild leukocytosis, urine abnormalities indicating nephrosis
5. ECG
6. Echocardiography—identification of vegetations and assessment of location and size of lesions

Patient Problems/Nursing Diagnoses

1. Reduction in cardiac output related to structural factors (incompetent valves).
2. Impaired tissue perfusion related to embolic lesions/vasculitis.
3. Inadequate nutritional intake related to anorexia.
4. Anxiety related to acute illness and hospitalization.
5. Potential for injury related to complications of disease and therapy.

Planning and Implementation

Treatment

Targeted at eradication of invading microorganism by parenteral antimicrobial therapy, treatment of symptoms of cardiac disease or failure, valve replacement relative to hemodynamic instability, and prevention of endocarditis in susceptible individuals.
1. Determine the causative organism by obtaining serial blood cultures.
2. Treat with bactericidal (capable of destroying bacteria) or other appropriate drugs based on proven sensitivity of causative agent and allergies the patient may have. Suggested drug therapy includes penicillin G, nafcillin, vancomycin, gentamicin, and rifampin, alone or in combination.
   Bactericidal serum levels of selected antibiotic are monitored by titering it against the causative organism; if the serum lacks adequate bactericidal activity, more antibiotic or a different antibiotic is given.
3. Obtain urine cultures before starting antibiotic regimen.
4. Obtain audiogram before starting antibiotic regimen.
5. Repeat blood cultures after 48 hours to assess efficacy of drug therapy (persistently positive blood cultures could indicate presence of metastatic infection, error in sensitivity tests, or error in drug administration).
6. Ensure daily physical examination by cardiologist.
7. Search and identify portal of entry of infection (usually difficult).
8. Supplement nutritional needs.
9. Follow up blood cultures at 1 month and 2 months after cessation of drug therapy to ensure early detection of relapse.

Nursing Interventions

A. Attaining hemodynamic stability
1. Auscultate heart to detect new murmur or change in existing murmur.
2. Monitor blood pressure and pulse.
3. Assess jugular venous distention.
4. Record intake and output.
5. Record daily weight.
6. Place the patient on cardiac monitor if arrhythmia is present.

B. Adequate tissue perfusion
1. Assess the patient for altered mentation, hemoptysis, hematuria, aphasia, loss of muscle strength, complaints of pain.
2. Observe for splinter hemorrhages of nailbeds, Osler's nodes, and Janeway lesions.
3. Notify physician of observed changes in the patient's status.

C. Improvement in nutritional status
1. Assess the patient's daily caloric intake.
2. Discuss food preferences with the patient.
3. Consult with a dietitian regarding nutritional needs of patient and food preferences.
4. Encourage small meals and snacks throughout the day.
5. Record daily caloric intake and weight.
6. Educate family members about the patient's caloric needs.
7. Encourage family members to assist the patient with meals and bring in the patient's favorite foods.

D. Reduction in anxiety
1. Encourage the patient to verbalize fears regarding illness and hospitalization.
2. Educate the patient about disease process and therapy needed.
3. Explain all procedures to patient before initiation.
4. Offer the patient literature, if available, about his disease.
5. Encourage diversional activities for the patient such as television, reading, and interaction with other patients.
6. Contact social worker to assist the patient with financial planning and home discharge arrangements if applicable.
7. Educate family members about the patient's disease and therapy.
8. Encourage family members to interact with the patient as frequently as possible.

E. Prevention of complications of disease
1. Observe basic principles of asepsis, good handwashing techniques, and continuity of patient care by primary nurse.
2. Employ meticulous IV care for long-term antibiotic therapy.
   a. Note the date of needle or cannula insertion on nursing care plan.
3. Develop chart for rotation of sites for intramuscular administration of antibiotic therapy.
4. Take the patient's temperature at least 2 times daily and mark on graph.
5. Auscultate for heart murmurs or change in heart murmurs.
6. Observe for side effects of long-term antibiotic therapy—ototoxicity, renal failure.
7. Monitor laboratory values—hematocrit, BUN, creatinine, WBC.

8. Observe for signs and symptoms of embolic phenomena (see IE, p. 314, Clinical Manifestations), congestive heart failure, mycotic aneurysms, and neurologic, hematologic, and renal complications.
9. Prepare for surgical intervention for:
   a. Acute destructive valvular lesion—excision of infected valves or removal of prosthetic valve
   b. Hemodynamic impairment
   c. Recurrent emboli
   d. Infection that cannot be eliminated with antimicrobial therapy
   e. Drainage of abscess/empyema—for patient with localized abscess or empyema
   f. Repair of peripheral or cerebral mycotic aneurysm

Health Education

1. Develop in-depth formal program to educate individuals at risk regarding disease process, pathologic manifestations, therapy, and preventions.
   a. Discuss anatomy of heart and changes that occur during endocarditis, using diagrams of the heart.
   b. Give the patient written literature on early signs and symptoms of disease; review these with the patient.
   c. Discuss with individual the mode of entry of infection.
   d. Antibiotic prophylaxis is recommended for persons at risk who are undergoing procedures most likely to cause bacteremia (dental procedures causing gingival bleeding, surgery on or instrumentation of GI tract, certain genitourinary procedures, etc.).*
   e. Identify individual steps necessary to prevent infection.
      (1) Good oral hygiene, regular tooth brushing and flossing.
      (2) Notification to health-care personnel of any history of congenital heart disease or valvular disease.
      (3) Discuss importance of carrying emergency identification with information of medical history at all times.
      (4) Take temperature if infection is suspected and notify physician of elevation.
      (5) Teach individual to inspect soles of feet for Janeway lesions indicative of possible relapse.
      (6) Educate persons at risk to look for and treat symptoms of illness indicating bacteremia—injuries, sore throats, furuncles, etc.
   f. Discuss antibiotic prophylaxis—what it means and what individual must do to ensure his safety.
   g. Encourage susceptible individuals to receive pneumococcal vaccine and influenza vaccines.
      Teach that vaccines reduce the risk of severe infections that could precipitate heart failure.
   h. Teach women in childbearing years the risks of utilizing IUDs for birth control (source of infection) and that antibiotic therapy is not necessary for individuals having normal deliveries.
2. Educate individuals who have had endocarditis regarding possible relapse.

* From statement prepared by the Committee on Prevention of Rheumatic Fever and Bacterial Endocarditis of the American Heart Association. Circulation 1977 July; 56:139A–143A.

a. Discuss importance of keeping follow-up appointments after hospital discharge (infection can recur in 1–2 months).
b. Review the tests that will be performed after hospital discharge—blood cultures, physical examination.

Evaluation
Expected Outcomes

1. Maintains hemodynamic stability—exhibits no symptoms of heart failure
2. Maintains satisfactory tissue perfusion—lack of signs/symptoms of embolic phenomena
3. Demonstrates decrease in anxiety
4. Achieves improved nutritional status—increases daily caloric intake compatible with height/weight/age
5. Remains free of complications—normal temperature, negative blood cultures, normal WBC count, BUN, and creatinine, no hearing impairments

Rheumatic Endocarditis
(Rheumatic Heart Disease)

Rheumatic endocarditis is damage done to the heart, particularly the valves, resulting in valve leakage (regurgitation) and/or obstruction (narrowing or stenosis). There are associated compensatory changes in the size of the heart's chambers and the thickness of chamber walls.

Role of Streptococcal Infection in Rheumatic Fever and Rheumatic Endocarditis

Rheumatic fever is a sequela to group A streptococcal infection. It is a preventable disease through the detection and adequate treatment of streptococcal pharyngitis.

A. Symptoms of Streptococcal Pharyngitis

1. Sudden onset of sore throat; throat reddened with exudate
2. Swollen, tender lymph nodes at angle of jaw
3. Headache and fever 38.9°–40°C. (101°–104°F.)
4. Abdominal pain (children)

▶ **NURSING ALERT:** Some cases of streptococcal throat infection are relatively asymptomatic.

Clinical Manifestations of Rheumatic Fever

1. Polyarthritis; warm and swollen joints
2. Carditis
3. Chorea (irregular, jerky, involuntary, unpredictable muscular movements)
4. Erythema marginatum (wavy, thin red-line skin rash on trunk and extremities)
5. Subcutaneous nodules
6. Fever
7. Prolonged PR interval demonstrated by ECG
8. Heart murmurs; pleural and pericardial rubs

Diagnostic Evaluation

1. Throat culture—to determine presence of streptococcal organisms
2. Increased sedimentation rate; WBC count and differential and C-reactive protein—increase during acute phase of infection
3. Elevated antistreptolysin titer

Treatment

The objectives of treatment are targeted toward eradicating the involved microorganism through antimicrobial therapy, maintaining optimal cardiac function through rest, controlling fever and pain with salicylates, and preventing recurrent episodes of rheumatic fever in susceptible individuals.

Nursing Management

1. Limit physical activity during the acute phase—patient should rest in bed as long as there is fever or signs of active carditis.
2. Administer penicillin therapy—to eradicate hemolytic streptococcus; erythromycin may be used if the patient is allergic to penicillin.
3. Give salicylates to suppress rheumatic activity by controlling toxic manifestations, to reduce fever, and to relieve joint pain.
4. Assess for effectiveness of drug therapy.
   a. Take and record temperature every 3 hours.
   b. Evaluate the patient's comfort level every 3 hours.
5. Monitor the patient's dietary intake (symptoms of disease inhibit the patient's ability to take in nutrients).
   a. Record the patient's daily caloric intake.
   b. Supplement diet with high-carbohydrate liquids if indicated.
6. Assess for signs/symptoms of acute rheumatic carditis.
   a. Be alert to the patient's complaints of chest pain, palpitations, and/or precordial "tightness."
   b. Monitor for tachycardia (usually persistent when the patient sleeps) or bradycardia.
   c. Be alert to development of second degree heart block or Wenckebach syndrome (acute rheumatic carditis causes PR interval prolongation).
7. Auscultate heart sounds every 4 hours.
   a. Document presence of murmur or pericardial friction rub (see Endocarditis, p. 314; Pericarditis, p. 319).
   b. Document extra heart sounds (S_3 gallop, S_4 gallop; see Congestive Heart Failure, p. 323).
8. See Treatment of Rheumatic Fever in Children, page 1308.
9. Be aware of the possible complication of chronic rheumatic endocarditis. Chronic rheumatic endocarditis is a complication of rheumatic fever, which frequently produces progressive disability and a shortened life span. Every structural component of the heart is likely to be the site of an inflammatory reaction.
   a. Although the patient is symptom-free for a time, the damage to the valves (rigidity and deformity, thickening and fusion of the commissures, or shortening and fusion of chordae tendinae) will produce heart sounds that are characteristic of valvular stenosis, regurgitation, or both.
   b. The myocardium will compensate for these valvular defects for a while, but in time it fails to compensate, and the patient develops symptoms of congestive heart failure.
   c. See page 321 for treatment of valvular heart disease and page 324 for treatment of congestive heart failure.

Health Education

1. Teach the patient the importance and ways of preventing a recurrence of rheumatic heart disease.
   a. Counsel the patient to maintain good nutrition.
      (1) Provide teaching on basic food groups.
      (2) Assist with planning several daily meal plans.
      (3) Discuss proper preparation of food (clean utensils and kitchen area) and proper storage of food.
      (4) Discuss with the patient his financial situation and home facilities relative to nutritional health maintenance. If appropriate, contact social services for the patient.
   b. Counsel the patient on hygienic practices.
      (1) Discuss proper handwashing, disposal of tissues, laundering of handkerchiefs (decrease chance of exposure to microbes).
      (2) Discuss importance of using patient's own toothbrush, soap, and wash cloths when living in group situations.
   c. Counsel the patient on importance of receiving adequate rest.
   d. Counsel the patient to seek treatment immediately should sore throat occur.
      (1) Explore with patient his ability to pay for medical treatment. If appropriate, contact social services for the patient. (Financial difficulties may inhibit the patient from seeking early treatment of symptoms.)
2. Instruct the patient to utilize prophylactic penicillin therapy before undergoing surgery of genitourinary tract, lower intestinal tract, and respiratory tract.
3. See Health Education, Endocarditis, page 316.

Myocarditis

Myocarditis is an inflammatory process involving the myocardium.

Etiology

1. Infectious process—viral (particularly Coxsackie group B, and may develop after influenza A or B, herpes simplex), bacterial, mycotic, parasitic, protozoal, rickettsial, and spirochetal infections.
2. Following drug administration (doxorubicin [Adriamycin]).
3. Other conditions—sarcoidosis, collagen diseases (rheumatic fever).
4. Immunosuppressive therapy.

Assessment
Clinical Manifestations

A. **Symptoms**

1. Depend on type of infection, degree of myocardial damage, capacity of myocardium to recover, and host resistance. Can be acute or chronic and occur at any age. Symptoms may be minor and go unnoticed.
   a. Fatigue and dyspnea
   b. Palpitations
   c. Occasional precordial discomfort

B. **Clinical Findings**

1. Cardiac enlargement
2. Cardiac murmur—abnormal heart sound; sounds like

fluid passing an obstruction (due to papillary muscle dysfunction)
3. Pericardial friction rub
4. Gallop rhythm—a tripling or quadrupling of heart sounds (resembling the galloping of a horse) heard upon auscultation
5. Pulsus alternans—a pulse in which there is a regular alternation of weak and strong beats
6. Fever with tachycardia
7. Evidence of development of congestive heart failure

Diagnostic Evaluation

1. History of recent infection
2. Transient ECG changes—ST segment flattened, T wave inversion, conduction defects, extrasystoles, supraventricular and ventricular ectopic beats
3. Elevated WBC count and sedimentation rate
4. Chest x-ray—may show heart enlargement and lung congestion
5. Elevated antibody titers (antistreptolysin-o [ASO titer] as in rheumatic fever)
6. Stool and throat cultures isolating bacteria or a virus

Patient Problems/Nursing Diagnoses

1. Potential complications of disease—congestive heart failure and arrhythmias.
2. Activity intolerance related to myocardial tissue damage.
3. Potential for ineffective coping (individual) related to life-threatening illness and hospitalization.

Planning and Implementation
Treatment

Treatment objectives are targeted toward management of complications.
1. Diuretic and digoxin therapy for congestive heart failure and atrial fibrillation
2. Antiarrhythmic therapy (usually quinidine or procainamide)
3. Strict bed rest to promote healing of damaged myocardium
4. Antimicrobial therapy if causative bacteria is isolated

Nursing Interventions

A. Maintaining hemodynamic stability

1. Evaluate for clinical evidence that disease is subsiding—monitor pulse, auscultate for abnormal heart sounds (murmur or change in existing murmur), check temperature, auscultate lung fields, monitor respirations.
2. Record daily intake and output.
3. Record weight daily.
4. Check for peripheral edema.
5. Elevate head of bed, if necessary, to enhance respiration.
6. Treat the symptoms of congestive heart failure (see p. 323).
   a. Give digitalis—augments myocardial contractility and slows heart rate.
   b. Administer diuretics—to control pulmonary or systemic congestion.

▶ **NURSING ALERT:** Patients with myocarditis may be sensitive to digitalis—assess for toxic symptoms (see p. 325).

7. Evaluate the patient's pulse and apical rate for signs of tachycardia and gallop rhythm—indications that congestive heart failure is recurring.
8. Evaluate for evidences of arrhythmias—*patients with myocarditis are prone to develop arrhythmias.*
   a. Place patient in unit with continuous cardiac monitoring if evidences of an arrhythmia develop.
   b. See page 296 for management of arrhythmias.
   c. Have equipment for resuscitation, cardiac defibrillation, and cardiac pacing available in event of life-threatening arrhythmia.

B. Strict bed rest

1. Place patient on bed rest to reduce heart rate, stroke volume, blood pressure, and heart contractility; also helps to decrease residual damage and complications of myocarditis, and promotes healing.
   Prolonged bed rest may be required—until there is reduction in heart size and improvement of function.
2. Provide diversional activities for patient.
3. Allow the patient to use bedside commode rather than bedpan (reduces cardiovascular workload).

C. Effective coping with illness

1. Explore with the patient his fears, anxieties, and concerns regarding illness and hospitalization.
2. Answer questions with a straightforward approach.
3. Discuss with the patient activities that can be continued after discharge.
   a. Discuss need to modify activities in immediate future.
   b. Explore with the patient life-style modifications and discuss adequacy of self-concept.
4. Emphasize the patient's strengths rather than limitations.
5. Encourage family members to support the patient and learn about his illness.
6. Discuss with family members their fears and anxieties relative to the patient's illness so that they will be able to communicate positively with the patient.

Health Education

Instruct the patient as follows:
1. There is usually some residual heart enlargement; physical activity may be *slowly* increased; begin with chair rest for increasing periods of time; follow with walking in the room and then outdoors.
2. Report any symptom involving rapidly beating heart.
3. Avoid competitive sports, alcohol, and other myocardial toxins (doxorubicin).
4. Pregnancy is not advisable for women with cardiomyopathies (diseases that affect structure and function of myocardium).
5. Prevention—prevent infectious diseases by means of appropriate immunizations.

Evaluation
Expected Outcomes

1. Maintains hemodynamic stability—respirations within range of 14–20, lung sounds clear on auscultation, normal sinus rhythm
2. Adheres to strict bed rest
3. Copes adaptively to illness—expresses ability to adapt to change in life-style imposed by illness, participates in self-care activities and health education program, avoids maladaptive coping mechanisms such as strong denial, inappropriate grief, anger, depression

Pericarditis

Pericarditis is an inflammation of the pericardium, the membranous sac enveloping the heart. It is often a manifestation of a more generalized disease.

Pericardial effusion is an outpouring of fluid into the pericardial cavity.

Constrictive pericarditis is a condition in which a chronic inflammatory thickening of the pericardium compresses the heart so that it is unable to fill normally during diastole.

Etiology

1. Acute idiopathic—most common and typical form; etiology unknown
2. Infection
   a. Viral (influenza; Coxsackie virus)
   b. Bacterial—staphylococcus, meningococcus, streptococcus, pneumococcus, gonococcus, *Mycobacterium tuberculosis*
   c. Fungal
   d. Parasitic
3. Disorders of connective tissues and allergies—lupus erythematosus, periarteritis nodosa
4. Myocardial infarction; early, 24–72 hours; or late, 1 week to 2 years (Dressler's syndrome)
5. Malignant disease; thoracic irradiation
6. Chest trauma, heart surgery, including pacemaker implantation
7. Drug induced (procainamide; phenytoin)

Assessment

Clinical Manifestations

1. Pain in anterior chest, aggravated by thoracic motion—may vary from mild to sharp and severe; located in precordial area (may be felt beneath clavicle, neck, scapular region)—may be relieved by leaning forward.
2. Pericardial friction rub—scratchy, grating, or creaking sound occurring in the presence of pericardial inflammation.
3. Dyspnea—from compression of heart and surrounding thoracic structures.
4. Fever, sweating, chills—due to inflammation of pericardium.
5. Arrhythmias.

Diagnostic Evaluation

1. Echocardiogram—most sensitive method for detecting pericardial effusion
2. Chest x-ray—may show heart enlargement

▶ **NURSING ALERT:** Normal pericardial sac contains less than 25–30 ml. of fluid; pericardial fluid may accumulate slowly without noticeable symptoms. However, a rapidly developing effusion can produce serious hemodynamic alterations.

3. ECG—to evaluate for myocardial infarction
4. WBC and differential
5. Antinuclear antibody serologic tests and lupus erythematosus cell preparation—to rule out lupus erythematosus
6. PPD test—for tuberculosis; ASO titers—for rheumatic fever
7. Pericardiocentesis—for examination of pericardial fluid for etiologic diagnosis
8. Serum urea nitrogen (BUN)—to evaluate for uremia

Treatment

The objectives of treatment are targeted toward determining the etiology of the problem, administering pharmacologic therapy for specified etiology, when known, and being alert to the possible complication of cardiac tamponade.

Patient Problems/Nursing Diagnoses

1. Chest pain related to pericardial inflammation.
2. Potential for complications—cardiac tamponade and constrictive pericarditis.

Planning and Implementation

Nursing Interventions

A. Reducing discomfort

1. Evaluate the patient's complaint of chest pain.
   a. Ask the patient if pain is aggravated by breathing, turning in bed, twisting body, coughing, yawning, or swallowing.
   b. Elevate head of bed; position pillow on over-the-bed table so that the patient can lean on it.
      (1) Assess if above intervention relieves the patient's chest pain (associated pleuritic pain of pericarditis is usually relieved by sitting up and/or leaning forward).
      (2) Be alert to the patient's medical diagnoses when assessing pain. Postmyocardial infarction patients may experience a dull, crushing pain radiating to neck, arm, and shoulders, mimicking an extension of infarction (Dressler's syndrome).
2. Auscultate for friction rub.
   a. Place the diaphragm of the stethoscope firmly on the chest wall along the mid-to-lower left sternal border or at the apex. Listen to the heart with patient in different positions.
      (1) Listen carefully; friction rub may appear intermittently and briefly with respiratory movement.
      (2) Confirm ausculatory findings with another staff nurse.
3. Give prescribed drug regimen for pain and symptomatic relief.
   a. Nonsteroid anti-inflammatory drugs (aspirin, indomethacin)—suppress inflammatory symptoms of acute pericarditis.
   b. Corticosteroids—for more severe symptoms.
4. Give specific therapy when the cause is known.
   a. Bacterial pericarditis—penicillin or other antimicrobial agents
   b. Rheumatic fever—procaine penicillin, prednisone
   c. Tuberculosis—antituberculosis chemotherapy (see p. 876)
      (There is a high incidence of constriction in tuberculosis pericarditis)
   d. Fungal pericarditis—amphotericin B
   e. Disseminated lupus erythematosus—adrenal steroids
   f. Uremic pericarditis—dialysis, indomethacin, biochemical control of uremia
   g. Neoplastic pericarditis—intrapericardial instillation of chemotherapy; radiotherapy

h. Postmyocardial infarction syndrome—bed rest, aspirin, prednisone
   (1) Relieve anxiety of the patient and family by explaining the difference between pain of pericarditis and pain of recurrent myocardial infarction (patients may fear extension of myocardial tissue damage).
   (2) Explain to the patient and family that pericarditis does not indicate further heart damage.
i. Postpericardiotomy syndrome (after open heart surgery)—treat symptomatically
5. Encourage the patient to remain on bed rest when chest pain, fever, and friction rub occur.

B. Avoiding complications

1. Be alert to the possibility of cardiac tamponade (see Pericardiocentesis, p. 289).
   a. Assess for distant heart sounds, falling arterial pressures, and rising venous pressure.
   b. Note presence of paradoxical pulse.
   c. Prepare the patient for immediate pericardiocentesis (see Pericardiocentesis, p. 289).
2. Be cognizant of other complications of pericarditis—congestive heart failure, arrhythmias, hemopericardium (complication in post myocardial infarction patients on anticoagulation therapy).

3. Be alert for signs/symptoms of pericarditis when administering procainamide or phenytoin (agents may induce a lupus-like syndrome with pericarditis).
4. Prepare the patient for surgical intervention (direct pericardial decompression)—for patient with cardiac embarrassment associated with constrictive pericarditis.

Health Education

1. Teach patient the etiology of pericarditis.
2. Instruct patient about signs/symptoms of pericarditis and the need for long-term medication therapy to help relieve symptoms.
3. Review all medications with the patient—purpose, side effects, dosage, and special precautions.
4. Evaluate the patient's understanding by asking the patient to define pericarditis, the medications necessary for therapy, and the side effects and correct dosage of medications.

Evaluation
Expected Outcomes

1. Experiences minimal discomfort—no chest pain
2. Experiences no complications—respirations 14–18 times per minute, no dyspnea, no apprehension or acute anxiety

Acquired Valvular Disease of the Heart

Altered Physiology

1. The function of normal heart valves is to maintain the forward flow of blood from the atria to the ventricles and from the ventricles to the great vessels.
2. Valvular damage may interfere with valvular function by stenosis or by impaired closure that allows backward leakage of blood (valvular insufficiency, regurgitation, or incompetence).
3. Acquired valvular heart disease is often the result of previous rheumatic fever, which has damaged one or more heart valves; mitral valve is most commonly involved, followed by aortic, tricuspid, and pulmonary valves.
4. Patients with valvular disease usually develop congestive heart failure in time.

Types of Valvular Disease

1. Mitral stenosis
2. Mitral insufficiency
3. Aortic stenosis
4. Aortic insufficiency
5. Tricuspid stenosis
6. Tricuspid insufficiency

Nursing Process Overview

Assessment
Physical Assessment Data

1. Assess patient as often as necessary for complications and progression of valvular dysfunction (see Congestive Heart Failure, p. 323, Infective Endocarditis, p. 314, and Rheumatic Heart Disease, p. 316).
2. Auscultate for extra heart sounds and murmurs every tour of duty.

a. *Mitral stenosis*
   (1) Auscultate for accentuated first heart sound, usually accompanied with an "opening snap" (due to sudden tensing of valve leaflets) at apex with diaphragm of stethoscope.
   (2) Place the patient in left lateral recumbent position. With bell of stethoscope at apex, auscultate for a low-pitched diastolic murmur (rumbling murmur). Note duration of murmur (long duration indicative of significant stenosis).
b. *Mitral insufficiency*
   (1) Auscultate for diminished first heart sound.
   (2) Auscultate for systolic murmur (prominent finding), commencing immediately after first heart sound at apex, and note radiation of sound to axilla and left intrascapular area.
   (3) Mild insufficiency may produce a pansystolic murmur (little connection between severity of mitral insufficiency and intensity of murmur auscultated).
c. *Aortic stenosis*
   (1) Auscultate for prominent fourth heart sound and possible paradoxical splitting of second heart sound (suggestive of associated left ventricular dysfunction). First heart sound is normal.
   (2) Auscultate for a midsystolic murmur at the base of the heart (heard best) and at the apex of heart. Note harsh and rasping quality at base of heart and a higher pitch at apex of heart.
d. *Aortic insufficiency*
   (1) Auscultate for soft first heart sound.
   (2) Place the patient in sitting position leaning forward.

(3) Place diaphragm of stethoscope along left sternal border at the third and fourth intercostal space and then along the right sternal border. Auscultate for a high-pitched diastolic murmur. To increase audibility of murmur, ask the patient to hold his breath at end of deep expiration. Re-auscultate for murmur.

e. *Tricuspid stenosis*
   (1) Auscultate for a third heart sound (may be accentuated by inspiration).
   (2) Auscultate for a pansystolic murmur in the parasternal region at the fourth intercostal space. Murmur is usually high-pitched.

Patient Problems/Nursing Diagnoses

1. Decreased cardiac output related to mechanical factors (preload, afterload, contractility).
2. Activity intolerance related to reduced oxygen available for energy.
3. Potential for ineffective coping related to acute and chronic illness.

Planning and Implementation
Nursing Interventions

A. Maintaining adequate cardiac output

1. Assess the patient for possible complications that would compromise cardiac function. Implement treatment protocols for these complications (congestive heart failure, infective endocarditis, rheumatic heart disease).
2. Prepare the patient for surgical intervention, if indicated (see Management of Patient for Heart Surgery, p. 328).

B. Improvement in coping ability

1. Instruct the patient regarding specific valvular dysfunction, possible etiology, and therapies implemented to relieve symptoms.
   a. Include family members in discussions with the patient.
   b. Stress the importance of adapting life-style to cope with illness.
   c. Discuss with the patient surgical intervention as the treatment modality, if applicable (see Heart Surgery, p. 328).
2. Assess the patient's use of appropriate coping mechanisms to deal with illness.
      Spend some time daily with the patient, allowing him to express concerns and ask questions.
3. Refer the patient to appropriate counseling services, if indicated (vocational, social work, cardiac rehabilitation).

Health Education

See Health Education, Congestive Heart Failure, page 326; Infective Endocarditis, page 316; and Rheumatic Endocarditis, page 317.

Evaluation
Expected Outcomes

1. Maintains adequate cardiac output—blood pressure and heart rate within normal limits for patient, respirations unlabored on exertion at 14–18 per minute, no cough or sputum production, no chest pain, fatigue minimal (rests between activities of daily living, verbalizes that fatigue has not worsened)
2. Copes adaptively to illness

Mitral Stenosis

Mitral stenosis is the progressive thickening and contracture of valve cusps with narrowing of the orifice and progressive obstruction to blood flow. It is the most common of the late lesions produced by rheumatic fever.

Altered Physiology

1. Acute rheumatic valvulitis has "glued" the mitral valve flaps (commissures) together, thus shortening the chordae tendinae, so that the flap edges are pulled down, greatly narrowing the mitral orifice.
2. The left atrium has difficulty in emptying itself through the narrow orifice into the left ventricle; therefore, it dilates and hypertrophies. Pulmonary circulation becomes congested.
3. As a result of the abnormally high pulmonary arterial pressure that must be maintained, the right ventricle is subjected to a pressure overload and may eventually fail.

Clinical Manifestations

1. Progressive fatigue—result of low cardiac output
2. Dyspnea on exertion, cough, repeated respiratory infections, emotional stress
3. Hemoptysis—from pulmonary venous hypertension
4. Weak, irregular pulse; atrial fibrillation
5. Characteristic murmurs—increased first heart sound, opening snap, and low-pitched rumbling diastolic murmur heard at the apex
6. Chest pain (infrequent)
7. Hoarseness (due to compression of left recurrent laryngeal nerve)

Diagnostic Evaluation

1. ECG
2. Echocardiography—can demonstrate mitral valve thickening, calcification, and abnormal, slowed diastolic valve excursion
3. Cardiac catheterization and angiocardiography
4. Medical history, physical examination

Treatment

1. Medical treatment
   a. Prevent rheumatic recurrences with antimicrobial therapy.
   b. Treat the developing congestive failure—vasodilators, digitalis, sodium restriction, limitation of activity (see p. 324).
   c. Control arrhythmias (especially atrial fibrillation).
2. Surgical intervention may be accomplished by:
   a. Closed mitral valvotomy—introduction of a dilator through the mitral valve to split its commissures.
   b. Open mitral valvotomy—direct incision of the commissures.
   c. Mitral valve replacement.
   d. See page 328 for the management of the patient undergoing heart surgery.

Mitral Insufficiency

Mitral insufficiency (*regurgitation*) is the result of incompetence and distortion of the mitral valve so that the free margins can no longer come into apposition during systole. The chordae tendinae may become shortened, preventing complete closure of the leaflets.

   Mitral insufficiency may be caused by mitral valve prolapse, chronic rheumatic heart disease, postinfarction mitral regurgitation, infective endocarditis, and penetrating and nonpenetrating trauma.

Clinical Manifestations

(Mild mitral regurgitation may produce no symptoms.)
1. Palpitations; arrhythmias.
2. Shortness of breath on exertion; cough—due to pulmonary congestion.
3. Murmur—soft first heart sound and a blowing pansystolic murmur heard at the apex and transmitted to the axilla. (Characteristic of mild regurgitation due to papillary muscle dysfunction of mitral prolapse.)
4. Weakness/fatigue—result of low cardiac output.

Diagnostic Evaluation

(Same as for mitral stenosis)

Treatment

1. Prophylaxis for infective endocarditis and rheumatic heart disease (see Infective Endocarditis, p. 316, and Rheumatic Endocarditis, p. 317).
2. Treat developing congestive heart failure (see Congestive Heart Failure, p. 323).
3. Surgical intervention—mitral valve replacement or annuloplasty (retailoring of the valve ring).

Aortic Stenosis

Aortic stenosis is a narrowing of the orifice between the left ventricle and the aorta. The obstruction to the aortic outflow places a pressure load on the left ventricle that results in hypertrophy and failure. In adults it may be congenital or from cusp calcification.

Clinical Manifestations

1. Loud, rough systolic murmur over aortic area; often associated with a palpable thrill.
2. Exertional dyspnea and fatigue.
3. Dizziness and fainting—from reduced blood supply to brain.
4. Angina pectoris.
5. Low blood pressure and low pulse pressure—from diminished blood flow, precipitating syncopal episodes.
6. Arrhythmias.
7. Symptoms of congestive heart failure.
8. Emboli.

Diagnostic Evaluation

1. Chest x-ray—usually shows left ventricular enlargement
2. Cardiac catheterization ⎫
3. Angiocardiography ⎬ will reveal the pressures in the left ventricle and aorta
4. Echocardiography ⎭

Treatment

1. Surgical replacement of aortic valve—prosthetic or tissue valve.
   See page 328 for care of patient undergoing heart surgery.
2. Treat angina and congestive heart failure as dictated by the patient's condition. (Digitalis not indicated for treatment unless evidence of increased ventricular volume or decreased ejection fraction (see Angina, p. 302, and Congestive Heart Failure, p. 324).

Aortic Insufficiency

Aortic insufficiency (*regurgitation*) is caused by inflammatory lesions that deform the flaps so that they fail to completely seal the aortic orifice during diastole and thus permit a backflow of blood from the aorta into the left ventricle and by trauma.

It may be caused by rheumatic endocarditis, infective endocarditis, or congenital malformation or by diseases that cause dilation or tearing of the ascending aorta (syphilitic disease, rheumatoid spondylitis, dissecting aneurysm).

Clinical Manifestations

1. Awareness of increased force of heartbeat, especially when lying down
   a. Arterial pulsations visible and palpable over precordium
   b. Arterial pulsations visible in neck
2. Exertional dyspnea; easy fatigability, progressing to paroxysmal nocturnal dyspnea and orthopnea
3. Widened pulse pressure
4. Water-hammer (Corrigan's) pulse—pulse strikes palpating finger with a quick, sharp stroke and then suddenly collapses
5. Murmur—high-pitched blowing decrescendo diastolic murmur audible along the left sternal edge
6. Nocturnal angina with diaphoresis
7. Tachycardia with exertion

Diagnostic Evaluation

1. ECG—shows pattern of left ventricular hypertrophy
2. Chest x-ray—reveals varying degrees of cardiomegaly from left ventricular enlargement
3. Echocardiography—estimates size and thickness of left ventricle
4. Cardiac catheterization and angiography

Treatment

1. *Surgical intervention*—replacement of damaged aortic valve. See page 328 for nursing management of patient undergoing heart surgery.
2. Prophylaxis for Infective Endocarditis and Rheumatic Heart Disease (see Infective Endocarditis, p. 316, and Rheumatic Heart Disease, p. 317).

Tricuspid Stenosis

Tricuspid stenosis is restriction of the tricuspid valve orifice due to commissural fusion and fibrosis, usually following rheumatic fever. It is commonly associated with diseases of the mitral valve.

Clinical Manifestations

1. Dyspnea, nocturnal dyspnea, orthopnea
2. Visible pulsations of neck veins (may cause fluttering sensation)
3. Murmurs—similar to those of rheumatic mitral disease; blowing diastolic murmur along left sternal border
4. Symptoms of right-sided heart failure (late)—hepatomegaly, abdominal swelling, anasarca

Diagnostic Evaluation

1. ECG—may reveal atrial fibrillation
2. Cardiac catheterization and angiocardiography—to confirm diagnosis

3. Echocardiography—useful in estimating size of tricuspid orifice
4. Chest x-ray—marked cardiomegaly, enlarged right atrium

Treatment

1. The patient may have mitral and aortic disease, which must be corrected.
2. Surgical treatment of accompanying tricuspid valve disease may be carried out at the time of operation after correction of mitral valve disease.
3. Diuretics and sodium restriction to diminish hypervolemic symptoms

Tricuspid Insufficiency (Regurgitation)

Tricuspid insufficiency allows the regurgitation of blood from the right ventricle into the right atrium during ventricular systole. Common cause is dilation of right ventricle.

Clinical Manifestations

1. Right-sided heart failure—from overload of right ventricle
2. Edema—with congestion of liver and hepatic malfunction, ascites, hydrothorax
3. Elevated venous pressure
4. Pansystolic murmur in tricuspid area
5. Weakness, fatigue
6. Atrial fibrillation
7. Jugular venous distention

Diagnostic Evaluation

1. Chest x-ray—marked cardiomegaly
2. ECG—atrial fibrillation
3. Echocardiography

Treatment

Surgical treatment of associated mitral valve disease, tricuspid valvuloplasty, or tricuspid valve replacement.

Congestive Heart Failure

Heart failure is the inability of the heart to pump the amount of oxygenated blood necessary to effect venous return and to meet the metabolic requirements of the body.

Congestive heart failure is the occurrence of circulatory congestion due to decreased myocardial contractility; as a result, cardiac output is inadequate to maintain the blood flow to body organs and tissues. This ultimately causes sodium and water retention and elevation of left atrial pressure, which results in pulmonary vascular congestion.

Causes

1. Disorders of heart muscle resulting in decreased contractile properties of the heart; coronary heart disease leading to myocardial infarction; hypertension; valvular heart disease; congenital heart disease; cardiomyopathies; arrhythmias
2. Pulmonary embolism; chronic lung disease
3. Hemorrhage and anemia
4. Anesthesia and surgery
5. Transfusions or infusions
6. Increased body demands (fever, infection, pregnancy, arteriovenous fistula)
7. Drug-induced (doxorubicin)
8. Physical and emotional stress
9. Excessive sodium intake

Assessment
Clinical Manifestations

Initially there may be isolated left ventricular failure, but in time, the right ventricle fails because of the additional workload. Combined left and right ventricular failure is usual.

A. Left-sided Heart Failure (forward failure)

1. Congestion occurs mainly in the lungs from backing up of blood into pulmonary veins and capillaries
   a. Shortness of breath, dyspnea on exertion, paroxysmal nocturnal dyspnea (due to reabsorption of dependent edema that has developed during day), orthopnea, pulmonary edema
   b. Cough—may be dry, unproductive; often occurs at night
2. Fatigability—from low cardiac output, nocturia, insomnia, dyspnea, catabolic effect of chronic failure
3. Insomnia
4. Tachycardia—S_3 ventricular gallop
5. Restlessness

B. Right-sided Heart Failure (backward failure)

Signs and symptoms of elevated pressures and congestion in systemic veins and capillaries:

1. Edema of ankles; unexplained weight gain
   Pitting edema—is obvious only after retention of at least 4.5 kg. (10 pounds) of fluid
2. Liver congestion—may produce upper abdominal pain
3. Distended neck veins
4. Abnormal fluid in body cavities (pleural space, abdominal cavity)
5. Anorexia and nausea—from hepatic and visceral engorgement
6. Nocturia—diuresis occurs at night with rest and improved cardiac output
7. Weakness

Complications

1. Intractable or refractory heart failure—patient becomes progressively refractory to therapy (not yielding to treatment)
2. Cardiac arrhythmias
3. Myocardial failure
4. Digitalis toxicity—from decreased renal function, potassium depletion, etc.
5. Pulmonary infarction; pneumonia; emboli

Diagnostic Evaluation

1. Cardiovascular findings
   a. Cardiomegaly (enlargement of the heart)—detected by physical examination and chest x-ray

b. Ventricular gallop—evident on auscultation; ECG
c. Rapid heart rate
d. Development of pulsus alternans (alternation in strength of beat)
e. Distended neck veins
f. Hepatomegaly (enlargement of the liver)
2. ECG, echocardiography
3. Chest x-ray—to evaluate heart size, show lung fields (for pleural effusion) and vascular congestion
4. Arterial blood gas studies
5. Liver function studies—may be altered because of hepatic congestion

Patient Problems/Nursing Diagnoses

1. Decreased cardiac output related to mechanical factors (contractility, preload, afterload)
2. Impaired gas exchange related to inadequate ventilation/perfusion ratio
3. Body fluid excess related to continued sodium and water retention
4. Activity intolerance related to inability of heart to deliver adequate oxygen supply to muscle
5. Disturbance in sleep pattern related to anxiety and restlessness

Planning and Implementation
Treatment

The objectives of treatment are targeted toward reducing the work of the heart through promotion of rest, increasing the force and efficiency of myocardial contraction through administration of pharmacologic agents, and eliminating excessive accumulation of body water by use of diuretics and sodium restriction.

Nursing Interventions

A. Maintaining adequate cardiac output

1. Place patient at physical and emotional rest to reduce work of heart.
   a. Provide rest in semirecumbent position or in armchair in air-conditioned environment—reduces work of heart, increases heart reserve, reduces blood pressure, decreases work of respiratory muscles and oxygen utilization, improves efficiency of heart contraction; recumbency promotes diuresis by improving renal perfusion.
   b. Provide bedside commode—to reduce work of getting to bathroom and for defecation.
   c. Provide for psychological rest—emotional stress produces vasoconstriction, elevates arterial pressure, and speeds the heart.
      (1) Promote physical comfort.
      (2) Avoid situations that tend to promote anxiety/agitation.
      (3) Offer careful explanations and answers to the patient's questions.
   d. Assess the patient's response to rest; are his symptoms alleviated?
2. Evaluate frequently for progression of left ventricular failure.
   a. Take frequent blood pressure readings.
      (1) Observe for lowering of systolic pressure.
      (2) Note narrowing of pulse pressure.
   b. Assess peripheral arterial pulses frequently.
      (1) Note alternations in strong and weak pulsations (pulsus alternans).
      (2) Document findings of assessment.

c. Auscultate heart sounds every 4 hours.
   (1) Note for presence of S_3 or S_4 gallop (S_3 gallop is a significant indicator of congestive heart failure).
   (2) Observe precordium for lateral displacement of point of maximum impulse.
   (3) Monitor for premature ventricular beats.
   d. Observe for signs/symptoms of reduced peripheral tissue perfusion—cool temperature of skin, facial pallor, poor capillary refill of nailbeds.
3. Administer pharmacotherapy as described below.

B. Digitalis therapy

Administer digitalis (a cardiac glycoside) as prescribed—to increase the force of myocardial contraction and produce a stronger systolic contraction of the heart and to slow the heart rate. This results in increased cardiac output; decreased heart size, venous pressure, and blood volume; diuresis and relief of edema. Digitalis is also used to slow the ventricular rate in the setting of supraventricular arrhythmias.

1. A loading (digitalizing) dose may be given in order to induce the full therapeutic effect of the drug when rapid digitalization is necessary.
2. Otherwise, the patient is started without a loading dose. The patient is then given a daily dose just adequate to replace the drug that is destroyed or excreted—to maintain digitalis effect without toxicity.
3. *Digitalis preparations* (Choice of drug depends on speed of onset and duration of action required and on individual patient response.)

Oral

Digoxin
Digitalis
Digitoxin
Lanatoside C (Cedilanid)
Acetyldigitoxin (Acylanid)
Gitalin (Gitalgin)

Parenteral

Digoxin
Ouabain
Deslanoside (Cedilanid-D)
Digitoxin

4. Be alert to factors that may cause increased sensitivity to digitalis:
   a. Myocardial infarction, particularly ischemia
   b. Potassium depletion
   c. Kidney or hepatic disease
   d. Diuretic therapy
   e. Diarrhea
   f. Loss of appetite
   g. Advancing age
   h. Hypoxia and hypercapnia in pulmonary disease
   i. Acidosis; alkalosis
5. Monitor serum concentration of digitalis. Digitalis assay may be measured by laboratory for therapeutic guidance and to assess for toxicity.
6. Monitor serum potassium levels and ECGs, especially in patients receiving digitalis and diuretics. *There is a predisposition to arrhythmias if the state of potassium balance is not evaluated and corrected.*
7. Assess clinical response of patient with respect to relief of symptoms (lessening dyspnea and orthopnea, decrease in crackles, relief of peripheral edema).
8. Watch for toxic effects—*arrhythmias* (most important toxic effect), *anorexia,* nausea, vomiting, diarrhea,

bradycardia, headache, malaise, behavioral changes, increasing congestive failure.

▶ **NURSING ALERT:** The incidence of digitalis toxicity is high because of the narrow margin between therapeutic and toxic doses. Toxic effects do not always appear in a predictable manner. Digitalis toxicity has a high mortality rate.

9. Take pulse and apical heart rate before administering each dose of digitalis.
   Withhold digitalis and notify physician if following is noted:
   a. Slowing of rate
   b. Change in rhythm—bradycardia, premature ventricular contraction, bigeminy (2 pulse beats following in rapid succession), atrial fibrillation*
   c. Dangerous cardiac arrhythmias require immediate treatment (see p. 339).

C. **Vasodilator therapy and inotropic agents** (for heart failure unresponsive to usual therapy)

1. *Rationale:* Vasodilators are used to increase cardiac output by dilating the peripheral vascular vessels and reducing impedance (resistance) to left ventricular outflow.
   a. By relaxing capacitance vessels (veins and venules), vasodilators reduce ventricular filling pressures (preload) and volumes.
   b. By relaxing resistance vessels (arterioles), vasodilators can reduce impedance to left ventricular ejection and improve stroke volume.

2. Vasodilators used in congestive heart failure:
   a. Nitrates (nitroglycerin, isosorbide dinitrate, nitroglycerin ointment)—predominantly dilates systemic veins
   b. Nitroprusside—dilator effect in both arterial and venous beds
   c. Hydralazine—predominantly affects arterioles; reduces arteriolar tone
   d. Prazosin—balanced effects on both arterial and venous circulation

3. Invasive hemodynamic monitoring is often used to guide drug administration (see p. 282).

▶ **NURSING ALERT:** Watch for sudden unexpected hypotension, which can cause myocardial ischemia and decrease perfusion to vital organs.

4. Inotropic agents
   a. Dobutamine—directly increases myocardial contractility
   b. Digitalis
5. Combinations of above drugs used

D. **Achieving an improved ventilation/perfusion ratio**

1. Raise head of bed 20–30 cm. (8–10 inches)—reduces venous return to heart and lungs; alleviates pulmonary congestion.
   a. Support lower arms with pillows—to eliminate pull of their weight on shoulder muscles.
   b. Sit orthopneic patient on side of bed with feet supported by a chair, head and arms resting on

---

* Regularization of the rate in a patient with chronic atrial fibrillation should be a warning that digitalis intoxication may be present.

an over-the-bed table, and lumbosacral area supported with pillows.

2. Auscultate lung fields every 4 hours for crackles and wheezes in dependent lung fields (fluid accumulates in areas affected by gravity).
   a. Mark with water-soluble ink the level on the patient's back where adventitious breath sounds are heard.
   b. Use markings for comparative assessment during changes in tours of duty with other nursing personnel.

3. Observe for increased rate of respirations (could be indicative of falling arterial pH).

4. Observe for Cheyne–Stokes respirations (may occur in elderly because of a decrease in cerebral perfusion stimulating a neurogenic response).

5. Position the patient every 2 hours (or encourage the patient to change position frequently)—to help prevent atelectasis and pneumonia.

6. Encourage deep breathing exercises every 1 to 2 hours—to avoid atelectasis.

7. Offer small, frequent feedings—to avoid excessive gastric filling and abdominal distention with subsequent elevation of diaphragm that causes decrease in lung capacity.

E. **Decreasing excessive body fluid**

Administer prescribed diuretic (agent that increases the rate of urine flow).

1. Type and dosage of diuretic administered depends on degree of heart failure and state of renal function.

2. Give diuretic early in the morning—nighttime diuresis disturbs sleep.

3. Keep input and output record—the patient may lose large volume of fluid after a single dose of diuretic.

4. Weigh the patient daily—to determine if edema is being controlled; weight loss should not exceed 0.45–0.9 kg. (1–2 pounds) per day.

5. Assess for weakness, malaise, muscle cramps—diuretic therapy may produce hypovolemia and electrolyte depletion, namely *hypokalemia*.
   Hypokalemia may cause weakening of cardiac contractions and may precipitate digitalis toxicity in the form of arrhythmias.

6. Give oral potassium as prescribed.

7. Be aware that problems associated with diuretic administration include disorders of potassium balance, hyperuricemia, volume depletion and hyponatremia, magnesium depletion, hyperglycemia, and diabetes mellitus.

8. Watch for signs of bladder distention in the elderly male with prostatic hyperplasia.

9. Assess for symptoms of electrolyte depletion—lassitude, apathy, mental confusion, anorexia, decreasing urinary output, azotemia.

10. Limit intravenous fluid administration through use of heparin lock (allows for periodic drug administration without increasing excessive fluid intake).

11. Assess for pitting edema of lower extremities and sacral area.
    Utilize "egg crate" mattress and sheepskin to prevent pressure sores (poor blood flow and edema increase susceptibility).

12. Observe for the complications of bed rest—pressure sores (especially in edematous patients), phlebothrombosis, pulmonary embolism.

13. Be alert to complaints of right upper quadrant abdominal pain, poor appetite, nausea, and abdominal

distention (may indicate hepatic and visceral engorgement).

14. Monitor the patient's diet. Diet may be limited in sodium—to prevent, control, or eliminate edema; may also be limited in calories.
    a. Patients on diuretics may not be on sodium-restricted diet.
    b. Caution patients to avoid added salt in food and foods with high sodium content.

F. Establishing a balance between oxygen supply and demand

1. Increase the patient's activities gradually.
    Alter or modify the patient's activities—to keep within the limits of his cardiac reserve.
    a. Assist the patient with self-care activities early in the day (fatigue sets in as day progresses).
    b. Be alert to complaints of chest pain or skeletal pain during or after activities.
2. Observe the pulse, symptoms, and behavioral response to increased activity.
    a. Monitor the patient's heart rate during self-care activities.
    b. Allow heart rate to decrease to preactivity level before initiating a new activity.
        (1) Note time lapse between cessation of activity and decrease in heart rate (decreased stroke volume causes immediate rise in heart rate).
        (2) Document time lapse and revise patient care plan as appropriate (progressive increase in time lapse may be indicative of increased left ventricular failure).
    c. Ask the patient about degree of fatigue experienced during and after activities.

G. Achieving adequate rest

1. Relieve nighttime anxiety and provide for rest and sleep—patients with congestive heart failure have a tendency to be restless at night because of cerebral hypoxia with superimposed nitrogen retention.
    a. Give oxygen during acute stage—to diminish work of breathing and increase the comfort of the patient.
    b. Give appropriate sedation—to relieve insomnia and restlessness.
        (1) Give small doses of morphine as prescribed for extreme dyspnea.
        (2) Give mild sedation as needed for sleep. Use sedation carefully to prevent respiratory depression; detoxification of drugs is delayed because of hepatic congestion and immobility of patient.
    c. Keep a night light on in the room; the presence of a family member provides reassurance to some persons.
    d. Avoid restraints—resistance to restraints increases cardiac load.

Health Education

1. Explain the disease process to the patient; the term "failure" may have terrifying implications.
    a. Explain the pumping action of the heart—"to move blood through the body to provide nutrients and aid in the removal of waste material."
    b. Explain the difference between "heart attack" and congestive heart failure.
2. Teach the signs and symptoms of recurrence.
    a. Ask patient to recall how he felt when he first became ill.
    b. Watch for:

        (1) Gain in weight—report weight gain of more than 2–3 pounds (0.9–1.4 kg.) in a few days. Weigh at same time daily to detect any tendency toward fluid retention.
        (2) Swelling of ankles, feet, or abdomen
        (3) Persistent cough
        (4) Tiredness; loss of appetite
        (5) Frequent urination at night
3. Review medication regimen.
    a. Label all medications.
    b. Give written instructions concerning digitalis and diuretic therapy.
    c. Inform patient not to substitute another brand of digitalis for the one he is taking.
        (1) Make sure the patient has a check-off system that will show that he has taken his medications.
        (2) Teach the patient to take and record his pulse rate.
        (3) Inform the patient of the signs and symptoms of digitalis toxicity and potassium depletion.
        (4) If the patient is taking oral potassium solution, it may be diluted with juice and taken after a meal.
    d. Tell the patient to weigh himself daily and log his weight if he is on diuretic therapy.
4. Review activity program.
    Instruct the patient as follows:
    a. Increase walking and other activities gradually, provided they do not cause fatigue and dyspnea.
    b. In general, continue at whatever activity level can be maintained without the appearance of symptoms.
    c. Avoid excesses in eating and drinking.
    d. Undertake a weight reduction program until optimal weight is reached.
    e. Avoid extremes in heat and cold—which increase the work of the heart; air conditioning may be essential in a hot, humid environment.
    f. Keep *regular* appointment with physician or clinic.
5. Restrict sodium as directed.
    a. Give patient a booklet containing sodium content of common foods from local chapter of American Heart Association.
    b. Give patient a written diet plan with list of permitted and restricted foods.
    c. Advise patient to look at all labels to ascertain sodium content (antacids, laxatives, cough remedies, etc.).
        (1) Teach the patient to rinse the mouth well after using tooth cleansers and mouthwashes—some of these contain large amounts of sodium. Water softeners are to be avoided.
        (2) Teach the patient that sodium is present in alkalizers, cough remedies, laxatives, pain relievers, estrogens, etc.
    d. Ascertain the amount of sodium in the local drinking water through inquiry to local department of health.
6. Advise the patient to accept the fact that restricting sodium and taking digitalis will be a permanent part of his life-style.
7. Teach the patient the importance of adhering to the low-sodium diet.
    Sodium is present in many types of natural foods and in varying amounts in processed foods.
    Make the diet as palatable as possible.

(1) Use flavorings, spices, herbs, and lemon juice.
(2) Avoid salt substitutes in the presence of renal disease.

Evaluation
Expected Outcomes
1. Maintains adequate cardiac output—normal blood pressure and heart rate (no hypotension, tachycardia, or cool clammy skin)
2. Exhibits improved ventilation/perfusion ratio—respiratory rate 16–20, arterial blood gases within normal limits, no signs of crackles or wheezes in lung fields
3. Demonstrates a decrease in body fluid—weight decrease of 1 pound (2.2 kg.) daily, no pitting edema of lower extremities and sacral area
4. Maintains balance between oxygen supply and demand—heart rate within normal limits, rests between activities—checks heart rate after activities, if elevated more than 10 beats above preactivity heart rate, waits until heart rate decreases before next activity

Acute Pulmonary Edema

Acute pulmonary edema refers to the presence of excess fluid in the lung, either in the interstitial spaces or in the alveoli. It usually follows acute left ventricular failure.

▶ **NURSING ALERT:** Acute pulmonary edema is a true medical emergency, since it is a life-threatening condition.

Causes
1. Heart disease—acute left ventricular failure, myocardial infarction, aortic stenosis, severe mitral valve disease, hypertension, congestive heart failure
2. Circulatory overload—transfusions and infusions
3. Drug hypersensitivity; allergy; poisoning
4. Lung injuries—smoke inhalation, shock lung, pulmonary embolism or infarct
5. Central nervous system injuries—stroke, head trauma
6. Infection and fever—infectious pneumonia (viral, bacterial, parasitic)
7. Postcardioversion, postanesthesia, postcardiopulmonary bypass
8. Narcotic overdose

Assessment
Clinical Manifestations
1. Coughing and restlessness during sleep (premonitory symptoms)
2. Extreme dyspnea and orthopnea—patient usually uses accessory muscles of respiration with retraction of intercostal spaces and supraclavicular areas
3. Cough with varying amounts of white- or pink-tinged frothy sputum
4. Extreme anxiety and panic
5. Noisy breathing—inspiratory and expiratory wheezing and bubbling sounds
6. Cyanosis with profuse perspiration
7. Distended neck veins
8. Tachycardia
9. Precordial pain (if pulmonary edema secondary to myocardial infarction)

Diagnostic Evaluation
1. Medical history, physical examination
2. Chest x-ray
3. Echocardiogram (suspected valvular disease)
4. Measurement of pulmonary artery wedge pressure by Swan–Ganz catheter (differentiates etiology of pulmonary edema—cardiogenic or altered alveolar–capillary membrane)
5. Blood cultures (suspected infection)
6. Cardiac enzymes (suspected myocardial infarction)

Patient Problems/Nursing Diagnoses
1. Impaired gas exchange related to inadequate ventilation/perfusion ratio
2. Altered breathing patterns (dyspnea, orthopnea, wheezing) related to excess fluid in the lungs
3. Anxiety related to sensation of suffocation

Planning and Implementation
Treatment
The objective of treatment is to improve ventilation and oxygenation and to reduce pulmonary congestion. Strategy for management is initiation of nonspecific measures* (i.e., oxygen therapy, morphine sulfate administration, patient in upright position), identification of precipitating factors (i.e., myocardial infarction, infection), and correction of factors contributing to underlying condition.

Nursing Interventions
A. Improved Oxygenation
1. Auscultate lung fields frequently.
    a. Note inspiratory and expiratory wheezes, rhonchi, moist fine crackles appearing initially in lung bases and extending upward.
2. Auscultate for extra heart sounds.
    a. Note presence of third heart sound (may be difficult to hear because of respiratory sounds).
3. Give oxygen in high concentration—to relieve hypoxia and dyspnea.
    a. Oxygen may be given with high enough pressure to provide blood oxygenation and to overcome the pressure barrier of the edema fluid.
    b. This is accomplished by giving oxygen by intermittent or continuous pressure.
4. *Take steps to reduce venous return to the heart.*
    Place patient in upright position; head and shoulders up, feet and legs hanging down—to favor pooling of blood in dependent portions of body by gravitational forces; to decrease venous return.
5. Give morphine in small titrated intermittent doses (IV) until dyspnea lessens—to allay acute anxiety and decrease respiratory effort, allowing better oxygen exchange; this also decreases peripheral resistance so that blood can be redistributed from the pulmonary circulation to the periphery.

* Many of the nonspecific measures are implemented simultaneously.

a. Morphine is *not* given if pulmonary edema is caused by cerebral vascular accident or occurs in the presence of chronic pulmonary disease or cardiogenic shock.
b. Watch for excessive respiratory depression.
c. Monitor blood pressure, since morphine may intensify hypotension.
d. Have morphine antagonist available—naloxone hydrochloride (Narcan).

6. Give injections of diuretic (ethacrynic acid; furosemide) IV—to reduce blood volume and pulmonary congestion by producing prompt diuresis.
   a. Insert an indwelling catheter—large urinary volume will accumulate rapidly.
   b. *Watch for falling blood pressure, increasing heart rate, and decreasing urinary output—indications that the total circulation is not tolerating diuresis and that hypovolemia may develop.*
   c. Check electrolyte levels, since potassium loss may be significant.
   d. Watch for signs of urinary obstruction in men with prostatic hyperplasia.

7. Use rotating tourniquets or automatic inflating cuffs on extremities (p. 294)—to decrease venous return and right ventricular output and thus aid in decongesting lungs.

8. Administer vasodilator if patient fails to respond to therapy—to reduce impedance (resistance) to left ventricular ejection of blood; allows more complete ventricular emptying and increases venous capacity so that left ventricular filling pressure is reduced. Patient monitored by measuring pulmonary artery pressure and cardiac output.

   Nitroprusside or sublingual nitroglycerin usually prescribed by physician (see Congestive Heart Failure, p. 325).

9. Assist physician with phlebotomy if indicated for treatment.
   a. *Phlebotomy* is the rapid withdrawal of approximately 500 ml. of blood from peripheral vein.
   b. Phlebotomy aids in decreasing venous return and produces a corresponding decline in right ventricular output.
   c. Phlebotomy is usually done to reduce intravascular pressure when attack is precipitated by overadministration of blood or infusion fluids.

10. Administer dobutamine as prescribed by physician.
11. Aminophylline may be given when indicated to relieve bronchospasm.
    a. Monitor blood levels of drug.

b. Assess the patient for side effects of drug—ventricular arrhythmias, hypotension, headache.
12. Administer cardiac glycosides (digitalis) per physician request (usually prescribed in treating pulmonary edema secondary to myocardial infarction).
13. Assist with cardioversion if indicated (pulmonary edema precipitates tachycardias).
14. Give appropriate drugs for severe, sustained hypertension.
15. Continually evaluate the patient's response to therapy. Reevaluate lung fields and cardiac status (see Intervention, #1).

B. Decrease in Anxiety

1. Stay with the patient and display a confident attitude—the presence of another person is therapeutic, since the acute anxiety of the patient may tend to intensify the severity of his condition. (Arterial vasoconstriction diminishes as anxiety is relieved.)
2. Explain to the patient in a calm manner all therapies administered and the reason for their use.
   a. Give brief explanations related to goal of therapies (i.e., "Morphine will help you relax and ease your work of breathing").
   b. Explain to the patient importance of wearing oxygen mask. Assure the patient that mask will not increase sensation of suffocation.
3. Inform the patient and family of progress toward resolution of pulmonary edema.
4. Allow time for the patient and family to ventilate concerns and fears.

Health Education

During convalescence, instruct the patient as follows in order to prevent recurrences of pulmonary edema:
1. Ask: What symptoms did you have before the attack? (He should be aware of these.)
2. If coughing develops (a wet cough), sit with legs dangling over side of bed.
3. See Health Education, Congestive Heart Failure, page 326.

Evaluation
Expected Outcomes

1. Attains improved oxygenation—unlabored respirations at 14–18 times per minute, lungs clear on auscultation, blood gases within normal limits for patient, no cough or sputum
2. Achieves decrease in anxiety—appears calm; rests comfortably

Heart Surgery

Nursing Process Overview

Assessment
Health History

1. Review the patient's record to learn past history and present condition, paying close attention to pulmonary, renal, hepatic, hematologic, and metabolic systems.
   a. Cardiac history; *history of cardiac arrhythmias.*
   b. Pulmonary health—patients with COPD may require prolonged postoperative respiratory support.
   c. Depression—can produce a serious postoperative depressive state and can affect postoperative morbidity and mortality.
   d. Ask about previous / present alcohol intake; smoking history.
2. Assess laboratory studies.
   a. Complete blood count; serum electrolytes; lipid profile; and nose, throat, sputum, and urine cultures

b. Antibody screen
c. Preoperative coagulation survey (platelet count, prothrombin time, partial thromboplastin time)—extracorporeal circulation will affect certain coagulation factors.
d. Renal and hepatic function tests
3. Assess the patient's reactions to medications—these patients are usually on multiple drugs.
    a. Digitalis
        (1) Patient may be receiving large doses to improve myocardial contractility.
        (2) Drug may be stopped several days before surgery—to avoid digitoxic arrhythmias from cardiopulmonary bypass.
    b. Diuretics
        (1) Assess the patient for potassium depletion and volume depletion (weakness, postural hypotension)—diuretics may produce potassium loss, and severe diuresis may cause a decrease in blood volume.
        (2) Give potassium supplement if the patient is on prolonged diuretic therapy—to replenish body stores.
        (3) Diuretics may be omitted several days preoperatively to avoid electrolyte imbalance and consequent arrhythmias postoperatively. Salt and water restriction may be advised.
    c. Beta-adrenergic blockers (propranolol)—continue as directed.
    d. Psychotropic drugs (diazepam; chlordiazepoxide)—postoperative withdrawal may cause extreme agitation.
    e. Antihypertensives (reserpine)—omitted as far in advance of procedure as possible to allow norepinephrine repletion.
    f. Alcohol—sudden withdrawal may produce delirium.
    g. Anticoagulant drugs—discontinued several days before operation to allow coagulation mechanism to return to normal.
    h. Determine if the patient has taken corticosteroids within the year prior to surgery—patients on steroids are given supplemental doses to cover stress of surgery.
    i. Prophylactic antibiotics may be given preoperatively.
    j. Determine whether the patient has any drug sensitivities.
4. Be aware of the preoperative conditions that predispose to postoperative respiratory complications.
    a. Pulmonary hypertension
    b. Pulmonary congestion or edema
    c. Preexisting lung disease
    d. Pulmonary sepsis
    e. Elderly or debilitated patient
5. Encourage the patient to stop smoking—smoking increases incidence of postoperative respiratory complications.
6. Surgical preparation:
    a. Shave anterior and lateral surfaces of trunk and neck; shave entire body down to ankles (for coronary bypass).
    b. Shower/bathe with Betadine soap.

Patient Problems/Nursing Diagnoses

1. Anxiety related to fear of unknown, fear of death, and fear of pain.
2. Potential for impaired gas exchange related to inadequate ventilation/perfusion ratio.
3. Potential for decreased cardiac output related to manipulation of heart during surgery.
4. Potential for fluid and electrolyte disturbances related to heart–lung machine.
5. Potential for sensory overload related to excessive environmental stimuli.
6. Potential for complications—arrhythmias, cardiac tamponade, myocardial infarction, hypovolemia, and embolization.
7. Pain related to sternotomy and leg incisions.

Planning and Implementation
Preoperative Nursing Interventions
A. Decrease in Anxiety

1. Evaluate the patient's emotional state and try to reduce his anxieties—patients undergoing heart surgery are more anxious and fearful than other surgical patients. (Moderate anxiety assists patient to cope with stresses of surgery. Low anxiety level may indicate that the patient is in denial. High anxiety may impair the patient's ability to learn and listen.)
    a. Offer support to patients in low or high anxiety states. Give support by being present, by listening, and by showing interest—patient is called upon to deal with a stressful and life-threatening crisis.
    b. Encourage the patient to express what he feels and thinks—ventilation of feelings and fantasies relieves sense of isolation and facilitates a growing and supportive relationship.
        (1) Try to elicit special concerns.
        (2) Patients with unusual degree of anxiety and history of mental illness may require psychiatric consultation.
        (3) Patients with low levels of anxiety may have stormy postoperative course—have not prepared themselves for stress of surgery.
        (4) Patients with characteristics of type A personality (competitive striving for achievement, sense of time urgency, aggressiveness, and hostility) may be extremely anxious because of sudden role reversal; attempt to meet needs with explanations of objectives of surgery and probable postoperative experience.
    c. Help the patient and family to mobilize defenses and cope with fears.
    d. Clarify the information given the patient previously by the cardiovascular surgeon.
        (1) Ask the patient to state why surgery is necessary.
        (2) Give the patient pamphlet on heart surgery to reinforce discussions with health-team members and to review with family members.
    e. Anticipate and answer the patient's questions.
        (1) Ask the patient what he wants to know.
        (2) Establish a relationship of trust.
    f. Support the patient undergoing diagnostic studies to determine type and severity of specific lesions; tests also provide a baseline for postoperative evaluation.
        (1) Cardiac catheterization and angiography
        (2) Pulmonary function studies
        (3) ECG, echocardiogram, phonocardiogram

      (4) Exercise stress testing

      (5) Chest x-ray

   g. Expect some patients to have psychological and psychiatric problems from prolonged illness.

B. Preoperative Teaching

1. Prepare the patient for events in the postoperative period.

   a. Take the patient and family on tour of ICU—lessens anxiety about being in ICU.

      (1) Introduce the patient to staff personnel who will be caring for him.

      (2) Give family a schedule of visiting hours and times for phone contact.

   b. Teach chest physical therapy procedures—to optimize pulmonary function.

      (1) Have the patient practice with incentive spirometer.

      (2) Show and practice diaphragmatic breathing techniques.

      (3) Have the patient practice effective coughing, leg exercises.

   c. Prepare patient for presence of monitors, chest tubes, IVs, blood transfusion, endotracheal tube, nasogastric tube, pacing wires, arterial line, indwelling catheter.

      (1) Explain to the patient that two chest tubes will be inserted below incision into chest cavity for drainage and maintenance of negative pressure.

      (2) Explain to the patient that endotrachial tube will prevent speaking, but that he will be able to communicate through writing until tube is removed (usually within 24 hours).

      (3) Explain to the patient that his diet will consist of liquids until 24 hours after surgery.

      (4) Explain to the patient that monitoring equipment and intravenous lines will restrict movement, and nursing staff will position the patient comfortably every 2 hours and as necessary.

   d. Discuss with the patient the need to monitor vital signs frequently and the likelihood of frequent disturbances of the patient's rest.

   e. Discuss pain management with the patient.

      (1) Explain to the patient that median sternotomies require one-third as much analgesia for relief of the patient's pain than do abdominal incisions.

      (2) Assure the patient that analgesics will be administered as necessary to control pain.

2. Tell the patient that both hands may be loosely restrained for a number of hours after surgery to eliminate possibility of pulling out tubes and intravenous lines inadvertently.

3. Discuss with the patient surgical preparation for the day of scheduled surgery and the night prior.

   a. Shave anterior and lateral surfaces of trunk and neck. (Shave entire body down to ankles for coronary bypass.)

   b. Explain to the patient that sedatives will be given before he goes to the operating room.

4. Encourage the patient to stop smoking—smoking increases chance of postoperative respiratory complications.

5. Document preoperative teaching done and the patient's behavior and level of understanding before and after teaching. Record specifically what the patient was taught.

Postoperative Nursing Interventions

1. Orient the patient to surroundings as soon as he awakens from surgical procedure. Tell the patient that operation is over, where he is, the time of day, and your name.

2. Allow family members to visit the patient as soon as his condition stabilizes. Encourage family members to talk to and touch the patient (family members may be overwhelmed by critical care environment).

3. As the patient becomes more alert, remind him of the purpose of all the equipment in his environment. Continually orient the patient to time and place (let the patient know if it is day or night).

A. Adequate Oxygenation

1. Secure all connections for lines and tubes (arterial, Swan–Ganz, CVP, chest tubes, urinary catheter to collecting bottle, endotracheal tube to ventilator, ECG to monitoring system, pacing wires, etc.).

2. Provide for tissue oxygenation and assess respiratory status. Ensure adequate oxygenation in early postoperative period; respiratory insufficiency is common following open heart surgery.

   a. Employ assisted or controlled ventilation (see p. 227)—respiratory support is used during first 24 hours to provide airway in the event of cardiac arrest, to decrease work of heart, to maintain effective ventilation.

      (1) Adequacy of ventilation is assessed by the patient's clinical status and by direct measurement of tidal volume and arterial blood gases.

      (2) Check endotracheal tube placement.

      (3) Auscultate chest for breath sounds—crackles indicate pulmonary congestion; decreased or absent breath sounds indicate pneumothorax.

      (4) Arterial blood gas analysis (see p. 143) is usually performed during first hour postoperatively and prn thereafter.

      (5) Sedate patient adequately—to help him tolerate endotracheal tube and cope with ventilatory sensations.

      (6) Utilize chest physiotherapy for patients with lung congestion to prevent retention of secretions and atelectasis.

         (a) Check chest x-ray and auscultate chest to determine problem areas.

         (b) Use percussion and vibrating techniques to loosen secretions.

         (c) Promote coughing, deep breathing, and turning—to keep airway patent, prevent atelectasis, and facilitate lung expansion.

      (7) Suction tracheobronchial secretions carefully (see p. 222)—prolonged aspiration leads to hypoxia and possible cardiac arrest.

      (8) Restrict fluids (per request) for first few days—danger of pulmonary congestion from excessive fluid intake.

      (9) Chest x-ray taken immediately after surgery and daily therafter—to evaluate state of lung expansion and to detect atelectasis; to demonstrate heart size and contour, confirm

placement of central line, endotracheal tube, and chest drains.

(10) See page 230 for weaning process and endotracheal tube removal.

B. Adequate Cardiac Output

1. Employ hemodynamic monitoring* during immediate postoperative period, especially for cardiovascular and respiratory status and fluid and electrolyte balance—to prevent complications or to recognize them as early as possible.

2. Monitor cardiovascular status to determine effectiveness of cardiac output with hemodynamic monitoring. Serial readings of blood pressure and arterial pressure, heart rate, CVP and left atrial or pulmonary artery pressure from monitor modules are observed, correlated with the patient's condition, and recorded.

   a. Assess arterial pressure every 15 minutes until stable and as directed thereafter—blood pressure is one of the most important physiologic parameters to follow.

   Take direct measurement (arterial line, transducer)—most accurate blood pressure. Extreme vasoconstriction following extracorporeal circulation makes auscultatory blood pressure unobtainable.

   b. Check peripheral pulses (pedal, tibial, radial) as a further check on heart action.

   Palpate the carotid, brachial, popliteal, and femoral pulses; absence of these pulses may be due to recent catheterization of the extremity.

   c. Measure left atrial pressure or pulmonary artery wedge pressure—to determine the left ventricular end-diastolic volume and to assess cardiac output (see p. 282).

   Rising pressures may indicate congestive heart failure or pulmonary edema.

   d. Take central venous pressure readings hourly (see p. 286)—indicate blood volume, vascular tone, and pumping effectiveness of the heart.

   (1) High CVP reading may result from hypervolemia, heart failure, cardiac tamponade. Ventilator may elevate CVP.

   (2) If blood pressure drop is due to low blood volume, CVP will show corresponding drop.

   (3) *Changes* in values are more important than isolated readings.

3. Check urine output every ½ to 1 hour (from indwelling catheter)—urine output is an index of cardiac output and renal perfusion. Continue with ongoing patient assessment.

   a. Observe buccal mucosa, nail beds, lips, ear lobes, and extremities for duskiness/cyanosis—signs of low cardiac output.

   b. Feel the skin; cool, moist skin reveals lowered cardiac output. Note temperature and color of extremities.

   c. Note fullness and tone of superficial veins of feet; evaluate pedal and femoral pulses.

   d. Assess for venous distention of neck veins or veins of dorsal surface of hands (raised above

level of heart)—may signal a changing demand or diminishing capacity of heart.

   e. Evaluate temperature.

4. Assess neurologic status—the brain is dependent on a continuous supply of oxygenated blood and must rely on adequate and continuous perfusion by the heart.

   a. Hypoperfusion or microemboli (air debris) may produce CNS damage after heart surgery.

   b. Observe for symptoms of hypoxia—restlessness, headache, confusion, dyspnea, hypotension, and cyanosis.

   c. Assess the patient's neurologic status hourly in terms of:

   (1) Level of responsiveness

   (2) Response to verbal commands and painful stimuli

   (3) Pupillary size and reaction to light

   (4) Movement of extremities; handgrasp ability

   d. Treat postoperative convulsive seizures. Give medications according to therapeutic directives—coronary vasodilators, antibiotics, analgesics, anticoagulants (patients with prosthetic valves).

C. Fluid and Electrolyte Balance

1. Maintain fluid and electrolyte balance—adequate circulating blood volume is necessary for optimal cellular activity; metabolic acidosis and electrolyte imbalance can occur after use of pump oxygenator.

   a. Fluids may be limited to avoid overloading.

   b. Keep intake and output flow sheet—as a method of determining positive or negative fluid balance and the patient's fluid requirements.

   (1) IV fluids (including flush solutions through arterial and venous lines) considered intake.

   (2) Assess hydration status of patient—evaluation of pulmonary wedge, left atrial pressure, and CVP readings; weight, electrolyte levels, hematocrit readings, distention of neck veins, tissue edema, liver size, breath sounds.

   (3) Record urine output every ½ to 1 hour.

   (4) Measure postoperative chest drainage—should not exceed 200 ml./hour for first 4–6 hours.

   (a) Watch for sudden cessation of chest drainage—from kinked or blocked chest tube.

   (b) See page 183 for management of patient with water-seal drainage.

2. Be alert to changes in serum electrolytes—a specific concentration of electrolytes is necessary in both extracellular and intracellular body fluids in order to sustain life.

   a. *Hypokalemia* (low potassium level)

   (1) May be caused by inadequate intake, diuretics, vomiting, excessive nasogastric drainage, stress from surgery.

   (2) Effects of low potassium level—arrhythmias, digitalis toxicity, metabolic alkalosis, weakened myocardium, cardiac arrest.

   (3) Watch for specific ECG changes.

   (4) Give IV potassium replacement as directed.

   b. *Hyperkalemia* (high potassium level)

   (1) May be caused by increased intake, red cell breakdown from the pump, acidosis, renal insufficiency, tissue necrosis, and adrenal cortical insufficiency.

---

* Monitoring equipment is valuable only when it is understood and used correctly. The clinical assessment of the patient by the nurse is indispensable to patient care.

(2) Effects of high potassium level—mental confusion, restlessness, nausea, weakness, and paresthesia of extremities.

(3) Be prepared to administer an ion-exchange resin, sodium polystyrene sulfonate (Kayexalate), which binds the potassium, or give IV sodium bicarbonate or IV insulin and glucose to drive the potassium back into the cells from the extracellular fluid.

c. *Hyponatremia* (low sodium)

(1) May be due to reduction of total body sodium or to an increased water intake causing a dilution of body sodium.

(2) Assess for weakness, fatigue, confusion, convulsions, and coma.

d. *Hypocalcemia* (low calcium level)

(1) May be due to alkalosis (which reduces the amount of Ca^{++} in the extracellular fluid) and multiple blood transfusions.

(2) Signs and symptoms of reduced calcium levels—numbness and tingling in the fingertips, toes, ear, and nose, carpopedal spasm, muscle cramps, and tetany.

(3) Give replacement therapy as directed.

e. *Hypercalcemia* (high calcium level)

(1) May cause arrhythmias imitating those caused by digitalis toxicity.

(2) Assess for signs of digitalis toxicity.

(3) Institute treatment as directed—this condition may lead to asystole and death.

D. Decrease in Discomfort

1. Examine sternotomy incision and leg dressings.
2. Relieve the patient's pain—cardiac surgical patients experience pain caused by sternotomy incision and irritation of pleura by chest tubes.

a. Record nature, type, location, and duration of pain—pain and anxiety increase pulse rate, oxygen consumption, and cardiac work.

b. Differentiate between incisional pain and anginal pain.

c. Watch for restlessness and apprehension—may be from hypoxia or a low-output state; analgesics or sedatives do not correct this problem.

d. Administer medication as often as prescribed—to reduce amount of pain and to aid the patient in performing deep breathing and coughing exercises more effectively.

(1) Reassure the patient that staff understands that treatment is painful and that it is "OK to be angry."

(2) Allow the patient to talk about his experience.

E. Mental and Psychological Orientation

Postcardiotomy delirium—may appear after a brief lucid period.

1. Symptoms

a. Psychic disturbances are more frequent after heart operations with extracorporeal circulation than after general surgery.

b. Signs and symptoms include delirium (impairment of orientation, memory, intellectual function, judgment), transient perceptual distortions, visual and auditory hallucinations, disorientation, and paranoid delusions.

c. Symptoms may be related to sleep deprivation, increased sensory input, disorientation to night and day, prolonged inability to speak because of

endotracheal intubation, age, preoperative cardiac status, etc.

2. Keep the patient oriented to time and place; notify the patient of procedures and expectations of his cooperation. Give repeated explanations of what is happening.

3. Encourage family to come in at regular times—helps the patient regain sense of reality.

4. Plan care to allow rest periods, day–night pattern, and uninterrupted sleep.

5. Encourage mobility as soon as possible. Keep environment as free as possible of excessive auditory and sensory input. Prevent bodily injury.

6. Reassure the patient and his family that psychiatric disorders following cardiac surgery are usually transient.

7. Remove the patient from ICU as soon as possible. Allow patient to *ventilate* events of his psychotic episode—helps him deal with and assimilate experience.

F. Avoidance of Complications

1. *Cardiac arrhythmias*

a. Watch ECG monitor—cardiac arrhythmias frequently occur after heart surgery.

(1) Premature ventricular contractions occur most frequently following aortic valve replacement and coronary bypass surgery. May be treated with pacing, lidocaine, potassium.

(2) Arrhythmias also apt to occur with ischemia, hypoxia, alterations in serum potassium, edema, bleeding, acid–base or electrolyte disturbances, digitalis toxicity, myocardial failure.

(3) Observe other parameters in correlation with monitor information—a low serum potassium level makes the heart susceptible to ventricular arrhythmias.

(4) See page 339 for discussion of cardiac arrhythmias.

2. *Cardiac tamponade*—results from bleeding into the pericardial sac or accumulation of fluids in the sac, which compresses the heart and prevents adequate filling of the ventricles.

a. Assess for signs of tamponade—arterial hypotension, rising CVP, rising left atrial pressure, muffled heart sounds, weak, thready pulse, neck vein distention, falling urinary output.

b. Check for diminished amount of drainage in the chest-collection bottle; may indicate that fluid is accumulating elsewhere.

c. Prepare for pericardiocentesis (see p. 289).

3. *Myocardial infarction*

a. Check cardiac enzymes daily—elevations may indicate myocardial infarction.

b. Symptoms may be masked by the usual postoperative discomfort.

(1) Watch for decreased cardiac output in the presence of normal circulating volume and filling pressure.

(2) Obtain serial ECGs and isoenzymes to determine extent of myocardial injury.

(3) Assess pain to differentiate myocardial pain from incisional pain.

c. Treatment is individualized. Postoperative activity level may be reduced to allow heart adequate time for healing.

4. *Cardiac failure* (low-output syndrome)—causes deficient blood perfusion to different organs.

Observe for falling mean arterial pressure, rising filling pressures (CVP, PCW, or LAP), and increasing tachycardia; the patient may exhibit signs of restlessness and agitation, cold and blue extremities, venous distention, labored respirations, tissue edema, and ascites.

5. *Persistent bleeding*—from cardiac incision, tissue fragility, trauma to tissues, clotting defects; blood clotting disturbances usually transitory following cardiopulmonary bypass; however, a significant platelet deficiency may be present.
   a. Watch for steady and continuous drainage of blood; watch CVP and left atrial pressures.
   b. Treatment—protamine sulfate, vitamin K, or blood components.
   c. Prepare for potential return to surgery for bleeding persisting (over 300 ml. per hour) for 4–6 hours.

6. *Hypovolemia* (decreased circulating blood volume)
   a. Low central venous pressure is an indication of hypovolemia.
   b. Assess for arterial hypotension, low CVP, increasing pulse rate, and low left atrial and pulmonary artery wedge pressures.
   c. Prepare to administer blood, IV solutions.

7. *Renal failure*—urine output depends on cardiac output, blood volume, state of hydration, and condition of kidneys.
   a. Renal injury may be caused by deficient perfusion, hemolysis, low cardiac output prior to and following open heart surgery; use of vasopressor agents to increase blood pressure.
   b. Measure urine volume; less than 20 ml./hour can indicate decreased renal function.
   c. Carry out specific gravity tests to determine kidneys' ability to concentrate urine in renal tubules.
   d. Watch BUN and serum creatinine levels, as well as urine and serum electrolyte levels.
   e. Give rapid-acting diuretics and/or inotropic drugs (dopamine, dobutamine) to increase cardiac output and renal blood flow.
   f. Prepare the patient for peritoneal dialysis or hemodialysis if indicated. (Renal insufficiency may produce serious cardiac arrhythmias.)

8. *Hypotension*—may be caused by inadequate cardiac contractility and reduction in blood volume or by mechanical ventilation (when the patient "fights" the ventilator, or PEEP is used), all of which can produce a reduction in cardiac output.
   a. Monitor vital signs, left atrial pressure, CVP and arterial pressure.
   b. Note chest tube drainage—hypotension may be caused by excessive bleeding.
   c. Give blood as directed to maintain left atrial pressure at a level which will provide an adequate circulating volume for good tissue perfusion.

9. *Embolization*—may result from injury to the intima of the blood vessels, dislodgement of a clot from a damaged valve, venous stasis aggravated by certain arrhythmias, loosening of mural thrombi, and coagulation problems.
   a. Common embolic sites are lungs, coronary arteries, mesentery, extremities, kidneys, spleen, and brain.
   b. Symptoms of embolization (vary according to site)—Midabdominal or midback pain; pain, cessation of pulses, blanching, numbness, coldness of extremity; chest pain and respiratory distress with pulmonary embolus or myocardial infarction; and, one-sided weakness, pupil changes, as in stroke.
   c. Initiate preventive measures — antiembolic stockings; omit pressure on popliteal space (leg crossing, raising knee gatch); start passive and active exercises.

10. *Postpericardiotomy syndrome*—a group of symptoms occurring following cardiac and pericardial trauma and myocardial infarction.
    a. Cause is not certain—may be from anticardiac antibodies, viral etiology, etc.
    b. Manifestations—fever, malaise, arthralgias, dyspnea, pericardial effusion, pleural effusion, friction rub.
    c. Treatment is symptomatic (bed rest, aspirin), since condition is self-limiting but recurrence is not uncommon.

11. *Postperfusion syndrome*
    a. Signs and symptoms—fever, splenomegaly, lymphocytosis.
    b. Draw blood for culture—postperfusion syndrome can mimic bacterial endocarditis or hepatitis.
    c. Treatment is symptomatic, since syndrome is self-limiting.
    d. Reassure patient that this is only a temporary setback in his convalescence.

12. *Febrile complications*—probably from body's reaction to tissue trauma or accumulation of blood and serum in pleural and pericardial spaces.
    a. Control higher degrees of fever by use of hypothermia mattress.
    b. Evaluate for atelectasis, pleural effusion, or pneumonia if fever persists.
    c. Evaluate for urinary tract infection/wound infection.
    d. Bear in mind the possibility of infective endocarditis if fever persists (see p. 314).

13. *Hepatitis*

Health Education, Discharge Planning, and Rehabilitation Following Cardiac Surgery

Goal:
Assume a normal life as promptly as possible.

1. Begin discussing long-range plans with patient during convalescence in order to help him make modifications in his life-style.
2. Give written guidelines:
   a. *Activities*
      (1) Increase activities gradually within limits. Avoid strenuous activities until after exercise stress testing.
      (2) Take short rest periods.
      (3) Avoid lifting more than 20 pounds.
      (4) Participate in activities that do not cause pain or discomfort.
      (5) Increase walking time and distance each day.
      (6) Stairs (1–2 times daily) the first week; increase as tolerated.
      (7) Avoid large crowds at first.
      (8) Driving—avoid driving until after first postoperative checkup. At this time ask physician when you may drive.
      (9) Sexual relations—resumption of sexual relations parallels ability to participate in other activities. Usually may resume sexual activi-

ties 2 weeks after surgery. Avoid if tired or after heavy meal. Consult physician if chest discomfort, difficult breathing, or palpitations occur and last longer than 15 minutes after intercourse.

   (10) Return to work—after first postoperative checkup, as advised by physician.

   (11) Expect some chest discomfort.

  b. *Diet*

   (1) Some patients are placed on minimum salt restriction (e.g., no salt added at table); cholesterol may be limited.

   (2) Weigh daily and report weight gain of more than 5 pounds per week.

  c. *Medications*

   (1) Label all medications; give purposes and side effects.

   (2) Patients with prosthetic valves may continue warfarin regimen indefinitely.

3. Patients with prosthetic valves:

  a. Pregnancy usually discouraged in women with prosthetic valves.

  b. Caution patient about need for antibiotic coverage following dental and surgical procedures.

  c. Patients on anticoagulants should watch for bleeding and should avoid use of aspirin (and many other drugs)—interferes with action of warfarin.

4. Advise the patient to carry an identification card stating cardiac condition and medications being taken.

5. The patient may be placed on rehabilitation and exercise program after exercise stress testing.

6. Inform the patient whom to contact (and how) in case of an emergency.

7. See also Health Education After MI, page 309 and Health Education, Infective Endocarditis.

Evaluation

Expected Outcomes

1. Experiences a decrease in anxiety—verbalizes a lessening of anxiety, listens to and learns preoperative content taught (states reasons for operation, events to occur prior to and after surgery, need for follow-up rehabilitation after surgery)

2. Maintains adequate oxygenation—arterial blood gases within normal limits for patient, extubated 24 hours after surgery, spontaneous, unlabored respirations 14–18 per minute

3. Demonstrates adequate cardiac output—blood pressure and heart rate within normal limits for patient, skin warm and dry, urine output greater than 50 ml. per hour

4. Achieves fluid and electrolyte balance—serum electrolytes normal, lungs clear on auscultation, absence of edema

5. Adapts to intensive care environment—no hallucinations, oriented to time and place consistently when asked, sleeps 5 hours without interruption.

6. Remains free of complications—absence of life-threatening arrhythmias, heart sounds normal, cardiac enzymes normal, temperature within normal limits for patient, absence of bleeding

7. Experiences minimal discomfort; absence of incisional pain

2: Fundamentals of Electrocardiography

The Electrocardiogram (ECG) and Heart Dynamics

Heart Anatomy and Physiology (Fig. 9-11)

1. Heart tissue is highly specialized muscle mass, which possesses the special properties of automaticity, rhythmicity, conductivity, and excitability.

2. The above properties make it possible for the heart to initiate a rhythmic wave of impulse with the subsequent conduction of that impulse resulting in a single heart contraction.

3. The site of normal impulse origin is referred to as the *sinoatrial node* and is located in the right atrium. The sinus node is the natural pacemaker of the heart because it possesses the fastest intrinsic rate above all other heart muscle. The SA node paces between 60 and 100 times per minute. The AV node has an intrinsic rate of between 40 and 60 times per minute; the ventricles' intrinsic rate is 20 to 40 times per minute.

4. Once excited by the sinoatrial node, the wave of impulse spreads over the thin walls of the atria to the atrioventricular node. The impulse is physiologically delayed at the AV node to allow for ventricular filling.

5. The AV node, as the name implies, lies at the junction of the atria and ventricles.

6. The wave of impulse then traverses the bundle of His and the left and right bundle branches of the ventricles and finally terminates in the Purkinje fibers

of the ventricles. This electrical activity results in a single heart contraction and is referred to as *depolarization of the ventricles* (see Fig. 9-11).

7. The conduction system of the heart is under the control of the autonomic nervous system.

  a. Sympathetic—speeds the heart rate

  b. Parasympathetic—slows the heart rate (Vagus nerve)

8. The relaxation phase, which follows contraction, is referred to as *repolarization*.

The ECG

1. Machine capable of transcribing to graph paper the electrical activity of the heart.

2. Electrical activity is generated by the cells of the heart as ions are exchanged across cell membranes.

3. Electrodes that are capable of conducting electrical activity from the heart to the ECG machine are placed at strategic positions on the extremities and chest precordium.

4. The electrical energy sensed is then converted to a graphic display by the ECG machine. This display is referred to as the electrocardiogram (Fig. 9-12).

Clinical Uses of ECG

The ECG is a useful tool in the diagnosis of those conditions that may cause aberrations in the electrical

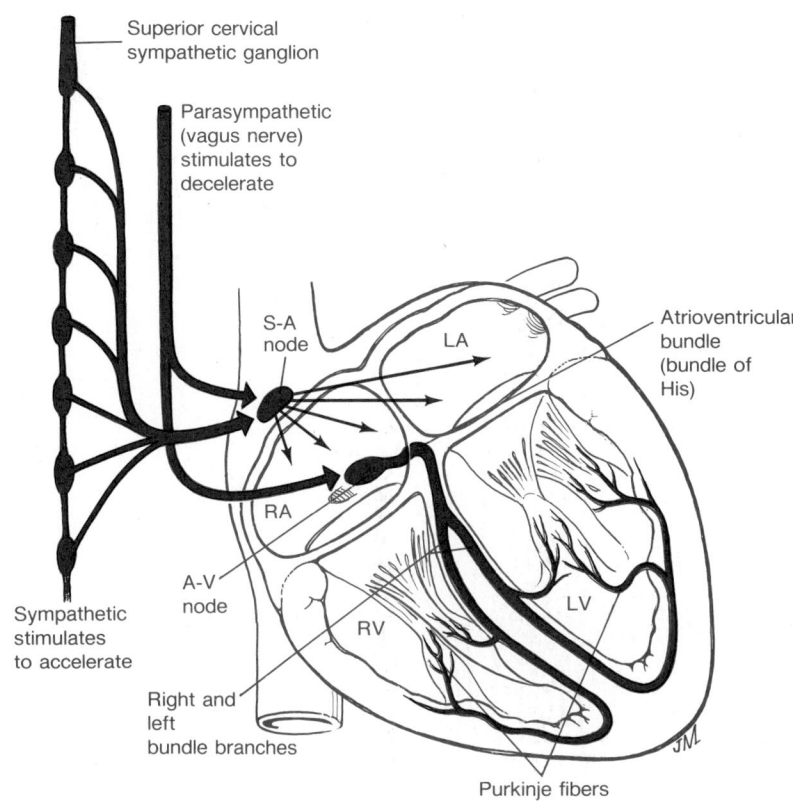

Superior cervical sympathetic ganglion

Parasympathetic (vagus nerve) stimulates to decelerate

S-A node

LA

Atrioventricular bundle (bundle of His)

RA

A-V node

RV

LV

Sympathetic stimulates to accelerate

Right and left bundle branches

Purkinje fibers

Figure 9-11. Heart dynamics or wave of depolarization. Schematically represented is the pathway followed by a normal electrical impulse initiated at the sinus node. The electrical event is followed by a mechanical event which results in heart contraction. The influence of the autonomic nervous system is also depicted.

activity of the heart. Examples of these conditions are as follows:
1. Myocardial infarction and other types of coronary artery diseases, such as angina
2. Cardiac arrhythmias
3. Cardiac enlargement
4. Electrolyte disturbances, especially of calcium and potassium levels.
5. Inflammatory diseases of the heart
6. Drug effect

The Normal ECG

1. Figure 9-13 represents the lead II of the normal ECG.
2. A heart contraction is represented by wave forms on the graph paper that are arbitrarily designated P, Q, R, S, and T waves.
3. Wave forms are referred to as deflections relative to an isoelectric line (e.g., a line that expresses no energy). The isoelectric line can be determined by looking at the T to P interval.
4. The P wave is the first positive deflection.
   a. The Q wave is the first negative deflection after the P wave; the R wave is the first positive deflection after the Q wave.
   b. The S wave is the negative deflection after the R wave.
   c. The T wave follows the S wave and is joined to the QRS complex by the ST segment.
   d. The QT interval is the time between the Q wave and the T wave.

5. The P wave represents atrial depolarization; the configuration of the P wave is useful in determining the source of impulse formation as being sinus node versus atrial muscle.
6. The QRS wave form is generally regarded as a unit and represents ventricular depolarization.
7. The T wave represents relaxation of the muscle fibers and is referred to as repolarization of the ventricles.

ECG Paper (Fig. 9-14)

1. ECG paper is graph paper with horizontal and vertical axes.
2. Time is measured on the horizontal axis. There are 1,500 1-mm. blocks in 60 seconds; therefore a 1-mm. square equals 0.04 second (e.g., 1,500 ÷ 60 = 0.04 second).
3. The superior margin of the ECG paper is marked by small vertical lines at 3-second intervals.
4. Amplitude is measured on the vertical axis; 1 small square equals 1 mm. of voltage.
5. Cardiac rate may be determined in a variety of ways using the time interval measurements.
6. The most expedient method for rate determination is to count the number of QRS complexes within a 6-second time interval (use the superior margin of ECG paper) and multiply the complexes by a factor of 10. (The factor of 10 is determined by dividing the 6-second interval into 60 seconds or 1 minute.) A gross estimate of rate may be determined in this manner.
   a. One must be cautioned that this method is

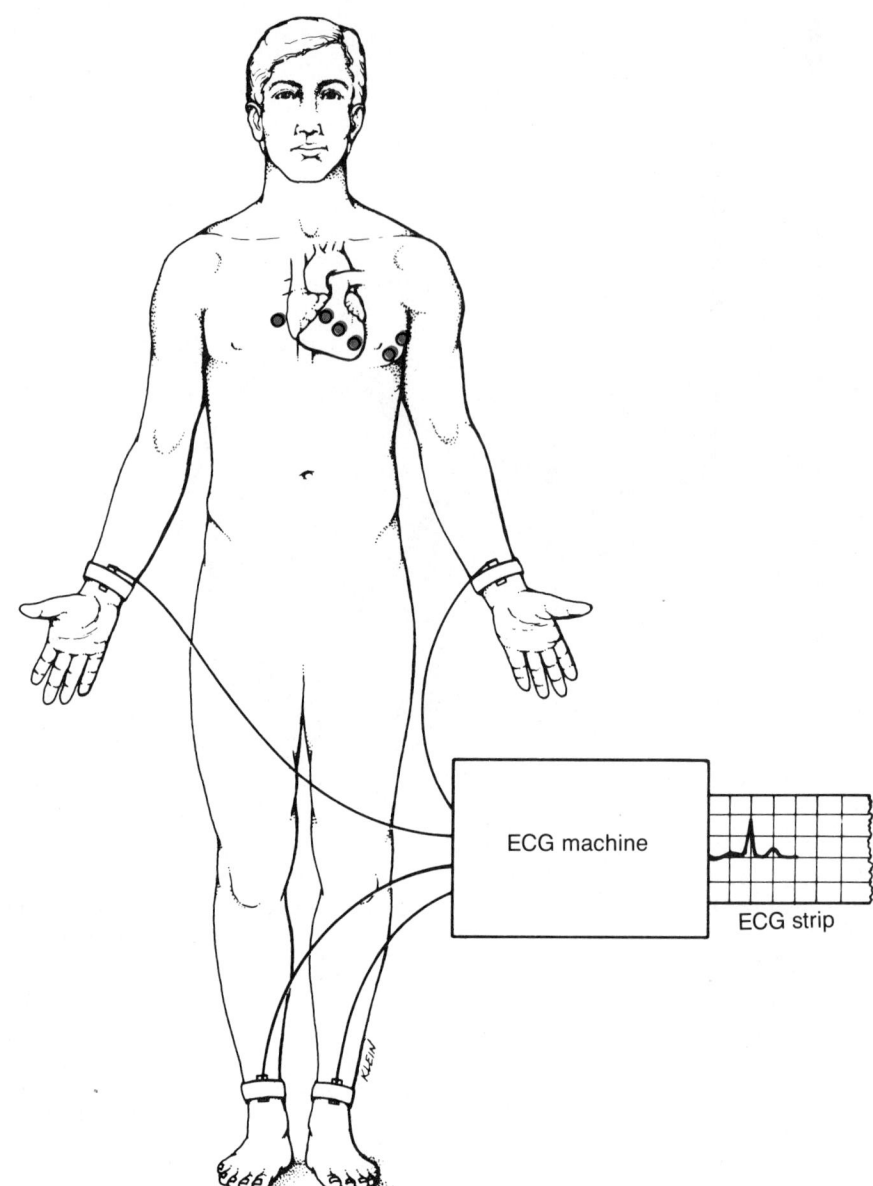

Figure 9-12. Transmission of heart's impulse to a graphic display by ECG machine. The electrodes that are capable of conducting electrical activity from the heart to the ECG machine are placed at strategic positions on the extremities and chest precordium.

accurate only for rhythms that are occurring at normal intervals and should not be used for determining rates in irregular rhythms.

    b. Irregular rhythms *are always* counted for 1 full minute for accuracy.

7. Another means of obtaining rate is to divide the number of large 5-square blocks between each two complexes into 300. Three hundred large blocks represent 1 minute on the ECG paper.
   Example: In Figure 9-13 the number of large square blocks between complexes #3 and #4 equals 5, or a rate of 60.

ECG Leads

1. The standard ECG consists of 12 leads (I, II, IH, AVR, AVL, AVF, V_1, V_2, V_3, V_4, V_5, V_6).

2. Each lead records the heart's electrical activity from a different anatomical position.

3. Experience has rendered data that confirm that certain leads give information about specific surfaces of the heart.

4. Identification of specific myocardial changes on certain leads assists in defining pathologic conditions.

Wave Form Analysis (Fig. 9-15)

A. P Wave

1. The P wave represents atrial depolarization.

2. The normal amplitude of the P wave is 3 mm. or less; the normal duration of the P wave is 0.04 to 0.11 seconds. P waves that exceed these measurements are considered to be a deviation from normal.

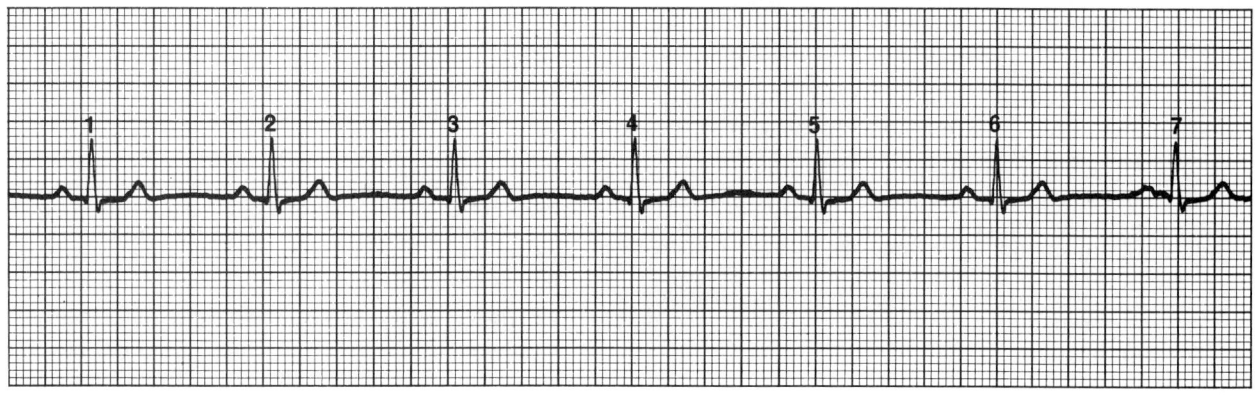

Figure 9-13. Lead II normal sinus rhythm.

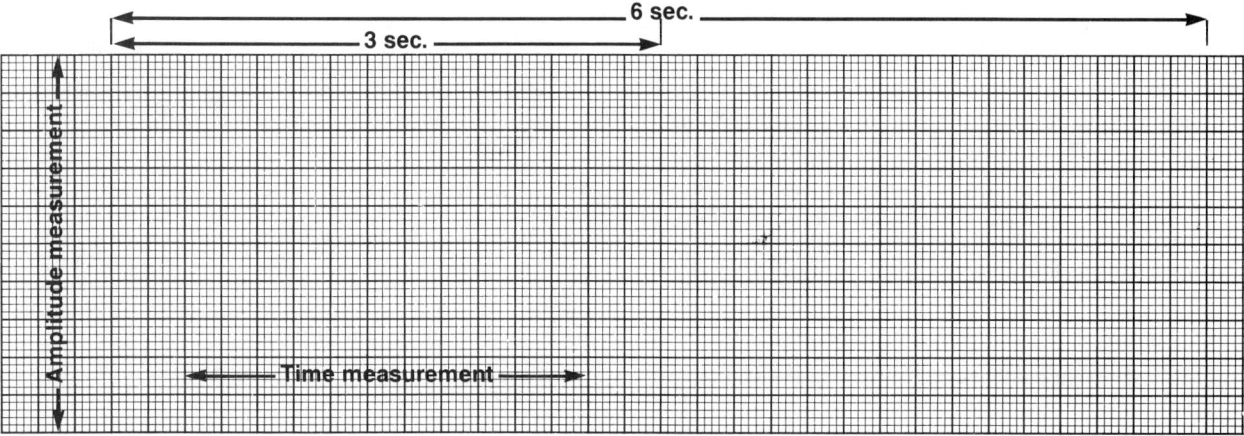

Figure 9-14. Plain ECG paper.

3. Since the P wave represents atrial depolarization, enlargement of the atria may be inferred from ECG findings that exceed the normal limits. For example, atrioventricular valvular stenosis may cause atrial enlargement. The increase in workload imposed on the atria when mitral or tricuspid stenosis is present may cause the atria to enlarge. Pulmonary diseases may also cause P wave abnormality.

B. P–R Interval

1. Is measured from the upstroke of the P wave to the QR junction.
2. The P–R interval is widely accepted to be between 0.12 and 0.20 seconds.
   a. The P–R interval represents the time of impulse transmission from the SA node to the AV node.
   b. There is a built-in delay in time at the AV node to allow for adequate ventricular filling to maintain normal stroke volume (the amount of blood ejected with each contraction).

C. Prolongation of the P–R Interval—may be a precursor to a variety of heart blocks; the causes

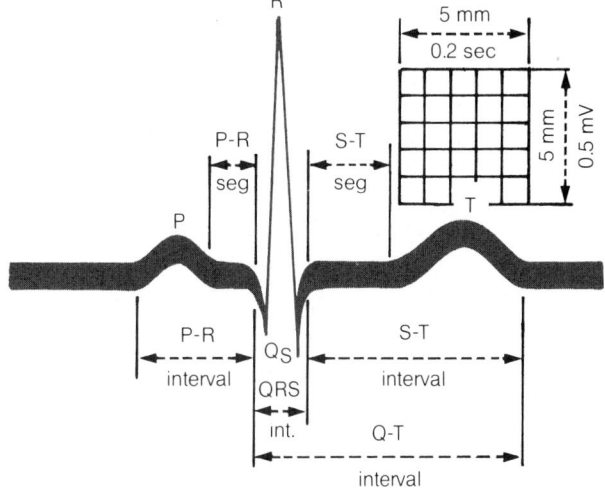

Figure 9-15. Wave form analysis.

may be drug therapy and myocardial disease or ischemia.

D. The QRS Complex

1. First downward stroke after the P wave. A Q wave of significant deflection is not normally present in the healthy heart. A pathologic Q wave usually indicates an old myocardial infarction.
2. The R wave is the first positive deflection after the Q wave, normally 5 to 10 mm. in height. Increases and decreases in amplitude become significant in certain disease states. Ventricular hypertrophy produces very high R waves because the hypertrophied muscle requires a longer time to depolarize.

E. The S–T Segment

1. Begins at the end of the S wave, the first negative deflection after the R wave, and terminates at the upstroke of the T wave.
2. The S–T segment is elevated in states of acute injury; the S–T segment is depressed in ischemic states. Hypocalcemia will lengthen the S–T segment, whereas hypercalcemia will shorten the S–T segment. The S–T segment is also influenced by changes in potassium level.

F. The T Wave

1. Represents the repolarization of myocardial fibers or provides the resting state of myocardial work; the T wave should always be present.
2. Normally, the T wave should not exceed a 5-mm. amplitude in all leads except the precordial (V_1–V_6) leads, where it may be as high as 10 mm.
3. May invert during the evolution of myocardial infarction but will usually return to normal after the MI is resolved.
4. Is sensitive to potassium level changes.

ECG Interpretation of Myocardial Infarction
(Fig. 9-16)

Note: The ECG is but one tool in diagnosing heart disease. The patient's history and serum enzymes are important for diagnosis of acute myocardial infarction. The newer noninvasive radionuclide studies are making it unnecessary to use the ECG beyond the initial onset of illness.

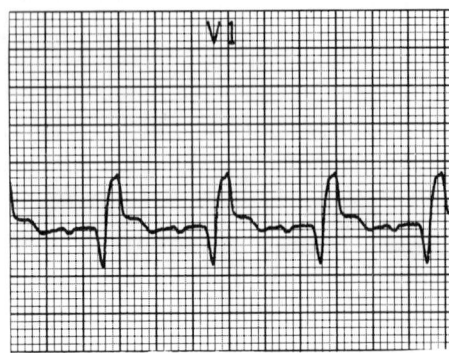

Figure 9-16. Abnormal Q wave.

1. Elevation of the S–T segment heralds a pattern of injury and usually occurs as an initial change in acute MI.
2. T wave inversion may occur as the MI evolves. The T waves will return to the upright position after the MI resolves.
3. A pathologic Q wave will evolve as the patient's R waves diminish in amplitude or disappear. The evolution of Q waves is permanent. A pathologic Q wave is one that is greater than 0.04 seconds in time and greater than 3 mm. in depth or greater than ⅓ the height of the R wave.

ECG Interpretation of Cardiac Dysrhythmias

1. Dysrhythmias (irregular rhythms) are a symptom of an underlying process and should be regarded as a symptom, not a diagnosis.
   Note: All heart muscle tissue is capable of exciting impulses when the normal pacemaker is compromised. This fact serves as the basis for dysrhythmia formation.
2. Dysrhythmias are generally evaluated continuously by placing at-risk patients on a bedside monitor.
3. The rhythm strips obtained from the monitor should not be used for diagnostic purposes.
4. If a question should arise regarding a rhythm that requires diagnostic data, a standard 12-lead ECG is always done.

▶ **NURSING ALERT:** Cardiac output, which is defined as the volume of blood ejected from the ventricle with each heart beat, is a function of heart rate times the stroke volume. Dysrhythmias, which are alterations in rate or rhythm of heart contraction, can seriously alter cardiac output. This concept must be considered each time a patient experiences a dysrhythmia.

Format for Assessment and Interpretation of Dysrhythmias

When reviewing a dysrhythmia, one should develop a systematic approach to assist in accurate interpretation. There is a variety of approaches that may be taken. One format that is particularly helpful is as follows:

1. Determine the rate. Is it fast, slow, or normal?
2. Determine the rhythm. Is it regular, irregular, regularly irregular, or irregularly irregular?
3. Find the P waves. Is one present for each QRS complex? Are they absent? Are they replaced by other wave forms? What is the configuration like? Are they identical, well-formed, or do they change shape?
4. Measure the P–R interval. The normal interval should be between 0.12 and 0.20 seconds.
5. Measure the QRS complex. The normal QRS complex should be between 0.06 and 0.10 seconds. Are they identical in configuration? Do they fall early? Does the configuration vary?
6. Look at the T wave. Is it positively or negatively deflected? Is it peaked?
7. Measure the Q–T interval. The normal Q–T interval should be less than ½ the R to R interval.

By following a format, one can, through deductive reasoning, arrive at a correct interpretation by associating each part of the format with anatomical and physiologic function of the heart.

Commonly Encountered Dysrhythmias

Dysrhythmias may be classified as disturbances in impulse formation or disturbances in conduction (heart blocks). The following dysrhythmias are considered disturbances of impulse formation. Heart blocks are treated in a separate section (see p. 347).

Sinus Tachycardia

Sinus tachycardia is a dysrhythmia that is normal, except that the rate exceeds 100 beats per minute.

A. Etiology

The SA node is under the influence of the autonomic nervous system. The sympathetic fibers, which act to speed up excitation of the SA node, are stimulated by underlying causes.

B. Underlying Causes

1. Anxiety
2. Exercise
3. Fever
4. Shock
5. Drugs
6. Altered metabolic states, such as hyperthyroidism
7. Electrolyte disturbances

C. Mechanism of Sinus Tachycardia

The wave of impulse is transmitted through the normal conduction pathways; the rate of sinus stimulation is simply greater than normal.

D. Analysis of Rhythm Strip Depicting Sinus Tachycardia (Fig. 9-17)

Rate—130
Rhythm—R–R intervals are regular
P wave—present for each QRS complex, normal configuration, and each P wave is identical
P–R interval—falls between 0.12 and 0.20, or 0.16 seconds

QRS complex—normal in appearance, one follows each P wave
QRS interval—0.06 seconds
T wave follows each QRS complex and is positively conducted

E. Treatment

1. The urgency of treatment of sinus tachycardia is dependent on the effect of the rapid rate on the maintenance of adequate cardiac output. For example, sinus tachycardia is much more life-threatening to the individual with a new acute MI than it is to the person who experiences the dysrhythmia secondary to a fever.
2. Digitalis preparations may be required if the effect on cardiac output is negative; otherwise, treatment is directed to the cause of the tachycardia.

Sinus Bradycardia (Fig. 9-18)

Sinus bradycardia is a dysrhythmia that is normal, except that the rate falls below 60 beats per minute.

A. Etiology

The parasympathetic fibers (vagal tone) are stimulated and cause the sinus node to slow.

B. Underlying Causes

1. Can be expected in the well-trained athlete
2. Drugs
3. Altered metabolic states, such as hypothyroidism
4. The process of aging, which causes increasing fibrotic tissue and scarring of the SA node
5. Certain cardiac diseases, such as acute MI

C. Mechanism of Sinus Bradycardia

The wave of impulse is transmitted through the normal conduction pathways; the rate of sinus stimulation is simply less than normal.

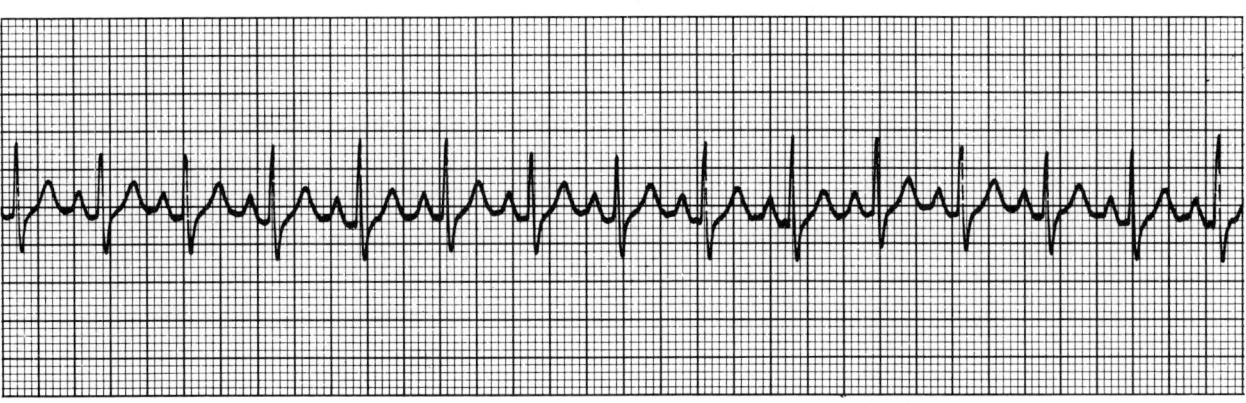

Figure 9-17. Sinus tachycardia.

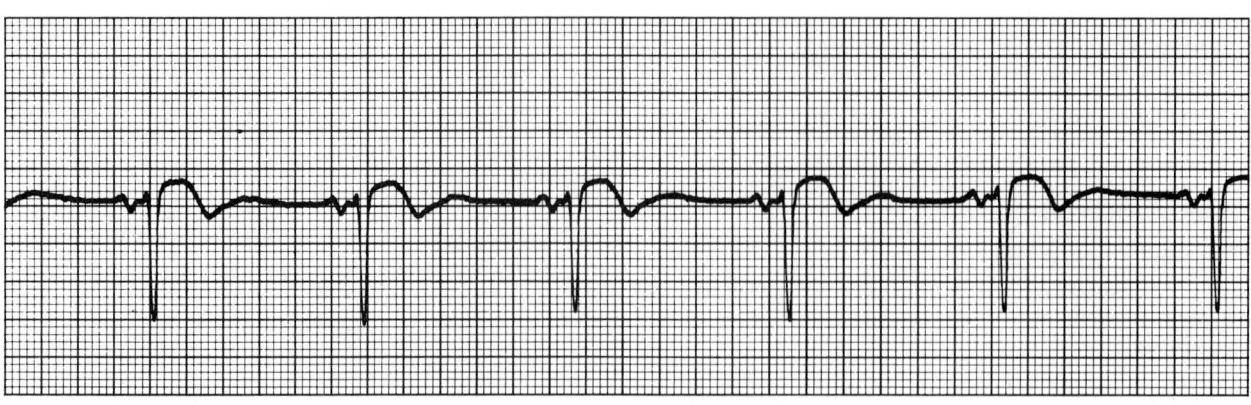

Figure 9-18. Sinus bradycardia.

D. Analysis of Sinus Bradycardia

Rate—55
Rhythm—R–R interval is regular
P wave—present for each QRS complex, normal configuration, and each P wave is identical
P–R interval—falls between 0.12 and 0.20, or 0.18
QRS—normal in appearance, one follows each P wave
QRS interval—0.06
T wave follows each QRS and is positively conducted

E. Treatment

1. The urgency of treatment of sinus bradycardia is dependent on the effect of the slow rate on maintenance of cardiac output.
2. Atropine 0.5–1.0 mg. IV push blocks vagal stimulation to the SA node and therefore accelerates heart rate.
3. Isoproterenol hydrochloride may be used as a sympathetic stimulator if atropine is ineffective or contraindicated. (The accepted dilution is isoproterenol 1 mg./500 ml. D₅W.) The solution may be titrated to control the rate within parameters prescribed by the physician. Isoproterenol has a propensity for causing ventricular dysrhythmias and should be discontinued if this occurs.

4. If the bradycardia persists, a pacemaker may be required.

Sinus Arrhythmia

Sinus arrhythmia is a dysrhythmia that is conducted normally but presents a regular irregularity in rhythm that is related to respiratory exchange. During inspiration the rate increases, and during expiration the rate decreases; therefore, it is not considered pathologic.

A. Etiology

1. Generally found in children and young adults.
2. There is a varying effect on the vagus nerve, believed to be related to respiratory exchange. This causes the vagus nerve to alternate its stimulation to the sinus node, causing the variance in rate between fast and slow.

B. Mechanism of Sinus Arrhythmia

The wave of impulse is transmitted through the normal conduction pathways; the rate of sinus stimulation varies, causing the R–R intervals to vary in a pattern that is described as a regular irregularity.

C. Analysis of Sinus Arrhythmia (Fig. 9-19)

Rate—varies between a fast rate and a slow rate
Rhythm—is irregular in a regular pattern; for example,

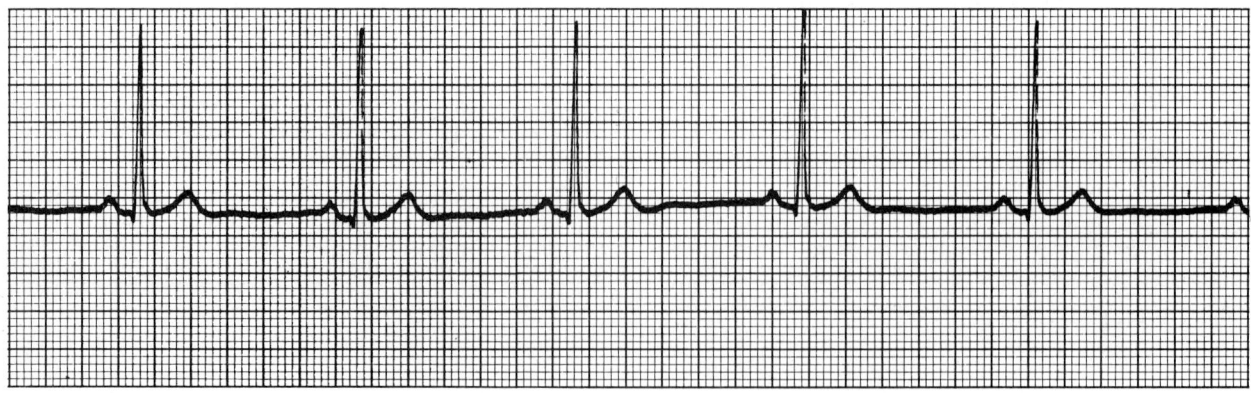

Figure 9-19. Sinus arrhythmia.

4 beats may occur at a rate of 80, then 4 beats may occur at a rate of 72. During observation of the patient's chest movements, a relationship between the fast rate and inspiration and between the slow rate and expiration may be obvious.

P wave—present for each QRS complex, normal configuration, and each P wave is identical

P–R interval—falls between 0.12 and 0.20 seconds

QRS complex—normal in appearance, one follows each P wave

QRS interval—T wave follows each QRS complex and is positively conducted

E. Treatment

None

Sick Sinus Syndrome (Fig. 9-20)

Sick sinus syndrome is a dysrhythmia that is caused by a diseased sinus node. The sinus node conducts at a slow rate or may fail to conduct at all, producing sinus block or pauses. Sometimes there is a related tachycardia, thus causing some to refer to this syndrome as "brady-tachy-cardia syndrome." If the related tachycardia should stop abruptly, and the sinus node does not fire, all heart activity will cease (asystole).

A. Etiology

1. Arteriosclerotic heart disease
2. Acute MI

B. Mechanism of Sick Sinus Syndrome

1. When the sinus node fails to fire for whatever reason, the end result is a lack of impulse conducted to the atria or ventricles. Thus, there is a long pause before another impulse is discharged.
2. Whether or not the patient is affected depends on the length of the pause.
3. Ischemia is a common cause of sick sinus syndrome.

C. Analysis of Sick Sinus Syndrome

Rate—may be slow or within normal limits. Rhythm will be regular except when a pause occurs; when the rhythm resumes, it will be regular.

P wave—present before each QRS complex; normal configuration and identical, the P wave will suddenly not appear when expected. No QRS complex will follow.

P–R interval—within normal limits

QRS complex—follow each QRS except where there is no P wave. The QRS will also be absent.

T wave—normally conducted in the normal complexes

D. Treatment

A pacemaker will be required if the sick sinus syndrome does not abate with the treatment of ischemia.

Premature Atrial Contraction (PAC)

A *premature atrial contraction (PAC)* is an ectopic beat that originates in the atria and is discharged at a rate faster than that of the sinus node. The atrial beat occurs sooner than the next normal beat and is said to be early or premature.

A. Etiology

1. May occur in the healthy or diseased heart. It is of no particular significance in the healthy heart. In the diseased heart, it may represent ischemia and a resultant irritability.
2. The PAC may increase in frequency and be the precursor of more serious arrhythmias in the diseased heart.

B. Mechanism of Premature Atrial Contraction

1. The wave of impulse of the PAC originates within the atria and outside the sinus node, hence the name ectopic beat.
2. Because the impulse originates within the atria, the P wave will be present, but it will be different in appearance as compared with those beats originating within the sinus node.
3. The impulse traverses the remainder of the conduction system in a normal pattern; thus the QRS complex is identical in configuration to the normal sinus beats.

C. Analysis of a PAC (Fig. 9-21)

Rate—may be slow or fast

Rhythm—will be irregular; this is caused by the early occurrence of the PAC.

P wave—will be present for each normal QRS complex; the P wave of the premature contraction will be distorted in shape.

P–R interval—may be normal but can also be shortened, depending on where in the atria the impulse originated. The closer the site of atrial

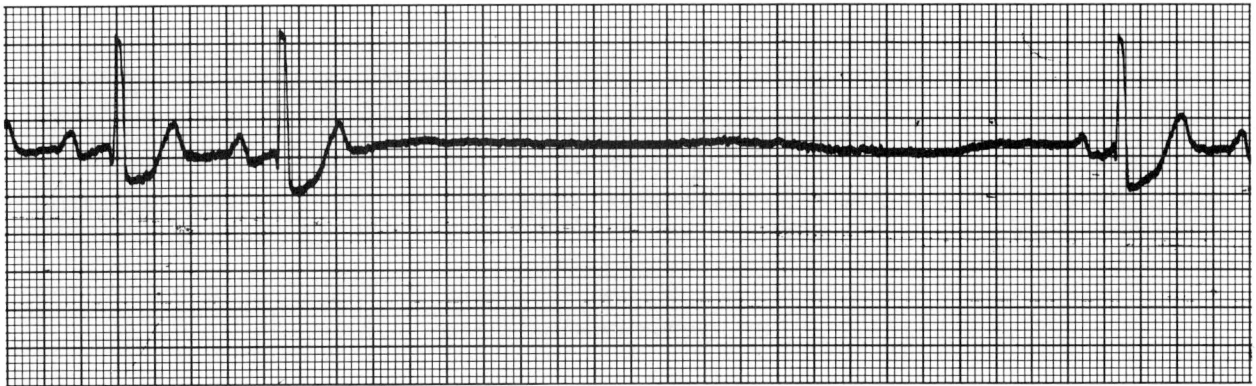

Figure 9-20. Block or pause seen in sick sinus syndrome.

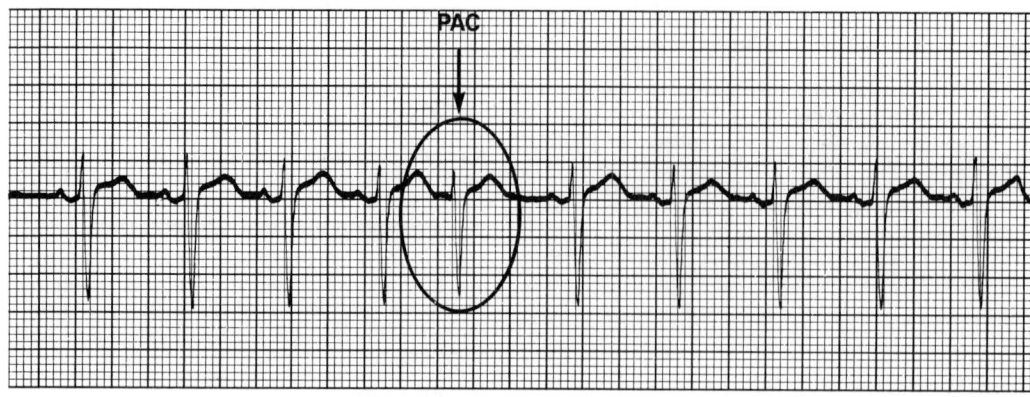

Figure 9-21. Normal sinus rhythm with premature atrial contraction.

impuse formation to the AV node, the shorter the P–R interval will be.

QRS complex—within normal limits because all conduction below the atria is normal.

T wave—normally conducted

D. Treatment

1. Generally requires no treatment.
2. PACs should be monitored for increasing frequency.
3. If treatment is required, quinidine or a calcium-channel blocker may be used.

Paroxysmal Atrial Tachycardia (PAT)

Paroxysmal atrial tachycardia (PAT) is a sudden onset of an atrial tachycardia with rates that vary between 140 and 250 beats per minute.

A. Etiology

1. Syndromes of accelerated pathways (e.g., Wolff–Parkinson–White syndrome
2. Syndrome of mitral valve prolapse
3. Ischemic coronary artery diseases
4. Excessive use of alcohol, cigarettes, caffeine
5. Drugs

B. Mechanism of PAT

An ectopic atrial focus captures the rhythm of the heart and is stimulated at a very rapid rate; the impulse is conducted normally through the conduction system so that the QRS complex usually appears within normal limits. The rate is often so rapid that P waves are not obvious but may be "buried" in the preceding T wave.

C. Analysis of PAT (Fig. 9-22)

Rate—between 140 and 250 beats per minute

Rhythm—regular

P waves—are present before each QRS complex; however, the faster the rate, the more difficult it becomes to visualize P waves. The P waves can frequently be measured with calipers by observing the varying configuration of the preceding T wave.

P–R interval—usually not measurable

QRS complexes—will appear normal in configuration and within 0.06–0.10 seconds

T wave—will be distorted in appearance as a result of P waves being buried in them

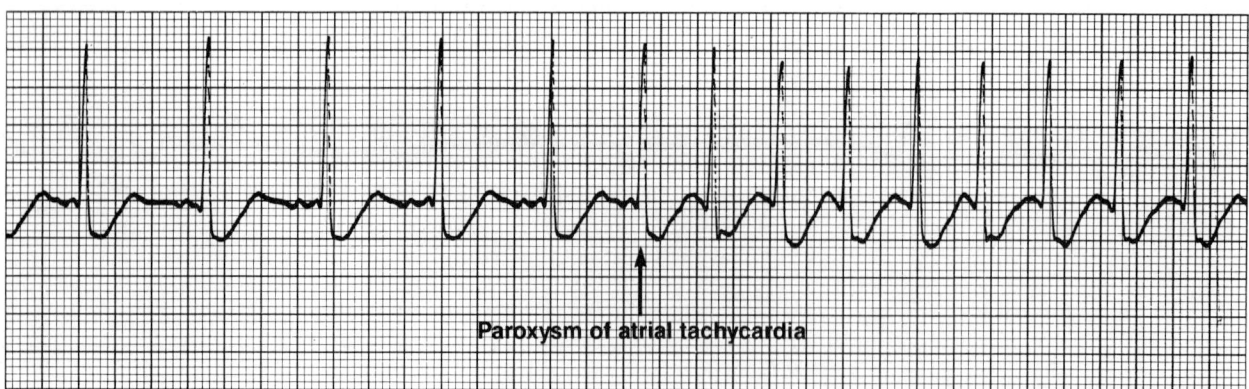

Figure 9-22. Paroxysmal atrial tachycardia.

D. Treatment

1. Treatment is directed to first slowing the rate and second, reverting the dysrhythmia to a normal sinus rhythm.
2. Reducing the rate may be accomplished by having the patient perform a Valsalva maneuver. This stimulates the vagus nerve to slow the heart. A Valsalva maneuver may be done by having the patient gag himself or "bear down," as though attempting to have a bowel movement. The physician may choose to perform carotid massage. This should be performed by a *physician,* and only one side of the neck should be massaged at a time.
3. Digitalis preparations may also be used in varying doses as prescribed.
4. A family of drugs referred to as beta-adrenergic blockers may also be used. Propranolol (by IV push) is an example of a commonly used beta-adrenergic blocker.
5. The calcium ion antagonists (e.g., verapamil) are effective in reverting this dysrhythmia.
6. If drug therapy is ineffective, electrical cardioversion can be used.
7. Other, less common, drugs that may be used include morphine sulfate and diazepam.

Atrial Flutter

Atrial flutter is a dysrhythmia in which an ectopic atrial focus captures the heart rhythm and discharges impulses at a rate of between 200 and 400 times per minute.

A. Etiology

1. Atrial stretching or enlargement, as occurs in diseases of the atrioventricular valves
2. Myocardial infarction
3. Congestive heart failure

B. Mechanism of Atrial Flutter

1. An ectopic atrial focus captures the rhythm in atrial flutter and fires at an extremely rapid rate, with regularity.
2. Conduction of the impulse through the conduction system is normal; thus, the QRS complex is unaffected.
3. An important feature of this dysrhythmia is that the AV node for some reason sets up a therapeutic block, which disallows some impulse transmission.

a. This can produce a varying block or a fixed block; that is to say, sometimes the AV node will transmit every second flutter wave, producing a 2:1 block, or the rhythm can be 3:1 or 4:1.
b. This is an important feature of this rhythm; if the AV node conducted 1:1, then the outcome would be ventricular flutter, a life-threatening dysrhythmia.

C. Analysis of Atrial Flutter (Fig. 9-23)

Rate—atrial rate between 200 and 400 beats per minute; ventricular rate will depend on degree of block
Rhythm—regular or irregular, depending on kind of block (e.g., 2:1, 3:1, or a combination)
P wave—not present; instead, it is replaced by a saw-toothed pattern that is produced by the rapid firing of the atrial focus. These waves are also referred to as "F" waves.
P–R interval—not measurable
QRS complex—normal configuration and normal conduction time
T wave—present but may be obscured by flutter waves

D. Treatment

1. The standard treatment for atrial flutter is a digitalis preparation. This enhances the block at the AV node, thus slowing the rate.
2. Quinidine may also be given to control the ectopic focus. The concomitant use of digitalis and quinidine usually reverts the rhythm to sinus rhythm.
3. The calcium-channel blockers are being used for this dysrhythmia.
4. A beta-adrenergic blocking drug such as propranolol (Inderal) may also be used.
5. If drug therapy is unsuccessful, atrial flutter will often respond to electrical cardioversion. Small doses of electrical current are often successful.

Atrial Fibrillation

Atrial fibrillation is a dysrhythmia that is caused by the rapid and chaotic firing of atrial impulses by a multitude of foci. The AV node establishes a physiologic block so that only random foci are conducted to the ventricles. The rhythm of atrial fibrillation is a classic irregular irregularity.

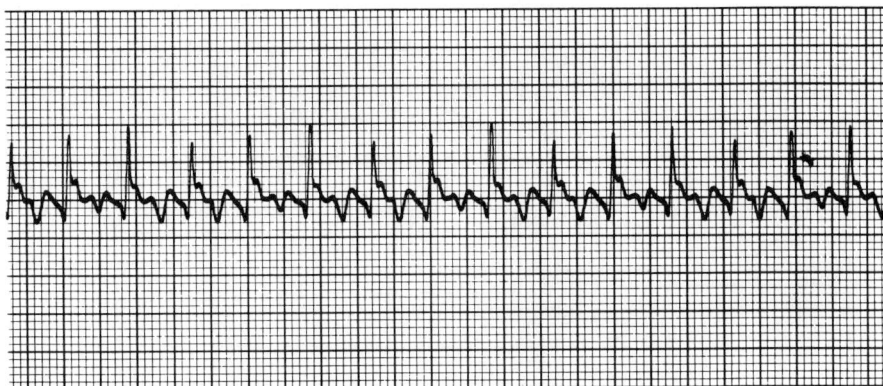

Figure 9-23. Atrial flutter.

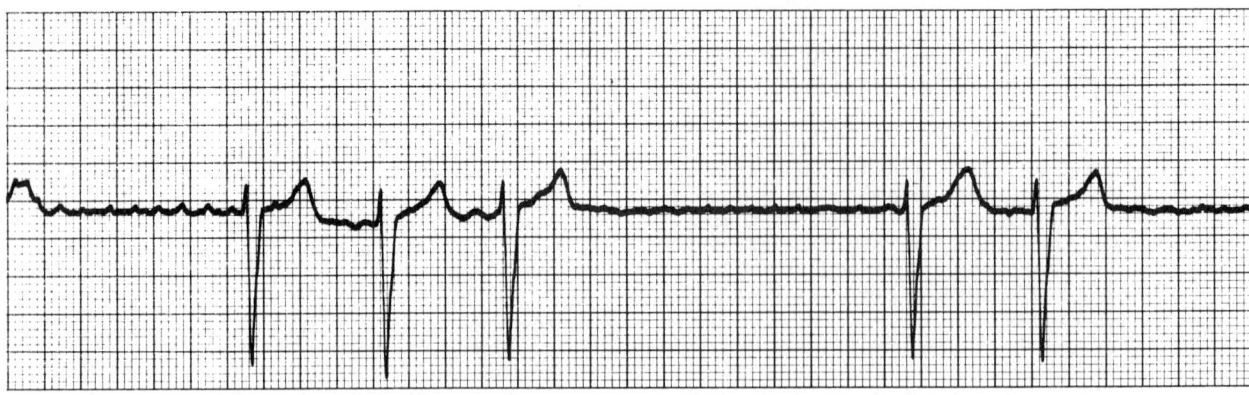

Figure 9-24. Atrial fibrillation with slow ventricular response (controlled).

A. Etiology

1. Fibrotic changes associated with the aging process
2. Acute MI
3. Valvular diseases
4. Digitalis preparations

B. Mechanism of Atrial Fibrillation

1. The atria fire impulses at rapid and disorganized rates.
2. The atria are not depolarized effectively; hence there are no well-formed P waves.
3. Instead, the baseline between QRS complexes is filled with a "wiggly" line that is described as fine or coarse.
4. If the atrial rate is rapid enough, the line will appear almost flat. The atria are said to be firing at rates of between 300 and 500 times per minute.
5. The conduction of a QRS complex is so random that the rhythm is extremely irregular.
6. Atrial fibrillation may be described as *controlled* if the ventricular response is 100 beats per minute or less; the dysrhythmia is *uncontrolled* if the rate is above 100 beats per minute.

C. Analysis of Atrial Fibrillation (Fig. 9-24 and Fig. 9-25)

Rate—atrial fibrillation is usually immeasurable because fibrillatory waves replace P waves; ventricular rate may vary from bradycardia to tachycardia.

Rhythm—classically described as an "irregular irregularity"

P wave—replaced by fibrillatory waves, sometimes called "little F" waves

P–R interval—immeasurable

QRS complex—a normally conducted complex

T wave—normally conducted

D. Treatment

1. Controlled atrial fibrillation of long-standing duration requires no treatment as long as the patient is experiencing no untoward effects. Most cardiologists agree that reversion of long-standing atrial fibrillation is hazardous because of the potential for a thrombus to be dislodged from the atria at the time of reversion.
2. Uncontrolled atrial fibrillation (ventricular responses of 100 beats per minute or greater) is treated with digitalis preparations. If the atrial fibrillation is of

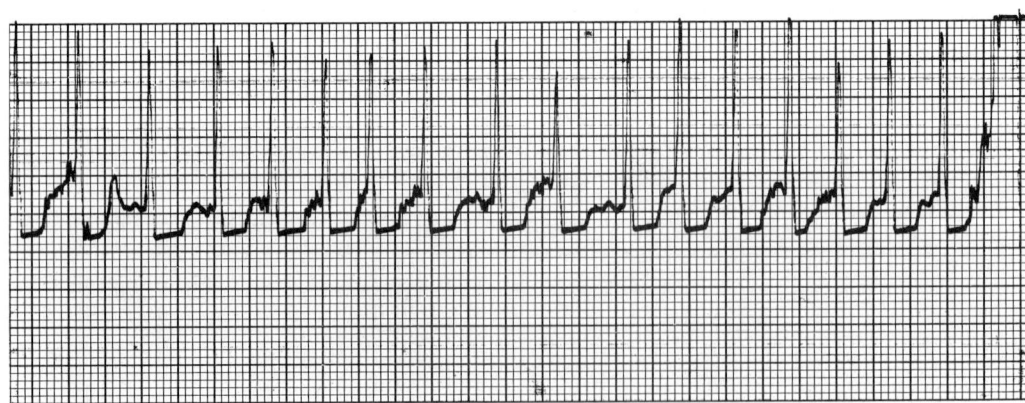

Figure 9-25. Atrial fibrillation with a rapid ventricular response (uncontrolled).

recent onset, the cardiologist may choose to revert the rhythm to a sinus rhythm.

3. Quinidine may be used in conjunction with digitalis if the rhythm is reverted to sinus. Quinidine is used to suppress ectopic foci.
4. Atrial fibrillation is treated less frequently with electrical cardioversion.
5. The beta-adrenergic blocking drugs may also be used if digitalis and quinidine prove ineffective.

Digitalis Toxicity

Digitalis toxicity is a dysrhythmia that results from excessive levels of serum digitalis. The two dysrhythmias that are most frequently associated with digitalis toxicity are ventricular bigeminy (every other beat is a ventricular complex) and PAT with block although any dysrhythmia may occur.

Note: Digitalis effect, in contrast to toxicity, is a characteristic pattern of S–T depression. Digitalis toxicity and digitalis effect are not synonymous.

A. Analysis of Digitalis Effect

1. Therapeutic levels of digitalis will frequently be manifested by ECG.
2. A "drooping" of the S–T segment is apparent. The S–T segment depression that is manifest in myocardial ischemia is flatter in appearance. These wave form features are sometimes not distinguishing.
3. Measurement of the Q–T interval may be helpful.
   a. The Q–T interval in digitalis effect will be shortened.
   b. The Q–T interval in digitalis toxicity will be lengthened.

B. Analysis of Digitalis Toxicity

1. Digitalis toxicity should always be considered when the patient who has been taking the drug has a new onset of dysrhythmia, has excessive slowing of the heart rate, and complains of malaise, anorexia, and nausea and vomiting. This syndrome is frequently found in the poorly nourished population. Potassium level in the diet may be low, and hypokalemia tends to exaggerate the effect of digitalis.
2. Digitalis may be administered concomitantly with diuretics, which may contribute to potassium loss.
3. The dysrhythmias most commonly associated with digitalis are the ventricular ectopic beats; these usu-

ally, but not always, appear as bigeminy. Multifocal ventricular premature beats may also occur.
4. The next most common dysrhythmia is PAT with block.

C. Treatment

1. Obtain serum levels of digitalis and potassium.
2. Discontinue digitalis until excretion can take place and administer potassium if indicated by hypokalemia. This treatment usually resolves the problem.
3. Administer phenytoin (Dilantin) in a single dose as prescribed; this may be done as prophylaxis for ventricular dysrhythmia.
4. In more serious situations, when the patient may be hemodynamically threatened (cardiac output is severely compromised), a pacemaker may be required until the crisis is passed.
5. Cardioversion is extremely risky because of the potential for converting this dysrhythmia to a more lethal one; it is seldom done and only because no other therapies have been of benefit.

Premature Ventricular Contraction (PVC)

A *premature ventricular contraction (PVC)* is a dysrhythmia that is produced by an ectopic beat originating in the ventricle and being discharged at a rate faster than that of the next normally occurring beat. The PVC is, by far, the most common dysrhythmia seen in the acute hospital setting.

A. Etiology

1. Acute MI
2. All other forms of heart disease
3. Pulmonary diseases
4. Electrolyte disturbances
5. Metabolic instability

B. Mechanism of PVC

1. The wave of impulse originates within the ventricles.
2. Because the normal conduction pathway is bypassed, the configuration of the PVC is wider than normal and is distorted in appearance.
3. The PVC occurs early, and the P wave is absent.

C. Analysis of PVC (Fig. 9-26)

Rate—may be slow or fast
Rhythm—will be irregular because of the premature firing of the ventricular ectopic focus

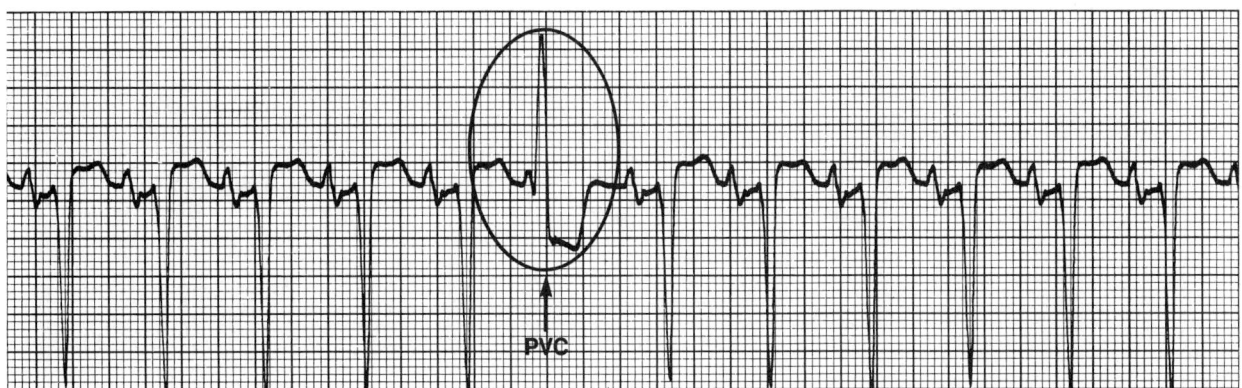

Figure 9-26. Normal sinus rhythm with premature ventricular contraction.

P wave—will be absent, since the impulse originates in the ventricle, bypassing the atria and AV node.

P–R interval—immeasurable

QRS complex—the QRS of the PVC will be widened greater than 0.12 seconds, bizarre in appearance when compared to the normal QRS complex. The QRS of a PVC is often referred to as having a "sore thumb" appearance.

T wave—the T wave of the PVC is usually deflected opposite to the QRS.

D. Treatment

1. PVCs are usually the precursors of more serious ventricular dysrhythmias. The following conditions involving PVCs require prompt and vigorous treatment:
    a. PVCs occurring at a rate exceeding 6 per minute.
    b. Occur 2 together (couplet).
    c. Occur 3 together (a salvo or ventricular tachycardia).
    d. Occur in a patterned sequence with the normal rhythm (e.g., every other beat is a PVC [bigeminy]). (Fig. 9-27)
    e. PVCs fall on the peak or down slope of the T wave.
    f. Are of varying configurations, indicating a multiplicity of foci.
2. The standard treatment of PVCs is with lidocaine hydrochloride by IV push.
    a. For effective treatment of PVCs, it is important to raise the serum level of lidocaine as rapidly as possible without causing toxic effects.
    b. An initial bolus of 75–100 mg. may be administered, followed by continuous drip of lidocaine in D_5W in a 4:1 concentration.
    c. The dosage may vary between 1 and 4 mg. per minute.
    d. If the dysrhythmia continues to "break through," another 50–100 mg. bolus of lidocaine may be given within 10–15 minutes.
3. Be alert to the development of confusion, slurring of speech, and diminished mentation, since lidocaine toxicity affects the central nervous system. Should these symptoms appear, slowing the lidocaine may cause them to abate.
4. If ventricular ectopy occurs concomitantly with a bradycardia, use lidocaine with caution, if at all. The ectopy may be compensation for the bradycardia. If lidocaine abolishes compensatory beats, the cardiac output may be seriously compromised, to the patient's detriment.
5. If ventricular premature beats occur in conjunction with a bradydysrhythmia, the physician may choose to use atropine to accelerate the heart rate and eliminate the need for ectopic beats.
6. Atropine should be used with caution in the acute MI. The injured myocardium may not be able to tolerate the accelerated rate.
7. If lidocaine proves to be ineffective in controlling PVCs, procainamide may be given (IV push), followed by a continuous drip. The average bolus dose is 300 mg. Procainamide may cause hypotension.
8. If lidocaine and procainamide prove ineffective, either alone or in combination therapy, bretylium tosylate may be used. Bretylium is administered in a continuous infusion.

Ventricular Tachycardia

Ventricular tachycardia is a life-threatening dysrhythmia that originates from an irritable focus within the ventricle. It is an ineffective rhythm for maintaining cardiac output.

A. Etiology

1. Acute MI
2. Syndromes of accelerated rhythm that deteriorate (e.g., Wolff–Parkinson–White syndrome)
3. Metabolic acidosis, especially lactic acidosis
4. Electrolyte disturbances
5. Toxicity to certain drugs, such as digitalis or Isuprel

B. Mechanism of Ventricular Tachycardia

The wave of impulse originates within the ventricles, firing at a very rapid rate. Because the ventricles are capable of an inherent rate of 40 beats per minute or less, a ventricular rhythm at a rate of 100 beats per minute may be considered tachycardia.

C. Analysis of Ventricular Tachycardia (Fig. 9-28)

Rate—usually between 140 and 220 beats per minute

Rhythm—usually regular but may be irregular

P wave—not present

P–R interval—immeasurable

QRS complex—broad, bizarre in configuration, widened greater than 0.12 seconds

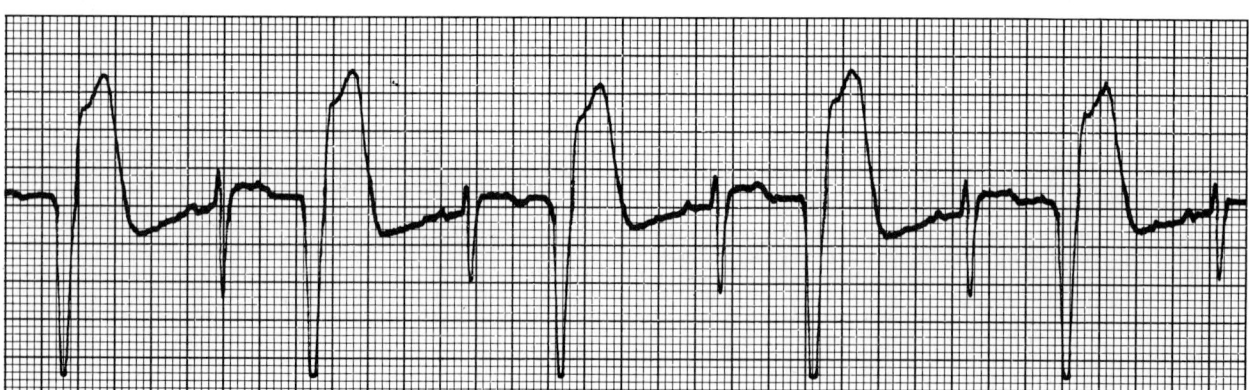

Figure 9-27. Ventricular bigeminy.

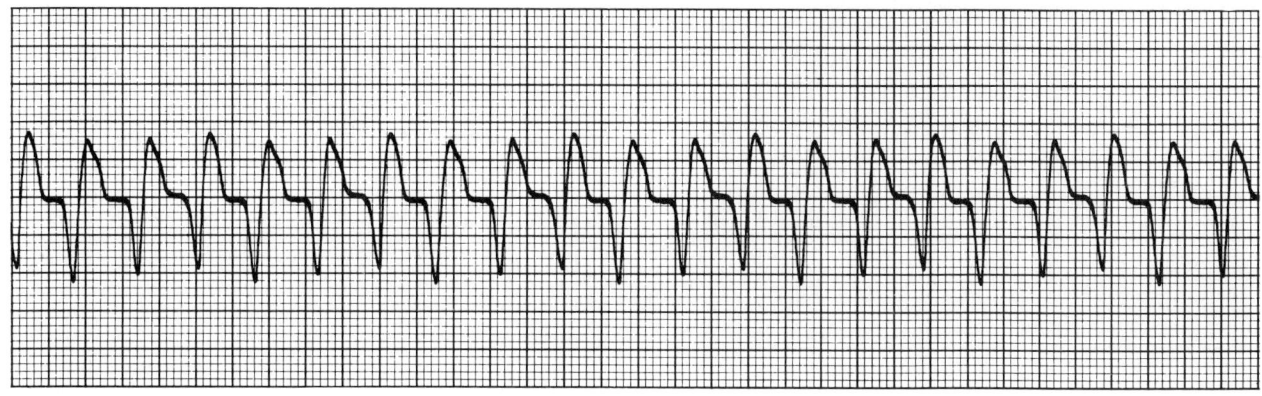

Figure 9-28. Ventricular tachycardia.

T wave—usually deflected opposite to the QRS complex.

D. Treatment

Ventricular tachycardia is life-threatening, and its presentation calls for immediate intervention by the nurse.

1. If the patient is alert and not hemodynamically decompensating, lidocaine hydrochloride is administered as a bolus. This is followed by continuous lidocaine infusion 4:1 drip from 1–4 mg./minute.
2. If the patient loses consciousness, immediate electrical defibrillation is indicated.
3. If the patient remains alert and drug therapy is not working, then synchronized defibrillation or cardioversion is applied. The purpose of electrical cardioversion is to abolish all cardiac rhythm and allow the normal pacemaker the opportunity to capture the rhythm.

▶ NURSING ALERT: An atypical form of ventricular tachycardia, referred to as polymorphous ventricular tachycardia or Torsades de Pointes, can result as a consequence of quinidine therapy. It is important to differentiate this atypical form because its therapy differs from that of the more typical ventricular tachycardia.

1. Torsades de Pointes is characterized by a Q–T interval prolonged to greater than 0.60 seconds, varying R–R intervals, and polymorphous QRS complexes.
2. The treatment of choice is administration of isoproterenol, which shortens the Q–T interval. Propranolol and phenytoin may also be used if isoproterenol is ineffective.
3. Ventricular pacing to override the ventricular rate and hence capture the rhythm is also an acceptable treatment.
4. Lidocaine and procainamide should be avoided, since their effect is to prolong the Q–T interval.

Ventricular Fibrillation

Ventricular fibrillation is a dysrhythmia that is characterized by the random and chaotic discharging of impulses within the ventricle at rates that exceed 300 beats per minute. Ventricular fibrillation produces clinical death and must be reversed immediately, or the patient will succumb.

A. Etiology

1. Deteriorating ventricular rhythms
2. Acute MI

3. Acidosis
4. Electrolyte disturbances

B. Mechanism of Ventricular Fibrillation

The ventricles are firing chaotically and so do not allow for effective impulse conduction. Cardiac output ceases, and the patient loses pulse, blood pressure, and consciousness.

C. Analysis of Ventricular Fibrillation (Fig. 9-29)

Rate—immeasurable because of absence of well-formed QRS complexes
Rhythm—chaotic
P wave—not present
P–R interval—not present
QRS complex—bizarre, chaotic, no definite contour
T wave—not apparent

D. Treatment

1. The only treatment for ventricular fibrillation is *immediate* electrical defibrillation. The current used may vary from 200–400 watt/second.
2. Successful defibrillation will stop the heart and allow the heart to restart, controlled by the normal sinus pacemaker.
3. Unsuccessful defibrillation may be a result of lactic acidosis; therefore, it is important to administer sodium bicarbonate.
4. Epinephrine hydrochloride may also make the fibrillation more vulnerable to defibrillation.

The Heart Blocks

AV block implies that the transmission of the wave of impulse from the sinus node through the normal conduction pathway is altered at the level of the AV node. The altered state does not allow the impulse to be conducted "on time" or at all.

A. Types of AV Block

1. First-degree
2. Second-degree
3. Third-degree

B. Mechanisms of AV Blocks

1. Impaired tissue at the level of the AV node prevents the timely passage of the wave of impulse through the conduction system.

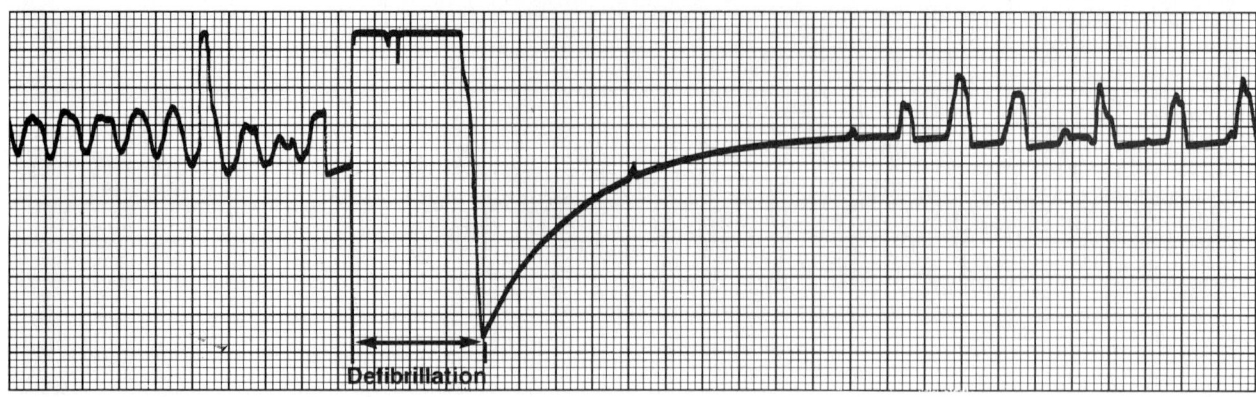

Figure 9-29. Ventricular fibrillation with defibrillation.

2. In first-degree AV block, the impulse is transmitted normally, but it is delayed longer at the level of the AV node. The P–R interval exceeds 0.20 seconds.
3. In second-degree AV block, the AV node becomes selective about which impulses are conducted to the ventricles.
4. In third-degree AV block, there is no relationship between the atrial activity recorded on the monitor and the ventricular activity. Both chambers are discharging impulses, but activity of the atria and activity of the ventricles bear no relationship to each other.

C. Analysis of First-Degree AV Block (Fig. 9-30)

Rate—usually normal but may be slow
Rhythm—regular
P wave—present for each QRS complex, identical in configuration
P–R interval—prolonged to greater than 0.20 seconds
QRS complex—normal in appearance and between 0.06 and 0.10 seconds
T wave—normally conducted

D. Analysis of Second-Degree AV Block (Fig. 9-31)

Rate—usually normal
Rhythm—may be regular or irregular
P wave—present but some may not be followed by a QRS complex. A ratio of 2, 3, or 4 P waves to one QRS complex may exist.
P–R interval—may be normal or prolonged
QRS complex—normally conducted
T wave—normally conducted

E. Analysis of Third-Degree AV Block (complete heart block) (Fig. 9-32)

Rate—atrial rate is measured independently of the ventricular rate. The ventricular rate is usually very slow.
Rhythm—each independent rhythm will be regular, but they will bear no relationship to each other
P wave—present before some QRS complexes; other P waves will fall at random
P–R interval—not really measurable
QRS complex—will be widened and distorted in appearance but are usually all identical
T wave—normally conducted.

F. Treatment of AV Blocks

Like that of other dysrhythmias, the treatment of heart blocks depends on the effect the rate is having on cardiac output.

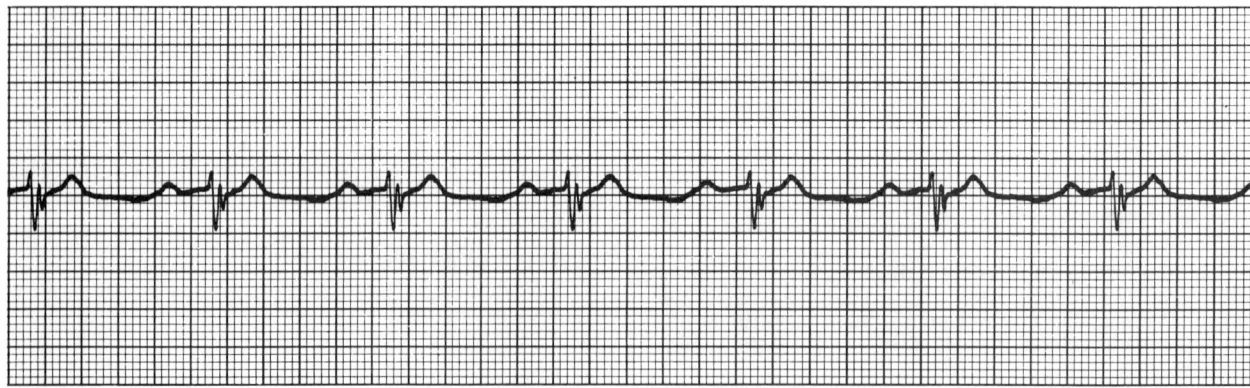

Figure 9-30. First-degree AV block.

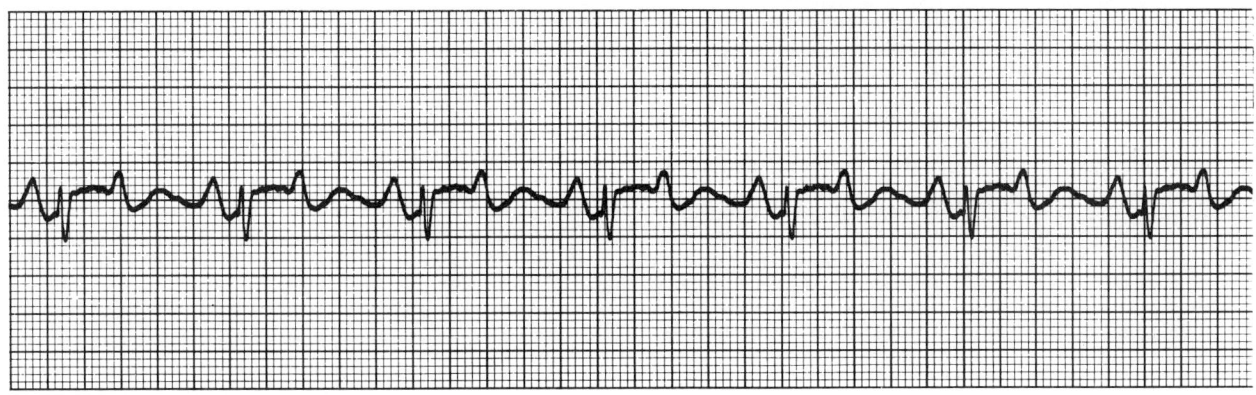

Figure 9-31. Second-degree AV block.

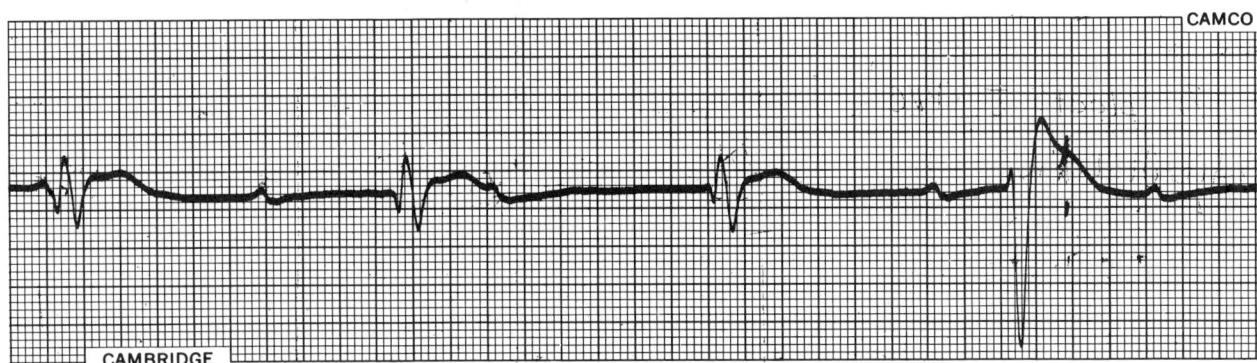

Figure 9-32. Third-degree AV block.

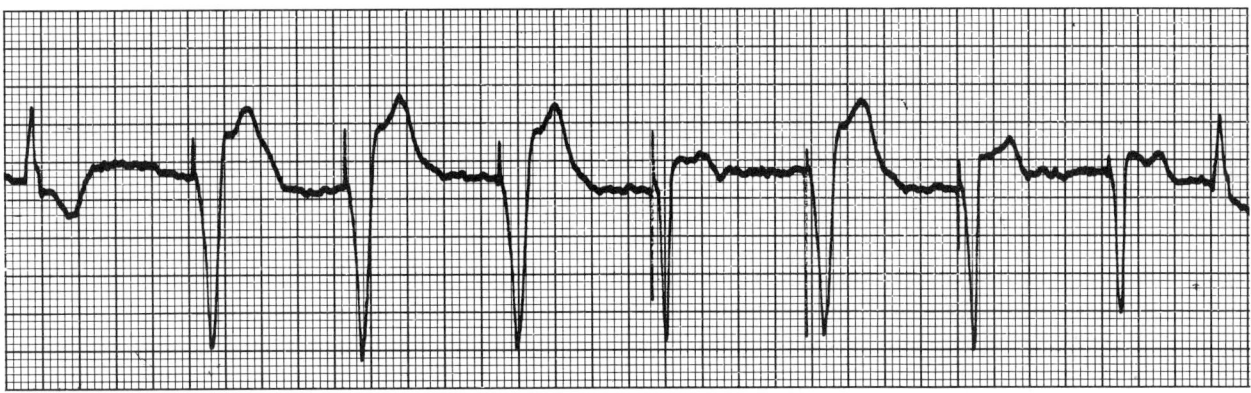

Figure 9-33. Ventricular pacemaker.

1. First-degree AV block requires no treatment.
2. Second-degree AV block may require treatment if the ventricular rate falls too low to maintain effective cardiac output.
3. Third-degree AV block may require treatment if cardiac output is compromised.
4. A ventricular pacemaker is the treatment of choice for an AV block requiring intervention.
5. Atropine may be given while awaiting the pacemaker, but it must be remembered that the effect of atropine is to block vagal tone, and the vagus acts on the sinus node. Since the AV node is the culprit in heart block, atropine may not be helpful.
6. A continuous infusion of isoproterenol 1 mg. in 500 ml. D₅W may also be attempted; however, the consequence of using isoproterenol may be ventricular tachycardia.

7. Persistent third-degree AV block will require a ventricular pacemaker. As in second-degree AV block, atropine and isoproterenol may be used, but their efficacy is questionable.

The Artificial Pacemaker

A. Ventricular Pacemaker (Fig. 9-33)

1. A *ventricular pacemaker* writes a pacing spike on the ECG paper just prior to the conduction of the QRS complex.
2. A QRS complex should follow each pacing spike.
3. On some occasions, a pacing catheter will fail to function normally.
4. The malfunctioning of a pacemaker can be caused by mechanical or electrical events.

Guidelines: Synchronized Cardioversion

Synchronized cardioversion is a *timed* electrical shock to the heart for the purpose of terminating certain arrhythmias. Asynchronized cardioversion is the same as defibrillation and is used principally for ventricular fibrillation.

Both types of cardioversion use the same type of electricity, but timed shock is not needed in ventricular fibrillation because there are no T waves. (Synchronized cardioversion is timed *not* to hit the T wave, since an electrical discharge during this phase of the cardiac cycle may cause ventricular fibrillation.)

Purpose   To stop the abnormal electrical activity of the heart and allow the SA node (heart's natural pacemaker) to resume normal sinus rhythm.

Contraindications

Synchronized cardioversion is relatively *contraindicated* when a patient has been taking a significant amount of *digitalis*, since more lethal arrhythmias may ensue after electrical discharge.

Equipment

Cardioverter and ECG machine
Conduction jelly and cardiac medications
Resuscitative equipment, including:
    Endotracheal tubes
    Laryngoscopes
    Suctioning equipment
    Manual breathing bag
    Pacing equipment

Procedure

Nursing Action	Rationale/Amplification

1. If the procedure is elective, it is advisable to have the patient "NPO" 12 hours before the cardioversion.
  a. Reassure the patient and see that informed consent has been obtained.
  b. Make sure the patient has not been taking digitalis and that the serum potassium is normal.
	1. During sedation or the procedure, the patient may vomit and aspirate if the stomach is full.
	  a. Do not use word "shock" since this will increase the patient's apprehension.
	  b. Low potassium may precipitate post-shock arrhythmias.

2. Make sure IV line is secure.	2. An IV line may be necessary for medications such as lidocaine and atropine.
3. Obtain a 12-lead ECG before and after cardioversion with the ECG machine. The ECG machine wires are best left on the patient, since the ECG printout is of much better quality than that of the monitor. This fact is especially important when one is trying to dissect complicated arrhythmias.	3. An ECG is taken to ensure that the patient has not had a recent myocardial infarction (either just before or after the cardioversion).

4. a. Allow the patient to receive oxygen before and after cardioversion.
  b. Do *not* give oxygen during the procedure.
	4. a. Oxygen will help prevent unwanted arrhythmias after cardioversion.
	  b. An explosion could occur if a spark from the paddles should ignite the oxygen during the procedure.

Procedure
(Cont.)

Nursing Action	Rationale/Amplification

5. Place the paddles in one of the following 2 positions:
  a. *Anterior–posterior position*
    One paddle—left infrascapular area
    Other paddle—upper sternum at 3rd interspace
  b. *Anterior position*
    One paddle—just to right of sternum at 2nd interspace
    Other paddle—just under left nipple	

6. Determine if the machine's synchronization mechanism is working before applying the paddles.
  a. The discharge should hit near the peak of the R wave.
  b. The R wave usually must be of substantial height; if it is not, adjust the gain (sensitivity) or change the lead. On many machines, the R wave must be upright before there is synchronization.
	a. If the electrical discharge hits the T wave, ventricular fibrillation may occur.
	b. Synchronization is not used for ventricular fibrillation. (The machine will not work for *defibrillation* if the synchronization mode is on.)

7. Apply electrode paste to all of the paddle surface, but make sure there is no excess around the edges of the paddles.
  a. The paste should be rubbed into the skin very thoroughly, since this allows more electricity to penetrate the body surface.
  b. Make sure paddles are clean because surface material will interfere with the flow of electricity.
  c. Apply firm pressure to the paddle.
	7. If there is excess paste around the paddles, the discharge may run onto the skin, causing a burn. If there is not firm contact between the paddle and skin, a burn may occur, also, electricity is lost from the heart.

8. Set dial for lowest level of electrical energy that can be expected to convert the arrhythmia. Some arrhythmias (such as atrial flutter) can be converted with very low energies, such as 25 watt-seconds (joules).	8. Excessive energies may cause unnecessary discomfort to the patient.
9. Valium or a short-acting barbiturate should be given if the patient is conscious.	9. This helps produce amnesia concerning the cardioversion.
10. After the patient is in a light sleep from the IV medication and when no one is touching the bed or patient, discharge the cardioverter. If cardioversion does not occur, proceed to a higher energy level.	
11. Monitor the ECG after conversion occurs. Blood pressures should be recorded about every 15 minutes until the preshock blood pressure is reached.	11. The patient may revert to his previous arrhythmia after conversion.

3: Vascular Disorders

Vascular disorders is a term that refers to conditions of the blood vessels.

    Peripheral vascular disease (PVD) refers to disease affecting the blood vessels that supply the extremities: veins, arteries, and lymphatics.

Nature of the Disorder

1. Long-term—often discouraging to the patient: treatment may be painful and tedious; healing is slow.
2. Appears minor, but disability may last for months before healing takes place.
    Patient may have financial concerns and may worry about loss of job and community responsibilities.
3. Older people are especially prone to peripheral vascular disease.
4. This condition is often compounded by other medical problems, such as diabetes.
5. If lesions heal, recurrence of the condition, with concomitant incapacitation, is frequent.

Thrombus and Embolus Formation

1. *Thrombus*—a blood clot that partially or completely occludes a blood vessel.
    a. Thrombosed vessel—an occluded vessel
    b. Thrombosis—the condition of having a thrombosed vessel
2. Spontaneous clotting of the blood will usually not occur unless there is damage to the intimal surface of the vessel wall.
    a. Injury by trauma
    b. Inflammation
    c. Degenerative changes due to arteriosclerosis
3. Injured intima—causes platelets to collect, fibrin to form, and thrombus to develop.
4. *Embolus*—a fragment of a thrombus or a thrombus that has broken away from the point of formation.
    a. *Embolism*—occurs when an embolus moving through a blood vessel arrives at a narrowing of the vessel and thus occludes it.
    b. Air embolism—a bubble of air in the bloodstream
    c. Fat embolism—multiple droplets of fat in the bloodstream

Ischemia

Ischemia is a lack of blood supply sufficient to meet tissue needs. This can develop as a result of:

1. Gradual occlusion of the lumen of the artery by encroachment of the thickened wall (atherosclerosis).

2. More rapid development of ischemia because of formation of a blood clot (thrombus) at the atherosclerotic site.
3. Rapid occlusion of an artery when a free-flowing clot (embolus) lodges at a bifurcation or narrowing of the vessel.

Assessment and Pathophysiologic Manifestations of Vascular Disorders

Assessment begins with a history and physical examination. More specifically for manifestations of vascular disorders, the following conditions are noted:

Skin Color and Temperature

Objective determination of skin temperature—differences between 2 extremities are observed when individual is placed in a new environment; coolness of 1 extremity.

A. Coldness

1. Due to deficient blood supply to a part even though the environment is warm.
2. One extremity may be compared with another to note the difference.
3. The patient notices that the part feels uncomfortably cold.

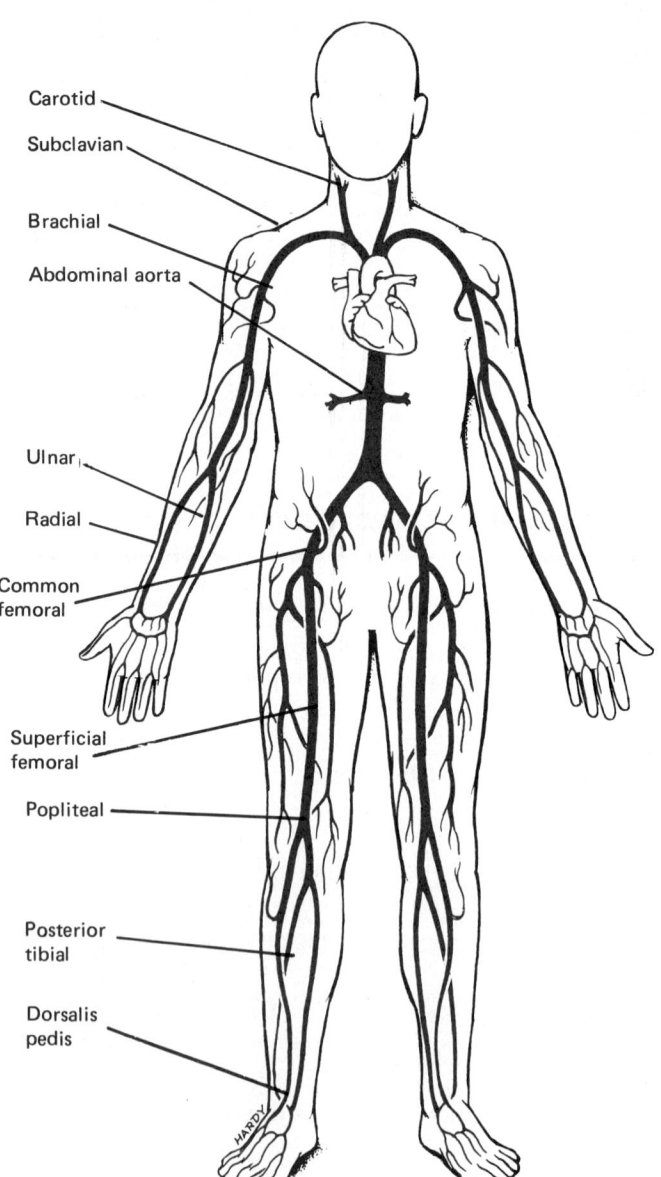

Figure 9-34. Salient points in evaluating peripheral arterial insufficiency. Look for bruits over the carotid, subclavian, femoral, superficial femoral, and popliteal arteries as well as the aorta. (*a*) Reduced or absent femoral pulses indicate aortoiliac disease. (*b*) Absent popliteal pulses indicate superficial femoral occlusion. (*c*) Pulse deficits in one extremity, with normal pulses in contralateral extremity, suggest acute arterial embolus. (*d*) Absent pedal pulses indicate tibioperoneal artery involvement.

B. Pallor (Paleness)

1. Normally, the pink hue of the skin is due to adequate superficial circulation.
2. Diminished blood supply produces paleness, or lack of color.
3. Blanching occurs when the part is elevated above the level of the heart and the arterial pressure in that part is lower than normal.

C. Rubor (Redness)

1. Instead of a normal rosy-pink, the part may be red or reddish-blue. This is due to injury of superficial capillaries, which causes them to remain dilated; it may also occur with chronic ischemia.
2. Circulation is impaired.
3. Anoxia or coldness may be the cause of rubor.

D. Cyanosis (Blueness)

1. Indicates that less than a normal amount of oxygen is in the blood.
2. When localized, it implies very slow circulation in that part.

Other Signs

A. Pain

1. Due to inadequate blood supply.
2. This is common, but varies with the condition.
   May be constant and severe (e.g., ulceration).
3. When it occurs only after a certain amount of exercise, it is called *intermittent claudication*. (This disappears after rest, but returns with exercise.)
4. When it occurs at rest (rest pain), it indicates a more severe degree of ischemia.

B. Necrosis

1. Loss of viability of tissue.
2. Noted first in most distal parts of the extremity.

C. Atrophy

1. The muscle shrinks, and there is loss of strength and joint mobility.
2. Due to chronic ischemia.

Exercise Tolerance

Measurement of the amount of exercise the involved part can tolerate before pain is experienced.

Pulse Volume

A useful method for recording peripheral pulse volume, based on a scale from zero to +4, follows:

0	Not palpable—absent pulsations
+1	Thready, weak, fades in and out—marked impairment of pulsations
+2	Difficult to palpate; stronger than +1—moderate impairment
+3	Easily palpable, not easily obliterated with pressure—slight impairment
+4	Strong and bounding—normal pulsations

Bruits

1. An abnormal sound heard on auscultation as blood flows through a stenotic area of the artery (Fig. 9-34).
2. This is heard most easily during systole; pitch is higher as stenosis becomes more marked.

Capillary Refill Time

The capillary bed contains arterial blood and is called *microcirculation*. Capillary refill time is an indicator of peripheral perfusion and cardiac output.

1. This test can be done at the same time that arterial pulses are checked.
2. Depress finger or toe nailbed until skin blanches.
3. Release pressure and note how rapidly color returns to the original appearance.
   a. Normally, capillaries fill within a fraction of a second.
   (1) Acceptable—less than 3 seconds
   (2) Abnormal or sluggish—more than 3 seconds

Blood Pressure (See p. 20 and p. 380)

Serial blood pressure readings are taken with Doppler Ultrasound, see below.

See Assessment of Acute Arterial Occlusion vs. Deep Vein Thrombosis (see below).

Diagnostic Evaluation of Vascular Conditions

A. Doppler Ultrasound—a noninvasive test used to detect blood flow.

1. A beam of ultrasound is sent into the tissues through an acoustic gel on the skin. Reflected sound from moving blood cells is detected, amplified as audible sound, and recorded; velocity of blood flow has a direct effect on the waveforms (Figs. 9-35 and 9-36).
2. Usually, the posterior tibial, calf, popliteal, and common femoral veins are examined. Arterial flow can be detected by the pulsatile nature of the flow.
3. Signals are assessed for venous patency and valvular competence. Arterial flow is used as an indicator of

Assessment of Acute Arterial Occlusion vs. Deep Vein Thrombosis

	Acute Arterial Occlusion	Deep Vein Thrombosis
Onset	Sudden	Gradual
Color	Pale; later—mottled, cyanotic	Slightly cyanotic; rubescent
Skin temperature	Cold	Warm
Leg size—diameter	May be reduced from normal	Enlarged
Superficial veins	Collapsed	Appear enlarged and prominent
Arterial pulsation	Pulse deficit noted	Normal and palpable (except in marked edema)
Effect of elevating leg	Condition worsens	Condition improves

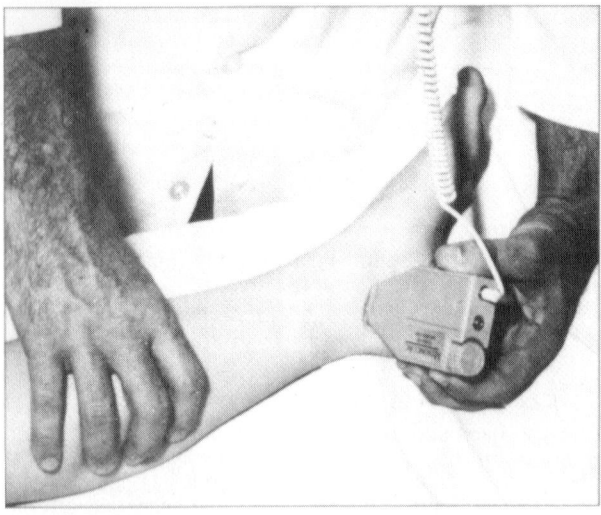

Figure 9-35. Doppler ultrasound transducer being used in screening for major deep-vein thrombosis.

patency, and the cuff pressure required to stop it indicates arterial pressure at that point.

4. Entire test takes about 5–10 minutes.
5. This technique, when checked with arteriography, has a reliability factor of 95% and thus qualifies as a simple, inexpensive, highly reliable, and noninvasive diagnostic tool.

B. Plethysmography (pulse volume recording, PVR)—a noninvasive measurement of changes in calf volume corresponding to changes in blood volume brought about by temporary venous occlusion with a high pneumatic cuff.

1. Variations of the above test are practiced in various clinics; some use a strain-gauge placed around the calf.
2. Temporary venous occlusion with a pneumatic cuff (50 mm. Hg) applied to the thigh results in an increase in circumference of the calf.
3. Sudden cuff deflation results in a decrease in calf circumference; this is proportional to rate of venous outflow from extremity.
4. Ocular pneumoplethysmography (OPG)—some clinics use this modality to measure indirectly carotid

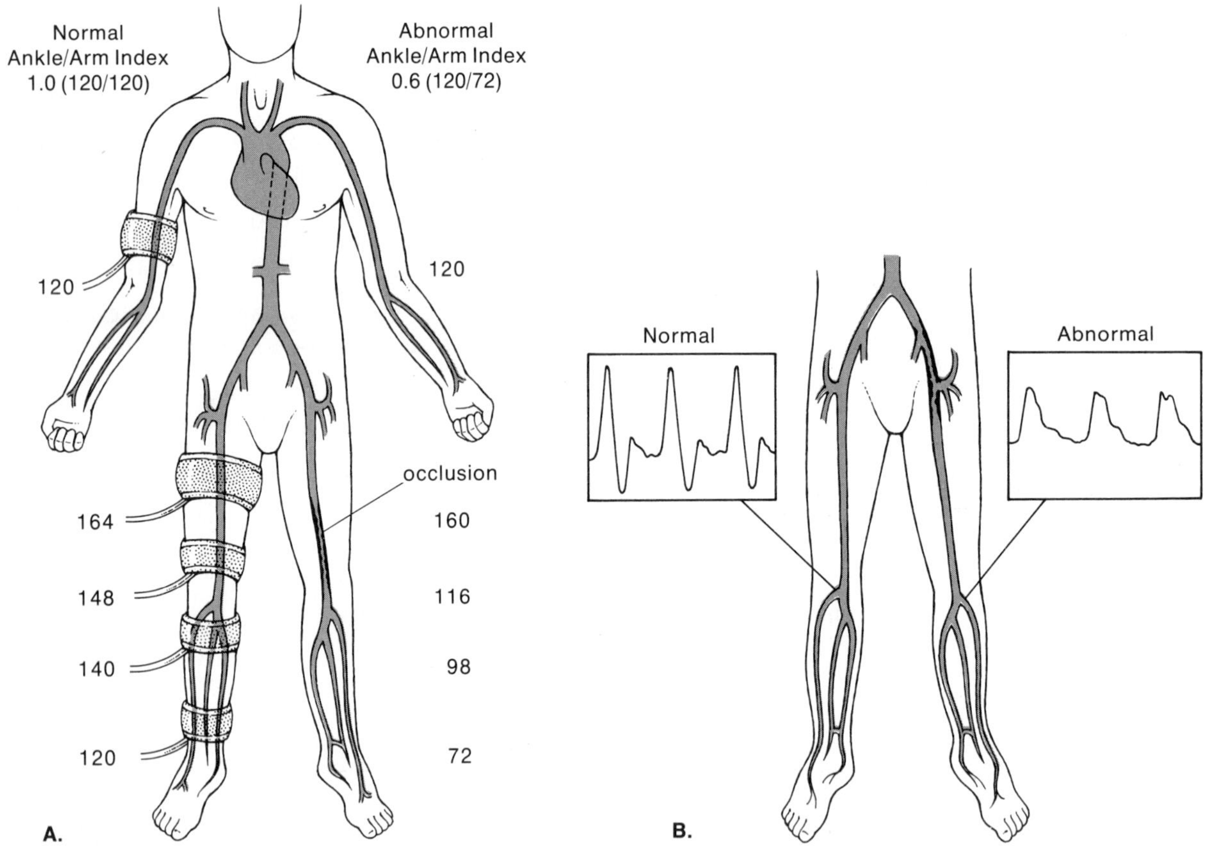

Normal
Ankle/Arm Index
1.0 (120/120)

Abnormal
Ankle/Arm Index
0.6 (120/72)

120

120

164

160

148

116

140

98

120

72

occlusion

A.

Normal

Abnormal

B.

Figure 9-36. (A) The Doppler probe determines pressures over the brachial and posterior tibial or dorsalis pedis arteries. The cuff is inflated until the arterial segment disappears; the cuff is then slowly deflated until the arterial velocity signal returns at systolic pressure. NOTE: Normally, ankle pressure is equal to or slightly above arm pressure. In the presence of occlusive arterial disease (right side of diagrammed person), ankle and lower leg pressures are lower by an amount proportional to the degree of circulatory impairment.
(B) Diagram comparing the analogue wave tracings in a normal (*left*) and a diseased extremity (*right*). Note the lack of diastolic deflection and the protracted systolic components in the tracing of the abnormal extremity. (AbuRahma et al: Doppler testing in peripheral vascular occlusive disease. Surg Gynecol Obstet 1980 Jan; 150[1]:27)

artery blood flow; this is done by the application of pneumatic pressure on the eye to measure ophthalmic eye pressure.

C. Oscillometry

1. Degree of arterial occlusion may be measured by an oscillometer, which measures pulse volume. One extremity may be compared with the other.
2. An inflatable cuff is wrapped around the extremity, and the *oscillometric index* is determined by inflating the cuff and reading the dial.
3. Normal readings (points of pressure at which circulation ceases):
   a. Lower extremity

Midthigh	4–16 mm./Hg
Upper third of leg	3–12 mm./Hg
Above ankle	1–18 mm./Hg
Foot	0.2–1.0 mm./Hg

   b. Upper extremity

Upper arm	4–16 mm./Hg
Elbow	3–12 mm./Hg
Wrist	1–10 mm./Hg
Hand	0.2–2.0 mm./Hg

D. Phlebography (Venography)—an x-ray
visualization of the vascular tree after the injection of a contrast medium (renografin).

1. Inform the patient that he may experience an intense burning sensation in the vessel where the solution is injected. This will last for only a few seconds.
2. Note any evidence of allergic reaction to the contrast medium; this may occur as soon as the contrast medium is injected, or it may be delayed and occur when the patient reaches his room.
   a. Perspiring, dyspnea, nausea, vomiting
   b. Rapid heart rate, numbness of extremities
   c. Hives
   d. Management
      (1) Notify physician.
      (2) Have adrenalin available for injection, as well as antihistamine drugs and oxygen.
3. Nursing management
   a. Observe injection site for the following:
      (1) Signs of redness, swelling, bleeding; signs of thrombosis (loss of distal pulses)
         If above signs occur, notify physician.
      (2) Evidence of bleeding
         (a) Apply pressure dressing.
         (b) Notify physician.
   b. Check for arterial occlusion.
      (1) Note extremity pulses; check for quality.
      (2) Observe color (pallor or cyanosis).
      (3) Ask the patient about sensation of pain, numbness.
4. Chief disadvantages: It is an expensive and invasive diagnostic method and may cause painful side effects.

E. Treadmill Test

1. At 1½ mph on a 10%–12% incline, the patient walks for 5 minutes; he is stopped if:
   a. Symptoms of claudication occur
   b. Other signs of intolerance, such as shortness of breath, develop
2. Following the exercise, he is returned to the examining table, where ankle pressures, pulse volumes, and brachial systolic pressures are taken.
3. Normally, there is an increase in total extremity blood flow.

F. Intermittent Claudication Determination

1. At rest, blood supply is adequate—but an exercised muscle may require 10 times more blood.

2. Following exercise such as walking, running, or climbing stairs, a severe cramping pain or sensation of tiredness develops in those muscle areas not receiving an adequate blood supply.
3. Upon resting, pain is relieved; metabolites are carried away and normal blood-to-tissue demand ratio is restored.
4. Measurement
   a. Have the patient walk up steps, counting number of steps taken before pain occurs.
   b. Use a foot-pedal device, which lifts a weight when pressed.
      (1) Normally, fatigue occurs in 5–10 minutes.
      (2) The person with arterial occlusion usually complains of pain in less than a minute.

G. Carotid Phonoangiogram (CPG)—a noninvasive
diagnostic test of the carotid artery.

1. Sound is greatly amplified, and the instrument permits localization of the source of the bruit and provides a method of photographing the oscillographic tracing from which one can estimate the degree of stenosis.

H. ^{125}I Fibrinogen Uptake Test—an invasive
radioactive test in which labeled fibrinogen, given before a thrombus forms, will be concentrated in the area of clot formation. Formation of clots may be detected with serial scanning and by comparing one leg with the other.

1. Advantages
   a. The most sensitive method to screen for acute calf vein thrombosis
   b. Preferred in detecting recurrent *active* venous thrombosis
2. Disadvantages
   a. Not sensitive to thrombi high in the iliofemoral region or to inactive thrombosis
   b. Costly and time-consuming

I. Digital Subtraction Angiography (DSA), or digital intravenous angiography

A radiologic technique that uses an image-intensifier video system to display vessels on a television monitor. The images are received by a computer that translates them into numbers. By this conversion, it is possible to subtract the image obtained (before the injection of contrast medium) from the later images. Therefore, after computer subtraction, an enhanced image of the arterial system is presented.

1. Advantages
   a. Low risk for vascular injury and stroke
   b. Cost-effective, since it may be done as an outpatient procedure
   c. Rare reaction may be allergy to iodine-containing contrast medium (nausea, vomiting, dizziness)
   d. Enhanced image
2. Disadvantages
   a. Low resolution of contrast medium
   b. Nonselectivity; interpretation may be difficult when all vessels in an area are opacified
   c. Not useful for coronary arteries
   d. Slight movement (even peristalsis, respiration) may alter image
   e. Resuscitation facilities must be available, as with any injection of contrast medium
3. Patient preparation
   a. No food intake within 2 hours of the test to prevent vomiting if there is a reaction to the contrast medium.
   b. The patient must be able to hold his breath and lie very still when directed.

c. The patient is placed in supine position (appropriately centered) on a radiographic table.
d. Brachial vein is prepared, and a large sterile drape is positioned to accommodate the guidewire and catheter (No. 16 gauge Angiocath).
e. Fluoroscopy aids in moving the catheter properly; No. 7 French 65-cm. pigtail catheter is moved over the guidewire and positioned near the superior vena cava/right atrial junction.

f. The radiologist positions the area of interest under fluoroscopy.
g. Study takes 20–40 minutes.
h. Upon completion, the catheter is removed and pressure is applied to the puncture site for about 5 minutes; a sterile dressing is applied.
i. The patient is instructed to increase fluid intake over next 24 hours (1,500–2,000 ml.) to aid in excretion of contrast medium.

Nursing Management of Patients with Vascular Disorders

Nursing Process Overview
Assessment
Clinical Manifestations
1. Details concerning the signs of vascular disorders can be found in the preceding pages.
2. Included in the main list of manifestations are skin color and temperature, pain on walking (intermittent claudication), exercise intolerance, capillary refill time, blood pressure, and chest sounds.

Diagnostic Evaluations
Doppler ultrasound, plethysmography, oscillometry, phlebography, treadmill test, etc. These tests and others are discussed in detail in the preceding section.

Patient Problems/Nursing Diagnoses
1. Pain related to reduced blood supply.
2. Ischemia related to impaired blood flow.
3. Potential alterations in tissue perfusion related to ischemia.
4. Impaired physical mobility related to reduced blood supply to extremities.
5. Knowledge deficit of rehabilitation program.
6. Potential nonadherence related to unwillingness or demands of life-style changes.

Planning and Implementation
Nursing Interventions
A. **Activities to enhance arterial blood supply to tissues and to decrease venous congestion**
1. *Walking*—a simple but very effective exercise.
   a. A level surface is preferred.
   b. Encourage the patient to set realistic goals; each week these goals may be extended in keeping with his tolerance.
   c. Use assistive devices as necessary—walker, cane, etc.
   d. Evaluate the patient's ability to climb stairs.
2. *Jogging*—a means of stimulating collateral blood flow not only to legs, but also to the myocardium.
   May be practiced as long as it is comfortable and pleasurable.
3. *Buerger's exercises*—prescribed according to condition of extremities and condition of patient.
   a. Elevate extremity for a minute.
   b. Place extremities in a dependent position until cyanosis or rubor becomes maximal.
   c. Lie with extremities horizontal for a minute.
   d. See Buerger–Allen exercises below.
4. *Buerger–Allen exercises*—exercises by which gravity alternately fills and empties the blood vessels (Fig. 9-37).

a. Procedure
   (1) Begin with the patient lying flat in bed. Elevate legs to above level of heart—2 minutes or until blanching takes place.
   (2) Allow legs to be dependent; exercise feet—3 minutes or until legs are pink.
   (3) Instruct the patient to lie flat—5 minutes.
   (4) Repeat a, b, and c 5 times; do entire set 3 times a day.
b. Tolerance and proper pacing
   (1) Advise the patient to rest when he feels pain.
   (2) Avoid chilly environment, since it causes vasoconstriction, which in turn further diminishes flow.
   (3) Maintain stability, particularly if postural hypotension is a problem.
c. Comfort
   (1) Improvise equipment that will provide comfortable support for the patient in the leg-elevated position.
   (2) Well-padded straight-back chair can be placed on the bed so that the back of the chair supports the leg—top of chair is toward the top of the thigh.
   (3) Overbed table may be used with a pillow.
5. *Oscillating bed*—provides postural exercises using a passive method.
   a. Aids indirectly in prevention of pressure areas—pressure sores.
   b. Prescribed according to the patient's needs.
   c. Explain to the patient that the bed will assist in relieving his circulatory difficulty.
      (1) Explain how the bed is turned on, regulated, and stopped.
      (2) Advise the patient whether he can stop for meals, treatments, rest periods, etc.
   d. Introduce motion of bed gradually in order to eliminate the possibility of headache, dizziness, or nausea.
   e. Follow prescribed cycle for the individual patient. Cycle: Degree of angle and the length of time to be elevated
      Degree of angle and the length of time to be lowered
   f. Prevent the patient from slipping downward by providing a padded footboard.

B. **Thermotherapy to promote vasodilatation**

▶ **NURSING ALERT:** When heat is applied externally to an extremity—demand for circulation is increased. When applied to diseased tissues—sensations are impaired; may result in damaging burn and necrosis.

POSITION 1
Place legs on a pillow-cushioned chair
for one minute to drain blood.

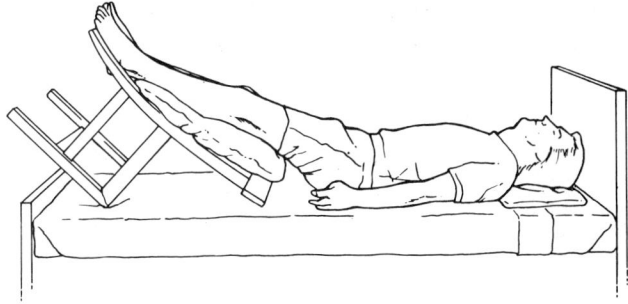

POSITION 2
Hold each of these
stretching positions
for 30 seconds
to enhance blood return.

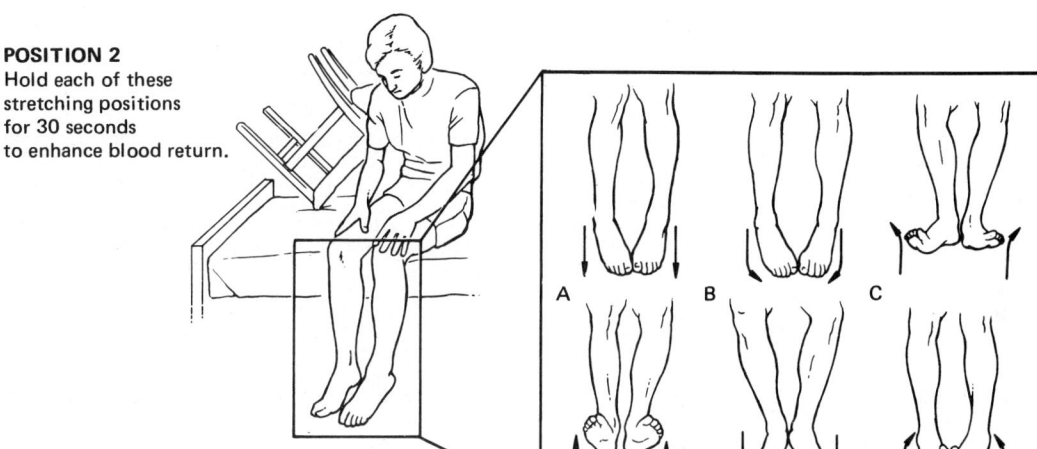

POSITION 3
Lie flat on back, with legs straight.
Hold position for one minute.

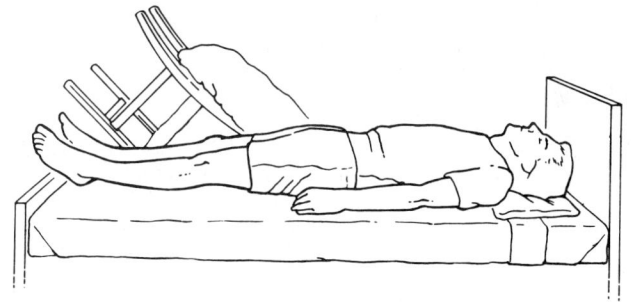

Figure 9-37. Buerger-Allen exercises. Do exercise series 6 times, 4 times a day. (Forshee T and Minckley B: Lumbar sympathectomy. RN Vol. 39[2])

1. *Dry heat*
   a. Warm water bottles
      (1) Check temperature of water before filling bottle—not to exceed 48.8°C. (120°F.).
      (2) Apply cover to bottle so that it does not come in direct contact with skin.
   b. Heat cradle (thermostatically controlled or regulated with electric bulbs)
      (1) Pad metal edges of cradle to prevent injury to extremities.
      (2) Control temperature so that it will not exceed 32.2°C. (90°F.).
      (3) Ensure that bulbs are not likely to be touched by extremity (usually legs and feet).
      (4) Higher temperatures would stimulate metabolism (not desired).
      (5) Reduce temperature if patient complains of pain in extremity.
   c. Ultrasound (acoustic vibration with frequencies beyond human ear perception)
      (1) Useful in small areas where deeper penetration of heat is desired and where circulation needs to be stimulated.
      (2) Application time is under 10 minutes.
      (3) Avoid areas where metal sutures may be present.
   d. Paraffin bath
2. *Moist heat*
   a. Hydrotherapy
      (1) Sitz bath—used for perineal therapy.
      (2) Basin—for hands or feet, with prescribed temperatures and for prescribed times.

Put on supports early in the morning, before swelling occurs.

Always begin with supports "inside-out" . . . as they are when you receive them.

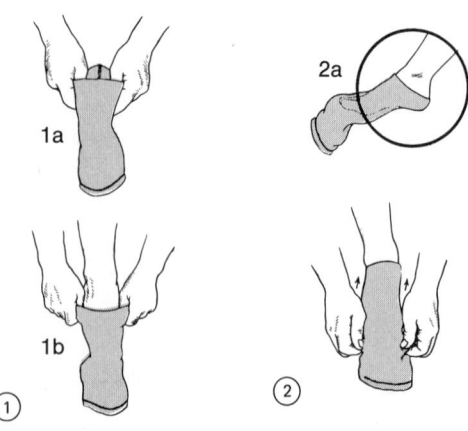

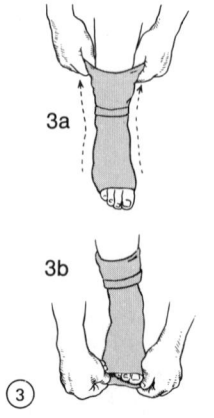

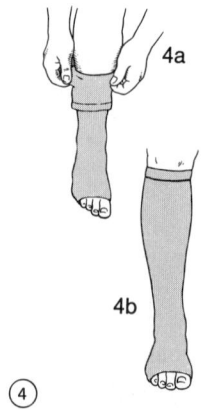

Sit with feet in easy reach. Support must be "inside out," with its foot inverted back to heel. Seam faces down (sketch 1a). Grasp each side firmly and pull onto foot (sketch 1b).

Pull past midpoint of heel (sketch 2a), so support will not slip back. Then, reach just beyond toes and grasp fabric between fingers and start pulling over foot. Pull from sides . . . never by seams.

Pull all the way up past ankle (sketch 3a). Seat heel in place. Pull foot portion of support out toward tips of toes (sketch 3b) to set fabric evenly on foot. Allow to settle back normally.

Using short (2 inches at a time) snappy pulls (sketch 4a) pull support up to point it was measured to end (sketch 4b). Smooth evenly down leg. **Never allow top to roll or turn down.**

Figure 9-38. Method of applying supporting hose. (Courtesy of Jobst)

b. Whirlpool bath
   (1) In addition to moist heat, the effect of agitated water provides hydromassage.
   (2) May be used for 1 or 2 extremities or the whole body.
c. Warm compresses
   (1) Applied directly to the skin.
   (2) When hot, apply over toweling.

C. Pressure gradient therapy to promote vasodilatation (compression devices and garments)

1. *Cuffs, sleeves, or boots*
   a. Circulator—electrically produced air pressure alternately inflates and deflates a boot in which the extremity is encased. Rhythm of occlusion and release as well as pressure can be regulated to correspond to pulse.
   b. Pressor sleeve or boot—a plastic tube filled with air.
      (1) Can be maintained at low pressure for several hours.
      (2) Can be regulated to function intermittently. (Useful in lymphedema of arm following mastectomy; see p. 597.)
2. *Elastic garments*
   a. Support for an extremity can be tailor-made: A unique measuring tape was devised by Jobst* so that exact "fabric pressures" are produced with their custom-made venous pressure gradient supports.
   b. Method of applying supporting hose is demonstrated in Figure 9-38.
   c. Any type of support hose, if applied incorrectly (such as permitting rolling at the top), can act as a tourniquet. This will produce stasis, rather than prevent it.

* The Jobst Institute, Box 653, Toledo, OH 43694.

d. Many question the effectiveness of elastic stockings; the nurse will be guided by the preferences of the patient's physician.
e. Elastic stockings with inflatable pneumatic bladders connected to an automatic air pump are available to help prevent deep-vein thrombi from forming in the calf and lower leg.
   (1) The bladders in this device, called the *Pulsatile Anti-Embolism System,* expand and contract and are designed to stimulate circulation.

D. Prevention of vasoconstriction in the vessels of the extremities

1. Impress the patient with the *dangers of smoking,* especially inhaling.
2. Promote an atmosphere that is devoid of emotional tension; restrict those visitors who appear to upset the patient.
3. Advise the patient against wearing constrictive garments, such as panty girdles, garters, belts, jeans, and tight panty hose.

E. Hygienic measures and activities to increase the blood flow to the extremities

1. Maintain a warm and properly humidified environment.
2. Put on warm clothing before going out into cool air; protect hands and feet with lamb's wool lining in gloves and boots to prevent vasoconstriction.
3. Take a warm bath to offset chilling; replace vigorous rubbing of the skin after a bath with gentle patting.
4. Avoid excessive heat to extremities (using hot water bottle, electric pad, etc.)—increases metabolism, so that more oxygenated blood is demanded.
5. Sleep with the head of the bed elevated about 20.3 cm. (8 inches)—if patient has pain at rest; wear bedsocks to keep feet warm if necessary.
6. Walking is the best form of exercise; otherwise,

active or passive exercise of the extremities is recommended.

7. Utilize analgesic and tranquilizing medications as required to keep comfortable.
8. Take prescribed vasodilating medications even though they may not appear to help; at times, they maintain the status quo and keep the problem from worsening.
9. Take prescribed antilipidic drugs to retard progress of concomitant atherosclerotic disease by reducing serum lipids.
10. Wear properly fitting and repaired hose and shoes.

Health Education

Teach the patient the following:

A. Signs and symptoms of circulatory disturbances affecting peripheral tissues

1. Pain in the extremity—(Note whether this occurs at rest, with limited activity, or with more pronounced exercise.)
2. Color changes of the skin or nails—pallor, pinkness, rubor, cyanosis
3. Impaired or peculiar growth of nails
4. Shiny, taut skin
5. Discrepancy in size of one extremity when compared to contralateral (opposite) extremity
6. Enlarged veins or abnormal pulsations of veins
7. Temperature variations—abnormally cold or abnormally warm
8. Ulcerations, necrosis, or gangrene

B. Methods for reducing metabolic demands on the body

1. Take precautions to prevent injury and infection, particularly of the extremities.
2. Practice daily hygienic cleanliness and care of the feet: trim nails properly, avoid strong medications, utilize lamb's wool for pressure areas, wear shoes and hosiery that fit correctly.
3. Avoid exposure to cold or excessive heat.
4. Exercise within recognized limits; set up a reasonable rest plan.
5. Remain in bed if there is evidence of necrosis, ulceration, or gangrene; consult physician.

C. Foot care

1. Keep the feet clean to prevent irritation and infection.
   a. Wash daily with a bland soap and warm water.
   b. Dry thoroughly, paying particular attention to areas between the toes; pat rather than rub dry.
   c. Apply lanolin or petrolatum to prevent drying and cracking of skin.
   d. Wear clean hose daily: woolen socks for winter, cotton for summer.
2. Avoid injury, excessive pressure, or other irritants to the feet.
   a. Shoes
      (1) Wear properly fitting shoes with a comfortable heel.
      (2) Check inside of shoe; avoid wearing shoes with protruding seams, torn lining, piercing nails, or faulty lumps.
      (3) Wear shoes when out of bed; avoid going barefoot.
      (4) Break in new shoes gradually; alternate with an older pair.
      (5) Leather is preferred to rubber or synthetics because the latter interfere with proper circulation of air.
      (6) Allow wet or damp shoes to dry slowly on shoe trees to prevent misshaping.
   b. Hose
      (1) Wear proper length and size—if too short, toes are compressed; if too long, wrinkles form and exert pressure on skin.
      (2) Avoid seams, holes, or lumpy darned areas.
      (3) Use bedsocks rather than hot water bottle or heating pad if feet are cold in bed.
      (4) Use woolen or cotton hose; they absorb moisture; nylon is not as absorbent.
      (5) Avoid constricting garments—foundation garments, garters, and even support hose unless they are specifically prescribed.
   c. Pedicure
      (1) Trim toenails straight across after soaking the feet in warm water.
      (2) Place wisps of cotton under corner of great toenail if there is a tendency toward ingrown toenails.
      (3) Have a podiatrist cut corns and calluses; do not use corn pads or strong medications.
   d. Heat and cold
      (1) Keep feet warm; avoid exposure to cold for long periods of time.
      (2) Use heating devices only on advice of physician; excessive heat can be as damaging as insufficient warmth.
      (3) Rely on warm socks, fleece-lined boots or mitts, lightweight blankets, etc. rather than on heating extremities near a fire, oven, or radiator.
   e. General measures
      (1) Avoid areas where injury to feet is likely, e.g., crowded subways, construction areas, sports shows, etc.
      (2) Prevent sunburn in the summer and avoid wading in very cold water.
3. Prevent pressure on feet; rest and exercise in moderation.
   a. Place a pillow under covers at end of bed to provide a footrest and prevent weight of top bedding from exerting pressure on toes.
   b. Avoid remaining in one position for long periods of time.
   c. Do not cross legs when sitting because of pressure on nerves and blood vessels.
   d. Elevate feet on a chair or footstool with proper support of leg; do this about 15 minutes every 2 hours.
4. If damage or injury occurs to any part of foot or leg, report to physician.
   a. Redness, swelling, irritation, blistering
   b. Itching, burning—athlete's foot
   c. Bruises, cuts, unusual appearance of skin

D. A second opinion if lower-extremity amputation is suggested

1. Major vascular centers are reporting commendable results in vascular surgery as an alternative to amputation.
2. Various synthetic graft materials are available for very specific vascular needs.
3. Microsurgery is adding a new dimension to very fine surgical repair.

Evaluation

Expected Outcomes

1. Demonstrates increased arterial blood supply to extremities—palpable pulses, warm extremities, reduced pain, normal color

2. Exhibits decreased venous congestion—reduced swelling and pain
3. Promotes vasodilatation by adhering to proper hygienic practices
4. Has no pain; avoids practices that cause vasoconstriction/injury
5. Attains/maintains tissue integrity; avoids injury
6. Adheres to the rehabilitation program

Anticoagulant Therapy

Anticoagulant therapy is the administration of medications to achieve the following:

Goals:
1. Disrupt the blood's natural clotting mechanism.
2. Prevent formation of a thrombus in postoperative patients.
3. Intercept the extension of a thrombus once it has formed.

Types of Anticoagulants
Oral

Coumarin derivatives: dicumarol, phenprocoumon, warfarin sodium, and warfarin potassium
Indandione derivatives: anisindione and phenindione

Parenteral

Heparin sodium

▶ **NURSING ALERT: Anticoagulants cannot dissolve a thrombus that has already formed. Precise nursing assessment is required because of the delicate balance sought between too much clotting (thrombus formation) and too little clotting (hemorrhage).**

Clinical Indications
(Authorities disagree about the justification of long-term use of anticoagulants in various disease entities.)
1. *Venous thrombosis*—because of the danger of extension and the danger of emboli.
2. *Pulmonary embolism*—prophylactically, if patient is known to be suspect; also indicated during recovery phase to prevent further clot formation.
3. *Patient susceptible to embolism*—such as a surgical patient who has rheumatic heart disease, one who has had valve surgery.
4. *Coronary occlusion with myocardial infarction.*
5. *Cerebral vascular accident caused by emboli or cerebral thrombi*—to reduce sludging of blood: useful in prevention and treatment of strokes.

Highest Risk
1. Patients whose prothrombin time has been difficult to control from the outset.
2. Men (not women) with aortic valve prostheses.
3. Patients treated with anticoagulants for more than 3 years.

Contraindications
1. May cause spontaneous bleeding—therefore not used when there is likelihood of bleeding because of increased capillary fragility or an aneurysm.
2. Individuals with peptic ulcer and chronic ulcerative diseases are considered poor risks, because of the possibility of bleeding.
3. Should not be given following neurosurgery because of danger of hemorrhage in brain or spinal cord.
4. Liver disease may present a problem because of interference with plasma protein clotting factors.

5. Liver and kidney insufficiency diseases because of difficulty in metabolizing and eliminating them—resulting in toxicity and difficulty in responding to antidotal medication (not true of heparin).
6. Poor follow-up by patients; unless the patient cooperates by reporting for blood tests, etc., he should not be on anticoagulants.
7. Severe diabetes, infections, or severe traumatic conditions are circumstances in which anticoagulant therapy may be contraindicated.

Nursing Interventions
1. The preferred method of heparin administration is continuous infusion (using a pump) because of the low incidence of hemorrhagic complications.
2. Check patient's weight, since dosage is calculated on the basis of weight.
3. Be sure clotting profiles are obtained before treatment is initiated, to detect hidden bleeding tendencies.
4. Place pump out of reach of patient to prevent interference with its proper functioning.
   a. Check frequently to ensure that system is working properly: exact dosage, no leaks, no kinks.
5. Note that periodic coagulation tests are done; these include hematocrit and partial thromboplastin time (PTT).
6. Recognize that heparin may be given by *intermittent intravenous injection.* This may be facilitated by the use of a "heparin-lock" (see p. 109).
7. *Minidose heparin* is used in certain patients preoperatively to reduce postoperative thromboembolism (see p. 80).
8. Since heparin may be given along with longer lasting hypoprothrombinemic agents, for the first few days of treatment, each day's medication orders should be checked *after* reports of daily prothrombin time tests are known.
9. Have on hand the antidotes to anticoagulants being used:
   > Heparin—protamine sulfate
   > Coumarin—phytonadione (vitamin K₁, Aquamephyton, Konakion, Mephyton)
10. Note that the relatively long duration of action of oral anticoagulants makes it easier to maintain low prothrombin levels for long periods.
11. Observe carefully for any possible signs of bleeding and report immediately so that anticoagulant dosage may be reviewed and altered if necessary:
    a. Urine—note evidence of hematuria; indandione derivatives may turn alkaline urine a red orange color—acidifying this urine causes this color to disappear.
    b. Stool—check for tarry color; use Hemoccult test tape for easy rapid checking.
    c. Emesis basin following tooth brushing—note any pink or bloody return.
12. Be aware of the following with regard to sensitivity to coumarin derivatives:

May be intensified by	*May be decreased by*
Antibiotics	Antacids
Mineral oil	Barbiturates
Quinidine	Oral contraceptives
Salicylates	Adrenal corticosteroids
Tolbutamide (Orinase)	

▶ **NURSING ALERT: Drug interactions can alter the effect of anticoagulants. Review with the physician the effect of other medications the patient may be taking during anticoagulant therapy.**

Guidelines: Subcutaneous Injection of Heparin

Purpose   When prolonged therapy is indicated, heparin may be given subcutaneously into fatty tissues.

Equipment

1- or 2-ml. syringe or disposable tuberculin syringe
Fine sharp needle, No. 27, 1.6-cm. (⅝ inch) long (or premeasured Tubex cartridge-needle unit)
Skin antiseptic

Considerations

1. Most convenient sites are along lower abdominal fat pad—to avoid inadvertent intramuscular injection and hematoma formation.
    a. A common location site is the fatty area anterior to either iliac crest.
    b. Avoid injection sites within 5 cm. (2 inches) of the umbilicus because of possibility of entering a larger blood vessel.
2. Areas where subcutaneous layer is thin should be avoided.

Procedure

Nursing Action	Rationale/Amplification
Performance Phase	
1. Sponge the area gently with alcohol. Do not rub!	1. Rubbing or pinching skin might initiate damage to the tissue; heparin would aggravate any bleeding.
2. Attempt to stretch skin out, using palm of left hand. Some prefer to (gently) pick up a well-defined fold of skin.	2. Try to empty blood vessels in local area to lessen likelihood of their being pierced by needle—with subsequent hematoma formation.
3. Holding the shaft of the syringe in dart fashion, insert needle directly through the skin at a right angle just into the subcutaneous fatty layer.	
4. Move right hand into position to direct plunger. a. Do not move needle tip once it is inserted. b. Do not pull back plunger for testing.	4. Aspiration in a forcible manner can damage small blood vessels and frequently lead to bleeding and hematoma formation, especially in the presence of high local concentration of heparin.
5. Firmly push plunger down as far as it will go.	5. This ensures administration of total dose of heparin.
6. When injection has been made, withdraw needle gently at the same angle at which it entered, releasing skin roll upon withdrawal of needle.	6. To minimize tissue damage.
7. Press an alcohol sponge to the site for a few seconds.	7. To minimize oozing or bleeding.
Follow-up Care	
1. *Do not rub the area. Instruct patient not to rub area.*	1. Rubbing would increase the likelihood of bleeding.
2. *Site of injection* a. Change site of injection each time heparin is administered. b. A chart can be marked with time, date, and measured dosage so that rotation of sites can be ensured. **Note:** Low dose heparin (5,000 units subcutaneously q 8 hours or 12 hours) may be used to prevent deep vein thrombosis postoperatively.	

Health Education

1. Information to be relayed to the physician before anticoagulant therapy is initiated:
    a. What medications are currently being taken? Note that barbiturates increase metabolism of coumarin medications—therefore an increased dose of anticoagulants is in order.
    b. What treatments are being done for problems other than circulatory problems?
    c. If female, whether a pregnancy is planned or confirmed?
    d. If other treatments are anticipated, such as major dental work, hemorrhoidectomy?
2. During anticoagulant therapy:
    a. Follow instructions carefully and take medications exactly as prescribed.
    b. Take medications at the same time each day and do not stop taking them even though symptomless.
    c. Wear a bracelet or carry a card indicating that anticoagulants are being taken; include name, address, and phone number of physician.
3. Notify the physician:
    a. In case of accident, infection, or other significant illness that may affect blood clotting.
    b. If surgical care by another physician or dentist is needed. Inform him that anticoagulants are being taken.
    c. If a dose of anticoagulant is forgotten. Do not take extra pills to make up for a skipped dose.
    d. In case of diarrhea, upset stomach, high fever.
4. Avoid:
    a. Taking any other medications without first checking with physician, particularly
        (1) Vitamins

(2) Aspirin
(3) Mineral oil
(4) Cold medicines
(5) Antibiotics
(6) Phenylbutazone (Butazolidin)
    b. Excessive use of alcohol, since alcohol may affect clotting capacity; check on acceptable limits for social drinking.
    c. Participation in activities in which there is high risk or injury.
    d. Foods that may cause diarrhea or upset stomach.
  5. Be alert for these warning signs:
    a. Excessive bleeding that does not stop quickly (such as following shaving, a small cut, teeth brushing with gum injury, nose bleed)
    b. Excessive menstrual bleeding

c. Skin discoloration or bruises that appear suddenly
d. Black or bloody bowel movements; for questionable stool discoloration, use Hemoccult test tape
e. Blood in urine

▶ **NURSING ALERT:** Patients taking phenindione produce orange or beige-colored urine; when the urine is acidified, this coloration disappears. With true hematuria, acid does not affect color.

    f. Faintness, dizziness, or unusual weakness
  6. A reminder:
      Later, when anticoagulant medication is stabilized, the patient must be reminded to keep prothrombin test appointments as scheduled—once a week or however often they are required.

Conditions of the Veins

Phlebitis, Thrombophlebitis, Phlebothrombosis

Note: While the terms do not necessarily represent identical pathologies, for clinical purposes they are used interchangeably when discussing the same process.

Phlebothrombosis is the formation of a thrombus or thrombi in a vein; in general, the clotting is related to (1) stasis, (2) abnormality of the walls of the vein(s), and (3) abnormality of clotting mechanism. Deep veins of the lower extremities are most commonly involved.

Deep vein thrombosis (*DVT*) is the thrombosis of deep rather than superficial veins. Two serious complications are pulmonary embolism (p. 168) and postphlebitic syndrome (p. 365).

Phlebitis is an inflammation of the walls of a vein.

Thrombophlebitis is a condition in which a clot forms in a vein secondary to phlebitis or because of partial obstruction of the vein.

Etiology

1. Venous stasis—following operations, childbirth, or bed rest for any chronic illness
2. Prolonged sitting or as a complication of varicose veins
3. Injury (bruise) to a vein; may result from direct trauma to veins from IV injections, indwelling catheters
4. Extension of an infection of tissues surrounding the vessel
5. Continuous pressure of a tumor, aneurysm, heavy pregnancy
6. Unusual activity in a person who has been sedentary
7. Hypercoagulability associated with malignant disease, blood dyscrasias
Basically, there are 3 causes: stasis, injury to a vessel wall, and hypercoagulability (or a combination of these factors).

High-Risk Factors

1. Hip fracture
2. Prosthetic joint replacement
3. Malignancy
4. Major surgery after age 40
5. Acute myocardial infarction
6. Thrombotic cerebrovascular accident
7. Previous venous insufficiency
8. Contraceptives (oral)

Assessment
Clinical Manifestations

1. For phlebothrombosis, there are no clinical signs, since there is no inflammation.
2. Slight swelling around ankle; obvious prominence of leg veins in affected leg.
3. Calf pain may be aggravated when foot is dorsiflexed with the knee flexed. Unfortunately, this is no clear sign of early or positive thrombosis. In some patients with obvious thrombophlebitis, this sign is not present, and in other kinds of involvement (irritation of sciatic nerve roots and myositis), the sign may be positive.
4. Muscle ache—may be falsely assumed to result from wearing flat bedroom slippers postoperatively (Fig. 9-39A).

Nursing Assessment

1. Inspect the lower extremities by removing top bedding from foot end up to the patient's groin (remove any temperature-controlling devices such as heavy wool socks, ice bag, at least 10 minutes before clinical inspection).
2. Note symmetry or asymmetry
      Measure and record leg circumferences daily (see Guidelines: Obtaining Leg Measurements to Detect Early Swelling)—mark on skin with felt-tip pen where the measuring tape is used so that the same area is measured each time.
3. Observe for evidence of venous distention or edema, puffiness, stretched skin, hardness to touch.
4. Hand test extremities for temperature variations.
    a. The examiner's hands should be placed in cold water and then dried.
    b. Hands are then placed simultaneously on each leg—first compare ankles, then move to the calf and up to the knee.
5. Examine for signs of obstruction due to occluding thrombus—swelling, particularly in loose connective tissue of popliteal space, ankle, or suprapubic area.

Patient Problems/Nursing Diagnosis

1. Ischemia and pain related to impaired circulation
2. Possible alteration in tissue perfusion related to ischemia
3. Impaired physical mobility related to pathophysio-

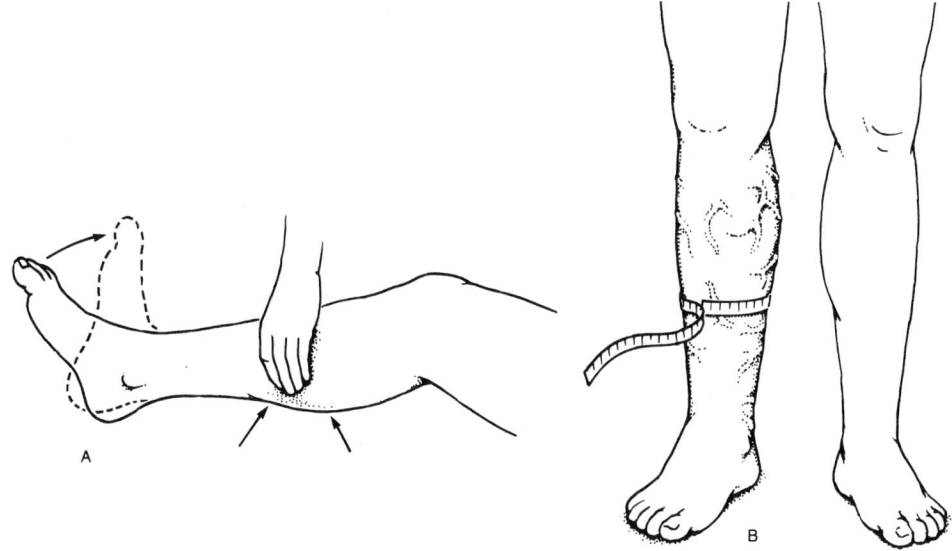

Figure 9-39. Assessment of signs and symptoms of phlebothrombosis. (A) With the knee flexed, the patient may complain of pain in the calf on dorsiflexion of foot (Homans' sign)—this was considered an unmistakable sign of early and subclinical thrombosis; it may or may not be present. Gentle compression reveals tenderness of the calf muscles (note arrow). (B) The affected leg may swell; veins are more prominent and may be palpated easily.

logic problem causing reduced blood supply to the extremities.

4. Potential nonadherence to the rehabilitation program related to lack of understanding and nonacceptance of required lifestyle changes.

Planning and Implementation
Nursing Intervention

A. Early resolution of thrombi and prevention of sequelae

1. Avoid massaging or rubbing calf because of the danger of breaking up the clot, which can then circulate as an embolus.
2. Consult physician concerning proper position of the extremity, since there may be differences of opinion.
   a. Some recommend elevation—reduces venous congestion and edema.
   b. Others do not recommend elevation—because of the possibility of releasing emboli.
3. If prescribed, apply heat in the form of hot, wet dressings or a heat cradle to promote circulation and comfort.
4. Place the patient on anticoagulant therapy (see p. 360).

▶ **NURSING ALERT:** This may not be done preoperatively because of fear of increasing possibility of hemorrhage during operation. Mini-doses of heparin may be prescribed.

5. Encourage early ambulation of surgical patients— encourage leg exercises for the bedridden patient, to prevent venous stasis.
6. Suggest deep-breathing exercises that produce increased negative pressure in the thorax, which in turn assists in emptying large veins.
7. Recommend properly applied pressure gradient stockings to increase deep venous blood circulation. (Remove twice daily and check for skin changes or calf tenderness.)
8. Utilize electrical stimulation of calf and pneumatic compression of leg if prescribed.

Guidelines: Obtaining Leg Measurements to Detect Early Swelling

Purpose   To obtain leg measurements for serial data compilation that may detect early swelling and thus indicate onset of thrombophlebitis.

Equipment

Flexible tape measure in centimeters/inches
Black felt-tip pen

Procedure

Preparatory Phase

1. Instruct patient to lie in dorsal recumbent position

(continued)

Guidelines: Obtaining Leg Measurements to Detect Early Swelling (continued)

Procedure
(Cont.)

Nursing Action	Rationale/Amplification
Performance Phase	
1. On admission of the patient, measure the circumference of the ankle, calf, and thigh.	1. This will provide baseline data.
2. Obtain measurements at the widest part of the ankle, calf, and thigh.	2. To provide a consistent anatomical place of measurement; some clinics have a predetermined starting point, such as 15 or 20 cm. from the knee cap.
3. Mark the leg with a black felt-tip pen.	3. To promote accuracy of measurements.
4. Thereafter, when measuring, place the measuring tape on the marked line.	
5. Repeat measurements taken on admission the next morning before any patient activity.	5. Otherwise, later measurements may give a false reading because of gravitational edema.
6. Thereafter, obtain measurements weekly unless there is evidence of swelling, in which case it is done daily.	6. Weekly—to detect swelling. Daily—to monitor swelling and its response to treatment.
7. Record measurements:	

Leg Measurements

Date:

Time: Right   Left

Ankle _____	cm/inches	Ankle _____	cm/inches
Calf _____	cm/inches	Calf _____	cm/inches
Thigh _____	cm/inches	Thigh _____	cm/inches

Nursing Action	Rationale/Amplification
8. Compare measurements: a. Check one leg with the other. b. Check each leg with baseline data.	*Significant Findings:* 1.5 cm. (males) difference between legs or compared with baseline 1.2 cm. (females) difference between legs or compared with baseline

9. Practice prophylactic measures for bedridden patients who are prone to develop thrombosis:
   a. Lie in bed in the slightly reversed Trendelenburg position because it is better for the veins to be full of blood than empty.
   b. Place a footboard across the foot of the bed.
   c. Instruct the patient to press the balls of the feet against the footboard, just as if he were rising up on his toes.
   d. Then have the patient relax the foot.
   e. Request that the patient do this many times a day.

Health Education

Teach the patient as follows:

A. Increase venous return from lower extremities

1. Prevent venous stasis by proper positioning in bed.
   a. Support full length of legs when they are to be elevated (Fig. 9-40).
   b. Prevent bony prominence of one leg from pressing on soft tissue of other leg (in side-lying position, place a soft pillow between legs).
   c. Avoid hyperflexion at knee as in jackknife position (head up, knees up, pelvis and legs down); this promotes stasis in pelvis and extremities.
2. Initiate active exercises, *unless contraindicated,* in which case use passive exercises.
   a. If the patient is on bed rest:
      (1) Simulate walking if lying on back—5 minutes every 2 hours.

   (2) Simulate bicycle pedaling if lying on side— 5 minutes every 2 hours.
   b. If contraindicated, resort to passive exercises— 5 minutes every 2 hours.
   c. If permissible, have the patient sit up and move to side of bed in sitting position.
      Provide a foot support (stool or chair)—dangling of feet is not desirable, since pressure may be exerted against popliteal vessels and may cause obstruction to blood flow.
   d. If the patient is permitted out of bed, encourage him to walk 10 minutes each hour; otherwise, carry out passive exercises.
   e. Discourage crossing of legs because compression of vessels can restrict blood flow.

B. Avoid further injury to damaged vessel walls

1. Promote circulation and prevent stasis by applying elastic hose.
   Apply elastic hose or elastic bandage from the toes up the leg; support must be consistent along entire leg.

▶ **NURSING ALERT: Elastic hose have no role in the management of the acute phase of deep venous thrombosis, but are of value once ambulation has begun. Their use will minimize or delay the development of the postphlebitic syndrome.**

2. Avoid straining or any maneuver that increases venous pressure in the leg. Eliminate the necessity to strain

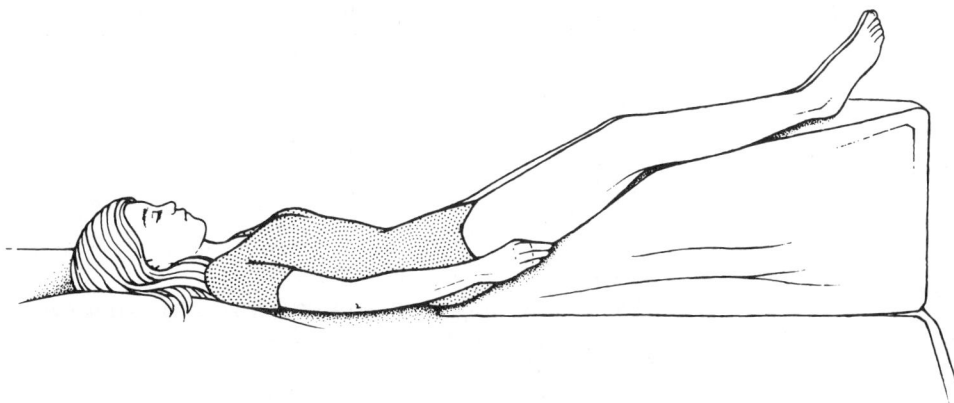

Figure 9-40. This leg elevator is of foam construction with a removable cotton cover that may be machine washed. It is clamped to the lower end of the mattress. This position is anatomically correct and provides adequate support to all parts of the leg. Edema and stasis of the lower extremities can be controlled. (Courtesy of Jobst)

at stool by providing increased fiber in the diet and administer stool softeners if necessary.
3. Also follow Planning and Implementation—Vascular Disorders, p. 356.

Evaluation
Expected Outcomes

1. Achieves resolution of thrombi; avoids rubbing calf; performs exercises
2. Avoids trauma or injury to extremities; practices prescribed exercises, does not cross legs, takes stool softeners, wears proper footwear, reports injuries to leg

Chronic Venous Insufficiency
(Postphlebitic Syndrome)

Postphlebitic syndrome is a form of chronic venous stasis; it may be a residual effect of phlebitis. It results from chronic occlusion of the veins or destruction of the valves.

Etiology

1. Smaller vessels have dilated because main channel for returning blood from the leg to the heart was blocked by a thrombus.
2. Valves of diseased veins can no longer prevent backflow, thereby leading to → chronic venous stasis → swelling and edema → superficial varicose veins.
3. Lower leg becomes discolored because of venous stasis and pigmentation ulceration (postphlebitis).

Altered Physiology and Clinical Manifestations

1. Pressure in veins at ankle is much greater than normal when leg is dependent—leads to transudation of fluid from intravascular to interstitial space.
2. Stasis, intractable induration, chronic edema, discoloration, pain, venous congestion, ulceration, recurrent thrombosis → cellulitis.
3. The medial malleolus is the most common site.

Diagnostic Evaluation

1. Noninvasive screening—Doppler, plethysmography (see pp. 353–356).

Treatment and Nursing Management

1. Best treatment is prevention of phlebitis and constant use of compression if phlebitis has occurred.
2. After this syndrome has developed, only palliative and symptomatic treatment is possible because the damage is irreparable.
3. *Health Education*
   Instruct the patient as follows:
   a. Wear elastic stockings to prevent edema.
   b. Avoid sitting or standing for long periods of time.
   c. Elevate legs on a chair for 5 minutes every 2 hours.
   d. Elevate legs above level of head by lying down (2–3 times daily).
   e. Raise foot of bed 15–20 cm. (6–8 inches) at night to allow venous drainage by gravity.
   f. Apply bland, oily lotions to prevent scaling and dryness of skin.
   g. Avoid constricting bandages.
   h. Prevent injury, bruising, scratching, or other trauma to skin of leg and foot.

Varicose Veins

Primary varicose veins—bilateral dilatation and elongation of saphenous veins; deeper veins are normal. As the condition progresses, because of hydrostatic pressure and vein weakness, the vein walls become distended, with asymmetrical dilatation, and some of the valves become incompetent. The process is irreversible.

Incidence

This is a common venous disorder of the lower extremity; over the age of 40, 20% of women and 7% of men develop varicose veins.

Etiology

1. Dilatation of the vein prevents the valve cusps from meeting; this results in increased back-up pressure, which is passed into the next lower segment of the vein. The combination of vein dilatation and valve incompetence produces the varicosity (Fig. 9-41).
2. Varicosities may occur elsewhere in the body (esoph-

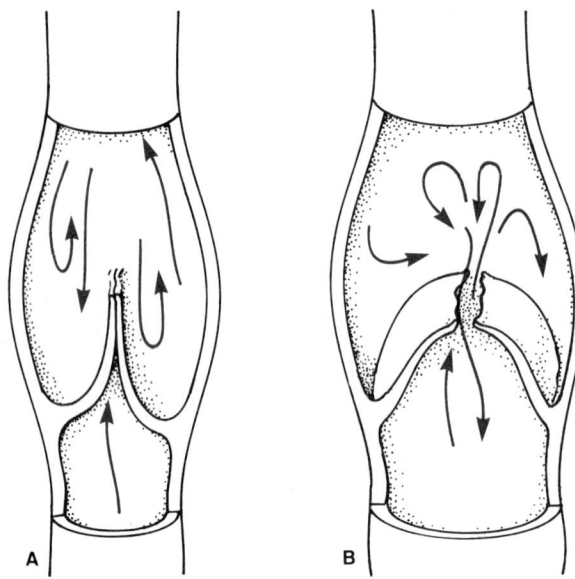

Figure 9-41. Valve incompetence develops as dilatation of a vessel prevents effective approximation of valve cusps. (A) Closed venous valve. (B) Incompetent venous valve.

ageal and hemorrhoidal veins) when flow or pressure is abnormally high.
3. Predisposing factors
    a. Hereditary weakness of vein wall or valves
    b. Long-standing distention of veins brought about by pregnancy, obesity, or prolonged standing
    c. Old age—loss of tissue elasticity

Assessment

Clinical Manifestations

1. Disfigurement due to large, discolored, tortuous leg veins
2. Easy leg fatigue, cramps in leg, heavy feeling, increased pain during menstruation, nocturnal muscle cramps

Diagnostic Evaluation

1. *Walking tourniquet test*—to demonstrate presence or absence of valvular incompetence of communicating veins.
    a. A penrose drain is snugly fastened around the lower extremity just above the highest noted varicosities.
    b. The patient is directed to walk briskly for 2 minutes.
    c. Failure of varicosities to empty suggests valvular incompetence of communicating veins distal to Penrose drain.
2. *Photoplethysmography*—a noninvasive technique to observe venous flow hemodynamics by noting changes in the blood content of the skin. It can be done rapidly, is inexpensive and highly reproducible.
3. *Doppler ultrasound*—can detect accurately and rapidly the presence or absence of venous reflux in deep or superficial vessels.
4. *Venous outflow and reflux plethysmography*—able to detect deep venous occlusion.
5. *Ascending and descending venography*—an invasive

technique that can also demonstrate venous occlusion and patterns of collateral flow.
   This test is expensive; it may not be required if a careful history, physical examination, and laboratory testing are done.

Complications

1. Leg edema, pain from superficial thrombosis
2. Hemorrhage due to the weakening of the vein wall and pressure upon it
3. Skin infection and breakdown, producing ulcers (rare in primary varices)

Patient Problems/Nursing Diagnoses

1. Pain related to venous insufficiency and venous stasis
2. Edema related to chronic venous insufficiency
3. Potential for injury and infection of extremities related to impaired venous return
4. Impaired physical mobility related to pain and chronic swelling

Planning and Implementation

Medical Management and Nursing Interventions

The patient is instructed to:
1. Avoid activities that cause venous stasis by obstructing venous flow.
    a. Wearing tight garters, tight girdle
    b. Sitting or standing for prolonged periods of time
    c. Crossing the legs at knees for prolonged periods while sitting (reduces circulation by 15%)
2. Control excessive weight gain.
3. Wear firm elastic support as prescribed, from toe to thigh when in upright position.
    a. Put elastic stockings on in bed before getting up.
    b. Waist-high elastic support hose are available and may be useful.
4. Elevate foot of bed 15–20 cm. (6–8 inches) for night sleeping.
5. Avoid injuring legs.

Surgical Management and Nursing Implementation

1. Indications
    a. Progressively advancing varicosities
    b. Stasis ulceration
    c. Cosmetic needs
2. Modalities—A single method or combination of methods is tailored to meet the needs of the individual:
    a. *Sclerosing injection*—not used as frequently today; may be combined with ligation or limited to treatment of isolated varicosities. The affected vessel may be sclerosed by injecting sodium tetradecyl sulfate or similar sclerosing agent. Compression bandage is then applied without interruption for 6 weeks; inflamed endothelial surfaces adhere by direct contact.
    b. *Multiple vein ligation.*
    c. *Ligation and stripping* of the greater and/or lesser saphenous systems. This is the most effective procedure.
    d. Some physicians are using the *laser* beam to treat varicosities.
3. Preoperative patient care
    a. Prepare the skin at least 12 hours prior to surgery by thoroughly cleansing the lower abdomen and

legs with a detergent–germicidal soap. This may be done by shower or local scrub.

b. Hair removal may be by depilatory or shave according to surgeon's request.

c. Have the patient prepared on the day before surgery (and after his daily skin cleansing) for the surgeon to mark his skin with a felt-tip pen (indelible). Usually, the patient stands on a chair in good light so that the incision site, paths of veins, dilated tributaries, etc. can be marked to aid the surgeon during the operation.

4. Postoperative nursing care and patient support

a. At first, the legs are encased in pressure bandages from the toes to the groin; this is followed by knee-level elastic stockings for 3–4 weeks after surgery.

b. Elevate the legs about 30 degrees and provide adequate support of the entire leg.

c. Observe the patient for complaints of pain in specific areas of the foot or ankle; if the elastic bandage is too tight, loosen the bandage—later, have it reapplied.

d. Observe circulation to detect constriction or hemorrhage.

e. Activate the individualized therapeutic plan for the following:

(1) Permit ambulation according to the preoperative condition of the skin and subcutaneous tissues; if skin is healthy, bathroom privileges are usually permitted the day after surgery.

(2) Discourage dangling of the legs because it causes stasis of blood in the lower leg.

(3) Encourage the patient to walk with a normal gait; offer support if necessary; this activity should be progressive, depending on tolerance.

f. If there are significant trophic changes in the leg, due to long-term varicosities (past history), postoperative care requires more bed rest and slow ambulation; in this event, leg and foot exercises in bed are helpful.

g. Note that complaints of patchy numbness can be expected but should disappear in less than a year.

h. Recognize that varicosities may recur; therefore, conservative measures, learned preoperatively, should be continued.

i. Follow-up visits every 6 months are urged.

Evaluation
Expected Outcomes

1. Reduces leg fatigue and cramps by limiting standing, avoiding restricting garments that impede leg circulation, and maintaining proper weight

2. Recovers from surgical treatment, if indicated—demonstrates improved circulation, performs exercises, and gradually ambulates as tolerated

3. Adheres to the safeguards as taught and plans to have follow-up visits every 6 months

Stasis Ulcers

Stasis ulcer is an excavation of the skin surface produced by sloughing of inflammatory necrotic tissue, usually caused by vascular insufficiency in the lower extremity.

Incidence

1. Occurrence is increasing, particularly in the older age-group.

2. Postphlebitic syndrome and stasis account for most leg ulcers.

3. Other causes include obstruction of one of the main veins by pregnancy or abdominal tumor, incompetency of valves of the ileofemoral vein, burns, sickle cell anemia, neurogenic disorders.

4. Hereditary factors also play a role in the predisposition of certain individuals.

Prevention

1. Prevent edema—in stasis dermatitis, pruritus and scaling pigmentation may be the only manifestations; bed rest and a 30-degree elevation of the lower extremity may alleviate the edema.

2. Avoid trauma.

Assessment
Diagnostic Evaluation

1. Noninvasive screening—Doppler and plethysmography (see pp. 353–354).

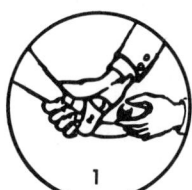 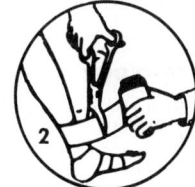 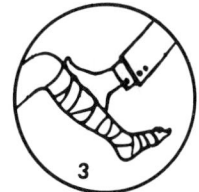 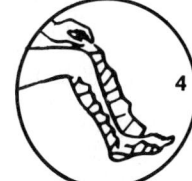

1. Apply right from can. Hold knee in slight flexion. Pad instep and ankle with cotton wad. Start at inner ankle. Make overlapping turns. Figure of eight turn around ankle joint. Use firm equal compression up to the knee.

2. If a turn does not fit snugly, nip the edges with scissors or cut bandage off and start a new turn.

3. Mold cast during application with free hand until cast appears even and smooth. Make a cut 5 cm. (2″) long below knee to avoid constriction. Cover cast with loosely woven gauze bandage.

4. Patient can be fully ambulatory. Boot is usually changed once a week. Remove by cutting with scissors.

Figure 9-42. Application of gelatin compression boot. (Manufactured by Graham-Field Surgical Co., Inc., New Hyde Park, NY)

Patient Problems/Nursing Diagnoses

1. Impaired skin integrity related to vascular insufficiency
2. Pain related to inflamed leg ulcer

Planning and Implementation

Nursing Interventions

A. Reducing inflammation

1. Elevate the leg and maintain bed rest.
2. Initiate proper cleansing routine.
   a. Handle leg very gently.
   b. Use mild soap, warm water, and cotton balls.
3. Remove devitalized tissue.
   a. Flush out necrotic materials with hydrogen peroxide.
   b. Apply enzymatic ointments such as fibrinolysin and desoxyribonuclease (Elase), and proteolytic enzymes with neomycin (Biozyme; prescribed in some clinics).

B. Promoting healing

1. Again, elevation of the extremity is most important.
2. Participate in physiotherapy and maintain a regular exercise program.
3. Control excess weight and provide proper vitamin and protein dietary supplements.
4. Apply gold leaf (done in some clinics) directly over ulcer site to stimulate formation of granulation tissue.
5. Check with individual physician for specific therapy; treatment varies from clinic to clinic.

6. Use sterile saline compresses if area is inflamed or oozing.
7. Apply compression bandages to the leg (gelatin compression boot—Fig. 9-42).
8. Some clinics prefer moist dressings using aqueous solution of aluminum subacetate 0.25% because it is inexpensive, bacteriostatic, and nonmacerating to adjacent skin.

Health Education

1. Stress the importance of following explicitly the recommendations of the physician–nurse team.
2. Explain the hazards of trying other remedies on his own at home.
3. Indicate that the treatment may be long but that patience is an important aspect.
4. Maintain healthy tissue when the ulcer is healed by continuing with the safeguards practiced before, because breakdown of healthy tissue, unfortunately, frequently occurs.

Evaluation

Expected Outcome

1. Relates that pain is relieved
2. Promotes healing by elevating the extremity as prescribed, participates in physiotherapy, and maintains prescribed diet
3. Controls infections by using aseptic technique when changing dressings; wears gelatin compression boot as prescribed.

Conditions of the Arteries

Arterial Embolism

Etiology

1. Arterial emboli usually (about 85%) originate from thrombi in the heart chambers.
2. Arteriosclerosis may cause roughening or ulceration of atheromatous plaques, which can lead to emboli.

Clinical Manifestations

May vary from:
1. The patient's being totally unaware of the event, to
2. Acute pain—severe, to
3. Loss of function—motor and sensory
   a. Paralysis of part ⎫ Due to embolic block of
   b. Anesthesia of part ⎬ artery
   c. Pallor and coldness ⎭ Due to associated vasomotor reflex

Also see Table on Acute Arterial Occlusion, p. 369.

Treatment

Note: This is an emergency and is life-threatening; it requires immediate operative intervention if the embolus has major effect.

1. Heparin should be administered intravenously to reduce tendency of emboli to form or expand—useful in smaller arteries.
2. Protect the extremity by keeping it at or below the horizontal plane; protect leg from hard surfaces and tight or heavy overlying bed linens.
3. Administer analgesics as prescribed for relief of pain.
4. Prepare the patient for surgery; surgical intervention (embolectomy) is essential when an embolus blocks a large artery, such as the iliac (Fig. 9-43).

Arteriosclerosis and Atherosclerosis

Arteriosclerosis is an arterial disease manifested by a loss of elasticity and a hardening of the vessel wall.

Atherosclerosis is the most common type of arteriosclerosis, manifested by the formation of atheromas (patchy lipoidal degeneration of the intima).

Significance

1. Arteriosclerosis is the chief cause of death in the US.
2. One of the major clinical manifestations of arteriosclerosis is coronary heart disease (CHD).
3. Studies indicate that arteriosclerotic heart disease is partially preventable if attention is paid to "risk" factors.

Etiology

(A combination of many factors)
1. Predisposition to arteriosclerosis is thought by many authorities to be inheritable (genetics).
2. Other etiologic factors include metabolic disturbances, arterial hypertension, platelet capability of initiating formation of atherosclerotic lesions.

Risk Factors

1. Age—death rate in white males, ages 25–34, is 10 per 100,000
   death rate in white males, ages 55–64, is 1,000 per 100,000
2. Sex—death rate (ages 35–44) is 6 times greater in white males than in females
3. Impaired glucose tolerance (diabetes mellitus)

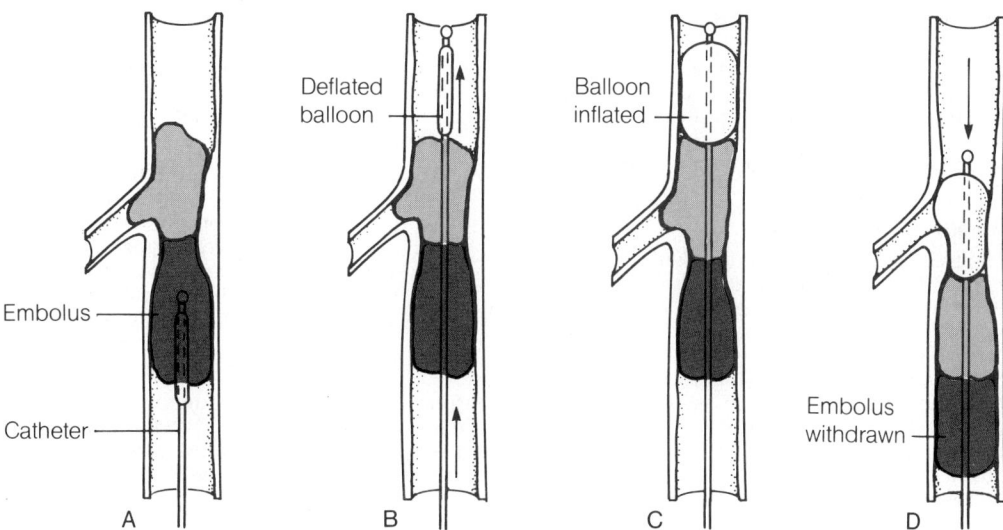

Figure 9-43. Extracting an embolus from a vessel can be done with the use of a Fogarty embolectomy catheter. The catheter with a soft deflated balloon near the tip is threaded through the artery via an arteriotomy. (*A&B*) It is passed through the embolus and its thrombus; (*C*) it is then inflated. (*D*) A steady pull downward withdraws the embolus along with the catheter.

Differential Diagnosis of Acute Iliofemoral Venous Thrombosis, Acute Arterial Occlusion, and Acute Lymphangitis and Cellulitis

Manifestation	Acute Iliofemoral Venous Thrombosis	Acute Arterial Occlusion	Acute Lymphangitis and Cellulitis
Size of limb	Enlarged	Shrunken	Enlarged
Color of limb	Normal or cyanotic	Pale at onset; later may be mottled, cyanotic	Red
Skin temperature of limb	Usually normal	Low	High
Superficial veins	Prominent and distended	Collapsed	Usually not affected
Arterial pulsations	Usually normal	Lacking	Normal
Chills	Rare	Lacking	Frequent at onset
Fever	Slight to moderate, rarely more than 39°C (102°F)	Usually lacking	Usually high, 39.5 to 40.5°C. (103–105°F.)

(From Kazmier FI, and Juergens JL. Venous thrombosis and obstructive diseases of the veins. In Juergens JL, Spittell JA Jr and Fairbairn JF II [eds]. Peripheral Vascular Disease, 5th ed., Philadelphia, WB Saunders, 1980)

4. Hypertension
5. A relatively large amount of cholesterol in the low-density lipoprotein fraction (serum)
6. Obesity
7. Cigarette smoking
8. Physical inactivity—since substantial collateral circulation is not established
9. Emotional tension
10. High salt intake

Altered Physiology

1. Arteriosclerosis → narrowing of arterial vessels → malnutrition of tissue cells → ischemic necrosis → fibrosis → sclerosis.
2. Sclerosis → degeneration of major organs because of lack of blood supply (nutrition): brain, myocardium, kidney.
3. Fatty streaks develop in the subintimal region.
4. Fibrous plaques of cholesterol, fatty acids, and often

calcium form on intima of arterial vessels (atherosclerosis).

5. Dislodging of plaque may occur, or a thrombus may be formed near the plaque; subsequent embolus may cause arterial occlusion and infarction in distant body sites.
6. After menopause, women are no longer protected by estrogen.

General Patient Assessment

1. Arteriosclerosis is a generalized vascular disease; however, it varies from patient to patient in that it may affect one area more than another.
2. Often, it limits itself to a segment of the vascular tree.
3. Five areas that are the most dangerous and cause disturbing symptoms are:
   a. Brain—cerebroarteriosclerosis
   b. Heart—coronary artery disease
   c. Gastrointestinal tract
   d. Kidneys
   e. Extremities
4. Prognosis depends on extent of pathology and area of involvement.

Treatment

1. Since arteriosclerosis and atherosclerosis affect many different parts of the body, treatment is described where the major condition occurs. For example: angina pectoris and myocardial infarction are brought about by atherosclerosis of coronary arteries; treatment is discussed under the disease entity.
2. Operative reconstruction of involved vessels.

Health Education

Attention is directed to reducing risk factors by avoiding tension, reducing excess weight, giving up cigarette smoking, controlling diabetes, and adjusting diet to reduce cholesterol intake (Table 9-2).

Table 9-2   Fat- and Cholesterol-Controlled Diet

A variety of foods may be selected from each of the Basic Four Food Groups. Emphasize those foods listed in the "Suggested" column.

Meat, Poultry, Fish, Dried Beans and Peas, Eggs

Suggested	Avoid or Use Infrequently
For 100-mg. cholesterol diet, limit flesh foods to 3 oz. daily. For 200-mg. cholesterol diet, limit flesh foods to 6–8 oz daily	Duck, goose, shrimp
Most often: chicken, turkey, or cornish game hen (no skin), veal, fish, shellfish (except shrimp)	Fatty meats (e.g., heavily marbled beef, spare ribs, frankfurters, sausage, bacon, bologna and other lunch meats, regular hamburger, canned corn beef)
A few times a week: very lean beef, lamb, pork, ham if all visible meat fat is discarded	Organ meats
*Dried peas, beans, lentils—prepared with allowed ingredients	Beans prepared with salt pork or bacon
*Peanut butter (count as a fat choice)	Egg yolks, whole eggs
*Egg whites as desired	
*Egg substitute (e.g., Egg Beaters)	

Vegetables and Fruit—At Least 4 Servings Daily, Including Sources of Vitamins C and A

Suggested	Avoid or Use Infrequently
All types of fruits and vegetables may be used (unless prepared with restricted ingredients): fresh, frozen, canned, dried	Vegetables in butter, cream, or cheese sauce
	Vegetables fried in saturated fat

Bread and Cereals (Whole Grain, Enriched, or Fortified)—At Least 4 Servings Daily

Suggested	Avoid or Use Infrequently
*Breads: whole wheat, rye, pumpernickel, oatmeal, white enriched, French, Italian, raisin, English muffins, bagels, hard rolls	Egg bread, cheese bread, egg bagels
*Cereal (hot or cold), rice, bulghur, barley	Commercial biscuits, muffins, doughnuts, butter rolls, sweet rolls
*Pasta: spaghetti, macaroni, ziti, and so forth	Commercial granola, Cracklin' Bran
*Melba toast, matzo, pretzels	Egg noodles
Biscuits, muffins, and so forth, made at home using allowed ingredients, in moderation (a source of fat)	Snack crackers
	Commercial mixes containing dried eggs, whole milk, and/or shortening

Milk Products—Adults Should Use 500 ml. (2 or more cups) or the Equivalent Daily

Suggested	Avoid or Use Infrequently
Skim milk dairy products: fortified skim (nonfat) milk or milk powder, buttermilk, evaporated skim milk, chocolate-flavored skim milk, yogurt made with skim milk	Whole milk and whole milk products: chocolate milk, canned evaporated whole milk, ice cream, cream of any type, whole milk yogurt
Cheeses made from skim milk: cottage cheese (rinsed regular cottage cheese may be substituted), farmer's, baker's or hoop cheese; sapsago cheese	Most nondairy cream substitutes
Cheese substitutes made with corn oil, in moderation	Cheeses made from cream or whole milk

Table 9-2 Fat- and Cholesterol-Controlled Diet (continued)

Fats and Oils (Polyunsaturated)—Limit total amount used, including that used in cooking, so that fat content of diet does not exceed prescribed amount (e.g., 20% or 30% of calories)

Suggested	Avoid or Use Infrequently
*Polyunsaturated vegetable oils: corn oil, cottonseed oil, safflower oil, sesame seed oil, soybean oil, sunflower seed oil, walnut oil	Solid fats and shortenings: butter, hard margarine and vegetable shortening with a low P/S ratio (i.e., 3:2 or lower), lard, salt pork, meat fat, coconut oil, palm oil
*Margarines and liquid oil shortenings made with an allowed oil and having a high P/S ratio (i.e., about 2:1 or above)	(Peanut oil and olive oil are not saturated or polyunsaturated. They may be used occasionally for flavor.)
Salad dressings made with allowed ingredients, mayonnaise (omitted on 100-mg. cholesterol diet)	Creamy and cheese salad dressings
Soups and sauces: clear fat-free broth, fat-free vegetable soup, chicken noodle, and rice soup (fat removed)	Cream soup, commercial chowder

Desserts, Beverages, Snacks, Condiments

Acceptable If Calories Allow	Avoid or Use Infrequently
*Cocoa powder, fruit whip, gelatin, puddings made with nonfat milk, water ice	Chocolate, whole milk puddings, ice cream (ice milk is sometimes allowed)
*Jelly, jam, marmalade, honey, hard candy, angel food cake, most types of nuts	Chocolate candy, caramels, butterscotch
Homemade baked desserts using allowed ingredients	Coconut, macadamia nuts, cashews
*Carbonated beverages, fruit drinks, wine,† beer,† whisky†	Commercial cakes, pies, cookies, and mixes
	Potato chips and other commercial fried snacks

Negligible Calorie Content

*Tea, herb tea, coffee, decaffeinated coffee

Herbs, spices, vinegar, mustard, small amounts of ketchup and barbecue sauce, horseradish, meat sauce, soy sauce

* Free of cholesterol.
† With approval of physician.
(Suitor CW and Hunter MF. Nutrition: Principles and Application in Health Promotion, 2nd ed, pp. 608–609. Philadelphia, JB Lippincott, 1984)

Percutaneous Transluminal Angioplasty (PTA)

Percutaneous transluminal angioplasty (PTA) is a non-invasive technique designed to relieve arterial stenosis when lesions are accessible, as in superficial femoral and iliac arteries, through the use of special inflatable catheters (Gruntzig balloon).

A. Procedure

1. A balloon catheter is passed, usually via the common femoral artery, after a guidewire and angiographic catheter have been inserted under fluoroscopy. The balloon is then properly positioned.
2. The balloon is dilated with contrast material and inflated to exert pressure against the stenosed lesions of the arterial wall, thereby dilating the artery.
3. The catheter is then removed; heparin is injected through the angiographic catheter to prevent clots. Pressure is maintained at catheter entry site for 10 to 20 minutes.
4. The patient is instructed to lie flat for several hours.
5. After 8 hours, all restrictions are removed; aspirin and dipyridamole (Persantine) may be prescribed to reduce the possibility of recurrence by its vasodilating action.

B. Advantages

1. Short-term procedure under local anesthesia; the patient is able to resume normal activities the following day. Note the effect on vessel wall.
2. Useful in poor-risk (surgery) patients.
3. Cost-effective; causes minimal discomfort.

C. Disadvantages

1. Many lesions not suitable for this treatment modality.
2. Requires high-quality x-ray equipment and well-trained angiographic personnel.
3. Durability of treatment may be less than that of surgical intervention.

Occlusive Arterial Disease

Occlusive arterial disease is a form of arteriosclerosis in which the vascular system of the leg becomes blocked. Chronic occlusive arterial diseases occurs much more frequently than does acute (which is the sudden and complete blocking of a vessel by a thrombus or embolus).

Incidence

Parallels that of arteriosclerotic heart disease.

Clinical Manifestations

Symptoms appear gradually:
1. Intermittent claudication (see p. 353)
2. Coldness of extremity
3. Color change—pallor
4. Decrease in size of leg
5. Tingling, numbness of toes
6. Later—pain, even when leg is at rest; occurs at night, requiring patient to get out of bed to walk to relieve pain
7. Cramp-like excruciating pain in calf muscles
8. Ulcers of toes and feet develop

Diagnostic Evaluation

1. Vascular physical examination, including brachial and ankle systolic pressures, before and after exercise
2. Doppler ultrasound probe
3. Segmental plethysmography
4. Angiography

Treatment and Nursing Management

Goals:
1. Preserve the extremity.
2. Relieve the intermittent claudication.

See page 356, Nursing Management of Patients with Vascular Problems.

1. Where conservative measures clearly are not enough, constructive arterial surgery (endarterectomy, arterial bypass grafting, or a combination) may be required.
2. Percutaneous transluminal angioplasty (PTA) may be used alone or with reconstructive surgery for dilatation of localized noncalcified segments of narrowed arteries (see Procedure, p. 371).
3. Microvascular surgery may be required for small-artery occlusive disease.
4. Following any surgery, a conservative program to manage intermittent claudication may be initiated (walking, weight reduction, no smoking, control of other conditions such as hypertension, diabetes mellitus).

Vasospastic Disorder—Raynaud's Phenomenon

Raynaud's phenomenon is a general term to describe a condition in which there is an increased or unusual sensitivity to cold or emotional factors, and it occurs primarily in the hands, rarely in the feet.

Etiology

1. Unknown; there appears to be a hereditary predisposition.
2. Vasoconstriction appears to be mediated through release of catecholamines at the neuroarteriole junction.
3. An underlying problem such as a collagen vascular disease may exist.

Assessment

Clinical Manifestations and Diagnostic Evaluation

1. Intermittent arteriolar vasoconstriction resulting in coldness, pain, pallor.
2. Occasionally, there is ulceration of the finger tips.
3. The condition occurs most commonly in females between the age 16 and 40 years.
4. It occurs more frequently in cold climates and during winter months.
5. Involvement of the fingers appears to be asymmetric; thumbs are less often involved.
6. Characteristic color changes: blue–white–red
   a. Blue—cyanotic, relatively stagnant blood flow
   b. White—blanching, dead-white appearance if spasm is severe
   c. Red—a reactive hyperemia upon rewarming
7. The Allen test may provide clues to circulatory problems (Fig. 9-44).

Patient Problems/Nursing Diagnoses

1. Impairment of skin integrity (potential) related to the possibility of finger-tip ulceration

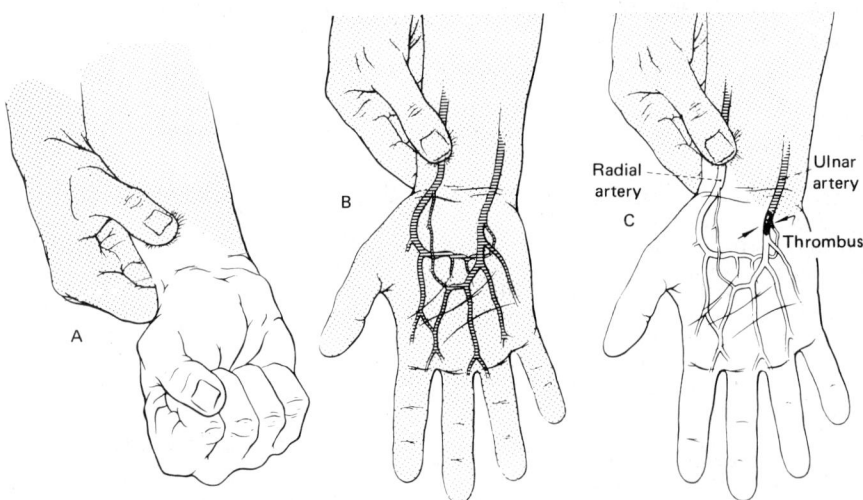

Figure 9-44. Allen test: Diagrammatic representation of the procedure (*A*) for determining patency of occlusion of the ulnar artery distal to the wrist.
(*B*) The ulnar artery is patent as determined by the prompt return of color to the skin of the hand while the radial artery is still compressed.
(*C*) Occlusion of the ulnar artery is demonstrated by persistence of pallor as long as the radial arterial inflow is blocked by the examiner's finger. (Modified from Juergens and Fairbairn: Arteriosclerosis Obliterans. Heart Bulletin 8:22–24. By permission of the American Heart Association)

2. Impaired physical mobility of hands related to intermittent arteriolar vasoconstriction
3. Knowledge deficit related to misunderstanding about precautions necessary to minimize discomfort, as well as to avoid precipitating factors

Planning and Implementation
Health Education

1. Avoid whatever provokes vasoconstriction of vessels of hands.
2. Prevent injury to hands, which can aggravate vasoconstriction and lead to ulceration.
3. Minimize exposure to cold, since this precipitates a reaction.
4. Wear warm clothing—boots, gloves, hooded jackets, when going out in cold weather.
   a. Turn heat on in automobile during travel.
   b. Shop in heated stores; avoid unheated buildings.
5. Avoid placing hands in cold water, the freezer, or the refrigerator unless protective gloves are worn.
6. Use extra precautions to avoid injuries to fingers and hands from needle pricks, knife cuts.
7. Varying benefits are reported with such medications as reserpine, methyldopa, tolazoline (Tazol), and phenoxybenzamine (Dibenzyline).

Medication	Adverse Effects
1. Phenoxybenzamine hydrochloride (Dibenzyline)	Headache, tachycardia, nasal congestion, orthostatic hypotension
2. Cyclandelate (Cyclospasmol)	Headache, nausea, heavier than usual perspiration, vertigo, flushing, tingling
3. Tolazoline hydrochloride (Tazol, Tolzol)	Gastrointestinal upset, orthostatic hypotension, chilliness, tachycardia, palpitations
4. Nifedipine (Procardia)	None apparent

Evaluation
Expected Outcomes

1. Avoids injury to hands
2. Follows prescribed therapy to avoid vasoconstriction of hands—especially careful about protecting hands in cold weather
3. Adheres to pharmacotherapy as prescribed.

Diseases of the Aorta*

Aortic Aneurysm

Aneurysm is a distention of an artery brought about by a weakening/destruction of the media of the arterial wall. It tends to enlarge, thereby producing serious complications by compressing surrounding structures or rupturing, causing a fatal hemorrhage.

Types of Aneurysms

Morphologically, they may be classified as follows:
1. Saccular—distention of a vessel projecting from one side
2. Fusiform—distention of the whole artery (i.e., entire circumference is involved)
3. Dissecting—hemorrhagic or intramural hematoma, separating the medial layers of the aortic wall

Etiology

1. Local infection, pyogenic or fungal (mycotic aneurysm)
2. Congenital weakness of vessels
3. Arteriosclerosis
4. Syphilis
5. Trauma

Aneurysm of the Thoracoabdominal Aorta

(Lower descending thoracic aorta and upper abdominal aorta)

A. Clinical Manifestations

1. Subjective symptoms
   a. At first no symptoms; later symptoms may come from congestive heart failure or a pulsating tumor mass in the chest.

   b. Pain and pressure symptoms
      (1) Constant, boring pain because of pressure, or
      (2) Intermittent and neuralgic pain because of infringement on nerves
   c. Dyspnea, causing pressure against trachea
   d. Cough, often paroxysmal and brassy in sound
   e. Hoarseness, voice weakness, or complete aphonia, resulting from pressure against recurrent laryngeal nerve
   f. Dysphagia due to impingement on esophagus
2. Objective signs
   a. Edema of chest wall—infrequent
   b. Dilated superficial veins on chest
   c. Cyanosis because of vein compression of chest vessels
   d. Ipsilateral dilatation of pupils due to pressure against cervical sympathetic chain
   e. Pulse difference in 2 wrists if aneurysm interferes with circulation in left subclavian artery
   f. Abnormal pulsation may be apparent on chest wall—due to erosion of aneurysm through rib cage—in syphilis

B. Management

1. The prognosis is poor for untreated patients.
2. Surgical—remove aneurysm and restore vascular continuity.
   Aortic arch aneurysms are the most difficult to treat.

Abdominal Aneurysm

A. Clinical Manifestations

1. Many of these patients are asymptomatic; most are males (9:1) in their 6th or 7th decade.
2. Abdominal pain is most common; persistent or inter-

* For aortic stenosis and aortic insufficiency, see page 322.

mittent—often localized in middle or lower abdomen to the left of midline.

3. Low back pain.
4. Feeling of an abdominal pulsating mass.
5. Hypertension may be in evidence.

B. Diagnostic Evaluation

1. Ordinarily the systolic blood pressure of the thigh exceeds that in the arm; in many of these patients, the opposite is true.
2. A palpable pulsating abdominal mass; fluoroscopy will reveal pulsating tumor.
3. Angioaortogram allows visualization of vessels and aneurysm.
4. Ultrasound allows visualization of vessels and aneurysm. This is the best test to confirm the presence of and check the size of abdominal aortic aneurysms. It is less expensive than other tests.
5. Computed tomography allows visualization of vessels and aneurysm.

C. Management

1. If untreated, the prognosis is poor.
2. Types of surgical intervention

   a. Excision of area affected
   b. Replacement of excised segment by a bypass (synthetic) graft

Dissecting Aneurysm of the Aorta

1. This is a type of aneurysm in which there is a tear in the intima of the aorta; as a result of pressure, blood splits the wall and may produce a large hematoma or may continue to rip the wall.
2. Symptoms may resemble coronary occlusion; diagnosis is confirmed by aortography.
3. Prognosis is poor, but surgical removal of involved aneurysm and replacement of segment with a graft may be effective.

Peripheral Vessel Aneurysms

1. May involve renal artery, subclavian artery, popliteal artery (knee) or any major artery.
2. These produce a pulsating mass and may cause pain or pressure on surrounding structures.
3. Replacement grafts are used to repair these aneurysms.

Hypertension

Hypertension is a disease of regulation in which the mechanisms that control arterial pressure within the normal range are deranged. Predominant mechanisms are the central nervous system, the renal pressor system (renin–angiotensin–aldosterone system), and extracellular fluid volume. Why these mechanisms fail is not known. The basic explanation is that blood pressure is elevated when there is increased cardiac output plus peripheral vessel resistance.

Essential (primary) hypertension refers to patients (over 90%) with high blood pressure of undetermined cause.

Community Health Concern

The cardiovascular mortality decline between 1972 and 1982 in the US can be attributed to improved high blood pressure control.

1. Undetected and uncontrolled hypertension can lead to heart attacks, heart failure, strokes, and renal failure.
2. Few patients with hypertension need to be hospitalized.
3. Most patients with hypertension do not have symptoms.
4. Most patients with hypertension need life-long treatment.
5. Early recognition and management of hypertension are essential in preventing end organ damage (brain, eye, heart, kidney).
6. The nurse is a prime agent in early detection of hypertension and patient education.

Normal Physiology

(See p. 380 for Blood Pressure Determination.)

1. *Normal blood pressure* (normotension) is the pressure of the blood within the systemic arterial system. It ranges from 100/60 to 140/90.
2. *Systolic pressure* represents the greatest pressure of

the blood against the wall of the vessel following ventricular contraction.
3. *Diastolic pressure* represents the least pressure of the blood against the wall of the vessel following closure of the aortic valve.
4. *Pulse pressure* represents the difference between the systolic and diastolic readings—the range of pressure in the arteries.
5. The *mean arterial pressure* is the average pressure attempting to push blood through the circulatory system.

   This can be determined electronically or mathematically, as well as by using an intra-arterial catheter and mercury manometer.
   Mathematical determination (slightly less than average of systolic and diastolic)
   Example: for a blood pressure of 130/85
   Mean arterial pressure is roughly 100 mm. Hg
   Kidney function requires a minimum of 70 mm. Hg (mean arterial pressure).
6. *Basal blood pressure* is the lowest blood pressure taken in supine position after several days of hospitalization without treatment.*

   Basal sitting pressure and basal standing pressure are often taken for later comparison.

---

* Most hypertensive patients admitted to the hospital are admitted for non–hypertension-related problems (i.e., breast surgery, total hip replacement, etc.). These patients are not routinely taken off their antihypertensive medications.

If the patient is admitted for evaluation of secondary hypertension or refractory hypertension, then all antihypertensive medications are cancelled, and basal pressures are obtained.

All patients going onto investigational antihypertensive medication are, if possible, "washed out" (medications cancelled for several days); most studies are done with these persons as outpatients.

Factors Affecting Pressure of Blood

Blood volume, peripheral resistance, blood viscosity, cardiac output.

1. Blood pressure = cardiac output × total peripheral resistance.
   a. Pressure varies with exercise, emotional reaction, sleep, digestion, time of day.
   b. Renal, adrenal, vascular, and neurogenic functions affect blood pressure.
2. Higher blood pressure = increased cardiac output × greater total peripheral resistance (circulatory overload).
3. Lower blood pressure = lessened cardiac output × lesser total peripheral resistance.
4. Increased diastolic pressure due to peripheral resistance indicates decrease in diameter of arterioles: These are affected by sympathetic stimulation, hereditary factors, more vasopressor hormones in the blood.
5. Increased systolic pressure indicates increased cardiac output and systolic hypertension, which is always secondary.

Etiology and the Significance of Blood Pressure Elevation

1. Cause of essential hypertension is unknown; however, there are several areas of investigation:
   a. Hyperactivity of sympathetic vasoconstricting nerves
   b. Presence of blood component containing a vasoconstrictor that acts on smooth muscle, sensitizing it to constrictor substances
   c. Increased cardiac output, followed by arteriole constriction
   d. Prostaglandins affect regulatory mechanisms, which include the renin–angiotensin system, renal sodium and water excretion, and vascular smooth muscle tone
   e. Familial (genetic) tendency
   f. Hypertensive vascular disease—modifications of both large elastic arteries (macroangiopathy) and small muscular arteries and arterioles (microangiopathy)
2. Individual tolerance of increased blood pressure varies; however, there is a direct correlation between increase in blood pressure and the rate at which atherosclerosis and arteriosclerosis develop.
3. Rising blood pressure adversely affects the brain, the heart, and the kidneys.
   a. Heart—myocardial infarction, congestive heart failure
   b. Kidney—nephrosclerosis, kidney failure
   c. Brain—headache (in some persons), encephalopathy, cerebral hemorrhage, cerebrovascular accident
   d. Eye—papilledema, swelling of optic disc
4. Emotional stress affects the central nervous system, and there may be increased cardiac output; increased catecholamines, etc. may account for increased peripheral vascular resistance.
5. Obesity and diabetes mellitus are associated with hypertension.

Prevalence and Risk Factors

1. Hypertension is one of the most prevalent chronic diseases for which treatment is available.
2. There is a higher incidence among blacks (2:1 ratio).
3. It appears that a high sodium intake is related to the development of hypertension; when sodium intake is decreased, blood pressure often decreases.
4. Increase in incidence is associated with the following risk factors:
   a. Age—between 30 and 70
   b. Race—black
   c. Birth control pills and estrogen supplements
   d. Overweight
   e. Medications with sodium-retaining properties
   f. History of smoking
   g. Lack of activity
5. Possible risk factors under investigation:
   a. Sodium intake/chloride intake
   b. Caffeine intake
   c. Stress
   d. Industrialized societies
   e. Genetic factors

Prevention of Hypertension

1. *Sodium restriction* is important in the treatment of some hypertensive patients, but whether limiting sodium intake will prevent the disease is not known. Some researchers believe that chloride may also be implicated—perhaps it enhances the action of sodium (under investigation). Until more facts are available, it is recommended that restraint be exercised in sodium consumption. Recommendations include:
   a. Not using the salt shaker at the table
   b. Cooking with only small amounts of salt
   c. Avoiding salted prepared foods
   d. Reducing the amount of sodium added to baby foods
2. In the U.S. as persons age, they gain weight; arterial pressure rises with age. Excess body fat must work, through some mechanisms, to elevate arterial pressure. Although it is very difficult, attempts should be made to *keep weight under control*—behavior modification, group therapy programs.
3. There is increased prevalence of hypertension among subjects with poor physical fitness. Considering the benefits of exercise for weight control and general health, *emphasis on physical fitness* should be increased.

Classification of Hypertension

A. Primary or Essential Hypertension
(Approximately 90% of patients with hypertension)

1. When the diastole pressure is 90 mm. Hg or higher and other causes of hypertension are absent, the condition is said to be *primary hypertension.*
   More specifically, an individual is considered hypertensive when the average of 3 or more blood pressure readings taken at rest several days apart exceeds the upper limits of the following chart:

Classification of Hypertension

Classification (Strata)		Diastolic Pressure (mm. Hg)	Percentage of Individuals
Mild	Stratum I	90–104	70%
Moderate	Stratum II	105–114	20%
Severe	Stratum III	115	10%

2. "Mild" is labeled such because of common usage; however, even for persons with so-called mild hy-

pertension, the cardiovascular risk is twice that for individuals with normal blood pressure.

3. With the presence of target organ damage, the overall risk is increased.

4. Genetic factors appear to contribute to this condition; patterns of the patient indicate that he is hypersensitive to internal and external stimuli.

5. Hypertension may be present for years *without any symptoms.*

6. *Labile* is a term used to indicate intermittently elevated blood pressure.

7. *Accelerated* refers to a sudden and severe escalation in arterial pressure, producing many symptoms and vascular damage.

8. *Resistant* is a reference to hypertension that is not responsive to usual treatment.

B. Secondary Hypertension

1. Occurs in approximately 5%–10% of patients with hypertension.

2. Apparently follows other pathology.
    a. *Renal pathology*—may lead to hypertension
        (1) Congenital anomalies, pyelonephritis, renal artery obstruction, acute and chronic glomerulonephritis
        (2) Reduced blood flow to kidney (such as atherosclerotic plaque)—release of *renin*
            (a) Renin reacts with serum protein in liver (alpha-2-globulin) → angiotensin I; this plus an enzyme → angiotensin II → leads to increased blood pressure.
            (b) Symptoms—proteinuria, polyuria, elevated blood pressure.
            (c) Therapy—endarterectomy, bypass graft, nephrectomy; blood pressure may be reduced if the initial problem is corrected.
    b. *Coarctation of aorta* (stenosis of aorta)
        (1) Blood flow to upper extremities is greater than flow to lower extremities—hypertension of upper part of body.
        (2) Correction—removal of stenosed section of vessel; anastomosis or graft to eliminate area.
    c. *Endocrine disturbance*—elevated blood pressure may be due to pheochromocytoma.
        (1) Pheochromocytoma—causes release of epinephrine and norepinephrine and a rise in blood pressure
        (2) Adrenal cortex tumors lead to an increase in aldosterone secretion and an elevated blood pressure
        (3) Cushing's syndrome leads to an increase in adrenocortical steroids and hypertension
        (4) Hyperthyroidism

C. Accelerated Hypertension—A Hypertensive Emergency (formerly called ''malignant''; Fig. 9-45)

1. Blood pressure may elevate very rapidly, with serious damage to vital organs.
    a. Hypertensive encephalopathy or cerebrovascular accident
       Progressive headache—stupor—convulsions
    b. Eye effect—visual impairment, hemorrhage, papilledema, exudates
    c. Kidney effect
        (1) Blood flow decreased, vasoconstriction
        (2) BUN more than 100 mg./dl.
        (3) Plasma renin activity
        (4) Specific gravity lowered
        (5) Proteinuria
    d. Epigastric pain
    e. Left ventricular failure
    f. Morning headache, nausea, and vomiting.

2. Onset of complications
    a. Pathology
        (1) Elevated diastolic pressure → strain on arterial wall → thickening and calcification of arterial media (sclerosis) → narrowed blood vessel lumen.
        (2) Sclerosis of vessels → increased wall per-

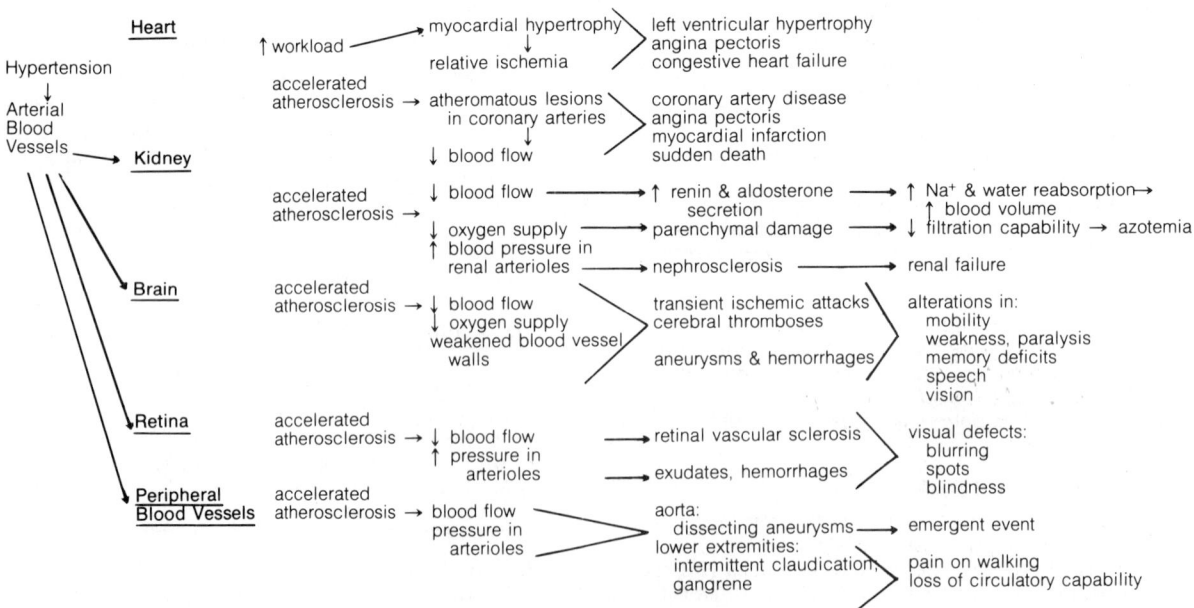

Figure 9-45. Pathologic effects of sustained hypertension. (Massachusetts Nurse. Hypertension: The Scope of the Problem and the Role of the Nurse, MNA Bulletin, Special Edition, rev. 1980)

meability → deposits placed on intima and media of vessels → cerebral, myocardial, or renal ischemia.
  b. Cerebrovascular manifestations
  Changes are determined by the type of onset of symptoms
    (1) *Rapid*
      (a) Cerebral hemorrhage → headache, increase in cerebrospinal pressure → papilledema → retinal hemorrhages → hemiplegia → coma
      (b) Cerebral thrombosis → tingling sensations → numbness, paresis of extremity → aphasia
      (c) Subarachnoid hemorrhage → stiffness of neck → pupil dilatation on side of hemorrhage → blood cells in cerebrospinal fluid → unconsciousness
    (2) *Slow*—gradual vascular insufficiency
    (3) Neurologic changes with recovery in a few hours ("TIA"—transient ischemic attacks) → cerebrovascular spasms
  c. Therapy
    (1) If exceeding 130 mm. Hg (diastole), hospital rest is recommended.
    (2) Immediate treatment if the following are present:
      (a) Convulsive movements
      (b) Abnormal neurologic signs
      (c) Severe occipital headache
      (d) Pulmonary edema
    (3) Monitor blood pressure; reduce gradually and avoid wide pressure variations—note that bringing pressure down to the usual normal may not be tolerated.
    (4) Measure and record urinary output.

Medical and Pharmacotherapeutic "Stepped Care"

Goal:
Prevent morbidity and reduce mortality that usually results from high blood pressure.

"Stepped care" is an approach (applied on an individual basis) in which initial therapy is nonpharmacologic; however, if this is unsuccessful, it is followed with a pharmacotherapeutic approach beginning with the mildest medication and progresses with additional drugs as determined by the needs of the patient.

A. Initial Conservative Nonpharmacotherapy

1. Reduce weight if one is overweight, since there is a correlation between increases in body weight and increases in blood pressure.

2. Reduce dietary sodium to a level of 70 to 90 mEq/day. Blood pressure response should be monitored to determine individual sensitivity to sodium restriction.
3. Imbibe moderately, since heavy alcohol consumption may elevate arterial blood pressure.
4. Reduce abnormal levels of blood cholesterol by reducing dietary saturated fat.
5. Avoid smoking to reduce cardiovascular risk.
6. Develop an exercise program after appropriate evaluation.
7. Consider relaxation and biofeedback therapies, since such behavioral modification methods may produce significant blood pressure reduction.

B. "Stepped Care" Regimen

Step 1
  a. Thiazide-type diuretics are drugs of choice.
    1. Favored for those over 50 years of age, black patients, those with peripheral vascular disease, asthma, or other chronic pulmonary disease.
    2. Use smallest effective dose to minimize side effects.
    3. Avoid hypokalemia by administering potassium supplement.
  b. Beta-adrenergic blockers
    1. Favored for those under 50 years of age.
    2. May produce side effects.
    3. Sexual dysfunction may be experienced by patients taking this or other antihypertensive agents.
Step 2—Adrenergic inhibiting agents
  1. If step 1 does not produce a response, small doses of adrenergic inhibiting agent should be added.
  2. There are several drugs in this category, and it may be necessary to shift from one drug to another to find the best drug for a particular patient.
  3. If necessary, it may require an angiotensin-converting enzyme inhibitor to be added.
Step 3—Hydralazine hydrochloride/minoxidil
  1. This is an effective peripheral vasodilator.
    a. May increase heart rate and myocardial contractility.
    b. Use cautiously in patients with angina pectoris.
    c. Usually used in combination with an adrenergic inhibiting agent plus a diuretic.
  2. If dosages are increased too rapidly, the side effects may be headache, tachycardia, and palpitations.
  3. Minoxidil—more potent than hydralazine.
    Disadvantage—may cause hypertrichosis and fluid retention.
Step 4—Guanethidine
  1. Used when first 3 steps are ineffective
  2. May cause orthostatic hypotension, diarrhea, and retrograde ejaculation.

Pharmacotherapy for Hypertension

Goal: Maintain blood pressure within normal ranges by the simplest and safest means possible with the fewest side effects for each individual patient.

Medication	Major Action	Advantages	Contraindications	Effects and Nursing Considerations
I. Diuretics and related drugs				
A. Chlorthalidone (Hygroton) Quinethazone (Hydromox) Chlorothiazide (Diuril)	At beginning of therapy: Decrease of blood volume, renal blood flow, and cardiac output	Effective orally Effective during long-term administration Mild side effects Enhance other antihypertensive drugs	Gout Known sensitivity to sulfonamide-derived drugs Severely impaired kidney function	Dry mouth, thirst, weakness, drowsiness, lethargy, muscle aches, muscular fatigue, tachycardia, GI disturbance Orthostatic hypotension may

(continued)

Medication	Major Action	Advantages	Contraindications	Effects and Nursing Considerations
Hydrochlorothiazide (Esidrix; Hydro-DIURIL) Metolazone (Diulo; Zaroxolyn)	Depletion of extracellular fluid Negative sodium balance (from natriuresis), mild hypokalemia Directly affects vascular smooth muscle	Counter sodium-retention effect of other antihypertensive drugs		be potentiated by alcohol, barbiturates, or narcotics Because thiazides cause sodium loss, patient is instructed to watch for postural hypotension in the summer Administer supplementary potassium
B. Loop diuretics Furosemide (Lasix) Ethacrynic acid (Edecrin) Bumetanide (Bumex)	Volume depletion Blocks reabsorption of sodium and water in kidney Antagonizes action of aldosterone	Action is rapid Potent blocks To be used only when thiazides fail	Same as for thiazides Hepatic coma	Volume depletion is rapid—profound diuresis Electrolyte depletion—replacement is required Thirst, nausea, vomiting, skin rash, postural hypotension Sweet taste noted; oral and gastric burning Ototoxicity (especially with IV use)
C. Potassium-sparing diuretics Spironolactone (Aldactone) Triamterene (Dyrenium) Amiloride (Moduretic) (Midamor)	Competitive inhibitor of aldosterone Acts on distal tubule independently of aldosterone	Spironolactone effective in treating hypertension accompanying primary aldosteronism Both spironolactone and triamterene retain potassium	Renal disease Azotemia Severe hepatic disease Give with potassium supplements only with extreme caution (hyperkalemia likely)	Drowsiness, lethargy, headache—decrease the dosage Diarrhea and other GI symptoms—give drug after meals Skin eruptions, urticaria Mental confusion, ataxia—perhaps dosage needs to be reduced Gynecomastia (not for triamterene or amiloride)
II. Peripheral antiadrenergic agents	Decrease in sympathetic tone results in ↓ heart rate, ↓ peripheral vascular resistance. (Note: This means that reflex responses to positional changes are blocked to varying degrees by each of these agents.) Decreases renal blood flow	Block reflex tachycardia caused by vasodilators		Inhibit sexual function (arousal, erection, ejaculation) Na^+ and H_2O retention usually necessitates concurrent diuretic use Orthostatic hypotension common May exacerbate peptic ulcer Sedation Headache
A. Guanethidine (Ismelin)	Depletes stores of norepinephrine Initial release of norepinephrine may cause hypertension Hypotensive effects delayed for days or weeks while stores are being depleted	High potency	CHF not due to hypertension Pheochromocytoma	Tolerance develops, requiring increased dosage Effects continue for days after discontinuance while stores are depleted Diarrhea Effects blocked by tricyclic antidepressants, phenothiazines
B. Guanadrel (Hylorel)	Like guanethidine but onset is faster (several hours), duration shorter (12 hours)			As for guanethidine
C. Reserpine and derivatives	Impairs intracellular storage of norepinephrine		History of depression or psychosis Chronic sinusitis Peptic ulcer Pheochromocytoma	Assess mental status—suicides have occurred because of depression Nasal stuffiness—may require topical vasoconstrictor Increased appetite—may require stricter diet
D. Prazosin (Minipress)	Blockade of postsynaptic alpha-adrenergic receptors causes arteriolar and venous dilation	Unlike older alpha blockers, does not cause reflex tachycardia Cardiac "unloading" effect is helpful in CHF		May cause syncope, especially with first dose or rapid increases in dose
III. Central antiadrenergic agents	Probably act by stimulating central adrenergic receptors, resulting in decreased sympa-	Less likely to cause orthostatic hypotension Does not decrease renal blood flow		Sedating Dry mouth May cause sexual dysfunction Sleep disturbances (nightmares), memory loss,

Medication	Major Action	Advantages	Contraindications	Effects and Nursing Considerations
	thetic outflow to the heart, vasculature, and kidneys	Blocks reflex tachycardia due to vasodilators		depression, and other CNS changes possible
A. Clonidine (Catapres)		Less sodium and water from retention than methyldopa		Use with caution in patients with severe coronary insufficiency, recent myocardial infarction, cerebrovascular disease, chronic renal failure, Raynaud's disease Rebound hypertension possible with abrupt withdrawal (taper dose over 2–4 days) Dry mouth
B. Guanabenz (Wytensin)		Sodium and water retention unlikely No decrease in cardiac output		Use with caution in patients with severe vascular insufficiency Dry mouth or sedation are prominent
C. Methyldopa (Aldomet)		Parenteral dosage form available Useful for hypertensive emergencies	Active liver disease Previous hypersensitivity reaction to methyldopa (hemolytic anemia, liver dysfunction)	Sedation is prominent Hemolytic anemia Hepatic toxicity Drug fever
IV. Direct-acting vasodilators	Peripheral resistance is lowered via a relaxant effect on vascular smooth muscle	Increase cardiac output Particularly effective in combination with a beta blocker to inhibit reflex tachycardia Minimal orthostatic hypotension	Relative contraindication in recent myocardial infarct or severe angina	Reflex tachycardia limits effectiveness and may cause palpitations, worsen angina, cause MI Sodium and water retention are prominent (must use with diuretic) May increase pulmonary artery pressure Vasodilation may cause headache
A. Hydralazine (Apresoline)		Parenteral dosage form available—useful for hypertensive emergencies Increases renal blood flow		May cause lupus-like syndrome, or arthritis
B. Minoxidil (Loniten)	Limited to patients unresponsive to less toxic drugs	High potency		Pericardial effusion with tamponade Hypertrichosis Monitor for fluid retention even if given with diuretic
V. Beta-adrenergic blocking agents Propranolol (Inderal) Atenolol (Tenormin) Metoprolol (Lopressor) Nadolol (Corgard) Timolol (Blocadren)	Blockage of beta-adrenergic receptors decreases cardiac output and inhibits vasoconstriction Other effects may contribute to antihypertensive effect	No fluid retention No orthostatic effects Blocks reflex tachycardia due to vasodilators Often effective as a single agent	Asthma Allergic rhinitis Sinus bradycardia Heart block greater than first-degree Right ventricular failure secondary to pulmonary hypertension	May cause bronchoconstriction (caution with COPD) (metoprolol and atenolol may cause less bronchoconstriction than others) May block symptoms of hypoglycemia May worsen congestive heart failure Abrupt withdrawal may precipitate or worsen angina, may induce myocardial infarction
VI. Captopril (Capoten)	Angiotensin-converting enzyme inhibitor—blocks formation of angiotensin II, which is a potent vasoconstrictor	High potency Infrequent tachycardia Infrequent orthostatic effects		Proteinuria with possible nephrotic syndrome Neutropenia with possible agranulocytosis Use with caution in patients with autoimmune disease such as SLE May cause severe hypotension with concurrent diuretic therapy May increase serum potassium Rash is common but usually disappears without discontinuation of medication Loss of taste in 7% of patients but usually disappears without discontinuence

Table 9-3 Recommended Bladder Dimensions for Blood Pressure Cuff

Arm Circumference at Midpoint* (cm.)	Cuff Name	Bladder Width (cm.)	Bladder Length (cm.)
17–26	Small adult	11	17
24–32	Adult	13	24
32–42	Large adult	17	32
42–50†	Thigh	20	42

* Midpoint of arm is defined as half the distance from the acromion to the olecranon.

† In persons with very large limbs, the indirect blood pressure should be measured in the leg or forearm.

Recommendations for Human Blood Pressure Determination by Sphygmomanometers. Am Heart Assoc, 1980)

Assessment

▶ **NURSING ALERT:** The actual blood pressure reading by itself is not the sole criterion for determining the severity or urgency of the person's condition. The patient/client must be assessed in terms of what, if any, evidence there is of end organ damage. For example: a person with a blood pressure of 140/105 and papilledema is at far greater risk than one with a reading of 170/115 with no evidence of papilledema. The nurse will respond accordingly.

Blood Pressure Determination

Measure the blood pressure of the patient under the same conditions each time. Individuals should not have blood pressure readings taken immediately after experiencing stressful or taxing situations.

1. Place the patient in the desired position (sitting, standing, etc.) according to the routine of the agency or the preferences of the physician.
2. Support the bared arm (an unsupported arm may cause the reading to be higher and lead to a false diagnosis of hypertension). Avoid constriction of arm by a rolled sleeve.
3. Use a blood pressure cuff of the correct size (Table 9-3).
4. Record precisely the systolic and diastolic pressures:
   a. Systolic—the pressure within the pressure cuff indicated by the level of the mercury column at the moment when the first of two consecutive Korotkoff sounds is first heard (Fig. 9-46).
   b. Phase 4 (first diastolic)—the pressure within the compression cuff indicated by the level of the mercury column at the moment when the sound suddenly becomes muffled (beginning of phase 4).
   c. Phase 5 (second diastolic)—the pressure within

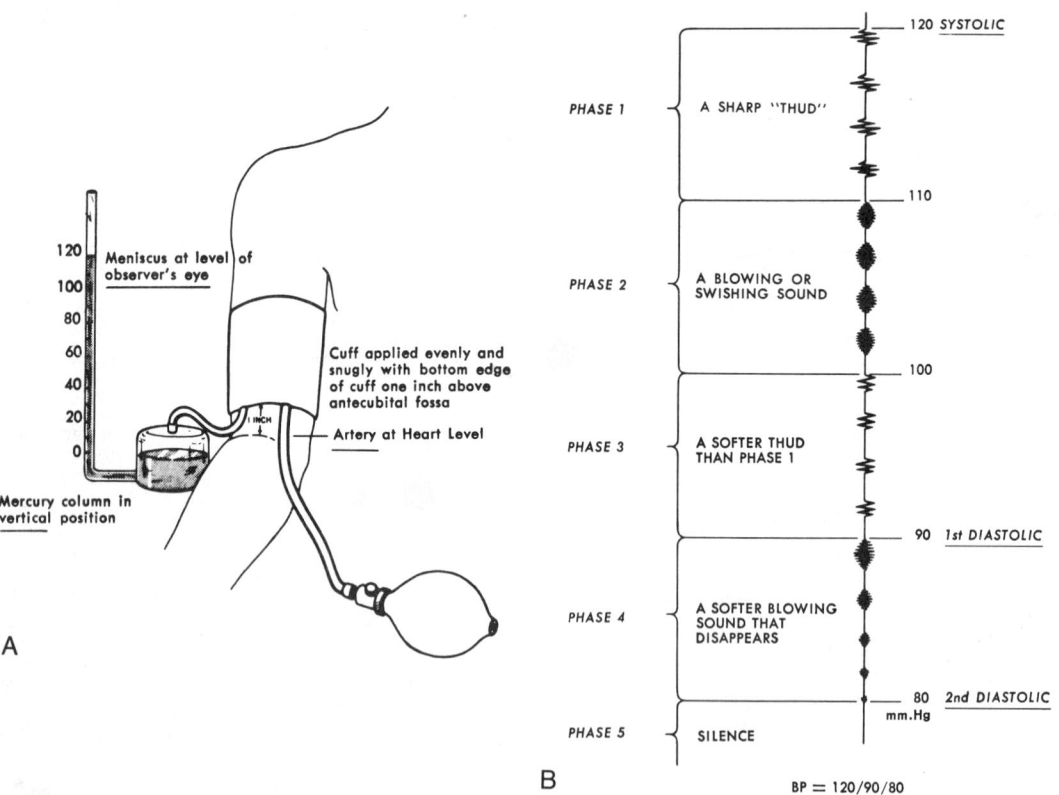

Figure 9-46. (A) Important "rules" for accurate recording of arterial blood pressure. (B) The various phases of the Korotkoff sounds. Consult text for details. (Burch GE and DePasquale NP: Primer of Clinical Measurement of Blood Pressure. St. Louis, CV Mosby)

the compression cuff at the moment when the sound finally disappears (beginning of phase 5), that is, the onset of silence.

5. If required, document the blood pressure reading to indicate the patient's position and the arm used:
   L (lying)
   St (standing)
   Sit (sitting)
   RA (Right Arm)
   LA (Left Arm)
   Example: LA 152/78/68 St

6. Average 2 readings or the second and third of 3 readings, if procedure requires. Mancia noted that most patients' blood pressure rises immediately and significantly when the physician is present. Remeasurement is recommended after about 10 minutes.

7. Compare present reading with several previous readings to note differences and detect trends.

8. Alert physician if significant changes are apparent.

General Detection, Confirmation, and Referral of Patients with High Blood Pressure*

When there is group screening and measurement of blood pressure, resources for referral, confirmation, and follow-up should be provided.

1. Prior to blood pressure determination, ask the patient whether he has been or is currently under treatment for hypertension.
   a. Urge him to continue treatment even if blood pressure is normal.
   b. Urge the patient to report an elevated blood pressure to his physician.

2. Take blood pressure as described above.

3. Discuss with the patient/client:
   a. Previous treatment for high blood pressure
   b. Numerical value of current blood pressure
   c. Need for periodic remeasurement
   d. Desirability of blood pressure control and the potential dangers of uncontrolled hypertension
   e. Vital need to seek promptly and maintain antihypertensive therapy

4. Referral or confirmation cutoff levels are arbitrary; they may be modified by presence of risk factors:
   a. Smoking
   b. Hyperlipemia
   c. Coronary or cerebrovascular disease
   d. Cardiac or renal failure
   e. Diabetes

5. The higher the blood pressure, the greater the urgency for follow-up management. (Early initial follow-up improves adherence to treatment plan.)

6. Adults with a diastolic blood pressure of 95 mm. Hg or higher at screening or first visit should have the elevation confirmed promptly (within 1 month).
   a. Those with diastolic blood pressures of 90–95 mm. Hg should be remeasured within three months.
   b. A diastolic blood pressure of 115 mm. Hg or greater warrants immediate referral.

7. Adults with a systolic blood pressure over 160 mm. Hg should have reading confirmed promptly.
   Those under age 35 years should have systolic elevations greater than 150 mm. Hg confirmed.

* Based on the 1984 Report of the Joint National Committee on Detection, Evaluation and Treatment of High Blood Pressure. Arch Intern Med 1984 May; 144(5):1045–1057.

8. *Confirmation*—Purpose is to determine whether initial elevations
   a. Remain high or require closer observation and evaluation, or
   b. Have returned to normal and require only remeasurement within 1 year

Note: Two or more measurements should be taken at each visit. The diagnosis of hypertension is *confirmed* when the average of multiple blood pressure measurements made on at least two subsequent visits is 90 mm. Hg or higher (diastolic) or when the average of multiple systolic blood pressures on two or more subsequent visits is consistently high.

Diagnostic Assessment of Patient

1. Careful nursing and medical history (including family history of hypertension); note any previous history of hypertension, excessive salt intake, lipid abnormalities, cigarette smoking, and history of headache, weakness, muscle cramps, palpitation, sweating.
   a. Take a complete history of all medications taken, including:
      (1) Oral contraceptives, steroids
      (2) Nonsteroids, anti-inflammatory agents
      (3) Nasal decongestants, appetite suppressants, tricyclic antidepressants

2. Blood pressure—supine and standing; also assess vital signs and evaluate function of vital organs.

3. Physical assessment and examination (Fig. 9-47).

4. Fundoscopic examination of the eye to detect vascular changes in the capillaries—note edema, spasm, hemorrhage.

5. Careful examination of the heart; examination of peripheral pulse disparities, and evidence of edema.

6. Listen for bruits over all peripheral arteries to determine presence of atherosclerosis; also listen for bruits in abdomen to note signs of renal arterial stenosis.

7. Chest x-ray to determine cardiac size; auscultation of lungs.

8. Neurologic tests to detect cerebral damage, neurologic deficits.

9. Laboratory studies
   a. Hematocrit reading; hemoglobin
   b. Urinalysis for blood, protein, and glucose to determine renal parenchymal disease
   c. BUN to determine renal excretory function
   d. Serum potassium concentration to determine hyperaldosteronism, serum cholesterol and creatinine levels
   e. Electrocardiogram to establish a baseline
   f. Total and high-density lipoprotein cholesterol

10. If the patient has:
    a. Gout or diabetes—serum glucose and uric acid need to be determined
    b. Asthma—no beta blockers are given
    c. Peptic ulcer—no reserpine is given.

11. If the patient has confirmed hypertension:
    a. Is target organ involvement present?
    b. Are cardiovascular risk factors other than hypertension present?
    c. Does the patient have primary or secondary hypertension?

Patient Problems/Nursing Diagnoses

1. Potential complications of underlying pathology, including increased cardiac workload, kidney dysfunc-

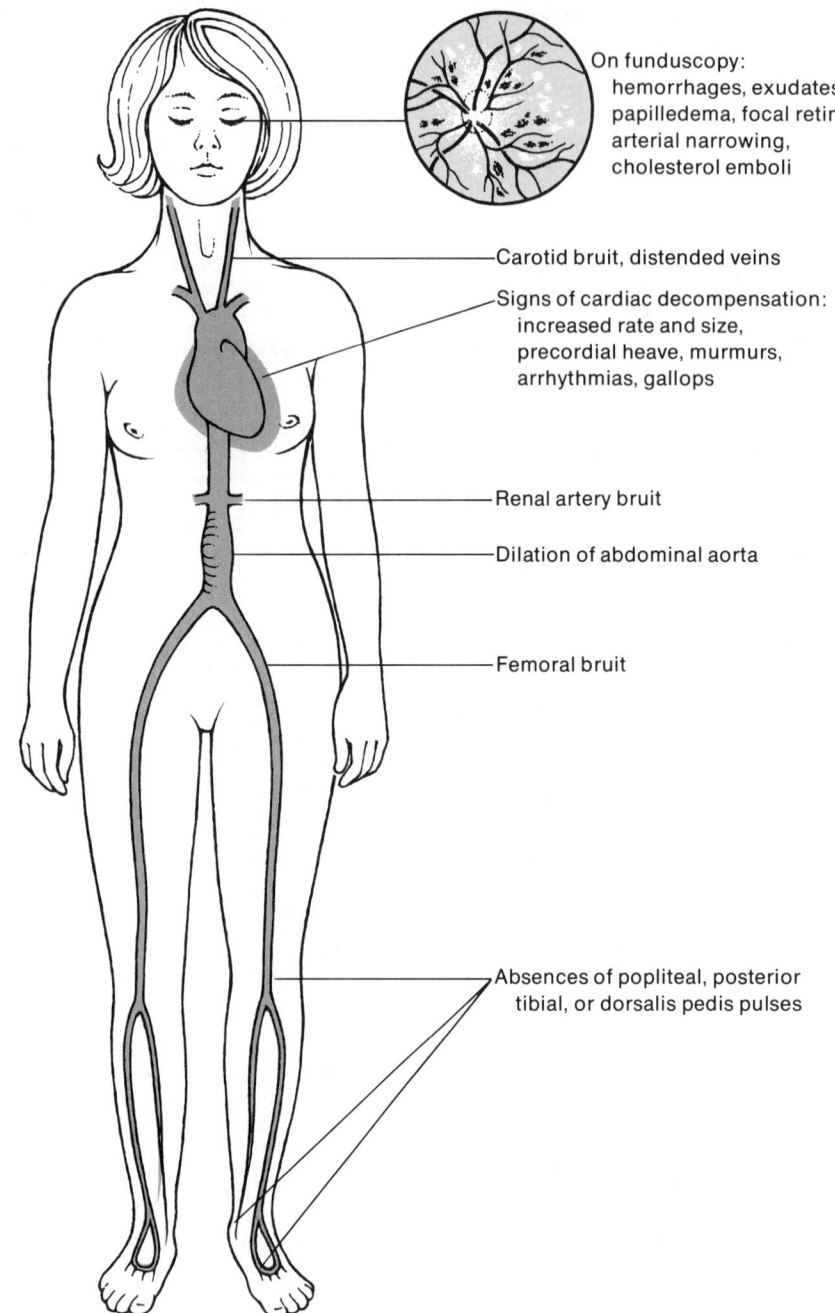

On funduscopy:
hemorrhages, exudates,
papilledema, focal retinal
arterial narrowing,
cholesterol emboli

Carotid bruit, distended veins

Signs of cardiac decompensation:
increased rate and size,
precordial heave, murmurs,
arrhythmias, gallops

Renal artery bruit

Dilation of abdominal aorta

Femoral bruit

Absences of popliteal, posterior
tibial, or dorsalis pedis pulses

Figure 9-47. Physical assessment for hypertension. In addition to assessment of the central nervous system and a complete physical examination, the above specific observations are significant in detection of high blood pressure.

tion, mobility impairment, weakness, lethargy, memory deficit, confusion, speech difficulties, visual defects, and pain on walking.
2. Possible nonadherence to therapeutic regimen related to length of treatment and life-style changes.
3. Knowledge deficit—of basic problem, treatment protocols, negative effects of disease.

Planning and Implementation
Nursing Interventions (Ambulatory/Outpatient)

A. Follow-up Care for Monitoring Progress and for Relieving Stress

1. Measure the patient's blood pressure under the same conditions each day.

Place the patient in the desired position, sitting, standing, etc., according to the preference of the physician.

2. If elevated blood pressure can be brought down to normal range, there is very clear evidence that congestive heart failure, strokes, and renal failure can be almost completely prevented; therefore treatment should continue in spite of medication cost or inconvenience.

3. Practice supportive psychotherapy by observing the patient's reactions, appearance, and personality as he relates to the professional staff, visitors, ancillary personnel, etc.
   a. Permit the patient to express his feelings; promote positive reactions; analyze negative reactions in an attempt to avoid their recurrence.
   b. Note side reactions, which can be easily missed; investigate these.
      (1) Failure to make eye contact in conversation
      (2) Suggestion of uneasiness, nervousness, restlessness
      (3) Side remarks or "under-the-breath" comments

Note: In the US, only 24% of the 60 million individuals with high blood pressure are effectively treated. Of those under treatment, only 50% to 60% are fully compliant (Reichgott).

B. Awareness of Pharmacotherapeutic Side Effects

1. Assist the patient in coping with the side effects of the therapeutic medications.
   a. Recognize that the drugs used for effective control of elevated blood pressure will very likely produce side effects.
   b. Warn the patient of the possibility that hypotension may occur following the intake of certain drugs.
      (1) Instruct the patient to get up slowly to offset the feeling of dizziness.
      (2) Encourage the patient to lie down immediately if he feels faint.
   c. Alert the patient to expect effects such as nasal congestion, asthenia (loss of strength), anorexia (loss of appetite), orthostatic hypotension (dizziness on changing position).
   d. Inform the patient that the goal of treatment is to control his blood pressure, reduce the possibility of complications, and utilize the minimum number of drugs with lowest dosage necessary to accomplish this.
2. Educate the patient to be aware of toxic manifestations and report them so that adjustments can be made in his individual pharmacotherapy.
   a. Note that dosages are individualized; therefore, they may need to be adjusted, since it is often impossible to predict reactions.
   b. Remember that certain circumstances produce vasodilatation—a hot bath, hot weather, febrile illness, consumption of alcohol.
   c. Be aware that blood pressure is decreased when circulating blood volume is reduced—dehydration, diarrhea, hemorrhage.
   d. Suspect the presence of edema as a reportable symptom, particularly when guanethidine is taken; these medications are less effective in the presence of edema.

C. Adherence to the Therapeutic Regimen

1. Explain the meaning of hypertension, risk factors, and their influences on the cardiovascular system; hypertension is a life-long problem.
2. Usually, there can never be total cure, only control of essential hypertension; emphasize the consequences of uncontrolled hypertension.
3. Stress the fact that there may be no correlation between high blood pressure and symptoms; the patient cannot tell by the way he feels whether his blood pressure is normal or elevated.
4. Have the patient recognize that hypertension is chronic and requires persistent therapy and periodic evaluation; effective treatment improves life expectancy, therefore, follow-up visits to the physician are mandatory.
5. Present a coordinated and complementary plan of guidance.
   a. Be available when the physician visits the patient so that his approach and instructions to the patient are known.
   b. Inform the patient of the meaning of the various diagnostic and therapeutic activities to minimize his anxiety and to obtain his cooperation.
   c. Solicit the assistance of the patient's spouse—provide information regarding the total treatment plan.
   d. Be aware of the dietary plan developed for this particular patient.
8. Develop a plan of instruction to be practiced by the patient at home.
   a. Instruct the patient regarding proper method of taking his blood pressure at home and at work if his physician so desires. (Some authorities recommend this practice.) Inform him of the readings that are to be reported to the physician.
   b. Plan the patient's medication schedule so that the many medications are given at proper and convenient times; set up a daily checklist on which he can record the medication he has taken.
   c. Determine recommended dietary plans (e.g., extent of salt restriction, exchange foods, etc.).

D. Life-style Adjustments

1. Recognize the various effects of certain factors on symptoms of a patient with primary hypertension.
   a. Age, sex, occupation, race, environment, emotional response of the individual, etc.
   b. Understanding of his problem and his rapport with physician, nurse, etc.
   c. Ability to adapt and adjust his activities in line with the prescribed therapeutic regimen.
2. Enlist the patient's cooperation in redirecting his life-style in keeping with the guidelines of therapy.
   a. Present an instructional pattern to fit individual requirements.
   b. Reassure the patient when encouragement is needed; the modifications required must appear meaningful to him.

Hypertensive Crisis—Inpatient Care

A. Pharmacotherapy and Nursing Intervention

1. Use parenteral medications in hypertensive emergencies.
   a. Diastolic blood pressure over 150 mm. Hg
   b. Pulmonary edema, cerebral hemorrhage, en-

cephalopathy in combination with diastolic pressure over 120 or 130

2. The patient must be hospitalized and monitored constantly.
   a. Record blood pressure frequently.
      Some drugs such as trimethaphan, nitroprusside, and pentolinium necessitate the taking of blood pressure readings every 5 minutes.
   b. Measure urine output accurately.
   c. Be prepared to administer vasopressors if severe hypotension develops.
   d. Administer diuretics such as furosemide and ethacrynic acid as adjuncts, when prescribed. They serve to maintain sodium diuresis when the arterial pressure falls.
   e. Administer spironolactone, when prescribed, if hypokalemia is a problem.
3. Observe the patient for signs of cerebral nervous system complications.
   a. Note signs of confusion, irritability, lethargy, disorientation.
   b. Listen for complaints of headache, difficulty with vision; be alert for evidence of nausea or vomiting.
   c. Be prepared to offer protection to the patient if he exhibits seizures—padded bed sides, nonrestrictive garments, anticonvulsive medications.
4. Prevent those reactions or activities that will increase arterial pressure.
   a. Avoid situations that might engender feelings of anxiety, anger, or annoyance in the patient. Psychological stress has a direct effect on physiologic function.
   b. Prevent alterations in the ordinary functions of eating, sleeping, or elimination that might lead to discomfort or annoyance—physiologic disturbance may increase stress reaction.
   c. Provide rest period and maintain a pleasant, comfortable environment.
      (1) Advise the patient to rest for a short time before and after eating.
      (2) Remind the patient to rest during the waking hours for a full hour.
   d. Serve food frequently and in small quantities rather than in 3 heavier meals.

   (1) Cardiac output increases with food intake.
   (2) Blood pressure is elevated with large intake of fluids.
   (3) Sodium intake may be restricted, depending on severity of hypertension.
5. Pharmacotherapy
   a. Drugs that act in a few minutes but are not satisfactory for long-term management:
      (1) Diazoxide
      (2) Nitroprusside
      (3) Trimethaphan
      (4) Pentolinium
   b. Drugs that require 30 minutes or more to obtain full effects; they can later be used orally for long-term management of hypertension:
      (1) Methyldopa
      (2) Hydralazine

Health Education

Instruct the patient as follows:

1. Recognize when blood pressure is above normal values.
2. Realize that long-term therapy and follow-up are essential for control.
3. Understand that an elevated blood pressure is usually asymptomatic.
4. Recognize that therapy will not cure but should control hypertension.
5. Expect that by following the suggested therapeutic regimen, the prognosis is good, and normal life-style can be experienced.

Evaluation
Expected Outcomes

1. Exhibits stabilized blood pressure as shown on personal daily charts and confirmed by health-care personnel
2. Corrects controllable risk factors—reduces weight, stops smoking, adheres to daily exercise program, reduces stress
3. Enumerates side effects of drugs that necessitate contacting a member of the health-care team
4. Adheres to therapeutic regimen by limiting sodium intake, exercising, conscientiously taking medications, and keeping follow-up appointments

The Lymphatic System

The *lymphatic system* is a network of vessels and nodes that are interrelated with the circulatory system. It removes tissue fluid from intercellular spaces and protects the body from bacterial invasion. Lymph nodes are located along the course of the lymphatic vessels and filter lymph before it is returned to the bloodstream.

Significance of Lymphangiography
   Radiologic visualization of the lymphatic system is possible when a contrast medium is injected into a lymphatic vessel of the hands or feet.
   It is a means of detecting lymph node involvement due to metastatic carcinoma, lymphoma, or infection in otherwise inaccessible sites (except by surgery) such as the pelvis, retroperitoneum, deep axilla.

Lymphangitis

Lymphangitis is an acute inflammation of lymphatic channels.

Etiology

Arises most commonly from a focus of infection in an extremity.

Clinical Manifestations

1. Displays characteristic red streaks that extend up an arm or leg from an infection that is not localized and that can lead to septicemia.
2. Produces general symptoms—high fever, chills.

Produces local symptoms—local pain, tenderness, swelling along involved lymphatics.

Produces local lymph node symptoms—enlarged, red, tender (acute lymphadenitis).

Produces an abscess—necrotic, pus-producing (suppurative lymphadenitis).

Treatment of Nursing Management

1. Administer antimicrobial agents, since causative organisms usually are streptococci and staphylococci.
2. Treat affected part by rest, elevation, and the application of hot, moist dressings.
3. Incise and drain if necrosis and abscess formation take place.

Lymphedema

Lymphedema is a swelling of the tissues (particularly in the dependent position), produced by an obstruction to the lymph flow in an extremity.

Clinical Manifestations

1. Edema may be massive and is often firm.
2. Obstruction may be in lymph nodes, as well as in the lymphatic vessels.

   Observed in arm following radical mastectomy (see pp. 597, 598)

Treatment and Nursing Management

1. Apply elastic bandages or stocking.
2. Keep the patient at rest, with affected part elevated, each joint higher than the preceding one.
3. Administer diuretics to control excess fluid.
4. Give antimicrobials as prescribed.
5. Recommend isometric exercises with extremity elevated.
6. Suggest moderate sodium restriction in diet.
7. Advise the patient to avoid infection and trauma and to practice good hygiene to avoid superimposed infections.

Bibliography

Heart Disorders

Books

Alpert JS and Francis GS. Manual of Coronary Care. Boston, Little, Brown & Co, 1980

Andreoli K et al. Comprehensive Cardiac Care, 5th ed. St Louis, CV Mosby, 1984

Blocker WP and Cardus D. Rehabilitation in Ischemic Heart Disease. New York, Medical and Scientific Books, 1983

Boden WS and Capona RJ. Coronary Care. Philadelphia, WB Saunders, 1984

Braunwald E. Heart Disease: A Textbook of Cardiovascular Disease. Philadelphia, WB Saunders, 1984

Cooley D. Techniques in Cardiac Surgery. Philadelphia, WB Saunders, 1984

Holloway N. Nursing the Critically Ill Adult, 2nd ed. Menlo Park, CA, Addison Wesley, 1984

Hurst JW (ed). The Heart, 5th ed. New York, McGraw-Hill, 1982

Kinny M et al. AACN's Clinical Reference for Critical Care Nursing. New York, McGraw-Hill, 1981

Malasanos L et al. Health Assessment. St Louis, CV Mosby, 1981

McGurn WC. People with Cardiac Problems. Philadelphia, JB Lippincott, 1981

McIntyre K and Lewis AJ (ed). Textbook of Cardiac Life Support. Dallas, American Heart Assoc, April, 1983

Meltzer LE, Pinneo R, and Kitchell JR. Intensive Coronary Care: A Manual for Nurses. Bowie, MD, Prentice-Hall, 1983

Morse D, Skirer RM and Parsonnet V. A Guide to Cardiac Pacemakers. Philadelphia, FA Davis, 1983

Neal MC, Cohen PF and Cooper PG. Nurse Care Planning Guide: Set I and II, 2nd ed. California, Nurseco, 1981

Quaal SJ. Comprehensive Intra-aortic Balloon Pumping. St Louis, CV Mosby, 1984

Shoemaker WC, Thompson WL and Halbrook PR. Textbook of Critical Care. Philadelphia, WB Saunders, 1984

Sprung CL. The Pulmonary Artery Catheter: Methodology and Clinical Applications. Baltimore, University Park Press, 1983

Underhill S et al. Cardiac Nursing, Philadelphia, JB Lippincott, 1982

Vinsant MO and Spence MI. Commonsense Approach to Coronary Care: A Program. St Louis, CV Mosby, 1981

Articles

Assessment/Diagnosis/Manifestations

Carlson E. Noncardiac origins of chest pain. Occup Health Nurs 1981 Dec; 29(12):39–40

Huebsch JA. Health assessment of the cardiovascular patient. Occup Health Nurs 1981 Dec; 29(12):11–17

Pantaleo N et al. The noninvasive evaluation of left ventricular function by performance of equilibrium radionuclide ventriculography. Crit Care Q 1981 Sept; 4(2):55–65

Verani MS. Noninvasive diagnostic techniques in cardiology. Compr Ther 1983 Oct; 9(10):27–36

Hemodynamic Monitoring

Abbott N, Walrath JM and Scanlon-Trump J. Infection related to physiologic monitoring: Venous and arterial catheters. Heart Lung 1983 Jan; 12(1):28–34

Bodai BI and Holcroft JW. Use of pulmonary arterial catheter in the critically ill patient. Heart Lung 1982 Sept–Oct; 11(5):406–416

Grabenkort RW. A cardiopulmonary physiologic profile for use with the

Swan–Ganz catheter. Resident Staff Physician 1983 July; 29(7):80–85

Hedges J. Preload and afterload revisited. J Emerg Nurs 1983 Sept–Oct; 9(5):262–267

Kaye W. Invasive monitoring techniques: Arterial cannulation, bedside pulmonary artery catheterization, and arterial puncture. Heart Lung 1983 July; 12(4):395–427

Palmer PN. Advanced hemodynamic assessment. DCCN 1982 May–June; 1(3):139–144

Runkel R and Burke L. Troubleshooting Swan–Ganz catheters. Heart Lung 1983 Nov; 12(6):591–596

Cardiopulmonary Resuscitation/Defibrillation

Cronin K, Haagsma JL and Lane GH. Defibrillation. Crit Care Nurse 1982 Nov–Dec; 2(6):32–35

Arrhythmias

Baily JC. The electrophysiologic basis for cardiac electrical activity: Normal and abnormal. Heart Lung 1981 May–June; 10(3):455–464

McCarthy C. Hemodynamic effects and clinical assessment of arrhythmias. Crit Care Q 1981 Sept; 4(2):9–15

Shepard N, Vaughn P and Rice B. A guide to arrhythmia interpretation and management. Crit Care Nurse 1982 Sept–Oct; 2(5):57–85

Williams ES. Supraventricular tachycardias. Heart Lung 1981 Aug; 10(4):634–643

Cardiac Pacing

Beeler B. Infections of permanent transvenous and epicardial pacemakers in adults. Heart Lung 1982 Mar–Apr; 11(2):152–156

Gage A. Implantable cardiac pacemakers: Current techniques and clinical concerns. Compr Ther 1983 Oct; 9(10):37–45

Gotsman MS et al. Atrial pacing in the diagnosis of ischemic heart disease. Heart Lung 1983 July; 12(4):372–381

Klein LR. Temporary AV sequential pacing. Crit Care Nurs 1983 May–June; 3(3):36–41

Lasche PA. Permanent cardiac pacing. Focus Crit Care 1983 Oct; 19(5):28–36

Owen PM. The effects of external defibrillation on permanent pacemakers. Heart Lung 1983 May; 12(3):274–277

Parsonnet V and Bernstein AD. Cardiac pacing in the 1980's: Treatment and techniques in transition. J Am Coll Cardiol 1983 Jan; 1(1):339–354

Patros R. Pulse counting and the pacemaker patient. DCCN 1983 May–June; 2(3):180–182

Angina

Alyn IB. Chest pain due to angina. Occup Health Nurs 1981 Dec; 29(12):35–38

Bourget C. Verapamil: A calcium channel blocker. DCCN 1982 May–June; 1(3):134–138

Braun LT. Calcium channel blockers for the treatment of coronary artery spasm: Rationale, effects, and nursing responsibilities. Heart Lung 1983 May; 12(3):226–232

Crevey B. Mechanism of action of the calcium channel blockers. Cardiovas Rev Rep 1983 Nov; 4(11):1419–1425

Franciosa J. The role of vasodilators. Postgrad Med 1980 Jan; 67(1):87–98

Gould L and Gopalaswamy C. Vasodilator drugs. Compr Ther 1984 Feb; 10(2):38–45

Hartshorn JC. Administering calcium-channel blocking agents. DCCN 1983 Mar–Apr; 2(2):70–73

Hummelgard AB and Esrig BC. Calcium and calcium slow channel blockers: An overview. Crit Care Q 1981 Sept; 4(2):17–28

Klein DM. Angina: Physiology, signs, and symptoms. Nursing '84 1984 Feb; 14(2):44–46

Matheuson M. Current vasodilator therapy. Focus Crit Care 1983 Feb; 10(1):49–53

McGregor M. The nitrates and myocardial ischemia. Circulation 1982; 66(4):689–692

Trifiletti P. Nitroglycerin ointment: Application and use. Crit Care Nurse 1982 Sept–Oct; 2(5):46–48

Percutaneous Transluminal Coronary Angioplasty

Allen JA and Thom LA. Percutaneous transluminal coronary angioplasty: A new alternative for ischemic heart disease. Crit Care Nurs 1982 Sept–Oct; 2(5):24–29

Cowley MJ, Vetrovec GW and Wolfgang TC. Efficacy of PCTA: Technique, patient selection, salutary results, limitations, and complications. Am Heart J 1981 Mar; 101(3):272–280

Doran KA and Hansen C. PTCA: Patient education. DCCN 1983 Jan–Feb; 2(1):56–64

Gershan JA and Jiricka MK. PCTA: Implications for nursing. Focus Crit Care 1984 Aug; 2(4):28–35

McCarthy CL. Percutaneous transluminal coronary angioplasty: Therapeutic intervention in the cardiac catheterization laboratory. Heart Lung 1982 Nov–Dec; 11(6):499–504

Partridge SA. The nurse's role in percutaneous transluminal coronary angioplasty. Heart Lung 1982 Nov–Dec; 11(6):505–511

Quint RA. Percutaneous transluminal coronary angioplasty: Pre- and post-procedural care. Crit Care Q 1981 Sept; 4(2):35–42

Shillinger FL. Percutaneous transluminal coronary angioplasty. Heart Lung 1983 Jan; 12(1):45–51

Myocardial Infarction

Braunwald E et al. Role of beta-adrenergic blockade in therapy of patients with myocardial infarction. Am J Med 1983 Jan; 74(1):113–123

Corday E and Corday S. Advances in clinical management of acute myocardial infarction in the past 25 years. J Am Coll Cardiol 1983 Jan; 1(1):126–132

Gawlinski A. Current approaches for the complicated myocardial infarction patient: A case study. Crit Care Q 1981 Sept; 4(2):97–103

Papenhausen JL. Data based criteria for cardiovascular nursing intervention. Crit Care Q 1981 Sept; 4(2):1–7

Sommers MS and Russell A. Location of myocardial infarction: Assessing the patient's response. DCCN 1984 Jan–Feb; 3(1):8–16

Stratton M. Use of nitrates in patients with acute myocardial infarction. Clin Phar 1984 Jan–Feb; 3:32–38

University of Washington Critical Care Unit. Nursing care plan for MI patients. Crit Care Nurse 1982 July–Aug; 2(4):78–84

Vaughan P. Bedside assessment of the myocardial infarction patient. Crit Care Nurse 1984 Mar–Apr; 4(2):60–77

Vaughn P and Rice B. Complications of myocardial infarction. Crit Care Nurse 1982 May–June; 2(3):44–51

Counterpulsation Therapy

Angerpointner TA, Jackson PG and Williams BT. The long term effect of intra-aortic balloon counterpulsation on left ventricular performance. J Cardiovas Surg 1980 July–Aug; 21(4):399–404

Bitran B et al. Intra-aortic balloon counterpulsation in acute mycardial infarction. Heart Lung 1981 Nov–Dec; 10(6):1021–1027

Bricker PL. The intense nursing demands of the intra-aortic balloon pump. RN 1980 July; 43(7):23–29

Bullas JB. Care of the patient on the percutaneous intra-aortic counterpulsation balloon. Crit Care Nurse 1982 July–Aug; 2(4):40–52

Gould KA. Hemodynamic assessment of IABP timing. DCCN 1983 July–Aug; 2(4):206–211

Haak SW. Intra-aortic balloon pump techniques. DCCN 1983 July–Aug; 2(4):196–204

Lorente P et al. Multivariate statistical evaluation of intra-aortic counterpulsation in pump failure complicating acute myocardial infarction. Am J Cardiol 1980 July; 46:124–134

Pollack LC. Mechanical cardiac assist devices: The efficacy of external counterpulsation. Crit Care Q 1981 Sept; 4(2):89–95

Purcell JA, Pippin L and Mitchell M. Intra-aortic balloon pump therapy. Am J Nurs 1983 May; 83(5):775–796

Shively M. The physiologic principles of intra-aortic balloon counterpulsation. Crit Care Q 1981 Sept; 4(2):83–88

Rheumatic Heart Disease/Endocarditis/Myocarditis/Pericarditis

Barry J and Dieter G. Endocarditis: An overview. Heart Lung 1982 Mar–Apr; 11(2):138–145

Cantrell M and Yoshikaawa TT. Aging and infective endocarditis. J Am Geriatr Soc 1983 Apr; 31(4):216–221

Coakly LD and Capasso VC. Trauma to the heart. J Emerg Nurs 1981 Nov–Dec; 7(6):255–261

Committee on Rheumatic Fever and Infective Endocarditis of the Council on Cardiovascular Disease in the Young. Prevention of bacterial endocarditis. A statement for health professionals. Circulation 1984 Dec; 70(6):1123–1127

Duffy KF et al. A severe case of viral myocarditis. Am J Nurs 1981 Jun; 1148–1151

Fenoglio JJ. Diagnosis and classification of myocarditis by endomyocardial biopsy. N Engl J Med 1983 Jan 6; 308(1):12–18

Hermans PE. The clinical manifestations of infective endocarditis. Mayo Clin Proc 1982 Feb; 47(7):15–21

Himes VJ. Traumatic cardiac tamponade. J Emerg Nurs 1980 Mar–Apr; 6(2):28–32

Hunan DG, Hill ID and Fraser CB. Treatment of choice in acute rheumatic carditis. Arch Dis Child 1984 May; 59(5):410–413

Kaye W. Invasive therapeutic techniques: Emergency cardiac pacing, pericardiocentesis, intracardiac injection, and emergency treatment of tension pneumothorax. Heart Lung 1983 May; 12(3):300–319

Leirisalo M et al. Rheumatic fever and its sequels in children. J Rheumatol 1980 July–Aug; 7(4):506–514

Long G. Myocarditis. Nursing '82 1982 Dec; 12(12):59

Lowes JA et al. 10 years of infective endocarditis at St. Bartholomew's hospital: Analysis of clinical features and treatments in relation to prognosis and mortality. Lancet 1980 Jan 19; 1(8160):133–136

Macek L. Acute rheumatic fever. Nurse Pract 1983 May; 8(5):17–19

Moles KW, Morton P and McKeown F. Valvulitis—Bacterial or rheumatic?

Arch Dis Child 1982 Oct; 57(1):783–785

Proudfet WL. Skin signs of infective endocarditis. Am Heart J 1983 Dec; 106(6):1451–1453

Pursley P. Acute cardiac tamponade. Am J Nurs 1983 Oct; 83(10):1414–1418

Rahimtoola S. Surgery for infective endocarditis. Crit Care Q 1981 Dec; 4(3):51–55

Reynolds SF. Cardiac trauma and tamponade. Crit Care Q 1981 Dec; 4(3):27–36

Thompson RL. Staphylococcal infective endocarditis. Mayo Clin Proc 1982 Feb; 57(2):106–114

Wilkowske CJ. Enterococcal endocarditis. Mayo Clin Proc 1982 Feb; 57(2):101–105

Williams RC Jr. Host factors in rheumatic fever and heart disease. Hosp Pract 1982 Aug; 17(8):125–129, 135–138

Wilson WR et al. General considerations in the diagnosis and treatment of infective endocarditis. Mayo Clin Proc 1982 Feb; 57(2):81–85

Wilson WR et al. Management of complications of infective endocarditis. Mayo Clin Proc 1982 Mar; 57(3):162–170

Wilson WR et al. Prosthetic valve endocarditis. Mayo Clin Proc 1982 Mar; 57(3):155–161

Valvular Disease

Cannobbio MM and Perloff JK. Critical care of adults with congenital heart disease. Crit Care Q 1981 Dec; 4(3): 39–50

Clark DB, McAnulty J and Rahimtoola SH. Valve replacement in aortic insufficiency with left ventricular dysfunction. Circulation 1980 Feb; 61(2):411–421

Ng L. Nursing aspects of the surgical treatment of idiopathic hypertrophic subaortic stenosis. Heart Lung 1982 July/Aug; 11(4):364–373

Partridge SA. Cardiac auscultation. DCCN 1982 May–June; 1(3):152–164

Rahimtoola SH. Valvular heart disease: A perspective. J Am Coll Cardiol 1983 Jan; 1(1):199–215

Saul L. Heart sounds and common murmurs. Am J Nurs 1983 Dec; 83(12):1681–1689

Stuart EM et al. Nursing rounds: Care of the patient with a mitral commissurotomy. Am J Nurs 1980 Sept; 80(9):1611–1632

Congestive Heart Failure/Pulmonary Edema

Bohachick P and Rongaus AM. Hypertrophic cardiomyopathy. Am J Nurs 1984 Mar; 84(3):320–326

Chatterjee K. Digitalis versus newer inotropic agents: Which to use. Drug Ther 1982 Jan; 12(1):83–96

Chatterjee K, Doule B and Avakian D. Vasodilator therapy for heart failure. Crit Care Q 1981 Dec; 4(3):13–24

Chyron D. Intravenous nitroglycerin in ischemic heart disease. DCCN 1983 Jan–Feb; 2(1):10–17

Cohen S. New concepts in understanding congestive heart failure: Part I How the clinical features arise. Am J Nurs 1981 Jan; 81(1):119–142

Cohen S. New concepts in understanding congestive heart failure: Part II How the therapeutic approaches work. Am J Nurs 1981 Feb; 81(2):357–380

Conley SK and Small RE. Administering IV nitroglycerin: Nursing implications. DCCN 1983 Jan–Feb; 2(1):18–22

Fenster PE and Bressler R. Treating cardiovascular disease in the elderly: Part II Antiarrhythmics, diuretics, and calcium channel blockers. Drug Ther 1984 Mar; 14(3):209–216

Frye R. Chronic congestive heart failure. Postgrad Med 1981 Mar; 69(3):165–174

Goldberger A. Congestive heart failure in adults: Six considerations in systematic diagnosis. Postgrad Med 1981 Mar; 69(3):151–160

Iseri L and Benvenuti D. Pathogenesis and management of congestive heart failure—Revisited. Am Heart J 1983 Feb 1; 105(2):346–349

Michaelson C. Bedside assessment and diagnosis of acute left ventricular failure. Crit Care Q 1981 Dec; 4(3):1–11

Quinlan M. Edema: What really causes it—How to control it. RN 1984 Apr; 47(4):55–57

Wold B. Dilated (congestive) cardiomyopathy: Considerations for the coronary care unit nurse. Heart Lung 1983 Sept; 12(5):545–553

Cardiovascular Surgery

Brown GL. Heart disease requiring surgical intervention: A continuum of nursing care. Occup Health Nurse 1981 Dec; 29(12):28–34

Cisar NS and Morpheu SF. Preoperative teaching: Aortocoronary bypass patients. Focus Crit Care 1983 Feb; 10(1):21–23

Finkelmeier BA and O'Mara SR. Temporary pacing in the cardiac surgical patient. Crit Care Nurse 1984 Jan–Feb; 4(1):108–114

Waggoner PC. Postoperative care of the patient undergoing cardiac valve replacement: A nursing perspective. Crit Care Q 1981 Dec; 4(3):57–65

Rehabilitation

Beglinger JE. Coping tasks in critical care. DCCN 1983 Mar–Apr; 2(2):80–89

Bille DA. Process oriented patient education. DCCN 1983 Mar–Apr; 2(2): 108–115

Budan LJ. Cardiac patient learning in the hospital setting. Focus Crit Care 1983 Oct; 10(5):18–22

Dion WF. Medical problems and physiologic responses during supervised inpatient cardiac rehabilitation: The patient after coronary artery bypass grafting. Heart Lung 1982 May–June; 11(3):248–255

Milhorn HT. Prescribing a cardiovascular fitness program. Compr Ther 1984 Feb; 10(2):46–53

Thomas SA et al. Denial in coronary

care patients—An objective reassessment. Heart Lung 1983 Jan; 12(1):74–80

Electrocardiology

Books

Andreoli K et al. Comprehensive Cardiac Care, 5th ed. St Louis, CV Mosby, 1984

Castellanos A. Cardiac Arrhythmias: Mechanisms and Management. Cardiovascular Clinics. Philadelphia, FA Davis, 1980

Chung E. Electrocardiography. Hagerstown, Harper & Row, 1980

Chung E. Principles of Cardiac Arrhythmias, 3rd ed. Baltimore, Williams & Wilkins, 1983

Conover M. Understanding Electrocardiography, 3rd ed. St Louis, CV Mosby Company, 1980

Grauer K. Problem Solving in Cardiac Arrest. St Louis, CV Mosby, 1984

Holloway N. Nursing the Critically Ill Adult. Menlo Park, CA, Addison Wesley, 1984

Hurst W. The Heart, 5th ed. New York, McGraw-Hill, 1982

Kinny M et al. AACN's Clinical Reference for Critical Care Nursing. New York, McGraw-Hill, 1981

Mangiola S and Ritota M. Cardiac Arrhythmias, 2nd ed. Philadelphia, JB Lippincott, 1982

Marriott H. Practical Electrocardiography, 7th ed. Baltimore, Williams & Wilkins, 1983

Meltzer L, Pinneo R and Kitchell J. Intensive Coronary Care, 4th ed. Bowie, Charles Press, 1983

Underhill S et al. Cardiac Nursing. Philadelphia, JB Lippincott, 1982

Articles

Barnaby PF, Barret PA and Lvoff R. Routine prophylactic lidocaine in acute myocardial infarction. Heart Lung 1983 July–Aug; 12(4):362–365

Bourget C. Verapamil: A calcium-channel blocker. DCCN 1982 May–June; 1(3):134–138

Burke LJ. Dealing with Bretylium-induced hypotension. DCCN 1983 Sept–Oct; 2(5):285–286

Butler JD and Harrison BL. Keeping pace with calcium channel blockers. Nurs 1983 July; 13(7):38–43

Cantwell R, Hollis R and Rogers M. Think fast—What do you know about cardiac drugs for a code? Nursing '82 1982 Oct; 12(10):34–41

Hartshorn J. Administering calcium-channel blocking agents. DCCN 1983 Mar–Apr; 2(2):70–74

Jacobs ML and Schamroth L. A study in atrioventricular block. Heart Lung 1982 May–June; 11(3):278–279

Johnson GP and Johanson BC. Beta blockers. Am J Nurs 1983 July; 83(7): 1034–1043.

Kesten KS, Reuter N and Swisher J. Diltiazem: The latest calcium-channel blocker. DCCN 1984 May–June; 3(3): 154–160

Kupper NS et al. Tachycardia—Stay a

step ahead of your patient's racing heart. Nursing '84 1984 Aug; 14(8): 34-41

Lasche P. Permanent cardiac pacing. Focus 1983 Oct; 10(5):28-36

Marriott HJL and Gozensky C. Arrhythmias in coronary care: A renewed plea. Heart Lung 1982 Jan-Feb; 11(1):33-39

McFadden EA, Zaloga GP and Chernow B. Hypocalcemia: A medical emergency. Am J Nurse 1983 Feb; 83(2):226-230

Nikolic G. Lidocaine bradycardia. Heart Lung 1984 May-June; 13(3):290-291

Parker M and Lemberg L. Pacemaker update 1984. Part I, Introduction to electrocardiographic analysis of pacing function and site. Heart Lung 1984 May; 13(3):315-318

Patros RJ. Temporary ventricular pacemakers demonstrating bipolar and unipolar modes. Heart Lung 1983 May; 12(3):177-180

Purcell J and Haynes L. Using the ECG to detect MI. Am J Nurs 1984 May-June; 84(5):627-642

Rossi LP and Antman EM. Calcium channel blockers: New treatment for cardiovascular disease. Am J Nurs 1983 Mar; 83(3):382-387

Rowe M and Sears G. Experimental antiarrhythmic drugs. DCCN 1983 Sept-Oct; 2(5):285-286

Scordo KA. Taming the cardiac monitor, part II. Nursing '82 1982 Sept; 12(9): 61-69

Selzer A. Quinidine in perspective: The rise and fall of quinidine. Heart Lung 1982 Jan-Feb; 11(1):33-39

Slusarczk S and Hicks FD. Helping your patient to live with a permanent pacemaker. Nursing '83 1983 Apr; 13(4):58-63

Trevino S and Massey JA. Risk factors for arrhythmias after myocardial infarction. Heart Lung 1983 May; 12(3):240-247

Vascular Disorders

Books

Bergan JJ and Yao JST. Aneurysms. Diagnosis and Treatment. New York, Grune & Stratton, 1982

Epstein M. Hypertension. Philadelphia, FA Davis, 1984

Goodfriend T. Hypertension Essentials. New York, Grune & Stratton, 1983

Hallet J. Manual of Patient Care in Vascular Surgery. Boston, Little, Brown & Co, 1982

Hobson R. Venous Trauma. Mt Kisco, NY, Futura, 1983

Najarian J (ed). Advances in Vascular Surgery. Chicago, Year Book Medical Publisher, 1983

Rutherford RB. Vascular Surgery. Philadelphia, WB Saunders, 1984

Savage P. Problems in Peripheral Vascular Disease. Philadelphia, FA Davis, 1983

Thompson DA. Cardiovascular Assessment: Guide for Nurses and Other Health Professionals. St Louis, CV Mosby, 1981

Articles

Diagnostic Evaluation

Barnes RW. Current status of noninvasive tests in the diagnosis of venous disease. Surg Clin North Am 1982 June; 62(3):489-500

Bastaroche MM et al. Assessing peripheral vascular disease at the bedside. Noninvasive testing. Am J Nurs 1983 Nov; 83(11):1552-1556

Bell DD and Gaspar MR. Routine aortography before abdominal aortic aneurysmectomy. Am J Surg 1982 Aug; 144(2):191-193

Bernstein EF and Fronek A. Current status of noninvasive tests in the diagnosis of peripheral arterial disease. Surg Clin North Am 1982 June; 62(3):473-487

Brady WR et al. Intravenous arteriography using digital subtraction techniques. JAMA 1982 Aug 13; 248(6):671-674

Criss E. Digital subtraction angiography. Am J Nurs 1982 Nov; 82(11):1706-1707

Crummy AB, Levy JM and White RI Jr. Using digital subtraction angiography. Patient Care 1983 Sept 15; 17(15):16-38

Cudworth-Bergin KL. Detecting arterial problems with a Doppler probe. RN 1984 Jan; 47(1):38-41

Doubilet P and Abrams HL. The cost of under-utilization (percutaneous transluminal angioplasty for peripheral vascular disease). New Engl J Med 1984 Jan 12; 310(2):95-102

Durbin N. The application of Doppler techniques in critical care. Focus Crit Care 1983 June; 10(3):44-46

Gibbs GE. How to improve your blood pressure measurement technique. Today's OR Nurse 1982 May; 4(3):12-15

Hudson B. Sharpen your vascular assessment skills with the Doppler ultrasound stethoscope. Nursing '83 1983 May; 13(5):55-57

Intravenous digital subtraction angiography. Med Lett 1983 Nov 25; 25(649):107-108

Messerli FH. Continuous noninvasive automatic blood pressure recording. Postgrad Med 1984 Mar; 75(4):115-124

Nuno IN. Should aortography be used routinely in the elective management of abdominal aortic aneurysm? Am J Surg 1982 July; 144(1):53-57

White RA et al. Noninvasive evaluation of peripheral vascular disease using transcutaneous oxygen tension. Am J Surg 1982 July; 144(1):68-75

General Vascular Problems

Ansel AL and Johnson JM. Prevention and management of polytetra fluorethylene (PTFE) graft complications in peripheral vascular reconstruction. Am J Surg 1982 Aug; 144(2):228-230

Babu SC, Shah PM and Clauss RH. Unappreciated causes of ischemia in the leg. Am J Surg 1982 Aug; 144(2): 225-227

Callow AD. Current status of vascular grafts. Surg Clin North Am 1982 June; 62(3):501-513

Cox G. Capillaries—A microexplanation. NITA 1983 May-June; 6(3):171-174

de Toledo LW. How vasodilators backfire. RN 1982 July; 45(7):41-45

Drury DA. Foot care for the high-risk patient. RN 1982 Nov; 45(11):46-49

Ekers MA and Satiani B. EAB (extra-anatomic bypass). A new route for vascular rehabilitation. Nursing '82 1982 Nov; 82(11):34-41

Ells L. We had to help Katie adjust her expectations (amputation). Nursing '82 1982 June; 12(6):60-63

Pearce WH, Yao JST and Bergan JJ. Noninvasive vascular diagnostic testing. Curr Prob Surg 1983 Aug; 20(8):464-537

Peterson FY. Assessing peripheral vascular disease at the bedside. Am J Nurs 1983 Nov; 83(11):1549-1551

Roberts B and Ring EJ. Current status of percutaneous transluminal angioplasty. Surg Clin North Am 1982 June; 62(3): 357

Scordo K. Using radial artery palpation to monitor blood pressure. DCCN 1983 Mar/Apr; 2(2):75-79

Evidence lacking that exercise improves lower-extremity circulation (letter). Postgrad Med 1984 Feb 1; 75(2):33

Gever LN. Streptokinase and urokinase. Nursing '83 1983 Jan; 13(1):76

Grundy SM. Atherosclerosis: Pathology, pathogenesis, and role of risk factors. Disease-a-Month 1983 June; 29(9):3-58

Hathaway D and Giden EA. Energy expenditure during leg exercise programs. Nurs Res 1983 May/June; 32(3):147-150

Katz P. Hypersensitivity vasculitis. Am Fam Physician 1982 July; 26(1):171-175

King SL. Patient care in vascular surgery. AORN J 1981 April; 33(5):843-848

Lennihan R Jr et al. Easing intermittent claudication. Patient Care 1983 Aug 15; 17(14):123-129

Menzoian JO. Management of vascular injuries to the leg. Am J Surg 1982 Aug; 144(2):231-234

Moake JL and Funicella T. Common bleeding problems. Clinical Symposia Summit, NJ, CIBA 1983; 35(3):2-32

Sparacino J. Blood pressure, stress, and mental health. Nurs Res 1982 Mar/Apr; 31(2):89-94

Sparacino J et al. Psychological correlates of blood pressure: A closer examination of hostility, anxiety and engagement. Nurs Res 1982 May/June; 31(3):143-149

Tolins SH. Treatment of varicose veins. Am J Surg 1983 Feb; 145(2):248-252

Vasodilators. Nursing '83 1983 Nov; 13(11):64a-65a

Winston TR, Henly WS and Geis RC. Surgery for peripheral vascular disease. AORN J 1981 April; 33(5): 849-853

Anticoagulant Therapy

Cheng TC. Thrombocytopenia associated with minidose heparin therapy. Postgrad Med 1981 Dec; 70(6):73-78

Hyll R. Adjusted subcutaneous heparin vs warfarin sodium in the long-term treatment of venous thrombosis. New Engl J Med 1982 Jan 28; 306(4):189–194

Kirschenbaun HL and Rosenberg JM. Coumarin. RN 1982 Oct; 42(10):54–56

McConnell EA. The subtle art of really good injections. RN 1982 Feb; 45(2):25–34

Pierson S et al. Efficacy of graded elastic compression in the lower leg. JAMA 1983 Jan 14; 249(2):242–243

Sohn CA. Rescind the risks in administering anticoagulants. Nursing '81 1981 Oct; 11(10):34–41

Thompson DA. Teaching the client about anticoagulants. Am J Nurs 1982 Feb; 82(2):278–281

Thrombolytic enzymes. Nursing '83 1983 May; 13(5):64

Winston E et al. Nifedipine as a therapeutic modality for Raynaud's phenomenon. Arth Rheum 1983; 26:1177–1180

Conditions of the Veins

Bergan JJ, Flinn WR and Yao JST. Venous reconstructive surgery. Surg Clin North Am 1982 June; 62(3):399–410

Byrne P et al. The role of intraoperative heparin in reducing the incidence of postoperative deep venous thrombosis. Surg Gynecol Obstet 1984 May; 158(5):419–422

Chobanian AV. The influence of hypertension and other hemodynamic factors in atherogenesis. Prog Cardiovas Dis 1983 Nov/Dec; 26(3):177–196

Dale WA. Venous bypass surgery. Surg Clin North Am 1982 June; 62(3):391–398

Doyle JE. All leg ulcers are not alike; managing and preventing arterial and venous ulcers. Nursing '83 1983 Jan; 13(1):58–63

Fahey VA. Deep vein thrombosis. Nursing '84 1984 March; 14(3):34–41

Grundy SM et al. Atherosclerosis: Pathology, pathogenesis, and role of risk factors. Disease-a-Month 1983 June; 29(9):3–58

Hardin WD et al. Management of traumatic peripheral vein injuries. Am J Surg 1982 Aug; 144(2):215–238

Hessler K and Kenny M. Using humans umbilical vein grafts. AORN J 1981 Apr; 33(5):862–866

Hinnant JR and Stallworth JM. Simplified surgery for varicose veins. AORN J 1981 July; 34(1):135–150

Hirsh J and Hull R. Difficulties in diagnosing and treating venous thrombosis. Emerg Med Rep 1983 July; 4(14):81–87

Hull R et al. Cost effectiveness of clinical diagnosis, venography, and noninvasive testing in patients with symptomatic deep-vein thrombosis. New Engl J Med 1981 June 25; 304(26):1561–1567

Jones ER. Relationship between pH of intravenous medications and phlebitis: An experimental study. NITA 1982 July/Aug; 5(4):273–276

Keith LM and Smead WL. Saphenous vein stripping and its complications. Surg Clin North Am 1983 Dec; 63(6):1303–1311

Larson E, Lunche S and Tran JT. Correlates of IV phlebitis. NITA 1984 May–June; 7(3):203–205

Mathewson M. A Homan's sign is an effective method of diagnosing thrombophlebitis in bedridden patients. Crit Care Nurs 1983 July/Aug; 3(4):64–65

Menzoian JO. Management of vascular injuries to the leg. Am J Surg 1982 Aug; 144(2):231–234

Niewiarowski S and Koneti Rao A. Contribution of thrombogenic factors to the pathogenesis of atherosclerosis. Prog Cardiovas Dis 1983 Nov/Dec; 26(3):197–222

Rosen T and Mills JM. From simple plaque to necrotic ulcer. RN 1983 Nov; 46(11):42–43

Satiani B. Management of acute deep vein thrombosis. Am Fam Physician 1982 Apr; 75(4):103–109

Svedman P. Irrigation treatment of leg ulcers. Lancet 1983 Sept 3; 2(8349):532–534

Taheri SA et al. Surgical treatment of postphlebitic syndrome with vein valve transplant. Am J Surg 1982 Aug; 144(2):221–224

Taylor DL. Thrombophlebitis. Nursing '83 1983 July; 13(7):52–53

Tyson RR and Derrick BM. Vascular prostheses today. Med Times 1983 Dec; 3(12):45–49

Varicose Veins and Leg Ulcers

Keith L and Smead WF. Saphenous vein stripping and its complications. Surg Clin North Am 1983 Dec; 63(6):1303–1312

Lofgren ER. Leg ulcers. Postgrad Med 1984 Sept 15; 76(4):51

When the complaint is varicose veins. Patient Care 1984 Mar 30; 18(6):22–54

Which therapy and when for varicose veins? Patient Care 1984 Mar 30; 18(6):63–73

Conditions of the Arteries

Antilipemics. Nursing '84 1984 March; 14(3):57

Baum PL. Abdominal aortic aneurysm? Nursing '82 1982 Dec; 12(12):34–41

Blumenberg RM and Gelfand ML. Application of intestinal staplers to aortoiliac surgery. Am J Surg 1982 Aug; 144(2):198–202

Boozer M and Craven RF. Nursing care of the patient with chronic occlusive peripheral artery disease. Cardiovasc Nurs 1981 July–Aug; 15(4):13–17

Claus PL et al. Am J Surg 1982 July; 144(1):180–185

Craven RF and Curry TD. When the diagnosis is Raynaud's. Am J Nurs 1981 May; 81(5):1007–1009

Cudworth-Bergin KL. Detecting arterial problems with a Doppler probe. RN 1984 Jan; 47(1):38–41

DeLuca SA and Rhea JT. Aortic aneurysm with duodenal obstruction. Am Fam Physician Jan; 29(1):143–144

Doyle JE. Arterial insufficiency. Nursing '81 1981 April; 11(4):74–79

Doyle JE. Bypass graft surgery. Am J Nurs 1982 Oct; 82(10):1559–1562

Doyle JE and Sequeira JC. Renal artery dilation (treating renovascular hypertension). Am J Nurs 1982 Oct; 82(10):1563–1564

Edwards WS. Thoracoabdominal aortic aneurysms. Surg Clin North Am 1982 June; 62(3):441–448

Fahey VA and Finkelmeier BA. Iatrogenic arterial injuries. Am J Nurs 1984 Apr; 84(4):448–451

Gomes MN. Diagnosis of abdominal aortic aneurysms. Am Fam Physician 1982 Mar; 25(3):167–176

Graor RA. Occlusive and aneurysmal aortoiliac disease. Postgrad Med 1984 May 15; 75(7):61–72

Hartshorn JC. Aneurysm: Keeping your patient alive until surgery. RN 1984 Jan; 47(1):30–33

Jasinkowski N. The unique needs of a distal bypass patient. RN 1982 Mar; 45(3):44–47, 122

Lennihan R Jr et al. Identifying arteriosclerosis obliterans. Patient Care 1983 Aug 15; 17(14):100–121

Lennihan R. When your patient has Raynaud's syndrome. Patient Care 1983 Nov 30; 17(20):70–97

Memon AS. Raynaud's vasospasm. Hosp Pract 1983 May; 18(5):141–150

Sauvage LR. Porous fabric arterial prosthesis. AORN J 1981 Apr; 33(5):854–861

Smith DC and McKendry RJR. Controlled trial of nifedipine in the treatment of Raynaud's phenomenon. Lancet 1982 Dec 11; 2(8311):1299–1301

Spittell JA. Occlusive peripheral arterial disease. Postgrad Med 1982 Feb; 71(2):137–151

Treiman RL et al. Aneurysmectomy in the octogenarian. Am J Surg 1982 Aug; 144(2):194–197

Hypertension

Joint National Committee on Detection, Evaluation, and Treatment of High Blood Pressure. The 1984 Report of the Joint National Committee on Detection, Evaluation, and Treatment of High Blood Pressure. Arch Intern Med 1984 May; 144(5):1045–1057

Black HR. Evaluation and treatment of the hypertensive patient. Prim Care 1983 Mar; 10(1):3–19

Chobanian AV. Hypertension. Clinical Symposia, Summit, NJ, CIBA 1982; 34(5):3–32

Comparison of propranolol and hydrochlorothiazide for the initial treatment of hypertension. JAMA 1982 Part 1, Oct 22/29; 248(16):1996–2003; Part 2, 2004–2011

Cunningham S and Hill M. Current status of high blood pressure control. 1982 March; 7(3):37–44

Daniels LM and Kochar MS. Monitoring and facilitating adherence to hypertension therapeutic regimens. Cardiovasc Nurs 1980; March–April; 16(2):7–12

Egan B and Julius S. Borderline hypertension. Prim Care 1983 Mar; 10(1):99–113

Freis ED. Mild hypertension. Postgrad Med 1983 Jan; 73(1):180–189

Gever LN. Thiazide diuretics—Minimizing their adverse effects. Nursing '84 1984 Feb; 14(2):72

Gifford RW. Mild hypertension—Should it be treated? Postgrad Med 1982 Apr; 71(4):19–21

Guanadrel (Hylorel)—a new antihypertensive drug. Med Lett 1983 Oct 14; 25(646):95–96

Hill MN and Foster SB. High blood pressure. Nursing '82 1982 Feb; 12(2): 72–75

Hill M and Fink JW. In hypertensive emergencies, act quickly but also act cautiously. Nursing '83 1983 Feb; 13(2):34–41

Kaplan NM. Newer anti-hypertensive agents. Postgrad Med 1983 Jan; 73(1): 213–222

Kelber MB Sr. Plasma renin activity. Nursing '82 1982 April; 12(4):140–144

Kirschenbaum HL and Rosenberg JM. Guanethidine and reserpine. RN 1984 Feb; 47(2):31–33

Kirschenbaum HL and Rosenberg JM. Hydralazine and minocidil. RN 1982 Dec; 45(12):42–43

Kirschenbaum HL and Rosenberg JM. Thiazides. RN 1983 July; 46(7):28–30

Langford HG. Potassium in hypertension. Postgrad Med 1983 Jan; 73(1):227–233

Larrabee PS and Hanna ND. Saralasin infusion test. Am J Nurs 1983 Dec; 83(12):1258–1259

Loustan A and Blair BJ. A key to compliance—Systematic teaching to help hypertensive patients follow through on treatment. Nursing '81 1981 Feb; 11(2):84–87

Lowther NB and Carter VD. How to increase compliance in hypertensives. Am J Nurs 1981 May; 81(5):963

Mancia G et al. Effects of blood-pressure measurement by the doctor on patient's blood pressure and heart rate. Lancet 1983 Sept 24; 2(8352):695

McCombs J, Fink J and Bandy P. Critical patient behaviors in high blood pressure control. Cardiovasc Nurs July–Aug; 16(4):19–23

Moore MA. Step-care approach to improving hypertensive patient compliance. Am Fam Practice 1982 July; 26(1):155–160

Moser M. Stepped care treatment of hypertension. Postgrad 1983 Jan; 73(1):199–210

Onesti G. Selection of drugs for hypertensive crisis. Am Fam Practice 1980 Dec; 22(6):141–142

Perez-Stable E. Mild hypertension: Patient Care. Treat all patients? 1983 Aug 15; 17(14):171–185

Pleuss J and Kochar MS. Dietary considerations in hypertension. Postgrad Med 1981 June; 69(6):34–43

Podell RN. Polyunsaturated fats and blood pressure control. Postgrad Med 1983 Nov; 74(5):327–332

Reichgott MJ and Simons-Morton BG. Strategies to improve patient compliance with antihypertensive therapy. Prim Care 1983 Mar; 10(1): 21–27

Rosenberg J and Kirschenbaum HL. Catopril. RN 1983 Feb; 42(2):56–57

Rosenberg J and Kirschenbaum HL. Alpha-adrenergic blocker. RN 1983 Dec; 46(12):46–47

Sandroff R. Blushing on the inside. A new look at hypertension. RN 1982 Feb; 45(2):40–41

Semple P. Hypertension. Nursing Mirror. Part 1, 1980 Oct 2; 151(14):18–21; Part 2, 1980 Oct 9; 151(15):24–26; Part 3, 1980 Oct 16; 151(16):30–32

Stress management in borderline hypertension. Am J Nurs 1983 Mar; 83(3):408

Stromborg MF and Stromborg P. Test your knowledge of managing the patient with hypertension. Nursing '81 1981 Mar; 11(3):56–59

Therapy for mild hypertension. JAMA 1983 Jan 21; 249(3):365–367

Thibodeau JA and Hebert P. Use of a nursing model to develop a hypertension protocol. Nurs Pract 1981 Mar–Apr; 6(2):21–27

Utz SW. Applying the Neuman model to nursing practice with hypertensive clients. Cardiovasc Nurs 1980 Nov–Dec; 16(6):29–34

Wartman SA. Sexual side effects of antihypertensive drugs. Postgrad Med 1983 Feb; 73(2):133–138

The Lymphatic System

Cohen DG. Metabolic complications of induction therapy for leukemia and lymphoma. CA Nurs 1983 Aug; 6(4): 307–310

King RC. Exploring the neck and lymphatics. RN 1982 June; 45(6):49–55, 99

Conditions of the Digestive System

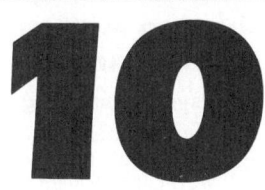

1: Conditions of the Mouth, Neck, and Esophagus

Mouth Conditions

Nursing Assessment for Effective Mouth Care

Psychosocial Significance

1. The person's comfort, good nutrition, and general well-being are promoted by maintaining clean and well-cared-for teeth and gums.
2. Personal attractiveness is enhanced.
3. Participation in community dental health programs promotes prevention, early detection, and correction of dental problems.

Self-Care Goals

1. Reduce bacterial count and prevent tissue infection by removing food and rinsing the mouth.
2. Prevent dental caries when plaque is removed periodically by the dentist.
3. Emphasize importance of regular periodic dental examination to maintain good mouth health.
4. Maintain healthy mouth structures by tooth brushing, flossing between teeth, and massaging gums.
5. Promote proper nutrition, since dentition and mouth tissue tone are directly affected.
6. Encourage topical application of fluoride, as well as fluoridation of water, since this chemical significantly reduces dental caries.
7. Recognize that fatigue, emotional upsets, and injury lower resistance of dental tissue to infection.
8. Examine soft tissues of the mouth frequently for evidences of irritation, unusual growths, discoloration, encrustation, and leukoplakia, since abnormal manifestations may herald malignancy and early detection may achieve early correction.

Causes of Trauma to Oral Structures

1. *Mechanical*—stiff-bristled toothbrush, hot pipe stem, ill-fitting dentures, carious or broken teeth, grinding of teeth, cheek and lower lip biting.
2. *Thermal*—smoking, hot liquids, hot foods.
3. *Chemical*—sucking hard candy, using full-strength antiseptic mouthwashes, chewing or smoking tobacco, drinking alcoholic beverages, chewing Aspergum, sucking mouth lozenges, using breath sweeteners, drinking citrus juices, drug reactions.
4. *Bacterial*—poor oral and nutritional attention that permits food to collect.
5. *Irradiation*—exposure to sun, ultraviolet rays, radium, and x-rays.
6. *Nutritional*—improper dietary habits.
7. Metabolic disorders, blood dyscrasias.

Assessment and Diagnostic Evaluation

A. Assessment

(See Physical Assessment of the Adult—Mouth, pp. 25.)

B. Oral Cell Smear for Cytologic Examination

1. Grasp the tongue with a 4″ × 4″ gauze square and gently move the tongue to expose the questionable area.
2. Using a moistened tongue depressor, scrape the area or lesion.

3. If a hyperkeratotic (hypertrophy of the stratum cornium layer of skin) lesion is present, scrape off surface keratin so that deeper epithelial cells are available for a specimen (these are usually involved in early malignant change).
4. Smear cells on a glass slide, immerse carefully in alcohol, and send to laboratory.

Lesions of the Mouth

Leukoplakia

See p. 394.

Lichen Planus

Lichen planus consists of minute white papules, which form a reticular or plaque pattern; it is often difficult to differentiate from leukoplakia. This condition may be related to a dermatologic problem.

1. Etiology—unknown
2. Assessment
   a. Usually asymptomatic
   b. Some complain of burning sensations, a metallic taste, or pain
   c. May last for weeks or years; if erosive, it is longer lasting
3. Management
   a. Asymptomatic—no treatment
   b. Topical steroids, topical anesthetics, and perhaps intralesional steroids.

Gingivitis

(Inflammation of gums)

1. The most common infection of oral tissues
2. *Clinical manifestations*
   a. Inflammation and slight swelling of superficial gingivae and interdental papillae
   b. With continued neglect, may advance to chronic degenerative gingivitis and eventually to periodontal disease
3. *Nursing management*
   a. Conscientious mouth hygiene
   b. Periodic professional dental cleaning

Acute Ulcerative Gingivitis

("Trench mouth," Vincent's gingivitis)

1. Pseudomembranous painful ulceration affecting gums, inner dental papillae, mouth mucosa, tonsils, and pharynx, especially in young adults and adolescents.
2. *Etiology*
   a. Thought to be caused by both a spirochete and a fusiform bacillus.
   b. May be due to poor oral hygiene, low tissue resistance, and infection from complex micro-organisms.
3. *Clinical manifestations*
   a. Painful bleeding gums, mild fever, swelling of lymph nodes of neck.
   b. If infection spreads to tonsils and pharynx, swallowing and talking may be painful.
4. *Treatment and nursing management*
   a. Encourage mouth irrigations with dilute hydrogen peroxide or 2% sodium perborate (to combat

anaerobic spirochetes) to treat infection, control fetid breath, and provide comfort.

b. Administer antibiotics as prescribed to curb infection; give analgesics for pain and discomfort.

c. Offer soft foods and liquids to reduce gum trauma.

d. Instruct the patient to avoid highly seasoned foods, alcoholic beverages, and smoking, all of which irritate infected oral tissues.

e. Teach the patient the importance of regular eating habits and sufficient rest.

Conditions of the Salivary Glands

Salivary Calculus

(Sialolithiasis)

1. Salivary stones may form in the submaxillary gland following glandular infection or ductal stricture due to trauma or inflammation.
2. Salivary stones are usually mostly calcium oxalate.
   a. Stones found in the gland are irregularly lobulated.
   b. Stones found in the duct are small and oval in shape.
3. *Diagnostic evaluation*—Sialogram (x-ray with contrast medium)
4. Clinical manifestations
   a. None unless there is an infection.
   b. If calculus obstructs gland, the following conditions may occur:
      (1) Sudden, local pain, which is suddenly relieved by a gush of saliva.
      (2) Gland is swollen and tender.
      (3) Stone may be palpable.
      (4) Stone is visible with x-ray studies.
5. *Treatment*
   a. Surgical extraction of stone.
   b. Gland may have to be removed if condition occurs repeatedly.

Maxillofacial Fractures

Fractures of the maxillofacial area usually include injury to the soft tissues and may occur as a result of a fall or if patient has been hit by a fist or a flying object.

Immediate Assessment and Management

1. Determine whether there is obstruction to the airway.
   a. Remove any obstruction from pharynx, such as broken teeth, dentures, blood clots, or broken bits of bone.
   b. Determine whether tongue has been displaced posteriorly; if so, insert index finger and pull tongue forward.
   c. Prepare for emergency tracheostomy if airway is obstructed.
2. Control hemorrhage by direct pressure on vessels supplying the area (see Fig. 23-4, p. 932).
   Prepare for fluid replacement.
3. Assess vital signs and note extent and involvement of other parts of the head and body.
4. Ascertain localization of pain to determine nerve injury.
5. Administer analgesics to relieve pain and anxiety but not to depress respirations.
6. Reassure the patient that he is being given the best possible care.

Mandibular Fractures

1. Two thirds of significant facial fractures in the US are of the mandible.
2. Most mandibular fractures can be treated with closed reduction and intermaxillary fixation.
3. Open reduction is preferred for certain patients:
   a. Aged, senile, edentulous, and debilitated
   b. Children and those who cannot tolerate intermaxillary fixation
   c. Professional athletes
   d. Patients who are psychotic or have a history of seizures
   e. The diabetic person with special nutritional needs

Assessment

Clinical Manifestations

1. Malocclusion, asymmetry, abnormal mobility, and crepitus (grating sound with movement).
2. Tissue injury; note extent and involvement.

Treatment

Mandibular fractures are reduced first; maxillary fractures follow in positioning.

Lower jaw is held tightly against upper jaw by crosswires or rubber bands placed around arch bars wired to the teeth (intermaxillary fixation).

Patient Problems/Nursing Diagnoses

1. Ineffective airway clearance related to malposition of mandible or jaw, and tissue edema related to injury.
2. Pain in lower face area and referred areas related to injury to tissues and fracture of mandible (maxilla).
3. Impaired verbal communication related to edema, pain, and fracture of jaw and subsequent intermaxillary fixation.
4. Alteration in nutrition related to limited or absent function of jaw (fracture) that interferes with normal eating.
5. Potential for mouth infection related to intermaxillary fixation and poor access to mouth for cleansing purposes.

Planning and Implementation

Nursing Interventions

A. Preoperative Preparation

1. Determine priorities for fracture reduction:
   a. Irrigate laceration with copious amounts of normal physiologic saline.
   b. Prepare for debridement and suturing of lacerations.
   c. Apply sterile pressure dressings to control swelling, prevent tension on stitches, and maintain an area that is as clean as possible to minimize or prevent infection.
   d. Administer tetanus prophylaxis as prescribed. Give antibiotics as prescribed.
2. Prepare the patient for roentgenograms to determine method of reducing and immobilizing fractures.

B. Postoperative Care

(Management of patient with intermaxillary fixation)

1. Immediately position patient on his side with head slightly elevated to facilitate breathing and for ease of suctioning.
2. Note wire cutter or scissors taped to bandages or in some other obvious place.
   a. These cutters or scissors are to cut wires or

rubber bands in the event the patient vomits; this will prevent aspiration.
   b. After the patient emerges from anesthesia, scissors or cutters must still be kept nearby for emergency use.
3. Suction drainage and stomach contents as required to lessen danger of aspiration.
   a. Connect nasogastric suction to low-pressure suction.
   b. If vomiting is anticipated, administer antiemetic medications as prescribed.
   c. Insert small catheter into nasopharyngeal area for suctioning if a nasogastric catheter has not been inserted during surgery.
   d. Aspirate oral cavity; this is facilitated by inserting a tongue blade to move cheek away from teeth.
   e. Insert oral catheter behind third molar (or where a tooth may be missing) to aspirate within the oropharynx.
4. Modify care as the patient emerges from anesthesia.
   a. Remind the patient that his jaw is wired but that he can breathe and swallow.
   b. Provide a means of communication such as a "magic slate" (or chalk and chalkboard) or signal system.
   c. Elevate the head of the bed for comfort and to facilitate breathing.
   d. Continue to administer parenteral intravenous fluids as prescribed until nourishment can be taken by mouth.
   e. Administer medications to control pain and restlessness, as well as to prevent nausea and infection.

C. Nutritional Considerations

Maintain adequate nutritional levels to promote healing:
1. Provide privacy for the patient to eat, since he might be sensitive to his appearance and to the noisy sounds he makes as he tries to eat and drink.
2. Provide a straw if the patient can manage it; the patient may suck soft foods from a demitasse spoon.
3. Serve food attractively and arrange an environment that is as pleasant as possible (music, television, view from window) to encourage nutritional intake.

D. Prevention of Infection

Promote a climate to prevent complications and to promote recovery:
1. Apply lubricant to the lips to prevent drying and cracking.
2. Provide frequent and careful attention to the mouth.
   a. Irrigate the mouth with tap water or normal saline after each feeding; use an Asepto syringe or irrigating set under low pressure.
   b. Use a Water Pik if available, since it is effective in a gentle way.
   c. Swab the area between teeth and cheek by using a tongue depressor to retract the cheek. Provide light with a flashlight.

Health Education

Set up a plan of instruction so that the patient will be able to manage at home even with the jaw wired.
1. Encourage exercise and proper diet to promote general good health and tissue healing, and to prevent constipation.
2. Develop a plan that is convenient for the patient to follow in maintaining oral cleanliness.

3. Work with the patient's family, if required, in determining interesting pursuits to counterbalance any worries he might have about appearance, cost of treatment, and other problems.
4. Remind the patient of follow-up visits to his physician.
5. Prepare the patient for possible reconstructive or orthodontic work if this is required.

Evaluation

Expected Outcomes

1. Patient is able to breathe easily; edema subsides once jaw has been positioned
2. Has no pain in the face—demonstrates fracture is healing
3. Able to communicate in an understandable manner
4. Receives adequate nourishment through a straw and via demitasse spoon
5. Demonstrates proper mouth hygiene—utilizes mouth rinses after feedings; swabs the area between his teeth and cheeks every morning and evening

Premalignant Mouth Lesions

Leukoplakia Buccalis

("Smoker's patch")
1. Characterized by the appearance of one or more small, often crinkled, pearly patches on the mucous membrane of tongue or mouth.
2. Due to the keratinization of the mucosa and sclerosis of the underlying tissues.
3. Health education
   a. If there are no symptoms other than appearance, emphasize importance of careful oral hygiene:
      (1) Recommend dental care and gingival treatment.
      (2) Advise the patient to avoid alcohol, tobacco, coffee, and tea.
      (3) Suggest mouth rinses of half-strength milk of magnesia after meals and at bedtime.
      (4) Encourage increased vitamin intake, particularly of vitamin C.
   b. If in addition to appearance of white patches there is pain, induration, and ulceration, do the following:
      (1) Suggest biopsy to rule out cancer.
      (2) Follow above regimen (3a).

Cancer of the Mouth

Incidence

1. Cancer of the mouth accounts for 3% of all male and 1% of all female cancer deaths in this country.
2. Males are afflicted more than twice as often as females.
3. Evidence suggests that the risk of cancer in the heavy smoker and drinker may be as much as 15 times greater than in those who neither smoke nor drink.

Preventive Measures

1. Eliminate causes of chronic irritation.
2. Practice good oral hygiene.
3. Obtain proper dental care—remove or repair jagged, carious, and infected teeth.
4. Reduce or eliminate smoking and smokeless tobacco (chewing tobacco and dipping snuff); also eliminate pipe smoking if it irritates the lip.
5. Restrict or eliminate ingestion of highly spiced foods and reduce alcohol consumption.

6. If sexually transmitted disease is suspected, seek treatment (see p. 863).

Treatment

1. Selection of treatment depends on size of lesion and how extensively surrounding tissues are involved.
2. Small lesions can be removed by wide excision or can be treated with radiotherapy or interstitial irradiation.
3. Large lesions may be excised widely or treated by external irradiation followed by radical neck dissection (see p. 397).
4. Advanced cancer (see p. 917)
   a. Radiation therapy can be palliative, providing it has not been given previously.
   b. Extensive surgical extirpation may be feasible but is done only with patient's full understanding that cure is not achievable.
   c. Intra-arterial chemotherapy has been done, but only with limited success. A brief regression in tumor size may be achieved.
   d. Thalamotomy may be a useful palliative procedure for the patient with advanced malignancy and severe pain.

Assessment
Clinical Manifestations

1. For precancerous mouth lesions—leukoplakia buccalis, keratosis labialis:
   a. Pearly patches—1 or 2 small thin, often crinkled areas on mucous membranes of the tongue, mouth, or both, due to
      (1) Keratinization of mucosa
      (2) Sclerosis of underlying tissue
   b. Later, most of tongue and mouth may become covered:
      (1) Creamy white, thick, fissured mucous membrane
      (2) Sometimes desquamates, leaving a beefy-red base
2. For cancerous lesions:
   a. White patchy area, sore spot or ulcer on lips, gums, or mouth, which fails to heal
   b. Swelling, numbness, or loss of feeling in the part
   c. An asymmetric, firm nodal enlargement or mass
   d. Erythroplakia—red plaques or well-defined velvety red patches, often with tiny areas of ulceration

Nursing History

1. Determine amount of patient discomfort, such as tenderness (where?), pain (type?), bleeding (where and when?), oozing or discharge?
2. Difficulty speaking? Eating? With what particular kinds of food?
3. Any referred pain? To where? Other parts of face, ear, head?

Diagnostic Evaluation

1. Roentgenogram of head and neck to determine involvement
2. Cytologic examination of sputum (see p. 141)
3. Biopsy of suspected tissue

Patient Problems/Nursing Diagnoses

1. Alteration in comfort (pain) related to malignant infiltration of oral tissues
2. Nutritional deficit related to inadequate fluid and food intake; caused by pain and difficulty in chewing and swallowing, excess salivation
3. Impaired verbal communication related to a tendency to inhibit movement of jaw and mouth because of painful lesions
4. Disturbance in self-concept related to changes occurring in facial image and contour
5. Fear and anxiety related to misinformation, suspected poor prognosis, and altered (postoperative) function

Planning and Implementation
Nursing Interventions

A. Preoperative Preparation

1. Provide optimal mouth care.
   a. Proper care of teeth because they are essential to mastication.
      (1) Stress regular dental care.
      (2) Promote good nutrition.
   b. Mouth cleanliness to reduce incidence of infectious disease such as mumps and surgical parotitis.
      (1) Brush teeth frequently.
      (2) Use oxygen-releasing and antimicrobial mouth-rinsing solutions.
      (3) Apply lanolin to dry and cracking lips.
      (4) Remove dentures and clean them frequently.
   c. Adequate fluid intake, particularly in debilitated patients who are prone to mouth infections.
   d. Stimulation of flow of saliva.
      (1) Offer chewing gum.
      (2) Encourage the patient to suck lemon sour balls, a fresh lemon, or orange slices.
      (3) Administer antibiotics as prescribed to assist in control of infection.

B. Postoperative Care

1. Maintain a patent airway.
   a. Recognize that the patient may have an airway, endotracheal tube, or tracheostomy to facilitate air exchange.
   b. Observe the patient closely for signs of respiratory embarrassment, such as changes in vital signs, dyspnea, and restlessness.
   c. Place the patient in a prone position, or in a supine position with head turned to side, or laterally; position should facilitate drainage and prevent aspiration.
   d. Suction as required; precautions are necessary to avoid injury to suture line and sensitive tissues.
   e. When the patient is out of anesthesia, elevate head of bed for comfort, to facilitate deep breathing and coughing up of secretions, and to lessen edema.
2. Monitor for bleeding.
   a. Take frequent vital sign readings.
   b. Observe tissues and dressings for evidence of oozing or bleeding.
   c. Inspect back of neck for accumulation of blood staining; observe patient for frequent swallowing.
3. Check pressure dressings that are used to control edema.
   a. Note whether dressings are hindering respirations.
   b. Observe surrounding tissues to determine whether dressings are constricting blood circulation.

c. If portable suction is used, pressure dressings may not be applied.
4. Control pain so that respirations are not depressed. Employ nursing measures to make the patient comfortable so that narcotics for pain relief are not used unless absolutely required.

C. Improved Nutritional Intake

1. Maintain nutritional and electrolyte levels.
   Following intravenous therapy, administer tube feedings by nasogastric tube or gastrostomy (see pp. 412 and 426).
2. Feeding problems may be handled in the following ways:
   a. Use straws, teaspoon, feeders, etc.
   b. Provide food that is soft, liquid, and nonirritating—not too hot or cold or highly seasoned.
   c. Serve small, frequent meals attractively.
3. Allow the patient to have his meals in privacy if he so desires.
4. Keep mouth clean for comfort and to assist in healing process.
   a. Mouth irrigations, using normal saline, diluted hydrogen peroxide, sodium bicarbonate, or alkaline mouthwashes
   b. Gentle lavaging, using a catheter between cheek and teeth to loosen mucus
   c. Power spray to clean inaccessible spaces
   d. Vaporizer to provide moisture to traumatized tissue and to discourage crusting
5. Excessive salivation and mouth odors may be handled as follows:
   a. Insert gauze wick in corner of mouth; place basin conveniently to catch drippings.
   b. Use small rubber catheter and suction.
   c. Encourage use of mouthwashes, particularly oxidizing agents such as half-strength hydrogen peroxide.
   d. Use power spray, if available.

D. Improvement in Communication Techniques

1. During preoperative period, prepare for postoperative communication, since the patient may not be able to talk for a few days after surgery.
   Practice lip reading, hand signals, magic slate, eye-blink codes, and flash cards (words or pictures).
2. Supply pad and pencil, magic slate, signal system (eye blinks or hand), so that the patient can express his needs and thoughts. Note that if the patient usually wears glasses to read and write, he may not be able to put his glasses on because of dressings, skin flaps, etc.
3. Refer the patient to a speech pathologist or therapist if the services of this specialist are indicated.

E. Psychosocial Adjustment

1. Promote optimal physical condition and psychological adjustment.

a. Assess the patient's reaction to his condition.
   (1) Evaluate the patient's apprehension and offer emotional support.
   (2) Correct any misinformation.
   (3) Determine therapeutic plan of care for the patient's rehabilitation.
2. Recognize that face and neck surgery can be disfiguring and the patient often is embarrassed, withdrawn, and depressed.
3. Encourage the patient's family and friends to visit so that he is aware others care for him.
4. Assist the patient in caring for his personal appearance.
5. Observe closely for indications of the patient's needs, which may be communicated in other ways.
6. Be consistent with emotional support.
7. Provide an environment conducive to the patient's recovery.
   a. Maintain proper humidification and aeration of room.
   b. Prevent odors by removing soiled dressings; use effective and pleasant deodorizers.
   c. Inform the patient that his general throat discomfort is due to endotracheal anesthesia and will improve in a few days.
8. Prepare the patient for convalescence and extended care at home.
   a. Provide detailed instructions to the patient and/or a member of his family.
   b. If suctioning is required, instruct as to method, type of equipment, and where it can be obtained.
   c. Emphasize adequate nutrition—proper consistency, proper seasoning, and right temperature. Suggest commercial baby foods or the use of a blender if available.
   d. Repeat the details of good mouth care and cleanliness of dressings.
   e. Review signs of obstruction, hemorrhage, infection, and depression and what to do about them if they are evident.

Evaluation

Expected Outcomes

1. Emerges from surgical treatment and radiation therapy with minimal problems
2. Maintains satisfactory nutritional status; controls mouth odors; utilizes a power spray and dilute hydrogen peroxide
3. Demonstrates proficiency in speaking clearly; when mouth is sore, uses a magic slate
4. Displays interest in personal appearance as manifested by attention to shaving daily and requesting the services of a barber, or applying make-up; looks forward to visits from family members
5. Voices optimism about the immediate future

Head and Neck Malignancy

Head and neck cancer refers to a group of malignant tumors that may occur at any one of a number of anatomic sites in the upper digestive tract.

Incidence

1. Usually occurs in individuals in their 6th or 7th decade; ratio of males to females is 3:1.

2. Approximately 35,000 to 40,000 will have this annually; mortality rate is near 15,000/year.

Assessment

Possible Clinical Manifestations

1. Pain, dysphagia, dysphonia, difficulty in breathing, hoarseness

2. Hemoptysis, excessive salivation, loosening of teeth, dentures no longer fitting
3. Earache, nasal bleeding, infection
4. Neck swelling, weight loss

Diagnostic Evaluation

1. Close scrutiny of head and neck structures during physical examination; neurologic examination of cranial nerves.
2. Examination of mouth by family dentist may disclose problems.
3. Use of nasal speculum, laryngoscope, and fiberoscope is necessary.
4. Biopsy and histologic examination of suspicious areas.
5. Roentgenogram of head and chest, tomogram, CAT scan, magnetic resonance imaging (MRI).

Treatment
Goal:

To remove all lymph-node-bearing tissue on the involved side of the neck.

1. Removal of all tissue under the skin from the ramus of the jaw down to the clavicle; from midline back to the angle of the jaw. This includes sternocleidomastoid muscle, other smaller muscles, jugular vein in the neck.
Concomitant surgery—tracheostomy (see p. 216)
2. In some clinics, surgical reconstruction is performed, utilizing a pectoral flap from the chest. In other clinics, a very conservative functional neck dissection is done.
3. Radiation therapy is often performed following surgery.
4. Radioactive isotopes or seeds may be used along with surgery.

Patient Problems/Nursing Diagnosis

1. Ineffective airway clearance related to obstruction by tumor or edema of tissues
2. Difficult swallowing related to impingement on oropharyngeal cavity by tumor pressure or extension, or edema
3. Possible hemorrhage related to surgical procedure
4. Infections related to difficulty in cleansing affected area because of inaccessibility or acute sensitivity of tissues
5. Weight loss related to growth of malignancy
6. Knowledge deficit of the effects of alcohol and tobacco abuse
7. Social isolation and ineffective coping related to sensitivity about possible disfigurement, malodor, tubes, and equipment

Planning and Implementation
Nursing Interventions

A. Preoperative Preparation

Preoperative care including diagnostic evaluation—see specific related condition, such as Cancer of Mouth, p. 394, Cancer of the Esophagus, p. 406, etc.

B. Postoperative Care—Immediate

1. Ensure effective breathing and oxygen exchange
   a. Place the patient in Fowler's position.
   b. Observe for signs of respiratory embarrassment, such as dyspnea, cyanosis, and edema.
   c. Provide supplemental oxygen by face mask if necessary; if tracheostomy is present, provide oxygen by collar or T-piece.

d. Auscultate for decreased breath sounds, wheezing, rhonchi.

C. Prevention of Complications of Hemorrhage and Infection

1. Evaluate vital signs that may suggest hemorrhage or onset of infection.
2. Note condition of dressings to detect early signs of hemorrhage.
3. Be aware of principal causes of sudden hemorrhage following surgery:
   a. Loose ligature around a large vessel
   b. Sudden distention of tied-off blood vessel followed by rupture
   c. Slipping of ligature that may occur in violent coughing spasm
   d. Rupture of a vessel due to trauma during surgery
   e. Rupture of a vessel weakened by erosion, tumor, or slough
   f. Sloughing associated with secondary infection
4. Institute immediate care if hemorrhage occurs
   a. Pressure over the common carotid and internal jugular vessels in the neck may be life-saving.
   b. Have someone notify the operating room immediately.
   c. Treat the patient for shock.
   d. Prepare the patient for surgical intervention to repair vessel defect.
      (1) Correct fluid and blood loss with proper replacement.
      (2) Initiate postoperative monitoring program until vital signs remain consistently normal.

D. Improved Swallowing and Coughing

1. Observe for throat irritation—edema, clearing of throat.
2. Note how the patient accepts liquids—refusal may mean difficulty in swallowing, which in turn may be indicative of superior laryngeal nerve damage.
3. Encourage the patient's intake of fluids in order to "thin" secretions.
4. Encourage coughing to remove secretions.
5. Allow the patient to assume sitting position to bring up secretions (the nurse should support his neck with her hands).
6. Suction secretions if the patient is unable to bring them up himself.

E. Improved Wound Healing

1. Reinforce pressure dressings from time to time to assist in obliterating dead spaces and providing immobilization.
2. Observe dressings for evidence of hemorrhage and constriction which may affect respiration.
3. If portable suction (Hemovac) is used, approximately 80–120 ml. of serosanguineous secretions are drawn off during the first postoperative day; this diminishes with each day.
4. Apply Aeroplast or other antiseptic plastic spray to protect the wound.
5. Cleanse skin area around drain exit using sterile saline or half-strength hydrogen peroxide.

F. Improved Communication Ability

1. Inform the patient that temporary hoarseness can be expected with extensive neck surgery and tracheostomy.
2. Encourage the patient to write messages for first few days; if writing is a problem, it may be due to denervation of the trapezius muscle.

3. Recognize that for this patient to nod "yes" or "no" may be difficult because of the neck dissection.
4. Place call bell and other articles within the patient's reach.
5. Recognize the need for support and encouragement, since this patient often is depressed and frustrated even during limited communication.

G. Psychosocial Adjustment

1. Respect the patient's desire for privacy during treatments, dressing change, and feedings.
2. Inform the patient's visitors of his appearance before they see him so that their expressions do not cause him to be upset.
3. Provide frequent aeration of the room and utilize deodorants to prevent unpleasant odors.
4. Observe for lower facial paralysis, since this may indicate facial nerve injury.
5. Watch for shoulder dysfunction, which may follow resection of spinal accessory nerves. See Rehabilitation Exercises in next column.
    a. Utilize postoperative muscle exercises and muscle reeducation.
    b. Work with the patient to obtain good functional range of motion.
6. Consult with the surgeon and patient in decisions on future cosmetic surgery or in use of a prosthetic device.
7. Encourage the patient to verbalize his concerns and feelings.
    a. Consult the physician to determine the nature and extent of explanation and prognosis he has given to the patient.
    b. Encourage the patient to seek confirmation of his personal philosophy and religious beliefs because this may provide answers for him.
    c. Accentuate the positive.
    d. Encourage the patient to participate in his plan of care.
    e. Recognize that a great effort has to be made in behavior modification to change a life-style that included alcohol consumption and cigarette smoking. It is difficult to do.

H. Provisions for Family Adjustments

1. Collaborate with the physician in informing the family of the nature and extent of the patient's disease and surgery.
2. Help them to understand that without surgery, the patient's condition would be worse.
3. Prepare them for the patient's postoperative appearance; how this will be done depends on the strengths and coping mechanisms of the family and the individual circumstances.
4. If there is difficulty with a spouse or person close to the patient in accepting his appearance, refer the person to the physician, social worker, psychiatrist, or whatever resource seems advisable.

Rehabilitation Exercises Following Head and Neck Surgery

Exercises are recommended when the neck incision is sufficiently healed inasmuch as the patient may experience limited range of shoulder motion, as well as neck and shoulder discomfort.

Goal:
Regain maximum shoulder function, as well as head and neck motion, following surgery.

1. Perform exercises morning and evening. At first, exercises are done only once; then the number is increased by one each day until each exercise is done ten times.
2. Following each exercise, the patient is instructed to relax.
3. For neck:
    a. Gently rotate head to each side as far as possible.
    b. Tilt head to the right side as far as possible; repeat for left side.
    c. Drop chin to chest and then raise chin as high as possible.
4. For shoulder:
    a. Standing beside bed, place hand from unoperated side on bed for support.
    b. Gradually swing arm on operated side up and back as far as is comfortable for the patient.
    c. Each day, work toward finishing a complete circle.

Evaluation
Expected Outcomes

1. Breathes easily following surgery, with subsequent drainage of neck area and reduction of edema
2. Demonstrates ability to swallow fluids and soft foods
3. Exhibits no sensitive areas, puffiness of tissue, or temperature elevation that would suggest infection
4. Maintains weight with no additional loss; relates that nutritional intake has been increased
5. Makes resolutions to reduce and possibly abolish intake of alcohol; smoking fewer cigarettes each day and plans to join a smoking cessation group
6. Demonstrates increasing sociability

Conditions of the Esophagus

Diagnostic Evaluation of the Esophagus

Nursing Assessment

During the taking of the nursing history, ask the following questions:

1. What problems or discomfort do you have when you eat? Do you have pain (odynophagia)? Where? Any pain along esophagus noted about 5 seconds after swallowing? Is there food sticking in your throat or chest? Are you nauseated? How long does the discomfort last? Is it daily or intermittent?
2. How is your appetite? Are there any signs of anorexia (loss of appetite)? Weight loss? Indigestion?
3. Do you have to restrict the kinds of food you eat as determined by size or consistency (meat for example), as determined by seasoning, or as determined by spiciness or acidity (citrus fruits)? Do you have to limit food because of temperature (hot or cold)?
4. Do you experience any nausea, heartburn (pyrosis), difficulty swallowing (dysphagia), regurgitation, re-

flux, or vomiting? Have you noticed bad breath (halitosis) or a disagreeable taste in your mouth? Water brash?

5. Does the position of your body (bending, stooping, lying down) affect the problem? Do you lie flat when sleeping or do you have the head of the bed elevated? Does assuming a particular position help or make the problem worse?
6. Do you have any gas formation? Eructation? Early satiety?
7. How has your weight been (stable, increasing, or decreasing)?
8. What relieves the discomfort?
9. Do you find food or saliva on your pillow in the morning on awakening?
10. How are your teeth? Do you have difficulty chewing?

Upper Gastrointestinal Roentgenography

(See p. 417)

Esophageal Endoscopy

This is the direct visualization of the entire mucosa of the esophagus utilizing a rigid esophagoscope or a flexible esophagogastroduodenoscope to detect inflammation, ulceration, masses (tumors), or varices, and to obtain specimens for cytologic studies or biopsy.

A. Nursing Management and Patient Instruction

1. Give the patient nothing by mouth for 6 hours prior to test. This is done to decrease the possibility of aspiration and to be sure the esophagus is clear of particles that would block visibility.
2. Explain the procedure to the patient before it is done, and explain the steps during the examination.
3. Administer diazepam (Valium) as a relaxant and meperidine (Demerol) as a narcotic as prescribed.
4. Spray the throat with local anesthetic (lidocaine spray) to dull the effects of passing the esophagoscope and to reduce gagging.
5. If the esophagus is dilated (fluid-filled esophagus was seen on x-ray) first pass Ewald tube and then evacuate and irrigate esophagus.

▶ **NURSING ALERT:** For *all* endoscopies, bouginage, and pneumatic dilatation procedures, have the following ready: oropharyngeal suction and emergency cardiopulmonary resuscitation equipment.

6. If a rigid scope is used, position the patient on his back. During insertion of esophagoscope, his neck is hyperextended and his head is tilted back and supported.
7. The flexible esophagofiberoscope is passed with the patient sitting; the examination is then completed with the patient lying on his left side.

B. Following Endoscopy

1. Withhold fluid and foods until the patient's gag reflex has returned (about 2 hours). Test the patient's swallowing with sips of water before foods or fluids are given.
2. Offer anesthetic lozenges or normal saline gargles for throat discomfort.
3. Observe the patient for 24 hours for symptoms such as bleeding, dysphagia, fever, and neck pain (cervical area) that are suggestive of perforation. Check also for substernal or epigastric pain (thoracic area); shoulder pain, dyspnea, abdominal pain (diaphragmatic area), and subcutaneous emphysema.

Esophageal Biopsy and Exfoliative Cytology

1. Biopsy of tissue may be taken during esophagoscopy: prepare tissue for laboratory examination.
2. Cytology
   a. Usually an overnight fast is required (no food or fluids).
   b. A No. 12 or No. 16 French nasogastric tube is passed to the cardioesophageal junction (45 cm.).
   c. Residual contents are aspirated.
   d. Physiologic saline (50 ml.) or Ringer's lactate solution is forcefully instilled with a syringe and is immediately aspirated below the cardia; this procedure is repeated at various levels of the esophagus (5-cm. intervals from 45 to 25 cm. from incisor teeth).
   e. Aspirated contents are collected in separate containers surrounded by ice; when all specimens are collected, they are to be taken *immediately* to the laboratory for analysis (must be centrifuged and pallet spread on slide as soon as possible after aspiration).

Esophageal Trauma

Esophageal trauma is injury to the esophagus caused by external or internal insult.

1. Externally—stab or bullet wounds, crush injuries, etc.
2. Internally—swallowed foreign bodies (i.e., metal objects, fishbones, dental appurtenances, poison—lye burn).

Treatment and Nursing Management

Goals:

Institute emergency life-saving treatment.
Restore continuity of esophagus.
Facilitate healing and prevent infection and constriction.

1. Assess condition of the patient to determine his physiologic needs.
2. Maintain open airway. Often, difficulty in respiration is due to edema of the throat or a collection of mucus in the pharynx.
3. Control hemorrhage if present.
4. Treat for pain and shock. (Shock may be due to hemorrhage, impairment of cardiorespiratory function.)
5. Provide high fluid intake; may require parenteral therapy.
6. For external wound:
   a. Initiate emergency first-aid wound care and prepare for surgery.
   b. Maintain feeding through nasogastric tube.
7. For internal chemical damage, give specific antidote. If lye or other caustic or organic solvent was swallowed, do NOT try to induce vomiting. (See also Swallowed Poisons, p. 944.)
   a. A gastrostomy may be performed, either as a temporary or a permanent means of feeding the patient (see p. 426).
   b. Resulting strictures may be relieved by dilating the narrow esophagus with bougies. (See Guidelines: Esophageal Dilatation Bougienage, p. 403, Pneumatic Dilatation p. 404.)
   c. Reconstructive surgery may be necessary to create a new passageway for food between pharynx and stomach.
8. For swallowed foreign bodies.

a. When foreign body is made of metal, such as bobby and safety pins, needles, jacks, nails, and other similar objects, it is not considered safe to allow object to make its way through the gastrointestinal tract.

b. These usually can be removed with the aid of an esophagoscope. A large-bore, rigid esophagoscope is best.

c. A skilled operator is required; magnets can be used on the end of a retrieving instrument passed through the esophagoscope.

Esophagitis

Esophagitis is an acute or chronic inflammation of the esophagus. Severity of symptoms may be unrelated to the degree of inflammation seen at endoscopy.

Causative Factors

1. Reflux of hydrochloric acid; gastric or duodenal contents (most common).
2. Fungal—*Candida*
3. Chemical—lye, ammonia, aerosols
4. Physical—alcohol, excessively hot liquids
5. Trauma—swallowing foreign body
   Medications (pills, capsules; see Nursing Alert below)
6. Reflux esophagitis due to incompetent lower esophageal sphincter; condition appears to have no relationship to hiatal hernia
7. Malignancy associated with achalasia
8. Prolonged nasogastric intubation
9. Following gastric or duodenal surgery
10. Repeated vomiting (common in alcoholics)
11. Bending, stooping, coughing, and straining at stool

▶ **NURSING ALERT:** When administering any solid medication (pills, capsules), have the individual sit or stand and follow drug with at least 100 ml. liquid. Otherwise, the patient should have liquid medication.

Clinical Manifestations

(Sudden or gradual in onset)
1. Hot burning pain (heartburn or pyrosis) behind xiphoid or sternum → spreading to throat, jaw, arms, and back.
2. Pain with eructation or regurgitation of acidic or bitter fluid (reflux).
3. Symptoms aggravated by recumbency.
4. Symptoms may be precipitated by increases in intra-abdominal pressure, such as when the patient bends over, lifts heavy objects, or has to strain to pass stool or urine (constipation or prostatism).
5. Dysphagia—worse at onset of meal. Food "sticking" in throat or chest—produced by spasm, edema, or narrow lumen. While swallowing bolus of food, the patient may require "washing down" of food with liquids.
6. Pain on drinking citrus liquids, alcohol, or hot or cold fluids. Coffee often aggravates the pain.
7. Bleeding—acute or chronic; melena or hematemesis also occurs.

Diagnostic Evaluation

(For all esophageal disorders)
1. Cineradiographic esophagograms
2. Esophagoscopy (see p. 399) with cytology and biopsy may differentiate esophagitis from carcinoma

3. Esophageal manometry
4. Acid perfusion test
5. Gastroesophageal scintiscanning

Medical and Nursing Management

A. Nutritional Considerations

1. Institute a feeding regimen similar to that for gastric ulcer (see p. 421).
   a. Frequent feedings, progressing to 5 meals—bland, low residue—no bedtime feedings.
   b. Avoid foods high in residue, very hot foods, spices, alcohol, tobacco, and coffee (even decaffeinated).
   c. Avoid salicylates, phenylbutazone (Butazolidin), and anticholinergics.
   d. Do not give food within 2 hours of retiring to avoid nocturnal reflux.
   e. Chew food well and eat slowly.
   f. Pain may be relieved by standing or walking, but aggravated in recumbent position.

▶ **NURSING ALERT:** Milk actually is contraindicated for ulcer or esophagitis because of high calcium content, which stimulates gastric acid secretion.

B. Relief of Pain

1. Administer antacids, especially at bedtime—administer cimetidine or ranitidine if prescribed to reduce gastric secretions.
2. Place 15–20 cm. (6–8 inch) bed blocks at head of bed. Be sure to remove wheels from bed.
3. Provide adequate mouth care and recommend appropriate dental attention.
4. Administer cholinergic agents.
5. Promote a relaxing environment during mealtime.
6. Avoid constricting abdominal garments.
7. Suggest a weight-reduction program if the patient is overweight.

C. Surgical Treatment

Dilatation therapy or surgery if necessary:
1. For strictures, dilatation therapy may be initiated; this is done several times weekly at first, then on a monthly basis.
2. Surgery is indicated when conservative measures fail.
   a. Fundoplication (Belsey or Nissen procedure) for reflux to throat—severe stricture.
   b. Combined with vagotomy–pyloroplasty if associated with gastroduodenal ulcer.
   c. Stricture may need to be resected, and an esophagogastrostomy may be required.

▶ **NURSING ALERT:** Anticholinergics are contraindicated because they may further impair competence of lower esophageal sphincter and interfere with cleansing action of esophageal peristalsis.

Achalasia

Achalasia refers to a benign spasm of the lower esophageal sphincter, often with marked dilatation of the esophagus. It is a neuromuscular disorder due to absent or defective nerves (of the myenteric plexus) going to the involuntary muscles in the esophagus.

Clinical Manifestations

1. Difficulty in swallowing both liquids *and* solids, substernal pressure, fullness and regurgitation, often heartburn appears.

2. Halitosis and inability to eructate may be noticed.
3. Secondary pulmonary complications due to spillover of esophageal contents (aspiration pneumonia).
4. Loss of peristaltic activity and failure of esophageal sphincter to relax during swallowing process (detected by x-ray or manometry) may occur.
5. Emotional upsets, sudden shock, or dietary indiscretion may aggravate this disorder.
6. Weight loss is eventually noticed inasmuch as the patient has a decreased intake in order to avoid discomfort; eventually this can lead to emaciation.
7. Increased risk of esophageal carcinoma (8%–10%) and suppurative lung disease.
8. The patient may also have carcinoma at cardia invading esophagus, simulating achalasia.

Diagnostic Evaluation

1. Cineroentgenogram of esophagus with barium; this reveals weak or absent peristaltic waves and failure of sphincter relaxation.
2. Esophagoscopy with cytologic studies and biopsy.
3. Esophageal manometry with perfused open-tip catheters and injection of methacholine.

Nursing Assessment

1. Determine what the patient can and cannot swallow.
2. Note location and kind of pain.
3. Determine how relief is obtained.
4. Ascertain what aggravates the problem.

Treatment and Nursing Management

Goals:
Enlarge the passageway so that contents pass more readily from esophagus to stomach
Pneumatic (Mosher) bag dilatation (see p. 404)
Surgical esophagomyotomy

A. Nursing Management—Medical Therapy or Minor Surgical Therapy

1. Direct patient to eat slowly, chew food thoroughly, and arch his back while swallowing to provide relief.
2. Suggest that the patient sleep with his head elevated to avoid reflux or aspiration.
3. Provide a bland diet and tell the patient to avoid alcohol, as well as spicy, very hot, and very cold foods, in order to minimize symptoms.
4. Administer pharmacologic agents such as urecholine to increase lower esophageal sphincter tone.

▶ **NURSING ALERT:** Anticholinergic drugs are contraindicated for achalasia because they further decrease esophageal peristalsis.

5. If pharmacotherapy fails, pneumatic dilatation is tried (see Guidelines: Pneumatic Dilatation, p. 404).

B. Nursing Management—Major Surgical Therapy
(Used only if pneumatic dilatation fails)

1. Esophagomyotomy—a division of muscular fibers enclosing the narrowed esophagus that permits mucosa to pouch out through the divided area in muscle layers.
2. Cardiomyotomy—when above operation is extended to include cardiac end of stomach.
3. Incisional approach determines nature of postoperative care; thus, an incision through chest implies nursing care similar to that given to a patient with a thoracotomy (see p. 179).

Diffuse Spasm of Esophagus

Diffuse esophageal spasm is a motor disorder of the esophagus. It is common in old age and may be an early stage of achalasia (see p. 400).

Clinical Manifestations

1. Pain on swallowing (odynophagia), dysphagia, chest or back pain.
2. Diffuse spasm may be associated with achalasia, obstruction of the cardia by tumor, precipitation by reflux acid.

Treatment and Nursing Management

A. Conservative

1. Administer sedatives for pain.
2. Avoid food and beverages that precipitate symptoms.
3. Eliminate source of tension as a precipitating factor producing stress during mealtime.
4. Administer nitroglycerin or long-acting nitrites if reflux is not a factor.

B. Later, If Necessary

Utilize pneumatic dilatation if manometric studies reveal increased lower esophageal sphincter pressure (providing gastroesophageal reflux is not part of the problem).

C. See Guidelines

1. Feeding the Patient with Dysphagia (see below)
2. Teaching a Patient with Dysphagia How to Swallow, p. 403
3. Esophageal Dilatation (Bougienage), p. 403
4. Pneumatic Dilatation, p. 404

Guidelines: Feeding the Patient with Dysphagia

Dysphagia—difficulty or discomfort in swallowing; a bolus of food becomes impeded in its movement between the mouth and stomach.

Causative Factors

1. Circulatory disturbances of brain (stroke, brain stem vascular accidents)
2. Cranial nerve disturbances
3. Trauma to neck
4. Radiation therapy/surgery for head and neck tumors
5. Presence of tumors, inflammation
6. Disturbances of laryngeal sphincter
7. Psychological pathology

(continued)

Guidelines: Feeding the Patient with Dysphagia (continued)

Clinical Manifestations

1. Patient complains of a sticking sensation behind sternum; relief is obtained by
   a. Retching
   b. Drinking liquids to dislodge bolus
2. Upper or thoracic esophageal discomfort noted in 3–5 seconds after attempting to swallow.
3. Lower thoracic discomfort noted in 5–15 seconds.

Nursing Assessment

1. Determine whether dysphagia occurs only with solid food. Does it occur with soft foods? liquids? Warm liquids or cold liquids? Saliva? Does it vary?
2. Has the patient lost weight? Evidence of cachexia?
3. Is hoarseness present? If so, it may be indicative of laryngeal lesion.
4. How long has the patient experienced this discomfort?
5. Did painful swallowing precede dysphagia? How long? Heartburn? How long? Hiccough?
6. Regurgitation—bringing up of undigested food or gastric acid into the mouth. Has this occurred?
7. In general, determine the patient's eating habits and their relevance to this problem.

Procedure

Nursing Action	Rationale/Amplification
1. Make a preliminary assessment of the patient's problem (see above, Assessment). a. Determine the swallowing limitation.	1. By individualizing the approach, a more effective plan to meet particular needs will be achieved.
2. Prepare environment so that it will be well ventilated, uncluttered, and cheerful without distractions.	2. This will make the patient's feeding experience more pleasant and easier.
3. Place the patient in an upright sitting position (90 degrees) for about 20 minutes before and after feeding. a. Provide adequate support and comfort.	3. This will provide time to adjust to this position, thereby eliminating postural change disturbances during feeding.

4. Explain what you plan to do; sit rather than stand, and encourage conversation. Face patient and proceed in an unhurried manner.
   a. Encourage eating; allow time for chewing.
   b. Remove tray when the patient is finished.
	4. This procedure will more likely secure cooperation.
	   a. Proceed slowly and give patient time to swallow.
	   b. Unclean or used tray may be psychologically distressing and may interfere with digestion.

5. If food is difficult to manage, begin with liquids; if he continues to have trouble:
   a. Place tip of irrigation syringe in the back of the mouth cavity on the better side; gently squeeze bulb.
   b. When he is ready, allow the patient to squeeze bulb himself.
   c. Frequent small feedings are offered initially.
	5. a. Proceed slowly and give the patient time to swallow.
	   b. Aim to involve the patient in his own care.
	   c. Blenderized or commercially prepared liquid formula supplements are available.

6. If the patient has difficulty chewing:
   a. Manipulate jaw in an upward and downward motion.
   b. Encourage the patient to close his lips after food is in his mouth, keep lips closed until the food is swallowed.
   c. If the patient does not swallow as soon as he should but appears to retain food in his mouth, place thumb on his chin and press downward toward his chest.
	6.
	   a. This not only stimulates jaw but will actually stimulate act of chewing.
	   b. It may be necessary to manually close the patient's lips, using your thumb and index finger. When lips are closed, the swallowing reflex is stimulated.
	   c. This maneuver moves his larynx superiorly and anteriorly, thereby facilitating swallowing.

7. In spoon-feeding, when one mouthful is swallowed, remove spoon at once. If the patient drools, wipe his mouth before the next mouthful is presented.	7. The patient is more comfortable without the sensation of food trickling down his chin.

Feeding the Patient with an Affected Side of the Mouth (Facial Paralysis, Hemiplegia, Hemilaryngectomy)

1. Turn the patient to his unaffected side.	1. This provides better head and neck support.
2. Place food on the strong side of mouth rather than in the middle of the mouth.	2. Permits food to be managed more effectively.
3. Encourage the patient to form a bolus by moving his tongue around inside of mouth.	3. This assists in placing food in a proper position for swallowing, rather than permitting food to collect near cheek.

Follow-up Care

1. Record the amount of intake, the patient's taste and food preferences, his progress, and any special tactics that were effective in helping him.	1. Progress notes will assist in moving the patient toward self-care.
2. Encourage family members to participate in the patient's feeding program.	

Guidelines: Teaching a Patient with Dysphagia How to Swallow

Purpose To assist the patient who has difficulty swallowing after injury/surgical correction of the oropharyngeal or upper esophagus, neurologic deficit, stroke.

Equipment

Baby bottle with nipple
Rubber glove for instructor's hand

Procedure

Nursing Action	Rationale/Amplification
1. Explain to the patient that you plan to work with him in developing the sensation of swallowing.	1. The patient's cooperation, concentration, and directed participation are essential to the success of this learning experience.
2. Demonstrate first how the lips pucker as you draw inward in sucking your gloved finger.	2. The patient's observation will assist him in imitating this action.
3. Wash your gloved hand and then put your gloved finger in the patient's mouth. When the patient demonstrates good sucking ability, proceed to the next step.	
4. The teacher redemonstrates the sucking maneuver with one hand while placing the other hand on her throat to feel the motions caused by sucking and swallowing.	4. It becomes apparent that after sucking, a need to move whatever is in the mouth causes the complex swallowing process to be initiated.
5. Ask the patient to duplicate these motions.	5. It may help to have the patient place his hand on the neck of the demonstrator to grasp the mechanisms of swallowing.
6. The swallowing function can be further stimulated as follows:	6.
a. Have the patient suck on a fresh lemon (if permissible), or use lemon glycerin swabs in his mouth; ice fruit popsicles may also help.	a. This will stimulate salivation reflexes.
b. If the sucking reflex is intact, a straw may be effective in initiating swallowing as he sucks on it. The straw may need to be placed further inside the mouth or patient's head may have to be tilted.	
c. Place a cup at corner of the lips and tilt slightly so that the patient can take liquid slowly. Encourage the patient to move toward cup.	c. This offers the patient more control as he moves forward; swallowing reflex occurs more easily.
7. Use a baby bottle if it appears that it might help.	7. Recognize the psychological effect this might have—will patient feel he is regressing?

Special Food Considerations for the Patient with Dysphagia

1. Avoid milk and milk products, since they stimulate production of thick saliva, which is difficult to swallow.
2. Serve liquids that are close to room temperature rather than cold or hot.
3. Diluted fruit juices are more palatable than concentrated juices.
4. Provide textured foods rather than foods that are too smooth (i.e., chopped cooked vegetables rather than pureed vegetables, baked rather than mashed potatoes).
5. Avoid strong-flavored foods, acids, or bitter-tasting foods—except lemon juice added to food.

Guidelines: Esophageal Dilatation (Bougienage)

Purpose To dilate the cardioesophageal sphincter so that food may pass from the esophagus into the stomach.

Equipment

Water-soluble lubricant
Bougies—flexible, woven silk-tipped or rubber, of various sizes
Dilators of the physician's preference

Procedure

Preparatory Phase

1. Cleanse dilators with povidone-iodine (Betadine) to prevent infection and bacteremia.
2. Explain the procedure to the patient and indicate why it is necessary for him to fast and drink no fluids for 12 hours beforehand.

(continued)

Guidelines: Esophageal Dilatation (Bougienage) (continued)

Procedure
(Cont.)

3. Administer sedative or narcotic as prescribed to allay apprehension and assist the patient in relaxation.
4. Have the patient in a sitting position in a chair or in bed elevated 30 to 45 degrees.
5. Place a drape bib-fashion around the patient's chest and over his shoulders to protect his clothing.
6. Provide the patient with an emesis basin; have suction equipment (oropharyngeal) available.
7. Remove dentures if present.

Nursing Action	Rationale/Amplification
Performance Phase	
1. Spray the patient's throat with a local anesthetic (gargle may be preferred).	1. The spray or gargle will desensitize local tissues.
2. Lubricate bougie with water-soluble lubricant (some bougies are weighted with mercury); remove excess lubricant.	2. Lubrication reduces friction between the mucous membrane and tube. Excess lubricant may be aspirated.
3. Assist the physician as he passes the tube and first dilator. Support the patient's head and encourage him to swallow.	3. The more relaxed the patient, the easier the bougie will descend to the cardiac sphincter.
4. Progressively larger bougies are passed until pain occurs. (For achalasia, a pneumatic or hydrostatic balloon is used with fluoroscopy.)	4. Sizes are increased to dilate the stricture progressively. By increasing the pressure of the balloon under fluoroscopy, the sphincter may be gradually dilated.

Note: If bougies do not pass the stricture, it will be necessary to pass a guide wire through the stricture via esophagoscope. The scope is then removed, and metallic olive dilators are passed down the guide wire, progressively increasing in size.

Nursing Action	Rationale/Amplification
Follow-up Phase	
1. Have the patient rest in bed following procedure.	1. Observe for 24 hours for evidence of esophageal perforation.
a. Give nothing by mouth for an hour after dilatation.	a. NPO to prevent aspiration.
b. Check pulse and temperature at least hourly for 6 hours.	b. Elevated pulse and temperature, plus chest pain and evidence of subcutaneous emphysema may indicate presence of air in the mediastinum.
c. Be attentive to complaints of chest pain.	c. It may be necessary to have x-ray verification.
d. Observe upper chest for signs of subcutaneous emphysema. Should any of the above abnormal signs occur, notify physician.	

Guidelines: Pneumatic Dilatation

Pneumatic dilatation is the introduction of a pneumatic dilator under fluoroscopic control to dilate a cardioesophageal sphincter (tightened by spasm), utilizing measured pressure control.

Equipment

Ewald tube (No. 34 French)
Pneumatic dilators (usually 3 balloon sizes: 1⅛, 1½, and 1⅞ inch)
Guide wire

Procedure

Preparatory Phase

1. Explain procedure to the patient; tell him that some discomfort may be experienced, but that he will be given medication to help combat this.
2. Intake is limited to fluids for at least 24 hours prior to dilatation.
   a. Give nothing by mouth after midnight prior to treatment.
   b. Medications are prescribed prior to treatment, usually meperidine (Demerol), atropine, and perhaps diazepam (Valium).
   c. The throat is sprayed with a local anesthetic, which may also be given in the form of a gargle (viscous lidocaine can be swallowed).
3. Procedure is done with fluoroscope control (x-ray department).

Medical Action	Rationale/Amplification/Nursing Support
1. Place the patient in sitting position and pass an Ewald tube.	1. Aspirates secretions and contents of esophagus.

Procedure
(Cont.)

Medical Action	Rationale/Amplification/Nursing Support
2. Remove tube following aspiration.	
3. Pass pneumatic dilator and position to straddle cardio-esophageal junction.	3. Done under fluoroscopic control.
4. Inflate balloon to 100 mm. Hg.	4. Keep at this pressure for 1 minute, still under fluoroscopic control.
5. Note slight constriction of sphincter.	5. The constriction should be positioned in center of balloon.
6. Inflate balloon to 200 mm. Hg.	6. Keep the balloon inflated for 2–3 minutes; nurse to observe the patient's response and provide support.
7. Inflate balloon to 300 mm. Hg.	7. The patient may experience moderate to moderately severe pain.
8. Release pressure and remove dilator.	8. A small amount of blood on balloon is frequently seen when it is deflated and removed.

(Procedure may be repeated over several days—gradually increasing pressure in balloon.)

Nursing Action	Rationale/Amplification
Follow-up Phase	
1. Continue to keep the patient fasting.	1. Done until the patient's condition is stabilized.
2. Monitor vital signs every 30 minutes for 2 hours.	2. When vital signs are stable, full fluids may be given.
3. Continue to monitor vital signs every 4 hours.	3. Monitor signs for an additional 16 hours.
4. Observe the patient for vital sign changes and complaints of severe pain. Should changes or complaints occur, notify physician and give the patient nothing by mouth.	4. May be indicative of bleeding or perforation; reassure the patient.
5. Be prepared for physician to request CBC, typing, cross matching, and chest x-ray.	5. These tests may be required to assist in assessing cardiovascular conditions.

Esophageal Diverticulum

An *esophageal diverticulum* is an outpouching of the wall, usually in the cervical posterior side.

Types
1. Pharyngoesophageal (pulsion)—also called Zenker's diverticulum; upper end of esophagus through cricopharyngeal muscle
2. Midesophageal (traction)—near tracheal bifurcation
3. Epiphrenic (traction–pulsion)—lower third of esophagus

Clinical Manifestations

A. Pharyngoesophageal
1. Difficulty in swallowing, fullness in neck, a feeling that food stops before it reaches the stomach, and regurgitation of undigested food.
2. Belching, gurgling, or nocturnal coughing brought about by diverticulum becoming filled with food or liquid, which is regurgitated and may irritate the trachea.
3. Halitosis and foul taste in mouth caused by decomposing of food in a pouch (diverticulum).
4. Hoarseness, asthma and pneumonitis may be the only signs in the very elderly.
5. Weight loss due to nutritional depletion.

B. Midesophageal
Generally no symptoms.

C. Epiphrenic
1. At times associated with achalasia or diffuse esophageal spasm (see p. 400).
2. No symptoms at first, but condition eventually may cause dysphagia, pain, and pulmonary complications.

Diagnostic Evaluation
1. Roentgenograms using barium should be taken.
2. Esophagoscopy is risky, because of danger of perforation of diverticulum, which may lead to mediastinitis.

Treatment
Surgery is usually recommended as soon as the diagnosis is made to prevent further nutritional deficit and complications.

A. Pharyngoesophageal
Usually a transverse cervical diverticulectomy and myotomy are done. Some surgeons use myotomy alone, and others do a diverticulopexy.
1. Caution is taken to avoid injury to common carotid artery and internal jugular vein.
2. Sac is dissected free and then excised flush with esophageal wall.
3. If transthoracic approach is used, nursing management is similar to that described for chest operations (see p. 178).

B. Midesophageal
Therapy is usually not required because of absence of symptoms and rareness of complications.

C. Epiphrenic
Underlying primary condition must be treated.

Nursing Management
1. Immediate postoperative care is as described on page 179.

2. If a nasogastric tube is in place, institute nasogastric feedings utilizing fluids.
   a. Irrigate tube carefully with water following each feeding.
   b. Record kind and amount of irrigating fluid.
3. Prepare the patient the morning after surgery for x-ray following ingestion of diatrizoate meglumine (Gastrografin) and diatrizoate sodium solution, or barium, to detect any leakage at mucosal closure site.
4. If no leakage occurs, liquid diet is started, with diet increased to regular in the next 72 hours.
5. Drains are shortened on third to fourth day.
6. Discharge when comfortable and able to resume activities.
7. If leakage occurs (rare), drains are left in place, and the patient will be maintained on parenteral feedings until repeat x-rays show adequate healing and closure.

Esophageal Varices

See page 479.

Esophageal Perforation

Esophageal perforation is an acute surgical emergency in which the esophagus is punctured by a swallowed foreign object (e.g., dental prosthesis, open safety pin), by gunshot, which results in trauma, or by an esophagoscope or stiff tube.

Clinical Manifestations

1. Chest pain, usually substernal—may be mild or severe.
2. Temperature elevation occurring within 24 hours.
3. Abdominal pain and tenderness, and epigastric muscle spasm.
4. Subcutaneous emphysema and crepitus of neck, face, and chest wall—noted in cervical and thoracic esophageal perforations.

Diagnostic Evaluation

1. History of recent esophageal trauma
2. Chest film to look for air in mediastinum
3. Esophagogram

Surgical Treatment and Nursing Measures

1. Utilize emergency resuscitative procedures.
2. Prepare for surgical intervention (may not be needed if diagnosed and treated early).
3. Administer parenteral fluids and antimicrobial agents as prescribed.
4. Pass nasogastric suction tubing to minimize pleural or mediastinal contamination. Give nothing by mouth.

Cancer of the Esophagus

Incidence

1. Benign tumors and sarcomas of esophagus are unusual, except for leiomyomas.
2. About 80% of cancers of the esophagus involve men, who are usually past age 60.
3. Middle third of esophagus is most involved with the lower third next most frequent.
4. Carcinoma of esophagus is responsible for 2% to 4% of all cancer deaths in the US.
   a. Usually this is a geriatric patient who also has pulmonary and cardiovascular disorders.
   b. Proximity of lesion to vital body structures (e.g.,

heart and lungs); lymph-node spread is easy and rapid.
   c. Before significant symptoms occur, the tumor may already have invaded surrounding structures.

Risk Factors

Causative factors have not been proved; the condition is associated with achalasia.
1. Chronic trauma—excessive use of alcohol, tobacco, spicy foods, hot liquid (tea) ingestion
2. Geographic—certain areas of Iran, Kenya, Honan Province in China, India, and Rhodesia show a higher incidence
3. Oral and pharyngeal cancer—probably related to smoking
4. Genetic predisposition—nonwhite male population
5. Nitrosamines
6. Lye ingestion

Clinical Manifestations

1. Progressively increasing difficulty in swallowing (dysphagia). At first, only solid foods give trouble; then, as growth progresses and obstruction becomes more complete, even liquids pass with difficulty into the stomach.
2. Pain on swallowing (odynophagia).
3. Possible hemorrhage—usually only occult bleeding.
4. Progressive loss of weight and strength due to starvation.
5. Later symptoms—vague substernal pain, hiccup, respiratory difficulty, foul breath, regurgitation of food and saliva.

Diagnostic Evaluation

1. Barium swallow; air contrast studies of esophagus
   A piece of bread or a marshmallow coated with barium may serve as a radiopaque bolus to locate the lesion.
2. Cineradiography
3. Endoscopy—inspection and photography
4. Biopsy, brush cytology
5. Computed tomography (CT) may be helpful in delineating the extent of the tumor, as well as in identifying presence of adjacent tissue invasion.

Treatment

1. The wide variety of treatments available reflects the overall poor results from any one approach. Palliation is usually the goal.
   a. Radiation alone; radiation with surgery
   b. Surgery and chemotherapy
   c. Chemotherapy alone
   d. Surgical removal of the involved segment
2. Lesions in middle and upper third, in particular, are not often suitable for excision.
   a. Irradiation is the preferred form of therapy.
   b. Some clinics report success with insertion of a prosthetic tube (Celestin or other plastic) through the mouth to bridge the involved area and to facilitate swallowing. This insertion may be done after dilatation of tumor-bearing portions of the esophagus.
3. Lesions of middle and lower esophagus are excised if there is no evidence of local or distant metastases.
   a. The portion of esophagus containing the tumor is removed.

b. Continuity of gastrointestinal tract is restored by bringing the stomach (or a tube in stomach, or a segment of colon) into the chest and implanting proximal end of esophagus into it. Some clinics prefer a side-to-side esophagogastrostomy.

c. Chest drainage of pleural cavity is carried out (see p. 183).

4. Gastrostomy is not recommended, since it provides little palliation and does not restore the swallowing mechanism. It is used only as a temporary measure.

Nursing Management

A. Preoperative

1. Preoperative preparation includes promoting the nutritional status with a diet high in calories, vitamins, and protein. This may have to be by mouth, intravenous infusion, or hyperalimentation.

2. To avoid aspiration, semi-Fowler's position is recommended for feeding.

3. A nasogastric tube may be inserted prior to surgery.

B. Postoperative

1. With Celestin tube (or other tube replacement), swallowing may be easier if small sips of water are offered at first.

2. Food is usually not given for several days and then in small quantities, leading to a soft diet.

3. Remind the patient to remain in the upright position after eating to promote digestion.

4. Monitor the patient for tube leakage; this may be manifested early by low-grade fever, fluid in the pleural space, or elevated pulse.

Nursing Principles for pre- and postoperative management are similar to those given for Radical Neck Dissection (p. 396) and Thoracic Surgery (p. 178).

2: Gastrointestinal Conditions

Nutritional Assessment

(See The Patient History, p. 13)

1. Interviewing is a convenient method of determining a patient's eating habits.

2. Determine the following factors, which are influential in affecting the patient's attitudes toward foods:
   a. Cultural heritage, religion, family background
   b. Socioeconomic status, education, current situation, effect of food fads and superstitions

3. Observation (see Table 10-1)

Questionnaire for Nutritional Assessment

Adults

Background Information
Name, age, sex, family, and occupational roles, general health status, dietary restrictions (past or present)

Food Purchase and Preparation
Who purchases and prepares food?
What factors influence kinds of foods purchased?
Is budgeting a matter of concern when buying food?
Where is food purchased?
How often do you shop?
What facilities are available for food storage and preparation?
What foods are served most frequently?
Do you participate in community food programs?

Relationship of Food to Life-style
Food likes and dislikes
Favorite foods when growing up
Special family foods for celebrations
Atmosphere at mealtime
Foods your body needs
Food supplements (vitamins, minerals)
Sources of information about nutrition
Eating away from home—frequency and location.

Adolescents

What is nutritious? Foods body needs?
Where are meals eaten? When is food eaten?
How much snacking?

4. *Anthropometric measurements* (of body size and composition)—necessary for assessment of nutritional status and for diet planning

Table 10-1 Physical Signs Indicative of Nutritional Status

Body Area	Signs of Good Nutrition	Signs of Poor Nutrition
Hair	Shiny, lustrous; firm, healthy scalp	Dull and dry, brittle, depigmented, easily plucked
Face	Skin color uniform; healthy appearance	Skin dark over cheeks and under eyes, skin flaky, face swollen
Eyes	Bright, clear, moist	Eye membranes pale, dry (xerophthalmia); Bitot's spots, increased vascularity, cornea soft (keratomalacia)
Lips	Good color (pink), smooth	Swollen and puffy (cheilosis), angular lesion at corners of mouth (angular fissures)
Tongue	Deep red in appearance, surface papillae present	Smooth appearance, swollen, beefy red, sores, atrophic papillae
Teeth	Straight, no crowding, no cavities, bright	Cavities, mottled appearance (fluorosis), malpositioned
Gums	Firm, good color (pink)	Spongy, bleed easily, marginal redness, recession
Glands	No enlargement of the thyroid	Thyroid enlargement (simple goiter)
Skin	Smooth, good color, moist	Rough, dry, flaky, swollen, pale, pigmented; lack of fat under skin
Nails	Firm, pink	Spoon shaped, ridged
Skeleton	Good posture, no malformation	Poor posture, beading of ribs, bowed legs or knock knees
Muscles	Well developed, firm	Flaccid, poor tone, wasted, underdeveloped
Extremities	No tenderness	Weak and tender; presence of edema
Abdomen	Flat	Swollen
Nervous system	Normal reflexes	Decrease in or loss of ankle and knee reflexes

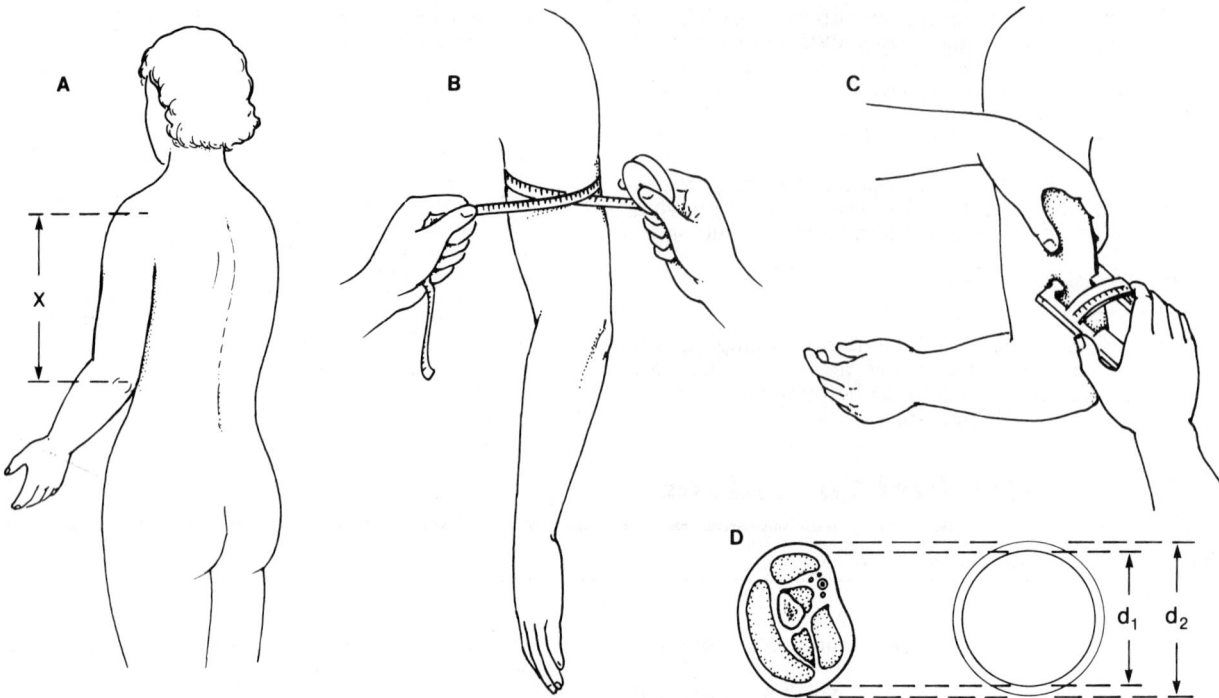

Figure 10-1. Proper positioning of the patient is required: (A) for measuring the mid-upper arm, (B) to determine mid-arm circumference (AC); this position is also used to measure (C) the triceps skinfold (TSF) thickness which is measured with a caliper; (D) shows the relation between d_1 (AMC—arm muscle circumference) and d_2 (AC—arm circumference). Arm muscle circumference is a significant measurement in determining protein–calorie malnutrition. Formula for calculation: AMC = AC − (0.314 × TSF). (Adapted from Blackburn GL and Harvey KB. Nutritional assessment as a routine in clinical medicine. Postgrad Med 1982 May; 71(5):51.)

a. *Height and weight* are determined upon patient admission and are used as a baseline for later comparisons.
b. *Triceps skinfold* (TSF) is a measurement used to estimate the degree of body fat. By itself, it may not be very significant; however, it is of value in calculating arm muscle circumference.
c. *Arm circumference* (AC) is mid-upper arm circumference. This measurement is necessary in determining AMC. See Figure 10-1 including caption.
d. *Arm muscle circumference* (AMC) is a significant calculation in determining prevalence of protein–calorie malnutrition (PCM).
5. Use of questionnaire to determine eating habits (see p. 407)

Major Manifestations of Gastrointestinal Disturbance

Anorexia, Nausea, and Vomiting

Normal Physiology

A. **Appetite**—a desire for food, or an agreeable attitude toward ingesting food, often specific kinds of food.
1. The frontal and parietal areas of the cerebrum, but especially the hypothalamus, are known to be associated with appetite.
2. Desire for food is acutely associated with increased rates of gastric hydrochloric acid secretion, with gastric hyperemia, and hypermotility.

B. **Hunger**—a strong sensation or urge to eat following a period of fasting.
1. Hunger is temporarily associated with rhythmic contractions of the stomach.
2. The precise mechanisms by which hunger is produced are unknown; it is related to a low blood sugar level.

C. **Satiety**—a condition following consumption of an amount of food sufficient to meet present requirements; a feeling that one has had enough to eat.

Anorexia

Lack of appetite for food; lack of interest in all food.
1. Associated with a disinterest in consumption of even those foods that one ordinarily likes to eat.
2. Associated with decreased secretion of gastric hydrochloric acid.
3. Possible causes:
   a. Unpleasant or upsetting experiences
   b. Apprehension, fear, and anxiety

c. Excitement, both pleasurable and undesirable
d. Systemic and local diseases, such as hepatic failure and uremia

Dyspepsia (Indigestion)

Painful, difficult, or disturbed digestion. The person suffers from several of a group of symptoms—nausea, regurgitation, vomiting, heartburn, bloating, and stomach discomfort.

Nausea

A most unpleasant sensation usually associated with a distinct revulsion toward the ingestion of food; it may or may not precede vomiting.

1. Very often, anorexia is succeeded by nausea and vomiting. However, either of these states may occur without the others.
2. Associated with decreased motor activity of the stomach, pallor of gastric mucosa, and contraction of proximal duodenum.
3. Frequently associated with evidence of diffuse autonomic discharge—profuse watery salivation, sudden drenching perspiration, tachycardia.
4. Many patients find it difficult to describe:
   a. Vague unpleasantness in epigastrium
   b. Distressing feelings in the throat
   c. Vague unpleasantness spread diffusely in abdomen (must be distinguished from mild visceral abdominal pain)

Vomiting

Sudden forceful expulsion of stomach contents through the mouth.

1. Vomiting center is located in the medulla.
2. May or may not be preceded by nausea and retching.
3. Exaggerated and often extreme vasomotor activities may immediately precede and accompany the vomiting act; watery salivation, sweating, pulse rate change, vasoconstriction, and pallor.
4. Tachycardia prior to vomiting becomes bradycardia during process.
5. Incited by neuromuscular "reverse peristalsis" or mechanical obstruction.

Nursing Management

1. Observe the preliminary symptoms.
   a. The patient is often lightheaded, weak, and dizzy.
   b. Irregularity of respiration before and during vomiting.
   c. Blood pressure may fall before and then fluctuate during vomiting.
2. Observe character and quantity of expectorated material.
   a. Note whether it has an odor, is sour-smelling, or is odorless.
   b. Is it liquid, containing mucus or pus, or food particles?
   c. Describe its color, taste, and consistency (see Nature of Vomitus).
3. Be aware of progression of events when there is a diminution of intake and output—weight loss, dehydration, fluid and electrolyte imbalance:
   a. Skin becomes dry and loses turgor
   b. Poor mouth hygiene leading to halitosis
4. Recognize progression of events that might lead to shock, tachycardia, hypotension, oliguria.

Nature of Vomitus

Color/Taste/Consistency	Possible Source
Yellowish or greenish	May contain bile Medication—senna
Bright red (arterial)	Hemorrhage, peptic ulcer
Dark red (venous)	Hemorrhage, esophageal or gastric varices
"Coffee grounds"	Digested blood from slowly bleeding gastric or duodenal ulcer
Undigested food	Gastric tumor? Ulcer obstruction?
"Bitter" taste	Bile
"Sour" or "acid"	Gastric contents
Fecal components	Intestinal obstruction

Disturbances Associated with Anorexia, Nausea, and Vomiting

A. Psychic and Neurologic Factors

1. Life situations that evoke subjective manifestations of fear, frustration, depression, and anxiety may be associated with these symptoms.
2. *Anorexia* is commonly a manifestation of a depressed state, which can lead to a profound impairment of food intake and possibly anorexia nervosa.
3. *Nausea and vomiting*
   a. Frequently occurs during or shortly after meals
   b. Often unaccompanied by nausea and retching
   c. Frequently does not empty stomach
   d. After vomiting, patient may desire to continue to eat
   e. No recurrence of vomiting occurs.
   f. Accompanying migraine headache
      (1) Hypoxemia affecting the vomiting center
      (2) Vascular changes
      (3) Associated visual disturbances
   g. Caused by unusual stimulation of labyrinth of the ear
   h. Projectile type associated with increasing intracranial pressure
      (1) Commonly not preceded by nausea
      (2) May indicate meningitis, internal hydrocephalus, space-occupying lesion, cerebellar lesions
   i. Associated with vertigo

B. Associated with Gastrointestinal and Biliary Conditions

1. Systemic diseases (e.g., liver failure, uremia)
2. Gastritis (alcohol, viruses, bacteria, or poisons)
3. Pyloric or intestinal obstruction
4. Cholecystitis, pancreatitis, or peptic ulcer
5. Mechanical obstruction in gastrointestinal tract

C. Drugs and Toxic Agents

1. Pathophysiologic effect
   a. Medullary chemoreceptor zone may be stimulated.
   b. Direct effect on gastrointestinal organs brought about by mercury.
   c. Stimulation of hypothalamus nuclei brought about

by alcohol, apomorphine, emetine, histamine, epinephrine.
2. Mucosal damage of upper gastrointestinal tract caused by mercury, ammonium chloride, copper sulfate, aminophylline, alcohol, aspirin.

D. Other Factors

1. Febrile illness
2. Chronic renal failure (see p. 517)
3. Motion sickness
4. Meniere's disease (see p. 750)
5. Hepatocellular disease

Nursing Interventions

1. Observe and assess status of the patient when he experiences anorexia, nausea, and vomiting. Note the general effect of these symptoms on the patient:
   a. Food and fluid intake
   b. Balance between intake and output
   c. Effect on body weight, indicating malnutrition
   d. Character and amount of vomitus—measure and record
   e. Effect on the patient's activity—malaise or apathy
   f. Changes in the patient's skin color and turgor and in mucous membranes
   g. Note other fluid losses—perspiration, feces, urine, fluid and electrolyte balance—which may result in dehydration
2. Improve psychological desire for food in order to overcome anorexia, nausea, and vomiting.
   a. Determine the patient's eating habits, cultural preferences, etc.
   b. Include the patient's family in soliciting information.
   c. Encourage adequate rest before, during, and after his meal; allay anxiety.
   d. Prepare the patient for his meals by being certain that he has had good oral hygiene, is comfortable, and has clean bedding and clothing.
   e. Promote the patient's physical comfort so that he may enjoy his food and not be distracted by discomfort during or after his meal.
   f. Protect the patient's environment from noise, foul odors, confusion, too many visitors, etc.
   g. Serve food with attractive appearance and in appropriate quantity.
   h. Be sure that food is served at proper temperature.
3. If the patient is nauseated but does not vomit:
   a. Reduce environmental stimuli.
      Visual—other "sick" patients; soiled dressings
      Olfactory—drainage bottle
      Sensory—colostomy; cauterization; bedpan
      Auditory—noise
   b. Encourage rest and deep breathing.
   c. Cater to the patient's preferences in food.
   d. Limit size of servings.
   e. Remove meal tray as soon as the patient is finished.
   f. If he does vomit, carefully observe vomitus and remove promptly; clean area and patient if necessary and offer mouthwash.
4. Provide opportunity for the patient to express his feelings.
   a. Keep channels of communication open.
   b. Provide time to allow patient to talk.
5. Correlate administration of medication with needs of the patient.
   a. If the patient has pain, analgesics may be administered.

b. If the patient is tired and exhausted, sedatives may be prescribed.
c. If the patient appears tense and worried, tranquilizers may be indicated.
d. Specific antiemetic agents.
6. If secondary to intestinal obstruction, nasogastric suction or the insertion of a Miller–Abbott tube is indicated.

Anorexia Nervosa and Bulimia

Anorexia nervosa is voluntary refusal to eat, usually occurring in a female between the ages of 12 and 18 years.
Bulimia nervosa is extreme overeating and subsequent attempts to rid the body of food by self-induced vomiting and laxative abuse.

Constipation and Diarrhea

Constipation

Constipation is a decrease in the frequency, volume, or ease of stool passage.
Obstipation is absence of intestinal output (no stool).
1. Constipation is usually caused by altered routine in dietary and activity patterns; by drugs such as morphine, codeine, and atropine; by mechanical obstruction or surgery; by psychological factors resulting from restricted use of toilet facilities; and by old age. It may also occur as a result of chronic, strong-laxative abuse.
2. Manifestations of constipation include changes in color, consistency, and ease of expulsion of stools, which may be darker, harder, and difficult or painful to pass.

Diarrhea

Diarrhea is an increase in frequency, fluidity, and/or volume of stools.
1. It is a leading cause of death in developing countries, where sanitation is poor and dietary deficiency widespread.
2. Acute diarrhea can be a serious problem in elderly and debilitated persons.
3. Chronic diarrhea is associated with malabsorption, malnutrition, anemia, and increased susceptibility to other diseases.

Assessment
Patient Problems/Nursing Diagnoses

1. Determine whether onset was sudden or gradual.
2. Find out how long the patient has had diarrhea—days? weeks? months?
3. Describe the character, consistency, and appearance of stools. Note that color changes are produced by presence of abnormal constituents.
   a. "Tarry" stools—may indicate digested blood that usually originates in upper gastrointestinal tract.
   b. Bloody stools—may indicate hemorrhage, usually from lower GI tract.
   c. Blood streaking on stool surface or on toilet paper—may indicate hemorrhoid or fissure.
   d. Pale, pasty (clay-colored) stools—indicate totally obstructed biliary tract.
   e. Foamy, foul-smelling stools—indicates malabsorption or malabsorption syndrome.
   f. Other color changes due to food or medication ingested indicates dietary excesses or effect of medication.

4. Learn when the bouts of diarrhea occur—in the daytime only, after meals, either day or night.
5. Determine whether diarrhea is associated with cramping or abdominal pain, fever, chills, nausea, weakness, travel exposure, etc.
6. Is pain in rectum or anus experienced at the time stools are passed? May be indicative of tumor, inflammation, hemorrhoids, or anal fissure.
7. Has the patient had any change in dietary habits, meals eaten away from home, etc?

▶ **NURSING ALERT:** Alteration in bowel habits (such as constipation, then diarrhea, then constipation, then diarrhea) may mean partial obstruction.

8. Determine degree of dehydration. Look for signs of dehydration—weakness, postural hypotension, tachycardia, mucosal dryness, lethargy, poor skin, turgor.
9. Expect the need for laboratory evaluation—serum electrolytes, BUN, creatinine, hemoglobin, serum albumin, blood gases and pH, stool cultures, and stool examination for ova and parasites.

Planning and Implementation
Nursing Management
A. Constipation and Diarrhea
1. Disturbances in elimination produce psychological discomfort; conversely psychologic deviation can produce elimination disturbances.
2. Assist the patient in overcoming correctable problems by:
   a. Affording privacy
   b. Helping the patient approach near-normal position during evacuation, as much as possible
   c. Providing comfort measures such as warmed bedpan
   d. Providing sufficient time and a schedule as close to the patient's own as possible.

B. Constipation
1. Correct dietary habits to include adequate fluids, fresh fruits, and vegetables, whole-grain cereal, bread
   a. Dried fruits such as prunes, apricots, and figs are high in fiber.
   b. Cut back on highly processed foods (sweets) and foods high in fat.
2. Suggest a small glass of prune juice or lemon juice in warm water each morning.
3. If possible, encourage the patient to participate in active daily exercise—brisk walking, swimming.
4. Encourage a regular time for evacuation each day.
5. Avoid taking laxatives if at all possible. If necessary, suggest a bulk-forming laxative, such as Metamucil, that does not irritate the bowel. One to two heaping teaspoonfuls in a glass of water, once or twice daily, followed by a second glass of water.
6. Do not expect to have a bowel movement every day or even every other day.

C. Diarrhea
1. Consider hospitalization if diarrhea continues unresolved and there is significant dehydration.
2. Perform rectal examination to check for fecal impaction (common in the elderly, in mental patients, and in patients with neurologic disorders). If found, manually disimpact (see p. 465). Then give enemas.
3. Remove such causative factors as stress and food until cause is determined.
4. Encourage patient to take fluids such as Gatorade.

juices, soups, and broths; avoid milk, fruits, and extreme roughage.
5. Prepare for fluid therapy administration if dehydration is suspected.
6. General measures
   a. Have required bathroom facilities readily available.
   b. Pay particular attention to proper hand and body hygiene, since diarrhea may be infectious.
   c. Use talcum powder or emollients to prevent skin excoriation.
   d. Provide dry and clean bed linen and clothing.
   e. Prepare for fluid therapy and electrolyte replacement if dehydration is suspected. Administer prescribed medications.
      (1) Kaolin-pectin (Kaopectate)—acts as an absorbent to bind gas and bacteria.
      (2) Diphenoxylate (Lomotil)—decreases intestinal motility by acting on gastrointestinal smooth muscle (contraindicated when etiologic agent is *Shigella* or invasive bowel disease).
      (3) Opiates—act to decrease bowel motility.

Gastrointestinal Problems in the Elderly
Types of Problems
A. Aberration of Taste
1. May be related to chronic smoking and frequent intake of hot beverages, causing thermal injury to taste buds.
2. Reduced capacity for drinking and eating.
3. Overindulgence can cause bloating and belching.
4. Greater reliance on antacids.

B. Lactose Intolerance
1. Orientals seem to be lactose-intolerant by age 40 years.
   Bloating, gas, and diarrhea develop from 1 to 3 hours after taking milk, cream, or ice cream.
2. This affects 30% to 65% of black Africans, black Americans, and Latin races.

C. Use of Sweeteners in Foods and Beverages
1. Symptoms produced are bloating, flatulence, and diarrhea.
2. Cause is fermentation of the nondigestible sweetener by colonic bacteria.

D. Belching and Flatus
1. Probably due to swallowed air.
2. May also be caused by methane and hydrogen produced by bacterial fermentation from indigestible carbohydrates from certain fruits and vegetables.
4. Odoriferous gases (Sketole, indole) may also be produced by bacterial fermentation in colon.
   Thought to result from incomplete digestion of wheat, barley, rye, oats, corn, and potatoes.

E. Indigestion and Heartburn
1. Often due to rich or greasy foods in combination with alcohol.
2. May be caused by carbonated beverages, tea, or coffee.
3. Excessive relaxation of lower esophageal sphincter may be caused by foods rich in fat or chocolate, as well as foods containing carminatives (onions, peppermint).

F. Hiatal Hernia

1. When lower esophageal sphincter mechanism becomes impaired, the problem often is aggravated in the presence of hiatal hernia.
   Symptoms:
   a. Fullness in upper abdomen, heartburn, regurgitation.
   b. Usually, eating less, taking antacids, and not reclining after eating will alleviate symptoms.

G. Esophageal Spasm

1. Symptoms—episodic, intermittent difficulty in swallowing while eating or drinking.
2. Pain under sternum may be caused by hot/cold beverages.
3. On occasion, a large piece of meat is swallowed too quickly, followed by retching and the urge to vomit.
4. Encourage complete chewing and eating slowly.

H. Diverticulosis

1. Occurs as a result of inherent weakness in colon wall; pressures within colon increase with colonic contractions.
2. Those with irritable bowel are prone to develop diverticulosis.
3. Maintain a high-fiber diet to increase bulk content of stool.

I. Cholelithiasis

1. Usually associated with females who have borne children.

2. A high-calorie diet seems related to increasing amounts of biliary cholesterol.
3. Only about 25% of patients who develop symptoms (abdominal pain, jaundice) require therapy.

J. Other Conditions

1. Incidence of gastric and duodenal ulcer increases in middle years.
2. Colitis and ileitis become less common.
3. Gastrointestinal cancers (stomach, pancreas, colon) increase in frequency after age 40.
4. Alcohol-related cirrhosis of liver increases.

Health Education

1. Practice moderation in eating and alcohol consumption.
2. Alcohol-induced damage requires an average daily intake of 150 g. for several years. This can be reached with the following daily intake:
   a. Ninety-proof whiskey—½ pint (4 strong drinks)
   b. Wine—25-oz. bottle contains 100 g. of alcohol
   c. Beer—6-pack of 12 oz. cans or bottles contains 120 g. of alcohol
3. Daily dietary calories to be regulated in three meals with foods from vegetables, fruits, starches, grains, protein, and dairy products.
4. Vitamin supplements are probably unnecessary.
5. Augment diet with fiber supplements—this appears to reduce incidence of diverticula and hemorrhoids.
6. Do not ignore these signs: change in bowel habits, unusual pain, weight loss, bleeding, or jaundice.

Intubation and Diagnostic Studies for Gastroduodenal Conditions

Guidelines: Nasogastric Intubation—Levin Tube (Short Tube) or Salem Sump Tube

Goals

1. Remove fluid and gas from the GI tract (decompression).
2. Prevent or relieve nausea and vomiting.
3. Determine the amount of pressure and motor activity in the GI tract (diagnostic studies).
4. Treat patients with mechanical obstruction and bleeding within the upper GI tract.
5. Administer medications and feeding (gavage) directly into the GI tract.
6. Obtain a specimen of gastric contents for laboratory studies (when pyloric or intestinal obstruction is suspected).

Equipment

Nasogastric tube—usually Levin (rubber or plastic, No. 12 to 18 French)—preferably disposable (plastic tubes are less irritating than rubber) or double-lumen Salem sump tube
Water-soluble lubricant
Clamp for tubing
Towel, tissues, and emesis basin
Glass of water and straw, or perhaps ice chips
Adhesive tape (hypoallergenic) ½″ and 1″
Irrigating set with 20-ml. syringe
Stethoscope
Penlight

Follow-up Equipment

Decongestant spray
Lip pomade
Mouth hygiene materials

Procedure

Preparatory Phase

1. Explain procedure to the patient and tell him how mouth breathing, panting, and swallowing can help in passing the tube.
2. Have the patient in a sitting or high Fowler's position; place a towel across his chest.
3. Determine with the patient what sign he might use, such as raising his index finger, to indicate "wait a few moments" because of gagging or discomfort.
4. Remove dentures; place emesis basin and tissues within the patient's reach.
5. Place rubber tubing in ice-chilled water, making tubing firmer. Plastic tubing may already be firm enough; if too stiff, dip in warm water.
6. Mark distance tube is to be passed by measuring as indicated in Figure 10-2. This will ensure the passage of the tubing into the stomach.

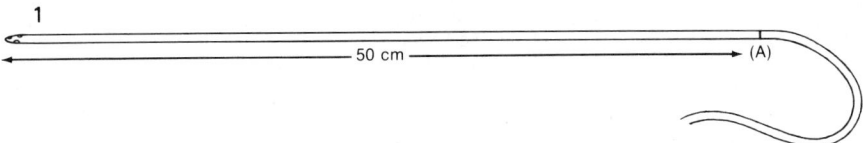

1. Mark the nasogastric tube at a point 50 cm. from the distal tip; call this point 'A'.

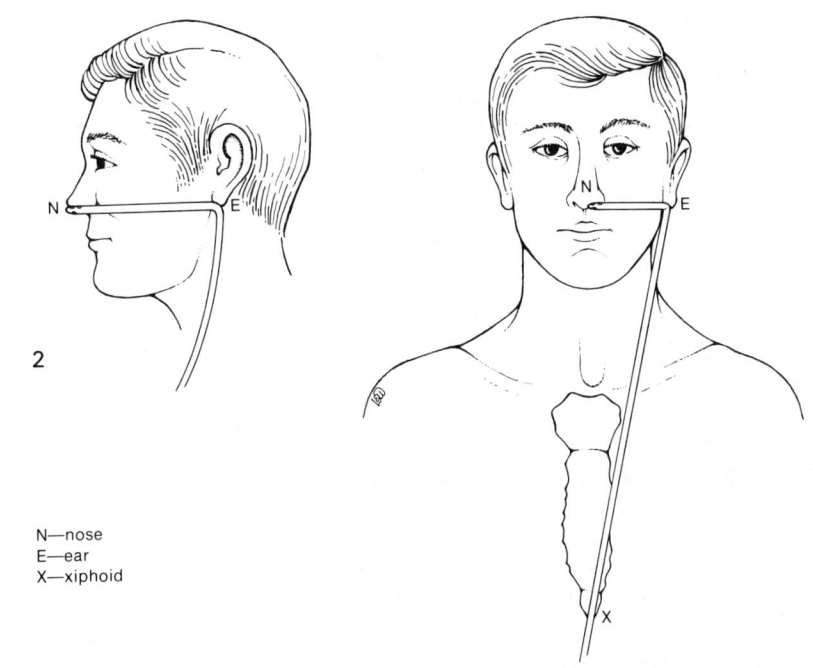

N—nose
E—ear
X—xiphoid

2. Have the patient sit in a neutral position with head facing forward. Place the distal tip of the tubing at the tip of the patient's nose (N); extend tube to the tragus (tip) of his ear (E), and then extend the tube straight down to the tip of his xiphoid (X). Mark this point 'B' on the tubing.

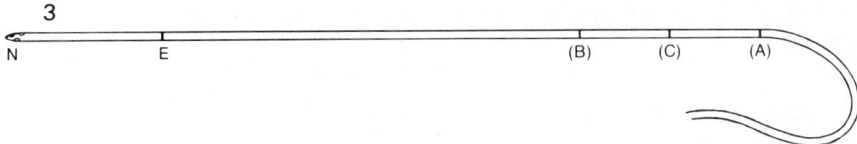

3. To locate point C on the tube, find the midpoint between points A and B. The nasogastric tube is passed to point C to ensure optimum placement in the stomach.

Figure 10-2. The above diagram and steps (*1, 2, 3*) indicate how far a nasogastric tube is passed for optimal placement in the stomach (Hanson RL. Predictive criteria for length of nasogastric tube insertion for tube feeding. J Parenteral Enteral Nutr 1979 May/June; 3 [3]. 160–163)

(continued)

Guidelines: Nasogastric Intubation—Levin Tube (Short Tube) or Salem Sump Tube (continued)

Procedure

Nursing Action	Rationale/Amplification
Performance Phase	
1. Lubricate tube for about 15–20 cm. (6–8 inches) with thin coat of water-soluble jelly.	1. Lubrication reduces friction between mucous membrane and tube.
2. Tilt back the patient's head before inserting tube into nostril and gently pass tube into the posterior nasopharynx, aiming downward and backward.	2. Passage of tube is facilitated by following the natural contours of the body.
3. When tube reaches the pharynx, the patient may gag; allow him to rest for a few moments.	3. Gag reflex is triggered by the presence of the tube.
4. Have the patient hold his head in a partially flexed position: offer him several sips of water sucked through a straw or permit him to suck on ice chips. Advance tube as he swallows.	4. Flexed head position makes swallowing easier and the tube less likely to enter trachea. Swallowing facilitates passage of tube. Actually, once the tube passes the cricopharyngeal sphincter into the esophagus, it can be slowly and steadily advanced, even if the patient does not swallow.
5. Continue to advance tube gently each time patient swallows.	
6. If obstruction appears to prevent tube from passing, do *not* use force. Rotating tube gently may help. If unsuccessful, remove tube and try other nostril.	6. Avoid discomfort and trauma to patient.
7. If there are signs of distress such as gasping, coughing, or cyanosis, immediately remove tube.	
8. To check whether the Levin tube is in the stomach:	
a. Aspirate contents of stomach with a 20-ml. syringe.	a. Aspirated stomach contents would indicate that the tube is in the stomach.
b. Place a stethoscope over epigastrium; inject 5 ml. of air into Levin tube.	b. Air can be detected by a "whooshing" sound entering stomach rather than the bronchus.
9. Adjust tubing after these tests to proper position in the stomach.	
After Tube Is Passed	
1. Anchor tube with hypoallergenic tape.	
a. Using 5 cm. (2 inches) hypoallergenic tape, split lengthwise and only halfway; attach upsplit end of tape to nose and cross split ends around tubing.	a. Prevent the patient's vision from being disturbed; prevent tubing from rubbing against nasal mucosa.
2. Anchor the tubing to the patient's gown.	2. To permit mobility of patient.
3. Clamp the tube until the purpose for inserting the tube is about to take place.	

▶ **NURSING ALERT:** All enteric tubes must be irrigated at regular intervals with small volumes of fluid to ensure patency.

4. Administer oral hygiene frequently. Cleanse tubing at nostril. Utilize a decongestant spray, if necessary.	4. To promote patient comfort.
5. Apply cream or lip pomade to lips and nostril to prevent encrustation.	5. To keep tissue soft.
6. If tube is to be in place for prolonged periods (beyond 12 hours), keep head of patient elevated at least 30 degrees.	6. To minimize gastroesophageal reflux.
7. Rotate tubing daily or more frequently.	7. To prevent adherence to mucosa.

Follow-up Phase

Before Removing Nasogastric Tubing

1. Be certain that gastric drainage is not excessive in volume nor from the small bowel.
2. Ensure, by auscultation, that audible peristalsis is present.
3. Determine whether the patient is passing flatus so that abdomen is not distended.

▶ **NURSING ALERT:** Recognize the potential for complications when intubation is prolonged—nasal erosion, sinusitis, esophagitis, and gastric ulceration. Pulmonary complications may occur postoperatively in patients with nasogastric intubation because of interference with coughing and clearing of the pharynx. (Fig. 10-3)

Removing Nasogastric Tubing

1. Place a towel across the patient's chest and inform him that the tube is to be withdrawn.	1. No doubt, the patient will be happy to have progressed to this stage.
2. Rotate tubing and inject about 10 ml. of saline before clamping tubing.	2. This will ensure its mobility. Tubing is clamped to prevent drainage within tube from being aspirated.

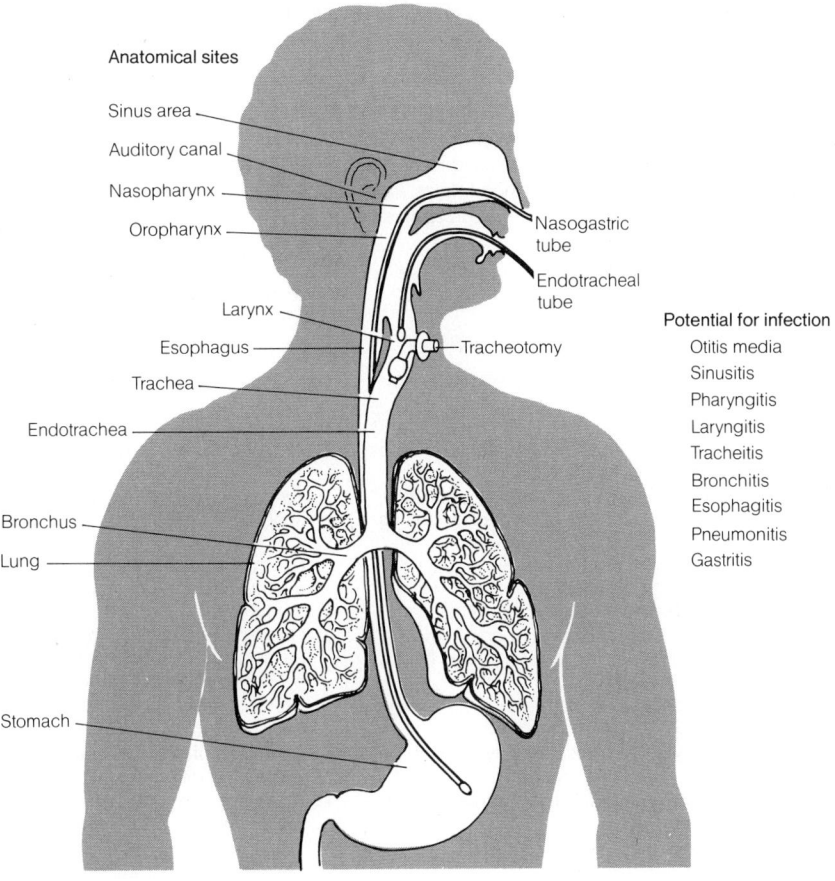

Anatomical sites

Sinus area
Auditory canal
Nasopharynx
Oropharynx
Nasogastric tube
Endotracheal tube
Larynx
Esophagus
Tracheotomy
Trachea
Endotrachea
Bronchus
Lung
Stomach

Potential for infection
Otitis media
Sinusitis
Pharyngitis
Laryngitis
Tracheitis
Bronchitis
Esophagitis
Pneumonitis
Gastritis

Figure 10-3. All along the upper respiratory tract and upper digestive system, there is the potential for abnormal areas of colonization (infection) when various tubes are in place (e.g., tracheostomy, nasogastric or endotracheal tube). In addition, there is the potential for aspiration of secretions that may cause bronchitis and/or pneumonitis.

Procedure
(Cont.)

Nursing Action	Rationale/Amplification
3. Instruct the patient to take a deep breath and exhale slowly.	3. Slow exhalation will relax the pharynx and facilitate withdrawal of tubing.
4. Slowly but evenly withdraw tubing and cover it with a towel as it emerges.	4. Covering the tubing should dispel the momentary feeling of nausea.
5. Provide the patient with materials for oral care and lubricant for nasal dryness.	5. Mouthwash and a nasal lubricant will be appreciated by the patient.
6. Document time of tube removal and the patient's reaction.	
7. Continue to monitor the patient for signs of GI difficulties; changes in vital signs may suggest infection (Fig. 10-3).	7. Recurrence of nausea, or vomiting may require re-insertion of nasogastric tube.

Guidelines: Gastric Analysis (Aspiration of Stomach Contents via Nasogastric Tube)

Goals

1. Determine secretory activity of the gastric mucosa because of diagnostic significance.
2. Study the secretory component, hydrochloric acid.
3. Analyze gastric contents in patients suspected of having pyloric or intestinal obstruction.
4. Remove poisons.

(continued)

Guidelines: Gastric Analysis (Aspiration of Stomach Contents via Nasogastric Tube) (continued)

Equipment

Rubber or plastic tube, No. 12–18 Fr. depending upon patient's size
Salem sump tube, Ewald, or Edlich—large single-lumen
Levacuator—double-lumen tube for aspiration and irrigation
Tube clamp; drape or towel; emesis basin and tissues
Syringe, 50-ml. or low-pressure intermittent suction apparatus
Water-soluble lubricant
Bowl of chipped ice for rubber tubing
Specimen containers

Procedure

Nursing Action	Rationale/Amplification
Preparatory Phase	
1. Instruct the patient to take no food or fluids and not to smoke for 8–10 hours prior to analysis.	1. An accurate sampling of stomach contents is ensured.
2. Withhold anticholinergics, antacids, alcohol, cimetidine, and adrenergic blockers, and any other medications as prescribed.	2. To permit normal emptying of the stomach and remove suppressive effect on gastric secretion.
3. Explain procedure to the patient; cover his upper body with a drape to protect his clothing and provide an emesis basin for spittle and emesis.	3. Patient's understanding of how to breathe through his mouth with occasional swallowing will assist in passing the tube.
4. Instruct the patient to sit in a back-supporting chair or to assume Fowler's position in bed with neck flexed, leaning forward from the waist.	4. Gravity and this anatomic position will facilitate tubes passing into esophagus. If neck is hyperextended, tube is more likely to enter trachea.
5. Establish with the patient a signal system to indicate when he wishes to rest for a few minutes.	5. Greater patient cooperation is obtained.
6. If dentures or bridges are present, they should be removed.	6. Dislodging of dentures could occur with risk of asphyxiation.
7. Chill tubing in ice water to make it firmer; if plastic tubing is too stiff, dip in warm water.	7. A manageable tube that droops naturally and is neither too stiff nor too limp is the objective.
Performance Phase	
Pass the nasogastric tube (see Guidelines, p. 412)	
1. Verify that the tube is in the stomach (for absolute assurance of tube position, fluoroscopic verification is required). Tip of the tube should be at least 50 cm. down from nose. When syringing air in and out, gurgling over stomach is audible with stethoscope.	1. Blue litmus turns pink in the presence of acid.
2. Place the patient semi-recumbent in left lateral decubitus position.	
3. Aspirate fasting stomach contents completely; then measure and record. If abnormal, notify physician before proceeding.	3. Normal—clear and watery; often contains green or yellow bile. Abnormal—see Nursing Alert
4. When tubing is properly positioned in the stomach, allow the patient to rest for 20–30 minutes and continuously aspirate contents. This procedure allows the patient to attain a basal state and to adjust to the tube in his throat.	4. Production of hydrochloric acid may be inhibited by the irritation of the tubing and by anxiety.
5. See below for types of analyses.	

▶ **NURSING ALERT:** In gastric analysis, note the following:
1. Residual of 100 ml. or more, including undigested food particles, may be indicative of gastric stasis or pyloric obstruction.
2. Fecal odor—suggests neoplasm or gastric fistula, intestinal obstruction.
3. Blood—indicates ulcerating lesion.
   Streaks of blood—suggest trauma from tubing.

Types of Gastric Analyses

A. Basal Analysis—A test to determine nature of secretions in the absence of stimuli.

1. For 12 hours preceding test—no food; for 8 hours preceding test—no fluids or smoking
2. Obtain specimens as follows:

1st specimen—label "residual"
2nd specimen (30 minutes later)—label as to amount and time of collection
Then 4 additional specimens must be collected at 15-minute intervals—label as to amount and time of collection.
   Continuous or frequent aspiration is required

(manually or with suction apparatus) to avoid losses through pylorus.

3. Normal ranges:
Female: 0.2–3.8 mEq./hour
Male: 1–5 mEq./hour

B. Stimulation Analysis (betazole hydrochloride or pentagastrin) usually performed following basal study.

1. Test of gastric secretion following injection of a stimulant
   a. Collect fasting specimen of gastric contents.
   b. Administer betazole hydrochloride (Histalog) or pentagastrin.
   c. Collect specimens every 15 minutes for 90 minutes, or longer if physician desires.
2. Significance
   a. In presence of gastric ulcer visualized radiologically or endoscopically, the absence of any acid after stimulation (pH never falls below 6.0) suggests that ulcer is malignant and that surgical treatment is indicated.

Note: In absence of an ulcer, achlorhydria does *not* have the same significance (present in 40% of adults over age 60 without ulcer or cancer).

   b. In presence of a duodenal ulcer, basal output is greater than 20 mEq./hour peak or maximal acid output greater than 50 mEq./hour. A basal/maximal ratio greater than 0.6 should strongly suggest Zollinger–Ellison syndrome.
   c. Otherwise, acid outputs, either basally or after stimulation, are of no diagnostic significance in peptic ulcer disease.

C. Hypoglycemic Analysis *(Hollander test)*, or "Insulin Gastric Analysis"—A test that shows the vagal stimulation of parietal cells following a blood sugar drop to a hypoglycemic level of less than 50 mg./ 100 ml. (Hypoglycemia stimulates the secretory activity of the vagus nerve: If the nerve is divided, secretion will not occur. This test may be done postsurgically to determine effectiveness of vagotomy.)

1. Collect fasting specimen of gastric contents; label "residual."
2. Collect specimens every 15 minutes for 1 hour; label "basal secretion."
3. Administer prescribed insulin intravenously (calculated according to body weight).
4. Collect gastric specimens every 15 minutes for next 2 hours. Concomitantly, collect blood specimens every 15 minutes for determination of blood sugar. Measure, note characteristics, and record.

▶ **NURSING ALERT:** Observe the patient for signs of hypoglycemia—weakness, vertigo, tremors, perspiration, convulsions, unconsciousness. Have 50% glucose ready for intravenous administration if blood glucose level drops too low.

Radiography

Roentgenography of the Gastrointestinal Tract (Upper GI Series)

1. The entire GI tract can be delineated by x-rays following the introduction of barium sulfate as the contrast medium. This procedure may be combined with cineradiography.

2. Barium is a tasteless, odorless, completely insoluble powder:
   a. It can be ingested in an aqueous suspension for upper gastrointestinal tract study (upper GI series), micronization of particles, as well as chocolate or strawberry flavoring, makes it more palatable.
   b. Effervescent fluids may also be administered to obtain air-contrast studies.
   c. Follow serially through small bowel over next 4–6 hours.
3. The fasting patient is required to swallow barium under direct fluoroscopic examination.
   a. Esophagus
      (1) Patency, caliber, and motility noted—may indicate anatomic and functional derangement.
      (2) Abnormally enlarged right atrium noted—indicates impingement on esophagus.
      (3) Esophageal varices noted—usually indicates liver cirrhosis.
   b. Stomach
      (1) Motility and thickness of gastric wall noted.
      (2) Spasms, ulcerations, malignant infiltrates, and anatomic abnormalities noted.

▶ **NURSING ALERT:** If the patient stands when drinking barium, transit time may be too rapid through the esophagus; if this is a problem, consider supine position with the head somewhat elevated.

      (3) Pressure from outside of stomach detected.
      (4) Patency of pyloric valve observed.
   c. Small intestine
      Barium swallow or a continuous infusion of a thin barium sulfate suspension via duodenal tube may be done to visualize jejunum and ileum.
4. During fluoroscopic examination, roentgenograms or video tapes are taken for permanent records.

Implementation
Nursing Management and Health Education

A careful nursing history may suggest that a patient is at high risk for reactions to contrast medium. (See chart below.)

▶ **NURSING ALERT:** For patients receiving radiographic contrast agents intravenously—observe closely for a delayed reaction during the next 30–60 minutes.

1. The patient is to be on a low-residue diet for preceding 2–3 days and is to receive nothing by mouth after midnight prior to the test.
2. During this interim, the patient is to receive no purgative, however mild, and no other medication unless specifically prescribed.
3. The patient remains in a fasting state until the last roentgenogram is taken.
4. Barium from prior barium enema must be fully evacuated before GI series, or it will interfere with visualization of stomach and upper intestine. Cleansing enema is of particular value here.
5. Since this test takes 5–6 hours, and much time is spent waiting, encourage the patient to take some reading material with him.

Lower GI Series—see p. 435.

Reactions to Radiographic Contrast Material and Their Management

Reaction	Incidence	Manifestations	Medical and Nursing Management
Vasomotor	Up to 50% of patients	Mild flushing Warmth Tingling sensations Slight giddiness Metallic taste Nausea	Because these manifestations are mild and transient, treatment or pre-x-ray medication is not required
Anaphylactoid	Up to 4% of persons with history of allergy, hay fever, or bronchial asthma	Hives Sneezing Chest tightness Wheezing Angioedema Bronchoconstriction Hypotension Compensatory tachycardia	Check pulse frequently Vasopressors IV fluids Oxygen Antihistamines Steroids Pretreatment medication may help: Steroids (oral prednisone) 3 times prior to x-ray Antihistamine (Benadryl) 1 hour before examination
Vagus		Apprehension Restlessness Hypotension Bradycardia—50 beats/minute or less	Atropine—high doses IV fluids Monitor pulse rate, since this indicates response to atropine Pretreatment—some recommend atropine

Upper Gastrointestinal Endoscopy

Upper gastrointestinal fiberoscopy is the direct visualization of the gastric mucosa through a lighted endoscope (gastroscope). Endoscopes are flexible scopes equipped with a fiberoptic lens through which colored photographs or motion pictures can be taken.

Primary diagnostic gastrointestinal endoscopy (PRIDGE) is a rapid accurate, and safe method of examining the upper GI tract in selected patients and is an excellent initial examination.

Nursing Interventions

1. Explain the following to the patient:
    a. What is about to happen.
    b. That he must fast before the examination to prevent aspiration of gastric contents and to permit complete visualization of the stomach.
    c. That dentures must be removed to facilitate passing the scope and to prevent injury.
    d. That a sedative or tranquilizer may be given to help him to relax.
    e. That a topical anesthetic may be used for local comfort and to prevent gagging.
    f. That air will be pumped into the stomach during the procedure to permit visualization of the stomach.
2. Following a gastric examination:
    a. Check the gag reflex before offering food or fluids.
        (1) Tickle the back of the patient's throat with a tongue depressor or cotton swab; usually 2–4 hours after the examination, the reflex functions return to normal.
        (2) If fluids are handled normally, the patient may then be offered food.
    b. Check for signs of perforation—abdominal pain, subcutaneous emphysema, dyspnea, cyanosis, back pain, temperature elevation, hydrothorax, rigid abdomen.
    c. Offer throat lozenges or warm saline gargles to relieve throat soreness.
    d. Inform the patient that because of air pumped into the stomach he may pass gas by belching or passing flatus.

Comparison of Computed Tomography and Ultrasonography

	Computed Tomography	Ultrasound
Availability	Fixed central location	Easily available and possibly portable
Imaging ability	Transverse only	Multiple plane
Image limitations	Limited by patient motion Limited in thin patients	Patient able to move Limited in obese patients
Penetration	Excellent	Cannot penetrate air or bone
Length of time	Longer	Short
Invasiveness	May require contrast medium	None
Radiation risk	Utilizes ionizing radiation	None
Cost	Expensive	Relatively inexpensive

Gastric Biopsy

Obtaining a piece of gastric mucosa can be done through a gastroscope during endoscopy or fiberoscopy. Forceps extended through the scope may be used to bite tissue, or tissue may be obtained via suction as it pulls mucosa to excising blades within the scope. Tissue in one area may be representative of tissue in all sections of the stomach; however, by looking through the scope, the physician can be discriminating in selection of specific tissue.

Nursing management is similar to that for gastric endoscopy (see above).

Computed Tomography (CT Scan) and Ultrasonography (Ultrasound)

A. **Computed Tomography** (CT) is accomplished using a scanner that operates by detecting x-rays from a finely focused beam that rotates around a patient.

The subtle differences in x-ray absorption by various tissues are then assembled by a computer and displayed on a screen as a radiologic image.
1. It provides precise anatomic and pathologic information for a wide array of intra-abdominal and other conditions.
2. Abscesses can be drained using CT as a guide for catheter placement (obviating need for surgery).
3. By exactly noting the full extent (staging) of a malignancy, surgical intervention can be more precise.
4. In abdominal trauma, multiple organ involvement can be noted by CT, thereby reducing number of diagnostic tests.
5. Invasive vascular techniques may be reduced utilizing CT scanner.

B. **Ultrasonography** is the focusing of a beam of high-frequency sound waves over an abdominal organ. This creates waves that vary with changes in tissue density (see also Biliary Conditions, p. 484.)

Gastroduodenal Conditions and Management

Gastrointestinal Bleeding

Bleeding is a symptom of a digestive or vascular problem or problems. It may be obvious in emesis or stool, or it may be *occult* (hidden).

Etiology and Causative Factors
1. Trauma anywhere along the gastrointestinal tract
2. Erosion of a blood vessel due to an ulcer, benign tumor, or malignancy
3. Rupture of an enlarged vein, such as a varicosity (esophageal varices, hemorrhoid)
4. Inflammation such as esophagitis, caused by acid or bile, gastritis, small intestine (Crohn's disease), polyps
5. Irritation of mucous membrane due to certain drugs—alcohol, aspirin, aspirin-containing compounds, other drugs
6. Infection, such as intestinal (ulcerative colitis)
7. Diverticulosis

Clinical Manifestations
1. Signs of blood
   a. Bright red—vomited from high in esophagus; from rectum or distal colon (coating stool)
   b. Mixed with dark red—higher up in colon and small intestine; mixed with stool
   c. Shades of black ("coffee ground")—esophagus, stomach, and duodenum; vomitus from these areas
2. Symptoms of massive bleeding
   a. Weakness, dizziness, faintness, short of breath, crampy abdominal pain, diarrhea
   b. Rapid pulse, drop in blood pressure, shock
   c. Pale appearance, fatigue, lethargy

Diagnostic Evaluation
1. It is not difficult to diagnose bleeding, but it may be a problem to locate source of bleeding.
2. History—change in bowel pattern, presence of pain or tenderness, recent intake of food and what kind (red beets?)
3. Complete blood count; occult test of stool
4. Endoscopy
5. Radioactive scanning

Treatment
1. Depends on cause and whether bleeding is acute or chronic
   a. If aspirin, eliminate aspirin and treat bleeding.
   b. If ulcer, an anti-ulcer drug is prescribed, along with life-style change and dietary change.
   c. If cancer, tumor to be removed (see Mouth Cancer, p. 394, Esophageal Cancer, p. 406, Gastric Cancer, p. 424, Colon Cancer, p. 458).
2. May require skilled endoscopist with a well-prepared diagnostic team.
   a. Intravenous lines and oxygen therapy equipment to be available
   b. If life-threatening bleeding occurs, treat shock, administer blood replacement
      (1) Equipment—large-bore irrigation tube, Pitressin, irrigating equipment of physician's preference
      (2) Cardiac monitor, pulse/blood pressure monitor, emergency cart
      (3) Surgery if conservative measures fail
3. Electrocoagulation and photocoagulation (laser) may be the treatment of choice.
   a. Postlaser treatment requires careful monitoring for bleeding recurrence, nasogastric intubation, dependent drainage.

Peptic Ulcer

A *peptic ulcer* is an excavation found in the mucosal wall of the esophagus, the stomach, the pylorus, or the duodenum because of the erosion of a circumscribed area of its mucous membrane. Basically, the problem is too much secretion of hydrochloric acid in relation to the degree of protection afforded by both mucous secretion and the neutralization of gastric acid by duodenal, biliary, and pancreatic fluid.

Predisposing Factors

1. Emotional stress—anxiety, anger, resentment
2. Intake of methylxanthines (tea, coffee, cola, chocolate) and cigarette smoking are associated with increased risk of ulcer development
3. Drugs (salicylates, aspirin, reserpine, phenylbutazone, aminophylline, and others) may be irritating to the mucous lining of the stomach, pylorus, and duodenum
4. Genetic susceptibility
5. A combination of the above factors

Incidence

1. Duodenal ulcer is found most frequently in the 25–40 age-group and in males 4 times more than in females.
2. Gastric ulcer occurs most frequently in the 40–55 age-group and in males 2½ times more often than in females.
3. Five percent to 15% of population in US have ulcers; only one half the cases are recognized.
4. Duodenal ulcers occur 10 times more frequently than gastric ulcers (Fig. 10-4).
5. Peptic ulcer occurs 2–2½ times more frequently among siblings with ulcers as among the general population.

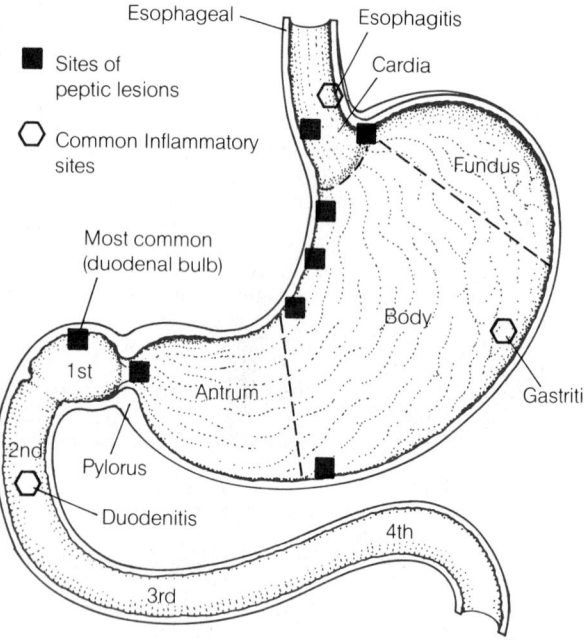

Figure 10-4. The stomach is divided on the basis of its physiologic functions into two main portions. The proximal two thirds, the fundic gland area, acts as a receptacle for ingested food and secretes acid and pepsin. The distal third, the pyloric gland area, mixes and propels food into the duodenum and produces the hormone gastrin. "Peptic" lesions may occur in the esophagus (esophagitis), stomach (gastritis), or duodenum (duodenitis). Note peptic ulcer sites and common inflammatory sites.

6. Duodenal ulcer occurs more frequently in patients with type O blood.

Altered Physiology

(Duodenal ulcer)

1. Increased mass of gastric mucosa and more parietal and peptic cells
2. Increased sensitivity to gastrin (peptide hormone secreted by gastric antrum stimulates gastric secretion)
3. Increased vagal stimulation, which in turn releases gastrin
4. Increased release of gastrin in response to a meal
5. More rapid gastric emptying
6. Increased acid load to duodenum

Assessment

Clinical Manifestations

A. Underlying Observations

1. Peptic ulcers are more likely to be in the duodenum than in the stomach (ratio of 10:1).
2. A peptic ulcer occurs only in the areas of the GI tract that are exposed to hydrochloric acid and pepsin (see Fig. 10-4).
3. A small percentage of patients will have no symptoms and will first be diagnosed during a bleeding episode (more common in teenagers).

B. Pain

1. Types
   a. Pain or discomfort—quality usually not well described; may be sharply localized in midepigastrium. Description may be "hunger-like," burning, gnawing.
   b. Pyrosis (heartburn, substernal burning) is associated with peptic ulcer in many patients; this may occur with sour eructation.
   c. Pain may radiate to the back if the duodenal ulcer has begun to penetrate the pancreas.
2. Time of occurrence
   a. Pain is worse when stomach is empty—usually ½ to 2 hours after meals; it may waken the patient in early AM hours (12–3 AM).
   b. Pain is seldom present when the patient first wakens, because gastric secretion is lowest at this time.
   c. Periodicity occurs in clusters—the patient may have trouble for days to weeks, then experience long symptom-free intervals.
3. Relief—obtained by ingesting food or taking antacids; if truly effective, this occurs within 5–10 minutes.

C. Eructation

Belching is due to increased air swallowing. (This is a nonspecific symptom and is most common in persons with *no* organic GI disease.)

D. Nausea and Vomiting

Reflex vomiting occurs in 10%–20% of patients, with some retching; it is associated with ulcer pain and also is seen with duodenal obstruction in chronic ulcer disease, when it usually occurs with or just after evening meal.

Diagnostic Evaluation

1. Observation, nursing history, and assessment include the following:
   a. Determine location of pain, whether it is localized, whether it radiates, how long it lasts, and when it occurs.

b. Find out if pain is relieved by food, alkalies, vomiting.

c. Determine eating patterns—regularity, type of food, conditions for eating, such as relaxed atmosphere, standing at quick-lunch counter, while driving a truck, etc.

d. Learn if there is a history of tension, problematic situations, fears, or anxiety.

e. Determine whether the patient ingested drug irritants.

f. Determine whether the patient smokes or consumes alcohol.

2. Fiberoptic panendoscopy, which permits visualization of entire stomach and proximal duodenum, is most accurate.

3. Upper GI series (see p. 417).

4. Gastric secretory studies (p. 416) are of value mainly to check for possible Zollinger–Ellison syndrome.

5. Stool specimen to detect occult blood, which indicates bleeding.

Patient Problems/Nursing Diagnoses

1. Pain and epigastric distress related to gastric hyperactivity, mucosal erosion

2. Fear and anxiety related to possibility of developing a complication (hemorrhage, perforation)

3. Ineffective rest/activity pattern related to type A personality or lack of understanding

4. Knowledge deficit related to misunderstanding of biological, dietary, and pharmaceutical limitations

5. Potential for development of complications

Medical Management

1. The patient is advised to reduce stressful activities and to provide for rest and relaxation; sedation/tranquilizers may be prescribed.

2. Antacids, anticholinergics, and ulcer-healing medications may be prescribed as required.

3. Fluid, electrolyte, and blood needs are monitored; intravenous replacement is prescribed.

4. Dietary intake may consist of frequent, small feedings—soft, bland foods at first, then diet as tolerated.

5. Vital signs and clinical manifestations are monitored for progress.

Planning and Implementation

Nursing Interventions

A. Relief of pain and discomfort

1. Administer antacid medications to neutralize hydrochloric acid and relieve pain.

a. Liquid antacids are more effective than tablets.

b. Increasing aluminum in antacids leads to constipation; increasing magnesium leads to diarrhea.

c. Antacids are given 1 hour after meals, at bedtime, and during the night as required for pain.

d. Look for antacids that effectively neutralize stomach acid, leave low sodium content, require about 5 ml. to swallow at a time, and are least expensive (Maalox therapeutic concentrate).

e. Antacids with calcium may produce hypercalcemia.

f. Magaldrate is the antacid containing the least amount of salt and is useful for patients on restricted salt diet.

2. Administer anticholinergic drugs to suppress gastric

secretions and delay gastric emptying. This is most useful at night.

a. Anticholinergics are contraindicated in patients with glaucoma, urinary retention, gastric retention, and possibly arrhythmia.

b. Encourage hydration to minimize side effects of anticholinergic medications.

3. If ulcer problems persist after first being treated with antacids, it may be necessary to administer cimetidine (Tagamet), ranitidine (Zantac), or sucralfate (Carafate).

a. Cimetidine (Tagamet) owes its effectiveness to its H_2-receptor blocking action in inhibiting gastric acid secretion; to its potency (superior to that of cholinergics); and to its failure to produce acute side effects.

b. Cimetidine is administered with meals because it is rapidly absorbed and its blood concentration peaks about 75 minutes after ingestion.

c. Between 60% and 90% of patients with duodenal ulcers heal within 4 weeks.

d. About 85% of patients with duodenal ulcers suffer acute episodes, which can be managed effectively without surgery.

e. During short-term therapy, side effects are most unusual.

f. Symptoms of misuse of Tagamet should be noted: diarrhea, dizziness, gynecomastia, decreased sperm count, hallucinations, bradycardia.

g. Cimetidine is effective only in preventing bleeding from starting, not in stopping bleeding once it has started.

h. See Table 10-2 for comparative analysis of cimetidine, ranitidine, and sucralfate.

B. Dietary considerations

1. Eliminate foods that the patient says cause him pain or distress; otherwise the diet is unrestricted.

2. Offer regular milk, since the fat in milk decreases secretion. (Skim milk is usually not given, because the calcium in milk increases secretion.)

3. Give small servings to decrease distention and release of gastrin.

4. Provide frequent feedings to neutralize gastric secretions and to dilute stomach contents.

5. Advise the patient to avoid coffee and other caffeinated beverages and cola drinks.

6. Advise the patient to avoid hot or cold foods and fluids, to chew food thoroughly, and to eat in a leisurely fashion.

C. Modification in life-style to promote physical and mental rest

1. Encourage bed rest to reduce physical activity and to separate patient from usual environment.

2. Offer sedatives or tranquilizers to lessen the response to stimuli and to promote relaxation and sleep.

3. Provide frequent feedings, antacids, and other medications given on time.

4. Inform visitors to avoid upsetting conversation.

5. Emphasize the need to avoid anxiety-producing situations.

6. Alert the patient to the irritating effects on the gastric mucosa of certain drugs—especially aspirin and aspirin-containing drugs such as Alka-Seltzer.

7. Review the reasons for smaller meals and midmeal snacks.

8. Suggest that he cut down on smoking; suggest

Table 10-2 **Comparison of Cimetidine (Tagamet), Ranitidine (Zantac), and Sucralfate (Carafate)**
Purpose of these medications: Treat active peptic ulcer

	Cimetidine	Ranitidine	Sucralfate
Effectiveness	←————————————→	Equally effective	←————————————→
Duration or rate of action	Action peaks in 60–90 minutes	Basal action—up to 4 hours Nocturnal—up to 12 hours	5 hours
Potency		Three times more potent than cimetidine	
Reaction with other drugs	Oxidatively metabolized by liver, e.g., reacts with propranolol (Inderal), Warfarin, theophylline, diazepam (Valium), phenytoin	None reported	Antacids may interfere with its effectiveness Absorption of oral tetracyclines may be decreased May interfere with absorption of fat-soluble vitamins A, D, E, K
Adverse reaction	Confusion (especially in elderly and/or with decreased renal function) Practically none In young men, reduced sperm count	Rarely, hepatotoxicity	Constipation may be noted
Dose	300 mg. qid (ac plus hs)	150 mg. bid until ulcer heals, or 4–8 weeks	1 g. given 1 hour before meals and at bedtime
Safety at high doses	Lesser	Greater	(Not given)
Serum creatinine concentration	Increased	Does not increase, therefore preferred when renal function is significantly impaired	(Not reported)
Penetration of CNS	Somewhat? Elderly patients may develop CNS toxicity	Poor penetration No problems in elderly	
Complications		No hematologic toxicity No anti-androgenic action and gynecomastia	Occasional constipation rare
Rate of absorption from GI tract	Rapidly—60%–70%	About 50% slowly absorbed from GI Low bioavailability, which permits a single dose to last longer; therefore, taken only bid	Up to 5% absorbed from GI tract
Action	Gastric acid secretion inhibitor Histamine H_2-receptor antagonist	Same as cimetidine	Appears to form an ulcer-adherent complex that covers ulcer site; this protects site against action by acid, pepsin, bile salts

switching from coffee and cola to caffeine-free beverages such as ginger ale, 7-Up, and Postum.

D. Prevention of complications

1. Prevent complications by following therapeutic regimen.
2. Treat epigastric or ''warning'' pain by taking an antacid.
3. Renew the taking of anti-ulcer medication if indiscretions have been ''unavoidable''—limited rest because of studying for tests, excess partying with alcohol consumption, etc.
4. Practice coping measures to reduce stress.
5. Rest and notify physician if black, tarry stool is noted; prepare for possible hospital admission.

Health Education

1. Modify life-style to incorporate health practices that will prevent recurrences of ulcer pain, bleeding, and distress.
2. Plan for rest periods and avoidance of stressful situations.
3. Chew food thoroughly and eat in leisurely manner on a regular schedule.
4. Avoid large meals, since they tend to overstimulate acid secretion.
5. Avoid irritating substances such as alcohol, coffee, cola, highly spiced foods, tart fresh fruits, and rich pastries.
6. Avoid specific foods that cause this particular patient distress.
7. Assume responsibility for rejecting ulcerogenic drugs—aspirin, steroids.
8. Monitor one's practices—avoid fatigue, recognize signs of potential problems (mid-epigastric pain), walk away from stress-producing situations, reinstitute anti-ulcer medication if necessary.

Evaluation
Expected Outcomes

1. Obtains relief from discomfort and pain of duodenal ulcer by following therapeutic regimen
2. Reviews activity schedule and allocates time for rest periods to offset fatigue and tension
3. Describes the therapeutic regimen to be followed to prevent recurrence of ulcers—such as avoiding caffeine, heavily spiced and fried food, stressful situations, irritating drugs (such as aspirin)
4. Lists signs that indicate potential complications and what to do about them, such as treating epigastric

pain with an antacid and avoiding intake of aspirin or Indocin

Complications of Peptic Ulcer

Hemorrhage → Shock
Perforation → Peritonitis
Pyloric Obstruction → Dehydration
Intractability → Incapacitation—Surgery

A. Hemorrhage

1. Experienced by 15%–25% of patients with duodenal ulcer; accounts for 40% of deaths from peptic ulcer.
2. Manifestations
   a. Giddiness, faintness, breathlessness with slight exertion
   b. Tachycardia, sweating, and coldness of extremities
   c. Black, tarry stool (melena)—test for occult blood
   d. Vomiting of blood (hematemesis)
3. Medical and nursing interventions
   a. Encourage bed rest and check vital signs frequently.
   b. Give medication for restlessness or pain, but be on alert for shock.
   c. Employ nasogastric suction to empty stomach of clots and to monitor rate of bleeding.
   d. Give whole blood or blood component therapy to keep circulating blood volume at a safe level. (This is not needed if hematocrit is greater than 30 and vital signs are stable, with no orthostatic drop in blood pressure or rise in pulse.)
   e. Note color, consistency, and volume of stools and vomitus.
   f. Provide treatment if the patient goes into oligemic shock (see p. 90).

B. Perforation

1. Clinical manifestations
   a. Severe upper abdominal pain, persisting and increasing in intensity and often spreading from upper to lower abdomen
   b. Vomiting suddenly
   c. Referring of pain to top of shoulders (phrenic nerve irritation)
   d. Abdomen—extremely tender and rigid
   e. X-ray of abdomen—50%–75% free air visible
   f. Shock, tachypnea
   g. Patient lying still in bed, afraid to move; pain increased by the patient's coughing or jostling the bed
2. Surgical intervention
   a. Repair fluid deficit (peritoneal "burn").
   b. Close perforation; plication of ulcers is performed (see Postoperative Care, p. 435) if chronic symptoms preceded perforation.

C. Pyloric Obstruction

1. Etiology—area around pyloric sphincter becomes narrowed from spasm, edema, or scar tissue formed when ulcer alternately heals and breaks down. Inflammation, muscle spasm, or edema may cause a temporary obstruction.
2. Assessment and major manifestations—nausea, vomiting of retained food, constipation, weight loss, cramping, epigastric pain after meals.
3. Medical and nursing intervention
   a. Gastric decompression and intravenous fluids.
   b. Later, test emptying with fluid load and then with solid bolus.

   c. Surgery may follow if clinical course is prolonged and obstruction is unrelieved.

D. Intractability

The failure of medical management to accomplish healing of the ulcer—usually a calloused posterior ulcer that penetrates into the pancreas.
1. Manifestations—pain continues without adequate relief from milk or antacid.
2. Surgical intervention
   a. Vagotomy and gastrojejunostomy or pyloroplasty—to abolish cephalic phase of secretion
   b. Vagotomy and hemigastrectomy—to abolish cephalic and gastric phase of secretion
   c. Gastric resection—to abolish acid-secreting parietal cells

Surgical Treatment

Surgery is required in only about 15%–20% of ulcer patients; operation is individualized, based on patient's age, ability to withstand procedure, preoperative nutritional status, and particular indications.

Goal:
Relieve complications.
   a. Perforation (described in B, above)
   b. Hemorrhage (described in A, above)
   c. Pyloric obstruction (described in C, above)
   d. Intractability (described in D, above)
Treat the tendency to ulcer formation.

A. Types of Gastric Operations

1. Gastrojejunostomy and vagotomy (Fig. 10-5)—the jejunum is anastomosed to the stomach to provide a second outlet of gastric contents. The severed vagus nerve reduces secretions and movements of the stomach (90% good results).
2. Antrectomy and vagotomy (Fig. 10-6)—the resected portion includes a small cuff of duodenum, the pylorus, and the antrum (about one half of the stomach). The stump of the duodenum is closed by suture, and the side of the jejunum is anastomosed to the cut end of the stomach.
3. Subtotal gastrectomy (Fig. 10-7)—the resected portion includes a small cuff of the duodenum, the pylorus, and from two thirds to three quarters of the stomach. The duodenum or side of the jejunum is anastomosed to the remaining portion of the stomach.

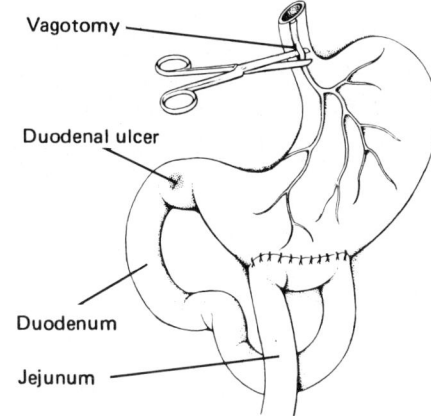

Figure 10-5. Gastrojejunostomy and vagotomy.

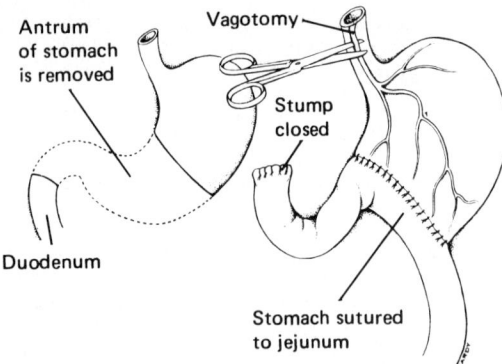

Figure 10-6. Antrectomy and vagotomy.

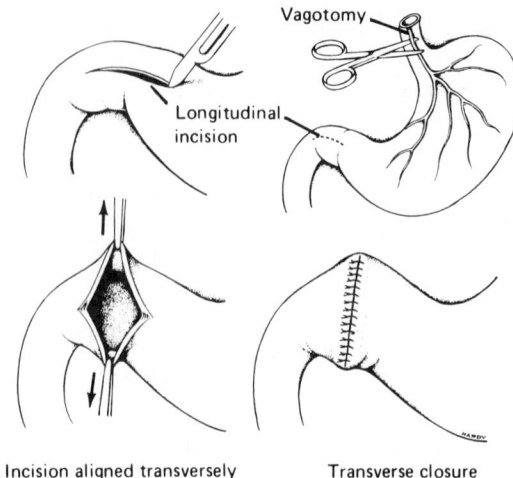

Incision aligned transversely   Transverse closure

Figure 10-8. Vagotomy and pyloroplasty.

4. Vagotomy and pyloroplasty (Fig. 10-8)—a longitudinal incision is made in the pylorus, and it is closed transversely to permit the muscle to relax and to establish an enlarged outlet. This compensates for the impaired gastric emptying produced by vagotomy.

B. Nursing Management

(See below, for management of the patient undergoing a gastric resection.)

Gastric Cancer

Cancer of the stomach accounts for about 14,000 deaths annually in the US—usually males of middle age. For unknown reasons, there has been a decrease in incidence in the US over the last 2 decades.

Clinical Manifestations

A. Early Manifestations

(Most often, patient presents with same symptoms as gastric ulcer; later, on evaluation, the lesion is found to be malignant.)
1. Progressive loss of appetite
2. Noticeable change in, or appearance of, gastrointestinal symptoms—gastric fullness (early satiety), dyspepsia lasting more than 4 weeks
3. Blood (usually occult) in the stools
4. Vomiting, which may indicate pyloric obstruction or cardiac-orifice obstruction

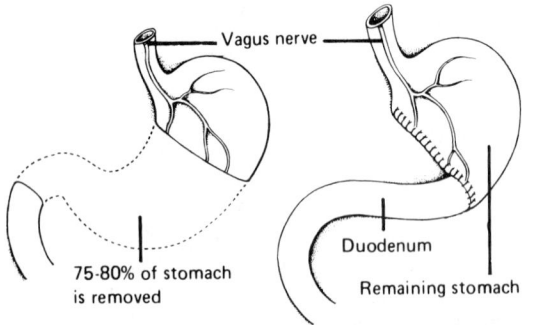

Figure 10-7. Subtotal gastrectomy. It is also possible to do the Billroth II procedure by suturing the gastric stump to the side of the jejunum.

5. Occasionally, vomiting that has a coffee-ground appearance because of slow leaks of blood from ulceration of the cancer

B. Later Manifestations

1. Pain is a late symptom, often induced by eating and relieved by vomiting.
2. Weight loss, loss of strength, anemia, metastasis (usually to liver), hemorrhage, obstruction.

Diagnostic Evaluation

1. Nursing history—weight loss and loss of strength over several months.
2. Cytologic examination of gastric juice, which may show cancer cells.
3. Palpable unusual abdominal mass.
4. Suspicion of metastasis by palpable lymph nodes—surface of liver, skin at umbilicus, supraclavicular nodes, etc.
5. Gastric analysis—absence of acid after maximal stimulation (Histalog, gastrin) indicates that ulcer is malignant.
6. Roentgenologic studies, fluoroscopy, and gastroscopy; also cytologic studies and biopsy-fiberoscopy.
7. Stool examination and tests for occult blood may be indicated.
8. Ultrasonography and computed tomography may be required. These are usually reserved for questionable diagnoses, since they are more costly tests.

Treatment

1. The only successful treatment of gastric cancer is surgical removal.
2. If tumor is localized to stomach and can be removed, chances are still poor that the patient can be cured.
3. If tumor has spread beyond the area that can be excised surgically, cure cannot be accomplished. Palliative surgery such as subtotal gastrectomy with or without gastroenterostomy may be performed to maintain continuity of the gastrointestinal tract. Surgery may be combined with chemotherapy to provide palliation and prolong life.

Gastric Resection

Gastric resection is the surgical removal of part of the stomach.

Treatment and Nursing Management

A. **Promote comfort and wound healing by relieving the patient of pain and discomfort.**

1. Frequently turn the patient and encourage deep-breathing to prevent vascular and pulmonary complications.
2. Institute nasogastric suction to remove fluids and gas in the stomach.
3. Provide conscientious mouth care to prevent mouth dryness and ulceration.
4. Administer parenteral antibiotics to prevent infection.
5. See that the patient has nothing by mouth until prescribed (to promote gastric wound healing).

B. **Meet nutritional needs of the patient.**

1. Give intravenous fluids to prevent shock and to provide adequate fluid and electrolytes.
2. Give fluids by mouth when audible bowel signs are present.
3. Increase fluids according to the patient's tolerance.
4. Offer a diet with vitamin supplements when the patient's condition permits.
5. Give protein–vitamin supplements to foster wound repair and tissue building.
6. Avoid high-carbohydrate foods, such as milk, that may trigger "dumping syndrome."

C. **Anticipate complications in order to prevent them.**

1. Shock and hemorrhage
   a. Evaluate status of blood pressure, pulse, and respiration.
   b. Observe the patient for evidence of apathy, apprehension, air hunger, pallor, or clammy skin.
   c. Check the dressings and drainage bottle frequently for evidence of bleeding.
   d. Administer fluid and blood as prescribed.
2. Cardiopulmonary complications
   a. Encourage the patient to cough and take deep breaths to produce ventilatory exchange and enhance circulation.
   b. Assist the patient to turn and move, thereby mobilizing secretions.
   c. Promote ambulation as prescribed to increase respiratory exchange.
3. Thrombosis and embolism
   a. Initiate a plan of self-care activities to promote circulation.
   b. Encourage early ambulation to stimulate circulation.
   c. Prevent venous stasis by use of elastic stockings if indicated.
   d. Check for tight dressings or binder that might restrict circulation.
   e. See also page 362.
4. "Dumping syndrome"—a complex reaction, which may occur because of excessively rapid emptying of gastric contents.
   Manifestations—nausea, weakness, perspiration, palpitation, some syncope, and possibly diarrhea.
   Instruct the patient as follows:
   a. Eat small, frequent meals rather than three large meals.
   b. Suggest a diet high in protein and fat and low in carbohydrates, and avoid meals high in sugars, milk, chocolate, salt.
   c. Reduce fluids with meals but take them between meals.
   d. Take anticholinergic medication before meals (if prescribed) to lessen gastrointestinal activity.
   e. Relax when eating; eat slowly and regularly.
   f. Take a rest after meals.
5. Phytobezoar formation (formation of a gastric concretion composed of vegetable matter)
   a. Avoid fibrous foods such as citrus fruits (skins and seeds), because they tend to form phytobezoars.
      (1) Following a gastric resection, the remaining gastric tissue is not able to disintegrate and digest fibrous foods.
      (2) This undigested fiber congeals to form masses that become coated by mucous secretions of the stomach.
   b. Stress the importance of adequate mastication.

Health Education

(Adjustment to self-care and return to the community)

1. Emphasize the importance of coping with stressful situations.
2. Review nutritional requirements and regimen with the patient (Table 10-3).
3. Stress the importance of vitamin B_{12} supplements.
4. Encourage follow-up visits with the physician.
5. Recommend annual blood studies and medical checkups for any evidence of pernicious anemia or other problems.
6. See above, C-4 "Dumping Syndrome."

Table 10-3 Diet Guidelines Following Gastric Surgery*

Foods Usually Well Tolerated

Meat, fish, poultry, eggs, cheese, refined breads and cereals (unsweetened)

Unsweetened canned fruits and juices

Cooked mild vegetables, including potatoes

Fats and oils

Foods to Add as Tolerance Improves

Sweetened canned fruits*

Whole grains

Foods That Often Cause Symptoms of Dumping*

Sugar, candy, syrup, sweetened desserts (cake, cookies, pie, pudding, ice cream)

Foods and Beverages to Avoid

Cold high-carbohydrate items such as milkshakes, slush, fruit ice

Coffee and tea (unless allowed by physician)

Special Considerations

Begin with *very* small portions; eat five to six times daily

Take most liquids between rather than with meals

Milk—include in early stages unless poorly tolerated

Fresh fruits and vegetables—gradually include after 2 to 3 weeks; chew thoroughly

* Add gradually to diet if desired unless bothered by symptoms of dumping or unless weight loss is a desirable goal.
(Suitor CW and Crowley MF. Nutrition, 2nd ed. Philadelphia, JB Lippincott, 1984)

Gastrostomy

A *gastrostomy* is an opening into the stomach performed for the purpose of administering food and fluids when a complete obstruction of the esophagus exists. The obstruction may be due to scar-tissue contracture such as may result from a lye burn or a carcinomatous growth. A gastrostomy may also be done occasionally in the unconscious or debilitated patient for prolonged nutritional support.

Preoperative Patient Care

1. Explain the nature of the problem and the recommended treatment to the patient; use simple line drawings for clarification.
2. Achieve adequate fluid, electrolyte, and nutritional balance by administering the required foods and fluids.
3. Immediate preoperative care is similar to that described on page 84.

Surgery

1. Frequently performed under local anesthesia.
2. The anterior gastric wall is incised through a left rectus incision.
3. A tube is inserted and held in place in the stomach wall with several purse-string sutures. The tube may be a rubber tube or a Foley catheter inflated with 5–8 ml. of water or air and pulled taut to the abdominal wall.
4. The skin is closed close to the tube to prevent leakage.
5. The tube is clamped at all times except for feedings.

Guidelines: Assisting the Patient with Gastrostomy Feedings

Purpose To provide a means of alimentation when the oral route is inaccessible.

Types of Feedings

1. Powdered feedings that are easily liquefied are commercially available.
2. Avoid milk in excess in blacks or other lactate-deficient patients.

Procedure

Preparatory Phase

1. Food blender is very useful in preparing a normal diet; blended food is physiologically more acceptable, since fiber and residue content are retained and good bowel function is promoted.
2. Prepare a tray containing a funnel, tubing and adapter, and water at room temperature.
3. Pour feeding into a graduated container; warm to 37.8°C. (100°F.) in a basin of water.
4. Begin feeding the patient when peristalsis has returned.
5. Place the patient in high Fowler's position unless contraindicated.
6. Place a half-sheet or bath towel over upper half of patient; fold top bedding down to cover the patient from the waist downward. This permits a space for gastrostomy tube exposure.

Nursing Action	Rationale/Amplification
Performance Phase	
1. Connect funnel to tubing and connecting tube.	
2. Uncover opening of gastrostomy (or jejunostomy) tube and insert connecting tube.	2. Provides a receptacle for feeding that will lead into gastrostomy tube.
3. Pour feeding into tilted funnel, unclamp tubing, and allow fluid to flow into the stomach by gravity.	3. Tilting the funnel allows air bubbles to escape; when tubing is unclamped, air bubbles will not enter stomach.
4. Regulate flow by raising or lowering receptacle.	4. Raising increases pressure; lowering decreases pressure.

▶ **NURSING ALERT:** Force should not be used nor should feeding be given directly from the refrigerator; such action would cause abdominal discomfort to the patient. If there appears to be an obstruction, stop feeding and report the problem.

Nursing Action	Rationale/Amplification
5. After each feeding, the tube is irrigated with water (room temperature) and clamped.	5. A water flush prevents the tube from clogging and assists in keeping it clean.
6. Apply a small dressing over the tube opening, using a rubber band to keep it in place.	6. This keeps the tube opening clean for the next feeding.
7. Twist a thin strip of adhesive around tube and attach firmly to abdomen, or coil the tubing on a dressing.	7. Prevents the tubing from being accidentally pulled out of the stomach.
8. Cover tubing with a dressing and apply a firm abdominal binder to hold in place.	8. Provides maximum mobility for the patient.

Gastric Gavage (Tube Feeding)

Gastric gavage is the introduction of liquid feedings directly into the stomach.

Purpose

1. Effective in persons who have difficulty swallowing (dysphagia), prolonged unconsciousness, or anorexia.

2. Useful when there is oral or esophageal obstruction or trauma.
3. Life-saving in one who is debilitated or who has had surgery on some part of the GI tract that does not permit normal ingestion of food.

Avenues (Fig. 10-9)

These vary with the patient and circumstances.
1. Nasogastric—orogastric—see Guidelines, page 412
2. Esophagotomy—a stoma (temporary or permanent) may be created at one of several sites along the esophagus.
   a. The feeding tube is introduced through the skin directly into the esophagus.
   b. The tube is usually removed between meals, making this method easy to manage.
3. Gastrostomy—see page 426 and Guidelines, page 426
4. Jejunostomy—an abdominal stoma is constructed providing direct access to the jejunum.
   a. This is advantageous when the stomach must be bypassed.
   b. Disadvantages are the high incidence of diarrhea and dumping syndrome.

Feeding Elements

1. Formulae may be prepared or purchased commercially—"elemental" diets.
2. Physician orders type, amount, and frequency.

Feeding Methods

1. Gravity—a funnel or Asepto syringe (minus bulb) is used as the receptacle for feedings. The rate of flow is affected by raising or lowering receptacle.
2. Drip-regulated
   a. A Murphy drip is connected by tubing to a receptacle (Kelly flask), which hangs on an IV pole.
   b. From the other end of the Murphy drip, tubing is connected to the feeding tube.
   c. The rate of flow of liquid can be adjusted.
   d. Requires thorough cleaning or may be disposable. Consider cost.
3. Motor pump—feeding is delivered at a preset rate.

Continuous Nursing Assessment

1. Recognize that even though some nutritional deficits are corrected, other problems may arise, such as fluid

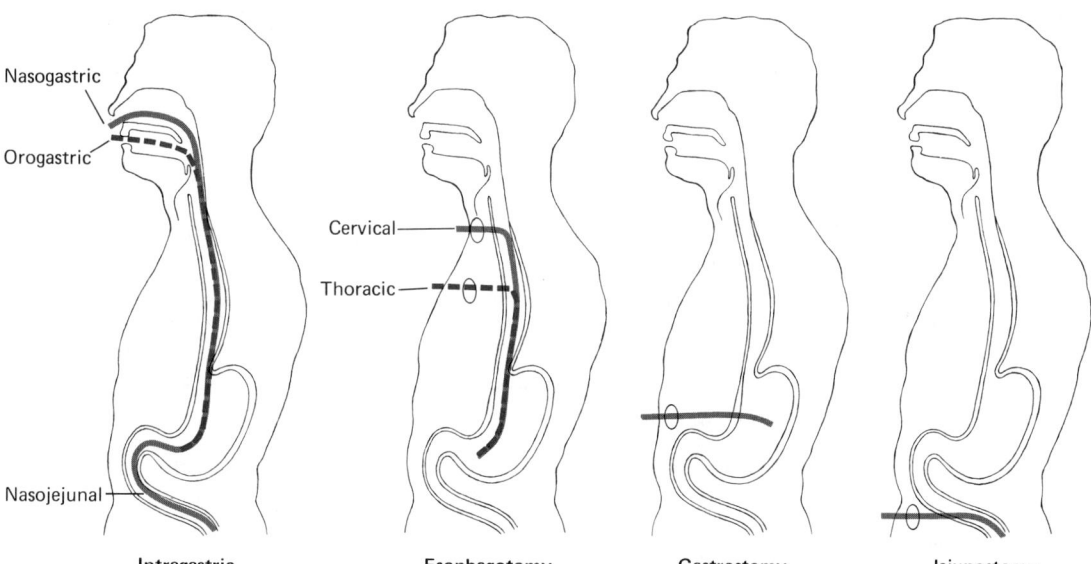

Figure 10-9. Types and sites of gastric feeding.

Intragastric (nasogastric, NG): A tube is passed through the nose or mouth into the stomach and secured in place. (A tube passed through the mouth is more correctly called an orogastric tube. An orogastric tube is ordinarily inserted at mealtime and removed following the meal.) Intragastric tube preferred for short-term gavage feeding; easily inserted by physician or nurse, remains in place between feedings. (Some clients are taught to insert their own tube; they may remove the tube between meals.) Variations include nasopharyngeal and nasojejunal feeding tubes.

Esophagotomy: A temporary or permanent opening (stoma) is constructed at one of several sites to allow a tube to be introduced through the skin into the esophagus. Feeding tube is usually removed between meals. Advantages—dependable for long-term feeding, allows concealment of apparatus, easy to handle.

Gastrostomy: A temporary or permanent stoma is constructed, allowing food to be introduced through the skin directly into the stomach. Preferred for long-term gavage feeding of children and for long-term feeding of adults when use of esophagus is contraindicated. Disadvantages—partial undressing necessary at mealtime, skin care may pose problems.

Jejunostomy: A stoma is constructed to give direct access to the jejunum. This method of feeding may be used when the stomach must be bypassed. Disadvantages—high incidence of dumping syndrome and diarrhea; adequate nutrient intake difficult to maintain. (Suitor CW and Crowley MF. Nutrition. Principles and Application in Health Promotion, p. 391. Philadelphia, JB Lippincott, 1984)

deficit, electrolyte imbalance, diarrhea, esophageal reflux.

2. Cleanse all containers and tubing thoroughly; formulae and feedings make excellent media for bacterial growth.
3. Aspirate the tubing prior to feeding to verify that the tube is in place.
4. Avoid air bubbles in the system, which could cause distention.
5. Provide oral and nasal hygiene before and after orogastric and nasogastric feedings for comfort and to prevent infection.
6. Follow last amount of each feeding with water to flush tubing for cleansing and to promote fluid balance.
7. Monitor the patient for signs of fluid and electrolyte imbalance.
8. Record amount of feeding and water; indicate the patient's participation and acceptance.
9. See Table 10-4 regarding problems that may be encountered and examples of corrective measures.

Health Education

1. Since the tube should be changed every 2 or 3 days, the patient may be taught how to do it. (The tube should be clean but not necessarily sterile.)
2. The patient should learn how to feed himself. (He can learn what foods may be taken.)
3. Skin requires special care.
   a. It can be irritated by action of gastric juices that leak out.
   b. Daily dressing of wound averts skin maceration.
   c. Bland ointment, such as zinc oxide or petrolatum, can be applied to area around the tube.
4. After several weeks, the tube may be removed and inserted only for feedings.
5. For problems that may be encountered in tube-fed clients and corrective measures, see Table 10-4.

Table 10-4 Potential Problems in Tube-fed Clients and Examples of Corrective Measures

Factors to Assess	Possible Causes of Problems	Corrective Measures
Gastrointestinal Function		
Vomiting	Feeding too soon after intubation	Allow patient time to relax and rest after tube is inserted.
	Improper location of tip of feeding tube	Qualifed health professional should reposition tube.
	Rapid rate of infusion	Administer slowly.
	Excessive volume	
	Air	Be sure tube feeding container does not run dry before feeding is completed.
	Formula	Check with physician regarding number and size of feedings.
	Position of patient	Position on right side for 30 minutes following feeding—reverse Trendelenburg or semi-Fowler's position.
Applies to both vomiting and diarrhea	{ Food infection or poisoning	Check sanitation of formula and equipment.
	{ Anxiety	Explain procedures. Provide reassurance and other needed types of support. Provide privacy.
Diarrhea	Rapid rate of infusion	Administer slowly—very slowly if formula is cold.
	High osmolarity of formula or high concentration of formula	Adapt the patient to formula gradually.
	Lactose intolerance	Contact physician regarding change of formula.
Constipation	Lack of fiber	Contact physician regarding:
	Inadequate fluid intake	Change in formula
		Laxatives
		Increasing fluid
Fluid and Electrolyte Balance		
Dehydration	Rapid infusion of carbohydrate → hyperglycemia → osmotic diuresis → dehydration	Administer slowly. Exogeneous insulin is sometimes needed.
	Excess protein and electrolytes in formula	Change formula and/or increase fluid according to physician's requests.
	Inadequate fluid intake	
Edema	Excessive sodium in formula	Check with physician about change in formula
Nutritional Adequacy		
Undernutrition (gradual weight loss)	Inadequate number of calories to meet energy requirements	Check to see if the patient is receiving prescribed amount of formula. Estimate the patient's caloric intake.
		Check with physician regarding increasing the volume, concentration, or number of feedings given.
Overnutrition (gradual, undesirable gain of weight)	Excessive caloric intake	Check with physician regarding decreasing the volume, concentration, or number of feedings given.
Undernutrition (inadequate intake of protein and/or micronutrients leading to biochemical or clinical signs of deficiency)	Amount of standard formula needed to maintain weight is too low to meet requirements for essential nutrients.	Check with physician regarding providing appropriate nutrient supplements.

(Suitor CW and Crowley MF. Nutrition, 2nd ed. Philadelphia, JB Lippincott, 1984)

Guidelines: Intravenous Hyperalimentation (IVH) (Total Parenteral Nutrition [TPN] Hyperalimentation)

Intravenous hyperalimentation (IVH) is a means of providing body nutrients by way of the intravenous route when it is impossible or inadvisable to use the normal digestive routes.

Physiological Basis

1. The intravenous route has heretofore not provided adequate nutrition; caloric and nitrogen deficiencies occurred.
2. Because of nutritional deficiencies, the process of *gluconeogenesis* takes place; this is the body's conversion of protein to carbohydrate.
3. Approximately 1,500 calories/day are required by the average adult postoperative patient to prevent body protein from being utilized.
4. Body needs are increased when the patient has a hypermetabolic disease, a fever, or injury—these needs may require up to 10,000 calories daily.
5. To meet the fluid volume necessary to provide so many additional calories would exceed fluid tolerance and lead to pulmonary edema or congestive heart failure.
6. This process (IVH) provides desired calories in concentration directly into the intravenous system, which rapidly dilutes incoming nutrients to satisfactory levels of body tolerance.
   a. Hypertonic glucose → fulfills caloric requirement → permits amino acids to be released for protein synthesis (not energy).
   b. Potassium → provides proper electrolyte balance → transports glucose and amino acids across cell membranes.
   c. Calcium, magnesium, and sodium chloride → meet cell requirements as determined by serum electrolyte needs.
   d. Other trace elements whose function is not known may be deficient in IVH, since they are not included.

Clinical Indications

1. As a substitute for oral or nasogastric intubation when these are not effective, undesirable, or even hazardous. Use TPN under the following conditions:
   a. Chronic vomiting
   b. Cancer, chemotherapy, or radiotherapy
   c. Cerebrovascular accident
   d. Anorexia nervosa
2. As a supplement for patients demonstrating large nitrogen losses (e.g., burn patients, those with metastatic cancer, and those who are receiving radiation and chemotherapy).
3. As a means of putting the gastrointestinal tract at rest.
   a. When there is evidence of gastrointestinal fistula
   b. With severe and extensive inflammatory bowel disease
   c. Following major intestinal resection
   d. Instances of intestinal obstruction

Equipment

Skin detergent–germicide	Connecting tubing and adapters
Sterile drapes and gloves	250-ml. flask, 50% D/W
20-ml. syringe	3 × 3 dressings—adhesive for occlusive dressing
No. 14 (5 cm.) needle	Suture material
No. 16 gauge 20-cm. radiopaque catheter	Antimicrobial ointment
Tincture of benzoin spray	

Procedure

(for subclavian vein catheterization)

Nursing Action/Physician Action	Rationale/Amplification
Preparatory Phase—Nurse	
1. Explain the procedure to the patient and why it is important for him not to touch the area where the catheter is inserted.	1. To provide reassurance; to prevent dislodging and contaminating catheter.
2. Tell the patient that he will probably be ambulatory during the extended time of therapy.	2. In the absence of other conditions requiring bed rest, ambulation is possible.
3. Place patient in head-low position.	3. This position permits dilatation of neck and shoulder vessels, which makes catheter entry easier and prevents air embolus.
4. Suggest that the patient turn his face away from the area selected.	4. To prevent contamination of TPN site.

(continued)

Guidelines: Intravenous Hyperalimentation (IVH) (Total Parenteral Nutrition [TPN] Hyperalimentation) (continued)

Procedure
(Cont.)

Nursing Action/Physician Action	Rationale/Amplification
5. Support the patient in proper position to permit hyper-extension of shoulder.	5. This position can be facilitated by placing a rolled sheet or towel vertically along spinal column.
6. Use depilatory or shave area if necessary and remove surface oils with acetone or ether.	6. To reduce probability of contamination to the barest minimum.
7. Instruct the patient to be still during insertion of catheter.	7. To prevent the possibility of dislodging of catheter and perforation of subclavian vein.

Performance Phase (by physician)

1. Prepare area with detergent–germicide and place sterile drape in proper position.	1. To prevent infection.
2. Inject local anesthesia to skin and underlying tissues.	2. To promote comfort of patient and prevent patient movement.
3. Using a No. 14 (5 cm.) needle with syringe, insert needle beneath the clavicle and into subclavian vein.	3. Subclavian vein is selected because it leads into the superior vena cava, which has a large volume of blood flow, and provides rapid dilution of hypertonic solution.
4. Instruct the patient to perform Valsalva maneuver.	4. By the patient's bearing down with mouth closed, positive pressure is produced when syringe and needle are replaced by catheter.
5. Detach syringe and insert a No. 16 gauge 20-cm. radiopaque catheter through the needle into the vein; withdraw needle.	5. This permits the more flexible catheter to remain in position during subsequent feedings.
6. Attach Intra-Cath to tubing from a flask of 5% dextrose in water.	6. To keep tube patent between feedings and to provide calories.
7. Prepare the patient for x-ray.	7. To ensure that tip of catheter is in proper location.

▶ **NURSING ALERT AND PRIORITIES OF CARE**

Patients receiving hyperalimentation are particularly susceptible to catheter-related infections. To minimize these complications:

1. Solutions are to be prepared under a laminar flow hood.
2. Solutions are prepared fresh daily and refrigerated until used.

Maintain sterility during entire IVH procedure to prevent sepsis.
Maintain consistent infusion rate, which is calculated on a 24-hour basis.
Monitor patient carefully—including vital signs.
Record data accurately.
Provide emotional support to the patient.

Nursing Action	Rationale/Amplification
Follow-up Phase	
1. Remind the patient not to touch dressings.	1. Permit the patient to turn in bed or to ambulate, but caution him against handling dressings, which would cause contamination.
2. Check infusion rate every 30 minutes. Adjust infusion rate to not more than 10% of the original rate if too fast or too slow.	2. If too rapid → hypermolar diuresis occurs → excess sugar is excreted → intractable seizures occur → coma → death. If too slow → inadequate nutritional intake.
3. Weigh the patient daily and keep accurate intake and output records.	3. Accurate comparison of daily weight change is noted.
4. Check vital signs every 4 hours.	4. Note temperature rise, which could signify a complication.
5. Change dressings every 48–72 hours and as required.	5. Strict aseptic technique must be followed.
6. IV tubing and filters must be changed daily.	6. Procedure is done by a nurse especially trained to do this.
7. Encourage diversional therapy and activity during ex-tended therapy.	7. This distracts the patient from the procedure and pro-motes assimilation of nutrients.

Guidelines: Intravenous Fat Emulsion

Intravenous fat emulsion is a form of essential fatty acids that can be administered to the patient intravenously when these essential nutrients are needed and cannot be acquired in any other way. Lipid emulsions (10% and 20%) may be "piggybacked" onto the hyperalimentation solution and administered by this central line.

Chief Advantage

A concentrated amount of essential fatty acids and calories can be supplied in a relatively small volume of liquid.

Clinical Indications

Treatment or prevention of essential fatty acid deficiencies that may be due to:

1. Severe nutritional disorders and inability to take nourishment by mouth
2. Malignancies, burns, ulcerative colitis, severe renal disorders, nonfunctional gastrointestinal tracts
3. Extended semiconsciousness or unconsciousness
4. Specific preoperative and postoperative patients in whom it is necessary to increase caloric intake
5. Essential fatty acid deficiencies—characterized by sparse hair growth, eczematous scaly skin lesions, thrombocytopenia, and poor wound healing

Action

1. Lipid emulsion is introduced into the blood; protein in the blood acts as emulsifier (lipid–protein complex).
2. The lipid–protein complex carries nutrients to the liver, adipose tissue, etc., where they are degraded, synthesized, stored, mobilized, and oxidized for energy.
3. It is delivered with amino acid dextrose solution in order not to deplete the patient's protein resources.

Equipment

1. Amino acid dextrose solution
2. Fat emulsion
3. Y-type nonphthalate administration set:
   Vented line for fat emulsion
   Nonvented line (with filter) for amino acid dextrose solution

▶ **NURSING ALERT:** Use the administration set as recommended by the manufacturer, since some plastics in combination with lipids cause leaching of diethylhexyl phthalate (DEHP).

Procedure

Nursing Action	Rationale/Amplification
Preparatory Phase	
1. Do not shake emulsion flask.	1. Agitation of emulsion may cause fat globules to aggregate.
2. Inspect flask of fat emulsion.	2. Look for signs of altered stability: a. Inconsistency in texture and color b. Separation of oil
3. Connect tubing to emulsion flask and clear tubing of all air (do not use the pump to prime tubing but use gravity only).	3. Air in system may cause an air embolus in the patient.
4. Connect IV tubing to Y-tube connection closest to insertion site; insert tubing primed with IV fat emulsion directly into this site.	4. This reduces length of time emulsion comes in contact with substances that may affect its stability.
5. Do not use in-line filters.	5. Particles are too large to go through a filter.
6. If infusion is to be administered by gravity drip, hang fat emulsion flask higher than flask of amino acid solution.	6. This will prevent backflow of fat emulsion (less density) into other amino acid flask (higher density).*
7. Explain procedure to the patient; tell him that the milk-white solution is unlike other solutions he has received intravenously. Remind him that he is not to leave the unit while this emulsion is running.	7. Patient will have a better understanding of the reason for more frequent vital signs and other observations.
8. Document the patient's vital signs.	8. These will be used as a baseline comparison for later evaluation.
Performance Phase	
1. Start flow rate at 1 ml./minute for first 30 minutes; monitor vital signs every 10 minutes during this time.	1. Provides opportunity to assess patient for chills, fever, headache, dizziness, sleepiness, allergic reactions, back pain, chest pain, nausea, vomiting, pressure over eyes, etc.
2. If untoward signs occur, stop infusion and notify physician.	
3. If problems occur, physician may prescribe heparin.	3. Heparin will hasten clearing of lipids from the patient's plasma.
4. If no complications occur, infusion rate may be increased—a good gauge is to administer 500 ml. in 4–6 hours.	4. Continue constant observation; monitor vital signs hourly.
5. At conclusion of infusion, detach emulsion flask and attach flask of 5% dextrose as per physician request.	5. Dextrose flushes out remaining fat emulsion from tubing.

* Pennington and Richards. Three-liter bags containing Intralipid for parenteral nutrition (letter). J Parent Enter Nutr 1983; 7(3):304 suggest combining Intralipid in parenteral nutrition formulations.

(continued)

Guidelines: Intravenous Fat Emulsion (continued)

Nursing Action	Rationale/Amplification
Follow-up Phase	
1. When dextrose has run in, clamp tubing securely until next lipid emulsion is to be given. If this is final treatment, disconnect as with any IV.	
2. Continue to be alert for delayed adverse reactions.	2. Fat overload syndrome manifestations—headache, low-grade fever, nausea, abdominal pain, irritability.†
3. Record the nature of lipid emulsion given, amount, time, patient reactions, time of termination of procedure.	3. Include documentation of vital signs.
4. Request periodic serum triglyceride levels and liver function studies.	4. These will provide indicators of the patient's ability to metabolize and clear the emulsion from the bloodstream.
5. Monitor the patient for effectiveness of this treatment. Observe for changes in his clinical status.	5. This would determine effectiveness in treating an essential fatty acid (EFA) deficiency.

† This may be indicative of splenomegaly, hepatomegaly, hyperlipemia, thrombocytopenia, jaundice, gastroduodenal ulcer.

Guidelines: Duodenal Drainage

Purposes
1. To detect abnormal constituents of bile, pancreatic juice, or duodenal fluid.
2. To assist in diagnosis of cholelithiasis (gallstones), choledocholithiasis (common duct stones), pancreatitis, and pancreatic carcinoma.
3. To assist in diagnosing gallbladder problems when x-rays prove inadequate.
4. To assist in parasitologic studies, especially in detection of *Giardia intestinalis*.

Equipment

Rehfuss' tube (metal tip) with markings: 45, 60, 65, 70, and 90 cm. (or rubber tubing with mercury-weighted bag), or Abbott–Rawson tube with mercury-weighted tip
Clamp for tubing
Towel and emesis basin
Glass of water; straw
Container for specimen
30 g. of magnesium sulfate in 50 ml. of water
Optional: Clear plastic tubing (7.5 cm.) to use as a sleeve over rubber tubing; this can be slipped over tubing and kept near patient's teeth to prevent biting of rubber tubing

Procedure

Action	Rationale/Amplification
Preparatory Phase	
1. Explain procedure to the patient and tell him how to breathe through mouth and swallow.	1. This can help in passing the tube.
2. Have the patient in a chair or high Fowler's position in bed, with neck flexed; place a towel across his chest.	2. This position will facilitate passing of tube utilizing gravity.
3. Determine with the patient what sign he might use to indicate gagging or discomfort.	3. Such as raising his index finger to indicate "wait a few moments."
4. Remove dentures.	4. To prevent their becoming dislodged during procedure and even obstructing airway.
Performance Phase (by the physician assisted by nurse)	
1. Ask the patient to open his mouth and breathe through it.	1. Mouth-breathing facilitates the relaxation process.
2. Place the tube's metal tip or the tubing with the mercury bag on the back of the tongue.	2. Proper positioning of the tip encourages and promotes swallowing.
3. Ask the patient to close his mouth (without biting the tubing) and swallow.	
4. Permit the patient to drink water through a straw as he swallows tubing until the 45-cm. mark is reached. It is even better to have him suck on ice chips.	4. Water aids in lubricating and swallowing. However, avoid administering more than 100 ml. in volume.
5. Instruct the patient to sit in chair or on edge of bed and to lean forward with elbows on his knees. The tube is slowly advanced to the 60-cm. mark.	5. These are all maneuvers that have been found helpful in permitting the tube to pass through.

Procedure
(Cont.)

Action	Rationale/Amplification
6. Next have the patient curl up on his *right* side with hips on a pillow and shoulders low. Advance tube to the 70-cm. mark.	6. The tube tip should be in the second portion of the duodenum (Fig. 10-10). Check to see if bile can be aspirated and if the pH is greater than 7.0.

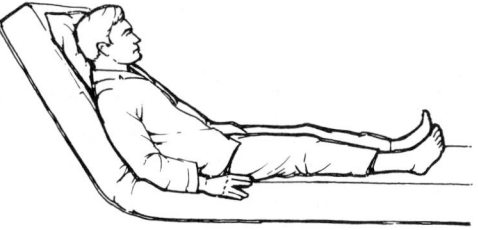

A. With patient in sitting position pass tube to 45 cm. mark.

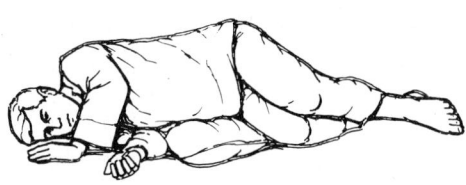

C. Then have patient curl up on right side with hips on a pillow and shoulder low. Tube is advanced to 70 cm. mark.

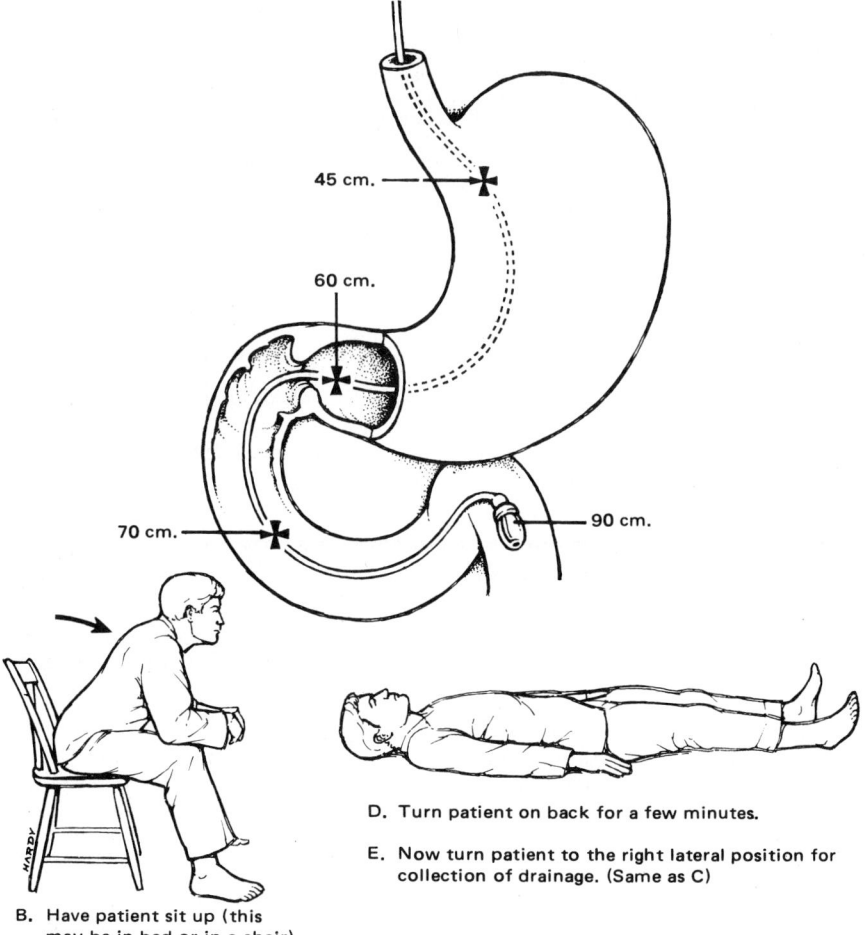

B. Have patient sit up (this may be in bed or in a chair), leaning forward, sway back, with elbows on knees. Slowly advance tube to 60 cm. mark.

D. Turn patient on back for a few minutes.

E. Now turn patient to the right lateral position for collection of drainage. (Same as C)

Figure 10-10. Positions to be assumed by the patient in passing a duodenal drainage tube. Note on the central diagram how the tubing is advanced by each position change.

(continued)

Guidelines: Duodenal Drainage (continued)

Procedure
(Cont.)

Action	Rationale/Amplification
7. The patient is then rolled over on his back for 5 minutes.	
8. Drainage procedure may now take place with the patient in right lateral position. Following are the ways of testing to see if tube is in duodenum:	
a. Aspirate gently—inspect fluid; instill 30 ml. water.	a. Record color, amount, and consistency of bile, as well as duration of flow (normal—clear, golden brown).
b. Instill 30 ml. air rapidly and aspirate immediately; if as much as 5 ml. can be recovered, the tip is probably in the stomach.	b. Usually no air can be recovered from the duodenum.
c. Use a stethoscope to locate tube's tip as air is slowly injected through tubing by syringe.	c. A bubbling sound is substantially louder than elsewhere. The spot should be small and well to the right of the midline. If bubbling can be heard over an area as large as the hand, the tip is in the stomach.
d. To be absolutely sure of position of tube, check position fluoroscopically.	
9. Anchor tube by using plastic guard.	9. To prevent the patient's biting rubber tube.
10. Collect specimens as directed by gravity drainage or by low-pressure intermittent suction with container on floor. If the tube is determined to be in the duodenum, an appropriate stimulant is injected and collection begins.	
a. Administer magnesium sulfate solution to stimulate relaxation of sphincter of Oddi and contraction of gallbladder.	a. Done if gallbladder function is to be evaluated.
b. Administer secretin or secretin-CCK to stimulate pancreatic secretion. Measure volume, bicarbonate concentration, and amylase content.	b. Done if pancreatic function is to be evaluated.

Follow-up Phase

1. At conclusion of test, slowly withdraw tubing.	1. Rapid withdrawal may be injurious to mucous lining because of metal tip; teeth also may be injured by metal tip.
2. As tube emerges from the patient's mouth, cover it immediately with a towel.	2. Covering the mouth will help prevent the urge to vomit.
3. Offer toothbrush and paste or mouthwash.	3. To freshen mouth.
4. Record test and patient's reaction.	

Intestinal Conditions and Treatment

Diagnostic Studies

Stool Specimen

1. The stool is examined for its amount, consistency, and color; a screening test for occult blood is also done. Normal color varies from light to dark brown. Special tests may be made for fecal urobilinogen, fat, nitrogen, parasites, food residue, and other substances.
2. Various foods affect stool color.
   a. Meat protein—dark brown
   b. Spinach—green
   c. Beets—red
   d. Cocoa—dark red or brown
   e. Licorice—black
3. Various medications affect stool color.
   a. Phenylbutazone (Butazolidin, Azolid)—black
   b. Oxyphenbutazone (Tandearil, Oxalid)—black
      Phenazopyridine (Pyridium)—orange-black
   c. Aluminum hydroxide—gray-white
   d. Pyrvinium pamoate (Povan)—red-orange
   e. Bismuth compounds—black
   f. Senna laxatives—yellow-green
   g. Hematinics (iron salts)—black
   h. Barium—white
4. Hemoglobin and bleeding affect the stool in the following way:
   a. Considerable quantities of hemoglobin—occult blood (not visible to naked eye); use "Hemoccult Stool" testing packet
   b. Upper GI bleeding—tarry black (melena)
   c. Lower GI bleeding—bright red blood
   d. Lower rectal or anal bleeding—blood streaking on surface of stool or on toilet paper
5. Characteristic clinical entities related to characteristics of stool:
   a. Bulky, greasy, foamy, foul in odor, gray in color with silvery sheen—steatorrhea
   b. Light gray "clay-colored" (due to absence of "acholic" bile pigments)—biliary obstruction
   c. Mucus or pus visible—chronic ulcerative colitis, shigellosis
   d. Small, dry, rocky-hard masses—constipation, obstipation, fecal obstruction

e. Marble sized stool pellets—spastic colon syndrome

Nursing Management

1. Use a tongue blade to place a small amount of stool in a disposable waxed container.
2. Save a sample of any fecal material if it is unusual in appearance, contains worms or blood, is blood-streaked, has unusual color or much mucus.
3. Send specimen to be examined for parasites to the laboratory immediately so that the parasites may be observed under microscope while viable, fresh, and warm.
4. Test for occult blood or to confirm grossly visible melena or blood—hemoccult guaiac slide test.

Hemoccult Guaiac Slide Test

Commercially available guaiac-impregnated slides present a simple, inexpensive, and esthetically acceptable method of testing feces for blood.

A. Patient Preparation

(Preparation varies; therefore, check with physician.) Common practices are:
1. Diet should be high-residue during 48–72 hours before specimen is collected.
2. Similar diet is followed for next 3 days:
   a. Vegetables—particularly lettuce, spinach, and corn; cooked and raw
   b. Fruits—particularly prunes, grapes, plums, and apples
   c. Any product that is "all bran" for daily cereal
3. Any foods that cause severe diarrhea or severe abdominal pain are to be avoided.

B. Procedure

1. A wooden applicator is used to apply a stool specimen to the slide (for 3 successive days). Three samples are taken because:
   a. There may be intermittent bleeding.
   b. There is the possibility of false-negative results.
2. Slides inside a packet can be brought or mailed to the physician.
3. When hydrogen peroxide (denatured alcohol-stabilizing mixture) is added to samples, any blood cells present liberate their hemoglobin, and a bluish ring appears on the electrophoretic paper. Read *precisely* at 30 seconds, no more or less.
4. A single positive test is an indication for further diagnostic research for gastrointestinal lesions.
   a. False-positive results occur in about 10% of tests.
   b. Tests may become false-negative in 10% of specimens tested 4 or more days after streaking on paper.

Roentgenography of the Colon— Barium Enema

The fasting patient receives a rectal instillation of a barium sulfate suspension, which is viewed in the fluoroscope and then filmed. If the patient is adequately prepared, fluoroscope will reveal:
   a. Colon—contour of entire colon is visible.
   b. Cecum and appendix—contour and motility observed.

Note: Air may be induced to give air contrast studies.

Nursing Management and Patient Instruction

1. Explain to the patient:
   a. What the x-ray procedure involves
   b. That proper preparation provides a more accurate view of the tract
   c. That it is important to retain the barium so that all surfaces of the tract are coated with opaque solution
2. Two days before the examination, the patient may be given a minimal-residue diet.
3. The day before the examination, some physicians limit food intake to liquids; others advise liquids for the evening meal only.
4. The day before the examination, a cathartic may be prescribed.
5. The evening before and on the morning of the examination, a cleansing enema may be given. Food and fluids are restricted for the examination.
6. The above preparation varies, but the objective remains the same: to have the large intestine as clear of fecal material as possible.

▶ **NURSING ALERT:** Use nursing judgment regarding the administration of cathartics or enemata in the presence of acute abdominal pain or obstruction. For the patient with ulcerative colitis, cathartics or cleansing enemas may be too rigorous, and can possibly cause bleeding.

7. Administer an oil-retention enema or a cathartic following the barium enema to completely evacuate the barium.
8. Encourage the patient to eat following the examination, since he has been fasting and is undoubtedly hungry.

Visualization Measures

1. Two visualization measures are sigmoidoscopy and colonoscopy.
2. The details of these two procedures are presented in the Guidelines on pages 436 and 438.

Guidelines: Nasointestinal Intubation (Long Tube)

Purposes
1. To remove fluid and flatus from the intestinal tract (decompression).
2. To assess gastrointestinal bleeding.

Equipment

(Choice made by physician)
1. Type of tube
   Single-lumen tube:

   Harris, Cantor
   Distal end has a small rubber bag weighted with mercury; suction openings are proximal to bag.
   Some single-lumen tubes use air to inflate balloon or have a metal bulb at distal end.

(continued)

Guidelines: Nasointestinal Intubation (Long Tube) (continued)

Equipment
(Cont.)

Double-lumen tube: Miller–Abbott
a. One outlet is for drainage.
b. The other outlet is for filling the small rubber bag near the distal end.

2. Tube selection
  a. Miller–Abbott tube is used in presence of mechanical bowel obstruction with hyperactive bowel sounds.
  b. Other tubes are used for adynamic ileus (absent bowel sounds).

Procedure

Preparatory and Performance Phases

▶ **NURSING ALERT:** All tubes and endoscopes should be routinely pretested for patency and function *before* passage.

Physician Action—Nurse Assisted	Rationale / Amplification
1. Similar to passing a short nasogastric tube (p. 412). Exception: Miller–Abbott. Carry out the procedure as follows:	
a. Pretest the bag volume; the proper amount of air will fill the bag to just less than fully distended (slightly compressible).	a. This will ensure that the bag is not leaky.
b. Place 1 ml. mercury in the bag after it is in the stomach.	b. This helps to pass tubing through the pylorus.
c. After duodenum has been entered, instill 20–50 ml. air in bag according to pretested volume; place other opening on suction.	c. This position checked by x-ray. Air-filled bag acts as a bolus and is carried distally by peristaltic action as suction evacuates retained air and fluid just ahead of bag.
2. After the tubing enters the stomach, it passes by peristalsis and gravity into the small intestine.	
a. Change position from Fowler's to a position in which the patient is leaning forward.	a. This will assist in advancing the tubing to and through the pylorus; tilting to the right is helpful.
3. Upon x-ray confirmation that the tubing is past the pylorus, permit the patient to ambulate.	3. Passing the tube through the pylorus and into the duodenum under fluoroscopic guidance allows the entire procedure to be completed in less than 15 minutes with little patient discomfort.

Nursing Action

4. At specified time intervals, advance tubing 5–10 cm. (2–4 inches).	4. Physician may prescribe or suggest these times.
5. Tubing may be taped to the face, and suction may be applied when the tubing tip has reached its destination.	
6. Measure drainage; record its characteristics every 8 hours.	

▶ **NURSING ALERT:** If drainage is clear and up to 3,000 ml. obtained/day, there is complete intestinal obstruction. If drainage is yellow with a fecal odor, the patient may have an obstruction of the small intestine.

Follow-up Phase

1. Similar to short nasogastric tube.	1. See page 414.
2. Exception: in removing tubing, patient may feel tube resistance and become nauseated.	2. Due to action of sphincters through which the tube is withdrawn.
3. As tubing is drawn through posterior nasopharynx, have the patient open his mouth so that balloon or bag can be grasped with a clamp. Withdraw remaining tubing through the nose.	3. This permits balloon or bag to be removed through the mouth.
4. If tubing has advanced beyond the ileocecal valve, the physician may release it so that it can pass through the gastrointestinal tract. Peristalsis aids in passing the tubing.	4. After distal tube has been retrieved at the rectum, the proximal end can be released at the nose.

Guidelines: Sigmoidoscopy

A *sigmoidoscopy* is the viewing of the lumen of the sigmoid and rectum by means of a sigmoidoscope, a tubular instrument that can be illuminated.

Equipment

Fleet-type enema—used at least 1 hour before the sigmoidoscopy
Water-soluble lubricant

Equipment
(Cont.)

Sigmoidoscope—a 2-part instrument (obturator and cannula)
a long, thin metal tube with light bulb at one end
Glass eyepiece to fit on scope during insufflation of air
Inflation bulb
Long applicator sticks (cotton)
Disposable gloves for preliminary digital examination

Procedure

Preparatory Phase
1. An hour before the sigmoidoscopy, a Fleet enema may be administered by the nurse (or by the patient himself).
2. The enema is retained for 5 minutes before being evacuated.
3. Some physicians request that the patient be on a light diet the evening before and the breakfast before the examination. Others prefer a cathartic the evening prior to the examination.

Nursing Action	Rationale/Amplification
Performance Phase	

1. Have the patient assume the knee–chest or Sims' lateral position.
  a. Knee–chest position
    (1) Knees are spread comfortably apart.
    (2) Thighs are perpendicular to table.
    (3) Feet are extended over the edge.
    (4) Head is turned sideways to right (head shares pillow with chest).
    (5) Left arm is flexed to side of chest.
    (6) Right arm may rest above head.
  b. Sims' lateral position
    (1) Place patient on left side with left leg partially flexed at hip and knees; right leg should be fully flexed.
    (2) Pelvis to be perpendicular to table.
	1. The position used depends on physician preference, patient condition, and nature of examining table (or bed).
	  a. This position permits the sigmoid to hang forward, diminishing the angle at the rectosigmoid junction.
	
	  b. Used for elderly, ill, or arthritic patients or those who are reluctant to assume the knee-chest position.

2. Drape the patient so that only the perineum is visible.	2. A disposable large sheet with a circular opening is practical.
3. Check scope lights after connecting cord to battery.	
4. Physician first examines anal and perianal region. Digital examination indicates the direction of the anal canal, its patency, and the presence of any abnormality.	4. The purpose is to note inflammation, fistula, and ulceration. Digital examination also promotes anal relaxation and helps to lubricate orifice.
5. Warm sigmoidoscope in tap water or sterilizer to slightly above body temperature; lubricate tip of scope.	5. A cold scope would cause discomfort and promote contraction rather than relaxation of perianal muscles. Water-soluble lubricant permits easier passage of scope.
6. Physician spreads buttocks and anal margins with left hand and inserts instrument with right hand (or vice versa).	6. Keep instrument out of view of patient.
7. Nurse encourages relaxation and explains each step in advance.	7. Reassuring patient promotes relaxation.
8. Physician may use a glass eyepiece over viewing end of scope; an insufflation bulb and tubing are attached. He may proceed to pump a small quantity of air into the bowel.	8. The purpose of inflating lower bowel with air is to expand the area viewed so that vision is not obstructed by mucosal folds.
9. The nurse should relay to the physician, expressions or complaints of pain by the patient.	9. Tenderness and pain may be experienced by the patient with a history of abdominal surgery; procedure may have to be terminated in order not to risk perforation.
10. As the scope advances, it may be necessary to attach suction to remove secretions, exudate, blood, or excreta.	10. Connect tubing to suction equipment and turn to lowest degree at first.
Follow-up Phase	
1. Upon withdrawal of scope, assist patient in gradually assuming a relaxed position.	1. Wipe the perineal area to prevent soilage of garments and to promote comfort.
2. If disposable scope is used, rinse scope and discard in proper receptacle. Reusable scopes are thoroughly cleaned in soap and water.	2. Sterilizable parts are sterilized before scope is stored.
3. Record the procedure and the reaction of the patient.	

Guidelines: Colonoscopy

Colonoscopy is the direct visual inspection of the large intestine by means of the colonoscope.

Purposes
1. As a diagnostic aid to view and assess the status of the large intestine (Fig. 10-11).
2. As an operative instrument to remove polyps, to obtain tissue for biopsy, and to remove foreign bodies.

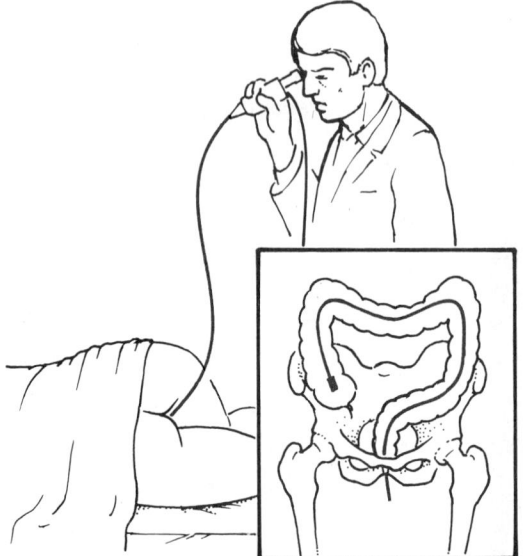

Figure 10-11. Technique of colonoscopy. The patient is turned from one side to the other to take advantage of gravity as the scope is being advanced. Insert shows path of flexible scope from rectum through sigmoid colon and descending, transverse, and ascending colon. If the physician desires to check scope position with fluoroscopy, he should don a lead apron.

Equipment

Complete colonoscope, possibly with sidearm second observer scope
Water-soluble lubricant
Suction apparatus
Air-insufflating equipment
Snares
Drapes
Fluoroscope
The Colonoscope
The colonoscope is an instrument consisting of a flexible 4-mm. glass bundle (containing about 250,000 glass fibers).
1. There is a lens at both ends equipped to focus and magnify.
2. Light is transmitted from an external source by way of a fiberoptic bundle to the tip of the scope; an image is transmitted regardless of the looping or twisting of the flexible bundle.
3. Accessory channels provide for
   a. Suction of fluid, blood, and mucus
   b. Insufflation of air or water
   c. Biopsy
4. There are two kinds of colonoscopes:
   a. To visualize left side of colon—105 cm.
   b. To visualize entire colon—165–185 cm.

Procedure

Preparatory Phase

1. Explain procedure to patient; his understanding and cooperation will promote his relaxation and facilitate his comfort during examination.
2. Limit the patient's intake to liquids for 24–48 hours prior to the procedure (as directed by the endoscopist).
3. Serve the patient a cathartic as prescribed, in the evening for 2 days before the examination.
4. Give tap water or saline enemas approximately 3 hours prior to the colonoscopy until the returns are clear.

Alternate Preparation (G.R. Davis)
   a. *Golytely* (''go-lightly'') is a modified electrolyte solution containing sodium, potassium, sulfate, bicarbonate, chloride, and, lastly, polyethylene glycol (prevents transfer of electrolytes into or out of solution).

Procedure
(Cont.)

    b. The chilled, slightly salty solution is taken orally (average: 4 liters in 2–4 hours).

    c. The preparation time is greatly reduced from usual procedure; the patient must understand the procedure and keep record of his intake, output, and any symptoms during this time.

    d. Diarrhea is to be expected; mild cramps and transient feeling of fullness may be experienced.

5. Administer sedative or analgesic as prescribed; sedation is desirable, but the patient must be sensitive to any pain during the examination so that his response can be relayed to the endoscopist.

6. Preferably, this procedure is performed where fluoroscopy is available.

Nursing Action (As Assistant)	Rationale/Amplification
Performance Phase (by endoscopist)	
1. Place patient in the left lateral position.	1. This position is assumed to follow the location of the sigmoid-rectum anatomically.
2. The lubricated scope is inserted and passed through the rectum.	2. This procedure is done under direct visualization; valvulae are prominent throughout the colon.
3. At apex of rectosigmoid area, there is a red "blur-out."	3. Blur-out occurs because the tip of the colonoscope touches the sigmoid colon wall.
4. The instrument is steadily inserted, rotated, and flexed.	4. This will promote the sliding of the tip along the greater curvature of any loops in the sigmoid colon.
5. If mucosa does not appear red, but seems to blanch or become white, the scope is withdrawn until red mucosa appears.	5. Whitening or blanching is indicative of compression of bowel wall with danger of perforation.
6. The endoscopist utilizes "maneuvers" to straighten difficult curves. A fluoroscope can also be used.	6. By various maneuvers, such as "alpha," "hooking," or "lifting," the endoscopist is able to continue with the insertion and examination of the walls of the colon. Fluoroscopy assists in monitoring position and direction.
7. Maneuvers are resorted to at sharp turns such as the sigmoid-descending colon, the splenic flexure, the transverse colon, and the hepatic flexure.	7. Occasional withdrawal and appearance of a triangular configuration or a bluish color are techniques and observations to assist in advancing the scope.
8. As the scope is advanced into the ascending colon, the nurse can position the patient on his back or on his right side.	8. This permits the maneuvering of the colonoscope into the cecum. It takes about 20–45 minutes to reach this point in the examination.
9. Observation and close inspection is accomplished during insertion and withdrawal of scope.	

Polypectomy and Postcare

1. Prepare intestinal tract meticulously; if there is any fecal matter in the field near the polyp, the procedure will be postponed and bowel preparation will have to be repeated.

2. Skill is required to remove the optimum amount of polyp, to avoid burning the bowel wall, and to prevent cutting the base too close to the bowel wall.

3. When the tissue has been cut by cauterization, the snare-cautery device is removed, and the polyp tissue is withdrawn by suction.

4. Following polypectomy, the colonoscope may be reinserted, the inner bowel insufflated with air, and the operated area carefully examined for possible hemorrhage.

5. Postpolypectomy care depends on size of the polyps removed and the general condition of the patient. Usually the ambulatory patient can be discharged with no medication and no dietary restriction.

6. For in-hospital patients, vital signs are checked for several hours, full liquid diet is given the day of surgery, and soft, low-residue diet is given for 2 weeks thereafter.

7. Follow-up by complete colonoscopic examination usually is scheduled for 6–8 weeks later.

▶   **NURSING ALERT:** If polypectomy is done through sigmoidoscope or colonoscope, barium enema should not be done until 7–10 days thereafter because of risk of perforation at the polypectomy site.

Management of the Patient Undergoing Major Intestinal Surgery

Nursing Process Overview

Patient Problems/Nursing Diagnoses

1. Alteration in bowel elimination related to surgical intervention

2. Impairment of skin integrity related to surgical wound and possible stoma placement

3. Possible infection related to surgical wound

4. Alteration in nutrition related to dietary modification following surgery

5. Knowledge deficit of special care and function of possible ileostomy or colostomy

Planning and Implementation
Preoperative Nursing Interventions
A. Physical Preparation

1 Administer parenteral therapy to correct fluid and electrolyte imbalance.
2. Correct nutritional deficiencies—protein supplements, between-meal feedings.
3. Provide blood replacement to overcome losses sustained by bleeding, infection, and neoplasm.
4. Assist with diagnostic studies as they relate to the evaluation of the cardiopulmonary, hepatorenal bodily functions.
5. Give the patient psychological support as he encounters the stresses of accepting the diagnosis, surgery, and possibly a colostomy.
6. Insert an indwelling urinary catheter immediately prior to the patient's going to the operating room.
7. Oversee general personal cleanliness to minimize skin and wound infection postoperatively.

B. Preoperative Measures to Prevent Infection

1. Administer antibiotic agents to suppress aerobic colon microflora. Combinations of kanamycin or neomycin with tetracycline, erythromycin, or lincomycin.

Note: Evidence that administration of antibiotic agents is preferable to a good intestinal cleansing is lacking.

2. Reduce content of colon.
   a. Give low-residue diet and, when required, change to liquid diet.
   b. Offer laxatives as prescribed. Saline catharsis may be preferred.
   c. Administer enemas or colonic irrigations.
3. Decompress gastrointestinal tract by means of indwelling gastrointestinal tube to control distention and vomiting, if necessary.
   Miller–Abbott or Cantor tube (see p. 435).

Postoperative Nursing Interventions
A. Nutritional Requirements

1. Utilize intravenous catheter if intravenous therapy is to continue several days. Observe tissue for infiltration of fluid.
2. Maintain meticulous mouth hygiene while the patient is on parenteral therapy.

B. Nasogastric Decompression and Increased Comfort

1. Observe and record quality and quantity of aspirated material.
2. Lubricate nostrils with water-soluble lubricant.
3. Humidify room to prevent dryness of mucous membranes.
4. Turn the patient frequently to minimize discomfort.
5. Remove tube (when required) upon reestablishment of peristalsis (determined by auscultation, passage of flatus rectally).
6. Administer analgesics according to needs.
7. Promote restfulness with appropriate nursing measures prior to giving sedation or hypnotics.

C. Prevention of Complications

1. Evaluate vital signs and recognize patterns of development that may suggest hemorrhage, infection, shock, obstruction, etc.

2. Stress preventive measures, such as turning frequently, maintaining fluid balance, encouraging coughing, emphasizing cleanliness and movement of legs.

D. Convalescence and Follow-up Care

1. Encourage the patient to express concerns and questions. (See Colostomy and Ileostomy Management if these are pertinent, pp. 460 and 447.)
2. Encourage ambulation and self-care activities.
3. Stimulate appetite by promoting those measures that will make the patient want to eat what he should eat.
4. Help patient set goals toward which he can progress.
5. Emphasize the importance of follow-up visits to evaluate healing process, general physical and psychological adjustment.

Evaluation
Expected Outcomes

1. Regains normal pattern of elimination or learns to accommodate any intestinal diversion surgery such as colostomy or ileostomy
2. Recovers from surgery with proper wound healing and no signs of infection
3. Modifies diet if need be in accordance with aftereffects of surgery (colostomy, ileostomy)
4. Demonstrates ability to carry out stoma care if diversional surgery was performed

Appendicitis

Acute appendicitis is an inflammation of the appendix due to an infection. It is almost always a surgical problem.

Incidence

1. Occurs most frequently in young adults but may occur in any age-group.
2. Incidence of appendicitis in US has been decreasing during the past decade.

Clinical Manifestations

1. Begins with a progressively severe abdominal pain, beginning in midabdomen (periumbilical) and moving to right lower quadrant after 6–12 hours.
2. An effective early assessment of the patient for acute appendicitis is to have him rise on his toes and then drop down on his heels with a thump or to have him cough. If he has an acute inflammation, he will feel localized pain in the inflamed area.
3. Within a few hours, the acute tenderness becomes localized in the right lower quadrant (McBurney's point).
4. Anorexia, slight or moderate temperature elevation, mild change in bowel habit (usually constipation), and perhaps nausea and vomiting occur.

Note: If these clinical manifestations occur in any person, encourage him to see a physician immediately. There is a tendency in the aging person to ignore aches and pains and to delay seeing a physician. Consequently, mortality in elderly persons with inflammatory bowel lesions is as high as 20%.

Diagnostic Evaluation

1. Physical examination noting especially location and localization of pain, rebound tenderness, etc.
2. Blood studies, with particular attention to white blood cell count; urinalysis.
   A white blood cell count reveals a moderate leukocytosis.

3. Careful history to rule out other possibilities.
4. In some medical centers, when appendicitis is difficult to diagnose, laparoscopy may be utilized.

Treatment and Nursing Management

A. Palliative Preoperative Care

1. Place the patient in a comfortable position to relieve abdominal pain and tension—usually Fowler's position.
2. See that the patient takes nothing by mouth—to decrease peristalsis and to allow stomach to empty before going to surgery. Note time and nature of last meal.
3. Place ice bag to right lower quadrant—*never heat* because of the possibility of causing a rupture of appendix and peritonitis.
4. Do not administer cathartics—may cause rupture.
5. Evaluate vital signs frequently—to assess progression of infection.
6. When diagnosis of acute appendicitis is made, administer chemotherapy and/or antibiotics.

Note: If there is evidence that perforation has occurred recently and a generalized peritonitis has developed, operative urgency is increased (see below).

B. Operative

1. If diagnosis of acute appendicitis is established, a simple appendectomy is performed.
2. Because the patient will obtain relief from pain, he usually accepts surgery very willingly, which affords a smooth recovery.
3. Anesthetic may be general or spinal.
4. Incision may be McBurney, muscle-splitting or gridiron, or right rectus.

C. Postoperative Care (see also p. 85).

1. Without drainage
   a. Following recovery from anesthetic, Fowler's position is maintained, analgesic is given every 3 or 4 hours as needed, and fluids and food are given as tolerated.
   b. Stitches removed between 5th and 7th day (usually in physician's office).
2. With drainage—treat same as for peritonitis (see below).

Peritonitis

Peritonitis is an inflammation of the peritoneal cavity.

Etiology

Peritonitis indicates transgression of peritoneum by trauma (blunt or penetrating) or inflammatory or neoplastic disease. The point of origin may be the gastrointestinal tract, the ovaries, the uterus, or extraperitoneal organs (i.e., inflammation of the kidney).

A. Primary Peritonitis—acute, diffuse

1. Occurs primarily in young females; often due to pathogenic bacteria (streptococci, pneumococci, gonococci) introduced through uterine tubes or through hematogenous spread.
2. In patients with nephrosis or cirrhosis, the offending organism is most often *E. coli.*

B. Secondary Peritonitis

1. Commonly seen in surgical patients; caused by appendicitis, peptic ulceration, biliary tract disease, colonic inflammation.
2. May occur following gunshot wound, stab wounds, and motor vehicle accidents.

C. Postoperative

1. Theoretically preventable.
2. Noted following poor preoperative preparation—inadequate nutrition and fluid and blood replacement, and technical problems.
3. May occur in compromised patients who are diabetic, have malignancy, or are taking steroids.

Altered Physiology

1. Any irritant, such as blood, bile, or pancreatic enzymes, causes an exudation of plasma-like, protein-rich fluid—"internal burn."
2. Secondary peritonitis often presents mixed flora, which include *E. coli,* as well as the enterococci, *Clostridium, Klebsiella, Pseudomonas,* and *Bacteroides.*
3. If there is failure to seal the source of contamination (i.e., perforation along gastrointestinal tract), peritonitis will become progressively worse.
4. When offended, the surface of the peritoneal cavity begins to exude a plasma-like fluid. This process can account for losses of as much as 5 liters/day.
5. Paralytic ileus is usual, with fluid loss into dilated intestinal loops and stomach.
6. Individual is compromised because of fluid loss, abdominal distention with respiratory embarrassment; nutrients are not absorbed, leading to progressive rapid catabolism.

Assessment

Clinical Features

(Dependent on location and extension of inflammation)
1. Initially, local type of abdominal pain tends to become constant, diffuse, and more intense.
2. Abdomen becomes extremely tender, and muscles become rigid; rebound tenderness and ileus may be present; patient lies very still, usually with legs drawn up.
3. Nausea and vomiting often occur; peristalsis diminishes; anorexia is present.
4. Elevation of temperature and pulse as well as leukocyte count.
5. Fever and thirst occur.
6. Percussion—resonance and tympany due to paralytic ileus; loss of liver dullness may indicate free air in abdomen.
7. Auscultation—decreased bowel sounds.

Diagnostic Evaluation

1. Blood studies—to show leukocytosis (leukopenia, if severe).
2. Urinalysis—may indicate urinary tract problems as primary source.
3. Peritoneal aspiration—to demonstrate blood, pus, bile, bacteria (gram staining), amylase.
4. X-ray of abdomen—may indicate free air in abdomen under diaphragm; of thorax—to rule out unexpected pneumonia.

Patient Problems/Nursing Diagnoses

1. Increasing abdominal pain related to the spread of an infection.
2. Generalized discomfort (malaise, nausea, vomiting, abdominal pain, elevated temperature, thirst) related

to elevated temperature, paralytic ileus, fluid loss, and other effects of infection.

3. Anxiety concerning spread of infection and possible death.

Medical Treatment

1. If localized:
   a. If acutely inflamed appendix—an appendectomy is necessary.
   b. If ruptured duodenal ulcer—ulcer closed or plicated.
   c. Resection of diseased bowel; decompression (gastrostomy, colostomy, ileostomy).
2. If not localized, the patient is acutely ill, and surgery is not performed until after distention and electrolyte and fluid problems are treated.

Planning and Implementation

Nursing Interventions

A. General Prevention Measures

1. Encourage the individual who has early signs and symptoms of appendicitis to see his physician.
2. Instruct the patient to avoid taking a laxative or applying heat to abdomen when abdominal pain of unknown cause is experienced.
3. Practice meticulous aseptic technique during abdominal surgery.

B. Ongoing Assessment

1. Monitor for central venous pressure (see p. 286).
2. Record urinary output hourly.
3. Note and record blood pressure every other hour.
4. Check vital signs frequently.
5. Obtain baseline and take frequent analyses of hematocrit, blood gases, and electrolytes.

C. Prevention of Infection and Promotion of Comfort

1. Give nothing by mouth—to reduce peristalsis; ensure meticulous oral hygiene.
2. Provide fluids by vein to establish adequate fluid level and to promote adequate urinary output.
3. Record accurately intake and output, including the measurement of vomitus.
4. Administer antibiotics as prescribed.
5. Observe and describe symptoms accurately—pain and tenderness have a tendency to shift and must be reported precisely.
6. Reassure the patient and gain his confidence because he usually realizes the seriousness of his condition.

D. Prevention of Complications

1. Following recovery from anesthetic, place the patient in Fowler's position to facilitate drainage.
2. Administer fluids by vein, since nothing is given by mouth initially.
3. Prevent nausea, vomiting, and distention by use of nasogastric suction; institute proper nursing measures for nasal and oral comfort.
4. Reduce parenteral fluids and give oral food and fluids when the following occur:
   a. Temperature and pulse return to normal.
   b. Abdomen becomes soft.
   c. Peristaltic sounds return (determined by abdominal auscultation).
   d. Flatus is passed and patient has bowel movements.
5. Be alert for possibility of complications—*report immediately:*

a. Wound evisceration—"It feels as if something just gave way."
b. Abscess formation—an area of abdomen is tender or painful, and fever increases.

Evaluation

Expected Outcomes

1. Reports little or no pain or discomfort—is out of bed and has no complaints of physical discomfort
2. Recovers from surgery with little or no complications—is not nauseated; has no abdominal pain, has normal vital signs
3. Demonstrates lessening of anxiety.

Abdominal Hernia

A *hernia* is a protrusion of viscus through the wall of the cavity in which it is normally contained. It is often called a "rupture."

Incidence

1. Occurs 3 times more frequently in men than women; may occur at any age.
2. Results from congenital or acquired weakness of the abdominal wall.
3. Tends to increase in size and occurrence with increase of intra-abdominal pressure brought about by coughing, straining, or pressure from a nearby tumor.

Classification

A. According to Area

1. Inguinal
   a. In male—due to weakness in abdominal wall where spermatic cord emerges; enters inguinal canal and then scrotum.
   b. In female—due to weakness in abdominal wall where round ligament is located; enters inguinal canal and then labia.
      (1) Direct inguinal
          Medial-to-deep epigastric artery
          Majority are acquired
      (2) Indirect inguinal
          Lateral-to-deep epigastric artery
          Majority are congenital
2. Femoral
   a. Occurs most often in women.
   b. Located below Poupart's ligament (below groin).
3. Umbilical
   a. Results from failure of umbilical orifice to close.
   b. Occurs most often in obese women and children and in patients with cirrhosis and ascites.
4. Ventral or incisional
   a. Due to weakness in abdominal wall.
   b. May occur following impaired healing of incision because of drainage, infection, etc.

B. According to Severity

1. *Reducible*—the protruding mass can be replaced in abdomen.
2. *Irreducible*—the protruding mass cannot be moved back into abdomen.
3. *Incarcerated*—an irreducible hernia in which the intestinal flow is completely obstructed.
4. *Strangulated*—an irreducible hernia in which the blood and intestinal flow are completely obstructed. Symptoms—pain, vomiting, swelling of hernial sac, fever, lower abdominal signs of peritoneal irritation.

Treatment

A. Mechanical

(Reducible hernia only)

A *truss* is an appliance having a pad that is held snugly in the hernial orifice.

1. Does not cure a hernia—it prevents abdominal contents from entering hernial sac.
2. May be used in treatment of hernia in adults when, because of disease or age, it is inadvisable to perform surgery. In general, surgical treatment is preferred.

B. Surgical

Surgical treatment is recommended to correct the hernia before a strangulation occurs, in which case an emergency situation ensues.

1. Hernial sac is dissected free.
2. Contents of sac are replaced in abdominal cavity.
3. Neck of sac is ligated.
4. Muscle and fascial layers are sewed together firmly to prevent a recurrence. If this is not possible, synthetic mesh may be sutured over area.
5. Strangulated hernia requires resection of ischemic bowel in addition to hernia repair.

Nursing Management

A. Preoperative

1. If hernia is strangulated, emergency conditions prevail (see Intestinal Obstruction, p. 456).
2. If surgery is elective, the patient is usually in good physical condition.
3. Use depilatory or shave suprapubic region and anterior surface of upper thigh.
4. Observe for upper respiratory infection—if present, surgery will be postponed because coughing or sneezing postoperatively may break the sutures.
5. Surgery may be done with patient admitted to the hospital or it may be performed in the day surgery clinic.

B. Postoperative

1. Take the following measures for scrotal edema or swelling:
   a. Bed rest
   b. Ice pack and scrotal suspensory for support
2. Observe for urinary retention.
3. Ambulate patient in a day or two, or sooner if permissible.

C. Patient Education

1. Athletics and extremes of exertion are not permitted for 8–12 weeks postoperatively.

Ulcerative Colitis

Ulcerative colitis is an inflammatory disease of the mucosa and less frequently, the submucosa, of the colon and rectum. Occasionally it involves the distal ileum as well.

Etiology and Incidence

1. Unknown (idiopathic); however, there are several unproven possibilities:
   a. Emotional response alters blood supply to colon mucosa, but there is question as to whether stress is a cause or effect of the disease process.
   b. Unidentifiable organisms cause pathology.
   c. A combination of causative factors—infection, stress, allergy, autoimmunity.
2. Most common in young adulthood and middle life; almost equal between sexes (slightly more in females); more prevalent among Jews; highest in 3rd and 4th decades, familial incidence.

Assessment

Clinical Manifestations

1. Diarrhea (may be bloody), tenesmus (painful straining), sense of urgency, and cramping.
2. Multiple crypt abscesses of intestinal mucosa that may become necrotic and lead to ulceration.
3. Increased bowel sounds; abdomen may appear flat but as condition continues, abdomen may become distended.
4. There often is weight loss, fever, dehydration, hypokalemia, anorexia, nausea and vomiting, iron deficiency anemia, and cachexia.

Note: See differences between Regional Enteritis and Ulcerative Colitis, p. 446.

5. May appear depressed and show difficulty in getting along with others.

Clinical Features

1. Involvement extends proximally from rectum and is mainly of left colon.
2. The disease usually begins in the rectum and sigmoid and spreads upward, eventually involving the entire colon. Anal area may be excoriated and reddened; left lower abdomen may be tender on palpation.
3. There is a tendency for the patient to experience remissions and exacerbations.
4. Very high frequency of secondary and often multiple colon cancer.
5. It is a serious disease accompanied by systemic complications (see Complications below) and high mortality rate.

Diagnostic Evaluation

1. Stool examination to rule out bacillary or amebic dysentery
2. Sigmoidoscopy; proctoscopy to reveal petechiae, hyperemia, and ulcerations
3. Barium enema x-ray

▶ **NURSING ALERT:** If disease is in acute stage, cathartic may be contraindicated because it may cause exacerbation and lead to toxic megacolon.

4. Review of nursing history for patterns of fatigue and overwork, tension, family problems.
5. Assessment of behavioral manifestations indicative of emotional concerns.
6. Assessment of food habits that may have a bearing on triggering symptoms (milk intake may be a problem).
7. Careful clinical assessment to rule out diverticulitis, cancer, etc.
8. Complete blood studies if they appear to be warranted.
9. Fecal analysis if blood and mucus are evident.

Complications

1. Skin ulcers
2. Arthritis
3. Malnutrition
4. Anemia
5. Abscess formation
6. Stricture, anal fistula

7. Erythema nodosum
8. Amyloidosis
9. Electrolyte imbalance
10. Malignancy (colonic cancer)
11. Toxic megacolon
12. Ankylosing spondylitis

Patient Problems/Nursing Diagnoses

1. Alteration in comfort (cramp-like pain in lower abdomen, especially prior to defecation) related to disease process
2. Inadequate nutrition and alteration in fluid and electrolyte balance related to effects of diarrhea, nausea and vomiting
3. Diarrhea, dehydration, anorexia related to course of disease
4. Impaired mobility related to fatigue, anorexia, and anemia
5. Compromised coping related to fatigue, feeling of helplessness, and lack of support systems (friends and family)

Note: There is no cure for ulcerative colitis because the cause is unknown; the prime goal is to control the disease to achieve patient comfort and improve the quality of life.

This can be done by:
1. Initiating early, effective management of exacerbations.
2. Prolonging remissions with appropriate therapy.
3. Subjecting the patient to surgery only when judiciously necessary.

Planning and Implementation
Nursing Interventions

A. Comfort Measures to Rest and Relax the Intestinal Tract

1. It may be necessary to reduce or eliminate food and fluid and then to resort to parenteral feeding or to low-residue diets.
2. Give sedatives and tranquilizers not only to provide general rest but also to allow peristalsis to slow down and afford rest to the inflamed bowel.
3. Be aware of the possibility of pressure sores in this patient because of malnourishment and enforced inactivity, especially if he is thin.
   Cleanse the skin gently after each (or every other) bowel movement. Apply a protective emollient such as petrolatum jelly, karaya gel, A&D ointment, Desitin, or a similar agent.
4. Administer tincture of belladonna, atropine, or diphenoxylate (Lomotil), as prescribed, to lessen intestinal motility. Sulfasalazine (Azulfidine) is effective for antidiarrheal effect even though it is an antibiotic. Some patients experience side effects (epigastric distress, headache, dizziness); discontinue medication for 2–3 days and gradually introduce it again.
5. Relieve painful rectal spasms (produced by frequent diarrheal stools) with anodyne suppositories.
6. Report any evidence of sudden abdominal distention, since it may indicate toxic megacolon.
7. Reduce physical activity to a minimum or provide frequent rest periods.
8. Provide commode or bathroom next to bed, since urgency of movements may be a problem.

B. Interventions to Combat Infection and Toxicity

1. Give sulfa drugs as prescribed—nonabsorbable sulfasalazine (Azulfidine) may be prescribed as an oral medication.

2. Administer corticosteroids as prescribed—the type depends on the condition of patient, mode of administration may be oral, intravenous, or rectal. Rectal administration may be in the form of hydrocortisone-retention enemas.
3. Provide conscientious skin care because excoriation is common following severe diarrhea.
4. For severe proctitis, nightly instillations of steroids as prescribed (dissolved in tap water, or as suppositories) may produce a remission of symptoms. Belladonna suppositories also may help.

C. Nutritional and Fluid Requirements

1. If the patient is acutely ill, maintain him on parenteral replacement of vitamins, fluids, and electrolytes (potassium is very important).
2. When resuming oral fluids and foods, select those that are nonirritating to the mucosa (mechanically, thermally, and chemically). If this fails, an elemental diet (such as Precision LR) may be prescribed; the purpose of this diet is to provide low residue, which can rest the lower intestinal tract.
3. Consider a milk-free diet, since studies have shown that fewer relapses occur on a milk-free diet; the incidence of lactase deficiency is more frequent in patients having attacks than in those in remission.
4. Provide a well-balanced, low-residue, high-protein diet to correct malnutrition.
5. Determine which foods agree with this patient and which do not. Modify diet plan accordingly.
6. Bolster with supplemental vitamin therapy, including vitamin C, B complex, and K.
7. Avoid cold fluids because they increase intestinal motility.
8. Administer appropriate electrolytes, which have been lost in diarrheal bouts, especially potassium.
9. Administer diphenoxylate (Lomotil) as prescribed for symptomatic relief of diarrhea.
10. Prohibit smoking because it also increases intestinal motility.

▶ **NURSING ALERT:** Since opiates may precipitate toxic megacolon, use only for brief periods, if at all, in acutely ill patients.

11. Administer prescribed therapy to correct existing anemia.
12. Carefully note fluid intake and output and character of bowel movements.
13. Weigh the patient frequently and record weight; rapid increase or decrease may relate to fluid imbalance.

D. Coping and Psychological Adjustment

1. Offer psychological support.
2. Educate the patient to accept and learn to live with this chronic disease. This is done on a long-range basis, and the patient should participate in the evaluation and planning of his care.
3. Plan all aspects of the patient's care in conference so that a team effort promotes the nursing process and ensures continuity of care, communication, and periodic evaluation.
4. Indicate by actions and expressions that you, the nurse, are responsible for and care for him. A good nurse–patient relationship enables him to satisfy his dependency needs.
5. Solicit the assistance of the family in helping to understand the patient; assist the family in understanding the patient.

6. If the patient is to have an ileostomy, before surgery it is helpful to have the patient visited by someone who has had a similar operation and has made a good adjustment. After surgery, these persons can also help with management problems. (Ostomy Clubs exist in most major cities.)

Note: Impotence occurs in males rather frequently after a colectomy because of damage to pudendal nerves.

E. Prevention of Complications

1. Observe for signs of colonic perforation and hemorrhage.
2. Assess carefully the patient's behavior and all his complaints.

Surgical Treatment and Nursing Management

A. Indications and Contemplated Surgery

1. Approximately 20% of patients with ulcerative colitis in the US require surgical intervention.
2. Recommended when no improvement occurs through conservative means—evidenced by impending perforation, actual perforation, deteriorating clinical course after 24–48 hours of maximum medical regimen, severe hemorrhage, or persistent colonic dilation for longer than 1 week.
3. Total proctocolectomy and permanent ileostomy are frequently used. Becoming more popular is an ileoanal abdominal colectomy with mucosal proctectomy and construction of an ileoanal reservoir (see p. 454).

B. Preoperative Physical and Psychological Preparation

1. Institute an intensive program of fluid, blood, and protein replacement.
2. Administer chemotherapy and antimicrobials to reduce intestinal organisms.
3. Recognize psychological needs of this patient:
   a. Fear, anxiety, and discouragement accompany diarrhea.
   b. Hypersensitivity may be evident.
   c. Let the patient know that his complaints are understood.
4. Encourage the patient to talk; listen to what he says is bothering him.
5. Answer his questions about the permanent ileostomy he is about to have.

C. Postoperative Care Including Ileostomy Management

(See Management of Patient having Major Intestinal Surgery, p. 439.)
(See Conditions—Caring for a Patient with an Ileostomy, p. 447.)

Health Education

1. It is important to involve the patient in understanding chronic ulcerative colitis and each component of care prescribed; he should be made to feel that he is sharing responsibility for maintaining his health.
2. This patient needs encouragement and support postoperatively even though surgery is considered curative; there may be problems with skin care; there may also be aesthetic difficulties, surgical revisions.
3. When early indications of relapse are noted, such as bleeding or increased diarrhea, the patient should report these findings early so that steroid treatment may be initiated.
4. Monitoring of the patient's condition should continue when new symptoms develop and on a regular annual basis.

5. Let the patient know that he has a valuable resource person in the enterostomal therapist and that he should not hesitate to call this person about his ileostomy problems.

Evaluation
Expected Outcomes

1. Reports a lessening of pain; functions well without analgesics
2. Demonstrates improved food and fluid intake; avoids roughage intake
3. Tolerates moderate activity, such as short walks or visits, without becoming fatigued
4. Shows improved psychological outlook; appears to enjoy visits from friends and family

Regional Enteritis (Crohn's Disease, Granulomatous Colitis, Transmural Colitis)

Regional enteritis is a chronic inflammatory disease of the small intestine, usually affecting the terminal ileum at the region just before the ileum joins the colon. The etiology is unknown.

Incidence

1. Affects both sexes equally.
2. Appears more often in Jewish persons of Eastern European origin.
3. A familial tendency exists.
4. May occur at any age, but occurs mostly in those between 15 and 35 years of age.

Clinical Features

1. Intestinal tissue thickens first by edema and later by formation of scar tissues and granulomas.
2. At times, "skip lesions" occur with normal intestine in between.
3. This condition interferes with the ability of the intestine to transport the contents of upper intestine through the constricted lumen; this causes crampy pains after meals.
4. Inflammation and ulcers form in the lining membrane, producing a constant irritating discharge.
5. In some patients, the inflamed intestine may perforate and form intra-abdominal and anal abscesses.

Assessment
Clinical Manifestations

These are characterized by exacerbations and remissions—may be abrupt or insidious:
1. Crampy pain after meals; this causes the patient to eat in small amounts or even to avoid eating, which then results in malnutrition, weight loss, and possibly anemia (hypochromic or macrocytic).
2. Chronic diarrhea due to irritating discharge may occur; usual consistency is soft or semi-liquid.
3. Milk products and chemically or mechanically irritating food may aggravate the problem.
4. Melena and malabsorption syndrome may occur; occult blood may appear in stool.
5. Low-grade fever occurs if abscesses are present.
6. Lymphadenitis occurs in mesenteric nodes.
7. Abdominal tenderness, especially in right lower quadrant.

Diagnostic Evaluation

1. Regional enteritis may simulate acute appendicitis.
2. Upper gastrointestinal barium studies—classic "string

sign" is noted at terminal ileum that suggests a constriction of a segment of intestine.
3. Barium enema to permit visualization of lesions of large intestine and terminal ileum.
4. Proctosigmoidoscopy to note ulceration.

Clinical Complications

1. Stricture and fistulae formation (ischiorectal, perianal—even to bladder or vagina).
2. Hemorrhage, bowel perforation, mechanical intestinal obstruction.
3. Incidence of colorectal cancer is higher in these patients.

Patient Problems/Nursing Diagnoses

1. Reduced nutritional intake related to postprandial pain
2. Abdominal pain related to the inflammatory disease of the small intestine
3. Ineffective coping mechanisms related to feelings of dejection and embarrassment
4. Knowledge deficit related to insufficient information about regional enteritis

Planning and Implementation
Nursing Interventions

A. Promotion of comfort, adequate nutrition, and fluid intake

1. Administer a diet low in residue, fiber, and fat, and high in calories, protein, and carbohydrates, with vitamin supplements (especially vitamin K).
   Prepare for hyperalimentation if the patient is debilitated.
2. Provide iron medications if anemia is present.
3. Treat pain and diarrhea symptomatically; encourage the patient to rest.

B. Prevention of transmission of pathogenic organisms

1. Practice conscientious handwashing before and after patient care.
2. Dispose of soiled linen according to hospital policy.
3. Maintain good hygienic practices and instruct the patient in this regard.

C. Pharmacotherapy

1. Consider antimicrobials and sulfonamides such as sulfasalazine (SAS; Azulfidine) for control of inflammatory process.
2. Some clinics treat this patient with sulfasalazine, steroids, prednisone, and mercaptopurine (Purinethol).
3. If the patient does not respond to conservative medical and pharmacotherapy, surgery may be necessary to relieve segmental obstruction.
   a. Surgery is determined specifically for each patient.
   b. The involved segment may be resected with anastomosis; bypass procedures may be done.
4. Unfortunately, recurrence of the disease is possible following surgery.

D. Psychosocial considerations

1. The nurse can offer understanding, concern, and help in encouraging this person, who is often dejected, debilitated, embarrassed about frequent and malodorous stools, and even fearful of eating.

Evaluation
Expected Outcomes

1. Achieves relief of pain after several days of dietary, pharmacologic, and psychological therapy
2. Maintains proper nutritional intake and adequate fluid intake

Differences Between Regional Enteritis and Ulcerative Colitis

	Regional Enteritis	Ulcerative Colitis
Pathology		
Early	Transmural thickening	Mucosal ulceration
Later	Deep, penetrating granulomas	Mucosal minute ulcerations
Involvement		
Rectum	Approximately 50%	Over 90%
Right Colon	Frequently	Occasionally
Small Intestine	Yes	Usually not
Disease Distribution	Segmental	Continuous
Clinical Manifestations		
Bleeding	Generally no, but may occur	Common
Perianal disease	Common	Rare
Fistula	Common	Rare
Perforation	Common	Rare
Disease Course	Slowly Progressive	Remissions and Relapses
X-ray—Barium Studies		
Stricture	Common	Rare
Distribution	Segmental	Continuous
Associated with malignancy	Not common	Common

3. Verbalizes improved mental attitude toward ways to live with the disease and methods for socializing with others
4. Demonstrates an understanding of the need for life-style changes

Ileostomy

An *ileostomy* is an opening in the ileum for the purpose of treating intractable granulomatous or ulcerative colitis or of diverting intestinal contents in colon cancer, familial polyposis, congenital defects, or trauma. The opening (*stoma*) is brought out through the abdominal wall, usually the lower right section of the abdomen. This stoma becomes the outlet for discharge of intestinal contents.

Implications for the Patient

(See also Colostomy for Pre- and Postoperative Nursing Management, p. 459)
1. Some patients welcome the ileostomy, since it means the removal of a long-standing incapacitating disease process; in general, however, many patients experience psychological problems that are often overwhelming. Preoperative counseling by the medical and nursing team, as well as by a trained visitor from the local chapter of the United Ostomy Association, is most helpful.
2. The patient appreciates that now he has the prospect of enjoying a normal diet, instead of the low-residue diet to which he was restricted.
3. The patient wears a soft vinyl or rubber pouch with an open-end bottom; a clamp fitted on the bottom of the pouch permits emptying. He empties the pouch 4–5 times a day, usually when he goes to the bathroom to urinate.
4. The ileostomate requires instruction—first from the nurse in the hospital or an enterostomal therapist* and then from the community nurse.
5. Appliances may be reusable or disposable. They are held in place in several ways—cement, double-faced adhesive discs, karaya rings.
6. Waterproof tape is effective in anchoring the appliance when the patient showers or swims.
7. At first the discharge will be liquid, but later the small intestine will begin to take on its water-absorbing function to permit a more semisolid, pasty discharge.
8. Because the discharge is rich in enzymes, it may cause skin irritation; therefore optimal skin care becomes a top priority consideration for the patient. Cleanse the skin thoroughly with mild soap and water; rinse well. Take baths or showers as soon after surgery as possible. Dry area thoroughly. For elderly patients, soap may be too drying for the skin; however, oil base soaps may prevent adhesives from adhering.

*An *enterostomal therapist* (ET) is a health care professional with special training in the rehabilitation of persons with ostomies and related problems. Enterostomal therapists are certified by the IAET (below).

The *International Association for Enterostomal Therapy* (IAET) is the professional association for enterostomal therapists. Its address is 505 N. Tustin, Suite 219, Santa Ana, CA 92705.

The *Journal of Enterostomal Therapy* is the official publication of the IAET and is published 6 times yearly by AMC Publishers, 2506 Gross Point Road, Evanston, IL 60201.

The *United Ostomy Association* (UOA) is a self-help group for ostomates and other interested persons. Its address is 2001 W. Beverly Boulevard, Los Angeles, CA 90057.

Guidelines: Changing an Ileostomy Appliance

Goals:
1. Prevent leakage (bag is usually changed every 2–4 days).
2. Permit examination of skin around stoma.
3. Assist in controlling odor if this presents a problem.

Time
1. Early in morning, before breakfast or 2–4 hours after a meal, when the bowel is least active.
2. Immediately, if patient is complaining of burning or itching underneath the disc or has pain around the stoma.

Equipment

Duplicate ileostomy appliance with or without belt (Fig. 10-12); pouch-closing device
Soap, water, and washcloth
Appropriate skin barrier (karaya powder, karaya paste, and/or karaya ring, Stomahesive™, ReliaSeal™, Skin Prep™ or other)
Gauze
Emesis basin
Tape (hypoallergenic)

Procedure

Nursing Action	Rationale/Amplification
Preparatory Phase	
1. Have the patient assume a relaxed position. Provide privacy.	1. Encourage patient participation and understanding so that eventually he will be able to change appliance himself.
2. Explain details of this activity to the patient.	2. Encourage questions.
3. Expose ileostomy area; remove ileostomy belt (if worn).	
4. Position lamp; wash hands.	

(continued)

Guidelines: Changing an Ileostomy Appliance (continued)

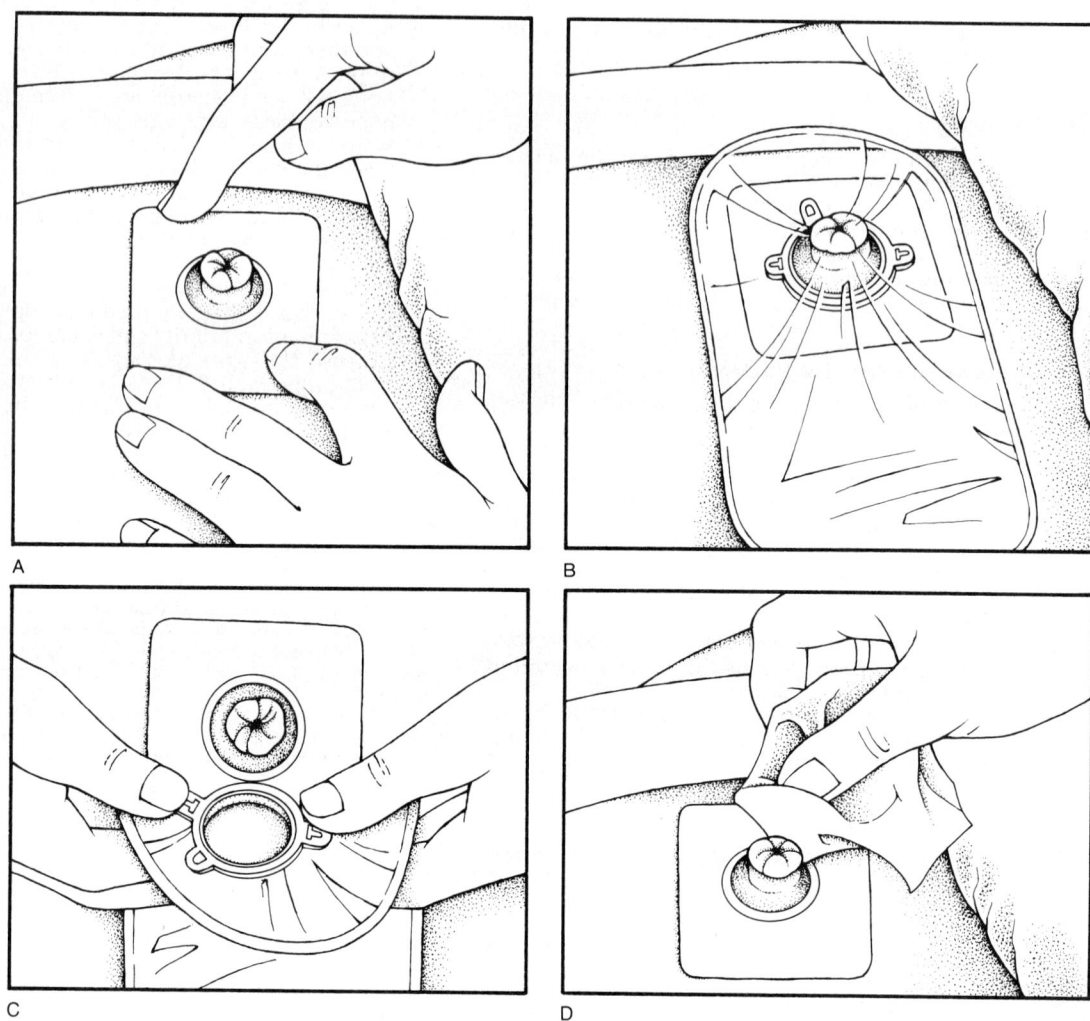

Figure 10-12. Ileostomy care. (*A*) A Stomahesive wafer with flange (1½″, 1¾″, 2¼″, 2¾″) can be applied directly to the peristomal area after it has been thoroughly cleaned and dried. (*B*) An opaque or transparent drainable pouch is positioned at desired angle over stoma. (*C*) Pouch may be removed without removing water. (*D*) Stoma may be assessed without removing wafer. (Adapted by permission from ConvaTec, a Division of ER Squibb & Sons, Inc.)

Procedure
(Cont.)

Nursing Action	Rationale/Amplification
Performance Phase	
1. *To remove appliance:*	
a. Sit or stand in a comfortable position.	a. Have the patient sit on toilet or on a chair facing toilet. If standing, face toilet.
b. Fill a container with prescribed solvent, then fill medicine dropper with solvent; apply a few drops of solvent between disc of appliance and skin. *Do not pull off appliance!*	b. As solvent works, pouch loosens and pulling is unnecessary. Solvent is often unnecessary when skin cement is not used. Pouch can be removed by gently pushing skin away from adhesive.
c. If adhesive residue builds up on skin, use very small amount of adhesive remover on gauze.	c. Do not use acetone, ether, or benzene because they are irritating to skin.

Procedure
(Cont.)

Nursing Action	Rationale/Amplification
2. *To cleanse skin:* a. Remove any excess karaya with dry toilet tissue. b. Wash skin gently with soft cloth moistened with *tepid* water and mild soap, or bathe before putting on clean appliance. c. Rinse and dry skin thoroughly after cleansing.	a. During this time, a gauze dressing or pieces of tissue may be used to cover the stoma to absorb excess drainage while skin is being cleaned. b. The patient may shower before removing appliance. Micropore or waterproof tape applied to sides of disc will keep it secure while bathing. c. Moisture or soap residue will interfere with appliance adhesion.
3. *To put on appliance if no skin irritation:* a. An appropriate skin barrier should be applied to peristomal skin before the pouch is applied. b. It is optional to apply Tr. Benzoin or one of the many specially formulated skin preparations to help protect peristomal skin. c. Remove cover from adherent surface of disc of disposable plastic pouch and apply directly to skin. d. Press firmly in place for 30 seconds.	a. Stomahesive™ (Fig. 10-12) or karaya preparation (powder, paste, or rings) may be used. Many disposable pouches have a built-in skin barrier. b. *Note:* Do not confuse with Tr. benzoin comp., which is too irritating. c. Be sure skin is thoroughly dry. d. To ensure adherence.

4. *To put on appliance if there is skin irritation:*
a. Cleanse skin thoroughly but gently; pat dry.
b. Apply Kenalog spray; blot excess moisture with a cotton pledget and dust lightly with nystatin (Mycostatin) powder.
 	
  (1) An alternate effective measure is to apply a wafer of Stomahesive (Squibb), which is available in 10 × 10 cm. (4″ × 4″) and 20 × 20 cm. (8″ × 8″) pieces. The stomal opening should be cut the same size as the stoma; use a cutting guide (supplied with Stomahesive). The wafer is applied directly to the skin.
  (2) A second alternative is to moisten a karaya gum washer and apply when it is tacky. If skin is "weepy," karaya powder may be applied first and any excess dusted off gently.
c. The pouch is then applied to the treated skin.
	a. To remove debris.
	b. The steroid preparation (Kenalog) helps decrease inflammation. The antifungal (nystatin) treats those types of infections that are common around stomas. A prescription is required for both medications.
	  (1) Stomahesive is a substance that facilitates healing of excoriated skin. It adheres well even to "weepy" irritated skin.
	
	  (2) Karaya also facilitates skin healing. Tackiness promotes adherence.
	
	c. This will allow skin to heal while appliance is in place.

5. Check the pouch bottom for closure; use rubber band or clip provided.	5. Proper closure controls leakage.
Follow-up Phase 1. Dispose of waste materials. 2. Clean reusable ileostomy pouch by washing in soap and water. 3. Soak pouch in deodorant solution and hang to dry.	 2. Preserves life of appliance and controls odor. 3. Deodorizing agents should be effective but not destructive to rubber or vinyl.

Nutritional Management of the Ileostomate
Nutritional needs of the patient with an ileostomy are similar to those of a healthy individual. With adequate diet, additional vitamins or food supplements are unnecessary. These are the exceptions:

Health Education
Discharge from hospital for patient with ileostomy or colostomy

A. Clothing
1. A girdle is permissible—a size larger is recommended to accommodate the pouch.
2. Swim suits (even 2-piece) can be worn; men prefer boxer-styled trunks; women may prefer a swim suit with a skirt.
3. For swimming, a rubber belt is preferred to elastic cloth which sometimes loses elasticity when wet.

B. Medications
1. The ileostomate should not have laxatives, irrigations, enteric-coated or time-release capsules.

C. Travel
1. Travel by plane or any other vehicle is not contraindicated.
2. If traveling by plane, it is suggested that patient carry his ostomy kit with him (in the event that there is a delay in retrieving baggage).
3. Colostomates who irrigate should use only water suitable for drinking.
4. Ileostomates should bring along a suitable antidiarrheal medication.

D. Sports
1. All kinds of sports may be participated in, as reported by ostomates—tennis, water surfing, skin diving, water skiing, ice skating, horseback riding.

Patient Problems/Nursing Diagnoses	Interventions
Negative nutritional balance during or immediately after surgery	Offer diet high in calories and protein, and additional vitamin and mineral supplements.
Fluid and electrolyte depletion related to vomiting, diarrhea, and excessive perspiration	Avoid salt tablets, which may act as cathartics. Supplement fluids with beverages containing electrolytes and glucose (Gatorade, Sportade).
Inadequate absorption of nutrients	Continue diet high in protein with vitamin and mineral supplements; fat restriction may be necessary. Consider use of elemental diets (diet preparations already broken down to simple, easily digested forms) until ileum adapts to new shortened length. (e.g., Vivonex [Eaton], Flexical [Mead–Johnson]).
Weight loss or gain	Weigh and record weight daily. Explain to the patient that ileostomy will continue to function even if oral intake is limited and that adequate nutritional intake is essential for healing to occur. Dietary supplements are appropriate (Ensure [Ross], Isocal, Sustacal [Mead–Johnson].
Loss of specific absorptive site for vitamin B_{12} and bile salts related to resection of terminal ileus	Check blood for B_{12} levels. Give replacements by injection. Restrict fat, since the patient may not be able to digest and absorb fats because of bile salt deficiency. This must be monitored carefully because, on a fat-restricted diet the patient may lose weight and be unable to absorb fat-soluble vitamins: A, D, E, and K. Also, with bile salt deficiency, this patient may be more susceptible to formation of gallstones.
Excessively watery effluent	Restrict fibrous foods: whole-grain bread and cereals, fresh fruit skins, fresh vegetables, beans, corn, and nuts.
Excessively dry effluent	Increase salt intake. Note: *increased intake of water does not increase effluent because excess water is excreted in urine.*
Stomal obstruction	Restrict fibrous foods; be alert to offenders such as celery, cabbage, nuts and corn. Instruct the patient to chew food thoroughly.

Problems Encountered by the Patient with an Ileostomy

Problem/Nursing Diagnoses		Interventions: Prevention/Management
Skin excoriation	related to 1. Irritating intestinal effluent 2. Materials used to hold appliance in place 3. Allergies	Evaluate for proper fit of appliance. Karaya protects skin—it comes as powder, paste, rings, and sheets. Good substitutes for karaya are Stomahesive (Squibb) or ReliaSeal (Davol). An appropriate skin barrier should always be used between skin and appliance.
	4. Fungal or bacterial growth	Avoid products to which the patient may be sensitive. Patch test any new or suspect problems on patient's inner arm.
	5. Belt applied too tightly	If large areas of skin are involved or ulcerated, avoid rubber cement-type adhesive.
	6. Poor stoma location—peristomal skin folds or scars	Severe problems due to poor stoma location necessitate surgical revision.
Minor stomal bleeding	related to irritation This may occur following wiping the stoma.	Mucosa is friable and easily injured. However, when handled gently, these tissues heal readily because of the rich blood supply.

Problems Encountered by the Patient with an Ileostomy (continued)

Problem/Nursing Diagnoses		Interventions: Prevention/Management
Prolapsed stoma	related to an oversized opening resulting from 1. Excessive bowel shrinkage 2. Abdominal pressure due to coughing 3. Failure of opposing layers of bowel to adhere in the turnback suture procedure	Remove appliance. Observe bowel for signs of compromised circulation (pale or dark color). Apply cold pads or packs to control edema. Notify surgeon. He will manually replace bowel into abdomen (medical treatment) or suggest surgical correction.
Odor	related to 1. A reusable appliance that is not changed frequently enough or not cleaned properly 2. An appliance that is not odor-proof 3. Certain foods: onions, cabbage, eggs, fish 4. Obstruction or dysfunction of ostomy 5. Certain medications; vitamins, penicillin, estrogens	Be meticulous in cleaning procedure. Alternate reusable pouches; when not in use, allow pouch to hang in fresh air (not sun). If using disposable pouches, select odor-proof materials. Change medications when one is found to be odor-producing. Use oral deodorants: chlorophyll derivatives, bismuth subcarbonate, or bismuth subgallate. Insert deodorizer in appliance: charcoal, Banish (TM-United), or baking soda. Encourage foods such as spinach and parsley that act on the intestinal tract as deodorizers.
Expulsion of intestinal flatus	related to lack of sphincter control. Because of this the patient often feels everyone around him is aware of gas passage.	Limit gas-producing foods such as beans, cabbage, onions, beer. Try to avoid air-swallowing, which may occur during smoking, talking, eating, emotional upset.
Potential for obstruction	This is suggested by the following signs: 1. Abdominal cramping, distention 2. Malodor, along with liquid projectile effluent 3. Vomiting 4. Signs of dehydration	Obstruction or stenosis may be due to edema or lymphatic blockage. More commonly, it is due to food blockage brought about by poor chewing habits and high-cellulose foods. *Nursing intervention:* 1. Remove appliance. 2. Have the patient lie down in bed and apply hot compresses to abdomen, or have the patient relax in tub of warm water. 3. Offer hot tea drinks. If this does not help within 2–3 hours, check with physician; it may be necessary to gently irrigate the ileostomy (physician prescribed) with a small volume of saline.
Obstruction due to adhesions or volvulus		This may require surgical correction.
Potential for kidney stones	related to 1. Dehydration—increases formation of urate crystals because of loss of bicarbonate in intestine 2. Increased absorption of oxalates after ileal resection—oxalate stones form	Increase the patient's fluid intake. If stones are urate crystals, sodium bicarbonate may be required to alkalinize urine. If stones are calcium, ascorbic acid may be prescribed to acidify urine.

(continued)

Problems Encountered by the Patient with an Ileostomy (continued)

Problem/Nursing Diagnoses		Interventions: Prevention/Management
Diarrhea	Observe whether there is an increase in the number of times the patient needs to empty pouch. Normal output is about 750 ml./day. Check for food poisoning, mechanical obstruction, stomal stenosis. Assess for signs of dehydration.	Electrolyte imbalance may easily occur. Treat with clear liquids and antidiarrheal medications. Water, salts and fluids can be replaced with commercial preparations such as Gatorade, Quick Kick. Another suggestion is to alternate a cup of salted broth and a cup of sweetened tea each hour. Water-absorbing drugs (hydrophilic colloids) such as Metamucil Powder are sometimes effective. If diarrhea does not resolve in 24 hours, the patient should seek medical care. IV fluids and electrolytic therapy may be necessary.
Medication difficulties	1. Drug action can be affected by the absence of the colon and altered transit time through small intestine. 2. Suggest taking uncoated tablets or liquids for oral medication. 3. Have the patient check effluent to be sure pills are not being passed undissolved. 4. Do not use time-release tablets or sustained-release capsules. 5. Administer vitamin B_{12} subcutaneously if distal ileum has been removed.	1. The various functions of the small and large bowel are interrupted or absent. 2. Coated tablets may pass undissolved through bowel into ileostomy appliance. 3. If they do pass undissolved, thereafter crush them and take them with water or applesauce. 4. They may not be absorbed. 5. The terminal ileum is where the absorptive site for B_{12} is located.

2. Problems may arise if the ostomate participates in contact sports such as football, ice hockey.

E. Sexual Functioning

1. Approximately 10%–20% of male ileostomates experience impaired sexual function; in many individuals this is only temporary.
2. Male colostomates vary from being fully potent to impotent.
3. Most males who have urinary surgery for malignancy as adults are impotent—may be candidates for penile implant.
4. In many instances, potency is regained, but this may take up to 2 years.

F. Pregnancy

1. An ostomy is not a contraindication to a successful pregnancy.

2. Careful medical supervision during pregnancy is required for a female ostomate. The ostomy opening may change in size (stretch) as the pregnancy continues; thereafter, changes in the size of the appliance opening may be required. Change in abdominal contour may necessitate the use of a very flexible appliance or faceplate.

G. Sleeping

1. Almost any position of comfort can be assumed if the pouch is properly fitted.
2. Sleeping on the stomach is comfortable when a small cushion is placed under the hip on the side of the stoma.

H. Obstruction or Blockage

1. Know signs and symptoms; notify enterostomal therapist or physician if necessary.

Guidelines: Continent Ileostomy (Kock Pouch)

A *continent ileostomy* is the surgical creation of a pouch of small intestine that can act as an internal receptacle for fecal discharge; a nipple valve is constructed at the outlet to permit drainage from the abdomen. This kind of ileostomy may be done initially for selected patients when they present for an ileostomy, or it may be constructed from the conventional ileostomy (Fig. 10-13).

Preoperative Management

This is essentially the same as for the patient having a traditional ileostomy.

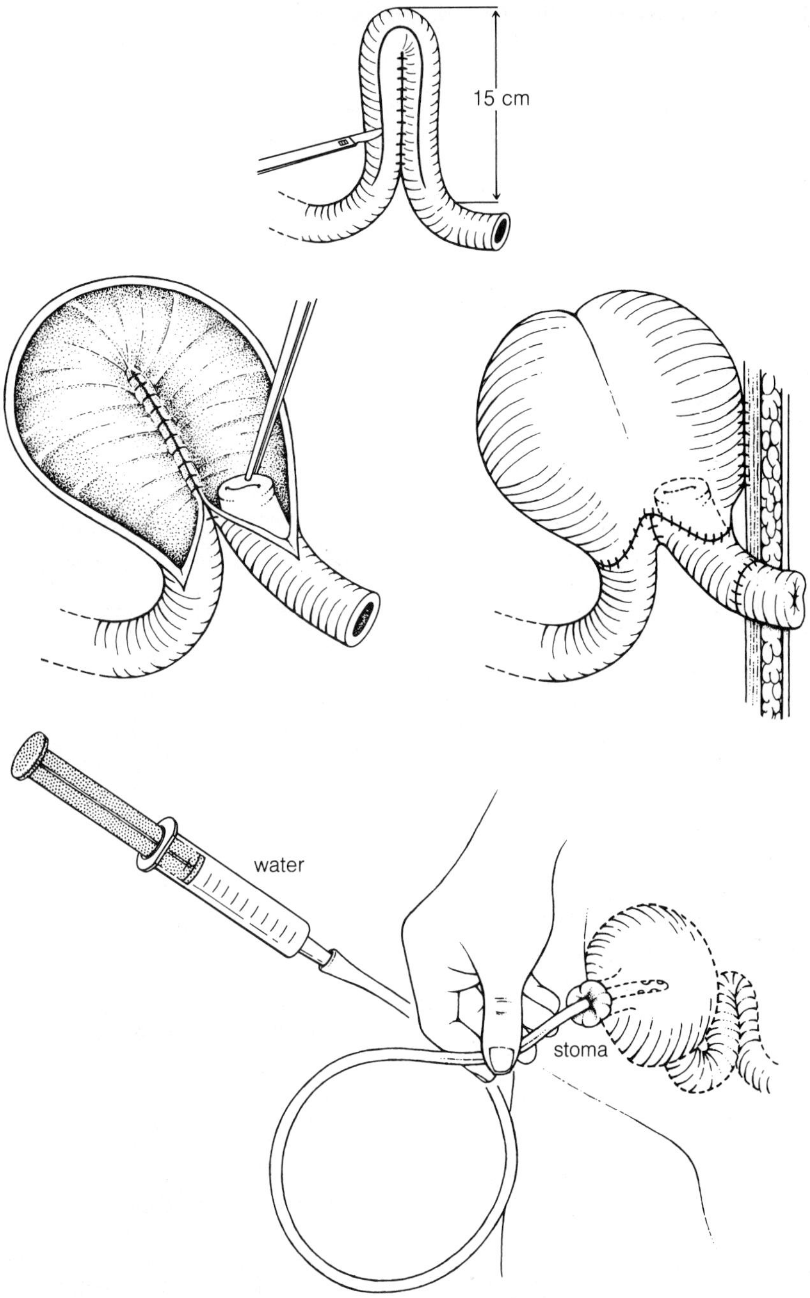

Figure 10-13. Continent ileostomy (Kock pouch). *1.* About 30 cm of ileum will become an ileal pouch. By looping the ileum, there are about 15 cm. on each side as shown. The 2 sides are stitched together in the center. The surgeon then makes a U-shaped incision. *2.* The ileum is opened, and the inner section is stitched, much like a seam, to make a smooth inner surface. After this, a valve or ''nipple'' is constructed on the right between pouch and stoma. Then the top of the ileum is folded to the bottom and stitched closed, as illustrated in part 3. This pouch is stitched to the inner wall for immobilization; likewise, the stoma is fixed to the abdominal wall. In part 4 a lubricated catheter is being gently inserted about 5 cm. into the ileal pouch for drainage. (Brunner LS, Suddarth DS. Textbook of Medical and Surgical Nursing. Philadelphia, JB Lippincott, 1980)

(continued)

Guidelines: Continent Ileostomy (Kock Pouch) (continued)

Postoperative Management

1. A catheter will extend from the stoma and be attached to closed suction; drainage will be maintained about 10 days.
2. Catheter irrigation is done usually every 2 hours with a 20–30 ml. saline to ensure patency; return flow is by gravity.
3. Nasogastric suction is used to relieve pressure on suture line by preventing a buildup of gastric contents.
4. Parenteral fluids are administered for 4–5 days; thereafter, clear liquids and diet as tolerated.
5. Monitor for nausea and abdominal distention.
6. Pain medication is given as required; early ambulation is encouraged.
7. In about 10–14 days, the catheter is removed from the stoma and the patient participates in the management of his ileostomy.

Equipment

Catheter
Water-soluble lubricant
Gauze squares
Syringe
Irrigating solution in a bowl, emesis, or receiving basin

Nursing Action	Rationale / Amplification
1. Lubricate catheter and gently insert about 5 cm. (2 inches).	1. Resistance may be felt at valve or "nipple."
2. If much resistance, fill syringe with 20 ml. air or water and inject through catheter—gently exert pressure on catheter.	2. This will permit catheter to enter pouch.
3. Place end of catheter in drainage basin (below level of stoma); later this can be done at toilet bowl.	3. Gravity facilitates drainage. Drainage may include flatus as well as effluent.
4. Following drainage, remove catheter. Wash area around stoma; dry and apply absorbent pad. Fasten with hypoallergenic tape.	4. Entire procedure requires about 5–10 minutes. At first, irrigation is done every 2 hours, then gradually extended to 3 times daily. If feces are not too thick, drainage through catheter may occur successfully without irrigation.

Ileo-Anal Abdominal Colectomy with Mucosal Proctectomy and Construction of an Ileo-Anal Reservoir

Patient Screening

Eliminate patients
1. With Crohn's disease
2. Acutely ill with ulcerative colitis
3. Who are nutritionally depleted and steroid-dependent
4. With frequent episodes of diarrhea

Surgical Intervention

This may be performed in two stages (first performing a temporary ileostomy); or two teams may work together doing the abdominal and perineal surgery.

The S-shaped reservoir is one type; a J-shaped or side-to-side reservoir may be done.

Postoperative Management

1. General postoperative abdominal care is applicable (see p. 85).
2. Assess for potential complications—partial obstruction of small intestine, pelvic sepsis due to leakage from reservoir.
3. Diarrhea, which frequently occurs with permanent ileostomy, is eliminated with this procedure.
4. Long-term follow-up studies need to be done for proper evaluation, since this procedure has been done only relatively recently.

Diverticulosis and Diverticulitis

A *diverticulum* is a pouch or saccular dilatation leading out from a tube or main cavity (Fig. 10-14).

Diverticulitis is an inflammation of diverticula.

Diverticulosis is the condition in which an individual has multiple diverticula.

Predisposing Factors

1. Probable congenital predisposition
2. Weakening and degeneration of muscular wall of the intestine, causing herniation of the lining mucous membrane through a muscle at site of artery penetration
3. Increased mechanical pressure due to abnormal high-pressure contractions of sigmoid colon in response to neurohumoral stimuli
4. Chronic overdistention of the large bowel

Incidence

1. Diverticulosis usually occurs in about 10% of individuals over 40 years of age and nearly 50% of persons over age 60; only a small percentage develop diverticulitis.
2. The condition is most common in sigmoid colon.

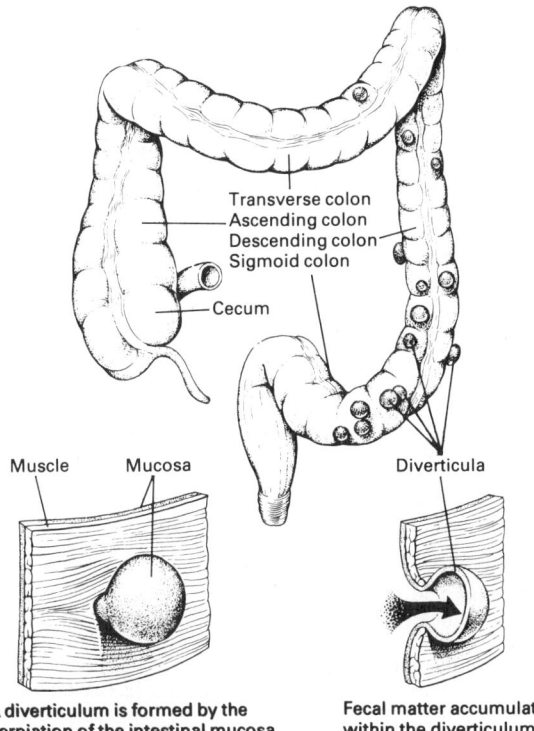

Muscle   Mucosa   Diverticula

A diverticulum is formed by the herniation of the intestinal mucosa through the weakened muscular wall usually at site of arterial penetration on the mesenteric border of the colon.

Fecal matter accumulates within the diverticulum

Figure 10-14. Diverticula are most common in the sigmoid colon; they diminish in number and size as the colon approaches the cecum. Diverticula are rarely found in the rectum.

3. Small-bowel diverticula are unusual, but when they occur they are often multiple. They may act as areas of stasis and bacterial overgrowth, leading to malabsorption of fat and vitamin B_{12}.

Altered Physiology

(Colon diverticulosis and diverticulitis)
Constipation from spastic colon syndrome often precedes the development of diverticulosis by many years.
1. Following local inflammation of the diverticula, there may be narrowing of the colon with fibrotic stricture, which then leads to narrowed stools, cramps, and increasing constipation.
2. With the development of granulation tissue, occult bleeding may occur, producing iron deficiency anemia; fatigue and weakness are then evident. However, massive bleeding is more common.
3. Abscess development causes a tender palpable mass; fever and leukocytosis also occur.
4. If the diverticulum perforates, local abscess or peritonitis results; peritonitis causes rigidity, abdominal pain, loss of bowel sounds, and eventually shock.
5. Uninflamed or minimally inflamed diverticula may erode adjacent arterial branches, causing acute massive rectal bleeding.

Assessment
Clinical Manifestations

A. **General Clinical Signs**
1. May occur in acute attacks or may persist as a long, drawn-out smoldering infection.
2. Tends to spread into surrounding bowel wall, increasing the irritability and spasticity of the colon.
3. When infections are severe, perforation of the colon can occur, leading to peritonitis.
4. When infection is less acute but slowly progressive, extensive scarring and abscess formation involving the bowel wall may occur, with the possibility of lower bowel obstruction. Sometimes, fistulae form with the bladder, the adjacent small bowel, the vagina, or even the skin.
5. Sepsis may spread via portal vein to liver, causing liver abscesses.

B. **Specific Clinical Signs**
1. Diverticulosis
   a. Bowel irregularity, constipation, and diarrhea
   b. Sudden massive hemorrhage (occurs in 10%–20% of patients)
2. Milder forms of diverticulitis
   a. Bouts of soreness, mild lower abdominal cramps
   b. Bowel irregularity, constipation, and diarrhea
3. Moderately severe acute diverticulitis
   a. Crampy pain in lower left quadrant of abdomen
   b. Low-grade fever, chills, leukocytosis

Diagnostic Evaluation

1. Sigmoidoscopy; possibly colonoscopy
2. Fluoroscopy and x-ray with barium enema

Patient Problems/Nursing Diagnoses

1. Intestinal discomfort, diarrhea, or constipation related to bowel irregularity
2. Alteration in nutrition related to uncertainty as to appropriate diet to follow
3. Anxiety related to concern about the possibility of malignancy
4. Knowledge deficit related to lack of understanding of the relation between diet and diverticulosis

Planning and Implementation
Nursing Interventions

A. **Provide rest for the intestinal tract and alleviate constipation.**
1. During acute episode, maintain fluid and nutritional requirements with intravenous therapy; give nothing by mouth.
2. Maintain antimicrobial therapy as prescribed to reduce infection.
3. For pain, meperidine (Demerol) is the analgesic of choice because it is less spasmogenic than other analgesics.
4. When indicated, employ stool softeners such as docusate sodium (Colace, Bu-Lax, Surfak).
5. Administer bulk additives to counteract tendency toward constipation; a frequently prescribed smooth bulk laxative is psyllium hydrophilic mucilloid (Metamucil).
6. Warm-oil-retention enemas may be prescribed to treat inflammation locally by softening fecal mass.

▶ **NURSING ALERT:** Ordinary enemas and laxatives may be harmful and should not be used.

Note: In some patients, an increase in mass results in an increase in symptoms.

7. Check with physician as to type of diet to be followed. Some authorities prefer fiber content in the diet rather than a low-residue diet. With increased fiber, more bulk is added to give the stool proper consistency. With a low-residue diet, the colon may work harder to propel contents, thereby producing high pressure on the intestinal wall, which in turn promotes diverticula formation.

Surgical Treatment

1. If there is little response to medical treatment, or if complications such as hemorrhage, obstruction, or perforation occur, surgery is necessary.
2. Preparation for surgery:
   a. Low-residue diet or nothing by mouth.
   b. Antimicrobials, systemic and intestinal surface-acting, to reduce bowel bacterial flora, diminish bulk of stool, and soften fecal mass for easier movement.
   c. Cleansing enemas may be prescribed.
3. Resection of segment of intestine involved with diverticula, reuniting (anastomosing) two ends to maintain continuity.
4. Temporary colostomy is sometimes performed to divert fecal stream (see p. 459), with continuity restored in later second-stage procedure.

Health Education

Goal:
Prevent recurrence of diverticular disease.

1. Maintain a diet that is high in soft residue and low in sugar; obtain lists of these foods in order to be familiar with proper dietary control; how well the intestinal tract functions in great measure depends on proper food intake.
2. Bran products will add bulk to the stool and can be taken with milk or sprinkled over cereal.
3. Establish regular bowel habits to promote regular and complete evacuation; mineral oil can be used nightly if necessary, but dependence on it should be discouraged.
4. Have the patient continue periodic medical supervision and follow-up; report problems and untoward symptoms.

Evaluation

Expected Outcomes

1. The patient reports near-normal bowel function; no diarrhea or constipation
2. Consumes a prescribed diet and can relate what foods to include or avoid
3. Expresses relief that diagnostic studies revealed no malignancy
4. Delineates the general nature of diverticulosis and can list what helps or aggravates the condition

Intestinal Obstruction

Intestinal obstruction is an interruption in the normal flow of intestinal contents along the intestinal tract.

The block may occur in the small or large intestine, may be complete or incomplete, may be mechanical or paralytic, and may or may not compromise the vascular supply. Obstruction most frequently occurs in the very young and the very old.

Types of Obstruction

1. Mechanical—a physical block to passage of intestinal contents without disturbing blood supply of bowel
   a. Location
      Extrinsic (e.g., adhesion, hernia, intussusception)
      Intrinsic (e.g., hematoma, tumor)
      Intraluminal (e.g., foreign body, fecal or barium impaction, polyp)
   b. Clinical pattern
      High small-bowel (jejunal) or low small-bowel (ileal) occurs 4 times more frequently than colonic obstruction.
2. Paralytic (adynamic, neurogenic) ileus
   Peristalsis is ineffective (diminished motor activity perhaps because of toxic or traumatic disturbance of the autonomic nervous system); there is no physical obstruction and no interrupted blood supply.
3. Strangulation
   Obstruction also compromises blood supply, leading to gangrene of the intestine.

Causes

1. Mechanical (extramural)
   a. Adhesions—postoperative
   b. Hernia
   c. Malignancy
   d. Volvulus (loop of intestine that has twisted)
2. Mechanical (intramural)
   a. Carcinoma
   b. Hematoma
   c. Intussusception (telescoping of intestine)
   d. Stricture or stenosis (scarring)
3. Paralytic
   a. Spinal cord injuries, vertebral fractures
   b. Postoperatively after any abdominal surgery
   c. Peritonitis, pneumonia
   d. Wound dehiscence (breakdown)
   e. Gastrointestinal tract surgery

NOTE:

1. In postoperative patients, approximately 90% of mechanical obstructions are due to adhesions.
2. In nonsurgical patients, hernia (most often inguinal) is the most common cause of mechanical obstruction.

Altered Physiology

1. Disturbed physiologic responses as a result of mechanical small-intestine obstruction results in increased peristalsis, distention by fluid and gas, and increased bacterial growth proximal to obstruction. The intestine empties distally.
2. Increased secretions into the intestine are associated with diminution in the bowel's absorptive capacity.
3. The accumulation of gases, secretions, and oral intake above the obstruction causes increasing intraluminal pressure.
4. Venous pressure in the affected area increases, and circulatory stasis and edema result.
5. Bowel necrosis may occur because of anoxia and compression of the terminal branches of the mesenteric artery.
6. Bacteria and toxins pass across the intestinal membranes into the abdominal cavity, thereby leading to peritonitis.
7. "Closed-loop" obstruction is a condition in which the intestinal segment is occluded at both ends,

preventing either the downward passage or the regurgitation of intestinal contents.

Assessment

Clinical Manifestations

Fever, peritoneal irritation, increased white blood cell count, toxicity and shock may develop with all types of intestinal obstruction.

1. Simple mechanical—high small bowel
   Colic (cramps) mid to upper abdomen, some distention, early bilious vomiting, increased bowel sounds (high-pitched tinkling heard at brief intervals), minimal diffuse tenderness
2. Simple mechanical—low small-bowel
   Significant colic (cramps) midabdominal, considerable distention, vomiting—slight or absent—later feculent, increased bowel sounds and "hush" sounds, minimal diffuse tenderness
3. Simple mechanical—colon
   Cramps (mid-to-lower abdomen), later-appearing distention, then vomiting may develop (feculent), increase in bowel sounds, minimal diffuse tenderness
4. Partial chronic mechanical obstruction—may occur with granulomatous bowel (Crohn's) disease.
   Symptoms are cramping abdominal pain, mild distention, and diarrhea.
5. Strangulation
   Symptoms are initially those of mechanical obstruction but later progress rapidly: Pain is severe, continuous and localized. There is moderate distention, persistent vomiting, usually decreased bowel sounds and marked localized tenderness. Stools or vomitus become melenous or bloody or contain occult blood.
6. Paralytic ileus
   Gaseous distention is prominent; abdomen is tense; pain is dull, continuous, and diffuse; obstipation (intractable constipation) is rarely complete, since small amounts of flatus may be passed; peristalsis is usually depressed, and bowel sounds are infrequent or absent; vomiting occurs only after eating (vomiting may later become fecal).

Nursing Assessment

▶ **NURSING ALERT:** Because of loss of water, sodium, and chloride, signs of dehydration become evident—intense thirst, drowsiness, general malaise, aching; tongue becomes parched, face appears pinched, abdomen becomes distended. Shock may result (pulse increasingly rapid and weak, temperature and blood pressure lowered, skin pale, cold, clammy) ending in death.

1. In the nursing history, describe accurately the nature and location of the patient's pain, the presence of distention, the absence of flatus or defecation.
2. The overview of symptoms is important in differentiating intestinal obstruction from other more benign conditions.
3. Monitor and record vital signs (including blood pressure) every 4 hours.
4. Elderly patients with poor bowel tonus who often remain in the recumbent position for extended periods are likely to experience air–fluid lock syndrome, which is described below:
   a. Fluid collects in dependent bowel loops.
   b. Peristalsis is too weak to push fluid "uphill."

c. Obstruction occurs primarily in the large bowel.
   d. Management consists simply of alternately turning the patient from supine to prone position every 10 minutes until enough flatus is passed to decompress the abdomen. A rectal tube may help.
5. Measure and record accurately all intake and output.
6. Save any stool that may be passed; this is to be tested for occult blood.
7. Anticipate physician's request for urinalysis, hemoglobin determination, and blood cell counts.
8. Frequently, determine the patient's level of consciousness; decreasing responsiveness may offer a clue to an increasing electrolyte imbalance.
9. Observe for evidence of postural hypotension as patient is moved from a low Fowler's position to an upright position; this may suggest circulatory insufficiency.
10. Compare the patient's state of orientation with his admission status; a lessening awareness of his environment may suggest his going into shock.

Patient Problems/Nursing Diagnoses

1. Alteration in bowel elimination related to an obstruction, whatever the cause
2. Abdominal pain (colicky, continuous, sometimes severe and localized) related to distention/strangulation of a segment of intestine
3. Respiratory impairment related to abdominal distention that interferes with proper lung expansion
4. Compromised fluid balance related to impaired fluid intake, fluid lost by vomiting and diarrhea resulting from an intestinal obstruction; potential for hypovolemia
5. Alteration in nutritional status related to intestinal obstruction, which prevents normal food intake
6. Anxiety and fear of death related to life-threatening symptoms of intestinal obstruction

Planning and Implementation

Nursing Interventions

A. Relief of Pain

1. Administer prescribed analgesics.
2. Institute long-tube decompression of intestine proximal to block (p. 435); this can be passed more effectively with the patient lying on his right side; begin decompression to remove gas and fluid.
3. Provide supportive care during nasoenteral intubation, since this will help in relieving discomfort.

B. Relief of Anxiety and Fears

1. Recognize the patient's concern and initiate measures to secure his cooperation and confidence in the staff.
2. Ascertain the patient's specific anxieties and provide him with therapeutic responses.

C. Fluid Therapy

1. Correct fluid imbalance by initiating the following:
   a. Na^+, K^+, blood component therapy
   b. Ringer's lactate to correct interstitial fluid deficit
   c. Dextrose/water to correct intracellular fluid deficit
2. Minimize those factors that would enhance gastric secretions in order to prevent fluid loss (via nasogastric suction); avoid conversation about enticing meals and eliminate meals being served within his range of seeing or smelling.

D. Ongoing Assessment to Monitor Progress

1. Prevent infarction by carefully assessing the patient's status; if pain increases in intensity, localizes, or becomes continuous, it may herald strangulation.
2. Detect early signs of peritonitis, such as rigidity and tenderness, in an effort to minimize this complication.
3. Recognize that giving an enema may distort an x-ray picture by introducing gas into the tract distal to the obstruction. An enema may make a partial obstruction worse; hence it is contraindicated.

Surgical Correction

A. Preoperative Nursing Interventions

1. Undertake measures to prepare the patient for surgery, since most problems of mechanical obstruction require surgical correction.
2. Complete small-bowel obstruction and colon obstruction require an operation for relief. When tube suction therapy does not help after 12 hours, surgery is indicated.
   a. *Resection* of obstructing lesion and end-to-end anastomosis is done when no evidence of peritonitis and only minimal edema exist; this requires a proximal colostomy to decompress new anastomosis.
   b. Resection of all necrotic intestine is necessary.
   c. A tube *enterostomy* may be done by introducing a catheter into distended bowel; the other end of catheter is brought out through the abdominal wall via a separate incision. This is a palliative measure.
   d. A *loop colostomy* is done when relief is sought by drawing a proximal loop or segment of colon up to the skin surface and opening it as a colostomy; the distal portion of colon is treated later.

B. Postoperative Nursing Care

1. To meet fluid, electrolyte, and nutritional needs, administer prescribed amounts of fluids; keep accurate intake and output records.
2. For an enterostomy, connect tube to drainage bottle at side of bed; expect considerable amount of fecal drainage during the first 12–15 hours (500–1,000 ml.).
   a. Observe frequently the patency of drainage equipment.
   b. If there is difficulty with drainage, it may be necessary to inject 15 ml. of warm saline into the enterostomy tube every 2–4 hours, with approval of physician.
   c. Protect skin around enterostomy tube with a skin barrier such as Stomahesive or karaya preparations.
3. Follow additional postoperative management described in Major Intestinal Surgery on page 440.

Evaluation

Expected Outcomes

1. Demonstrates relief of bowel obstruction—passes flatus, has first bowel movement
2. Demonstrates improved breathing ability
3. Takes food and fluid orally
4. Exhibits no vomiting or diarrhea
5. Experiences minimal pain
6. Appears relaxed and reports he is "feeling better"

Cancer of the Colon

Incidence

1. Cancer of the colon and rectum will account for over 60,000 deaths annually—the second highest overall death rate in the US for any type of cancer.
2. Males are affected slightly more often than females.
3. The highest incidence occurs in patients about 50 years old.
4. Five-year survival is 40%–50% (best of visceral cancers).

Etiology and Risk Factors

1. Familial polyposis (numerous pedunculated growths arising from mucosa and extending into lumen of intestine).
2. Chronic ulcerative colitis—definite risk of colon cancer (up to 20% after 20 years of age with active disease).
3. Diverticulosis and cancer may be found together and simulate each other—no definite evidence that the presence of diverticula is significant in the development of cancer.
4. Cancer of the colon occurs much more frequently in developed countries and rarely in underdeveloped countries. The increased incidence of colon cancer in developed countries is probably related to the relatively lower fiber content of diet in these areas.
5. Unabsorbable fiber deficit appears to be related to intestinal transit time, stool bulk, and consistency.
6. The effect of diet on the colon bacterial flora is a factor possibly contributing to cancer.

Risk Reduction

Studies (Burkitt) indicate that high risk populations should:
1. Double daily intake of starch and fiber
2. Reduce sugar and salt intake by one half
3. Reduce dietary fat by one third

Assessment

Clinical Manifestations

1. Distribution of cancer in the colon is shown in Figure 10-15.
2. Most common symptoms:
   a. Blood in stools (usually occult)—causing anemia
   b. Partial obstruction—causing constipation alternating with diarrhea, lower abdominal pains (crampy), distention
   c. Additional signs—progressive weakness, anorexia, weight loss, shortness of breath, anginal pain, anemia

Diagnostic Evaluation

1. Digital rectal examination—half of all colon and rectal cancers are found this way.
2. Endoscopy (fiberoptic sigmoidoscopy/colonoscopy)—two thirds of all colon and rectal cancer can be seen and biopsied via proctoscope alone.
3. Stool examination for blood—often reveals evidence of carcinoma when the patient is otherwise asymptomatic.

▶ **NURSING ALERT:** Giving a guaiac-impregnated slide kit to individuals over age 40 is an *effective way of screening for colorectal cancer*. Diet preparation prior to use of 3 slides is optional:

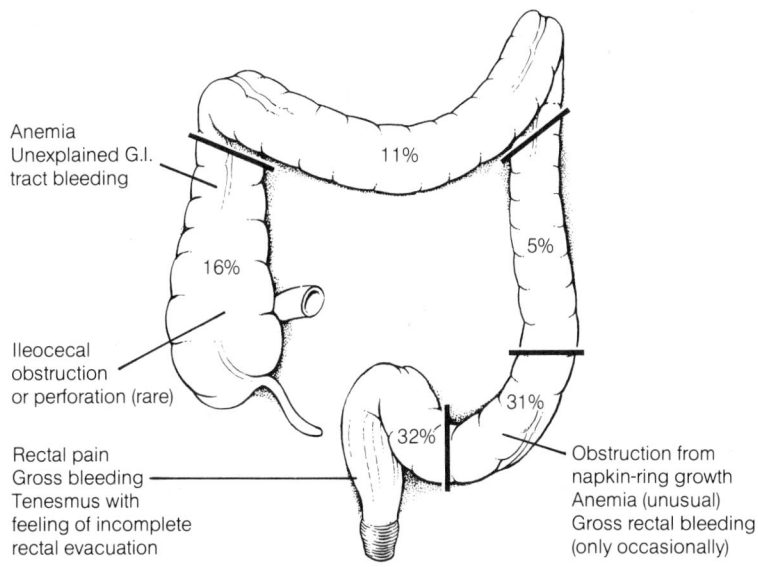

Anemia
Unexplained G.I.
tract bleeding

11%

5%

16%

Ileocecal
obstruction
or perforation (rare)

31%

32%

Rectal pain
Gross bleeding
Tenesmus with
feeling of incomplete
rectal evacuation

Obstruction from
napkin-ring growth
Anemia (unusual)
Gross rectal bleeding
(only occasionally)

Figure 10-15. Distribution of colorectal cancer.

a. Some recommend meat-free, high-residue diet with avoidance of peroxidase-producing vegetables (horse-radish, turnips, and rutabagas), which produce false-positive results.

b. Some prefer no dietary restriction except retesting those who have a positive test result.

4. Blood hemoglobin determination for anemia.

5. Barium enema—especially significant in unexplained abdominal mass.
Napkin-ring-type outline clearly indicates obstruction and possible tumor.

6. Intravenous pyelography and possible cystoscopy may be indicated to assess whether malignancy has spread locally to involve ureter or bladder.

Treatment

A. Diagnosis confirmed by

1. Removing rectosigmoid polyps through sigmoido-scope for histologic study.

2. Removing polyps above rectosigmoid by colonoscopy or laparotomy (if other symptoms are present) to verify diagnosis.

B. Surgical therapeutic plan

1. Recommend total colectomy for patient with familial history of polyposis or prolonged, universal, chronically active colitis, even before cancer is confirmed.

2. Most common operative procedures:
   a. Wide segmental resection of colon and mesentery with anastomosis, or
   b. Abdominoperineal resection with colostomy (if lesion is in rectum). See Colostomy below.
   c. Even more extensive surgery involving removal of other organs if cancer has spread—such as to the bladder, uterus, small intestine, groin, etc.
   d. If cancer is extensive and it may not be in the patient's best interest to do radical surgery, palliative treatment may be done using radon seed implantation (combined surgery and preoperative radiation therapy is being done in several clinics)

or local fulguration via colonoscope or procto-scope.

3. *Colostomy*—This is a temporary or permanent opening of the colon through the abdominal wall. The placement of the colostomy will influence the nature of the discharge (Fig. 10-16). The *stoma* is that part of the colon that is brought above the abdominal wall in a colostomy and becomes the outlet for discharge of intestinal contents. Purposes are as follows:
   a. It may be part of an abdominoperineal resection for cure or palliation of cancer.
   b. It may be palliative when unresectable malignancy is present.
   c. It can be a temporary measure to protect an anastomosis, such as after abdominal trauma.
   d. It may be temporary to divert fecal stream during radiation or other therapy.

Patient Problems/Nursing Diagnoses

1. Nutritional deficit and weight loss related to malignant tumor

2. Pain/discomfort related to spread of malignancy, inflammation, and possible obstruction of intestinal tract

3. Worry and fear related to anesthesia, results of surgery, and potential for complications

Planning and Implementation
Preoperative Nursing Interventions

A. When colostomy is not anticipated

1. Meet the patient's nutritional needs by serving a high-calorie, low-residue diet for several days prior to surgery, if condition permits.

2. Observe and record fluid losses, such as may be sustained by vomiting and diarrhea.

3. Maintain hydration by assisting with intravenous infusion, and observing and recording urinary output.

4. Reduce bacterial count of colon by mechanical cleansing and administering antimicrobials as prescribed—orally and systemically. Whatever the choice,

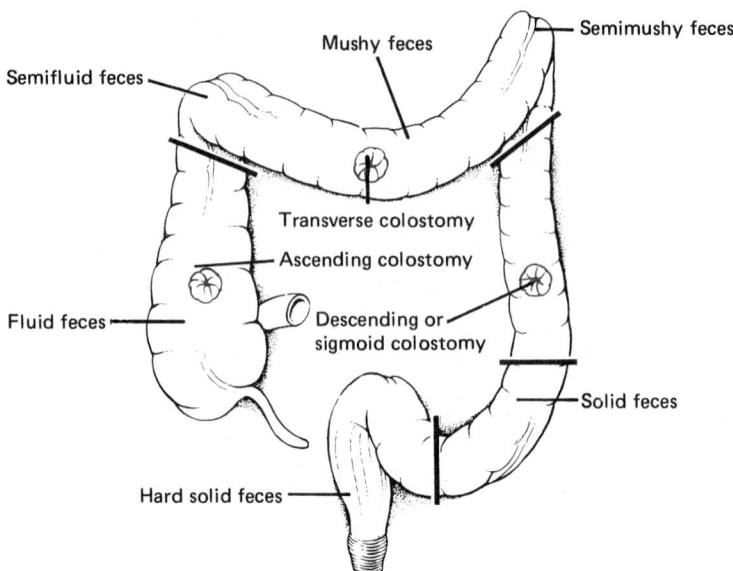

Figure 10-16. A diagrammatic representation of the placement of permanent colostomies and the nature of the discharge at these sites.

it should be effective against the full spectrum of aerobic and anaerobic fecal microbes. The degree of obstruction, acuteness, inflammation—all have a bearing on the nature of antimicrobial administration.
5. Assist the patient during nasoenteral intubation for decompression of intestinal tract.

B. In preparation for colostomy

1. Determine the nature of anticipated surgery; the colostomy must be positioned where the patient can see and care for it (this is determined by the surgeon or enterostomal therapist).
   a. The colostomy should not be placed in the laparotomy incision.
   b. It should be placed where it will not interfere with proper fitting and comfortable wearing of an appliance—away from iliac crest, costal margin, umbilicus, scars, deep folds.
2. Make specific plans for the patient's understanding and acceptance of a colostomy.
   a. Collaborate with the surgeon in ascertaining the nature of communication and information exchanged between surgeon and patient, including initial patient contact, in-hospital experience, plans for rehabilitation.
   b. Reinforce the patient's hope for a future that will be manageable and will lead to independent functioning.
   c. If possible, show the patient the intended appliance and have him try it on.
   d. Arrange a preoperative visit by a trained visitor from the local chapter of the United Ostomy Association.
   e. Develop a plan with the enterostomal therapist and patient to include short-term and long-term goals. Provide the patient with literature and information according to his level of understanding. Take care not to overwhelm the patient with too much information.

3. Preparation for surgery—follow usual preoperative procedures and modify to meet individual needs.

Postoperative Nursing Interventions

A. See also General Postoperative Care, p. 85.

B. Initial Care of the Colostomy

1. Apply a temporary plastic colostomy bag to control odors and soiling.
   Tactfully try to have the patient look at his colostomy, and encourage him to participate in caring for it. Psychosocial skills and understanding are required. Evaluate learning readiness; never force independence.
2. Begin to irrigate when the immediate postoperative period is past and bowel function has resumed (usually 5th or 6th day) (see Guidelines, p. 462).
3. Utilize the treatment time of irrigating the colostomy as the learning time for the patient to begin to master the art of managing his colostomy independently.
   Recognize that some patients are learning to control their colostomy without irrigation.
4. Although irrigation is widely used, recognize that there are some persons who cannot control the colostomy this way (i.e., the patient with an "irritable" colon or unpredictable bowel movements). Also, because of the nature of the contents in various parts of the colon, only colostomies in the descending or sigmoid colon can be expected to be controlled by irrigation. Ascending and transverse colostomies have outputs that are too frequent and too liquid to facilitate control.
5. Often the recognition of a bowel movement occurs when the patient's pouch or dressing is checked; for others, it may be the awareness of the escape of flatus or the contact of stool on the skin.
6. For some there is an awareness of motility, which enables them to get to the bathroom in time for discharging stool into the toilet.

7. Frequency and number of movements vary from person to person.
8. Irrigations for most persons are done every other day.
9. The cone-tip is excellent to prevent insertion of a catheter into insensitive mucosa with risk of perforating the bowel wall. The cone-tip is plugged into the stoma for about 2.5 cm. and permits irrigation without perforation or leakage.
10. Regulation is enhanced when there is systematic planning, balanced meals eaten at regular intervals, and a regular time for irrigation and evacuation.

Discharge Planning/Health Education

A. See also Health Education (Discharge from Hospital), **p. 449.**

B. Irrigation of Colostomy (see p. 462).

C. Skin Care

1. One group of effective skin barriers is made of karaya gum. Karaya is available in powder form, discs, or rings, which can be placed on excoriated peristomal skin (i.e., new skin can grow under them). Karaya paste and rings are excellent for preventing skin irritation immediately around the stoma.
2. Hypoallergenic skin shields include Stomahesive (Squibb), ReliaSeal (Davol), and Hollihesive (Hollister). These tend to deteriorate less quickly than the karaya washers and often can be worn in areas where there are creases and wrinkles.
   a. Stomahesive and Hollihesive can be used as 4″ × 4″ sheets or can be cut into washer size. Stomahesive and Hollihesive adhere well on weepy irritated skin and allow healing to occur.
   b. ReliaSeal comes as a round shield (3¾″ in diameter) or as an oval barrier; it is most effective on reddened peristomal skin but not on ulcerated, weepy skin.
3. Coverings over the stoma may be a disposable pouch, gauze, facial tissue covered with petrolatum, Saran Wrap, or wax paper over a dressing. Hypoallergenic tape may be used.
4. For peristomal excoriation, corticosteroid aerosol sprays or nystatin powders are useful when used sparingly.
5. For allergic reactions, try other products until a compatible one is found; antacid suspensions are found to be practical for some patients.

C. Odor Control

1. Avoid foods known to cause odors—for example, onions, members of the cabbage family, eggs, fish, and beans.
2. Note that fecal odors are lessened with yogurt, cranberry juice, and buttermilk.
3. Odors can be controlled by taking one or two tablets of bismuth subcarbonate or bismuth subgallate at mealtimes and bedtime.

D. Control of Gas

1. Most gas is due to swallowed air (often taken in while chewing gum), highly spiced foods, and carbonated beverages, including beer.
2. Avoid gas-forming foods: beans, cabbage family, onions, radishes, cucumbers, and highly seasoned foods.

E. Diet

1. Avoid overeating and eating irregularly; chew food well.
2. Individualize the diet so that it is balanced and will not cause diarrhea and constipation. A daily diary is effective in determining what foods cause difficulty and can then be eliminated from the diet.
3. Note that fruits, fruit juices, and tomatoes may cause frequent bowel movements. Beer may be a laxative, as well as a gas-producer.

F. Enhanced Life-style

1. According to the United Ostomy Association, approximately 10%–12% of male ostomates suffer impairment of sexual function and potency; fortunately, this impairment is temporary in most cases. Male colostomates vary in degree of potency from full potency to complete impotence. Some patients take up to 2 years to regain potency.
2. An ostomy in a woman does not preclude a successful pregnancy; close medical care is required.
3. There is no contraindication to any form of travel, including horseback riding.
4. Participation in any type of sport is possible.
5. Showering is possible with or without the appliance.
6. Girdles, swim trunks, and panty hose may all be worn, provided there is neither discomfort nor too much constriction.
7. Promote the patient's acceptance of the colostomy by building up self-esteem; encourage the family to assist the patient during the period of adjustment.
8. Contact the community nurse, who will serve as a liaison among hospital, physician, and home as a follow-up when the patient continues to adjust to the colostomy at home.
9. Inform the patient about the United Ostomy Association and enroll him in the local group so that he may obtain information and exchange ideas with other ostomates.
10. Provide the patient with literature, addresses, and telephone numbers of the following organizations:
    Community Nursing Agencies.
    American Cancer Society.
    a. Journal of the Colostomy/Ileostomy Rehabilitation Association, PO Box 121, Philadelphia, PA 19105
    b. *Ostomy Quarterly*—Official Publication of the United Ostomy Association, 2001 W. Beverly Boulevard, Los Angeles, CA 90057
    c. The United Ostomy Association also has available many excellent booklets.
    d. Many manufacturers of ostomy supplies have free booklets available covering a wide variety of ostomy-related topics.

Evaluation
Expected Outcomes

1. Exhibits weight gain trend and improved nutritional status as demonstrated by adequate dietary intake
2. Has no pain and minimal discomfort following surgery for removal of colon cancer
3. Is adjusting to changed life-style following surgery; no evidence of complications
4. Demonstrates ability to care for colostomy

Guidelines: Irrigating a Colostomy

Purposes
1. To empty the colon of its contents: feces, gas, mucus.
2. To cleanse the lower intestinal tract.
3. To establish a regular pattern of evacuation so that normal life activities may be pursued.

Equipment

Reservoir for irrigating fluids; enema bag, irrigating can
Irrigating fluid: 500–1,500 ml. lukewarm tap water or other solution if prescribed by physician
Tubing, connecting tubes, and clamp; preferable clamp—one that can be operated with 1 hand
Irrigating tip: soft rubber catheter—No. 22 or No. 24 with some type of shield to prevent backflow of irrigating solution (or soft rubber or plastic cone irrigating tip)
Irrigating sleeve or sheath: self-adhering (adhesive) or held in place with a belt (a plastic or rubber sheet can be used as a trough in place of a sheath)
Newspaper or plastic bag: to collect soiled dressings and disposable pouch
Toilet tissues and water-soluble lubricant

Procedure

Preparatory Phase
1. Select a suitable time, preferably after a meal, so that this hour fits into the patient's posthospital pattern of activity. Irrigation should be done at the same time each day.
2. Hang irrigating reservoir with solution 45–50 cm. (18–20 inches) above stoma (shoulder height with patient seated).
3. Have the patient sit in front of toilet commode on chair or on commode itself.
4. Remove dressings or pouch and place in bag.

Nursing Action	Rationale/Amplification
Performance Phase	
1. Apply irrigating sleeve or sheath to stoma. Place end in commode.	1. Helps control odor and splashing. Allows feces and water to flow directly into commode.
2. Allow some of solution to flow through tubing and catheter/cone.	2. To release air bubbles in the setup so that air is not introduced into the colon, which would cause crampy pain.
3. Lubricate catheter/cone and gently insert into stoma. Insert catheter no more than 8 cm. (3 inches). Hold shield/cone gently, but firmly, against stoma to prevent backflow of water.	3. These steps are necessary to prevent intestinal perforation.
4. If catheter does not advance easily, allow water to flow slowly while advancing catheter. *NEVER FORCE CATHETER!*	4. Slow rate of flow helps relax bowel and facilitates passage of catheter.
5. Allow fluid to enter colon slowly. If cramping occurs, clamp off tubing and allow the patient to rest before progressing. Water should flow in over a 5–10-minute period.	5. Painful cramps are usually caused by too-rapid flow or too much solution. 500 ml. is usually sufficient for initial postoperative irrigation. Volume may be increased with subsequent irrigations to 1,000 or 1,500 ml., as patient needs for effective results.
6. Hold shield/cone in place 10 seconds after water has been instilled, then gently remove.	
7. Allow 10–15 minutes for most of return, then dry bottom of sleeve/sheath and attach it to top, or apply appropriate clamp to bottom of sleeve.	7. Most of water, feces, and flatus will be expelled in 10–15 minutes.
8. Leave sleeve/sheath in place about 20 minutes while patient gets up and moves around.	8. Ambulation stimulates peristalsis and completion of irrigation return.
Follow-up Phase	
1. Cleanse area with mild soap and water; pat dry.	1. Cleanliness and dryness will provide the patient with hours of comfort.
2. Apply a karaya preparation or other peristomal skin barrier; replace colostomy dressing or pouch.	2. The patient should use pouch until colostomy is sufficiently controlled. Karaya will protect skin from irritation.
3. Clean equipment with soap and water; dry before storing in well-ventilated area.	3. This will control odor and prolong life of equipment.

Anorectal Conditions and Treatments

Nursing Process Overview

Assessment

Nursing History

1. Observe the stool for evidence of bleeding. Is stool mixed or coated with blood?
2. Determine presence of pain during and after evacuation. Is there associated abdominal pain? How long does it last?
3. When recording, describe the problem in the patient's words.
4. Note presence of a discharge. Is it purulent, bloody?

Patient Problems/Nursing Diagnoses

1. Pain in rectal region related to pathology, infection, or surgery
2. Alteration in bowel elimination related to discomfort during defecation
3. Psychosocial and diversional activity deficit related to discomfort
4. Self-care deficits (hygiene, toileting) related to difficulty in seeing or reaching anal area
5. Knowledge deficit of how to keep rectal area clean and reasons why this is important

Planning and Implementation

Preoperative Nursing Interventions

1. Be an understanding and concerned listener when this patient relates problems of a personal nature.
2. Ensure and respect the patient's privacy when attending to personal hygiene, examinations, and treatments.
3. Do not minimize complaints of discomfort.

Postoperative Nursing Interventions

A. Comfort and Wound Healing

1. Be gentle in changing dressings, shaving, irrigating, or administering perineal care.
2. Use petrolatum gauze in protecting edges of wounds (e.g., following incision and drainage of ischiorectal abscess, excision of pilonidal sinus) to prevent crusting and the dressings from sticking to wound.
3. Provide sitz baths when recommended; adjust temperature of solution and provide a comfortable position for the patient.
4. Use caution in applying analgesic or anesthetic ointments, since this often leads to secondary skin rashes from allergy.
5. Keep the perineal area clean to minimize or eliminate infection; presence of *E. coli* demands meticulous cleanliness to prevent infection and promote healing.
6. Change the patient's position from side to side to prevent added discomfort of pressure areas; use air ring properly inflated—not too full.
7. Prevent constipation by proper attention to diet needs of patient; give mineral oil or mild cathartic only as prescribed; use stool softeners.
8. Encourage voluntary voiding to avoid catheterization; this may be facilitated by getting patient out of bed.

9. Observe vital signs and dressings for evidence of hemorrhage, particularly following hemorrhoidectomy.
10. Daily rectal sphincter dilatation may be needed to relieve pain from spasm, to ensure granulation of incisional wounds from bottom out, and to prevent postoperative stricture.

Health Education

(To prepare patient for posthospital convalescence)
1. Instruct the patient on perianal hygiene to minimize the possibility of infection; avoid rubbing area with toilet tissue; instead, pat the area dry.
2. Apply wet dressings (equal parts of witch hazel and water) to relieve edema.
3. Advise the patient regarding the effect of diet on stool formation; plant fibers of leafy vegetables and the roughage of bran flakes, whole grains, and whole wheat bread add roughage to the diet to form cellulose. Cellulose absorbs water, swells, and softens stool, thereby stimulating peristalsis and aiding in intestinal elimination. Encourage the patient to eat fresh fruits, fruit juice, and fresh vegetables except for seeds, skins, corn, and nuts.
4. Avoid cathartics so that stool is formed rather than being soft or liquid.
5. Recommend hot sitz baths or hot compresses to relieve painful sphincter spasm.
6. Suggest adequate fluid intake and daily exercise to prevent constipation; encourage the patient to have a regular time each day for having a bowel movement.
7. Stool softeners are often given until good bowel habits are established.
   a. "Wetting agents" contain dioctyl sodium sulfosuccinate, a substance that penetrates, moistens, and softens hard, dry stool.
   b. "Bulk producers" such as psyllium and agar preparations absorb water, add bulk, and add moisture to stool.
   c. Mineral oil tends to destroy oil-soluble vitamins A, D, E, and K and interferes with absorption of calcium and phosphorus. It should be given at least 3 hours after the evening meal. (Do not give mineral oil to elderly patients because of possible aspiration pneumonia.)
8. Administer enemas only when absolutely necessary; rectal suppositories may be helpful.

Evaluation

Expected Outcomes

1. Describes the dietary modification to be practiced to ensure regular and moderately soft stool
2. Experiences decreased discomfort in rectal area
3. Is mobile and active as a result of decrease or elimination of pain and discomfort
4. Practices hygienic health measures and uses special comfort cushion when sitting
5. Increases social contacts
6. States explicitly how to clean perineal area after defecation/voiding

Perianal Abscess/Fistula in Ano/Fissure in Ano

Condition	Description	Management
Perianal abscess	Localized infection in fatty tissue near rectum. Pain increases. Condition should raise suspicion of granulomatous bowel disease.	Incision and drainage
Fistula in ano	Abnormal opening from the skin near the anus that winds tortuously into the anal canal. Because it is an infectious area, pus leaks outward. Condition should raise suspicion of granulomatous bowel disease.	1. Surgical identification of the path of a fistula. 2. Fistulotomy or partial sphincterotomy.
Fissure in ano	Longitudinal ulcer (a crack that does not heal in the anal canal) frequently associated with constipation, as well as excruciating pain and blood streaking on defecation.	1. Stool softener (dioctyl sodium sulfosuccinate) or psyllium seed. 2. If failure to heal with nonoperative therapy, dilatation of anal sphincter and sphincterotomy or fissurotomy.

Hemorrhoids

Hemorrhoids are varicosities in the lower rectum or anus resulting from congestion in the veins of the hemorrhoidal plexus; *external* hemorrhoids appear outside the external sphincter, whereas *internal* hemorrhoids appear above the internal sphincter. When blood within the hemorrhoids becomes clotted and infected, the hemorrhoids are referred to as *thrombosed.*

Predisposing Factors

1. Pregnancy
2. Straining at stool
3. Chronic constipation
4. Prolonged sitting
5. Anal infection
6. Hereditary factor
7. Portal hypertension (cirrhosis)

Clinical Manifestations

1. Sensation of incomplete fecal evacuation
2. Protrusion
3. Constipation
4. Bleeding during defecation
5. Infection or ulceration
6. Pain noted more in external hemorrhoids
7. Mucus discharge
8. Cosmetic deformity

Diagnostic Evaluation

1. History and visualization by external examination and the use of an anoscope or proctoscope.
2. Barium enema also should be performed, since hemorrhoids are often warning signs of more serious colonic lesions, which may be the actual source of observed rectal bleeding.

Treatment and Nursing Intervention

Hemorrhoids appear to be normal; asymptomatic hemorrhoids require no treatment.

A. Medical

1. Patient should adhere to a low-roughage, high-fiber diet to keep stool soft. Some authorities suggest a diet that includes 30 g. miller's bran per day or replacing white bread with whole wheat.
2. Bowel habits should be regulated with nonirritating stool softeners (e.g., mineral oil or milk of magnesia) to keep stools soft.
3. Frequent hot sitz baths.
4. Insertion of soothing anal suppository 2–3 times daily; topical hydrocortisone foam is comforting.
5. Application of witch hazel compresses for comfort.
6. Control of itching by placement of a cotton pledget on folded soft tissue between the buttocks against the anus to absorb moisture.
7. Do not use topical anesthetics chronically on hemorrhoids or fissures, since they often produce hypersensitivity (allergic) perianal skin rashes with severe itching.
8. If hemorrhoids are prolapsed and the patient is unable to reduce them himself, the nurse may have to reduce them manually:
   a. Apply cold compresses to anal area.
   b. Gently apply anesthetic ointment with a gloved finger.
   c. Very gently manipulate hemorrhoids back through rectal sphincter.
   d. Apply an anesthetic ointment on a dressing to rectal area.
9. Surgery may be indicated when the following conditions exist:
   a. Prolonged bleeding
   b. Disabling pain
   c. Intolerable itching
   d. General unrelieved discomfort

B. Surgical

1. Barron ligation with a rubber band is considered "ideal" treatment.
   a. A large anoscope is used; the apex of the internal hemorrhoid is grasped and drawn through a double-sleeved cylinder.
   b. An elastic band is loaded on the inner cylinder

and released by a trigger device so that the band encircles the base of the hemorrhoid.

c. After a period of time, the hemorrhoid sloughs away.

2. Cryodestruction—freezing of hemorrhoids.

It is claimed to be less painful; some patients have a foul-smelling discharge for about a week to 10 days following cryosurgery.

3. Dilatation—forced dilatation of the anal canal and lower rectum under general anesthesia is another advocated treatment.

This procedure is not advocated for patients whose main complaints are prolapse or inconti-nence. It also is not recommended for aging patients with weak sphincters.

4. Incision and removal of clot from acutely thrombosed hemorrhoid.

5. Excision of hemorrhoids includes the following pro-cedures:

a. Dilatation of rectal sphincter

b. Ligation and excision of hemorrhoid under local or spinal anesthesia

c. Insertion of drainage tube to permit escape of flatus and blood

d. Application of Gelfoam or oxycel gauze to control bleeding, if necessary

Guidelines: Manual Removal of Fecal Impaction

A *fecal impaction* is the retention of hardened feces in the rectum or lower sigmoid.

Manifestations and Occurrence

1. The patient may say he is constipated; often he has a desire to defecate but is unable to do so.
2. Diarrhea or liquid fecal seepage may occur around the obstructing impaction.
3. The patient may complain of rectal pain.
4. This condition may occur in elderly persons following chronic constipation, insufficient hydration, or ingestion of fibrous foods.
5. Orthopedic patients who have been in traction or in body casts may develop an impaction.
6. Occasionally, impaction occurs in patients following rectal surgery or when barium has not been adequately removed following radiologic examination.
7. Impaction is also common in patients with neurologic or psychotic disorders.

Purpose of Fecal Disimpaction

To remove hardened feces in the rectum or lower sigmoid*

Equipment

Clean (not necessarily sterile) rubber or plastic glove
Water-soluble lubricant
Bedpan
Plastic or rubber sheet with cloth protection
Soap, water, washcloth

Procedure

Nursing Action	Rationale/Amplification
Preparatory Phase	
1. Explain procedure to the patient.	
2. Position the patient on left side with upper knee flexed.	2. To permit access to rectum and lower sigmoid.
3. Drape the patient and place protecting pad under but-tocks.	3. To prevent chilling and undue exposure.
4. Place bedpan in a convenient place.	4. To serve as receptacle.
5. Put on glove and lubricate index finger generously (some prefer the middle finger because it is longer).	
Performance Phase (Fig. 10-17)	
1. Insert gloved finger *gently* into rectum until impaction is felt.	1. This stimulation may increase peristalsis.
2. *Gently* remove or break fecal material within reach and deposit in bedpan; work finger around and into mass to break it up if possible.	2. The emphasis is on *gentleness,* since this may be painful.
3. Gently stimulate rectal sphincter by making a circular motion once or twice.	3. This may stimulate peristalsis and relax the sphincter.

* Some health-care personnel use a lubricated impaction evictor (Max Woeher & Sons, Cincinnati, OH).

(continued)

Guidelines: Manual Removal of Fecal Impaction (continued)

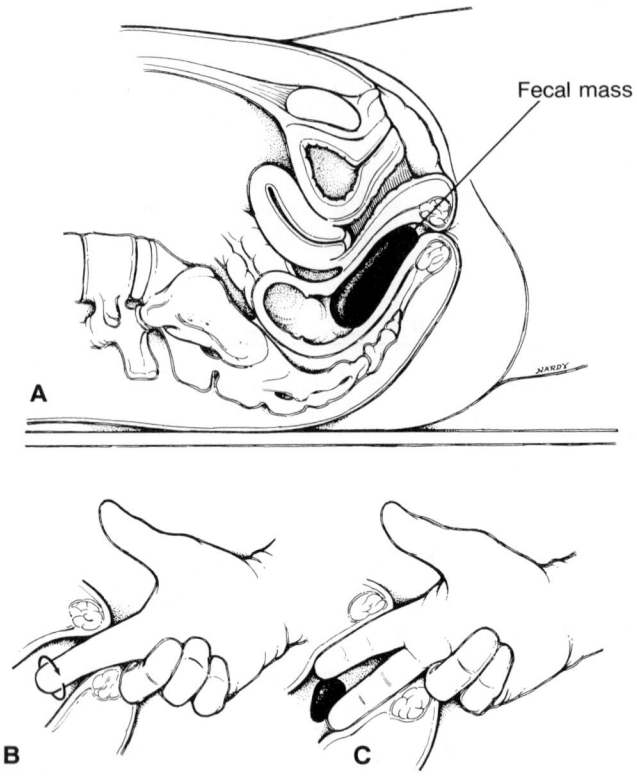

Fecal mass

A

B   C

Figure 10-17. Fecal impaction. (*A*) Note shaded area inside rectal sphincter—this indicates fecal impaction. (*B*) By gently stimulating the rectal wall with a gloved index finger, and using a circular motion, it is possible to loosen fecal material. (*C*) It may be necessary to gently insert 2 fingers in an attempt to crush the fecal mass. A scissor-like motion is used.

Procedure
(Cont.)

Nursing Action	Rationale/Amplification
4. If step 3 does not result in removal of the impaction, it may be necessary to *gently* insert the middle and index finger and attempt to break up the mass by a scissorlike movement of the fingers. Repeat steps 2 or 4 until all easily reachable fecal masses are removed.	4. Greater leverage is afforded, and the mass may be more easily broken.
5. Note any bleeding or pain; observe the patient for shortness of breath or perspiration.	5. Should any of these responses occur, stop the procedure.

Follow-up Phase

1. Gently wash and dry the rectal area; make the patient comfortable and have him rest.	1. Drying the area prevents skin excoriation and promotes comfort.
2. Note bedpan contents and then empty.	
3. Record color, consistency, and odor of stool.	3. These characteristics may provide clues to the nature of the problem.
4. Plan health instruction measures in an effort to prevent a recurrence. Explore nutritional and fluid needs of the patient; determine activity level and encourage suitable exercises to promote adequate elimination.	4. Investigate the possibility of using stool softeners; suggest periodic use of Fleet's enema.

3: Conditions of the Hepatic and Biliary System

Manifestations of Disorders of the Liver

Pathophysiology

Disorders of the liver result from direct damage to the liver cells (hepatocytes) or indirectly as a result of alterations in bile or blood flow through the liver.

Etiology

1. Viral infections and the effects of toxins may lead to hepatocellular dysfunction.
2. Chronic alcohol consumption, along with malnutrition, may cause toxic liver damage (cirrhosis).
3. Impairment of liver function may occur when flow of bile into the intestine is impeded (i.e., obstruction of the biliary tract by gallstones or a tumor).

General Assessment, Which May Indicate Liver Dysfunction

(Also see Physical Assessment of Liver, below)

Physical Assessment of Liver

1. Begin by placing the left hand under the patient's back at the level of the 11–12th rib. The liver border, if felt, should be firm and smooth.
   Place the right hand, with fingers angled and slightly facing the costal margin, just below the percussed lower border of the liver.
2. During palpation with the right hand, press upward with the left hand to move the liver anteriorly (to facilitate palpation).
3. Have the patient inspire, and on expiration press the fingers of the right hand inward. On deep inspiration by the patient, do not change the position of the right hand, feel for the liver edge moving over the fingers. If nothing is felt on inspiration, palpate more deeply, then on each subsequent inspiration, move the finger upward toward the costal margin. With each new position of the fingers, have the patient breathe deeply and feel for the liver.

Clinical Manifestations

A. Altered Skin Integrity Related to Jaundice and Edema

Jaundice is present when all tissues, including the sclerae and skin, assume a yellow or greenish-yellow tinge because of an increased concentration of bilirubin. (See p. 470 for types of jaundice.) Edema occurs when the liver is no longer able to synthesize adequate amounts of albumin. These changes impair normal skin integrity.

1. Normal bilirubin concentration in blood is 0.1–1.0 mg./100 ml. of blood.
2. Over 3.0 mg./100 ml. of blood—jaundice can be detected.
3. Normal albumin level is 3.5–5.5 gm./dl.
4. An albumin level below 3.0 gm./dl., with an increased serum globulin level, occurs with liver disease.

B. Bleeding Tendencies Related to Altered Clotting Mechanisms and Portal Hypertension

1. Because of blood coagulation defects, gastrointestinal hemorrhage, as well as bleeding gums, blood in urine, rectal bleeding, and tarry stool, may occur
2. Minor skin trauma may produce ecchymosis (bruising).
3. Following all types of intramuscular and intravenous injections and arterial punctures, it is necessary to apply pressure for longer than usual and to observe for hematoma.

C. Altered Fluid and Electrolyte Balance

1. Tissue edema and intra-abdominal fluid (ascites) are manifestations of sodium and water retention, combined with potassium excretion.
2. Hypoproteinemia, iron-decreased hepatic synthesis, and disturbed kidney function also contribute to fluid retention.

D. Altered Mental and Neurologic States Related to Deterioration of Liver Function

1. Pyridoxine deficiency can result in nervous irritability and convulsive seizures.
2. Thiamine deficiency may lead to polyneuritis and Wernicke–Korsakoff psychosis.
3. Failure to metabolize ammonia arriving from intestine in portal venous system and impaired metabolism of sedative drugs produce range of symptoms from irritability and confusion to stupor, somnolence, and coma.

Diagnostic Evaluation of Liver Disease

Liver Diagnostic Studies

Test and Purpose	Normal	Clinical and Nursing Significance
Bile Formation and Secretion 1. *Serum bilirubin (van den Bergh reaction)* Measures bilirubin in the blood; this determines the ability of the		

(continued)

Liver Diagnostic Studies (continued)

Test and Purpose	Normal	Clinical and Nursing Significance
liver to take up, conjugate, and excrete bilirubin. Bilirubin is a product of the breakdown of hemoglobin.		
Direct (conjugated)—soluble in water	0.1–0.2 mg./dl.	Abnormal in biliary and liver disease causing jaundice clinically.
Indirect (unconjugated)—insoluble in water	0.1–0.8 mg./dl.	Abnormal in hemolysis and in functional disorders of uptake or conjugation.
Total serum bilirubin	0.1–1.0 mg./dl.	
2. *Urine bilirubin* Not normally found in urine, but if direct serum bilirubin is elevated, some spills into urine.	None	Mahogany-colored urine; when specimen is shaken, yellow tint to foam can be observed. Confirm with Ictotest tablet or Dipstick. If phenazopyridine (Pyridium) is being taken, there may be a false-positive bilirubin result. (Mark laboratory slip if this medication is being taken.)
3. *Urobilinogen* Formed in small intestine by action of bacteria on bilirubin. Related to amount of bilirubin excreted into bile.	Urine urobilinogen up to 1–4 mg./24 hr. Fecal urobilinogen 40–280 mg./24 hr.	Urine specimen is collected over 2-hr. period after lunch. Place specimen in dark brown container and send it to laboratory immediately to prevent decomposition. If the patient is receiving antimicrobials, mark laboratory slip to this effect, since production of urobilinogen can be falsely reduced.
Protein Studies		
1. *Albumin and globulin measurement* Is of greater significance than total protein measurement.		As one increases, the other decreases; hence,
Albumin—produced by liver cells	3.5–5.5 gm./dl.	Albumin ↓ cirrhosis chronic hepatitis
Globulin—produced in lymph nodes, spleen, and bone marrow and Kupffer's cells of liver	1.5–3.0 gm./dl.	Globulin ↑ cirrhosis chronic obstructive jaundice
Total serum protein	6.0–8.0 mg./dl.	viral hepatitis
2. *Prothrombin time (PT)* Prothrombin and other clotting factors are manufactured in the liver; its rate is influenced by the supply of vitamin K.	60%–100% of control	Prothrombin time may be prolonged in liver disease, in which case it will not return to normal with vitamin K. It may also be prolonged in malabsorption of fat and fat-soluble vitamins, in which case it will not return to normal with vitamin K.
Fat Metabolism		
1. *Cholesterol* It is possible to measure lipid metabolism by determining serum cholesterol levels.	150–270 mg./100 ml. (depends on age and diet) Esters = 60% of total	Serum cholesterol level is decreased in parenchymal liver disease. Serum lipid level is increased in biliary obstruction.
Liver Detoxification		
1. *Serum alkaline phosphatase* Since bile disposes this enzyme, any impairment of liver cell ex-	Varies with method: 2–5 Bodansky units, 30–85 I.U./ml.	*Abnormalities:* The level is elevated to more than 3 times normal in obstructive jaundice, intrahepatic

Liver Diagnostic Studies (continued)

Test and Purpose	Normal	Clinical Nursing Significance
cretory function will cause an elevation. In cholestasis or obstruction, increased synthesis of enzyme causes very high levels in blood.		cholestasis, liver metastasis, or granulomas. Also elevated in osteoblastic diseases, Paget's disease, and hyperparathyroidism.
Enzyme Production		
Transaminase (SGOT) (Aspartate aminotransferase or AST)	7–40 mU./ml.	An elevation in these enzymes indicates liver cell damage.
Transaminase (SGPT) (Alanine aminotransferase or ALT)	10–40 mU./ml.	**NOTE:** Opiates may also cause a rise in SGOT and SGPT. Aspirin may cause an increase or decrease in SGOT and SGPT.
Other ''Liver Profile'' Tests		
GGT (gamma glutamyl transpeptidase) (See Appendix for laboratory values) Bile acids radioimmunoassay are replacing BSP tests.		

Guidelines: Assisting with Liver Biopsy

Liver biopsy is the sampling of liver tissue by needle aspiration.

Purpose To establish a diagnosis of liver disease by histologic study of liver tissue.

Equipment

Sterile aspiration syringe and biopsy needle (Silverman)
Local anesthetic
Skin antiseptics, sterile fenestrated towel, gloves
Glass slides, specimen bottles containing fixative and/or test tubes

Procedure

Preparatory Phase

1. See that consent form is signed.
2. Verify that the patient has had prothrombin tests and blood typing by checking the chart.
3. Determine availability of compatible blood, since these patients often have clotting defects.
4. Determine and record patient's pulse, respiration, arterial pressure, and prothrombin time immediately before the biopsy in order to have a baseline of comparison with the postbiopsy condition of the patient.
5. Explain the steps of this procedure to the patient to reduce his concerns and gain his cooperation.

Nursing Action	Rationale/Amplification
Performance Phase	
1. Place the patient flat in bed with right arm under head and face turned left.	
2. Expose the upper abdomen in readiness for skin disinfection and local anesthetic injection.	2. For optimal exposure and comfort of patient, the right hypochondriac region is treated as a surgical area, to minimize danger of infection.
3. Physician will determine biopsy site—one interspace below upper border of liver dullness 2 cm. behind anterior axillary line.	
4. Physician anesthetizes the skin, intercostal tissues, and liver capsule with local anesthetic.	4. To promote local comfort.
5. Physician introduces biopsy needle into intercostal tissues but not into liver.	5. To prevent tearing of diaphragm or liver.

(continued)

Guidelines: Assisting with Liver Biopsy (continued)

Procedure
(Cont.)

Nursing Action	Rationale/Amplification
6. Instruct the patient to inhale and exhale deeply 3 or 4 times, then to exhale and hold his breath.	6. Holding one's breath immobilizes the chest wall and diaphragm; this helps to prevent the needle from tearing the diaphragm or the liver.
7. The physician rapidly introduces biopsy needle into the liver, aspirates tissue, and withdraws.	
8. As soon as needle is withdrawn, inform the patient to resume normal breathing.	8. Actual insertion and withdrawal of needle takes about 10 seconds.

Follow-up Phase

1. Following biopsy, assist the patient to turn on his right side, place a pillow under his lower rib cage and instruct him to remain in this position for several hours.	1. Compressing the liver against the chest wall near the biopsy site reduces the possibility of bleeding.
2. Determine and record the patient's pulse and respiratory rates and his blood pressure at frequent intervals until they stabilize. Observe biopsy site for bleeding or drainage.	2. The nurse needs to be aware of the possible complications of liver biopsy; hemorrhage and bile peritonitis. Anticipatory nursing includes early recognition of symptoms.
3. Recognize that an increasing pulse and decreasing blood pressure may be indicative of hemorrhage; note any indication of pain.	

Jaundice

Jaundice is a *symptom* of dysfunction or disease and not a disease itself. Dysfunction of several body organs or systems may be implicated when jaundice occurs.

Hemolytic Jaundice

Hemolytic jaundice is attributable to an abnormally high concentration of bilirubin in blood exceeding the capacity of liver cells to excrete it. This form is also referred to as *prehepatic jaundice;* liver function is usually normal.

1. Most common cause is massive hemolysis seen in hemolytic transfusion reactions, hereditary spherocytosis, autoimmune hemolytic anemia, erythroblastosis fetalis, and other hemolytic disorders.
2. Bilirubin in the blood is unconjugated (indirect-reacting).
3. In feces and urine, urobilinogen is increased; urine is free of bilirubin.
4. Prolonged jaundice leads to formation of "pigment stones" in gallbladder.
5. Extremely severe jaundice (unconjugated bilirubin elevated: 20–25 mg./100 ml.) causes brain stem damage in neonates.

Hepatocellular Jaundice

Hepatocellular or *hepatic jaundice* is due to an inability of diseased liver cells to clear the normal amount of bilirubin from the blood.

A. Causes

1. Infection—hepatitis A, hepatitis B, or hepatitis non-A, non-B
2. Drug or chemical toxicity—carbon tetrachloride, chloroform, phosphorus, arsenicals, ethanol, halothane, isoniazid, acetaminophen, mushroom poisoning

B. Clinical Manifestations

1. Mildly or severely ill patient.
2. Lack of appetite, nausea, loss of vigor and strength, weight loss.

3. Elevated aspartate aminotransferase (AST, transaminase or SGOT) and alanine aminotransferase (ALT, SGPT)—2 enzymes that are liberated with cellular necrosis.
4. Rise in bromsulphalein (BSP) and bilirubin. Alkaline phosphatase mildly elevated.
5. Abnormal serum proteins in prolonged illness; prothrombin time increased.
6. Headache and chills possible in infectious condition.
7. Bile acids radioimmunoassay are replacing BSP tests.

Cholestatic Jaundice (posthepatic or obstructive jaundice)

A. Causes

1. Extrahepatic obstruction—blockage of bile ducts by gallstone(s), tumor(s), an inflammatory process, or an enlarged pancreas pressing on the duct.
2. Intrahepatic cholestasis—caused by injury to bile canaliculi or blockage of intrahepatic ducts due to tumors or granulomas.
   Certain drugs may cause this, for example, "cholepulmonarystatic" agents: phenothiazine derivatives (Thorazine), perphenazine (Trilafon), sulfonamides, tolbutamide (Orinase) and other antidiabetic drugs, thiouracil, and aminobenzoic acid (previously named para-aminobenzoic acid [PABA]).

B. Clinical Manifestations

Because of damming back of bile, it is reabsorbed by blood. The following responses may be noted:

1. Jaundice of skin and sclerae
2. Deep orange-colored urine
3. White or clay-colored stools
4. Itchy skin and dyspepsia due to impaired bile acid excretion
5. SGOT and SGPT (AST and ALT) rise only moderately.
6. Bilirubin and BSP are increased.
7. Alkaline phosphatase is strikingly elevated.
8. Cholesterol is elevated.

Patient Problems/Nursing Diagnoses

Although the clinical manifestations and treatment depend on the type and outcome of the dysfunction, the patient with jaundice is likely to experience the following problems:

1. Altered skin integrity related to pruritis
2. Altered self-esteem related to change in appearance
3. Bleeding tendencies related to altered clotting mechanism and portal hypertension
4. Altered fluid and electrolyte balance related to fluid deficit
5. Altered mental and neurologic status related to deterioration of liver function

Planning and Implementation
Nursing Interventions

A. **Relief of pruritus and maintenance of skin integrity**

1. Use starch or baking soda baths, soothing lotions such as calamine.
2. Administer antihistamines, tranquilizers, and sedatives if prescribed.
3. Administer cholestyramine (Questran) to promote fecal excretion of bile salts to decrease itching.
4. Assist the patient in reducing the strong tendency to scratch his skin:
   a. Encourage activities to divert the patient's attention.
   b. Keep nails trimmed and clean.
   c. Avoid excessive top bedding.
   d. Give soothing massages, particularly at night in preparing the patient for sleep, since this is a time when he is especially likely to scratch.
   e. Provide clean white gloves to use at night if the patient scratches during sleep.

B. **Increase in self-esteem**

1. Encourage the patient to discuss his concerns; accept the patient's concerns without minimizing them.
2. Instruct staff and the patient's visitors to avoid remarks or behaviors that indicate rejection or fear of the patient's altered appearance.
3. Explain cause of jaundice and altered appearance.
4. Reinforce the fact that change in appearance is usually temporary.
5. Place the patient's bed in a position where he cannot look at himself in a mirror.

Evaluation
Expected Outcomes

1. Demonstrates improved skin integrity—does not scratch or complain of itching; no signs of excoriation or infection of skin
2. Demonstrates improved self-esteem by verbalizing own reactions to altered appearance and by interacting with others

Hepatitis

Hepatitis is a diffuse inflammation of the liver parenchyma.

Etiology

Hepatitis is usually caused by one or more viruses; however, a less common form is toxic or drug-induced hepatitis.

Types of Hepatitis

1. Hepatitis A virus; HAV, infectious hepatitis, IH virus, short-incubation hepatitis
2. Hepatitis B virus; HBV, serum hepatitis, SH virus, homologous serum hepatitis, long-incubation hepatitis
3. Hepatitis non-A non-B; NANB
   Features of HAV, HBV, and NANB hepatitis are summarized in Table 10-5.

Significance

1. Community health—concern with ease of disease transmission and morbidity.
2. Socioeconomic—prolonged loss of time from school and employment.

Treatment

1. Management is largely devoted to treatment of symptoms and support of the patient during the acute and convalescent phases.
2. Treatment consists of nutritional support and moderate restriction of activity, depending on the severity of the patient's fatigue, anorexia, and abdominal discomfort.
3. The patient is monitored closely for deterioration of liver function or the occurrence of complications.

General Preventive Measures

1. Stress importance of proper public and home sanitation.
2. Recognize merits of conscientious surveillance in the proper and safe preparation and dispensation of food.
3. Promote effective health supervision in schools, dormitories, and camps.
4. Initiate and support health education programs.
5. Identify individuals or groups of individuals at high risk.
6. Encourage administration of appropriate immune globulin or vaccine when indicated.
7. Protect self through use of appropriate measures and precautions (gloves, etc.) when indicated in care of patients with known or suspected hepatitis.
8. Instruct the patient and family members about transmission and prevention of transmission.

Assessment
Diagnostic Evaluation

1. SGPT (or ALT) levels rise 1–2 weeks before clinical jaundice appears.
2. The presence of HAV/IgM indicates antibody to hepatitis A virus and an acute stage of hepatitis A infection.
3. The presence of hepatitis B antigen (HB_sAg) is detected in individuals who have hepatitis B. The antigen can be detected before the onset of symptoms.
4. The absence of markers for hepatitis A or B leads to the diagnosis of non-A, non-B hepatitis, hepatic toxicity, or some other viral infection.

Table 10-5 Quick Summary of Hepatitis

	Hepatitis A Virus (HAV)	Hepatitis B Virus (HBV)	Non-A, Non-B Hepatitis Virus (NANBH)
Other Names	Type A hepatitis, infectious or epidemic hepatitis, IH virus	Type B hepatitis, serum hepatitis, SH virus, Dane particle	Hepatitis "C"; "D"; type C
Epidemiology			
Cause	Hepatitis A virus	Hepatitis B virus	Another virus; more than 1 virus
Method of transmission	Fecal-oral; poor sanitation Person-to-person Waterborne, foodborne—shellfish Rarely, if at all, by blood transfusion	Parenterally or by intimate contact with carriers or those with acute disease; male homosexuals. Vertical transmission from mothers to babies Contaminated instruments, syringes, needles; renal dialysis*	Transfusion of blood or blood products Personnel in renal transplant and dialysis units Parenteral drug abusers Blood transfusion products Institutions with long-term residents* Male homosexuals
Source of virus/antigen	Blood, feces, saliva	Blood Saliva Semen, vaginal secretions	Appears to be bloodborne Sexual contact
Distribution by age	Young adults (15–29) and middle-aged who have escaped childhood infection	Affects all ages, but mostly young adults	Same as HBV
Incubation period	3–5 weeks Mean, 30 days	2–5 months Mean, 90 days	Variable; 2–6 months Mean, 50 days
Occurrence	Worldwide	Worldwide	Worldwide Accounts for 20% of sporadic cases
Antibody	Anti-HAV Present in convalescent sera and immune serum globulin (ISG)	Anti-HB$_c$ (core antigen) Anti-HB$_s$ (surface antigen)	
Immunity	Homologous	Homologous	
Severity	Most anicteric and asymptomatic	More severe than HAV	Wide spectrum of severity resembling HAV or HBV. Often prolonged illness—months May progress to chronic hepatitis*
Nature of Disease			
Signs and Symptoms	May occur with or without symptoms; flu-like illness Preicteric phase: Headache, malaise, fatigue, anorexia, lassitude, fever Icteric phase: Dark urine, scleral icterus, jaundice, liver tenderness, and perhaps enlargement	May occur without symptoms 1,000 I.U./liter serum transaminase level May develop antibodies to virus Similar to HAV, but more severe Fever and respiratory symptoms rare, but may have arthralgias, rash	Similar to HBV Less severe and anicteric
Diagnosis and method	Elevated serum transaminase Complement fixation rate Radioimmunoassay	Check serum for HB$_s$Ag, HB$_e$Ag, anti-HB$_c$ in absence of anti-HB$_s$ (obtainable as panel) Elevated serum transaminase Radioimmunoassay—hemagglutination	Diagnosed by excluding HAV and HBV
Severity	Usually mild Fatality rate 0–1%	Variable, may be severe Fatality rate varies, 1%–10%	Variable, usually mild Fatality rate 1%–2%
Specific treatment	Adequate fluids, rest, nutrition Avoid alcohol; use drugs with caution	Same as HAV In research, vaccine antiviral chemotherapy to eliminate chronic HBV carrier state (being tested)	Same as HAV
Prevention	Good sanitation Proper personal hygiene Effective sterilization procedures Careful screening of food handlers Immune serum globulin (ISG) given within a few days of exposure	Specific hepatitis B immune globulin (HBIG) probably useful after exposure by ingestion, inoculation, or splash involving hepatitis B surface antigen (HB$_s$Ag) Hepatitis B vaccine recommended for pre-exposure immunization of those at high risk.	Mandatory screening of blood donors: 1) for HB$_s$Ag, 20% 2) for non-A, non-B, 80%

* Probably the same for HBV and NANBH, recent intensive research suggests.

Patient Problems/Nursing Diagnoses

1. Alteration in nutritional status related to anorexia, nausea, and vomiting
2. Impaired skin integrity related to pruritus
3. Activity intolerance related to fatigue and generalized malaise
4. Abdominal pain related to tender, enlarged liver

Planning and Implementation
Nursing Interventions

A. Improved nutritional status

1. Provide balanced meals consistent with the patient's food preferences.
2. Provide pleasant environment for meals.

3. Encourage the patient to eat in a sitting position to decrease abdominal tenderness and feeling of fullness.
4. Provide frequent, small meals if anorexia is severe.
5. Instruct the patient about the importance of a balanced diet and the need to avoid alcohol during illness.

B. Relief of pruritus and improvement in skin integrity

(See p. 471)

C. Increase in ability to carry out activities

1. Encourage the patient to limit activity when fatigued.
2. Assist the patient in planning periods of rest and activity when symptoms begin to subside.
3. Encourage gradual resumption of activities and mild exercise during recovery.

D. Decrease in abdominal pain/tenderness

1. Assess and record presence or absence of abdominal pain or tenderness, hepatomegaly, and splenomegaly.
2. Encourage the patient to maintain bed rest or restricted activities if abdominal pain or tenderness is present.
3. Administer analgesics as prescribed.
4. Notify the physician of sudden occurrence of or increase in pain or tenderness.

Evaluation

Expected Outcomes

1. Maintains adequate nutritional intake, avoids alcohol during illness, maintains weight, and identifies features of a balanced diet
2. Reports decrease in anorexia, nausea, and vomiting
3. Demonstrates improved skin integrity—intact skin with no evidence of excoriation for infection; decreased scratching, no pruritus
4. Exhibits increased ability to carry out desired activities and allows sufficient periods for rest and relaxation
5. Reports a decrease or absence of abdominal pain and tenderness; restricts activities if pain recurs; participates in planned activities when free of pain; takes prescribed analgesics if necessary

Type A Hepatitis (HAV)

Epidemiology

1. HAV is probably an RNA virus of the enterovirus family.
2. Mode of transmission
   a. Fecal–oral route
   b. Poor sanitation; person-to-person (epidemic-type prevalent in camps and overcrowded residences)
   c. Contaminated food, milk, polluted water, or shellfish
   d. Sexual contact
   e. Blood transfusion (rarely)
3. Incubation: 3–7 weeks; average, 4 weeks
4. Occurrence
   a. Worldwide
   b. Usually in children and young adults
5. Mortality—0.3% develop fulminating disease, which has a mortality rate of 75%–80%.

Assessment and Clinical Manifestations

1. Preicteric phase (prior to period of jaundice)
   a. Most patients are anicteric and symptomless. Highly contagious during preicteric phase.

   b. Initial symptoms—headache, fatigue, anorexia, fever, flu-like upper respiratory infection
2. Icteric phase—jaundice, dark urine, vague epigastric symptoms, anorexia, flatulence. When jaundice reaches its peak, symptoms tend to subside. Liver is tender and perhaps enlarged.

Nursing Management

1. Promote rest during acute or symptomatic stage.
2. Encourage an adequate diet. The patient may have severe anorexia, which may hinder ordinary efforts to promote an adequate dietary intake.
3. Utilize appropriate measures to minimize spread of the disease.

Preventive Measures and Health Education

1. Encourage optimum sanitation practices.
2. Instruct the patient to practice good personal hygiene.
3. Employ proper safeguards to prevent use of blood and its components from infected donors.
4. Screen food handlers carefully.
5. Practice safe preparation and serving of food.
6. Administer immune globulin intramuscularly or subcutaneously within a few days of exposure.
7. Use disposable needles and syringes; dispose of these carefully.
8. Wear gloves when handling bedpans and fecal-contaminated linens.

Type B Hepatitis (HBV)

Hepatitis B virus is a double-shelled particle containing DNA.

Epidemiology

1. Causative agent—this particle is composed of:
   a. Antigenic material in an outer coat—hepatitis B surface antigen (HB_sAg)
   b. Antigenic material in an inner coat—hepatitis B core antigen (HB_cAg)
   c. An independent protein circulating in the blood—HB_eAg
2. Antibody—each antigen elicits a specific antibody:
   a. Anti-HB_s (produced early after hepatitis B infection). Its presence indicates immunity. Therefore, it is present if the patient has received hepatitis B vaccine.
   b. Anti-HB_c (noted late in acute phase or in convalescence)
   c. Anti-HB_e (noted later in convalescence)
3. Significance:
   a. HB_sAg—may be detected transiently in blood of 80%–90% of infected persons; may be noted in blood for months and years, indicating that the patient has acute or chronic hepatitis B or is a carrier.
   b. HB_cAg—found only in liver cells, not serum.
   c. HB_eAg—if absent, the patient is an asymptomatic carrier. If present, it indicates highly infectious period of acute, active hepatitis. If it persists, indicates progression to chronic state.
4. Modes of transmission (percutaneous or permucosal routes):
   a. Oral—via saliva (i.e., mother to child via breast feeding)
   b. Parenterally, or by intimate contact with carriers. (Susceptible persons are surgeons, clinical laboratory workers, nurses, respiratory therapists.)

c. Male homosexuals
d. Blood, saliva, semen, vaginal secretions
5. Incubation—2–5 months
6. Occurrence—affects all ages but mostly young adults; worldwide

Assessment and Clinical Manifestations
1. Resembles hepatitis A clinically.
2. Symptoms insidious and variable.
3. Arthralgias and rashes may be observed; fever and respiratory symptoms are rare.
4. Jaundice may or may not be present.
5. Anorexia, abdominal pain, generalized malaise may be noted.

Treatment and Nursing Management
1. Provide adequate fluids, nutrition, and bed rest.
2. Administer alkalies, belladonna, and antiemetics if these agents are required to control dyspepsia and malaise.
3. Recognize that recovery and convalescence are slow and prolonged, sometimes taking 3–4 months; provide psychosocial support and diversional activities.

Preventive Measures and Health Education
1. Screening of blood donors to exclude carriers.
2. Caution in giving care to patients with known or suspected HBV. Use gloves when starting intravenous infusions or handling blood-contaminated articles from patients with known or suspected hepatitis.
3. Hepatitis B vaccine is recommended for those individuals at high risk for hepatitis B.
4. Hepatitis B immune globulin (HBIG) should be administered within 72 hours to those exposed directly to hepatitis B virus by accidental needle stick or splashing with blood products of patients with HBV.
5. Transfuse a patient only when justified.
6. Use blood substitutes when feasible.

7. Use disposable needles and syringes; dispose of these carefully.
8. Instruct *all* patients who have received a blood transfusion to refrain from donating blood for 6 months. This is necessary because of the long incubation period of hepatitis B.

Hepatitis non-A non-B

This type of hepatitis is a viral infection that at present does not have an identified agent or antigenic markers. Therefore, it is diagnosed by excluding HAV and HBV.

Epidemiology
1. Over 80% of post-transfusion hepatitis fall into this category.
2. Mode of transmission
   a. Associated with blood transfusions
   b. Personnel in renal dialysis units
   c. Parenteral drug abusers
   d. Appears to be bloodborne
3. Incubation—2–6 months
4. Occurrence—same as Hepatitis B

Assessment and Clinical Manifestations
Same as that of hepatitis B; less severe and anicteric

Treatment and Nursing Management
(Similar to that for Hepatitis B)
1. Non-A non-B hepatitis waxes and wanes over many months. There is probably a chronic carrier state.
2. Gamma globulin significantly reduces the incidence of this type of hepatitis and reduces the incidence of chronic active liver disease.

Preventive Measures and Health Teaching
Same as that for hepatitis B, although there is no vaccine available for protection against non-B non-B hepatitis

Hepatic Cirrhosis

Cirrhosis of the liver is a chronic disease in which there has been diffuse destruction of parenchymal cells followed by liver cell regeneration and an increase in connective tissue. These processes result in disorganization of the lobular architecture and obstruction of the hepatic venous and sinusoidal channels, causing portal hypertension.

Classification of Hepatic Cirrhosis
1. Laennec's cirrhosis of the alcoholic (micronodular)
   a. Fibrosis—mainly around central veins and portal areas
   b. Most commonly due to chronic alcoholism and malnutrition
2. Postnecrotic (macronodular)
   a. Broad bands of scar tissue—due to collapse of necrotic lobules and confluence of portal areas
   b. Due to previous acute viral hepatitis or drug-induced massive hepatic necrosis
3. Biliary
   a. Scarring around bile ducts and lobes of liver
   b. Results from chronic biliary obstruction (with or without infection)

   c. Much more rare than Laennec's and postnecrotic cirrhosis

Etiology
1. Cirrhosis of the liver is characterized by repeated occurrences of death of the liver cells, replacement with scar tissue, and regeneration of liver cells.
2. Onset is insidious; it may be developing and progressing over many years.
3. Major causes in the US are excessive consumption of alcohol with nutritional deficiencies and chronic viral hepatitis.
4. Twice as many men as women are affected; age-group most often affected is from 40–60 years.

Pathophysiology
1. Early in disease—gastrointestinal disturbances, fever and liver enlargement due to deposits of fats in the liver cells; as tissue is replaced, scars contract and become smaller, the surface becomes rough and has a hobnail appearance.
2. Anorexia, weight loss, weakness, and fatigability occur;

jaundice and fever may be present in the active stage. There are signs of portal hypertension and estrogen–androgen imbalance.
3. Later—chronic failure of liver function and obstruction of portal circulation.
   a. Obstruction of portal circulation, causing portal hypertension with congestion of spleen, pancreas, and gastrointestinal tract.
      (1) Chronic dyspepsia, change in bowel habits—diarrhea, constipation
      (2) Esophageal varices, dilated cutaneous veins around the umbilicus, internal hemorrhoids, ascites, splenomegaly, pancytopenia, and caput medusae
   b. Chronic failure of liver function
      (1) Plasma albumin is reduced, thereby leading to edema and contributing to ascites.
      (2) Weakness increases, leading to depression, wasting, delirium, coma, and eventually death.
      (3) Estrogen–androgen imbalance, causing spider angiomata and palmar erythema, amenorrhea develops in females; testicular and prostatic atrophy, gynecomastia, loss of libido, and impotence develop in males.
      (4) Bleeding tendencies may be evident.

Treatment

Medical management is directed toward minimizing further deterioration of liver function, correction of nutritional deficiencies and fluid and electrolyte imbalances, and relief of the patient's symptoms.
1. Prevent further damage to the liver by withdrawing toxic substances, alcohol, and drugs.
2. Offer supportive care of the patient.
3. Maintain adequate nutritional levels.
   a. Provide protein within ability of liver to handle it. Normal nutritious diet with vitamin supplements, especially B, C, and K and folate.
   b. Eliminate alcohol consumption.
4. Restrict salt intake when fluid retention occurs.
5. Protect the patient from infections and toxic agents.
6. Treat ascites with diuretics gently and only when acute activity of liver damage has subsided. (Potassium-sparing diuretics are frequently prescribed.)
   a. Although rarely the treatment of choice, portacaval shunt may be tried to control ascites; however, operative mortality is high.
   b. Abdominal paracentesis is to be avoided if possible (if necessary, see Procedure, p. 476).
   c. LeVeen peritoneovenous shunt may be performed; this is used only in patients with "intractable" ascites, circulatory failure of cirrhosis, or abdominal hernia with severe ascites.
      (1) Complications:
         (a) Coagulopathy (bleeding); requires monitoring of clotting factors
         (b) Shunt malfunction
7. Treat hepatic coma as necessary (see p. 478).
8. Provide multivitamin supplements and thiamine to compensate for liver's inability to store or activate them and folic acid to correct folic acid deficiency anemia.

Assessment
Diagnostic Evaluation

1. Liver biopsy—high risk of massive bleeding in presence of clotting defects (see p. 470 for precautions)
2. Esophagoscopy
3. Barium-contrast esophagography (only about 50% accurate) to check for esophageal varices
4. Radioisotopic liver scans—increased splenic and vertebral uptake of radioactive technetium (^{99}Tc) sulfur colloid
5. Paracentesis to examine ascitic fluid, for cell count, for protein content, and for bacterial count

Patient Problems/Nursing Diagnoses

1. Potential bleeding related to altered clotting mechanism and portal hypertension
2. Altered nutritional status related to inadequate dietary intake, anorexia, and gastrointestinal distress
3. Altered skin integrity related to edema, jaundice, and altered immune response
4. Activity intolerance related to fatigue, muscle wasting, and general disability

Planning and Implementation
Nursing Interventions

A. Decrease in the Risk of Bleeding

1. Anticipate manifestations of hemorrhage, such as ecchymosis, petechiae, and epistaxis; and initiate preventive measures.
2. Maintain a safe environment to prevent injury.
3. Avoid trauma such as forceful nose blowing, use of hard toothbrush, large-gauge needles for injection.
4. Apply prolonged pressure after arterial and venous punctures, and all injections.
5. Note and report signs of hematemesis and melena.
   a. Assess for anxiety, weakness, restlessness, and epigastric fullness as possibly heralding hemorrhage.
   b. Take and record vital signs frequently.
   c. Administer vitamin C as prescribed.
   d. Observe each stool for color, consistency, and amount. Test for occult blood.
   e. Record nature, amount, and time of vomiting.

B. Improvement in Nutritional Status

1. Evaluate nutritional status and needs.
2. Assist the patient in overcoming anorexia, weight loss, and fatigue.
   a. Encourage him to eat all meals and supplementary feedings by serving them with eye-catching appeal, in small servings, and in small frequent meals.
   b. Recognize the effect of esthetic factors—control odors, disturbing conversations, unpleasant situations.
   c. Eliminate alcohol but encourage high caloric intake.
   d. Give supplementary vitamins (A, B complex, C, and K) and folate.
   e. Conserve the patient's energy so that total food intake is not expended to replace energy requirements.
   f. Provide special mouth care if the patient has bleeding from gums.
   g. Offer small, frequent meals rather than 3 large meals.
   h. Consider the patient's preferences in food.
   i. If the patient is severely anorexic or nauseated and eating poorly, tube feeding may be necessary; include milk and starch hydrolysate. Do not increase dietary protein if serum ammonia level is increased.

j. Give pancreatin (if diarrhea and steatorrhea are present) to permit better tolerance of diet.

3. Monitor intake and output accurately; weigh carefully.

4. Adjust nutritional offerings if the patient has ascites or edema.
   a. Restrict sodium intake to 200–500 mg. daily (less than 10 mEq. daily).
   b. Maintain caloric and vitamin intake; give protein as tolerated.
   c. Avoid table salt, salty foods, salted margarine, and butter, as well as all ordinary frozen and canned foods, mouthwash, baking soda, and all other products containing large quantities of salt.
   d. Use "salt" substitutes such as lemon juice, oregano, thyme to enhance flavor; commercial salt substitute should be approved by physician.
   e. Encourage use of powdered low-sodium milk and milk products.
   f. If water accumulation is not controlled on above regimen, resort to the following:
      (1) Limit sodium allowance to 200 mg. daily.
      (2) Restrict fluids if serum sodium is low.
      (3) Administer oral diuretics—hydrochlorothiazide (HydroDiuril) furosemide (Lasix).
      (4) Administer spironolactone (Aldactone) if prescribed—this is an aldosterone-blocking agent used to reinforce the actions of diuretics and prevent undue potassium loss.
      (5) Promote slow diuresis to avoid renal failure.
   g. Measure and record abdominal girth daily.

C. Improvement in Skin Integrity

1. Observe skin and control pruritus.
   a. Provide good skin care; bathe without soap; apply soothing lotions.
   b. Keep the patient's fingernails short to prevent him from scratching his skin.
   c. Administer medications as prescribed for pruritus; be alert for side effects of nausea, diarrhea or constipation, and vitamin K depletion, which leads to bleeding.

2. Turn the patient frequently to prevent pressure sores.

3. Avoid trauma to skin through gentle handling and prevention of falls.

4. Encourage intake of foods high in vitamin C.

D. Promotion of Rest and Balanced Activities

1. Promote rest during acute episodes to decrease demands on the liver.

2. Limit visitors.

3. Encourage the patient to limit activity when fatigued.

4. Assist the patient in planning activities to limit exertion.

5. Encourage gradual resumption of activities.

Health Education

Instruct the patient regarding precautions and regimen to follow upon discharge from the hospital.

1. Stress the necessity of giving up alcohol completely; urge acceptance of skillful assistance from psychiatrist, Alcoholics Anonymous, or the alcohol treatment unit in the hospital.

2. Provide written dietary instructions, emphasizing the restriction of sodium (and protein, if necessary).

3. Emphasize the significance of rest, a sensible lifestyle, and an adequate, well-balanced diet.

4. Involve the person closest to the patient (usually spouse) because recovery often is not easy and relapses are common; a close, trusted helper can help patient over the rough spots.

Evaluation

Expected Outcomes

1. Experiences decreased risk of bleeding
   a. No episodes of hemorrhage or frank bleeding (absence of melena, hematemesis and epistaxis; no petechiae, hematoma formation, or ecchymosis)
   b. Minimizes risk of trauma (blows nose gently, uses soft toothbrush, avoids straining during defecation, avoids falls by following safety measures)

2. Increases nutritional intake—consumes diet based on specific nutritional and vitamin needs; eliminates alcohol from diet; gains weight without increased edema or ascites

3. Skin intact, with no evidence of excoriation or infection; decreased scratching; normal skin turgor without edema
   a. Applies soothing lotions to skin to avoid itching
   b. Changes position frequently to relieve pressure and avoids trauma to skin

4. Demonstrates increased activity tolerance with periods of rest and relaxation as needed; shows increased strength and sense of well-being; carries out own self-care as capable; plans activities to avoid undue exertion

Guidelines: Assisting with Abdominal Paracentesis

Paracentesis is the withdrawal of fluid from the abdominal or peritoneal cavity.

Purposes
1. To withdraw fluid for diagnostic examination.
2. To remove ascitic fluid when large accumulation of fluid causes severe symptoms and is resistant to other therapy.
3. To prepare for other procedures (peritoneal dialysis, ascitic fluid reinfusion, surgery, etc.).

Danger and Complications
1. In chronic liver disease, paracentesis may precipitate hepatic coma.
2. Shock and hypovolemia can occur if fluid from general circulation shifts to abdomen to replace withdrawn fluid; this can be minimized if no more than 1 liter of paracentesis fluid is withdrawn, or if lost fluid is replaced by parenteral administration of salt-poor human albumin.

Equipment

Sterile paracentesis tray and gloves
Procaine hydrochloride 1%
Drape or cotton blankets
Collection bottle (vacuum bottle)
Skin preparation tray with antiseptic
Specimen bottles and laboratory forms

Procedure

Nursing Action	Rationale/Amplification
Preparatory Phase	
1. Explain procedure to the patient.	1. This may reduce the patient's fear and anxiety.
2. Record the patient's vital signs.	2. Provides baseline values for later comparison.
3. Have the patient void before treatment is begun. See that consent form has been signed.	3. This will lessen the danger of accidentally piercing the bladder with the needle or trocar.
4. Position the patient in Fowler's position with back, arms, and feet supported (sitting on the side of the bed is a frequently used position).	4. The patient is more comfortable, and a steady position can be maintained.
5. Drape the patient with sheet exposing abdomen.	5. Minimizes exposure of patient and keeps him warm.
Performance Phase	
1. Assist physician in preparing skin with antiseptic solution.	1. This is considered a minor surgical procedure, requiring aseptic precautions.
2. Open sterile tray and package of sterile gloves; provide anesthetic solution.	
3. Have collection bottle and tubing available.	
4. Assess pulse and respiratory status frequently during procedure; watch for pallor, cyanosis, or syncope (faintness).	4. Preliminary indications of shock must be watched for. Keep emergency stimulants available.
5. Physician administers local anesthesia and introduces No. 20 needle or trocar.	
6. Needle or trocar is connected to tubing and vacuum bottle or syringe; fluid is drained from peritoneal cavity.	6. Drainage is usually limited to 1–2 liters to relieve acute symptoms and minimize risk of hypovolemia and shock.
7. Apply dressing when needle is withdrawn.	7. Elasticized adhesive patch is effective, serving as waterproof adhering dressing.
Follow-up Phase	
1. Assist the patient to be comfortable after treatment.	
2. Record amount and kind of fluid removed, number of specimens sent to laboratory, the patient's condition through treatment.	
3. Check blood pressure and vital signs every half hour for 2 hours, every hour for 4 hours, and every 4 hours for 24 hours.	3. Close observation will detect poor circulatory adjustment and possible development of shock.
4. Usually, a dressing is sufficient; however, if the trocar wound appears large, the physician may close the incision with sutures.	
5. Watch for leakage or scrotal edema after paracentesis.	5. If seen, notify physician at once.

Hepatic Coma/Hepatic Encephalopathy

Two Major Types

1. Fulminant—due to acute massive liver cell necrosis, usually in previously healthy liver. Mortality in adults is 50%–60%, but it is lower in younger age-groups.
2. Subacute—due to acute metabolic insult in a cirrhotic patient with borderline compensation of hepatic function. Mortality is 10%–20% and usually reversible if the precipitating cause is withdrawn (see below).

Causes

1. Incomplete metabolism of nitrogenous compounds by the diseased liver—manifestation of profound liver failure.
2. Biochemical abnormalities responsible are not known; however, significant accumulation of nitrogenous substances, particularly ammonia, in the blood is believed to be highly suspect.

3. Shunting of portal blood that contains ammonia and other bacterial metabolites of protein around the damaged liver.

Precipitating Factors

1. Progressive hepatocellular diseases not associated with any acute irritation of the liver
2. Increased sources of ammonia in the blood; azotemia, high-protein diet, gastrointestinal bleeding, following administration of ammonium chloride, thiazides
3. Infections, paracentesis, acute alcoholism, hypotension, shock, general anesthesia, minor surgery, hypokalemia, alkalosis, administration of sedatives or narcotics
4. Portacaval shunts, especially if protein in the diet is not restricted postoperatively

Pathophysiology

A. Cellular changes

1. Disruption of enzymatic function in liver cells, muscle, and brain
2. Failure of liver cells to detoxify the ammonia (by converting it to urea)
3. Accumulation of sympathomimetic amines (false neurotransmitters) from abnormal metabolism of aromatic amino acids

B. Sources of ammonia—it comes from the bloodstream as a result of the following:

1. Its absorption from the *gastrointestinal tract* (largest source)
   Enzymatic and bacterial digestion of ingested protein and of urea passing from blood into the gastrointestinal tract increases blood ammonia.
   Increases result from:
   a. Gastrointestinal bleeding
   b. High-protein diet
   c. Ingestion of ammonium salts (diuretic—ammonium chloride)
   d. Bacterial overgrowth in small bowel (infection)
   e. Uremia
2. Its production by metabolizing *kidney* tissue (deamination of various amino acids, especially glutamine). Increases with:
   a. Diuretics (steroids, chlorothiazide)
   b. Restriction of dietary sodium (hyponatremia)
   c. Potassium depletion (hypokalemia)
   d. Alkalosis
3. Its liberation from contracting *muscle* cells. Increases during exercise.

Treatment/Management

A. The precipitating causes are identified and treated if possible. Nitrogen load and ammonia production and absorption from gastrointestinal tract are decreased.

1. Arrest gastrointestinal bleeding and reduce intraintestinal nitrogen.
   a. If there is upper gastrointestinal bleeding, constant gastric aspiration may be required.
   b. If bleeding has ceased, administer a cathartic or enema to clear blood from intestine.
   c. Cancel requests for ammonium products, sedatives, tranquilizers, and narcotics.
   d. Greatly reduce dietary protein—if patient begins to improve, gradually increase protein intake; provide sufficient calories in absorbable form (i.e., IV glucose or lipid emulsion).
   e. Cleanse the intestinal tract of nitrogenous substrates by administering prescribed purgatives such as magnesium citrate or sorbitol, or enemas.
   f. Administer oral lactulose, if prescribed, to reduce intestinal absorption of ammonia.
   g. Give neomycin, a nonabsorbable antibiotic, if prescribed, to suppress urea-splitting enteric bacteria.
   h. Administer lactulose (Cephulac) to reduce blood ammonia if neomycin is contraindicated.
   i. Reduce and eliminate all unnecessary sedatives and analgesics. Administer only those specifically prescribed.
   j. Weigh the patient daily and keep an accurate intake and output record; record frequency and characteristics of feces.

B. Prevention and treatment of complications. Underlying liver disease is treated if possible.

1. Correct preexisting complicating diseases—cardiovascular, renal, and pulmonary.
2. Treat any infections, including respiratory infections, since these can become severe in this patient.
3. Administer antacids to reduce gastric acid and to protect against peptic ulceration. Prophylactic use of intravenous cimetidine to keep gastric pH above 5.0 is helpful.
4. Monitor blood glucose every 8 hours or whenever level of consciousness deteriorates; administer intravenous glucose.
5. Monitor status of hydration and correct any electrolyte, acid–base, or fluid imbalance.

C. Supportive therapy

1. Correct electrolyte abnormalities, especially hypokalemia.
2. Provide adequate nutrition.

Assessment

Clinical Manifestations

Five stages:
1. Minor mental aberrations—the patient is slightly confused, untidy, and displaying inappropriate behavior and defective abstract thinking.
2. Motor disturbance—coarse or "flapping" tremor (*asterixis*), especially of hands, hyper-reflexia.
3. Progression to gross disturbances of consciousness—somnolence or stupor, hepatic encephalopathy (HE).
4. Complete disorientation to time and place; eventual coma.
5. Decerebrate rigidity, hypoventilation → apnea.

Patient Problems/Nursing Diagnoses

1. Risk of bleeding
2. Impaired skin integrity
3. Altered nutritional status related to inadequate dietary intake, anorexia, and gastrointestinal distress
4. Impaired thought processes related to rising blood ammonia levels
5. Impaired ability to carry out activities of daily living related to deterioration of neurologic function and rising blood ammonia levels

Planning and Implementation

Nursing Interventions

A. Improvement in Neurologic Status and Thought Processes

1. Evaluate neurologic function
   a. Assess the patient's neurologic status (i.e., his ability to do handwriting and perform simple

arithmetic calculations). Keep daily record and note differences.
   b. Observe and record the extent and magnitude of characteristic tremor.
   c. Note and record state of consciousness, including slight drowsiness, slight confusion, drowsy, confused, or disoriented.
   d. Note response to painful stimuli.
   e. When the patient does not respond, note sucking and grasping abilities; check corneal reflex.
2. Recognize signs of increasing stupor, notify physician, and initiate nursing measures as follows:
   a. Be alert for evidence of mental changes, lethargy, hallucinations.
   b. Avoid giving the patient narcotics and barbiturates.
   c. Restrict dietary protein; offer small high-calorie feedings frequently.
   d. Protect the patient by keeping him in bed; pad siderails.
   e. Arouse the patient at intervals; orient to time, place, and person.
   f. Limit visitors.
   g. Provide constant nursing surveillance and emphasize sensitivity to the patient's changes and needs.
3. Remove factors that precipitate hepatic coma.
   a. Administer intestinal antibiotics (neomycin) as prescribed to reduce serum ammonia absorption from gastrointestinal tract.
   b. Administer medications with caution.
   c. Promote bowel evacuation to reduce intestinal nitrogen load.

   d. Prevent complications that increase metabolic rate and severity of hepatic coma (e.g., infection, sepsis, aspiration, hypovolemia)

B. Promotion of Rest and Activity as Indicated

1. Eliminate unnecessary stimuli to promote rest when indicated.
   a. Group nursing activities together to minimize disruption of the patient's rest.
   b. Limit visitors.
   c. Eliminate or reduce environmental noise and light.
2. Assist the patient in planning periods of rest and activity when symptoms begin to subside.
3. Encourage gradual resumption of activities during recovery.

Evaluation
Expected Outcomes

1. Demonstrates improved thought processes—identifies time, place, person correctly; initiates conversation and responds appropriately to others' conversations; shows no signs of hallucinating or periods of confusion
2. Shows improved mental status—performs simple arithmetic calculations, responds normally to painful (and other) stimuli
3. Demonstrates return of normal neurologic reflexes and responses.
4. Participates in appropriate schedule of rest and activity—carries out own hygiene and self-care activities as capable, reports increased strength and well-being; gradually resumes activities and mild activity

Bleeding Esophageal Varices

Esophageal varices are dilated tortuous veins found in the submucosa of the lower esophagus; they may extend up in the esophagus and down into the stomach.

Pathophysiology

1. Increasing portal vein obstruction—venous blood returning to right atrium from intestinal tract and spleen seeks new pathways, through enlarging collateral esophageal veins.
2. Usually no symptoms are produced by dilated veins unless mucosa becomes ulcerated.
3. Hematemesis and melena, plus a history of alcoholism, tend to suggest esophageal varices; however, bleeding may result from associated gastritis or duodenal ulcer in 25% of patients with varices.
4. The strain of coughing or vomiting may precipitate variceal rupture, hemorrhage, and death.
5. Irritation of vessels by gastroesophageal reflux may cause esophagitis, esophageal rupture, hemorrhage, and death.
6. Has a high mortality rate due to further deterioration of liver function (hepatic coma) and complications (e.g., aspiration pneumonia, sepsis, renal failure).

Etiology

1. Nearly always due to portal hypertension, which may result from obstruction of the portal venous circulation and cirrhosis of the liver.

2. Abnormalities of the circulation in splenic vein or superior vena cava.

Treatment

A. Control of Hemorrhage

1. Purpose
   a. To lessen transfusion requirements.
   b. To reduce large amounts of blood in gastrointestinal tract.
   c. To avoid hepatic coma.
2. Methods
   a. Administer vasopressin systemically to reduce portal pressure and to initiate hemostasis. Intraarterial infusion into the superior mesenteric artery may be used after angiography, but offers no definitive advantage.
   b. Ice-water lavage of stomach (gastric hypothermia) may temporarily control bleeding.
   c. Aspirate blood from the stomach.
   d. Esophageal tamponade—pressure is exerted on the cardiac portion of the stomach and against the bleeding varices by a double balloon tamponade (Sengstaken–Blakemore tube).
   e. Treat bleeding by complete rest of the esophagus (parenteral feedings); avoid straining and vomiting and continue gastric suction.
   f. Initiate vitamin K therapy; administer multiple blood transfusions.

g. Avoid sedation, since it may lead to coma.
h. Administer saline cathartic (magnesium citrate) plus enemata to remove blood.

B. Injection Sclerotherapy

This method of controlling bleeding from esophageal varices has been used recently to treat patients who are poor surgical risks.

1. A sclerosing agent is injected through a fiberoptic endoscope into the bleeding varices to promote thrombosis and sclerosis.
2. May be used as prophylactic measure to treat varices before bleeding has occurred.
3. The patient may require repeated treatments if bleeding recurs.
4. The patient must be observed after treatment for bleeding, perforation of the esophagus, and aspiration pneumonia.

C. Surgical Intervention

If bleeding of esophageal varices is not controlled by conservative measures, surgical procedures may be employed:

1. Surgical Procedures
   a. Direct ligation of varices.
   b. Surgical by-pass (*portacaval anastomosis*)—by shunting portal blood into the vena cava, pressure in the portal system is reduced.
   c. Splenorenal shunt—a shunt is made between the splenic vein and the left renal vein; this is done when the portal vein cannot be used because of thrombosis or for other reasons.
2. Evaluation of Surgery
   a. Varying degrees of success are reported with shunting procedures.
   b. The success depends mainly on the condition of the patient; it is used as an emergency procedure following bleeding. Most common use is to prevent recurrence after the patient recovers from an initial variceal bleed.
   c. Complications are acute hepatic failure and chronic portal systemic encephalopathy (PSE).
   d. Postoperative care is similar to postabdominal surgery complicated by care required for a patient with severe cirrhotic liver.

Assessment

Clinical Manifestations

1. Blood loss may be sudden and massive; frank hemorrhage from upper gastrointestinal tract may occur.
2. Hematemesis, melena, or rectal bleeding (bright red blood).
3. May develop signs of hypovolemia and shock.
4. Should be suspected in all patients with signs of portal hypertension (e.g., ascites, dilated abdominal veins) or any occurrence of upper gastrointestinal hemorrhage.

Diagnostic Evaluation

1. The patient's history, physical examination, and neurologic examination will assist in identifying any evidence of hepatic encephalopathy.
2. Fiberoptic endoscopy may be used if bleeding is controlled. It is essential to exclude other causes of bleeding.
3. If bleeding is massive, arteriography or umbilical venous catheterization to visualize portal collaterals; by placement of a catheter in the portal vein via recanalized umbilical vein, direct venous pressure and portovenography can be done in 75% of patients.
4. Splenoportography using diodrast can be effective when studied as a series of x-ray plates or done as a segmental roentgenogram; extensive collateral circulation of esophageal vessels may be indicative of varices.
5. Portal vein pressure above 250 mm. of water is abnormal; this can be measured in the operating room by introducing a needle into spleen or via umbilical vein catheter.
6. Liver function tests include bromsulphalein retention, serum transaminase, bilirubin, serum proteins, alkaline phosphatase, serum ammonia levels.

Patient Problems/Nursing Diagnoses

1. The patient who experiences bleeding esophageal varices has severe liver disease and, as a result, is subject to the problems encountered in cirrhosis and hepatic coma (see p. 478 for discussion). In addition, this critically ill patient experiences the following problems:
2. Potential hypovolemia related to blood loss
3. Potential impaired gas exchange related to asphyxiation and aspiration pneumonia
4. Increased risk of bleeding related to erosion of gastric and esophageal mucosa, portal hypertension, and abnormal clotting mechanism
5. Fear related to possibility of massive hemorrhage and possibly impending death

Planning and Implementation

Nursing Interventions

A. Maintaining Adequate Fluid Volume

1. Assess for signs of potential hypovolemia:
   a. Monitor blood pressure; arterial catheter may be inserted to monitor blood pressure directly. Use CVP monitoring for fluid replacement.
   b. Assess urinary output; indwelling catheter may be required.
   c. Check blood gases to assess oxygenation of blood. An endotracheal tube may be inserted to protect, control and manage the patient's airway.
2. Initiate measures to overcome blood loss.
   a. Replace blood with *fresh* whole blood.
      (1) Ammonia content is lower than in stored blood
      (2) Coagulation effect is greater, particularly if the patient has severe liver disease.
   b. Administer vitamin K intramuscularly.

B. Improving Gas Exchange

1. Assess respirations and blood gases frequently.
2. Note and report occurrence of signs of obstructed airway or ruptured esophagus from Sengstaken–Blakemore tube (e.g., changes in skin color, respirations, breath sounds, level of consciousness, presence of chest pain, vital signs, etc.)
3. Check location and inflation of balloons of Sengstaken–Blakemore tube frequently.
4. Have scissors readily available. Cut tubing and remove Sengstaken–Blakemore tube immediately if the patient develops acute respiratory distress.
5. Keep head of bed elevated to avoid gastric regurgitation and aspiration of gastric contents.

C. Reducing Fear and Apprehension

1. Explain all procedures to the patient.
2. Remain with patient; place call bell within patient's reach.
3. Maintain close surveillance of the patient.
4. Avoid discussing the patient's condition or unrelated matters in the patient's vicinity.
5. Provide alternate means of communication if tubes or other equipment interfere with patient's ability to talk.
6. Use touch and other tactile stimuli to provide reassurance to patient.
7. Use protective restraints to prevent dislodging of Sengstaken–Blakemore tube in confused, combative patient.
8. Aspirate the patient's airway if indicated.

D. Reducing the Risk of Bleeding

1. Observe the patient for straining, gagging, or vomiting; these increase pressure in portal system and increase risk of further bleeding.
2. Note and report signs of hematemesis and melena. Check all gastrointestinal secretions and feces for occult and frank blood.
3. Observe for signs of hypovolemia and shock.

4. Remove blood from gastrointestinal tract to reduce possibility of hepatic encephalopathy (hepatic coma).
5. Perform gavage with iced saline if bleeding recurs.
6. Have extra Sengstaken–Blakemore tube available for reinsertion if bleeding occurs or recurs.
7. When bleeding has ceased, introduce nonirritating, soothing foods and fluids gradually.
8. Reinforce need for the patient to avoid alcohol.

Evaluation

Expected Outcomes

1. Experiences decreased risk of bleeding—no episodes of straining, gagging, or vomiting; no hematemesis or melena; blood-free gastrointestinal secretions and stools; no recurrence of bleeding, hypovolemia or shock
2. Demonstrates improved gas exchange—normal respiratory rate and pattern, normal breath sounds, adequate blood gases; absence of chest pain, dyspnea, or shortness of breath; appropriate cough, clear sputum
3. Demonstrates lessening of fear and apprehension
4. Uses alternate means of communication when necessary.

Guidelines: Using the Sengstaken–Blakemore Tube to Control Esophageal Bleeding

Purposes
1. To exert pressure on the cardiac portion of the stomach and against bleeding varices by a double balloon tamponade.
2. To reduce transfusion requirements.
3. To prevent blood accumulation in the gastrointestinal tract, which could precipitate hepatic coma.

Equipment

Sengstaken–Blakemore tube
Basin with cracked ice
Clamp for tubing
Towel and emesis basin
Glass of water and straw
Flashlight

Procedure (Fig. 10-18)

Preparatory Phase

1. Provide nursing support by reassuring the patient that this procedure will help to control his bleeding.
2. Explain procedure to the patient and tell him how breathing through the mouth and swallowing can help in passing the tube.
3. Elevate head of bed slightly unless the patient is in shock.

Nursing Action	Rationale/Amplification
Performance Phase	
1. Check balloons by trial inflation to detect leaks.	1. This is best done under water because it is easier to see escaping air bubbles.
2. Chill the tube, then lubricate it before physician passes it via mouth or nose (preferable).	2. Chilling will make the tube more firm and lubrication will lessen friction.
3. After the tube has entered the stomach, gavage stomach and aspirate all clots.	
4. After obtaining an x-ray of the lower chest and upper abdomen to check position of the balloon, it is fully inflated (200–250 ml.) of air and then pulled back gently.	4. This is to exert force against cardia. The triple-lumen tube provides 2 channels to inflate compression balloons, one in the stomach and one in the esophagus. Balloons are inflated using a manometer to measure pressure to 25 or 30 mm. Hg.

(continued)

Guidelines: Using the Sengstaken-Blakemore Tube to Control Esophageal Bleeding (continued)

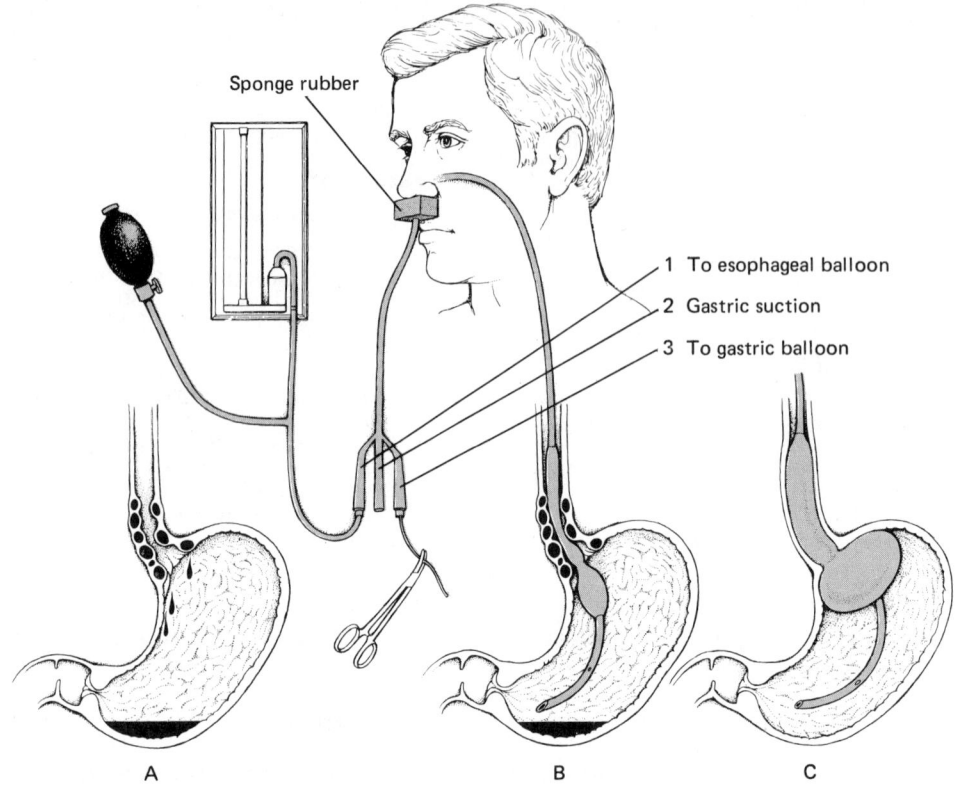

Sponge rubber

1 To esophageal balloon
2 Gastric suction
3 To gastric balloon

A   B   C

Figure 10-18. Diagram showing esophageal varices and their treatment by a compressing balloon tube (Sengstaken–Blakemore). (*A*) Dilated veins of the lower esophagus. (*B*) The tube is in place in the stomach and the lower esophagus but is not inflated. (*C*) Inflation of the tube and compression of the veins, which can be obtained by inflation of the balloon. In some instances, it may be necessary to pass an additional tube through the other nostril for the purpose of aspirating secretions.
Note: The Minnesota four-lumen esophagogastric tamponade tube has an additional outlet for aspiration of the esophagus.

Procedure
(Cont.)

Nursing Action	Rationale / Amplification
5. Traction is placed on tubing where it enters the patient's nose. Then the esophageal bag is inflated to 35–40 mm. Hg. This is tied with double ties to prevent leakage (Fig. 10-19).	5. This keeps balloons in position and assists in exerting proper pressure.
6. Gastric suction may be attached to the 3rd outlet of the catheter.	6. By using suction and irrigating the tubing hourly, it is possible to tell how well the bleeding is controlled by the appearance of the drainage.
7. A second nasogastric (Levin) tube is passed into the lower esophagus.*	7. To aspirate saliva and to check for bleeding *above* the esophageal balloon.
8. Deflate esophageal balloon for 5 minutes at 8- or 12-hour intervals. Do not deflate gastric balloon under traction.	8. To prevent erosion and necrosis of the esophagus or stomach. If the gastric balloon is deflated or ruptures while traction on the tube is applied, the inflated esophageal balloon will be pulled upward and obstruct the patient's airway.
9. Pressure on tubes and traction is released in 2–4 days.	9. If bleeding remains controlled, the tubing is removed in 24 hours.

* If the Minnesota four-lumen esophagogastric tube is used, this will not be necessary.

Nursing Responsibilities

1. Maintain *constant* vigilance while balloons are inflated in the patient.
2. Keep balloon pressures at required level to control bleeding. (Hemostats are utilized as clamps.)
3. Observe and record vital signs frequently—bleeding, shock, etc.
4. Be alert for chest pain—may indicate injury or rupture of esophagus.
5. Irrigate suction tube as prescribed; observe and record nature and color of aspirated material.
6. Keep head of bed elevated to avoid gastric regurgitation and to diminish nausea and a sensation of gagging.
7. Maintain nutritional and electrolyte levels parenterally.
8. Maintain nasogastric suction to aspirate saliva through an accessory nasogastric tube.
9. Note nature of breathing; if counterweight pulls the tube into oropharynx, the patient may be asphyxiated.

▶ **NURSING ALERT:** Keep a pair of scissors taped to the head of the bed. In the event of *acute respiratory distress*, use the scissors to cut across tubing (to deflate both balloons) and remove tubing.

Note: This procedure should be reserved for patients who are known, without a doubt, to be bleeding from esophageal varices, and in whom all forms of conservative therapy have failed.

Chief Hazard: Vomiting with an inflated esophageal balloon tamponade in place, which results in massive pulmonary aspiration. Manage this problem by inserting a nasogastric tube in the free nostril to drain the esophagus above the esophageal balloon, thereby preventing aspiration. The Minnesota four-lumen esophagogastric tamponade tube has the additional outlet for aspiration of the esophagus.

Diseases of the Biliary (Gallbladder) System

Incidence

1. About 500,000 persons a year in the US are hospitalized for gallbladder disease; two thirds of these are treated surgically.
2. Women develop the disease more frequently than men: 4 to 1.
3. Patients are most often past 40, multiparous, and overweight; however, the condition can also occur in younger patients.
4. Postmenopausal women on estrogen therapy are at greater risk for gallbladder disease; likewise, women on birth control pills are at greater risk than nonusers of these pills.
5. Malabsorption of bile salts in patients with gastrointestinal disease or T-tube fistula or those who have had ileal resection increases the risk of gallstones and gallbladder disease.

Pathophysiology

1. Ninety-five percent of patients with acute cholecystitis have gallstones; however, a majority of the 15 million Americans with gallstones have no pain and are unaware of the presence of stones.
2. There are two types of gallstones: those composed of pigment and those composed of cholesterol.
3. Pigment stones form when unconjugated pigments in the bile precipitate to form stones, which must be removed surgically.
4. Cholesterol stones account for most gallbladder disease in the US; these stones form in the presence of cholesterol-saturated bile, which is low in bile acid synthesis.
5. Cholesterol-saturated bile acts as an irritant and produces inflammatory changes in the gallbladder.

Types of Gallbladder Disease

("Chole"—gallbladder)
Cholecystitis—inflammation of the gallbladder
Cholelithiasis—stones in the gallbladder
Choledocholithiasis—stones in the common duct

Diagnostic Evaluation of Biliary Conditions

Overall assessment of the patient should include detection of associated disease processes (cardiovascular, pulmonary, and renal); diabetes status; and realization of increased surgical risk if patient is over age 65.

A. Flat Plate of Abdomen—used to visualize the 25% of stones that are radiopaque.

B. Cholecystography—used to visualize the shape and position of the gallbladder.

Note: This test is effective only if the liver cells are functioning properly and are capable of excreting the radiopaque contrast medium into the bile.

1. Purpose
   a. To detect gallstones
   b. To estimate ability of gallbladder to fill, concentrate its contents, contract, and empty in a normal manner
2. Method
   a. Because gallstones are usually radiolucent, it is necessary to fill the gallbladder with a radiopaque contrast medium, which permits stones to show up as clear areas.
   b. Iodide-containing contrast medium is excreted into bile by the liver and concentrated in the gallbladder. Caution: Prior to administration of iodide, determine whether patient is sensitive to iodine.
      (1) Orally
         (a) Contrast media may be given by mouth (e.g., Telepaque, Monophen).
         (b) Iodide preparation is usually given in oral doses of 3.6 gm. approximately 10–12 hours before x-ray. If there is no visualization the next morning, repeat dose of 3.6 gm. the following evening.
         (c) Administer nothing by mouth from the time of iodide administration to the time of x-ray to prevent contraction of

gallbladder and expulsion of contrast medium.
  (2) Intravenously
      Intravenous cholecystography involves giving an iodide preparation (e.g., Cholografin) about 10 minutes before x-ray.
3. Patient preparation
  a. At least 1 hour after the evening meal, the patient takes the prescribed tablets or capsules of iodide preparation by mouth.
  b. These tablets are taken one at a time at 3- to 5-minute intervals with at least 8 oz. of water.
  c. From this time until bedtime, nothing is taken by mouth except water; from midnight on, water is also excluded. (If nausea, vomiting, or diarrhea occurs, notify physician; test may be postponed.)
  d. No laxatives are given during this time; however, a saline enema may be required on the morning of the x-ray.
  e. Breakfast is withheld, and the patient goes to x-ray.
  f. Right upper abdominal quadrant is x-rayed.
  g. The patient is fed a fatty meal containing cream, butter, or eggs to test contractility of the gallbladder.
  h. X-ray examination is repeated at intervals until gallbladder has expelled contrast medium.

▶ **NURSING ALERT:** Cholecystography is ineffective in the jaundiced patient, since the liver cells in this situation cannot transport contrast medium to the biliary tract.

  C. **Cholangiography**—(contrast medium is injected directly into biliary tree)
  1. Advantages
    a. Procedure is best way to visualize biliary tree in the patient after cholecystectomy.
    b. All components of the biliary tree can be observed—hepatic ducts within liver, common hepatic duct, and cystic duct, but the gallbladder is often not well visualized.
  2. Clinical usefulness
    a. In differentiating hepatocellular jaundice from jaundice due to biliary obstruction

  b. In locating stones within bile ducts
  c. In detecting and diagnosing cancer of the biliary system.
  d. In investigating gastrointestinal symptoms of patients who had cholecystectomy.
  3. Patient preparation
    a. The patient is dehydrated by restricting his fluid intake.
    b. Enema is given early in morning of test.
    c. A sedative is given at least 1 hour before the x-ray.
    d. Contrast medium (e.g., Cholografin sodium) is injected either intravenously (results not as conclusive) or directly into the common duct.
      (1) Operatively; this can be done during surgery.
      (2) Postoperatively, by injecting contrast medium into the common duct drain.
      (3) Via retrograde endoscopic cannulation of duct via duodenum.
    e. Following the x-ray, regardless of method of contrast medium injection, as much as possible of the contrast medium and bile is aspirated to prevent leakage into the peritoneal cavity, thus avoiding a possible bile peritonitis.

  Note: Operative cholangiography may be done during gallbladder surgery in the operating room.

  D. **Ultrasound Examination (Echogram)**—B scanner and transducer

  This test can be used to demonstrate gallbladder distention, bile duct distention, and calculi.

  E. **Liver Scan**

  1. In the jaundiced patient, this scan may show evidence of hepatocellular disease or metastatic lesions.
  2. With radioactive rose bengal, which is excreted by the liver-like gallbladder dyes, obstructive pathology of the biliary tree may be revealed.

  F. **Endoscopic Retrograde Cholangiopancreatography** (ERCP)

  See Guidelines, below.

Guidelines: Endoscopic Retrograde Cholangiopancreatography (ERCP)

A fiberoptic endoscope (a side-viewing instrument) is placed in the descending duodenum so that the ampulla of Vater can be located and cannulated (Fig. 10-19).
  In this examination, both the common and pancreatic ducts may be injected with contrast media to visualize the hepatobiliary tree and pancreatic ducts radiologically.
  The clinician is able to diagnose abnormalities of the ductal system, detect disease processes, and obtain direct secretory information, as well as cells for cytologic examination.

Indications

1. Biliary disease
2. Pancreatic disease
3. To diagnose:
   Cancer of the papilla
   Obstructive jaundice
   Calculus disease, pre- and postcholecystectomy

   Carcinoma of biliary ducts
   Carcinoma of pancreas
   Pancreatitis

Contraindications

1. Acute cardiorespiratory disease
2. Acute recent attack of pancreatitis (within 3 weeks) because of risk of inducing another attack
3. Stricture or obstruction of esophagus or duodenum
4. Acute cholangitis

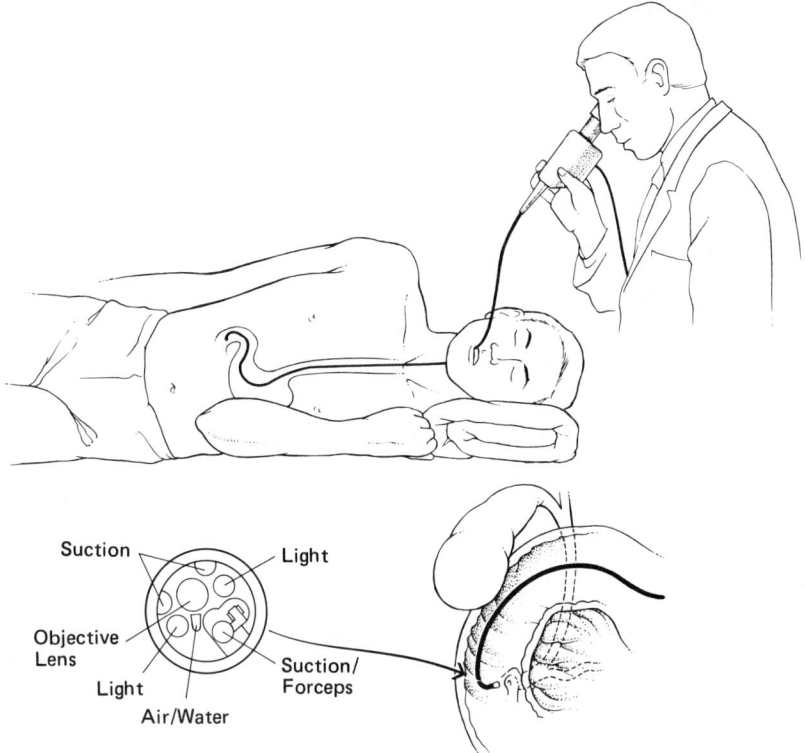

Figure 10-19. Endoscopic retrograde cholangiopancreatography (ERCP). The patient is moved from left lateral to prone position as the flexible scope is passed. The circle on the left shows the tip of the scope; the objective lens is the viewing section assisted by two side lights. Air or water may be directed to an area, and suction is available. If a biopsy is to be taken, a separate channel is available.

The lower right diagram shows the scope nearing the ampulla of Vater; the scope is in the duodenum; gallbladder is the topmost sac—note the biliary and common bile ducts.

Equipment

A side-viewing duodenoscope* (to be sterilized after use with suspected infectious patients)

Sterilized cannula

This duodenoscope is 125 cm. long and 1 cm. in diameter. Visual fields are oriented 90 degrees to its long axis. It includes a channel through which a cannula or biopsy forceps can be passed under direct vision.

Considerations

1. ERCP is not a simple endoscopic procedure; it must be done by a skillful, well-trained physician.
2. There are certain risks, described below:
   a. After ERCP, a very small percentage of patients develop clinical pancreatitis, which may last 1–3 days.
   b. The patient may retain contrast material injected proximal to an obstructed duct; this may result in cholangitis or pancreatitis. Such a patient should be given broad-spectrum antibiotics; surgical drainage may be indicated.
   c. A very few patients are sensitive to iodinated compounds.
   d. The more experienced the team in performing ERCPs, the fewer the complications and the better the success rate.

Procedure

Nursing Action	Physician's Role	Rationale / Amplification
Preparatory Phase		
1. Be sure that consent form is signed and noted on the patient's chart.	1. Obtain informed consent.	
2. Remind the patient to take nothing by mouth after midnight.	2. Collaborate with nurse in patient preparation.	2. Limited intake produces a basal condition with reduced body secretions; this permits better visualization of tissues.

(continued)

Guidelines: Endoscopic Retrograde Cholangiopancreatography (ERCP) (continued)

Procedure
(Cont.)

Nursing Action	Physician's Role	Rationale/Amplification
3. Explain contemplated examination to patient; discuss possibilities of aftereffects.		
4. Determine the patient's sensitivity to iodine (or fish, which contains iodine) or any other medication.		4. A few patients are sensitive to iodine preparations (Hypaque sodium).
5. Take and record vital signs.		5. This information becomes a baseline for later comparison.
6. Offer the patient 3 ml. of tetracaine (Pontocaine) to be used as a gargle and swallow.		6. Tetracaine is an oropharyngeal topical anesthetic.
7. Intravenous infusion may be started, for administration of medications.	7. Start an intravenous infusion with normal saline.	7. This becomes the avenue for direct intravenous medications such as diazepam (Valium) and meperidine (Demerol) to promote relaxation prior to insertion of duodenoscope.
8. Instruct the patient to remove dentures; a mouthpiece is inserted.		8. To facilitate insertion of scope.

Performance Phase

1. Place the patient in left lateral position.	1. Scope is passed through the patient's mouth into esophagus and stomach.	1. Anatomy is carefully examined as the scope advances.
2. Administer IV medication, which may include Demerol, Valium, atropine, or glucagon.	2. Gently advance tip through pyloric ring into duodenal bulb and into descending duodenum.	2. Atropine will produce a hypotonic duodenum and relaxed sphincter at ampulla of Vater; secretion will be reduced.
	3. Minimal air insufflation used to search for the ampulla of Vater.	3. Unless this is obstructed by tumor, it can usually be identified with careful search.
4. Place the patient in prone position. (This provides the radiologist with a better position for fluoroscopy and radiography.)	4. Administer glucagon.	4. Glucagon is given to further reduce duodenal motility.
5. Prepare a special radiopaque Teflon cannulation tube by filling it with contrast medium (to eliminate air).	5. When cannulation tubing is in correct position, contrast medium is slowly injected: 3–5 ml. for pancreatic ductal system; 15–20 ml. for biliary ductal system.	5. Cannulation tube is passed through biopsy channel of scope. Contrast medium is warmed to body temperature. Tube is advanced under fluoroscopy. X-ray pictures are taken while patient is in prone position following injection of contrast medium.
6. Upon completion of film-taking, turn patient to lateral position. Draw blood sample for serum amylase determination. Use suction to remove oropharyngeal secretions.	6. Keep scope and cannula in place and patient in prone position until films are completed. If films are satisfactory, scope is carefully removed.	6. Await return and reading of films.

Follow-up Phase

1. Check vital signs every 4 hours. Notify family as to when the patient will return to his room.		1. Postcannulation patient may experience a temperature rise, chills, abdominal pain. Report these responses to physician.
2. In the absence of complications, permit the patient to eat in 2–4 hours (light diet); permit a full diet the next day.		2. A mild rise in serum amylase is observed in a high percentage of patients.
3. Watch for palpitations related to atropine sulfate injection. Also watch for respiratory depression and transient hypotension.		3. Some patients experience mild to severe epigastric pain, nausea, and vomiting. These discomforts are usually transitory.

A. Chronic Cholecystitis with Cholelithiasis

1. Assessment and clinical manifestations
   a. History of episodic, usually colicky epigastric or right upper quadrant (RUQ) pain, often associated with nausea and vomiting
   b. Jaundice due to choledocholithiasis
2. Treatment
   a. Surgery is advised if gallstones are present with typical pain attacks and/or jaundice. Whether asymptomatic stones should be removed surgically is still open to debate.
   b. In the older patient, the risk of surgery must be evaluated in relation to other disease conditions present.
   c. Chenodeoxycholic acid, chenodiol, can decrease the size of existing stones, dissolve small ones, and prevent new stones from forming.
      (1) The major adverse effects appear to be mild diarrhea and cramps and SGOT elevation; with dose regulation these disappear.
      (2) Stones may recur; therefore, long-term therapy may be required.
      (3) Useful only in treatment or prevention of stones composed chiefly of cholesterol
      (4) Should be used with caution in patients at risk from elevated serum cholesterol levels.
      (5) Indicated in patients at high risk from gallbladder surgery because of systemic disease or age.

B. Acute Cholecystitis

1. Clinical manifestations
   a. RUQ pain, fever, nausea, and vomiting.
   b. The condition may occur at any age, but it is most common in patients over the age of 50.
   c. The chief hazard is perforation with local or generalized peritonitis.
2. Treatment
   a. Provide hospitalization, bed rest, withholding of oral fluids, and insertion of nasogastric tube with suction.
   b. Administer IV fluids to correct electrolyte imbalance, to maintain adequate urinary output, and to provide nutritional needs.
   c. Administer medication for pain and antimicrobials for infection control.
   d. Prepare patient for laboratory studies, chest x-ray, ECG, and possibly intravenous cholangiogram.
   e. Record vital signs every 4 hours.
   f. Evaluate and prepare the patient for surgery, if indicated. (Most patients achieve remission with rest, intravenous fluids, nasogastric suction, analgesia, and antibiotic administration. Surgery is usually delayed until the acute symptoms subside; however, deterioration of the patient's condition mandates surgical intervention.)

Nonsurgical Management

Patient Problems/Nursing Diagnoses

1. Pain and discomfort related to obstruction of biliary system and inflammation and obstruction of the gallbladder
2. Altered nutritional status related to dietary intolerance and medical therapy (withholding of food and fluids and nasogastric suctioning)
3. Impaired skin integrity related to jaundice (a rare occurrence)

Planning and Implementation
Nursing Interventions

A. Relief of Pain and Increase in Comfort Level

1. Assess level, location, and severity of pain.
2. Administer meperidine hydrochloride as prescribed for pain relief.
3. Avoid use of morphine sulfate, which is thought to increase spasm of the sphincter of Oddi and thus increase pain.
4. Assist the patient to assume position of comfort.
5. Assess and record response to pain medication.
6. Assist the patient to cough and breathe deeply to avoid respiratory complications secondary to upper abdominal pain.

B. Improved Nutritional Status

1. Maintain intravenous infusion and withhold oral fluids during acute episode of cholecystitis.
2. Introduce foods and fluids gradually after acute symptoms subside.
3. Provide high protein and carbohydrate diet that is low in fat content.
4. Instruct the patient to avoid foods that may initiate pain and gas-forming foods.

Evaluation
Expected Outcomes

1. Demonstrates decreased pain and abdominal distention—normal respiratory rate and pattern; reports increased comfort, uses analgesics as prescribed
2. Maintains adequate dietary intake—consumes diet low in fat, high in protein and carbohydrates during recovery period, and identifies food to be avoided
3. Indicates fewer episodes of nausea, vomiting, food intolerance, and abdominal discomfort after meals

Surgical Management

Types of Gallbladder Surgery

1. Cholecystostomy

Simple opening of gallbladder to remove stones, bile, or pus; a tube is then sutured into the gallbladder for drainage.

Note: When the patient returns to the recovery unit, this drainage tube is connected to a drainage bottle.

2. Cholecystectomy

Removal of the gallbladder after ligation of the cystic duct and vessels; done in most situations of acute or chronic cholecystitis. A drain (Penrose type) may be inserted in the gallbladder bed to permit drainage into dressings.

3. Choledochostomy

An opening into the common duct for the purpose of removing obstructing stones; a drainage T-tube is inserted into the duct and is connected to a drainage bottle. Usually a cholecystectomy is done at this time because the gallbladder often contains stones also.

Preoperative Nursing Management

1. Diagnostic evaluation
   a. Gallbladder x-rays (p. 483)
   b. Chest roentgenogram
   c. Examination of urine and stool
   d. Blood studies including liver function tests (see p. 467)
2. Vitamin K and fresh blood may be administered to correct a low prothrombin level.
3. Supplements of protein hydrolysate may be required to maintain proper nutrition, to aid in wound healing, and to prevent liver damage.
4. An operative consent form is obtained after the operative procedure is described to the patient.
5. Adequate instruction regarding immediate postoperative requirements such as turning, deep-breathing, and use of incentive spirometry to prevent hypostatic pneumonia, a common postoperative complication.

Patient Problems/Nursing Diagnoses

1. Pain and discomfort related to surgical procedure
2. Altered respiratory pattern and potential for inadequate gas exchange related to the high surgical incision and its effects on breathing
3. Nutritional alterations related to dietary restrictions
4. Potential complications from biliary drainage

Planning and Implementation
Nursing Interventions

A. Improvement in Gas Exchange and Prevention of Respiratory Complications

To prevent respiratory complications, which are common in obese patients and in those having upper abdominal incisions.

1. Encourage the patient to take 10 deep breaths hourly and to turn frequently.
2. Administer analgesics as prescribed to permit the patient to take deep breaths comfortably (may be painful otherwise).
3. Splint abdominal incision with hands or pillow when the patient coughs.
4. Place the patient in low Fowler's position to facilitate lung expansion.
5. Activate and ambulate as early as permissible; apply a scultetus or appropriate abdominal binder if it will make the patient more comfortable.
6. Since he may still have a drainage bottle, place it in a below-the-waist pocket or fasten so that it is at a desired level.

B. Prevention of Complications from Biliary Drainage

To promote drainage from T-tube or cholecystostomy tube until normal flow of bile is established.

1. Place the patient in low-Fowler's position and later in semi-Fowler's position, as tolerated, to facilitate drainage.
2. Connect drainage tube to drainage bottle at side of bed; observe for kinking, twisting, and blockage of tubes.
3. Check postoperative orders regarding positioning of drainage bottle; often, the bottle or tubing is elevated so that bile drains through the apparatus only if pressure develops in the system. This is done to prevent total bile loss and to promote normal bile flow through the common bile duct.
4. Allow enough tubing leeway to permit the patient to be turned without dislodging tubes.
5. Observe, describe, and record amount and character of drainage frequently.
6. After 5 or 6 days of drainage, the T-tube may be clamped 1 hour before and after each meal to allow bile to flow into duodenum to aid in digestion. (Done with physician's permission.)
7. T-tube drain may be removed in 1–2 weeks. Cholecystostomy tube is removed in 6 weeks to 6 months. Drainage tube from gallbladder bed may be removed in 5–6 days.
8. Observe color changes in skin, sclerae, and stool, which will indicate whether bile pigment is disappearing from blood and draining again into the duodenum.
   a. Note color and consistency of all stools; chart an accurate description.
   b. Send specimens of urine and stool to the laboratory at frequent intervals for examination of bile pigments.
   c. Observe skin and sclerae for yellowish color, which would indicate bile-flow obstruction.
9. Protect skin around incision site from bile seepage.
   a. Change the outer dressings frequently to provide for absorption of drainage; Montgomery straps may facilitate dressing changes.
   b. Apply skin pastes of zinc oxide or petrolatum to prevent the bile drainage from attacking and digesting the skin.

Health Education
Goal:
Stress elements in posthospital care that will assist the patient in his convalescence.

1. It is not unusual after cholecystectomy for the patient to have "looseness of the bowel," consisting of 1–3 movements a day. This diminishes over a period of a few weeks to several months; within a year, the bowel habit is normal.
2. Usually there are no dietary instructions except to maintain a nutritious diet and to restrict fats for 4–6 weeks. (Otherwise, flatulence may occur.) Thereafter, adequate bile will be released into the digestive tract to emulsify fats and permit their digestion.
3. Review medications and their purpose—vitamins, anticholinergics, antispasmodics.
4. Be aware of reportable symptoms—jaundice, dark urine, pale-colored stools, pruritus, pain, or fever.
5. Emphasize the importance of follow-up visits to the physician.

Evaluation
Expected Outcomes

1. Is free of respiratory complications—normal respiratory rate and pattern, no fever, full respiratory excursion with normal breath sounds, effective cough
2. Is free of complications related to biliary drainage—no fever, no abdominal pain, normal vital signs, no drainage around tubes, normal color of skin, sclerae, urine, and stool

3. Maintains skin integrity—area around tube or drainage tube is intact and free of excoriation

4. Identifies signs and symptoms of complications to be reported

4: Conditions of the Pancreas*

Acute Pancreatitis

Acute pancreatitis is an inflammation of the pancreas brought about by the digestion of this organ by enzymes, particularly trypsin, an enzyme that it produces.

Etiology

1. Autodigestion of the pancreas by its own enzymes, although the exact mechanism is unknown.
2. Alcohol causes secretory and, eventually, structural changes in the pancreas; excessive alcohol intake is most common cause in the US.
3. Also associated with gallstones, which block ampulla of Vater, causing reflux of bile into pancreatic duct and activation of pancreatic enzymes in the pancreas itself.
4. Less commonly associated with mumps, bacterial disease, blunt trauma to the abdomen, use of oral contraceptives, and congenital hyperlipidemias.

Pathophysiology

1. There is a broad spectrum of pathologic changes in acute pancreatitis, ranging from edema and inflammation of the pancreas to necrosis and hemorrhage.
2. Pancreatic enzymes, normally activated in the gastrointestinal tract following dietary stimulation, are activated in the pancreas in acute pancreatitis and begin to digest the pancreas itself.
3. Kinins are activated, altering the permeability of cell membranes and producing loss of protein-rich fluid into the tissues and peritoneal cavity, and hypovolemia.

Treatment

1. Medical management is focused on alleviation of symptoms and support of the patient to prevent hypovolemia, shock, and death.
2. Includes medications and gastric suction to relieve pain and decrease stimulation of pancreatic enzymes, and fluid maintenance to prevent hypovolemia and shock.
3. Surgical intervention
   a. There is considerable disagreement about the place of surgery in treating acute pancreatitis. It is considered only if all other therapy has failed.
   b. Laparotomy may reveal an alternate problem, which can be corrected:
      (1) Tense gallbadder—cholecystostomy
      (2) Stones in ductal system—establish common duct patency
      (3) Necrotic material and fluid removed by peritoneal lavage

* For discussion of diabetes mellitus, see pages 696-708.

Assessment
Clinical Manifestations
A. Acute Interstitial or Edematous Pancreatitis

1. Pancreatic edema and escape of enzyme into nearby tissues and peritoneal cavity
2. Fat necrosis of omentum caused by pancreatic lipase
3. Increase in peritoneal fluid
4. Abdominal and back pain
5. Nausea, vomiting; fever
6. Tenderness across upper abdomen—often minimal
7. Elevated blood lipase and amylase
8. May be self-limiting if intense medical and nursing supportive care is provided

B. Acute Hemorrhagic Pancreatitis

1. A more advanced, severe form of acute pancreatitis with mortality rate greater than 30%.
2. Enzymatic digestion of gland more widespread.
3. Tissue becomes necrotic—blood escapes into pancreas and retroperitoneally, producing bloody ascites.
4. Severe abdominal and back pain; tenderness is often present in epigastrium, but rigidity is often absent.
5. Symptoms similar to acute interstitial pancreatitis, only more severe.
6. Blood lipase and amylase are elevated.
7. Respiratory distress may occur.
8. With severe pancreatitis, there is often psychic disturbance manifested in restlessness, hallucinations, coarse tremor.
9. Severe leakage of exudate from plasma into peritoneum (large 3rd-space loss).
10. Shock, due to activation of kinins.
11. Hypokalemic alkalosis and hypocalcemia usually present.
12. Pancreatic cysts and abscesses are late complications.

Diagnostic Evaluation

1. Determination of serum amylase. If serum amylase is elevated, and there is clinical evidence, pancreatitis is likely.
2. An elevated serum lipase level may also be present and persists longer than elevation of amylase levels.
3. Ultrasonography and computed tomography (CT) scan may be indicated to identify pancreatic cysts or pseudocysts in acute pancreatitis.

Patient Problems/Nursing Diagnoses

1. Pain and discomfort related to edema and inflammation of the pancreas and to peritoneal irritation
2. Potential alteration in gas exchange related to immobility, pain, and pulmonary infiltrates
3. Altered fluid and nutritional intake related to vomiting, long-standing malnutrition, gastric intubation, sepsis, fluid shifts, and paralytic ileus

Planning and Implementation
Nursing Interventions
A. Relief of Pain and Discomfort

1. Relieve discomfort and pain to control restlessness, which increases body metabolism, causing stimulation of enzyme secretions.
   a. Give meperidine (Demerol); this is preferred because it depresses the central nervous system. (Opiates, on the other hand, may produce spasm of biliary–pancreatic ducts.)
   b. Encourage the patient to assume position of comfort.
2. Remove stimulus to secretion of pancreatic enzymes.
   a. Give nothing by mouth, to eliminate chief stimulus to enzyme secretion.
   b. Offer anticholinergic medications as prescribed to assist in reducing pancreatic secretions by suppressing vagal mechanisms.
   c. Initiate nasogastric suction to remove hydrochloric acid from stomach, thus preventing release of secretin; adynamic ileus is also treated.
      (1) Record color and nature of gastric secretions.
      (2) Measure secretions at periodic intervals.
   d. Maintain the comfort of the intubated patient.
      (1) Assist the patient in cleansing and refreshing mouth care.
      (2) Apply lubricant to external nares to prevent irritation of mucous membrane and skin.
      (3) Alternate side-positioning to prevent esophageal and gastric irritation by tube.
      (4) Provide cool-mist vapor therapy to increase humidity and control drying of mucous membrane.

B. Improvement in Gas Exchange

1. Monitor blood gases to detect early signs of respiratory failure.
2. Perform pulmonary assessment frequently to observe for changes in respiratory status (anticholinergic medications, given to decrease pancreatic secretions, also predispose the patient to respiratory complications by drying the mucous membranes of the respiratory tract).
3. Position the patient in semi-Fowler's position to decrease pressure on the diaphragm from the distended abdomen and to allow full respiratory excursion.
4. Turn the patient frequently to prevent pulmonary–vascular complications.
5. Teach and assist the patient to cough and take deep breaths.
6. Decrease oxygen requirements by keeping the patient's body metabolism low.
   a. Administer oxygen therapy if breathing is labored.
   b. Keep the patient in bed to control overexertion.
   c. Turn on air-conditioning to keep body heat under control.

C. Adequate Fluid and Nutritional Intake

1. Maintain the patient's fluid volume and prevent hypovolemia.
   a. Maintain surveillance of vital signs.
   b. Monitor hematocrit (if it rises in first 24–48 hours, volume replacement was inadequate).
   c. Monitor central venous pressure (keep to 8–10 cm. of water above baseline).
   d. Monitor urinary output (keep to 50–100 ml./hr.).
   e. Provide blood, balanced electrolytes to maintain blood volume; limit solutions containing glucose because this patient is often hyperglycemic.
   f. Monitor blood sugar every 4 hours; administer IV insulin to keep blood sugar levels under 200 mg./100 ml.
   g. If marked hyperglycemia occurs, give insulin in small doses (crystalline insulin at 6-hour intervals) rather than long-acting insulin.
2. Provide fluids and medications to correct deficiencies and prevent complications.
   a. Give parenteral fluids—electrolytes and blood to meet body's nutritional needs, replace losses, and combat shock. Keep accurate intake and output record.
   b. Administer antimicrobials to ward off secondary infection or abscess formation. (Use of antibiotics remains controversial. Some physicians suggest intravenous administration of cephalothin every 6 hours.)
   c. Monitor serum calcium; it may be necessary to administer calcium gluconate if calcium level falls low enough to produce symptoms.
3. Control nausea and vomiting.
   a. Administer antiemetics as prescribed.
   b. Maintain gastric suction and monitor closely.
4. Instruct the patient about normal, adequate nutrition and importance of avoiding alcohol during recovery.
   a. Provide diet high in carbohydrate, low in fat, proteins, and stimulants.
   b. Instruct the patient to avoid alcohol and heavy meals.

Health Education and Discharge Planning

Manage recovery phase and offer guidelines to the patient to prevent future attacks of pancreatitis.
1. When the patient's condition permits, offer the following:
   a. Small amounts of fat-free liquids
   b. Anticholinergics, parenterally or orally
   c. Nonabsorbable antacids hourly
2. Instruct the patient as follows:
   a. Gradually resume normal diet.
   b. Alcohol use and excessive use of coffee are prohibited, since they increase pancreatic secretion.
3. Urge follow-up visits with physician. (Biliary tract studies and surveillance may uncover the cause of the pancreatitis.)

Evaluation
Expected Outcomes

1. Experiences relief of pain and discomfort—indicates less discomfort, describes self as feeling better, ambulates and participates in mild forms of activity without complaints of pain
2. Shows no signs of respiratory complications—normal blood gases, normal respiratory rate and pattern, normal breath sounds, adequate cough and frequent deep breaths, adequate fluid intake to liquefy secretions
3. Attains adequate fluid and nutritional intake—regular body weight without increase in ascites or edema; normal blood glucose levels and urine glucose levels; eating prescribed diet; no complaints of gastric distress, vomiting, or nausea

Chronic Pancreatitis

Chronic pancreatitis is a chronic fibrosis and calcification of the pancreas with obstruction of its ducts and destruction of its secreting acinar cells.

Incidence

1. Occurs most often in men between 45 and 60.
2. Follows repeated attacks of acute interstitial pancreatitis.
3. Usually occurs in patients having a history of prolonged use of alcohol.
4. Gallstones, hyperparathyroidism, and hyperlipidemia are occasionally associated with chronic pancreatitis.

Pathophysiology

1. Alcohol exerts direct toxic effect on cells of the pancreas; the likelihood of chronic pancreatitis is increased by genetic predisposition.
2. Alcohol may also stimulate pancreatic secretion at the same time it induces spasm of the sphincter of Oddi, causing pain.
3. Repeated episodes of acute pancreatitis and alcohol ingestion produces fibrosis, cyst formation, and distortion of pancreatic tissue.

Clinical Manifestations

1. Recurrent episodes of severe upper abdominal and back pain (morphine often does not relieve pain), vomiting, and low-grade fever. Drug addiction is often a secondary problem.
2. Protein and fat digestion is disturbed because of deficient pancreatic secretion.
3. Steatorrhea—stools that are frequent, frothy, and foul-smelling with high fat content because of faulty fat digestion.
4. Later formation of calcium stones in the duct as calcification develops.
5. Weight loss.
6. Jaundice may occur because of constriction of common bile duct as it passes through head of pancreas.

Diagnostic Evaluation

1. Determine whether levels of serum amylase and lipase are elevated. Levels often are not elevated in chronic pancreatitis.
2. Examine stool to measure fecal fat and trypsin content.
3. Arteriography and x-ray may show fibrous tissue and calcification.
4. Diabetes or abnormal glucose tolerance may be detectable.

Treatment and Nursing Management

1. The treatment measures indicated depend on the nature and severity of the patient's symptoms, which may be similar to those of acute pancreatitis.
   a. The patient is often drug dependent because of recurring episodes of severe pain requiring careful assessment and management of pain.
   b. The long-term nature of chronic pancreatitis often results in an acutely ill patient who is malnourished, emaciated, and at risk of multiple complications.
   c. The patient is frequently a poor surgical risk.
2. Offer the patient bland, low-fat diet in 6 feedings daily.
3. Give antacids and anticholinergic medication to reduce acid, which would stimulate the release of secretin and enhance pancreatic activity.
4. Pancreatic insufficiency is controlled by giving medication containing amylase, lipase, and trypsin—Pancreatin, Cotazym, Viokase.
   Medication may need to be administered with antacids or bicarbonates.
   Note: Steatorrhea should be present before enzyme replacement therapy is initiated.
5. Since these patients often develop diabetes, be alert for symptoms such as polydipsia, polyuria, weakness, polyphagia (excessive eating), or weight loss and report these to the physician.
6. The use of alcohol should be discouraged, since this will aggravate the pancreatitis; treatment of alcoholism must be done if this is a problem, as it usually is.
7. If hyperparathyroidism or hyperlipemia is diagnosed, these certainly must be treated.
8. Surgical aspects are similar to those of biliary tract surgery (see p. 488).
9. Nature of surgery is determined by identifying the cause; surgery usually fails if alcoholism or drug addiction persists.
   a. With gallbladder disease—biliary tract surgery to explore common bile duct, choledocholectomy (removing stones in duct) and cholecystectomy (removing gallbladder).
   b. Sphincteroplasty or sphincterotomy may be done to divide sphincter of Oddi to improve drainage of common bile duct, or
   c. Selective or generalized drainage of dilated ducts via pancreaticojejunostomy.
   d. Pancreatectomy may be done when pancreas is severely diseased or when persistent pain is a major problem.

Pseudocysts and Pancreatic Abscesses

Pseudocysts of the pancreas are collections of inflammatory fluid walled off by fibrous tissue in the pancreas, usually resulting from local necrosis at the time of acute pancreatitis.

Clinical Manifestations and Diagnosis

1. Cysts may attain considerable size; they develop rapidly or slowly (within 72 hours or over several weeks or months).

2. Because they occur in the posterior peritoneum, they may exert pressure against the stomach or colon, visible on barium studies.
3. Persistent elevation of amylase (serum or urine) is the most common finding. Pain and vomiting may occur.
4. Leukocytosis and fever are common but are usually mild with pseudocysts; these responses are more striking with abscess formation.
5. Sonography has been found useful in confirming the diagnosis.

Treatment

1. Pseudocysts may occasionally subside spontaneously.

2. Symptoms of secondary infection may require surgery for drainage.
3. Drainage may be established into gastrointestinal tract (internal) or through skin surface (external); this latter method is controversial because it presents the risk of the patient developing pancreatic fistulae.

Nursing Management

1. Should external drainage be done, recognize the irritating qualities of the pancreatic enzyme; meticulous skin care is required.
2. Maintain adequate drainage, avoiding tube dislodgment (See discussion on p. 488).

Pancreatic Cancer

Cancer may arise in the head, body, or tail of the pancreas; insulin-secreting pancreatic islet cells may or may not be involved.

Treatment

Surgical only. Although surgical cures are possible, 5-year survival is about 25%. Tumor is removed if it has not invaded important surrounding structures.

1. Whipple resection—removal of head (and sometimes neck) of pancreas; removal of adjacent stomach, distal portion of common duct, and duodenum. Patient has severe malabsorption afterward.
2. If Whipple procedure cannot be done, jaundice may be relieved by diverting bile from gallbladder into the jejunum (cholecystojejunostomy). If duodenum is invaded, gastrojejunostomy should be done to bypass duodenal obstruction.
3. For cancer of the body and tail of the pancreas, distal pancreatectomy and splenectomy are the most commonly employed procedures.
4. Total pancreatectomy—en bloc resection of the common bile duct, stomach, duodenum, pancreas, and spleen.

Assessment
Clinical Manifestations

The "big three" are *weight loss, pain,* and *jaundice.*

1. Initial symptoms of cancer of the pancreas are often vague, thereby accounting for a reported 4–9 months' delay from onset of symptoms to diagnosis.
2. Disease usually occurs in older men; alcoholism may be a contributing cause.
3. Weight loss, anorexia, dyspepsia, nausea, some bowel disturbance, and occasionally chills and fever develop.
4. Intermittent, dull-to-severe, vague, epigastric, or back pain, often aggravated by eating or associated with fullness and bloating after meals.
   a. Right upper quadrant pain suggests involvement of the head of the pancreas.
   b. Left upper quadrant pain suggests involvement of the body or tail of the pancreas.
   c. Pain often radiates to the back or is exclusively in back.
   d. Pain is often worse at night, aggravated in recumbent position and relieved by lying with legs drawn up or by walking bent over.
   e. Fear of eating may take place.

5. The patient may experience depression and lethargy, combined with a feeling of anxiety and premonition of serious illness.
6. Obstruction of the common bile duct produces jaundice, clay-colored stools, dark urine, and itching (due to cancer of the head of pancreas).
   Differentiation must be made between jaundice from biliary obstruction (due to a stone in the common duct) and jaundice from hepatic metastases.

Diagnostic Evaluation

1. Blood studies, including serum bilirubin, alkaline phosphatase, SGOT, and prothrombin time
2. Secretin studies and radiologic procedures—UGI series, gallbladder studies, and possibly fiberoptic duodenoscopy with cannulation of papilla and pancreatic ductography, or transhepatic cholangiography
3. Scanning—radioactive selenomethionine (^{75}Se); note that frequent false-positive findings occur
4. Angiography
5. Ultrasonography
6. Computed tomography

Patient Problems/Nursing Diagnoses

1. Altered nutritional status related to anorexia and increased gastrointestinal disturbances after eating
2. Pain and discomfort related to tumor involvement of the pancreas
3. Impaired skin integrity related to jaundice and debilitation
4. Altered self-concept related to change in role function
5. Inability to cope related to depression over diagnosis of cancer

Planning and Implementation
Nursing Interventions

A. Appropriate Fluid and Nutrient Intake to Meet Body Needs

1. Because of the patient's poor nutritional state, it is a challenge to maintain adequate calorie levels. A bland, low-fat diet is recommended, plus whatever he can tolerate without overeating.
2. Medium-chain triglycerides are better tolerated, since they cause less fat excretion.
3. Alcohol to be avoided.
4. Anticholinergics used.

5. Provide small, frequent meals.
6. Determine and provide foods preferred by the patient.
7. Provide supplements of high-calorie foods between meals.
8. Encourage the patient to drink adequate fluids to prevent complications (e.g., urinary tract infection, etc.).

B. Relief of Pain and Promotion of Comfort

1. Administer analgesic medication for pain as prescribed.
2. Assist the patient to assume positions of comfort.
3. Assess quality, severity, and location of the patient's pain.
4. Assess and record the patient's response to analgesia.
5. Provide additional means of pain relief (e.g., distraction, massage, etc.).

C. Improved Skin Integrity

1. Assist the patient to change position frequently to prevent pressure sores.
2. Massage bony prominences frequently.
3. Note appearance of reddened areas of skin.
4. Apply sheepskin or foam rubber to bed; use "eggcrate" or special mattress to relieve pressure on the skin.
5. Provide soothing lotions and baths to alleviate pruritus and scratching.
6. Administer medications prescribed for pruritus.
7. Keep the patient's fingernails short to prevent scratching of skin.

8. Avoid trauma to skin through gentle handling and prevention of falls.

D. Promotion of Coping Abilities

1. Assist the patient in recognizing and verbalizing feelings and reactions to current situation.
2. Identify tasks and activities that the patient can accomplish.
3. Assist the patient in identifying his own priorities of tasks.
4. Assist the patient in planning achievable goals and activities.
5. Assist the patient in confronting his future with dignity (e.g., major surgical procedure, persistent pain, increasing disability, or impending death).

Evaluation
Expected Outcomes

1. Maintains adequate fluid and nutritional intake—good appetite; meals are consumed when delivered; weight is maintained without edema; urine output is normal
2. Achieves pain relief or increased comfort via pharmacologic and nonpharmacologic methods (mental distraction, mental imagery, proper positioning)
3. Maintains skin integrity—no redness, breakdown, excoriation, or infection; normal skin turgor, no complaints of pruritus; uses precautions to prevent trauma
4. Demonstrates improved coping abilities—verbalizes feelings and participates in own care

Bibliography

Books
Gastrointestinal Conditions
Beck ML. Caring for the Gastrointestinal Patient. Photobook. Ensuring Intensive Care. Springhouse, PA, Intermed Communication, 1981
Bolt RJ et al (eds). The Digestive System. Somerset, NJ, John Wiley & Sons, 1983
Bongiovanni G. Manual of Clinical Gastroenterology. New York, McGraw-Hill, 1982
Broadwell DC and Jackson BS. Principles of Ostomy Care. St Louis, CV Mosby, 1982
Given BA and Simmons SJ. Gastroenterology in Clinical Nursing, 4th ed. St Louis, CV Mosby, 1984
Grant JP. Handbook of Total Parenteral Nutrition. Philadelphia, WB Saunders, 1980
Greenberger NJ and Winship DH. Gastrointestinal Disorders, 2nd ed. Chicago, Year Book Medical Publishers, 1981
Latimer PE. Functional Gastrointestinal Disorders: A Behavioral Medicine Approach. New York, Springer-Verlag, 1983
Michigan Nurses Association. Reducing Diarrhea in Tube-Fed Patients: A CURN Project. New York, Grune & Stratton, 1981
Nord JH and Brady PG. Critical Care

Gastroenterology. New York, Churchill Livingstone, 1982
Nursing Photobook. Performing Gastrointestinal Procedures. Springhouse, PA, Intermed Communications, 1982
Ryan WJ. The Nurse and the Communicatively Impaired Adult. New York, Springer-Verlag, 1982
Silberman H. Parenteral and Enteral Nutrition for the Hospitalized Patient. New York, Appleton-Century-Crofts, 1982
Simko MD, Cowell C and Gilbride JA. Nutrition Assessment. Germantown, MD, Aspen Systems, 1983
Sleisenger MH and Fordtran JS. Gastrointestinal Disease: Pathophysiology Diagnosis Management, 3rd ed. Philadelphia, WB Saunders, 1983
Spiro HM. Clinical Gastroenterology 3rd ed. New York, Macmillan, 1982
Steefel JS. Dysphagia Rehabilitation for Neurologically Impaired Adults. Springfield, IL, Charles C Thomas, 1981

Conditions of the Hepatic and Biliary System
Fischbach FA. Manual of Laboratory Diagnostic Tests. Philadelphia, JB Lippincott, 1984
Kim MJ, McFarland GK and McLane AM.

Pocket Guide to Nursing Diagnosis. St Louis, CV Mosby, 1984
Koff RS. Liver Disease in Primary Care Medicine. New York, Appleton-Century-Crofts, 1980
Schiff L and Schiff ER. Diseases of the Liver. Philadelphia, JB Lippincott, 1982
Stephens GJ. Pathophysiology for Health Practitioners. New York, Macmillan, 1980

Articles
General
Danovitch SH. Gastrointestinal function after forty. Am Fam Physician 1984 Feb; 29(2):205–210
Gever LN. Antidiarrheals, Ensuring their safe use. Nurs '83 1983 Oct; 13(10):17
Intestinal bypass patients show long-term complications. AORN J 1982 Jan; 35(1):96–99
Kadas N. The dysphagic patient: Everyday care really counts. RN 1983 Nov; 46(11):38–41
Kornguth ML. Weight problems: Nursing management. Am J Nurs 1981 Mar; 81(3):533–554
Myers S et al. Quality of life after surgery for Crohn's disease: A psychosocial survey. Gastroenterology 1980 Jan; 78(1):1–6
Nivatvongs S and Hooks VH. Chronic

constipation. Postgrad Med 1983 Nov; 74(5):313–323

Delaney R et al. Nutritional support of the acutely ill patient. Heart & Lung 1983 Sept; 12(5):477–480

Stratton JW and Mackeigan JM. Treating constipation. Am Fam Physician 1982 June; 25(6):139–142

Tuttobene SA. A bowel prep that's easy to swallow. RN 1984 Mar; 47(3):52

Nutrition

Carino CM and Chmelko P. Disorders of eating in adolescence: Anorexia nervosa and bulimia. Nurs Clin North Am 1983 June; 18(2):343–352

Grant JP, Custer PB and Thurlow J. Current techniques of nutritional assessment. Surg Clin North Am 1981 June; 61(3):437

Gray DS and Kaminski MV. Nutritional support of the hospitalized patient. Am Fam Physician 1983 Sept; 26(3): 143–150

Handler S. Dietary fiber. Postgrad Med 1983 Feb; 73(2):301–307

Hill GJ. Surgically created nutritional problems. Surg Clin North Am 1981 June; 61(3):721–728

Johnson PK. Getting enough to grow on. Am J Nurs 1984 March; 84(3):336–339

Kolars JC et al. Yogurt—an autodigesting source of lactose. N Engl J Med 1984 Jan 4; 310(1):1–3

Levine GM. Nutritional support in gastrointestinal disease. Surg Clin North Am 1981 June; 61(3):701–708

Marks RG. Anorexia and bulimia: Eating habits that can kill. RN 1984 Jan; 47(1):44–47

Meeroff JC. Etiologic evaluation and treatment of malabsorption syndrome. Hosp Pract 1984 Apr; 19(4):88x–88BB

Newcomer AD and McGill DB. Clinical importance of lactase deficiency. N Engl J Med 1984 Jan 4; 310(1):42–43

Smith GP. The peripheral control of appetite. Lancet 1983 July 9; 2(8352): 88–89

Diagnostic Evaluation of the Gastrointestinal Tract

Amis AS Jr et al. Role of abdominal computed tomography. Postgrad Med 1982 July; 72(1):131–136

Beck ML. Preparing your patient psychologically for an esophagogastroduodenoscopy. Nursing '81 1981 Jan; 11(1):28–30

Beck ML. Preparing your patient physically for an esophagogastroduodenoscopy. Nursing '81 1981; Feb 11(2):88–96

Beck ML. Three common gastrointestinal tests and how to help your patient through each. Nursing '81 1981 Apr; 11(4):44–47

Beck ML. Three more gastrointestinal tests—and how to help your patient through each. Nursing '81 1981 May; 11(5):22–27

Dardick KR. Hematuria and false-positive tests for stool occult blood. Am Fam Physician 1984 Feb; 29(2): 201–202

Davis GR et al. Development of a lavage solution associated with minimal water and electrolyte absorption or

secretion. Gastroenterology 1980 May; 78(5):991–995

Didich JM. Gauging abdominal girth accurately. Nursing '81 1981 Aug; 11(8):32–33

Fisher RS and Kaplan W. The role of gastrointestinal endoscopy. Med Times 1983 Feb; 111(2):31–37

Get the most from abdominal sonography. Patient Care 1984 Feb 15; 18(3):17–61

Haughey CW. Understanding ultrasonography. Nursing '81 1981 Apr; 11(4):100–104

Hocutt JE et al. Flexible fiberoptic sigmoidoscopy. Am Fam Physician 1982 Nov; 26(5):133–141

Katerndahl DA. Ultrasonic examination of the abdomen. Postgrad Med 1982 Mar 71(3):227–237

Malkiewicz J. For a really thorough abdominal examination. RN 1982 Oct; 45(10):59–64

Munro-Black J. The ABCs of total parenteral nutrition. Nursing '84 1984 Feb; 14(2):50–56

Nelson RS. Proctosigmoidoscopy. Hosp Med 1984 Feb; 20(2):67–78

Smith CE. Abdominal assessment. Nursing '81 1981 Feb; 11(2):42–49

Stiklorius C. Gastrointestinal studies. RN 1982 Mar; 45(3):64–65

Stiklorius C. When patient preparation is the key to success. RN 1982 Apr; 45(4):64–65

Stiklorius C. Two diagnostic procedures that demand your all-out care. RN 1982 Aug; 45(8):64

Stiklorius C. Preparing for two uncomfortable tests: Gastric analysis and liver biopsy. RN 1982 Sept; 45(9): 64

Thomas G et al. Patient acceptance and effectiveness of a balanced lavage solution (Golytely) versus the standard preparation for colonoscopy. Gastroenterology 1982 March; 82(3): 435–437

Intubation

Amato EJ. Gastrointestinal tubes and drains. Part II. Esophageal tubes. Crit Care Nurse 1983 Jan/Feb; 3(1):46–48

Aspiration with nasogastric feeding. See Ann Intern Med 1981 July; 95(1):67

Beck ML. Tests: What to do when they call for inserting gastrointestinal tubes. Nursing '81 1981; 11(3):74–76

Knodel AR and Beekman JF. Unexplained fevers in patients with nasotracheal intubation. JAMA 1982; Aug 20; 248(7):868–870

Mangieri D. Looking at the tube . . . and we don't mean T.V. Nursing '83 1983 Apr; 13(4):47–49

Strange JM. An expert's guide to tubes and drains. RN 1983 Apr; 46(4):35–42

Thompkins T. Capsulizing small tube placement. Patient Care 1981 May 30; 15:65

Wilson JM et al. Silicone catheters (patient teaching pamphlet). NITA 1984 May/June; 7(3):169–172

Parenteral and Enteral Nutrition

Appleby L. Initiation, maintenance, and termination of total parenteral

nutrition. NITA 1983 Jan–Feb; 6(1): 31–35

Bower RH. Metabolic complications of parenteral nutrition therapy. NITA 1983 Jan–Feb; 6(1):37–39

Colley R. TPN nursing. NITA 1983 Jan–Feb; 6(1):44–47

Contamination of enteral feeding products during clinical usage, Proceedings of the Ross Laboratories Workshop, Columbus, OH, Ross Laboratories, 1983

Curtiss FR. Third-party reimbursement for home parenteral nutrition and IV therapy. NITA 1983 May–June; 6(3): 193–197

Daly JM and Long JM III. Intravenous hyperalimentation: Techniques and potential complications. Surg Clin North Am 1981 June; 61(3):583–592

Davis J, Jedlicka L and Johnson F. Sure-fire asepsis for your TPN patients. RN 1982 Dec; 45(12):39–41, 91

Duval A and Hennessy K. Care of the Broviac catheter. NITA 1983 Jan–Feb; 6(1):40–42

Gordon AM. Enteral nutritional support. Postgrad Med 1982 July; 72(1):72–82

Henderson DK, Myers RF and Laniak JM. Catheter-acquired infection in total parenteral nutrition. NITA 1982 Jan/Feb; 5(1):62–68

Hennessy K. HHNK dehydration. Am J Nurs 1983 Oct; 83(10):1425–1426

Hushen SC. Questioning TPN as the answer. Am J Nurs 1982 May; 82(5): 852–854

Johnstone JD. Infrequent infections associated with Hickman catheters. CA Nurs 1982 Apr; 5(2):125–129

Kennedy G. Total parenteral nutrition down to the basics. Can Nurse 1981 March; 77(3):32–35

Lees CS et al. Home parenteral nutrition. Surg Clin North Am 1981 June; 61(3):621–633

Maker VK. Applications of central vs peripheral TPN. NITA 1983 Sept/Oct; 6(5):357–365

Masoorli ST. Tips for trouble-free subclavian lines. RN 1984 Feb; 47(2): 38–39

Meador B. If your "continuous" tube feeding stops. RN 1983 July; 46(7):27

Munro-Black J. The ABC's of total parenteral nutrition. Nursing '84 1984 Feb; 14(2):50–56

Nonkin R. The Broviac catheter: OR technique. AORN J 1982 Feb; 35(2): 25

Pennington CR and Richards JM. Three-liter bags containing intralipid for parenteral nutrition. J Parenter Enter Nutr 1983 May/June; 7(3):304–305

Persons C. Why risk TPN when tube feeding will do? RN 1981 Jan; 44(1): 35–41

Rombeau JL and Barot LR. Enteral nutritional therapy. Surg Clin North Am 1981 June; 61(3):605–620

Ryan JA and Gough J. Complication of central venous catheterization for total parenteral nutrition. NITA 1984 Jan/Feb; 7(1):29–35

Schmidt A and Williams D. The Hickman catheter. RN 1982 Feb; 45(2):57–61

Schwartz-Fulton J et al. Hyperalimentation dressings and skin flora. NITA 1981 Sept/Oct; 5(1):354–357

Stamm WE. Infections related to medical devices. Ann Intern Med 1978 Nov; 89(5)Part 2:764–769

Teitell BC and Strickland A. Evaluating methods of administering antibiotics and TPN when using a pump system. NITA 1982 July/Aug; 5(4):270–272

Watters JM and Freeman JB. Parenteral nutrition by peripheral vein. Surg Clin North Am 1981 June; 61(3):593–604

Wilson SE et al. Current status of vascular access techniques. Surg Clin North Am 1982 June; 62(3):531–551

Mouth

Arthur JD, Bass JW and York WB. How is suspected streptococcal pharyngitis managed? Postgrad Med 1984 Mar; 75(4):241–248

Attie JN and Sciubba JJ. Tumors of major and minor salivary glands: Clinical and pathologic features. Curr Prob Surg 1981 Feb; 18(2):68–155

Berrani G and Carl W. Oral care for cancer patients. Am J Nurs 1983 April; 83(4):533–536

Chase DC et al. "Doctor, my jaw aches" (Roundtable). Patient Care 1983 Dec 15; 17(21):108–136

Common sense management for TMJ. Patient Care 1984 Jan 15; 18(1):129–157

Denning DC. Head and neck cancer: Our reactions. CA Nurs 1982 Aug; 5(4):269–273

Dreizen S. Systemic significance of glossitis. Postgrad Med 1984 Mar; 75(4):207–215

Dworkin SF. Benign chronic orofacial pain. Postgrad Med 1983 Sept; 74(3):239–248

Glossectomy and Maxillectomy. Chapt. 5 Ryan WJ. The Nurse and the Communicatively Impaired Adult. New York. Springer-Verlag, 1982, pp. 78–92

Gonzalez ER. Stressed whites especially prone to trench mouth. JAMA 1983 Jan 14; 242(2):157

Geisler J. Tips for your fractured-jaw patient. RN 1981 Jan; 44(1):33, 114

Help for the patient with dry mouth. Patient Care 1984 Feb 29; 18(4):42–76

Ketoconazole (Nizoral) for oral thrush. RN 1982 Mar; 45(3):74

King RC. A systematic plan for assessing the head and face. RN 1982 Jan; 45(1):55–58

Luce EA. Maxillofacial trauma. Curr Prob Surg 1984 Feb; 21(2):6–68

Lynch DP. Ulcerations of the tongue. Postgrad Med 1984 Mar; 75(4):152–163

MacMillan KM. New goals for oral hygiene. Can Nurse 1981 March; 77(3):40–43

Malkiewicz J. What assessing the mouth can tell you, RN 1982 May; 45(5):65–69

McLoy DG. Hecht SS and Wynder EL. The roles of tobacco, alcohol, and diet in the etiology of upper alimentary and respiratory tract cancers. Prev Med 1980 Sept; 9(5):622–629

Miller GW. Acute epiglottitis in adults. Am Fam Physician 1982 Aug; 26(2):183–185

Sessions DG. Surgical resection and reconstruction for cancer of the base of the tongue. Surg Clin North Am 1983 May; 126(2):309–329

World Health Information Services. Herpes simplex infections. NITA 1983 Jan Feb; 6(1):58–60

Yonkers AJ and Mercurio GA. Tracheostomal stenosis following total laryngectomy. Surg Clin North Am 1983 May; 16(2):391–405

Head and Neck Problems

Baker HW. Staging of cancer of the head and neck: Oral cavity, pharynx, larynx and paranasal sinuses. CA 1983 May/June; 33(3):130–144

Clark WD and Bailey BJ. Diagnosis: Evaluation of neck masses. Hosp Med 1983 Aug; 19(8):57–70

Carter SK. Head and neck cancer: Etiology, prevention, diagnosis, and staging. Curr Conc Oncol 1982 Fall; 4(3):3–16

Grace MP and Mauirer LH. Early diagnosis of head and neck cancer. Hosp Med 1982 July; 18(7)40A–40EE

Jacobs C. Chemotherapy and combined-modality treatment of head and neck cancer. Curr Conc Oncology 1982 Fall; 4(3):17–21

Petrogallo A. Caring for the patient who has undergone radical neck dissection. 1983 Point of View (Ethicon) 20(4):14–15

Esophagus

Beauchamp G and Durancian AC. Diagnostic and therapeutic esophagoscopy. Surg Clin North Am 1983 Aug; 63(4):801–813

Bremner CG. Benign strictures of the esophagus. Curr Prob Surg 1982 Aug; 19(8):406–489

Channer K and Virjee J. Effect of posture and drink volume on the swallowing of capsules. Br Med J 1982 Dec 11; 285(6356):1702

DiPalma JA and Perucca PJ. An approach to the diagnosis and management of reflux esophagitis. Med Times 1984 Apr; 112(4):29–33

Goldenberg DA. Management of bleeding esophageal varices. Crit Care Q 1982 Sept; 5(2):33–46

Ellis FH. Cancer of the esophagus and cardia. Postgrad Med 1984 Feb 15; 75(3):139–147

Mannell A. Carcinoma of the esophagus. Curr Prob Surg 1982 Oct; 19(10):557–647

Payne WJ and King RM. Pharyngoesophageal (Zenker's) diverticulum. Surg Clin North Am 1983 Aug; 63(4):815–824

Rajan RK. Esophageal diverticula. Am Fam Physician 1979; March 19; 19(3):119–122

Stiklorius C. "Fair warnings" for patients facing esophagoscopy and gastroscopy. RN 1982 June; 45(6):64–65

Also see SCNA August 1983

Stomach and Duodenum

Anderson J, Poklis A and Slavin R. A fatal case of theophylline intoxication. Arch Intern Med 1983 Mar; 143(3):559–560

Bachman BA. Gastroesophageal reflux. Postgrad Med 1983 Nov; 74(5):133–141

Burnstein AV. Peptic ulcer disease: Medical and surgical considerations. Crit Care Q 1982 Sept; 5(2):1–7

Collen MJ et al. Comparison of ranitidine and cimetidine in the treatment of gastric hypersecretion. Ann Intern Med 1984 Jan; 100(1):52–57

Drake D and Hollander D. Neutralizing capacity and cost effectiveness of antacids. Ann Intern Med 1981 Feb; 94(2):215–217

Fierst SM. Axioms on gastric carcinoma. Hosp Med 1982 Apr; 18(4):36e–36v

Fisher RS. Modern concepts of peptic ulcer disease: Advances in treatment; Med Times 1983 Jan; 111(1):111–121

Johnston IDA. The adverse effects of gastric surgery for peptic ulceration. Med Times 1984 May; 112(5):63–69

Kraft RO. Long-term results of vagotomy and pyloroplasty in the treatment of gastric ulcer disease. Ann Surg 1984 April; 95(4):460

Messer J et al. Association of adrenocorticosteroid therapy and peptic ulcer disease. N Engl J Med 1983 July 7; 309(1):21–24

"Nursing Grand Rounds" Gastric bypass for morbid obesity. Nursing '81 1981 Jan; 11(1):55–59

Rogers AI. Milk and ulcer therapy. Postgrad Med 1983 Mar; 73(3):58

Rosenberg JM and Kirschenbaum HL. Antacids. RN 1982 Sept; 45(9):54–56

Schumacker HB Jr. Little used surgical techniques of value (gastrostomy: 186–187) Am J Surg 1982 Aug; 144(2):186–190

Stabile BE and Passaro E. Duodenal ulcer; A disease in evolution. Curr Prob Surg 1984 Jan; 21(1):6–79

Steinberg WM, Lewis JH and Katz DM. Antacids inhibit absorption of cimetidine. N Engl J Med 1982 Aug 12; 307(7):400–404

Strickland RG. Acute and chronic gastritis. Hosp Med 1983 June; 19(6):148–176

Sucralfate for peptic ulcer—a reappraisal. Med Lett 1984 Apr 27; 26(660):43–44

Velasco N et al. Gastric emptying and gastroesophageal reflux. Am J Surg 1982 July; 144(1):58–62

Wilson SE. Modern management of anastomotic leak after esophagogastrectomy. Am J Surg 1982 July; 144(2):95–101

Small Intestine

Berne TV et al. Antibiotic management of surgically treated gangrenous or perforated appendicitis. Am J Surg 1982 July; 144(1):8–13

Cassell BL. The new trend in ileostomy surgery. RN 1984 Jan; 47(1):48–51

Sisley J and Wagner C. Barium appendicitis. South Med J 1982 Apr; 75(4):498–499

Hernia

Ropka ME. Hiatal hernia. Nursing '82 1982 Apr; 12(4):126–131

Sweet K. Hiatal hernia. Nursing '83 1983 Dec; 13(12):38–45

Intestinal Problems

Barber JM. Gastrointestinal trauma: A review of delayed complications for the critical care nurse. Crit Care Q 1982 Sept; 5(2):69–80

Burkitt D. Fiber as protective against gastrointestinal diseases. Am J Gastroenterol 1984 April; 79(4):249–252

Burns TW. Parasitic bowel disease. Postgrad Med 1982 May; 71(5):130–139

Condon RE. Preoperative antibiotic bowel preparation. Drug Ther 1983 Jan; 83(1):29–37

Das KM. Pharmacotherapy of inflammatory bowel disease. Part 1. Sulfasalazine. Postgrad Med 1983 Dec; 74(6):141–151

Fazio VW. Regional enteritis (Crohn's disease). Surg Clin North Am 1983 Feb; 63(1):27–48

Frank MS, Brandt LJ and Bernstein LH. Pharmacotherapy of inflammatory bowel disease. Part 2. Metronidazole. Postgrad Med 1983 Dec; 74(6):155–160

Greenburg JL. Diagnosis of inflammatory bowel disease. Postgrad Med 1983 Dec; 74(6):112–121

Korelitz BI. Pharmacotherapy of inflammatory bowel disease. Part 3. 6-Mercaptopurine. Postgrad Med 1983 Dec; 74(6):165–172

Latimer PR. A behavioral approach to irritable bowel syndrome. Med Times 1983 July; 3(7):95–99

Managing a lower G.I. bleed. Patient Care 1984 Mar 30; 18(6):118–133

Marshall JB. Management of acute upper gastrointestinal bleeding. Postgrad Med 1982 May; 71(5):149–157

Perkel MS. Acute inflammatory bowel disease. Crit Care Q 1982 Sept; 5(2):21–27

Petlin AM and Carolan JM. Getting your patient through a lower gastrointestinal bleed. RN 1982 Feb; 45(2):42–45

Riepe SP. Acute lower gastrointestinal bleeding. Crit Care Q 1982 Sept; 5(2):29–32

Schwarz T. Is it 'acute abdomen?' RN 1982 July; 45(7):29–31; 94–96

Sherlock P. Cancer surveillance in inflammatory bowel disease. Postgrad Med 1983 Dec; 74(6):191–205

Simmons MA. Using the nursing process in treating inflammatory bowel disease. Nurs Clin North Am 1984 Mar; 19(1):11–25

Sparacino LL. Psychosocial considerations for the adolescent and young adult with inflammatory bowel disease. Nurs Clin North Am 1984 Mar; 19(1):41–49

Stotts NA et al. Care of the patient critically ill with inflammatory bowel disease. Nurs Clin North Am 1984 Mar; 19(1):61–70

Strange JM. The riddle of abdominal trauma. RN 1983 March; 46(3):43–46, 98–100

Tracking the cause of lower G.I. bleeding. Patient Care 1984 Mar 30; 18(6):76–117

Thomson NA. Abdominal trauma. Nursing '83 1983 July; 13(7):26–33

Ostomy Considerations

Cassell BL. The new trend in ileostomy surgery. RN 1984 Jan; 4(7):48–51

Click C. Chemotherapy and the ostomy patient. J Enterostomal Ther 1980 Sept–Oct; 7(5):10–12, 16

Nortridge JAS. Helpful hints for addressing the ostomate. Nursing '82 1982 Apr; 12(4):72–77

Simmons KN. Sexuality and the female ostomate. Am J Nurs 1983 Mar; 83(3):409–411

Trainor MA. Acceptance of ostomy and the visitor role in a self-help group for ostomy patients. Nurs Res 1982 Mar/Apr; 31(2):102–106

Watson PG. The effects of short-term postoperative counseling on cancer/ostomy patients. Ca Nurs 1983 Feb; 6(1):21–29

Wilkins L and Reeves K. The cuff-link flatus filter. Nurs Times 1984 May 31–June 5; 80(22):24–27

Zierath M. We'd made Gene more comfortable (ileostomy). Nursing '82 1982 Apr; 12(4):43–45

Colon and Rectum

Brils JG and Goldberg SM. Surgical options in ulcerative colitis. Postgrad Med 1983 Dec; 74(6):175–189

Burkett DP. Etiology and prevention of colorectal cancer. Hosp Pract 1984 Feb; 19(2):67–77

Fonkalsrud EW. Endorectal ileal pullthrough with ileal reservoir for ulcerative colitis and polyposis. Am J Surg 1982 July; 144(1):81–87

Gilman CJ. Improving survival in patients with rectal cancer. Am Fam Physician 1984 Jan; 29(1):165–169

Gramse CA. Diverticular disease. Nursing '83 1983 June; 13(6):56–57

Harary AM and Rogers AI. Gastroduodenal Crohn's disease. Postgrad Med 1983 Dec; 74(6):129–133, 137

Hocutt JE et al. Flexible fiberoptic sigmoidoscopy. Am Fam Physician 1982 Nov; 26(5):133–141

Ivarsson L et al. Short-term systemic prophylaxis with cefoxitin and doxycycline in colorectal surgery. Am J Surg 1982 Aug; 144(2):257–261

Mager-O'Connor E. How to identify and remove fecal impactions. Geriatr Nurs 1984; May/June; 5(3):158–161

Meyers S et al. Quality of life after surgery for Crohn's disease: A psychosocial survey. J Enterostomal Ther 1980 Sept–Oct; 7(5):25–31

Miskovitz PF and Steinberg H. Diverticula of the gastrointestinal tract. DM 1982 Dec; 29(3):1–61

Nursing Grand Rounds. Supporting the patient with Crohn's disease. Nursing '83 1983 Nov; 13(11):46–51

Scheotz DJ, Coller JA and Veidenheimer MC. Procto-colectomy with ileoanal reservoir, Postgrad Med 1984 Feb 15; 75(3):123–127

Sohn N, Weinstein MA and Robbins RD. Anorectal disorders. Curr Probl Surg 1983 Jan; 20(1):8–66

Stiklorius C. Large bowel diagnostics challenge your stress-reduction skills. RN 1982 May; 45(5):56–57

Sugarbaker PH. Carcinoma of the colon—prognosis and operative choices. Curr Probl Surg 1981 Dec; 18(12):757–801

Supporting the patient with Crohn's disease (Nursing Grand Rounds). Nursing '83 1983 Nov; 13(11):46–51

Weakley FL. Cancer of the rectum. Surg Clin North Am 1983 Feb; 63(1):129–135

Diagnostic Evaluation of the Liver

Dougherty WM. Serum bilirubin. Nursing '82 1982 Nov; 12(11):138–139

Frey CF. Endoscopic retrograde cholangiopancreatography. Amer J Surg 1982 July; 144(1):109–114

Horwitz CA. Laboratory diagnosis of viral hepatitis. Postgrad Med 1981 Nov; 70(5):105–117

Percutaneous transhepatic cholangiography. Postgrad Med 1981 Oct; 70(4):70–72

Winzelberg GG. Radionuclide evaluation of the hepatobiliary system. Am Fam Physician 1982 Oct; 26(4):203–207

Liver Dysfunction

Bullas J and Pfister S. Are you listening: Case Study. Crit Care Nurse 1983 Nov–Dec; 3(6):113–116

Balasegaram M. Management of hepatic abscess. Curr Probl Surg 1981 May; 18(5):285–340

Blendis LM. Status report on peritoneovenous shunting. Med Times 1984 May; 112(5):94–100

Bryan JA. Viral hepatitis. 1. Clinical and laboratory aspects and epidemiology. Postgrad Med 1980 Nov; 68(5):66–76

Bryan JA. Viral hepatitis. 2. Prevention and control. Postgrad Med 1980 Nov; 68(5):81–86

Can you carry hepatitis home? RN 1982 Feb; 45(2):91

DeVore NE, Jackson VM and Piening SL. TORCH infections. Am J Nurs 1983 Dec; 83(12):1660–1665

Dong B, Barton EC and Mancini BA. Viral hepatitis. Nurse Pract 1984 March; 9(3):27–32, 79

Dzik WH and Aller HHJ. Hepatitis B viral infection: Part 1—Clinical features. Am Fam Physician 1982 Aug; 26(2):119–126

Dzik WH and Aller HHJ. Hepatitis B viral infection: Part 2—Public health aspects. Am Fam Physician 1982 Sept; 26(3):135–142

Fredette SL. When the liver fails. Am J Nurs 1984 Jan; 84(1):64–67

Garvey EC and Manganaro M. Nursing implications of hepatic artery infusion. Cancer Nurs 1982 Feb; 5(1):51–55

Gever LN. Preventing hepatitis B with a new vaccine. Nursing '83 1983 Apr; 13(4):106

Gregory DH II. Hepatitis B vaccine. Postgrad Med 1984 Jan; 75(1):199–211

Gullatte MM and Foltz AT. Hepatic chemotherapy via implantable pump. Am J Nurs 1983 Dec; 83(12):1674–1676

Gurevich I. Viral hepatitis. Am J Nurs 1983 Apr; 83(4):571–586

Hepatitis B vaccine. Med Lett 1982 Aug 20; 24(616):75–76

Klopp A. Shunting malignant ascites. Am J Nurs 1984 Feb; 84(2):212–213

Leu MM. Hepatitis B: *You* are at highest risk. RN 1981 Sept; 44(9):74–79, 128, 130, 132

Maletic-Staschak S. Orthotopic liver transplantation. AORN J 1984 Jan; 39(1):35–39

Mar DD. Drug-induced hepatotoxicity. Am J Nurs 1982 Jan; 82(1):124–126

Misra P. Hepatic encephalopathy. Med Clin North Am 1981 Jan; 65(1):209–226

New hepatitis B vaccine: A breakthrough in hepatitis prevention. Am J Nurs 1982 Feb; 82(2):306–307

Pimstone NR and French SW. Alcoholic liver disease. Med Clin North Am 1984 Jan; 68(1):39–55

Resnick RH. Treatment of bleeding varices: controversy and opportunity. Hosp Pract 1984 Apr; 19(4):54a–54p

Schaal PG and Slemenda MB. Nurse's response to transplants. AORN J 1984 Jan; 39(1):42–45

Skelley L. Organ donation process. Focus Crit Care 1983 Aug; 10(4):44–46

Stever K. Liver carcinoma. AORN J 1984 Apr; 39(5):787–792

Traiger GL and Bohacheck P. Liver transplantation. Care of the patient in the acute postoperative period. Crit Care Nurse 1983 Sept/Oct; 3(5):96–103

West MJ. Liver transplantation. AORN J 1984 Jan; 39(1):40–41

Williams A. Hepatitis B virus vaccine. Nurse Pract 1983 Oct; 8(9):30, 32

Bleeding Esophageal Varices

Gruber M and Nuwer N. Treating esophageal varices with injection sclerotherapy. Am J Nurs 1982 Aug; 82(8):1214–1216

Gusberg R. Shunts for variceal hemorrhage: Why? when? what? Surg Clin North Am 1980 Oct; 60(5):1265–1272

King DE. Portal shunts: A fighting chance for your patient. RN 1983 July; 46(7):31–37

Martin F. How to salvage a bleeding cirrhosis patient. RN 1980 Jan; 43(1):59–65

Quinless, F. Portal hypertension—physiology, signs, and symptoms. Nursing '84 1984 Jan; 14(1):52–53

Gallbladder

Brown M. New internal bile drain prolongs lives. RN 1982 Jan; 45(1):46–47

Clearfield HR. Drug dissolution of gallstones. Am Fam Physician 1982 Jan; 25(1):202–204

Gannon RB and Pickett K. Jaundice. Am J Nurs 1983 March; 83(3):404–407

Heiss FW et al. Common bile duct calculi. 1. Surgical therapy. Postgrad Med 1984 Feb 15; 75(2):88–104

Heiss FW et al. Common bile duct calculi. 2. Nonsurgical therapy. Postgrad Med 1984 Feb 15; 75(2):109–117

Henry ML and Carey LC. Complications of cholecystectomy. Surg Clin North Am 1983 Dec; 63(6):1191–1204

Jordan GL. Choledocholithiasis. Curr Probl Surg 1982 Dec; 19(12):723–798

Kozarek RA. Endoscopically placed biliary drains and stents. Am Fam Physician 1983 Aug; 26(2):189–192

Quinless F. Teaching tips for T tube care at home. Nursing '84 1984 May; 14(5):62–64

Schoenfield LJ. Gallstones and other biliary diseases. Clin Symp (CIBA) 1982; 34(4):2–32

Stiklorius C. Getting ready for gallbladder studies. RN 1982 July; 45(7):64–65

Tangedahl TN. Management of gallstones. Postgrad Med 1983 Nov; 74(5):115–121

Taylor DL. Jaundice. Nursing '83 1983 Aug; 13(8):52–54

Taylor DL. Gallstones. Nursing '83 1983 June; 13(6):44–45

Thomas MJ, Pellegrini CA and Way LW. Usefulness of diagnostic tests for biliary obstruction. Am J Surg 1982 July; 144(1):102–108

Conditions of the Pancreas

Cooperman AM. Chronic pancreatitis. Surg Clin North Am 1981 Feb; 61(1):71–83

Geokas MC. Ethanol and the pancreas. Med Clin North Am 1984 Jan; 68(1):57–75

Gotch PM. Are you ready for a total pancreatectomy patient? RN 1981 Nov; 44(11):54–57

Kelber Sr MB. Pancreatic enzymes. Nursing '82 1982 Dec; 12(12):65–67

Kosel K et al. Total pancreatectomy and islet cell autotransplantation. Am J Nurs 1982 April; 82(4):568–571

Levine CD. Preventing complications in the pancreatoduodenectomy patient. DCCN 1983 Mar/Apr; 2(2):90–97

McFadden EA, Zaloga GP and Chernow B. Hypocalcemia: A medical emergency. Am J Nurs 1983 Feb; 83(2):227–230

Moossa AR and Altorki N. Pancreatic biopsy. Surg Clin North Am 1983 Dec; 63(6):1205–1214

Nasrallah SM. The management of acute pancreatitis. Crit Care Q 1982 Sept; 5(2):15–20

Ropka ME. Pancreatic insufficiency in the person with cancer. Cancer Nurs 1981 Feb; 4(1):37–41

Sigmon HD. Helping your long-term trauma patient travel the road to recovery. Nursing '84 1984 Jan; 4(1):58–63

Toskes PP and Greenberger NJ. Acute and chronic pancreatitis. DM 1983 Mar; 29(6):5–81

Van Hurden JA. First encounters with pheochromocytoma. Am J Surg 1982 Aug; 144(2):277–279

Renal and Genitourinary Conditions

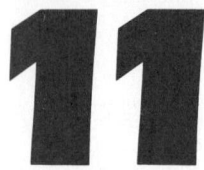

Clinical Manifestations of Urinary Dysfunction

Changes in Micturition (Voiding)

1. Hematuria (red blood cells in urine)
   a. Hematuria is considered a serious sign and requires evaluation.
   b. Color of bloody urine dependent on pH of urine and amount of blood present.
      (1) Acid urine is dark, smoky color.
      (2) Alkaline urine is red color.
   c. Hematuria may be due to systemic cause such as blood dyscrasias, anticoagulant therapy, neoplasms, trauma, extreme exercise.
   d. Painless hematuria may indicate neoplasm in the urinary tract.
   e. Hematuria from renal colic (stones in kidney).
   f. Bloody spotting reveals bleeding from urethra, bladder neoplasms.
   g. Hematuria also seen in renal tuberculosis, polycystic disease of kidneys, septic pyelonephritis, thrombosis and embolism involving renal artery or vein.
2. Proteinuria (albuminuria)
   a. Normal urine does not contain persistent protein in significant quantities.
   b. Proteinuria characteristically seen in all forms of acute and chronic renal disease (more characteristic of glomerulonephritis than pyelonephritis).
      (1) The protein is mainly albumin, but globulin is also present.
      (2) Albumin and globulin escape through damaged glomerular capillaries in a greater amount than can be reabsorbed by the tubules, or damaged tubules fail to reabsorb normal amount filtered.
   c. Proteinuria occurs in systemic diseases where there are varying degrees of renal anoxia, as in cardiac decompensation, diabetic glomerulosclerosis.
   d. Mild proteinuria may occur from other sources—urethritis, prostatitis, cystitis.
3. Dysuria (painful or difficult voiding)—seen in wide variety of pathologic conditions.
4. Frequency—voiding occurs more often than usual, when compared with the patient's usual pattern (or with a generally accepted norm of once every 3–6 hours).
   a. Determine if habits governing fluid intake have been altered; it is essential to know normal voiding pattern in order to evaluate frequency.
   b. Increasing frequency can result from a variety of conditions—such as infection and diseases of urinary tract, metabolic disease, hypertension, medications (diuretics).

5. Urgency (strong desire to urinate)—due to inflammatory lesions in bladder, prostate, or urethra, acute bacterial infections, chronic prostatitis in men, and chronic posterior urethrotrigonitis in women.
6. Burning upon urination—seen in urethral irritation or bladder infections.
7. Pneumaturia (passage of gas in urine during voiding)—caused by fistulous connection between bowel and bladder, rectosigmoid cancer, regional ileitis, sigmoid diverticulitis (most common), and gas-forming urinary tract infections.
8. Strangury (slow and painful urination); only small amounts of urine voided; blood staining may be noted—seen in severe cystitis.
9. Hesitancy (undue delay and difficulty in initiating voiding)—may indicate compression of urethra, outlet obstruction, neurogenic bladder.
10. Nocturia (excessive urination at night)—suggests decreased renal concentrating ability or heart failure, diabetes mellitus, poor bladder emptying.
11. Urinary incontinence (involuntary loss of urine)—may be due to injury to external urinary sphincter, acquired neurogenic disease, severe urgency, etc.
12. Stress incontinence (intermittent leakage of urine due to sudden strain)—indicates weakness of sphincteric mechanism.
13. Polyuria (large volume of urine voided in given time)—demonstrated in diabetes mellitus, diabetes insipidus.
14. Oliguria (small volume of urine; output between 100–500 ml./24 hours)—may result from acute renal failure, shock, dehydration, fluid–ion imbalance.
15. Anuria (absence of urine in the bladder; output less than 50 ml./24 hours)—indicates serious renal dysfunction requiring immediate medical intervention.
16. Enuresis (involuntary voiding during sleep)—may be physiologic to age of 3 years; thereafter, may be functional or symptomatic of obstructive disease (usually of lower urinary tract).

Urinary Tract Pain

1. Genitourinary pain is not always present in renal disease, but is generally seen in the more acute conditions.
2. Pain of renal disease is caused by sudden distention of the renal capsule; severity is related to how quickly the distention develops.
3. Kidney pain—may be felt as a dull ache in costovertebral angle; may spread to umbilicus.
4. Ureteral pain—felt in the back and radiates to the abdomen, upper thighs, testes, or labia.
5. Flank pain (side area between ribs and ilium)—radiates to lower abdomen or epigastrium and often is associated with nausea, vomiting, and paralytic ileus; most commonly secondary to a renal lesion (stone, tumor, or infection).
6. Bladder pain (low abdominal pain or pain over suprapubic area)—may be due to bladder infection or overdistended bladder.
7. Urethral pain from irritation of bladder neck, from foreign body in canal, or from urethritis due to infection or trauma.
8. Pain in scrotal area from inflammatory swelling of epididymis or testicle, or torsion of the testicle.
9. Testicular pain due to injury, mumps orchitis, torsion of spermatic cord.
10. Perineal or rectal discomfort from acute prostatitis, prostatic abscess.
11. Back and leg pain from cancer of prostate with metastases to pelvic bones.
12. Pain in glans penis is usually from prostatitis; penile shaft pain is from urethral problems.

Related Gastrointestinal Symptoms

Gastrointestinal symptoms related to urologic conditions include nausea, vomiting, diarrhea, abdominal discomfort, paralytic ileus, and gastrointestinal hemorrhage with uremia.

Assessment of Urologic Function

Health History

Seek the following information related to urinary and renal function:

1. What is the patient's chief concern? Why is he seeking help?
2. What is (are) the patient's present and past occupation(s)? (Look for occupational hazards related to the urinary tract—contact with chemicals, plastics, pitch, tar, rubber.)
3. What is the patient's smoking history?
4. What is the past history, especially in relation to urinary problems?
5. Is there any family history of renal disease?
6. What childhood diseases did the patient have?
7. Is there a history of urinary infections?
8. Did enuresis continue beyond the usual age (past 3 years of age)?
9. Are there any voiding disorders?
   a. Dysuria? When does it occur? Where is it felt? Initial or terminal dysuria?
   b. Hesitancy? Straining? Pain during or after urination?
   c. Changes in color of urine? Diminished urine output?
   d. Incontinence? Stress incontinence? Urgency incontinence?
   e. Any history of hematuria?
   f. How often does the patient get up to void during the night? How much urine is passed?
10. Is pain present?
    Location? Character? Radiation? Duration? Related to voiding? What brings it on? What relieves it?
11. Has the patient had fever? Chills? Passage of stones?
12. Any history of genital lesions or sexually transmitted diseases?
13. For the female patient:
    What is the number of children? Their ages? Any forceps deliveries? Catheterizations? When? Any signs of vaginal discharge? Vaginal/vulvar itch or irritation?
14. Does the patient have diabetes mellitus? Hypertension? Allergies?
15. Has the patient ever been hospitalized with a urinary tract infection?
    Urinary tract infection before the age of 12? Ever

cystoscoped? Catheterized with an indwelling catheter? Kidney x-ray procedures?

Diagnostic Tests

Radiologic Techniques

A. **Roentgenogram**—flat plate, KUB (x-ray of kidney, ureters, bladder) is used to delineate size, shape, and position of kidneys, but includes organs up to the level of symphysis pubis.

1. Gives a baseline reference for subsequent films.
2. Reveals any deviations, such as stones, hydronephrosis, cysts, tumors, or kidney displacement by abnormalities in the surrounding tissues.

B. **Computed Tomography**—provides a cross-sectional view of kidney and urinary tract to detect the presence and extent of urologic disease; a computer measures small changes in x-ray absorption and magnifies the differences from tissue to tissue so a display can be made and read. No preparation needed; noninvasive.

C. **Nephrotomogram**—body section roentgenograms, which bring into focus the different layers of the kidney and the diffuse structures in that layer; done also as part of intravenous pyelogram study.

D. **Infusion Drip Pyelography**—an intravenous infusion of a large volume of dilute solution of contrast material to produce opacification of the renal parenchyma and complete filling of urinary tract. Films taken at intervals to demonstrate the filled and distended collecting system.

1. Patient preparation is same as for excretory urography *except that the patient is not dehydrated* (see below).
2. Infusion drip pyelography has almost replaced standard intravenous pyelography; it is used when regular urographic techniques fail to show drainage structures satisfactorily.

E. **Excretory Urography** (intravenous urogram [IVU] or intravenous pyelogram [IVP])—introduction (IV) of a radiopaque contrast medium, which concentrates in the urine and thus facilitates visualization of the kidneys, ureter, and bladder. The contrast medium is cleared from the bloodstream by renal excretion.

1. Excretory urography is used in the following:
   a. Initial investigation of any suspected urologic problem, especially in diagnosis of lesions in kidneys and ureters.
   b. To provide a rough estimate of renal function.
2. Patient preparation
   a. See that the patient is not overhydrated—will dilute contrast material and thus cause inadequate visualization (except in patients with myeloma).
   b. Remove obstructing intestinal content, if possible, to minimize intestinal gas; enema not usually given, since it may increase gas in the gastrointestinal tract.
   c. It is customary to take no liquids for 8–10 hours before this test, although good films are often obtained in the hydrated patient.

▶ **NURSING ALERT:** Elderly patients with poor renal reserve or those with multiple myeloma may not tolerate dehydrating procedures and should be given water to drink. Persons with uncontrolled diabetes may be sensitive to fluid restriction.

d. Give laxative the night before the test to eliminate feces and gas in the intestinal tract.
e. Ascertain if the patient has history of allergies—to find the high-risk patient.
   See pages 660–662.

F. **Retrograde Pyelography**—injection of opaque material through ureteral catheters, which have been passed up ureters into renal pelvis by means of cystoscopic manipulation. The opaque solution is introduced by gravity or syringe.

1. Retrograde pyelography usually done when nonfunctioning kidney is suspected or if the patient is allergic to intravenous contrast material.
2. Performed with decreasing frequency because of improvement of IVP techniques.

G. **Renal Angiography**—visualization of renal arterial supply. Contrast medium is injected through a catheter (which is placed under fluoroscope control) via the femoral and iliac arteries into the aorta or renal artery.

1. Angiography evaluates blood flow dynamics, demonstrates abnormal vasculature, and differentiates renal cysts from renal tumors.
2. *Nursing responsibilities before procedure*
   a. Give cathartic or enema as prescribed to eliminate fecal material and gas from colon and to ensure unobstructed radiographs.
   b. Shave proposed injection sites—groin (for femoral approach) or axilla (for axillary approach).
   c. Locate and mark peripheral pulses to facilitate postprocedure nursing evaluation.
   d. Inform the patient what to expect during procedure.
      (1) Procedure is done under local anesthesia; the patient will probably be given preoperative medication.
      (2) The procedure may take from 30 minutes to 2 hours.
      (3) There may be a transient feeling of heat along the course of the vessel upon injection of contrast material.
3. *Nursing responsibilities following procedure*
   a. Take vital signs until stabilized; take blood pressure readings on opposite arm if axillary artery was punctured.
   b. Assess puncture site for swelling and development of hematoma.
   c. Palpate peripheral pulses (radial, femoral, dorsalis pedis).
   d. Note color and temperature of involved extremity, comparing it with the uninvolved extremity.
   e. Apply cold compresses to puncture site—to decrease edema and pain.

H. **Radionuclide Techniques** (noninvasive procedures that do not interfere with normal physiologic processes and require no specific patient preparation)

1. Radiopharmaceuticals (^{99}Tc-labeled compound or ^{131}I–hippurate) are injected intravenously.
2. Studies obtained with a scintillation camera placed posterior to the kidney with the patient in a supine, prone, or sitting position.
3. The resultant image (scan) indicates the distribution of the radiopharmaceutical within the kidney.

I. **Ultrasonic Scan** (echogram, sonography)—scanning by ultrasound is a noninvasive technique for investigation of renal disease. The kidneys produce a characteristic ultrasonic pattern, making abnormalities readily identifiable. Also used in assessing retroperitoneal disease and in staging malignancies of urinary bladder and prostate. Noninvasive test; no special patient preparation is necessary.

Endourology *(urologic endoscopic procedures)*

A. Cystoscopic Examination—involves direct visualization of the urethra, prostatic urethra, and bladder by means of a tubular, lighted, telescopic lens.

1. *Uses*
   a. To inspect bladder wall directly for tumor, stone, or ulcer and to inspect urethra, especially the prostatic urethra prior to surgery.
   b. To allow insertion of catheters into the ureters to obtain a separate specimen from each kidney and evaluate renal function separately.
   c. To see configuration and position of ureteral orifices.
   d. To remove calculi from urethra, bladder, and ureter.
   e. To treat lesions of bladder, urethra, and prostate.
2. *Patient preparation*
   a. Preparation depends on type of anesthesia to be used (general or local).
   b. Give information about the examination, prescribed oral fluids, and preoperative medication.
3. *Nursing support following procedure*
   a. Expect the patient to have some burning upon voiding, blood-tinged urine, and urinary frequency from trauma to mucous membrane.
   b. Watch patients with prostatic hypertrophy for urinary retention due to edema from instrumentation.
   c. If the patient complains of pain, give warm sitz baths.
   d. Use indwelling catheter if urinary retention persists.
4. *Complications following cystoscopy*
   (More apt to occur in patients with obstructive pathology)

a. Urinary retention
b. Urinary tract hemorrhage
c. Infection within prostate or bladder

B. Renal and Ureteral Brush Biopsy—introduction of catheter followed by a biopsy brush, which is passed through the catheter; suspected lesion is brushed back and forth to obtain cells and surface tissue fragments for histologic diagnosis.

C. Renal Endoscopy, Nephroscopy—introduction of fiberoptic scope into the renal pelvis during an open renal operation (pyelotomy) or percutaneously to view interior of renal pelvis, remove calculi, biopsy small lesions, and diagnose renal hematuria and selected renal tumors.

Needle Biopsy of Kidney

Needle biopsy of the kidney is performed by percutaneous needle biopsy through renal tissue (Fig. 11-1*A*) or by open biopsy through a small flank incision. It is useful in evaluating the course of renal disease and in securing specimens for electron and immunofluorescent microscopy.

A. Prebiopsy Management

1. Coagulation studies are carried out to identify the patient at risk for postbiopsy bleeding; serum creatinine and urinalysis are done.
2. The patient may be placed on a fasting regimen for 3 hours before the procedure. An IV line may be established.
3. Secure and save a voided specimen before biopsy—for comparison with postbiopsy specimen.
4. Instruct the patient that he may be asked to hold his breath (to stop movement of the kidney) while the biopsy needle is inserted.

B. Postbiopsy Nursing Management
   Goal:
   Observe the patient for evidences of bleeding.

1. Keep the patient supine as long as directed.
2. Take the vital signs every 5–15 minutes for first hour

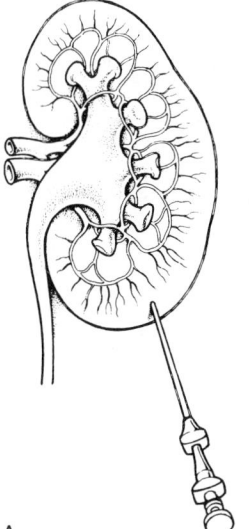
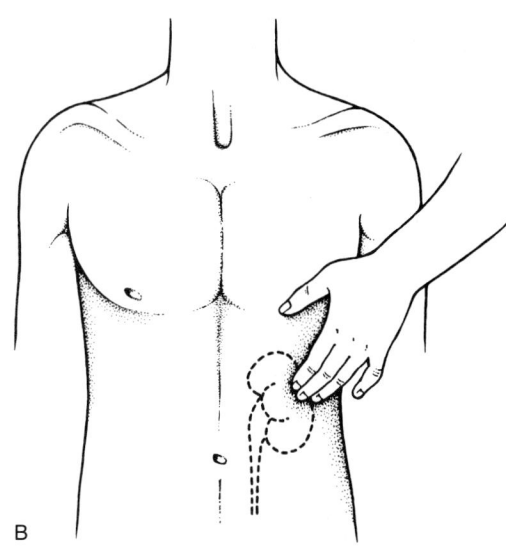

Figure 11-1. *(A)* Percutaneous needle biopsy of the kidney. *(B)* Examining for enlarging hematoma.

A   B

and then with decreasing frequency if stable to assess for hemorrhage, which is a major complication.
  a. Watch for rise or fall in blood pressure, anorexia, vomiting, or development of a dull, aching discomfort in abdomen.
  b. Assess for flank pain (usually represents bleeding into the muscle) or colicky pain (clot in the ureter).
  c. Assess for backache, shoulder pain, or dysuria.
  d. Persistent bleeding may be suspected when there is an enlarging hematoma, which is palpable (Fig. 11-1*B*).
  e. If perirenal bleeding develops, avoid palpating or manipulating the abdomen after the first examination has determined that a hematoma exists.
3. Measure each voiding and inspect for bleeding. Compare samples with each other and with prebiopsy specimen.
4. Assess for any patient complaints, especially frequency and urgency.
5. Keep the fluid level at 3,000 ml. daily if tolerated, unless the patient has renal insufficiency.
6. A hematocrit and hemoglobin study may be done within 8 hours to assess for anemia.
7. Prepare for transfusion and surgical intervention for control of hemorrhage, which may necessitate surgical drainage or nephrectomy (removal of kidney).

C. Discharge Planning and Patient Education

Instruct the patient as follows:
1. Avoid strenuous activity, strenuous sports, and heavy lifting for at least 2 weeks.
2. Notify physician if any of the following occur: flank pain, hematuria, light-headedness and fainting, rapid pulse, or any other signs and symptoms of bleeding.
3. Report for follow-up 1–2 months after biopsy; the patient is checked for hypertension, and the biopsy area is auscultated for a bruit.

Urodynamic Studies

A. Urodynamic studies—provide physiologic and structural tests to evaluate bladder and urethral function by measuring the (1) rate of urine flow, (2) bladder pressures during voiding and at rest, (3) internal urethral resistance, and (4) bladder contraction and relaxation.

B. Uroflowmetry (flow rate)—record of the volume of urine passing through the urethra per unit of time (ml./second).

C. Cystometrogram—graphic recording of the pressures exerted at varying phases of filling of the urinary bladder. Intermittent filling of the bladder can be recorded and compared with changes in intravesical pressure.
1. The patient is requested to void. Physician observes the time it takes to initiate voiding; size, force, and continuity of urinary stream; degree of straining, hesitancy, intermittency of urination, presence of terminal dribbling.
2. The patient is then placed in lithotomy position, and a retention catheter is placed through urethra and into bladder. The residual volume is measured, and the catheter is left in place.
3. The urethral catheter is connected to a water manometer, and water is allowed to flow into bladder, usually at the rate of 1 ml./second.
  a. The patient informs examiner when he feels the

first desire to void and again when the bladder feels full. The degree of bladder filling at these points is recorded.
  b. The pressures above the zero level at the symphysis pubis are measured, and the pressures and volumes within the bladder are plotted and recorded.

D. Urethral pressure profile—graphic recording of the pressure within the urethra at each point along its length. Gas and fluid are instilled through a catheter that is withdrawn while pressures along the urethral wall are obtained.

E. Cystourethrogram—visualization of urethra and bladder either by retrograde injection or by voiding of contrast material.
1. Bladder is filled with radiopaque medium, and the patient then voids while rapid spot films are taken.
2. With the image intensifier, the presence or absence of vesicoureteral reflux and/or congenital abnormalities in the lower urinary tract can be demonstrated. Also used to investigate difficulty in bladder emptying and incontinence.

F. Electromyography—uses placement of electrodes into the anus or insertion of fine needle probes through the perineum into the periurethral or perianal musculature.

Tests of Renal Function

1. Renal function tests are used to determine effectiveness of the kidneys' excretory functioning, to evaluate the severity of kidney disease, and to follow the patient's progress.
2. Renal function may be within normal limits until about 50% of renal function has been lost.
3. Best results are obtained by combining a number of clinical tests. Table 11-1 lists the more common tests of renal function.

Urine Examination

Factors Affecting Composition of the Urine
1. Nutritional status
2. Metabolic processes
3. Status of kidney function

Amount
1. 1,200–1,500 ml./24 hours; less than 500 ml. is considered *oliguria*.
2. Day volume 2 to 3 times more than night volume.

Appearance
1. Normal urine is clear.
2. Turbid (cloudy) urine is not always pathologic. Normal urine may develop turbidity on refrigeration or from standing at room temperature; bacteria ferment urine quickly at room temperature.
3. Abnormally cloudy urine—due to pus, blood, epithelial cells, bacteria, fat, colloidal particles, phosphate, urates.

Odor
1. Normal—faint aromatic odor.
2. Characteristic odors produced by ingestion of asparagus, thymol.
3. Cloudy urine with ammonia odor—urea-splitting

Table 11-1   Tests of Renal Function

1. **There is no single test of renal function; renal function is variable from time to time.**
2. **The rate of change of renal function is more important than the result of a single test.**

Test	Purpose/Rationale	Test Protocol

Renal concentration test
  Specific gravity
  Refractive index
  Osmolality of urine
	Evaluates the ability to concentrate solutes in the urine.
	Concentration ability is lost early in kidney disease; hence, this test detects early defects in renal function.
		Fluids may be withheld 12–24 hours to evaluate the concentrating ability of the tubules under controlled conditions. Specific gravity measurements of urine are taken at specific times to determine urine concentration.

Phenolsulfonphthalein excretion test (PSP)	A diagnostic agent (phenolsulfonphthalein) is given to determine the functional capacity of the kidney. (PSP test can also be used as a measure to assess residual urine.) Delayed excretion is seen in renal disease, cardiac failure, primary vascular disease.	Encourage fluids 1–1½ hours before the test. Phenolsulfonphthalein is given IV. (1) Record exact time dye is administered. (2) Collect urine in 15 minutes, 30 minutes, and 1 hour.
Creatinine clearance* (endogenous creatinine clearance)	Provides a reasonable approximation of rate of glomerular filtration. Measures volume of blood cleared of creatinine in 1 minute. Most sensitive indication of early renal disease. Useful to follow progress of the patient's renal status.	Collect all urine over 24-hour period. Draw one sample of blood within the period.
Serum creatinine	A test of renal function reflecting the balance between production and filtration by renal glomerulus. Most sensitive test of renal function.	Do test on blood serum.
Serum urea nitrogen (blood urea nitrogen [BUN])	Serves as index of renal excretory capacity. Serum urea nitrogen is dependent on the body's urea production and on urine flow. (Urea is the nitrogenous end-product of protein metabolism.) Affected by protein intake, tissue breakdown.	Do test on blood serum.

* Clearance is the amount of blood cleansed of a constituent per unit of time.

bacteria such as *Proteus,* causing urinary tract infections.

4. Offensive odor—bacterial action in presence of pus.

Color

1. Color shows degree of concentration and depends on amount voided.
2. Normal urine is clear yellow or amber because of the pigment urochrome.
3. Color varies with specific gravity:
   a. Dilute urine is straw-colored.
   b. Concentrated urine is highly colored; a sign of insufficient fluid intake.
4. Abnormally colored urine
   a. Turbid or smoky colored—may be from hematuria, spermatozoa, prostatic fluid, fat droplets, chyle.
   b. Red or red-brown—due to blood pigments, porphyria, transfusion reaction, bleeding lesions in urogenital tract, some drugs.
   c. Yellow-brown or green-brown—may reveal obstructive lesion of bile duct system or obstructive jaundice.
   d. Orange-red or orange-brown—from urobilin or from Pyridium, a urinary antiseptic.
   e. Dark brown or black—due to malignant melanoma, leukemia.

Reaction (pH)

1. Reflects the ability of kidney to maintain normal hydrogen ion concentration in plasma and extracellular fluid; indicates *acidity* or *alkalinity* of urine.
2. The pH should be measured in fresh urine, since the breakdown of urine to ammonia causes urine to become alkaline.
3. Normal pH is around 6 (acid); may normally vary from 4.6 to 7.5.
4. Urine acidity or alkalinity has relatively little clinical significance unless the patient is on special diet or therapeutic program or is being treated for renal calculous disease.
5. Alkaline urine is often cloudy because of phosphate crystals.

Specific Gravity

1. Reflects the kidney's ability to concentrate or dilute urine; may reflect degree of hydration or dehydration.
2. Normal specific gravity ranges from 1.005–1.025.
3. Specific gravity is fixed at 1.010 in chronic renal failure.
4. In a person eating a normal diet, inability to concentrate or dilute urine indicates disease.

Osmolality

1. *Osmolality* is an indication of the amount of osmotically active particles in urine (specifically, it is the number of particles per unit volume of *water*). It is similar to specific gravity, but is considered a more precise test; it is also easy to do—only 1–2 ml. of urine are required.
2. The unit of osmotic measure is the *osmole.*
   Average values:
   Females: 300–1,090 mOsm./kg.
   Males: 390–1,090 mOsm./kg.

Abnormal Urine Constituents

1. *Proteinuria* (albuminuria)—characteristically seen in all forms of acute and chronic renal disease.
   a. Normal urine does not have persistent protein in significant quantities.
   b. Proteinuria also occurs in systemic diseases where there are varying degrees of renal anoxia, cardiac decompensation, diabetic glomerulosclerosis, etc.
2. *Glucosuria*—glucose in the urine; seen most frequently in diabetes mellitus.
3. *Ketonuria*—the presence of ketone bodies (acetone, acetoacetic acid, and beta-hydroxybutyric acid). Ketonuria indicates incomplete fat metabolism (diabetic ketoacidosis), dehydration, starvation; also seen after aspirin ingestion.
4. *Hematuria*—red blood cells in the urine.
5. *Pyuria*—white blood cells in the urine.
6. *Bacteriuria*—bacteria in the urine.
7. *Crystalluria*—excretion of crystals in the urine.

Dipstick Tests (Reagent Tests)

Strips that have been impregnated with chemicals are dipped quickly in urine and "read" as a means of testing urine.
1. When dipped in urine, the chemicals react with abnormal substances in the urine by changing color.
2. Some dipsticks can test for only one substance, whereas others can test several substances simultaneously.

Basic Principles for Collecting Urine Specimens

1. The first morning urine specimen is most concentrated and more likely to reveal abnormalities.
2. Urine should not be left standing at room temperature, since it becomes alkaline because of contamination of urea-splitting bacteria from the environment.
3. All specimens should be refrigerated as soon as possible after they are voided.
4. Microscopic examination should be done within ½ hour after collection—standing causes dissolution of cellular elements and casts, and bacterial overgrowth unless obtained by sterile methods.
5. Urine specimens should be collected from the patient by means of the clean-catch midstream technique using a wide-mouth container (see below and Fig. 11-2).
6. Collection of 24-hour specimen:
   a. Ensure that the patient understands the procedure. *All* urine must be collected within a 24-hour period via clean-catch technique.
   b. Have the patient empty the bladder at specified time (e.g., 8:00 AM). *Discard urine.*
   c. Collect all urine voided during the next 24 hours.
   d. Collect last specimen at 8:00 AM on following day (or 24 hours after collection was started).
   e. Keep collected urine in the refrigerator in a clean bottle; a suitable preservative/stabilizer may be required.
   f. Start with an empty bladder and finish with an empty bladder.

Guidelines: Technique for Obtaining Clean-Catch Midstream Voided Specimen

A *clean-catch midstream specimen* is the best clinically effective method of securing a voided specimen for urinalysis. It is not a simple procedure and requires patient education and active assistance of the female patient.

Equipment

Antiseptic solution or liquid soap solution
Sterile water
4 × 4 sponges
Disposable gloves for nurse assisting female patient
Sterile specimen container

Procedure

Nursing Action	Rationale/Amplification
Male Patient	
1. Instruct the patient to expose glans and cleanse area around meatus. Wash area with mild antiseptic solution or liquid soap. *Rinse thoroughly.*	1. The urethral orifice is colonized by bacteria. Urine readily becomes contaminated during voiding. Rinse antiseptic solution or soap solution thoroughly because these agents can inhibit bacterial growth in a urine culture.
2. Allow the initial urinary flow to escape.	2. The first portion of urine washes out the urethra and contains debris.
3. Collect the midstream urine specimen in a sterile container.	
4. Avoid collecting the last few drops of urine.	4. Prostatic secretions may be introduced into urine at the end of the urinary stream.
5. Send specimen to laboratory immediately.	

Procedure
(Cont.)

Nursing Action	Rationale/Amplification
Female Patient	
1. Ask the patient to separate her labia to expose the urethral orifice. If no one is available to assist the patient, she may sit backwards on the toilet seat facing the water tank or sit on (straddle) the wide part of the bedpan.	1. Keeping the labia separated prevents labial or vaginal contamination of the urine specimen. By straddling the toilet seat/bedpan, the patient's labia are spread apart for cleansing.
2. Cleanse the area around the urinary meatus with sponges soaked with antiseptic/soap solution. Rinse thoroughly. a. Wipe the perineum from the front to the back. b. Do not use sponges more than once.	2. The urethral orifice is colonized by bacteria. Urine readily becomes contaminated during voiding.
3. While the patient keeps the labia separated (Fig. 11-2), instruct her to void forcibly.	3. This helps wash away urethral contaminants.

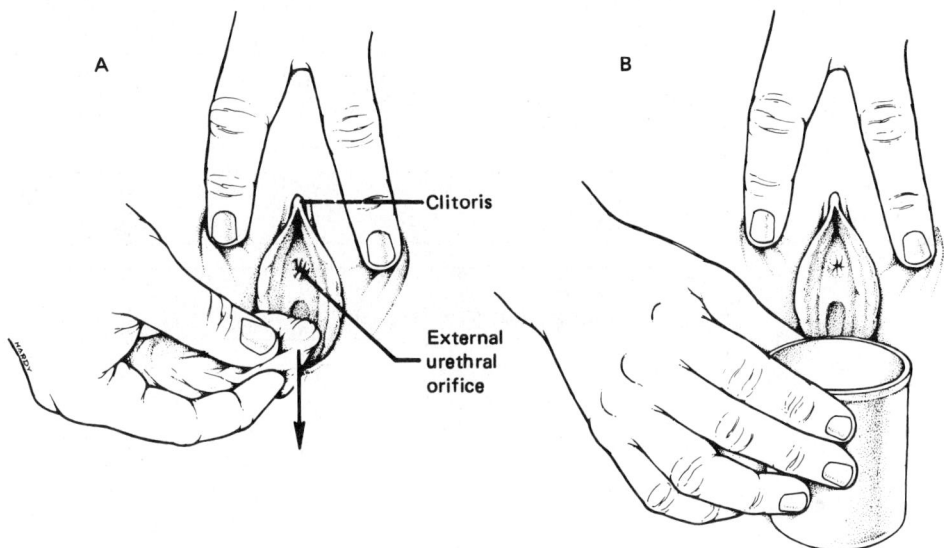

Figure 11-2. Obtaining a clean-catch midstream urine specimen in the female. (A) Instruct the patient to hold the labia apart and wash from high up front toward the back with gauze soaked in soap. (B) The collection cup is held so that it does not touch the body, and the sample is obtained only while the patient is voiding with the labia held apart.

Nursing Action	Rationale/Amplification
4. Allow initial urinary flow to drain into bedpan (toilet) and then catch the midstream specimen in a sterile container, making sure that the container does not come in contact with the genitalia.	4. The first portion of urine washes out the urethra. Have the patient remove the container from the stream while she is still voiding.
5. Send the specimen to the laboratory immediately.	5. Too long an interval between collection and analysis produces unreliable results.

Catheterization

Guidelines: Catheterization of the Urinary Bladder

Purpose
1. To relieve acute or chronic urinary retention.
2. For preoperative and postoperative urinary drainage.
3. To determine amount of residual urine after voiding.

(continued)

Guidelines: Catheterization of the Urinary Bladder (continued)

Equipment

        Sterile gloves
        Disposable sterile catheter set with single-use packet of lubricant
        Antiseptic solution for periurethral cleansing (sterile)
        Gloves, drape, sponges
        Sterile container for culture
        Bath blanket/sheet for draping
        Standing lamp (preferred) or flashlight

Selection of Catheter Size

Use the smallest size catheter capable of providing adequate drainage (Fig. 11-3)

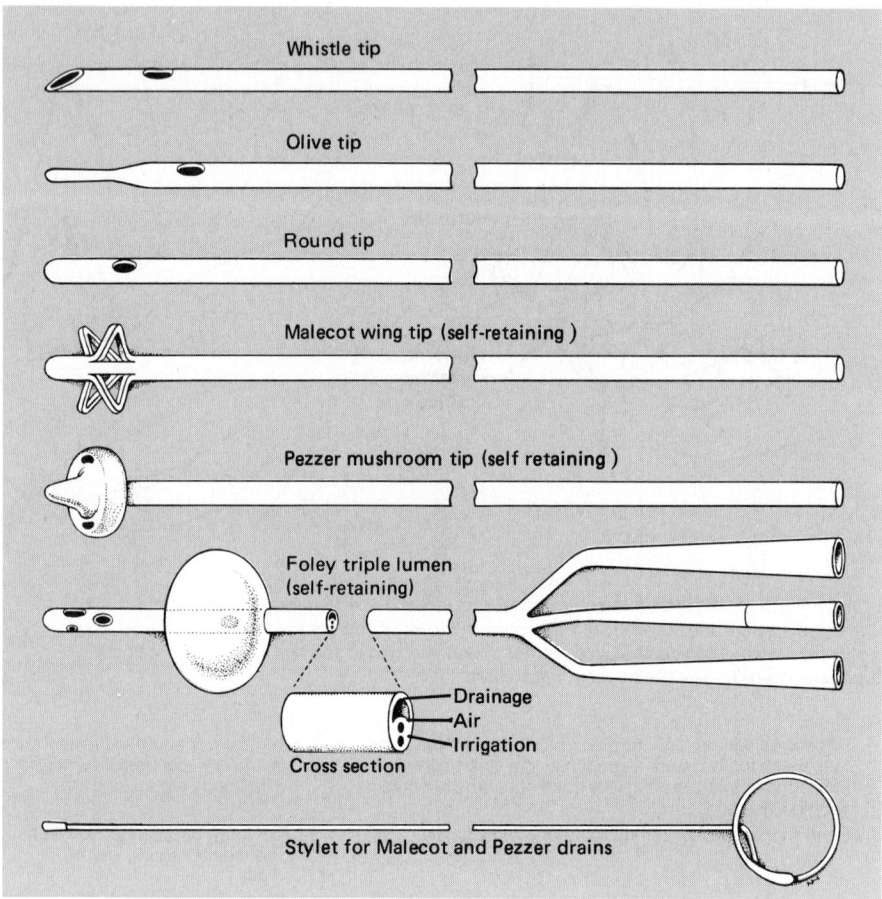

Figure 11-3. Types of catheters.

Procedure

Nursing Action	Rationale/Amplification
Female Patient	
Preparatory Phase	
1. Put the patient at ease.	1. The patient will feel reassured if the procedure is explained and if she is handled gently and considerately.
2. Open catheter tray using aseptic technique. Place waste receptacle in accessible place.	2. Catheterization requires the same aseptic precautions as a surgical procedure.

Procedure
(Cont.)

Nursing Action	Rationale/Amplification

Nursing Action

3. Direct light for visualization of genital area.
4. Place the patient in a supine position with knees bent, hips flexed, and feet resting on bed about 0.6 m. (2 feet) apart. Drape the patient.
5. Position moisture-proof pad under the patient's buttocks.
6. Wash hands. Put on sterile gloves.

Performance Phase

1. Separate labia minora so that urethral meatus is visualized; one hand is to maintain separation of the labia until catheterization is finished.

Rationale/Amplification

1. This maneuver helps prevent labial contamination of the catheter (Fig. 11-4).

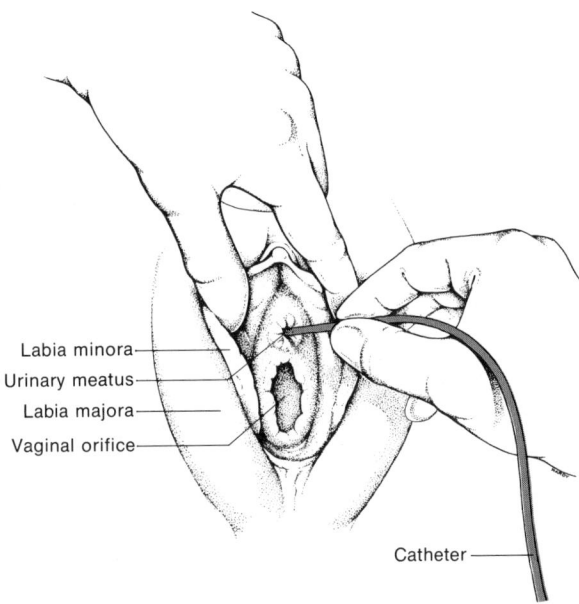

Labia minora
Urinary meatus
Labia majora
Vaginal orifice

Catheter

Figure 11-4. Catheterization of urinary bladder in female.

2. Cleanse around the urethral meatus with a povidone-iodine solution.
   a. Manipulate cleansing sponges with forceps, cleansing with downward strokes from anterior to posterior.
   b. Dispose of cotton sponge after each use.
   c. If the patient is sensitive to iodine, benzalkonium chloride or other cleansing agent is used.
3. Introduce well-lubricated catheter 5–7.5 cm. (2–3 inches) into urethral meatus using strict aseptic technique.
   a. Avoid contaminating surface of catheter.
   b. Ensure that catheter is not too large or too tight at urethral meatus.
4. Pinch off catheter and remove gently when urine ceases to flow.

Follow-up Phase

1. Dry area; make patient comfortable.
2. Measure urine and dispose of equipment.
3. Send specimen to laboratory as indicated.
4. Record time, procedure, amount, and appearance of urine.

2. Microorganisms inhabiting the distal urethra may be introduced into the bladder during or immediately after catheter insertion. Inadequate preparation of the urethral meatus is a major cause of infection.

3. A well-lubricated catheter reduces friction and trauma to the meatus. The female urethra is a relatively short canal, measuring 3.0–4 cm. in length.
   b. Too large a catheter may cause painful distention of the meatus.

4. Pinching off the catheter prevents air from entering the bladder as the catheter is removed.

(continued)

Guidelines: Catheterization of the Urinary Bladder (continued)

Procedure
(Cont.)

Nursing Action	Rationale/Amplification

Male Patient

1. Carry out all of "preparatory phase" as for female patient except:
2. Place the patient in supine position with legs extended. Place the moisture-proof pad across upper thighs.
3. Position the perineal drape.
4. Lubricate the catheter well.

    4. A well-lubricated catheter prevents urethral trauma (decreasing the opportunity for bacterial invasion).

5. Wash off glans penis around urinary meatus with an iodophor solution (Betadine) using forceps to hold cleansing sponges. Keep the foreskin retracted. Maintain sterility of right hand.

    5. Cleanse urethral meatus from tip to foreskin with downward stroke on one side. Discard sponge. Repeat as required.

6. Grasp shaft of penis (with left hand) raising it almost straight up (Fig. 11-5). Maintain grasp on penis until procedure is ended.

    6. This maneuver straightens the penile urethra and facilitates catheterization. Maintaining a grasp of the penis prevents contamination and retraction of penis.

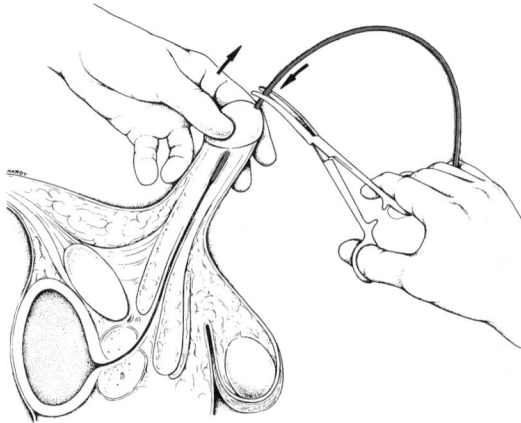

Figure 11-5. Technique for catheterization in male.

7. Using sterile gloves or forceps, insert catheter into the urethra; advance catheter 15–25 cm. (6–10 inches) until urine flows.

    7. The male urethra is a canal extending from the bladder to the end of the glans penis. The length varies within wide limits; the average length is about 21 cm.

8. If resistance is felt at the external sphincter, slightly increase the traction on the penis and apply steady, gentle pressure on the catheter.
Ask patient to strain gently (as if passing urine) to help relax sphincter.

    8. Some resistance may be due to spasm of external sphincter. Inability to pass the catheter may mean that a urethral stricture or other forms of urethral pathology exist. The urethra may have to be dilated with sounds by a urologist.

9. When urine begins to flow, advance the catheter another 2.5 cm. (1 inch).

    9. Advancing the catheter ensures its position in the bladder.

10. Reduce (or reposition) the foreskin.

    10. Paraphimosis (retraction and constriction of the foreskin behind the glans penis), secondary to catheterization, may occur if the foreskin is not reduced.

Follow-up Phase

Same as for female patient.

Guidelines: Management of the Patient with an Indwelling (Self-Retaining) Catheter and Closed Drainage System

Purpose

1. To empty urine from the bladder following bladder, prostate, or vaginal surgery.
2. To relieve urinary tract obstruction.
3. To permit urinary drainage in patients with neurogenic bladder dysfunction/urinary retention.
4. To determine accurate measurement of urinary drainage in critically ill patients.

Equipment

Completely closed system of urinary drainage (Fig. 11-6)
Catheter tray with triple-lumen catheter
Antibacterial solution for cleansing
Gauze squares
Single-use packet of lubricant

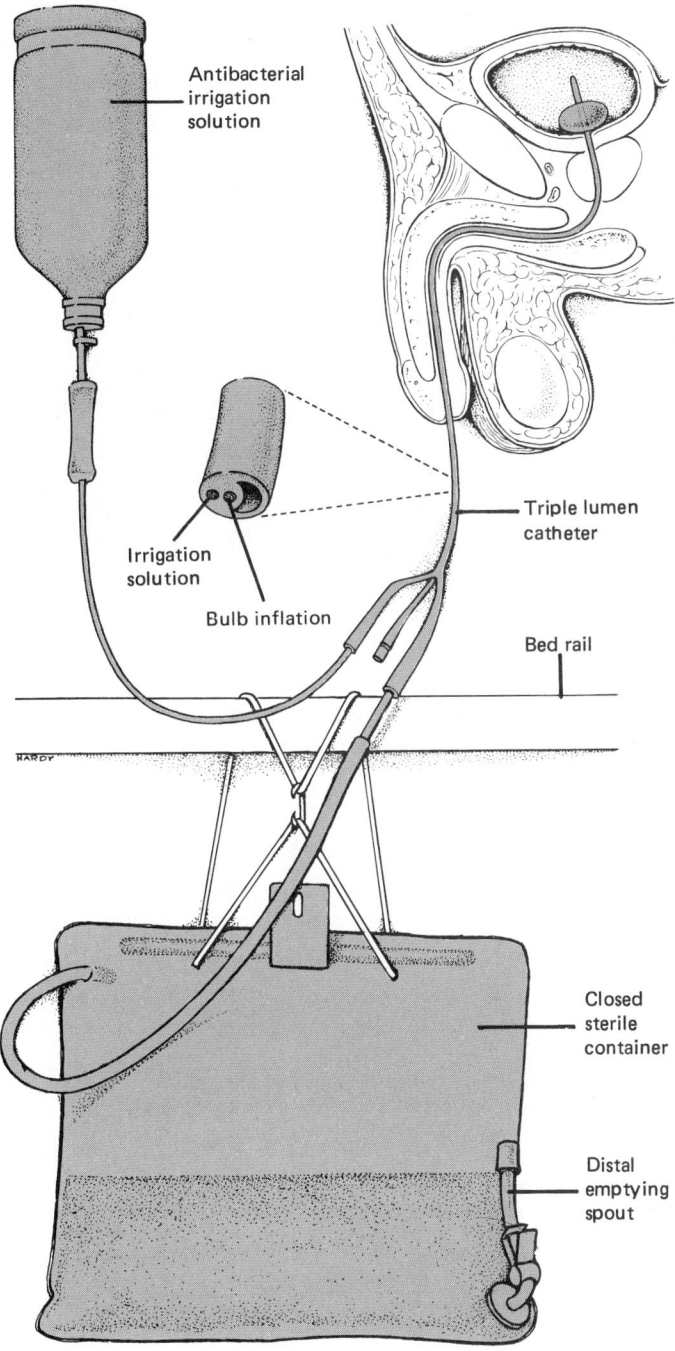

Figure 11-6. Closed sterile drainage system.

(continued)

Guidelines: Management of the Patient with an Indwelling (Self-Retaining) Catheter and Closed Drainage System (continued)

Procedure

Nursing Action	Rationale/Amplification

General Considerations

1. Catheterize the patient (p. 505), using a catheter that is preconnected to a closed drainage system.
   a. Advance catheter almost to its bifurcation (for male patient).
   b. Inflate the balloon according to manufacturer's directions. Be sure catheter is draining properly before inflating balloon, then withdraw catheter slightly.

2. Secure the indwelling catheter.

   a. Female: Tape the catheter and drainage tubing to the thigh.
      Male: Tape the catheter to the lower abdomen and the tubing to the shaved thigh (Fig. 11-7).

   b. Allow some slack of the tubing to accommodate the patient's movements.
   c. Keep the tubing over the patient's leg.

1. A closed drainage system is one that is closed to outside air. This prevents the balloon from becoming trapped in the urethra.
   a.
   b. Inadvertent inflation of the balloon within the urethra is painful and causes urethral trauma.

2. Properly securing the catheter prevents catheter movement and traction on the urethra.

   This smooths out urethral curve and eliminates pressure on the urethra at the penoscrotal junction, which can eventually lead to the formation of a urethrocutaneous fistula.

   c. This tubing position helps prevent kinking or forming loops of stagnant urine.

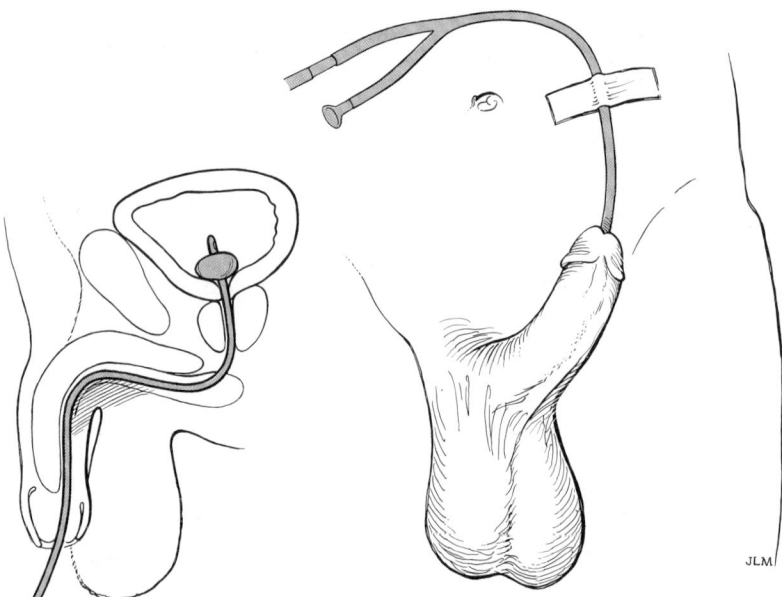

Figure 11-7. In the male patient, the indwelling catheter is taped to the abdomen to straighten the angulation of the penoscrotal junction, thus reducing pressure on the urethra exerted by the catheter.

Care of the indwelling catheter

1. Cleanse around the area where catheter enters urethral meatus (meatal-catheter junction) with soap and water during the daily bath to remove debris.
2. Avoid using powders and sprays on the perineal area.
3. Avoid pulling on the catheter during cleansing.

1. Suppurative drainage and encrustation occur at the exit of any tube. Infectious organisms can migrate to the bladder along the outside of any indwelling catheter.
2. This helps prevent infection.
3. This action may introduce new organisms into the urethra.

To obtain urine for culture

1. Clamp the drainage tubing below the aspiration (sampling) port for a *few minutes* to allow urine to collect.

2. Cleanse the aspiration port with povidone-iodine or 70% alcohol.

1. Avoid separating catheter and connecting tube. Disconnection of the catheter and tubing is a major cause of urinary tract infection.

Procedure
(Cont.)

Nursing Action	Rationale/Amplification
3. Insert a sterile No. 25-gauge needle (attached to a sterile syringe) into the aspiration port or hub of the catheter.	3. Avoid inserting needle into the shaft of the catheter because this may cause balloon deflation.
4. Aspirate a small volume of urine for culture.	
5. Remove needle from syringe and release urine carefully into sterile specimen container.	
6. *Unclamp the drainage tube.*	

To irrigate the catheter

Note: This is not done unless obstruction is anticipated (bleeding following bladder/prostate surgery).

Nursing Action	Rationale/Amplification
1. Wash hands. Don gloves.	
2. Using aseptic technique, pour sterile irrigating solution into sterile container.	
3. Cleanse around catheter/drainage tubing connection with sterile gauze pads soaked in povidone-iodine solution.	3. If frequent irrigations are necessary to keep the catheter open, change the catheter as the catheter itself is probably contributing to the problem.
4. Disconnect catheter from drainage tubing. Cover tubing with a sterile cap or drainage-tubing adapter bag (sleeve).	
5. Place a sterile drainage basin under the catheter.	
6. Irrigate catheter using a large volume syringe and prescribed amount of sterile irrigant.	6. Instill about 30 ml. irrigating solution at a time. Avoid instilling the solution forcibly to prevent bladder irritation and spasms.
7. Remove syringe and place end of catheter over drainage basin, allowing returning fluid to drain into basin.	7. This provides gravitational flow.
8. Repeat irrigation procedure until fluid is clear or according to physician's directives.	
9. Disinfect the distal end of the catheter and end of drainage tubing; reconnect the catheter and tubing. Remove gloves. Wash hands.	
10. Document type and amount of irrigating solution, color and character of returning fluid, presence of sediment/blood clots, and patient's reaction.	10. Use irrigating equipment one time and then discard.

Changing the catheter

Nursing Action	Rationale/Amplification
Change catheter according to the needs of the patient.	An indwelling catheter should *not* be changed at arbitrarily fixed intervals.

Principles of care when managing a closed drainage system

Nursing Action	Rationale/Amplification
1. Wash hands immediately before and after handling any part of the system. Wear clean disposable gloves when handling the drainage system.	1. Hands are the major route of transmission of gram-negative bacteria.
2. Maintain unobstructed urine flow.	2. Urine flow must be downhill.
a. Keep the drainage bag below the level of the bladder.	a. Raising the bag will cause reflux of contaminated urine from the bag into the patient's bladder.
b. Urine should not be allowed to collect in the tubing, since a free flow of urine must be maintained to prevent infection.	b. Improper drainage occurs when the tubing is kinked or twisted, allowing pools of drainage to collect in the loops of tubing.
3. To empty the drainage bag.	
a. Wash hands; don gloves.	a. Empty the bag at regular intervals, taking care to see that the drainage valve/spout is not contaminated.
b. Disinfect spigot. Empty the bag in a separate collecting receptacle for each patient. Disinfect spigot again.	b. Each patient should have his own collecting receptacle that is labeled with his name and kept in his bathroom, not on the floor.
c. Avoid letting the drainage bag touch the floor.	
d. Change the drainage bag if contamination occurs, if the urine flow becomes obstructed, or if the connecting junctions start to leak.	

Measures to prevent cross-contamination

Nursing Action	Rationale/Amplification
1. Wash hands before and after handling the catheter/drainage system and between patients.	1. Many urinary tract infections are due to extrinsically acquired organisms transmitted by cross-contamination.
2. Assign only one patient with an indwelling catheter to a room. If this is not possible, separate the infected patient with an indwelling catheter from an uninfected patient.	2. There appears to be a greater risk of microbial transmission between catheterized patients.
3. Know the patients at risk.	3. Female, elderly, debilitated, and critically ill patients, those in the postpartum state, and patients with obstructed or neurologically impaired bladders are at risk for infection.

(continued)

Guidelines: Management of the Patient with an Indwelling (Self-Retaining) Catheter and Closed Drainage System (continued)

Health Education (Self-Care of Catheter at Home)

1. Wash hands before and after handling the catheter.
2. Wash around urinary opening and then up the catheter with soap and water daily, taking care to avoid pulling on the catheter during cleansing.
3. Drink 8–12 glasses of fluids daily; increase fluid intake if urine becomes dark and concentrated.
4. Wipe all connecting junctions with alcohol before changing from leg-bag drainage to overnight bottle drainage.
5. Call physician/clinic if fever, cloudy, bloody or odoriferous urine develops.

Guidelines: Assisting the Patient Undergoing Suprapubic Drainage (Cystostomy)

Suprapubic bladder drainage is a method of establishing drainage from the bladder by inserting a catheter or tube through the suprapubic area into the bladder by either a stab incision or puncture with a needle or trocar.

Purpose

1. To drain the bladder via a tube placed in the bladder through the suprapubic area.
2. To divert the flow of urine from the urethra.
3. To obtain a urine specimen for culture.

Clinical Usefulness

1. When urethral route is impassable—urethral stricture, injuries
2. Following gynecologic operations—vaginal hysterectomy, vaginal repair
3. Following bladder surgery
4. Pelvic fractures

Equipment

Sterile suprapubic drainage system package (disposable)
Skin germicide for suprapubic skin preparation
Local anesthetic agent if needed

Procedure

Nursing Action	Rationale/Amplification
Preparatory Phase	
1. Place the patient in a supine position with one pillow under head.	
2. Expose the abdomen.	
Performance Phase (by physician)	
1. The bladder is distended with 300–500 ml. of sterile saline via an urethral catheter, which is removed, or the patient is given fluids (oral or IV) before the procedure.	1. Distention of the bladder makes the bladder easier to locate by the suprapubic route.
2. The suprapubic area is surgically prepared. After the skin is dried, the needle entry point is located.	2. The needle entry point is approximately 5 cm. (2 inches) above the symphysis.
3. The procedure may be performed in several ways:	
a. By open operation (incision of the bladder)	
b. By puncture with a trocar/cannula assembly	
(1) The trocar/cannula is passed in a slightly caudal direction.)	(1) Entrance into the bladder is usually felt and can be verified by reflux of urine through a hole in the trocar/cannula.
(2) After the bladder has been entered, the trocar is removed, leaving the outer cannula in place.	(2) Usually, a 3-way stopcock is attached to the proximal end of the catheter and connected to a siphon drainage system.
(3) The catheter is threaded through the cannula and well into the bladder (Fig. 11-8A).	
(4) The cannula is slowly withdrawn, leaving the catheter in position.	
(5) The catheter is secured with sutures, tape, or a body-seal system (Fig. 11-8B).	(5) Aseptic technique is employed in the area around the cystostomy tube.
(6) Cover the area around the catheter with a sterile dressing.	
(7) Attach the drainage tubing to a closed sterile system.	
c. By needle puncture into bladder to secure a specimen for culture.	c. Avoid ''forcing fluids'' before a urine culture is obtained, since this will produce a low density of organisms.

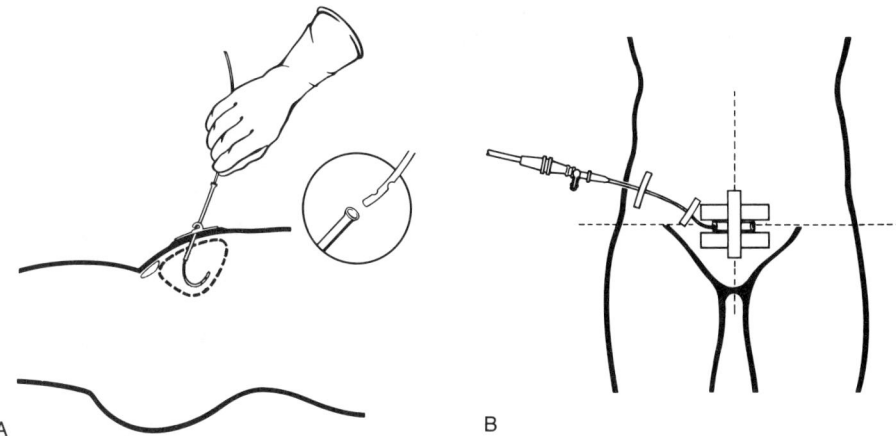

Figure 11-8. (A) Introduction of suprapubic catheter. (B) The body seal and catheter are taped to the abdomen. (Courtesy of Dow Corning Corporation)

Procedure
(Cont.)

Nursing Action	Rationale/Amplification
4. Secure drainage tubing to lateral abdomen with tape (Fig. 11-8B).	4. Prevents undue tension on the catheter.
5. If the catheter is not draining properly, withdraw the catheter 2.5 cm. (1 inch) at a time until urine begins to flow. Do not dislodge catheter from bladder.	
6. The drainage is maintained continuously for several days.	
7. If a "trial of voiding" is requested, the catheter is clamped for 4 hours.	7. Usually, patients will void earlier after surgery with suprapubic drainage than with indwelling catheters.
a. Have the patient attempt to void while the catheter is clamped.	
b. After the patient voids, unclamp the catheter and measure residual urine.	
c. Usually, if the amount of residual urine is less than 100 ml. on 2 separate occasions (AM and PM), the catheter may be removed.	
d. If the patient complains of pain or discomfort, or if the residual urine is over the prescribed amount, the catheter is usually left open.	
8. The catheter is removed upon request, and a sterile dressing is placed over the site.	8. Suprapubic drainage is considered more comfortable than an indwelling urethral catheter; it allows greater patient mobility, and there is less risk of bladder infection.

Urinary Retention

Urinary retention is the inability to urinate despite a desire to do so. Retention may be acute or chronic. Chronic retention will often lead to overflow incontinence or residual urine (urine that remains in the bladder after voiding).

Etiology
Males
1. Benign prostatic hyperplasia
2. Stricture of urethra, calculus or foreign body in urethra, urethritis, tumor
3. Phimosis

Females
1. Urethral obstruction secondary to stricture, stones, vaginal cysts, carcinoma, edema
2. Retroverted gravid uterus

Either Male or Female
1. Following any operation, particularly on anal or perineal region—due to reflex spasm of sphincters
2. Trauma
3. Neurogenic bladder dysfunction—spinal cord tumor, trauma, herniated intervertebral disc, multiple sclerosis

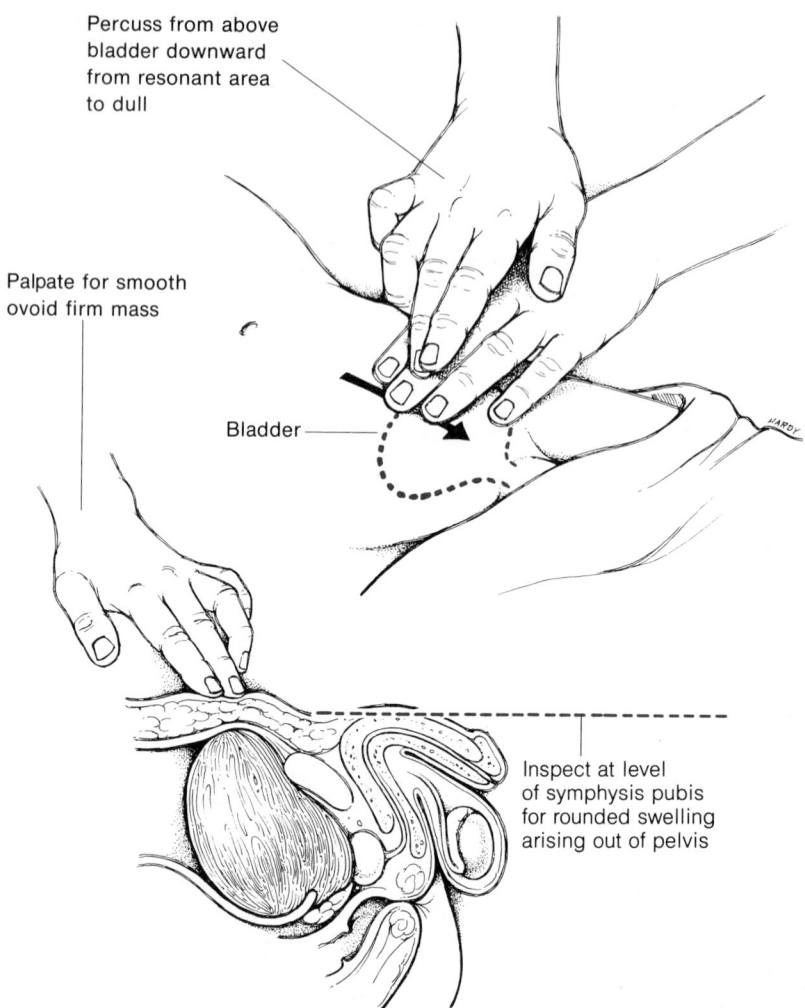

Percuss from above
bladder downward
from resonant area
to dull

Palpate for smooth
ovoid firm mass

Bladder

Inspect at level
of symphysis pubis
for rounded swelling
arising out of pelvis

Figure 11-9. Nursing assessment for urinary retention.

4. Certain drugs (anticholinergics, antihistamines)
5. Fecal impaction
6. Psychogenic urinary retention

Clinical Manifestations (See Fig. 11-9)

1. History of no voiding or frequent passing of small amounts of urine without relief.
2. Progressive slowing of urinary stream; hesitancy.
3. Lower abdominal discomfort and distress; severe pain. The patient may have little or no discomfort if bladder distends slowly.
4. Smooth, firm, oval-shaped mass that is palpable over bladder area.
5. Dullness to percussion above symphysis pubis (residual urine below 130 ml. is not usually percussible).
6. Visualization of a rounded swelling arising out of the pelvis.
7. Urine-stained clothing.

Treatment and Nursing Management

Goal:
The patient empties his bladder completely.

1. Use nursing measures to help patient void.
   a. Transport the patient to bathroom (or bedside commode) or allow to stand beside bed if possible—many patients are unable to void while lying in bed.
   b. Use warmth to relax sphincters—sitz bath, warm compresses to perineum, warm shower.
   c. Give hot tea to drink.
   d. Have patient listen to sound of running water; place hands in warm water.
   e. Administer bethanechol chloride (Urecholine) only if directed.
   f. Give psychological reassurance and support.
2. Give prescribed analgesic medication postoperatively.
   a. Voiding may be difficult because of pain in incisional area, especially in anterior vaginal operations.
   b. Sphincter spasm is generally present in patients with acute urinary retention.
3. Decompress bladder before overdistention occurs—bladder mucosa that has been stretched from urinary retention is readily infected.
   a. Utilize indwelling catheter and closed drainage.
      (1) It may be advisable to decompress the bladder gradually if the patient is elderly or hypertensive or has diminished renal reserve,

or if retention of large amounts of urine has persisted for several weeks.

(2) Call urologist if unable to pass catheter easily; he will use special instruments (or operation may be necessary).

(3) Blood pressure may fluctuate and renal function decline the first few days after bladder drainage is instituted.

b. Suprapubic cystostomy may be required if it is impossible to pass urethral catheter (p. 512).

4. Assist in determining the underlying cause.

a. Carry out blood urea nitrogen tests and other renal function tests.

b. Assist in carrying out diagnostic tests if obstructive uropathy (pathologic change in urinary tract from obstruction) is suspected.

Nursing Assessment for Fluid and Electrolyte Imbalance

The following signs and symptoms tend to occur in patients with renal disease.

Clinical Manifestations

Signs and Symptoms	Possible Indication
Acute weight loss (in excess of 5%), drop in body temperature, dry skin and mucous membranes, longitudinal wrinkles or furrows of tongue, oliguria or anuria	Volume deficit of extracellular fluid
Abdominal cramps, apprehension, convulsions, finger-printing on sternum, oliguria or anuria	Sodium deficit of extracellular fluid
Dry sticky mucous membranes, flushed skin, oliguria or anuria, thirst, rough and dry tongue	Sodium excess of extracellular fluid
Anorexia, gaseous distention of intestines, silent intestinal ileus, weakness, soft, flabby muscles	Potassium deficit of extracellular fluid
Diarrhea, intestinal colic, irritability, nausea	Potassium excess of extracellular fluid
Abdominal cramps, carpopedal spasm, muscle cramps, tetany, tingling of ends of fingers	Calcium deficit of extracellular fluid
Deep bone pain, flank pain, and muscle hypotonicity	Calcium excess of extracellular fluid
Deep, rapid breathing (Kussmaul), shortness of breath on exertion, stupor, weakness	Primary base bicarbonate deficit of extracellular fluid
Depressed respiration, muscle hypertonicity, tetany	Primary base bicarbonate excess of extracellular fluid
Chronic weight loss, emotional depression, pallor, ready fatigue, soft, flabby muscles	Protein deficit of extracellular fluid
Positive Chvostek's sign, convulsions, disorientation, hyperactive deep reflexes, tremor	Magnesium deficit of extracellular fluid

Nursing Interventions

1. Observe the clinical course of the patient; record the data collected.
2. Keep an accurate intake and output record.
3. Check the vital signs every 4 hours. Weigh the patient daily.
4. Support the patient having repeated blood examinations for the surveillance of electrolyte balance.

Acute Renal Failure

Acute renal failure is a sudden decline in renal function caused by failure of the renal circulation or by glomerular or tubular damage. The substances normally eliminated in the urine accumulate in the body fluids as a result of impaired renal excretion and lead to a disruption in homeostatic, endocrine, and metabolic functions. Renal failure is a disease affecting the entire body.

Precipitating Factors

1. Reduction in renal blood flow—volume depletion, hypotension, shock, trauma, burns, hemorrhage
2. Sepsis
3. Dehydration; trauma
4. Obstructive lesions—vascular lesions, bladder outlet obstruction, calculi
5. Nephrotoxic drugs
6. Multiple blood transfusions and mismatched blood
7. Cardiopulmonary bypass
8. Surgery of aorta, renal vessels, biliary tree
9. Extensive surgery in the elderly

Preventive Measures

1. Initiate adequate hydration before, during, and after operative procedures.

2. Avoid exposure to various nephrotoxins. Be aware that the majority of drugs or their metabolites are excreted by the kidneys.
3. Avoid chronic analgesic abuse—causes interstitial nephritis and papillary necrosis.
4. Prevent and treat shock with blood and fluid replacement. Prevent prolonged periods of hypotension.
5. Monitor urinary output and central venous pressure hourly in critically ill patients to detect onset of renal failure at the earliest moment.
6. Schedule diagnostic studies requiring dehydration so that there are "rest days," especially in aged who may not have adequate renal reserve.
7. Avoid infections, which may produce progressive renal damage.
8. Pay special attention to draining wounds, burns, etc., which can lead to sepsis.
9. To avoid infection, give meticulous care to patients with indwelling catheters and intravenous lines.
10. Take every precaution to ensure that the right person receives the right blood—to avoid severe transfusion reactions, which can precipitate renal complications.

Assessment

Clinical Phases and Clinical Manifestations

A. Period of oliguria (urine volume less than 400 ml./24 hours)

1. However, there can be a decrease in renal function with increasing nitrogen retention even when the patient is excreting more than 2–3 liters of urine daily—called high output failure.
2. Accompanied by rise in serum concentration of elements usually excreted by kidney (urea, creatinine, uric acid, organic acids, and the intracellular cations—potassium and magnesium).
3. Clinical manifestations—scant, bloody urine, lethargy, nausea, vomiting, diarrhea, dryness of skin and mucous membranes.
   a. Central nervous system (CNS) manifestations—drowsiness, headache, muscle twitching and convulsions.
   b. Period of oliguria lasts approximately 10 days–3 weeks.

B. Period of diuresis
Gradually increasing urinary output, which doubles daily until relatively fixed volume is attained—glomerular filtration has started to recover, but renal function is still abnormal. With dialysis, the diuretic phase may not occur.

C. Period of recovery
Signals the improvement of renal function and may take from 3–12 months; usually there is a permanent partial loss of some glomerular filtration rate and concentrating ability.

Diagnostic Evaluation

1. Urinalysis—reveals proteinuria, hematuria, casts
2. Rising blood urea nitrogen and serum creatinine concentrations
3. Abnormalities in fluid and electrolyte homeostasis

Patient Problems/Nursing Diagnoses

1. Alteration in urinary elimination related to impaired renal function
2. Retention of metabolic wastes related to impaired renal function
3. Fluid and electrolyte imbalance

4. Potential for complications (infection, gastrointestinal, and central nervous system complications) related to buildup of toxic wastes in system

Planning and Implementation
Nursing Interventions

A. Restoration of normal homeostasis to allow repair of renal tissue

1. Assist in removing the cause of renal failure if possible.
2. Implement prescribed treatment for underlying condition.
3. Prepare for peritoneal dialysis or hemodialysis to prevent metabolic deterioration (see p. 519 and p. 522).
   a. Dialysis produces a more sustained correction of biochemical abnormalities.
   b. Allows for liberalization of fluid, protein, and sodium intake; helps wound healing; diminishes bleeding tendencies and predisposition to infection.

B. Establishment of fluid and electrolyte balance

1. Carry out biochemical and urinary studies as prescribed. (Electrolyte administration is guided by serial measurements of central venous pressure, serum and urine electrolyte concentrations, fluid losses, and the clinical status of the patient.)
   a. Record these parameters on a flowchart to indicate rate and trend of biochemical improvement/deterioration.
   b. Weigh the patient daily to provide an index of fluid balance—expected weight loss 0.25–0.5 kg. (½–1 lb.) daily.
   c. Monitor the urinary output and urine specific gravity. Measure and record intake and output (include urine, gastric suction, stools, wound drainage, perspiration, etc.).
   d. Observe fluid excess by assessing the patient's clinical status—dyspnea, tachycardia, distended neck veins, crackles, peripheral edema, pulmonary edema.
2. Give only enough fluids to replace losses during oliguric phase (usually 400–500 ml./24 hours, plus measured fluid losses associated with gastrointestinal drainage, fever, surgical drainage, or other routes).
3. Measure and replace sodium losses, especially if large losses occur from the gastrointestinal tract via suction, vomiting, or diarrhea.
   a. Monitor arterial blood gases and institute ventilatory measures if severe acidosis is present and respiratory problems develop.
   b. Prepare for sodium bicarbonate therapy or dialysis if necessary.
4. Control potassium balance (protein catabolism causes release of cellular potassium into body fluids, resulting in serious potassium intoxication).
   a. Sources of potassium are diet, tissue breakdown, blood in the gastrointestinal tract, blood transfusion, other sources (intravenous infusions, potassium penicillin), and extracellular shift in response to metabolic acidosis.
   b. Evaluate for hyperkalemia (potassium intoxication) by assessment of serum potassium levels (potassium value above 6.0 mEq./liter) correlated with ECG changes (peaked T waves) and patient evaluation.
   c. Give cation exchange resins—sodium polystyrene

sulfonate (Kayexalate); provides for more prolonged correction of elevated potassium.
  (1) Orally (laxative may be given concurrently to avoid fecal impaction), or
  (2) By retention enema, since the colon is the principal site for potassium exchange
    (a) Use catheter with balloon to facilitate retention if necessary.
    (b) Assist the patient to retain the resin 30–45 minutes to remove the potassium.
  (3) Sorbitol (induces water loss in GI tract) may be given orally.
  d. Intravenous glucose and insulin or calcium gluconate sometimes used as emergency (and temporary) measure for potassium intoxication; causes potassium to enter cells.
  e. Give sodium bicarbonate as directed—promotes elevation of plasma pH; when available sodium ions are provided, there is a migration of potassium into the cell and a lowering of potassium in the plasma; this is short-term therapy and is used along with other, long-term, measures.
  f. Watch for cardiac arrhythmias (cardiac arrest) and congestive heart failure from hyperkalemia, electrolyte imbalance, and/or fluid overload.
5. Assess for an increase in serum phosphate concentrations (hyperphosphatemia)—occurs because of failure of glomerular filtration. Give phosphate-binding antacid (aluminum hydroxide) to keep phosphate from being absorbed into bloodstream and to help prevent a continuing rise in serum phosphate levels.

C. **Sufficient nutritional intake to preserve protein stores of the body until renal function returns**
1. Limit dietary protein during oliguric phase to minimize accumulation of toxic end-products, etc., that result from digestion and metabolism of dietary protein.
  a. Offer high-carbohydrate feedings, since carbohydrates have a greater protein-sparing power.
  b. Restrict foods and fluids containing potassium and phosphorus (bananas, citrus fruits/juices, coffee).
  c. Restrict sodium intake as directed.
  d. Prepare for hyperalimentation (see p. 429) when adequate nutrition cannot be taken through the gastrointestinal tract.

D. **Prevention of complications**
1. Watch for signs and symptoms of dehydration or hypovolemia—regulating capacity of kidneys is usually still inadequate.
2. Monitor for reduction in body weight, poor skin turgor, dryness of mucous membranes, hypotension, tachycardia.
3. Prevent and forestall the following if possible:
  a. Infection
  b. Gastrointestinal complications (bleeding; sepsis)
  c. CNS complications (drowsiness to acute psychoses, delirium, and coma)
  d. Metabolic acidosis
  e. Circulatory overload (dyspnea, orthopnea, pulmonary congestion, pulmonary edema)
  f. Hypertension, hypertensive crisis, convulsions
  g. Neurologic complications—abnormalities of mental status.

Evaluation
Expected Outcomes

1. Excretes metabolic wastes; is in acid–base equilibrium
2. Attains fluid and electrolyte balance
3. Is free of complications

Chronic Renal Failure

Chronic renal failure is a progressive deterioration of renal function, which ends fatally in uremia (an excess of urea and other nitrogenous wastes in the blood) and its complications unless dialysis or a kidney transplant is performed.

Reversible Causes

1. Urinary tract obstruction and infection
2. Infectious diseases, which cause increased catabolism with retention of metabolites and hyperkalemia
3. Hypertension
4. Metabolic disease
5. Nephrotoxic (poisonous to kidney cells) agents
6. Dehydration

Stages of Chronic Renal Failure

Decreased renal reserve → renal insufficiency → renal failure → uremia

Assessment
Clinical Manifestations

1. Gastrointestinal manifestations—anorexia, nausea, vomiting, hiccoughs, ulceration of gastrointestinal tract, and hemorrhage.
2. Cardiopulmonary manifestations—hypertension, fibrinous pericarditis, pleuritis.
3. Neuromuscular disturbances—fatigue, sleep disorders, headache, lethargy, muscular irritability, peripheral neuropathy, seizures, coma.
4. Fluid and electrolyte disturbances.
5. Metabolic and endocrine alterations—glucose intolerance, hyperlipidemia, sex hormone disturbances.
6. Personality changes—emotional dullness, lability with impatient, demanding behavior.
7. Dermatologic disturbances—pallor, hyperpigmentation, pruritus, ecchymoses, uremic frost.
8. Anemia

Diagnostic Evaluation

1. Anemia (a characteristic sign)
2. Elevated serum creatinine or BUN
3. Elevated serum phosphorus
4. Decreased serum calcium
5. Low serum proteins, especially albumin
6. Usually, low CO_2 and acidosis (low blood pH)

Patient Problems/Nursing Diagnoses

1. Alteration in urinary elimination related to disturbance of renal function
2. Electrolyte abnormalities related to biochemical derangements due to renal failure.
3. Acute fluid volume deficit or overhydration related

to impaired concentrating and diluting mechanisms of the kidneys.

4. Potential for complications of every organ system related to biochemical and physiologic disturbances from progressive destruction of neurons.

5. Alteration in thought processes (shortened attention span, diminished cognitive ability, irritability, personality changes) related to altered CNS function and declining renal function.

6. Potential alteration in skin integrity related to itching and hyperpigmentation.

7. Powerlessness and ineffective coping related to restrictions imposed by disease and treatment.

8. Potential for nonadherence with the therapeutic regimen related to feelings of hopelessness

Planning and Implementation
Nursing Interventions

A. Maintenance of homeostasis and conservation of renal function as long as possible

1. Detect and treat reversible causes of chronic renal failure (see previous Reversible Causes).

2. Offer diet according to blood chemistry levels and clinical status of the patient.
   a. Regulate protein intake according to impairment of renal function, since metabolites that accumulate in the blood derive almost entirely from protein catabolism.
      (1) Protein should be of high biologic value, rich in essential amino acids (dairy products, eggs, meat), so that the patient does not rely on tissue catabolism for essential amino acids.
      (2) Low-protein diet may be supplemented with essential amino acids and vitamins.
      (3) As renal function declines, protein intake may be restricted proportionally.
      (4) Protein will be increased if the patient is on a dialysis program to allow for loss of amino acids occurring during dialysis.
   b. Ensure high calorie intake—essential to spare protein for its own work, to provide energy, and to prevent wasting.
      Encourage intake of hard candy, jelly beans, jellies, flavored carbohydrate powders.

B. Achieving fluid and electrolyte balance

1. Weigh the patient daily to assess fluid overload or depletion—weight should not increase or decrease more than 0.45 kg. (1 lb.) per day.

2. Treat acidosis if the patient is symptomatic; acidosis commonly appears in chronic renal failure.
   a. Assess the patient for stupor, deep, rapid breathing of Kussmaul type, shortness of breath on exertion, weakness, unconsciousness.
   b. Replace bicarbonate stores by infusion or oral administration of sodium bicarbonate.

3. Adjust sodium requirements as required (determined by serum and urine measurements and daily weights)—patients with chronic renal diseases cannot tolerate severe restriction or marked excess in sodium intake.

4. Restrict dietary potassium and administer potassium-binding agents (Kayexalate) if decreasing renal function results in hyperkalemia.

5. The following measures may or may not be employed:
   a. Decrease phosphorus intake (restrict meat, milk, legumes, carbonated beverages)—phosphate retention contributes to development of secondary hyperparathyroidism and development of uremic bone disease (renal osteodystrophy).
   b. Reduce elevated levels of phosphorus with phosphate-binding agents (aluminum hydroxide compounds), since they bind phosphorus in the intestinal tract.
      (1) Phosphate binders cause constipation, which *cannot* be managed with the usual interventions.
      (2) Employ emollient stool softeners (Surfak®; Colace®) and bulk laxatives (Metamucil®).
      (3) Avoid laxatives and cathartics which cause electrolyte toxicities (compounds containing magnesium or phosphorus).

C. Adjustment of fluid intake to maintain adequate urinary volume and to avoid dehydration

1. Fluid restriction is not usually initiated until renal function is quite low.

2. Fluid allowance should be distributed throughout the day.

3. Avoid restricting fluids for prolonged periods for laboratory and radiologic examinations, since dehydrating procedures are hazardous to those patients who cannot produce concentrated urine.

4. Restrict salt and water intake if there is evidence of extracellular excess (congestive heart failure, pulmonary edema, hypertension).

D. Prevention of complications

1. Treat associated cardiac conditions with digitalis, diuretics, and antiarrhythmic agents to reverse congestive heart failure and to improve renal hemodynamics.
   a. Patients with chronic renal failure may also have a variety of other conditions—hypertension, neuropathy, bone disease, infection, anemia—that require pharmacologic therapy.
   b. Patients with renal failure have increased sensitivity to drugs because of impaired metabolism and renal excretion.

▶ **NURSING ALERT:** Patients with impaired renal function may require major adjustments of common therapeutic agents. Give medications with caution.

2. Monitor blood pressure. Hypertension increases rate of renal deterioration and adversely affects the vascular system.

3. Observe for other complications.
   a. Anemia—has many causes and is invariably found in patients with advanced renal failure.
   b. Renal osteodystrophy—uremia is associated with abnormal calcium metabolism, which causes bone pathology.
   c. Infection
   d. Paresthesias—neurologic abnormalities (dysarthria, myoclonus, muscle twitching, tremulousness; asterixis, disorientation, stupor, seizures, coma).
   e. Hyperkalemia

E. Prevention or reduction of cognitive distortions

1. Speak to the patient in simple orienting statements, using repetition when necessary.

2. Maintain predictable routine and keep change to a minimum.

3. Correct cognitive distortions.
4. Anticipate psychiatric intervention for acute changes in personality and cognition.

F. Maintenance of skin integrity

1. Use measures to produce vasoconstriction; cool environment, removal of excessive bedding.
2. Provide tepid, cooling baths or cool wet dressings—gradual evaporation of water from dressings cools skin and relieves pruritus.
3. Eliminate irritants; apply emollient lotions.

G. Preparation for dialysis or kidney transplant

1. Offer hope tempered by reality.
2. Advent of chronic dialysis and renal transplantation have revolutionized treatment and prognosis of patient with chronic renal failure (see Dialysis, below, and Renal Transplantation, p. 526).

Evaluation

Expected Outcomes

1. Maintains homeostasis
2. Attains improved electrolyte measurements
3. Attains adequate fluid balance
4. Is free of "new" complications
5. Is oriented to time, place, and person
6. Achieves some relief of itching
7. Verbalizes interest in dialysis/renal transplantation

Dialysis

Dialysis refers to the diffusion of solute molecules through a semipermeable membrane, passing from the side of higher concentration to that of lower concentration. The purpose of dialysis is to maintain the life and well-being of the patient until kidney function is restored. It is a substitute for some kidney excretory functions but does not replace the kidneys' endocrine and metabolic functions.

Methods

1. Peritoneal dialysis
   a. Intermittent peritoneal dialysis (short-term [see below] or chronic)
   b. Continuous ambulatory peritoneal dialysis (see p. 522)
   c. Continuous cycling peritoneal dialysis—uses automated peritoneal dialysis machine overnight with prolonged dwell time during day.
      (1) The patient is connected to cycler machine every evening, receiving 3–5 exchanges during night. In the morning, after infusing fresh dialysate, the catheter is capped.
      (2) Permits freedom from exchanges during day.
2. Hemodialysis (see p. 522)

Guidelines: Assisting the Patient Undergoing (Acute) Peritoneal Dialysis*

Peritoneal dialysis is a substitute for kidney function during renal failure. The peritoneum acts as a dialyzing membrane, and dialysate is delivered into the peritoneal cavity.

Purposes
1. Aid in the removal of toxic substances and metabolic wastes.
2. Establish electrolyte balance.
3. Remove excessive body fluid.
4. Assist in regulating the fluid balance of the body.
5. Control blood pressure.
6. Control severe, intractable heart failure when diuretics no longer promote elimination of water and sodium.

Equipment

Dialysis administration set (disposable, closed system)
Peritoneal dialysis solution as requested
Supplemental drugs as requested
Local anesthesia
Central venous pressure monitoring equipment
ECG
Suture set
Sterile gloves
Skin antiseptic

* Automated closed-system peritoneal cycling machines are available.

(continued)

Guidelines: Assisting the Patient Undergoing (Acute) Peritoneal Dialysis (continued)

Procedure

Nursing Action	Rationale/Amplification
1. Prepare the patient emotionally and physically for the procedure.	1. Nursing support is offered by explaining procedure mechanics, providing opportunities for the patient to ask questions, allowing him to verbalize his feelings, and giving expert physical care.
2. See that the consent form has been signed.	
3. Weigh the patient before dialysis and every 24 hours thereafter, preferably on an in-bed scale.	3. The weight at the beginning of the procedure serves as a baseline of information. Daily weight is helpful in assessing the state of hydration.
4. Take temperature, pulse, respiration, and blood pressure readings prior to dialysis.	4. Measurement of vital signs at the beginning of dialysis is necessary for comparing subsequent changes in vital signs.
5. Have the patient empty his bladder.	5. If the bladder is empty, there is less likelihood of perforating it when the trocar is introduced into the peritoneum.
6. Assist with insertion of central venous pressure (CVP) catheter; ECG monitoring may also be employed.	6. CVP measurements may be carried out to assess fluid volume changes. Cardiac arrhythmias may occur because of serum potassium changes and vagal stimulation.
7. Flush the tubing with dialysis solution.	7. The tubing is flushed to prevent air from entering the peritoneal cavity. Air causes abdominal discomfort and drainage difficulties.
8. Make the patient comfortable in a supine position. Have the patient and health-care personnel wear masks.	8. This helps protect the patient from airborne contamination.

Performance Phase (by the physician)

The following is a brief summary of the method of insertion of a temporary peritoneal catheter (*done under strict asepsis*).

1. The abdomen is prepared surgically, and the skin and subcutaneous tissues are infiltrated with a local anesthetic.	1. Surgical preparation of the skin minimizes or eliminates surface bacteria and decreases the possibility of wound contamination and infection.
2. A small midline stab wound is made 3–5 cm. below the umbilicus.	
3. The trocar is inserted through the incision with the stylet in place, or a thin stylet cannula may be inserted percutaneously.	
4. The patient is requested to raise his head from the pillow after the trocar is introduced.	4. This maneuver tightens the abdominal muscles and permits easier penetration of the trocar without danger of injury to the intra-abdominal organs.
5. When the peritoneum is punctured, the trocar is directed toward the left side of the pelvis. The stylet is removed, and the catheter is inserted through the trocar and maneuvered into position.	
a. Dialysis fluid is allowed to run through the catheter while it is being positioned.	a. This prevents the omentum from adhering to the catheter, impeding its advancement or occluding its opening.
6. After the trocar is removed, the skin may be closed with a purse-string suture. (This is not always done.) A sterile dressing is placed around the catheter.	6. The catheter is attached to the skin to prevent loss of the catheter in the abdomen.
7. Attach the catheter connector to the administration set, which has been previously connected to the container of dialysis solution (warmed to body temperature, 37°C.)	7. The solution is warmed to body temperature for patient comfort and to prevent abdominal pain. Heating also causes dilatation of the peritoneal vessels and increases urea clearance.
8. Drugs (heparin, potassium, antibiotic) are added in advance.	8. The addition of heparin prevents fibrin clots from occluding the catheter. Potassium chloride may be added on request unless patient has hyperkalemia. Antibiotics are added for the treatment of peritonitis.
9. Permit the dialyzing solution to flow unrestricted into the peritoneal cavity (usually takes 5–10 minutes for completion). If the patient experiences pain, slow down the infusion.	9. The inflow solution should flow in a steady stream. If the fluid flows in too slowly, the catheter may need to be repositioned, since its tip may be buried in the omentum, or it may be occluded by a blood clot. Flushing may help.
10. Allow the fluid to remain in the peritoneal cavity for the prescribed time period (15 minutes–4 hours). Prepare the next exchange while the fluid is in the peritoneal cavity.	10. In order for potassium, urea, and other waste materials to be removed, the solution must remain in the peritoneal cavity for the prescribed time (dwell or equilibration time). The maximum concentration gradient takes place in the first 5–10 minutes for small molecules, such as urea and creatinine.

Procedure
(Cont.)

Nursing Action	Rationale/Amplification
11. Unclamp the outflow tube. Drainage should take approximately 10–30 minutes, although the time varies with each patient.	11. The abdomen is drained by a siphon effect through the closed system. Gravity drainage should occur fairly rapidly, and steady streams of fluid should be observed entering the drainage container. The drainage is usually straw-colored.
12. If the fluid is not draining properly, move the patient from side to side to facilitate the removal of peritoneal drainage. The head of the bed may also be elevated. Ascertain if the catheter is patent. Check for closed clamp, kinked tubing, or air lock. *Never push the catheter in.*	12. If the drainage stops, or starts to drip before the dialyzing fluid has run out, the catheter tip may be buried in the omentum. Rotating the patient may be helpful (or it may be necessary for the physician to reposition the catheter). Pushing in the catheter introduces bacteria into the peritoneal cavity.
13. When the outflow drainage ceases to run, clamp off the drainage tube and infuse the next exchange, using strict aseptic technique.	
14. Take blood pressure and pulse every 15 minutes during the first exchange and every hour thereafter. Monitor the heart rate for signs of arrhythmia.	14. A drop in blood pressure may indicate excessive fluid loss from glucose concentrations of the dialyzing solutions. Changes in the vital signs may indicate impending shock or overhydration.
15. Take the patient's temperature every 4 hours (especially after catheter removal).	15. An infection is more apt to become evident after dialysis has been discontinued.
16. The procedure is repeated until the blood chemistry levels improve. The usual duration for short-term dialysis is 36–48 hours. Depending on the patient's condition, he will receive 24–48 exchanges.	16. The duration of dialysis depends on the severity of the condition and on the size and weight of the patient.

17. Keep an exact record of the patient's fluid balance during the treatment.
  a. Know the status of the patient's loss or gain of fluid at the end of each exchange. Check dressing for leakage and weigh on gram scale if significant.
  b. The fluid balance should be about even or should show slight fluid loss or gain, depending on the patient's fluid status.
	17. Complications (circulatory collapse, hypotension, shock, and death) may occur if the patient loses too much fluid through peritoneal drainage. Large fluid losses around the catheter may not be noted unless the dressings are checked carefully.

18. Promote patient comfort during dialysis.
  a. Provide frequent back care and massage pressure areas.
  b. Have the patient turn from side to side.
  c. Elevate head of bed at intervals.
  d. Allow the patient to sit in chair for brief periods if condition permits (only with surgically implanted catheter; with trocar, patient is usually on bed rest).
	18. The dialysis period is lengthy, and the patient becomes fatigued.

19. Observe for the following:
  a. Respiratory difficulty
    (1) Slow the inflow rate.
    (2) Make sure tubing is not kinked.
    (3) Prevent air from entering peritoneum by keeping drip chamber of tubing three-fourths full of fluid.
 	
    (4) Elevate head of bed; encourage coughing and breathing exercises.
    (5) Turn patient from side to side.
  b. Abdominal pain
    (1) Encourage the patient to move about.
 	
  c. Leakage
    (1) Change the dressings frequently, being careful not to dislodge the catheter.
    (2) Use sterile plastic drapes to prevent contamination.
	19.
	  a. This is caused by pressure from the fluid in the peritoneal cavity and the upward displacement of the diaphragm—producing shallow respirations.
	    (3) In severe respiratory difficulty, the fluid from the peritoneal cavity should be drained immediately and the physician notified.
	
	  b. Pain may be caused by the dialyzing solution's not being at body temperature, incomplete drainage of the solution, chemical irritation, pressure by the catheter, peritonitis, or air pressing on the diaphragm, causing referred shoulder pain.
	  c. Leakage around the catheter predisposes the patient to peritonitis.

20. Keep accurate records.
  a. Exact time of beginning and end of each exchange: starting and finishing time of drainage
  b. Amount of solution infused and recovered
  c. Fluid balance
  d. Number of exchanges
  e. Medications added to dialyzing solution
  f. Pre- and postdialysis weight, plus daily weight
  g. Level of responsiveness at beginning, throughout, and at end of treatment
  h. Assessment of vital signs and patient's condition	

(continued)

Guidelines: Assisting the Patient Undergoing Acute) **Peritoneal Dialysis** (continued)

Procedure
(Cont.)

Nursing Action	Rationale / Amplification
Complications	

1. Peritonitis
  a. Watch for nausea and vomiting, anorexia, abdominal pain, tenderness, rigidity, and cloudy dialysate drainage.
  b. Send specimen of dialysate for WBC count and full set of cultures.
	1. Peritonitis is the most common complication. Antibiotics may be added to dialysate and also given systemically.

2. Bleeding a. A hematocrit of the drainage fluid may be taken to determine the amount of bleeding.	2. A small amount of bleeding around the catheter is not significant if it does not persist. During the first few exchanges, blood-tinged fluid from subcutaneous bleeding is not uncommon. Small amounts of heparin may be added to inflow solution to prevent the catheter from becoming clogged.
3. Low serum albumin level	3. Small amounts of albumin are lost with each exchange, resulting in a lowered serum albumin level. Edema may occur, with possible hypotension.
4. Constipation	4. Inactivity, altered nutrition, phosphate binders, and the presence of fluid in the abdomen tend to cause constipation.

Continuous Ambulatory Peritoneal Dialysis
(CAPD) (Fig. 11-10)

Continuous ambulatory peritoneal dialysis is a practical self-dialysis method that involves almost constant peritoneal contact with a dialysis solution for patients with end-stage renal disease.

1. A permanent indwelling catheter is implanted into the peritoneum; the internal cuff of the catheter becomes embedded by fibrous ingrowth, which stabilizes it and minimizes leakage.
2. A connecting tube is attached to the external end of the peritoneal catheter, and the distal end of the tube is inserted into a sterile plastic bag of dialysate solution.
3. The dialysate bag is raised to shoulder level and infused by gravity into the peritoneal cavity.
4. Then the plastic bag attached to the connecting tube is folded and placed in a pouch at the waist, under the patient's clothing.
5. At the end of the dwell time (approximately 4 hours) the bag is removed from the pouch, unfolded, and placed near the floor to allow the dialysate to drain by gravity over a 20- to 40-minute period.
6. After the dialysate is drained, a fresh bag of dialysate solution is attached under aseptic conditions, and the procedure is repeated.
7. The patient performs 4–5 exchanges daily, 7 days/week with an overnight dwell time allowing uninterrupted sleep; most patients become unaware of fluid in the peritoneal cavity.
8. Advantages
   a. Physical and psychological freedom and independence
   b. Free dietary intake; improvement of nutritional status
   c. Relatively simple and easy to use
   d. Satisfactory biochemical control of uremia
   e. Least expensive form of dialysis therapy
   f. Eliminates need for complicated machines/dialyzers
9. Complications
   a. Peritonitis and damage to peritoneal membrane

   b. Pain (decreases with repeated treatments)
   c. Orthostatic hypotension
10. Patient education
   a. The use of CAPD as a long-term treatment depends on prevention of recurring peritonitis.
      (1) Use strict sterile techniques while caring for catheter.
      (2) Report signs and symptoms of peritonitis—cloudy peritoneal fluid, abdominal pain or tenderness, malaise, fever.
      (3) Send sample of peritoneal fluid to laboratory for culture and stain.
      (4) Expect some type of treatment with intraperitoneal antibiotics at home or in hospital.
   b. Do not omit bag changes—this will cause inadequate control of renal failure.
   c. Some weight gain may accompany CAPD; the dialysate fluid contains a significant amount of dextrose, which adds calories to daily intake.

Hemodialysis

Hemodialysis is a process of cleansing the blood of accumulated waste products. It is used for patients with end-stage renal failure or for acutely ill patients who require short-term dialysis.

Underlying Principles

1. Heparinized blood passes down a concentration gradient through a semipermeable membrane by dialysis to the dialysate fluid.
2. The dialysate is composed of all of the important electrolytes in their ideal extracellular concentrations.
3. Through the process of diffusion, the blood components equilibrate with those in the dialysate. By appropriate adjustment of the dialysate bath composition, noxious substances (urea, creatinine, uric acid, phosphate, and other metabolites) are transferred from the blood into the dialysate so that they can be discarded. Small pores of the membrane hold back desirable blood components.

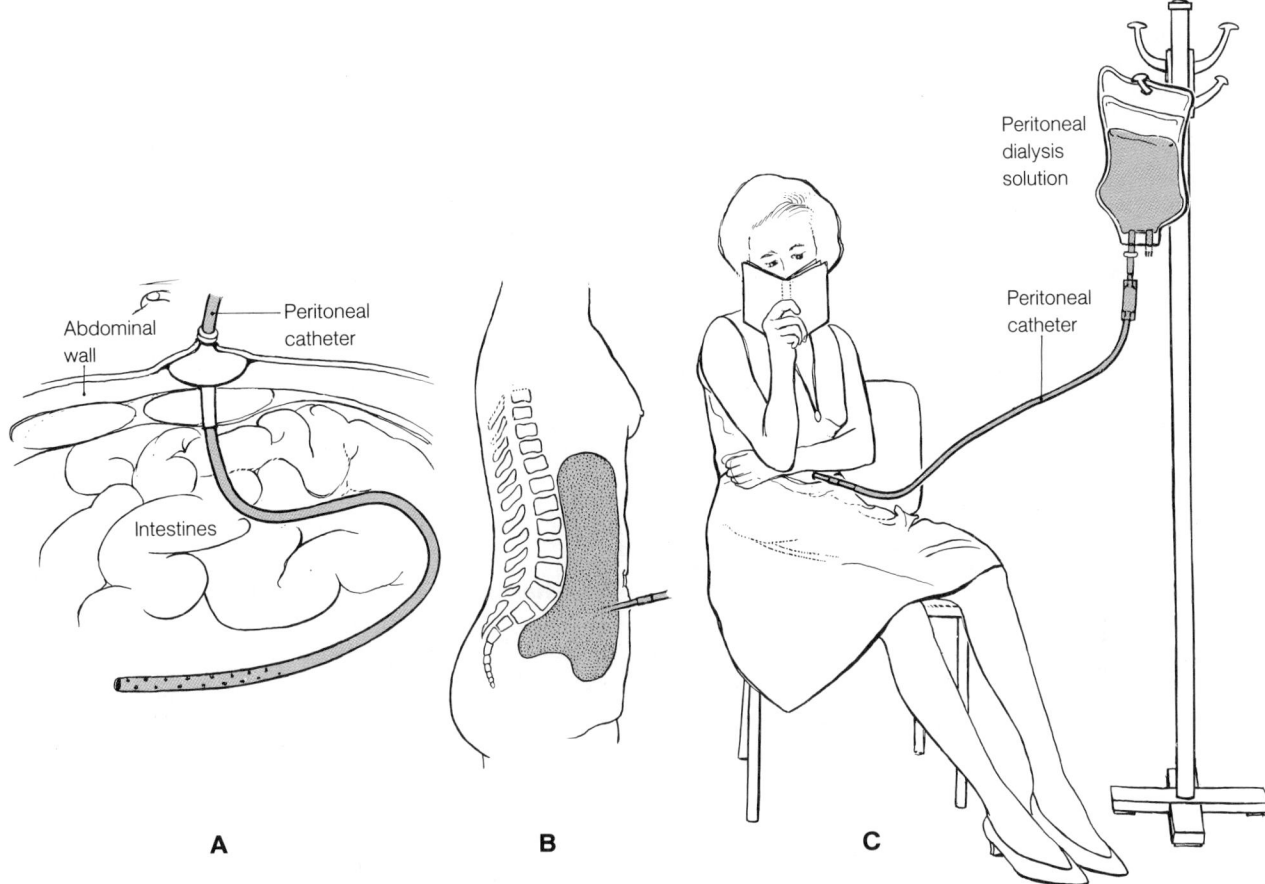

Figure 11-10. Continuous ambulatory peritoneal dialysis. *(A)* The peritoneal catheter is implanted through the abdominal wall. *(B)* Fluid infusing into the peritoneal cavity. *(C)* The patient allows for the prescribed dwell time and then drains the peritoneal cavity by gravity.

4. Excess water is removed from the blood (ultrafiltration).
5. The body's buffer system is maintained by the addition and diffusion of acetate from the dialysate into the patient; it is metabolized to form bicarbonate.
6. Purified blood is returned to the body through one of the patient's veins.
7. At the end of the treatment, most poisonous wastes have been removed, electrolyte and water balances have been restored, and the buffer system has been replenished.

Requirements for Hemodialysis

1. Access to the patient's circulation
2. Dialyzer with semipermeable membrane
3. Appropriate dialysate bath
4. Time—approximately 4 hours, 3 times weekly, for a total of 12 hours
5. Place—home (if feasible) or at a dialysis center

Methods of Access to the Patient's Circulation

1. Arteriovenous fistula (AVF)—creation of a vascular communication by suturing a vein directly to an artery.

a. Usually, radial artery and cephalic vein are anastomosed in nondominant arm; vessels in leg may also be used.
b. Following the procedure, the superficial venous system of the arm dilates.
c. By means of 2 large-bore needles inserted into the dilated venous system, blood may be obtained and passed through the dialyzer. The arterial end is used for arterial flow and the distal end for reinfusion of dialyzed blood.
d. Healing of AVF requires several weeks; an external shunt (see below) is used in the interim.
e. Problems
   (1) Infection; thrombosis; aneurysm formation
   (2) Disadvantage of being injected with large-bore needles before each dialysis treatment
   (3) Average life expectancy of fistula—5 years
2. Prosthetic arteriovenous fistula—vascular prosthesis (bovine; human umbilical vein; polytetrafluoroethylene [PTFE])
3. External arteriovenous shunt (cannula)
   a. Teflon–Silastic cannula sewn into radial artery and a forearm vein (or placed in leg). The 2 are connected by a Teflon bridge.
   b. During dialysis, the bridge is removed and the

arterial and venous ends are connected to the flow lines of the artificial kidney.
  c. Currently used while AVF is healing.
  d. Problems
    (1) Clotting and infection; chronic erosion of the skin
    (2) Limited shunt life—must be surgically revised every few months
    (3) Dislodgement with hemorrhage
    (4) Visible reminder to the patient of his disability
  4. Direct cannulation of vessels (femoral or subclavian vein)

Types of Dialyzers

Many varieties of artificial kidneys have been described, but most conform to one of the following types:
  1. Coil dialyzer
  2. Flat plate or parallel flow dialyzer
  3. Hollow-fiber kidney

Monitoring During Dialysis

The management of the patient on a dialyzer is a complex subject beyond the scope of this discussion. The reader is referred to the written protocol for the machine being used.

▶ **NURSING ALERT:** Nurses attending patients undergoing hemodialysis are at risk of acquiring hepatitis B.

Dietary Management of the Patient on Long-term Hemodialysis

  1. The individual patient's dietary regimen is adjusted according to the extent of his residual renal function to avoid wide fluctuation in body chemistry.
  2. Dietary management involves restriction or adjustment of protein, sodium, potassium, and/or fluid intake.
    a. Protein—protein of highest biologic quality is given to prevent poor protein utilization, to maintain positive nitrogen balance, and replace amino acids lost during each dialysis.
      (1) Usually 1–1.2 gm. of protein/kg. body weight is given; additional supplement given when stress situations (bleeding, infection) occur.
      (2) Calories (35 kcal./kg. body weight) are supplied from carbohydrates and fats to provide energy and to spare tissue breakdown.
    b. Sodium
      (1) The patient may not excrete the necessary amount of sodium to maintain balance.
      (2) Observe for fluid overload—hypertension, edema.
      (3) Or the patient may be a "salt loser," unable to conserve salt; he thus loses large amounts of sodium in the urine and will require sodium replacement by pharmacologic and dietary means.
    c. Potassium—a mineral found in the body cells.
      (1) Ability to eliminate excessive amounts of potassium is decreased in chronic renal failure.
      (2) Accumulation of potassium in body can be toxic to heart and cause serious arrhythmias.
      (3) Potassium is found in practically all foods—fruit juices, salt substitutes, bananas, chocolate, and baked potatoes are rich sources of potassium.
    d. Fluid limitations
      (1) Fluid is restricted according to output; usually between 500 and 800 ml., depending on renal function, losses, activity, environmental temperature.
      (2) The patient should be able to adjust his fluid intake according to the weight he has gained between dialysis treatments.
      (3) "Sourballs" are satisfactory to use as thirst quenchers.
    e. Calcium and phosphorus intake may have to be adjusted.

Nutrition—Health Education

Instruct the patient as follows:
  1. Avoid eating frequently in places where salt-free cooking cannot be obtained consistently.
  2. Read food labels carefully; avoid commercially prepared foods that have added sodium.
  3. Avoid "salt substitutes"—may contain potassium chloride, which should be avoided.
  4. Eat fresh vegetables and fruits within dietary prescription.

Pharmacologic Management

  1. Phosphate-binding gels (Amphojel, Aludrox, Basaljel)
    a. Phosphorus tends to accumulate, resulting in hyperparathyroidism and osteodystrophy.
    b. These medications bind phosphate in the intestine and may help maintain proper calcium and phosphorus levels in the blood.
  2. Potassium-binders (Kayexalate)—binds potassium in intestine to prevent dangerous elevations in blood.
  3. Multivitamins—necessary because of significant nutrient losses during dialysis (especially of ascorbic acid and folic acid).

Health Problems of Patients on Long-Term Hemodialysis

Although hemodialysis can prolong life indefinitely, it does not completely control uremia or halt the natural course of the underlying kidney disease. There are various abnormalities, syndromes, discomforts, and long-term metabolic complications associated with hemodialysis.
  1. Arteriosclerotic cardiovascular disease—leading cause of death and major factor limiting long-term survival.
    a. Disturbances of lipid metabolism (hypertriglyceridemia) appear to be accentuated by hemodialysis.
    b. Congestive heart failure, coronary heart disease with anginal pain, stroke, peripheral vascular insufficiency may incapacitate the patient.
  2. Intercurrent infection—patient has reduced resistance to infection.
    a. Exposure of blood to blood products and foreign material—may cause infection and gram-negative and gram-positive bacteremia
    b. Local infection of shunt site and in fistulas
    c. Hemodialysis-associated hepatitis
    d. Immunosuppression—facilitates opportunistic infection
  3. Anemia and fatigue—may be caused by accelerated red cell loss (from hemolysis and bleeding) and impaired erythropoietin production.
    a. Sleeplessness, fatigue, and malaise may be persistent

b. Diminution of physical and emotional well-being—lack of energy, drive, loss of interest
4. Intractable pruritus (itching)
5. Bleeding
   a. Bleeding from heparin rebound
   b. Gastrointestinal bleeding
   c. Subdural hematoma
   d. Hemorrhagic pericarditis
   e. Menorrhagia
6. Hypertension
7. Bone problems
   a. Renal osteodystrophy (leading to bone pain and fractures)—pathogenesis obscure, but excessive parathyroid hormone secretion and vitamin D resistance may be causal factors.
   b. Aseptic necrosis of hip
   c. Vascular calcification
8. Chronic ascites—may be due to fluid overload associated with congestive heart failure, malnutrition (hypoalbuminemia), and inadequate dialysis.
9. Disequilibrium syndrome—from rapid fluid and electrolyte changes, may produce increased intracranial pressure, hypertension, headache, vomiting, convulsions, coma, and psychiatric problems.
10. Dialysis dementia—progressive, irreversible, and fatal neurologic syndrome thought to be due to aluminum intoxication (from aluminum-containing dialysate fluid) or prolonged oral administration of aluminum hydroxide.

Psychosocial Problems

Long-term hemodialysis has unpredictable and uneven results. The impact of renal disease and the stresses of dialysis can be destructive to the ego and can place patients and families under severe mental and emotional stress.
1. Depression—an expected occurrence; most common psychological manifestation seen in patients on hemodialysis. Depression occurs from multiple causes—losses of bodily functions, working capability, and sexual drive; impotence, other physical complications, chronic illness, feelings of deprivation from diet and fluid restriction, limited capacity to compete, fear of death and dying, unpredictable medical status.
2. Dependence–independence conflict
   a. Although the patient is dependent on the dialysis machine, personnel, and treatment regimen, he is at the same time encouraged to be independent, work, and lead a "normal" life.
   b. Dependence may create aggressive feelings that cannot be expressed.
   c. The patient may repress hostility toward medical and nursing staff.
   d. The highly dependent patient may "enjoy" hemodialysis.
3. Anxiety—a normal reaction to stress and threat.
   a. The patient is anxious because of constant changes in his clinical status and unpredictability of his health.
   b. The patient may use denial, fantasy, repression, rejection, etc., as defense mechanisms to deal with anxiety.
   c. Try to clarify the nature of the patient's anxiety before attempts at reassurance.
4. Suicidal behavior—usually an act that stems from depression—suicide rate is more than 100 times that of general population.
   a. Allow the patient to express his feelings about self-destruction.
   b. Point out the patient's positive coping mechanisms and emphasize his capabilities.
   c. Psychiatric referral may be necessary.
5. Denial—a common response to a shift in health status.
   a. Denial may be protective and useful to a certain extent—may protect the patient from emotional decompensation (denial has both adaptive and maladaptive functions).
   b. Failure of this defense may lead to depression.
6. Stress from dietary restrictions—patient may "act out" conflicts by binges of overeating/drinking.
7. Sexual dysfunctions—diminished interest and ability due to biologic, pharmacologic, and psychological reasons.

Impact of Dialysis on Family

1. Altered family life-style
   a. Social activities may be decreased because of the large amount of time spent on dialysis.
   b. Close confinement to home (if the patient is on home dialysis) may create conflicts, frustration, and depression in some families.
   c. Role changes—traditional roles altered.
   d. The patient and family may impose unnecessary limitations on their own activities.
2. Decreasing sexual activity may lead to marital problems.
3. Feelings of resentment (revealed or hidden)—due to personal sacrifices made by family.
4. Feeling that patient is a "marginal" person with limited life expectancy can be transmitted to the patient.
5. Developmental/social problems of family members
6. Difficulties in communication between the patient and spouse—difficult to express anger, negative feelings, and fear of death.
   a. Fear that expressed anger will cause something to happen to the patient.
   b. Expressions of anger may be displaced or covered up by anxiety.

Health Education

1. Encourage the patient to assume the management and control of his therapeutic regimen.
   a. Determine the patient's own value system and ego strengths; use these to help him adapt to a different life-style.
   b. Emphasize the patient's capabilities.
   c. Teach the patient about his condition and treatment in "small doses."
   d. Deemphasize the patient's image of himself as "sick."
   e. Help the patient develop a sense of independence from the machine.
   f. Encourage the patient to interact with his surroundings during dialysis.
2. Encourage the patient to set realistic goals.
   a. Work activities should be introduced gradually—returning to work may not be a realistic goal for some patients.
   b. Modify attitudes in direction of permissiveness in area of productivity.
3. Encourage the patient to express his angry feelings (pain, discomfort, frustration)—helps to reduce level

of emotional tension and will help prevent depression.
4. Let family have an opportunity (away from the patient) to express their feelings of anger, helplessness, etc.
   a. Help family to accept their negative feelings.
   b. Teach family what is involved in chronic hemodialysis.
5. Organizations helpful to patients on chronic dialysis:

National Association of Patients on Hemodialysis and Transplantation, Inc.
505 Northern Boulevard
Great Neck, NY 11021

National Kidney Foundation
116 East 27th Street
New York, NY 10016

Kidney Transplantation

Kidney transplantation is the transplantation of a kidney from a living donor or human cadaver donor to a recipient with end-stage renal failure who requires support from dialysis in order to maintain life.

Kidney transplants from well-matched related living donors are more successful than those from cadaver donors.

Transplantation Procedure

1. The donor kidney is transplanted retroperitoneally in either iliac fossa.
2. The ureter of the newly transplanted kidney is transplanted into the bladder or anastomosed to the ureter of the recipient.

Potential Problems

1. Infection—leading cause of death after transplant.
2. Renal graft failure and renal graft rejection. Except when the donor is a twin, the immunologic defense of the recipient tends to reject (and destroy) a foreign substance, e.g., the kidney graft.
3. Possibility of recurrence of original disease in the graft (e.g., rapidly progressive glomerulonephritis)
4. Death from complications

Procedures Done Before Transplantation

1. Bilateral nephrectomy—for uncontrolled hypertension (renin variety), for removal of potential source of infection, if present, and for patients with obstructed kidneys or vesicoureteral reflux, rapidly progressive glomerulonephritis, polycystic renal disease.
2. Immunosuppressive drugs given in order to minimize or overcome body's defense mechanism:
Azathioprine (Imuran) and prednisone administration is usually begun 48 hours preoperatively for a scheduled transplant patient.
3. Donor-specific blood transfusion may be given—appears to improve graft survival.
4. Hemodialysis (see p. 522) is usually done 24 hours preoperatively.
5. Preoperative skin preparation is meticulous to decrease bacterial count on the skin. Preoperative shaving done in operating room—inadvertent scratches and nicks from shaving serve as nidi for bacterial colonization.

Assessment

Diagnostic Evaluation

(In addition to the usual preoperative preparation)
1. Tissue typing done to determine histocompatibility of donor and recipient.
2. Antibody screening for red and white cell antibodies.
3. Blood counts, chemistries, coagulation profiles, liver function tests, required cultures, ECG, state of hydration, blood pressure, temperature, pulse, respiration, and weight are corrected and documented.

Patient Problems/Nursing Diagnoses

1. Potential for infection
2. Fear related to threat of rejection and loss of kidney
3. Disturbance in self-concept (moon facies, acne, hirsutism, etc.) related to steroid medications
4. Potential for complications
5. See Patient Problems, Chronic Renal Failure, page 517

Planning and Implementation

Postoperative Nursing Interventions

A. Monitoring for threatened rejection

1. Watch for signs of rejection—progressive enlargement, pain and tenderness of graft, elevated blood pressure, diminished urine volume, increased serum creatinine, weight gain, apprehension, and fever.
   a. Acute rejection is common and usually reversible; often occurs in first weeks or months following transplant.
   b. If rejection is inevitable or when excessive immunosuppression is required, transplanted kidney is removed.
   c. The patient is placed back on maintenance dialysis; will require understanding and supportive emotional care.
2. Assist with various test systems used to monitor graft recipient immune status; tissue injury monitoring may be predictive of a rejection episode.
3. Give prescribed combinations of immunosuppressive agents; azathioprine, corticosteroids, cyclosporine, total lymphoid irradiation are given.
4. Be aware of complications of immunosuppressive protocols—infection or incomplete control of rejection.

B. Prevention of infection

1. Monitor and protect the patient from infection—kidney recipient is susceptible to faulty healing and infection because of both immunosuppressive therapy, which suppresses the immune response, and complications of renal failure.
   a. Infection may be masked or confused with symptoms of rejection since impaired renal function and fever are evidences of both infection and rejection.
   b. Immunosuppressive drugs render the transplant recipient more vulnerable to infection, permitting opportunistic infections to occur (fungal, viral, bacterial infections).
2. Carry out protective isolation as required; health team members and family may wear masks until immunosuppressive drug dosages are lowered.

3. Give aseptic care to wounds and puncture sites (central venous pressure [CVP] and IV lines, draining sites, etc.).
   a. Wound healing may be delayed because of effects of renal disease and immunosuppressive drugs.
   b. Change dressings promptly if drainage is present—drainage is an excellent culture medium for bacteria.
   c. Carry out bacteriologic testing of urine and all exit wounds. Catheter and drain tips are cultured on removal.
      (1) Before removing catheter, disinfect skin around entry site of catheter (or drain). Remove.
      (2) Using aseptic technique, cut off tip of catheter or drain and place in sterile container for laboratory culture.
4. Monitor vascular access to hemodialysis to ensure patency and watch for evidence of infection.
5. Give oral mycostatin mouthwash—to prevent mucosal candidiasis (fungal colonization occurs secondarily to steroid and antibiotic administration).
6. Give regular skin hygiene.

C. Maintenance of fluid and electrolyte balance

After kidney transplant, the following may occur:
1. A few donor kidneys function immediately after grafting.
   a. May produce large quantities of dilute urine (10–15 liters in first 24 hours)—due partly to tubular dysfunction or overhydrated state found in some dialyzed patients.
      Give IV fluid replacement to balance losses.
   b. Cadaver kidney (because of period of ischemia following donor's death) may undergo tubular necrosis and not function for 2–3 weeks. This is common in early postoperative period.
      Restrict fluid intake—usually approximately 600 ml./24 hours, plus amount of fluid losses from drainage, etc.
   c. Or kidney may produce amounts of urine varying from extremes of no urine to large volumes of urine.
2. Monitor CVP, ECG, and skin temperature frequently to guard against occult blood volume depletion and electrolyte imbalance.
   a. CVP readings observed and recorded hourly or more frequently as necessary.
   b. Avoid using dialysis access extremity for IV lines, intra-arterial monitoring, or restraints.
3. Monitor output from indwelling catheter, which has been connected to a closed drainage system.
   a. Measure urine every 30 minutes–1 hour.
   b. Irrigate catheter only on direct request.
   c. Palpate bladder to detect presence of distention.
   d. Instruct the patient to void frequently after catheter removal to avoid stressing the bladder closure.
4. Monitor serum and urine electrolytes to determine the patient's chemical balance.
   a. Anticipate adjustment of fluid replacement.
   b. Give IV fluids according to urine volume and serum electrolyte levels; serum and urine chemistries are measured at specified intervals.
   c. Notify physician immediately if arrhythmias or other cardiac symptoms develop.
5. Prepare for hemodialysis in postoperative period until transplanted kidney is functioning well.

D. Prevention of complications

1. Acute renal failure—from ischemia, renal artery thrombosis, hyperacute rejection
2. Gastrointestinal complications
   a. GI ulceration and bleeding; perforation; sepsis.
      (1) Steroids mask symptoms of ulceration.
      (2) GI hemorrhage associated with high mortality rate.
      (3) Give antacids frequently as directed until steroid doses are lowered—as a means of protection against GI ulceration.
   b. Fungal colonization of GI tract—occurs secondarily to steroid and antibiotic administration.
   c. Fecal impaction—decrease in colonic motility may occur from steroid effect.
3. Other late complications; some may be the cause of death.
   a. Infection, diabetes, GI bleeding, thrombosis, osteoporosis, psychosis, disorders of calcium metabolism, cushingoid facies, glaucoma, cataracts, acne—from prolonged steroid administration
   b. Bone marrow depression—from immunosuppressive therapy
   c. Vascular complications—hemorrhage and thrombosis
   d. Grafted ureter—stricture, fistula (also fistula of bladder)
   e. Viral hepatitis; liver failure
   f. Hypertension—from renal artery stenosis in allograft, from steroids, from renal–vascular disease
   g. Cardiovascular complications—myocardial infarction; stroke.
   h. Bone complications—aseptic necrosis due to secondary hyperparathyroidism
   i. Suicide
   j. Cancer—persons on long-term immunosuppressive therapy develop cancer more frequently than does the general population

E. Psychosocial support

1. Be aware of the stresses associated with renal transplantation—difficulty in planning for uncertain future, fear of organ rejection, problems associated with immunosuppressants and steroids.
2. Keep the patient informed of his progress, proposed treatment plans, and short- and long-term goals.
3. Observe for changes in behavior, altered thought and feeling processes.
4. See page 525 for other aspects of psychological support.

Health Education

1. The hospitalization period for a kidney transplant may be prolonged.
2. The patient receives individualized instruction about the following:
   a. Diet
   b. Medications (immunosuppressive drugs, antacids, vitamins, iron)
      (1) Review medications in detail, including color identification of pills, dose schedules, side effects, and the necessity for taking the medication.
   c. Fluids
   d. Daily weight
   e. Daily measurement of urine

f. Management of intake and output
g. Stool test for occult blood twice weekly
h. Prevention of infection
i. Resumption of activity; exercise
3. Instruct the patient to report to the physician immediately if any of the following occur:
   a. Decrease in urinary output
   b. Weight gain (detectable edema means excess fluid)
   c. Malaise
   d. Fever
   e. Graft swelling and tenderness
   f. Changes in blood pressure readings
   g. Respiratory distress
   h. Anxiety, depression, changes in eating, drinking, or other habit patterns
4. Advise the patient to avoid strenuous contact sports after surgery.

5. The patient should know that follow-up care after transplantation is a lifelong necessity.
6. Encourage the patient to become active in renal self-help group:
   National Association of Patients on Hemodialysis and Transplantation, Inc.
   505 Northern Boulevard
   Great Neck, NY 11021
   Publication: NAPHT NEWS

Evaluation
Expected Outcomes

1. Is free of infection
2. Shows no signs of rejection or renal failure
3. Copes with fear of graft rejection—communicates feelings and concerns; takes responsibility for health monitoring
4. Adapts to changes in self-concept and appearance

Nursing Management of the Patient Undergoing Renal/Urologic Surgery

Nursing Process Overview

Preoperative Assessment

Note: Surgical approaches to the kidney predispose the patient to respiratory complications and paralytic ileus.

1. Support the patient undergoing diagnostic examination of the urinary tract.
2. Determine history of patient's ability to engage in physical activity without distress. Observe for dyspnea, productive cough, other cardiac symptoms.
3. Do an electrocardiogram on all patients over 50. The preoperative cardiogram also serves as a baseline reference in event of postoperative cardiopulmonary complications.
4. Secure a chest x-ray.
5. Carry out pulmonary function studies and blood gas analysis in patients with impaired respiratory function.
6. Assess status of vascular system of lower extremities (especially varicosities).
   a. Elevate the patient's leg and apply elastic stockings to minimize stasis in superficial veins.
   b. Encourage patients to do leg exercises.
7. Inquire if the patient has any bleeding tendencies.
8. Assess fluid and electrolyte status.
   a. Weigh the patient daily to determine status of fluid balance.
   b. Assess status of mucous membranes and skin turgor; maintain the hematocrit at optimal level.
   c. Measure and record intake and output as an index of hydration.

Preoperative Nursing Interventions

1. Encourage liberal intake of fluids to promote excretion of waste products before surgery and to ensure that the patient is well-hydrated.
2. Give antimicrobial therapy as directed; kidney infection may be present preoperatively.
3. Teach the patient deep-breathing exercises and an effective cough routine.
4. Encourage the patient to express his feelings and concerns about impending surgery.
   a. Keep in mind that most patients entering the hospital with urologic conditions have pain, fever, hematuria, difficulty in voiding, etc.
   b. Obtain the patient's confidence by establishing a relationship of trust and by giving gentle and considerate care.
   c. Increase the patient's understanding of what to expect during the pre- and postoperative periods.
   d. Assess for alertness, appetite, and general well-being of the patient.
   e. Avoid physical inactivity.
   f. Give preoperative medications as prescribed to allay worry and fear.
5. See page 75 for general preoperative preparation.

Patient Problems/Nursing Diagnoses

1. Potential for complications related to the site of incision and nature of surgery
2. Pain and discomfort related to the surgical procedure(s) and presence of drainage tubes/catheters
3. Anxiety related to uncertainty of surgical outcome.

Planning and Implementation
Nursing Interventions

A. Prevention of Complications

1. Employ frequent and close observation of blood pressure, pulse, and respiration in order to recognize hemorrhage (and shock)—chief danger after renal surgery.
   a. Watch for pain, blood loss from drain site, mass over flank, shock.
   b. Prepare for reoperation; see management of hemorrhage, page 92.
2. Assess for pulmonary complications; postoperative atelectasis, page 93, pneumothorax, page 174, and pneumonia, page 155.
3. Be alert for symptoms of postoperative ileus (fairly common following renal surgery).
   a. Assess for abdominal distention, pain, and lack of intestinal peristalsis (determined by stethoscope auscultation).
   b. Avoid oral intake for patient until active bowel sounds are heard (auscultation) or passage of flatus is noted.

c. Give adequate and appropriate fluid and electrolyte replacement intravenously.
d. Assist with decompression via nasogastric tube for relief of abdominal distention (p. 412). See page 456 for treatment of paralytic ileus.
e. Keep record of fluid status.
4. Monitor for thromboembolic episodes.
a. Employ early ambulation as an aid in preventing thromboembolic episodes and improving patient endurance.

Note: Ambulation is contraindicated in prostatic patients with bleeding and with some types of reconstructive surgery.

b. Encourage the patient to do leg exercises in bed.
5. Watch for elevation of temperature and monitor the drainage tube sites and urine output for evidences of infection.

B. Relief of Pain and Discomfort

1. Give postoperative sedation and pain control on an individual basis to reduce splinting of respiratory movements and to permit coughing, since incision is close to diaphragm; the patient will voluntarily tend to splint chest while breathing.
a. Use narcotics at proper intervals—to help the patient perform deep breathing and coughing more effectively.
b. Use moist heat, massage, and analgesics for muscular aches and pain resulting from position on operating table.
c. Assess for pain similar to renal colic—caused by passage of clotted blood down the ureter; requires adequate doses of narcotic for relief.
d. Use incentive spirometer (p. 208) to help maximize lung inflation; encourage coughing after each deep breath to loosen secretions.

C. Management of Drainage Tubes and Catheters

1. Make certain that drainage tubes are functioning, since almost all urologic patients have drains, tubes, or catheters.
a. Make sure indwelling catheter is dependent and draining.
(1) Tape tubing to thigh to relieve traction on bladder. In supine male patient, tape catheter to lower abdomen. In women, anchor catheter to thigh, allowing enough slack for movement.
(2) Give meticulous catheter care.
b. Change dressings as indicated when the patient has profuse drainage.
c. Employ care with the patient with nephrostomy tube drainage (insertion of tube directly into kidney for temporary or permanent urinary diversion). It is attached to closed gravity drainage or to a urostomy appliance. A self-retaining U-tube or circular nephrostomy tube may be used.
(1) Purpose of nephrostomy drainage:
(a) To provide drainage from kidney after surgery.

(b) To conserve and permit physiologic restoration of renal tissue that has been traumatized by obstruction.
(c) To provide drainage when ureter is no longer functioning.
(2) Evaluate for bleeding from nephrostomy site (main complication of nephrostomy).
(3) Ensure that the nephrostomy tube is draining freely—plugging of the tube causes pain, trauma, bursting of suture lines, and infection.
(a) Call surgeon *immediately* if tube is inadvertently dislodged.
(b) Do not clamp the nephrostomy tube.
(c) Irrigate nephrostomy tube only by direct physician request. Use 10 ml. warm sterile saline solution—to avoid mechanical damage to kidney or infection from pyelorenal backflow.
(d) Encourage adequate fluid intake—to produce effective mechanical flushing and to dilute urinary elements that cause calculous formation.
(e) If there is a nephrostomy tube in each kidney, keep separate output records for each nephrostomy tube.
2. Assess the patient with indwelling ureteral catheter or stent (utilized to permit drainage from affected kidney).
a. Ureteral catheters are inserted through a cystoscope and left in place for a period of time; they are taped to the indwelling urethral catheter to hold them in place.
b. Tape catheter to thigh to reduce pulling on catheter.
c. Make notation on nursing care plan that catheter is an *ureteral* catheter.
d. Do not irrigate an ureteral catheter; this is done by the urologist.
3. Watch for complications from ureteral stent; infection (from foreign body in genitourinary tract) bleeding or clot obstruction within the stent, dislodgement of the stent.

Health Education

1. Teach the patient/family about care of catheters/tubes and management of dressings if the patient is to return home with indwelling tubes.
2. Continue a liberal intake of fluids.
3. Take frequent short rest periods and increase activities gradually.
4. Avoid straining or lifting heavy objects until permitted.

Evaluation
Expected Outcomes

1. Remains free of complications
2. Achieves relief of pain and discomfort; requests pain medication; moves freely
3. Discusses fears; making post discharge plans

Infections of the Urinary Tract

A *urinary tract infection* (UTI) is caused by the presence of pathogenic microorganisms in the urinary tract with or without signs and symptoms. Infection may predominate at the bladder (cystitis), urethra (urethritis), prostate (prostatitis), or kidney (pyelonephritis). Unfortunately, noninfectious conditions may generate symptoms that mimic those of urinary tract infection.

Bacteriuria refers to the presence of bacteria in the

urine (10^5 bacteria/ml. of urine or greater generally indicates infection).

In *asymptomatic bacteriuria,* organisms are found in urine, but the patient has no symptoms.

Recurrent urinary tract infections may indicate the following:
1. Relapse—recurrence of bacteriuria with same infecting microorganism
2. Reinfection—recurrence of bacteriuria with a microorganism different from that of the original infection (i.e., a "new" infection)

▶ **NURSING ALERT:** Infections in any part of the urinary tract may persist for months or years without symptoms and eventually cause serious kidney damage.

Predisposing Factors
1. Urinary stasis and obstruction (ureteral stenosis, stone, tumor)—slowing of urinary flow causes kidney to be more susceptible to bacterial infection.
2. Increasing intraluminal pressure or overdistended bladder
3. Reflux
   a. Urethrovesical reflux—flowing back of urine from urethra into bladder
   b. Vesicoureteral reflux (ureterovesical reflux)—flowing back of urine from bladder into one or both ureters
4. Fecal soiling of urethral meatus
5. Instrumentation—catheter, cystoscope
6. Metabolic disorders (diabetes mellitus) and diseases of blood vessels (arteriosclerosis) may diminish blood supply to organs of urinary tract.
7. Neurologic abnormalities (neurogenic bladder dysfunction)
8. Renal disease increases susceptibility of kidney to infection.

Pathways of Infection Within Urinary Tract
Bacteria invade and spread within tract by the ascending (most common), bloodstream, and/or lymphatic pathways.
1. Urethra—from ascending bacteria
2. Bladder—from bacteria ascending from urethra (or, less commonly, descending from kidney)
3. Kidney—from ureterovesical reflux (incompetence of ureterovesical valve, which allows urine to regurgitate into ureters, usually at time of voiding); bloodborne
4. Prostate—from ascending urethral flora
5. Epididymis—from infected prostate
6. Testis—from bacteria via the bloodstream

Lower Urinary Tract Infection
(Cystitis, Acute Urethral Syndrome)

Cystitis is an inflammation of the urinary bladder; it is usually a superficial infection that does not extend to the bladder mucosa.

Acute urethral syndrome is symptomatic urinary tract infection in women whose urine is either sterile or contains less than 10^5 bacteria/ml.

Etiology
1. Ascending infection after entry via the urinary meatus.
   a. Women seem to be more apt to develop acute cystitis because of shorter length of urethra, anatomic proximity to vagina, periurethral glands, and rectum (fecal contamination), and the mechanical effect of coitus.
   b. Women with recurrent urinary tract infections often have gram-negative organisms at the vaginal introitus; there may be some defect of the mucosa of the urethra, vagina, or external genitalia of these patients that allows enteric organisms to invade the bladder.
   c. Poor/abnormal voiding patterns cause decrease in blood supply to bladder.
   d. Acute infection in women most often from organisms of the patient's own intestinal flora (*Escherichia coli*).
2. In males, obstructive abnormalities (strictures, prostatism)—most frequent cause.
3. Upper urinary tract disease may occasionally cause recurrent bladder infection.

Assessment
Clinical Manifestation
1. Frequency, urgency, burning, and pain on urination
2. Nocturia
3. Bearing-down sensation in region of bladder; suprapubic pain
4. Changes in composition of urine (bacteria and red blood cells)

Diagnostic Evaluation
Urine culture is done to detect presence of bacteria and for antimicrobial susceptibility testing.

Patient Problems/Nursing Diagnoses
1. Urinary frequency and dysuria related to presence of bacterial infection
2. Potential for recurrence of infection

Planning and Implementation
Nursing Interventions
A. Eradicating the Causative Pathogen
1. Obtain uncontaminated urine specimen for smears, culture, and antimicrobial sensitivity studies to determine pathogen so that appropriate drug may be selected.
2. Give prescribed antimicrobial medication, since urinary infections usually respond to drugs that are excreted in the urine in high concentrations; a potentially effective drug should rapidly sterilize the urine and thus relieve the patient's symptoms.
   a. For uncomplicated infection:
      (1) Single-dose antimicrobial therapy (amoxicillin; sulfisoxazole; trimethoprim–sulfamethoxazole) is currently being administered to nonpregnant women, along with follow-up cultures to prove treatment effectiveness.
      (2) Side effects are nausea, diarrhea, drug-related rash, and vaginal candidiasis.
   b. For acute urethral syndrome:
      (1) Antimicrobial therapy for 10 days.
      (2) Repeat urine culture in 7–10 days to ensure elimination of infection.
   c. For recurrent infections with closely spaced episodes:
      (1) The patient may require treatment for 6 months or more.
      (2) Patients with recurring infections should have periodic urine cultures, since most recurrences are new infections with different

organisms; relapses may occur with same organism.

3. Maintain an appropriate urine pH—efficacy of certain antimicrobial drugs is affected by the reaction (pH) of the urine. Sodium bicarbonate alkalinizes urine; ascorbic acid acidifies urine.

B. Increasing the Body's Normal Defense Mechanisms

1. Encourage the patient to drink fluids sufficient to promote renal blood flow and to flush out bacteria in urinary tract.
2. Encourage the patient to void frequently (every 2–3 hours) and to empty bladder completely, since this enhances bacterial clearance, reduces urine stasis, and prevents reinfection. Infrequent voiding overstretches the bladder wall, leading to hypoxia of bladder mucosa, which is then susceptible to bacterial invasion.
3. Promote patient comfort.
   a. Give analgesics and antispasmodics and apply heat to perineum to relieve pain, spasm, and urgency.
   b. Encourage bed rest during the acute phase.

Health Education

1. Encourage the patient to have follow-up urine studies to determine if there is resolution of infection or if asymptomatic infection is present; there is a marked tendency for infection to recur.
2. For women with repeated urinary tract infections, give the following instructions:
   a. Reduce vaginal introital concentration of pathogens by hygienic measures.
      (1) Wash in shower or while standing in bathtub—bacteria in bath water may gain entrance into urethra.
      (2) Cleanse around the perineum and urethral meatus after each bowel movement, with front to back cleansing to minimize fecal contamination of periurethral area.
   b. Drink liberal amounts of fluid to flush out bacteria.
   c. Avoid irritants—coffee, tea, alcohol, cola drinks.
   d. Void every 2–3 hours during day and completely empty bladder.
   e. In certain women, sexual intercourse is the initiating event for the development of bacteriuria—urethral massage associated with intercourse facilitates entry of microorganisms into the bladder.
      (1) Void immediately after sexual intercourse.
      (2) A single dose of an oral antimicrobial agent may be prescribed following sexual intercourse.
   f. Avoid external irritants such as bubble baths and perfumed vaginal cleansers or deodorants.
   g. An antibacterial vaginal suppository may be prescribed to reduce concentration of bacteria in introitus.
   h. Patients with persistent bacteria may require long-term antimicrobial therapy to prevent colonization of periurethral area and recurrence of urinary tract infection.
      (1) Take drug the last thing at night after emptying bladder to ensure adequate concentration of drug during overnight period, since low rates of urine flow and infrequent bladder emptying predispose to multiplication of bacteria.

(2) Use self-monitoring kit* at home to monitor urinary tract infection.
   (a) Perform the test on the first urination of the morning for 3 consecutive days.
   (b) Wash around urethral meatus several times.
   (c) Collect midstream specimen.
   (d) Remove the plastic strip from its container, dip the test area urine sample, and remove it immediately.
   (e) Read the results by comparing test area with the the color chart.
   (f) Consult physician if the reagent test on the plastic strip gives a positive result.
3. Instruct patients who have had urinary tract infections during pregnancy to have follow-up studies.
4. Teach the patient that bacteriuria in young girls (under 5 years) increases the risk of developing a urinary tract infection as an adult.

Evaluation
Expected Outcomes

1. Is free of urinary frequency, dysuria, and bacteriuria
2. Demonstrates no evidence of recurrence

Bacterial Pyelonephritis

Bacterial pyelonephritis is an acute inflammatory renal disease caused by bacteria.

Causes

1. Enteric bacteria (*E. coli*)
2. Secondary to vesicoureteral reflux (incompetence of ureterovesical valve, which allows urine to regurgitate into ureters, usually at time of voiding)
3. Urinary obstruction/infection
4. Trauma
5. Blood-borne infection
6. Renal disease
7. Pregnancy
8. Metabolic disorders

Clinical Manifestations

Flank pain; tenderness in the costovertebral angle, dysuria, fever, urgency, and frequency.

Diagnostic Evaluation

1. Identification of antibody-coated bacteria (ACB) in urine; bacteria invading kidney induce an antibody response that coats the bacteria—differentiates renal infection from bladder infection.
2. Identification of pyuria, bacteriuria, and casts in urinary sediment.
3. Other radiologic/urinary tests as directed.

Nursing Interventions

A. Eradication of bacteria from the urinary tract

1. Assist with carrying out intravenous urogram and other diagnostic tests—relief of obstructions is essential to save kidney from rapid destruction.
2. Obtain urine specimen (under aseptic conditions) for culture and sensitivity studies, since choice of drug is based on sensitivity studies.
3. Give organism-specific antimicrobial therapy. Anti-

* Microstix-Nitrite (Ames Company, Division of Miles Laboratories, Inc.)

bacterial agent is maintained in urine for a long enough period to prevent reseeding of residual foci of infection.

   a. Acute pyelonephritis usually caused by *E. coli,* which is sensitive to many antimicrobial drugs.

   b. A minimum of 14 days of treatment with an appropriate antimicrobial is needed for bacteriuria of renal origin.

     (1) The patient is admitted to hospital if he is toxic and cannot tolerate oral antimicrobial medication; bacteremia is common.

     (2) Parenteral antimicrobial therapy may be necessary.

4. Obtain urine for repeated cultures to determine the patient's response to treatment, to search for secondary organisms, and to determine clinical and microbiologic resolution of infection.

B. For the patient with chronic or recurring infections—Preservation of renal function

1. Employ continuous treatment with urine-sterilizing agents after initial antibiotic treatment has been employed.
2. Advise the patient to continue this regimen for months to years until (1) there is no evidence of inflammation, (2) causative factors have been treated or controlled, and (3) there is evidence of stability of renal function.
3. Emphasize to the patient that serial urine cultures and evaluation studies must be done for an indefinite period of time.
4. Encourage the patient to have blood counts and serum creatinine determinations if he is on long-term therapy.

Genitourinary Tuberculosis

Genitourinary tuberculosis is caused by the organism *Mycobacterium tuberculosis* and is usually disseminated from the lungs via the bloodstream to one or both of the kidneys and to other organs of the genitourinary tract.

Clinical Manifestations

1. Hematuria (microscopic or gross)
2. Bladder irritation—burning on urination, frequency, nocturia
3. Manifestations from infection of prostate and epididymis
4. Slight afternoon fever, loss of weight, anorexia

Diagnostic Evaluation

1. Urine culture for tubercle bacilli (smears of urinary sediment also stained for acid-fast bacilli).
2. Excretory urogram—to reveal renal and ureteral lesions.
3. Cystoscopic examination—to determine extent of bladder involvement, for biopsy purposes, and for ureteral catheterization of each kidney to determine if one or both kidneys are affected.

▶ **NURSING ALERT:** A search for tuberculosis elsewhere in the body must be conducted when tuberculosis of the kidney or urinary tract is found.

Be alert for patient who has had previous contact with tuberculosis.

Management

1. Combination of the following drugs usually given: rifampin, isoniazid, ethambutol.
   a. Multiple drug regimen appears to delay the emergence of resistant organisms.
   b. Many centers are using short-term chemotherapy for initial treatment of genitourinary tuberculosis.
2. Surgical intervention may be necessary to prevent obstructive problems and to remove severely infected organ. However emphasis is on medical treatment.

Health Education

Instruct the patient as follows:
1. Follow-up examinations, including periodic urine examinations and excretory urograms are necessary to detect reactivation of disease.
2. Report for cystoscopic examination as directed to detect ureteral stricture formation, which is a complication of genitourinary tuberculosis.
3. Adhere to medication regimen.
4. Maintain good health practices since genitourinary tuberculosis is a manifestation of a systemic disease.
5. For other aspects of health teaching, see page 875.

Acute Glomerulonephritis

Acute glomerulonephritis refers to a group of kidney diseases in which there is an inflammatory reaction in the glomeruli. It is not an infection of the kidney per se, but rather the result of untoward side effects of the defense mechanisms of the body. It is thought to involve an antigen–antibody reaction, which produces damage to the glomeruli, the filtering bed of the kidney.

Altered Physiology

Cellular proliferation, infiltration of glomerulus by leukocytes → glomerular trapping of circulating immune complexes → thickening of glomerular filtration membrane → scarring and loss of filtering surface → renal failure.

Assessment
Clinical Manifestations

1. The disease may be so mild that it is discovered accidentally through a routine urinalysis.
2. History of preceding pharyngitis or tonsillitis with fever (2–3 weeks previously); majority of cases caused by streptococci.
3. Dark or smoky urine; oliguria
4. Facial edema; edema of extremities
5. Fatigue and anorexia
6. Hypertension (mild, moderate, or severe); headache
7. Tenderness over costovertebral angle
8. Anemia from loss of red blood cells into the urine

Diagnostic Evaluation

1. Urinalysis—hematuria (microscopic or gross), proteinuria (500 mg.–3 gm./day), red cell casts, white cells, renal epithelial cells, and various casts in the sediment.
2. Blood—elevated blood urea nitrogen (BUN) and serum creatinine levels, low total serum protein level, increased antistreptolysin titre (from reaction to streptococcal organism).

3. Needle biopsy of the kidney reveals obstruction of glomerular capillaries from proliferation of endothelial cells.

Clinical Course

1. Diuresis usually starts 1–2 weeks after onset of symptoms.
    a. Renal clearances and blood urea concentration return to normal.
    b. Edema decreases and hypertension lessens.
    c. Microscopic proteinuria or hematuria may persist many months.
2. Recovery is usual in children and young adults; in an older person, the disease may progress to chronic glomerulonephritis.

Patient Problems/Nursing Diagnoses

1. Altered urinary elimination patterns
2. Severe protein loss related to glomerular damage
3. Fluid imbalance
4. Potential for renal failure
5. Fatigue and anorexia related to underlying disease

Planning and Implementation
Nursing Interventions

A. Promotion of kidney function

1. Encourage bed rest during the acute phase until the urine clears and BUN, creatinine, and blood pressure normalize. (Rest also facilitates diuresis.)
2. Restrict dietary protein moderately if there is oliguria and the BUN is elevated.
    a. Give carbohydrates liberally to provide energy and reduce catabolism of protein.
    b. Restrict protein more drastically if acute renal failure develops (see p. 515).
    c. Restrict sodium intake in presence of edema or signs of congestive heart failure.
3. Measure and record intake and output.
4. Give fluids according to the patient's fluid losses (urine, respiration, feces) and daily body weight.

B. Prevention of complications

1. Recognize and treat any intercurrent infections promptly.
2. Watch for symptoms of renal failure—nausea, fatigue, vomiting, diminished urinary output (see p. 516).
3. Evaluate the patient for:
    a. Hypertensive encephalopathy
    b. Cardiac failure and pulmonary edema
4. Dialysis may be considered if uremia and fluid retention cannot be controlled.

Health Education

Instruct the patient as follows:
1. Explain that the patient must have follow-up evaluations of blood pressure, urinary protein, and BUN concentrations to determine if there is exacerbation of disease activity.
2. Treat any infection promptly.
3. Call physician/clinic if symptoms of renal failure occur.

Evaluation
Expected Outcomes

1. Shows no signs of proteinuria
2. Achieves stabilization of renal function—normal urine/blood evaluations; normal blood pressure

Nephrotic Syndrome

Nephrotic syndrome is a clinical disorder characterized by (1) marked proteinuria, (2) hypoalbuminemia, (3) edema, and (4) hyperlipidemia as a consequence of excessive leakage of plasma proteins into the urine because of increased permeability of the glomerular capillary membrane to protein.

Etiology

In any condition that seriously damages the glomerular capillary membrane, any of the following etiologies are possible.
1. Chronic glomerulonephritis
2. Diabetes mellitus with intercapillary glomerulosclerosis
3. Amyloidosis of kidney
4. Systemic lupus erythematosus
5. Renal vein thrombosis
6. Secondary to malignancy (older adults)

Assessment
Clinical Manifestations

1. Insidious onset of edema; easily pitting edema.
2. Marked proteinuria—leads to negative nitrogen balance.
3. Extensive depletion of body proteins (hypoalbuminemia) from extensive urinary protein losses.
4. Hyperlipidemia—may lead to accelerated atherosclerosis.

Diagnostic Evaluation

1. Needle biopsy of kidney—for histologic examination of renal tissue to confirm diagnosis
2. Serum electrolyte evaluations (protein, albumin, etc.)
3. Triglyceride profile—to evaluate degree of hyperlipidemia
4. Urinary tests—for microscopic hematuria, proteinuria, RBCs, WBCs, casts, fat bodies
5. Renal function tests

Patient Problems/Nursing Diagnoses

1. Edema related to renal retention of salt and water
2. Potential for infection
3. See also Acute Glomerulonephritis

Planning and Implementation
Medical Management

1. Sodium restriction
2. Diuretics, if renal insufficiency is not severe
3. Steroids (prednisone)—to reduce edema and proteinuria
4. Immunosuppressive agents—may be effective when nephrosis is associated with autoimmune disease

Nursing Interventions

1. Keep on bed rest for a few days to mobilize edema.
2. Utilize dietary treatment to replace protein losses.
    a. High protein diet to replenish wasted tissues and restore body proteins
    b. Mild to moderate sodium restriction to control severe edema
    c. High calorie diet (25–50 cal./kg. body weight/day)
3. Protect patient from infection—thought to be due to loss of serum immune globulins into the urine.

4. Evaluate for thromboembolism (renal vein thrombosis, pulmonary emboli, thrombophlebitis)—increased incidence in patients with nephrotic syndrome.
5. See page 533 for nursing the patient with acute glomerulonephritis and page 518 for care of the patient with chronic renal failure.

Evaluation

Expected Outcomes

1. Is free of edema
2. Shows no signs of proteinuria or infection
3. Adheres to diet to replace protein loss
4. Is free of complications

Hydronephrosis

Hydronephrosis is distention of the pelvis and calyces by urine due to obstruction of the ureter.

Causes

1. Congenital causes—stenosis of ureteropelvic junction, urethral valves
2. Progressive changes in bladder, ureters, and kidneys from obstruction anywhere in urinary tract
   a. Obstruction from enlarged prostate
   b. Obstructing calculus
   c. Malignant lesion (cancer of prostate, bladder, or cervix)
   d. Obstruction of ureter—from calculus, stricture, etc.
3. Neurogenic causes
4. Vesicoureteral reflux

Altered Physiology

Interference with passage of urine from kidney → chronic infection → increasing pressure → distention of renal pelvis and calyces → decreased renal blood flow → atrophy of renal parenchyma (as one kidney undergoes gradual destruction, the contralateral kidney gradually enlarges [compensatory hypertrophy]) → impairment of renal function.

Assessment

Clinical Manifestations

1. Often asymptomatic and insidious onset
2. Aching in flank and back (present with acute obstruction)
3. Bladder irritability—fever and dysuria if infection is present
4. Gastrointestinal disturbances
5. Chills, fever, tenderness, pyuria—from infection
6. Hematuria—hydronephrotic kidney may bleed from congestion
7. Uremia—if condition is advanced

Diagnostic Evaluation

Complete urographic survey.

Patient Problems/Nursing Diagnoses

1. Alteration in urinary elimination (reduced urinary output, hematuria) related to obstruction of ureters
2. Pain and discomfort related to obstruction of urinary flow
3. Potential for infection

Planning and Implementation

Nursing Interventions

1. Relieve obstruction, etc.
   Urine may have to be diverted by nephrostomy or other types of diversion.
   a. Ureteral catheter may be inserted by urologist to decompress kidney if the patient is having severe flank pain.
   b. See page 529 for care of the patient having a nephrostomy.
2. Give antimicrobial as directed to eradicate infection, since residual urine in calyces produces infection and pyelonephritis.
3. Prepare for surgical intervention to correct obstruction (see p. 528).
   a. Removal of obstructive lesions (calculus, tumor, obstruction of ureter)
   b. Operations to improve drainage of kidney; plastic reconstruction procedures
   c. Nephrectomy—if one kidney is severely damaged

Health Education

Report for urinalysis follow-up every 2–3 weeks and excretory urography as directed to determine if satisfactory progress is being made.

Evaluation

Expected Outcomes

1. Demonstrates normal urinary output without signs of hematuria
2. Is free of infection

Urolithiasis

Urolithiasis refers to the presence of stones in the urinary system. Stones are formed in the urinary tract by the deposit of crystalline substances (calcium phosphate, oxalate, uric acid) excreted in the urine. They may be found anywhere in the urinary system and vary in size from mere granular deposits (called sand or gravel), to bladder stones the size of an orange.

Factors Favoring Stone Formation

1. Obstruction and urinary stasis facilitating precipitation of salts from the urine
2. Infection—particularly of urea-splitting organisms (*Proteus vulgaris*)
3. Dehydration and urine concentration—encourages precipitation of solids

4. Immobilization—produces slowing of renal drainage and altered calcium metabolism
5. Metabolic disorders
    a. Hypercalcemia (abnormally high concentration of blood calcium compounds) and hypercalciuria (abnormally large amounts of calcium in urine) from dissolution of bone, excessive ingestion or excessive absorption of calcium from GI tract, or faulty renal reabsorption of calcium
    b. Hyperparathyroidism
    c. Excessive intake of vitamin D
    d. Excessive intake of milk and alkali
    e. Myeloproliferative disorders (leukemia, polycythemia vera) and chemotherapy for cancer—patients excrete increased amounts of uric acid
6. Excessive excretion of uric acid
7. Vitamin deficiency (especially vitamin A)
8. Foreign bodies in urinary tract
9. High intake of protein, calcium, excessive consumption of tea and fruit juices
10. Small bowel disease or small bowel surgery
11. Heredity—plays a part in calcium oxalate stones (most common type), cystine, and uric acid stones
12. Idiopathic—no cause can be found

Clinical Features

1. The problem occurs predominantly in the 3rd to 5th decade, affecting men more than women.
2. The majority of stones are composed of calcium oxalate with or without apatite, uric acid, or (rarely) cystine.
3. Infection and obstruction may cause destruction of renal tissue and subsequent loss of a kidney.
4. Most renal stones migrate downward (causing severe, colicky pain) and are discovered in the lower ureter.
5. People who have had 2 stones tend to have recurrences.

Medical Management

(Dictated by size, shape, position and likely chemical composition of stone[s])
Specific therapy—regimen depends on stone type/metabolic abnormality.
1. *Calcium stones* (calcium oxalate and calcium phosphate; most prevalent)
    a. Moderate dietary intake of calcium and phosphorus; restrict oxalate-containing beverages (cola, tea).
    b. Administer drugs, depending on classification of hypercalciuria—orthophosphates, thiazides, magnesium oxide, sodium cellulose phosphate, potassium citrate.
    c. Round-the-clock intake of fluid to maintain a high urine flow rate.
2. *Uric acid stones* (develop in highly acidic and concentrated urine)
    a. Alkalinize the urine to enhance urate solubility.
    b. Limit protein and purine intake; encourage high fluid intake.
    c. Administer allopurinol to lower serum and urinary acid levels and inhibit uric acid synthesis.
    d. Amenable to dissolution techniques.
3. *Cystine stones* (rare)
    a. Increase fluid intake; exclude excess dietary animal protein.
    b. Administer penicillamine—decreases stone formation and sometimes results in stone dissolution.
4. *Struvite stones* (infection-related stones)—associated with urinary tract infections with urea-splitting bacteria (*Proteus* species, *Klebsiella, Pseudomonas, Staphylococcus*). May occur as a large staghorn calculi and cause significant renal damage from infection and obstruction.
    a. Acidify urine.
    b. Give appropriate antimicrobial therapy—may be given continuous antimicrobial therapy to keep urine sterile if surgery is not possible.
    c. Stone dissolution may be an alternative to surgery for selected patients.

Interventional Procedures

A. **Percutaneous Stone Removal Procedures** (Fig. 11-11)

1. *Percutaneous nephrostomy/nephrolithotomy* (radiologic placement of tube into collection system of kidney). Under fluoroscopic or ultrasound guidance, needle is advanced into collecting system; guide wire is advanced into kidney pelvis (or ureter). On the

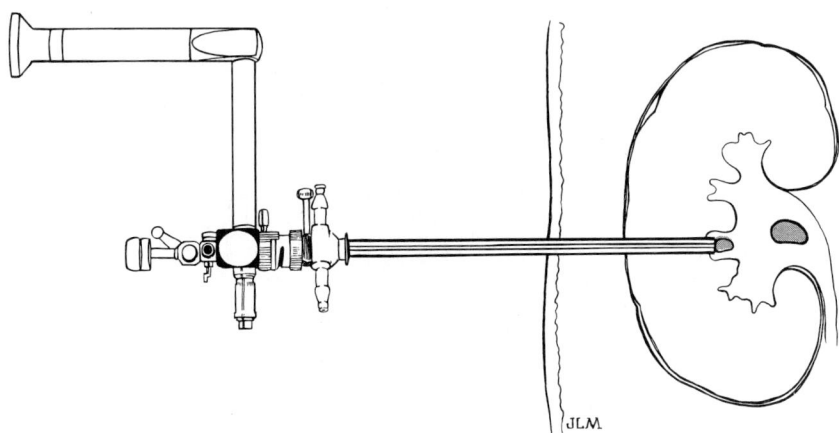

Figure 11-11. A percutaneous nephrostomy tract permits access to the collecting system of the kidney for removal of kidney stones under direct vision via a nephroscope.

following day, dilators are passed over guide wire for dilatation, tract is established through the renal parenchyma, and catheter placed in renal pelvis.

  a. After 24 hours, endoscope is passed down through established tract to visualize interior of collecting system.

  b. Small stones may be retrieved through forceps, snared with a basket extractor under vision, or washed out.

  c. Larger or impacted stones require fragmentation (by ultrasound, electrohydraulic shock waves, or lasers).

  d. Offers shorter hospital stay, less patient morbidity, and earlier return to employment.

2. *Percutaneous stone dissolution* (chemolysis, dissolution by chemical agents). A multiholed nephrostomy tube (catheter) is placed in kidney; offers a pathway for introduction of solvent (depending on chemical composition of stone) to be infused into stone. A second catheter may be used for drainage.

  a. Used for struvite, uric acid, and cystine stones.

  b. May be used to shrink large stones before using other retrieval methods or to irrigate debris after lithotripsy procedures (see below).

    (1) Irrigating solution introduced at a continuous rate that patient can tolerate without flank pain or elevation of intrarenal pressure above 25 cm. H_2O.

    (2) The patient receives antimicrobial agents before, during, and after procedure to maintain sterile urine.

    (3) Complications include infection (renal and perirenal abscesses, pyelonephritis, septic shock) and thrombophlebitis and pulmonary embolism (associated with immobilization).

B. Surgical Procedures

1. *Pyelolithotomy*—removal of stones from kidney pelvis. *Coagulum pyelolithotomy*—intraoperative injection of certain coagulation factors into the renal pelvis, producing a coagulum that entraps the stones and expedites their removal (Fig. 11-12).

2. *Nephrolithotomy*—incision into kidney for removal of stone.

3. *Nephrectomy*—removal of kidney; indicated when kidney is extensively and irreparably damaged and is no longer a functioning organ; partial nephrectomy sometimes done.

4. *Ureterolithotomy*—removal of stone in ureter.

5. *Cystolithotomy*—removal of stone from bladder.

C. Stone destruction (by energy in various wave forms)**—allows endoscopic removal of stones too large to pass.**

1. *Ultrasonic lithotripsy*—introduction of an ultrasonic probe through a nephrostomy tube to shatter the stone into fragments.

  a. The portion of the stone in contact with vibrating tip of probe is reduced to dust/small fragments, which are continuously removed by suction.

  b. Remaining stone fragments are retrieved by forceps or stone basket (residual calculi may present a problem).

2. *Electrohydraulic lithotripsy*—disintegration of stone by creating an electrical discharge in a fluid.

  a. The patient is placed in tank of water through which are propagated shock waves that break up the stone.

  b. Considered investigational.

3. Stone disruption by laser impulse (investigational).

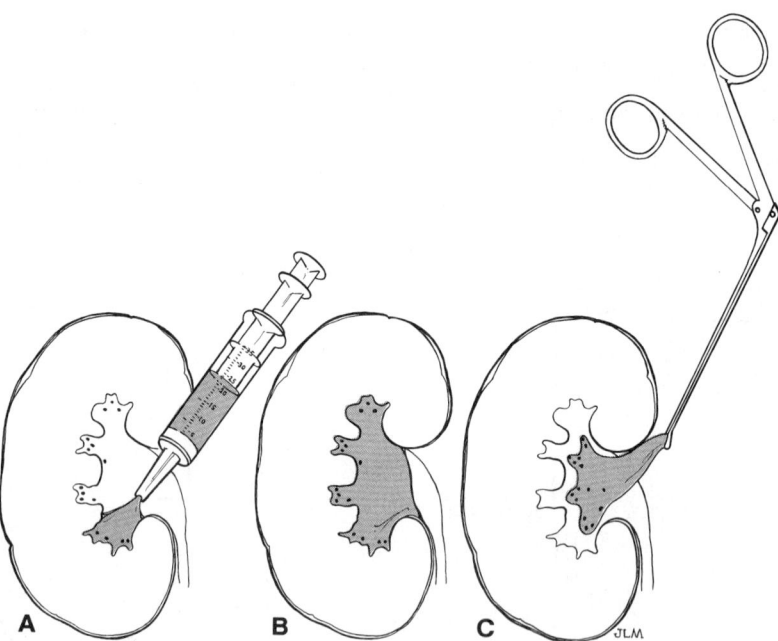

Figure 11-12. The procedure, coagulum pyelolithotomy, is useful for removal of multiple kidney stones. (A) Components of coagulum are instilled into the renal pelvis (B) to produce a jelly-like clot. (C) The stones are entrapped in the clot and extracted with forceps.

Assessment
Clinical Manifestations

Dependent on presence of obstruction, infection, edema.
1. Stones blocking flow of urine produce symptoms of urinary tract infection—chills, fever, dysuria.
2. Renal stones—produce an increase in hydrostatic pressure and distention of the renal pelvis and proximal ureter, causing:
    a. Pain in renal area—radiates anteriorly and downward toward bladder in female and toward testicle in male.
    b. Renal colic—acute pain with tenderness over loin; nausea and vomiting.
3. Ureteral stones
    a. Acute colicky pain, referring down the thigh and to genitalia (ureteral colic).
    b. Frequent desire to void, but little urine is passed.
4. Gastrointestinal symptoms
    a. Due to renal–intestinal reflexes and anatomic relation of kidneys to stomach, pancreas, colon, etc.
    b. Include nausea, vomiting, diarrhea, abdominal discomfort.

Diagnostic Evaluation

1. Intravenous urography
2. Laboratory screening studies—complete blood count, urinalysis/culture, serum chemistry survey; 24-hour urine study for calcium, phosphorus, uric acid, creatinine, sodium oxalate

Patient Problems/Nursing Diagnoses

1. Pain and discomfort related to location/migration of stone(s)
2. Alteration in urinary elimination related to blockage of urine flow by stones
3. Potential for infection and obstruction related to obstruction of urine flow
4. Nausea, vomiting, diarrhea related to intestinal reaction to urinary disturbance
5. Potential for stone recurrence

Planning and Implementation
Nursing Interventions

A. Relief of pain

1. Initiate treatment for renal and ureteral colic; relieve pain until its cause can be removed—administration of morphine or meperidine hydrochloride, hot baths or moist heat applied to flank areas.
2. Strain all urine through gauze for stone analysis—crystallographic studies and x-ray diffraction are useful in obtaining data about the amount and distribution of chemical components of the stone.
3. Give specific therapy as directed—regimen depends on stone type (see Management).
4. Maintain proper urine reaction (pH); give appropriate drugs to acidify or alkalinize urine (depending on stone type).
    a. Phosphate, oxalate, and carbonate stones form in alkaline urine.
    Drugs used to acidify urine include ammonium chloride and methenamine mandelate (Mandelamine) and vitamin C.
    b. Uric acid, urate, and cystine stones form in acid urine.
    Drugs used for alkalinizing the urine include potassium acetate or citrate, sodium bicarbonate.

B. Prevention of infection and obstruction

1. Encourage the patient to maintain a high round-the-clock fluid intake (250–300 ml. of fluid hourly when awake) to reduce concentration of urinary crystalloids and to ensure a high urinary output; also lowers specific gravity of urine.
2. Treat infection (if present) with appropriate drugs—infection may accelerate stone growth and be difficult to eradicate.
3. Correct obstructive process to prevent impairment of tubular function, atrophy of nephrons, reduced renal blood flow, and increased susceptibility to infection.
4. Treat and correct metabolic problems (hyperparathyroidism, renal tubular acidosis).
5. Prepare for surgical intervention if the patient's condition indicates that the stone:
    a. Is too large to pass, or
    b. Is producing obstruction, unremitting pain, infection that does not respond to treatment, or is causing progressive renal damage

C. Prevention of stone recurrence

1. Employ principles of diet therapy if stone composition is known—to control urine pH, supply proper vitamins, and eliminate stone-forming substances.
2. See Health Education (below).

Health Education

Instruct the patient as follows:
1. Maintain a high fluid intake over a 24-hour period, since stones form more readily in concentrated urine.
    a. Drink enough fluids to achieve a urinary volume of 2000–3000 ml. or more/24 hours.
    b. Drink larger amounts during periods of strenuous exercise, if you perspire freely.
    c. Take fluids in evening to guarantee a high urine flow during the night.
    d. Set the alarm clock in order to drink water in middle of night.
    e. Avoid sudden increases in environmental temperatures that may cause a drop in urinary volume.
    f. Increase fluid intake when engaging in activities that produce excessive perspiration.
2. For patients who form stones because of excessive absorption of dietary calcium:
    a. Stay on low-calcium diet; avoid dairy products.
    b. Avoid excessive salt and vitamin C intake.
3. Avoid prolonged periods of recumbency—slows renal drainage and alters calcium metabolism.
4. Avoid excessive ingestion of vitamins and minerals, especially vitamin D.
5. Test urine pH with a pH indicator if urine pH is a factor in causing particular type of stone.
6. Follow a healthy eating pattern.
    a. Avoid excessive sugar and animal protein, which can cause changes in chemical composition of urine.
    b. Increase consumption of fiber.

Evaluation
Expected Outcomes

1. Achieves relief of pain/discomfort; passes stone
2. Is free of infection and obstruction; excretes clear urine without burning or discomfort
3. Participates in educational program to avoid stone recurrence

Renal Tumors

General Considerations

1. All renal tumors should be considered malignant until proved otherwise.
2. Renal cell carcinoma is the most common malignant renal tumor; occurs more frequently in males and metastasizes early to the lungs, bone, liver, brain, and contralateral kidney.

Clinical Manifestations

1. Many renal tumors produce no symptoms and are discovered on routine physical examination as a palpable abdominal mass.
2. Classic triad (late symptoms)
   a. Hematuria (intermittent, microscopic, or gross)—may be initial, terminal, or total, depending on location of tumor.
   b. Pain—from distention of renal capsule, invasion of surrounding structures.
   c. Palpable mass in flank.
3. Low-grade fever, anemia, weight loss—systemic effects common to most tumors.
4. Gastrointestinal symptoms—due to reflex action or encroachment on intraperitoneal organs.

Diagnostic Evaluation

1. Plain film of abdomen—often shows kidney enlargement.
2. Intravenous urography—usually initial screening procedure.
3. Cystoscopic examination—for visualization of tumor by retrograde pyelography.
4. Assessment of urinary lactic dehydrogenase activity; this enzyme may be elevated in carcinoma of the kidney, bladder, prostate, in infection, etc.
5. Ultrasonography—helpful in differentiating renal cyst from renal tumor.
6. Renal angiogram
7. Computed tomography—used in assessing solid renal masses and to detect invasion of perirenal structures; contributes to staging of renal cell carcinoma.

Management
Goal:
To eradicate the tumor and prevent metastasis.
(The following treatment options may be done singly or in combination.)

1. Radical nephrectomy (en bloc removal of kidney, perirenal fat, adrenal gland, Gerota's fascia, and possibly regional lymph nodes
2. Chemotherapy
3. Hormonal therapy (progesterone) may exert an antitumor effect
4. Interferons (glycoproteins produced by human cells in response to viral infections/other inducers)—have antitumor effects; can induce regression of metastatic tumors
5. Immunotherapy—to stimulate host's own immune system
6. Renal artery embolization—for the patient with metastatic renal cancer
   a. Catheter is advanced into renal artery.
   b. Embolizing material (Gelfoam, steel coils, blood clot) is injected into artery and carried with arterial blood flow to occlude the tumor vessels.
   c. Procedure usually followed by nephrectomy.
   d. Tumor embolization decreases tumor vascularity, relieves pain and bleeding, and may slow tumor growth, thus allowing time for chemotherapy to achieve greater effect on neoplastic cells; may stimulate host immune response and enhance prognosis.
   e. Monitor and treat postinfarction syndrome—severe abdominal pain, nausea, vomiting, diarrhea, fever.
   f. Complications—arterial obstruction, bleeding, diminution of renal function.
7. Symptomatic management to promote comfort
   a. Radiation of skeletal lesions
   b. Internal fixation for large-bone lesions
   c. Nutritional support
   d. Psychologic support

Health Education
Have a yearly physical examination and x-ray examination of chest.

Injuries to the Kidney

Trauma to abdomen, flank, or back may produce renal injury. Suspicion is high in a patient with multiple injuries.

Types of Injuries

1. Contusion
2. Laceration
3. Rupture
4. Renal pedicle injury

Major Problems Following Kidney Trauma

1. Control of hemorrhage—may be persistent or recurring
2. Injuries to other organs
3. Late complications are significant

Clinical Manifestations

1. Hematuria—amount shows no correlation with extent of injury
2. Pain—costovertebral, flank, upper abdomen
3. Nausea, vomiting, abdominal rigidity—from ileus (seen when there is retroperitoneal bleeding)
4. Shock—from severe/multiple injuries

Diagnostic Evaluation

1. History of injury—determine if injury was caused by blunt or penetrating trauma (stab/gunshot wounds)
2. Serial urine studies for hematuria
3. Plain film of abdomen—to determine presence of

other fractures (pelvis, ribs, transverse processes of lumbar vertebrae)
4. Excretory urography (IVP)—to define extent of injury to involved kidney and function of contralateral kidney
5. Renal angiography—to assess vascular integrity, outline renal parenchyma

Treatment and Nursing Management

A. Prevention of hemorrhage and infection

▶ **NURSING ALERT:** Excessive bleeding may occur several days after renal injury. Perirenal abscess or infection may occur 2–4 weeks following injury.

1. Place the patient on bed rest to minimize bleeding.
2. Monitor blood pressure and pulse—to assess for bleeding and impending shock; perirenal hemorrhage may cause rapid exsanguination.
3. Save, inspect, and compare each urine specimen—to follow the course and degree of hematuria.
4. Carry out serial hematocrit and hemoglobin determinations—to assess degree of anemia, since progressive anemia indicates hemorrhage.
5. Evaluate the patient frequently during the first few days following injury.
   a. Assess for flank and abdominal pain, muscle spasm, and swelling over flank—suggests renal hemorrhage and extravasation.
   b. Outline original mass with marking pencil for future comparisons.
   c. Examine renal area for development of bruising and/or swelling.
   d. Watch for any *sudden* change in the patient's condition. This may indicate hemorrhage, which require surgical intervention.
6. Avoid narcotic analgesia—may mask accompanying abdominal symptoms.
7. Give antibiotics as directed to discourage infection—from perirenal hematoma and/or urinoma (cyst containing urine).
8. Maintain urinary drainage.

B. Restoration or maintenance of renal function

1. Monitor for complications—hemorrhage, infection, stone formation, thrombosis of major/minor arteries of kidneys, eventually leading to hypertension, loss of renal function.
2. Prepare for surgical exploration if the patient has penetrating injury (laceration, rupture, pedicle injury), palpable mass and tenderness in flank or shock.

Health Education

1. Activity should be restricted for about 1 month following trauma to minimize incidence of delayed/secondary bleeding.
2. Encourage the patient to have follow-up examinations after discharge—to detect late-developing complications (post-traumatic hypertension, decreasing renal function).

Neurogenic Bladder

Neurogenic bladder refers to a bladder disturbance due to dysfunctions related to lack of neural control of voiding.

Normal Physiology

1. Normal bladder action depends on intact sensory and motor nerve supply.
2. The bladder fills to approximately 300–500 ml.—triggers an emptying reflex.
3. This reflex initiates a contraction of the musculature inside the bladder wall, which forces urine out through the urethra until the bladder is empty.

Causes

1. Spinal cord injury; spinal tumor; herniated intervertebral disc
2. Disease—multiple sclerosis, diabetes mellitus, syphilis
3. Certain congenital anomalies (spina bifida, myelomeningocele)
4. Infection

Types of Neurogenic Bladder

A. Spastic (reflex or automatic)

1. A bladder disorder caused by any lesion of the cord above the voiding reflex arc (upper motor neuron lesion); most common type.
2. There is loss of conscious sensations and cerebral motor control.
3. The patient has reduced bladder capacity and marked hypertrophy of bladder wall.
4. Bladder behaves in reflex fashion with minimal or no controlling influence to regulate its activity (spontaneous uncontrolled voidings).

B. Flaccid (atonic, nonreflex or areflexic, or autonomous)

1. A bladder disorder caused by a lower motor neuron lesion.
2. Bladder continues to fill until it becomes greatly distended—bladder musculature does not contract forcefully at any time.
3. When pressure reaches a breakthrough point, small amounts of urine dribble from urethra as bladder continues to fill (overflow incontinence).
4. Sensory loss may accompany flaccid bladder; the patient is not aware of discomfort.
5. Extensive distention causes damage to bladder musculature, infection of stagnant urine, and infection of kidneys by back pressure of urine.

C. Mixed (spastic/flaccid)

1. Generally associated with injuries occurring at the conus–cauda equina junctions.
2. Leads to a combination of upper motor neuron/lower motor neuron dysfunction.

Complications

1. *Infection*—from stasis of urine and subsequent catheterization.
2. *Hydronephrosis*—hypertrophy of bladder wall leads ultimately to vesicoureteral reflux.
3. *Urolithiasis*—from demineralization of bone from bed rest; urinary stasis and infection.
4. *Renal failure*—major cause of death of patients with neurologic impairment of the bladder.

Assessment

Diagnostic Evaluation

1. Measurement of residual urine volume
2. Measurement of fluid intake and urinary output
3. Evaluation of urine (color, odor, concentration, pH, protein content, specific gravity)
4. Assessment of sensory awareness (bladder fullness) and motor control
5. Urodynamic studies (see p. 502)

Patient Problems/Nursing Diagnoses

1. Alteration in patterns of urinary elimination (partial or complete, temporary or permanent loss of control of bladder function) related to lack of neural control of bladder.
2. Disturbance in self concept (social isolation, lack of self-esteem) related to potential/actual loss of bladder control.
3. Potential for infection and renal failure related to urinary retention.

Planning and Implementation

Nursing Interventions for Initial Phase

A. **Catheterization to reduce bladder distention**— Following spinal cord injury, the syndrome of spinal shock is reflected in the bladder; sensation is not perceived, and the bladder usually cannot contract and empty itself. The bladder must be decompressed by either intermittent or continuous catheterization.

1. Intermittent catheterization (preferred)
   a. Bladder catheterized at designated intervals (4, 6, or 8 hours) with a small-caliber catheter; this intermittent emptying approximates physiologic function; circumvents complications usually seen with indwelling catheter.
      (1) Hourly fluid intake and output record is kept to assess individual output patterns.
      (2) Catheterization technique requires strict asepsis and skilled personnel.
      (3) Patients with upper extremity function may be taught to catheterize themselves.
2. Continuous catheterization
   a. Bladder is catheterized using continuous drainage and irrigation system (p. 508) to avoid overdistention and risk of contracture from being constantly empty.
      (1) Tape catheter to abdomen (male) to remove sharp angulation and pressure at penoscrotal angle (see Fig. 11-7).
      (2) Maintain a high fluid intake.

B. **Assist with evaluation studies** (as soon as the patient's condition permits)—to assess for bladder and bladder neck problems. Do initial studies to provide a baseline against which later changes can be measured.

1. Serial studies of BUN, serum creatinine, creatinine clearance—to determine status of renal function
2. Cystogram—to determine presence of vesicoureteral reflux
3. Urethrogram—for presence of urethral complications
4. IV urogram—to outline upper urinary tract
5. Pressure and flow studies
6. Cystoscopy—to assess for loss of muscle fibers and elastic tissues; gives opportunity for biopsy

Nursing Interventions for Chronic Phase

Each person with neurogenic bladder disease has a particular type of problem(s); it is difficult to assess what

the rehabilitation potential and eventual urologic disability may be.

A. **Establishing an effective spontaneous reflex voiding**

1. Have the patient drink a measured amount of fluid from 8 AM–8 PM; no fluids (except sips) taken after 8 PM to avoid bladder overdistention.
2. At specified time, the patient attempts to void by using pressure over bladder or stimulates reflex voiding by abdominal tapping or digital stretch of anal sphincter to trigger the bladder.
3. Estimate residual urine by comparing intake and output; palpate and percuss over bladder.
4. Palpate the bladder at repeated intervals to determine if bladder is being emptied (see Fig. 11-9).
5. Immediately following voiding attempt, catheterize the patient to determine urine residual.
   a. Measure all urine, voided and catheterized.
   b. Avoid *overdistention* of bladder.
   c. Caution patient to be alert for any sign that his bladder is full—perspiration, coldness of hands or feet, feelings of anxiety, etc.
6. *Intervals between catheterizations.* Catheterization intervals are lengthened and program is moved forward as less and less urine is retained; catheterization checks are usually discontinued when the volume of residual urine is at an acceptable level compatible with urine sterility and radiologic normalcy of the upper urinary tract.
7. Encourage liberal fluid intake—to reduce urinary bacterial count, reduce stasis, decrease the concentration of calcium in urine, and minimize the precipitation of urinary crystals and stone formation.
8. Keep the patient as mobile as possible—to reduce incidence of calculosis (presence of calculi).
   a. Turn, move, and exercise the patient.
   b. Get the patient up on tilt table (p. 64) or in wheelchair as soon as possible.
   c. Give low-calcium diet—to prevent calculosis.

Nursing Interventions for Flaccid Bladder

A. **Establishing complete and regular emptying of bladder**

1. The patient may be placed on bladder routine (outlined above); the fluid intake and output are adjusted to prevent bladder overdistention.
   The patient may be given orally administered doses of parasympathomimetic drugs (bethanechol chloride) to facilitate detrusor contraction.
2. *Or,* if no reflex or only a partial reflex can be induced, the patient is maintained on intermittent catheterization until he develops spontaneous reflex voiding; or surgical intervention may be required.
   a. Male patient—may use condom collecting device if bladder empties well and no residual remains.
   b. Female patient—may use pads, waterproof pants; or urinary diversion procedure may be required.
3. Electrical stimulation—application of electrical stimulation to bladder or reflex voiding center in spinal cord.

B. **Surgical intervention to correct condition**—Surgical intervention may be carried out to correct bladder neck contractures, correct vesicoureteral reflux, or perform urinary diversion procedures (p. 544).

1. Tubeless cystostomy (continent vesicostomy)—tube is formed from bladder wall and brought to abdominal

surface; external valve is created by intussusception of the proximal portion of the tube into the bladder; procedure appears useful in patients with neurogenic bladder.

    a. Bladder emptied by intermittent transabdominal catheterization.

    b. Urinary collection device not necessary.

    c. Complications—bladder stone formation, stricture of cutaneous stoma, incontinence (urinary flooding of vesicostomy).

2. Ileal conduit (see p. 541).

Health Education

1. Instruct the patient to do vaginal and rectal contractions to strengthen periurethral tissue.

    a. Tighten the rectum or vaginal vault.

    b. Hold the contraction while counting slowly to 6; relax.

    c. Continue relaxing and tightening for a 5-minute period.

    d. Perform these exercises twice daily for 5 minutes over a 6- to 8-week period—success or failure of exercise program is then evaluated.

2. Bladder rehabilitation may take weeks to months.

3. The patient with chronic problem should have kidney function studies and intravenous urogram annually.

Evaluation

Expected Outcomes

1. Achieves bladder control—no signs of overdistention, fever, concentrated cloudy, or odoriferous urine

2. Assumes responsibility for bladder care and regulates fluid intake

---

Guidelines: Intermittent Self-Catheterization—Clean (Nonsterile) Technique

Intermittent self-catheterization is the periodic drainage of urine from the bladder by the patient via catheterization; it is necessitated by temporary or permanent inability to empty the bladder (vesical dysfunction, neurogenic disease, obstructive uropathy, decompensated bladder).

Underlying Considerations

1. Intermittent catheterization is the treatment of choice following spinal cord injury. It is done under aseptic conditions by qualified health professionals until the patient is able to catheterize himself. After discharge from the hospital, the patient may be able to use a ''clean'' (nonsterile) technique.

2. The patient should be medically followed at regular intervals to prevent complications—reflux, hydronephrosis, external sphincter spasm, infection.

3. Advantages of self-catheterization: Better patient acceptance; promotes independence; fewer complications; permits more normal sexual relations.

4. Goal: to decrease morbidity associated with long-term use of indwelling catheter and to achieve a catheter-free status, if possible.

Equipment

No. 14 Fr. catheter (several to be kept in reserve); lubricant
Mirror (female patient)
Shallow pan
Irrigation tip syringe
Clear plastic bag or case—for carrying catheter

Procedure

Action (By Patient)	Rationale/Amplification
1. The patient must understand the importance of frequent catheterization and emptying of bladder at prescribed time regardless of circumstances.	1. An overdistended bladder slows the circulation of blood through the bladder walls and weakens its resistance to infection.
2. Try to void before catheterizing self using reflex triggering mechanisms—pressure on abdomen, thigh stroking, etc.	2. This may help to develop voluntary voiding without catheterization.
3. Wash hands with soap and water.	3. Do not forgo catheterization if soap and water are not available.
Female	
1. Position mirror in line of vision with urinary meatus. Assume modified dorsal recumbent position with feet on bed, legs flexed, and knees apart; later, the patient may sit on toilet seat if physical condition permits.	1. This position helps to expose the urethral meatus.
a. The nurse points out the location of the clitoris, urethral meatus, and vaginal outlet (in the mirror).	a. The patient is taught to confirm the position of the clitoris, urethral meatus, and vaginal outlet by palpation so that eventually a mirror will not be necessary.
b. Expose the urinary meatus and cleanse.	

(continued)

Guidelines: Intermittent Self-Catheterization—Clean (Nonsterile) Technique (continued)

Procedure
(Cont.)

Action (By Patient)	Rationale / Amplification
2. Lubricate the catheter with water or water-soluble jelly. Hold the catheter 7.5 cm. (3 inches) from its tip and insert it 5–7.5 cm. (2–3 inches) in a downward and backward direction into the urethra. Allow urine to flow into a shallow pan/toilet or into a disposable plastic urine bag.	
3. Remove catheter when urine stops flowing.	3. Measure or estimate volume of residual urine.
Male Patient	
1. Assume sitting position until technique is learned.	
2. Lubricate the catheter.	2. A well-lubricated catheter is particularly necessary in the male to avoid traumatic urethritis.
3. Retract foreskin of penis with one hand; then grasp penis and hold it at right angle to body.	3. This maneuver straightens the urethra and facilitates ease of catheter insertion.
4. Insert the catheter 15–25 cm. (6–10 inches) until urine begins to flow.	
5. Then advance catheter about 2.5 cm. (1 more inch) and allow urine to flow into shallow pan/toilet. When urine stops flowing, remove catheter.	5. Measure or estimate volume of residual urine.
Follow-up Phase	
1. Wash catheter in warm, soapy water. Rinse.	
2. Wrap catheter in clean towel/paper towel.	2. The catheter may be carried in a clean plastic bag or case. The emphasis should be on availability and cleanliness.

Injuries to the Bladder (And Urethra)

Types of Bladder Injuries

1. Contusion of bladder
2. Intraperitoneal rupture
3. Extraperitoneal rupture } or combination of both
4. Injury to urethra

Types of Urethral Injuries

1. Contusion
2. Partial or complete rupture

Problems Associated with Bladder Injury

1. Injuries to the bladder and urethra are commonly associated with pelvic fractures and multiple trauma. Certain surgical procedures (hysterectomy, surgery of lower colon and rectum) also carry a risk to the bladder.
2. With injury, there is a rise in intravesical (within bladder) pressure, which produces extravasation of urine into the peritoneal cavity or perivesical space.
3. Rupture of the bladder requires immediate treatment.

Clinical Manifestations

1. Failure to void
2. Hematuria; presence of blood at urinary meatus
3. Shock and hemorrhage—pallor, rapid and increasing pulse rate
4. Suprapubic pain and soreness
5. Rigid abdomen—indicates intraperitoneal rupture
6. Swelling/discoloration of penis, scrotum and anterior perineum

Diagnostic Evaluation

1. Retrograde urethrogram—to detect any rupture of urethra. *Do first* (before catheterization).
2. Cystogram—to detect and localize perforation/rupture of bladder.
3. Plain film of abdomen—may show associated pelvic fracture.
4. Excretory urogram—to survey the kidneys for injury.

Treatment and Nursing Management

1. Treat for shock and hemorrhage.
2. Carry out retrograde urethrography in suspected injuries involving lower urinary tract.
3. Catheterize the patient only after urethrogram is done.
   a. Indwelling catheter serves as a means of continuous urinary drainage.
   b. Catheter also serves as a splint to urethra if urethra has been injured, but it may complete a partial rupture if urethral injury is not recognized with a urethrogram.
4. Prepare for surgical intervention for bladder rupture:
   a. Extravasated blood and urine will be drained and urine diverted with suprapubic cystostomy and indwelling catheter.
   b. Bladder tears will be sutured; urethral repairs may be postponed.
5. Observe drainage systems after surgery.
   a. Suprapubic cystostomy drainage—until healing of bladder is complete.
   b. Indwelling urethral catheter drainage—to divert urine drainage and permit suprapubic incision to heal.

c. Perivesical areas drained with Penrose drain (will be brought out through suprapubic incision).

For Urethral Injury (treatment is controversial)

1. Assist with cystostomy drainage (p. 512)—to provide urine drainage until reconstructive surgery is done.

2. Treatment modalities determined by level of urethral injury and its effect on bladder continence.

Health Education

Urethral stricture, incontinence, and impotence may follow urethral injury.

Cancer of the Bladder

Etiology

It appears that multiple agents are responsible for the development of cancer of the bladder. The specific etiology is unknown.

1. Cigarette smoking
2. Prolonged exposure to aromatic amines or their metabolites—generally dyes manufactured by the chemical industry and used by other industries.
3. Causal relationship may exist between excessive coffee drinking and consumption of excessive amounts of analgesics and bladder cancer.
4. Chronic infection and irritation
5. Bladder schistosomiasis (rare in US)
6. Cyclophosphamide (Cytoxan®)—causes bladder tumors after a variable period.
7. Secondary metastasis from prostate, colon, rectum (males), and lower gynecologic tract (females)

▶ **NURSING ALERT:** High-risk persons should have annual cytologic examinations of the urine.

Clinical Features

1. Bladder cancer is a highly malignant condition; it occurs 3 times more frequently in males, particularly after the 5th decade.
2. Large numbers of these tumors occur in the lateral and posterior bladder wall and near the trigone.
3. Metastases appear in vesical, hypogastric, common iliac, and lumbar lymph nodes; in liver, lungs, vertebrae, pelvis.
4. Recurrences may occur years after last known tumor is treated.
5. Small bladder tumors are seeded from tumors of renal pelvis.

Clinical Manifestations

1. Painless hematuria, either gross or microscopic—most characteristic sign
2. Dysuria, frequency, urgency—symptoms of bladder irritability
3. Flank pain, chills, fever—from progressive tumor growth, infiltration of bladder wall, ureteral obstruction, and bladder infection
4. Pelvic or back pain—from distant metastasis
5. Leg edema—from invasion of pelvic lymph nodes

Diagnostic Evaluation

1. Intravenous urography (IVU)—to rule out ureteral obstruction or presence of renal pelvic tumor
2. Cystourethroscopy—for visualization and biopsy of lesion
3. Bimanual examination of pelvis—to determine degree of mobility, fixation of tumor, and degree of extravesical extension
4. Retrograde pyelography—to define presence/absence of upper urinary tract pathology

5. Computed tomography (CT scan) and ultrasonography—to assess disease status and measure tumor responsiveness
6. Cytologic study of fresh urinary sediment to assess for malignant transitional cells shed from tumor
7. Chest x-ray and bone scan—to demonstrate distant metastases

Management

A. Underlying Rationale

1. There is no single effective method of treatment. The surgical procedure of choice depends on the characteristics of the tumor and whether or not bladder wall infiltration and local or distant metastasis has occurred. The patient's age and physical, mental, and emotional status are considered.
2. The patient is usually considered incurable if gross extension of the tumor beyond the bladder wall has occurred; in such cases, adjuvant modalities such as radiotherapy and chemotherapy may be somewhat palliative.

B. Modalities of Treatment

1. Surgery
   a. Transurethral resection or fulguration—for superficial tumors; usually combined with intravesical chemotherapy (see below).
   b. Cystectomy (removal of bladder) or radical cystectomy for invasive or poorly differentiated tumors; may be combined with radiation therapy.
      (1) Radical cystectomy in male—removal of bladder, pelvic peritoneum, prostate, and seminal vesicles, and possible regional node dissection and removal of the urethra to the meatus.
      (2) Radical cystectomy in female—removal of bladder, pelvic peritoneum, urethra, uterus, broad ligaments, vagina, tubes, and ovaries, and regional lymphadenectomy (iliac and pelvic nodes).
      (3) Cystectomy requires diversion of the urinary stream.
         (a) Early complications include wound infection (wound dehiscence or evisceration), pneumonitis, ileus, peritonitis, intestinal obstruction, urine leakage, ureterointestinal obstruction, rectal fistula.
         (b) Long-term complications include pyelonephritis, calculi, stomal stenosis, conduit fibrosis, progressive loss of renal function.
   c. Urinary diversion procedures (see below) to relieve frequency and hemorrhage in patients with inoperable disease.
   d. Hydrostatic pressure therapy—placement of wa-

ter-filled balloon within the bladder to produce tumor necrosis by reducing blood circulation in the bladder wall.
2. Radiation therapy—may be internal or external.
3. Chemotherapy
   a. Topical chemotherapy—places a high concentration of drug in contact with neoplastic cells
   b. Systemic chemotherapy
4. Combinations of surgery, radiation, and chemotherapy
5. Immunotherapy—bacille Calmette Guérin (BCG) vaccine given intravesically as well as intradermally to improve immune competence of patient (controversial).

Nursing Interventions

1. Emphasize the positive aspects of the treatment to the patient.
2. See nursing management of the patient undergoing chemotherapy, page 905, radiation therapy, page 912, and urinary diversion, below.
3. Support the patient undergoing intravesical chemo-

therapy (instillation of antineoplastic agent into the bladder, allowing a high concentration of drug to come into contact with the tumor with minimal systemic toxicity).
   a. Instruct the patient as follows:
      (1) Do not take fluids during instillation period (about 2 hours) to prevent excessive diuresis and to promote retention of drug in the bladder.
      (2) Change position every ½ hour during instillation.
      (3) Wash hands and perineal area after voiding the medication to prevent contact dermatitis.
      (4) Void frequently after procedure to avoid chemical cystitis from residual drug in the bladder.
      (5) Drink fluids liberally after procedure is completed.
   b. Monitor the patient for allergic reaction during instillation period.
   c. Monitor the patient for signs and symptoms of urinary infection.

Urinary Diversion

Urinary diversion refers to diverting the urinary stream from the bladder so that it exits via a new avenue. There are a large number of operative procedures.

Clinical Conditions Requiring Urinary Diversion

1. Malignancy of bladder or ureters; pelvic malignancy
2. Congenital abnormality of lower urinary tract
3. Stricture and trauma to ureters and urethra
4. Neurogenic bladder
5. Severe ureteral and renal damage due to vesicoureteral reflux or chronic infection
6. Injuries

Methods of Urinary Diversion (Fig. 11-13)

The most common methods of urinary diversion are:
1. *Ileal conduit*—transplanting the ureters to an isolated section of the terminal ileum and bringing one end to the abdominal wall as an ileostomy. The ureter may also be transplanted into the transverse colon (colon conduit) or proximal jejunum (jejunal conduit).
2. *Ureterosigmoidostomy*—implantation of the ureter(s) into the sigmoid, thereby allowing urine to flow through the colon and out of the rectum.
3. *Cutaneous ureterostomy*—bringing the detached

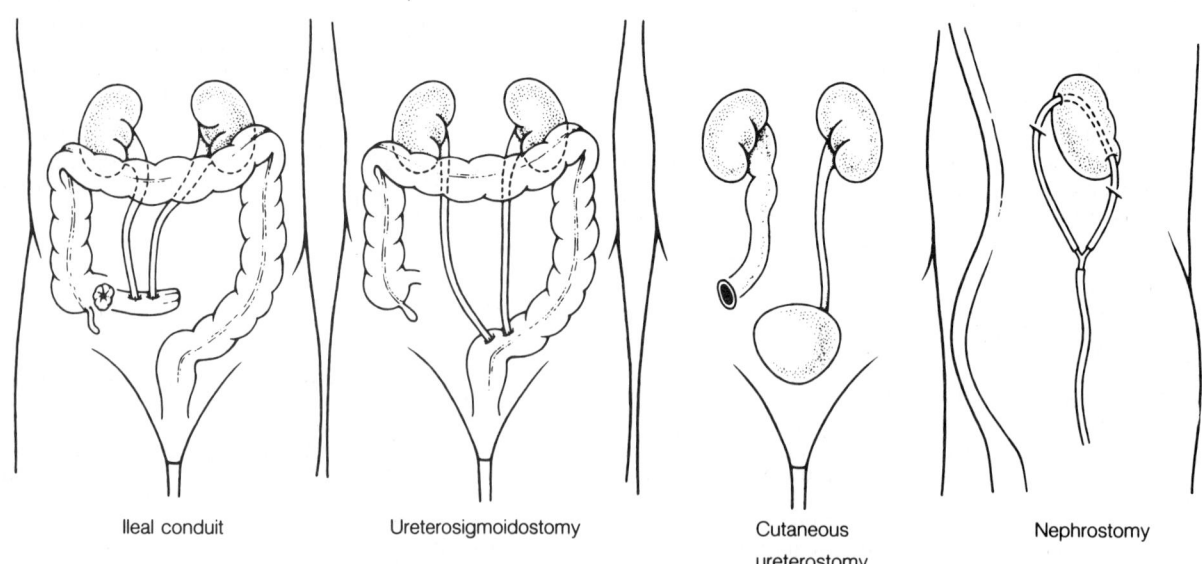

Ileal conduit   Ureterosigmoidostomy   Cutaneous ureterostomy   Nephrostomy

Figure 11-13. Methods of urinary diversion.

ureters through the abdominal wall and attaching them to an opening in the skin.

4. *Suprapubic cystostomy* (vesicostomy)—draining the bladder through an abdominal wound.
5. *Nephrostomy*—inserting a catheter via an incision into the flank or by percutaneous catheter placement into the kidney.

Patient Problems/Nursing Diagnoses

1. Disturbances in body image related to change in toileting habits, presence of external stoma and collecting device, fear of urine leakage
2. Fear (of recurring disease, sexual impotency) related to diagnosis of genitourinary cancer
3. Potential for morbidity and complications related to nature of surgery and tumor effects

Planning and Implementation

Preoperative Nursing Interventions

A. Preoperative evaluation to correct physiologic abnormalities

1. For the patient undergoing renal surgery, see page 528 for general aspects of preoperative care.
2. Pay careful attention to cardiopulmonary status, since the patient is probably older and undergoing a lengthy, complex procedure.
3. Prepare the patient for sigmoidoscopy and barium enema if ureterosigmoidostomy is to be performed.
   a. Enemas are given (increasing in amount of fluid) to help develop sphincter control.
   b. Assess the patient's ability to retain enema as a means of evaluating adequacy of rectal sphincter.
4. Prepare the bowel for surgical intervention to minimize fecal stasis and postoperative ileus.
   a. Give clear liquids.
   b. Administer antimicrobial agents (neomycin)—for bowel disinfection to reduce pathogenic bacterial flora, since bowel contents frequently spill with transection of intestine.
   c. Give enemas as directed for mechanical cleansing of lower bowel.
5. Employ adequate hydration procedures, including intravenous infusions, to ensure urine flow during surgery and to prevent hypovolemia during the prolonged operative procedure.
6. Reinforce the surgeon's explanations of the surgical procedures.
   a. The stoma site is planned preoperatively with the patient standing, sitting, and lying—to place the stoma away from bony prominences, skin creases, and scars, and where the patient can see it.
   b. Apply several types of skin adhesives or cement to abdomen preoperatively to determine contact allergies and to facilitate management of ostomy appliance postoperatively.
   c. Have the patient wear the intended appliance preoperatively.
7. Assist with enteral or intravenous hyperalimentation—to give nutritional support, minimize toxicity, promote healing, and improve response to treatment.
8. Assist the patient undergoing nasogastric intubation before surgery (p. 412), or, temporary gastrostomy may be done during surgery to facilitate gastric decompression.

B. Enhancing coping abilities to adapt to altered body state

1. Encourage the patient to express his feelings about his situation; reflect and amplify the patient's insights and judgments.
2. Help the patient talk about his support network.
3. Include the family in caring for the patient; allow for verbalization of fear and anxiety.
4. Encourage membership in a self-help group (United Ostomy Association) and visits by an ostomy association visitor.
5. Help the patient and family gain a positive attitude and hope.

Postoperative Nursing Interventions

1. See page 440 for nursing management of patient following intestinal surgery and page 528 for nursing management of the patient following urologic surgery.
2. Watch for any abnormal signs and symptoms (wound infections, leaking at anastomosis site, peritonitis, paralytic ileus, intestinal obstruction, stenosis of stoma). These operations are extremely taxing, and patients have little or no reserve.
3. Ensure adequate circulating volume with intravenous fluids and blood as directed.
4. Keep nasogastric tube in place until the patient passes gas via rectum.
5. Monitor total parenteral nutrition (p. 429) if the patient is unable to return to oral feeding.
6. Accept the patient's depression, which usually follows any surgery that interferes with body integrity.
   a. Accept the patient's irritability and lack of motivation to learn.
   b. Give extra support until the patient can cope with his situation.
   c. Counsel the patient to take 1 day at a time.

Nursing Interventions Following Ilial Conduit

1. The patient wears a transparent disposable urinary drainage bag cemented to the abdominal wall until edema subsides and stoma shrinks to normal size. (Some patients prefer using disposable bags thereafter.)
2. The patient with an ileal conduit wears a cemented-on appliance day and night. The ileal bladder drains urine (but not feces) constantly.
   a. Appliance is connected to a drainage tube and bag; urinary volume is recorded hourly.
   b. Appliance remains in place as long as it is watertight; it is changed as necessary.
3. Inspect stoma for congestion and cyanosis, bleeding and friability of stomal mucosa—during first few postoperative weeks, the stoma appears swollen and edematous.
4. Examine skin around stoma for signs of irritation, alkaline encrustation with peristomal dermatitis (from alkaline urine coming in contact with exposed skin), and wound infections.
   a. Alkaline urine is usually a result of bacteria; assess for odorous, cloudy-appearing urine.
   b. Keep urine pH below 6.5; test the urine dribbling from the stoma with pH indicator (Nitrazine paper [Squibb]).
   c. Ascorbic acid may be given to acidify urine.
   d. Encourage high fluid intake—to flush ileal conduit and prevent mucus from congealing.

Health Education for Stoma Care

A. **Appliance**—The urinary appliance may consist of 1 or 2 pieces and may be disposable, semidisposable, or reusable (choice determined by location of stoma, patient activity, body build, and economic status).

1. Reusable appliance—has a faceplate that is attached to the body with cement or adhesive.
2. Semidisposable appliance—has a reusable faceplate to which disposable pouches are attached.
3. Disposable appliance—discarded after each change.

B. **Determining Stoma Size** (for ordering correct ostomy appliance)

1. The stoma will shrink considerably as edema subsides, and the opening is recalibrated every 3–6 weeks for the first few months postoperatively.
2. Measure the widest part of the stoma with a ruler. The inside diameter of the faceplate should not be more than $\frac{1}{16}$ to $\frac{1}{8}$ of an inch larger than the diameter of the stoma.
3. The patient is taught to dilate stoma himself with a finger in a plastic glove (usually weekly).

C. **Changing the Appliance** (every 5–7 days)

1. Change appliance early in morning, before taking fluids.
2. Assemble all equipment needed for the type used.
3. Prepare the appliance according to the manufacturer's directives.
4. Moisten the edge of the faceplate with adhesive solvent or soap and water and gently remove it by pushing the skin down and away from the appliance. Adhesive solvent is not used if skin barriers (ReliaSeal or Stomahesive) are used.
5. Instruct the patient to bend over quickly and remain in that position for a minute to allow conduit to empty before the skin is washed and dried.
6. Clean all cement from the skin with adhesive solvent; use a soft cloth. Wash skin with non-cream-based soap and water. Pat dry. *The skin must be dry or appliance will not adhere.*
   a. Inspect skin for signs of irritation.
   b. Keep the skin free from direct contact with urine.
   c. A gauze or tissue wick may be applied over the stoma to absorb urine while the appliance is being changed.
7. Center the appliance directly over the stoma and apply it carefully. Apply gentle pressure around appliance for secure adherence and to remove air bubbles and creases.
8. Apply hypoallergenic tape in a picture-frame effect around the pouch.
9. The skin under the appliance may be dusted with pure talcum powder and a cotton cover used to absorb perspiration and eliminate warmth from the pouch.
10. The use of a belt is optional, but follow manufacturer's directions, since an ill-fitting belt can cause abrasion of the stoma.

D. **Odor Control**

1. Instruct the patient to avoid foods and medication that produce strong odors.
2. Drink liberal amounts of fluids to flush the conduit free of mucus and reduce possibility of urinary infection.
3. Introduce a few drops of liquid deodorizer or diluted white vinegar through the drain spout into the bottom of the pouch with a syringe or eye dropper.

E. **Managing the Ostomy Appliance**

1. Empty the appliance when it is $\frac{1}{3}$–$\frac{1}{2}$ full to prevent weight of urine from loosening adhesive seal—urinary ostomy appliances are closed with a drain valve (spigot) for periodic emptying.
2. Some patients prefer wearing a leg bag attached with an adapter to the drainage apparatus.
3. Attach outlet on appliance to a collecting bottle with plastic tubing for nighttime drainage; have at least 1.5 m. (5 ft.) of tubing to allow patient to turn in bed. The tubing may be threaded down the pajama leg to prevent kinking.
4. Position the drainage bottle lower than the level of the bed—to enhance flow by gravity.

F. **Securing a Urine Specimen for Culture from an Ileal Conduit**

1. Open catheter set.
2. Remove the bag from the stoma. Place a 4×4 gauze sponge over the stoma to absorb the urine.
3. Don sterile gloves.
4. Using a sterile surgical forceps and cotton balls, cleanse the area around the stoma from the center outward.
5. Insert a catheter 5 cm. (2 inches) into the stoma and wait for the urine flow.

G. **Cleaning and Deodorizing the Appliance**

1. Clean faceplate with solvent and remove all adhesive; rinse in clear water.
2. Clean appliance with a brush and detergent solution; rinse and soak in a solution of water and white vinegar, washing soda solution, a few drops of bleach, or any commercial deodorizing solution.
3. After soaking (5–10 minutes) hang it up to air-dry away from direct sunlight.
4. Discard equipment that can no longer be cleaned adequately.

H. **General Patient Instructions**

1. Urinary stoma care is not difficult or complicated and should be regarded as part of personal grooming and dressing routine.
2. The stoma is normally red in color; it may protrude or be flush with the skin. It may bleed if it is bumped or rubbed. Report to your physician if it continues bleeding for several hours.
3. Mucus shreds in the urine are normal following an ileal conduit operation.
4. Choose an appliance that fits your needs. Successful urinary ostomy requires a well-fitting appliance, meticulous skin care, and control of urinary odor.
5. Always carry spare pouches and cement in a small case in handbag or pocket.
6. The wearing time of an appliance varies. Experiment with your appliance; usually an appliance may be worn 5–7 days. See above for changing, cleaning, and management of appliance.
7. Before changing to a new skin adhesive, apply a test patch to the other side of the abdomen of forearm.
8. Wear cotton (rather than nylon) underwear. Avoid a heavy girdle because it may cause chafing of the stoma and leakage from pressure on the pouch.
9. Avoid heavy lifting for 6 weeks. Sexual activities, driving the car, returning to work, etc., may be resumed when energy level increases.

10. Get in touch with local medical supply distributor or enterostomal therapist or consult *Ostomy Quarterly* (address below) for manufacturer's advertisements of appliances, deodorizers, skin barriers, and other new products.
11. Call your physician for instructions if skin problems develop or if one or more of the following symptoms of kidney complications occur: fever, chills, pain, change in color of urine (cloudy, bloody), diminishing urine output.
12. Contact local ostomy association for visits, reassurance, and practical information from ostomy visitor.
13. For further information and valuable periodical materials:
    United Ostomy Association, Inc.
    2001 W. Beverly Boulevard
    Los Angeles, CA 90057

Nursing Interventions Following Ureterosigmoidostomy

1. Patient will have rectal tube (or mushroom catheter) draining urine postoperatively—to ensure drainage and prevent reflux of urine into ureters and kidneys.
   a. Tape the tube to the buttocks.
   b. If the tube must be removed for defecation, reinsert the tube approximately 10 cm. (4 inches) into rectum to prevent trauma to site of ureteral anastomosis.
2. Give special skin care around anus to prevent skin erythema and excoriation.
3. Following removal of the tube, the patient voids through his rectum.
   a. Encourage the patient to empty rectum every 2–3 hours (or more often) to keep rectal pressure low and to minimize the absorption of urinary constituents from the colon.
   b. In time, the patient will be able to differentiate between the sensation to void and the urge to defecate.
   c. Reinsert the tube (catheter) at night (attached to drainage bottle) to permit uninterrupted sleep.
   d. Do not give enemas or cathartics.
   e. If irrigations are requested, avoid using force because of danger of introducing an infection into newly implanted ureters.
4. Evaluate for electrolyte imbalance and acidosis—potassium and magnesium imbalances may occur from presence of urine in the bowel, which stimulates diarrhea.
   a. Maintain fluid and electrolyte balance in immediate postoperative period by serum chemical determinations and intravenous infusions.
   b. Low-chloride diet supplemented with sodium potassium citrate—to prevent acidosis.

5. Health education
   a. Give specific diet instructions when the patient can tolerate oral intake.
      (1) Avoid gas-forming foods, since flatus can cause stress incontinence, socially embarrassing offensive odor, and discomfort.
      (2) Watch for air swallowing (chewing gum, smoking, carbonated beverages) to avoid gas.
      (3) Reduce salt intake to prevent hyperchloremic acidosis.
      (4) Increase potassium intake through medication and foods, since potassium may be lost in acidosis.
   b. Take prophylactic antimicrobials as directed—pyelonephritis (due to reflux of bacteria from colon) can occur in some patients.
   c. Report for frequent follow-up studies (incidence of carcinoma of colon is significant); watch for changes in bowel patterns.

Nursing Intervention Following Other Diversionary Procedures

A. Following Cutaneous Ureterostomy

1. A urinary appliance is fitted immediately following surgery and is worn at all times.
2. Ureteral dilatation with sterile catheter is performed at regular intervals to ensure patency and prevent ureteral stricture.
3. See page 545, nursing considerations for patient having ileal conduit—for general aspects of care.

B. Following Cystostomy (temporary or permanent)

1. Usually done on the patient with an obstruction below bladder (prostatic obstruction) when it is not possible to insert urethral catheter.
2. Encourage liberal amounts of fluid to avoid encrustation around catheter.
3. See also page 512.

C. Following Nephrostomy (temporary or permanent)

1. May be performed rapidly under local anesthesia when other procedures are not technically possible.
2. See page 529 for care of the patient.

Evaluation
Expected Outcomes

1. Adapts to change in body image—takes responsibility for care of stoma and appliance
2. Discusses fears and feelings
3. Is free of complications—excretes urine freely; maintains healthy appearing stoma and skin; has no signs of wound or urinary infection

Problems Affecting the Urethra

Urethritis

Urethritis is inflammation of the urethra.

Etiology

1. Nongonococcal urethritis—urethritis not caused by gonococcus. However, a large number of cases are sexually transmitted by:
   a. *Chlamydia*—a virus-like intracellular bacterium
   b. *Trichomonas vaginalis*
   c. *Herpes simplex* virus
   d. *Candida*
   e. *Ureaplasma urealyticum*
   f. Mycoplasms
   g. Unknown organisms

2. Nonsexually transmitted:
   a. Bacterial urethritis—may be associated with urinary tract infection
   b. From trauma—secondary to passage of urethral sounds, repeated cystoscopy, indwelling catheter
3. These agents can cause either mucosal urogenital tract infection (urethritis, cervicitis) or spread contiguously or hematogenously to produce epididymitis, endometritis, pelvic inflammatory disease (PID), or disseminated gonococcal infection.
4. Reiter's syndrome—urethritis, conjunctivitis, arthritis of unknown etiology

Clinical Manifestations

1. Itching and burning around area of urethra
2. Dysuria and frequency
3. Urethral discharge; may be scant or profuse; thin, clear, or mucoid; or thick and purulent
4. Penile pain

Diagnostic Evaluation

1. Study of stained urethral smear
2. Culture for gonorrhea
3. Blood test for syphilis
4. History and physical findings (interview to elicit past history of gonorrhea)

Treatment

1. Antimicrobial (tetracyclines are usually effective for nongonococcal urethritis)
2. Metronidazole (Flagyl) may be administered for *Trichomonas* infection
3. Treatment of associated prostatitis (see p. 549)

Nursing Management

1. Encourage the patient to stay on the antimicrobial regimen for the prescribed time period.
2. Advise the patient to temporarily discontinue sexual activity and ingestion of alcohol—these activities may prolong the acute phase of urethritis.
3. Urge treatment for sexual partner—in event of treatment failure and recurrence.
4. Support and reassure patient—nongonococcal urethritis is usually self-limited and is not a serious health threat.

Urethritis From Gonorrhea

Etiology

1. *Neisseria gonorrhoeae*—the specific organism.
2. Transmitted through sexual contact.
3. More and more asymptomatic carriers are being recognized.

Clinical Manifestations

Male

1. Inflammation of meatal orifice; burning on urination; *may be asymptomatic*
2. Urethral discharge—scant and serous to thick, yellowish pus (4–10 days or longer after sexual exposure)

Female

1. Purulent urethral discharge
2. Frequency, urgency, nocturia
3. Red, swollen urinary meatus
4. Pelvic infection accompanied by abdominal pain
5. Often is asymptomatic

Complications (local)

1. Male—periurethritis, prostatitis, epididymitis, urethral stricture, sterility due to vasoepididymal duct obstruction
2. Female—pelvic infection, abscess of greater vestibular glands (Bartholin's glands), urethral stricture

Treatment and Health Education

1. See page 867 for treatment of gonorrhea.
2. Instruct the patient to avoid sexual activity with untreated previous sexual partners until they have been treated and examined to prevent reinfection.
3. Emphasize that the patient must return in 4–7 days to assess results and determine if there is need for further treatment and tests.
4. Urge the patient to have any sexual contacts present themselves for treatment.

Urethral Stricture

Urethral stricture is a narrowing of the lumen and loss of distensibility of the urethra caused by scar tissue formation and contraction.

Etiology

1. Urethral injury
   a. Urethral instrumentation—transurethral surgical procedures, indwelling catheters, cystoscopic procedures
   b. Straddle injuries, automobile accidents, pelvic fractures, direct trauma to urethra
2. Untreated gonorrheal urethritis
3. Congenital abnormalities

Clinical Manifestations

1. Diminution in force and size of urinary stream
2. Urinary infection and retention—dysuria and urgency
3. Symptoms of complication from stricture—back pressure produces cystitis, prostatitis, pyelonephritis, etc.

Diagnostic Evaluation

1. Urethrogram and voiding cystogram—to locate site and degree of stricture
2. Elevated WBC count, pus and bacteria in urine—if urinary tract infection present
3. Passing of catheter or sounds (bougies)—to determine the diameter and location of urethral narrowings
4. Residual urine measurement

Prevention

1. Treat urethral infections promptly.
2. Utilize utmost care in urethral instrumentation (catheterization, etc.).
3. Avoid prolonged urethral catheter drainage.

Treatment

1. Dilatation of urethra with urethral sounds.
   a. Sounds of increasing size are used.
   b. Sounds are passed at lengthening intervals (2 weeks, 1 month, 3 months) for an indefinite period, depending on how long the strictured lumen is patent.
   c. Hot sitz baths and nonnarcotic analgesics—to control pain after instrumentation.
   d. Antimicrobials may be given several days after dilatation—lessens discomfort and minimizes infectious reaction.
2. Surgical excision, urethroplasty, or suprapubic cystostomy may be necessary for severe strictures.

Conditions of the Prostate

Benign Prostatic Hyperplasia
(Hypertrophy)

Benign prostatic hyperplasia is enlargement of the prostate. The etiology is uncertain but is presumably related to endocrine changes associated with aging that initiate hyperplasia of both glandular and cellular tissue of the prostate.

Clinical Manifestations

1. In early or gradual prostatic enlargement, there may be no symptoms, since the bladder can compensate for increased peripheral resistance.
2. Obstructive symptoms—hesitancy, diminution in size and force of urinary stream, postvoiding dribbling, sensation of incomplete emptying of the bladder.
3. Symptoms of recurring urinary infection and stasis—frequency, nocturia, chills, fever.
4. Renal symptoms (prolonged obstruction)—ureteral dilatation, hydronephrosis, renal infection, azotemia, uremia.

Diagnostic Evaluation

1. Rectal examination—allows rough estimate of size of gland.
2. Cystourethroscopy—to inspect urethra and bladder and evaluate prostatic size.
3. Catheterization after voiding—to determine amount of residual urine.
4. Excretory urogram—to document upper urinary tract obstruction.
5. Serum creatinine and BUN—to evaluate renal function.

Management

(The plan of treatment depends on the cause, the severity of obstruction, and the condition of the patient.)
1. Conservative treatment if no symptoms of urinary impairment—intermittent catheterization, urethral dilation, prostatic massage—to relieve symptoms of acute obstruction.
2. Prepare the patient for surgery (enucleation or removal of hyperplastic prostatic tissue) when obstructive symptoms occur. See page 551 for nursing management of the patient having a prostatectomy.
3. Cystostomy drainage of bladder—for the poor-risk patient or one acutely ill with retention, uremia, etc.

Health Education

1. Surgical procedures for benign enlargement usually do not result in impotence, but may cause retrograde ejaculation (passing back of fluid into the bladder during sexual intercourse).
2. See page 553.

Prostatitis

Prostatitis is an inflammation of the prostate gland.

Classification

Bacterial prostatitis (acute or chronic), nonbacterial prostatitis, prostatodynia.

Etiology (bacterial prostatitis)

1. Bacterial invasion of prostate
   a. From hematogenous (bloodstream) origin (tonsils, GI tract, GU tract)
   b. From ascent of bacteria from urethra
   c. Secondary to urethritis
2. Descending infection from kidneys

Clinical Manifestations

(From infection and local inflammation)
1. Sudden chills and fever (moderate to high fever)
2. Bladder irritability—frequency, dysuria, urgency, hematuria
3. Pain in perineum, rectum, lower back, lower abdomen, and penile head

Diagnostic Evaluation

1. Culture and sensitivity tests of urethral and prostatic fluid and urine.
   a. The pathogens in each specimen are identified by collection of divided urine specimens and expressed prostatic fluid (obtained by prostatic massage).
   b. The pH of the prostatic fluid is usually elevated.
2. Rectal examination—frequently reveals exquisitely tender, painful, swollen prostate, warm to the touch.

Treatment

A. Acute Bacterial Prostatitis—antimicrobial therapy (10–14 days) based on drug-sensitivity studies of the organisms

B. Chronic Bacterial Prostatitis

1. Specific therapy (doxycycline, trimethoprim)—chronic bacterial prostatitis is difficult to cure because many antibacterial agents diffuse poorly into prostatic fluid.
   a. Prolonged therapy (3–6 months) may be necessary to effect a cure.
   b. Chlamydia now frequently identified as sole pathogen or may be present with other common bacterial uropathogens.

C. Nonbacterial Prostatitis

1. Most common type; etiology obscure.
2. Therapy is directed toward control of symptoms and is individualized to meet specific needs; acute symptoms may be controlled with anticholinergic or anti-inflammatory drugs, hot sitz baths, etc.

D. Prostatodynia—the patient has symptoms of urinary irritation but no evidence of bacteria or inflamed prostatic fluid or tissue.

Treatment is symptomatic.

Nursing Management

1. Give supportive care.
   a. Bed rest—to relieve perineal and suprapubic pain.
   b. Hot sitz baths—to promote muscular relaxation of pelvic floor and reduce potential for urinary retention.
   c. Antipyretics, analgesics, stool softeners, as necessary.

2. Watch for urinary retention—due to edema of prostatic tissue; suprapubic catheter may be required.
3. Monitor for persistence of fever, perineal pain or difficulty in voiding—may indicate presence of prostatic abscess, which may require surgical drainage.
4. Be aware of other complications—urinary retention (from swelling of gland), recurring urinary tract infection, relapsing infection, epididymitis, bacteremia, septicemia.

Health Education

Instruct the patient as follows:
1. Take antibiotic for the full time period.
2. Use hot sitz baths (10–20 minutes) several times daily.
3. Drink fluids to satisfy thirst, but avoid "forcing fluids," since an effective level of drug must be maintained in the urine.
4. Avoid food and drinks that have diuretic action or are prostatic irritants and increase prostatic secretions (alcohol, coffee, tea, chocolate, cola, spices).
5. Avoid sexual arousal/intercourse during period of acute inflammation; sexual intercourse may be beneficial in the treatment of chronic prostatitis; chronic prostatic infection is *not* sexually transmissible.
6. Be assured that the causative agent of prostatitis is not the type that causes venereal disease. (This may be an unspoken fear.)
7. Avoid sitting for long periods of time.
8. Prolonged follow-up is necessary, since recurrence of prostatitis due to the same or different organisms can occur.

Cancer of the Prostate

Cancer of the prostate is a malignant tumor of the prostate gland. It arises from the parenchyma of the prostate, usually in the most posterior part; therefore most prostatic cancers are palpable on rectal examination.

Clinical Features

1. Cancer of the prostate is the 2nd leading cause of cancer death among American men and is the most common carcinoma in men over 65 years of age.
2. It can spread by local extension, by lymphatics, or via the bloodstream.
3. Prostatic cancer is potentially curable at an early stage; however, the majority of patients present with obstructive symptoms or metastatic lesions.

▶ **NURSING ALERT:** Annual rectal examination of males over 40 is important for early diagnosis of prostatic cancer.

Medical and Surgical Management

A. Curative (depends on stage)
1. Radiation
   a. Megavoltage radiation therapy (cobalt, high-energy linear accelerator)—delivers tumorcidal doses to prostate without undue damage to normal structures.
      (1) Some degree of proctitis, diarrhea, and dysuria may be seen toward end of treatment.
      (2) Impotence may occur.
   b. Interstitial implantation of ^{125}I radioactive seeds in the prostate combined with bilateral pelvic lymphadenectomy.

2. Surgical interventions
   a. Transurethral resection or open enucleation of prostate—for patients with stage A disease.
   b. Radical prostatectomy—removal of prostate and its capsule, prostatic urethra, and seminal vesicles; may include regional lymphadenectomy
      (1) Done by retropubic or perineal approach.
      (2) Sexual impotence follows radical procedure, but urinary control is usually normal.
      (3) See page 551 for care of the patient undergoing prostatectomy.

B. Palliative
1. Radiation therapy for palliation and to relieve bone pain from metastases (bone metastases are almost always multiple).
2. Hormonal manipulation—the aim of hormonal treatment is to suppress or eliminate the main sources of androgen production (most prostatic cancers are androgen dependent) and thereby to alleviate symptoms and retard progress of disease.
   a. Bilateral orchiectomy (removal of testes)—removes major source of androgen production, since 95% of circulating plasma testosterone originates from testes. Or,
   b. Estrogen therapy (diethylstilbestrol)—thought to inhibit the gonadotropins (responsible for testicular androgenic activity), thus removing androgenic hormone upon which the tumor growth depends.
      (1) Therapy with estrogens leads to cardiovascular side effects and gynecomastia (soreness and enlargement of breasts).
      (2) Low-dose breast irradiation administered prior to diethylstilbestrol administration to reduce gynecomastia.
      (3) Synthetic gonadotropin-releasing hormone agonist (leuprolide acetate)—acts by inhibiting production of testosterone (investigational).
   c. Orchiectomy (removal of the testes)—lowers plasma testosterone, resulting in removing the testicular stimulus required for continued prostatic growth.
   d. Both orchiectomy and estrogen administration may be used in treatment of metastatic prostatic cancer.
3. Chemotherapy (singly or in combination) appears to be beneficial in advanced prostatic cancer.
   a. Estramustine phosphate (Emcyt [nitrogen mustard linked to estradiol])—given to destroy prostate tumor tissue.
   b. Nonhormonal cytotoxic chemotherapy may be administered.
4. *Transsphenoidal hypophysectomy*—gives prompt pain relief, but mechanisms of action for pain relief not understood (see p. 696).
5. Treatment of bone pain
   a. After hormonal therapy is established, chemotherapy, systemic bone-seeking radioactive materials or radiation may be used.
   b. Prevent pathologic fractures.
6. Transurethral resection to remove obstructing tissue.

Assessment
Clinical Manifestations

1. Symptoms due to obstruction of urinary flow
   a. Hesitancy and straining on voiding, frequency, nocturia
   b. Diminution in size and force of urinary stream

2. Symptoms due to metastases
    a. Pain in lumbosacral area radiating to hips and down legs (from bone metastases)
    b. Perineal and rectal discomfort
    c. Anemia, weight loss, weakness, nausea, oliguria (from uremia)
    d. Hematuria—from urethral or bladder invasion, or both

Diagnostic Evaluation

1. Digital rectal examination—reveals "stony hard" fixed gland if lesion is advanced (there are indurated lumps without fixation if condition is found earlier)
2. Prostatic biopsy
3. Cystoscopy—helps evaluate local extent of disease
4. Radioimmunoassay for prostatic acid phosphatase—levels frequently become elevated with progression of disease
5. Radionuclide bone scan—to detect metastases
6. Skeletal roentgenograms—to reveal osteoblastic metastases
7. Excretory urogram—to demonstrate changes from ureteral obstruction
8. Lymphangiography—to determine the presence and extent of lymph node involvement
9. Pelvic lymphadenectomy and biopsy—for staging and to determine spread to lymph nodes

Patient Problems/Nursing Diagnoses

1. Urinary dysfunction (frequency, nocturia, incontinence, hematuria) related to prostate tumor and sequelae of surgical intervention
2. Potential for sexual dysfunction related to radical surgery and external radiation therapy
3. Weight loss, fatigue, activity intolerance related to effects of cancer

Planning and Intervention
Nursing Interventions
A. Relief from symptoms of urinary dysfunction

1. Support the patient undergoing radiation therapy (see p. 912) and prostatic surgery (next column).
2. See nursing management of the patient with pain, page 917, and care of the patient with late-stage cancer, page 917.
3. Monitor catheter drainage (see p. 552; either via suprapubic or urethral) when maintaining patency of the urethral passage becomes difficult.

B. Sexual rehabilitation

1. Be aware that the patient may be in ill health and suffering from pain, weight loss, and the effects of endocrine therapy or chemotherapy; in this event, the patient may not be much concerned with sexuality.
2. Give the patient permission to communicate his concerns and sexual needs.
3. Understand the stages (shock and denial, mourning, resolution) the patient goes through concerning sexual dysfunction.
4. Expect some patient feelings of depression, anxiety, anger, and regression.
5. Help the patient to use positive coping strategies (sexual counseling, learning other options of sexual expression, consideration of penile implant).

Health Education

Be alert for neurologic changes in lower extremities (prostatic cancer can lead to paraplegia); a decompressive laminectomy may be required as an emergency procedure.

Evaluation
Expected Outcomes

1. Achieves relief of urinary dysfunction
2. Verbalizes coping strategies in dealing with fears, sexual dysfunction, and anxiety

Management of the Patient Undergoing Prostatic Surgery

Surgical Procedures
A. Four Approaches for Prostatectomy

1. Transurethral removal of prostatic tissue by an instrument introduced through urethra.
2. Open surgical removal of prostate (procedures used are named for area of incision).
    a. Perineal
    b. Retropubic
    c. Suprapubic

B. Factors Influencing Choice of Surgical Approach

1. Size of gland and severity of obstruction
2. Age and condition of the patient
3. Presence of associated disease(s)

Preoperative Management
A. Establishing optimal kidney function

1. Maintain adequate bladder drainage via indwelling catheter or suprapubic cystostomy—renal function usually improves with reestablishment of drainage.
    a. Introduce indwelling catheter if the patient has continuing retention, if residual urine is more than 75–100 ml., or if renal function has been impaired by back pressure of urine into the upper tract.
    b. Utilize cystostomy if the patient cannot tolerate urethral catheter.
    c. Give antibiotics (according to culture and sensitivity tests)—to combat and control infection.
    d. Watch the patient closely after drainage is instituted—blood pressure fluctuates and renal function may decline first few days after drainage is established.
    e. Ensure adequate hydration—the patient is frequently dehydrated from self-limitation of fluids because of frequency.
        (1) Encourage fluid intake of 2,500–3,000 ml. daily (if cardiac reserve is adequate)—to help in overcoming azotemia.
        (2) Weigh the patient daily and monitor fluid intake and output.
        (3) Give intravenous fluids according to need as indicated by clinical status and serum electrolyte determinations.
2. Carry out prescribed renal function studies—to determine if there is renal impairment from prostatic back pressure and to evaluate renal reserve.

B. Ensuring optimal preoperative condition

1. Carry out complete hematologic investigation—to ascertain specific clotting defects, since hemorrhage is a major postoperative complication.
2. Correct nutritional deficiencies, hypoproteinemia, vitamin deficiencies and anemia.
3. Give cardiac supporting drugs when indicated—helps alleviate renal symptoms.
4. Prepare the patient with pulmonary emphysema with antibacterial agent, tracheobronchial cleansing, and

incentive spirometry. The patient should stop smoking at least 2 days before surgery.
5. Teach active leg exercises; apply graded antiembolism stockings to prevent deep vein thrombosis.
6. Type and cross match for blood transfusion(s).

Postoperative Patient Problems/Nursing Diagnoses

1. Potential complications (hemorrhage, urinary infection, urethral stricture) related to the surgical procedure
2. Urinary elimination dysfunction related to problems with indwelling catheter, bladder spasms, and the nature of the surgery
3. Pain and discomfort related to bladder spasms and surgical procedure
4. Anxiety concerning incontinence and sexual function
5. Knowledge deficit of postoperative self-care, and after effects of surgery

Planning and Implementation
Nursing Interventions
A. Prevention of Complications

1. Evaluate for shock and hemorrhage.
   a. Watch for evidence of hemorrhage in drainage bag, on dressings, and at incision site.
   b. Take blood pressure, pulse, and respiration as frequently as clinical condition indicates. Compare with preoperative vital sign readings to assess degree of hypotension present.
      (1) Observe for cold, sweating skin, pallor, restlessness, fall in blood pressure, increasing pulse rate.
      (2) Apply manual traction on the urethral catheter as directed to help stop bleeding; release traction intermittently and reassess the bleeding.
      (3) Prepare for surgical intervention if bleeding persists (suturing of bleeders or transurethral coagulation of bleeders).
   c. Give blood transfusion as indicated.
2. Monitor for other postoperative complications.
   a. Urinary infection, septic shock, urethritis (from catheter), urinary fistula
   b. Epididymitis
   c. Late complications—urethral stricture, internal meatal stenosis

B. Establishing Adequate Drainage of the Bladder

1. Utilize a closed sterile gravity system of drainage—3-way system is useful in controlling bleeding; irrigating system keeps clots from forming (does not correct the *cause* of bleeding).
2. Watch drainage for evidence of increased bleeding—bright red urine indicates arterial bleeding; dark red urine suggests venous bleeding.
3. Irrigate bladder (amount and time prescribed by urologist) to avoid clot formation in the bladder.
   a. Frequency of bladder irrigation determined by amount of bleeding.
   b. Irrigation is adjusted to keep urine a light pink to straw color, free of clots, and transparent in appearance.
   c. Irrigate catheter *gently* if it is occluded—catheter opening may be obstructed by blood clot, tissue remnant, or by being in contact with the bladder wall.

(1) Rotate catheter to move drainage eye of catheter away from bladder wall/clot.
(2) Irrigate catheter with small amount of sterile fluid; too much force or fluid may damage recently operated area.
(3) Apply *gentle* suction; strong suction on a recently occluded vessel can cause bleeding.
(4) Avoid overdistending bladder—may produce secondary hemorrhage by stretching the coagulated vessels in the prostatic capsule.
4. Maintain an input and output record, including the amount of fluid used for irrigation.
5. Tape the drainage tubing (not the catheter) to shaved inner thigh—to prevent traction on bladder. (However, traction on the catheter by the urologist may control bleeding.)
6. Tape cystostomy catheter to lateral abdomen.
7. Note time and amount of each voiding after removal of catheter.
   a. May be urinary leakage around wound several days after removal of catheter in perineal, suprapubic, and retropubic surgery.
   b. Cystostomy tube may be removed before or after removal of urethral catheter.

C. Relief of Pain and Discomfort

1. Keep the patient quiet and comfortable during *immediate* postoperative period to prevent episodes of bleeding.
   When a patient experiences pain following prostatectomy, it may cause him to strain (from bladder irritability); this causes pelvic vein engorgement and promotes venous hemorrhage and clot formation.
2. Use tranquilizers, sedatives, antispasmodics, and appropriate analgesics for pain control.
   a. Elderly patients do not usually tolerate barbiturates.
   b. Take blood pressure before administering tranquilizers and analgesics.
   c. Give pain medication before irrigation if bladder spasms are severe.
3. Explain again to the patient the purpose of the catheter.
   a. Tell the patient that the urge to void is caused by the presence of the catheter and bladder spasm (painful contractions of muscles of bladder wall and neck).
      (1) Watch catheter tubing; a column of urine moving between pain episodes or when patient coughs may indicate bladder spasms.
      (2) A frequent cause of spasm is the catheter touching (and stimulating) the posterior bladder wall.
      (3) Gently draw catheter back toward external meatus; adjust catheter so that only its tip projects into the bladder.
   b. Give antispasmodics (propantheline bromide) as directed.
   c. Encourage him to refrain from pulling on catheter—will cause bleeding, clots, plugging of catheter, and distention.
   d. Tape catheter to lower abdomen (see Fig. 11-6) to prevent pressure on penoscrotal junction.
   e. Wash urethral meatus adjacent to catheter with soap and water; rinse and apply an antibacterial ointment as directed.
4. Be alert for blockage of urinary drainage tube by kinking, mucous plugs, and blood clots.

5. Give antibiotics as directed—to promote urinary antisepsis.
6. Avoid rectal instrumentation (thermometers, rectal tubes, enemas) following prostatic surgery. Because the rectum is close to the prostatic fossa, instrumentation may be dangerous until healing has taken place.
7. Help the patient to ambulate as quickly as possible; avoid sitting for prolonged periods, since this increases intra-abdominal pressure and increases the possibility of bleeding.
8. Promote the comfort of the patient with perineal sutures.
   a. Wash perineum with surgical soap as directed.
   b. Use heat lamp to perineal area (cover scrotum with towel)—to promote healing.
   c. Assist the patient with sitz bath as directed—to promote healing.

Discharge Planning and Health Education

Instruct the patient as follows:

A. Urinary Control

1. After the catheter is removed, there may be some burning on urination and/or frequent desire to void. These symptoms will disappear in a few weeks.
2. Expect urinary dribbling for a period of time (especially after catheter removal). Urinary incontinence may follow any type of prostatic surgery.
3. Exercises to gain urinary control.
   a. Perineal exercises
      (1) Tense the perineal muscles by pressing the buttocks together. Hold this position as long as possible; relax.
      (2) Perform this exercise 10–20 times each hour.
      (3) Continue with perineal exercises until full urinary control is gained.
   b. When starting to void
      (1) Shut off the stream for a few seconds.
      (2) Continue with full voiding.
      (3) Continue this exercise with each urination until control improves; may take many weeks.
4. Urinate as soon as the first desire to do so is felt.
5. The urine may be cloudy for several weeks after surgery. As the prostate area heals, the cloudiness will disappear.
6. Avoid long automobile trips, which increase tendency to bleed.

7. Avoid alcohol, which increases urinary burning.
8. Drink adequate fluids (8 glasses/day), since dehydration increases tendency for clot obstruction.
9. Do not take anticholinergics and diuretics unless by direct prescription of the physician.

B. Sexual Functioning

1. Prostatectomy does not usually cause impotence—penile erection depends on intact spinal cord, intact autonomic nerves to penis, normal erectile tissue/adequate blood supply and psychological well-being; a simple prostatectomy does not affect these factors.
   a. Total prostatectomy (removal of entire prostatic contents and capsule) results in impotence, since the nerves and muscular tissue surrounding the capsule (which have a function in penile erection) have been severed.
   b. Penile prosthesis (inflatable, semi-rigid, and flexible types) may be surgically implanted—used to make the penis rigid for sexual intercourse.
2. In most instances sexual activity may be resumed in 6–8 weeks; this is the time required for healing of the prostatic fossa to take place.
3. Do not be alarmed if no fluid appears on ejaculation; following ejaculation, the fluid goes into the bladder and is voided at the next urination.
   a. This does not reduce the level of sexual performance or satisfaction.
   b. The urine voided after intercourse may have a milky appearance.

C. Other Considerations

1. Avoid straining and strenuous exercises.
2. Report to the physician any bleeding or a decrease in the size of the urinary stream.

Evaluation

Expected Outcomes

1. Shows no signs of complications—no evidence of hemorrhage or infection
2. Achieves bladder drainage; no clots; urine becoming clear
3. Reports diminished discomfort and pain; taking minimal amount of analgesics
4. Ventilates feelings about urinary control and sexual functioning; performing perineal exercises; gaining urinary control

Hydrocele

Hydrocele is a collection of fluid generally in the tunica vaginalis of the testicle, although it may also occur within the spermatic cord.

Causes

(Caused by defective or inadequate reabsorption of normally produced hydrocele fluid)
1. Secondary to local injury, including hernia operation
2. Secondary to infection
3. Following epididymitis or orchitis

4. As a complication of tumor of testicle
5. In edematous states such as congestive heart failure, cirrhosis of the liver
6. Idiopathic

Clinical Manifestations

1. Enlargement of the scrotum
2. Usually painless until fluid accumulation is large enough to cause pressure
3. Transmits light when transilluminated

Treatment

1. No treatment is required unless complications are present.
   a. Circulatory complications involving testicle
   b. Painful large hydrocele, which is uncomfortable and cosmetically unacceptable to the patient
2. Surgical intervention—hydrocelectomy (excision of tunica vaginalis of testis) for removal of fluid and control of swelling.

   a. Periodic aspiration of hydrocele fluid in poor-risk patient
   b. Open operation for eversion of hydrocele sac or removal of hydrocele sac
3. See below, Postoperative Nursing Support (Varicocele).
4. Complication—formation of a hematoma in the loose tissues of the scrotum.

Varicocele

Varicocele is a mass of varicose veins in the scrotum, usually part of the spermatic cord.

Clinical Manifestations

1. Subfertility may occur with varicocele—may suppress spermatogenesis due to vascular and temperature changes or more likely to reflux of left adrenal corticosteroids to both testes because of intercommunication of their venous circulations.
2. A dragging sensation in the scrotum is usually the patient's chief complaint.
3. Varicocele on the right may indicate retroperitoneal tumor.

Diagnostic Evaluation

Palpation of intrascrotal mass (with patient in upright position) that disappears in a short time after he has been lying down.

Management

1. Scrotal support to relieve discomfort
2. Surgical intervention—ligation and excision of veins (varicocelectomy)

Postoperative Nursing Support

1. Apply ice bag for first few hours postoperatively to relieve edema.
2. Apply scrotal support for comfort.

The etiology of testicular tumors is unknown, but cryptorchidism (see p. 1353), infections, and genetic and endocrine factors appear to play a role in their development.

Clinical Features

1. Tumors of the testicle are usually malignant; they occur primarily in men between the ages of 20 and 40.
2. Most testicular tumors metastasize early to the peri-aortic and pericaval lymph nodes, lungs, and liver.
3. A patient with a history of 1 testis tumor is more apt to develop another than is the random patient to develop a first testis tumor.
4. Testicular germ cell tumors are now considered curable.

Clinical Manifestations

1. Mass in scrotum; painless enlargement of the testis, accompanied by feeling of heaviness in scrotum.
2. Pain in the testis (if patient has epididymitis or bleeding into tumor).
3. Gynecomastia (enlargement of the breasts) from elaboration of chorionic gonadotropins from testicular tumor.
4. Symptoms of metastases
   a. Left supraclavicular or abdominal mass
   b. Abdominal pain
   c. Cough (lung metastases)

Diagnostic Evaluation

1. Testicular tumor markers—radioimmunoassay of human chorionic gonadotropins (HCG) and alpha-fetoprotein (AFP)—serologic and cellular markers used for diagnosis, detection of early recurrence, staging, and monitoring treatment.
2. Intravenous urogram to evaluate presence of enlarged lymph nodes as manifested by ureteral displacement.
3. Chest film to seek pulmonary or mediastinal metastases.
4. Lymphangiography—to assess extent of lymphatic spread of tumor.
5. Computed tomography—to identify lesions in retroperitoneum and to follow the patient's course during/ after treatment.
6. Ultrasound examination—noninvasive method of identifying scrotal masses.

Treatment

1. *Surgery*—orchiectomy (removal of testis and its tunica and spermatic cord)
   a. Usually done through an inguinal incision.
   b. Retroperitoneal lymphadenectomy usually performed after orchiectomy.
      (1) Orchiectomy (unilateral) usually has no adverse effects on sexual potency or fertility. Gel-filled prosthesis can be implanted at time of orchiectomy or electively thereafter to offset absence of one testis.
      (2) Possible postoperative complication is ejaculation without emission (loss of ejaculation due to interruption of sympathetic ganglia at L2–L4 level, since they are in close proximity to involved nodes).
         Patient will not be fertile, but normal libido and orgasm will be unimpaired.

2. *Radiation therapy* to lymphatic drainage pathways is used in most patients with testicular cancer; may be curative or palliative, depending on circumstances. Treatment of choice for seminoma.
3. *Chemotherapy*—used in the treatment of primary tumor and regional lymphatic metastases and in managing distant metastatic disease; usually given in combination.
   a. Cyclophosphamide, vinblastine, actinomycin-D, bleomycin, cisplatin—induce a high percentage of durable complete remissions (metastatic testicular cancer is potentially curable).
   b. These regimens are toxic and require intensive therapeutic support; require high degree of patient commitment and cooperation.
   c. May be used as adjuvant to surgery and/or radiation in advanced disease.
   d. Etoposide—has proved effective when combined with other antineoplastic agents for intensive second-line treatment of patients who have failed initial chemotherapy.

Nursing Interventions

1. See page 85 for care of the patient following surgery, page 912 for care of the patient undergoing radiation therapy, and page 905 for care of the patient undergoing chemotherapy.

2. Teach the patient that one testis is expendable.
3. Make it clear that an orchiectomy will not diminish potency, fertility, or virility.
4. Give the adolescent male or younger patient the opportunity to discuss depositing sperm in sperm bank, particularly if he is to receive radiation therapy. (However, he may be ineligible for sperm-banking because of disease-impaired sperm production.)
5. Inform the patient of the following:
   a. Genital cancer is not "punishment" for real/imagined sexual activity.
   b. Radiotherapy to the abdomen will cause no change in sexual performance but may diminish semen volume.
   c. Refer the patient to social worker as required; frequent hospitalization may be necessary with interruption of work/personal life.

Health Education

Instruct the patient as follows:
1. Follow-up evaluation includes chest films, excretory urography and radioimmunoassay of HCG and AFP, examination of lymph nodes—to monitor success of therapy and to detect recurrence of malignancy.
2. Carry out periodic self-examinations of the testes (see Guidelines, below).

Guidelines: Self-Examination for Testicular Tumor

1. The testis is easily accessible for self-examination. Most tumors are palpable and can be detected by self-examination.
2. The hormonally active years (15–35) are the tumor-prone years.

Procedure

Action by Patient	Explanation
1. Examine for testicular tumor periodically, preferably while showering/bathing.	1. Detection of abnormalities is more readily accomplished after or during a warm shower or bath, when the scrotum wall is relaxed.
2. Use both hands to palpate (feel). Carefully examine all scrotal contents.	2. A small lump (nodule) can slip away from one hand. You can feel differences in weight between the testicles by using both hands.
3. Locate the epididymis; this is the cord-like structure at the back of the testis.	3. It is important to know what the epididymis feels like so you will not confuse it with an abnormality.
4. The spermatic cord (and vas) extends upward from the epididymis.	
5. Feel each testis between the thumb and first 2 fingers of each hand.	5. The testes lie freely in the scrotum, are oval shaped, and measure 4–5 cm. in length, 3 cm. in width, and about 2 cm. in thickness.
6. Note size, shape, abnormal tenderness.	6. An abnormality may be felt as a firm area on the front or side of the testicle.
7. Stand in front of mirror and look for changes in size/shape of scrotum.	7. Tumors or cystic masses tend to involve only 1 side.

Epididymitis

Epididymitis is an infection of the epididymis that usually descends from an infected prostate or urinary tract.

Causes

1. Prostatic infection (most common cause); complication of infected urine containing pyogenic bacteria
2. Trauma; urethral stricture
3. Postoperative epididymitis—complication of prostatectomy and urethral catheterization
4. Specific causes—gonorrhea, syphilis, tuberculosis, *Chlamydia trachomatis* infection, *Ureaplasma urealyticum* infection

Clinical Manifestations

1. Localized scrotal pain and tenderness
2. Edema, redness, and tenderness of scrotum
3. Chills and fever
4. Pyuria and bacteriuria

Diagnostic Evaluation

1. Examination of initial and midstream urine sample for pyuria
2. Elevated white blood count (may be as high as 20,000–30,000/cu. ml.)
3. Epididymal aspiration
4. Staining of urethral discharge if preceded by urethritis (either nonspecific or gonorrheal); usually no discharge is present with epididymitis

Treatment and Nursing Management

1. Give specific antimicrobial therapy until all evidence of acute inflammatory reaction has subsided.
2. Encourage bed rest during the acute phase.
3. Apply scrotal support for enlarged testicle (scrotal bridge; rolled towel under scrotum)—to relieve edema and discomfort, to improve venous drainage, and to take the tension off the cord. A cotton-lined athletic supporter may promote comfort.
4. Assist with infiltration of spermatic cord with local anesthetic agent (procaine hydrochloride)—for pain relief if patient is seen within 24 hours after onset.
5. Give analgesics for pain relief—this gives pain relief while more specific therapy begins to work.
6. Apply intermittent cold compresses to scrotum during initial period—for pain relief.
7. Use local heat or sitz bath later—to hasten resolution of inflammatory process.
8. Offer stool softeners.
9. Observe for possible abscess formation.

Health Education

Instruct the patient as follows:
1. Avoid straining (lifting, defecation) and sexual excitement until infection is under control.
2. It may take 4 weeks or longer for epididymis to return to normal.
3. Sex partners of patients with chlamydial urethritis or epididymitis should be examined and treated.
4. Reassure the patient that sexual performance should not be affected after the inflammation has subsided.

Vasectomy

Vasectomy is the ligation and transection of a section of the vas deferens; a bilateral vasectomy is a sterilization procedure for males.

Clinical Indications

1. Performed as a sterilization procedure.
2. Performed if the patient has recurrent acute epididymitis (see above).

Underlying Considerations

1. A vasectomy interrupts the transportation of the sperm. This procedure has no effect on sexual potency, erection, ejaculation, or production of male hormones.
2. Seminal fluid is mostly manufactured in the seminal vesicles and prostate, which are unaffected by vasectomy.
   a. There will be no noticeable decrease in the amount of ejaculated fluid; the sperm accounts for less than 5% of the volume. The sperm cells are reabsorbed into the body.
   b. Psychological problems have been noted in an occasional patient following this procedure.
3. A vasectomy can be done on an outpatient basis with local anesthesia.
4. A legal consent form must be obtained, usually from the patient and his partner.
5. The patient should be advised that he will be sterile but that potency will not be altered following a bilateral vasectomy. Rarely is there a spontaneous reanastomosis resulting in pregnancy.
6. A vasectomy may not be reversible and should be considered permanent; microsurgical techniques are being used for vasectomy reversal (vasovasotomy); success rates are promising.

Complications

1. Sperm granuloma—due to extravasation of sperm
2. Infection; scrotal abscess
3. Recanalization of vas deferens (very rare)
4. Bleeding and hematoma

Treatment and Nursing Interventions

1. Place patient on bed rest for several hours.
2. Apply ice bags intermittently to the scrotum for several hours after surgery to reduce swelling and relieve discomfort.
3. Reassure the patient that discoloration of scrotal skin, swelling, and edema are to be expected.
4. Advise the patient to wear scrotal support for added comfort and support.

Health Education

Instruct the patient as follows:
1. The primary function of the testicle(s) is the production of hormones and of sperm. A vasectomy will not interfere with these functions, but it will interrupt the descent of sperm from the testicle to the ejaculatory ducts.
2. Rest for 48 hours after surgery to prevent discomfort.
3. Avoid strenuous activities for several days.
4. Sexual intercourse may be resumed as desired.
5. Contraceptives should be used until the sperm stored distal to the point of interruption of the vas is evacuated; (2 negative semen specimens 1 month apart). *The patient is still fertile for a variable period of time after vasectomy.*
6. Absence of sperm must be demonstrated microscopically; laboratory tests confirm that no sperm are present in the seminal fluid.
7. A vasectomy does not prevent venereal disease.

Conditions Affecting the Penis

Infections

1. *Chancre*—venereal ulceration caused by *Treponema pallidum* (see Syphilis, p. 870)
2. *Chancroid*—a sexually transmitted disease caused by *Haemophilus ducreyi;* usually 1 or several penile ulcers are present, as well as enlarged lymph nodes
3. *Genital herpes* (herpes simplex virus [HSV])—a sexually transmitted disease that produces multiple bilaterally distributed vesicles on or near the penis.
4. *Gonorrhea*—see pages 863–868.

Clinical Manifestations

Ulceration of the penis should be suspected as being venereal in origin until proved otherwise.

Diagnostic Evaluation

1. Dark field microscopic examination of smear for spirochetes
2. Serologic (blood) test for syphilis

Treatment

Varies greatly, depending on the cause of ulceration

Other Conditions

Phimosis

A condition in which the foreskin is constricted so that it cannot be retracted over the glans. The treatment is circumcision.

Paraphimosis

A condition in which the foreskin is retracted behind the glans, and because of narrowness and subsequent edema, cannot be reduced back to its normal position.

Priapism

An uncontrolled persistent erection of the penis occurring from neural or vascular causes, including sickle cell thrombosis, spinal cord tumors, and tumor invasion of the penis or its vessels. This condition is considered a urologic emergency. Treatment includes bed rest, sedation, and/or surgery.

Carcinoma of the Penis

Carcinoma of the penis occurs in the skin of the penis; appears as a painless, wart-like growth or ulcer on the glans or coronal sulcus under the prepuce. Treatment is radiation or surgical intervention.

Circumcision

Circumcision is the excision of the foreskin (prepuce) of the glans penis.

Clinical Indications

1. Usually done in infancy for hygienic purposes
2. In adults—phimosis; paraphimosis; recurrent infection of the glans and foreskin; personal desire of the patient
3. Circumcision is thought to be a preventive measure against carcinoma of the penis.

Postoperative Nursing Management

1. Watch for bleeding.
2. Change petrolatum (Vaseline) gauze dressing as directed.
3. Give analgesia as the patient's condition indicates; circumcision can be quite painful in the adult male.

Bibliography

Books

Ashken MH (ed). Urinary Diversion. New York, Springer-Verlag, 1982

Avram MM (ed). Prevention of Kidney Disease and Long-Term Survival. New York, Plenum, 1982

Barrett DM and Wein AJ. Controversies in Neuro-Urology. New York, Churchill Livingstone, 1984

Brenner BM and Lazarus JM (eds). Acute Renal Failure. Philadelphia, WB Saunders, 1983

Bricker NS and Kirschenbaum MA (eds). The Kidney: Diagnosis and Management. New York, John Wiley & Sons, 1984

Brooks D and Mallick N. Renal Medicine and Urology. New York, Churchill Livingstone, 1982

Brown RD. Clinical Urology Illustrated. York, ADIS Press, 1982

Castro JE (ed). The Treatment of Renal Failure. Lancaster, MTP Press, 1982

Chaussy C et al (eds). Extracorporeal Shock Wave Lithotripsy: New Aspects in the Treatment of Kidney Stone Disease. New York, Karger, 1982

Dalton JR. Basic Clinical Urology. Philadelphia, Harper & Row, 1983

Finkbeiner AE, Barbour GL and Bissada NK. Pharmacology of the Urinary Tract and the Male Reproductive System. New York, Appleton-Century-Crofts, 1982

First MR. Chronic Renal Failure: Pathophysiology, Clinical Manifestations, and Management. Garden City, NY, Medical Examination Publishers, 1982

Flamenbaum W and Hamburger RJ. Nephrology. Philadelphia, JB Lippincott, 1982

Glenn JF. Urologic Surgery, 3rd ed. Philadelphia, JB Lippincott, 1983

Heptinstall RH. Pathology of the Kidney, vols 1–3. Boston, Little, Brown & Co, 1983

Herman JR. Handbook of Urology. Philadelphia, Harper & Row, 1983

Horsely JA et al (eds). Closed Urinary Drainage Systems. New York, Grune & Stratton, 1981

Horsely JA, Crane J and Reynolds M. Clean Intermittent Catheterization. New York, Grune and Stratton, 1982

Javadpour N (ed). Principles and Management of Urologic Cancer, 2nd ed. Baltimore, Williams & Wilkins, 1983

Jones JMD, Briggs JD and Hargreave TB. Diagnosis and Management of Renal and Urinary Diseases. Boston, Blackwell Scientific, 1982

Klahr S (ed). The Kidney and Body Fluids in Health and Disease. New York, Plenum, 1983

Lattimer JK et al (eds). Urology and Psychosocial aspects of Chronic, Critical and Terminal Illness. Springfield, Charles C Thomas, 1983

Lerner J and Khan Z. Mosby's Manual of Urologic Nursing. St Louis, CV Mosby, 1982

Martinez-Maldonado M (ed). Handbook

of Renal Therapeutics. New York, Plenum, 1983

Mauermayer W. Trans-Urethral Surgery. New York, Springer-Verlag, 1983

McConnell EA and Zimmerman MF. Care of Patients with Urologic Problems. Philadelphia, JB Lippincott, 1983

Nursing Photobooks. Implementing Urologic Procedures. Horsham, PA, Nursing Photobooks, 1981

Oberley ET and Oberley JH. Understanding Your New Life with Dialysis. Springfield, IL, Charles C Thomas, 1983

Raz S. Female Urology. Philadelphia, WB Saunders, 1983

Resnick MI and Older RA (eds). Diagnosis of Genitourinary Disease. New York, Thieme Stratton, 1982

Roth RA and Finlayson B. Stones: Clinical Management of Urolithiasis. Baltimore, Williams & Wilkins, 1983

Scott R, Deane RF and Callander R. Urology Illustrated, 2nd ed. New York, Churchill Livingstone, 1982

Spiers ASD (ed). Chemotherapy and Urological Malignancy. New York, Springer-Verlag, 1982

Stone WJ and Rabin PL. End-Stage Renal Disease. New York, Academic Press, 1983

Tilney NL and Lazarus JM (eds). Surgical Care of the Patient with Renal Failure. Philadelphia, WB Saunders, 1982

VanStone JC et al. Dialysis and the Treatment of Renal Insufficiency. New York, Grune & Stratton, 1983

vonEschenbach AC and Rodriguez DB (eds). Sexual Rehabilitation of the Urologic Cancer Patient. Boston, GK Hall, 1981

Wickham JEA and Miller RA. Percutaneous Renal Surgery. New York, Churchill Livingstone, 1983

Articles

Diagnosis

Engram BW. Do's and don't's of urologic nursing. Nursing '83 1983 Oct; 13(10):49

Fischbach F. Analyzing urinalysis results. DCCN 1983 Jul–Aug; 2(4):225–232

Gault MH and Muehrcke RC. Renal biopsy: Current views and controversies. Nephron 1983 May; 34(1):1–34

Googe MCS and Mook TM. The inflatable penile prosthesis: New developments. Am J Nurs 1983 Jul; 83(7):1044–1047

McConnell EA. Urinalysis: A common test, but never routine. Nursing '82 1982 Feb; 12(2):108–111

Cancer: Bladder/Kidney

Barrett N. Cancer of the bladder: A case history. Am J Nurs 1981 Dec; 81(12):2192–2195

DeKernion JB. Treatment of advanced renal cell carcinoma—traditional methods and innovative approaches. J Urol 1983 Jul; 130(1):2–7

Javadpour N. Recent advances in urologic cancer. Int Perspectives Urol 1982; 2:entire volume

Lang N. Advanced renal cell carcinoma: Treatment by transcatheter embolization with inert material and radioactive particles. Prog Clin Cancer 1982; 8:299–310

Malek RS, Rosen JS and O'Dea MJ. Adenocarcinoma of bladder. Urology 1983 Apr; 21(4):357–359

Mather DG. Ileal conduit surgery: How to help a terrified patient. RN 1981 Oct; 44(10):29–31

Montie JE et al. Unresectable carcinoma of the bladder. Cancer 1983 June; 51(12):2351–2355

Nakano H, Nihira H and Toge T. Treatment of renal cancer patients by transcatheter embolization and its effects on lymphocyte proliferative responses. J Urol 1983 July; 130(1):24–27

Pontes JE. Adjunctive treatment of renal cell carcinoma. Int Adv Surg Oncol 1983; 6:309–322

Princenthal RA et al. Ureterosigmoidostomy: The development of tumors, diagnosis, and pitfalls. AJR 1983 Jul; 141(1):77–81

Quesada JR et al. Renal cell carcinoma: Antitumor effects of leukocyte interferon. Cancer Res 1983 Feb; 43(2):940–947

Radriguez DB. Urinary stomas. Part 2: Stoma care. Clin Gastroenterol 1982 May; 11(2):318–326

Shehata WM, Meyer RI, and Costandi YT. Curative and palliative radiotherapy of bladder cancer. A retrospective study of 11 years experience. Radiology 1983 Feb; 146(2):523–526

Simmons KN. Sexuality and the female ostomate: Patient-to-patient advice. Am J Nurs 1983 Mar; 83(3):409–411

Soloway MS. Bladder cancer. Management of an increasingly common tumor. Postgrad Med 1983 Mar; 73(3):139–151

Sufrin G. The challenges of renal adenocarcinoma. Surg Clin North Am 1982 Dec; 62(6):1101–1118

Torti FM (ed). Urologic cancer: Chemotherapeutic principles and management. Rec Res Cancer Res 1983; 85:entire volume

Weinberg DM et al. Bladder cancer etiology. A different perspective. Cancer 1983 Feb 15; 51(4):675–680

Glomerulonephritis/Nephrotic Syndrome

Cameron JS. Glomerulonephritis: Current problems and understanding. J Lab Clin Med 1982 Jun; 99(6):755–787

Madaio MP and Harrington JT. Current concepts. The diagnosis of acute glomerulonephritis. N Engl J Med 1983 Nov 24; 309(21):1299–1302

Zech P et al. The nephrotic syndrome in adults aged over 60: Etiology, evolution and treatment of 76 cases. Clin Nephrol 1982 May; 17(5):232–236.

Male Urologic Conditions

Bates P. Three post-op perils of prostate surgery. RN 1984 Feb; 47(2):40–43

Bennett AH (ed). Management of male impotence. Int Perspect Urol 1982; 5: entire volume

Blick KE, Dick TT and Webb TA. Radioimmunoassay for prostatic acid phosphatase helps discriminate patients with prostatic cancer. Clin Chem 1982 Dec; 28(1):2373–2377

Brunner H, Weidner W and Schiefer HG. Studies on the role of ureaplasma urealyticum and mycoplasma hominis in prostatitis. J Infect Dis 1983 May; 147(5):807–813

Chartham R. Ante- and post-prostatectomy supportive therapy. Practitioner 1982 Nov; 226(1373): 1965–1967

Clark N and O'Connell P. Prostatectomy: A guide to answering your patient's unspoken questions. Nursing '84 1984 Apr; 14(4):48–51

Donohue JP. Testis tumors. Int Perspect Urol 1983; 7:entire volume

Franchimont P et al. Radioimmunoassay of prostatic acid phosphatase: Validation and clinical application. Int J Cancer 1983 Feb 15; 31(2):149–155

Gault-Catarrinho PL. Testicular cancer. Crit Care Update 1983 Mar; 10(3):32–35

Henahan J. New prostate cancer drugs: Few CV effects? JAMA 1983 Oct 28; 250(16):2097–2099

Hoeft RT and Jones AG. Cancer of the prostate: Treating metastasis with estramustine phosphate. Am J Nurs 1982 May; 82(5):828–830

Jacobs SC. Spread of prostatic cancer to bone. Urology 1983 Apr; 21(4):337–344

Jewett HJ. Prostatic cancer: A personal view of the problem. J Urol 1984 May; 131(5):845–849

Jonas P, Lindner A and Ohrv A. Postprostatectomy impotence in elderly patients. Geriatrics 1983 Sep; 38(9):113, 117

Jones AG and Hoeft RT. Cancer of the prostate. Am J Nurs 1982 May; 82(5): 826–828

Kaempfer SH, Hoffman DJ and Wiley FM. Sperm banking: A reproductive option in cancer therapy. Cancer Nurs 1983 Feb; 6(1):31–38

Kessler R. Vasectomy and vasovasostomy. Surg Clin North Am 1982 Dec; 62(6):971–980

Nickel CJ and Morales A. Estramustine phosphate versus stilbestrol as primary treatment for metastatic cancer of the prostate. Can J Surg 1983 Sept; 26(5): 434–438

Ristuccia AM and Cunha BN. Current concepts in antimicrobial therapy of prostatitis. Urology 1982 Sept; 20(3): 338–345

VanArsdalen KN et al. Deep vein thrombosis and prostatectomy. Urology 1983 May; 21(5):461–463

Renal Failure/Dialysis/Transplantation

Chambers JK. Bowel management in dialysis patients. Am J Nurs 1983 July; 83(7):1051–1052

FDA OKs cyclosporine for transplants. Am J Nurs 1984 Jan; 84(1):9

Fleming LM and Kane J. Step-by-step

guide to safe peritoneal dialysis. RN 1984 Feb; 47(2):44–47

Goldstein MB. Acute renal failure. Med Clin North Am 1983 Nov; 67(6):1325–1341

Murphy LM and Cole MJ. Renal disease: Nutritional implications. Nurs Clin North Am 1983 Mar; 18(1):57–70

Novick AC (ed). Symposium on renal transplantation. Urol Clin North Am 1983 May; 10(2):205–370

Reckling JB. Safeguarding the renal transplant patient. Nursing '82 1982 Feb; 12(2):46–49

Reed SB. Giving more than dialysis. Nursing '82 1982 Apr; 12(4):58–63

Rosansky SJ. Choosing therapy for end-stage renal disease. Am Fam Physician 1983 July; 28(1):115–124.

Schrier RW. Acute renal failure. JAMA 1982 May 14; 247(18):2518–2525

Stark JL. How to succeed against acute renal failure. Nursing '82 1982 July; 12(7):26–33

Stark JL and Hunt V. Helping your patient with chronic renal failure. Nursing '83 1983 Sept; 13(9):56–63

Starzl TE et al. Steps in immunosuppression for renal transplantation. Kidney Int (Suppl) 1983 May; (14):S-60–65

Strom TB and Carpenter CB. Transplantation: Immunogenetic and clinical aspects—Part II. Hosp Pract 1983 Jan; 18(1):135–150

Tilney NL and Lazarus JM. Acute renal failure in surgical patients. Surg Clin North Am 1983 Apr; 63(2):357–377

Waltzer WC. Acute renal failure. Am Fam Physician 1982 Sept; 26(3):173–178

Washer GF et al. Causes of death after kidney transplantation. JAMA 1983 Jul 1; 250(1):49–54

Surgery/Trauma

Bergquist D et al. Blunt renal trauma. Analysis of 417 patients. Eur Urol 1983; 9(1):1–5

Cain L and Bigongiari LR. The percutaneous nephrostomy tube. Am J Nurs 1982 Feb; 82(2):296–298

McConnell JD, Wilkerson DD and Peters PC. Rupture of the bladder. Urol Clin North Am 1982 June; 9(2):293–296

MacMahon R, Hoskins D and Ramsey EW. Management of blunt injury to the lower urinary tract. Can J Surg 1983 Sept; 26(5):415–418

Mitty HA, Train JS and Dan SJ. Antegrade ureteral stenting in the management of fistulas, strictures, and calculi. Radiology 1983 Nov; 149(2):433–438

Morehouse DD. Emergency management of urethral trauma. Urol Clin North Am 1982 June; 9(2):251–254

Webster GD, Mathes GL and Selli C. Prostatomembranous urethral injuries: A review of the literature and a rational approach to their management. J Urol 1983 Nov; 130(5):898–902

Yoonessi M and Sanchez F. Self-retaining ureteral stent catheters in the management of urologic complications of gynecologic malignancies. J Surg Oncol 1982 Jun; 20(2):95–98

Urinary Tract Infection

Bates P. A troubleshooter's guide to indwelling catheters. RN 1981 Mar; 44(3):62–68

Drach GW. Bacterial prostatitis: Diagnosis and treatment. Ariz Med 1983 May; 40(5):329–332

Farrar WE Jr. Infections of the urinary tract. Med Clin North Am 1983 Jan; 67(1):187–201

Gleckman RA. Urinary tract infection in women. New perspectives on office management. Postgrad Med 1983 May; 73(5):277–280, 282

Kennedy AP. The nursing management of patients with long-term indwelling catheters. J Adv Nurs 1982 Sep; 7(5):411–417

Kennedy AP, Brocklehurst JC and Lye MDW. Factors related to the problems of long-term catheterization. J Adv Nurs 1983 May; 8(3):207–212

Keys TF and Edson RS. Antimicrobial agents in urinary tract infections. Mayo Clin Proc 1983 Mar; 58(3):165–168

Killion A. Reducing the risk of infection from indwelling catheters. Nursing '82 1982 May; 12(5):84–88

Kunin CM. Duration of treatment of urinary tract infections. Am J Med 1981 Nov; 71(5):849

Kunin CM. Genitourinary infections in the patient at risk: Extrinsic risk factors. Am J Med 1984 May 15; 76(5A):131–139

Neu HC and Parry M. Urinary tract infections: 1982—use of new concepts to guide therapy. Bull NY Acad Med 1983 Apr; 59(3):288–300

Pien FD and Landers JQ Jr. Indwelling urinary catheter infections in small community hospital. Urology 1983 Sept; 22(3):255–258

Plantemoli LV. When the patient has a Foley. RN 1984 Mar; 47(3):42–43

Platt R. Quantitative definition of bacteriuria. Am J Med 1983 Jul 28; 75(1B):44–52

Pollock HM. Laboratory techniques for detection of urinary tract infections. Am J Med 1983 Jul 28; 75:79–84

Quinlan MW. UTI: Helping your patient control it once and for all. RN 1984 Mar; 47(3):38–42

Roberts JA. Pathogenesis of pyelonephritis. J Urol 1983 Jun; 129(6):1102–1106

Seal DV and Ward K. Catheterization and urinary tract infection. Basic techniques for aseptic catheterization of the urinary tract. Nursing (Oxford) 1983 May; 2(13):5–6

Stamm WE. Measurement of pyuria and its relation to bacteriuria. Am J Med 1983 Jul 28; 75(1B):53–58

Stamm WE and Turck M. Urinary tract infection. Adv Intern Med 1983; 28:141–159

West KH. Infection control. Foley catheters: Problems and management. J Oper Room Res Inst 1983 May; 3(5):13–23

Wong ES. Guideline for prevention of catheter-associated urinary tract infections. Am J Infect Control 1983 Feb; 11(1):28–36

Wong ES and Stamm WE. Urethral infections in men and women. Annu Rev Med 1983; 34:337–358

Urolithiasis

Blume E. Sound, shock waves shatter kidney stones. JAMA 1983 May 13; 249(18):2434–2435

Clayman RV et al. Percutaneous nephrolithotomy. JAMA 1983 Jul 1; 250(1):73–75

Dillon MJ. Coagulum pyelolithotomy to remove multiple stones. AORN J 1982 Oct; 36(4):680–689

Dretler SP and Pfister RC. Percutaneous dissolution of renal calculi. Annu Rev Med 1983; 34:359–366

Huffman JL et al. Transurethral removal of large ureteral and renal pelvic calculi using ureteroscopic ultrasonic lithotripsy. J Urol 1983 July; 130(1):31–34

Lang EK and Price ET. Redefinitions of indications for percutaneous nephrostomy. Radiology 1983 May; 147(2):419–426

Lytton B. Intraoperative ultrasound for nephrolithotomy. J Urol 1983 Aug; 130(2):213–217

Marberger M. Disintegration of renal and ureteral calculi with ultrasound. Urol Clin North Am 1983 Nov; 10(4):729–742

Marwick C. New drugs selectively inhibit kidney stone formation. JAMA 1983 July 15; 250(3):321–322

Menon M and Krishnan CS. Evaluation and medical management of the patient with calcium stone disease. Urol Clin North Am 1983 Nov; 10(4):595–615

Noble M and Mebust WK. Management of recurrent renal calculi. Compr Ther 1983 Aug; 9(8):15–26

Rao PN et al. Dietary management of urinary risk factors in renal stone formers. Br J Urol 1982 Dec; 54(6):578–583

Sherrard DJ. Metabolic causes of nephrolithiasis. West J Med 1983 Apr; 138(4):541–545

Silverman DE and Stamey TA. Management of infection stones: The Stanford experience. Medicine (Baltimore) 1983 Jan; 62(1):44–51

Agencies

National Association of Patients on Hemodialysis and Transplantation
156 William Street
New York, NY 10038

National Kidney Foundation
Two Park Avenue
New York, NY 10016

United Ostomy Association
2001 W. Beverly Boulevard
Los Angeles, CA 90057

National Institute of Arthritis, Diabetes, and Digestive and Kidney Diseases
National Institutes of Health
Bethesda, MD 20205

Gynecologic and Breast Conditions

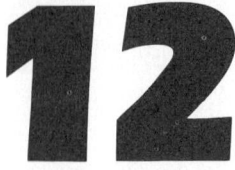

12

1: Gynecologic Conditions

1: Gynecologic Conditions

Ovulation and Menstruation

Ovulation refers to the expulsion of an ovum from the ovary 14 days before the onset of the next menstrual period.

As the endometrium is being shed, the process of repair and regrowth starts again—preparing once more for the reception of a fertilized ovum.

1. If conception does not occur, the ovum dies; tissue lining the endometrial cavity, which has become thickened and congested, becomes hemorrhagic.
2. Tissue lining the uterus, blood cells, and breakdown-products slough off and are discharged through the cervix into the vagina.
3. This cyclic process is called *menstruation*

Disturbances of Menstruation

A relationship with feedback mechanism exists between the hormonal secretions of the ovary, adrenal, thyroid,

and pituitary glands. An increase or decrease in the activity of one or more glands can cause a disturbance in menstruation.

Dysmenorrhea

Dysmenorrhea is painful menstruation.

A. Occurrence

Common in unmarried women and women who have not borne children.

B. Types

1. Primary—due to unknown factors; thought to be intrinsic to uterus; extrinsic pathology such as polyp and fibroids may be a factor. May involve emotional and psychological factors.
2. Secondary—due to factors such as endometriosis, pelvic infection, or intrauterine device.

C. Symptoms

1. Pain may be due to uterine spasm caused by a narrowing of the cervical canal (exaggerated uterine contractility).
2. Pain—colicky, cyclic, nagging, dull ache; usually in lower abdomen, may radiate down back of legs. May be severe enough to require bed rest for a day or two.
3. Severe dysmenorrhea may be experienced—with chills, headache, diarrhea, nausea, vomiting, and syncope.

Menstruation

Characteristics	Range	Average
Menarche (onset)	9–17 years of age	12.5 years
Cycle length	24–32 days	29 days
Flow—duration	1–8 days	3–5 days
Flow—amount	10–75 ml.	35 ml.
Menopause—onset	45–55 years of age	47–50

D. Etiology

1. Endocrine
   Some investigators believe there is a relation between release of prostaglandin from the endometrium and the symptoms of dysmenorrhea; this has not been proved.
2. Anatomic
   a. Some discomfort results from the passing of a cervical sound or from dilatation of the cervix; a pathologic growth could produce the same symptoms.
   b. An infantile or small uterus may contribute to dysmenorrhea, but this has not been proved.
3. Constitutional
   Chronic illnesses and general debilitation seem to be associated with a high incidence of dysmenorrhea (anemia, fatigue, diabetes, tuberculosis).
4. Psychogenic
   Most studies indicate that strong underlying psychological factors cause dysmenorrhea. Parental instruction and a healthy emotional environment for the growing young girl, in a setting where realistic family relations are cultivated, almost preclude primary dysmenorrhea.

E. Treatment and Nursing Management

Since there is no single treatment for dysmenorrhea, a three-pronged approach seems best to relieve symptoms: Combine therapies as they relate to constitutional, hormonal, and psychological factors.

1. Be selective, according to needs of individual and severity of problem.
   a. Proper psychological preparation of girls for menarche.
   b. Good posture; use special exercises to improve posture and correct weak musculature and imbalance.
2. Since emotional makeup may accentuate discomfort, psychotherapy or pharmacotherapy may be necessary.
3. Complete physical examination to rule out other physical abnormalities.
4. Instructions to patient:
   a. Usual activity is possible—should be encouraged.
   b. Mild analgesics for discomfort are permissible.
   c. Avoid use of habit-forming drugs such as narcotics and alcohol.
5. Dysmenorrhea can usually be eliminated by oral contraceptives which block ovulation.
6. Regular exercises (as well as physical activity) are recommended.
7. Administration of a prostaglandin inhibitor such as ibuprofen (Motrin), mefenamic acid (Ponstel), or naproxen sodium (Anaprox) are recommended in relieving primary dysmenorrhea.
   a. Medications are to be taken with water; milk may be used if the medication causes an upset stomach.
   b. If medication causes drowsiness or sleepiness, do not drive a car or operate machinery.
8. If the above are unsuccessful, surgery may be necessary. Presacral and ovarian neurectomy (cutting nerve fibers) may be done.
9. Psychological counseling may also benefit some individuals.

Premenstrual Syndrome (PMS)

Premenstrual syndrome (PMS) is a condition related to neuroendocrine events within the hypothalamus–pituitary axis that modulate neurotransmitter function.

1. It differs from dysmenorrhea in that it has no relation to ovulation.
2. Some women accept these symptoms as normal.
3. When symptoms are severe, medical relief is sought.

A. Clinical Manifestations

1. Symptoms may begin 10 days or more prior to menstrual flow onset; they diminish 1 or 2 days after menses begin.
2. Edema, breast swelling, abdominal distention—transitory because of increase in water content in tissues.
3. Behavioral—irritability, sleep disturbance, lethargy, depression.
4. Neurologic—headache, vertigo, paresthesia of hands or feet.
5. Respiratory—colds, hoarseness, allergies (asthma) usually worse.
6. Miscellaneous—palpitation, backache, skin problems, eye complaints.

B. Treatment and Nursing Interventions

1. Many forms of therapy have been tried, but research fails to support consistent success.
2. Medications prescribed—progesterone (injection, suppository), oral contraceptives, diuretics, monamine oxidase inhibitors.
3. Placebo/tranquilizers may be helpful.
4. Encourage women with PMS to explore ways and means to avoid stress in the premenstruum; relaxation techniques may be helpful.
5. Restrict sodium intake and limit use of caffeine, tobacco, and alcohol.
6. Try a modified hypoglycemic diet with small, frequent feedings; this often alleviates irritability.
7. Suggest contacting a premenstrual tension center for supportive services and recent research-substantiated treatment recommendations.*

Amenorrhea

Amenorrhea is absence of menstrual flow.

A. Primary—when a girl is 16 or 17 and has not menstruated.

1. May be caused by embryonic maldevelopment.
2. Treatment is according to etiology.

B. Secondary—menstruation has begun (initial menarche) but stops.

1. Criteria
   a. No bleeding for 6 months after having regular cyclic bleeding
   b. No bleeding for 12 months after a history of irregular bleeding
2. Causes
   a. Normal pregnancy and lactation
   b. Psychogenic (minor emotional upsets) Hypothalamic disturbances (autonomic nervous

* National Center for PMS and Menstrual Distress
15 Smith Road
Bedford, NH 03102

The National PMS Society
Box 11467
Durham, NC 27703

PMS Action, Inc.
PO Box 9326
Madison, WI 53715

Rocky Mountain PMS Society
PO Box 16453
Salt Lake City, UT 84116

system) may also be the cause (e.g., anorexia nervosa).
  c. Constitutional
     Any disturbance of metabolism and nutrition (e.g., diabetes, tuberculosis, obesity).
  d. Exercise-related—rigorous involvement
3. Assessment
  a. Progesterone challenge test
     (1) Positive—if bleeding (or even "spotting"); anovulation is most likely
     (2) Negative—no bleeding occurs; indication of end organ failure. Other tests are indicated.
4. Treatment—directed at cause—constitutional therapy, psychotherapy, hormone therapy, surgery.

Oligomenorrhea

Oligomenorrhea is markedly diminished menstrual flow—nearing amenorrhea.

Menorrhagia

Menorrhagia is excessive bleeding during regular menstruation.

A. Causes

1. Endocrine disturbances
2. Inflammatory diseases; benign or malignant pelvic tumors
3. Emotional stress

B. Treatment

1. Search for underlying cause.
2. Correct blood deficiency.

Metrorrhagia

Metrorrhagia is bleeding from uterus between regular menstrual periods. It is significant because it is usually a symptom of some disease—often cancer or benign tumors of uterus and adnexa.

Polymenorrhea

Polymenorrhea is frequent menstruation occurring at intervals of less than 3 weeks.

Menopause

Menopause is the stage of female life when there is physiologic cessation of the menses along with progressive ovarian failure.
  Climacteric is the transition period (perimenopausal period: premenopause, menopause, and postmenopause) during which the woman's reproductive function gradually diminishes and disappears. It usually occurs between the ages of 49 and 55 (mean, 51.4).

Clinical Manifestations

1. The monthly menstrual flow becomes smaller in amount, then becomes irregular, and finally ceases.
2. Hot or warm flashes and other vascular disturbances may be in evidence and are of endocrinologic origin.
3. Additional physical signs
  a. Manifestations of atrophy—sagging structures, atrophic vaginitis
  b. Evidence of stress incontinence on occasion
  c. Skin dryness; weight gain
  d. Calcium deficiency (which may lead to osteoporotic changes)
4. Psychological manifestations
  a. Dizziness, weakness, nervousness, insomnia
  b. Headaches; inability to concentrate
  c. A feeling of being unneeded
  d. Fear of growing old; depression

Treatment and Nursing Interventions

1. Most women respond favorably to a regimen of education and modification of life-style. Adherence to habits that promote good health is desirable.
   In the past, this time in a woman's life was regarded as the onset of old age; a realistic and helpful approach is to realize that the menopausal woman can expect to live another 25 or 30 years.
2. Mild sedatives and tranquilizers may be required by some to relieve nervousness and tension.
3. For persistent or severe hot flashes, it may be necessary to resort to estrogen therapy: diethylstilbestrol,

Premarin, or ethinyl estradiol (Estinyl). Close medical supervision is required.
4. Continued use of estrogens to prevent widespread degenerative changes continues to be controversial; however, long-term use of estrogens has been linked with cancer.
  a. Indications for estrogen replacement therapy include psychomotor complaints, urogenital atrophy, prevention of osteoporosis, and prevention of coronary heart disease.
  b. Future research needs to be directed toward identifying postmenopausal women at risk for osteoporosis and/or coronary heart disease.
  c. Estrogen replacement should not be withheld from women who need it (less than one fourth of menopausal women). Indiscriminate use of estrogens is strongly discouraged.

Health Education

1. "Change of life" is not abnormal nor need it be limiting.
2. Sex life is by no means terminated; in many instances, it is enhanced.
3. Avoid overfatigue and stress situations, since these exaggerate minor problems.
4. Encourage a nutritious diet and keep weight under control.
5. Develop outside interests that help to absorb anxieties and lessen tension.
6. Continue to exercise and develop self-fulfilling and enriching activities.
7. Recognize that the expected life span after menopause is 30–35 years.
8. To alleviate vaginal dryness and pain on intercourse (due to estrogen deficiency), it is safer to use a water-based lubricant (K-Y Jelly or Lubafax) than an estrogen cream.
   Topical estrogens produce systemic effects; therefore, it cannot be assumed that their action has limited local effects.

Diagnostic Studies for Gynecologic Conditions

Pelvic Examination

A *pelvic examination* is an inspection of the external genitalia for signs of inflammation, swelling, bleeding, discharge, or local skin and epithelial changes. A speculum is inserted to permit the examiner to visualize the vagina and cervix.
(For Guidelines: Vaginal Examination by the Nurse, see below.)

A. Patient Preparation

1. Provide psychological support—the patient needs reassurance, understanding, and skillful consideration of her emotional as well as physical problems.
2. Instruct the patient to avoid douching for 24 hours before examination; cellular deposits might wash away.
3. Encourage the patient to void and evacuate the bowels before examination—provides more relaxation of perineal tissues.
4. Advise the patient to remove sufficient clothing to permit adequate exposure of genitalia and allow for examination of the abdomen.
5. Avoid undue exposure of the patient.

B. Positioning of Patient (best done on an examining table but can be achieved on a bed)

1. *Lithotomy*—knees and hips flexed; heels resting on foot rests.
   a. Drape sheet diagonally over the patient so that corner may be grasped and pulled upward to expose perineal area.
   b. When examination is done in bed, the patient is positioned across the bed with hips extending slightly over the edge (dorsal supine position); feet are placed on examiner's knees or on 2 chairs placed next to the bed.
2. *Sims' position*—the patient lies on one side, usually the left, with the left arm behind her back. The right (uppermost) thigh and knee are flexed as much as possible; left leg is partially flexed.
3. *Knee–chest*—the patient kneels on a table with feet extending over the end.
   a. Separate the patient's knees and maintain thighs at right angles to the table.

b. Turn the patient's head to one side and allow face and chest to rest on a soft pillow.
   c. The patient's arms may grasp sides of table.
4. *Semi-sitting*—the patient is placed in a position similar to the lithotomy position with the exception that instead of lying supine, she is in a semi-sitting position.*
Advantages:
   a. Greater patient comfort physically.
   b. Enhanced eye and spoken communication.
   c. Easier bimanual examination for examiner.
   d. With hand-held mirror, the patient is able to see anatomy, lesions, etc.
   e. More effective patient teaching concerning anatomy, pathology, contraceptive information, etc.

C. Procedure for Examining the Pelvis

1. A speculum is inserted so that the vaginal tissues and condition of cervix can be visualized.
2. *Cytology smear* (Papanicolaou, or Pap) is best made by scraping cervix directly (see Fig. 12-1).
3. *Bimanual examination*—by inserting 1 or 2 gloved fingers of the left hand in the vagina and palpating the abdomen with the right hand, it is possible to further examine the uterus and adnexa.
4. *Rectal examination*—to detect abnormalities of contour, motility, and placement of adjacent structures and tissues.

D. Nursing Intervention and Support

1. Attend and support the patient by encouraging her to relax, by holding her hand, etc.
2. Focus the light and uncover examining tray with speculum, swabs, cytology necessities, etc.
3. Assist physician by providing gloves, lubricant, etc.
4. At conclusion of examination, wipe discharge from the patient before assisting her from the table.
5. Have the patient slide up on table before removing feet from stirrups.
6. Allow time for the older patient to adjust to sitting position before helping her off the table.
7. Answer any questions the patient may have; elaborate on physician's instructions.
8. Assist the patient with dressing if necessary.

   * Study done by WH Swartz, MD: JAMA 1984 Mar 2; 251 (9):1163.

Guidelines: Vaginal Examination by the Nurse

Purposes   1. To inspect the vaginal canal and cervix.
2. To obtain tissue specimen for cervical cytology and other tests.

Equipment

Perineal drape
Vaginal specula
Water-soluble lubricant
Sterile gloves

Long swab sticks
Pap smear equipment
Adequate lighting

(continued)

Guidelines: Vaginal Examination by the Nurse (continued)

Procedure

Preparatory Phase

1. Have the patient void before assistant positions her on examining table.
2. Position the patient on examining table (slip may be kept on, but other clothing from waist to knees is removed).
   a. Have buttocks at edge of table.
   b. Position feet in stirrups to assume dorsal lithotomy position.
   c. Make the patient as comfortable as possible with a small pillow under her head.
   d. Drape the patient to permit minimal exposure (but adequate for examiner).
3. Encourage the patient to relax; tell her what you are doing and what she may feel.
4. Adjust light for maximum focus.

Nursing Action	Rationale / Amplification
Performance Phase	
1. Be gentle and take your time; don sterile gloves; lubricate fingers.	1. This promotes relaxation of the patient, making the procedure easier for both.
2. Observe external genitalia for apparent abnormalities, gently separate labia and continue visual inspection.	2. Note any evidence of irritation, infection, or abnormalities.
3. To encourage relaxation in the patient, gently place the tip of 1 or 2 fingers into introitus.	3. Say to the patient, "Tighten your muscles and squeeze my fingers—try hard—then relax."
4. Identify cervix manually and depress the perineum downward with your fingers.	4. Downward pressure is away from the more sensitive anterior structures.
5. Gently insert warm speculum horizontally, passing it over your fingers and aiming it toward the cervix.	5. If it is preferred not to initially insert gloved fingers, the speculum is introduced vertically using a downward pressure; after entering the vestibule, the speculum is slowly rotated to the horizontal position.
6. Slowly open the speculum and lock into position. With slow manipulation, the speculum can be turned to permit visualization of the vaginal walls.	6. Walls normally are pink and moist. A pale white secretion may be noted.
7. Inspect the cervix, which should be pink. Normally, the os is a dent, unless the woman has had children, in which case a slit is noted.	7. If woman is taking an oral contraceptive, the cervix may be deep pink to red. A thread coming out of the cervix would suggest presence of an intrauterine device (IUD).
8. If Pap test is to be done, follow procedure in Figure 12-1. For a Schiller test, see p. 565.	
9. When removing speculum, hold it open until cervix is cleared, then withdraw speculum, allowing it to close.	9. By the time speculum is completely withdrawn, it will be closed.
10. For palpation (bimanual examination) see above.	
Follow-up Phase	
1. Gently wipe the perineal area with soft tissue or gauze, using firm strokes from the pubic area back to beyond the rectum.	1. This will remove secretions and liquid lubricant.
2. Instruct assistant in carefully helping the patient to remove feet from stirrups.	2. Both feet must be removed at the same time to reduce strain.
3. Elevate the lower third of the examining table to receive legs. Keep the patient covered with a sheet.	3. This permits the patient to assume dorsal recumbent position.
4. Assist the patient in sliding toward head end of table; provide a wide-based stool for her to step on as she gets off table.	4. Do not rush the patient as she is getting off the table, since sudden shifting from recumbent to sitting position may cause a feeling of dizziness.
5. Assist the patient in dressing (closing zippers, etc.) if necessary. Answer any queries she may have.	

Other Diagnostic Tests

Cytology Test for Cancer (Papanicolaou)

A. **Purpose**—To screen for cervical dysplasia and/or cervical cancer. Occasionally, adenocarcinoma of the endometrium will also be discovered.

B. **Procedure**—see Figure 12-1

1. Examination and interpretation of cytologic smear is done by the pathologist.
2. Classification of cytologic findings (after Papanicolaou):

Class 1—absence of atypical or abnormal cells.
Class 2—atypical cytology but no evidence of malignancy.
Class 3—cytology suggestive of, but not conclusive for, malignancy.
Class 4—cytology strongly suggestive of malignancy.
Class 5—cytology conclusive for malignancy.

3. If the patient has an abnormal smear of class 2, 3, or 4, explain to her that this is not conclusive but requires additional testing such as biopsy and conization.

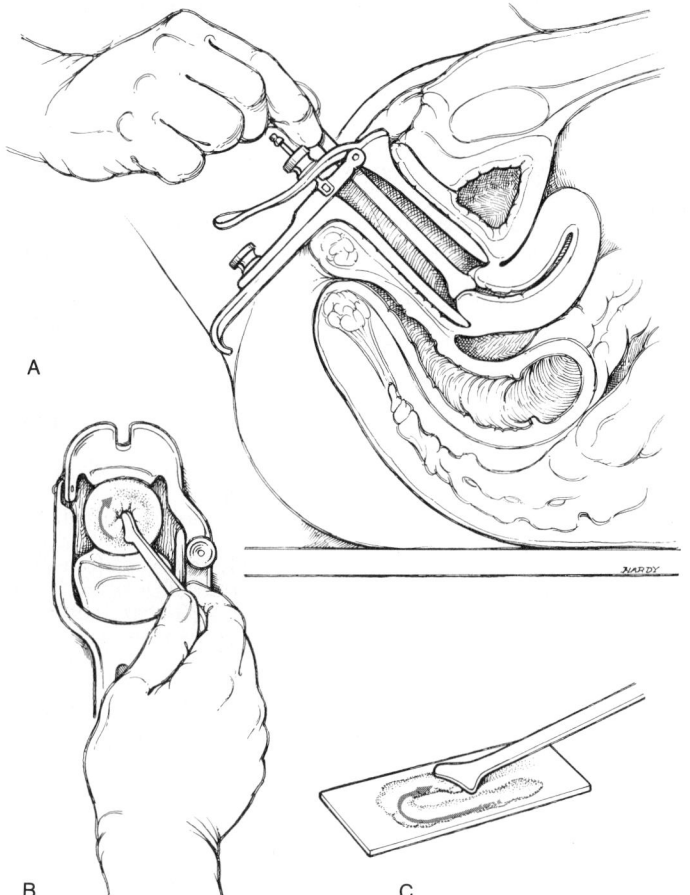

A

B

C

Figure 12-1. A cervical scrape of secretions for cytology is obtained by using a wooden Ayre spatula. (*A*) Shows the speculum in place: the Ayre spatula is inserted so that the longer end is placed snugly in the os. (*B*) A representative sample of secretions is obtained by rotating the spatula. (*C*) Cervical secretions are gently smeared on a glass slide in a single circular motion. The slide is placed in the appropriate fixative. Using a cotton-tipped applicator, also obtain a smear from the floor of the vagina below the cervix and preserve in the same manner.

Schiller's Iodine Test

(A simple test to outline unhealthy epithelium)

A. Rationale—Cancer epithelium contains no glycogen, whereas normal cervical epithelial cells do contain glycogen; glycogen has the ability to absorb iodine stain.

Note: Schiller's test is unreliable for cancer and only suggests some epithelial change.

B. Procedure—A long applicator stick is used to paint the cervix with Schiller's 2% iodine solution.

1. Negative result—a mahogany brown color covering entire surface indicates a reaction between iodine and glycogen of normal cells.
2. Positive result—tissues are not stained brown; this indicates that immature cells are present and suggests the need for a biopsy.

Cervical Biopsy and Cauterization

A. Purpose—To remove cervical tissue for laboratory study.

B. Patient Preparation

1. To be done preferably at a time when cervix is least vascular (usually a week after the end of the menstrual flow).
2. Explain the nature of the procedure to the patient.

3. Place the patient in lithotomy position and drape her properly.
4. Explain to the patient that no anesthesia is required, since the cervix does not have pain receptors.

C. Procedure

1. After the speculum is positioned in the vagina and the cervix properly exposed, the surgeon, under colposcopic guidance, uses a biopsy forceps to obtain bits of cervical tissues.
2. Tissue is preserved in 10% formalin, labeled, and sent to the laboratory.
3. If bleeding occurs, suturing and packing may be necessary.

D. Aftercare of Patient

1. A brief rest after the procedure is usually necessary before the patient leaves.
2. Discharge instructions/health education—instruct the patient as follows:
   a. Avoid heavy lifting for 24 hours.
   b. Packing will remain in place for 12–24 hours, depending on physician's preference.
   c. There may be some bleeding; however, more than that of a normal period must be reported to the physician.
   d. Obtain physician's instructions regarding douching and sexual relations.

Uterotubal Insufflation (Rubin's Test)

Carbon dioxide is injected under pressure through a special cannula into the cervical canal. If 1 or both tubes are patent, the gas will pass through the uterine tubes into the peritoneal cavity.

1. The patient is prepared as for a vaginal examination.
2. A Graves speculum is positioned in the vagina.
3. Special cannula is passed through intrauterine canal; cervix is held tightly with a tenaculum against a rubber stopper to prevent gas leakage.
4. Tubing is connected to a machine that measures and records pressure.

Findings

1. Normal—if pressure is below 180 mm. Hg, and gas is heard (with a stethoscope) passing through the tubes
2. Partial obstruction—180–200 mm. Hg
3. Complete obstruction—200 mm. Hg and above

Culdoscopy

A *culdoscopy* is an uncommon operative, diagnostic procedure in which an incision is made into the posterior vaginal cul-de-sac so that a culdoscope can be inserted for the purpose of visualizing the uterus, tubes, broad ligaments, uterosacral ligaments, rectal wall, sigmoid, and even the small intestines.

1. The patient is prepared as for any vaginal operation.
2. Anesthesia may be local, general, or regional.
3. The knee–chest position is best for a culdoscopy.
4. Following the examination, the scope is withdrawn and sutures placed; the patient is returned to her room.

Hysteroscopy

Hysteroscopy is the endoscopic visualization of the uterine cavity by means of a hysteroscope.

1. Earlier attempts were usually unsuccessful because uterine bleeding obscured the view.
2. Today, fiberoptic lighting and the distention of the uterine cavity with dextran solution permits optimal visualization.

A. Indications—primarily to complement other diagnostic procedures, chiefly the staging of endometrial cancer.

1. Problem of infertility
2. When the cause of uterine bleeding is unknown
3. To view lesions that can be photographed and, in some instances, removed

4. To diagnose and manage intrauterine adhesions
5. For transuterine tubal sterilization

B. Contraindications

1. Pelvic infection
2. Recurrent upper genital tract infection
3. Uterine perforation
4. Pregnancy, because of possible disturbance of pregnancy and risk of infection

C. Patient Preparation and Examination

1. Administer the prescribed sedative and mild tranquilizer prior to the examination. Explanation is similar to that for dilatation and curettage (D&C).
2. Place the patient in the lithotomy position as for a D&C.
3. Cleanse the perineum and vagina immediately prior to sterile draping.
4. The examiner performs a bimanual palpation of the uterus.
5. Inject local anesthesia into the cervix, which is positioned with a tenaculum forceps.
6. Insert sounds into the cervical canal for dilatation prior to insertion of endoscope.
7. With endoscope in place, slowly infuse endometrial cavity with a concentrated solution of dextran.
8. Uterine walls are visualized with a 30-degree oblique lens rather than with the 180-degree system.

D. Follow-up

1. Following removal of instruments, the patient is encouraged to rest.
2. The patient may be discharged later the same day.

X-Ray Studies—Hysterosalpingogram

A *hysterosalpingogram* is an x-ray study of the uterus and uterine tubes following the injection of a contrast medium.

A. Purpose

1. To study sterility problems
2. To determine extent of tubal patency
3. To note the presence of pathology in the uterine cavity

B. Procedure

1. The patient is placed in lithotomy position on a fluoroscopic x-ray table.
2. The bivalve speculum is introduced to expose cervix.
3. Contrast medium is injected into uterine cavity.
4. X-rays are taken to determine configuration of pelvic area.

Guidelines: Colposcopy

Colposcopy is a stereoscopic examination of the cervix using a binocular instrument with strong light illumination.

Purposes
1. To determine distribution of abnormal squamous epithelium.
2. To pinpoint areas from which biopsy tissue can be taken.

Indications

1. Following atypical vaginal or cervical cytology (in Pap smear).
2. When suspicious cervical lesions are present.
3. Previous treatment for dysplasia or cancer of the cervix.

Advantage: Colposcopy may spare the patient a conization or D&C.

Procedure

Preparatory Phase

1. Identical to that for preparation of patient having pelvic examination (see p. 564).
2. Additional explanation may be required so that the patient will know what to expect.

Nursing Action	Rationale/Amplification
Performance Phase	
1. Use a long cotton applicator stick to dry cervix.	1. This will clear away mucus and other secretions.
2. Swab cervix with saline, using long cotton applicator.	2. Moistening of cervical epithelium allows vascular patterns and squamous columnar junction to be visualized.
3. Examine tissue with colposcope, utilizing green filter illuminator.	
4. Paint cervix with 3% acetic acid.	4. This acts as a mucolytic agent and accentuates epithelial topography.
5. Note colposcopic patterns—particularly the transformation area (where columnar epithelium is replaced by squamous epithelium).	5. Acetic acid tends to draw moisture from tissues of high nuclear density—this accounts for color changes in the cervical epithelium.
6. Biopsy (using a fine biopsy forceps) any questionable area; endocervical curettage should also be done.	6. Since the cervical os has few nerve endings, the patient will experience minimal discomfort.
7. If bleeding occurs, direct pressure or application of silver nitrate stick will usually stop it. Some clinicians prefer to apply ferric subsulfate (Monsel's solution) via applicator stick for hemostasis.	7. Measures to prevent or control bleeding.
8. Insert a vaginal tampon following examination.	8. To absorb discharge; may be removed after 5–6 hours.

Follow-up Phase

Similar to that following pelvic examination, see p. 564.

Dilatation and Curettage (D&C)

Dilatation and curettage is a widening of the cervical canal with a dilator and the scraping of the uterine canal with a curette. The cervix is scraped first without dilatation.

Goals:

1. Control abnormal uterine bleeding.
2. Secure endometrial and endocervical tissue for tissue study.
3. Serve as a therapeutic measure for incomplete abortion.

Nursing Management

A. Preoperative Care

1. Inform the patient of the nature of the operation to be done (usually done by a gynecologist).
2. Ascertain what the patient has been told about postoperative discomfort and drainage following the D&C.
3. Answer questions the patient has about the procedure and aftercare.
4. Request the patient to void.

B. Postoperative Care

1. Check that perineal pad is in place with a sanitary belt.
2. Replace each perineal pad with a sterile pad as required during the time packing is in place.
3. Report excessive bleeding.
4. Recommend bed rest for the remainder of the day, with bathroom privileges.
5. Offer mild analgesics for low back pain and pelvic discomfort.
6. Offer meals as desired.

Conditions of the External Genitalia and Vagina

Pruritus (Itching) and Contact Dermatitis (Vulva)

Assessment

Nursing history and physical examination. Itching is often more acute at night; aggravated by warmth and scratching.

Causative Factors

1. Faulty perineal hygiene followed by itching
2. Itching causes scratching, which presents an open lesion subject to many irritants:
   a. Vaginal discharge, skin secretions, menstrual discharge
   b. Urine, feces
3. Mechanical irritation
   a. Close-fitting, synthetic fabrics
4. Chemical irritation
   a. Laundry detergent (washed clothing not completely rinsed)
   b. Vaginal sprays, deodorants, perfumes
5. Chronic infections, such as
   a. Trichomonas, gonorrhea, yeast
   b. Systemic—diabetes mellitus
6. Allergy or sensitivity reactions

Health Education

1. Cleanliness must be scrupulous.
   a. Use cotton pledgets that have been moistened in a warm, bland soap solution.

b. Always wipe from front to back.
c. Pat dry.
d. Dust lightly with nonirritating powder (cornstarch).
2. Do not use sprays, perfumed soaps, or topical anesthetic agents—they may compound the problem.
3. Replace synthetic-fabric undergarments with loose cotton underclothing.
4. Avoid wearing tight garments over the cotton undergarments.
5. Take prescribed pharmacotherapeutic agents.
a. Utilize cool compresses.
b. Apply soothing lotions and ointments (hydrocortisone).
c. Take sedatives to promote sleep at night.
6. Control allergies if this is a cause.
7. Control glucosuria and incontinence.

Vulvitis and Abscess of Greater Vestibular Gland (Bartholin's Gland)

Vulvitis is an inflammation of the vulva; the cause may be infection, possibly caused by uncleanliness. Common offending organisms are *Escherichia coli,* staphylococcus, streptococcus, gonococcus, and *Trichomonas vaginalis.*

Clinical Manifestations

1. Burning pain, which is worse with intercourse.
2. Red and edematous tissue with profuse purulent exudate.
3. Acute throbbing pain and swelling between labia, indicating vulvovaginal abscess (infection of Bartholin's glands).
4. When the acute infection subsides, the problem tends to become chronic.

Treatment and Nursing Interventions

1. Advise the patient to remain in bed; administer analgesics for the relief of pain.
2. Employ thermotherapy in the form of hot packs and sitz baths for comfort.
3. Administer broad-spectrum antibacterial agents to combat infection.
4. Prepare the patient for incision and drainage of the abscess, which will afford immediate relief.
5. Marsupialization (creation of a pouch), with or without biopsy, is indicated when there are painful recurrences or obstruction at introitus.
a. Ice packs are applied intermittently for 24 hours to reduce edema and provide comfort.
b. Thereafter, warm sitz baths or a perineal heat lamp are comforting.

Guidelines: Vaginal Irrigation

Purpose
1. To cleanse or disinfect the vagina and adjacent tissues.
2. To soothe inflamed tissue.

Equipment
1. Sterile reservoir for irrigating fluid—can or bag.
2. Sterile irrigating fluid as prescribed (1,000–4,000 ml.) at 40.5°–43.3° C. (105°–110° F.)
3. Tubing, connecting tubes, and clamp (sterile)
4. Irrigating vaginal nozzle (sterile)
5. Bedpan or douche pan
6. Plastic or rubber sheet with cloth protection
7. Sterile cotton balls, cleansing solution
8. Sterile disposable gloves

Procedure (Fig. 12-2)

Nursing Action	Rationale/Amplification
Preparatory Phase	
1. Have the patient void before beginning irrigation.	1. A full bladder would prevent adequate distention of vagina by solution.
2. Place the patient in dorsal recumbent position.	2. To permit gravity to assist in allowing fluid to reach distal areas of vagina.
3. Drape the patient.	3. To prevent chilling and undue exposure.
4. Arrange irrigating receptacle at a level just above the patient's hips (not more than ⅔ meter, i.e., 2 feet, above hips) so that fluid flows easily but gently.	4. The higher the fluid source, the greater the pressure.
Performance Phase	
1. Cleanse vulva by separating labia and allowing solution to flow over area; if insufficient, use cotton balls saturated in soap solution, cleanse from front toward anal area.	1. Materials found around vaginal meatus may be introduced into vagina and cervix. This is to be avoided.
2. Allow some solution to flow through tubing and out over nozzle to lubricate it.	2. Moisture provides lubrication and less resistance when one surface is moved against another.
3. Insert nozzle gently into vagina in a downward and backward direction.	3. When the patient is in a dorsal recumbent position, the natural anatomical position of the vagina is in the downward-backward direction.

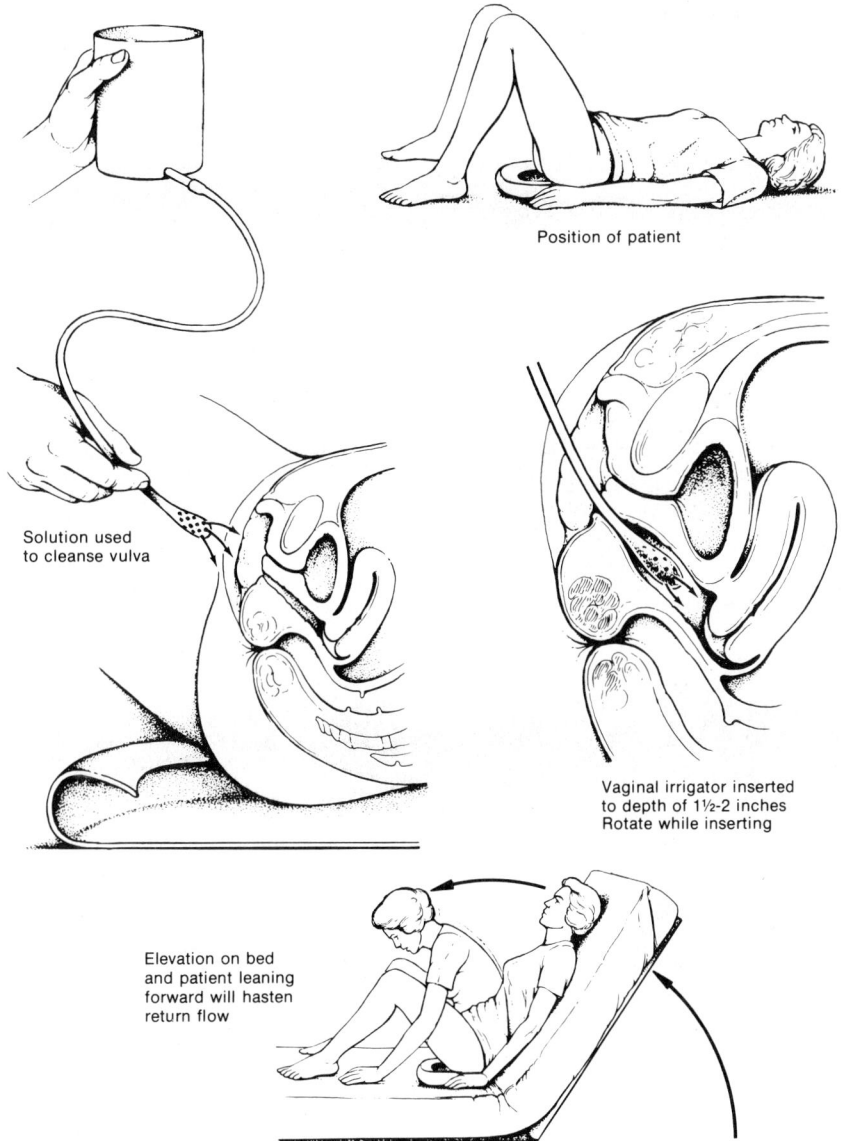

Position of patient

Solution used to cleanse vulva

Vaginal irrigator inserted to depth of 1½-2 inches Rotate while inserting

Elevation on bed and patient leaning forward will hasten return flow

Figure 12-2. Vaginal irrigation.

Procedure
(Cont.)

Nursing Action	**Rationale/Amplification**
4. Rotate nozzle gently in the vagina during inflow.	4. All surfaces are irrigated when nozzle is rotated.
5. Clamp tubing when solution is almost all used, remove nozzle and permit the patient to sit on bedpan for return flow.	5. Gravity will assist in allowing return flow to drain from vaginal tract.

Follow-up Phase

1. Wipe the patient dry, using cotton balls in a front-to-back direction.	1. Drying the area prevents skin excoriation and promotes comfort.
2. Remove bedpan from the patient and apply sterile perineal pad.	
3. Cleanse equipment with soap and water, dry before storing in well-ventilated area.	3. This will prolong life of equipment.

Guidelines: Vulvar Irrigation

Purpose   To cleanse the perineal area after urination or a bowel movement in order to minimize infection.

Equipment

Sterile pitcher with irrigating fluid (300–500 ml.) 40.5°–43.3° C. (105°–110° F.)

Sterile sponge forceps and cotton pledgets

Bedpan

Plastic or rubber sheet with cloth protection

Paper bag for cotton pledget disposal

Procedure (Fig. 12-3)

Preparatory Phase

1. Place patient in dorsal recumbent position with knees flexed and separated.
2. Place protecting sheet under patient.

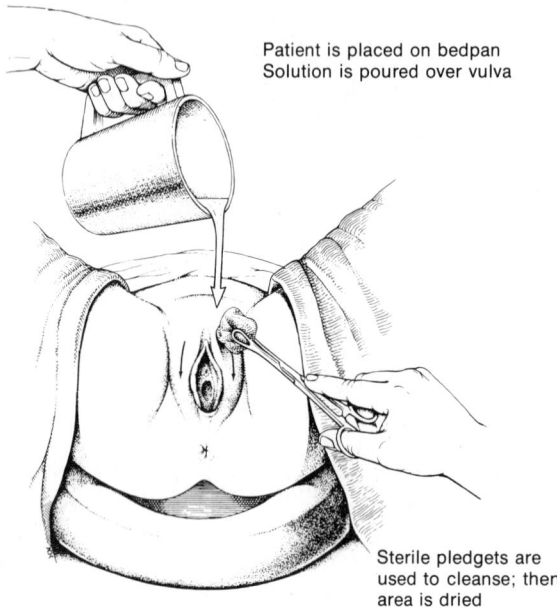

Patient is placed on bedpan
Solution is poured over vulva

Sterile pledgets are used to cleanse; then area is dried

The bedpan is removed
The posterior area is dried

Figure 12-3. Perineal care.

Nursing Action	Rationale/Amplification
Performance Phase	
1. Pour warmed irrigating solution gently over vulva from a sterile pitcher.	1. Materials will be flushed from perineal area into bedpan.
2. Cleanse perineal area with cotton pledget held in a sponge holder, use a top-down direction and discard each sponge in a plastic or paper bag after one use.	2. Friction facilitates cleansing process and the removal of soil.
3. Dry perineal area using dry cotton pledgets in same fashion as for cleansing.	3. Cleansing from front to back assists in preventing intestinal organisms from entering vaginal area.
Follow-up Phase	
1. Apply sterile perineal pad.	1. To maintain cleanliness and provide comfort for patient.

Vaginal Fistula

A *fistula* is an abnormal, tortuous opening between 2 internal hollow organs, or between an internal hollow organ and the exterior of the body.

Ureterovaginal fistula is an opening between the ureter and vagina.

Vesicovaginal fistula is an opening between the bladder and vagina.

Rectovaginal fistula is an opening between the rectum and vagina.

Causes

Vaginal fistula may result from
1. Obstetric injury
2. Pelvic surgery (hysterectomy or vaginal reconstructive procedures are most common)

3. Extension of carcinoma or a complication of treatment for carcinoma

Clinical Manifestations

1. Patient with vesicovaginal fistula will experience continuous trickling of urine into vagina.
2. Patient with rectovaginal fistula will experience fecal incontinence and flatus passed through vagina, a malodorous condition.

Diagnostic Aids in Locating Fistula Site

1. Methylene blue test—following instillation of this dye in the bladder
   a. Methylene blue appears in vagina in vesicovaginal fistula.
   b. Methylene blue does not appear in vagina in ureterovaginal fistula.
2. Indigo carmine test—following a negative methylene blue test, indigo carmine is injected intravenously. If dye appears in vagina, this indicates a ureteral fistula.
3. Intravenous pyelogram—(see p. 500) a valuable test for determining presence of hydroureter or hydronephrosis, and position or location of the fistula.
4. Cystoscopy—performed to determine number and location of fistulas.

Treatment

1. In rare cases, a fistula will heal without surgical intervention.
2. Fistulas recognized at time of delivery should be corrected immediately.
3. Treatment of postoperative fistulas is delayed, sometimes for 2 or 3 months, to allow for treatment of inflammation.
4. Surgery is recommended if tissues are healthy.

Nursing Interventions

A. Promotion of Healing

1. Maintain cleanliness · by encouraging frequent, soothing sitz baths and deodorizing douches.
2. Use perineal pads and plastic or rubber pants if required.
3. Provide optimal skin care to prevent excoriation; bland creams or a light dusting of cornstarch may be soothing.
4. Recognize value of meeting psychosocial needs, such as feminine morale boosters (attractive hairdo, nail polish, perfume, new bed jacket, etc.); encourage visitors, diversion, recreation, activities, etc.

B. Preoperative

1. Maintain adequate nutrition; increase intake of vitamins and protein content of meals.
2. Promote local cleanliness by vaginal flushing and rectal enemas.
3. Administer chemotherapeutic agents to reduce pathogenic flora in intestine.
4. If the patient is postmenopausal, oral estrogen may be given to promote healthier, more viable tissue in the operative area.

C. Postoperative

1. Rectovaginal fistula
   a. Limit bowel activity by keeping patient on clear fluids for several days; progress to a low residue, then a full diet.
   b. Give warm perineal irrigations and perhaps controlled heat lamp treatments to assist the healing process.
   c. Encourage rest because of the high degree of debilitation.
2. Vesicovaginal fistula
   a. Maintain proper drainage from indwelling catheter—otherwise, pressure may build up and be exerted against newly sutured tissues.
   b. Employ gentleness in administering bladder or vaginal irrigations because of tenderness of the operative site.
   c. Pay particular attention to urinary output.

Vaginal Infections

Normal Vaginal Condition

1. The vaginal secretions are acid (pH 3.5–4.5); acidity is produced by the conversion of cellular glycogen to lactic acid by Döderlein's bacilli, which normally inhabit the vagina.
2. When estrogen production is low (before menarche and after menopause) the epithelium is inactive; the cells contain no glycogen; lactobacilli (Döderlein's bacilli) are absent, and the pH is between 6 and 7.
3. *Leukorrhea* is a whitish vaginal discharge; it is considered normal to have a slight discharge at the time of ovulation or just before menstruation.

Assessment

History and Physical Examination

1. Health history including questions specific to the condition:
   a. Nature of discharge: Cheese-like, frothy, pus-like, thick or thin, scant? When was it first noticed? Character, color, odor? Other symptoms: dysuria, itching, dyspareunia?
   b. Menstrual history: Age at menarche, menopause; length of cycles, duration and amount of flow, dysmenorrhea, amenorrhea, dysfunctional bleeding?
   c. Disease history: Presence of diabetes mellitus in patient or family? Other debilitating diseases? Control of these? Previous vaginal infections? Sexually transmitted diseases?
   d. Pregnancy history
   e. Sexual history: Partner(s), how active sexually? Its nature? Urogenital infections in partner? Nature of contraceptives?
   f. Medications being taken: Purpose?
   g. Vaginal hygiene: Use of douches, deodorants, sprays, ointments; type of tampons, bubble bath, shower/bath, nature of clothing (tight-fitting)?
   h. Concerns, stresses, anxieties, any questions?
2. Physical examination, including vaginal examination

Diagnostic Tests

1. Laboratory tests, including wet smear for microscopic examination
   a. Saline slide—discharge mixed with saline; useful in detecting *Gardnerella* and *Trichomonas*.
   b. Potassium hydroxide (KOH)—discharge mixed with 10% KOH; useful in detecting *C. albicans*. If fishy odor is noted, suspect *Gardnerella*.
2. Culture—significant when purulent discharge is present; used to detect gonorrhea.
3. Vaginal pH—use Nitrazine paper
   Normal pH—4.0–4.5

Gardnerella—5.0–5.5
Trichomonas—5.5+
4. Pap test

Patient Problems/Nursing Diagnoses

(For vaginal infections)
1. Discomfort and pain related to abnormal discharge
2. Irritation of vaginal mucous membrane and perineum related to infection and invasion of pathogenic organisms
3. Knowledge deficit of adequate vaginal hygiene
4. Fear related to possible acquisition of an "incurable" sexually transmitted disease
5. Potential for altered pH and growth of pathogens related to excess carbohydrate intake
6. Sexual dysfunction related to discomfort and abnormal discharge

Planning and Implementation
Nursing Interventions

A. Relief of pain and correction of abnormal discharge

1. Reduce local irritation and discomfort by applying prescribed medication to affected area as recommended.
2. Foster cleanliness by meticulous care after voiding and defecation.
3. Initiate chemotherapy and/or antibiotics as prescribed to control infectious organisms.

B. Treatment regimen for abnormal vaginal condition

1. Tell why the perineal area must be clean before applying prescribed ointments, etc.
2. Demonstrate how medication is applied locally, depending on its nature (ointment, suppository, or tube-full of vaginal gel).
3. Stress the importance of following the recommended time frame for taking medication.
4. Emphasize the importance of keeping follow-up appointments.

C. Practice of proper hygienic vaginal care

1. Encourage correct procedure of wiping from front to back following urination and/or defecation.
2. Suggest a daily shower rather than tub bathing, since the latter may cause reinfection of the genital area.
3. Discuss the problem of irritation of tissues that results when tight-fitting garments are worn.
4. Explain the importance of changing sanitary pads and tampons frequently.

D. Coping abilities to overcome fear of "incurable illness"

1. Discuss the nature of the infecting organisms and its preference for the "warm, dark, undisturbed" cavity (vagina).
2. Explain the effect of prescribed local or systemic medication on the offending organism.

E. Modification of dietary intake of carbohydrates

1. Explain the effect of a high-carbohydrate diet on maintaining an optimal pH in the vaginal vault to prevent growth of undesirable organisms.
2. Describe what foods (that the patient enjoys) should be eliminated.
3. Suggest alternate kinds of equally satisfying foods.

F. Promotion of satisfactory sexual relations with partner

1. Recommend that the partner be checked medically if he has a discharge or other symptoms suggestive of an infection.
2. Discuss interim sexual habits that can be enjoyed without intercourse.

Health Education

1. Avoid irritating douches, bubble bath, and deodorant sprays.
2. Following urination and defecation, wipe from front to back.
3. Wear comfortably fitting undergarments; white cotton is safer than other fabrics during the treatment period.
4. Avoid intercourse during active infection of vagina.
5. Encourage partner to seek treatment if he has a discharge or infection.
6. Vaginal infections increase with multiple sex partners.
7. Recommend partner wear a condom if intercourse is resumed before treatment is completed.

Evaluation
Expected Outcomes

1. Enjoys relief of pain and absence of abnormal discharge.
2. Accepts treatment regimen and can verbalize what is to be done if there is a recurrence of the problem.
3. Recites the proper practice for maintaining adequate vaginal hygiene.
4. Demonstrates lessening of fear; can discuss difference between malignancy and vaginal infection.
5. Prepares a dietary plan to show how carbohydrate intake is reduced.
6. Indicates to what extent sexual relations may be resumed.

Kinds of Vaginitis

Description	Manifestations	Treatment
Simple Vaginitis		
An inflammation of the vagina, with discharge; this may be due to invading organisms, irritation, poor hygiene. *Urethritis* often accompanies vaginitis because of the proximity of the urethra to the vagina.	1. Increased vaginal discharge with itching, redness, burning, and edema. 2. Voiding and defecation aggravate the above symptoms.	1. Enhance the natural vaginal flora by administering a weak acid douche, 15 ml. of vinegar to 1,000 ml. water, (1 T. white vinegar to 1 qt. water). 2. Stimulate the growth of lactobacilli (Döderlein's bacilli) by ad-

Description	Manifestations	Treatment
Predisposing factors: *Trichomonas vaginalis, Candida* or *Monilia, Gardnerella vaginalis, Pediculosis pubis,* contact allergens, excessive perspiration, poor hygiene, foreign bodies (tampons, condoms, diaphragms that have been left in too long)		ministering beta-lactose vaginal suppository; this dissolves with body heat, and the sugar then acts. 3. Foster cleanliness by meticulous care after voiding and defecation. 4. Control infection by initiating chemotherapy: Insert medication into vagina via applicator or by using a chemotherapeutic cream locally as prescribed.
Gardnerella Vaginitis An inflammation of the vagina heretofore referred to as "nonspecific vaginitis," since it is not caused by *Trichomonas, Candida,* or gonorrhea. It is considered a sexually transmitted disease.	1. Vaginal discharge with odor. 2. Itching and burning may suggest concomitant organisms present. 3. It is benign in that when the discharge is wiped away, underlying tissue is healthy and pink. 4. Vaginal pH is between 5.0 and 5.5.	1. Metronidazole (Flagyl) taken 3 times daily for 7 days. 2. Alcohol intake should be avoided during Flagyl treatment to avoid nausea and vertigo. 3. Centers for Disease Control does not recommend treating partners with Flagyl unless the condition is recurrent.
Trichomonas Vaginalis A condition produced by a protozoan that infects the vagina and that is evident as a bubbly, greenish-yellow, irritating leukorrhea and as a red, speckled ("strawberry") punctate hemorrhages on the cervix.	1. Caused by a pear-shaped mobile flagellate that thrives in an alkaline medium. 2. *Trichomonas vaginalis* is persistent and resistant. 3. Vulvar edema, dysuria, and hyperemia occur secondary to irritation of discharge. 4. Remissions may occur; the organism meanwhile remains inaccessible to treatment in the urinary tract. 5. The male may carry the organism in his urogenital tract and reinfect his partner.	1. Destroy infective protozoa by taking metronidazole (Flagyl) for 10 days (orally). NOTE: Flagyl is contraindicated in the first trimester of pregnancy. 2. Prevent reinfection by treating male concurrently with Flagyl.
Candida Albicans A fungal infection caused by *Candida albicans.* *Incidence*—several factors have been found to be significantly associated with the incidence of *Candida albicans:* 1. Drug addiction 2. Obesity 3. Pregnancy 4. Antibiotic therapy 5. Diabetes mellitus 6. Oral contraceptives 7. Frequent douching 8. Chronic debilitative diseases Characteristics 1. *Candida albicans* is a normal inhabitant of the intestinal tract and therefore a frequent contaminant of the vagina.	1. Vaginal discharge is thick and irritating; white or yellow patchy, cheese-like particles adhere to vaginal walls. 2. Itching is common; dyspareunia, frequency, and dysuria. 3. Appearance of vulva and vagina varies from normal to that of an acute inflammation.	1. Eradicate the fungus by applying miconazole nitrate (Monistat 7) vaginal cream, 1 application daily at bedtime for 7 days; and clotrimazole (Gyne-Lotrimin Vaginal Cream) one applicator-full intravaginally nightly for 1 week. 2. Treat the symptomatic or uncircumcised partner by applying antifungal cream under the foreskin nightly for 7 nights.

(continued)

Description	Manifestations	Treatment

2. Since this fungus thrives in an environment rich in carbohydrates, it is seen commonly in patients with poorly controlled diabetes.

3. This infection is observed in patients who have been on antibiotic or steroid therapy for a while (reduces natural protective organisms in vagina).

Atrophic (Postmenopausal) Vaginitis

This is a common postmenopausal occurrence. Because of atrophy of vaginal mucosa, the woman is prone to postmenopausal dyspareunia (painful intercourse due to a tight vagina).

Vesicovaginal itching, burning, dyspareunia, and vulvar irritation.

▶ **Nursing Alert:** In the postmenopausal woman, if vaginal bleeding occurs, encourage the patient to see her physician immediately, because cancer may be suspected.

Since this is a manifestation of general body estrogenic depletion, the patient should be treated with oral, water-soluble, natural, conjugated estrogen (Premarin).

The condition reverses itself under treatment, which must be maintained.

If infection is also present, this is treated.

Estrogenic or cortisone vaginal cream may be prescribed.

Herpes Virus Type 2 Infection (Herpes Genitalis, Herpes Simplex Virus [HSV])

Herpes genitalis is a viral infection that causes herpetic lesions on the cervix, vagina, and external genitalia; it is primarily acquired by sexual transmission. It is also possible to acquire the infection by sitting on a plastic surface in a health spa that was previously occupied by a person who had the infection.

1. It is estimated that 10–20 million Americans have genital herpes.
2. At least 300,000 new cases occur annually.
3. A striking representation of the rapid spread of this condition is noted in Figure 12-4, which is based on the number of patient visits to the offices of private physicians from 1966–1983.

Health Implications

1. Babies delivered vaginally may become infected with the virus; there is significant fetal morbidity and mortality. In the early pregnancy, there is increased incidence of spontaneous abortion.
2. Incidence of cervical cancer is higher in women who have had genital herpes.

Assessment

History, Nursing and Medical

1. A sexual history is taken to reveal frequency and types of sexual activity and kinds of discomforts noted.
2. Urogenital history to suggest nature of problems—pruritus, burning, tenderness, urinary symptoms, and unusual discharge.
3. Psychosocial concerns—stigmas, fears, misinformation.

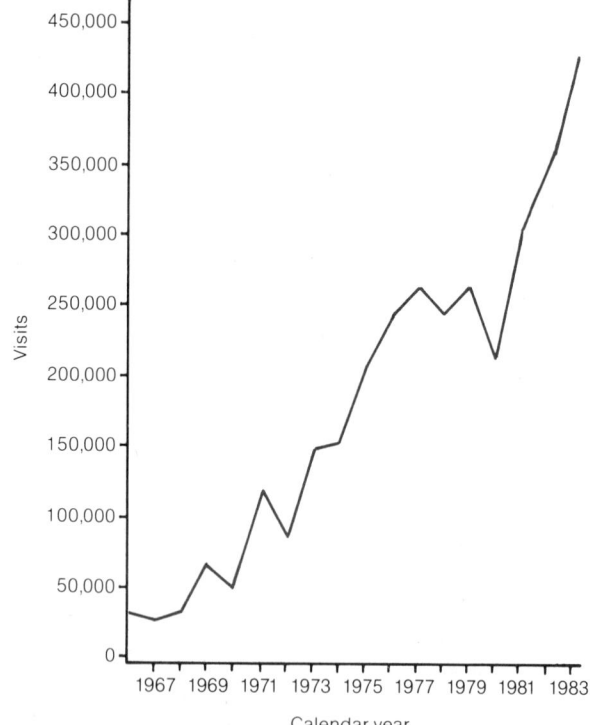

Figure 12-4. Herpes genitalis (number of visits to private physicians' offices, United States, calendar years 1966–1981. (Adapted from CUTIS, 33 (1):75, Jan 1984; with permission. Original graph and update, courtesy NDTI, IMS, Inc., Ambler, PA)

Clinical Manifestations

1. Herpes genitalis is manifested within 3–7 days and is most prevalent in young adults.
2. Multiple vesicles appear on the vulva; surrounding area is inflamed and edematous.
3. Itching may be intense and even painful; scratching may further aggravate the problem.
4. Lesions appear on the vulva, and in most patients, the cervix is also involved; it, too, may be inflamed and edematous, and bleeds easily when touched. Lesions may develop into painful ulcers.
5. A profuse watery discharge may be present.
6. Fever, malaise, and headache may accompany the acute flare-up.
7. A sensation of burning may develop along with dysuria.
8. Within 1–4 weeks, the sores disappear; however, the virus remains in the body, and recurrences are common with leukorrhea, abnormal bleeding, vaginal pain, and dyspareunia.

Diagnostic Evaluation

1. Usually can be made by inspection.
2. To determine true causative agent, cell cultures are taken; 1–3 days required for results.
3. Pap smear—if herpes infection is present, multinucleated giant cells are noted.
4. Tzanck smear
   a. Scrapings from base of a vesicle are obtained.
   b. If herpetic, multinucleated giant cells containing viral inclusion bodies are noted.
   c. Note: Other herpetic disease such as "shingles" or chickenpox will also yield positive findings.
5. Immunofluorescence

Patient Problems/Nursing Diagnoses

1. Pain and discomfort related to herpetic lesions/ulcers of the genitalia
2. Distorted self-image related to the "stigma" of having genital herpes, and possibly a feeling of being betrayed by the partner
3. Sexual dysfunction and social isolation related to the effects of a sexually transmitted condition, including guilt and embarrassment
4. Lesions and ulcer of the genitalia
5. Knowledge deficit of the nature of genital herpes

Planning and Implementation

Treatment

1. Acyclovir (Zovirax) ointment reduces pain and shortens time the herpetic patient can infect others.
2. Oral acyclovir (investigational) given in capsule form interferes with the reproductive process of the virus, thereby reducing recurrences. Recommended for those who had had repeated recurrences.
3. A gel of 2-deoxy-D-glucose (2-DDG) in miconazole nitrate (2%) cream or in miconazole alone has been effective in providing relief of pain and dysuria in 12–72 hours.
4. Other investigational drugs are FIAC, cyclaradine, bromovinyl-dioxyuridine, ribavarin, body's own antiviral agent—interferon, and vaccines.
5. Support and understanding are parts of the therapeutic regimen.

Nursing Interventions

A. Healing of Genital Tissue with Relief of Pain and Discomfort

1. Recommend that the patient take the prescribed analgesics and apply the proper topical medications.
2. Take sitz baths 3 times a day to increase blood supply to the genital area and facilitate tissue healing.
3. Keep genital area dry; remind the patient to wear fresh, clean, loose-fitting undergarments daily.
4. Apply acyclovir ointment as prescribed.
5. Take drying agents and antibiotics if prescribed.
6. Avoid sexual relations during healing process.

B. Coping Strategies and Psychological Support

1. Encourage the patient to verbalize whatever psychological disturbance she is experiencing.
2. Ensure the patient of the confidentiality of information.
3. Suggest that the patient join a support group such as HELP (located in most cities—check telephone book).
4. Reiterate that when she is feeling better physically, her feelings about self and others will improve.
5. Advise the patient to tell new partner that she/he has been/is a victim of herpes.
   a. During active stages of disease, suggest sexual abstinence.
   b. Consider developing noncoital aspects of sexual relationship.
   c. When symptom-free, recommend use of lambskin condom for male.

Health Education

1. Provide information about the management of the infection; sexual activity should be avoided until the infection is cleared; recognize that this person is a potential transmitter of the disease.
2. Encourage the patient to describe the nature of the condition and what can be done to avoid/treat it.
3. Assist the patient in recognizing precipitating factors.
4. Review the necessary hygienic measures that discourage infection.
   a. Health-spa bathers can place clean, dry towels on seats to avoid inadvertently picking up herpes virus.
   b. Towel sharing should be avoided.

Evaluation
Expected Outcomes

1. Is pain-free with an absence of discomfort and no draining lesions
2. Is at ease while verbalizing the impact such a disease can have on one emotionally and mentally.
3. Demonstrates clean, healed, normal genital tissue; reports no burning sensation on urination and no unusual vaginal discharge
4. Describes a new life-style that is optimistic, wholesome, and knowledgeable with regard to sexual encounters with partner(s)
5. Recalls essential information about the nature of herpes genitalis and lists adequate health measures to manage any future situation

Toxic Shock Syndrome (TSS)

Toxic shock syndrome (TSS) is a condition caused by a bacterial toxin (*Staphylococcus aureus*) in the bloodstream; it can be life-threatening. This condition, first identified in 1975, came to public attention in 1980 because of increased incidence.

1. Over 90% of patients are women under 30 years of age.
2. The disorder is almost always associated with menstruation; women using high-absorbency tampons are at greatest risk.
3. Research studies suggest that magnesium-absorbing fibers in tampons may account for lower levels of magnesium in the body; this contributes to providing an ideal condition for toxin production by the bacteria.
4. TSS has been observed in nonmenstruating individuals with conditions such as cellulitis, surgical wound infection, vaginal infections, and subcutaneous abscesses.

Clinical Manifestations

1. Sudden onset of high fever <39°C. (102°F.)
2. Vomiting and profuse watery diarrhea
3. Rapid progression to hypotension and shock within 72 hours of onset
4. Mucous membrane hyperemia
5. Sometimes, sore throat, headache, and myalgia are experienced
6. Rash (similar to sunburn) that develops 1–2 weeks after onset of illness and is followed by desquamation, particularly of the palms and soles

Diagnostic Evaluation

1. Determine whether the female patient has used tampons recently.
2. Take blood and urine samples and throat cultures, and where appropriate, cerebrospinal fluid, vaginal and/or cervical specimens.
3. Perform blood and urine studies.
4. Rule out other illnesses—sepsis, Rocky Mountain spotted fever, etc.
5. Determine whether there is a history of recent skin infection.

Treatment and Nursing Interventions

1. Fluid replacement is instituted to replace fluid and electrolyte deficits.
2. Medications to raise the blood pressure are given.
3. Because of the need to administer large fluid volumes, edema becomes a problem, and even respiratory distress syndrome may result. This can be managed with endotracheal intubation and continuous positive airway pressure.
4. Administer antibiotics to control infection.
   a. Patients at risk but having only mild symptoms—oral dicloxacillin (Dycill, Dynapen), cloxacillin (Cloxapen, Tegopen), cephalexin (Keflex)
   b. These are given for 10 days–2 weeks
   c. For severely ill—antistaphylococci nafcillin (Nafcil, Unipen) or methicillin (Celbenin, Staphcillin)
5. The use of antibiotics, switching to sanitary napkins, and avoidance of using tampons for the next 3 menstrual cycles will reduce recurrence significantly.
6. The use of steroid therapy is still controversial.
7. After a bout with TSS, recommend close follow-up with pelvic examination and repeat cultures.

Health Education

1. Until more definitive research provides answers to this puzzling problem, women are advised to:

a. Alternate use of pads with tampons.
   b. Be alert to the symptoms of TSS.
   c. Change tampons frequently and not wear one longer than 8 hours; 4 hours is maximum for heavy discharge times.
   d. Be careful of vaginal abrasions that can be caused by some applicators.
   e. Avoid using super-absorbent tampons.
2. Since the risk is low (1/1000 over age 30, 4/1000 under age 30), it seems unwarranted to recommend that the use of tampons be discontinued.
3. Cases of TSS are to be reported to State Health departments and to the Centers for Disease Control (CDC)* so that additional data can be accumulated.

Cancer of the Vulva

Incidence

1. Most common in elderly women; cancer of the vulva represents 3%–4% of all malignancies of the female reproductive system.
2. Women seem reluctant to seek medical attention in early phases when ulcer is small and on the skin surface; they tend to delay until the ulcer becomes infected and painful.

Clinical Manifestations

1. In orderly progression, symptoms are severe vulvar pruritus, reddened, pigmented, whitish, or slightly elevated lesions with ulceration.
2. Frequent site
   a. Labia majora—mid or anterior portion
   b. Clitoris
   c. Encroachment upon urethra in larger lesions
3. Less frequent sites—fourchette and posterior labial areas.
4. As disease progresses, tissues become edematous, and lymphadenopathy is apparent.
5. Secondary infection is responsible for foul-smelling discharge.

Diagnostic Evaluation

1. A biopsy is taken after procaine is injected. The entire lesion, when it is small, may be excised; but final treatment is reserved until laboratory studies are completed.
2. Superficial lymph nodes on both sides are palpated for metastasis.
3. Pelvic examination is necessary to determine the extent of the cancer (clinical stage) and to rule out other pelvic neoplastic disease.

Treatment

This depends on type and extent of malignancy:
1. Basal cell carcinoma requires superficial hemivulvectomy.
2. Carcinoma in situ (noninvasive carcinoma) is treated by simple vulvectomy.
3. Invasive carcinoma calls for a radical vulvectomy and bilateral lymph node resection—often requiring removal of the deep pelvic (retroperitoneal) nodes.
4. Early radical vulvectomy with complete node dissection is curative. If the lesion is large and treatment late, cures are unlikely.

* Attn: Meningitis and Special Pathogens Branch, Division of Bacterial Diseases, Atlanta, GA 30333. Phone: (404) 329-3687.

Preoperative Preparation

A. Physical Preparation

1. Shave a wide area to include perineal, pubic, and inguinal areas.
2. Cleanse vulva thoroughly 2 or 3 days prior to surgery by using sitz baths twice daily.
3. Evacuate the intestinal tract before surgery to provide the advantage of no bowel movements for 2–3 days postoperatively.
4. Adhere to protocol for preoperative care as described on page 75.

B. Psychosocial Support

1. Have the patient describe what her understanding is regarding her problem.
2. Emphasize the positive outcomes of the prescribed treatment plan; reinforce what the physician has discussed with her.
3. Answer her questions tactfully; utilize available resources for those questions about which assistance is needed.
4. Encourage her to talk about her concerns regarding fear of mutilation and loss of sexual function.

Postoperative Patient Problems/ Nursing Diagnoses

1. Pain and discomfort related to nature of the surgery
2. Potential postoperative complications—infection, abdominal distention, bowel and bladder problems
3. Inadequate coping, poor self-image, related to fear of effects of surgery on sexual functioning

Planning and Implementation
Nursing Interventions

1. Maintain proper drainage and compression of tissues, connect drains to suction.

2. Promote comfort; place patient in low Fowler's position with knees slightly elevated with a pillow to lessen tension on sutures.
3. Minimize postoperative complications; mobilize the patient on the day of surgery.
4. Prevent infection of wound and bladder, clean the wound daily with warm sterile solutions as prescribed (dilute hydrogen peroxide, saline, antibacterial solution) and follow with a warm water spray. Later, after the stitches are removed, a heat lamp to the vulva for 5 minutes twice a day may be required.
5. Facilitate wound healing; some physicians prefer dry heat such as that provided by a heating lamp until the stitches are removed; this is followed by perineal packs or soaks.
6. Prevent straining on defecation and wound contamination; offer a low-residue diet.
7. Prevent bladder infection, give meticulous care to the vagina and urethral orifice.
8. Promote tissue repair, sitz baths of pHisoHex solution may be prescribed after the 10th day.
9. Encourage social adjustment, maintain a relationship conducive to allowing the patient to voice her concerns.

Evaluation
Expected Outcomes

1. Free of discomfort following surgery
2. Absence of complications
3. Adjusts to altered physical status; discusses life-style changes
4. Understands and can relate what to watch for regarding future problems:
   a. Possible metastasis
   b. Adhesions
   c. Other complications

Problems Resulting from Relaxed Pelvic Muscles

Cystocele and Urethrocele

Cystocele is a downward displacement (protrusion) of the bladder into the vagina.

Urethrocele is a downward displacement of the urethra into the vagina.

Etiology

1. Associated with obstetrical trauma to fascia, muscle, and ligaments during childbirth (results in poor support).
2. Often becomes apparent years later, when genital atrophy associated with aging occurs.

Clinical Manifestations

No early symptoms.
1. Later, fatigue, and pelvic pressure "like sitting on a ball"
2. Urinary symptoms—urgency, frequency, incontinence
3. Aggravated with vigorous activity such as coughing, sneezing—relieved by resting or lying down

Prevention

A. Medical

1. Kegel's pelvic floor exercises are useful and may prove beneficial in some women.

   a. Conscious contraction of the pelvic floor or levator ani muscles.
   b. This can be done many times during the day, as one sits, stands, or lies in bed.
2. Voluntarily stopping the flow of urine during micturition is a good exercise.
3. Estrogen therapy after menopause may be of some effectiveness.
4. A vaginal pessary may be used temporarily. Prolonged use may lead to pressure necrosis and vaginal ulceration.

B. Surgical

Done when cystocele is large and interferes with proper bladder functioning—anterior vaginal colporrhaphy. This is often combined with vaginal hysterectomy and posterior colpoperineorrhaphy.

Rectocele/Enterocele

Rectocele is displacement (protrusion) of the rectum into the vagina. *Enterocele* is displacement of intestine into vagina.

Etiology

Similar to cystocele; however, posterior vaginal wall is weakened in a rectocele.

Clinical Manifestations

1. Disturbance of bowel function—constipation.
2. A "bearing down" feeling—as though the "pelvic organs were going to fall out."
3. Difficulty in fecal evacuation; some patients state that "they must put their fingers in the vagina to push the mass up" so that defecation can take place.
4. Symptoms disappear in the recumbent position.
5. Incontinence of gas and feces (in patients with a complete tear between rectum and vagina).

Treatment

Surgery is done only when rectocele becomes so large that fecal evacuation is impaired or difficult. Posterior colpoplasty (perineorrhaphy)—repair of posterior vaginal wall.

Nursing Interventions

A. Preoperative Care

1. Promote rest, particularly in a patient who has been working hard.
2. Suggest low Fowler's position in bed to lessen edema and congestion.
3. Recognize that this problem often occurs in older women.
4. Prepare intestinal tract by administering a cathartic and enema.

B. Postoperative Care

1. Encourage voiding every 4–8 hours to reduce pressure so that no more than 150 ml. will accumulate in bladder—catheterization or use of an indwelling catheter may be required.
2. Administer perineal care to the patient after each voiding and defecation.
3. Employ a heat lamp to help dry the incision line and enhance the healing process.
4. Utilize available sprays for anesthetic and antiseptic effects.
5. Apply an ice pack locally to relieve congestion and discomfort.
6. Administer analgesics as prescribed for relief of pain.

Malposition of the Uterus

When the uterus is in a normal position, the cervix lies in the axis of the vagina with the corpus inclined forward on the bladder.

Twenty-five percent of women have, to some degree, the reverse position (retroversion).

Retroversion and Retroflexion

In *retroversion,* the cervix remains in the normal axis, but body is directed to hollow of the sacrum.

In *retroflexion,* angulation of the corpus on the cervix is extreme.

A. Clinical Manifestations

1. There may be none.
2. With significant uterine displacement—pelvic pain, backache, menstrual aberration, possibly infertility.

B. Treatment

1. A pessary may be required to temporarily treat symptoms.
2. Uterine suspension may be done surgically.

Prolapse and Procidentia

Uterine prolapse is a herniation of the uterus through the pelvic floor with a resultant protrusion into the vagina (prolapse) and at times even beyond the introitus (*procidentia*).

Prolapse

1st degree—cervix, without straining or traction, is at the introitus (spread the labia and it is visible).
2nd degree—the cervix extends over the perineum.
3rd degree—the entire uterus (or most of it) protrudes.

Procidentia

The uterus, vaginal vault, rectum, and bladder (and in some cases the posterior cul-de-sac) protrude.

A. Factors Aggravating the Condition

1. Obstetrical trauma
2. Overstretching of the musculofascial supports
3. Standing, straining, coughing, lifting a heavy object

B. Treatment

1. A vaginal pessary may be used temporarily or for palliation.
2. Surgical correction is recommended treatment. This usually is a vaginal hysterectomy—combined with anterior and posterior repair.

Tumors of the Uterus

Incidence and the Importance of Health Education

1. In the US, malignant tumors of the uterus (cervix and endometrium) rank 3rd highest among cancers in women (breast, colon–rectum, uterine, lung).
2. The death rate for uterine cancer has been showing a steady decline; this is attributed to the unremitting education of women, which stresses the importance of annual checkups, including the cytology smear.
3. Nurses need to seek out the reasons why millions of women have not had Pap tests—lack of information, no transportation, inconvenient schedules of clinics, fear of results, and general lack of motivation.

Cancer of the Cervix

Etiology

1. It is most common between the ages of 35 and 55, but it can occur at any age.
2. Early cancer of the cervix is usually asymptomatic; it is almost always curable in its preinvasive stage.
3. Early sexual activity and multiple sexual partners appear to be related to the incidence of this cancer.
4. Viral and chronic infections, as well as erosions of the cervix, appear to be significant in the development of cancer.
5. Incidence of cancer of the cervix is higher in groups

with low socioeconomic status; occurs more often in black women than in white.
6. In developing countries, cancer of the cervix is the most frequent malignancy among females.

Clinical Manifestations

1. There are no symptoms of early cervical carcinoma.
2. Initial symptoms of carcinoma of the cervix.
   a. Posttraumatic bleeding (coitus)
   b. Irregular vaginal bleeding or spotting—between periods (metrorrhagia) or after the menopause; at first it may be very slight, but as disease progresses, bleeding becomes more constant
   c. Leukorrhea—increases in amount, becomes dark and foul-smelling because of necrosis and infection of tumor mass
3. With advanced cancer, there is excruciating pain in back and legs, relieved only by large doses of narcotics.
4. Later, extreme emaciation and anemia; occasionally there is irregular fever due to secondary infection, peritonitis, and abscesses in ulcerating mass.

Diagnostic Evaluation

1. Physical, including pelvic examination, plus a complete history are done initially.
2. Laboratory studies include cytology smear, routine blood examinations, plus fasting blood sugar to detect diabetes, total plasma proteins for nutritional status evaluation, and bleeding and clotting times.
3. Colposcopy, Schiller's test, biopsy (cone and punch), and proctosigmoidoscopic examination are essential diagnostic aids.
4. Roentgen studies should include chest x-ray, intravenous pyelogram, barium enema, and bone studies.
5. Electrocardiogram

Treatment

1. Hysterectomy (see p. 581)—depending on stage of lesion
   a. Cervical amputation, wide conization, cryosurgery are alternatives to hysterectomy, but there is less assurance of complete removal of the lesion.
2. Invasive carcinoma
   a. Treatment is individualized, depending on the stage of the disease, age of the patient, and general physical condition.
   b. Most often, invasive carcinoma is treated by radiation; radical operations (exenteration) are performed on some patients.

Health Education and Follow-up Emphasis

Regardless of the treatment, the nurse must emphasize the necessity of follow-up visits for this patient, since they will be required for the rest of her life:
1. To determine the patient's response to treatment
2. To detect spread of cancer (metastasis)
3. To take regular cytologic smears
4. To maintain the best health possible

Cancer of the Corpus Uteri

Incidence

1. Carcinoma of the body and carcinoma of the cervix of the uterus occurred in the ratio of 4:1 a few years ago; at present the ratio is 2:1.
2. Endometrial cancer is most common in women past 50 (peaks at age 55).
3. Seventy-five percent of women with cancer of the corpus uteri are postmenopausal.
4. Often this malignancy occurs when the patient is also affected by obesity, hypertensive cardiovascular disease, and diabetes.
5. Forty years of statistical and laboratory experimentation have failed to show a definite relationship between estrogen and cancer.

Clinical Manifestations

1. The first evidence is usually a serous, malodorous leukorrhea—often this is disregarded by the patient.
2. This is followed by a bloody discharge—it may be spotty, or it may be steady.
3. Pain is not a symptom until the late stages.
4. Anemia may result if there is considerable bleeding.

Diagnostic Evaluation

1. Determine source of bleeding; even if it is coming from the cervical canal, it could be caused by a condition other than carcinoma.
   (If a tampon is inserted in the vagina overnight, the place where blood is noted on the dressing may offer a clue to bleeding source [i.e., near the string could suggest bladder source, but near the tip of the tampon would suggest cervix as source]).
2. Endometrial biopsy—positive test result indicates cancer, whereas a negative test result does not necessarily exclude carcinoma.
3. Fractional curettage is the most effective and accurate diagnostic aid.

Treatment

1. Hysterectomy (p. 581)—depending on stage of lesion.
2. Radiation therapy (p. 580)—depending on stage of lesion.

Myoma of the Uterus

Myomas are benign tumors of the uterus; (they are also called fibromyomas, "fibroids," and leiomyomas).

Incidence and Characteristics

1. Such tumors occur in about 20% of women past age 30.
2. Myomas rarely develop after menopause; tumors that developed earlier may regress slightly after menopause—but the significant ones do not disappear.
3. Incidence is higher in black women than in white.
4. These tumors tend to be of dense musculofibrous structure; they are encapsulated and tend to form small or large nodules.

Clinical Manifestations

1. Small myomas do not cause symptoms.
2. After myomas (or myomata) grow, the first indication of the presence of a tumor is a palpable mass.
3. Excessive or prolonged menstruation is usually the chief symptom (with little or no change in the menstrual interval); intermenstrual or postmenopausal bleeding may also occur.
4. Pain comes from pressure on adjacent organs. As myomas grow, there may be a sensation of weight—a heavy feeling.
5. Secondary symptoms may be a feeling of lassitude, general weakness, anemia, and lower abdominal discomfort.

Diagnostic Measures

1. These are done primarily to rule out cancer—cytology, dilatation and curettage, cervical biopsy.
2. Diagnosis is made by abdominal and bimanual palpation.

Treatment

1. If the patient is of childbearing age and desires children, treatment is conservative.
   a. If small tumor—myomectomy
   b. If large tumor—hysterectomy
   c. Ovaries are preserved
   d. If tumor is large with excessive bleeding—hysteromyomectomy (tumor and uterus removed)
2. For medical and nursing management, see page 581.

Nursing Care of the Patient Receiving Radiation Therapy of the Uterus

Radiation Therapy (see also p. 912)

1. Radium, cesium-137, or radioactive cobalt is introduced into the endocervical canal and vagina for a prescribed time; radium (or cesium) is placed in tubes designed to filter out most alpha and beta rays while allowing gamma rays to penetrate into the tumor.
2. Such therapy may be supplemented by external radiation (supervoltage x-ray, telecobalt, or linear accelerator sources) directed over the pelvis in an effort to eliminate cancer spread via lymphatic system; energy may be delivered via anterior or posterior portals over lower abdomen or back, or by means of rotational therapy permitting more uniform exposure of pelvis.
3. Therapy is individualized according to stage of disease and the patient's response to and tolerance of radiation.
4. A popular method of treatment involves using radiation therapy externally, then shifting to radium application, and then returning to radiation therapy. Total treatment time is 5–6 weeks.

Patient Preparation for Radium (Cesium) Implantation

1. Physician explains to the patient the reason why such therapy is advocated; nurse can amplify or answer any questions patient may later raise.
2. Prepare the patient for various preliminary tests (may be done on an outpatient basis)—blood studies, biopsies (endometrial and cervical), chest x-ray, electrocardiogram, cystoscopy.
3. Be available for questions and conversation with the patient regarding any phase of the preliminary studies or treatment.
4. Following admission to the hospital, prepare the patient for surgery and, in addition, prepare the intestinal tract by enemas and the vaginal tract by a cleansing douche.

Radium Application

After-loading technique using an applicator:
1. In surgery, the tandem and ovoids are positioned (without radium or cesium).
2. Upon recovery from anesthesia, x-rays are taken in various positions in the x-ray department.
3. Therapeutic radiologist then inserts radium (cesium) into prepositioned apparatus.

Nursing Management

▶ **NURSING ALERT:** It is imperative to keep the radiation applicator in the uterine canal and to prevent its changing position. Adjust all nursing measures to meet this.

A. While Radium Is in Place

1. Maintain the patient on a low-residue diet to prevent bowel movements, which might dislodge apparatus.
2. Inspect catheter frequently to ensure straight drainage—a distended bladder may cause severe radiation burns.
3. Observe for symptoms of radiation sickness—nausea, vomiting, elevated temperature.
4. Encourage the patient to eat by offering a variety of small rather than large servings and present meals attractively to offset poor appetite.
5. Offer citrus fruit juices because vitamin C is essential in tissue repair.
6. The patient must lie on her back; head of bed may be elevated 30 degrees.
7. Provide back care but spend a minimum amount of time at the bedside.
8. Relieve the patient of anxiety and fear by utilizing wisely the contact time with the patient—engage in profitable conversation about her interests and health problems.

B. Radium Removal

1. Notify surgeon when it is time to remove radium (or cesium).
2. Provide sterile gloves, long forceps, and a large waste basin.
3. Note on the chart the number of tubes applied so that this number is accounted for on removal.
4. Practice radium precautions in handling and returning radium (cesium) to the radiotherapy department.
5. Administer a cleansing enema before the patient gets out of bed.

C. Postirradiation Patient Care

1. Keep the patient's skin (exposed to radiation) dry; avoid use of soap since it irritates.
2. Apply a soothing, nonmedicated powder such as cornstarch to relieve itching and discomfort.
3. For erythematous areas, apply a bland ointment such as A&D ointment to relieve irritation.
4. Nausea or vomiting may occur with large doses of radiation.

▶ **NURSING ALERT:** Do not tell the patient nausea and vomiting may occur, since the power of suggestion may initiate these symptoms.

5. Observe for any symptoms that might suggest radiation injury to the intestine—diarrhea, tenesmus; report these if they occur.
6. Tell the patient the importance of monthly follow-up visits to her physician for the first 6 months—to assess effects of radiation on tumor.

a. Cytologic smears are taken; if positive, surgery may be indicated.
b. If cytology smear is negative and tissue looks satisfactory, follow-up visits after 6 months may be further apart (on a semiannual basis).

▶ **NURSING ALERT:** Recognize that 5%–8% of women who are followed for the treatment of a particular cancer may develop other primary cancers. Therefore, such follow-up visits are essential even though the woman is symptomless.

Hysterectomy

Hysterectomy is the surgical removal of the uterus.

Possible Indications

1. Malignant and nonmalignant growth on uterus, cervix, and adnexa that should be removed
2. Control of uterine bleeding and/or hemorrhage
3. Severe (life-threatening) pelvic infection
4. Correction of problems associated with pelvic floor relaxation—cystocele, rectocele
5. Treatment of endometriosis when conservative measures have failed
6. Irreparable rupture or perforation of uterus

Qualifying Considerations

1. Woman's age
2. Woman's desire to have children
3. Possible effectiveness of alternative treatment
4. Degree of dysfunction
5. Woman's willingness to endure dysfunction in order to retain her uterus

Types of Abdominal Hysterectomy

(Approximately 70% done abdominally)
1. *Subtotal hysterectomy*—corpus of uterus is removed, but cervical stump remains.
2. *Total hysterectomy*—entire uterus is removed, including cervix; tubes and ovaries remain.
3. *Total hysterectomy with bilateral salpingo-oophorectomy*—entire uterus, tubes, and ovaries are removed.

Vaginal Hysterectomy

Preferred approach for:
1. Repair of pelvic relaxation (uterine descensus, urinary stress incontinence, cystocele/rectocele) is more easily managed vaginally than abdominally.
2. High-risk patients, very obese patients, or those unable to withstand prolonged anesthesia.

Advantages

1. Less likelihood of paralytic ileus, postoperative pain, and intestinal adhesions
2. Less chance of pulmonary complications and thrombophlebitis
3. Wound dehiscence possibility is less; shorter hospitalization
4. No abdominal scar

Disadvantages

1. More limited surgical field; inability to examine intrapelvic and intra-abdominal organs
2. May be increased risk of bleeding and postoperative infection

Postoperative Patient Problems/ Nursing Diagnoses

1. Potential bladder problems related to proximity of bladder to surgical site
2. Pain and discomfort related to surgical procedure and abdominal distention
3. Potential complications following surgery
4. Fear and anxiety related to fear of cancer, loss of reproductive function and sexual concerns

Planning and Implementation
Nursing Interventions

A. Resolution of Bladder Problems

1. Monitor and record intake and output; administer parenteral fluids as prescribed.
2. Insert an indwelling catheter, if prescribed, because edema or nerve trauma may cause temporary bladder atony. A suprapubic catheter may be used (see p. 572).
3. Remove catheter as soon as feasible (as directed).
4. Catheterize the patient if no catheter is in place and the patient has not voided after 8 hours, or is uncomfortable.
5. Determine whether there is residual urine; catheterize the patient after each voiding; otherwise, bladder infection may develop.

B. Relief of Pain, Discomfort, and Abdominal Distention

1. A nasogastric tube may be inserted while the patient is in the operating room.
2. Fluids and food may be restricted until peristalsis has resumed.
3. Auscultate abdomen for bowel sounds to determine onset of peristalsis.
   a. Apply heat to the abdomen and insert a rectal tube to relieve abdominal flatus.
   b. Permit the patient to sit on edge of bed with feet supported and to get out of bed and walk.
   c. Serve additional fluids and soft diet as peristalsis returns.

C. Prevention of Complications

1. Assist the patient in turning every 2 hours and encourage her to take deep breaths.
2. Avoid high Fowler's position and pressure under the knees, which might cause stasis and pooling of the blood.
3. Assess dressings or vaginal pad for amount and nature of discharge.
   a. Color of stain; wetness or dryness
   b. Size of stain—record in centimeters; note odor or its absence.
   c. Document observation, as well as time of assessment, so that differences can be noted at the next observation.
4. Measure amount of blood loss by weighing each pad when removed (before evaporation takes place); compare weight of saturated pad with that of a dry pad (the difference will be weight of blood loss).

5. Evaluate legs for positive Homans' sign (tenderness, pain in calf upon dorsiflexion of foot).
6. Observe legs for the presence of varicosities; promote circulation with special leg exercises.
7. Apply antiembolic stockings as a precautionary measure to promote peripheral circulation.
8. Attempt to counteract effects resulting from removal of a large tumor or unusual blood loss.
    a. Administer high-protein diet with iron supplement to combat anemia.
    b. Recommend a girdle or apply an abdominal binder following removal of a large tumor to provide support for relaxed abdominal muscles.

D. Reduction in Fear and Anxiety

1. Patient may have deep-seated fears that cancer or a sexually transmitted disease may be discovered.
2. There may be a conflict between recommended medical treatment and her personal religious beliefs.
3. Concerns may be raised regarding the possibility that all phases of her reproductive process may be disturbed.
4. She may be disappointed, particularly if she never had children.
5. The patient may feel that she will no longer be able to fulfill her role and needs as a woman.
6. Depression and heightened emotional sensitivity to people and situations may have to be assessed.
7. The complexity of problems that are a mixture of physical, emotional, and social factors needs to be considered by the nurse as she assists this patient.
8. Questions arise about how a hysterectomy will affect the patient's participation in sexual activities.
9. The relationship of this woman to her partner and family should be determined.

Discharge Planning/Health Education

1. A total hysterectomy produces a surgical menopause (if the adnexa were also removed).
2. Explain to the patient the importance of hormonal replacement (prescribed) if she has had a total hysterectomy with oophorectomy/salpingectomy.
3. Advise her against sitting too long at one time, as in driving long distances, because of the possibility of pooling of blood in the pelvis and of thromboembolism.
4. Suggest that the patient delay driving a car until the 3rd postoperative week, since even pressing the brake pedal may initiate slight discomfort in the lower abdomen.

5. Tell the patient to expect a "tired feeling" for the first few days at home and, therefore, not to plan too many activities for the first week.
6. Assist her in planning a flexible schedule so that she will be able to perform most of her usual household activities within a month; within 2 months, she will feel her "normal" self.
7. Stress that the patient should assume employment outside the home only when her physician indicates; this will depend on the type of work, etc.
8. Tell the patient not to feel discouraged if at times during convalescence she experiences depression, feels like crying, and seems unusually nervous. This is common, but will not last.
9. Remind her to ask her physician regarding resumption of various preferred physical activities; note that some of the most strenuous tasks are hanging clothes on a line and using the vacuum cleaner. These tasks should be delayed for several weeks. The patient should not lift heavy objects for at least a month to 6 weeks.
10. Determine what the physician has told the patient regarding resumption of intercourse; reinforce this and explain that too-enthusiastic genital sex may injure the incision site and produce bleeding. In other words, she is to "go easy" at first. Suggest coital position variation.
    Usually sexual relations, douching, or use of tampons is discouraged for 4–6 weeks, unless otherwise specified by the physician.
11. Showers are permitted, but tub bathing is deferred until the physician indicates that tissues are sufficiently healed.
12. Emphasize the importance of follow-up physical and gynecological examinations, not only for peace of mind, but also to detect any beginning pathology. Temperature elevation over 37.8°C. (100°F.), heavy vaginal bleeding, drainage, and foul odor of discharge are reportable.

Evaluation
Expected Outcomes

1. Reports no difficulties with urinary control or output
2. Asserts that pain is gone; discomfort is lessening each day postoperatively
3. Recognizes the signs that suggest possible complications; none noted
4. Presents an optimistic outlook regarding general state of health, reproduction, and sexual activity

Endometriosis

Endometriosis is a disease characterized by displaced groups of cells (resembling the cells that line the uterus) growing aberrantly in the pelvic cavity outside of the uterus.

Incidence

1. Frequency of occurrence is about 25%–30% in white women.
2. It is rarely encountered in women of the black race.
3. Usually this condition becomes evident in the 3rd or 4th decade of a woman's life.

Characteristics

1. Pelvic endometriosis attacks many areas. Order of frequency is the ovary, ureterosacral ligaments, the cul-de-sac, ureterovesical peritoneum, cervix, umbilicus, laparotomy scars, hernial sacs, and appendix.
2. Misplaced endometrium responds to ovarian hormonal stimulation and even depends on this for survival.
    a. When the uterus goes through the process of menstruation, this misplaced tissue also bleeds;

because there is no outlet for accumulated blood, pain and adhesions result.

b. At surgery, concealed bleeding is in evidence because lesions are brown or blue-black.

c. Ovarian cysts in which such bleeding has occurred are referred to as "chocolate cysts," but all such cysts are not indicative of endometriosis.

Etiology

1. Embryonic tissue remnants may cover pelvic peritoneum and ovaries and may differentiate as a result of hormonal stimulation.
2. Such tissue may be spread via lymphatic or venous channels.
3. Endometrial tissue, during surgery, may accidentally be transferred by way of instruments (uncommon).

Clinical Manifestations

1. Persistent infertility in an otherwise healthy married woman.
2. Lower abdominal and pelvic pain or discomfort, rectal pain, increasing dyspareunia (painful intercourse), and abnormal uterine bleeding and hematuria.
3. Symptoms are more acute during menstruation and subside after menstruation.
4. When a cyst ruptures, symptoms mimic acute appendicitis or ruptured ectopic pregnancy—an acute abdomen is apparent.

Diagnostic Evaluation

1. Manual rectal and pelvic examinations reveal fixed, tender nodular structures, ovarian abnormalities, and the uterus fixed by restraining adhesions.
2. X-ray studies, such as barium enema, may demonstrate constrictions suggestive of endometriosis.
3. Laparoscopy is an effective diagnostic aid because tissue can be visualized.

Treatment

1. If the patient is pain-free and does not desire pregnancy, no treatment is prescribed.

2. For discomfort, analgesics/antiprostaglandin drugs are prescribed for dysmenorrhea.
3. Endocrine therapy utilizing hormones to produce pseudopregnancy (such as Ovral, Demulen, and Norlestrin) may be prescribed.
   A combination-type oral contraceptive may be used—with the least amount of estrogen necessary to suppress ovulation and the maximum amount of progestogen to induce a decidual reaction in the implants.
4. Surgical intervention may be required—laparoscopic surgery, laparotomy, presacral neurectomy, laser surgery, or more radical definitive surgery, such as hysterectomy, bilateral salpingo-oophorectomy.

Nursing Interventions

A. Relief of Discomfort

1. Administer hormonal therapy as prescribed—estrogen–progestogen, "pseudopregnancy"
2. Explain to the patient why such medications as Ovral are prescribed.
3. Prepare the patient for surgery when indicated; this is directed toward the resection of cysts and lysis of adhesions. Perhaps other, more involved, surgery may be indicated.
4. Describe why radical surgery may be necessary.
5. Tell the patient that menopause also improves or cures endometriosis; this is only of value to the older patient.

B. Psychosocial Considerations

1. Include the patient in the treatment plans so that she knows why a particular method of treatment has been selected and how her role is a vital one in its success.
2. Encourage the patient to express her concerns; false ideas often emerge—such as, "Perhaps I have endometriosis because I used tampons."
3. Monitor the reaction of the patient to the various treatments prescribed.
4. Encourage the patient to continue the therapeutic drug program even though she is beginning to feel little discomfort.

Ovarian Cancer

Ovarian cancer is high-risk cancer of the ovary.

Incidence

1. Barber states that ovarian cancer accounts for about 25% of all gynecologic cancers; it also accounts for about 47% of all genital cancer deaths.
2. Cancer of the ovary is the leading cause of death from gynecological cancer; it is the third most frequent gynecological cancer.

Clinical Manifestations

1. Earliest manifestations—insidious and vague
   a. Some abdominal discomfort
   b. Indigestion
   c. Flatulence
   d. Slight anorexia
2. These gastrointestinal symptoms may be due to an acid reaction of the peritoneal fluid in ovarian cancer.

3. Advanced cancer—abdominal swelling, pain, and a mass in the abdomen

Diagnostic Evaluation

1. Because of the high-risk nature of ovarian cancer, it is important that every effort be made to diagnose the condition early.
2. The nurse should recognize those conditions in a woman that collectively place her in a high-risk category. Individuals at high risk include women who are
   a. Infertile
   b. Anovulatory
   c. Nulliparous
   d. Habitual aborters
3. If only *one* of the above conditions is present, along with *three* of the following symptoms, the patient should be labeled as "high risk."

a. Increasing premenstrual tension
b. Irregular menses
c. Menorrhagia with breast tenderness
d. An early menopause
4. Semiannual gynecological examination and cervical cytology.
5. Investigate any ovarian enlargement by laparoscopy or laparotomy. This is particularly true of postmenopausal women whose ovaries should not be palpable.

Treatment

1. Surgical removal of diseased area—extensiveness depends on the malignancy.
2. Treatment may be ovariectomy, hysterectomy, bilateral salpingo-oophorectomy, omentectomy, appendectomy.
3. Modalities may be surgery first, radiation and chemotherapy, and finally immunotherapy. The effectiveness of combination therapy is being studied.
4. Chemotherapy is frequently used following surgery.

Pelvic Infection

All structures in the pelvic cavity can become infected. Two types can be roughly distinguished according to the site of the infection and its spread.

Etiology
Nongonococcal Infections

Chlamydia trachomatis is a genital tract infection in women that is similar to gonorrhea; the incidence is increasing.
1. This condition may occur with or without a gonorrheal infection.
2. It may be mild enough to be ignored or severe enough to cause symptoms.
   Mucopurulent cervical exudate with erythema, edema, and congestion; in addition, there may be friability (easily crumbled) of the cervix.

Gonoccocal and Mixed Infection

1. Gonococcal infection originates in the urethra, cervix, and/or rectum.
2. If reinfection does occur following proper treatment, the disease is self-limiting.
3. Most frequently, women are reinfected, and the secondary invaders (streptococcus, staphylococcus, *Escherichia coli,* etc.) take over. Accordingly, as a rule, what started as a self-limiting salpingitis becomes a chronic process. The disease is spread by way of the uterine canal into the tube and through the fimbria.
4. As a rule, the endometritis resulting from gonorrhea is shortlived.
5. The largest group of infections are created by pelvic cellulitis (i.e., endometritis from a complication of pregnancy or an intrauterine device).
6. Here all the cervical and vaginal pathogens are offenders. They spread by way of the lymphatics and blood vessels.
7. Cellulitis tends to be unilateral, whereas gonorrhea is a bilateral process.
8. Tuberculous endometritis—uncommon in the US and common in Israel—is a likely cause of infertility.

Risk Factors

1. Higher occurrence in sexually active women; especially if they or their mates or partners have more than one sexual partner.
2. The use of an intrauterine contraceptive device (IUD).

Assessment
Clinical Manifestations

1. Abdominal pain, nausea and vomiting, temperature elevation, malaise

2. Leukocytosis
3. Malodorous, purulent vaginal discharge

Diagnostic Evaluation

1. Nursing history, pelvic and physical examination
2. Culture of endocervix
3. Laparoscopy

Patient Problems/Nursing Diagnosis

1. Pain and discomfort related to presence of pelvic infection
2. Potential for spread of infection
3. Potential for complications

Planning and Implementation
Nursing Interventions

A. Control of Discomfort and Improvement in Fluid and Nutritional Status

1. Provide prescribed analgesics to control abdominal discomfort.
2. Support patient nutritionally. Review principles of nutrition with patient.
3. Recognize the depressing nature of the disease and that the patient needs support and understanding, particularly when she has discomfort and vague symptoms.
4. Apply heat to the abdomen externally and warm douches vaginally as prescribed to improve circulation.

B. Control of Infection

1. Administer appropriate antibiotics and chemotherapeutic agents as prescribed.
   a. Nongonococcal (chlamydiae)—tetracycline regimen
   b. Gonococcal—penicillin G, ampicillin, spectinomycin
2. Place the patient in a semi-Fowler's position to facilitate drainage.
3. Avoid use of tampons.
4. Instruct the patient to protect herself and others from reinfection by careful handwashing and proper hygienic measures.
5. Document the patient's progress. Record vital signs, patient responses (physical and mental) to therapy, and nature and amount of vaginal discharge.
6. Control spread of infection by the following safeguards:
   a. Handle perineal pads with extreme precautions:
      (1) Use an instrument or gloves.
      (2) Deposit pad in paper bag for proper disposal.
   b. Wash hands carefully before and after patient contacts.

c. Disinfect utensils, bedpans, toilet seats, and linen. Adopt procedure appropriate for specific organism.
7. Encourage use of barrier methods of contraception (condom, diaphragm with foam or jelly, birth control pills after completion of treatment.

C. Prevention of Complications from Untreated or Recurrent Infection

1. Chronic pelvic discomfort; disease becomes rampant.
2. Sterility occurs because of closing of uterine tubes with scar tissue.

3. Ectopic pregnancy is possible if fertilized egg is unable to pass stricture.
4. Inflammatory masses may develop, eventually requiring removal of uterus, tubes, and ovaries.

Evaluation

Expected Outcomes

1. Absence of discomfort
2. No evidence of infection
3. Relates what signs and symptoms are reportable that may suggest the development of a complication(s)

Fertility Control

Basic Principles

1. The nurse should be familiar with the application, advantages and disadvantages of the various methods of contraception available.
2. The most effective method is the one a woman selects for herself and will use consistently.
3. Women are entitled to contraceptive advice as part of good health care without the burden of moral judgment.

Contraceptive Methods

Note: Failure rate (pregnancy) is determined by the experience of 100 women for 1 year and is expressed as *pregnancies per 100 woman years.*

A. Periodic Abstinence

Abstention from sexual intercourse during the fertile period of each cycle.
1. This depends on:
   a. Identification of fertile period—usually about 14 days before next menstrual period.
   b. Abstaining for about 7–18 days.

B. Natural Family Planning (NFP)

1. Cervical mucus method—abstain when mucus is present and also during menstruation.
2. Symptothermal method (STM)—based on rise in basal body temperature, as well as changes in cervical mucus.

C. Coitus Interruptus

This is the withdrawal of the penis from the vagina when ejaculation is imminent.
1. Indications—effective when mechanical devices are unavailable.
2. Contraindications
   a. When male is not able to exert self-control.
   b. Ineffective when premature ejaculation occurs—this is true of almost 50% of males.
3. Undesirable effects
   a. Failure rate is between 35%–40%.
   b. Psychological ill effects for both male and female.
   c. Subsequent prostatitis has been substantiated.

D. Condom

Application of a rubber sheath worn over the penis by the male during coitus.
1. Procedure for use and precautions
   a. Place condom over erect penis.
   b. Leave a dead space at the tip of the condom (from which air has been expelled) to allow room for ejaculate.

c. Lubricate (spermicidal) exterior of condom—as an added precaution.
   d. Avoid leaving condom in vagina during withdrawal; this is facilitated by grasping ring around top of condom at time of withdrawal.
2. Advantages
   a. Inexpensive and easy to use; available without a prescription.
   b. Protects against pregnancy and offers some protection against sexually transmitted diseases.
   c. May lessen premature ejaculation.
   d. Ensures male's involvement in the contraceptive process.
3. Disadvantages
   a. May dull sensation somewhat for male and female.
   b. Requires an erect penis for application.
   c. Condom may tear or rupture and thus be ineffective.
   d. May cause a contact dermatitis.
4. Failure rate (pregnancy)
   Varies from 15 to 35 (various authorities) undesired pregnancies per 100 woman years.

Note: If condom ruptures, the female should see her gynecologist immediately to obtain "morning after pill" (high estrogen) for pregnancy interception.

E. Diaphragm

A rubber, dome-shaped device with a flexible wire rim, which is inserted in the vagina to fit snugly behind the pubic bone and over the cervix into the posterior fornix. It is used to prevent sperm from reaching the cervical os. Spermicidal jelly is often used on both sides of the diaphragm.
1. Indications—preferred by women who
   a. Object to a device in utero
   b. Object to hormonal or chemical contraceptives
   c. Do not object to insertion of the diaphragm immediately prior to intercourse
2. Procedure for insertion and follow-up
   a. Bimanual pelvic examination and cytology smear are preliminary to measurement for a diaphragm.
   b. Measure depth of vagina; select largest diaphragm that can be retained comfortably; if too small, the device will be displaced during intercourse.
   c. Teach the patient how to insert diaphragm behind lower edge of pubic bone; use spermicidal jelly or cream for additional contraceptive action.
   d. Instruct her to retain diaphragm for 6–8 hours after intercourse.

e. Remind the patient of annual gynecological examination.

f. Inform the patient that a larger diaphragm may be necessary after a pregnancy.

3. Failure rate (pregnancy)
15 undesired pregnancies per 100 woman years of using diaphragm.

F. Vaginal Foam

This is a spermicidal cushioning foam that is available in cream, gel, aerosol, or tablet form. All except the tablet are effective immediately—tablets require 5–10 minutes to dissolve.

1. Advantages
   a. Requires little instruction; a favorite method with lower socioeconomic groups.
   b. May be used to advantage with coitus interruptus.
2. Disadvantage
   Higher failure rate than other contraceptive methods.
3. Failure rate (pregnancy)
   Between 35 and 45 per 100 woman years.

G. Intrauterine Device (IUD)

The IUD is a device made of metal or plastic that fits inside the uterus; it may be in the shape of a spiral, loop, shield, or ring.

▶ **NURSING ALERT:** It is now apparent that the IUD is more dangerous than ever anticipated. Endometritis, ovarian abscesses, ruptured uteri, and their consequences have resulted in pelvic surgery and permanent crippling that cannot be ignored.

1. Indications
   a. When hormonal medications appear to be contraindicated.
   b. When motivation and other resources are lacking; as a last resort.
2. Contraindications
   a. Inflammation or infection of cervix, uterus, or uterine tubes.
   b. Objections on the part of the woman to a foreign device in her uterus.
   c. Severe dysmenorrhea.
3. Advantages
   a. Effectiveness listed as 97%–99%
   b. Convenient; permits spontaneity of intercourse
4. Disadvantages
   a. Increased dysmenorrhea and amount of menstrual flow
   b. Some discomfort with insertion of IUD
   c. Increased risk of pelvic inflammatory disease
   d. In prolonged use (over 3 years without IUD having been removed) there is increasing risk of pelvic actinomycosis
5. Procedure for insertion
   a. Nursing history is obtained to determine contraceptive history and pertinent health information such as abnormal vaginal bleeding, pelvic infections, past surgery on reproductive organs, pregnancy history, nature of menses, presence of other diseases.
   b. Client is counseled as recommended by the US Food and Drug Administration:
      (1) Preinsertion
          What you should know about the IUD
          Use-effectiveness
          What you should tell your physician: adverse reactions

(2) Postinsertion
    Description of the IUD
    Directions for use
    Side effects
    Warnings
    Special warning about pregnancy with an IUD in place

c. A pelvic examination and a (Pap) cytology smear is done.

d. Calibre of interior of the uterus is determined by means of sounding.

e. Insertion of IUD with the aid of a plastic inserter at time of menstruation is done by a physician (or one specifically trained). Menstruation ensures dilatation of cervix and that the patient is not pregnant.

f. A nylon string attached to the IUD dangles from the cervix and can be detected during vaginal examination.

▶ **NURSING ALERT:** If the patient is pregnant when an IUD is inserted, she may suffer septic abortion and possibly fatal septicemic shock; hence the wisdom of having the device inserted during menstruation.

6. Patient education
   a. Inform the client how to check for IUD nylon string.
   b. Instruct the patient to avoid intercourse for 5 days (time to permit IUD to induce endometrial changes).
   c. Recommend follow-up visits as directed.
   d. Suggest that the patient promptly seek assistance if any of the following occurs:
      (1) Unusually heavy or prolonged bleeding
      (2) Bleeding between periods
      (3) Pain; unusual vaginal discharge
      (4) Infection signs—chills/fever
      (5) Inability to locate string
      (6) Signs of pregnancy
      (7) Suspected or obvious expulsion of IUD
   e. Provide the patient with a wallet card showing IUD insertion date, clinic, and emergency telephone numbers.
   f. Suggest that the woman consult her physician as to how long her particular IUD can be worn before being removed. It should be removed and replaced every 2 to 3 years.

H. Hormonal Control—the "Pill"

1. Basis of operation of oral contraceptives (OC)
   Oral synthetic preparations of estrogens and progesterone are used. It is believed that in the presence of sufficient amounts of these synthetic compounds, the hypothalamus fails to secrete the usual luteinizing hormone (LH) releasing factor and its stimulating product LH, which normally occurs about 12–14 days after the onset of the monthly menstrual cycle and is essential to ovulation.
2. Indications
   a. For those desirous of a highly effective contraceptive with no special preparation immediately before intercourse.
   b. For women who will conscientiously adhere to a daily plan of pill-taking.
3. Methods
   a. Combined steroid therapy
      A pill with an estrogen and progestogen, usually

taken 20 days during each month, beginning on the 5th day after the onset of menstruation.
   b. Microprogestational therapy
   Low dosage of progestational drug given continuously:
   Androgens—19-carbon compounds
   Progesterone—21-carbon compounds
   Estrogens—Ethinyl estradiol
4. Protective effects
   a. Minimizes menstrual blood loss
   b. Decreases dysmenorrhea
   c. Decreased incidence of first attacks of rheumatoid arthritis
   d. Lower incidence of pelvic infection
   e. Appears to have protective effect against ovarian and endometrial cancer
5. Risk factors and possible contraindications

▶ **NURSING ALERT:** Cigarette smoking increases risk of serious cardiovascular side effects from oral contraceptives. Women who use the pill should be strongly advised not to smoke.

   a. Women over 40 years of age
   b. History of migraine, hypertension, epilepsy
   c. Leiomyomas of the uterus
   d. Past history of cardiovascular disease
   e. Known or suspected breast carcinoma
   f. Known or suspected estrogen-dependent neoplasia of uterus (endometrium or cervix)
   g. Liver disease or impaired liver function
   h. Known or suspected pregnancy
   i. Genital bleeding—undiagnosed
   j. Obesity, diabetes mellitus, and hypercholesterolemia
6. Management
   a. Monitored carefully with physical examination and Pap test at least annually.
   b. The lowest effective dose of estrogen and progestin (compatible with low failure rate and needs of individual patient) is used.
7. Disadvantages
   a. Interference with laboratory diagnostic procedures; sedimentation rate, thyroid test for protein-bound iodine or thyroxine, cervical smears, and biopsy.
   b. FDA 1984 revised labeling includes a warning that oral contraceptive use may be associated with an increased risk of cervical carcinoma.
8. Side effects
   Occur in approximately 1%–3% of women on low-dose pill
9. Failure rate (pregnancy)
   Combined—less than 1 pregnancy per 100 woman years.
I. Topical Spermicide—chemically active substance that incapacitates spermatozoa; when used properly, it is estimated to be 95% effective, and even when used improperly, it is considered about 85% effective. *Sponge* (Today*) is a soft, disposable, polyurethane contraceptive permeated with spermicide.
1. To use:
   a. Moisten sponge with water; fold between thumb and forefinger.

* VLI Corp., Irvine, CA

   b. Insert with concave side over the cervix.
   c. Upper walls of vagina hold sponge in place.
   d. A flat polyester ribbon serves as a "handle" for removal.
   e. A spermicide (nonoxynol-9) kills sperm on contact; sponge blocks path of sperm and absorbs them.
   f. May be worn up to 30 hours; leave in place for 6 hours after intercourse, then discard.
2. Advantages
   a. One size fits all; it is comfortable and easy to use.
   b. No prescription required.
   c. As effective as diaphragm.
3. Disadvantages
   a. Some find it expensive.
   b. Others believe the effectiveness rate is too low.

J. Other Contraceptives
Depo-Provera (injectable depot progestin, medroxyprogesterone) for long-acting contraception—investigational

Sterilization Procedures
A. Indications
1. The patient's desire
   a. Socioeconomic reasons
   b. Therapeutic or eugenic reasons to prevent a pregnancy that might endanger the mother's life
2. Legal considerations
   a. Laws much less rigid than those governing therapeutic abortion
   b. Written consent required from a legally responsible and informed person
   c. Must be compatible with state laws
3. Incidence and indications
   a. Increasing numbers are performed annually in US
   b. Done for multiparity, 2 or more previous cesarean sections, hypertensive cardiovascular disease
   c. Done for other reasons—vaginal plastic procedures, for inheritable life-threatening disease

B. Tubal Sterilization
1. Types
   a. Tubal ligation with or without resection
   b. Tubal ligation with or without crushing
   c. Tubal transection and burying of stumps
   d. Cornual resection
   e. Cornual occlusion utilizing cautery
2. Approaches
   a. Abdominal
   b. After a cesarean section
   c. Vaginally
3. Evaluation
   a. There are advantages and disadvantages to each of the above—the individual situation must be considered.
   b. Reversible methods of tubal occlusion or semi-permanent sterilization using metal clips or chemical injections are still investigational.
4. Laparoscopy
   a. A procedure in which coagulation and transection of the isthmic tubal segments are done through a laparoscope (an electrical current is passed for 3–5 seconds to cut and coagulate tube).
   b. The procedure is considered rapid, safe, and effective.

c. Effectiveness
  (1) Hysterosalpingography done 12 weeks post-operatively confirms tubal occlusion in 98% of patients.
  (2) No adverse effects occur in sex relations, menstrual function, or outward bodily appearance.
d. Hazards
  (1) Pulmonary embolism, hemorrhage, infection

  (2) Tubal pregnancy
  (3) Some women are disturbed emotionally by procedure; however, 90% of patients who request this have no subsequent regret.

C. Vasectomy (see p. 556)

Source of Information: American Fertility Society, 1801 Ninth Avenue, South, Birmingham, AL 35205

D. Abortion (see p. 1013)

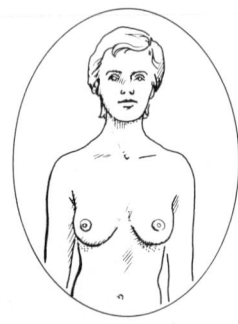

1. Careful examination of the breasts before a mirror for symmetry in size and shape, noting any puckering or dimpling of the skin or retraction of the nipple.

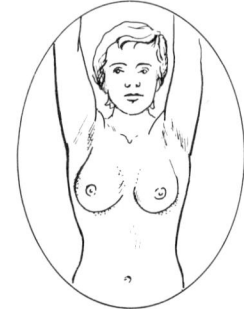

2. Arms raised over head, again studying the breasts in the mirror for the same signs.

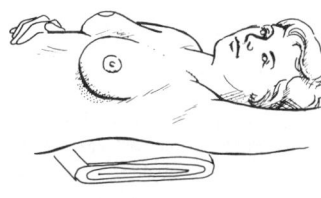

3. Reclining on bed with flat pillow or folded bath towel under the shoulder on the same side as breast to be examined.

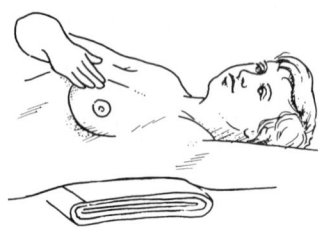

4. To examine the inner half of the breast, the arm is raised over the head. Beginning at the breastbone and, in a series of steps, the inner half of the breast is palpated.

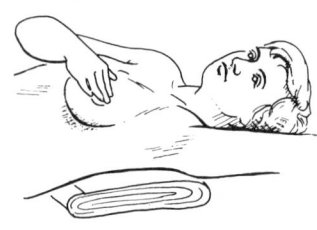

5. The area over the nipple is carefully palpated with the flat part of the fingers.

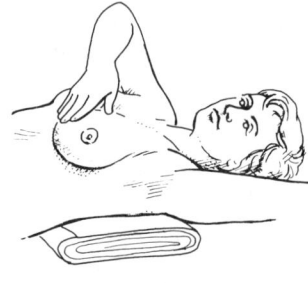

6. Examination of the lower inner half of the breast is completed.

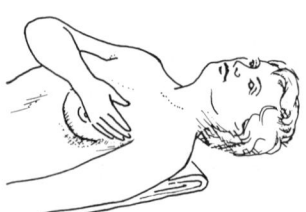

7. With arm down at side, self examination of breasts continues by carefully feeling the tissues which extend to the armpit.

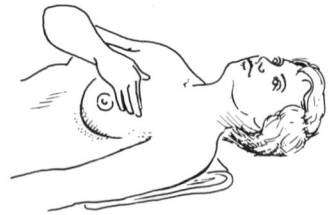

8. The upper outer quadrant of the breast is examined with the flat part of the fingers.

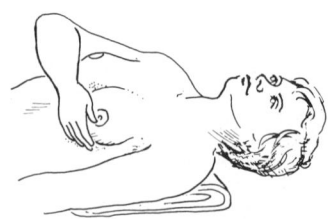

9. The lower outer quadrant of the breast is examined in successive stages with flat part of the fingers.

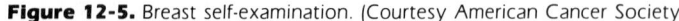

Figure 12-5. Breast self-examination. (Courtesy American Cancer Society)

2: Breast Conditions

Assessment and Diagnostic Evaluation

Breast Self-Examination (BSE)

A. Clinical Value

1. Experience has verified that more than 90% of breast cancers are found by women themselves.
2. When women discover lumps in their breasts at a very early stage, surgery can save 70%–80% of proved cases.

B. Health Education

1. Encourage women to examine their breasts once a month, just after the menstrual period, because breasts are less engorged at this time and a tumor is easier to detect, and at regular monthly intervals after the cessation of menses (Fig. 12-5).
2. The breast can be examined in the sitting or standing position, noting in a mirror any contour changes, asymmetry, nipple discharge, or eczematoid scaling around the nipple.
3. Then the breast is examined in the supine position with the breast spread out on the chest wall; use the flattened, more sensitive surface of the fingers to gently knead breast tissue in the search for abnormalities.
4. Since most of the lesions occur in the upper outer quadrant (see Fig. 12-8B), an effective pattern to follow is to start the examination in the upper outer quadrant, proceed around the breast, and repeat (at the end) the upper outer quadrant. (In this manner, five fourths of the breast are examined.)
5. When in doubt, compare findings with opposite breast.
6. Differences in the adolescent (11–18 years)
   a. Gynecomastia in the male occurs in 1 of 3 young men; these signs regress in 1–2 years.
   b. Thelarche (breast development in young female) commonly occurs unilaterally.
   c. The areola enlarges and forms a contour separate from the rest of the breast; the areola later becomes part of the normal contour.

C. Suggestions for Patients Who Find Self-Examination Difficult or Impossible To Do:

1. Determine the problem:
   a. If the patient complains of tenderness, gentle self-examination may be more effective and less painful than examination by someone else.
   b. For the woman who has cysts or lumps, recommend professional examination annually and instruct her in detecting changes from one month to the next.
   c. If the patient has large, pendulous breasts, encourage her to lie on her back and perform self-examination slowly and in a specific pattern or order.
2. Recommend other diagnostic aids periodically—mammography, thermography (below) as condition indicates.

D. Community Health Education

1. Tell women's organizations about the breast self-examination film and advise them to see it.
2. Arrange for local showings of the film.
3. Take part in the discussion of the film. Be prepared—know the signs that may mean breast cancer.
4. Help to create healthy psychological attitudes.
5. Know the resources within the community where medical help is available: physicians and nurse practitioners, cancer clinics, or cancer hospitals.

Guidelines: Examination of the Breast by the Nurse

Purpose
1. To detect abnormalities in the breasts
2. To teach a woman how to perform breast self-examination

Equipment
A good lamp and privacy

Procedure

Nursing Action	Rationale/Amplification
Preparatory Phase and Superficial Examination	
1. Have the woman strip to her waist and sit comfortably, facing the examiner.	1. This provides an opportunity to observe breasts visually for lack of symmetry and for gross signs such as redness, irritated nipple, dimpling, orange-peel skin.
2. Wash your hands under warm water and dry them; powder if they feel "sticky."	2. The breast is sensitive to cold.
Examination	
1. Palpate supraclavicular area.	1. Note whether lymph nodes are enlarged, fixed, movable, or difficult to locate.

(continued)

Guidelines: Examination of the Breast by the Nurse (continued)

Procedure
(Cont.)

Nursing Action	Rationale/Amplification
2. Palpate axillary nodes; hold the woman's forearm in your left palm while you check nodes with your right fingertips. Repeat on other side.	2. Same as 1 above.
3. Instruct the patient to lie down with her right arm under her head. Place a small pillow under the right shoulder.	3. This will spread breast tissue evenly over chest wall.
4. With the flattened surface of 2 or 3 fingers, gently palpate breast tissue, beginning at the upper outer quadrant. a. Proceed in an orderly pattern around the breast and repeat the first quarter examined. b. Repeat procedure for other breast.	4. The sensitive fingers, proceeding in a kneading fashion, can detect thickened, lumpy, or "buckshot" tissue between the patient's skin and chest wall. Since the majority of breast lesions are in the upper outer quadrant, this segment is double checked.
5. Recognize that there is a prolongation of the axillary extension of normal breast tissue, which may extend high into axilla.	5. This is normal if symmetrical and abnormal if asymmetrical.
6. Check the areolar area for crustiness, nipple discharge, signs of infection.	6. Prepare to collect a discharge specimen for cytology if indicated (see Fig. 12-7, p. 592).
7. Record findings and report abnormalities to the physician.	
8. Instruct the patient in performing self-examination on her own (Fig. 12-5). Encourage her to ask any questions; provide her with appropriate literature.	8. Ninety-five percent of women discover their own abnormalities.

Physical Examination

1. Annual physical checkup should include breast examination and palpation.
2. Twice-a-year examination recommended for women with a family history of cancer.

Diagnostic Tests

A. **Mammography**—roentgenography of breast without injection of contrast medium; 2 views: (1) caudal and (2) mediolateral.

1. Indications: Greatest value is in detecting suspicious area before a "lump" is felt.
2. Guidelines for use of mammography for breast cancer screening:
   a. In women under 35, no mammography.
   b. In women 35–39, use only if patient has had breast cancer.
   c. Women in their 40s, use annually if there is a history of breast cancer in immediate family.
   d. Offer annually to women over age 50.
3. Use other than for cancer screening:
   a. Breast disease evident in the form of a questionable lump.
   b. Lumpy or very large breasts, which are difficult to examine.
   c. Screening the opposite breast in a woman with a mass on one side.
   d. Cancerophobia (fear of cancer).

B. **Thermography**—infrared photography gives a pictorial representation of heat patterns on the surface of the breast, which may indicate signs of abnormality. This is recognized by either graphic or thermal asymmetry.

1. Heat-sensing equipment is used to detect minute amounts of heat generated in and around areas of increased blood supply.
2. Thermography is a complementary diagnostic tool that may be useful in the evaluation of breast disease when combined with both physical examination under the supervision of a qualified physician and mammography by a trained radiologist.
3. An advantage is that there is no radiation exposure.

C. **Telethermometry**

1. Heat emissions are measured by an infrared sensor.
2. These are then recorded by camera.

D. **Ultrasonography**—sensitive to differentiating a solid from a cystic lesion.

1. Can detect hidden lesions
2. Painless and noninvasive

E. **Diaphanography**—a combination of transillumination, visual inspection, and documented film-recording with nonionizing radiation. It is similar in value to spot-filming in fluoroscopy.

F. **Computed Tomography**

1. May be useful in detecting cancer in small, dense breasts, which are difficult to examine by mammography.
2. It is unsuitable for routine screening and diagnostic studies.

In summary, none of the techniques described above are used as a substitute for mammography. None of the above techniques eliminates the need for surgical biopsy or breast aspiration if clinically indicated.

Biopsy

A. **Aspiration** (needle)

Purpose: This is a simple, rapid, and accurate procedure to detect breast cancer.

1. Tumor or cyst is immobilized between 2 fingers to stabilize it during needle insertion (Fig. 12-6).
2. Gently create a vacuum in syringe by pulling back and forth on plunger; allow pressure to equalize before withdrawing needle.
3. Spread needle contents on glass slide; further spread specimen with a 2nd glass slide held at an angle.

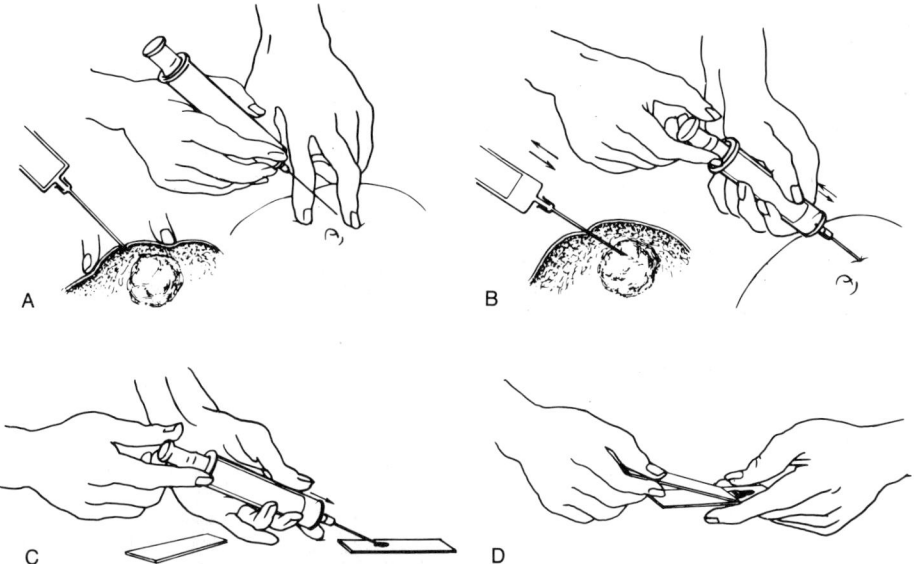

Figure 12-6. Aspiration cytology. (*A*) Tumor is immobilized with two fingers before the needle is inserted. (*B*) A vacuum is created by withdrawing the plunger slowly but forcefully several times. Before the needle is removed, the pressure is allowed to equalize. (*C*) Contents of the needle are placed on a glass slide. (*D*) The smear is spread forward gently with a glass slide inclined at an angle of about 35°, with an up-and-down movement. (Zajdela A. The value of aspiration cytology in the diagnosis of breast cancer. Cancer 35)

Note: Positive results are significant. Negative results are ignored; other clinical evaluations must be done.

B. Incisional (Surgical)

A specimen of tissue is obtained in the operating room and sent to the laboratory for frozen section, which is then stained and examined under the microscope. It is desirable to allow at least a day or two between the biopsy and definitive treatment.

C. Excisional

Following an incision into the breast, the entire lump is removed for microscopic study.

D. Estrogen-Receptor and Progesterone-Receptor Assay—A test of tumor tissue to determine whether or not the cancer cells have receptor sites. If such sites are present, the patient is more likely to respond to hormonal manipulation.

Conditions of the Nipple

Fissures and Bleeding

	Fissure of Nipple	Bleeding from Nipple

Assessment and clinical manifestations	A *fissure* of the nipple is a longitudinal type of ulcer that occasionally develops in the breast of a nursing mother.
	  a. Nipple appears sore and irritated
	  b. Bleeding from nipple
		Bloody discharge—usually on edge of areola.

Causes	1. Lack of preparation of nipples in prenatal period. 2. Condition aggravated by sucking infant.	1. Most commonly due to wart-like papilloma in one of larger collecting ducts at edge of areola. 2. Occasionally a malignancy is responsible (Fig. 12-7, cytology examination).
Health education	1. Keep nipple clean by washing and drying after each nursing period (see p. 999).	

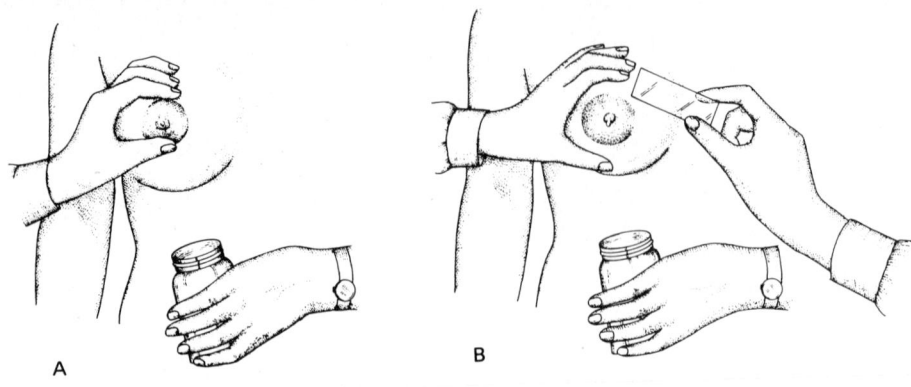

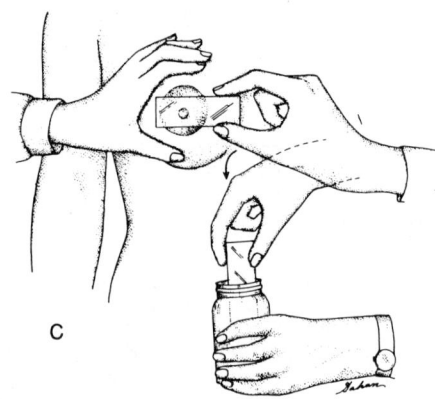

Figure 12-7. Obtaining nipple discharge specimen for cytologic examination.
1. Wash nipple gently with cotton pledget; pat dry.
2. Gently strip duct and express fluid only until a small pea-sized drop appears on nipple.
3. Obtain assistance of the patient in holding container of fixative solution near breast to receive the prepared slide.
4. Stabilize breast with fingers and thumb of one hand (*A*).
5. Gently place one end of slide on nipple (*B*); rapidly draw slide across nipple and immediately drop into fixative solution (*C*).
6. This may be repeated to secure additional specimens if necessary.
NOTE: 1. Positive results are significant.
    2. Negative results may be "false-negatives." This test is never used alone but in conjunction with other diagnostic tests.

	Fissure of Nipple	Bleeding from Nipple

Treatment and nursing interventions	2. In prenatal period, wash, dry, and lubricate nipples in preparation for nursing.
	1. Wash nipples with sterile saline solution.
	2. Use artificial nipple for nursing.
	3. If above does not initiate healing process, stop nursing and use breast pump.
		1. Surgery for palpable mass.
		  a. Duct is identified.
		  b. Papilloma is excised (or a wedge of breast from area producing the bleeding is excised if no gross papilloma is identified) through a small periareolar incision—send for laboratory analysis.
		  c. Sterile dressings applied.
		2. If no palpable mass, mammography and xerography.

Inflammation of the Breast

Acute Mastitis and Mammary Abscess

	Acute Mastitis	Mammary Abscess
Incidence	May occur at beginning or end of lactation.	Often follows acute mastitis.
Source of infection	1. Hands of patient 2. Personnel caring for the patient 3. Infection from baby 4. Blood-borne	Same
Assessment and clinical manifestations	1. Infection attacks duct, causing stagnation of milk in lobules. 2. Dull pain occurs in the area affected. 3. Breast feels doughy and tough. 4. May also have a discharging nipple.	1. Area is very sensitive, appears dusky red. 2. Pus may be expressed from nipple (see Fig. 12-7, nipple discharge for cytology). 3. Mass is palpable.
Treatment and nursing interventions	1. Have the patient stop breast-feeding. 2. Apply heat or cold (depending on stage of infection). 3. Administer chemotherapeutic agents as prescribed. 4. Give progesterone to relieve congestion. 5. Have the patient wear firm breast support. 6. Encourage the patient to practice meticulous personal hygiene.	1. Administer antibiotics and chemotherapy as prescribed. 2. Incise and drain. 3. Apply hot, wet dressings to increase drainage and hasten resolution.

Fibrocystic Disease

Fibrocystic disease is mammary dysplasia characterized by increased formation of fibrous tissue, hyperplasia of the epithelial cells of the ducts and breast glands, and dilatation of the ducts. It is related to the cyclic stimulation of the breast by estrogen, but represents a departure from the normal stimulation and regression pattern of this process.

Incidence

1. The most common lesion of the female breast; 3 to 4 times more prevalent than cancer.
2. Overgrowth of fibrous tissue around ducts; dilatation of the ducts to form cysts; epithelial hyperplasia of the ducts.
3. Occurs usually in women between 35 and 50 and is endocrine related.

Clinical Manifestations

1. The patient complains of an uncomfortable feeling in the breast.
2. Cysts or lumps are usually firm, single or multiple, smooth, round masses; bilateral.
3. They are tender on palpation or pressure and slightly mobile.
4. Pain may be of the "shooting" type and may be aggravated by congestion before a menstrual period.

Treatment and Nursing Interventions

1. Aspiration
   a. The patient is placed in supine position. Under aseptic precautions, skin area is cleansed with a skin antiseptic.
   b. Local anesthesia is given.
   c. The physician immobilizes cyst with thumb and index finger of one hand.
   d. Using a 20-ml. syringe and No. 16 or 18 gauge needle, the cyst is penetrated and aspirated.
2. Excision
   If cyst refills within a week or 2, excisional biopsy is usually performed.
3. The nurse emphasizes the importance of frequent reexaminations.
   a. Individuals with fibrocystic disease have an increased incidence of subsequent malignancy.
   b. Self-examination is difficult in the markedly fibrotic breast.
4. Avoidance of methylxanthines (coffee, tea, cola, and chocolate) tends to resolve these cysts.

Note: The palpable changes of fibrocystic disease may mask an underlying cancer.

Tumors of the Breast

Fibroadenomata

Clinical Manifestations

1. Firm, round, movable, benign tumors of the breast.
2. Appear in breasts of girls in their late teens or early twenties.
3. No pain or tenderness.

Treatment

Removal through a small incision

Prognosis

No malignant potential

Cancer of the Breast

Incidence

1. Breast cancer is the leading cause of cancer incidence and death in American women today.
2. One of every 4 women having an initial breast biopsy will have a malignancy.
3. About 119,000 new cases are predicted yearly, and it is estimated that there will be 38,000 deaths.
4. Despite all efforts to date, the breast cancer death rate remains high.
5. Over 90% of patients discover their condition themselves through breast self-examination.
6. Survival rates
   a. For all women: 5-year survival rate is about 68%.
   b. Localized in breast: 5-year survival rate is 88%.

Risk Factors in Breast Cancer

A. **Major Risk Factors** (Also see Table 12-1)

1. Sex—99% occur in females.
2. Age—more than 85% of women with breast cancer are over age 45.

Table 12-1   Major Risk Factors—Breast Cancer

Characteristic	Risk	
	High	Low
Sex—female	High	
Age		
Early 40s	Yes	No
45–55 (past menopause)	Yes	No
Genetics—women whose mother and sisters had breast cancer are twice as likely to develop cancer.	Yes	No
Race	Caucasian	Oriental
Menarche	Early	Late
Parity	Nulliparous	Parous
Unmarried	Higher	Lower
Infertile	Higher	Lower
Women who have had first child after 34	Yes	No
Menopause		
Natural	Late	Early
Artificial	No	Yes
History of severe constipation (2 or fewer bowel movements/week)	Yes	No

3. Genetics—women whose mothers and sisters have had breast cancer are twice as likely to develop cancer.
4. Parity—decreased risk threefold to fourfold if first birth is before 18 years of age. Decrease in risk continues, but at a declining rate up to age 25 for first parity. Increased risks in unmarried women, infertile women, women with fewer than 3 children, and women who have first child after 34.
5. If breast cancer appears in one breast, the likelihood of cancer in the other breast is greater.
6. Benign cystic breast is considered to be a precursor to cancer; likelihood of cancer is about 4 times greater in women who have cystic disease.
7. Severely constipated women (2 or fewer bowel movements a week) demonstrate a fourfold increase in risk of breast cancer.

B. **Prominent Risk Factors**

1. Prolonged total menstrual activity. Increased incidence under the following circumstances:
   a. When menarche occurs before 12 years of age
   b. In those with 30 or more years menstrual activity
   c. When menopause occurs after 55
2. Other organ cancers such as ovary, colon, endometrium
3. Wet-type cerumen (earwax)—genetic predisposition

C. **Possible Risk Factors**

1. Heavy radiation exposure
2. Immunodeficiency
3. Exogenous estrogen administration
4. Excessive intake of dietary fat

Treatment

Goals:
Preserve the life of the woman.
Achieve permanent local control of the disease.
Minimize the possibility of recurrence.
Provide the best cosmetic result.

These may be accomplished by surgical removal of the cancer. Radiation, chemotherapy, and immunotherapy are other treatment modalities that may be employed independently or in combination with surgery for the purpose of helping to cure, control growth, alleviate pain, and/or prevent recurrence (Table 12-2).

Prognosis

1. When malignancy is confined to breast: 5-year survival—85%
2. When malignancy has spread to axilla: 5-year survival—55%

A. **Types of Surgical Interventions:**

1. *Lumpectomy* (tylectomy, tumorectomy)—removal of circumscribed area around and including tumor.
2. *Quadrantectomy*—removal of a breast quadrant that includes the tumor area followed by radiotherapy of the breast and the lymph drainage paths.
3. *Partial mastectomy* (segmental mastectomy)—removal of the tumor plus 2–3-cm. wedge of normal tissue surrounding it as well as a portion of the overlying skin and underlying fascia that envelop breast and chest muscle. Augmental surgery may be done later, since this operation may be disfiguring.
4. *Modified radical*—entire breast is removed, as is the

Table 12-2   Classification of Breast Tumor and Preferred Method of Treatment

Clinical Anatomic Observation	Treatment

Stage I	Variable—tylectomy (p. 594)
	    Some prefer simple mastectomy plus irradiation. Others prefer simple mastectomy
	        without irradiation.

Breast mass localized; all nodes negative	Modified radical mastectomy
Stage II	
Breast mass localized; axillary nodes positive	Radical mastectomy preferred with or without postoperative irradiation.
Stage III	
	This is considered inoperable for cure. Variable depending on extensiveness:
Breast mass locally extensive; axillary, supraclavicular, and internal	1. Simple mastectomy with radiation, chemotherapy, and
mammary nodes positive	2. Radiation therapy, chemotherapy, and endocrine manipulation
Stage IV	

	Variable, depending on location of metastasis (bone, soft tissue, etc.)
	1. Radiation therapy for primary lesion or metastasis
	2. Endocrine manipulation
	    a. Systemic—estrogens, androgens, or steroids
	    b. Ablation—oophorectomy, adrenalectomy, hypophysectomy

Distant metastasis	3. Chemotherapy

pectoralis minor muscle; some or most of axillary lymph nodes are removed.
5. *Total mastectomy*—entire breast is removed, but pectoralis muscles left intact; most or all of axillary lymph nodes are left intact.
6. *Classical radical mastectomy (Halsted)*—removal of breast and underlying muscles down to chest wall; also removal of nodules and lymphatics of axilla. This is rapidly being replaced.

B. Radiation
1. Radiation is effective in damaging and preventing cell reproduction. Cancer cells are especially susceptible to radiation.
2. Utilization in breast cancer
    a. As adjuvant therapy with surgery
    b. To shrink a large tumor to operable size
    c. To alleviate pain caused by metastasis
    d. As primary therapy
3. Method—following tumor and lymph node excision, a series of external radiation treatments are begun:
    a. Usually 4–5 treatments a week for 4–5 weeks (a total of approximately 5,000 rads)
    b. Radiation directed to chest wall, remaining lymph nodes
    c. Side effects—mild fatigue; later, skin will look and feel sunburned and eventually the breast becomes more firm.
    d. A "booster" or second phase of treatment may be given:
        (1) electron beam or (2) radioactive implant.

C. Adjuvant Therapy
This is therapy used to supplement surgery or primary radiation therapy.
1. Local or regional adjuvant therapy—radiotherapy. Value is controversial.
2. Systemic adjuvant therapy—this includes chemotherapy, hormonal therapy, or immunotherapy.

Assessment
Clinical Manifestations (Fig. 12-8)
1. Early signs are insidious.
2. A nontender lump appears in the breast, most frequently in the upper outer quadrant; it may be movable and isolated.
3. Pain usually is absent except in the late stages. A recent study indicated that 13% of patients described

pain as a primary symptom; 7% indicated that it was the first clue that led them to probe and examine the breast. Pain was described as a "hurt" or "funny feeling" rather than acute or sharp.
4. Retraction or dimpling of the skin over the mass may be noted.
5. On mirror examination, asymmetry may be observed—the affected breast appears more elevated than the other.
6. Nipple retraction or nipple bleeding may be apparent.
7. Later, the nodule becomes more fixed to the chest wall.
8. Nodular axillary masses may appear.
9. Ulceration appears in late stages.

Patient Problems/Nursing Diagnoses
1. Anxiety and fear related to possibility of mutilation, disturbance of patient's marriage, and the termination of life.
2. Impairment in skin integrity related to breast surgery, wound drainage, and radiation.
3. Knowledge deficit related to inadequate information of preoperative and postoperative care and the many support services available.
4. Grieving about lost femininity and a coveted body part as well as alteration in self-concept related to breast removal for cancer.
5. Potential physical and sexual dysfunction related to loss of a breast.

Planning and Implementation
Preoperative Nursing Interventions
A. Psychosocial Preoperative Preparation
1. Begin emotional support when the patient is told that biopsy and hospitalization may be required.
2. Dispel fear by
    a. Listening to the patient's concerns and dispelling misconceptions.
    b. Collaborating with physician on a unified approach to informing the patient.
    c. Emphasizing successful program of rehabilitation, use of prosthesis, and possibly reconstruction.
    d. Having a patient who made a satisfactory postoperative adjustment visit present patient.
    e. Soliciting support of the husband and/or significant others.
    f. Providing encouragement and reassurance.

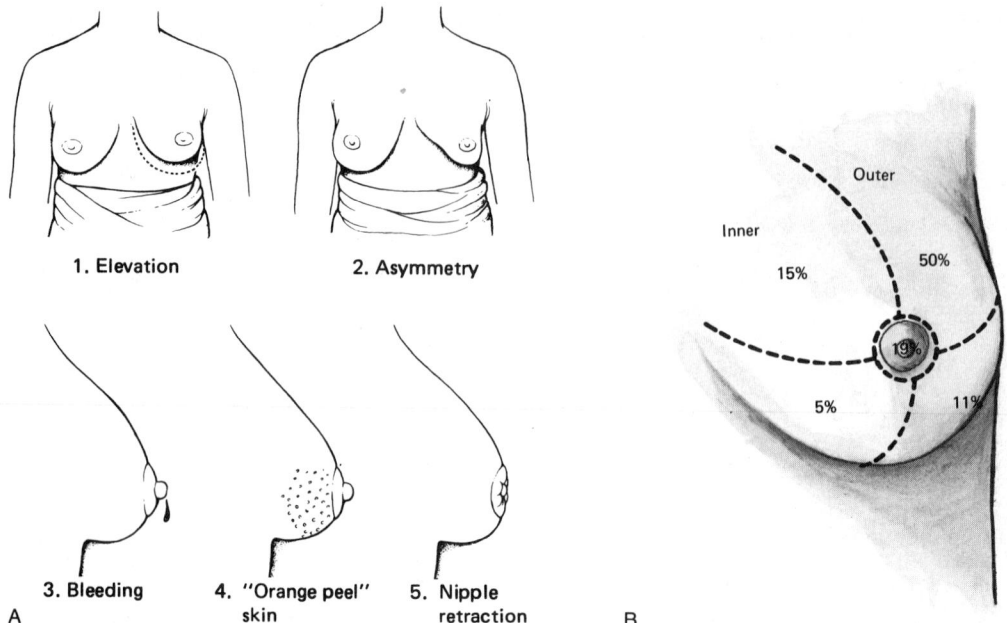

1. Elevation   2. Asymmetry

3. Bleeding   4. "Orange peel" skin   5. Nipple retraction

A

B

Outer
Inner
15%   50%
19%
5%   11%

Figure 12-8. (A) Signs of cancer of the breast. (B) Distribution of carcinomas in different areas of breast.

3. Minimize delay before operation.
   Determine physical, nutritional, and emotional needs.
4. Include the patient's husband/partner by keeping him informed of the treatment plan and its progress.
5. Administer hypnotic to block the patient's concerns.
6. Relay any positive verified information related to the successful removal of all tumors, limited spread, etc.; this can accelerate recovery.
7. Support the surgeon's plan to remove malignancy, minimize disfigurement, and prevent spread of cancer cells.
8. Work with the patient in preparation for anesthesia and surgery; describe each activity to the patient.
   Note: Protocols for preoperative and postoperative care are given in detail on pp. 84–87.

B. Preoperative Physical Preparation

1. Instruct the patient to wash operative area with a detergent–germicide for several days before admission.
2. When skin graft is anticipated, shave and clean donor area (usually anterior aspect of thigh).
3. If radical surgery is anticipated, have blood replacement available.

Postoperative Nursing Interventions

A. General Care

1. See Chapter 6 for detailed discussion of postoperative care.
2. Upon the patient's return from the recovery room, promote comfort and rest; administer analgesics for pain.
3. Encourage fluid and nutritional support as tolerated and desired.
4. Position the patient comfortably in semi-Fowler's position; if arm is free, elevate on a pillow; the most

distal part (hand) is placed higher to permit gravity to aid in removal of fluid via lymphatics and venous pathways.
5. Check dressings for undue constriction, signs of hemorrhage, etc.; ensure that portable suction or other drainage devices are operating properly.

B. Exercises and Ambulation

1. Encourage mobility of arm on the affected side as recommended by the surgeon, to prevent such complications as lymphedema and frozen shoulder:
   a. Initiate bed exercises after 24 hours, such as wrist and elbow flexion and extension, hourly.
   b. Encourage the patient to use her arm in self-care: washing face, applying lipstick, combing hair.
   c. See Table 12-3, page 597, for activities to be resumed eventually.
2. Ambulate the patient early, as determined by the individual patient.

C. Other Treatment Modalities

1. Radiation therapy
   a. Primary treatment when surgery has been ruled out by advanced age, inoperable condition, other complications.
   b. Adjunct therapy to surgery.
   c. To reduce tumor size; as palliation for pain.
   When radiation therapy is used, follow principles of care, page 913.
2. Chemotherapy—also see pp. 905–912.
   a. Used as adjunct therapy to surgery and/or radiotherapy.
   b. Usually various combinations of drugs are preferred.
   c. Four major types of drugs are alkylating, antimetabolite, antibiotic, and mitotic inhibitor.

3. Immunotherapy (unproved)
   a. Theory is that immunologic response could destroy invading cancer cells while sparing normal cells.
   b. Bacille Calmette Guérin (BCG) and levamisole have shown promise of being able to destroy cancer cells.

D. Coping Measures

1. Permit the patient to view incision line when psychologically appropriate; have her assist in keeping the wound clean; have her use a mirror if necessary to view the area adequately; instruct her in the proper technique to use in applying dressings and fixing them properly.
2. Familiarize the patient with "Reach to Recovery" program of the American Cancer Society:
   a. Combine this with visits by helpful persons who have had a successful mastectomy rehabilitation.
   b. Acquaint the patient with prosthetic possibilities as determined feasible by the surgeon.
   c. Suggest clothing adjustments and possibilities.
3. Encourage the patient to "talk out" and express her feelings—provide support, including psychospiritual if required.
4. Assist the patient in addressing psychosocial adjustment problems, including sexual problems; include her husband or important others as required.

Complication: *Lymphedema of the Arm*

Lymphedema is an obstruction of the lymph flow in the arm on the operated side, producing a chronic swelling of the part, particularly if it is in a dependent position. Lymphedema is due to lymph node removal and compression of axillary vein by tumor or scar.

Table 12-3 Exercises for the Rehabilitation of the Patient Following Mastectomy

Exercise	Equivalent Daily Activities
1. Stand erect. Lean forward from waist. Allow arms to hang. Swing arms from side to side together; then in opposite direction. Next: swing arms from front to back together; then in opposite direction.	Broom sweeping Vacuum cleaning Mopping floor Pulling out and pushing in drawers Weaving Playing golf
2. Stand erect facing wall with palms of hand flat against wall; arms extended. Relax arms and shoulders and allow upper part of body to lean forward against hands. Push away to original position; repeat.	Pushing self out of bath tub Kneading bread Breast stroke—swimming Sawing or cutting types of crafts
3. Stand erect facing wall with palms of hands flat against wall. Climb the wall with the fingers; descend, repeat.	Raising windows Washing windows Hanging clothes on line Reaching to an upper shelf
4. Stand erect and clasp hands at small of back; raise hands; lower; repeat. Clasp hands back of neck; reach downward; upward; repeat.	Fastening brassiere Buttoning blouse or dress Pulling up a dress zipper Fastening beads Washing the back
5. Toss a rope over the shower curtain rod. Hold the ends of the rope (knotted) in each hand and raise arms sideways. Using a see-saw motion and with arms outstretched slide the rope up and down over the rod.	Drying the back with a bath towel Raising and lowering a window blind Closing and opening window drapes
6. Flex and extend each finger in turn	Sewing, knitting, crocheting Typing, painting, playing piano or other musical instrument

Hand Care*

After a radical mastectomy, an arm may swell because lymph nodes and lymph vessels were necessarily removed and the body is therefore less able to combat infection in this extremity.

Make every effort to avoid all cuts, scratches, pin pricks, hangnails, insect bites, burns, and the use of strong detergents, since these can lead to serious infection with increased swelling.

Some "DO NOT'S":
DO NOT hold a cigarette in this hand

DO NOT carry your purse or anything heavy with this arm
DO NOT wear a wristwatch or other jewelry on this arm
DO NOT cut or pick at cuticles or hangnails on this hand

DO NOT work near thorny plants or dig in the garden

DO NOT reach into a hot oven with this arm
DO NOT permit injection in this arm
DO NOT permit blood to be drawn from this arm
DO NOT allow your blood pressure to be taken on this arm

Some "DO'S":
DO wear a loose rubber glove on this hand when washing dishes
DO wear a thimble when sewing

DO apply a good lanolin hand cream several times daily
DO wear your "Life-Guard Medical Aid" tag engraved with "CAUTION—LYMPHEDEMA ARM—NO TESTS—NO HYPOS"
DO contact your doctor if your arm gets red, warm, or unusually hard or swollen
DO return for a check-up and re-measurement for a new sleeve in two months
DO show this Hand Care Sheet to your surgeon

* Reprinted through the courtesy of the CLEVELAND CLINIC Department of Physical Medicine and Rehabilitation.

A. Prevention

1. Exercises indicated in Table 12-3 should be done.
2. The affected arm should be massaged 3 or 4 months postoperatively to increase circulation and lessen edema.
3. The affected arm is elevated frequently to prevent dependent edema.
4. The arm and operative site is kept scrupulously clean to prevent infection.
5. Nonconstrictive clothing is worn to permit adequate circulation.
6. The suggestions in the hand care chart below should be followed diligently.

B. Treatment

1. May include a diuretic.
2. An intermittent compression unit with pressurized sleeve may be used to force fluid back into venous system.

Health Education

1. Talk to and listen to patient; encourage questions and provide helpful answers.
2. Prepare the husband for his role in providing the necessary emotional support.
3. Initiate active exercise on the affected side 24 hours postoperatively for hand and elbow. Check with physician on extent of exercise for each individual patient. Exercises will increase daily, and the patient will do more of her own activities, such as hair combing, teeth brushing, etc. (Table 12-3).

Note: Be cautious in exercising the shoulder during the first week after surgery. Excessive abduction of the arm at the shoulder can lift skin flaps from chest wall and increase serous formation.

    a. Exercise should not be painful.
    b. Bilateral activity is emphasized.
    c. Proper posture should be maintained.
    d. If the patient has had a skin graft or if the skin was approximated under tension, exercises will be limited.

4. Care of Wound
    a. Explain how the wound will gradually change.
    b. Note that the newly healed wound may have less sensation due to severed nerves.
    c. Bathe gently and blot carefully to dry.
    d. Recognize signs of infection—pain, tenderness, redness, swelling; if these are present, report to physician.
    e. Massage gently the healed incision with cocoa butter to encourage circulation and increase skin elasticity. This is initiated with physician approval.

5. Use of a prosthesis—sponge rubber, air-filled, or fluid-filled.
    a. Type and style are suggested on an individual basis; skilled fitters from reliable companies are most helpful.
    b. Observe effect of prosthesis on incision; to prevent irritation, lamb's wool padding may be used.
    c. A prosthesis should not be worn unless authorized by the physician.

Importance of Follow-up Visit

1. Incision healing evaluated
2. Rehabilitative effort assessed
3. Effectiveness of prosthesis determined
4. Patient's psychosocial adjustment evaluated
5. Possible recurrence detected

Evaluation
Expected Outcomes

1. Accepts diagnosis of breast cancer and adjusts positively
2. Experiences acceptable wound closure and adapts to rehabilitation program
3. Utilizes various support services as required
4. Moves through the grieving process and exhibits a satisfactorily optimistic outlook
5. Adjusts to physical and sexual dysfunction and proceeds with positive alternate plans

Prophylactic Mastectomy

Removal of breast tissue (leaving skin and nipple area), followed by insertion of a mammary implant in *carefully selected patients who are in the high-risk group for developing breast cancer.* Implants may be inserted immediately or at a later date.

Postoperative Nursing Goal:
Maintain skin viability and survival over implant area.

    a. Keep head of bed elevated about 30 degrees to promote drainage.
    b. Instruct the patient to keep elbows at her side to prevent stretching of breast skin (3–4 weeks); soft wristlet restraints may be necessary at night.
    c. Check dressings and suction drains frequently for evidence of bleeding.
    d. Eliminate any pressure on dressings which might restrict circulation.
    e. Encourage intake of fluid to prevent dehydration.
    f. Advise the patient not to turn on her side or abdomen for at least a month to avoid trauma to operated area.
    g. Encourage the patient to take deep breaths and cough at prescribed intervals to aerate lungs that may otherwise develop complications because of limited movement.

Breast Mammaplasty
(Breast Reconstruction)

Breast mammaplasty is the reconstruction of the breast by using prosthetic implants or fashioning a flap from the patient's own tissues; an areola–nipple reconstruction may also be performed.

A. Prevalence and Indications

1. The possibility of breast reconstruction is receiving more attention for several reasons:
    a. Breast surgery is less radical
    b. Recent advances in plastic surgery
    c. Greater acceptance of cosmetic surgery
2. Reconstruction is performed usually 3 months to a year after a mastectomy; there is no maximum time limit.
3. Reconstruction is not recommended for women under the following circumstances:
    a. Presence of large tumors or extensive nodular involvement; recent history of breast abscess or history of diffuse, painful cystic mastitis
    b. Presence of other diseases that might impair the healing process
    c. Radiation therapy or chest skin grafts
    d. Marked obesity
    e. Advanced age
    f. Previous radical mastectomy

B. Implants—flexible plastic sacs filled with silicone gel (greater firmness) or saline solution (lesser firmness). Some can be subtly adjusted by inflation with air or injection of additional saline solution (Fig. 12-9).

1. This pouch can be inserted through a small incision at the base-fold area and positioned underneath breast skin.
2. The tightness of the skin often determines the size of the implant; this may require alteration of the remaining breast to match the reconstructed breast.

Health Education

1. The patient is instructed to keep her elbow close to her side for several days to a week.
2. Full use of the patient's arm is achieved in about a month; however, strenuous arm use in tennis, golf, or swimming may be delayed.
3. A well-fitted brassiere worn day and night for 3 months may assist the breast(s) in taking on the desired shape.
4. Instruct the patient to report thinning or discoloration of skin over the implant area.
5. The patient is instructed in how to distinguish the prosthesis from normal or abnormal breast tissue during self-examination for breast cancer.

C. Flap Graft

This is the transfer of skin from another part of the body, usually in stages, to the mastectomy site (see Grafts, pp. 628). This requires several hospitalizations, is costly and not as cosmetically effective as implants.

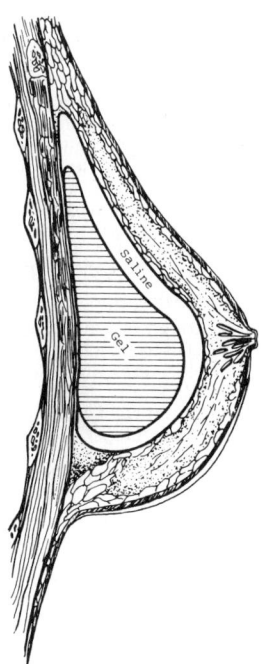

Figure 12-9. The diagrammatic sketch shows the placement of a mammary implant—in this case, one featuring a sealed inner gel implant surrounded by an inflatable outer saline implant. (Courtesy American Heyer-Schulte Corporation, Goleta, CA 1980)

D. Areola–Nipple Reconstruction

The nipple and areola are saved during mastectomy and banked (suturing to a temporary site, usually thigh or abdomen) until the breast reconstruction is done.

1. If banking is not possible, tissue from the other breast, labia, or ear lobe may be grafted.

Recurrent or Metastatic Breast Cancer

Modalities of Endocrine Manipulation

Theory and Goal:

Malignant tumor cells depend on hormonal function in the host; deprivation of hormones reduces tumor's growth. Currently, tumor removed at operation is tested for estrogen receptors. If positive, the use of hormonal therapy or ablation can be carried out on a more rational basis than heretofore, with an anticipated good response.

A. Ablative Procedures

1. Bilateral salpingo-ovariectomy
   a. This is often the initial treatment of choice for premenopausal patients with metastatic breast cancer.
   b. Remission lasts from 3 months to several years (median—1 year).
   c. If signs of reactivation of tumor growth occur, further endocrine therapy may be done (hypophysectomy or adrenalectomy).
2. Hypophysectomy—done microsurgically (transnasal or transsphenoidal)
   a. This is done for postmenopausal patients with metastatic breast cancer.
   b. Remission lasts from 6 months to several years (median—1½ years).
   c. Upon signs of reactivation of tumor growth, cytotoxic chemotherapy is initiated.
3. Adrenalectomy
   a. Bilateral adrenalectomy is usually combined with bilateral salpingo-ovariectomy.
   b. This is often recommended for postmenopausal patients with metastatic breast cancer.
   c. Remission lasts from 6 months to several years (median—1 year).
   d. Women who have had ovariectomy and adrenalectomy and who show signs of recurrence are given cytotoxic chemotherapy.

B. Hormones

1. Estrogens
   a. Most commonly used in women who are 5 or more years postmenopausal with recurrent breast carcinoma.
   b. Diethylstilbestrol or ethinyl estradiol are the estrogens used.
   c. Remissions last 3 months to several years (median—1 year).
   d. With initial exacerbation of the disease, hormone therapy is immediately terminated.
   e. Recurrence of this disease following remission is treated with hypophysectomy or adrenalectomy.

▶ **NURSING ALERT:** Observe for fluid retention following estrogen therapy; this can be prevented with dietary sodium restriction and use of diuretics.

2. Progestins (medroxyprogesterone acetate)
   a. Useful in about 30% of postmenopausal women with metastatic carcinoma.
   b. Remission is about 8 months.
   c. Failure with progestins suggests a change to other modalities of endocrine therapy.
3. Androgens (fluoxymesterone)
   a. Useful in about 20% of postmenopausal women.
   b. Remissions last about 6 months.
   c. When no longer effective, other kinds of endocrine therapy may be useful.
   d. Side effects
      (1) Fluid retention, which can be prevented by restricting sodium and using diuretics
      (2) Virilization (development of secondary male characteristics)
4. Corticosteroids (prednisone, dexamethasone)
   a. Not usually used in primary management of postmenopausal women with metastatic breast cancer because of the possibility of Cushing's syndrome.
   b. Useful as
      (1) An adjunct to radiation therapy in patients with cerebral metastasis
      (2) An adjunct to cytotoxic chemotherapy in patients with advanced liver and pulmonary metastasis
5. Tamoxifen—synthetic anti-estrogen
   a. Administered orally twice a day

b. Causes tumor to regress in 6–17 months
   (1) Effective in about ⅓ of all patients
   (2) Effective in about ⅔ of women who are estrogen receptor-positive
c. Incidence of side effects is very low; hypercalcemia in about 3% of patients.
6. Aminoglutethimide (investigational)—suppresses estrogen production
   a. Administered with hydrocortisone
   b. Best responses in women with metastasis to bone and soft tissues
   c. Side effects—lethargy, unstable gait, dizziness, transient rash

C. Cytotoxic Chemotherapy

Alkylating agents: 5-fluorouracil, methotrexate, vincristine

1. Remission lasts about 6 months (in 20% of patients).
2. Five-drug combination can boost remission rate to about 9 months (in 65% of patients)—5-fluorouracil, methotrexate, vincristine, cyclophosphamide, prednisone.
3. Recommended for patients who have metastasis to liver or lungs and are poor surgical risks for endocrine ablative surgery.
4. Recommended for premenopausal patients who are not benefitting from ovariectomy or hypophysectomy.
5. Doxorubicin hydrochloride (Adriamycin) usually used when 5-drug chemotherapy fails.

Bibliography

Gynecologic Conditions

Books

Barber HRK. Manual of Gynecologic Oncology. Philadelphia, JB Lippincott, 1980

Barwin NB and Belisle S. Adolescent Gynecology and Sexuality. New York, Masson, 1982

Beacham DW and Beacham WD. Synopsis of Gynecology, 10th ed. St Louis, CV Mosby, 1982

Benson RC (ed). Current Obstetric and Gynecologic Diagnosis and Treatment. Los Altos, CA, Lange Medical Publisher, 1984

Blaustein A (ed). Pathology of the Female Genital Tract, 2nd ed. New York, Springer-Verlag, 1981

Budoff PW. No More Menstrual Cramps and Other Good News. New York, GP Putnam's Sons, 1980

Danforth DN. Obstetrics and Gynecology, 4th ed. Philadelphia, JB Lippincott, 1982

Delgado G and Smith JP. Management of Complications in Gynecologic Oncology, New York, John Wiley & Sons, 1982

Edlund BJ and McKenzie CA. Symposium on Women's Health Issues. Nurs Clin North Am, Philadelphia, WB Saunders, 1982

Fogel CI and Woods NF. Health Care of Women: A Nursing Perspective. St Louis, CV Mosby, 1981

Griffith H et al. Instructions for Obstetric and Gynecologic Patients. Philadelphia, WB Saunders, 1984

Hawkins DF. Gynecological Therapeutics. New York, Macmillan, 1981

Main D and Main E. Obstetrics and Gynecology. Chicago, Year Book Medical Publisher, 1984

Morgan S. Coping with a Hysterectomy. New York, Dial Press, 1982

Nursing Photobook. Attending Ob/Gyn Patients. Springhouse, PA, Intermed Publications, 1982

Porter CW et al. Contraception: The Health Provider's Guide. Orlando, FL, Grune & Stratton, 1984

Sonstegard L, Korvalski KM and Jennings B (eds). Womens' Health: Ambulatory Care, vol 1. New York, Grune & Stratton, 1982

Wynn RM. Obstetrics and Gynecology. New York, Appleton-Century-Crofts, 1984

Articles

General

Chihal HJ. Office gynecologic endocrinology. Postgrad Med 1982 Apr; 71(4):73–83

Gelein JH. Aging women and health. Top Clin Nurs 1983 Jan; 4(4):56–68

Glebatis DM and Janerich DT. A statewide approach to diethylstilbestrol—the New York program. N Engl J Med 1981 Jan 1; 304(1):47–50

Mishel MH et al. Predictors of psychosocial adjustment in patients newly diagnosed with gynecological cancer. Cancer Nurs 1984 Aug; 7(4): 291–300

Mulligan JE. Some effects of the women's health movement. Top Clin Nurs 1983 Jan; 4(4):1–9

Rosser WW. Benzodiazepine prescription to middle-aged women. Postgrad Med 1982 Apr; 71(4):115–124

Sherman KO. The battered women. DCCN 1983 Jan/Feb; 2(1):30–35

Menstruation

Clough DH and Higgins PG. Discrepancies in estimating blood loss. Am J Nurs 1981 Feb; 81(2):331–333

Cooper SL. Dysmenorrhea. Can Nurse 1981 Oct; 77(9):50–52

Evaluating menstrual dysfunction. Patient Care 1982 Sept 15; 16(15): 12–48

Gibbons WE. Diagnosis: Amenorrhea. Hosp Med 1983 Dec; 19(12):57–69

Hansen AM, Immordino KF and Farber M. The diagnostic evaluation and therapy of secondary amenorrhea. JOGN Nurs 1984 May/June; 13(3): 180–184

Laughlin M and Johnson RE. Premenstrual syndrome. Am Fam Physician 1984 March; 29(3):265–269

McFarland KF. Amenorrhea. Am Fam Physician 1980 Dec; 22(6):95–101

Roberts SJ and Garling J. The menstrual myth revisited. Nurs Forum 1981; 20(3):267–273

Tampon—absorbency testing questioned. Am J Nurs 1984 May; 84(5):589–590

Wilson MA. Menstrual disorders: Premenstrual syndrome, dysmenorrhea, amenorrhea. JOGN Nurs 1984 (supplement) Mar/Apr; 13(23):11s–19s

Menopause

Beauchamp PJ and Held B. Estrogen replacement therapy. Postgrad Med 1984 May 15; 75(7):42–49

Carroll JS. Middle age does not mean menopause. Top Clin Nurs 1983 Jan; 4(4):38–44

Council on Scientific Affairs. Estrogen replacement in the menopause. JAMA 1983 Jan 21; 249(3):359–361

Cutick R. Special needs of premenopausal and menopausal women. JOGN Nurs 1984 (Supplement) Mar/Apr; 13(2):68s–73s

Hotchner B. Menopause and sexuality: Gearing up or down? Top Clin Nurs 1980 Jan; 1(4):45–52

Moore PG. Assessment of the effects of menopause on individual women: A review of literature. Issues Health Care Women 1983 Nov/Dec; 4(6): 341–350

Muhlenkamp AF, Waller MM and Bourne AE. Attitudes toward women in menopause: A vignette approach. Nurs Res 1983 Jan/Feb; 32(1):20–23

Rosenthal MB. Psychological aspects of menopause. Primary Care 1979 June; 6(2):357–364

Sedlack TV. Postmenopausal estrogen therapy. Am Fam Physician 1983 July; 28(1):207–208

Semmens JP and Wagner G. Estrogen deprivation and vaginal function in postmenopausal women. JAMA 1982 July 23/30; 248(4):445–448

Pelvic Examination and Diagnostic Assessment

Aretz HT et al. Fine-needle aspiration. Postgrad Med 1984 Feb 15; 75(3): 49–56

Cavanaugh RM. Pelvic examination of adolescent girls. Am Fam Physician 1982 Oct; 26(4):105–108

Hoffer EP (ed). Tricks of the trade: Exam without pain (vaginal examination). Emerg Med 1983 Oct 30; 15(18):137

Katernadahl DA. Obstetric and gynecologic applications of ultrasound. Postgrad Med 1982 Apr; 71(4):177–182

Koeckeritz JL. Assessing the genitalia. RN 1983 Jan; 46(1):53–59

Paritzky JF and Overby BA. Preoperative teaching on a gynecology unit. JOGN Nurs 1982 Nov/Dec; 11(6):384–386

Patterson JE. Colposcopy. JOGN Nurs 1983 Jan/Feb; 12(1):11–15

Pelvic sonography: When to order it. Patient Care 1984 Mar 15; 18(5):65–97

Primrose RB. Taking the tension out of pelvic exams. Am J Nurs 1984 Jan; 84(1):72–74

Prolonged lithotomy position results in compartment syndrome. AORN J 1984 June; 39(7):1219

Rood SR and Johnson JT. Examination for cervical masses. Postgrad Med 1982 Apr; 71(4):189–194

Swartz WH (letter). The semi-sitting position for pelvic examination. JAMA 1984 Mar 2; 251(9):1163

Vulva and Vagina

Ervin CT et al. Behavioral factors and vaginitis. Nurs Pract 1982 Feb; 7(2): 20–21

Friedrich EG Jr. Vaginitis. Am Fam Physician 1983 Nov; 28(5):238–242

Gerbie MV. Malignant tumors of the vagina. Postgrad Med 1983 Feb; 73(2): 271–282

Gorline LL and Stegbauer CC. What every nurse should know about vaginitis. Am J Nurs 1982 Dec; 12(12): 1851–1855

Huffman JW. Dyspareunia of vulvo-vaginal origin. Postgrad Med 1983 Feb; 73(2):287–296

Hurley M, Meyer-Ruppel A and Evans E. Emma needed more than standard teaching (vulvectomy). Nursing '83 1983 Mar; 13(3):63–64

Jick H et al. Vaginal spermicides and gonorrhea. JAMA 1982 Oct 1; 248(13): 1619–1621

King J. Vaginitis. JOGN Nurs 1984 (supplement) Mar/Apr; 13(2):41s–48s

Larson E. Intransigent genital infection? Suspect chlamydiae. RN 1984 Jan; 47(1):42–43

Piver MS. Early diagnosis and treatment of vulvar cancer. Hosp Med 1984 Feb; 20(2):163

Polk BF et al. PID: How to track down its cause. Patient Care 1983 June 30; 17(12):81–109

Schachter J et al. Chlamydia trachomatis and cervical neoplasia. JAMA 1982 Nov 5; 248(17):2134–2138

Schneider GT. Vaginal infections. Postgrad Med 1983 Feb; 73(2):255–262

Woodruff JD. Vulvar disease. Postgrad Med 1983 Feb; 73(2):232–245

Infections—Herpes Genitalis

Bean B. Acyclovir in the treatment of herpes virus infections. Postgrad Med 1983 Mar; 73(3):297–303

Corey L et al. Intravenous acyclovir for the treatment of primary genital herpes. Ann Intern Med 1983 June; 98(6):914–921

Corey L. The diagnosis and treatment of genital herpes. JAMA 1982 Sept 3; 248(9):1041–1049

Couch RB et al. Genital herpes: An epidemic disease. Heart Lung 1983 May; 12(5):320–324

Genital herpes and acyclovir. Harvard Med Sch Health Letter 1982 Sept; 7(11):3

IV and oral acyclovir surpass topical use. JAMA 1982 Dec 10; 248(22):2942–2943; 2948

Kellum MD and Loucks A. Genital herpes infections: Diagnosis and management. Nurse Pract 1982 Feb; 7(2):14–21

Klein RJ et al. Herpes simplex virus infections. Hosp Med Part 1, 1983 Nov; 19(11):169–193; Part 2, 1983 Dec; 19(12):33–46

Moore JA and Duke HM. Acyclovir for herpes simplex infections. Am Fam Physician 1984 Feb; 29(2):187–190

Pallasch TJ, Joseph CE and Gill CJ. Acyclovir and herpes virus infections: A review. Oral Surg 1984 Jan; 57(1): 41–44

Skinner G. Herpes simplex virus infections: A cure for some ills. Nurs Mirror 1980 Oct 2; 151(14):38–39

US Department of Health & Human Services. Genital Herpes. NIH Pub. 84-2005, Sept 1983

Warmbrodt L. Herpes. RN 1983 May; 46(5):47–49

Toxic Shock Syndrome

Davis JP et al. Toxic shock syndrome. N Engl J Med 1980 Dec 18; 303(25): 1429–1439

Hulka BS. Tampons and toxic shock syndrome. JAMA 1982 Aug 20; 248(7): 872–873

Morrison VA and Oldfield EC. Postoperative toxic shock syndrome. Arch Surg 1983 July; 118(7):791–794

Schlech WF et al. Risk factors for development of toxic shock syndrome. JAMA 1982 Aug 20; 248(7): 835–839

Shands KN et al. Toxic shock syndrome in menstruating women. N Engl J Med 1980 Dec 18; 303(25):1436–1442

Smirniotopoulos TT. Update on toxic shock syndrome. Postgrad Med 1983 Oct; 74(4):369–372

Tofte RW and Williams DN. Toxic shock syndrome. Postgrad Med 1983 Jan; 73(1):275–288

Wheltam J. Update on toxic shock: How to spot it and treat it. RN 1984 Feb; 47(2):55–60

Wiesenthal AM. Toxic shock syndrome—an update. Drug Ther 1983 Mar; 83(3):33–39

Ovary and Uterus

Alcoff JM. Estrogen replacement therapy. Amer Fam Physician 1982 June; 25(6): 183–186

Baram A and Schachter A. Cervical carcinoma: Disease of the future for Jewish women. Lancet 1982 Mar 27; 1(8273):747–748

Cali RW. Estrogen replacement therapy—boom or bane? Postgrad Med 1984 Mar; 75(4):279–286

Cramer DW. Epidemiology of the gynecologic cancers. Med Times 1983 Aug; 3(8):67–69

Devesa SS. Descriptive epidemiology of cancer of the uterine cervix. Obstet Gynecol 1984 May; 63(5):605–612

Dicker RC et al. Hysterectomy among women of reproductive age. JAMA 1982 July 16; 248(3):323–327

Fayez JA. Dysfunctional uterine bleeding. Am Fam Physician 1982 Mar; 25(3):109–115

Lauver D. Irregular bleeding in women: Causes and nursing intervention. Am J Nurs 1983 Mar; 83(3):396–401

Lunt R. Worldwide early detection of

cervical cancer. Obstet Gynecol 1984 May; 63(5):708–713

Parmley TH. Diagnosis: Endometriosis. Hosp Med 1983 Oct; 19(10):152–167

Schachter J et al. Chlamydia trachomatis and cervical neoplasia. JAMA 1982 Nov 5; 248(17):2134–2138

Shapiro M et al. Risk factors for infection at the operative site after abdominal or vaginal hysterectomy. N Engl J Med 1982 Dec 30; 307(27): 1662–1665

Pelvic Infections

Blount JH, Reynolds GH and Rice RJ. Pelvic inflammatory disease: Evidence and trends in private practice. MMWR 1983; 32(4ss):27ss–34ss

Gordon M. Pelvic inflammatory disease. Hosp Med 1982 June; 16(6):60A–60J

Hager WD. Pelvic inflammatory disease. Hosp Med 1982 Apr; 18(4):69–77

Fertility Control

A pill for males. Harvard Med Sch Health Letter 1981 Dec; 7(2):6

Boosting fertility with a cervical cup. Am J Nurs 1984 Mar; 84(3):298

Contraception sponge selling despite opposition. Am J Nurs 1983 Oct; 83(10):1372

Cupit LG. Contraception. JOGN 1984 (supplement) Mar/Apr; 13(2):23s–29s

Dickerson J. The pill, a closer look. Am J Nurs 1983 Oct; 83(10):1392–1398

Dilating the cervix with a mag sulfate sponge. Am J Nurs 1983 Dec; 83(12): 1645

Goldzieher JW. Hormonal contraceptives. Postgrad Med 1984 Apr; 75(5):75–86

Jick H et al. Vaginal spermicides and gonorrhea. JAMA 1982 Oct 1; 248(13): 1619–1621

Kelaghan J et al. Barrier-method contraceptives and pelvic inflammatory disease. JAMA 1982 July 9; 248(2): 184–187

Lane C and Kemp J. Family planning needs of adolescents. JOGN Nurs 1984 (supplement) Mar/Apr; 13(2): 61s–65s

Litt IF. Adolescent contraception. Med Times 1983 June; 111(6):37–40

Longstreth WT Jr and Swanson PD. Oral contraceptives and stroke. Curr Concepts Cerebrovasc Dis 1984 Jan–Feb; 19(1):1–6

Marks RG, Fuentes RJ and Rosenberg JM. How drugs can change fertility. RN 1983 March; 46(3):61–63

Nagel TC. Intrauterine contraceptive devices. Postgrad Med 1983 Mar; 73(3):155–194

Ollivier S, Lesser C and Bell KB. Providing infertility care. JOGN Nurs 1984 (supplement) Mar/Apr; 13(2): 85s–89s

Oral contraceptives and cancer. FDA Drug Bull 1984 April; 14(1):2–3

Pelvic infections and the IUD. Am J Nurs 1983 Oct; 83(10):1374

Periodic abstinence. Population Reports—1981 Sept; 1(4):1–35 to 1–70

Redmond MA. Couple-directed contraceptive counseling. Can Nurse 1982 Sept; 78(8):38–39

Weiss BP. The Majzlin spring revisited. Am Fam Physician 1982 Dec; 26(6): 123–124

Sexual Considerations

Bachman R. Homosexuality. The cost of being different. Can Nurse 1981 Feb; 77(2):20–23

Coleman E. The relational cause of sexual dysfunction. Top Clin Nurs 1980 Jan; 1(4):33–37

Lewis D. The gynecologic consideration of the sexual act. JAMA 1983 July 8; 250(2):222–229

Ramsey P. Adolescent morality—a theologian's viewpoint. Postgrad Med 1982 July; 72(1):233–236

Romanowski B and Harris JRW. Sexually transmitted diseases. Clin Sym 1984; 36(1):2–32

Satterfield SB and Stayton WR. Understanding sexual function and dysfunction. Top Clin Nurs 1980 Jan; 1(4):21–32

Schachter J. Sexually transmitted chlamydia trachomatic infection. Postgrad Med 1982 Oct; 72(4):60–69

Shen JT. Adolescent sexual behavior. Postgrad Med 1982 Apr; 71(4):46–55

Walbroehl GS. Sexuality and aging. Am Fam Physician 1984 Feb; 29(2):239–242

Breast Conditions

Books

Bassett L. Mammography, Thermography, and Ultrasound in Breast Cancer Detection. Orlando, FL, Grune & Stratton, 1982

Casseleth BR and Casseleth PA. Clinical Care of the Terminal Cancer Patient. Philadelphia, Lea & Febiger, 1982

D'Orsi CJ and Wilson RE. Carcinoma of the Breast. Boston, Little, Brown & Co, 1983

Feig SA and McLelland R (eds). Breast Carcinoma: Current Diagnosis and Treatment. New York, Am College of Radiology, Masson, 1983

Gant TD and Vasconez LO. Post-Mastectomy Reconstruction. Baltimore, Williams & Wilkins, 1981

Graham J. In the Company of Others. New York, Harcourt, Brace, Jovanovich, 1982

Haagensen CD, Bodian C and Haagensen DE Jr. Breast Carcinoma. Philadelphia, WB Saunders, 1981

Haagensen CD, Haagensen BE and Bodian C. Risk and Detection of Breast Carcinoma. Philadelphia, WB Saunders, 1981

Harris JR et al. Conservative Management of Breast Cancer. Philadelphia, JB Lippincott, 1984

Hawkins JW and Higgins LP. Maternity and Gynecological Nursing. Philadelphia, JB Lippincott, 1981

Lewison E (ed). Diagnosis and Treatment of Breast Cancer. Baltimore. Williams & Wilkins, 1981

US Department of Health and Human Services. The Breast Cancer Digest, 2nd ed. PHS. NIH Pub. #84-1691. National Cancer Institute, Bethesda, MD, 1984

Articles

Etiology and Risk Factors

Chronic anovulation may increase postmenopausal breast cancer risk. JAMA 1983 Jan 28; 249(4):445–446

Groveman HD and Norcross WA. Adolescent breast masses. Hosp Med 1982 May; 18(5):65–84

Hildreth NG et al. Risk of breast cancer among women receiving radiation treatment in infancy for thymic enlargement. Lancet 1983 July 30; 2(8344):273

Larson E. Epidemiological correlates of breast, endometrial, and ovarian cancers. CA Nurs 1983 Aug; 6(4):295

Rosenberg L et al. Breast cancer and cigarette smoking. N Engl J Med 1984 Jan 12; 310(2):92–94

Senie RT, Rosen PP and Kinne DW. Epidemiologic factors associated with breast cancer. Can Nurs 1983 Oct; 6(5):367–371

Webster LA et al. Alcohol consumption and risk of breast cancer. Lancet 1983 Sept 24; 2(8352):724–726

Breast Self-Examination and Diagnostic Evaluation

Baines CJ. Breast self-examination: The doctor's role. Hosp Pract 1984 Mar; 19(3):120–127

Bennett SE et al. Profile of women practicing breast self-examination. JAMA 1983 Jan 28; 249(4):488–491

Bolsen B. Ultrasound breast scanning: (Only) a complement to mammography? JAMA 1982 Sept 3; 248(9):1015–1027

Boosting better breast exams. Am J Nurs 1983 Nov; 83(11):1534

Detailed guidelines for a thorough examination of the breast. RN 1982 July; 45(7):57–63

Hallal JC. The relationship for health beliefs, health locus of control, and self concept to the practice of breast self-examination in adult women. Nurs Res 1982 May/June 31(3):137–142

King RC et al. An assessment of three alternative formats for promoting breast self-examination. CA Nurs 1983 June; 6(3):207–211

Oberst MT. Testing approaches to teaching breast self-examination. CA Nurs 1981 June; 4(3):246

Petrakis NL and King EB. Cytological abnormalities in nipple aspirates of breast fluid for women with severe constipation. Lancet 1981 Nov 28; 2(8257):1203–1205

Scott D. Anxiety, critical thinking and information processing during and after breast biopsy. Nurs Res 1983 Feb; 32(1):24–28

Benign Breast Disease

Love SM, Gelman RS and Silen W. Fibrocystic "disease" of the breast—a non disease? N Engl J Med 1982 Oct 14; 16(307):1010–1014

Schydlower M. Breast masses in adolescents. Am Fam Physician 1982 Feb; 25(2):141–145

Breast Cancer

Bullough B. Nurses as teachers and support persons for breast cancer patients. CA Nurs 1981 June; 4(3): 221–225

Dulcey MP. Addressing breast cancer's assault on female sexuality. Top Clin Nurs 1980 Jan; 1(4):61–68

Ferguson DJ. Staging of breast cancer and survival rates. JAMA 1982 Sept 17; 248(11):1337–1341

Gilliland MD et al. The implications of local recurrence of breast cancer as the first site of therapeutic failure. Ann Surg 1983 March; 197(3):284–287

Greiner L and Weiler C. Early-stage breast cancer. What do women know about treatment choices. Am J Nurs 1983 Nov; 83(11):1570

Gristina AG et al. Intraosseous metastatic breast cancer treatment with internal fixation and study of survival. Ann Surg 1983 Feb; 197(2): 128–134

Holleb AI (interview): Progress against breast cancer. Cancer News 1984 Spring/Summer; 38(2):7

McGuire WL. Steroid hormone receptors in breast cancer. Drug Ther 1982 Sept; 82(8):56–62

Meyerowitz BE, Watkins IK and Sparks FG. Quality of life for breast cancer patients receiving adjuvant chemotherapy. Am J Nurs 1983 Feb; 83(2):232–235

Mitchell MS. Breast cancer treatment—

adjuvant therapy. Postgrad Med 1983 Sept; 74(3):161–175

Moetzinger CA and Dauber LG. The management of the patient with breast cancer. CA Nurs 1982 Aug; 5(4):287–292

Moskowitz M. How can we decrease breast cancer mortality? CA 1980 Sept/Oct; 30(5):272–277

O'Brien RL. Breast cancer treatment—current status. Postgrad Med 1983 Sept; 74(3):124–125

Pilch YH. Breast cancer treatment—Mastectomy, standard surgical approach. Postgrad Med 1983 Sept; 74(3):126–134

Pilch YH. Breast cancer treatment—segmental mastectomy, alternative to total breast excision? Postgrad Med 1983 Sept; 74(3):139–146

Scott DW. Quality of life following the diagnosis of breast cancer. Top Clin Nurs 1983 Jan; 4(4):20–37

Wilson JF. Breast cancer treatment—simple excision with irradiation. Postgrad Med 1983 Sept; 74(5):151–158

Postmastectomy

Aitken DR and Minton JP. Complications associated with mastectomy. Surg Clin North Am 1983 Dec; 63(6):1331–1352

Northouse LL. Mastectomy patients and

the fear of cancer recurrence. CA Nurs 1981 June; 4(3):213–220

Reich SD. Estrogen receptors and advanced breast cancer. CA Nurs 1981 June; 4(3):247–248

Chemotherapy and Radiation Therapy

Carter SK. Adjuvant chemotherapy of breast cancer. N Engl J Med 1981 Jan 1; 304(1):45–47

Decker DA et al. Complete responders to chemotherapy in metastatic breast cancer. JAMA 1979 Nov 9; 242(19): 2075–2079

Gilman CJ. Primary radiotherapy in early breast cancer. Am Fam Physician 1982 Apr; 25(4):113–117

Hassey KM, Bloom LS and Burgess SL. Radiation—alternative to mastectomy. Am J Nurs 1983 Nov; 83(11):1567–1569

Hicks MJ et al. Sensitivity of mammography and physician examination of the breast cancer. JAMA 1979 Nov 9; 242(19):2080–2083

Reconstructive Surgery

Koch AJ. Augmentation mammaplasty. Am J Nurs 1980 Aug; 80(8):1480–1484

Rutledge DN. Nurse's knowledge of breast reconstruction: A catalyst for earlier treatment of breast cancer? CA Nurs 1982 Dec; 5(6):469–474

Skin Problems

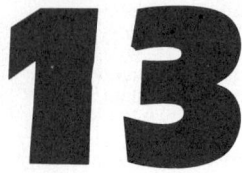

1: Dermatologic Conditions

1: Dermatologic Conditions

Nursing Patients with Dermatologic Conditions

Psychological Considerations

1. Patients with dermatological problems can see and feel their problems and are more disturbed by their complaints than many patients with other conditions.
2. Skin eruptions evoke feelings of shame, disgust, avoidance, withdrawal, and anger that compound the problems of management of patients with skin conditions. Touching the patient reduces his sense of isolation.
3. Irritation is a constant feature of skin disease and produces loss of sleep, anxiety, and depression, which in turn reinforce discomfort and fatigue.
4. Cosmetic needs constitute the underlying motive that brings the patient to treatment.
5. Nursing support requires understanding, unending patience, and continuing encouragement for these patients.

Assessment

Nursing Assessment

1. Be aware that many systemic conditions may be accompanied by dermatologic manifestations.
2. The skin may be a portal of entry for locally invasive and disseminated infection.

A. History

1. Obtain a dermatologic history.
   a. Where is the rash? When did it start?
   b. How long has the patient had the skin condition?
   c. Has it occurred previously?
   d. Were there any other symptoms besides the rash?
   e. What did the rash/lesion look like when it first appeared?
   f. How did it spread?
   g. Are there itching, burning, tingling, or crawling sensations? Loss of sensation?
   h. Is it worse at a particular time? Season?
   i. Does the patient have any idea how it started?
   j. Is there personal history of hay fever, asthma, urticaria? Eczema? Allergies? Is there family history (some skin conditions are hereditary)?
   k. Was the appearance of the eruption related to the intake of food?
   l. Was there a relationship between a specific event and the outbreak of the rash/lesion?
   m. What medications is the patient taking? What medications (salves, ointments, cream) have been applied to the lesion? (Include over-the-counter medications.)
   n. What is the patient's occupation?
   o. What is in his immediate environment (plants,

animals) that might be precipitating the problem? Anything new or any changes in the environment?

p. Ask if there is anything else the patient wishes to talk about in regard to this problem.

B. Examination of the Skin

1. Ask the patient to undress; the entire skin must be examined.
2. Have good lighting available. Use a hand magnifying lens to inspect for fine detail (altered skin markings, loss of skin lines, etc.).
3. Inspect the skin in an orderly sequence: hair, scalp, nails, buccal mucosa, skin surface.
4. Assess the general appearance of the skin, observing temperature, moisture, dryness, skin texture (rough or smooth).
5. Look at the distribution, arrangement, and grouping of the rash/lesions. Compare the left and right sides of the body.
6. Note the shape, border, color, texture, and surface of the lesion.
7. Palpate the shape, border, texture, and surface of the lesion.
8. Use a metric ruler to measure the size of lesions— to compare extension of lesions from baseline measurements.

C. Assessment of Patients with Dark or Black Skin

1. Healthy dark skin has a reddish undertone; buccal mucosa, tongue, lips, and nails normally appear pink.
2. Lightening, darkening, or blotching of the skin are very noticeable and can cause emotional distress.
   a. Hyperpigmentation of the mouth is normal in some individuals.
   b. Some blacks have pigmented streaks on nails; usually normal.
3. The degree of pigmentation of the black patient may affect the appearance of a lesion; lesions may be black, purple or gray (instead of tan or red color that is seen in the white patient).
4. Certain procedures (freezing, topical peeling and drying agents, or diseases) can cause hypopigmentation (loss or decrease in skin color) or hyperpigmentation (increase in color). These changes are more apparent in dark-skinned patients.

D. Examination of Black Skin

1. Have good lighting; look in mouth and nail beds as well as entire skin area.
2. Palpate all suspicious areas.
3. For rash:
   a. Ask the patient if he has an area of itching.
   b. Stretch the skin gently to decrease the reddish tone and make the rash stand out.
   c. Palpate by running fingertips lightly over the skin—to feel the differences in skin temperature and to feel the borders of the rash.
   d. Palpate the lymph nodes; take the patient's temperature.
4. For erythema:
   a. Inspect for a purplish–grayish cast of skin.
   b. Palpate for increase in warmth and for signs of smoothness (edema) or hardness—to detect possible infection.
5. For cyanosis:
   a. Look for a gray cast of the skin.
   b. Inspect areas around the mouth, lips, over cheek bones, and earlobes.
   c. Evaluate for the usual signs of shock (see p. 90).

6. Describe and document the dermatosis (abnormal condition of the skin) clearly and in detail.
   a. What is (are) the color(s) of the lesion?
   b. Is there redness, heat, pain, or swelling?
   c. How large an area is involved; where is it?
   d. Is the eruption macular, papular, scaling, oozing, discrete, confluent?
   e. What is the distribution of the lesion—symmetrical, linear, circular?

Description of Skin Lesions

A. Primary Lesions (initial lesions)

1. *Macule*—nonelevated discoloration of the skin; of various sizes, shapes, and colors
2. *Papule*—a solid, elevated lesion less than 1 cm. (0.4 inch) in diameter
3. *Nodule*—a raised lesion that is deeper than a papule
4. *Vesicle*—a small elevation of the skin that is filled with clear fluid less than 1 cm. in diameter
5. *Bulla*—a large blister, larger than 1 cm. (0.4 inch) in diameter
6. *Pustule*—vesicle or bulla that contains pus; may form as a result of purulent changes in a vesicle
7. *Wheal*—transient elevation of the skin caused by edema of the dermis and surrounding capillary dilatation
8. *Plaque*—a large papule, greater than 1 cm. in diameter
9. *Cyst*—a tumor that contains semisolid or liquid material

B. Secondary Lesions (changes that take place in primary lesions and possibly modify them)

1. *Scales*—heaped-up, horny layers of dead epidermis; may develop as a result of inflammatory changes
2. *Crusts*—a covering formed by the drying of serum, blood, or pus on the skin
3. *Excoriations*—linear scratch marks or traumatized area of skin
4. *Fissures*—cracks in the skin, usually from marked drying and long-standing inflammation
5. *Ulcer*—lesion formed by local destruction of the epidermis and part or all of the underlying dermis
6. *Lichenification*—thickening of skin accompanied by accentuation of skin markings
7. *Scar*—a fibrotic change in the skin following a destructive process
8. *Atrophy*—loss of substance

Selected Dermatologic Diagnostic Tests

1. Wood's light examination—a special long-wave ultraviolet light produced by a Wood's lamp induces visible fluorescence in certain skin lesions; best seen in a darkened room.
2. Skin biopsy—performed to obtain tissues for examination.
3. Patch testing
   a. Used to document contact sensitivity or allergy.
   b. Suspected allergens are placed on normal skin beneath patches of tape.
   c. Patches are removed and the skin under the patches is examined at specified intervals.
4. Fungal scraping—scales from a lesion are scraped with a scalpel and placed on a glass slide, covered with potassium hydroxide (KOH), and examined.
5. Tzanck smear
   a. Used for cytologic evaluation of blistering diseases of the skin.
   b. Suspected vesicle or pustule is opened, and

contents applied to a glass slide and examined after staining.

6. Clinical photographs—reveal nature and extent of skin condition and show progress or improvement from treatment.

Nursing Process Overview— Patients with Dermatoses
(Abnormal Skin Conditions)

Assessment

For details of data collection, see pages 604–605.

Patient Problems/Nursing Diagnoses

1. Potential alteration in skin integrity related to change in barrier function of skin
2. Potential nonadherence to treatment regimen related to length of treatment or the life-style adjustments required
3. Knowledge deficit of underlying cause of ailment and methods of treating
4. Potential for infection related to entry of organisms through break in skin
5. Potential fluid and electrolyte imbalance related to loss of tissue fluids and serum from denuded skin
6. Pain and discomfort related to irritated nerve endings in open lesions
7. Disturbance in self-concept related to unsightly skin appearance
8. Ineffective coping related to emotional drain of dealing with painful, unsightly skin condition

Planning and Implementation
Nursing Interventions
A. Reduction in Pain and Discomfort and Pruritus

1. Examine area of involvement
    a. Attempt to discover the cause of discomfort.
    b. Record observations in detail, using descriptive terminology.
    c. Be aware that *sudden* onset of a generalized rash may indicate a drug allergy.
2. Advise the patient to employ measures that produce vasoconstriction
    a. Maintain cool, humid environment—itching is aggravated by heat, chemicals, and physical irritants.
    b. Eliminate irritants and strong soaps.
    c. Reduce excess clothing or bedding.
    d. Provide tepid, cooling baths or cool, wet dressings—gradual evaporation of water from dressings cools the skin and relieves pruritus.
3. Treat dryness (xerosis) as prescribed.

▶ **NURSING ALERT:** Xerosis (dry skin) is a common skin problem of the elderly, resulting from diminished sebaceous secretion and a slower rate of perspiration.

    a. Keep humidity above 40%; use a humidifier
    b. Avoid excessive bathing and excessive exposure to soaps, solvents, etc.
    c. Apply emollient to moist skin frequently, especially after baths or compresses.
4. Apply prescribed lotions or ointments.
5. Supply analgesic and antipruritic medications as prescribed.
6. Administer tranquilizing agents or sedatives as prescribed and as necessary.

7. Instruct the patient to refrain from self-medication with salves or lotions that are commercially advertised.

B. Reduction in Inflammation

1. Instruct the patient clearly and in detail to ensure that treatments are carried out as prescribed.
2. Apply continuous or intermittent wet dressings to reduce intensity of inflammation.
3. Remove crusts and scales before applying topical medications.
4. Use topical medications containing corticosteroids as prescribed and as indicated.
    a. Observe lesion periodically for changes in response to therapy.
    b. Instruct the patient about possible ill effects of long-term use of fluorinated topical steroids.

C. Removal of Crust Formation and Management of Oozing

1. Provide tub baths and wet dressings to loosen exudates and scales.
2. Remove medications with mineral oil before reapplying fresh medication.
3. Use mildly astringent solutions to precipitate proteins and decrease oozing.
4. Supply a high-protein diet if oozing is voluminous and serum loss is substantial.
5. Administer antibiotics as prescribed and indicated.

D. Protection of Skin from Trauma and Infection

1. Protect healthy skin from maceration when applying wet dressings.
2. Remove moisture from skin by blotting gently and avoiding friction.
3. Guard carefully against risk of thermal injury from excessively hot wet dressings.
4. Advise the patient to use sun-screening agents to prevent actinic damage (chemical changes from ultralight).

E. Coping Mechanisms to Deal with Skin Condition

1. Help the patient to accept the prolonged treatment that some skin conditions require.
2. Listen empathetically to expressions of grief about changes in body image.
3. Assist the anxious patient to improve his insight and to identify and cope with his problems.
4. Mobilize the patient's support systems.
5. Advise the patient of available cosmetic measures to conceal disfiguring conditions.

Evaluation
Expected Outcomes

1. Obtains relief of itching and pain—states that itching is relieved; no excoriation or scratch marks; no complaints of discomfort; skin begins to regain healthy appearance
2. Follows treatment as prescribed and understands rationale for measures taken—carries out the prescribed baths, application of lotions, and wet dressings; dries skin carefully after washing; takes medication if prescribed
3. Avoids infection or adheres to treatment if infection occurs; takes care to avoid trauma or maceration to skin; applies antibiotic ointments or takes antibiotic medication as prescribed
4. Demonstrates an improved self-image and coping abilities—appears less self-conscious; is not afraid to socialize or be seen by others; uses concealing and high-lighting techniques to enhance appearance

Dermatologic Therapy

Open Wet Dressings

Open wet dressings are wet compresses applied to skin areas. They may be either sterile or unsterile, depending on the condition being treated.

Purposes

1. To reduce inflammation by producing vasoconstriction—thus decreasing vasodilatation and the local blood flow present in inflammation.

Solution and Material	Desired Effect	Nursing Interventions
Solution Room-temperature tapwater Physiologic saline solution Aluminum acetate solution Magnesium sulfate **Material** Soft toweling Diapers Soft cotton sheeting Kerlix (Bauer and Black)	Effective in treating oozing dermatosis or swollen, infected dermatitis (furunculitis, cellulitis). Relieves inflammation, burning, and itching. Has cooling effect.	Wash hands thoroughly before applying dressings. Protect areas of normal skin with petrolatum jelly or a silicone oil or zinc oxide paste to avoid skin maceration. Keep dressing at room temperature. Moisten compress to the point of slight dripping. Compresses may be remoistened using an asepto syringe. Add ice cubes to solution if coolness is desired. Apply for 15 minutes every 2–3 hours unless otherwise indicated. Reapply every 5 minutes or so since compresses reach body temperature rather quickly. Keep the patient warm if extensive areas are to have compresses. Do not treat more than 1/3 of the body at one time because chilling and hypothermia may result. Discard dressing material daily. CAUTION: Avoid burns.

Baths (Balneotherapy)

Baths are useful in treating widespread eruptions of the skin, removing crusts, scales, and old medications, and relieving inflammation and itching.

Bath Solution and Medication	Desired Effect	Nursing Action
Water	Same effects as wet dressings	Fill the tub half full.
Saline	Used for widely disseminated lesions	Keep the water at a comfortable temperature.
Colloidal—oatmeal or Aveeno	Antipruritic and drying	
Sodium bicarbonate	Cooling	Do not allow the water to cool excessively.
Starch		Use a bath mat—*medications may cause tub to be slippery.*
Medicated tars (follow package directions) Alma-Tar, Balnetar	Tar baths are used for psoriasis and chronic eczematous conditions.	Apply a lubricating agent to wet skin after bath if emollient action is desired—increases hydration. Since tars are volatile, the bath area should be well ventilated. Dry by blotting with a towel.
Bath oils Alpha-Keri, Lubath, Nutraderm Bath Oil	Bath oils are used for antipruritic and emollient actions. Used for acute and subacute eczematous eruptions.	Keep room warm to minimize temperature fluctuations. May be applied to wet skin after bathing. Encourage the patient to wear light, loose clothing after the bath.

Medications for Skin Conditions

Type of Medication	Desired Effect	Nursing Action
Lotions Liquid vehicles for carrying medication	Cool through water evaporation. May be protective antipruritic, and drying; may act as sunscreen.	May be applied with cotton gauze or soft paintbrush or by hand, using a firm stroke for a thin, even coat. Not usually washed off between applications.
Creams (suspensions of oil and water) Have greasy, nongreasy, or penetrating base, depending on nature of lesion and drug applied	Lubricate. Protect the skin. Serve as vehicle for medications.	Creams are rubbed into the skin by hand. Teach the patient to apply his own cream.
Gels Semi-solid emulsions that become liquid when applied to skin	Dries as a thin, greaseless nonocclusive, nonstaining film; some topical steroids are prescribed in gel form.	See corticosteroid agents below.
Ointments	Usually used when inflammation becomes chronic and skin is dry, with scaling and lichenification (leathery thickening of the skin). Retard water loss and lubricate and protect the skin.	Applied by hand or wooden tongue depressor. Ointments may have to be covered with a dressing to prevent soiling of clothing.
Pastes Mixtures of a powder in an ointment base	Used in inflammatory conditions.	May need to be removed with a cotton ball soaked in mineral oil or vegetable oil.
Topical corticosteroid agents (many preparations available)	Have anti-inflammatory action, thus relieving pain and itching. Some of the newer, more potent steroids have time and volume limitations to prevent systemic effects.	Apply to localized area requiring medication. Use only a small amount and rub in thoroughly. Use with occlusive dressing as directed—enhances penetration. Prolonged or excessive use may produce thinning of the skin, stretch marks, and susceptibility to bruising. Apply with caution around the eyes—chronic use around the eyes may cause glaucoma, cataracts, and viral and fungal infections.
Powders (usually with a talc, zinc oxide, bentonite or cornstarch base)	Act as hygroscopic agents (take up moisture). Absorb perspiration. Provide antipruritic and cooling sensations.	Be sure area is thoroughly dry to prevent caking. Dispense with shaker top. Avoid accumulating powder in intertriginous areas.

Other Skin Medications

Intralesional therapy Injection of sterile suspension of medication (usually suspension of corticosteroid) into lesion	Has anti-inflammatory action. Skin lesions treated with intralesional therapy include psoriasis, keloids, and cystic acne.	Be aware that local atrophy may result if injection is made into subcutaneous fat.

Systemic medications
Corticosteroids
Antibiotics
Antifungals
Sedatives and tranquilizers
Analgesics
Antineoplastics

Type of Medication	Desired Effect	Nursing Action

Health Education

1. Use topical medication *only* as directed.
2. Wash hands thoroughly before applying.
3. Avoid reapplying prescribed topical agent at frequent intervals to improve appearance or for cosmetic purposes; may cause further irritation or impede healing.
4. Do not use over-the-counter hydrocortisone preparations indiscriminantly because chronic abuse can produce steroid rosacea and thinning of the skin.

2. To cleanse skin of exudates, crusts, scales—thus making a cleaner and drier surface.
3. To maintain drainage of infected areas.

Clinical Uses

1. Vesicular, bullous, pustular, and ulcerative disorders
2. Acute inflammatory conditions
3. Erosions and exudative, crusted surfaces.

Dressings for Skin Conditions

A. Occlusive Dressing—an airtight plastic film is applied to cover medicated skin (usually corticosteroid)
   1. Purposes
      a. Enhances absorption of topically applied medication
      b. Increases penetration of corticosteroids into the skin, thus enhancing anti-inflammatory effect
      c. Produces moisture retention; permits medication from evaporating

▶ **NURSING ALERT:** Prolonged use of occlusive dressings may cause skin atrophy, striae, telangiectasia, folliculitis, nonhealing ulceration, erythema, or systemic absorption of corticosteroids. Dressings should be removed for 12 out of 24 hours to prevent some of these complications.

2. Plastic surgical tape containing corticosteroid is available and can be cut to size.

B. Other Dressings

1. Fingers and toes—gauze or cotton cloth; held in place with small size tubular material (Surgitube, Tubegauze)
2. Hands—disposable polyethylene gloves; sealed at wrists
3. Feet—cotton socks or disposable plastic bags
4. Extremities (arms and legs)—cotton cloth covered with tubular material
5. Groin, perineum—disposable diapers; cotton cloth folded in diaper fashion
6. Axillae—cotton cloth taped in place or held by commercial dress shields
7. Trunk—cotton or light flannel pajamas
8. Scalp—turban or plastic shower cap
9. Face—mask made from gauze with holes cut out for eyes, nose, mouth

Seborrheic Dermatoses

Dermatoses refers to abnormal skin conditions.
   Seborrhea is excessive production of sebum (secretion of sebaceous glands) in those areas where glands are normally found in large numbers (face, scalp, scrotum).
   Seborrheic dermatitis is a chronic, inflammatory, scaling eruption with a predilection for areas that are well supplied with sebaceous glands or that lie between folds of skin where the bacterial count is high.

Clinical Features

1. Characteristic lesion (remarkably varied)
   a. Dry, moist, or greasy scales
   b. Crusted pinkish-yellow or yellowish patches of varying shapes and sizes
   c. Possible erythema (redness), fissuring (cracking), and secondary infection
   d. Dry, flaky desquamation on scalp with profuse amount of fine, powdery scales (dandruff); itching may be mild or intense
2. Sites—scalp (dandruff), eyebrows, eyelids, nasolabial crease, lips, ears, axillae, under breast, groin, gluteal crease
3. Seborrheic dermatitis is associated with genetic predisposition and aggravated by physical or emotional stress.
4. There is a tendency to lifelong recurrences lasting for weeks, months, or years.

Nursing Interventions

1. Advise the patient to remove external irritants and avoid excess heat and perspiration—rubbing and scratching will prolong the disorder.
2. Suggest local remedies.
   a. For scalp—to control dandruff
      (1) Give the hair an initial cleansing shampoo to remove accumulated scale.
      (2) Use shampoo with selenium sulfide suspension (Selsun) 2–3 times a week.
      (3) Shampoos containing tar are also effective, but may cause irritation and may alter the color of blonde or gray hair.
      CAUTION: Observe precautions on container.
      (4) Other shampoos, based on detergents, zinc pyrithione, or antimicrobial agents, are often effective.
   b. Seborrheic dermatitis of the body and face
      (1) May respond to a topically applied cortico-

steroid cream—allays secondary inflammation.

   (2) Use with extreme caution on the eyelids, since it can induce glaucoma in predisposed individuals.

   (3) Prolonged use of fluorinated steroids on the face can produce acne. Prolonged use can produce disfiguring telangiectasia and atrophy. Therefore, plain hydrocortisone is used.

3. Use antibacterial measures if exudation and crusting occur.

   a. Systemic antibiotic may be required for a spreading infection.

   b. Topical antibiotics (cream or lotion) may be applied.

4. Watch for occurrence of secondary candidiasis that may occur in body creases or folds.

   a. Advise the patient to cleanse intertriginous areas carefully; ensure maximum aeration of skin.

   b. Patient with coincidental candidiasis should be evaluated for diabetes mellitus.

Health Education

1. Advise the patient to avoid aggravating systemic factors—overwork, lack of sleep, infection, emotional stress.
2. Seborrheic dermatitis may be made worse by conditions that increase perspiration.
3. Sunlight may be beneficial.
4. Seborrheic dermatitis does recur, and treatment should be reinstituted. .

Acne Vulgaris

Acne vulgaris is a common disorder of the sebaceous (oil) glands and their follicles (pilosebaceous follicles), characterized by the presence of closed comedones (whiteheads), open comedones (blackheads), papules, pustules, nodules, and cysts. The primary sites are the face, chest, upper back, and shoulders.

Predisposing Factors

1. Genetic predisposition—strong genetic overtones
2. Hormonal changes of adolescence—from androgenic stimulation of sebum production
3. Cutaneous flora—high concentration of *Propionibacterium acnes* found in acne-susceptible individuals
4. External irritants—climate, chemical, mechanical irritants, cosmetics, pharmacologic agents

Altered Physiology

Stimulation of androgenic hormones → increase in amount and thickness of oil secretion → lipids arising in the sebaceous glands → follicular bacteria (*P. acnes*) → obstruction of sebaceous glands by blackheads (comedones) → disruption of the follicular epithelium, allowing discharge of the follicular contents into the dermis → inflammatory reaction → papules → pustules → nodules → cysts.

Treatment and Nursing Management

A. Prevent Obstruction of the Oil Glands.

1. Wash face gently 1–2 times daily with mild soap and water.
Mild abrasive soaps and drying preparations may be used for mild involvement (mainly comedones)—to eliminate the oil feeling.
Avoid excessive abrasion, since it makes acne worse.

2. Shampoo scalp nightly or twice weekly with medicated shampoo.
3. Use bath brush if back is involved.
4. Advise the patient to have blackheads removed manually with a comedone extractor.
5. Removal of superficial skin cells may be done mechanically by use of a polyester sponge pad (Buf-Puf).

B. Topical Agents for More Severe Involvement— to clear keratin plugs from follicular ducts and to suppress *P. acnes* in the follicles. The therapeutic regimen depends on the type of lesion (comedonal, papular, pustular, or cystic).

1. Topical benzoyl peroxide—exerts antibacterial effects, suppresses *P. acnes,* reduces concentration of surface free fatty acids, and is a comedolytic.

   a. Apply sparingly to completely dry skin; adjusted to point of tolerance.

   b. Advise patient that he may not see improvement for 1–2 or up to 6 weeks.

2. Topical vitamin A acid, (tretinoin [Retin-A])—speeds up the cellular turnover, which forces out the comedones and prevents occurrence of new comedones. Instruct the patient as follows:

   a. The symptoms may worsen during the early weeks of treatment because of action of medication on previously unseen comedones; there is a possibility of some erythema and peeling. Improvement may take 4–8 weeks.

   b. Read the product-information brochure.

   c. Apply vitamin A acid to thoroughly dry skin—wet skin enhances penetration and increases the potential for irritation.

   d. Keep medication away from eyes, nasolabial folds, corners of mouth—likely to pool in these areas, causing local irritation.

   e. Apply as tolerated; the concentration of the preparation used and the frequency of its application are adjusted according to the reactivity of the skin to vitamin A acid.

   f. Wash hands thoroughly after applying vitamin A acid.

   g. Be cautious during first few weeks about exposure to sun (including sunlamps)—antikeratinizing effect of tretinoin makes patient more sensitive to sunburn.

   h. Avoid other irritants, such as strong soaps.

3. Topical antibiotic therapy—suppresses growth of *P. acnes* and produces decrease in comedones, papules, and pustules without systemic side effects.

   a. Topical tetracycline, clindamycin, and erythromycin are available.

   b. Used alone or in combination with other agents.

C. Systemic Therapy

1. *Systemic antibiotics* appear to reduce *P. acnes* in pilosebaceous follicles and inhibit sebum production, and are used for the more inflammatory and extensive lesions.

   a. Tetracycline, erythromycin, or minocycline is given and adjusted according to therapeutic response.

   b. Long-term, low-dose antibiotic may be given.

   c. May take several weeks for effect of antibiotics to show.

   d. Instruct the patient to take tetracycline at least 1 hour before or 2 hours after mealtime; avoid taking any dairy products (milk, ice cream) within

2 hours before or after taking medication—tetracycline is poorly absorbed with food.

    e. Side effects of tetracycline include nausea, diarrhea, superinfection, and candidiasis (vaginitis in women; cutaneous infection in either sex, but more often in men).

2. *Retinoid therapy*—oral retinoids (isotretinoin), synthetic derivatives, are being used to treat severe, recalcitrant, nodular–cystic acne that is unresponsive to conventional therapy; appears to have an inhibitory effect on sebum production and sebaceous gland secretion.

    a. Adverse effects, comparable to hypervitaminosis (mucocutaneous and systemic), are frequently encountered.

        (1) Mucocutaneous effects—cheilitis, facial dermatitis, dry nose and mouth, dry eyes, conjunctivitis, pruritus, epistaxis.

        (2) Systemic effects—headache, thirst, arthralgia, fatigue, elevation of triglyceride and cholesterol levels, and lowering of high-density lipoproteins.

        (3) Headache is a serious symptom. It may be associated with increased intracranial pressure, papilledema, projectile vomiting, and other signs of pseudotumor cerebri. Persistent headache should be evaluated by the physician.

    b. Health education for patients receiving retinoid therapy:

        (1) Have careful monitoring of lipid status.

        (2) Women of childbearing potential should be counseled about risks to fetus and advised to use an effective form of contraception. Some physicians advocate pregnancy tests before beginning drug therapy in women of childbearing age.

        (3) Avoid vitamin supplements containing vitamin A because of possible additive toxic effects.

3. *Estrogen therapy* (usually in form of oral contraceptive)—suppresses the androgenic stimulation of sebum production.
Usually reserved for young women with severe cystic acne; not given to males because of undesirable side effects (symptoms and signs of feminization).

D. Surgical Treatment

1. Comedo extraction (see following Guidelines).
2. Intralesional injection of steroids (triamcinolone acetonide). Diluted steroid suspension is injected into inflamed lesions—leads to rapid resolution.
3. Incision and drainage of cysts and pustular lesions—may be required in large, fluctuant, nodular–cystic lesions.
4. Cryosurgery (freezing with liquid nitrogen)—for nodular and cystic forms of acne.
5. Dermabrasion—surgical planing of skin to reduce surface configuration of old scars and give smooth appearance.

Health Education

1. Gain the patient's confidence. Outline the therapy—try to relieve unspoken fear and guilt.

    a. Acne is not caused by dirt and cannot be washed away; it is a chemical imbalance that causes the oil in the skin to form blackheads.

    b. Acne is *not* related to sexual activity.

2. Keep hands away from face.
3. Do not squeeze pimples or blackheads—squeezing the skin makes acne worse. The majority of blackheads are pushed down into the skin by squeezing. This may cause the follicle to be ruptured.
4. Eat a healthful diet; eliminate any food that you feel worsens your acne.
5. Keep hair off the face; wash hair daily if necessary.
6. Avoid friction and trauma.

    a. Do not prop your hands against your face.

    b. Avoid overzealous washing of face, rubbing the face, pressure from tight collars/helmets.

    c. Avoid perspiration around the face.

7. Avoid cosmetics (including cleansing creams), shaving creams and lotions—they may contain chemicals that can aggravate acne.
8. Continue treatment even though your skin clears.
9. Be able to talk over your problems with an understanding person—acne may become a source of power struggle between teenager and parent. Emotional stress may worsen acne in certain individuals.

Guidelines: Comedo Extraction*

A *comedo* (blackhead) is a mass composed of lipids, keratin, and entrapped follicular bacteria that forms a solid plug in a dilated follicular opening (pore).

Underlying Considerations

1. Blackheads are approximately 4 mm. deep and cannot be washed away.
2. Comedones are considered end-stage lesions and their removal is only of temporary benefit. However, removal reduces the chance of their evolving into papules, pustules, and cysts.

Equipment

Light
Magnifying loupe
Alcohol and sponges

Instruments:
    Comedo extractor
    Scalpel blade No. 11
    No. 18 gauge needle

* This procedure must be performed with skill by a prepared person.

(continued)

Guidelines: Comedo Extraction (continued)

Procedure

Nursing Action	Rationale/Amplification
1. Wipe off the site with an alcohol sponge.	1. For antisepsis and to allow visualization of lesions.
2. Nick the overlying skin of the comedo with No. 18 gauge sterile needle or tip of scalpel blade.	2. This widens the port and facilitates comedo removal.
3. Place opening of the extractor over the lesion and apply firm downward pressure directly on the lesion.	3. This causes extrusion of the plug through the expressor. Overly vigorous attempts to express comedones may result in an increased inflammatory response.
4. Wipe off the site with a fresh alcohol sponge.	
5. Inform the patient that removal of comedones may leave areas of erythema which may take several weeks to subside.	

Infections and Infestations of the Skin

Bacterial Infections (Pyodermas)

Bacterial infections of the skin may be primary, originating in previously normal-appearing skin and usually caused by a single organism, or secondary, arising from a preexisting skin disorder in which several microorganisms may be implicated. The most common primary bacterial skin infections are *impetigo* and *folliculitis.*

Impetigo

Impetigo is a superficial infection of the skin caused by streptococci, but staphylococci and streptococci or multiple bacteria can usually be recovered on routine culture.

Bullous impetigo is a superficial infection of the skin caused by *S. aureus,* characterized by the formation of bullae from original vesicles, which rupture, leaving a raw area.

Clinical Features

1. Lesions begin as small red macules, which rapidly become thin-walled vesicles that rupture and become covered with a loosely adherent, honey-yellow crust.
2. Crusts are easily removed and reveal a smooth, red, moist surface on which new crusts soon develop.
3. Areas affected—exposed parts of body (face, hands, neck, and extremities).
4. Impetigo is a contagious disease. It is seen in all ages, but is particularly common among children living in poor hygienic conditions.
5. Sources of infection—children's pets, dirty fingernails, other children, adults, barber shops, beauty parlors, swimming pools, contaminated clothing, bedding, towels.
6. May be secondary to pediculosis capitis, scabies, herpes simplex, insect bites, poison ivy, eczema.

Treatment and Nursing Management

1. Give systemic antibiotic (depending on infective organism and its sensitivity) for nonbullous impetigo. Glomerulonephritis is a complication of impetigo, depending on the strain of streptococcus found. However, this therapy has not been proved to prevent nephritis.
2. Give penicillinase-resistant penicillin (oxacillin, cloxacillin, dicloxacillin) for bullous impetigo.
3. Soak lesions in warm tapwater, saline solution, or soap solution (or wash with antibacterial soap and apply warm compresses at least 3 times a day) to aid in the removal of the crusts.
4. Apply a topical antibiotic cream (neomycin, bacitracin, polymyxin B) after crust removal to treat existing lesions and to help prevent local spread of infection.
5. Wear gloves while treating the patient.

Health Education

1. Avoid close contact with other people because impetigo is transmissible when there is oozing and crusting.
   a. Use separate towels and washcloths for each person in family; launder bed linens after first day of treatment; launder clothing daily during crusting or oozing stages.
   b. Dispose of tissues and materials that come in contact with lesion.
2. Encourage good hygienic practices to prevent spread of disease from one skin area to another and from one person to another—handwashing, keeping the fingernails short.
3. The patient and family should bathe at least once daily with bactericidal soap as recommended.

Folliculitis and Furuncles

Folliculitis is a staphylococcal infection that arises within the hair follicle.
1. Lesions may be superficial or deep; single or multiple papules or pustules appear close to the hair follicle.
2. Folliculitis commonly seen in the hair area of men who shave and on women's legs.
   Pseudofolliculitis barbae (shaving bumps)—an inflammatory reaction on face of curly haired males caused by ingrowing hairs that pierce the skin, causing an irritative reaction.
   a. Common problems in black males.
   b. Management
      (1) Avoid shaving; grow a beard or use a handbrush over facial area to mechanically dislodge hairs.
      (2) A depilatory cream may be used if the patient must shave.
Furuncle (boil) is an acute inflammation arising deep within one or more hair follicles and spreading into

surrounding dermis (a deeper form of folliculitis); the causative agent is almost always *Staphylococcus aureus*.

Clinical Manifestations

1. Tenderness, pain, and surrounding cellulitis; after furuncle localizes, the center becomes boggy and fluctuant, and a soft yellow or white head appears on the surface.
2. Sites of predilection—back of neck, axillae, buttocks.

Treatment and Nursing Management

1. Protect area from irritation, squeezing, and trauma.
2. Apply hot wet compresses—to increase vascularization and hasten resolution.
3. Cleanse surrounding skin with antibacterial soap.
4. Apply antibacterial ointment to surrounding skin—to prevent spillage and seeding of the bacteria when furuncle ruptures or is incised.
5. Prepare for surgical drainage when furuncle has become localized and shows fluctuation (wave-like motion upon palpation); furuncle may rupture spontaneously.
6. Give systemic antibiotic therapy (selected by sensitivity study) if spreading still occurs or if area of involvement poses a risk of complications.
7. See Health Education section under Carbuncle.

▶ **NURSING ALERT:** Take special precautions with boil on face, since the skin area drains directly into the cranial venous sinuses.
1. Place the patient with boils on nose, lip, groin, or perineal or perianal region on bed rest.
2. Give course of systemic antibiotic therapy as prescribed—to control spread of infection.

Carbuncles

Carbuncle is a multiloculated abscess produced by infection of 2 or more follicles; usually caused by staphylococcal infection.

Clinical Features

1. Seen most frequently within the thick, fibrous, inelastic skin of the back of the neck and upper back.

2. More apt to occur in older and debilitated persons; especially frequent in diabetics.

▶ **NURSING ALERT:** Every patient past middle age with a carbuncle should be suspected of having diabetes.

3. Symptoms
   a. Fever, leukocytosis, extreme pain, and prostration.
   b. Bacteremia is common because the extensive inflammation makes it difficult to completely wall off the infection, so that absorption of toxins takes place; extension of infection to bloodstream may take place.

Treatment and Nursing Management

1. Administer antibiotic (based on sensitivity studies)—antibiotic is continued until infective process is controlled.
2. Determine whether there is an underlying disease condition (diabetes, hematologic disease, etc.).
3. Prepare for surgical incision and drainage when definite fluctuance occurs. (Local surgical incision is usually necessary.)
4. Use supportive modalities (infusions, fever sponges, etc.) for the toxic patient.

Health Education

Instruct the patient as follows:
1. Wash hands thoroughly before and after caring for lesion.
2. Avoid excessive manipulation of the lesion, since this may cause dispersion of the bacteria.
3. Keep draining lesion covered with a dressing.
4. Wrap soiled dressings in paper and burn; discard razor blades after each use.
5. Use disposable tissues for wiping the nose—to reduce skin contamination.
6. A boil may be infectious; do not work in health-care facility or in food-service occupation until boil has healed.
7. If boil does not improve after treatment, report to the physician/clinic as a different antibiotic or treatment is indicated.

Mycotic (Fungal) Infections

Fungi are plant-like organisms that feed on organic matter; they are responsible for a variety of common skin infections. The mycoses affecting primarily the skin may be divided into 3 groups: dermatophyte (*Trichophyton, Epidermophyton,* and *Microsporum* genera), candida (*Candida albicans*), and *Malassezia furfur*.

Tinea Pedis (Athlete's Foot) Or Ringworm of the Feet

Tinea pedis (athlete's foot) is a superficial fungal infection due to *Trichophyton rubrum,* which may manifest itself as an acute, inflammatory, vesicular process or as a chronic rash involving the soles of the feet and the interdigital web spaces.

Clinical Features

1. Tinea pedis is the most common fungal infection.
2. Causes intense itching, burning, and erythema.
3. Lymphangitis and cellulitis may occur when bacterial superinfection is present.

Diagnostic Evaluation

1. Direct examination of scrapings (skin, nails, hair)
2. Isolation of the organism in culture

Management of Cutaneous Mycotic Infections

A. **Types of Agents**

1. *Topical agents*—have antidermatophyte and anticandidal activity.

  a. Haloprogin   c. Clotrimazole
  b. Miconazole   d. Econazole; ciclopirox olamine
2. *Griseofulvin*—for dermatophyte infections. Side effects include nausea, headache, blood dyscrasias, and liver toxicity.

B. Interventions

1. Use soaks (potassium permanganate, Burow's solution, saline solution) to remove scales, crusts, debris, and residual medications; also for mild anti-inflammatory effect.
   For the vesicular–bullous type of painful infection, elevation of the feet is necessary.
2. Apply topical antifungal agent such as tolnaftate (Tinactin), haloprogin (Halotex), miconazole (MicaTin), or clotrimazole (Lotrimin) to involved skin.
3. Continue with topical therapy for several weeks—there is a high rate of recurrence.
4. Give systemic antifungal agent (griseofulvin or ketoconazole) if there is extension of the infection or resistance to topical therapy.

Preventive Measures and Health Education

Instruct the patient to keep feet dry—moisture encourages the growth of fungi.
1. Dry carefully between the toes.
2. Alternate shoes—to permit adequate drying of shoes between wearings.
3. Wear cotton socks or stockings with cotton feet—synthetic material does not absorb perspiration as well as cotton.
4. Change socks frequently.
5. Wear perforated shoes if feet perspire excessively—to permit aeration of feet.
6. Apply talcum powder or antifungal powder twice daily—to keep feet dry.
7. Use small pieces of cotton between toes at night—to absorb moisture.
8. Avoid plastic or rubber-soled footwear.

Tinea Corporis or Tinea Circinata

Tinea corporis or *tinea circinata* is ringworm of the body.

Clinical Features

1. Appearance—begins as erythematous macule advancing to rings of vesicles with central clearing; lesions appear in clusters.
2. Lesions usually appear on exposed areas of body; may extend to scalp, hair, or nails.

3. An infected pet is a common source of infection.
4. Ringworm of the body causes intense itching.

Treatment

1. Apply topical antifungal medication to small areas (clotrimazole, miconazole, tolnaftate, haloprogin).
2. Griseofulvin may be used in very extensive cases in which the skin is broken, weeping, or oozing or for noninflammatory ringworm that is of the chronic, extensive, scaling type.
3. Ketoconazole (an alternate oral treatment) is effective in the griseofulvin-resistant patient.

Health Education

Instruct the patient as follows:
1. Wear clean cotton clothing next to skin.
2. Use a clean towel daily; dry thoroughly all areas and skin folds that retain moisture, since fungi thrive in a warm, moist environment.
3. Use self-monitoring for signs of reinfection after a course of oral therapy for chronic tinea corporis.

Tinea Cruris

Tinea cruris ("jock itch") is a superficial fungal infection of the groin, which may extend to the inner thighs and buttock area and is commonly associated with tinea pedis.

Clinical Features

1. Appears as a dull-red to red-brown eruption of the upper thighs; then advances outward from the crural (thigh) creases and extends to form circular plaques with elevated scaly or vesicular borders. Itching is usually present.
2. Seen most frequently in joggers, obese individuals, and those wearing tight underclothing.

Management

1. Topical therapy (miconazole cream or lotion; clotrimazole cream and lotion).
2. Griseofulvin (orally) for extensive eruption.
3. Treat concomitant tinea pedis to minimize reinfection.

Health Education

1. Avoid excessive washing/scrubbing.
2. Avoid nylon underclothing, tight-fitting underwear, and prolonged wearing of a wet bathing suit.
3. Wear cotton underwear.

Tinea Capitis (Ringworm of the Scalp)

Tinea capitis (ringworm of the scalp) is a fungal disease of the scalp. See page 1369.

Parasitic Skin Diseases

Three varieties of lice infest humans; their itching bites are the cause of many skin problems. Lice bite the skin to obtain the blood on which they feed. They leave their eggs and excrement on the skin; lice are passed from person to person.

Pediculosis Capitis

Pediculosis capitis is an infestation of the scalp by the head louse, *Pediculus humanus,* var. capitis.

Clinical Features

1. Appearance—minute white nits (eggs) attached to hair shaft in series: usually on scalp and hair at back of head and behind ears. Look at hair 2–5 cm. (¾–2 inches) away from scalp; unlike dandruff, lice/nits cannot be brushed off.
2. Most often found in children and persons having long hair.
3. The bite of the insect causes intense itching, and the

scratching may lead to complications such as impetigo, furuncles, and enlarged cervical lymph nodes.
4. May be transmitted by direct physical contact or contact with infested combs, brushes, wigs, hats, and bedding.

Management

1. Instruct the patient as follows:
   a. The following treatments are used for head lice:
      (1) Lindane shampoo (Kwell)
      (2) Pyrethrins with piperonyl butoxide (RID®)
      (3) Malathion (Prioderm lotion)
   b. Use the product as directed.
   c. Comb hair, while wet, with a fine-tooth comb dipped in vinegar—to remove remaining dead lice and nits.
   d. Disinfect comb and brushes with Kwell shampoo; sterilize all washable fomites.
   e. Put on clean clothing and machine wash clothing and bed linen.
   f. Delouse unwashable clothing by sealing in plastic bag for 10 days.
2. Treat all family members and close contacts who are infested.
3. Treat complications—severe pruritus, pyoderma (pus-forming infection of the skin), and dermatitis—with antipruritics, systemic antibiotics, and topical corticosteroids.

Health Education

1. Head lice infestation may happen to anyone; it is not a sign of being dirty. Head lice do not carry other diseases.
2. Treatment should be started immediately, since the condition spreads rapidly.
3. Control of school epidemics may be helped by having all of the students shampoo their hair on the same night.

Pediculosis Corporis

Pediculosis corporis is an infestation of the body by the body louse, *Pediculus humanus,* var. corporis.

Clinical Features

1. The body louse lives chiefly in the seams of undergarments and other clothing to which it clings.
2. Its bite causes characteristic minute hemorrhagic points.
   a. Purpuric macule at site of the bite is the primary lesion.
   b. Widespread excoriations may appear on the shoulders, trunk, and buttocks.
   c. May produce secondary lesions—hyperemia, parallel linear scratches, and hyperpigmentation in persistent cases.
3. Areas of skin involved are those that come in closest contact with the undergarments (axillae, neck, trunk, thighs).
4. The lice and nits may be seen in the seams of clothing. They move to the skin for blood feedings and then return to the clothing.

Treatment and Nursing Management

1. Instruct the patient as follows:
   a. Treatment consists of fumigation of the clothing and linens.
      (1) Machine wash on hot cycle and press with

hot iron, paying special attention to the seams (lice adhere to the seams); or dry clean clothing.
      (2) Or store the clothes in plastic bags for 2 weeks.
   b. Bathe with soap and water.
   c. Put on clean clothing.
2. Examine and treat all family members and contacts.
3. Treat pruritus, secondary bacterial infections, and dermatitis.

Pediculosis Pubis

Pediculosis pubis is an infestation by *Phthirus pubis* (crab louse); it is transmitted chiefly by sexual contact and is generally localized to the genital region.

Clinical Manifestations

1. Chief symptom is itching.
2. Black or rust-colored dots clinging to the base of the hairs.
3. Lice may infest hairs of chest, axillary hair, beard, and eyelashes.
4. Gray-blue macules (1–3 cm. in diameter) may be seen on the trunk, thighs, and axillae as a result of the action of the insects' saliva on bilirubin—converts it to biliverdin.
5. Itching of eyelid margins, blepharitis, and conjunctival inflammation—associated with *Phthirus pubis* palpebrarum (Figs. 13-1 and 13-2).

Management and Health Education

1. Instruct the patient as follows:
   a. Bathe with soap and water.
   b. Apply lindane lotion or shampoo or pyrethrin (RID®) to areas of involvement.
      (1) Leave on for specified time period.
      (2) Do not apply lindane to eyebrows, eyelids, or eyelashes—may cause eye irritation.
         (a) Apply ophthalmic petrolatum to eyelashes and eyebrows—smothers the lice and allows easier removal of nits and lice.
         (b) Remove nits manually from eyelashes and eyebrows with cotton-tipped applicator, toothpick, or fine tweezers.
         (c) Physostigmine ophthalmic ointment may then be applied to lid margins as directed.
   c. Machine wash all clothing and bedding with hot water; a temperature of 50°C (122°F) kills both lice and eggs in 30 minutes.
2. Treat all sexual contacts, family members, and close companions.
3. Schedule the patient for workup for coexisting sexually transmitted disease.
4. Treat secondary bacterial infection, itching, and dermatitis.
5. Be sure to follow directions; do not misuse product. Persistent itching is not uncommon even after infestation has been effectively controlled.

Scabies

Scabies is an infestation of the skin by *Sarcoptes scabiei* (itch mite). Scabies is transmitted by close personal contact.

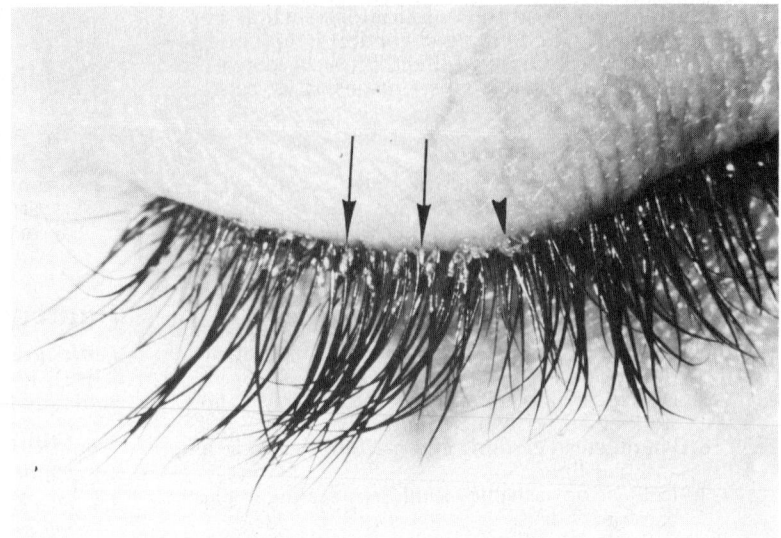

Figure 13-1. *Phthirus pubis* palpebrarum (crab lice on eyelids). Numerous nits (*arrows*) and crusty, granular material (*arrowhead*) are shown at lid margin. (Courtesy of W. Richard Green, MD, from Couch JM, Green WR et al. Diagnosing and treating *Phthirus Pubis* Palpebrarum. Surv Ophthalmol 1982 Jan–Feb; 26[4]:220; used by permission.)

Clinical Features

1. Primary lesion
   a. Adult female burrows into superficial layer of skin after fertilization has occurred on skin surface; burrows are short, wavy, brownish or blackish, thread-like lesions.
   b. She extends the burrow, laying 2–3 eggs daily for approximately 30 days. The eggs progress through larval and nymphal stages to form adult mites in 10 days.
   c. Male mites die shortly after mating; average number of adult female mites on an infested patient is 11.
2. Ask the patient where itch is most severe at the time you are examining him; look for burrows (short, wavy, dirty-appearing lines) with a magnifying glass (may or may not be visible). See below for procedure for obtaining skin scrapings for mite.
3. Look for small erythematous papules—scabies can imitate almost all pruritic dermatoses.
4. Secondary lesions include vesicles, papules, pustules, excoriations, and crusts; bacterial superinfection or eczematization may complicate the picture.
5. Sites—between fingers, on flexor surfaces of wrists and palms, around nipples, umbilicus, in axillary folds, under pendulous breasts, in or near groin or gluteal fold, penis, scrotum.
6. Symptoms—intense itching, more pronounced at night; usually occurs 1 month after initial infection.

Laboratory Evaluation

Examination of the epidermal scrapings microscopically.

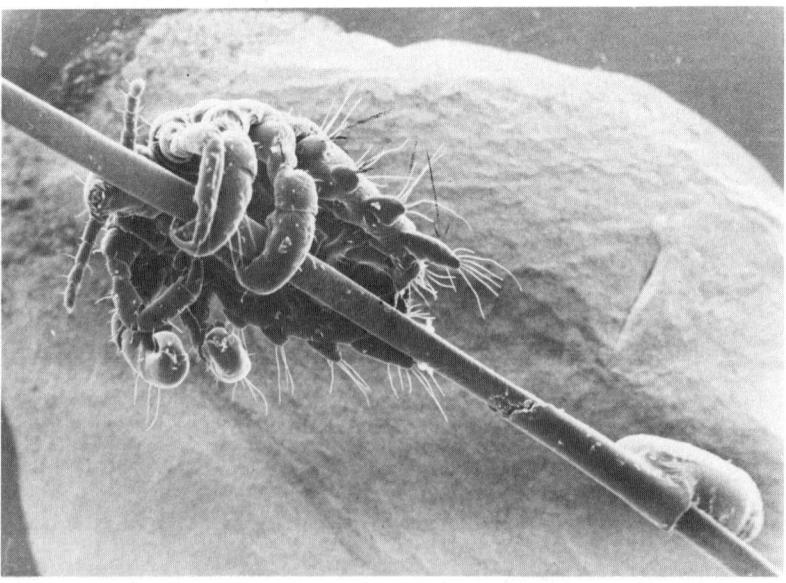

Figure 13-2. Scanning electron-micrograph of louse firmly grasping cilium (eyelash) with stout hind legs. Below the *Phthirus pubis* is an oval nit (egg) that adheres to the cilium by means of the cement secreted by the louse. (Courtesy of W. Richard Green, MD, from Couch JM, Green WR et al. Diagnosing and treating *Phthirus Pubis* Palpebrarum. Surv Ophthalmol 1982 Feb; 26[4]:221, used by permission.)

Treatment and Health Education

Instruct the patient as follows:

1. Apply scabicide such as lindane lotion or cream (Kwell) or crotamiton lotion or cream (Eurax).
   a. Apply thin layer from neck downward with particular attention to hands, feet and intertriginous areas; every inch of skin must be treated because mites are migrating. Apply to dry skin. (Wet skin allows more penetration and the possibility of toxicity.)
   b. Leave medication on for specified time period but no longer, since this will irritate the skin. Then wash thoroughly. The patient is no longer able to transmit the disease 24 hours after effective treatment.
   c. Machine wash and dry clothing and bed linens using the hot cycle.
   d. A bland ointment may be applied to the skin after the completion of treatment.
   e. Do not apply medication unless specifically prescribed by physician.
2. All family members and sexual contacts are treated simultaneously to eliminate the mites.
3. The animal with scabies is treated by a veterinarian.
4. Advise the patient that he may be uncomfortable and that itching may persist for days or weeks (this is from an allergic reaction to the mites); do *not* apply more mite-killing medicine but go to clinic/physician for special treatment if itching and rash persist (postscabies pruritus).
5. It is unnecessary to disinfect or fumigate the house/furnishings.

Guidelines: Skin Scraping for Scabies

Purpose	To demonstrate the mite *Sarcoptes scabiei* (or ova or feces) in skin scrapings removed from burrows or papules (Fig. 13-3).

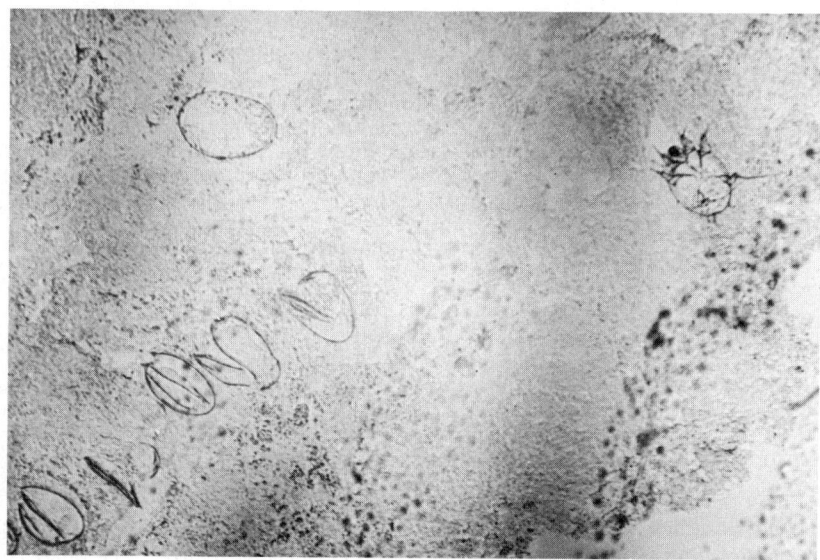

Figure 13-3. Scabies; scraping from a burrow. (*Lower left*) Hatched eggs. (*Upper left*) Intact egg. (*Upper right*) Newly hatched organism. (Courtesy Mervyn L. Elgart, MD)

Equipment

Hand lens
Mineral oil in dropper bottle
Scalpel and scalpel blade, No. 15
Glass slide/cover slip
Microscope

Procedure

Nursing Action	Rationale/Amplification
Preparatory Phase	
1. Place a small drop of oil in the middle of a glass slide.	

(continued)

Guidelines: Skin Scraping for Scabies (continued)

Procedure
(Cont.)

Nursing Action	Rationale / Amplification
Performance Phase	
1. Inspect for the burrows of *Sarcoptes scabiei* on webs of fingers, lower abdomen, pubic and axillary areas, legs, arms.	1. The female scabies mite, ova, and fecal deposits may be found in burrows on the skin.
2. Apply a small amount of mineral oil on unexcoriated burrows or papule.	2. The mineral oil causes the mite to float and enhances visualization.
3. Scrape the involved skin with the scalpel blade.	
4. Transfer the scrapings to the prepared glass slide and apply coverslip; or pick out the mite with a disposable needle and transfer it to a glass slide.	4. To avoid air bubble.
5. Examine the slide with a scanning lens of the microscope.	5. Look for the mites, eggs, and fecal pellets (which outnumber living organisms).

Viral Infection: Herpes Zoster

Herpes zoster (shingles) is an inflammatory condition in which a virus produces a painful vesicular eruption along the distribution of the nerves from one or more posterior ganglia.

Etiology

Caused by a varicella virus, commonly known as a varicella-zoster virus, which is a member of a group of DNA viruses.

Virus appears to be identical to the causative agent of varicella (chickenpox). After the primary infection, the varicella-zoster virus may persist in a dormant state in the dorsal nerve root ganglia. The virus may emerge from this site in later years, either spontaneously or in association with immunosuppression, to cause herpes zoster.

Clinical Manifestations

1. Eruption usually accompanied or preceded by malaise, itching, tenderness, and pain, which may radiate over entire region supplied by the nerves.
   a. Inflammation is usually unilateral, involving one or two nerve roots in a band-like configuration.
   b. Pain may be burning, lancinating, stabbing, or aching.
2. Vesicles appear in 3–4 days.
   a. Characteristic patches of grouped vesicles on erythematous and edematous skin.
   b. Early vesicles contain serum—they become cloudy (secondary to inflammatory response).
   c. The lesions dry, crust, and clear; scarring may occur.
3. Eruption appears posteriorly and progresses to the anterior and peripheral distribution of the nerves from one or more posterior ganglia.
4. Clinical course varies from 1–3 weeks; healing time varies from 7–26 days.
5. A susceptible person can acquire chickenpox if he comes in contact with the infective vesicular fluid of a zoster patient. A person with a previous history of chickenpox is immune and hence is not at risk from infection after exposure to zoster patients.

▶ **NURSING ALERT:** Varicella-zoster virus may be a life-threatening condition to the patient who is immunosuppressed or is receiving cytotoxic therapy.

Diagnostic Evaluation

Culture of varicella-zoster virus from lesions or detection by fluorescent antibody techniques.

Treatment and Nursing Management

1. The lesions usually clear spontaneously in healthy adults.
2. Place immunosuppressed patient or patients with disseminated disease on strict isolation.
3. The following treatment regimen may be given.
   a. Give systemic corticosteroids as directed for patients with severe and complicated herpes—given for anti-inflammatory effect, relief of pain, and prevention of complications.
   b. For the immunocompromised patient:
      (1) *Antiviral drugs*
         (a) Acyclovir—prevents progressive cutaneous dissemination and development of visceral zoster; reduces pain, prevents new lesion formation, and heals skin faster.
         (b) Vidarabine—reduces severity of acute pain, new vesicle formation, cutaneous dissemination, and visceral complications if given early.
      (2) Interferons (broad-spectrum antiviral proteins)—act directly to induce other antiviral enzymes to modulate host response (investigational).
4. Give analgesics to control pain—it is thought that effective pain control at the time of appearance of lesions may decrease incidence and severity of postherpetic neuralgia.

▶ **NURSING ALERT:** In older persons, the pain from herpes zoster may persist as postherpetic neuralgia for months after disappearance of the skin lesions.

5. Apply local treatment to skin lesions.
   a. Apply cool, wet dressings to pruritic lesions.
   b. Apply topical steroid—triamcinolone acetonide (Kenalog) etc.—to give relief and promote healing.
   c. Do not apply topical steroids if secondary infection is present.

6. Treat secondary bacterial infection of skin lesions—culture and sensitivity studies will indicate appropriate antibiotic.
7. Support the patient undergoing diagnostic studies to investigate the possibility of underlying disease.
8. Reassure the patient and employ stress-reduction techniques.
9. Monitor for complications—higher incidence in patients over 60.
   a. Postherpetic neuralgia—persistent pain of affected nerve following healing.
   b. Ophthalmic herpes zoster—(involvement of ophthalmic branch of trigeminal nerve with keratitis, uveitis, corneal ulceration, and possibly blindness). Patients with ophthalmic herpes zoster should be examined by an ophthalmologist to avoid serious ocular complications.
   c. Facial and acoustic nerve involvement (facial paralysis, vertigo, tinnitus, hearing loss).
   d. Visceral dissemination

Patient Education

1. Shingles is a viral infection of the nerves; "nervousness" does not cause shingles.
2. Do not open blisters.

Contact Dermatitis

Contact dermatitis is a common inflammatory, often eczematous, condition caused by a skin reaction from contact with a variety of irritating or allergenic materials. There is damage to the epidermis by repeated physical and chemical insults.
1. *Primary irritant contact dermatitis* is a nonallergic reaction caused by exposure to an irritating substance.
2. *Allergic contact dermatitis* results from exposure of sensitized individuals to contact allergens.

Causes

1. Poison ivy
2. Cosmetics
3. Soaps, detergents, and scouring compounds
4. Industrial chemicals
5. Hair dye, metals, rubber, chemicals

Predisposing Factors

1. Preexisting irritant dermatitis
2. Extremes of heat and cold—low humidity favors irritant contact dermatitis; high humidity favors allergic contact dermatitis
3. Frequent immersion in soap and water
4. Friction; occlusion

Clinical Manifestations

(Skin eruptions begin at point of contact with causative agent.)
1. Itching, burning, erythema, vesiculation, and eczema.
2. Weeping, crusting, drying, fissuring, and peeling.
3. Thickening of skin (lichenification) and pigmentation changes, if repeated reactions occur or if there is continual scratching by the patient.
4. Secondary bacterial invasion may occur—prevention of normal sweating produces vesicles, itching, and inflammation.

Treatment and Nursing Management

1. Inspect the entire body for a distribution pattern—helps to narrow down possible causes, which may be irritant or allergic.
2. Obtain a detailed history including the *site* of the *initial* eruption.
3. Instruct the patient as follows:
   a. Identify and remove the causative agent and contributing factors.
      (1) Avoid the use of soap until healing occurs.
      (2) Avoid exposing skin to the causative agent after recovery.
      (3) Wear protective gloves (thin white cotton gloves under rubber gloves) when using soap and water.
   b. Topical treatment
      (1) Use cool, wet dressings 15–20 minutes, 3–4 times daily for small areas of acute, vesicular dermatitis—for soothing and to help stop oozing.
      (2) Cleanse away softened crusts and other debris.
      (3) Use bland, unmedicated lotion for small patches of erythema.
      (4) Apply a thin layer of cream or ointment containing one of the steroids, as directed—usually not as beneficial when blisters are present, although some authorities feel it is helpful in these instances if used more frequently (i.e., at least 5 times daily).
      (5) Use medicated baths at room temperature (see p. 607) for larger areas of dermatitis.
4. Give sedatives and antihistamines if necessary to relieve itching and burning.
5. Give systemic antibiotics if secondary bacterial infection is present—purulent exudate and systemic symptoms (fever, lymphadenopathy, etc.).
6. Administer short course of systemic steroids if a more widespread and disabling condition is involved—can shorten the course of a severe disease; allays inflammation.
7. See also the patient with a dermatosis, p. 606.

Health Education

Instruct the patient as follows:
1. Avoid heat, soap, rubbing—all are external irritants.
2. Avoid topical medications except when specifically prescribed; avoid overtreatment.
3. Wash thoroughly immediately after exposure to antigens.
4. Protect the skin from trauma, excessive sunlight, wind, and rapid temperature changes while the dermatitis is active.

Poison Ivy Dermatitis

Poison ivy grows in the form either of climbing vines or of upright shrubs; the leaves grow in clusters of 3, one at the end of the stalk and the other 2 opposite one another. Poison ivy has a sticky sap that contains an active ingredient known as *urushiol,* an oleoresin (a combination of plant resin and volatile oil). This urushiol can cause an allergic skin reaction (contact dermatitis).

Exposure to Urushiol

1. Urushiol must make contact with the skin—contact is usually made by touching the plant leaves or stems.
2. Contact with urushiol may be made indirectly—clothing, tools, or pets touching the plant can pick up the sap and pass it to a person indirectly.
3. Urushiol is present in all parts of the plant, including dead stems and roots.
4. Smoke from burning plants carries droplets containing urushiol, which can get on the skin or enter the nose, throat, and lungs.

Clinical Manifestations

1. Eruption may develop in hours or days after contact.
   a. Reddened area will be noted, followed by rash and edema.
   b. Eruption occurs in a streak or line; it burns and itches.
   c. Small weeping areas may form (papules, vesicles, blisters)—in more severe cases, large blistered areas with inflammation and swelling may appear.
2. Secondary infection may give lesion the appearance of pyoderma (purulent skin disease) or plaque of eczema.

Treatment and Nursing Management

A. Mild to Moderate Eruption

1. Apply cold or tepid compresses or use tub baths if rash is diffuse.
2. Apply calamine lotion for soothing effect or
3. Apply topical cortisone cream or ointment.

a. If applied before blistering, a gel steroid may stop or ease reaction.
b. May also be helpful after vesicular stage has resolved to relieve itching, drying, and scaling.

B. Severe Eruption

Give systemic corticosteroid (prednisone) as directed—to control rash and itching.

1. Dosage is adjusted according to severity of reaction and then tapered off gradually.
2. Buffer the drug with milk or antacid if the patient has history of peptic ulcer.

Health Education

1. Advise the patient as follows to recognize and avoid contact with urushiol (poison ivy, poison oak, or poison sumac).
   a. Do not pull, chop, or burn vines and brush—sap-carrying smoke may produce outbreak in a sensitive person.
   b. Wear protective clothing (long sleeves, gloves, slacks) in heavily wooded areas—to guard against exposure.
   c. Apply protective ointments before working in the vicinity of the plants.
   d. Take off contaminated clothing carefully and wash clothing immediately—urushiol on clothing can cause outbreak of poison ivy.
   e. Wash skin *immediately* with nonirritating soap and rinse well—to remove the plant juice.
2. Avoid overtreatment.
3. Reassure the patient that poison ivy rash is not contagious.

Noninfectious Inflammatory Dermatoses

Psoriasis

Psoriasis is a chronic skin disorder in which there is an abnormally rapid multiplication of the cells of the epidermis. It appears as an eruption of circular patches of all sizes, sharply defined against the normal skin and covered with heavy, dry, silvery scales (Fig. 13-4). In time, the patches coalesce, forming extensive, irregularly shaped patches.

Clinical Features

1. In psoriasis, the rate of production of the epidermis of the skin is about 9 times faster than normal; this abnormal process does not allow for formation of normal protective layers of skin.
2. There appears to be a loss of normal regulatory mechanisms of cell division.
3. Onset is usually before the age of 20, but all age groups are affected.

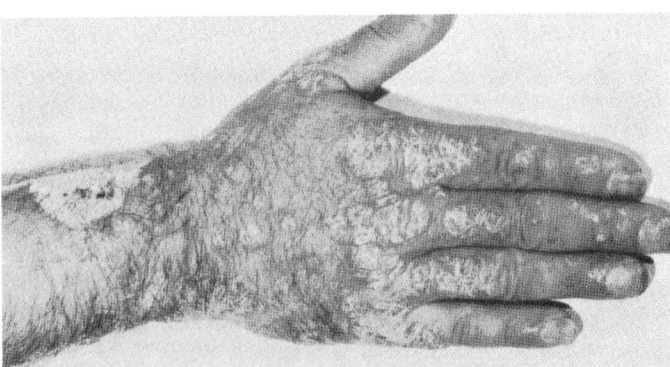

Figure 13-4. Psoriasis. (Sauer G. Manual of Skin Diseases, 4th ed. Philadelphia, JB Lippincott, 1980)

4. Psoriasis may be coupled with polyarthritis and cause crippling disability.
5. Sites (bilateral symmetry)
   a. Bony prominences (knees, elbows, sacrum), scalp, external ears, genitalia, perianal area, nails and dorsa of hands
   b. Psoriasis of the ears—scaling and dryness
   c. Psoriasis of palms and soles—scaly and pustular pruritic lesions
   d. Psoriasis of nails—thickening, discoloration, crumbling beneath free edges; pitting of nails
   e. Psoriasis between skin folds—smooth, shiny red lesions, easily fissured
6. The disease may range from a benign cosmetic source of annoyance to a physically disabling and disfiguring affliction with significant morbidity. It may be life-ruining—physically, emotionally, and economically.

Treatment and Nursing Management

A. Daily Skin Care

Instruct patient to take daily tub bath—to help soak off scales.
1. Gently remove excess scales with a soft brush while bathing.
2. Apply prescribed ointment after removal of scales.

B. Topical Therapy (includes corticosteroids, coal tar, anthralin, salicylic acid, etc.)

1. Coal tar preparations (ointments/baths)—retard and inhibit the rapid growth of psoriatic tissue
   a. Coal tar is applied for a period of time; may then be removed; this treatment is followed by carefully graded doses of ultraviolet radiation.
   b. Begin ultraviolet radiation with low doses (10 seconds) and build up dosage time gradually. Advise the patient to wear goggles to protect the eyes.
   c. Ultraviolet produces mild redness and slight desquamation.
   d. Tar gel preparations may be used for scalp lesions.
2. Anthralin preparations (a distillate of crude coal tar)—numerous variations in treatment approaches)
   a. Useful for especially thick and resistant psoriatic plaques.
   b. Instruct the patient to apply anthralin medication as directed with a tongue blade or gloved fingers; do not apply to normal skin.
   c. Wash hands thoroughly after application—medication can produce a chemical conjunctivitis.
   d. Anthralin stains badly and should be covered in some way (gauze dressings, stockinette, old pajamas).
   e. After prescribed time period, anthralin is removed with mineral oil and a tar bath is given; the patient is then exposed to conventional ultraviolet B (UVB) followed by application of a cream.
3. Topical steroids
   a. Apply wet dressings to irritated areas of psoriasis.
   b. Apply corticosteroid preparations (triamcinolone) to skin.
   c. Hold dressings in place with occlusive film (traps heat and moisture, softens scaly plaques and enhances transepidermal penetration).
      (1) Occlusive dressings over the entire body may be held in place with a large plastic bag with holes cut out for the head and arms; another bag may be used for the legs; extremities (arms) may be wrapped in plastic film.
      Caution the patient not to smoke while wrapped in these dressings.
      (2) In patients being treated at home, a plastic vinyl jogging suit may be used; hands can be wrapped in gloves, the feet in plastic bags, and the head in a shower cap.
   d. Caution the patient that skin atrophy may occur from long-term use, and rebound worsening of psoriasis can occur when steroid is discontinued.

C. Intralesional Therapy (triamcinolone acetonide)—may be injected directly into psoriatic plaques.

D. For More Resistant and Severe Psoriasis

1. Methotrexate—inhibits DNA synthesis and hence has a marked suppressive effect on the reproduction of rapidly proliferating cells.
2. Is hepatotoxic and requires pretreatment and follow-up liver biopsies, liver function tests, and blood counts. Birth control measures are necessary.
3. The patient should avoid alcohol intake while on methotrexate—increases possibility of liver damage.
4. Hydroxyurea may be used in patients with liver toxicity.

E. Photochemotherapy (PUVA Therapy)

1. Oral psoralen tablets (methoxsalen or 8-MOP, a photosensitizing chemical) followed by exposure to long-wave ultraviolet light (UVA)—in the presence of ultraviolet light, methoxsalen binds to DNA and leads to temporary inhibition of DNA synthesis (inhibits abnormally rapid multiplication of cells).
2. Long-term concerns include skin cancer, cataracts, aging effect, and systemic effects on other organs.
3. Methoxsalen capsules taken with milk or food 2 hours before scheduled UVA exposure in a UVA irradiation chamber; exposure is determined by the patient's skin type.
4. An average of 25 treatments given 2–3 times per week is required for clearing; maintenance treatments are usually necessary.
5. Patient education
   a. Since PUVA treatment produces photosensitization, the patient is sensitive to sunlight the entire day of treatment; he must wear protective clothing and use a sunscreen on the face and exposed areas of the body.
   b. Wraparound gray- or green-tinted glasses must be worn for a 24-hour period following ingestion of methoxsalen, for exposure to direct or indirect sunlight in the open or through a window glass—to prevent irreversible binding of methoxsalen to the proteins and DNA components of the lens.
   c. Initial blood tests and urinalysis are done, and eye examinations are required at specified times.
   d. PUVA may cause irreversible or slowly reversible clinical and histologic skin changes; loss of elasticity; irreversible solar damage; carcinogenesis.

Health Education

1. Psoriasis is thought to have multifactorial etiology, involving genetic, environmental, and systemic considerations.

2. Psoriasis is a disease of the entire skin, but it is not infectious or contagious.
3. Have an awareness of factors that may precipitate flare-ups.
    a. Know inciting factors—illness, certain drugs (propranolol, lithium, etc.).
    b. Develop insight and determine what life events may worsen the condition.
4. Avoid injury to the skin (patches of psoriasis bleed after minor trauma).
    a. Keep skin, especially on the hands, as pliable and soft as possible by applying appropriate creams.
    b. Wear heavy gloves when doing gardening, etc.
    c. Report to physician if severe injury to skin has occurred; injection of intralesional steroids may prevent untoward response.
5. Consider learning stress-reduction techniques.
6. Find another person with psoriasis to exchange ideas.
7. Learn to live with psoriasis and accept that it is a chronic disease, often requiring continuous therapy; treatment can be time-consuming and expensive.
8. Try to schedule exposure to sunlight on a regular basis. Avoid sunburn, since it can cause a generalized flare-up.

Exfoliative Dermatitis
(Generalized Erythroderma)

Exfoliative dermatitis is a serious condition characterized by progressive inflammation in which erythema and scaling often occur in a more or less generalized distribution. It may be associated with chills, fever, prostration, severe toxicity, and an itchy scaling of the skin.

Clinical Manifestations

A. Appearance

1. Starts acutely as either a patchy or generalized erythematous eruption accompanied by fever, malaise, and occasionally gastrointestinal symptoms.
2. The skin color changes from pink to dark red; then after a week, the characteristic exfoliation (scaling) begins, usually in the form of thin flakes which leave the underlying skin smooth and red, new scales forming as the older ones exfoliate (cast off).
3. Hair loss and nail shedding may accompany the disorder.

B. Systemic Effects

Exfoliative dermatitis has a marked effect on the entire body.

1. There is a profound loss of stratum corneum (outermost layer of the skin)—causes capillary leakage, hypoproteinemia, and negative nitrogen balance.
2. Iron loss from the skin produces anemia.

C. Multiplicity of Causes

1. May follow a previous skin condition (eczema, psoriasis) that had become generalized.
2. May arise as a primary condition.
3. May appear as a part of the lymphoma group of diseases and may precede the appearance of lymphoma or leukemia.
4. Also appears as a severe reaction to a wide number of drugs, including antimicrobial agents (sulfonamides, penicillins), anticonvulsants, and analgesics.
5. In many patients, cause is never found.

Treatment and Nursing Management

1. Discontinue all possibly offending drugs; early recognition of offending agent will shorten disease course and prevent severe consequences.
2. Hospitalize the patient and place him on bed rest. Maintain comfortable room temperature—patient does not have normal thermoregulatory control because of temperature fluctuations from vasodilation and evaporative water loss.
3. Monitor and correct deficits in fluid and electrolyte balance. Offer a high protein diet.
4. Give systemic corticosteroids as directed—for antiinflammatory action; may be a life-saving procedure.
5. Use compresses, soothing baths, and lubrication—to treat acute extensive dermatitis and give symptomatic relief.
6. Watch for symptoms of heart failure (p. 323)—hyperemia and increased cutaneous blood flow can produce a cardiac failure of high-output origin.
7. Maintain nursing surveillance for intercurrent or cutaneous infection; the erythematous, moist skin is receptive to infection and becomes colonized with pathogenic organisms, which produce more inflammation.
Antibiotics are given if infection is present; selected by culture and sensitivity.

Health Education

Advise the patient to avoid all irritants, particularly drugs.

Pemphigus

Pemphigus is a serious autoimmune disease of the skin and mucous membranes characterized by the appearance of blisters (bullae) of various sizes on apparently normal skin and mucous membranes (mouth, vagina) (Fig. 13-5). The cause is unknown.

Familial benign chronic pemphigus (Hailey–Hailey disease) is a familial type of pemphigus appearing in adult life affecting particularly the axillae and groin. There are other variants of the disease.

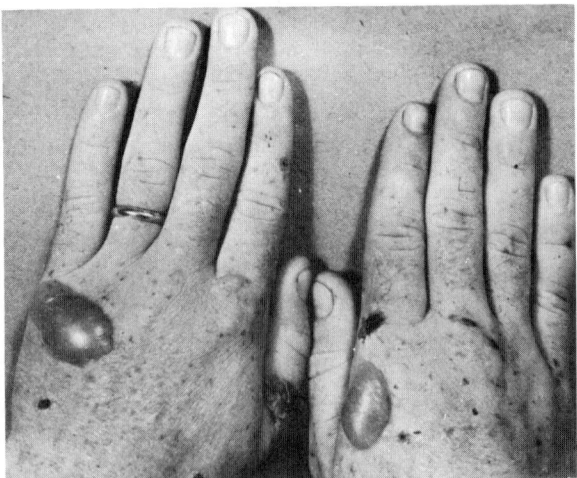

Figure 13-5. Pemphigus; bullous dermatitis of hand (vesicles). (Courtesy Armed Forces Institute of Pathology)

Clinical Manifestations

1. Appearance
    a. The bullae enlarge and rupture, forming painful raw and denuded areas that eventually become crusted.
    b. The eroded skin heals slowly; eventually, huge areas of the body are involved.
    c. In the mouth, the blisters are usually multiple, of varying size and irregular shape, painful, and persistent.
    Oral lesions may appear *initially;* may also affect mucous membranes of pharynx, esophagus, conjunctivae, larynx, urethra, cervix, and rectum.
2. An offensive odor emanates from the bullae.
3. Positive Nikolsky's sign—production of a blister upon rubbing adjacent normal skin.

Diagnostic Evaluation

1. Laboratory evaluation
2. Immunofluorescent studies of skin and serum
3. Skin biopsies of blisters or margins of erosion

Management

1. Corticosteroids (prednisone) in large doses, as prescribed—to control the disease.
    a. High dosage level is maintained until remission is apparent.
    b. Dosage is reduced to minimum daily maintenance dose as soon as possible.
    c. Give medication with or immediately after a meal; may be accompanied by an antacid as prophylaxis against gastric complications.
2. Immunosuppressive agents (cyclophosphamide, azathioprine [employed alone or in combination with steroids])—for immunosuppressive or anti-inflammatory treatment, which will supplement steroid action and enable reduction of steroids.
3. Treatment of denuded skin.

Nursing Interventions

A. Fluid and Electrolyte Balance

1. Evaluate for fluid and electrolyte imbalance—extensive denudation of the skin leads to fluid and electrolyte imbalance.
    a. Monitor serum albumin and protein levels.
    b. Monitor vital signs.
    c. Take measurements of body weight; test urine for glucose.
    d. Administer saline infusions as directed—significant loss of tissue fluids and therefore of sodium chloride occur through the skin.
    e. Encourage the patient to maintain adequate fluid intake.
    f. Give soft, high-protein, high-calorie diet—patients with painful oral involvement have difficulty maintaining nutrition.
    g. See nursing management of the patient with extensive burns, page 634 (large amounts of serum may be lost through denuded skin).
    h. Monitor for problems related to high-dose steroid therapy (steroid-induced diabetes, steroid-induced psychosis, bleeding ulcers, edema and fluid retention, secondary infection from opportunistic agents [may be fatal]).

B. Relief of Skin Discomfort

1. Keep skin clean and eliminate debris and dead skin—the bullae will clear if epithelium at the base is clean and not infected.

2. Culture skin frequently—most common organism is *Staphylococcus aureus.*
3. Give systemic antimicrobials as prescribed.
4. Administer cool, wet dressings and/or baths—patients with large areas of blistering have a characteristic odor that is lessened when secondary infection is under control.
    a. Potassium permanganate baths help keep areas from becoming infected and to some extent precipitate some of the protein that oozes through open skin.
        (1) Dissolve potassium permanganate crystals thoroughly in small container; then pour into bathtub.
        (2) Undissolved crystals may be irritating if patient sits on them.
    b. Following the bath, dry the patient and cover him with talcum powder as directed—enables the patient to move more freely in bed. Fairly large amounts are necessary to keep patient from sticking to sheets.
5. The nursing management of patients with blistering or bullous skin conditions is similar to that of the patient with extensive burns (see p. 634).

C. Adequate Oral Intake

1. Keep oral mucosa clean and allow regrowth of epithelium—secondary infection may be associated with offensive odor from oral lesions. *Candida albicans* infection of the mouth frequently seen in patients on high-dose steroid therapy.
2. Give topical oral therapy as directed—lesions in mouth are painful and slow to heal.
3. Offer a high-protein, pureed diet.
4. Encourage the patient to drink fluids.
5. Consider parenteral nutrition if the patient is unable to eat.

D. Resolution of Infection

1. Assess the patient for evidence of local and systemic infection—bullae are susceptible to infection, and septicemia may follow. Combinations of steroids and immunosuppressives predispose the patient to severe infection.
2. Observe for psychiatric problems caused by high-dose steroids.

Health Education

Instruct the patient as follows:
    Monitor skin/mouth for recurrence of pemphigus activity.

Toxic Epidermal Necrolysis (TEN)

Toxic epidermal necrolysis (TEN) is a severe, potentially fatal skin disease most commonly related to drug exposure in adults, although it is occasionally induced by staphylococcus. The drugs most commonly implicated are the sulfonamides, phenytoin, allopurinol, phenylbutazone, salicylates, penicillins, and barbiturates.

Clinical Manifestations

1. Fever
2. Erythema, involving much of skin surface
3. Appearance of large, flaccid bullae
4. Wide, sheet-like peeling and denudation of the skin—appearance is that of a second-degree burn with a moist, blistered, and tender surface (Fig. 13-6).
5. Skin necrosis; ulcerations of lips and oral pharynx

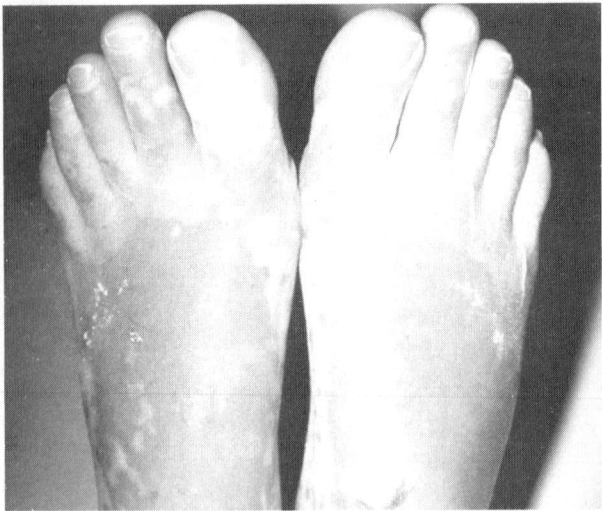

Figure 13-6. Toxic epidermal necrolysis showing denudation of the skin of the feet. (Courtesy of Mervyn L. Elgart, MD)

6. Positive Nikolsky's sign (desquamation of skin in sheets upon light digital pressure)

Diagnostic Evaluation

Microscopic examination of skin biopsy specimens obtained from lesions; may be done as a frozen section because prompt diagnosis is important.

Treatment and Nursing Management

A. Fluid and Electrolyte Balance

1. Transfer the patient to unit (burn unit) equipped to handle long-term management of extensive dermal loss—the principles of *burn wound management* with its associated hemodynamic problems apply to this condition (see p. 634).

2. Stop all administration of nonessential drugs immediately.
3. Start intravenous (IV) fluid resuscitation in volumes required to maintain urine output of 50 ml./hour; start on oral fluid intake when the patient demonstrates tolerance.
4. Monitor serum electrolytes and osmolarity.
5. Keep room warm.

B. Avoidance of Infectious Complications

1. Use strict isolation precautions (as with a second-degree burn) and wear a mask and sterile gloves.
2. Take cultures of nasopharynx, eyes, ears, blood, urine, skin, and unruptured bullae as directed to determine presence of pathogenic organisms.
3. Monitor IV sites for infection, which may result in septicemia.
4. Give parenteral steroids as directed—may be given in an attempt to abort skin necrosis and denudation.
5. Administer antibiotics as directed.
6. Apply warm compresses of aqueous silver nitrate *gently* to raw areas to reduce bacterial population.
7. Employ meticulous oral hygiene.
8. Use extreme care in handling the patient, since skin fragility is a problem.
   a. Place the patient on a turning frame.
   b. Secure services of several health-care personnel to support an extremity evenly when the patient moves—to reduce trauma and shearing of the superficial epidermis.
   c. Use indwelling arterial line with pressure transducer giving a constant readout of blood and pulse; avoid using a cuff sphygmomanometer because of skin trauma.
   d. Give analgesics for the patient experiencing pain from raw areas.

C. Nutritional Balance

1. Consider parenteral nutrition because the patient may have perioral lesions.
2. Monitor nutritional status, with measurement of nitrogen excretion because this provides a guide to adequacy of protein intake; collect urine for assay of nitrogen excretion.

Ulcers and Tumors of the Skin

Ulcers of the Skin

Ulceration is a superficial loss of surface tissue from the death of cells.

Causes

Ulcers of the skin usually arise from (1) infection or (2) an interference with the blood supply.
1. Infection as cause of skin ulcers.
   a. Usually develop from an infection with anaerobic streptococci or from combination of infections (hemolytic streptococci and staphylococci).
   b. Tend to progress peripherally—characterized by an overhanging edge.
2. Deficient circulation as cause of skin ulcers—see page 367.
3. Pressure sores (see p. 59).

Tumors of the Skin

Cysts

Epidermal cysts are common, slow-growing, firm, elevated tumors consisting of a mass of epidermal cells; frequently found on the back.
Pilar cyst (sebaceous cysts) are cysts that arise from the isthmus (middle) part of the hair follicle. They are common on the face and scalp.

Benign Tumors

A. Seborrheic Keratoses—tumors are benign wartlike lesions of varying size and color, ranging from light tan to black; most common skin tumors in middle-age and elderly persons.

B. Actinic Keratoses—premalignant skin lesions appearing as rough, scaly patches with underlying erythema.

1. Develop in chronic sun-exposed areas of the body.
2. Many available treatments; liquid nitrogen cryosurgery, or currettage, or biopsy.

C. Verrucae (warts)—common, benign skin tumors caused by viruses.

1. Many times warts do not need treatment, since they tend to disappear spontaneously.
2. Treatment (remedies are legion)
   a. Freezing with liquid nitrogen—liquid nitrogen has a somewhat destructive action, although it tends to spare the epidermis.
   b. Area may be treated locally with salicylic acid plasters, electrodesiccation, application of cantharidin, topical fluorouracil, topical vitamin A acid, etc.

D. Angiomas (birthmarks)—benign vascular tumors involving the skin and subcutaneous tissues.

1. May occur as flat, violet-red patches (port-wine angiomas) or as raised, bright-red nodular lesions (strawberry angiomas). Strawberry angiomas may involute spontaneously, whereas port-wine angiomas usually persist indefinitely.
2. Most patients use masking cosmetics (Covermark) to camouflage the defect.

E. Pigmented Nevi (moles)—common skin tumors of various sizes and shapes ranging from yellowish to brown to black.

1. May be flat, macular lesions or elevated papules or nodules that occasionally contain hair.
2. Majority of pigmented nevi are harmless; however, in rare cases, malignant changes supervene and a melanoma develops at the site of the nevus.
3. Treatment
   a. Nevi at sites subject to repeated irritation from clothing, etc., should be removed—for comfort.
   b. Nevi that show change in size or color, or become symptomatic (itch or bleed) should be removed—to determine if malignancy has occurred. This is especially true for nevi with irregular borders or variations of blue, red, and/or white color.
   c. Excised nevi should be examined histologically.

F. Keloids—benign overgrowths of fibrous tissue at site of scar or trauma in predisposed individuals.

1. More prevalent among black race.
2. Usually asymptomatic—may cause disfigurement and cosmetic concern.
3. Treatment—irradiation or intralesional injection with corticosteroids.

Cancer of the Skin

Clinical Features

1. Skin cancer is the most common malignancy; the number of cases is increasing yearly.
2. There is a 95% cure rate because of early diagnosis, the slow progression of most skin cancers, and the effective methods of treatment available.

Causes

1. Exposure to sun over a period of time. *Sun damage is cumulative.*

2. Persons who do not produce sufficient pigment to protect underlying tissue are susceptible to sun damage—fair, blue-eyed, red-haired persons of Celtic ancestry or those with ruddy or light complexions; those who sunburn and do not tan.
3. Exposure to irradiation (history of x-ray treatment of benign skin lesions).
4. Exposure to certain chemical agents (arsenic, nitrates, tar and pitch, oils and paraffins).
5. Burn scars, areas of chronic osteomyelitis, fistulae of chronic nature.
6. Immunosuppressive therapy.
7. Genetic susceptibility.

Nursing Assessment

Look for:
1. Chronic sunburn
2. Actinic damage—pigment change, splotches, wrinkling, leathery complexion
3. Precancerous lesions (keratosis, leukoplakia)
4. Change in a skin lesion

▶ **NURSING ALERT:** Any skin lesion that changes in size or color, bleeds, ulcerates, or becomes infected may be skin cancer.

Diagnostic Evaluation

1. Biopsy
2. Histologic evaluation

Types of Skin Cancer

A. Basal Cell Carcinoma

1. Most common skin cancer; higher incidence in regions where population is subjected to intense and extensive exposure to sun.
2. Lesions are small nodules with a rolled, pearly, translucent border with telangiectasia (dilatation of end blood vessels), crusting, and occasionally ulceration (Fig. 13-7).
3. These tumors may be pigmented, multiple, superficial, or cystic.
   a. Characterized by invasion and erosion of continuous tissues—rarely metastasizes.

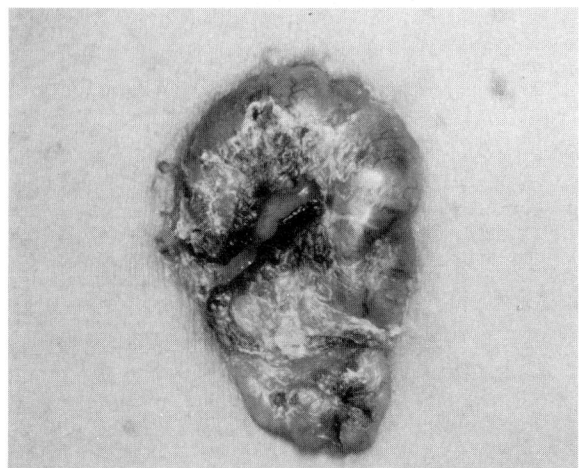

Figure 13-7. Basal cell carcinoma. (Courtesy of Mervyn L. Elgart, MD)

b. Lesions appear most frequently on sun-exposed skin, principally on the head and neck.

B. Squamous Cell (Epidermoid) Carcinoma

1. A malignancy that arises on sun-exposed areas of skin and mucous membrane and is considered a truly invasive carcinoma.
2. Appears as a solitary rough, thickened, scaly tumor with an inflamed base and an indistinct margin.
3. May be preceded by leukoplakia (premalignant lesion of mucous membrane), actinic keratoses, scarred or ulcerated lesions.
4. Seen most commonly on lower lip, rims of ears, head, neck, and dorsa of hands.
5. Requires more aggressive approach (wider margin of normal skin included in excision)—greater chance of metastases from squamous cell carcinoma and significantly lower cure rate.

Management

1. Method of treatment depends on tumor location, cell type (location and depth), history of previous treatment, and whether or not it is invasive and metastatic nodes are present.
   Usual modes of treatment are (1) curettage and electrodesiccation and (2) surgical excision.
2. *Curettage followed by electrodesiccation*—usually done on small tumors (less than 1–2 cm.).
   a. Curettage—excision of skin tumor by scraping with a curette; electrodesiccation (alternating high-frequency current, which results in death of cell) is used to achieve hemostasis and to destroy any viable malignant cells in margins or in base of wound.
   b. This form of treatment takes advantage of the fact that the tumor, in each instance, is softer than surrounding skin and can be outlined by curette, which "feels" the extent of the tumor.
   c. Tumor is removed and the base cauterized; process is repeated a number of times.
3. *Surgical excision*
   a. Wide surgical excision—adequacy of excision verified by microscopic study of sections of the specimen.
   b. Histologic study of excised tissue allows determination of whether or not margins are free of tumor.
   c. Skin grafting may be necessary.
4. *X-ray or irradiation therapy*—usually done for cancer of eyelid, tip of nose, in or near vital structures (facial nerve) where tissue sparing is difficult with other forms of treatment; used for extensive malignancies when goal is palliation or when other medical conditions contraindicate other forms of therapy.
   a. Explain to the patient that he may experience skin reddening and swelling about the time of the third treatment; may progress to blistering.
   b. Apply bland skin ointment as prescribed—to relieve discomfort.
   c. Stress importance of follow-up care—there is always the possibility of recurrence or a new primary lesion.
   d. Caution the patient against exposure to the sun.
5. *Cryosurgery*—deep freezing to destroy tumor tissue selectively.
   a. Liquid nitrogen is applied by cryospray or cryoprobe technique.

b. Site thaws naturally and then becomes gelatinous and heals spontaneously.
6. *Microcontrolled surgery*—fresh tissue is sequentially excised in layers and immediate microscopic examination of each tissue layer is made. More extensive carcinomas are examined with a fixed tissue technique (chemosurgery).

Health Education

Instruct the patient as follows:
1. *Sunlight permanently damages the skin.* Most skin cancer can be prevented by avoidance of and protection from direct exposure to sun.
2. Avoid unnecessary exposure to the sun, especially during times when ultraviolet radiation is most intense (10 A.M.–2 P.M.).
3. Apply a protective sunscreen with recommended sun protection factor if an activity requires a long period of exposure.
   a. Sun protection factor (SPF) ranges from 2 (minimal protection) to 15 (ultra- or superprotection).
   b. Specific SPF number is selected according to skin sensitivity ("burns easily" to "never burns"). Use a sunscreen with SPF 15 *routinely.* Apply evenly to all exposed areas of body.
   c. Sunscreen selected should not come off easily; those which contain 5% para-aminobenzoic acid in 55%–70% alcohol do not come off easily.
   d. Periodically reapply more sunscreen, especially after swimming/bathing.
   e. Protect your lips—use darker shades of lipstick or ultraviolet-absorbing lip pomade.
4. Wear protective clothing (long sleeves, broad-brimmed hat, etc.)—however, damaging radiation to skin still occurs from ground radiation.
5. Have moles removed that are accessible to repeated friction and irritation.
6. Watch for indications of potential malignancy in moles (e.g., change in color, increase in size, ulceration, bleeding, or serous exudation).
7. Skin cancers tend to be multiple—watch your skin for development of new or changing lesions. Have follow-up evaluation throughout lifetime.
8. Caution your children and grandchildren, especially those with fair skin, to avoid excessive exposure to the sun to prevent later skin cancers.

Malignant Melanoma

Malignant melanoma is a malignant tumor developing from the melanocytes (cells with capability of manufacturing melanin) that occurs in several forms (see Classification, p. 627).

Malignant melanoma may arise in apparently normal skin or may arise in association with preexisting acquired and congenital melanocytic nevi.

Risk Factors

1. Skin pigmentation—fair-skinned, light-colored eyes, light-colored hair; persons who sunburn readily and do not tan
2. Ultraviolet radiation from the sun
3. Certain preexisting pigmented skin lesions
4. Dysplastic nevi—acquired abnormal moles present both in general population and in certain melanoma-prone families:
   a. Larger than common nevi

b. Variegated color; irregular and frequently ill-defined borders; frequently occur on covered areas of body

5. Congenital nevi (a melanocytic nevus present at birth)

Classification

A. Superficial Spreading Melanoma (most common)

1. Occurs anywhere on body; usually affects middle-aged persons.
2. Tends to be circular, with portion of its outline irregular (either protruding or indenting).
3. Has combination of colors—hues of tan, brown, and black admixed with gray, bluish-black, or white.
4. May be dull pink-rose color in a small area within the lesion.

B. Nodular Melanoma

1. Spherical blueberry-like nodule with relatively smooth surface and relatively uniform blue-black, blue-gray, or reddish-blue color; occurs commonly on back, head, and neck.
2. May be polypoidal, with smooth surface of rose-gray or black color; may be present as elevated, irregular plaque.
3. Least favorable prognosis.

C. Lentigo-maligna Melanoma

1. Slowly evolving pigment lesions; occur on exposed skin surfaces of persons in the 5th or 6th decade.
2. First appears as tan, flat macule—malignant degeneration is manifested by changes in size, color, and topography.

D. Acral-lentiginous Melanoma

1. A tumor occurring on hands and feet with predilection for fingers and toes, subungual areas, and heels.
2. Predominates in blacks, Asians, and some dark-skinned Caucasians; may be deeply invasive.

Clinical Manifestations (Fig. 13-8)

1. Have a penlight to view lesions with oblique lighting and use a magnifying lens.
2. Signs that suggest malignant change:
   a. *Variegated color*
      (1) Colors that may indicate malignancy in a brown or black lesion are shades of red, white, and blue; shades of blue are considered ominous.
      (2) White areas within a pigmented lesion are suspicious.
      (3) Some malignant melanomas are not variegated but are uniformly colored (bluish-black, bluish-gray, bluish-red).
   b. *Irregular border*—look for angular indentation or notch present in the border of a malignant melanoma.
   c. *Irregular surface*
      (1) Look for uneven elevations of the surface; irregular topography may be palpable or visible; change in the surface (smooth to scaly).
      (2) Some nodular melanomas have a smooth surface.
   d. *Change in color, size, symmetry, surface characteristics, symptoms (itching, tingling, tenderness, pain), and shape.*
3. Common sites of melanoma—skin of back, legs (of

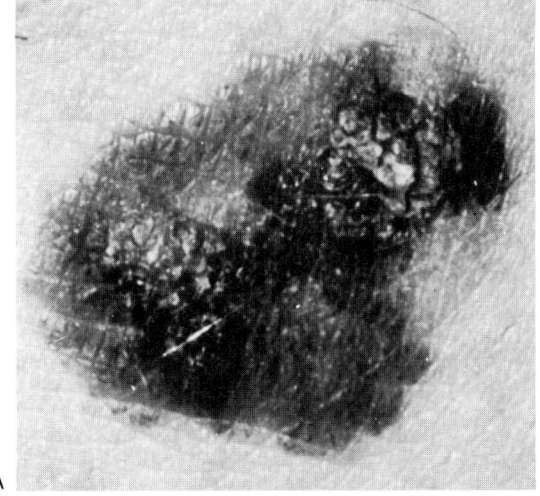

A

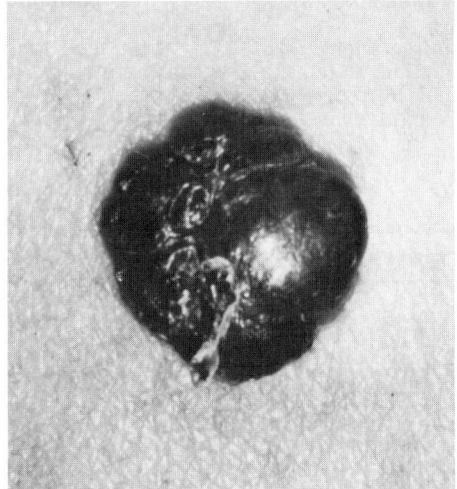

B

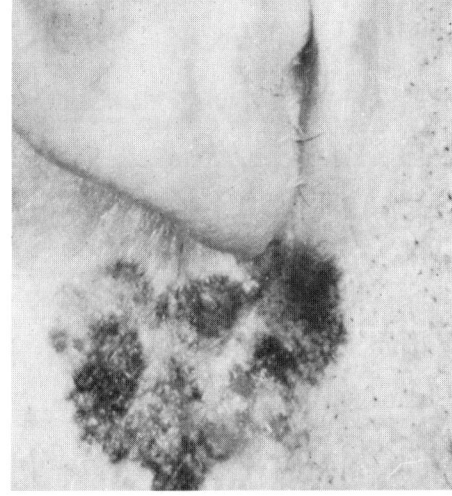

C

Figure 13-8. (*A*) Superficial spreading melanoma; note irregular border. (*B*) Nodular melanoma. (*C*) Lentigo-maligna melanoma; note irregular pigment pattern. (Courtesy of Arthur J. Sober, MD)

women), between toes, and on feet, face, scalp, fingernails, back of hands.

Diagnostic Evaluation

1. Appearance of lesion (see above) with consideration of history of recent changes within lesion.
2. Excision biopsy (for histopathologic diagnosis) and microstaging determination of thickness.

Treatment

The therapeutic approach depends on the type, level, thickness, and location of the lesion, and the stage of disease.

1. Wide surgical excision of tumor, sometimes followed by plastic repair or skin grafting. The role of regional node dissection is in dispute.
2. Regional isolation perfusion as an adjuvant to surgery; specific area is isolated by mechanically controlling its arterial inflow and venous outflow. This allows high concentration of cytotoxic drugs to be delivered to cancer-bearing sites with less systemic toxicity (see p. 906).
3. Immunotherapy (BCG)—to stimulate the patient's immune system to produce antibodies (investigational).
4. Chemotherapy (dacarbazine [DTIC])—generally used

for recurrence of metastasis or as palliation; may be combined with autologous bone marrow transplantation.

Health Education

Instruct the patient as follows:

1. Examine your skin monthly in an orderly manner; include scalp examination.
   a. Use a full-length mirror and a small hand mirror to aid in examination.
   b. Learn where moles/birthmarks are located.
   c. Inspect all moles and other pigmented lesions; report to the physician/clinic immediately moles that *change* colors, enlarge, become raised or thicker, itch, or bleed.
   d. Have physician examine your skin at least twice yearly. A patient with malignant melanoma should have lifelong follow-up.
2. Large congenital moles are recognized as precursors of melanoma and should be carefully monitored. Some clinicians advocate removal.
3. One key factor in development of malignant melanoma is exposure to sunlight. See page 626 for preventive aspects.
4. A person developing a malignant melanoma has a higher risk of developing a second primary malignant melanoma.

Dermatologic Surgery

Plastic Reconstructive Surgery

Reconstructive surgery (plastic surgery) is performed to repair extravisceral defects and malformations, both congenital and acquired, and to restore function as well as prevent further loss of function.

Cosmetic surgery involves reconstruction of the cutaneous tissues around the neck and face; done to restore function, correct defects, and remove the marks of time (Table 13-1).

Skin Grafting

Definitions

1. *Skin graft* (free graft)—a section of skin tissue that is separated from its blood supply and transferred as a free section of tissue to the recipient site.
2. *Skin flap* (pedicle graft)—a section of skin tissue used to cover or fill a defect; it is lifted from its bed but still has partial attachment by a pedicle from

Table 13-1 Common Cosmetic Plastic Operations

Operation	Purpose	Surgery	Postoperative expectations
Rhinoplasty (nose)	To improve the shape of the nose in relation to the rest of the face	1–1½ hours; excess bone or cartilage is removed; nose is reshaped	Nasal splint; soft intranasal packing; foam rubber dressings
Chin augmentation	To improve the profile, as is necessary with a receding chin	Incision approach is within the mouth, inorganic (Silastic) implant is positioned	Healing complete in 1 week
Rhytidoplasty (face-lifting)	To remove excess skin due to elastosis and to tighten remaining skin	Incision is anterior to ear and extended down to nasolabial fold to the mental foramen near the chin and to the midline in the upper neck; the stretched subcutaneous tissues and fascia of the face are folded to provide a basic firmness	Improvement lasts up to 10 years
Glabellar rhytidoplasty	To remove 2 vertical furrows between eyebrows	Dermabrasion and excision; skin graft may be required	
Otoplasty (ear)	To correct deformed, flattened, or protruding ears	1–1½ hours, silicone or plastic implant may be used	Ear bandaged for 1 week; protection during sleep required for 3 weeks
Blepharoplasty (eyelid)	To remove wrinkles and bulges caused by herniation of fat, aging, or inheritance	1–1½ hours, two incisions, one on upper lid and one on lower lid	Neosporin ointment applied around eyes and lids; individual eye dressings are applied; swelling and discoloration subside in about 10 days

which it receives its blood supply until healing takes place in its new location. Flaps are used to cover defects in which there is poor vascularity; for reconstruction of eyelids, ears, nose, and cheeks.

3. *Autograft*—transfers or transplants from same person.
4. *Allograft*—transfer or transplants between two individuals of same species.
5. *Isografts*—grafts between identical twins.
6. *Xenografts*—grafts between two animals of different species (e.g., rabbit to mouse, baboon to man).
7. *Split-thickness skin graft* (Thiersch's graft)—graft of approximately one-half the thickness of skin, which is removed by a knife or dermatome; deeper layers of dermis are left behind. (Used for coverage and closure of skin defects.)
8. *Full-thickness skin graft*—contains the epidermis and all of the dermis.
   a. Used frequently for reconstruction of facial defects, for it neither contracts nor develops unsightly pigmentation.
   b. Grafts may be further subdivided into thin and thick:
      (1) Thin (0.010–0.015 inch thick)—used to resurface contaminated granulations or recipient sites in which blood supply is jeopardized.
      (2) Thick (0.015–0.020 inch thick)—used where durability is the important factor.
9. *Pinch graft*—a small piece of skin graft obtained by elevating the skin with a needle or forceps and cutting it off with scissors or knife.
10. *Take*—refers to the appearance of the graft between the 3rd and 5th day after transfer, signifying that the vascular connections have developed between the recipient bed and the transplant.

Causes of Graft Failure

1. Fluid beneath the graft
2. Hematoma—avoid by early inspection and removal of clots
3. Infection

Patient Problems/Nursing Diagnoses

1. Impairment in skin integrity related to movement of skin graft from one site to another
2. Social isolation related to embarrassment about appearance, possible malodor, and slow healing process
3. Potential for infection related to disruption of an intact skin, inadequate dermal nutrition, and ideal conditions for growth of pathogenic organisms
4. Knowledge deficit related to maintaining aseptic wound conditions, changing appearance of skin as it heals, and restrictive movement required

Planning and Implementation
Preoperative Nursing Interventions
A. Establishing Optimal Grafting Procedure

1. Prepare the patient psychologically.
   a. Attempt to establish the reasons why the patient seeks surgery.
      (1) The patient's attitudes toward his disfigurement, his motivations for seeking surgery, and his assessment of how his disfigurement has influenced his life and his psychosocial relationships are taken into consideration before surgery is considered.
      (2) Desirable to have unimpaired body image and realistic acceptance of surgical limitations.
      (3) Poor candidate for cosmetic surgery is one who has delusions concerning his deformity, unhealthy psychological responses, and unrealistic expectations of results.
   b. Explain the limitations of the contemplated procedure, the possibility of complications, and the unpredictability of the result (responsibility of the surgeon).
2. Assess for nutritional status.
   a. Give vitamins and increase protein intake as directed—to facilitate healing.
   b. Note hemoglobin level and clotting time—these levels can affect healing process.
3. Prepare donor and recipient sites for surgical excision.
4. Inform the patient of what to expect postoperatively.
   a. Appearance of the wound—redness, distortion, swelling, and unattractive suture lines are characteristics that will change with time.
   b. Pressure dressings, immobilization devices, etc.

Postoperative Nursing Interventions
A. Care of Recipient Site

1. Inspect graft under dressing daily, using a good light—to be sure that edema, blistering, or hematoma has not formed and is not jeopardizing success of graft.
   a. Surgeon carefully teases dressing away from wound—changing dressing may cause avulsion (tearing away) of recent graft around margin of wound.
   b. Surgeon will nick graft to evacuate blood clots.
      (1) Fluid may be rolled out of graft with cotton-tipped applicator or by aspirating with needle and syringe.
      (2) Seromas or hematomas may impede healing.
2. Apply mittens to the patient if he is inadvertently scratching the graft during sleep—to protect graft and donor site from inadvertent scratching.
3. Apply wet dressings to infected graft as directed.
4. Use prophylactic antibiotic therapy for the patient with infected graft. Utilize sensitivity testing to identify organism.
5. Elevate grafted extremity for 7–10 days.
   a. Immobilize part—movement of body areas beneath graft may predispose to loss of graft.
   b. Apply cast or immobilizing bandages to restrict all regional movements of the extremity.
   c. Begin ambulation activities very gradually.

B. Care of the Donor Site

1. The donor site is usually covered with a layer of nonadherent gauze (Xeroform) and held in place with a gauze dressing (Kerlix) without cotton to absorb blood and serum from the wound.
   a. The outer dressings may be removed in 24 hours down to the first layer (Xeroform).
   b. Area may be left exposed after 1st or 2nd postoperative day.
   c. A hair dryer may be employed until dry coagulum is formed.
   d. Xeroform gauze is not disturbed until it separates spontaneously (about 10 days).
2. Prevent area from coming in contact with clothing or bedding—to provide adequate circulation of air to the donor site.

3. Apply wet dressing as directed (silver nitrate solution or acetic acid) if donor site becomes infected.
4. Lubricate donor site with lanolin or cocoa butter after healing—to keep it soft and pliable.
5. Donor sites heal by re-epithelialization; healing should be complete in 2 weeks' time.

Health Education

1. Inform the patient of the changing hues of the graft—to help him accept his situation.
   a. Free graft is at first pale, then pink and red—it then fades and appears similar to neighboring skin.
   b. Full-thickness grafts may remain deeply red for months.
   c. Anticipate skin scaling in full-thickness grafts.
   d. Teach the patient that the graft is vulnerable to sun; avoid overexposure to the sun.
2. Instruct the patient to apply a thin coating of mineral oil or lanolin on wound after 2nd or 3rd week—to remove superficial crusts, moisten the graft, and stimulate circulation to the wound area.

Evaluation

1. Skin-grafted area healing in a desirable manner—absence of inflammatory signs such as puffiness, redness, tenderness
2. Moves body part where graft has taken place with caution to avoid breaking down newly healed tissue
3. Indicates signs that would suggest wound disruption by infection, trauma, extremes in temperature—tells what he should do under these conditions
4. Appears pleased with results and verbalizes this feeling

Dermabrasion

Dermabrasion is surgical planing of the superficial portion of the skin.

Clinical Indications

1. Done on selected patients with facial disfigurements from scars due to acne, trauma, nevi, freckles, chickenpox or smallpox, benign tumors, tattoos.
2. Removal of precancerous lesions (keratosis).
3. To smooth and improve color of transplanted or grafted skin.

Treatment and Nursing Management

Preoperative

1. Wash the part to be treated with pHisoHex for several days before surgery.
2. Administer adequate preoperative sedation as prescribed.

Operative

The epidermis and some superficial dermis are removed, but enough of the dermis is preserved to allow re-epithelialization of the dermabraded areas.
1. The patient is anesthetized.

2. The skin may be sprayed with a topical anesthetic to stabilize and stiffen the skin.
3. The superficial layer of skin is removed by an abrasive machine (Dermabrader) or by sandpapering.
4. Copious saline irrigations are carried out during and after the planing procedure.
5. At the conclusion of surgical planing:
   a. The surgeon may apply a layer of Xeroform or Telfa, followed by fluffed gauze and a pressure dressing.
   b. Another method is to apply a thick paste of thrombin (mixture of thrombin powder and saline) to the abraded areas. This controls bleeding and oozing, which dries to form a protective eschar.

Postoperative

1. Mild oozing may be expected for 24 hours. Crusts then form; are shed in 7–10 days. Skin remains pink for 6–12 weeks.
2. The patient may be discharged from the hospital the day after surgery.
3. Techniques vary—some surgeons prefer to leave bulky dressings in place for several days, others prefer the exposure method.
4. When dressings are removed, the patient experiences a "recent sunburn" experience.
5. Caution the patient to avoid exposure to direct sunlight for 3–4 months—planed area may become darker or lighter than surrounding skin as a result of exposure.

Health Education

1. In the later stages of healing, Neosporin, bacitracin, or hypoallergenic cold cream may be applied; these aid in the removal of coagulum (crusts). Coagulum should never be forcibly removed because this would injure new epithelium and delay healing.
2. Advise the patient to avoid exposure to direct or reflected sunlight.
   Suggest applying an effective sun-screening cream to the affected area; reapply frequently and use for about 3 months postoperatively.
3. Should hyperpigmentation occur, it regresses in 3 to 18 months. Hypopigmentation occurs occasionally but also regresses. Meanwhile, effective cover-up cosmetics are recommended.

Chemical Planing

Chemical planing (chemosurgery, chemabrasion, chemical face-lifting) is the application of a cauterant (caustic material) to the skin for the purpose of superficially destroying epidermis and upper levels of dermis.
1. Phenol combined with other agents and trichloracetic acid are the agents commonly used.
2. *Salabrasion* is a combination of chemical and mechanical action occasionally used for tattoo removal.
3. Chemical planing is painful; meticulous care is required over a period of time. It is not corrective surgery but may supplement it. It should be done by a skilled plastic surgeon.

2: Burns

Etiology and Physiology of Burns

Burns are a form of traumatic injury caused by thermal, electrical, chemical, or radioactive agents.
   Inhalation injury and associated pulmonary compli-
cations are a significant factor in mortality and morbidity from burn injury (50%–60% of fire deaths are secondary to inhalation injury).

Etiology and Incidence

1. Over 2 million injuries and 9,000 deaths occur as a result of fire and burns each year in the US.
2. The home is most frequently the place where burn injuries occur.
3. Smoking, often combined with alcohol intake, is associated with at least half of major fire injuries and deaths.
4. The very young and the elderly are at greatest risk for burn injuries.
5. Infants and toddlers are especially prone to scald injuries.
6. School-age children may incur flame burns as a result of playing with matches and gasoline.
7. Teenage boys have a high incidence of electrical injuries.
8. Women are more commonly injured by burns than are men.

Severity

Severity of burn injury is related to:
1. Depth
2. Extent (percentage of body surface burned)
3. Age (the elderly and the very young have a poorer prognosis)
4. Parts of body burned
5. Past medical history
6. Concomitant injuries and illnesses
7. Presence of inhalation injury

Pathophysiology

A. Burn Injury

Burn injury usually results from energy transfer from a heat source to the body. It can occur by direct conduction or electromagnetic radiation. Many factors alter the response of body tissues to these sources of heat:
1. Conductivity of local tissues—nerves and blood vessels conduct heat with greatest ease, whereas bone is most resistant
2. Peripheral circulation
3. Surface pigmentation; presence of insulating material or clothing
4. Water content of tissue

B. Inhalation Injury

Carbon monoxide poisoning, smoke toxicity, upper airway trauma, and restrictive defects are the four major types of pulmonary injury associated with burn injury.
1. Carbon monoxide (CO) is a colorless, odorless, tasteless, and nonirritating gas produced from incomplete combustion of carbon-containing materials.
2. Affinity of hemoglobin for CO is 200 times greater than for oxygen.
3. Toxicity will depend on concentration of CO in inspired air and the length of time of exposure.
4. Inhalation of hot, dry air ($148.9°C.$ [$300°F.$] or higher) appears not to have much effect on the lower respiratory tract because a sudden closing of the glottis and reflex apnea occur.
5. From fire in a closed space, most particles of soot are filtered through upper airway, but because they may be superheated and may cause direct damage to mucosa.
6. Sulfur dioxide (SO_2) and nitrous oxide (N_2O) (toxic agents) most likely are clinging to soot; in the presence of water, they form corrosive acids and alkalies that are extremely toxic.
7. Toxic fumes from burning plastic are more dangerous than smoke; noxious gases include hydrogen cyanide, hydrochloric acid, sulfuric acid, halogens, and perhaps phosgene.
8. Upper airway obstruction may occur during the first 48 hours postburn due to pharyngeal and laryngeal edema resulting from superficial burn of the upper airway. Edema of the neck may also decrease tracheal patency.
9. Restrictive pulmonary complications can occur because of the tourniquet effect of edema seen with circumferential chest burns. Lung compliance and alveolar gas exchange can also be decreased because of pulmonary edema.

Local Effects of Burns

1. The depth of injury is directly related to the temperature of the burning agent and the duration of contact with body tissue.
2. Below $44°C.$ ($112°F.$), no local damage occurs unless exposure is for a protracted period.
3. Between $44°C.$ ($112°F.$) and $51°C.$ ($124°F.$), the rate of cellular destruction doubles with each 1-degree rise in temperature. Only limited exposure is necessary for tissue destruction.
4. A full-thickness burn may occur in as little as 1 second of exposure at $70°C.$ ($158°F.$).
   a. *Partial-thickness* burn injuries involve the epidermis and upper portions of the dermis. Some of the dermal appendages remain, from which the wound can spontaneously re-epithelialize.
   b. In *full-thickness injuries,* all layers of the skin and sometimes underlying tissues are destroyed. Grafting usually is required to close the wound (see Fig. 13-9).
5. Physiologic reaction
   a. When skin is burned, adjacent intact vessels dilate.
   b. Platelets and leukocytes begin to adhere to the vascular endothelium as an early event in the inflammatory process.
   c. Increased capillary permeability produces wound edema.
   d. An influx of polymorphonuclear leukocytes and monocytes occurs at the injury site.
   e. Eventually, new capillaries, immature fibroblasts, and newly formed collagen fibrils appear within the wound. This supports the regenerating epithelium or forms a granulating tissue bed to accept a skin graft.

Systemic Changes in Major Burn

A. Fluid Shifts

1. In addition to changes in the local burned area, there are alterations and disruptions in the vascular and other systems of the body.
2. The water-vapor barrier for the body is the outermost layer of epidermis. When it is rendered nonfunctioning, severe systemic reactions from fluid losses can occur.
3. Blanching of the skin following burn injury is caused by contraction of skin capillaries; redness occurs when arterioles and capillaries dilate.
4. Fluid volume deficit is directly proportional to extent and depth of burn injury.
5. Capillary permeability increases, permitting fluid and protein to move from vascular to interstitial spaces (edema results). Protein-rich fluid is lost in blebs of the burned tissues, as well as by weeping of second-degree wounds and surface of full-thickness wounds. With reduced vascular volume, the patient will go into shock if untreated.

Assessment of Burn Injury

Extent or Degree	Assessment of Extent	Reparative Process
Superficial partial thickness (first degree)	Pink to red: slight edema, which subsides quickly. Pain may last up to 48 hours; relieved by cooling.	In about 5 days, epidermis peels, heals spontaneously. Itching and pink skin persist for about a week. No scarring.
Deep partial thickness (second degree)	*Superficial:* Pink or red; blisters form (vesicles); weeping, edematous, elastic. Superficial layers of skin are destroyed; wound moist and painful.	Heals spontaneously if it does not become infected within 10 days–2 weeks.
	Deep dermal: Mottled white and red; edematous reddened areas blanch on pressure. May be yellowish but soft and elastic—may or may not be sensitive to touch; sensitive to cold air. Hair does not pull out easily.	Takes several weeks to heal. Scarring may occur.
Full thickness (third degree)	Destruction of epithelial cells—epidermis and dermis destroyed. Reddened areas do not blanch with pressure. Not painful; inelastic; coloration varies from waxy white to brown; leathery devitalized tissue is called *eschar.*	Eschar must be removed. Granulation tissue forms to nearest epithelium from wound margins or support graft. For areas larger than 7–8 cm., grafting is required. Expect scarring and loss of skin function
Fourth degree	Destruction of epithelium, fat, muscles, and bone.	Area requires debridement, formation of granulation tissue, and grafting.

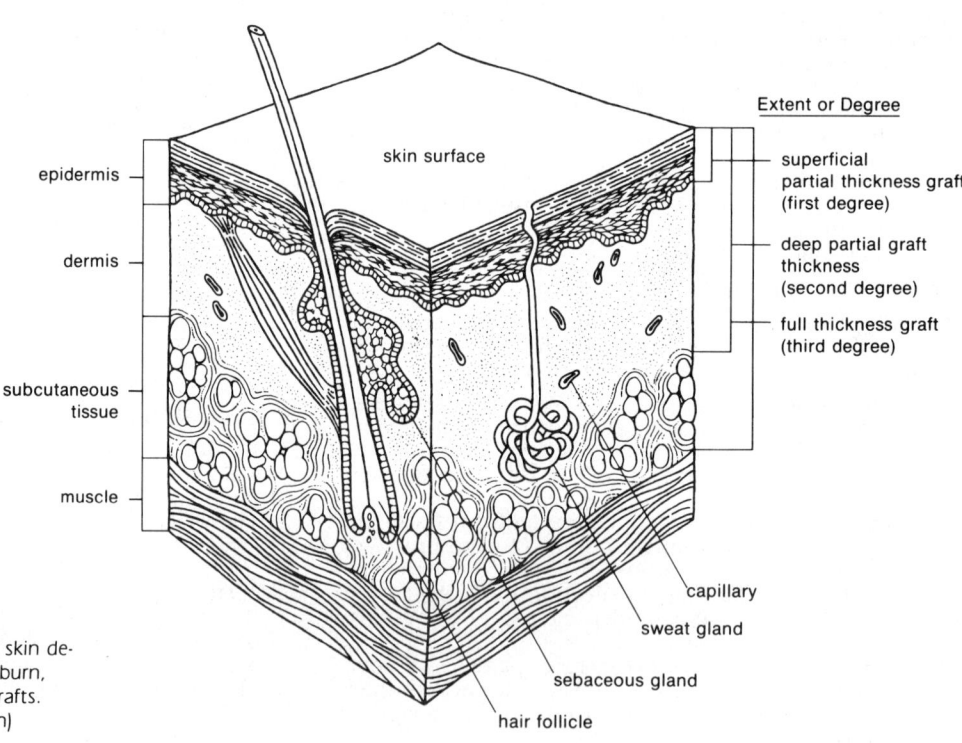

Figure 13-9. Cross section of skin depicting blood supply, depth of burn, and relative thickness of skin grafts. (From The Burn Patient, Ethicon)

6. Vascular fluid loss occurs rapidly and peaks at 12 hours postburn.
7. Capillary permeability returns to near normal in about 48 hours—but protein lost in interstitial spaces remains there for 5 days–2 weeks, before returning to the vascular system.
   a. When fluid mobilizes (moves from interstitial spaces back to vascular compartment) patients with good cardiac and renal function will diurese.
   b. Observe carefully for fluid overload and pulmonary edema; patient requires decreased fluid intake, frequent observation of vital signs, CVP, and urine output.
8. Red cell mass is also diminished, because of thrombosis sludging, and red cell death from thermal injury; as fluid escapes from capillary walls, blood concentrates, and the flow is sluggish—hematocrit rises.
9. Capillary stasis may cause ischemia and even necrosis.
10. The body attempts to compensate for losses of plasma volume.
    a. Constriction of vessels
    b. Withdrawal of fluid from undamaged extracellular space
    c. Patient is thirsty. (Oral fluids are not given until bowel sounds are heard.)

Fluid Loss

Adult	Amount per Hour per Square Meter of Body Surface
Normal unburned individual	15–20 ml.
Average adult with a flame burn of 40% of his body	100 ml.

B. Hemodynamics

1. Lessened circulating blood volume results in decreased cardiac output initially and increased pulse rate.
2. There is a decreased stroke volume, as well as a marked rise in peripheral resistance (due to constriction of arterioles and increased hemo-viscosity).
3. This results in inadequate tissue perfusion, which may in turn cause acidosis, renal failure, and irreversible burn shock.
4. A burn injury often upsets the acid–base balance; therefore, careful monitoring of arterial blood gases, serum electrolytes, and urine volume is needed for proper fluid therapy; this will allow one to replace fluid loss and prevent dilatation and paralytic ileus.

C. Metabolic Demands

1. Immediately following an extensive burn, there is a breakdown of cells (catabolism), resulting in a marked outpouring of potassium and nitrogen.
2. Healing a large surface area requires much energy; glucose is the primary metabolic fuel.
3. Because total body glucose stores are limited and liver and muscle glycogen is exhausted within the first few days postburn, hepatic glucose synthesis increases.

4. When adequately treated, an extensively burned patient will probably increase his weight the first 3–4 days, because of collection of fluid in the interstitial spaces; thereafter, weight loss will be progressive, at the rate of about 1 pound a day in a young adult, for about a month, depending on nutritional support. *Adequate nutritional therapy* can reduce this loss to no more than 5%–10% of preburn body weight before weight stabilizes.
5. In spite of all nutritional support, it is almost impossible to counteract a negative nitrogen balance; the sooner a burn wound is closed, the more rapidly a positive nitrogen balance is reached.
6. The postburn adult may require 4,000–6,000 calories a day; high calories, high protein may be given orally and in some instances by intravenous hyperalimentation or by nasogastric feeding along with normal meals and snacks.

D. Renal Activity

1. Glomerular filtration may be decreased in extensive injury.
2. Without resuscitation or with delay, decreased renal blood flow may lead to high output or oliguric renal failure and decreased creatinine clearance.
3. Hemoglobin and myoglobin, present in the urine of patients with deep muscle damage, often associated with electrical injury, may cause acute tubular necrosis and calls for a greater amount of initial fluid therapy and osmotic diuresis.

E. Pulmonary Changes

1. Hyperventilation and increased oxygen consumption are associated with major burns.
2. The majority of deaths from fire are due to smoke inhalation. See page 631 for discussion of inhalation injury.
3. Fluid resuscitation may cause pulmonary edema, contributing to decreased alveolar exchange.
4. Initial respiratory alkalosis resulting from hyperventilation may change to respiratory acidosis associated with pulmonary insufficiency as a result of major burn trauma.

F. Hematologic Changes

1. Thrombocytopenia, abnormal platelet function, depressed fibrinogen levels, inhibition of fibrinolysis and a deficit in several plasma clotting factors occurs postburn.
2. Anemia results from the direct effect of destruction of erythrocytes due to burn injury, reduced life span of surviving red cells, overt or (more commonly) occult blood loss from duodenal or gastric ulcers, and blood loss during diagnostic and therapeutic procedures.

G. Immunologic Activity

1. The loss of the skin barrier and presence of eschar favor bacterial growth.
2. Granulation tissue, richly vascular, resists bacteria.
3. Abnormal inflammatory response after burn injury causes a decreased delivery of antibodies, white blood cells, and oxygen to the injured area.
4. Hypoxia, acidosis, and thrombosis of vessels in the wound area impair host resistance to pathogenic bacteria.
5. Several major immunoglobulins, complement, and

serum albumin are decreased soon after the burn occurs.

6. Depressed cellular immunity is reflected by lymphocytopenia, impaired delayed skin sensitivity, decreased allograft rejection potential, depletion of thymus-dependent lymphoid tissue, and increased susceptibility to fungi, viruses, and gram-negative organisms.

7. Burn wound sepsis
   a. Following colonization of the burn wound surface by bacteria, subeschar and intrafollicular colonization develop. Intraeschar and subeschar colonization may progress to invasion of subadjacent, nonburned, previously viable tissue.

   b. A bacterial count of 10/gram of tissue as determined by burn wound biopsy indicates burn wound sepsis.

8. Seeding of bacteria from the wound may give rise to systemic septicemia.

H. Gastrointestinal

1. As a result of sympathetic nervous system response to trauma, peristalsis decreases and gastric distention, nausea, vomiting, and paralytic ileus may occur.

2. Ischemia of the gastric mucosa and other etiologic factors put the burn patient at risk for duodenal and gastric ulcer manifested by occult bleeding, and, in some cases, life-threatening hemorrhage.

Methods of Treating Burns

Overview

1. Treatment of burn injury includes hemodynamic stabilization, metabolic support, wound debridement, use of topical antibacterial therapy and biologic dressings, and wound closure.

2. Prevention and treatment of complications, including infection and pulmonary damage and rehabilitation, are also of major importance.

Intravenous Therapy and Metabolic Support

Hemodynamic Stabilization; Prevention of Burn Shock

A. Intravenous Fluid Therapy

1. Immediate intravenous fluid resuscitation is indicated for:
   a. Adults with burns over greater than 15%–20% of body surface area
   b. Children with burns involving more than 10% of body surface area
   c. Patients with electrical injury, the elderly, or anyone with cardiac or pulmonary disease and compromised response to burn injury.

2. The goal is to give sufficient fluid to allow perfusion of vital organs without overhydrating the patient and risking later complications and circulatory overload.

3. Generally, a crystalloid (electrolyte) solution is used initially.
   a. Usually, 2–4 ml./kg./% burn surface area is required in the first 24 hours postinjury.
   b. One-half of the total calculated amount should be given in the first 8 hours postburn, and the other half over the next 16 hours.

4. Use formula as a guide only.
   Patient parameters, including urine output, vital signs, central venous pressure, and hematocrit, are the best indicators of fluid requirements and response.

5. A large-bore central venous catheter is recommended for large-volume replacement.

6. Fluids may be titrated to achieve a urine output of 30–50 ml./hour (0.5 ml./kg./hour) in an adult and 1.0 ml./kg./hour in a child.

7. An indwelling urinary catheter is needed to monitor response to fluid therapy.

8. Weigh the patient on admission and then daily.
9. Elevate extremities.
10. Monitor peripheral pulses.
11. Administer humidified oxygen.

Metabolic Support

1. Initially, keep the patient NPO until bowel sounds return (1–2 days).

2. Reduce metabolic stress by allaying pain, fear, and anxiety and maintaining a warm environment.

3. Nutritional management must be aggressive to combat acute nutritional deficiency and weight loss; a positive nitrogen balance should be the goal throughout the postburn course.

4. When bowel sounds return, administer oral fluids and advance diet as tolerated.

5. Offer more solid food after 2–3 days postburn as tolerance for food improves.
   a. Build up daily caloric intake to match daily caloric expenditure.
   b. Provide 3 gm. protein/kg. body weight; 20% of needed calories in form of fats; remainder in carbohydrates.

6. When caloric requirements cannot be met by enteral feedings, it may be necessary to initiate intravenous hyperalimentation (amino acids, carbohydrates) and fat emulsions.

7. Provide potassium and vitamin supplements.

Wound Care

Wound Cleansing and Debridement

1. Burn wounds must be cleansed initially and usually daily with a mild antibacterial cleansing agent and saline solution or water.
   a. This may be done in the hydrotherapy tub, in the bath tub, or at the bedside.
   b. See chart on Hydrotherapy, page 635.

2. Nonviable tissue (eschar) may be removed through natural, enzymatic, mechanical, and/or surgical debridement.

3. Burn eschar will begin to separate from the underlying viable tissue by a natural process of bacterial growth, which causes a lysis of protein at viable–nonviable tissue interface.

4. Eschar can be removed through daily or twice-daily

Hydrotherapy *Hydrotherapy* ("tubbing" or "tanking") is the bathing of the burn patient in a tub or tank of water to facilitate cleansing of the burn area (removal of dead tissue and topical medications).

Advantages:
1. Topical medications, adherent dressings, and eschar are more easily removed.
2. Provides an opportunity for the patient to practice range-of-motion exercises.
3. Total assessment of the burn area is facilitated; total body cleansing can be achieved.

Disadvantages:
1. Loss of body heat; sodium loss also occurs in tub water.
2. Uncomfortable to the patient and at times painful.
3. Maintenance of IV lines, ventilation care may be difficult during tubbing.

Nursing Plan and Interventions:
1. Describe the procedure to the patient who is experiencing hydrotherapy for the first time.
2. Select the time for future tubbings in collaboration with the patient; administer a pain-control medication, if prescribed, before the treatment so that maximum benefit is realized. Use nursing activities to assist patient with his pain experience.
3. If the patient has an indwelling catheter, drain and plug it, or maintain a closed system to avoid contamination.
4. Isolation and aseptic technique are adhered to rigidly in preparing the patient for hydrotherapy, during hydrotherapy, and then in redressing wounds of the patient following therapy.
5. During hydrotherapy, following cleansing of the wounds, shave and debride as required.
6. Limit therapy to no more than 30 minutes.
7. Never leave the patient unattended in the tub.
8. Respect the patient's feelings and expressions of stress, pain, cold, fatigue.
9. Following treatment, the patient may be weighed before being carefully dressed and returned to his unit.
10. Document significant data, including status of the wound.

dressing changes and use of forceps and scissors at time of wound cleansing.
5. Enzymatic agents applied to the burn wound may be used for more rapid debridement of eschar.
6. In surgical excision, primary or tangential, all non-viable tissue is removed down to a viable base, which is covered with biologic dressings: heterograft, homograft (both temporary), or autograft.

Topical Antimicrobials

Topical medications are used to cover burn areas and to reduce the number of organisms.
1. They are applied directly to the burn area as ointments, creams, or solutions, or they may be incorporated in single-layer dressings that do not stick to the wound but permit drainage (Fig. 13-10).

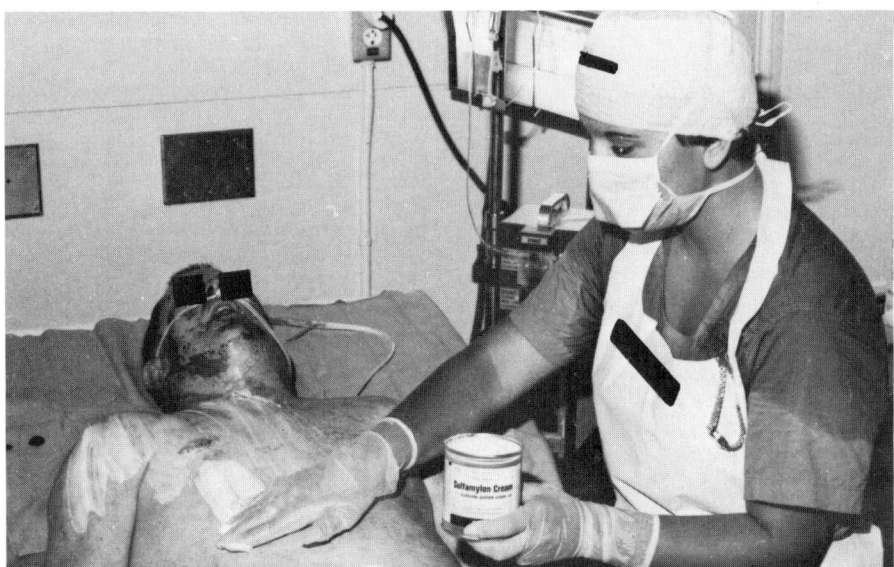

Figure 13-10. Nurse applying a topical agent to protect the patient from infections. The topical agent is applied with sterile gloves. A nasogastric tube is inserted to prevent abdominal distention and for the administration of antacids to prevent Curling's ulcers. (Courtesy of the US Army Institute of Surgical Research, Fort Sam Houston, TX)

2. On top of the fine mesh gauze are placed bulky dry dressings to permit drainage to enter dressing but not come through.
3. Usually, these dressings are held in place by a single layer of stretch bandage or by net tube dressings (Surgifix).
4. When the patient is lying in bed, fluffy absorbent dressings or pads are placed on the bed where the burn area will make contact.
5. Desired characteristics in a topical antimicrobial:
   a. Demonstrate action against gram-negative aerobic intestinal bacteria *Pseudomonas aeruginosa* and *Staphylococcus aureus.*
   b. Ability to diffuse through the wound and penetrate the eschar.
   c. Nontoxic and noninjurious to body tissue.
   d. Inexpensive, pleasant to use, odorless or has pleasant odor; will not stain skin or clothing.
   e. Will not cause resistant strains of pathogenic organisms to develop.
6. To date there is no "ideal" topical antimicrobial.

Silver Sulfadiazine 1% (Silvadene)

In a hydrophilic (readily absorbing moisture) water-soluble cream base.

A. Advantages and Mode of Action

1. Chlorides of the body are not readily precipitated, as with silver nitrate. Therefore, no electrolyte abnormality occurs and no acidosis develops.
2. Applied as a cream with tongue blades or in impregnated gauze.
3. Little pain experienced with application of cream.
4. Viscous dressings are easily and painlessly removed.
5. Silver sulfadiazine is odorless; absorption of silver is minimal, and toxicity is rare.
6. Action occurs by oligodynamic action (active in minute quantities) of silver and is dependent on chloride and other anions in the wound exudate.
7. It utilizes the special antibacterial action of sulfonamide; it is particularly effective against infections due to gram-negative and gram-positive microorganisms and to *Candida albicans.*
8. It can be bactericidal up to 48 hours; however, when wounds are not clean, dressings are changed 2–3 times daily.

B. Disadvantages

1. Some patients develop a skin rash, probably due to sensitivity to sulfonamides.
2. When dressings are removed, they often have a gray-green appearance—this does not necessarily mean a gross infection.
3. Because sulfa drugs are known to increase possibility of kernicterus, silver sulfadiazine should not be used in infants through the first month of life or in pregnant women near term.
4. If topical proteolytic enzymes are used in debriding, silver sulfadiazine may inactivate them.
5. Lately it has been suggested that with protracted use, gram-negative bacilli, particularly *Enterobacteriaceae,* can become highly resistant.
6. Because isolated incidences of leukopenia have occurred following use of Silvadene, it is suggested that blood counts be carefully monitored.

C. Mode of Application

1. Silver sulfadiazine can be applied directly to the burn wound, spread thinly (2–4 mm.), and left exposed; wound should be so covered that no part is visible.

2. Some surgeons prefer that after ointment or cream is applied, it should be covered with a single layer of mesh gauze; others apply ointment to gauze and then apply the medicated gauze to the burn. Cover with stockinette or Surgifix.
3. Reapply as it rubs off (remove all old cream before applying new); if occlusive dressings are used, change every 48 hours.

Cerium Nitrate—Silver Sulfadiazine

Modification of silver sulfadiazine with cerium nitrate enhances its clinical effectiveness.

A. Advantages and Mode of Action

1. Cerium (a lanthanide element) has a broad antibacterial and antifungal effect.
2. Cerium has low toxicity, is readily available and poorly absorbed from open wounds.
3. Gram-negative bacilli are rarely present when wound is treated by cerium nitrate; however, gram-positive bacteria are more effectively treated by silver nitrate or silver sulfadiazine. When combined as cerium nitrate 2.2% with silver sulfadiazine 1% in a cream, results showed promise.
4. Appear to provide more efficient prophylaxis against gram-negative bacteria than other medications did heretofore.

B. Disadvantage

An occasional methemoglobinemia has occurred.

Silver Nitrate (0.5%) Solution

(Silver nitrate is being used less because of its disadvantages)

A. Advantages and Mode of Action

1. Silver nitrate is a bacterostatic chemical and is effective in reducing colonization.
   a. Above 1% concentration produces tissue necrosis.
   b. Below 0.5% solution is ineffective as an antiseptic.
2. Cap, gown, and mask are not required.
3. An effective method for treating large numbers of burns, as during war; is relatively inexpensive.
4. Several layers of 4-ply gauze dressings *must be thoroughly wet every 2–4 hours with silver nitrate solution* to be effective. It is held close to the wound by stretch bandage or net tube dressings.
5. Silver nitrate can be used over grafted areas and donor sites, as well as burn surfaces.
6. Bacterial flora with which it is principally effective are gram-negative.

B. Disadvantages

1. Since silver nitrate solution penetrates only 1–2 mm. of burn eschar, only surface contaminants can be controlled.
2. The wound must be completely free of oil or grease for silver nitrate solution to be effective.
3. Hyponatremia (loss of sodium ions), hypokalemia (loss of potassium ions) and hypochloremia (loss of chlorine ions) may occur. (For this reason, it should not be used for children.)
4. Frequent blood samples are required to determine sodium, potassium, and calcium ion levels.
5. It is necessary to replace electrolytes that are lost.
6. Methemoglobinemia (a modified form of oxyhemoglobin) may be caused by the reduction of nitrates to nitrites, resulting in cyanosis.
7. Silver nitrate turns black in sunlight.

a. Clothes, hands, floor, etc. are stained black.
b. Gloves must be worn by the nurse and assistants.
8. It is a costly agent to use because of the number of dressings required.

Mafenide Acetate (Sulfamylon Acetate)

A. Mode of Action and Advantages

1. Accumulated experience with mafenide acetate suggests that use of this agent probably should be limited to treatment of invasive burn wound sepsis, especially when relatively localized.
2. It will penetrate the eschar (slough) to reduce the number of infecting organisms.
3. In cream form, mafenide acetate diffuses rapidly through the burned skin; this agent must be reapplied at 12-hour intervals.

▶ **NURSING ALERT: Careful monitoring of acid–base balance and pulmonary function is essential.**

B. Disadvantages

1. Causes a burning pain within ½ hour following application.
2. Has a tendency to cake; tubbing permits easy removal.
3. Inhibits carbonic anhydrase activity in the renal tubules and may cause metabolic acidosis.
4. Usually not recommended for patients with pulmonary disease, since they cannot use respiratory mechanism sufficiently to maintain acid–base balance in most instances.
5. Some patients are allergic to sulfa drugs.
6. Never use under an occlusive dressing because it will cause severe maceration and contact dermatitis.
7. Appears to inhibit spontaneous epithelial regeneration.
8. Reports of superinfection have been noted, especially by antibiotic-resistant *Providencia stuartii;* fungal infections have also been reported.

Povidone-Iodine Ointment 10% and Betadine Solution

A. Advantages

1. This agent appears to be effective against a wide variety of gram-negative and gram-positive organisms as well as yeasts, fungi, and viruses.
2. It can be applied as an ointment (similar to Sulfamylon), the solution can be sprayed on, or it can be incorporated into mesh-gauze dressings.
3. The dressings usually are changed every 6 hours, during tubbing; however, it may be more convenient merely to remove outer dressings and rewet inner layer of dressings with Betadine solution.

B. Disadvantages

1. This agent tends to cause crusting—this may be helpful in some situations, a hindrance in others.
2. Materials may be stained, but stain can be removed by laundering immediately.
3. Some stinging is noted by patients, but it soon disappears.
4. Some patients are allergic to iodine preparations. Although povidone-iodine is recommended for moderate and major burns, more documentation is needed to recommend it for extensive burns.

Gentamicin Sulfate (Garamycin Cream) **0.1%**

A. Advantages and Mode of Action

1. Useful against a wide variety of gram-negative and gram-positive organisms (even effective against *Providencia stuartii*).
2. Application and use are similar to Sulfamylon acetate (see opposite column).
3. Ointment spreads easily and tends to become invisible.
4. No pain is associated with this cream.
5. It is useful for brief periods when applied to small areas of invasive infection; monitor blood levels of drug carefully.

B. Disadvantages

1. Since this drug has a tendency to promote the emergence of gentamicin-resistant organisms that may spread to other patients in the burn unit, it is usually reserved for life-threatening situations.
2. Is nephrotoxic—monitor creatinine levels.
3. With long-term use, superinfection with resistant bacterial strains can occur rapidly.

Biologic Dressings

Biologic dressings are used to cover large denuded surfaces of the body. Usually they are split-thickness grafts harvested either from human cadavers or other mammalian donors such as pigs. Human amnion may also be used.

An *allograft* is a graft of skin taken from a person other than the burn victim and applied to a burn wound temporarily (a cadaver is the most common source).

A *xenograft* or *heterograft* is a segment of skin taken from an animal such as a pig or dog. It is useful in preparing debrided area for grafting and is really a biologic dressing (see p. 628 for Skin Grafting).

Donor Criteria

1. Skin color unimportant, since it is only a temporary graft.
2. Donor should be an adult free of infection.

Purpose and Benefits

1. Decreases heat, fluid, and protein losses
2. Reduces bacterial proliferation
3. Closes wound temporarily; enhances production and protection of granulation tissue
4. Protects exposed neurovascular and muscle tissue as well as tendons
5. Reduces pain and facilitates patient comfort
6. Acts as a test-graft to determine when granulating wounds will accept autograft successfully
7. Provides an effective donor-site dressing

Clinical Procedure

1. Porcine skin grafts (xenografts) are the most popular temporary biologic dressings.
2. Devitalized tissue is first removed surgically or enzymatically.
3. Porcine graft is applied directly (epidermis side up) to the denuded area; it may be trimmed to adhere to wound contour. Before applying, it may be dipped in saline solution.
4. Grafts are usually left exposed except when applied to circumferential wounds; stretch gauze (Surgifix) is applied to prevent adherence to and malpositioning by bed sheets.
5. The first xenograft dressing may have to be changed

in 24 hours to permit more intimate adherence to granulating wound bed.
6. Thereafter, grafts may be left in place 2–5 days between changes; inspect wound daily to detect early signs of suppuration.
7. After good xenograft adherence is achieved, the wound is ready for autografting.

Wound Closure

1. Skin grafting is usually required or preferred with full-thickness burns greater than 2 cm. in diameter or in deep partial-thickness wounds.
2. Following gradual eschar removal and development of a base of granulating tissue, or in the presence of viable tissue following excision, grafts of the patient's own skin (autografts) are applied.
3. Sheet grafts or meshed grafts, providing wider expansion from donor sites, may be used.
4. Blood flow is established by the 3rd or 4th day, and by the 7th–10th day postgrafting, vascular continuity and wound closure have been established.
5. Many partial-thickness burn wounds will heal spontaneously within a few weeks, provided they are protected from infection (see the following).

Prevention and Treatment of Complications

Primary causes of morbidity and mortality in burn victims are those related to infection and pulmonary problems.

1. Intravenous antibiotics may be given prophylactically to prevent gram-positive infection.
2. Topical antibacterial agents help to retard the proliferation of pathogenic organisms until wound closure occurs spontaneously or through surgical intervention.
3. Broad-spectrum antibiotics may be necessary to treat systemic gram-positive and gram-negative infections and sometimes fungal infection.
4. Critical diagnostic parameters include observing for signs of burn-wound sepsis, including quantitative and qualitative wound biopsy and observing for signs of systemic septicemia and taking blood for cultures (Table 13-2).

Assessment

Note: As with all trauma victims, a primary and secondary trauma survey, including assessment of airway, breathing, and circulation as well as vital signs are done. Other assessment parameters specific to the burn injury are included in the following:

Assessment for Inhalation Injury

1. If victim was burned in closed area, there should be a high index of suspicion that smoke inhalation has occurred (Fig. 13-11).
2. Evaluate all patients in closed space fires for presence of symptoms of carbon monoxide poisoning: headache, visual changes, confusion, irritability, decreased judgment, nausea, ataxia, collapse.
3. Question the patient about types of things that burned in this room—type of carpet, vinyl articles, synthetics.
4. Observe for upper body burns, erythema or blistering of lips, buccal mucosa, or pharynx, singed nares hair, soot in oropharynx, dark gray or black sputum.
5. Listen for hoarseness and crackles.
6. Obtain blood gases and carboxyhemoglobin levels.
7. Prepare the patient for bronchoscopy to confirm presence of mucosal erythema, hemorrhage, ulceration, edema, carbonaceous particles.
8. Obtain chest x-ray for baseline data.

Signs and Symptoms of Toxicity From Carbon Monoxide

CO Blood Level	Manifestations
0–10%	None Smokers may normally have 10% CO level
10%–20%	Headache, visual disturbance, angina in patients with cardiovascular disease, slowed mental function
20%–40%	Tight feeling in head, rapid fatigue from muscular effort, decreased muscular coordination, confusion, irritability, ataxia, nausea, vomiting, increased pulse rate, decreased blood pressure, arrhythmias
40%–60%	Pulmonary and cardiac dysfunction, collapse, coma, convulsions
Over 60%	Often fatal

Extent of Body Surface Burned

1. Anatomic location—burns affecting hands, feet, face, and perineum require specialized care.
2. Determination is based on the use of tables for this purpose, such as the "rule of nines" chart (Fig. 13-12) and the burn evaluation chart (Fig. 13-13). Calculation of the percent of burn surface area also serves as a guide for fluid therapy.
3. Repeat assessment on 2nd and 3rd day to verify demarcation of burned areas.

Depth of Burn and Triage Criteria

1. See Figure 13-9 (Assessment of Burn Injury).
2. It may be difficult to differentiate between partial-

Table 13-2 Methods for Bacteriological Assessment of the Burn Wound*

Method	Advantage	Disadvantage
Gauze capillarity surface culture	Noninvasive, simple, reproducible, quantitative	Samples surface flora only
Wound-biopsy culture (with histologic examination)	Quantitative, samples cross-section of wound	Most expensive, invasive, unsuitable for frequent multiple cultures
Swab culture	Simplest, noninvasive, painless	False negatives, no quantitation, speculation may be incomplete
Rapid slide technique for quantitation of bacteria in specimens	Quantitates specimen bacterial density within a few hours	None if rapid quantitation desirable

* Modified from Edlich RE, Rodeheaver GT, Spengler M et al. Practical bacteriologic monitoring of the burn victim. Clin Plast Surg 1977; 4:561–569

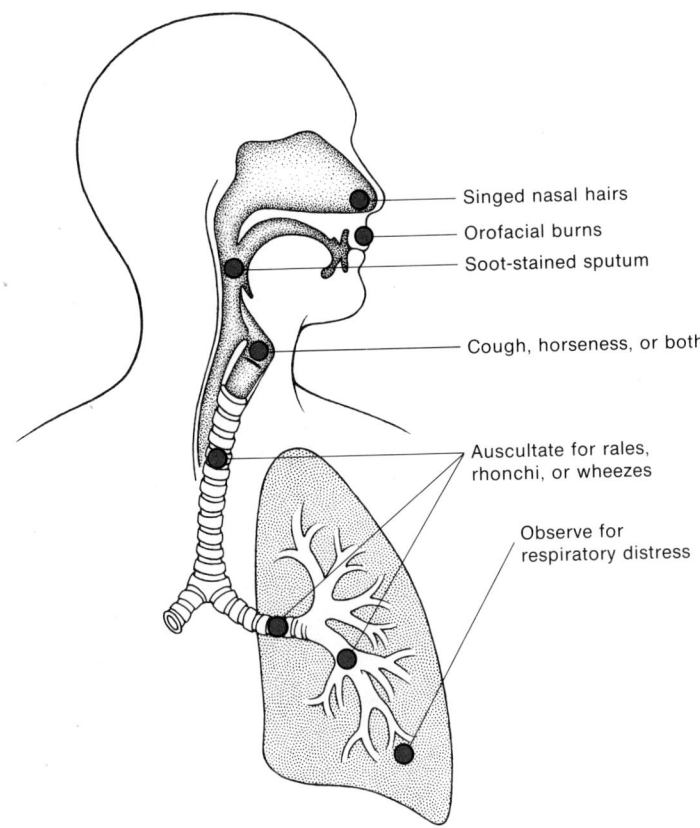

- Singed nasal hairs
- Orofacial burns
- Soot-stained sputum

- Cough, horseness, or both

Auscultate for rales, rhonchi, or wheezes

Observe for respiratory distress

Figure 13-11. In the nursing history, determine whether the victim was in a closed area during the fire and whether he lost consciousness. If any of the above physical findings are noted in addition to the nursing history data, the victim should be taken to a health center for further evaluation. Baseline arterial blood gas measurements (to detect hypoxemia) should be taken immediately upon admission.

and full-thickness wounds initially; if hair can be pulled out easily, there is likelihood of full-thickness injury.

3. Cleanse wounds and reassess daily for first several days.
4. Triage criteria—Table 13-3 presents triage criteria for determining when it is advisable to admit a burn victim to the hospital or transfer to a burn center.

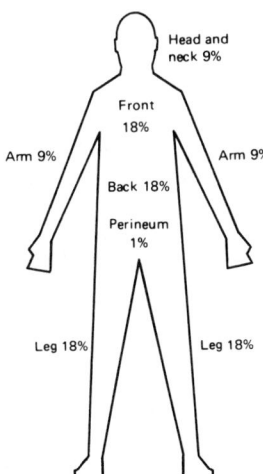

Head and neck 9%

Front 18%

Arm 9%   Arm 9%

Back 18%

Perineum 1%

Leg 18%   Leg 18%

Figure 13-12. "Rule of nine" chart.

Other Factors to Assess

1. Causative agent—hot water, chemical, gasoline, flame, etc.
2. Duration of exposure
3. Circumstances of injury, including whether in closed or open space
4. Age
5. Initial treatment, including first aid
6. Preexisting medical problems—heart disease, diabetes, ulcers, alcoholism, COPD, epilepsy, psychosis
7. Current medications
8. Concomitant injuries (e.g., from fall or explosion)
9. Evidence of inhalation injury (p. 631)
10. Allergies
11. Tetanus immunization status
12. Height and weight
13. Take photograph of burned area (with patient permission) for medical record of extent of burn

Patient Problems/Nursing Diagnoses

1. Impaired gas exchange related to carbon monoxide poisoning, upper airway obstruction, smoke inhalation, and/or edema of lung parenchyma
2. Impaired ventilation related to circumferential edema of chest
3. Decreased cardiac output related to fluid changes and hypovolemic shock
4. Inadequate tissue perfusion related to peripheral burn-wound edema, generalized edema, and circumferential full-thickness burn

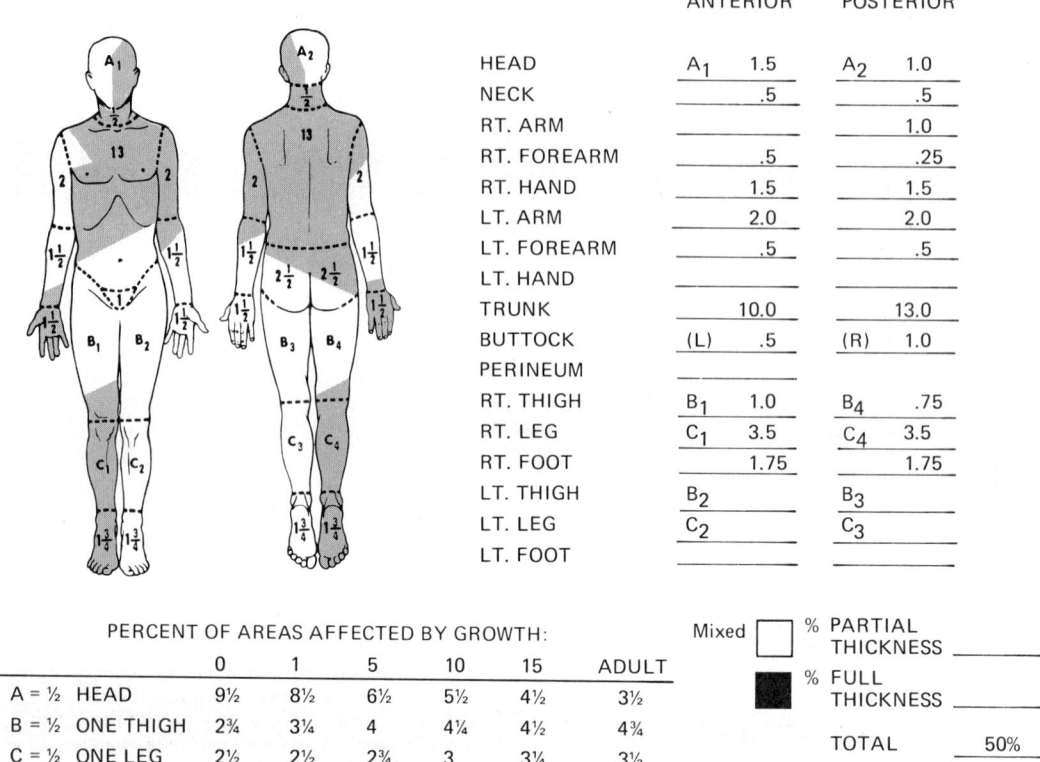

	ANTERIOR		POSTERIOR	
HEAD	A_1	1.5	A_2	1.0
NECK		.5		.5
RT. ARM				1.0
RT. FOREARM		.5		.25
RT. HAND		1.5		1.5
LT. ARM		2.0		2.0
LT. FOREARM		.5		.5
LT. HAND				
TRUNK		10.0		13.0
BUTTOCK	(L)	.5	(R)	1.0
PERINEUM				
RT. THIGH	B_1	1.0	B_4	.75
RT. LEG	C_1	3.5	C_4	3.5
RT. FOOT		1.75		1.75
LT. THIGH	B_2		B_3	
LT. LEG	C_2		C_3	
LT. FOOT				

PERCENT OF AREAS AFFECTED BY GROWTH:

	0	1	5	10	15	ADULT
A = ½ HEAD	9½	8½	6½	5½	4½	3½
B = ½ ONE THIGH	2¾	3¼	4	4¼	4½	4¾
C = ½ ONE LEG	2½	2½	2¾	3	3¼	3½

Mixed ☐ % PARTIAL THICKNESS _____

■ % FULL THICKNESS _____

TOTAL ____50%____

Figure 13-13. Burn evaluation chart—estimation of percent of body burns. (Crozer-Chester Medical Center)

5. Fluid volume deficit related to increased capillary permeability and evaporative fluid loss from burn wound
6. Potential for fluid volume excess related to fluid mobilization 3–5 days postburn
7. Impaired skin integrity related to burn injury and surgical interventions (donor sites)
8. Altered urinary elimination related to indwelling catheter

9. Hypothermia related to loss of skin and microcirculatory regulation
10. Potential for infection related to loss of skin barrier and altered immune response
11. Impaired physical mobility related to edema, pain, skin and joint contractures
12. Ineffective rest–activity pattern related to burn wound discomfort and treatment priorities
13. Activity intolerance related to long periods of immobility
14. Alterations in nutrition—less than body requirements—related to hypermetabolic response to burn injury
15. Alteration in gastric function related to stress response
16. Alteration in comfort (skin tightness, dryness, and itching) related to loss of skin lubricants, wound contraction in healing, altered nerve function
17. Pain related to injured nerves in burn wound
18. Ineffective individual coping related to fear and anxiety
19. Knowledge deficit related to inexperience with burn injury and subsequent related health-care needs
20. Self-care deficit related to functional sequelae of burn injury
21. Disturbance in self-concept related to altered body image
22. Anticipatory/dysfunctional grieving related to biological, psychological, and social losses resulting from burn injury

Table 13-3. Triage Criteria*

Criteria	Consider admission to hospital	Consider transfer to burn center
Burned area 2° and 3°	>15%	>20%
Burned area 3° only	>2%	>10%
Age	<5 or >60	<5 or >60
Airway or inhalation injury	Present	Severe
Electrical injury	Present	Present
Significant associated injury or pre-existing disease	Present	Present
Burns of face, hands, feet, or perineum	Present	Present
Suspected child abuse	Present	Present

* These guidelines should be modified by the judgment and experience of the responsible physician. (Courtesy of the Burn Foundation, Philadelphia, PA)

Planning and Implementation
Nursing Interventions

A. Establishing adequate tissue oxygenation and respiratory function

1. Provide humidified 100% oxygen until carbon monoxide level is known. (CAUTION: Adjust oxygen flow rate for patient with COPD as prescribed.)
2. Assess for signs of hypoxemia and differentiate this from pain.
3. Note history of injury; suspect respiratory injury if burn occurred in an enclosed space.
4. Observe for erythema or blistering of buccal mucosa, singed nares, burns of lips, face, or neck, increasing hoarseness.
5. Monitor respiratory rate, depth, rhythm, cough.
6. Auscultate chest and note breath sounds.
7. Note character and amount of respiratory secretions. Report carbonaceous sputum, tracheal tissue.
8. Observe for signs of inadequate ventilation and include monitoring of arterial blood gases.
9. Provide mechanical ventilation, continuous positive airway pressure or positive end-expiratory pressure if requested.
10. Keep intubation equipment at bedside and be alert for signs of respiratory obstruction.
11. In mild inhalation injury:
    a. Provide humidification of inspired air.
    b. Encourage coughing and deep breathing.
    c. Maintain pulmonary toilet.
12. In moderate to severe inhalation injury:
    a. Initiate more frequent bronchial suctioning.
    b. Monitor vital signs, urinary output, and blood gases.
    c. Judiciously administer bronchodilators.
    d. For additional respiratory problems, it may be necessary to have patient intubated and placed on mechanical ventilation.

B. Maintaining adequate tidal volume and unrestricted chest movement

1. Observe rate and quality of breathing; if progressively more rapid and shallow, notify physician.
2. Assess tidal volume; report decreasing volume to physician.
3. Encourage deep-breathing and incentive spirometry (or hyperinflation with Ambu-bag for artificial airway) hourly.
4. Place patient in semi-Fowler's position to permit maximal chest excursion.
5. Ensure that chest dressings are not constricting.
6. Document and report respiratory changes, including dyspnea, shortness of breath.
7. Prepare the patient for escharotomy and assist physician as indicated.

C. Restoration of normal hemodynamic status with slightly elevated cardiac output

1. Position the patient to increase venous return.
2. Give digoxin per physician's request.
3. Give fluids as prescribed.
4. Monitor vital signs, including apical pulse, respirations, central venous pressure, pulmonary artery pressures, and urine output, at least hourly.
5. Determine cardiac output as requested.
6. Monitor sensorium.
7. Document all observations and particularly note trends in vital-sign changes (Fig. 13-14).

| | VITAL SIGNS | | | | | INTAKE | | | | OUTPUT | | |
	B.P.	V.P.	T.	P.	R.	TYPE I.V. FLUID & MEDICATION ADDED	READING ON BOTTLE	AMOUNT ABSORBED	ORAL	URINE	SP. GR.	GASTRIC & STOOL
7:00 AM												
8:00												
9:00												
10:00												
11:00												
12:00 N												
1:00 PM												
2:00												
8 Hr. Total												
3:00 PM												
4:00												
5:00												
6:00												
7:00												
8:00												
9:00												
10:00												
8 Hr. Total												
11:00 PM												
12:00 M												
1:00 AM												
2:00												
3:00												
4:00												
5:00												
6:00												
8 Hr. Total												
24 Hr. Totals												

I.V. MEDICATION AND FLUID THERAPY

Figure 13-14. Twenty-four-hour flow sheet for monitoring burn patients during initial treatment. (From The Burn Patient, Ethicon)

D. Maintaining adequate circulation to all areas, including extremities

1. Monitor peripheral pulses hourly.
2. Elevate extremities.
3. Remove all constricting jewelry and clothing. Loosen dressings if necessary.
4. Prepare the patient for escharotomy (surgical procedure to relieve constricting effect of edematous circumferential burns and permit adequate circulation to underlying tissues).
5. Monitor signs of adequate tissue perfusion, including renal status; appraise mental reactions and responses.

E. Maintaining fluid and electrolyte balance within a normal range

1. Titrate fluid intake as prescribed.
2. Maintain accurate intake and output records.
3. Weigh the patient daily.
4. Provide potassium replacement after fluid resuscitation is completed.
5. Be alert to signs of fluid overload and congestive heart failure during period of fluid mobilization, 3–5 days postburn.

F. Reestablishing skin integrity

1. Cleanse wounds daily with antibacterial solution or mild soap and water; pat dry. This may be done in the hydrotherapy tank, in the bath tub, or at bedside.
2. Debride eschar using scissors and forceps. Limit time to 20 minutes; stop if there is pain or bleeding.
3. Apply topical bacteriostatic agents as directed (see p. 635).
4. Dress wounds with coarse mesh gauze for new wounds requiring debridement; use fine-mesh gauze on granulating and healing wounds. (Many commercial dressings are available for special wound situations and may be used in consultation with the physician.)
5. For grafted areas, use extreme caution in removing dressings; observe for serous or sanguineous blebs or purulent drainage; report to physician. Redress grafted areas per physician's protocol.
6. Observe all wounds daily and document wound status on the patient's record.
7. Promote healing of donor sites by:
   a. Preventing contamination of donor sites that are clean wounds.
   b. Opening to air for drying 24 hours postoperatively if gauze or impregnated gauze dressing is used.
   c. Following physician's or manufacturer's instructions for care of sites dressed with synthetic materials.
   d. Allowing dressing to peel off spontaneously.
   e. Cleansing healing donor site with mild soap and water once dressings are removed; lubricating site twice daily when healed.

G. Avoiding bladder infection

1. Maintain closed urinary drainage system.
2. Ensure a patent urinary catheter.
3. Observe color, quality, amount of urine every 8 hours.
4. Empty drainage bag at least frequently.
5. Provide catheter-care protocol.
6. Encourage removal of catheter and use of urinal, bedpan, or commode as soon as frequent urine-output determinations are not required.

H. Maintaining normal or only slightly elevated body temperature

1. Be efficient in care; do not expose wounds unnecessarily.
2. Maintain warm ambient temperature.
3. Use heat lamps, radiant warmers, space blankets to keep the patient warm.
4. Provide a dry top layer for wet dressings to reduce evaporative heat loss.
5. Warm wound cleansing and dressing solutions to body temperature.
6. Use dry dressings and blankets in transporting patient outside of hospital.

I. Avoiding wound or systemic infection

1. Wash hands before and after all patient contact with antibacterial cleansing agent.
2. Use barrier garments—isolation gown or plastic apron—for all care requiring contact with the patient or the patient's bed.
3. Be sure nurse covers hair and wears mask when wounds are exposed or when performing a sterile procedure.
4. Use clean examination gloves for all care involving patient contact.
5. Maintain proper concentration of topical antibacterial agents used in wound care.
6. Be alert for reservoirs of infection and sources of cross-contamination in equipment, assignment of personnel, etc.
7. Check history of tetanus immunization and provide passive and/or active range tetanus prophylaxis as prescribed.
8. Change intravenous (IV) lines every 24–48 hours; change IV tubing every 24–48 hours.
9. Administer antibiotics as prescribed and be alert for toxic effects and incompatibilities.
10. Assess wounds daily for local signs of infection—swelling and redness around wound edges, purulent drainage, discoloration, loss of grafts, etc.
11. Be alert for early signs of septicemia, including changes in mentation, tachypnea, and decreased peristalsis, as well as later signs, such as increased pulse, decreased blood pressure, increased or decreased urine output, facial flushing, increased temperature, malaise; report promptly to physician.
12. Promote optimal personal hygiene for the patient, including daily cleansing of unburned areas, meticulous care of teeth and mouth, shampooing of hair every other day, shaving of hair in or near burned areas, meticulous care of IV and urinary catheter sites.
13. Inspect skin carefully for signs of pressure and breakdown.
14. Observe for and report signs of thrombophlebitis or catheter-induced infections.
15. Prevent atelectasis and pneumonia through physical therapy, postural drainage, meticulous pulmonary technique, and, if indicated, tracheostomy care.

J. Enhancing range of joint motion and ability to perform activities of daily living

1. Obtain consultation from physical and occupational therapists.
2. Assist the patient with prescribed exercise regimen, passive and active range-of-motion exercises, ambulation (Fig. 13-15).

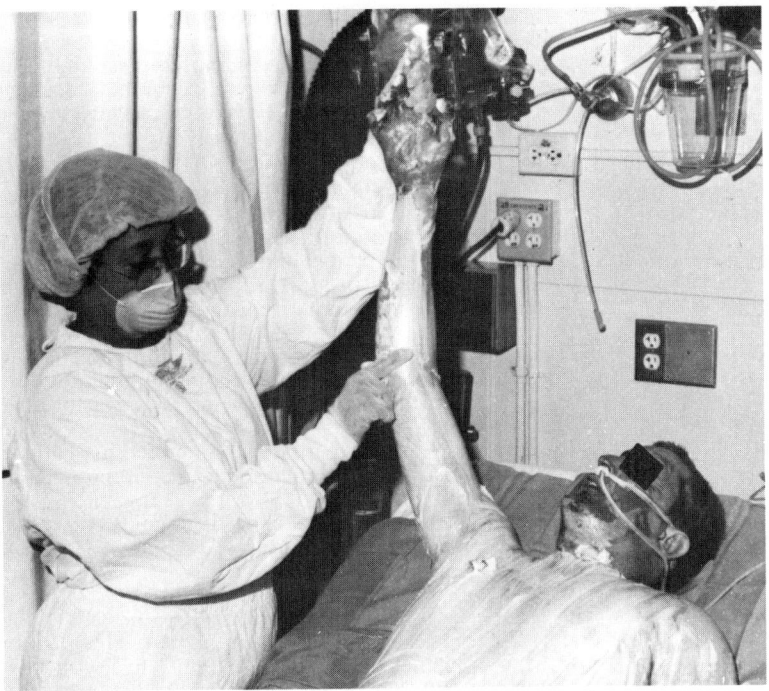

Figure 13-15. The patient is put through full range-of-motion exercises at least twice daily to prevent contractures. (Courtesy of the US Army Institute of Surgical Research, Fort Sam Houston, TX)

3. Maintain splints in proper position as prescribed by occupational therapist; remove splints on regular schedule and observe for signs of skin irritation before reapplying.
4. Position the patient to decrease edema and avoid flexion of burned joints.
5. Coordinate pain management and other care to allow optimal effort during periods of physical exercise.
6. Encourage independence in activities that afford motion of burned joints.
7. Initiate passive and active range-of-motion and breathing exercises during early postburn period.
8. Plan with physical, occupational, and respiratory therapists for a conditioning regimen that gradually increases energy expenditure and tolerance for activity.
9. Coordinate plan for rest, nutritional intake, and pain minimization to maximize physical and mental energy available for increasing activities.
10. Contract with the patient to assist him to meet goals for type and level of activity desired.
11. Act as advocate for the patient's need for rest by coordinating the patient's therapeutic and social activities and prioritizing interventions and visits.
12. Assess preburn sleep pattern and determine what helps the patient achieve relaxation and sleep; implement to the extent possible.
13. Provide sleep medication as prescribed.

K. Augmenting nutritional intake

1. Weigh the patient daily with dressings removed.
2. Obtain consultation from dietitian for calculation of nutritional needs based on age, weight, height, and burn size.
3. Administer vitamins and mineral supplements as prescribed.

4. Minimize metabolic stress by allaying fears, pain, and anxiety and by maintaining a warm environmental temperature.
5. When bowel sounds return, administer oral fluids slowly, so that patient tolerance can be observed. If there are no problems, advance diet to the patient's usual diet, as tolerated.
6. Provide nasogastric tube feedings as prescribed, using caution to prevent aspiration by checking tube placement prior to each feeding and checking amount of gastric aspirate.
7. Administer IV hyperalimentation and fat emulsions prescribed with usual nursing precautions (see p. 429).
8. Keep record of caloric intake.
9. Encourage the patient to feed self.
10. Supplement meals with between-meal high-protein, high-caloric snacks, including appropriate foods brought from home.

L. Resumption of normal gastric motility and function

1. Keep NPO until bowel sounds resume.
2. Assess bowel sounds every 2–4 hours while acutely ill. (Decreased peristalsis may be an early sign of septicemia.)
3. Decompress stomach with nasogastric tube on low intermittent suction until bowel sounds resume.
4. Check amount and pH of gastric drainage or aspirate and report as requested.
5. Administer antacids as prescribed.
6. Heed complaints of nausea while intubated by checking for abdominal distention, tube placement.
7. Provide mouth care every 4 hours while intubated.
8. Test stools for occult bleeding.

M. Reducing pain and enhancing relaxation

1. Assess the patient for pain periodically.
2. Teach relaxation, imagery, breathing exercises, or other techniques to help the patient cope with pain.
3. Determine previous experience with pain, the patient's response and coping mechanisms.
4. Offer analgesics prior to wound care or before particularly painful treatments.
5. Change the patient's position when possible, supporting extremities with pillows.
6. Reduce anxiety by approaches such as sensory-oriented explanations of procedures.

N. Care of concomitant illnesses and injuries

1. Obtain complete nursing data base, including history of events surrounding the burn injury, past health/illness, physical assessment, and laboratory results.
2. Observe for fractures, spinal, head, or internal organ damage in victims of electrical burns, explosions, or history of falling or jumping from a fire.
3. Obtain ophthalmologic consultation if face is burned.
4. Observe for signs and symptoms of chronic illness heightened by stress of burn injury.
5. Implement appropriate independent and dependent nursing activities related to above findings.

O. Promoting an understanding of consequences of burn injury, required therapy, and rationale

1. Develop an individualized teaching plan that includes explanations of pathophysiologic changes resulting from burn injury, both immediate and long-term, treatments, and rationale.
2. Include aspects of care provided by all burn-team members.
3. Periodically "test" the patient's understanding.
4. Provide time for and encouragement of questions related to care, both in hospital and projected home setting.

P. Enhancing coping strategies

1. Assess the patient's coping mechanisms from past history and current behavior.
2. Provide opportunities for the patient to express his thoughts and feelings, and fears and anxieties regarding his injury.
3. Explore with the patient alternative mechanisms for coping with the burn injury and its consequences.
4. Assure the patient of the normality of his responses and the effect that time and healing will likely have on his current concerns.
5. Interpret patient behavior to concerned family and significant others.
6. Respect current coping mechanisms and remove them only when an appropriate alternative can be provided.
7. Support family and friends' communications and visits if this is noted to help the patient.
8. Assess need for psychiatric nursing consultation/medical (psychiatric) intervention.
9. Offer antianxiety medications as prescribed.
10. Assist the patient to adapt to altered body image or life-style resulting from burn injury.
    a. Gather data on the patient's preburn self-image and life-style.
    b. When the patient is ready, encourage him to express his concerns regarding changes in self-image or life-style that may result from burn injury.
    c. Be honest, but positive, in responding to the patient and family.
    d. Positively reinforce appropriate, effective coping mechanisms.
    e. Utilize hospital and community resources, including psychologists, counselors, teachers, clergy, and significant others to provide support for the patient.
11. Assist the patient to resolve grief related to burn injury in an appropriate manner.
    a. Recognize the patient's need to grieve over losses related to the burn injury.
    b. Support the patient and significant others through the grieving process, recognizing that each individual may move through this at a different pace.
    c. Differentiate between normal depression following traumatic injury and depression that requires medication or psychiatric intervention for amelioration.
    d. Arrange for the patient to talk with other patients who have had a similar injury and are progressing satisfactorily.
    e. Help the patient set short-term goals and reflect on progress in small steps.

Health Education

Health education is closely related to the rehabilitation of the burn patient as he prepares to return to a productive place in society. Functional and cosmetic reconstruction is accomplished, and the patient attempts to integrate a new self-concept into social realities. Broadly viewed, health education focuses on biological, psychological, and social parameters.

1. Assist the patient in transition from dependence on the health team to independence by helping him develop methods of communicating his needs and functioning abilities to others.
2. Guide the patient in thinking positively about himself. Promote ability to redirect others' attention from the scarred body to the self within.
3. Demonstrate and explain wound care procedures to be continued after discharge:
   a. Wash hands.
   b. Cleanse small open wounds with mild soap in tub or shower.
   c. Rinse well with tap water.
   d. Pat dry with clean towel.
   e. Apply prescribed topical agent and/or dressing.
4. Observe for local signs of wound infection:
   a. Increased redness of normal skin around burn area
   b. Increased cloudy yellow pus or drainage
   c. Increased pain, foul odor in burn area
   d. Elevated body temperature
5. Instruct the patient in measures to lubricate and enhance comfort of healing skin:
   a. Cleanse skin with mild soap and rinse well daily.
   b. Apply lubricant such as cocoa butter or Nivea to healed areas twice daily.
   c. Wear clean, white underwear and clothing free of irritating dyes.
   d. Take antipruritics as prescribed.
   e. Stay in a cool environment if itching occurs.
   f. Protect skin from further trauma, including sunburn (use sunblock containing PABA).
6. Develop a schedule to incorporate exercise regimen as prescribed by physical therapist:

a. Assist the patient and family to practice exercises.
b. Suggest scheduling exercises immediately after wound cleansing and application of topical agent, since skin may be more pliable and less sensitive to stretching then.

7. Instruct the patient in use and care of splints and pressure garments:
    a. Cleanse with mild soap and rinse well daily.
    b. Keep away from heat; dry garment by laying it flat on towels.
    c. Wear garment on schedule prescribed by therapist.
    d. Pad open wounds with light dressing under splints or pressure garments.
    e. Observe for signs of skin breakdown.
    f. Wear/bring splints and pressure garments to follow-up visits to be checked for proper fit.

8. Acquaint patient and family with resources, including support groups for recovering burn victims, family group meetings in burn center, community resources as required.

9. Review with the patient and family common emotional responses during convalescence (depression, withdrawal, grieving, dreaming, anxiety, guilt, excessive sensitivity, emotional lability, insomnia, fear of future) and discuss usual temporary nature of these and effective coping mechanisms.

10. Arrange for return visit for follow-up care and home health-care services, as needed in interim.

11. Provide written instructions regarding all care required on discharge.

Evaluation

Expected Outcomes

1. Achieves normal respiratory function (e.g., CO < 10, ABGs within normal limits, respiratory rate 12–20)
2. Achieves normal cardiovascular function (e.g., pulse 60–100, peripheral tissues adequately perfused)
3. Maintains fluid and electrolyte parameters in healthy balance
4. Demonstrates adequate wound healing—small open wound areas are clean
5. Skin is soft, comfortable; scars flat
6. Has normal urinary elimination
7. Demonstrates normal body temperature
8. Is free of pathogenic organisms
9. Achieves normal range of motion and can perform activities of daily living with necessary endurance
10. Achieves positive nitrogen balance; regains optimal weight
11. Regains normal integrity and function of gastrointestinal system
12. Reports minimal pain in burn area and joints; explains use of analgesics and other pain-reduction techniques
13. Uses appropriate coping mechanisms to deal with stress of burn injury and its sequelae
14. Adapts to losses and alterations in body image and to life-style resulting from the burn injury
15. Explains rationale of required self-care related to burn injury. Demonstrates ability to carry out wound and skin care, exercises, splint and pressure garment application

Bibliography

Dermatologic Conditions

Books

General

Adams RM. Occupational Skin Disease. New York, Grune & Stratton, 1983

Arndt KA. Manual of Dermatologic Therapeutics: With Essentials of Diagnosis, 3rd ed. Boston, Little, Brown & Co, 1983

Binnick SA. Skin Diseases—Diagnosis and Management in Clinical Practice. Menlo Park, CA, Addison-Wesley, 1982

Domonkos AN, Arnold HL and Odom RB. Andrews' Diseases of the Skin. Philadelphia, WB Saunders, 1982

Emmett AJJ and O'Rourke MGE (eds). Malignant Skin Tumours. New York, Churchill Livingstone, 1982

Epstein E. Common Skin Disorders: A Physician's Illustrated Manual, With Patient Instruction Sheets, 2nd ed. Oradell, NJ, Medical Economics Books, 1983

Epstein E. Controversies in Dermatology. Philadelphia, WB Saunders, 1984

Epstein E and Epstein E Jr (eds). Skin Surgery, 5th ed. Springfield, IL, Charles C Thomas, 1982

Fitzpatrick TB, Polano MK and Suurmond D. Color Atlas and Synopsis of Clinical Dermatology. New York, McGraw-Hill, 1983

Maddin S (ed). Current Dermatologic Therapy. Philadelphia, WB Saunders, 1982

Maiback HI and Gellin GA (eds). Occupational and Industrial Dermatology. Chicago, Year Book Medical Publishers, 1982

Marks R. Psoriasis. New York, Arco, 1981

Masters R. Psyche and skin. In Soter NA and Baden HP. Pathophysiology of Dermatologic Diseases, pp. 441–453. New York, McGraw-Hill, 1984

Nasemann T, Sauerbrey W and Burgdorf WHC. Fundamentals of Dermatology. New York, Springer-Verlag, 1983

Parish LC, Nutting WB and Schwartzman RM (eds). Cutaneous Infestations of Man and Animal. New York, Praeger, 1983

Pilch YH. Malignant melanoma. In Pilch YH (ed). Surgical Oncology, pp. 861–887. New York, McGraw-Hill, 1984

Robinson TWE and Heath RB. Virus Diseases and the Skin. New York, Churchill Livingstone, 1983

Vasarinsh P. Clinical Dermatology. Boston, Butterworths, 1982

Plastic and Reconstructive Surgery

Chang WHI. Fundamentals of Plastic and Reconstructive Surgery. Baltimore. Williams & Wilkins 1980

Articles

Assessment and Treatment

Anders JE. Topicals. RN 1982 Sept; 45(9):32–42

Delancy VL and North C. Skin assessment. Top Clin Nurs 1983 Jul; 5(2):5–10

Dotz W and Berman B. The facts about treatment of dry skin. Geriatrics 1983 Sept; 38(9):93–100

Engels WD. Dermatologic disorders. Psychosomatics 1982 Dec; 23(12): 1209–1211, 1214–1219

Hughes JE et al. Psychiatric symptoms in dermatology patients. Br J Psychiatry 1983 Jul; 143:51–54

Kannangara DW, Smith B and Cohen K. Exfoliative dermatitis during cefoxitin therapy. Arch Intern Med 1982 May; 142(5):1031–1032

McKay M. Topical dermatologic therapy. Primary Care 1983 Sept; 10(3):513–524

McLaurin CI. Unusual patterns of common dermatoses in blacks. Cutis 1983 Oct; 32(4):352–355, 358–360

Malkiewicz J. The integumentary system. RN 1981 Dec; 44(12):54–60

Solomon AR et al. Tzanck smear in the diagnosis of cutaneous herpes simplex. JAMA 1984 Feb 31; 251(5): 633–635

Weston WL. Topical corticosteroids in dermatologic disorders. Hosp Pract 1984 Jan; 19(1):159–178

Acne

Eady EA, Holland KT and Cunliffe WJ. The use of antibiotics in acne therapy: Oral or topical administration? J Antimicrob Chemother 1982 Aug; 10(2):89–115

Hansen RC. Use and abuse of Accutane. Ariz Med 1983 Jul; 40(7):459–462

Oral medication for cystic acne. FDA Drug Bull 1982 Aug; 12(2):12–13

Pochi PE. Hormones, retinoids, and acne. N Engl J Med 1983 Apr 28; 308(17):1024–1025

Shalita AR et al. Isotretinoin treatment of acne and related disorders: An update. J Am Acad Dermatol 1983 Oct; 9(4):629–638

Shalita AR (ed). Symposium on acne. Dermatologic Clinics 1983 July; 1(3): entire volume

Update on isotretinoin (Accutane) for acne. Med Lett Drugs Ther 1983 Nov 25; 25(649):105–106

Ward A et al. Etretinate. A review of its pharmacological properties and therapeutic efficacy in psoriasis and other skin disorders. Drugs 1983 Jul; 26(1):9–43

Infections/Infestations

Adler MW. Genital infestations. Br Med J (Clin Res) 1984 Jan 28; 288(6413): 311–313

Becker LE and Tschen E. Common bacterial infections of the skin. Primary Care 1983 Sept; 10(3):397–409

Burkhart CG. Scabies—an epidemiologic reassessment. Ann Intern Med 1983 Apr; 98(4):498–503

Couch JM et al. Diagnosing and treating *Phthirus pubis* palpebrarum. Surv Ophthalmol 1982 Jan–Feb; 26(4):219–225

East M, Henderson JT and Jevons S. Ticonazole in the treatment of fungal infections of skin. Dermatologica 1983; 166(Suppl 1):20–33

Fragola LA and Watson PE. Common groin eruptions: Diagnosis and treatment. Postgrad Med 1981 May; 69(5):159–172

Hazen PG. Use of ketoconazole in the management of common cutaneous mycoses. Ohio State Med J 1984 Jan; 80(1):63–65

Jolly HW et al. A multicenter double-blind evaluation of ketoconazole in the treatment of dermatomycoses. Cutis 1983 Feb; 31(2):208–210, 212–213

Jones HE. Therapy of superficial fungal infection. Med Clin North Am 1982 Jul; 66(4):873–893

Malathion for treatment of head lice. Med Lett Drugs Ther 1983 Mar 18; 25(631):30–31

Orkin M and Maibach HI. Current views of scabies and *Pediculosis pubis*. Cutis 1984 Jan; 33(1):85–88, 90, 92

Ortiz JE, Horn MS and Peterson HD. Toxic epidermal necrolysis—case report and review of the literature. Ann Plast Surg 1982 Sep; 9(3):249–253

Parish LC, Witkowski JA and Kucirka SA. Lindane resistance and *Pediculosis capitis*. Int J Dermatol 1983 Dec; 22(10):572–574

Shelley WB and Shelley ED. Common causes of treatment failure in scabies. IMJ 1983 Feb; 163(2):112–114

Taplin D. Malathion for treatment of *Pediculus humanus* var capitis infestation. JAMA 1982 Jun 11; 247(22):3103–3105

Tschen E. What treatment for skin infestations in the elderly? Geriatrics 1982 Aug; 37(8):38–44

Witkowski JA and Parish LC. Bacterial skin infections. Postgrad Med 1982 Oct; 72(4):166–168, 171–173, 176–178

Herpes Zoster

Adams HG. Herpes: A problem in older age groups. Geriatrics 1983 Jul; 38(7): 91–100

Balfour HH Jr et al. Acyclovir halts progression of herpes zoster in immunocompromised patients. N Engl J Med 1983 Jun 16; 308(24):1448–1453

Bean B, Aeppli D and Balfour HH. Acyclovir in shingles. J Antimicrob Chemother 1983 Sept; 12(Suppl B): 123–127

Brigden D, Keeney RE and King DH. The present and future for acyclovir. J Antimicrob Chemother 1983 Sept; 12(Suppl B):195–199

Hirsch MS and Schooley RT. Drug therapy. Treatment of herpesvirus infections. N Engl J Med 1983 Oct 20; 309(16):963–970

Truesdell ML. The scourge of the aged: Herpes zoster. Gerontol Nurs 1983 Apr; 9(4):221–223, 226, 245

Weller TH. Varicella and herpes zoster. Changing concepts of the natural history, control, and importance of a not-so-benign virus. N Engl J Med 1983 Dec 1; 309(22):1362–1368

Yardley DE, Schwartz RA and Adams HG. Herpes zoster. Am Fam Physician 1983 Dec; 28(6):138–144

Psoriasis

Boer J et al. Comparison of phototherapy (UV-B) and photochemotherapy (PUVA) for clearing and maintenance therapy of psoriasis. Arch Dermatol 1984 Jan; 120(1):52–57

Ingraham DM et al. Long-term and short-term histopathologic changes in the skin after PUVA therapy. Cleve Clin Q 1983 Summer; 50(2):133–139

Langnor A, Wolska H and Hebborn P. Treatment of psoriasis of the scalp with coal tar gel and shampoo preparations. Cutis 1983 Sept; 32(3): 290–291, 295–296

Pemphigus

Ahmed AR and Moy R. Death in pemphigus. J Am Acad Dermatol 1982 Aug; 7(2):221–228

Levene GM. The treatment of pemphigus and pemphigoid. Clin Exp Dermatol 1982 Nov; 7(6):643–652

Lever WF and Schaumburg-Lever G. Treatment of pemphigus vulgaris. Arch Dermatol 1984 Jan; 120(1):44–47

Lorenzen KM. Pemphigus: A review of current concepts. SD J Med 1983 Nov; 36(11):19–25

Patel HP et al. Bullous pemphigoid and pemphigus vulgaris. Ann Allerg 1983 Mar; 50(3):144–150

Skin Cancer/Malignant Melanoma

Adam YG and Efron G. Cutaneous malignant melanoma: Current views on pathogenesis, diagnosis, and surgical management. Surgery 1983 Apr; 93(4):481–494

Aigner K et al. Regional perfusion with cis-platinum and dacarbazine. Recent Results Cancer Res 1983; 86:239–245

Anders JE and Leach EE. Sun versus skin. Am J Nurs 1983 Jul; 83(7):1015–1020

Consensus Conference. Precursors to malignant melanoma. JAMA 1984 Apr 13; 251(14):1864–1866

Epstein JH. Photocarcinogenesis, skin cancer, and aging. J Am Acad Dermatol 1983 Oct; 9(4):487–502

Fitzpatrick TB. Early recognition of primary cutaneous melanoma. Hosp Pract 1982 Jan; 17(1):67–75

Fraser MC. The role of the nurse in the prevention and early detection of malignant melanoma. Cancer Nurs 1982 Oct; 5(5):351–360

Gussack GS. Cutaneous melanoma of the head and neck: A review of 399 cases. Arch Otolaryngol 1983 Dec; 109(12):803–808

Robinson JK. Mohs' surgery for skin cancer. Am J Nurs 1982 Feb; 82(2): 282–283

Roses DF, Harris MN and Ackerman AB. Diagnosis and management of cutaneous malignant melanoma. Maj Prob Clin Surg 1983; 27:entire issue

Schulmeister L. Screening for skin cancer: A necessary part of your assessment routine. Nursing '81 1981 Oct; 11(10):42–45

Swanson NA. Basal cell carcinoma. Primary Care 1983 Sept; 10(3):443–458

Swanson NA. Mohs surgery. Arch Dermatol 1983 Sept; 119(9):761–773

Thomas MR et al. Treatment of advanced malignant melanoma with high-dose chemotherapy and autologous bone marrow transplantation. Preliminary results—Phase I study. Am J Clin Oncol 1982 Dec; 5(6):611–622

Warshaver DM and Steinbaugh JR. Sunlight and protection of the skin. Am Fam Physician 1983 Jun; 27(6): 109–115

Young KJ and Longman AJ. Quality of life and persons with melanoma: A pilot study. Cancer Nurs 1983 Jun; 6(3):219

Plastic and Reconstructive Surgery

Atnip RG and Burke J. Skin coverage. Curr Prob Surg 1983 Oct; 20(10):623–683

Fanoris N. Correction of thin lips: "Lip lift." Plast Reconstr Surg 1984 July; 74(1):33–41

Fitzsimmons VM. The aging integument: A sensitive and complex system. Top Clin Nurs 1983 July; 5(2):32–38

Hutton B and Hutton J. Living with a facial prosthesis. Am J Nurs 1984 Jan; 84(1):50–52

McCray MK and Roenigk HH. Cosmetic correction of alopecia. Am Fam Physician 1983 Oct; 28(4):207–214

Sheretz EF and Flowers FP. Rational use of topical corticosteroids. Am Fam Physician 1984 Jan; 29(1):262–266

Stucker FJ Jr, Shockley WW and Byarly RC Jr. Modifications of facial flaps.

Surg Clin North Am 1983 May; 16(2): 457–465

Yarrington CT Jr and Larrabee WF Jr. Reconstruction following lip resection. Surg Clin North Am 1983 May; 16(2):407–408

Agencies

American Cancer Society
777 Third Avenue
New York, NY 10017

National Psoriasis Foundation
6415 S.W. Canyon Court
Portland, OR 97221

Skin Cancer Foundation
575 Park Avenue, South
New York, NY 10016

National Institute of Arthritis, Diabetes, and Digestive and Kidney Diseases
Arthritis, Musculoskeletal, and Skin Diseases Division
National Institutes of Health
Bethesda, MD 20205

Burns

Books

Artz CP, Moncrief JA and Pruitt BA. Burns: A Team Approach. Philadelphia, WB Saunders, 1979

Bernstein N. Emotional Care of the Burned and Facially Disfigured. Boston, Little, Brown & Co, 1976

Bowden ML, Jones CA and Feller I. Psycho-Social Aspects of Burns: A Review of the Literature. Ann Arbor, National Institute of Burn Medicine, 1979

A Curriculum for Basic Burn Nursing Practice. Rochester: University of Rochester School of Nursing, vol. 1. Health Services Administration Contract No. 240-77-0162. US Department of Health and Human Services, 1980

Feller I and Grabb VC. Reconstruction and Rehabilitation of the Burned Patient. Ann Arbor, National Institute for Burn Medicine, 1981

Hummel RP (ed). Clinical Burn Therapy: A Management and Prevention Guide, Boston, John Wright, 1982

Johnson CL, O'Shaughnessey EJ and Ostergren G. Burn Management. New York, Raven Press, 1981

MacMillan BG. The Surgical and Medical Support of Burn Patients. Boston, John Wright, 1982

Nicosia JE and Petro JA (eds). Manual of Burn Care. New York, Raven Press, 1983

Salisbury RE, Newman NM and Dingeldein GP. Manual of Burn Therapeutics. Boston, Little, Brown & Co, 1983

Wachtel TL, Frank HA and Kahn V (eds). Current Topics in Burn Care. Rockville, MD, Aspen Systems, 1983

Articles

Bartlett RH. Skin substitutes. J Trauma 1981 Aug; 21(8 Suppl):731–732

Baxter CR. Controversies in the resuscitation of burn shock. Curr Concepts Trauma Care 1982; 5(1)

Bayley EW and Moore DA. Group meetings for families of burn victims. Top Clin Nurs 1980 July; 2(2):67–76

Brandenburg J. Inhalation injury: Carbon monoxide poisoning. Am J Nurs 1980 Jan; 80(1):98–100

Budassi SA. Smoke inhalation. J Emerg Nurs 1982 May/June; 8(3):156–157

Burke JF. Early excision of the burn wound. J Trauma 1981 Aug; 21(8 Suppl):726–727

Conrad FL. Tips for treating corrosive burns. Nursing '83 1983 Feb; 13(2):55–57

Cuono CB. Early management of severe thermal injury. Surg Clin North Am 1980; 60(5):1021–1033

DeCrosta T. What burn centers want you to know. Nursing Life 1984 Jan/Feb; 4(1):45–49

Gaston SF and Schumann LL. Inhalation injury: Smoke inhalation. Am J Nurs 1980 Jan; 80(1):94–97

Gray DT et al. Early surgical excision versus conventional therapy in patients with 20 to 40 per cent burns. Am J Surg 1982 July; 144(1):76–80

Hartford CE. The bequests of Moncrief and Moyer: An appraisal of topical therapy of burns. J Trauma 1981 Oct; 21(10):827–834

Helm PA, Kevorkian CG and Lushbaugh M. Burn injury: Rehabilitation management in 1982. Arch Phys Med Rehab 1982 Jan; 63(1):6–16

Kenner C and Manning S. Emergency care of the burned patient. Crit Care Update 1980 Oct; 7(10):24

Knudson-Cooper MS. Emotional care of the hospitalized burned child. J Burn Care Rehab 1982 Mar/Apr; 3(2):109–117

Kudsk KA, Stone JM and Sheldon GF. Nutrition in trauma and burns. Surg Clin North Am 1982 Jan; 62(1):183–92

Lushbaugh MA. Critical care of the child with burns. Nurs Clin North Am 1981 Dec; 16(4):635–646

Luterman A, Kraft E and Bookless S. Biologic Dressings: An appraisal of current practices. J Burn Care Rehab 1980 Sept/Oct; 1(1):18–22

Marvin JA. Planning home care for burn patients. Nursing '83 1983 Aug; 13(8):65–67

Marvin JA and Einfeldt LE. Infection control for the burn patient. Nurs Clin North Am 1980 Dec; 15(4):833–842

Moylan, JA. Inhalation injury. J Burn Care Rehab 1982 Jan/Feb; 3(1):51–53

Moylan JA. Outpatient treatment of burns. Postgrad Med 1983 Mar; 73(3):235–242

Ninneman JL. Immunologic defenses against infection: Alterations following thermal injuries. J Burn Care Rehab 1982 Nov/Dec; 3(6):355–366

Oss SV. Emergency burn care. RN 1982 Oct; 42(10):44–49

Perry S, Heidrich G and Ramos E. Assessment of pain by burn patients. J Burn Care Rehab 1981 Nov/Dec; 2(6):322–326

Philbin P and Marvin JA. Management of the pediatric patient with a major burn. J Burn Care Rehab 1982 Mar/Apr; 3(2):118–125

Second Conference on Supportive Therapy in Burn Care. J Trauma (Suppl) 1981 Aug; 21(8):entire issue

Severely burned patients: Anticipating their emotional needs. Nursing '80 1980 Sept; 10(9):47–50

Stoddard FJ. Coping with pain: A developmental approach to treatment of burned children. Am J Psychiatry 1982 Jun; 139(6):736–740

Surveyor JA and Halpern J. Age-related burn injuries and their prevention. Pediatric Nurs 1981 May; 7(5):29–34

Surveyor JA. Smoke inhalation injuries. Heart Lung 1980 Sept/Oct; 9(5):823–832

Surveyor JA and Clougherty DM. Burn scars: Fighting the effects. Am J Nurs 1983 May; 83(5):746–751

Wooldridge-King M and Surveyor JA. Skin grafting for full-thickness burn injury. Am J Nurs 1980 Nov; 80(11):200–204

Wooldridge-King M. Nursing consideration of the burn patient during the emergent period. Heart Lung 1982 July/Aug; 11(4):353–361

Connective Tissue Disorders

Rheumatoid Arthritis

Rheumatoid arthritis is a chronic, systemic, progressive disease of unknown cause, characterized most prominently by recurrent inflammation involving the synovium or lining of the joints, leading to destructive changes in the joints. Any or every organ or system may be involved by the connective tissue disease, which occurs most often in women (3:1).

Pathophysiology Underlying Joint Destruction

Inflammation of joint (synovitis) → synovial effusion → granulation tissue covering articular cartilage (pannus) → joint capsular and subchondral bone destruction → pain → loss of mobility of joint → muscular weakness about the joint → damage to tendons and ligaments → joint instability and deformity → joint malfunction and disuse → muscular atrophy and contracture deformity.

Assessment
Clinical Manifestations

1. Inflammation of the synovial joints characterized by pain, stiffness, swelling, heat, redness, and limitation of function and deformity
2. Subcutaneous nodules over bony prominences, bursae, and tendon sheaths; may appear in myocardium, aorta, and lung
3. Constitutional symptoms (may accompany or precede arthropathy):
   a. Fatigue
   b. Anemia
   c. Weight loss
   d. Fever
4. Late or severe stage symptoms:
   a. Osteoporosis
   b. Vasculitis (blood vessel inflammation)
   c. Sjögren's syndrome (dry eyes and mouth)

Diagnostic Evaluation

1. History (onset of symptoms, areas and patterns of involvement, associated constitutional symptoms) and physical examination
2. Laboratory tests
   a. Complete blood tests—most patients have mild anemia
   b. Erythrocyte sedimentation rate—elevated during periods of active arthritis
   c. Tests for rheumatoid factor in the serum—positive in 70%–80% of patients with rheumatoid arthritis (Rose and Latex)
   d. Documentation of presence of antinuclear antibodies—positive fluorescent antinuclear antibody test (FANA)
   e. Serum protein electrophoresis—increased globulins (gamma and alpha globulins); decreased albumin
3. Roentgenograms of involved joints—to determine extent, rate of progress, and structural changes within bones; reveals swelling of soft tissue, erosion of bone at articular margins, narrowing of joint space
4. Thermography—pinpoints areas of inflammation and increased metabolic activity in the body by pictorially recording (mapping) the heat emitted from the skin over the affected areas
5. Synovial fluid analysis—to distinguish between inflammatory, traumatic, or degenerative arthritis
6. Arthroscopy—endoscopic examination of knee joint; allows observation of synovial lining, articular cartilage, and minisci; permits examination of knee during passive movements and allows biopsy under direct vision; detects pathology earlier than other methods

Patient Problems/Nursing Diagnoses

1. Pain and stiffness related to joint and muscle inflammation, degeneration, and deformity
2. Impaired physical mobility related to pain, deformity, and muscle atrophy
3. Self-care deficits (feeding, bathing/hygiene, dressing/grooming, toileting) related to fatigue, pain, and deformity
4. Weight loss, anorexia related to reduced nutritional intake
5. Disturbance in self-concept and alteration in body image related to deformity and loss of independence

Planning and Implementation
Nursing Interventions

A. Relief of Pain and Discomfort

1. Regular rest at specified periods is needed to relieve pain and control fatigue—arthritis affects the whole body.
   a. Complete bed rest for patients with active widespread inflammatory disease.
   b. Have the patient rest in a recumbent position (one pillow under head) on a firm mattress—to take the weight off the joints.
   c. Advise the patient to establish one or more daytime rest periods of 30–60 minutes.

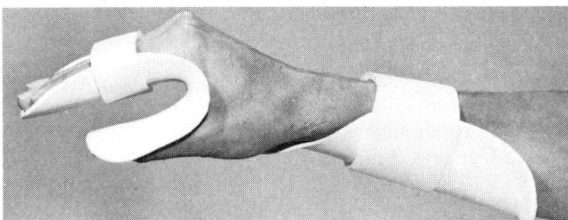

Figure 14-1. Rest splint for hand. Rest of the hand is important when soft tissues are acutely inflamed. Instruct the patient to maintain full range of motion of all joints and maintain tendon excursion while wearing a rest splint to prevent loss of important hand function. (Courtesy of The Western Pennsylvania Hospital, Pittsburgh, PA)

    d. Encourage the patient to rest in bed 8–9 hours at night.
    e. Instruct the patient to lie in prone position twice daily to prevent hip flexion and knee contractures.
    f. Pillows should not be placed under painful joints—promotes flexion contractures.
  2. Painful inflamed joints may be rested with splints—to locally decrease synovitis; to reduce pain, stiffness, and swelling (in wrists and fingers); and to rest inflamed joints in optimum position and to prevent/correct deformities (Fig. 14-1).
    a. Use correctly designed splints: a "working" splint (Fig. 14-2) for daytime, to allow continuing function despite a painful joint, and a "resting" splint for nighttime may be indicated.
      (1) A resting splint is used at night to keep knee in extension.
      (2) The wrist is splinted with slight dorsiflexion—useful in patients with carpal tunnel syndrome (compression of median nerve within carpal canal).
    b. Splints may need modifications as joint structures change.
    c. Metatarsal bars or pads (for shoes), inserts, or custom-made shoes may be used to decrease pressure on painful arthritic feet.

    d. Cervical collar to prevent cervical motion may help if patient has painful neck.
    e. Exercise is usually prescribed with splinting—to prevent joint deterioration and muscle weakness.
  3. Use of transcutaneous electrical nerve stimulation (TENS).
  4. Hot and/or cold applications reduce joint pain and swelling.
    a. Apply moist heat (15–30 minutes) to reduce muscle spasm and postrest stiffness; provide as much relief from pain as possible so that exercise program can be carried out.
      (1) Take warm bath or shower upon arising—shortens period of morning stiffness.
      (2) Use hot paraffin baths for fingers, hands.
    b. Use cold packs or ice when indicated for hot, swollen, acutely inflamed joints; heat is sometimes contraindicated when a joint is acutely inflamed. Cold will relieve swelling and pain and help restore function. (Keep commercial cold packs in freezer.)
    c. Employ gentle massage to relax muscles.
    d. Take joints through range of motion after heat treatments.
  5. Anti-inflammatory/analgesic medication as prescribed (see p. 651).

B. Increased Physical Mobility and Muscle Strength

  1. Regular exercises to maintain function of all joints, to strengthen muscles that support the joints, to improve circulation, and to promote endurance.
    a. Encourage the patient to follow a prescribed *daily* program of exercise composed of conditioning exercises and specific exercises for particular joint problems (after inflammatory process is controlled).
      (1) Avoid *excessive* exercise.
      (2) Stop exercise before tiring.
      (3) Pain lasting more than ½ hour after activity indicates that exercise is too vigorous; decrease, but do not stop activity.
      (4) Exercise slowly and smoothly in short, frequent sessions.

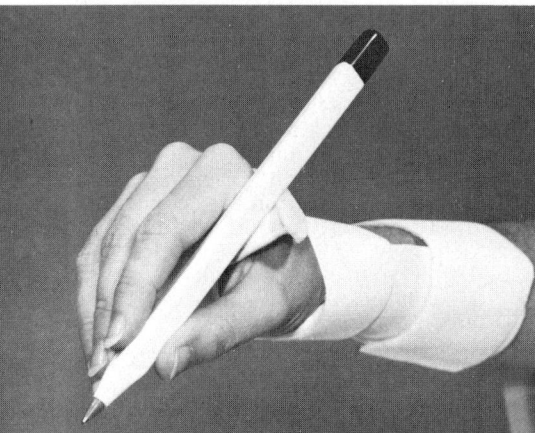
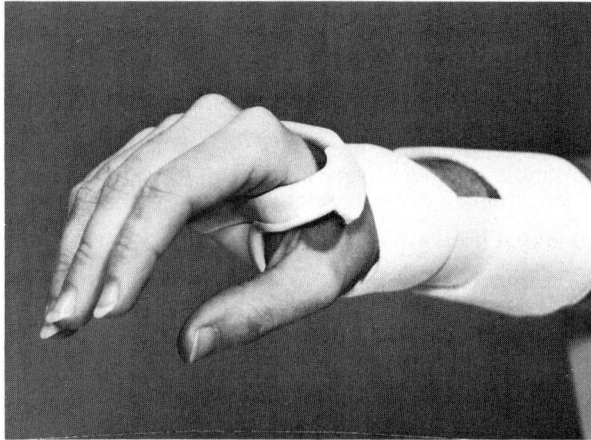

Figure 14-2. Arthritic cock-up splint is a type of working splint that allows continuing function despite a painful joint. (Courtesy of The Western Pennsylvania Hospital, Pittsburgh, PA)

b. See that the patient performs isometric exercises—to help prevent muscle atrophy, which contributes to joint instability.

c. Have the patient move joints through full range of motion 1–2 times daily to prevent loss of joint motion.

(1) Assist the patient in performing required joint motion if necessary.

(2) Avoid grasping painful joints; grasp belly of muscle.

d. Have the patient do progressive resistive exercises—for muscle building, after joint inflammation has been controlled.

2. Crutches or cane held in hand opposite affected knee/hip can be used—to reduce the load on the affected knee/hip.

3. Proper positioning to prevent flexion contractures of hips, knees, neck.

C. Optimal Independence in Activities of Daily Living (ADLs)

1. Self-help devices can be used to help with daily activities.
   a. Eating utensils with built-up handles
   b. Raised chair seats, toilet seats
   c. Special fastenings on clothing
   d. Dressing sticks, extended shoe horns

2. Allow extra time for the patient to perform activities, assisting only if necessary.

D. Improved Nutritional Intake

1. Offer well-balanced diet to include foods high in protein, iron, and vitamin C.

2. Encourage weight loss, if the patient is obese, to prevent excess stress on weight-bearing joints (hips and knees).

E. Positive Self-concept

1. Maintain a supportive relationship—successful management usually requires a long period of treatment.

2. Discuss nature of disease and positive expectations of treatment; encourage the patient to set goals.

3. Adopt a positive but realistic attitude.

4. Emphasize that something can and will be done to relieve the patient's pain and mobilize his joints.
   a. Encourage him to express his feelings—the patient becomes hostile and angry because of chronic pain, stiffness, and loss of mobility.
   b. Let the patient know that you are aware of his fears and that his future is important to the health team.

5. Try to modify or adapt to stress-producing situations.

6. Promote independence in ADLs (see above).

7. Encourage the patient to participate in social activities, hobbies, and family activities.

8. Allow the patient to participate in decision-making concerning treatment plan.

Health Education

1. Understand the disease, accept the realities of arthritis, and live within the limits imposed by it.
   a. Learn the nature of the disease and its treatment.
   b. Have confidence in your physician and treatment program.
   c. Avoid "miracle cures," dietary fads, drugs not prescribed by your physician, and other forms of "quackery."
   d. Report to the physician or clinic *regularly* for evaluation; have regular medical and functional reevaluation to determine if there is any loss of joint function.

2. Maintain independence.
   a. Rely on your own capabilities.
   b. Participate in as many activities as possible without producing fatigue.
   c. Conserve energy and simplify daily activities using self-help devices, work simplification methods, and energy-saving methods.
   d. Work at an even pace.
   e. Alternate periods of work, exercise, and rest. Avoid overdoing on good days.
   f. Alternate sitting and standing tasks; do not remain seated too long.

3. Take the medication exactly as prescribed, on a regular schedule.
   a. Aspirin is the primary drug (used for its anti-inflammatory effect). It must be taken over a long period and at high doses to achieve desired response. Long-term use does *not* lead to addiction.
   b. Report ringing in the ears or decreased hearing, since this is a guide in controlling dosage.
   c. Watch for symptoms of gastric irritation.
   d. Take with food (a buffering agent).
   e. Do not substitute acetaminophen (Tylenol), etc., for aspirin—this drug possesses no anti-inflammatory properties but is a pain reliever.

4. Use prescribed heat or cold treatments for muscle relaxation and relief of pain.
   a. Take a warm shower or tub bath upon arising to relieve morning stiffness; rest in bed 20–30 minutes after warm bath.
   b. If heat or cold treatment intensifies pain, discontinue and notify physician.
   c. Try an electric blanket to ascertain its usefulness in relieving morning stiffness.

5. Do the prescribed exercises to preserve joint motion and to gain muscular strength and coordination.
   a. Exercise also in water (pool; bathtub)—water provides buoyancy, support, and relaxation; muscles are exercised while joints are supported by water.
   b. Review publications from The Arthritis Foundation, 1314 Spring Street, N.W., Atlanta, GA 30309.

6. Conserve energy.
   a. Pace yourself when doing activities.
   b. Delegate jobs to others when possible.
   c. Avoid rushing.
   d. Organize and arrange materials, utensils, and tools.
   e. Simplify all activities.
   f. Perform any activity lasting more than 10 minutes in a seated position.

7. Protect joints from further damage.
   a. Consciously maintain correct posture—pain and swelling cause one to assume a position of deformity, which makes muscles work harder.
   b. Lower yourself gently into a chair, using the sidearms. Collapsing into a chair produces knee and hip joint trauma.
   c. Use an elevated chair if knee and hip joints are affected.
   d. Straighten up before walking.
   e. Avoid tension and stress on fingers and thumb joints.
   f. Avoid obesity, which places greater strain on weight-bearing joints.

g. Use a cane—to reduce load and impact on diseased joint.
h. Always use large joints to perform activities.
i. Slide objects instead of lifting them.
j. Respect pain—do on "good" days, don't do on "bad" days.

8. Seek sexual counseling (position and techniques) if arthritic involvement is a barrier to sexual performance.
9. Surgical procedures are available for relief of pain and deformity (when recommended by physician).
   a. Osteotomy
   b. Synovectomy
   c. Total joint replacement (see p. 841–844 for discussion).
10. The therapeutic program must be maintained for a lifetime; there is no cure at this time.

Evaluation

Expected Outcomes

1. Achieves relief of joint pain and stiffness; no overt evidence of joint inflammation; can move joint with ease
2. Demonstrates increased mobility and muscle strength; ambulates without manual assistance
3. Achieves independence in self-care activities, including transporting self outside of home environment
4. Maintains optimal nutrition, keeping body weight between ideal and 10% over ideal body weight
5. Develops and maintains a positive self-concept, expressing feelings and socializing with family and friends
6. Describes disease and treatment plan, adhering to plan as prescribed

Drugs Used in Connective Tissue Disease

Drug	Action	Adverse Effects
Anti-inflammatory Agents *Salicylates* Aspirin (may be buffered or enteric coated)	Has anti-inflammatory, antipyretic, and analgesic effects Aspirin is the cornerstone of treatment, especially in early phase of diseases such as rheumatoid arthritis	Tinnitus, gastric intolerance, or GI bleeding and purpuric tendencies
Other Nonsteroidal anti-inflammatory agents Ibuprofen (Motrin) Fenoprofen (Nalfon) Naproxen (Naprosyn) Tolmetin (Tolectin) Sulindac (Clinoril) Piroxicam (Feldene) Indomethacin (Indocin)	Anti-inflammatory, analgesic, antipyretic action Mechanism of action may be related to inhibition of prostaglandin synthesis (prostaglandins have a role in inflammatory process, pain and fever).	

Phenylbutazone (Butazolidin)
Oxyphenbutazone (Tandearil)
	Nonsteroidal antirheumatic agents for adjunctive treatment of rheumatoid arthritis
	Sometimes remarkably effective in control of articular symptoms
		Gastrointestinal effects:
		  Nausea, vomiting, epigastric distress, precipitation and reactivation of peptic ulcer
		Hematologic:
		  Bone marrow depression, anemia, leukopenia, agranulocytosis, thrombocytopenia purpura
		  Irreversible blood element depression may occur rapidly despite careful supervision and frequent testing.
		Sodium and water retention

Antimalarial Compounds Hydroxychloroquine sulfate (Plaquenil)	Anti-inflammatory, exact mechanism unknown Used primarily in discoid lupus and rheumatoid arthritis	Headache, dizziness, GI complaints, ocular toxicity, and retinopathy
Gold Therapy (Chrysotherapy) Gold sodium thiomalate (Myochrysine) (water-based) Aurothioglucose (Solganal) (oil-based) **Note:** Oral form of gold being made available	Gold salts may be useful when rheumatoid activity is uncontrolled by nonsteroidal therapy Anti-inflammatory; exact mechanism unknown Gold therapy is cumulative, with slow onset of beneficial effects	Dermatitis, stomatitis, nephropathy, blood dyscrasias Local irritation/necrosis at injection site

Drug	Action	Adverse Effects
Corticosteroids Prednisone (Deltasone) Prednisolone	Anti-inflammatory and immunosuppressive actions Corticosteroids used in treatment of incapacitating active rheumatoid arthritis, systemic lupus erythematosus, progressive systemic sclerosis, necrotizing arteritis	Osteoporosis, fractures, avascular necrosis Gastric ulcers, psychiatric problems, infection susceptibility Hirsutism, acne, moon facies, abnormal fat deposition, edema, emotional disorders, menstrual disorders Hyperglycemia, hypokalemia Hypertension Cataracts and glaucoma
Immunosuppressive Drugs Cyclophosphamide (Cytoxan) Azathioprine (Imuran)	Mechanisms underlying action of these drugs not known; thought to affect the production of antibodies at the cellular level Suppress autoimmune mechanism Used in advanced rheumatoid arthritis or systemic lupus erythematosus that is unresponsive to conventional therapy	Bone marrow depression, GI ulcerations Skin rashes, alopecia Bladder toxicity *Reduces the patient's resistance to infections*

Degenerative Joint Disease (Osteoarthritis)

Degenerative joint disease, the most common of all joint diseases, is the degeneration of the articular cartilage in the joints. It is characterized by bony spur formation at the edges of the joint surfaces, thickening of the capsule and the synovial membrane, and thinning of articular cartilage.

Although the exact underlying mechanism is not known, there appears to be a biochemical abnormality of cartilage.

Predisposing Factors

1. Aging
2. Anatomic abnormality; malalignment
3. Trauma (acute or repetitive)
4. Excessive joint use/abuse; obesity
5. Systemic diseases
6. Genetic influences

Assessment
Clinical Manifestations

1. Pain and swelling in one, two, or more joints, particularly after activity
2. Stiffness (occurs less frequently than in rheumatoid arthritis)
3. Limitation of joint motion and muscle spasm; particularly in weight-bearing and finger joints
4. Heberden's nodes—nodular bony enlargements that occur on the distal joints of some or all of the fingers
5. Bouchard's nodes—nodular bony enlargements that occur on the proximal joints of some or all of the fingers
6. Crepitus—audible, grating sound produced by bony irregularities within joint
7. Primary joints involved—hips, knees, vertebrae, and fingers

Diagnostic Evaluation

Radiographic examination demonstrates bony hypertrophy, spur formation, and cartilage disruption.

Patient Problems/Nursing Diagnoses

1. Pain related to joint degeneration and muscle spasm
2. Impaired physical mobility related to pain and limited joint movement
3. Self-care deficits (feeding, bathing/hygiene, dressing/grooming, toileting) related to pain and limited joint movement

Planning and Implementation
Nursing Interventions

A. Relief of Pain and Discomfort

1. Give anti-inflammatory agents as prescribed when synovial inflammation is present; also used for analgesic effect.
2. Give analgesics for pain control.
3. Provide rest for involved joints—excessive use aggravates the symptoms and accelerates degeneration.
   a. Use splints, braces, cervical collars, traction, lumbosacral corsets as necessary.
   b. Have prescribed rest periods in recumbent position.
4. Advise the patient to avoid activities that precipitate pain.
5. Use heat—relieves pain, muscle spasm, and stiffness and allows a more effective follow-up exercise program.
6. Support the patient undergoing intra-articular (into the joint) injections of long-acting steroids.
7. Teach the patient to use correct posture and body mechanics.

8. Advise the patient to sleep with a rolled terry towel under the neck—for relief of cervical osteoarthritis.
9. Have the patient use crutches, braces, or cane when indicated—to reduce weight-bearing stress on hips and knees.
Hold cane in hand on side opposite that of involved hip/knee.
10. Encourage the use of postural exercises to correct poor posture.
11. Have the patient wear corrective shoes and metatarsal supports for foot disorders—also helps in the treatment of arthritis of the knee.
12. Stress the importance of a weight reduction program under nursing and medical supervision—to decrease stress on weight-bearing joints.
13. Teach the patient to avoid engaging in excessive activity and unusual exercise or effort.
14. Support the patient undergoing orthopedic surgery for unremitting pain and disabling arthritis of joints.
   a. Repair of joint-supporting structures (tendon repairs)
   b. Debridement of loose bodies (cartilage, bone, large spurs)
   c. Osteotomy to redistribute joint forces; arthrodesis (fusion of joint)
   d. Joint replacement (hip, knee, ankle, shoulder, elbow)
15. Use transcutaneous electrical nerve stimulation (TENS) as prescribed.

B. Increased Physical Mobility

1. Keep active as much as possible without causing pain; avoid activities that cause pain.
2. Use range-of-motion exercises to maintain joint mobility and muscle tone for joint support, to prevent capsular and tendon tightening, and to prevent deformities.
3. Avoid flexion and adduction deformities—if deformities are avoided, pain is more likely to disappear.
4. Use isometric exercises and graded exercises to improve muscle strength around the involved joint.

C. Optimal Independence in Activities of Daily Living (ADLs)

See Rheumatoid Arthritis, page 650.

Evaluation

Expected Outcomes

1. Achieves relief of joint pain; prn analgesic not necessary
2. Demonstrates increased mobility; ambulates without manual assistance
3. Achieves independence in self-care activities, including transporting self outside of home environment
4. Describes disease and treatment plan, adhering to plan as prescribed

Gout

Gout is a disease manifested by an acute inflammation of a joint; it is caused by the deposit of uric acid crystals in joints and connective tissues.
1. *Uric acid*—end-product of purine metabolism derived from both dietary sources and endogenous synthesis.
2. *Hyperuricemia*—persistent elevation of urates in the blood usually found in gout patients. It is caused by overproduction or underexcretion of uric acid.
3. *Tophi*—deposits of urates in the tissues about the joints or on the ear; development of tophi related to duration of disease, degree of hyperuricemia, and renal function status.

Types of Gout

1. *Primary gout*—due to a genetic defect of purine metabolism; occurs most often in men over 40.
2. *Secondary gout* (an acquired disease)—hyperuricemia occurs in conditions in which there is an increase in cell turnover (leukemia, multiple myeloma, psoriasis) and in cell breakdown, or because of impaired renal excretion of uric acid.
May be precipitated by prolonged ingestion of diuretic agents, aspirin, trauma, treatment of myeloproliferative diseases, alcohol.

Assessment
Clinical Manifestations
A. Acute Gout

1. Sudden onset of severe pain in one or more peripheral joints—may be accompanied by intense inflammation, swelling, and tenderness.
   a. First joint of great toe is susceptible; later, other joints of foot are affected.

   b. Joints of feet, ankles, knees, wrist, and elbow commonly affected.
2. Fever 38.3°–39.4°C. (101°–103°F.)
3. Attacks involving the same joints tend to recur; variable lengths of time between attacks.

B. Chronic Gout

1. Development of tophi, external (skin) and/or internal—may become ulcerated and infected
2. Renal complications—40% of gout patients develop urate renal calculi
3. Joint deformity

Diagnostic Evaluation

1. Clinical history
2. Therapeutic response to colchicine
3. Serial elevations of serum uric acid
4. Identification of uric acid crystals in synovial fluid—obtained by arthrocentesis (aspiration of fluid from a joint cavity)
5. Marked increase in urinary uric acid levels

Patient Problems/Nursing Diagnoses

1. Severe pain related to joint inflammation
2. Alteration in pattern of urinary elimination related to renal calculi
3. Alteration in skin integrity related to tophi formation

Planning and Implementation
Nursing Interventions
A. Relief of Joint Pain

1. Immobilize and elevate affected joint(s); encourage the patient to rest, since early ambulation may precipitate a recurrence.

2. Give colchicine *early* in attack—suppresses inflammatory manifestations of acute gout; useful in establishing diagnosis, since it gives dramatic relief if patient has gout.
   a. An initial dose of colchicine is given and is followed by doses every 1–2 hours until the pain disappears and gastrointestinal symptoms develop (nausea, vomiting, abdominal cramping, diarrhea).
   b. Colchicine produces diarrhea—stop drug temporarily until diarrhea subsides. Drug may be given intravenously.
   c. A maintenance dose of colchicine may be given as soon as diarrhea stops; it is given as a prophylactic agent against recurrent gouty arthritis.
   d. Colchicine may be given before and after surgery to patients with gout—reduces the incidence of acute attacks of gouty arthritis precipitated by operative procedures.
3. Alternative forms of therapy
   a. Phenylbutazone (Butazolidin) or oxyphenbutazone or indomethacin (Indocin) are other drugs given during the acute stage of gout—these drugs reduce the fever and have an anti-inflammatory and analgesic effect (Indocin preferred).
   b. Fenoprofen, naproxen, ibuprofen (nonsteroidal anti-inflammatory agents)—also effective in acute gout (see p. 651).
4. Give additional analgesic for severe pain if necessary.

B. Adequate Urinary Elimination

1. Encourage large fluid intake (at least 3,000 ml./day) to maintain high urinary volume and promote urinary urate excretion.
2. Monitor intake and output.
3. Avoid foods high in purine content—sardines, anchovies, shellfish, organ meats.
4. Maintain an alkaline urine to prevent uric acid precipitation in the urinary system.
   a. Eat alkaline-ash foods, such as milk, potatoes, citrus fruits.
   b. Give sodium bicarbonate or citrate solution to maintain high urinary pH.

C. Skin Integrity

1. Provide adequate skin hygienic measures.
2. Prevent trauma to tophaceous areas.
3. Cover draining tophi and apply topical antibiotic ointment as directed.
4. Avoid restrictive clothing around tophi.
5. Tophi may be surgically removed.

Health Education

1. Take medications as prescribed for acute gouty attacks.
2. Take medications for chronic gout, even if asymptomatic, to lower uric acid level.
   a. Allopurinol (Zyloprim), a xanthine oxidase inhibitor—interferes with final stages of conversion of purines to uric acid, thus inhibiting production of uric acid.

(1) Dosage based on serum uric acid levels.
(2) Is drug of choice for chronic gout.
(3) Takes several weeks before therapeutic effect is noted.
(4) Side effects—rash, bone marrow depression, gastrointestinal disturbances.
   b. Give uricosuric agents for urate-lowering therapy—acts on renal tubule to inhibit urate reabsorption and thereby increases urinary excretion of urate and lowers the serum urate level; prevents formation of new tophi and reduces size of those already present. Drug selection depends on the mechanism of hyperuricemia.
   (1) Probenecid (Benemid)
       Side effects—headache, gastrointestinal disturbances, skin rash
   (2) Sulfinpyrazone (Anturane)
       Side effects—gastrointestinal disturbances (including peptic ulcer), skin rash, hematologic side effects
   (3) Give after meals or with antacids if there are gastric side effects.
3. Avoid foods rich in purine content; avoid excessive alcohol content. Eat foods high in alkaline-ash content.
4. Maintain a high fluid intake to sustain high urinary volume—minimizes urate precipitation in urinary tract.
5. Avoid fasting (to lose weight or when on alcoholic spree)—fasting has been found to increase the serum uric acid level.
6. Avoid crash diets—rapid reduction of weight may increase the serum uric acid level; slow weight reduction reduces the serum urate level without inducing an acute attack.
7. Avoid aspirin, diuretics, and other drugs that interfere with uric acid excretion.
8. Avoid or cope with stress—emotional, physical (e.g., trauma, surgery).
9. Seek medical attention and begin prompt treatment early during an acute attack. Repeated attacks lead to joint deformity and immobility.

Evaluation

Expected Outcomes

1. Achieves relief of pain by following comfort measures and adhering to drug regimen for acute gout
2. Maintains adequate renal function by increasing fluids—no evidence of renal calculi; adequate intake and output
3. Prevents recurrence of attacks by avoiding certain drugs, lowering food purines, and avoiding stress
4. Complies with treatment regimen in the absence of acute attacks
5. Maintains skin integrity; tophi, if present, are not ulcerated or infected
6. Describes disease stages (acute and chronic) and appropriate treatment for each stage

Systemic Lupus Erythematosus

Systemic lupus erythematosus (SLE) is a chronic, inflammatory, autoimmune disease involving multiple organ systems and producing widespread damage to connective tissues, blood vessels, serosal surfaces, and mucous membranes.

Discoid lupus erythematosus (DLE) is a chronic

eruption of the skin, which, although often disfiguring, does not pose a threat to life. DLE may later become systemic.

Clinical Features

1. Etiology is not understood—evidence indicates that immune, genetic, and viral factors play a role. There is also a drug-induced form of SLE (procainamide and hydralazine are most common offenders).
2. Most frequently found in young women with signs and symptoms referable to the joints and skin.
3. Is characterized by spontaneous remissions and exacerbations.
4. Often difficult to validate diagnosis.

Assessment

Clinical Manifestations

(Multiple organ involvement is explained by the deposit of antigen–antibody complexes throughout the body—kidneys, skin, brain, heart, and joints.)

1. Vary greatly, since they can affect any or every organ system; mimic many other diseases
2. Arthritis and arthralgia, fever, skin rash, alopecia, and involvement of serosal surfaces (pleurisy and pericarditis)
3. Skin manifestations
   a. Malar rash, alopecia, dermal vasculitis, Raynaud's phenomenon, purpura
   b. Facial rash with butterfly distribution over bridge of nose and malar bone prominences
   c. Similar lesions over neck, chest, upper and lower extremities—may become pruritic and scaly
   d. Brittleness or loss of scalp hair
   e. Photosensitivity with rashes developing after sun exposure
4. Generalized lymphadenopathy, anemia, leukopenia, thrombocytopenia
5. Long-continued low-grade fever
6. Cardiopulmonary involvement (pericarditis, myocarditis, pleural effusion)
7. Renal involvement (proteinuria, hematuria, renal insufficiency and failure)—leading cause of death
8. Central nervous system involvement (convulsive disorders, abnormalities in mental function and cranial nerves, depression, emotional lability, neurosis, psychosis)

Diagnostic Evaluation

(Many laboratory abnormalities may be found)
1. Clinically documented multisystem disease
2. Documentation of presence of antinuclear antibodies—positive fluorescent antinuclear antibody test (FANA)
3. Tests for complement (decrease) and antibodies to DNA
4. Erythrocyte sedimentation rate—elevated during exacerbation
5. Tests for serum rheumatoid factor (Rose and Latex)—often elevated during exacerbation
6. Complete blood and renal function studies

Patient Problems/Nursing Diagnoses

1. Alteration in skin and mucous membrane integrity related to rash and vascular lesions
2. Alteration in metabolism related to fever, fatigue, and anorexia
3. Disturbance in self-concept related to skin rash, fatigue, or joint deformity
4. Alteration in comfort—pain and stiffness related to joint and muscle inflammation
5. Anticipatory grieving related to unpredictability of chronic, potentially fatal disease
6. Self-care deficit related to fatigue, weakness, pain, and joint deformity
7. Alteration in nutrition related to anorexia, weight loss, and anemia

If multiple organ involvement is present, additional diagnoses would be identified (e.g., alteration in urinary elimination, cardiac output, etc.)

Planning and Implementation

Nursing Interventions

A. Skin Integrity

1. Keep skin clean; avoid powders and other irritants.
2. Avoid sunlight and ultraviolet lighting by wearing a hat, sunglasses, and long-sleeved clothing; use sunscreens (sun can precipitate exacerbation).
3. Topical corticosteroid creams or ointments may be prescribed for use as necessary to decrease inflammation.
4. Antimalarials (hydroxychloroquine [Plaquenil]) may be used to control skin manifestations.
   Patient should be examined by ophthalmologist at least twice yearly because drug may cause retinal degeneration, resulting in visual impairment.
5. Provide meticulous mouth care to prevent or care for oral and mucous lesions.

B. Decreased Fatigue and Anorexia, and Normal Body Temperature

1. Provide frequent rest periods combined with a 10- to 12-hour sleep period each night.
2. Utilize principles of energy conservation (see discussion under Rheumatoid Arthritis, p. 650).
3. Give antipyretics as needed to reduce fever.

C. Positive Self-concept

1. Provide emotional support—use realistic but optimistic approach.
2. Refer to cosmetologist for skin make-up to cover lesions.
3. Patient may require psychiatric intervention if severe depression persists.

D. Relief of Joint Pain and Discomfort

1. Daily exercise regimen balanced with frequent rest periods.
2. Salicylates or nonsteroidal anti-inflammatory agents—for arthritis and arthralgia
   a. Patient should take salicylates on a regular schedule so that adequate blood levels are maintained.
   b. See treatment of arthritis, page 648.
3. Corticosteroids (prednisone)—used for suppressing inflammation and thus relieving severe symptoms
   a. Observe patient carefully—may be difficult to distinguish between drug effects and those of SLE.
   b. See page 692 for discussion of side effects of steroids.

E. Psychosocial Adjustment

1. Allow the patient to ventilate feelings.
2. Identify and use support systems—family, friends, etc.
3. See Positive Self-concept, above.

F. Optimal Independence in ADLs

See Rheumatoid Arthritis, page 650.

G. Improved Nutritional Intake

1. Eat well-balanced meals, including foods high in iron, protein, and vitamin C unless otherwise contraindicated (as in renal complications).
2. Supplemental vitamin and iron therapy may be prescribed.

Health Education

1. Obtain physical and emotional rest; fatigue and depression are fairly common.
2. Eat a well-balanced diet.
3. Avoid whatever you know may aggravate the condition.
   a. Avoid sun exposure—sunlight may worsen dermal lesions and precipitate a flare-up of the disease. Use a sunscreen when exposure to sun is necessary.
   b. Avoid any drugs except those prescribed by physician; avoid using hair sprays and hair coloring agents.
   c. Avoid taking contraceptive pills—anovulatory drugs may precipitate lupus syndrome in susceptible person.
4. Use positive coping mechanisms or seek counseling to deal with stress—emotional turmoil may precipitate a flare-up.
5. The make-up Covermark® may conceal facial lesions and scarring.
6. Report to the physician immediately any worsening of symptoms—fever, cough, skin rash, increasing joint pain, etc. SLE also compromises the ability to fight infection.
7. Report onset of new signs and symptoms that may indicate additional complications of nephritis, congestive heart failure, central nervous system involvement, etc.
8. Seek medical attention for any concurrent illness (e.g., upper respiratory infection, urinary tract infection, etc.). Any illness, surgery, pregnancy, trauma may precipitate an exacerbation.
9. Observe for and report side effects of drugs—salicylates, nonsteroidal anti-inflammatory agents, corticosteroids, immunosuppressive agents (given as last resort to decrease SLE manifestation) (e.g., azathioprine [Imuran], cyclophosphamide [Cytoxan]).
10. See also Health Education, Rheumatoid Arthritis, page 650.
11. Support groups:
    Arthritis Foundation
    1314 Spring Street
    Atlanta, GA 30309

    Lupus Foundation of America, Inc.
    11921A Olive Drive
    St. Louis, MO 63141

    American Lupus Society
    23751 Madison Street
    Torrance, CA 90505

Evaluation
Expected Outcomes

1. Maintains skin integrity; no skin breakdown or scarring
2. Achieves decreased fatigue and increased appetite; maintains body temperature within normal range
3. Develops and maintains a positive self-concept, expressing feelings and socializing with family and friends
4. Achieves relief of joint pain and discomfort; no overt evidence of joint inflammation
5. Accepts the course of disease, adhering to treatment plan as prescribed
6. Avoids stress-producing situations, thus preventing exacerbations and additional complications of SLE
7. Maintains optimal nutrition, eating well-balanced diet; hemoglobin and hematocrit within low-normal range
8. Achieves independence in self-care activities, including transporting self outside of home environment
9. Describes variable course of disease and treatment regimen

Progressive Systemic Sclerosis

Progressive systemic sclerosis (PSS) is a disease of unknown etiology characterized by hardening and/or thickening of the skin (scleroderma) and fibrotic, degenerative, and inflammatory changes with vascular insufficiency resulting in joint changes and dysfunction of certain internal organs (gastrointestinal tract, heart, lungs, kidneys). There are several forms of localized scleroderma.

Clinical Features

1. Thought to be an autoimmune disease.
2. Affects women more often than men, usually between the ages of 30 and 50.
3. Has a variable course, with spontaneous remissions and exacerbations.
4. Prognosis not as good as for lupus or other connective tissue diseases.

Assessment
Clinical Manifestations

1. The disease usually starts insidiously on hands and face:
   a. Painless pitting edema of fingers, hands, feet, legs, face; edema gradually replaced by thickening and tightening of skin, which acquires a tense, wrinkle-free, bound-down appearance.
   b. Wrinkles and lines are obliterated.
   c. Skin is dry—sweat secretion over involved area is suppressed.
   d. Face appears mask-like, immobile, and expressionless; mouth becomes rigid ("bird mouth").
   e. Condition spreads slowly; extremities become stiff and immobile; the fingers semiflexed, immobile, and useless, and the hands claw-like.
2. Detectable clinical changes may occur in the internal organs (treated symptomatically).
   a. Heart becomes fibrotic—causing congestive heart failure, arrhythmias and conduction disturbances, angina.
   b. Esophagus is hardened, with disruption of normal esophageal peristalsis—gastroesophageal reflux, with heartburn and dysphagia.
   c. Pulmonary fibrosis/pulmonary hypertension.

d. Intestines become hardened—digestive disturbances.
e. Progressive renal failure may occur (leading cause of death).
f. Variety of other disturbances develop, including Raynaud's phenomenon, arthritis, and polymyositis (inflammation of skeletal muscle).
3. C-R-E-S-T syndrome is common:
Çalcinosis
Ŗaynaud's
Ȩsophagitis
Ṣclerodactyly
Ṭelangiectasias

Patient Problems/Nursing Diagnoses

See problems of patient with lupus erythematosus, page 655.

In addition, the following major problems may occur:
1. Alteration in nutrition (less than body requirements) related to difficulty in swallowing from esophagitis
2. Alteration in skin integrity related to scleroderma
3. Alteration in tissue perfusion related to Raynaud's phenomenon

Planning and Implementation

Nursing Interventions

A. Improved Nutritional Intake

1. Elevate head of bed while eating and at least 1 hour after eating.
2. Give antacids before or after meals and at bedtime to decrease dyspepsia.
3. Provide foods that are soft, yet form a bolus (e.g., mashed potatoes, puddings).
4. Offer well-balanced diet with supplement of protein, iron, and vitamin C.

5. Provide nutritional counseling if severe bowel involvement or evidence of malabsorption is present.

B. Skin Integrity

1. Lubricate skin with topical creams and petrolatum lubricants to prevent fissuring and ulceration.
2. Avoid soap and other drying agents.
3. Monitor body temperature carefully as sweat secretion is decreased.

C. Optimum Tissue Perfusion to Skin and Body Organs

1. Avoid exposure to cold and trauma to hand (aggravates Raynaud's phenomenon).
2. Vasoactive drugs and anti-inflammatory agents may be helpful in increasing blood flow.

D. See Also Discussion Under Systemic Lupus Erythematosus, page 655.

Health Education

Support group:
United Scleroderma Foundation
P.O. Box 350
Watsonville, CA 95077

Evaluation

Expected Outcomes

1. Maintains optimal nutrition, keeping body weight within normal range for age and body build
2. Avoids reflux from esophagitis by compliance with treatment regimen
3. Maintains skin integrity; no evidence of fissures or ulcerations from dryness
4. Complies with health instruction to prevent exacerbation of Raynaud's phenomenon, thus increasing tissue perfusion

Polyarteritis (Periarteritis Nodosa)

Polyarteritis (periarteritis nodosa or PAN) is a disease of unknown cause (probably autoimmune) characterized by inflammation and necrosis of medium-sized and small vessels, especially arteries, which results in altered function of the organ system in which the arterial supply has been impaired.

Clinical Features/Manifestations

1. The walls of the vessels are involved; spotty inflammation causes changes in circulation and tissue damage.
2. Occurs most often in men.
3. Clinical manifestations vary according to organ(s) involved and amount of necrosis produced by obstructing vascular lesion.
   a. Prolonged fever; myalgia and arthralgia; renal involvement; gastrointestinal manifestations (abdominal pain, nausea, vomiting, diarrhea); cardiovascular manifestations (coronary insufficiency, myocardial infarction); palpable nodules along the arterial trunks—may occur.
   b. Ocular manifestations (retinal exudates and hemorrhages) are fairly common.
   c. Skin lesions are usually in the form of painful nodules that may ulcerate.
      (1) Subcutaneous nodules vary in size and may be located in any part of the body.
      (2) Overlying skin may be reddened or ulcerated.
      (3) Purpuric papules may be present.
4. Periarteritis is apt to run a course of a few years' duration; recovery is unpredictable—death may ensue from renal decompensation, congestive failure, etc.

Bibliography

Books

General

Arthritis Foundation. Arthritis, Living, and Loving: Information About Sex. Atlanta, Arthritis Foundation, 1982

Arthritis Foundation. Primer on the Rheumatic Diseases. Atlanta, Arthritis Foundation, 1983
Bluestone R. Rheumatology. Boston, Houghton Mifflin, 1980
Currey H. An Introduction to Clinical Rheumatology. Philadelphia, JB Lippincott, 1980
Giansiracusa DF and Kantrowitz FG. Rheumatic and Metabolic Bone Diseases in the Elderly. Lexington, MA, DC Heath, 1982

Kelley WN et al. Textbook of Rheumatology, vols. 1 and 2. Philadelphia, WB Saunders, 1981

Melvin JL. Rheumatic Disease: Occupational Therapy and Rehabilitation. Philadelphia, FA Davis, 1982

Moll JMH. Management of Rheumatic Disorders. New York, Raven Press, 1983

Porter SF. Arthritis Care: A Guide for Patient Education. Norwalk, CT, Appleton-Century-Crofts, 1984

Riggs GK and Gall EP. Rheumatic Diseases: Rehabilitation and Management. Boston, Butterworth, 1984

Roth SH. New Directions in Arthritis Therapy. Littleton, MA, PSG Publishing, 1980

Rothschild BM. Rheumatology: A Primary Care Approach. New York, Yorke Medical Books, 1982

Systemic Lupus Erythematosus

Hayslett JP and Hardin JA. Advances in Systemic Lupus Erythematosus. New York, Grune & Stratton, 1983

Schur PH. The Clinical Management of Systemic Lupus Erythematosus. New York, Grune & Stratton, 1983

Articles
General

Adult arthritis. Am J Nurs 1983 Feb; 83(2):254–278

Gotch PM. Teaching patients about adrenal corticosteroids. Am J Nurs 1981 Jan; 81(1):78–81

Lanham J et al. The place of antimalarials in rheumatology. Ann Rheum Dis 1981 Mar; 40(3):323–324

Simon LS et al. Nonsteroidal anti-inflammatory drugs. N Engl J Med 1980 May 22; 302(21):1179–1185

Rheumatoid Arthritis

Bunch TW et al. Disease-modifying drugs for progressive rheumatoid arthritis. Mayo Clin Proc 1980 Mar; 55(1):161–179

Feinberg J et al. Use of resting splints by patients with rheumatoid arthritis. J Occup Ther 1981 Mar; 35(3):173–178

Hajiroussou VJ et al. Prolonged low-dose corticosteroid therapy and osteoporosis in rheumatoid arthritis. Ann Rheum Dis 1984 Feb; 43(1):24–27

Hunder GG and Bunch TW. Treatment of rheumatoid arthritis. Bull Rheum Dis 1982; 32(1):1–6

Liang MH et al. The psychosocial impact of systemic lupus erythematosus and rheumatoid arthritis. Arthritis Rheum 1984 Jan; 27(1):13–19

Lipsky PE. Remission-inducing therapy in rheumatoid arthritis. Am J Med 1983 Oct 31; 75(4B):40–49

Neustadt DH. Recent strategies in the use of corticosteroids in rheumatoid arthritis. Clin Rheum Practice 1983 Sep/Oct; 1(5):196–204

Scott DL et al. Progression of radiological changes in rheumatoid arthritis. Ann Rheum Dis 1984 Feb; 43(1):8–17

Degenerative Joint Disease

Altman RD et al. Degenerative joint disease. Clin Rheum Dis 1983 Dec; 9(3):681–693

Lewis D et al. Transcutaneous electrical nerve stimulation in osteoarthritis: A therapeutic alternative? Ann Rheum Dis 1984 Feb; 43(1):47–49

Weiss TE and Quinet RJ. Clinical concepts of osteoarthritis: Part I. Clin Rheum Practice 1983 Nov/Dec; 1(6):269–284

Gout

Delaney P. Gouty neuropathy. Arch Neurol 1983 Dec; 40(13):823–824

Diamond HS. The kidney in hyperuricemia and gout. Clin Rheum Practice 1983 Sep/Oct; 1(5):205–220

Edwards NL. The diagnosis and management of gouty arthritis. Compr Ther 1983 Sep; 9(9):14–19

Gibson T et al. Renal impairment and gout. Ann Rheum Dis 1980 Oct; 39(5):417–423

Nakayama DA et al. Tophaceous gout: A clinical and radiographic assessment. Arthritis Rheum 1984 Apr; 27(4):468–471

Lupus Erythematosus

Calabrese LH. Diagnosis of systemic lupus erythematosus. Postgrad Med 1984 May 15; 75(7):103–105, 108–112

Catoggio LJ et al. Systemic lupus erythematosus in the elderly: Clinical and serological characteristics. J Rheum 1984 Feb; 11(2):175–181

Hess E. Introduction to drug related lupus. Arthritis Rheum 1981 Aug; 24(8):vi–ix

Liang MH et al. The psychosocial impact of systemic lupus erythematosus and rheumatoid arthritis. Arthritis Rheum 1984 Jan; 27(1):13–19

Podell RN. Systemic lupus erythematosus. Postgrad Med 1984 Jan; 75(1):251–254

Systemic lupus erythematosus. Clin Rheum Dis 1982 Apr; 8(1):1–323

SLE: "Wolf" in sheep's clothing. Patient Care 1984 Mar 30; 18(6):134–174

Progressive Systemic Sclerosis and Polyarteritis

Beckett VL. Scleroderma. Minn Med 1984 Feb; 67(2):105–106

Lee EB et al. Pathogenesis of scleroderma: Current concepts. Int J Dermatol 1984 Mar; 23(2):85–89

Mackel SE. Treatment of vasculitis. Med Clin North Am 1982 Jul; 66(4):941–954

Steen VD et al. Factors predicting development of renal involvement in progressive systemic sclerosis. Am J Med 1984 May; 76(5):779–786

Allergy Problems

15

The Allergic Reaction

Definitions

1. *Antigen*—a substance that, when repeatedly in contact with the body, stimulates production of a counteracting substance, a globulin "antibody."
2. *Antibody*—an immunoglobulin produced by the lymphoid cells as a result of stimulation of these cells by an antigen; the antibody is capable of combining with the antigen in a very specific manner.
3. *Immunity*—a state of increased resistance to a particular substance.
   a. *Active-acquired immunization*—resistance brought about by the injection of an antigenic substance (e.g., tetanus toxoid).
   b. *Passive-acquired immunization*—resistance brought about by the transfer of antibody-containing serum from an immunized donor to a normal recipient (e.g., tetanus antitoxin).
4. *Allergic reaction*—a manifestation of tissue injury resulting from an interaction between an antigen and an antibody.

Immunoglobulins

Antibodies that are formed by lymphocytes and plasma cells in response to an immunogenic stimulus comprise a group of serum proteins called *immunoglobulins.*
1. The abbreviation for immunoglobulin is "Ig."
2. Antibodies combine with antigens in very special ways (lock-and-key style).
3. There are 5 major classes of immunoglobulins:
   a. IgM ("gamma-M")—largest molecule; tends to stay in bloodstream and is primarily engaged in defense in intravascular compartment.
   b. IgG ("gamma-G")—most abundant and one of the smallest; readily diffuses into tissue spaces to assist in combating tissue infection.
   c. IgA ("gamma-A")—circulates in the blood, but its role here is uncertain; it is produced in external secretions (saliva, tears) where it provides a primary defense mechanism.
   d. IgD—function has not yet been fully determined.
   e. IgE ("gamma-E")—responsible for most of the immediate types of allergic reactions; has property of attaching to human epithelial cells.

Antibody–Antigen Reaction

1. Consists of:
   a. Those that are protective and beneficial to the body (*immunogen*).
   b. Those that are not always protective and beneficial to the body (*allergen*).
      (1) May cause tissue damage
      (2) May produce discomfort to the patient
2. Under certain circumstances, an antibody is produced that reacts not only to a noxious agent but also to another harmless agent of similar chemical composition.

Products of Antigen-antibody Union

(Chemical Mediator Products)
1. *Histamine*—released from tissue mast cells by the interaction of an antigen and its corresponding antibody.
   a. Causes contraction of smooth muscle of bronchioles, uterus, intestines
   b. Dilates and causes increased permeability of capillaries of skin and mucous membrane
   c. Lowers blood pressure
   d. Stimulates secretion of nasal, lacrimal, salivary, and gastrointestinal glands
   e. Produces itching of skin and mucous membrane
2. *Serotonin*—an amine released at the same time as histamine.
3. *Bradykinin*—acts chiefly by increasing capillary permeability and contractility of smooth muscle.
4. *Acetylcholine*—acts to stimulate autonomic nervous system.
5. *SRS-A*—slow-reacting substance of anaphylaxis.

Hypersensitivity Phenomena

1. "Sensitivity" is said to exist when the body reacts against substances in the environment that elicit no response from most persons.
2. Some authorities consider that
   a. "Immunity" is produced when antigen and antibody are beneficial to the individual.
   b. "Allergy" is produced when antigen and antibody are harmful to the individual.
3. Inhaled allergens
   a. Plant pollens—ragweed, grasses, tree pollens
   b. Molds, fungi, spores, animal danders, house dust
4. Ingested allergens—cow's milk, egg white, fish, nuts, chocolate, certain fruits
5. Contact allergens—contact dermatitis (see p. 619)
6. Sensitivity reactions
   a. Local or systemic
   b. Mediated by sensitized cells, not circulating globulins

659

c. Mediated by circulating immunoglobulin E (IgE) (see Immunoglobulins)

Delayed Hypersensitivity

1. Term for a reaction that reaches its peak 24–48 hours after an antigen is brought into contact with the skin surface of a sensitized individual.

2. The reaction usually consists of erythema and induration.
3. Delayed hypersensitivity is mediated by sensitized "T" (thymus-dependent) lymphocytes (not by immunoglobulins).
4. Examples—tuberculin skin test, contact dermatitis such as poison ivy

Anaphylaxis

Anaphylaxis is an unusual systemic allergic reaction (hypersensitivity) to a foreign protein or other substance. It is usually precipitated by the injection of a medication or by an insect sting. The reaction occurs rapidly and may cause death because of respiratory obstruction or vascular collapse.

▶ **NURSING ALERT:** With injection of allergenic extracts, the risk of systemic reaction is always present.

Skin testing, usually of the intradermal type, has resulted in systemic reactions to pollen, penicillin, and food antigens.

Have epinephrine 1:1000 on hand during skin testing (with syringe and tourniquet).

Early Manifestations

1. Feeling of uneasiness or apprehension, weakness, perspiration, sneezing, or nasal pruritus
2. Generalized pruritus, urticaria, angioedema
3. Dyspnea, wheezing, dysphagia, vomiting, abdominal pain
4. Pulse—may be rapid, weak, irregular, or unobtainable
5. Syncope or shock—may follow rapidly; potentially fatal
6. Possible urgency, fecal and urinary incontinence, convulsions, and coma

Treatment

Administer epinephrine—the pharmacologic antagonist of the action of chemical mediators on smooth muscle and other effector cells.

A. Immediate

(Anticipate physician's need of the following)
1. Inject 0.3–0.5 ml. of 1:1000 aqueous epinephrine IM into upper arm; massage.
2. Apply tourniquet above site of antigen injection (allergy injection, insect sting, etc.).
3. Inject 0.3 ml. of 1:1000 aqueous epinephrine into site of previous antigen injection.

B. If Reaction Is Not Reversed by Epinephrine

(Physician administration)
1. Diphenhydramine chloride is given IV to help prevent development of laryngeal edema.
2. Bronchospasm—aminophylline IV, intravenous fluids
3. Hypotension—vasopressors, volume repletion, isoproterenol
4. Laryngeal obstruction—tracheostomy and oxygen
5. Cardiac arrest—CPR, sodium bicarbonate
6. Corticosteroids may be helpful for laryngeal edema and hypotension; however, it must be emphasized that steriods are not helpful in immediate anaphylaxis, since they take at least 1 hour and probably several hours to act even if given intravenously.

C. Ongoing Monitoring

1. Evaluate patient reaction.
2. Repeat aqueous epinephrine, if necessary.
3. Remove tourniquet if reaction seems to be under control.
4. Monitor vital signs as required.
5. Assess for hypotension and respiratory distress.

Allergy Survey Sheet*

Name _____ Age _____ Sex _____ Date _____

  I. Chief complaint:

 II. Present illness:

III. Collateral allergic symptoms:

Eyes:	Pruritus _____	Burning _____	Lacrimation _____
	Swelling _____	Injection _____	Discharge _____
Ears:	Pruritus _____	Fullness _____	Popping _____
	Frequent infections _____		
Nose:	Sneezing _____	Rhinorrhea _____	Obstruction _____
	Pruritus _____	Mouth breathing _____	
	Purulent discharge _____		
Throat:	Soreness _____	Post-nasal discharge _____	
	Palatal pruritus _____	Mucus in the morning _____	

* From Patterson R. *Allergic Diseases,* 3rd ed. Philadelphia, JB Lippincott, 1985

Allergy Survey Sheet (cont.)

Chest:	Cough _____	Pain _____		Wheezing _____
	Sputum _____	Dyspnea _____		
	Color _____	Rest _____		
	Amount _____	Exertion _____		
Skin:	Dermatitis _____	Eczema _____		Urticaria _____

IV. Family Allergies:

V. Previous allergic treatment or testing:

Prior skin testing:

Drugs:	Antihistamines	Improved _____	Unimproved _____
	Bronchodilators	Improved _____	Unimproved _____
	Nose drops	Improved _____	Unimproved _____
	Hyposensitization	Improved _____	Unimporved _____
	Duration _____		
	Antigens _____		
	Reactions _____		
	Antibiotics	Improved _____	Unimproved _____
	Steroids	Improved _____	Unimproved _____

VI. Physical agents and habits:

Bothered by:

Tobacco for _____ years
Cigarettes _____ packs/day
Cigars _____ per day
Pipe _____ per day
Never smoked _____
Bothered by smoke _____

Alcohol _____
Heat _____
Cold _____
Perfumes _____
Paints _____
Insecticides _____
Cosmetics _____

Air cond. _____
Muggy weather _____
Weather changes _____
Chemicals _____
Hair spray _____
Newspapers _____

VII. When symptoms occur:
Time and circumstances of 1st episode:
Prior health:
Course of illness over decades: Progressing _____ regressing _____
Time of year:
   Perennial _____
   Seasonal _____
   Seasonally exacerbated _____
Monthly variations (menses, occupation):
Time of week (weekends vs weekdays):
Time of day or night:
After insect stings:

VIII. Where symptoms occur:
Living where at onset:
Living where since onset:
Effect of vacation or major geographic change:
Symptoms better indoors or outdoors:
Effect of school or work:
Effect of staying elsewhere nearby:
Effect of hospitalization
Effect of specific environments:
Do symptoms occur around:
old leaves _____ hay _____ lakeside _____ barns _____
summer homes _____ damp basement _____ dry attic _____
lawnmowing _____ animals _____ other _____
Do symptoms occur after eating:
cheese _____ mushrooms _____ beer _____ melons _____
bananas _____ fish _____ nuts _____ citrus fruits _____
other foods (list) _____
Home: city _____ rural _____
      house _____ age _____
      apartment _____ basement _____ damp _____ dry _____
      heating system _____
      pets (how long) _____ dog _____ cat _____ other _____

Allergy Survey Sheet (cont.)

Bedroom:	Type	Age	*Living Room:*	Type	Age
Pillow	————	————	Rug	————	————
Mattress	————	————	Matting	————	————
Blankets	————	————	Furniture	————	————
Quilts	————	————			
Furniture	————	————			

Anywhere in home symptoms are worse: ————————————————————

IX.   What does patient think makes him worse: ————————————————

 X.   Under what circumstances is he free of symptoms: ————————————

XI.   Summary and additional comments: ——————————————————

Sensitivity Tests and Immunotherapy (Hyposensitization)

Immunotherapy is a procedure designed to increase a person's resistance to offending antigens by administration of small, gradually increasing amounts of a specific antigen over a period of time. Immunotherapy is preceded by skin testing.

RAST (radioallergosorbent test) is a technique for laboratory determination of IgE antibodies in serum. It is useful in corroborating skin test findings in questionable situations. It is also a useful substitute when skin testing is contraindicated (e.g., patient objection, generalized dermatitis).

Guidelines: Skin Testing

Skin testing is the introduction of an antigen (bacterial, fungal, chemical) to the skin surface or directly beneath the skin to determine body sensitivity and reaction to the antigen.

Purpose
1. Diagnosis
2. Desensitization
3. Immunization

Methods
1. *Patch test*—application of test material either directly to skin or to skin immediately covered with a small gauze dressing (or gauze part of a Band-Aid).
2. *Scratch (prick or tine)*—antigen is applied to a superficial scratch that pentrates the outer layer of skin.
3. *Intradermal*—injection of a small amount of antigen into the superficial layers of skin.

Reactions
1. *Positive*
   a. Indicates antibody response to previous contact with the antigen.
   b. Does not prove presence of active infection.
2. *Negative*
   a. Indicates antibodies have been formed against the antigen.
   b. In presence of active infection, it means that not enough time has elapsed to build antibodies.
   c. May mean that antigen has been injected too deeply.
   d. Patient may be anergic (abnormal inactivity).
3. *Suppressed reaction*—may occur if the patient:
   a. Is on corticosteroids.
   b. Is on immunosuppressive drugs.
   c. Is on antihistaminics.
   d. Has received (within 3 weeks) live virus immunizations (e.g., smallpox, measles).
   e. Feels faint or is cold.

Sites
1. Volar or anterior surface of the upper third of the forearm or upper arm (over muscle belly).
2. Back, below top of scapula (Fig. 15-1) (useful for scratch or tine test).
3. Anterior thigh (scratch or tine test).

1. Approximately 10 cm. (4 inches) below bend of elbow or 10 cm. above bend of elbow.
2. Avoid spine.

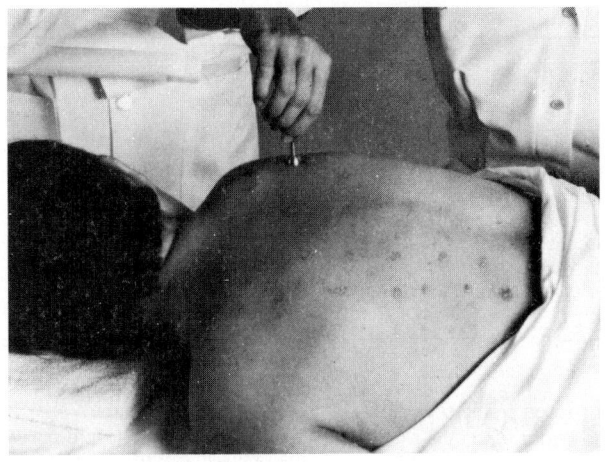

Figure 15-1. Skin testing from the top of the scapula to the lower rib cage and from the posterior axillary line to 5 or 10 cm. (2 or 4 inches) from the spine. Most scarifications should be at least 5 cm. (2 inches) apart; however, pollen tests should be as much as 10 cm. (4 inches) apart to prevent one reaction from overlapping another.

Side Effects

Symptom	Treatment
1. Itching, discomfort, pain.	1. Apply cold packs. Apply topical steroids.
2. Vesiculation, ulceration.	2. Keep dry—expose to air.

3. Bleeding
  a. Wheal type—bleeding is of no consequence.
  b. Tine test—bleeding can wash away antigen.
	3. Apply pressure if bleeding is excessive.
	
	  b. Apply pressure if bleeding is excessive.
	    Repeat test in another area.

4. Allergic reaction to preservatives or stabilizers.	4. Discontinue use.
5. Anaphylactic shock.	5. Administer epinephrine (see p. 660).

Procedure

1. Place tests approximately 10 cm. (2 inches) apart.	1. To prevent results of one test from coalescing with those of another.
2. Avoid hairy area.	2. Will interfere with reading.
3. Avoid areas near bone or tendons or areas without adequate subcutaneous tissue.	

Preparation of Patient

1. Explain to the patient what is being done and why.
2. Provide adequate lighting.
3. Thoroughly cleanse testing area with alcohol or ether and allow the area to dry.

Patch Test

Advantage:
    Effective in cases involving contact hypersensitivity to topically applied substance.
Disadvantage:
    Not as accurate as other methods.

Nursing Action	Rationale/Amplification
Technique	
1. Apply test material directly to skin for purpose of producing a small area of allergic dermatitis (e.g., plant oils, hair tonic, shaving cream).	1. Leave area exposed, OR Cover with a small gauze dressing and adhesive or use a Band-Aid.
Reaction	
1. Remove patch after 48 hours.	1. Usually site itches.
2. Wait for 20–30 min. to allow any unrelated reaction to subside.	2. A true allergic reaction persists for several days.

3. Observe reaction and describe:
    + erythema
    ++ erythema, papules
    +++ erythema, papules, vesicles
    ++++ erythema, papules, vesicles, and severe edema
	3. Positive patch test reactions often show an increase in severity in next 24 hours. Reexamine in 72 hours.

4. Record nature of sensitizers and reactions.	

(continued)

Guidelines: Skin Testing (continued)

Preparation of Patient
(Cont.)

Scratch Test (Prick or Tine)

Equipment:
   Sterile "darning" needle, 4-prong tine scarifier, such as Von Pirquet, Robinson
   (A needle pricks the skin through a drop of antigen.)
Advantage:
   Relatively little risk of a general constitutional reaction.
Disadvantage:
   May not be sufficiently sensitive unless a very strong antigen is used.

Nursing Action	Rationale/Amplification
1. Place a drop of glycerin–saline solution on the skin.	1. This serves as a control.
2. Place a drop of each antigen to be tested on the skin; drops should be spaced about 4 cm. (2 inches) apart.	2. Spacing is required to prevent the coalescing of one reaction with another. Skin-marking pencil may be used to number each antigen.
3. Scratch the skin about 2 mm. through each drop of antigen; the skin should be lightly abraded. If a 4-prong tine is used, grasp forearm firmly and stretch skin tightly.	3. A sterile darning needle or commercially available scarifying instrument may be used. This is to prevent undue movement of the arm when the tine is applied; if the arm moves, a larger scratch results.
4. Apply tine with pressure; hold 1 second.	4. Pressure is applied to produce 4 puncture sites. (A circular depression made by the disc is also visible.)
5. Remove disc and release skin; discard disc.	5. Discs are never reused.

▶ **NURSING ALERT:** Do not wipe the skin following a scratch or tine test, since this may remove the antigen.

6. Record site, type of antigen, and time when it is to be read.	6. Read in about 30–40 minutes.

Intradermal Test

Limit number of intradermal tests to no more than 20.
Advantage:
   More dilute solutions of antigen are required.
Disadvantage:
   There is risk of systemic reaction unless this test follows a scratch test.
Equipment:
   Sterile tuberculin syringe with gradations of 1/100 of a ml.
   Intradermal needle or No. 26 or No. 27 gauge ¾- or ½-inch needle
   Separate syringe and needle (preferably disposable) for each antigen

Technique

1. Eject all air from syringe and needle.	1. Air injected will affect reading.
2. Hold forearm with one hand and use thumb to stretch skin.	2. Left hand can be used if syringe is to be held in right hand (or vice versa).
3. Hold syringe between thumb and forefinger and place plunger against heel of hand.	3. If necessary, air can be expelled by contracting thumb and forefinger.
4. Position bevel upward and place needle and syringe almost parallel along long axis of arm.	4. With bevel upward, needle can penetrate superficial layer of skin; sensitizer can be deposited directly under skin surface.
5. Depress needle into arm and advance until bevel just disappears into corium.	
6. Contract hand and advance plunger, injecting amount needed to raise a bleb of 1 cm. (¾ inch, or 10 mm.)	
7. Remove needle.	7. Transient bleeding is of no significance.
8. Repeat for additional testing.	
9. Record what was given, where it was given, and time it is to be read.	9. Draw pattern on chart. Usually read in 30–40 minutes.
10. Grading of reactions from negative to positive (intracutaneous tests)* (Fig. 15-2)	

   − no reaction
   + erythema smaller than a nickel in diameter
   ++ erythema larger than a nickel in diameter (21 mm.)
   +++ erythema and a wheal without pseudopod formation
   ++++ erythema and a wheal with pseudopod formation

* Patterson R. Allergic Diseases, 3rd ed. Philadelphia, JB Lippincott, 1985

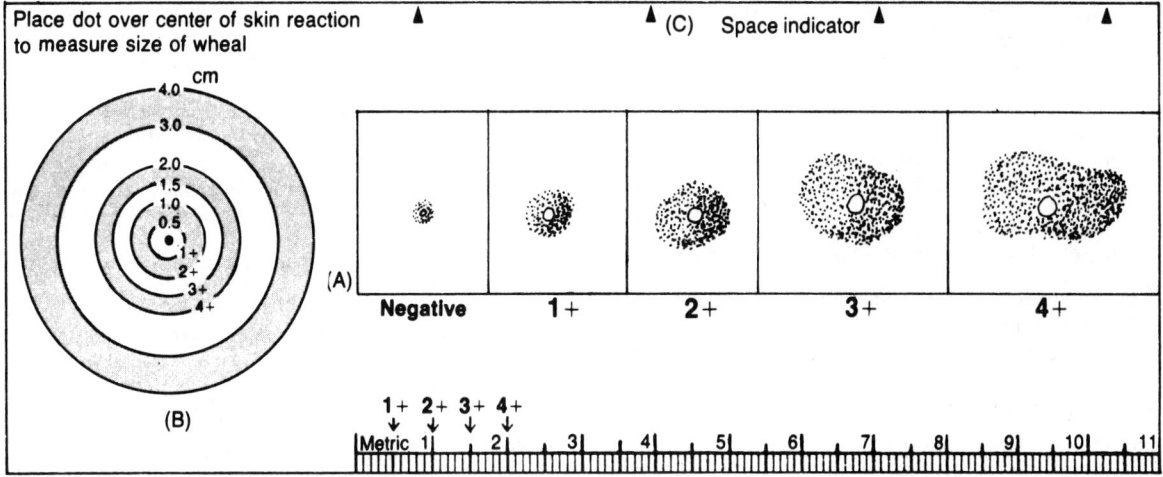

Figure 15-2. (*A*) These series of reactions indicate the sizes of wheals when the allergist refers to them as 1+, 2+, etc. A negative reaction is shown at the left. (*B*) The target wheal guide can be traced on a transparent sheet (acetate or x-ray film) and then placed over the wheal to measure the size in centimeters or according to plus-size. The relationship between the two is indicated on the lower metric scale. (*C*) Showing placement of test sites spaced uniformly. (Patient Care Sept. 15, 1973. Copyright © 1973, Patient Care Publications, Inc.; Darien, CT. All rights reserved.)

Management of the Person With an Allergy

Goals:

1. To encourage the person with an allergy to find out to which antigens he is sensitive.
2. To assist the patient in recognizing the importance of avoiding offending antigens whenever possible.
3. To seek relief for the patient when he has been exposed to an offending antigen.
4. To direct the patient to seek assistance in increasing his resistance to the offending antigen.

Measures to Control the Environment

A. Respiratory Allergies

1. Encourage the patient to modify his environment as much as he can, but not to the point of developing such a rigid regimen that his activities are unduly restricted.
2. In the hospital unit
   a. Restrict flowers and plants in the patient's room, since they introduce antigens or irritating vapors to which he may be sensitive.
   b. Avoid dry-dusting and mopping while the patient is in the room.
   c. Do not flourish sheets or plump pillows excessively during bed-making.
   d. Recommend cake face powder rather than loose powder; limit the use of talcums.
   e. Replace feather pillows with Dacron-filled or hypoallergenic pillows.
   f. Attempt to find acceptable replacements for items removed from the patient's environment so that his surroundings will still be psychologically therapeutic.
3. In the home (primarily the bedroom)
   Advise the patient as follows:
   a. Use hypoallergenic materials for bedding (blankets, comforters, bedpad, pillows).
   b. Enclose the mattress and box springs in plastic airtight covers.
   c. Avoid keeping the window open at night if allergy is due to sensitivity to pollens and grasses.
   d. Replace carpeting with washable throw rugs; heavy draperies with easily laundered light curtains.
   e. Limit the number of dust-catching articles in the room.
4. Room air
   Advise the patient as follows:
   a. Utilize a system of heating or cooling that can both humidify and filter the air.
   b. Avoid rapid changes in room temperature or variations in humidity that can aggravate or stimulate allergy symptoms.
   c. Weigh the benefits of air conditioning:
      (1) If it tends to circulate dust, it may be a source of irritation.
      (2) If it causes a marked change in temperature when the person moves from one part of the room to another, then it may be undesirable.
      (3) If it provides evenness of temperature, humidity, etc., it may be most desirable.
5. Smoking
   Encourage the patient as follows:
   a. Avoid smoking, since the smoker is exposed to pollutants likely to aggravate the respiratory passages.
   b. Make an effort to avoid areas where others are smoking.

B. Dietary Allergies

Advise the patient as follows:

1. Recognize the difficulties in trying to determine which foods cause allergic reactions.

2. Develop a pattern of eliminating a certain food for a period of time.
    a. Keep a diary, indicating when food was eliminated from the diet.
    b. Record any allergic reactions or the fact that none occurred.
3. Begin with those foods commonly found to cause reactions—nuts, chocolate, milk, strawberries, eggs, etc.
4. Remember to note contents of prepared foods, canned foods, etc. for the specific ingredients one may wish to avoid.
5. In a restaurant, order those foods which are certain not to include the offending ingredients.

    Note: Foods are considered a very rare cause of respiratory allergic symptoms.

C. Contact Allergies

Instruct the patient as follows:

1. Exert extra effort to avoid household items likely to bring on allergic reactions.
    a. Use gloves to avoid skin contact with detergents, fabric dyes, strong soap powders, etc.
    b. Use liquid soaps rather than granules that might permeate the air breathed.
2. Avoid cosmetics unless they are known to be hypoallergenic.
3. Do not rub or scratch itchy skin. (Mild doses of barbiturate or tranquilizers may be necessary if this will assist the patient in such control.)
4. Eliminate items of wearing apparel that irritate the skin, such as those made of wool or nylon. Note that permanent press cottons may be a cause of dermatitis.
5. Avoid overexertion, which causes perspiration and itchiness.

Administration of Medications

1. Warn the patient that it may be dangerous for him to drive during the first few days of antihistaminic therapy, since these medications may cause drowsiness.
2. Advise the patient to keep antihistamines out of reach of children—may cause serious accidental poisoning.
3. Utilize corticosteroids with caution because of side effects when administered over a long period of time.
    a. For short-term use, apply drops or ointment form of eye medication effective in relieving conjunctivitis and swollen eyelids.
    b. Avoid long-term use of eye corticosteroids because they may cause an increase in intraocular pressure.
4. When instilling nosedrops, have the patient lie on his back across the bed with his head hanging down; instill drops and have him remain in this position for 1 or 2 minutes; then have the patient turn over for another minute or 2 as though he were trying to look under the bed.
5. Caution the patient about the possibility of recurrent congestion when decongestants are used repeatedly; in such a situation, topical decongestant administration should be stopped.

Respiratory Hypersensitivity

Allergic Rhinitis (Hay Fever–Pollinosis)

Allergic rhinitis is induced by airborne pollens (seasonal); the body reacts by releasing histamine, which produces related symptoms.

Classification

(According to Season)
1. *Spring type*—March to early May
   Stimulated by pollens of certain trees (oak, elm, poplar)
2. *Summer type*—May to early July
   Stimulated by pollens of certain grasses (timothy, red top)
3. *Fall type*—August to the first frost
   Stimulated by pollens of ragweed family

Clinical Manifestations

1. Edematous, closed nostrils
2. Nasal mucous membranes—itch, burn, and secrete thin, irritating discharge
3. Sneezing—violent paroxysms
4. Eyes—red, burning, lacrimating

Diagnostic Evaluation

Sensitivity Tests

Skin tests confirm the patient's hypersensitivity to pollens.

Nursing Interventions

A. Maintaining effective breathing patterns

1. Use antihistamines; this will not only control symptoms in 4 of 5 patients but will also have an atropine-like drying effect.
   Be alert for individual reactions to antihistamines, since they are variable—sedation, depression, somnolence, incoordination.
2. If nasal obstruction is a persistent problem, a sympathomimetic may be given (effective for short-term but not long-term therapy).
   Pseudoephedrine hydrochloride (Sudafed), ephedrine sulfate, phenylpropanolamine (Propadrine), also combination products (Actifed, Dimetapp Extentabs)
3. Treat sinusitis and other otolaryngologic infections during symptom-free seasons.
4. Administer prophylactic injections of extract of pollens (specific for the individual); begin several months before the attacks and administer once a week throughout the peak season.
5. Resort to oral corticosteroids when antihistamines are not effective; these act by reducing the responsiveness of mucous membranes to histamine.

B. Preventing social isolation from attempts to avoid offending allergens

1. Advise the patient to consider moving to an area where pollen count is low; this, however, is often impractical.
2. Control indoor environment by removing irritating substances (e.g., pets, stuffed toys, feather pillows).
3. Avoid outside allergens by remaining indoors as much as possible, using air conditioning.

Health Education

1. See Nursing Interventions above.
2. If avoidance therapy is unsuccessful, hyposensitization may be used; also known as immunotherapy—in-

creases threshold level toward offending allergens (see p. 662).

Bronchial Asthma

Bronchial asthma is a reversible condition that manifests itself clinically by intermittent episodes of wheezing and dyspnea; it is generally associated with a hyperresponsive state of the bronchi, which may be antigen-mediated (allergic).

The main characteristic differentiating bronchial asthma from other pulmonary conditions is that the former is reversible.

Pathophysiology

1. Autonomic nerves are stimulated by irritants; this triggers mucous secretion and capillary dilatation.
   a. There appears to be a defect in the sympathetic nerves (beta-adrenergic end plates) in the bronchi.
   b. When exposed to stimulants to which they are particularly hypersensitive, these nerves fail to induce smooth muscle relaxation but instead cause contraction; they fail to decrease mucous secretion, and produce edema of bronchial mucosa.
2. Antibody-antigen reaction
   a. Susceptible individuals form abnormally large amounts of IgE when exposed to certain allergens.
   b. This immunoglobulin (IgE) fixes itself to the mast cells of the bronchial mucosa.
   c. When the individual is exposed to certain allergens, the resulting antigen combines with the cell-bound IgE molecules, causing the mast cell to degranulate and release chemical mediators.
   d. These chemical mediators, primarily histamine and slow reacting substance of anaphylaxis (SRS-A) are known to produce bronchospasm.
3. Other factors can precipitate an asthmatic attack.
   a. Respiratory tract infection
   b. Intolerance to certain drugs, such as aspirin, indomethacin
   c. Cold and sudden barometric changes
   d. Exercise
   e. Emotional upset
   f. Air pollutants—industrial chemicals

Classification

(Also see Table 15-1)

A. Extrinsic Bronchial Asthma

1. Cause
   a. Hypersensitivity reaction to inhalant allergens
   b. Mediated by immunoglobulin E (IgE-mediated)

2. Diagnostic evaluation
   a. Correlation with exposure to aeroallergens
   b. Positive skin tests
3. Major inhalant allergens
   House dust, mold spores, pollens, feathers, animal danders
4. Prognosis
   Favorable, with avoidance of offending allergens; good response to bronchodilators and specific therapy

B. Intrinsic Bronchial Asthma

1. Cause
   a. Nothing definite
   b. Infection—often present
   c. Skin tests of common inhalant antigens and foods are usually negative (non IgE-mediated)
2. Occurrence
   Primary onset before age 5 or after age 35
3. Prognosis
   a. Remission of intrinsic asthma is variable
   b. Control may be difficult

C. Mixed Asthma—immediate type appears to combine allergic reaction and infection

D. Aspirin-induced Asthma (ASA Sensitive)

(A type of intrinsic asthma induced by ingestion of aspirin and related compounds.)

1. Clinical manifestations spread over a period of time have been described as a "triad":
   a. Bronchial asthma
   b. Nasal polyposis
   c. Severe reactions to aspirin
2. Onset of symptoms after aspirin ingestion (20 min.–2 hrs)
   a. Watery rhinorrhea, followed by marked flushing of upper part of body
   b. Nausea, vomiting
   c. Wheezing, dyspnea, and cyanosis

Precipitating Factors

Any one of these may trigger an asthmatic attack in person with intrinsic bronchial asthma.

1. Strong odors (fumes)—turpentine, paints, chemicals, sprays, heavily scented flowers, perfumes, tobacco smoke
2. Cold air; sudden barometric changes
3. Air pollutants
4. Emotion-triggering situations

Assessment
Clinical Manifestations

1. There are symptom-free intervals.
2. During an attack of asthma, the amount of airway

Table 15-1 Suggested Clinical Grading of Asthma Severity*

Class	Description of Symptoms	Number of Attacks	Total Duration of Attacks	Restricted Activity or Work-loss Days	Bed Disability Days
Minimal	Annoying, but no marked discomfort	1–2/month	4 hours	1–2/month	0
Moderate	Marked discomfort, but not interfering with usual activities	2/week	4–10 hours	2/week	0
Severe	Some interference with sleep, but not incapacitating	Daily	11–20 hours	3 or more/week	Occasional
Severe (refractory)	Intolerable, diet and fluid restriction, unable to perform ordinary daily activities	Daily	Continuous	Total	2 or more/week

* Bernstein IL. Asthma in adults. In Conn HF (ed). Current Therapy, p. 584. Philadelphia, WB Saunders, 1980.

obstruction determines the degree of severity of symptoms.
   a. During early or mild episodes—dry cough, mild chest tightness
   b. As asthmatic episode becomes more severe—wheezing, coughing, shortness of breath; expiration more prolonged and laborious than inspiration.
   c. Dyspnea may become apparent; inspiratory wheezing and use of accessory respiratory muscles (bronchospasm).
   d. Weak pulse, sweating; cough becomes productive.
   e. As severity of attack increases, the patient becomes more anxious, restless, and apprehensive.
   f. A fatigue state may follow—respirations are less labored and there is less audible wheezing.
   g. This may lead to respiratory failure with hypercapnia, respiratory acidosis, and hypoxemia.
3. Rhinitis (swollen nasal mucosa) if extrinsic asthma.

Diagnostic Evaluation
1. Observation of an attack.
2. Pulmonary function studies usually show marked improvement after administration of a bronchodilator.
3. Bronchoprovocation techniques may be performed in a pulmonary function laboratory.
4. Sputum tests
   a. Mild asthma—foamy, clear, white
   b. More severe asthma—thicker and more tenacious
   c. Asthma with infection—purulent greenish, yellow
5. To establish baseline data, blood gas evaluation and simple spirometry may be required.
6. Increased eosinophil count for extrinsic allergic asthma.

Patient Problems/Nursing Diagnoses
1. Ineffective airway clearance related to bronchial constriction
2. Dyspnea and possible respiratory failure related to bronchial spasm and obstruction
3. Inadequate tissue perfusion related to reduction in oxygen intake
4. Anxiety related to severe dyspnea
5. Potential for secondary infection

Planning and Implementation
Treatment
Pharmacotherapy—This phase of management should be integrated with environmental control and immunotherapy; medications are administered in a stepwise approach—one drug is added at a time, and dosage is adjusted to achieve maximum benefit (Table 15-2).
General considerations:
1. Bronchodilators are used as follows:
   a. Short-term use to reverse asthmatic attacks.
   b. Long-term use to maintain ventilatory capacity as close to normal as possible.
2. The majority of patients with asthma will be well controlled with oral bronchodilators.
3. Sympathomimetics that are available as aerosols are epinephrine (least active), isoproterenol, metaproterenol.
4. There is limited use for sympathomimetic aerosols; they are used primarily to abort an attack or provide some breathing time before an oral medication takes effect (½–2 hours).

5. Subcutaneous and/or intravenous bronchodilators may be indicated for severe asthmatic attacks. Epinephrine and terbutaline are equally effective.
6. The great hazard associated with these medications is that they may be overused; this leads to excessive drying of the tracheobronchial tree and serious cardiac arrhythmias (see also Table 7-3, p. 188).

Nursing Interventions
A. Establishing optimum airway clearance and breathing
1. Administer pharmacotherapy as prescribed.
2. Administer oxygen during acute attack.
3. Elevate head of bed; use additional pillows.
4. Regulate temperature and humidity to comfortable levels.
5. Increase fluid intake to thin bronchial secretions.
6. Use chest physiotherapy to remove mucous plugs.

B. Relieving anxiety
1. Act calmly, reassuring patient during attack.
2. Administer mild sedatives and tranquilizers as prescribed.
3. Stay with patient until attack subsides.

C. Avoiding respiratory infection secondary to asthma
1. Give antibiotics prophylactically as prescribed.
2. Avoid crowds and sources of infection.

Health Education
1. Control the environment as much as possible to reduce number of allergens.
   a. Particularly in bedroom—eliminate dust (loose carpeting, draperies); remove feather pillows, wool blankets, dust-collecting articles.
   b. Exclude house pets, to eliminate dander.
   c. Exclude plants, to eliminate mold spores.
2. Promote optimal health practices—good nutrition, liberal fluids intake, adequate rest, sleep, and exercise.
3. Provide adequate hydration to keep secretions from thickening.
4. Avoid outdoors on high-humidity days.
5. Check Air Quality Index—stay indoors when index is poor, indicating high-pollution day.
6. Practice breathing exercises (may not be helpful).
7. Avoid cigarette smoking.
8. Do not overuse nebulizers; side/toxic effects may occur.
9. See physician promptly if respiratory or other infection suspected.
10. See also Nursing Interventions for Allergic Rhinitis.
11. There is no cure for asthma, but asthma can be controlled.

Evaluation
Outcome Criteria
1. Controls environment to prevent asthmatic attack
2. Monitors uncontrollable environmental factors which may precipitate attack, such as pollution index
3. Complies with treatment plan, including cautious use of pharmacotherapeutic agent
4. Utilizes coping mechanisms to control anxiety about condition
5. Maintains optimal health by adequate rest, exercise, fluids, and nutrition

Table 15-2 Commonly Used Medications: Bronchial Asthma

Drug	Action	Side Effects
1. Adrenergics		
A. Catecholamines		
Epinephrine (Adrenalin)	Stimulates alpha- and beta-adrenergic receptors of autonomic nervous system: alpha—vasoconstriction beta—bronchodilation A drug of choice because of its potent bronchodilating effect and rapidity of action	Pallor, tremulousness, tachycardia, arrhythmia, headache, nausea and vomiting
B. Noncatecholamines		
Isoproterenol (Isuprel)	Stimulates beta receptors found in smooth muscles of heart, bronchial wall and its capillaries—relaxes muscles and dilates blood vessels Duration of action is relatively short	Similar to those of epinephrine
Ephedrine	Stimulates beta receptors found in smooth muscles of heart, bronchial wall and its capillaries—relaxes muscles and dilates blood vessels Less potent than epinephrine and isoproterenol but can be given by mouth; also, duration of action is longer (3–6 hours)	Similar to epinephrine and isoproterenol
Metaproterenol (Metaprel, Alupent)	A potent, fast-acting beta-adrenergic stimulator Given orally or via metered dose inhaler Less active than terbutaline but superior to ephedrine as bronchodilator	Tachycardia, hypertension, palpitation, nervousness, tremor, nausea and vomiting, bad taste Less likely to cause peripheral muscle tremor than terbutaline
Terbutaline sulfate (Brethine, Bricanyl)	Of sympathomimetic amines, this drug has the least B_1 (cardiogenic) and most B_2 (bronchial smooth muscle) receptor action (oral therapy use) Bronchodilation is provided for 4–6 hours	Peripheral muscle tremor; tachycardia, decreased diastolic blood pressure
2. Methylxanthines		
Theophylline	Relaxes bronchial smooth muscles May be given orally or rectally	Nausea, vomiting, headache, epigastric pain, palpitation; agitation, insomnia, seizures
Aminophylline	Relaxes bronchial smooth muscles May be administered orally, rectally, or intravenously	Nausea, vomiting, epigastric distress

▶ **NURSING ALERT:** Guidelines for initiation and subsequent levels of aminophylline (theophylline products) have been set by FDA. Check drug package inserts. (Selected patients are monitored by measurement of serum theophylline concentration.)

Drug	Action	Side Effects
3. Cromolyn sodium (Intal)	Inhibits allergic reaction if inhaled *before* challenged by antigen. *Ineffective for acute bronchial asthmatic attacks.* Appears to act directly on mast cell and hinders release of chemical mediators (bronchoconstriction). Has no bronchodilator, anti-inflammatory, or antihistamine action.	Cough, hoarseness, rash, hypersensitivity, pneumonitis
4. Corticosteroids—*Use with caution*		
Oral, parenteral (Prednisone)	Indicated for severe symptoms with full therapy Effective inhibitor of asthmatic reaction	Fluid retention, weight gain, acne, hypertension, cushingoid state, gastritis, gastric ulcers, adrenal suppression, hypokalemia, psychosis
Inhalation Beclomethasone dipropionate (Beclovent, Vanceril)	Only small proportion is systemically absorbed	Local irritation from spray Short-term: Occasional growth of yeast organisms (*Monilia*) in mouth and pharynx Rinsing or gargling with water or half-strength hydrogen peroxide after inhalation usually prevents this. If unsuccessful, try topical nystatin. Long-term: Same side effects as listed above for oral administration
5. Anticholinergics		
(Atropine)	Most commonly given by inhalation Relaxes bronchial smooth muscles, causing bronchodilation	Mucosal drying, pulse changes, headache (uncommon)

Status Asthmaticus

Status asthmaticus is that state of severe bronchial asthma in which there is no response to conventional therapy (epinephrine, theophylline).
1. Alveolar hypoventilation has progressed to ventilatory failure—arterial pCO_2 is greater than 44 mm. Hg.
2. This is a medical emergency and requires extraordinary therapeutic measures.

Contributing Factors

1. CO_2 retention, followed by acidosis
2. Infection
3. Dehydration
4. Overuse of sedation

Clinical Manifestations

1. Hypoxia causes changes in the central nervous system—fatigue, headache, irritability, dizziness, impaired mental functioning.
2. With continued carbon dioxide retention—muscle twitching, somnolence, asterixis (intermittent lapse of an assumed posture—flapping tremor) diaphoresis.
3. Tachycardia, elevated blood pressure.
4. At very low oxygen levels and high carbon dioxide levels, sudden hypotension may occur.
5. Pulmonary vasoconstriction $\rightarrow$ heart failure, death from suffocation.

Treatment and Nursing Management

Requires team effort—including allergist, chest physician, anesthesiologist, and respiratory intensive care nurse.
1. Careful monitoring of pH, pCO_2, pO_2, in order to evaluate serially the changes in gas exchange and the patient's response to therapy.

Note: In early status asthmaticus, low pO_2 is followed by increased respiratory effort; this leads to low pCO_2 (hyperventilation). Then follow fatigue, reduced ventilation, and increasing pCO_2.

▶ **NURSING ALERT:** In status asthmaticus, the return to a normal or increasing pCO_2 does not necessarily mean that the asthmatic patient is improving—it may indicate a fatigue state that develops just before the patient slips into respiratory failure.

2. Correction of derangement of blood gases (hypoxemia) and hemoconcentration.
3. Rapid mobilization and removal of bronchial and bronchiolar secretions.
   a. Provide adequate hydration orally and intravenously; give humidified oxygen as prescribed.
   b. Administer expectorant and mucolytic drugs.
   c. Remove secretions by coughing, suctioning, or bronchoscopy and lavage.
4. Alleviate the patient's anxiety and fear with reassurance and the proper use of adequate doses of tranquilizers.
5. When intravenous fluids are administered, aminophylline may be prescribed and administered by constant infusion; the clinician must be constantly alert for signs of theophylline toxicity.
6. Many physicians administer corticosteroids, and since these act slowly, their beneficial effects may not be apparent for several hours.

Bibliography

Books

Altman LC. Clinical Allergy and Immunology. Boston, GK Hall, 1984

Dawson A and Simon RA. The Practical Management of Asthma. Orlando, FL, Grune & Stratton, 1984

Klaustermeyer WB. Practical Allergy and Immunology. New York, John Wiley & Sons, 1983

Lawlor GJ Jr and Fischer TJ. Manual of Allergy and Immunology. Boston, Little, Brown & Co, 1981

Lieberman PL and Crawford LV. Management of the Allergic Patient. New York, Appleton-Century-Crofts, 1982

Middleton E Jr et al. Allergy: Principles and Practice. St Louis, CV Mosby, 1983

Patterson R. Allergic Diseases. Philadelphia, JB Lippincott, 1980

Speer F. Handbook of Clinical Allergy. Littleton, MA, Wright PSG, 1982

Articles

Allergic Reaction

Adkinson NF Jr et al. Keeping current on allergy treatment. Patient Care 1984 Feb 15; 18(3):137–173

Buckley RH et al. Common "allergic" skin diseases. JAMA 1982 Nov 26; 248(20):2611–2621

Corn M. Assessment and control of environmental exposure. J Allergy Clin Immunol 1983 Mar; 72(3):231–241

Dolan B. A rapid desensitization. Am J Nurs 1982 Oct; 82(10):1532–1534

Elenhaas RM. Anaphylactic shock. Crit Care Q 1980 Mar; 2(4):77–84

Georgitis JW et al. Local intranasal immunotherapy for grass-allergic rhinitis. J Allergy Clin Immunol 1983 Jan; 71(1):71–76

Mathews KP. Urticaria and angioedema. J Allergy Clin Immunol 1983 Jan; 72(1):1–13

Metcalfe DD. Food hypersensitivity. J Allergy Clin Immunol 1984 Jun; 73(6):749–776

Wasserman SI. Mediators of immediate hypersensitivity. J Allergy Clin Immunol 1983 Feb; 72(2):101–114

Bronchial Asthma/Status Asthmaticus

Cherniak RM. Chronic and acute asthma. Postgrad Med 1984 Feb 1; 75(2):87–98

Fuchs PL. Asthma: Physiology, signs, and symptoms. Nursing '83 1983 Dec; 13(12):36–37

Griffin MP et al. Short- and long-term effects of cromolyn sodium on the airway reactivity of asthmatics. J Allergy Clin Immunol 1983 Mar; 71(3):331–338

Hudgel DW and Madsen LA. Acute and chronic asthma: A guide to intervention. Am J Nurs 1980 Oct; 80(10):1791–1795

Kirilloff LH and Tibbals SC. Drugs for asthma: A complete guide. Am J Nurs 1983 Jan; 83(1):55–61

McFadden ER Jr. Pathogenesis of asthma. J Allergy Clin Immunol 1984 Apr; 73(4):413–424

Mathews KP. Respiratory atopic disease. JAMA 1982 Nov 26; 248(20):2587–2610

Nursing Grand Rounds. Fighting the frustrations of status asthmaticus. Nursing '82 1982 Mar; 12(3):58–63

Raffen T and Roberts P. The prevention and treatment of status asthmaticus. Hosp Pract 1982 Feb; 17(2):80a–80z

Refas EM. Teaching patients to manage acute asthma. Nursing '83 1983 Apr; 13(4):77–82

Rogers TR. Clinical problems in the adult with asthma. Hosp Pract 1981 Feb; 16(2):293–297

Weinberger M. The pharmacology and therapeutic use of theophylline. J Allergy Clin Immunol 1984 May; 73(5):525–540

Agency

Asthma and Allergy Foundation of America
1302 18th Street NW
Washington, DC 20036

Metabolic and Endocrine Disorders

16

1: Disorders of the Thyroid Gland

The Thyroid Gland and Tests of Thyroid Function

Physiology

1. The thyroid gland affects the rate at which all tissues metabolize.
   a. Speed of chemical reactions
   b. Volume of oxygen consumed
   c. Amount of heat produced
2. The stimulating effect is through the production and distribution of 2 hormones:
   a. Levothyroxine (T_4)—contains 4 iodine atoms; maintains body's metabolism in a steady state; it is believed that T_4 serves as a precursor of T_3.
   b. Triiodothyronine (T_3)—contains 3 iodine atoms; is approximately 5 times as potent as thyroxine; has a more rapid metabolic action and utilization than thyroxine. Most conversion of T_4 to T_3 occurs at the cellular level in the periphery. Some T_3 is produced in the thyroid gland.

Diagnostic Evaluation

See also Physical Assessment, p. 27.

A. Serum Thyroxine (T_4)

1. It is a direct measurement of the concentration of total thyroxine in the blood; a good index of thyroid function when thyroxine-binding globulin (TBG) is normal.
2. Normal values: 4.5–11.5 μg./dl.
3. Normally elevated in pregnancy and with estrogen therapy.
4. Used to diagnose hypo- and hyperfunction of thyroid and to guide and evaluate therapy.

B. Serum Triiodothyronine (T_3)

1. Directly measures concentration of triiodothyronine in the blood; T_3 is much less stable than T_4 and occurs in minute quantities in the active form.
2. Useful to rule out T_3 thyrotoxicosis, hypo- and hyperfunction of the thyroid, to determine thyroid gland status, and to evaluate effects of thyroid replacement therapy.
3. Normal values: 110–130 ng./dl.
4. When the T_3 level is low, the patient is usually hypothyroid.

C. T_3 Resin Uptake

1. Is an indirect measure of thyroid function based on the available protein-binding sites in a serum sample that can bind to radioactive T_3.
2. The radioactive triiodothyronine is added to the serum sample in the test tube.
3. The effect of estrogen and pregnancy is to produce an increase in binding sites, causing a lowered percentage of binding by the available thyroid hormones.

4. Rates
   a. Normal binding: 25%–35%
   b. High T_3 is associated with hyperthyroidism
   c. Low T_3 is associated with hypothyroidism
5. This test is often used in conjunction with serum thyroxine (T_4).
6. Results may be altered if this patient has been taking estrogens, androgens, salicylates, or phenytoin.

D. Radioiodine (^{131}I) (^{99m}Tc)

1. ^{131}I uptake
   a. A solution of sodium iodide-131 is administered orally to the fasting patient.
   b. After a prescribed interval (anywhere from 2–48 hours, but frequently by 24 hours), measurements are taken with a scintillator of radioactive counts per minute that are detected above the isthmus of the thyroid gland.
   c. Normal thyroid will remove 15%–50% of the iodine from the bloodstream.
   d. Hyperthyroidism may result in the removal of as much as 90% of the iodine from the bloodstream.
2. Thyroidal iodide clearance
   a. Radioiodine clearance test measures the amount of circulating blood that is completely cleared of iodide per unit of time.
   b. Radioiodine is injected intravenously; radioactivity over the thyroid gland is measured continuously for 30–60 minutes—total amount of ^{131}I concentrated in the gland per minute is computed.
   c. Also, plasma ^{131}I content is measured in samples of blood collected 45–70 minutes after injection; these values are averaged.
   d. Thyroid ^{131}I divided by the mean plasma ^{131}I equals thyroid clearance (i.e., ml. of plasma cleared of iodide per minute).
   e. Normal   25 ml./minute
      Hyperthyroidism   250 ml./minute
      Hypothyroidism   1.6 ml./minute
3. ^{131}I excretion
   a. Urinary output of radioiodine is measured during 6-hour and 24-hour periods after ingestion.
   b. Normal   40%–80% of ingested
                          iodine in 24 hours
      Hyperthyroidism   less than 40%
      Hypothyroidism   greater than 80%
4. Thyroid "scan" ^{131}I
   a. The patient ingests sodium iodide-131 and is scanned the next day; if medium is given intravenously, the patient may be scanned within ½ to 1 hour.
   b. The patient is supine; the detector head of the scintillation camera is centered over the patient's neck.
   c. The thyroid images from the oscilloscope of the camera are recorded on film.
   d. Benign adenomas may be visualized as "hot" nodules, indicating increased uptake of iodine, or as "cold" nodules, indicating decreased uptake. Malignant nodules usually take the form of "cold" nodules.

5. Triiodothyronine (T_3) suppression test
   a. Measure 24-hour radioactive iodine uptake.
   b. Place the patient on T_3 for 7 days.
   c. Again measure 24-hour radioactive iodine uptake.
   d. Normal: suppression to a radioactive iodine uptake below 20% at 24 hours (half original value)
      Graves disease: no suppression

▶ **NURSING ALERT:** The use of radioactive substances is contraindicated in pregnancy. During pregnancy, thyroid testing is limited to blood testing.

Thyroid tests must be scheduled carefully so that thyroid-blocking contrast agents for other x-rays, diagnostic tests, and medications do not interfere with interpretation of tests of thyroid function.

E. Thyrotropin Radioimmunoassay (TSH)

1. Useful in differentiating between thyroid disorders due to disease of the thyroid gland itself and disorders due to disease of the pituitary or hypothalamus.
2. In patients with primary hypothyroidism, TSH levels are elevated.
   In secondary hypothyroidism (failure of the pituitary gland), TSH levels are low.
3. In patients with hyperthyroidism, TSH levels are low.
4. Blood sample is analyzed by radioimmunoassay.

F. Thyrotropin-releasing Hormone (TRH)

1. Have the patient fast overnight.
2. Fifteen minutes prior to TRH injection, draw a blood specimen.
3. Physician injects into arterial system 500 μg. synthetic TRH; draw blood specimen for thyroid-stimulating hormone (TSH).
4. Draw blood specimens at 15, 30, 45, 60, 90, and 120 minutes.

G. Protein-bound Iodine (PBI)—A conjugated molecule formed when thyroxine becomes attached to certain plasma protein fractions.

1. A reasonably accurate index of thyroid function is the concentration of PBI in the blood, but it is affected by many medications and conditions.
2. Normal values: 3.5–8.0 μg. (0.0035–0.0080 mg./100 ml. of plasma)
   a. Over 8.0—thyroid overactivity
   b. Under 3.5—hypothyroidism
3. In many health-care facilities, this test has been replaced by tests for serum T_3 and serum T_4.

▶ **NURSING ALERT:** Certain factors impair the PBI test:
1. Use of iodine skin antiseptic at venipuncture site
2. Ingestion of drugs or administration of dyes containing iodine
   a. Expectorants, cough syrups, etc.
   b. Dyes used in arteriogram, bronchogram, etc.
3. Mercurial diuretics, estrogens, sulfonamides, steroids, phenylbutazone, thiocyanates
4. Pregnancy

Hypothyroidism

Hypothyroidism may be classified as primary, secondary, or tertiary. *Primary hypothyroidism* is a condition resulting from the inability of the thyroid gland to secrete a sufficient amount of hormone. *Secondary hypothyroidism* is caused by a failure of the pituitary gland to secrete an adequate amount of TSH (thyroid-stimulating hormone).

Tertiary hypothyroidism results from failure of the hypothalamus to release thyroid-releasing hormone (TRH).

Cretinism is a severe form of hypothyroidism resulting from deficiency of thyroid function during fetal life or shortly after birth. The mother has usually had deficiency of thyroid hormone function during pregnancy.

Etiology

1. Primary hypothyroidism is the most common form of this condition and is generally due to
   a. Removal, destruction, or suppression of all or some of the thyroid tissue by thyroidectomy
   b. Use of radioactive iodine
   c. Overtreatment with antithyroid drugs
2. Hypothyroidism may also be idiopathic in origin or a result of chronic immunological dysfunction, as in Hashimoto's thyroiditis.

Pathophysiology

1. Inadequate secretion of thyroid hormone leads to a general slowing of all physical and mental processes.
2. There is a general depression of most cellular enzyme systems and oxidative processes.
3. The metabolic activity of all cells of the body decreases, reducing oxygen consumption, decreasing oxidation of nutrients for energy, and producing less body heat.
4. The signs and symptoms of the disorder range from vague, nonspecific complaints that make diagnosis difficult, to severe symptoms that may be life-threatening if unrecognized and untreated.

Assessment
Clinical Manifestations

1. Fatigue and lethargy.
2. Temperature and pulse become subnormal; unable to tolerate cold and desires room temperature increased.
3. Complains of cold hands and feet.
4. Menorrhagia or amenorrhea; may have difficulty conceiving or experiences spontaneous abortion.
5. Mental processes become dulled; develops loss of memory.
6. Gain weight.
7. Hair thins and falls out; skin becomes thickened and dry.
8. Develops severe constipation.
9. Neurologic signs develop (polyneuropathy, cerebellar ataxia); muscle aches or weakness, clumsiness.
10. Facial expression becomes solid and mask-like; later, facial bloating and pallor develop.
11. In severe hypothyroidism, hypotension, unresponsiveness, bradycardia, hypoventilation, hyponatremia, (possibly) convulsions, hypothermia, cerebral hypoxia, and myxedema may occur.
12. Accelerated atherosclerosis and coronary artery disease may occur because of deposits of mucopolysaccharides in myocardium.
13. Increased susceptibility to all hypnotic and sedative drugs and anesthetic agents.
14. Has a mortality rate of 50%.

Diagnostic Evaluation

1. T_3 and T_4 levels are low.
2. Thyroid-stimulating hormone levels are elevated in primary hypothyroidism.
3. Elevation of serum cholesterol.
4. ECG—sinus bradycardia, low-voltage of QRS complexes, and flat or inverted T waves.

5. Prolonged deep tendon reflex response, especially ankle jerk.
6. The patient's past medical history may reveal previous treatment with radioactive iodine.
7. Complete physical examination may reveal subtle signs of hypothyroidism or a general suppression and depression of organs and systems.

Patient Problems/Nursing Diagnoses

The patient with severe hypothyroidism experiences multiple systemic problems, including:

1. Potential alteration in cardiac output related to decreased metabolic rate, decreased cardiac conduction, elevated cholesterol levels, atherosclerosis, and coronary artery disease
2. Activity intolerance related to lethargy and fatigue, depressed neuromuscular status
3. Alterations in fluid and nutritional status related to decreased metabolic rate, poor appetite, and depressed gastrointestinal function.

Planning and Implementation
Treatment

A. Approach

1. The medical management depends on the severity of the patient's symptoms and may necessitate replacement therapy in mild cases or life-saving support and treatment for the patient with severe hypothyroidism and myxedema coma.
2. As the patient's thyroid hormone levels are gradually returned to normal, the patient is also monitored closely to prevent complications resulting from sudden increases in metabolic rate and oxygen requirements.

B. Objective of Medical Management: to restore a normal metabolic state (euthyroid) **as rapidly and safely as possible.**

1. Administer thyroid hormone—levothyroxine (Synthroid, Levothroid), thyroglobulin (Proloid), liotrix (Euthroid, Thyrolar). Give once a day.
   a. Because triiodothyronine acts more quickly than thyroxine, give this initially; if the patient is unconscious, give via stomach tube.
   b. Administer sodium levothyroxine (Synthroid) parenterally (until consciousness is restored) to restore thyroxine level; continue daily.
   c. Later, continue the patient on oral thyroid hormone therapy.
   d. Recognize that with rapid administration of thyroid hormone, plasma thyroxine levels may initiate adrenal insufficiency—hence, steroid therapy may be initiated.
2. Monitor the patient carefully to anticipate such effects of treatment as:
   a. Diuresis, decreased puffiness
   b. Improved reflexes and muscle tone
   c. Accelerated pulse rate
   d. A slightly higher level of total serum thyroxine

Nursing Interventions

A. Improved cardiac output

1. Control factors that increase metabolic rate and threaten cardiovascular status
   a. Monitor vital signs frequently to detect changes in the patient's cardiovascular status and ability to respond to stress.
   b. Monitor ECG tracings to detect arrhythmias and deterioration of cardiovascular status.

   c. Prevent and treat factors that increase metabolic rate (infection, stress, trauma).

   d. Prevent chilling to avoid increasing metabolic rate, which, in turn, places strain on the heart. Provide bed socks, bed jacket, warm environment.

   e. Even though hypothermia exists, do not apply external heat, since the resulting increased oxygen requirements and decreased peripheral vascular tone may compound the existing cardiac failure.

   f. Administer fluids cautiously even though hyponatremia is present.

   g. Give glucose in concentrated amounts to prevent fluid overload if hypoglycemia is in evidence.

2. Administer all drugs with caution before and after thyroid replacement begins.

   a. Before treatment with thyroid hormone, the patient is susceptible to the effects of sedatives, narcotics, anesthetics, and other medications.

   b. After thyroid replacement is initiated, the thyroid hormones may increase the effects of digitalis and anticoagulants.

3. Report occurrence of angina, and the signs and symptoms of myocardial infarction and cardiac failure.

4. Monitor arterial blood gases to assess cardiopulmonary function.

5. Instruct the patient how and when to take medications.

6. Instruct the patient about signs and symptoms of insufficient and excessive medication.

B. Increased activity tolerance and a balance of rest and activity

1. Limit visitors during acute stage to prevent excessive stimulation

2. Carry out activities, hygiene, and care for the patient during acute stage of illness.

3. Prevent pulmonary complications of immobility during acute stage by turning, and encouraging the patient to cough and take deep breaths.
Provide assisted ventilation if needed to combat hypoventilation.

4. Encourage very gradual resumption of activities as severe symptoms begin to subside and the patient begins to improve.

5. Assist the patient in planning activities to limit exertion and provide ample periods of rest.

6. Identify for the patient signs and symptoms indicating excessive exertion.

7. Provide good skin care to prevent skin breakdown secondary to immobility.

   a. Apply lubricant to the skin, since it is usually dry and scaly.

   b. Observe for pressure areas and initiate measures to stimulate circulation to these areas.

C. Improved Fluid and Nutritional Status

1. Administer prescribed foods and fluids cautiously during acute stage.

2. Offer oral fluids and food gradually and carefully.

3. Assess the patient's dietary preferences.

4. Serve attractive, low-calorie meals; this patient is usually overweight, although his appetite is poor.

5. Offer fluids frequently and include dietary fiber to prevent constipation.

6. Assess return and gradual increase of gastrointestinal function (return of bowel sounds, absence of abdominal distention, occurrence and frequency of bowel movements).

7. Administer stool softeners if necessary.

8. Discourage straining at stool because of increased strain on the heart.

Evaluation
Expected Outcomes

1. Experiences/demonstrates improved cardiac status and output—normal blood pressure and pulse rate; normal ECG tracing (normal amplitude and return of normal T wave)

2. Avoids factors and events that increase metabolic rate (trauma, respiratory or other infections, stressful situations)

3. Reports absence of chest pain, dyspnea, or palpitations

4. Reports increased sense of warmth to a comfortable level (decreased sensitivity or intolerance to cold)

5. Identifies appropriate schedule of medications and takes medications as prescribed

6. Identifies signs and symptoms of hypo- and hyperthyroidism that should be reported

7. Demonstrates increased activity tolerance:

   a. Plans activities and exercise to allow adequate periods of rest and relaxation

   b. Ceases activities if signs and symptoms of cardiac dysfunction develop

   c. Reports increased strength and well-being; decreased fatigue and lethargy

   d. Participates in own care and hygiene

8. Takes measures to prevent respiratory complications and skin breakdown—turns frequently when in bed; coughs and takes deep breaths

9. Reports absence of respiratory complications or infections

10. Demonstrates adequate fluid and nutritional intake:

   a. Identifies foods encouraged in diet; consumes low-calorie meals

   b. Avoids foods restricted in diet

   c. Reports loss of weight and absence of edema

   d. Drinks adequate fluids daily

11. Reports return of normal bowel function and decrease in gastrointestinal disturbances and constipation

Hyperthyroidism

Hyperthyroidism (diffuse toxic goiter) is excessive activity of the thyroid gland.

Incidence

More common in women than in men; occurs in about 2% of the female population.

Types

1. Graves' disease (most prevalent)—diffuse hyperfunction of the thyroid gland associated with ophthalmopathy; most common in younger women; may subside spontaneously.

2. Toxic nodular goiter (single or multiple)—more

common in older females with preexisting goiter; will continue to be overactive unless eradicated or kept under suppressive therapy.

Etiology

1. Unknown; immunologic origin is likely
2. Possible causes
   a. Thyroid-stimulating antibody (TSA$_b$; formerly LATS—long-acting thyroid stimulator) correlates very closely with the clinical course of Graves' disease.
   b. TSA$_b$, an immunoglobulin found in the blood of patients with Graves' disease, is capable of reacting with the receptor for TSH on the thyroid plasma membrane and stimulating glandular function.
   c. May appear after an emotional shock, infection, or emotional stress.
   d. Genetic predisposition, female sex.
   e. B and T lymphocytes (immunologic factors) have been implicated.

Pathophysiology

1. Hyperthyroidism is characterized by hypertrophy and hyperplasia of the thyroid gland, which is accompanied by increased vascularity and blood flow and enlargement of the gland.
2. A hypermetabolic condition results from the excessive secretion of thyroid hormone, resulting in exaggeration of all metabolic processes.
3. The majority of cases of hyperthyroidism are thought to be due to an autoimmune reaction in which circulating autoantibodies mimic the action of TSH and increase the secretion of thyroid hormone.
4. Most of the clinical manifestations result from increased metabolic rate, excessive heat production, increased neuromuscular and cardiovascular activity, and hyperactivity of the sympathetic nervous system.
5. Hyperthyroidism ranges from a mild increase in metabolic rate to the severe hyperactivity known as thyrotoxicosis, thyroid storm, or thyroid crisis.
6. A patient with mild hyperthyroidism is not usually admitted to the hospital unless admitted for another problem and the hyperthyroidism is initially unsuspected.
7. The patient with severe thyrotoxicosis or thyroid crisis, however, is admitted to control the hypermetabolic state, prevent cardiac failure, or prepare for surgery.

Assessment

Diagnostic Evaluation

1. T$_3$ and T$_4$ are elevated.
2. T$_3$ resin uptake; hyperthyroidism is suspected if elevated.
3. PBI is elevated in hyperthyroidism.
4. Complete physical examination reveals a hypermetabolic state.
5. A bruit or thrill over the thyroid can often be detected because of the increased blood flow.
6. Thyroid gland may be palpable on examination.

Clinical Course and Manifestations

1. Nervousness, emotional hyperexcitability, irritability, apprehension
2. Difficulty in sitting quietly
3. Rapid pulse, at rest as well as on exertion (ranges between 90 and 160); palpitation
4. Low heat tolerance; profuse perspiration; flushed skin (e.g., hands may be warm, soft, moist)
5. Fine tremor of hands; change in bowel habits—constipation or diarrhea
6. Increased appetite and progressive weight loss
7. Muscle fatigability and weakness; amenorrhea
8. Atrial fibrillation possible (cardiac decompensation common in elderly patients)
9. Bulging eyes (exophthalmos)—produces a startled expression
10. Course may be mild, characterized by remissions and exacerbations
11. It may progress to emaciation, extreme nervousness, delirium, disorientation, thyroid storm or crisis, and death
12. *Thyroid storm or crisis,* an extreme form of hyperthyroidism, is characterized by hyperpyrexia, diarrhea, dehydration, tachycardia, arrhythmias, extreme irritation, delirium, coma, shock, and death if not adequately treated (Fig. 16-1).
13. Thyroid storm may be precipitated by stress (surgery, infection, etc.) or inadequate preparation for surgery in a patient with known hyperthyroidism.

Medical Management/Treatment

Immediate Treatment

For severe hyperthyroidism or thyroid storm

A. Restoring and maintaining vital functions

1. The patient is hospitalized if thyroid storm or other complications, such as heart failure, are imminent.
2. Sedatives such as phenobarbital or tranquilizers such as chlordiazepoxide (Librium) are given to combat nervousness, hyperactivity, and irritability.
   Intravenous barbiturates may be necessary to control agitation.
3. Temperature may be lowered with a hypothermia blanket or cooling mattress and salicylates.
4. Phenothiazines in large doses may be prescribed for hyperpyrexia, but watch for hypotension.
5. Administer fluids, electrolytes, and vasopressor agents to treat dehydration, electrolyte imbalance, and hypotension.
6. Administer digitalis if heart failure or atrial fibrillation occurs.
7. Give propranolol for sinus tachycardia and other supraventricular arrhythmias.
8. Give steroids because of possibility of a relative adrenal insufficiency state.
9. Sustain nutritional requirements with glucose administered intravenously; administer vitamin B.
   Guard against infection; treat if infection is likely.
10. Give vitamin supplements to offset demands of appetite which may continue after hyperthyroidism is controlled.

B. Controlling synthesis and release of thyroid hormone

1. Administer sodium iodide intravenously—inhibits release of hormone from thyroid.
2. Give methimazole or propylthiouracil orally or by nasogastric tube to prevent accumulation of hormone stores.

C. Diminishing metabolic effects of thyroid agents and reversing peripheral effects of hyperthyroidism

Administer propranolol, reserpine, or guanethidine.

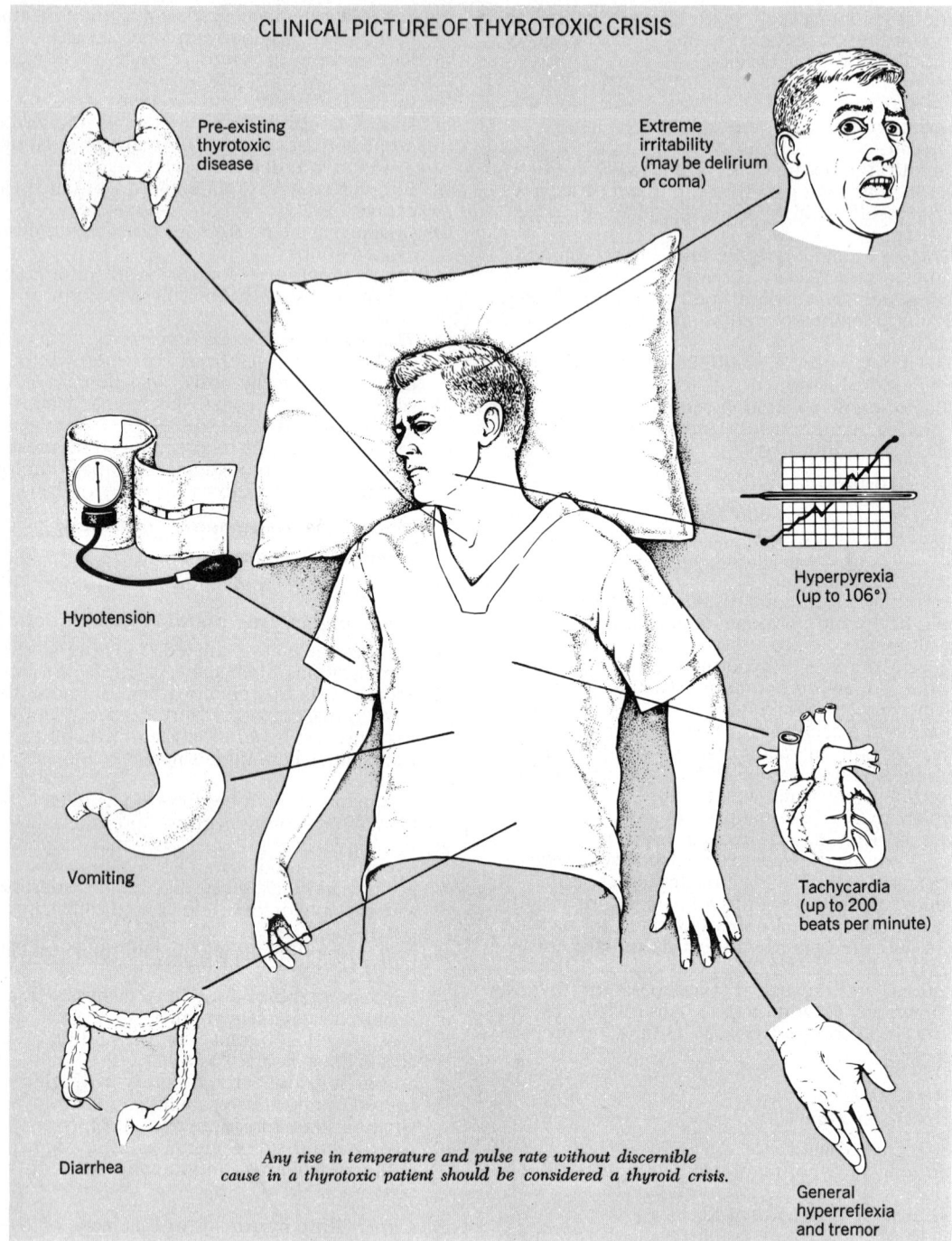

Figure 16-1. Thyrotoxic crisis. (From Hospital Medicine 3[1]:39, by permission; © Hospital Publications, Inc.)

Other Modalities of Treatment

1. General considerations
   a. Types of treatment—pharmacology, radiation, and surgery.
   b. Treatment depends on causes, age of patient, severity of disease, and complications.
2. According to causes
   a. Remission of hyperthyroidism (Graves' disease) occurs spontaneously within 1–2 years; however, relapse can be expected in half of the patients. All 3 forms of therapy are appropriate.
   b. Nodular toxic goiter—excessive amounts of thyroid hormone secreted.
      Surgery or use of radioiodine is preferred.
   c. Thyroid carcinoma.
      Surgery or radiation.

3. According to age of patient
    a. Radioiodine therapy may be used in all patients, regardless of age, when other forms of therapy are contraindicated.
    b. Use radioiodine in older patients for whom surgery is contraindicated.
    c. Radioiodine therapy is contraindicated in pregnancy and in women of childbearing age.
4. According to severity
    Administer drug therapy before proceeding with use of radioiodine or surgery.
5. According to patient preference
    a. Radioiodine or surgery is suggested to the patient who does not take medication regularly.
    b. Surgery is recommended to those who prefer it.

Pharmacotherapy—Drugs That Inhibit Hormone Formation

Goal:
To bring the metabolic rate to normal as soon as possible and maintain it at this level.

Anticipated Results
1. Diagnosis can be confirmed if the patient responds to antithyroid therapy.
2. Autonomic nervous system is brought into balance and the patient is more comfortable.
3. Opportunity is provided for getting to know the patient.

A. Thionamides
1. Preparations
    a. Propylthiouracil
    b. Methimazole (Tapazole)
       (1) Carbimazole—a derivative of methimazole
2. Action
    a. Depresses the synthesis of thyroid hormone by inhibiting peroxidase.
    b. It has been standard practice to give these medications in divided daily doses (every 8 hours); experimental evidence appears to indicate that once-a-day dosage is effective for 24 hours or longer. Patient compliance is better with this latter medication schedule.
3. Assessment and duration of treatment determined by clinical criteria
    a. Observe clinical course—thyroid gland usually gets smaller.
    b. Measure T_4 and T_3 uptake to determine adequacy of dose.
    c. Continue treatment until patient becomes clinically euthyroid; this varies from 3 months to 1–2 years; if euthyroidism cannot be maintained without therapy, then another form of therapy (i.e., RAI or surgery) should be recommended.
    d. Withdraw therapy gradually to prevent exacerbation.
    e. For relapses, recommend radioiodine or surgery.
4. Toxicity
    a. Agranulocytosis is a most serious toxic condition, occurring with a sudden onset—therefore, the patient should be apprised of this possibility and urged to report any signs of infection, such as fever, sore throat, upper respiratory infection.
    b. Skin rashes, fever, urticaria, granulopenia, inflammation of the salivary glands are other possible side effects.
    c. Substitute an alternate drug if there are toxic manifestations.

Pharmacotherapy—Drugs That Control Peripheral Manifestations of Hyperthyroidism

Propranolol (Inderal)
1. Acts as a beta-adrenergic blocking agent
2. Abolishes tachycardia, tremor, excess sweating, nervousness
3. Controls hyperthyroid symptoms until antithyroid drugs or radioiodine can take effect

Radioactive Iodine
1. Action
    a. Limits secretion of thyroid hormone by destroying thyroid tissue.
    b. Control dosage so that hypothyroidism does not occur.
2. Advantages and disadvantages
    a. Chief advantage of radioiodine over thionamides is that a lasting remission can be achieved.
    b. Chief disadvantage is that permanent hypothyroidism can be produced in patients treated with radioiodine.
3. Considerations in use
    a. Radiation thyroiditis, a transient exacerbation of hyperthyroidism, may occur as a result of leakage of thyroid hormone into the circulation from damaged follicles.
    b. Iodide should not be given prior to radioiodine, since it interferes with the uptake of ^{131}I.
    c. Vigilance is required during and after treatment to detect occurrence of hypothyroidism.
    d. Use during pregnancy can cause fetal death or hypothyroidism (cretinism) in the infant.

Psychotherapy
1. Greater emphasis is being placed on the effect that psychogenic factors have on the severity of this disease.
2. A determination needs to be made in caring for each patient about whether psychotherapy would be of value in preventing exacerbations.
3. The patient and family may require psychological support because of the disturbance caused by the irritability and outbursts related to the patient's hypermetabolic state.

Surgery
Surgery is an effective treatment modality in selected patients, those with very large goiters or those for whom the use of radioiodine or thionamides is contraindicated.

A. Subtotal Thyroidectomy
Effective in treating hyperthyroidism; involves removal of most of the thyroid gland.

B. Preparation for Surgery
1. The patient must be euthyroid at time of surgery.
2. Administer thionamides to control hyperthyroidism.
3. Give iodide to increase firmness of thyroid gland and reduce its vascularity.

▶ **NURSING ALERT:** Observe the patient for evidence of iodine toxicity—swelling of buccal mucosa, excessive salivation, coryza, skin eruptions. If these occur, discontinue iodides.

C. Complications
1. Damage to recurrent laryngeal nerve may occur (1%–4%).

a. Unilateral damage—results in minimal voice change.
b. Bilateral damage—serious airway obstruction develops.

2. Hypothyroidism
Occurs in 5% of patients in first postoperative year; increases at rate of 2%–3%/year

3. Hypoparathyroidism
a. About 4% occurrence.
b. Usually is mild and transient.
c. Requires calcium supplements intravenously and orally when more severe.

D. Nursing Management—see page 679

Patient Problems/Nursing Diagnoses

The patient problems encountered in hyperthyroidism depend on the severity of the disorder and occur in varying degrees. In general, the patient could be expected to experience:

1. Alterations in fluid, electrolyte, and nutritional balance related to hypermetabolic state, increased fluid and calorie requirement, and fluid loss through diaphoresis

2. Potential impaired skin integrity related to extreme diaphoresis, pyrexia, excessive restlessness, movement and tremor, and rapid weight loss

3. Altered thought processes related to insomnia, decreased attention span, and irritability

4. Apprehension and anxiety related to concern about upcoming surgery

Planning and Implementation
Nursing Interventions

A. Improved Fluid, Electrolyte, and Nutritional Intake

1. Assess the patient's fluid, electrolyte, and nutritional requirements.
2. Determine the patient's food and fluid preferences.
3. Provide high-calorie foods and fluids consistent with the patient's requirements.
4. Provide a quiet, calm environment at meals.
5. Restrict stimulants (tea, coffee, alcohol).
6. Explain rationale of requirements and restrictions to patient.
7. Encourage/permit the patient to eat alone if embarrassed or otherwise disturbed by voracious appetite.
8. Maintain intravenous infusion if indicated to maintain fluid, nutritional, and electrolyte balance.
9. Monitor fluid and nutritional status by weighing the patient daily and keeping accurate intake and output records.
10. Monitor vital signs to detect changes in fluid volume status.
11. Assess skin turgor, mucous membranes, and neck veins for signs of increased or decreased fluid volume.
12. Provide supplementary vitamins, particularly thiamine chloride and ascorbic acid.

B. Improved Skin Integrity

1. Assess skin frequently to detect diaphoresis.
2. Bathe frequently with cool water; change linens when damp.
3. Provide cool environment to prevent pyrexia; use fans or air conditioning.
4. Use hypothermia unit, antipyretics, cool water, ice packs, or alcohol baths to reduce body temperature; avoid shivering.
5. Protect and massage bony prominences while immobilized or while hypothermia unit/mattress is in use.
6. Monitor rectal temperature frequently; report elevations in temperature.

C. Promotion of Normal Thought Processes

1. Explain procedures to patient in an unhurried, calm manner.
2. Limit visitors; avoid stimulating conversations or television programs.
3. Reduce stressors in the environment; reduce noise and lights.
4. Promote sleep and relaxation through use of prescribed medications, massage, and relaxation exercises; draw the blinds for nap times.
5. Minimize disruption of the patient's sleep or rest by clustering nursing activities.
6. Employ safety measures to reduce risk of trauma or falls (padded side rails, maintain bed in low position).
7. Encourage the patient to verbalize concerns and fears about illness, treatment, and possible surgery.
8. Be selective in placing a suitable roommate with the patient (preferably one who is convalescing).
9. Gain the patient's confidence and attempt to uncover anything that might cause aggravation or unhappiness; if a disturbance exists, it could thwart treatment efforts.

Evaluation
Expected Outcomes

1. Achieves adequate fluid, electrolyte, and nutritional intake
2. Maintains normal fluid and electrolyte balance as measured by serum electrolyte levels and vital signs
3. Demonstrates normal skin turgor, moist mucous membranes, and normal neck vein distention
4. Reports and records balance of urine output and fluid intake
5. Demonstrates skin integrity—skin is dry, cool and intact without reddened, excoriated or infected areas
6. Reports improved tolerance to heat or warmth; normal rectal temperature
7. Demonstrates improved thought processes:
a. Maintains concentration, follows conversation and responds appropriately
b. Verbalizes concerns and fears about illness, treatment, and possible surgery
c. Interacts with family members and visitors
8. Uses medications as prescribed and relaxation techniques to promote sleep and relaxation
9. Reports increased sense of well-being, decreased fatigue and lethargy

Ophthalmopathy in Hyperthyroidism

Exophthalmos is abnormal protrusion of the eyeball, probably due to an autoimmune phenomenon.

Proptosis—a forward bulging (displacement) of the eye.

Ophthalmoplegia—paralysis of the eye muscle.

Goal:
Protect eyes from irritation.

A. Mild

1. Recommend wearing sunglasses.
2. Instill methylcellulose eyedrops 0.5%–1% (Tearisol) for comfort; relief from pain and burning.
3. Advise the patient to elevate his head while sleeping to improve drainage.

B. Rapidly Progressive or Severe (chemosis, conjunctivitis, proptosis, visual impairment)

1. Tarsorrhaphy (suturing eyelids together) may be required to extend lid when proptosis is so marked that lid does not close during sleep. Operation will prevent corneal ulceration.
2. Administer corticosteroids in high doses to help arrest rapid progression of exophthalmos; with improvement, reduce dose.

C. Muscle Surgery

1. Correction of imbalance of extraocular muscles.
2. Lysis of adhesions.

D. Orbital Decompression Procedures

(Performed only if vision is threatened.)

1. Decompression of orbit into ethmoid sinus and maxillary antrum (Ogura procedure).
2. Removal of lateral orbital wall (Krönlein operation).
3. Decompression of orbit into cranial cavity (Naffziger operation).

Medical and Nursing Management of the Patient Undergoing Thyroidectomy

Preoperative Care

A. Provide a restful and therapeutic environment (see discussion, p. 76)

B. Promote adequate nutritional intake (see discussion, p. 79)

C. Support the patient undergoing various diagnostic tests to determine nature of the endocrine problem or to ensure a euthyroid state prior to surgery

1. Explain the purpose and requirements of each prescribed test.
2. Inform the patient and visitors of safeguards required during radioisotope tests.
3. Remind the patient that he must remain in his room until tests are completed, if indicated.
4. Explain results of tests if unclear to the patient or questions arise.

D. Prepare the patient for surgery

1. Shave the upper chest, neck (bedline to bedline), up to chin edge.
2. Make a special effort to ensure that this patient has a good night's rest preceding surgery.
3. Explain to the patient that speaking is to be minimized immediately postoperatively and that oxygen may be administered to facilitate breathing.
4. Explain that postoperatively, fluids may be given intravenously to maintain fluid, electrolyte, and nutritional needs; glucose may also be given intravenously in the hours before the administration of anesthesia.
5. Proceed with usual preoperative preparation (see pp. 75, 84).

Postoperative Care

A. Provide optimum immediate postoperative care to avoid complications

1. Move the patient carefully; provide adequate support to the head, so that no tension is placed on the sutures.
2. Place the patient in semi-Fowler's position with the head elevated and supported by pillows; avoid flexion of neck.
3. Administer humidified oxygen if breathing is labored.
4. Check the infusion for prescribed flow rate.
5. Avoid administration of epinephrine, norepinephrine, cholinergic depressants (atropine) because of the patient's sensitivity to these drugs.
6. Discontinue antithyroid drugs as a metabolic rate closer to normal is attained (to continue such medication might cause hypometabolism–hypothyroidism).

B. Assess the patient's condition as he emerges from anesthesia

1. Damage of laryngeal nerve
   a. Observe for hoarseness or "whispery" voice suggesting possible nerve damage.
   b. Encourage voice rest except when assessing for hoarseness or other change.
   c. Recognize that a bilateral flaccid paralysis may lead to cord paralysis → closure of glottis → suffocation, months after operation.
2. Hemorrhage
   a. Be alert for this possibility between 12 and 24 hours postoperatively.
   b. Observe for bleeding at sides and back of the neck, as well as anteriorly, when the patient is in dorsal position.
   c. Reinforce dressing if indicated.
   d. Note and report hypotension, tachycardia, and other signs of hypovolemia and shock.
   e. Watch for signs of irregular breathing, swelling, and choking—signs pointing to the possibility of hemorrhage (see p. 92) and tracheal compression.
   f. Keep a tracheostomy set in the patient's room for 48 hours for emergency use.
3. Tetany
   a. The likelihood that tetany may develop depends on the number of parathyroid glands that have been removed or disturbed:
      1—no clinical tetany
      2—tetany mild and transient
      4—tetany within 24 hours and worsening within the next 24 hours
   b. Progression of signs
      (1) First—tingling of toes and fingers and around the mouth; apprehension
      (2) Second—positive Chvostek's sign (tapping the cheek over the facial nerve causes a twitch of the lip or facial muscles)
      (3) Third—Trousseau's sign (carpopedal spasm induced by occluding circulation in the arm with a blood pressure cuff)

C. Medical and nursing management of tetany

1. Position the patient for optimal ventilation; pillow removed to prevent head from bending forward and compressing trachea.
2. Keep siderails in position and position the patient to prevent injury if a seizure occurs; do not use restraints, since they only aggravate the patient and may result in muscle strain or fractures.
3. Have equipment available to treat respiratory difficulties; provide tracheostomy and cardiac arrest equipment.
4. Determine calcium levels: If in 48 hours, level falls below 7½ mg./100 ml. (3 mEq.), replacement of calcium (gluconate, lactate) is done intravenously.
5. Use caution in intravenous administration of calcium to the patient who has renal disease or who is receiving digitalis preparations.

Other Thyroid-Related Conditions

Subacute Thyroiditis

Subacute thyroiditis is usually a self-limiting inflammation of the thyroid gland.

Incidence

Affects younger women predominantly.

Clinical Manifestations

1. Pain, swelling, thyroid tenderness, which lasts several weeks or months, then disappears
2. Temperature elevation, sore throat
3. Pain referred to the ear, making swallowing difficult and uncomfortable
4. Fever, malaise, chills
5. May develop clinical manifestations of hyperthyroidism (irritability, nervousness, insomnia, and weight loss) or hypothyroidism.

Management

1. Administer analgesics and mild sedatives; encourage activities that will promote psychosocial comfort.
2. The patient may be placed on thyroid medications to maintain a normal level of circulating thyroid hormone.
3. Steroids may be administered in active inflammatory stage.
4. Aspirin may be indicated in mild cases to treat the symptoms of inflammation.

▶ **NURSING ALERT: Aspirin should be avoided if the patient exhibits signs of hyperthyroidism; because it displaces thyroid hormone from its binding sites, it increases the amount of circulating hormone and the degree and severity of the symptoms of hyperthyroidism.**

Lymphocytic Thyroiditis
(Hashimoto's Thyroiditis)

Lymphocytic thyroiditis (*Hashimoto's thyroiditis*) is a chronic progressive disease of the thyroid gland caused by infiltration of lymphocytes and resulting in progressive destruction of the parenchyma and hypothyroidism if untreated.

Cause

Unknown; believed to be an autoimmune disease, genetically transmitted and perhaps related to Graves' disease.

Incidence

1. Ninety-five percent of the cases affect women in their 40s or 50s.
2. Possibly the most common cause of adult hypothyroidism.
3. Appears to be increasing in incidence since first described in 1912.

Clinical Manifestations

1. Marked by a slowly developing, firm enlargement of the thyroid gland.
2. Usually no gross nodules.
3. Basal metabolic rate usually low.

4. Normal or high concentration of protein-bound iodine.

Diagnostic Testing

1. Twenty-four-hour radioactive iodine (RAI) uptake
2. Thyroid scan
3. Resin T_3 uptake determination
4. Thyroid needle biopsy
5. T_3 and T_4 usually become subnormal as the disease progresses

Treatment and Nursing Management

1. The patient should be placed on thyroid medications to maintain a normal level of circulating thyroid hormone; this is done to suppress production of thyrotropin, to prevent enlargement of the thyroid and/or to maintain a euthyroid state.
2. Propranolol is often prescribed to control symptoms of thyrotoxicosis if they occur.
3. Firm nodular thyroid enlargement may at times be associated with tracheal compression, cough, hoarseness. Resection of the isthmus can produce relief of symptoms (see discussion, p. 679).
4. The patient is followed closely to detect and treat hypothyroidism and myxedema.

Cancer of the Thyroid

Incidence

1. It has been estimated that of the thyroid lumps that occur in 40,000 of 1,000,000 persons in any 1 year, only 25 will be cancerous; this is a relatively rare disease but one that is increasing in incidence.
2. It occurs twice as frequently in females as in males and more frequently in whites than in blacks; incidence increases with age. The average age at time of diagnosis is 45.
3. It appears well-established that an association exists between external radiation to the head and neck in infancy and childhood and subsequent development of thyroid carcinoma. (Between 1949 and 1960 radiation therapy was often given to shrink enlarged tonsil and adenoid tissue, to treat acne, or to reduce an enlarged thymus.)
The American Thyroid Association emphasizes that these individuals should:
   a. Consult a physician
   b. Request an isotope thyroid scan as part of the evaluation
   c. Submit to surgical thyroidectomy or take thyroid hormones if abnormalities of the glands are present
   d. Continue with annual checkups if all is normal

Types

1. Papillary and well-differentiated adenocarcinoma (most common)
   a. Growth is slow, and spread is confined to lymph nodes that surround thyroid area.
   b. Cure rate is excellent after removal of involved areas.
2. Follicular (rapidly growing, widely metastasizing type)

a. Occurs predominantly in middle-age and elderly persons.
b. Brief encouraging response may occur with x-ray irradiation.
c. Progression of disease is rapid; high mortality rate.

3. Parafollicular—medullary thyroid carcinoma (MTC)
   a. Rare, inheritable type of thyroid malignancy, which can be detected early by a radioimmunoassay for the hormone, calcitonin.
   b. Screening of familial MTC suspects is done by measuring circulating plasma calcitonin levels.

Diagnostic Evaluation

1. History and physical examination are important. On palpation of the thyroid, there may be a firm, irregular, fixed, painless mass or nodule.
2. The occurrence of signs and symptoms of hyperthyroidism is rare.

3. If a thyroid scan is to be done, ^{99m}technetium pertechnetate is preferred, since it delivers a much lower radiation than ^{131}I. ^{123}I is even better.
4. Needle biopsy is recommended only for the very skilled performer and for the experienced pathologist. Needle aspiration may induce metastasis by seeding of other tissues.
5. Surgical exploration.

Treatment

1. Surgical removal is extensive, as required.
2. Thyroid replacement
   a. Thyroid hormone is administered to suppress secretion of TSH.
   b. Such treatment is continued indefinitely and requires annual checkups.
3. For unresectable cancer, patient is referred to a thyroid specialist for consideration of treatment with ^{131}I, chemotherapy, or radiation therapy.

2: Disorders of the Parathyroid Glands

The Parathyroid Glands

The *parathyroid glands* are small, bean-sized structures embedded in the posterior section of the thyroid gland.

Functions

1. Produce, store and secrete parathormone in response to the serum level of ionized calcium.

2. Increase plasma calcium ions by acting on:
   a. The kidney—to decrease elimination of calcium ions in the urine
   b. The gastrointestinal tract—to increase absorption of calcium ions from chyme
   c. Bone—to increase its contributions of calcium ions to the plasma

Hyperparathyroidism

Hyperparathyroidism is overactivity of the parathyroids.

Cause

1. An overgrowth or hypertrophy of parathyroid glands, as a primary disorder of the parathyroid glands or as a secondary condition occurring with renal failure as a result of renal retention of phosphorus.
2. Carcinoma of the parathyroid or secretion of parathyroid hormone by ectopic tissue in malignancy may produce manifestations of hyperparathyroidism.

Assessment
Clinical Manifestations

1. Decalcification of bones
   a. Skeletal pain, backache, pain on weight-bearing, pathologic fractures, deformities, formation of bony cysts
   b. Formation of bone tumors—overgrowth of osteoclasts
2. Depression of neuromuscular function
   a. The patient may trip, drop objects, show general fatigue, emotional instability, changes in level of consciousness with stupor and coma
   b. Cardiac arrhythmias, hypertension, cardiac standstill
   c. Formation of calcium-containing stones in the kidneys

Diagnostic Evaluation

1. Persistently elevated serum calcium (11 mg./100 ml.); test is performed 3 times to determine consistency of results
2. Exclusion of other causes of hypercalcemia—malignancy, vitamin D excess, multiple myeloma, sarcoidosis, milk-alkali syndrome, drugs such as thiazides, Cushing's disease, hyperthyroidism
3. Serum calcium and alkaline phosphatase levels are elevated and serum phosphorus levels are decreased with increased parathyroid activity.
4. Parathyroid hormone (PTH) levels are increased with hyperactivity of the parathyroid glands.
5. Skeletal changes are revealed by x-ray.
6. Diagnosis often extremely difficult (complications may occur before this condition is diagnosed).
7. Cineradiography will disclose parathyroid tumors more readily than x-ray.

Complications

1. Kidney disturbances
   a. Formation of renal stones
   b. Calcification of kidney parenchyma
   c. Renal shutdown
2. Gastrointestinal complications
   Ulceration of upper gastrointestinal tract (stomach, duodenum) leading to hemorrhage and perforation

3. Skeletal problems
   a. Simple demineralization
   b. Cysts and fibrosis of marrow—leading to fractures
   c. Fractures of vertebral bodies and fractures of the ribs

Patient Problems/Nursing Diagnoses

1. Alterations in fluid and electrolyte balance related to effects of elevated serum calcium levels
2. Potential alteration of urinary elimination related to renal calculi and calcium deposits in the kidneys
3. Alterations in musculoskeletal status related to abnormal bone formation, weakness, bone pain, and pathologic fractures
4. Potential complications of surgery and hypocalcemia

Planning and Implementation
Nursing Interventions

A. **Establishment of normal fluid and electrolyte balance to prevent or counteract life-threatening effects of hypercalcemia**

1. Assess fluid intake and output.
2. Provide adequate hydration—administer water, glucose, and electrolytes by mouth or intravenously.

▶ **NURSING ALERT:** A low specific gravity for urine does not necessarily mean adequate hydration.

3. Administer diuretic—furosemide (Lasix).

▶ **NURSING ALERT:** Thiazide diuretics should not be administered to the patient with hyperparathyroidism, since they decrease the renal excretion of calcium, thereby causing hypercalcemia.

4. Administer phosphate therapy as prescribed to control hypercalcemia.
5. Obtain daily serum calcium and BUN determinations.
6. Monitor ECG to detect changes secondary to hypercalcemia. (During moderate elevations of serum calcium, Q–T interval is shortened; with extreme hypercalcemia, widening of the T wave is seen.)
7. Administer glucocorticoids, calcitonin, or mithramycin (cytotoxic agent that inhibits bone resorption) cautiously in severe hypercalcemia.
8. Prevent or promptly treat dehydration; report vomiting or other sources of fluid loss promptly.
9. Avoid dietary sources of calcium.

B. **Improved urinary elimination**

1. Assess urinary output; strain all urine to observe for kidney stones (renal calculi).
2. Increase fluid intake to 3,000 ml./day to maintain hydration and prevent precipitation of calcium and formation of stones.
3. Encourage high intake of cranberry juice to promote low urine pH (acidic urine) and reduce stone formation.
4. Provide diet low in calcium; eliminate milk and milk products.
5. Instruct the patient about dietary recommendations.
6. Observe the patient for signs of urinary tract infection, hematuria, and renal colic.
7. Instruct the patient to avoid medications containing calcium (some antacids).
8. Assess renal function through serum creatinine and BUN levels.

C. **Normal musculoskeletal function**

1. Assist the patient in hygiene and activities if bone pain is severe or if the patient experiences musculoskeletal weakness.
2. Protect the patient from falls or injury.
3. Turn the patient cautiously and handle extremities gently to avoid fractures.
4. Administer analgesia as prescribed.
5. Assess level of pain and the patient's response to analgesia.
6. Encourage the patient to participate in mild exercise gradually as symptoms subside.
7. Instruct and demonstrate correct body mechanics to reduce strain, backache, and injury.
8. Ensure early diagnosis and treatment of fractures.
   a. Treatment for vertebral body fractures (see p. 824)
   b. Treatment for rib fractures, page 174
   c. Fixation of other long bones
   d. Continued hydration of the patient
   e. Earliest mobilization of fracture areas

D. **Postoperative recovery without complications or manifestations of hypocalcemia**

1. See page 679 as postoperative care is similar to that after thyroidectomy.
2. Recognize that the patient will retain some fluid postoperatively.
   a. This will be manifested by a low urinary output.
   b. Therefore, avoid overhydration for first day or two.
3. Avoid giving calcium until the patient's calcium level is determined.
4. Evaluate signs and symptoms of hypocalcemia and onset of tetany.
   a. Observe calcium levels—if well below normal and if decline continues into the 2nd week, the skeletal system is absorbing calcium.
      If some involvement was noted preoperatively (elevated alkaline phosphatase level), calcium should be administered.
   b. Administer calcium—usually lactate or gluconate. When gastrointestinal tract cannot absorb large amount, administer intramuscularly as gluconate, or intravenously in emergency situation.
   c. Give vitamin D to increase absorption of calcium.
5. Reassure the patient about skeletal recovery.
   a. Bone pain diminishes fairly quickly.
   b. Cysts, bone tumors, and osteoporosis resolve themselves.
   c. Fractures are cared for by usual orthopedic procedures.

Evaluation
Expected Outcomes

1. Achieves/maintains adequate fluid and electrolyte balance
   a. Balance of urine output and fluid intake
   b. Normal skin turgor, moist mucous membranes, and no thirst
   c. Normal calcium levels and BUN levels
   d. No ECG changes; normal sinus rhythm
2. Maintains high fluid intake with low calcium intake and uses phosphate therapy as prescribed
3. Uses prescribed diuretics
4. Attains/maintains improved urinary elimination
   a. Adequate urine output without signs of kidney stones
   b. Urine is acidic (low pH), dilute, and clear.

c. No signs and symptoms of urinary tract infection, hematuria, or renal colic
d. Normal kidney function as indicated by normal serum creatinine and BUN levels

5. Achieves normal musculoskeletal function
   a. Decreased bone and joint pain
   b. Increased strength and well-being
   c. Analgesia taken as prescribed
   d. Mild exercise as musculoskeletal symptoms subside
   e. Uses correct body mechanics to move, turn, and carry out activities

6. Recovers from surgery without complications or manifestations of hypocalcemia
   a. Normal fluid balance postoperatively without manifestations of hypervolemia (distended neck veins)
   b. Normal calcium balance as indicated by normal serum calcium levels
   c. No manifestations of hypocalcemia and tetany
   d. No numbness and tingling in extremities or around mouth (circumoral paresthesias)

7. Uses calcium and vitamin D if indicated and prescribed

Hypoparathyroidism

Hypoparathyroidism results from a deficiency of parathyroid hormone and is characterized by hypocalcemia and neuromuscular hyperexcitability.

Etiology

1. The most common cause is accidental removal or destruction of parathyroid tissue or its blood supply during thyroidectomy or radical neck dissection for malignancy.
2. Decrease in gland function (idiopathic hypoparathyroidism); may be autoimmune or familial in origin.
3. Malignancy or metastasis from a cancer to the parathyroid glands.
4. Resistance to parathyroid hormone action.

Pathophysiology

1. With inadequate parathyroid hormone (PTH) secretion, there is decreased resorption of calcium from the renal tubules, decreased absorption of calcium in the gastrointestinal tract, and decreased resorption of calcium from bone.
2. Blood calcium falls to a low level, causing symptoms of muscular hyperirritability, uncontrolled spasms, and hypocalcemic tetany.
3. In response to decreased serum calcium levels and in the absence of parathyroid hormone, there is a rise in serum phosphate level and decreased phosphate excretion by the kidneys.
4. If onset of hypocalcemia is acute, the major concerns are laryngeal spasm, acute airway obstruction, and cardiovascular failure.
5. Long-term effects of persistent hypoparathyroidism include calcium deposits in tissues.

Assessment
Diagnosis and Clinical Signs

1. Due to deficiency of parathormone
   a. Accumulation of phosphorus in blood
   b. Decrease in serum calcium level to a low level (7.5 mg./100 ml. or less)
2. *Tetany*—general muscular hypertonia; attempts at voluntary movement result in tremors and spasmodic or uncoordinated movements; fingers assume classic position.
   a. *Chvostek's sign*—a spasm of facial muscles that occurs when muscles or branches of facial nerve are tapped.
   b. *Trousseau's sign*—carpopedal spasm within 3 minutes after a blood pressure cuff is inflated 20 mm. Hg above the patient's systolic pressure.
   c. Laryngeal spasm
3. Anxiety and apprehension are very marked.

4. Renal colic is often present if the patient has had stones; preexisting stones loosen and migrate into the ureter.

Patient Problems/Nursing Diagnosis

1. Altered electrolyte balance related to decreased serum calcium level
2. Anxiety related to impending sense of disaster
3. Altered urinary elimination related to presence of kidney stones
4. Pain related to passage of kidney stones

Planning and Implementation
Treatment

1. Administer calcium.
   a. A syringe and an ampule of a calcium solution are to be kept at the bedside at all times.
   b. Most rapidly effective calcium solution is ionized calcium chloride (10%).
   c. For rapid use to relieve severe tetany, infuse every 10 minutes.
      (1) Administer ionized calcium chloride (10%) slowly. It is highly irritating, stings, and causes thrombosis; patient experiences unpleasant burning flush of skin and, more particularly, of the tongue. Too rapid calcium administration may cause cardiac arrest.
      (2) Give calcium intravenously; calcium carbohydrate combination may also be used—gluconate or heptonate (10%) are not irritating.
   d. Continue a slow drip of intravenous saline containing calcium gluconate until control of tetany is ensured; then switch to intramuscular or oral administration of calcium.
   e. Later, add vitamin D to calcium intake—increases absorption of calcium and also induces a high level of calcium in the bloodstream.
2. Control anxiety.
   a. It is difficult to reassure this patient since he has a strong feeling of impending disaster.
   b. Administration of intravenous calcium seems to bring about rapid relief of anxiety.
3. Relieve renal colic.
   Stone may have to be removed cystoscopically or by surgery.
4. Monitor for hypercalciuria. Recommend periodic 24-hour urinary calcium determinations.
5. Monitor blood calcium periodically; variations in vitamin D may affect calcium levels.
6. Inform the patient about symptoms of hypocalcemia

and hypercalcemia; should these occur, he is to notify his physician.

Nursing Interventions

A. Establishment of normal electrolyte balance

1. Assess neuromuscular status in patients at risk for hypocalcemia (patients in the immediate postoperative period following thyroidectomy, parathyroidectomy, radical neck dissection).
2. Check for positive Trousseau's or Chvostek's sign.
3. Assess respiratory status frequently in postoperative recovery phase.
4. Monitor serum calcium and phosphorus levels.
5. Administer infusions of calcium salts with caution.
6. Observe and report response to infusion of calcium salts.
7. Have tracheostomy set available at the patient's bedside.
8. Report indications of respiratory distress, laryngeal stridor, or cardiovascular failure.
9. Instruct the patient about signs and symptoms of hypo- and hypercalcemia that should be reported.
10. Use caution in administering other drugs to the patient with hypocalcemia.
    a. The hypocalcemic patient is insensitive to digoxin; as hypocalcemia is reversed, the patient may rapidly develop digitalis toxicity.
    b. Cimetidine (Tagamet) interferes with normal parathyroid function, especially in the patient with renal failure, which increases the risk of hypocalcemia.
11. Institute seizure precautions (airway at bedside, padded siderails).

Evaluation

Expected Outcomes

1. Demonstrates normal neuromuscular status without evidence of tremor or neuromuscular excitability
2. Demonstrates negative Trousseau's and Chvostek's signs
3. Demonstrates and reports absence of respiratory distress; respiratory rate and pattern normal
4. Demonstrates normal serum calcium and phosphorus levels
5. Identifies symptoms of respiratory distress and cardiovascular changes that should be reported
6. Demonstrates absence of seizures
7. Identifies reportable signs and symptoms of hypo- and hypercalcemia
8. Uses calcium salts and consumes high-calcium diet if prescribed
9. Identifies importance of avoiding other medications unless checking first with nurse or physician

3: Disorders of the Adrenal Glands

The Adrenal Glands

Composition

A. Medulla

1. Is not necessary to maintain life but enables a person to cope with stress
2. Secretes 2 hormones:
   a. Epinephrine (adrenalin)
      (1) Acts on alpha and beta receptors
      (2) Increases contractility and excitability of heart muscle, leading to increased cardiac output
      (3) Facilitates blood flow to muscles, brain, and viscera
      (4) Enhances blood sugar—by stimulating conversion of glycogen to glucose in liver
      (5) Inhibits smooth muscle contraction
   b. Norepinephrine (noradrenalin, arterenol)
      (1) Acts primarily on alpha receptors
      (2) Increases peripheral vascular resistance, leading to increases in diastolic and systolic blood pressure

B. Cortex

1. Is essential to life
2. Secretes adrenocortical hormones—synthesized from cholesterol
   a. Glucocorticoids; cortisone and hydrocortisone
      (1) Enhance protein catabolism and inhibit protein synthesis
      (2) Antagonize action of insulin
      (3) Increase synthesis of glucose by liver
      (4) Influence defense mechanism of body and its reaction to stress
      (5) Influence emotional reaction
   b. Mineralocorticoids
      (1) Aldosterone—supplied by adrenal cortex
      (2) Desoxycorticosterone—usually not present in significant amounts
      (3) Regulate reabsorption of sodium cation
      (4) Regulate excretion of potassium cation by renal tubules
   c. Adrenosterones (adrenal androgens)

Adrenal Hyperfunction

Pheochromocytoma

Pheochromocytoma is a catecholamine-secreting neoplasm associated with hyperfunction of the adrenal medulla. It may appear wherever chromaffin cells are located; however, most are found in the adrenal medulla. Pheochromocytoma can occur at any age but is most common between the ages of 30 and 60; it is uncommon in individuals over age 65.

Pathophysiology

1. Pheochromocytoma, a tumor of epinephrine- and norepinephrine-producing tissue, usually occurs in the adrenal gland; ectopic tumors can occur in other

locations, including spleen, urinary bladder, kidneys, etc.

2. Most pheochromocytoma tumors are benign; 10% are malignant with metastasis.
3. These tumors produce increased secretion of epinephrine and norepinephrine; tumors located in the adrenal medulla produce both epinephrine and norepinephrine and those located outside the adrenal gland tend to produce epinephrine only.
4. The excessive secretion of norepinephrine and epinephrine produces hypertension, hypermetabolism, and hyperglycemia.
5. Variation in symptoms depends on the predominance of norepinephrine or epinephrine secretion and on whether the hormones are secreted continuously or intermittently.
6. Hypertension may be paroxysmal (intermittent) or persistent (chronic).

    Chronic form may be difficult to differentiate from "essential hypertension"; however, drugs effective for essential hypertension are not effective in this patient.

7. The hypermetabolic and hyperglycemic effects of pheochromocytoma produce tachycardia, excessive perspiration, tremor, pallor, or face flushing, nervousness, elevated blood glucose levels, polyuria, nausea, vomiting, diarrhea and abdominal pain, paresthesia in extremities.
8. Symptoms are often triggered by allergic reactions, physical exertion, emotional upset; they can also occur without identifiable stimulus.

Diagnostic Evaluation

1. If there is sympathetic overactivity, along with marked elevation of blood pressure, pheochromocytoma is strongly suspected.
2. Administration of certain drugs produces certain changes in arterial pressure.

▶ **NURSING ALERT:** If these tests are performed, have emergency equipment and medication available in case of sudden increase or decrease in blood pressure.

3. Twenty-four-hour urine tests
    a. Vanillylmandelic acid (VMA) and metanephrine determinations in urine. (VMA and metanephrine are metabolites of epinephrine and norepinephrine.)
    b. Determinations of catecholamines in urine and blood offer an effective test for overactivity of adrenal medulla.
    c. Normal urinary values:
    VMA, 0.7–6.8 mg./24 hours
    Metanephrines, less than 1.3 mg./24 hours
    Catecholamines, 0–275 μg./24 hours
4. Other tests—computed tomography (CT scan) of the adrenal glands, abdominal arteriograms and intravenous pyelogram (IVP) or x-ray examination may help in identifying the location of tumor.

Patient Problems/Nursing Diagnoses

1. Potential alterations of the vascular system related to severe hypermetabolism during the preoperative and intraoperative period and to hypotension during the postoperative period
2. Fear related to the systemic effects of norepinephrine and epinephrine and preoperative anxiety

Planning and Implementation

Treatment

Goals:
Control blood pressure
Diagnose the condition accurately
Prepare the patient adequately for surgery
Remove the cause surgically

A. Preoperative Care

1. To accomplish blood pressure control, administer alpha-adrenergic blocking agents such as phentolamine (Regitine) or phenoxybenzamine hydrochloride (Dibenzylene) to inhibit the effects of catecholamines. (Effective control of blood pressure and blood volume may take 1 or 2 weeks.)
2. Catecholamines synthesis inhibitors may also be used—metyrosine (Demser).
3. Propranolol is helpful in controlling cardiac arrhythmias, if present.
4. Plasma volume is determined, since these patients are very sensitive to blood loss and therefore may benefit from preoperative volume expansion.
5. Adequate hydration is essential to minimize risk of intraoperative and postoperative hypotension.
6. For long-term maintenance of patients with inoperable tumors, metyrosine may be given.
    a. Moderate to severe sedation is a side effect when therapy is initiated; patients are cautioned against driving or participating in activities requiring alertness.
    b. Avoid concurrent use of alcohol or other CNS depressants.
    c. Maintain fluid intake as a precaution against crystalluria; maintain daily urinary output of at least 2,000 ml.

B. Postoperative Care (see p. 690)

1. Maintain adequate fluid intake and blood volume
2. Evaluation and documentation of 24-hour urine specimens. The patient is considered surgically cured when 24-hour urine specimens are evaluated as "normal" when tested for catecholamines or catecholamine metabolites.

C. Familial Pheochromocytoma

Evaluation of the patient's family for pheochromocytoma and medullary carcinoma of the thyroid (p. 681) should be done.

Nursing Interventions

A. Establishment of normal vascular status

1. Monitor cardiovascular, neurologic, and renal function closely.
2. Assess and record blood pressure, pulse, respiratory rate, intake and output, neurologic signs, and serum creatinine and BUN levels.
3. Report changes in neurologic, cardiovascular, and renal status and elevations in blood pressure.
4. Administer an alpha-adrenergic blocking agent such as phentolamine (Regitine) or antihypertensive agents (nitroprusside) as prescribed for controlling acute hypertensive episodes.
5. Enforce bed rest and elevate the head of the bed to 45 degrees during episodes of severe hypertension.
6. Stay with the patient during acute episode of hypertension and restrict visitors.
7. Reduce environmental stressors by providing calm, quiet environment.
8. Explain all tests, procedures, and events to the patient.

9. Use sedatives as prescribed to promote relaxation and rest.
10. Eliminate stimulants (coffee, tea, cola) from the patient's diet.
11. Reduce events that precipitate episodes of severe hypertension—palpation of the tumor, physical exertion, emotional upset, anesthesia induction, and surgical intervention without adequate physical and emotional preparation.
12. Monitor ECG and arterial pressures postoperatively to detect cardiovascular changes and hyper- or hypotension.
13. Maintain intravenous infusion postoperatively.
14. Use vasopressors postoperatively as prescribed to maintain vascular tone and perfusion.
15. Administer corticosteroids postoperatively if bilateral adrenalectomy was performed.
16. Explain rationale for medications and necessity of taking medications for the rest of life if prescribed.

B. **Control of fear and anxiety**

1. Encourage the patient to verbalize fears and feelings about events and upcoming surgery.
2. Remain with the patient during stressful tests and procedures.
3. Explain tests, procedures, and events to the patient.
4. Remain with the patient during acute episodes of hypertension.
5. Carry out tasks and procedures in calm, unhurried manner when with the patient.
6. Instruct the patient about use of relaxation exercises.

Evaluation
Expected Outcomes

1. Demonstrates normal vascular tone as evidenced by normal blood pressure readings
2. Demonstrates absence of neurologic, cardiovascular, and renal dysfunction as evidenced by normal vital signs, normal neurologic signs, adequate urine output, and normal serum creatinine and BUN levels
3. Identifies reportable symptoms of neurologic, cardiovascular, and renal dysfunction
4. Remains on bed rest with head of the bed elevated to 45 degrees during acute episodes of hypertension
5. Reports feelings of rest and relaxation
6. Consumes diet without stimulants (coffee, tea, cola)
7. Uses antihypertensives or pressor agents, and corticosteroids as prescribed and indicated
8. The patient achieves control of fear and anxiety

Primary Aldosteronism

Primary aldosteronism refers to excessive secretion of aldosterone by the adrenal cortex. Primary aldosteronism is usually caused by a cortical adenoma; secondary aldosteronism occurs in conjunction with heart failure, renal dysfunction, or cirrhosis of the liver.

Diagnostic Evaluation and Clinical Manifestations

1. Hypertension (1%–2% of cases of hypertension are a result of primary aldosteronism, which can usually be treated successfully by surgical removal of the adenoma)
2. A profound decline in blood levels of potassium (hypokalemia) and hydrogen ions (alkalosis)—results in muscle weakness and inability of kidneys to acidify or concentrate urine, leading to excess volume of urine (polyuria)
   a. Increase in pH
   b. Increase in CO_2-combining power
3. A decline in hydrogen ions (alkalosis)—results in tetany, paresthesias
4. An elevation in blood sodium (hypernatremia)—results in excessive thirst (polydipsia) and arterial hypertension

Treatment
Primary Aldosteronism

Removal of adrenal tumor—adrenalectomy (see p. 690)

Secondary Aldosteronism

Management is dependent on treatment of the underlying disorder.

Cushing's Syndrome

Cushing's syndrome is a condition in which the plasma cortisol levels are elevated, causing signs and symptoms of hypercortisolism.

Etiology

1. Pituitary Cushing's syndrome (Cushing's disease)—65% of all patients with Cushing's; mostly women in childbearing age range
   Hyperplasia of both glands due to overstimulation of the adrenal cortex by ACTH
   Pituitary tumors
2. Adrenal Cushing's syndrome—associated with tumors of the adrenal cortex
   A neoplasm of the adrenal cortex—adenoma or carcinoma
3. Ectopic—results from autonomous ACTH secretion by extrapituitary neoplasms
   Tumors elsewhere in body producing excess ACTH

Pathophysiology

1. The normal feedback mechanisms that control adrenal cortical function are ineffective, resulting in secretion of adrenal cortical hormones despite adequate amounts of these hormones in the circulation.
2. The manifestations of Cushing's syndrome are the result of excess hormones (glucocorticoids, mineralocorticoids, and sex hormones).
3. Excess of one hormone or all the hormones can occur; the predominant hormone secreted in excess (usually glucocorticoids) determines the predominant symptoms.

Treatment
See Table 16-1.

A. **Establishing the diagnosis and identify etiology of Cushing's syndrome and appropriate treatment**

1. Overnight dexamethasone suppression test
   a. Dexamethasone is administered the night before in the amount equivalent to the amount of cortisol normally produced by the patient in a day.
   b. Dexamethasone will normally suppress ACTH secretion and stop cortisol production.
   c. The next day, blood studies will be done; patients with Cushing's syndrome will not show suppression below a certain level.
2. If above test does not rule out the possibility of Cushing's syndrome, specific urinary excretion tests are performed with dexamethasone suppression.
3. Additional tests are done to determine whether the problem is due to hyperplasia or adrenocortical tumor.

Table 16-1 **Current Therapeutic Options for Three Distinct Etiologies of Cushing's Syndrome**

Treatment	Indication	Prognosis
Surgery		
Transsphenoidal (microresection)	Pituitary Cushing's syndrome	90%–95% remission rates after removal of pituitary microadenoma. Temporary cortisol replacement may be required.
Transfrontal (hypophysectomy)	Pituitary Cushing's syndrome	Panhypopituitarism; permanent replacement therapy.
Adrenalectomy	Adrenal Cushing's syndrome	Temporary cortisol replacement therapy required if unilateral; lifelong if bilateral.
	Pituitary Cushing's syndrome	Mortality 4%–10%; recurrent hypercortisolism 10%; Nelson's syndrome 10%–20%: lifelong adrenal hormone replacement required if bilateral.
Irradiation		
External high-voltage x-ray (cobalt-60)	Pituitary Cushing's syndrome	80% remission in patients under 20 years of age; 20% remission in adults.
Cyclotron (α-particle, proton beam)	Pituitary Cushing's syndrome	60% remission in adults; morbidity 7%–8%
Internal yttrium-90, gold-198 (implants)	Pituitary Cushing's syndrome	Requires transsphenoidal surgery; seldom used in US.
Drugs		
CNS-active cyproheptadine (24 mg./day orally in 3–4 divided doses)	Pituitary Cushing's syndrome	Remission in 60%–65% after 6–8 weeks of cyproheptadine; relapse if treatment is discontinued.
CNS-active bromocriptine (10 mg./day orally)		
Adrenal-active o,p'-DDD (mitotane) (60 gm./day)	Ectopic Cushing's syndrome; inoperable adrenal Cushing's syndrome; pituitary Cushing's syndrome treated with irradiation	Remission of hypercortisolism in up to 90%; adrenocorticolytic; may require gluco- and mineralocorticoid replacement.
Metyrapone (1.0 gm./day)	Same as for o,p'-DDD (above); preoperative buildup of patients who are poor surgical risks because of metabolic effects of hypercortisolism	Not adrenocorticolytic; minor side effects; may require cortisol replacement during therapy; relapse if discontinued.
Aminoglutethimide (1.0 gm./day)		
Trilostane (0.5 gm./day)		

(Gold EM. Cushing's syndrome: A tripartite entity. Hospital Practice 1979 June; 14:72).

4. Computed tomography (CT scan) and ultrasonography may be requested to detect the exact location of the tumor.

B. Removing the causative factor surgically

1. Tumor (adrenal or pituitary)—should be removed or treated with irradiation.
   The most recent development in the management of pituitary Cushing's syndrome in adults is transsphenoidal hypophysectomy (see p. 696).
   This procedure requires skilled neurosurgical and radiological teams.
2. Hyperplasia of adrenals—adrenalectomy

C. Administering replacement therapy postoperatively

1. Adrenalectomy patients require lifelong replacement therapy with the following:
   a. A glucocorticoid—cortisone
   b. A mineralocorticoid—fludrocortisone (Florinef)
2. Following pituitary irradiation or hypophysectomy, patients may require adrenal replacement plus thyroid and gonadal replacement therapy.
3. Following transsphenoidal adenomectomy, patients require hydrocortisone replacement therapy for periods of 12–18 months.
4. Protein anabolic steroids may facilitate protein replacement; potassium stores are usually depleted rapidly and may require replacement.

D. Considering medical treatment in patients unable to undergo surgery (e.g., because of myocardial infarction)

1. The physician may prescribe:
   a. Mitotane, an agent toxic to the adrenal cortex (DDT derivative)—"medical adrenalectomy"; serious side effects accompany this drug;

   b. Metyrapone (Metopirone) to inhibit steroid biosynthesis; this is used for temporary control.

Assessment
Clinical Manifestations
A. Children

1. Precocious puberty—due to excess of sex hormones
2. Affected growth rate—due to excess glucocorticoids and altered metabolism

B. Adult ("central-type obesity")

1. Manifestations due to excess glucocorticoids:
   a. "Buffalo hump" in neck and supraclavicular area
   b. Heavy trunk; thin extremities
   c. Skin—fragile and thin; striae and ecchymosis, acne
   d. Face—rounded, plethoric, oily
   e. Muscles—wasted due to excessive catabolism
   f. Osteoporosis—characteristic kyphosis, backache
   g. Mental disturbances—mood changes, psychosis
   h. Increased susceptibility to infections
2. Manifestations due to excess mineralocorticoids:
   a. Hypertension
   b. Edema
3. Manifestations due to excess sex hormones
   a. *Females* (Cushing's syndrome occurs 10 times more frequently in females than in males.)
      (1) "Virilism" or masculinization
         (a) Hirsutism—excessive growth of hair on the face and midline of trunk
         (b) Breasts—atrophy
         (c) Clitoris—enlarges
         (d) Voice—masculine
         (e) Loss of libido
      (2) In utero—possible hermaphrodite
   b. *Males*—loss of libido

Diagnostic Evaluation

1. Excessive plasma cortisol levels
2. An increase in blood glucose levels and glucose tolerance curve of diabetes mellitus
3. A decrease in serum potassium level
4. A reduction in the number of blood eosinophils
5. Elevation in the urine level of 17-hydroxycorticoids and 17-ketogenic steroids
6. Elevation of plasma ACTH in patients with pituitary tumors
7. Very low plasma ACTH levels in a patient with hypercortisolism are characteristic of an adrenal tumor
8. Loss of diurnal variation of cortisol secretion
9. X-rays of the skull to detect erosion of the sella turcica by a pituitary tumor
10. Adrenal angiography (procedure and preparation of the patient are similar to that of renal angiography, but the inferior adrenal artery, a branch of the renal artery, is injected with contrast medium for visualization)

Patient Problems/Nursing Diagnoses

1. Altered skin integrity related to impaired healing, thin, fragile skin, and increased susceptibility to infection and edema
2. Impaired ability to carry out activities of daily living related to muscle wasting, osteoporosis, weakness, and fatigue
3. Altered body image and self-esteem related to altered physical appearance, and emotional instability and role change

Planning and Implementation
Nursing Interventions
A. Improved skin integrity

1. Assess skin frequently to detect reddened areas, breakdown or tearing of skin, excoriation, infection, or edema.
2. Handle skin and extremities gently to prevent trauma; protect from falls by use of siderails.
3. Avoid use of adhesive tape to reduce risk of trauma to skin upon its removal.
4. Assist the patient to turn in bed frequently or ambulate to reduce pressure on bony prominences and areas of edema.
5. Use meticulous skin care to reduce injury and breakdown.
6. Provide foods low in sodium to minimize edema formation.
7. Assess intake and output and daily weights to evaluate fluid retention.

B. Increased participation in activities of daily living

1. Assist the patient with ambulation and hygiene when weak and fatigued.
2. Assist the patient in planning schedule to permit exercise and rest.
3. Encourage the patient to rest when fatigued.

4. Encourage gradual resumption of activities as the patient gains strength.
5. Identify for the patient signs and symptoms indicating excessive exertion.
6. Instruct the patient in correct body mechanics to avoid pain or injury during activities.
7. Utilize assistive devices during ambulation to prevent falls and fractures.
8. Provide foods high in potassium to counteract weakness related to hypokalemia.

C. Improved body image and increased self-esteem

1. Encourage the patient to verbalize concerns about illness, changes in appearance, and altered role functions.
2. Identify those situations that are disturbing to the patient; record these on the nursing care plan as situations to be avoided.
3. Be alert for evidence of depression; in some instances this has progressed to suicide; therefore, mood changes are most important.
4. Report if depression continues after surgery.
5. Recognize and accept the emotional stress in the female patient who manifests masculinization tendencies.
6. Explain to the patient who has benign adenoma or hyperplasia that, with proper treatment, evidence of masculinization can be reversed.
7. Recognize that weakness is a frustrating experience in a patient who heretofore has been active.
8. Provide a low-calorie, low-carbohydrate diet to reduce hyperglycemia and prevent obesity.

Evaluation
Expected Outcomes

1. Demonstrates intact skin without evidence of breakdown or excoriation, infection, or evidence of trauma
2. Utilizes handrails or walks with assistance only
3. Consumes low-sodium diet and identifies foods high in sodium that are restricted and describes rationale for restrictions
4. Demonstrates balance of fluid intake and output
5. Returns to ideal body weight without fluid retention or increased body mass
6. Participates safely in activities of daily living
   a. Assists in own hygiene care
   b. Plans schedule to permit rest periods and gradual participation in mild exercise
7. Experiences improved body image and increased self esteem
   a. Verbalizes concerns about illness, appearance, and altered role function
   b. Interacts appropriately with others
   c. Identifies reasons for change in appearance and verbalizes expectation that appearance will return to normal gradually as treatment becomes more effective

Adrenal Hypofunction

Adrenocortical Insufficiency

Adrenocortical insufficiency occurs when there is inadequate secretion of the hormones of the adrenal cortex, primarily the glucocorticoids and mineralocorticoids.

Etiology

Primary adrenocortical insufficiency (or Addison's disease) occurs with destruction and subsequent hypofunction of the adrenal cortex resulting in deficient production of adrenal steroids:

1. Glucocorticoids (principally cortisol)
2. Mineralocorticoids (principally aldosterone)
   Secondary adrenocortical insufficiency is a result of ACTH deficiency from:
1. Pituitary disease with atrophy of adrenal cortex (a result of pituitary hypofunction)
2. Suppression or atrophy of hypothalamic–pituitary axis by corticosteroids (used in treating nonendocrine disorders)

Pathophysiology

1. The majority of the clinical manifestations of adrenocortical insufficiency result from deficiency of aldosterone, the chief mineralocorticoid, and cortisol deficiency; few symptoms related to deficiency of sex hormones, or androgens, occur.
2. Inadequate aldosterone produces disturbances of sodium, potassium, and water metabolism.
3. Cortisol deficiency produces abnormal fat, protein, and carbohydrate metabolism; absence of cortisol during a period of stress can precipitate addisonian crisis, an exaggerated state of adrenal cortical insufficiency, and lead to death.

Treatment

1. Restore normal fluid and electrolyte balance.
   a. Administer high-sodium, low-potassium diet and fluids.
   b. Treat glucocorticoid deficiency with cortisone, cortisol, or prednisone. Treat mineralocorticoid deficiency with fludrocortisone.
   Overtreatment may be manifested by hypertension, edema from sodium and water retention, weakness due to sodium loss.
2. Initiate treatment immediately if addisonian crisis or circulatory collapse is imminent.
   a. Administer blood transfusions to replace blood volume.
   b. Start intravenous flow of sodium chloride solution to replace sodium ions.
   c. Give hydrocortisone.
   d. Inject circulatory stimulants.
3. Diagnose and treat underlying cause of adrenocorticol insufficiency or addisonian crisis (e.g., antibiotic therapy to treat infection if this is a factor in crisis).
4. Provide cardiovascular support if indicated.

Assessment
Clinical Manifestations

1. Increased sodium loss and increased potassium loss by the renal tubules.
2. Water loss, dehydration, and hypovolemia.
3. Muscular weakness, fatigue, weight loss
4. Gastrointestinal problems—anorexia, nausea, vomiting, diarrhea, constipation, abdominal pain
5. Low blood pressure, low blood sugar, low basal metabolism rate (BMR)
6. After a while, symptoms worsen, and the patient is forced to go to bed.
   a. Skin color changes to tan, bronze, or brown—diffuse or patchy, freckling.
   b. Mucous membranes also discolor—bluish black or gray.
   c. Mental changes occur—depression, irritability, anxiety, apprehension due to hypoglycemia and hypovolemia.
7. Normal responses to stress are lacking.

Diagnostic Evaluation
A. Blood Studies

1. Hypoglycemia—decrease in serum glucose level
2. Hyponatremia—decrease in sodium concentration
3. Hyperkalemia—increase in potassium concentration
4. Lymphoid hyperplasia
5. Low fasting plasma cortisol levels; low aldosterone levels

B. Urine Studies

Twenty-four-hour specimen for 17-ketosteroids, 17-hydroxycorticoids, and 17-ketogenic steroids—all values decreased

C. Injection of a Potent Pituitary Adrenocorticotropic Hormone to Artificially Stimulate Adrenals

1. Normal response—normal rise in plasma cortisol and urinary 17-ketosteroids
2. In Addison's disease
   a. Decrease in circulating eosinophils
   b. Increase in uric acid excretion in about 4 hours
   c. No rise in plasma cortisol and urinary 17-ketosteroids

Patient Problems/Nursing Diagnoses

1. Altered fluid and electrolyte balance related to renal losses of sodium and water and renal retention of potassium, gastrointestinal losses of fluid and electrolytes, and inadequate dietary intake
2. Inadequate physiologic response to stressors related to decreased secretion of glucocorticoids and aldosterone
3. Activity intolerance related to fatigue
4. Anorexia, nausea, vomiting, diarrhea related to effects of endocrine imbalance

Planning and Implementation
Nursing Interventions
A. Normal fluid and electrolyte balance

1. Assess circulatory status by frequent measurements of fluid intake and output and serial daily weights.
2. Assess vital signs frequently for deviation.
   a. Monitor vital signs and blood pressure; a drop in blood pressure may suggest impending crisis.
   b. Record the temperature hourly, since an elevation may easily be precipitated.
3. Assess skin turgor and status of mucous membranes frequently.
4. Collect 24-hour urine specimens to aid in monitoring fluid and electrolyte status. (Inform the patient's family, as well as all nursing personnel who come in contact with this patient, that all urine must be saved for a 24-hour urine specimen.)
5. Assess serum levels of sodium and potassium frequently.
6. Provide diet high in sodium and fluid content; administer potassium supplements if prescribed.
7. Administer prescribed glucocorticoids and mineralocorticoids; report response of patient.
8. Administer intravenous infusions of sodium, water, and glucose if prescribed and indicated by the patient's condition.

B. Normal response to stressors

1. Minimize stressful situations in the patient with altered response to stressors.
2. Protect the patient from infection.
   a. Control the patient's contacts so that infectious organisms are not transmitted.

b. Protect the patient from drafts, dampness, exposure to cold.
c. Prevent overexertion.
3. Administer optimum physical nursing care.
   a. Do not allow the patient who is in adrenal crisis to do anything for himself.
   b. Assist the patient in moving and turning, in feeding, and in providing mouth care.
   c. Limit conversation to what is essential to the patient's care.
4. Observe carefully the emotional status of the patient.
   a. Promote rest periods to avoid overexertion.
   b. Control the temperature of the room to avoid sharp deviations in the patient's temperature.
   c. Maintain a quiet, peaceful environment; avoid loud talking and noisy radios.
5. Assess frequently for early signs of *addisonian crisis*.
   a. Nausea, vomiting, cyanosis
   b. Sudden drop in blood pressure
   c. Very high temperature
6. Recognize that circulatory collapse may result from the following:
   a. Overexertion
   b. Exposure to cold
   c. Acute infection
   d. Decrease in salt intake
   e. Excessive diarrhea
   f. Surgery in the patient with marginal adrenal cortical function
7. Assess for delayed or later signs of addisonian crisis.
   a. Fall in systolic pressure to 40–50 mm. Hg
   b. Weak pulse and cold clammy skin
8. Instruct the patient about reportable symptoms of addisonian crisis.

Health Teaching

1. Instruct the patient about the necessity for long-term therapy for adrenocortical insufficiency and medical follow-up.

a. Inform the patient that therapy must be continued for the rest of his life.
b. Emphasize the importance of taking more hormones when the patient is under stress.
c. Suggest that the patient carry an identification card on which are indicated the type of medication he is receiving and the telephone number of his physician.
2. Instruct the patient about manifestations of excessive use of medications and reportable symptoms.

Evaluation

Expected Outcomes

1. Demonstrates adequate circulatory status by normal vital signs
2. Maintains balance of fluid intake and output; maintains weight at normal level without signs and symptoms of fluid overload
3. Demonstrates normal skin turgor and moist mucous membranes
4. Demonstrates normal serum sodium and potassium levels
5. Consumes foods high in sodium and with normal potassium content
6. Uses glucocorticoids and mineralocorticoids as prescribed
7. Demonstrates normal response to stressful situations as evidenced by normal vital signs
8. Plans rest and activity to avoid overexertion
9. Identifies actions to take to avoid factors that may precipitate addisonian crisis (infection, extremes of temperature, etc.)
10. Carries identification card with information about condition, and emergency treatment with him at all times

Management of the Patient Having an Adrenalectomy

Preoperative

1. Correct hyperglycemia by proper diet and insulin.
2. Administer high-protein diet to correct protein deficiency.
3. See page 75—Care of patient is similar to that for general surgery of abdomen.

Postoperative

1. Similar to that for an abdominal operation (see p. 85).
2. Will require administration of hydrocortisone or similar compounds in large amounts; this should begin prior to surgery. If bilateral adrenalectomy is performed, lifelong replacement is necessary.
3. For removal of pheochromocytoma:
   a. Because of manipulation of tumor during surgery, there may be extreme fluctuations of blood pressure.

b. Upon ligation of vessels from tumor, an abrupt fall of blood pressure may result. Administer large amounts of epinephrine intravenously.

▶ **NURSING ALERT:** Be prepared to monitor blood pressure frequently for 24–48 hours and to regulate vasopressor intravenous medications in order to stabilize the blood pressure.

4. Monitor vital signs, including blood pressure and central venous pressure, up to 48 hours—to detect early changes that may indicate impending cardiovascular collapse.
5. Anticipate stressful situations for the patient and avoid them; provide rest periods, anticipate the patient's needs, provide comfort measures.

Steroid Therapy

Classification of Steroids
(By major metabolic effects on body)
1. Mineralocorticoids
   a. Concerned with sodium and water retention and potassium excretion
   b. Example—aldosterone and 11-desoxycorticosterone
2. Glucocorticoids
   a. Concerned with metabolic effects, including carbohydrate metabolism
   b. Example—cortisol
3. Sex hormones
   a. Important when secreted in large amounts or when the growth of hormone-sensitive cancers is stimulated
   b. Examples:
      Androgens—dehydroepiandrosterone, testosterone
      Estrogens—estradiol
      Progestins—progesterone

Effects of Glucocorticoids
(corticosteroids, steroids)

1. Antagonize action of insulin—promote gluconeogenesis, which provides glucose.
2. Increase breakdown of protein (inhibit protein synthesis).
3. Increase breakdown of fatty acids.
4. Suppress inflammation, inhibit scar formation, block allergic responses.
5. Decrease number of circulating eosinophils and leukocytes; decrease size of lymphatic tissue.
6. Exert a permissive action (allow full expression of effects of another hormone) on all effects caused by catecholamines.
7. Exert a permissive action on functioning of central nervous system.
8. Inhibit release of adrenocorticotropin.
   IN SUMMARY: Glucocorticoids are necessary to resist noxious stimuli and environmental change.

Uses of Steroids
1. Physiologically—to correct deficiencies or malfunction of a particular endocrine organ or system (e.g., Addison's disease).
2. Diagnostically—to determine proper functioning of the endocrine system.
3. Pharmacologically—to treat the following:
   a. Rheumatoid arthritis
   b. Acute rheumatic fever
   c. Blood conditions
      (1) Idiopathic thrombocytopenic purpura
      (2) Leukemia
      (3) Hemolytic anemia
   d. Allergic conditions—bronchial asthma, allergic rhinitis
   e. Dermatologic problems—drug rashes, giant hives, atopic dermatitis
   f. Ocular diseases—conjunctivitis, uveitis
   g. Connective tissue disorders—lupus erythematosus, periarteritis nodosa
   h. Gastrointestinal problems—ulcerative colitis
   i. Organ-transplant recipients—as an immunosuppressive agent

   j. Neurologic—cerebral edema
   k. Other conditions—gout, multiple sclerosis
4. Emergency conditions
   a. Status asthmaticus
   b. Acute adrenal insufficiency
   c. Anaphylactic reaction (only after epinephrine has been given)

Preparing the Patient to Receive Steroid Therapy

1. Perform a thorough physical examination and medical history.
2. Determine contraindications for such therapy.
   a. Peptic ulcer
   b. Diabetes mellitus
   c. Viral infections
3. Administer a tuberculin test to determine need for antituberculin drugs.
   If this is not done prior to steroid therapy, the patient's hypersensitivity to tuberculin and response to the tubercle bacillus are suppressed.
4. Assess the patient's own level of steroid secretion, if possible.
5. Explain the nature of the therapy, what is required of the patient, how long he is to be on steroid medications, what adverse signs to watch for, and answer any of his questions.

Choice of Steroid and Method of Administration

1. Determined on an individual basis by physician.
2. May be given for local effects or systemic effects.
3. May be given by a wide variety of methods—orally, parenterally, sublingually, rectally, by inhalation, or by direct application to skin or mucous membrane.
4. Combinations of steroids with other drugs should be avoided.
5. To help avoid steroid side effects, alternate-day therapy should be used if at all possible but is not always feasible.
6. Sometimes steroids are given in extremely high doses, then sharply reduced; if the patient has been taking steroids for a while, doses must be tapered gradually to prevent addisonian crisis.

Potential Side Effects of Steroid Therapy
See Chart, page 692.

A. Classification

1. Mineralocorticoid
   a. Sodium and water retention
      Edema, weight gain, elevated blood pressure
   b. Potassium depletion
      Weakness, tiredness, alkalosis
2. Glucocorticoid
   a. Masking of infections
   b. Osteoporosis
   c. Steroid diabetes
   d. Exacerbation of tuberculosis

B. Control or Avoidance of Side Effects

1. Mineralocorticoid
   Use triamcinolone or newer synthetic steroids. (Some of the newer synthetics cause less sodium retention but have other side effects.)

The Patient on Steroid Therapy

Acceptable and Expected Side Effects*

Nature of Effect	Action
Facial mooning (Cushing's syndrome)	May be minimized by restricted calorie intake.
Weight gain	Restrict calorie intake; may require a change in steroid medication; may require a diuretic.
Edema	May require diuretics and potassium.
Potassium loss	Prescribe diuretics and potassium.
	May require addition of a fluorinated synthetic.
	Administer potassium supplement.
Acne	Treat with topical medications.
Urinary frequency and nocturia	Check for evidence of genitourinary infection or diabetes mellitus; urinalysis.
Insomnia, headache, fatigue, euphoria	Treat symptomatically.
Glucosuria, leukocytosis	

Undesirable and Unacceptable Side Effects

Nature of Effect	Action (Report to Physician)
Allergic reaction to ACTH or steroid	Withdraw drug promptly.
	Substitute steroid or synthetic ACTH.
Cardiovascular system effects:	
Hypertension	Suggest reduction in dosage of steroids.
Thromboembolic complications	
Arteritis	
Infection	Suggest antimicrobial medications as indicated.
Eye complications:	
Glaucoma	Refer to ophthalmologist.
Corneal lesions	
Subcapsular cataract	
Musculoskeletal effects:	
Osteoporosis	Suggest sex hormones—synthetic estrogens and/or androgens.
Pathologic fractures	Suggest calcium supplement.
Growth suppression	
Myopathies	
Central nervous system:	
Seizures	Refer to neurologist.
Neuritis	
Psychotic reactions	
Adrenal insufficiency (after steroid withdrawal) manifested by peripheral circulatory collapse—in upright position.	Administer hydrocortisone promptly (intravenously). The following day give steroid replacement.

Counseling of Patients on Long-term Steroids

1. Recognize that steroids are valuable and useful medications, but if taken longer than 2 weeks, they may produce certain side effects.
2. "Acceptable" side effects may include weight gain (perhaps due to water retention), acne, headaches, fatigue, and increased urinary frequency (see above).
3. "Unacceptable" side effects which are to be reported to the physician: dizziness when rising from chair or bed (postural hypotension indicative of adrenal insufficiency), nausea, vomiting, thirst, abdominal pain, or pain of any type (see above).
4. Additional side effects that are reportable are convulsive seizures, feelings of depression or nervousness, or development of an infection (see above).
5. Patient and/or family member is/are instructed about the rationale for and side effects of steroid medication.
6. If the patient has a fall or is in an automobile accident, his condition may precipitate adrenal failure. He requires an immediate injection of hydrocortisone phosphate. (Long-term patients should wear a Medic-Alert tag and carry a kit with hydrocortisone.)
7. The patient is instructed to inform any physician, dentist, or nurse in future contacts that he is on steroid therapy.
8. See physician on a regular follow-up basis.

   * These side effects may be acceptable in terms of therapeutic goals, but unacceptable to the patient.

2. Glucocorticoid
Difficult to separate anti-inflammatory effects from sodium-retaining effects.

Nursing Management of Patients Receiving Steroid Therapy

1. Know the routes by which steroids are given.
   a. Ascertain advantages of the method chosen for the particular patient.
   b. Determine what is expected of the medication in a particular situation.
   c. Be informed about side effects and untoward manifestations.
   d. NOTE:
      (1) Local application of steroid medications to the skin (to a large area, over a prolonged period, using occlusive dressings) leads to adrenal suppression.
      (2) Local administration to the eye over a prolonged period leads to increased eye pressure, corneal ulceration.
      (3) Long-term systemic corticosteroid therapy may produce manifestations of Cushing's syndrome (skin atrophy, impaired wound healing, and development of petechiae and ecchymoses in the extremities).
   e. Recognize that it is necessary to understand pharmacologic action of a particular steroid before planning the scheduled doses. Be aware of the following:
      (1) How frequently it can be given.
      (2) How late in the day it may be administered.
      (3) Whether every other day is sufficient, etc. Patients on intermittent therapy have few side effects.
2. Be aware of the problems encountered during periods when steroids are being withdrawn or lowered in dosage: precipitation of addisonian crisis.
   a. Associate symptoms of tiredness, muscular weakness, and lethargy with drug withdrawal.
   b. Report any stress situations during this time, such as surgery, a family crisis, etc.
   c. Instruct the patient why it may be necessary to save all urine for 24 hours (for determination of 11-hydroxycorticosteroid level).
3. Monitor carefully the patient who is on intravenous corticosteroid therapy.
   a. Determine the flow rate of fluids necessary to give a precise amount of medication.
   b. Observe the tissues, catheter site, flow rate, fluid level, and patient's response at frequent intervals to be sure the system is functioning well.
   c. Note signs and symptoms indicative of adrenal crisis—restlessness, weakness, headache, nausea, vomiting, diarrhea, and falling blood pressure.

Guidelines: The Patient Receiving Steroid Therapy— Clinical Assessment, Surveillance, and Health Education

Goal:
To detect early signs of side effects from steroid therapy.

Nursing Action	Rationale
Infection Control	
1. Encourage the patient to avoid crowds and the possibility of exposure to infection.	Steroids may affect the circulating blood—resulting in decreased eosinophils and lymphocytes, increased red cells, and increased incidence of thrombophlebitis and infection.
2. Utilize exercise schedules to prevent stasis.	
3. Be aware that cardinal symptoms of inflammation may be masked.	
4. Instruct all personnel coming in contact with this patient to wash hands thoroughly and practice meticulous asepsis.	
Diet and Metabolism Considerations	
1. Determine whether the patient needs assistance in dietary control.	1. Steroids may cause weight gain and an increase in appetite.
2. Administer a high protein, high carbohydrate diet.	2. Steroids affect protein metabolism; there may be negative nitrogen balance.
3. Encourage the patient to take steroids with milk or food.	3. Steroids cause an increase in secretion of gastric hydrochloric acid and have an inhibiting effect on secretion of mucus in the stomach; they may aggravate an existing peptic ulcer.
4. Be on guard for early evidence of gastric hemorrhage such as melena, blood in vomitus.	
5. Check urine for evidence of glucose.	5. Steroids precipitate gluconeogenesis and insulin antagonism, which results in hyperglycemia, glucosuria, decreased carbohydrate tolerance.

(continued)

Guidelines: The Patient Receiving Steroid Therapy—
Clinical Assessment, Surveillance, and Health Education (continued)

Nursing Action	Rationale
Possible Bone Complications	
1. Be on the alert for the possibility of pathologic fractures. Stress safety measures to prevent injury.	Steroids affect the musculoskeletal system, causing potassium depletion and muscular weakness. Steroids cause increased output of calcium and phosphorus, which may lead to osteoporosis.
2. Administer a diet high in calcium and protein.	
3. Recommend a program of activities of daily living; normal range of motion for the bedridden.	
Electrolyte Disturbance	

1. Restrict sodium intake and increase potassium intake.
  a. Lemon juice is high in potassium and low in sodium.
  b. Avoid saline as a diluent in preparing injectable medications.
	Mineralocorticoid differs from other steroids, resulting in sodium retention and potassium depletion: edema, weight gain.

2. Check blood pressure frequently and weigh the patient daily.	
3. Observe for evidence of edema.	
Behavioral Reactions	
1. Watch for convulsive seizures (especially in children).	Steroids may alter behavior patterns, increase excitability, and affect the central nervous system.
2. Avoid overstimulating situations.	
3. Recognize and report any mood deviating from the usual behavior patterns.	
4. Report unusual behavior, haunting dreams, withdrawal, or suicidal tendencies.	
Stress Reactions	
1. Recommend that the patient carry at all times an identification card indicating that he is on steroid therapy and including the name of his physician and instructions for emergency care.	Steroids affect the hypothalmic–pituitary–adrenal system, this in turn affects the individual's ability to respond to stress.
2. Advise the patient to avoid extremes of temperature, as well as infections and upsetting situations.	
Safety Measures	
1. Instruct the patient to avoid injury; stress safety precautions.	Steroids interfere with fibroblasts and granulation tissue, there is altered response to injury, resulting in impaired growth and delayed healing.
2. Observe daily the healing process of wounds, particularly surgical wounds, in order to recognize the potential for wound dehiscence.	

4: Disorders of the Pituitary Gland

Diabetes Insipidus

Diabetes insipidus is a disorder of water metabolism caused by deficiency of vasopressin, the antidiuretic hormone (ADH) secreted by the posterior pituitary.

Etiology
1. Primary; idiopathic
2. Secondary; head trauma, neurosurgery tumors (intra-cranial or metastatic) vascular disease (aneurysms, infarct) infection (meningitis, encephalitis)

Clinical Manifestations
1. Marked polyuria—daily output of 5–20 liters of very dilute urine; appearance of urine like that of water,

with a specific gravity of 1.001–1.005, corresponding to a urine osmolality of 50–200 mOsm./kg.

2. Polydipsia (intense thirst); 4–40 liters of fluid daily; patient has a craving for cold water.

Diagnostic Evaluation

1. Fluid deprivation test

Objective:

Restrict water intake and observe changes in urine volume and concentration.

   a. Fluids withheld for 8–12 hours or until 5% of body weight is lost.
   b. Plasma and urine osmolality studies are determined at beginning and end of test—inability to increase specific gravity and osmolality of urine is characteristic of diabetes insipidus.
   c. Some form of vasopressin is administered—to determine the response of kidneys to hormone administration.
   d. The patient is weighed frequently while fluid is withheld.

2. Measurement of urinary ADH by radioimmunoassay.

Treatment and Nursing Management

1. Assist in diagnostic testing to search for and correct underlying pathology; diabetes insipidus may occur in the course of many forms of intracranial pathology and systemic cancer.

2. Administer antidiuretic hormone (ADH) or its derivative, the principal hormone controlling water balance. Available ADH preparations include:
   a. Vasopressin tannate (Pitressin tannate in oil)—effective for 24–72 hours.
      (1) Administered by IM injection.
      (2) Warm vial and shake vigorously before administering—to ensure uniform dispersion, since active component settles at bottom of vial.
   b. Lypressin (Diapid nasal spray)—drug absorbed through nasal mucosa into blood.
      (1) Duration of action only a few hours.
      (2) May cause chronic nasal irritation.
   c. Desmopressin acetate (DDAVP)—a synthetic vasopressin derivative administered into the nose through a soft, flexible nasal tube.

3. For patients who have some residual hypothalamic vasopressin:
   a. Chlorpropamide (Diabinese)—potentiates action of vasopressin on renal-concentrating mechanism.
   b. Clofibrate (Atromid-S.)—probably acts by augmenting ADH secretion from neurohypophysis.
   c. Carbamazepine (Tegretol)—stimulates endogenous ADH release.

Health Education

1. Inform the patient that long-term monitoring of his metabolic state is essential because the severity of diabetes insipidus changes from time to time.
2. Avoid limiting fluids to decrease urinary output; thirst is a protective function.
3. Wear an alerting device stating that the wearer has diabetes insipidus.
4. Weigh daily to monitor fluid retention/fluid loss.
5. Consider eliminating coffee and tea from diet—may have an exaggerated diuretic effect.
6. Give written instruction on vasopressin administration. Have the patient demonstrate injection technique.

Pituitary Tumors

Types of Pituitary Tumors

1. *Chromophobe adenoma*—tumor of the anterior pituitary gland of adults.
   a. Most common pituitary tumor; does not secrete clinically significant amounts of hormones but can destroy rest of pituitary gland.
   b. Produces failing vision, optic atrophy, bitemporal hemianopsia, enlargement of sella turcica, and endocrine disturbances.

2. *Eosinophilic adenoma*—endocrine secretion of tumor produces gigantism in children and acromegaly in adults.

3. *Basophilic adenoma*—gives rise to so-called Cushing's syndrome with features largely attributable to hyperadrenalism—masculinization and amenorrhea in females, girdle obesity, hypertension, osteoporosis, and polycythemia.

Hypophysectomy

Hypophysectomy is removal of the pituitary gland.

Indications

1. Primary neoplasms (tumors) of the pituitary gland
2. Diabetic retinopathy
   a. Used to halt progress of hemorrhagic diabetic retinopathy and to prevent blindness
   b. Also reduces insulin requirements
3. Palliative measure for relief of bone pain secondary to metastasis of malignant lesions of breast and prostate; alters hormonal milieu of body to create a hormonal environment hostile to continued growth of neoplasm

Methods of Pituitary Ablation (Removal)

1. Surgery—done by transsphenoidal or frontal craniotomy approach
2. Cryogenic destruction or stereotaxic radiofrequency coagulation

3. Radiation therapy
4. Drug therapy

Management

The absence of the pituitary gland alters the function of many parts of the body.
1. The patient may need substitution therapy with adrenal steroids (hydrocortisone) and thyroid hormone.
2. Menstruation ceases and infertility occurs almost always after total or nearly total ablation.
3. See page 695 for treatment of diabetes insipidus; transient or permanent diabetes insipidus may follow surgery of pituitary gland.
4. See page 770 for nursing management of the patient undergoing cranial surgery and below for nursing management of the patient undergoing transsphenoidal hypophysectomy.

Transsphenoidal Microsurgical Approach for Pituitary Surgery

Preoperative Management

1. See Nursing Management of Patient Undergoing Intracranial Surgery, page 770.
2. Assist the patient undergoing diagnostic and preoperative preparation, endocrinologic tests, neuroradiologic evaluation, rhinologic evaluation, or visual field examination.
3. Physical preparation
   a. Take preoperative swabs of nasal and oral mucous membranes for bacterial culture and sensitivity studies.
   b. Administer prescribed antimicrobial nose drops.
   c. Give frequent oral hygiene with half-strength hydrogen peroxide.
   d. Inform the patient that he will have nasal packing in place following surgery.
      (1) Practice mouth-breathing.
      (2) Avoid nose blowing/coughing postoperatively—may disrupt muscle graft and cause cerebrospinal leak.

Postoperative Management

1. Carry out usual neurologic evaluation until the patient's condition stabilizes.
2. Maintain fluid therapy at basal replacement levels (approximately 75 ml./hour).
   a. Monitor intake, output, and specific gravity determinations of each voided specimen.
   b. Monitor daily electrolyte measurements.
   c. Take daily weight.
3. Monitor for postoperative complications.
   a. *Diabetes insipidus* (usually transitory)
      (1) Give adequate fluid replacement in *early*
      postoperative course if diabetes insipidus is encountered.
      (2) Encourage the patient to drink in response to his thirst sensation.
      (3) Give intravenous fluids when indicated, taking care not to overhydrate the patient.
      (4) Give aqueous vasopressin as directed during transient phase of diabetes insipidus.
   b. *Cerebrospinal leak*
      (1) See page 772 for assessing for rhinorrhea.
      (2) Prepare for lumbar cerebrospinal fluid (CSF) drainage or for surgical intervention if leak is persistent.
   c. *Meningitis*
      (1) Monitor for elevated temperature, nuchal rigidity, and headache.
      (2) Administer prescribed antimicrobial agents, antipyretics, and analgesics.
   d. *Hemorrhage*
      (1) Monitor for evidences of bleeding especially on "moustache" dressing.
      (2) Conduct visual field examination as soon as possible to determine if significant changes in vision are occurring.
4. Carry out nursing activities to increase the patient's comfort.
   a. Elevate head of bed.
   b. Administer medication for paranasal pain (from surgical manipulation and nasal packing) and headache (from loss of CSF during surgery).
   c. Use measures to alleviate dry mouth (from nasal packing and subsequent mouth-breathing)—cool-mist therapy, oral hygiene, fluid replacement.
   d. Assist with removal of nasal packing and nasal stents.
5. Monitor studies for hormone imbalance/replacement—degree of hormonal imbalance depends on whether there has been partial or complete removal of anterior and/or posterior lobe or transsection of the pituitary stalk.
   a. Monitor for signs and symptoms of adrenal insufficiency; low-grade fever, tachycardia.
   b. Give ACTH or cortisone preparations as prescribed—to prevent sodium excretion, potassium retention, extracellular fluid volume loss, hypotension, hypoglycemia, and stress intolerance.
   c. Give thyroid replacement as prescribed.

Health Education

1. Report for review of endocrine and visual status as directed.
2. Patient with invasive tumor may require course in radiation therapy.

5: Diabetes Mellitus (Pancreatic Disorders)

Diabetes Mellitus*

Diabetes mellitus is a heterogeneous group of clinical syndromes characterized by hyperglycemia. There may be either a relative or absolute deficiency of insulin or ineffective insulin secretion. There are several types of diabetes with different causes, different clinical courses, and different treatment regimens; the common denominator is hyperglycemia.

Altered Physiology

1. In diabetes mellitus, there is excessive output of glucose from the liver via glycogenolysis and gluco-

* See page 1376 for diabetes mellitus in children and page 1021 for diabetes during pregnancy.

neogenesis, and inadequate utilization of glucose by skeletal muscle, adipose tissue, and liver. Triglycerides are transported from the fat cells to the liver, where they are converted into ketones that can be utilized by the muscles for energy.

2. *Insulin* is a hormone secreted, when blood glucose rises, by the beta cells of the islets of Langerhans located in the pancreas.
   a. Insulin increases glycogen storage in the liver and the transport of glucose through the cell membrane of muscle and fat cells. Glucose passes into endothelial and nerve cells without the aid of insulin.
   b. The increased secretion of insulin following meals helps maintain the blood glucose at a normal level.
   c. The decreased secretion of insulin between meals facilitates the conversion of glycogen, amino acids, and triglycerides into glucose in the liver (gluconeogenesis).

3. In insulin-dependent diabetes mellitus (IDDM, type I), little or no insulin is secreted. In non–insulin-dependent diabetes mellitus (NIDDM, type II), there is an insensitivity of the glucose-sensing mechanism of the beta cells, and in obese patients with NIDDM, there is a decrease in the number of insulin receptors on the cell membrane of muscle and fat cells. Obese patients secrete an excessive amount of insulin, but it is ineffective because of the decreased number of receptors.

4. When blood glucose is sufficiently high, the renal tubules are unable to reabsorb all of the glucose in the glomerulo-filtrate, and glucosuria occurs. This causes an osmotic diuresis accompanied by the loss of water, sodium, chloride, potassium, and phosphate.

5. Diabetic ketoacidosis is due to an absence of effective insulin. The ketone bodies are organic acids and cause acidemia. The patient compensates by hyperventilating and by excreting more water and salt in the urine.

6. Decompensated diabetes mellitus causes loss of fat stores, liver glycogen, cellular protein, electrolytes, and water, eventually resulting in death from ketoacidosis.

7. The sequelae of long-term poorly controlled diabetes (persistent hyperglycemia) are accelerated atherosclerosis in the larger arteries, thickened capillary basement membranes throughout the body, and degenerative changes in the peripheral nerves. These may lead to such complications as coronary thrombosis, stroke, gangrene of the feet, blindness, renal failure, and neuropathy.

Classification of Diabetes

A. Insulin-dependent diabetes mellitus
(IDDM, type I)

1. These patients are unable to produce endogenous insulin. They require injections of insulin to prevent ketoacidosis and to stay alive.
2. Only 5%–10% of all diabetic patients have IDDM. There may be a hereditary predisposition to this disease, but current evidence suggests that autoimmunity, viruses, and certain histocompatibility (HLA) antigens play a major role in the development of this type of diabetes. It may occur at any age but is most commonly seen in young people and generally has a sudden onset.

B. Non–insulin-dependent diabetes mellitus
(NIDDM, type II)

1. There may be a defect in insulin release from the beta cells of the islets of Langerhans, but most commonly there is resistance to the action of insulin in the peripheral tissues.
2. This type usually develops after age 40 but may be seen in obese children.
3. Eighty percent of these individuals are obese.
4. This type has an almost exclusive hereditary component, and the onset may be prevented or postponed by calorie restriction and weight loss.

C. Diabetes associated with other conditions

1. When the pancreas is damaged by inflammation or degeneration it may be unable to produce sufficient insulin.
2. Several drugs, chemicals, hormones, and genetic syndromes are associated with decreased insulin activity and hyperglycemia.

D. Impaired glucose tolerance (IGT)

1. This stage of glucose intolerance was previously referred to as "latent diabetes" or "chemical diabetes."
2. Chief characteristic of the stage of glucose intolerance is a normal fasting glucose value with an abnormally high postprandial glucose or postglucose load value.
3. It is an asymptomatic stage of glucose intolerance, which may go on to overt diabetes or never progress to overt diabetes.
4. IGT that does not progress to overt diabetes rarely leads to microvascular complications, but there is a significant increase in atherosclerotic disease, a higher prevalence of ECG abnormalities and hypertension.
5. The boundaries of this stage are not well-defined, but need to be so that proper recommendations can be made to these persons regarding treatment.

E. Gestational diabetes (GDM)

This type of diabetes will be discussed in the section on diabetes in pregnancy, see page 1022.

Clinical Manifestations

A. Insulin-dependent diabetes mellitus
(IDDM, type I)

1. The onset is usually abrupt, with polyuria (excessive urine), polydipsia (excessive thirst), and polyphagia (excessive ingestion of food), followed by weight loss, weakness, and fatigue.
2. The insulin deficiency causes hyperglycemia, which in turn causes glucosuria, osmotic diuresis, and the loss of water and electrolytes.
3. Increased gluconeogenesis from the mobilization of protein and fat stores results in weight loss and muscle wasting.
4. Excess ketogenesis leads to ketonemia and acidosis. Excessive diuresis leads to dehydration and hypovolemia (decreased blood volume).

B. Non-insulin-dependent diabetes mellitus
(NIDDM, type II)

1. In the early stages there are no symptoms.
2. Later symptoms include any of those for type I diabetes, as well as the slow healing of cuts, fatigue, blurred vision, cramps in the legs, feet and fingers, itching, and drowsiness.
   a. The symptoms often are so obscure that the

diagnosis is not made until a routine health examination or screening test reveals it.

b. Frequently, a person presents with one of the long-term complications of diabetes (e.g., impotence resulting in a diagnosis of diabetes).

Diagnostic Evaluation

1. In the presence of classic symptoms (polydipsia, polyuria, polyphagia, and weight loss) a random glucose value over 200 mg./dl. is sufficient for diagnosis or
2. Fasting venous plasma glucose over 140 mg./dl. on two occasions or
3. Fasting plasma glucose level under 140 mg./dl. and a 2-hour plasma glucose value over 200 mg./dl. with one intervening value over 200 mg./dl. following a 75-gm. glucose load (oral glucose tolerance test— OGTT).
4. When unsuspected glucosuria is found, the plasma glucose should be determined immediately.
5. Impaired glucose tolerance—fasting plasma glucose level under 140 mg./dl. and 2-hour plasma glucose value between 140 mg./dl. and 200 mg./dl. with one intervening value over 200 mg./dl. following a 75-gm. glucose load.
6. Glucose tolerance test is rarely needed for diagnosis and is not accurate unless it is done properly:
   a. The patient should be on an unrestricted high-carbohydrate diet (150–300 gm. of carbohydrate) and participate in unrestricted physical activity for 3 days.
   b. The test is done in the morning after a 10- to 14-hour fast.
   c. A 75-gm. glucose load is given in adults; 100-gm. glucose load is given in pregnant women.
   d. The patient should remain seated and not smoke during the test; he should take no medication that affects blood glucose.
   e. Blood is drawn before the glucose is administered and every 30 minutes afterwards for 2 hours or more.

Treatment

Treatment will correct biochemical and metabolic abnormalities, attain and maintain the ideal body weight, and postpone the progression of the complications of diabetes by maintaining the plasma glucose level as close to normal as possible. *Every new patient requires intensive and extensive education in order to learn to eat properly, take prescribed insulin or oral agents, test blood and urine, and exercise adequately. Reinforcement of diabetes education at every opportunity is an important part of the nursing management of the patient with diabetes mellitus.*

A. Dietary Management

Goal:

The purpose of dietary management is to attain or maintain ideal body weight and ensure normal growth

1. The meal plan is designed to contain adequate calories, protein, vitamins, and minerals. Most adults require 30 calories/kg. of ideal body weight.
   a. This may be increased to 35–40 calories/kg. for children or adults who are extremely active.
   b. This may be reduced to 15–25 calories/kg. for obese patients and sedentary adults.
2. For most patients the meal plan is calculated to give protein 0.5–1.2 gm./kg. (12%–20% of total calories) and carbohydrates 2–4 gm./kg. (55%–60% of total calories).
3. Fat is added to make up the difference and varies from 0.5–1.5 gm./kg. to give 20%–30% of the total calories. Saturated fats are decreased and polysaturated fats increased as much as possible.
4. An effort is made to use high-fiber food and add more fiber to the meal plan in order to lower glucose absorption. High fiber levels should be added gradually. Intake (40 gm.) should be maintained daily because of possible fluctuations in blood glucose levels. High fiber content may cause abdominal fullness, nausea, vomiting, increased flatulence, increased bowel movements, and vitamin/mineral deficiencies.
5. Use of complex rather than simple carbohydrates should be used because of their effect on glycemia. Not all complex carbohydrates produce the same degree of glycemic response. The effect depends not just on the food itself, but how it is prepared, when it is eaten, what is eaten with, when the last meal was eaten and what it contained, as well as the physiology of the person eating it.
6. The menu should be varied according to the patient's ethnic and cultural background, life-style, food preferences, exercise routine, and eating habits. The emphasis should be on what is allowed rather than on what is forbidden. The meal plan should be adapted to the diabetic, not the diabetic to the meal plan.
7. When insulin is taken, special consideration must be given to ensure adequate carbohydrate intake to correspond to the time when insulin is most effective and less carbohydrate when insulin is least effective.
8. Obese diabetics should be on a strict weight-control program. Many will have a normal plasma glucose after they lose weight. (Remember that obese patients have an excessive amount of circulating insulin but are insulin resistant because of obesity).
9. The American Diabetes Association and American Dietetic Association have prepared exchange lists for patients that reflect these recommendations.
   EXCHANGE LISTS FOR MEAL PLANNING:
   American Diabetes Association, Inc.
   2 Park Avenue
   New York, NY 10016

   American Dietetic Association
   430 North Michigan Avenue
   Chicago, IL 60611
   A GUIDE FOR PROFESSIONALS: The Application of "Exchange Lists for Meal Planning" is also available to those health professionals who provide dietary counseling to individuals with diabetes and their families.
10. Each individual patient must be taught how to measure the correct portions at each meal and how to exchange one item for another on the list.
11. Routine blood glucose testing before each meal and at bedtime is necessary during initial control, in unstable patients, and during illness. Well-controlled, stabilized patients may be followed with fewer tests daily (see p. 702).
12. Intensive nutritional counseling by a professional diet counselor should be done initially and repeated several times with every patient.

B. Exercise

Exercise promotes the utilization of carbohydrates and enhances the action of insulin.

1. Insulin-treated patients may develop hypoglycemia after exercise unless they take extra carbohydrate beforehand.
2. Patients should be encouraged to exercise on a regular basis each day.
3. Because insulin is absorbed more quickly from an exercised extremity, many patients are more stable when injections are given in the abdomen on days when arms or legs are exercised.
4. The rate of insulin absorption varies with the site used—deltoid > anterior thigh > abdomen > buttocks. Site rotation should consist of rotation within a site and then use of another site, instead of daily rotation from one site to another.
5. Diabetics with blood glucose levels over 250 mg./dl., or who have ketones in their urine should not begin exercising until their blood glucose levels are in the normal range. Exercising with elevated blood glucose levels will cause increased secretions of glucagon, growth hormone, and catecholamines, resulting in high blood glucose levels.
6. Exercise in the diabetic with microangiopathy should be discussed with the physician because of potential harmful effects.

C. Insulin Therapy

1. When the patient cannot produce an adequate amount of insulin, it is necessary to give it by injection.
2. Insulin lowers the blood glucose by decreasing the release of glucose from the liver and increasing the utilization of glucose by muscle and fat cells.
3. One or more insulin injections each day is required for patients with insulin-dependent diabetes.
4. Patients with non–insulin-dependent diabetes may require insulin during an acute illness, infection, stress, surgery, or pregnancy.
5. Obese patients can usually achieve a normal blood glucose by calorie restriction and weight loss.

Insulin Preparations

1. Insulin is extracted from the pancreas of slaughtered pigs and cows or is produced synthetically by amino acid substitution or by recombinant DNA techniques in bacteria. The latter two insulin production techniques result in an insulin identical in amino acid sequence to human insulin.
2. Indications for human insulin use include newly diagnosed insulin-dependent diabetes, diabetics using insulin temporarily (e.g., surgery, pregnancy), insulin allergy, and insulin resistance because of the likelihood of producing few if any insulin antibodies.
3. The available preparations vary in onset of action, time of peak effect, and duration of action (Table 16-2). It is important to know the action curve for each type of insulin in order to treat the patient properly.
4. Insulin is prescribed in units. U-100 insulin contains 100 units per milliliter.

Insulin Syringes and Needles

1. The insulin syringe is calibrated according to units (e.g., U-100 insulin should be given with a U-100 syringe).
2. Needles are numbered according to diameter; the higher the number the thinner the needle.
3. No. 27 or No. 28 needles are usually used; 1.2–2.5 cm. (½ to 1 inch).

Regulation of Insulin Doses

1. The dose of insulin is adjusted to maintain the blood glucose within normal range (65–130 mg./dl.) before

Table 16-2 Insulins Available in the United States

Type*	Product Name—Manufacturer†	Appearance
Short Acting		
Onset 0.25–1 hour Peak 2–4 hour Duration 5–7 hour	Regular (Lilly; Squibb–Novo) Actrapid (Squibb–Novo) Velosulin (Nordisk) Humulin R (Lilly)† Actrapid Human (Squibb–Novo)‡	Clear
Intermediate Acting		
Onset 1–4 hour Peak 2–15 hour Duration 12–28 hour	Semilente (Lilly; Squibb–Novo) Semitard (Squibb–Novo) Protophane NPH (Squibb–Novo) NPH (Lilly, Squibb–Novo) Monotard (Squibb–Novo) Insulatard (Nordisk) Lente (Lilly; Squibb–Novo) Lentard (Squibb–Novo) Humulin N (Lilly)‡ Monotard Human (Squibb–Novo)‡	Turbid
Long Acting		
Onset 4–6 hour Peak 10–30 hour Duration 36+ hour	PZI (Lilly; Squibb–Novo) Ultralente (Lilly; Squibb–Novo) Ultratard (Squibb–Novo) Mixtard (Nordisk)	Turbid

* Consult individual manufacturer for exact time of onset, peak, and duration. Values given are approximate ranges.

† Some insulins are available in pure beef, pure pork, beef-pork, or human. Consult individual manufacturer for source.

‡ Lilly's human insulin is of recombinant DNA (biosynthetic) origin, while Squibb-Novo's human insulin is of semi-synthetic origin.

Note: Many insulins are available in either a standard or a purified form.

each meal and at bedtime. Blood glucose tests obtained at this time give the blood glucose value.
2. Insulin activity curves vary from patient to patient and with the site of injection.
   a. Insulin acts more quickly when injected in the upper extremities than in the lower extremities.
   b. Insulin acts more quickly when injected intramuscularly than when injected subcutaneously.
   c. Insulin acts more quickly if there is vigorous exercise of the extremity that received the injection.
3. New patients with IDDM may be started on 20 units of Lente or NPH given before breakfast.
   a. The dose is increased each day until the blood glucose and urine glucose values are normal.
   b. When insulin requirements are changing rapidly, supplemental injections of regular insulin (crystalline zinc insulin) are given before each meal.

▶ **NURSING ALERT:** There is a narrow margin between the amount of insulin needed to make the blood glucose normal and the amount that will cause hypoglycemia. Exercise and delayed meals decrease the need for insulin, whereas illness and emotional stress increase the need for insulin.

    c. The nurse should know when hypoglycemia is most likely to occur with the type of insulin that is being used.

4. Patients are instructed to test blood for sugar before each meal and at bedtime.
5. The patient should keep a record of the blood tests and note on this record any changes in insulin dose, diet, or activities.
6. If blood glucose levels are elevated, urine should be tested for the presence of ketones.

Insulin Administration

See page 703.

Hypoglycemic Reactions to Insulin

1. *Hypoglycemia* is an abnormally low blood glucose (usually below 50 mg./dl.).
2. Hypoglycemia results from too much insulin, not enough food, and/or excessive physical activity.
3. Hypoglycemia may occur 1–3 hours after regular (crystalline zinc) insulin, 4–18 hours after NPH or Lente insulin, or 18–30 hours after Protamine Zinc or Ultra-lente insulin.
4. Hypoglycemia may occur at any time, but it is most commonly seen before meals.
5. Patients at high risk for hypoglycemia are those with deficits of counterregulatory hormones.

Evaluation of Signs and Symptoms of Hypoglycemia

1. Sweating, tremor, pallor, tachycardia, palpitation, nervousness—from release of adrenalin from the central nervous system when the blood glucose falls rapidly.
2. Headache, lightheadedness, confusion, emotional changes, memory lapses, numbness of lips and tongue, slurred speech, lack of coordination, staggering gait, double vision, drowsiness, convulsions, coma—from depression of the central nervous system when the blood glucose level falls slowly.

▶ **NURSING ALERT:** Patients with long-standing diabetes complicated by autonomic neuropathy may develop hypoglycemia without warning, as well as patients taking certain beta blockers. Severe and prolonged hypoglycemia may cause brain damage and death. Any abnormal behavior in a patient taking insulin should be considered as resulting from hypoglycemia until proven otherwise.

Management of Hypoglycemia

1. Give some form of sugar orally if the patient is conscious and can swallow—orange juice, candy, lump sugar, or corn syrup.
2. Give glucagon (subcutaneously or IM) if the patient cannot take sugar by mouth—this causes glycogenolysis in the liver if adequate glycogen stores are present.

3. As soon as the patient regains consciousness, he should be given carbohydrate by mouth.
4. If the patient does not respond to the above measures, he is given 50 ml. of 50% glucose intravenously (IV) or 1000 ml. of 5%–10% glucose in water IV. The recovery will be slow in patients who have had severe and prolonged hypoglycemia.

Preventing Hypoglycemic Reactions Due to Insulin

Instruct the patient as follows:
1. Hypoglycemia may be prevented by maintaining a regular regimen of diet, insulin, and exercise.
2. The early symptoms of hypoglycemia should be recognized and treated.
3. Some form of simple carbohydrate should be carried at all times and taken at the first symptom of hypoglycemia.
4. Between-meal and bedtime snacks may be necessary to maintain a normal glucose level.
5. Extra food should be taken before unusual physical exertion.
6. Frequent blood tests may be necessary, especially in patients with fluctuating blood glucose levels.
7. An identification card or bracelet should be worn.
    a. Identification bracelet may be obtained from Medic-Alert Foundation, International, 2323 Colorado, Turlock, CA 95380.
    b. The card may be obtained from the American Diabetes Association, 2 Park Avenue, New York, NY 10016.

Somogyi Phenomenon

Hypoglycemia is followed by compensatory rebound hyperglycemia that lasts 12–72 hours or longer and is usually caused by an excessive dose of insulin.
1. The patient will have transient hypoglycemia, but most urine specimens will contain glucose.
2. Gradual reduction of the insulin dose and increase of the diet at the time of the hypoglycemia will help to stabilize the patient.

Local Allergic Reactions to Insulin

A. Local reactions

Cause redness, stinging, and induration at the injection site.
1. The reaction may occur within 1 hour but may be delayed for 24 hours.
2. The reaction is usually seen in the early stages of therapy and disappears after a few weeks.
3. If local reactions persist, changing to purified pork insulin or human insulin will usually correct this problem.
4. A few patients have insulin resistance due to insulin allergy. These should be referred to a medical center for antibody testing and treatment.

B. Insulin lipodystrophy

Causes either lipoatrophy (a loss of fat) or lipohypertrophy (an indurated fatty tumor) to appear at the site of insulin injection.
1. Insulin lipoatrophy causes pitting at the site of injection. It previously occurred in 25% of the women and children taking insulin but now occurs in only 2% or less of those who use purified pork or human U-100 insulin.

2. Lipohypertrophy can also be prevented by changing to either a purified pork insulin or human insulin.

C. Insulin edema

Results from fluid retention after the sudden correction of prolonged hyperglycemia.

D. Insulin resistant

Term applied to patients whose requirements exceed 200 units of insulin each day. This condition is rarely seen.

Oral Hypoglycemic Agents (Table 16-3)

1. Oral hypoglycemic agents may be effective for older, non–insulin-dependent (NIDDM), nonketotic patients who are normal in weight and have persistent hyperglycemia after treatment by only diet adjustment.
2. In the US, 6 sulfonylurea drugs are available as oral hypoglycemic agents. The initial effect of these drugs is to increase insulin release from the pancreas. There is a long-term effect of increasing the number of insulin receptors. (See package information for side effects and drug interactions.)
3. Patients usually are treated by diet and exercise alone before oral hypoglycemic drugs are used.
4. Insulin is required when ketosis or severe infection is present, or during surgery or periods of extreme stress.

Patient Problems/Nursing Diagnoses

1. Hyperglycemia related to inadequate metabolism of glucose
2. Potential for development of hypoglycemia related to imbalance between insulin need and insulin dose
3. Potential for development of ketosis/ketoacidosis related to insulin deficiency and faulty fat metabolism
4. Potential development of long-term complications related to persistent hyperglycemia and accelerated atherosclerotic changes in blood vessels (macroangiopathy of the heart and peripheral circulation; microangiopathy of the kidney and retina; peripheral neuropathy and increased susceptibility to infections)
5. Potential nonadherence to the therapeutic regimen related to nonacceptance of disease and regimen or to lack of understanding (dietary regimen, weight control, insulin therapy, exercise program)
6. Anxiety related to diabetes and its prognosis

Nursing Interventions

A. Establishment of normoglycemia

1. Encourage patient to eat regularly spaced meals and snacks within prescribed caloric requirements.
2. Emphasize the importance of a daily exercise program in order to:
   a. Decrease blood glucose levels
   b. Increase levels of high-density lipoproteins (HDL)
   c. Lower cholesterol and triglyceride levels
   d. Reduce stress
   e. Create a feeling of well-being
3. Advise the patient to take insulin and/or oral hypoglycemic agents in the dose and time prescribed and using the appropriate method.
4. Encourage early treatment for hypoglycemia or ketoacidosis.
5. Advise the patient to contact physician if signs of a

Table 16-3 Oral Hypoglycemic Agents Sulfonylurea Compounds

Agent	Duration of action (hr.)	How given
"First Generation"		
Tolbutamide (Orinase)	6–10 hr.	Divided doses
Chorpropamide (Diabinese)	36–60 hr.	Single dose
Acetohexamide (Dymelor)	10–20 hr.	Single or divided doses
Tolazamide (Tolinase)	12–24 hr.	Single or divided doses
"Second Generation" (as of April 1984)		
Glyburide (Micronase or Diabeta)	12–24 hr.	Single or divided doses
Glipizide (Glucotrol)	10–18 hr.	Single or divided doses

local insulin allergy, lipodystrophy, insulin edema, or insulin resistance appear.
6. Encourage the patient to monitor blood glucose levels and urine ketone levels if symptoms of hypoglycemia/hyperglycemia occur.
7. Seek immediate advice from physician if unable to eat or if vomiting or diarrhea occur, and follow sick day rules regarding insulin, diet, and blood/urine glucose monitoring.

B. Prevention or prompt treatment of episodes of hypoglycemia

1. Encourage the patient to:
   a. Eat prescribed meal plan/snacks as scheduled
   b. Eat extra food before periods of vigorous exercise
   c. Take the prescribed insulin dose at same time each day
   d. Monitor blood glucose levels daily
2. Emphasize early treatment of hypoglycemia with a simple sugar.

C. Prevention of or immediate action to counter ketosis/ketoacidosis

1. Encourage the patient to:
   a. Avoid overeating
   b. Take prescribed insulin dose at scheduled times
   c. Continue daily exercise levels
   d. Monitor blood glucose levels daily
   e. Monitor urine for ketones if blood glucose levels are elevated
2. Emphasize early recognition and treatment of hyperglycemia to avoid ketosis.
3. Advise the patient to contact physician for change in insulin dosage or additional insulin as indicated by elevated blood glucose and/or presence of urinary ketones.

Expected Outcomes

1. Achieves/maintains normoglycemia
2. Prevents or reduces incidences of ketosis/ketoacidosis
3. Prevents or reduces incidences of hypoglycemia
4. Delays or prevents the development of long-term complications
5. Adheres to the prescribed regimen

Principles of Health Education: Managing Self-Care

The person with diabetes mellitus must accept a major role in the management of his disease. His education must be amplified, reinforced, and updated continually, since diabetes is a lifelong disease.

Goal:
Maintain the best possible control of diabetes.

The Patient's Goals

A. Become familiar with diabetes and how it affects the body

1. Visit the physician on a regular basis.
2. Study and review available literature from reputable sources.
3. Secure booklets and pamphlets from the American Diabetes Association, Inc, 2 Park Avenue, New York, NY 10016.
4. Attend available classes.

B. Maintain health at an optimal level

1. Maintain a consistent daily routine.
2. Get adequate rest and sleep.
3. Exercise regularly and consistently.
   a. Avoid "spurts" of arduous exercise before meals.
   b. Exercise 1½ hours after meals.
   c. Keep some form of carbohydrate (sugar, candy, orange juice) available during exercise periods.
4. Seek employment with regular hours.

C. Follow the prescribed dietary regimen

1. Eat 3 or more measured meals each day. Plan ahead for prescribed meals and snacks.
2. Become thoroughly familiar with the food exchange lists.
3. Learn how to follow a calculated diet.
4. Know the caloric value of foods frequently eaten.
5. Use household measures or a gram scale until serving sizes can be judged accurately.
6. Avoid concentrated carbohydrates.
7. Avoid periods of fasting and feasting.
8. Keep weight at optimal level; normalize body weight.
   a. Weigh weekly.
   b. Keep a weight record.
9. If taking insulin, eat extra calories when unusual physical activity is anticipated.
10. Eat a bedtime snack when taking insulin (if permissible).

D. Be aware of the degree of diabetes control

1. Test blood for sugar.
2. Test blood before each meal and at bedtime while control is being attained or during periods of illness.
3. Test urine when blood sugar levels are high.
4. Keep a daily record of blood sugar tests (date, hour, value).
5. Test only freshly voided urine.
6. Take the record of blood tests to physician at appointed times.
7. Know that acetone in the urine indicates need for *more insulin.*
8. Protect all urine- and blood-testing equipment from light, moisture, and heat (to prevent false interpretation due to deterioration of test materials).
9. Monitor blood glucose when insulin requirements vary and during illness.
   a. Capillary blood is obtained from finger puncture and spread on enzyme strip.

b. Reaction may be quantitated visually or with the use of a meter.

E. Become familiar with all aspects of insulin usage (see p. 703 for guidelines for teaching self-injection of insulin)

1. Know when the prescribed insulin is having its peak action.
2. Adjust insulin dosage according to blood sugar tests as prescribed.
3. Rotate the sites of insulin injections in a systematic manner within sites and with attention to rates of insulin absorption.
4. Keep the syringe and needle in one particular place.
5. Keep a reserve supply of insulin in the refrigerator.
   a. Keep bottle in current use at *room temperature.*
   b. Avoid injecting cold insulin because it may contribute to tissue reaction.
6. Have an extra insulin syringe available.
7. Know the conditions that produce insulin reactions.
   a. Omission of a meal
   b. Unaccustomed or strenuous exercise
   c. Too much insulin
8. Know the symptoms of an insulin reaction.
   a. Any unfamiliar or peculiar sensation
   b. Hunger, perspiration, palpitation, tachycardia, weakness, tremor, pallor
9. Know how to treat an impending insulin reaction.
   a. Eat carbohydrates (orange juice, sugar, candy) when symptoms first occur.
   b. Test blood sugar.
   c. Carry extra carbohydrate at all times (sugar lumps, candy).
   d. Eat extra carbohydrate before strenuous exercise and during periods of prolonged exercise, or reduce insulin dosage.
   e. Eat a snack at bedtime.
10. Keep a check-off system to ensure taking insulin.
11. Wear identification bracelet or necklace. Carry more detailed information about insulin, etc., in wallet.
12. When traveling, carry diabetic supplies in hand luggage.
    a. Have letter from physician stating that you are a diabetic, as well as a prescription for insulin syringes and other medications.
    b. Keep your watch at the time of departure point until arrival at destination; do not change diabetic regimen en route.

F. Take prescribed oral hypoglycemic medication

1. Adhere faithfully to the prescribed diet.
2. Test urine or blood daily.
3. Take the medication exactly as directed.

G. Appreciate the importance of proper foot care to prevent infection, ischemia, and neuropathy, which may lead to amputation and death

1. Inspect the feet carefully and daily for calluses, corns, blisters, abrasions, redness, and nail abnormalities.
   a. Use a small mirror to check bottom of each foot.
   b. Use a magnifying glass under good light if eyesight is poor, or have someone else check feet.
2. Bathe the feet daily in warm (never hot) water.
   a. Do not soak the feet for prolonged periods. (Soaking is defatting.)
   b. Dry feet carefully, especially between the toes.

3. Massage the feet with an absorbable agent (vegetable oil, lanolin, Nivea cream) except between the toes—autonomically denervated foot loses its ability to sweat, and dries and cracks easily.

4. Prevent moisture between the toes to prevent maceration of the skin.
   a. Insert lamb's wool between overlapping toes.
   b. Use powder in the web spaces, especially if feet perspire.

5. Wear well-fitting, noncompressive shoes and socks—long enough, wide enough, soft, supple, and low-heeled.
   a. Buy shoes in the afternoon—feet are larger in the afternoon than in the morning.
   b. Have each foot measured before buying shoes—feet enlarge with age.
   c. Have the measurement taken while standing, since foot is larger in the standing position.
   d. Do not "break in" shoes all at one time.
   e. Avoid rubber- or plastic-soled shoes, or vinyl shoes, which cause the feet to perspire and aggravate fungal infections.
   f. Avoid working in bedroom slippers or other casual footwear.

6. Go to a podiatrist on a regular basis if corns, calluses, and ingrown toenails are present.
   a. Cut toenails straight across to prevent ingrown toenails.

7. Avoid heat, chemicals, and injuries to the feet—do not go barefoot or expose feet to hot-water bottles, heating pads, caustic solutions, etc. Heat increases demand for blood, which cannot be met because of the reduction of vascular reserve. Diabetic neuropathy causes loss of cutaneous sensation, so that the patient may suffer burns or pressure lesions without being aware of them.
   a. Switch off electric blanket before going to bed; wear socks at night to keep feet warm if necessary.
   b. Avoid overheated baths and sitting too close to a fire.

8. Inspect inside of shoes for foreign objects, etc.

9. If an injury occurs to the foot:
   a. Wash the area with mild soap and water.
   b. Cover with a dry sterile dressing *without* adhesive.
   c. Wear white cotton socks; dye in colored socks and wool may serve as irritants when skin is already irritated.
   d. Call the physician.

H. Maintain diabetes control during periods of illness or stress

1. Call physician immediately when any unusual symptoms become evident; *do not allow diabetes to get out of control.*

2. Make dietary adjustments during illness according to physician's directions.

3. Continue taking insulin; physician may increase dosage during illness.

4. Test blood for sugar and urine for acetone more frequently; keep records.

5. Monitor blood glucose.

6. Know the conditions that bring about diabetic acidosis.
   a. Nausea and vomiting
   b. Failure to increase insulin when blood sugar is increasing
   c. Failure to take insulin
   d. Stress
   e. Infections
   f. Menstrual periods

7. Know how to treat impending diabetic acidosis.
   a. Examine blood for sugar and urine for acetone and report results to physician.
   b. Take additional insulin as advised by physician.
   c. Go to bed and keep warm.
   d. Alert someone to be in attendance.
   e. Drink a glass of liquid hourly if possible. Replace calories needed with carbohydrate containing liquids.

I. Follow other health directives

1. Avoid tobacco—nicotine constricts blood vessels, causing reduction in blood flow to feet.

2. Take only medications prescribed by physician—many drugs enhance effect of insulin and oral antidiabetic agents.

Guidelines: Teaching Self-Injection of Insulin

Underlying Considerations

1. Insulin injection should be taught as soon as the need for insulin treatment has been established.
2. A member of the patient's family should also be taught how to administer insulin.
3. An optimistic approach will offer the patient encouragement.
4. Teach insulin injection *first,* since this is the patient's major concern; then teach loading the syringe.

Equipment

Prescribed bottle of insulin
Disposable insulin syringe and needles
Absorbent cotton and alcohol or prepackaged alcohol swabs

Procedure

Teaching Action	Rationale/Amplification
1. Give the patient the prepared syringe containing the prescribed dose of insulin.	
2. Have patient wipe the skin with alcohol.	
3. Instruct the patient to hold the syringe as he would a pencil.	

(continued)

Guidelines: Teaching Self-Injection of Insulin (continued)

Procedure
(Cont.)

Teaching Action	Rationale/Amplification
4. Show the patient how to spread the skin taut on the anterior thigh (Fig. 16-2A). or Form a skin fold by picking up subcutaneous tissue between the thumb and forefinger if the patient is thin (Fig. 16-2B).	4. Either of the techniques ensures that the needle tip is inserted into subcutaneous tissue and outside the muscle. Avoid pressing the skin *tightly* between the fingers, since this is a common cause of local induration and infection.

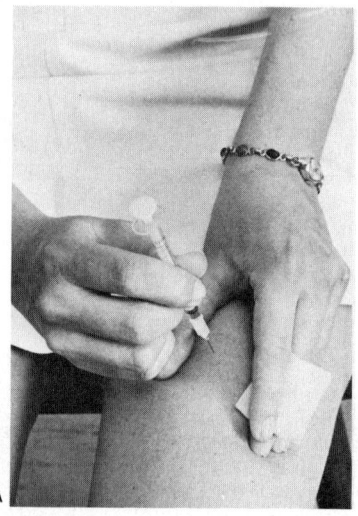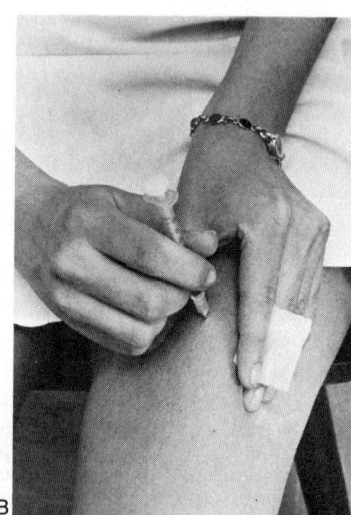

Figure 16-2. Self-injection of insulin. *(A) The insulin syringe is held perpendicular to the stretched skin before the needle is thrust into the subcutaneous tissues. (B) Alternate method: If the patient has only a thin layer of subcutaneous fat, a fold of skin is pinched between the fingers to keep the needle from penetrating into the muscle.*

Teaching Action	Rationale/Amplification
5. Select areas of upper arms, thighs, flanks, and upper buttocks for injection after patient becomes proficient with needle insertion.	5. The skin is loose and there is more subcutaneous fat in these areas.
6. Assist the patient to insert needle with a quick thrust to the hub at a right angle to the skin surface (Fig. 16-2B).	6. The insulin is injected into deep subcutaneous tissue.
7. Instruct the patient to release the skin fold.	
8. Hold the alcohol sponge against the needle and gently withdraw the needle. Wipe area with alcohol sponge.	8. This maneuver prevents painful pulling of the skin as the needle is withdrawn.
9. Develop a systematic plan for insulin administration (e.g., rotation of sites in a clockwise fashion [Fig. 16-3]).	9. Systematic rotation of sites will keep the skin supple, and will favor uniform absorption of insulin.

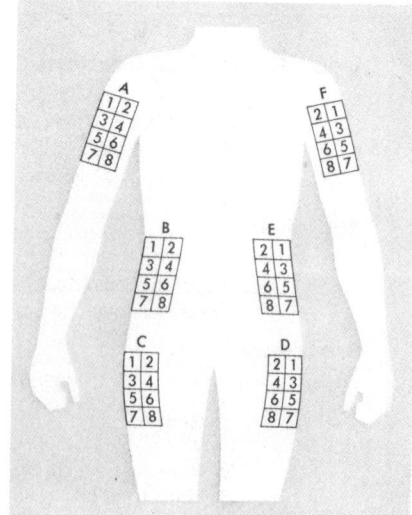

Figure 16-3. *Rotate within each site and keep in mind the various rates of absorption in different sites. Exercising an injected site will hasten insulin absorption also. (From ADA Forecast—the Diabetics' Own Magazine. vol 4[1]. Courtesy of Becton, Dickinson.)*

Procedure
(Cont.)

Teaching Action	Rationale/Amplification

To Load the Syringe:

1. Roll the bottle of insulin (Protamine Zinc, NPH and Lente) between the palms of the hands.
2. Wipe off the top of the insulin vial with an alcohol sponge.
3. Inject approximately the same volume of air into the insulin vial as the volume of insulin to be withdrawn.

1. The rolling action mixes the insulin.

3. Air is injected into the vial to keep its contents under slight positive pressure and to make it easier to withdraw the insulin.

To Fill a Syringe with Long- and Short-Acting Insulin Mixture:

1. Wipe off the vial tops with an alcohol swab.
2. Inject air equal to the number of units to be injected into long-acting insulin first; withdraw needle.
3. Inject air into short-acting insulin bottle and withdraw prescribed amount of insulin.
4. Then withdraw prescribed amount of insulin from long-acting insulin bottle.

Rapid Methods of Urine Testing for Glucose (Sugar) and Ketones (Acetone)

Underlying Considerations

1. Sugar appears in the urine when the glucose in the blood rises over 170 mg./dl. In most people but especially older people, the renal threshold rises above this level.
2. Urinary sugar (glucosuria) may appear when:
   a. More insulin or sulfonylurea is needed.
   b. The patient is eating more than he should.
   c. Exercise is inadequate.
   d. Infection is present.
3. Incorrect tests occur because:
   a. Deteriorated reagent tablets are used.
   b. The directions are not followed accurately.
   c. The patient is taking medication that gives false-positive or false-negative results.

Instructions to the Patient

The first-voided urine is the preferable urine specimen to use (if it has not been in the bladder for hours) for screening the urine for sugar. Second-voided specimens were thought to correlate better with blood glucose values than the first-voided specimens, but this has since been disproved.

Tests for Glucose (Sugar)

Copper Reduction Test

A. Clinitest*—uses a reagent tablet

1. *Two-drop method*—allows estimation of concentration of sugar in the urine up to 5%
   a. Hold dropper vertically and place 2 drops (0.1 ml.) of urine in test tube.
   b. Rinse dropper. Add 10 drops (0.5 ml.) of water to test tube.
   c. Add 1 Clinitest reagent tablet. *Do not shake test tube.*
   d. Wait 15 seconds after boiling stops and shake test tube gently to mix contents.
   e. Compare color of urine with appropriate color chart. (Use only the 2-drop method color scale,

which has 7 colors, ranging in value from 0–5%.)
2. *Five-drop method*
   a. Hold dropper vertically and place 5 drops of urine in test tube.
   b. Rinse dropper. Add 10 drops of water to test tube.
   c. Put 1 Clinitest tablet in test tube.
      (1) Watch while reaction takes place.
      (2) Do not shake test tube during reaction or for 15 seconds after boiling inside test tube has stopped.
   d. Observe the solution in the test tube *while the reaction takes place and during the 15-second waiting period to detect pass-through color changes caused by glucosuria over 2%.*
      (1) If the solution passes through orange and dark shades of green-brown, it indicates more than 2% (4+) urine sugar is present.
      (2) Record as such without reference to color scale.
   e. After 15-second waiting period, shake test tube gently and compare with the color scale.
   f. Record results.

Enzyme Methods

B. Diastix*—reagent strip

1. Dip reagent end of strip in urine specimen for 2 seconds and remove (or wet end of strip for 2 seconds by passing through urine stream).
2. Tap edge of strip against side of urine container or sink to remove excess urine.
3. Exactly 30 seconds after removing from urine, compare reagent side of strip to closest matching color block on package label.

C. Tes-Tape†—reagent tape

1. Dip part of the Tes-Tape into the urine.
2. Expose to air 60 seconds—the enzyme requires oxygen for color development.
3. Compare the darkest area with the color chart. If tape indicates ½% or higher, wait 1 additional minute and make final comparison.

---

* Clinitest, Diastix, Acetest, Ketostix, and Keto-Diastix are products of Ames Company, Division of Miles Laboratories, Inc., Elkhart, IN 46514.

† Tes-Tape is a product of Eli Lilly and Company, Indianapolis, IN 46225.

Tests for Acetone (Ketone bodies)

A. Acetest*—reagent tablets

1. Use freshly voided specimen—prolonged standing of urine specimen encourages bacterial growth which can decrease the number of ketone bodies.
2. Place tablet on a piece of white paper.
3. Place 1 drop of urine on tablet.
4. Compare urine ketone test results to color chart at 30 seconds after application of specimen.
5. Acetest* may also give semi-quantitative determinations of ketones in serum, plasma, or whole blood.

B. Ketostix*—reagent strips

1. Dip test strip in freshly voided specimen or pass it briefly through the urinary stream.
2. Remove immediately. Draw edge of strip against urine container to remove excess urine.
3. Wait 15 seconds. Compare color of test strip with the color chart.
4. See package directions for testing serum and plasma.

Combined (Ketone–Glucose) **Reagent Strip**

Keto-Diastix—combined ketone–glucose reagent strip

1. Dip reagent end of strip in urine specimen and remove immediately.
2. Tap edge of strip against side of container to remove excess urine.
3. Compare reagent side of test areas with corresponding color charts at the time specified on the charts. (Glucose is read exactly at 30 seconds, and ketone is read at exactly 15 seconds.)

Acute Complications of Diabetes

The diabetic may become comatose because of hypoglycemia (see p. 700), diabetic ketoacidosis, and hyperosmolar–nonketotic coma, in addition to all of the conditions that can produce coma in the nondiabetic.

Diabetic Ketoacidosis

Diabetic ketoacidosis results from the absence of effective insulin, which causes hyperglycemia, ketonuria, dehydration, and acidosis. Glucose no longer enters muscle cells, and fat is metabolized to produce energy. Free fatty acids are converted to ketone bodies in the liver. The ketone bodies are organic acids that cause metabolic acidosis.

Precipitating Causes

1. Failure to take an adequate amount of insulin
2. Failure to increase the dose of insulin in the presence of acute infection
3. Failure to increase insulin to compensate for pregnancy, injury, surgery, or emotional stress

Clinical Manifestations

A. Early Manifestations

1. Polyuria, polydipsia, fatigue, malaise, drowsiness
2. Anorexia, headache, abdominal pains
3. Muscle cramps, nausea, vomiting, constipation

B. Later Manifestations

1. Kussmaul breathing—very deep respiratory movements
2. Sweetish odor of the breath due to ketonemia
3. Hypotension and weak, thready pulse
4. Stupor and coma

Laboratory Evaluation

A. Blood

Glucose elevated, bicarbonate decreased, arterial pH decreased, strongly positive plasma ketone

B. Urine

Strongly positive for sugar and ketone, and moderately positive for protein

Goals:
Restore normal metabolism.
Correct hypovolemia.

Reduce hyperglycemia and correct electrolyte imbalance.

1. Obtain blood and urine samples immediately:
   a. Test blood for glucose, ketone, BUN, electrolytes, complete blood count, arterial pH, PO_2, and PCO_2.
   b. Obtain urine specimen at prescribed time and measure sugar, acetone, and volume. Catheterize only if a voided specimen cannot be obtained.
   c. Start a flow chart that includes vital signs, clinical manifestations, laboratory data, and therapy arranged in a chronological manner.
2. Carry out a rapid physical examination to look for infection, myocardial infarction, stroke, etc.
   a. Record vital signs, state of hydration, and mental status.
3. Start intravenous infusion of isotonic saline solution at a rate of about 500 ml. per hour to rehydrate the patient. Later the type of fluid and rate of administration are changed.
4. Give insulin as directed—to increase glucose utilization and decrease lipolysis. Insulin may be given by:
   a. Continuous infusion low-dose therapy. An infusion pump may be used, or insulin may be put into the bottle containing the intravenous solution. Because ⅓ of the solution sticks to the bottle and tubing, it is necessary to increase the dose as directed.
   b. Deep intramuscular injections of regular insulin into the deltoid may be used instead.
   c. Insulin may be administered via a bedside closed-loop insulin pump, which has a glucose sensor and an insulin reservoir. Only available in large medical centers. Used until the ketoacidosis has been resolved.
5. As the serum glucose falls, glucose is added to the infusion, and the insulin dose is reduced as directed.
6. Determinations of serum glucose, ketone, bicarbonate, and potassium are done every 3–6 hours.
7. One or more ECG tracings may be needed to rule out silent myocardial infarction, and to monitor intracellular potassium levels.
8. The rapid utilization of glucose under the influence of insulin causes potassium to migrate into the cells,

and results in hypokalemia after 4–8 hours of treatment.

   a. This is corrected by administering buffered potassium phosphate (or chloride) at a rate of no more than 20 mEq. per hour. This is usually added to the infusion after 3 or 4 hours.

9. Hypotension will usually respond to adequate saline infusion.
10. If the patient is given nothing by mouth for 3 hours while rehydration takes place, nausea usually subsides, and the patient can usually be given clear liquids.
11. The recurrence of diabetic ketoacidosis can be prevented by adequate patient education. The patient should increase the dose of insulin when there is glucosuria and ketonuria, and seek medical advice when there are symptoms of diabetic ketoacidosis.

Nonketotic Hyperosmolar Coma

Nonketotic hyperosmolar coma is characterized by hyperglycemia, hyperosmolarity, severe dehydration, and stupor or coma, but there is no ketonemia or acidosis.

Altered Physiology

1. There is some, but not enough, insulin present. This condition occurs in older people who do not have diabetes but who have been given excessive carbohydrate without adequate fluid administration.
2. Hyperglycemia causes osmotic diuresis, resulting in severe loss of water and electrolytes.
3. Water shifts from the intracellular to the extracellular fluid and causes intracellular dehydration.

Clinical Manifestations

1. History of precipitating event—severe burns, pancreatitis, hemodialysis, hyperalimentation, and excessive use of diuretics may be factors.
2. Severe hyperglycemia with a negative serum acetone and a normal serum bicarbonate.
3. Severe dehydration with poor skin turgor, hypotension, fever, and decreased brain activity. Seizures may occur.
4. Serum osmolarity is greatly elevated.

Treatment

Goal:

Correct the volume depletion and hyperosmolar state.

1. Isotonic saline solution and low-dose insulin infusion is the primary treatment.

2. Potassium and glucose are added later as indicated by results of the blood chemistry tests.
3. As soon as the patient regains consciousness, liquids are given orally.

Infections

Underlying Considerations

Infections are more protracted and serious in diabetics for the following reasons:

1. Hyperglycemia causes decreased leukocyte phagocytosis. Ketonemia causes decreased leukocyte migration.
2. Diabetes becomes more severe in the presence of infection.
3. Ketoacidosis may be precipitated by infection and inadequate insulin.

Types of Infection

1. Infections of the urinary tract may follow incomplete emptying of the bladder due to diabetic neuropathy or urethral obstruction. Bladder infections may spread to the kidney and cause pyelonephritis.
2. Infections of the extremities due to local injury may occur in patients with diabetic neuropathy who cannot recognize pain. If the skin is dry and cracked, bacteria may penetrate the protective envelope and cause infection.
   a. Inflammation due to infection causes edema of the tissue, decreased blood supply, and decreased resistance to infection.
   b. Atherosclerosis may also cause ischemic injury to the tissue.
3. Dermatologic infections:
   a. Infections of the skin and vagina frequently found in poorly controlled diabetes.
   b. Furuncles and carbuncles due to staphylococcus.
   c. Gas-forming infections under the skin and in the genitourinary tract.

Treatment

1. The dose of insulin is increased enough to correct the ketonemia and hyperglycemia.
2. The blood is tested frequently for sugar to adjust the insulin dose.
3. Cultures of blood, urine, sputum, and pus are essential for determining the responsible organism and for selecting the correct antibiotic.

Long-Term Complications of Diabetes

Underlying Considerations

1. Diabetes is the most common cause of new blindness and new cases of end-stage renal disease in the US. Accelerated atherosclerosis causes an increased incidence of myocardial infarction, stroke, and gangrene.
2. Because diabetics are living longer, these complications are becoming more common.

Vascular Complications

1. The specific pathologic lesion (microangiopathy) of long-standing diabetes is thickening of the capillary basement membrane in every organ.

2. The prevalence of microangiopathy parallels the duration and severity of hyperglycemia.
3. Intercapillary glomerulosclerosis (Kimmelstiel–Wilson syndrome), the specific renal disease of diabetes, results from the thickening of the capillary basement membrane in the glomeruli.
4. Microangiopathy of the vessels supplying the skin, peripheral nerves, and walls of large arteries may be a factor in skin diseases, neuropathy, and atherosclerosis.
5. Major vessel occlusion (macroangiopathy) resulting from atherosclerosis causes stroke, myocardial infarction, intermittent claudication, and gangrene. The progress of atherosclerosis is accelerated in diabetics.

Diabetic Retinopathy

Diabetic retinopathy is a progressive impairment of retinal circulation that causes vitreous hemorrhage and loss of vision.

1. Incidence and severity of retinopathy is related to the duration and degree of control of diabetes; half of the patients who have had diabetes for more than 10 years have some evidence of retinopathy.
2. Impaired vision and blindness are caused by hemorrhage and neovascularization into the vitreous with the formation of scar tissue and eventual detachment of the retina.
3. *Treatment*
   a. Photocoagulation—produced when a narrow, intensive beam of light is directed into the eye and focused on the retina; the absorption of light produces heat, which coagulates the treated vessel and prevents it from bleeding.
      (1) Used when there are areas of newly formed blood vessels and proliferative retinopathy.
      (2) Photocoagulation must be done when proliferative changes first occur so that bleeding can be prevented.
   b. Vitrectomy—removal of blood and fibrous tissue through a small opening on the side of the eye and replacement with clear fluid that maintains the shape of the eye; may be tried for patients whose blindness is due to vitreous hemorrhage.

Diabetic Neuropathy

Diabetic neuropathy affects the peripheral and autonomic nervous system and produces a wide variety of syndromes.

1. Clinical manifestations
   a. Peripheral neuropathy—pain (dull, aching, burning, lancinating, or crushing), paresthesia (sensations of tingling or burning or coldness and numbness).
   b. Involvement of autonomic nervous system—orthostatic hypotension, sexual impotency, retrograde ejaculation, pupillary changes, abnormal sweating, bladder paralysis, nocturnal diarrhea.
2. Assessment of the feet of diabetic patients
   (The complications of neuropathy and vascular disease are most evident in the feet. Most amputations, other than those occurring from trauma, occur in diabetics.)
   a. Watch for lesions of the feet that do not heal.
   b. Compare the skin color of both feet and ankles. A blue-gray color is caused by diminution of the blood supply.
   c. Change the position of the extremity and note the color change. Pallor on elevation and dusky cyanosis on dependency indicate vascular insufficiency.
   d. Feel the temperature of the skin with the back of your hand and notice decreased temperature.
   e. Examine the toenails. Thick, ridged nails suggest circulatory impairment or fungus infection.
   f. Look for athlete's foot between the toes (epidermophytosis), and fungus infection of the nails (onycomycosis). Fungal infection is more serious in the diabetic and requires treatment.
   g. Look for calluses, corns, blisters, cracks, and abrasions; look between the toes and on the soles of the feet.
   h. Palpate the dorsalis pedis and posterior tibial arterial pulses; absence of a discernible pulse or diminution of the pulses indicate atherosclerosis.

Management of the Diabetic Patient Undergoing Surgery

Underlying Considerations

The diabetic patient must be followed closely at the time of surgery because stress, infection, and missed meals change insulin requirements.
1. The trauma of surgery causes hyperglycemia.
2. Infection causes the insulin requirements to rise.
3. Anesthesia may cause hyperglycemia and ketosis.
4. The patient's normal schedule of food intake is usually interrupted.

Treatment
Goal:
Achieve the best nutritional balance and best possible metabolic control of the diabetes preoperatively.

A. Preoperative Preparation
1. Essential preoperative evaluation studies are urinalysis, blood glucose, BUN, electrolyte, and CBC.
2. The usual diet is given, but the insulin dose may be reduced the day before surgery.

B. Day of Surgery
1. A fasting blood glucose is drawn and an intravenous infusion of 1,000 ml. of 5% glucose may be given over a 4-hour period for each meal that is missed.
2. The patient is usually given ½ to ¾ his usual dose of insulin.

C. Postoperative management
1. Maintain nutrition with intravenous glucose until patient is able to tolerate food by mouth.
2. Give insulin as directed. The usual dose of intermediate-acting insulin is started the day after surgery, and supplemental regular insulin may be given on a sliding scale according to blood glucose tests.

Bibliography

Disorders of the Thyroid Gland

Books

Fischbach F. A Manual of Laboratory Diagnostic Tests. Philadelphia, JB Lippincott, 1984

Kim MJ, McFarland GK and McLane AM.

Pocket Guide to Nursing Diagnosis. St Louis, CV Mosby, 1984

Muthe NC. Endocrinology: A Nursing Approach. Boston, Little, Brown & Co, 1981

Nurse's Clinical Library. Endocrine Disorders. Springhouse, PA, Springhouse Corp, 1984

Stephens GJ. Pathophysiology for Health

Practitioners. New York, Macmillan, 1980

Williams RH. Textbook of Endocrinology. Philadelphia, WB Saunders, 1981

Articles

Arcangelo VP. Simple goiter. Nursing '83 1983 March; 13(3):47

Brown JS and Steiner AL. Medullary thyroid carcinoma and the syndromes of multiple endocrine adenomas. DM 1982 Aug; 28(11):1–37

Comments on thyrotoxicosis treatment. Patient Care 1983 Dec 15; 17(21):26

DeGroot LJ. Differentiating the forms of thyroiditis. Patient Care 1983 June 30; 17(12):127–144

Evangelisti JT and Thorpe CJ. Thyroid storm—a nursing crisis. Heart Lung 1983 Mar; 12(2):184–193

Farrar WB. Complications of thyroidectomy. Surg Clin North Am 1983 Dec; 63(6):1353–1361

Flaherty RJ. Postpartum thyroiditis. Am Fam Physician 1984 Feb; 29(2):195–197

Gambert SR and Brensinger JF. Assessing thyroid function in the elderly. Nurse Practitioner. 1983 July/Aug; 8(7):38–43

Gilliland PF. Endocrine emergencies. Postgrad Med 1983 Nov; 74(5):215–227

Gresham DG and Wool MS. Hypothyroidism after radioiodine therapy for Graves' disease. Postgrad Med 1984 Mar; 75(4):299–305

Hilyard N. Solitary thyroid nodules in adults. Nurse Practitioner 1983 Feb; 8(2):14–15

Hollingsworth DR. Graves' disease. Clin Obstet Gynecol 1983 Sept; 26(3):615–634

Honigman RE. Thyroid function tests. Nursing '82 1982 Apr; 12(4):68–71

Jackson I. That thyroid nodule: Is it cancer? Mod Med 1984 Apr; 52(4):88–91, 94

Johnson D. Pathophysiology of thyroid storm: Nursing implications. Crit Care Nurse 1983 Nov/Dec; 2:80–86

Kabadi UM. Laboratory evaluation of anatomic disorder of the thyroid. Am Fam Physician 1983 Nov; 28(5):195–203

Martyn PA. If you guessed cardiovascular disease, guess again (Thyroid). Am J Nurs 1982 Aug; 82(8):1238–1241

Molitch ME. Role of nutritional status on thyroid function. Nutrition and the MD 1982 Sept; 8(9):1–2

Morley JE. The aging endocrine system. Postgrad Med 1983 Mar; 73(3):107–120

Roman SH and Davies TF. Thyroid antibody titers: How can they help you? Mod Med 1984 Jan; 52(1):131–141

Trence D. Thyroid replacement therapy. Postgrad Med 1983 Feb; 73(2):367

Volpe R. Autoimmune thyroid disease. Hosp Pract 1984 Jan; 19(1):141–158

Disorders of the Parathyroid Glands

Falko JM et al. Primary hyperparathyroidism: Analysis of 220 patients with special emphasis on familial hypocalciuric hypercalcemia. Heart Lung 1984 Mar; 13(2):124–131

Hoffman JTT and Mewby TB. Hypercalcemia in primary hyperparathyroidism. Nurs Clin North Am 1980 Sept; 15(3):469–480

Jordan RM. Endocrine emergencies.

Med Clin North Am 1983 Nov; 67(6):1193–1213

McFadden EA, Zaloga GP and Chernow B. Hypocalcemia: A medical emergency. Am J Nurs 1983 Feb; 83(2):227–230

Stoffer SS, Szpunar WE and Block M. Hyperparathyroidism and thyroid disease. Postgrad Med 1982 June; 71(6):91–94

Disorders of the Adrenal Glands

Camunas C. Pheochromocytoma. Am J Nurs 1983 June; 83(6):887–891

Didonato K. High dose, short-term steroid therapy (40 days). CA Nurs 1984 June; 7(3):251–256

Harris RB and DelaRoca RR. Pheochromocytoma: A medical review. Heart Lung 1984 Jan; 13(1):73–81

Harris RB and Heany G. Comprehensive nursing care of the patient with pheochromocytoma. Heart Lung 1984 Jan; 13(1):82–88

Jones SG. Adrenal patient. Proceed with caution. RN 1982 Jan; 45(1):66–68, 70, 72

Miller PH. Primary aldosteronism: A challenging case. DCCN 1984 Mar/Apr; 3(2):84–90

Sanford SJ. Dysfunction of the adrenal gland: Physiologic considerations and nursing problems. Nurs Clin North Am 1980 Sept; 15(3):481–498

Shapiro GG. Corticosteroids in the treatment of allergic disease: Principles and practice. Ped Clin North Am 1983 Oct; 30(5):955–971

Pituitary Disorders
Books

Laws ER Jr et al (eds). The Management of Pituitary Adenomas and Related Lesions with Emphasis on Transsphenoidal Microsurgery. New York, Appleton-Century-Crofts, 1982

Odell WD and Nelson DH. Pituitary Tumors. Mt Kisco, Futura Publishing, 1984

Articles

Houston C. Transsphenoidal pituitary microsurgery. Today's OR Nurse 1983 Nov; 5(9):23–28

Tindall GT and Tindall SC. Surgery of the pituitary gland. Curr Probl Surg 1981 Oct; 18(10):610–679(entire volume)

Diabetes Mellitus
Books

A Guide for Professionals: The Effective Application of Exchange Lists for Meal Planning. New York, American Diabetes Association and Chicago, the American Dietetic Association, 1977

Diabetes in the Family. Bowie, Robert J Brady, 1982

Feet First. A booklet about foot care for older people and people who have diabetes. US Department of Health, Education and Welfare, 1970

Guidelines for Diabetes Care. New York, American Diabetes Association and

Chicago, American Association of Diabetes Educators, 1981

Guthrie D and Guthrie R (eds). Nursing Management of Diabetes. St Louis, CV Mosby, 1982

Hamburg B et al (eds). Behavioral and Psychosocial Issues in Diabetes. Proceedings of the National Conference. US Department of Health and Human Services, NIH Publication No. 80-1993, 1979

Kozak G. Clinical Diabetes Mellitus. Philadelphia, WB Saunders, 1982

Marble A et al (eds). Joslin's Diabetes Mellitus. Philadelphia, Lea & Febiger, 1985

Podolsky S (ed). Clinical Diabetes: Modern Management. New York, Appleton-Century-Crofts, 1980

Rifkin H and Raskin P (eds). Diabetes Mellitus. Bowie, Robert J Brady, 1981

Sims DF (ed). Diabetes: Reach for Health and Freedom. St Louis, CV Mosby, 1984

Van Son A (ed). Diabetes and Patient Education: A Daily Nursing Challenge. New York, Appleton-Century-Crofts, 1982

Articles
Comas

Murray P. When hyperglycemia goes critical. RN 1983 Mar; 46(3):56–60, 106

Shade D and Eaton RP. Pathogenesis of diabetic ketoacidosis: A reappraisal. Diabetes Care 1979 May–Jun; 2(3):296–306

Complications

Blankenship GW and Skyler JS. Diabetic retinopathy: A general survey Diabetes Care. 1978 Mar–Apr; 1(2):127–137

Block AM. Sexual dysfunction of the male with diabetes mellitus. Nurse Pract 1982 Sep; 7(8):19–25

Bodansky HJ et al. Risk factors associated with severe proliferative retinopathy in insulin-dependent diabetes mellitus. Diabetes Care 1982 Mar–Apr; 5(2)97–100

Colwell J et al. Pathogenesis of atherosclerosis in diabetes mellitus. Diabetes Care 1981 Jan–Feb; 4(1):121–133

Diabetic neuropathy—where are we now? (editorial) Lancet 1983 Jun 18; 1(8338):1366–1367

Diabetic Retinopathy Study Research Group. Four risk factors for severe visual loss in diabetic retinopathy. Third report from the Diabetic Retinopathy Study. Arch Ophthalmol 1979 Apr; 97(4):654–655

Ellenberg M. Sexual aspects of the female diabetic. J Mt Sinai Hosp 1977 Jul/Aug; 44(4):495–500

Ellenberg M. Sex and diabetes. A comparison between men and women. Diabetes Care 1979 Jan–Feb; 2(1):4–8

L'Esperance FA Jr et al. Long-term retention of vision following vetrectomy in diabetic patients. Diabetes Care 1981 Nov–Dec; 4(6):631–633

Manouchehr-Pour M et al. Periodontal disease in juvenile and adult diabetic patients: A review of the literature. J

Am Dent Assoc 1983 Nov; 107(5):766–770

Medalie J. Risk factors other than hyperglycemia in diabetic macrovascular disease. Diabetes Care 1979 Mar–Apr; 2(2):77–84

Nemchik R. Diabetes retinopathy: The current status of therapy (pictorial). RN 1983 Jun; 46(6):34–37, 40, 63

Nemchik R. Diabetes today: Facing up to the long-term complications. RN 1983 Jul; 46(7):38–45

Oehler JW. Self-management of diabetes mellitus following vision loss. J Ophthalm Nurs Technol 1982 Nov; 1(3):20–27

Patz A. Management of patients with severe disc neovascularization in diabetic retinopathy. Trans New Orleans Acad Ophthalmol 1983; 366–371

Pirart Jean. Diabetes mellitus and its degenerative complications: A prospective study of 4,400 patients observed between 1947 and 1973. Part 2. Diabetes Care. 1978 Jul–Aug; 1(4):252–263

Porte D. Diabetic neuropathy and plasma glucose control. Am J Med 1981 Jan; 70(1):195–200

Riblett B. Diabetes mellitus: The undiscussed side effect: Sexual dysfunction. RN 1983 Jul; 46(7):40–41

Ruhland F. The diabetic with visual impairment. In Steiner G and Lawrence P (eds). Educating Diabetic Patients. New York, Springer Publishing Co, 1981; pp. 242–243

Tamborlane WV et al. Longterm improvement of metabolic control with the insulin pump does not reverse diabetic microangiopathy. Diabetes Care 1982 May–Jun; 5 suppl 1:58–64

Taub S et al. Review: Gastrointestinal manifestations of diabetes mellitus. Diabetes Care 1979 Sep/Oct; 2(5):437–447

Villeneuve ME. Self-care for the totally blind diabetic: It is possible. RN 1983 Jun; 46(6):38–39

Diagnosis

National Diabetes Data Group. Classification of diabetes mellitus and other categories of glucose intolerance. Bethesda, MD, National Institutes of Health, 1978; see also Diabetes 1979 Dec; 28(12):1039–1057

Diet/Nutrition

American Diabetes Association and The American Dietetic Association. Exchange List for Meal Planning. New York, 1976

Anderson J et al. Review: Fiber and diabetes. Diabetes Care 1979 Jul/Aug; 2(4):369–379

Crapo P. A survey of sweeteners. Clin Diabetes 1983 Nov/Dec; 1(6):21

Crapo P. The nutritional therapy of non-insulin dependent (type II) diabetes. Diabetes Educ 1983 Fall; 9(3):13–18, 59

McDonald J. Alcohol and diabetes. Diabetes Care 1980 Sep/Oct; 3(5):629–637

National Diabetes Information Clearinghouse. Nutrition for the Diabetic Patient. Selected annotations. 805 15th Street, NW, Suite 500, Washington, DC 20005

Nemchik R. A very different diet; a new generation of oral drugs. RN 1982 Nov; 41–45, 97–99

Nuttal FQ and Brunzell JD. Principles of nutrition and dietary recommendations for individuals with diabetes mellitus. Diabetes 1979 Nov; 28(11):1027–1030

West KM. Diet therapy of diabetes: An analysis of failure. Ann Intern Med 1973 Sep; 79(3):425

Etiology

Barbosa J et al. Do genetic factors play a role in the pathogenesis of diabetic microangiopathy? Diabetologia 1984 Nov; 27(5):487–492

Greenberg DA et al. The search for heterogeneity in insulin-dependent diabetes mellitus: Evidence for familial and nonfamilial forms. Am J Med Genet 1983 Mar; 14(3):487–499

Rotter J et al. Diabetes mellitus: The search for genetic markers. Diabetes Care 1979 Mar/Apr; 2(2):215–226

Stiller CR et al. Effects of cyclosporine immunosuppression in insulin-dependent diabetes mellitus of recent onset. Science 1984 Mar 30; 223(4643):1362–1367

Yoon JW. Viruses in the pathogenesis of type I diabetes. Curr Prob Clin Biochem 1983; 12:11–44

Exercise

Beeken R. Initiating exercise programs for patients with non–insulin-dependent diabetes. Diabetes Care 1980 Sep/Oct; 3(5):627–628

Koivisto VA and Felig P. Effects of leg exercise on insulin absorption in diabetic patients. N Engl J Med 1978 Jan; 298(2):79–83

Skyler JS. Diabetes and exercise: Clinical implications. Diabetes Care 1979 May/Jun; 2(3):307–311

General

Alogna M. Perception of severity of disease and health locus of control in compliant and noncompliant diabetic patients. Diabetes Care 1980 Jul/Aug; 3(4):533–534

Cianciola LJ et al. Prevalence of periodontal disease in insulin-dependent diabetes mellitus (juvenile diabetes). J Am Dent Assoc 1982 May; 104(5):653–660

DeFronzo R. Glucose intolerance and aging. Diabetes Care 1981 Jul/Aug; 4(4):493–501

Ganda OP. Morbidity and mortality from diabetes mellitus: A look at preventable aspects (editorial). Am J Pub Health 1983 Oct; 73(10):1156–1158

Hauser S and Pollets D. Psychological aspects of diabetes: A critical review. Diabetes Care 1979 Mar/Apr; 2(2):227–232

Hoover JW. Patient burnout, and other reasons for noncompliance . . . the constant stress and frustration of diabetes management. Diabetes Educ 1983 Fall; 9(3):41–43

Hopper SV. Meeting the needs of the economically deprived diabetic. Nurs Clin North Am 1983 Dec; 18(4):813–825

Madsbad S et al. Influence of smoking on insulin requirement and metabolic status in diabetes mellitus. Diabetes Care 1980 Jan/Feb; 3(1):41–43

Nemchik R. Diabetes today: A startling new body of knowledge. RN 1982 Oct; 31–37

Schmidt MI et al. The dawn phenomenon, an early morning glucose rise: Implications for diabetic intraday blood glucose variation. Diabetes Care 1982 Nov–Dec; 4(6):579–585

Unger R. Meticulous control of diabetes: Benefits, risks, and precautions. Diabetes 1982 Jun; 31:479–483

Wheat JL. Infection and diabetes mellitus. Diabetes Care 1980 Jan/Feb; 3(1):187–197

Insulin/Insulin Delivery

Barbosa J et al. Long-term, ambulatory, subcutaneous insulin infusion versus multiple daily injections in brittle diabetic patients. Diabetes Care 1981 Mar/Apr; 4(2):269–274

Crouch M et al. Reuse of disposable syringe-needle units in the diabetic patient. Diabetes Care 1979 Sep/Oct; 2(5):418–420

Grammer LC et al. Cutaneous allergy to human (recombinant DNA) insulin. JAMA 1984 Jan 12; 251(11):1459–1460

Koivisto VA and Felig P. Alterations in insulin absorption and in blood glucose control associated with varying insulin injection sites in diabetic patients. Ann Intern Med 1980 Jan; 92(1):59–65

Marliss EB et al. Present and future expectations regarding insulin infusion systems. Diabetes Care 1981 Mar–Apr; 4(2):325–327

Najarian JS et al. Pancreas and islet transplantation. Jpn J Surg 1982 Nov; 12(6):391–404

Nemchik R. The news about insulin. RN 1982 Dec; 45(12):49–54

Olson RL et al. Deaths among patients using continuous subcutaneous insulin infusion pumps—United States. MMWR 1982 Feb 26; 31(7):80–82, 87

Pietri A and Raskin P. Cutaneous complications of chronic continuous subcutaneous insulin infusion therapy. Diabetes Care 1981 Nov/Dec; 4(6):624–626

Reipp WM et al. The use of an implantable insulin pump in the treatment of type II diabetes. N Engl J Med 1982 Jul 29; 307(5):265–270

Rizza RA et al. Control of blood sugar in insulin-dependent diabetes: Comparison of an artificial endocrine pancreas, continuous subcutaneous insulin infusion, and intensified conventional insulin therapy. N Engl J Med 1980 Dec 4; 303(23):1313–1318

Salzman R et al. Intranasal aerosolized

insulin: Mixed meal studies and long-term use in type I diabetes. N Engl J Med 1985 Apr 25; 312(17):1078–1084

Schade D et al. Future therapy of the insulin-dependent diabetic patient—the implantable insulin delivery system. Diabetes Care 1981 Mar/Apr; 4(2):319–327

Schade DS and Easton RP. Insulin delivery: How, when and where. N Engl J Med 1985 Apr 25; 312(17): 1120–1121

Schiffrin A and Belmonte MM. Comparison between continuous subcutaneous insulin infusion and multiple injections of insulin: A one-year prospective study. Diabetes 1982 Mar; 31(3):255–264

Skyler J et al. Algorithms for adjustment of insulin dosage by patients who monitor blood glucose. Diabetes Care 1981 Mar/Apr; 4(2):311–318

Skyler JS et al. Optimizing pumped insulin delivery. Diabetes Care 1982 Mar/Apr; 5(2):135–139

Sutherland D et al. Pancreas transplantation—an historical overview and its current status. Diabetes Educ 1982 Spring; 8(1):11–13

Wong DL. The significance of dead space in syringes. Am J Nurs 1982; 82(8):1237

Monitoring

Cox DJ et al. Symptoms and blood glucose levels in diabetes (letter to editor). JAMA 1985 Mar 15; 253(11): 1558

Gonen B and Rubenstein A. Glycosylated hemoglobins in diabetes: A reappraisal. Diabetes Care 1979 Sep/Oct; 2(5):451–452

Guthrie D et al. Single-voided vs double-voided urine testing. Diabetes Care 1979 May/Jun; 2(3):269–271

Joyce MA et al. Those new blood glucose tests . . . self blood glucose monitoring. RN 1983 Apr; 46(4):46–52, 120

Walford S et al. The influence of renal threshold on the interpretation of urine tests for glucose in diabetic patients. Diabetes Care 1980 Nov/Dec; 3(6):672–678

Policy Statements

Policy Statement. Dietary goals for the United States, Second Edition, 1977: A reaction statement by the American Dietetic Association. Diabetes Care 1979 May/Jun; 2(3):286

Policy Statement 1980: Fast Food Restaurants. Diabetes Care 1980; 3(2): 389

Policy Statement 1979: Saccharin. Diabetes Care 1979; 2(4):380

Policy Statement 1979: U.G.D.P. Controversy. Diabetes Care 1979; 2(1):1–3

Policy Statement: Indications for use of continuous insulin delivery systems and self measurement of blood glucose. Diabetes Care 1982 Mar–Apr; 5(2):140–141

Surgery

Bovington MM et al. Management of the patient with diabetes mellitus during surgery or illness. Nurs Clin North Am 1983 Dec; 18(4):661–671

Busick EJ. The medical management of diabetic patients during surgery. Diabetes Educ 1982 Fall; 8(3):24–25

Nyberg K. When diabetes complicates your pre- and post-op care. RN 1983 Jan; 46(1):42–47

Walts LF. Managing diabetics during surgery. AORN J 1983 Apr; 37(5):928–930, 939–941

Sensory Disorders

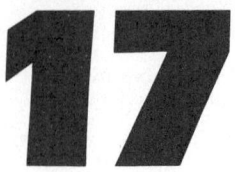

1: Eye Problems

Eye Care Specialists*

Definitions

1. An *ophthalmologist* or *oculist* is a physician (M.D.) who specializes in diagnosis and treatment of defects and diseases of the eye, performing surgery when necessary or prescribing other types of treatment, including glasses.
2. An *optometrist,* a licensed, nonmedical practitioner, measures refractive errors (irregularities in the size or shape of the eyeball or surface of the cornea) and eye muscle disturbances. In his treatment, the optometrist uses glasses, prisms, and exercises only.
3. An *optician* grinds lenses, fits them into frames, and adjusts the frames to the wearer and/or teaches the patient to use contact lens.

Normal Vision and Refractive Errors

Vision

Vision is the passage of rays of light from an object through the cornea, aqueous humor, lens, and vitreous humor to the retina, and its appreciation in the cerebral cortex.

  A. Normal—emmetropia

Rays coming from an object at a distance of 6 meters (20 feet) or more are brought to a focus on the retina by the lens.

  * Definitions from US Department of Health and Human Services.

  B. Abnormal—ametropia

1. Nearsightedness (myopia)
    a. Rays of light coming from an object at a distance of 6 meters (20 feet) or more are brought to a focus in front of the retina.
    b. Correction—concave lens.
2. Farsightedness (hyperopia)
    a. Rays of light coming from an object at a distance of 6 meters (20 feet) or more are brought to a focus in back of the retina.
    b. Correction—convex lens.

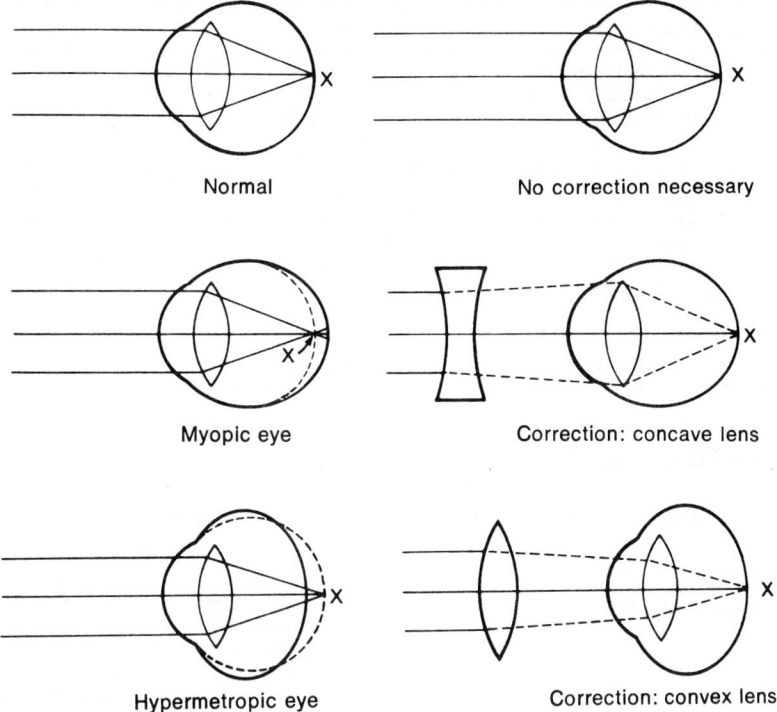

Normal	No correction necessary
Myopic eye	Correction: concave lens
Hypermetropic eye	Correction: convex lens

Accommodation

In *accommodation,* the focusing apparatus of the eye adjusts to objects at different distances by means of increasing the convexity of the lens (brought about by contraction of ciliary muscles).

Presbyopia—the elasticity of the lens decreases with increasing age; an emmetropic person with presbyopia will read a paper at arm's length and requires prescription lenses to correct the problem.

Curvature of Cornea

A. Normal—equal curvature of cornea

B. Abnormal—astigmatism

1. Uneven curvature of the cornea, causing the patient to be unable to focus horizontal and vertical rays on the retina at the same time
2. Correction—cylinder lenses

Vision Correction

Option	Durability	Advantages	Disadvantages
Spectacles	Excellent, but frames go out of style	Ease of care; excellent vision correction in most people	Cosmetic drawbacks; fogging in cool weather; inconvenient in athletics; may require more frequent replacement than some contact lenses
Hard contact lenses	As long as 20 years wearing time is possible with care	Excellent vision correction; best choice for some with astigmatism or need for bifocals; usually less expensive	Discomfort in sensitive eyes; period of adaptation; can "pop out" of eye; intolerance may develop in time
Soft contact lenses	Replace every 1 to 3 years. Deposits on lens may require more frequent replacement.	Greater comfort than hard lenses; longer wear during the day may be possible; less likely to "pop out," intermittent wear possible	Daily sterilization routine; greater risk of eye irritation and infection; may not correct vision as well as hard lenses in some with astigmatism; intolerance may develop in time

(continued)

Option	Durability	Advantages	Disadvantages
Gas permeable lenses	Last longer than soft, not as long as hard contact lenses	Better comfort than hard lenses; better vision correction than soft lenses (for some)	May be more expensive; intolerance may develop in time
Extended-wear lenses	More fragile than soft lenses; some patients need new lenses every 6 months or even more frequently	Left in place for 2 weeks at a time; vision correction 24 hours a day	Risk of corneal injury; significant expense; multiple office visits; vision may not be corrected as well; deposits on lenses more of a problem than with other soft lenses; intolerance may develop in time

(Weinstock FJ. Choosing contact lenses. America's Health 1983; 5(3):6–7)

Examination and Diagnostic Procedures

(For history, physical examination, and assessment see pages 15 and 21–23.)

External Examination

Includes examination of eye and adnexa without the aid of special apparatus.

A. Visual Acuity

Snellen Chart and other methods.
1. Each eye is tested separately, with and without glasses.
2. Letters or objects are of a size that can be seen by the normal eye at a distance of 6 meters (20 feet) from the chart.
3. Letters appear in rows and are arranged so that the normal eye can see them at distances of 9, 12, 15 meters (30, 40, 50 feet), etc.
4. When a person can identify letters of the size 6 at 6 meters (20 at 20 feet), his eye is said to have 6/6 (20/20) vision.
5. Additionally, if vision is less than 6/60 (20/200), test may be recorded as follows:

Counting fingers at _____
meters (feet): C.F.
Hand motion—ability to detect hand movement at a certain distance: H.M.
Light perception: L.P.

	meters	feet
Visual Acuity	6/6	20/20
	6/9	20/30
	6/12	20/40
	6/15	20/50
	6/21	20/70
	6/30	20/100
	6/60	20/200
Then:	C.F.@ _____	meters (feet)
	H.M.	Hand motion
	L.P. & P.	Light perception and projection
	L.P.	Light perception only
	N.L.P.	No light perception

B. Visual Fields

To determine function of retina, optic nerve, and optic pathways.
1. Equipment—perimeter, tangent screen, light source, and test objects.
2. Fields
   a. *Peripheral*—useful in detecting disorders that cause constriction of peripheral vision in one or both eyes.
      (1) Patient is seated at a "perimeter."
      (2) The left eye is covered while the patient focuses with the right eye on a spot in the central portion of the perimeter, about 1 ft. (0.33 meters) from the eye.
      (3) A test object (white) is brought in from the side at 15-degree intervals, through 360 degrees.
      (4) The patient is asked to signal when he sees the test object.
      (5) The object is passed along the same meridian from the seeing to the nonseeing segment and the patient is asked to signal when it disappears.
   b. *Central*
      (1) The patient is seated 1–2 meters from a 2–3 meter (6–8 foot) black felt tangent screen.
      (2) Each eye is covered, and central field vision is tested—including a determination of blind spots and scotomas (visual field defects).

C. Color Vision Tests

These tests are done to determine the person's ability to perceive primary colors and shades of colors; it is particularly significant for individuals whose occupation requires color perception: transportation workers, surgeons, nurses, artists, interior decorators.
1. Equipment
   a. Polychromatic plates; these are dots of primary colors printed on a background of similar dots in a confusion of colors.
   b. Individual colored discs; each disc is matched to its next closest color.
2. Procedure
   a. Various polychromatic plates are presented to the patient under specified illumination.
   b. The patterns may be letters or numbers that the

normal eye can perceive instantly, but that are confusing to the person with a perception defect.
3. Outcome
   a. Color-blindness—person is unable to perceive the figures
   b. Red–green blindness—8.0% of males; 0.4% of females
   c. Blue–yellow blindness—extremely rare

D. Refraction

Refraction is a clinical measurement of the error of focus in an eye.
1. Usually this is accomplished by instilling a cycloplegic (atropine or cyclopentolate) into the conjunctival sac.
2. The ciliary muscle is relaxed.
3. Accommodative power is lowered (cycloplegia).
4. The pupil is dilated (mydriasis), which facilitates the examination.
5. The refractive state of the eye can be determined as follows:
   a. Objectively—via retinoscopy
   b. Subjectively—trial of lenses to arrive at the best visual image

   Note: *Auto-Refractor*—in eye clinic centers, this device provides automatic refraction of an individual's eyes as he sits in front of the special instrument. Findings are transferred by computer directly onto a printout sheet.

Internal Examination

A. Ophthalmoscopic Examination

The interior of the eye is examined when a beam of light is reflected through the pupil while the examiner looks through an ophthalmoscope.
1. Defects in the clarity of the media (e.g., cataracts, vitreous opacities, corneal scars) may be detected.
2. The retinal blood vessels may be examined closely for the pathologic changes of diabetes, hypertension, etc.
3. The choroid can be examined for tumors, inflammation.
4. The retina can be examined for retinal detachment, scars, diabetes, etc.

B. Gonioscopy

Direct visualization of the junction of the iris and cornea (angle of anterior chamber).
1. *Equipment*—Local anesthetic solutions, goniolens, biomicroscope (slit lamp)
2. Procedure
   a. A local anesthetic is instilled into the eye.
   b. The goniolens is placed over the cornea; sterile methylcellulose solution is injected between the cornea and the lens.
   c. The patient fixes his gaze as the examiner views the anterior chamber, through the biomicroscope, through a circumference of 360 degrees.

C. Tonometry

Measurement of intraocular tension or pressure.
1. Schiøtz tonometry
   a. After instillation of topical anesthesia, the Schiøtz tonometer is gently rested on the eyeball (Fig. 17-1).
   b. The indicator measures the ocular tension in mm. Hg.
   c. Normal tension is approximately 11–22 mm. Hg.

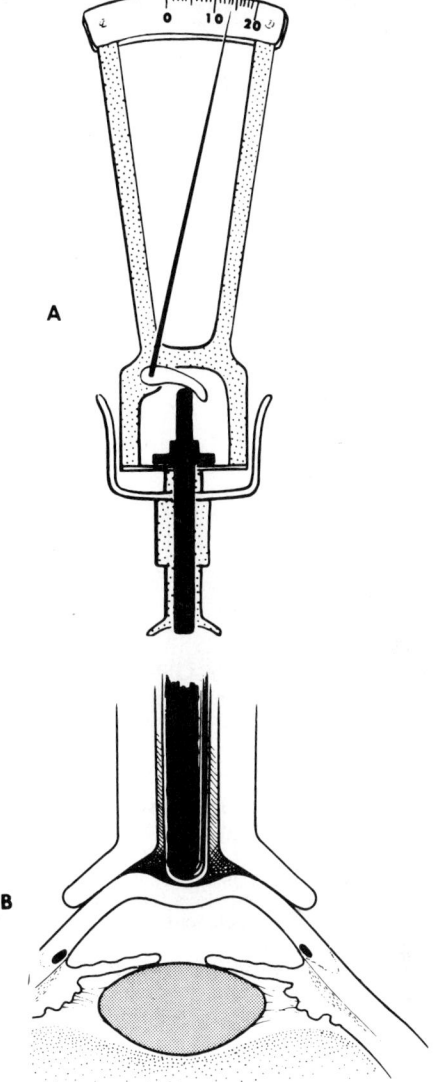

Figure 17-1. *(A)* Schiøtz tonometer in which the plunger, in black, measures the ease of indentation of cornea. *(B)* Indentation of the anesthetized cornea by the plunger of the tonometer in order to measure ocular tension. (Newell Frank W. Ophthalmology: Principles and Concepts, ed. 4. St Louis, CV Mosby)

2. Applanation tonometry
   a. This is the most effective measuring method for determining intraocular pressure; however, it requires a biomicroscope and a trained interpreter.
   b. After instillation of topical anesthesia, the cornea is flattened by a known amount (3.14 mm.).
   c. The pressure necessary to produce this flattening is equal to the intraocular pressure, counterbalancing the tonometer.
3. Air applanation tonometry
   This requires no topical anesthesia and measures tension by sensing deformation of the cornea in reaction to a puff of pressurized air.

Guidelines: Assisting the Patient Undergoing Tonometry

Tonometry is the measurement of intraocular pressure by means of placing a sensitive instrument (tonometer, Fig. 17-2) directly on the partially anesthetized eyeball. Normal reading: 11–22 mm. Hg.

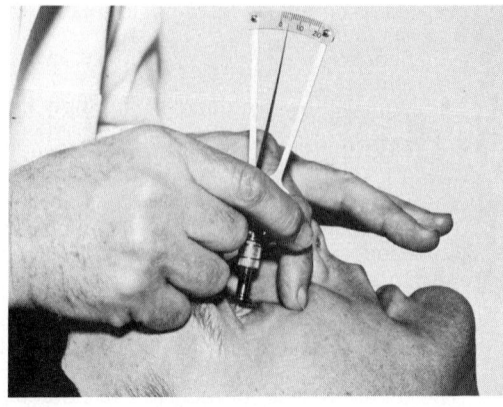

Figure 17-2. *The Schiøtz tonometer measures the ocular tension in mm. Hg. (Courtesy of FH Roy, MD)*

Purpose   To measure one of the diagnostic criteria of glaucoma

Procedure

Preparatory Phase

1. The patient is placed in a tilt-type chair, tilted back and instructed to look upward.

Action	Rational/Amplification
Performance Phase	
1. Physician:	
a. Instills a drop of proparacaine 0.5% in each eye.	a. This will produce corneal anesthesia within a minute.
b. Places a sterile tonometer gently on the center of the cornea for a few seconds.	b. Pressure from the eyeball will be transferred to the sensitive measuring indicator.
c. Repeats for second eye.	
2. Nurse:	
a. Offers the patient an absorbent tissue.	
b. Instructs the patient to pat the *closed* eyes dry.	
c. Cautions the patient against rubbing his eyes.	c. The cornea is still anesthetized; painful abrasions can result from the natural tendency to rub the eyes because of the unusual numb sensation.

Follow-up Phase

1. Remind patient to have an eye-pressure check at least every 2 years if his pressure is normal.

Guidelines: Instillation of Eyedrops

Purposes   1. To dilate or contract the pupil.
2. To relieve pain and discomfort.
3. To act as an antiseptic in cleansing the eye.
4. To combat infection; to relieve inflammation.

Equipment

Sterile solution or medication
2 × 2-inch gauze squares or cotton balls
Sterile eyedropper (Most medications come in plastic bottles with built-in dropper.)

Procedure

Preparatory Phase
1. Inform the patient of the need and reason for instilling eyedrops.
2. Allow the patient to sit with head tilted slightly backward or to lie in the dorsal recumbent position.
3. Check visual acuity and record: This can be used as a base line to determine subsequent change in condition.

Nursing Action	Rationale/Amplification

Performance Phase

Nursing Action	Rationale/Amplification
1. Check the patient's name.	1. For proper patient identification.
2. Check orders and bottle or vial for correct medication and correct concentration.	2. To avoid medication error.
3. Check orders designating which eye requires medication: O.D. (oculis dexter)—right eye O.S. (oculis sinister)—left eye O.U. (oculis uterque)—both eyes	
4. Wash hands prior to instilling medication.	4. Good hygiene.
5. Check glass eyedropper for defects. If plastic disposable dropper is used, squeeze plastic to allow medication to come to the tip.	5. Provides an effective and safe vehicle for transmission of medication.
6. Prevent medication from flowing back into bulb end.	6. Loose particles of rubber may slip into medication.
7. Using forefinger, pull lower lid down gently (see Fig. 17-3A).	7. To expose inner surface of lid and cul-de-sac.
8. Instruct patient to look upward (see Fig. 17-3B).	8. Prevents medication from hitting sensitive cornea.
9. Drop medication into center of lower lid (cul-de-sac).	
10. Instruct the patient to close eyes slowly but not to squeeze them (Fig. 17-3C). Open eye (Fig. 17-3D).	10. Squeezing would express medication; closing allows medication to be distributed evenly over eye.
11. Wipe off excess solution with a gauze square.	11. Instruct the patient not to rub his eye.
12. Wash hands after instilling medication.	12. To prevent transferring microorganisms to self or other patients.

Note: Eye ointments are frequently used—procedure is similar to instillation of eyedrops. Ointment from tube is gently squeezed as a ribbon of medication along inner lower lid with care taken not to touch eye with end of tube.

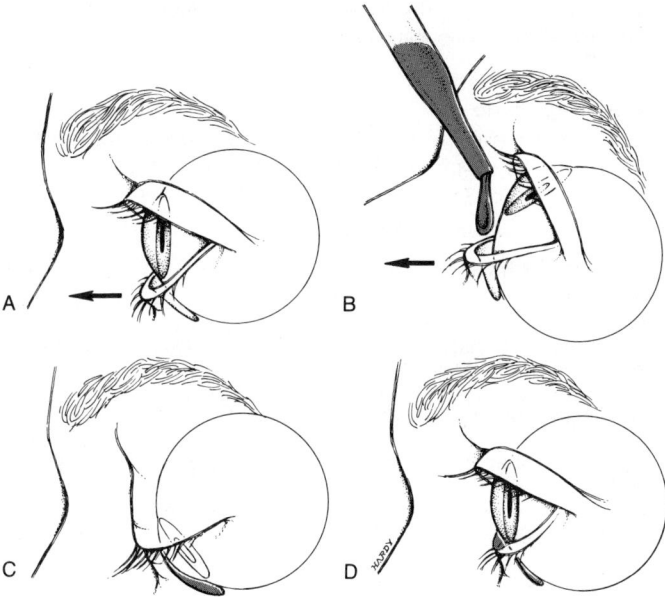

Figure 17-3. Instillation of eyedrops.

(continued)

Guidelines: Instillation of Eyedrops (continued)

Procedure
(Cont.)

Nursing Action	Rationale/Amplification

Follow-up Phase

Record time; type, strength, and amount of medication; and the eye into which medication was instilled.

Nursing Action	Rationale/Amplification
Self-Instillation of Eyedrops	
1. Tilt head back.	1. This places eye and lower lid in a horizontal position.
2. Using forefinger, pull lower lid downward.	2. This presents inner lower lid ready to receive medication drop.
3. With other hand, hold dropper horizontally and facing top of head.	3. This positions dropper outlet above receiving lid.
4. Look upward and instill one drop onto lower lid.	
(Continue with items 10, 11, and 12 above.)	

Guidelines: Irrigating the Eye (Conjunctival Irrigation)

Purposes
1. To remove secretions from the conjunctival sac.
2. To treat infections, using a prescribed solution.
3. To relieve itching.
4. To provide moisture on the surface of the eyes of an unconscious patient.
5. To irrigate chemicals or foreign bodies from the eye.

Sterile

Equipment

For small amount of solution—an eyedropper
For larger amount of solution—asepto bulb syringe or plastic bottle with prescribed solution
For copious use (chemical burns)—IV set with sterile normal saline
For continuous lavage—The Morgan Therapeutic Lens*
    Molded scleral lens with directional fins (polymethylmethacrylate)
    Attached silicone tubing with polypropylene adapter

Procedure

Preparatory Phase
1. Verify that you have the right patient; check chart, address the patient by name.
2. The patient may sit or lie in the dorsal recumbent (supine) position.
3. Have the patient tilt head toward the side of the affected eye.

Nursing Action	Rationale/Amplification
Performance Phase	
A. General	
1. Wash eyelashes and lids with prescribed solution at room temperature; placed a curved basin on the affected side of the face to catch the outflow.	1. Any materials on the lids or lashes can be washed off before exposing conjunctiva.
2. Evert the lower conjunctival sac. (If feasible, have the patient pull down lower lid with his index finger.)	2. The inner part of the lower lid is less sensitive than the cornea. (This involves the patient and gives him a sense of control.)
3. Instruct the patient to look up; avoid touching eye with dropper.	3. To prevent eye injury—never touch cornea.
4. Allow irrigating fluid to flow from the inner canthus to the outer canthus along the conjunctival sac.	4. This prevents the solution from flowing toward the lacrimal sac, duct, and nose (which would aid in transmitting the infection).
5. Use only enough force to flush secretions from conjunctiva. (Allow the patient to hold towel or sponges near the eye to catch fluid.)	5. Too much force may be injurious to eye tissues. (Involve the patient in his treatment.)
6. Occasionally have patient close his eyes.	6. This allows upper lid to meet lower lid with the possibility of dislodging additional particles.

* Mor-Tan Inc., Torrington, WY 82240.

Procedure
(Cont.)

Nursing Action	Rationale/Amplification
B. Using The Morgan Therapeutic Lens (Fig. 17-4)	
1. Instill topical anesthetic.	1. For patient comfort.
2. Place an absorbent pad under the patient's head.	2. To absorb excess fluid.
3. For lavage, attach syringe or IV tubing to silicone short tubing.	3. Solution source is thus made available.
4. Instruct the patient to look down; insert edge of lens under upper lid.	4. This positions plastic lens in place over cornea and sclera.
5. Have the patient look up and retract lower lid; release lower lid over lens and continue fluid flow.	5. Fixes lens in place.
6. Tape tubing to the patient's forehead with hypoallergenic tape.	6. To prevent accidental lens removal.
7. Regulate fluid flow.	7. The patient is able to sleep, rest, or ambulate with lens in place.

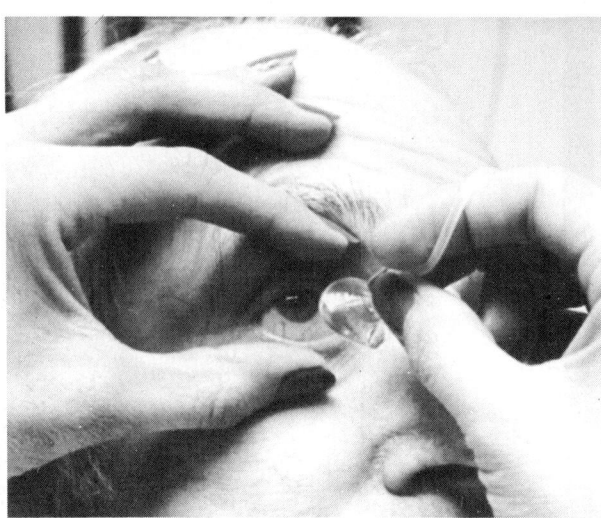

Figure 17-4. The Morgan Therapeutic Lens.

C. Removal of lens	
1. Instruct the patient to look up; retract lower lid behind inferior border of lens—hold position.	1. This dislodges lower segment of lens.
2. Have the patient look down, retract upper lid, and slide lens out.	2. Lens becomes disengaged from contact with eye.
3. Both eyes may be irrigated at same time, using a second irrigation set.	
4. Remove wet towel and pad; dry the patient's face.	4. For patient comfort.
Follow-up Phase	
1. Pat eye dry and dry the patient's face with gauze or cotton ball.	1. Makes patient comfortable.
2. Record kind and amount of fluid used, as well as its effect on the patient.	

Guidelines: Application of an Eye Patch, Eye Shield, and Pressure Dressings to the Eye

Purposes
1. To keep an eye at rest, thereby promoting healing (patch).
2. To prevent the patient from touching his eye (patch, shield, dressings).
3. To absorb secretions (patch and pressure dressing).
4. To protect the eye (patch, shield, dressing).
5. To control or lessen edema (pressure dressing).

(continued)

Guidelines: Application of an Eye Patch, Eye Shield, and Pressure Dressings to the Eye (continued)

Procedure

Nursing Action	Rationale/Amplification
Eye Patch (Fig. 17-5 A, B, C)	
1. Instruct the patient to close both eyes.	1. It is too difficult to close only the affected eye.
2. Place patch over the affected eye.	
3. Secure the patch with 3 or more strips of special transparent tape; tape from mid-forehead to below ear.	3. Adhesive tape (Scotch) is easy to remove—use hypoallergenic type if patient is allergic to tape.
4. For the unconscious patient, moisten the eye patch.	4. Dry patch can irritate cornea
Eye Shield (Plastic or Metal, Fig. 17-5D)	
1. Apply over dressings or directly over the eye (without dressings).	1. Used primarily to protect the eye. Place tab or irregular extension toward the patient's ear.
2. Fasten with special transparent tape; use 2 strips.	
3. For metal eye shields, a guard can be placed around flanged edges before use:	
a. Cut 1.2–2.5-cm. (½″ × 1″) piece of latex rubber from a glove finger.	a. This eliminates the need for adhesive tape around edge.
b. Stretch it around perimeter of shield.	b. Two such pieces will add cushioning and provide comfort to the patient.
Pressure Dressings (Fig. 17-5E, F)	
1. Prepare 8–10 adhesive strips by cutting 2.5-cm. (1-inch) adhesive tape in 35-cm. (9-inch) lengths. Stretch tape (3M) may also be used.	1. Use of a warming tray for strips will improve their adhesiveness.

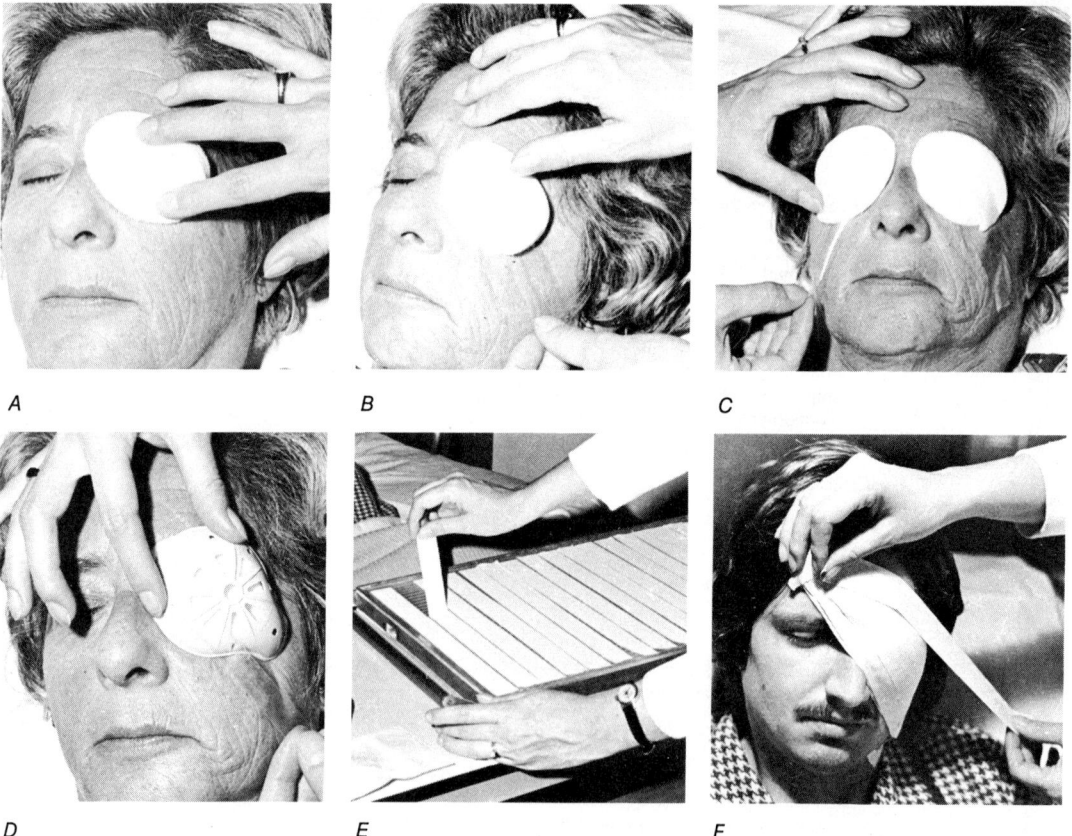

A   B   C

D   E   F

Figure 17-5. Application of an eye patch, eye shield, and pressure dressings to the eye. (Nursing '75, 5[6]:54) pp 54–55)

Procedure
(Cont.)

Nursing Action	Rationale/Amplification
2. Paint forehead and cheeks with tincture of benzoin compound.	2. To promote adherence of tape and prevent excoriation of skin.
3. Apply two eye patches to the affected eye.	3. For pressure dressing bulk.
4. Apply strips from forehead over unpatched eye across dressings to the cheek bone (maxillary prominence).	4. This is a secure dressing which accomplishes its purpose while permitting freedom of movement of the head.

Eye Injuries

Assumptions

1. Recognize that all ocular injuries are potentially serious.
2. Protect the integrity of the visual system and prevent further damage to the injured part.
3. Evaluate the extent of injury; either refer the patient to an ophthalmologist or provide immediate treatment that will not extend damage.
4. Suspect a penetrating ocular injury with every eye wound until suspicion is proved incorrect.
5. Record visual acuity as soon as possible on every eye patient; this is a reflection of the basic integrity of the eye.

▶ **NURSING ALERT:** All eye emergency patients should have visual acuity checked in each eye, both with and without glasses, as a part of history-taking and preliminary examination and *prior to any* form of treatment.

Emergency Management

A. Corneal abrasion—an injury to the cornea which goes no deeper than the epithelium. A common occurrence as a result of inadvertent contact with objects such as fingernails or tree branches, or over-wearing of contact lenses (non-oxygen permeable)

1. Instill tetracaine (Pontocaine) solution as requested—to relieve pain and facilitate eye examination. Some ophthalmologists prefer systemic analgesics only.
2. Stain the cornea with fluorescein—to detect existence of an abrasion and its extent (Fig. 17-6).
   a. Gently touch conjunctiva of lower lid with edge of fluorescein paper strip.
   b. The exposed (damaged) layers of epithelium will take the stain and turn green; undamaged areas remain unstained.
   c. Following use of fluorescein, flush the eye well since some patients react to fluorescein as an allergen.
   d. Instill a drop of antibiotic since subsequent patching creates a good environment for flora growth.
3. Apply pressure bandage firmly but gently over eye (see Fig. 17-5)—to put eye at rest and to prevent movement of the eyelid, with resultant irritation of abraded corneal area.
4. Give oral analgesic as necessary—abrasions of the cornea are painful.
5. Advise the patient to rest his eyes for 24 hours for greater comfort; the corneal epithelium usually heals in 24–48 hours.
6. Instruct the patient to return to the ophthalmologist the following day for dressing change and inspection of eye for evidence of infection or ulcer formation.

7. Corneal ulcer is a complication to be guarded against (see p. 726).

B. Contusion

Black eye; hemorrhage into the orbit from trauma.
1. Contusions usually clear slowly and without treatment.
   a. Apply cold compresses intermittently for first 24 hours to control pain and swelling.
   b. Apply warm compresses (after 24 hours) intermittently.
2. Place the patient on bed rest with both eyes bandaged for hyphema.
3. To rule out orbital fracture or hyphema (hemorrhage into anterior chamber of eye), consult an ophthalmologist if hemorrhage is severe or if pain and double vision are noted.

C. Foreign Bodies Lodged in Cornea

Treatment by ophthalmologist or emergency department physician.

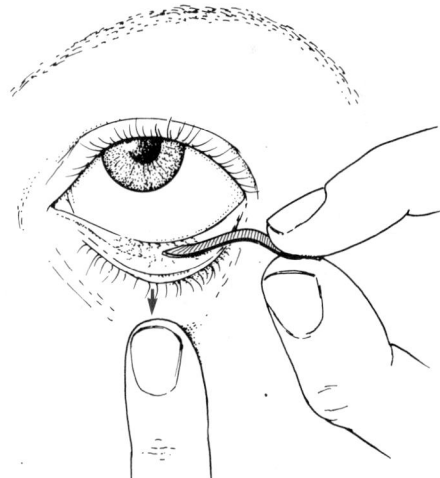

Figure 17-6. Staining cornea with fluorescein strip.
1. After informing the patient what you plan to do, wet the distal end of a fluorescein strip with sterile normal saline solution (use sterile, individually wrapped, fluorescein strip).
2. Pull lower eyelid down; gently touch the inner segment of the lower lid with the strip; a green stain will coat area of abrasion.
3. Have the patient blink several times to distribute the fluorescein dye.
4. The eye is now ready for examination.

1. Instill sterile anesthetic into the conjunctival sac—to facilitate examination.
2. Ophthalmologist will remove superficial particles with a moist cotton-tipped applicator; foreign body removed with a spud or similar instrument, using a slit lamp for magnification.
3. Apply eye patch and reinforce instruction to return to ophthalmologist the following day to determine if healing is underway.

D. Penetrating Injuries to the Eye

1. Cover eye with sterile dressing and call ophthalmologist.
   a. Intraocular foreign bodies should be removed as soon as possible; they cause damage by disintegration or become encapsulated by fibrous tissue.
   b. Apply eye patch lightly—pressure of pad may cause further penetration.
2. Give sedative–analgesic combination as directed; have the patient lie quietly until ophthalmologist arrives.
3. Give tetanus prophylaxis for any penetrating eye injury.
4. Give oral antimicrobials in high doses as directed—blood aqueous barrier resists penetration.
5. Aside from direct trauma, metallic foreign bodies may also release ions and cause toxicity.
6. Powerful magnets are still used; however, intraocular surgery through the posterior part of the ciliary body may be less traumatic.

E. Burns of the Eye

Cause drying of the cornea with resulting chronic conjunctivitis and corneal ulceration.
1. *Thermal burns* (associated with face or body burns).
   a. Call ophthalmologist.
   b. Thermal burns are treated in the same way as burns of skin structures.
2. *Actinic trauma*
   a. Excessive sunlight (or other strong light such as a sun lamp, bright sun or snow) can cause ultraviolet-ray (UV) damage to cornea.
   b. Damage may be superficial and resolve in 48 hours; however, punctate keratitis may develop.
   c. An ophthalmologist should be consulted immediately.
   d. Treatment
      (1) Reassure the patient.
      (2) Apply patch to both eyes.
      (3) Report to an ophthalmologist.

   (4) Instill anesthetic drops.
   (5) Instill mydriatic–cycloplegic to relax ciliary muscles and iris sphincter spasm.
   (6) Instill emollient antibiotic ointment.
3. *Chemical burns*—may be either acid or alkali in nature. Both cause intense pain and inflammation.
   a. *Irrigate eye with copious amounts of water*—holding the patient's eye directly under running water with lids retracted by gauze flats is the best way to irrigate the eye when immediate irrigation is required.
   b. Irrigate for at least 5 minutes.
   c. Repeat irrigation in 15–20 minutes (using eye irrigation equipment) until the patient is seen by the ophthalmologist.
   d. Instill topical anesthetic for pain and control severe pain thereafter with systemic analgesics as prescribed.
   e. Check pH of tears with litmus paper and continue irrigations until pH is neutral.
   f. Measure vision and intraocular pressure to determine status.
   g. Alkali eye burns are more severe than acid burns; long-term management may require lavage, cycloplegics, and even collagenase inhibitors; contact lenses may be used to prevent ulceration.

Health Education and Preventive Measures

1. Appropriate glasses should be used for protection against very bright light, sun shining on snow, fumes of sprays or chemicals, etc.
2. Goggles should be worn if there is danger of flying gravel (power-mower lawn cutting), flying wood chips (while chopping wood), flying metal or glass bits (in a machine factory).
3. Children should be reminded of dangers of sling shots, BB guns, "sparklers," darts, arrows, etc.
4. Eyeglasses and sunglasses should have impact-resistant lenses.
5. Many states have school eye safety laws that require all students to use industrial-quality safety eyewear in shops and laboratories.
6. Anhydrous ammonia used as agricultural fertilizer is a very destructive agent. Goggles must be worn when handling this chemical. Sufficient water for irrigation should always be present.
7. Protective lenses or goggles should be worn when using a hammer, mowing the lawn, etc. They are also highly recommended in various sports—hockey, tennis, handball, racquet ball, hunting, etc.

Guidelines: Removing a Particle from the Eye

Equipment

Local anesthesia	Cotton applicator sticks or tongue depressor
Hand lens	Saline (Irrigating)
Sterile fluorescein strips	Antibiotic solution

Procedure

Nursing Action	Rationale/Amplification
1. As patient looks upward, evert lower lid to expose the conjunctival sac (see Fig. 17-7A).	1. Dust particles are often washed downward by the upper lid.

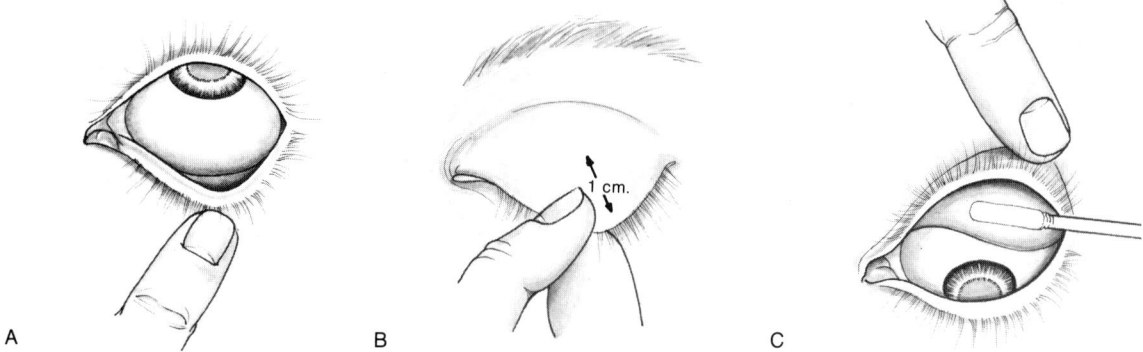

Figure 17-7. Examining the eye for a foreign particle. *(A)* Evert lower lid. *(B & C)* Evert upper lid.

Procedure
(Cont.)

Nursing Action	Rationale / Amplification
2. With small cotton applicator dipped in saline, gently remove particle.	2. Wipe gently across lid—inner to outer. Use hand magnifying lens if necessary.
3. If offending particle is not found, proceed to examine upper lid.	
4. Have the patient look downward while you stand in front of him.	4. Serves as a safety measure since cornea is away from area of activity. Looking downward relaxes the levator muscle, which is attached to the upper border of the tarsal plate.
5. Encourage the patient to relax; move slowly and reassure him that you will not hurt him.	5. This will prevent squeezing the lids shut, a maneuver that contracts the obicularis muscle, making eversion of lid impossible.
6. Place cotton applicator stick or tongue blade horizontally on outer surface of upper lid. Apply pressure about 1 cm. above lid margin (see Fig. 17-7*B*).	6. Since the upper tarsal plate extends 10–12 mm. above the lid margin, pressure must be applied at least 1 cm. above lid margin for easy eversion of lid.
7. Grasp upper eyelashes with fingers of other hand and pull the upper lid outward and upward over cotton stick.	7. Particles may be washed under the lid; visual exposure assists in detection. Eyelid will remain everted by itself.
8. With a cotton applicator moistened with saline, gently remove particle (see Fig. 17-7*C*).	
9. Use fluorescein strip to detect corneal abrasion.	9. Green stain will so indicate if abrasion is present.

▶ **NURSING ALERT:** It is very important to take a history. Determine what the nature of the particle is—wood? (Fungus infection may result.) Metal? What kind—magnetic? copper? Was it projectile?

　　If particle cannot be removed by the method described above, it may have become imbedded in lens or vitreous, in which case an ophthalmologist is required.

Guidelines: Removing Contact Lenses

Purpose　Since most contact lenses are designed to be worn while awake, if a person is injured and incapacitated because of an accident, sickness, or other cause, the lenses should be removed.

▶ **NURSING ALERT:**
1. If the injured person is unconscious or unable to remove his lenses, an optometrist or ophthalmologist is called.
2. If professional help is not available and the lenses must be removed:
　a. Determine the type of lens.
　　(1) Small *corneal lenses* are most widely used. The diameter is less than the colored part of the eye (smaller than a dime).
　b. *When Not to Remove Lenses:* If the colored part of the eye is not visible upon opening the eyelids, await the arrival of an optometrist or ophthalmologist.

(continued)

Guidelines: Removing Contact Lenses (continued)

Procedure

Preparatory Phase

1. Since the patient will undoubtedly be in the recumbent position, it is acceptable to remove the lens while he is in this position.
2. Wash your hands thoroughly.

Nursing Action	Rationale/Amplification

Performance Phase

Corneal Lens (Hard Type)

If an eye suction cup is available (as in emergency department) simply separate eyelids to expose lens fully; then place cup over lens and apply slight pressure to cup. The suction produced will permit cup to lift lens from cornea.

1. For right eye, stand on right side of patient so hands will have easier access to eye.
2. Lightly place left thumb on upper eyelid; right thumb on lower eyelid close to the edge and parallel with lids (Fig. 17-8A). Thumbs are placed in a leverage position on the eyelids.
3. Gently pull lids apart and observe if contact lens is visible (Fig. 17-8B). If contact lens is not visible wait for an experienced practitioner.
4. If lens is visible, it should slide with the movement of the eyelids while thumbs are still kept at the edges of the eyelids.
5. Gently open the lids wider beyond the edge of the lens and maintain this position.
6. Press gently downward with right thumb on eyeball (Fig. 17-8C). This should cause the contact lens to tip up on one edge.
7. Then slide the eyelids and thumbs together gently (Fig. 17-8D). The lens should slide out between the lids where it can be taken off.
8. FORCE SHOULD NOT BE USED!
   Cornea may be irreparably damaged.
9. If lens can be seen but cannot be removed, gently slide it to the white sclera.
10. For left eye, move to left side of patient and repeat.

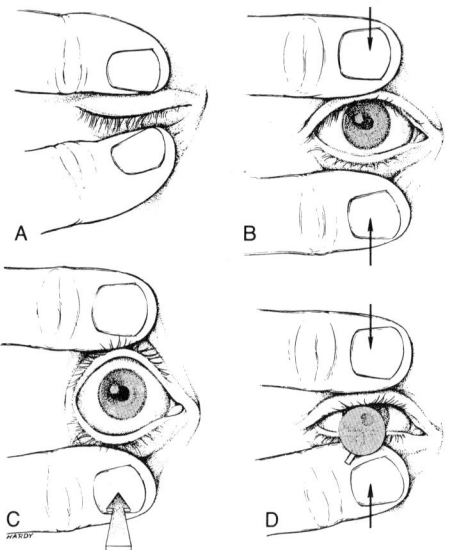

Figure 17-8. Removing corneal contact lens.

Soft Contact Lenses

May be removed by gently grasping and pinching lens between thumb and forefinger. This is rarely necessary, since soft contact lens may remain on the eye for many hours without harm. An ophthalmologist can be called to remove lenses if the patient is unable to do so. Also note, if a contact lens cannot be removed with relative ease, discontinue efforts and wait for the ophthalmologist to remove it.

Disposition of Lenses

1. When lenses are found and removed, place in a case or bottle; label "right" and "left."

2. Store in normal saline solution to prevent drying.

1. Since right and left lenses are often different, storing them with proper labels will be appreciated by the patient.

2. Soft lenses must be kept moist.

Inflammation of the Eye

Superficial Lid Infections

Blepharitis—infection of eyelids, with crusting lids, redness, irritation, and mucopurulent secretion.
Hordeolum (sty)—infection of eyelash follicle.
Chalazion—infection of the meibomian gland.

Treatment

1. Cleanse lid margins by applying warm, moist compresses for 5 minutes 3 or 4 times daily.
2. Carefully wipe loose crusts away from lashes; apply ophthalmic antibacterial ointment and/or drops.
3. Continue for several days until infection clears.
4. Keep the patient's hands away from eyes and wash hands after eye care.
5. Chronic chalazion may require incision and curettage.

Conjunctivitis

Conjunctivitis is an inflammation of the conjunctiva resulting from an allergy, from a bacterial, viral, or chlamydial infection, or from physical or chemical trauma. The infection is often referred to as "pinkeye."

Clinical Manifestations

1. Redness, pain, swelling, lacrimation; lids are frequently stuck together with crusting upon awakening
2. Discharge according to offending organisms
   a. Abundant purulence indicates infection caused by pneumococcus or gonococcus
   b. In this country, chlamydia cause a subacute follicular conjunctivitis
   c. Also see Trachoma, below (chronic keratoconjunctivitis) caused by chlamydial agent

Treatment and Nursing Management

1. Administer frequent saline irrigations—to remove discharge.
2. Apply warm or cold compresses—for 15 minutes, 3 or 4 times a day for comfort.
3. Prevent dissemination of infection to the other eye or other persons.
   a. Wash hands before and after treating eye.
   b. Restrict washcloth and towel to infected eye and change frequently.
4. Instill chemotherapeutic ointments as prescribed following Gram stain for specific organism—to clear infection in 1–3 days. (Without treatment first, followed by chemotherapy, infection subsides in 7–10 days.)
5. Trifluridine (Viroptic) is an antiviral agent used in the treatment of keratoconjunctivitis and recurrent epithelial keratitis due to herpes simplex virus.

Trachoma

Trachoma is a type of chlamydial keratoconjunctivitis.
1. It is particularly severe in developing countries—a serious medical, social, and economic problem.
2. Leading cause of preventable blindness.
3. *Chlamydia trachomatis* is an intracellular parasite with a bacterial cell wall.

Pathology

1. Follicular conjunctivitis (elevated, grayish granules 0.2–2 mm. in diameter).
2. This proceeds to papillary hypertrophy, engorgement, and inflammation of conjunctiva.

Complications

3. Then conjunctival scarring takes place.
4. In mild trachoma—linear scars are noted.
   In severe trachoma—epithelium atrophies and broader synechial scars are seen.
5. The scarred conjunctiva contracts, inverting the tarsal plate of eyelid; this leads to *entropion* (eyelid turns inward); these eyelashes rub against the cornea, causing discomfort and pain; this, in turn, causes corneal erosion and scarring.

Clinical Manifestations

1. Onset is insidious—minimal discomfort.
2. Chemosis (swelling of conjunctiva), redness, velvety appearance of palpebral conjunctiva.
3. Later, photophobia, pain, and tearing.
4. By 3rd week, follicles appear, and conjunctiva becomes congested.
5. If treated, symptoms subside; if not treated, conjunctival scars appear in about 2 months.

Treatment

1. Medical—tetracycline topically (1% ointment).
2. With corneal ulceration, topical gentamicin and systemic penicillin are prescribed.
3. For an isolated case, tetracycline may be prescribed twice a day for 2–3 months.
4. The World Health Organization (WHO) has designed a scoring system to facilitate measurement of intensity of trachoma in any given area—personal hygiene and health education are very important.
5. A vaccine for prophylactic use is being investigated.

Uveitis

Uveitis is an inflammation of the uveal tract (iris, ciliary body, choroid).

Classification

1. Location
   a. Anterior uveitis → iritis, iridocyclitis
   b. Posterior uveitis → choroiditis, chorioretinitis
   c. Panuveitis → entire uveal tract
2. Granulomatous or nongranulomatous

Complications

	Granulomatous	Nongranulomatous
Location	Any portion, mostly posterior	Anterior
Onset	Insidious	Acute
Pain	None or minimal	Marked
Circumcorneal flush	Minimal	Present
Course	Chronic	Acute
Complications	Adhesions impede aqueous flow from posterior to anterior uvea—metabolic disturbance of lens, leading to cataract	Adhesions impede aqueous outflow leading to glaucoma; may cause cataracts
Prognosis	Fair to poor	Good

Treatment

Goals:
Patient comfort
Preservation of good vision.
1. Infectious uveitis responds to specific antibodies.
2. Mydriatic–cycloplegics
   Atropine, scopolamine, or homatropine to relieve discomfort caused by contraction of ciliary muscles
3. Anti-inflammatory agents to relieve inflammation
   a. Corticosteroids in lowest effective dose.

b. Topical steroids in high dosages is effective in anterior uveitis.

Sympathetic Ophthalmia

Sympathetic ophthalmia is a severe granulomatous bilateral uveitis that may occur after any surgical or traumatic perforation involving the uveal tract. A severe infection that appears to be an autoimmune reaction to uveal tissue may rarely occur.

Clinical Manifestations

Photophobia, blurring vision, and injection of conjunctiva ("bloodshot"); injured (exciting) eye becomes inflamed, then the other eye (sympathizing) follows with an inflammation.

Treatment

1. Administer corticosteroids, locally and systemically, to reduce the amount of intraocular scarring.
2. Instill atropine (mydriatic) locally to prevent adhesions between the iris and lens.
3. Possibility of preventive enucleation of originally injured eye before sympathetic ophthalmia occurs.

Nursing Interventions

1. Understand the patient's condition and the goals desired for him.
2. Recognize the difficult decision facing the patient if enucleation approach is suggested.
3. Assess the psychosocial implications of the individual situation, offer sustaining support, and collaborate in planning immediate and long-term goals.

Corneal Ulcer

Keratitis is an inflammation of the cornea, which when combined with a loss of substance, results in *corneal ulcer.*

Clinical Manifestations

1. Pain, marked photophobia, and increased lacrimation
2. Injected ("bloodshot") eye
3. When a corneal ulcer progresses deeper to involve the iris, iritis develops; pus forms in the anterior chamber and collects as a white or yellow deposit (hypopyon) behind the cornea.
4. If corneal ulcer perforates, iris may prolapse through the cornea.

Treatment and Nursing Interventions

1. Prevention is much easier than treatment.
   a. Foreign bodies must be removed quickly.
   b. Corneal abrasions must be treated promptly.

2. Suggest the wearing of dark glasses to relieve photophobia.
3. Explain to the patient that physician may administer mydriatics preparatory to examining the eye and will instill topical anesthetic to relieve pain, and fluorescein to outline ulcer.
4. Administer antibiotic or chemotherapeutic agent as prescribed for specific type of infection.
5. Apply warm compresses for comfort as prescribed.
6. Administer systemic antibiotics when prescribed.

▶ **NURSING ALERT:** Always question the patient about allergies to medications, whether topical or systemic, prior to institution of therapy.

Eye Conditions Possibly Requiring Surgery

Nursing Process Overview

Patient Problems/Nursing Diagnoses

1. Alteration in visual sensory perception related to disease/trauma or postoperative condition (eye)
2. Fear of blindness related to diminishing vision caused by trauma/disease
3. Disturbance in self-concept related to exaggerated feelings of inadequacy because of limited vision
4. Social isolation related to reduced contacts with people because of impaired vision
5. Self-care deficit related to reduced vision
6. Activity limitation related to concern and fear of physical injury because of impaired vision
7. Knowledge deficit of physical and psychological preparation for eye surgery
8. Potential for injury related to limited vision

Planning and Implementation
Nursing Interventions

A. Reduction in Anxiety

1. Recognize that dependence on sight is exaggerated when one faces a possible diminution or loss of sight.

2. Observe that the concern of the patient may be manifested as fear, depression, tension, resentment, anger, and even rejection.
3. Encourage the patient to express his feelings in order to determine the underlying problems.
4. Provide diversional and occupational therapy to keep the patient occupied mentally within the limits of his decreased vision so as not to accentuate his feelings of depression or despair over loss of vision.
5. Demonstrate interest, empathy, and understanding, but try not to be oversolicitous.
6. Recognize individual differences that affect the method of dealing with anxiety.
7. Reassure the patient that rehabilitative programs and personnel are available if his condition requires them.

B. Increase in Self-Care Activities

1. Always orient the new patient who has diminished vision to his surroundings—his room and the people in his immediate environment.
2. Encourage the patient to care for himself so that he will be self-sufficient and not feel that he is a burden.
3. Supervise him as he attempts to feed himself so that he does not become discouraged.

4. Promote proper elimination by an adequate diet, laxatives, or an enema as required.
5. Provide a rest period daily if the patient is ambulatory.
6. For safety reasons, discourage the patient's reading, smoking, or shaving (done by members of the health team).
7. Caution the patient against rubbing his eyes or wiping them with a soiled tissue or handkerchief.
8. Instruct the patient to wear dark glasses if he has had atropine instilled.
9. Maintain a safe environment that is free of obstacles such as footstools or loose rugs.
10. Doors should be completely open or closed.

C. Preoperative Preparation: General Anesthesia

1. In preparation for general anesthesia, evacuate lower bowel (enema) in the morning of the day of surgery; offer liquid diet only after this. (This is unnecessary for local anesthesia.)
2. Arrange long hair of female patients (braiding) so that it will be conveniently out of the way.
3. Cut eyelashes of the affected eye, using small, curved, blunt scissors covered with petrolatum so that lashes will adhere to it and not drop into the patient's eye. This is done to reduce the possibility of infection. Lashes will grow back in about 3 weeks.
4. Check local hospital policy regarding preoperative skin preparation; in many hospitals, this is done in the operating room.
5. Remove dentures or artificial eye before the patient goes to the operating room.
6. Instruct the patient regarding postoperative restrictions (these will be specific for each type of surgery). Tell him he will have a patch and shield on eye when he returns from the OR.
7. Make sure the eye specified on the operative permit and eye to be operated on are the same.
8. Instill proper preoperative medications in the proper eye.

D. Preoperative Preparation: Local Anesthesia

1. Instruct the patient to wash his hair the day before surgery.
2. Orient the patient to his environment and introduce him to those who will be sharing the room with him.
3. Have the patient use antibacterial soap, particularly around the eyes on day of surgery; caution him about getting soap in his eyes.
4. Let the patient know if his eyes will be bandaged after surgery.
5. Brief the patient on the procedure during operative and postoperative phases—remind him to hold his head still during surgery.
6. Be available to the patient for any questions he might think of relating to his surgery or immediate postoperative care.
7. Administer analgesics and tranquilizer(s) as prescribed.

E. Postoperative Recovery

1. Place the patient in the dorsal recumbent position with a small pillow under his head, or permit him to lie on unoperated side.
2. Position bed rails to offer the patient a sense of security.
3. Place a call bell within reach of the patient; have him call the nurse rather than risk stress or strain in an attempt to be self-sufficient.
4. Direct anyone who enters the patient's room to announce himself; also, let the patient know when you are leaving the room. Otherwise he may be left talking to himself.
5. Avoid disturbing the patient's head with such activities as combing the hair; delay combing the hair until the patient is allowed out of bed.

▶ **NURSING ALERT:** For eye patients requiring bed rest (e.g., following keratoplasty, injury, retinal detachment surgery) measures should be taken to prevent pulmonary and/or circulatory complications. This may include passive range of motion activities, antiembolism stockings, special positioning, etc.

Health Teaching

1. Consult ophthalmologist before recommending diversional or recreational therapy that is not fatiguing to the eyes—no reading; television in moderation; radio.
2. Recognize the soothing and relaxing effect of soft pastels for the wall and ceiling colors.
3. Regulate lights so that they are not too bright and do not produce a glare.
4. Inform the patient before he leaves the hospital regarding medications, eye glasses, follow-up visits, type of work he can do, and when he can do it.
5. Instruct the patient or family as follows on instillation of eye medications and proper cleansing of eyes:
   a. Wash hands before and after treating eyes.
   b. To clean around the eye, use sterile, wet gauze and wipe gently across lid from inner corner to outer corner.
   c. To apply eye medications, pull down lower lid and place eye drop in cul-de-sac, place ribbon of ointment along the entire length of the conjunctiva of lower lid.
   d. Apply protective shield over the operated eye at bedtime.
6. Inform the patient of "Talking Book" records, machines, and tapes that are available from most public libraries without charge.
7. Initiate follow-up visits with ophthalmologist. The nurse can make the first appointment for the patient.
8. Check the following with patient/family:
   a. Does the patient have a return appointment date with physician confirmed?
   b. Does the patient have his medication properly identified and labeled? Does he (or a responsible member of the family) know how to use his prescribed medications?
   c. Does the patient understand the restrictions placed on him and the reasons for them?

Evaluation
Expected Outcomes

1. Demonstrates improved vision in accordance with expectations of the surgery
2. Shows no signs of infection or other postoperative complications
3. Experiences no discomforts; does not complain of pain
4. Manages self-care with minimum of assistance
5. Carries cane to prevent possible falls. (With increasing age, walking unescorted may not be possible.)
6. Describes precautions that must be taken as safety measures and enumerates symptoms that may occur if complications develop
7. Appears relaxed and positive concerning outcome of surgery

Corneal Transplantation (Keratoplasty)

Keratoplasty is the transplantation of a donor cornea, usually obtained at autopsy, to repair a corneal scar, burn, or deformed cornea, as in keratoconus (cone-shaped deformity of cornea).

Types of Grafts

1. Full-thickness (6.5–8 mm.)—most common
2. Partial-thickness—lamellar

Corneal Graft

1. Fresh cornea is the preferred tissue; it is removed from the donor within 8–12 hours after death and used within 24 hours.
2. Special solution for storage of fresh cornea is available (M-K medium), which may extend storage up to 3 days.
3. *Cryopreservation* is the care and handling of corneal graft by freezing to retain its transparency.
   a. Because an intact endothelium is required for ultimate transparency of the corneal graft, it is necessary in the preservation process to freeze properly, defrost, and quickly use the graft to reduce the likelihood of damage to the graft.
   b. Eye Bank laboratories* cut the cornea from the enucleated eye and place it in several solutions before freezing.
   c. During defrosting, the cornea is gently rotated in a glass tube at a certain temperature for a certain period of time. When only a small ice ball adheres to the cornea, it is allowed to melt without shaking the vial.
   d. Fluid from the vial is decanted and is replaced with fresh, diluted human albumin for several prescribed minutes before using immediately.
   e. The technique described above requires trained personnel.

Preoperative Care

1. Psychological preparation for surgery may be simplified because the patient is usually optimistic about the imminent transplant.
2. If cultural and spiritual concerns need to be voiced by the patient, the nurse, and possibly the hospital chaplain, should be available so that the patient faces surgery in the best frame of mind possible.
3. Soon after admission, the patient will have a thorough face cleansing with a detergent germicide; eyelashes may be clipped (use petrolatum so that lashes adhere to scissors and do not enter the patient's eye).
4. Instruct the patient who will have local anesthesia that most discomfort will be alleviated with preoperative medication.
   a. Miotics and osmotic agents may be prescribed.
   b. Explain that momentary discomfort may be experienced during initial injection of local anesthesia. The patient needs to know the importance of remaining perfectly still during surgery.

* Function of Eye Banks:
1. Inform public of need of eye donations.
2. Procure eyes donated to the bank.
3. Assist in the optimum use of the tissue; either retain for local use or arrange for its transportation to the nearest Eye Bank with the greatest need.

Postoperative Care

A. Reducing postoperative anxiety

1. Following the procedure, an eye patch is applied with a shield for protection. This is changed daily at the time of examination.
2. Recognize that healing is slow because of the avascularity of the cornea.

B. Keeping eye pressure at safe level

This is to protect the eye from loss of aqueous humor or from injury because of the possibility of dislocating the newly transplanted cornea.
1. Prevent sudden turning of the head.
2. Minimize those activities or sources of irritants that may cause sneezing (dusting or sweeping, heavily scented flowers, sprays). (No pepper on trays.)
3. Avoid conversation that annoys or disturbs the patient; caution visitors not to upset the patient since emotional disturbances may increase his intraocular pressure.

C. Recognizing differences between care requirements of the patient having a full-thickness (penetrating) corneal transplant and those of the patient having a lamellar transplant

1. Full-thickness (penetrating) type—emphasize the need for longer recovery.
2. Lamellar type—activities resumed more rapidly.

D. Preventing complications

1. Avoid urinary retention by providing adequate fluids.
2. Prevent constipation or straining on defecation by avoiding constipating foods and maintaining adequate hydration.
3. Administer analgesics as necessary to relieve pain.
4. Report unrelieved pain since it may indicate that dressings are too tight, that graft has slipped, or that hemorrhage is occurring—or possible early infection, inflammation, or postoperative glaucoma.
5. Utilize measures that will prevent infection of the eye.
   a. Assist physician in practicing meticulous aseptic technique during dressing change to reduce the possibility of infection.
   b. Discourage the patient from touching the dressings.
6. If necessary, administer steroids, which will reduce likelihood of graft rejection (but often retards wound healing).
7. Introduce additional activities gradually each day, but continue to avoid those that will require straining.
8. Emphasize the importance of follow-up visits to the ophthalmologist.
9. Be alert for signs of graft rejection (about 10–14 days postoperatively); decreased vision, ocular irritation, corneal edema, redness of sclera.
10. Instruct the patient to assess his eye for graft rejection; this becomes a daily activity because graft rejection may occur months after the operation.
    a. Recommend doing this the same time each day in order to make comparisons of changes.
    b. Vision varies with individuals. Functional vision does not return until sutures are removed: Interrupted sutures removed in 6 weeks–3 months
    Continuous sutures removed in about a year.

Retinal Detachment

Retinal detachment is the detachment of the sensory retina (rods and cones) from the pigment epithelium of the retina.

Altered Physiology

1. The retina perceives light and transmits impulses from its nerve cells to the optic nerve.
2. Tears or holes in the retina may result rapidly from trauma or slowly from the aging process.
3. A tear in the retina allows vitreous humor and transudate from choroid vessels to seep behind the retina and separate it from the pigment epithelium.
4. That portion of the retina which is separated from its choroidal nutrition becomes blind. Early treatment is urged.
5. Detached retina may occur as a primary condition or secondary to other intraocular disorders.
6. Most common predisposing causes are aphakia (absence of lens) and myopia (retina may be thinner).

Clinical Manifestations

1. Retinal detachment occurs most commonly after age 40; it may occur slowly or suddenly.
2. The patient complains of flashes of light or blurred, "sooty" vision due to stimulation of the retina by vitreous pull.
3. The patient notes sensation of particles moving in his line of vision (normally most individuals can see floating filaments when looking at a light background).
4. Delineated areas of vision may be blank (a relative scotoma); there is no perception of pain.
5. A sensation of a veil-like coating coming down, coming up, or sideways in front of the eye may be present.
   a. This veil-like coating, or shadow, is often misinterpreted as a drooping eyelid or elevated cheek.
   b. Straight-ahead vision may remain good in early stages.
6. Unless the retinal holes are sealed, the retina will progressively detach, and ultimately there will be a loss of central vision as well as peripheral vision.
7. Retinal detachments do not cure themselves; they must be corrected surgically.

Diagnostic Evaluation

The diagnosis is confirmed by the patient's history and binocular ophthalmoscopy.

Treatment

Surgical intervention is the only treatment.

Goal:
Seal the retinal hole, thereby ensuring that the retina will adhere to the choroid.

A. Types of Surgery

1. *Electrodiathermy*—the passing of an electrode needle through the sclera to allow subretinal fluid to escape. An exudate forms from the pigment epithelium and adheres to the retina.
2. *Cryosurgery* or *retinal cryopexy*—a supercooled probe is touched to the sclera, causing minimal damage; as a result of scarring, the pigment epithelium adheres to the retina.
3. *Photocoagulation*—a light beam (either laser or xenon arc) is passed through the dilated pupil, causing a small burn and producing an exudate between the pigment epithelium and retina.
4. *Scleral buckling*—a technique whereby the sclera is shortened to allow a buckling to occur, which forces the pigment epithelium closer to the retina.

B. Prognosis

1. Untreated incomplete retinal detachment progresses to complete retinal detachment and legal blindness in that eye.
2. Surgical reattachment by scleral buckling, cryotherapy, or diathermy is successful in approximately 90%–95% of cases. Secondary operations may be required.
3. Return of visual acuity with a reattached retina depends on:
   a. Amount of retina detached prior to surgery
   b. Whether the macula was detached
   c. Length of time the retina was detached
   d. Amount of external distortion caused by the scleral buckle
   e. Possible macular damage as a result of diathermy or cryocoagulation
4. Retinal tears that may lead to retinal detachment may be present in the other eye. These often require surgical treatment by cryocoagulation, photocoagulation, or scleral buckling.
5. Two possible complications to watch for and guard against are glaucoma and infection.
6. If the retina remains attached for 2 months postoperatively, the condition is likely to be corrected and unlikely to recur.

Preoperative Nursing Interventions

1. Recognize the significance of emotional care during this time of stress and restriction.
2. Instruct the patient to remain quiet to prevent further detachment of the retina. Both eyes may be bandaged (according to physician's request).
3. Physician will determine proper position to be maintained, according to the area of detachment; such an area must be in a dependent position if adherence is to take place.
4. Explain what is to be expected before and after the operation. Tell the patient that:
   a. The circumorbital area may be black and blue, but this will gradually fade away in a few weeks.
   b. The patient will have a patch on his eye(s) after the operation.
5. Have patient wash his face preoperatively with a detergent–germicide to reduce possibility of eye infection; administer sedation and tranquilizing medications for comfort and relief of anxiety.

Postoperative Nursing Interventions

1. Proper positioning is important after the operation and is prescribed according to individual need. Usually the patient is permitted out of bed.
2. Take precautions to avoid bumping the patient's head, thus causing the retina to detach further.
3. Following general anesthesia, the patient is encouraged to breathe deeply but not to cough since this will increase eye pressure. Vomiting must be avoided.
4. Allow additional activity as type of treatment permits; for example, scleral buckling is less confining than diathermy.
5. Provide for diversional therapy, since this patient often becomes depressed.
   a. Moderate television viewing

b. No handwork or reading until physician's permission is obtained

c. "Talking books," radio, and visitors permitted

6. If local anesthesia is used, the patient is ambulatory postoperatively if condition permits (age, vision in other eye, other medical or physical problems).

7. Hospitalization is minimal unless the patient's condition requires additional attention.

Health Education and Discharge Planning

1. When the patient goes home, he is able to care for himself; he may care for all bodily needs in an unhurried manner, being careful to avoid falls, jerks, and bumps.

2. It is advisable to take precautions and moderate activities to avoid accidental injury.

3. Watching television, looking at friends, and using eyes in straight-line vision are harmless, but rapid eye movement, as in reading, should be avoided for several weeks.

4. For comfort of the eyes and eyelids, the use of a clean wash cloth, wrung out of hot water is most relaxing and soothing when applied several times during the day for 10 minutes.

5. Avoid straining and bending head below waist; driving is restricted.

6. Use meticulous cleanliness in giving eye medications.

7. The first follow-up visit to the ophthalmologist should take place in 2 weeks and other visits at longer intervals thereafter.

8. Within 3 weeks, light activities may be pursued; in 6 weeks, athletic and heavier activities are usually possible.

9. Acquaint the patient with the symptoms that indicate a recurrence of the detachment; floating spots, flashing light, progressive shadow.
   If they occur, recommend that the patient contact his physician.

Radial Keratotomy and Keratophakia

Radial keratotomy is an operation designed to provide correction of myopia (nearsightedness) by making a number of incisions on the outside of the cornea in order to flatten it. This permits images to fall on the retina instead of in front of it.

Assessment

In addition to the patient's general health assessment, he will undergo:

1. Visual acuity tests with and without glasses
2. Cycloplegic refraction
3. Slit-lamp examination, photographs, and epithelial cell count
4. Corneal thickness measurement, using an optical or ultrasonic pachymeter
5. Applanation tonometry
6. A-scan ultrasonography

Treatment

A. Operative Procedure

1. An operating microscope is used.
2. The cornea is anesthetized topically with proparacaine.
3. The surgeon marks the visual axis; utilizing a marking trephine, 8–16 radial incisions are made into the corneal surface.

4. Following an irrigation of basic saline solution to remove any foreign material, topical antibiotic, and a mydriatic are instilled.

5. The eye is patched for 24 hours.

B. Postoperative Course

1. Discomfort is felt for the first 10–18 hours and is aggravated by bright light. The pressure eye patch controls this problem.

2. Discomfort is almost gone in 24 hours and totally subsides in 2–3 days.

3. There is a persistence of foreign body sensation and photophobia.

4. There may be some temporary difference in visual refraction until the other eye is operated on.

5. Complications appear to be minimal.

C. Other Procedures

1. Prospective Evaluation of Radial Keratotomy Clinical Aspects (PERK) is a study being done by the National Eye Institute to determine the efficacy and safety of radial keratotomy as a means of reducing physiologic myopia (currently being done for 4 years).

2. *Keratophakia* (investigational surgery) is an operation designed to provide correction of hyperopia (farsightedness) by (1) temporarily removing a segment of cornea; (2) shaping a donor cornea to required shape; and (3) reinserting both pieces in an attempt to steepen or build up corneal curvature. This permits images to fall on the retina instead of in back of it.

Cataracts

A *cataract* is an opacity of the crystalline lens or its capsule; it is the leading cause of blindness in the United States.

Predisposing Factors

1. Most commonly, cataract occurs in adults past 70 years of age (senile cataract) as a result of the aging process.

2. A cataract may occur at birth (congenital cataract).

3. Occasionally a cataract occurs in young individuals as a result of disease or trauma.

Altered Physiology

1. Normally, the lens is a semisolid body of clear, gelatinous protein encased in a capsule lying behind the iris; the lens possesses great refractive powers (approximately $\frac{1}{5}$ of the total).

2. Chemical change in the lens protein may cause coagulation; as a result, the lens loses its pristine transparency and gradually becomes milky or whitish in color.

3. Physical changes result in a swelling of the fibers, which in turn causes a distortion of the image.

4. Although cataract may be readily diagnosed, the basic cause of senile cataract is unknown.

Clinical Manifestations

1. Alterations in vision are noted.
   a. Objects seem distorted and blurred.
   b. Glare annoys the patient when there are bright lights.
   c. Visual loss is gradual, but eventually the opacity becomes complete.

2. The pupil, usually black, becomes gray and later milky-white.

Nursing History

1. Determine patient's level of understanding of plan of treatment.
2. What type of cataract extraction is planned?
3. Will the patient require local or general anesthesia?
4. Does the patient have complicating conditions, such as diabetes, allergies, coronary heart disease, renal problems?
5. Will the patient be treated as an outpatient, or does he require hospitalization?
6. Determine the patient's ability to hear in order to assess level of communication (particularly significant if he is to have local anesthesia).
7. How is he reacting to the possibility of eye surgery? emotional status?

Management

1. Surgical removal of the lens is indicated.
2. Proper time for cataract removal is determined by the patient's eyesight, occupation, general health, and convenience.
3. Usually a patient with 1 cataract can manage without surgery.
4. If cataract occurs in both eyes, surgery is recommended when vision in the better eye causes problems in daily activities. Surgery is done on only 1 eye at a time.
5. Cataract surgery is usually done under local anesthesia, but occasionally general anesthesia is used. Preoperative medications produce decreased response to pain and lessened motor activity. Oral medications are given to reduce intraocular pressure.
6. Intraocular lens implants are usually implanted at the time of cataract extraction.
7. In some instances, following lens extraction and the healing process, the patient may have corrective refraction to replace the lens; he is later fitted with appropriate eyeglasses or contact lenses.

Intracapsular Extraction

In this surgery, which was the procedure of choice for cataract extraction, the lens as well as the capsule is removed through an 11-mm. incision.

Extracapsular Extraction

1. This surgery is conservative; it is simple to perform and is usually done under local anesthesia. It is the current procedure of choice.
2. The lens capsule is incised, and the nucleus, cortex, and anterior capsule are extracted by cryosurgery or phacoemulsification.
3. The posterior capsule is left in place. This is usually the base to which the intraocular lens (IOL) is implanted.

A. Cryosurgery

This is a special technique in which a pencil-like instrument with a metal probe is cooled to about −35°C; when the lens capsule is available after dissection, the cryosurgical instrument touches the lens and freezes to it so that the lens is easily pulled out.

B. Phacoemulsification (ultrasonic)

1. *Phacoemulsification* is the mechanical breaking up (emulsifying) of the lens by a hollow needle vibrating at 40,000 cycles per second (Fig. 17-9).
   a. The needle tip moves forward and backward (action similar to that of a jackhammer).
   b. It is powered by an ultrasound generator to produce the frequency necessary to emulsify the cataract.
   c. This action is coupled with simultaneous irrigation and aspiration of the emulsified particles from the anterior chamber through the needle tip.
   d. Only a 2–3 mm. incision is required, and the actual procedure takes from 20–30 minutes (performed by a specially trained ophthalmic surgeon).
   e. Normal activities may be resumed the day after surgery.
   f. Contact lenses can be used in about 3–6 weeks.
   g. Effective in management of soft cataracts in children and young adults.
2. Criteria to be met for this operation:
   a. Pupil must be able to dilate fully.
   b. Anterior chamber must be deep enough to accommodate the manipulation of the probe–aspirator.
   c. Cornea should be healthy.

C. Intraocular Lens

This is the implantation of a synthetic lens—designed for distance vision; the patient wears prescribed glasses for reading and near vision (Fig. 17-10).

1. Intraocular lens implant is an alternative to sight correction with glasses or contact lenses for the aphakic patient.
2. Sophisticated calculations are required to determine the prescription for lens:
   Corneal curvature
   Depth of anterior chamber
   Axial length of eyeball (by diagnostic ultrasound)
   a. *Unilateral cataract*—objective is to leave the patient slightly myopic (nearsighted).
      (1) Operated eye is used for reading.
      (2) Unoperated eye is used for distance vision.
   b. *Bilateral cataract*—objective is to leave the patient emmetropic (all rays of light focus perfectly on retina).
      (1) Vision is good for distance.
      (2) Glasses required for reading.
   c. Hyperopia (farsightedness) is avoided in implanting a lens because the image would be magnified and cause visual difficulty.
   d. Astigmatism is corrected with eyeglasses.
3. Insertion of intraocular lens
   a. There are a number of types of intraocular lens available.
   b. Polymethyl methacrylate is a common durable compound from which such lenses are made. Designs and material change as new developments occur. Extended-wear contact lenses may replace intraocular lens.
   c. Various methods of fixation are being used, including (1) fastening by sutures or clips; (2) holding in place in the way that a hub cap is fitted to the rim of a tire; and (3) sealing within the anterior and posterior capsule after extracapsular extraction (capsular fixation). The second method (no sutures) usually requires a miotic (pilocarpine) to keep the iris from dilating too widely—thereby causing displacement of the implant.
4. Advantages of intraocular lens

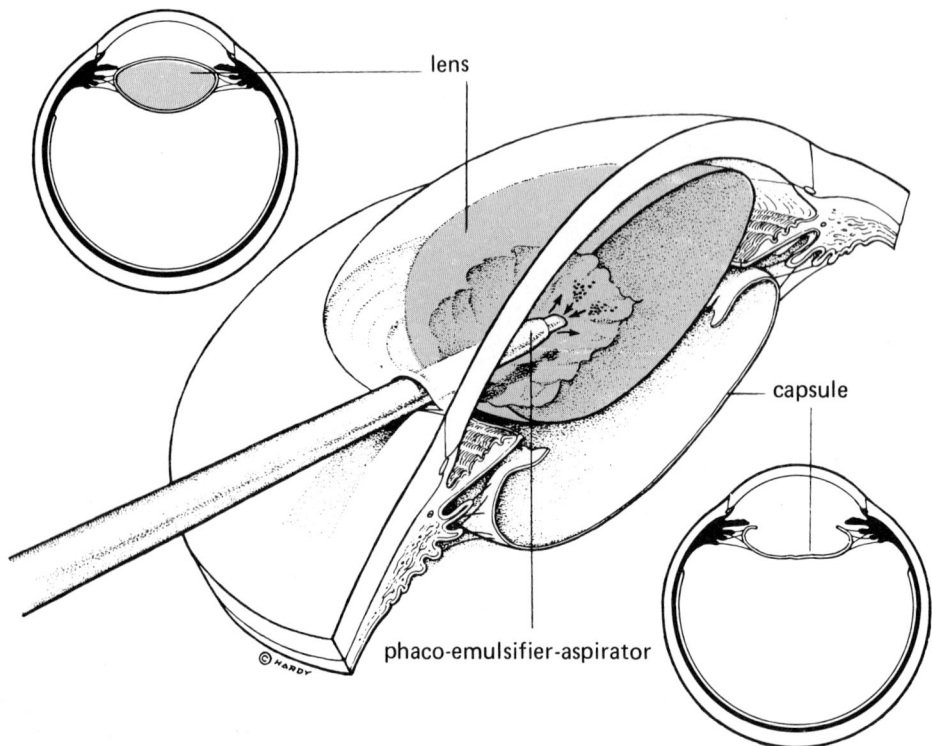

Figure 17-9. Cataract is shown in orb at upper left. Kelman ultrasonic needle (Cavitron Corp.) is inserted through 2- to 3-mm. incision at corneal–scleral junction to emulsify lens cortex and nucleus and aspirate them. Drawing at right shows cataract removed and posterior capsule intact. Cataract surgery requires a 19- to 20-mm. incision. (Copyright the American Journal of Nursing Co. Reproduced with permission from American Journal of Nursing, Vol. 75, No. 6.)

a. Provides an alternative to individuals who cannot wear cataract glasses or contact lenses.
b. Cannot be lost or misplaced like conventional glasses; does not need to be replaced.
c. Provides a permanent form of near normal vision.
5. Complications (specific to implantation)
   a. Iritis or vitritis—can be controlled with steroids.
   b. Rosy vision, due to keeping pupil from full constriction; excessive light enters pupil, causing a dazzling of macula.

c. Degeneration of cornea, chronic uveitis (see p. 725).
d. Malpositioning or dislocation of lens.

Preoperative Care

A. Relieve anxiety and ensure safety.

1. Explain the plan of care.
2. Escort the patient as he walks around the unit.
3. Provide bed rails if warranted/hospital policy.

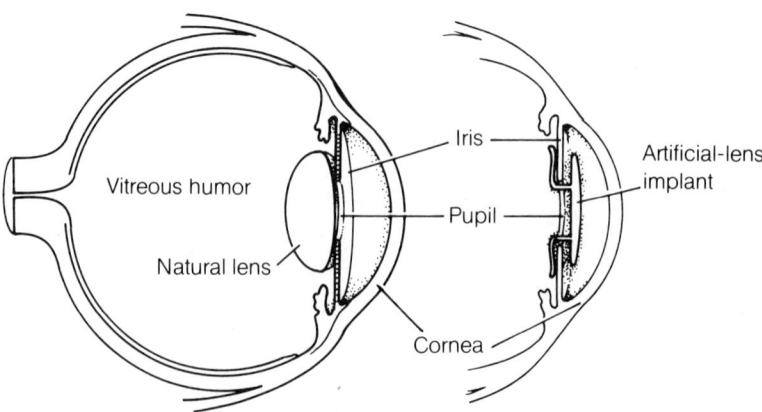

Figure 17-10. Illustration at left indicates position of natural lens; drawing on right shows artificial-lens implant following removal of cataract.

4. Determine how the patient feels about his operation.
5. Assess his knowledge level regarding the purpose of surgery and his expectations afterward.
6. Role play what the patient may expect in the operating room if he is to have local anesthesia; this will help him overcome anxiety.
7. Encourage the patient's questions and provide the answers.

B. Reduce the conjunctival bacterial count in order to minimize the chance of postoperative infection.

1. Obtain a conjunctival culture if requested.
2. Administer local antibiotics as prescribed.
3. Employ aseptic technique in any eye treatment or procedure.
4. Instruct the patient not to touch his eyes.

C. Preparation of the eye in the immediate preoperative period

1. Instill mydriatic if prescribed.
2. Note whether pupil dilates after instillation of mydriatic.

D. Preoperative medications

1. Tranquilizers—diazepam
2. Antiemetics—Compazine, Vistaril
3. Narcotics—meperidine for pain relief
4. Ocular hypotensive agents:
   a. Cholinesterase inhibitors—acetazolamide (Diamox)
   b. Osmotic hypotensives
      (1) Oral—glycerol (Glyrol)
      (2) Intravenous—mannitol

Postoperative Care

A. Prevent pressure build-up within eye (intraocular) **which may exert a stress on the fresh sutures.**

1. Caution the patient to refrain from coughing or sneezing.
2. Advise the patient to avoid rapid movement, but allow him to turn to the unoperated side or remain in the dorsal recumbent position.
3. Caution the patient not to bend from the waist.

B. Promote comfort and safety.

1. Allow the patient to turn on unoperated side or on his back.
2. Offer analgesics as prescribed to control pain.
3. Provide a pillow or permit head elevation if this is more comfortable.
4. Allow the patient to be ambulatory/go to bathroom, as soon as he has recovered from anesthesia.
5. Encourage the patient to wear eyeglasses during the day and the protective eye shield at night to ensure protection of his eye from injury.

C. Control and monitor signs/symptoms indicative of possible complications.

1. Sudden pain in the eye may be due to a ruptured vessel or suture and may lead to hemorrhage—notify physician immediately.
2. Restlessness and increasing pulse rate may suggest hemorrhage.
3. Nausea may lead to vomiting and increase intraocular pressure—administer antiemetic drugs as prescribed and perhaps an osmotic agent.

Health Education

A. Encourage the patient to become increasingly independent.

1. Assist the patient in getting around his room, locating needed personal items, using bathroom facilities.
2. Gradually increase the patient's activities each day.
3. Caution the patient to avoid any strain on the eye; this includes avoiding heavy lifting and straining on defecation.
4. Resumption of sexual activities may be discussed when the eye and suture line are examined.

B. Demonstrate to the patient and a responsible member of his family how to administer eye medications.

C. Promote the patient's interest in diversional activities as he recuperates.

Try to prevent his becoming uninterested and disengaged.

D. Acquaint the patient with the step-by-step requirements of a healthy convalescence.

1. Apply plastic shield over the eye at night to avoid accidental injury during sleep.
2. Fitting for temporary corrective lenses for the first 6 weeks will be done at this time.
3. Prescription for permanent lenses 6–12 weeks after surgery for intracapsular extraction.
4. Prescription for contact lenses about 3–6 weeks after phacoemulsification.
5. The use of dark glasses after eye dressings are removed may provide comfort.

E. Assist the patient in adjusting to the eyeglasses.

1. Stress the importance of patience in the coming weeks of adjustment—it is easy to become frustrated.
2. If spectacles are to be worn, they will cause the perceived image to be about ⅓ larger than that seen by the patient before cataract formation (glass is usually heavier and thicker than the more expensive plastic cataract eyeglass lenses).
3. Peripheral vision is markedly distorted; instruct the patient to look through the center of the corrective glasses; have him turn his head when looking to the side.
4. If only one eye is operated for cataract, the patient can use only one eye at a time, with spectacle (glasses) lenses, since the operated eye has a 30% increase in image size and the unoperated eye still has "normal" sized images, which cannot be superimposed.
5. It is necessary to relearn space judgment—walking, using stairs, reaching for articles on the table, such as a cup of coffee, pouring liquids. In walking, use handrails.

F. Familiarize the patient with contact lenses, if this is his choice.

1. With contact lenses, magnification is only about 5%–10%; peripheral vision is not distorted.
2. Since the image size difference between an aphakic eye with a contact lens and the unoperated eye is only 8%–10%, both eyes can be used together.
3. Space judgment presents little difficulty.
4. There may be problems if the patient has difficulty applying lenses, has a tremor of the hands, or if there are hygienic problems that could cause soiling and infection.

Extended wear lenses would be preferred because they can be worn for long periods of time without removal.

G. Recognize that with an intraocular lens, magnification problems are negligible.

Both the operated eye and the unoperated eye can work together after cataract surgery with lens implantation.
1. No eyeglasses may be required for distance but may be needed for reading and writing.
2. Again the caution—avoid straining of any type. If necessary to reach for something on the floor, keep head, neck, and back straight; bend knees only.
3. In bathing, a sponge bath is recommended. Avoid getting soap near or in eyes.
4. In shampooing of hair, it should be done with head tilted slightly backward and not with head forward over the sink. No vigorous shaking of the head is recommended.

H. Administer eye medications carefully

1. Wash hands before and after instilling eye medications.
2. Clean area around eye with sterile cotton balls or sterile gauze sponges moistened with sterile eye solution (Eye-Stream); wipe gently from inner corner to outer canthus.
3. Be seated while instilling eye drops (see Guidelines, p. 716).
4. When visiting the ophthalmologist, bring all eye medications to permit adjustments in dosage and medications. What will not be used can then be discarded to prevent confusion.

Glaucoma

Glaucoma is a condition in which the pressure within the eyeball is higher than normal; it is associated with progressive visual field loss. If allowed to proceed uncorrected, the problem may lead to atrophy of the optic nerve and eventual blindness. Early detection and treatment will prevent loss of eyesight.

Incidence

1. It is estimated that 1 million Americans have undiagnosed glaucoma.
2. Glaucoma is the cause of blindness in 1 of 10 persons who become blind.
3. Glaucoma is estimated to occur in 1.0%–2.5% of Americans aged 35 and over.
4. Persons with family history of glaucoma are more susceptible than others.

Altered Physiology

1. Pressure within the eye is determined by the rate of input of aqueous humor as produced by the ciliary body and the resistance to outflow of aqueous humor.
2. Inflow of aqueous humor is through the pupil; outflow is at the meshwork located at juncture of iris and cornea (canal of Schlemm). Clogging at the meshwork by blood, fibrin, or inflammatory cells accounts for the buildup of pressure, which produces secondary glaucoma.
3. Thickening of the meshwork appears spontaneously in those older individuals who appear to have a hereditary predisposition; chronic simple glaucoma results and is the most common type.
4. When the iris is abnormally anterior and exerts pressure against the meshwork, acute glaucoma results; this is the least frequent type.

Classification
1. Angle-closure (narrow angle)—acute or chronic
2. Open-angle (wide angle; simple; chronic simple)—chronic
3. Congenital
   Within these classifications, principal contributing factors may be *primary* or *secondary*
   Primary—genetically based
   Secondary—result of ocular disease, injury, neoplasia, or surgery

Diagnostic Evaluation

1. Because of the relative ease of developing glaucoma, unless a person past 40 has a complete physical examination periodically, including measurement of eye pressure (tonometry), the disease may not be discovered until it is considerably advanced (chronic simple type).
2. Tonometry (see Figs. 17-1, 17-2)
   A reading of 24–32 mm. Hg suggests glaucoma.
3. Tonography—application of tonometer, usually electronic, with a special device that records intraocular tension over a 4-minute period.
4. Gonioscopy—an examination to differentiate angle-closure glaucoma from open-angle type.
5. Examination of optic nerve and blood vessels by means of the ophthalmoscope.
6. Visual field examination—with either perimeter or tangent screen.

Acute (Angle-Closure) Glaucoma

Clinical Manifestations

1. As intraocular pressure increases rapidly (often above 75 mm. Hg), severe pain occurs in and around eye.
2. Artificial lights appear to have a rainbow of colors around them.
3. Vision becomes cloudy and blurred.
4. Pupils dilate; nausea and vomiting may occur.
5. Although onset may be insidious, severity of symptoms may progress within hours to include disturbances suggestive of gastrointestinal, sinus, neurologic and dental problems as well as eye pain.
6. If untreated, irreversible blindness may result.

Treatment/Pharmacotherapy

This will be initiated to control eye pressure before surgery. Medications listed below are prescribed at the discretion of the ophthalmologist according to the patient's condition and needs.

A. Parasympathomimetic Drugs Used as Miotic Drugs

Given as eye drops
1. Drug action—pupil contracts, iris is drawn away from cornea; aqueous humor may drain through lymph spaces (meshwork) into canal of Schlemm.
2. Types: (see chart below).

▶ **NURSING ALERT:** Dilatation of pupils is avoided if the anterior chamber is shallow. This is determined by oblique illumination of the anterior segment of the eye.

B. Sympathomimetic Drugs

Given as eyedrops (see chart, p. 735).

Medication	Action	Effect and Precautions
Parasympathomimetic Drugs		
Pilocarpine hydrochloride	Acts directly on myoneural junction	Action lasts 6–8 hours; may cause ciliary spasm (eye becomes more myopic).
Carbachol (Carbacel; Miostat)	Acts directly on myoneural junction	Used if pilocarpine is ineffective; prolongs pupillary constriction.
Physostigmine salicylate (eserine)	Cholinesterase inhibitor	Action lasts 6–8 hours; allergenic, unstable, short in action.
Echothiophate iodide (Phospholine Iodide)	Cholinesterase inhibitor	Water-soluble; produces less local irritation. Action lasts 24 hours. After instillation, apply finger pressure to tear duct to prevent drainage into nose and throat. Contraindicated in angle-closure glaucoma.
Isoflurophate (DFP; Floropryl; ophthalmic solution)	Cholinesterase inhibitor	Oil-soluble miotic. *Caution:* side effects—vomiting, diarrhea, tenesmus. Contraindicated in angle-closure glaucoma
Sympathomimetic Drugs		
Epinephrine	Decreases aqueous humor production rate	Contraindicated prior to iridectomy (may precipitate acute attack of glaucoma). Keep medication refrigerated to maintain effectiveness.
Carbonic Anhydrase Inhibitor		
Acetazolamide (Diamox) Methazolamide (Neptazane) Dichlorphenamide (Daranide)	Carbonic anhydrase inhibitor	Decreases production of aqueous humor. *Caution:* side effects—gastric distress, shortness of breath, dermatitis, tingling of extremities, general malaise, acidosis, ureteral stones.
		Stress importance of continuing with medications even if side effects occur.
		If diuresis occurs, supplement the patient's diet with potassium-containing foods.
Beta-blocker-nonselective		
Timolol (Timoptic)	Effectively lowers intraocular pressure in glaucoma with a minimum of side effects	May reduce production of aqueous humor. May facilitate outflow of aqueous humor.
	Mechanism of action not completely established	Use cautiously in patients who have bronchial asthma, congestive heart failure, or myasthenia gravis.
	No anesthetic action; has pH similar to that of eye (6.5–7.5)	Check pulse; do not administer if pulse is below 50 beats per minute.
Hyperosmotic Agents		
Intravenous (systemic) Mannitol Urea	Reduces intraocular pressure by increasing blood osmolality	Useful in treatment of acute attacks of pressure and preoperatively.
		May cause agitation and disorientation.
		Keep airway at bedside; use side rails; monitor fluids and vital signs.
Oral Glycerin (Osmoglyn, Glyrol) Isosorbide (Isonol)		Safer than intravenous medication for cardiac patients.
		May cause nausea, vomiting, headache; instruct the patient to lie down; bed in a flat position.
		Administer medication over cracked ice flavored with citrus juice to avoid nausea.

C. Carbonic Anhydrase Inhibitor

Given orally or intravenously
1. Drug action—restricts action of enzyme which is necessary to produce aqueous humor.
2. See chart below for type frequently used.

D. Beta blocker—nonselective

Given as eyedrops (see chart, p. 735).

E. Hyperosmotic Agents
   (See chart, p. 735.)

Surgical Management

Surgery is indicated if:
1. Intraocular pressure is not maintained within normal limits by medical regimen, and
2. There is progressive visual field loss with optic nerve damage.

Types

1. *Laser trabeculoplasty* (LTP)—an outpatient procedure
   a. After the eye is anesthetized with topical anesthetic, the patient sits at a slit-lamp microscope.
   b. A gonioscopic contact lens is placed on the eye to provide magnification of trabecular meshwork.
   c. Fifty superficial surface burns are placed evenly over 180 degrees of anterior meshwork. (If eye pressure is not lowered, this is repeated.)
   d. Outflow of aqueous humor is increased.
   e. Maximum decrease in IOP (intraocular pressure) is achieved in 2–3 months.
   f. This treatment is less effective in patients under the age of 40.
   g. Most patients require supplemental medical therapy to control glaucoma completely.
2. *Iridectomy*—an incision through cornea so that a portion of the iris may be drawn out and excised—peripheral or sector (keyhole).
   Result—iris is prevented from bulging forward and causing the angle at cornea and iris to be crowded. Consequently, drainage is facilitated and intraocular tension is reduced and there is relief of pupillary block.
3. *Iridencleisis*—an opening is created between anterior chamber and space beneath the conjunctiva; this bypasses the blocked meshwork, and aqueous fluid is absorbed into conjunctival tissues.
4. *Thermosclerectomy*—thermal cautery of posterior lip of corneoscleral wound combined with iridectomy.
5. *Trabeculectomy*—partial thickness scleral resection with 2–3 mm. removal of trabecular meshwork and iridectomy.

Chronic (Open-Angle) Glaucoma

Majority of patients with glaucoma have this type.

Clinical Manifestations

1. Insidious—mild discomfort (tired feeling in eye)
2. Slowly developing impairment of peripheral vision
3. Possible halos around lights
4. Progressive loss of visual field

Treatment/Pharmacotherapy

1. Often treated with a combination of miotic and carbonic anhydrase inhibitors (see p. 735).
2. Remission may occur; however, the patient should continue to see physician at 3- to 6-month intervals.

3. If medical treatment is not successful, surgery may be required.

Surgery
Goal:
Provide a filtering of fluid in order to decrease intraocular tension.

1. Corneoscleral trephine—making a permanent opening at the junction of the cornea and sclera through the anterior chamber so that aqueous humor can drain.
2. Iridencleisis—see above.
3. Sclerectomy—similar to trephining iridectomy except that a punch is used instead of a trephine.
4. Cyclocryotherapy—used when other methods fail. A 3-mm. cryoprobe is applied to the eye surface over the ciliary body; this freezes ciliary body and decreases its secretory function.
5. Laser trabeculoplasty—see treatment for Acute Glaucoma above.

Postsurgical Nursing Interventions

1. Patient usually not detained in the recovery room following local anesthesia.
   Operated eye will be covered by an eye patch.
2. Administer eyedrops, analgesic, or narcotic as prescribed and required.
3. Assist the patient in getting out of bed the first time following surgery; usually the patient is ambulatory following local anesthesia.
4. Following general anesthesia, the patient remains in recovery room until vital signs are stable and he is oriented to time and place; bathroom privileges usually permissible day of surgery.
5. Provide a liquid diet to eliminate straining on defecation. Change to regular diet as condition justifies.
6. Remind the patient of periodic eye check-up since pressure changes may occur.

Health Education

1. Even though glaucoma cannot be cured, it can be controlled.
2. Circumstances that may increase intraocular pressure are to be avoided, if possible.
   a. Emotional upsets—worry, fear, excitement, anger
   b. Constricting clothing such as tight collar, belt, or girdle
   c. Exertion such as snow shoveling, pushing, heavy lifting
   d. Upper respiratory infections
3. Recommended activities
   a. Exercise in moderation to maintain general well-being
   b. Moderate use of eyes for reading and watching television
   c. Maintenance of regular bowel habits (straining on defecation causes increased intraocular pressure)
   d. Continuous daily use of eye medications as prescribed
   e. Normal intake of fluids is not restricted even for alcohol or coffee unless these are known to increase eye pressure in the particular patient.
   f. Check-ups with ophthalmologist in order to keep condition under control
   g. Wearing a medical identification tag indicating the patient has glaucoma

Monocular Vision*

Each year more than 50,000 persons become "one-eyed" because of accidents, disease, or tumors. In addition to the usual postoperative care, the person with monocular vision will need specialized care in adjusting to his condition.

Psychological Adaptations

There are psychological "lows" intermingled with "highs." The support and understanding of family, friends, loved ones, and members of the health team are very important.

Physiological Adjustments

1. Depth perception is impaired and needs readjustment.
   a. Retinal disparity—each eye sees a slightly different image; to make one clear image, the brain notes the size and distance of each object and computes its position.
   b. Convergence—2 images are merged on the retina; this is useful only for objects at a distance of 7.6 meters (25 feet) or less.
   c. Accommodation—only effective in judging distances up to 1.8 meters (6 feet).

Note: All sighted persons are effectively one-eyed for distances greater than 6 meters (20 feet).

2. The horizontal field of vision is narrow because of the position of the nose (Fig. 17-11).

Guidelines For Making Necessary Adjustments and Adaptations

1. Relative motion
   a. By making a quick side movement of the head, one can get 2 slightly different views of an object. Retinal disparity can be overcome by this simple maneuver, and simulation of binocular vision can be created to give a sense of perspective, especially at close range.
2. Perspective
   a. Note that objects in the foreground are larger than similar objects at a distance (diminishing perspective).
   b. Colors are bolder and brighter in foreground (color perspective).
   c. Close objects are more clearly defined (vanishing perspective).
   d. If a distant object "just grows" in size but does not move, it is on a collision course with the viewer.
3. Coping with activities encountered daily:
   a. In reaching for an object (e.g., door knob or hand in a handshake), move hand in a direct line and keep moving hand until contact is made.
   b. When pouring, actually *touch* the receiving vessel with the one from which the liquid is being poured.
   c. Before making a turn to the deficient side, take a good look around by turning the head as far as possible.
   d. When dining, choose a place at the table that favors the good eye and is on the same side as the dinner partner; watch out for waiters serving on the sightless side.
   e. Watch the *last step* when going up or down steps; feel ahead with the toe and keep one hand on the handrail.
   f. In stepping off a curb, keep seeing eye on the edge of the curb so that one can observe its position relative to the backdrop of the street's surface (retinal disparity).
   g. Look both ways at the *very last moment* when crossing a street, especially to the side of limited vision.
   h. When participating in sports, motion that takes place in two dimensions (bowling, shuffleboard) rather than three dimensions (tennis, basketball) will be easier to master.
   i. Swimming is an attractive sport because the swimmer is virtually unaffected by the limits of monocular vision.
   j. In fishing, when casting, wear protective glasses with high-impact, shatter-resistant lenses to protect against accidental injury to the good eye.
   k. Bouncing a ball off a wall or playing catch (or tossing a Frisbee) with a friend can improve visual skills enormously.
   l. If an eyeglass is needed, wear impact-resistant glasses to protect the surviving eye. Wear thin-rimmed or rimless glasses, since heavy frames cut down on the visual field; use nonreflective coating to reduce distracting reflections and ghost images.

Note: To make emergency "glasses" to read a number in a telephone book when reading glasses are not available: Use a small piece of "cardboard" (size of a calling card) and punch a tiny hole in the cardboard with a pin or bent paper clip. Place eye against hole and hold 15 cm. (6") from page; read.

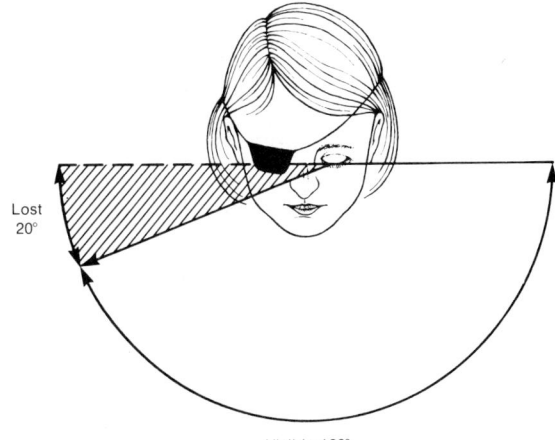

Figure 17-11. The normal field of vision for two eyes is 180 degrees. If a person's vision is limited to one eye, his field of vision encompasses up to 160 degrees, depending on the size of his nose.

---

* Adapted from Brady FB. A Singular View: The Art of Seeing With One Eye (revised edition). Oradell, Medical Economics, 1979

m. For driving, obtain a second external mirror mounted on right side of car; use curb feelers to assist in parking.

n. Remember that *loss of visual perception* is compensated for by an *increase in degree of alertness.*

o. A "swivel head" also compensates for limited vision.

p. Suggested reading: Brady, Frank B. *A Singular View: The Art of Seeing With One Eye,* revised edition. Oradell, Medical Economics, 1979

Nursing Care of the Nonseeing Patient

1. Upon entering the room of a nonseeing patient, address him by his name; use a clear, natural voice.
   a. Tell the patient your name and that you are a nurse.
   b. Indicate why you are there; do not touch the patient before he knows you are there.
   c. Inform the patient's family and visitors of this procedure for entering the patient's room so that he is not startled.
2. Acquaint the patient with his surroundings if he is in a room new to him.
   a. If the patient is in bed:
      (1) Take his hand and show him how to find the call bell and how to use it.
      (2) Help him in using his wash basin, soap, and towel; tell him you have drawn the curtains when he should have privacy.
   b. If the patient is out of bed:
      Assist him to acquaint himself with the room, chairs, bed, doors, bedside table, and place where his personal things are kept.
3. Guide the patient when walking:
   a. First, remember not to direct the visually handicapped person by steering him from behind—he may bump into things.
   b. Walk ahead of him and have him place his hand in the space at the bend of your elbow; walk normally, at an unhurried pace.
   c. Describe where you are walking and inform him when you are going through a narrow passage or are approaching a curb, steps, or an incline.
   d. Inform him that you are leading him to the bed, chair, or toilet and permit him to feel the front of the object with his knee or hands.

▶ **NURSING ALERT: Never** permit a nonseeing patient to smoke in bed unattended. If he insists on smoking, have some responsible person remain with him until the cigar or cigarette is extinguished.

4. Provide side rails in the "up" position for the sightless person who has both eyes bandaged for eye treatment or postoperatively.
   a. Hold the patient's hand as you direct him to feel the side rails.
   b. Tell the patient that the side rails are there to remind him not to attempt to get out of bed unassisted.
   c. Place the bell cord within easy reach and inform the patient that someone will answer his bell when he signals. If call light is multipurpose, place a piece of tape over the "nurse signal" area so that the patient can feel the proper switch.
5. Assist the patient so that he can enjoy his meals.
   a. Read the proposed menu and have him make his selections within his dietary prescription.
   b. Help him to assume a comfortable position when the tray arrives.
   c. Guide his hand to show him where the utensils, plate, cup, etc. are located. Describe food placement on the tray in terms of the face of a clock. If feeding the patient, describe the food: hot, cold, color, flavor.
   d. Plan to have the various items of food always arranged in the same pattern on the tray, so that he will know where the salad, coffee, and bread are. On his plate, the servings should be placed in a specific arrangement so that he knows that the meat is in a certain place, etc.
   e. Assist him by cutting the meat into bite-size pieces, buttering the bread, adding sugar and cream to the coffee. Permit him to do as much for himself as he can without embarrassing himself by spilling or knocking food onto the floor.
   f. Provide pleasant conversation or radio music to make mealtime a satisfying time.
6. Solicit the patient's cooperation when he is taking medications.
   a. Tell him you have his medication ready for him; indicate how many pills there are and that they are in a tiny medication cup.
   b. Offer him ½ glass of water to assist in swallowing the tablets.
   c. Tell him what the medication is for, if he asks.
   d. Prepare him for an injection so that he is not frightened by a "shot."
7. Attend to the psychological and sociological needs of the person with no vision.
   a. Recognize that time does not pass as rapidly when one is inactive.
   b. When giving care, mention day of week, date, and time. Radio and television are helpful here.
   c. Plan for him to have diversions that interest him—radio, braille books, talking books, visitors, television.
   d. Take time to stop and converse with him.

2: Ear Disorders

Hearing Problems and Ear Care Specialists

Problems with hearing rank high as a health disability. One of every 12 to 15 persons exhibits some degree of hearing loss.

Classification of Hearing Loss

1. *Conductive loss*—a hearing loss due to an impairment of the outer or middle ear or both. If causative

problem cannot be corrected, a hearing aid may help.

2. *Sensorineural (perceptive) loss*—a hearing loss due to disease of the inner ear or nerve pathways; sensitivity to and discrimination of sounds are impaired. Hearing aids usually are helpful.
3. *Combined hearing loss*—a combination of the above.
4. *Psychogenic hearing loss*—usually a manifestation of an emotional disturbance and unrelated to evident structural changes in the hearing mechanisms. Loss is often total, but without physical basis; thus the patient may suddenly recover.

Ear Care Specialists

1. *Otologist*—a physician who specializes in the diagnosis and treatment of problems of the ear.
2. *Otolaryngologist*—a physician who specializes in problems related to the ear, nose, and throat.
3. *Audiologist*—an individual who specializes in nonmedical evaluation and rehabilitation of hearing disorders (usually not a physician).

Ear Health Education

Self-Care/Hygienic Measures

1. Avoid putting bobby pins, matches, toothpicks, etc. into the external auditory canal (danger of possible infection and damage to the eardrum). Many physicians even object to the use of cotton-tipped applicators.
2. If it becomes necessary to remove wax deposits, instill 3 or 4 drops of Debrox twice a day for 3 or 4 days; after the 4th day, irrigate gently with warm water.
3. During an upper respiratory infection, avoid vigorous blowing of the nose, since middle ear infection can result.
4. In the presence of an ear infection, take precautions when swimming—either avoid this sport or insert a lamb's wool plug into the ear canal. It is preferable not to get the head wet.

Noise

1. Excessive noise is detrimental to health and decreases work efficiency; conversely, elimination of noise or substitution of pleasant soft music increases work efficiency.
2. The *decibel* (db) is the unit of measurement of sound intensity.
   a. Leaves rustling in a breeze—10 decibels
   b. Ordinary conversation—50 decibels
   c. Noisy subway—80 decibels
   d. Jet plane (100 feet away)—140 decibels
3. *Frequency*—number of sound waves emanating from a source per second. This is described as cycles per second (cps) or Herz (Hz).
4. *Pitch* is related to frequency.
   a. For example—100 cps or Hz is low pitch
   10,000 cps or Hz is high pitch
   b. A healthy young adult can distinguish frequencies from 16 cps to 20,000 cps.
5. Health implications
   a. Individuals react differently to noise.
   b. The noise level in the home should not exceed 35–40 decibels.
   c. Very loud electrical music can damage hearing.
   d. Protective muffs are recommended in work areas where the noise level exceeds 80–85 decibels.

Assessment and Diagnostic Procedures

Nursing History (Subjective Assessment)

1. Should include questions designed to reveal status of adult hearing.
2. A good example of an assessment tool is Figure 17-12.

Physical Examination (Objective Assessment)

Examination techniques: inspection, palpation, mechanical tests, tuning fork, and otoscopic examination.

▶ **NURSING ALERT:** In patients with ear pain, suggest examining the good ear first:

1. Otherwise, if sensitive ear is hurt during examination, examiner risks not getting a good look at it or the good ear.
2. If gentleness is demonstrated during examination of good ear, patient is more likely to submit to examination of painful ear.
3. Infection could be transmitted from painful ear to good ear.

Note: Tuning fork tests (Weber and Rinne tests) are used only for screening or confirmatory purposes. Mechanical tests include Weber Test and Rinne Test (see Table 17-1).

Audiometry

1. Pure-tone audiometry
   a. Sound stimulus consists of a pure (musical) tone.
   b. The louder the tone required before the patient hears it, the greater the hearing loss.
2. Speech audiometry
   a. Speech reception threshold (SRT), with masking* when appropriate
   b. Speech Discrimination Score (SDS), with masking when appropriate
   c. Acoustic impedance evaluation

* Masking is the introduction of noise into the nontested ear to aid in the elimination of assistance from the good ear (cross-hearing or interaural attenuation).

A. CHECK, (√) RIGHT, LEFT, OR BOTH, AND GIVE DURATION (Weeks, Months, Years)

	Right	Left	Both	Duration
Hearing loss?				
Ringing, roaring, or buzzing in ear?				
Fullness or pressure in ear?				
Pain or discomfort in ear?				
Itching in ear?				
Discharge or drainage from ear?				
Do you wear a hearing aid?				

B. ANSWER NO OR YES AND GIVE DATES AND DETAILS

	No	Yes	Dates and Details
Have you had dizzy spells, loss of balance or lightheadedness?			
Have you had any ear operations?			
Have you had tonsil, adenoid, or other nose or throat surgery?			
Have you consulted an ear specialist?			
Are you taking any medication?			
Are you allergic or sensitive to any drugs?			Which ones?
Have you ever taken large doses of aspirin, Anacin, Bufferin, Empirin, or quinine?			
Have you ever received antibiotic injections? (Coly-mycin, streptomycin, Kanamycin, or gentamicin?)			
Do you drink coffee and/or tea?			How much?
Do you smoke?			How much?
Have you been exposed to loud noises? (machinery, gunfire, rock music)			
Is there a history of hearing difficulties in your immediate family?			
Is your general health good?			

Figure 17-12. Status of adult hearing can be determined by a nursing history. (Goodhill V. Ear Diseases, Deafness, and Dizziness, p 99. Hagerstown, Harper & Row, 1979)

Table 17-1. Tuning Fork Tests

Ear Condition	Weber Test	Rinne Test
Normal, no hearing loss	No shifting of sounds laterally	Sound perceived longer by *air* conduction
Conductive loss	Shifting of sounds to poorer ear	Sound perceived as long or longer by *bone* conduction
Sensorineural loss	Shifting of sounds to better ear	Sound perceived longer by *air* conduction

Pure-Tone Testing—Audiometric Examination

A. Preliminary Requirements and Procedure

1. Air conduction and bone conduction pure-tone capabilities
2. A masking generator
3. A speech circuit to deliver speech materials (e.g., live voice, taped, or phonographic recording)
4. Acoustically shielded booth (soundproof)
5. Noise level controlled
6. Patient seated so that he cannot watch hand movement of audiologist during testing
7. Qualified audiologist, preferably certified in clinical competence by the American Speech and Hearing Association
8. The patient is instructed to put on earphones and to signal (1) when he hears the tone, and (2) when the tone disappears.
9. *Air conduction* is measured by applying tone directly to external auditory opening.
10. *Nerve conduction* is measured when stimulus is applied directly to the mastoid process.

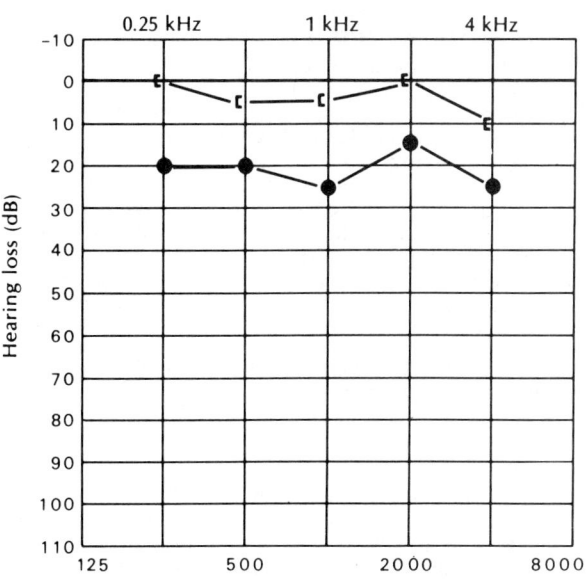

Figure 17-13. An audiogram with reduced air conduction (AC) levels (at least 15 decibels [DB] poorer than bone conduction [BC] levels) and essentially normal bone conduction levels is said to represent a *conductive hearing loss.*

AC ● —— ● unmasked RE (right ear)
BC [—— [masked RE

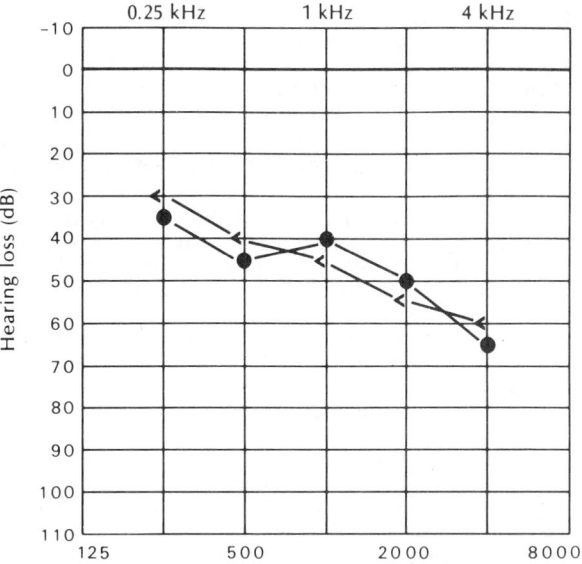

Figure 17-14. When AC = BC ± 10 db, the audiogram is reported to represent a *sensorineural hearing loss.*

AC ● —— ● unmasked RE (right ear)
BC <——< unmasked RE

B. Audiogram

1. The vertical lines represent the frequencies at which each ear is tested (25–8,000 Hz or cps) (Fig. 17-13).

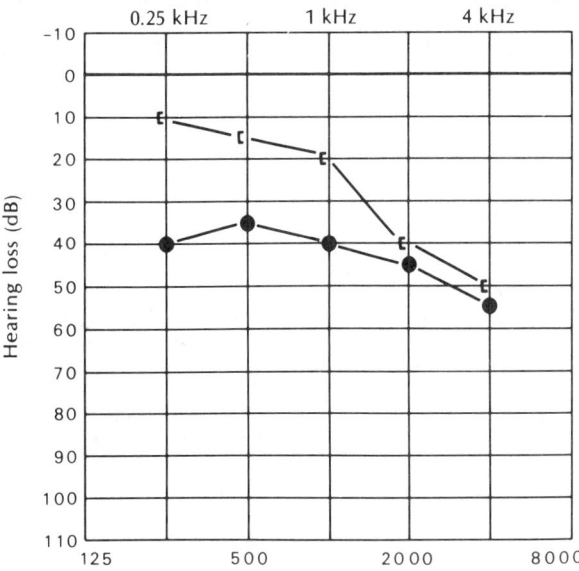

Figure 17-15. When air conduction and bone conduction levels are reduced from normal and the reduction for air conduction is greater than that for bone conduction, the audiogram is said to represent a *mixed hearing loss.*

AC ● —— ● unmasked RE
BC [—— [unmasked RE

(Figures 17-13, 17-14, 17-15: Goodhill V. Ear Diseases, Deafness, and Dizziness, pp 143–144. Hagerstown, Harper & Row, 1979)

2. The horizontal lines represent the degree of deviation from the norm in decibels.
3. Air conduction (AC) levels are plotted (obtained through pure-tone testing).
4. Bone conduction (BC) levels are plotted (obtained through vibrating oscillator placed in back of ear).

C. Examples of Impairment on an Audiogram

1. *Conductive hearing loss*
   A problem in the outer and middle ear may result in reduced sensitivity to tones received by air conduction. If the inner ear is unimpaired, bone conduction will be within normal range (see Fig. 17-13).
2. *Sensorineural hearing loss*
   A weakening of sound produced in some portion of the sensorineural mechanism (e.g., inner ear) results in reduced thresholds for air conduction. Usually it also causes a reduction in bone conduction (Fig. 17-14).
3. *Mixed hearing loss*
   As mentioned above, weakening of sound in some portion of the sensorineural mechanism results in reduced bone conduction and air conduction. When there is also a lesion in the external auditory canal or middle ear, there will be additional weakening in thresholds for air conduction (Fig. 17-15).

D. Evaluation

1. Normal human ear perception—20 cycles per second (cps) or 20 Herz (Hz) to 20,000.
2. Frequencies significant for speech range—500 to 2000 Hz.

Speech Audiometry

A. Speech Reception Threshold (SRT)

This is the softest hearing threshold level at which a person can correctly repeat approximately 50% of very familiar two-syllable words. This is not a test for discrimination but does provide a gross estimate of the patient's ability to recognize and respond to speech.

B. Speech Discrimination Score (SDS)

1. This is a supra-threshold measure of speech discrimination.
2. The tester presents phonetically balanced monosyllabic words, which the patient is asked to repeat. The percentage of correct responses is the SDS.

C. Acoustic Impedance Evaluation

1. An objective measurement (does not require direct patient response) relating to the function of the peripheral auditory mechanism:
   a. Tympanic membrane mobility
   b. Middle ear pressure
   c. Eustachian tube function
   d. Continuity and compliance of ossicular chain
   e. Abnormalities or functional hearing loss
2. The battery of acoustic impedance testing includes:
   a. Measurement of acoustic impedance (static compliance), hindrance, or resistance to passage of sound
   b. Tympanometry
   c. Measurement of acoustic reflex threshold

Hearing Impairment

Presbycusis

A progressive bilaterally symmetrical perceptive loss of hearing in the older individual that occurs with the aging process.

Treatment

There is no effective medical or surgical treatment.

Nursing Management

1. Hearing aids are usually unnecessary and may only serve to confuse and upset the patient. When indicated, the patient should be advised by an otologist in collaboration with an audiologist.
2. Helpful aids should be considered, such as a telephone amplifier, radio and television earphone attachments, buzzers instead of a door bell.
3. Understanding and help from family members is important.
4. "Cupping" the hand in back of the ear may help funnel sound toward the ear canal. See also Communicating with a Person who has Hearing Impairment (below).

Communicating With a Person Who Has a Hearing Impairment

(See Table 17-2, Degree of Hearing Loss and Relationship to Communicative Sequelae)

When the Person Is Able to Lip-Read

1. Face the person as directly as possible when speaking.
2. Place yourself in good light so that he can see your mouth.
3. Do not chew, smoke, or have anything in your mouth when speaking.
4. Speak slowly and enunciate distinctly.
5. Provide contextual clues that will assist him in following your speech. For example, point to a tray if you are talking about the food on it.
6. To verify that he understands your message, write it for him to read. (That is, if you doubt that he is understanding you.)

When It Is Difficult to Understand the Person When He Speaks

1. Pay attention when the person speaks; his facial and physical gestures may help you understand what he is saying.
2. Exchange conversation with him where it is possible to anticipate his replies—this is particularly helpful in your initial contact with him and may help you become familiar with his speech peculiarities.
3. Anticipate context of his speech to assist in interpreting what he is saying.
4. If unable to understand him, resort to writing or include in your conversation someone who does understand him; request that he repeat that which is not understood.

Table 17-2. Degree of Hearing Loss and Relationship to Communicative Sequelae

Pure-tone Average of the Better Ear	Effect of Hearing Loss on Communicative Skills	Aural Rehabilitation Requirements
27 to 40 db* (slight)	May only have difficulty with hearing faint speech	May benefit from a hearing aid when loss approaches 40 db Needs preferential seating and lighting May need lip-reading instructions
41 to 44 db (mild)	Understands conversational speech when face to face May miss as much as 50 per cent if voices are faint May exhibit anomalies in language and speech	Individual hearing aid evaluation and training in its use Needs preferential seating Attention to language skills Lip-reading instruction Speech conservation and correction Child should be referred to special education
56 to 70 db (marked)	Will only understand loud conversation Is likely to have defective speech Child is likely to be deficient in language usage and comprehension Will have limited vocabulary	Individual hearing aid evaluation and auditory training Lip-reading instruction Speech conservation and correction Special help in language development Child should be referred to special education
71 or more db (severe)	Will hear only very loud voices May be able to identify some loud environment sounds May be able to discriminate vowels but not all consonants Relies on vision rather than hearing as primary avenue for communication Speech and language defective and likely to deteriorate	Individual hearing aid evaluation Auditory training Child should be referred to full-time special program for deaf children with emphasis on all language skills, concept development, lip-reading and speech Continuous appraisal of needs in regard to oral and manual communication

* All decibel ranges according to American National Standards Institute, 1969 norm.

Harrison RJ. Current concepts in the management of hearing loss. Reprinted from January, 1979 issue of American Family Physician, published by the American Academy of Family Physicians.

Problems Affecting the External Ear

Otitis Externa

Otitis externa is an infection of the external ear canal that may occur 2–3 days after swimming and diving (swimmer's ear).

A. Prevention

1. Prevent or minimize by drying the ear canals after diving.
2. Shaking the head vigorously or jumping with head tilted to one side may be effective in removing trapped water in ear canal.
3. Fanning the ear may have a drying effect; a hair dryer held at a comfortable distance from the ear may be helpful.

▶ **NURSING ALERT:** Use of cotton-tipped applicators to dry the canal or remove ear wax should be avoided because:
a. Cerumen may be forced against tympanic membrane.
b. The canal lining may be abraded, making it more susceptible to infection.
c. Cerumen that coats and protects the canal may be removed.

4. Use of ear drops after swimming will assist in preventing swimmer's ear. Usually these medications contain several ingredients:
   a. Alcohol and glycerol to reduce moisture.
   b. Boric acid or acetic acid (vinegar) to limit growth of microorganisms and maintain normal acidity of the ear canal.

B. Treatment

1. Alcohol (dries moisture), acetic acid (restores acidity), and antibiotics (curb infection).
2. If canal is swollen and tender, insert cotton wick soaked with Burow's solution (aluminum acetate solution); wick is kept saturated until swelling recedes, usually in 24–48 hours.
3. When pain and swelling have subsided, a specially trained person can remove debris from ear canal.

Cerumen in Ear Canal

1. Accumulated cerumen (earwax) does not have to be removed unless it becomes impacted and interferes with hearing.
2. To irrigate ear canal, see Guidelines, below.

Foreign Bodies in External Canal

1. Inserted by young children or handicapped persons.
2. Insects
   Treat by instilling oil drops to smother insect, which then will float out.
3. Vegetable foreign bodies (peas)
   a. Irrigation is contraindicated because vegetable matter absorbs water, which would further wedge foreign body in ear canal.
   b. Unskilled persons should not attempt to remove a foreign body because:
      (1) It may be forced into bony portion of the canal.
      (2) The canal skin may be perforated.
      (3) The eardrum may be perforated.
   c. Removal should be done skillfully with instruments; if the victim is very young, general anesthesia is required.

Auricle Cancer

1. This is the most common (70%) ear malignancy; helix and postauricular regions are primary sites.

2. Basal cell cancer (40%) and malignant melanoma (30%) are the most common types.
3. Four fifths of all patients are male.

Management

Local excision and possibly radiation and/or chemotherapy.

Guidelines: Irrigating the External Auditory Canal

Purposes
1. To remove discharge from the canal.
2. To facilitate removal of cerumen or foreign bodies.
3. To apply heat to the tissues of the ear canal.

▶ **NURSING ALERT:** Ask the patient if he has a history of draining ears, or if he has ever had a perforation or other complications from a previous ear irrigation. If the reply is affirmative, check with the physician before proceeding with the irrigation.

Equipment and Solutions

Kind and amount of solution desired
Tray containing:
  Protective towels
  Cotton balls and cotton applicators
  Solution bowl and emesis basin
  Ear syringe or irrigating container with tubing, clamp, and irrigating catheter
  Paper bag for disposable cotton

Procedure

Preparatory Phase
1. After explaining procedure to the patient, place him in appropriate position (i.e., sitting or lying with head tilted toward affected ear).
2. Position protective toweling.

Nursing Action	Rationale/Amplification
Performance Phase	
1. Use a cotton applicator to remove any discharge on outer ear.	1. To prevent carrying discharge deeper into canal.
2. Place emesis basin close to the patient's head and under the ear.	2. To provide a receptable to receive irrigating solution.
3. Test temperature of solution by allowing some to run on inner aspect of wrist. Should be 35° to 40.6°C (95°–105°F.).	3. More comfortable for the patient; solutions that are hot or cold are most uncomfortable and may initiate a feeling of dizziness.
4. Ascertain whether impaction is due to a foreign hygroscopic (attracts or absorbs moisture) body before proceeding.	4. If water contacts such a substance, it may cause it to swell and produce intense pain.
5. Gently pull the outer ear upward and backward (adult); downward and backward (child).	5. To straighten ear canal.
6. Place tip of syringe or irrigating catheter at opening of ear; gently direct stream of fluid against sides of canal (Fig. 17-16).	6. To permit direction for inflow and outflow; if stream is directed forcefully against eardrum, it is possible to rupture it.
7. If an irrigating container is used, elevate not more than 15 cm. (6 inches).	7. To provide safe and effective pressure of fluid; if height is more than 6 inches, pressure will be too great and may damage tissue.
8. Observe for signs of pain or dizziness.	8. If they occur, discontinue treatment.
9. If irrigating does not dislodge the wax, instill several drops of glycerin, Debrox, or saturated solution of sodium bicarbonate, 2–3 times daily for 2–3 days.	9. To soften and loosen impaction.

Follow-Up Phase
1. Dry external ear with cotton pledgets.
2. Remove soiled towels, etc. and make the patient comfortable.
3. Record: Time of irrigation, kind and amount of solution used, nature of return flow, effect of treatment.

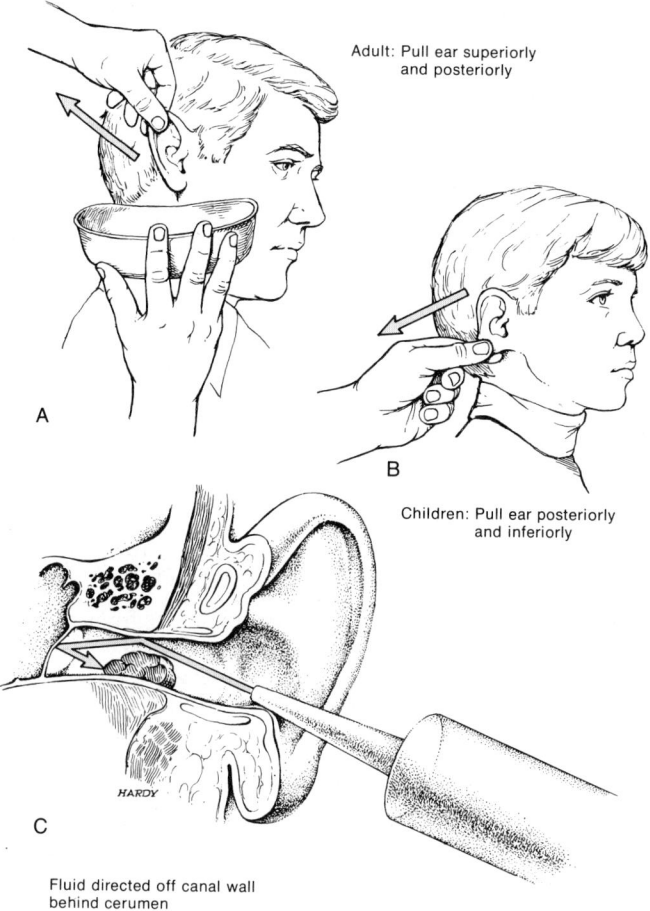

Adult: Pull ear superiorly
and posteriorly

A

B

Children: Pull ear posteriorly
and inferiorly

HARDY

C

Fluid directed off canal wall
behind cerumen

Figure 17-16. Ear irrigation. (*A*) The external auditory canal in the adult can best be exposed by pulling the earlobe upward and backward. (*B*) The same exposure can be achieved in the child by gently pulling the auricle of the ear downward and backward. (*C*) An enlarged diagram showing the direction of irrigating fluid against the side of the canal. NOTE: This is more effective in dislodging cerumen than if the flow of solution were directed straight into the canal.

Acute Otitis Media

Acute otitis media is an inflammation of the middle ear caused by the entrance of pathogenic organisms. Normally the middle ear is sterile in its environs.

Etiology

Hemolytic streptococcus, pneumococcus, staphylococcus, influenza bacillus.

Mode of Entry

1. Auditory canal—if drum is perforated.
2. Eustachian tube—during indiscriminate use of nasal drops or nasal douching, or as a result of forcibly sneezing or blowing the nose.
3. Rarely, following a fracture of the skull.

Assessment

Clinical Manifestations

1. Variable—may be mild or severe.
2. Pain is usually the first symptom—may be in and about the ear and may be intense.

May be relieved by spontaneous perforation of the drum or by myringotomy.

3. Fever—may be caused by a virus; in some patients, temperature may rise to 40.0°–40.6°C. (104°–105°F.).
4. Headache, difficulty hearing, ear and head noises, anorexia, nausea, and vomiting.

Diagnostic Evaluation

1. Nursing history may reveal the cause as upper respiratory infection, immunologic defect, head injury (fractured skull).
2. Pneumatic otoscopy (using a properly sealed otoscope)—the rubber bulb, when compressed, causes a normal tympanic membrane to flap in and out (total excursion 1–2 mm.).
   In otitis media, the membrane often moves inward to a greater extent than it moves outward.
3. Tympanometry—measures tympanic membrane mobility.
4. Cultures of discharge may suggest causative organism.

Patient Problems/Nursing Diagnoses

1. Pain and discomfort, possibly dizziness, related to inflammation of the mucous lining of the middle ear
2. Alteration in auditory sensory perception related to disease (infection) and hearing loss
3. Knowledge deficit related to preventive measures and treatment

Planning and Implementation
Treatment

1. Varies with virulence of bacteria, efficiency of therapy, and resistance of the patient.
2. Usually the drug of choice is penicillin; it may be necessary to employ wide-spectrum antibiotic therapy.
3. Some believe the most effective therapy is to administer decongestants along with self-inflation of the ear by the Valsalva maneuver.
   a. This is accomplished by having the patient try to exhale forcefully while holding his nose and mouth tightly—this forces air along the auditory canal into middle ear.
   b. When successful, the patient will experience a "pop" and an immediate (perhaps temporary) improvement.
   c. It should be performed 10–12 times daily.
4. Myringotomy may be required.
   Myringotomy—an incision made into the posterior inferior aspect of the tympanic membrane for draining purposes (to relieve pressure and drain pus from middle ear infection).
   a. The incision heals rapidly.
   b. Hearing is not adversely affected.
   c. This procedure is done less frequently now because antimicrobial therapy usually makes it unnecessary. However, it may be done because of failure to respond to antimicrobial therapy, for severe persistent pain, and for persistent conductive hearing loss.

Nursing Interventions

A. Relief of pain and pressure; preventing infection from spreading

1. Apply heat (moist or dry) to promote comfort and drainage.
2. Administer aspirin and other analgesics as prescribed. (Sedation is usually avoided because it may interfere with early detection of intracranial complications.)
3. Give penicillin/derivatives, or broad-spectrum antibiotics as prescribed; if the patient is allergic to penicillin, erythromycin may be the substitute. Be sure that the patient takes the medication on time and for the full time of therapy even though symptoms have disappeared.

▶ **NURSING ALERT:**
1. With wide-spectrum antibiotic therapy, acute otitis media may become subacute with continued purulent discharge.
2. Healing may take place, but the patient may be left with a residual deafness.
3. Recognize that symptoms such as headache, slow pulse, vomiting, and vertigo are significant and should be reported.
4. Secondary complications may involve the mastoid or even the brain, producing meningitis or brain abscess.

4. Administer decongestants (preferred by some physicians) along with inflation of the middle ear (Valsalva maneuver).
5. Prepare perioperative care plan if the patient is scheduled to have surgical treatment.

B. Safety measures to prevent falling if dizziness occurs

1. Utilize side rails when the patient is in bed.
2. Instruct the patient to call for assistance when getting out of bed or walking.
3. Tell the patient to move from one position to another slowly in order not to aggravate vertigo.

C. Pre- and postoperative care for patient undergoing myringotomy

1. Provide emotional support.
2. Keep the patient informed of the "next step" and how he can help.
3. Remind the patient not to touch ear or drainage because of its infectious nature.
4. Protect skin near the draining orifice with petrolatum.
5. Observe drainage and vital signs for possible evidence of bleeding.
6. Describe activities that are to be avoided until tympanic membrane heals (swimming, shampooing hair, showering).

Evaluation
Expected Outcomes

1. Remains free from any discomfort in the area of the ear—discomfort, pain, dizziness
2. Responds normally to sound and shows normal audiometric readings
3. Indicates hygienic practices that he is now aware of to prevent reinfection (ear-picking, inserting toothpick in ear to relieve itch, etc.)

Chronic Otitis Media and Mastoiditis

Chronic otitis media occurs as a result of repeated bouts of otitis media that cause inflammation and may lead to perforation of the eardrum. This condition often begins in childhood and continues into adult life.

Causes

1. A strain of organism that is resistant to the antibiotic used
2. A particularly virulent strain of organism

Altered Physiology

1. Marginal perforation of drum membrane
2. Presence of cholesteatoma (soft ball of dead skin) that erodes vital structures
   a. Caused by an ingrowth of skin from the perforated drum
   b. Fills area in the mastoid and middle ear; bacterial infection frequently develops

c. May encroach upon vital structures—facial nerve, labyrinth, and brain

3. If untreated, infection may spread to cause labyrinthitis, mastoiditis, and meningitis; end result is impaired hearing.

Clinical Manifestations

Symptoms are minimal: mild hearing loss, otorrhea (foul-smelling discharge); pain frequently means a CNS complication has occurred.

Diagnostic Evaluation

1. Nursing history will indicate several episodes of acute otitis media; possible rupture of tympanic membrane
2. Presence of above symptoms
3. X-rays to note mastoid pathology
4. Pneumatic otoscopy, tuning fork testing, audiometry
5. Audiometric test will possibly suggest air conduction hearing loss

Treatment

Goals:
Eradicate the disease.
Improve hearing.

A. Medical Therapy

1. Antibiotic and steroid eardrops may control infection and inflammation.
2. Frequent removal of epithelial debris and purulent drainage.
3. If advanced chronic ear disease is left untreated, inner-ear and life-threatening CNS complications may develop because of erosion of surrounding structures.

B. Surgery

1. Indicated when cholesteatoma is present.
2. Indicated when there is pain or complications—profound deafness, dizziness, sudden facial paralysis, stiff neck (may lead to meningitis or brain abscess).
3. *Simple mastoidectomy*—removal of mastoid cells—indicated when there is persistent tenderness, fever, discharge from ear, or headache.
4. *Radical mastoidectomy*—removal of all diseased tissue from mastoid area and middle ear.

5. *Posteroanterior mastoidectomy*—combines simple mastoidectomy with tympanoplasty.

Perioperative Nursing Interventions

1. Shaving depends on nature of the incision.
   a. Postaural (incision behind the ear)—clip hair and shave scalp for 3–4 cm. around ear (only if desired by surgeon).
   b. Endaural (incision through the ear canal)—shave is unnecessary.
2. Provide for relief of pain preoperatively.
   a. Give aspirin or codeine sulfate.
   b. Apply ice cap to area.
3. Postoperatively, administer sedatives for pain and restlessness.
4. Assist with dressing change since area is packed with gauze for drainage; this may be done daily or every other day—packing is removed on 3rd or 4th day.
5. Observe for possible complications:
   a. Facial paralysis may be indicative of facial nerve injury.
      (1) Immobility on side of face affected
      (2) Eye cannot close, mouth droops
      (3) Patient unable to whistle
      (4) Patient unable to drink without dripping from mouth
      (5) When the patient speaks or smiles, immobility of affected side is noticeable.
      (6) Administer cortisone preparation as prescribed to assist in restoration of nerve function. (Not used if paralysis is caused surgically.)
   b. Infection
      (1) Observe for clinical signs of inflammation.
      (2) Administer antibiotics.
   c. Vertigo—may be apparent following radical mastoidectomy due to inner ear disturbance.
   d. Spread of infection to brain.
      Unusual rise in temperature, chills, stiff neck, nausea and vomiting.
6. Note status of hearing.
   a. If stapes has been removed or dislodged, then hearing is lost.
   b. If stapes or cochlea have not been removed or disturbed, then hearing is regained; a hearing aid may be required.

Perforation of Eardrum

Etiology and Altered Physiology

1. Infection is the most frequent cause of permanent perforation of the tympanic membrane; often this is due to acute or chronic suppurative otitis media.
2. Trauma is the next cause of permanent perforation; may be due to:
   a. A severe blow on the ear
   b. Blast effect of high explosives
   c. Foreign objects
   d. Force of a stream of water
   e. Burns of face and head
   f. Postmyringotomy defects

Treatment

A. Medical

1. Most accidental perforations of the eardrum heal spontaneously.

2. Cauterization of the perforation with trichloroacetic acid at frequent intervals and application of a prosthesis will produce a healed membrane with scar tissue.

B. Surgical

Tympanoplasty, type I—myringoplasty—(simple patching of drum).

Tympanoplasty

Tympanoplasty is a reconstructive operation on the diseased or deformed components of the middle ear.

Goal:
Improve or preserve the conductive mechanisms in an effort to salvage or improve hearing.
Impetus for tympanoplasty has been aided by:

a. Illuminated binocular microscope
b. Use of antibiotics to prevent or control infection

Physiological Principles of Hearing

Why an intact drum is needed to hear:
1. Sound waves are transformed from airborne vibrations to mechanical stimulation of endolymphatic lymph; this is accomplished by the conductive ability of the eardrum and ossicles.
2. The ratio of the small oval window to the large tympanic membrane is 1:22; this, combined with the vibratory action of the ossicles, means a great increase in force from the air to the inner ear fluids.
3. When there is a disturbance in the above relationships, the result is a loss of hearing.
4. From the oval window, bordered by the annular ligament, impulses are received by the stapes footplate from the incus, malleus, and drum membrane.
5. A lag phase is normal after sound waves stimulate the oval window and before the final effect of the stimulus reaches the round window.

Altered Physiology

1. When there is a perforation of the eardrum, the lag phase (described above) disappears, with the result that sound waves hit the oval and round windows at the same time, causing diminished effect of labyrinth fluid motility → lessened stimulation of hair cells in the organ of Corti → diminished hearing.
2. Infections often produce fibrosis or necrosis of all or part of the ossicular chain.
3. Granuloma, polyps, and fibrous or bony plaques may resist normal function of the oval and round windows.
4. In addition to sequelae from otitis media, otosclerosis may exist.
5. Obstruction of tympanic orifice of the eustachian tube may produce dysfunction.

Types of Tympanoplasty (Table 17-3)

A. Type I (Myringoplasty)

1. *Purpose*—to close perforation by placing a graft over it in order to create a closed middle ear section, which in turn will improve hearing.
2. *Indications*—to avoid risk of contamination when the patient bathes, swims, or dives—this in turn prevents recurrence of chronic otitis media or mastoiditis.

3. *Contraindications*
   a. Ossicular involvement—prediction of surgical results can be made preoperatively by testing for improvement of hearing levels by placing a temporary patch over the defect. If no improvement is noticed in audiometric testing, the ossicular chain may be involved.
   b. Presence of active infection
   c. Presence of chronic middle ear infection, impairing or preventing drainage via eustachian tube
   d. Sinusitis or allergy that produces a chronic infectious discharge via nasopharynx
   e. History of acute exacerbations of otitis media
4. *Surgical repair*
   Perforation is closed using one of the following:
   a. Fascia from temporal muscle (in almost all cases)
   b. Vein grafts from hand or forearm (occasionally)
   c. Notify physician of any dizziness; medication will be prescribed as needed for vertigo and nausea.
   d. Caution the patient not to blow his nose with force and to avoid wetting dressings during bathing.
   e. Note that hearing improvement is achieved in inverse proportion to the amount of surgery required; the simpler the surgery, the better the chance for hearing to improve.
5. *Postoperative management*
   a. Administer antibiotics for several days postoperatively to ensure freedom from infection.
   b. Reinforce external dressings if they become soiled; otherwise leave dressings intact.
   c. Remove gauze packing in canal at end of week; do not apply suction or probe canal.
   d. Gentle capillary suction may be attempted by end of 2nd week to remove debris and crusts (Gelfoam remains).
   e. Do not use ear drops, because of danger of loosening graft.
   f. Dust lightly with antibiotic powder (Neosporin).

Health Education

A. General

1. Avoid shampooing or showering, which could cause contamination of ear canal, until permission is obtained from physician.

Table 17-3. **Types of Tympanoplasty**

Type	Middle Ear Damage		Repair Process
	Tympanic Membrane	Ossicles	
I	Perforated	Normal	Close–perforation–myringoplasty
II	Perforated	Erosion of malleus and/or incus	Close perforation; graft against incus or whatever remains of malleus
III	Tympanic membrane destroyed or widely perforated	Rest of ossicular chain destroyed BUT stapes are intact and mobile	Grafts implanted to contact the normal stapes Tympanostapedopexy
IV	Tympanic membrane destroyed or widely perforated	Ossicular chain destroyed. Head, neck, and crura of stapes destroyed. Stapes footplate mobile	Expose mobile stapes footplate—graft implanted. Air pocket between graft and round window provides protection The Cavum minor operation
V	Tympanic membrane destroyed or widely perforated	Ossicular chain destroyed. Head, neck, and crura of stapes destroyed. Stapes footplate fixed	Make opening in horizontal semicircular canal; graft seals off middle ear to give sound protection for round window Tympanoplasty and fenestration of lateral semi-circular canal

2. Continue with antibiotics beyond first week if there is evidence of infection.
3. Use antihistamine with an ephedrine derivative for at least 1 month postoperatively.
4. Continue using an antihistamine if the patient experiences rhinologic allergy.

B. Types II to V

1. *Purpose* (see Table 17-3). These procedures are modifications used to correct various middle ear problems.
2. *Preoperative and operative treatment*
   a. Topical and systemic antibiotics are administered when infection is present.
   b. Suitable replacement (polyethylene, stainless steel wire, bone, cartilage) is used to maintain continuity of conduction sound pathway.
   c. The necessity of a 2-stage procedure should be determined.
      (1) First stage—eradication of all diseased tissues; area is cleaned out to achieve a dry, healed middle ear.
      (2) Second stage—(performed 2–3 months after 1st stage) reconstruction, using grafts.
3. *Postoperative nursing management*
   a. Reinforce outer dressings as necessary but keep inner dressings intact.
   b. Assist the patient in getting out of bed for the first time because he may become dizzy.

Otosclerosis

Otosclerosis is a form of deafness caused by the formation of new spongy bone in the labyrinth, fixation of the stapes, and prevention of sound transmission through the ossicles to the inner fluids.

Incidence

1. Cause is unknown
2. Occurs more commonly in women than men; rare in the black race
3. Has a hereditary basis

Clinical Manifestations

1. Patient presents a history of slow, progressive hearing loss with no middle ear infection.
2. A frequent complaint is buzzing or ringing noises in the ears; both ears are usually affected equally.

Diagnostic Evaluation

1. Nursing history reveals gradual hearing loss.
2. Audiometry findings substantiate hearing loss.
3. Bone conduction is much better than air conduction.
4. Reduced tuning fork transmission by air, whereas there is intensification of bone conduction sound when tuning fork handle is placed over the mastoid bone.

Treatment

Goal:

Restore hearing and minimize hearing loss.

1. No known medical treatment for this form of deafness, but amplification with a hearing aid may be helpful.
2. Surgical treatment—stapedectomy

Stapedectomy

A *stapedectomy* involves removal of otosclerotic lesions at the footplate of stapes and the creation of a tissue implant with prosthesis to maintain suitable conduction. To perform such delicate surgery, the otologic binocular microscope is used.

Types of Prostheses

1. Steel wire and fat implant
2. Gelfoam and stainless steel wire
3. Metal or Teflon "piston"
4. Vein graft and polyethylene tubing (least frequent)

Preoperative and Postoperative Management

1. Observe for unusual symptoms, such as:
   a. Fever—may indicate infection, external otitis, otitis media
   b. Headache—may indicate infection, nerve encroachment
   c. Vertigo—may indicate labyrinthitis or inner ear reaction
   d. Ear pain—may indicate infection or irritation of auditory nerve
2. Position the patient postoperatively as desired by physician.
   a. Some surgeons prefer that the patient be positioned with operated ear uppermost to maintain position of graft and stability.
   b. Others prefer that the patient be lying on operated ear to permit drainage.
   c. Still others advocate that the patient assume the most comfortable position.
3. Administer antimotion medications and sedatives if the patient experiences vertigo, nystagmus, or nausea.
4. Assist the patient when he first tries to walk; he may feel dizzy for the first few days.
5. Instruct the patient not to blow his nose for a week; air may be forced up the auditory canal and disturb the operative site.
6. Encourage a restricted head position if the surgeon fears a misplacement of the prosthesis.
7. Replace soiled (bloody) cotton pledget in ear canal as necessary.
8. Administer meperidine or prescribed pain medication for first several hours.

Health Education

1. Advise the patient that it may be weeks before full effect of surgery is determined as far as hearing is concerned. At first, hearing may be impaired because of tissue edema, packing, etc.
2. Instruct the patient as follows:
   a. Do not smoke.
   b. Do not blow nose.
   c. Protect ears when going outdoors for the first week.
   d. Avoid crowds or exposure to colds so that upper respiratory infection is prevented.

Ménière's Disease (Endolymphatic Hydrops)

Ménière's disease involves the inner ear and causes a triad of symptoms: vertigo, hearing loss, and tinnitus.

Etiology

1. Ménière's disease stems from labyrinthine dysfunction.
2. Suggested theories of the cause of this syndrome:
   a. Increase in pressure of endolymph
   b. Emotional or endocrine disturbance
   c. Vasomotor changes causing a spasm of the internal auditory artery
   d. Allergic manifestation
   e. Adrenal pituitary insufficiency
   f. Congenital or acquired syphilis

Clinical Manifestations

A. During Attack

1. Dizziness, tinnitus, and reduced hearing occur on involved side.
2. The patient complains somewhat of headache, nausea, vomiting, incoordination.
3. Sudden attacks occur in which patient complains that room appears to spin around.
4. Sudden motion of the head may precipitate vomiting.
5. The patient often presents a history of ear trouble, vasomotor rhinitis, and allergies.
6. The most comfortable position for the patient is lying down.
7. Personality changes manifest themselves in irritability, depression, withdrawal, and refusal to eat.
8. Vertigo attacks may last several hours or all day.

B. After or Between Attacks

1. Patient behaves normally; may continue his work.
2. Only complaint may be tinnitus or impaired hearing.

Diagnostic Evaluation

1. Audiogram for pure tones and speech discrimination.
2. Caloric test/electronystagmography
   a. Useful in differentiating Ménière's syndrome from intracranial lesion.
   b. Fluid, which is above or below body temperature, is instilled into auditory canal.
   c. Reactions
      (1) Normal patient—complains of dizziness
      (2) The patient with acoustic neuroma—no reaction
      (3) The patient with Ménière's syndrome—severe attack (as described above)
   d. Nursing management
      (1) Anticipate possibility of the patient vomiting; have emesis basin and protective draping.
      (2) Support the patient as he walks after the test, since he may be dizzy.
3. Thyroid function tests, allergy history, and glucose tolerance tests are other diagnostic aids.

Medical Management

Goal:
1. Decrease or eliminate the occurrence of vertigo attacks.
2. Preserve hearing.

Conservative management has included:
1. Psychotherapy, allergic hyposensitization, diuretics, low-sodium diet, antihistamines, vasodilators, steroids

2. Administration of "vertigo sedatives" such as dimenhydrinate, meclizine, droperidol, fentanyl, diazepam
3. Diuretics to reduce fluids; antiemetics to reduce nausea, vomiting, and vertigo
4. Administration of aminoglycosides, gentamicin sulfate may control vertigo in many patients

Surgical Management

1. Conservative
   a. Simple sac decompression, vascular and muscular grafts to the sac, sac "shunts," sac obliteration (all conservative procedures but widely used).
   b. Ultrasound—semicircular canal reached through a mastoid incision; ultrasonic energy applied directly via a probe to the bone in the canal (may cause transient facial paralysis).
2. Destructive surgery
   a. Labyrinthectomy—recommended if the patient experiences progressive hearing loss and severe vertigo attacks so that he cannot perform normal tasks.
   b. Vestibular nerve section—neurosurgical suboccipital approach to the cerebellopontine angle for intracranial vestibular nerve neurectomy.
   c. Translabyrinthine or middle cranial fossa approach to Scarpa's ganglion.

Nursing Interventions

A. Protective Measures

1. Protect the patient who has an attack by placing him in a bed with side rails in position; if he is standing, help lower him to the floor to avoid injury.
2. Postoperatively, the patient may experience vertigo; therefore, he may be more comfortable in bed for the first 2 days.
3. Assist the patient when he gets out of bed since he may be unsteady; remind him to change his movements easily.
4. Provide a call bell for the patient should he need assistance; help him to recognize aura so that he has time to prepare for an attack.

B. Comfort Measures

1. Recognize the need for encouragement and understanding; this is particularly true when the patient experiences symptoms of a subjective nature.
2. Remind the patient to slow down his bodily movements since jerking or making sudden movement may precipitate an attack.
3. Provide a low-sodium diet and reduced fluid intake to reduce edema and the production of endolymphatic fluid.
4. Avoid noises and glaring, bright lights, which may initiate an attack.
5. Suggest pleasant, distracting sounds such as radio music to overcome tinnitus.

Health Education

1. Eliminate smoking and the intake of coffee, tea, alcohol, stimulating drugs.
2. Control environmental factors and personal habits that may cause stress or fatigue.

3. If there is a tendency to allergic reactions to foods, eliminate those that aggravate these responses (e.g., milk, eggs, chocolate, corn, pork, nuts).
4. Adhere to periodic use of diuretics, as prescribed, to relieve feeling of fullness in the ear, vertigo, and tinnitus.

5. Inform the patient that dizziness may persist as long as 4–6 weeks.
6. Note that a possible complication is Bell's palsy (a peripheral facial weakness with noticeable pain near the angle of the jaw or behind the ear (see p. 774) This will clear up eventually.

Cochlear Implant

Cochlear implant is a device that emits auditory signals for profoundly deaf individuals. The single-electrode system bypasses the damaged system of the cochlea (transduction) and stimulates the remaining auditory nerve fibers. This results in the perception of sound.

Components of Cochlear Implant (Fig. 17-17)

1. Microphone
   a. Mounted at ear level.
   b. Sensitive to environmental sound.
   c. Converts this sound to an electric current.
   d. Electric current is transmitted to an external stimulator.
2. External stimulator
   a. The signal undergoes amplification and modulation.
   b. The signal then is transmitted to an external coil behind the ear.
3. External coil
   a. Magnetic induction through the skin generates an electric signal to the internal system.

4. Internal coil
   a. Signal moves through electrode placed in scala tympani and then through the auditory canal (temporalis muscle).
   b. This produces sensation of sound—something resembling an electrical buzz.

Patient Criteria

1. Results of audiologic test—must show average hearing sensitivity at 500, 1000, 2000 Hz to be no better than 90–100 db hearing loss in either ear.
2. If the patient performs better with hearing aid than subjects with implants, participation in program is not recommended.
3. No evidence of brain impairment, psychoses, mental retardation.
4. Reasonable expectations and optimism; motivation must be present.

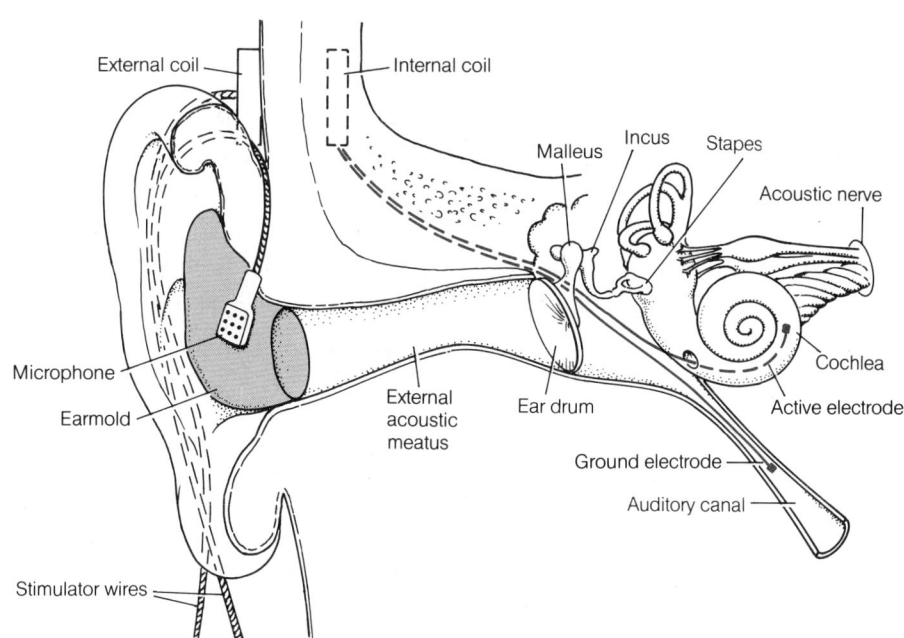

Figure 17-17. Cochlear implant.

Diagnostic Evaluation

1. General health history as well as otologic history
2. Electronystagmography, x-rays, and audiometric evaluation

Nursing Management

A. Preoperative and Intraoperative Management

1. Encourage the prospective patient to talk with one who is currently using an implant to learn the positive and negative results of a cochlear implant.
2. In addition to the usual preoperative preparation, shave a 15-cm. (3-inch) wide area around the ear.
3. Prepare the patient for general anesthesia.
4. A postauricular incision is made; using a drill, a "seat" is made in the bone to house an internal coil via a mastoidectomy.

B. Postoperative Management

1. Provide care similar to that for a postmastoidectomy patient (see p. 747).
2. Initiative rehabilitation—usually begun 2 months postsurgery.
   a. Adjustment of controls is accomplished.
   b. The patient is involved in operation and maintenance of stimulator unit.
   c. Patient learns and practices how to listen critically, and how to lip-read.
   d. Skills in item *c* must be combined with discrimination of sounds through the cochlear implant.

   Note: Understanding speech through cochlear implant is not possible with this device alone.

   e. Many individuals trained with such an implant can lip-read more easily, and can distinguish voices and environmental sounds.

Bibliography

Eye Problems

Books

Engelstein JM (ed). Cataract Surgery. New York, Grune & Stratton, 1984

Gittinger JW Jr. Ophthalmology. Boston, Little, Brown & Co, 1984

Koch DD et al. Adverse Effects of Contact Lens Wear: An Atlas for Ophthalmic Practitioners. Thorofare, NJ, Slack, 1983

Luntz MH, Harrison R and Schenker HI. Glaucoma Surgery. Baltimore, Williams & Wilkins, 1984

Mackety CJ. Perioperative Laser Nursing: A Practical Guide. Thorofare, NJ, Slack, 1984

Smith JF and Machazel DP. Ophthalmologic Nursing. Waltham, MA, Little, Brown & Co, 1980

Spoor TC (ed). Medical Management of Ocular Diseases. Thorofare, NJ, Slack, 1984

Trokel SL. YAG Laser Ophthalmic Microsurgery. Norwalk, CT, Appleton-Century-Crofts, 1983

Tuttle DW. Self-esteem and Adjusting with Blindness. Springfield, IL, Charles C Thomas, 1984

Vaughan D and Asbury T. General Ophthalmology. Los Altos, CA, Lange, 1983

Vogel TC. Managing head and neck problems (eye), pp. 18–28. In Nursing Photobook. Aiding Ambulatory Patients. Springhouse, PA, Intermed, 1983

Articles*

General

Brown GC. Retinal vascular diseases. Occup Health Nurs 1983 Aug; 31(8): 17–20

   * Note: JONT (Journal of Ophthalmology Nursing and Technology)

Fyfe J and Ellerbroek D. Colour vision defects and the school nurse. Nurs Times 1984 June 27; 80(26):48–49

Giarratana CM. Reach out . . . reach out and touch Henry. Nursing '84 1984 Feb; 14(2):47–48

Jeglum EL. Ocular therapeutics. Nurs Clin North Am 1981 Sept; 16(3):453–477

Roberts AM and Leibowitz HM. Corticosteroid therapy of ophthalmologic disease. Hosp Pract 1984 Feb; 19(2):181–196

Schneider HA and Easterlin MN. Trachoma: Ophthalmic crisis of the third world. JONT 1984 Jan/Feb; 3(1): 11–12

Smith JF. Why a single piece of advice may save your corneal transplant patient's sight. RN 1982; 45(8):66–68

Todd B. Using eye drops and ointments safely. Geriatr Nurs 1983 Jan–Feb; 4(1):53, 56–57

Assessment

Boyd-Monk H. Examining the external eye, Part 1. Nursing '80 1980 May; 10(5):58–63; Part 2. Nursing '80 1980 June; 10(8):58–63

Boyd-Monk H. How to use a direct ophthalmoscope. Occup Health Nurs 1983 Aug; 31(8):13–16

Budassi SA. Ophthalmic examinations. JEN (J Emerg Nurs) 1984 Mar/Apr; 10(2):112–114

King RC. Taking a close look at the eye. RN 1982 Feb; 45(2):49–56

Contact Lenses

Forstot SL and Ellis PP. Identifying and managing contact lens emergencies. ER Report 1982 April 5; 3(7):35–38

Horowitz TH and Kracher GP. Guidelines to observe in extended-wear lenses. JONT 1983 Aug; 2(3): 124–125

Rakow PL. Soft lens selection: The key

to success. JONT 1983 May; 2(2):89–90

Rakow PL. Using contact lenses as a tool for understanding. JONT 1983 Aug; 2(3):130–131

Rakow PL. A closer look at Septicon. JONT 1983 Nov; 2(4):182–183

Trauma

Born CP. Ocular injuries—treat or refer? Postgrad Med 1983 Feb; 73(2):311–317

Sanke RF. Blunt ocular trauma. Am Fam Physician 1984 Feb; 29(2):159–164

Tumulty G and Rester MM. Eye trauma. Am J Nurs 1984 June; 84(6):740–744

Infections

Boyd-Monk H. Conjunctivitis. Nursing '82 1982 Nov; 12(11):67

Schumann GB, Colon VF and Spinner PA. Eye cytology. Am Fam Physician 1980 Dec; 22(6):120–124

Whitman J and Cunningham RD. The red eye. Postgrad Med 1983 Nov; 74(5):65–71

Other Eye Conditions

Boyd-Monk H. A fortunate accident—Radial keratotomy. Today's OR Nurse 1984 Mar; 6(3):25–26, 31

Boyd-Monk H. Retinal detachment and vitrectomy. Nurs Clin North Am 1981 Sept; 16(3):433–451

Brown GC. Retinal vascular diseases. Occup Health Nurs 1983 Aug; 31(8): 17–20

Callahan A, Monheit GD and Callahan MA. Cancer excision from eyelids and ocular adnexa: The Mohs fresh tissue technique and reconstruction. CA 1982 Nov/Dec; 32(6):322–329

Hayes PL. Treatment and nursing care of corneal disease. Nurs Clin North Am 1981 Sept; 16(3):38–39

Laibovitz RA. The vitreous and vitreous

floaters. Postgrad Med April; 75(5):64–67

MacFadyen JS. Caring for the patient with a primary retinal detachment. Am J Nurs 1980 May; 80(5):920–921

Marta M. A guide to the posterior vitrectomy. Today's OR Nurse 1983 Mar; 5(1):26–29, 69

Shock D. Ischemic optic neuropathy. Postgrad Med 1983 Dec; 74(6):74–75

Whitton S. Penetrating keratoplasty—the gift of sight. Today's OR Nurse 1983 Mar; 5(1):20–22, 24, 72

Cataract

Allopurinol suspected of causing cataracts. Am J Nurs 1983 April 83(4):590

Burlew JA. The art of nursing a patient through the cataract experience. JONT 1983 Feb; 2(1):15–17

Cataract surgery. Nursing '83 1983 April; 13(4):65–69

Fraunfelder F et al. Cataracts associated with allopurinol therapy. Am J Ophthalmol 1982 Aug; 94(2):137–140

Hussey LCT. Intraocular lens implant. AORN J 1984 Apr; 39(5):880–891

Intraocular lens implantation for cataracts. Med Lett Drugs Ther 1982 Nov 12; 24(622):102

McCoy K. Cataracts and intraocular lenses: From cloudy to clear. Nurs Clin North Am 1981 Sept; 16(3):405–414

Melamed MA. Cataracts: Recognition and assessment. Hosp Med 1982 July; 18(7):73–82

Recommendations made for lens implant use. AORN J 1980 Jan; 31(1):33

Seale D. Intraocular injectable miotics. JONT 1983 Aug; 2(3):118–119

Smith JF. The patient having cataract surgery. JONT 1984 May/June; 3(3):124–126

Zack PL and Smirnow IH. IOL implantation. Today's OR Nurse. 1983 Mar; 5(1):12–16, 18, 68–69

Glaucoma

Bensinger RE. Precautions in dilating pupils. JONT 1984 Jan/Feb; 3(1):19–21

Easterline MN and Schneider HA. Acute angle closure glaucoma following surgery. AORN J 1984 May; 39(6):992–995

Glaucoma: Preventing diagnostic misses. Patient Care 1984 Sept 15; 18(15):16–51

Jindra LF. Closed-angle glaucoma: Diagnosis and management. Hosp Pract 1984 Mar; 19(3):114–119

Katz IM and Soll DB. Beta blockers and glaucoma. Am Fam Physician 1980 Apr; 21(4):150–151

Kilroy JL. Care and teaching of patients with glaucoma. Nurs Clin North Am 1981 Sept; 16(3):393–404

Laser trabeculoplasty for open-angle glaucoma. Med Lett Drugs Ther 1984 May 25; 26(662):52–53

McKenny M. Special tests (glaucoma), pp. 48–55. In Nursing Photobook. Carrying Out Special Procedures. Springhouse, PA, Intermed, 1983

Resler MM and Tumulty G. Glaucoma update. Am J Nurs 1983 May; 83(5):752–756

Vision Loss/Blindness

Blank HR. Sexuality in the blind. Med Aspects Human Sexuality 1982 June; 16(6):137–140

Margo C and Brown B. Adjustment to visual loss. JAMA 1982 Sept 10; 248(10):1231–1232

Stern EJ. Helping the person with low vision. Am J Nurs 1980 Oct; 80(10):1788–1790

Strickbine-VanReet P, Derman HS and Jackson D. Sudden blindness—transient and permanent. Heart Lung 1980 Sept–Oct; 9(5):898–904

Agencies

American Academy of Ophthalmology
P.O. Box 7424
1833 Fillmore Street
San Francisco, CA 94120

American Council of the Blind
1211 Connecticut Avenue, NW, Suite 506
Washington, DC 20036

American Foundation for the Blind
15 W 16th Street
New York, NY 10011

American Optometric Association
243 N. Lindbergh Blvd
St. Louis, MO 63141

Better Vision Institute Inc.
230 Park Avenue
New York, NY 10169

Contact Lens Society of America
301 First National Bldg
Lexington, KY 40507

Eye-Bank Association of America
6560 Fannin, Level 9
Houston, TX 77030

John Milton Society for the Blind
475 Riverside Drive
New York, NY 10115

Large Print Ltd
505 Pearl Street
Buffalo, NY 14204

Leader Dogs for the Blind
1039 Rochester Road
Rochester, MI 48063

National Association for the Visually Handicapped
305 E 24th Street
New York, NY 10010

National Braille Press
88 & Stephen Streets
Boston, MA 02111

National Society for the Prevention of Blindness
79 Madison Avenue
New York, NY 10016

Recording for the Blind
215 East 58th Street
New York, NY 10022

The New York Times, Large Type Weekly
Dept 0229, 220 West 43rd Street
New York, NY 10036

The Seeing Eye
Morristown, NJ 07960

Ear Disorders

Books

Ballengee JJ. Diseases of the Nose, Throat, Ear, Head and Neck, 13th ed. Philadelphia, Lea & Febiger, 1984

Chole R. A Color Atlas of Ear Disease. East Norwalk, CT, Appleton-Century-Crofts, 1982

Dayal VS. Clinical Otolaryngology. Philadelphia, JB Lippincott, 1981

Durrant JD and Lovrinic JH. Bases of Hearing Science. Baltimore, Williams & Wilkins, 1984

Gluckman JL. Medical Management of Common Problems of the Ear, Nose and Throat. Philadelphia, WB Saunders, 1984

Goode R and Levine P. Common Problems in Otolaryngology. Philadelphia, JB Lippincott, 1984

Hurvitz J and Carmen R. Special Devices for Hard of Hearing, Deaf, and Deaf–Blind Persons. Boston, Little, Brown & Co, 1981

Karmody CS. Textbook of Otolaryngology. Philadelphia, Lea & Febiger, 1983

Lucente FE and Sobol SM. Basic Otolaryngology. New York, Raven Press, 1983

Meyerhoff WL. Diagnosis and Management of Hearing Loss. Philadelphia, WB Saunders, 1984

Ryan WJ. The Nurse and the Communicatively Impaired Adult. New York, Springer Pub. Co, 1982

Wilson W and Nadol J. Quick Reference of Ear, Nose and Throat Disorders. Philadelphia, JB Lippincott, 1982

Articles
General—Ear Conditions

Brenman AK, Meltzer CR and Milner RM. Myringotomy and tube ventilation in adults. Am Fam Physician 1982 Oct; 26(4):181–184

Causse JB and Causse JR. Minimizing cochlear loss during and after stapedectomy. Otolaryngol Clin North Am 1982 Nov; 15(4):813–835

Christiansen TA. When to consider the PE tube. Postgrad Med 1984 Feb 1; 75(2):95–96

Crawford LV et al. Otitis media: Pinpointing the diagnosis. Patient Care 1983 Sept 15; 17(15):94–107

Crawford LV et al. Selecting the therapy. Patient Care 1983 Sept 15; 17(15):108–139

Crawford LV et al. When hearing impairment occurs. Patient Care 1983 Sept 15; 17(15):147–167

FDA approves use of artificial ear implants. AORN J 1984 June; 39(7):1228

Goldenberg RA. Evaluation of the dizzy

patient. Hosp Med 1982 Apr; 18(4): 140–158

Hough JVD. Experience in tympanoplasty—avoiding revision and complications. Otolaryngol Clin North Am 1982 Nov; 15(4):845–860

Lerner A et al. Randomised, controlled trial of the comparative efficacy, auditory toxicity, and nephrotoxicity of tobramycin and netilmicin. Lancet 1983 May 21; 9(8334):1123–1125

Lesinski SG. Complications of homograft tympanoplasty. Otolaryngol Clin North Am 1982 Nov; 15(4):795–811

Lovan WD. Motion sickness. Am Fam Physician 1984 June; 29(6):117–122

Malkiewicz J. How to assess the ears and test hearing acuity. RN 1982 Mar; 45(3):56–63

Middle ear infections. Harvard Med Sch Health Lett 1982 May; 7(8):1–2; 5

Morgan RH. Breaking through the sound barrier. Nursing '83 1983 Feb; 13(2): 112–114

Mowbry DB and Crayson DE. Motion sickness, ginger, and psychophysics. Lancet 1982 Mar 20; 1(8272):655–656

Olsen WD. Presbycusis. Postgrad Med 1984 Sept 1; 76(3):189–198

Physiology of the ear. Nurs Times 1984 Aug 15; 80(33):28–30

Saak AJ, Blackwelder WC and Kaslow RA. Treatment of acute otitis media. JAMA 1982 Sept 3; 248(9):1071–1072

Shambaugh GE Jr. Complications of the fenestration operation and their management. Otolaryngol Clin North Am 1982 Nov; 15(4):837–843

Vogel TC. Managing head and neck problems (ear), pp. 29–40. In Nursing Photobook. Aiding Ambulatory Patients. Springhouse, PA, Intermed, 1983

Wehrs RE. Homograft tympanoplasty. Otolaryngol Clin North Am 1982 Nov; 15(4):781–793

Hearing Loss

Anderson RG and Meyerhoff WL. Sudden sensorineural hearing loss. Otolaryngol Clin North Am 1983 Feb; 16(1):189–195

Austin DF. Avoiding failures in the restoration of hearing with ossiculoplasty and biocompatible implants. Surg Clin North Am 1982 Nov; 15(4):763–771

Bueche MN and Haxton DM. The student with a hearing loss: Coping strategies. Nurse Educ 1983 Winter; 8(4):7–11

Chasse PS. Hope of hearing. Today's OR Nurse 1983 Oct; 5(8):14–17

Chickadonz GH, Beach EK and Fox JA. Educating a deaf nursing student. Nurs Health Care 1983 June; 4(6):327–333

Guidotti TL and Novak RE. Hearing conservation and occupational exposure to noise. Am Fam Physician 1983 Oct; 128(4):181–186

Hansell HN. The behavioral effects of noises on man: The patient with "intensive care unit psychosis." Heart Lung 1984 Jan; 13(1):59–65

Hanawalt A and Troutman K. If your patient has a hearing aid. Am J Nurs 1984 July; 84(7):900–901

Holden L. Hearing aids. Nursing '82 1982 Apr; 12(4):64–67

Irvine PW. The hearing-impaired elderly patient. Postgrad Med 1982 Oct; 72(4):115–118

Koch KH. Hidden handicaps. The deaf and hard of hearing: Some hints. Nurs Times 1981 Aug 5–11; 77(32):19–20

Langham-Brown SJ. Problems in communication in patient care. Nurs Times 1981 June 11; 77(24):1035–1037

Ross T. Deafness: Breaking through the sound barrier. Nurs Mirror 1981 May 20; 152(21):20–23

Ménière's Syndrome

Best LG, Ferraro J and Arenberg IK. The clinical value of computerized sinusoidal harmonic acceleration testing in patients with endolymphatic hydrops. Otolaryngol Clin North Am 1983 Feb; 16(1):83–93

Gibson WPR. A study of endolymphatic sac surgery. Otolaryngol Clin North Am 1983 Feb; 16(1):181–188

Gibson WPR and Prasher DK. Electrocochleography and its role in the diagnosis and understanding of Ménière's disease. Otolaryngol Clin North Am 1983 Feb; 16(1):59–68

Goldenberg RA. Management of Ménière's disease. Postgrad Med 1984 Mar; 75(4):133–138

Imoto T and Stahle J. Glycerin and urea tests in Ménière's disease. Otolaryngol Clin North Am 1983 Feb; 16(1):37–48

Maddox HE. Medical treatment of Ménière's disease compared to early sac surgery. Otolaryngol Clin North Am 1983 Feb; 16(1):129–133

Pulec JL. Ménière's syndrome. Hosp Med 1983 June; 19(6):83–86

Van de Water SM and Arenberg IK. Auditory dehydration testing in the evaluation of hydrops: A comparison of glycerol and urea. Otolaryngol Clin North Am 1983 Feb; 16(1):49–58

Cochlear Implants

Berliner KI. Risk versus benefit in cochlear implantation. Ann Otolaryngol Rhinol Laryngol 1982 Mar–Apr: suppl (91. No. 2 Part 3):90–97

Chasse PS. Hope of hearing. Today's OR Nurse 1983 Oct; 5(8):14–16

House WF and Berliner KI. The cochlear implant. Otolaryngol Clin North Am 1982 Nov; 15(4):917–923

Maddox HE and Porter TH. Who is a candidate for cochlear implantation? Otolaryngol Clin North Am 1983 Feb; 16(1):249–255

Agencies

American Speech–Language–Hearing Association
10801 Rockville Pike
Rockville, MD 20852

American Academy of Otolaryngology, Head and Neck Surgery
1101 Vermont Avenue, NW, Suite 302
Washington, DC 20005

Alexander Graham Bell Association for the Deaf
3417 Volta Place NW
Washington, DC 20007

National Association of Hearing and Speech Action
10801 Rockville Pike
Rockville, MD 20852

National Association of the Deaf
814 Thayer Avenue
Silver Spring, MD 20910

National Hearing Aid Society
20361 Middlebelt Road
Livonia, MI 48152

(Toll-free for hearing impaired: 1-800-521-5247 [usable in all states except Michigan] 9 AM to 4 PM EST Monday through Friday. Hearing Aid Helpline sponsored by National Hearing Aid Society.)

Conditions of the Neurological System

18

Diagnostic Evaluation of Neurologic Disease

The neurologic examination involves history-taking, an assessment of the patient's mental status, speech, memory, and reasoning ability, as well as a physical examination in which special attention is given to examination of the nervous system. This involves testing of each cranial nerve, as well as assessment of functioning of peripheral nerves and the spinal cord.

Selected Radiologic Procedures

A. **Skull X-ray**—reveals configuration, density, vascular markings, and intracranial calcification and tumor.

B. **Computed Tomography** (CT)—(computerized axial tomography) an imaging method in which the head is scanned in successive layers by a narrow beam of x-ray. It provides a cross-sectional view of the brain and distinguishes differences in the densities of various brain tissues. A computer printout is obtained of the absorption values of the tissues in the plane that is being scanned. The data are transformed into an image through a series of complex equations. The image is displayed on an oscilloscope or television monitor and photographed.

1. Lesions are seen as variations in tissue density differing from the surrounding normal brain tissue.
2. Abnormalities of tissue density indicate possible tumor masses, brain infarction, ventricular displacement; useful in patients with head trauma, suspected brain tumor, hydrocephalus. CT is also used for diseases of the spinal column and spinal cord and is commonly used in the evaluation of patients with herniated discs.
3. More recently, CT-directed biopsies are being done.
4. May be done with IV contrast medium enhancement

to more accurately define boundaries of certain lesions and indicate presence of otherwise undetectable lesions.

5. *Patient preparation*
   a. Inquire about allergies and any previous adverse reaction to contrast agent.
   b. Be sure that a consent form has been signed.
   c. No special preparation is required; this is a noninvasive technique that can be done on an outpatient basis.
   d. Instruct the patient that he must lie perfectly still while the test is being carried out; he cannot talk or move his face as this distorts the picture.

C. **Positron Emission Tomography** (PET)—a computer-based imaging technique that permits study of the brain's metabolism and function; displays pictures of metabolic and biochemical activity within brain as thinking, speaking, hearing, and other activities occur.

D. **Magnetic Resonance Imaging** (MRI)—a diagnostic imaging modality that uses a magnetic field (rather than ionizing radiation) to produce images of the body. It is extremely sensitive in detecting abnormalities in the brain, especially biochemical assessment.

E. **Isotope Cisternography**—use of radioactive tracer injected into lumbar subarachnoid space. Useful in studying cerebrospinal fluid circulation, to locate cerebrospinal fluid leak, and to evaluate hydrocephalus, etc.

F. **Lumbar Epidural Venography**—percutaneous insertion of a catheter into the femoral vein; catheter is guided into ascending lumbar vein and/or internal iliac veins. Contrast medium is injected to opacify epidural venous plexus (fills epidural veins overlying disc spaces).

May reveal deviation or compression of the epidural veins due to herniated disc or tumor.

G. Discography—injection of radiopaque substance directly into the intervertebral disc. This study can be used in patients suspected of having herniated disc disease but is infrequently done.

Cerebral Angiography

The x-ray study of the cerebral circulation following the injection of contrast material into a selected artery.

A. General Procedure

1. Contrast material may be injected into femoral, common carotid, vertebral, or subclavian artery, or arch of the aorta.
2. After injection of selected artery, x-rays are made of arterial and venous phases of circulation through brain and head.
3. Useful in demonstrating position of arteries, intracranial aneurysms, presence or absence of abnormal vasculature, hematomas, or tumors, or to add specificity to a CT diagnosis.
4. Digital subtraction angiography—uses computerized radiographic techniques in the evaluation of vascular disease.
   a. Subtracts (masks out electronically) surrounding bony and soft tissue structures to give an unobstructed picture of blood vessels.
   b. Contrast material can be injected in a vein or artery.

B. Nursing Support: Before Angiogram

1. Withhold meal preceding test, but clear liquids are usually permitted up to the time of the study.
2. The patient may be given sedation before going to x-ray department—may help minimize intensity of burning sensation felt along course of injected vessel.
3. Mark the appropriate peripheral pulses with a felt-tipped pen.
4. Instruct the patient as follows:
   a. Try to lie quietly during injection.
   b. A burning sensation, lasting for a few seconds, may possibly be felt behind the eyes, or in jaw, teeth, tongue, and lips.

C. Nursing Support: Following Angiogram

1. Make repeated observations for neurologic sequelae—motor or sensory deterioration, alterations in level of responsiveness, weakness on one side, speech disturbances, arrhythmias, blood pressure fluctuation.
2. Observe injection site for hematoma formation; apply an ice cap intermittently—to relieve swelling and discomfort.
3. Evaluate peripheral pulses—changes may develop if there is hematoma formation at puncture site or embolization to a distant artery.
4. Note color and temperature of involved extremity—to detect possible embolism.

Myelography

Myelography is the injection of contrast medium into the spinal subarachnoid space by spinal puncture for radiologic examination; outlines the spinal subarachnoid space and shows distortion of the spinal cord or dural sac by tumors, cysts, herniated intervertebral discs, or other lesions.

A. General Points

1. Metrizamide (Amipaque) myelography is done with a water-soluble contrast agent that is reabsorbed and does not have to be removed.
   It can cause seizures and a transient encephalopathy if the patient's head is lowered below his trunk following the study.
2. Pantopaque myelography involves use of an oil-based contrast medium.
   a. After injection of the contrast medium, the head of the table is tilted down and the course of the contrast medium is observed radioscopically.
   b. Contrast material may be removed after test completion by syringe and needle aspiration; the patient may complain of sharp pain down leg during aspiration if a nerve root has been aspirated against a needle point—needle point is rotated or an adjustment in needle depth is made.
      With newer water-soluble contrast agents a smaller needle can be used (less likely to produce headache); material is reabsorbed and need not be removed.
   c. It may cause arachnoiditis (inflammation of the arachnoid layer of the dura).

B. Nursing Responsibilities: Before Test

1. Reinforce physician's explanation of procedure; explain that it is usually not painful and that the x-ray table will be tilted in varying positions during the study.
2. Omit the meal preceding myelography.
3. Patient may be given light sedative prior to test to help him cope.

C. Nursing Support Post Test

1. If water-soluble medium (metrizamide) has been used, the patient lies with the head of the bed elevated 15–30 degrees—to reduce the upward displacement of the medium.
2. If oil-based medium (Pantopaque) is used, the patient is instructed to lie in a recumbent position (12–24 hours) to reduce cerebrospinal fluid leakage and decrease the frequency of headache.
3. Encourage the patient to drink liberal quantities of fluid—for rehydration and replacement of cerebrospinal fluid and to decrease incidence of postlumbar puncture headache (thought to be due to escape of spinal fluid).
4. Assess neurologic and vital signs; note motor and sensory deviations from normal.
5. Check on patient's ability to void.
6. Watch for fever, stiff neck, photophobia, or other signs of chemical or bacterial meningitis.

Air Studies

A gaseous replacement of the fluid within the ventricles and subarachnoid systems serves as a contrast medium because air is less dense than fluid to roentgen rays. These studies are used infrequently since the advent of computed tomography and cerebral angiography.

A. Pneumoencephalogram

Withdrawal of cerebrospinal fluid and injection of air or other gas by means of a lumbar puncture.

1. Demonstrates ventricular system and subarachnoid space overlying the hemispheres and basal cisterns.
2. Useful in diagnosing degenerative cerebral atrophy and in detecting mass lesions at the base of the brain.

B. Fractional pneumoencephalogram

Withdrawal of small amounts of fluid and injection of small amounts of air to visualize the ventricular system.

C. Ventriculogram

Withdrawal of cerebrospinal fluid and injection of air or gas directly into the lateral ventricles through openings in the skull.

D. Nursing management following pneumoencephalogram or ventriculogram

1. Watch the patient for increasing intracranial pressure (see p. 763)
   a. Disturbances of intracranial pressure may cause serious complications.
   b. Prepare for ventricular tap and prompt decompression.
2. Take vital signs as frequently as clinical condition indicates and until stabilized.
3. Make frequent neurologic checks, especially of level of responsiveness.
4. Assess for complaints of headache and fever, and for signs of shock.
   a. Place ice cap on head intermittently.
   b. Give analgesics as directed—duration of headache depends on the speed with which the intracranial air is absorbed.
   c. Nausea and vomiting may follow air studies.
   d. Parenteral fluids may be necessary for first 24 hours.

Electroencephalography (EEG)

Records, by means of electrodes applied on the scalp surface (or by microelectrodes placed within brain tissue), the electrical activity which is generated in the brain.

1. Provides physiologic assessment of cerebral activity; useful in diagnosis of the epilepsies and as a screening procedure for coma and organic brain syndrome; also used as an indicator of brain death.
2. Electrodes are arranged on the scalp to permit the recording of activity in various head regions; the amplified activity of the neurons is recorded on a continuously moving paper sheet.
   a. For baseline recording, the patient lies quietly with his eyes closed.
   b. For activation procedures (done to elicit abnormal electrical discharges, especially seizure potentials), patient may be asked to hyperventilate for 3–4 minutes, look at a bright flashing light, or receive an injection of medication (Metrazol).
   c. EEG may also be made during sleep and upon awakening—some abnormal brain waves are seen only when patient is asleep.
3. Pharyngeal (electrode inserted through nose; rests on mucosa of pharyngeal roof) and sphenoidal (inserted transcutaneously with tips resting on sphenoid bone near foramen ovale) electrodes are used when epileptogenic area is inaccessible to conventional scalp preparation.
4. Patient preparation for routine recording
   a. Tranquilizers and stimulants may be withheld 24–48 hours before EEG—may alter EEG wave patterns.
   b. Omit coffee, tea, or cola drinks in meal before test; do not omit meal.
   c. Shampoo hair night before tests; omit hair sprays and hair dressings.
   d. Reassure the patient that he will not receive an electrical shock, that the EEG takes approximately 45–60 minutes (more for an EEG taken while sleeping), and that the EEG is *not* a form of treatment or a test of intelligence or insanity.

Evoked Potential Studies

These studies involve the changes and responses in brain waves recorded from scalp electrodes that are evoked (elicited) by the introduction of an external stimulus (visual, auditory, somatosensory).

1. These evoked changes are detected with the aid of computing devices, which extract, display, and store the signal.
2. These studies are based on the concept that any insult/dysfunction that can alter neuronal metabolism or disturb membrane function may change evoked electrical activity.
   a. Visual evoked responses—the patient looks at visual stimulus (flashing light); the average of several hundred stimuli are recorded by EEG leads over the occiput and the transit time from the retina to the occipital area is measured (in milliseconds), using computer averaging methods.
   b. Auditory evoked responses—auditory stimulus (repetitive auditory click) is presented, and its transit time up the brain stem into the cortex is measured. Specific lesions in auditory pathway will modify or delay the response.
   c. Somatosensory evoked response—peripheral nerves stimulated percutaneously. Transit time up the spinal cord to the sensory cortex of the brain is measured and recorded from scalp electrodes. Test is used to detect deficit in spinal cord, to measure conduction in spinal cord, and to monitor cord function during operative procedures.

Electromyography (EMG)

The introduction of needle electrodes into the skeletal muscles to study changes in electric potential of muscles and nerves leading to them. These are shown on an oscilloscope and amplified by a loudspeaker for simultaneous visual and auditory analysis and comparison.

1. Useful in determining the presence of a neuromuscular disorder; helps distinguish weakness due to neuropathy from that due to other causes. Useful in evaluation and follow-up of peripheral nerve injuries.
2. *Nursing responsibilities*
   a. No special patient preparation is required.
   b. Explain to the patient that he will experience a sensation similar to that of an IM injection as the needle is inserted into the muscle; muscles examined may ache slightly for a short time.

Other Neurologic Tests

A. **Nerve Conduction Studies**—performed by stimulating a peripheral nerve at several points along its course and recording the muscle action potential or the sensory action potential that results. This test assesses how well the nerve transmits its electrical impulses.

B. **Radionuclide Imaging Studies** (brain scan)—following intake (IV) of radiopharmaceutical, the radioactivity subsequently transmitted through the skull is scanned by a rectilinear scanner, which prints out a picture based on the number of counts received from the brain as it scans; (or a gamma camera, which prints out image without actually scanning, may be used). CT scanning is replacing traditional radioisotope scanning.

1. This test is based on the principle that a radiopharmaceutical may diffuse through a disrupted blood–brain barrier into the abnormal cerebral tissue or areas where there is new vascularization. (Normal brain tissue is relatively impermeable.) There is an increased uptake of radioactive material at the site of pathology.
2. Brain scanning is useful in early detection and evaluation of intracranial neoplasms, stroke, abscess, follow-up of surgical or radiation therapy of brain.
3. *Nursing responsibilities*
   a. Explain to the patient that he will be expected to lie quietly during the procedure.
   b. This is a noninvasive procedure.

C. Echoencephalography—the recording of echoes from the deep structures within the skull (generated by the transmission of ultrasound [high frequency] waves) to determine the position of midline structures of the brain and the distance from the midline to the lateral ventricular wall or the third ventricular wall.

1. Useful for detecting a shift of the cerebral midline structures caused by subdural hematoma, intracerebral hemorrhage, massive cerebral infarction, and neoplasms; can display dilation of ventricles; useful in evaluation of hydrocephalus.
2. Ultrasonic transducers are positioned over specified areas of the head; the echoes are imaged and stored on the oscilloscope.
3. *Nursing responsibilities*
   a. There is no special patient preparation.
   b. Explain that this is a noninvasive test and that some type of liquid may be used to eliminate the air gap between the transducer and the head.

Guidelines: Assisting the Patient Undergoing a Lumbar Puncture

Lumbar Puncture   Insertion of a needle into lumbar subarachnoid space and withdrawal of cerebrospinal fluid for diagnostic and therapeutic purposes.

Purposes
1. To obtain cerebrospinal fluid for examination (microbiologic, serologic, cytologic, or chemical analysis).*
2. To measure and relieve cerebrospinal pressure.
3. To determine the presence or absence of blood in the spinal fluid.
4. To detect spinal subarachnoid block.
5. To administer antibiotics intrathecally in certain cases of infection.
6. To administer anticancer drugs.

Equipment

Sterile lumbar puncture set   Skin antiseptic
Sterile gloves   Band-Aid
Xylocaine 1%–2%

Procedure

Nursing Action	Rationale/Amplification
Preparatory Phase	
1. Give a step-by-step summary of the procedure.	1. Reassures the patient and gains his cooperation.
For Lying Position: (Fig. 18-1).	
2. Position the patient on his side with a pillow under his head and a pillow between his legs. He should be lying on a firm surface.	2. The spine is maintained in a horizontal position. The pillow between the legs prevents the upper leg from rolling forward.
3. Instruct the patient to arch the lumbar segment of his back and draw his knees up to his abdomen, clasping his knees with his hands.	3. This posture offers maximal widening of the interspinous spaces and affords easier entry into the subarachnoid space.
4. Assist the patient in maintaining this position by supporting him behind the knees and neck. Assist the patient to maintain the posture throughout the examination.	4. Supporting the patient helps prevent sudden movements, which can produce a traumatic (bloody) tap and thus impede correct diagnosis.
For Sitting Position:	
5. Have the patient straddle a straight-back chair (facing the back) and rest his head against his arms, which are folded on the back of the chair.	5. In obese patients and those who have difficulty in assuming an arched side-lying position, this posture may allow more accurate identification of the spinous processes and interspaces.
Performance Phase (by the physician)	
1. The skin is prepared with antiseptic solution, and the skin and subcutaneous spaces are infiltrated with local anesthetic agent.	

* See Appendix for characteristics of normal cerebrospinal fluid.

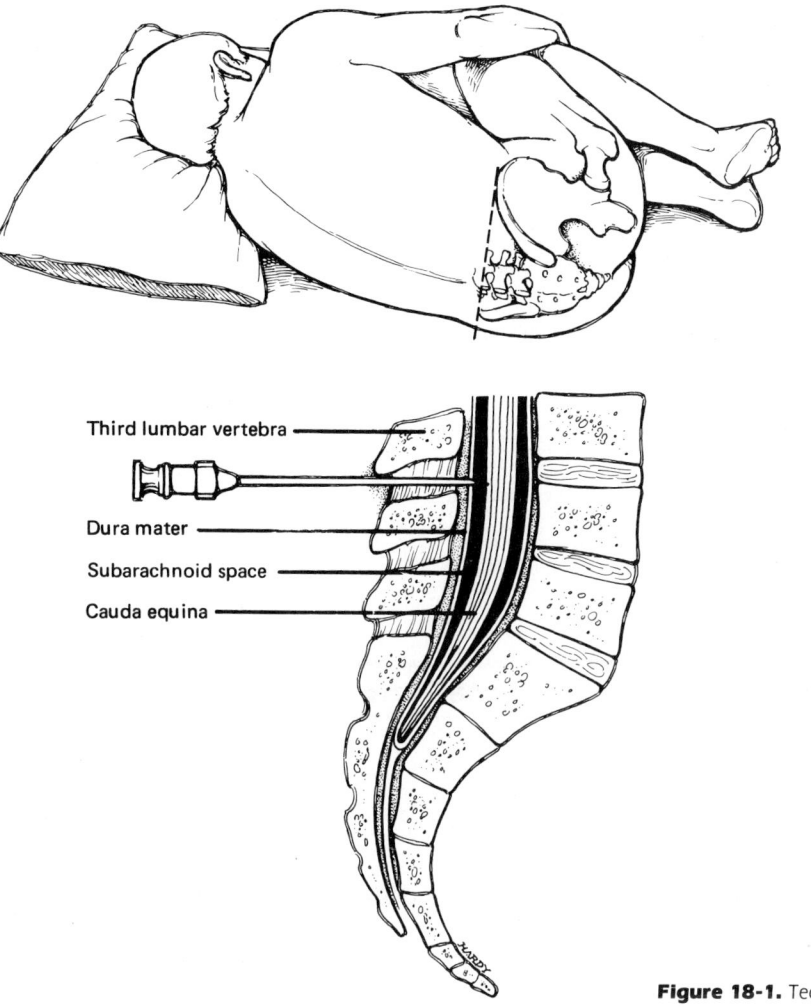

Third lumbar vertebra

Dura mater

Subarachnoid space

Cauda equina

Figure 18-1. Technique of lumbar puncture.

Procedure
(Cont.)

Action	**Rationale/Amplification**
2. A spinal puncture needle is introduced at the L3–L4 interspace. The needle is advanced until the "give" of the ligamentum flavum is felt and the needle enters the subarachnoid space. The manometer is attached to the spinal puncture needle.	2. L3–L4 interspace is *below* the level of the spinal cord.
3. After the needle enters the subarachnoid space, help the patient to slowly straighten his legs.	3. This maneuver prevents a false increase in intraspinal pressure. Muscle tension and compression of the abdomen give falsely high pressures.
4. Instruct the patient to breathe quietly (not to hold his breath or strain) and not to talk.	4. Hyperventilation may lower a truly elevated pressure. Talking can elevate CSF pressure.
5. The initial pressure reading is obtained by measuring the level of the fluid column after it comes to rest.	5. With respiration there is normally some fluctuation of spinal fluid in the manometer. Normal range of spinal fluid pressure with the patient in the lateral position is 70–180 mm. H$_2$O.
6. About 2–3 ml. of spinal fluid is placed in each of 3 test tubes for observation, comparison, and laboratory analysis.	6. Spinal fluid should be clear and colorless. Bloody spinal fluid may indicate cerebral contusion, laceration, subarachnoid hemorrhage, or a traumatic tap.

(continued)

Guidelines: Assisting the Patient Undergoing a Lumbar Puncture (continued)

Procedure
(Cont.)

Action	Rationale/Amplification
Lumbar Manometric Test (Queckenstedt Test) 1. A blood pressure cuff is placed around the patient's neck and inflated to a pressure of 20 mm. Hg (or an assistant compresses jugular vein or veins for 10 seconds). 2. Pressure readings are made at 10-second intervals. 3. After the needle is withdrawn, a Band-Aid is applied to the puncture site.	This test is made when a spinal subarachnoid block is suspected (tumor; vertebral fracture or dislocation). In normal persons there is a rapid rise in pressure of CSF in response to jugular compression with rapid return to normal when the compression is released. If the pressure fails to rise or rises and falls slowly, there is evidence of a block due to a lesion's compressing the spinal subarachnoid pathways. This test is not done if an intracranial lesion is suspected.
Follow-up Phase 1. Record (a) procedure, (b) appearance of spinal fluid, (c) whether or not specimens were sent to laboratory, (d) spinal pressure readings, and (e) condition and reaction of the patient. 2. Keep the patient horizontal (prone, supine, or on his side) for 6–12 hours. Encourage a liberal fluid intake.	Some patients suffer from postpuncture headache, which is thought to be caused by the leakage of spinal fluid at the puncture site.

Special Neurologic Nursing Considerations

Nursing Management of the Unconscious Patient

Clinical Problems

There are 2 major threats to the unconscious patient:
1. The disease or trauma that produced unconsciousness.
2. The threat of the unconscious state.

Assessment

Clinical Manifestations

Evaluate:
1. Responses to command or painful stimulus
   a. Eye opening
   b. Verbal responses
   c. Motor responses
2. Pupil reaction to light, size, equality; eye movement
3. Swallowing reflexes; deep tendon reflexes
4. Patterns of respiration (normal, Kussmaul, Cheyne–Stokes, apneic, etc.)
5. Neck stiffness
6. Head (for trauma); mouth, nose, ears for blood, CSF
7. Heart, lungs, abdomen

Diagnostic Evaluation

1. Computed tomography, angiogram
2. Drug screen
3. Infection screen
4. Other supportive investigations as patient's condition indicates

Patient Problems/Nursing Diagnoses

1. Ineffective airway clearance related to accumulation of secretions
2. Potential for deepening level of unconsciousness related to change in intracranial homeostasis
3. Alteration in fluid and electrolyte balance and reduced nutritional intake related to inability to take fluid and foods
4. Potential for complications related to the unconscious state

Planning and Implementation

Nursing Interventions (Fig. 18-2)

A. **Maintaining a patent airway, respiratory exchange, and circulation**

1. Place the patient in a three-fourths prone or semi-prone position or a lateral position—prevents the tongue from obstructing the airway, encourages drainage of respiratory secretions, and promotes oxygen and carbon dioxide exchange.
2. Keep the airway free of secretions with efficient suctioning—in the absence of the cough and swallowing reflexes, secretions rapidly accumulate in the posterior pharynx and upper trachea and can lead to fatal respiratory complications.
   a. See p. 153 for tracheal suctioning.
   b. Carry out periodic determinations of arterial PO_2 and PCO_2 to determine adequacy of treatment.
   c. Prepare for tracheostomy if coma is deepening and there are evidences of inadequate respiratory exchange. (See pages 218–220 for nursing management of patient with tracheostomy.)
3. Insert oral airway if tongue is paralyzed or is obstructing airway—an obstructed airway increases intracranial pressure. This is considered a short-term measure.
4. Employ oxygen therapy to deliver oxygenated blood to the CNS. (Care must be taken in oxygenating patient with COPD.)
5. Prepare for insertion of cuffed endotracheal tube if the patient's condition requires (see p. 213)—

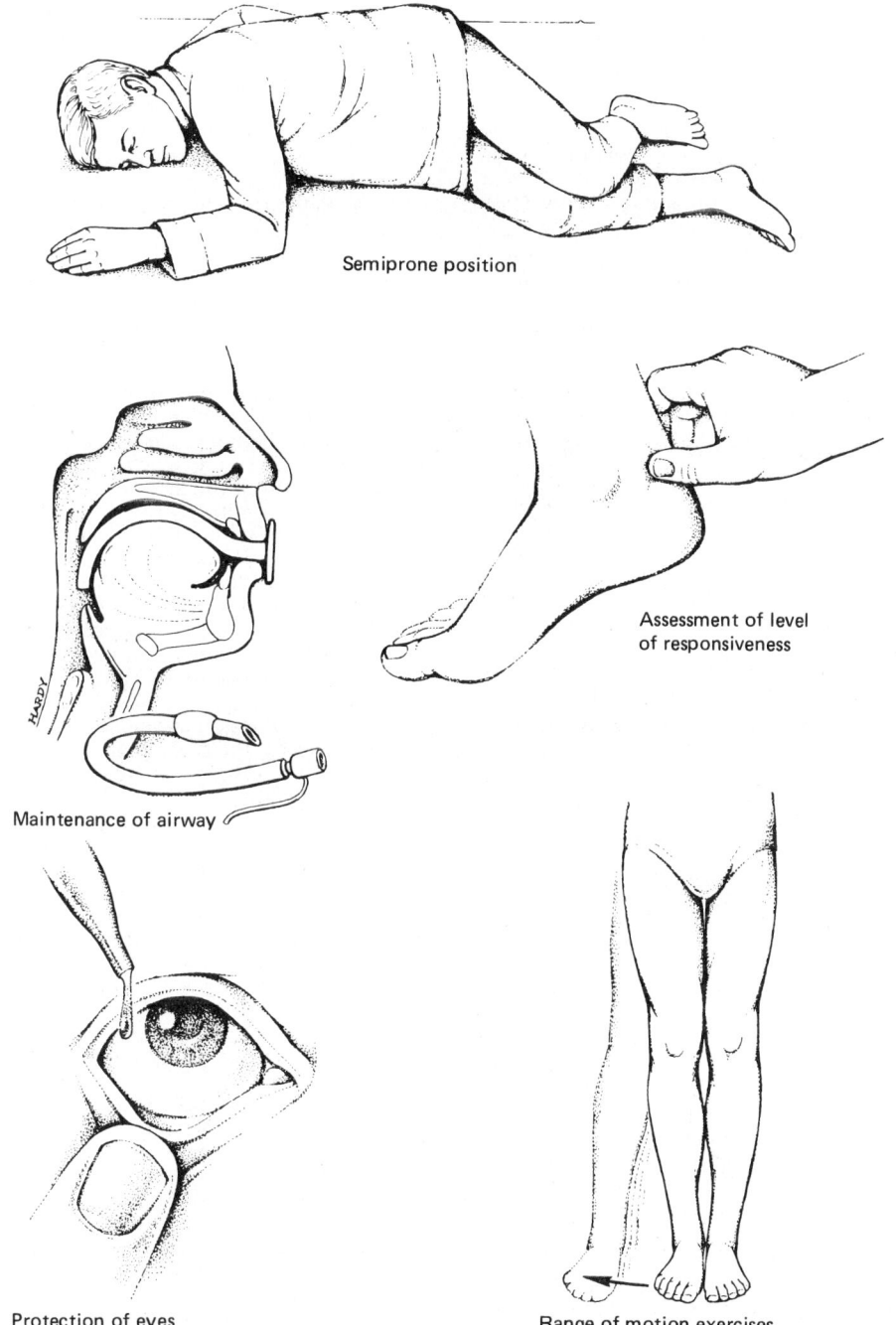

Semiprone position

Maintenance of airway

Assessment of level
of responsiveness

Protection of eyes

Range of motion exercises

Figure 18-2. Nursing priorities in the care of the unconscious patient.

endotracheal intubation is more effective in permitting positive pressure ventilation. The cuffed tube seals off the digestive tract, helping to prevent aspiration and allowing efficient removal of tracheobronchial secretions.
6. Maintain circulation; support the blood pressure and treat life-threatening cardiac arrhythmias.
7. Evaluate pulses (radial, carotid, apical, pedal); mea-sure blood pressure—these parameters are a measure of circulatory adequacy/inadequacy.
8. Give specific treatment when cause is known (hem-orrhage, infection, intoxication).

B. Assessing level of responsiveness
1. Carry out neurologic examination.
2. Maintain a constant assessment of the patient's level

of consciousness and changes in responsiveness—the level of consciousness is the most important measure of the patient's condition. Unconscious patients may deteriorate rapidly from numerous clinical causes.

3. Record the patient's *exact reactions,* eye opening, verbal response, movements, and quality of speech.
   a. Request the patient to speak.
   b. Ask the patient to perform some activity (raise arm, extend tongue, etc.).
   c. Apply painful stimuli if there is no response (pinching skin of arms or thighs) and assess the patient's perception of pain. No response or a delayed or unequal response is an unfavorable clinical sign.
   d. Use a neurologic rating scale to establish neurologic baseline; follow progress of the patient and effects of therapeutic measures.

C. Evaluating the progression of vital aigns

1. Know the patient's baseline vital signs and alert the physician if there are significant fluctuations of blood pressure and instability of the pulse and respiratory cycle—fluctuations of vital signs indicate a change in intracranial homeostasis; monitoring of vital signs is also essential to alert for hidden bleeding.
2. Take blood pressure readings, pulse and respiratory rates and temperature at frequently specified intervals until there is evidence of stabilization—temperature-regulating mechanisms may be disturbed.

D. Fluid and electrolyte and nutritional balance

1. Give intravenous fluids as indicated—serial laboratory electrolyte evaluations are made when the patient is maintained on intravenous fluids to ensure proper balance.
2. Or use hyperalimentation feedings.
3. Or initiate nasogastric feedings. Feeding through a gastric tube ensures better nutrition than does intravenous feeding. Paralytic ileus is fairly frequent in the unconscious patient, and a nasogastric tube assists in gastric decompression.
   a. Insert small gastric tube through nose into stomach.
   b. Aspirate stomach before each feeding. If aspirated residual exceeds 50 ml., the patient may be developing an ileus. Gastric distention and vomiting may result.
   c. Elevate the patient's head and thorax and slowly give 100–150 ml. of blenderized formula. Give small amount at first and gradually increase until 400–500 ml. are given at each feeding.
   d. Give 2,000–2,500 ml. of fluid (according to the patient's condition) through the tube daily. An unconscious patient requires adequate fluids since high protein feedings can produce a solute diuresis that will produce dehydration and hyperosmolar coma unless adequate fluid intake is ensured. Fever, excessive sweating, or fluid loss elsewhere in the body increases fluid requirements.
   e. Rinse the tube with water after each feeding. Keep tube feeding refrigerated.
   f. Measure urinary output and specific gravity.
   g. Prepare for gastrostomy if the patient's condition indicates.

E. Prevention of complications

1. Be aware of the varying phases of restlessness—a certain degree of restlessness may be favorable, since it may indicate the patient is regaining consciousness. However, restlessness is quite common in cerebral anoxia or when there is a partially obstructed airway, distended bladder, overlooked bleeding, or fracture; it may be a manifestation of brain injury.
   a. Have adequate lighting in the room to prevent hallucinations as the patient regains consciousness.
   b. Pad side rails, apply mitts or boxing gloves on hands, or use other devices to protect the patient.
   c. Avoid oversedating the patient—sedatives/narcotics depress level of responsiveness; certain drugs affect pupillary size and reaction, which is an important sign.
   d. Avoid restraints if at all possible.
   e. Speak softly to the patient, calling him by name.
   f. Touch him as gently as possible.
2. Keep the skin clean, dry, and free of pressure—comatose patients are susceptible to formation of pressure sores. Clip the patient's nails to prevent excoriation of the skin.
3. Put all extremities through range-of-motion exercises 4 times daily—contracture deformities develop early in unconscious patients.
4. Turn the patient from side to side at regular intervals—turning relieves pressure areas and helps keep lungs clear by mobilizing secretions. Prolonged pressure on extremities produces nerve palsies.
5. Observe the patient for indication of an overdistended bladder.
   a. Utilize external sheath catheter (condom catheter) for the male patient.
   b. If the patient is unable to void, insert 3-way indwelling catheter—infection invariably follows prolonged use of an indwelling catheter that is attached to straight drainage.
6. Observe the patient for constipation and diarrhea.
7. Carry out oral care (water, ice chips, and mouthwash solution).
8. Protect the eyes from corneal irritation—the cornea functions as a shield. If the eyes remain open for long periods, corneal drying, irritation, and ulceration are likely to result.
   a. Make sure the patient's eye is not rubbing against bedding if blinking and corneal reflexes are absent.
   b. Inspect the size of the pupils and condition of eyes with a flashlight.
   c. Remove contact lenses if worn (see p. 723).
   d. Irrigate eyes with sterile prescribed solution and instill ophthalmic ointment in each eye—prevents glazing and corneal ulceration.
   e. Prepare for temporary tarsorrhaphy (suturing of eyelids in closed position) if unconscious state is prolonged.
9. Protect the patient during convulsive seizures (see p. 769)—the patient with head trauma is a potential candidate for convulsive seizures.
   a. Protect the patient from self-injury.
   b. Observe the patient during the seizure and record observations.
   c. Give prescribed anticonvulsant medications through the nasogastric tube.
10. Be alert for the development of complications.
    a. Respiratory complications (infections, aspiration, obstruction, atelectasis)
    b. Fluid and electrolyte imbalance
    c. Infection (urinary, pressure sores, central nervous system)

d. Bladder and gastrointestinal distention
e. Convulsive seizures
f. Gastrointestinal bleeding

11. Provide for social contacts and environmental enrichment—introducing meaningful sounds (conversation, music, taped sound of patient's home and work environment) stimulates the cortical levels.

12. Be aware that the patient will feel uneasy concerning his period of unconsciousness when he gains awareness of what has happened.
    a. Give an explanation of what has happened during period of unconsciousness.
    b. Permit the patient to ask questions and talk about the experience of unconsciousness.

Evaluation
Expected Outcomes

1. Maintains clear airway—coughs up secretions; no crackles on lung auscultation; responds to appropriate stimuli
2. Attains/maintains adequate fluid, electrolyte, and nutritional status—swallowing reflexes normal; no clinical signs of dehydration; normal serum electrolyte values; bowel sound heard upon auscultation; minimal weight loss
3. Is free of preventable complications—absence of pressure sores, contractures, overdistended bladder, corneal irritation, etc.

Nursing Management of the Patient With Increasing Intracranial Pressure
(Intracranial Hypertension)

Intracranial pressure (ICP) is the pressure within the ventriculosubarachnoid space; in a "steady state," the intracranial compartments (blood, brain, cerebrospinal fluid [CSF]) are in a condition of pressure and volume equilibrium.

Causes

1. Head injury/hematoma
2. Cerebral edema; stroke
3. Abscess, infection
4. Hemorrhage; impending aneurysmal rupture
5. Brain tumor
6. Cranial surgery
7. Dialysis complication

▶ **NURSING ALERT: As intracranial pressure increases, the brain substance is compressed. A sudden increase may produce an emergency situation in a few minutes. This condition may lead rapidly to death or result in a vegetative existence for the patient.**

Assessment
Clinical Manifestations

1. Change in level of responsiveness (consciousness)
   a. *The level of responsiveness is the most important measure of the patient's condition.*
   b. Look for lethargy, delay in response to verbal suggestions, slowing of speech.
   c. Watch for sudden changes in condition—quietness to restlessness, orientation to confusion, increasing drowsiness, stupor, coma.
   d. *Progressive deterioration is a serious sign* that may necessitate immediate surgical intervention.

2. Changes in vital signs
   a. Rising blood pressure or widening pulse pressure (the difference between systolic and diastolic blood pressure).
   b. Pulse changes—bradycardia changing to tachycardia as intracranial pressure rises.
   c. Respiratory irregularities; slowing of rate with lengthening periods of apnea; Cheyne–Stokes or Kussmaul breathing.
   d. Moderately elevated temperature.

3. Headache—constant, increasing in intensity; aggravated by movement/straining.

4. Vomiting—recurrent with little or no nausea; may be projectile.

5. Subtle changes—restlessness, headache, forced breathing, purposeless movements, and mental cloudiness.

6. Papilledema

7. Pupillary changes—increasing pressure or an expanding clot can displace the brain against the oculomotor or optic nerve, producing pupillary changes.
   a. Inspect the pupils with a flashlight to evaluate size, configuration, and reaction to light. Compare both eyes for similarities/differences.
   b. Evaluate gaze to determine if it is conjugate (paired, working together) or if eye movements are abnormal.
   c. Evaluate ability of eyes to abduct and adduct.
   d. Inspect the retina and optic nerve for hemorrhage and papilledema.

Patient Problems/Nursing Diagnosis

1. Potential for loss of consciousness/death related to increased intracranial pressure
2. See Head Injury, page 766 for other patient problems/nursing diagnoses.

Planning and Implementation
Nursing Interventions

A. Reduction of intracranial pressure and prevention of irreversible brain damage

1. Provide continuing assessment of the patient's level of responsiveness (see p. 761).

2. Maintain a neurologic observation record.
   a. The Glascow Coma Scale (Fig. 18-3) is a tool for objectively assessing the consciousness level by determining the patient's best response to stimulation in terms of eye opening, motor response and verbal response.
   b. Know the patient's baseline (initial) condition; all observations should be compared with and evaluated accordingly.
   c. Carry out *repeated* nursing assessments—to determine clinical improvement or deterioration.
   d. Watch the patient carefully when changing his position; avoid compression of jugular veins (head falling to one side).

3. Use intracranial pressure monitoring when prescribed for sustained ICP; elevations (above 20 mm. Hg persisting 15 minutes or more or if there is a significant shift in pressure).

4. Employ hyperventilation with volume ventilator—hyperventilation leads to respiratory alkalosis, which causes cerebral vasoconstriction and decreased cerebral blood volume and results in reduction of intracranial pressure.
   a. Administer paralyzing agents (pancuronium bromide) or small doses of sedative if the patient

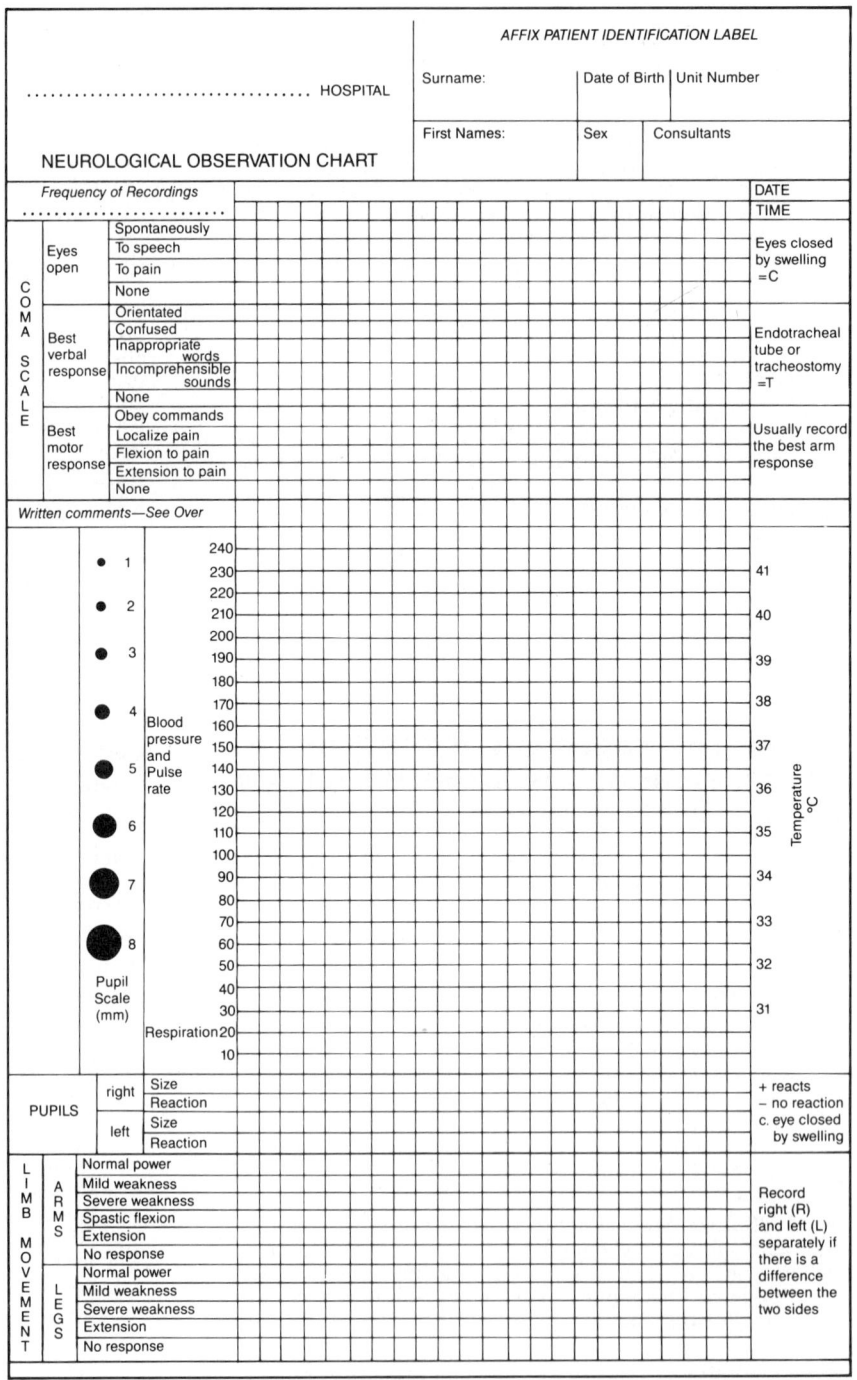

Figure 18-3. Example of observation chart that includes the Glasgow Coma Scale. (Reproduced by courtesy of Butterworth and Company, London, from Campkin and Turner, Neurosurgical Anaesthesia and Intensive Care)

is coughing, straining, or fighting the ventilator—to prevent unacceptable rises in pressure.
  b. Monitor arterial blood gases.
5. Administer pharmacologic agents as prescribed to reduce intracranial pressure.
  a. Hyperosmotic therapy (mannitol)—lowers cerebrospinal fluid pressure by reducing the volume of intracranial contents and rate of cerebrospinal fluid formation.
    (1) Evaluate for dehydration and electrolyte im-

balance since osmotherapy leads to dehydration
    (2) Insert indwelling urethral catheter since hyperosmolar solutions cause diuresis.
  b. Diuretics—act by removing sodium and water from edematous areas
  c. Steroids (dexamethasone)
  d. Barbiturates—reduce ICP; reduce brain metabolism and systemic blood pressure.
6. Closely monitor the systemic arterial pressure.

7. Prepare for CSF drainage to control pressure waves if ICP remains elevated.
   a. Via ventricular cannula used for ICP monitoring.
   b. Via needle inserted through burr hole.
8. Monitor the patient's temperature.
   a. Avoid elevation of temperature, since fever increases cerebral metabolism and the rate of cerebral edema formation.
   b. Monitor cardiac output with Swan–Ganz catheter if measures are taken to reduce the patient's temperature.
9. Avoid activities or positions that produce a rise in intracranial pressure.
   a. Keep the patient in a head-up posture with the head in a neutral plane with the body.
   b. Avoid turning the head from side to side or allowing the head to fall to one side (compresses jugular veins)—may markedly increase ICP.
   c. Avoid the prone position, flexion of the neck, extreme hip flexion, the Valsalva maneuver, isometric muscle contractions, coughing, and straining.
   d. Avoid any stimuli that can precipitate ICP.
      (1) Watch ICP monitor during endotracheal suctioning; discontinue procedure if ICP rises precipitously.
      (2) Give small amounts of sedation and mild manual hyperventilation before suctioning to blunt effects of noxious stimuli.
      (3) Discontinue chest physical therapy if ICP exceeds 30 mm. Hg; wait until pressure falls below 15 mm. Hg.
10. Prepare for high-dose barbiturate therapy when other treatment measures fail to control intracranial pressure; this requires ICP and intra-arterial monitoring and an experienced ICU team.
11. Prepare for surgical intervention if the patient's condition deteriorates.

Evaluation
Expected Outcomes
1. Becomes increasingly more responsive to environment
2. Responds to questions appropriately
3. Obeys simple commands
4. Oriented to time, place, and person
5. See Head Injury Evaluation, page 768.

Continuous Intracranial Pressure Monitoring

Intracranial pressure monitoring is the recording of the pressure exerted within the skull by the brain, cerebral blood, and cerebrospinal fluid. It gives a dynamic status of intracranial events.

Purpose
1. To provide immediate information for early detection and treatment of intracranial pressure to prevent brain deterioration
2. To guide therapy for control of intracranial pressure
3. To have access to cerebrospinal fluid for sampling and drainage
4. To serve as a prognostic indicator

Underlying Principles
1. Intracranial pressure is not in a steady state, but fluctuates; fluctuations are indicated by waves of high pressure and troughs of relatively normal pressure. These waves have been classified as A waves (plateau waves), B waves, and C waves.
2. The plateau (A) waves have clinical significance:
   a. They are characterized by rapid increases and decreases of pressure with recurring elevations of intracranial pressure that may last from 5–20 minutes and range in amplitude between 50–100 mm. Hg.
   b. Plateau waves are usually related to cerebral dysfunction and caused by brain shift or distortion.
   c. They may be accompanied by transient symptoms—headache, nausea, disturbances of consciousness.
3. B waves are of shorter duration ($^1/_2$–2 minutes) with smaller amplitude (up to 50 mm. Hg). They have less clinical significance than A waves, but B waves occurring in runs tend to be associated with pathologic depressions of consciousness and may precede the appearance of A waves.
4. C waves are small, rhythmic oscillations with frequencies of approximately 6 per minute at amplitudes up to 20 mm. Hg. They appear to be related to rhythmic variations of the systemic arterial blood pressure (Traube–Hering–Mayer waves).

Techniques for Measuring Intracranial Pressure*
1. *Intraventricular catheter*—placement of a catheter into the frontal horn of the lateral ventricle via a burr hole or twist drill hole; the intraventricular catheter is connected to an external pressure transducer by a fluid-filled manometer or a strain gauge. The output from the pressure transducer is displayed on a chart recorder.
2. *Subarachnoid screw (bolt)*—hollow screw that is inserted through a small twist-drill hole into the calvarium (dome of skull) to rest in the subarachnoid space; the external end of the screw is fitted to a 3-way stopcock connected to an external transducer for graphic and numerical recordings.
3. *Subdural cup catheter*—a barium-impregnated Silastic ribbon with a central lumen that is inserted via craniotomy or through burr holes; uses arachnoid surface of the brain as its sensing membrane.
4. *Epidural intracranial pressure monitoring*—implantation of miniature pressure sensor and transmitter in epidural space; a fiberoptic cable exits through the scalp and is attached to the bedside monitor.

Management
1. Watch for developing and increasing frequency of plateau wave. Normal ICP (as measured by any technique) will generally fluctuate around 10 torr (10 mm. Hg).
   a. Treatment is usually initiated when intracranial pressure is 15 torr to 20 torr.
   b. Start immediate measures to reduce intracranial pressure (see p. 763) since this signifies that the brain function may be in disequilibrium.
2. Monitor the patient's arterial blood gases—a high

---

* The direct measurement of intracranial pressure may be accomplished by a number of monitoring techniques that require complex sensors, transducers, recording devices, etc. The nurse needs a working knowledge of the system being used and its limitations. There is not a single ideal method of measuring ICP.

$PaCO_2$ will cause vasodilation of the cerebral vessels, an increase in cerebral blood flow, and a rise in intracranial pressure.

3. Monitor blood pressure and respirations—intracranial pressure wave forms correlate with changes in blood pressure and the respiratory cycle.
4. Keep connections tight and the system closed—any leakage of the fluid column produces a gradual drift from the baseline.
   a. Recalibrate the system according to manufacturer's directions at regular intervals.
   b. Realign the transducer and recalibrate if the level of the bed is changed—most systems require careful referencing of transducers.
   c. Use rigid sterile technique when opening a stopcock, changing a syringe, reconnecting tubing, etc.
5. Avoid activities that can initiate a rise in intracranial pressure.
   a. Avoid excessive rotation or flexion of the patient's head—interferes with the outflow of blood from the cranial cavity; temporary occlusion causes a rise in intracranial pressure.
   b. Avoid the Valsalva maneuver (straining at stool; coughing) which impedes venous return from brain.
6. Support the patient physically and emotionally—some monitoring systems limit patient mobility.
   a. Monitor site for infection—redness, swelling, leakage.
   b. Give meticulous care to catheter site.
   c. Change dressing as prescribed.
7. Watch for complications—infection, CSF leakage, blocked catheter, equipment malfunction.

Nursing Management of the Patient With a Head Injury

Assessment
Clinical Manifestations
1. Unconsciousness or disturbance in consciousness
2. Headache
3. Vertigo
4. Confusion or delirium
5. Restlessness
6. Changes in body temperature
7. Respiratory irregularities
8. Pupillary abnormalities
9. Sudden onset of neurologic deficit

Physical Assessment
1. Open brain injuries—recognized by inspection; patient taken to operating room
2. Depressed skull fracture—may/may not be recognized by gentle palpation
3. Basilar skull fracture—determined (in part) on basis of physical findings

Diagnostic Evaluation
1. CT scanning of head—reveals wide variety of lesions
2. Cerebral angiography—used when CT scans are not available
3. Skull films and cervical spine films—reveal bony abnormalities of skull and spine

▶ **NURSING ALERT:** Regard every patient who has a head injury as having a potential spinal cord injury. A

significant number of patients are under the influence of alcohol at the time of injury, which may mask the nature and severity of the injury.

Patient Problems/Nursing Diagnoses
1. Potential ineffective breathing pattern, ventilation, and brain oxygenation related to cerebral hypoxia
2. Alteration in consciousness related to head trauma
3. Alteration in fluid and electrolyte balance related to altered pathophysiology from head injury
4. Inadequate nutritional intake related to disturbance of consciousness
5. Potential for pressure sores related to disturbance of consciousness
6. Self-care deficits (feeding, bathing, hygiene, dressing, toileting) related to unconsciousness
7. Potential for physical and psychological complications related to brain injury

Planning and Implementation
Nursing Interventions
A. Immediate management in Emergency Department

See page 939.

B. Establishment of effective respiratory and ventilatory function

1. Prepare for endotracheal intubation or tracheostomy and ventilatory assistance as indicated—to optimize arterial oxygenation and allow hyperventilation.
   a. Controlled hyperventilation (which constricts blood vessels and reduces blood flow and oxygen to the brain) is helpful when brain blood flow is excessive; may be dangerous for the patient whose brain blood flow is abnormally low.
   b. Carry out arterial blood gas studies—to determine respiratory adequacy and evaluate effects of therapy.
   c. See page 227, managing the patient requiring mechanical ventilation.
2. Place the patient in a head-up position (with head in a neutral plane with the body) if the patient is not in shock or has a spinal cord injury—improves venous drainage, reduces jugular venous pressure, and lowers intracranial pressure. (See also the management of intracranial pressure.)
3. Maintain normothermia with fever sponges, hypothermia blanket, etc.—to lower metabolic requirements of the brain.

C. Evaluation of responses to external stimulation and improvement in level of consciousness

1. Observe, evaluate, and carry out repeated clinical examinations to determine minute-to-minute, hour-to-hour changes in the patient's status—pathologic events occurring as a result of head injury include (1) intracranial hemorrhage (extradural, subdural, intracerebral), which causes elevation of intracranial pressure, (2) edema, and (3) sepsis.

▶ **NURSING ALERT:** A change in the level of responsiveness is the most sensitive indicator of improvement or deterioration. The level of responsiveness may change from minute to minute.

   a. Make repeated and specific documentation of clinical findings, including state of responsiveness (consciousness), eye opening, verbal response,

motor response, quality of breathing, size and reaction of pupils—essential to assess whether the patient's condition is improving, worsening, or unchanged (see Neurologic Flow Record, p. 764).
  b. Describe stimuli administered and response obtained.
2. Start intracranial pressure (ICP) monitoring for patients with severe injuries, especially those with no eye opening, no verbal response, and nonpurposeful motor responses.
3. Obtain computed tomographic (CT) scan or angiogram as directed—to determine intracranial pathology.
  a. Prepare for surgical intervention if deteriorating level of consciousness or increasing focal neurologic deficit (or both)—for evacuation of a clot, placement of ICP monitoring device (see p. 765), resection of contused brain, etc.
  b. See page 763, the Patient with Increasing Intracranial Pressure.
4. Use intensive therapy to keep intracranial pressure at acceptable level.
  a. Hyperosmotic therapy (mannitol)—to dehydrate brain and reduce cerebral edema, thus lowering intracranial pressure.
  b. Steroids (dextramethasone)—to reduce brain edema (controversial); may have rebound effect.
    (1) Cimetidine may be given—to control gastric acid output.
    (2) Gastrointestinal hemorrhage is a common complication in head-injured patients on high-dose steroid therapy.
  c. Anticonvulsants (phenytoin)—usually given to patients with head injuries that produce coma.
  d. Barbiturates (pentobarbital)—to reduce cerebral metabolism and lower ICP.
  e. Muscle relaxants—to prevent coughing and straining while on ventilator, which raises ICP.
  f. Treat for shock—from associated fractures and injuries of chest, abdomen, pelvis.
  g. Monitor for systemic arterial hypertension.

D. Maintaining fluid, electrolyte, and nutritional balance

1. Give intravenous solutions fairly slowly—overhydration may lead to cerebral edema.
2. Restrict fluid intake in patients with severe cerebral contusion—to avoid increase in volume of extracellular space.
3. Weigh daily and keep records of intake and output and urinary specific gravity—to determine fluid loss and dehydration and to monitor for development of diabetes insipidus (especially in patients with hypothalamic involvement, craniofacial trauma, basilar skull fracture).
4. Carry out serial blood and urine electrolyte and osmolality studies—head injuries may be accompanied by disorders of sodium regulation, water retention, and decreased serum potassium levels; assess for apathy, headache, anorexia, nausea, vomiting, and in some instances, coma and convulsions.
5. Give nasogastric feedings (or gastrostomy feedings) if the patient is unable to swallow after several days, to maintain homeostasis.
6. Insert indwelling urethral catheter if the patient is unconscious—for assessment of urinary volume and to prevent restlessness from distended bladder.

E. Avoiding complications

1. Observe orifices for leakage of spinal fluid through the nose (rhinorrhea) or through the ear (otorrhea)—serious complication of head injury, which carries risk of meningitis.

▶ **NURSING ALERT:** Cerebrospinal fluid leakage may mask the usual clinical signs of an expanding intracranial hematoma without evidence of increased intracranial pressure, changes in vital signs, or alternations in state of consciousness.

  a. Tape sterile cotton pad under nose or loosely against ear to collect drainage.
  b. Elevate head of bed approximately 20–30 degrees as directed—to reduce intracraniai pressure and promote spontaneous closure of leak.
  c. Discourage the patient from blowing nose, sneezing, or straining.
  d. Persistence of spinal fluid otorrhea or rhinorrhea usually requires surgical intervention.
2. Support the patient during episodes of restlessness.
  a. Avoid restraints if at all possible; straining increases intracranial pressure.
  b. Give small doses of chloral hydrate, paraldehyde, or tranquilizing drugs; do not give narcotics and sedatives since these mask the level of responsiveness.
  c. Maintain as quiet an environment as possible.
  d. Be aware that restlessness may be caused by extradural hematoma, cerebral hypoxia, respiratory obstruction, pain from fractured extremities, tight cast or bandages, or distended bladder.
3. Watch for gastrointestinal complications—gastric acid hypersecretion is common in patients with head injuries and may result in ulceration and hemorrhage of stomach and upper intestinal tract (Cushing's ulcer—a potentially perforating ulcer of stomach or duodenum).

F. Preventing physical and psychological complications

1. See Nursing Management of the Unconscious Patient, page 760.
2. Carry out rehabilitation techniques.
  a. Position the patient correctly to prevent contractures.
  b. Put all extremities through range-of-motion exercises.
  c. Begin a program of graded exercises—exercise restores fitness and flagging motivation and assists in elevating the patient's mood to one of optimism.
  d. Keep the skin dry, clean, and free of pressure—to prevent pressure sores.
  e. Gradually increase physical and mental activity (including resumption of increasingly difficult mental tasks).
3. Be aware of aftereffects of head injury—usually related to coma duration, severity of injury, and age of patient.
  a. Post-traumatic syndrome
    (1) Headache
    (2) Dizziness and vertigo
    (3) Emotional instability or irritability, inability to concentrate, impaired memory
  b. Brain damage
  c. Post-traumatic epilepsy

d. Post-traumatic hydrocephalus
e. Late cerebrospinal fluid leaks
f. Cranial nerve dysfunction (anosmia, diplopia, facial palsy)
g. Post-traumatic neuroses and psychoses

Patient/Family Education

1. Reassure the patient that amnesia regarding injury impact is common.
2. Encourage the patient to continue his rehabilitation program following discharge; improvement in status may continue up to 3 or more years following injury.
3. Lessening of headache may be the most reliable guide to recovery; use a second pillow/backrest at night.
4. Encourage the patient to return gradually to usual activities.
5. Family may need information regarding cognitive and personality deficits and changes.
6. Family may need help in setting limits for the injured patient's impulses (anger, emotional lability, etc.) and in realistically evaluating his capabilities. Family may have difficulty in understanding and accepting alterations in patient's behavior.
   a. Some patients with severe trauma will be left with functional and psychological disabilities.
   b. The patient may require neuropsychological testing (IQ; tests of concentration, perception) to determine mental deficits.

7. If the patient is discharged from hospital in a relatively short time, tell the family to bring him to the emergency department *immediately* if the following signs occur: difficulty in awakening, difficulty in speaking, confusion, severe headache, vomiting, development of unequal pupils, or weakness of one side of body.

Evaluation

Expected Outcomes

1. Attains or maintains effective breathing, ventilation, and brain oxygenation—arterial blood gases within normal limits; normal breath sounds upon auscultation; spontaneous breathing without ventilatory assistance
2. Becomes increasingly more responsive and oriented to environment—opens eyes spontaneously; responds to questions appropriately; obeys simple commands; oriented to time, place, and person
3. Attains/maintains nutritional status—requests and takes fluids by mouth; maintains weight within expected limits
4. Demonstrates continuing progress toward recovery
5. Shows no evidence of physical or psychological complications—absence of seizures; less frequent outbursts of irritability or instability; beginning ability to remember names and recognize faces; reduced headache

Guidelines: Administering a Fever Sponge

Fever is an abnormal elevation of body temperature.

A *fever sponge* is the bathing of the body with tepid water (or alcohol and water) for a period of time to reduce fever. It is particularly effective in neurologic conditions in which there is a disturbance of the temperature-regulating center. Fever increases both intracranial pressure and the rate of development of cerebral edema.

Causes
1. Infection
2. Disturbance of temperature-regulating center (trauma, central nervous system hemorrhage)
3. Tumors; diseases of blood-forming organs
4. Heat stroke
5. Drug toxicity; allergens
6. Delirium tremens

Purpose To reduce body temperature when fever in itself may be deleterious.

Equipment

Basin of tepid water 21.1°–29.1°C. (70°–85°F.)	Hot water bottle with cover
or	Ice bag with cover
Basin of alcohol (25% saturated with tepid water)	Towels
Bath blanket/plastic sheet	7 Washcloths or wash mitts

▶ **NURSING ALERT:** Make certain that the patient is adequately hydrated; unrecognized dehydration can result in decreased circulating blood volume, causing peripheral vasoconstriction which prevents heat loss.

Procedure

Nursing Action	Rationale/Amplification
Preparatory Phase	
1. Place plastic sheet under patient and bath blanket over the patient.	
2. Remove top bedding.	
Performance Phase	
1. Take temperature, pulse, and respiration before starting sponge.	1. This serves as a baseline for determining effectiveness of treatment.

Procedure
(Cont.)

Nursing Action	Rationale/Amplification

2. Give antipyretic medication as directed 15–20 minutes before starting sponge.
  a. Acetaminophen
  b. Chlorpromazine
	2. There is a more rapid reduction of fever when sponging is combined with administration of antipyretic medication.
	  a. Has antipyretic and analgesic action
	  b. Controls shivering

3. Apply ice bag to head.	3. Relieves headache and promotes patient comfort.
4. Apply hot-water bottle to feet.	4. Aids in combating chilliness and shivering.
5. Use the same sequence for sponging as for giving a bed bath.	
6. Place a cold wet compress (washcloth) on neck and in each groin and axilla.	6. The application of cold over superficial large blood vessels aids in lowering body temperature.
7. Expose the body area to be sponged. Place a towel under area.	
8. Using 2 washcloths or mitts alternately, wet in water or alcohol and water solution; pat each area so that solution is uniform over skin surface.	8. Vaporization of water removes heat from the surface of the skin. Alcohol vaporizes at a lower temperature and removes heat from the skin more rapidly. Tepid water and alcohol are highly effective in producing vasodilation and evaporation of heat from skin.
9. If the patient's skin feels cold to the touch, apply skin friction to bring the blood to the surface.	
10. Bathe each extremity 5 minutes; bathe entire back and buttocks 5–10 minutes; bathe trunk and abdomen 5 minutes.	10. The fever sponge should not exceed 30 minutes.
11. Allow a fan to blow over the patient while sponging him if fever is high.	11. Increased air movement augments heat loss.
12. Watch for extreme shivering. Cover the patient and wait a few minutes before proceeding with sponge.	12. Shivering may raise heat production.
13. Stop sponge if cyanosis, mottling, chilling do not stop when friction (rubbing) is applied to the skin.	13. These symptoms indicate a change in vasomotor tone.

Follow-Up Phase

1. Remove bath blanket and plastic sheet. Place a dry gown on patient.	
2. Record TPR 30 minutes after sponge is finished.	2. Postsponge temperature indicates whether or not treatment has been effective.

Nursing Management of the Patient Having a Seizure

Seizures are episodes of abnormal motor, sensory, autonomic, or psychic activity (or a combination of these) as a consequence of sudden excessive discharge from cerebral neurons.

Nursing Interventions

A. Prevent injury to the patient

The following should be noted before and during the attack:

1. Description of the circumstances before the attack (visual stimuli, auditory stimuli, olfactory stimuli, tactile stimuli, emotional or psychic disturbances, sleep, hyperventilation).
2. The first thing the patient does in an attack—where the movements or the stiffness starts, position of the eyeballs and the head at the beginning of the attack. This information gives clues as to the location of the epileptogenic focus in the brain. (In recording, always state whether or not the beginning of the attack was observed.)
3. The type of movements of the part involved.
4. The parts involved. (Turn back bed covers and expose patient.)
5. The size of both pupils. Are the eyes open? Did the eyes/head turn to one side?
6. Whether or not automatisms (involuntary motor activity such as lip smacking or repeated swallowing) were observed.
7. Incontinence of urine or feces.
8. Did the patient bite his tongue?
9. Duration of each phase of the attack.
10. Unconsciousness, if present, and its duration.
11. Any obvious paralysis or weakness of arms or legs after the attack.
12. Inability to speak after the attack.
13. Movements at the end of the seizure.
14. Whether or not the patient sleeps afterward.
15. Whether or not the patient was confused following the attack.

B. Support the patient during the seizure

1. Ensure an adequate airway.
  a. When jaws are clenched in spasm, do not attempt to pry open to insert a mouth gag.
  b. If aura preceded seizure, insert a folded handkerchief between the teeth taking care not to injure your fingers as patient's jaw may go into spasm—to reduce possibility of tongue or cheek being bitten.
  c. When respiration returns following the seizure and the patient becomes flaccid, turn his head to the side to facilitate drainage of mucus and saliva and to prevent aspiration.
  d. Try to hold the lower jaw forward when the patient is in flaccid stage.

2. Try to protect the patient from injuring himself.
   a. Protect his head with a folded blanket/pad to prevent head injury.
   b. Loosen constrictive clothing.
   c. Push aside any furniture that the patient may strike during the seizure.
3. Give the patient privacy and protect him from curious onlookers; use a calm manner to defuse a potentially embarrassing event for the patient.
4. Stay with the patient until he is fully conscious.
5. Reorient him to his environment when he awakens.
6. Handle the patient with calm persuasion and gentle restraint when seizures are characterized by disturbed behavior.

Family Health Education

Instruct the family as follows:
1. Summon medical assistance if a second seizure follows before consciousness is regained. There is a risk of status epilepticus developing.
2. If the patient has severe postictal (following seizure) excitement, it may be necessary to bring him to the emergency department.

Nursing Management of the Patient Undergoing Intracranial Surgery

Craniotomy is the surgical opening of the skull to gain access to intracranial structures, remove a tumor, relieve intracranial pressure, evacuate a blood clot, or stop hemorrhage (Fig. 18-4).
   Craniectomy is excision of a portion of the skull.
   Cranioplasty is repair of a cranial defect by means of a plastic or metal plate.

Preoperative Management

Goal:
Determine the precise location of the lesion (clot, tumor, aneurysm).

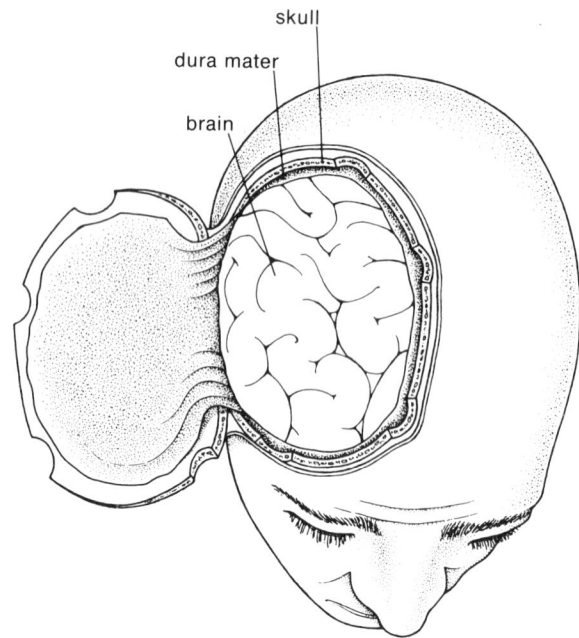

Figure 18-4. Craniotomy.

1. Assist the patient undergoing diagnostic tests and frequent neurologic examinations.
2. Evaluate and record the patient's symptoms and signs (paralysis, aphasia) preoperatively in order to make postoperative comparisons.
3. Explain the immediate postoperative care (monitoring devices, intubation, lines and catheters, dressings, and drains) and expected postoperative course.
4. Support the patient with neurologic motor and sensory defects.
   a. Position paralyzed extremities to prevent contracture deformities.
   b. Familiarize the blind patient with his environment.
      (1) Personnel entering room should announce themselves—helps the patient understand incoming stimuli.
      (2) Help patient to assume an active role in his care.
   c. Assist the aphasic patient to communicate by means of picture cards, writing materials, gestures, etc.
   d. Protect the confused patient.
      (1) Remove disturbing environmental stimuli.
      (2) Keep patient oriented to time and place; place wall calendar and clock where the patient can see them.
   e. Instruct and encourage the patient and family about the impending surgery—to relieve anxiety and tension.
5. Prepare the patient physically for surgery.
   a. Clip and shampoo the hair with bacteriostatic shampoo; shaving of the area of operation is usually done immediately prior to the surgery. Save the hair.
   b. Report any evidences of scalp infection.
   c. Give enemas only as directed—straining upon defecation raises intracranial pressure.
   d. Give medications and assist with treatments as indicated.
      (1) Steroids—to decrease brain edema.
      (2) Anticonvulsants—to prevent seizures.
      (3) Ventricular drainage—tumor may block ventricular fluid flow into the spinal canal, and the cerebrospinal fluid must be removed directly from the ventricles.
      (4) Parietal burr holes may be made immediately prior to posterior fossa surgery—to facilitate ventricular cannulation if cerebrospinal fluid drainage is necessary.
      (5) Indwelling urethral catheter—to assess urinary volume during dehydrating operative period.

Postoperative Patient Problems/Nursing Diagnoses

1. Impaired neurologic function related to brain pathology and postoperative cerebral edema.
2. Sensory perceptual alterations (visual, auditory, olfactory) related to head bandage, and postoperative orbital and cerebral edema.
3. Potential for complications related to nature of surgery.

Postoperative Nursing Interventions

Goals:
Watch for life-threatening complications, namely increasing intracranial pressure from edema and bleeding.
Improve the functional status of the patient.

A. Establish proper respiratory exchange—to eliminate systemic hypercarbia and anoxia which increase cerebral edema.

1. Keep the patient in a lateral or a semiprone position until consciousness returns.
2. Employ tracheopharyngeal aspiration carefully—to remove secretions; suctioning can raise intracranial pressure by an arousal response and by CO_2 accumulation during apnea.
3. Carry out arterial blood gas studies—to determine respiratory adequacy.
4. Employ hyperventilation when prescribed—to reduce cerebral blood flow and intracranial pressure.
5. Elevate the head of the bed 30 cm. (12 inches) after patient is conscious—to aid venous drainage of the brain.
6. See that the patient has nothing by mouth until an active coughing and swallowing reflex is demonstrated.
7. Monitor the patient's cardiovascular status.

B. Assess the patient's level of responsiveness.

1. Eye opening (spontaneous, to sound, to pain); pupil reactions to light.
2. Response to commands:
   a. Answers questions readily and correctly
   b. Can perform a complex maneuver
   c. Responds to simple command
   d. Gives delayed or unequal response
   e. Reacts only to loud voice
   f. Does not respond
3. Spinal motor reflexes (pinch Achilles tendon, arm, or other body site):
   a. Prompt, purposeful withdrawal
   b. Sluggish or nonpurposeful movement of extremities
   c. Facial grimace
   d. Involuntary voiding
   e. No response
4. Spontaneous activity:
   a. Verbal or other communication
   b. Changes in posture (frequency)
   c. Breathing pattern
   d. Retching, vomiting
   e. Restlessness, twitching, tremors, convulsions

C. Evaluate for signs and symptoms of increasing intracranial pressure.

1. Assess the patient (minute-by-minute, hour-by-hour) for:
   a. Diminished response to stimuli
   b. Fluctuations of vital signs
   c. Restlessness
   d. Weakness and paralysis of extremities
   e. Increasing headache
   f. Changes or disturbances of vision; pupillary changes
2. Control postoperative cerebral edema.
   a. Give osmotic dehydrating agents, and glycerol, when prescribed, in postoperative period to reduce brain swelling.
   b. Keep patient *slightly* underhydrated—to combat cerebral edema.
   c. Record urinary specific gravity at intervals—especially indicated for surgery of the pituitary and hypothalamus.
   d. Evaluate electrolyte status:
      (1) Early postoperative weight gain indicates fluid retention; a greater than estimated loss of weight indicates negative water balance.
      (2) Loss of sodium and chlorides will produce weakness, lethargy, and coma.
      (3) Low potassium will cause confusion and lower level of responsiveness.
   e. Give IV fluids with care—rate and composition depend on fluid deficit, urine output, and blood loss.
      Fluid input and fluid losses should remain relatively equal.
   f. Institute hypothermia procedures when indicated (see below) to decrease brain metabolism.
   g. Elevate head of bed 20–30 degrees to reduce intracranial pressure.
      Keep head in midline to prevent jugular compression and facilitate venous drainage.
   h. Avoid stimuli that may increase cerebral blood flow (CBF)—a rise in CBF may increase cerebral blood volume to dangerous levels.
   i. Use intracranial pressure monitoring (see p. 765) if the patient is at risk for intracranial hypertension.
   j. Monitor closely for blood pressure changes. Notify neurosurgeon if hypertension is present.

D. Keep the patient normothermic during the postoperative period—temperature control may be lost in certain neurologic states; a higher temperature increases the metabolic demands of the brain.

1. Take rectal temperature at specified intervals. Extremities may be cold and dry because of paralysis of heat-losing mechanisms (vasodilation and sweating).
2. Employ measures to reduce excessive fever when present.
   a. Remove blankets; place loin cloth over patient.
   b. Give aspirin if indicated. (High fever of central origin is less responsive to aspirin.)
   c. Apply ice bags to axilla and groin—application of cold over large superficial vessel helps lower body temperature.
   d. Give tepid water or alcohol sponge.
   e. Use a fan blowing on patient—to increase surface cooling.
   f. Use hypothermia blanket.
   g. Give chlorpromazine (IM)—prevents excessive shivering.
   h. Utilize ECG monitoring to detect arrhythmias during hypothermia procedures.

E. Perform supportive measures until the patient is able to care for himself.

1. Change position frequently since pain and pressure responses are variable.
2. Give analgesics that do not mask level of responsiveness—codeine, aspirin.
3. Support the patient if convulsive seizures occur (see p. 769).
4. Relieve signs of periocular edema.
   a. Lubricate eyelids and area around eyes with petrolatum.
   b. Apply light compresses in pliofilm (taped over eye) at specified intervals.
   c. Watch for signs of keratitis if cornea has no sensation.
5. Put extremities through range-of-motion exercises.
6. Use aseptic measures in management of indwelling 3-way urethral catheter (see p. 508).
7. Evaluate and support the patient during episodes of restlessness.

a. Evaluate for airway obstruction, distended bladder, meningeal irritation from bloody cerebrospinal fluid.

b. Pad the patient's hands and bed rails—to protect the patient from injury.

8. Watch for leakage of cerebrospinal fluid since there is ever present danger of meningitis.

a. Differentiate between cerebrospinal fluid (CSF) and mucus.

(1) Collect fluid on Dextrostix—if CSF is present, indicator will have positive reaction since cerebrospinal fluid contains sugar.

(2) Assess for moderate elevation of temperature and mild neck rigidity.

b. Keep cerebrospinal pressure low.

(1) Ventricular catheters may be inserted in patient undergoing surgery of posterior fossa (ventriculostomy); catheter(s) connected to a closed reservoir system.
Patency of the catheter can be noted by the pulsations of the fluid in the tubing.

(2) Elevate head of bed.

(3) Give antibiotics as indicated.

9. Reinforce bloodstained dressings with sterile dressing; blood-soaked dressings act as a culture medium for bacteria.

10. Evaluate the patient with hypophysectomy (surgery on pituitary) for diabetes insipidus.

a. Weigh daily.

b. Keep fluid input and output record.

F. Assess for complications.

1. Intracranial hemorrhage. (Postoperative bleeding may be intraventricular, intracerebral, intracerebellar, subdural, or extradural.)

a. Watch for progressive impairment of state of responsiveness, signs of increasing intracranial pressure, focal seizures.

b. Prepare the patient for CT scan; cerebral angiography.

c. Prepare the patient for reoperation and evacuation of hematoma.

2. Brain edema.

3. Postoperative meningitis.

4. Wound infections (scalp, bone flap)—wound may have to be reopened.

5. Pulmonary complications.

6. Cranial nerve dysfunction.

7. Epilepsy.

a. Give anticonvulsants on a long-term basis.

b. Watch for status epilepticus which may occur after any intracranial operation.

8. Gastrointestinal ulceration (signs and symptoms of hemorrhage and perforation or both).

Expected Outcomes

1. Demonstrates improved neurologic function

a. Opens eyes upon request—obeys commands with appropriate motor responses

b. Gradually participates in self-care activities; shows increasing alertness

2. Copes with postoperative sensory alterations

a. Makes needs known with gestures

b. Verbalizes that difficulties in seeing/hearing are temporary

3. Reveals minimal/absence of complications

a. No evidence of increased intracranial pressure

b. No evidence of rhinorrhea, otorrhea, or CSF seepage

c. Absence of fever or inflammation and infection around scalp incision

d. Absence of seizures

Neurosurgical Management of Intractable Pain

Intractable pain is pain that causes incapacitation of function and that cannot be relieved satisfactorily by drugs short of drug addiction or incapacitating sedation.

Therapeutic Goal:
Interrupt the pathways by which the painful sensations are perceived.

Causes

1. Malignant disease (especially of cervix, bladder, prostate, lower bowel)

2. Trigeminal neuralgia; spinal cord arachnoiditis

3. Uncontrollable ischemia or other forms of tissue destruction

Rhizotomy

1. *Posterior or spinal rhizotomy*—surgical interruption of selected posterior spinal nerve roots between the ganglion and the cord. This results in permanent loss of sensation and may be done at any spinal level.
Clinical uses—pain relief of lung cancer, head and neck malignancies.

2. *Percutaneous rhizotomy*—radio frequency current is used to deliver heat selectively to coagulate small pain fibers; the fibers concerned with touch and proprioception are preserved.

3. *Chemical rhizotomy*—injection of alcohol (phenol

or mixture of drugs) into the subarachnoid space; medication is maneuvered over affected nerve roots by tilting the patient to achieve desired level. The patient's perception of pain is absent but motor nerve root sensations are not.

Cordotomy

Surgical interruption of the anterolateral quadrant of the spinal cord for the relief of intractable pain.

1. Obliterates pain and temperature sense at some level below where the cord was sectioned, but leaves motor function intact.

2. May be done with a radiofrequency current applied through a needle electrode inserted percutaneously under x-ray guidance or by open cordotomy. Cordotomy is helpful for patients with unilateral pain of malignant origin, especially of thorax, abdomen, or lower extremities.

Nursing Management Following Cordotomy

A. Watch for complications

1. Respiratory (cervical cordotomy)

a. Observe for fatigue and weakening of voice.

b. Monitor arterial blood gases. Patients with reduced oxygen levels may require oxygen at night until blood gas levels return to normal. (Patient

may ventilate adequately while awake but may experience progressive hypercarbia and hypoxia while asleep.)
   c. Assisted mechanical ventilation may be required.
2. Urinary retention (usually transient)
3. Ipsilateral (on the same side) leg weakness from edema of the spinal cord—usually disappears in a few days
4. Hemorrhage—may produce motor and sensory loss; immediate surgical intervention is indicated.
   Test motion, strength, and sensation of each extremity every few hours during the first 48 hours.
5. See management of the patient following disc surgery, page 808, for principles of care also relevant to these operations.
6. Keep the patient flat as prescribed—less tension on incision.
7. For cervical incision, keep the neck in a neutral position.
8. Feel the patient's skin temperature at intervals to ascertain skin temperature changes.
9. Watch for development of pressure sores.
   a. Teach the patient to inspect his skin using a hand mirror to view hard-to-see areas.
   b. Place the patient on bladder-training program (see p. 70) if high cervical procedure has caused loss of bladder control.

B. Family and Patient Health Education

1. Protect the patient against external temperature changes and extremes of weather; he may not be aware of sunburn/frostbite; watch for skin lacerations due to unnoticed injury.
2. Test temperature of bath water before getting in tub.
3. Avoid constricting clothing that impairs circulation.
4. Sexual function may be impaired in males.

Sympathectomy

Interruption of afferent pathways in the sympathetic division of the autonomic nervous system; used to control pain from causalgia and peripheral vascular disorders (eliminates vasospasm and improves peripheral blood supply).

Transsphenoidal Hypophysectomy

Ablation of pituitary gland by transsphenoidal approach for relief of intractable pain (usually from metastatic cancer of breast or prostate gland). See page 696.

Psychosurgical Approaches

Procedures altering the patient's response to pain
1. *Thalamotomy*—destruction (unilaterally or bilaterally) of specific cell groups within thalamus. It is accomplished through burr holes—a lesion is produced by radio frequency current, cryosurgery, etc. This technique is useful for pain of central origin.
2. *Cingulumotomy*—unilateral or bilateral interruption of the anterior cingulate bundle in the frontal lobe of the brain.
   a. Accomplished by either open or stereotaxic approach.
   b. Tends to modify the patient's affective reaction to pain.

Suppression of Pain by Electrical Stimulation
(Neuromodulation)

Neuromodulation is a method of suppressing pain by applying an electronic device that stimulates the different parts of the nervous system for pain relief. It is accomplished by (1) transcutaneous electrical nerve stimulation (TENS), or (2) dorsal column stimulation.

A. Underlying Principles

1. This therapy is based on the theory (gate control theory) that nondestructive stimuli can interfere with the transmission of pain within the central nervous system. It is thought to relieve pain by preventing pain messages from reaching the brain. Another theory is that nerve stimulation enhances the release of endorphins, which relieves pain. The exact mechanics are not yet fully known.
2. It is nondestructive in nature and does not carry the potential risks of weakness, numbness, dysesthesia, bladder/bowel incontinence, impotence, or irreversibility, as do destructive surgical procedures for pain relief. However, long-term effectiveness of TENS is quite limited (see below).
3. The system consists of a pulse generator (containing the power source and electronics of the system), a pair of electric cables, and 2 flexible electrodes, which transfer the stimulating signal.
4. *Objective*—to help the patient live with his pain without permitting it to affect his life adversely.

B. Transcutaneous electrical nerve stimulation
(TENS)—controlled electrical stimulus is applied by electrodes taped to the skin.

1. Electrodes are placed over or around the patient's pain area or on any peripheral nerve pathway.
2. Procedure:
   a. The skin is washed with mild soap and water and dried thoroughly to reduce skin resistance.
   b. A conductive paste or jelly is applied to the electrodes, which are then placed over the nerves that serve the painful area. Electrodes are secured with hypoallergenic tape.
   c. The patient operates the amplitude control until stimulation is felt (buzzing or tingling sensation). The amplitude is increased until the sensation is strong but not uncomfortable.
   d. The patient is taught to adjust the wave amplitude, pulse width, and frequency.
3. Health education
   a. Give the patient the instruction booklet provided by the manufacturing company.
   b. Batteries must be replaced whenever levels of stimulation cannot be achieved.
   c. The electrodes are washed with alcohol and water after each use. The pulse generator and cables are wiped clean with a damp cloth moistened with alcohol/water solution.
   d. Apply talcum powder to the cables periodically to prevent tangling.
   e. Avoid getting the pulse generator wet; avoid pulling or kinking of the cable wire.
   f. Watch for skin irritation or soreness under the electrode.

C. Dorsal column stimulation

A method for the relief of chronic intractable pain that uses a surgically implanted device that allows the patient to apply pulsed electrical stimulation to the dorsal aspect of the spinal cord to block pain impulses.
1. The unit consists of a radio-frequency stimulation transmitter, a transmitter antenna, a radio-frequency receiver, and a stimulation electrode.
2. The battery-powered transmitter and antenna are

worn externally, and the receiver and electrode are implanted.

    a. A laminectomy is performed above the highest level of pain input and the electrode is placed in the epidural space over the posterior column of the spinal cord. (Placement of stimulating systems is varied.) A small subcutaneous pocket is constructed below the clavicle or upper abdomen (site may vary) for placement of receiver. The 2 are connected by a subcutaneous tunnel.

3. A careful preoperative evaluation is performed to select a patient who will benefit from dorsal column stimulation—history, physical examination, pain questionnaire, examination to determine areas of pain involvement, psychological and psychiatric evaluation, and a trial of transcutaneous stimulation.

    a. Trial of transcutaneous stimulation (see above) gives opportunity for the patient to receive stimulation sensation—to test his tolerance of the sensation, his ability to operate the system, and the efficiency of the system.

    b. It is essential that the patient understand that the stimulator will replace drugs and that it is implanted for a lifetime.

4. Postoperative nursing management

    a. See page 808 for the nursing management following disc surgery.

    b. Assess for paraplegia, quadriplegia, and urinary incontinence.

    c. Evaluate extremities for leg movement hourly. Report any decrease in movement immediately.

    d. Look for leakage of cerebrospinal fluid at operative site—dura is opened in surgery.

    e. Give medication as prescribed for relief of incisional pain.

    f. Withdraw narcotics as rapidly as possible.

    g. Help the patient to become independently involved with his activities of daily living as rapidly as possible—inactivity serves to compound his problems.

    h. Look for signs of infection at implantation site— dorsal column stimulator is a foreign body within the patient.

    i. The dorsal column stimulating system may be tested when the patient is fully alert; initial testing may not be accurate because of overlying bandage at receiver site.

5. Health education

    a. Give the patient the manufacturer's instruction booklet to acquaint him with the system.

        The stimulation transmitter has 4 basic controls: 2 for the patient to use during operation of the system and 2 for the physician to use when determining the voltage the patient will receive.

    b. The patient is taught method of attaching the antenna to the skin (and proper skin care), use of battery pack, and how to make and modify dorsal column stimulation setting.

        (1) Antenna is secured in place by an adhesive disc centered over the implanted receiver. (The antenna site is cleansed daily, and the adhesive discs are changed daily.)

        (2) Connect transmitter to antenna and adjust settings slowly to the point at which the patient first feels a definite sensation and the stimulation results in the desired effect.

        (3) Encourage the patient to try different stimulation frequencies to determine which frequency gives best pain relief.

        (4) Have the patient keep a record of stimulation use.

        (5) Instruct the patient that postural changes will cause changes in stimulation intensity.

        (6) Warn the patient not to adjust physician's controls.

        (7) Instruct the patient to keep several batteries in reserve; battery life depends on extent of use. Patient should be instructed in battery changing procedure.

        (8) Clean transmitter and antenna according to the manufacturer's directions.

D. Percutaneous epidural neurostimulation—a method of neuromodulation in which electrodes are inserted percutaneously into spinal epidural space. Effective in treating arachnoiditis and postamputation neuroma.

E. Brain (intracerebral) **stimulation**—implantation of stimulating electrodes stereotaxically into a target area deep within the brain. Used for patients with severe pain that is bilateral, deep midline, diffuse, from metastases, or of central origin. Allows self-stimulation of periventricular gray area to produce analgesia.

Cranial Nerve Involvement

Bell's Palsy

Bell's palsy (facial paralysis) is due to peripheral involvement of the 7th cranial nerve on one side, producing weakness or paralysis of the facial muscles.

Clinical Features

1. The etiology of Bell's palsy is unknown. The three theories of possible etiologic causes (and combinations thereof) are vascular ischemia, viral infection, and autoimmune disease.

2. The majority of patients have a viral prodome (upper respiratory infection) 1–3 weeks before onset of symptoms.

3. Bell's palsy can produce grotesque disfigurement with accompanying physical and emotional stress.

Clinical Manifestations

1. Distortion of face—from paralysis of facial muscles.

2. Paresthesia of face and tongue.

3. Eye problems:

    a. Epiphora (overflow of tears down the cheek)— from keratitis caused by drying of cornea and lack of blink reflex; laxity of lower eyelid may alter proper drainage of tears.

    b. Decreased tear production—may lead to a dry eye, which is predisposed to infection.

4. Painful sensations in face, behind ear, and in the eye.
5. Speech difficulties—from facial paralysis.

Diagnostic Evaluation

1. History of acute onset
2. Tests of cranial nerve function
3. Tests for lacrimation (Schirmer test)—measures the wetting of strip of filter paper placed in lower conjunctival fornix for 5 minutes.
4. Electrodiagnostic study of facial muscles through electromyography—electrodes placed over branches of facial nerve; facial muscles observed for movement

Treatment and Nursing Management

1. Protect the involved eye—facial paralysis may abolish the blinking reflex; eye is vulnerable to dust and foreign particles.

▶ **NURSING ALERT:** Keratitis is a major threat to a patient with Bell's palsy.

    a. Protect the cornea with a preparation of artificial tears.
    b. Apply tape to close lids in order to reduce the amount of ocular exposure.
    c. Use eye ointment at bedtime—helps to keep eyes closed during sleep by sticking the lashes together.
    d. Increase environmental humidity.
    e. Teach the patient to close his eye lids frequently with his residually functioning eye musculature or manually.
    f. See that the patient wears a protective patch, particularly at night.
       (1) Patch may eventually abrade cornea, as paretic (incompletely paralyzed) eyelids are difficult to keep closed.
       (2) Eyelids may have to be sutured together.
    g. Instruct the patient to use protective glasses (wraparound sunglasses or goggles) to decrease normal evaporation from eye.
2. Give steroid therapy (prednisone)—may be helpful in reducing inflammation and edema, and in turn reducing vascular compression and permitting restoration of blood circulation in the nerve; early administration appears to diminish severity of disease and mitigate pain.
3. Promote pain relief with aspirin or codeine and by applying heat to involved side of face.
4. Provide tape support of the affected side to prevent facial sagging.
5. Start facial massage (if no nerve tenderness present) as prescribed—to help maintain muscle tone.
6. Watch for complications.
    a. Corneal ulceration; blindness
    b. Facial weakness
    c. Facial spasm with contracture and synkinesis (unintentional movement)
7. Prepare for surgical intervention if necessary.
    a. Surgical decompression of facial nerve to decrease edema—may prevent or arrest degeneration.
    b. Surgical procedures to correct eyelid deformities and protect the eye.

Health Education

1. Reassure the patient that spontaneous recovery occurs in majority of patients; recovery usually takes place in 3–5 weeks.

2. Reinforce teaching concerning eye care (see above).
3. Keep the face warm and free from drafts.
4. Teach facial exercises—if prescribed—to prevent facial muscle atrophy and to improve strength of remaining innervated muscles. Do the following while looking in a mirror:
    a. Wrinkle forehead
    b. Close eyes
    c. Purse lips
    d. Move mouth from side to side
    e. Blow out cheeks
    f. Whistle

Trigeminal Neuralgia (Tic Douloureux)

Trigeminal neuralgia (tic douloureux) is a condition of the 5th cranial nerve, characterized by sudden paroxysms of lancinating or burning pain (alternating with periods of complete comfort) in the distribution of one or more branches of the trigeminal nerve.

Etiology

Unknown

Clinical Manifestations

1. Sudden and severe pain appearing without warning—in distribution of one or more branches of trigeminal nerve (Fig. 18-5).
2. Numerous individual flashes of pain, ending abruptly; usually on one side.
3. Attacks predicted by pressure on a trigger point, the terminals of the affected branches. (Movement of the face, talking, chewing, yawning, swallowing, shaving, cold wind, may precipitate an agonizing attack.)

Medical Treatment

Goal:
Relief of pain

1. Instruct the patient to avoid exposing affected cheek to sudden cold if this is known to trigger the nerve—iced drinks, cold wind, swimming in cold water.

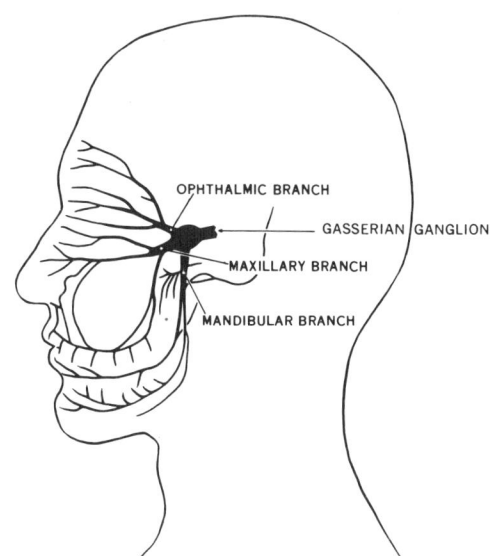

Figure 18-5. The main divisions of the trigeminal nerve are ophthalmic, maxillary, and mandibular. Sensory root fibers arise in the Gasserian ganglion.

2. Administer drug therapy as directed—to inhibit or reduce synaptic transmission and relieve pain.
   a. Carbamazepine (Tegretol), phenytoin (Dilantin), or baclofen; these drugs have anticonvulsant, muscle relaxant, and sedative properties.
   b. Serum levels of drug monitored to avoid drug toxicity.
   c. Observe for evidences of hematologic, hepatic, renal, and skin reactions.

Surgical Procedures

Surgical procedures—wide range used after medical treatment fails to give relief.
1. Alcohol and/or phenol block injection of ganglion of peripheral branches produces temporary chemical destruction of affected nerves.
   a. Usually produces complete anesthesia.
   b. Pain returns after nerve regeneration (8½–16 months).
2. Percutaneous radio-frequency rhizotomy—introduction of needle electrode through foramen ovale to the desired position of the trigeminal root; low-voltage stimulation applied to electrode, and a lesion is made. Carefully controlled electrical currents destroy enough of sensory portion of nerve to relieve pain without damaging touch sensation or motor function of face.
   a. Root selection is made by the conscious patient's response to electrical stimulation.
   b. Relief expected in most patients.
   c. Complications include reduced corneal sensation, dysesthesia/paresthesia, masseter weakness.

d. Instruct the patient to:
   (1) Place artificial tears on cornea every 4 hours if there is a marked loss of corneal sensation.
   (2) Restrict diet to soft foods for 2 weeks.
   (3) Chew on unaffected side of mouth until he becomes accustomed to numbness; avoid biting lips, tongue, or inside of mouth.
   (4) Do jaw-opening exercises as directed.
3. Percutaneous retrogasserian glycerol injection.
4. Microvascular decompression of trigeminal nerve—an intracranial approach (retromastoid craniectomy) using an operating microscope to decompress trigeminal nerve; postoperative management is the same as for any intracranial operation (see p. 770).
5. Peripheral neurectomy (excision of part of a nerve)
6. Open surgical retrogasserian rhizotomy (destruction of retrogasserian rootlets)
   a. Gasserian ganglion lies in the middle fossa and may be reached by a subtemporal, intradural, or extradural route.
   b. Following operation, the patient has a complete loss of sensation in the distribution of the divided nerve fibers.
   c. See nursing management following craniotomy, page 770.
   d. Complications—burning, stinging, numbness, discomfort in and around eye, herpetic lesions of the face, keratitis, and corneal ulceration.

Health Education

1. See Surgical Procedures, 2d above.
2. Report to dentist regularly—the patient may not have pain in the event of dental caries.

Cerebrovascular Disease

Cerebrovascular disease refers to any functional abnormality of the central nervous system caused by interference with normal blood supply to the brain. The pathology may involve an artery, a vein, or both, when the cerebral circulation becomes impaired as a result of partial or complete occlusion of a blood vessel or hemorrhage resulting from a tear in the vessel wall.

Cerebrovascular Disease From Impairment of Cerebral Circulation

A. Transient ischemic attacks (TIAs)

Transient episodes of cerebral dysfunction commonly manifested by a sudden loss of motor, sensory, or visual function, lasting minutes up to an hour or more, but no longer than 24 hours.
1. Causes—temporary impairment of blood flow to the brain from atherosclerosis of vessels supplying the brain, or obstruction of cerebral microcirculation by small embolus.
2. Therapy
   a. Antiplatelet aggregation drugs (aspirin)—when problem is related to platelet aggregation.
   b. Anticoagulant therapy (heparin, warfarin).
   c. Angiography—to identify surgically remediable lesions
   d. Surgical intervention—to increase blood flow to brain

   (1) Carotid endarterectomy (p. 777) or
   (2) Extracranial/intracranial anastomosis—provides revascularization of brain. (See p. 770 for care of patient undergoing intracranial surgery.)

B. Reversible ischemic neurological deficit (RIND)

Episode-producing neurologic deficits longer than 24 hours but followed by a return to the normal state.

C. Cerebral thrombosis (from cerebral arteriosclerosis and slowing of cerebral circulation) Usually produces transient loss of speech, visual disturbance, hemiplegia, or paresthesia in one half of the body, which may precede onset of severe paralysis. (See nursing management of the patient with a stroke.)

D. Cerebral embolism

Caused by heart disease (infective endocarditis, rheumatic heart disease, prosthetic heart valves, myocardial infarction), pulmonary emboli, arteriosclerotic plaque in carotid artery.
1. Embolism usually lodges in middle cerebral artery or its branches, where it disrupts circulation.
2. Symptoms—sudden onset of hemiparesis or hemiplegia, speech disturbances, visual disturbances.
3. See the nursing management of the patient with a stroke, in the discussion on page 778.

Cerebrovascular Disease from Hemorrhage

A. Extradural hemorrhage

Hemorrhage occurring outside the dura mater
1. This is considered a life-threatening emergency.
2. See care of the patient with head injury for principles of immediate care (p. 766).

B. Subdural hemorrhage

Hemorrhage occurring beneath the dura mater. See care of the patient with a head injury (p. 766).

C. Subarachnoid hemorrhage

Hemorrhage occurring in the subarachnoid space—may result from leaking aneurysm, congenital arteriovenous malformation, hypertension, tumor, or trauma. See treatment of subarachnoid hemorrhage, page 785.

D. Intracerebral hemorrhage

Hemorrhage occurring within the brain substance—usually from hypertension, cerebral atherosclerosis, aneurysm, etc.

Carotid Endarterectomy for Cerebrovascular Insufficiency

Carotid endarterectomy is the removal of atherosclerotic plaque(s) or thrombus from the carotid artery for the treatment of transient cerebral ischemic attacks, to prevent stroke, and/or bring relief of symptoms.

Assessment

Clinical Manifestations of Carotid Occlusive Disease

1. History of transient ischemic attacks; headache, dizziness, blackout spells; brief loss of vision of 1 eye (anaurosis fugax) or homonymous visual field defects; numbness or weakness of extremity; temporary speech impairment
2. Bruit heard over carotid artery
3. Absent/diminished carotid pulsation in neck

Diagnostic Evaluation

1. Carotid phonoangiography—auscultation, direct visualization, and photographic recording of carotid bruits using a microphone, oscilloscope, and camera.
2. Oculoplethysmography (OPG)—measures pulsation in blood flow through ophthalmic artery; gives comparative timing of simultaneously recorded ocular pulse wave forms (by corneal suction cups); light opacity sensors on the ear lobes provide timing of external carotid pulses; measures hemodynamic consequences of carotid stenosis.
3. Carotid angiography—to visualize intracranial and cervical vessels. Digital subtraction angiography— uses a computer to selectively eliminate background artifact and obtain view of carotid.
4. Doppler ultrasound techniques

Patient Problems/Nursing Diagnosis

1. Potential for neurologic deficit (stroke) related to insufficient cerebral perfusion/carotid endarterectomy.
2. Potential for complications related to carotid endarterectomy.

Planning and Implementation

Nursing Interventions

A. Prevention of neurologic deficit

1. Monitor for neurologic dysfunction and deficits— result of cerebral ischemia; emboli.
   a. Carry out frequent neurologic checks including assessment of equality, size, and reaction of pupils; handgrip; motor responses; speech; chewing; swallowing; altered mental status; symmetry of face; seizures; episodes of focal or sensory loss.
   b. Compare with preoperative status.
   c. Prepare for immediate reoperation to restore cerebral blood flow if stroke occurs.
2. Watch for respiratory insufficiency—resulting from edema due to operative manipulation or hematoma at operative site.
3. Maintain adequate blood pressure levels in immediate postoperative period—as postoperative blood pressure lability occurs frequently.
   a. Monitor for hypotension and bradycardia—may be result of increased pressure waves reaching carotid sinus receptors after removal of plaque.
   b. Give volume replacement to maintain CVP in range of 5–10 cm.
   c. Control postoperative hypertension—drug therapy (trimethaphan camsylate; sodium nitroprusside; nitroglycerin)—hypertension may precipitate a cerebral hemorrhage. Edema, hemorrhage in operative wound, or disruption of arterial reconstruction may also result from excessive hypertension.
   d. Assist the patient to assume upright posture cautiously—this activity can produce a significant drop in blood pressure.

B. Prevention of other postoperative complications

1. Watch for respiratory complications, neurologic deficits (stroke), vascular complications, carotid artery disruption, infection/hematoma of wound.
2. Observe neck size closely; measure girth.
3. Check for ability to swallow; check if cricoid cartilage is in midline—deviation may indicate impending tracheal obstruction from enlarging neck wound.
4. Palpate superficial temporal and facial arteries—to determine if external carotid artery is patent.

Evaluation

Expected Outcomes

1. Absence of retinal ischemia, speech deficits, sensory/motor deficits
2. Absence of dizziness, syncope, confusion, seizures
3. Absence of complications; no evidence of respiratory impairment, vascular complications, infection

Stroke or Cerebral Vascular Accident (CVA)

A stroke (*cerebral vascular accident*) is the onset of neurologic dysfunction resulting from disruption of the blood supply to the brain. It is brought on by: (1) thrombosis (blood clot within a blood vessel of the brain or neck); (2) cerebral embolism; (3) stenosis of an artery supplying the brain; and (4) cerebral hemorrhage (rupture of a cerebral blood vessel with bleeding or pressure into the brain substance).

Risk Factors

1. Hypertension
2. Previous transient ischemic attacks
3. Cardiac disease (atherosclerotic/valvular heart disease, arrhythmias)
4. Advanced age
5. Diabetes
6. Oral contraceptives
7. Cigarette smoking

Assessment

Clinical Manifestations

(Depend on size and site of lesion)
1. Motor loss (hemiplegia—paralysis on one side of body)
2. Communication loss
3. Visual field deficits (homonymous hemianopia—loss of half of the visual field)
4. Sensory loss
5. Bladder impairment
6. Impairment of mental activity and psychological effects

Diagnostic Evaluation

1. *Computed tomography*—distinguishes between hemorrhage and infarction
2. *Angiography*—demonstrates vascular pathology
3. *Positron scanning*—provides imaging of regional cerebral metabolism

Patient Problems/Nursing Diagnoses

1. Impaired physical mobility related to hemiplegia, weakness, and spasticity
2. Alteration in sensory perception (visual, tactile, proprioceptive, kinesthetic) related to cerebral dysfunction
3. Impaired communication related to aphasia, motor deficits, and/or generalized cognitive deficits
4. Urinary incontinence related to initial confusion, disinhibition, communication disorder, and flaccidity
5. Bowel incontinence related to immobility, alteration in nutrition, and unawareness of defecation impulse
6. Self-care deficits related to hemiplegia
7. Potential for ineffective family coping related to magnitude of the patient's neurologic deficits, prolonged illness, altered family life-style
8. Emotional and personality changes (depression, denial, anxiety, hostility) related to neurologic deficits from stroke, changes in body image, brain damage, and altered life-style

Planning and Implementation

Management During Acute Phase

1. Anti-edema agents (dehydrating agents, steroids)—to reduce brain swelling to prevent impairment of blood flow and brain herniation
2. Anticoagulation and antiplatelet aggregation drugs (heparin, aspirin and dipyridamole)—to retard the thrombotic process and prevent reembolization (may be contraindicated in stroke secondary to hemorrhage)
3. Therapies to improve cerebral blood flow and metabolism (vasodilators; vasopressors)—(clinical value unproven)

Nursing Interventions: Acute Phase
(Period of Altered Consciousness)

A. Monitor and preserve vital functions

1. See Nursing Management of the Unconscious Patient (p. 760).
2. Carry out a nursing assessment of the following: (Keep neurologic flow sheet.)
   a. A change in the level of responsiveness as evidenced by movement, resistance to changes of position, and response to stimulation.
   b. Presence or absence of voluntary or involuntary movements of the extremities; tone of the muscles; body posture and the position of the head.
   c. Stiffness or flaccidity of the neck.
   d. Comparison of pupils: size, reaction to light, and ocular position.
   e. Color of the face and extremities; temperature and moisture of the skin.
   f. Quality and rates of pulse and respiration; body temperature and arterial pressure.
   g. Ability to speak.
   h. Volume of fluids ingested or administered and volume of urine excreted each 24 hours.
   i. Serial arterial blood gas measurements.

B. Ensure an adequate perfusion pressure so that oxygenated blood can reach the brain.

1. Maintain blood pressure and cardiac output—to sustain cerebral blood flow.
2. Watch for evidence of myocardial infarction, arrhythmias, and congestive heart failure; arrhythmia may reduce cerebral blood flow and produce cardiac arrest.
3. Ensure hydration depending on clinical situation.
4. Use endotracheal intubation and mechanical ventilation for the patient with massive stroke; respiratory arrest is usually the life-threatening factor in this condition.
5. Prepare for surgical intervention (endarterectomy or extracranial–intracranial anastomosis) if necessary—to restore circulation and halt potential occlusive lesions.

C. Reorient the patient when he gains awareness/consciousness.

1. Expect some aphasia if the patient has right-sided hemiplegia.
2. Reassure the patient that he has not lost his mind and that he will receive help with communication (speech pathologist or therapist).
3. *Talk* to the patient while caring for him.
4. Make every effort to understand the patient.
5. Maintain a calm and accepting manner during periods of emotional lability.
6. Promote bladder and bowel control.
   a. Remove indwelling catheter as soon as the patient is able to sit up in bed.

b. Start the patient on bladder-training program (p. 70).

c. Initiate bowel program (p. 70).

d. Enhance bowel regularity with a high-fiber diet, adequate fluid intake, and stool softeners.

Nursing Interventions: Rehabilitation Phase

A. Prevent deformities, physical deterioration, and loss of range of motion.

1. Position the patient in bed correctly—to prevent contractures, relieve pressure, and maintain good body alignment. (These principles of positioning are also carried out during the phase of altered consciousness.) See Figure 18-6A.

   a. Place a board under the mattress—to give the body firm support.

   b. Encourage the patient to remain flat in bed except when engaged in activities of daily living—to prevent hip flexion deformities.

   c. Use a footboard during the flaccid period following a stroke to keep the feet dorsiflexed—prevents footdrop, heel cord shortening, and plantar flexion.

      (1) Avoid use of a footboard after spasticity develops—it will promote spasticity and increase plantar flexion.

      (2) Avoid excessive pressure on the ball of the foot after spasticity develops.

      (3) Do not allow top bedding to pull affected foot into plantar flexion.

   d. Use a padded posterior splint at night and keep the knee in a fully extended position; secure the posterior splint with an elastic compression bandage.

   e. Apply a trochanter roll from the crest of the ilium to the midthigh (Fig. 18-6*B*)—to prevent external rotation of the hip joint when the patient is in a dorsal position.

   f. Place a pillow in the axilla of the affected side when there is limited external rotation—to keep arm away from the chest and prevent adduction of the affected shoulder (Fig. 18-6).

   g. Place the affected upper extremity within its full range of motion (slightly flexed) on pillow supports with each joint positioned higher than the preceding one—to prevent edema and resultant fibrosis.

      (1) Alternate upper extremity position by allowing periods of elbow extension.

   h. Place the hand in slight supination with fingers slightly flexed; if upper extremity is flaccid, use a volar resting splint to support the wrist and hand in a functional position (Fig. 18-6*C*). If the upper extremity is spastic, use a dorsal cock-up splint to prevent pressure on the palm.

   i. Place the patient in a prone position for 15 minutes to ½ hour 2–3 times daily (Fig. 18-6*E*)—to prevent knee and hip flexion contractures.

B. Retraining of affected extremities

1. Exercise the affected extremities passively and carry out range of motion exercises 4–5 times daily—to

Figure 18-6. Positioning for a patient following a stroke during the flaccid period. (Dark side of pajamas represents affected or hemiplegic side.)

A. A pillow is placed in the axilla to prevent adduction of the affected shoulder. Pillows are placed under the arm, which is in a slightly flexed position with each joint positioned higher than the preceding one.

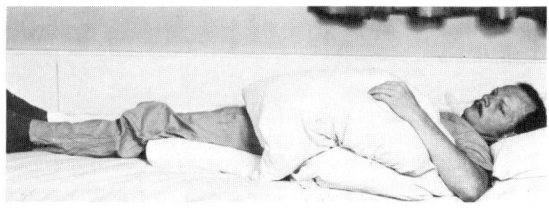

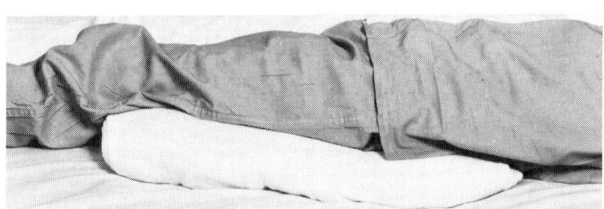

B. The trochanter roll should extend from the crest of the ilium to the midthigh, since the hip joint lies between these 2 points. The trochanter roll acts as a mechanical wedge under the projection of the greater trochanter and prevents the femur from rolling.

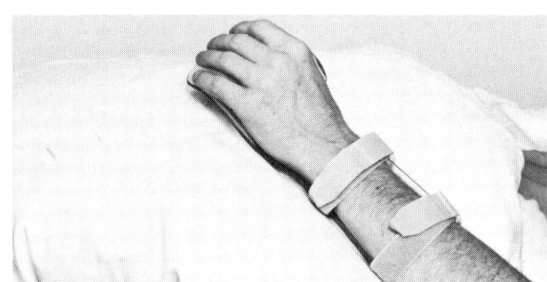

C. A volar resting splint may be used to support the wrist and hand if the upper extremity is flaccid.

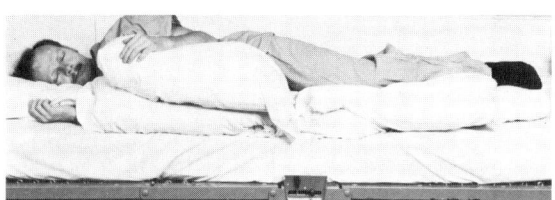

D. Lateral or side-lying position. The patient should be turned on his unaffected side. The upper thigh should not be acutely flexed.

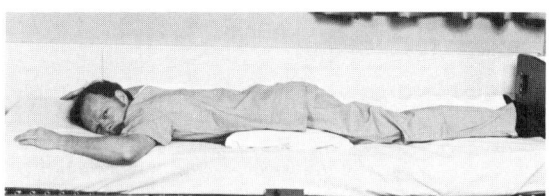

E. Prone position. A pillow is placed under the pelvis to help promote hyperextension of the hip joints, which is essential for normal gait. Note position of arms.

maintain joint mobility, to prevent contracture development in the paralyzed extremity, to prevent further deterioration of neuromuscular system, to regain motor control, and to enhance circulation.

2. Involve family in exercise program since care of a stroke patient requires time and effort.

3. Remind the patient to exercise unaffected extremities regularly at intervals throughout the day—to prevent contracture development in the normal extremities.

4. Teach the patient to put his unaffected leg under the affected one in order to move and turn himself.

5. Instruct the patient to move his affected arm (and hand) with his good hand (Fig. 18-7).

6. Teach quadriceps muscle setting and gluteal exercises (5 times daily for 10 minutes)—to improve the muscle strength needed for walking.

   a. *Quadriceps setting* (to each extremity)
    Instruct the patient as follows:

    (1) Contract the quadriceps muscle (anterior portion of thighs) while raising the heel and attempting to push the popliteal space against the mattress.

    (2) Hold the muscle contraction for the count of 5.
    Relax for the count of 5. Repeat.

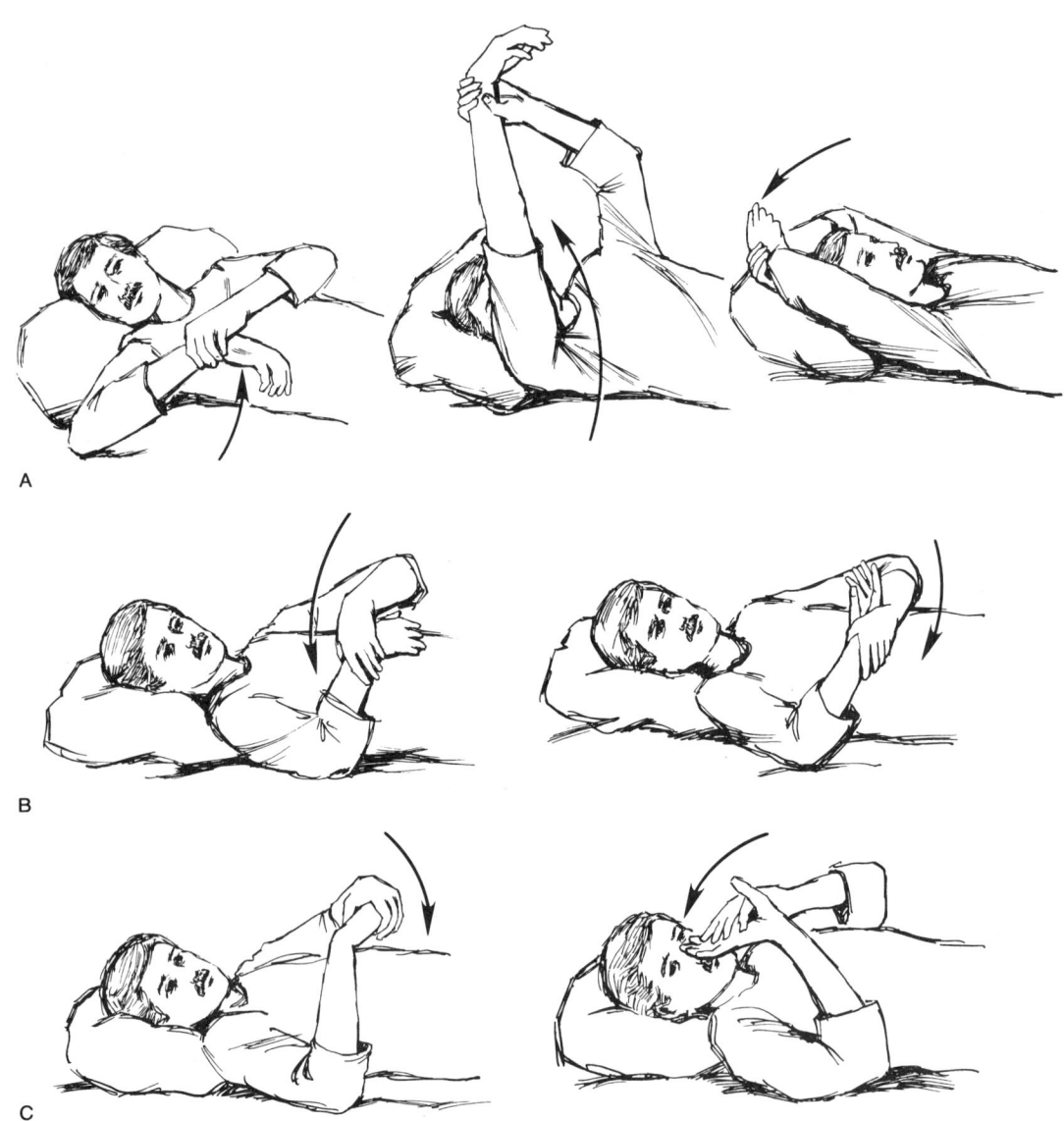

Figure 18-7. (*A*) Exercise to maintain range of motion of the involved shoulder and the elbow in hemiplegia. (*B*) Exercise to maintain range of motion of pronation and supination in affected hand. (*C*) Exercise to maintain range of motion of the wrist and the finger in hemiplegia. (Hirschberg G, Lewis L and Vaughan P. Rehabilitation, 2nd ed. Philadelphia, JB Lippincott, 1976)

b. *Gluteal setting*
Instruct the patient as follows:
(1) Contract or "pinch" the buttocks together for the count of 5.
(2) Relax for the count of 5. Repeat.
7. Biofeedback may be used to help the patient relearn control of activity of lower extremity muscles during early recovery period.
8. Maintain upper extremity joint mobility to prevent shoulder–hand syndrome.
a. Use a sling on the paralyzed arm when the patient is in upright position, if arm is flaccid, or if the patient complains of arm pain and heaviness. The sling is usually discarded when spasticity provides enough tone to prevent shoulder subluxation.
(1) Remove sling frequently and exercise arm.
(2) Instruct the patient to interlace his fingers, placing the palms together. With elbows extended, lift both arms above head repeatedly throughout day.
b. When seated, keep the affected arm and hand elevated with a pillow to prevent dependent edema of the hand.
c. Instruct the patient to flex and extend his wrist and fingers with unaffected hand at frequent intervals.
d. Watch for shoulder–hand syndrome—painful shoulder and generalized swelling and pain of hand—can cause atrophy of subcutaneous tissues and contractures.
9. Promote mobility to regain optimum function.
a. *To develop sitting balance*
(1) Raise the bed to a sitting position; instruct the patient to hold the bedrail with his good hand—helps to regain sense of balance.

(2) To sit on edge of bed
(a) Adjust the bed to the low position.
(b) Instruct the patient to place the strong leg beneath the weak leg and lift it toward the side of the bed.
(c) Instruct the patient to press the strong elbow (which is flexed to a 90-degree angle) into the mattress and come to a sitting position by transferring weight to the forearm and then to the hand, while lifting the affected leg with the strong leg over the edge of the bed. The force of gravity, set in motion by pushing against the hand and moving the legs, is sufficient to pivot the patient's torso on the buttocks.
(d) Extend the patient's strong arm with his hand flat on the bed behind him to assist in balancing.
(e) Stand in front of the patient to observe and, if necessary, help him to maintain this posture.
(f) A change in color, shortness of breath, increasing pulse rate, or profuse perspiration is an indication that the patient should be placed in bed again. The sitting time is increased as rapidly as the patient's condition permits.
b. *Develop standing balance* (Fig. 18-8)
(1) Put walking shoes with strong shank on the patient for all ambulation activities.
(2) Seat the patient on edge of bed and place a straight-back chair on each side of him.
(a) Tie affected hand to the chair if the patient lacks grasp strength.
(b) Assist the patient to a standing position

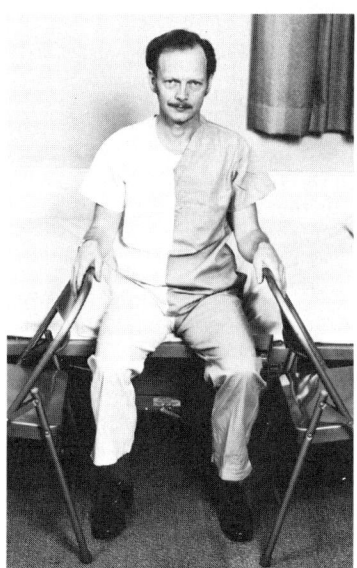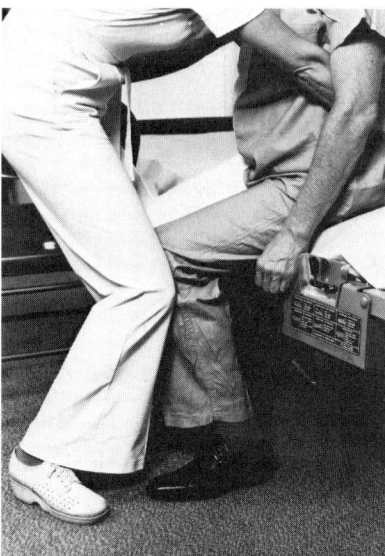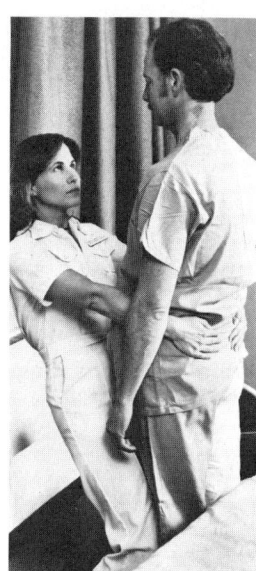

Figure 18-8. Getting the patient out of bed following a stroke. (*Left*) Place the bed in the low position so that the feet are resting on the floor. Observe the patient's reaction and increase the sitting time as rapidly as the patient's condition permits. (*Center*) Getting ready to arise to a standing position. Positioning the nurse's knees on the outside of the patient's knees will prevent the patient's knees from buckling. (*Right*) Stabilizing the patient as he assumes a standing position. Note that the nurse is (1) stabilizing the patient's lower back and knees and (2) assessing his reaction to standing. (Courtesy of Washington Adventist Hospital; Glenn Dalby, photographer)

by supporting his lower back with your hands and positioning your knees on the outside of the patient's knees.

  (c) Encourage the patient to look upward briefly—facilitates lower extremity extension.

  (3) Assess the patient for dizziness, pallor, and increasing pulse rate. Have the patient practice standing and shifting weight from one leg to the other.

  (4) Assist the patient to achieve standing balance at frequent intervals throughout the day.

  (5) Help the patient begin walking as soon as standing balance is achieved (using parallel bars). Stand behind patient and stabilize him at waist level.

  (6) Encourage the patient to look at his feet occasionally—proprioceptive loss may accompany hemiplegia.

10. Secure a wheelchair of the correct size with brakes that the patient can manage if he is unable to ambulate.

  a. Place wheelchair on the patient's unaffected side; allows him to see wheelchair and lead with the stronger leg.

  b. Lock wheelchair brake and lift pedals out of the way. To transfer from a chair to wheelchair, instruct the patient as follows:

    (1) Move forward in chair, placing weight over strong leg. Push up with strong arm and foot.

    (2) Place most of the weight on the strong leg while keeping weak knee locked.

    (3) Pivot in the direction of the stronger leg; bring weak leg over to stronger leg. Maintain standing position a few moments.

    (4) Lower body into chair gradually, using strong arm and leg.

    (5) Propel wheelchair by placing unaffected foot on floor (heel-to-toe) while simultaneously moving the wheel rim forward with the hand.

11. Assist in securing supportive devices if needed—most patients develop spasticity of lower extremity and will lack motor control.

  a. Secure posterior knee splint if the patient has a weakened or absent quadriceps muscle—gives better balance and helps prevent loss of position sense.

  b. Secure an adjustable aluminum cane (with 3-prong support if necessary) when the patient is able to walk alone.

C. Developing compensating skills for alterations in sensory perception

1. Test for hemianopia (defective vision in half of the visual field).

  a. Show the patient an object placed to one side and ask if he can identify it.

  b. Hemianopia is evident if the patient fails to see the object on the correct side, but responds by looking towards it on the other side. (Visual field is likely to be limited on the right if the patient has right hemiplegia.)

2. Place call light, bedside table, etc. on the side of his awareness.

3. Approach the bed from the uninvolved side.

4. Encourage the patient to turn his head from side to side to obtain the full view of a normal visual field.

5. Have the patient wear his eyeglasses.

6. Help the patient to relearn swallowing sequence (if capable of following instruction).

  a. Induce the sucking reflex.

    (1) Have the patient attempt to suck on gloved finger.

    (2) Place ice on tongue and encourage the patient to suck ice.

  b. Progress to popsicle, soft foods, and then regular diet.

  c. Give food and fluids from uninvolved side (if patient has droop of mouth).

  d. Remind the patient to chew on unaffected side.

  e. Inspect the patient's mouth for food collecting between cheek and gums on involved side; frequent oral hygiene is necessary.

D. Improving communication abilities

See page 783 for nursing management of the patient with aphasia.

E. Avoiding bladder and bowel incontinence

Continue with bladder and bowel program.

F. Promoting independence in self-care

1. Help set realistic goals and add a new task daily if possible.

2. Have the patient immediately transfer all self-care activities to the unaffected side. Teach one-handed methods and use adaptive equipment.

3. Encourage the patient to brush his teeth, comb his hair, and bathe and feed himself.

4. Be sure that the patient does not neglect his affected side.

5. Encourage the patient to dress himself for ambulatory activities.

  a. Instruct the family to bring clothing that is one size larger than usually worn.

  b. Have the patient dress himself (with assistance if necessary) while seated—to achieve better balance.

  c. Use clothing with front fasteners; stretch fabrics are preferable.

  d. Teach only one activity at a time.

G. Establishing family participation in the rehabilitation process

1. Involve family in care in order to develop and practice skills that help the patient reach his rehabilitation goals.

2. Help family adapt and adjust to the patient's residual function.

3. Provide some type of counseling and support system for family—need direction and support in coping with personality and intellectual impairment and psychiatric symptoms.

4. Prepare the patient for discharge to home, rehabilitation center, or extended-care facility.

  a. Give family as much information as possible about what the patient can do.

  b. Have equipment and adaptive devices ready.

  c. Consider day-care program or respite care arrangements with a nursing home to give family relief.

Family Health Education

Instruct the family as follows:

1. Expect some emotional lability and some degree of brain damage if the patient has had a more severe stroke.

  a. The patient may have episodes of inappropriate crying/laughing and temper outbursts.

(1) Change the subject; ask the patient to perform a motor act.

(2) Reassure the patient that this is not usually a permanent condition and gradually subsides.

b. Hemiplegic patients may be easily confused, forgetful, discouraged, hostile, uncooperative, withdrawn, and dependent.

c. Poststroke depression is *common* (especially those with left hemisphere lesions); use of tricyclic antidepressants and psychotherapy seems to be warranted.

d. Support the patient psychologically; hemiplegia has a tremendous psychological impact on the patient (and his family).

2. Explain that the patient becomes easily fatigued.
   a. See that the patient has scheduled rest periods.
   b. Promote sense of progress and improvement.
3. Avoid doing those things for the patient that he can do for himself.
4. Be supportive and optimistic but firm and direct.
5. Maintain constancy of the environment without too many distractions.
6. Install handrails by the toilet and tub or shower and put safety rails on the bed.
7. Obtain self-help devices to assist in activities of daily living; modify and adapt devices and "gadgets" to encourage independence.
8. Encourage the patient to keep active and adhere to exercise program, and to remain as self-sufficient as possible.
9. Set realistic goals; make the best of what remains.
10. Have the patient medically evaluated from time to time.

11. Take advantage of community service agencies and the local or regional branch of the State Office of Vocational Rehabilitation.

Evaluation
Expected Outcomes

1. Obtains optimum mobility
   a. Exercises affected/unaffected extremities; free of contractures
   b. Attains sitting balance and transfers to wheelchair
   c. Shows beginning ability to walk with reciprocal pattern
2. Compensates for sensory deficits—feeds self; turns head to compensate for visual field deficits; remembers to look at feet occasionally; achieves increasing ability in self-care
3. Communicates needs and wants to others—uses gestures when word-finding is difficult; able to make needs known; watches facial expression/body language for nonverbal communication; attends classes with speech–language pathologist
4. Attains/maintains bladder control—signals desire to urinate; transfers to bedside commode; absence of retention; absence of bacteriuria
5. Attains/maintains bowel control—signals desire to defecate; transfers to bedside commode; absence of fecal soiling/constipation
6. Acquires increasing independence in self-care
7. Copes with changes in life-style—uses cues and memory aids; has printed list of sequencing steps for activities; returns to some previous social interests/ activities
8. Demonstrates lessening emotional lability

Aphasia

Aphasia is a disturbance of language function resulting from injury or disease of the brain areas primarily responsible for language function. It may involve impairment of the ability to speak, understand the speech of others, read, write, and do arithmetic. The majority of aphasic individuals have difficulty with input (comprehension, reading) and output (speak, writing).

Causes

1. Stroke (present in about one third of immediate survivors)
2. Head injury
3. Brain tumor

Aphasic Syndromes

A. Fluent Aphasias—difficulty in comprehension of language

1. *Wernicke's aphasia*—the patient speaks readily, but speech lacks clear content, information, and direction; jargon frequently used.
2. *Anomic or amnesic aphasia*—speech is almost normal, but marred by word-finding difficulty.
3. *Conduction aphasia*—the patient's comprehension of language is good, but he has difficulty repeating spoken material.

B. Nonfluent Aphasia (motor aphasia, Broca's aphasia)—difficulty in production of language characterized by sparse verbal output produced with effort;

the patient usually can comprehend spoken/written word.

C. Global Aphasia—severe depression of language function in all modalities; fluent and nonfluent aphasia occur together, but one type may predominate; the predominant manifestation may be inability to speak, comprehend speech, repeat, or name; it results from injury to both Broca's and Wernicke's areas.

Patient Problems/Nursing Diagnoses

1. Impaired communicative behavior related to brain damage
2. Disturbance in self-concept related to inability to communicate
3. Ineffective coping related to frustration over communication deficit

Principle:

There are a variety of symptoms and disorders underlying aphasia. A speech and language pathologist determines the type of aphasia. Therefore, the treatment is individualized.

Nursing Interventions

A. Establishing improved communication

1. Determine the communication abilities of the patient—usually done by speech–language pathologist in cooperation with the neurologist.

2. Give the patient as much psychological security as possible.
3. Give the patient plenty of *time* to speak and respond; he cannot sort out incoming messages and formulate a response under pressure.
   a. Speak slowly while making eye contact with the patient.
   b. Face the patient on the uninvolved side.
   c. Avoid talking too fast, too loudly, or too much.
   d. Use short sentences; pause; see if the patient indicates that he understands.
   e. Repeat or rephrase sentence.
   f. Provide visual clues (gestures, demonstration, pictures) if the patient has comprehension problems.
   g. Supplement speech with gestures when indicated.
   h. Talk to the patient while caring for him. Know his former interests.
   i. Be consistent—by using the same wording each time instructions are given and questions are asked.
4. Keep the environment relaxed and permissive.
5. Keep distractions at a minimum—damaged input pathways cannot sort out distracting stimuli in the environment.
6. Use as many sensory channels as possible.
   a. Supplement auditory stimulation with visual stimulation.
   b. Use visual aids (pictures); ask the patient to point to and name what he sees.
   c. Use games to stimulate the patient's mind and help organize thoughts.
   d. Use television, tape recorders, audio cassettes, electronic learning games, etc. to stimulate the patient's interest.
   e. Encourage the patient to use any form of communication—gestures, writing, drawing, etc., until his speech begins to return.
   f. Elicit responses from the patient (e.g., "Please nod your head if you understand"). Reinforce every correct response.
   g. Restate what you think the patient has said from time to time.

B. Improving self concept

1. Give support by assuring the patient that there is nothing wrong with his intelligence.
   a. Treat the patient as an intelligent adult.

   b. Accept the patient as he is now; avoid artificial praise.
   c. Avoid forcing speech.
2. Maintain a calm, accepting, and deliberate manner, especially during periods of emotional lability.
3. Encourage the patient to socialize with his family and friends.
   a. Seek the help of other people to read aloud, play games, do puzzles.
   b. Have the patient's grandchildren visit and talk with him.
   c. Keep the patient in the social world.
   d. Be aware of support groups (stroke clubs) in the community.
4. Watch the patient for clues and gestures if his speech is unintelligible or jargon-like.
   a. Continue to listen to the patient.
   b. Nod and make neutral statements occasionally.
   c. Shift the topic when appropriate to provide another point of interest and frame of reference.
5. Observe the patient during the course of his daily schedule for clues to evaluate and assess his progress.

Family Health Education

1. See items A and B, above.
2. The patient's ability to speak may vary from day to day. Fatigue has an adverse effect on speech.
3. The patient is likely to become terribly frustrated by his inability to communicate; ignore swearing and abusive language.
4. Aphasia can also involve the patient's understanding. Some persons cannot express themselves but can comprehend the spoken or written word; others can speak but do not understand; while some who do neither may respond to gesture and actions.
5. Seek information about aphasia:
   American Speech–Language–Hearing Association, 10801 Rockville Pike, Rockville, MD 20852
6. Counsel family to continue life of their own and to seek counseling if necessary for dealing with frustration and pressures.
   a. Acknowledge the reality of the loss.

Expected Outcomes

1. Communicates with others (in accordance with his ability/disability)
2. Demonstrates improvement in self-concept
   a. Tries to reduce withdrawal/isolation by social interactions
   b. Returns to a few former activities

Rupture of Intracranial Aneurysm With Subarachnoid Hemorrhage

An *intracranial aneurysm* is a dilation of the walls of a cerebral artery.

Etiology

1. Atherosclerosis—reflects an acquired defect in vessel wall with subsequent weakness of wall
2. Intracranial arteriovenous malformation
3. Hypertensive vascular disease
4. Head trauma
5. Advanced age
6. Congenital
7. Unknown

Underlying Principles

1. Early recognition of warning signs should prompt early surgical intervention before major hemorrhage develops.
2. Rupture of an intracranial aneurysm leads to subarachnoid hemorrhage. Other causes of subarachnoid hemorrhage include arteriovenous malformation, tumors, blood dyscrasia.
3. The mortality rate corresponds to the level of consciousness and neurologic deficit. Many patients ultimately succumb to recurrence of bleeding.

Assessment
Clinical Manifestations

1. Due to compression of cranial nerves or brain substance
2. Due to leakage from or rupture of aneurysm causing subarachnoid hemorrhage
   a. Headache or head pain, often associated with pain in eye—abrupt onset, usually unilateral, frontal, recurrent, and severe; disturbances of consciousness
   b. Dizziness; nausea and vomiting
   c. Transient loss of consciousness
   d. Pain and rigidity in back of neck and spine—from meningeal irritation
   e. Visual disturbances—visual loss, diplopia (double vision), ptosis (drooping of upper eyelid)—when aneurysm is adjacent to oculomotor (III) nerve
   f. Tinnitus (ringing in the ears)
   g. Hemiparesis (muscular weakness affecting one side of body) or hemiplegia (paralysis of 1 side of body)
   h. Fever—due to meningeal or hypothalamic irritation

Diagnostic Evaluation

1. CT scan of head—to rule out other structural lesions and for presence of blood in the subarachnoid space
2. Lumbar puncture—to confirm subarachnoid hemorrhage
3. Cerebral angiography—to determine presence and location of aneurysm and cerebrovascular spasm

Patient Problems/Nursing Diagnoses

1. Potential for recurrent bleeding related to expansion of aneurysm or surrounding artery or bleeding into subarachnoid space
2. Potential for complications
3. Headache related to expansion of aneurysm, or bleeding into subarachnoid space, or ischemic symptoms

Planning and Implementation
Nursing Interventions
A. Modification of activities to prevent recurrent bleeding

▶ **NURSING ALERT:** There is a significant incidence of recurrent aneurysmal bleeding with a high mortality rate.

1. Place patient on immediate and absolute bed rest in a quiet, nonstressful setting—activity, pain, stress, anxiety may elevate blood pressure and potentiate bleeding.
   a. Restrict visitors except family who are counseled to ensure tranquility.
   b. Elevate head of bed 30–35 degrees—to facilitate venous drainage from brain and to lower intracranial arterial pressure.
   c. Dim lighting as photophobia is common.
   d. Avoid any activity that increases blood pressure or obstructs venous return (Valsalva maneuver, straining, sneezing, pulling up in bed, acute flexion/rotation of head and neck [compromises jugular veins], cigarette smoking).
   e. Instruct the patient to exhale through mouth during voiding/defecation to decrease strain.

   f. Give stool softeners to prevent straining.
   g. Eliminate coffee/tea (unless decaffeinated).
2. Use appropriate psychological intervention and reassurance to relieve fear and anxiety.

B. Prevention of complications

1. Monitor the patient continually to recognize neurologic deterioration (from recurrent bleeding, increasing intracranial pressure, vasospasm) and to determine optimum time for surgical intervention.
   a. Keep neurologic flow record; check blood pressure, pulse, and level of responsiveness hourly—level of responsiveness is an indicator of cerebral perfusion.
   b. Monitor respiratory status—reduction in PO_2 in brain areas with impaired autoregulation potentiates cerebral infarction.
   c. Use intracranial pressure monitoring (p. 765) for patients who are unconscious or showing progressive neurologic deterioration.
   d. Prepare for angiogram when patient is stable—to determine source of bleeding.
2. See Care of the Unconscious Patient, page 760.
3. Monitor for fluid and electrolyte disturbances—results from inappropriate secretion of antidiuretic hormone (common after subarachnoid hemorrhage).
4. Monitor for cerebral vasospasm (narrowing of cerebral blood vessels which reduces brain blood flow leading to ischemia and cerebral infarction).
   a. Usually occurs 4th–10th day following initial hemorrhage.
   b. May be treated by expanding the patient's blood volume and increasing blood pressure to increase perfusion through spastic cerebral vessels.
5. Monitor for other complications—hematoma (intracerebral and subdural), hydrocephalus (from blood in basal cisterns), brain edema, pituitary insufficiency.

C. Preservation of adequate cerebral perfusion

1. Use measures to maintain systemic blood pressure at a stable level and prevent rebleeding or to reduce systolic thrust on aneurysmal wall.
   a. Drugs
      (1) Sedatives (phenobarbital, diazepam)—for sedative and anticonvulsive effects.
      (2) Analgesics (codeine, acetaminophen)—for head and neck pain.
      (3) Antifibrinolytic agents (aminocaproic acid [Amicar])—to inhibit clot lysis and reduce likelihood of recurrent bleeding.
      (4) Stool softeners—to prevent straining because this elevates blood pressure.
      (5) Antihypertensive therapy (propranolol, hydralazine, methyldopa)—for elevated blood pressure. Avoid precipitous drop in blood pressure, which can produce brain ischemia.
      (6) Steroids (dexamethasone, methylprednisolone)—to combat cerebral edema (controversial). See also the patient with increased intracranial pressure, page 763.
      (7) Phenytoin—for seizure prophylaxis.
2. Prepare for surgical intervention when the patient is in suitable condition and his brain's reaction to hemorrhage subsides.
   a. Obliteration of aneurysm by clipping or ligation and removal of blood clot.
   b. Encasement or reinforcement techniques by wrapping aneurysm with plastic, muscle, muslin, or other material or applying a coating substance.

c. Extracranial–intracranial arterial bypass—to establish collateral blood supply in order to allow surgery on aneurysm.
Monitor for:
(1) Cerebral vasospasms—produce cerebral ischemia and stroke
(2) Psychological symptoms—disorientation, amnesia, Korsakoff's syndrome
(3) Motor disturbances, aphasia, water and electrolyte disturbances, gastrointestinal bleeding

(4) Major cause of death after first 6 months is rebleeding.

Evaluation

Expected Outcomes

1. Avoids recurrent bleeding; avoids doing Valsalva maneuver; complies with restrictions of bed rest
2. Absence of complications; vital signs within acceptable range
3. Experiences relief of headache

Brain Abscess

A *brain abscess* is a localized collection of pus within the brain substance. It exists as a mass lesion.

Etiology

1. By direct invasion of the brain (intracranial trauma or surgery)
2. By spread of infection from nearby sites (ear, sinus, mastoid)
3. By spread of infection from other organs (remote from the brain) by hematogenous or metastatic spread (lung infections, infective endocarditis)

▶ **NURSING ALERT: Have a high degree of suspicion of brain abscess when neurologic signs and symptoms develop in a person with a recent history of sinus or ear infection or lung abscess.**

Clinical Manifestations

Caused by major alterations of intracranial mass dynamics (edema, brain shift), by infection, or by location of the abscess.
1. Headache—may be from increased intracranial pressure; worse in morning
2. Focal neurologic signs (depending on site of abscess)—weakness of arm or leg, visual impairment, focal epileptic seizures, papilledema
3. Fever and leukocytosis; temperature may be subnormal when there is a thick-walled abscess
4. Change in the patient's mental alertness.

Nursing Interventions

1. Give antimicrobial therapy—to reduce the virulence of or to eliminate the organism. Large doses of the appropriate antimicrobial are given to penetrate the abscess cavity to help eradicate any existing septic focus.
2. Observe the patient for increased intracranial pressure (p. 763)—cerebral edema surrounds an acute brain abscess and may produce sudden increase of intracranial pressure.
   a. Secondary midbrain and brain stem compression can lead to rapid coma and death.
   b. The patient may be given dexamethasone for cerebral edema.
   c. Keep neurologic assessment record.
3. Assist in diagnostic studies for determining accurate localization of abscess; nursing assessments, laboratory studies, computed tomography, brain scanning, angiography, and repeated neurologic examinations.
4. Give anticonvulsants (phenytoin) as prescribed—risk of epilepsy is high during acute phase and is a common late complication.
5. Prepare for surgical intervention (the definitive treatment).
   a. Drainage of abscess through burr holes and instillation of appropriate antibiotics.
   b. Craniotomy with elevation of bone flap and radical excision of abscess (see nursing management of patient undergoing intracranial surgery, p. 770).
6. Support the patient during repeated computed tomographic (CT) brain scanning—used to diagnose and localize abscess, determine optimum timing of surgery, and diagnose postoperative complications.
   a. Relapse is common with high overall mortality and morbidity.
   b. Neurologic deficits following treatment of brain abscess include hemiparesis, seizures, visual defects, cranial nerve palsies, and learning problems in children.

Health Education

1. It is important that the anticonvulsant medication be taken on a daily basis as prescribed.
2. *Prevention:* Treat otitis media, mastoiditis, sinusitis, and other systemic infections to prevent brain abscess.

Brain Tumor

A *brain tumor* is a localized intracranial neoplasm which occupies space within the skull and tends to cause a rise in intracranial pressure.

Incidence

1. Tumors of the brain originate in the brain (including the roots of the cranial nerves and the meninges) in about 95% of all patients with this problem.
2. Tumors may be benign or malignant; however any mass within the closed cranial vault may be lethal.

3. The greatest incidence of brain tumors in adults occurs between the ages of 30 and 50 years.

Classification

A. Tumors Originating in the Brain Tissue

1. *Gliomas;* infiltrating tumors that may invade any portion of the brain; most common type of brain tumor
2. Classification according to cell type
   a. Astrocytomas (grades 1 and 2)

b. Glioblastomas (grades 3 and 4 astrocytomas)
c. Ependymomas
d. Medulloblastomas
e. Oligodendrogliomas
f. Colloid cysts

B. Tumors Arising from the Covering of the Brain

Meningioma; encapsulated, well-defined, growing outside the brain tissue; compresses rather than invades brain

C. Tumors Developing in or on the Cranial Nerves

1. Acoustic neuroma; derived from sheath of acoustic nerve
2. Optic nerve spongioblastoma polare

D. Metastatic Lesions (most commonly from lung and breast)

E. Tumors of the Ductless Glands

1. Pituitary
2. Pineal

F. Blood Vessel Tumors

1. Hemangioblastoma
2. Angioma

G. Congenital Tumors

Clinical Manifestations

A. General Symptoms

1. Brain tumor is usually characterized by a *progressive* course of symptoms over a period of time; signs and symptoms depend on tumor location and rate of growth.
2. Brain tumors manifest themselves by:
   a. *Symptoms due to increased intracranial pressure*
      (1) Headache—intensified by activity that increases intracranial pressure (stooping, straining); most common in morning.
      (2) Vomiting, unrelated to food intake (morning vomiting)—usually due to irritation of vagal centers in medulla
      (3) Papilledema (choked disc)—edema of optic nerve which can lead to impaired vision
      (4) Mental clouding, lethargy
   b. *Localized neurologic impairment due to local effects of tumor's interference with specific regions of the brain*
      (1) Motor abnormalities—weakness, paralysis, lack of coordination, convulsive seizures
      (2) Sensory abnormalities—aberrations in smell, vision, hearing, and touch

B. Manifestations According to Site

1. *Frontal lobe tumor*
   a. Mental changes (memory loss, euphoria, personality changes, loss of interest, moral laxity)
   b. Headache
   c. Focal seizures
   d. Hemiparesis or aphasia
   e. Failing or blurring vision
   f. Impairment of sphincter control
2. *Temporal lobe* (may be relatively silent)
   a. Focal epileptic seizures
   b. Dysphasia or aphasia
   c. Papilledema
   d. Headache
   e. Behavior disorders
3. *Parietal lobe tumors*
   a. Motor seizures
   b. Sensory loss or visual impairment
   c. Jacksonian convulsions

4. *Occipital tumors*
   a. Visual impairment; homonymous hemianopia
   b. Focal seizures
5. *Cerebellar tumors* (common brain tumors of childhood)
   a. Disturbances of equilibrium and coordination
   b. Early development of increasing intracranial pressure and papilledema
6. *Tumors of brain stem*
   Symptoms of cranial nerve palsies (dysphagia, dysphonia, nystagmus, ataxia in extremities)
7. *Tumors of the 3rd ventricle*
   Symptoms arise from increasing intracranial pressure

Diagnostic Evaluation

1. Clinical assessment of signs and symptoms
2. CT scanning (demonstrates location of tumor), specialized cerebral angiography, radionuclide scanning, electroencephalography
3. Stereotactic biopsy with CT scanning—tumor localized by CT scan with stereotactic apparatus employed to direct a needle/cannula to target area to obtain biopsy of lesion

Treatment

A. Problems Affecting Treatment

1. Effectiveness of treatment depends on type and site of tumor; many tumors are in vital or inaccessible areas (brain stem tumors); even biopsies in such locations can produce unacceptable disabilities.
2. Nonencapsulated and infiltrating tumors make complete removal almost impossible; resulting neurologic deficit (blindness, paralysis, mental impairment) would be too severe.
3. Cures may be obtained in certain tumors (meningiomas, acoustic neuromas, cystic astrocytomas of cerebellum, etc.) if treated early; complete removal of infiltrating gliomas not possible.

B. Principles of Treatment

1. Brain tumors require different therapeutic approaches, depending on cell type, tumor location, degree of invasiveness, and association with vital structures; and age and condition of the patient. Each patient (and his lesion) is evaluated individually, and the therapeutic program designed accordingly.
2. Treatment usually involves a multidisciplinary approach including surgery, radiation, and chemotherapy, or a combination of the three.

Management

A. Surgery

Goal:
To excise the tumor for potential cure or as an adjuvant treatment to radiation or chemotherapy.

1. Surgical approaches include total removal of tumor when possible, decompression and cerebrospinal fluid–vascular shunt procedures.
   a. New computer-monitored stereotactic system permits neurosurgeon to have a 3-dimensional orientation during removal of deeply seated or irregularly shaped tumors.
   b. Use of operating microscope, automated dissecting devices (carbon dioxide laser), ultrasonic aspirator, etc., have facilitated brain tumor removal.
2. Phenytoin usually given prophylactically; patients are at risk for seizures.
3. See page 770 for nursing management of the patient undergoing intracranial surgery.

B. Radiation Therapy

1. Give steroids (dexamethasone) as directed—to reduce cerebral edema associated with brain tumors, thus lowering intracranial pressure and reversing neurologic deficits (in some patients).
2. Administer antacids or cimetidine with steroids to prevent gastric upset or GI bleeding.
3. Steroids may be introduced prior to therapy and withdrawn gradually as soon as definitive local treatment (surgery/radiation) has demonstrated clinical results.
4. Repeat CT scanning may be used to increase accuracy and safety of radiotherapy.
5. Radiosensitive drugs may be given to increase radiosensitivity of neoplastic tissue.
6. Loss of hair may be expected; regrowth may be expected after several weeks.
7. Some headache and depression of mental status may appear after first week of radiation; nausea and fatigue may appear during latter part of course of radiation therapy.
8. Complications of whole brain radiation:
   a. Brain atrophy—may be correlated with a decrease in the patient's functional level
   b. Radiation necrosis
9. See page 913 for nursing management of the patient undergoing radiation therapy.

C. Chemotherapy (Neuro-oncology)

1. Chemotherapeutic drugs (BCNU, CCNU, procarbazine) may be given singly or in combination, or may be combined with surgery and radiation therapy.
   High-dose CCNU with marrow autotransplantation (bone marrow grafting) to assist hematologic recovery from risk of fatal marrow depression is being investigated.
2. Dosages of chemotherapeutic drugs may be limited by their toxicity.
3. See page 905 for nursing management of the patient undergoing chemotherapy.

D. Management of Patient with Brain Metastases From Systemic Cancer (lung, skin, breast)

1. Patients with systemic tumors may function well until tumor metastasizes to nervous system and rapidly produces frightening and disabling symptoms (motor loss, cranial neuropathies, intellectual impairment, convulsive seizures).
2. Metastases to brain are commonly multiple and often unresectable.
3. Therapeutic approach includes surgery, radiation, and chemotherapy; palliation more effective if treatment is started before major neurologic deficits develop.
4. Steroid doses may be increased in the patient with progression of tumor to decrease symptoms of increased intracranial pressure
5. Arrange for Nurse Clinician and/or Social Worker to meet with the patient and family to identify problems.
6. See page 905 for nursing management of the patient with cancer.

Health Education

1. Make the patient and family aware that discontinuing steroids may cause rapid deterioration and lapse into coma.
2. Encourage family to join a support group to provide psychological support, clarify attitudes and behaviors about the patient's illness, and provide education about the illness.

The Epilepsies

The *epilepsies* are a symptom-complex of several disorders of brain function characterized by recurrent seizures. There may be associated changes in behavior, mentation, and motor or sensory activity. The basic problem is thought to be an electrical disturbance (dysrhythmia) in the nerve cells in one section of the brain that causes them to give off abnormal, recurrent, uncontrolled electrical discharges.

Causes

The underlying disorder of the brain may be structural, chemical, or physiological, or a combination of all three.
1. Genetic factors
2. Trauma—head/brain
3. Brain tumor
4. Circulatory disorder (stroke, arteriovenous malformation)
5. Metabolic disorder (hypoglycemia, hypocalcemia, anoxia)
6. Toxicity (drugs and alcohol)
7. CNS infection (encephalitis, meningitis, abscess)

Assessment

Clinical Manifestations

1. Impaired consciousness
2. Disturbances of mental function
3. Excess or loss of muscle tone or movement
4. Disorders of sensation or special senses
5. Disturbances of the autonomic functions of the body

Diagnostic Evaluation

1. History of seizures (as noted by patient and observers)
2. Electroencephalograph (EEG)—finds and measures brain electrical discharge pattern; useful in locating the site where epileptic discharge begins, its spread, intensity, duration; helps classify seizure type (Fig. 18-9).
3. EEG and closed circuit television monitoring of patients—split screen techniques show the patient during a seizure with simultaneous EEG tracing (Fig. 18-9).
4. Telemetering computer equipment—the patient wears a device that holds electrodes on scalp and houses a small radio transmitter; EEG signals are picked up by receiver and tape-recorded; helps identify seizure patterns before and after they occur.
5. CT scan—to rule out slow-growing tumors, atrophic areas, cysts, and other pathologic processes.

Patient Problems/Nursing Diagnoses

1. Alteration in consciousness related to occurrence of seizures

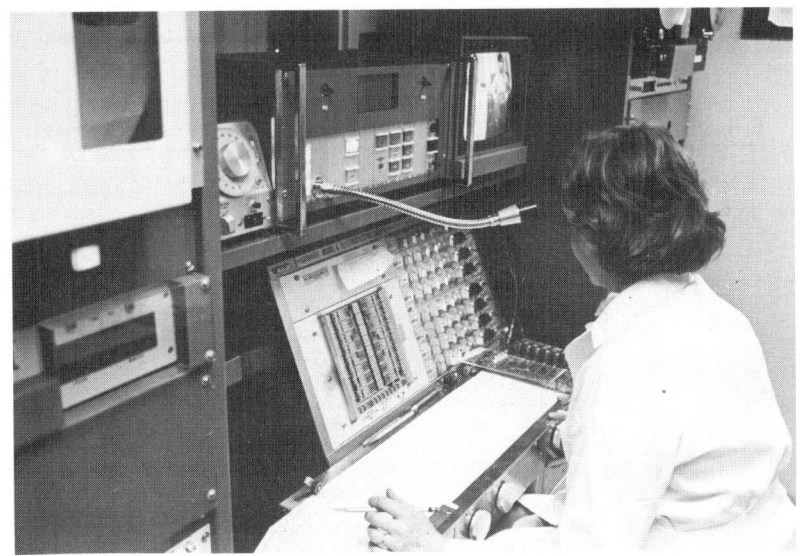

Figure 18-9. EEG and television monitoring of patient during a seizure. (Courtesy of National Institute of Neurological and Communicative Disorders and Stroke)

2. Fear related to occurrence of seizures and stress of having epilepsy
3. Ineffective individual coping related to psychosocial and economic stigma
4. Potential for injury related to sudden loss of consciousness

Planning and Implementation

Nursing Interventions

A. Control of seizures and prevention of recurrence

1. Emphasize the importance of *regularity* in taking the prescribed antiepileptic medication to reduce number and/or severity of seizures.
   a. Goal of drug therapy: to suppress seizure activity with fewest medication side effects.
   b. Drug therapy is regarded as a form of control; not a cure.
      (1) The choice of drug(s) is selected according to the type of seizure.
      (2) Treatment is usually started with one drug; the dosage is adjusted until seizures are controlled and effective serum concentration level of the drug is achieved and maintained or toxic symptoms develop: a second drug may be added if there is partial improvement.
      (3) See Table 18-1 for list of drugs of choice and alternative treatment of the most common types of epileptic seizures.
   c. Instruct the patient to keep a record of events surrounding his seizures (number, duration, time of occurrence, sleep/eating patterns)—to help determine proper therapy/patient compliance.

▶ **NURSING ALERT:** The patient should not stop taking his antiepileptic medication without medical supervision, since sudden withdrawal can cause an increase in seizure frequency or precipitate the development of status epilepticus.

   d. The patient should watch for toxic effects of antiepileptic medication—drowsiness, gingival hyperplasia, nervousness, visual difficulties, motor incoordination, staggering ataxia, bone marrow depression leading to blood dyscrasias.
      (1) Advise the patient to avoid taking medication on an empty stomach; gastritis is apt to occur, especially with phenytoin (Dilantin).
      (2) Instruct the patient to brush teeth frequently and massage gums to prevent gingival infection.
   e. Encourage the patient to have periodic blood evaluations when taking antiepileptic drugs that may depress hemopoiesis.
2. See nursing management of the patient with seizures, page 769.
3. Biofeedback training, in which the patient is taught to control his brain wave activity, is being used successfully.
4. Neurosurgical management of the epilepsies: Surgical procedures are performed when epilepsy results from intracranial tumors, abscess, cysts, vascular abnormalities, or when the patient has intractable seizures not responding to drug therapy. If the seizures originate in a reasonably well-circumscribed area of the brain that can be excised without producing significant neurologic deficits, the removal of the focus generating the seizures seems to give long-term control and improvement. See page 770 for postoperative care.

B. Maximizing coping resources to achieve improved quality of life

1. Use a multidisciplinary approach to cope with social, emotional, and vocational pressures.
2. See Health Education, below.

Health Education

1. Encourage the patient to study himself and his environment to determine what specific factors precipitate his seizures—illness, emotional stress, physical stress, hyperventilation, altered sleep patterns, photosensitivity, or other sensory stimuli, menses, etc.
2. The medication must be taken daily to prevent sei-

Table 18-1. Drugs Commonly Used in Epilepsy

Drug	Effective Plasma Level (μg./ml.)	High Effective Level (μg./ml.)*	Toxic Level (μg./ml.)	Seizure Types for Which Drug is Effective	Common Dose-Related Side Effects	Idiosyncratic Side Effects
Carbamazepine	4–10	7	>8	Partial Generalized tonic–clonic	Diplopia Ataxia Mild leukopenia	Skin rash Bone marrow depression (rare)
Primidone	5–15	10	>12	Partial Generalized tonic–clonic	Sedation Diplopia Ataxia	Skin rash
Phenytoin	10–20	18	>20	Partial Generalized tonic–clonic	Diplopia Ataxia Hirsutism Gingival hyperplasia	Skin rash Peripheral neuropathy
Phenobarbital	10–40	35	>40	Partial Generalized tonic–clonic	Sedation Diplopia Ataxia	Skin rash
Ethosuximide	50–100	80	>100	Absence	Nausea and vomiting	Skin rash
Valproate	50–100	80	>100	Absence Myoclonic Atonic Generalized tonic–clonic?	Nausea and vomiting Weight gain Hair loss Tremor	Skin rash Hepatotoxicity (rare)

* Level that should be achieved, if possible, in patients with refractory seizures, assuming that the blood samples are drawn before administration of the morning medication.
(Modified from Porter RJ. *Epilepsy: 100 Elementary Principles.* Philadelphia, WB Saunders Company, 1984, p. 69)

zures; medication may have to be adjusted because of recurrent illness, weight change, increase in stress, etc.
  a. Notify physician/clinic at the *first* sign of untoward medication reaction.
  b. Antiepileptic drugs can be withdrawn in 2–4 years in certain types of epilepsy.
3. Practice *regularity* and *moderation* in daily activities; diet, exercise, rest, avoidance of certain stimulating stresses.
  a. Have regular hours for sleep.
  b. Avoid emotional overstimulation (watching late television, etc.) or photic stimulation (flickering light).
  c. Eat a well-balanced diet—long-term antiepileptic therapy can cause deficiencies, particularly of vitamin D.
  d. Avoid alcohol when seizures are known to follow alcoholic intake.
  e. Avoid swimming alone or engaging in sports, occupations, or hobbies involving serious risks.
  f. Seek help and counseling (if necessary) during periods of crisis—death in family, divorce, etc.).
4. Report any changes in health status—easy bruising, purpura, bleeding gums, jaundice, fever, recurrent infections or dermatosis.
5. Have follow-up urinalysis and blood studies.
6. Stress the importance of activity, both physical and mental. Activity tends to inhibit, not stimulate, epileptic seizures.
7. Reorient the attitude of the patient and family to the disease.
  a. Help the family to understand that the patient has experienced rejection, anxiety (due to unpredictable seizure activity), feelings of being "different."
  b. Encourage the patient or family to discuss feelings and attitudes about epilepsy.

  (1) Family members frequently experience guilt (from unconscious rejection of patient) resulting in overprotection or scapegoating.
  (2) The patient/family may require psychological counseling if psychiatric problems are evident.
  c. Help the patient/family towards self-acceptance; reinforce areas of strength.
  d. Epilepsy can be *controlled;* it is not insanity or a supernatural condition.
8. Carry a wallet card and wear a medical-alert bracelet indicating that the wearer has epilepsy.
9. Learn of the services and publications of:
  a. Epilepsy Foundation of America, 4351 Garden City Drive, Landover, MD 20785
  b. Comprehensive Epilepsy Program (Epilepsy Research Program) National Institutes of Health Bethesda, MD 20892

Evaluation
Expected Outcomes
1. Maintains control of seizures; takes medication as prescribed
2. Copes with fears and achieves improved psychosocial adjustment
3. Demonstrates an understanding of the disorder
4. Identifies and avoids stressors that may increase susceptibility to seizures
5. Carries identification card or wears medical-alert bracelet indicating nature of disorder and possibility of seizures

Status Epilepticus

Status epilepticus (acute, prolonged, repetitive seizure activity) is a series of generalized seizures without return to consciousness between attacks. The term has been broadened to include continuous clinical and/or electrical seizures lasting at least 30 minutes, even without impairment of consciousness.

Underlying Considerations

1. Status epilepticus is considered a serious neurologic emergency. It has a high mortality and morbidity rate (permanent brain damage; severe neurologic deficits).
2. Common factors that precipitate status epilepticus include acute central nervous system insult (acute cerebral infarction, CNS infection, head trauma, cerebral neoplasm), and anticonvulsant drug withdrawal.

Patient Problems/Nursing Diagnoses

1. Alteration in consciousness related to prolonged seizure activity
2. Potential for complications (brain damage, cardiac arrhythmias) related to physiologic changes during generalized convulsive status

Nursing Interventions

A. Maintain an airway and restore homeostasis.

1. Give oxygen—there is some respiratory arrest at height of each seizure which produces venous congestion and hypoxia of the brain.
2. Draw blood for glucose, blood urea nitrogen, electrolytes, and anticonvulsant drug levels—to determine metabolic abnormalities and as a guide for maintenance of biochemical homeostasis.
3. Start intravenous infusions.
   a. Isotonic saline IV for maintenance of blood pressure.
   b. IV glucose—if hypoglycemia is the cause, the glucose infusion will stop the seizures.
   c. Thiamine is added to infusion if vitamin deficiency is suspected.

B. Stop the convulsive seizures as quickly as possible to prevent permanent brain damage and death.

1. Give intravenous anticonvulsant (diazepam, phenytoin, phenobarbital) *slowly*—to ensure effective brain tissue and serum concentrations.
   a. Give additional anticonvulsants as directed—effects of diazepam are of short duration.
   b. Obtain anticonvulsant blood levels.
   c. Employ mechanical ventilation as needed.
   d. If initial treatment is unsuccessful, general anesthesia (with a short-acting barbiturate) may be used.
   e. Monitor the patient continuously; depression of respiration and blood pressure induced by phenobarbital may be delayed.
2. Assist with diagnostic evaluation for causative factors.
   a. Monitor vital and neurologic signs on a continuing basis.
   b. Employ electroencephalographic monitoring—to determine nature and abolition (after diazepam administration) of epileptic activity.
   c. Determine (from family member) if there is a history of epilepsy, alcohol/drug use, trauma, recent infection.
   d. Assist with other studies (CT scan, CSF studies, biochemical and microbiological studies).

Evaluation
Expected Outcomes

1. Recovers from seizure episode with minimal side effects; no focal manifestations or tonic–clonic contractions
2. Becomes oriented to surroundings
3. Is free of complications
   a. Metabolic parameters within normal range
   b. Respiratory and blood pressure readings within preseizure range

Parkinson's Disease

Parkinson's disease is a progressive neurologic disorder affecting the brain centers responsible for control of movement. It is characterized by bradykinesia (slowness of movement), tremor, and muscle stiffness or rigidity.

Pathophysiology

The primary neurohumoral defect is deficiency of dopamine in the striatum of the basal ganglia.

Etiology

1. Unknown
2. Viruses, encephalitis, cerebrovascular disease, and poisoning or toxicity (manganese, carbon monoxide) have been suspected.
3. Theory advanced that there is an imbalance of 2 neurochemical systems, cholinergic and dopaminergic, and that the symptoms of parkinsonism are caused by overactivity or underactivity of one or the other of these systems.
4. Genetic susceptibility (positive family history)

Treatment

Treatment is based on a combination of drug therapy, physical therapy and rehabilitation techniques, and patient and family education.

Drug Therapy (decreases symptoms but does not halt progression of disease; regimen changes as disease progresses)

1. *Antihistamines* (diphenhydramine [Benadryl])—(given to the patient with minimal dysfunction) thought to help patients with tremor because of their anticholinergic properties.
2. *Anticholinergics* (block the action of acetylcholine)—given to relieve tremor and augment levodopa therapy.
   a. Frequently used anticholinergics include trihexyphenidyl (Artane and others); benztropine mesylate (Cogentin); ethopropazine (Parsidol); orphenadrine (Disipal).

   b. Assess for side effects of anticholinergic agents—dryness of mouth, blurred vision, urinary retention, constipation, confusion; forgetfulness.
3. *Tricyclic antidepressants* (amitriptyline [Elavil])—to control depression associated with parkinsonism.
4. *Amantadine* (Symmetrel)—an antiviral drug that may increase release of dopamine in the brain.
5. *Levodopa* (Dopar, Larodopa)
   a. Levodopa (an amino acid that is depleted in the substance of the brain involved in nerve transmission in patients with parkinsonism) is given in increasing doses until the patient's tolerance is reached; it relieves rigidity in majority of patients and usually improves tremor for a period of time. (The brain converts levodopa to dopamine.)
   b. Dosage is increased gradually until maximum therapeutic effect is achieved and side effects appear—nausea, vomiting, anorexia, postural hypotension, mental changes (confusion, agitation, mood alterations), cardiac arrhythmias, twitching.
   c. Beneficial effects most pronounced in first few years of treatment
   d. Adverse effects may increase with continued use.
      (1) Dyskinesias (abnormal involuntary movements)—facial grimacing, rhythmic jerking movements of hands progressing to head bobbing, chewing and smacking movements, jerking movements involving trunk and extremities
      (2) Progressive shortening of levodopa's effect (reduced "on" time)
         On–off phenomena—sudden episodes of immobility ("off effect") lasting minutes to hours, followed by sudden return of effectiveness ("on effect")
      (3) Psychiatric reactions—confusion, memory impairment, hallucinations, delusions
6. *Combination of levodopa and a decarboxylase inhibitor*—carbidopa, a decarboxylase inhibitor, slows down the peripheral metabolism of dopa.
   Sinemet (combination of carbidopa and levodopa)—potentiates therapeutic effects of levodopa; appears to achieve a therapeutic effect with much lower dose of levodopa and thus reduces incidence of side effects.
7. *Dopamine agonists*
   a. *Bromocriptine mesylate* (Parlodel)—crosses blood–brain barrier and stimulates dopaminergic receptors.
      (1) Given when the patient has intractable symptoms despite therapy with levodopa.
      (2) Adverse effects—confusion, delusions, hallucinations, gastrointestinal upset, abnormal involuntary movements.
   b. *Pergolide mesylate*—used in combination with levodopa in patients with advanced disease and with on–off phenomenon (investigational).

Assessment
Clinical Manifestations

1. Bradykinesia (dyskinesia, hypokinesia [gradual loss of spontaneous movement])—usually becomes the most disabling symptom
2. Tremor—tends to decrease or disappear on purposeful movement
3. Rigidity, particularly of large joints
4. Muscle weakness—affecting eating, chewing, swallowing, speaking, writing
5. Mask-like facial expression, unblinking eyes
6. Depression
7. Dementia

Patient Problems/Nursing Diagnoses

1. Impaired mobility related to bradykinesia, muscle rigidity
2. Inadequate nutritional intake related to muscle weakness, inability to swallow effectively, choking and saliva buildup
3. Impaired verbal communication related to reduced movement of muscles controlling respiration, phonation, articulation, and prosody (rhythm, intonation) and incoordination
4. Self-care deficits (feeding, hygiene, dressing, toileting) related to diminished motor function and tremor
5. Depression related to social withdrawal and dysfunction from progression of disease

Planning and Implementation
Nursing Interventions

A. Establishing optimum functioning capacity

1. Encourage the patient to continue on an exercise and physical therapy program to increase muscle strength, improve coordination and dexterity, treat muscular rigidity, prevent contractures, and compensate for lack of automatic movements.
2. Emphasize the importance of a *daily* exercise program (walk, ride stationary bike, swim, garden)—to maintain joint mobility.
   Instruct the patient to:
   a. Exercise each joint daily
   b. Lengthen stride when walking; swing arms while walking—loosens arms and shoulders and lessens fatigue
   c. Practice breathing exercises—to mobilize rib cage; helps transport oxygen to poorly aerated parts of lung
   d. Exercise facial muscles (grimace, make faces in front of mirror)—for facial mobility and facial expression
3. Advise the patient to do stretching exercises (stretch–hold–relax) to loosen the joint structures.
4. Teach postural exercises and walking techniques to offset shuffling gait and tendency to lean forward:
   a. Use a broad-based gait (feet wide apart).
   b. Make a conscious effort to swing arms, raise the feet while walking, use a heel–toe, heel–toe gait, and increase the width of the stride.
   c. Practice walking to marching music or sound of ticking metronome—provides sensory reinforcement.
5. Encourage the patient to take warm baths, massage, and passive and active exercises—to help relax muscles and relieve painful muscle spasms that accompany rigidity.
6. Advise the patient to have frequent rest periods—the patient becomes fatigued and frustrated by his symptoms.
7. Use assistive devices for help in activities of daily living.
8. Try to have the patient seen by a physical therapist

on a regular basis—reinforces his program; introduces new program of exercises.

B. Improving nutritional status

1. Help the patient think through swallowing sequence; close lips and with teeth together, place food on tongue, lift the tongue up—then back and swallow (up–back–swallow).
2. Encourage the patient to make a conscious effort to chew and to chew first on one side and then the other.
3. Control the buildup of saliva by holding head in an upright position and making a conscious effort to swallow saliva often.
4. Secure a stabilized plate, nonspill cup, built-up eating utensils and an electrical warming tray as assistive devices and to keep food hot and allow the patient to rest during prolonged eating time.
5. Encourage intake of foods with a moderate fiber content because a patient with parkinsonism has severe problems with constipation.
6. Place the patient on a bowel routine (p. 70).

C. Improving verbal communication

1. Advise the patient to take medication that improves speech disorders.
2. Refer to speech–language pathologist for assessment and therapy at an early stage.
   For list of approved speech and hearing centers and certified speech–language pathologists:
   > American Speech–Language-Hearing Association
   > 10801 Rockville Pike
   > Rockville, MD 20852
3. Remind the patient to face listener, exaggerate pronunciation, and speak in short sentences.
4. Advise the patient to practice reading aloud in front of mirror, exaggerating symbols, and enunciating deliberately.
5. Have the patient speak into tape-recorder to monitor progress.
6. Consider amplification devices for problem of weak voice (not beneficial for slurred speech, uneven speech rate).

D. Promoting independence in ADL

(See Health Education, this page, second column)

E. Establishing positive response to psychological support

1. Help the patient establish achievable goals (improvement of health and mobility, lessening of tremors).
2. Encourage the patient to be an *active* participant in his therapy and in social and recreational events—parkinsonism tends to lead to depression and withdrawal.
3. Have a planned program of activity throughout day—prevents daytime sleeping, disinterest, and apathy.
4. Reemphasize that disability can be prevented or delayed; offer realistic reassurance.
5. Try to dispel anxiety and fears of the patient that may be as disabling to him as his disease.
6. Provide caring and support for family who are vulnerable to emotional stresses and depression from living with a progressively disabled person.
   a. Allow expression of feelings of frustration, anger, depression, guilt, etc.
   b. Help family to identify problem areas and explore ways of coping and realistic alternatives.
   c. Avoid hurrying the patient.

Health Education

1. See A through C, pages 792–793.
2. Explain that sudden changes in disability are encountered in Parkinson's disease.
3. Try the following routine when feet and legs seem to be "glued" to the floor.
   a. Raise head.
   b. Raise toes (eliminates muscle spasm).
   c. Rock from one foot to the other while bending knees slightly.
   d. Or raise arms in a sudden, short motion.
   e. Or take a small step backward; then start forward.
   f. Or step sideways; then start forward.
   g. Instruct the family not to pull patient during episodes of "freezing"—this increases the problem and may cause falling.
4. For the patient who has difficulty rising up from a chair:
   a. Choose straight-back wooden chairs with armrests (captain's chair); raise rear legs of chair 10 cm. (2 inches) to give chair a slight forward tilt.
   b. Move toward edge of seat, placing heels as far back under chair as possible.
   c. Lean forward from hips so that center of gravity is above feet.
      Another person may hold the patient's hand while pushing forward gently and firmly on his head with the other hand.
   d. Rise to a standing posture.
5. Establish a regular bowel routine, consciously increase fluid intake, and eat foods with a moderate fiber content—patients with parkinsonism have trouble with constipation because of muscle weakness, lack of exercise, inadequate fluid intake, and drug effects.
6. Eat a well-balanced diet—nutritional problems develop from slowness of movement, difficulties in chewing and swallowing, and dry mouth from medications.
7. Report for blood evaluations and tonometry (screening test for glaucoma) because levodopa or Sinemet® can exacerbate blood disorders, GI bleeding, and glaucoma.
8. Avoid over-the-counter sedatives.
9. Learn all one can about Parkinson's disease. American Parkinson Disease Association, 116 John Street, New York, NY 10038, has illustrated booklets and a newsletter for patient education.

Evaluation

Expected Outcomes

1. Achieves improved physical mobility; exercises and walks daily
2. Maintains satisfactory nutritional status; eats slowly and without choking
3. Demonstrates improved verbal communication; practices speech exercises
4. Achieves self care; allows enough time to carry out activities and uses assistive devices when necessary
5. Can explain the purpose of drug therapy; adheres to the prescribed regimen

Multiple Sclerosis

Multiple sclerosis (MS) is a chronic, frequently progressive disease of the central nervous system characterized by the occurrence of small patches of demyelination of the central nervous system white matter, in association with inflammation and gliosis.

1. Demyelination results in disordered transmission of nerve impulses. (*Demyelination* refers to the destruction of myelin, the fatty and protein material that ensheathes certain nerve fibers in the brain and spinal cord.)
2. Although the cause and pathogenesis of MS are unknown, it is believed that immune abnormalities are related to the disease; infection by a slow virus, or a combination of these two have been postulated.

Incidence

Multiple sclerosis can be one of the most disabling of the neurologic diseases that strike young adults during their most productive years (20–40 years of age). It maximizes the medical, psychological, social, and economic problems encountered by the patient and his family. However, a number of these patients have little or no disability for many years after diagnosis.

Treatment

Although there is no specific treatment, the following is aimed at relieving symptoms and helping the patient function.

1. Immunosuppressive agents
   a. ACTH and adrenal corticosteroids during acute exacerbations—may ameliorate symptoms by preventing edema (edema may occur at margins of MS plaques during active phase of disease) and for its anti-inflammatory action
   b. Cyclophosphamide plus ACTH
   c. Azathioprine
2. Hyperbaric oxygen
3. Symptomatic treatment to manage complications
   a. Drugs for spasticity—baclofen, dantrolene sodium, diazepam
   b. Antidepressants—tricyclic antidepressant drugs
   c. Prophylactic antibiotic therapy in patients with recurring urinary infections
4. Treat the patient with appropriate therapy during periods of exacerbation—the residual effects of the disease may increase with each exacerbation.
   a. Give pharmacologic agents as prescribed.
   b. Encourage rest for a few days during acute exacerbation—continued activity appears to worsen attack.
   c. Try to have the patient avoid any known factor that causes exacerbation—activity (overexertion), stress, fever, and exposure to heat.
   d. Aim to prevent permanent damage; continue with range-of-motion exercises, specific muscle exercises, etc., as physical strength permits.
   e. Take corrective action for each new problem as it arises.
   f. Invent, adapt, and modify equipment that can be used for self-help devices so that the patient will not regress.

Assessment

Clinical Manifestations

Note: The signs and symptoms reflect the location and areas of demyelinization within the central nervous system. Patients with MS have a wide range of clinical symptoms; there is great variability in the course of the disease, with many relapses and remissions.

1. Fatigue and weakness
2. Abnormal reflexes, either absent or exaggerated
3. Visual disturbances; impaired vision, diplopia; optic neuritis
4. Tremor, ataxia, incoordination
5. Sensory disturbances; paresthesias
6. Bladder dysfunction with urinary frequency, nocturia, incontinence
7. Impaired vibration and position sense
8. Slurring, scanning speech (dysarthria)
9. Emotional lability; euphoria, depression

Patient Problems/Nursing Diagnoses

1. Progressive motor, sensory, and visual dysfunction related to demyelination
2. Bladder dysfunction (urgency, frequency, incontinence, urinary retention) related to detrusor hyperreflexia; detrusor areflexia
3. Bowel dysfunction related to spinal cord involvement
4. Impairment of skin integrity related to immobility, sensory loss, and spasticity
5. Self-care deficits related to general weakness, spasticity, and fatigue
6. Sexual dysfunction related to physical impairment, muscle weakness/spasticity, urinary/fecal incontinence
7. Compromised individual and family coping related to stresses of chronic illness, unpredictable course of disease

Planning and Nursing Implementation

Nursing Interventions

A. Improving functioning ability

1. Strengthen muscles and prevent and treat muscle spasticity—spasticity interferes with normal function.
   a. The patient should do muscle-stretching exercises daily—to minimize spasticity, joint contractures, and tightening and shortening of certain muscle groups.
   b. Give particular emphasis to hamstrings, gastrocnemius, hip adductors, biceps, wrist and finger flexors.
   c. Teach the patient's family passive exercises and range-of-motion exercises for patients with severe spasticity.
   d. Teach the stretch–hold–relax routine and encourage the patient to do it throughout the day for relaxation.
   e. Spasticity (increased tone) may also be treated with baclofen, dantrolene, and diazepam.
      Muscle relaxants may increase muscle weakness and prevent walking.
   f. Apply ice packs (30 minutes) and give slow

stretches to affected muscles; may reduce spasticity in early stages.

2. Advise the patient to avoid muscle fatigue; stop physical activity just short of fatigue and take frequent short rest periods, preferably lying down.
3. Encourage general body-strengthening exercises for correcting/preventing specific muscle weakness of disuse and for balance and coordination.
4. Prevent muscle contractures and loss of muscle power from lack of use—diminishing motor power is a significant problem in multiple sclerosis.
5. Encourage the patient to sleep prone—to minimize flexor spasm at knees and hips.
6. Advise the patient to participate in walking exercises—to improve gait affected by loss of position sense in legs.
7. Utilize braces, canes, crutches, walker when necessary—to keep the patient ambulatory.
8. Prepare patients with severe spasticity and contractures for surgical intervention—to prevent further contractures and disability.
9. Assist the patient to overcome effects of incoordination—caused by motor dysfunction.
   a. Teach the patient to walk with feet wider apart—to widen his base of support and increase his walking stability.
   b. Inform the patient to avoid abrupt change in position and to be careful in turning, sitting, and standing.
   c. Utilize weighted bracelets, wrist cuffs, eating utensils—to help overcome incoordination of upper extremities.
10. Help the patient with optic and speech defects—cranial nerves affecting sight and speech are affected by multiple sclerosis.
    a. Utilize eye patch, frosted lens—to block visual impulses of one eye when the patient has diplopia (double vision).
    b. Secure services of speech pathologist or therapist—to increase the coordination of phonation and prevent atrophy of the speech muscles.
    c. Prism glasses may be useful for the bedridden patient.
    d. For the patient who has impaired eyesight or who is unable to hold a book, turn pages, or read regular print, secure books and magazines recorded on discs, tape cassettes, and open reel magnetic tape provided free of charge by: Division for the Blind and Physically Handicapped, Library of Congress, Washington, DC 20542.

B. Establishing bladder control

1. See page 539 for management of the patient with a neurogenic bladder.
2. Assess for bladder infection.
3. Assess for urinary retention.
   a. Catheterize the patient; insert indwelling catheter only if absolutely necessary.
   b. Give urinary antiseptics—to reduce incidence of bacteriuria.
4. Ensure adequate fluid intake (3–5 liters daily)—to reduce urinary bacterial count, minimize precipitation of urinary crystals, stone formation, and encrustation of the lumen of the indwelling urethral catheter.
5. Support the patient who has urinary incontinence (or frequency and urgency).

Female patient
   a. Set up a voiding-time schedule; every 1½ to 2 hours initially, with lengthening time intervals if regimen is successful.
   b. Encourage the patient to drink a measured amount of fluid every 2 hours.
   c. Have the patient try to void 30 minutes after drinking.
   d. Teach self-catheterization technique.
   e. Use low fracture bedpan at night; set alarm clock for patient with diminished warning sensation.
   f. For permanent urinary incontinence, urine may have to be diverted by means of ileal conduit (see p. 544).
Male patient
   a. See a, b, c, and d under Female Patient, above.
   b. Use urinal at night.
   c. For permanent incontinence, the patient may wear external sheath or condom appliance for urine collection.

C. Achieving bowel control

1. Establish a program of *regularity*.
   a. Have the patient eat regularly scheduled meals; include high-fiber foods.
   b. Establish bowel evacuation at *same time each day*.
2. Encourage the patient to drink 120 ml. (4 ounces) of prune juice at bedtime (same time each night).
3. Insert a glycerin or Dulcolax suppository into the rectum 30 minutes before scheduled bowel evacuation time—*after* eating a meal (preferably after breakfast).
4. Advise the patient to attempt to have a bowel movement within 30 minutes of eating, using as normal a position for defecation as possible.
   a. Instruct the patient to bear down and contract abdominal muscles.
   b. Teach the patient to apply pressure to abdomen with his hands—to assist with defecation.
5. After this routine is established, mechanical stimulation with a suppository may not be necessary.

D. Preventing skin breakdown

1. Relieve pressure.
   a. Change position at least every 2 hours if the patient is in bed.
   b. Change position every 30 minutes if the patient is in a wheelchair.
   c. Use flotation pad, sheepskin, alternating air pressure mattress, and other modalities to distribute pressure away from bony points and over a wider area.
   d. Teach the patient to inspect pressure areas (using a long-handled mirror for posterior sites) for evidences of redness and heat.
2. Avoid skin trauma, heat, cold, and pressure.
3. Give careful attention to sacral and perineal hygiene.
4. See page 59 for discussion of prevention and treatment of pressure sores.

E. Striving toward increased independence in self-care and activities of daily living

1. Teach transfer activities (see p. 65).
2. Secure services of a knowledgeable wheelchair dealer to select correct wheelchair.
3. Use assistive and self-help devices.

a. Toilet facilities—raised toilet seat or bedside commode.
b. Bathing facilities—use shower hose and stool in shower or tub and hand rails to compensate for weakness and to prevent falls.
c. Self-care aids—prism glasses, telephone modifications, long-handled combs, tongs, and modified clothing.

F. Adapting to sexual dysfunction

See Sexuality: A Part of the Rehabilitation Process, page 53.

Discharge Planning and Health Education

1. Review A through F, pages 794–796.
2. Help the family (and patient) understand the stresses imposed by multiple sclerosis.
   a. There are embarrassing and humiliating symptoms to which the person may respond "inappropriately."
   b. The patient may be depressed, or have brain damage with resultant denial of his disease, euphoria, or depressive and paranoid behavior.
   c. MS patients are often forgetful and easily distracted.
3. Understand that patients adapt to illness in many ways—frustration, anger, denial, depression, withdrawal, inactivity, resentment, etc.
4. Support the defense mechanisms of the patient, according to the patient's time table, when feasible.
   a. Avoid confronting him with stark reality.
   b. Answer questions honestly.
   c. Help the patient remain in control.
   d. Offer services of mental health professionals when advisable.
5. The patient may have feelings of alienation from family, others, work, and social life; he feels that his personal worth is lessened.
   a. Give opportunities for the patient to vent his feelings; suppressed anger is destructive.
   b. Try to keep him in the mainstream of life as much as possible.
   c. Contact local chapter of the National Multiple Sclerosis Society* for services, publications, and contact with other MS patients.
   d. Encourage the patient to keep up social interests and activities.

6. Try to keep up the activities (physical, social, etc.) that the patient is able to do; once lost, certain abilities are almost impossible to regain.
   a. Physical abilities may vary from day to day.
   b. Devise modifications that will allow continuance of certain activities; obtain gadgets and adaptive devices for self-help (mail-order gift companies, medical supply catalogues, rehabilitation literature).
   c. Learn energy-conservation techniques.
   d. Follow short periods of exertion with periods of rest.
7. Try to avoid physical and emotional stresses—may worsen symptoms and impair performance.
   a. Exposure to heat/cold—appears to increase fatigue
      (1) Take tepid showers/baths.
      (2) Avoid becoming overheated, especially during summer months.
   b. Overexertion—lessens motor power
   c. Fever
   d. Emotional upsets
8. Assist the patient to accept his new identity as a handicapped person and cope with the disruption in his life.
9. Keep channels of communication open.
10. Encourage meaningful and realistic short-term goals—to achieve a sense of purpose.
11. Encourage family to have family therapy if conflicts, psychosomatic conditions, and exhaustion threaten family stability.

Evaluation

Expected Outcomes

1. Demonstrates improved neurologic functioning; has increased mobility; uses techniques to improve coordination
2. Copes with bladder dysfunction; has a workable voiding schedule; able to catheterize self
3. Attains bowel control
4. Demonstrates intact skin; changes position to relieve pressure
5. Achieves some independence in self-care
6. Verbalizes ways to adapt to sexual dysfunction
7. Uses coping strategies

Myasthenia Gravis

Myasthenia gravis is a disorder affecting the neuromuscular transmission of impulses in the voluntary muscles of the body; it is characterized by excessive fatigability of muscle function. Myasthenia gravis is considered to be an autoimmune disease in which acetylcholine receptor (AChR) antibodies are the principal factors interfering with neuromuscular transmission.

Altered Physiology

Defect in transmission of impulses from nerve to muscle cells due to loss of available or normal receptors on the postsynaptic side of neuromuscular junction.

* National Multiple Sclerosis Society, 205 E. 42nd Street, New York, NY 10017

Clinical Manifestations

1. Abnormal weakness and fatigability of skeletal muscle, characteristically worse after effort and improved by rest; may involve any striated muscle.
2. Diplopia (double vision), ptosis (drooping of one or both eyelids)—weakness of ocular motor muscles
3. Sleepy, mask-like expression—from involvement of facial muscles
4. Speech weakness (slurred and nasal speech), difficulty in swallowing, choking, aspiration of food—from weakness of laryngeal and pharyngeal muscles

Diagnostic Evaluation

1. Blood test for AChR antibody—positive in 80%–90% of patients.

2. Pharmacologic tests:
   Edrophonium (Tensilon) test—intravenous injection of edrophonium may relieve weakness markedly in 30 seconds; useful for patients with ocular, facial, or oropharyngeal weakness.
3. Electromyographic testing (EMG) to measure electrical potential of muscle cells and confirm the defect of neuromuscular transmission
4. Chest x-ray—to rule out thymoma (tumor of the thymus)
5. CT scan of chest—to rule out thymoma

Treatment

A. Primary Drug Therapy

1. *Anticholinesterase drugs*—will increase response of muscles to nerve impulses and improve strength; by temporarily inhibiting acetylcholinesterase at the neuromuscular junction, they enhance the action of acetylcholine there.
   a. Pyridostigmine bromide (Mestinon)
   b. Neostigmine bromide (Prostigmin)
   c. Ambenonium chloride (Mytelase)
2. Drug scheduling individualized; timed so that peak action coincides with patient activities.
3. Toxicity and side effects of anticholinesterase:
   a. Gastrointestinal—abdominal cramps, nausea, vomiting, diarrhea
      (1) Drug may be taken with small amount of milk, crackers, or other buffering substance or after meals.
      (2) Side effects may be ameliorated or prevented by addition of atropine or atropine-like drugs to regimen.
      (3) Give diphenoxylate hydrochloride (Lomotil) for diarrhea
   b. Skeletal—fasciculations (fine twitching), spasm, weakness.
   c. Central nervous system—irritability, anxiety, insomnia, headache, dysarthria, syncope, coma, convulsions.
   d. Other—increased salivation and lacrimation, increased bronchial secretions, moist skin.

▶ **NURSING ALERT:** Watch for increase in muscle weakness within 1 hour after taking anticholinesterase drug; be alert for signs of respiratory embarrassment.

4. After initial medication adjustment has been made, the patient learns to take his medication according to his needs. Individual doses may vary with physical or emotional stress, intercurrent infection, etc.
5. Anticholinesterase drugs are not to be taken with morphine, ether, quinine (commercial cold preparations), procainamide, and certain antibiotics.
6. Sedatives and tranquilizing drugs are given with caution; may aggravate hypoxia and hypercapnia and cause respiratory and cardiac depression.
7. Immunopharmacologic agents
   a. Corticosteroids
   b. Cytotoxic immunosuppressive drugs (azathioprine, cyclophosphamide)—watch for bone marrow depression and infection.

B. Surgical Intervention (Thymectomy)—may give improvement or remission of the disease, especially in patients with tumor or hyperplasia of the thymus gland.

1. May be carried out by transcervical or sternal-splitting procedure.
2. Preoperative evaluation includes assessment of respiratory status (tidal volume, vital capacity), muscular strength, and the patient's chewing, swallowing, and ocular movements.
3. Postoperative nursing management (in intensive care unit) includes:
   a. Monitoring and caring for the patient on mechanical ventilator, if needed
   b. Continuing assessment of ventilatory function
   c. Temporary cessation of anticholinesterase medications
   d. Reassuring the patient that any increase in weakness is usually temporary.

C. Plasmapheresis (plasma exchange)—removal of the plasma containing acetylcholine receptor antibodies to improve muscle strength temporarily in patients with severe symptoms who do not respond to other treatment; usually gives rapid clinical improvement.

Nursing Interventions

A. Prevent and treat respiratory weakness and myasthenic crisis

1. Watch for myasthenic crisis (decline in neuromuscular function leading to marked weakness of respiratory and bulbar musculature).
   Clinical manifestations of impending crisis:
   a. Sudden respiratory distress combined with varying signs of dysphagia (difficulty in swallowing), dysarthria (difficulty in speaking), eyelid ptosis, and diplopia
   b. Tachycardia; anxiety
   c. Rapidly increasing weakness of muscles of trunk and extremities
2. Types of crises in myasthenia gravis:
   a. Myasthenic crisis—may result from natural deterioration of disease, emotional upset, upper respiratory infection, surgery, or trauma; or may be brought about by ACTH therapy.
      The patient may be temporarily resistant to anticholinesterase drugs or may need increased dosage.
   b. Cholinergic crisis—from overmedication with anticholinergic drugs.
   c. Brittle crisis—occurs when the receptors at the neuromuscular junction become insensitive to anticholinesterase medication; not controlled by increasing or decreasing anticholinesterase therapy.
3. Nursing and medical management during crisis:
   a. Place the patient in intensive care unit for constant monitoring—myasthenia gravis is a disease of rapidly fluctuating intensity and the patient is on the verge of respiratory arrest.
   b. Provide ventilatory assistance when muscles of respiration and swallowing become involved; endotracheal intubation and mechanical ventilation may be needed.
      (1) Suction the patient as indicated—*aspiration is a common problem.*
      (2) See Chapter 7 for management of the patient requiring ventilatory support.
   c. Search for intercurrent infection—usually causes an exacerbation of myasthenic crisis.
   d. Determine the time of onset of symptoms in relation to the last dose of anticholinesterase—

may show whether patient is undermedicated or having a cholinergic reaction.

Edrophonium may be given to differentiate type of crisis; Edrophonium (IV) improves the condition of the patient in myasthenic crisis, temporarily worsens that of the patient in cholinergic crisis, and is unpredictable in brittle crisis.

e. Give appropriate drugs as determined by the patient's status:
   (1) For myasthenic crisis: neostigmine methylsulfate (Prostigmin) administered parenterally if the patient is in true myasthenic crisis.
   (2) For cholinergic crisis: all anticholinesterase drugs are withdrawn. Atropine may be given to reduce excessive secretions.

f. Administer fluids, medication, and food via nasogastric tube if the patient is unable to swallow.

g. Avoid giving enemas—may cause sudden respiratory problems.

h. Develop a communication system for the patient on ventilator (or if he is too weak to speak).
   (1) Try to read lips of the patient.
   (2) Use picture cards, hand signals, etc.
   (3) Give hand bell to the patient.

i. Give continuing psychological support since the patient is usually alert and anxious. Reassure him that the crisis will pass and that he will not be left alone.

Health Education

Instruct the patient as follows:
1. Know the basic facts about anticholinergic drugs: action, reason for and regulation of dose according to changing needs, importance of timing, dosage adjustment, symptoms of overdose, and toxic effects.
2. Know the drugs that interact with anticholinesterase drugs. Be aware that many drugs can aggravate the disease (antibiotics, antiarrhythmics, local and general anesthetics, muscle relaxants, analgesics).
3. Have mealtimes coincide with peak of anticholinesterase effect (when swallowing ability is best); have standby suction available in home if swallowing difficulties occur. (Use a blender when necessary.)
4. Wear an identification bracelet signifying that you have myasthenia gravis.
5. Try to prevent factors (emotional upset, infections) that may increase weakness and precipitate myasthenic crisis.
6. Wear an eyepatch over one eye (alternating from side to side) if diplopia occurs.
7. Avoid vigorous physical activity and other factors leading to fatigue.
8. Avoid contracting colds and influenza—respiratory infections are extremely dangerous to the myasthenic individual.
9. Avoid excessive heat and cold (hot baths, sun bathing); weak spells may follow long exposure to excessive heat/cold.
10. Advise the dentist that you are myasthenic, since Novocain is usually not well tolerated.
11. Rest before fatigue sets in; do not force yourself to continue with an activity.
12. Use adaptive and self-help devices to handle motion impairment problems.
13. Learn all you can about the condition; with good management, the patient should be able to live a relatively full life. The Myasthenia Gravis Foundation, Inc., 15 East 26th Street, Suite 1603, New York, NY 10010.

Amyotrophic Lateral Sclerosis

Amyotrophic lateral sclerosis (ALS) is a progressively incapacitating and fatal disease of unknown cause in which there is degeneration of upper motor neurons (nerves leading from brain to medulla or to spinal cord) and to the lower motor neurons (nerves leading from spinal cord to muscles of body).

There is usually progressive paralysis; 50% of patients with ALS succumb in approximately 3 years, usually from secondary causes.

Assessment

Clinical Manifestations

(Depends on location of affected motor neurons, since specific neurons activate specific muscle fibers.)
1. Progressive weakness and atrophy of muscles of arms, trunk, or legs—from loss of neurons of the spinal cord
2. Signs of spasticity, fasciculations (irregular twitching of muscles) and exaggerated reflexes
3. Progressive difficulty in speaking and swallowing; nasal and unintelligible speech—when bulbar muscles are affected

Diagnostic Evaluation

1. Electromyography—demonstrates presence of denervation, muscle wasting, atrophy
2. Nerve conduction studies
3. Elevated creatinine phosphokinase

Patient Problems/Nursing Diagnoses

1. Impaired physical mobility related to muscle wasting and weakness
2. Potential for aspiration related to difficulty in swallowing
3. Alteration in nutrition (less than body requirements) related to inability to swallow
4. Potential for respiratory failure related to impaired intercostal, thoracic, and diaphragmatic muscle function
5. Feelings of powerlessness, helplessness, and frustration related to paralysis and ultimate outcome

Planning and Implementation

Treatment

No specific treatment available at present time to arrest or alter course of disease.

Drug therapy for symptomatic relief:
1. Baclofen—for spasticity
2. Diazepam—for fasciculations
3. Quinine compounds—for leg cramps
4. Pyridostigmine—for patients with defect in transmission at neuromuscular junction

Nursing Interventions

A. Establishing techniques and devices to cope with lost function and impaired physical mobility

1. Teach the patient active exercises and range-of-motion exercises—to strengthen uninvolved muscles that can substitute for impaired ones; to prevent disuse weakness.
2. Instruct the patient to use energy conservation and work simplification methods; use self-help and assistive devices.
3. Use orthoses (braces; p. 69) to help the patient function as long as possible.
   a. Ankle-foot orthoses for weak dorsiflexors—help keep the patient mobile.
   b. Hand and wrist splints—for optimal joint position and to provide a stronger grip.
4. Help family to secure equipment to assist with care—hospital bed, mechanical lift, wheelchair, catapult spring seats.
   a. Teach family the technique of positioning, turning, and transfer techniques.
   b. Teach pressure sore prevention. See Rehabilitation Nursing Chapter, page 59.

B. Preventing aspiration (choking, difficulty in chewing, swallowing, excessive drooling, and speaking)

1. Have standby suction available—aspiration is a constant danger.
2. Have a glass of water available.
3. Place the patient in a bolt upright position with neck flexed (chin pointed toward chest) to eat and drink.
4. Use a soft cervical collar if the patient has difficulty holding his head up.
5. Give semi-solid foods.
   a. Avoid easily aspirated, pureed foods and mucus-producing foods (milk).
   b. Offer very warm or very cold (not room temperature) food/drinks—makes use of temperature receptors in the mouth that are in part responsible for swallowing.
   c. Use soft foods that hold together (casseroles, stews, food with gravy).
   d. Do not wash down solids with fluids—may cause choking and aspiration.

C. Maintaining nutritional status

1. Consider alternate feeding methods to maintain nutrition in patients with advanced dysphagia.
   a. Nasogastric tube
   b. Gastrostomy tube
   c. Cervical esophagostomy—opening into esophagus, which bypasses larynx and avoids aspiration; feeding tube placed into this opening.
2. See *5*, above.

D. Dealing with potential for respiratory failure

1. Watch for symptoms of respiratory failure—occurs late in the disease.
2. See page 185 for management of respiratory failure.
3. If the patient decides against using a ventilator, he may consider making a "living will" to preserve his autonomy (not going on life-support; discontinuing life support).

E. Enhancing coping abilities

1. Understand that the patient may have involuntary outbursts of forced laughing/crying unrelated to mood/surroundings (pseudobulbar affect).
2. Develop some form of a communication system.
   For patients with some speech:
   a. Consider speech therapy early while the patient has some control over speech musculature.
   b. Use hand-held or around-the-neck microphone—to amplify voice.
   c. Have amplifier installed in telephone.
   d. Try electrolarynx—for patients who can articulate but cannot phonate.
   When speech is lost:
   a. Communication board (ALS Association newsletter describes various communication devices)
   b. Use environmental control system—switch may be activated by slight movement of eyebrow, etc.
   c. Eye movement/eye blinks—may be the patient's only means of communication.
   d. Understand that the patient is alert and retains vision, ocular movement, intelligence, and consciousness, but he may be physically incapable of doing a solitary thing and cannot speak/swallow.
3. Give the patient and family compassionate and caring support; problems are ever-changing.
   a. Allow expressions of feelings (helplessness, desperation) and frustrations about losses and eventual outcome.
   b. Help the patient to know that something can be done to make his existence more comfortable.
   c. Use telephone, radio, television, tapes, talking books to help the patient maintain equilibrium.
   d. Include the patient in planning and decision making.
   e. Extend support and a sense of caring to the family; they may require intermittent psychotherapy.
   f. Advise the patient/family of helping services of The ALS Association, 15300 Ventura Blvd., Suite 315, Sherman Oaks, CA 91403 and 185 Madison Ave., New York, NY 10016 (pamphlets, newsletter, patient-care tips); and Muscular Dystrophy Association, 810 Seventh Avenue, New York, NY 10019 (services and equipment).

Evaluation

Expected Outcomes

1. Copes with lack of mobility; family assists patient in the use of mechanical lift, wheelchair, other aids
2. Avoids aspiration; chooses types of foods that he is able to swallow; has standby suction available
3. Attempts to maintain nutritional status; eats 6 small meals; avoids empty calories
4. Aware of danger of respiratory failure; can relate symptoms of respiratory dysfunction; seeks treatment information and options
5. Deals with feelings; makes his needs known through some form of communication

Polyradiculitis (Guillain–Barré Syndrome; Infectious Polyneuritis)

Polyradiculitis is a clinical syndrome of unknown cause involving the peripheral nervous system and cranial nerves; it is characterized by paresthesias of the extremities and by muscle weakness or paralysis. It may be due to an allergic or immunologic reaction and is frequently preceded by mild respiratory syndrome.

Assessment
Clinical Manifestations

1. Progressive muscle weakness—may progress to rapidly ascending paralysis involving the trunk, upper extremities, and facial muscles (complete paralysis)
2. Paresthesia (tingling and numbness) of toes and fingers
3. Difficulty in chewing, swallowing and talking—from cranial nerve involvement
4. Sensory distortion—pain, paresthesia
5. Diminished or absent tendon reflexes and decrease in position and vibratory sense
6. Autonomic dysfunction—tachycardia, bladder disturbances, orthostatic hypotension

Diagnostic Evaluation

1. CSF usually shows elevation in protein.
2. Electrophysiologic testing—nerve conduction tests show slowing of conduction.

Patient Problems/Nursing Diagnoses

1. Potential for ineffective breathing pattern related to weakness of respiratory muscles and paralysis
2. Impaired physical mobility related to paralysis
3. Potential for complications related to mechanical ventilation, lack of mobility, paralysis, prolonged illness

Planning and Implementation
Treatment

1. Endotracheal intubation and mechanical ventilation—to prevent respiratory failure and minimize chance of aspiration and pneumonia
2. Steroid therapy—may be of value if given early in course of disease
3. Plasmapheresis therapy (plasma exchange)—to remove postulated antibodies

Nursing Interventions

A. Support respiration when rapidly ascending paralysis develops.

1. Evaluate repeated measurements of vital capacity—gives warning that respiratory muscles are becoming weak.
2. Watch for breathlessness while talking, shallow and irregular breathing, increasing pulse rate, and *change* in the respiratory pattern.
3. Place the patient on mechanical ventilator when he shows signs of respiratory insufficiency (p. 185)—may require prolonged controlled mechanical ventilation.

B. Monitor for dysphagia resulting from respiratory paralysis—patient cannot cough normally and is at risk of choking to death.

1. Use nasogastric tube for feeding.
2. Offer oral intake when pharyngeal muscles are strong enough to prevent aspiration.

C. Monitor the patient for complications.

1. Evaluate for respiratory failure (see above).
2. Monitor for cardiac arrhythmias—cardiac arrest may occur if vagus nerve becomes affected.
3. Watch for urinary retention—thought to be due to involvement of autonomic fibers passing through the sacral nerve roots.
4. Position the patient to avoid nerve palsies—secondary effects of pressure can produce residual disabilities.
5. Assess for and prevent contractures and pressure sores (see Rehabilitation Nursing, Chapter 5).
6. Watch for hypotension, which is the usual manifestation of autonomic nervous system disturbances. Avoid sudden changes in position.

D. Use interventions to compensate for motor, sensory, and communication losses.

1. Establish some form of communication (eye blinking, lip reading)—patient is unable to talk, laugh, or cry because of paralysis, tracheostomy, intubation.
2. Maintain skin integrity.
   a. Monitor IV sites.
   b. Watch temperature of contact substance (bath water), environmental temperature.
   c. Evaluate for evidences of pressure sores.
3. Assess hydration status.
4. Monitor bowel sounds; evaluate for paralytic ileus, constipation/impaction.
5. Use measures to prevent pressure sores (see p. 59).
6. Put extremities through range of motion—to maintain tone, prevent contractures, and aid in muscle retraining.
7. Give continuing reassurance, explanations and high-level care—the patient is alert (and anxious) and has vision, hearing, and eye movements intact.

Health Education

There may be a rather lengthy convalescence; patients usually recover in 3 to 6 months; a few have sequelae lasting up to several years.
1. Reassure the patient that illness is self-limited and usually has a good prognosis.
2. Teach intermittent self-catheterization for the patient with protracted period of recovery of bladder function.

Evaluation
Expected Outcomes

1. Achieves effective breathing pattern; no signs of respiratory failure or aspiration
2. Swallows without choking
3. Demonstrates improved mobility; moves feet and legs and participates in reconditioning exercises
4. Is free of complications; shows normal skin integrity and is free of autonomic disturbances

Spinal Cord Injury

Spinal cord injury may vary from a mild cord concussion with transient numbness to immediate and permanent quadriplegia. The most common sites are the cervical areas C-5, C-6, and C-7 and the junction of the thoracic and lumbar vertebrae (T-12, L-1). Traumatic injury of the spinal cord may result in loss of function (paralysis) below the level of cord injury. There is usually a high frequency of associated injuries and medical complications. Ideally, patients should be admitted to regional spinal cord centers after condition has stabilized.

Pathogenesis of Spinal Cord Injury

1. Damage to the spinal cord ranges from transient concussion to contusion, laceration, and compression (either alone or in combination), to complete transection of the cord.
2. The cord's response to injury is ischemia, edema, and hemorrhage that lead to an irreversible cycle of progressive destruction unless there is appropriate intervention.

Causes

1. Trauma—automobile and motorcycle accidents, falls, diving and surfing injuries, gunshot wounds, hard contact sports—may cause compression, contusion, or laceration of the cord, hemorrhage into its substance, or compression of its vascular supply.

Management of the Patient With Cervical Spinal Injury

1. To manage a cervical spine injury, there must be immediate immobilization, early reduction, and stabilization of the vertebral column.
2. To reduce the fracture dislocation and maintain alignment of the cervical spine some form of skeletal traction (skeletal tongs/calipers; halo-vest technique) is used, or open reduction (surgery) may be required.

Cervical Traction (Fig. 18-10)

A. Skeletal Tongs

1. A variety of skeletal tongs are in use; spring-loaded Gardner–Wells and Heifitz tongs require no predrilled holes into the skull; Crutchfield and Vinke tongs are inserted through holes made with a special drill under local anesthesia.
2. Traction is applied to the tongs by weights (4.5–9 kg. [10–20 lbs.]) or more, depending on the patient's size.
3. The traction is gradually increased by addition of weights—as the amount of traction is increased, the spaces between the intervertebral discs widen, and the vertebrae slip back into position. Reduction will take place after correct alignment has been regained.
4. X-rays are taken after each addition of weight until reduction is obtained; monitor the patient carefully as weights are added.
5. When reduction is obtained, the weights are gradually removed until the amount of weight needed to maintain the alignment is obtained.
6. Keep traction tongs several inches from top of bed and allow weights to hang free—to prevent interference with traction.

B. Halo Devices

1. Halo devices consist of a stainless steel "halo ring," which is fixed to the skull by 4 pins. The ring is attached to a removable halo vest (lined with sheepskin or Kodel liner) which suspends the weight of the unit circumferentially around the chest. A metal frame connects the ring to the vest.
2. The halo ring may be used initially as a traction device or the ring and vest may be applied following removal of skull tongs/calipers.
3. Halo devices afford immobilization of the cervical spine while allowing early mobilization and participation in the rehabilitation program.

Assessment
Clinical Manifestations

1. Pain or tenderness in neck/back
2. Numbness, tingling, burning, muscle weakness, twitching, paralysis of arms and/or legs
3. Inadequate breathing
4. Lack of mobility
5. Marked reduction of blood pressure—from loss of peripheral and vascular resistance
6. Loss of bladder and bowel control; usually urinary retention and bladder distention
7. Loss of sweating and vasomotor tone below level of cord lesion

Patient Problems/Nursing Diagnoses
(Acute Stage)

1. Potential for respiratory paralysis related to paralysis of abdominal and intercostal muscles (cervical cord injury)
2. Potential for progressive neurologic deficits related to anoxemia, disruption of sympathetic pathways with loss of motor tone and hypotension
3. Potential for complications (shock, gastric distention, etc.) related to diminished visceral sensitivity and altered physiologic parameters from neurologic deficits
4. Impaired physical mobility related to paralysis of muscles
5. See also Paraplegia, page 805.

Planning and Implementation
Nursing Interventions

A. Implementing fracture reduction and spine immobilization

1. See Cervical Traction, this page, for application of tongs/halo devices.
2. Transfer the patient to a turning frame (Stryker) or continuous horizontal rotating bed. If none is available, place the patient on a firm mattress with a bedboard under the mattress.
   a. Keep the patient in an extended position—do not allow body to be twisted or turned.
   b. Place the patient (who is strapped to a transfer board) directly on the posterior frame of a Stryker frame.
   c. Place a blanket roll between the patient's legs.
   d. Place anterior frame in position. Secure frame straps.

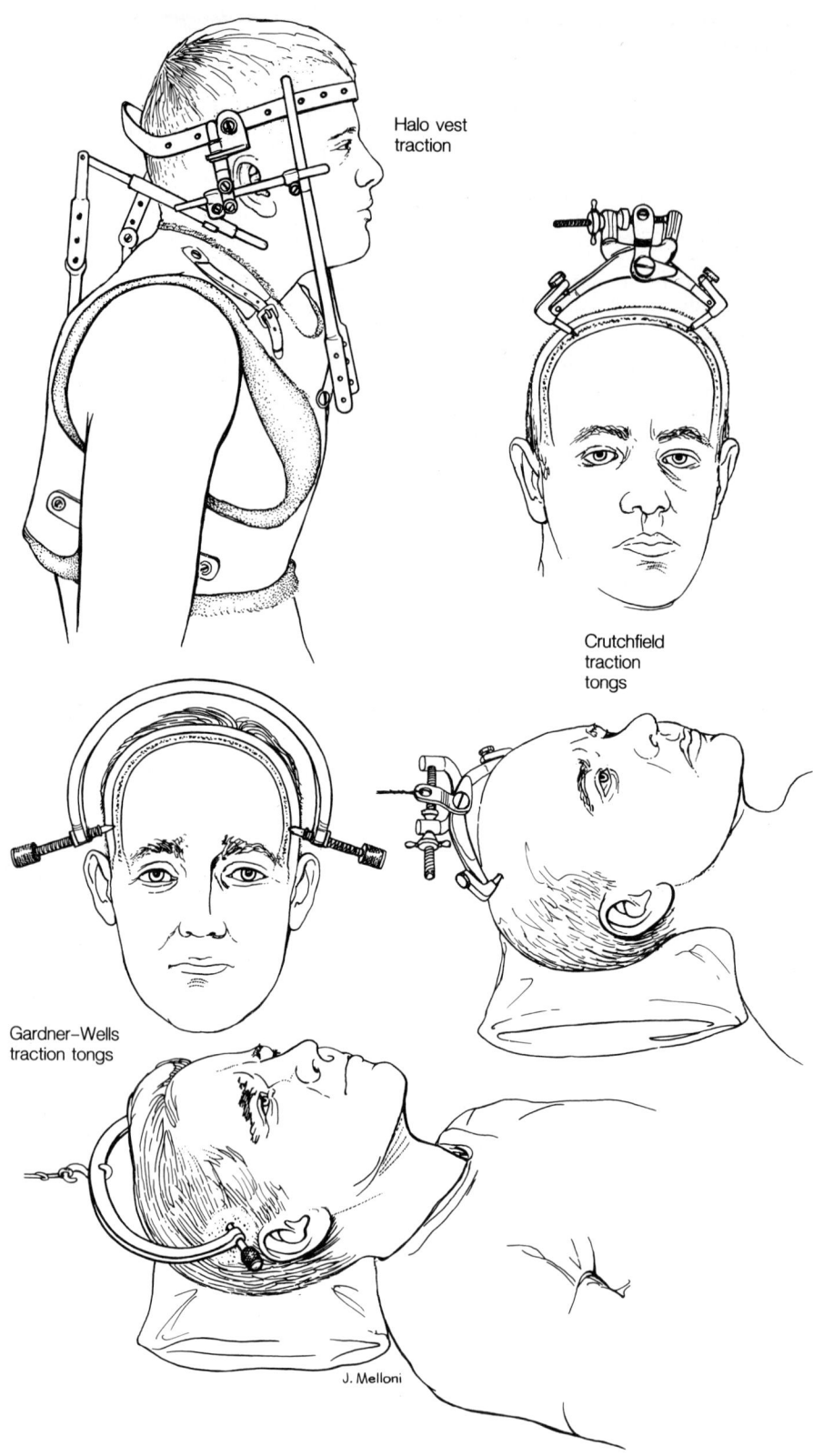

Halo vest
traction

Crutchfield
traction
tongs

Gardner–Wells
traction tongs

J. Melloni

Figure 18-10. Methods of cervical traction.

e. Turn the patient to the prone position.

f. Remove frame straps, head bandage, and posterior frame. Remove transfer board.

3. Maintain the patient in proper alignment to prevent deformities.

Position feet against padded footboard—to prevent footdrop.

Be sure there is a space between end of mattress and foot of bed—to allow for free suspension of the heels.

Apply trochanter rolls from crest of ilium to midthigh of both extremities—to prevent external rotation of the hip joints.

4. Employ care when placing the patient in the prone position—improper position on the headrest can cause pressure on the globe of the eye, resulting in retinal ischemia and blindness.

5. The patient may be placed on a kinetic treatment table, which rotates every 4–5 minutes, thus eliminating pressure on skin surface, providing access for patient care and maintaining correct body alignment.

B. Maintaining effective respiratory functioning

1. Assess the breathing pattern and maintain airway—patients with injuries at high levels are at risk for respiratory failure.

   a. Assess strength of cough.

   b. Measure vital capacity, tidal volume, and inspiratory force and arterial blood gases—these are guides to determine respiratory insufficiency.

   c. Start nasal oxygen to maintain a high arterial PO_2—anoxemia can create or worsen a neurologic deficit of the spinal cord.

   d. Consider diaphragm pacing (electrical stimulation of the phrenic nerve) for the patient with high cervical lesion.

2. Intubate the patient with extreme care; do not flex or extend his neck—can result in extension of the cord injury.

3. See page 227 for care of the patient on a ventilator.

4. For the halo patient, tape wrench to halo vest in case the vest must be removed for cardiopulmonary resuscitation.

C. Monitoring for progressive neurologic deficit

1. Evaluate the patient constantly for motor and sensory changes below the level of injury—motor and sensory loss occurs from cord edema, hemorrhage, etc., which may further compromise cord function. Document findings carefully.

   a. Test motor ability by requesting the patient to spread his fingers, squeeze examiner's hand, move toes, etc.

   b. Test sensation by pinching the skin, starting at shoulder level and progressing down the sides of all extremities. Ascertain when the patient feels pinching sensation.

   c. Note presence/absence of level of sweating.

2. Report immediately any decrease in neurologic function.

   a. Keep a neurologic assessment record (flow sheet).

   b. Observe for symptoms of progressive neurologic damage—symptoms of cord compression depend on level at which compression occurs. Clinical symptoms of cord compression are indistinguishable from those of cord edema.

   (1) Loss of sensation

   (2) Inability to move extremities

3. Prepare for laminectomy if progressive symptoms of cord compression occur—permits direct exploration and decompression of cord (p. 808).

4. Evaluate for presence of spinal shock—spinal shock represents a sudden loss of continuity between spinal cord and higher nerve centers. There is a complete loss of all reflex, motor, sensory, and autonomic activity below the level of the lesion.

   a. Falling blood pressure

   b. Paralysis and lack of sensation below level of cord injury

   c. Bladder distention—from paralysis of bladder

   d. Bowel distention—caused by depression of reflexes; retroperitoneal hemorrhage may occur with fracture of low back, producing paralytic ileus

   e. Hyperthermia—during periods of spinal shock, the patient does not perspire on the paralyzed portions of his body since sympathetic activity is blocked.

5. Give specific treatment as directed; theoretically, high doses of steroids counteract edema and possibly delay hemorrhage.

6. Employ continuous ECG monitoring—bradycardia and asystole are common in acute cervical injuries.

7. Support and maintain the patient's body defenses until shock remits and the system has recovered from the traumatic insult. (Spinal shock is temporary but may last several weeks.)

   a. Continue to support the airway, especially in cervical cord injury.

   b. Insert intravenous line(s) for fluid administration to avoid hypotension—from blood loss from associated injuries, vasomotor paralysis, from spinal cord injury (neurogenic hypotension); give blood transfusion as directed.

8. Avoid overdistention of bladder—after spinal injury, the bladder may lack functional nerve supply; overstretching of bladder may produce permanent damage. Urinary tract infection after spinal injury can cause death.

   a. Utilize intermittent catheterization early in acute phase, if possible, or insert indwelling catheter.

   b. See page 539 for management of neurogenic bladder.

9. Treat for acute gastric dilatation and ileus; gastrointestinal hemorrhage.

   a. Observe for abdominal distention and listen with stethoscope for presence or absence of peristaltic sounds.

   b. Initiate gastric suction to reduce distention and prevent vomiting and aspiration.

   c. Give neostigmine methylsulfate—for severe bowel distention.

   d. Administer rectal tube to relieve gaseous distention.

   e. Give intravenous infusions for fluid replacement; avoid overloading the labile cardiovascular system.

   f. Place the patient on bowel-training program to stimulate bowel function as soon as spinal shock has dissipated.

D. Preventing complications

1. Maintain nursing surveillance for complications.

   a. Pressure sores—inadequate peripheral circulation from spinal shock and immobility may cause pressure sores to develop within a few hours.

(1) Turn every 2 hours (using turning frame) if the patient can be turned to obtain complete pressure relief; patients with initial vasovagal instability, as well as associated injuries, may not be able to tolerate positional changes.

(2) Check back of head periodically for signs of pressure; massage back of head periodically.

(3) *For the patient in a halo device:*

   (a) Inspect under halo vest; look for excessive perspiration, redness, skin blistering, especially on bony prominences (scapulae, ribs, shoulders, spinous processes).

   (b) Have the patient lie prone for short periods to relieve pressure.

   (c) Wash skin under vest; dry with dry washcloth. Open vests at sides to wash and dry skin; do not allow liner to become wet because this will cause skin problems.
Avoid putting powder inside vest—may contribute to development of pressure sores.

   (d) Turn the patient and his brace as a unit; do not use the halo or vest to turn, lift, or reposition the patient.

(4) See page 59 for prevention and management of pressure sores.

2. Autonomic dysreflexia (autonomic hyperreflexia)—syndrome occurring in patients with spinal cord lesions at or above T-6. Characterized by exaggerated autonomic responses to local stimuli below the level of injury, distended bladder or bowel, stimulation of skin (tactile, pain, thermal stimuli), distention or contraction of visceral organs; may be accompanied by immediate and dangerous elevation of arterial blood pressure.

▶ **NURSING ALERT:** Autonomic dysreflexia (autonomic hyperreflexia) is considered an emergency.

  a. Syndrome characterized by pounding headache, profuse sweating, nasal congestion, piloerection (goose flesh), bradycardia, severe hypertension.

  b. Treatment—to remove the triggering stimulus and avoid possible serious complications.

   (1) Place patient in sitting position—to help lower the blood pressure.

   (2) Drain the bladder via catheter. (Do not irrigate catheter with more than 30 ml. of irrigating solution.)

   (3) Insert Nupercainal ointment in rectum if fecal mass is present. (Mass is removed manually *after* symptoms subside.)

   (4) Remove any other stimuli that may be triggering episodes: cold air, object on skin, etc.

   (5) Give ganglionic blocking agent slowly IV, if elevated blood pressure does not respond immediately to above measures. Monitor blood pressure.

   (6) Tag the patient's chart with an "Allergic" marker; the patient is apt to have another episode of hyperreflexia.

3. Respiratory complications (pneumonia).

4. *Infection*
Kidney and bladder—see management of the patient with indwelling catheter, page 508.
Pin site/tong site infections:
  a. Watch for inflammation and edema around pin sites—may indicate infection or *loose* pins (halo brace).

  b. Cleanse around pin sites (or tong insertion sites) daily with prescribed solution; avoid probing under crusting areas because this can cause infection; dry site with sterile applicator.

  c. Wash hair around pin site as needed.

  d. Monitor for loosening of pins; pain or discomfort at pin site, complaints of "something moving."

5. *Contractures*
  a. Initiate passive range-of-motion exercises for affected extremities within 48–72 hours *upon order*—to preserve joint motion.
  b. See Paraplegia, page 805.

6. Orthostatic hypotension

7. Vein thrombosis/pulmonary embolism

8. Depression

9. Stress ulcers

10. Endocrine, nutritional, and metabolic dysfunctions

E. Reestablishing mobility and independence

1. Participate in program designed according to the patient's neurologic deficit.

  a. An exercise conditioning regimen is started early.

  b. Muscle-strengthening exercises for shoulder depressors, maintenance of sitting balance, getting up and down from wheelchair (or whatever is possible for the individual patient).

  c. The period of immobilization is determined by the patient's condition. Mobilize only upon physician's request—if the patient has partial cord function, activity may produce further cord injury.

  d. For the halo patient:

   (1) Be aware that the patient may be initially distressed by bizarre appearance of the halo but usually adapts readily to device.

   (2) Anticipate that the patient may experience a slight headache or minor pain around the skull pins for several days following application.

   (3) Supervise the patient's activities (sitting, standing) initially because the weight of the halo may cause problems of balance, decreased peripheral field of vision, inability to see feet.

   (4) Have torque wrench available in the event that nuts/bolts on halo connections or vest need tightening.

  e. Anticipate that four-poster brace, neck brace, or molded collar is usually applied when the patient is mobilized after traction is removed.

2. Give ongoing support to enhance the patient's feelings of self-worth.

  a. See Paraplegia, page 805, for psychological support.

  b. See page 806 for sexual counseling.

Evaluation
Expected Outcomes

1. Maintains effective respiratory functioning; respiratory rate and arterial blood gases within acceptable limits

2. Shows no evidence of progressive neurologic damage/deficits

3. Absence of preventable complications; demonstrates intact skin; absence of respiratory, infectious complications

4. Demonstrates beginning adjustment to impaired physical mobility; performs exercises within limits of disability

5. See Paraplegia, page 806.

Paraplegia

Paraplegia is loss of motion and sensation in the lower extremities.

Quadriplegia (tetraplegia) is loss of motion and sensation involving both upper and lower extremities.

Causes

1. Trauma—accidents, gunshot wounds
2. Spinal cord lesions (intervertebral disc, tumor, vascular lesions)
3. Multiple sclerosis
4. Infections and abscesses of spinal cord
5. Congenital defects

Patient Problems/Nursing Diagnoses

1. Ineffective individual coping related to physical and psychologic sequelae of paraplegia
2. Compromised family coping related to care of permanently disabled member
3. Impaired physical mobility related to permanent neurologic deficits
4. Potential for pressure sores related to sensory deficits, lack of mobility, and spasticity
5. Urinary incontinence/retention related to spinal cord injury
6. Bowel incontinence related to effects of spinal cord injury
7. Potential for sexual dysfunction related to neurologic deficit

Nursing Interventions

See nursing management of the patient with spinal cord injuries for immediate management principles, page 801.

A. Promoting coping strategies

1. Allow the patient to work through his feelings about his disability at his own pace (unless his responses continue to be exaggerated or maladaptive).
   a. Realization of the finality of paraplegia or quadriplegia may prolong the grief process.
   b. Patient experiences a loss of self-esteem in areas of self-identity, sexual identity, and social and emotional roles.
2. Be aware that the patient may take 1 of 2 courses:
   a. Acceptance of disability, leading to development of realistic goals for the future.
   b. Rejection of disability—may exhibit self-destructive neglect, noncompliance with therapeutic program.
3. Assist the family in making adaptive changes.
   a. Family is faced with accepting the patient as "permanently different"; may cause frustration/isolation, feelings of alienation; resentment of changes in family's life-style, guilt-ridden death wishes for patient, overwhelmed and overburdened feelings.
   b. Assess developmental needs of family members. (At what developmental stage was each family member when patient became ill?)
   c. Focus on developmental issues and acquisition of strategies for long-term management of the patient.
   d. Allow expressions of anger.
   e. Be aware that the patient and family may require supportive psychotherapy and additional recreational therapy to prevent social and intellectual isolation.

B. Establishing optimum functioning

1. Prepare for weight-bearing activities—the patient with complete cord severance should start early weight bearing to decrease osteoporotic changes in long bones and to reduce incidence of urinary infections and the formation of renal calculi.
   a. Apply elastic hose from toes to thigh or a Jobst counterpressure leotard—to prevent pooling of blood in abdominal area; a patient with spinal cord paralysis lacks vasomotor tone in the lower extremities and will become hypotensive in the upright position.
   b. Use tilt table—to help the patient overcome vasomotor instability and tolerate upright posture (p. 63).
      (1) Start with elevation of 45 degrees and gradually increase angle of elevation over a period of days.
      (2) Take blood pressure immediately before and as soon as the patient is positioned on tilt table.
      (3) Observe for nausea and excessive perspiration, pallor, dizziness, or syncope; accommodation to the upright position may be a slow, gradual process.
   c. *Or* use high-back reclining wheelchair with extension leg rests; raise backrest slowly and lower leg rest gradually over a period of 7–10 days.
2. Build the unaffected part of body to optimal strength, endurance, and coordination—to prepare for transfer and mobilization activities.
   a. Weight lifting, manual resistance, etc., are employed.
   b. Encourage the patient to continue with muscle strengthening exercises for hands, arms, shoulders, chest, spine, abdomen, and neck—the patient must bear full weight on these muscles.
      (1) Do push-ups in prone position.
      (2) Do sit-ups in sitting position.
      (3) Extend and flex arms while holding weights.
      (4) Squeeze rubber ball to promote hand strength.
   c. Graded therapeutic exercises are supervised by physical therapist.
3. Use assistive devices to allow fuller patient participation.

C. Promoting bladder and bowel control

1. Continue with bladder-training program. See Neurogenic Bladder, page 539.
2. Start bowel-training program.
   a. Goal is to obtain reflex bowel evacuation by conditioning.
   b. Regular habit time, stool softeners, and digital stimulation are part of bowel management (see p. 70).

D. Preventing complications of paraplegic disorders

1. Infection of urinary tract; urinary calculi; urethrocutaneous fistula.
   a. Prevent overdistention of the bladder by intermittent catheterization.
   b. Do frequent urinalyses.
   c. Encourage fluid intake of at least 4,000 ml./24

hours; urinary output should be 2,000 ml./24 hours.
2. Pressure sores.

▶ **NURSING ALERT:** The threat of pressure sores persists throughout the patient's life.

    a. Emphasize that the patient is responsible for health of his skin.
    b. Teach the patient to:
      (1) Carry out regular skin inspection with a mirror.
      (2) Do push-ups for 15 seconds for pressure relief every 15–30 minutes.
    c. See page 59 for prevention of pressure sores.
3. Fecal impaction
    a. Ensure total evacuation of fecal material from lower bowel every day.
      (1) Employ regular digital examination of rectum—to determine presence of impacted fecal material.
      (2) Keep patient on bowel training program (see p. 70).
4. Spasticity
    a. Spasticity occurs 2 weeks–3 months after injury, starting with flexor activity, followed by extensor spasticity.
    b. Nursing interventions:
      (1) Provide relaxed and calm environment.
      (2) Correct any problems aggravating the spasticity (pressure sores; inadequate bladder/bowel emptying; apprehension). Teach the patient to search for cause of sudden increase of spasticity.
      (3) Allow time for transfers and positioning.
      (4) Maintain joint range of motion with slow, smooth movements.
      (5) Employ drug therapy (diazepam, baclofen); cold and hot applications, relaxation training; biofeedback when necessary.
    c. Surgical intervention:
      (1) Phenol blockade of muscle to inhibit spasticity.
      (2) Operative approaches for lengthening or release of contracted spastic muscles.
5. Autonomic dysreflexia (see p. 804)

6. Heterotrophic ossification of extra-articular tissues
7. Ankylosis of joints

Health Education

1. Support the counseling services provided for the patient and family.
    a. Rehabilitation engineering services—provide a greater range of self-help and mobility devices and environmental control systems.
    b. Occupational therapy—selects and utilizes devices that can aid the patient in mealtime, dressing, and other activities
    c. Vocational assessment and rehabilitation counseling
    d. Sexual counseling
      (1) Most cord-injured persons can have some form of meaningful sexual expression and relationship, but some modifications will have to be made to cope with anxiety.
      (2) Implantation of penile prosthesis may be considered.
      (3) The female patient may experience little sensation during intercourse, but fertility and ability to bear children are usually not affected.
      (4) Counseling and small group meetings provide an opportunity to share feelings, sexual concerns, give and receive information, and develop positive attitudes and adjustment.
      (5) See sexuality of the disabled, page 53.
    e. Family may require counseling and social services to help them cope with burden of spinal cord injury on their life-style and socioeconomic status.
2. Emphasize that patient must acquire life-long practice of preventive skin care.

Expected Outcomes

1. Copes with altered life-style; expresses feelings; seeks counseling
2. Achieves modified mobility—independence in self-care with appropriate adaptive equipment
3. Attains/maintains skin integrity
    a. Adheres to turning and positioning schedule
    b. Monitors self for evidence of pressure sores
    c. Does push-ups at intervals while seated
4. Attains/maintains bladder control and/or bowel control
5. Copes with changes in sexual function

Herniation of Intervertebral Disc (Ruptured Disc)

Herniation of the intervertebral disc is a protrusion of the nucleus of the disc into the annulus (fibrous ring around the disc), with subsequent nerve compression. The herniation may occur in any portion of the spine.

Types of Disc Herniation

1. Cervical
2. Lumbar
3. Thoracic (rare)

Causes

1. Degeneration
2. Trauma (accidents, strain, repeated minor stresses)
3. Congenital predisposition

Clinical Manifestations

Depend on location, size, rate of development (acute or chronic), and effect on surrounding structures

A. Cervical Disc

1. Pain and stiffness in neck, top of shoulders, and in region of scapulae
2. Pain in upper extremities and head
3. Paresthesia and numbness of upper extremities

B. Lumbar Disc

1. Low back pain accompanied by varying degrees of sensory and motor impairment
2. Pain in buttock and thigh, radiating to calf and

ankle—aggravated by actions that increase intraspinal pressure (sneezing, straining, lifting)
3. Postural deformity of lumbar spine
4. Pain induced by stretching sciatic nerve
   a. Place the patient on his back with his knees straight.
   b. Raise the unflexed leg (one at a time).
   c. This maneuver causes stretching of sciatic nerve that is transmitted to nerve roots, producing pain that radiates into the leg.
   d. The patient will experience little or no pain if leg is raised while bent at the knee since this relaxes tension on sciatic nerve.
   e. Lasègue's sign—pain with straight-leg raising and absence of pain with bent-leg raising.
5. Muscle weakness ⎱
6. Alterations in tendon reflexes ⎬ of lower extremities
7. Sensory loss ⎰

Diagnostic Evaluation

1. X-ray of spine—to rule out other lesions that cause similar signs and symptoms
2. Computed tomography
3. Myelogram—demonstrates area of pressure and localizes herniation of disc; disc protrusion is seen as indentation of contrast medium
4. Electromyography—localizes specific spinal nerve involved
5. Somatosensory evoked responses (p. 757).
6. Lumbar venogram

Nursing Interventions: Cervical Disc Dislocations

A. Promoting healing through rest and immobilization

1. Immobilize and rest the cervical spine by one of the following methods:
   a. Bed rest—reduces inflammation and edema in soft tissues around disc, relieving pressure on nerve roots; relieves cervical spine of supporting weight of head.
   b. Cervical collar—allows maximal opening of intervertebral foramina.
      (1) Collar should hold the head in a neutral or slightly flexed position.
      (2) Inspect under the collar at intervals for skin rash.
      (3) In acute herniation, the collar may have to be worn night and day until pain subsides (2–3 weeks).
      (4) Cervical isometric exercises are started when the patient is pain-free—to strengthen neck musculature in preparation for "weaning" from collar.
   c. Cervical traction (accomplished by head halter attached to a pulley and a weight)—increases vertebral separation and thus relieves pressure on the nerve roots.
      (1) Cervical traction should be comfortable.
      (2) Keep head of bed elevated and make sure that traction is in alignment.
      (3) Inspect for skin burns from cervical halter; pad under the halter as necessary.
      (4) Encourage male patient not to shave since beard offers a form of padding; shaving may cause irritation.
   d. Brace

B. Reducing inflammation

1. Administer anti-inflammatory medications (e.g., aspirin, phenylbutazone [Butazolidin], oxyphenbutazone [Tandearil], or steroids)—to treat inflammatory response.
   a. Give food or antacid with anti-inflammatory agents—to prevent gastrointestinal irritation.
   b. Take periodic blood counts—to watch for development of blood dyscrasias.
2. Give muscle relaxant—to interrupt cycle of muscle spasm and allow for patient comfort; to increase range of motion of cervical spine.
3. Give analgesics and sedatives—to control discomfort and anxiety often associated with cervical disc disease.
4. Apply moist hot compresses (10–20 minutes, several times daily) to back of neck—to increase blood flow to muscles and help relax the patient and his spastic muscles.
5. Prepare for surgical intervention if significant neurologic deficit from nerve root compression occurs, for unremitting and recurrent pain, or for signs of cord compression.

C. Discharge Planning and Health Education (Cervical Disc)

It may take 6 weeks to recuperate from significant disc herniation.
Instruct the patient as follows:
1. Avoid extreme flexion, extension, and rotation of the neck while working.
2. Keep head in a neutral position while sleeping.
   a. Pillow should be filled with feathers or down.
   b. Sleep on side or back; do not sleep prone.
   c. Avoid excessive neck flexion—do not prop up in bed with several pillows.
3. Avoid excessive automobile riding during acute phase—vibration has adverse effect on spine.

Nursing Interventions: Lumbar Disc Herniations

Majority of herniations occur at L4–L5 or L5–S1 interspace.

A. Reducing pain

1. Encourage the patient to remain on bed rest—disc is freed from stress and pressure when the patient is horizontal.
   a. Place the patient in position of comfort—usually semi-Fowler's with moderate hip and knee flexion.
   b. Place hinged bedboard under mattress—to limit spinal flexion.
   c. Help the patient to ambulate (usually after 2 weeks' bed rest) when inflammatory reaction and edema from disc herniation have subsided.
   d. Use corset or brace if necessary to mobilize the patient (for the obese patient with poor abdominal musculature).
2. Use appropriate drug therapy and physical therapy.
   a. Muscle relaxants—muscle spasm is prominent in acute phase.
   b. Anti-inflammatory drugs—to counter inflammation occurring in supporting tissues and nerve roots.
   c. Analgesic agents—to relieve the patient's acute pain.
   d. Utilize heat and massage—to relax muscle spasm; also provides analgesia.
3. Watch for development of neurologic deficit.

a. Muscle weakness and atrophy
b. Loss of sensory and motor function
c. Unrelieved acute pain
4. Have the patient increase activities gradually as his symptoms abate.

B. Surgical and postoperative interventions

1. Hemilaminectomy with removal of ruptured disc (see below).
   Indications for operative intervention include compression of cauda equina (motor and sensory paresis, loss of sphincter control), nerve root compression, and lack of response to conservative therapy.
   a. Patients with multilevel involvement may have recurrences of pain and disability and may require reoperation(s).
   b. Spinal fusion may be required on reoperation.
2. Chemonucleolysis—injection of chymopapain into herniated lumbar disc; has a proteolytic action that causes loss of water and proteoglycans from the disc; this reduces the size of the herniated material and relieves pressure on the nerve root.
   a. Usually performed in operating room or special procedures room of radiology department with IV line in place and with cardiac monitoring—anaphylactic reactions to injection occur in 0.5%–1.0% of patients.
   b. Postinjection nursing care includes bed rest for 24 hours, monitoring for neurologic dysfunction, adequate analgesia and muscle relaxants and gradual ambulation.
   c. Patient Education (after chemonucleolysis)
      (1) Expect some back stiffness and soreness, which are common after this procedure.

(2) Wear supportive shoes.
(3) Sit on a hard, straight chair.
(4) Restrict physical activity; lie down frequently during the first 3 weeks.
(5) Increase activity gradually during the next 3–6 weeks.

C. Health Education

1. Encourage the patient to do exercises after acute symptoms subside: (1) exercises to strengthen abdominal muscles and (2) gentle stretching exercises to improve the suppleness and elasticity of the paraspinal muscles and ligaments.
   a. Start exercises gently and gradually.
   b. Discontinue exercises if pain worsens.
2. Advise the patient to sleep on side with knees and hips flexed (pillow between knees).
   a. Do not sleep in prone position—hyperextends the spine.
   b. Pick up loads correctly (bend knees, keep back straight, avoid lifting anything above the elbows) and keep load close to body.
   c. Avoid lifting while back is in a flexed or rotated position.
3. Encourage proper posture while standing, sitting, walking, and working.
4. A lumbar sacral support (corset) may be necessary for persons with poor abdominal musculature—serves to pull in abdomen and alter lumbar-sacral curve, which relieves strain on ligaments.
5. Carry out weight control program—the obese patient with protruding abdomen and lordotic posture has chronic back strain.
6. See also health education, low back pain, page 851.

Management of the Patient Following Disc Surgery

Surgical excision of a herniated disc is done when there is evidence of a progressive neurologic deficit (muscle weakness and atrophy, loss of sensory and motor function, loss of sphincter control), and continuing pain and sciatica. Microsurgical techniques are now making it possible to remove a herniated nucleus pulposus through a small incision without a laminectomy.

Discectomy—removal of herniated disc tissue and related matter.

Laminectomy—removal of the lamina (arch of bone covering spinal cord) to expose the neural elements in the spinal canal. It allows inspection of the spinal canal and identification and removal of pathology and compression from the cord and roots.

Hemilaminectomy—half of arch removed.

Laminotomy—division of the lamina of a vertebra.

Spinal fusion—bone graft is used to fuse the vertebral spinous processes; the object of spinal fusion is to bridge over the defective disc to stabilize the spine.

Postoperative Nursing Management
Goal:
The patient achieves relief of pressure on nerve root in order to relieve pain.

(See also the postoperative principles for the patient undergoing orthopedic surgery, p. 840).

A. Cervical Disc

1. Check neurologic and vital signs at frequent intervals—there is always the possibility of respiratory compromise (from tracheal edema, pneumothorax, airway obstruction).
   a. Watch for hoarseness—from recurrent laryngeal nerve injury, resulting in inability to cough effectively and eliminate respiratory secretions.
   b. Observe for dysphagia (possibly from edema of the esophagus); offer a blenderized soft diet.
2. Promote patient comfort.
   a. Be aware that a sore throat will be a major complaint.
      (1) Give throat spray, throat lozenges as directed to relieve pain.
      (2) Do not give any spray or throat lozenges that numb the throat, since this may cause choking.
      (3) Humidify room air.
3. Protect bone graft (if fusion has been part of procedure).
   a. Prevent extremes of flexion and extension of neck.
   b. Use cervical collar to eliminate unnecessary movement.
4. Watch for sudden reappearance of radicular (root)

pain—indicative of nerve root compression from slipping of bone graft or collapsing of disc space (if bone grafting has not been done).

B. Lumbar Disc

1. Check vital signs and inspect wound for evidence of hemorrhage—vascular injury is a complication of disc surgery.
2. Assess sensation, motor power, color and temperature of lower extremities—postoperative neurologic deficits may result from nerve root injury.
3. Assess for signs of urinary retention.
4. Position the patient effectively.
   a. Use pillow under head and elevate the knee rest slightly—slight knee flexion relaxes muscles of the back.
   b. Encourage the patient to move and turn from side to side to relieve pressure.
      (1) Turn the patient as a unit (log rolling); place pillow between his legs while turning.
      (2) Place pillow between legs when the patient is lying on his side.
      (3) Avoid extreme knee flexion when the patient is on side.
      (4) Do not allow sitting except for defecation—to prevent compression.
5. Encourage early ambulation as soon as the patient is able. To get the patient out of bed:
   a. Raise head of bed as the patient lies on his side.
   b. Support the patient's head and shoulders as he pushes up to a sitting position while another person eases his legs over the side of the bed.
   c. Advise the patient to move from sitting to standing position in one smooth motion.

6. Give narcotics and sedatives to relieve pain and anxiety; discomfort in immediate postoperative period may vary from mild to severe pain.
7. Explain to the patient that there may be varying degrees of pain and sensory manifestations in the legs (sciatica type pain) due to temporary inflammatory changes, edema, and swelling of compressed nerve.

Discharge Planning and Health Education

1. It may take 6 weeks for ligamentous attachments of the muscles and skin to heal.
2. Instruct the patient as follows:
   a. Increase activities as tolerated—move up to the point of individual tolerance.
   b. Avoid activities that produce flexion strain on the spine—stair climbing, automobile riding, bending, sudden twisting of back.
   c. Reduce/restrict any activity that precipitates or aggravates discomfort.
   d. Have scheduled rest periods.
   e. Apply heat to back when indicated—helps absorb exudates in the tissues.
   f. Avoid heavy work for 2–3 months after surgery.
   g. Resume exercises to strengthen abdominal and erector spinae muscles as directed.
   h. A brace or corset may have to be worn if back pain persists.
   i. After the third week start a regular period of distance walking, increasing the length of walking as tolerance improves.
3. See health teaching for herniation of intervertebral disc, page 808, and management of low back pain, page 851.

Bibliography

Books

Albuquerque EX and Eldefrawi AT. Myasthenia Gravis. New York, Chapman & Hill, 1983

Anderson TP. Rehabilitation of patients with completed stroke. In Kottke FJ, Stillwell GK and Lehmann JF. Krusen's Handbook of Physical Medicine and Rehabilitation, 3rd ed, pp. 583–603. Philadelphia, WB Saunders, 1982

Austin GM (ed). The Spinal Cord, 3rd ed. New York, Igaku-Shoin, 1983

Bedbrook GM. The Care and Management of Spinal Cord Injuries. New York, Springer-Verlag, 1981

Belts TA. The psychological management of epilepsy. In Rose FC (ed). Research Progress in Epilepsy, pp. 315–322. London, Pitman, 1983

Bergan JJ and Yao JST. Cerebrovascular Insufficiency. New York, Grune & Stratton, 1983

Birkmayer W and Riederer P. Parkinson's Disease: Biochemistry, Clinical Pathology, and Treatment. New York, Springer-Verlag, 1983

Black RB, Hermann BP and Shope JT (eds). Nursing Management of Epilepsy. Rockville, MD, Aspen Systems Corp, 1982

Boller F and Frank E. Sexual Dysfunction in Neurological Disorders. New York, Raven Press, 1982

Brubaker SH. Sourcebook for Aphasia: A Guide to Family Activities and Community Resources. Detroit, Wayne State University Press, 1982

Caird FI. Neurological Disorders in the Elderly. Boston, Wright, 1982

Calenoff L (ed). Radiology of Spinal Cord Injury. St Louis, CV Mosby, 1981

Capildeo R and Maxwell A (eds). Multiple Sclerosis: Progress in Rehabilitation. London, Macmillan, 1982

Cooper PR. Head Injuries. Baltimore, Williams & Wilkins, 1982

Conway-Rutkowski BL. Carini and Owens' Neurological and Neurosurgical Nursing, 8th ed. St Louis, CV Mosby, 1982

Cottrell JE, Slivko B and Neufield P. Neurosurgical aspects of recovery room care, In Israel JS and DeKornfeld TJ. Recovery Room Care, pp. 234–266. Springfield, IL, Charles C Thomas, 1982

Davis GA. A Survey of Adult Aphasia. Englewood Cliffs, NJ, Prentice-Hall, 1983

Dorros S. Parkinson's, A Patient's View, 1st ed. Cabin John, MD, Seven Locks Press, 1981

Earnest MP. Neurologic Emergencies. New York, Churchill Livingstone, 1983

Gildenberg PL. Surgical management of brain tumors. In Copeland EM III (ed). Surgical Oncology, pp. 59–75. New York, John Wiley & Sons, 1983

Green B, Marshall LF and Gallagher TJ (eds). Intensive Care for Neurological Trauma and Disease. New York, Academic Press, 1982

Grob D (ed). Myasthenia Gravis: Pathophysiology and Management. New York, New York Academy of Sciences, 1981

Gumnit RJ. The Epilepsy Handbook: The Practical Management of Seizures. New York, Raven Press, 1983

Hallpike JF, Adams CWM and Tourtellotte WW (eds). Multiple Sclerosis: Pathology, Diagnosis and Management. London, Chapman & Hall, 1983

Hanak M and Scott A. Spinal Cord Injury, An Illustrated Guide for Health Care Professionals. New York, Springer-Verlag, 1983

Hardy RW Jr (ed). Lumbar Disc Disease. New York, Raven Press, 1982

Hartmann A and Brock M. Treatment of Cerebral Edema. New York, Springer-Verlag, 1982

Hopkins LN and Long DM. Clinical Management of Intracranial Aneurysms. New York, Raven Press, 1982

Horwitz NH and Rizzoli HV. Postoperative Complications of Intracranial Neurological Surgery. Baltimore, Williams & Wilkins, 1982

Howe JR. Manual of Patient Care in Neurosurgery, 2nd ed. Boston, Little, Brown & Co, 1983

Israel JS and DeKornfeld TJ. Recovery Room Care. Springfield, IL, Charles C Thomas, 1982

Ivan LP and Bruce DA. Coma. Physiopathology, Diagnosis, and Management. Springfield, Charles C Thomas, 1980

Laidlaw J and Richens A (eds). A Textbook of Epilepsy, 2nd ed. New York, Churchill Livingstone, 1982

Lisak RP and Barchi RL. Myasthenia Gravis. Philadelphia, WB Saunders, 1982

Logigian MK (ed). Adult Rehabilitation: A Team Approach for Therapists. Boston, Little, Brown & Co, 1982

Marsden CD and Fahn S (eds). Movement Disorders. Boston, Butterworth Scientific, 1982

McIntyre HB. The Primary Care of Seizure Disorders. Boston, Butterworths, 1982

Meyer JS and Shaw T. Diagnosis and Management of Stroke and TIAs. Menlo Park, CA, Addison-Wesley, 1982

Mulder DW. The Diagnosis and Treatment of Amyotrophic Lateral Sclerosis. Boston, Houghton Mifflin, 1980

Musselwhite CR and St. Louis KW. Communication Programming for the Severely Handicapped: Vocal and Non-vocal Strategies. Houston, College-Hill Press, 1982

Niedermeyer E. Epilepsy Guide: Diagnosis and Treatment of Epileptic Seizure Disorders. Baltimore, Urban & Schwarzenberg, 1983

Nursing Photobook. Coping With Neurologic Disorders. Springhouse, PA, Intermed Communications, 1981

Ojemann RG and Crowell RM. Surgical Management of Cerebrovascular Disease. Baltimore, Williams & Wilkins, 1983

Partain CL (ed). Nuclear Magnetic Resonance and Correlative Imaging Modalities. New York, Society of Nuclear Medicine, 1984

Russell RWR. Vascular Disease of the Central Nervous System. New York, Churchill Livingstone, 1983

Ropper AH, Kennedy SK and Zervas NT. Neurological and Neurosurgical Intensive Care. Baltimore, University Park Press, 1983

Ryan WJ. The Nurse and the Communicatively Impaired Adult. New York, Springer Publishing Co, 1982

Scheinberg LC. Multiple Sclerosis: A Guide for Patients and Their Families. New York, Raven Press, 1983

Schmidek HH and Sweet WH (eds). Operative Neurosurgical Techniques, Vol. 1 and 2. New York, Grune & Stratton, 1982

Schneider RC et al (eds). Correlative Neurosurgery, 3rd ed, Vol. I and II. Springfield, IL, Charles C Thomas, 1982

Sha'ked A (ed). Human Sexuality and Rehabilitation Medicine: Sexual Functioning Following Spinal Cord Injury. Baltimore, Williams & Wilkins, 1981

Shames GH and Wiig EH (eds). Human Communication Disorders: An Introduction. Columbus, OH, Merrill, 1982

Shanks SJ (ed). Nursing and the Management of Adult Communication Disorders. San Diego, College-Hill Press, 1983

Sharpless JW. Mossman's A Problem-Oriented Approach to Stroke Rehabilitation. Springfield, IL, Charles C Thomas, 1982

Snyder M (ed). A Guide to Neurological and Neurosurgical Nursing. New York, John Wiley & Sons, 1983

Stern G and Lees A. Parkinson's Disease: The Facts. New York, Oxford University Press, 1982

Swift-Bandini N. Manual of Neurological Nursing, 2nd ed. Boston, Little, Brown and Co, 1982

Tator CH (ed). Early Management of Acute Spinal Cord Injury. New York, Raven Press, 1982

Warlow C and Morris PJ (eds). Transient Ischemic Attacks. New York, Marcel Dekker, 1982

Widerholt WC (ed). Therapy for Neurologic Disorders. New York, John Wiley & Sons, 1982

Zejdlik CP. Management of Spinal Cord Injury. Monterey, Wadsworth Health Sciences, 1983

Articles

Assessment/Diagnosis

Forbes GS et al. Digital angiography. Mayo Clin Proc 1982 Nov; 57(11): 683–693

King RC. Checking the patient's neurological status. RN 1982 Dec; 45(12):56–62

Head Injury/Intracranial Pressure/Intracranial Pressure Monitoring

Bowers SA and Marshall LF. Severe head injury: Current treatment and research. J Neurosurg Nurs 1982 Oct; 14(5): 210–219

Bruya MA. Planned periods of rest in the intensive care unit: Nursing care activities and intracranial pressure. J Neurosurg Nurs 1981 Aug; 13(4):184–189

Caring for the patient with elevated intracranial pressure (ICP). Nursing '82 1982 Jan; 12(1):48–49

Cope DN and Hall K. Head injury rehabilitation: Benefit of early intervention. Arch Phys Med Rehabil 1982 Sep; 63(9):433–437

Crockard HA. Early management of head injuries. Br J Hosp Med 1982 Jun; 27(6):635–638, 641–644

Johnson LK. If your patient has increased intracranial pressure, your goal should be: No surprises. Nursing '83 1983 Jun; 13(6):58–63

Jones CC and Cayard CH. Care of ICP monitoring devices: A nursing responsibility. J Neurosurg Nurs 1982 Oct; 14(5):255–261

Mastrian KG. Of course you can manage head trauma patients. RN 1981 Aug; 44(8):44–51

Mirr MP, Jankowski K and Taylon MA. Nursing management for barbiturate therapy in acute head injury. Heart Lung 1983 Jan; 12(1):52

Mortara RW. Intracranial pressure monitoring in the emergency setting. Med Instrum 1982 Jul–Aug; 16(4): 197–198

Moss E et al. Intensive management of severe head injuries. Anaesthesia 1983 Mar; 38(3):214–225

Perry J. Rehabilitation of the neurologically disabled patient: Principles, practice, and scientific basis. J Neurosurg 1983 Jun; 58(6): 799–816

Pitts LH and Martin N. Head injuries. Surg Clin North Am 1982 Feb; 62(1): 47–60

Riley JM. Intracranial pressure monitoring made easy. RN 1981 Sep; 44(9):53–57

Rimel R. Head injury: A challenging future for neurosurgical nursing. J Neurosurg Nurs 1982 Oct; 14(5):207–209

Saul TG and Ducker TB. Intracranial pressure monitoring in patients with severe head injury. Am Surg 1982 Sep; 48(9):477–480

Schwartz ML. Head injury in multiple trauma. Can J Surg 1983 Jan; 26(1): 23–26

Pain/Neurosurgery

Avellanosa AM and West CR. Experience with transcutaneous electrical nerve stimulation for relief of intractable pain in cancer patients. J Med 1982; 13(3):203–213

Camp PE. The newer microsurgical techniques in neurosurgery. Head Neck Surg 1982 Jul–Aug; 4(6):514–517

DeJanovich JJ et al. Defining neurosurgical and neurological nursing practice: Establishing our clinical parameters. J Neurosurg 1983 Apr; 15(2):112–118

Garrido E and Bucheit W. Neurosurgical control of pain in cancer patient. Penn Med 1982 Jan; 85(1):25–28

Miller JD. Neurosurgery—triumphs and tragedies. J Roy Coll Surg (Edinb) 1983 Jan; 28(1):1–7

Nikas DL (ed). The critically ill neurosurgical patient. Contemp Issues Crit Care Nurs 1982; 3:1–168

Racz GB et al. Intractable pain therapy using a new epidural catheter. JAMA 1982 Aug 6; 248(5):579–581

Sutherland M. Informed consent—the informed neurosurgical patient and family. J Neuro Surg Nurs 1982 Aug; 14(4):195–202

Thiagarajah S. Postoperative care of neurosurgical patients. Int Anesthesiol Clin 1983 Spring; 21(1):139–156

Wallace KG and Hays J. Nursing management of chronic pain. J

Neurosurg Nurs 1982 Aug; 14(4):185–191

Cranial Nerve Involvement

Dalessio DJ. Tigeminal neuralgia: A practical approach to treatment. Drugs 1982 Sep; 24(3):248–255

Guin PR. Radiofrequency lesions—a treatment for trigeminal neuralgia. J Neurosurg Nurs 1982 Aug; 14(4):192–194

Kirkland J and Williams A. Trigeminal neuralgia: Approaches to nursing care. J Neurosurg Nurs 1983 Jun; 15(3):149–153

Lowe SS et al. Anaesthesia for trigeminal nerve thermocoagulation. Anaesthesia 1983 Feb; 38(2):152–154

Latchaw JP et al. Trigeminal neuralgia treated by radiofrequency coagulation. J Neurosurg 1983 Sep; 59(3):479–484

vanLoveren H et al. A 10-year experience in the treatment of trigeminal neuralgia. J Neurosurg 1982 Dec; 57(6):757–764

Cerebrovascular Disease

Anderson DC. Noninvasive carotid testing in threatened stroke. 1. Principles and techniques. Postgrad Med 1983 Aug; 74(2):239–245

Anderson DC. Noninvasive carotid testing in threatened stroke. 2. Predictive performance. Postgrad Med 1983 Aug; 74(2):254–256

Ball PM. Preventing stroke through non-invasive carotid artery assessment. J Neurosurg Nurs 1982 Aug; 14(4):182–184

Bashor PH. A nursing communication assessment guide. Rehabil Nurs 1983 Jan–Feb; 8(1):20–21, 30

Baum PL. Carotid endarterectomy: One strike against stroke. Nursing '83 1983 Mar; 13(3):50–58

Cranley JJ. Presidential address: Stroke—a perspective. Surgery 1982 May; 91(5):537–549

Delisa JA et al. Stroke rehabilitation: Part I-Cognitive deficits and prediction of outcome. Am Fam Physician 1982 Nov; 26(5):207–214

Delisa JA et al. Stroke rehabilitation: Part II. Recovery and complications. Am Fam Physician 1982 Dec; 26(6):143–151

Feibel JH and Springer CJ. Depression and failure to resume social activities after stroke. Arch Phys Med Rehabil 1982 Jun; 63(6):276–277

Fields WS. Aspirin for prevention of stroke: A review. Am J Med 1983 Jun 14; 74(6A):61–65

Gresham GE. Rehabilitation of the geriatric patient. Stroke rehabilitation, the rehabilitation team, and the usefulness of functional assessment. Primary Care 1982 Mar; 9(1):239–247

Heimlich HJ. Rehabilitation of swallowing after stroke. Ann Otol Rhinol Laryngol 1983 Jul–Aug; 92(4Pt1):357–359

Malone JM and Moore WS. Cerebrovascular disease in the elderly. Otolaryngol Clin North Am 1982 May; 15(2):405–419

Robinson RG and Price TR. Post-stroke depressive disorders: A follow-up study. Stroke 1982 Sep–Oct; 13(5):635–641

Smith DL, Akhtar AJ and Garraway WM. Proprioception and spatial neglect after stroke. Age Ageing 1983 Feb; 12(1):63–69

Smith-Brady R. Assessing adherence in stroke victims. Nurs Clin North Am 1982 Sep; 17(3):499–512

Stroker R. Impact of disability on families of stroke clients. J Neurosurg Nurs 1983 Dec; 15(6):360–365

Tilton CN and Maloof M. Diagnosing the problems in stroke. Am J Nurs 1982 Apr; 82(4):596–601

Treatment in the first 12 hours of stroke. Drug Ther Bull 1983 Mar 25; 21(6):21–24

Yatsu FM. Acute medical therapies of stroke. Clin Neurosurg 1982; 29:524–533

Cerebral Aneurysms

Asiddao CB et al. Factors associated with perioperative complications during carotid endarterectomy. Anesth Analg 1982 Aug; 61(8):631–637

Bardin JA and Bernstein EF. The current status of carotid artery surgery. Head Neck Surg 1982 May–Jun; 4(5):419–426

Carotid endarterectomy's value still uncertain (news). JAMA 1982 Apr 2; 247(13):1802–1803

Harrison MJG. Carotid endarterectomy. Top Rev Neurosurg 1982; 1:57–80

Imparato AM et al. Cerebral protection in carotid surgery. Arch Surg 1982 Aug; 117(8):1073–1078

Perdue GD. Management of postendarterectomy neurologic deficits. Arch Surg 1982 Aug; 117(8):1079–1081

Brain Abscess/Brain Tumor

Bloom HJG. Intracranial tumors: Response and resistance to therapeutic endeavors, 1970–1980. Int J Radiat Oncol Biol Phys 1982 July; 8(7):1083–1113

Burgess KE. Neurological disturbance in a patient with an intracerebral neoplasm: Sources and implications for nursing care. J Neurosurg Nurs 1983 Aug; 15(4):237–242

Cooper JS et al. Malignant glioma and results of combined modality therapy. JAMA 1982 Jul 2; 248(1):62–65

Dunn JH and Reynold AF. Management of primary brain tumors in adults. Ariz Med 1981 Jan; 38(1):26–28

Gamel-Bentzel C. Nursing management of the patient receiving high dose BCNU with autologous bone marrow harvest. J Neurosurg Nurs 1982 Apr; 14(2):98–102

Graham DC. Evaluation of the unconscious patient in the emergency department. J Am Osteopath Assoc 1983 Jan; 82(5):338–343

Greenberg DA and Simon RP. Flexor and extensor postures in sedative drug-induced coma. Neurology 1982 Apr; 32(4):448–451

Hahn AL. Stupor and coma: A clinical approach. Geriatrics 1983 July; 38(7):65–73

Kelly PJ, Alker GJ and Goerss S. Computer-assisted stereotactic laser microsurgery for the treatment of intracranial neoplasms. Neurosurgery 1982 Mar; 10(3):324–331

Magdinee M and Bay JM. The brain tumor clinic: Comprehensive, consistent, compassionate care. J Neurosurg Nurs 1983 Feb; 15(1):36–40

Neuwelt EA, Hill SA and Kikuchi K. Malignant and benign brain tumors: Current concepts and intervention. Compr Ther 1983 Jan; 9(1):24–32

Salcman M. Brain tumors and the geriatric patient. J Am Geriatr Soc 1982 Aug; 30(8):501–508

Thomas DGT. Brain tumors. Br J Hosp Med 1983 Feb; 29(2):148–158

Epilepsy

Beniak J. Patient education in epilepsy. J Neurosurg Nurs 1982 Feb; 14(1):19–22

Chuman CM. New developments in epilepsy. Compr Ther 1983 Jun; 9(6):40–47

Delgado-Escueta AV, Treiman DM and Walsh GO. The treatable epilepsies (Part I). N Engl J Med 1983 Jun 23; 308(25):1508–1514

Delgado-Escueta AV, Treiman DM and Walsh GO. The treatable epilepsies (Part II). N Engl J Med 1983 Jun 30; 308(26):1576–1578, 1579–1584

DeRienzo B. Nursing care in the evaluation of the epilepsy surgery candidate. J Neurosurg Nurs 1982 Dec; 14(6):285–289

Drugs for epilepsy. Med Lett Drugs Ther 1983 Sep 2; 25(643):81–84

Engel J Jr et al. Recent developments in the diagnosis and therapy of epilepsy. Ann Intern Med 1982 Oct; 97(4):584–598

Fountain AJ Jr, Lewis JA and Heck AF. Driving with epilepsy: A contemporary perspective. South Med J 1983 Apr; 76(4):481–484

Hall S. Status epilepticus. Am Fam Physician 1983 Sep; 28(3):117–121

Höppener RJ, Kuyer A and van der Lugt PJM. Epilepsy and alcohol: The influence of social alcohol intake on seizures and treatment in epilepsy. Epilepsia 1983 Aug; 24(4):459–471

Norman SE. Surgical treatment of epilepsy. Am J Nurs 1981 May; 81(5):994–996

Norman SE and Browne TR. Seizure disorders. Am J Nurs 1981 May; 81(5):984–994

Rosenbloom D and Upton ARM. Drug treatment of epilepsy: A review. Can Med Assoc J 1983 Feb 1; 128(3):261–270

Rowan AJ. Diagnosis and treatment of epilepsy. Hosp Community Psychiatry 1983 Jun; 34(6):540–547

Treiman DM. General principles of treatment: Responsive and intractable status epilepticus in adults. Adv Neurol 1983; 34:377–384

Waddell GH. Status epilepticus: Nursing management. Adv Neurol 1983; 34:405–409

Woodward ES. The total patient: Implications for nursing care of the epileptic. J Neurosurg Nurs 1982 Aug; 14(4):166–169

Multiple Sclerosis/Myasthenia Gravis/ Parkinson's Disease

Anchie T. Plasmapheresis as a treatment for myasthenia gravis. J Neurosurg Nurs 1981 Feb; 13(1):23–27

Arnason BGW. Multiple sclerosis: Current concepts and management. Hosp Pract 1982 Feb; 17(2):81–89

Barry L. The patient with myasthenia gravis really needs you. Nursing '82 1982 Jul; 12(7):50–53

Brooks NA and Matson RR. Social-psychological adjustment to multiple sclerosis. Soc Sci Med 1982; 16(24): 2129–2135

Catanzaro M and O'Shaughnessy EJ. Bladder dysfunction: A remedial social problem. J Fam Practitioner 1983 Mar; 16(3):517–520

Fischer BH, Marks M and Reich T. Hyperbaric-oxygen treatment of multiple sclerosis. N Engl J Med 1983 Jan 27; 308(4):181–186

Garrett EJ. Parkinsonism: Forgotten considerations in medical treatment and nursing care. J Neurosurg Nurs 1982 Feb; 14(1):13–18

Gould MT. Nursing diagnoses concurrent with multiple sclerosis. J Neurosurg Nurs 1983 Dec; 15(6):339–345

Hahn K. Management of Parkinson's disease. Nurse Pract 1982 Jan; 7(1): 13–25, 50

Hauser SL et al. Intensive immunosuppression in progressive multiple sclerosis. N Engl J Med 1983 Jan 27; 308(4):173–180

Lieberman AN et al. Bromocriptine and lisuride in Parkinson disease. Ann Neurol 1983 Jan; 13(1):44–47

Lieberman AN et al. Comparative efficacy of pergolide and bromocriptine in patients with advanced Parkinson's disease. Adv Neurol 1983; 37:95–108

Lieberman AN et al. The use of pergolide, a potent dopamine agonist in Parkinson's disease. Clin Pharmacol Ther 1982 Jul; 32(1):70–75

Lisak RP. Myasthenia gravis: Mechanisms and management. Hosp Pract 1983 Mar; 18(3):101–109

McFarlin DE. Treatment of multiple sclerosis. N Engl J Med 1983 Jan 27; 308(4):215–217

McFarlin DE and McFarland HF. Multiple sclerosis. Part I. N Engl J Med 1982 Nov 4; 307(19):1183–1188

McFarlin DE and McFarland HF. Multiple sclerosis: Part II. N Engl J Med 1982 Nov 11; 307(20):1246–1251

Nicholas J. Physiotherapy for multiple sclerosis. Physiotherapy 1982 May; 68(5):144–146

Reder AT and Antel JP. Clinical spectrum of multiple sclerosis. Neurologic Clin 1983 Aug; 1(3):573–599

Tanner CM and Klawans HL. Pergolide mesylate: New therapy for Parkinson disease. Ann Intern Med 1982 Apr; 96(4):522–523

Todes C. Inside parkinsonism . . . a psychiatrist's personal experience. Lancet 1983 Apr 30; 1(8331):977–978

Weiner M. Update on antiparkinsonism agents. Geriatrics 1982 Sep; 37(9):81–91

Weldon PR, Murray TJ and Quine DB. Hearing changes in multiple sclerosis. J Neurosurg Nurs 1983 Apr; 15(2):98–103

Amyotrophic Lateral Sclerosis

Bradley WG. Respirator support in amyotrophic lateral sclerosis (letter). Ann Neurol 1983 Apr; 13(4):466

Garfinkle TJ and Kimmelman CP. Neurologic disorders: Amyotrophic lateral sclerosis, myasthenia gravis, multiple sclerosis, and poliomyelitis. Am J Otolaryngol 1982 May–Jun; 3(3): 204–212

Hartley FD. A nurse's view: Amyotrophic lateral sclerosis. J Neurosurg Nurs 1981 Apr; 13(2):89–96

Olsen B. Motor neuron disease: Amyotrophic lateral sclerosis. J Neurosurg Nurs 1981 Apr; 13(2):83–88

Rabin D. Occasional notes. Compounding the ordeal of ALS: Isolation from my fellow physicians. N Engl J Med 1982 Aug 19; 307(8):506–509

Sivak ED, Gipson WT and Hanson MR. Long-term management of respiratory failure in amyotrophic lateral sclerosis. Ann Neurol 1982 Jul; 12(11):18–23

Wilson B. Battling with motor neurone disease. Br Med J 1982 Jan 2; 284(6308):34–35

Guillain–Barré Syndrome

Dyck PJ et al. Prednisone improves chronic inflammatory demyelinating polyradiculoneuropathy more than no treatment. Ann Neurol 1982 Feb; 11(2):136–141

Gracey DR et al. Respiratory failure in Guillain-Barré syndrome. Mayo Clin Proc 1982 Dec; 57(12):742–746

Kogan B, Solomon MH and Diokno AC. Urinary retention secondary to Landry–Guillain–Barré syndrome. J Urol 1981 Nov; 126(5):643–644

Osterman PO et al. Treatment of the Guillain-Barré syndrome by plasmapheresis. Arch Neurol 1982 Mar; 39(3):148–154

Poser CM. Criteria for the diagnosis of the Guillain-Barré syndrome. J Neurol Sci 1981 Nov–Dec; 52:(2–3):191–199

Spalding JMK. Guillain–Barré syndrome (editorial). Br Med J 1981 Oct 3; 283(6296):873–874

Tikkanen PL. Landry–Guillain–Barré–Strohn syndrome. J Neurosurg Nurs 1982 Apr; 14(2):74–81

Intervertebral Disc/Spinal Cord Injuries

Adelstein W and Watson P. Cervical spine injuries. J Neurosurg Nurs 1983 Apr; 15(2):65–71

Agee BL and Herman C. Cervical logrolling on a standard hospital bed. Am J Nurs 1984 Mar; 84(3):314–318

Andberg MM and Rudolph A. Improving skin care through patient and family training. Top Clin Nurs 1983 Jul; 5(2): 45

Barkin M et al. The urologic care of the spinal cord injury patient. J Urol 1983 Feb; 129(2):335–339

Benoist M et al. Treatment of lumbar disc herniation by chymopapain chemonucleolysis. Spine 1982 Nov–Dec; 7(6):613–617

Bosacco SJ and Berman AT. Surgical management of lumbar disc disease. Radiol Clin North Am 1983 Jun; 21(2):377–393

Brackett TO et al. The emotional care of a person with a spinal cord injury. JAMA 1984 Aug 10; 252(6):793–795

Devoti AL. Lumbar laminectomy: Diagnosis to discharge. J Neurosurg Nurs 1983 Jun; 15(3):140–143

Gunby P. What is intradiscal therapy, anyway? JAMA 1983 Mar 4; 249(9): 1120–1123

Hejna WF and Sinkora G. Chemonucleolysis of herniated lumbar discs. Am Fam Physician 1983 May; 27(5):97–103

Howard M and Corbo-Pelaia SA. The psychological afteraffects of halo traction and a review of acute care. Am J Nurs 1982 Dec; 82(12):1839–1843

Hummelgard A and Martin E. Management of the patient in a Halo brace. J Neurosurg Nurs 1982 Jun; 14(3):113–119

Javid MJ et al. Safety and efficacy of chymopapain (Chymodiactin) in herniated nucleus pulposus with sciatica. JAMA 1983 May 13; 249(18): 2489–2494

Maida MJ. Chymopapain for herniated lumbar disc disease. J Neurosurg Nurs 1983 Jun; 15(3):144–148

McGuire EJ and Savastano JA. Long-term followup of spinal cord injury patients managed by intermittent catheterization. J Urol 1983 Apr; 129(4):775–776

Mooney V (ed). Symposium on evaluation and care of lumbar spine problems. Orthop Clin North Am 1983 Jul; 14(3):entire volume

Musolf JM. Chemonucleolysis. A new approach for patients with herniated intervertebral disks. Am J Nurs 1983 Jun; 83(6):882–885

Parkinson D. Late results of treatment on intervertebral disc disease with chymopapain. J Neurosurg 1983 Dec; 59(6):990–993

Silver JR. Immediate management of spinal injury. Br J Hosp Med 1983 May; 29(5):412, 414, 417

Solomon J. Sex and the spinal cord injured patient. J Neurosurg Nurs 1982 Jun; 14(3):125–127

Sonntag VK. The early management of cervical spine injuries. Ariz Med 1982 Oct; 39(10):644–647

Steinglass P et al. Coping with spinal cord injury: The family perspective. Gen Hosp Psychiatry 1982 Dec; 4(4): 259–264

Sugarman B, Brown D and Musher D. Fever and infection in spinal cord injury patients. JAMA 1982 Jul 2; 248(1):66–70

Toth LL. Spasticity management in spinal cord injury. Rehab Nurs 1983 Jan–Feb; 8(1):14–17

Trafton PG. Spinal cord injuries. Surg Clin North Am 1982 Feb; 62(1):61–72

Weber H. Lumbar disc herniation. Spine 1983 Mar; 8(2):131–140

Weinberg JS. Human sexuality and spinal cord injury. Nurs Clin North Am 1982 Sep; 17(3):407–419

Musculoskeletal Conditions

19

Specific Problems Associated With Musculoskeletal Problems

Nursing Process Overview

Assessment

General observation—data on ability to move, existence of discomfort and gross abnormalities, and presence of involuntary movement
1. Observe gait and intentional movement for coordination and speed.
2. Note posture and body positions.
3. Identify use of assistive devices—canes, walker, prosthesis, etc.

Nursing History

The patient supplies data on primary problem and information indicating impact of problem on life-style.
1. Elicit information concerning chief complaint (e.g., onset of problem, how the patient has been handling the problem).
2. Assist the patient to describe symptoms such as pain, stiffness, and cramps.
3. Identify concurrent health problems, health maintenance practices (including medications), and allergies.
4. Note impact of musculoskeletal disorder on life-style, family interactions, family's economics, etc.
5. Assess the patient's perceptions and expectations related to health problems.
6. Estimate the patient's ability to learn (i.e., note language barriers).

Physical Assessment

Data on current system condition and functional abilities are secured through inspection, palpation, and measurement.

A. **Skeletal Component**
1. Note deviations from structural normal—bony deformities, length discrepancies, alignment, amputations.
2. Identify abnormal motion and *crepitus* (grating sensation) as found with fractures.

B. **Joint Component**
1. Identify swelling that may be due to inflammation or effusion
2. Note deformity associated with contractures or dislocations
3. Evaluate stability which may be altered
4. Estimate R.O.M. (range of motion) both actively and passively

C. **Muscle Component**
1. Inspect for size and contour of muscles.
2. Assess coordination of movement.
3. Palpate for muscle tone.
4. Estimate strength through cursory evaluation (i.e., handshake) or scaled criteria (i.e., 0 = no palpable contraction to 5 = normal range of motion against gravity with full resistance).
5. Measure girth to note increases due to swelling or bleeding into muscle or decreases due to atrophy (difference of more than 1 cm. is significant).
6. Identify abnormal *clonus* (rhythmic contraction and relaxation) or *fasciculation* (contractions of isolated muscle fibers).

D. **Neurovascular Component**
1. Assess circulatory status of involved extremities by noting skin color and temperature, peripheral pulses, capillary refill response, pain.

2. Assess neurologic status of involved extremities by the patient's ability to move distal muscles and description of sensation (e.g., paresthesia).
3. Test reflexes of extremities.
4. Note hair distribution and nail condition.

E. Skin Component

1. Inspect traumatic injuries (e.g., cuts, bruises, etc.).
2. Assess chronic conditions (e.g., dermatitis, stasis ulcers, etc.).

F. Subjective Component

Elicit data from patient concerning presence of pain, tenderness, abnormal sensation, or tightness during physical examination.

Diagnostic Evaluation

A. Radiologic and Imaging Studies

1. X-rays
   a. Of bone—to determine bone density, texture, erosion, changes in bone relationships
   b. Of cortex—to detect any widening, narrowing, irregularity
   c. Of medullary cavity—to detect any alteration in density
   d. Of involved joint—to show fluid, irregularity, spur formation, narrowing, changes in joint contour
2. Tomogram—special x-ray technique for detailed view of specific plane of bone
3. Computed tomogram—to identify tumors of the soft tissues or injuries to ligaments or tendons; to identify location/extent of fractures in difficult-to-define areas; to identify disc herniation
4. Bone scan—parenteral injection of bone-seeking radiopharmaceutical; concentration of isotope uptake revealed in primary skeletal disease (osteosarcoma), metastatic bone disease, inflammatory skeletal disease (osteomyelitis); fracture
5. Arthrogram—injection of radiopaque substance or air into joint cavity to outline soft tissue structures (e.g., meniscus) and contour of joint
6. Myelogram—injection of contrast medium into subarachnoid space at lumbar spine to determine level of disc herniation or site of tumor; see page 756
7. Discogram—injection of small amount of contrast medium into lumbar disc to visualize disc space

B. Joint Examinations

1. *Arthrocentesis*—insertion of needle into joint and aspiration of synovial fluid for purposes of examination.
2. *Arthroscopy*—endoscopic procedure that allows direct visualization of a joint, especially the knee. May be combined with arthrography.
   Technique
   a. Under local or general anesthesia, a large-bore needle is inserted into the suprapatellar pouch, and the joint is distended with saline.
   b. An arthroscope is introduced and the knee joint visualized, including the synovium, articular surfaces, and menisci.
   c. Patient may be advised to limit his activities for several days following the procedure, which is relatively painless.

C. Muscle and Nerve Studies—to differentiate nerve root compression, muscle disease (dystrophy, myositis, etc.), peripheral neuropathies, central nervous system–anterior horn cell neuropathies, neuromuscular-junction problems.

1. *Electromyography (EMG)*—measures electrical potential generated by the muscle during relaxation and contraction
2. *Nerve conduction velocities* (NCVs)—measures the rate of potential generation along specific nerves (speed of impulse conduction)

D. Laboratory Studies—baseline hematology, serum chemistry and urinalysis provide information on the general health of the patient. Few laboratory studies are specific for orthopedic conditions.

1. Clotting factors—evaluation prior to orthopedic surgery desirable; person with hemophilia prone to specific orthopedic problems; assessed in prophylactic and therapeutic anticoagulant regimens
2. Calcitonin—bone metabolism
3. Calcium—osteomalacia, parathyroid function
4. Creatine—trauma to muscle
5. Creatine phosphokinase (CPK)—skeletal muscle disease
6. Parathyroid hormone (PTH)—bone metabolism
7. Hyperkalemia—trauma with massive tissue damage
8. Phosphatase, alkaline—bone metabolism (osteoblastic activity), bone tumors, Paget's disease
9. Phosphorus, inorganic—parathyroid problems
10. Thyroid studies—bone metabolism
11. Transaminase (SGPT)—skeletal muscle disease
12. Vitamin D (1,25(OH)2D3)—bone metabolism
13. Urine: Bence–Jones protein—multiple myeloma
14. Urine: calcium—bone metabolism; parathyroid function
15. Urine: creatinine—muscular atrophy
16. Urine: phosphorus—rickets

E. Special Studies—bone biopsy, densitometry, total body calcium, etc.

Patient Problems/Nursing Diagnoses

(Associated with musculoskeletal conditions)
1. Pain related to muscular or skeletal dysfunction
2. Impaired mobility related to limitations imposed by underlying condition and treatment modalities such as casts, traction, or bed rest
3. Ineffective coping related to enforced immobility and altered life-style
4. Potential for injury (neuromuscular compromise such as compartment syndrome) related to constrictive dressings, crush injuries, ischemic swelling following arterial injury, etc.
5. Potential impairment of circulation and nerve function related to increased tissue pressure

Planning and Implementation
Nursing Interventions

A. Relief of pain

1. Secure data concerning pain.
   a. Have the patient describe the pain, location, characteristics (dull, sharp, continuous, throbbing, boring, radiating, aching, etc.)
   b. Ask the patient what causes the pain; makes the pain worse; relieves the pain, etc.
   c. Evaluate the patient for proper body alignment, pressure from equipment (casts, traction, splints, appliances)
   d. Recall pathophysiology related to different types of musculoskeletal pain

(1) Soreness and aching—muscular discomfort
(2) Associated with weather changes—chronic arthritic discomfort
(3) Associated with movement—joint sprain or muscle strain
(4) Sharp and piercing—fracture pain, muscle spasm
(5) Steady, increasing pain—osteomyelitis, tumor, vascular complication
(6) Radiating pain—pressure on nerve root
(7) Boring, night pain—bone pathology

2. Initiate activities to prevent or modify pain.
   a. Assist the patient with pain-reduction techniques—cutaneous stimulation, distraction, guided imagery, transcutaneous electrical nerve stimulation (TENS), biofeedback, etc.
   b. Position the patient in correct alignment.
   c. Move the patient slowly and steadily, providing adequate support to painful structure, and help of additional personnel as needed.
   d. Elevate painful extremity above the level of the heart.
   e. Apply heat or cold modalities as prescribed.
   f. Modify environment to facilitate rest and relaxation.
3. Administer pharmaceuticals as indicated and encourage use of less potent drugs as severity of discomfort decreases.
4. Encourage the patient to become an active participant in rehabilitative plans.

B. Establishing maximum physical mobility within limits of musculoskeletal problem and therapeutic regimen

1. Assess degree of physical mobility present.
   a. Identify use of mobility aids.
   b. Note ability to reposition self and ability to transfer from one place to another.
   c. Determine availability of assistants to facilitate mobility.
   d. Assess body systems (e.g., respiratory, gastrointestinal, etc.) for responses to limited activity.
   e. Evaluate short-term and long-term effects of chosen treatment modalities on mobility.
2. Identify true extent of imposed physical immobility.
3. Develop exercise regimen within prescribed physical activity limits.
4. Encourage weight-bearing and walking activities when possible.
5. Establish range-of-motion and isometric exercise (e.g., quadricep sets) plan in preparation for resumption of ambulation.
6. Encourage movement of all uninvolved bodily parts.
7. Teach proper and safe use of mobilization aids.

C. Avoiding neuromuscular compromise and ensuring optimum circulation, tissue perfusion, and nerve function

1. Assess for clinical manifestations of neuromuscular compromise.
   a. Complaint of deep, throbbing pain with persistent pressure sensation.
   b. Abnormal sensory evaluation (e.g., paresthesia, hypesthesia, loss of sensation)
   c. Pain with stretch of involved muscle
   d. Tight, tense muscle mass on palpation
   e. Elevation of tissue pressure indicated by direct needle measurement (above 30 mm. Hg)
   f. Paresis or weakness

▶ **NURSING ALERT:** Pulse and capillary refill may be present with inadequate tissue perfusion and can contribute to a false sense of security concerning impending compartment syndrome.

2. Elevate injured extremity above heart level, if possible, to minimize edema.
3. Apply ice pack to fresh injury if prescribed to control bleeding and swelling.
4. Inform the patient that frequent neurovascular assessments will be performed.
5. Have the patient move fingers or toes distal to injury.
6. Have the patient describe sensations in injured extremity.
7. Assess color, temperature, capillary refill, and pulses of involved extremity.
8. Notify physician immediately of compromised neurovascular status.
9. Release constrictive devices (e.g., bivalve cast).
10. If no improvement when external devices are released, a decompression fasciotomy (incision of tissue surrounding muscle) will be anticipated.
11. Give health education concerning preoperative and postoperative care.
12. Teach the patient to recognize and report increasing pain, tingling, and numbness.

D. Strengthening coping abilities

1. Nursing assessment
   a. Assess the patient and family for reactive behaviors of denial, anger, bargaining, depression, acceptance.
   b. Identify social isolation behaviors.
   c. Note expressions of diminished self-worth and self-concept.
   d. Assess degree of independence in self-care activites.
   e. Identify anxious behaviors.
2. Promote gradual acceptance of disabilities due to musculoskeletal problem.
   a. Assist the patient to recognize the impact of the musculoskeletal problem.
   b. Support the patient through the phases of acceptance.
   c. Recognize that the patient and family may be at different phases of coping/acceptance process.
   d. Accept the patient's behaviors as expressions of the coping process.
   e. Encourage the patient to focus on current abilities (instead of losses).
3. Reduce anxiety related to impact of musculoskeletal problem on life-style.
   a. Explore the patient's understanding of musculoskeletal problem and its therapeutic regimen.
   b. Identify areas for additional teaching.
   c. Clarify misconceptions.
   d. Encourage the patient to participate actively in planning and implementation of therapeutic regimen.
   e. Facilitate acceptance of abilities by the patient and family.
   f. Assist the patient to identify stress-producing situations.
4. Minimize social isolation related to hospitalization and decreased mobility.
   a. Plan frequent periods of interaction with the patient.
   b. Encourage contacts with family and friends.

c. Facilitate visits with children and other family members when feasible.
d. Involve the patient in personal and therapeutic decision-making processes.
e. Develop supportive relationships.

5. Initiate measures to cope with altered self-concept related to modified life role.
   a. Identify activities within treatment regimen where the patient can establish control.
   b. Provide genuine praise for self-care abilities.
   c. Encourage the patient to make own decisions within scheduled therapeutic regimen.
   d. Assist family in use of the patient's contributions to solve home problems.
   e. Promote feelings of independence.

6. Counter self-care deficits related to musculoskeletal problem or treatment modality.
   a. Assess residual abilities and utilize these in development of self-care regimens.
   b. Encourage the patient to assist in own care to fullest ability.
   c. Modify activities to facilitate maximum independence.
   d. Maximize time allotted for accomplishment of self-care activities
   e. Integrate physical therapy, occupational therapy, and other therapeutic approaches into nursing care activities.

Evaluation
Expected Outcomes

1. Achieves pain relief
   a. Participates in pain-reduction activities by elevating extremity, use of pain-reduction modality, accepting assistance in pain-producing situations
   b. Decreases use of pharmaceutical agents in the management of discomfort
2. Increases participation in rehabilitative activities by self-care activities, mobilization activities, planning for continuing care needs
3. Maintains adequate circulation and nerve function
   a. Minimal discomfort, normal sensations, and normal movement of fingers or toes of involved extremity.
   b. No extremity contracture or evidence of loss of function of extremity due to compromised circulation
4. Moves unaffected joints and extremities
5. Utilizes mobilization aids safely and effectively
6. Participates in rehabilitation program
7. Remains free of immobility complications
8. States modifications in life-style necessary to accommodate musculoskeletal disability

---

Musculoskeletal Trauma

Contusions

A *contusion* is an injury to the soft tissue produced by a blunt force (blow, kick, or fall).

Clinical Manifestations

1. Hemorrhage into injured part (ecchymosis)—from rupture of small blood vessels; also associated with fractures
2. Pain, swelling, and discoloration
3. Hyperkalemia may be present with extensive contusions resulting in destruction of body tissue and loss of blood.

Nursing Interventions

A. Relief of discomfort

1. Elevate the affected part.
2. Apply cold compresses for the first 24 hours (20–30 minutes at a time)—to produce vasoconstriction, decrease edema, and reduce discomfort.
3. Apply heat to affected area after 24 hours (20–30 minutes at a time) 4 times a day—to promote circulation and absorption.
4. Apply pressure bandage—to control bleeding and swelling.
5. Assess neurovascular status of contused extremity every hour to every 4 hours as the patient's condition indicates.

B. Activity schedule

1. Encourage range of motion of all joints.
2. Assist with activities as needed.
3. Teach the patient to avoid excessive exercise of injured part.
4. Teach the patient to avoid re-injury.

Strains and Sprains

A *strain* is a microscopic tearing of the muscle caused by excessive force, stretching, or overuse.

A *sprain* is an injury to ligamentous structures surrounding a joint; it is usually caused by a wrench or twist resulting in a decrease in the joint stability.

Clinical Manifestations

A. Strains

There is usually hemorrhage into the muscle, swelling, tenderness, and pain with isometric contraction of the muscle.

B. Sprains

1. Rapid swelling—due to extravasation of blood within tissues
2. Pain upon passive movement of joint
3. Increasing pain during first few hours due to continued swelling
4. X-ray of area reveals no bone injury.

Nursing Interventions

A. Relief of discomfort

1. Apply cold compresses (or ice bag) for 15–20 minutes intermittently for 12–36 hours—vasoconstricting effects of cold retard extravasation of blood and lymph (edema) and suppress pain.
2. After 24 hours, apply mild heat (15–30 minutes, 4 times daily)—to promote absorption.
3. Instruct the patient on use of pain medication as prescribed.

B. Immobilization of injured part to allow for healing

1. Splint and immobilize injured part.
2. Elevate injured extremity to minimize swelling.
3. Use elastic compressive dressing to support weakened joint structures and to control edema.
4. Severe sprains may require surgical repair and/or cast immobilization.

C. Resumption of self-care activities

1. Assist the patient in use of self-care and mobility aids to maintain independence within activity restrictions.
2. Participate in patient teaching on need to rest injured part for about a month to allow for healing.
3. Teach the patient to resume activities gradually.

Traumatic Joint Dislocation

A *dislocation of a joint* occurs when the surfaces of the bones forming the joint are no longer in anatomic contact—this is a medical emergency because of associated disruption of surrounding blood and nerve supplies.

Clinical Manifestations

1. Pain
2. Deformity
3. Change in the length of the extremity
4. Loss of normal movement
5. X-ray confirmation of dislocation without associated fracture.

Treatment

1. Immobilize part while the patient is transported to emergency department, x-ray department, or clinical unit.
2. Secure reduction of dislocation (bring displaced parts into normal position) as soon as possible; usually performed under anesthesia.
3. Stabilize reduction until joint structures are healed.
4. Monitor for development of sequelae (unstable joint, aseptic necrosis of bone, circulatory or nerve impairment).

Nursing Interventions

A. Promoting comfort

1. Secure the patient's permission to undergo reduction of dislocation under anesthesia if necessary.
2. Give medication to relieve discomfort.
3. Immobilize reduced joint.

B. Resumption of self-care activities

1. Assist the patient with activities of daily living as needed.
2. Initiate health teaching concerning need to comply with activity limitations, rehabilitation therapies, and long-term monitoring for sequelae.

Knee Injuries

Causes

1. Severe stresses are applied to the knee during many sport activities (e.g., soccer, skiing, running).
2. Injury to knee structures occur during rapid position changes involving flexing and twisting of the joint.
3. Torn cartilage (meniscus) causes pain, tenderness, joint effusion, clicking sensations, and decreased range of motion.

4. Knee ligaments may be torn, resulting in pain and joint instability. The patellar tendon may rupture.

Management

1. Arthroscopic meniscectomy
   Removal of cartilage fragments through operating arthroscope inserted through a small incision into the knee joint.
2. Open meniscectomy
   Direct surgical approach to knee joint structures for repair of disrupted structures.
3. Ligament injuries
   Treated with immobilization (i.e., elastic bandage, splint, cast) or suturing of ligament depending on severity of injury.
4. Rupture of tendon
   Must be sutured and immobilized during healing.

Patient Education

1. Elevate leg to minimize swelling.
2. Quadricep setting exercises and straight leg raising.
3. Weight-bearing and exercise program as prescribed.

Fractures

A *fracture* is a break in the continuity of bone. Although the bone is the part most directly affected, other structures may be involved, resulting in soft tissue edema, hemorrhage into muscles and joints, joint dislocations, ruptured tendons, severed nerves, damaged blood vessels, and injury to body organs.

Etiology

A fracture occurs when the stress placed on the bone is more than the bone can absorb. When a fracture occurs through an area of diseased bone (osteoporosis, bone cyst, bony metastasis) it is considered a *pathological fracture.*

Types of Fractures (Fig. 19-1)

1. *Complete*—a fracture involving the entire cross-section of the bone; usually displaced (not in normal position)
2. *Incomplete*—a fracture involving only a portion of the cross-section of bone; usually undisplaced
3. *Open*—break in the skin and underlying soft tissue, leading directly into the fracture
4. *Closed*—the fracture does not communicate with the outside area

Patterns of Fracture (Fig. 19-1)

1. *Greenstick*—a fracture in which one side of a bone is broken and the other side is bent
2. *Transverse*—the fracture is straight across the bone
3. *Oblique*—a fracture occurring at an angle across the bone
4. *Spiral*—a fracture twisting around the shaft of the bone
5. *Comminuted*—a fracture in which bone has splintered into several fragments
6. *Depressed*—a fracture in which fragment(s) is indriven (seen frequently in fractures of the skull and facial bones)
7. *Compression*—a fracture in which the bone collapses in on itself (seen frequently in vertebral fractures)
8. *Avulsion*—fragment of bone is pulled off by ligament or tendon attachment
9. *Impacted*—a fragment of bone·is wedged into other bone fragment

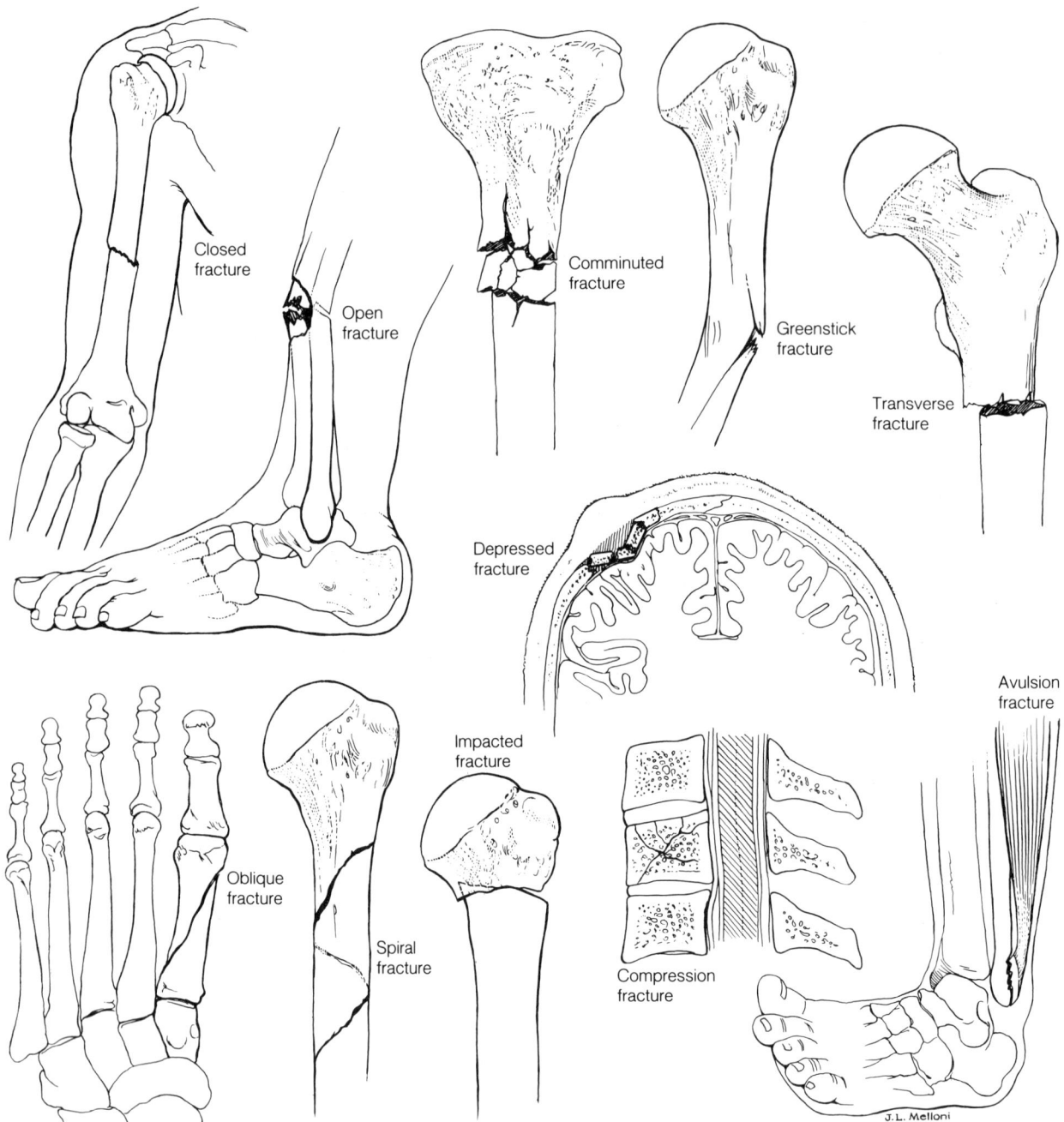

Figure 19-1. Types of fractures.

10. *Fracture dislocation*—a fracture complicated by the bone being out of the joint
11. Other—described according to anatomic location—epiphyseal, supracondylar, mid-shaft, intra-articular

Emergency Management

See page 941.

Fracture Treatment

There is no one solution in the management of fractures. Consideration is given to the severity of the fracture, damage to soft tissues, the age and condition of the patient, and economic factors before a specific form of treatment is selected.

A. Goals

1. To regain and maintain correct position and alignment
2. To regain the function of the involved part
3. To return the patient to his usual activities in the shortest time and at the least expense

B. Process

1. *Reduction*—setting the bone; refers to restoration of the fracture fragments into anatomic position and alignment
2. *Immobilization*—maintains reduction until bone healing occurs
3. *Rehabilitation*—regaining normal function of the affected part

C. Methods

1. *Closed reduction*—bony fragments are brought into *apposition* (ends in contact) by manipulation and manual traction—restores alignment
   a. May be done under anesthesia for pain relief and muscle relaxation
   b. Cast or splint applied to immobilize extremity and maintain reduction (see Casts, p. 828)
2. *Traction*—force applied to accomplish and maintain reduction and alignment (see Traction, p. 833)
   a. Frequently used for fractures of long bones
   b. Techniques—*Skin traction*—force applied to the skin using foam rubber, tapes, etc. *Skeletal traction*—force applied to the bony skeleton directly using wires, pins, or tongs placed into or through the bone
3. *Open reduction with internal fixation*—operative intervention to achieve reduction, alignment, and stabilization (see Orthopedic Surgery, Special Nursing Considerations, p. 840).
   a. Bone fragments are directly visualized.
   b. Internal fixation devices (metal pins, wires, screws, plates, nails, rods) may be used to hold bone fragments in position until solid bone healing occurs (may be removed when bone is healed).
   c. After closure of the wound, splints or casts may be used for additional stabilization and support
4. *Endoprosthetic replacement*—replacement of a fracture fragment with an implanted metal device; utilized when fracture disrupts nutrition of the bone or treatment of choice is bony replacement.
5. *External fixation device*—stabilization of complex and open fracture with use of a metal frame and pin system; permits active treatment of injured soft tissue
   a. Wound may be left open (delayed primary wound closure).
   b. Repair of damage to blood vessels, soft tissue, muscles, nerves, and tendons as indicated.
   c. Reconstructive surgery may be necessary.
   (See External Fixation for Complicated Fractures, p. 838.)

Nursing Process Overview (Fractures)

Assessment

Clinical Manifestations

1. Physical findings implicating fracture include:
   a. Pain at site of injury
   b. Swelling
   c. Tenderness
   d. False motion and crepitus (grating sensation)
   e. Deformity
   f. Loss of function
   g. Ecchymosis
   h. Paresthesia
2. X-ray and other imaging techniques demonstrating fracture
3. Signs and symptoms of shock
   a. Bone is very vascular; following trauma, large amounts of blood escape from circulating blood into soft tissues or through open wounds (especially in femoral and pelvic fractures).
   b. May be fatal within a few hours after injury.
4. Overt hemorrhage and covert blood loss (bleeding into the tissues)—note hemoglobin and hematocrit
5. *Fat embolism syndrome*—embolization of marrow or tissue fat or lipids with platelets and circulating free fatty acids within the pulmonary capillaries; pulmonary capillary leak may result, producing respiratory distress and central nervous system dysfunction.
   a. Onset may occur within 48 hours after injury.

▶ **NURSING ALERT:** Have a high degree of suspicion of fat embolism syndrome in patients with multiple fractures, and fractures of long bones and pelvis. Hypoxemia is an early manifestation and is detected by arterial blood gas analysis.

   b. Assess patient for:
      (1) Respiratory distress—tachypnea, dyspnea, hypoxemia, crackles, wheezing, acute pulmonary edema—lung filters and traps embolic material, producing disturbed ventilation, perfusion, and interstitial pneumonitis.
      (2) Mental disturbances—irritability, restlessness, confusion, disorientation, stupor, and coma—effects of systemic embolization and severe hypoxemia (may be first sign).
      (3) Fever
      (4) Petechiae—in buccal membranes, conjunctival sacs, on the hard palate, retina, chest, and anterior axillary folds—from occlusion of capillaries by fat and fibrin platelet particulate substances.
6. Neurovascular status—watch for neurovascular impairment in all patients with fractures—pain, decreased circulation, decreased sensation, and decreased motor activity.

Patient Problems/Nursing Diagnoses

1. Pain related to fractured bone, soft tissue injury and swelling, and muscle spasm
2. Inadequate tissue perfusion related to swelling of injured part and disrupted fluid circulation
3. Self-care deficits related to fracture immobility and therapeutic modality
4. Potential systemic problems (e.g., shock, fat emboli) related to injury and postinjury sequelae
5. Potential local fracture problems (i.e., compartment syndrome, nonunion, infection) related to disruption of healing sequence.
6. Ineffective coping and social isolation related to fracture event and ramifications

Planning and Implementation
Nursing Interventions

A. Relief of discomfort

1. See Pain related to musculoskeletal conditions, page 814.
2. Immobilize bone fragments—movement of fragments causes pain.
3. Support splinted fracture above and below fracture when repositioning or moving the patient.
4. Reposition patient with slow and steady motion; use additional personnel as needed.

B. Reduction in swelling associated with the injury

1. Elevate injured extremity above heart level.
2. Apply ice pack to injury if prescribed.
3. Assess neurovascular status of injured extremity.

C. Promotion of self-care activities within the limits of fracture treatment

1. Assist the patient with hygiene and nutrition activities as needed.
2. Encourage independence within immobility limits.
3. Modify activities to facilitate maximum independence.
4. Allow time for the patient to accomplish task.
5. Teach technique for safe use of mobility and other aids.

D. Prevention of systemic problems (e.g., shock [hemorrhagic or neurogenic]; fat emboli; pulmonary emboli)

1. Monitor vital signs.
2. Maintain arterial blood pressure—administer fluids/blood as needed.
3. Review laboratory reports for abnormal values.
4. Observe for signs and symptoms of fat embolism.
   a. Evaluate mental status.
   b. Maintain satisfactory pulmonary gas exchange and support the respiratory system.
      (1) Draw arterial blood for gas analysis—arterial hypoxia is present with fat emboli; cannot always be recognized clinically.
      (2) Administer oxygen as indicated by results of blood gas analysis (respiratory failure is the most common cause of death).
      (3) Assist with endotracheal intubation (for airway control); controlled volume ventilation and positive end-expiratory pressure (PEEP)—to obtain maximum aeration of lungs.
      (4) Administer steroids—to block chemical inflammation caused by free fatty acids; decreases endothelial damage (controversial).
      (5) See treatment of respiratory failure and insufficiency, page 186.
5. Assess for development of:
   a. Thromboembolism (particularly of fractures of lower extremities)
   b. Infection—all open fractures are considered contaminated. (See also gas gangrene, p. 882, and tetanus, p. 881)
   c. Disseminated intravascular coagulation (DIC)—a group of bleeding disorders with diverse causes (see p. 261)

E. Prevention of neurovascular and healing problems

1. See Neurovascular Compromise, page 815.

▶ **NURSING ALERT:** Monitoring the neurovascular integrity of the injured extremity is essential. Development of *compartment syndrome* (increased tissue pressure causing anoxia)—leads to permanent loss of function in 6–8 hours. This situation must be identified and managed promptly.

2. Support the patient if healing does not occur as projected because of inadequate immobilization, interposed tissue between bone fragments, or infection.
   a. Delayed union—signifies that a specific fracture has not healed in the time considered average for this type of fracture.
   b. Nonunion—failure of the ends of a fractured bone to unite (and union not expected to occur).
   c. Avascular necrosis of bone—may occur when the bone loses its blood supply following fracture or dislocation (notably in the hip) or in certain diseases.

F. Prevention of infection

1. Minimize chance of infection of wound, soft tissue, and bone.
2. Cleanse, debride, and irrigate the wound as soon as possible—to minimize chance of infection.
   a. Take swabs for culture and sensitivity of wound.
3. Protect the patient from tetanus.
   a. Determine the patient's status of immunization for tetanus.
   b. See page 881 for protocol of administration.
   c. Give antibiotics as directed (usually IV antibiotics are started quickly)—to avoid and treat serious infection; many open fractures are contaminated with bacteria at the time of admission.
4. Observe and record the patient's temperature at regular intervals—for septic complications.

G. Adjustment of life-style and responsibilities to accommodate limitations imposed by fracture.

See Psychological and social problems associated with musculoskeletal problems, page 815.

Health Education

1. Explain basis for fracture treatment and need for patient participation in therapeutic regimen.
2. Instruct the patient to actively exercise joints above and below the immobilized fracture at frequent intervals.
   a. Isometric exercises of muscles covered by cast—start exercise as soon as possible after cast application.
   b. Increase isometric exercises as fracture stabilizes.
3. After removal of immobilizing device (e.g., cast, splint), have the patient start active exercises and continue with isometric exercises.
4. Instruct the patient on exercises to strengthen upper extremity muscles if crutch walking is planned.
5. Instruct the patient in methods of safe ambulation—walker, crutches, cane.
6. Emphasize instructions concerning amount of weight bearing that will be permitted on fractured extremity.
7. Discuss prevention of recurrent fractures—safety considerations; avoidance of fatigue; proper footwear.
8. Discharge teaching—follow-up medical supervision; symptoms needing attention (e.g., numbness, decreased function, increased pain, elevated temperature); medication teaching.

Evaluation

Expected Outcomes

1. Achieves relief of discomforts related to fracture; elevates fractured extremity and uses pain-relief techniques
2. Experiences minimal swelling of injured part; applies ice pack as prescribed to fresh injury and demonstrates intact neurovascular status
3. Achieves self-care within limits of therapeutic regi-

men; participates in hygiene and nutritional care; uses assistive devices safely
4. Is free of potential systemic problems; maintains normal vital signs and laboratory values.
5. Shows no signs of potential local fracture problems; intact neurovascular status and fracture healing within anticipated period for particular type of fracture.
6. Demonstrates psychological adjustment to impact of therapeutic regimen on life-style; actively participates in therapeutic–rehabilitation program.

Fractures of Specific Site*

Fractures of the Upper Extremity

Fracture of the Clavicle (Collar Bone)

1. The clavicle helps to hold the shoulder upward, outward, and backward from the thorax.
2. Aim of reduction: to hold the shoulder in the position described above.
3. Most fractures of the clavicle are treated by closed reduction and immobilization accomplished by one of the following methods:
   a. Clavicular strap (Pad axilla to prevent nerve damage from pressure.)
   b. Sling
   c. Figure 8 bandage } Watch for tingling in hands; too tight a clavicular strap or figure 8 bandage may cause circulatory impairment.
   d. T-splint
4. Open reduction and internal fixation may be done for marked displacement and angulation of bone ends. Following surgery, the patient's arm is kept in a sling.

Health Education

1. Exercise elbow, wrist, and fingers as soon as possible.
2. Do shoulder exercises to obtain full shoulder motion as prescribed.

Fractures of the Surgical Neck of the Humerus (Fractures of the Proximal Humerus)

1. Most occur from falls in which the outstretched arm strikes the ground (impacted fracture). Osteoporosis is a predisposing factor.
2. Many impacted fractures of the surgical neck of the humerus do not require reduction. The weight of the arm helps to correct displacement.
   a. Place a soft pad under the axilla to prevent skin maceration.
   b. The arm is supported by a sling and swathe or Velpeau bandage for comfort (Fig. 19-2).
   c. Advise the patient that he will sleep more comfortably when supported in an upright position.
3. Displaced fractures are treated with reduction under x-ray control, open reduction, or replacement of humeral head with prosthesis.
   a. A program of exercises is started after a specified period of immobilization with emphasis on range of motion of the shoulder.

* For fracture of the skull see page 766, fracture of the cervical spine, page 801, and rib fractures, page 174.

Health Education

Goal:
To restore shoulder function and prevent adhesions.

1. Start active motion of shoulder joint early—to prevent limitation of motion and stiffness of shoulder.
2. Instruct the patient to lean forward and allow affected arm to abduct and rotate.

Fractures of the Shaft of the Humerus

1. Fractures of the shaft of the humerus are most frequently caused by direct violence—falls, blow to arm, auto injuries.
2. The radial nerve may be injured in this fracture because it lies immediately adjacent to the midportion of the humerus in the musculoskeletal groove.
3. Sling and swathe, splints, or hanging casts may be used.
4. Hanging cast is frequently applied to oblique, spiral, and displaced fractures with shortening of humeral shaft—the weight of the arm helps to correct displacement.

▶ **NURSING ALERT:** A hanging cast for treatment of fracture of the shaft of the humerus must be dependent (remain unsupported) to provide a traction force. Continuous traction on long axis of arm is affected by the weight of the cast. The patient must avoid supporting the elbow in the lap while seated.

5. See that the patient sleeps in a fairly upright position to maintain uninterrupted 24-hour traction.
6. Exercise fingers immediately after the application of the cast.
7. Start pendulum exercises as directed—provides active exercise of shoulder to prevent adhesions of the shoulder joint capsule after cast removal.
8. Open reduction and internal fixation (usually by compression plate) are performed when satisfactory alignment cannot be obtained with closed treatment, when there is associated vascular injury, and when the fracture is the result of a pathologic (malignant) lesion.

   Following a surgical procedure, the arm is placed in a sling and swathed until bone union has taken place at the fracture site.

Fractures and Dislocations about the Elbow

1. Dislocations or fractures about the elbow usually occur as the result of a fall on the elbow or the

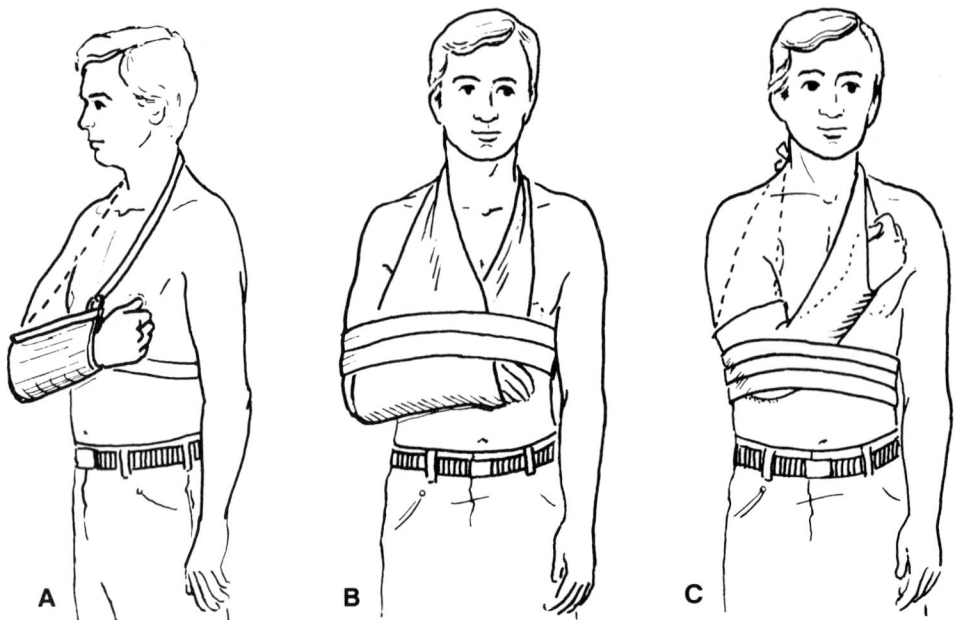

Figure 19-2. The types of immobilizing dressings used for upper humeral fractures. (*A*) A commercial sling and swathe that permits easy removal of the arm for exercises and is comfortable on the neck. (*B*) A conventional sling and swathe. (*C*) A stockinette Velpeau and swathe is used when there is an unstable surgical neck component, because this position relaxes the pectoralis major. (Redrawn from Rockwood CA and Green DP. Fractures. Philadelphia, JB Lippincott)

outstretched hand, or from a direct blow (sideswipe injury).
2. Each fracture is different, hence specific treatment cannot be described.
3. Treatment may be nonoperative (cast immobilization) or operative (open reduction and internal fixation; arthroplasty).

Nursing Management

1. Watch for signs of impaired circulation in forearm and hand.
   a. Observe hand for swelling, skin color (blueness or blanching of nailbeds), and temperature, comparing it with the unaffected hand.
   b. Evaluate radial pulse; if it weakens or disappears, call orthopedic surgeon *immediately* since irreversible ischemia may develop.
2. Assess for paresthesias (prickling and burning sensations) in the hand—indicate nerve injury or impending ischemia.
3. Encourage the patient to move his fingers frequently.
4. Exercises to increase range of motion are started when prescribed.

Fractures of the Head and Neck of the Radius

1. Usually produced by indirect trauma (fall on outstretched hand) or by direct trauma (blow).
2. *Undisplaced fracture*
   a. Aspiration of hemarthrosis (blood in joint) at the elbow may be done to relieve pain and allow earlier range of motion.
   b. Immobilization by plaster or sling.

3. *Displaced fracture*—open operation with excision of radial head when indicated.
   a. Postoperatively the arm is immobilized in a posterior plaster splint and sling and elevated.
   b. Early active motion of elbow and forearm is encouraged when prescribed.

Health Education

Encourage the patient to continue *daily* program of repetitive, progressive exercises (as prescribed). The exercise program is designed to restore full extension and supination.

Fractures of the Shafts of the Radius and Ulna

1. Objective of treatment is to preserve function of forearm.
2. *Undisplaced fractures*—treated by immobilizing arm in a long-arm cast with elbow flexed 90 degrees.
   a. Watch circulation and function of hand.
   b. Encourage active flexion and extension of fingers at frequent intervals to reduce edema. Encourage shoulder motion.
3. *Displaced fractures*—open operation with internal fixation accomplished by compression plate or some other fixation device.
   a. Postoperatively, a closed drainage system may be used to decrease hematoma and resultant swelling.
   b. The arm is usually immobilized in plaster splints or cast until there is evidence that fracture is healing.

Health Education

Encourage the patient to move his fingers and the shoulder of the involved extremity.

Fracture of the Wrist

1. Colles' fracture is a fracture of the radius 1.2–2.5 cm. (½–1 inch) above the wrist with dorsal displacement of the lower fragment.
   This fracture is frequently seen in patients with osteoporosis.
2. Treatment usually consists of closed reduction and plaster splint or cast support (or by skeletal pins incorporated in plaster).
   a. Elevate arm above level of heart for 48 hours after reduction.
   b. Watch for swelling of fingers—indicates decreased venous and lymphatic return. Check for constricting bandages or cast.

Health Education

Instruct the patient to do finger exercises to reduce swelling and prevent stiffness.
1. Hold hand above level of heart.
2. Move fingers from full extension to flexion (fist position). Hold and release.
3. Repeat at least 10 times every half hour when awake—as long as hand has a tendency to swell.

Fractures of the Hand

1. Numerous injuries to the hand require extensive reconstructive surgery which is beyond the scope of this book. The reader is referred to specialized texts on the hand.
2. Objective of treatment is to regain maximum function of the hand.
3. *Undisplaced fracture of the distal phalanx*
   a. Drainage of the hematoma under the fingernail may be necessary.
   b. Finger is splinted (to adjoining finger or by a dorsal or volar splint)—to relieve pain and to protect finger tip from further trauma.
4. *Open fractures* may be handled by Kirschner wire fixation following debridement and irrigation.

Fractures of the Lower Extremity

Fracture of the Shaft of the Femur

▶ **NURSING ALERT:** Fracture of the shaft of the femur may be accompanied by marked concealed blood loss.

1. Closed reduction
   a. Fracture reduced and stabilized by means of balanced skeletal traction, such as Thomas leg splint with a Pearson attachment (Fig. 19-7).
   b. Thomas splint suspends the thigh; Pearson attachment applied to the splint allows knee flexion and supports the leg below the knee. Examine skin under the ring on Thomas splint for signs of pressure.
   c. Skeletal traction in long axis of thigh is applied by means of a Kirschner wire or Steinman pin.
   d. May be supplemented with cast brace (for fractures of the shaft of femur—after a period of traction).
2. Open reduction with intramedullary (within the bone) fixation

   a. See nursing management following orthopedic surgery, page 840.
   b. A cast-brace may be used in conjunction with internal fixation of fractured femur.
3. See Rehabilitation and Health Education After Fracture of Lower Extremity, page 824.

Fractures at the Knee

1. Fractures at the knee may involve the distal shaft of femur (supracondylar fracture), the articular surfaces (femoral condyles and/or tibial plateau fracture), or the patella. Joint and ligamentous injury occur with these fractures.

Management

Management may include traction, internal fixation, and/or immobilization.
   Knee mobility is a concern in the overall treatment of these fractures.

Nursing Management

1. Elevate extremity; raise the gatch of the foot of the bed.
2. Evaluate for effusion of the knee—produces marked pain.
   a. Cut pressure dressing and reapply if pain is severe. Report to physician.
   b. Support the patient undergoing aspiration of fluid from knee joint.
3. Encourage quadriceps exercise to prevent atrophy of the thigh muscles; this also includes the unoperated leg.
4. Progressive exercises (straight leg raising, progressive resistive exercises) usually follow.
5. Weight-bearing is according to prescription. (Generally, full weight-bearing is not advised until 3 to 4 months postinjury.)

Fractures of the Tibia and Fibula

1. Treatment of tibial fractures represents a challenge; there is a high incidence of open infected fractures, since the tibia lies superficially beneath the skin.
2. These fractures may require prolonged immobilization—union is slow.
3. Tibial fractures generally heal in 12–16 weeks; open and comminuted fractures take longer.
4. *Treatment* (Broad range of opinion on treatment of these fractures):
   a. Closed fractures may be managed by simple manipulation and the reduction maintained by application of plaster cast (toe to groin).
      (1) In time, this long-leg cast may be replaced with a below-the-knee functional cast which permits weight-bearing and knee joint motion.
      (2) As an alternative, a functional cast-brace (fabricated with orthoplast-like material and special hinges) may be used.
   b. Or fracture may be treated by open reduction and fixation (plate, compression plate, intramedullary nails, or Hoffman external fixator) as indicated by etiology, type of trauma, and type of fracture.
   c. Pay special attention to ankle joint—may be problem of stiffness.

Fracture of the Ankle

1. Fracture may occur in the distal tibia and/or fibula, medial or lateral malleoli, or superior talus, and

include avulsion fracture. The fracture is generally the result of forceful twisting of the ankle and is associated with ligament disruption.
2. Treatment includes immobilization and possible open reduction and internal fixation with screws to reestablish joint function.
Weight-bearing is according to prescription.

Fracture of the Foot

Fractures of the metatarsals and phalanges result from crush injuries of the foot. They are generally treated by immobilization with cast, splint, or strapping. Partial weight-bearing is generally allowed.

Rehabilitation and Health Education After Fracture of Lower Extremity

1. Apply elastic stocking to uninvolved leg—maintains pressure on deeper leg veins, helps prevent stasis of blood, edema, and thrombophlebitis.
2. Elevate unaffected leg at intervals throughout day—to promote venous return.
3. Elevate affected extremity to promote venous return and relieve pain.
   a. The early reestablishment of venous return helps absorb blood and tissue fluid (edema from bleeding is a common cause of disability following fractures).
   b. Chronic edema predisposes extremity to fibrosis and ulceration.
   c. *It is desirable for the patient to lie down when elevating a leg cast.*
4. Exercise regularly all joints that do not move the bone fragments.
5. Avoid placing extremity in dependent positions for prolonged periods.
6. Mobilize the patient as soon as possible. Instruct in methods of ambulation—walker, crutches, and cane.

After immobilization device is removed,
1. Physical therapy procedures may be utilized (heat, cold, massage, exercise)—to restore joint mobility, increase muscle strength and endurance.
2. Instruct the patient to wear elastic bandage or hose to support venous circulation and to reduce edema.
3. Advise the patient to move feet up and down in pedaling motion to exercise calf muscles.
4. Recommend that the patient start moving affected extremity under water if necessary, since water supports the extremity and provides warmth which helps promote muscle relaxation.
5. Encourage adherence to weight-bearing prescription limits.

Fractures of the Lumbar and Dorsal Spine

Fractures of the vertebrae of the dorsal and lumbar spine may involve the vertebral body, lamina and articulating processes, and spinous processes or transverse processes. (Fractures of the cervical spine are discussed on p. 801.)

Clinical Manifestations

Severe pain in back—may radiate down legs or to the abdomen and chest.

Pathophysiology

1. Fractures of the vertebral bodies may be compression fractures; they are frequently multiple and comprise the most common types of fractures of the spine.
2. A spinal cord injury may occur with fracture or dislocation of a vertebra.

Etiology

1. Indirect trauma associated with excessive loading, motion beyond physiologic limits, severe muscle spasm
2. The majority of vertebral fractures seem to be related to osteoporosis

Treatment

A. For stable injuries to vertebrae

1. Treat symptomatically for pain, and encourage the patient to ambulate—or
2. Place the patient on a firm mattress and keep on bed rest until pain subsides.
3. Exercise to increase or maintain the strength of back muscles (2–3 weeks after fracture).
   a. Exercises that strengthen spinal extensor muscles are prescribed.
   b. Exercises that encourage spinal flexion are contraindicated.
4. Corset-type brace or cast may be used when ambulating.

B. For unstable fractures/displacement

1. The fracture may be reduced by postural positioning, protracted periods of immobilization, or open operation with internal fixation (Harrington rod).
2. The patient may then be placed in a body cast for immobilization.
3. Mobilize the patient when physical examinations and x-ray evaluations determine that there is no displacement or neurologic deficit.
4. Laminectomy (see p. 808) when indicated.

Assessment

1. Assess the patient for spinal cord injury (see p. 801).
2. Evaluate for paralytic ileus and difficulty in voiding—may occur the first few days after compression fracture of the lower dorsal or lumbar spine—may be from retroperitoneal hemorrhage.
   a. Assess anal sphincter tone.
   b. Observe for fecal retention.
3. Assess discomfort.

Patient Problems/Nursing Diagnoses

1. Potential spinal cord injury related to fracture and/or vertebral displacement (Rarely occurs with compression fractures related to osteoporosis.)
2. Pain related to vertebral fracture and associated muscle spasm
3. Potential complications related to fracture of spine and immobility
4. Impaired mobility related to pain of fracture
5. Constipation related to effects of pain medication, immobility, and paralytic ileus
6. Ineffective coping related to enforced immobility and inability to carry out activities of daily living
7. Nausea, vomiting related to pain medication and possibly paralytic ileus

Nursing Interventions

A. Avoiding spinal cord injury

1. Stabilize spine during diagnostic evaluation for fracture and displacement.

2. Monitor neurologic status (i.e., motion and sensations in extremities).
3. Provide nursing care according to the patient's condition and treatment regimen (e.g., laminectomy and fusion, internal fixation, casting).

B. Relieving pain

1. Encourage the patient to roll from side to side; the patient should not sit up during acute stage.
2. Give analgesics and muscle relaxants as required, since pain may be severe.
3. Assist the patient in application of brace or back support when he is ambulating; remove appliance while in bed.

C. Avoiding complications associated with spinal fracture and immobility

1. Use measures to prevent risk of thromboembolic complications—apply elastic stockings, encourage active ankle motion, give anticoagulant therapy as prescribed for patient at high risk.
2. Assist the patient to ambulate (wearing shoes) when discomfort subsides and when no neurologic deficits or vertebral displacement has been determined.
3. Encourage the patient to do the prescribed back exercises.
4. Monitor bowel and bladder function.

Health Education

1. Teach body mechanics for back conservation.
2. Encourage weight reduction, if applicable.
3. With fractures due to osteoporosis, teach the patient to be aware of safety factors necessary to avoid falls.

Expected Outcomes

1. Demonstrates normal neurologic function; normal sensations, motion, and strength in extremities
2. Achieves pain relief
3. Performs activities of daily living without complaint of pain and decreases use of analgesics
4. Maintains homeostasis; no evidence of paralytic ileus, urinary stasis, constipation, etc.

Fractures of the Pelvis

Etiology

Auto accidents, crush injuries, and falls cause most pelvic fractures. Injury to internal organs (i.e., bladder, urethra, liver, spleen) and blood vessels (e.g., iliac arteries and veins) frequently accompany these fractures. Bleeding from bone fragments occurs also.

Treatment

1. Emergency management of hemorrhage and shock includes:
   a. External compression suit (G-suit) (see Fig. 23-5) allows compression of pelvic area—provides tamponade for bleeding and immobilizes fracture.
   b. Angiographic visualization of pelvic vascular tree—for localization of bleeding points. Bleeding artery may be occluded by an injection of autologous clotted blood deposited proximal to bleeding vessel, by Gelfoam, or by balloon-tip catheter.
   c. Absence of peripheral pulses may indicate major vessel disruption (torn iliac arteries, veins, etc.).
2. Existence of internal organ injury is determined and treated according to problem (e.g., ruptured bladder requires surgical intervention and repair).
   a. Urine is examined for blood. A cystourethrogram and intravenous urogram are performed—to detect genitourinary injuries.
   b. Peritoneal lavage (p. 936) is carried out to diagnose intra-abdominal hemorrhage.
3. Definitive treatment of pelvic fractures
   a. Method of treatment depends on whether the pelvic ring has been disrupted and whether the fracture involves the weight-bearing portion of the pelvis.
   b. Pelvic fractures may be immobilized and stabilized by:
      (1) Bed rest
      (2) Pelvic slings
      (3) Skeletal traction
      (4) Bilateral hip spica cast
      (5) External fixation
      (6) Open reduction with or without internal fixation

Assessment

1. Determine the extent of internal injuries. Request the patient to void.
2. Palpate peripheral pulses.
3. Assess and evaluate for intra-abdominal hemorrhage—pelvic fractures may cause death from extraperitoneal and retroperitoneal hemorrhage.
4. Monitor stools and urine for blood.
5. Assess discomfort on movement and tenderness at fracture site.
6. Evaluate for other complications that are likely to develop as a result of shock, massive soft tissue injury, and multiple fractures—intravascular coagulation, thromboembolic complications, fat emboli, pulmonary complications, infection from large hematomas.

Patient Problems/Nursing Diagnoses

1. Potential life-threatening shock related to intra-abdominal hemorrhage and organ damage
2. Discomfort related to fracture and soft tissue trauma
3. Impaired mobility related to pelvic fracture and treatment regimen
4. Coping difficulties related to limited mobility

Nursing Interventions

A. Promoting adequate tissue perfusion

1. Monitor vital signs and level of consciousness.
2. Interpret laboratory data.
3. Support vital functions as needed and prescribed.

B. Ensuring abdominal-organ functioning

1. Monitor urine output for blood.
2. Monitor bowel function.
3. Assist the patient with therapeutic regimen prescribed for management of injury.

C. Relieving discomfort

See Pain (alteration in comfort) related to musculoskeletal conditions, page 814.

D. Promoting ambulation and activities of daily living

1. Assist the patient being treated with pelvic sling.
   a. Fold sling back over buttocks to enable the patient to use the bedpan.

b. Reach under sling to give skin care—sheepskin may be used to line sling to prevent pressure sores.
  c. Loosen the sling only upon physician request.
2. Turn the patient as a unit.
3. Encourage exercises (e.g., leg, breathing, isometric) and activities to minimize development of immobility-related problems.
4. Assist the patient with gradual resumption of activity and ambulation.
  Mobilization and weight-bearing are determined by x-ray and the patient's reaction to mobility.

Expected Outcomes

1. Maintains vital functions; vital signs stable, no evidence of bleeding, and normal bowel and bladder functioning
2. Achieves comfort; decreased use of analgesics and no complaint of pain
3. Achieves improved mobility; ambulates with assistance and uses cane or walker as needed

Fractures of the Hip

Types of Hip Fractures

Intracapsular—femur is fractured inside the joint (femoral neck fracture)
  Extracapsular—femur fractured outside the joint (intertrochanteric fracture)

Etiology

Hip fractures frequently occur in the aged and contribute to their mortality. They occur more frequently in women, often after insignificant injuries, and are associated with osteoporosis.

Treatment

1. Stable fractures are usually reduced and fixed with a nail, nail–plate combination, multiple pins, screw, sliding nails, etc., by replacement of the femoral head, or by a total hip procedure.
2. To ensure that the patient is in as favorable a condition as possible preoperatively:
   a. Assess cardiovascular, pulmonary, renal, and hematologic systems.
   b. Correct fluid and electrolyte disturbances. Give intravenous infusions *slowly*—older patients with limited cardiac reserve cannot tolerate additional circulatory loading.
   c. Prevent complications (e.g., thrombophlebitis, pneumonia, fat emboli, infection, pressure sores).

Assessment (Preoperative)

1. Note position of injured extremity—shortening and external rotation of affected leg.
2. Assess ability to move leg—usually unable to move leg but able to wiggle toes.
3. Assess pain—patients with fractured hip may complain of discomfort in the knee.
4. Coordinate preoperative diagnostic studies.
5. Determine if the patient is oriented to time, place, and person—mental confusion may be due to underlying systemic illness, particularly to cardiopulmonary disease with inadequate cerebral oxygen transport, stroke, etc.
6. Evaluate needs for posthospital care.
  Notify Social Services Department—to assist planning of postoperative care to avoid unnecessary prolonged hospital care.

Patient Problems/Nursing Diagnoses

1. Impaired mobility related to fracture
2. Alteration in comfort related to fracture
3. Knowledge deficit related to treatment regimen and expected patient participation

Nursing Interventions

A. Avoiding problems associated with immobility and fracture

1. Use anticipatory nursing techniques to avoid complications.

▶ **NURSING ALERT:** Thromboembolism is the most common complication following hip fractures, and it frequently occurs without clinical signs.

   a. Prevent thromboembolism with leg exercises, elastic stockings, early ambulation.
   b. Warfarin, low-molecular-weight dextran, aspirin, or low doses of heparin given subcutaneously may be effective in reducing the incidence of venous thrombi.
   c. Elevate foot of bed 25 degrees—to promote venous drainage.
   d. Use orienting activities to prevent confusion—clock, calendar, television, explanations and reassurance, same care-giver. (See p. 897 for care of the confused elderly patient.)
   e. Prepare the bed with a trapeze and flotation mattress.
2. Keep the skin dry and relieve pressure areas—pressure sores develop rapidly in the preoperative period. (See p. 59 for prevention of pressure sores.)
   a. Check the neurovascular status of the extremity.
   b. Inspect the heel *daily*—a patient with a painful hip tends to let weight of leg press the heel against the bed; area loses sensation when blood supply diminishes and nerve endings necrose.
   c. Support leg with pillow if permitted—distributes pressure more evenly.
   d. Place a sheepskin pad under the leg.
3. Encourage the patient to move by herself as much as possible to decrease the likelihood of complications (thromboembolism, diminished cerebral perfusion, aspiration of secretions and pneumonia, gastrointestinal stasis, urinary problems, increase in bone mineral loss, pressure sores).
4. Prevent urinary tract infection.
   a. Avoid the routine use of an indwelling catheter—infection almost always follows the use of an indwelling catheter. (A urinary tract infection can cause a prolonged period of morbidity, incontinence, and confusion in the elderly.)
   b. Watch the color, odor, and volume of urinary output.
   c. Maintain a liberal fluid intake (within limits of cardiorenal function).

B. Promoting comfort

1. Alleviate pain.
   a. Place a pillow between the legs—to keep affected leg in a secure position.
   b. With two nurses positioned at each side of the bed, use the sheet under the patient and lift the patient off the stretcher onto the bed.
   c. Turn the patient on the affected side while supporting the shoulder and thigh, and remove the sheet.

d. Position the patient supine. Place a pillow under the affected leg from mid-thigh to ankle and a sandbag under the pillow on the side of the patient's affected calf.
e. Raise the head of the bed slightly, no higher than 40 degrees.
f. The patient may be treated with either Buck's extension or pillow positioning.
 (1) Assist with the application of Buck's extension as indicated. Buck's extension is used to afford patient mobilization and to relieve pain until the operative procedure is performed. (Split–Russell's traction may be used.)
 (2) Check traction frequently, especially elastic bandages.
 (3) The patient with an intracapsular fracture will assume a flexed and externally rotated position. Support extremity in this position with pillows until surgery is performed.
g. Handle the affected extremity gently.
h. Give analgesics as the patient's condition indicates.
2. Watch for fat embolism—characterized by fever, tachycardia, dyspnea, and cough. (Fat embolism sometimes occurs after fractures of the long bones, particularly in elderly patients.)

Health Teaching

1. Teach the patient to assist with turning by having her grasp the trapeze or bedrails.
2. Encourage the patient to take deep breaths while turning.
3. Teach the use of incentive spirometer, coughing, deep-breathing, and exercises, especially quadriceps setting.
4. Clarify treatment plans and discuss the patient's participation.

Expected Outcomes

1. Shows no signs of problems related to immobility; lungs clear, skin intact, urine clear and adequate in amount
2. Achieves comfort; minimal complaint of discomfort at fracture; maintains positioning
3. Can explain planned treatment and participation regimen; follows directions to facilitate treatment and to prevent complications

Casts

A *cast* is an immobilizing device made up of layers of plaster or "fiberglass" (water-activated polyurethane resin) bandages molded to the body part that it encases.

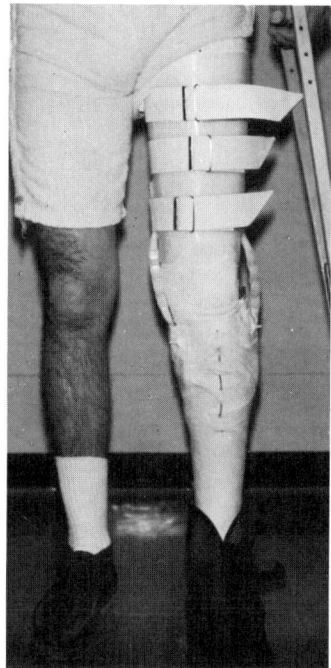

Figure 19-3. Cast-brace provides circumferential support to a segment of a fractured extremity while allowing mobility of nearby joints.

Purposes

1. To immobilize and hold bone fragments in reduction
2. To apply uniform compression of soft tissues
3. To permit early mobilization
4. To correct and prevent deformities
5. To support and stabilize weak joints

Types of Casts

1. *Short-arm cast*—extends from below the elbow to the proximal palmar crease
2. *Gauntlet cast*—extends from below the elbow to the proximal palmar crease, including the thumb (thumb spica)
3. *Long-arm cast*—extends from upper level of axillary fold to proximal palmar crease; elbow usually immobilized at right angle
4. *Short-leg cast*—extends from below knee to base of toes
5. *Long-leg cast*—extends from upper thigh to the base of toes; foot is at right angle in a neutral position
6. *Body cast*—encircles the trunk stabilizing the spine
7. *Spica cast*—incorporates the trunk and an extremity
 a. *Shoulder spica cast*—a body jacket that encloses trunk, shoulder, and elbow
 b. *Hip spica cast*—encloses trunk and a lower extremity
 (1) Single hip spica—extends from nipple line to include pelvis and 1 thigh
 (2) Double hip spica—extends from nipple line or upper abdomen to include pelvis and extends to include both thighs and lower legs
 (3) One and a half hip spica—extends from upper abdomen, includes 1 entire leg, and extends to the knee of the other
8. *Cast-brace* (Fig. 19-3)—external support about a

fracture that is constructed with hinges to permit early motion of joints, early mobilization, and independence

   a. Cast-bracing is based on the concept that some weight-bearing is physiologic and will promote the formation of bone and contain fluid within a tight compartment which compresses soft tissues, providing a distribution of forces across the fracture site.

   b. Cast-brace is applied after initial edema and pain have subsided and there is evidence of fracture stability.

Guidelines: Application of a Cast

Equipment

       Plaster or synthetic bandages in desired widths
  * Stockinette (tubular knitted material)
  * Cast padding (Webril cotton padding)
       Splints (for reinforcement)
  * Cotton, polyester, or polyurethane foam padding for bony prominences
       Knives, scissors, indelible pencil
       Polyethylene sheeting or newspaper—to protect floor
       Disposable gloves—to protect hands of operator
       Large, plastic-lined pail of water at room temperature—21°–24°C. (70°–75°F.)—or as recommended by cast material manufacturer
       Cast finishing hand cream for synthetic cast as needed

Underlying Considerations

1. The application of a cast requires 2–3 persons: one to apply the plaster (operator), one to dip and hand the plaster bandages to the operator, and a third person to hold the extremity in correct position. (Body spicas may require additional personnel.)
2. The time required for the cast to become rigid varies with the material used—generally 2–6 minutes.
3. There should be no movement of the extremity while the cast is being applied and set.
4. In general, the joints above and below the involved bone are immobilized.

Procedure

Action	Rationale / Amplification
Preparatory Phase	
1. Spread polyethylene sheeting or newspaper on floor.	
2. Explain to the patient that there will be a feeling of warmth as the plaster is applied.	2. Heat is produced by crystallization as plaster sets. The reaction of water with plaster of paris liberates heat.

3. Apply stockinette and roll cast padding on the extremity or part to be immobilized.
  a. Sheet wadding: Apply as smoothly and snugly as possible so that each turn overlaps the preceding turn by ½ the width of the roll.
  b. Extra pieces of padding may be placed over bony prominences: olecranon process, malleoli, patella.
	3. Padding is used to pad the sharp cast margins for patient comfort and to prevent pressure areas, minimize circulatory problems, and facilitate cast removal.
	  a. & b. Sheet wadding is applied from the distal to the proximal end of the extremity. When too much padding is used, it may shift and produce pressure areas under the cast.

4. While keeping the thumb under the forward edge of the bandage, submerge the plaster bandage vertically in water (room temperature) for a minute or so, or until bubbles cease to rise. Check directions on synthetic cast materials.	4. Water that is too warm will accelerate setting time, may cause a burn, and may result in excessive plaster loss by loosening the adhesive agents that bond the plaster to the fabric.
5. Expel excess water by squeezing (not wringing) towards the center of the bandage; hand bandage to operator with free end hanging loose.	5. The cast will dry more quickly (and thus will acquire maximum strength sooner) if a well-squeezed plaster bandage is used. Maximum strength is achieved by synthetic casts through chemical reaction.
Performance Phase (by operator)	
1. Starting at the distal end, roll the bandage gently and evenly on the extremity, overlapping the preceding turn by ½ the width of the roll.	1. Roll inward towards the patient's body for ease of control.
2. Keep the bandage moving and in constant contact with the surface of the extremity. Smooth and rub down successive layers or turns of each bandage into the	2. This keeps the cast uniformly thick. Rubbing the plaster as it is applied will form a smooth, solid and well-fused cast. Avoid indenting the cast with

---

* Material needs to be nonabsorbent if non-plaster cast is used.

Procedure
(Cont.)

Action	Rationale/Amplification
layers below with the thumbs and thenar eminences (mound on the palm) in circumferential and longitudinal directions.	the fingertips since this may produce pressure sores on underlying skin.
3. Take tucks in the lower border of the bandage by lifting the bandage off the surface (without tension) and overlapping it in a V-shaped fashion.	3. Tucking the bandage helps to contour the cast to the changing circumference of the extremity. Do not twist or reverse the bandage to change its direction since this produces sharp cutting edges.
4. Trim the cast to size with a sharp knife. Fold stockinette over edges of cast and anchor with cast material.	4. Stockinette produces smooth, comfortable edges on cast. Do not pull too vigorously on the stockinette since this may cause pressure on bony prominences.
5. Finish synthetic cast with cast hand cream as indicated.	5. Smooths rough exterior surface.
6. Ask the patient if there is any discomfort or pain.	6. If a patient complains of pain, it may be due to manipulation of fracture during setting; pain should subside rapidly. If it persists, the cast and encircling dressings are split to avoid constriction, circulatory problems, and pressure sores.

Follow-Up Phase

1. Write the diagnosis and date of injury and cast application with an indelible pencil on the cast.
2. Support the cast with the palm of the hand while moving the patient. Avoid indentations from tips of fingers.

   2. Finger indentation on a fresh cast can produce pressure sores.

3. Expose the cast to warm, circulating, dry air. Or blow air over cast with a circulating fan to increase the evaporation of water.

   3. Avoid covering the cast when it is drying as this delays drying time. Usually the plaster cast will reach its maximum temperature 5–15 minutes after it is applied and will then cool rapidly. The ultimate plaster cast strength is obtained after the cast is dry (up to 48 hours, depending on outside temperature and humidity).
The synthetic cast strength is maximum within 30 minutes of application and not dependent on being dry.

4. Clean equipment and store ready for use.

Guidelines: Removal of a Cast

Equipment

Cast cutter—an electric saw with circular blade that oscillates and is connected to a vacuum collector
Cast spreader
Surgical or plaster knife
Scissors

Procedure

Nursing Action	Rationale/Amplification
Preparatory Phase	
1. Describe to the patient how and where the cast cutter will be used and the expected sensations. Turn on the cutter and allow the patient to hear the motor.	1. Reassures the patient that the cutter produces vibrations but not pain.
2. Determine whether or not the cast is padded.	2. An electric plaster cast cutter should not be used on unpadded casts.
3. Determine where the cut will be made. Mark, with a felt pen, the area to be cut.	3. The line should be in front of the lateral malleolus and behind the medial malleolus on a lower extremity cast. An upper extremity cast is usually split along the ulnar or flexor surface.
Performance Phase	
1. Inform the patient to shield eyes.	1. Plaster dust may be irritating to the eyes.
2. Grasp the electric cutter as illustrated (Fig. 19-4A).	

(continued)

Guidelines: Removal of a Cast (continued)

Procedure
(Cont.)

Nursing Action	Rationale/Amplification
3. Rest the thumb on the cast.	3. The thumb serves as a depth gauge and acts as a guard in front of the blade.

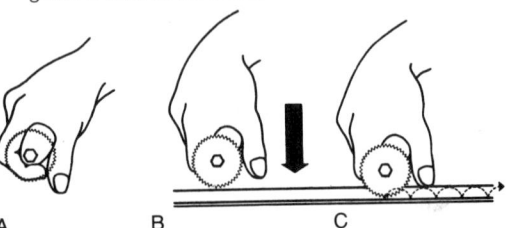

A   B   C

Figure 19-4. Operating a cast cutter. (Courtesy of Stryker Corporation)

Nursing Action	Rationale/Amplification
4. Turn on the electric cutter. Push the blade firmly and gently through the cast while holding the thumb against the cast to steady the blade while cutting through the cast.	
5. As the blade cuts through the plaster, a sudden lack of resistance is felt; plaster will "give" (or "dip") when the cut is completed.	
6. Lift the cutting blade up a degree (but not out of the cutting groove) and advance the blade at a slightly higher or lower level. The cast is cut by a series of alternating pressure and linear movements along the line of the cut (Fig. 19-5B, C).	
7. Avoid drawing the cutting blade along the extremity in a single motion.	7. This will cut the skin. If saw blade is in contact with padding too long, the patient will feel burning sensation on skin from rapidly oscillating blade.
8. Cut the cast on both sides. Then rock the anterior portion of the cast over the posterior portion.	8. This maneuver allows the operator to determine if the cast is completely cut.
9. Insert the blades of the cast spreader in the cut trough. Separate the 2 halves with the spreader at several sites along the cast split. Separate the cast with the hands.	
10. Cut through the padding and stockinette with scissors, keeping the scissor blade that is closest to the skin parallel to the skin.	10. Use bandage scissors; place the flat blade closest to the skin.
11. Lift the extremity carefully out of the posterior portion of the cast. Support the extremity so that it is maintained in the same position as when in the cast.	11. When the support of the cast has been removed, stresses and strain are placed on parts that have been at rest.

After Removal of Cast

Nursing Action	Rationale/Amplification
1. Cleanse the skin gently with bland soap and water. Blot dry. Apply a skin cream.	1. Explain to the patient that the skin will be scaly and the extremity will appear "thin" from disuse. Reassure him that it will take a few weeks to regain normal appearance and function.
2. Emphasize the importance of continuing the prescribed exercises, reporting for physical therapy, etc.	2. Exercises are necessary to redevelop and increase strength and function. Pain and stiffness may be expected after cast removal.

Nursing Process Overview
(The Patient with a Cast)

Assessment
Clinical Manifestations of Patient Problems

A. Neurovascular Problems

1. Trauma or surgery affecting an extremity will produce swelling (result of hemorrhage from bone and surrounding tissue and of tissue edema). Vascular insufficiency and nerve compression due to unrelieved swelling can cause a reduction in or obliteration of blood supply and peripheral nerve damage to an extremity.
2. Symptoms and signs
   a. Pain
   b. Swelling
   c. Discoloration—pale or blue
   d. Tingling or numbness
   e. Diminished or absent pulse
   f. Paralysis
   g. Pain on extension
   h. Cool extremity

B. Necrosis, Pressure Sores, and Nerve Palsies

1. Pressure of cast on neurovascular structures and bony structures causes necrosis, pressure sores, and nerve palsies.
2. Symptoms and signs
   a. Severe initial pain over bony prominences; this is a warning symptom of an impending pressure sore. *Pain decreases when ulceration occurs.*
   b. Odor
   c. Drainage on cast
3. Pressure sites (See Fig. 19-5)
   a. *Lower extremity*—heel, malleoli, dorsum of foot, head of fibula, anterior surface of patella
   b. *Upper extremity*—medial epicondyle of humerus, ulnar styloid
   c. Plaster jackets or body spica casts—sacrum, anterior and superior iliac spines, vertebral borders of scapulae

▶ **NURSING ALERT:** Do not ignore the complaint of pain of the patient in a cast. Suspect circulatory complications or a pressure sore.

Notify physician if symptoms persist. Cast may have to be split or removed.

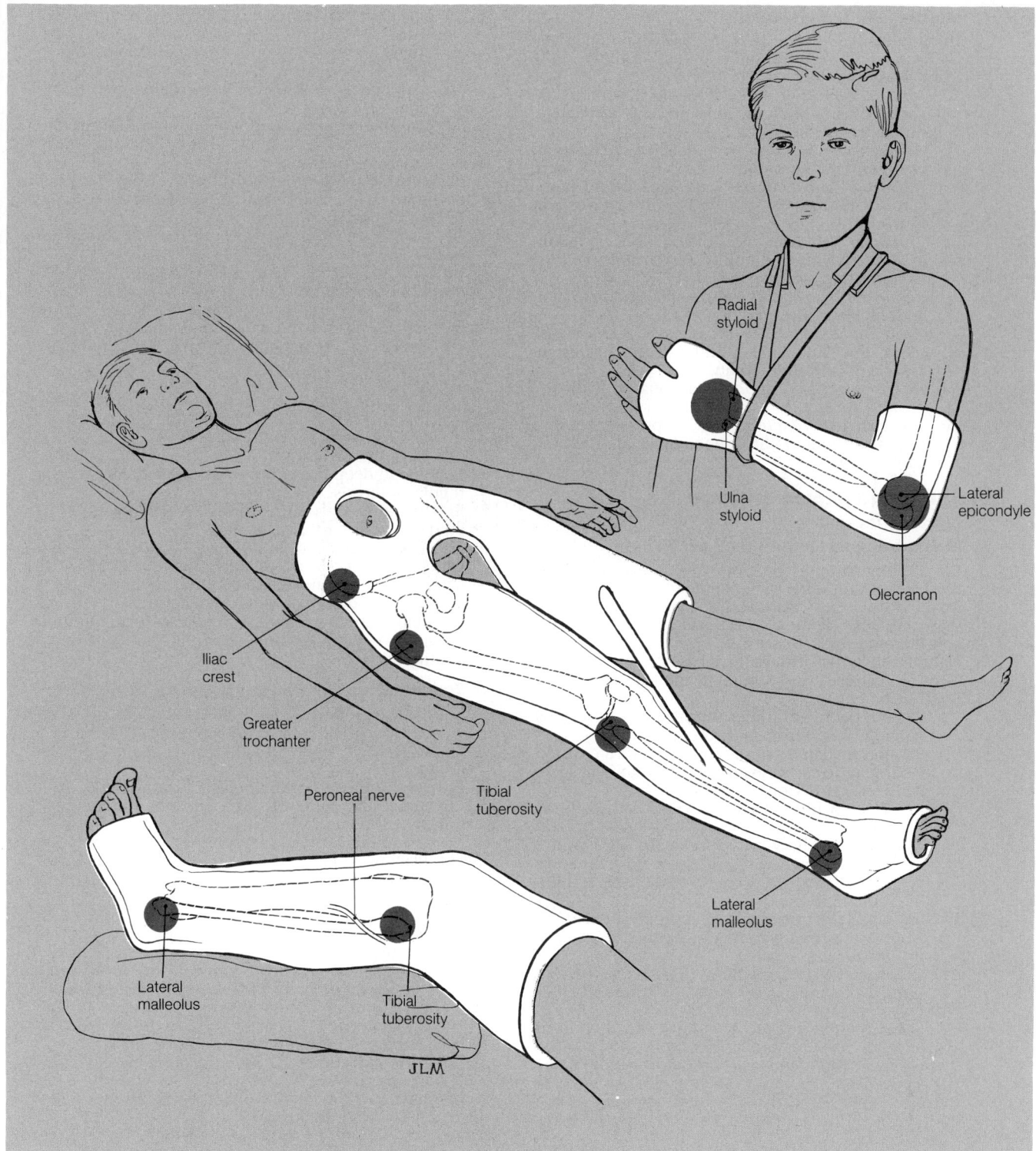

Figure 19-5. Pressure areas in different types of casts.

C. Multisystem Complications

1. Immobility and confinement in a cast—particularly a body cast—can result in multi-system problems.
2. Symptoms/signs/causes
   a. *Nausea, vomiting,* and abdominal distention associated with adynamic ileus and possible intestinal obstruction
   b. *Acute anxiety* reaction symptoms (i.e., behavioral changes and autonomic responses—increased respiratory and heart rate, elevated blood pressure, diaphoresis) associated with confinement in a space
   c. *Thrombophlebitis* and possible pulmonary emboli associated with immobility and ineffective circulation (e.g., venous stasis)
   d. *Respiratory atelectasis* and pneumonia associated with ineffective respiratory effort
   e. *Renal and bladder calculi* associated with urinary stasis, low fluid intake, and calcium excretion associated with immobility
   f. *Anorexia and constipation* associated with decreased activity
   g. *Psychological reaction* (e.g., depression) associated with immobility, dependence, and loss of control

Planning and Implementation
Nursing Interventions

A. Maintaining adequate tissue perfusion

1. Elevate the extremity on cloth-covered pillow above the level of the heart. Keep the heel off the mattress.
2. Avoid resting cast on hard surfaces or sharp edges that can cause denting or flattening of the cast and consequent pressure sores.
3. Handle moist cast with palms of hands.
4. Turn the patient every 2 hours while cast dries.
5. Spica or body cast
   a. Place a bedboard under the mattress—prevents sagging of bed from pressure of cast.
   b. Support the curves of the cast with cloth-covered flexible pillows—prevents cracking and flat spots while cast is drying.
      (1) Place 3 pillows crosswise on bed for body cast.
      (2) Place 1 pillow crosswise at the waist and 2 pillows lengthwise for affected leg for spica cast. If both legs are involved, use 2 additional pillows.
6. If symptoms of neurovascular compromise occur:
   a. Bivalve the cast: split cast on each side over its full length into 2 halves.
   b. Cut the underlying padding—blood-soaked padding may shrink and cause constriction of circulation.
   c. Spread cast sufficiently to relieve constriction.
7. If symptoms of pressure area occur, cast may be "windowed" (hole cut in it) so that the skin at the pain point can be examined and treated. The window must be replaced so that the tissue does not swell and cause additional pressure problems at window edge.

B. Countering immobility side effects

1. Monitor for development of symptoms associated with adynamic ileus.
   If symptoms occur:

   a. Place the patient prone to relieve pressure symptoms.
   b. Remove the cast from the patient if necessary.
   c. Employ nasogastric suction.
   d. Maintain normal electrolyte balance by intravenous replacement of fluid.
   Surgical intervention (duodenojejunostomy) may be necessary when conservative measures fail to relieve duodenal obstruction.
2. Encourage the patient to verbalize fears and concerns. Facilitate active participation in decision making. Encourage family support.
3. *Be alert for evidences of thromboembolic complications.*
   Individuals at high risk (increased age, previous thromboembolism, obesity, congestive heart failure, cancer of pancreas or lung, trauma) may require prophylaxis against thromboembolism.
   a. Encourage the patient to move about as normally as possible.
   b. Do prescribed exercises faithfully.
   c. Have the patient exercise the parts of the body that are not immobilized by the cast at regular and frequent intervals.
   d. Turn the patient.
4. Encourage deep-breathing exercises and coughing at regular intervals.
5. Encourage the patient to drink liberal quantities of fluid—to avoid urinary calculi.
6. Encourage balanced nutritional intake. Assess the patient's food preferences. Serve small meals. Provide natural bowel stimulants (e.g., fiber). Monitor bowels and utilize a bowel program if necessary.
7. Facilitate patient participation in care planning and activities. Encourage mobility within limits of therapeutic regimen.

Specific Care for Patient in Spica/Body Cast

1. Keep the cast level by elevating the lumbar sacral area with a small pillow when the head of the bed is elevated or when the patient is placed on the bedpan.
2. Protect the toes from the pressure of the bedding.
3. Encourage the patient to maintain physiologic position by:
   a. Using the overhead trapeze.
   b. Placing good foot flat on bed and pushing down while lifting himself up on the trapeze.
   c. Avoiding twisting motions.
   d. Avoiding positions that produce pressure on groin, back, chest, and abdomen.
4. Provide hygienic care of the patient.
   a. Cover perineum with a towel and apply spray (lacquer-type) to perineal area of cast. Tuck 10-cm. (4-inch) strips of thin polyethylene sheeting under perineal area of cast and tape to cast exterior. Replace when soiling occurs.
   b. Clean outside of cast with dry cleanser on almost-dry cloth.
   c. Pull stockinette taut, trim, and fasten to cast edges with adhesive.
   d. Inspect skin for signs of irritation:
      (1) Around cast edge
      (2) Under cast—pull skin taut and inspect under cast, using a flashlight for illumination.
   e. Reach up under cast and massage accessible skin.

f. Use a fracture bedpan. Roll the patient onto bedpan; place pillow in lumbosacral area.

5. Turn the patient in a body/spica cast.
   a. Move the patient to the side of the bed, using a steady, even, pulling motion.
   b. Place pillows along the other side of the bed; 1 for the chest and 2 (lengthwise) for the legs.
   c. Instruct the patient to place his arms at his side or above his head.
   d. Turn the patient as a unit. Avoid twisting the patient in the cast.
   e. Turn the patient toward the leg not encased in plaster or toward the unoperated side if both legs are in plaster.
      (1) One nurse stands at other side of bed to receive the patient's shoulders.
      (2) Second nurse supports leg in plaster while the third nurse supports the patient's back as he is turned.
      (3) *Do not grasp cross bar of spica cast to move the patient.* The purpose of the bar is to strengthen the cast.
      (4) Turn the patient in body cast to a prone position twice daily—provides postural drainage of bronchial tree; relieves pressure on back.

Health Education

1. Check neurovascular status. Watch for symptoms of circulatory disturbance.
   a. Watch for these danger signs (arm or leg cast): blueness or paleness of fingernails or toenails accompanied by pain and tightness, numbness, cold or tingling sensation.
   b. Elevate the affected limb above the heart and wiggle fingers/toes.
   c. Call the physician if condition persists.
2. Prevent or reduce swelling.
   a. Elevate the extremity in the cast above the level of the heart.
   b. Apply ice bags (⅓–½ full) to each side of the cast, making sure that they do not make indentations in plaster.
   c. After the patient begins ambulation, encourage him to elevate the cast when he is seated. Encourage the patient to lie down several times daily with cast elevated.
3. Prevent irritation at cast edge—pad edges of cast with moleskin or "petal" the cast edges with strips of adhesive tape.
4. Teach the patient to perform isometric exercises—

contracting the muscles without moving the joint, to maintain muscle strength and prevent atrophy (performed hourly when awake).

5. Exercise every joint that is not immobilized. Move the rest of the body.
6. Actively exercise joints that do not move bone fragments.
   a. Leg-cast—"Push down on the popliteal (knee) space, hold it, relax, repeat." Move toes back and forth; bend toes down, then pull them back.
   b. Arm cast—"Make a fist, hold it, relax, repeat." Move shoulders.
7. Avoid getting cast wet, especially padding under cast—causes skin breakdown.
8. Do not cover a leg cast with plastic or rubber boots since this causes condensation and wetting of the cast.
9. Avoid weight-bearing or stress on plaster cast for 24 hours.
10. Report to the physician if the cast cracks or breaks; instruct the patient not to try to fix it himself.
11. Avoid walking on wet floors or sidewalks.
12. Do not place sharp objects under the cast.
13. To clean the cast:
    a. Remove surface soil with slightly damp cloth.
    b. Rub soiled areas with household scouring powder.
    c. Wipe off residual moisture.
14. After cast is removed:
    a. Cleanse skin with mild soap and water.
    b. Apply emollient lotion to dry skin.
    c. Avoid scratching the skin.
    d. Gradually resume activities and exercise.
    e. Elevate extremity to control swelling.

Evaluation
Expected Outcomes

1. Maintains adequate tissue perfusion
   a. Minimal edema—no swelling or pressure
   b. Intact neurovascular status—normal pulse pressure, filling time, sensation
   c. Intact skin over bony prominences
2. Avoids immobility-related problems
   a. Normal body system functioning—normal bowel and urinary elimination pattern; vital signs normal; normal respiratory pattern; normal blood gases
3. Participates in self-care activities to optimum ability
4. Expresses feelings and fears, but maintains positive outlook and expectations

Traction

Traction is force applied in a specific direction. To apply the force needed to overcome the natural force or pull of muscle groups, a system of ropes, pulleys, and weights is used.

Running traction is a form of traction in which the pull is exerted in one plane. It may utilize either skin or skeletal traction, and it may be either unilateral or bilateral, for example, Buck's extension (Fig. 19-6).

Balanced suspension traction is produced by a coun-

terforce other than the patient's body weight. The extremity balances or floats in the traction apparatus. The line of traction on the extremity remains fairly constant despite changes in the patient's position (Figs. 19-7, 19-8).

Purposes of Traction

1. To reduce and immobilize fracture
2. To regain normal length and alignment of an injured extremity

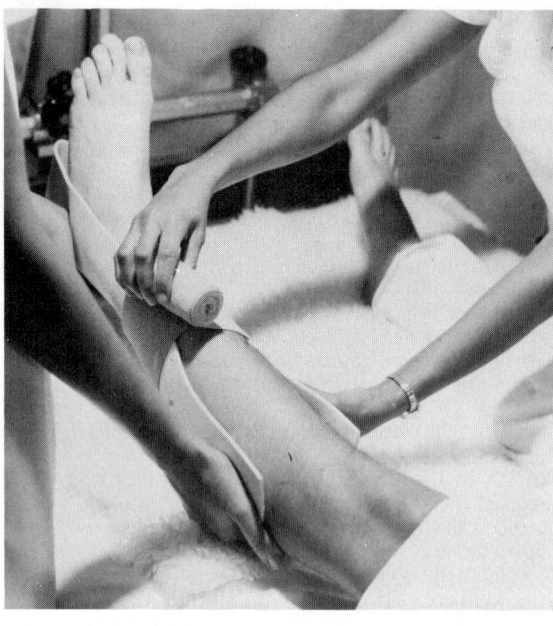

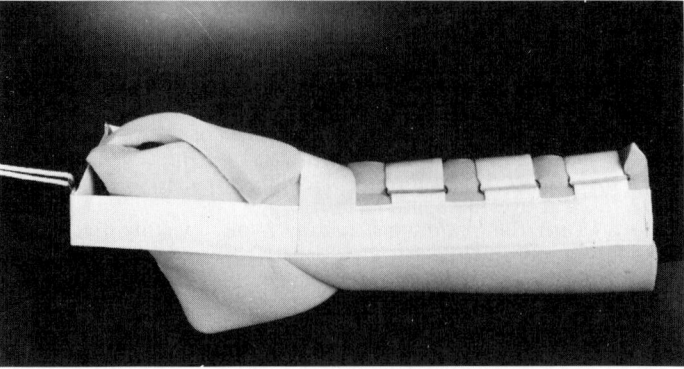

Figure 19-6. (*Left*) Applying elastic bandage for Buck's extension traction. (*Above*) Prepadded boot that may be used in Buck's extension. (Photo of boot courtesy of All Orthopedic Appliances)

3. To lessen or eliminate muscle spasm
4. To prevent deformity
5. To give the patient freedom for "in-bed" activities
6. To reduce pain

Application of Traction

Traction may be applied to the skin or to the skeletal system.

Skin traction is accomplished by a weight that pulls on tape, sponge rubber, or plastic materials attached to the skin or a special device (boots); traction on the skin transmits traction to the musculoskeletal structures.

Skin traction is used as a temporary measure in adults; used prior to surgery in treatment of intertrochanteric hip fracture (Buck's extension, see Guidelines, p. 835); Russell's traction is used for applying traction to the femoral shaft with the knee flexed. Pelvic traction is used for treatment of back disorders or injuries. Skin traction may be used definitively to treat fractures in children.

Skeletal traction is traction applied to bone using wires, pins, or tongs placed through bones; this is the most effective means of traction. It is applied by the orthopedic surgeon under aseptic conditions. Skeletal traction is used most frequently in treating fractures of the femur, humerus (supracondylar fractures), tibia, and cervical spine.

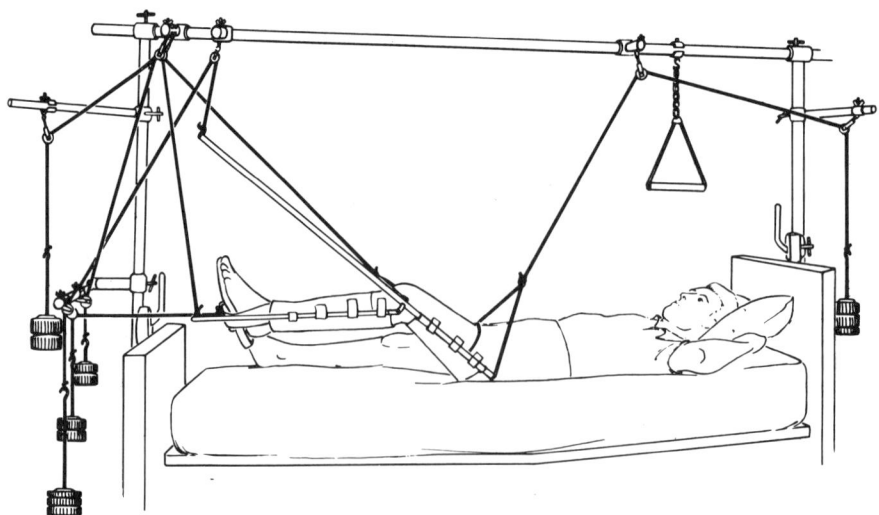

Figure 19-7. Balanced traction with Thomas leg splint with Pearson attachment.

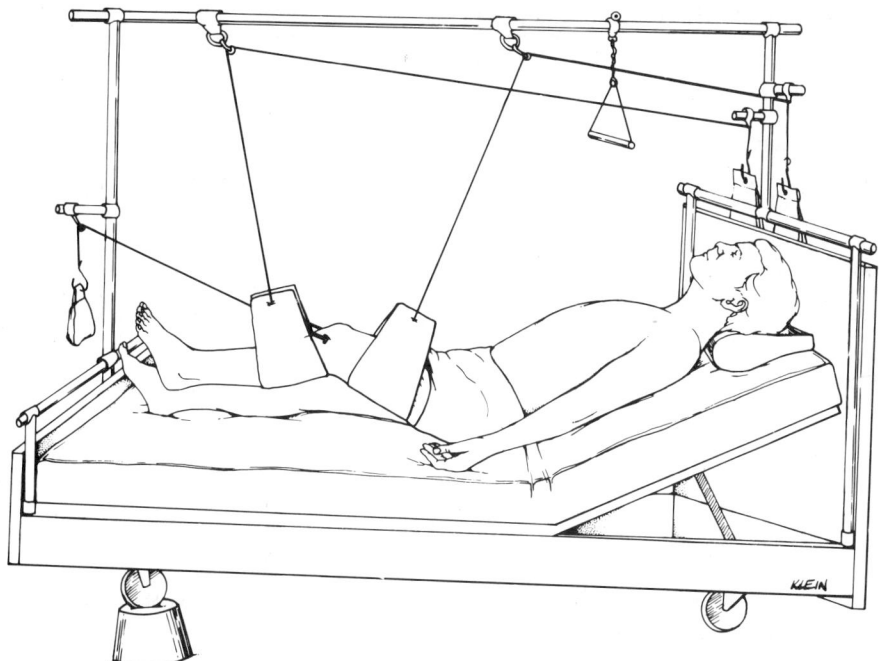

Figure 19-8. A type of balanced suspension traction with slings. (Brunner LS and Suddarth DS. Text-book of Medical–Surgical Nursing, 5th ed. Philadelphia, JB Lippincott, 1984)

Guidelines: Application of Buck's Extension Traction

Buck's extension (unilateral or bilateral skin traction) is a form of traction used as a temporary measure to provide support and comfort to a fractured extremity until definitive treatment is accomplished (Fig. 19-6).

Equipment

Foam Buck's traction boot or traction tape and 10-cm. (4-inch) elastic bandage
Spreader block or metal spreader
Pulley, nylon rope, and weights (2.3–3.1 kg. [5–7 lbs.] is usual; (amount of weight is prescribed by physician)
Sheepskin pad
Shock blocks or adjustable bed for Trendelenburg's position.

Procedure

Nursing Action	Rationale/Amplification
Preparatory Phase	
1. Place bedboard under the mattress. Bed position is flat or in Trendelenburg's position. This depends on the size of the patient and the weight applied.	1. Elevating the foot of the bed (countertraction) helps prevent the patient from sliding down toward the foot of the bed.
2. Question the patient to determine previous skin conditions (contact dermatitis). Inspect skin for evidences of atrophy, abrasions, and circulatory disturbances.	2. The skin must be in healthy condition to tolerate skin traction.
3. Make sure that the skin of the extremity is clean and dry.	3. A clean, dry skin helps traction tape adherence.
4. Document the neurovascular status of the extremity, any evidence of skin problems or varicosities.	
Performance Phase	
1. Position the patient in center of bed in good alignment.	1. For effective line of pull.
If traction tape is used:	
2. Apply continuous traction tape to medial and lateral aspects of lower leg (below knee and loosely around foot to allow for attachment of spreader).	2. Avoid pressure over malleoli and head of fibula. Pressure sores develop rapidly over bony prominences. Pressure over the region of the fibular head and common peroneal nerve may produce peroneal palsy and footdrop.

(continued)

Guidelines: Application of Buck's Extension Traction (continued)

Procedure
(Cont.)

Nursing Action	Rationale/Amplification
3. Have a second person elevate and support the extremity under the ankle and knee while the elastic bandage is applied. Beginning at the ankle, wrap the elastic bandage snugly over the tape up to the tibial tubercle.	3. The elastic bandage improves adherence of tape to the skin and helps prevent slipping.
4. Attach a spreader block (or metal spreader) to the distal end of the tape. Attach a rope to the spreader block and pass it over a pulley fastened to the end of the bed.	4. The spreader block prevents pressure along the side of the foot. The spreader should not be too narrow (causes pressure sores on ankle) or too wide (pulls traction tape away from the heel).
If foam boot is used:	
1. Place leg in foam boot, adjusting it so that the heel is in the heel of the boot.	1. Preventing sore heels is a primary concern.
2. Secure Velcro bootstraps, avoiding excessive pressure on malleoli and fibular head.	2. Pressure over bony prominences causes skin breakdown and pressure on peroneal nerve may result in footdrop.
3. Attach rope to built-in spreader plate.	

Follow-up Phase

Nursing Action	Rationale/Amplification
1. Make sure knots are tied securely. Gently attach the traction weight. Release gradually.	1. The rope should be unobstructed; the weight should hang free of the bed and should not touch the floor.
2. Place a sheepskin pad under the leg (or use a commercial heel protector).	2. Sheepskin is used to reduce friction of the heel against the bed.
3. Assess the patient to ensure that he is in proper alignment.	3. The part of the body in traction should be in line with the pull of the weight.
4. Provide skin care at regular intervals.	4. Foam boot tends to make the leg sweat and moisture contributes to skin breakdown.

Nursing Assessment of the Patient Following Application of Buck's Extension

1. Palpate over area of traction tapes daily. If area is tender to palpation, suspect skin irritation and report it immediately. The traction bandage may have to be removed.
2. Inspect for skin irritation and pressure on:
   a. Achilles tendon
   b. Heel (keep heel off bed!)
   c. Malleoli
   d. Peroneal nerve (as it passes around the neck of the fibula just below the knee)
3. Evaluate dorsum of foot for loss of sensation, weakness of dorsiflexors of foot and toes, inversion of foot—may be caused by tight traction tape and pressure on the common peroneal nerve.
4. Unwrap the elastic bandage periodically and assess neurovascular status; check for evidence of slipping of traction tape.
   Have second person stabilize leg in position, applying manual traction when inspecting skin or when giving skin care. Slipping of dressing or boot causes pressure on bony prominences.
5. Assess for complaints of persistent itching and burning.
6. Maintain the extremity in a neutral position. Avoid external rotation.
7. The patient may not turn from side to side because the position of the leg on the bed will cause the bony fragments to move against each other.
8. Inspect and bathe back. To give back care instruct the patient to:
   a. Place hands on overhead trapeze.
   b. Bend the knee of unaffected extremity and place foot flat on bed.
   c. Push down on the uninvolved foot and at the same time pull up on the trapeze—allows the entire body and trunk to rise off the bed.
   The shoulders, back, and buttocks must move as a single, straight unit.

Nursing Process Overview
(The Patient in Traction)

Assessment

1. Determine pathologic basis for traction (e.g., muscle spasm, fracture, deformity).
2. Assess the patient's physiologic and psychological status.
   a. Pain
   b. Deformity
   c. Swelling
   d. Neurovascular status—paralysis, paresthesia, pulse, color
   e. Emotional reactions
   f. Understanding of treatment regimen
   g. Skin condition—examined frequently for evidences of pressure or friction over bony prominences.
3. Examine traction equipment for safety and effectiveness.
   a. The patient is placed on a firm mattress, often with a hinged bedboard beneath it.

b. The ropes and the pulleys should be in straight alignment.
c. The pull should be in line with the long axis of the bone.
d. Any factor that might reduce the pull or alter its direction must be eliminated.
   (1) Weights should hang freely.
   (2) Ropes should be unobstructed and not in contact with the bed or equipment.
   (3) Help the patient to pull himself up in bed at frequent intervals. Traction is *not* accomplished if the knot in the rope or the footplate is touching the pulley or the foot of the bed, or if the weights are resting on the floor.
e. The amount of weight applied in skin traction must not exceed the tolerance of the skin. The condition of the skin must be inspected frequently.
4. Evaluate the patient in skeletal traction for the possible development of infection.
Check the patient for odor and signs of infection.
5. Review body systems for possible immobility-related problems (e.g., pneumonia, constipation, thrombophlebitis, depression).

Patient Problems/Nursing Diagnoses

1. Potential for problems of immobility (musculoskeletal weakness, respiratory dysfunction, constipation) related to traction therapy
2. Potential neurovascular compromise related to injury or traction therapy
3. Potential skin breakdown related to pressure on soft tissue
4. Potential infection related to bacterial invasion at skeletal traction site.

Nursing Interventions

A. Maintaining effective traction therapy

1. Check traction apparatus at repeated intervals to see that the direction of pull is correct and the ropes are unobstructed; that weights are in proper position; and that the patient is comfortable.
2. The ropes and the pulleys should be freely movable.
3. The traction must be continuous to be effective unless prescribed as intermittent, as with pelvic traction.
4. Maintain adequate countertraction by adjustment of bed position.
5. *With running traction,* the patient may not be turned without disrupting the line of pull.
6. *With balanced suspension traction,* the patient may be elevated, turned slightly, and moved as desired.

▶ **NURSING ALERT:** *Every complaint of the patient in traction should be investigated immediately.*

B. Maintaining normal body system functions

1. Encourage deep breathing hourly to facilitate expansion of lungs and movement of respiratory secretions.
2. Auscultate lung fields twice a day.
3. Encourage fluid intake of 2,000–2,500 ml. daily.
4. Provide balanced high fiber diet rich in protein; avoid excessive calcium intake.
5. Establish bowel routine through use of diet and/or stool softeners, laxatives, and enemas as prescribed.
6. Encourage active exercise of uninvolved muscles and joints to maintain strength and function. Dorsiflex feet hourly to avoid development of footdrop.
7. Encourage patient participation in planning and care activities.
8. Provide diversional activities.
9. Examine the patient for development of thrombophlebitis (e.g., calf tenderness).

C. Retaining intact neurovascular status of immobilized extremity

1. See Neurovascular Compromise, page 815.
2. Assess specific nerve functioning of peroneal nerve
   a. Have patient point great toe towards his nose
   b. Question about abnormal sensations
   c. Observe for footdrop
3. Assess other nerves (e.g., ulnar, median, radial) that may be compressed.
4. Determine adequacy of circulation (e.g., color, temperature, motion, capillary refill of peripheral fingers or toes).
   a. With Buck's traction the foot should be inspected for circulatory difficulties within a few minutes and then periodically after the elastic bandage has been applied.
5. Notify physician promptly if change in neurovascular status is identified.

D. Maintaining intact skin without development of pressure areas

1. Examine bony prominences frequently for evidence of pressure or friction irritation.
2. Observe for skin irritation around the traction bandage.
3. Observe for pressure under the sling at the popliteal space.
4. Any complaint or burning sensation under the traction bandage should be reported immediately.
5. Special care must be given to the back at regular intervals, because the patient maintains a supine position.
6. Relieve pressure without disrupting traction effectiveness.

E. Avoiding infection at pin site

1. Monitor vital signs.
2. Watch for signs of infection, especially around the pin tract.
   a. The pin should be immobile in the bone and the skin wound should be dry. Small amount of serous oozing from pin site may occur.
   b. If infection is suspected, percuss gently over the tibia; this may elicit pain if infection is developing.
   c. Assess for other signs of infection: heat, redness, fever.
If directed, clean the pin tract with sterile applicators and prescribed medication/ointment—to clear drainage at the entrance of tract and around the pin, since plugging at this site can predispose to bacterial invasion of the tract and bone.
3. Apply a cork or adhesive over the sharp edges of the pin to protect patient and care-givers from injury.

Health Education

1. Teach the patient the purpose of traction therapy.
2. Delineate limitations of activity necessary to maintain effective traction.

3. Teach use of patient aids (e.g., trapeze).
4. Instruct the patient not to adjust or modify traction apparatus.
5. Instruct the patient in activities designed to minimize effects of immobility on body systems.
6. Teach the patient necessity for reporting changes in sensations, pain, movement, etc.

Expected Outcomes

1. Achieves effective traction therapy, immobilization and comfort

    a. Maintains normal respiratory pattern; normal blood gases, vital signs and lung sounds
    b. Maintains muscular strength and joint mobility; participates in exercise program and activities of daily living
2. Maintains normal neurovascular functioning—normal sensations, movement, and circulatory parameters
3. Shows no evidence of skin breakdown; no reddened skin from pressure
4. Experiences no infection at pin site—tissue at pin site is not inflamed, red, or tender beyond normal expectations; no fever

External Fixation for Complicated Fractures

External fixation is a technique of fracture immobilization in which a series of transfixing pins is inserted through bone and attached to a rigid external metal frame (Fig. 19-9). The method is used mainly in the management of open fractures with severe soft tissue damage.

Advantages

1. Permits rigid support of severely comminuted open fractures, infected nonunions, and infected unstable joints.

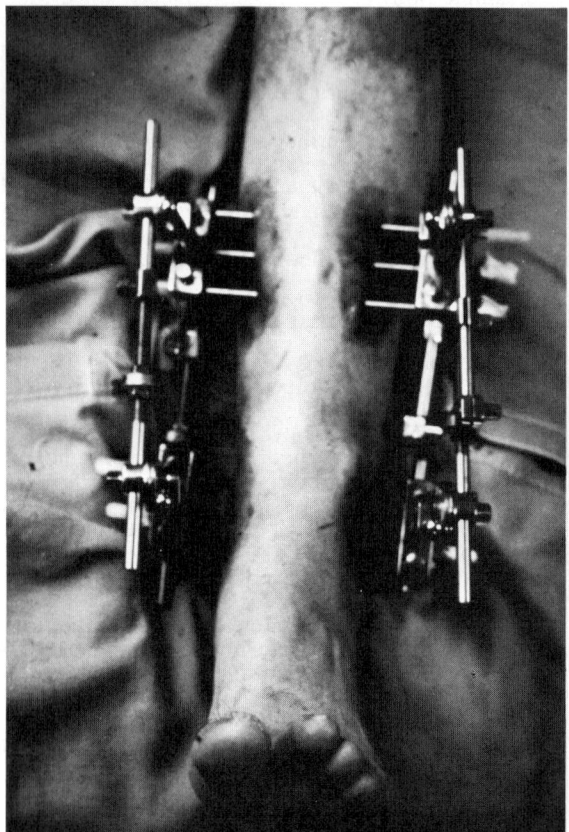

Figure 19-9. External fixation. (Courtesy of University of Texas Health and Science Center at Dallas)

2. Facilitates wound care (frequent debridements, irrigations, dressing changes) and soft tissue reconstruction (delayed wound closure, muscle flaps, skin grafts).
3. Allows early function of muscles and joints.
4. Allows early patient comfort.

Procedure

Under general anesthesia the skin is cleansed and transfixing pins are inserted through small incisions above and below the fracture and drilled through the bony cortex. Following reduction of the fracture, the appliance is tightened by adjusting and tightening the bars connecting the sets of pins.

The sharp pin heads are covered with plastic covers or cork or rubber plugs—to protect other extremity and bed linens.

Nursing Assessment

1. Determine the patient's understanding of procedure and fixation device.
2. Evaluate neurovascular status of involved body part.
3. Inspect each pin site for redness, drainage, tenderness, pain, and loosening of the pin.
4. Inspect open wounds for healing, infection, or devitalized tissue.
5. Assess functioning of other body systems.

Patient Problems/Nursing Diagnoses

1. Anxiety and ineffective coping related to appearance of external fixation device
2. Potential inadequate tissue perfusion and neurovascular compromise related to injury
3. Potential infection related to open injury and skeletal pin insertion
4. Impaired mobility and ability to perform activities of daily living related to restrictions imposed by injury and external fixator

Nursing Interventions

A. Relieving anxiety and fear related to the external fixation device

1. If possible before placement of the device, reassure the patient that although the fixator appears clumsy and cumbersome, it should not hurt once it is in place.
2. Emphasize the positive aspects of this device in treating complex musculoskeletal problems.
3. Encourage the patient to verbalize reaction to the

device, thereby minimizing the development of other system problems.

4. Inform the patient that he will achieve greater mobility with an external fixation device, thereby minimizing the development of other system problems.
5. Involve the patient in his care and in the management of external fixator.

B. Maintaining intact neurovascular status

1. See Neurovascular Compromise, page 815.
2. Establish baseline of functioning for comparative monitoring. Complex musculoskeletal injuries frequently result in disruption of soft tissue functioning.

▶ **NURSING ALERT:** Assess neurovascular status frequently and *record findings*.

3. Elevate extremity in balanced suspension traction to reduce swelling.
   a. Extremity can be suspended by hanging the fixator directly to the traction frame.
   b. Suspension is for control of edema and not for application of traction force.
4. Notify physician of change in neurovascular status.

C. Avoiding infection

1. Pin site and fixator care:
   a. Cleanse pin sites and remove crusts with sterile cotton applicator dipped in hydrogen peroxide or as directed 2–3 times daily—crusts formed by serous drainage can prevent fluid from draining and cause infection.
   b. Apply nonocclusive antimicrobial agent around pin sites as directed.
   c. Wipe off fixator with sterile cloth dampened with sterile water.
   d. Avoid shortcuts. Meticulous technique is important.
2. Wound care:
   a. The open wounds at the fracture site are usually treated by daily dressing changes.
   b. Use sterile technique.
   c. Change dressings around pins first and those underneath fixator rods last.
3. Monitor for local and systemic indicators of infection.

D. Promoting self-care activities

1. Encourage the patient to participate in care activities. Patient may become the "authority" for routine care activities (e.g., pin care).
2. Assure the patient that pain associated with injury will diminish as tissue reactions to injury and manipulation resolve and healing progresses.
3. Inform the patient that the external fixator maintains the fracture in a very stable position and that the extremity can be moved. Adjustment of the fixator is done by the physician.
4. To move the extremity, grasp the frame and assist the patient to move. Reassure the patient that the fixator can withstand normal movement.
5. Quadriceps exercises and range-of-motion for joints are usually started on first postoperative day.
6. Patient ambulates on crutches when soft tissue swelling has diminished; weight-bearing is done only as prescribed.

Health Education

1. Inspect around each pin site daily for signs of infection and loosening of pins. Watch for pain, soft tissue swelling, and drainage.

2. Cleanse around each pin tract daily, using aseptic technique. *Do not touch wound with hands*.
3. Clean fixator regularly—to keep it free of dust and contamination.
4. *Do not tamper with clamps or nuts*—can alter compression and misalign fracture.
5. Review weight-bearing and other restrictions associated with injury and treatment regimen.
6. Encourage the patient to follow rehabilitation regimen.

Expected Outcomes

1. Overcomes any anxiety about the external fixation device—does not appear worried about it; handles and cares for equipment with ease
2. Maintains normal neurovascular functioning—normal sensations, movement, circulation, and tissue perfusion
3. Shows no signs of infection at pin sites or at site of open injury—no inflammation at pin site; tissue not overly tender; healing progresses as anticipated; no temperature rise or other systemic signs of infection
4. Performs activities of daily living within limits of restrictions and uses ambulatory aids safely

Internal Fixation Device

General Considerations

1. Some fractures may be reduced under anesthesia and stabilized with the surgical implantation of metal nails, nail–plate combinations, compression screw devices, and intramedullary nails.
2. Surgical procedure is usually carried out as soon as possible after full medical assessment since these patients are usually elderly, for whom prolonged bed rest is detrimental.
3. Surgical fixation of a fracture permits early mobilization of the patient thereby decreasing the adverse effects of immobilization. The metal hardware is not strong enough to permit full function of the extremity, but does facilitate maintenance of muscle strength, joint mobility, and development of bony union.

Assessment

1. Carry out neurovascular check of affected extremity.
2. Monitor drainage from portable suction.

Patient Problems/Nursing Diagnoses

1. Potential for injury from dislocation or loosening of fixation device related to malalignment and adverse stresses
2. Impaired mobility related to injury and presence of fixation device
3. Potential complications (constipation, contractures, neurovascular and respiratory problems) related to immobility
4. Ineffective coping related to the limitations imposed by the treatment

Nursing Interventions

For hip fracture treated with internal fixation

A. Maintaining proper alignment of extremity

1. Position affected leg as directed—usually on a pillow with mild abduction.
2. Place pillow between legs—to maintain alignment.
3. Using two persons, gently pull the patient onto

affected side; when lying on unoperated side, keep the affected extremity in position of abduction.

B. Achieving ambulation as soon as possible

1. Wrap the lower extremities with elastic compression bandages or elastic hose—increases venous velocity in legs and helps minimize dependent edema.
2. Use the tilt table as soon as the patient's condition permits (p. 63). With the use of the tilt table the patient becomes accustomed to the upright position, and circulation and respiratory functioning improve.
3. Assist the patient into a wheelchair several times daily as prescribed—helps avoid arterial hypotension, helps maintain strength, aids pulmonary function, and is beneficial psychologically.
   a. With the aid of the overhead trapeze, encourage the patient to move into the dangle position. (Use a Hi-Lo bed.)
   b. Assist the patient to stand on the *unaffected extremity* and transfer to the chair.
   c. If weight-bearing is permitted, the patient may be encouraged to ambulate with walker, applying as much weight to extremity as is comfortable.
   d. Certain types of fractures must be supported and protected until bone union is secure and displacement of fractures unlikely. If this is the case, the patient may have to be lifted into the chair.
   e. Allow the patient to get up at her own pace; avoid hurrying.
4. Encourage the patient to participate in activities of daily living (eating, bathing, hair care)—to condition the patient for future ambulation activities and to help maintain a degree of independence.

C. Promoting active exercises

1. Encourage quadriceps-setting exercises hourly—the quadriceps femoris muscle extends the leg and is one of the major muscles necessary for ambulation.

2. Do heel-cord stretching of both legs and abdominal and gluteal contractions (isometric contractions). Isometric muscle contractions strengthen the muscle but do not move the joint.
3. Avoid knee contractures.
   a. Maintain the knee in a position of extension while the patient is in bed.
   b. Flex the knee in a 90-degree angle while the patient is in the chair. Avoid extending the knee for long periods when the patient is in a sitting position because extension produces undue strain on the fractured hip.
   c. Move the knee through assisted range-of-motion exercises.
4. Assist the patient to perform arm strengthening exercises (flexion and extension of the arms). The muscles in the shoulder girdle and upper extremities must be strong enough to bear the patient's weight while she is using the walker.
5. Assist the patient to learn to use the walker—ambulating with a non–weight-bearing (or partial weight-bearing depending on the fracture and its fixation) technique.
6. Remind the patient *not* to bear weight on the affected extremity until the orthopedist gives permission and the x-rays reveal sufficient healing. Early weight-bearing before bony union occurs exerts too much stress and may cause bending or breaking of the pin, crushing of the bone, or loss of fixation due to the device's cutting through the bone.

Expected Outcomes

1. Maintains alignment—bony fusion occurs
2. Transfers from bed with ease; out of bed in chair that provides good support several times a day.
3. Participates in active exercises and mobility activities; does prescribed exercises and uses ambulatory aids safely

Orthopedic Surgery

Special Nursing Considerations

Preoperative Nursing Management

A. Assessment

1. Carry out normal assessment standards for a person undergoing surgery (see p. 75).
2. Assess nutritional status. Ensure adequate protein and calorie intake.
3. Question the patient to determine whether he has had previous therapy with corticosteroids (especially with patients with arthritis).
   a. Steroid therapy (current or past) may adversely affect the patient's response to anesthesia.
   b. Steroids should be administered per request to cover stress of surgery.

B. Patient Education

1. Teach patients about the following: tests and routines, coughing and deep-breathing, and immediate postoperative activities.
2. Have the patient practice voiding in bedpan or urinal in recumbent position before surgery. This helps reduce the need for postoperative catheterization.

3. Acquaint the patient with traction apparatus and the need for splints and casts—to familiarize him with postoperative environment.

Postoperative Assessment

A. Immediate Postoperative Period

1. Evaluate the blood pressure and pulse rates frequently—rising pulse rate or slowly falling blood pressure indicates persistent bleeding or development of a state of shock.
2. Assess changes in respiratory rate or in the patient's color—may indicate obstruction of respiratory exchange or pulmonary or cardiac complications.
3. Carry out neurovascular checks (nerve function and circulation) of affected extremity. Watch circulation distal to the part where cast, bandage, or splint has been applied.
   a. Prevent constriction leading to interference with blood or nerve supply.
   b. Watch toes and fingers for healthy color.
   c. Check pulses of affected extremity; compare with unaffected extremity.

d. Note skin temperature—raised skin temperature may indicate bleeding or infection.

▶ **NURSING ALERT:** Abnormal coolness of skin, cyanosis, rubor, or pallor indicates interference with circulation.

4. Watch for excessive bleeding—orthopedic wounds have a tendency to ooze more than other surgical wounds.
   a. Measure suction drainage if used.
   b. Anticipate up to 200–500 ml. of drainage in the first 24 hours, decreasing to less than 30 ml. per 8 hours within 48 hours, depending on surgical procedure.
5. Assess for pain related to musculoskeletal surgery (see p. 814).
6. Watch for urinary retention—elderly men with some degree of prostatism may have difficulty in voiding.
7. Evaluate orthopedic apparatus for safety and effectiveness.

B. Later Postoperative Period

1. Watch for development of pressure sores. See page 59 for prevention and management.
2. Watch for complications due to prolonged disability. Venous thrombosis—see page 362 for clinical manifestations.
3. Assess fluid and nutritional status.
4. Watch for signs and symptoms of anemia—especially after fracture of long bones.
Hemoglobin determination usually done on 3rd postoperative day or sooner.

Patient Problems/Nursing Diagnoses

1. Pain related to musculoskeletal surgery
2. Potential complications related to systemic responses to stresses of surgery, orthopedic injury, or immobility
3. Potential infection related to break in skin integrity

Nursing Interventions

A. Relief of Pain

1. See Pain related to musculoskeletal disorder, page 814.
2. Administer prescribed parenteral medications to control pain during the first few postoperative days.
   a. Avoid injection sites near operative site.
   b. Rotate injection sites.
   c. Muscle spasms may contribute to pain experience.

B. Prevention of Complications

1. Monitor vital signs frequently.
2. Assess neurovascular status of involved extremity.
   a. See Neurovascular compromise, page 815.
   b. Document observations.
   c. Elevate affected extremity and apply ice packs as directed.
   d. If neurovascular problems are identified, notify surgeon and loosen cast or dressing at once.
3. Maintain sufficient pulmonary ventilation.
   a. Avoid or give respiratory depressant drugs in minimal doses.
   b. Change position every 2 hours—mobilizes secretions and helps prevent bronchial obstruction.
4. Encourage early resumption of activity.
5. Prevent venous complications.
   a. Encourage the patient to exercise by himself with a planned program of exercise as soon as possible after surgery.
   b. Have the patient flex his knee, extend the knee with hip still flexed, and then lower the extremity to the bed.
   c. Encourage the patient to move fingers and toes periodically.
   d. Advise the patient to move joints that are not fixed by traction or appliance through their range of motion as fully as possible.
   e. Suggest muscle-setting exercises (quadriceps setting) if active motion is contraindicated.
   f. Wrap lower extremities with elastic bandages or apply elastic hose.
   g. Give prophylactic anticoagulants as directed (heparin, warfarin, aspirin, etc.).
6. Provide a normal balanced diet.
   a. Give supplemental vitamins (B and C) to elderly patients or those with chronic disease as prescribed.
   b. Avoid giving large amounts of milk to orthopedic patients on bed rest—adds to calcium pool in the body and demands more calcium excretion by the kidneys, predisposing to the formation of urinary calculi.
   c. Give iron supplements as directed.
7. Maintain urinary output by maintaining adequate fluid intake.
8. Monitor for signs and symptoms of infection.
   a. Monitor vital signs.
   b. Examine incision for redness, increased temperature, and swelling.
   c. Note character of drainage.
   d. Evaluate complaints of recurrent or increasing pain.
   e. Administer antibiotic therapy as prescribed.

Health Education

1. Teach the patient activities that will minimize the development of complications (e.g., turning, coughing, and deep-breathing).
2. Instruct the patient in dietary considerations to facilitate healing and minimize development of constipation and renal calculi.
3. Inform the patient of techniques that facilitate moving while minimizing associated discomforts (e.g., supporting injured area and practicing smooth, gentle position changes).

Expected Outcomes

1. Achieves pain relief; utilizes pain-reduction measures and states achievement of comfort
2. Demonstrates homeostasis; vital signs within normal limits and no evidence of thrombophlebitis, pressure sores, etc.
3. Achieves wound healing; no drainage and no signs of infection

Arthroplasty and Total Joint Replacement

Arthroplasty is an operation to restore motion to a joint and function to the structures (muscles, ligaments, soft tissues) that control it. It may involve either replacement of the joint by a prosthesis or surgical reshaping of the bones of the joint.

Total hip replacement (total joint arthroplasty) is the replacement of a severely damaged hip with an artificial

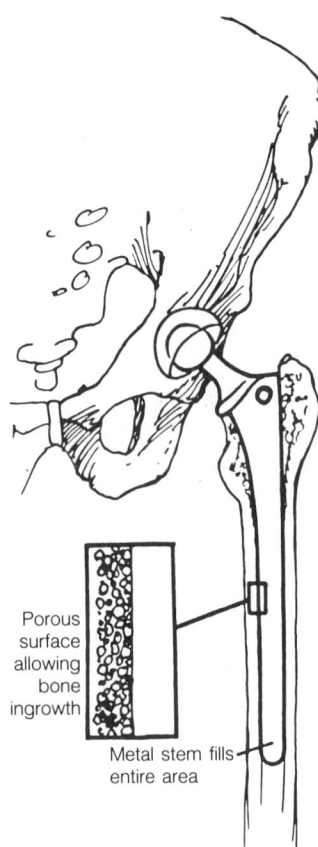

Figure 19-10. Total hip replacement using ingrowth porous-coated prosthesis. (Courtesy of Dr. Charles Engh, Arlington, VA)

joint. Although a large number of implants are available, most consist of a metal femoral component topped by a spherical ball fitted into a plastic acetabular socket (Fig. 19-10).

A *total knee arthroplasty* is an implant procedure in which tibial, femoral, and patellar joint surfaces are replaced because of destroyed knee joint(s). Different types of implants are used, depending on degree of destruction and stability of joint (Fig. 19-11).

Total joint arthroplasty is an exacting and meticulous procedure.

Bone ingrowth prosthesis designs allow for cementless fixation of the components in selected patients. Some patients require cement fixation of the components because of bone structure or condition (see Fig. 19-10).

Clinical Indications

1. For patients with unremitting pain, irreversibly damaged joints
    Primary degenerative arthritis (osteoarthritis)
    Rheumatoid arthritis
2. Selected fractures (e.g., femoral neck fracture)
3. Failure of previous reconstructive surgery (osteotomy, cup arthroplasty, femoral head replacement for complications of nonunion and avascular necrosis)
4. Problems resulting from congenital hip disease

5. Pathologic fractures from metastatic cancer
6. Joint instability

Treatment

Goals:
Reduce or eliminate pain.
Restore, improve, or maintain joint function.
Provide greater stability of the joint.
Avoid complications.

Prevention of Infection

1. Operative area is scrubbed twice daily—microorganisms of the skin are potential cause of infection.
2. Give "on-call" preoperative medication into opposite (uninvolved) extremity.
3. Special precautions carried out in OR (impermeable OR attire, clean air system) to reduce particulate matter and bacterial count of air.
4. Antimicrobials usually given immediately preoperatively, intraoperatively, and postoperatively to reduce incidence of infection.

Preoperative Nursing Interventions

1. Give meticulous skin preparation.
2. Administer antibiotic as prescribed.

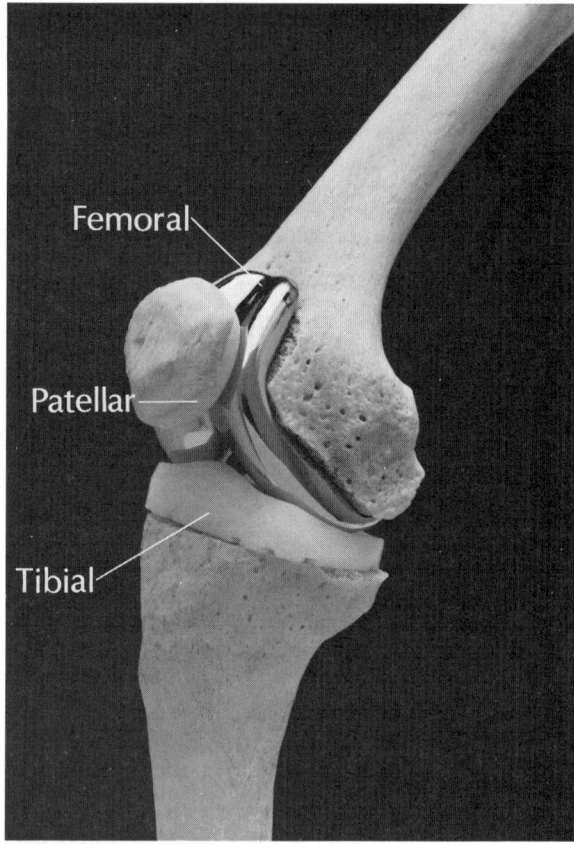

Figure 19-11. Total knee replacement. (Courtesy of Richards Manufacturing Co., Inc.)

3. Use elastic stockings to minimize development of thrombophlebitis.
4. Provide preoperative patient teaching.
   a. Educate the patient concerning his postoperative regimen (e.g., extended exercise program will be carried out after surgery—atrophied muscles must be reeducated and strengthened).
   b. Teach isometric exercises (muscle setting) of quadriceps and gluteal muscles; teach active ankle motion.
   c. Fit with crutches and instruct the patient to walk without weight-bearing (if prescribed)—to develop crutch-walking ability and facilitate the patient's postoperative ambulation.
   d. Teach bed-to-wheelchair transfer without going beyond the hip flexion limits (usually 45 degrees).
   e. Show balanced suspension apparatus, abduction splint, overhead traction frame, and trapeze—to acquaint the patient with postoperative environment.
   f. Demonstrate continuous passive motion equipment if it will be used postoperatively (see Fig. 19-12).

Postoperative Nursing Interventions

A. Postoperative assessment

1. Assess the patient's position for compliance with positioning prescription.
   a. Following hip arthroplasty, the patient is usually positioned flat in bed with the affected extremity held in slight abduction by either an abduction splint or pillows (may or may not be in Buck's extension)—to prevent dislocation of the prosthesis until soft tissue healing has occurred.
   b. Following knee arthroplasty, the knee may be immobilized in extension with a firm compression dressing and an adjustable soft extension splint or long-leg plaster cast.

Leg may be elevated on pillows above the level of patient's heart.
Alternatively, continuous passive motion may be started.

Note: There are numerous modifications with differing requirements in the postoperative positioning of these patients.

2. Monitor the patient for signs of joint dislocation (i.e., shortened extremity, increasing discomfort, inability to move joint).
3. Assess the patient for the development of complications.
   a. Early—infection, thromboembolic complications, peroneal nerve palsy
   b. Late—deep infection, loosening of prosthetic components, implant wear and dislocation, fracture of components

B. Proper positioning and turning activities

1. Position the patient as prescribed—generally with hip arthroplasty the leg is in abduction with the use of an abduction splint or pillows.
2. Avoid acute flexion of the hip.

▶ **NURSING ALERT:** The patient must not adduct or flex operated hip—may produce dislocation.

2. Turn the patient (as required by his prosthesis and condition) when indicated by surgeon.
   Following hip arthroplasty:
   a. Two nurses turn the patient on unoperated side while supporting operated hip securely in an abducted position; the entire length of leg is supported by two pillows.
   Use pillows to keep the leg abducted; place pillow at back for comfort.
   b. Keep bed flat except during prescribed intervals (meals)—to prevent hip flexion contraction.

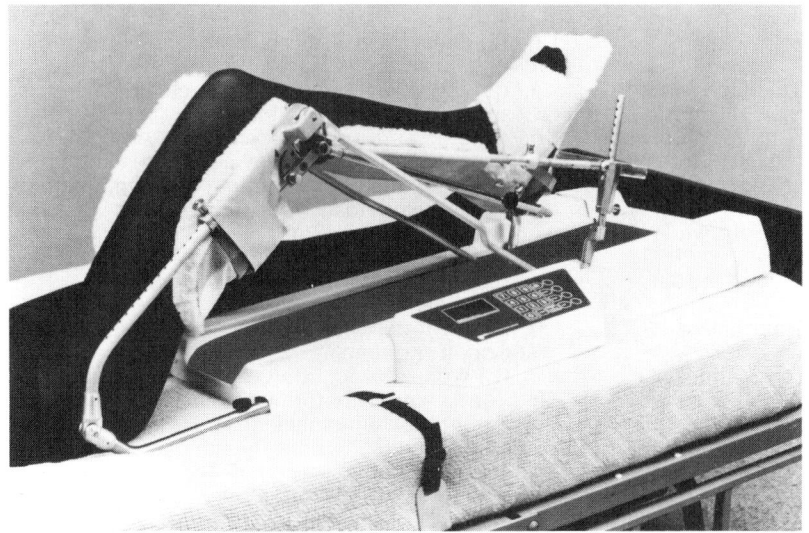

Figure 19-12. Continuous passive motion device used for postoperative total knee arthroplasty patients to facilitate joint range of motion. (Courtesy of Sutter Biomedical Inc.)

(1) The bed is usually not elevated more than 45 degrees; placing the patient in an upright sitting position puts a strain on the hip joint and may cause dislocation.

(2) Support the low back with a small pillow or towel when the patient is supine—to relieve strain placed on muscles by the flat position.

c. As the patient becomes familiar with the turning routine, assist him to change position by using overhead trapeze.

C. Transfer and ambulation

1. Assist in use of the fracture bed pan—instruct the patient to flex the unoperated hip and knee and pull up on the trapeze to lift buttocks onto pan. Instruct the patient *NOT* to bear down on the operated hip in flexion when getting off the pan.

2. Assist in transfer from bed.
   a. *Following hip arthroplasty:*
      (1) Use an abduction splint or pillows while assisting the patient to get out of bed.
         (a) Keep the hip at maximum extension.
         (b) Instruct the patient to pivot on unoperated extremity.
         (c) Assess the patient for orthostatic hypotension.
      (2) When the patient is ready to ambulate, teach him to advance the walker and then advance the operated extremity to the walker, bearing most of the weight on the hands.
      (3) The patient progresses to use of crutches as directed, to prevent excessive use of hip abductors before healing occurs.
   b. *Following knee arthroplasty,* the patient may transfer out of bed into wheelchair with extension splint in place; no weight-bearing is permitted at this time.

D. Prevention of complications

1. Assess neurovascular status of operated extremity—check sensation, pulses, color, and skin temperature and compare with unoperated leg.

2. Monitor blood loss—portable suction is used to decrease incidence of wound hematoma, which is a possible focus of infection.

3. Give narcotics as required the first 24 hours postoperatively and then taper to nonnarcotic analgesia thereafter.

4. Encourage the patient to carry out prescribed exercise program, usually under direction of physical therapist.
   a. Pain medication is usually given $\frac{1}{2}$ hour before exercise session as required.
   b. Instruct the patient to think about the motion required to contract the appropriate muscles.
   c. Encourage the patient to breathe deeply while exercising.
   d. Exercise activities depend on procedure and on condition of the patient.
      (1) Active motion of affected foot and ankle is started on the first postoperative day.
      (2) Isometric exercise of quadriceps, gluteals, abductors is started on direction of orthopedic surgeon.
      (3) Flexion, extension, abduction, rotation exercises, and ambulation are started upon direction of surgeon.
   e. Assist and encourage the patient during exercise.

5. Assist the patient in use of continuous passive motion equipment. Early postoperative passive exercise of joint facilitates joint healing and restoration of joint range of motion.

6. Use anticipatory nursing measures to prevent complications.
   a. Thromboembolism (major threat following reconstructive hip operations).
      (1) Continue to exercise ankles and legs—accelerates blood flow and prevents venous stasis.
      (2) Antiembolic stockings for uninvolved extremity—to increase venous velocity; elastic stocking applied to operated extremity when elastic compression dressing is removed.
      (3) Check for calf edema, tenderness, local pain.
      (4) Heparin, warfarin, aspirin—may be used for thromboembolic prophylaxis.
   b. Infection
      (1) Give antimicrobials as directed.
      (2) Watch for elevation of temperature and inspect wound at intervals.
      (3) Infection may not become apparent until months or years after surgery.
      (4) Deep infection almost always requires removal of implant.
   c. Complicating medical conditions (cardiac, gastrointestinal, genitourinary).
   d. Dislocation of prosthesis, fatigue fracture of metal component, avascular necrosis or dead bone caused by loss of blood supply, heterotrophic ossification (formation of bone in periprosthetic space).

Health Education

Instruct the patient as follows:

1. Continue to wear elastic stockings after going home until full activities are resumed.

2. Avoid excessive hip adduction, flexion, and rotation.
   a. Avoid sitting in low chair/toilet seat.
   b. Keep knees apart; do *not* cross legs.
   c. Limit sitting to 30 minutes at a time—to minimize hip flexion and the risk of prosthetic dislocation and to prevent hip stiffness and flexion contracture.

3. Continue quadriceps setting and range-of-motion exercises as directed.
   a. Have a *daily* program of stretching, exercise, and rest throughout lifetime.
   b. Acquire a stationary bicycle if possible.
   c. Do not participate in any activity placing undue or sudden stress on joint (jogging, jumping, lifting heavy loads, becoming obese, excessive bending and twisting).
   d. Use a cane when taking fairly long walks.

4. Use self-help and energy-saving devices.
   a. Handrails by toilet
   b. Raised toilet seat if there is some residual hip flexion problem
   c. Bar-type stool for shower and kitchen work

5. Lie prone twice daily for 30 minutes.

6. Report for follow-up evaluation and testing; supportive equipment (crutches, cane) is modified as needed.

7. Take prophylactic antibiotic if undergoing any procedure known to cause bacteremia (tooth extraction, manipulation of genitourinary tract).

Amputation

Lower Extremity Amputation

General Considerations

A. Conditions warranting amputation

1. Inadequate tissue perfusion as a result of diabetes mellitus or other vascular disease
2. Trauma
3. Malignant tumor
4. Congenital deformities

B. Treatment

1. Level of amputation is determined by estimation of maximum viable tissue and development of a functional stump.
2. Modern trend is toward selecting most distal amputation level consistent with wound healing.

Preoperative Assessment

1. Hemodynamic evaluation—arterial blood flow evaluated by Doppler pressure measurements and xenon-[133] flow studies—for accurate and optimum amputation level determination.
2. Culture and sensitivity tests of draining wounds. Control of gangrene or advancing infection preoperatively is sought.
3. Evaluation of sound (contralateral) extremity.
4. Evaluation of cardiovascular, respiratory, renal, and other body systems to determine preoperative condition of the patient.
5. Evaluation of the patient's and family's emotional response to amputation.
    a. Anticipation of relief of pain related to amputation is frequent.
    b. Distress at anticipated loss of body part exhibited by patient and family.

Patient Problems/Nursing Diagnoses

1. Anxiety related to proposed amputation
2. Alteration in comfort related to primary condition requiring amputation
3. Alteration in mobility related to general muscle weakness and projected use of ambulatory aids
4. Health and nutritional deficits related to chronic condition and impending major surgery
5. Knowledge deficit related to expected participation in projected rehabilitation program

Nursing Interventions

A. Reduction of anxiety

1. Support the patient psychologically. Knowing what to expect helps reduce anxiety.
2. Amputation may be viewed as a surgical reconstructive procedure and as the first step in rehabilitation for the patient who has had prolonged periods of disability from peripheral vascular disease.
3. Avoid unrealistic and misleading reassurance—management of a prosthesis can be slow and painful.

B. Relief of pain

1. Instruct patient on use of pain-modifying techniques (see p. 815).

2. Inform the patient of the availability of postoperative pain medication
3. Explain to the patient that he will continue to "feel" the foot for a time; this sensation may be helpful for the placement of the prosthetic foot while he is learning to use the prosthesis.

C. Incorporation of effective position changes and ambulation with use of ambulatory aids

1. Encourage the patient to reposition self every 1–2 hours with an awareness of body positioning to avoid contractures.
2. Have the patient strengthen the muscles of the upper extremity, trunk, and abdomen as a preparation for crutch walking. (Develop arm extensors and shoulder depressors, which are the muscle groups needed for crutch walking.) Instruct the patient as follows:
    a. Flex and extend arms while holding traction weights.
    b. Do push-ups from a prone position.
    c. Do sit-ups from a seated position.
3. Teach the patient to use ambulatory aids preoperatively—prepares for postoperative mobility, maintains mobility and arm function, and instills confidence.

D. Establishing maximal health status prior to surgery

1. Assess laboratory reports for optimal values (e.g., hematology, urinalysis, and blood chemistries are within normal limits).
2. Encourage balanced diet with adequate protein to enhance wound healing.
3. Evaluate each body system for adequacy of function.

E. Preoperative activities to enhance recovery

1. Clarify plans for management of perioperative and postoperative periods as outlined by the physician.
2. Address concerns expressed about the possibilities of obtaining and using a prosthesis—not all amputees can benefit from a prosthesis.
    a. Diabetes mellitus, heart disease, infection, CVA, COPD, peripheral vascular disease, and increasing age are factors limiting full rehabilitation.
    b. Wound breakdown, infection, and delay in healing of amputation stump are significant limiting factors.
3. Introduce the patient to physical therapist.
4. Encourage the patient to attain his highest physical and emotional level in preparation for wearing a prosthesis (artificial extremity) and/or attaining mobility by other means.
5. Explain various phases of rehabilitation involved—active participation in rehabilitation is essential for a successful outcome.
6. Teach postoperative routines (i.e., turn, cough, deep-breathe, etc.).

Treatment

1. The surgeon creates a residual limb (stump) which is functional (with stability), nontender, pressure tolerant, and not susceptible to tissue breakdown. The skin, soft tissue, and scar placement are considered.

2. A closed, rigid plaster dressing applied immediately after surgery provides for the attachment of a prosthetic extension (pylon) and a prosthetic foot immediately or within 10–30 days.
3. The rigid dressing controls edema, supports circulation, minimizes pain on movement, helps shape the residual limb, and promotes healing. It allows earlier fitting of the prosthesis, shortens the interval between amputation and walking, and is of tremendous psychological value to the patient.
4. Although the rigid dressing is used, early weight-bearing is not always desirable in patients with severe peripheral vascular disease.
5. A soft dressing permits wound inspection and may be used with compression dressings or external splints.
6. Prevention of complications associated with a major operation and facilitation of early rehabilitation are essential to prevent prolonged disability.

▶ **NURSING ALERT:** Amputation of the lower extremity can be a life-threatening procedure, especially in patients over 60 with peripheral vascular disease. Significant morbidity accompanies above-knee amputations because of associated poor health and disease as well as the complications of sepsis and malnutrition and the physiological insult of amputation.

Postoperative Assessment

1. Watch for signs and symptoms of hemorrhage.
   a. Keep tourniquet (in view) attached to end of bed—to apply to residual limb (stump) if excessive bleeding occurs.
   b. Monitor suction drainage.
2. Monitor the patient's general physiologic response to anesthesia, surgery, and immobility.
3. Evaluate the patient's pain (see page 814).
   a. Anticipate complaint of pain and sensation located in the missing limb ("phantom pain").
   b. Narcotics may not relieve these sensations; physical modalities (e.g., wrapping, temperature changes) and TENS may be useful.

Patient Problems/Nursing Diagnoses

1. Potential hemorrhage related to inadequate/disrupted surgical hemostasis
2. Ineffective coping related to change in body image and alteration in mobility
3. Potential contracture deformity related to positioning and inactivity
4. Alteration in ambulatory stability related to muscle weakness and change in body-weight distribution
5. Residual limb conditioning related to edema and postoperative tissue responses
6. Knowledge deficit related to management of residual limb (stump) and prosthesis

Nursing Interventions

A. Minimal blood loss

1. Raise foot of bed slightly to elevate residual limb. Do not flex the patient's hips by elevating stump on pillow since this will produce a hip flexion contracture.
2. Monitor the patient for systemic symptoms of excessive blood loss.

3. Maintain accurate record of bloody drainage on dressings and in drainage system.
4. Reinforce dressing as required using aseptic technique.

B. Body image adjustment

1. Accept the frustrations and behavior of the patient.
   a. The patient views amputation as death of part of his body; expect some depression and withdrawal.
   b. The self-image has to be adjusted after amputation. It will take time for the patient to make this modification.
2. Exhibit a positive approach combined with physical therapy; this helps improve the patient's outlook on his potential.

C. Prevention of contractures

1. Prevent deformities in the immediate postoperative period. Contracture of the next joint above an amputation is a frequent complication.
   Deformities include:
   (1) Flexion deformities
   (2) Abduction deformities
   a. Avoid pillows under stump, hips, or between legs.
   b. Encourage the patient to turn from side to side.
   c. Place the patient in prone position twice daily—to stretch the flexor muscles and prevent flexion contracture of the hip.
      (1) Keep the patient's legs close together—to prevent abduction deformity.
      (2) Place pillow under abdomen and residual limb while the patient is prone.
2. Encourage the patient to move residual limb—to avoid contractures.
3. Start range-of-motion exercises—contracture deformities develop rapidly and cause serious problems in management of prosthesis.

D. Pre-ambulation training

1. Start the patient on standing and ambulation activities.
   a. The timing depends on age, general physical status, condition of remaining foot, etc.
   b. The patient may stand by his bed (or on tilt table) within 48 hours postoperatively with rigid dressing attached and the prosthetic foot touching down (no weight-bearing)—helps minimize fear of pain and promotes confidence of the patient in his ability to handle himself.
2. Muscle-strengthening and balancing exercises—to strengthen muscles, mobilize joints, and increase balance sense.
   Instruct the patient as follows (stand behind the patient and stabilize him at the waist, if necessary):
   a. Arise from chair and stand.
   b. Stand on toes while holding on to a chair.
   c. Bend the knee while holding on to a chair.
   d. Balance on one leg without support.
   e. Hop on one foot while holding on to a chair.

E. Residual limb conditioning

1. Wrap residual limb with elastic bandage to control edema and to form a firm, conical shape for prosthesis fitting.
   a. Wrapping generally begins 1–3 days after surgery.
   b. Use 2- to 6-inch elastic bandages for above-knee

amputation and 2- to 4-inch bandages for below-knee amputation.

c. Use diagonal figure 8 bandaging technique (Fig. 19-13).

d. Wrap distal to proximal to maintain pressure gradient and to control edema.

e. Begin wrapping with minimal tension and increase as wound heals and sutures are removed.

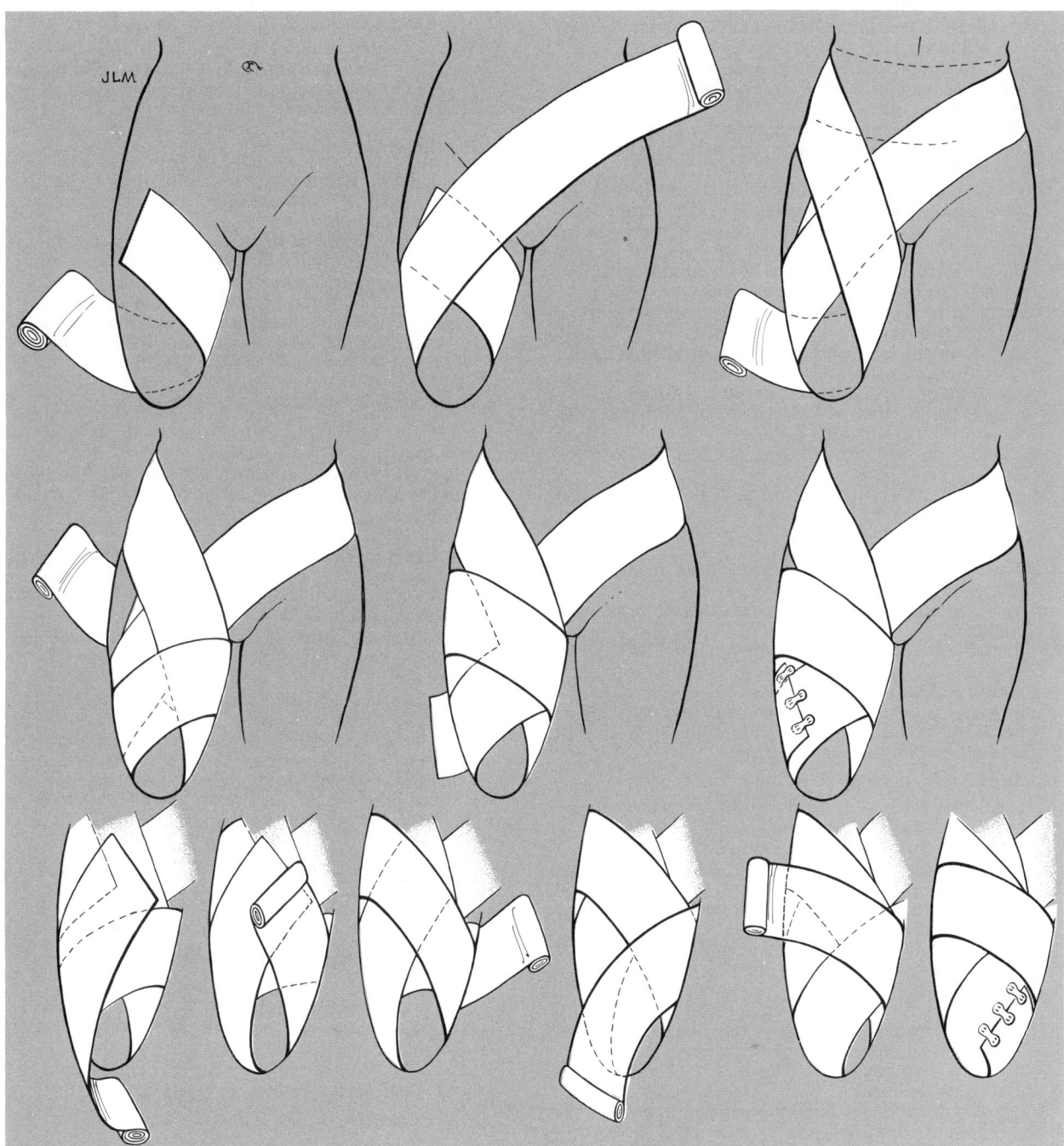

Figure 19-13. Wrapping above-knee residual limb. Elastic bandaging reduces edema and shapes the residual limb in a firm conical form for the prosthesis.

f. Flatten skin at ends of incision to ensure conical stump shape.

g. Apply bandages snugly to adductor area to prevent formation of adductor roll.

h. Rewrap if the patient complains of more pain—dressing is probably too tight.

i. Keep residual limb wrapped at all times except when bathing.

j. Prosthesis is measured and fitted when maximum shrinkage occurs.

2. Include the patient in stump-wrapping activities.

3. Air splint may be applied to residual limb to control edema.

4. Encourage exercises to strengthen muscles necessary for ambulation—hip flexion, abduction, adduction, and extension.

5. Teach the patient to avoid long periods of sitting with limb flexed—minimizes the development of dependent edema, flexion contractures, and pressure areas.

6. Have the patient do residual limb-conditioning exercises—to harden the residual limb.
   a. The patient pushes the residual limb against a soft pillow.
   b. Gradually he pushes residual limb against harder surfaces.
   c. Teach the patient to massage the residual limb to soften the scar, decrease tenderness, and improve vascularity.
      (1) Massage is usually started when healing takes place.
      (2) Initially, massage is usually done by physical therapist.

F. Self-care of residual limb

1. Wash healed residual limb daily with soap and water, removing all soap residue.

2. Avoid soaking residual limb because it results in edema.

3. Inspect residual limb daily for potential and actual skin breakdown.

4. Wrap residual limb at all times.

5. Rewrap residual limb a couple of times a day and as necessary demonstrating skillful ability, resulting in smooth, graded tension dressing.

G. Avoidance of complications

1. Make sure that the residual limb remains in the plaster cast socket during the patient's hospitalization; if the socket inadvertently comes off, excessive edema will form very rapidly, causing a delay in rehabilitation.
   a. Rewrap the residual limb immediately with elastic compression bandage (see Fig. 19-13).
   b. Prepare for immediate reapplication of cast socket.

2. Control pain.
   Assess for development of complications: increasing residual limb pain, hematoma, odor emanating from cast, infection, residual limb necrosis.
   Keep the patient active—decreases occurrence of phantom-limb pain.
   a. If the patient is not a candidate for prosthesis/ambulation, teach him to participate in self-care activities in a special wheelchair designed for amputees.
   b. Reassure the patient that phantom-limb sensation

(painful sensation that amputated foot is still there) will soon pass.

3. Protect the residual limb from infection.
   a. Use plastic material to protect dressing if the patient is incontinent.
   b. Wash residual limb with mild soap and water.

4. Observe and protect the remaining foot from injury.
   a. Examine remaining foot and malleoli daily.
   b. Keep pressure (bedclothes) off foot.

5. Watch for deterioration of remaining leg—from disuse, poor vascular supply, foot trauma. (Obliterative arteriosclerotic vascular disease may necessitate *bilateral* lower extremity amputation.)

Health Education

1. The patient will require rehabilitation services to learn mobility skills, transfers, wheelchair or automobile locomotion, etc.

2. Progressive ambulation following first change of dressing is carried out under the supervision of physical therapist or nurse. Gait training is continued under the direction of physical therapist.

3. A going-home prosthesis is fitted as soon as possible following surgery. The permanent prosthesis is fitted when the residual limb is fully conditioned.

Expected Outcomes

1. Avoids excessive blood loss following surgery; hematology values in normal range

2. Exhibits behavior indicating self-esteem and adjustment to altered mobility patterns; participates in self-care activities; learns use of mobility aids; has realistic future orientation

3. Avoids development of contractures; exercises residual limb; avoids positions that encourage contracture development; spends increasing time prone to inhibit flexion contracture

4. Demonstrates standing balance and ambulatory stability; increase in muscle strength, increased ambulatory ability

5. Participates in residual limb conditioning; wraps stump with elastic dressing skillfully

6. Demonstrates ability to care for residual limb and prosthesis; washes residual limb daily, inspects residual limb for skin pressure or breakdown, keeps residual limb wrapped at all times, works with physical therapist and orthotist to obtain optimal fit and function

Upper Extremity Amputation

General Considerations

A. Reasons for upper extremity amputation

1. Trauma (acute injury, electrical burns, frostbite)
2. Congenital malformations
3. Malignant tumors

B. Treatment

See Lower Extremity Amputation, page 845.

Postoperative Assessment

1. Assess the patient's response to surgery and potential hemorrhage. Monitor drainage.

2. Evaluate the patient's pain (see p. 814).

Patient Problems/Nursing Diagnoses

1. Potential problems related to surgery (e.g., hemorrhage, infection)
2. Ineffective coping related to change in body image and decreased independence
3. Potential contracture deformity related to joint immobility
4. Knowledge deficit related to management of residual limb, one-handed aids, and prosthesis

Nursing Interventions

A. Avoiding postoperative complications

1. When the patient returns from the operating room he will have either a rigid plaster of paris socket with provision for the application of a temporary prosthesis or a conventional compression bandage in place.
2. Monitor the amount and character of the suction drainage—used to eliminate hematoma and approximate the tissues.

B. Adaptation to altered body image

1. Give the patient psychological support to help him adapt to changes in his life-style.
   Listen to his fears and concerns. The patient will have impaired personal body image, loss of sensory input, and inadequate motor output.
2. Psychological problems (denial, withdrawal)—responses influenced by support and encouragement of rehabilitation team, by early introduction of one-handed activities, and by discussion of prosthetic options and capabilities.
3. Start the patient on one-handed self-care activities as soon as possible—to promote independence. Occupational therapist teaches self-feeding, bathing, grooming, etc.

C. Prevention of contractures

1. Encourage active motion of residual limb after mobility restrictions have been removed.
   Exercises are carried out to prevent contracture, obtain full range of motion, combat muscle atrophy, increase muscle strength, and prepare residual limb for prosthesis.
   a. Muscle setting, joint mobilizing, range-of-motion exercises are performed as soon as tolerated—to strengthen muscles and joints (under direction of physical therapist).
   b. Exercise muscles of both shoulders—an upper extremity amputee uses both shoulders to operate prosthesis.
   c. Carry out postural exercises—loss of weight of amputated extremity may produce postural abnormality.
2. Assess for residual limb contraction or residual limb contour problems.

D. Residual limb care (upper extremity)

1. Assist with dressing change and inspect wound.
   a. *Rigid dressing*
      A plaster socket with temporary prosthetic device is applied—increases the patient's endurance, allows early prosthetic training and fitting of permanent prosthetic device.
   b. *Compression dressing* (Fig. 19-14)
      (1) Rewrap the residual limb 3–4 times daily—to maintain proper tension in the bandage and to reduce the fluid and shape the residual limb so that a prosthesis may be fitted.
      (2) Keep residual limb snugly wrapped with elastic bandage for 24-hour period except for periods of bathing and exercise.
      (3) Teach the patient and his family the correct technique of application since residual limb wrapping will be continued until the permanent prosthesis is fitted (6 weeks–1 year).

E. Self-care activities

1. Discuss the available prosthetic replacement (by orthotist, physical therapist).
   The fitting of the prosthesis depends on the level of amputation, age of the patient, and whether weakness or limitation of range of motion of joints proximal to amputation site is present.
   a. The patient will require instruction in putting on and removing prosthesis, control of prosthesis, etc.
   b. Ultimate patient rehabilitation ideally requires the services and supervision of rehabilitation team at a comprehensive medical rehabilitation unit or center.
2. Demonstrate aids to independence (one-handed knife for cutting, elastic shoelaces, one-handed methods of functioning)—usually done in cooperation with occupational therapist.
3. Teach how to assess for skin problems—from irritants in prosthetic components, lack of ventilation.

Health Education

Instruct the patient to maintain careful residual limb hygiene to prevent skin irritation and infection.
1. Wash and dry residual limb thoroughly at least twice daily.
2. Wear residual limb sock. Change daily (and wash immediately)—to absorb perspiration and avoid direct contact between prosthetic socket and skin.
3. Avoid wrinkles in residual limb sock—may irritate skin.
4. Wipe the socket of prosthesis with damp cloth upon removal in evening.
5. Wear cotton tee shirt—to prevent contact between skin and shoulder harness and to absorb perspiration. Change daily.
6. Inspect the skin under harness for pressure, irritation, and abrasion.
7. Launder the washable portions of the harness as often as necessary; if practical, have two harnesses so that one can be laundered while the other is worn.
8. Have prosthesis checked periodically.

Expected Outcomes

1. Avoids problems related to amputation; hematology values normal; residual limb heals without infection
2. Exhibits adjustment to change in body image and functions independently; uses residual limb, uses one arm aids as necessary
3. Avoids development of joint contracture; exercises joint routinely, obtains full range of motion, maintains muscle strength
4. Demonstrates ability to care for residual limb, prosthesis, and self; washes residual limb daily, wraps residual limb to shrink and shape it, uses self-help aids as needed

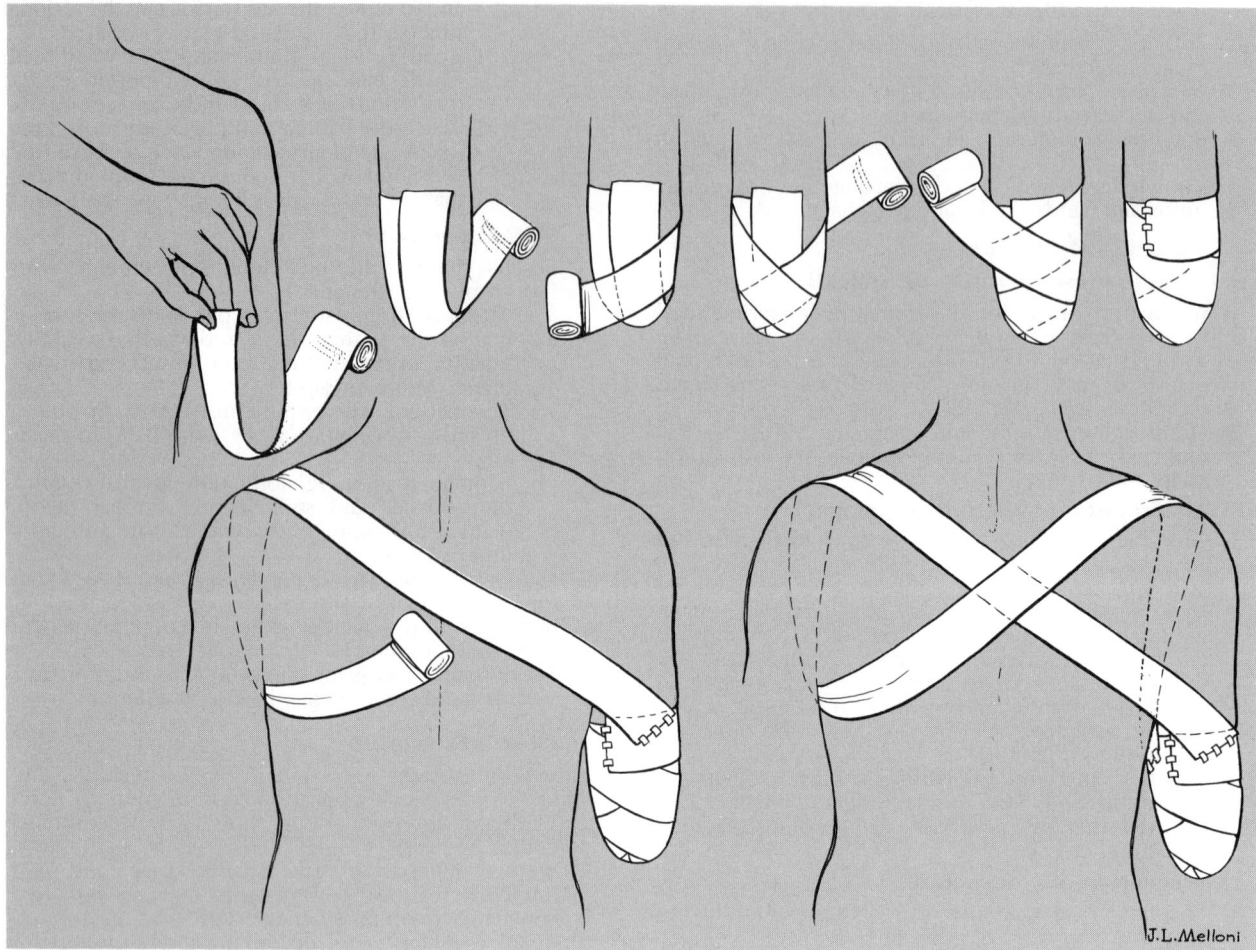

Figure 19-14. Wrapping above-elbow residual limb. An elastic bandage wrapping for an above-the-elbow residual limb minimizes edema and shapes it for a prosthesis. The bandage may need to be secured by wrapping across the back and shoulders.

Low Back Pain

Low back pain is characterized by an uncomfortable or acute pain in the lumbosacral area associated with severe spasm of the paraspinal muscles, often with radiating pain.

Muscle spasm is a condition in which muscles are painfully contracted.

Etiology

(Multiple causes)
1. Mechanical (joint, muscular, or ligamentous sprain)
2. Congenital disorders
3. Degenerative disc disease; acute herniation of disc(s)
4. Lack of physical activity and exercise; weakness of musculature
5. Arthritic conditions
6. Predisposing endocrine and systemic diseases
7. Diseases of bone (Paget's disease, metastatic carcinoma)
8. Infections of disc spaces or vertebrae
9. Spinal cord tumors
10. Referred pain from other areas

Treatment

1. Advise the patient to rest in bed in a semi-Fowler's position (hips and knees flexed)—to relieve painful muscle and ligament sprain, heal soft tissue injury, remove stress from lumbar sacral area, relieve tension on sciatic nerves, and open the posterior part of the intervertebral spaces
   a. Acute spasm should subside in 3–7 days if there is no nerve involvement or other serious underlying disease.
   b. Do prescribed isometric exercises hourly while on bed rest if possible.
2. Use heat or ice to relax muscle spasm and relieve discomfort. Follow heat by massage.

3. Medications
   a. Give oral pain medication and muscle relaxants.
   b. Inject painful trigger points with hydrocortisone/ xylocaine for pain relief (by physician).
   c. Use parenteral pain medication in acute severe pain syndromes.
4. Pelvic traction and manipulation may be used.
5. Lumbosacral support may be used—provides abdominal compression and decreases load on lumbar intervertebral discs.
6. Transcutaneous nerve stimulation (TENS) may be helpful.
7. Psychiatric intervention may be needed for the patient with chronic depression, anxiety, and low back syndrome.
   a. The patient may undergo psychological testing (Minnesota Multiphasic Personality Inventory [MMPI])
   b. Psychotropic medication may be used for treatment of depression and anxiety, which potentiate pain.
8. Myelogram if patient shows no improvement after 7–10 days of conservative treatment, when there is a neurologic deficit, intractable pain, loss of bowel or bladder control; operative intervention may be necessary. (See page 807 for treatment of herniated nucleus pulposus.)

Assessment

1. History—to determine when, where, and how the pain occurs, aggravating or relieving factors, relationship of pain to specific activities, presence of numbness or paresthesia.
2. Neurologic evaluation—to spot localized weakness of extremities and reflex and sensory loss; to exclude neurogenic disease.
3. Evaluation of muscular system—for changes in strength, tone, and flexibility of key posture muscles.
4. Diagnostic studies may be conducted
   a. Electromyography—to record changes in electric potential of muscle and of nerve leading to it.
   b. X-ray—of lumbar spine (anteroposterior, lateral, and oblique)
   c. Myelography; computed tomography

Nursing Interventions

A. Relief of discomfort

See Pain (alteration in comfort) related to musculoskeletal disorders, page 814.
1. Advise the patient to rest in bed. (Rest in bed may eliminate the need for pain medications.)
2. Keep pillow between flexed knees while in side-lying position.
3. Apply moist warm heat (moist towels, hydrocolator packs) as prescribed.
4. Administer pain medications and muscle relaxants as prescribed.

B. Resumption of activities

See Psychological and Social Problems related to musculoskeletal problems, page 815.
1. Encourage the patient to discuss problems that may be contributing to his backache.
2. Advise the patient to start activity as soon as possible— activity speeds recovery and helps prevent loss of muscle function.
3. Encourage the patient to do prescribed back exercises (Fig. 19-15). Exercise keeps postural muscles strong, helps recondition the back and abdominal musculature, and serves as an outlet for emotional tension.

Health Education

Instruct the patient to avoid recurrences as follows:
1. Standing, sitting, lying, and lifting properly are necessary for a healthy back.
2. Pace yourself. Keep *moving* and *active,* alternating periods of activity with periods of rest.
   a. Avoid prolonged *sitting* (intradiscal pressure in lumbar spine is higher during sitting), standing, and driving.

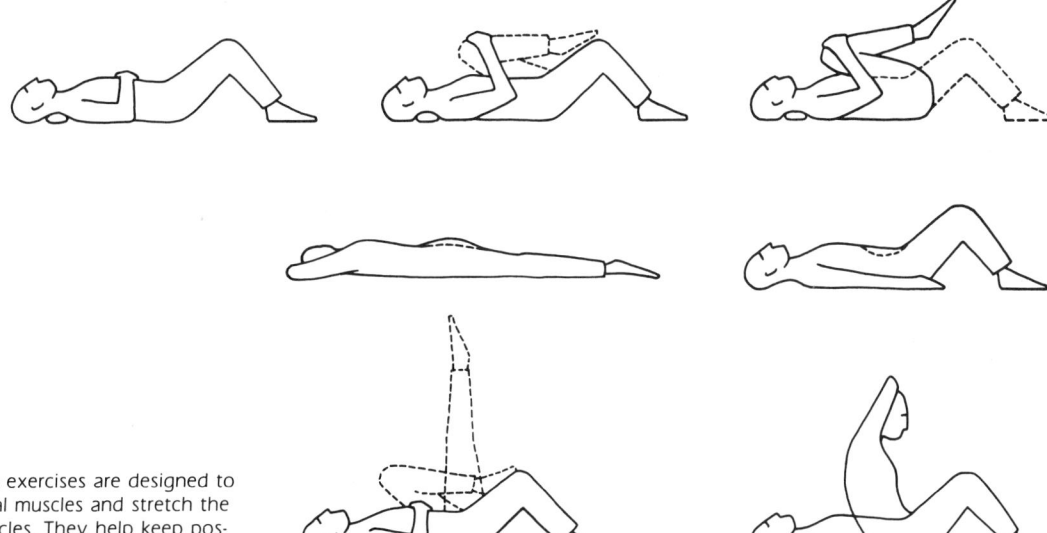

Figure 19-15. Back exercises are designed to strengthen abdominal muscles and stretch the contracted back muscles. They help keep posture muscles strong and flexible.

b. Avoid assuming tense, cramped positions.
c. Sit in a straight back, fairly high-seated chair. Sit with the knees higher than the hips. Use a footstool.
d. Flatten the hollow of the back by sitting with the buttocks "tucked under."
Pelvic tilt (small of back is pressed against a flat surface)—decreases lordosis.
e. Avoid knee and hip extension. When driving a car, have the seat pushed forward as necessary for comfort. Place a cushion in the small of the back for support.
3. When standing for any length of time, rest one foot on a small stool or wooden box to relieve lumbar lordosis.
4. When lying on the side, place a pillow under the head and one between the legs, which should be flexed at the knees.

a. Rest at short intervals—fatigue contributes to spasm of the back muscles.
b. Avoid sleeping in a prone position.
c. Use a firm mattress.
5. Pick up objects or loads correctly.
a. Maintain a straight spine.
b. Flex knees and hips while stooping.
c. Keep load close to body.
d. Lift with the legs. Avoid twisting trunk while lifting.
e. Avoid lifting above waist level and reaching up for any length of time.
6. *Daily exercise is important in the prevention of back problems.*
a. Do prescribed back exercises twice daily.
b. Walking outdoors (progressively increasing distance and pace) is recommended.
c. Reduce weight if necessary.

Osteoporosis

Osteoporosis is a condition in which the bone matrix is lost, thereby weakening the bones and making them more susceptible to fracture.

Etiology

1. Osteoporosis is a condition of the elderly, particularly the postmenopausal woman.
2. The demineralization is a silent process, causing no apparent problem until a fracture occurs.
3. Factors associated with the bone mass loss include decrease in estrogen level, calcium deficiency, insufficient vitamin D intake, and lack of exercise.

Treatment

Major effort is aimed at *prevention* of the condition.
1. Adequate intake of calcium
2. Adequate intake of vitamin D and exposure to sunlight
3. Weight-bearing exercise (walking) throughout life
4. Use of estrogen therapy for the menopausal woman
5. Treatment of fracture when it occurs—most frequently fractures of the distal radius, vertebral bodies, proximal humerus, pelvis, and proximal femur (hip)
6. Prevention of falls in the elderly

Assessment

1. Identify patients at risk—middle-aged to elderly patients, particularly inactive white females.
2. Review the patient's dietary patterns—assess for adequate calcium and vitamin D intake.
3. Determine use of estrogens in menopausal and postmenopausal women.

4. Note fractures associated with osteoporosis. Fracture occurs after minor trauma.
5. Review x-ray reports for evidence of osteoporosis.
6. Assess symptoms associated with vertebral compression fracture—local back pain, loss of body height, kyphosis, respiratory (e.g., hypoventilation, episodic pneumonia) and abdominal (e.g., bloating, constipation) symptoms.

Health Education

1. Encourage exercise for all. Teach the value of walking daily throughout life to provide stress required for strong bone remodeling.
2. Give dietary education in relation to adequate calcium intake. Daily intake of 1,000–1,500 mg. of calcium a day may decrease the development of osteoporosis. Anyone with a history of urinary tract stones should consult with the physician before increasing calcium intake.
3. Participate in dietary education related to vitamin D intake. Vitamin D is required for calcium absorption and utilization. Vitamin D requirements increase with age, especially when the person is not exposed to the sun.
4. Teach strategies to prevent falls. Assess home for hazards (e.g., scatter rugs, slippery floors, extension cords, adequate lighting). Encourage use of walking aids when balance is poor and muscle strength weakens.

Bone Tumors

Pathophysiology

A. Benign Bone Tumors

Osteochondroma, chondroma, and osteoclastoma (benign giant cell tumor) are examples of some benign bone tumors. Malignant transformation occurs with some.

B. Malignant Bone Tumors

1. Chondrosarcoma and osteosarcoma are examples of primary malignant bone tumors. Hematogenous spread to the lung occurs.
2. Multiple myeloma is a malignant neoplasm arising from the bone marrow.

C. Metastatic Bone Tumors

Metastatic bone tumors are most frequently associated with cancers of the breast, the prostate, and the lung (primary malignancy site).

Treatment

1. Treatment depends on the type of tumor.
2. A multidisciplinary approach in a cancer center is often preferred.
3. The basic objective is to halt the progression of the tumor by destroying or removing the lesion.
   a. Tumor curettement or resection with bone grafting may be used.
   b. Surgical ablation of the tumor may require amputation or disarticulation of affected extremity. See nursing management following amputation, page 846.
      (1) Some centers are performing limb-salvaging procedures (resection of affected bone and surrounding normal muscle tissue and reconstruction using metallic prostheses or allografts for bone/joint replacement).
   c. Chemotherapy—to eradicate micrometastatic lesions.
      (1) Chemotherapy used in combination to achieve a greater patient response at a lower toxicity rate and to minimize potential problems of drug resistance.
      (2) Chemotherapy may be administered before and after surgery.
      (3) Combinations of chemotherapeutic agents may be given in varying courses separated by rest periods.
         (a) Vincristine, high dose methotrexate with citrovorum factor, doxorubicin and cyclophosphamide in various combinations.
            (i) Vincristine—given IV before methotrexate infusion—may promote methotrexate uptake by tumor cells
            (ii) High-dose methotrexate—given by infusion to destroy malignant cells
            (iii) Citrovorum factor—"rescue" of the patient from methotrexate by allowing larger doses of methotrexate; prevents excess toxicity
         (b) Doxorubicin (antitumor antibiotic) given in high doses; may be given alone or in combination with other agents.
         (c) Chemotherapy may be used in combination with radiation therapy.
   d. Tumor irradiation may be used.
   e. Immunotherapeutic approach may be selected.
   f. Hormone therapy may be used with metastatic tumors of the breast and prostate.
4. Prophylactic lung irradiation may be carried out—to suppress metastases.
   Thoracotomy (pulmonary resection)—for treatment of pulmonary metastases.
5. If pathologic fracture occurs, the fracture is managed with open reduction and internal fixation or other fracture treatment method.

Assessment

1. Assess for pain in the involved bone—from effects of tumor (destruction, erosion, and expansion of bone)
   a. Generally mild to constant pain which may be worse at night or with activity.
   b. Pain will be acute with fracture.
   c. Neurologic symptoms may present with nerve root compression.
2. Note swelling and limitation of motion and joint effusion
3. *Physical findings*
   a. Palpable, tender, fixed bony mass
   b. Increase in skin temperature over mass
   c. Superficial veins dilated and prominent
4. Note diagnostic test findings.
   a. X-ray will usually reveal bone tumor; may show increased or decreased bone density
   b. Bone scan—helpful in detecting initial extent of malignancy, planning therapy, defining level of amputation, and following course of radiation/chemotherapy
   c. Serum alkaline phosphatase—usually increased
   d. Biopsy of bone—to confirm suspected diagnosis
   e. Chest x-ray and lung scan—to determine if metastases are present
   f. Arteriography—to assess soft tissue involvement
5. Assess psychological status of the patient for coping mechanisms.
6. Determine understanding of condition and treatment regimen.

Patient Problems/Nursing Diagnoses

1. Alteration in comfort related to bone tumor
2. Potential for pathologic fracture related to bone tumor and immobility
3. Alteration in emotional status related to diagnosis and treatment regimen
4. Alteration in ability to perform self-care activities related to pathology

Nursing Interventions

A. Relief of pain

See Pain (alteration in comfort) related to musculoskeletal problems, page 814.
1. Administer pain medications $\frac{1}{2}$ hour before ambulation or other uncomfortable movement.
2. Support painful extremities on pillows.

B. Prevention of pathological fractures

1. Assist the patient in movement with gentleness and patience.
2. Avoid jarring the patient or bed.
3. Support joints when repositioning the patient.
4. Guard the patient to avoid falls.
5. Create a hazard-free environment.

C. Strengthening of coping abilities

See Psychological and social problems associated with musculoskeletal problems, page 815.
1. Create a supportive environment.
2. Utilize psychological support services as needed.

D. Promotion of self-care activities

1. Encourage the patient to help self.
2. Allow sufficient time for the patient to complete tasks.
3. Space activities to avoid fatigue.
4. Assist the patient as needed.

Expected Outcomes

1. Achieves comfort; uses medications and/or other modalities to reduce discomfort and states increased comfort

2. Avoids pathologic fracture; uses safety precautions to prevent falls and moves slowly and carefully.
3. Demonstrates ability to cope with demands of condition and treatment regimen; explores responses to

medical problem and participates in decision making process
4. Participates in self-care activities; feeds self and performs hygiene care

Bibliography

Books

American Academy of Orthopedic Surgeons. Symposium on Trauma to the Legs and its Sequelae. St Louis, CV Mosby, 1981

Apley AF and Solomon L. Apley's System of Orthopaedics and Fractures, London, Butterworth Scientific, 1982

Avioli LV (ed). The Osteoporotic Syndrome. New York, Grune & Stratton, 1983

Banerjee SN and Basmajian JV. Rehabilitation Management of Amputees. Baltimore, Williams & Wilkins, 1982

Brantley P and Analla M. The Nurse and Orthopedic Surgery. Rutherford, NJ, Orthopedic Nurses' Assoc, 1980

Brunner N. Orthopedic Nursing, A Programmed Approach, 4th ed. St Louis, CV Mosby, 1983

Cyriax J and Cyriax P. Illustrated Manual of Orthopaedic Medicine. London, Butterworth Scientific, 1983

Donahoo C and Spickler L. Core Curriculum of Orthopedic Nursing. Atlanta, Ga. Orthopedic Nurses' Assoc, 1980

Duthie RB and Bentley G. Mercer's Orthopedic Surgery, 8th ed. London, Edward Arnold, 1983

Edmonson A and Crenshaw A. Campbell's Operative Orthopedics, 6th ed. St Louis, CV Mosby, 1980

Farrell J. Illustrated Guide to Orthopedic Nursing, 2nd ed. Philadelphia, JB Lippincott, 1982

Finneson B. Low Back Pain, 2nd ed. Philadelphia, JB Lippincott, 1980

Hilt N. Manual of Orthopedics. St Louis, CV Mosby, 1980

Kane W. Current Orthopaedic Management. New York, Churchill Livingstone, 1981

Kostuik J and Gillespie R. Amputation Surgery and Rehabilitation: The Toronto Experience. New York, Churchill Livingstone, 1981

McRae R. Clinical Orthopaedic Examination, 2nd ed. Edinburgh, Churchill Livingstone, 1983

McWilliams N. Manual of Orthopedic Surgery for Nurses. Bowie, MD, Robert J Brady, 1982

Mears D. External Skeletal Fixation. Baltimore, Williams & Wilkins, 1983

Minor M and Minor S. Patient Care Skills. Reston, VA, Reston Publishing Co, 1984

Nickel VL. Orthopedic Rehabilitation. New York, Churchill Livingstone, 1983

Nursing Photobook. Working with Orthopedic Patients: Nursing Skillbook. Springhouse, PA, Intermed Communications, 1982

Pinney E and Stone E. Orthopaedic Nursing, 6th ed. London, Bailliere Tindall, 1983

Powell M. Orthopaedic Nursing and Rehabilitation, 8th ed. Edinburgh, Churchill Livingstone, 1982

Roaf R and Hodkinson L. Textbook of Orthopaedic Nursing, 3rd ed. Oxford, Blackwell Scientific Publications, 1980

Salter R. Textbook of Disorders and Injuries of the Musculoskeletal System, 2nd ed. Baltimore, Williams & Wilkins, 1983

Stanton-Hicks M and Boas RA (eds). Chronic Low Back Pain. New York, Raven Press, 1982

Stewart JD and Hallett JP. Traction and Orthopaedic Appliances, 2nd ed. Edinburgh, Churchill Livingstone, 1983

Straub L and Wilson P. Clinical Trends in Orthopaedics. New York, Thieme-Stratton, 1982

Turek SL. Orthopaedics: Principles and their Application, 4th ed, Vol. 1 & 2. Philadelphia, JB Lippincott, 1984

Turner RH and Scheller A. Revision Total Hip Arthroplasty. New York, Grune & Stratton, 1982

Wilkinson HA. The Failed Back Syndrome: Etiology and Therapy. Philadelphia, Harper & Row, 1983

Articles
Assessment/Diagnostic Procedures

Arthroscopy of the knee (monograph). National Association of Orthopaedic Nurses, 1983

Derscheid G. Rehabilitation of common orthopedic problems. Nurs Clin North Am 1981 Dec; 16(4):709–720

Farrell J. Arthroscopy. Nursing '82 1982 May; 12(5):73–75

Herndon J: Orthopedic surgery. Surg Clin North Am 1983 Jun; 63(3):513–578

Hirsch P: Office orthopedic practice. Orthop Clin North Am 1982 Jul; 13(3):427–586

Jensen J et al: Nutrition in orthopaedic surgery. J Bone Joint Surg (Am) 1982 Dec; 64-A(9):1263–1272

Policoff LD. Effective use of physical modalities. Orthop Clin North Am 1982 Jul; 13:579–586

Smith C. Orthopaedics and the elderly. Nurs Times 1984 Apr 11–17; 80(15): 46–49

Tepperman P and Devlin M: Therapeutic heat and cold. Postgrad Med 1983 Jan; 73(1):69–76

Nursing Assessment

Duetsch S and Gandsman E. Diagnosis and management of musculo-skeletal trauma. Surg Clin North Am 1983 Jun; 63(3):580–583

Dunn B. Components of the musculoskeletal examination. Orthop Nurs 1982 Nov/Dec; 1(6):33–36

Dunn B. Musculoskeletal assessment (Gait assessment). Orthop Nurs 1982 May/Jun; 1(3):33–37

Farrell J. The human side of assessment. Nursing '80 1980 Apr; 10(4):10–14

Hackett C. Limbering up your neurovascular assessment technique. Nursing '83 1983 Mar; 13(3):40–43

Hilt N. Musculoskeletal assessment (Screening for congenital dislocation of the hip). Orthop Nurs 1982 Mar/Apr; 1(2):22–24

Jobes R. Musculoskeletal assessment (Cranial nerve assessment with halo traction). Orthop Nurs 1982 Jul/Aug; 1(4):11–15

Laughlin R and Clancey G. Musculoskeletal assessment (Neurovascular examination of the injured extremity). Orthop Nurs 1982 Jan/Feb; 1(1):43–48

Malkiewicz J. A pragmatic approach to musculoskeletal assessment. RN 1982 Nov; 45(11):57–62

Rodts MF. An orthopedic assessment you can do in 15 minutes. Nursing '83 1983 May; 13(5):65–73

Ross D. Musculoskeletal assessment (Range of motion of the fingers and hand). Orthop Nurs 1982 Sep/Oct; 1(5):11–17

Ross D. Musculoskeletal assessment: the knee. Orthop Nurs 1983 Sep/Oct; 2(5):23–28

Taylor S. Musculoskeletal assessment (Low back pain assessment: Part I—History taking). Orthop Nurs 1983 Jul/Aug; 2(4):11–16

Taylor S. Musculoskeletal assessment (Low back pain assessment: Part II—Defining range of motion and terminology). Orthop Nurs 1983 Sep/Oct; 2(5):39–44

Taylor S. Musculoskeletal assessment (Low back pain assessment: Part III—The physical examination). Orthop Nurs 1983 Nov/Dec; 2(6):21–27

Wassel A. Nursing assessment of injuries to the lower extremity. Nurs Clin North Am 1981 Dec; 16(4):739–748

Common Problems

Aaron RK and Ciombor D. Venous thromboembolism in the orthopedic patient. Surg Clin North Am 1983 Jun; 63(3):529–537

Brighton C: Electrically induced osteogenesis. Ortho Clin North Am 1984 Jan; 15(1):1–174

Cardona V: Trauma post-op: The real nursing challenge. RN 1982 Mar; 45(3):23–29

Ceccio C: Postoperative pain relief

through relaxation in elderly patients with fractured hips. Orthop Nurs 1984 May/Jun; 3(3):11–19

DiPiro J et al: The prophylactic use of antimicrobials in surgery. Curr Prob Surg 1983 Feb; 20(2):109–112

Fahey VA: An indepth look at deep vein thrombosis. Nursing '84 1984 Mar; 14(3):34–41

Farrell J: Orthopedic pain: what does it mean? Am J Nurs 1984 Apr; 84(4): 466–469

Fitzgerald R and Thompson R: Cephalosporin antibiotics in the prevention and treatment of musculoskeletal sepsis. J Bone Joint Surg (Am) 1983 Oct; 65-A(8):1201–1205

Gates S. Helping your patient on bedrest cope with perceptual–sensory deprivation. Orthop Nurs 1984 Mar/Apr; 3(2):35–38

Hayden JW. Compartment syndromes. Postgrad Med 1983 Jul; 74(1):191–202

Jensen JE et al. Nutrition in orthopedic surgery. J Bone Joint Surg [Am] 1982 Dec; 64(9):1263–1272

Lentz M. Selected aspects of deconditioning secondary to immobility. Nurs Clin North Am 1981 Dec; 16(4):729–737

Martin S. Fat embolism syndrome. DCCN 1983 May/Jun; 2(3):158–161

Meyer TM: TENS—relieving pain through electricity. Nursing '82 1982 Sep; 12(9):57–59

Moore DE and Blacker HM: How effective is TENS for chronic pain? Am J Nurs 1983 Aug; 83(8):1175–1177

Mubarak S and Hargens A: Acute compartment syndromes. Surg Clin North Am 1983 Jun; 63(3):539–565

Schutt RC Jr, Winter WG and Kempczinski RF. The management of orthopedic patients with arterial insufficiency. Clin Orthop 1982 Jun; (166):212–218

Sigmon HD. Helping your long-term trauma patient travel the road to recovery. Nursing '84 1984 Jan; 14(1): 58–63

Taylor AG et al: How effective is TENS for acute pain? Am J Nurs 1983 Aug; 83(8):1171–1174

Turner P. Caring for emotional needs of orthopedic trauma patients. AORN J 1982 Oct; 36(4):566–570

Injuries and Fractures

Bailey M. Emergency! first aid for fractures. Nursing '82 1982 Nov; 12(11):72–81

Brown SL. Avoiding postop pitfalls with hip fracture patients. RN 1982 May; 45(5):48–54

Duerksen J. Hip fractures: Special considerations for the elderly patient. Orthop Nurs 1982 Jan/Feb; 1(1):11–22

Keene JS and Anderson CA. Hip fractures in the elderly. JAMA 1982 Aug 6; 248(5):564–567

Meyers M. Pitfalls in simple fracture care. Postgrad Med 1982 Jun; 71(6): 181–192

Spickler LL. Knee injuries of the athlete. Orthop Nurs 1983 Sep/Oct; 2(5):11–19

Wassel A. Sports medicine: Acute and overuse injuries. Orthop Nurs 1984 Mar/Apr; 3(2):29–33

Casts/Traction/External Fixation Devices

Brooker A. New techniques in fracture management. Surg Clin North Am 1983 Jun; 63(3):607–629

Cass AS et al. Bladder problems in pelvic injuries treated with external fixator and direct urethral drainage. J Trauma 1983 Jan; 23(1):50–53

Coppola AJ Jr and Anzel SH. Use of the Hoffmann external fixator in the treatment of femoral fractures. Clin Orthop 1983 Nov; (180):78–82

Gill KP and Laflamme D. External fixation: the erector sets of orthopedic nursing. Can Nurse 1984 May; 80(5): 29–31

Hankin FM, Gragg AJ and Kaufer H. Bleeding beneath postoperative plaster casts. Orthop Nurs 1983 Jan/Feb; 2(1):27–31

Howard M and Corbo-Pelaia SA. The psychological after-effects of halo traction and a review of acute care. Am J Nurs 1982 Dec; 82(12):1839–1843

Kelly D. The use of fiberglass as reinforcement with plaster cast. Orthop Nurs 1983 Nov/Dec; 2(6):33–38

Lane P and Lee M. New synthetic casts: What nurses need to know. Orthop Nurs 1982 Nov/Dec; 1(6):13–20

Lane P and Lee M. Special care for special casts. Nursing '83 1983 Jul; 13(7):50–51

McFarland M. Encircling cast drainage: Is it valuable? Orthop Nurs 1984 Mar/Apr; 3(2):29–33

Milazzo V. An exercise class for patients in traction. Am J Nurs 1981 Oct; 81(10):1842–1844

Miller MC. Nursing care of the patient with external fixation therapy. Orthop Nurs 1983 Jan/Feb; 2(1):11–15

Trigueiro M. Pin site care protocol. Can Nurse 1983 Sep; 79(8):24–26

Vidal J et al. Guidelines for treatment of open fractures and infected pseudarthroses by external fixation. Clin Orthop 1983 Nov; (180):83–95

Arthroplasty and Total Joint Replacement

Aaron RK. Total joint arthroplasty. Surg Clin North Am 1983 Jun; 63(3):697–715

Ceder L, Thorngren K and Walden B. Prognostic indicators and early home rehabilitation in elderly patients with hip fractures. Clin Orthop 1980 Oct; (152):173–184

Ceder L, Svensson K and Thorngren K. Statistical prediction of rehabilitation in elderly patients with hip fracture. Clin Orthop 1980 Oct; (152):185–190

Coutts J et al. The role of continuous passive motion in the postoperative rehabilitation of the total knee patient. Orthop Trans 1982 Summer; 6(2): 277–278

Dorr L, Taker G and Conaty J. Total hip arthroplasties in patients less than

forty-five years old. J Bone Joint Surg (Am) 1983 Apr; 65-A(4):474–479

Engh C. Hip arthroplasty with a Moore prosthesis with porous coating: A five year study. Clin Orthop 1983 Jun; (176):52–66

Frank C et al. Physiology and therapeutic value of passive joint motion. Clin Orthop 1984 May; (185): 113–125

Greene WB. The role of continuous passive slow motion in the postoperative rehabilitation of difficult pediatric knee and elbow problems. J Pediatr Ortho 1983 Sep; 3(4):419–423

Harrold AJ: Outlook for hip replacement (letter). Br Med J (Clin Res) 1982 Feb 13; 284(6314):509

Hecht PJ et al. Effects of thermal therapy on rehabilitation after total knee arthroplasty. Clin Orthop 1983 Sep; (178):198–201

Herndon JH and Hubbard LF. Total joint replacement in the upper extremity. Surg Clin North Am 1983 Jun; 63(3): 715–736

Jensen JE et al. Nutritional assessment of orthopaedic patients undergoing total hip replacement surgery. Hip 1981; 123–135

Jolley MN, Salvati EA and Brown GC. Early results and complications of surface replacement of the hip. J Bone Joint Surg (Am) 1982 Mar; 64(3):366–377

Korcok M. Motion, not immobility, advocated for healing synovial joints. (Medical News). JAMA 1981 Nov 6; 246(18):2005–2006

Mattix MW. Preoperative education for the total hip patient. ONA J 1979 Jun; 6(6):251–252

Nelson JP et al. The effects of previous surgery, operating environment, and preventive antibiotics on post operative infection following total hip arthroplasty. Clin Orthop 1980 Mar/Apr; (147):167–169

Papademetriou T. Joint replacement in the lower extremities of the elderly. Primary Care 1982 Mar; 9(1):197–208

Ratliff AH. Vascular and neurologic complications following total hip replacement. Hip 1981; 276–292

Scott WN (ed). Total knee arthroplasty. Orthop Clin North Am 1982 Jan; 13(1):1–249

Spindler C. Audiovisual preoperative teaching for the total hip patient. Orthop Nurs 1984 Jan/Feb; 3(1):30–40

Amputation

Burgess E. Amputation. Surg Clin North Am 1983 Jun; 63(3):749–770

Clark MW. Consultations. Orthop Nurs 1982 May/Jun; 1(3):19

Farrell J. Helping the new amputee. Orthop Nurs 1982 May/Jun; 1(3):18–19

Gandy ED. Help the amputee stand on his own again. Nursing '84 1984 Jul; 14(7):46–49

Littlefield C and Strube P. Care and wrapping of a below-knee stump. (Videorecording). Chapel Hill, NC, University of South Carolina, 1979

Littlefield C and Smith I. Care and wrapping of an above-knee stump. (Videorecording). Chapel Hill, NC, University of South Carolina, 1984

Moye CR. Nursing care of the amputee: an overview. Orthop Nurs 1982 May/Jun; 1(3):11–13

Rutan FM. Preprosthetic program for the amputee. Orthop Nurs 1982; 1(3):14–17

Smith A. Common problems of lower extremity amputees. Orthop Clin North Am 1982 Jul; 13(3):569–578

Stratmann D and Donnelly L. Determination of ideal body weight and nutritional requirements post-amputation. Orthop Nurs 1984 May/Jun; 3(2):37–40

Walters J. Coping with a leg amputation. Am J Nurs 1981 Jul; 81(7):1349–1352

Low Back Pain

Burton C. Conservative management of low back pain. Postgrad Med 1981 Nov; 70(5):168–183

Howden L. Basic back care: it doesn't have to hurt. Can Nurse 1981 Jul/Aug; 77(4):46–50

Jones A et al. Treating chronic low back pain. Phys Ther 1980 Jan; 60(1):58–63

Keim H and Kirkaldy-Willis W. Low back pain. Clin Symp 1980; 32(6):entire issue

McCarthy R. Coping with low back pain through behavioral change. Orthop Nurs 1984 May/Jun; 3(3):30–35

Mulford E. Degenerative disease or slipped disc? . . . assessment of low back pain. RN 1981 Feb; 44(2):44–49

Myofascial origins of low back pain: 1. Principles of diagnosis and treatment. Postgrad Med 1983 Feb; 73(2):66, 68–70, 73

O'Keeffe MC. Long term back clients: a review of multidisciplinary evaluations of Federal workers' compensation clients. Orthop Nurs 1983 Jan/Feb; 2(1):33–35

Petty NE and Mastria MA. Management of compliance to progressive relaxation and orthopedic exercises in treatment of chronic back pain. Psychol Rep 1983 Feb; 52(1):35–38

Selby D. Conservative care of nonspecific low back pain. Orthop Clin North Am 1982 Jul; 13(3):427–438

Osteoporosis

Aloia JF. Exercise and skeletal health. J Am Geriatr Soc 1981 Mar; 29(3):104–107

Aloia JF. Estrogen and exercise in prevention and treatment of osteoporosis. Geriatrics 1982 Jun; 37(6):81–85

Breaking news on osteoporosis (clinical news). Am J Nurs 1984 Jun; 84(6):708–710

Deni L. Osteoporosis: the unnecessary crippler of women. J Nurs Care 1981 Jan; 14(1):10–13

Dickenson RP, Hutton WC and Stott JR. The mechanical properties of bone in osteoporosis. J Bone Joint Surg (Br) 1981 Aug; 63-B(2):233–238

Faehnrick J. When pathological fractures threaten. RN 1983 Nov; 46(11):34–37

Frost HM (ed). Symposium on osteoporosis. Orthop Clin North Am 1981 July; 12(3):entire issue

Gonzales ER. Premature bone loss found in some nonmenstruating sportswomen (news) JAMA 1982 Aug 6; 249(5):513–514

Gregory CA. Possible influence of physical activity on musculoskeletal symptoms of menopausal and postmenopausal women. JOGN Nurs 1982 Mar/Apr; 11(2):103–107

Gruber HE and Baylink DJ. The diagnosis of osteoporosis. J Am Geriatr Soc 1981 Nov; 29(11):490–497

Handy RC. Osteoporosis: aetiology and management. Practitioner 1983 Jul; 227(1381):1127–1136

Kanis JA. Treatment of osteoporotic fracture. Lancet 1984 Jan 7; 1(8367):27–33

Korcok M. Adding exercise to calcium in osteoporosis prevention. JAMA 1982 Feb 26; 247(8):1106, 1112

Krolner B and Toft B. Vertebral bone loss: An unheeded side effect of therapeutic bed rest. Clin Sci 1983 May; 64(5):537–540

Kruse HP and Kuhlencordt F. Pathogenesis and natural course of primary osteoporosis. Lancet 1980 Feb 9; (8163):280–282

Lane JM and Vigorita VJ. Osteoporosis. J Bone Joint Surg (Am) 1983 Feb; 62(2):247–278

Lukert BP. Osteoporosis—a review and update. Arch Phys Med Rehabil 1982 Oct; 63(10):480–487

Mallette LE. Osteoporosis. Approaching treatment with optimism. Postgrad Med 1982 Nov; 72(5):271–278

Palma LF. Family practice grand rounds. Postmenopausal osteoporosis and estrogen therapy: Who should be treated? J Fam Pract 1982 Feb; 14(2):355–359

Parfitt AM. Dietary risk factors for age-related bone loss and fractures. Lancet 1983 Nov 19; 2(8360):1181–1185

Raisz LG. Osteoporosis. J Am Geriatr Soc 1982 Feb; 30(2):127–138

Richards M. Osteoporosis. Geriatr Nurs 1982 Mar/Apr; 3(2):98–102

Riggs BL and Melton LJ 3rd. Evidence for two distinct syndromes of involutional osteoporosis. Am J Med 1983 Dec; 75(6):899–901

Seeman E and Riggs BL. Dietary prevention of bone loss in the elderly. Geriatrics 1981 Sep; 36(9):71–73, 75, 79

Spencer H. Osteoporosis: goals of therapy. Hosp Pract 1982 Mar; 17(3):131–138, 143–148

Strom BL. Are estrogens effective in preventing fractures from postmenopausal osteoporosis? Drug Ther 1982; 67–80

Bone Tumors

Bhardwaj S and Holland JF. Chemotherapy of metastatic cancer in bone. Clin Orthop 1982 Sep; (169):28–35

Greditzer HG 3rd et al. Bone sarcomas in Paget disease. Radiology 1983 Feb; 142(2):327–333

Hays K and Rafferty DC. Care of the patient with malignant lymphoma. Nurs Clin North Am 1982 Dec; 17(4):677–695

Hubbard LF. Computed tomography in orthopedics. Surg Clin North Am 1983 Jun; 63(3):591–593

Kerns LL and Simon MA. Musculoskeletal sarcomas. Surg Clin North Am 1983 Jun; 63(3):671–695

Kofoed H and Solgaard S. Resection alloplasty in the treatment of certain malignant bone tumors. Cancer 1983 Dec 1; 52(11):2180–2184

Malkawi H, Shannak A and Amr S. Surgical treatment of pathological subtrochanteric fractures due to benign lesions in children and adolescents. J Pediatr Orthop 1984 Jan; 4(1):63–69

Mankin HJ, Lange TA and Spanier SS. The hazards of biopsy in patients with malignant primary bone and soft-tissue tumors. J Bone Joint Surg (Am) 1982 Oct; 64(8):1121–1127

Schajowicz F. Current trends in the diagnosis and treatment of malignant bone tumors. Clin Orthop 1983 Nov; (180):220–252

Sherry AS, Levy RN and Siffert R. Metastatic disease of bone in orthopedic surgery. Clin Orthop 1982 Sep; (169):44–52

Infectious Diseases

20

The Infection Process

Causative Agent

Type: Bacterium, virus, fungus, parasite, rickettsia, chlamydia, etc.
1. Pathogenicity (ability to cause disease)
2. Virulence (disease severity) and invasiveness (ability to enter and move through tissue)
3. Infective dose (number of organisms needed to initiate infection)
4. Organism specificity (host preference), antigenic variations
5. Elaboration of toxins

Reservoir

(The environment in which the agent is found)
1. Human–man is the reservoir of diseases that are more dangerous to humans than to other species
2. Animal—responsible for infestations with trophozoites, worms, etc.
3. Nonanimal—street dust, garden soil, lint from bedding

Mode of Escape from Reservoir

1. Respiratory tract (most common in man)
2. Gastrointestinal tract
3. Genitourinary tract
4. Open lesions
5. Mechanical escape (includes bites of insects)
6. Blood

Mode of Transmission

There are 4 main routes of transmission:

A. By Contact Transmission

1. Direct contact (person to person)
2. Indirect contact (usually an inanimate object)
3. Droplet contact (from coughing, sneezing, or talking by an infected person)

B. By Vehicle Route (through contaminated items)

1. Food—salmonellosis
2. Water—shigellosis, legionellosis
3. Drugs—bacteremia resulting from infusion of a contaminated infusion product
4. Blood—hepatitis B, or non-A non-B hepatitis

C. Airborne Transmission

1. Droplet nuclei (residue of evaporated droplets that remain suspended in air)
2. Dust particles in the air containing the infectious agent
3. Organisms shed into environment from skin, hair, wounds, or perineal area

D. Vectorborne Transmission

Via contaminated or infected arthropods such as flies, mosquitoes, ticks, and others

Mode of Entry of Organisms into Human Body

1. Respiratory tract
2. Gastrointestinal tract
3. Genitourinary tract
4. Direct infection of mucous membranes/skin

Host Factors

Illness following entrance of infection into the body depends on:
1. Age, sex, genetic constitution of host
2. Nutritional status, fitness, environmental factors
3. General physical, mental, and emotional health
4. Absent or abnormal immunoglobulins
5. Status of hematopoietic system; efficacy of reticuloendothelial system
6. Presence of underlying disease (diabetes mellitus; lymphoma, leukemia, neoplasia, granulocytopenia, or uremia)

7. Patients treated with certain antimicrobials, corticosteroids, irradiation, or immunosuppressive agents

Epidemiology, Therapy, and Control of Communicable Infections

See Table 20-1, page 860.

Emerging Problems in Infectious Diseases

1. Increase in number of different organisms that are developing resistance to increasing numbers of available antimicrobials.

2. Increasing number of persons in state of immunosuppression. These persons, who would formerly have died from cancer, leukemia, etc., are now surviving but are susceptible to invasion by any type of organism, including those usually considered non-pathogenic.
3. Persons with serious diseases are living longer and are exposed to more aggressive surgical procedures.
4. The use of indwelling lines and implanted foreign bodies have increased, thus rendering these patients more susceptible to infections.

Control and Management of Infectious Disease

Nursing Process Overview

Assessment

History

Points to emphasize in the history:
1. Local or systemic infection?
2. History of travel?
3. Any contact with animals or animal products?
4. Any animal or insect bite? Cat scratch, exposure to birds?
5. Any illness that compromises body defenses?
6. What medications taken?
7. Vaccination history?

Clinical Manifestations

1. Assess for manifestation of infection—productive cough, skin and mucous membrane lesions, fever, diarrhea, dysuria, vomiting, purulent drainage.
2. Obtain specimens of blood, urine, stools, sputum, throat swabbings, nasal secretions, and pyogenic exudates for bacteriologic study.
3. Secure or assist in securing smears of blood and other materials for microscopic examination.
4. Assist with aspirations of spinal fluid, bone marrow, and other body fluids or tissues for cytologic, serologic, and bacteriologic tests.
5. Carry out appropriate skin tests for specific diagnostic reactions as directed.

Patient Problems/Nursing Diagnoses

1. Fluid and electrolyte imbalance related to fever, nausea, vomiting, and excessive sweating
2. Fever related to body's defense reaction to invading organism
3. Potential for spread of infection
4. Alteration in comfort (generalized aching, malaise, headache) related to effects of infection
5. Potential respiratory insufficiency related to lung congestion (if infection has effect on respiratory system)
6. Potential alteration in elimination (diarrhea, urinary frequency, burning on urination) related to underlying pathophysiology of infection
7. Potential for serious systemic complications related to progression of unabated infection
8. Ineffective coping and social isolation related to isolation techniques
9. Knowledge deficit of causes of infection, treatment, and preventive measures

Planning and Implementation

Nursing Interventions

A. Implementation of therapeutic plan to treat infection

1. Administer the appropriate antimicrobial agents as directed.
2. Assist in administering specific immune therapy, if prescribed (i.e., immune globulins, etc.).
3. Observe the patient carefully for evidence of drug or serum sensitivity.
4. Avoid damage to body barriers.
   a. Avoid invasive procedures as much as possible.
   b. Give special care to intravenous and arterial puncture sites, etc.

B. Ensuring adequate homeostasis

1. Ensure adequate hydration in the event of excessive fluid loss through vomiting, diarrhea, or excessive sweating.
   a. Encourage liberal fluid intake.
   b. Prepare for the administration of intravenous fluids as required.
2. Reduce the fever when indicated (it is often important to watch temperature curve).
   a. Administer antipyretic drugs as prescribed.
   b. Employ cool sponges cautiously as indicated (see p. 768).
3. Measure and record body temperature, pulse, and respiratory rates frequently.
4. Measure arterial pressure at regular intervals if the patient exhibits a tendency to vascular collapse.
5. Weigh the patient periodically, preferably at same hour of the day, on the same scale.

C. Measures to prevent spread of infection to others

1. *Wash hands immediately after contact with each patient and after every contact with material that may be contaminated and potentially infectious.*
   a. Wash hands even if sterile gloves are used.
   b. Wear gloves for direct exposure to blood, drainage, or secretions.
2. Plan what you are going to do *before* the initial patient contact.
3. Carry out isolation precautions as required to prevent spread of microorganisms among patients, personnel, and visitors.
4. Observe asepsis as indicated.

5. Use high-efficiency disposable mask, covering nose and mouth, when indicated.
   a. Use mask only once and discard in appropriate receptacle.
   b. Refrain from handling mask while in use.
6. Use gown when required to prevent soiling of clothing.
   a. Use gown once and discard in appropriate receptacle.
   b. Use sterile gown in certain instances (extensive burns; wounds).
   c. Collect linen in water-soluble bags; double-bag and mark "Isolation."
7. Use gloves when indicated by the patient's condition.
   a. Disposable, single-use gloves should be worn.
   b. Use once and discard in appropriate receptacle.
8. Handle needles and syringes with *extreme* care because it is usually not known which patient's blood is contaminated with hepatitis virus or other micro-organisms.
   a. Place used needles in a labeled, puncture-resistant container; do not bend or break by hand.
   b. Blood spills should be cleaned up promptly with a solution of 5.25% sodium hypochlorite solution diluted 1:10 with water.
9. Disinfect and handle wastes with all due precautions.
10. Handle bed linens and fomites with care.
11. Carry out concurrent disinfection of fomites.
12. Control dissemination of infectious droplets.
    a. Encourage the patient to cover nose and mouth when coughing or sneezing.
    b. Wrap contaminated tissues and articles in paper before disposal.
13. Control dust.
    a. Avoid creating aerosols (e.g., shaking bedlinens).
    b. Require damp dusting of furniture and wet vacuum cleaning of floors.
    c. Maintain cleanliness of surroundings; wash soil from walls as soon as it appears.
    d. Reduce to a minimum the activity of personnel in the patient's room.
14. Ventilate the patient's room properly with a system that directs room air to the outside.
    Keep the door to the room closed.

D. Prevention of overwhelming infection in the immunosuppressed patient

1. Use meticulous hand-washing techniques before each patient contact as well as between patient-care activities to different body sites.
2. Tell the patient to request all personnel/visitors to wash their hands before touching him.
3. Give *prompt* attention to fever.
4. Use a private room; persons with known infections should not enter.
5. Do not use invasive devices unless absolutely necessary; use only under aseptic conditions.
6. Control water supplies (pitcher, sink) and ice machine. Dispose of open containers on a periodic basis; remember that every item in the room is potentially dangerous.
7. Teach the patient about personal hygiene and the signs and symptoms of infection.
8. Bathe the patient with antiseptic solution paying special attention to axillary and perineal areas.
9. Give attention to proper house-keeping procedures.
10. Offer low microbial foods and beverages when indicated—fresh fruits and vegetables, cold sliced meat/rare meat can increase bacterial colonization.
11. Be aware of the patient's emotional state.

E. Relief of symptoms of infection

1. Combat generalized aching and malaise.
   a. Utilize warm applications and massage as indicated.
   b. Apply cold compresses for headache.
   c. Administer analgesic medications as prescribed.
   d. Attend to oral hygiene.
   e. Limit physical activity.
2. Relieve cough.
   a. Humidify inspired air.
   b. Administer hot gargles and throat irrigations.
   c. Supply expectorants or cough depressants as indicated and prescribed.

F. Enhancement of coping mechanisms to promote adaptation

1. Develop a trusting relationship with the patient and family.
   a. Spend unhurried time with the patient.
   b. Show sensitivity to the patient's feelings; avoid showing repulsion.
   c. Employ a nonjudgmental approach to the patient with sexually transmitted disease.
   d. Lend encouragement to the patient faced with prospect of prolonged convalescence.
2. Relieve anxiety and depression of patient/family.
   a. Recognize loneliness of the isolated patient.
   b. Employ active listening without interruption; accept the patient's feelings and thoughts without judgment.
   c. Give appropriate feedback.
   d. Include the patient in decision making.
   e. Encourage family to communicate feelings, expressions of support and affection.

Health Education

1. Make available, facilitate, or perform whatever vaccination procedures are known to be effective and are indicated for the stimulation of active immunity in exposed and susceptible individuals (see p. 860).
2. Furnish specific immune serum (heterologous or human convalescent) or human gamma globulin if indicated, to provide passive immunity and temporary protection to contacts who are particularly vulnerable.
3. Give the patient/family instruction in handwashing and personal hygiene measures as well as in isolation and precaution techniques.
4. Isolate patients with communicable infections, as well as known carriers and contacts, when required.
5. Educate the public with respect to:
   a. Availability and importance of prophylactic immunization
   b. Manner in which infectious illnesses are spread and methods of avoiding spread
   c. Importance of seeking medical advice in the event of a febrile illness or skin eruption
   d. Importance of environmental cleanliness and personal hygiene
   e. Importance of adequate housing and nutrition
   f. Means of preventing the contamination of food and water supplies:
      (1) Supervision, cleanliness, and inspection of food handlers
      (2) Dangers of "perishable" foods; the identity

(Text continues on p. 862)

Table 20-1 Epidemiology, Therapy, and Control of Communicable Infections

Disease	Infective Organism	Infectious Sources	Entry Site	Method of Spread	Incubation Period	Chemotherapy*	Prophylaxis
Amebiasis	*Entamoeba histolytica*	Contaminated water and food	Gastrointestinal tract	Patients and carriers; fecal–oral route; oral and sexual contact	Variable	Metronidazole; diloxanide furoate; iodoquinol	Detection of carriers and their removal from food handling; plumbing safeguards
Bacillary dysentery (shigellosis)	*Shigella* group	Contaminated water and food	Gastrointestinal tract	Patients and carriers; fecal–oral route	24–48 hours	Ampicillin; chloramphenicol; tetracycline; Sulfatrimethoprim	Detection and control of carriers; inspection of food handlers; decontamination of water supplies
Brucellosis	*Brucella melitensis* and related organisms	Milk, meat, tissues, blood, and absorbed fetuses and placentas from infected cattle, goats, horses, and pigs	Gastrointestinal tract	Ingestion of or contact with infective material	5–30 days (variable)	Tetracycline and streptomycin or chloramphenicol	Milk pasteurization; control of infection in animals
Chancroid	*Haemophilus ducreyi*	Human cases and carriers	Genitalia	Direct sexual contact	3–5 days	Erythromycin or trimethoprim–sulfamethoxazole	Effective case-finding and treatment of infection
Chickenpox (varicella)	Varicella-zoster (V-Z) virus	Human cases	Probably nasopharynx	Probably respiratory droplets	14–16 days	Acyclovir (?)	Varicella-zoster immune globulin (VZIG) primarily for immunocompromised children and certain neonates exposed in utero
Diphtheria	*Corynebacterium diphtheriae*	Human cases and carriers; fomites; raw milk	Nasopharynx	Nasal and oral secretions; respiratory droplets	2–5 days	Penicillin; or erythromycin	Active immunization with diphtheria toxoid
Encephalitis, epidemic (eastern and western equine)	Viruses	Chicken and wildbird mites; horses; hibernating garter snakes	Skin	Mosquitoes	Variable	None	Eastern equine encephalitis vaccine, dried
Gonorrhea	*Neisseria gonorrhoeae*	Urethral and vaginal secretions	Urethral or vaginal mucosa; pharynx; rectum	Sexual activity	2–7 days	Aqueous procaine penicillin G, preceded by probenecid or alternative regimen outlined by Public Health Service	Examination culture; treatment of sexual partners
Granuloma inguinale	*Calymmatobacterium granulomatis*	Infectious exudate	External genitalia; cervix	Sexual intercourse	Unknown, presumably 8–80 days	Tetracyclines; trimethoprim–sulfamethoxazole	Chemotherapy of carriers and contacts; case-finding and treatment of patients
Infectious mononucleosis	Epstein–Barr virus	Human cases and carriers	Mouth	Probably oral–pharyngeal route; via blood transfusion in susceptible recipients	2–6 weeks	None	None
Influenza	Virus	Human cases	Respiratory tract	Respiratory	24–72 hours	Amantadine; rimantadine	Influenza virus vaccine
Lymphogranuloma venereum	*Chlamydia trachomatis*	Human cases	External genitalia; urethral or vaginal mucosa	Sexual intercourse; indirect contact with contaminated articles/clothing	5–21 days	Tetracyclines	Case-finding and treatment of infection
Malaria	*Plasmodium vivax, falciparum, malariae,* and *ovale*	Human cases	Skin	Mosquitoes (*Anopheles*)	Variable, depending on strain	Chloroquine; primaquine; amodiaquine; quinine; proguanil	Coordinated measures for wide-scale mosquito control; prompt detection and effective treatment of cases; suppressive drugs in malarious areas
Measles	Virus	Human cases	Respiratory mucosa	Nasopharyngeal secretions	8–13 days	None	Measles vaccine

Disease	Causative organism	Reservoir	Portal of entry	Mode of transmission	Incubation period	Treatment	Control and prevention
Meningococcal meningitis	Neisseria meningitidis	Human cases and carriers	Nasopharynx; tonsils	Respiratory droplets	2–10 days	Penicillin; chloramphenicol	Meningococcal polysaccharide vaccine to persons at risk; rifampin/sulfadiazine for carriers or contacts
Mumps	Virus	Human cases (early)	Upper respiratory tract	Respiratory droplets	12–26 days (avg. 18 days)	None	Live mumps vaccine
Paratyphoid fever	Salmonella paratyphi A and B and related organisms	Contaminated food, milk, water; rectal tubes; barium enemas	Gastrointestinal tract	Infected urine and feces	7–24 days	Chloramphenicol; ampicillin; sulfatrimethoprim	Control of public water sources, food vendors, food handlers; treatment of carriers
Pneumococcal pneumonia	Streptococcus pneumoniae	Human carriers; patient's own pharynx	Respiratory mucosa	Respiratory droplets	Variable	Penicillin	Polyvalent pneumococcal vaccine; control of upper respiratory infections; avoidance of alcoholic intoxication
Poliomyelitis	Polioviruses (types I, II, III)	Human cases and carriers	Gastrointestinal tract	Infected feces; pharyngeal secretions	7–12 days	None	Oral polio vaccine (OPV), the live attenuated vaccine containing all three strains of poliovirus—produces long-lasting immunity in most recipients
Rocky Mountain spotted fever	Rickettsia rickettsii	Infected wild rodents, dogs, wood ticks, dog ticks	Skin	Tick bites	3–10 days	Tetracyclines; chloramphenicol	Avoidance of tick-infected areas, or wearing of protective clothing in such areas; frequent search for, and prompt removal of, ticks from body
Rubella (German measles)	Virus	Human cases	Respiratory mucosa	Nasopharyngeal secretions	14–21 days	None	Rubella virus vaccine; immune serum globulin (human) given to contacts of rubella; rubella in early stages of pregnancy legally recognized as indication for abortion
Scarlet fever	Group A streptococcus	Human cases; infected food	Pharynx	Nasal and oral secretions	3–5 days	Penicillin	Isolation; prophylactic chemotherapy with penicillin; asepsis during obstetric procedures; specific chemoprophylaxis for persons with rheumatic fever
Syphilis	Treponema pallidum	Infected exudate or blood	External genitalia; cervix; mucosal surfaces; placenta	Sexual activity; contact with open lesions; blood transfusion; transplacental inoculation	10–70 days	Penicillin; erythromycin; tetracycline	Case-finding by means of routine serologic testing and other methods; adequate treatment of infected individuals
Tetanus	Clostridium tetani	Contaminated soil	Penetrating and crush wounds	Horse and cattle feces	4–21 days (avg. 10 days)	Tetanus immune globulin (human; TIG) and penicillin	Wound debridement; toxoid booster injections for patients previously immunized; tetanus toxoid and tetanus immune globulin (separate sites and separate syringes) for nonimmune persons
Trichinosis	Trichinella spiralis	Infected pigs	Gastrointestinal tract	Ingestion of infected pork, undercooked	2–28 days	Steroids; thiabendazole	Regulation of hog breeders; adequate meat inspection; thorough cooking of pork

(continued)

Table 20-1 Epidemiology, Therapy, and Control of Communicable Infections (continued)

Disease	Infective Organism	Infectious Sources	Entry Site	Method of Spread	Incubation Period	Chemotherapy*	Prophylaxis
Tuberculosis	*Mycobacterium tuberculosis*	Sputum from human cases; milk from infected cows (rare in US)	Respiratory mucosa	Sputum; respiratory droplets	Variable	Isoniazid; ethambutol; rifampin; streptomycin; pyrazinamide	Early discovery and adequate treatment of active cases; milk pasteurization
Tularemia	*Francisella tularensis*	Wild rodents and rabbits	Eyes; skin; gastrointestinal tract	Handling infected animals; ingestion of undercooked, infected meat; drinking contaminated water; bites from infected flies, ticks	1–10 days	Streptomycin; tetracyclines; chloramphenicol	Use of rubber gloves when skinning/handling potentially infectious wild animals; avoidance of contact with potentially infected rodents; adequate cooking of wild rabbit dishes; vaccination of hunters, butchers, laboratory workers risking heavy exposure
Typhoid Fever	*Salmonella typhi*	Contaminated food and water	Gastrointestinal tract	Infected urine and feces	1–3 weeks	Chloramphenicol; ampicillin; sulfatrimethoprim	Decontamination of water sources; milk pasteurization; individual vaccination of high-risk persons; control of carriers
Typhus, endemic	*Rickettsia typhi (mooseri)*	Infected rodents	Skin	Flea bites	1–2 weeks	Tetracyclines; chloramphenicol	Delousing procedures; case quarantine
Whooping cough (pertussis)	*Bordetella pertussis*	Human cases	Respiratory tract	Infected bronchial secretions	Commonly 7 days	Erythromycin; ampicillin	Active immunization with vaccine; case isolation

* Research developments produce changes in drug therapy. The reader is referred to drug brochures and digests to keep abreast of changing dosages and uses.

of foods that tend to promote bacterial growth; and methods of food preservation

(3) Significance of milk pasteurization
(4) Indications for and methods of sterilizing food by means of heat
(5) Importance of meat inspection

g. Knowledge of insect, rodent, and other animal vectors and reservoirs of human infections and the importance of eliminating them.

Evaluation
Expected Outcomes

1. Takes prescribed antimicrobials as directed and adheres to other aspects of treatment program
2. Achieves normal fluid and electrolyte balance; normal skin turgor, moist mucous membranes, lowering of temperature to near normal; adequate intake of fluids; fewer episodes of vomiting and diarrhea, etc.
3. Shows signs of recovering from infection—temperature begins to decline; breathing patterns return to near normal; sense of well-being returns
4. Protects self and others from spread of infection—adheres to any isolation and hygiene measures that are implemented; reminds personnel and visitors to wash hands when entering and leaving room
5. Regains more normal elimination patterns as diarrhea or urinary frequency abates
6. Maintains proper rest schedule to conserve energy and strengthen body's defenses
7. Uses effective coping strategies
   a. Interacts with health personnel and visitors
   b. Expresses feelings, and works out any anxiety or concerns
   c. Acts interested in surroundings
   d. Participates in ADLs and maintains control over certain activities
8. Becomes informed of infectious disease process; how to avoid such a disease and measures to take when symptoms appear; recounts this information as indication of cognitive awareness

Isolation Precautions

Isolation precautions are used to prevent the spread of microorganisms among patients, personnel, and visitors.

1. There are several systems for isolation:
   a. Category-specific isolation precautions
   b. Disease-specific isolation precautions
   c. One designed by an individual health agency
2. The infection control committee of the individual agency makes the decision regarding which of the alternative systems of isolation precautions is to be used. Standards of practice are evaluated in the face of new information and changing situations.
3. See CDC Guideline for Isolation Precautions in Hospitals and CDC Guideline for Infection Control in Hospital Personnel, 1983, National Technical Information Service, U.S. Department of Commerce, Springfield, VA 22161.

Immunization

Immunity is the resistance that an individual has against disease.

1. Specific immunity to a particular organism implies that an individual has either generated the appropriate antibody in his own body or received ready-made antibodies from another source.

2. Immunization may be natural (not acquired through previous contact with the infectious agent) or acquired.
3. Acquired immunity may be *passive* or *active*.

Active Immunization

Active immunization is immunization that has been produced by natural or acquired stimulation so that the body produces its own antibodies.

1. It may be produced by clinical or subclinical infection (the person gets the disease); by vaccination with live or killed microorganisms or their antigens; or by inactivated vaccines and toxoids.
2. The organisms have been treated by heating or by chemical inactivation to destroy their harmful properties without destroying their ability to stimulate antibody protection.
3. Active immunizations that are available for adults include tetanus and diphtheria toxoid, adult-type tetanus toxoid, and vaccines for influenza, mumps, poliovirus, measles, rubella, hepatitis B and pneumococcal pneumonia.

4. Vaccines are also available for cholera, plague, rabies, typhoid, typhus, yellow fever, and smallpox.
5. Immunization recommendations are made by the US Public Health Service Immunization Practices Advisory Committee (ACIP), Centers for Disease Control, Atlanta, GA 30333, and are published periodically in the *Morbidity and Mortality Weekly Report* (MMWR).

Passive Immunity

Passive immunity to a disease is a state of relative temporary protection produced by the injection of serum containing antibodies which have formed in another host.
Types of preparations for passive immunity:
1. Immune globulin (IG); see p. 267
2. Specific immune globulins (for specific illnesses—rabies immune globulin, varicella-zoster immune globulin; hepatitis B immune globulin; tetanus immune globulin)
3. Human immune serum globulin with a known antibody content (for specific illnesses)
4. Animal antiserum or antitoxins

Sexually Transmitted Diseases (STD)

Sexually transmitted diseases are transmitted by sexual activity and include venereal diseases as well as nonspecific urethral and genital infections, enteric infections, and parasitic infestations (Table 20-2).

1. Sexually transmitted diseases are the most common infections in the US; patients present with physical symptoms, urethral/vaginal discharge, lesions, and rashes. Gonorrhea (p. 863) and syphilis (p. 870) are the most important STD because their prevalence constitutes a world-wide health problem.
   The incidence of acquired immunodeficiency syndrome (AIDS) continues to increase (p. 886).
2. Persons at high risk are those who frequently change partners and homosexuals with multiple sex partners.
3. STDs are increasing in prevalence because of
   a. Early behavioral maturity
   b. Increased use of alcohol and drugs contributing to decrease in inhibitions concerning sex
   c. Changing sexual mores
   d. Contraceptive practices that allow more sexual freedom
   e. Development of antibiotics
   f. Male homosexuality
   g. More travel opportunities

Nursing History

1. Foster a nonjudgmental attitude and atmosphere because this is an emotionally laden area.
   a. Convey an attitude of acceptance
   b. Explain why the following questions are relevant.
2. Ask or discuss the following:
   a. The patient's sexual orientation (heterosexual, bisexual, homosexual) Use nongender terms (i.e., "person," "individual").
   b. Is the patient involved primarily with one individual or different individuals?
   c. How many sexual contacts over a defined length of time?
   d. Where is the place of sexual encounter? Singles bars? Gay bars? Bath house? (Risk of disease transmission is higher in certain places.)

   e. Sexual practices? What orifices are used for sexual activities?
   f. What other sexual behaviors are practiced? (Behaviors that cause trauma, abrasions, etc. increase risk of systemic access to infection.)
3. Permit the patient to carry discussion further.
4. Know the disease spectrum in the area; there are geographic differences in incidence and types of STDs.
5. Identify the patient's chief complaint.
   a. When?
   b. Character of complaint? Location?
   c. Related to sexual activity?
   d. Any previous episode of STD? What was the treatment?
   e. Have you a sex partner with a known STD?
   f. Any history of drug allergies?
   g. For women: Any abortions? Miscarriages?
6. Inform the patient that the major STDs are reportable; the health department is notified when the diagnosis is confirmed.

Gonorrhea

Gonorrhea is an infection involving the mucosal surface of the genitourinary tract, rectum, and pharynx; it is caused by the gonococcus *Neisseria gonorrhoeae*. It is an infectious disease that is transmitted sexually, the exception being gonococcal ophthalmia of the newborn. It may be acquired by sexual intercourse, orogenital, and/or anogenital contacts between members of opposite sexes as well as members of the same sex.

Epidemiology

1. Changes in sexual behavior; liberalization of attitudes
2. Sexual contact at earlier ages
3. Greater personal mobility

Clinical Problems

1. Gonorrhea is the most common reportable communicable disease in the US.

(Text continues on p. 866)

Table 20-2 Sexually Transmitted Diseases Summary*

	Etiology	Prevalence	Clinical Presentation
Gonorrhea	*Neisseria gonorrhoeae* A nonmotile, gram-negative diplococcus; 0.6–1.0 μ in diameter	1,013,436 (468.3/100,000) cases reported in 1978. Highest reported case rates are in age-groups 20–24 and 15–19.	Men have dysuria, frequency, and urethral discharge that is usually purulent and often more severe in the morning. Women experience vaginal discharge and cystitis, 5%–20% of men and about 60% of women have no symptoms.
Syphilis	*Treponema pallidum* A motile spirochete with 6–14 spirals and ends pointed with finely spiral terminal filaments; 6–15 μ in length.	21,656 (10/100,000) infectious cases reported in 1978. Highest reported case rates are in age-groups 20–24 and 25–29.	*Primary syphilis:* Classical chancre is a painless, eroded papule with a raised, indurated border. Atypical lesions are common; multiple lesions may occur. Extragenital chancres may appear on any part of body. Unilateral or bilateral lymphadenopathy may accompany. *Secondary syphilis:* Various cutaneous and mucous membrane lesions, alopecia, generalized lymphadenopathy, mild constitutional symptoms.
Nongonococcal urethritis (NGU)	1. *Chlamydia trachomatis*—estimated to cause NGU in about 50% of cases. An obligate intracellular parasite. Diameter 250–500 nm. 2. *Ureaplasma urealyticum*—estimated by some workers to cause NGU in about 30% of cases. A mycoplasma of the T strain, less than 150 nm. in diameter. 3. *Other etiologic agents*—estimated to cause NGU in 10%–20% of cases: *Trichomonas vaginalis* *Candida albicans* Herpes simplex Coliform bacteria	Age distribution of nongonococcal urethritis parallels that of other sexually transmitted diseases, notably gonorrhea. Recurrences are very common.	Urethral discharge varies from profusely purulent to slightly mucoid. Dysuria may or may not be present. In half of the cases, the incubation period appears to exceed 10 days. Some men may have asymptomatic infection.
Trichomoniasis	*Trichomonas vaginalis* A motile protozoan with 4 anterior flagella and a short, undulating membrane; 5–15 μm. in length.	Prevalence ranges from as low as 5% of private gynecologic patients to as high as 50%–75% of prostitutes. Colonization rates are higher among women than men.	From no signs or symptoms to erythema and edema of external genitalia and frothy greenish-gray vaginal discharge. Granular vaginitis may include punctuate hemorrhages and may involve the cervix. Most men are asymptomatic, though some may present with urethritis.
Genital herpes infection	Herpes virus—type 2 A spherical DNA virus, enveloped, with cubic symmetry; 150 nm.	Prevalent among adolescents, young adults, and the sexually active.	Vesicular lesions on vulva, perineum, vagina, and cervix in women; lesions on penile shaft, prepuce, glans penis, and (less frequently) scrotum and perineum in men. Recurrent infections. Tender adenopathy, dysuria, and constitutional signs more common with primary infections than those recurring.
Vulvovaginal candidiasis	*Candida albicans* A dimorphic gram-positive fungus that appears as oval, budding yeast cells, has hyphae and pseudohyphae; 3 × 6 μm.	Saprophytic in the oropharyngeal and gastrointestinal tracts in 50% of the population and in the vagina in 20% of nonpregnant women.	Vulva is usually erythematous and edematous. Vaginal discharge, when present, may be thick and white, resembling cottage cheese. Occasionally discharge is thin and watery. Satellite lesions may spread to the groin. Many women have no symptoms. Sexual partners may develop balanitis or cutaneous lesions on penis.
Corynebacterium vaginale vaginitis or *Hemophilus vaginalis* vaginitis	*Corynebacterium vaginale* Or *Hemophilus vaginalis* Gram-negative pleomorphic coccobacillus, precise taxonomy not decided. Measures 1–3 μm. × 0.4–0.7 μm.	Cultured from 23%–96% of women with vaginitis. Recovered from 0–52% of asymptomatic women.	Homogenous, relatively thin, occasionally frothy vaginal discharge, usually gray-white. Punctate hemorrhages and vulvar irritation are occasionally seen. Between 10% and 40% of culture-positive patients have no symptoms.
Pediculosis pubis	*Phthirus pubis* Pubic louse, an oval, grayish insect which becomes reddish-brown when engorged with blood, 1–4 mm. in length.	Age-group of patients affected by pubic lice parallels that of patients with gonorrhea. Transmitted during sexual intercourse, very rarely by bedding or clothing.	Erythematous, itching papules. Nits or adult lice adhering to pubic hair or hair around the anus, abdomen, and thighs.

* US Department of Health and Human Services.

Diagnosis	Therapy	Complications
Presumptive identification— Microscopic identification of typical gram-negative, intracellular diplococci on smear of urethral exudate from men or endocervical material from women, OR positive oxidase reaction of typical colonies from specimen obtained from anterior urethra, endocervix or anal canal, and inoculated on Modified Thayer–Martin Medium.	Aqueous procaine penicillin G, 4.8 million units IM at 2 sites with 1 g. of probenecid orally, OR tetracycline HCl, 0.5 g. orally q.i.d. for 5 days, 10 g. total, OR ampicillin, 3.5 g. or amoxicillin, 3 g., either with 1 g. of probenecid orally.	Epididymitis Pharyngitis Meningitis Septicemia Arthritis Endocarditis Conjunctivitis in newborn Pelvic inflammatory disease (PID)
Demonstration of *T. pallidum* from exudate of primary or secondary lesions by darkfield microscopy. Typical lesions, reactive reagin test for syphilis (VDRL or RPR), and FAT/ABS will confirm except in early primary cases.	Benzathine penicillin G, 2.4 million units IM at 1 visit, OR Aqueous procaine penicillin G, 4.8 million units total: 600,000 units IM daily for 8 days, OR tetracycline HCl, 500 mg. orally q.i.d. for 15 days.	Late syphilis Congenital syphilis
Clinical picture of dysuria and/or urethral discharge; discharge on examination; polymorphonuclear leukocytes or urethral smear negative for *Neisseria gonorrhoeae* and negative culture for gonorrhea on Modified Thayer–Martin Medium.	Tetracycline, 500 mg. q.i.d. for 7–21 days. Many clinicians recommend similar therapy for sexual consorts.	Epididymitis Prostatitis Proctitis Cervicitis Salpingitis Reiter's disease Ophthalmia neonatorum
Microscopic examination of wet mount of vaginal discharge. Papanicolaou smears may show the parasite. Culture methods are available.	Oral metronidazole 2 g.p.o. STAT, OR 250 mg. t.i.d. for 7 days. Advise patient against consuming alcohol. Treat steady sex partners.	Rare Epididymitis Prostatitis
Clinical appearance of herpetic lesions. Papanicolaou smears from lesions, stained to show multinucleated giant cells with intranuclear inclusion bodies. Tissue culture.	No specific therapy is available. Symptoms may be relieved by warm baths.	Keratitis Encephalitis Neonatal herpes infection
Microscopic examination of gram-stained smears of introital or vaginal wall scrapings. Microscopic examination of wet mount of vaginal discharge. Culture on Sabouraud's modified agar.	Nystatin vaginal suppositories b.i.d. for 7–14 days, OR miconazole vaginal cream qd. for 7 days. Discuss with patient predisposing factors and means of avoiding a recurrence.	Nil
Clinical picture, microscopic examination, and culture. Gram stain of vaginal exudate may show tiny, gram-negative coccobacilli ("clue cells") adhering to vaginal epithelial cells, although specificity of this finding is low. Wet mount far less sensitive than gram stain.	Oral ampicillin 500 mg. q.i.d. for 7–10 days (Examine patient for syphilis or gonorrhea before prescribing this regimen, because ampicillin may mask symptoms), OR oral metronidazole 250 mg. t.i.d. for 7 days.	Nil
Clinical observation of lice OR microscopically, by identification of nits at base of hair.	1% Y-benzene hexachloride lotion 25% benzyl benzoate lotion. Combine with appropriate antimicrobials if secondary infection is noted.	Rare Impetigo Furunculosis Pustular eczema

(continued)

Table 20-2   Sexually Transmitted Diseases Summary (continued)

	Etiology	Prevalence	Clinical Presentation
Scabies	*Scarcoptes scabiei* The adult female mite is 300–400 μm. long and has 4 pairs of short legs. Posterior legs end in long bristles. Male is 100–200 μm. in length.	Transmitted via close bodily contact, often incidental to coitus, infested bedding and clothing.	Linear burrows 1–10 mm. in length, often with a red papule which contains the mite. Scratching may produce excoriation. Most common sites are finger webs, wrists, elbows, ankles, penis. Nighttime itching is characteristic.
Genital warts (*Condyloma acuminata*)	Human papillomavirus. A small DNA virus, icosahedral, of the papovavirus group.	Age distribution of venereal papillomatous lesions parallels that of patients with gonorrhea.	Flesh-colored to pinkish papillary or sessile growths which occur around the vulva, introitus, vagina, cervix, perineum, anus, anal canal, urethra, and glans penis.
Chancroid	*Hemophilus ducreyi* A coccobacillus that is nonmotile, non–acid-fast, gram-negative. Size 1–1.5 μm. × 0.6 μm.	May occur in conjunction with other genital infections, particularly genital herpes and syphilis.	A ragged, tender ulcer that is not indurated ("soft chancre"), its base covered with gray or yellow necrotic exudate. May be multiple ulcers. Tender inguinal adenopathy, usually unilateral. Women contacts are usually asymptomatic.
Lymphogranuloma venereum	*Chlamydia trachomatis* An obligate intracellular parasite. Diameter 250–500 nm.	Occurs frequently in tropical and semi-tropical regions, although 348 cases (0.2 per 100,000) were reported in the US in 1977.	Primary lesion is an evanescent, painless vesicle or superficial nonindurated ulcer on the genitalia. Adenopathy of the regional lymph nodes is common. A frank purulent proctocolitis may signal rectal involvement. Rare.
Granuloma inguinale	*Calymmatobacterium granulomatis* A nonmotile coccobacillus that is gram-negative. Size 2 μm. × 0.8 μm.	Though fairly common in a few underdeveloped nations, frequency has declined from a high of 2611 cases reported in 1949 to 75 in 1977 in the US. More common among men than women, and in Southern states.	Single or multiple subcutaneous nodules may erode through the skin, producing clean granulomatous, beefy-red lesions (usually painless).
Hepatitis B infection	Hepatitis virus—type B A virus of probable DNA nucleic acid content, 26 μm. or less.	Common among homosexuals and prostitutes.	Onset is usually insidious, with vague abdominal discomfort, anorexia, nausea, arthralgia, which often progresses to jaundice. Fever may be absent or mild. Asymptomatic, anicteric hepatitis may occur.

2. Gonorrhea has a short incubation period which permits rapid spread; a high percentage of infected females are symptom-free.
3. Syphilis and gonorrhea are frequently observed in the same patient.
4. Gonorrhea is becoming increasingly resistant to penicillin.

Clinical Manifestations

A. Women (small percentage)

1. Vaginal discharge; abnormal uterine bleeding
2. Urinary frequency and pain
3. Pelvic infection when gonococcus spreads through uterine (fallopian) tubes (salpingitis)
   a. Fever
   b. Nausea and vomiting
   c. Abdominal pain/tenderness
4. Disseminated gonococcal infection

B. Men (incubation period 3–5 days or longer)

1. Acute anterior urethritis—purulent discharge followed by painful urination
2. Spread of infection to posterior urethra, prostate, seminal vesicles, and epididymis
3. Prostatitis
4. Pelvic pain and fever

5. Epididymitis
   Severe scrotal pain, tenderness, and swelling
6. Postgonococcal urethritis and urethral stricture become major problems in males

C. Anorectal Manifestations

Anal and rectal burning, itching, bleeding, mucopurulent discharge or painful defecation; may be asymptomatic

D. Pharyngeal Manifestations

Sore throat, but may be asymptomatic

E. Adult Gonococcal Conjunctivitis

Gonococci usually reach the eye via the fingers.

Diagnostic Evaluation

Diagnosis is made by identification of the organism by gram-stained smear, by culture, or by the direct fluorescent antibody test. See Guidelines: Obtaining Culture Specimen for Diagnosis of Gonorrhea, page 868.

A. Women

Culture specimens obtained from cervix and anal canal and inoculated on selected media such as modified Thayer–Martin (T–M) medium. (T–M medium contains antibiotics to inhibit growth of other bacteria.)

Diagnosis	Therapy	Complications
Identifying the burrows and microscopic identification of the mites.	25% benzyl benzoate emulsion. Y-benzene hexachloride crotomiton. Combine with appropriate antimicrobials if secondary infection is noted. Trace and treat family, domestic, and sex contacts.	Impetigo Pustular eczema
Clinical appearance. Histology. Electron microscopy.	Podophylin 10%–25% in tincture of benzoin, applied weekly. Electrocautery. Curettage. Cryotherapy.	Rare Malignant change
Clinical appearance. Exclude possibility of syphilis through absence of indurated lesions and negative darkfield. Gram-stained exudate from lesion or aspirates from nodes may reveal short, gram-negative rods, OR culture on blood agar or media with blood derivatives.	Sulfasoxazole 1 gm. orally q.i.d. OR Tetracycline 500 mg. q.i.d. for 10–14 days OR Kanamycin 500 mg. IM b.i.d. for 10–14 days, or streptomycin 500 mg. IM b.i.d. for 10–14 days. Fluctuating gland masses will call for aspiration.	Chronic fistulas of gland masses in groin.
Clinical picture. Complement fixation test (CFT), significantly positive with a titer of 1:16 or higher in more than 80% of cases. Material for Frei skin test is no longer available.	Tetracycline 500 mg-orally q.i.d. for 2–3 weeks OR sulfasoxazole 4 g. orally, followed by 500 mg. q.i.d. for 3 weeks. Fluctuating gland masses indicate a need for aspiration.	Rare Elephantiasis Rectal strictures producing tenesmus, pain, and constipation. Men: Ulcerative and fistular lesions of urethra, penis, scrotum Women: Ulcerative genital lesions
Clinical picture. Intracytoplasmic rods ("Donovan's bodies") in large mononuclear cell from biopsy material stained with Giemsa or Wright's stain.	Tetracycline 500 mg. orally q.i.d. for 2–3 weeks OR gentamicin 40 mg. IM b.i.d. for 2 weeks.	Rare Elephantiasis Urethral, vaginal, or rectal stricture from cicatrix following healing. Massed pelvic glands; occasional bony involvement.
Detection of hepatitis B surface antigen (HBsAg) in blood by radioimmunoassay, passive hemagglutination, or other techniques.	Symptomatic	Death Carriers (rare) Cirrhosis (late and rare)

B. Men

Smear of urethral exudate for microscopic examination (see Fig. 20-1*C*).

C. The pharyngeal and rectal site should be cultured in persons engaging in oral and/or rectal sex.

D. Obtain serologic test for syphilis also.

Treatment and Nursing Management

1. *Recommended regimens** (the order of presentation does *not* indicate preference)
   a. Tetracycline HCl—500 mg. by mouth, 4 times a day for 7 days
   OR
   b. Amoxicillin/ampicillin—Amoxicillin, 3.0 g., or ampicillin, 3.5 g., either with 1.0 g. probenecid by mouth
   OR
   c. Aqueous procaine penicillin G—4.8 million units injected intramuscularly at 2 sites, with 1.0 g. of probenecid by mouth.

* Sexually Transmitted Diseases Treatment Guidelines 1982, Public Health Service, Centers for Disease Control.

d. Other treatment schedules are used for patients with coexisting chlamydial infection.
2. Treatment of sexual partners—examined, cultured, and treated with one of the above regimens.
3. Follow-up cultures should be obtained from infected sites within 4–7 days after completion of treatment. In addition, cultures should be obtained from the rectum of all women who have been treated for gonorrhea.
4. Patients with gonorrhea who also have syphilis must be given additional treatment depending on stage of syphilis.
5. Patients with proven penicillinase-producing *Neisseria gonorrhoeae* (PPNG) infection and their partners are treated with spectinomycin.
6. Pharyngeal gonococcal infection is treated with tetracycline or aqueous procaine penicillin G.
7. Treatment failures are likely due to reinfection, but infection with PPNG should be ruled out.
8. Treatment of complications of gonorrhea (endocarditis, bacteremia, arthritis, etc.) is individualized.

Principles of Control

1. Gonorrhea is a reportable disease; public health authorities are notified so that sexual contacts can be found and treated.

2. Each patient should be interviewed for names of contacts. Conduct interview and record history in nonjudgmental, empathetic manner.
3. Contacts of known gonorrhea cases should be investigated; known contacts should be treated within 10 days.
4. The patient should be instructed to avoid reinfection by sexual activity with untreated previous sexual partners until they have been tested and treated.

Complications

1. Sterility and pelvic infection in women; postgonococcal urethritis in men
2. Secondary foci of infection may develop in any organ system—disseminated gonorrhea, gonococcal arthritis, tenosynovitis, bursitis, endocarditis, pelvic infection, meningitis, lesions of the skin, severe proctitis

Health Education

1. Sexually transmitted disease is acquired by sexual contact (vaginal sexual intercourse, anal intercourse, oral intercourse) and by close and direct contact with an infected person.
2. A person who thinks that he or she may have a sexually transmitted disease or who has been exposed to someone who might have it should have a checkup.

Immediate treatment should be sought if symptoms develop.
3. Anyone who is sexually active with a number of sexual partners should have regular checkups.
4. Washing the sex organs (before and after sexual contact) and the use of a condom may give limited protection against sexually transmitted disease.
5. Birth control pills and IUDs give no protection against sexually transmitted disease.
6. Gonorrhea and syphilis are different diseases, caused by different germs; they attack the body in different ways but are spread in the same manner. A person may have both gonorrhea and syphilis as well as other sexually transmitted diseases at the same time.
7. There appears to be no natural or acquired immunity to gonorrhea and syphilis. A person can get gonorrhea and syphilis again and again.
8. Pregnant women may pass infection of syphilis to the unborn child. Pregnant women may pass gonorrhea to the baby during the birthing process.
9. Bacteria from gonorrhea may enter the bloodstream and affect joints, joint linings, heart valves, etc.
10. VD National Hotline: 800-227-8922 or 8923 (nationwide); 800-982-5883 (California); provides toll-free information and referral services for sexually transmitted diseases.

Guidelines: Obtaining Culture Specimen for the Diagnosis of Gonorrhea*

Purpose To obtain specimens from the cervix (women), anal canal (men and women), urethral specimen (men), or oropharynx specimen (men and women) for culture for *N. gonorrhoeae*.

Equipment

Vaginal speculum
Ring forceps
Cotton balls
Sterile, cotton-tipped swabs
Sterile calcium alginate urethral swabs
Sterile wire loop
Sterile disposable gloves
Selective medium—Martin–Lewis (ML), modified Thayer–Martin (MTM), or New York City (NYC) (for isolation of *N. gonorrhoeae*)

Procedure

Nursing Action	Rationale/Amplification
Preparatory Phase	
1. Place patient in dorsal lithotomy position with adequate draping.	
2. Put on sterile disposable gloves.	
Performance Phase	
For Female Patient:	
Cervical Culture	
1. Moisten vaginal speculum with warm water. Do not use any other lubricant.	
2. Separate labia. Depress the perineum and posterior vaginal wall with the finger of one hand.	2. This maneuver helps avoid uncomfortable pressure against the more sensitive anteriorly placed structures.
3. Gently insert a bivalve vaginal speculum.	3. The speculum is made self-retaining by adjusting one or more screws. The short blade should be uppermost. The tip of the posterior blade is pushed down into the posterior fornix.
4. Remove excessive cervical mucus with a cotton ball held in ring forceps.	

* Adapted from Criteria and Techniques for the Diagnosis of Gonorrhea, U.S. Public Health Service, Centers for Disease Control.

For Female Patient

Oropharynx Culture

Swab the posterior pharynx and tonsillar crypts with a cotton-tipped applicator.

Cervical Culture

1. Moisten vaginal speculum with warm water. Do not use any other lubricant.
2. Separate labia. Depress the perineum and posterior vaginal wall with the finger of one hand.
3. Gently insert a bivalve vaginal speculum.
4. Remove excessive cervical mucus with a cotton ball held in ring forceps.
5. Insert sterile cotton-tipped swab into endocervical canal (Fig. 20-1A).
   a. Move from side to side in cervix.
   b. Allow 30 seconds for absorption of organisms by the swab.

Anal Canal Culture (Rectal Culture)

1. Obtain anal specimen *after* getting cervical specimen.
2. Insert sterile cotton-tipped swab approximately 2.5 cm. (1 inch) into the anal canal (Fig. 20-1B).
3. Move swab from side to side in anal canal.
4. Allow 10–30 seconds for absorption of organism by the swab.

For Male Patient

Oropharynx Culture

(Same as in women)

Urethral Culture

Use a sterile bacteriologic wire loop or a sterile calcium alginate urethral swab to obtain a specimen from the anterior urethra by gently scraping the mucosa (Fig. 20-1C). Do not insert loop or swab more than 2 cm.

Anal Canal Culture

(Same as in women)

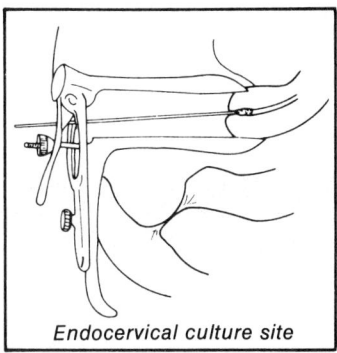

A   *Endocervical culture site*

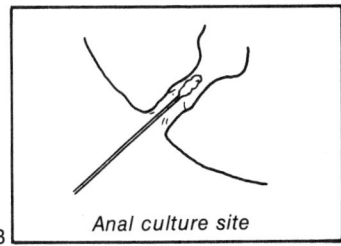

B   *Anal culture site*

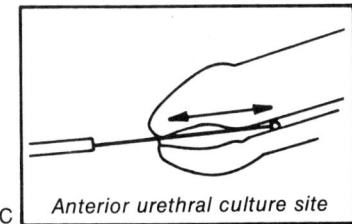

C   *Anterior urethral culture site*

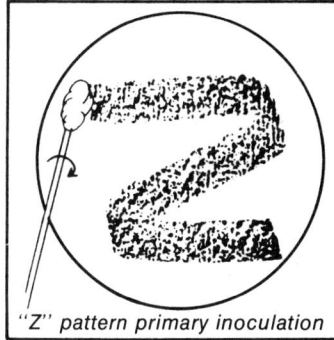

D   *"Z" pattern primary inoculation*

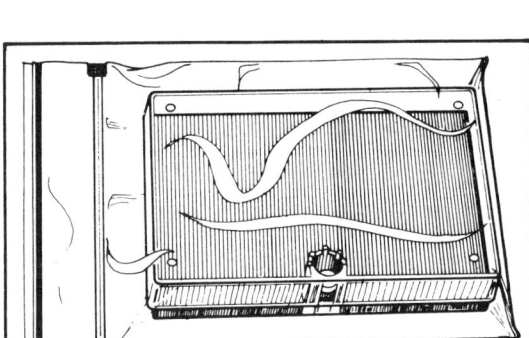

E   *Biological environmental chamber*

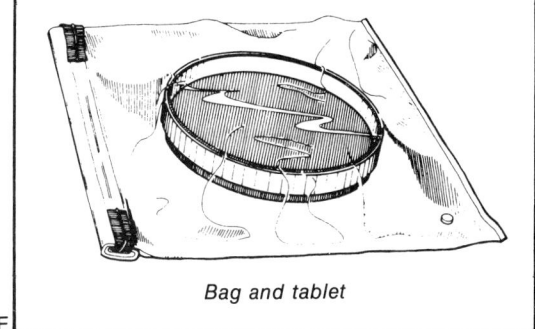

F   *Bag and tablet*

Figure 20-1. Obtaining culture for specimen in diagnosis of gonorrhea. (Criteria and Techniques for the Diagnosis of Gonorrhea. US Public Health Service, Centers for Disease Control)

(continued)

Guidelines: Obtaining Culture Specimen for the Diagnosis of Gonorrhea (continued)

Procedure
(Cont.)

Nursing Action	Rationale/Amplification

5. Insert sterile cotton-tipped swab into endocervical canal (Fig. 20-1*A*).
  a. Move from side to side in cervix.
  b. Allow 30 seconds for absorption of organisms by the swab.
	5. The endocervical canal is considered the best culture site. Movement of the cotton swab ensures adequate sampling.

Anal Canal Culture (Rectal Culture) 1. Obtain anal specimen *after* getting cervical specimen.	1. The anal canal is the most likely site to be positive when the cervix is negative.
2. Insert sterile cotton-tipped swab approximately 2.5 cm. (1 inch) into the anal canal (Fig. 20-1*B*).	2. Use another swab to obtain specimen if swab is inadvertently pushed into feces.
3. Move swab from side to side in anal canal.	3. Movement of the swab in anal canal permits specimen to be secured from anal crypts.
4. Allow 10–30 seconds for absorption of organism by the swab. *Oropharynx Culture* 1. Swab the posterior pharynx and tonsillar crypts with a cotton-tipped applicator.	1. Oropharyngeal specimens should be obtained from patients suspected of having disseminated gonococcal infection.
For Male Patient: *Urethral Culture* 1. Use sterile bacteriologic wire loop or a sterile calcium alginate urethral swab to obtain a specimen from the anterior urethra by gently scraping the mucosa (Fig. 20-1*C*). Do not insert loop or swab more than 2 cm. into urethra.	1. A urethral culture of the male is indicated when the gram stain of urethral exudate is not positive, in tests-of-cure, or as a test for asymptomatic urethral infection. Avoid using a standard cotton-tipped swab because it is too large.
Anal Canal Culture (Same as in women) *Oropharynx Culture* (Same as in women)	
To Inoculate Selective Medium in Plates: Candle Jar System 1. Roll swab in a large "**Z**" pattern on selective medium (Fig. 20-1*D*). If a second specimen is collected, inoculate on a separate part of medium.	1. This pattern provides adequate exposure of swab to plate for transfer of organisms.
2. Cross streak immediately with a sterile wire loop or tip of swab (in the clinical facility).	2. Streaking with a wire loop isolates colonies of *N. gonorrhoeae* from the few contaminants that occasionally grow on selective medium.
3. Place the culture plate in a CO_2-enriched atmosphere (candle jar) within 15 minutes of inoculation.	3. Successful recovery of *N. gonorrhoeae* requires an atmosphere enriched with carbon dioxide.
4. Incubate plates within 1–2 hours at 35°–36° C. (95°F–96.8°F).	
CO_2 Tablet/Plastic Bag System 1. After the medium is inoculated, place the CO_2-generating tablet in a special well of the plate (biological environmental chamber), *not* on the medium surface (Fig. 20-1*E*). Use forceps to handle the tablets. Secure the top of the plate tightly.	1. Read the package inserts on the handling and storing of CO_2 tablets.
2. Another method is to drop a CO_2-generating tablet into the plastic bag (Fig. 20-1*F*).	2. The tablet and plastic bag system is easy to use, safe, and economical.
3. Place plate in plastic bag. Expel excess air from the bag and seal it tightly. No portion of the bag is to be left open.	3. Moisture from the medium will activate the CO_2-generating tablet.
4. Incubate plates within 1–2 hours at 35°–36°C. (95°–96.8°F.).	

Syphilis

Syphilis is a chronic infectious multisystem disease caused by *Treponema pallidum* (a spirochete). It is acquired by sexual contact or may be congenital in origin.

Epidemiology

Trace the source and spread of infections by interviewing known patients for sex contacts.

1. Interviewing and reinterviewing every reported patient with syphilis for sex contacts.
2. Rapid investigation to identify contacts for examination within a minimal time period.
3. Identifying and conducting blood tests of other persons who by definition (suspect or associate) are possibly involved sexually in an infectious chain (cluster procedure).

4. Epidemiologic (preventive or prophylactic) treatment of sexual contacts and infectious syphilis cases.
5. More than 50% of reported cases of syphilis in the US occur in homosexual men.

Nursing History

History of rash on body? Sores, particularly on genitals? History of sexually transmitted disease?

Clinical Manifestations

Syphilis is capable of destroying tissue in almost any organ in the body; it thus produces a wide variety of clinical manifestations.

Stages of Untreated Syphilis

A. Incubation Period

1. 10–90 days; average 21 days
2. No symptoms or lesions
3. Spirochetemia is present; the patient's blood is infective

B. Primary (early) Syphilis

1. Most infectious stage; lasting 1–6 weeks
2. Manifestations include:
   a. Chancre or primary sore, a painless ulcer with heaped-up firm edges, appears at the site where the treponema enters the body (genitalia, anorectal area, lips, oral cavity, fingers); generally related to pattern of sexual behavior.
   b. Chancre becomes eroded and heals after 4–6 weeks, leaving a small scar; in some patients, no primary sore can be found.
   c. Enlargement of regional lymph nodes.

▶ **NURSING ALERT:** Syphilis should be suspected when an indolent, painless ulceration appears on the body.

C. Secondary Syphilis

1. Secondary stage follows onset of chancre by 9–90 days.
2. Signs and symptoms of secondary syphilis:
   a. Influenza-like syndrome—headaches, lacrimation, nasal discharge, sore throat, generalized arthralgia
      (1) Rise in temperature
      (2) *Generalized lymphadenopathy*
   b. Generalized skin eruption—maculopapular rash, etc.; bilaterally symmetrical in distribution, polymorphous (macular, papular, follicular, pustular)
   c. Moist papules occur most frequently in anogenital region (condylomata) and in mouth.
   d. Lesions of mouth, throat, and cervix (mucous patches) frequently occur in secondary stage; lesions highly infectious.
   e. Generalized patchy hair loss on scalp.
3. Arthritic and bone pain
4. Acute iritis
5. Hoarseness, chronic sore throat

D. Late Syphilis (clinically destructive stage after latent period)—manifestations may occur 10–30 years after exposure; recovery unpredictable.

1. Granulomatous lesions appear in skin, bones, liver, cardiovascular system, and central nervous system.
2. Syphilis will mainly affect cardiovascular system (aneurysm of ascending aorta, aortic insufficiency), central nervous system, and skeletal system.

Diagnostic Evaluation

There are 2 types of serologic tests:

A. Nontreponemal or reagin tests—screening tests to detect antibody-like substances, called reagin, found in serum of infected patient.

1. Venereal Disease Research Laboratory (VDRL) slide test.
2. Rapid Plasma Reagin Circle Card (RPR-CT) test

B. Treponemal tests—measure specific antibodies to *Treponema pallidum;* recommended for patients who have reactive reagin tests and atypical signs of primary or secondary syphilis and for diagnosis of late syphilis.

1. Fluorescent treponemal antibody absorption test (FTA-ABS)
2. *Treponema pallidum* hemagglutination (TPHA) test

Treatment and Nursing Management (early syphilis)

A. Recommended Regimen*

1. Benzathine penicillin G: 2.4 million units total, IM at a single session. Patients who are allergic to penicillin are treated with tetracycline HCl: 500 mg. by mouth, 4 times a day for 14 days.
   a. Screen for history of previous reaction to penicillin; reaction can occur in a patient with negative history.
   b. Patient should be detained 30 minutes after administration of parenteral penicillin in case of development of anaphylactoid reaction.
2. Patients with syphilis of more than 1 year's duration are treated with a different regimen.
3. Post-treatment follow-up is essential—treatment failures do occur, and retreatment is required, followed by nontreponemal tests at least 3, 6, and 12 months after treatment.
4. Jarisch–Herxheimer reaction—a reaction appearing within hours after initiating treatment of syphilis (particularly in the secondary stage) and subsiding within 24 hours; consists of transient fever and flulike symptoms of malaise, chills, headache, and myalgia. It may involve release of endotoxin-killed treponemes or from an allergic phenomenon.
   a. Managed by bed rest and aspirin.
   b. Warn the patient that this reaction may be expected.

Prevention and Health Education

1. Patients who have been exposed to infectious syphilis within the preceding 3 months should be treated as for early syphilis.
2. All patients with early syphilis should return for repeat nontreponemal tests 3, 6, and 12 months after treatment. Patients with syphilis of more than 1 year's duration should, in addition, have a serologic test 24 months after treatment. (Spinal tap may be necessary.)
3. Instruct the patient to refrain from sexual contact with previous partners who are not under treatment.
4. A program of sex education and epidemiologic screening should be ongoing. Mass screening of special groups with a known high incidence of sexually transmitted disease should be conducted.
5. VD National Hotline: 800-227-8922 or 8923—toll-free telephone numbers, provides information and referral services about sexually transmitted diseases.
6. See Health Education, Gonorrhea, page 868.

* Sexually Transmitted Diseases Treatment Guidelines, 1982, Public Health Service, Centers for Disease Control.

Bacterial Infections

Nosocomial (Hospital-Associated) Infections

Nosocomial infections are infections acquired in a health care facility during hospitalization; infection is neither present nor incubating at the time of admission unless it is related to a previous hospitalization. The major cause of hospital-associated infections in the United States is gram-negative bacteria, although in other countries, gram-positive pathogens are on the rise.

Gram-negative Infections

Gram-negative infections are bacterial infections caused most frequently by *Escherichia coli, Enterobacter* species, *Staphylococcus aureus, Klebsiellae, Pseudomonas aeruginosa, Proteus–Providencia* species, and *Serratia marcescens.*

Related Terms (bacterial shock; toxic shock)

Septic shock—circulatory shock occurring as a complication of a severe infection (usually by gram-negative enteric bacilli, although gram-positive cocci can cause bacterial shock)
Bacteremia—bacterial invasion of the bloodstream

Predisposing Events

1. Most gram-negative bacilli are not invasive in normal hosts; they are opportunistic bacteria that become invasive in persons with diminishing defense mechanisms and in persons with serious underlying disorders.
2. Diagnostic and treatment procedures (tubes, catheters, etc.) result in disruption of usual protective barriers normally provided by the skin and mucous membranes.
3. The advent of potent immunosuppressive drugs, cytotoxic drugs, steroids, radiation therapy, and previous splenectomy contribute to diminishing the defense mechanisms of the patient.

▶ **NURSING ALERT:** Persons over 70 are at high-risk of acquiring a nosocomial infection.

4. Patients in intensive care units are at risk because of underlying conditions that compromise host defenses, frequent exposure to invasive procedures, close proximity to other susceptible/at-risk patients that allows opportunity for cross-infection, and resistant microorganisms in ICU environment.
5. The following contribute to the development of gram-negative infections:
   a. Genitourinary tract—indwelling catheters, instrumentation, urinary obstruction
   b. Gastrointestinal tract—from obstruction, perforation, neoplasia, abscesses, diverticuli
   c. Biliary tract—cholangitis, obstruction (stones), surgical procedures
   d. Prolonged hospitalization
   e. Changing microbial flora
   f. Emergence of antibiotic-resistant bacteria
   g. Reproductive system—abortion, instrumentation, postpartum period
   h. Vascular system—venous cutdowns, intravenous catheters, intracardiac pacemakers, prosthetic heart valves, total parenteral nutrition, indwelling arterial lines, pressure-monitoring devices, surgical procedures
   i. Skin—wound infections, burns, pressure sores
   j. Respiratory tract—aspiration, tracheostomy, mechanical ventilation.

Prevention

1. *Handwashing by personnel and patient—fundamental to the control of all infections*
2. Isolation precautions for immunosuppressed patients
3. Strict aseptic technique for all diagnostic/therapeutic procedures—wounds, tracheostomies, tube drainage, catheters, intravenous therapy, cardiac pacing, ventilatory equipment
   a. Avoid invasive procedures as much as possible.
   b. Anchor IV catheter securely to prevent movement in vein; avoid prolonged IV therapy.
4. Use nursing surveillance to prevent cross-infection.
5. Monitoring sterilization procedures and cleaning practices.
6. Try to avoid housing 2 patients with indwelling catheters in the same room.
   a. Use closed urinary drainage system if an indwelling catheter is required.
   b. Regard outside of catheter and drainage bag as highly contaminated.

Clinical Manifestations of Bacteremia

1. Shaking chill and rapid rise in temperature

▶ **NURSING ALERT:** Fever may be absent in the compromised or elderly patient.

2. Warm, dry, flushed skin (during early stage)
3. Deteriorating mental status—due to reduction in cerebral blood flow
4. *Hypotension and shock*
   a. Tachycardia/tachypnea
   b. Cool, clammy skin/peripheral cyanosis
   c. Decreasing pulse pressure
   d. Oliguria
   e. Vascular collapse—death may occur as a result of vascular collapse
5. Intravascular coagulation

Nursing Interventions

A. Instituting appropriate treatment of bacteremia

1. Examine the patient carefully to identify source of sepsis.
   a. Assist with collection of blood culture—to identify etiologic agent and for sensitivity testing.
   b. Obtain other smears and cultures as indicated.
2. Administer appropriate antimicrobial agent—give promptly when the patient is too ill to await result of culture.
   a. Therapy is usually started before bacteriological diagnosis is made because of seriousness of illness.
   b. The choice of antimicrobial therapy also depends on the patterns of resistance in the patient's environment.
      Each health agency should monitor the susceptibility pattern of the most commonly occurring isolates.

3. Remove any foreign source of possible infection (when possible)—venous or bladder catheters.
4. Assist with surgical drainage of localized infection (abscesses, infected sites).

B. **Establishing tissue and organ perfusion and recovery from shock**

1. Monitor the state of responsiveness; skin temperature, moisture, color, turgor; appearance of mucous membranes and nails; pulse and respiration; input and output; blood pressure, heart and lung sounds; peripheral pulses.
   Focus assessment on *trends* and patterns of change.
2. Administer adequate volume of fluid and blood to correct fluid and electrolyte disturbances.
   a. Insert 2 or 3 large IV catheters—for rapid fluid and blood replacement, to ensure perfusion of vital organs.
   b. Administer blood, low-molecular-weight dextran, or saline as directed for volume expansion and to combat vascular collapse.
   c. Follow central venous pressure measurements—provides gauge for restoration of volume replacement (rate and amount).
   d. Follow measurements of left ventricular filling pressure (Swan–Ganz, see p. 282).
   e. Monitor serum electrolytes every several hours.
   f. Monitor for reduced urinary output—when shock ensues, kidney function deteriorates.
   g. Monitor for deteriorating mental status.
3. Administer oxygen to keep arterial PO_2 at desired level.
   a. Follow blood gas and pH measurements (p. 143) to assess the patient's need for assisted ventilation. Inadequate respiratory exchange is a frequent cause of death in gram-negative shock.
   b. The patient is usually hypoxic from increased AV shunting and from hypermetabolism from high fever.
   c. Administer sodium bicarbonate if severe acidosis exists—after initial hypoxemia and respiratory alkalosis, acidosis supervenes because of reduced kidney and lung function and accumulation of lactic acid.
4. Administer dopamine or isoproterenol, digitalis, diuretics, and other pharmacologic agents as directed to treat heart failure.
5. Treat disseminated intravascular coagulation (p. 261)—abnormalities of the coagulation system may accompany bacteremia.
6. See also Control and Management of Infectious Disease, Nursing Process Overview, page 858.

Staphylococcal Infections

Staphylococci are responsible for a wide variety of infections. They cause most superficial infections, but they also produce serious infections of the lungs, pleural space, bones, kidneys, and surgical wounds.

Examples of Staphylococcal Disease

1. *Skin and soft tissue infections*—furuncles (boils), impetigo, carbuncles, cellulitis, abscesses, infected lacerations
2. *Invasion of lymphatics*—axillary, cervical, mediastinal, retroperitoneal, and subdiaphragmatic abscesses
3. *Invasion of bloodstream*—endocarditis, pneumonitis, empyema, perinephritic abscess, hepatic abscess, splenic abscess, staphylococcal enteritis, septic arthritis, meningitis, osteomyelitis, generalized septicemia

Infectious Agent

Various strains of coagulase-positive staphylococci (*Staphylococcus aureus*)

Modes of Transmission

1. Direct hand transfer
2. Ingestion of food
3. Nasal secretions, draining wound, asymptomatic carrier
4. Break in skin/mucous membrane
5. Aerosolization during dressing changes
6. Vascular access sites (intravenous lines, drug abusers)

Hospital Staphylococcal Infections

(Include all of the above infections)

A. **Susceptible Hospital Patients**

1. Chronically ill or debilitated patients
2. Patients receiving systemic steroids or cancer chemotherapy
3. Patients undergoing major or prolonged surgery
4. Infants in the nursery
5. Patients with impairment of skin integrity (dermatoses, burns, abrasions)

B. **Prevention and Control**

1. All hospitals and extended-care facilities should enforce aseptic techniques supervised by infection control committee of the individual health agency.
2. Personnel with staphylococcal lesions should not work in the health agency until healing has occurred or cultures have become negative after treatment.
3. Patients with staphylococcal infections should be placed under strict isolation precautions until antibiotic treatment has rendered cultures negative for staphylococci.
4. Reduce cross traffic between hospital areas housing infected patients and those in which noninfected patients are located.

Specific Therapy for Staphylococcal Infections (Systemic)

1. Penicillinase-resistant penicillins (oxacillin, methicillin, nafcillin) and the cephalosporins (cephalothin) are antistaphylococcal drugs and are selected according to sensitivity studies.
   a. Intravenous administration is usually selected because of the large doses of drug required.
   b. Serious staphylococcal infections may require 4–6 weeks of treatment.
2. Provide supportive care—surgical measures, pain relief, treatment of fever, etc.

Preventive Measures and Health Education

1. Public should be educated concerning personal hygiene.
2. Persons with draining lesions should be isolated from their group and treated.

Streptococcal Infections

Most *streptococcal infections* in humans are caused by group A streptococci. Streptococci gain entrance to the body primarily through the upper respiratory tract or skin;

transmission is by persons with streptococcal infections or by asymptomatic carriers.

Beta Hemolytic Streptococcal Infections

1. Streptococcal pharyngitis ("strep" sore throat, p. 131)
2. Wound and skin infections—impetigo, puerperal infections, cellulitis, erysipelas
3. Scarlet fever (streptococcal throat with a rash which occurs if infectious agent produces erythrogenic toxin to which patient is not immune)
4. Sinusitis, otitis media, mastoiditis, peritonsillar abscess
5. Pericarditis, arthritis, peritonitis, meningitis
6. Pneumonia and empyema

Poststreptococcal Diseases (sequelae of Hemolytic Streptococci)

1. Rheumatic fever
2. Acute glomerulonephritis

Diagnostic Evaluation

1. Throat culture and sensitivity test
2. Culture from wounds

Treatment

1. Penicillin is the drug of choice in streptococcal infections (except enterococcal streptococci group D infections).
   a. Therapy should be continued for at least 10 days—to eliminate the organism, reduce frequency of suppurative complications, prevent the majority of cases of rheumatic fever (and to a lesser extent acute glomerulonephritis) and help prevent further spread of streptococci.
   b. Cephalosporins, erythromycin, or clindamycin may be used for penicillin-sensitive patients.
2. Make sure that the patient understands the importance of *completing* the course of antimicrobial treatment.

Preventive Measures and Health Education

1. Public should be educated concerning the relationship of streptococcal infections to heart disease and glomerulonephritis.
2. Long-term penicillin prophylaxis may be used for high-risk individuals (rheumatic heart disease)—to prevent a repeat attack.
3. Obstetrical patients should be protected from personnel or visitors with respiratory or skin infections.
4. Food handlers should be instructed about and monitored for hygienic procedures.

Pulmonary Tuberculosis

Tuberculosis is an infectious disease caused by the tubercle bacillus, *Mycobacterium tuberculosis*. It usually invades the lungs, but it also involves and sometimes produces gross lesions in other organs and tissues.

Transmission

1. The term *mycobacterium* is descriptive of the organism, which is a bacterium that resembles a fungus. The organisms multiply slowly and are characterized as acid-fast aerobic organisms which can be killed by heat, sunshine, drying, and ultraviolet light.
2. Tuberculosis is an airborne disease transmitted by droplet nuclei, usually from within the respiratory tract of an infected person who expels them during coughing, talking, sneezing, or singing.

3. When an uninfected susceptible person inhales the droplet-containing air, the organism is carried into the lung to the pulmonary alveoli.

Pathology

1. Tubercle bacilli infect the lung, forming a tubercle (lesion).
2. The tubercle
   a. May heal, leaving scar tissue.
   b. May continue as a granuloma:
      (1) May heal.
      (2) May be reactivated.
   c. May eventually proceed to necrosis (death), liquefaction, sloughing, and cavitation.
3. The initial lesion may disseminate tubercle bacilli:
   a. By extension to adjacent tissues
   b. Via bloodstream
   c. Via lymphatic system
   d. Through the bronchi

Risk Factors for Activation of Tuberculosis

Persons at risk:

1. Adults whose initial infection was acquired many years previously; these persons harbor live dormant bacilli that at any time may reactivate and spread disease.
2. Persons in close contact with someone who has infectious tuberculosis.
3. Persons whose tuberculin skin tests have recently converted to a significant reaction.
4. Persons with lowered resistance because of alcoholism
5. Elderly persons living in extended care facilities who have healed dormant lesions.
6. Patients receiving corticosteroid therapy; patients with chronic renal failure who are undergoing hemodialysis; patients with cancer or organ transplants who are receiving immunosuppressive therapy; patients who have had intestinal bypass surgery for obesity.
7. Persons with silicosis, diabetes mellitus, postgastrectomy state.

Clinical Manifestations

Patient may be asymptomatic or may have insidious symptoms that are ignored.

1. Generalized systemic signs and symptoms
   a. Fatigue, anorexia, weight loss, low-grade fever, night sweats, indigestion
   b. Some patients have acute febrile illness, chills, generalized influenza-like symptoms
2. Pulmonary signs and symptoms
   a. Cough (insidious onset) progressing in frequency and producing mucoid or mucopurulent sputum
   b. Hemoptysis; chest pain; dyspnea (indicates extensive involvement)
3. Extrapulmonary tuberculosis: *Mycobacterium* can infect any organ in the body (pleurae, lymph nodes, genitourinary tract, bones/joints, peritoneum, central nervous system)

Diagnostic Evaluation

1. Sputum smear and culture—diagnosis made by finding the acid-fast bacilli in sputum obtained by coughing and expectoration, induced by inhaled aerosols, bronchoscopic aspiration, transtracheal aspiration, gastric aspiration (swallowed sputum in aspirate is cultured).

2. Confirmation by sputum culture that the organisms are *Mycobacterium tuberculosis.*
3. Chest x-ray—to determine presence and extent of disease.
4. Tuberculin skin test (Mantoux test)—inoculation of tubercle bacillus extract (tuberculin) into the intradermal layer of the inner aspect of the forearm (see p. 877).
5. Screening tests—multiple puncture tests—introduces tuberculin into the skin either by puncture with a device with points coated with dried tuberculin or by puncturing through a film of liquid tuberculin.
   a. Used for screening large groups since there is no way to standardize the amount of tuberculin introduced and does not allow precise interpretation of test results.
   b. Test read 48–72 hours after administration (see p. 877).
   c. See product information sheet for reading and interpretation.
   d. All reactors should be retested with the Mantoux test and have a chest x-ray.

Nursing Interventions

1. Administer prescribed antituberculosis drugs (see Table 20-3).
   a. A combination of two or more drugs to which organisms are susceptible is given to destroy viable microbial organisms as rapidly as possible and to minimize the emergence of drug-resistant mutants. (Isoniazid and rifampin are usually included in the initial treatment regimen.)
   b. Treatment is continued until x-rays demonstrate improvement and negative sputum cultures are obtained.
   c. Then the patient is placed on continuing drug therapy for an additional period of time; total treatment time varies from 9–24 months.
2. Expect the majority of patients to improve rapidly after antituberculosis therapy is begun.

Health Teaching

1. Educate the patient about his disease. He must understand the importance of continuing to take his medicine for the prescribed time.
2. Secure the booklet *Understanding Tuberculosis Today: A Handbook for Patients* from the local Lung Association to give insight into and knowledge of the disease.
3. Review the side effects of the drug therapy with the patient (p. 877); he should report to the clinic if any of these occur.
4. Review possible complications with the patient and family: hemorrhage, pleurisy, symptoms of recurrence (persistent cough, fever, or hemoptysis).
5. Educate the patient to control propagation of secretions while coughing.
   a. Cover mouth and nose with double-ply tissue when coughing/sneezing. Do not sneeze into bare hand.
   b. Wash hands after coughing/sneezing.
6. Encourage the patient to eat a nutritious diet.
7. Patients with problems of alcoholism should be referred to an alcoholic clinic or other appropriate health agency.
8. Avoid job-related exposure to excessive amounts of silicone (working in foundry, rock quarry, sand blasting).
9. Encourage the patient to report to clinic/physician at specified intervals for bacteriologic (smear) examination of sputum to monitor therapeutic response and patient compliance.

▶ **NURSING ALERT:** Patient compliance remains a major problem in eradicating tuberculosis.

Preventive Treatment (Chemoprophylaxis)

Prevention of tuberculosis by prophylactic use of chemotherapeutic agent.

Goal:
Identify infected persons and give preventive therapy to those at risk of developing disease and becoming transmitters.

Most cases occur in persons known to be positive tuberculin reactors. These patients are the source of infection in 80%–90% of future cases of active tuberculous disease.

A. Isoniazid Therapy

1. The following high-risk groups are recommended for preventive (isoniazid [INH]) therapy*:
   a. Household members/close associates of newly diagnosed persons
   b. Newly infected persons
   c. Significant tuberculin test reactors with abnormal chest x-rays
   d. Significant tuberculin skin test reactors with special clinical situations (steroid therapy, diabetes, silicosis, gastrectomy)
   e. Other significant tuberculin skin test reactors up to age 35
   f. Other significant tuberculin skin test reactors over 35 only in special epidemiologic situations
2. Complication of isoniazid therapy
   a. Liver dysfunction (hepatitis)
      (1) Question the patient who is receiving isoniazid: Do you have loss of appetite? fatigue? joint pain? fever? dark urine?
      (2) Monitor serum transaminase values for persons at risk of developing hepatitis—over 35, daily drinkers, those taking potentially hepatotoxic drugs, history of liver disease.

B. BCG Vaccine

1. BCG vaccine (bacille Calmette Guérin)—produces a high level of immunity; may be given to populations with excessive/unavoidable exposure to tuberculosis.
2. In developing countries, BCG is considered the first line of tuberculosis control because it is inexpensive and easy to administer, and rarely results in serious side effects.
3. The vaccine is infrequently used in the US because of the relatively low rate of new infections, availability of low-cost isoniazid prophylaxis for persons exposed to tuberculosis, and effectiveness of short-term combination treatment which rapidly renders patients noncontagious and cures them of tuberculosis.

Health Education

(See above)

(Text continues on p. 878)

* Joint statement of the American Thoracic Society, American Lung Association, and the Centers for Disease Control.

Table 20-3 **Treatment of Mycobacterial Disease in Adults and Children**

	Dosage*		Most Common Side Effects*	Tests for Side Effects*	Drug Interactions†	Remarks*
	Daily Dose	Twice Weekly Dosage				
Commonly Used Agents						
Isoniazid	5 to 10 mg./kg. up to 300 mg. PO or IM	15 mg./kg. PO or IM	Peripheral neuritis, hepatitis, hypersensitivity	SGOT/SGPT (not as a routine)	Phenytoin—synergistic Antabuse	Bactericidal to both extracellular and intracellular organisms. Pyridoxine 10 mg. as prophylaxis for neuritis; 50 to 100 mg. as treatment.
Rifampin	10 mg./kg. up to 600 mg PO	10 mg./kg. up to 600 mg PO	Hepatitis, febrile reaction, purpura (rare)	SGOT/SGPT (not as a routine)	Rifampin inhibits the effect of oral contraceptives, quinidine, corticosteroids, coumarin drugs and methadone; digoxin, oral hypoglycemics; PAS may interfere with absorption of rifampin.	Bactericidal to all populations of organisms. Orange urine and other body secretions. Discoloring of contact lens.
Streptomycin	15 to 20 mg./kg. up to 1 g. IM	25 to 30 mg./kg.	8th nerve damage, nephrotoxicity	Vestibular function, audiograms‡; BUN and creatinine	Neuromuscular blocking agents—may be potentiated to cause prolonged paralysis	Bactericidal to extracellular organisms. Use with caution in older patients or those with renal disease.
Pyrazinamide	15 to 30 mg./kg. up to 2 g. PO	50 to 70 mg./kg.	Hyperuricemia, hepatotoxicity	Uric acid, SGOT/SGPT		Bactericidal to intracellular organisms. Combination with an aminoglycoside is bactericidal.
Ethambutol	15 to 25 mg./kg.	50 mg./kg. PO	Optic neuritis (reversible with discontinuation of drug; very rare at 15 mg./kg.), skin rash	Red–green color discrimination and visual acuity;‡ Difficult to test in a child under 3 years.		Bacteriostatic to both intracellular and extracellular organisms, primarily used to inhibit development of resistant mutants. Use with caution with renal disease or when eye testing is not feasible.
Less Commonly Used Agents						
Capreomycin	15 to 30 mg./kg. up to 1 g. IM		8th nerve damage, nephrotoxicity	Vestibular function, audiograms‡; BUN and creatinine	Neuromuscular blocking agents—may be potentiated to cause prolonged paralysis.	Bactericidal to extracellular organisms in cavities. Use with caution in older patients. Rarely used with renal diseases.
Kanamycin	15 to 30 mg./kg. up to 1 g. IM		Auditory toxicity nephrotoxicity, vestibular toxicity (rare)	Vestibular function, audiograms‡; BUN and creatinine.	Neuromuscular blocking agents—may be potentiated to cause prolonged paralysis.	Bactericidal to extracellular organisms. Use with caution in older patients. Rarely used with renal disease.
Ethionamide	15 to 30 mg./kg. up to 1 g. PO		GI disturbance, hepatotoxicity, hypersensitivity	SGOT/SGPT		Bacteriostatic to both intracellular and extracellular organisms. Divided dose may help GI side effects; has a metallic taste. Avoid use during pregnancy.
Para-aminosalicylic acid (aminosalicylic acid)	150 mg./kg. up to 12 g. PO		GI disturbance, hypersensitivity, hepatotoxicity, sodium load	SGOT/SGPT		Bacteriostatic to extracellular organisms only. GI side effects very frequent making cooperation difficult.
Cycloserine	10 to 20 mg./kg. up to 1 g. PO		Psychosis, personality changes, convulsions, rash	Psychologic testing	Alcohol—may aggravate or precipitate psychiatric problems.	Bacteriostatic to both intracellular and extracellular organisms. Alcohol may aggravate psychiatric problems. Very difficult drug to use. Side effects may be blocked by pyridoxine, ataractic agents, or anticonvulsant drugs.

* Check product labeling for detailed information on dose, contraindications, drug interaction, adverse reactions, and monitoring.
† Reference should be made to current literature, particularly on rifampin, because it induces hepatic microenzymes and therefore interacts with many drugs.
‡ Initial examination should be done at start of treatment.
(American Review of Respiratory Disease 1983 June; 127[6]:791).

Guidelines: Tuberculin Skin Test

The *tuberculosis intradermal skin test* is used to detect tuberculosis infection.

Purposes
1. To detect infection, either past or present, with *Mycobacterium* tuberculosis.
2. To serve as a diagnostic procedure in selected patients.

Equipment

PPD (purified protein derivative) tuberculin antigen
Tuberculin syringe
Short 1.25 cm. (½ inch) 26 or 27 gauge steel needle
Alcohol sponge

Procedure

Nursing Action	Rationale/Amplification
1. Determine if the patient has ever had BCG vaccine, recent viral disease, immunosuppression by disease, drugs, or steroids.	
2. Draw up PPD-tuberculin into tuberculin syringe.	2. Follow the manufacturer's directions. Each 0.1-ml. dose should contain 5 TU (tuberculin units of PPD-tuberculin). Use the antigen immediately to avoid absorption onto the plastic/glass syringe.
3. Cleanse the skin of the inner aspect of forearm with alcohol. Allow to dry.	
4. Stretch the skin taut.	
5. Hold the tuberculin syringe close to the skin so that the hub of the needle touches it as the needle is introduced, bevel up.	5. This reduces the needle angle at the skin surface and facilitates the injection of tuberculin just beneath the surface of the skin.
6. Inject the tuberculin into the superficial layer of the skin to form a wheal 6 mm. to 10 mm. in diameter.	6. If no wheal appears (because the injection was made too deep), inject again at another site at least 5 cm. (2 inches) away.

To Read the Test:

1. Read the test within 48–72 hours when the induration is most evident.	1. Tuberculin skin tests are tests of *delayed* hypersensitivity.
2. Have a good light available. Flex the forearm slightly at the elbow.	
3. Inspect for the presence of *induration.* Inspect from a side view against the light. Inspect by direct light.	3. Induration refers to hardening or thickening of tissues.
4. Palpate: Lightly rub the finger across the injection site from the area of normal skin to the area of induration. Outline the diameter of induration.	4. Erythema (redness) without induration is generally considered to be of no significance.
5. Measure the maximum transverse diameter of induration (not erythema) in millimeters with a flexible ruler.	

Interpretation:

1. Significant reaction: Induration 10 mm. or more in diameter.	1. A significant reaction indicates that a patient has had contact with tubercle bacillus. It does not necessarily mean that active disease is present in the body.
2. Reaction not significant: Induration less than 10 mm. in diameter.	2. This is considered "not significant" in persons who are not tuberculosis suspects or who are not close contacts of someone whose sputum is or was recently positive for *M. tuberculosis.*

NOTE: A tuberculin converter is a person whose tuberculin reaction changes from less than 10 mm. in diameter to 10 or more mm. in diameter, with the increase measuring at least 6 mm. (American Lung Association).

Follow-up Phase

Record:
1. Size of induration.
2. Name of antigen, strength of antigen, lot number, date of testing, date of reading.

Salmonella Infections (Salmonellosis)

Salmonellosis refers to infections caused by the genus *Salmonella*. Salmonellosis is seen in four forms: gastroenteritis (the most common); enteric fever (typhoid [p. 879]; paratyphoid disease); bacteremia with and without focal extraintestinal infection; and asymptomatic carrier state.

Although there are approximately 2,000 serotypes known, *Salmonella typhimurium* is the most commonly reported in the US.

The patient is infected by ingesting the organism in food contaminated by infected feces of man or animal, in eggs/egg products, in meat/meat products, in poultry, and in pharmaceuticals of animal origin.

Clinical Manifestations

(Usually 8–48 hours after ingestion of contaminated food)
1. Diarrhea—sudden onset of frequent, bulky stools followed by profuse, watery diarrhea; may lead to marked dehydration
2. Abdominal pain
3. Nausea and vomiting
4. Fever
5. Other manifestations due to infectious agent localizing in any body tissue—abscesses, cholecystitis, arthritis, endocarditis, meningitis, pericarditis, pneumonia, pyelonephritis

Diagnostic Evaluation

Isolation of organism from feces and blood.

Treatment and Nursing Management
Goal:
Prevent dehydration and electrolyte imbalance.

Treatment is supportive:
1. Restrict food until nausea and vomiting subside.
2. Offer clear liquids as tolerated.
3. Correct fluid and electrolyte depletion with intravenous infusions.
4. Avoid giving antimotility drugs (anticholinergics; paregoric) since a slowed peristaltic activity may extend the period of infection by interfering with cleansing mechanism of diarrhea.
5. Treatment is similar to that for typhoid fever (p. 879) if patient has focal (abscess) or systemic infection; parenteral antibiotic is given.

Preventive Measures and Health Education

1. Food service workers should have training courses and ongoing in-service training in facts about foodborne illnesses, avoidance of food contamination, food storage methods, cleaning of food preparation and service areas, and maintenance of good personal hygiene.
2. Raw eggs or egg drinks should not be ingested, nor should cracked or dirty eggs be used.
3. All foods from animal sources, especially fowl, egg products, and meat dishes, should be thoroughly cooked.
4. Foods should be refrigerated during storage and should be protected against insects/rodents.
5. Any person handling food should be instructed to wash hands after toilet use, before and after food preparation.
6. Chicks, ducklings, and turtles (as well as other domestic animals and pets) are sources of infection.
7. The patient must wash his hands after toilet use, particularly during illness and carrier state—to prevent infection of others.

Shigellosis (Bacillary Dysentery)

Shigellosis, an acute bacterial disease of the intestinal tract, includes a group of enteric infections caused by bacilli of the *Shigella* group of which there are 4 types: *S. sonnei, S. flexneri, S. boydii,* and *S. dysenteriae.* The source of infection is feces from an infected person. The route of spread is fecal–oral. Foodborne outbreaks can almost always be traced to contamination of food by a food handler. Shigellosis may also be of sexual origin (anal–oral contact).

Clinical Manifestations

1. Fever and headache
2. Cramping and abdominal pain
3. Persistent diarrhea—passage of varying amounts of blood, mucus, and pus
4. Profound prostration

Diagnostic Evaluation

Culture of freshly passed stool
Goals:
Maintain fluid and electrolyte balance.
Prevent the spread of shigellosis to the patient's contacts (i.e., to eliminate the carrier state).

1. Determine the type of shigella—organism is recovered from the patient's stool.
2. Do sensitivity testing for selection of antibiotic—resistance to antibiotics is common.
3. Give antibiotics that are absorbed from intestinal tract (trimethoprim-sulfamethoxazole; ampicillin) and to which the shigellae are sensitive; initial therapy is guided by susceptibility pattern of *Shigella* species in the community. May shorten duration of illness and decrease the duration of excretion of organisms.
4. Maintain fluid and electrolyte balance—to prevent profound dehydration resulting from an excessive loss of salts in the diarrheal stools.
   a. Assess weight loss, skin turgor, dryness of mucous membranes, urinary volume, vital signs.
   b. Weigh daily and measure urinary volume.
   c. Give intravenous fluids as required.
   d. Offer clear fluids during acute stage of illness; supplementary potassium may be required.
5. Avoid giving antimotility drugs (Lomotil)—may abolish antibiotic effectiveness.
6. Carry out epidemiology studies of every patient in whom the organism is found.
   a. Question the patient about travel to underdeveloped countries, exposure to crowded institutions, swimming in contaminated rivers. Inquire about water supplies, food eaten at home/restaurant.
   b. Inform the patient that infected individuals for whom anal–oral contact is a sexual practice should be treated.
   c. Notify local and state authorities.

Preventive Measures and Health Education

1. See Health Education for typhoid fever, page 879
2. Program of fly control
3. Surveillance of water sanitation; adequate sewage disposal
4. Detection and treatment of carriers

5. Handwashing after defecation
6. Untreated sexual partners, particularly those of homosexual men, may reinfect the patient

Typhoid Fever

Typhoid fever is a bacterial infection transmitted by contaminated water, milk, shellfish, or other foods. It is caused by *Salmonella typhi,* which is harbored in human excreta. Today it is spread chiefly by carriers, patients who have recovered from the fever, but whose stools or urine may spread these bacilli for years. The ingestion of infected oysters or shellfish taken from waters contaminated by offshore sewage disposal depots is another common source of infection. There is an increased incidence of typhoid acquired during foreign travel (certain areas of the developing world) and in microbiology laboratories.

Altered Physiology

The organism enters the body via the gastrointestinal tract; it invades the walls of the gastrointestinal tract, leading to bacteremia which localizes in mesenteric lymph nodes, in the masses of lymphatic tissue in the mucous membrane of the intestinal wall (Peyer's patches), and in small, solitary lymph follicles in the ileum and colon; ulceration of the intestines may ensue.

Clinical Manifestations

A. Gradual Onset

1. Severe headache, malaise, muscle pains, nonproductive cough.
2. Chills and fever; temperature rises slowly, reaching highest level in 3–7 days (40°–41°C. [104°–105°F.]).
3. Pulse is full and slow in comparison to height of fever; may have distinct dicrotic wave.
4. Skin eruption—irregularly spaced small rose spots on abdomen, chest, back. Each spot fades over a period of 3–4 days.

B. Second Week

1. Fever remains consistently high.
2. Abdominal distention and tenderness; constipation or diarrhea.
3. Delirium in severe infections—from severe toxemia.

C. Third Week

Gradual decline in fever and subsidence of symptoms

Diagnostic Evaluation

1. White blood count—leukopenia is a distinctive hematologic feature but is not always present
2. Blood culture—positive for organism after 1st week
3. Stool culture—positive for organism after 1st week
4. Urine culture—organism may or may not be present
5. Blood serum agglutination test usually becomes positive by end of 2nd week

Treatment and Nursing Interventions

1. Give specific treatment for typhoid.
   a. Chloramphenicol as directed. Monitor blood count to detect chloramphenicol toxicity.
   b. Combination of sulfamethoxazole and trimethoprim may be given for chloramphenicol-resistant strains of typhoid.
   c. Ampicillin or amoxicillin are also in use.
2. Give supportive care—typhoid fever is a nursing challenge.
   a. Support the patient during period of toxemia—the patient may be drowsy, partially incontinent, or delirious.
   b. Position the patient to prevent aspiration.
   c. Give steroids if prescribed for toxic or delirious patients.
   d. Take rectal temperature every 2–4 hours.
      (1) Give fever sponge (p. 768) for temperature of 40°C. (104°F.) or higher.
      (2) Encourage a high fluid intake—the patient may become dehydrated from high insensible water loss, vomiting, and/or diarrhea and poor oral intake.
   e. Watch for bladder distention—the patient may lose the urge to void during toxic state. Keep input and output record.
   f. Observe for retention of feces.
      (1) Enemas are given under *low* pressure to diminish chance of intestinal perforation.
      (2) Relieve distention with rectal tube, inserted for a short time.
   g. Give a high-calorie, low-residue diet during febrile stage.
3. Watch for complications which can occur after an apparent clinical cure.
   a. *Perforation of intestine*—from erosion of one of the ulcers; most common during 3rd week.
      (1) Symptoms
         Sudden, sharp abdominal pain—may stop suddenly
         Abdominal rigidity
         Shock
      (2) Treatment
         Prepare for intestinal decompression procedure, intravenous fluids, and surgical intervention if conservative measures do not produce clinical improvement.
   b. *Intestinal hemorrhage*—from erosion of blood vessel in ulcerated small intestine (occurs in 10% of patients).
      (1) Clinical manifestations
         Apprehension, sweating, pallor
         Weak, rapid pulse; narrowing pulse pressure
         Hypotension
         Bloody or tarry stools
      (2) Treatment
         Withhold food
         Give blood transfusions
   c. Other complications—thrombophlebitis, urinary infections, cholecystitis, meningitis, osteomyelitis

Prevention and Health Education

1. *Prevention*—typhoid vaccine, 1 subcutaneous injection followed by second injection 4 or more weeks later; booster injection every 3 years for selected individuals. (See recommendations of the Public Health Service Advisory Committee on Immunization Practices.)
2. *Maintain environmental hygiene in endemic areas.*
   a. Protect and purify water supplies.
   b. Employ sanitary waste disposal techniques.
   c. Pasteurize milk and dairy products; refrigerate while transporting.
   d. Avoid eating fresh, uncooked vegetables or unpeeled fruits (in endemic areas) that have not been washed in iodinated or chlorinated water.

e. Ensure that food handlers use handwashing facilities.
3. The patient must be followed with routine stool culture after recovery to detect the development of the carrier state—approximately 2%–5% of typhoid patients become permanent carriers, harboring the organism and excreting it in their urine and stools.
   a. Carriers may be given ampicillin or amoxicillin—to attempt to abolish carrier state (there is evidence that treating certain patients with salmonella in their stools may prolong the carrier state).
   b. Positive chronic carrier state—documented evidence of *S. typhi* in stool or urine for 1 year or more.
   c. Carriers must not become food or milk handlers.

Bacterial Meningitis
(Meningococcal Meningitis)

Meningitis—inflammation of the membranes surrounding the brain and spinal cord. (Encephalitis is inflammation of the brain itself).

Bacterial meningitis is most frequently caused by *Neisseria meningitidis, Streptococcus pneumoniae* (in adults), and *Haemophilus influenzae* (in young children). It starts as an infection of the oropharynx and is followed by meningococcal septicemia, which extends to the meninges of the brain and the upper region of the spinal cord. There are several distinct immunologic strains of the meningococcus, but groups B and C account for the majority of cases; recently, serologic groups Y and W-135 have become more important.

Clinical Features

1. Human cases and carriers are sources of infection; transmission is by contact or droplet infection.
2. Meningococcus may localize in the brain, skin, or joint synovia.
3. Predisposing factors include otitis media, mastoiditis, sickle cell anemia (or other hemoglobinopathies), recent neurosurgical procedures, head trauma, respiratory infection, immunologic defects.
4. The disease occurs in winter and spring months; epidemics are most apt to occur when people live in crowded quarters.

Clinical Manifestations

Symptoms result first from infection and then from increased intracranial pressure.
1. High fever
2. Nausea and vomiting
3. Sudden severe headache, irritability, confusion, delirium, convulsions
4. Neck, shoulder, and back stiffness—from spasms of extensor muscles due to meningeal irritation
5. Appearance of petechiae (usually on trunk and legs); may progress to large ecchymotic or purpuric lesions
6. Resistance to neck flexion
   a. *Positive Kernig's sign*—when lying with the thigh flexed on the abdomen, patient cannot completely extend his leg (a sign of meningeal irritation).
   b. *Positive Brudzinski's sign*—when the patient's neck is flexed on the chest, flexion of the knees and hips is produced. When passive flexion of the lower extremity on one side is made, a

similar movement will be seen on the contralateral (opposite) extremity.
7. Sudden confusion—focal abnormalities in the CNS—often exhibited by older patients.

Diagnostic Evaluation

Organism usually demonstrated by smear and culture of cerebrospinal fluid and blood.

Treatment and Nursing Interventions

1. Give specific drug therapy, depending on culture and sensitivity tests.
   a. Penicillin G (drug of choice); chloramphenicol or ampicillin given in high IV doses—to achieve high blood concentrations.
   b. Most antimicrobials enter cerebrospinal fluid and central nervous system inefficiently, and thus IV drug therapy is essential.
2. Maintain a clear airway—altered consciousness may lead to airway obstruction.
   a. Carry out arterial blood gas determinations.
   b. Provide oral airway or cuffed endotracheal tube or tracheostomy as the patient's condition indicates.
   c. Administer oxygen to maintain arterial PO_2 at desired levels.
3. Provide monitoring procedures and care for the patient with fulminating (coming on suddenly, with severity) disease. Death may occur within the first few hours after recognition of the disease.
   a. Assess the patient for shock, widespread vasoconstriction, circumoral cyanosis, cold extremities—may lead to coma.
   b. Keep a flow sheet of vital signs, signs and symptoms, medications, number of petechial lesions, etc.
   c. Monitor blood pressure continuously.
   d. Monitor the central venous pressure—to assess for incipient shock (which precedes cardiac or respiratory failure) and to estimate adequacy of fluid therapy.
   e. Monitor input and output.
4. Provide for rapid intravenous replacement of fluids, electrolytes, blood, and plasma.
5. Encourage a liberal fluid intake; the patient becomes readily dehydrated from fever.
6. Give diazepam (Valium) or phenytoin (Dilantin) to control seizures. See page 769 for care of the patient having seizures.
7. Employ measures to reduce temperature in the patient with high fever—to decrease the load on the heart and the oxygen demand of the brain.
8. Be on constant alert for complications—disseminated intravascular coagulation, shock, heart failure, pericarditis, pneumonia, and neurologic sequelae.

Health Education

1. Antimicrobial (rifampin) prophylaxis is indicated for persons who have intensive direct contact with the infected patient and who do not use proper precautions.
2. Meningococcal vaccine (types A and C) may be used for epidemic control or as an adjunct to antimicrobial prophylaxis for close contacts of patients with meningococcal disease.
3. Close contacts should be observed and immediately evaluated if fever or other signs and symptoms of meningococcal meningitis develop.

4. Prevent overcrowding of living quarters.
5. Improve practices of personal hygiene, particularly control of droplet infection.

Tetanus (Lockjaw)

Tetanus is an acute disease caused by the tetanus bacillus *Clostridium tetani,* whose spores are introduced into the body when an injury becomes contaminated with soil, street dust, or animal or human feces. The bacillus is an anaerobe (cannot live in presence of oxygen).

Assessment

Clinical Manifestations

(Caused by potent neurotoxins elaborated by *C. tetani* which have a special affinity for nervous tissue.)
1. Hyperirritability; restlessness, headache, low-grade fever
2. Rigidity of muscles, muscle spasms of both flexor and extensor muscle groups
   a. *Trismus*—painful spasms of masticatory muscles; difficulty in opening the mouth (lockjaw); neck rigidity, stiffness, dysphagia
   b. *Risus sardonicus*—distorted grin produced by spasm of facial muscles
   c. Recurrent painful reflex spasms of almost every muscle group in body—involvement of respiratory muscles may lead to respiratory failure; fractures of the vertebral bodies can occur during severe spasms.
   d. *Opisthotonus*—arching of the trunk (from spasms)

▶ **NURSING ALERT:** In recent years, approximately two thirds of the patients with tetanus have been over 50 years old.

A. Prevention of respiratory and cardiovascular complications

1. Maintain an adequate airway—tetanic spasm of larynx, pharynx, and respiratory muscles usually occurs during convulsions and may lead to hypoxia, asphyxia, and death.
   a. Place patient in an intensive care unit—requires expert respiratory management with early endotracheal intubation and mechanical ventilation.
   b. See page 225 for management of the patient requiring respiratory intensive care.

▶ **NURSING ALERT:** The hearing of the patient with respiratory paralysis may be acute. Do not make unguarded comments in his presence.

2. Provide cardiac monitoring—overactivity of sympathetic nervous system may lead to "sympathetic crisis" and death.
   a. Watch for isolated unexplained tachycardia, temporary hypertension, premature ventricular contractions, sweating.
   b. Requires aggressive physiologic monitoring and pharmacologic treatment (propranolol to control tachycardia; phentolamine to control hypertensive episodes).
3. Keep vein open—for infusions and in the event of respiratory/cardiac arrest.

B. Wound and systemic care

1. Give tetanus immune globulin (human) (TIG) in an effort to neutralize the toxins and to ensure that appropriate circulating levels will be present when the wound is debrided; prevents neurotoxins released into circulation during debridement from being attached to nerve endings.
2. Carry out effective wound care; debride all necrotic tissue—necrotic tissue favors growth of tetanus bacillus. Irrigate wound copiously to wash out tissue fragments and foreign bodies; immune globulin may also be infiltrated into wound site.
3. Give antimicrobials (penicillin)—to eradicate persisting *C. tetani* and other pathogens from the wound and stop the production of new toxin.
4. Give active immunization with tetanus toxoid according to immune status of the patient. When tetanus toxoid and TIG are given concurrently, use separate syringes and separate sites.

C. Ongoing assessment and support

1. Support the patient during tetanic spasm and convulsions—caused by the action of toxins in the cells of central nervous system; mortality rate of patients with frequent and severe spasms is high.
   a. Give diazepam, as directed, and sedatives to treat muscle rigidity and reflex spasms.
   b. Give neuromuscular blocking agents (metocurine iodide) for reflex spasms and to prevent seizures.
2. Plan nursing management during periods when sedation has maximum effect for minimal patient disturbance—tactile stimulation may promote spasms.
   a. Place the patient in a quiet, semi-dark environment—to avoid stimulating reflex spasms.
   b. Avoid sudden stimuli and light—slightest stimulation may trigger paroxysmal spasms.
3. Maintain fluid and electrolyte balance. Parenteral nutrition may be required—aspiration is a constant threat.
4. Avoid contractures and pressure sores—from prolonged immobility.
5. Watch for urinary retention—occurs when perineal muscles are affected.
6. Be alert for the development of fractures of the vertebral bodies which may occur with severe spasm.
7. See page 769 for management of the patient with convulsive seizures and page 760 for management of the unconscious patient.

Prevention of Tetanus and Health Education

1. Tetanus has occurred almost exclusively in persons who are unimmunized or inadequately immunized, or whose immunization history is unknown.
2. The primary immunization series for tetanus consists of a combination of tetanus and diphtheria toxoids, adult type (Td), of three doses given IM; the second dose is given 4–8 weeks after the first, and the third dose 6–12 months after the second. Booster immunization with Td every 10 years is recommended.
3. Consider every break in the skin a potential portal of entry for *C. tetani.*
   a. Tetanus-prone wounds—compound fractures; gunshot injuries; burns; foreign bodies; wounds contaminated with soil or feces; wounds neglected for more than 24 hours; puncture wounds; wounds infected with other microorganisms; wounds from induced abortions; wounds made by dirty hypodermic needles (drug addicts).

▶ **NURSING ALERT:** Tetanus-prone wounds are those in which there has been an invasion of soil or feces or those involving a severe traumatic injury. Tetanus may develop from an insignificant wound contaminated by soil. Deep necrotic pressure sores are tetanus-prone.

4. The most important step in the prevention of tetanus is the thorough washing and cleansing of the wound, with removal of all foreign material and devitalized tissue—helps eliminate tetanus bacilli from wounds and removes the material that forms a focus in which tetanus spores can develop.
5. Following injury, the immunization status of the patient will determine whether or not to provide active immunization with tetanus toxoid and passive immunization with tetanus immune globulin; the nature and age of the wound, the conditions under which it was incurred, and the treatment are considered on an individual basis.
6. Encourage the patient to keep an up-to-date record of his immunization status.

Clostridial Myonecrosis (Gas Gangrene)

Gas gangrene is a severe infection of skeletal muscle and surrounding tissue caused by gram-positive clostridia which may complicate compound fractures and contused or lacerated wounds by producing exotoxins that destroy tissue. Several species of clostridia (*C. perfringens, C. septicum, C. histolyticum, C. sporogenes,* and others) may produce gas gangrene. These organisms are putrefactive, gram-positive, spore-forming, encapsulated bacilli. They are normally found in the intestinal tract of man and in soil.

Altered Physiology

Injury → bacteria (*Clostridia*) invade devitalized tissue, especially where blood supply is compromised, lowering of oxygen tension of surrounding tissue and rapid spread of necrotizing process → bacteria multiply and produce toxins → toxins cause hemolysis, vessel thrombosis, and damage to organs, especially brain and kidneys.

Clinical Manifestations

1. Sudden and severe pain at site of injury—caused by gas and edema in the tissues.
2. Appearance of wound:
   a. Skin is white and tense initially; then progresses to bronze, brown, or black color.
   b. Soft tissue crepitus (crackling)—produced by gas in the tissue.
   c. Vesicles appear; are filled with red, watery fluid.
   d. Muscle is dark red or black and edematous, contains red, watery, foul-smelling fluid.
   e. Gas bubbles seen emanating from tissues—toxins ferment muscle sugar; produce acid and gas, which digest muscle protein. (Obvious gangrene is present.)
3. Rapid, feeble pulse progressing to circulatory collapse—death from toxemia is frequent.
4. Anemia and jaundice (from hemolysis); prostration; apprehension.
5. Delirium and stupor.

Diagnostic Evaluation
Clinical Assessment

Gram-stain of wound drainage shows gram-positive rods.

Treatment and Nursing Interventions

1. Prepare the patient for surgical removal and debridement of necrotic tissue—this is preventive as well as curative.
   a. Early excision of all devitalized and infected tissue with wide incisions will render wound unsuitable for growth of clostridium; also diminishes intracompartmental pressure, thereby reducing muscular necrosis.
   b. Extensive incisions (once infection has developed) in affected part allow air to inhibit growth of anaerobic organisms.
2. Give antimicrobial therapy (penicillin is the drug of choice for prophylaxis and treatment of gas gangrene; chloramphenicol may be given to penicillin-allergic individuals).
3. Prepare the patient for transfer to facility with a hyperbaric oxygen chamber—increases the dissolved oxygen in the arterial system by increasing the partial pressure of the oxygen breathed by the patient; stops the production of exotoxins.
4. Support the patient with toxemic manifestations— gas bacillus infection produces an intense toxemia.
   a. Monitor central venous pressure, pulmonary capillary wedge pressure; and urinary output (patient at risk for developing renal failure).
   b. Give IV fluids to support cardiovascular system; maintain fluid and electrolyte balance; give transfusions to maintain adequate hematocrit levels.
   c. Monitor potassium levels—hemolysis and tissue destruction may lead to hyperkalemia.

Health Education/Prevention

Use effective cleansing/care for wounds/trauma.

Botulism*

Botulism is a type of poisoning that affects the central nervous system; it is caused by eating food in which *Clostridium botulinum* has grown and produced toxins. The organism is widely distributed in soil. Human intoxication usually follows ingestion of contaminated foods: home-canned, dried, or smoked foods; or poorly processed foods.

Course

1. Variable; illness may be prolonged with a high risk of superinfection and fatal outcome.
2. Recovery in survivors may be prolonged.

Clinical Manifestations

(Usually begin 12–36 hours after ingestion of contaminated food)

The toxins elaborated by *C. botulinum* are extremely potent and are rapidly absorbed by the GI tract; they become bound to neural tissues and produce a neuroparalytic syndrome.
1. Nausea and vomiting
2. Blurred vision; diplopia
3. Dizziness
4. Severe dryness of mouth and throat
5. Difficulty in speaking and swallowing

* Botulism is an intoxication, not an infection. The Centers for Disease Control, Atlanta, GA 30333, offers diagnostic consultation and laboratory testing services and support for epidemiological studies of botulism.

6. Symmetrical descending weakness and paralysis
7. Progressive respiratory weakness and paralysis with normal mental status

Diagnostic Evaluation

1. Electromyography—to document electrophysiologic abnormalities
2. Mouse-toxin neutralization test—for detection of botulinal toxin; the patient's serum sent to laboratory that has capacity for performing this test
3. Examination of fecal samples, serum, gastric contents, incriminated food, for botulinal toxin
4. Suspected cases should be reported to public health authorities in order to identify and treat patients *early* in the course of illness.

Treatment and Nursing Interventions

1. Give intensive respiratory support—death is frequently due to onset of respiratory failure.
   a. Measure vital capacity and inspiratory force—for indication of ventilatory impairment.
   b. Carry out arterial blood gas evaluations—may show only minor abnormalities despite substantial loss of ventilatory reserve.
   c. Monitor for aspiration pneumonia.
   d. Prepare for endotracheal intubation and mechanical ventilation.
2. Administer trivalent ABE botulinal antitoxin as directed to neutralize any toxin that may be in the circulation.
   a. Determine if there is a history of allergy, asthma, hay fever—high rate of untoward reaction to antitoxin.
   b. Perform a skin test for sensitivity; read package insert.
   c. Have ventilatory equipment and emergency drugs ready in event of life-threatening reaction.
3. Give cathartics, enemas, and gastric lavage (when these can be safely administered)—to eliminate unabsorbed toxin and *C. botulinum* from the gastrointestinal tract.
4. Guanidine hydrochloride may be administered—enhances the release of acetylcholine from the nerve terminals; not as effective in overcoming respiratory paralysis as it is in combating paralysis of extremities and extraocular muscles.
5. Treat superimposed infections with antibiotics if necessary.
6. Provide ECG monitoring—to detect signs of cardiac arrest.
7. Inform family (during the patient's convalescence) that there is a high prevalence of persistent symptoms (tiredness, weakness, dyspnea) 1 year or more after onset of illness.

Prevention and Health Education

1. Home canners should be taught how to prevent botulism; use proper containers and adhere to time and temperature guidelines for processing.
2. Home-canned foods should be inspected before being eaten—foods contaminated with *Clostridium botulinum* may look soft, contain gas bubbles, and give off an odor of decay. However, contaminated food items may have a normal appearance and taste.
3. Discard any rusty or swollen canned food; do not taste contents.
4. Canned foods should be heated at temperature over 80°C. (176°F.) for 30 minutes or boiled for 10 minutes—toxins are heat-labile and destroyed by proper cooking of foods.
5. Be careful in preparing food for canning at high altitudes since it is difficult to provide a temperature high enough to destroy the spores of *Clostridium botulinum.* Use pressure cooker method of canning at high altitudes.

Actinomycosis

Actinomycosis is a chronic, suppurating, granulomatous disease. The usual pathogen in man is an anaerobic, gram-positive, branching, filamentous bacterium, *Actinomyces israelii,* a normal commensal that may be found in the tonsillar crypts, dental caries, and colon of apparently healthy people. Minor trauma, aspiration, or surgical manipulation may initiate the infectious process.

Pathology

1. The characteristic lesions are firmly indurated granulomas which spread slowly to adjacent tissues and break down focally to form multiple sinus tracts which penetrate to the surface.
2. The exudate from the sinus tracts contains the characteristic sulfur granules which are visible masses of the organisms.

Clinical Manifestations

Actinomycosis involves 3 major forms of infection:
1. *Cervicofacial type*—swelling about the teeth, submaxillary region, and neck producing a flat, hard, painless tumor mass which is fixed firmly to the jawbone. Granuloma ultimately breaks down and becomes riddled with abscesses which perforate externally.
2. *Abdominal type*—soft tissue mass or draining sinus in the abdominal wall or flank; the ileocecal area is the most common site of gastrointestinal involvement with sinus tracts and extension to bone, muscles, and other intra-abdominal structures.
3. *Thoracic type*—acute and chronic inflammatory reaction may involve lungs, pleura, mediastinum, chest wall, and pericardium, producing chest pain, fever, cough, and hemoptysis.

Diagnostic Evaluation

Culture and histologic identification of affected tissue.

Treatment

1. Give penicillin (drug of choice)—therapy should be continued for weeks to months to prevent recurrence; alternative antimicrobials are given if the patient is allergic to penicillin.
2. Surgical drainage, resection of damaged tissue, and excision of sinuses and fistulous tracts may be required.

Health Education

1. Encourage good dental hygiene to reduce infection around teeth.
2. There appears to be a relationship between intrauterine device use and colonization or infection of the genital tract with *Actinomyces,* especially when pelvic infection is present.

Viral Infections

Influenza

Influenza is an acute infectious disease caused by an RNA-containing myxovirus. It is characterized by respiratory and constitutional symptoms. Epidemics of influenza develop rapidly; there is a fairly high mortality rate among the elderly and those debilitated by chronic disease.

Etiology

1. The primary factor in the etiology of influenza is a filtrable virus of which 3 major strains have been isolated, designated types A, B, and C.
2. The numerous variants within a given type are called subtypes.
3. Three subtypes of hemagglutin (H_1, H_2, H_3) and two subtypes of neuraminidase (N_1, N_2) are among influenza A viruses that have caused widespread human disease.
4. Influenza appears to become epidemic when new strains appear against which most of the population lacks immunity.
5. Transmission is by close contact or by droplets from the respiratory tract of an infected person.

Clinical Course

1. The virus is airborne and multiplies in the upper respiratory tract—selected invasion of nasal, tracheal, and bronchial mucosal cells.
2. Influenza virus damages the ciliated epithelium of the tracheobronchial tree, rendering the patient vulnerable to the development of secondary invaders such as pneumococci or staphylococci, *Haemophilus influenzae,* streptococci, and other organisms.

Clinical Manifestations

1. Sudden onset of fever (39°–40°C. [102°–104°F.]), malaise, sore throat, cough, rhinorrhea, headache, myalgia.
2. Gastrointestinal symptoms—nausea, vomiting, abdominal pain, diarrhea.

Treatment and Nursing Interventions

1. Give aspirin or acetaminophen every 4 hours for fever, headache, and myalgia—take regularly to avoid marked swings of temperature with sweating and chills.
2. Offer cough syrup for dry, hacking cough.
3. Use a vaporizer—to reduce irritation to respiratory mucosa.
4. Encourage liberal fluid intake.
5. Give antiviral therapy (amantadine hydrochloride [Symmetrel]) as directed (used for prevention and therapy)—appears to interfere with the uncoating step in the virus replication cycle and also reduces virus shedding.
6. Watch for complications; persons at risk include those over 65, persons with underlying disorders of the cardiovascular, pulmonary, and/or renal systems as well as those with metabolic diseases, severe anemia, and/or compromised immune function.
   a. Pneumonia—watch for dyspnea early in course of illness.
   b. Neurologic complications—meningoencephalitis, cranial nerve palsies.

c. Myocarditis, heart block, peripheral vasoconstriction.

Prevention

1. *Vaccination*
   a. Active immunization consists of a single dose of vaccine (influenza virus vaccine) for either primary or annual booster vaccination.
   b. Influenza vaccine should be given by mid-November.
2. Annual vaccination with inactivated influenza vaccine is recommended for the following:
   a. Persons at high-risk (i.e., the elderly, persons with chronic disorders of cardiovascular, pulmonary and/or renal system, metabolic disease, severe anemia, and/or compromised immune function)
   b. Individuals who wish to reduce their chances of acquiring influenza or to reduce severity of disease
3. *Antiviral therapy*
   a. Amantadine hydrochloride (Symmetrel)—used for *prevention and treatment* of respiratory tract infection caused by influenza A viruses.
      (1) Chemoprophylaxis for unvaccinated high-risk persons exposed to influenza—used immediately after exposure to influenza because virus replication occurs early in disease.
      (2) Treatment for high-risk persons who have influenza (those with chronic heart/lung, metabolic, neuromuscular, immunodeficiency disease; elderly in extended care facilities) may reduce severity and duration of symptoms.
   b. Side effects—dizziness, nervousness, insomnia.

Health Education

1. The risk of developing influenza is related to crowding and close contacts of groups of individuals.
2. Restrict visiting privileges within health care facilities during epidemics—to minimize chance of introducing influenza.
3. It appears wise to humidify home and office air and to discourage cigarette smoking for high-risk persons.
4. See Prevention (above).

Infectious Mononucleosis

Infectious mononucleosis ("mono") is an acute infectious disease of the lymphatic system caused by the Epstein–Barr virus (EBV), a DNA virus of the herpes virus group. Cytomegalovirus infection can produce a clinical picture closely resembling that of infectious mononucleosis. Infectious mononucleosis occurs in individuals without antibodies to EBV.

Incidence and Transmission

1. Occurs mainly between ages of 14 and 30; high frequency of occurrence in college students and military population.
2. The virus is excreted in the saliva of patients with active disease or of those who are carriers, and is spread by intimate personal contact. It can also be transmitted by blood transfusion.

Clinical Manifestations

(May be vague and masquerade as those of leukemia, streptococcal sore throat, hepatitis, drug rash)
1. Sore throat, fever, lymphadenopathy (particularly in anterior and posterior cervical lymph nodes, producing neck pain)
2. Periorbital edema, headache, malaise, muscle aches
3. Skin rash, petechiae on hard palate
4. Enlargement of spleen

Diagnostic Evaluation

1. Blood smears—show lymphocytosis and atypical lymphocytes
2. Heterophil antibody agglutination test—increase in titer
3. EBV specific antibody test (positive)
4. Abnormal liver function tests

Treatment

1. The treatment is symptomatic and supportive.
    a. Encourage the patient to obtain additional rest and to tailor activity to individual tolerance.
    b. Give analgesics for headache, muscle pains, and fever.
2. Steroids may be helpful in severe cases; EBV infection can be fatal.
3. Observe for complications—rupture of spleen, Guillain–Barré syndrome (p. 800) causing respiratory failure, glottic edema, hepatic failure, renal failure.

Health Education

Inform the patient as follows:
1. Avoid constipation and straining—increases pressure on an enlarged spleen.
2. Avoid heavy lifting, strenuous exercise and competitive sports until recovery is complete—exertion or trauma may cause rupture of the spleen.
3. The need for increased sleep and rest may continue for a period of time.
4. Observe for abdominal and upper quadrant pain radiating to shoulder with signs of peritoneal irritation—evidence of splenic rupture.

Rabies (Hydrophobia)

Rabies is a severe viral infection of the central nervous system that is communicated to humans in the saliva of infected animals, especially wildlife (skunks, raccoons, foxes, bats) and cattle. The infection is transmitted by a bite or by contact of the animal's saliva with mucous membranes or with open wounds such as cuts, scratches, or abrasions.

Incubation Period

1. Varies from 10 days–1 year (average 20–60 days).
2. Influenced by viral dose, location of bite, type of exposure, and host response; bites on the head and neck are most dangerous.

Prevention

Rabies in humans can be prevented by eliminating exposure to rabid animals and by promptly treating local wounds and immunizing when exposed.

Prophylactic Management of the Patient

A. Local Treatment of Wound

1. Immediately wash wound and surrounding skin area with soap and water—to remove saliva from area.

2. Take victim to emergency department for further cleansing and flushing of wound.
3. Provide tetanus prophylaxis and antibacterial therapy as required.

B. Rabies Postexposure Prophylaxis of the Patient

A combination of passive and active immunization is recommended when postexposure treatment is deemed necessary. Two types of immunizing products are used concurrently:

1. *Vaccine,* which induces an active immune response that develops more slowly:
    a. Human diploid cell rabies vaccine (HDCV [Imovax]) is given at the same time a single injection of rabies immune globulin is given.
    b. See product information sheet for drug data and schedule; vaccine is administered IM on days 0, 3, 7, 14, and 28.
    c. Antirabies treatment is discontinued if fluorescent antibody tests of the animal's brain are negative.
2. *Globulin,* providing rapid protection.
    a. Rabies immune globulin (human) (RIG [Hyperab]); part of the RIG is infiltrated around the wound and the rest is administered IM in the patient's buttock.
    b. Do not give at same site as rabies vaccine is given.

Management of Biting Animal

1. Capture the dog or animal that inflicted the bite and keep under veterinary surveillance—this may enable the bitten person to avoid undergoing rabies vaccination unnecessarily.
    a. If animal remains healthy for 10 days, it is assumed that it was not infective.
    b. If animal becomes ill or dies, notify local health department; animal is humanely killed and brain examined for characteristic Negri bodies.
2. Kill wild animal (or stray dog/cat) that bites a person and send head to health department—brain examined for rabies.
3. If the biting animal escapes or is unknown, determination of the degree of risk is judged by the following factors:
    a. Prevalence of rabies in the area
    b. Species of biting animal
    c. Severity of wound(s)
    d. Whether attack was provoked or unprovoked
4. Any domestic animal that is bitten or scratched by a bat or by a wild carniverous mammal that is not available for testing should be regarded as having been exposed to a rabid animal.

Clinical Course and Clinical Manifestations

A. Prodromal Stage

1. Headache and nausea
2. Fever
3. Malaise; loss of appetite; mental depression
4. Sore throat
5. Pain and paresthesia of bitten areas
6. Unusual sensitivity to sound, light, and changes in temperature
7. Dilation of pupils; increased salivation

B. Stage of Excitement

1. Episodes of irrational excitement alternating with periods of alert calm
2. Convulsions

3. Severe and painful throat spasms when the patient attempts to swallow (or even views) liquids (hydrophobia); violent spasms of inspiratory muscles
4. Death usually occurs in this stage from cardiac or respiratory failure.

C. Paralytic Stage
Fatal progressive paralysis

Diagnostic Evaluation

1. History of exposure and development of characteristic symptoms
2. Demonstration of rabies antibodies in the patient's blood
3. Demonstration of characteristic *Negri bodies* in samples of brain tissue of infected animal

Treatment of Rabies in Man

1. No specific treatment; the care of the patient is symptomatic and supportive in the intensive care unit.
2. Employ continuing cardiac and pulmonary monitoring.

▶ **NURSING ALERT:** The rabies virus is contained in the saliva of patient with this disease, constituting a distinct hazard to personnel caring for him.

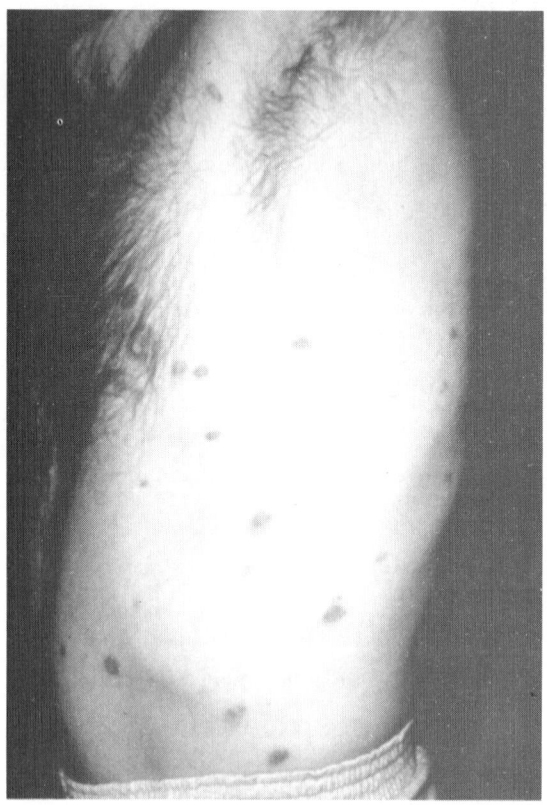

Figure 20-2. Lesions from Kaposi's sarcoma of a patient with acquired immunodeficiency syndrome. (Photo courtesy of Henry Masur, MD, Clinical Center, National Institutes of Health)

Acquired Immunodeficiency Syndrome (AIDS)

Acquired immunodeficiency syndrome is a severe disorder of immunoregulation whose underlying defect is impairment of cell-mediated immunity (abnormal regulation of the immune system) occurring in persons with no known cause of diminished resistance to disease. The disease is characterized by multiple opportunistic infections and is associated with malignancy.

Etiology

Evidence has shown that a newly recognized retrovirus is the cause of AIDS. The virus has been given several names but is commonly referred to as HTLV-III (human T-lymphotropic virus type III). It appears that AIDS can be transmitted through sexual contact and exposure to various blood products.

At Risk

1. Sexually active homosexual and bisexual men with multiple partners
2. Intravenous drug abusers
3. Persons with hemophilia
4. Sexual partners of individuals at risk for AIDS
5. Persons with symptoms and signs suggestive of the prodrome (see below)

Clinical Manifestations

A. Prodrome

1. Fatigue; malaise
2. Fever (weeks–months)
3. Weight loss
4. Lymphadenopathy; may be present before, during, and after prodrome
5. Persistent diarrhea; copious liquid stools many times daily associated with significant weight loss and malnutrition
6. Recurrent oral thrush, extensive herpes of mucous membranes, prolonged episodes of folliculitis
7. Blue or brown spots on skin—may indicate Kaposi's sarcoma (Fig. 20-2).

B. Appearance of Disease (usually from opportunistic infections)

1. Pulmonary syndrome—dyspnea, hypoxemia, chest pain, diffuse pulmonary infiltration—from *Pneumocystis, Legionella,* cytomegalovirus infection
2. CNS syndrome—dementia, confusion, headaches, neurologic symptoms—from opportunistic infections
3. Gastrointestinal syndrome—diarrhea, weight loss, colitis—from *Toxoplasma gondii,* cryptococcus, *Candida albicans, Cryptosporidium* species
4. Fever of unknown origin—from *Mycobacterium avium-intracellulare* infection with acid-fast bacilli invading bone marrow, lymph nodes
5. Malignancies—Kaposi's sarcoma (rare and aggressive tumor involving skin, lymph nodes, and gastrointestinal tract)

Diagnostic Evaluation

1. No previous history of immunosuppressive disease or therapy
2. Immunologic evaluation—reveals profound defect in cell-mediated function; degree of immunodeficiency

is predictive of prognosis and may determine specific diagnostic and therapeutic approaches
3. Skin test—to determine if cellular immune system is working
4. Serologic alterations
5. Stool evaluation—may reveal enteric pathogens

Treatment and Nursing Interventions

A. Combating Infection and Providing Physiologic Support

1. Give prescribed treatment for opportunistic pathogens; some infections are not treatable with currently available regimens.
2. Have a high index of suspicion for infection even when clinical manifestations are hazy or subtle; most patients recovering from an infectious episode develop subsequent opportunistic infections.
3. Monitor blood and bone marrow studies; monitor for adverse reactions.
4. Monitor for relapse after therapy is discontinued.
5. Search for other potentially treatable concurrent illnesses.
6. Participate in attempts to bring the patient's immune system back into balance with immunomodulating therapy. The following may be tried:
   a. Interferon—a protein existing in minute quantities in the body; known for its antiviral and antitumor activity; different types of interferon are being evaluated.
   b. Thymic hormones
   c. Transfer factor
   d. Interleukin II—stimulates gamma interferon production; also has a role in proliferation and differentiation of T-lymphocytes
   e. Plasmapheresis and bone marrow transplant
7. Participate and support the patient undergoing treatment of malignancies
   a. Kaposi's sarcoma
      (1) Radiation therapy for patients with limited disease
      (2) Chemotherapy; single chemotherapy for patients with slowly progressive disease and combination chemotherapy for patients with more rapid disease dissemination
      (a) Chemotherapy may need to be prolonged
      (b) Toxicity of chemotherapy may be more profound than expected
   b. Other malignancies treated symptomatically

B. Providing Psychosocial Support

1. Explore your own prejudices toward homosexuals/addicts; most are fearful of the health care system.
2. Approach the patient with compassion; many patients have lost family ties.
3. Know the resources available: Gay Men's Health Crisis, Red Cross, etc.
4. Arrange for the patient to have crisis counseling to help him through the initial reaction to his illness; psychological consequences of having AIDS are severe.
5. Answer queries simply; explore anxieties that prompt questions.
6. Offer consultation with a therapist to ameliorate emotional upheaval, social isolation and anxiety.
7. Be available to provide emotional and moral support.

Prevention/Health Education

1. Persons with symptoms suggestive of AIDS and those at increased risk for AIDS should refrain from donating blood.
2. Modify sexual behaviors:
   a. Avoid anonymous sex
   b. Have sexual relations with only one person, known to be in good health; use condoms.
   c. Refrain from oral and anal sex.
   d. Avoid persons with known infection.
3. Practice meticulous personal hygiene.
4. Avoid taking drugs that suppress the immune system.
5. Know the signs and symptoms of infection, *particularly elevation of temperature.*
6. Optimize immune system function by sound dietary practices, exercise, and regular periods of sleep.
7. Promote changes in the direction of more healthful living.
8. Toll-free line established by the U.S. Department of Health and Human Services provides the *latest* health information on AIDS:
   1-800-342-AIDS (nationwide)

Rickettsial Infections

Rocky Mountain Spotted Fever

Rocky Mountain spotted fever (tick-borne typhus fever) is characterized by continuous fever and headache. It is caused by the bite of an infected tick, by crushing an infected tick on the skin, or via conjunctival contamination with infected tick secretions.

Etiology

1. The organism responsible for Rocky Mountain spotted fever is *Rickettsia rickettsii.*
2. A large number of wild animals are hosts for the tick, but dogs appear to be an important source of risk for tick acquisition. The American dog tick and the Lone Star tick are important vectors of *R. rickettsii.*
3. Most prevalent in South Atlantic and South Central states.

Clinical Manifestations

During infection, *R. rickettsii* localize and proliferate in the vascular endothelium of small and medium-size blood vessels, producing widespread swelling and degeneration. This generalized vasculitis accounts for the manifestations of the disease and may involve virtually every organ.
1. Severe headache, malaise, anorexia, photophobia, muscle and joint pain.
2. High fever—up to 42°C. (107°F.) in severe cases—subsides by lysis.
3. Rash—appears in 3–7 days (discrete maculopapular rose lesions appearing on distal parts of body (wrists, ankles, soles, and palms) and spreading to central parts of the body may progress to petechial or purpuric stages; large subcutaneous hemorrhages may appear. *The rash is sometimes absent.*

a. Areas of skin necrosis may appear as a result of endarteritis—necrosis may involve ear lobes, fingers, toes, and scrotum.
b. Generalized edema—from generalized vascular involvement and resulting escape of serum.
4. Abdominal pain, rigidity, rebound tenderness—from vasculitis in the small abdominal vessels.
5. Restlessness, insomnia, hyperesthesia, and stupor and delirium
6. Thrombocytopenia

Diagnostic Evaluation

1. *History of exposure to ticks; typical clinical picture*
2. Serologic confirmation (complement fixation tests; tests for indirect fluorescent antibodies, indirect hemagglutination, latex agglutination or microagglutination)
3. Skin biopsy (from macular portion of rash)

Treatment and Nursing Interventions

1. Administer one of the tetracyclines or chloramphenicol as directed—effective if given in the *early* stages of the disease.
2. Give sedatives and analgesics as required for restlessness, insomnia, and pain.
3. Utilize supportive nursing measures for combating fever and promoting patient comfort.
   a. Turn frequently and give skin care; position patient carefully—disease can cause vasculitis (inflammation of a vessel) with severe edema and necrosis.
4. Measure circumference of abdomen, arms, and legs—to determine extent of edema.
5. Keep input and output records for determination of oliguria—the patient may develop renal failure because of poor tissue perfusion from vascular degeneration.
6. Watch for signs and symptoms of disseminated intravascular coagulation, circulatory collapse, hypotension, oliguria, azotemia, hypoproteinemia, myocarditis, and pulmonary complications—Rocky Mountain

spotted fever is an infectious vasculitis and can produce marked physiologic disturbances.
a. Support vital functions.
b. Central venous pressure measurements are used to guide fluid and electrolyte replacement because myocarditis is present in some patients and there is a risk of congestive heart failure.
c. Packed red cells and platelets may be given.
d. Monitor for thrombocytopenia—patients may succumb from hemorrhagic complications.

Prevention and Health Education

1. Clean weeds and cut brush and grass in recreational areas. Spray heavily infested areas (chemical control of recreation sites).
2. Exterminate rodents—serve as hosts for immature ticks.
3. Avoid sitting on grass/logs in infested areas.
4. In a tick-infested area:
   a. Tick repellent should be applied to exposed parts of body and clothing.
   b. Body and clothing should be examined for ticks 2–3 times daily. Ticks must be attached several hours for infection to occur.
   c. Tick should be removed by grasping with tweezers as close as possible to the point of attachment and pulling gently but firmly without crushing the tick. If tweezers are not available, use fingers protected with paper tissue.
   d. Or to lessen tick's hold on the skin, apply kerosene, gasoline, lighter fluid, alcohol, a drop of mineral oil or Vaseline on the tick.
   e. Do not crush the tick, thus avoiding contamination of the broken skin with infectious tick secretions.
   f. Hands should be protected with gloves or paper tissue while tick is removed. Wash hands immediately with soap and water.
   g. The bite should be disinfected immediately.
   h. Examine household pets for ticks on a regular basis; if infested, shampoo or dust with an appropriate insecticide.

Protozoan Infections

Malaria

Malaria is an acute and chronic infectious disease caused by protozoa plasmodia. Transmission is by way of an intermediate host (the bite of an infective female *Anopheles* mosquito). Malaria has also been transmitted via blood transfusions and from the use of shared contaminated needles and syringes by narcotic addicts.

Etiology

1. Four species of malaria parasites—grouped under genus *Plasmodium,* each causing a different type of malaria: *P. falciparum, P. vivax, P. malariae, P. ovale.*
2. The parasite has a complicated life cycle. Not all patients demonstrate classical cycles of fever and chills.
3. *P. falciparum* causes the most serious type of malaria because of the development of high parasitic densities in blood; infected red cells tend to agglutinate and form microemboli.

Clinical Problems

1. Malaria causes more disability and a heavier economic burden than any other parasitic disease.
2. In parts of Southeast Asia, Africa, South America, Panama, and Oceania, *P. falciparum* infections are increasingly drug-resistant.
3. Mosquitoes evolve resistance against insecticides.
4. There has been an increased number of cases imported into the US from Indochinese refugees and from US citizens traveling to endemic areas.

Clinical Manifestations

1. Paroxysms of shaking chills; rapidly rising fever followed by profuse sweating
2. Headache, muscle aches
3. Splenomegaly, hepatomegaly, orthostatic hypotension, anemia
4. Paroxysms may last about 12 hours, after which the cycle may be repeated daily, every other day, or every third day.

Diagnostic Evaluation

1. Demonstration of malaria parasites in blood smears by microscopic examination—confirms presence, species, and density of parasites.
2. Travel in an endemic area is an important diagnostic clue.

Treatment and Nursing Interventions

1. Determine the species of parasite infecting the patient (by blood smear). The most favorable time for discovery of the parasite is during and 12–18 hours after a chill.
2. Give specific therapy. The use of antimalarial drugs depends on the stage of the life cycle of the parasite that is involved; malarial parasites can evolve drug-resistant forms.
   a. Chloroquine is given for infections due to sensitive strains of *P. falciparum, P. vivax,* or *P. ovale.*
   b. Relapses of vivax or ovale malaria can be eradicated/prevented with daily doses of primaquine.
   c. Sulfadoxine (Fansidar) for resistant *P. falciparum* strains; since *P. falciparum* develops resistance to antimalarials, the longevity of this regimen is uncertain.
   d. An erythrocyte exchange transfusion may be carried out for rapid reduction of high levels of parasites in the treatment of overwhelming falciparum malaria.
3. Give supportive nursing care.
   a. Have the patient under close monitoring and nursing surveillance.
   b. Keep input and output records to prevent pulmonary edema and to evaluate for development of renal failure; dialysis may be lifesaving.
   c. Take a sample of venous blood daily for estimating serum quinine, bilirubin, blood urea nitrogen concentrations, parasite count, and packed red cells.
   d. Determine arterial blood gases and plasma electrolytes if respiratory or renal symptoms occur.
   e. Consider the patient with severe falciparum malaria as a medical emergency.
      (1) Administer IV quinine as directed—given in intermittent IV infusions.
      (2) Watch for neurologic toxicity (from quinine infusion)—twitching, delirium, confusion, convulsions, and coma.
      (3) Oxygen may be administered—tissue anoxia is thought to be common in this disease.
      (4) Watch for jaundice—related to density of the falciparum parasitemia (presence of malarial parasites in the blood); abnormalities of hepatic function are also common in falciparum malaria.
      (5) Evaluate degree of anemia—related to severity of infection.
      (6) Watch for abnormal bleeding (nose bleeds, oozing of blood from venipuncture sites, passage of blood in the stool)—may be due either to decreased production of clotting factors by a damaged liver or to disseminated intravascular coagulation (DIC).

Preventive Measures and Health Education

1. Eliminate anopheline mosquito vectors.
2. Advise travelers of risk in areas where malaria is endemic—Centers for Disease Control (CDC) booklet

Health Information for International Travel annually updates the current status of malaria in each country and advises of the most recent prophylactic recommendations.
   a. Limit dusk-to-dawn outdoor exposure, wear protective clothing, live in screened quarters, sleep under mosquito netting, and use topical repellents.
   b. Advise malaria chemoprophylaxis when traveling to areas where malaria is endemic. Malaria prophylaxis should start *before* a person enters an endemic area.
   c. Advise the traveler to seek prompt health care if he develops fever after stopping prophylaxis.
   d. Travelers to malarious areas should not donate blood for up to 3 years.

Amebiasis (Amebic Dysentery)

Amebiasis is a worldwide parasitic disease which is responsible for multiple medical–surgical problems. It is caused by the protozoa *Entamoeba histolytica* and is acquired by ingestion of the cyst stage of *E. histolytica* in food or water contaminated by infected human feces. It is also acquired by person-to-person transmission of enteric pathogens by orogenital, oroanal, or proctogenital sexual activity, particularly among homosexuals.

Incidence

1. Occurs as an endemic infection of man in most regions of the world.
2. In the US, found in rural areas or in patients who have lived or traveled in the tropics. Generally limited to warmer regions.

Pathological Insights

1. *E. histolytica* lives in the large intestine and feeds mainly on bacteria.
2. Amebas may be located in the bowel lumen and intestinal wall or outside the gastrointestinal tract.
   a. Trophozoites develop from viable cysts in the small intestine.
   b. Trophozoites may erode intestinal mucosa, invade the bloodstream, and travel to the liver via the portal circulation.
   c. Amebas can produce abscesses and other serious complications.

Clinical Manifestations

(May be symptomatic or asymptomatic)
1. Colicky abdominal pain
2. Diarrhea—watery, foul-smelling stools, often containing blood-streaked mucus

Diagnostic Evaluation

1. Stool specimen for *E. histolytica.* (Trophozoites or cysts may be found in the feces.)
   a. Three specimens of stool on different days should be examined either fresh or after fixation.
2. Scraping of lesions obtained during sigmoidoscopy/colonoscopy examined for amebic forms.
3. Positive serologic tests (indirect hemagglutination test and indirect fluorescent antibody test).
4. Examination of exudate from liver abscess for trophozoites.

Complications

1. Liver abscess
2. Thoracic complications—secondary to rupture of amebic liver abscess through diaphragm

3. Meningoencephalitis
4. Intestinal obstruction, rupture of colon; peritonitis
5. Ameboma (amebic granuloma found in cecum, rectum, transverse colon, sigmoid)

Management

1. Treatment consists of a systemic drug plus a lumenal amebicide: metronidazole (Flagyl) plus either iodoquinol or diloxanide furoate—produces cessation of diarrhea and eradicates encysted organisms in most patients.
   a. Caution the patient not to drink alcohol when taking Flagyl; may cause severe reaction.
   b. Serial follow-up of stools is necessary—relapses are common.
2. Keep the patient on bed rest if diarrhea is acute.
3. Give intravenous infusions as indicated to correct fluid and electrolyte imbalance resulting from severe diarrhea.
4. Prepare for aspiration of liver abscess; metronidazole plus chloroquine phosphate may be given for liver abscess.

Prevention and Health Education

1. Prevent contamination of food and water with human feces.
2. Carry out health education in personal hygiene—hand washing after defecation, before food preparation and eating.
3. Avoid ground-grown vegetables (lettuce, etc.) and local water supply when traveling in areas where amebiasis is endemic.
4. Examine contacts of recently diagnosed patients.
5. Advise male homosexuals of person-to-person transmission of enteric pathogens by sexual activity.

Systemic Mycotic Infections (Fungal Infections)

Mycoses and Histoplasmosis

Fungi are primitive organisms that take their nourishment from living plants and animals and from decaying organic material. The 3 main types of mycoses (fungal infections), determined by the tissue level at which the fungus settles, are:
1. Systemic or deep mycoses—primarily involve the internal organs, usually centering in the lungs.
2. Subcutaneous mycoses—involve the skin, subcutaneous tissue, and sometimes the bone.
3. Superficial or cutaneous mycoses—grow in outer layer of skin (epidermis), in hair, and in nails.

Histoplasmosis is a chronic systemic fungus infection caused by a spore-bearing mold called *Histoplasma capsulatum*. This highly infectious mycosis is transmitted by airborne dust which contains *H. capsulatum* spores. (Partially decayed droppings of pigeons, chickens, birds offer an excellent medium for growth of this fungus.)

Clinical Manifestations

(Fungal infections mimic symptoms of other diseases.)
1. Closely resembles pulmonary tuberculosis, including symptoms of fever, cough, dyspnea, anorexia, and loss of weight and strength.
2. The patient may present findings of malignant lymphoma, including anemia, thrombocytopenia, splenomegaly, hepatomegaly.
3. Other patients may develop ulcerations at mucocutaneous junctions (e.g., lip margins and perianal area).
4. Histoplasmosis may produce bleeding gastrointestinal ulcers and the syndrome of Addison's disease.

Diagnostic Evaluation

1. X-ray—appearance of lesions scattered throughout the lung fields
2. Positive sputum culture of *H. capsulatum*
3. Skin test with histoplasmin—shows hypersensitive reaction; of limited value in endemic areas where most of population is already positive
4. Histoplasma latex agglutination test
5. Complement fixation titers for histoplasma yeast

Treatment

Most patients do not require treatment.
1. Amphotericin B is the mainstay of therapy for disseminated or acute pulmonary disease.
   a. Dosage is controlled by blood level studies. (The patient is assessed for renal toxicity, manifested by rising blood urea nitrogen, decreased creatinine clearance, and other laboratory tests.)
   b. Severe toxic reactions to amphotericin B include nausea and vomiting, chills, fever, diarrhea, hypokalemia, phlebitis; pretreatment with meperidine may control chills.
2. Ketoconazole, a newer antifungal agent that is orally absorbable, is also effective. Monitor the patient for hepatic toxicity; anaphylaxis has been reported after a single oral dose.
3. Surgery may be done for persistent lung cavitation.

Health Education

1. Avoid stirring up dust around bird-roosting sites (raking and sweeping, etc.).
2. Minimize exposure to dust in a contained closed environment; spray area with water to reduce dust.

Helminthic Infestations

It is estimated that approximately one quarter of the world's population suffers from infestation by 2 common helminths: hookworms and roundworms.

Hookworm Disease

Hookworm disease (ancylostomiasis; "ground itch") is the result of infestation of the small intestine by quite similar hookworms about 1.2 cm. (½ inch) long. Three species of hookworms infect humans:

Necator americanus (predominant species in U.S.)
Ancylostoma duodenale
Ancylostoma ceylonicum

The infection is usually contracted by penetration of the skin by infected larvae in the soil.

Incidence

1. Southeastern US
2. Endemic in tropical and subtropical countries

Clinical Course

1. Hookworm eggs are passed in human feces onto the ground (indiscriminate defecation habits). Eggs develop into infective larvae.
2. The larvae *bore through the skin of bare feet* ("ground itch"). Infection with *Ancylostoma duodenale* can be by both percutaneous and the oral route.
3. After gaining access to the blood or lymph vessels, they are carried via the blood to the lungs, migrate from the pulmonary capillaries into the alveoli, reach the pharynx, and are swallowed, maturing to adult forms in the bowel.

Clinical Manifestations

1. Dermatitis ("ground itch")—occurs at site where larvae penetrate skin.
2. *Gastrointestinal symptoms*—maturation of worms in the intestine is usually marked by epigastric/abdominal pain, diarrhea, and other gastrointestinal symptoms.
3. Low-grade fever and malaise.
4. Coryza, pharyngitis, laryngitis, sensation of obstruction in throat, cough—from larval migration to upper respiratory tract.
5. *Severe anemia* and hypoproteinemia—the worms attach to intestinal mucosa and suck blood; a single adult worm can extract 0.03 ml. of blood daily. The patient's iron stores become depleted. A low level of serum protein often develops (protein malnutrition).

Diagnostic Evaluation

1. History of anemia and malnutrition
2. Recovery and identification of the eggs in feces

Treatment

1. Mebendazole—specific therapy of choice.
2. Ensure that the patient is eating a nutritious diet—hookworm disease occurs in persons suffering from malnutrition.
   a. Correct anemia prior to therapy for worms in patients with severe anemia.
   b. Give protein and iron supplementation—to aid in correction of anemia.

Prevention and Health Education

1. Treat infected individuals; an estimated one fourth of the world's people are hookworm infected.
2. Dispose of fecal wastes in a sanitary manner; this is an important facet of health education.
3. Instruct the patient to wear shoes at all times. However, half the world's population cannot afford shoes.
4. "Night soil" (human excrement used as fertilizer) and sewage effluents should not be used for fertilizer unless there is chemical disinfection of feces.

Ascariasis (Roundworm Infestation)

Ascariasis is an infection caused by *Ascaris lumbricoides* (intestinal roundworm). It is characterized by an early pulmonary invasion from larval migration and a later more prolonged intestinal phase.

Incidence

Occurs throughout the world in both temperate and tropical areas, particularly in areas of poor sanitation.

Clinical Course

1. Indiscriminate defecation in streets, fields, and doorways provides a major source of infective eggs.
2. Infection may be contracted from eating raw vegetables when night soil is used for fertilizer; water pollution may cause water transmission.
3. Eggs containing embryonated larvae are swallowed; the latter hatch out in the lumen of the small intestine.
4. Larvae penetrate the intestinal mucosa and enter lymphatics and blood vessels.
5. After reaching the lungs, they pierce the capillary wall, crawl up the trachea, are swallowed, and are returned to the small intestine where they grow, mature, and mate.

Clinical Manifestations

1. *Pulmonary phase*—cough, fever, and blood-tinged sputum—from tissue damage.
2. *Intestinal phase*—masses of worms cause gastrointestinal discomfort, colicky and epigastric pain.

▶ **NURSING ALERT:** Large masses of worms may migrate into various organs of the body and cause obstruction (to trachea, bronchi, bile duct, appendix, pancreatic duct).

Diagnostic Evaluation

1. Stool specimen—for detection of eggs in the feces.
2. Patient occasionally vomits a worm.
3. Malnutrition—from high protein requirements and damage to intestinal mucosa impairing the absorption of protein and other nutrients.

Treatment

1. Mebendazole or piperazine citrate.
2. Follow-up stool examination should be done 1–2 weeks after treatment.

Preventive Measures and Health Education

1. All patients with infestations should be treated.
2. Adequate toilet facilities should be provided.
3. The importance of personal hygiene should be explained.

Trichinosis

Trichinosis is infestation by the parasite *Trichinella spiralis,* one of the roundworms. It is acquired by consuming infected meat, usually pork.

Clinical Course

1. Tiny embryos of the parasite *Trichinella spiralis* become encysted in the muscle fibers of an infected pig.
2. These calcified cysts appear in meat (chiefly pork); resemble tiny grains of sand.
3. If insufficiently cooked pork is eaten, the embryos are set free by the gastric juice and develop in the intestine during the following week, becoming adult worms 3–4 mm. long.
4. These worms make their way into the mucous membranes and there produce myriad embryos (larvae) (period of invasion).
5. The larvae, carried by the bloodstream and their own activity, migrate to all parts of the body (period of migration).
6. The larvae gradually become encysted in striated skeletal muscle.

Clinical Manifestations

Intestinal Stage

1. Malaise
2. Gastrointestinal complaints, diarrhea, abdominal pain
3. Mild fever—progresses to high and spiking by 3rd week
4. Nausea and vomiting

Muscular Invasion (symptoms derive from inflammatory process developing in the muscles)

1. Edema of the eyelids; scleral hemorrhages; pain on eye motion
2. Generalized pain and soreness in the muscles (myalgia)
3. Cardiac irregularities (occasional)—from trichinae in the heart muscle; may be fatal
4. Difficulty in breathing, masticating, swallowing, speaking
5. Evidence of myocardial and CNS involvement

Diagnostic Evaluation

1. Biopsy specimen of muscle—reveals larvae. (Deltoid, biceps, gastrocnemius muscles are sites of biopsy.)
2. Positive serologic tests (precipitin, complement-fixation, bentonite–flocculation, fluorescent–antibody)—demonstrable titers 3–4 weeks after infection.
3. Rising eosinophil count—appears in 2nd week.

Treatment and Nursing Management

The treatment is symptomatic; there is no satisfactory treatment.

1. Thiabendazole (Mintezol)—may produce clinical improvement and prevent or minimize effects of illness.
   Adverse effects—nausea, vertigo, vomiting, rash
2. Corticosteroid agents may be given to relieve symptoms in the acute stage (when myocarditis or CNS involvement are complications).
3. Keep the patient on bed rest until he experiences some relief of symptoms.
4. Give analgesics to relieve muscle pain.
5. Carry out ECG evaluations to determine evidence of myocarditis.

Prevention and Health Education

1. The public should be educated about the importance of thoroughly cooking all pork and pork products, especially sausage. There should be no trace of pink in cooked pork.
2. Smoking, pickling, seasoning, and spicing do not

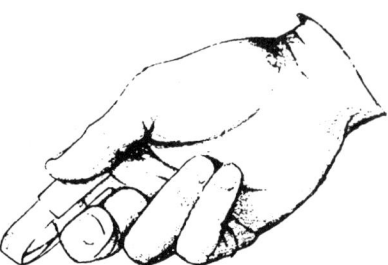

Figure 20-3. Most suitable method of finding eggs in perianal area: Bend cellophane tape back over index finger with sticky part out. (Courtesy of "Forum on Infection")

make pork safe unless it is thoroughly cooked (especially homemade sausage).
3. Beef hamburger may be contaminated by a meat grinder that has been used for pork.
4. Garbage intended for feed for hogs should be cooked.
5. Pork should be inspected to determine if disease is present (not always reliable).

Enterobiasis (Pinworm Disease; Oxyuriasis)

The pinworm or seatworm (*Enterobius vermicularis*) causes the most common form of intestinal roundworm infestation in the US and is most prevalent in children. It is caused by swallowing infective eggs.

Clinical Problems

1. One pinworm may produce 11,000–15,000 eggs.
2. Ingested eggs hatch in the small intestine; embryos reach adulthood in the cecum.
3. The gravid female worm migrates down the large intestine and deposits eggs on the skin of the perianal area.
4. The eggs that survive are ingested and reach maturity in 2–6 weeks in the gastrointestinal tract.
5. Scratching leads to contamination of the hands and nails; hand to mouth transmission results in reinfection.
6. Infective eggs may contaminate food and drink, bed linen, dust, etc.

Clinical Manifestations

(Pinworm-infected person may be asymptomatic.)

1. Intense itching (nocturnal) around the anus—from nocturnal migration of gravid females from anus and deposition of eggs in perianal folds of skin.
2. Restlessness; nervousness
3. Vaginitis—from pinworm migration into the vagina

Diagnostic Evaluation

1. Anal impressions on cellophane tape taken in morning before going to toilet or bathing, so that ova deposited during the night will not be removed (Fig. 20-3).
   a. A family member may be taught the method so that the test may be carried out first thing in the morning.
   b. Wash hands thoroughly.
2. Detection (inspection) of characteristic eggs about the anus or on the feces.

Treatment

1. Mebendazole in a single oral dose usually results in cure.

Prevention of Reinfection; Health Education

1. All members of the family should be treated, or reinfection is apt to occur. Treat on the same day to eliminate cross-infection.
2. To prevent reinfection:
   a. Cut fingernails short—eggs may be obtained from beneath the nails of infected person.
      (1) Avoid nail biting.
      (2) Wash hands frequently during treatment period.
      (3) Scrub nails with a brush, especially before going to bed.
   b. Wash hands with soap and water after using toilet and before meals.

c. Wash around anal area upon arising (after diagnostic test).

d. Apply salve or ointment to anal area—to prevent dispersal of eggs.

e. Infected child should wear snug-fitting cotton pants—to discourage contact of hands with perianal region and contamination of bed linen.

f. Use a shower since the bathtub may be a source of infection.

g. See that the infected person sleeps alone.

h. Handle bedding and nightwear carefully—there are large numbers of infective eggs in a contaminated house that cause reinfection.

i. Clean sleeping quarters frequently.

j. Reassure mother and family members that pinworms are not a sign of poor hygiene or housekeeping.

Bibliography

Books

Axnick KJ and Yarbrough M. Infection Control: An Integrated Approach. St Louis, CV Mosby, 1984

Bannister BA. Infectious Diseases. London, Bailliere Tindall, 1983

Brown HW and Neva FA. Basic Clinical Parasitology, 5th ed. Norwalk, CT, Appleton-Century-Crofts, 1983

Case LG (ed). Guide to the Management of Infectious Disease. New York, Grune & Stratton, 1983

Emmerson AM. The Microbiology and Treatment of Life-threatening Infections. New York, RSCH Studies Press, 1982

Evans AS and Feldman HA. Bacterial Infections of Humans. New York, Plenum Press, 1982

Fulginiti VA. Immunization in Clinical Practice. Philadelphia, JB Lippincott, 1982

Gleckman RA and Gantz NM (eds). Infections in the Elderly, 1st ed. Boston, Little, Brown & Co, 1983

Hoeprich PD (ed). Infectious Diseases: A Modern Treatise of Infectious Processes, 3rd ed. Philadelphia, Harper & Row, 1983

Howe BH. Stressors and behavioral responses of patients with infectious processes, In Mill JF. Coping with Chronic Illness, pages 177–194. Philadelphia, FA Davis, 1982

Kassler J. Gay Men's Health. New York, Harper & Row, 1983

Ma P and Armstrong D. The Acquired Immune Deficiency Syndrome and Infections of Homosexual Men. New York, Yorke Medical Books, 1984

Marr JJ. Infectious Diseases in General Medical Practice. Menlo Park, CA, Addison-Wesley, 1982

McCormack WM (ed). Diagnosis and Treatment of Sexually Transmitted Diseases. Boston, John Wright, 1983

Meyer RD (ed). Practical Infectious Diseases. New York, John Wiley & Sons, 1983

Myerowitz RL. The Pathology of Opportunistic Infections. New York, Raven Press, 1983

Ostrow DG, Sandholzer TA and Felman YM. Sexually Transmitted Diseases in Homosexual Men. New York, Plenum Press, 1983

Strickland GT. Hunter's Tropical Medicine, 6th ed. Philadelphia, WB Saunders, 1984

Waldman RH and Kluge RM (eds). Textbook of Infectious Diseases. New York, Medical Examination Publishing Co, 1984

Articles

Control of Infectious Diseases

Campbell B. The nursing process and infection control. Dimens Health Serv 1983 Sep; 60(9):26–27

Goodman RA, Orenstein WA and Hinman AR. Vaccination and disease prevention for adults. JAMA 1982 Oct 1; 248(13):1607–1610

Gordon EK, Brill JC and Geiderman JM. Immunoprophylaxis in the emergency department. Top Emeg Med 1982 Apr; 4(1):82–94

Hargiss CO and Larson E. Infection control: Guidelines for prevention of hospital acquired infections. Am J Nurs 1981 Dec; 81(12):2175–2183

Jackson MM and Lynch P. Infection control: Too much or too little? Am J Nurs 1984 Feb; 84(2):208–210

Lang WR and Kreider SD. Immunization. Around the world in 80 shots. Postgrad Med 1983 Feb; 73(2):219–226

Moree NA and Garner JS. New infection control guideline. Am J Nurs 1984 Feb; 84(2):210–211

Nieman RE. Immunization for adults. Med Times 1984 Mar; 112(3):39–42

Pizzo PA and Schimpff SC. Strategies for the prevention of infection in the myelosuppressed or immunosuppressed cancer patient. Cancer Treat Rep 1983 Mar; 67(3):223–234

Williams WW. Guidelines for infection control in hospital personnel. Ann J Infect Control 1984 Feb; 12(1):34–57

Sexually Transmitted Diseases

Apuzzo-Berger D. A.I.D.S: Could you be at risk? RN 1983 Feb; 46(2):67–78

Bone JR. Transfusion-associated AIDS—a cause for concern. N Engl J Med 1984 Jan 12; 310(2):115–116

Campbell CE and Herten RJ. VD to STD: Redefining venereal disease. Am J Nurs 1981 Sep; 81(9):1629–1635

Conte JE et al. The acquired immune deficiency syndrome (AIDS)—a multidisciplinary enigma. West J Med 1984 Jan; 140(1):81

Curran JW et al. Acquired immunodeficiency syndrome (AIDS) associated with transfusions. N Engl J Med 1984 Jan 12; 310(2):69–75

Curran JW and Barker LF. The acquired immunodeficiency syndrome associated with transfusions: The evolving perspective. Ann Intern Med 1984 Feb; 100(2):298–300

Daul CB and deShazo RD. Acquired immune deficiency syndrome: An update and interpretation. Ann Allergy 1983 Sep; 51(3):351–361

Fauci AS. The acquired immune deficiency syndrome. JAMA 1983 May 6; 249(17):2375–2376

Fauci AS et al. Acquired immunodeficiency syndrome: Epidemiologic, clinical, immunologic, and therapeutic considerations. Ann Inter Med 1984 Jan; 100(1):92–106

Gremminger RA. Taking a sexual history. Wis Med J 1983 Nov; 82(11):20–24

Howard DR. Acquired immune deficiency syndrome. Compr Ther 1983 Aug; 9(8):3–5

Jemison-Smith P. Understanding the acquired immune deficiency syndrome. NITA 1984 Mar–Apr; 7(2):114–116

Marx JL. Strong new candidate for AIDS agent. Science 1984 May 4; 224(4648):475

Masur H. The acquired immunodeficiency syndrome. DM 1983 Oct; 30(1):1–48

Memon AS. Acquired immune deficiency syndrome: A diagnostic update. Med Times 1984 Apr; 112(4):91–94, 99

Nichols SE Jr. Psychiatric aspects of AIDS. Psychosomatics 1983 Dec; 24(12):1083–1089

Popkin B et al. Caring for the AIDS patient—fearlessly. Nursing '83 1983 Sep; 13(9):50–55

Popovic M et al. Detection, isolation, and continuous production of cytopathic retroviruses (HTLV-III) from patients with AIDS and pre-AIDS. Science 1984 May 4; 224(4648):497–500

Ratner J and Thomas A. Opportunistic infections in homosexual men. South Med J 1984 Feb; 77(2):227–228

Sarngadharan MG et al. Antibodies reactive with human T-lymphotropic retroviruses (HTLV-III) in the serum of patients with AIDS. Science 1984 May 4; 224(4648):506–508

Sonnabend J, Witkin SS and Purtilo DT. Acquired immunodeficiency syndrome, opportunistic infections and malignancies in male homosexuals. JAMA 1983 May 6; 249(17):2370–2374

Weller, I. ABC of sexually transmitted diseases. Acquired immune deficiency syndrome. Br Med J (Clin Res) 1984 Jan 14; 288(6411):136–137

Wong ES and Stamm WE. Urethral

infections in men and women. Annu Rev Med 1983; 34:337–358

Bacterial Infections

Barclay WR. BCG: An effective immunizing agent. JAMA 1983 May 6; 249(17):2376 ·

Clemens JD, Chuong JJH and Feinstein AR. The BCG controversy. JAMA 1983 May 6; 249(17):2362–2369

Craig CP. Gram-negative septicemia and shock. Compr Therapy 1982 Feb; 8(2):13–18

Cross A et al. Nosocomial infections due to *Pseudomonas aeruginosa:* Review of recent trends. Rev Infect Dis 1983 Nov–Dec; 5(Suppl 5):S837–S845

Crow S. Nursing care of the immunosuppressed patient. Infect Control 1983 Nov–Dec; 4(6):465–467

de la Monte SM, Gupta PK and White CL. Systemic *Actinomyces* infection. A potential complication of intrauterine contraceptive devices. JAMA 1982 Oct 15; 248(15):1876–1877

DeVoe IW. The meningococcus and mechanisms of pathogenicity. Microbiol Rev 1982 Jun; 46(2):162–190

Eustache JM and Kreis DJ Jr. Typhoid perforation of the intestine. Arch Surg 1983 Nov; 118(11):1269–1271

Fernsebner B. Patients at risk for nosocomial infections. AORN J 1983 Oct; 38(4):613–620

Gransden WR, Eykyn S and Phillips I. *Staphylococcus aureus* bacteraemia: 400 episodes in St. Thomas's Hospital. Br Med J 1984 Jan 28; 288(6413):300–303

Hart GR, Lamb RC and Strauss MB. Gas gangrene. J Trauma 1983 Nov; 23(11):991–1000

Hughes JM and Tackett CO. "Sausage poisoning" revisited. Arch Intern Med 1983 Mar; 143(3):425–427

Jay SJ. Nosocomial infections. Med Clin North Am 1983 Nov; 67(6):1251–1277

Johnson ET. Nosocomial infection: Update. J Natl Med Assoc 1983 Feb; 75(2):147–154

Kalager T and Solberg CO. Diagnosis and treatment of septicaemia. Trop Gastroenterol 1983 Jul–Aug; 4(3):121–128

Kim TC et al. Acid–fast bacilli in sputum smears of patients with pulmonary tuberculosis. Am Rev Respir Dis 1984 Feb; 129(2):264–268

Klotz SA et al. Typhoid fever. Arch Intern Med 1984 Mar; 144(3):533–537

Lamb LS. Think you know septic shock? Read this. Nursing '82 1982 Jan; 12(1):34–43

Lambert HP. Management problems in meningitis. Br J Hosp Med 1983 Feb; 29(2):128–133

Larson E. Current handwashing issues. Infect Control 1984 Jan; 5(1):15–17

Lefrock JL and Smith BR. Tuberculosis therapy. Am Fam Physician 1983 Mar; 27(3):261–264

Lepow ML and Cold R. Meningococcal A and other polysaccharide vaccines. A five-year progress report. N Engl J Med 1983 May 12; 308(19):1158–1160

Maloney JJ and Cho SR. Pelvic actinomycosis. Radiology 1983 Aug; 148(2):388

McGowan JE Jr. Whence come nosocomial infections? N Engl J Med 1982 Dec 16; 307(25):1576–1577

McHenry MC and Weinstein AJ. Symposium on infections in office practice. Med Clin North Am 1983 Jan; 67(1):entire volume

Neu HC. The emergence of bacterial resistance and its influence on empiric therapy. Rev Infect Dis 1983 Mar–Apr; 5(Suppl 1):S9–S20

Overturf GD. Meningitis. Top Emerg Med 1982 Apr; 4(1):16–25

Satterwhite TK and DuPont HL. Infectious diarrhea in office practice. Med Clin North Am 1983 Jan; 67(1):203–220

Schlech WF 3rd et al. Medical management of visceral actinomycosis. South Med J 1983 Jul; 76(7):921–922

Schmidt-Nowara WW, Samet JM and Rosario PA. Early and late pulmonary complications of botulism. Arch Intern Med 1983 Mar; 143(3):451–456

Scully RE, Mark EJ and McNeely BU (eds). A young man with a mass involving the lung, pleura, and chest wall. N Engl J Med 1983 Nov 10; 309(19):1171–1178

Simmons BP. CDC guidelines for the prevention and control of nosocomial infections. Guideline for hospital environmental control. Am J Infect Control 1983 Jun; 11(3):97–120

Snider DE Jr et al. Six-months isoniazid–rifampin therapy for pulmonary tuberculosis. Am Rev Respir Dis 1984 Apr; 129(4):573–579

Sommers HM. Recent developments in the diagnosis and management of mycobacterial infections. Clin Lab Med 1982 Jun; 2(2):305–319

Täuber MG and Sande MA. The impact of penicillin on the treatment of meningitis. JAMA 1984 Apr 13; 251(14):1877–1880

Taylor DN, Pollard RA and Blake PA. Typhoid in the United States and the risk to the international traveler. J Infect Dis 1983 Sep; 148(3):599–602

Unsworth IP and Sharp PA. Gas gangrene. An 11-year review of 73 cases managed with hyperbaric oxygen. Med J Aust 1984 Mar 3; 140(5):256–260

Wenzel RP (ed). First international symposium on hospital-acquired infections. Proceedings. Infect Control 1983 Sep–Oct; 4(5):363–397

Viral Infections

Collins TR and Burridge MJ. Rabies prophylaxis. Am Fam Physician 1984 Mar; 29(3):295–300

Coward DD. The other herpesviruses: Epstein–Burr and cytomegalovirus. Nurse Pract 1983 Apr; 8(4):13–18

Crespin FH Jr and Gordon RC. Infectious mononucleosis in the community hospital. J Fam Pract 1983 Apr; 16(4):703–708

Douglas RG Jr. Antiviral drugs 1983. Med Clin North Am 1983 Sep; 67(5):1163–1172

Heggie J and Chang M. What to do about flu. RN 1983 Jan; 46(1):60–63

Heldrich FJ and Sainz D. Infectious mononucleosis with splenic rupture. MD State Med J 1984 Jan; 33(1):40–41

Immunization Practices Advisory Committee. Prevention and control of influenza. MMWR 1984 May 18; 33(19):253–266

Immunization Practices Advisory Committee: Varicella-zoster immune globulin for the prevention of chickenpox. MMWR 1984 Feb 24; 33(7):84–100

Nichols AO. Taking the fear out of rabies treatment. Nursing '83 1983 Jun; 13(6):42–43

Riddiough MA et al. Influenza vaccination. JAMA 1983 Jun 17; 249(23):3189–3195

Rickettsial Infections

Kaplowitz LG et al. Correlation of rickettsial titers, circulating endotoxin, and clinical features in Rocky Mountain spotted fever. Arch Intern Med 1983 Jun; 143(6):1149–1151

Kossmann CE. Rocky Mountain spotted fever. J Tenn Med Assoc 1983 Nov; 76(11):730–736

Marx RS. Rocky Mountain spotted fever. Compr Ther 1983 May 9(5):43–48

Purgason TJ. Rocky Mountain spotted fever. A case presentation with discussion of fatal complications. J Okla State Med Assoc 1982 Aug; 75(8):263–266

Rocky Mountain Spotted Fever—United States, 1983. MMWR 1984 Apr 13; 33(14):188–195

Strickland AL, Darby CP and Corbett B. Rocky Mountain spotted fever. J SC Med Assoc 1983 Aug; 79(8):431–434

Thompson S. Summertime and ticks. Am J Nurs 1983 May; 83(5):768–769

Protozoan Infections

Files JC, Case CJ and Morrison FS. Automated erythrocyte exchange in fulminant falciparum malaria. Ann Intern Med 1984 Mar; 100(3):396

Lobel HD and Campbell CC. Trends in imported malaria, United States. MMWR Surveill Summ 1983 Aug; 32(3SS):15SS–18SS

Most H. Treatment of parasitic infections of travelers and immigrants. N Engl J Med 1984 Feb 2; 310(5):298–304

Wyler DJ. The ascent and decline of chloroquine. JAMA 1984 May 11; 251(18):2420–2422

Wyler DJ. Malaria—resurgence, resistance and research, Part I. N Engl J Med 1983 Apr 14; 308(15):875–878

Wyler DJ. Malaria—resurgence, resistance and research, Part II. N Engl J Med 1983 Apr 21; 308(16):934–940

Fungal Infections

Comer JB. Amphotericin B; Ten common questions. Am J Nurs 1981 Jun; 81(6):1166–1167

Rees PL and Dixon DM. Opportunistic mycoses. Am J Nurs 1981 Jun; 81(6):1160–1165

Helminthic and Parasitic Infections

Gilman RH. Hookworm disease: Host-pathogen biology. Rev Infect Dis 1982 Jul–Aug; 4(4):824–829

Sharma P. Broad-action anthelminthics against intestinal helminthiases. Trop Gastroenterol 1984 Jul–Aug; 4(3):137–154

Weller PF. Parasitic infections of concern to primary care practice. Med Times 1983 Aug; 111(8):32–36

Care of the Aging Person

21

Definitions

Aging—a normal process of time-related changes that occur throughout life; old age is a normal part of human development and is the final phase of the life cycle.

Geriatrics—branch of health science concerned with the study and treatment of problems and diseases associated with aging.

Gerontology—study of the aging process and its effects on older persons.

Health Maintenance and Preventive Care

Goals:
Maintain health and function.
Detect disease at an early stage.
Prevent deterioration of an existing condition.

A. Maintaining health and function.

1. Promote positive feelings about the health of the aged.
   a. Stress that physiologic changes of aging are normal and a natural phase of life; life-style and personality play an important role in health and longevity.
   b. Encourage efforts to maintain activities, wellness, and control of health during later years.
2. Educate the older person on ways to conserve his health.
3. Encourage periodic health appraisal and counseling to give attention to health before illness develops and to prevent deterioration of an existing condition. Health assessment techniques utilize automated procedures, computer analysis, and read-out results to obtain baseline health information and determine state of wellness.
4. Promote accident prevention among the elderly and their families.
   a. High incidence of falls due to age, pathologic conditions, locomotor disabilities, decline of postural control, environmental risks, and fear of falling.
   b. Maintain physical and mental activities—to improve confidence and mobility.
   c. Rise to an upright posture *slowly* from a supine position.
5. Protect the patient against infectious diseases by immunization (especially against influenza and pneumonia).
6. Promote socialization to prevent mental deterioration and depression and to preserve a reason for living.
   a. Know risk factors—living alone, recently bereaved, mobility problems, recent discharge from hospital, sudden life change, social isolation.
   b. Encourage the aged to continue to take on intellectual challenges.
   c. Encourage a variety of interests and activities.
   d. See that the patient has sensory input from the outside world.
7. Schedule and coordinate preventive, therapeutic, and restorative health services.

B. Detecting disease at an early stage

1. Explain diagnostic tests available for early detection of problems; provide support and encouragment.
   a. Electrocardiogram—to show subtle heart abnormalities.
   b. Chest x-ray—for tuberculosis, lung cancer, heart size, changes in large blood vessels and bony structure of the chest.
   c. Pulmonary function tests—to rule out chronic bronchitis and emphysema.
   d. Tonometer test—to measure intraocular pressure for glaucoma.
   e. Blood glucose test—to detect diabetes mellitus.
   f. Papanicolaou smear—to detect cancer of the cervix.
   g. Blood and urine tests.
   h. Hearing and vision tests—sensory deprivation can cause a downhill course.
   i. Assessment for alcoholism.
2. Emphasize accident prevention and control of the environment.

C. Preventing deterioration of an existing condition

Assess the patient's health habits and knowledge of disease.
1. Advise the patient to avoid temperature extremes.
2. Encourage the patient to stop smoking.
3. Educate about proper foot care.
4. Ensure proper nutrition and monitor weight.
5. Educate the patient to avoid undesirable effects of drugs.

6. Provide education programs on specific health problems of the elderly.

D. Community resources

1. Include preretirement counseling.
2. Every person over 70 who is living alone should be visited regularly by a health visitor (nurse, social worker, volunteer health aid).

3. Use comprehensive services available for elderly: (diagnostic centers, extended care facilities, home care programs, homemaker services, friendly visitors, "Meals on Wheels," daily telephone calls ["buddy system"], day care centers, mental health services, vocational projects, continuing education, foster grandparents, social service).

Health Problems of the Aged

Underlying Considerations

1. Although aging is not synonymous with illness, the aged are vulnerable to disease because of decreased physiologic reserve, less flexible homeostatic processes, and less effective defense mechanisms of the body.
2. An estimated 85% of elderly have some form of chronic illness. More than one disease may be present.
3. Disease in the aged does not always present classic signs and symptoms; the usual clinical manifestations may be absent, attenuated, or disguised; and atypical signs and symptoms may be present.
4. Depression and dementia often worsen health problems.
5. Resistance to stress is diminished—one major illness lowers resistance and allows other illnesses to appear.
6. Illnesses tend to cluster during closing years of the very old person's life—chain reaction of one degenerative process leading to another and finally to death.

Disease Aspects

(Consult index for specific disease.)

Mental Health Aspects

Psychological Needs

1. Basic psychological needs of all people include respect, security, self-esteem, and the need to feel appreciated and valued by others.
2. The maintenance of "self" (self-continuity, integrity, identity) is important to the psychological survival of the elderly.
3. The elderly person is vulnerable to emotional and mental stress from many losses.
   a. Losses through death of spouse, children, other "significant persons."
   b. Loss of social roles and resources—affects status and prestige; person may withdraw and disengage himself from the mainstream of life.
   c. Socioeconomic losses—decreased income; inflation.
      Affect quality of health care, self-esteem, and position in society.
   d. Loss of work role—produces sense of uselessness, feelings of nonparticipation.
   e. Loss of health—includes loss of self-esteem.

Psychiatric and Cognitive Disorders

The psychiatric disorders of late life are a major cause of chronic ill health and disability. Incidence increases with age; disorders include depression, paranoid reactions, and dementias.

A. Depression (disorder of mood)—most common emotional disorder of the aged occurring in 20%–30% of elderly.

1. Characterized in late life by apathy, sense of hopelessness, and exhaustion; loss of interest and somatic complaints. It may result from accumulation of many unavoidable and real losses (see above).
2. Depression may be masked as a cognitive disturbance in the elderly.
3. Older people (who make up 11% of population) account for about 25% of reported suicides.

Assessment

1. Look for physical signs and symptoms that may be the cause of depression.
2. Take a drug (including alcohol) history; many drugs can cause depression in the elderly.

Nursing Interventions

1. Have an awareness that the depressed elderly may be mislabeled as "demented."
2. Allow the patient to release anger, guilt, and grief.
3. Treatment consists of psychotherapy, drugs, and occasionally, electroconvulsive therapy.

B. Paranoia—characterized by suspicion and ideas of persecution (second most common psychiatric disturbance among elderly).

1. More common among elderly with sensory deficits and those who are "loners."
2. Management—appropriate medication, supportive therapeutic relationships, hearing aid/glasses to decrease sensory isolation, and development of social network.

C. Dementias—progressive deterioration of intellectual functioning. (Refer to a psychiatric nursing textbook for discussion of the types of dementias.)

Senile Dementia of the Alzheimer's Type (Alzheimer's Disease)

Alzheimer's disease is a chronic, progressive and deteriorative brain disorder accompanied by profound effects on memory, cognition, and ability for self-care. Its cause remains unknown.

Alzheimer's disease is the most common form of dementia among the aged, affecting some 2 million elderly Americans, many of whom are in nursing homes at a total cost of 25 billion dollars per year.

Pathophysiology

1. Changes occur in the proteins of the nerve cells of the cerebral cortex and lead to accumulation of

neurofibrillary tangles (abnormal tangled fibers), granulovacuolar degeneration, and characteristic senile plaques (degenerated nerve cell pieces which form around a fibrous core in the cerebral cortex).
2. Research scientists report there is evidence of a significant and progressive decrease in the activity of the enzyme, choline acetyltransferase (ChAT) in the brain tissue. Choline acetyltransferase is a crucial ingredient in the chemical process that produces acetylcholine, a neurotransmitter involved in learning and memory.
3. There is also a marked loss of nerve cells in part of the base of the brain (nucleus basalis).

Assessment
Clinical Manifestations

1. Significant forgetfulness
2. Deterioration of higher cognitive function with loss of ability to read, to write, to calculate, and eventually to speak intelligently
3. Personality changes
4. Disorders of motor function, including disorder of gait; incontinence

Diagnostic Evaluation

Probable Alzheimer's disease diagnosis based on clinically determined dementia confirmed by:
1. Neuropsychologic tests
2. Two or more cognitive deficits
3. Progressive worsening of memory and other cognitive functions
4. No disturbances of consciousness
5. Onset between ages 40 and 90 (most often after age 65)
6. Absence of systemic disorders or other brain disorders that could cause progressive deficits in memory and cognition

Management
A. Maintaining the patient's current abilities in optimal state

1. No treatment presently known to prevent or arrest underlying pathologic process
2. Management of concomitant physical health problems to prevent excess disability/worsening of behavior
3. Behavioral interventions are used to manage memory problems and intellectual dysfunction
4. Continuing monitoring for signs and symptoms of illness

Patient Problems/Nursing Diagnoses

1. Ineffective family coping related to burdens imposed by Alzheimer's disease
2. Loss of cognitive function and memory related to physiologic alterations in brain tissue
3. Catastrophic behavior related to cognitive, intellectual, and memory dysfunction
4. Alterations in sleep/rest patterns related to effects of disease
5. Incontinence related to cognitive deterioration
6. Impaired communication (verbal) related to loss of word recognition or meaning
7. Diversional activity deficit related to lack of awareness
8. Self-care deficit related to loss of memory function and cognitive awareness
9. Ineffective coping related to awareness in early stages of disease that memory is fading

Planning and Implementation
Nursing Interventions

Goal:
The family receives knowledge and support and acquires skill in handling their loved one and in coping with stresses imposed by Alzheimer's disease.

A. Teaching and supporting the family

1. Encourage family to become part of a support group that functions to educate about latest developments in Alzheimer's disease; this helps them to know, anticipate, and plan for changes.
2. Tell family what to expect.
   a. Encourage family to do legal and financial planning.
   b. Keep them informed about changes in the patient.
3. Help caregiver to maintain own physical and mental well-being.
   a. Encourage scheduling of *regular* respite care from the demands of a "36-hour day."
   b. Discuss with caregiver the need to plan for personal fulfillment outside the relationship with the patient.
4. Assist the caregiver/family to identify and work through their feelings.
   a. Encourage expressions of grief, frustration, anger, loss—helps the family to know that these feelings are normal.
   b. Acknowledge problem behaviors ("shadowing" caretaker, combativeness, accusations, excessive demands, frequent somatic complaints) before they exist.
   c. Talk about skills needed to prevent or moderate catastrophic reactions of patient (see below).
5. Support family's decision to place the patient in an extended care facility; problems that are especially difficult for family are aggression, delusions, hallucinations, confusion, and inability to provide self-care. Help the family cope with inevitable feelings of grief.

B. Enhancing, preserving, or compensating for loss of cognitive function

1. See that the patient has sufficient sensory input that is recognized as friendly.
   a. Be sure that all sensory deficits are corrected; eye glasses and hearing aid on; teeth in.
   b. Approach in front of patient; avoid suddenly appearing from behind.
   c. Gain eye contact; speak slowly and in short sentences.
   d. Keep the patient oriented to time, place, and person *repeatedly*.
      (1) Speak the patient's name; then touch his hand or arm.
      (2) Introduce yourself (again and again); show your name tag.
   e. Keep conversation at close range.
      (1) Do not move around while talking to the patient.
      (2) Make short, frequent contacts.
      (3) Pay attention to what the patient is saying—much of what he is saying makes sense.
   f. Use nonverbal (body language) communication: gestures, eye contact, smiles, friendliness, gentle touch.

2. Provide aids to help maintain or stimulate cognitive functioning.
   a. Keep frequently used articles in a definite place.
   b. Keep a calendar and clock, both with easily readable numbers, within range of vision.
   c. Give written information; use lists; mark calendar.
   d. Use pictures plus written communication.
   e. Label frequently used items.
3. Extend the person's life space.
   a. Encourage family to bring in pictures, family album, etc. since familiar objects promote a sense of continuity, aid memory, and provide security and comfort.
   b. Use pictures, music, color, indoor gardens, etc. to enhance the environment.
   c. Read newspaper headlines. Discuss current events.
   d. Take the patient outdoors; encourage family to take him to a restaurant, shopping center, etc.
   e. Use sensory retraining (seeing, tasting, touching, smelling, hearing).
4. Maintain activities as close to normal as possible.
   a. Keep environment ordered, predictable and fail-ure-free.
   b. Assist the patient to continue daily routine, physical activities, and social contacts.
   c. Arrange for visits from others to counteract isolation.
      (1) Use services of a volunteer who can visit regularly if no family is available.
      (2) Work with family toward specific goals.

C. **Maintaining consistent environment and avoiding threatening situations**

1. Keep the environment consistent and failure-free.
   a. Respect the patient's territorial rights.
   b. Do not move the patient's personal belongings.
   c. Avoid changing rooms—difficult for marginally oriented person to cope with change.
   d. Have the patient's personal belongings where he can see and use them.
   e. Allow the patient to "hoard" a few things; do not dispose of them.
2. Avoid overestimating the patient's ability; mental and physical tasks beyond his capacity produce anxiety, frustration, and anger.
3. Reassure the patient that he is safe; remind him that you are caring for him when he repeatedly calls out, asks for "Mother," etc.
4. Study individual to recognize tolerance level to stimulation.
   a. Avoid excessive stimulation that precipitates a reaction.
   b. Avoid telling the patient to "try harder," "try to remember," etc.
   c. Remove tasks that precipitate frustration.
   d. Give positive directions.
5. Remain calm when the patient becomes upset.
   a. Expect some anger, passivity, frustration, and dependency.
   b. Change focus of interaction; *use distraction.*
   c. Avoid restricting movement—may lead to agitation.
6. Help the patient maintain dignity and self-respect.
   a. Avoid talking about confused person in his presence.
   b. Explain what is happening and when it will happen.
   c. Encourage independence as much as possible.

D. **Promoting safety and reducing anxiety**

1. Attempt to deal positively with wandering behavior.
   a. Evaluate for underlying pathology (cardiac decompensation).
   b. Ascertain if the patient is trying to satisfy a need (hunger, warmth).
   c. Study environment and identify potential threats to safety because patient is at risk for falls, burns, and accidents.
   d. Restructure environment to improve well-being.
   e. Allow the patient mobility without jeopardizing safety.
   f. Try to engage the patient in a more stimulating activity because boredom and tension may be the basis of wandering.
   g. Give directions or suggestions if the patient appears lost.
   h. Have the patient wear identification bracelet (name, address, telephone number).
   i. Have an alarm system/special locks to prevent wandering away from home.
2. Attempt to alleviate the patient's anxiety and restlessness.
   a. Try "laying on of hands"—touching, stroking, hugging; many aged persons have no one to touch them.
   b. Use warm milk, warm baths, back massage, and also understanding and compassion as therapeutic modalities.
   c. Give the patient gentle and constant reassurance.
   d. Schedule the patient's daily activities and adhere to the schedule—order and predictability reduce anxiety and promote security.
   e. Be consistent. Each member of the health care team should know the patient's goals and use the same approach.
   f. Give "permission" to express grief, anger, and hostility.
3. Maintain a normal day and night pattern.
   a. Encourage the patient to dress in clean, attractive (color-coordinated) clothes daily—the wearing of nightwear during the day confuses the concepts of day and night.
   b. See that the patient wears shoes—not slippers.
   c. Encourage the patient to *walk* and not use the wheelchair, which limits his environment.
   d. Encourage the patient to eat at a table and not at the bedside.
   e. Encourage the patient to stay awake during the day. Keep him physically active.
   f. Keep the room well-lighted to reduce confusion and fear; use a night-light to reduce risk of "sundowning" (worsening of a condition at night).
   g. Reorient the patient during periods of sleeplessness.

E. **Managing bladder and bowel incontinence.**

1. See page 70 for discussion of how to prevent bladder and bowel incontinence.
2. Keep a record of the patient's voiding and defecation patterns.
3. Maintain the patient on a *regular* voiding and defecation schedule.
   a. Color code or mark the bathroom door.
   b. Take the patient to the bathroom on schedule.
   c. Keep bathroom light on at night.
   d. Avoid long-acting sedatives or hypnotics—may prevent the patient from awakening at night.

4. Provide special disposable undergarments that trap wetness away from the skin if incontinence cannot be managed by above measures.

Evaluation
Expected Outcomes

1. Family uses positive coping mechanisms while living with a patient with Alzheimer's disease; belongs to a support group; verbalizes that they may have to place the patient in an extended-care facility

2. Patient uses some compensatory mechanisms for loss of cognitive function
3. Family tries to avoid situations that precipitate catastrophic behavior
4. Family attempts to prevent alterations in sleep and rest patterns and wandering behavior; has made the patient's environment "safe"; demonstrates ability to calm the patient during periods of agitation
5. Family adheres to a bladder and bowel training schedule; the patient is free of bladder and bowel incontinence

Approach to the Aged Patient

Assessment of the Elderly Patient

In addition to the health history and physical examination, the nursing assessment involves an attempt to determine the functioning ability, strengths, and limitations of the patient.

Physiologic Assessment

1. How does the patient describe the activities of a "typical" day? (Assess for the usual level of functioning.)
2. How does he view his health?
3. How effective is the patient at self-care?
4. How much physical capacity does the patient have?
5. How much muscle strength and coordination does the patient have?
6. How well does the patient see and hear?
7. What are the patient's usual eating, sleeping, elimination, and activity patterns? What constitutes a "normal" bowel movement?
8. How does the patient handle his sexual feelings?
9. Does the patient have any sexual concerns or problems?
10. Are there any changes in bodily functions?
11. What will the patient have to do to regain or maintain functioning ability?

Socioeconomic Assessment

1. What is the patient's background? Early history?
2. How many person-to-person contacts does the patient have in a day?
3. Who is the patient's "significant other"? (Include pet.) Are there good social supports (friends, family)?
4. Who visits the patient?
5. What is the patient's religion?
6. What are the patient's living arrangements?
7. Is the patient in proximity to relatives or helping neighbors?
8. Are the patient's activities limited because of transportation problems? High-crime environment?
9. How much independence does the patient possess?
10. What are the patient's feelings about living at home?
11. Does the patient participate in any phase of community life?
12. How can the environment be adjusted to maintain independence?

Psychological Assessment

1. Is the patient alert and optimistic in outlook?
2. What does the patient identify as his major concerns and problems?

3. What are the patient's attitudes toward aging?
4. What are the patient's attitudes toward himself? Is there a feeling of being needed? useful?
5. What psychological defenses does the patient use?
6. What are the patient's activities, interests, and hobbies?
7. What ego strengths and coping skills did the patient use in the past?
8. Are there any disturbances in experiencing pleasure?
9. What are the patient's plans and hopes?

Management of Special Needs and Problems

Nutritional Considerations for the Aged

1. Nutritional requirements of the elderly are similar to those of adults except that calorie intake should be reduced. Older persons need a *variety* of foods.
   a. Energy needs diminish with age—both metabolic rate and activity decrease, so that calorie requirements of the aged are reduced.
   b. The calorie intake is adjusted on an individual basis to maintain normal weight.
   c. Protein requirements are not reduced but protein utilization may be less efficient in old age.
   d. High-nutrient-density foods should be consumed to obtain adequate intake.
2. The elderly are at risk for malnutrition. Nutritional deficiencies frequently seen in independently living elderly, include dietary iron, folic acid, vitamins A, B_{12} (and other B vitamins), and C, and calcium.
   a. Vitamin C and vitamin K deficiency—ecchymoses due to capillary fragility.
   b. Vitamin A deficiency—fissuring of skin around mouth; reduced visual sensitivity.
   c. Vitamin B deficiency—changes in mucous membranes of tongue and lips.
   d. Mineral deficiencies—demineralization of bone.
3. Factors affecting nutritional habits of the elderly.
   a. Food habits of a lifetime
   b. Social factors (eating alone)
   c. Susceptibility to food fads
   d. Dental problems
   e. Shopping problems
   f. Reduced income
   g. Lack of motivation for meal planning and food preparation
   h. Decreased appeal of food—loss of taste buds; less acute sense of smell
   i. Drug-induced malnutrition
   j. Alcohol abuse

4. Assistance programs
   a. Community-based meals
   b. Multipurpose senior centers
   c. Supplemental security income
   d. Home-delivered meals; "Meals on Wheels"
   e. Friendly visitor program
   f. Nutritional counseling
   g. Food stamps
   h. Day-care for the elderly
   i. Self-help eating devices

Drug Therapy and the Aged

A. Factors Altering Drug Response in Elderly

1. Age-related changes in body function (decline in lean body mass and renal competency) predispose elderly to problems with medication side effects.
2. Absorption, distribution, metabolism, and excretion of many drugs are affected by aging.
   a. *Absorption*—affected by gastric pH, rate of gastric emptying, reduction in intestinal blood flow.
   b. *Distribution*—affected by alterations in body composition, protein binding, tissue permeability.
   c. *Metabolism*—decreased metabolic capacity for detoxifying drugs and decreased number of receptors at which drug may act; diminished cardiac output.
   d. *Excretion*—renal clearance may be limiting factor.

B. Nursing Strategies to Improve Medication Use

1. Be aware that drug effect is more pronounced in old persons. The potential for adverse reactions, interactions and medication-induced disease is greater.
   a. Older persons may not be able to handle multiple medications.
   b. They appear to be more sensitive to digoxin, diuretics, aspirin, oral antidiabetic drugs, sedatives, analgesics, psychotropic agents, etc.
   c. The more medications the patient takes, the greater is the risk for drug interactions and adverse reactions.
2. Obtain a nursing and drug history.
   a. Check nutritional status.
   b. Find out if the patient is taking drugs not currently prescribed.
   c. Ask what over-the-counter medications the patient is taking (laxatives, antacids, aspirin)—the elderly use twice as many nonprescription preparations as those that are prescribed.
   d. Assess for alcohol usage.
3. Usually the physician will hold the dosage to lowest effective amount; doses may be given further apart.
   a. Reinforce verbal instructions with *written* instructions.
   b. Have the patient repeat the instructions.
   c. Give instructions also to a relative/friend to reinforce patient education.
   d. Write what the drug is used for (e.g., "to thin the blood.").
   e. Explain possible side effects.

   f. Be sure that the drug name and instructions for taking it are typed in large letters on the label. Bottles may have color-coded strips.
   g. Make sure that the patient can open medication container; child-proof container may not be appropriate.
   h. Arrange drug schedule to coincide with a regular activity (arising, eating, retiring)—helps the patient to remember to take drug.
   i. Arrange some sort of check-off system.
   j. List all medications the patient is taking; tape list to refrigerator or other special place.
4. Carry out periodic drug review.
   a. Ask the patient to bring all medication on next visit to physician or clinic.
   b. Assess for patient compliance, response to therapy, possible side effects, drug interactions—rate of noncompliance is high in elderly.
   c. Have the patient ask pharmacist to keep his drug profile on computer—used as a safeguard to detect potential drug interactions.
   d. Give the patient friendly support.

Hygienic Care

A. Skin Care

1. Aging skin is dry, thin, and inelastic; sweat gland and sebaceous gland activity and water binding capacity of skin are decreased.
2. Bathe every other day using a mild, superfatted soap.
3. After damp-drying the skin, use a nonocclusive emollient (a petrolatum- or lanolin-based preparation) to prevent transepidermal water loss.
4. Consult dermatologist if redness and pruritus occur.

B. Oral Care

1. Common oral complaints include loss of teeth, dry mouth, abnormal taste, and burning sensations in mouth.
2. Components of dental/oral care include proper diet, maintaining health of oral and denture-bearing structures, and using available dental services.
   a. Use electric toothbrush and WaterPic® to remove retained food particles between teeth.
   b. Encourage increased fluid intake in persons with decreased salivary flow.

C. Elimination Problems (See p. 70)

D. Foot Care

1. One third of the elderly have foot disorders. Degenerative and systemic diseases, trauma, neglect, and misuse cause foot problems in the elderly.
2. Systemic diseases such as diabetes mellitus, arterial insufficiency, and the arthritides often are compounded by loss of sensation, abnormal gait patterns, and impaired vision; thus the assessment made by the nurse is of prime importance.
3. Nail disorders account for about one fourth of foot complaints.
4. See pages 702 for assessment of feet.

Summary of Principles Underlying the Nursing Management of the Elderly Patient

1. Growth and adaptation continue to occur when the individual's strengths and potential are recognized and reinforced.

2. Nursing care must be individualized, taking into consideration the patient's past experiences, needs, and individual goals.

3. Assess the data to determine the older person's health status; establish a nursing diagnosis/nursing diagnoses.
4. Realistic and attainable goals, which are understood by the patient, are set to help him gain a sense of accomplishment and purpose.
   a. Have an optimistic view of aging and the older person.
   b. Engage in mutual goal-setting.
   c. The underlying goal is independence or partial independence in activities of daily living.
   d. Keep communicating to the patient and family the planned goals of his care.
   e. Support his belief in his own inner resources.
   f. Prepare the older individual (especially women) to meet own needs after leaving the hospital.
5. The patient should be an active participant in his own plan of care.
   a. Learn something about the patient before the initial encounter; find out the patient's strengths.
   b. Consult the patient's preferences.
   c. Concentrate on what the patient can do.
   d. Ask the patient's opinions.
   e. Encourage the patient to keep control over his life and to make choices and decisions.
   f. Avoid making decisions for him; this promotes low self-esteem, dependency, and depression.
   g. Praise even minimal achievements.
   h. Support the patient during periods of anxiety; allow expression of troubles and difficulties.
   i. Urge the patient to remain active. Direct attention to gains being made and on the controls the patient still retains.
6. Nursing activities should be done *with* the patient rather than *for* him.
7. Necessary modifications and compromises imposed by the physiological limits of aging must be made in the medical and nursing management of the patient.
8. The individuality of the patient should be encouraged—to preserve his identity and sense of control.
   a. Respect the patient's personal space or territorial boundaries.
   b. Encourage the patient to have and use personal possessions that help bridge the gap between past and present.
   c. Respect the right to self-direction.
   d. Allow the person to take some risks (i.e., live alone) when benefits can outweigh risks.
   e. Give the patient *time* to express his feelings.
   f. Help him retain the social graces.
   g. Help him cope with thoughts of death.
9. Elderly persons should be kept in the mainstream of life to prevent physical, emotional, and mental deterioration.
   a. Avoid removing the element of challenge. Encourage contact with others.
   b. Give dignity and privacy for personal relationships with opposite sex and expression of sexual needs.
   c. Work out a "buddy system" to prevent loneliness and isolation.
   d. Stimulate mental acuity and sensory input—minimizes preoccupation with body monitoring.
   e. Encourage physical activity.
   f. Share your world with the patient.
   g. Remember the patient's preferences; accept his idiosyncracies.
   h. Provide opportunities for him to do some tasks of daily living.
   i. Encourage the patient to feed/help other residents.
   j. Provide meaningful diversional activity.
   k. Give the patient something to look forward to.
10. The patient's potentialities should be utilized.
    a. Select activities that are in keeping with lifelong interests.
    b. Do not attempt to alter lifelong character and behavior patterns.
    c. Give the patient time to listen, to learn, and to adapt.
    d. Help the patient to learn new ways to maintain independence.
11. Act as an advocate of the elderly.
12. Evaluate the patient's progress toward attainment of goals.

Bibliography

Books

Alford BB and Bogle ML. Nutrition During the Life Cycle. Englewood Cliffs, NJ, Prentice-Hall, 1982

Alzheimer's Disease: An Information Paper. Washington, DC: G.P.O., January 1984, Comm Pub No 98-402

American Nurses' Association Division on Gerontological Nursing Practice. A Challenge for Change: The Role of Gerontological Nursing. Kansas City, MO, American Nurses' Association, 1982

Anderson F and Williams B. Practical Management of the Elderly, 4th ed. St Louis, Blackwell Scientific Publications, 1983

Aronson MK, Bennett R and Gurland B. The Acting-Out Elderly. New York, Haworth Press, 1983

Beaver ML. Human Service Practice With the Elderly. Englewood Cliffs, NJ, Prentice-Hall, 1983

Belsky JK. The Psychology of Aging. Monterey, CA, Brooks/Cole, 1984

Blumenthal HT. Handbook of Diseases of Aging. New York, Van Nostrand Reinhold, 1983

Burnside I. Working With the Elderly, 2nd ed. Monterey, CA, Wadsworth Health Services Division, 1984

Butler RN and Lewis MF. Aging and Mental Health. St Louis, CV Mosby, 1983

Cape RDT, Coe RM and Russman I (eds). Fundamentals of Geriatric Medicine. New York, Raven Press, 1983

Carotenuto R and Bullock J. Physical Assessment of the Gerontologic Client. Philadelphia, FA Davis, 1981

Covington TR and Walker JI. Current Geriatric Therapy. Philadelphia, WB Saunders, 1984

Cox H. Later Life: The Realities of Aging. Englewood Cliffs, NJ, Prentice-Hall, 1984

Cummings JL and Benson DF. Dementia: A Clinical Approach. Woburn, MA, Butterworths, 1983

Elipoulos C (ed). Health Assessment of the Older Adult. Menlo Park, CA, Addison-Wesley, 1984

Fromer MJ. Aging. In Community Health Care, The Nursing Process, 2nd ed, pages 432–456. St Louis, CV Mosby, 1983

Gardner K and Halamandaris VJ. Elder Abuse (An Examination of a Hidden Problem). Washington, DC, Government Printing Office, 1981

Gonda TA and Ruark JE. Dying Dignified. Menlo Park, CA, Addison-Wesley, 1984

Gress LD and Bahr RT. The Aging Person: A Holistic Perspective. St Louis, CV Mosby, 1984

Hall BA (ed). Mental Health and the

Elderly. Orlando, FL, Grune & Stratton, 1984

Heston LL and White JA. Dementia, A Practical Guide to Alzheimer's Disease and Related Illnesses. New York, WH Freeman, 1983

Holden UP and Woods RT. Reality Orientation: Psychological Approaches to the "Confused" Elderly. New York, Churchill Livingstone, 1982

Katzman R (ed). Biological Aspects of Alzheimer's Disease. Cold Spring Harbor Laboratory, NY, Cold Spring Harbor Laboratory, 1983

Kelly WE (ed). Alzheimer's Disease and Related Disorders: Research and Management. Springfield, IL, Charles C Thomas, 1984

Lieberman MA and Tobin SS. The Experience of Old Age: Stress, Coping, and Survival. New York, Basic Books, 1983

Mace NL and Rabins PV. The 36-Hour Day. Baltimore, University Park Press, 1981

Miller JF. Powerlessness in the elderly: Preventing hopelessness. In Coping with Chronic Illness: Overcoming Powerlessness, pages 109–131. Philadelphia, FA Davis, 1983

Murray RB, Huelskoetter MMW and O'Driscoll DL. The Nursing Process in Later Maturity. Englewood Cliffs, NJ, Prentice-Hall, 1980

O'Hara-Devereaux M, Andrus LH and Scott CD (eds). Eldercare. New York, Grune & Stratton, 1981

Reichel W (ed). Clinical Aspects of Aging: A Comprehensive Text, 2nd ed. Baltimore, Williams & Wilkins, 1983

Reisberg B (ed). Alzheimer's Disease. New York, Free Press, 1983

Reisberg B. Brain Failure: An Introduction to Current Concepts of Senility. New York, Free Press, 1981

Roe DA. Geriatric Nutrition. Englewood Cliffs, NJ, Prentice-Hall, 1983

Rothschild H (ed). Risk Factors for Senility. New York, Oxford University Press, 1984

Schrier RW (ed). Clinical Internal Medicine in the Aged. Philadelphia, WB Saunders, 1982

Simonson W. Medications and the Elderly: A Guide for Promoting Proper Use. Rockville, MD, Aspen, 1984

Steinberg FU (ed). Care of the Geriatric Patient, 6th ed. St Louis, CV Mosby, 1983

Task Force on Scope of Gerontological Nursing Practice. A Statement on the Scope of Gerontological Nursing Practice. Kansas City, MO, American Nurses' Association, 1981

Williams TF (ed). Rehabilitation in the Aging. New York, Raven Press, 1984

Wolanin MO and Phillips LRF. Confusion: Prevention and Care. St Louis, CV Mosby, 1981

Woodruff DS and Birren JE (eds). Aging: Scientific Perspectives and Social Issues, 2nd ed. Monterey, CA, Brooks Cole, 1983

Yurick AG et al. The Aged Person and the Nursing Process, 2nd ed. Norwalk, CT, Appleton-Century-Crofts, 1984

Articles

Alfin-Slater RB. Aging: A condition or a disease? Aging 1984; 26:323–330

Archibald JW and Ullman MA. Is it really senility—or just depression? RN 1983 Nov; 46(11):49–51

Bartol MA. Reaching the patient. Geriatric Nurs 1983 Jul/Aug; 4(4): 234–236

Beam IM. Alzheimer's disease: Helping families survive. Am J Nurs 1984 Feb; 84(2):228–232

Coyle JT, Price DL and DeLong MR. Brain mechanisms in Alzheimer's disease. Hosp Pract 1982 Nov; 17(11): 55–63

Delapp TD. Helping the elderly live longer—and better. Nursing '83 1983 Nov; 13(11):61–63

Dugan JS. Winning the battle against incontinence. Nursing '84 1984 Jun; 14(6):59

Emr M. Facets of dementia. J Gerontol Nurs 1984 Apr; 10(4):38–39

Forgan Morle KM. Patient satisfaction: Care of the elderly. J Adv Nurs 1984 Jan; 9(1):71–76

Gwyther LP and Matteson MA. Care for the caregiver. J Gerontol Nurs 1983 Feb; 9(2):92–95, 110

Gwyther LP and Blazer DG. Family therapy and the dementia patient. Am Fam Physician 1984 May; 29(5):149–156

Herst LD. Emergency psychiatry for the elderly. Psychiatr Clin North Am 1983 Jun; 6(2):271–280

Hudson MF. Safeguard your elderly patient's health through accurate physical assessment. Nursing '83 1983 Nov; 13(11):58–64

Jernigan JA. Update on drugs and the elderly. Am Fam Physician 1984 Apr; 29(4):238–247

Kahn R. Alzheimer's disease: Theories and therapies. Am J Nurs 1984 Feb; 84(2):223–224

Kopac CA. Sensory loss in the aged: The role of the nurse and the family. Nurs Clin North Am 1983 Jun; 18(2):373–384

Lamy PP. Hazards of drug use in the elderly. Commonsense measures to reduce them. Postgrad Med 1984 Jul; 76(1):50–53, 56–57, 60–61

Lederer A et al. Confusion: Recognition and remedy. Geriatric Nurs 1983 Jul–Aug; 4(4):224–248

Lederer A. Notes on a nursing home. Geriatric Nurs 1983 Jul–Aug; 4(4): 224–227

Lipsky JG. Saving the elderly from the killing cold. Nursing '84 1984 Feb; 14(2):42–43

Mayeux R and Rosen WG. The dementias. Adv Neurol 1983; 38:1–263(entire volume)

O'Malley TA et al. Identifying and preventing family-mediated abuse and neglect of elderly persons. Ann Intern Med 1983 Jun; 98(6):998–1005

Pajk M. Alzheimer's disease: Inpatient care. Am J Nurs 1984 Feb; 84(2):216–222

Panicucci CL. Functional assessment of the older adult in the acute care setting. Nurs Clin North Am 1983 Jun; 18(2):355–363

Parker C and Somers C. Reality orientation on a geropsychiatric unit. Geriatric Nurs 1983 May/Jun; 4(3): 163–165

Porth C and Kapke K. Aging and the skin. Geriatric Nurs 1983 May/Jun; 4(3):158–162

Raskind M. Nutrition and cognitive function in the elderly. JAMA 1983 June 3; 249(21):2939–2940

Reisberg B. Alzheimer's disease: Stages of cognitive decline. Am J Nurs 1984 Feb; 84(2):225–228

Salisbury S and Goehner P. Separation of the confused or integration with the lucid? Geriatric Nurs 1983 Jul/Aug; 4(4):231–233

Samiy AH (ed). Symposium on clinical geriatric medicine. Med Clin North Am 1983 Mar; 67(2):entire volume

Schirmer MS. When sleep won't come. J Gerontol Nurs 1983 Jan; 9(1):16–21

Shine MS. Discharge planning for the elderly patient in the acute care setting. Nurs Clin North Am 1983 Jun; 18(2):403–410

Stelle RE and Mills J. Ambulation of the institutionalized elderly. Am Fam Physician 1983 Sep; 28(3):163–167

Tavon E. Tips to trigger memory. Geriatric Nurs 1984 Jan–Feb; 5(1):26–27

Tyler KL and Tyler HR. Differentiating organic dementia. Geriatrics 1984 Mar; 39(3):38–43, 46–49, 52, 131–132

Turner ML. Skin changes after forty. Am Fam Physician 1984 Jun; 29(6):173–181

Wells CE. Diagnosis of dementia: A reassessment. Psychosomatics 1984 Mar; 25(3):183–187

Zimberg S. Alcoholism in the elderly. Postgrad Med 1983 Jul; 74(1):165–173

Selected Agencies

Alzheimer's Disease and Related Disorders Association
360 North Michigan Avenue
Chicago, IL 60601

American Association of Retired Persons
1909 K Street, N.W.
Washington, DC 20049

National Council of Senior Citizens
925 15th Street, N.W.
Washington, DC 20005

National Institute on Aging
National Institute of Mental Health
National Institute of Neurological and Communicative Disorders and Stroke
National Institutes of Health
Bethesda, MD 20892

U.S. Department of Health and Human Services
Office of Human Development Services
Administration on Aging (AOA)
Federal Council on the Aging
H.H.H. Building
200 Independence Avenue, S.W.
Washington, DC 20201

Nursing the Person with Cancer

22

General Considerations

The Optimistic Side of Cancer

1. One third of all cancer patients are cured.
2. Improved treatment modalities enable patients with cancer to live longer, more comfortably, and more productively.
3. Most cancer patients spend almost all their time away from hospitals and only come to the hospital intermittently for treatment.
4. More intense efforts at patient rehabilitation are proving effective.
5. Forty-eight percent of all patients with cancer can now be cured according to the National Cancer Institute's Surveillance, Epidemiology, and End Results (SEER) Program (Fig. 22-1).
6. Research continues unabated, and, as findings accumulate, prospects for specific cures are encouraging.

Cancer's Warning Signals

C hange in bowel or bladder habits
A sore that does not heal
U nusual bleeding or discharge
T hickening or lump in breast or elsewhere
I ndigestion or difficulty in swallowing
O bvious change in wart or mole
N agging cough or hoarseness

Early Detection of Cancer

Early detection provides a very effective way to reduce the morbidity and mortality of several cancers.

Benign and Malignant Tumors

	Benign	Malignant
Type of cell	Adult cell	Young cell
Nature	Closely resembles parent tissue	Tends to be anaplastic (reverting to primitive cells)
Growth	Slow	Rapid, usually
Encapsulated	Often	Never
Effect on surrounding tissue	Never invades	Invades widely
Localization	Remains at original site	Nonlocalized—forms secondary growths by metastasis
Recurrence after removal	Does not tend to recur	Tends to recur

Metastasis

Metastasis is the transfer of disease cells from one organ or part to another not directly connected with it.

1. *Extension and invasion*—because they are not encapsulated, it is easy for cancer cells to invade other tissues and extend themselves rapidly via lymphatic and blood circulatory systems; cancer may also recur in treated areas.
2. *Lymph*—secondary growths of tumor cells are often caught in the lymph filter, the lymph node.
3. *Blood*—by invasion, tumor cells enter the blood vessels and are carried to organs where the venous blood passes through a capillary bed.

Incidence

1. The annual death toll from malignancy in the US is at least 450,000.
2. Cancer ranks second as the leading cause of death in the US.
3. Cancer strikes at any age. It affects children as well as adults, but it strikes with increasing frequency with advancing age.
4. There will be about 870,000 new cancer cases this year (diagnosed for the first time).
5. No organ of the body is exempt. (See Fig. 22-2 for cancer death rates by site.)

Treatment

1. Modalities of treatment include surgery, radiotherapy, radioactive substances (including radioisotopes), var-

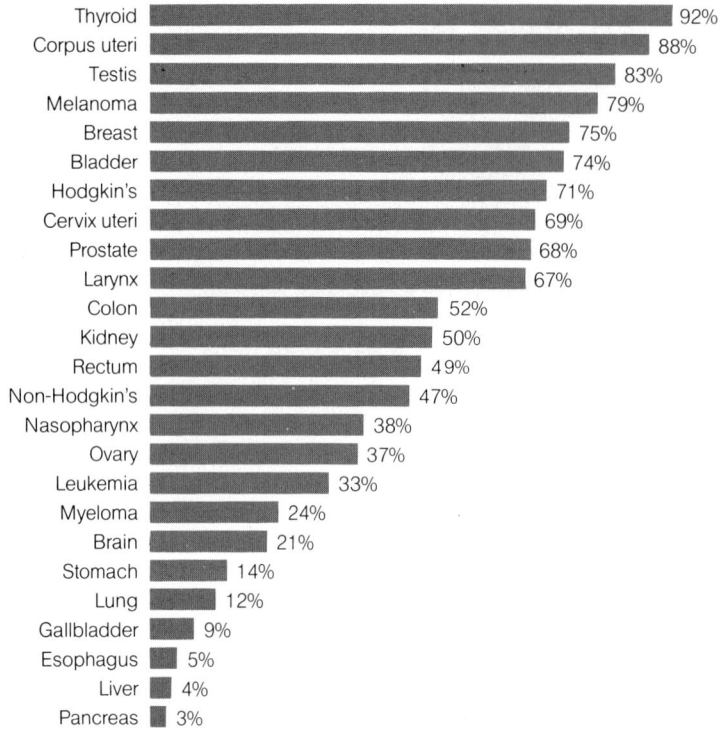

Figure 22-1. Five-year survival rates for patients diagnosed between 1973 and 1981 show that more than two thirds of patients with certain major types of cancer can be cured. Forty-eight percent of all patients with cancer can now be cured. (National Cancer Institute's Surveillance, Epidemiology, and End-Results [SEER] Program. Updated by VT DeVita, Jr, MD, Director, National Cancer Institute, November 26, 1984)

ious drugs (pharmaceuticals and hormones), and immunotherapy (see pp. 916–917).
2. Method of treatment will depend on the type of malignancy, precise staging, localization or spread, condition of patient, and the physician; the use of more than one kind of therapy, often in combination, is frequently utilized.

Nutrition and Cancer

1. No concrete dietary advice can be given that will guarantee prevention of any specific human cancer.
2. There is sufficient information to make recommendations that are likely to provide some measure of reducing cancer risk.
3. The following nutritional guidelines approved by the American Cancer Society are in general similar to those issued by the National Research Council of the National Academy of Sciences, and the National Cancer Institute.
   a. Avoid obesity.
   b. Cut down on total fat intake.
   c. Eat more high-fiber foods, such as whole grain cereals, fruits, and vegetables.
   d. Include foods rich in vitamins A and C in the daily diet.
   e. Include cruciferous vegetables, such as cabbage, broccoli, brussels sprouts, kohlrabi, and cauliflower in the diet.
   f. Be moderate in consumption of alcoholic beverages.
   g. Be moderate in consumption of salt-cured, smoked, and nitrite-cured foods.

Surgery

Definitions

1. *Biopsy*—surgical removal of a piece of tissue from the questionable area; the tissue sample is sent to the pathology laboratory for diagnostic verification.
2. *Preventive or prophylactic surgery*—removal of lesions which, if left in the body, are apt to develop into cancer. Example: polyps in rectum may lead to cancer of the colon.
3. *Palliative surgery*—a type of surgery which attempts to relieve the complications of cancer (e.g., obstruc-

tion of the gastrointestinal tract, pain produced by tumor extension into surrounding nerves).
4. *Curative surgery*—the removal of the primary site of malignancy and any lymph nodes to which the neoplasm has extended. Such surgery may be all that is required.

5. *Surgery combined with radiation, chemotherapy, or immunotherapy*—combinations of treatment required to halt the spread of a malignancy.

Note: Details of surgical treatment are given in the sections relating to specific disease entities.

Chemotherapy for Cancer

Value of Chemotherapy in Treating a Malignancy

1. As yet no drugs are available to cure most malignant tumors. Chemotherapy is used successfully in treating choriocarcinoma, lymphoma, and leukemia.
2. Effects of chemotherapy:
   a. May produce a regression of the tumor or of its metastases.
   b. May reduce or slow the appearance of secondary growths.
   c. May relieve pain and other symptoms, such as pleural effusion, ascites, for a time.
   d. May improve quality of survival.
3. Cancer chemotherapy offers some relief to patients for whom surgery and irradiation are no longer beneficial.
4. Chemotherapeutic agents are useful in treatment of leukemias, Hodgkin's disease, lymphomas, Ewing's tumor, Wilms's tumor, testicular tumors, and retinoblastomas. Can lead to remissions—sometimes for many years.
5. Combinations of chemotherapeutic agents are often more effective and no more toxic than single agents.
6. Chemotherapy may be effective in patients who have been treated successfully by surgery and/or radiotherapy but in whom the recurrence risk may be high.
7. Combination with immunotherapy appears promising.
8. Precise scheduling of dosages is necessary to achieve effective results.
9. Many chemotherapeutic agents have unpleasant systemic effects in addition to their effect on malignant tissue; therefore, it is imperative that these be recognized by the nurse.

Pharmacologic Action (Table 22-1)

1. These drugs are capable of destroying young, rapidly multiplying cells, such as malignant cells.
2. They interfere with manufacture of nucleic acids (inhibit the chain of synthesis or function of DNA and RNA) so that cellular growth and reproduction are inhibited.
3. Since many normal cells in the body also grow rapidly and have short life spans (e.g., bone marrow, gastrointestinal tract lining, hair follicles), many chemotherapeutic agents directly attack these normal cells. Herein lies the challenge.

Method of Administration

Drugs may be given orally, intravenously, intramuscularly, or intra-arterially, depending on the drug.

A. Intravenous Administration

1. See page 96 for principles of intravenous therapy. Additional specific concerns related to administration of chemotherapeutic agents include the following:
   a. In general, avoid venipuncture in an arm where:

   (1) Dissection of the axillary nodes has been performed
   (2) Radiotherapy has caused marked fibrosis in the axillary area
   b. Avoid areas of sclerosis, thrombosis, or scar formation.
2. If a small focal hematoma develops during insertion of needle into a vein, do not use this avenue for administration of toxic chemotherapeutic agents because of the danger of extravasation.
3. Maintain constant supervision during administration of potentially locally toxic chemotherapeutic agents.
4. If any doubt exists regarding vein patency or safety of drug administration, discontinue administration.
5. It is better to prevent *extravasation* than to treat it.
   a. Symptoms
      Pain (severe enough to cause the patient to cry out); area may appear red, mottled, and/or swollen—often leading to necrosis.
   b. Treatment
      (1) Apply cold compresses to slow down local tissue metabolism.
      (2) Some physicians recommend local infiltration of the involved area with an anti-inflammatory agent.
      (3) Later, warm compresses may be applied; local management as indicated.
   c. If only a small amount of drug is extravasated and frank necrosis does not occur, phlebitis may still result causing pain for several days and/or induration at the site that may last for weeks or months.
   d. For one agent, Mustargen, the specific antidote is sodium thiosulfate, which should be injected immediately (subcutaneously or intradermally) into the area of extravasation.
6. Observe for occurrences other than extravasation:
   a. Intraluminal
      (1) Symptoms
         (a) Patient may describe sensations of pain, stretching, or pressure within the vessel, originating near venipuncture site or 7.5–12.5 cm. (3–5 inches) along vein course.
         (b) Discoloration—deep blue or purple 5–10 cm. (2–4 inches) proximal to venipuncture site.
      (2) Treatment
         Wait and observe; change puncture site or discontinue administration of drug.
   b. Subcutaneous tissue
      (1) Symptoms
         Itching, muscle cramp, pressure within arm, possible urticaria
      (2) Treatment
         (a) Wait and observe; change puncture site, or discontinue administration of drug.

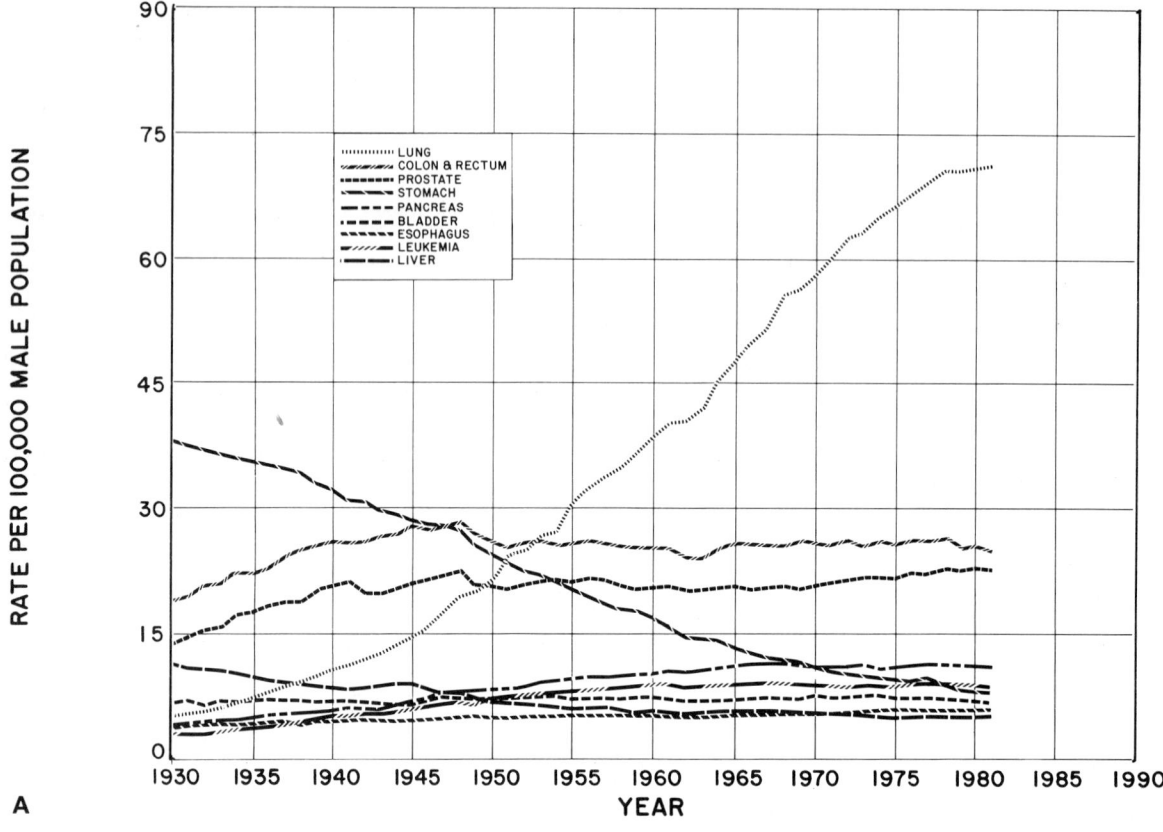

Figure 22-2. (A) Male and (B) female cancer death rates by site, United States, 1930–1981. Rates for male and female populations standardized for age on the 1970 US population. (Epidemiology & Statistics Department, American Cancer Society, Aug 1984; data from National Vital Statistics Division and Bureau of the Census, United States)

    (b) Notify physician if systemic effects are observed.

B. Isolation-Perfusion—administration of large doses of extremely toxic drugs to an isolated extremity, organ, or region of the body (excluding systemic circulation). Usually such a dose cannot be tolerated by the entire body. By this means, short, intensive recirculation of high doses of antineoplastic drugs is used.

1. Areas
  a. Lower extremity—iliac, femoral, popliteal arteries and veins
  b. Pelvis—abdominal aorta, vena cava
2. Patient preparation
  a. Weigh the patient since drug dosage is calculated on basis of kilograms of body weight.
  b. Obtain results of blood, urine, and x-ray studies.
  c. Explain to the patient the nature of the procedure and the reason for applying tourniquets.
3. Operative procedure
  a. A totally occlusive tourniquet may be applied to an extremity in order to separate this area from systemic circulation.
  b. A pump oxygenator is used to circulate the patient's blood in a closed system for the involved part of the body.

  c. Concentrated doses of the chemotherapeutic agent are injected.
  d. Duration of perfusion depends on drug and on extent and location of growth.
  e. Oxygenated blood is pumped into the artery; it passes through the extremity affected by the tumor and out through the vein, where the blood is reoxygenated and recirculated.
  f. For an abdominal or lower pelvic tumor, a laparotomy may be done.
    (1) Blood supply to the tumor area is blocked from systemic circulation by means of pneumatic tourniquets on the legs and special clamps on the inferior mesentery artery and vein.
    (2) Catheters are inserted into the major vessels near the tumor site.
    (3) The desired drug is injected into the artery; venous blood is conveyed to an oxygenator for oxygenation, and is then pumped back into the arterial system.
    (4) Upon completion of treatment, fresh blood may be transfused if necessary; clamps and tourniquets are removed, and the surgical wound is closed.

C. Intra-arterial Infusion—the introduction percutaneously of a catheter into a major artery under

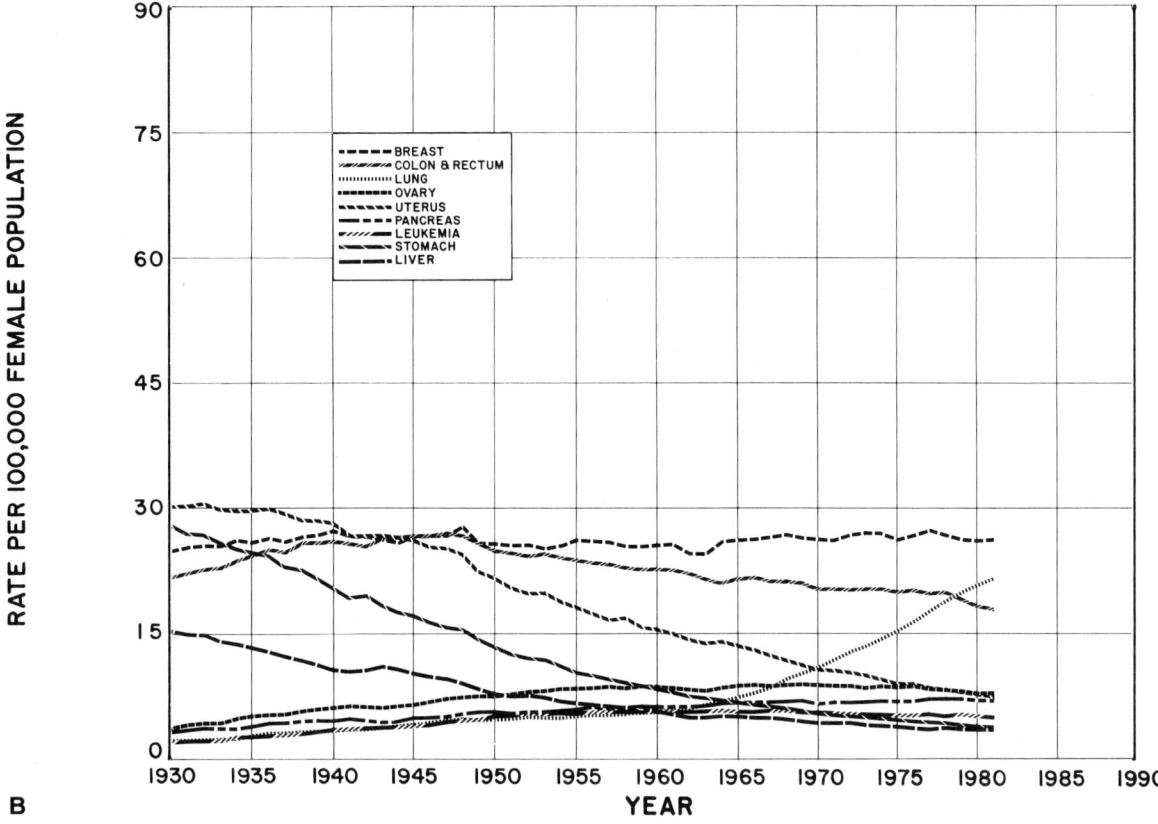

Figure 22-2. (continued)

fluoroscopic guidance. This does not require major surgery and can be repeated at intervals. The continuous administration of the chemotherapeutic agent into the artery leading to the tumor may last for several days or several weeks.

1. Routes
   Brachial, axillary, carotid, or femoral artery—determined by location of tumors.
2. Uses and advantages
   a. This method is used preferably when the tumor is completely encompassed by the vessels in question: to check this, fluoroscein may be injected into the catheter and the tumor observed under a special lamp for fluorescence.
   b. Arterial infusion acts on the tumor over a longer period of time than is possible with isolation perfusion.
   c. By increasing regional concentrations and using minimal systemic drug concentrations, systemic toxicity is limited.
3. This treatment is still considered investigational.
D. Adjunct Chemotherapy—administration of a chemotherapeutic agent at the time of surgery to kill any tumor cells which may spill into the bloodstream when the tumor is manipulated.
E. Combined Chemotherapy and Irradiation—permits drug to enhance the effect of irradiation. This has been particularly effective in treating head and neck lesions.

Medical and Nursing Care of Patients Receiving Perfusion or Arterial Infusion

Before Special Treatment

1. The patient needs concerned care; these are procedures (perfusion and arterial infusion) which are tried because the disease is advanced, although limited to an anatomic area.
2. Provide encouragement and enough information to acquaint the patient with the possible benefits as well as dangers of the procedure.
3. Give emotional support since the unpleasant side effects of chemotherapy can cause depression.

During Chemotherapy

1. Be familiar with the nature of the chemotherapeutic agent being used (toxic manifestations, etc.).
2. Observe arterial injection site to see that catheter is properly positioned. Guard against hemorrhage, leakage, sepsis, and tissue irritation.
3. Note any signs of malaise, nausea, vomiting, diarrhea, temperature elevation, changes in blood pressure and pulse.
4. Report intake and output accurately.
5. If necessary, administer fluids intravenously for first 48 hours to maintain general hydration as well as dilution of posttreatment antineoplastic drugs.

(Text continues on p. 910)

Table 22-1 Commercially Available Cancer Chemotherapeutic Drugs*
Note: major or dose-limiting effects are in bold type

Drug	Acute Toxicity	Delayed Toxicity
Alkylating Agents		
Busulfan (*Myleran*—Burroughs Wellcome)	Nausea and vomiting; rare diarrhea	**Bone marrow depression;** pulmonary fibrosis; hyperpigmentation; cutaneous reactions; alopecia; gynecomastia; amenorrhea; menopausal symptoms; sterility; azospermia; leukemia; chromosome aberrations; cataracts; addisonian syndrome
Chlorambucil (*Leukeran*—Burroughs Wellcome)		**Bone marrow depression;** pulmonary fibrosis; leukemia; hepatic toxicity
Cyclophosphamide (*Cytoxan*—Mead Johnson)	**Nausea and vomiting**	**Bone marrow depression;** alopecia; hemorrhagic cystitis; sterility (may be temporary); pulmonary fibrosis; hyperpigmentation; secondary malignancies; nonspecific dermatitis; hyponatremia
Estramustine phosphate sodium (estracyt; *Emcyt*—Roche)	Nausea and vomiting, diarrhea	Mild gynecomastia; increased frequency vascular accidents; myelosuppression (uncommon); edema; dyspnea
Mechlorethamine (nitrogen mustard; HN2; *Mustargen*—Merck)	Nausea and vomiting; local reaction and phlebitis	Bone marrow depression; alopecia; diarrhea; oral ulcers
Melphalan (1-phenylalanine mustard; *Alkeran*—Burroughs Wellcome)	Mild nausea; hypersensitivity reactions	**Bone marrow depression** (especially platelets); possible pulmonary fibrosis; interstitial pneumonitis; leukemia
Thiotepa (triethylenethiophosphoramide; *Thiotepa*—Lederle)	**Nausea and vomiting;** local pain	**Bone marrow depression;** menstrual dysfunction; interference with spermatogenesis
Antimetabolites		
Cytarabine HCl (cytosine arabinoside; *Cytosar-U*—Upjohn)	**Nausea and vomiting;** diarrhea; anaphylaxis	**Bone marrow depression;** megaloblastosis; oral ulceration; hepatic damage; fever; iritis, conjunctivitis; pulmonary edema (at very high doses)
Floxuridine (*FUDR*—Roche)	**Nausea and vomiting;** diarrhea	**Oral and gastrointestinal ulceration; bone marrow depression;** pigmentation; alopecia; dermatitis
Fluorouracil (5-FU; *Fluorouracil*—Roche; *Adrucil*—Adria)	**Nausea and vomiting;** diarrhea	**Oral and GI ulcers; bone marrow depression;** increased lacrimation; neurological defects, usually cerebellar; pigmentation; alopecia; dermatitis
Mercaptopurine (6-MP; *Purinethol*—Burroughs Wellcome)	**Nausea and vomiting;** diarrhea	**Bone marrow depression; cholestasis and rarely hepatic necrosis; oral and intestinal ulcers;** anorexia
Methotrexate (MTX; *Methotrexate*—Lederle; *Mexate*—Bristol)	**Nausea and vomiting:** diarrhea; fever; anaphylaxis	Oral and gastrointestinal ulceration, perforation may occur; **bone marrow depression;** hepatic toxicity including cirrhosis and acute hepatic necrosis; renal toxicity; pulmonary infiltrates; osteoporosis; chills, fever; alopecia; depigmentation; cutaneous reactions; infertility; menstrual dysfunction
Thioguanine (6-TG; *Tabloid Brand Thioguanine*—Burroughs Wellcome)	**Occasional nausea and vomiting**	**Bone marrow depression;** hepatic damage; stomatitis
Natural Products		
Asparaginase (*Elspar*—Merck)	**Nausea and vomiting; fever,** chills; headache; **hypersensitivity,** anaphylaxis; abdominal pain; hyperglycemia leading to coma	CNS depression or hyperexcitability; acute hemorrhagic pancreatitis; coagulation defects; renal damage; hepatic damage
Bleomycin (*Blenoxane*—Bristol)	**Nausea and vomiting; fever;** anaphylaxis and other allergic reactions	**Pneumonitis and pulmonary fibrosis; cutaneous reactions;** stomatitis; alopecia; hyperpigmentation; Raynaud's phenomenon
Dactinomycin (actinomycin D; *Cosmegen*—Merck)	**Nausea and vomiting;** diarrhea; local reaction and phlebitis	**Stomatitis; oral ulceration; bone marrow depression;** alopecia; folliculitis
Daunorubicin (Daunomycin; *Cerubidine*—Ives)	**Nausea and vomiting;** diarrhea; red urine (not hematuria); severe local tissue damage and necrosis on extravasation; transient EKG changes	**Bone marrow depression; cardiotoxicity** (may be irreversible); alopecia; stomatitis; cutaneous toxicity; anorexia; diarrhea; fever and chills
Doxorubicin (*Adriamycin*—Adria)	**Nausea and vomiting;** red urine (not hematuria); severe local tissue damage and necrosis on extravasation; diarrhea; transient EKG changes; ventricular arrhythmia	**Bone marrow depression; cardiotoxicity** (may be irreversible); alopecia; stomatitis; cutaneous toxicity; anorexia; diarrhea; fever, chills; urticaria; anaphylaxis; conjunctivitis; lacrimation
Mithramycin (*Mithracin*—Miles)	**Nausea and vomiting;** diarrhea; fever	**Hemorrhagic diathesis; bone marrow depression** (thrombocytopenia); coagulation abnormalities; hepatic damage; hypocalcemia and hypokalemia; stomatitis; cutaneous reactions
Mitomycin (*Mutamycin*—Bristol)	**Nausea and vomiting;** local reaction if extravasation; fever	**Bone marrow depression** (cumulative); stomatitis; alopecia; pulmonary fibrosis; hepatotoxicity and renal toxicity at high doses
Vinblastine sulfate (*Velban*—Lilly)	**Nausea and vomiting;** local reaction and phlebitis if extravasation	**Bone marrow depression;** alopecia; stomatitis; loss of deep tendon reflexes; jaw pain; paralytic ileus; inappropriate ADH secretion

* The Medical Letter, Issue 626, January 7, 1983.

Table 22-1   Commercially Available Cancer Chemotherapeutic Drugs (continued)

Drug	Acute Toxicity	Delayed Toxicity
Vincristine sulfate (*Oncovin*—Lilly)	Local reaction if extravasation	**Peripheral neuropathy** (loss of deep tendon reflexes, numbness, tingling and muscle weakness); neuritic pain; alopecia; mild bone marrow depression; constipation; paralytic ileus; inappropriate ADH secretion

Other Synthetic Agents

Drug	Acute Toxicity	Delayed Toxicity
Carmustine (BCNU; *BiCNU*—Bristol)	**Nausea and vomiting;** local phlebitis	**Delayed leukopenia and thrombocytopenia** (may be prolonged); pulmonary fibrosis (may be irreversible); delayed renal damage; gynecomastia; reversible liver damage
Cisplatin (Cis-Diammine-dichloroplatinum; Cis-DDP; *Platinol*—Bristol)	**Nausea and vomiting;** anaphylactic reactions; fever	**Renal damage;** bone marrow depression; ototoxicity; hemolysis; hypomagnesemia; peripheral neuropathy; hypocalcemia; hypokalemia
Dacarbazine (DTIC; DIC; *DTIC–Dome*—Miles)	**Nausea and vomiting;** diarrhea; anaphylaxis; pain on administration; flu-like syndrome	**Bone marrow depression;** alopecia; renal impairment; hepatic necrosis; facial flushing, paresthesia; rash; photosensitivity
Hydroxyurea (*Hydrea*—Squibb)	**Nausea and vomiting;** allergic reactions to tartrazine dye	**Bone marrow depression;** hyperkeratosis and hyperpigmentation; stomatitis; dysuria; alopecia; rare neurologic disturbances
Lomustine (CCNU; *CeeNU*—Bristol)	**Nausea and vomiting**	**Delayed (4–6 weeks) leukopenia and thrombocytopenia** (may be prolonged); transient elevation of transaminase activity; neurologic reactions; pulmonary fibrosis
Mitotane (o,p′-DDD; *Lysodren*—Bristol)	**Nausea and vomiting;** diarrhea	**CNS depression;** dermatitis; visual disturbances; adrenal insufficiency; brain damage with long-term high dosage; hematuria, hemorrhagic cystitis, albuminuria; hypertension; orthostatic hypotension
Procarbazine HCl (*Matulane*—Roche)	**Nausea and vomiting;** CNS depression; Antabuse-like effect with alcohol	**Bone marrow depression;** stomatitis; dermatitis; peripheral neuropathy; pneumonitis; secondary malignancies
Streptozocin (streptozotocin; *Zanosar*—Upjohn)	Nausea and vomiting; local pain; chills	Renal damage; hypoglycemia; hyperglycemia; liver damage; diarrhea; bone marrow depression (uncommon); fever; eosinophilia

Hormones

Estrogens

Drug	Acute Toxicity	Delayed Toxicity
Diethylstilbestrol (DES; many manyfacturers)	**Nausea and vomiting;** cramps	**Fluid retention;** hypercalcemia; feminization; uterine bleeding; if given during pregnancy, may cause vaginal carcinoma in offspring; increased frequency of vascular accidents
Ethinyl estradiol (*Estinyl*—Schering; others)		**Fluid retention;** hypercalcemia; feminization; uterine bleeding; increased incidence of vascular accidents

Androgens

Drug	Acute Toxicity	Delayed Toxicity
Dromostanolone propionate (*Drolban*—Lilly)		**Fluid retention; masculinization;** hypercalcemia
Fluoxymesterone (*Android-F*—Brown; *Halotestin*—Upjohn)		**Fluid retention; masculinization;** cholestatic jaundice; hypercalcemia; painful hypertrophy of clitoris; hirsutism
Testolactone (*Teslac*—Squibb)	Local pain, inflammation at injection site	Hypercalcemia; rare alopecia; masculinization (minimal)
Testosterone propionate (many manufacturers)		**Fluid retention; masculinization;** hypercalcemia

Progestins

Drug	Acute Toxicity	Delayed Toxicity
Hydroxyprogesterone caproate (*Delalutin*—Squibb; others)	Local abscess, pain	Hypercalcemia; cholestatic jaundice
Medroxyprogesterone acetate (*Provera*—Upjohn; others)	Orally; nausea (rare); IM: local pain, abscess at injection site	Fluid retention; hypercalcemia
Megestrol acetate (*Megace*—Mead Johnson; *Pallace*—Bristol)	Allergic reactions to tartrazine dye	Fluid retention; thromboembolism; alopecia; carpal tunnel syndrome

Corticosteroids

Drug	Acute Toxicity	Delayed Toxicity
Prednisone or prednisolone		Mental aberrations; gastric ulcers; glucose intolerance; osteoporosis; hypertension; cataract formation; Cushingoid features; metabolic abnormalities; myopathy

Antiestrogen

Drug	Acute Toxicity	Delayed Toxicity
Tamoxifen citrate (*Nolvadex*—Stuart))	Nausea and vomiting; hot flashes; transient increased bone or tumor pain	Vaginal bleeding and discharge; rash; hypercalcemia; retinopathy; corneal changes; decreased visual acuity; peripheral edema; depression; dizziness; headache

Adrenal suppressant

Drug	Acute Toxicity	Delayed Toxicity
Aminoglutethimide (*Cytadren*—Ciba)	Skin rash; drowsiness; nausea; dizziness	Hypothyroidism (rare); bone marrow depression; fever; hypotension; masculinization

6. Record local or systemic changes in detail (e.g., diarrhea or melena).
7. Observe skin tissue in local area for reaction—erythema, blistering, edema, petechiae.
8. Check mucous membranes for signs of tissue breakdown, hemorrhage, or infection.
9. Turn the patient frequently because of increased possibility of pressure area breakdown.

Management of Complications

A. Blood Difficulties

1. Withdraw drugs if leukocyte or platelet counts fall to dangerous levels.
2. If leukocyte count is below 1,200, obtain a culture to assist in determining specific treatment.
3. Practice reverse isolation when leukocyte count falls to low levels, or discharge the patient.
4. Administer packed cells if anemia occurs.
5. Treat for thrombocytopenia (decrease in number of blood platelets) if it is severe; steroids may also be used.

B. Other Problems

Difficulties such as nausea and vomiting, diarrhea, mucositis, infection, alopecia (hair loss) are discussed in the next section: *Nursing Care of the Patient Receiving Chemotherapeutic Agents for Neoplastic Disease.*

Nursing Precautions in Handling Cytotoxic Anticancer Drugs

Most cytotoxic anticancer drugs are irritating to the skin, eyes, and mucous membranes. If mishandled, these drugs can result in local toxic or allergic reactions.

Personal Safety

Purpose:
Protect skin and eyes.

1. Wash hands thoroughly before and after admixing.
2. Wear long-sleeved gown and disposable polyvinyl gloves.
3. Wear a mask and safety glasses in absence of a vertical flow hood.

(Vertical laminar air-flow hood is recommended for areas where large volumes of drugs are prepared. A glass plate in front of hood protects eyes and face).

Note: A hood is not a substitute for meticulous technique.

4. Hold drug ampules away from the face when they are being opened to remove contents. Cover ampule completely with a gauze pad prior to breaking.
5. Wash contaminated skin and surfaces with copious amounts of soap and water.

Environmental Safety

Purpose:
Minimize surface and atmospheric contamination by containing drugs.

1. Vials
   a. Drugs are reconstituted by slowly adding diluent down side of vial.
   b. Never place needle of syringe containing diluent into reconstituted diluent solution.
   c. Allow air pressure to equalize back into the syringe.
   d. Place an alcohol swab over needle as it is withdrawn from vial to prevent aerolization.
   e. Expel excess air into a separated sealed waste bottle (vented with hydrophilic filter).
   f. Affix a new needle to syringe (after dilution and mixing) and draw a volume of air less than the desired amount of drug solution, introduce into vial (to allow withdrawal of correct dose without aspiration of air into syringe).
   g. If transferring from syringe to infusion or piggyback bottle, use an injection cap to avoid multiple punctures in rubber cap.
2. Wear gloves, a face mask, and eye protection when cleaning up spills of cytotoxic material:
   a. Wipe up spills with a damp cloth or paper towels.
   b. Place all of the material in a plastic bag, seal it, place in a second plastic bag, and seal.
   c. Mark outer bag "Dangerous Material" and send to incinerator.
   d. Needles are not clipped from syringes after use to prevent aerosol formation.

Special Precautions with Certain Anticancer Drugs:

Anticancer Drug	Problem	Nursing Action
Actinomycin D (Cosmegen)	Contact with skin	Rinse area with water for 10 minutes Rinse finally with buffered phosphate solution
Methotrexate (MTX)	Contact with skin	Wash skin thoroughly; apply bland ointment to relieve stinging
Actinomycin D Azathioprine (Imuran) Carmustine (BCNU) Lomustine (CCNU) Melphalan (Alkeran) Nitrogen mustard (Mustargen)	Especially irritating to eyes	Protect eyes well by using goggles or other protective device

The Patient Receiving Chemotherapeutic Agents for Neoplastic Disease

Assessment and Interventions

1. Recognize that side effects and/or toxicity may be anticipated.

   Side effects are usually not life-threatening but can be annoying (e.g., alopecia, change in taste sensation, skin reaction).

   Toxic effects usually refers to a life-threatening reaction such as nephrotoxicity, severe bone marrow depression, or anemia. Medication dosage may have to be reduced or therapy may be postponed/discontinued.

   a. Note that signs vary from patient to patient.

   b. Utilize combative measures to offset disturbances, such as antiemetics for nausea.

   c. Anticipate that the patient will experience discomforts, but avoid suggesting to him that they might occur, since this might act psychologically to hasten their occurrence.

2. Assess status of *oral mucosa* and utilize measures to minimize *mucosal trauma* and *stomatitis.*

   a. Initiate a program of oral hygiene so that the mouth does not become a breeding place for bacteria.

   b. Cleanse the mouth with nonabrasive, soft materials, such as a very soft toothbrush or finger wrapped with a layer of gauze and dipped in a cleansing solution.

   c. Use mouthwash of 3 parts saline to 1 part hydrogen peroxide (dilute further if this is irritating).

   d. Avoid commercial mouthwashes which may irritate sensitive tissue.

   e. If mouth is sore, avoid spicy, hot, and acid foods; avoid irritating foods and fluids such as toast and citrus fruit juices.

   f. Suggest and serve ice cream, ice milk, and Popsicles for a refreshing change.

3. Be alert for evidence of *gastrointestinal tract disturbances: nausea and vomiting.*

   a. Nausea

   (1) Administer antiemetic about ½ hour before or immediately after chemotherapy.

   (2) Offer ice chips or a fruit Popsicle at onset of nausea.

   (3) Try giving the patient a cup of tea and crackers.

   (4) Encourage good mouth hygiene before and after meals.

   (5) Have the patient eat small meals frequently and chew food thoroughly.

   (6) If no stomatitis is present, some patients find lemons or dill pickles enjoyable.

   (7) In situations where antiemetics do not help, some patients have obtained relief from delta-9-tetrahydrocannabinol (THC)—the main active ingredient of marihuana.

   (8) Provide distraction such as television or some diversion.

   b. Vomiting

   (1) Provide emesis basin and tissues; empty and clean basin after use.

   (2) Apply a cool, wrung-out washcloth to forehead, face, and neck.

   (3) Administer an antiemetic; assess for dehydration.

   (4) Offer items for oral care after vomiting: mouthwash, toothbrush, and toothpaste.

4. Assess for *fluid retention and diarrhea,* which are common problems.

   a. Note evidence of superficial edema and signs of congestive heart failure (see p. 323).

   b. Prevent undue pressure on bony prominences since retained fluid stretches and weakens skin; turn the patient frequently, massage and lubricate pressure points.

   c. Be alert for signs of hypokalemia and modify diet to increase potassium.

   d. Diarrhea

   (1) Place the patient on a diet low in roughage and higher in constipating foods.

   (2) Administer antidiarrheal medication.

   (3) Assess for signs of dehydration; monitor fluids and electrolytes.

5. Maintain adequate *nutritional levels,* recognizing that there may be nausea, vomiting, anorexia, stomatitis, and oral mucositis.

   a. Regulate temperature of fluids and foods coming in contact with the oral mucosa; avoid temperature extremes (too hot or too cold).

   b. Serve high-protein and high-carbohydrate food; allow the patient to choose his foods; guide his selection so that a well-balanced diet of nutritionally desirable foods is served.

   c. Present food as attractively as possible and serve it in a pleasant setting.

   d. Ensure that the patient is physically comfortable; encourage having friends or family provide company during mealtime if this helps.

   e. Encourage fluids because tissue metabolic rate is elevated and the patient needs to clear wastes from his body.

   f. Entice the anorexic patient with refreshing mouth care before serving meals; a bad taste in the mouth discourages eating.

   (1) Try giving the patient high-protein, high-calorie foods.

   (2) Monitor weight loss.

   g. Modify chemical and mechanical factors in an effort to avoid tissue trauma to the mouth—use a soft toothbrush and soothing dentifrices and mouthwash; avoid ill-fitting dentures.

   h. Avoid highly seasoned foods, even if the patient ordinarily thrives on such foods.

   i. Discourage smoking and use of alcoholic beverages since these irritate the mucous membranes.

   j. Recognize that occasionally cancer and/or treatment may cause an alteration of taste perception, such as a keener taste of bitterness and loss of ability to detect sweet tastes.

6. Note the manifestations of *bone marrow depression.*

   a. Check for reduction in number of leukocytes, erythrocytes, and platelets; report abnormal findings.

   b. Note any swelling or redness of any body part.

c. Observe for evidence of infection and bleeding tendencies.

d. Explain to the patient that he is susceptible to infection; caution him to guard against exposure to upper respiratory infections and other infections.

e. Instruct the patient to avoid cuts, bruises, or trauma; give injections only if absolutely necessary.

f. Apply site pressure (if an injection must be given) to avoid prolonged bleeding.

g. Stress importance of cleanliness and hand washing.

7. Anticipate possible signs of *anemia.*
   a. Caution the patient about physical overexertion; encourage him to rest frequently and to expect a tired feeling.
   b. Explain that blood transfusions, if given, are a part of therapy and not necessarily an indication of a setback.
   c. Observe skin color; monitor laboratory results (Hb, RBC).

8. Inspect body for signs of *nasal infections, eye infection, rectal abscesses.*
   a. Teach the patient how to keep these vulnerable areas clean to avoid infection.
   b. Alert the patient to the importance of avoiding persons who have infections.
   c. Recognize that with an altered blood count, the patient may be easily fatigued and therefore requires daily rest periods.

9. Promote patient comfort and administer analgesics if he is experiencing *pain.*
   a. Administer acetaminophen instead of aspirin for general or local discomfort; aspirin may be irritating to the stomach.
   b. Offer viscous Xylocaine to use as a mouthwash and gargle; this acts as a topical anesthetic agent to relieve pain.

10. Expect that with some chemotherapeutic agents (doxorubicin, cyclophosphamide, vincristine) and with certain methods of administration, there may be *alopecia (hair loss).*
    a. Reassure the patient that hair will usually grow back.
    b. Suggest wearing a turban or head scarf.
    c. Temporary use of a hair piece or wig may be suitable; have wig fitted before chemotherapy is started.
    d. Scalp tourniquet and hypothermia (ice packs) may be used to control alopecia; results are variable.

11. Attend to the *psychosocial needs* of the patient receiving chemotherapeutic agents.
    a. When there is hair loss, recognize that this change in physical appearance may result in antisocial behavior and depression (see *10,* above).
    b. Utilize any and all measures that will tend to distract the patient from himself; provide diversional and recreational therapy.
    c. Provide rest periods that are conducive to rest— quiet, relaxing backrubs, soft music, comfortable surroundings.
    d. Be honest with the patient about all aspects of his therapy and condition. To promote self-sufficiency and self-esteem, encourage him to be a participant in the planning of his care.
    e. Encourage the patient to stay on the therapeutic program.
    f. Provide the patient with stimuli to combat sensory deprivation if he is on reverse isolation.

Radiation in Diagnosis and Therapy

Radiation is frequently used in diagnosing and treating cancer. Newer modalities are being added: ultrasonography, computed tomography, digital radiology, and magnetic resonance imaging.

Sources of Radiation

1. Naturally occurring radioactivity—radium radon
2. Radiopharmaceuticals
   a. Internal application (brachytherapy)
Technetium	^{99m}Tc
Xenon	^{133}Xe
Thallous chloride	^{201}Tl
Iodine	^{123}I
	^{131}I
Gallium citrate	^{67}Ga
b. External application (teletherapy)
Cobalt	^{60}Co
Cesium	^{137}Cs
3. Megavoltage and supervoltage beams
   a. Betatron
   b. Cyclotron
   c. Linear accelerator

Definitions

1. *Nuclide*—any atomic entity capable of existing for a measurable lifetime, usually more than 10^{-9} seconds.

2. *Radionuclide* (radioactive nuclide)—one that disintegrates with the emission of particulate or electromagnetic radiations.

3. *Radioactivity*—the disintegration of the atom which gives up energy in the form of rays or particles.

4. *Isotope*—an element whose nucleus contains a fixed number of protons but has a differing number of neutrons, thereby changing its weight.
   a. Optimal ratio between proton and neutron is stable.
   b. By using nuclear reactors, it is possible to bombard a stable isotope with additional free neutrons.
   c. Most radioisotopes emit:
      (1) Particulate radiation—small fragments of the nucleus having mass and size (alpha and beta particles).
      (2) Electromagnetic radiation—rays that have no mass (x-rays).

5. *Radioactive decay or disintegration*
   a. The rate of decay varies from isotope to isotope.
   b. "Half-life" or decay rate is the time required to reduce a particular radioactive substance by one half of its atoms, thereby reducing it to half of its initial activity.
   Example: ^{225}Radium—half-life of over 1,600 years

c. A radioisotope administered to a patient in unsealed form has a relatively short life and is essentially inactive after therapeutic use has been completed.

Examples: ^{131}Iodine—half-life about 8 days
^{123}Iodine—half-life about 13 hours
^{99m}Technetium—half-life 6 hours

d. Longer-lasting isotopes are implanted temporarily in the patient in a sealed container.

Example: ^{60}Co—half-life about 5 years

6. *Units of measurement (Activity)*
   a. Curie (c.)—basic unit for measuring amount of activity in a radioactive sample
   b. Millicurie (mc.)—one thousandth of a curie
   c. Microcurie (μc.)—one millionth of a curie
   d. Picocurie (pc.)—one billionth of a curie

7. *Units for measuring radiation exposure or absorption*
   a. Roentgen (r.)—a standard unit of exposure (usually applied to x-ray or gamma rays)
   b. Milliroentgen (mr.)—one thousandth of a roentgen
   c. Rad—a unit to measure absorbed dose
      (1 rad = amount of radiation required to deposit 100 ergs of energy per gram of irradiated material)
   d. Rem—a unit of measure of radiation-dose equivalent which relates to biological effectiveness (roentgen equivalent man)
      Standards have been established by the International Committee on Radiation Protection (ICRP) that the maximum permissible dose (MPD) for radiation workers is 5 rems for persons over age 18.
   e. Grays (Gy.)—1 Gy. equals 100 rads, or 1 rad equals 0.01 Gy.

Biological Aspects and Clinical Application

A. Nature and Indications for Use

1. Individualized to produce effective ionization within a tumor while avoiding unnecessary irradiation of normal structures
2. Tissues most likely to respond to radiation exposure—those originating from reticuloendothelial tissues (leukemia, lymphomas) and those from embryonal tissues (teratomas)
3. Tissues least likely to respond—bone and muscle

B. Factors Affecting the Benefit of Radiation Exposure vs. Risk of Tissue Damage

1. *Dose rate*—a prescribed dose causes less tissue destruction if given in small amounts over a long period of time than given all at once.
2. *Area of body exposure*—the larger the area exposed, the greater the effect.
3. *Cell susceptibility*
   a. Greater susceptibility—rapidly dividing cells with no specialized function (e.g., lymphocytes and germ cells)
   b. Lesser susceptibility—nondividing cells and highly differentiated cells (e.g., nerve or muscle cells)
4. *Biological variability*—individual differences play a role in human susceptibility.
   a. Healthy person more responsive than malnourished individual.
   b. Skin is especially vulnerable to radiation injury.
   c. Bone marrow is very radiosensitive; therefore, such damage is potentially the most lethal.

d. Radiation cataracts result from excessive eye exposure.
e. Lung fibrosis may occur following radiation of chest.

C. Symptoms of Radiation Syndrome—High Level

(Major portion of body exposed to large doses of irradiation [*over 100 rems*] in a short period of time.)
1. Prodromal—nausea, vomiting, malaise
2. Latent—symptoms subside
3. Illness—general malaise, epilation (hair loss), hemorrhage (petechiae, nosebleed), pallor, diarrhea, inflammation of mouth and throat, leukopenia
4. Recovery or death

D. Symptoms of Radiation Syndrome—Low Level

(Low levels of radiation over a long period of time)
Examples:
1. Radiologists—may acquire leukemia
2. Clock dial painters—may develop sarcomas (from radium-containing luminizing paint)
3. Gonad exposure to radiation—may affect progeny

E. Roentgenologic Precautions During Radiography, Imaging, Fluoroscopy, or Radiotherapy

1. No one permitted in the room where the patient is undergoing x-ray therapy.
2. Equipment should not leak radiation.
3. Fluoroscopy room attendants should be protected from scattered radiation by wearing lead aprons and, if necessary, lead-impregnated gloves.
4. Appropriate lead shielding should be available to protect the patient's gonads during radiation exposure.

Diagnostic Radiology (See Table 22-2)

Ultrasonography—sound waves are reflected off points of variation in acoustic impedance.
Sonoendoscopy—utilizing high-frequency ultrasound transducers incorporated near tip of a flexible endoscope, such as for visualization of upper and lower gastrointestinal tract.
Computed tomography (CT)—density differences are revealed by passing a very narrow x-ray beam over tiny cubes of tissue. A computer reconstructs a transverse section of the body and displays the image on a television monitor.
Magnetic resonance imaging (MRI)—combines advantages of CT scan with ultrasound in using nonionizing radiation and providing tomography in any desired plane.
Digital radiography

Nursing Support and Interventions in Radiation Therapy

A. Physical and Psychological Preparation of the Patient

1. Provide psychological support to this patient because radiation therapy is associated with fears of:
   a. Being burned
   b. Being disfigured
   c. Dying and death
   d. Inability to perform normal bodily functions
   e. Pain
   f. Sterility and loss of sexual function
2. Recognize systemic responses to fear:

Table 22-2 Comparison of Newer Imaging Techniques

	Radionuclide Imaging	Ultrasound	CT Scan	Digital Radiography	Nuclear Magnetic Resonance Imaging
Equipment cost	Low	Low	High	High	Very high
Portability (bedside)	Yes	Yes	No	No	No
Radiation exposure	Lower, generalized	None	Higher, localized	Higher, localized	None
Invasive	No	No	No	Maybe	No
Hypertonic contrast agent	No	No	Often	Always	No
Air obstructs	No	Yes	No	No	No
Tissue specificity	High	None	None	None	Low

(Reproduced with permission, from Way LW [ed]. Current Surgical Diagnosis and Treatment, 6th ed. Copyright 1983 by Lange Medical Publications, Los Altos, CA).

    a. Mouth dryness, pupillary dilatation
    b. Hand tremor, vomiting, severe palpitations
3. If above signs are noted, initiate open discussion, since this often relieves anxiety.
4. Remove all opaque objects such as pins, buttons, and hairpins, and replace clothing with a gown for body x-rays.
5. Have the patient remain perfectly still; maintain position with use of sandbags, etc. if required.
6. Tell the patient that there will be no sensation or pain accompanying either picture-taking or penetration of x-rays.
7. Advise the patient that he will be alone in the room for the protection of the technician but that he will be in voice contact.
8. Determine from the physician what he has told the patient about radiotherapy, particularly in the case of the patient with advanced cancer.
9. If a series of treatments is to be given, include the patient in the planning phase.
10. Give special attention to diet and medications; administer antinauseants, analgesics, specific medications for diarrhea, proctitis, and cystitis.
11. Explain the need for routine blood counts.

B. Skin Manifestations and Precautions

1. Inform the patient that some skin reaction can be expected but that it varies from patient to patient. Example: dry erythema, desquamation, moist erythema, healing, epilation, tanning, telangiectasis.
2. Apply no lotions, ointments, cosmetics, etc. to the site of radiation unless prescribed by the physician; avoid talcum powder because it contains heavy metals that can be irritating.
3. Discourage vigorous rubbing, friction, or scratching because it can destroy skin cells; apply a bland ointment (containing vitamins A and D).
4. Take precautions against irritation from friction, exposure to sunlight, and extremes in temperature.
5. Do not apply adhesive or other tape to the skin.
6. Avoid shaving the skin in the treatment area.
7. Avoid wearing tight-fitting clothing over treatment field; prevent irritation by not using rough cloth such as wool and corduroy.

C. Mucous Membrane Effects

1. Oral mucosa
    a. There may be a change in or loss of taste.
    b. There may be various degrees of soreness and inability to swallow.
    c. Avoid smoking and such irritants as hot, spicy foods or alcohol.
    d. Maintain good oral hygiene; use mild cleansing agents in the mouth.
    e. Apply topical anesthetics such as viscous Xylocaine.
    f. Encourage oral liquid intake; moisten lips with small amounts of petrolatum, lip pomade, or baby oil.
2. Digestive tract
    a. Diarrhea is a common symptom if large areas are irradiated or if colon is significantly affected.
    b. Treat diarrhea with simple measures such as Kaopectate or opiate-like agents (Lomotil); it may be necessary to suspend radiotherapy for a few days.

D. Dietary Disturbances

1. Provide dietary restrictions to relieve symptoms of chronic radiation enteritis:
Administer diet free of gluten, protein, and lactose to overcome or avoid absorptive problems resulting from atrophy of intestinal villi.
2. Maintain high level of nutrition but eliminate those foods that irritate the mucous membrane; this may preclude the need for nasogastric feeding.
3. Consider parenteral hyperalimentation (p. 429).

E. Systemic Reactions

Nausea, vomiting, fever, loss of appetite, malaise.
1. Administer antiemetics and/or sedatives for greater comfort.
2. Select fluids and foods that will not induce or aggravate nausea.
3. Provide small, frequent meals rather than 3 larger meals.
4. Suggest time for rest and relaxation; avoid noise, confusion.
5. Recognize that the patient needs encouragement and understanding.

Radioisotope Therapy

Types of Radioisotope Therapy
A. Teletherapy—utilizes gamma rays from a radioactive source which is kept in a shielded unit placed at a distance from the patient.

1. Radioisotope Cobalt-60 (^{60}Co) and Cesium-137 (^{137}Ce) deliver radiation similar to that produced by supervoltage x-ray apparatus.
2. ^{60}Co therapy unit requires extra shielding because

rays are being emitted constantly. Because gamma rays cannot be entirely absorbed, personnel are advised to spend minimum time in this room.

3. *Advantages of ^{60}Co over conventional x-ray*
   a. Skin problems are significantly reduced.
   b. Bone or cartilage involvement is lessened.
   c. Electronic circuits are not required.
4. *Disadvantages of ^{60}Co*
   a. Because it has a half-life of 5 years, it is necessary to replace the ^{60}Co.
   b. Radiation energy cannot be varied.
   c. Cost of room shielding is high.

B. External Molds—a packaged and screened container in which a radioisotope can be placed and applied directly to the skin surface.

Examples:
1. ^{60}Co can be applied in this manner to small areas, as in the treatment of carcinoma of the lip, larynx, ear, etc.
2. ^{182}Ta (radioactive tantalum) can be applied in a flexible wire mold (e.g., to the external surface of a retinoblastoma involving eyeball and optic nerve).
3. ^{90}Sr (radioactive strontium) and ^{90}Y (radioactive yttrium) as in external molds used for shallow irradiation of eye neoplasms.

C. Intracavitary Isotope Therapy

Examples:
   Liquid radioisotopes:
   ^{198}Au (radioactive colloidal gold)
   ^{20}Na (radioactive sodium)
   ^{82}Br (radioactive bromine)
   Used in the balloon of a catheter inside the bladder for internal bladder radiation of a few millimeters.

D. Interstitial Isotope Therapy

Examples:
1. Radioactive needles, seeds, tubes, or wires can be implanted directly into tumor tissue: ^{60}Co, ^{137}Ce, ^{198}Au, ^{222}Rn, ^{182}Ta, ^{125}I.
2. Implants may be temporary or permanent; they may be supplementary to surgery or to external beam irradiation.
3. Radioactive solutions may be injected directly into the tumor or surrounding tissue. Colloidal solution of radioactive colloidal gold (^{198}Au) is one of the most commonly used solutions.

E. Internal Irradiation

Examples:
1. Oral ingestion of solutions of radioiodine (^{131}I)—administered to patients with hyperthyroidism.
2. Intravenous injection of sodium phosphate (^{32}P)—used in the treatment of polycythemia vera.

Clinical action:
   In above instances, the target tissue has an affinity for the therapeutic agent; the isotope concentrates within the substance.

Nursing Management of Patients Receiving Radioisotopes

A. Identification of the Patient as a Radiation Source

1. Have patient wear a wristband with a radioactive symbol.
2. Identify the chart cover, doctor's and nurse's order sheets, and special radiation instruction sheet with the radioactive symbol.
3. For patients receiving the most minute quantities of tracer radioisotopes, such identification (see above) is not necessary.

4. Personnel who may be exposed to penetrating radiation (x-ray or gamma rays) should wear film badges on front of the body.

B. Radiation Instruction Sheet

1. Type of radioactivity used
2. Time of insertion
3. Anticipated time of removal
4. Precautions to follow
5. Whom to notify when in doubt or in an emergency

C. Factors Affecting the Amount of Radiation

1. *Amount* of radioactivity present, 10 mc., 20 mc., 30 mc., etc.
2. The *distance* of the nurse from the patient

   Note: The inverse square law applies: doubling the distance from a radiation source cuts intensity received to one fourth.

3. Amount of *time* spent in actual contact with the patient
4. Degree of *shielding* utilized
   Chosen according to type of radiation—alpha, beta, gamma (Fig. 22-3).
5. Amount of *body area exposed* to radiation

▶ **NURSING ALERT:** During the period of greatest radioactivity (24–72 hours), limit amount of time spent with the patient to that required for essential care. Require the patient to remain in his bed or room during course of treatment.

D. Vital Nursing Measures in Caring for the Patient with Internal Radiation

1. Be acquainted with the nomenclature describing dissipation of radioisotopes.
   a. *Physical half-life*—a constant rate in which one half of radioactivity is dissipated in a given time.
   b. *Biologic half-life*—the time it takes for a radioisotope to disappear from the body via normal metabolic processes.
   c. *Effective half-life*—a combination of physical half-life and biologic half-life.
2. Recognize that an isotope that is completely dispersed throughout the body (or a major portion of it) is less hazardous to an organ or tissue than an isotope concentrated by the body into a limited area.
3. Recognize that an isotope that is excreted rapidly is less hazardous than radium, which may be kept in the body for long periods.
4. Take appropriate measures associated with *sealed sources of radiation* implanted within a patient (sealed internal radiation).
   a. Follow directives on precaution sheet which is placed on chart of all patients receiving radiotherapy.
   b. Do not remain within 1 meter (3 feet) of the patient any longer than required to give essential care.

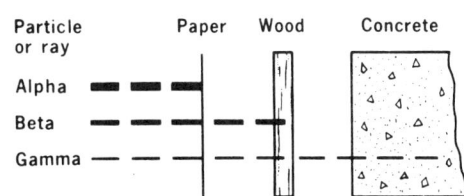

Figure 22-3. Relative penetration of alpha, beta and gamma radiation. (U.S. Atomic Energy Commission.)

c. Know that the casing material absorbs all alpha radiation and most beta radiation, but that a hazard concerning gamma radiation may exist.

d. Do not linger longer than necessary in giving patient care, even though all precautions are followed.

e. Be alert for implants that may have become loosened (those inserted in cavities that have access to the exterior), for example, check the emesis basin following mouth care for a patient with an oral implant.

f. Notify the radiologist of any implant that has moved out of position.

g. Utilize long-handled forceps or tongs and hold at arm's length when picking up any accidentally dislodged radium needle, seeds, tubes, etc., that may appear on dressings, bed, or floor. *Never pick up a radioactive source with your hands.*

h. Do not discard any dressings or linens unless sure that no radioactive source is present.

i. Wash hands with soap and water after caring for a patient who is being treated with a radioisotope. When wearing gloves, wash them with soap and water before removing them.

Note: This is not necessary for sealed sources.

j. Encourage patients who are ambulatory to remain in their own rooms.

k. Upon discharge of a patient, it is a good policy for the radiologist to check the room with a radiograph or survey meter to be certain that all radioactive materials have been removed.

l. Continue radiation precautions when a patient has a permanent implant, until the radiologist declares precautions unnecessary. (See p. 913 for nursing care of the patient receiving radiation therapy.)

5. Take appropriate measures associated with *unsealed sources;* radioactivity may be (1) widely spread in the body, (2) localized, or (3) present in any body tissue or fluid.

Examples:

a. *Radioactive iodine*
   (1) Circulates in bloodstream, excreted by kidneys—urine and blood contain radioactive material.
   (2) Can be secreted by sweat glands.
   (3) May be found in vomitus of a patient who recently took an oral dose.

b. *Radioactive colloidal gold*
   (1) May be noted in wound seepage as pink, red, or purple stain following intracavitary injection.
   (2) May be noted in small amounts in urine.

c. *Radioactive phosphorus solution*
   Be alert for contamination from excreta (urine and feces) and vomitus.

Immunotherapy

The *immune system* of the body has the ability to recognize and to defend itself against infection and invasion by foreign cells such as those of cancer. The immune system may be weakened or overwhelmed by the invasion of foreign cells so that it cannot function effectively.

Immunotherapy employs the immune mechanism of the body to combat cancer and overcome it. The immunotherapeutic approach to cancer is based on the fact that most tumors provoke an immune response (such as antitumor activity, production of tumor antigens) in the patient (host).

Although it is still considered investigational, significant research in immunotherapy is going on and progress is being made.

Goals of Immunotherapy

1. Successfully treat the cancer patient.
2. Challenge and induce mobilization of the patient's immune defenses by utilizing a chemical or microbial agent to which the patient has previously been sensitized.
   a. This produces a delayed hypersensitivity response that can be employed against the cancer.
   b. Once developed in this way, immunocompetence (either alone or in combination with radiation, chemotherapy, or surgery) can fight the cancer.

Various Approaches of Immunotherapy

A. Active Specific Immunotherapy

1. Utilization of the patient's own immune mechanisms to reject or control his own malignant cells.

2. To date, active immunization, used alone, appears incapable of boosting the immune mechanism in the patient with advanced disseminated cancer.

B. Active Nonspecific Immunotherapy

1. Primarily activates macrophages and enhances delayed hypersensitivity of cellular immunity.
2. Utilization of bacteria or bacterial products as an immunologic adjuvant to enhance the immune response.
   a. *BCG* is a live attenuated strain of tubercle bacillus
   b. *MER* (methanol extraction residue) is a more highly refined, nonviable component of BCG
   c. *C. parvum* is a killed anaerobe
3. These agents are easy to distribute widely, and the responses achieved in patients with melanoma and several other solid tumors, as well as acute leukemia, make them attractive for a large number of therapy protocols.

C. Passive-Adoptive Immunotherapy

1. Utilization of the immunity of a competent donor.
2. The use of hyperimmune serum for rubella (passive) or for immunodeficiency diseases (adoptive) appears possible.
   Example: Immune RNA and lymphocyte transfer factor (LTF)
3. Again, further study is needed.

D. Adjunctive Immunotherapy

Because the above immunotherapeutic approaches appear inadequate, immunotherapy may be best utilized as an adjunct to other modalities (and even following curative methods, to eliminate the few remaining malignant cells).

1. *Immunotherapy and surgery*
   a. Following surgical removal of the bulk of a tumor, immunotherapy may be effective in attacking small foci of cancer cells.
   b. Whereas surgery is directed toward larger primary tumors, immunotherapy can control small foci of metastatic disease at distant sites.
2. *Immunochemotherapy*
   a. Timing is critical in successfully combining immunotherapy with chemotherapy.
   b. Cancer chemotherapeutic drugs are often immunosuppressive, but certain chemotherapeutic

agents actually stimulate the immune response to some antigens.
3. *Immunoradiotherapy*
   a. A problem associated with chemotherapy and radiation therapy is that they attack normal cells as well as cancer cells; because of the selectivity of immunotherapy, it could logically be combined with these other modalities.
   b. If the patient is given tumor-specific antibodies that are attached to isotopes, large doses of radiation could be directed to tumor cells; this would combine the destructive effects of radiation with the specificity of immunotherapy.

Care of the Patient with Advanced Cancer

Nursing Process Overview

Patient Problems/Nursing Diagnoses

1. Pain/discomfort related to invasion of normal tissue by malignant cells
2. Fear/emotional disturbance related to the pronouncement of having a diagnosis of "cancer"
3. Nutritional deprivation related to accelerated nutritional needs of cancer cells and anorexic effects of cancer/treatment modalities
4. Discomfort of side effects related to radiation and/or chemotherapy therapy
5. Impaired skin integrity related to effects of radiation therapy
6. Potential for hemorrhage related to invasion of malignancy into large blood vessels.
7. Potential for bladder and bowel disturbances related to tissue breakdown and cancer spread

Planning and Implementation

Nursing Interventions

A. Achieving comfort and relief of pain

1. Assist the patient in bathing and with personal hygiene; personal cleanliness is a comfort measure.
2. Provide warmth when required; in cool seasons the debilitated patient is more sensitive to chilling.
3. Assist the patient as required in moving, turning, getting out of bed, walking, etc., in an effort to promote maximum activity and minimum amount of pain.

4. Evaluate objectively the nature of his pain (location, duration, quality) and manner in which the patient tolerates or accepts it.
5. Convey the impression that his pain is understood and that relief is forthcoming.
6. Ascertain pain source—is it carcinoma-related? Is there some other physical source? Is it psychological?
7. Administer medications as specifically required:
   a. Sedative and hypnotics—to induce and promote sleep
      Assist the patient in controlling his pain by allowing him a degree of independence in use of pain "cocktails," such as Brompton's cocktail.
   b. Local anesthetics—for localized pain
   c. Ataractic drugs—for fear and apprehension
   d. Specific medications—for nausea and vomiting

   e. Muscle relaxant and antispasmodic drugs—to relieve tenseness
   f. Tranquilizers—to promote a sense of well-being
   g. Analgesics—for discomfort or pain
   h. Narcotics—for more intense pain
8. Prepare the patient for the prescribed modality of treatment: surgery, chemotherapy, or radiation.
9. Assist with diagnostic evaluation in an attempt to determine precise location(s) of involvement or spread.
10. Control local and generalized infections.

▶ **NURSING ALERT:** Recognize that elderly debilitated patients have increased sensitivity. Avoid this cycle: a narcotic → drowsiness → less food and fluid → dehydration → nausea and vomiting → increased pain → more narcotic (and a resumption of the cycle).

11. Prepare the patient for surgical pain-relieving interventions.
    a. Percutaneous procedures: intrathecal alcohol injection, nerve block
    b. Localized radiotherapy
    c. Presacral neurectomy for visceral pain
    d. Sacral rhizotomy
    e. Midline myelotomy
    f. Hypophysectomy—transsphenoidal route
    g. Cordotomy for intractable pain
    h. Neurosurgical nerve interruption

B. Enhancing coping abilities

1. Provide the patient with psychosociological support.
   a. Listen to his concerns.
   b. Observe and support his reactions where appropriate.
   c. Explain the aspect of treatment that is pertinent at that time.
2. Allow the patient to verbalize his feelings, thoughts; provide unhurried time for listening.
3. Maintain an optimistic atmosphere; limit the time plans to hour by hour or day by day (not week by week, month by month, or year by year).
4. Invite the patient to participate socially, visit with other individuals, etc.
5. Provide opportunities for communication and mind-occupying activities.
6. Accept the patient as an individual with natural defense mechanisms; encourage him to talk about

himself, his concerns, his understanding, his future—even the possibility of dying.

7. Support the patient as he taps his spiritual resources.
8. Understand his alteration(s) in behavior, even when socially unacceptable; when the episode passes, assist in restoring his self-esteem.
9. Empathize with him in an effort to show concern and understanding.
10. Include the patient's family in planning with him meaningful day-to-day activities.
11. Promote physical activities as much as possible; encourage rest periods.
12. Change the patient's environment if possible by encouraging him to walk and go outdoors.

C. Meeting nutritional requirements

1. Promote optimum nutritional, fluid, and electrolyte levels by correcting deficiencies.
2. Provide a high-calorie and high-vitamin diet; cater to his personal food likes.
3. Offer between-meal feedings.

D. Countering side effects from radiation therapy

1. Radiation sickness
   a. Administer sedatives, antiemetics, and antihistamines as prescribed.
   b. Encourage adequate fluid intake.
   c. Tempt the patient with small, frequent, high calorie, high-protein feedings.
   d. Record his reactions.
2. Skin reactions
   a. Offer regular back and body massages; these can stimulate circulation and promote relaxation as well.
   b. Ensure wrinkle-free, dry bedding—helps prevent skin breakdown in debilitated patients. Special mattress pads can be used.
   c. Observe skin for dryness, tautness, erythema, desquamation.
   d. Apply bland cream or oil to radiation site as directed.
   e. Cleanse skin gently with bland soaps (Neutrogena) and lukewarm water.
   f. Protect skin from sunlight, heat, trauma, constricting clothing.
   g. Note change such as telangiectasis (small network of dilated arterioles).
   h. Offer medicated mouthwashes to soothe oral mucosa.
   i. Maintain an exercise program utilizing range-of-motion activities.
   j. Control edema of extremities by elevating the part as well as supporting it.
   k. Initiate measures to prevent pressure sores (see p. 59).
3. Control of odors that may emanate from affected tissues
   a. Promote an esthetically comfortable environment.
   b. Encourage good personal hygiene.
   c. Irrigate external wounds with saline solution and use mechanical cleansers as prescribed (half-strength hydrogen peroxide, diluted antiseptic detergents, etc.).
   d. Remove soiled dressings promptly and change all soiled linens frequently—wrap dressings in paper and place in covered container immediately.
   e. Provide fresh circulating air—use aerosol deodorants when necessary.
   f. Change packing or pads frequently; irrigate thoroughly any affected body cavities and shave

where hair presents a problem—mouth, nasal area, vagina, rectum.
   g. Avoid dressing changes at inopportune times—visiting hours, meal times, etc.

E. Recognizing and handling complications

1. Recognize the potential for blood cell depression.
   a. Protect the patient from injury and infection.
   b. Observe for evidences of bleeding or infection and take measures to correct.
2. Anticipate and control hemorrhage.
   a. Monitor vital signs to detect increase in pulse rate and respiration and decrease in blood pressure.
   b. Apply pressure, if active bleeding occurs, at convenient pressure points between the site and heart.
   c. Employ emergency hemorrhage-control measures.
   d. Note and record amount and nature of bleeding; notify physician.
   e. Reassure and comfort the patient.
   f. Use packing if bleeding involves accessible cavity (e.g., rectum, vagina).
   g. Administer platelet or whole-blood transfusion.
   h. Prepare the patient for cauterization and ligation if necessary.

F. Assist in overcoming bladder and bowel disturbances.

1. Bladder frequency or incontinence
   a. Keep an accurate input and output record.
   b. Establish a bladder control program (see p. 70).
   c. Maintain perineal cleanliness.
   d. Insert an indwelling catheter if other measures fail.
2. Constipation
   a. Maintain an adequate fluid level.
   b. Omit constipating foods from diet—ensure adequate fruits and vegetables.
   c. Administer glycerin suppository or mild laxative as prescribed.

▶ **NURSING ALERT:** Avoid giving enemas when the patient has leukopenia or is taking drugs that irritate the intestinal tract (e.g., 5-fluorouracil).

3. Diarrhea
   a. Give antidiarrhea medications as prescribed.
   b. Avoid serving foods that aggravate the problem, such as stewed prunes.
   c. Provide suppositories as suggested.
   d. Keep diet restricted to low residue or bland foods.

Evaluation
Expected Outcomes

1. Is pain-free and fairly comfortable—receives medication as needed or prescribed
2. Shows beginning acceptance of the diagnosis of cancer; expresses the philosophy of "living fully for each day"
3. Maintains weight; arranges menus for personal preference so that nutritional input is adequate
4. Abides by recommendations to keep radiation side effects to their minimum
5. Protects skin to avoid injury; assists with wound care
6. Relates signs/symptoms suggestive of possible hemorrhage
7. Follows bladder and bowel program; is continent of urine and feces

Psychosocial Support of the Dying Patient

Reactions of the Patient to Dying*

A. Stage of Denial

1. Period of denial allows the patient to mobilize his defenses.
2. The patient will exhibit withdrawal and avoidance of subject of death.
3. Usually a temporary defense to be replaced in time by partial acceptance.
4. The patient may talk of death and then change topic abruptly.
5. The patient may be in a temporary state of shock.

B. Stage of Anger

1. Denial may be replaced by anger, rage, envy, and resentment.
2. Anger may be displaced and projected into environment.
   a. Anger frequently directed at health care personnel. (Avoid reacting personally to this anger.)
   b. Try to tolerate rational and irrational anger. The patient may experience considerable relief in expressing anger.

C. Stage of Bargaining

Bargaining is an attempt to postpone the inevitable and to extend life.

D. Stage of Depression

1. This is a stage in which the patient is preparing himself to accept the loss of everything and everyone he loves.
2. The patient may be undergoing anticipatory grief to prepare himself for the final separation; may mourn the loss of meaningful people in his life.
   a. Allow the patient to express his sorrow—helps make the final acceptance easier.
   b. Sit with the patient.
   c. Use touch therapy if appropriate.

E. Stage of Acceptance

1. The patient is neither depressed nor angry about his impending death; he bows to the sentence.
2. May contemplate his demise with quiet acceptance and expectation—detachment may make death easier.
3. During this stage, the patient may be almost devoid of feelings—his circle of interest diminishes.
4. The patient will sleep and rest more—does not desire news or visitors from outside world.
5. The patient may just wish someone to hold his hand—reassures him that he is not forgotten.
6. The patient may reach the point where death comes as a relief.
7. Family may require more support during this stage.

Supportive Attitudes and Actions to the Patient, Family, and Health Team

Goals:
Allow the patient to live as fully as possible.
Relieve his discomfort and distress.
Be attuned to the special needs of the dying.
Help the patient achieve death with dignity.

A. Physical Support of the Dying Patient

See page 917.

* Adapted from Kübler-Ross E. On Death and Dying. New York, Macmillan, 1970.

B. Emotional Support of the Dying Patient

1. Make sure that the patient has continuing, personal, and caring contacts—gives comfort and reassurance.
   a. Avoid changing personnel.
   b. Be willing to become involved with the patient—personal involvement is necessary if human interaction is to be supportive.
   c. Make sure the nursing approach reflects the mutuality of human interaction.
   d. Take *time* with the patient—gives him the feeling that he is being cared for.
   e. Do not withdraw from the presence of death.
2. Give the patient an opportunity to talk about himself, his illness, and his dying.
   a. Accept the patient as he is now.
   b. Be able to accept the patient's anger—whether overt anger or that expressed as depression.
   c. Encourage the patient to talk about changes made by his illness.
   d. Demonstrate interest in the patient's total lifestyle.
      (1) Learn what supports his ego and self-esteem.
      (2) Be accessible.
3. Allow the patient to act out his feelings without judgment.
   a. Understand that the patient is increasingly overwhelmed by feelings of rage, anger, fear, guilt, futility, despondency, and pain.
      (1) Understand the patient rather than judge him.
      (2) Demonstrate patience, tolerance, and support.
   b. Allow the patient to keep his hold on *hope*—hope is therapeutic and will help maintain the patient through his suffering.
      (1) Maintain hope with the patient.
      (2) Avoid reinforcing hope after the patient has given up (stage of acceptance).
   c. Understand the patient's dread of being deserted.
4. Be alert for behavioral changes—patient may be trying to communicate something.
   Anticipate that the patient's behavior will be altered by his deteriorating physical condition.
      (1) Withdrawal from customary interests
      (2) Impairment of self-esteem
5. Encourage the patient to retain confidence in his health team.
   a. Emphasize to the patient that he and the health team are in the battle together—the patient will not be as fearful of loneliness, rejection, deceit.
   b. Reassure him that everything possible will be done for him.
   c. Let the patient know that he is respected and understood; treat him as a fellow human being.
   d. Seek the opinions of the patient—bolsters his self-esteem.
   e. Encourage the patient to take some initiative in his care.
   f. Keep the room neat and confusion at a minimum.
6. Help the patient who must undergo the "business" of dying.
   a. Settling of affairs, settling problems in human relationships, planning future for children, parent, spouse.
   b. Utilize services of chaplain, legal counselor, social worker, etc.

7. Pay attention to the patient's day-to-day complaints.
   a. Recognize the wide variety of symptoms accompanying anxiety—palpitation, nausea, insomnia, diarrhea, irritability.
   b. Be aware of the symptoms of depression—fatigue, lethargy, disturbances of sleep and appetite, inability to concentrate, psychomotor retardation.
   c. Try to alleviate each symptom.
   d. Reassure the patient that his pain will be relieved—helps the patient to cope with his discomfort.
   e. Give appropriate drugs to help the dying patient face death, cope with his anxiety and depression, and alter his sensitivity to pain.
   f. Help make each day as good a day as possible.

C. Support of the Family of the Dying Patient

Anticipatory grief—mourning that occurs over an extended period of time before actual death:

   Bereavement starts when one realizes that loss is inevitable.
   Family experiences awareness of loss and depression.
   Family may begin to adapt, physically and psychologically, to the consequences of death.

1. Understand that the family may be undergoing anticipatory mourning and reacting to anticipated loss.
   a. Recognize that various family members behave differently while working out their anticipatory grief.
      (1) Avoid showing disapproval of the behavior of others—may produce feelings of shame, guilt, and inadequacy.
      (2) Understand that family members may feel guilty when they are unable to demonstrate grief—there may be little or no feeling at actual time of death because family members have worked through their grief during the anticipatory period.
      (3) Family may withdraw emotional investment from the patient as they perceive he has no future.
   b. Be alert for untoward reactions to death—family

member may need supportive therapy and counseling.
2. Accept the feelings and attitudes of the family—helps avoid mutual hostility and recriminations. Feelings include:
   (1) Fear and anxiety
   (2) Sorrow and grief
   (3) Overt or suppressed hostility interwoven with guilt feelings; self blame
   (4) Ambivalent feelings toward dying member
   (5) Overprotective attitude
   (6) Depersonalization
   (7) Projection of guilt to health care personnel
   (8) Submission or excessive courtesy—may mask hostility
3. Realize the problems faced by the family—anticipated separation of loved one, financial problems, disruption of family life, problems of communication.
4. Demonstrate concern for the family.
   a. Inform them of practical help—financial assistance, social worker, other supporting services of local helping agencies.
   b. Reassure family that they will not be left alone.
   c. Provide opportunity for family member to ventilate his conflicts—anger, depression, victimization by illness.

D. Support of the Health Team

1. Examine your own attitudes and ability to face terminal illness and death.
   a. Look at possessions and relationships in context of inevitability of death.
   b. Plan for disaster and death.
2. Monitor your own feelings.
   a. Accept the ideas of denial, fear, and guilt.
   b. Assess and correct one's own biases and fears.
   c. Watch emotional responses to challenges of incurable disease and "difficult" families.
3. Do not withdraw from the presence of death.
   a. Face the reality of the dying patient.
   b. Become skilled and sensitive in the art of human interaction.

Bibliography

Books

Becker TM. Cancer Chemotherapy: A Manual for Nurses. Boston, Little, Brown & Co, 1981

Beyers M, Durburg S and Werner J (eds). Complete Guide to Cancer Nursing. Oradell, NJ, Medical Economics Books, 1984

Billings A. Outpatient Management of Advanced Cancer. Philadelphia, JB Lippincott, 1985

Bouchard-Kurtz R and Speese-Owens N. Nursing Care of the Cancer Patient, 4th ed. St Louis, CV Mosby, 1981

Brager BL and Yasko JM. Care of the Client Receiving Chemotherapy. Reston, VA, Reston Publishing Co, 1984

Cancer. The Health Consequences of Smoking. A Report of the Surgeon General. USDHHS, PHS, 1982

Cassileth BR and Cassileth PA. Clinical Care of the Terminal Cancer Patient. Philadelphia, Lea & Febiger, 1982

Cohen J, Cullen JW and Martin LR. Psychosocial Aspects of Cancer. New York, Raven Press, 1982

del Regato JA and Spjut HJ. Cancer: Diagnosis, Treatment and Prognosis, 6th ed. St Louis, CV Mosby, 1984

Donoghue M, Mennally C and Yasko JM. Nutritional Aspects of Cancer Care. Reston, VA. Reston Publishing Co, 1982

Dorr RT and Fritz WL. Cancer-Chemotherapy Handbook. New York, Elsevier North Holland, 1980

Gonda TA and Ruark JE. Dying Dignified. Menlo Park, CA, Addison-Wesley, 1984

Marino LB. Cancer Nursing. St Louis, CV Mosby, 1981

Morra M and Potts E. Choices: Realistic Alternatives in Cancer Treatment. New York, Avon Books, 1980

Vredevoe DL et al. Concepts of Oncology Nursing. Englewood Cliffs, NJ, Prentice-Hall, 1981

Williams C. All About Cancer. Somerset, NJ, John Wiley & Sons, 1983

Yasko JM. Guidelines for Cancer Care. Symptoms Managements. Reston, VA, Respon Publishing Co, 1983

Articles

General

Adams J and Guido G. The adolescent coping with cancer. DCCN 1984 March/Apr; 3(2):70–75

American Cancer Society Special Report. Nutrition and Cancer: Cause and Prevention. 1984 Mar/Apr; 34(2):121–126

Bagley CS et al. Pain management: A pilot project. Cancer Nurs 1982 June; 5(3):191–199

Baird SB. Economic realities in the treatment and care of the cancer patient. Top Clin Nurs 1981 Jan; 2(4): 67–80

Browder JP and Tomsick RS. Basal cell

epithelioma. Postgrad Med 1983 Feb; 73(2):161–168

Cancer survival rates up over past decade. Am Fam Physician 1984 Jan; 29(1):363–364

Craytor JK and Fass ML. Changing nurses' perceptions of cancer and cancer care. Cancer Nurs 1982 Feb; 5(1):43–49

Davis AJ. Whom can you tell? Am J Nurs 1981 Nov; 81(11):2078

Derdiarian AK. Dependence–independence behavioral changes in cancer surgical patients. Cancer Nurs 1983 Dec; 6(6):453–462

Doogan RA. Hypercalcemia of malignancy. Cancer Nurs 1981 Oct; 4(5):299–304

Driever MJ and McCorkle R. Patient concerns at 3 and 6 months postdiagnosis (cancer). Cancer Nurs 1984 June; 7(3):235–241

Faulkenberry JE. Cancer prevention and detection—risk assessment: The medical history (programmed instruction). Cancer Nurs 1983 Oct; 6(5): 389–401

Foltz AT. Nursing care of ulcerating metastatic lesions. Oncol Nurs Forum 1980 Spring; 7(2):8–13

Gallagher P and Tweedle DE. Taste threshold and acceptability of commerical diets in cancer patients. J Parent Enter Nutrition 1983 Apr; 7(4): 361–363

Goodman LS et al. Nitrogen mustard therapy. JAMA 1984 May 4; 251(17): 2255–2261

Heinrich RL and Schag CC. A behavioral medicine approach to coping with cancer: A case report. Cancer Nurs 1984 June; 7(3):243–247

Hoffman RS et al (roundtable). Helping the elderly live with cancer. Patient Care 1983 Dec 15; 17(21):61–107

Hoffman RS et al. Pinpointing cancer in the elderly. Patient Care 1983 Oct 15; 17(17):24–57

Hoffman RS. Cancer: Giving the elderly long-term care. Patient Care 1983 Nov 30; 17(20):105–142

Kane NE. How to make cancer nursing more bearable. RN 1984 July; 47(7): 45–47

Kaplan M. Viewpoint: The cancer patient. Cancer Nurs 1983 Apr; 6(2): 103–107

Karlin DA. Anorexia and taste abnormalities in cancer patients. Med Times 1983 Jan; 111(1):71–78

Karsell PR. Sheedy PF and O'Connell MJ. Computed tomography in search of cancer of unknown origin. JAMA 1982 July 16; 248(3):340–343

Kelley SL and Meyer TJ. Carcinoma of unknown primary site. Postgrad Med 1983 Oct; 74(4):269–280

Klopp A. Shunting malignant ascites. Am J Nurs 1984 Feb; 84(2):212–213

Krouse HJ and Krouse JH. Cancer as crisis. The critical elements of adjustment. Nurs Res 1982 March/April; 31(2):96–101

Lane B and Forgay M. Upgrading your oral hygiene protocol for the patient with cancer. Can Nurse 1981 Dec; 77(11):27–29

Lauer P, Murphy SP and Powers MJ.

Learning needs of cancer patients: A comparison of nurse and patient perceptions. Nurs Res 1982 Jan/Feb; 31(1):11–16

Lee A. Common problems, uncommon solutions. RN 1983 June; 46(6):55–56

Levine ME. Bioethics of cancer nursing. Rehab Nurse 1982 Mar/Apr; 7(2):27–31; 47

Lewis FM. Family level services for the cancer patient: Critical distinctions, fallacies, and assessment. Cancer Nurs 1983 June; 6(3):193–200

Long DM. Relief of cancer pain by surgical and nerve blocking procedures. JAMA 1980 Dec 19; 244(24):2759–2761

Luther SL, Price JH and Rose CA. The public's knowledge about cancer. Cancer Nurs 1982 Apr; 5(2):109–116

Lym LLQ and Gallagher-Allred CR. Nutrition and the cancer patient: A cooperative effort by nursing and dietetics to overcome problems. Cancer Nurs 1984 Dec; 2(6):469–474

Maher MM, Henderson DK and Brennan MF. Central venous catheter exchange in cancer patients during total parenteral nutrition. NITA 1982 Jan/Feb; 5(1):54–60

Manchester PB. The adolescent with cancer: Concerns for care. Top Clin Nurs 1981 Jan; 2(4):31–37

Maxwell MB. The use of social networks to help cancer patients maximize support. Cancer Nurs 1982 Aug; 5(4): 275–281

Maxwell MB. Pedal edema in the cancer patient. Am J Nurs 1982 Aug; 82(8): 1225–1228

McLoughlin WJ. Cancer rehabilitation: People investing in people. Hosp Pract 1984 June; 19(6):177–183

McNaull FW. The costs of cancer: A challenge to health care providers. Cancer Nurs 1981 June; 4(3):207–212

Miaskowski C. Potential and actual impairments in skin integrity related to cancer and cancer treatment. Top Clin Nurs 1983 July; 5(2):64–71

Miller DG. Susceptibility to cancer. Med Times 1983 Jan; 111(1):61–65

Moore K and Altmaier EM. Stress inoculation training with cancer patients. Cancer Nurs 1981 Oct; 4(5): 389–393

Muller RA and Pelczynski L. You can control cancer pain with drugs. Nursing '82 1982 June; 12(6):50–57

Northouse LL. Living with cancer. Am J Nurs 1981 May; 81(5):960–962

O'Connor RB. Emotional aspects of oncology nursing. NITA 1983 Mar/Apr; 6(2):102–103

Oleski D. Questions about cancer: Indicators for patient education. Top Clin Nurs 1981 Jan; 2(4):1–8

Ostchega Y and Jacob JG. Providing "safe conduct." Helping your patient cope with cancer. Nursing '84 1984 April; 14(4):42–47

Perez K. Nursing management of the Hickman–Broviac catheter. NITA 1982 May/June; 5(3):210–212

Pruyn JFA. Coping with stress in cancer patients. Patient Ed Counsel 1983; 5(2):63–67

Rankin M. The progressive pain of

cancer. Top Clin Nurs 1980 Apr; 2(1): 57–73

Rankin MA. Use of drugs for pain with cancer patients. Cancer Nurs 1982 June; 5(3):181–190

Reich SD. Choice of a strong analgesic for cancer patients. Cancer Nurs 1982 Feb; 5(1):67–69

Ryan LS. Nursing assessment of the ambulatory patient with brain metastases. Cancer Nurs 1981 Oct; 4(5):281–291

Serpick AA. Cancer in the aged. Am Fam Physician 1982 Oct; 26(4):113–117

Shipes E and Lehr S. Sexuality and the male cancer patient. Cancer Nurs 1982 Oct; 5(5):375–381

Taddeine L and Rotschafer JC. Pain syndromes associated with cancer. Postgrad Med 1984 Jan; 75(1):101–108

Wabrek AJ and Gunn JL. Sexual and psychological implications of gynecologic malignancy. JOGN Nurs 1984 Nov/Dec; 13(6):371–376

Watson S and Hickey P. Cancer surgery. Help for the family in waiting. Am J Nurs 1984 May; 84(5):604–607

Welch D. Planning nursing interventions for family members of adult cancer patient. Cancer Nurs 1981 Oct; 4(5): 365–370

Welch-McCaffrey D. When it comes to cancer, think family. Nursing '83 1983 Dec; 13(12):32–35

Wellisch DK and Yager J. Is there a cancer-prone personality? CA 1983 May/June; 33(3):145–153

Chemotherapy

Anderson M and Faulkner N. Amphotericin B: Effective management of adverse reactions. Cancer Nurs 1982 Dec; 5(6):461–464

Antineoplastic drugs. Am J Nurs 1981 Sept; 81(9):1680–1683

Barber HRK. Fetal and neonatal effects of cytotoxic agents. Obstet Gynecol 1981 Nov; 58(5)(supplement):41S–47S

Berry-Oppersteny D and Heusinkveld KB. Prophylactic antiemetics for chemotherapy-associated nausea and vomiting. Cancer Nurs 1983 Apr; 6(2): 117–123

Besharah A. Guidelines for safe handling of cytotoxic agents. Can Nurse 1982 Jan; 78(1):46–47

Bledsoe L. Antineoplastic agents. Management of health risk for the I.V. nurse. NITA 1983 Sept/Oct; 6(5):332–333

Bubela N. Technical and psychological problems and concerns arising from the outpatient treatment of cancer with direct intraarterial infusion. Cancer Nurs 1981 Oct; 4(5):305–309

Buckalew PG. On the opposite side of the bed: A nurse clinician's experiences with anxiety during chemotherapy. Cancer Nurs 1982 Dec; 5(6):435–439

Butler MC. Families' responses to chemotherapy by an ambulatory infusion pump. Nurs Clin North Am 1984 Mar; 19(1):139–144

Campbell S et al. Chemotherapy drug administration. A beginning survey of chemotherapy as a workload index. Cancer Nurs 1984 June; 7(3):213–220

Cline BW. Prevention of chemotherapy-induced alopecia: A review of the literature. Cancer Nurs 1984 June; 7(3):221–228

Cohen MR. Use particular caution when administering cancer drugs. Nursing '84 1984 Aug; 84(8):66

Cotanch PH. Relaxation training for control of nausea and vomiting in patients receiving chemotherapy. Cancer Nurs 1983 Aug; 6(4):277–283

Cozzi E et al. Nursing management of patients receiving hepatic arterial chemotherapy through an implanted infusion pump. Cancer Nurs 1984 June; 7(3):229–234

Crudi CB, Stephens BL and Maier P. Possible occupational hazards associated with the preparation/administration of antineoplastic agents. NITA 1982 July/Aug; 5(4):264–269

Dodd MJ and Mood DW. Chemotherapy: Helping patients to know the drugs they are receiving and their possible side effects. Cancer Nurs 1981 Aug; 4(4):311–318

Dodd MJ. Assessing patient self-care for side effects of cancer chemotherapy. Part I. Cancer Nurs 1982 Dec; 5(6):447–451

Dodd MJ. Self-care for side effects in cancer chemotherapy: An assessment of nursing interventions. Part II. Cancer Nurs 1983 Feb; 6(1):63–67

Engelking CH and Steele NE. A model for pretreatment nursing assessment of patients receiving cancer chemotherapy. Cancer Nurs 1984 June; 7(3):203–212

Fredette SL and Gloriant FS. Nursing diagnosis in cancer chemotherapy in theory. Am J Nurs 1981 Nov; 81(11):2013–2020 (in practice: 2021–2022)

Garvey E and Kramer R. Improving cancer patients' adjustment to infusion chemotherapy: Evaluation of a patient education program. Cancer Nurs 1983 Oct; 6(5):373–378

Goldie JH. New thoughts on resistance to chemotherapy. Hosp Pract 1983 May; 18(5):165–177

Hedrick C. Patient teaching—side effects of chemotherapy. NITA 1984 May/June; 7(3):178–180

Hennessy K and Duval A. Chemotherapy waste disposal: A safe and practical method. NITA 1982 Sept/Oct; 5(5):311–312

Hunt JM, Anderson JE and Smith IE. Scalp hypothermia to prevent adriamycin-induced hair loss. Cancer Nurs 1982 Feb; 5(1):25–31

Johnson BL and Gross J. Handling methotrexate—a safety problem? Am J Nurs 1982 Oct; 82(10):1531

Jones RB, Frank R and Mass T. Safe handling of chemotherapeutic agents: A report from the Mount Sinai Medical Center. CA 1983 Sept/Oct; 33(5):258–262

Koza CM. Principles and practices of cancer chemotherapy. NITA 1983 Sept/Oct; 6(5):326–328

Markman M. Newer techniques in cancer chemotherapy. DM 1984 July; 30(10):6–47

Mattia MA and Blake SL. Hospital hazard cancer drugs. Am J Nurs 1983 May; 83(5):759–762

Mayer D et al. Weight loss in patients receiving recombinant leukocyte A interferon (IFLrA): A brief report. Cancer Nurs 1984 Feb; 7(1):53–56

Neilan BA. Cancer chemotherapy. Postgrad Med 1983 Jan; 73(1):125–130

Petton S. Easing the complications of chemotherapy. Nursing '84 1984 Feb; 14(2):58–63

Redd WH. Control of nausea and vomiting in chemotherapy patients. Postgrad Med 1984 Apr; 75(5):105–113

Reich SD. Mechlorethamine (nitrogen mustard). Cancer Nurs 1981 April; 4(2):147–148

Reich SD. Rationale for anticancer drug dosing schedules. Cancer Nurs 1983 Dec; 6(6):465–467

Rhodes VA, Watson PM and Johnson MYH. Development of reliable and valid measures of nausea and vomiting. Cancer Nurs 1984 Feb; 7(1):33–41

Rose-Williamson K. Cisplatin: Delivering a safe infusion. Am J Nurs 1981 Feb; 81(2):320–323

Rovinski CA. Therapeutic use of noninvestigational marijuana in cancer care. Cancer Nurs 1983 Apr; 6(2):141–144

Schaffner A. Safety precautions in home chemotherapy. Am J Nurs 1984 Mar; 84(3):346–347

Schulmeister L. Vascular access grafts in cancer chemotherapy. Am J Nurs 1982 Sept; 82(9):1388–1389

Smith FP and McCabe MS. Preventing chemotherapy-induced alopecia. Am Fam Physician 1983 July; 28(1):182–184

Strohl RA. Nursing management of the patient with cancer experiencing taste changes. Cancer Nurs 1983 Oct; 6(5):353–359

Treating cancer with a toxic form of oxygen. Am J Nurs 1983 Dec; 83(12):1643–1644

Trester AK. Nursing management of patients receiving cancer chemotherapy. Cancer Nurs 1982 June; 5(3):201–210

"When toxic drugs infiltrate." Am J Nurs 1982 Apr; 82(4):562

Williams LT, Peterson DE and Overholser CD. Acute periodontal infection in myelosuppressed oncology patients: Evaluation and nursing care. Cancer Nurs 1982 Dec; 5(6):465–467

Wroblewski SS and Wroblewski SH. Caring for the patient with chemotherapy-induced thrombocytopenia. Am J Nurs 1981 Apr; 81(4):746–749

Radiation

Brady LW. The changing role of radiation oncology in cancer management. CA 1983 Mar/Apr; 33(2):66–73

del Regato JA and Brady LW. Therapeutic radiology. JAMA 1984 Oct 26; 252(16):2265–2269

Hunter OB. Nuclear medicine. JAMA 1984 Oct 26; 252(16):2269–2271

Jacobson HG and Leeds NE. Diagnostic radiology. JAMA 1984 Oct 26; 252(16):2256–2271

Johnson CM et al. Digital subtraction angiography. Surg Clin North Am 1984 Feb; 64(1):151–172

Kelly PP and Tinsley C. Planning care for the patient receiving external radiation. Am J Nurs 1981 Feb; 81(2):338–342

Upon AC. Low-dose radiation. Postgrad Med 1981 Dec; 70(6):34–47

Immunotherapy

Coral FS. Immunologic approaches to the diagnosis and treatment of malignant disease. NITA 1982 July/Aug; 5(4):256–261

Couillard-Getreuer DL. Herpes zoster in the immunocompromised patient. Cancer Nurs 1982 Oct; 5(5):361–370

Garvey ED, Matutat RJ and Bolten D. Care of the patient undergoing interferon therapy. Cancer Nurs 1983 Aug; 6(4):303–306

Jeffs C and Laqszlo J. A coordinating role for the nurse clinician in a Phase I interferon study. Cancer Nurs 1983 Oct; 6(5):379–386

Koren ME and Herrmann CS. Cancer immunotherapy. What, why, when, how? Nursing '81 1981 Jan; 11(1):34–41

Advanced Cancer

Arsenault L. Metastatic cancer and the nervous system. Focus Crit Care 1984 Dec; 11(6):39–47

Baldwin PD. Epidural spinal cord compression secondary to metastatic disease; A review of the literature. Cancer Nurs 1983 Dec; 6(6):441–446

Borkovic SP and Schwartz RA. Kapoli's sarcoma. Am Fam Physician 1982 Oct; 26(4):133–137

Davis AJ. To make live or let die. Am J Nurs 1981 March; 81(3):582

Gargaro WJ. Criminal prosecution for the discontinuance of life support. Part I. Cancer Nurs 1983 Apr; 6(2):145–146. Part II. Cancer Nurs 1983 June; 6(3):227–228. Part III. Cancer Nurs 1983 Aug; 6(4):311–312.

Kaiko R et al. Central nervous system excitatory effects of meperidine in cancer patients. Ann Neurol 1983 Feb; 13:180–185

Lewis FM. Experienced personal control and quality of life in late-stage cancer patients. Nurs Res 1982 Mar/Apr; 31(2):113–119

Liaschenko JM. Assessment of anxiety and depression in the dying patient. Top Clin Nurs 1981 Jan; 2(4):39–45

McGivney WT and Crooks GM. The care of patients with severe chronic pain in terminal illness. JAMA 1984 Mar 2; 251(9):1182–1188

McNairn N. Helping the patient who wants to die at home. Nursing '81 1981 Feb; 11(2):66

Murray ME. Palliative care. Can Nurse 1981 May; 77(5):16–17

Presant CA, Klahr C and Hogan L. Evaluating quality-of-life in oncology patients: Pilot observations. Cancer Nurs Forum 1981 Summer; 8(3):26–30

Rodek CF and Jacob S. Perspectives on hospice. Cancer Nurs 1983 June; 6(3):181–185

Emergency Nursing

Emergency Management*

Emergency management has traditionally referred to the care given to patients with urgent and critical needs. However, the philosophy of emergency care has broadened to include the concept that an emergency is whatever the patient or his family considers it to be.

Principles of Assessment and Emergency Management

Underlying consideration: Injuries or conditions interfering with vital physiologic function take precedence.

A. **Treat the potentially life-threatening problems first.**

   Goals:
   Preserve life.
   Prevent deterioration before definitive treatment can be given.
   Restore patient to useful living.

B. **Stabilize the pulmonary cardiovascular and central nervous systems.**

   1. Maintain a patent airway and provide adequate ventilation, employing resuscitation measures when necessary.
   Assess for chest injuries with subsequent airway obstruction.

---

* This section will deal mainly with emergency management of trauma and other conditions not found elsewhere in this book. Management of acute heart conditions is found on page 277 and management of acute respiratory problems on page 185.

   2. Control hemorrhage and its consequences.
   3. Evaluate and restore cardiac output.
   4. Prevent and treat shock; maintain or restore effective circulation.
   5. Carry out a rapid initial and ongoing physical examination; the clinical course of the injured or seriously ill patient is not static.
   6. Assess whether or not the patient can follow commands: evaluate the size and reactivity of the pupils and motor responses.
   7. Start ECG monitoring if appropriate.
   8. Splint suspected fractures, including fractures of cervical spine in patients with head injuries.
   9. Protect wounds with sterile dressings.
   10. Check to see if patient has a Medic Alert or similar identification designating allergies, etc.
   11. Start a flow sheet of the patient's vital signs, blood pressure, etc., to guide decision making.

Obtaining Data (History)

If possible, a brief history of the accident/illness is taken from the patient or the person accompanying him—relative, emergency medical technician.
   1. What were the circumstances, forces, location, and time of injury?
   2. When did the symptoms appear?
   3. Was the patient unconscious after the accident?
   4. How did the patient reach the hospital?
   5. What was the health status of the patient before the accident or illness?
   6. Is there a past history of illness? of past admissions?

7. Is the patient currently taking any medications—especially hormones, insulin, digitalis, anticoagulants?
8. Does the patient have any allergies?
9. Does the patient have any bleeding tendencies?
10. Is the patient under a physician's care? (Name of physician)
11. When was the last meal eaten? (Important if an anesthetic is to be given.)
12. What was the date of the patient's most recent tetanus immunization?

Psychological Management of Patients and Families in Emergencies

Underlying Consideration: Body trauma is an insult to physiological and psychological homeostasis; it requires both physiologic and psychologic healing.

A. Approach to the Patient

1. Understand and accept the basic anxieties of the acutely traumatized patient. Be aware of the patient's fear of death, mutilation, and isolation.
   a. Personalize the situation as much as possible—speak, react, and respond in a warm manner.
   b. Give explanations on a level that the patient can grasp—an informed patient can cope with psychologic/physiologic stress in a more positive manner.
   c. Accept the rights of the patient and family to have and display their own feelings.
   d. Maintain a calm and reassuring manner—helps the emotionally distressed patient or family to mobilize their psychological resources.
2. Understand and support the patient's feelings concerning his loss of control (emotional, physical, and intellectual).
3. Treat the unconscious patient as if he were conscious—touch him, call him by name, and explain every procedure that is done. Avoid making negative comments about the patient's condition.
   a. Orient the patient to person, time, and place as soon as he is conscious; reinforce by repeating this information.
   b. Bring the patient back to reality in a calm and reassuring way.
   c. Encourage the family, when possible, to orient the patient to reality.
4. Be prepared to handle all aspects of acute trauma; know what to expect and what to do—alleviates the nurse's anxieties and increases the patient's confidence.

B. Approach to the Family

1. Inform the family where the patient is and give as much information as possible about the treatment he is receiving.
2. Recognize the anxiety of the family and allow them to talk about their feelings—allow expressions of remorse, anger, guilt, and criticism.
3. Allow the family to relive the events, actions, and feelings preceding admission to the emergency department.
4. Deal with reality as gently and quickly as possible; avoid encouraging and supporting denial.
5. Assist the family to cope with sudden and unexpected death. Some helpful measures include the following:
   a. Take the family to a private place.
   b. Talk to all of the family together—so that they can mourn together.
   c. Assure family that everything possible was done; inform them of the treatment rendered.
   d. Avoid using euphemisms such as "passed on," etc. Show the family that you care by touching, offering coffee, etc.
   e. Allow family to talk about the deceased and what he meant to them—permits ventilation of feelings of loss. Encourage family to talk about events preceding admission to the emergency department.
   f. Encourage family to support each other and to express emotions freely: grief, loss, anger, helplessness, tears, disbelief.
   g. Avoid volunteering unnecessary information (patient was drinking, etc.).
   h. Avoid giving sedation to family members—may mask or delay the grieving process which is necessary to achieve emotional equilibrium and prevent prolonged depression.
   i. Encourage family members to view the body if they wish to do so—helps to integrate the loss (cover mutilated areas).
      (1) Go with family to see the body.
      (2) Show acceptance of the body—by touching—to give family "permission" to touch, talk to, etc. the body.
      (3) Spend a few minutes with the family, listening to them.
6. Encourage the emergency department staff to discuss among themselves their reaction to the event—to share intense feelings, for review, and for group support.

Cardiopulmonary Resuscitation and Airway Management

Cardiopulmonary resuscitation is described in the Guidelines that follow. Artificial ventilation is also accomplished by a bag–mask unit (p. 204) or endotracheal intubation (p. 213). Cricothyroidotomy (p. 929) and esophageal obturator airway (p. 930) are used in certain emergencies for resuscitation. The management of foreign-body obstruction is included on pages 927–929. Airway management and artificial ventilation are discussed in detail under Respiratory Failure and Insufficiency, Chapter 6, page 185.

Guidelines: Cardiopulmonary Resuscitation for Cardiac or Respiratory Arrest*

Cardiac arrest is a sudden and unexpected cessation of the heartbeat and effective circulation that results in inadequate delivery of oxygenated blood to vital organs.

Causes

1. Cardiac arrest
   Ventricular fibrillation
   Ventricular standstill
   Cardiovascular collapse

2. Respiratory arrest
   Drowning
   Stroke
   Heart attack
   Airway obstruction
   Drug overdose
   Electrocution
   Suffocation
   Accident/injury
   Head trauma

Signs and Symptoms

1. Absence of palpable carotid or femoral pulse; pulselessness in large arteries
2. Immediate loss of consciousness
3. Absence of breath sounds or air movement through nose or mouth
4. Ashen gray color

Purpose

1. To establish effective circulation and respiration promptly for a victim of cardiac or respiratory arrest through cardio-pulmonary resuscitation.
2. To prevent irreversible cerebral anoxic damage.

Equipment

Trained personnel
Arrest board
Oral airway
Bag and mask device

IV setup
Defibrillator
Emergency cardiac drugs
ECG machine

ABCs of CPR*

1. Airway
   Open the airway
   Determine whether patient is breathing (look, listen, feel)
2. Breathing
   Rescue breathing (mouth to mouth)
   Foreign-body airway obstruction
3. Circulation
   Establish presence or absence of pulse
   Active emergency medical services (EMS)
   Begin chest compression (if pulse absent)

Procedure

Nursing Action	Rationale/Amplification
Performance Phase	
1. Note the time as soon as the cardiac/respiratory arrest is determined. Summon help immediately. Place the patient in a horizontal position on a firm surface.	▶ **NURSING ALERT:** Lack of effective circulation to the central nervous system for more than 3–5 minutes may result in irreversible brain damage.
2. When a monitored patient undergoes cardiac arrest, deliver a precordial thump (a single, sharp blow over the mid-portion of the sternum) using the fleshy part of the fist and striking from a distance of 20.3–30.5 cm. (8–12 inches) above the chest. Then proceed with defibrillation, intubation, etc., as required.	2. The precordial thump is useful when the pulse cannot be detected following a witnessed cardiac arrest or when dealing with a patient who is being monitored or is being paced for a known AV block. The precordial thump should be administered within the first minute after cardiac arrest; it produces a small electrical stimulus.
Artificial Ventilation	
1. Open the airway. Move the lower jaw forward; this is done as follows:	1. Moving the lower jaw forward lifts the tongue off the back wall of the pharynx and opens the airway.

* Adapted from "Standards and Guidelines for Cardiopulmonary Resuscitation (CPR) and Emergency Cardiac Care (ECC)." JAMA 1980 Aug 1; 244(5), pp. 453–509.

(continued)

Guidelines: Cardiopulmonary Resuscitation for Cardiac or Respiratory Arrest (continued)

Procedure
(Cont.)

<table>
<tr><td align="center">Nursing Action</td><td align="center">Rationale/Amplification</td></tr>
<tr><td>

a. *Head Tilt*
  (1) Place one hand on the victim's forehead and apply firm, backward pressure with the palm
         OR

b. *Head Tilt–Neck Lift*
  (1) Place one hand on the victim's forehead (to apply backward pressure) and the other hand beneath the neck close to the back of the head to lift and support it upward.
         OR

c. *Head Tilt–Chin Lift*
  (1) Place tips of fingers of one hand under bony part of the lower jaw bringing the chin forward while pressing on the forehead with the other hand to tilt the head back.

2. Check for breathlessness. Place ear over the victim's mouth and nose, looking toward the victim's mouth and stomach. Watch to see if the victim's chest is rising.

3. Ventilate the patient if necessary. Inflate the patient's lungs by 4 quick, full breaths without allowing for full lung deflation between beats.

  a. Pinch the nostrils closed with the thumb and index finger of the hand that is on the forehead.
  b. Take a deep breath, open mouth wide; and place it outside of the victim's mouth, making a tight seal.

</td><td>

(1) This maneuver produces maximal backward tipping of the head.

2. If the chest is rising; the lungs are being ventilated.

3. Forceful ventilation helps maintain positive pressure in the airway and helps overcome airway obstruction by increasing the pressure gradient of air movement and dilating the upper airway.
  a. To prevent air from escaping.

  b. Adequate ventilation is determined by:
    (1) Seeing the chest rise and fall.
    (2) Feeling in your own airway the resistance and compliance of the victim's lungs as they expand.
    (3) Hearing and feeling the air escape during exhalation.

</td></tr>
</table>

4. Check the carotid pulse.
5. Start external cardiac compression immediately if carotid pulse is absent or questionable.

External Cardiac Compression—the rhythmic application of pressure over the lower half of the sternum (must be accompanied by artificial ventilation).

<table>
<tr><td>

1. Kneel as close to side of the patient's chest as possible. Place the heel of one hand on the lower half of the sternum 3.8 cm. (1½ inches) from the tip of the xiphoid.

2. Place the other hand on top of the first one, with the fingers of both hands directed away from the rescuer.

3. Using your weight while keeping the arms straight and elbows locked, quickly and forcefully depress the lower half of the sternum 4–5 cm. (1½–2 inches) toward the spine, and then release the sternal pressure; allowing the chest to return to its normal position.
  a. Do not allow the hands to lose contact with the sternum.
  b. The body weight should be carried by the arm muscles.
  c. The time allowed for release should be equal to the time required for compression.

4. Use 60 compressions per minute for 2 persons performing CPR.* Compressions should be regular, smooth, and uninterrupted.

</td><td>

1. Proper placement of the hands reduces possible complications of fractured ribs or injury to adjacent abdominal organs. The heart is located to the left of the middle of the chest between the lower sternum and spine.

2. The fingers may be either extended or interlaced but should not touch the chest wall.

3. Each compression forces the blood from the heart into the arterial system. Release following compression allows the heart to rest.

4. If done correctly, this rate can maintain adequate blood flow and pressure and allows cardiac refill.

</td></tr>
</table>

    * This procedure is done best by 2 persons. If only 1 person is available, he must perform both artificial ventilation and external cardiac compression, using a 15:2 ratio consisting of 2 quick lung inflations after each 15 chest compressions. The single rescuer must perform each series of chest compressions at a faster rate of 80 compressions per minute because of interruptions for lung inflation.

Procedure
(Cont.)

Nursing Action	Rationale/Amplification
5. The second person delivers 1 deep breath during the upstroke of the fifth chest compression.	5. If only 1 person is available, he must give 2 quick, full breaths after each cycle of 15 compressions.
6. Palpate for carotid pulse periodically and note size of pupils as an indication of response.	6. The presence of a palpable carotid pulse and constriction of pupils are evidence of effective circulation and oxygenated blood. If pupils remain widely dilated and do not react to light, and if the patient is deeply unconscious with absence of spontaneous respirations, serious brain damage is imminent or has occurred.
7. Insert an artificial airway, endotracheal tube, or esophageal airway as soon as possible.	7. This keeps the airway patent and prevents aspiration.

Definitive Therapy

Nursing Action	Rationale/Amplification
1. While resuscitation proceeds, simultaneous efforts are made to start an intravenous infusion. Have suction ready and attach ECG electrodes to the patient.	1. An IV line provides access to the circulation for drugs/solutions.
2. Continue to assess status of pulses (palpable carotid pulse/femoral pulse) and spontaneous respiratory movement.	
3. Initiate hemodynamic monitoring.	
4. Monitor ECG. Stabilize rhythm.	
5. Draw arterial blood gases.	5. To determine oxygenation and acid–base status.
6. Correct electrolyte and acid–base abnormalities.	6. Tissue anoxia from cardiac arrest leads to metabolic acidosis. Sodium bicarbonate (IV) will correct acidosis.
7. The decision to terminate resuscitation is a medical one and takes into consideration the cerebral and cardiac status. Cardiac compression should continue until the patient can maintain blood pressure, etc., or the situation becomes hopeless.	7. If ventricular fibrillation occurs, conversion to a normal sinus rhythm must be effected by electric countershock delivered by a defibrillator.
8. Place the patient in an intensive care unit.	

▶ **NURSING ALERT:** The patient who has been resuscitated is at risk for another episode of cardiac arrest.

Guidelines: Management of Foreign-Body Airway Obstruction*

Foreign-body obstruction of the airway may be either partial or complete.

Assessment of Clinical Manifestations

Weak, ineffective cough; high-pitched noises on inspiration
Respiratory distress
Inability to speak or breathe
Cyanosis; collapse

Emergency Management

Nursing Action	Rationale/Amplification
1. Carry out a sequence of back blows, manual thrusts, and finger sweeps (see below).	
Back Blows	
a. Administer 4 sharp blows with the heel of the hand over the spine between the shoulder blades while supporting the patient with the other hand on the sternum.	a. A back blow raises pressure in the thorax distal to the obstructing object.

* Adapted from Standards and Guidelines for Cardiopulmonary Resuscitation (CPR) and Emergency Cardiac Care (ECC). JAMA 1980 Aug 1; 244(5):464–467.

(continued)

Guidelines: Management of Foreign-Body Airway Obstruction (continued)

Emergency Management
(Cont.)

Nursing Action	Rationale/Amplification
b. Apply the back blows forcefully in rapid succession; they may be administered with the victim sitting, standing, or lying.	
c. If possible, have patient's head lower than his chest.	

Manual Thrusts

Abdominal thrust for standing patient:

a. Stand behind the patient and wrap your arms around his waist. The rescuer's arms should be just above the belt line.

a. Manual thrusts to the upper abdomen (abdominal thrust) or lower chest (chest thrust) force air out of the lungs and create an artificial cough intended to remove the foreign body.

b. Make a fist with one hand and grasp the fist with your other hand. Place thumb side of your fist against the patient's abdomen between the waist and the rib cage (Fig. 23-1).

c. Press your fist 4 times into the patient's abdomen with a quick inward–upward thrust.

c. A combination of back blows and manual thrusts may be effective in removing obstruction.

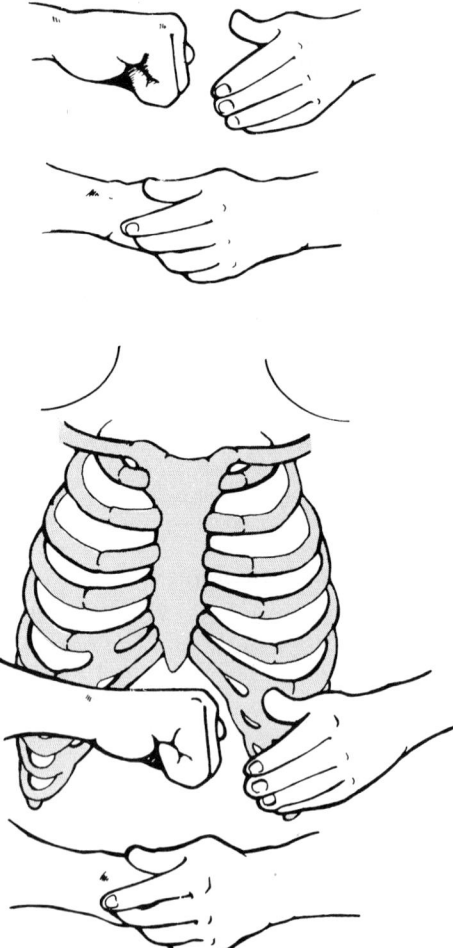

Figure 23-1. Hand placement for abdominal thrusts. (Reprinted from the Supplement to Journal of the American Medical Association, August 1, 1980. Copyright 1980, the American Medical Association. Reprinted with permission from the American Heart Association.)

Emergency Management
(Cont.)

Nursing Action	Rationale/Amplification

For lying (unconscious) patient:
a. Position the patient on his back.
b. Sit astride the patient's hips, facing his head; with one of your hands on top of the other, place the heel of the bottom hand on the patient's abdomen between the waist and rib cage.
c. Press into the abdomen with an inward and upward thrust.

b. Spleen or liver injury may result from sudden increase of abdominal pressure.

Chest Thrust (An Alternate Technique)
a. Stand behind the victim with your arms under his axillae and encircling his chest.
b. Place the thumb side of your fist on the middle of his breast bone.
c. Grasp your fist with your other hand and exert 4 backward thrusts.

a. Chest thrust is an alternate technique.
b. Avoid the xiphoid process and the margins of the rib cage.
c. Each thrust is performed with the intent of relieving the obstruction without having to complete the full series.

2. Apply the finger sweep.
a. Open the patient's mouth by grasping both the tongue and lower jaw between your thumb and fingers and lift the tongue and jaw.
b. Sweep your index finger inside the patient's mouth using a hooking action to dislodge and remove foreign body.
c. If the patient is still unconscious, attempt to ventilate with mouth-to-mouth ventilation; repeat back blows, manual thrusts, and finger sweep.

a. This maneuver draws the tongue away from the back of the pharynx and the obstructing foreign body.
b. The finger probe technique can worsen the situation and should probably be used only under direct visualization or as a last resort.
c. During unconsciousness, muscles relax and these maneuvers may become more effective.

Guidelines: Cricothyroidotomy

Cricothyroidotomy is the puncture or incision of the cricothyroid membrane to establish an emergency airway in certain emergency conditions when endotracheal intubation or tracheostomy cannot be accomplished.

Equipment
No. 11 gauge needle or No. 11 scalpel blade

Procedure

Nursing Action	Rationale/Amplification

1. Extend the neck.
2. Identify the prominent thyroid cartilage (Adam's apple) and allow your finger to descend in the midline to the depression between the lower border of the thyroid cartilage and the upper border of the cricoid cartilage (Fig. 23-2).
3. Insert a needle or any sharp instrument at a 10- to 30-degree caudal direction in the midline just above the upper part of the cricoid cartilage.
4. Listen for air passing back and forth through the needle synchronously with the patient's respirations.
5. Direct the needle downward and posteriorly.
6. Tape the needle with adhesive.
7. An alternate method is to make a transverse incision overlying the cricothyroid membrane and a similar incision through the membrane itself.
The membrane incision is spread and a tracheostomy tube is advanced caudally into the trachea.
8. Prepare for endotracheal intubation/tracheostomy.
9. Potential complications; vocal cord injury, subcutaneous emphysema, bleeding.

1. So that the cricothyroid membrane can be palpated readily.
2. This depression represents the cricothyroid membrane.
5. To avoid injury to the vocal cords (located cephalad to the cricothyroid membrane).
6. To prevent laceration or perforation of the posterior tracheal wall.

(continued)

Guidelines: Cricothyroidotomy (continued)

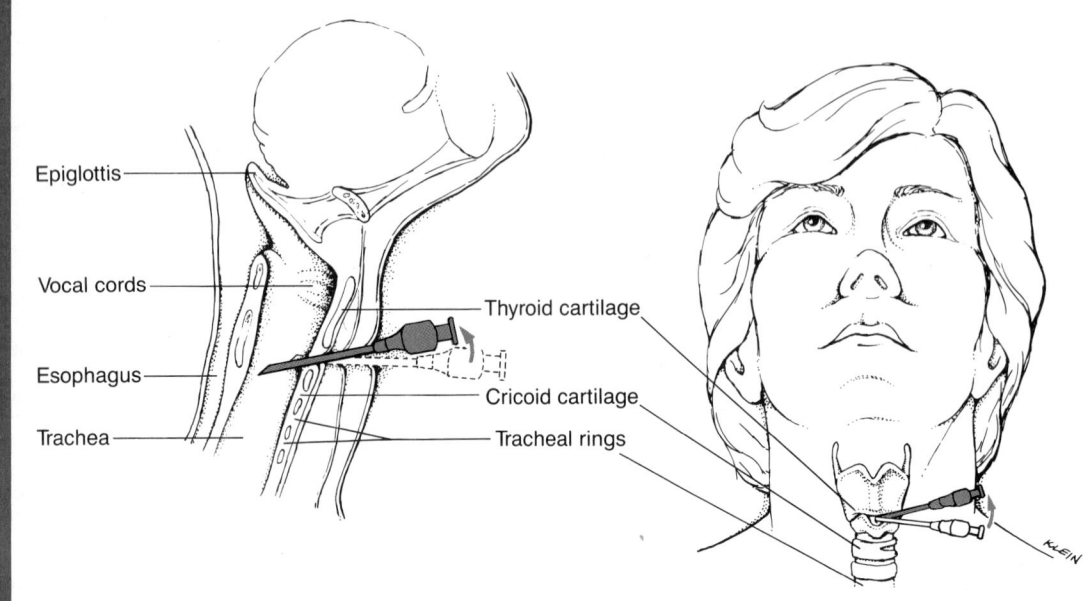

Figure 23-2. Crycothyroidotomy, or cricothyroid membrane puncture.

Guidelines: Esophageal Obturator Airway (EOA)

The *esophageal obturator airway* is a ventilatory device used in respiratory emergencies for resuscitation. It consists of (1) a face mask—to seal off the nose and mouth and anchor the airway; (2) a flexible tube with openings at the level of the pharynx—to permit ventilation of the lungs; and (3) a balloon on the distal end of the tube—to block the esophagus, thus reducing the possibility of aspirating gastric contents.

Purpose   To ventilate an apneic, unconscious patient when endotracheal intubation is not feasible.

Equipment

Esophageal obturator airway   Water-soluble gel
50-ml. syringe   Bag and mask unit

Procedure

Nursing Action	Rationale/Amplification
Preparatory Phase	
Lubricate the tube and attach the mask to the tube by the snap lock.	This procedure is contraindicated in conscious or semi-conscious patients or in those with corrosive poisoning, esophageal disease, or a foreign body in the trachea.
Performance Phase	
1. Using the left hand, insert the thumb as deeply as possible over the patient's tongue, pulling on it while using the fingers to lift the jaw upward and away from the posterior pharyngeal wall.	
2. Insert the esophageal obturator airway into the mouth, carefully guiding the tube over the tongue and past the pharynx; rotate the tube 180 degrees into the esophagus.	2. Maintain the patient's head in a neutral position.
3. Stop advancing the tube when the mask reaches the face; press the mask firmly against the face.	
4. Ventilate the patient by blowing a few breaths through the tube or by attaching a bag mask to it.	4. *If the tube is in the esophagus, the chest will rise.*
If the chest does not rise or no breath sounds are heard, withdraw the tube immediately.	Inadvertent tracheal intubation is a complication associated with the use of the EOA.
Continue ventilating the patient (by bag–mask ventilation) and prepare for and proceed with second attempt at insertion.	

Procedure
(Cont.)

Nursing Action

5. Auscultate over both lung fields to check that *both* lungs are receiving adequate ventilation and that the airway is in the esophagus and *not* in the trachea.
6. Inflate the cuff (balloon) with approximately 30 ml. of air.
7. Connect the end of the esophageal obturator to a bag–mask or mechanical ventilator, or continue mouth-to-tube ventilation.
8. One type of EOA unit has a central lumen that allows passage of a nasogastric tube (Fig. 23-3).

Rationale / Amplification

6. Inflating the balloon prevents air from entering the stomach and prevents regurgitation/vomiting.
7. Air or oxygen is blown into the sealed mask and exits through the holes at the hypopharynx, passing into the trachea and lungs.
8. This allows suctioning and decompression of the stomach.

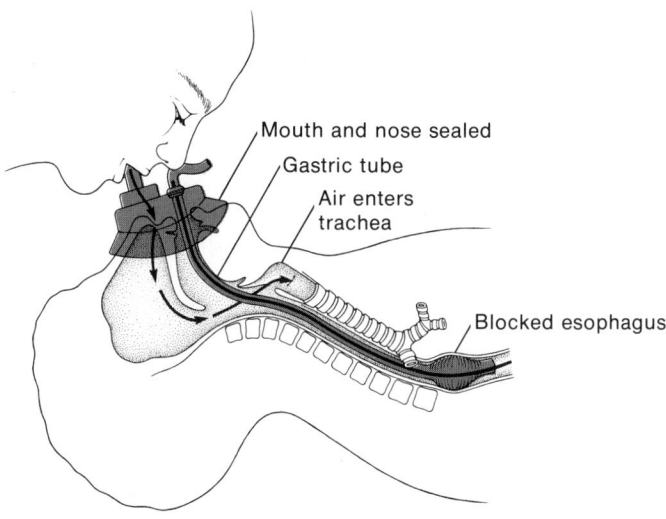

Mouth and nose sealed
Gastric tube
Air enters trachea
Blocked esophagus

Figure 23-3. The Esophageal (Gastric Tube) Airway®. Courtesy of Brunswick Mfg. Co., Inc. (Redrawn)

9. Do not remove the EOA until the patient regains consciousness or has a gag reflex *OR* until endotracheal intubation has been accomplished.
   a. To remove tube: Have suction available. Turn the patient's head to side; deflate cuff and remove.

9. If the tube is taken out prematurely, regurgitation and aspiration are almost inevitable. The EOA tube must be deflated before it is removed.

Hemorrhage

Goals:
Control bleeding.
Maintain an adequate circulating blood volume for tissue oxygenation.
Prevent shock.

Assessment
(Signs and symptoms of shock occur.)
1. Cool, moist skin—from poor peripheral perfusion
2. Falling blood pressure
3. Increasing heart rate
4. Decreasing urine volume

Emergency Management
1. Cut the patient's clothing away quickly and carry out a rapid physical examination.
2. Apply firm pressure over the bleeding area or the artery involved (Fig. 23-4); almost all bleeding can be stopped by direct pressure. Unchecked arterial bleeding results in death.
3. Apply a firm pressure dressing. Elevate the injured part to stop venous and capillary bleeding. Immobilize an injured extremity to control blood loss.
4. Insert intravenous cannula to provide means of blood replacement.
   a. Withdraw blood samples for analysis, typing, and cross-matching.
   b. Give replacement fluids, including isotonic electrolyte solutions, or plasma protein fraction or blood (depending on clinical estimates of type and volume of fluids lost).
      (1) Fresh blood is infused when there is massive blood loss—to prevent loss of platelets and coagulation factors.

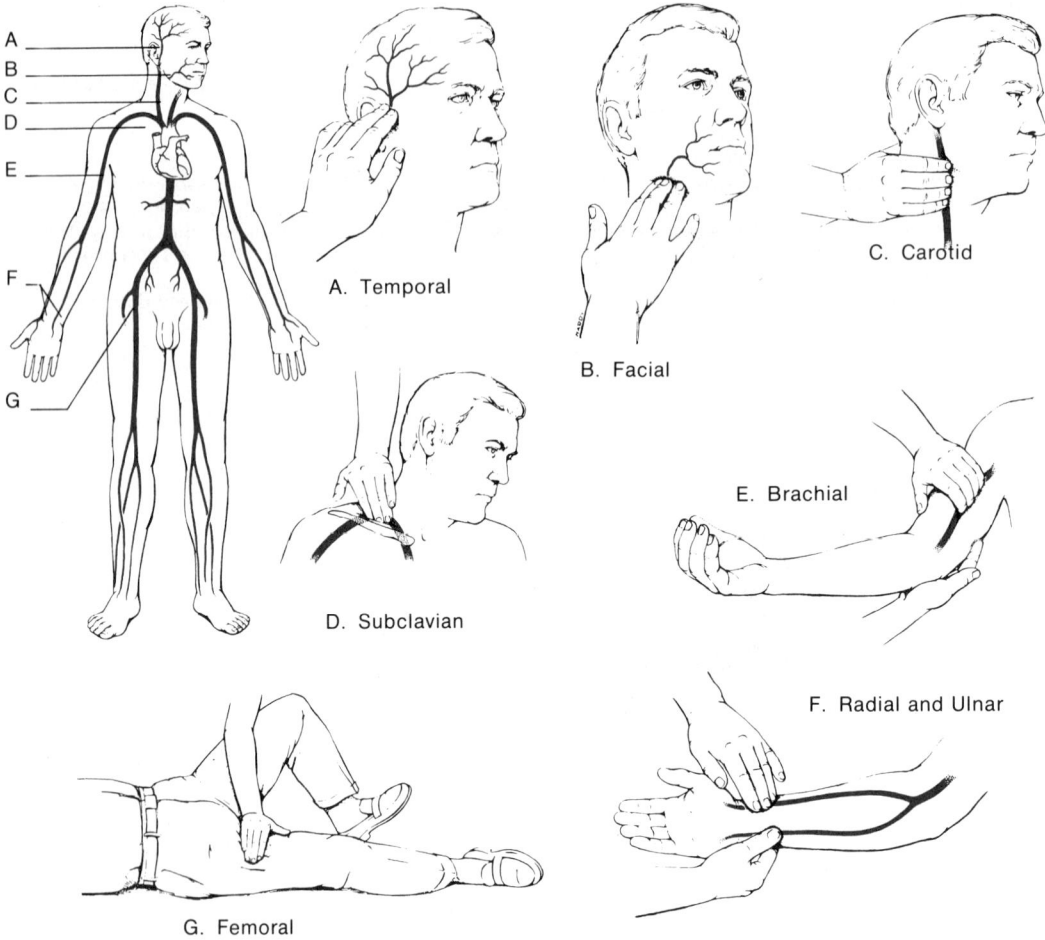

A. Temporal
B. Facial
C. Carotid
D. Subclavian
E. Brachial
F. Radial and Ulnar
G. Femoral

Figure 23-4. Pressure points for control of hemorrhage.

(2) Additional platelets and clotting factors are given when large amounts of blood are needed, since replacement blood is deficient in clotting factors.

(3) Warm the blood (commercial warmer or basin of warm water)—massive blood replacement has a cooling effect that can cause cardiac arrest.

c. Rate of infusion depends on severity of blood loss and clinical evidence of hypovolemia.

5. Take the following steps for internal bleeding:

a. Suspect internal bleeding in patients with hypovolemic shock with no external signs of bleeding: rising pulse rate; falling blood pressure; thirst; apprehension; cool, moist skin.

b. Give whole blood or plasma expanders at the rate of blood loss.

c. Prepare the patient immediately for surgical intervention.

d. Apply pneumatic counterpressure device if available—to control internal bleeding and to facilitate blood flow to vital areas (Fig. 23-5).

e. Obtain blood gas determinations; establish central venous pressure monitoring as an index of

the amount of replacement fluid the patient can tolerate.

6. Apply a tourniquet only as a *last resort* when the hemorrhage cannot be controlled by any other method. Anticipate loss of an extremity if tourniquet is applied.

a. Apply the tourniquet as close as is feasible to the wound; tie it tightly enough to control arterial blood flow.

b. Tag the patient (with a skin-marking pencil or on adhesive tape on his forehead) with a "T" stating the location of the tourniquet and the time applied.

c. Loosen the tourniquet as directed to prevent irreparable vascular or neurologic damage if the patient is in an emergency facility. If there is no arterial bleeding, remove the tourniquet and again try pressure dressing.

d. In the event of a traumatic amputation, leave the tourniquet in place until the patient is in the operating room.

7. Watch for cardiac arrest; patients who hemorrhage are candidates for cardiac arrest caused by hypovolemia with secondary anoxia.

8. See page 92 for further discussion of hemorrhage.

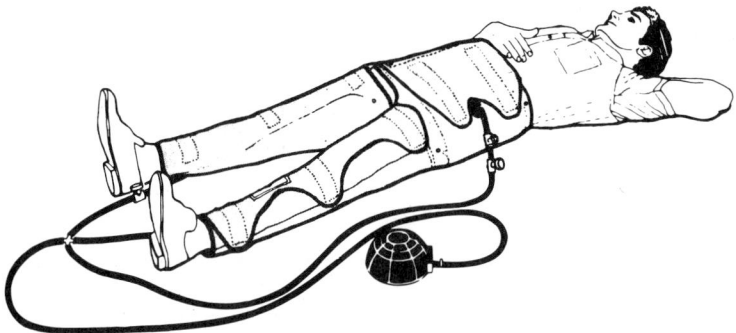

Figure 23-5. The Medical Anti-Shock Trouser (MAST) is a garment designed to correct internal bleeding and hypovolemia by the application of counter pressure around the legs and abdomen. This creates an artificial peripheral resistance and helps sustain coronary perfusion. It should be applied as soon as possible after injury, preferably before the patient is transferred to the emergency department. (Courtesy of David Clark Co., Inc., 360 Franklin Street, Worcester, MA 01604.)

Control of Hypovolemic Shock

Shock is a condition in which there is loss of effective circulating blood volume; inadequate organ and tissue perfusion result, ultimately causing cellular metabolic derangements.

Clinical Manifestations

1. Decrease in systolic blood pressure
2. Increasing pulse rate; tachycardia
3. Cold, clammy skin; prostration
4. Pallor; circumoral pallor
5. Thirst
6. Alterations of mental status
7. Decrease in urine output

Emergency Management

Goals:
Restore and maintain tissue perfusion.
Correct physiologic abnormalities.

1. Establish and maintain an airway; start resuscitation procedures if necessary.
   a. Administer oxygen to augment oxygen-carrying capacity of arterial blood.
   b. Give additional ventilatory assistance as required.
2. Stop any blood loss.
3. Restore circulating blood volume with rapid fluid and blood replacement to correct hypotension and maintain tissue perfusion.
   a. Insert central venous catheter in or near right atrium (p. 286)—to serve as a guide for fluid replacement. (Continuing CVP reading gives direction and degree of change from baseline reading; also is a vehicle for emergency fluid volume replacement.)
   b. Insert large-gauge intravenous needles or catheters into peripheral vein(s); 2 or more catheters may be necessary for rapid replacement and reversal of hemodynamic instability. The emphasis is on volume replacement.

   (1) Establish IV lines in both upper and lower extremities if there is suspicion that a major vessel in the chest or abdomen has been disrupted.
   (2) Withdraw blood for specimens, arterial blood gases (arterial blood), chemistry studies, typing and cross-matching, and hematocrit.
4. Start intravenous infusion at a rapid rate until CVP rises to a satisfactory level above baseline measurement or until there is improvement in clinical condition.
   a. Infusion of lactated Ringer's solution is effective initially to restore circulation.
   b. Start transfusion of blood component therapy, especially when blood loss has been severe or when patient continues to hemorrhage.
   c. Carry out serial hematocrit examinations if continued bleeding is suspected. Hemorrhage will compound the shock state.
   d. Maintain the systolic blood pressure at a satisfactory level by administering IV fluids and blood.
5. Insert an indwelling urinary catheter; record urinary output every 15–30 minutes. Urinary volume reveals adequacy of kidney and visceral perfusion.
6. Carry out a rapid physical assessment to determine cause of shock.
7. Maintain ongoing nursing surveillance of *total patient*—blood pressure, heart, and respiratory rates; skin temperature, color; CVP, arterial blood gases, urinary output, ECG, hematocrit, hemoglobin, coagulation profiles, and electrolytes—to assess patient response to treatment. Keep a flow sheet of these parameters—trend analysis reveals improvement or deterioration of patient.
8. Elevate the feet slightly to assist venous return from lower extremities (also helps prevent air embolism during insertion of subclavian catheter). *(This position is contraindicated in patients with head injuries.)*

9. Give specific pharmacologic agents (sodium bicarbonate, dopamine, etc.) when indicated by the patient's condition.
10. Support the defense mechanisms of the body.
    a. Reassure and comfort the patient; sedation may be necessary to relieve apprehension.
    b. Relieve pain by *cautious* use of analgesics or narcotics.

c. Maintain the body temperature.
   (1) Too much heat produces vasodilatation, which counteracts the body's compensatory mechanism of vasoconstriction and also increases fluid loss by perspiration.
   (2) A patient who is in septic shock should be kept cool, since high fever will increase the cellular metabolic effects of shock.

Wounds

Wounds (injury to tissues) vary from minor lacerations to severe crushing injuries.
Underlying Considerations
Life-threatening problems such as airway obstruction, hemorrhage, and shock must be dealt with before the wound is treated.

Emergency Management

Goals:
Avoid complications.
Promote rapid healing.
Minimize scarring and prevent deformity.

1. Ask the patient *when* as well as *how* the wound occurred; a delay of more than 3 hours in treatment increases the risk of infection developing.
2. Inspect the wound using aseptic technique—to determine the extent of damage to underlying structures.
   a. Shave around wound (with exception of eyebrows) only if directed.
   b. Cleanse skin around wound with antimicrobial agent. Do not allow cleansing solution to get into wound, since it may be injurious to exposed tissues.
   c. Infiltrate with local anesthetic intradermally through the wound margins or by regional block.
3. Cleanse and debride the wound.
   a. Irrigate gently and copiously with isotonic sterile saline solution—to remove surface dirt.

b. Remove devitalized tissue and foreign matter—impairs wound's ability to resist infection.
c. Clamp and tie small bleeding vessels (or achieve hemostasis with a cautery).
4. Suture wound if primary closure is indicated (depends on nature of wound, length of time since injury was sustained, degree of contamination, vascularity of tissues). (Usually done by physician.)
   a. Subcutaneous fat is approximated loosely with a few sutures to close off dead space.
   b. Subcuticular layer or dermis is then closed.
   c. Epidermis is closed; sutures placed close to wound edge with skin edges carefully leveled to prevent uneven scar surfaces.
   d. Sterile strips of reinforced microporous tape may be used to close clean superficial wounds.
5. Apply nonadherent dressing—to protect the wound; may serve as a splint and as a reminder to the patient that he has sustained an injury.
6. For delayed primary closure (when wound cannot be sutured because of tissue loss):
   a. A thin layer of gauze covered by occlusive dressing (to ensure drainage and prevent pooling of exudate) may be used, or split-thickness cadaver or porcine xenografts may be used since they simulate the function of epithelium.
   b. Splint the wound in position of rest—to prevent motion.
   c. Close the wound (using local anesthesia) when there are no signs of suppuration.
7. Give antimicrobial treatment as directed—depends on how injury occurred, age of wound, presence of soil-infection potential, etc.
8. Elevate site to limit accumulation of fluid in wound interstitial spaces.
9. Give tetanus prophylaxis as indicated.
10. Inform the patient to contact physician if there is sudden onset/persistent pain, fever/chills, bleeding, rapid swelling, foul odor, profuse drainage, or redness surrounding the wound.

Tetanus Prophylaxis in Wound Management*
Underlying Considerations

1. Available evidence shows that complete primary immunization with tetanus toxoid provides long-lasting protective antitoxin levels.
   a. Additionally, protective antitoxin develops rapidly in response to a booster dose in persons who have previously received at least 2 doses of tetanus-toxoid.

Summary guide to tetanus prophylaxis in routine wound management, 1981*

History of tetanus immunization (doses)	Clean, minor wounds		All other wounds	
	Td[1]	TIG	Td[1]	TIG
Uncertain	Yes	No	Yes	Yes
0–1	Yes	No	Yes	Yes
2	Yes	No	Yes	No[2]
3 or more	No[3]	No	No[4]	No

[1] For children less than 7 years old DTP (DT, if pertussis vaccine is contraindicated) is preferred to tetanus toxoid alone. For persons 7 years old and older, Td is preferred to tetanus toxoid alone.
[2] Yes, if wound more than 24 hours old.
[3] Yes, if more than 10 years since last dose.
[4] Yes, if more than 5 years since last dose. (More frequent boosters are not needed and can accentuate side effects.)
Td = Tetanus and Diphtheria Toxoids Adsorbed (for adult use)
TIG = Tetanus Immune Globulin

* Morbidity & Mortality Weekly Report, Vol 30/Number 32 Aug 21, 1981.

b. Therefore, passive protection with TIG (tetanus immune globulin) or antitoxin need be considered only when the patient has had less than 2 previous injections of tetanus toxoid or when the wound has been untended for more than 24 hours.

2. A summary guide to tetanus prophylaxis is on page 934. It assumes a reliable knowledge of the patient's immunization history.
3. When tetanus toxoid and TIG are given concurrently, separate syringes and separate sites should be used.
4. See also p. 881.

Intra-abdominal Injuries

Intra-abdominal injuries may be either penetrating or blunt.

Penetrating Abdominal Injuries

Persons with *penetrating abdominal injuries* (gunshot wounds, stab wounds, etc.) should be treated like critically ill patients.

High-velocity missiles (bullets) create extensive tissue damage; such damage usually requires surgical exploration.

Stab wounds may be managed more conservatively.

Assessment

1. Assess the patient for progression of distention, tenderness, pain, muscular rigidity or rebound tenderness, diminished bowel sounds, hypotension, and shock.
2. Auscultate for bowel sounds because the absence of bowel sounds is an early sign of intraperitoneal involvement. If signs of peritoneal irritation are present, an immediate exploratory celiotomy (surgical incision into the abdominal cavity) is usually performed.
3. Record all physical signs as the patient is examined.
4. Look for chest injuries, which frequently accompany intra-abdominal injuries.

Emergency Management

Goals:
Control the bleeding.
Maintain blood volume.

1. Keep the patient on the stretcher, since movement may fragment or dislodge a clot in a large vessel and produce massive hemorrhage.
   a. Ensure patency of the airway and stability of the respiratory, circulatory, and nervous systems.
   b. Cut the clothing away from the wound.
   c. Tabulate the number of wounds.
   d. Look for entrance and exit wounds.
   e. If the patient is comatose, splint the neck until after cervical films are made.
2. Assess for signs and symptoms of hemorrhage. Hemorrhage frequently accompanies abdominal injury, especially if the liver and spleen have been traumatized.
3. Control the bleeding and maintain the blood volume until surgery can be performed.
   a. Apply compression to external bleeding wounds.
   b. Insert indwelling intravenous catheter(s) for rapid fluid replacement to restore circulatory dynamics.
   c. Watch for occurrence of shock after an initial positive response to transfusion therapy; this is often the first sign of internal hemorrhage.
4. Aspirate the stomach contents with a nasogastric tube—also helps detect gastric wounds and prevents lung complications from aspiration.
5. Cover protruding abdominal viscera with sterile saline dressings to protect viscera from drying.
   a. Flex the patient's knees, since this position will prevent further protrusion.
   b. Withhold oral fluids to prevent increased peristalsis and vomiting.
6. Insert indwelling urethral catheter to ascertain the presence of hematuria and to monitor the urinary output.
7. Keep an ongoing flow sheet of the patient's vital signs, urinary output, central venous pressure readings, hematocrit values, and neurologic status.
8. Prepare for paracentesis or peritoneal lavage (see p. 936) when there is uncertainty about intraperitoneal bleeding.
9. For stab wounds, prepare for sinography to determine whether there is peritoneal penetration.
   a. Purse string suture is placed around wound.
   b. A small catheter is introduced through the wound.
   c. Contrast medium is introduced through catheter; x-rays are made and will reveal whether peritoneal penetration has taken place.
10. Carry out tetanus prophylaxis as directed.
11. Give broad-spectrum antimicrobial as directed to prevent infection, since bacterial contamination is a frequent complication (depending on history and nature of wound).
12. Prepare for surgery if the patient shows evidence of shock, blood loss, free air, evisceration, hematuria, etc.

Blunt Abdominal Trauma

Underlying Considerations

1. Trauma to the abdomen is frequently associated with extra-abdominal injuries—chest, head, and extremities.
2. The incidence of delayed trauma-related complications is greater than that associated with penetrating injuries; this is especially true of blunt injuries involving the liver, spleen, or blood vessels, which can lead to substantial blood loss into the peritoneal cavity.

Clinical Manifestations

1. Pain; pain on movement
2. Rebound and maximal point tenderness
3. Muscle guarding
4. Diminishing or absent bowel sounds

Emergency Management

1. Begin resuscitation procedures and evaluation of the patient simultaneously.
2. Take a detailed history (frequently unobtainable, inaccurate, and misleading); obtain all possible data about the following:
   a. Method of injury
   b. Time of onset of symptoms
   c. Passenger location (driver frequently sustains spleen/liver rupture)
   d. Time of last food/fluid intake
   e. Bleeding tendencies
   f. Concurrent disease
   g. Immunization history, with attention to tetanus
   h. Allergies
3. Carry out ongoing examination (inspection, palpation, auscultation, and percussion of the abdomen). The changes noted in subsequent examinations may reveal an undetected abdominal injury.
   a. Avoid moving the patient until initial assessment is done—movement may fragment a clot in a large vessel and produce massive hemorrhage.
   b. Look for chest injuries, especially fracture of lower ribs.
   c. Inspect the front, flanks, and back for bluish discoloration, asymmetry, abrasions, contusions.
   d. Evaluate for signs and symptoms of hemorrhage—frequently accompanies abdominal injury, especially if the liver and spleen have been traumatized.
   e. Note tenderness, rebound tenderness, guarding, rigidity, and spasm.
      (1) Press the area of maximal tenderness (let the patient point to the area).
      (2) Remove the fingers quickly; pain at suspected point indicates peritoneal irritation.
   f. Look for increasing abdominal distention.

Measure abdominal girth at umbilical level upon admission—serves as a baseline from which changes can be determined.
   g. Auscultate for bowel sounds; a silent abdomen accompanies peritoneal irritation.
   h. Note loss of dullness over solid organs (liver; spleen)—indicates presence of free air; dullness over regions normally containing gas may indicate presence of blood.
   i. Assist with rectal examination/vaginal examination—for diagnosis of injury to pelvis, bladder, and intestinal wall.
4. Avoid giving narcotics during observation period—may mask clinical picture.
5. Monitor vital signs frequently and carefully—may be the only clue to intra-abdominal bleeding.
6. Obtain baseline laboratory studies.
   a. Urinalysis—as a guide to possible urinary tract injury; to monitor urine output.
   b. Serial hemoglobin and hematocrit levels—their trend reflects presence or absence of bleeding.
   c. CBC—white blood cell count may be elevated with rupture of spleen.
   d. Serum amylase—elevation usually indicates pancreatic injury or trauma to bowel.
7. Obtain abdominal and chest x-rays—may reveal free air beneath diaphragm, indicating ruptured hollow viscus.
8. Assist with peritoneal lavage—to test for intraperitoneal bleeding (see below), especially if the patient is obtunded.
9. Assist with insertion of a nasogastric tube—to prevent vomiting and subsequent aspiration; helpful in decompressing (removing fluid/air) from gastrointestinal tract.
10. Patient may be admitted for observation or exploratory laparotomy.

Guidelines: Peritoneal Lavage

Peritoneal lavage is a technique of irrigation of the peritoneum and examination of the irrigating fluid to evaluate the effects of trauma to the abdomen.

Purposes
1. To test for intra-abdominal bleeding.
2. To look for injuries requiring surgical treatment.
3. To test patients with equivocal abdominal findings.
4. To avoid unnecessary operation, especially in patients with altered states of consciousness (from head injuries, drugs, alcohol) and when physical findings are unreliable (spinal cord injuries).

Equipment

Peritoneal dialysis tray
Sterile solution (lactated Ringer's solution)
IV tubing; IV pole
Peritoneal dialysis catheter (multiple perforations)
Local skin anesthetic; sterile gloves

Procedure

Nursing Action	Rationale/Amplification
Preparatory Phase	
1. Explain the procedure to the patient; see that the consent form has been signed.	
2. Empty the bladder (by catheter if necessary).	2. To prevent puncture of urinary bladder.
3. Shave the lower abdomen from umbilicus to pubic area. Prepare the abdomen as for surgery.	3. To minimize or eliminate surface bacteria and decrease the possibility of wound contamination and infection.

Procedure
(Cont.)

Nursing Action	Rationale/Amplification
4. Place the patient in a supine position.	
5. Fill the IV tubing with solution using aseptic technique.	

Performance Phase (by the physician)

Nursing Action	Rationale/Amplification
1. The skin is infiltrated 2–3 cm. (.7–1.2 inches) below the umbilicus in the midline with local anesthetic.	1. The midline area is relatively avascular. Epinephrine may be injected with local anesthetic to produce capillary constriction and prevent a false-positive tap.
2. A small vertical incision is made at the chosen site.	2. There are various methods (open or percutaneous) of introducing the catheter into the peritoneal space.
3. Bleeding vessels are carefully ligated.	3. Ligation of vessels helps avoid a false-positive lavage.
4. The peritoneum is brought upward between 2 hemostats and is punctured under direct vision. The peritoneum is opened, and a peritoneal dialysis catheter is directed into the incision and advanced toward the pelvis.	
5. A gauze sponge is packed into the subcutaneous tissue.	5. To absorb minor bleeding.
6. A syringe is attached to the catheter, and the peritoneal cavity is aspirated.	6. If more than 10 ml. of blood is obtained, the test is considered positive and the patient is prepared for immediate celiotomy (incision into abdominal cavity).
7. If no blood (or less than 10 ml.) is present, the catheter is attached to the IV tubing; 500–1000 ml. of solution is infused into the peritoneal cavity through the intravenous tubing attached to the dialysis catheter.	7. If not contraindicated by the patient's condition, he may be turned from side to side to ensure that the solution reaches all parts of the abdominal cavity.
8. Remove the empty IV bottle from the pole and lower the bottle near the floor.	8. Lowering the bottle creates a siphon effect to drain the excess fluid. As much of the fluid as possible is siphoned out of the peritoneal cavity by gravity.
9. The peritoneal dialysis catheter is removed, and the wound is closed (unless laparotomy is necessary).	
10. The fluid recovered from the peritoneal cavity is examined visually and is usually sent to the laboratory for cell counts and microscopic inspection of spun down sediment.	

Interpretation of Lavage Fluid

Nursing Action	Rationale/Amplification
Clear fluid indicates a lack of significant intraperitoneal bleeding.	This indicates a negative test.
1. *Gross examination (visual)* Inability to read newsprint through the intravenous tubing with the retained lavage tube usually means that the amount of blood is sufficient to consider laparotomy.	
2. *Laboratory evaluation* (positive tests) RBC count greater than 100,000 per ml.; 50,000–100,000 per ml. equivocal.	2. If the test is positive, a laparotomy is usually done. Indeterminate or equivocal results merit monitoring and investigation.

Follow-up Phase

Nursing Action	Rationale/Amplification
1. Assess the patient for complications.	1. Complications include visceral perforation, wound hematoma, perforated bowel, puncture of bladder, laceration of major vessels, and lack of fluid return.
2. Watch the patient closely for any type of deterioration.	2. Repeated physical examinations of the abdomen should be carried out when intra-abdominal injury is suspected.

Head Injuries

Head injuries are classified as open or closed injuries. About 15%–20% of all patients who come to emergency departments for treatment have some form of head trauma. (See p. 766 for a more complete discussion of treatment of head injuries.)

Emergency Management

▶ **NURSING ALERT:** Exercise care when moving the patient's head and neck. Fracture of the cervical spine frequently accompanies a head injury.

1. Maintain the airway and ventilation—hypoxia and hypercapnia can increase brain swelling and cell damage.
   a. Keep the patient supine with his neck in a neutral position. Immobilize cervical spine.
   b. Clear the respiratory passages by means of suctioning.
   c. Ensure adequate oxygenation and humidification. (Hypoxia of the brain, which leads to increased intracranial pressure, is the most frequent cause of death following head injury.)
   d. Obtain a portable x-ray of lateral cervical spine before intubation, to rule out cervical spine fracture. A cricothyroidotomy may be considered if the patient is in acute respiratory distress.
   e. Assist with endotracheal intubation if the patient is comatose (after determining that a cervical neck injury is not present).
   f. Utilize assisted ventilation if necessary. (The brain is very sensitive to lack of oxygen.)
2. Control hemorrhage and shock.
   a. Shock is rarely the result of head injury—look for an extracranial source of bleeding (abdomen, thorax, long bone fracture).
   b. Marked intracranial bleeding in an adult usually produces hypertension.
   c. Profound hypotension may be secondary to acute scalp blood loss.
3. Determine the baseline condition of the patient— serves as a basis for comparison as the patient's condition changes.
   a. Assess level of responsiveness (consciousness) (see p. 761). Record exactly what the patient does and can do on command and to verbal and painful stimuli.
   b. Determine the presence of headache, double vision, nausea, vomiting, papilledema, retinal hemorrhage.
   c. Evaluate pupil size and reaction to light and ocular movements.
   d. Measure blood pressure, pulse, respirations.
   e. Evaluate for signs of rising intracranial pressure— deterioration in level of responsiveness, slowing of pulse, rising systolic pressure, increasing pulse pressure, changes in pattern of respiration, dilating, nonreacting pupils.
   f. Evaluate motion and strength of extremities.
   g. Assess for injuries to other organ systems.
4. Evaluate for changes in the patient's condition. *(Change in level of responsiveness is the most sensitive sign of improvement or deterioration.)*
5. Prepare for computed tomography or angiography— to diagnose type of pathology and plan definitive care.
6. Utilize intracranial monitoring (if available)—for recognition of increased intracranial hypertension and to help guide therapy.
7. See page 766 for definitive therapy of head trauma.

Crush Injuries

Crush injuries occur when a person is crushed beneath debris, run over, or compressed by machinery.

Clinical Manifestations

1. Oligemic shock—due to extravasation of blood and plasma into injured tissues after compression has been released.
2. Paralysis of part, erythema and blistering of skin— damaged part (usually an extremity) becomes swollen, tense, hard.
3. Renal dysfunction—prolonged hypotension causes kidney damage and acute renal insufficiency.

Emergency Management

1. Control shock.
2. Observe carefully for acute renal insufficiency (see p. 515)—injury to back may cause severe kidney damage.
3. Splint major soft tissue injuries to control bleeding and pain.
4. Elevate the extremity. Incise fascia if the blood supply is blocked to relieve the pressure of extravasated fluid.
5. Administer medication for pain and anxiety.

Spinal Cord Injury

Spinal cord injury may vary from a mild cord concussion with transient numbness to an immediate and permanent quadriplegia.

Any person with a head, neck, or back injury should be suspected of having a potential spinal cord injury until the suspicion is proved groundless.

Clinical Manifestations

1. Intercostal paralysis with diaphragmatic breathing— indicates cervical spinal cord injury.
2. Total sensory loss and motor paralysis below level of injury.
3. Loss of bowel and bladder control; usually urinary retention and bladder distention.
4. Loss of sweating and vasomotor tone below level of cord lesion.
5. Marked reduction of blood pressure—from loss of peripheral and vascular resistance.
6. Neck pain.
7. Priapism—persistent erection of penis.

Emergency Management

1. Immobilize the patient. Keep him on the transfer board or on a hard, flat stretcher.

▶ **NURSING ALERT:** A spinal cord injury can be made worse during the acute phase of injury. Proper handling is an immediate priority.

a. Keep the head and neck in a straight line with the long axis of the body. Do not move the spine; avoid flexion or rotation of the head and neck or flexing, extending, or twisting the spine.

b. Keep the head and neck in a neutral position while applying a cervical collar to maintain stability.

c. Move the patient on a firm transfer board; at least 4–5 persons are needed to move the patient as one unit to the board.

d. Apply continuous, gentle traction to the head.

e. Transport to a spinal cord center (if available) or special care unit as rapidly as possible.

f. Upon admission to the hospital, radiological studies are carried out while the patient is on the board.

g. Transfer to a special frame (Stryker) after initial evaluation.

2. Evaluate the patient's respiratory exchange—death may occur from respiratory failure in cervical cord victims.

3. Evaluate and examine the patient for level of spinal cord injury and associated injuries; the presence of spinal shock (p. 803) may make assessment difficult.

a. Test for strength and motion of extremities.

(1) Request the patient to flex and extend elbows and to squeeze fingers of examiner.

(2) Request the patient to move hips, knees, ankles, toes.

(3) Observe pattern of respirations—intercostal muscle paralysis causes paradoxical movement of chest and abdomen.

(4) Observe for priapism (persistent erection of penis)—a sign of spinal cord injury.

b. Test for sensory impairment—prick the skin with a pin.

c. Test the biceps, triceps, quadriceps, and Achilles reflexes.

d. Evaluate vital signs.

e. Look for the presence of associated injuries.

4. Continue with repeated neurologic examinations to determine if there is deterioration in the spinal cord lesion.

5. Evaluate the patient's respiratory exchange. Prepare for tracheostomy if there is a high cervical lesion.

6. Introduce a nasogastric tube—to prevent and treat adynamic ileus, gastric and intestinal distention.

7. Catheterize the patient—patient with spinal cord injury cannot empty his bladder.

8. Start intravenous infusion.

9. Administer dexamethasone—has been found empirically to help diminish or prevent swelling.

10. See page 801 for definitive management of spinal cord injury.

Multiple Injuries

Underlying Considerations

1. The patient with multiple injuries requires a team approach with one person responsible for coordinating the treatment.

2. *Evidence* of gross trauma may be slight or may be completely absent. The injury regarded as the least significant may be the most lethal.

3. Any injury interfering with a vital physiologic function is an immediate threat to life and has highest priority for immediate treatment (obstructed airway, hemorrhage).

4. The patient should be completely undressed and a rapid physical examination should be carried out as quickly as possible after the airway has been established.

5. Mortality in patients with multiple injuries is related to the severity of the injuries and the number of systems and organs involved.

Emergency Management (Fig. 23-6)

Goals:

Determine the extent of injuries.
Establish priorities of treatment.

Carry out a *rapid* physical examination to determine if patient is breathing, bleeding, or in shock; determine the status of his responsiveness and if he has severe wounds or fracture deformities.

1. Establish an open airway and maintain ventilation.*

a. Note the character and symmetry of chest wall motion and pattern of breathing.

b. Ask the conscious patient if he is having difficulty in breathing. Ask if he has chest pain.

* Imperative lifesaving procedures are performed simultaneously by the emergency team.

c. Apply suction to clear the trachea and bronchial tree.

d. Insert oropharyngeal airway—to prevent occlusion by tongue.

e. Ventilate the patient (bag–mask system) to alleviate hypoxia—see page 204.

f. Prepare for endotracheal intubation (p. 213) if adequate airway cannot be maintained.

g. Suspect serious intrathoracic injuries if respiratory distress continues after adequate airway has been established. See pages 173–175 for management of chest injuries.

2. Assess cardiac function and treat cardiac arrest—hypoxia, metabolic acidosis, and chest trauma may precipitate cardiac arrest.*

a. For cardiac arrest, start closed chest compression and ventilation (p. 925).

b. If chest wall is unstable (flail chest), emergency thoracotomy and manual compression may be necessary.

c. Be prepared to give sodium bicarbonate (IV) to compensate for acidosis if indicated—severely traumatized patients with respiratory and circulatory embarrassment will have some degree of metabolic acidosis.

3. Control hemorrhage.*

a. Apply pressure over bleeding points if hemorrhage is overt.

b. Expect significant blood loss in patient with fracture of shaft of femur, with multiple fractures, or with major pelvic trauma.

c. Use tourniquet(s) for massive arterial bleeding from extremities which cannot be halted with pressure.

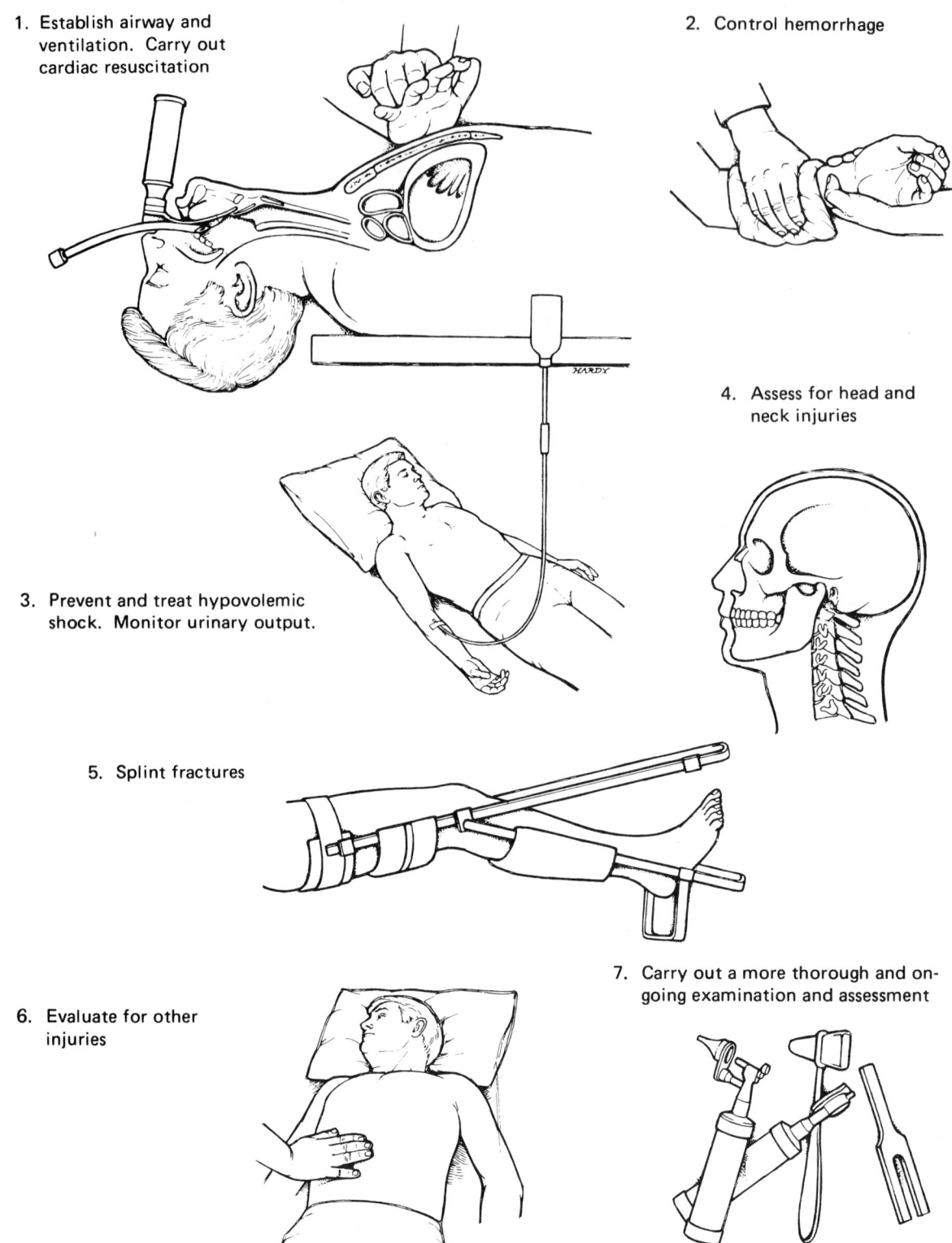

1. Establish airway and ventilation. Carry out cardiac resuscitation

2. Control hemorrhage

3. Prevent and treat hypovolemic shock. Monitor urinary output.

4. Assess for head and neck injuries

5. Splint fractures

6. Evaluate for other injuries

7. Carry out a more thorough and on-going examination and assessment

Figure 23-6. The patient with multiple injuries. Any injury that interferes with vital physiologic function and poses an immediate threat to life takes priority for immediate treatment. Imperative lifesaving procedures are performed simultaneously by the emergency team.

d. Prepare for immediate surgical intervention if patient is bleeding internally.

4. Prevent and treat hypovolemic shock.*
   a. Insert at least 2 (sometimes 4) IV lines, one above diaphragm and one below. Use venous cutdown if necessary.
   b. Draw blood for laboratory studies as directed (typing and cross-matching, baseline CBC, electrolytes, blood urea nitrogen, glucose, prothrombin time).
   c. Introduce central venous catheter ro monitor the patient's response to fluid infusion, to prevent fluid overload and as a route for fluid infusion.
   d. Start intravenous infusions.
      (1) Balanced saline solution (lactated Ringer's solution) is given for volume replacement until blood is available.
      (2) Give blood as directed—massive transfusions have a cooling effect which can cause cardiac irritability and arrest; blood should be warmed.
   e. Give intravenous infusions rapidly enough to keep central venous pressure readings at 5–15 cm. H_2O (see p. 286); monitor rate and direction of change (important parameters).
   f. Insert indwelling urethral catheter and monitor urinary output to aid in diagnosis of shock and monitors effectiveness of resuscitation. Do not force the catheter—the patient may have a ruptured urethra.
   g. Monitor ECG—to detect changes.
   h. Carry out ongoing clinical evaluation to observe for improvement or deterioration; changes in vital signs, improvement in level of responsiveness, skin warmth, speed of capillary filling, etc., shows reversal of shock state.
   i. Prepare for immediate surgical intervention if the patient does not respond to fluids or blood. Inability to restore blood pressure and circulatory volume in the patient usually indicates major internal bleeding.

5. Assess for head and neck injuries.
   a. Make definite statements concerning baseline neurologic status of the patient (level of responsiveness, size and reactivity of pupils, motor power, reflexes).
   b. Neck (and chest) films may be taken; apply cervical collar until x-rays preclude possibility of cervical spine injury.
   c. Intracranial pressure monitoring (see p. 765) may be instituted.
6. Administer dexamethasone as directed—corticosteroids appear to protect pulmonary function in patients with multiple injuries and help prevent posttraumatic pulmonary insufficiency. (However, this is considered a controversial issue.)
7. Splint fractures to prevent further trauma to soft tissues and blood vessels and to relieve pain; note presence or absence of pulses in fractured extremities.
8. Assess the patient for gastrointestinal injuries.
   a. Examine the patient repeatedly for abdominal pain, muscular rigidity, tenderness, rebound tenderness, diminished bowel sounds, hypotension, and shock.
   b. Prepare for peritoneal lavage to assess for intraperitoneal bleeding.
   c. Assist with insertion of nasogastric tube if upper gastrointestinal bleeding is suspected or if gaseous distention of stomach develops—will decrease incidence of vomiting and aspiration.
   d. Prepare for laparotomy if the patients shows continuing signs of hemorrhage and deterioration.
9. Continue to monitor urinary output hourly—reflects cardiac output and state of perfusion of visceral organs.
   a. Assess for hematuria and oliguria.
   b. Record measurements on a flow sheet.
10. Evaluate the patient for other injuries and institute appropriate treatment including tetanus immunization.
11. Carry out a more thorough physical examination after resuscitation and management of above priorities.

Fractures

A *fracture* is a break in the continuity of the bone.

Emergency Management

1. Give immediate attention to the patient's general condition. If there is any question of multiple injury, the patient needs to be completely undressed, draped, and examined periodically.
   a. Evaluate for respiratory difficulties—caused by edema due to facial and neck injuries, accumulation of secretions in respiratory tract, etc.
      (1) Examine chest for evidences of sucking chest wounds, pneumothorax, flail chest, etc.
      (2) Prepare for tracheal intubation or emergency tracheostomy.

   b. Control hemorrhage.
      (1) Control venous bleeding by direct pressure along with digital pressure over artery closest to bleeding area.
      (2) Suspect internal hemorrhage (pleural, pericardial, or abdominal) in the event of continuing shock and in the presence of injuries to chest and abdomen.
   c. Treat for shock—usually the result of blood loss in patients with fractures.
      (1) Assess for falling blood pressure, cold and clammy skin, and rapid, thready pulse.
      (2) Keep in mind that a large amount of blood loss may accompany fractures of the femur and pelvis.
      (3) Maintain the blood pressure with intravenous infusions.
      (4) Give blood transfusion(s) or blood component therapy as soon as blood is available.

---

* Imperative lifesaving procedures are performed simultaneously by the emergency team.

(5) Administer oxygen—cardiopulmonary embarrassment produces decreased oxygen supply to the tissues and circulatory collapse.

(6) Give analgesic to control pain. (Splinting the extremity and controlling pain are essential in treating shock accompanying fractures.)

(7) Look for evidence of head, chest, and other injuries—patients with multiple fractures may have other serious injuries.

2. Inspect the fractured part(s).
   a. Cut away clothing if necessary.
   b. Observe the entire body using a methodical head-to-toe physical examination—inspect for lacerations, swelling, and deformities.
   c. Look for *angulation* (bending), *shortening,* and *rotation.*
   d. Feel the pulse distal to the extremity fracture. Check all peripheral pulses.
   e. Assess for coolness, blanching, decreased sensation and motor function, diminished or absent pulses—indicate injury to the blood supply.
   f. Handle the part gently and as little as possible.

3. Apply the splint before the patient is moved since splinting relieves pain, improves circulation, prevents further tissue injury, and prevents a closed fracture from becoming an open one.
   a. Immobilize the joint above and below the fracture; place one hand distal to the fracture and apply some traction while placing the other hand beneath the fracture for support.
   b. Extend the splints well beyond the joints adjacent to the fracture.
      (1) Use the patient's clothing for padding (tie, shirt) if nothing else is available.
      (2) Use newspapers, magazines, pillows, tree limbs, and boards for splints if necessary. (Specialized splints and traction are used in the hospital.)
      (3) Splint joints in functional positions.
   c. Check the vascular status of the extremity after splinting; check color, temperature, pulse, blanching of nail bed.

4. Evaluate for neurologic deficits caused by the fracture.
5. Apply a sterile dressing if the fracture is an open one.
6. Investigate any complaint of pain or pressure.
7. Transport the patient gently and carefully.
8. See pages 821–828 for a complete discussion of the treatment of fractures at specific sites.

Temperature Emergencies

Heat Stroke

Heat stroke is a medical emergency caused by failure of the heat-regulating mechanisms of the body when the temperature–humidity index is high. The following are particularly vulnerable: persons who (1) are not acclimatized to heat exposure, (2) are at the extremes of age, (3) are unable to care for themselves, (4) have chronic and debilitating diseases, and (5) are taking certain medications (major tranquilizers, anticholinergics, diuretics, propranolol). Exertional heat stroke is a leading cause of death in athletes in this country.

Clinical Manifestations

1. History of exposure to elevated ambient temperature and/or excessive exercise
2. High fever (40.6°C. [105°F.]) and above
3. Central nervous system dysfunction (manifested by confusion, delirium, bizarre behavior, coma)
4. Hot dry skin; usually absence of sweating

Emergency Management

Goal:
Reduce high temperature as rapidly as possible.

1. Reduce the core (internal) temperature to 39°C. (102°F. rectally) as *rapidly* as possible. Monitor the rectal temperature by a rectal thermistor probe (if available) left in place. One or more of the following temperature-lowering methods may be used.
   a. Immerse the patient in ice-water bath or cover naked patient with towel or sheet wetted with ice water and ice chips; provide air circulation with fans.
      (1) Massage immersed patient—promotes circulation and maintains cutaneous vasodilation and stimulates exchange of heat from skin.
   b. Place the patient on a hypothermia blanket if available.
   c. Sponge the patient continuously with cold water; place electric fan so that it blows on patient, since air movement increases evaporation.

2. Monitor the patient carefully; vital signs (electronic rectal thermometer) ECG, CVP, and level of responsiveness change with rapid alterations in body temperature.

3. Start intravenous infusions as directed to replace fluid losses and maintain adequate circulation and urine output; give slowly because of danger of myocardial injury due to high body temperature or poor renal function.

4. Administer oxygen to supply tissue needs exaggerated by hypermetabolic condition. Intubate patient with cuffed endotracheal tube and attach to ventilator if necessary to support failing cardiorespiratory systems.

5. Give supportive care as directed. Monitor for hypotension, convulsions, acidosis, hypocalcemia, and hypokalemia.

6. Measure urinary output—acute tubular necrosis is a complication of heat stroke.

7. Continue to monitor ECG because atrial and ventricular arrhythmias are common.

8. Carry out serial testing for bleeding diatheses (disseminated intravascular coagulation) and serum enzymes to estimate thermal hypoxic injury to the liver and muscle.

9. Admit to intensive care unit—permanent liver, heart, and central nervous system damage may occur.

Health Education

1. Advise the patient to avoid immediate reexposure to high temperatures; the patient may remain hypersensitive to high temperatures for a considerable length of time.
2. Emphasize the importance of maintaining an adequate fluid intake, wearing loose clothing, and reducing activity in hot weather.
3. Athletes should monitor fluid losses, replace fluids and use a gradual approach to physical conditioning, allowing sufficient time for acclimatization.

Cold Injuries to Extremities (Frostbite)

Frostbite is trauma due to exposure to freezing temperatures that cause actual freezing of the tissue fluids in the cell and intracellular spaces, resulting in vascular damage.

Underlying Considerations

1. The extent of injury from exposure to cold is not always known when the patient is seen initially.
2. A frozen extremity may be hard, cold, and insensitive to touch and appear white or mottled blue–white.

Emergency Management

Goal:
Restore normal body temperature.

1. Do not allow the patient to walk if lower extremities are involved.
2. Remove all constrictive clothing.
3. Rewarm extremity by controlled and rapid rewarming, 38°–42°C. (100°–108°F.), usually in a whirlpool, until the tips of the injured part flush (about 20 minutes)—flush indicates that maximum circulatory flow and vasodilatation have been accomplished; early thawing appears to decrease the amount of tissue loss.
   a. Administer analgesic for pain—thawing process may be very painful.
   b. Handle part gently to avoid further mechanical injury.
   c. Protect thawed part; do not rupture blebs that develop from 1 hour to a few days after rewarming.
   d. Place sterile gauze/cotton between affected fingers/toes to prevent maceration.
   e. Elevate the part periodically to promote circulation.
   f. Use a protective cradle to prevent contact with bedding if the feet are involved.
4. Carry out physical examination—to look for concomitant injury (soft tissue injury, fracture, dehydration, alcoholic coma, fat embolism).
5. Restore electrolyte balance; dehydration and hypovolemia occur frequently in frostbite victims.
6. Use sterile sheets, gowns, gloves, and masks when caring for an open wound—frostbite injuries make the patient susceptible to infection.
7. Give tetanus prophylaxis if indicated by associated trauma.
8. The following may be carried out when appropriate:
   a. Whirlpool bath (with disinfectant) for the affected extremity—to aid circulation, debride dead tissue, and help prevent infection.
   b. Escharotomy—to prevent further tissue damage, allow for normal circulation, and permit joint motion.
   c. Fasciotomy—to treat compression syndrome.
   d. Sympathectomy—if the cold injury is severe enough to produce necrosis.
9. Encourage hourly active motion of the affected digits to promote maximum restoration of function and to prevent contractures.
10. Prohibit the use of tobacco because of its vasoconstrictive effect.

Accidental Hypothermia

Accidental hypothermia is a condition in which the core (internal) temperature of the body is less than 35°C. (95°F.) as a result of exposure to cold.

Underlying Considerations and Clinical Manifestations

1. There is progressive deterioration marked by apathy, poor judgment, ataxia, dysarthria, drowsiness, and eventually coma. Shivering may be suppressed below a temperature of 32.2°C. (90°F.).
2. Below this temperature, the body's self-warming mechanisms become ineffective. The heartbeat and the blood pressure may be so weak that the peripheral pulsations become undetectable. Cardiac irregularities also may occur. Other physiological abnormalities include hypoxemia and acidosis.
3. Those at risk include the *elderly,* the very young, and persons with concurrent illnesses.

Emergency Management

Management consists of continuous monitoring, rewarming, and supportive care.
1. Monitor the patient—vital signs, CVP, urinary output, arterial blood gases, blood chemistry determinations (BUN, creatinine, glucose, electrolytes), chest x-ray.
   a. Monitor body temperature with rectal thermometer or probe.
   b. Employ continuous ECG monitoring. Cold-induced myocardial irritability leads to conduction disturbances, especially ventricular fibrillation.
   c. Maintain arterial line for recording blood pressure and to facilitate blood sampling.
2. Rewarm the patient: rewarming methods include active core (internal) rewarming, active external rewarming, and passive or spontaneous rewarming. There are different opinions about which method is best.
3. Supportive care during rewarming includes:
   a. External cardiac massage if indicated; electrical cardioversion of ventricular fibrillation.
   b. Mechanical ventilation and heated humidified oxygen—to maintain tissue oxygenation.
   c. IV fluids (warmed)—to correct hypotension and maintain urinary output.
   d. Sodium bicarbonate—to correct metabolic acidosis.
   e. Antiarrhythmic drugs as necessary.
   f. Indwelling urethral catheter—to monitor fluid status.
   g. Careful handling to prevent cardiac arrhythmias.

Poisoning

Poison is any substance that when ingested, inhaled, absorbed, applied to the skin, injected into or developed within the body, in relatively small amounts, produces injury to the body by its chemical action. (See p. 1487 for prevention of poisoning.)

Swallowed Poisons

Goals of Emergency Management

1. Remove or inactivate the poison before it is absorbed.
2. Give supportive care to maintain vital organ systems.
3. Use the specific antidote to neutralize the poison.
4. Give treatment to hasten the elimination of the absorbed poison.

General Aspects of Management

1. Maintain the airway and adequacy of respirations.
   a. Administer artificial respiration if respiration is depressed; positive expiratory pressure applied to airway may help keep alveoli inflated (bag–mask).
   b. Administer oxygen for respiratory depression, unconsciousness, cyanosis, shock.
   c. Take arterial blood samples to measure pH and blood gas tensions.
   d. Prevent aspiration of gastric contents by positioning, use of oropharyngeal airway, and suctioning.
   e. Stabilize cardiovascular function.
   f. Insert indwelling catheter to monitor kidney function.
   g. Assess for central nervous system depression.
3. Give supportive care—there is multisystem involvement from many agents.
   a. Treat shock appropriately.
   b. Monitor ECG—some agents cause cardiovascular toxicity.
4. Consider gastric lavage or induce emesis as the clinical situation dictates to prevent absorption of orally ingested substances; save gastric aspirate for toxicology screens.
5. Support the patient having convulsions; many poisons excite the central nervous system; the patient may convulse because of oxygen deprivation.
6. Give specific therapy. Administer special chemical antidote (if indicated) or specific pharmacologic antagonists as early as possible (if indicated).
7. Monitor central venous pressure as indicated.
8. Monitor fluid and electrolyte balance.
9. Reduce elevated temperature.
10. Give analgesics for pain with caution; severe pain causes vasomotor collapse and reflex inhibition of normal physiologic function.
11. Provide constant nursing surveillance and attention to the patient in a coma (p. 760); coma from poisoning results from interference with brain cell function or metabolism.
12. Assist in carrying out procedures to enhance removal of the ingested substance (forced diuresis, alteration of urine pH, dialysis).
13. Assist in securing specimens of blood, urine, stomach contents, or vomitus for laboratory analysis and drug screen.
14. Refer for psychiatric consultation if suicide attempt or drug abuse is involved.

Corrosive Poisons

A. Types of Corrosive Poisons

1. Acid and acid-like substances; sodium acid sulfate (toilet bowl cleaners), acetic acid, sulfuric acid, nitric acid, oxalic acid, hydrofluoric acid (rust removers), iodine, silver nitrate.
2. Alkali corrosives—most common are sodium hydroxide (lye; drain cleaners), dishwasher detergents, sodium carbonate (washing soda), ammonia water, sodium hypochlorite (household bleach).

B. Clinical Manifestations

1. Severe pain; burning sensation in mouth and throat
2. Painful swallowing or inability to swallow
3. Vomiting; drooling
4. Destruction of oral mucosa, esophageal burns

C. Emergency Management

1. If the patient can swallow after ingestion of a *corrosive poison,* he may be offered milk as an emollient agent (controversial). Do not induce vomiting if the patient has consumed a strong acid, alkali, or other corrosive substance.
2. Esophagoscopy may be performed (early) to assess for presence of esophageal stricture.

Noncorrosive Poisons

Emergency Management

1. *Remove poison from the patient's stomach immediately by inducing vomiting.*

▶ **NURSING ALERT:** Do not induce vomiting if the victim has consumed a strong acid, alkali, or other corrosive or hydrocarbon solvent. Do not induce vomiting if the patient is in a coma, is unconscious, or is having convulsions.

   a. Give 3–4 glassfuls of milk or water to drink—to dilute poison.
   b. Induce vomiting by giving syrup of ipecac or by inserting the index finger or blunt end of a spoon at the back of the patient's throat.
2. Carry out gastric lavage procedure (see below) to remove any unabsorbed poison. This procedure is *not* done if corrosives or hydrocarbon solvents have been ingested (e.g., turpentine, gasoline, kerosene, liquid wax, charcoal fluid lighter, etc.).
   A patient who has ingested hydrocarbons should have a chest film done to evaluate for chemical pneumonia.
3. Instruct family to bring unused poison to hospital for identification.
4. Know the poison control center in the area; call the center if an unknown toxic agent has been taken or if it is necessary to identify an antidote for a known toxic agent.

Guidelines: Assisting with Gastric Lavage

Gastric lavage is the aspiration of the stomach contents and washing out of the stomach by means of a gastric tube.

Purposes
1. To remove unabsorbed poison after poison ingestion.
2. To diagnose gastric hemorrhage and for the arrest of hemorrhage.
3. To cleanse the stomach before endoscopic procedures.
4. To remove liquid or small particles of material from the stomach.

▶ **NURSING ALERT:** Gastric lavage may be dangerous (1) after the ingestion of acids, alkalis, hydrocarbons, or petroleum distillates and (2) in the presence of convulsions. It is dangerous after the ingestion of strong corrosive agents.

Equipment

Large-bore orogastric tubes or large-bore Ewald tube
Large irrigating syringe with adapter
Large plastic funnel with adapter to fit stomach tube
Water-soluble lubricant
Tap water or appropriate antidote (milk, saline solution, sodium bicarbonate solution, fruit juice, activated charcoal*)
Bucket for aspirate
Mouth gag; nasotracheal or endotracheal tubes with inflatable cuffs
Containers for specimens

Procedure

Nursing Action	Rationale/Amplification
1. Remove dental appliances and inspect oral cavity for loose teeth.	
2. Measure the distance between the bridge of the nose and the xiphoid process. Mark with indelible pencil or tape.	
3. Lubricate the tube with water soluble lubricant.	
4. If the patient is comatose, he is intubated with a cuffed nasotracheal or endotracheal tube.	4. A cuffed endotracheal tube prevents aspiration of gastric contents.
5. Place the unconscious patient in a left lateral position with the head, neck, and trunk forming a straight line.	5. This position prevents fluid from running into the trachea and keeps reflux vomitus from being aspirated.
6. Pass the tube via the oral (or nasal) route while keeping the head in a neutral position. Pass the tube to the adhesive marking or about 50 cm. (20 inches). After the lavage tube is passed, the head of the table is lowered. Have standby suction available.	6. The depth of insertion of the tube will vary with the height of the patient. If the tube enters the larynx instead of the esophagus, the patient will experience coughing and dyspnea.
7. Submerge free end of tube below water level at the moment of the patient's exhalation.	7. If tube is inadvertently in the lungs, the water will bubble with each exhalation.
8. Aspirate the stomach contents with syringe attached to the tube before instilling water or antidote. Save the specimen for analysis.	8. Aspiration is carried out to remove the stomach contents.
9. Remove syringe. Attach funnel to the stomach tube or use 50-ml. syringe to put lavage solution in gastric tube. Volume of fluid placed in the stomach should be small.	9. Overfilling of the stomach may cause regurgitation and aspiration, or force the stomach contents through the pylorus.
10. Elevate funnel above the patient's head and pour approximately 150–200 ml. of solution into funnel.	
11. Lower the funnel and siphon the gastric contents into the bucket.	
12. Save samples of first 2 washings.	12. Keep first washings isolated from other washings for toxicologic analysis (pill particles; occult blood). Keep track of fluid input/output to be sure that most of fluid is being removed.

* Activated charcoal adsorbs (binds) many drugs in the gastrointestinal tract and prevents their absorption in the bloodstream.

(continued)

Guidelines: Assisting with Gastric Lavage (continued)

Procedure
(Cont.)

Nursing Action	Rationale/Amplification
13. Repeat lavage procedure until the returns are relatively clear and no particulate matter is seen.	
14. At the completion of lavage:	
a. Stomach may be left empty.	a. This is done to diminish subsequent absorption of certain poisons.
b. An absorbent (powder form of activated charcoal mixed with water to form a slurry, the consistency of thick soup) may be instilled in the tube and allowed to remain in the stomach.	
c. A saline cathartic may be instilled in the tube.	c. A cathartic facilitates the transit of the charcoal and remains of the ingested substance through the intestinal tract.
15. Pinch off tube during removal or maintain suction while tube is being withdrawn.	15. Pinching off the tube prevents aspiration and the initiation of the gag reflex. Keeping the patient's head lower than the body also gives this protection.
16. Give the patient a cathartic if prescribed.	16. A cathartic may be given if the poison has no corrosive action on the bowel. The cathartic will help remove unabsorbed material from the intestine.

Inhaled Poisons

Carbon Monoxide Poisoning

May occur as an industrial or household accident or as an attempted suicide.

A. Underlying Principles

1. Carbon monoxide exerts its toxic effect by binding to circulating hemoglobin to reduce the oxygen-carrying capacity of the blood.
2. The affinity between carbon monoxide and hemoglobin is 200–300 times that between oxygen and hemoglobin. (Carbon monoxide combines with hemoglobin to form carboxyhemoglobin.) As a result, tissue anoxia occurs.
3. Clinical manifestations:
   a. The patient may appear intoxicated (result of cerebral hypoxia).
   b. Headache, muscular weakness, palpitation, dizziness, mental confusion—may progress rapidly to coma.
   c. Skin may be pink, cherry red, or cyanotic and pale—*skin color is not a reliable sign.*
4. History of exposure to carbon monoxide should justify immediate treatment.

B. Emergency Management

Goals:
Reverse cerebral and myocardial hypoxia.
Hasten carbon monoxide elimination.

1. Give 100% oxygen at atmospheric or hyperbaric pressures to reverse hypoxia and accelerate elimination of carbon monoxide.
2. Draw blood for carboxyhemoglobin levels.
3. Employ continuous ECG monitoring; treat arrhythmias and correct acid–base and electrolyte abnormalities.
4. Observe the patient constantly—psychoses, spastic paralysis, visual disturbances, and deterioration of personality may persist following resuscitation and may be symptoms of permanent central nervous system damage.

Injected Poisons

Stinging Insects

(Bee, yellow jacket, hornet, wasp)

▶ **NURSING ALERT:** A patient may have an extreme sensitivity to *Hymenoptera* stings (yellow jackets, bees, hornets, wasps, and some ants). This constitutes an acute emergency. Stings of the head and neck are especially serious, although stings in any area of the body can result in anaphylaxis.

A. Clinical Manifestations

Anaphylactic reaction (p. 660)
1. Severe fall in blood pressure
2. Difficult breathing
3. Edema of face, lips
4. Urticaria
5. Itching
6. Bronchial constriction
7. Diarrhea, abdominal cramps

B. Emergency Management and Health Education

1. Give epinephrine as requested. Massage the site to hasten absorption.
2. See page 660 for treatment of anaphylactic reaction.
3. Patients known to be sensitive to *Hymenoptera* venom should carry an emergency self-treatment kit containing a syringe prefilled with epinephrine.
   a. Instruct the patient to take epinephrine immediately if he is stung.
   b. Remove stinger with one quick scrape of fingernail.
   c. Do not squeeze venom sac—may cause additional venom to be injected.
   d. Report to nearest health care facility for observation.
4. Instruct the patient to limit exposure to stinging insects by:

a. Avoiding locales with stinging insects (camp and picnic sites).
b. Staying away from insect feeding areas—flower beds, ripe fruit orchards, garbage, fields of clover.
c. Not going barefoot outdoors—yellow jackets may nest on ground.
d. Avoiding perfumes, scented soaps, bright colors—attract bees.
e. Keeping car windows closed.
f. Spraying garbage cans with rapid-acting insecticide, and keeping areas meticulously clean.
g. Securing a professional exterminator to dispose of wasp/hornet nests or bee hives in home area.
h. Using electric hedge clippers and power mowers with extreme caution (or not at all)—mowing over a yellow jacket's nest will infuriate these insects and cause them to swarm.

5. Hypersensitive persons should not be alone when involved in outdoor activities since they may need immediate help in initiating emergency treatment measures.
6. A person with this allergy should consider undergoing immunotherapy with a venom preparation—given in gradually stronger doses to stimulate the patient's immune system to become increasingly more resistant to insect sting.
7. All allergic individuals should wear medical warning bracelets indicating hypersensitivity.

Chemical Injuries to Skin

Emergency Management

1. Drench skin with water (shower, hose, faucet)—burning continues as long as agent is on the skin.
2. Apply stream of water on skin while removing clothing.
3. Continue to cleanse skin thoroughly with water for at least 15 minutes; rapidity in washing is most important in reducing extent of injury.
   a. Personnel should wear gloves, gowns, and masks if the offending agent is considered to be toxic.
   b. Apply topical antimicrobial ointment, and give tetanus immunization.
   c. Arrange for follow-up because there is a risk of underestimating extent of burn.

Food Poisoning*

Food poisoning is a sudden, explosive illness which may occur after the ingestion of food or drink.

* Botulism is discussed on pages 882–883 since the treatment differs.

Emergency Management

1. Determine the source and type of food poisoning.
   a. Have family bring suspected food to medical facility.
   b. Take the history:
      (1) How soon after eating did the symptoms occur? Immediate onset suggests chemical, plant, or animal poisoning.
      (2) What was eaten in the previous meal? Did the food have any unusual odor or taste? Most foods causing bacterial poisoning do not have unusual odor or taste.
      (3) Did anyone else eating the same food become ill?
      (4) Did vomiting occur? What was the appearance of the vomitus?
      (5) Did diarrhea occur? Diarrhea is usually absent with botulism or with shell-fish or other fish poisoning.
      (6) Are any neurologic symptoms present? These occur in botulism, chemical, plant, and animal poisoning.
      (7) Does the patient have a fever? Fever is seen in salmonella, favism (ingestion of fava beans), and some fish poisoning.
      (8) What is the patient's appearance?
2. Collect food, gastric contents, vomitus, serum, and feces for examination.
3. Monitor vital signs on a continual basis.
   a. Assess respiration, blood pressure, sensorium, central venous pressure (if indicated), and muscular activity.
   b. Weigh the patient for future comparisons.
4. Support the respiratory system. Death from respiratory paralysis can occur with botulism, fish poisoning, etc.
5. Maintain fluid and electrolyte balance; severe vomiting produces alkalosis; large amounts of electrolytes and water are lost by vomiting and diarrhea.
   a. Watch for oligemic shock from severe fluid and electrolyte losses.
   b. Evaluate for apathy, rapid pulse, fever, oliguria, anuria, hypotension, and delirium.
   c. Carry out blood electrolyte studies.
6. Correct and control hypoglycemia.
7. Control the nausea.
   a. Give antiemetic drug parenterally if the patient cannot tolerate fluids or medications by mouth.
   b. Give sips of weak tea, carbonated drinks, and tap water for mild nausea.
   c. Give clear liquids 12–24 hours after nausea and vomiting subside.
   d. Graduate to a low-residue, bland diet.

Substance Abuse

Substance abuse includes the use of specific substances that are intended to alter mood or behavior.

Drug Abuse

Drug abuse is the use of drugs for other than legitimate medical purposes. There is a growing tendency among drug users to take a variety of drugs simultaneously, including alcohol, barbiturates, tranquilizers, and sedatives, which may have additive effects. The clinical manifestations may vary with the drug used, but the underlying principles of management are essentially the same.

Emergency Management

Goals:
Support the respiratory and cardiovascular functions.
Give definitive treatment for drug overdose.

Prevent further absorption, enhance drug elimination, and reduce its toxicity.

1. Assess the presence and adequacy of respirations. Attain control of the airway, ventilation, and oxygenation.
    a. Use a cuffed endotracheal tube and provide assisted ventilation in a severely depressed patient lacking gag or cough reflexes.
    b. Measure arterial blood gases—for hypoxia due to hypoventilation, acid–base derangements, etc.
    c. Administer oxygen.
2. Stabilize the cardiovascular system (this is done simultaneously with airway management).
    a. Begin external cardiac compression and ventilation in the absence of heartbeat.
    b. Start ECG monitoring.
    c. Draw blood samples for testing glucose, electrolytes, BUN, creatinine, and appropriate toxicologic screen.
    d. Start intravenous fluids.
3. Give specific drug antagonist if drug is known; naloxone hydrochloride (Narcan) is frequently used. Fifty-percent glucose in water is also used.
4. Remove the drug from the stomach as soon as possible (if drug has been ingested).
    a. Induce vomiting if the patient is seen *early* after ingestion; save vomitus for toxicologic study.
    b. Use gastric lavage if the patient is unconscious or if there is no way to determine when the drug was ingested; save gastric aspirate.
       (1) In patients lacking gag or cough reflexes, carry out this procedure only after intubation with cuffed endotracheal tube to prevent aspiration of stomach contents.
       (2) Activated charcoal may be a useful adjunct to therapy and is used after emesis or lavage.
5. Give supportive care.
    a. Take rectal temperature—extremes of thermoregulation (hyperthermia/hypothermia) must be recognized and treated.
    b. Treat convulsions.
    c. Assist with hemodialysis/peritoneal dialysis for potentially lethal poisoning.
    d. Try to maintain a free urine flow since the drug or metabolites are excreted by the urine.
6. Do a thorough physical examination to rule out insulin shock, meningitis, subdural hematoma, stroke, trauma.
    a. Look for needle marks and external evidence of trauma.
    b. Carry out a rapid neurologic survey (level of responsiveness [depressed or stimulated], pupil size and reactivity, reflexes, focal neurologic findings).
    c. Keep in mind that many drug abusers take multiple drugs simultaneously.
    d. Be aware that there is a high incidence of infectious hepatitis among drug users, which is thought to be the result of communal use of unsterile needles and syringes.
    e. Examine the patient's breath for characteristic odor of alcohol, acetone, etc.
7. Try to obtain a history of the drug experiences (from the person accompanying the patient or from the patient himself).
    a. Adapt a supportive, empathetic, and realistic relationship with the patient.
    b. Do not leave the patient alone; there is a potential for the patient to harm himself or emergency department staff.
8. Admit the patient to the ICU if he remains unconscious; if the patient has deliberately taken a drug overdose, psychiatric consultation is necessary.
9. Make every effort to enroll the patient in a drug treatment program (detoxification and rehabilitation) to intervene in a life-style that fosters addiction.
10. Arrange consultation with a psychiatrist/social worker to explore the intent of poisoning (suicide?).

Narcotic Abuse

Examples

Heroin (most frequently involved)
Opium or paregoric
Morphine, codeine, synthetic narcotics (methadone)

Clinical Manifestations

Acute intoxication:
1. Pinpoint pupils (may be dilated with severe hypoxia)
2. Marked respiratory depression
3. Stupor → coma
4. Fresh needle marks along course of any superficial vein

Emergency Management

1. Support respiratory and cardiovascular functions.
2. Give narcotic antagonist (naloxone hydrochloride [Narcan]; nalorphine hydrochloride [Nalline]) to reverse severe respiratory depression and coma.
3. Continue to monitor the level of responsiveness and respirations, pulse, and blood pressure—duration of action of naloxone hydrochloride is shorter than that of heroin, etc., and repeated dose(s) may be necessary.
   Do not leave the patient alone—may lapse back into coma rapidly; clinical status may change from minute to minute.
4. Establish an intravenous line—the patient may be given a bolus of glucose to eliminate possibility of hypoglycemia.
5. Send urine to laboratory for analysis—opiates can be detected in urine.
6. Secure blood for chemical and toxicologic analysis; also for baseline studies.
7. Secure an ECG.
8. Hemodialysis may be indicated for severe drug intoxication.
9. Monitor for pulmonary edema which is frequently seen in patients who abuse/overdose narcotics.

Heroin Withdrawal Syndrome

A. Clinical Manifestations

1. Lethargy; yawning
2. Perspiration, lacrimation, runny nose
3. Dilated pupils, poorly reactive to light
4. Gooseflesh, muscular aches
5. Twitching, anorexia, nausea, vomiting, abdominal pain
6. Chills and fever

B. Management

1. Methadone may be prescribed if the patient is receiving treatment at a methadone center, or substitution therapy should be given in a hospital setting.
2. Give intravenous fluids since the patient is dehydrated from vomiting; may progress to toxic delirium.

3. Assess for concomitant medical problems (hepatitis, pneumonia, severe diarrhea).
4. Place the patient in protected environment under proper medical supervision.
5. Make every effort to enroll the patient in a narcotics treatment program—to intervene in a life-style that fosters addiction.

Hallucinogens or Psychedelic-Type Drugs

Common Forms
1. Lysergic acid diethylamide (LSD)
2. Phencyclidine HCl (PCP)
3. Mescaline, psilocybin
4. Jimson weed seeds

Clinical Manifestations
1. Marked anxiety bordering on panic
2. Confusion, incoherence, hyperactivity
3. Hallucinations
4. Hazardous behavior (delirium, mania, self-injury)
5. Flashback (return of the drug experience after acute effects have worn off—can occur months or even years after initial drug use)
6. Convulsions, coma, circulatory collapse, death

Emergency Management
1. Determine if the patient has ingested a hallucinogenic drug or has a toxic psychosis.
2. Try to communicate with the patient—use "vocal anesthesia" to reassure him (except for PCP abusers).
   a. "Talking down" involves understanding the process through which the patient is proceeding and helping him overcome his fears while establishing contact with reality.
   b. Remind the patient that fear is common with this problem.
   c. Reassure the patient that he is not losing his mind; that he is experiencing effect of drugs and that this will wear off.
   d. Instruct the patient to keep his eyes open— reduces intensity of reaction.
   e. *Reduce sensory stimuli*—minimize noise, lights, movement, tactile stimulation.
   f. Do not leave the patient alone.
3. Sedate the patient if his hyperactivity cannot be controlled—diazepam (Valium) or a barbiturate may be given.
4. Search for evidences of trauma—hallucinogenic users have a tendency to "act out" their hallucinations.
5. Manage convulsions; place the patient in the intensive care unit.
6. Watch the patient closely—his behavior may become hazardous.
7. Monitor for hypertensive crisis if the patient has prolonged psychosis due to drug ingestion.
8. Place the patient in a protected environment under proper medical supervision to prevent self-inflicted bodily harm.

Management for Phencyclidine Abusers
1. Protect from self-injury—patients frequently have recurring delusions of superhuman strength.
2. Place the patient in a calm, supportive environment to minimize stimuli.
3. Approach with great caution.

4. Avoid "talking down"—may increase agitation and belligerence.
5. Treat symptoms as they occur.
   a. Drug effects are unpredictable and prolonged.
   b. Symptoms are likely to exacerbate; the patient becomes out of control.
6. Refer the patient to drug treatment center.

Amphetamine-Type Drugs
(Pep pills, "uppers," "speed")

Examples
Amphetamine (Benzedrine)
Dextroamphetamine (Dexedrine)
Methamphetamine (Desoxyn)

Clinical Manifestations
Abrupt or insidious development of behavioral disturbances
1. Aggressive type of behavior
2. Irritability, insomnia
3. Visual misperceptions; auditory hallucinations
4. Fearful anxiety/depression; cold, distant hostility
5. Hyperactivity, stereotyped activities; rapid speech, euphoria
6. Paranoid suspiciousness
7. Increasing pulse rate and blood pressure
8. Hallucinosis; high temperature
9. Convulsions → coma → death

Emergency Management
1. Try to communicate with the patient—amphetamine paranoid psychosis is frequently seen.
   a. The patient may have delusions of persecution, ideas of reference, visual and auditory hallucinations, changes in body image, hyperactivity, excitation.
   b. Maintain verbal contact.
2. Use specific drug therapy to alleviate agitative state.
   a. Usually within 24 hours after last dose of amphetamine, the patient will begin to spend increasing amounts of time sleeping.
   b. Keep the patient relatively quiet and reassured; the patient may become aggressive/assaultive and reach a state of panic.
3. Carry out urine checks for amphetamines.
4. Place the patient in protective environment—observe for suicide attempts.
   a. Use techniques of dealing with acutely paranoid individuals; do not move close to the patient or behind him.
   b. Avoid physical and pharmacologic restraints.
   c. Avoid confined spaces; refer to a psychiatric nursing textbook.

Barbiturates—Acute Intoxication

Examples
Pentobarbital (Nembutal)
Secobarbital (Seconal)
Amobarbital (Amytal)

Clinical Manifestations
Acute intoxication
1. Flushed face
2. Decreased pulse rate
3. Increasing nystagmus

4. Depressed tendon reflexes
5. Decreasing mental alertness
6. Difficulty in speaking
7. Poor motor coordination
8. Dilated, nonreacting pupils
9. Coma; death

Emergency Management

1. Maintain airway and give respiratory support.
2. Consider endotracheal intubation or tracheostomy if there is any doubt about the adequacy of airway exchange.
   a. Check airway frequently.
   b. Perform *regular* suctioning.
3. Support cardiovascular and respiratory functions—most deaths result from depression of these systems.
4. Evacuate stomach with emesis or lavage as soon as possible.
5. Start intravenous infusion through large-gauge needle or intravenous catheter to support blood pressure—coma and dehydration result in hypotension and respond to infusion of intravenous fluids with elevation of blood pressure.
6. Sodium bicarbonate may be given to alkalinize urine—increases excretion of phenobarbital.
7. Assist with hemodialysis—for high blood levels.
8. Maintain neurologic and vital sign flow sheet.
9. The patient awakening from overdose may demonstrate hostility; this can stimulate automatic angry responses by health care personnel.
10. Refer for psychiatric consultation to evaluate suicide potential, drug abuse, etc.

Barbiturate Withdrawal Syndrome

A. Clinical Manifestations

1. Shakiness, anxiety, muscular irritability
2. Orthostatic hypotension, tachycardia
3. Seizures; withdrawal psychosis
4. Hyperpyrexia; death

▶ **NURSING ALERT:** Symptoms of barbiturate withdrawal are serious because abrupt withdrawal from the drug may be life-threatening and may begin when the patient is recovering from an overdose.

B. Emergency Management

1. Maintain airway and stimulate depressed respiration.
2. Administer phenobarbital according to level of patient's tolerance; gradually reduce dosage of barbiturates until drug-free state is achieved.
3. Give oxygen, antibiotics, and intravenous fluids as required.
4. Watch for excessive agitation, confusion, and convulsions.
5. Consider treatment in residential treatment center.

Nonbarbiturate Tranquilizers

Examples

Glutethimide (Doriden)
Methyprylon (Noludar)
Ethchlorvynol (Placidyl)
Ethinamate (Valmid)

Meprobamate (Miltown, Equanil)
Chlordiazepoxide (Librium)
Diazepam (Valium)

Clinical Manifestations

1. Decreasing mental alertness
2. Confusion
3. Slurred speech
4. Ataxia
5. Pulmonary edema
6. Coma, possible death

Emergency Management

1. Insert endotracheal tube as a precaution; utilize assisted ventilation.
   Watch for sudden apnea and laryngeal spasm (especially in patients habituated to Doriden).
2. Start ECG monitoring.
   Watch for cardiovascular instability with arrhythmia.
3. Assess for hypotension—may appear rapidly and become persistent.
   a. Insert indwelling catheter for comatose patient—decreased urinary volume is an index of reduced renal flow associated with reduced intravascular volume or vascular collapse.
   b. Start volume expansion with saline, or dextrose as required.
4. Assist with gastric lavage.
5. Use hemodialysis therapy if needed.

Aspirin and Other Salicylate Poisoning

Clinical Manifestations

1. Tinnitus and some degree of deafness
2. Profuse perspiration; flushing
3. Bounding pulses
4. Hyperventilation with rate and depth of respiration increased
5. Agitation; restlessness
6. Acid–base abnormalities

Emergency Management

1. Treat respiratory depression.
2. Carry out gastric lavage—will remove significant amounts of salicylates up to 12 hours following ingestion, or give ipecac as directed.
3. Give water, milk, or activated charcoal—to diminish absorption of ingested poison after emesis or lavage.
4. Support the patient with intravenous infusions to correct electrolyte imbalance and maintain hydration.
5. Correct acid–base disturbances; monitor electrolytes.
6. Administer blood transfusion if indicated.
7. Enhance the elimination of salicylates from the body.
   a. Forced alkaline diuresis—diuresis induced by IV administration of isotonic dextrose and saline solution alone or combined with an osmotic diuretic.
      (1) Urine is alkalized (sodium bicarbonate).
   b. Hemodialysis is used to eliminate salicylate from circulation of the patient with severe intoxication.
8. Give vitamin K for bleeding—salicylates lower plasma prothrombin by interfering with vitamin K utilization in the liver.

Alcohol Abuse

Acute Alcoholism

Clinical Manifestations

(Caused by depressant action of alcohol on nervous system)
1. Drowsiness, incoordination, slurring of speech—or
2. Belligerency, grandiosity, uninhibited behavior
3. Odor of alcohol on breath or clothing
4. Stupor—hypoventilation, hypotension

Emergency Management

The treatment involves (1) detoxification of acute poisoning; (2) recovery, or "drying out"; and (3) rehabilitation.
1. Approach the patient in a nonjudgmental manner. (Alcoholic patients have a tendency to stimulate rejecting behavior in health care personnel.)
   a. Expect the patient to use mechanisms of denial and defensiveness.
   b. Adapt a firm, consistent, accepting, and reasonable attitude.
   c. Speak calmly.
   d. If the patient appears drunk, he is probably drunk even though he denies any alcohol intake.
2. Take a blood alcohol test as directed.
3. Allow the drowsy patient to "sleep off" the state of alcoholic intoxication; it takes time for the liver to metabolize the excess alcohol.
   a. Observe for symptoms of CNS depression; keep the patient under observation.
   b. Protect the airway.
   c. Undress the patient and cover him with a blanket.
4. Sedate the belligerent, noisy patient as directed.
   a. Monitor the patient carefully.
   b. Check vital signs and monitor heart rate and blood pressure.
5. Examine the patient for injuries and organic disease which can easily be masked by alcoholic intoxication; chronic alcohol abusers suffer more injuries and illnesses than the general population.
   a. Look for symptoms of head injury. Assess the neurologic status of the patient.
   b. Assess for alcoholic coma—a medical emergency.
   c. Evaluate for pulmonary infection.
      (1) Pulmonary infections are more common in alcoholic individuals because of an impaired defense system and a tendency toward gastric aspiration.
      (2) The patient may show little increase in temperature or white blood cell count.
   d. Watch for hypoglycemia.
6. Hospitalize if necessary, or admit to detoxification center; an effort should be made to examine the problems underlying substance abuse.

Delirium Tremens
(Alcoholic Hallucinosis)

Delirium tremens is an acute toxic state that follows a prolonged bout of steady drinking or the diminution or cessation of alcoholic intake. It may be precipitated by acute injury or infection.

▶ **NURSING ALERT:** Delirium tremens is a serious complication and poses a threat to the life of the alcoholic patient.

Clinical Manifestations

1. Anxiety; uncontrollable fear
2. Tremulousness, restlessness and agitation, irritability, insomnia
3. Talkativeness; preoccupation
4. Visual, tactile, and auditory hallucinations (usually of a frightening nature)
5. Autonomic overactivity—tachycardia, dilated pupils, profuse perspiration, fever

Emergency Management

Goal:

Give proper sedation and support to enable the patient to rest and recover without the danger of injury or exhaustion.

1. Take the blood pressure since the patient's subsequent medication may depend on his blood pressure readings.
2. Carry out physical examination to identify preexisting or contributing illnesses or injuries (head injury, pneumonia, etc.).
3. Sedate the patient with sufficient dosage of medication to produce adequate relaxation—to reduce his agitation, prevent exhaustion, and promote sleep.
   a. A variety of drugs and combinations of drugs are used—chloral hydrate, diazepam (Valium), hydroxyzine (Vistaril), etc.
   b. The dosage is adjusted according to the patient's symptoms and blood pressure response.
4. Place the patient in a private room where he can be observed closely.
   a. Keep room lighted—to reduce incidence of visual hallucinations.
   b. Close closet and bathroom doors to eliminate shadows.
   c. Keep environment calm and nonstressful; shut out loud noises; call the patient by name.
   d. Observe the patient closely—he may become homicidal or suicidal in response to his hallucinations if he is having alcoholic hallucinations.
   e. Have someone stay with the patient as much as possible—presence of another person has a reassuring and quieting effect and helps the patient maintain contact with reality.
   f. Explain visual misinterpretations (illusions)—strengthens link with reality.
   g. Explain every procedure done to the patient in detail.
   h. Take the patient to the bathroom if permitted.
   i. Use restraints if the patient is not under direct and constant observation.
5. Maintain electrolyte balance and hydration via oral or intravenous route—fluid losses may be extreme because of profuse perspiration and agitation.
6. Record temperature, pulse, respiration, and blood

pressure frequently (every 30 minutes in severe forms of delirium)—in anticipation of peripheral circulatory collapse and/or hyperthermia (the 2 most common lethal complications).

7. Administer phenytoin (Dilantin) or other anticonvulsant drugs as prescribed to prevent or control alcoholic or epileptic convulsions.

8. Assess respiratory, hepatic, and cardiovascular status of patient—pneumonia, liver disease, and cardiac failure are complications.
   a. Hypoglycemia may accompany alcoholic withdrawal because alcohol depletes liver glycogen

stores and impairs gluconeogenesis; many patients also suffer from malnutrition.
   b. Administer parenteral dextrose if liver glycogen is depleted.
   c. Give orange juice, Gatorade, or other carbohydrates to stabilize blood sugar and to counteract tremulousness.

9. Give supplemental vitamin therapy and a high-carbohydrate diet; these patients are usually vitamin deficient.

10. Refer to alcoholic treatment center for subsequent follow-up and rehabilitation.

Psychiatric Emergency

A *psychiatric emergency* is an urgent, serious disturbance of behavior, affect, or thought which makes the patient unable to cope with his life situation and interpersonal relationships.

Behavioral Manifestations

A. Overactive (or violent)

1. Disturbed, uncooperative, unpredictable paranoid behavior
2. Anxiety and panic-like state
3. Assaultive and destructive impulses and behavior (patient may be noisy or disturbed from acute alcohol or drug intoxication)
4. Crying, depression, intense nervousness

B. Underactive (or depressed)

1. Depression
2. Fearfulness, detached attitude
3. Slowing of responses
4. Sad facial expression

C. Suicidal

Emergency Management

Goal:
Maintain the patient's self-esteem (and life, if necessary), while carrying out assessment and intervention.

A. Overactive Patient

1. Determine (from family, ambulance driver, etc.) if the patient has had past mental illness, hospitalizations, injuries or serious illnesses, uses alcohol or drugs, or has experienced crises in interpersonal relationships or intrapsychic conflicts.
2. Be aware that abnormal thought and behavior may be manifestations of an underlying physical disorder (hypoglycemia, stroke, epilepsy) and drug toxicity, including alcohol toxicity.
3. Try to gain control of the situation.
   a. Approach the patient with a calm, confident, and firm manner—this attitude is therapeutic and will help calm the patient.
   b. Introduce yourself by name.
   c. Tell the patient, "I am here to help you."
   d. Repeat the patient's name from time to time.
   e. Speak in one-thought sentences. Be consistent.
   f. Give the patient space. Let him slow down by himself and allow him to become compliant.
   g. Be interested in and listen to the patient—encourage him to talk of his thoughts and *feelings*.
   h. Offer appropriate explanations. Tell the truth.
4. Give tranquilizer or psychotropic agent for emergency management of functional psychosis. Chlorpromazine (Thorazine) or haloperidol (Haldol) act specifically against psychotic symptoms of thought fragmentation and perceptual and behavioral aberrations.
   a. Initial dosage depends on body weight and severity of symptoms.
   b. Observe the patient for 1 hour after initial dose to determine degree of change in psychotic behavior.
   c. Subsequent dosages depend on the patient's reaction.
   d. If behavior is caused by hallucinogens (LSD, etc.), psychotropic drugs (exerting an effect on the mind) are not used.
5. Use restraints only as a last resort.
6. Admit to psychiatric unit or arrange for psychiatric outpatient treatment.

B. Violent Patient

Violent and aggressive behavior is usually episodic and is a means of expressing feelings of anger, fear, or hopelessness about a situation. Persons with a tendency to violence frequently lose control when intoxicated with alcohol or drugs.

Emergency Management:

Goal:
Protect the patient and staff from harm.

1. If possible, have 2 persons see the patient initially; a specially designated room with at least 2 exits should be used, in which no objects that could be used as weapons are in sight.
2. Keep the door of the room open and be in clear view of the staff. Do not block the patient's exit to the door; the patient may feel closed in and threatened.
3. Give the patient space. Do not make any sudden movement. If the patient is carrying a weapon, ask him to place it in a neutral area.
4. Adopt a calm, noncritical approach and remain in control of the situation. External calm and structure may help the patient to gain control.
5. Talk and listen to the patient.
   a. Crisis intervention is best done with an attitude of interest in the patient's well-being and with

an attempt to "tune in" to the patient while at the same time remaining firm.

b. Acknowledge the patient's state of agitation: "I want to work with you to relieve your distress," etc. Ask if he is thinking of hurting someone.

c. Give the patient the opportunity to ventilate his anger verbally.

d. Try to hear what the patient is saying.

e. Convey an expectation of appropriate behavior and make the patient aware that help is available for him to gain control.
   (1) Let the patient know that his behavior may be frightening to those around him and that violence is not acceptable.
   (2) Describe the help available in crisis situations—clinic, emergency department, mental health facility.
   (3) Offer the patient something to eat or drink if talking does not defuse the situation.

6. Allow the security personnel/police to intervene if the patient does not become calm.
   a. Offer protection of hospitalization—usually welcomed by the patient who fears his loss of control.
   b. Offer medication as prescribed (rapid tranquilization [haloperidol; diazepam; chlorpromazine]) if the above fails to attenuate the patient's tension—to reduce tension, anxiety, and hyperactivity.
   c. Use restraints when necessary but with minimum of force.
      (1) Have enough personnel available when applying restraints.
      (2) Talk reassuringly to the patient while applying restraints.
   d. Refer the patient for further mental health treatment after combativeness, agitation, and fear have cooled.

C. Underactive or Depressed Patient

The underactive or depressed patient will be fearful, depressed, and slow to respond, will be plagued by feelings of worthlessness, guilt, ambivalence, and indecision, and will be prone to insomnia, a worsening mood in the morning, sad facial expression, and feelings of isolation.

Emergency Management:

1. Listen to the patient in a calm, unhurried manner.
   a. The patient will benefit from ventilation of feelings.

b. Give the patient an opportunity to talk about his problems.

c. Anticipate that the patient may be suicidal.

d. Attempt to find out if the patient has thought about or attempted suicide.
   (1) "Have you ever thought about taking your own life?"
   (2) The patient is generally relieved because of the opportunity to discuss his feelings.

e. Find out if there is an illness, perceived or real.

f. Assess whether there has been sudden worsening of depression.

g. Notify relatives about a seriously depressed patient. Do not leave the patient alone since suicide is usually an act committed in solitude.

2. Give antidepressant and antianxiety agents as prescribed.

3. Point out to the patient that depression is treatable.

4. Be aware of crisis and supportive services in the community; telephone counseling and referral, suicide prevention centers, group therapy, marital and family counseling, drug/alcohol counseling, adolescent counseling, befriending programs.

5. Refer the patient for psychiatric consultation or to psychiatric unit.

D. Suicidal Patient

Suicide is an act that stems from depression (the loss of a loved one, the loss of body integrity or status, poor self-image) and can be viewed as a cry for help and intervention.

Persons at Risk:

Older person, male, unusual loss or stress, unemployed, divorced, living alone, showing significant depression (weight loss, sleep disturbances, somatic complaints, suicidal preoccupation), history of previous suicidal attempts, psychiatric illness.

Emergency Management:

1. Treat the consequences of the suicide attempt (gunshot wound, drug overdose, etc.).

2. Prevent further self-injury—a patient who has made a suicide gesture may do so again.

3. Employ crisis intervention (a form of brief psychotherapy)—to determine suicide potential; discover areas of depression and conflict; find out about the patient's support system; and determine whether hospitalization, psychiatric referral, etc. is warranted.

4. Admit to intensive care unit (if condition warrants), arrange follow-up care, or admit to psychiatric unit, depending on assessment of suicide potential.

Sexual Assault

Rape is defined as unlawful carnal knowledge of a woman by a man by force or the threat of force against her will. The patient should be seen immediately upon entrance into the emergency department.

Emergency Management

Goals:

Provide physical care and emotional support.
Reduce the emotional trauma of the patient.
Gather available evidence for possible legal proceedings.

A. Respect the privacy and sensitivity of the patient; be kind and supportive.

1. The manner in which the patient is received and treated in the emergency department is important to the future psychological well-being of the patient. Crisis intervention should begin when the patient enters the health facility.
   a. Emotional trauma may be present for weeks, months, years. The patient's reaction to rape has been called the "rape trauma syndrome." Patient may go through phases of psychological reactions:
      (1) Acute phase (disorganization)—shock,

disbelief, fear, guilt, humiliation, anger, self-blame

(2) Long-term process (reorganization; putting incident into perspective)—may have sleep disturbances, phobias, sexual fears

b. Reassure the patient that anxiety is natural and that appropriate support is available from professional and community resources.

2. Accept the emotional reactions of the patient (hysteria, stoicism, overwhelmed feeling, etc.).

3. Do not leave the patient alone.

B. Assist with the physical examination.

1. Secure written, witnessed informed consent from the patient (or parent/guardian if patient is a minor) for examination and for the taking of photographs if necessary and for release of findings to police.

2. Take history *only* if the patient has not already talked to police officer, social worker, crisis intervention worker, etc. Do not ask the patient to repeat the history.

   a. Record history of event in the patient's own words.

3. Ask if the patient has bathed, douched, brushed teeth, changed clothes, urinated or defecated since attack—may alter interpretation of subsequent findings.

4. Record time of admission, time of examination, date and time of alleged rape, and the general appearance of the patient.

   a. Document any evidence of trauma—discoloration, bruises, lacerations, secretions, torn and bloody clothing.

   b. Record emotional state.

5. Assist the patient to undress; drape properly.

   a. Save clothing; label. Note tears/holes in clothing and indicate on label.

   b. Ask the patient to place each item of clothing in a separate paper bag (plastic bags may promote molding of seminal stains and blood which destroys evidence).

   c. Give to appropriate law enforcement authorites.

6. Examine the patient (from head to toe) for injuries, especially to the head, neck, breasts and thighs, back, and buttocks.

   a. Assess for external evidence of trauma (bruises, contusions, lacerations, stab wounds).

   b. Assess for dried semen stains (appearing as crusted, flaking areas) on the patient's body.

   c. Inspect fingers for broken nails and tissue and foreign materials under nails.

   d. Assist in conducting oral examination; secure a specimen of saliva on sterile gauze pads; take prescribed cultures of gum–teeth areas.

   e. Document evidence of trauma with body diagrams/photographs.

C. Assist with pelvic and rectal examinations.

1. Advise the patient of the nature and necessity of each procedure; give the rationale for each question asked.

   a. Examine perineum (and other areas) with a Wood light (prostatic secretions are fluorescent).

   b. Note color and consistency of any discharge present.

   c. Use water-moistened vaginal speculum for examination; do not use lubricant (contain chemicals and may affect the acid phosphatase test).

2. Assist with securing laboratory specimens.

   a. Collect vaginal aspirate, which is examined for presence or absence of motile/nonmotile sperm.

   b. Use sterile swab to draw from vaginal pool for acid phosphatase, blood group antigen of semen, and precipitin test against human sperm and blood.

   c. Obtain separate smears from the oral, vaginal, and anal areas.

   d. Obtain culture of body orifices for gonorrhea (see p. 868).

   e. Obtain cultures for *C. trachomatis* from any potentially infected sites.

   f. Obtain blood serum for syphilis; a sample of serum may be frozen and saved for future testing.

   g. Conduct test for pregnancy if there is a possibility that the patient may be pregnant.

   h. Collect foreign material (leaves, grass, dirt) and place in a clean envelope.

   i. Comb the pubic hairs with prepackaged, clean comb; cut off a few pubic hairs and save; place in separate container.

   j. Label all specimens with name of patient, date, time of collection, body area from which specimen was obtained, and names of personnel collecting specimens to preserve chain of evidence; give to designated person (crime laboratory, etc.) and obtain an itemized receipt.

   k. Photographs are taken by designated person.

D. Treat associated injuries as indicated.

E. Give the patient option of prophylaxis against sexually transmitted disease.

1. Tetracycline: 500 mg. by mouth, 4 times a day for at least 7 days; OR
   Doxycycline: 100 mg. by mouth, twice a day for at least 7 days

2. Patients who are allergic to tetracycline and pregnant women should be treated with:
   Amoxicillin/ampicillin: amoxicillin 3.0 g. or ampicillin 3.5 g., each given with 1.0 g. of probenecid as a single oral dose

F. Offer antipregnancy measures if the patient is of childbearing age, is using no contraceptives, and is at high risk in menstrual cycle.

1. Inform the patient that if she misses a menstrual period she has the option of having menstrual extraction or abortion.

2. Postcoital contraceptive drugs may be given after obtaining negative result from pregnancy tests (conjugated estrogen; ethinyl estradiol). These preparations may cause nausea and vomiting and an antiemetic may be given to decrease discomfort from side effects.

G. Offer cleansing douche, mouthwash, and fresh clothing.

H. Provide for follow-up services.

1. Make appointment for follow-up examinations for pregnancy and sexually transmitted disease; the patient should be seen in 7 days for follow-up and the aforementioned studies, except for serologic test for syphilis, repeated. A serologic test for syphilis is done 6 weeks after incident.

2. Inform the patient of counseling services to prevent long-term psychological effects; counseling services should be made available to the family.

3. Encourage the patient to return to previous level of functioning as soon as possible.

4. The patient should be accompanied by family/friend when leaving health care facility.

Bibliography

Books

Bennett G, Vourakis C and Woolf DS (eds). Substance Abuse. New York, John Wiley & Sons, 1983

Budassi SA and Barber J. Mosby's Manual of Emergency Care, 2nd ed. St Louis, CV Mosby, 1984

Campbell J and Humphreys J. Nursing Care of Victims of Family Violence. Reston, Reston Publishing, 1984

Chafetz ME. The Alcoholic Patient: Diagnosis and Management. Oradell, NJ, Medical Economics Books, 1983

Cosgriff JH Jr and Anderson DL (eds). The Practice of Emergency Care, 2nd ed. Philadelphia, JB Lippincott, 1984

Cowley RA and Dunham CM. Shock Trauma/Critical Care Manual. Baltimore, University Park Press, 1982

Eliastam M, Sternbach GL and Bresler MJ. Manual of Emergency Medicine. Chicago, Year Book Medical Publisher, 1983

Emergency Department Nurses Association. Standards of Emergency Nursing Practice. St Louis, CV Mosby, 1983

Estes NJ, Smith-Dijulio K and Heinemann ME. Nursing Diagnosis of the Alcoholic Person. St Louis, CV Mosby, 1980

Foley TS and Davies MA. Rape: Nursing Care of Victims. St. Louis: CV Mosby, 1983.

Giannini AJ, Slaby AE and Giannini MC. Handbook of Overdose and Detoxification Emergencies. New Hyde Park, NY, Medical Examination Pub, 1982

Greenfield LJ (ed). Complications in Surgery and Trauma. Philadelphia, JB Lippincott, 1984

Guthrie MM. Shock, vol. 2. New York, Churchill Livingstone, 1982

Haddad LM and Winchester JR (eds). Clinical Management of Poisoning and Drug Overdose. Philadelphia, WB Saunders, 1983

Hammon BB and Lee G. Quick Reference to Emergency Nursing. Philadelphia, JB Lippincott, 1984

Hoff LA. People in Crisis: Understanding and Helping, 2nd ed. Menlo Park, CA, Addison-Wesley, 1984

Hofmann FG. A Handbook on Drug and Alcohol Abuse, 2nd ed. New York, Oxford University Press, 1983

Kravis TC and Warner CG. Emergency Medicine, A Comprehensive Review. Rockville, MD, Aspen Systems, 1983

Lamphier TA. Guidelines for Medical and Surgical Emergencies. New York, Masson, 1983

Lanros NE. Assessment and Intervention in Emergency Nursing, 2nd ed. Bowie, MD, Robert J Brady, 1983

May HL (ed). Emergency Medical Procedures. New York, John Wiley & Sons, 1984

May HL (ed). Emergency Medicine. New York, John Wiley & Sons, 1984

Mills J, Ho MT and Trunkey DD. Current Emergency Diagnosis and Treatment. Los Altos, CA, Lange Medical Publications, 1983

Mills K, Morton R and Page G. A Colour Atlas of Accidents and Emergencies. London, Wolfe Medical Publications, 1984

Moore EE, Eiseman B and VanWay CW III. Critical Decisions in Trauma. St Louis, CV Mosby, 1984

Moser KM and Spragg RG. Respiratory Emergencies, 2nd ed. St Louis, CV Mosby, 1982

Rosen P et al. Emergency Medicine: Concepts and Clinical Practice, Vol 1 & 2. St Louis, CV Mosby, 1983

Sahn SA. Pulmonary Emergencies. New York, Churchill Livingstone, 1982

Shoemaker WC, Thompson WL and Holbrook PR. Textbook of Critical Care. Philadelphia, WB Saunders, 1984

Simon RR. Procedures and Techniques in Emergency Medicine. Baltimore, Williams & Wilkins, 1982

Tinker J and Rapin M. Care of the Critically Ill Patient. New York, Springer-Verlag, 1983

Walker JA. Psychiatric Emergencies: Intervention and Resolution. Philadelphia, JB Lippincott, 1983

Walt AJ et al (eds). Early Care of the Injured Patient, 3rd ed. Philadelphia, WB Saunders, 1982

Warner CG. Emergency Care: Assessment and Intervention, 3rd ed. St Louis, CV Mosby, 1983

Wilkins EW Jr. MGH Textbook of Emergency Medicine. Baltimore, Williams & Wilkins, 1983

Wilson L, Simson SP and Baxter CR. Handbook of Geriatric Emergency Care. Baltimore, University Park Press, 1984

Worth MH Jr (ed). Principles and Practice of Trauma Care. Baltimore, Williams & Wilkins, 1982

Articles

Approach to Patient/Family

Beglinger JE. Coping tasks in critical care. DCCN 1983 Mar–Apr; 2(2):80–89

Billings CV. Providing better emergency care when behaviors bar the way. Nursing '82 1982 May; 12(5):57

Curtis NM. Caring for families during the "unknown" period. DCCN 1983 Jul–Aug; 2(4):248–254

Daley L. The perceived immediate needs of families with relatives in the intensive care setting. Heart Lung 1984 May; 13(3):231–237

Elliott FC. A nursing protocol for anxiety following catastrophic injury. Rehab Nurs 1983 May–Jun; 8(3):18–20; 38

Hickey M. Nursing diagnosis in the critical care unit. DCCN 1984 Mar–Apr; 3(2):91–97

Trauma

Berry TK et al. Diagnostic peritoneal lavage in blunt trauma patients with coagulopathy. Ann Emerg Med 1984 Oct; 13(10):879–880

Butson ARC. The clinical use of antishock trousers. Can Med Assoc J 1983 Jan 15; 128(12):1428–1430

Brand DA et al. Adequacy of antitetanus prophylaxis in six hospital emergency rooms. N Engl J Med 1983 Sept 15; 309(11):636–640

Cardona VD. Trauma post-op: The real nursing challenge. RN 1982 Mar; 45(3):22–29

Cowan BN et al. The relative prognostic value of lactate and haemodynamic measurements in early shock. Anaesthesia 1984 Aug; 39(8):750–755

Cox EF and Dunham CM. A safe technique for diagnostic peritoneal lavage. J Trauma 1983 Feb; 23(2):152–154

Frye TA and Deluca SA. Splenic trauma 1984 Jun; 29(6):149–150

George JE. Missed trauma in the emergency department. JEN 1984 Jul–Aug; 10(4):228–229

Gruenberg JC et al. The diagnostic usefulness of peritoneal lavage in penetrating trauma. Am Surg 1982 Aug; 48(8):402–407

King RC. Emergency! Dealing with abrasions and lacerations. RN 1984 Jun; 47(6):53–56

McSwain NE Jr. Resuscitation of the trauma patient. Clin Emerg Med 1983 2:113–120

Nowak RM (ed). Cardiopulmonary-cerebral resuscitation: State of the art. Ann Emerg Med 1984 Sept; 13(9 Pt 2):756–875(entire volume)

O'Mara K and Mavichak V. Trauma and oral anticoagulants. Ann Emerg Med 1983 Nov; 12(11):700–703

Rogove HJ. Hypovolemic shock: The need for early intervention. JAOA 1983 Jan; 82(5):321–325

Shaftan GW. The initial evaluation of the multiple trauma patient. World Surg 1983 Jan; 7(1):19–25

Sigmon HD. Helping your long-term trauma patient travel the road to recovery. Nursing '84 1984 Jan; 14(1): 58–63

Siskind J. Handling hemorrhage wisely. Nursing '84 1984 Jan; 14(1):34–61

Smith JP et al. The esophageal obturator airway. A review. JAMA 1983 Jan 26; 250(8):1081–1084

Soballe PW. Peritoneal lavage in blunt abdominal trauma. Am Fam Physician 1984 Mar; 29(3):193–198

Strange JM. The riddle of abdominal trauma: How much damage—and *where?* RN 1983 Mar; 46(3):42–46, 98–100

Stuzin J, Engrav L and Buehler P. Care of open wounds. Compr Ther 1982 Feb; 8(2):32–34

Thomson NA. Convert your assessment into a lifesaving care plan for the patient with abdominal trauma. Nursing '83 1983 Jul; 13(7):26–33

Temperature Emergencies

Anerson RJ et al. Early Assessment and management. Heat injuries. Emerg Med Ann 1982; 1:117–140

Bristow G. Accidental hypothermia. Can Anaesth Soc J 1984 May; 31(3 Pt 2): S52–S55

Clochesy JM. Profound hypothermia. Focus Crit Care 1984 Feb; 11(1):19–21

DeLapp TD. Accidental hypothermia. Am J Nurs 1983 Jan; 83(1):62–67

Feenaghty DA. Atropine poisoning: Jimsonweed. JEN 1982 May–Jun; 8(3): 139–141

MacFarlane P. Recognizing and treating heat stroke and exhaustion in the road runner. Can Nurse 1983 Apr; 79(4): 21–23

Okada M. The cardiac rhythm in accidental hypothermia. J Electrocardiol 1984 Apr; 17(2):123–128

Smith DS. Living death: Don't let hypothermia fool you into a fatal mistake. RN 1983 Jan; 46(1):48–51

Stadnyk AN and Glezos JD. Drug-induced heat stroke. Can Med Assoc J 1983 Apr 15; 128(8):957–959

Poisoning

McCarron MM. The use of toxicology tests in emergency room diagnosis. J Anal Toxicol 1983 May–Jun; 7(3):131–135

Saxena K. The basic principles in the treatment of the poisoned patient. Med Times 1983 Sept; 111(9):43–48; 51

Spyker DA et al. A user-oriented information system for emergency medicine. Compr Ther 1984 May; 10(5):42–47

Substance Abuse

Armen K, Kanel G and Reynolds T. Phencyclidine-induced malignant hyperthermia causing submassive liver necrosis. Am J Med 1984 Jul; 77(1): 167–172.

Carter JH Jr. Health promotion and disease prevention. Combating substance abuse with health life-styles. Ala J Med Sci 1984 Apr; 21(2):165–169

Chychula NM. Screening for substance abuse in a primary care setting. Nurse Pract 1984 Jul; 9(7):15–24

Einstein S. Drug misuse/abuse intervention: a schematic tool for decision making and planning. Int J Addict 1984 May; 19(3):355–366

Khansari N, Whitten HD and Fudenberg HH. Phencyclidine-induced immunodepression. Science 1984 Jul 6; 225(4657):76–78

Lamy PP. Alcohol misuse and abuse among the elderly. Drug Intell Clin Pharm 1984 Jul–Aug; 18(7–8):649–651

Leckman AL, Umland BE and Blay M. Prevalence of alcoholism in a family practice center. J Fam Pract 1984 Jun; 18(6):867–870

Mittleman RE and Wetli CV. Death caused by recreational cocaine use. An update. JAMA 1984 Oct 12; 252(14): 1889–1893

Rector CS and Foster ME. Assessment and care of the patient experiencing alcohol withdrawal syndrome. Crit Care Nurse 1984 Jul–Aug; 4(4):64–68

West LJ et al. Alcoholism. Ann Intern Med 1984 Mar; 100(3):405–416

Psychiatric Emergencies

Barash DA. Defusing the violent patient—before he explodes. RN 1984 Mar; 47(3):34–37

Carmack BJ. Suspect a suicide? Don't be afraid to act. RN 1983 Apr; 46(4):43–45, 90

Jacobs D. Evaluation and management of the violent patient in emergency settings. Psychiatr Clin North Am 1983 Jun; 6(2):259–269

Locke AM and Gaffey GK. Managing psychological disturbances in critical care. DCCN 1983 Sept–Oct; 2(5):314–320

Maagdenberg AM. The "violent" patient. Am J Nurs 1983 Mar; 83(3):402–403

Pasternack SA. Suicide: The cry of the depressed patient. South Med J 1983 Oct; 76(10):1290–1293

Soreff SM (ed). Emergency psychiatry. Psychiatr Clin North Am 1983 Jun; 6(2):211–362(entire vol)

Velente S. Stalking patient depression. Nursing '84 1984 Aug; 14(8):62–64

Sexual Assault

Frank E and Stewart BD. Depressive symptoms in rape victims. A revisit. J Affective Disord 1984 Aug; 7(1):77–85

Martin, CA, Warfield MC and Braen GR. Physician's management of the psychological aspects of rape. JAMA 1983 Jan 28; 249(4):501

Mittleman RE, Goldberg HS and Waksman DM. Preserving evidence in the emergency department. Am J Nurs 1983 Dec; 83(12):1652–1656

Modlin HC. Traumatic neurosis and other injuries. Psychiatr Clin North Am 1983 Dec; 6(4):661–682

Ruch LO and Leon JJ. Sexual assault trauma and trauma change. Women Health 1983 Winter; 8(4):5–21

STD and the management of rape victims and sexually abused children. MMWR 1982 Aug 20; 31(2S):59S–60S

Maternity Nursing

Maternal and Fetal Health

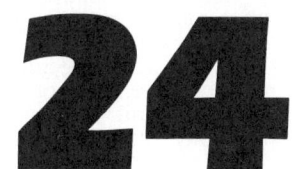

Introduction to Maternity Nursing

Providing care to childbearing families is aimed at the ideal of having every pregnancy result in a healthy mother, baby, and family unit. In the last 15–20 years, care provided to childbearing families has changed dramatically. Advances such as in vitro fertilization, embryo transplants, and intrauterine fetal surgery have just begun. Technological advances in fetal monitoring, sonography, and neonatal intensive care units are now providing the means to save fetuses and infants who would not have survived 15–20 years ago.

Regionalization of obstetrical services so that childbearing families have access to the technological advances and skilled personnel capable of managing pregnancy or neonatal complications is being implemented. At the same time, childbearing families opposed to the use of advanced technology are demanding and receiving alternate types of care in birthing centers, birthing rooms in hospitals, home deliveries, alternate methods used during delivery, and changes in hospital policies such as 24 hour discharge following delivery and having children present during their mother's labor and delivery.

These changes in the delivery of care and advances in technology have also required changes in the delivery of nursing care, requiring advanced knowledge for nursing practice and additional educational preparation for many nurses. Currently *nurse–midwives,* nurses who have completed additional education in caring for childbearing women, normal newborns, and gynecologic problems of women, are providing more care to childbearing families. Other nurses specializing in care of high-risk pregnant women and in care of high-risk neonates are providing the link between advanced technology and more personal and human systems of health care.

Current Problems Affecting Maternal and Infant Morbidity and Mortality

1. Higher maternal and infant mortality among the nonwhite and rural populations
2. Higher mortality rate for fetuses of teenagers, women over 35 years of age, women in lower socioeconomic groups
3. Continued steady rate of low-birth-weight infants born annually
4. Infant deaths due to congenital malformations, sudden infant death syndrome, low birth weight and its resulting sequelae

Terminology

Gravida—a woman who is or has been pregnant, without regard to pregnancy outcome

Nulligravida—a woman who is not now and never has been pregnant

Primigravida—a woman pregnant for the first time

Multigravida—a women who has been pregnant several times

Para—refers to past pregnancies that have reached viability

Nullipara—a woman who has never completed a pregnancy to the period of viability. The woman may or may not have experienced an abortion.

Primipara—refers to a woman who had completed 1 pregnancy to the period of viability regardless of the number of infants delivered (the birth of twins or triplets increases parity by 1) and regardless of the infant being live or stillborn

Multipara—refers to a woman who has completed 2 or more pregnancies to the stage of viability

A woman pregnant for the first time is a primigravida and is described as Gravida 1, Para 0.

A woman who delivered one fetus to the period of viability and who is pregnant again is described as Gravida 2, Para 1.

A woman with 2 abortions and no viable children is Gravida 2, Para 0.

In some obstetrical services, a woman's past obstetric history is summarized by a series of 4 digits, such as 5-1-2-5. The first digit refers to the number of term infants, the second to the number of premature infants, the third to the number of abortions and the fourth to the number of children currently alive.

The Expectant Mother

Manifestations of Pregnancy

Presumptive Signs and Symptoms

1. Cessation of menses—pregnancy is suspected if more than 10 days have elapsed since the time of the expected onset. Suggestive of pregnancy in a woman with a previously spontaneous, cyclic, and predictable menses.
2. Breast changes
   a. Breasts enlarge and become tender. Veins in breast become increasingly visible.
   b. Nipples become larger and more pigmented.

c. Colostrum, a thin, milky fluid, may be expressed in the 2nd half of pregnancy.
d. Montgomery glands, small elevations on the areolae, may appear.
3. Vaginal color changes (*Chadwick's sign*)—a bluish discoloration and congestion of vaginal wall.
4. Abdominal striae (*striae gravidarum*)—sometimes appear on the breasts, abdomen, and thighs because of the stretching, rupture, and atrophy of the deep connective tissue of the skin.
5. Nausea and vomiting (morning sickness)—occurs mainly in the morning, but may occur at any time of the day, lasting a few hours. Usually disappears spontaneously near the end of the 1st trimester.
6. *Quickening* (sensations of fetal movement in the abdomen)—occurs between 16th and 20th week after the onset of the last menses.
7. Frequency of urination
   a. Caused by pressure of the expanding uterus on the bladder
   b. Decreases when the uterus rises out of the pelvis
   c. Reappears when the fetal head engages in the pelvis at the end of pregnancy
8. Fatigue—characteristic of early pregnancy.

Probable Signs and Symptoms

1. Enlargement of abdomen—near the end of the 3rd month, the uterus can be felt through the abdominal wall, just above the symphysis.
2. Changes in shape, size, and consistency of the uterus
   a. Uterus enlarges, elongates, and decreases in thickness as pregnancy progresses.
   b. *Hegar's sign*—lower uterine segment softens 6–8 weeks after the onset of the last menstrual period.
3. Changes in cervix
   a. At 6–8 weeks of gestation, the cervix often becomes considerably softened.
   b. *Goodell's sign*—softening of the cervix.
   c. With inflammation and carcinoma during pregnancy, the cervix may remain firm.
4. Intermittent contractions of the uterus (*Braxton Hicks contractions*)—painless, palpable contractions occurring at irregular intervals.
5. *Ballottement*—a sinking and rebounding of the fetus in its surrounding amniotic fluid in response to a sudden tap on the uterus (occurs near mid-pregnancy).
6. Outlining of the fetal body through the maternal abdomen by palpation in the second half of pregnancy.
7. Positive hormonal tests for pregnancy (test reactions produced by the presence of gonadotropin in maternal plasma and urine).

Positive Signs and Symptoms

1. Fetal heartbeat (separate and distinct from that of the mother)—usually heard between 16th and 20th week of gestation
2. Fetal movements felt by the examiner (after about 20 weeks' gestation).
3. X-ray visualization of the fetus (after 16 weeks' gestation).
4. Sonographic evidence (after 8 weeks' gestation).

Maternal Physiology During Pregnancy

Duration of Pregnancy

1. Averages 280 days or 40 weeks from the first day of the last normal menstrual period.

2. Duration may also be divided into 3 equal parts, or trimesters, of slightly more than 13 weeks or 3 calendar months each.
3. *Estimated date of confinement* (EDC) is calculated by adding 7 days to the date of the 1st day of the last menstrual period and counting back 3 months (*Nägele's rule*).
   a. For example, if a woman's last menstrual period began on 9/10/86, her EDC would be 9/10/86 plus 7 days = 9/17/86, minus 3 months = 6/17/87.

Changes in Reproductive Tract

A. Uterus

1. Enlargement during pregnancy involves stretching and marked hypertrophy of existing muscle cells.
2. In addition to an increase in the size of the uterine muscle cells, there is an increase in fibrous tissue, elastic tissue, blood vessels, and lymphatics.
3. Enlargement and thickening of the uterine wall is most marked in the fundus.
4. By the end of the 3rd month, the uterus is too large to be contained wholly within the pelvic cavity—it can now be palpated suprapubically.
5. As the uterus rises out of the pelvis it rotates somewhat to the right because of the presence of the rectosigmoid on the left side of the pelvis.
6. By 20 weeks' gestation, the fundus has reached the level of the umbilicus.
7. By 36 weeks, the fundus has reached the xiphoid.
8. During the last 3 weeks, the uterus descends slightly—because of fetal descent into pelvis. Walls of uterus become thinner.
9. Changes in contractility occur—from the 1st trimester, irregular painless contractions occur (Braxton Hicks contractions). In latter weeks of pregnancy, these contractions become stronger and more regular.
10. There is a progressive increase in uteroplacental blood flow during pregnancy.

B. Cervix

1. Pronounced softening and cyanosis—due to increased vascularity, edema, hypertrophy, and hyperplasia of the cervical glands.
2. Clot of very thick mucus obstructs the cervical canal.
3. Erosions of cervix, common during pregnancy, represent an extension of proliferating endocervical glands and columnar endocervical epithelium.

C. Ovaries

1. Ovulation ceases during pregnancy; maturation of new follicles is suspended.
2. One corpus luteum functions during early pregnancy (first 8 weeks), producing mainly progesterone.

D. Vagina and Outlet

1. Increased vascularity, hyperemia, and softening of connective tissue in skin and muscles of perineum and vulva.
2. Chadwick's sign noted—characteristic violet color due to increased vascularity and hyperemia.
3. Vaginal walls prepare for labor: mucosa increases in thickness, connective tissue loosens, and small-muscle cells hypertrophy.
4. Vaginal secretions increase; pH is 3.5–6—because of increased production of lactic acid from glycogen in the vaginal epithelium by *Lactobacillus acidophilus*. (Acid pH probably aids in keeping vagina relatively free of pathogenic bacteria.)

Changes in the Abdominal Wall

1. Striae gravidarum often develop—reddish, slightly depressed streaks in the skin of abdomen, breast, and thighs. (Become glistening silvery lines after pregnancy.)
2. *Linea nigra* may form a line of dark pigment extending from the umbilicus down the midline to the symphysis.
3. *Diastasis recti* may occur as muscles (rectus) separate. If severe, a part of the anterior uterine wall may be covered only by a layer of skin, fascia peritoneum.

Breast Changes

1. Are tender and tingle in early weeks of pregnancy.
2. Increase in size by 2nd month—hypertrophy of mammary alveoli.
3. Nipples become larger, more deeply pigmented, and more erectile early in pregnancy.
4. Colostrum may be expressed by 2nd trimester.
5. Areolae become broader and more deeply pigmented. The depth of pigmentation varies with the individual's complexion.
6. Scattered through the areola are a number of small elevations (glands of Montgomery) which are hypertrophic sebaceous glands.

Metabolic Changes

Are numerous and intensive—response to rapidly growing fetus and placenta.

A. Weight Gain Averages 10.896 kg. (24 lbs.)

1. Fetus, 3.4 kg. (7½ lbs.)
2. Placenta, 0.681 kg. (1½ lbs.)
3. Amniotic fluid, 0.91 kg. (2 lbs.)
4. Hypertrophy of uterus, 1.137 kg. (2½ lbs.)
5. Breasts, 0.454 kg. (1 lb.)
6. Increase in blood volume, 1.60 kg. (3½ lbs.)
7. Water retention; fat and protein deposition, 2.724 kg. (6 lbs.)

B. Water Metabolism

1. Average woman retains 6.5 liters of extra water during pregnancy.
2. Fetus, placenta, and amniotic fluid total 3.5 liters.
3. The uterus, maternal blood volume, and breast tissue total 3 liters.
4. Many pregnant women experience edema of the legs and ankles at the end of the day.

C. Protein Metabolism

1. Fetus, uterus, and maternal blood are rich in protein rather than in fat or carbohydrates.
2. At term, fetus and placenta contain 500 gm. of protein or approximately ½ of the total protein increase of pregnancy.
3. Approximately 500 gm. more of protein are added to the uterus, breasts, and maternal blood in the form of hemoglobin and plasma proteins.

D. Carbohydrate Metabolism

1. Pregnancy, potentially, can initiate diabetes.
2. Diabetes mellitus may be aggravated by pregnancy.
3. Clinical diabetes appears in some women only during pregnancy.
4. During pregnancy, there is a "sparing" of glucose used by maternal tissues and a shunting of glucose to the placenta for use by the fetus.
5. Human placental lactogen (placental hormone) promotes lipolysis, increases plasma free fatty acids, and thereby provides alternative fuel sources for the mother.

6. Human placental lactogen, estrogen, progesterone, and an insulinase produced by the placenta oppose the action of insulin during pregnancy.

E. Fat Metabolism

Plasma lipids increase during the latter half of pregnancy.

F. Iron Metabolism

1. Iron requirements increase—often exceed amounts available.
2. Total volume of circulating red blood cells increases by about 450 ml. during pregnancy; iron requirement is therefore increased.
3. Supplemental iron is valuable during the latter half of pregnancy and for several weeks after pregnancy.

Changes in Cardiovascular System

A. Heart

1. Diaphragm is progressively elevated during pregnancy; heart is displaced to the left and upward, with the apex moved laterally.
2. Heart sounds—an exaggerated splitting of the first heart sound, a loud, easily heard 3rd sound.
3. Heart murmurs—systolic murmurs are common and usually disappear following delivery.

B. Circulation

1. Cardiac volume increases by 10% from the beginning to the end of pregnancy, causing slight hypertrophy of the heart and increased cardiac output.
2. In the supine position, the large uterus compresses the venous return from the lower half of the body to the heart. This may cause arterial hypotension, referred to as the *supine hypotensive syndrome.* Cardiac output increases when the woman turns from her back to her left side.
3. Femoral venous pressure increases—because of retardation of blood flow from lower extremities as a result of pressure of enlarged uterus on pelvic veins and inferior vena cava.
4. Pulse rate usually increases 10–15 beats/minute during pregnancy.
5. Increased cutaneous blood flow dissipates excess heat caused by increased metabolism of pregnancy.

C. Hematologic Changes

1. Total volume of circulating red blood cells increases; hemoglobin concentration at term averages 12 gm./dl.
2. Leukocyte count is elevated to 25,000 or more during labor—cause unknown; probably represents the reappearance in the circulation of leukocytes previously shunted out of active circulation.
3. Blood coagulation—fibrinogen levels increase 50%. Other clotting factors that increase include: factor VII (proconvertin), factor VIII (antihemophiliac globulin), factor IX (plasma thromboplastin component), and factor X (Stuart factor). Factor II (prothrombin) increases slightly, while factors XI (plasma thromboplastin antecedent) and XIII (fibrin-stabilizing factor) are decreased during pregnancy. There is no significant change in the number, appearance, or function of platelets.

Changes in Respiratory Tract

1. Hyperventilation occurs—increase in respiratory rate, tidal volume (45%), and minute volume (40%).
2. Increased total volume lowers blood PCO_2, causing mild respiratory alkalosis which is compensated for by lowering of the bicarbonate concentration.
3. Increased respiratory rate and reduced PCO_2 are

probably induced by progesterone and estrogen to a lesser degree on the respiratory center.

4. Diaphragm is elevated during pregnancy—chiefly by the enlarging uterus.
5. Thoracic cage expands by means of flaring of the ribs—result of increased mobility of rib attachments.

Changes in Urinary Tract

1. Ureters become dilated and elongated during pregnancy because of mechanical pressure and perhaps the effects of progesterone. When the uterus rises out of the uterine cavity, it rests on the ureters, compressing them at the pelvic brim. Dilation is greater on the right side—left side is cushioned by the sigmoid colon.
2. Glomerular filtration (GF) increases early in pregnancy, and the increase persists almost to term. Renal plasma flow (RPF) increases early in pregnancy and decreases to nonpregnant levels in the 3rd trimester. These changes may be due to placental lactogen.
3. Glucosuria may be evident—because of the increase in glomerular filtration without increase in tubular resorptive capacity for filtered glucose.
4. Proteinuria does not occur normally, except for slight amounts during or just after vigorous labor.
5. Toward the end of pregnancy, pressure of the presenting part impedes drainage of blood and lymph from the bladder base, often leaving the area edematous, easily traumatized, and more susceptible to infection.

Changes in Gastrointestinal Tract

1. Gums may become hyperemic and softened and may bleed easily.
2. A localized vascular swelling of the gums may appear—called *epulis of pregnancy.*
3. Stomach and intestines are displaced upward and laterally by the enlarging uterus. Heartburn is common, caused by reflux of acid secretions in the lower esophagus.
4. Tone and motility of gastrointestinal tract decreases, leading to prolongation of gastric emptying due to large amount of progesterone produced by the placenta.
5. Hemorrhoids are common because of elevated pressure in veins below the level of the large uterus and constipation.
6. Bile is thickened; pregnancy predisposes women to gallstones.
7. Liver function tests yield significantly different results during pregnancy.

Changes in Endocrine System

1. Pituitary gland enlarges slightly.
2. Thyroid is moderately enlarged because of hyperplasia of glandular tissue and increased vascularity.
   a. Basal metabolic rate increases progressively during normal pregnancy (as much as 25%)—because of metabolic activity of fetus.
   b. Level of protein-bound iodine and thyroxin rises sharply and is maintained until after delivery—because of increased circulatory estrogen.
3. Adrenal secretions considerably increased—amounts of aldosterone increase as early as 15th week.

Changes in Integumentary System

1. Pigmentary changes occur because of melanocyte-stimulating hormone, level of which is elevated from the 2nd month of pregnancy until term.
2. Striae gravidarum appear in latter months of pregnancy as reddish, slightly depressed streaks in the skin of the abdomen and occasionally over the breasts and thighs.
3. A brownish black line of pigment is often formed in the midline of the abdominal skin—known as *linea nigra.*
4. Brownish patches of pigment may form on the face—known as *chloasma* or "mask of pregnancy."
5. Angiomas (vascular spiders), minute red elevations commonly on the skin of the face, neck, upper chest, and arms—may develop.
6. Reddening of the palms (*palmar erythema*) may also occur.

Changes in Musculoskeletal System

1. The increasing mobility of sacroiliac, sacrococcygeal, and pelvic joints during pregnancy is a result of hormonal changes.
2. This mobility contributes to alteration of maternal posture and to back pain.
3. Late in pregnancy, aching, numbness, and weakness in the upper extremities may occur because of lordosis which ultimately produces traction on the ulnar and median nerves.
4. Separation of the rectus muscles due to pressure of the growing uterus creates a diastasis recti. If this is severe, a portion of the anterior uterine wall is covered by only a layer of skin, fascia, and peritoneum.

Pelvis

A. Bones of the Pelvis

Pelvis is composed of 4 bones:
1. 2 Innominate bones (hip bones) form sides and front
2. Sacrum and coccyx form the back

Pelvic bones are held together by fibrocartilage of the symphysis pubis and several ligaments.

B. Pelvis is Divided into 2 Parts—false pelvis and true pelvis.

1. False pelvis—lies above an imaginary line called the *linea terminalis* (Fig. 24-1). Function of the false pelvis is to support the enlarged uterus.
2. True pelvis lies below the pelvic brim or linea terminalis; it is the bony canal through which the infant must pass. It is divided into 3 parts: the inlet, the midpelvis, and the outlet.

C. Inlet

1. Upper boundary of true pelvis; bounded by upper margin of symphysis pubis in front, linea terminalis on sides, and sacral promontory (1st sacral vertebra) in back.
2. Largest diameter of inlet is transverse (Fig. 24-2).
3. Smallest diameter of inlet is anteroposterior (AP).
4. AP diameter is most important diameter of inlet; measured clinically by *diagonal conjugate*—distance from lower margin of symphysis to the sacral promontory (usually 12.5 cm.) (Fig. 24-3).
5. *Obstetrical conjugate*—distance between inner surface of symphysis and sacral promontory measured by subtracting 1.5–2 cm. (thickness of symphysis) from the diagonal conjugate. It is usually 11 cm.

D. Midpelvis

1. Bounded by inlet above and outlet below, a true bony cavity.
2. Diameters cannot be measured clinically.
3. Clinical evaluation of adequacy is made by noting

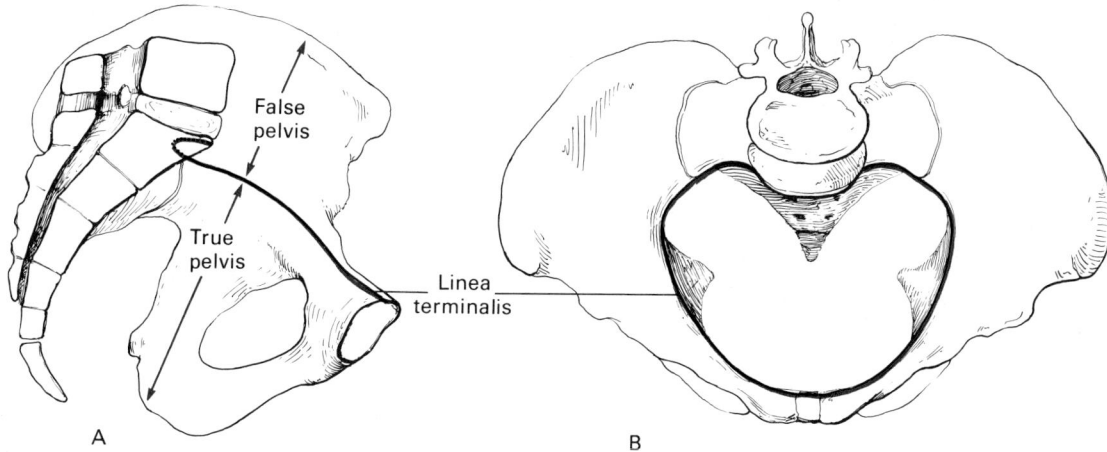

Figure 24-1. (A) Side view of true and false pelvis. (B) Front view showing linea terminalis (pelvic brim).

the ischial spines. Prominent spines that protrude into the cavity indicate a contracted midpelvic space.

E. Outlet
1. Lowest boundary of the true pelvis.
2. Bounded by lower margin of symphysis in front, ischial tuberosities on sides, tip of sacrum posteriorly.
3. Most important diameter clinically is distance between the tuberosities (usually 9 cm.).

F. Pelvic Shapes
There are 4 main types of pelvic shapes (Fig. 24-4):
1. Gynecoid (normal female pelvis)
2. Android
3. Anthropoid
4. Platypelloid

Assessment

Health History
1. Age—increased risk of anemia, preeclampsia and prematurity in very young women; risk of hypertension in older women.

2. Family history—congenital disorders; hereditary diseases; multiple pregnancies; diabetes; heart disease; hypertension; mental retardation.
3. Woman's medical history—childhood disease; major illnesses; surgery; blood transfusions; drug sensitivities; urinary infections; heart disease; diabetes; hypertension; endocrine disorders; anemias; use of oral or other contraceptives; menstrual history (menarche; length and regularity of menstrual periods); use of medications, other drugs; alcohol; tobacco.
4. Woman's past obstetrical history—problems of infertility; data of previous pregnancies and deliveries—dates; infant weights; length of labors; types of deliveries; multiple births; abortions; maternal, fetal, and neonatal complications. Woman's perception of past pregnancy, labor, and delivery for herself and impact on her family.
5. Woman's present obstetric history
   a. Gravidity; parity
   b. Date of last menstrual period (LMP)

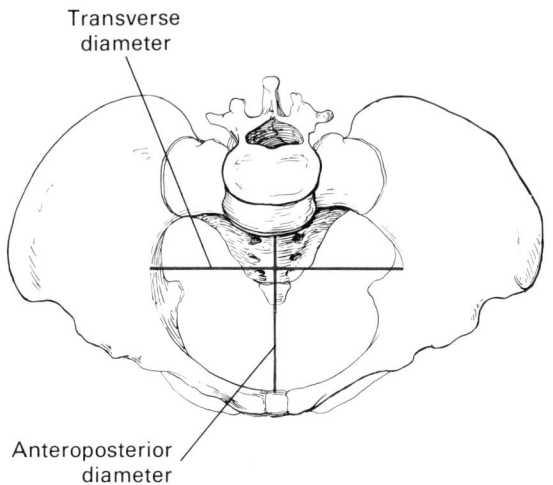

Figure 24-2. Inlet of normal female pelvis showing transverse and anteroposterior diameters.

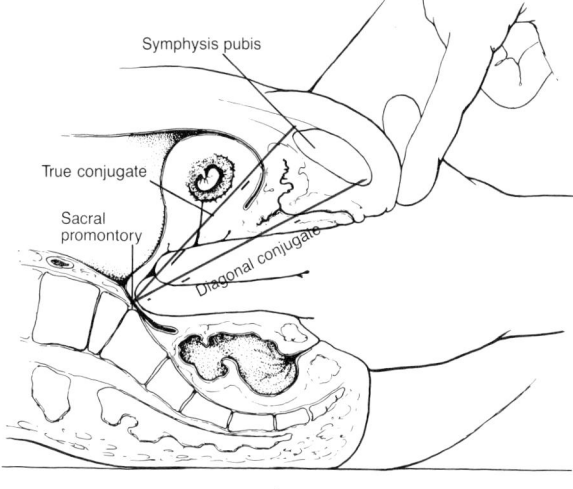

Figure 24-3. Method of obtaining diagonal conjugate diameter.

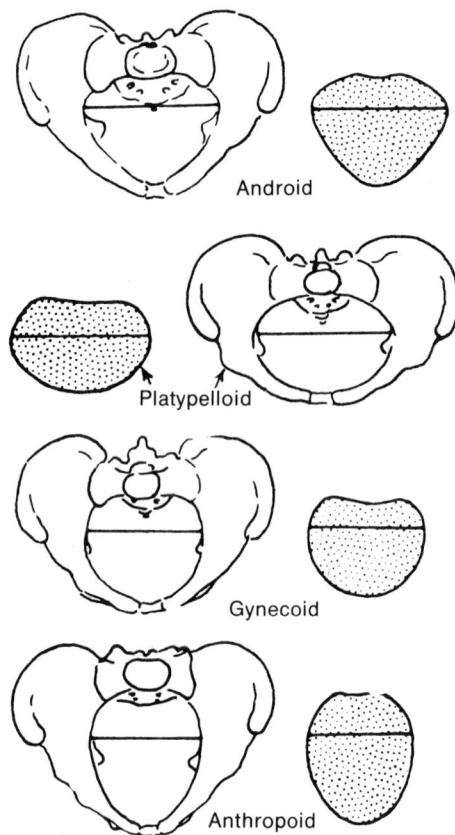

Figure 24-4. The four types of female pelvis. *Android*—male-type pelvis. *Platypelloid*—broad pelvis with shortened anteroposterior diameter and flattened, oval, transverse shape. *Gynecoid*—typical female pelvis in which inlet is round instead of oval. *Anthropoid*—pelvis in which anteroposterior diameter is equal to or greater than the transverse diameter.

c. Estimated date of birth—expected date of confinement (EDC) is calculated by counting back 3 calendar months from the first day of the last menstrual period and adding 7 days.

d. Signs and symptoms of pregnancy—amenorrhea, breast changes, nausea and vomiting, fetal movement, fatigue, urinary frequency, skin pigmentary changes. For possible presumptive and positive signs of pregnancy, see page 959. What are her expectations for her present pregnancy, labor, and delivery?

e. Rest and sleep patterns—length, quality, and regularity of rest and sleep.

f. Activity and employment—exercise patterns, type and hours of employment; plans for continued employment.

g. Sexual activity—sexual satisfaction; frequency and positions during intercourse; alternative practices used to achieve sexual satisfaction.

h. Diet history—weight gain; eating patterns (times and frequency of eating daily); social or cultural dietary habits; number of servings of food from 5 food groups (see Table 24-1); calories, protein, vitamins, and minerals consumed daily.

i. Psychosocial status—emotional changes she is experiencing; woman's and family's reactions to present pregnancy; support system—family's and friends' willingness to provide support; woman's present coping with life-style changes caused by the pregnancy.

Laboratory Data

1. Urinalysis
    a. Urine is tested for glucose and protein.
    b. Glucose may be present in small amounts since the glomerular filtration rate is increased without the same increase in kidney tubular reabsorption.
    c. Protein in the urine should be reported since it may be a sign of a hypertensive disorder of pregnancy or renal problems.
    d. If the urine is cloudy and bacteria or leukocytes are present, a urine culture is done.
2. Blood—determination of hematocrit and hemoglobin levels, and description of the morphology of the red blood cells in an effort to find evidence of anemias such as sickle cell or Mediterranean anemia. Hemoglobin levels average 12 gm./dl.
3. Biochemical determinations—usually only glucose and urea nitrogen done; however, women with renal disorders may require estimation of total protein with albumin and globulin ratios.
4. Serologic tests
    a. Tests for syphilis (STS or VDRL) are usually done twice during pregnancy, on initial visit and at the beginning of the 3rd trimester.
    b. Rubella titre—immunity can be measured by a positive hemagglutination inhibition test.
    c. Blood type and Rh factor—if the woman is found to be Rh negative, the father's blood is typed; if he has Rh-positive blood, an antibody titre of the mother's blood is indicated.

Physical Examination

1. Ask the woman to empty her bladder before the examination so that during vaginal examination her uterus and pelvic organs may be readily palpated
2. Evaluate the woman's weight gain and blood pressure.
3. Examination of eyes, ears, and nose—nasal congestion during pregnancy may occur as a result of peripheral vasodilation.
4. Examination of the mouth, teeth, throat, and thyroid—gums may be hyperemic and softened because of increased progesterone.
5. Inspection of breasts and nipples—breasts may be enlarged and tender; nipple and areolar pigment may be darkened.
6. Auscultation of heart
7. Auscultation and percussion of the lungs
8. Abdominal examination
    a. Examination for scars or striations, diastasis (separation of the rectus muscle), or umbilical hernia.
    b. Palpation of the abdomen for height of the fundus (palpable after 13 weeks of pregnancy); measurement recorded and used as guideline for subsequent calculations (Fig. 24-5).
    c. Palpation of the abdomen for fetal outline and position—3rd trimester (see Fig. 25-5, p. 984).
    d. Fetal heart tone checked (heard by fetoscope at 20–24 weeks of gestation, earlier if a Doptone is used).
    e. Fetal position, presentation, and heart rate are recorded.

9. Pelvic examination
   a. Woman in lithotomy position.
   b. External genitalia inspected.
   c. Vaginal examination done to rule out abnormalities of the birth canal and to obtain cytologic smear (Papanicolaou and, if indicated, smears for gonorrhea, vaginal trichomoniasis, or candidiasis).
   d. Examination of the cervix for position, size, mobility, and consistency. Cervix is softened and bluish (increased vascularity) during pregnancy.
   e. Identification of the ovaries (size, shape, and position).
   f. Rectovaginal exploration to identify hemorrhoids, fissures, herniation, or masses.
   g. Evaluation of pelvic inlet—anteroposterior diameter by measuring the diagonal conjugate (see Fig. 24-3).
   h. Evaluation of midpelvis—prominence of the ischial spines.
   i. Evaluation of pelvic outlet—distance between ischial tuberosities and mobility of coccyx.

Subsequent Prenatal Assessments

Monthly visits are made for the first 7 months, then every 2 weeks, and weekly during the last month, providing that the woman's pregnancy is healthy.
1. Uterine growth and estimated fetal growth (Fig. 24-6).
   a. Fundus at symphysis pubis = 12 weeks' gestation
   b. Fundus at umbilicus = 20 weeks' gestation
   c. Fundus 28 cm. from top of symphysis pubis = 28 weeks' gestation
   d. Fundus at lower border of rib cage = 36 weeks' gestation

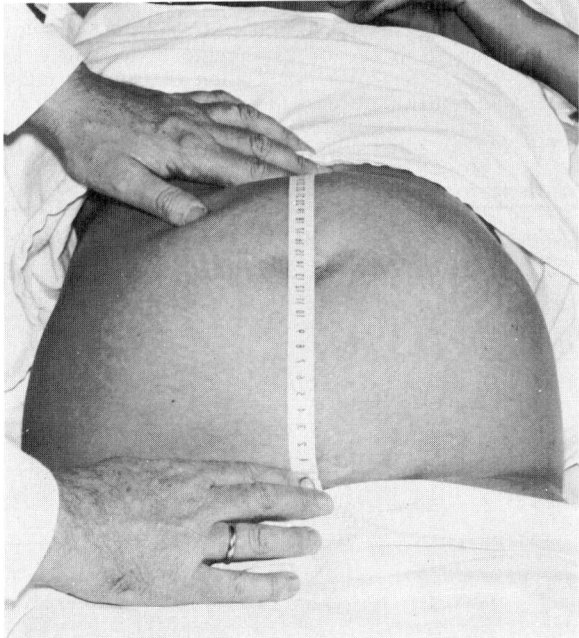

Figure 24-5. Measuring fundus-to-symphysis distance by McDonald's method. (Danforth DN [ed]. Obstetrics and Gynecology, 4th ed. Philadelphia, Harper & Row, 1982)

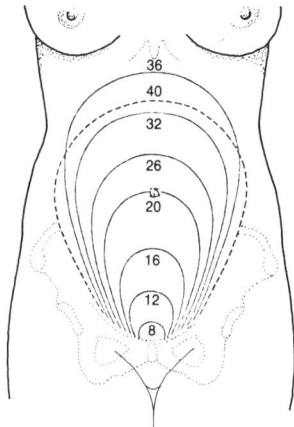

Figure 24-6. Height of fundus. (From Danforth DN [ed]. Obstetrics and Gynecology, 4th ed. Philadelphia, Harper and Row, 1982)

   e. Uterus becomes globular and drops = 40 weeks' gestation
2. A greater fundal height suggests:
   a. Multiple pregnancy
   b. Miscalculated due date
   c. Polyhydramnios (excessive amniotic fluid)
   d. Hydatidiform mole (degeneration of villi into grape-like clusters; fetus does not usually develop)
3. A lesser fundal height suggests:
   a. Intrauterine fetal growth retardation
   b. Error in estimating gestation
   c. Fetal or amniotic fluid abnormalities
   d. Intrauterine fetal death
4. Fetal heart tones—palpate abdomen for fetal position
   a. Normal—120–160 beats/minute
5. Weight—major increase in weight occurs during 2nd half of pregnancy; usually between 0.22 kg. (½ lb.)/week and 0.44 kg. (1 lb.)/week. Greater weight gain may indicate fluid retention and hypertensive disorder.
6. Blood pressure—should remain near woman's normal baseline.
7. Hemoglobin—checked at beginning of 3rd trimester.
8. Serology and smear or culture for gonorrhea at 36 weeks.
9. Urinalysis—for protein and glucose.
10. Edema—check for pretibial, facial, and hand edema.
11. Discomforts of pregnancy—fatigue, heartburn, hemorrhoids, backache.
12. Evaluate eating and sleeping patterns and general adjustment and coping with the pregnancy.
13. Evaluate concerns of the woman and her family.
14. Evaluate preparation for labor, delivery, and parenting.
15. Unusual reportable signs—have the woman report these at any time:
    a. Signs of hypertensive disorder—edema of face, hands, or fingers, persistent headache, fainting, blurred or double vision
    b. Signs of infection—chills, fever, pain when urinating
    c. Signs of possible abortion or labor—abdominal pain or cramps, bleeding or fluid loss from vagina
    d. Persistent vomiting

Patient Problems/Nursing Diagnoses

1. Problems related to physical alterations of pregnancy—fatigue, discomfort, nutritional intake, urinary frequency, mobility, constipation.
2. Problems related to psychosocial–sexual factors of pregnancy—body image, sexual functioning, life-style changes, coping, anxiety.
3. Knowledge deficit related to physical and psychosocial changes of pregnancy and preparation for parenthood.
4. Anxiety related to uncertainty about labor and delivery.

Planning and Implementation

Nursing Interventions: Health Teaching

A. Dealing with physical, psychosocial, and life-style changes

1. Teach the woman reasons for fatigue and have her plan a schedule for adequate rest.
   a. Fatigue in the 1st trimester is due to increased progesterone and its effects on the sleep center.
   b. Fatigue in the last trimester is due mainly to carrying increased weight of the pregnancy.
   c. About 8 hours of rest is needed at night.
   d. Inability to sleep may be due to excessive fatigue during day.
   e. In the latter months of pregnancy, sleeping on the side with a small pillow under the abdomen may enhance comfort.
   f. Frequent 15- to 30-minute rest periods during the day are important to avoid overfatigue.
   g. Whenever possible, the woman should work while sitting with her legs elevated.
   h. The woman should avoid standing for prolonged periods of time, especially during the 3rd trimester.
2. Help the woman plan for adequate exercise.
   a. In general, exercise during pregnancy should be in keeping with the woman's prepregnancy pattern and type of exercise.
   b. Activities or sports that have a risk of bodily harm (skiing, snowmobiling) should be avoided.

   c. During pregnancy, endurance during exercise may be decreased.
   d. Exercise classes for pregnant women that concentrate on toning and stretching have resulted in enhanced physical condition, increased self-esteem, and greater social support as a result of being in the exercise group.
3. Teach the woman the importance of good nutrition for herself and her fetus; have her plan good daily nutrition.
   a. Pregnancy increases the need for protein, vitamins A, D, E, and B complex, calcium, phosphorus, and iron (see Table 24-1).
   b. Review Table 24-2 with the mother, emphasizing the important function of these nutrients for her body and the fetus during pregnancy.
   c. Daily calorie requirements are approximately 300 calories in addition to the prepregnancy maintenance calories.
   d. According to her life-style, culture, income, and eating patterns, have the woman plan daily menus that include the following:
      (1) 4 Servings of protein foods
      (2) 4 Servings of milk or milk products
      (3) 3 Servings of grain products
      (4) 1 Serving of vitamin C-rich fruits and vegetables
      (5) 2 Servings of leafy green vegetables
      (6) 1 Serving of other fruits and vegetables
   e. Average weight gain in pregnancy is 24 lbs.: approximately 2 lbs. in 1st trimester, 11 lbs. in 2nd trimester, and 11 lbs. in 3rd trimester.
   f. Women in their teens need additional nutrients to meet their own growth needs as well as those imposed by pregnancy.
   g. Carefully evaluate the dietary intake of overweight or underweight women, as well as those of vegetarians.
   h. Caffeine intake should be limited to about 3 cups of coffee or its caffeine equivalent daily. Research on the association of caffeine intake and birth defects is inconclusive to date.

Table 24-1   Recommended Dietary Allowances of Selected Nutrients for Pregnancy and Lactation

Nutrients	11–14 Years (101 lb.—62 in.)	15–18 Years (120 lb.—64 in.)	19–22 Years (120 lb.—64 in.)	23–50 Years (120 lb.—64 in.)	Added for Pregnancy	Added for Lactation
Protein (gm.)	46	46	44	44	+30	+20
Fat-soluble vitamins						
Vitamin A (μg. RE)	800	800	800	800	+200	+400
Vitamin D (μg.)	10	10	7.5	5	+5	+5
Vitamin E (mg. αTE)	8	8	8	8	+2	+3
Water-soluble vitamins						
Vitamin C (mg.)	50	60	60	60	+20	+40
Thiamine (mg.)	1.1	1.1	1.1	1.0	+0.4	+0.5
Riboflavin (mg.)	1.3	1.3	1.3	1.2	+0.3	+0.5
Niacin mg NE	15	14	14	13	+2	+5
Vitamin B_6 (mg.)	1.8	2.0	2.0	2.0	+0.6	+0.5
Folacin (μg.)	400	400	400	400	+400	+100
Vitamin B_{12} (μg.)	3.0	3.0	3.0	3.0	+1.0	+1.0
Minerals						
Calcium (mg.)	1,200	1,200	800	800	+400	+400
Phosphorus (mg.)	1,200	1,200	800	800	+400	+400
Magnesium (mg.)	300	300	300	300	+150	+150
Iron (mg.)	18	18	18	18	30 to 60 mg. of supplemental iron is recommended	
Zinc (mg.)	15	15	15	15	+5	+10
Iodine (μg.)	150	150	150	150	+25	+50

(From Food and Nutrition Board, National Academy of Sciences—National Research Council, 1980)

i. Alcohol intake should be limited; no safe level of alcohol intake has been established; March of Dimes organization recommends eliminating alcohol during pregnancy.

j. Smoking should be eliminated or severely reduced during pregnancy; risk of spontaneous abortion, fetal death, birth of a low-birth-weight infant, and neonatal death increases directly with increasing levels of maternal smoking during pregnancy.

4. Discuss methods of achieving sexual satisfaction during pregnancy.
   a. There are no contraindications to intercourse or masturbation to orgasm provided the woman's membranes are intact, she has no history of premature labor, and the present pregnancy is uncomplicated. There are reports of orgasm resulting in the initiation of labor if the woman is within 3 weeks of term.
   b. Sexual activity may change in frequency because of maternal fatigue, physical discomfort, loss of interest, or difficulty finding comfortable positions for intercourse. Some women experience heightened sexual activity during the second trimester.
   c. The woman may find deep penile penetration uncomfortable.
   d. Female superior or side-lying positions are often more comfortable in the latter half of pregnancy.

5. Assist the woman in her employment planning.
   a. Generally there is no reason to stop working unless complications arise or there are hazards to the fetus in the work place.
   b. It is desirable to avoid severe physical strain and get adequate periods of rest.
   c. Use good body mechanics.
   d. Avoid toxic substances such as chlorinated hydrocarbons, lead, benzene, toluene, pesticides, mercury, and radioactive substances.
   e. Investigate policy on pregnancy and childbirth furloughs and benefits.
   f. Begin childcare planning if employment after birth is planned.

B. Minimizing common discomforts of pregnancy

1. Morning sickness—nausea, sometimes accompanied by vomiting, occurs frequently in the morning but may occur at any time.
   a. Cause unknown—hormonal changes believed to be a causative factor. Duration of morning sickness mirrors duration of elevated human chorionic gonadotropin (HCG) production. Emotional upsets and hypoglycemia also seen as contributing factors; self-limited to 1st trimester.
   b. Eating dry carbohydrates such as toast or crackers often helps.
   c. Eating frequent, small meals is helpful.
   d. Avoid heard-to-digest, greasy, pungent foods and odors.

2. Urinary frequency
   a. Cause—pressure of enlarging uterus on bladder.
   b. Course—usually subsides spontaneously by the 2nd or 3rd month when the uterus rises into the abdominal cavity; returns in the last weeks of pregnancy when the vertex drops into the pelvic cavity (engagement).

3. Heartburn
   a. Cause—pressure on stomach from enlarged uterus and decreased gastric motility results in a reflux of stomach contents in lower esophagus and a feeling of heartburn.
   b. Smaller, more frequent meals of foods easy to digest are helpful.
   c. Local antacids such as aluminum hydroxide gels soothe the mucosa and neutralize acid reflux.
   d. Avoid sodium bicarbonate since it results in absorption of excessive sodium and fluid retention.

4. Backache
   a. Cause—pregnant woman's center of gravity changes; as compensation she walks with head and shoulders backward, chest forward. This posture may produce lordosis and backache. Late in pregnancy, relaxation of pelvic joints exaggerates the problem.
   b. Standing tall, good posture, avoiding fatigue, and good body mechanics help.
   c. Wear comfortable, low-heeled shoes with good arch supports.
   d. Maternity girdle may help.
   e. Pelvic rocking exercises can provide relief.

5. Constipation
   a. Cause—decreased intestinal peristalsis due to pressure of gravid uterus and effects of progesterone.
   b. Additional fluid and dietary roughage will help.
   c. Adequate daily exercise is an aid.
   d. Establish regular patterns of elimination.
   e. If a laxative is necessary, prune juice, bulk-forming agents, stool softeners, or milk of magnesia are usually prescribed. Mineral oil interferes with absorption of fat-soluble vitamins.

6. Respiratory discomfort
   a. Cause—pressure of enlarged uterus on diaphragm.
   b. Spontaneous relief occurs with "lightening" (sensation of decreased abdominal distention caused by descent of fetus into pelvis) or with the birth of the baby.
   c. Provide relief by semi-Fowler's position arranged with pillow.
   d. Some relief obtained with good posture and standing tall.
   e. Eating small, frequent meals prevents increased pressure from full stomach.

7. Varicose veins—may affect lower extremities, vulva, pelvis, and anus.
   a. Cause—hereditary predisposition; pressure of gravid uterus on large veins; prolonged standing may be contributing factors.
   b. Rest frequently by sitting or lying with legs elevated.
   c. For leg varicosities, wear support hose and avoid constricting clothing.
   d. For vulvar varicosities, rest periodically with small pillow under buttocks to elevate pelvis.
   e. For anal varicosities (hemorrhoids)
      (1) Avoid constipation
      (2) Apply cold compresses with or without witch hazel
      (3) Avoid standing or sitting for prolonged periods—rest lying down
   f. Varicosities are totally or greatly resolved after delivery.

8. Leg cramps ("Charley horse")
   a. Cause unknown—fatigue, impaired circulation because of gravid uterus, impaired calcium absorption.

Table 24-2 Summary of Major Functions and Sources of Nutrients

	Function	Source	

Protein	Growth of fetus and accessory tissues
	Production of breast milk
		Animal protein
		  Meat
		  Fish
		  Poultry
		  Eggs
		  Milk
		  Cheese
			Vegetable protein
			  Dried beans
			  Dried peas
			  Lentils
			  Nuts
			  Peanut butter

Iron	Maintains hemoglobin level of mother
	Maintains mother's stores of iron
	Provides iron for fetal development
	Furnishes infant with iron stores needed for blood formation during neonatal period before food sources of iron are added to diet
		Good sources
		  Pork liver
		  Kidney
		  Beef liver
		  Oysters
		  Clams
		  Canned dried beans
		  Prune juice
		  Liverwurst
		  Heart
		  Lean pork
		  Lean beef
		  Raisins
		  Cooked dried beans
		  Cooked dried peaches
		  Cooked dried apricots
		  Cooked dried prunes
		  Canned green peas
			Fair sources
			  Enriched pastas
			  Spinach
			  Canned mackerel
			  Enriched white bread
			  Kale
			  Mustard greens
			  Whole wheat bread
			  Canned string beans
			  Eggs
			  Brussels sprouts
			  Broccoli

Calcium	Skeletal structures of the fetus
	Production of breast milk
	Blood coagulation, neuromuscular irritability, and muscle contractility
		Good sources
		  Skim milk
		  Buttermilk
		  Whole milk
		  Nonfat dry milk
		  Cheese
		  Ice milk
		  Ice cream
			Fair sources
			  Dark green leafy vegetables
			  Dried beans
			  Broccoli
			  Cottage cheese
			  Canned fish—including bones
			  Oranges

Vitamin A	Tooth formation
	Normal bone growth
	Healthy skin
	Vision—light/dark adaptation
		Vitamin A
		  Butter
		  Egg yolk
		  Fortified margarine
		  Kidney
		  Liver
		  Whole milk
		  Cream
			Carotenes
			  Dark green and deep yellow vegetables and a few fruits
			  Apricots
			  Broccoli
			  Cantaloupe
			  Carrots
			  Chard
			  Collards
			  Kale
			  Mustard greens
			  Persimmons
			  Spinach
			  Pumpkin
			  Sweet potatoes
			  Turnip greens
			  Winter squash

Riboflavin	Functions in number of enzyme systems in tissue respiration
	Metabolism of amino acids and carbohydrates
		Good sources
		  Heart
		  Kidney
		  Liver
		  Milk
		  Ice milk
			Fair sources
			  Broccoli
			  Cheese
			  Dark green leafy vegetables
			  Eggs
			  Ice cream
			  Lean meat
			  Poultry

Thiamine	Maintains normal appetite and digestion
	Maintains health of nervous system
	Completion of carbohydrates
		Good sources
		  Whole grain and enriched bread
		  Whole grain and enriched cereals
		  Dried peas
		  Dried beans
		  Oranges
		  Liver
		  Heart
		  Kidney
		  Lean pork
		  Nuts
		  Potatoes
		  Peas
		  Wheat germ
			Fair sources
			  Eggs
			  Fish
			  Meat
			  Poultry
			  Milk
			  Many vegetables

Niacin	Helps translate sources of energy into usable form	Good sources
		  Fish
		  Heart
		  Lean meat
		  Liver
		  Peanuts
		  Peanut butter
		  Poultry
			Fair sources
			  Milk
			  Potatoes
			  Whole grain and enriched bread
			  Whole grain and enriched cereal

Table 24-2 Summary of Major Functions and Sources of Nutrients (continued)

	Function	Source	

Ascorbic acid	Production of intercellular substances necessary for the development and maintenance of normal connective tissue in bones, cartilage, and muscles
	Improves health of bones and teeth
	Increases absorption of iron
		Good sources
		  Citrus fruits or juice
		  Broccoli
		  Brussels sprouts
		  Cantaloupe
		  Greens—collards, mustard, turnip
		  Peppers
			Fair sources
			  Asparagus
			  Cabbage, raw
			  Cauliflower
			  Chile, fresh or canned
			  Kale
			  Liver
			  Other melons
			  Potatoes or sweet potatoes in jackets
			  Spinach
			  Tomatoes or prunes

Vitamin D	Promotes absorption and retention of calcium and phosphorus necessary for growth and formation of bones and teeth	Butter Egg yolk Fish oils Liver Milk fortified with Vitamin D Other foods may contain added vitamin D—check labels	

(Cross AT and Walsh HE. Prenatal diet counseling. J Reproductive Med)

b. Frequent rest periods with legs elevated may be helpful.
c. Adequate calcium intake may decrease the incidence.
d. For immediate relief, push toes upward while applying pressure to the knee to straighten the leg.

9. Leg and ankle edema
   a. Cause—pressure of gravid uterus impeding venous and lymphatic return.
   b. Rest frequently with legs elevated.
   c. Combined with facial and finger edema may be signs of hypertensive disorder of pregnancy.

10. Vaginal discharge
    a. Increased vaginal discharge is common in pregnancy. Increased hygiene (washing) is important.
    b. Green, yellow, foul-smelling, or bloody discharge may indicate infection or other complication—see midwife or physician.

11. Tender breasts and nipple irritation
    a. Wear well-fitting supporting brassiere.
    b. Wash breasts and nipples with water only.
    c. Nipple rolling 3 times a day (between thumb and forefingers) and drying nipples with a rough towel daily may toughen nipples for breast-feeding.
    d. Lanolin creams applied to nipples help minimize irritations from colostrum and clothing.

C. **Reducing anxiety and preparing for upcoming labor and delivery**

a. Have the woman/couple discuss perceptions and expectations of labor and delivery process.
   a. Labor coach and/or family members present during labor and delivery
   b. Use of birthing room
   c. Position for delivery
   d. Type of anesthesia, if needed
2. Encourage the couple to attend childbirth education classes.
3. Have the woman/couple tour labor and delivery area and meet staff.
4. Discuss value of breathing exercises as another tool for coping with labor—encourage their practice and use (see p. 990).

5. Have the woman identify when to come to the birthing center or hospital (primigravida—when contractions are 5–10 minutes apart; multigravida—when contractions have established a regular pattern).
6. The woman also knows signs of complications during pregnancy (see p. 965).

D. **Preparing for parenthood**
1. Have the woman/couple discuss perceptions and expectations of new parenthood.
   a. Perceptions of their "idealized child"
   b. Perceptions and expectations of infant's sleeping, eating, activity, and response patterns
   c. Expectations of returning to work and child-care arrangements when appropriate; babysitters for evenings or hours out.
2. Physical preparations for the newborn—crib or other place to sleep, clothing, blankets, bathing equipment, feeding equipment
3. Help the woman/couple plan for time for themselves and each other apart from the newborn.

Evaluation

Expected Outcomes
1. Understands reason for fatigue, establishes and follows a schedule for adequate rest, and avoids tiring activities such as standing for long periods
2. Engages in prescribed program of exercise
3. Understands the essentials of good nutrition during pregnancy; follows adequate diet for self and fetus, including proper intake of protein, milk products, grains, vegetables, and fruits
4. Avoids potentially harmful substances such as alcohol, cigarettes, and excessive caffeine
5. Is aware of impact of pregnancy on sexual functioning and becomes informed of means of achieving sexual satisfaction
6. Learns and practices means of dealing with physical discomforts of pregnancy—morning sickness, urinary frequency, backache, constipation, varicosities, leg cramps, edema, breast tenderness
7. Couple prepares for upcoming labor and delivery by discussing expectation of labor and delivery, attending childbirth classes, and preparing for life-style changes to result from presence of new baby in the home

The Fetus

In the past, methods used to determine how well the fetus was growing and maturing consisted of evaluating uterine growth and listening to fetal heart sounds. During the last 25 years, advances in knowledge and technology have provided newer methods for assessing fetal well-being, including ultrasound, amniocentesis, additional laboratory tests, and fetal monitoring. These advances have made possible the diagnosis of abnormalities and multiple pregnancies, and interventions such as intrauterine blood transfusions and fetal surgery.

Fetal Growth and Development (Fig. 24-7)

A. 1st Lunar Month (fertilization—2 weeks of embryonic growth)

1. Implantation is complete.
2. Primary chorionic villi forming.
3. Embryo develops into 2 cell layers (bilaminar embryonic disc).
4. Amniotic cavity appears.

B. 2nd Lunar Month (3–6 weeks of embryonic growth)

1. At the end of 6 weeks of growth, the embryo is approximately 12 mm. long.
2. Arm and leg buds are visible; arm buds are more developed with finger ridges beginning to appear.
3. Rudiments of the eyes, ears, and nose appear.
4. Lung buds are developing.
5. Primitive intestinal tract is developing.
6. Primitive cardiovascular system is functioning.
7. Neural tube, which forms the brain and spinal cord, closes by the 4th week.

C. 3rd Lunar Month (7–10 weeks of growth)

1. At the end of 10 weeks of growth, the fetus is 61 mm. from crown to rump and weighs 14 gm.
2. The middle of this period (8 weeks) marks the end of the embryonic period and the beginning of the fetal period.
3. Appearance of external genitalia.
4. By the middle of this month, all major organ systems have formed.
5. The membrane over the anus has broken down.
6. The heart has formed 4 chambers (by 7th week).
7. The fetus assumes a human appearance.
8. Bone ossification begins.
9. Rudimentary kidney begins to secrete urine.

D. 4th Lunar Month (11- to 14-week-old fetus)

1. At the end of 14 weeks of growth, the fetus is 120 mm. crown–rump length and 110 gm.
2. Head erect; lower extremities well developed.
3. Hard palate and nasal septum have fused.
4. External genitalia of male and female can now be differentiated.
5. Eyelids are sealed.

E. 5th Lunar Month (15- to 18-week-old fetus)

1. At the end of 18 weeks of growth, the fetus is 160 mm. crown–rump length and 320 gm.
2. Ossification of fetal skeleton can be seen on x-ray.
3. Ears stand out from head.
4. Meconium is present in the intestinal tract.
5. Fetus makes sucking motions and swallows amniotic fluid.

6. Fetal movements may be felt by the mother (end of month).

F. 6th Lunar Month (19- to 22-week-old fetus)

1. At the end of 22 weeks of growth, the fetus is 210 mm. crown–rump length and 630 gm.
2. Vernix caseosa covers the skin.
3. Head and body (lanugo) hair visible.
4. Skin is wrinkled and red.
5. Brown fat, an important site of heat production, is present in neck and sternal area.
6. Nipples are apparent on the breasts.

G. 7th Lunar Month (23- to 26-week-old fetus)

1. At the end of 26 weeks of growth, the fetus is 250 mm. crown–rump length and 1,000 gm.
2. Fingernails present.
3. Lean body.
4. Eyes partially open; eyelashes present.
5. Bronchioles are present; primitive alveoli are forming.
6. Skin begins to thicken on hands and feet.
7. Startle reflex present; grasp reflex is strong.

H. 8th Lunar Month (27- to 30-week-old fetus)

1. At the end of 30 weeks of growth, the fetus is 280 mm. crown–rump length and 1,700 gm.
2. Eyes open.
3. Ample hair on head; lanugo begins to fade.
4. Skin slightly wrinkled.
5. Toenails present.
6. Testes in inguinal canal, begin descent to scrotal sac.
7. Surfactant coats much of the alveolar epithelium.

I. 9th Lunar Month (31- to 34-week-old fetus)

1. At the end of 34 weeks of growth, the fetus is about 320 mm. crown–rump length and 2,500 gm.
2. Fingernails reach fingertips.
3. Skin pink and smooth.
4. Testes in scrotal sac.

J. 10th Lunar Month (35- to 38-week-old fetus; end of this month is also 40 weeks from onset of last menstrual period)

1. End of 38 weeks of growth, fetus is about 360 mm. crown–rump length and 3,400 gm.
2. Ample subcutaneous fat.
3. Lanugo almost absent.
4. Toenails reach toe tips.
5. Testes in scrotum.
6. Vernix caseosa mainly on the back.
7. Breasts are firm.

Alternate Means of Fertilization

A. In Vitro Fertilization

Used when a woman's uterine tubes are damaged or obstructed and transport of a fertilized egg to the uterus is not possible.

1. The woman is often given infertility drugs such as clomiphene citrate (Clomid) or menotropins (Pergonal) to stimulate ovulation.
2. The ovary is punctured via laparoscopy and mature follicles are removed by suction.
3. Each egg is placed in a mixture of salts, sugars, and proteins designed to simulate the maternal fluids found in the uterine tubes.

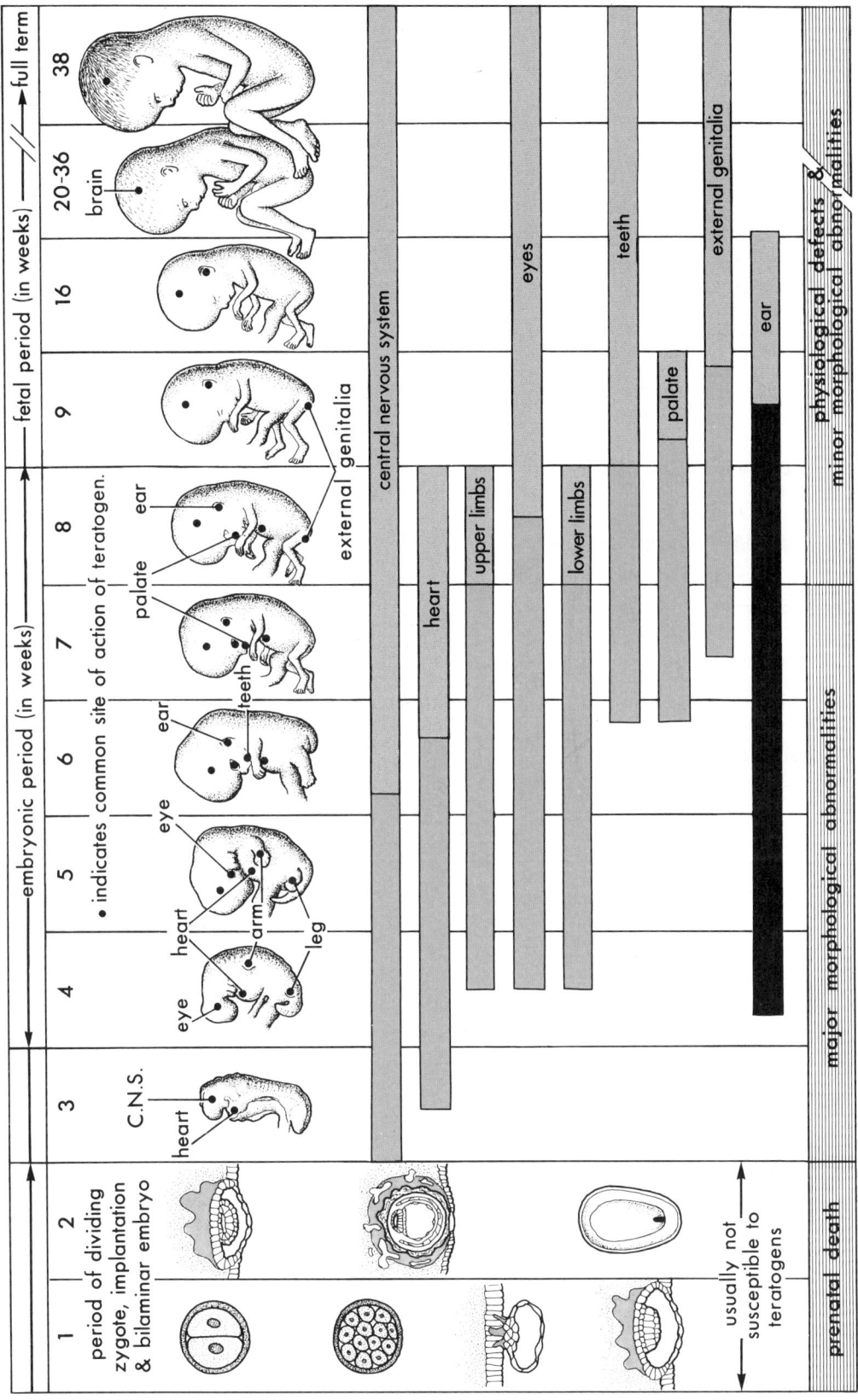

Figure 24-7. Schematic illustration of the sensitive or critical periods in human development. During the first 2 weeks of development, the embryo is usually not susceptible to teratogens. During these predifferentiation stages, a substance either damages all or most of the cells of the embryo, resulting in its death, or damages only a few cells, allowing the embryo to recover without developing defects. The left (shaded) sides of the bars denote highly sensitive periods; the right sides indicate stages that are less sensitive to teratogens. (From Moore KL. The Developing Human: Clinically Oriented Embryology. 3rd ed. Philadelphia, WB Saunders, 1982)

4. Following several hours of incubation to maturity, semen is added and the egg and fluids are again incubated for several hours. If the egg is fertilized, it is incubated further until it begins division. At this stage, the fertilized egg is deposited in the woman's uterus via a thin plastic catheter.

B. Embryo Transplants

Used when the woman is not capable of producing normal mature follicles, but the male partner is fertile.

1. Through hormonal therapy, the menstrual cycles of the donor woman and the recipient woman are synchronized.
2. Sperm of the fertile husband is artificially inseminated in a fertile donor woman following her normal ovulation.
3. If fertilization occurs, several days later the fertilized egg is washed from the donor woman's uterus.
4. The fertilized egg is then deposited in the uterus of the wife who was incapable of producing a normal mature follicle. If successful, implantation occurs soon afterward.

Fetal Circulation—Before and After Birth

(See chart below and Fig. 24-8.)

Assessment of Fetal Maturity and Well-Being

Maternal History and Exam

A. History

1. The woman's general health
2. History of current pregnancy and identified risk factors
3. Health during previous pregnancies
4. Outcome of previous pregnancies

Estimation of Fundal Height

(See p. 965).

Fetal Heart Tones

1. Can be heard using a fetal stethoscope (fetoscope) after 20 weeks' fetal gestation
2. Can be heard using techniques that amplify sounds (Doppler) at approximately 10 weeks' fetal gestation
3. Rate—between 120 and 160 beats/minute
4. In latter months of pregnancy, fetal heart sounds found:
   a. Near the woman's midline in fetal occipitoanterior positions
   b. Lateral to midline in fetal occipitotransverse positions
   c. In the woman's flank in fetal occipitoposterior positions
   d. Below the woman's umbilicus in cephalic presentations
   e. At or above the woman's umbilicus in breech presentations
5. Failure to hear fetal heart sounds may be due to maternal obesity, polyhydramnios (excessive amniotic fluid), miscalculated EDC (expected date of confinement) or fetal death.

Ultrasound

1. Uses reflected soundwaves as they travel in tissue to produce a picture.
2. Can identify a pregnancy as early as 5 weeks of embryonic growth; at 7 weeks, fetal parts can be recognized.
3. Used also to detect multiple pregnancy, fetal abnormalities, hydatiform mole, fetal death, fetal presentation, placental position, and fetal weight.
4. Used to determine fetal maturity using biparietal diameter (BPD) of fetal head. BPD of >0.92 cm. has been correlated with mature fetal lungs.
5. Since fetal head growth can vary, ultrasound is used to determine BPD of fetal head and thoracic diameter; in times of stress, head growth is spared and body

Structure	Before Birth	After Birth
Unique to Fetal Circulation		
Umbilical vein	Brings arterial blood to liver and heart	Obliterated; becomes the ligamentum teres
Umbilical arteries	Brings arteriovenous blood to the placenta	Intra-abdominal portion becomes medial umbilical ligaments; proximal portion persists as superior vesical arteries
Ductus venosus	Shunts arterial blood into inferior vena cava	Obliterated; becomes ligamentum venosum
Ductus arteriosus	Shunts arterial and some venous blood from the pulmonary artery to the aorta	Obliterated; becomes ligamentum arteriosum
Foramen ovale	Opening between right and left atrium	Closes
General Structures		
Lungs	Contain no air and very little blood	Filled with air and well-supplied with blood
Pulmonary arteries	Bring little blood to lungs	Bring much blood to lungs
Aorta	Receives blood from both ventricles	Receives blood from left ventricle only
Inferior vena cava	Because of ductus arteriosus, contains only venous blood from body and arterial blood from placenta	Contains venous only blood, which passes to right atrium

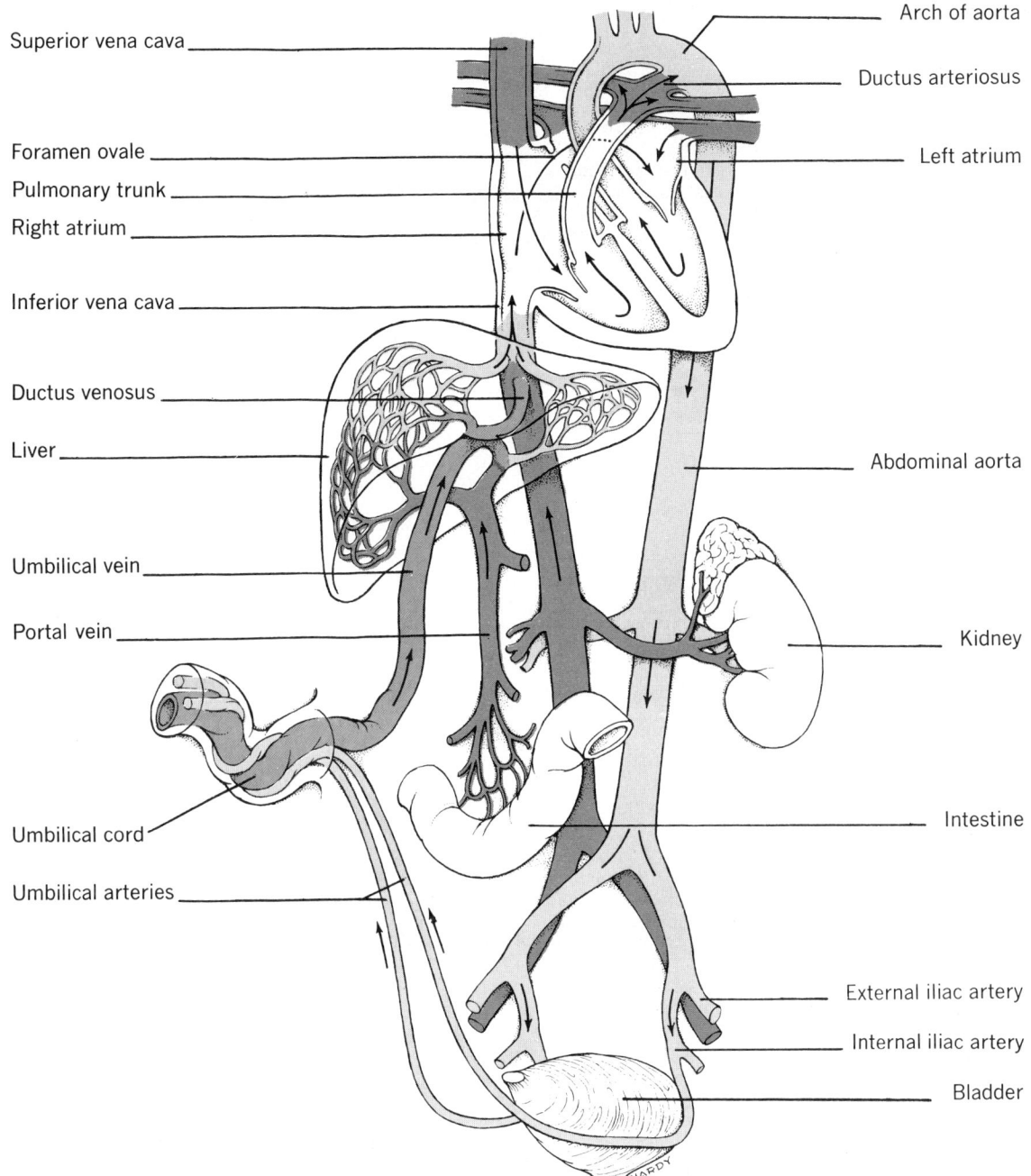

Superior vena cava

Foramen ovale

Pulmonary trunk

Right atrium

Inferior vena cava

Ductus venosus

Liver

Umbilical vein

Portal vein

Umbilical cord

Umbilical arteries

Arch of aorta

Ductus arteriosus

Left atrium

Abdominal aorta

Kidney

Intestine

External iliac artery

Internal iliac artery

Bladder

Figure 24-8. Diagram of the fetal circulation shortly before birth. Course of blood is indicated by arrows.

wasting occurs, therefore abdominal transverse diameter or abdominal circumference is an important measure. Head/abdomen (H/A) ratios are also used. An H/A ratio below 1.0 has been correlated with gestations greater than 36 weeks.

6. Portable ultrasound (real-time imaging) can be used to visualize the fetus in motion (e.g., breathing movements, cardiac activity including activity of the heart valves and chambers, swallowing, and fetal motion).

Amniotic Fluid Studies (Amniocentesis)

Amniocentesis is a procedure in which amniotic fluid is removed from the uterine cavity by insertion of a needle through the abdominal and uterine walls and into the amniotic sac.

A. Determination of Fetal Maturity

1. Lecithin/sphingomyelin (L/S) ratio measures the maturity of the fetal lung.
   a. When the ratio of lecithin to sphingomyelin is 2:1 or greater, the fetal lung is considered mature and the incidence of respiratory distress syndrome in the newborn is low.
   b. May have false mature L/S ratios in some maternal conditions such as maternal diabetes.
   c. A rapid foam test, mixing amniotic fluid and ethanol, is also used to determine the presence of mature L/S ratios. Adequate amounts of lecithin are present when a stable foam ring forms and remains on top of the solution after vigorous shaking.
2. Presence of phosphatidyl glycerol (PG) indicates fetal lung maturity.
   a. PG is an important phospholipid which functions to stabilize lecithin in the fetal alveoli of the lung.
   b. The presence of PG may be a more accurate predictor of lung function than the L/S ratio.
3. Creatinine
   a. Used in conjunction with other measures such as L/S ratio to indicate fetal maturity.
   b. Levels increase after 34 weeks' gestation; levels in excess of 2.0 mg./100 ml. correlate with gestational ages over 37 weeks.
   c. Concentration depends on fetal muscle mass, kidney excretion, amniotic fluid volume, and maternal serum levels. Misleadingly high levels are found in women with impaired renal function.
4. Fat cells
   A 20% fat cell count has been used to indicate fetal maturity. Fat cells increase in amniotic fluid after 36 weeks' gestation.

B. Determination of Fetal Well-Being

1. Bilirubin—generally very little bilirubin is found after 36 weeks' gestation. An increase in bilirubin levels occurs with hemolytic disease. When used to determine fetal maturity, optical density (OD) measure of OD 650 ≥ 0.15 have been correlated with mature fetuses and low incidence of respiratory distress syndrome.
2. Alpha-fetoprotein—major plasma protein of early fetuses; levels decrease rapidly in amniotic fluid after 13 weeks' gestation; increased levels are found in fetuses with spina bifida, anencephaly, and other neural tube defects.
3. Estriol—levels increase as pregnancy progresses. Levels that drop 40%–50% or more in 1 week signify danger to the fetus. Serum determination or 24-hour urinary levels can be used.
4. Karyotyping and cell enzyme studies—used to determine sex of the fetus, normalcy of the chromosomes, and presence or lack of enzymes found in some inherited disorders. Sex determination is important in sex-linked disorders such as hemophilia and severe immune deficiencies. Evaluation of chromosomes is important when trisomy 21 (Down's syndrome), trisomy 18, and other chromosomal problems are suspected. Enzyme evaluation is important when galactosemia, Lesch–Nyhan syndrome, Tay–Sachs disease, and other conditions are suspected.

C. Nursing Interventions During Amniocentesis

1. Reduce anxiety related to the procedure.
   a. Reduce the parents' anxiety by determining their understanding of the procedure and the meaning it holds for them.
   b. Explain the procedure before it begins and answer any questions they have.
   c. Provide explanations during the procedure; correct misinformation they may have; make sure they know when the results will be available and how they may obtain the results as soon as possible.
2. Reduce pain and discomfort related to the procedure.
   a. Reduce discomfort by having the mother lie comfortably on her back with her hands and a pillow under her head. Relaxation breathing may help.
   b. Ensure adequate time between infiltration of local anesthetic and introduction of needle into the amniotic sac.
3. Reduce potential for traumatic injury to fetus, placenta, or maternal structures.
   a. Have the woman empty her bladder if the fetus is more than 20 weeks' gestation to avoid injury to the woman's bladder. If the fetus is less than 20 weeks' gestation, the woman's full bladder will hold the uterus steady and out of the pelvis. The placenta is localized via ultrasound.
   b. Obtain vital signs, including fetal heart rate to serve as a baseline to evaluate possible complications.
   c. Monitor the woman during and following the procedure for signs of premature labor or bleeding.
   d. Tell the woman to report signs of bleeding, unusual fetal activity or abdominal pain, cramping, or fever while at home following the procedure.

Chorionic Villus Biopsy

Used to obtain samples of chorionic villi (tissue of fetal origin) to test for genetic disorders in the fetus.
1. Using an ultrasound picture, a catheter is passed vaginally into the woman's uterus, where a sample of chorionic villous tissue is snipped off or obtained by suction.
2. Samples can be obtained earlier in pregnancy than can fetal cells obtained via amniocentesis. Biopsy is performed between 8 and 12 weeks of pregnancy.

Assay of Maternal Urine

1. Estriol levels (24-hour urine specimens)
   a. Provide information on fetal, placental, and maternal-renal function. The biosynthesis of estriol by the placenta depends on precursor substances produced in the fetal adrenal gland.
   b. Levels found in a 24-hour urine specimen are influenced by length of gestation, fetal and placental size, multiple pregnancy, maternal renal function, and adequacy of urine collection.
   c. Since there is considerable variation in amount of excretion by different women, serial testing is done rather than a single 24-hour sample.
   d. Levels of estriol that drop between 40% and 50% within 1 week signify danger to the fetus.

Assay of Maternal Serum

1. Plasma estriol levels may be measured.
2. Maternal serum may be analyzed for alpha-fetoprotein levels. Increased levels are associated with Rh and ABO maternal immunization, fetoplacental dysfunction, and fetal neural tube defects.

Nonstress Test (NST)

1. Used to evaluate fetal heart rate accelerations that normally occur in response to fetal activity in a fetus in good condition.
2. *Indications*—women with prolonged pregnancies, diabetes, hypertensive disorders, abnormal estriol levels, a history of stillbirths, or poor pregnancy outcomes.
3. Nursing Interventions
   a. Place woman in semi-Fowler's position in bed; external fetal and uterine monitoring is performed.
   b. Make mark on monitoring paper each time fetal movement is felt.
   c. Evaluate response of fetal heart rate immediately following fetal activity.
   d. Monitor mother's blood pressure and uterine activity for deviations during procedure.
4. *Interpretation*—test period should be a minimum of 40 minutes to allow for fetal rest cycle patterns.
   a. *Reactive*—fetal heart rate increased by 15 beats/minute above baseline in response to fetal activity. To label fetal heart rate reactive, 5 such responses should be obtained during a 20-minute recording.
   b. *Nonreactive*—fetal heart rate does not increase with fetal movements, or fewer than 5 such responses are found within a 20-minute recording. Test period is usually extended to allow for fetal rest cycles.

Oxytocin Challenge Test (OCT) or Contraction Stress Test (CST)

1. Used to evaluate the ability of the fetus to withstand the stress of uterine contractions as would occur during labor. The test is generally used after 34 weeks' gestation; used with decreasing frequency since it may stress an already stressed fetus.
2. *Indications*—usually used when a woman has a nonreactive or abnormal nonstress test. In this situation, should a woman have a positive OCT, it indicates placental dysfunction placing the fetus at risk. Used with women who have diabetes, prolonged pregnancy, hypertensive disorders, history of previous stillbirth, abnormal estriol values, or other evidence of potential fetal distress.
3. *Contraindications*—women with previous cesarean birth, 3rd trimester bleeding, multiple gestations, incompetent cervix, or premature rupture of membranes.
4. Nursing Interventions
   a. Place the woman in semi-Fowler's position.
   b. Conduct external fetal and uterine monitoring for 30 minutes to establish baselines of fetal and uterine activity.
   c. Intravenous dilute oxytocin is administered via an infusion pump.
   d. The dose of oxytocin is increased every 15 minutes until the woman has 3 uterine contractions within a 10-minute period.
5. *Interpretation*
   a. Negative test—three contractions of good quality and duration without late decelerations or other ominous responses of the fetal heart rate. Indicates adequate placental sufficiency.
   b. Positive test—occurrence of late or other ominous responses of the fetal heart rate in response to the uterine contraction; indicates placental insufficiency in response to the stress of a uterine contraction.

Fetoscopy

The insertion of a fiberoptic instrument into the uterine cavity to visually examine the fetus or to obtain blood, placental or tissue samples for identification and diagnosis of:

1. Congenital anomalies or teratogenic-induced malformations
2. Hemoglobinopathies such as sickle cell anemia and beta-thalassemia
3. Sex-linked autosomal abnormalities or neural tube disorders
4. Metabolic disorders

Other Studies

A. Amnioscopy

The insertion of a fiberoptic instrument into the woman's cervical canal to visualize the amniotic fluid for the presence of blood or meconium.

B. X-Ray

Has been used to determine fetal maturity based on epiphyseal centers of ossification, the size of the fetal skull, fetal length, multiple pregnancy, fetal death, hydrocephalus, and fetal edema found in hydrops fetalis. Currently the use of x-ray to determine fetal maturity has been largely replaced by the use of ultrasound, thus avoiding exposure to radiation for fetus and mother.

In Utero Fetal Surgery

1. Used to correct malformations through hysterotomy in which the fetus may be brought partially out of the uterus, operated upon, and replaced in the uterus, or through fetoscopy in utero.
2. Used to correct malformations such as congenital hydronephrosis, obstructive hydrocephalus, and neural tube defects.
3. Used when delivery of the fetus or other treatment is not yet possible and further normal growth and development is not possible.
4. Complications include uterine damage, hemorrhage, and premature delivery.

Assessment of Fetal Presentation and Position

As pregnancy progresses, it becomes important to determine the presentation and position of the fetus in relation to the mother's pelvis (Fig. 24-9). In approximately 95% of all births, the fetal head presents first, making its landmarks very important.

General Terms

1. *Lie*—a comparison of the long axis of the fetus with the long axis of the mother. Fetal lie is either longitudinal or transverse. In a longitudinal lie either the fetal head presents (cephalic) or the buttocks presents (breech). In a transverse lie, the shoulder presents.
2. *Presentation*—the part of the fetus deepest in the birth canal. Presentation may be vertex, face, brow, breech, or shoulder.
3. *Presenting part*—portion of the fetus deepest in the birth canal and felt on vaginal examination.

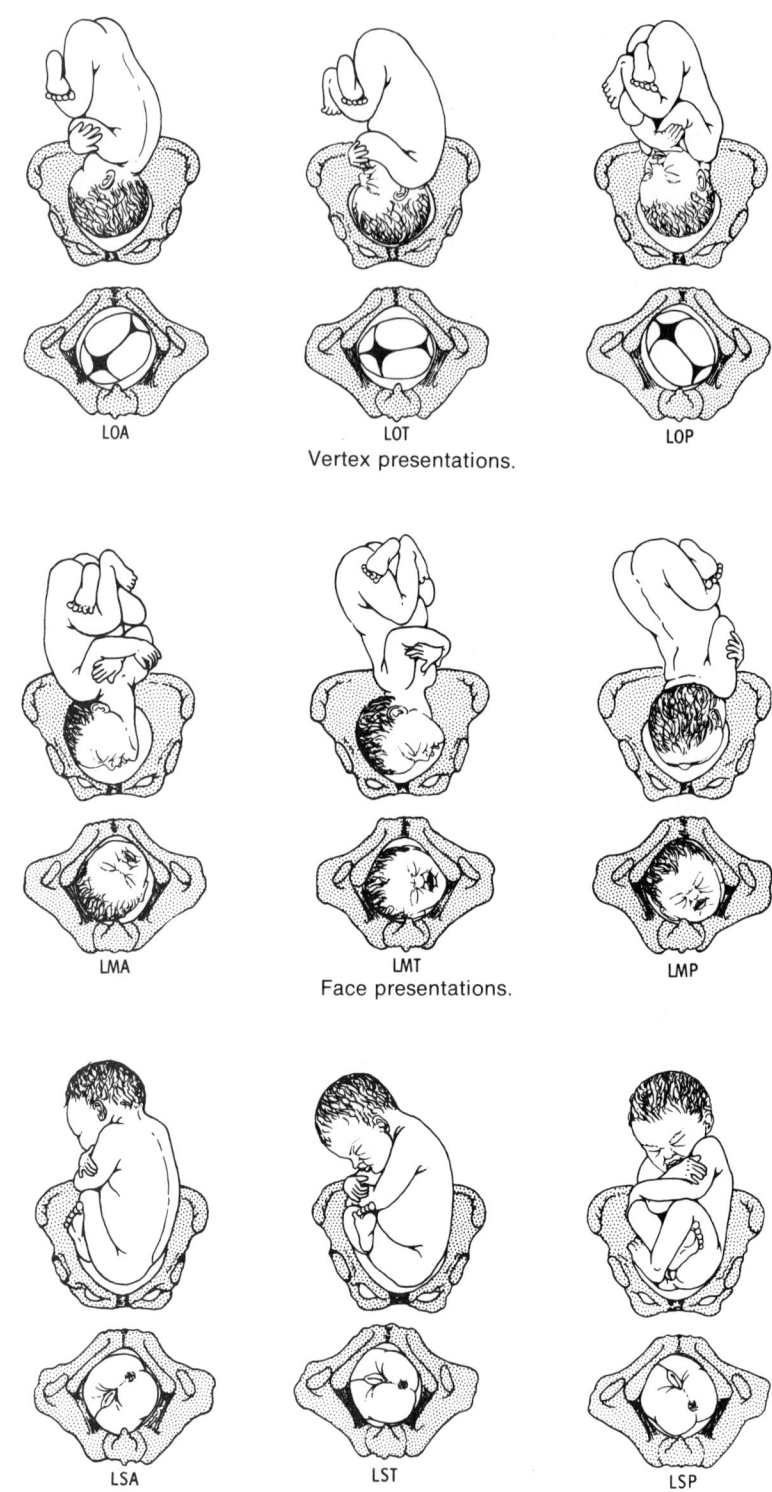

Figure 24-9. Fetal presentations. (From Benson RC. Handbook of Obstetrics and Gynecology. Los Altos, CA, Lange Medical Publications)

4. *Attitude*—relationship of fetal parts to each other.
5. *Position*—relationship of landmark on the fetal presenting part to the front (anterior = A), back (posterior = P), or side (transverse = T) of the mother's pelvis.

Landmarks on the fetal presenting parts include head = occiput (O); buttocks = sacrum (S); shoulder = scapula or acromion (A); face = chin or mentum (m).

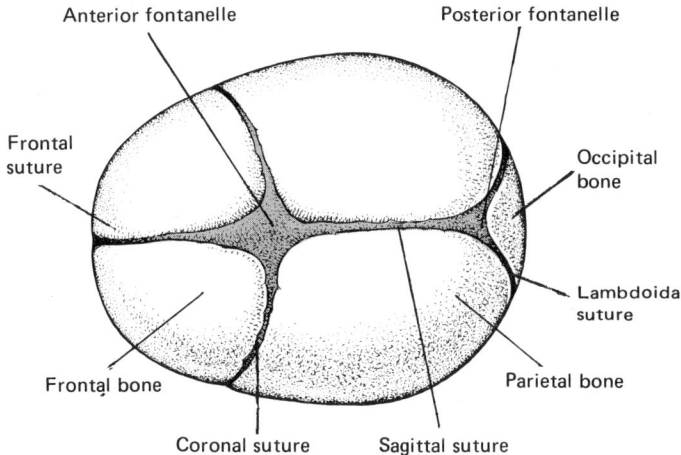

Anterior fontanelle

Posterior fontanelle

Frontal
suture

Occipital
bone

Lambdoidal
suture

Frontal bone

Parietal bone

Coronal suture

Sagittal suture

FIGURE 29-8. *Fetal skull.*

Figure 24-10. *Fetal skull.*

Fetal Head

(See Fig. 24-10)

A. Bones of the Fetal Skull

1. Occipital bone posteriorly
2. 2 Parietal bones on the sides
3. 2 Temporal bones anteriorly
4. 2 Frontal bones anteriorly

B. Sututes of the Fetal Skull—membranous spaces between the bones of the fetal skull

1. Frontal suture—between the 2 frontal bones
2. Sagittal—between the 2 parietal bones

3. Coronal—between the frontal and parietal bones
4. Lambdoid—between the back of the parietal bones and the margin of the occipital bone

C. Fontanelles—irregular spaces formed where 2 or more sutures meet. Sutures and fontanelles allow fetal skull bones to overlap in order to pass through the maternal pelvis.

1. Anterior fontanelle—junction of the sagittal, frontal, and coronal sutures—closes by 18 months of age.
2. Posterior fontanelle—located where the sagittal suture meets the lambdoidal (smaller than anterior)—closes at 6–8 weeks of age.

Bibliography

Books

Pregnancy

Alouf FE and Barglow P. Sexual counseling for the pregnant and postpartum patient. In JJ Sciarra et al (ed). Gynecology and Obstetrics, Vol. 2. Hagerstown, Harper & Row, 1981

Berkowitz RL, Couston DR and Mochizuki TK. Handbook for Prescribing Medications During Pregnancy. Boston, Little, Brown & Co, 1981

Bradley RA. Husband-Coached Childbirth, 3rd ed. New York, Harper & Row, 1981

Bullough VL and Bullough B. Health Care of the Other Americans. New York, Appleton-Century-Crofts, 1982

Butnarescu GF, Tillotson DM and Villarreal PP. Assessment of Reproductive Risk in Perinatal Nursing, Vol. 2. New York, John Wiley & Sons, 1980

Danforth DH (ed). Obstetrics and Gynecology, 4th ed. Philadelphia, Harper & Row, 1982

Evaneshko V. Tonawanda Seneca childbearing culture. In MA Kay (ed). Anthropology of Human Birth. Philadelphia, FA Davis, 1982

Food and Nutrition Board. Recommended Dietary Allowances. Washington, DC, National Academy of Sciences, National Research Council, 1980

Friedman MM. Family Nursing Theory and Assessment. New York, Appleton-Century-Crofts, 1981

Horn BM. Northwest coast Indians: The Muckleshoot. In MA Kay (ed). Anthropology of Human Birth. Philadelphia, FA Davis, Company, 1982

Lion EM (ed). Human Sexuality in Nursing Process. New York, John Wiley & Sons, 1982

Pritchard J and MacDonald P. Williams Obstetrics, 16th ed. New York, Appleton-Century-Crofts, 1980

Quilligan E and Kretchmer N. Fetal and Maternal Medicine. New York, John Wiley & Sons, 1980

The Alan Guttmacher Institute. 1981. Teen Pregnancy: The Problem That Hasn't Gone Away. New York, 1981

The Fetus

Babson S, et al. Diagnosis and Management of the Fetus and Neonate at Risk. St Louis, CV Mosby, 1980

Burrow G, and Ferris T. Medical Complications During Pregnancy. Philadelphia, WB Saunders, 1982

Korones S. High-Risk Newborn Infants. St Louis, CV Mosby, 1981

Moore K. The Developing Human: Clinically Oriented Embryology, 3rd ed. Philadelphia, WB Saunders, 1982

Niswander K. Obstetrics. Boston, Little, Brown & Co, 1981

Pritchard J and MacDonald P. Williams Obstetrics, 16th ed. New York, Appleton-Century-Crofts, 1980

Quilligan E and Kretchmer N. Fetal and Maternal Medicine. New York, John Wiley & Sons, 1980

Schuster C and Ashburn S. The Process of Human Development. Boston, Little, Brown & Co, 1980

Articles

Pregnancy

Alley N. Morning sickness: The client's perspective. JOGN Nurs 1984 May–Jun; 13(3):185–189

Andersen R et al. Access to medical care among the Hispanic population of Southwestern United States. J Health Soc Behav 1981 Mar; 22(1):78–89

Artinian B. Collaborative planning of patient care in the prenatal, labor and delivery, and neonatal setting. JOGN Nurs 1984 Mar–Apr; 13(2):105–110

Ashley MJ. Alcohol use during pregnancy: A challenge for the 80's. Can Med Assoc J 1981 Jul 15; 125(2): 141–143

Baldwin W. Adolescent pregnancy and childbearing: An overview. Semin Perinatol 1981 Jan; 5(1):1–8

Balser M. Acute fatty liver disease of pregnancy. MCN 1984 May–Jun; 9(3): 188–191

Bash DM. Jewish religious practices related to childbearing. J Nurse Midwife 1980 Sep–Oct; 25(5):39–42

Blum RW and Goldhagen J. Teenage pregnancy in perspective. Clin Pediat (Phila) 1981 May; 20(5):335–340

Brooten D and Jordan C. Caffeine and pregnancy: A research review and recommendations for clinical practice. JOGN Nurs 1983 May–Jun; 12(3):190–195 (34 ref)

Carr KC. Obstetric practices which protect against neonatal morbidity: Focus on maternal position in labor and birth. Birth Fam J 1980 Winter; 7(4):249–254

Calandra C, Abell DA and Beischer NA. Maternal obesity in pregnancy. Obstet Gynecol 1981 Jan; 57(1):8–12

Creasy R. Prevention of preterm birth. Birth Defects 1983; 19(5):97–102

Dunn P. Reduction of teenage pregnancy as a rationale for sex education: A position paper. J Sch Health 1982 Dec; 52(10):611–613

Earls F and Siegel B. Precocious fathers. Am J Orthopsychiatry 1980 Jul; 50(3): 469–480

Ebrahim GJ. Cross-cultural aspects of pregnancy and breast feeding. Prac Nutr Soc 1980 Feb; 39(1):13–15

Elster A. Medical and psychosocial risks of pregnancy and childbearing during adolescence. Pediatr Ann 1980 Mar; 9(3):89–94

Elster A. Teenage Fathers: Stesses during Gestation and Early Parenthood. Clin Pediatr 1983 Oct; 22(10):700–703

Grace J. Does a mother's knowledge of fetal gender affect attachment? MCN 1984 Jan–Feb; 9(1):42–45

Harris RE et al. Cystitis during pregnancy: A distinctive clinical entity. Obstet Gynecol 1981 May 57(5):578–580

Haworth JC et al. Fetal growth retardation in cigarette smoking mothers is not due to decreased maternal food intake. Am J Obstet Gynecol 1980 Jul 15; 137(6):719–723

Heggenhougen HK. Father and childbirth: An anthropological perspective. J Nurse Midwife 1980 Nov–Dec; 25(6):21–26

Hollingsworth AO, Brown LP and Brooten DA. The refugees and childbearing: What to expect. RN 1980 Nov; 43(11):45–48

Horan M. Discomfort and pain during pregnancy. MCN 1984 Jul–Aug; 9(4) 267–269

Horn M and Manion J. Creative grandparenting: bonding the generations. JOGN Nurs 1985 May–Jun; 14(3):233–236

Horon I et al. Birth weights among infants born to adolescent and young adult women. American J Obstet Gynecol 1983 Jun 15; 146(4):444–449

Johnsen N and Gaspard M. Theoretical foundations of a prepared sibling class. JOGN Nurs 1985 May–Jun; 14(3):237–242

Kelley M. Maternal position and blood pressure during pregnancy and delivery. Am J Nurs 1982 May; 82(5): 809–812

Ketter D and Shelton B. Pregnant and physically fit, too. MCN 1984 Mar–Apr; 9(2):120–122

Kirkinen P et al. The effect of caffeine on placental and fetal blood flow in human pregnancy. Am J Obstet Gynecol 1983 Dec 15; 147(8):939–942

Leader A, Wong KH and Deitel M. Maternal nutrition in pregnancy. Part I. A review. Can Med Assoc J 1981 Sept; 125(6):545–549

Ledger W. Identification of the high risk mother and fetus. Clin Perinatol 1980 Mar; 7(1):125–134 (22 ref)

Luke B, Hawkins MM and Petrie RH. Influence of smoking: Weight gain and pregravid weight for height on intra-uterine growth. Am J Clin Nutr 1981 Jul; 34(7):1410–1417

Maloney R. Childbirth education classes: Expectant parents' expectations. JOGN Nurs 1985 May–Jun, 14(3):245–248

Manderino M and Bydek V. Effects of modeling and information on reactions to pain: A childbirth preparation analogue. Nurs Res 1984 Jan–Feb; 33(1):9–14

Manderson L. Roasting, smoking and dieting in response to birth: Malay confinement in cross-cultural perspective. Soc Sci Med 1981 Oct; 15(4):509–520

Mann JM et al. Assessing risk of rubella infection during pregnancy: A standardized approach. JAMA 1981 Apr 24; 245(16):1647–1652

Marrs RP and Mishell DR. Placental trophic hormones. Clin Obstet Gynecol 1980 Sep; 23(3):721–735 (42 ref)

McKay SR. Smoking during the childbearing year. MCN 1980 Jan–Feb; 5(1):46–50

Mercer RT. Assessing and counseling teenage mothers during the perinatal period. Nurs Clin North Am 1983 Jun; 18(2):293–301

Messer E. Hot-cold classification: Theoretical and practical implications of a Mexican study. Soc Sci Med 1981 Apr; 15(2):133–145

Mocarski V. Asymptomatic bacteruria—a silent problem of pregnant women. MCN 1980 Jul–Aug; 5(4):238–241

Moore DS, Bingham PE and Kessling O. Nursing care of the pregnant woman with diabetes mellitus. JOGN Nurs 1981 May–Jun; 10(3):188–194

Naeye RL. Influence of maternal cigarette smoking during pregnancy on fetal and childhood growth. Obstet Gynecol 1981 Jan; 57(1):18–21

Olson ML. Fitting grandparents into new

families. MCN 1981 Nov–Dec; 6(6): 419–421

Osborne N and Pratson L. Sexually transmitted diseases and pregnancy. JOGN Nurs 1984 Jan–Feb; 13(1):9–12

Platt LD et al. Exercise in pregnancy II. Fetal responses. Am J Obstet Gynecol 1983 Nov; 147(5):487–490

Rao JM and Arulappu R. Drug use in pregnancy: How to avoid problems. Drugs 1981 Nov; 22(5):409–414

Rauramo I et al. Antepartum fetal heart rate variability and intervillous placental blood flow in association with smoking. Am J Obstet Gynecol 1983 Aug 15; 146(8):967–969

Rosett HL, Weiner L and Edelin KC. Strategies for prevention of fetal alcohol effects. Obstet Gynecol 1981 Jan; 57(1):1–7

Socol M et al. Maternal smoking causes fetal hypoxia. Am J Obstet Gynecol 1982 Jan 15; 142(2):214–218

Szlachter BN et al. Relaxing in normal and pathogenic pregnancy. Obstet Gynecol 1982 Feb; 59(2):167–170

Tamez EG. Familism, machismo, and childbearing practices among Mexican Americans. J Psychiatr Nurs 1981 Sep; 19(9):21–25

Tilden V. The relationship of selected psychosocial variables to single status of adult women during pregnancy. Nurs Res 1984 Mar–Apr; 33(2):102–107

Tyson JE. Changing role of placental lactogen and prolactin in human gestation. Clin Obstet Gynecol 1980 Sep; 23(3):737–747

Vernon MEL et al. Teenage pregnancy: A prospective study of self-esteem and other sociodemographic factors. Pediatrics 1983 Nov; 72(5):632–635

Wiles L. The effect of prenatal breastfeeding education on breastfeeding success and maternal perception of the infant. JOGN Nurs 1984 Jul–Aug; 13(4):253–257

Wieser M and Castiglia P. Assessing early father–infant attachment. MCN 1984 Mar–Apr; 9(2):104–106

Zacharias JF. Childbirth education classes: Effects on attitudes toward childbirth in high risk indigent women. JOGN Nurs 1981 Jul–Aug; 10(4):265–267

Zellman GL. Public school programs for adolescent pregnancy and parenthood. Fam Plan Perspect 1982 Jan–Feb; 14(1):15–21

The Fetus

Adamson S. Ultrasonic measurement of rate and depth of human fetal breathing: Effect of glucose. Am J Obstet Gynecol 1983 Oct 1; 147(3): 288–295

Barnico L and Cullinane M. Maternal phenylketonuria: An unexpected challenge. MCN 1985 Mar–Apr; 10(2): 108–110

Beeson D. Prenatal diagnosis of fetal disorders Part I: Technological capabilities. Birth 1983 Winter; 10(4): 227–232

Beeson D. Prenatal diagnosis of fetal

disorders Part II: Issues and implications. Birth 1983 Winter; 10(4): 233–241

Bishop E. Acceleration of fetal pulmonary maturity. Obstet Gynecol 1981 Nov; 58(5 suppl):485–515

Council on Scientific Affairs. In utero fetal surgery. JAMA 1983 Sep 16; 250(11):1443–1444

Cruikshank D. Amniocenesis for determination of fetal maturity. Clin Obstet Gynecol 1982 Dec; 25(4):773–785 (59 ref)

Eik-Nes S and Andersson N. Estimation of fetal weight by ultrasound measurement. Acta Obstet Gynecol Scand 1982; 61(4):299–305

Fuchs F. Genetic amniocentesis. Sci Am 1980 Jun; 242(6):47–53

Gaffney S. Intrauterine fetal surgery: The ramifications for nurses. 1985 Jul–Aug; 10(4):250–254

Grace J. Does a mother's knowledge of fetal gender affect attachment? MCN Jan/Feb 1984 Jan–Feb; 9(1):42–45

Hamilton P et al. Comparison of lecithin:sphingomyelin ratio, fluorescence polarization, and phospholidylglycerol in the amniotic fluid in the prediction of respiratory distress syndrome. Obstet Gynecol 1984 Jan; 63(1):52–56

Herschel M et al. Survival of infants born at 24 to 28 weeks gestation. Obstet Gynecol 1982 Aug; 60(2):154–158

Johnson M, Hattan R and Rees G. The normal fetus. Semin Roentgenol 1982 Jul; 17(3):182–189

Kopta M, May R and Crane J. A comparison of the reliability of the estimated date of confinement predicted by crown–rump length and biparietal diameter. Am J Obstet Gynecol 1983 Mar 1; 145(5):562–565

Kurjak A and Kirkinen P. Ultrasonic growth pattern of fetuses with chromosomal abberations. Acta Obstet Gynecol Scand 1982 61(3):223–225

Lessick ML. Genetic counseling of families with endocrine disorders. Issues Compr Pediatr Nurs 1980 Apr; 4(2):27–40

Levine A and Imai P. Intrauterine treatment of fetal hydronephrosis. AORN J 1982 Mar; 35(4):655–662

Lieber M. Nonstress antepartal monitoring. MCN 1980 Sep–Oct; 5(5): 335–339

Lipshitz J, Anderson G and Whybrew W. Accelerated pulmonary maturity as measured by the lumodex-foam stability index test. Obstet Gynecol 1983 Jul; 62(1):31–36

Liston R et al. Antepartum fetal evaluation by maternal perception of fetal movement. Obstet Gynecol 1982 Oct; 60(4):424–426

Mennutti MT. Antenatal diagnosis of neural tube defects. Clin Perinatol Sept 1980 Sep; 7(2):227–242

Newton E, Cetrulo C and Kosa D.

Biparietal diameter as a predictor of fetal lung maturity. J Reprod Med 1983 Jul; 28(7):480–484

Patterson P. Fetal therapy: Issues we face. AORN J 1982 Mar; 35(4):663–668

Pedersen J. Fetal crown–rump length measurement by ultrasound in normal pregnancy. Br J Obstet Gynecol 1982 Nov; 89(11):926–930

Sabbagha R, Tamura R and Socol, M. The use of ultrasound in obstetrics. Clin Obstet Gynecol 1982 Dec; 25(4): 735–752

Sabbagha R, Tamura R and Dal Compo S. Fetal dating by ultrasound. Semin Roentgenol 1982 Jul; 17(3):190–197

Sabbagha R. Ultrasonic evaluation of fetal congential anomalies. Clin OB/GYN 1980 Apr; 7(1):103–21

Selbing A. Gestational age and ultrasonic measurement of gestational sac, crown–rump length and biparietal diameter during first 15 weeks of pregnancy. Acta Obstet Gynecol Scand 1982; 61(3):233–235

Sorokin Y and Dieker L. Fetal movement. Clin Obstet Gynecol 1982 Dec; 25(4):719–734

Strassner H and Nochimson D. Determination of fetal maturity. Clin Perinatol 1982 Jun; 9(2):297–312

Venes J. Management of intrauterine hydrocephalus. Neurosurg 1983 May; 58(5):793–794

Weingold A, Yonekura M and O'Kieffe J. Nonstress testing. Am J Obstet Gynecol 1980 Sep 15; 138(2):195–202

Nursing Management During Labor and Delivery

25

The Labor Process

Initiation of Labor

The exact mechanism that initiates labor is unknown. Theories include:

1. Uterine stretch theory—uterus becomes stretched, pressure increases causing physiologic changes that initiate labor.
2. As pregnancy advances, the uterus becomes more sensitive to oxytocin.
3. As pregnancy advances, progesterone is less effective in controlling rhythmic uterine contractions that occur normally throughout pregnancy.
4. There is increased production of prostaglandins by fetal membranes and uterine decidua as pregnancy advances.
5. In later pregnancy, the fetus produces increased levels of cortisol which inhibit progesterone production from the placenta.

Factors Affecting Labor

Successful labor and delivery depend on adequate pelvic dimensions, adequate fetal dimensions and presentation, and adequate uterine contractions.

A. Pelvic Dimensions

1. Adequate pelvic inlet (anteroposterior diameter; normal shape)
2. Adequate midpelvis (ischial spines do not protrude into bony canal)
3. Adequate outlet (adequate distance between tuberosities; mobile coccyx)
4. Adequacy of pelvic dimensions determined by pelvic examination during pregnancy (see p. 965) and again with the onset of labor

B. Fetal Dimensions—important fetal dimensions influenced by fetal size, posture, lie, and presentation. Fetal position is also an important factor in successful labor.

1. *Fetal size*—with excessive size, fetal skull bones may not be able to override enough to be accommodated in the bony pelvic cavity.
2. *Fetal posture*—fetus assumes a characteristic posture in later pregnancy to accommodate to the uterine cavity. The fetal head is flexed, back is bent, and extremities are flexed. Flexed head allows smallest diameter of fetal head to present and pass through the birth canal (Fig. 25-1).
3. *Fetal lie*—fetus assumes a lie (comparison of the fetal long axis to the long axis of the woman) that is either transverse or longitudinal. In a longitudinal lie (99% of all births) the fetal head will present (cephalic presentation) or the buttocks or feet will present (breech presentation). In a transverse lie, the shoulder presents.
4. *Fetal presentation*—whichever portion of the infant is deepest in the birth canal and is felt on vaginal examination is referred to as the *presenting part;* this determines fetal presentation.
5. *Fetal position*—designation of landmark of fetal presenting part (occiput, mentum, sacrum, acronium) to right or left, and anterior, posterior, or transverse portion of the woman's pelvis. For example, a fetus presenting by the vertex with his occiput on the left antertior part of the woman's pelvis would have his presentation and position described as LOA, or left occiput anterior (see Fig. 24-9, p. 976).

C. Uterine Contractions

Successful labor also depends on uterine contractions occurring at regular intervals and having adequate intensity.

1. Uterine contractions are involuntary.
2. During uterine contractions, the active upper portion of the uterus becomes thicker, while the lower uterine segment stretches and becomes thinner.
3. At the completion of a contraction, the upper uterine segment retains its shortened, thickened cell size and with each succeeding contraction becomes thicker and shorter. Cells of lower uterine segment become thinner and longer with each contraction. This mechanism is greatly responsible for the progress of the fetus through the birth canal.

Events Preliminary to Labor

1. *Lightening* (the settling of the fetus in the lower uterine segment) occurs 2–3 weeks before term in the primigravida and later, during labor in the multigravida.
   a. The woman's breathing becomes easier as the fetus falls away from the diaphragm.
   b. Lordosis of the spine is increased for the woman as the fetus enters the pelvis and falls forward. Walking may become more difficult; leg cramping may increase.
   c. Urinary frequency occurs because of pressure on the bladder.
2. Vaginal secretions may increase.

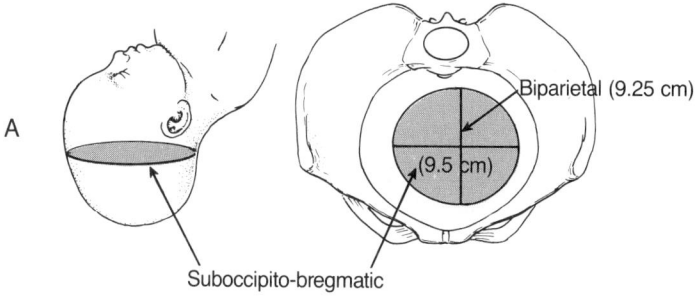

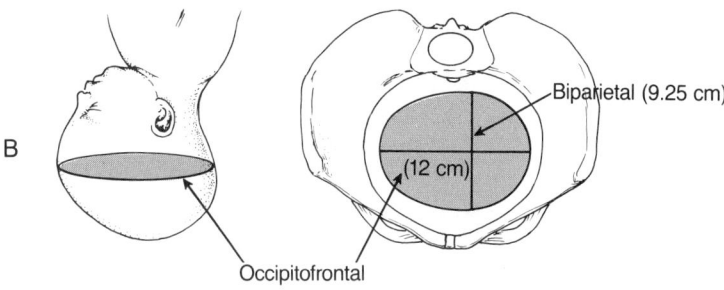

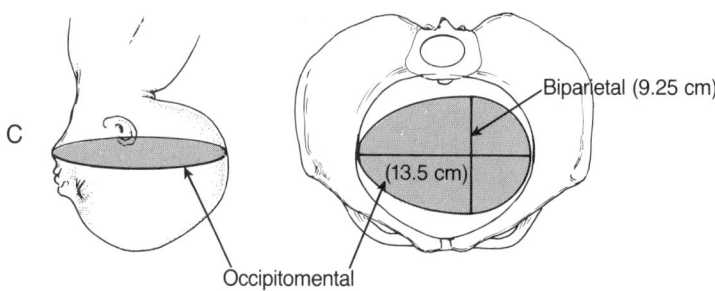

Figure 25-1. (*A*) Complete flexion allows smallest diameter of head to enter pelvis. (*B*) Moderate extension causes larger diameter to enter pelvis. (*C*) Marked extension forces largest diameter against pelvic brim, but head is too large to enter pelvis.

3. Mucous plug is discharged from the cervix along with a small amount of blood from surrounding capillaries—referred to as "show" ("bloody show").
4. Cervix becomes soft and effaced (thinned).
5. Membranes may rupture.
6. False labor contractions may occur (Table 25-1).
7. Backache may increase.

Stages of Labor

1. *First stage of labor,* or stage of cervical dilation, begins with first true labor contractions and ends with complete dilation of the cervix (10 cm. dilation).
   a. Latent phase—0–4 cm.
   b. Active phase—4–7 cm.
   c. Transitional phase—7–10 cm.
2. *Second stage of labor,* or stage of expulsion, begins with complete dilation and ends with birth of the baby.
3. *Third stage of labor,* or placental stage, begins with delivery of the baby and ends with delivery of the placenta.
4. *Fourth stage* lasts from delivery of the placenta until the postpartum condition of the woman has become stabilized (usually 1 hour after delivery).

Mechanisms of Labor

If the woman's pelvis is adequate, size and position of the fetus are adequate, and uterine contractions are regular and of adequate intensity, the fetus will move through the birth canal. The position and rotational changes of the fetus as he moves down the birth canal will be

Table 25-1   True and False Labor Contractions

True Labor Contractions	False Labor Contractions
Result in progressive cervical dilation and effacement	Do not result in progressive cervical dilation and effacement
Occur at regular intervals	Occur at irregular intervals
Interval between contractions decreases	Interval between contractions remains the same or increases
Intensity increases	Intensity decreases or remains the same
Located mainly in back and abdomen	Located mainly in lower abdomen and groin
Generally intensified by walking	Generally unaffected by walking
Not affected by mild sedation	Generally relieved by mild sedation

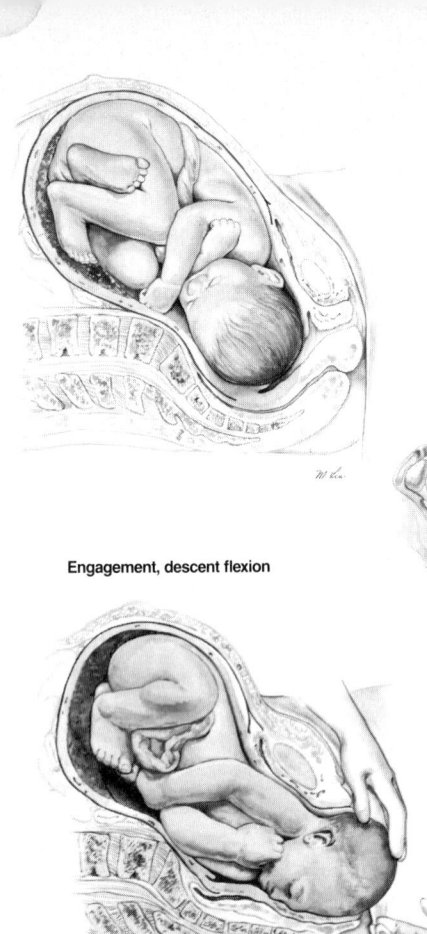
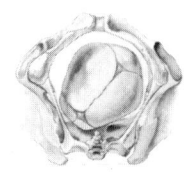

Engagement, descent flexion

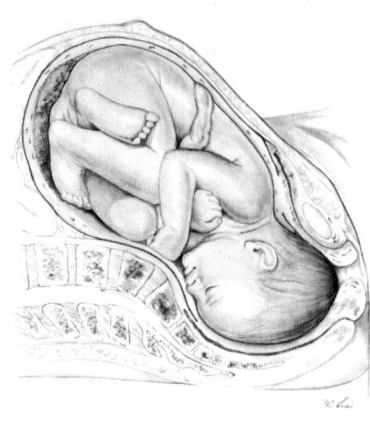
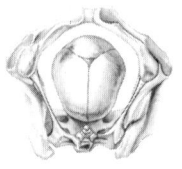

Internal rotation

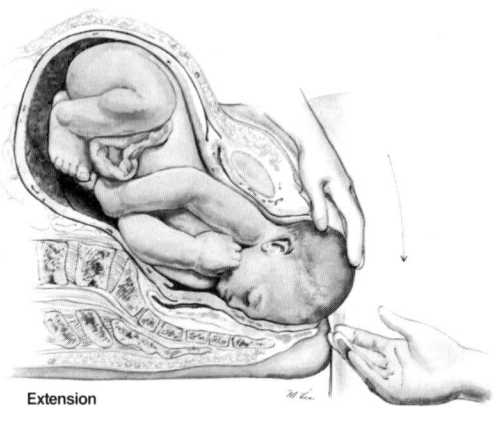
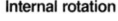

Extension

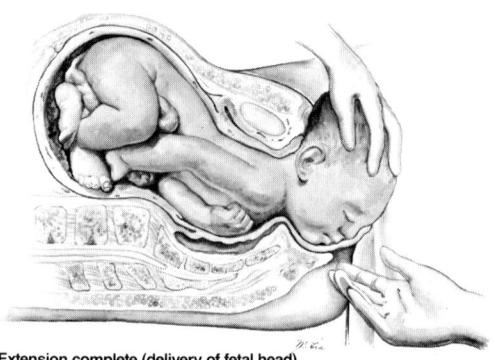

Extension complete (delivery of fetal head)

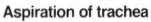

Aspiration of trachea

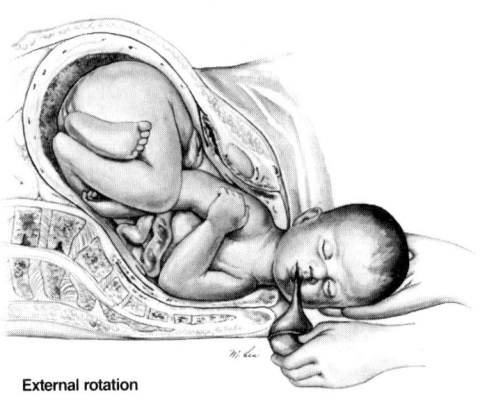

External rotation

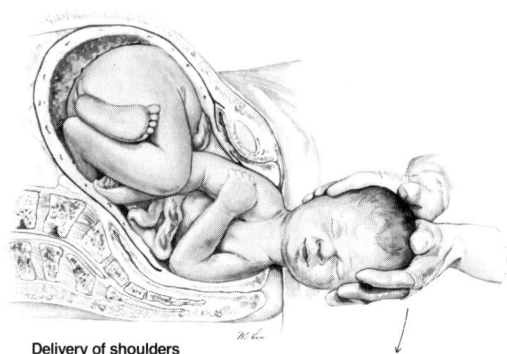

Delivery of shoulders

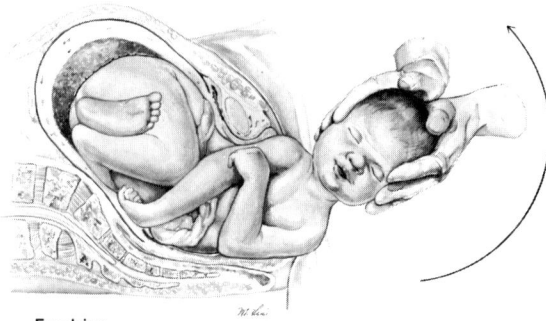

Expulsion

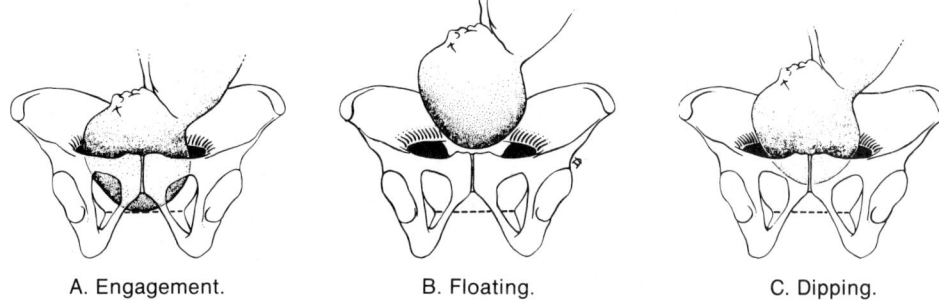

A. Engagement.   B. Floating.   C. Dipping.

Figure 25-3. Engagement, floating, and dipping. (From Oxom H and Foote WR. *Human Labor and Birth.* New York, Appleton-Century-Crofts)

affected by resistance offered by the woman's bony pelvis, cervix, and surrounding tissues. The events of engagement, descent, flexion, internal rotation, extension, external rotation, and expulsion overlap in time (Fig. 25-2).

A. Engagement

When biparietal diameter of fetal head has passed through pelvic inlet:
1. Primigravidas—occurs up to 2 weeks before onset of labor
2. Multigravidas—usually occurs with onset of labor
3. Since biparietal diameter is narrowest diameter of fetal head, and anteroposterior diameter is narrowest of pelvic inlet, the fetal head usually enters pelvis in a transverse position

B. Descent

Occurs throughout labor and is essential for fetal rotations prior to birth.
1. Accomplished by force of uterine contractions on fetal portion in fundus; during second stage of labor, bearing down increases intra-abdominal pressure, thus augmenting effects of uterine contractions.
2. Degree of descent described as:
    a. Floating—fetal presenting part is not engaged in pelvic inlet (Fig. 25-3).
    b. Fixed—fetal presenting part has entered pelvis.
    c. Engagement—fetal presenting part (usually biparietal diameter of fetal head) has passed through pelvic inlet
    d. Station 0—presenting part has reached level of ischial spines
    e. Stations −1, −2, −3, −4—presenting part is 1, 2, 3, 4 cm. *above* the level of ischial spines (Fig. 25-4).
    f. Station +1, +2, +3, +4—presenting part is 1, 2, 3, 4 cm. *below* level of ischial spines. A station

of +4 indicates that presenting part is on the pelvic floor.

C. Flexion

Resistance to descent causes head to flex so that the chin is close to the chest; this causes the smallest fetal head diameter, the suboccipitobregmatic (9.5 cm.) to present through the canal.

D. Internal Rotation

In accommodating to the birth canal, the fetal occiput rotates anteriorly from its original position toward the symphysis. This movement results from the shape of the fetal head, space available in the midpelvis, and contour of the perineal muscles. The ischial spines project into the midpelvis causing the fetal head to rotate anteriorly to accommodate to the available space.

E. Extension

As the fetal head descends further, it meets resistance from the perineal muscles and is forced to extend. The fetal head becomes visible at the vulvovaginal ring; its largest diameter is encircled (*crowning*), and the head then emerges from the vagina.

F. External Rotation

When the head emerges, the shoulders are undergoing internal rotation as they turn in the midpelvis to accommodate to the projection of the ischial spines. The head, now born, rotates as the shoulders undergo this internal rotation.

G. Expulsion

Following delivery of the infant's head and internal rotation of the shoulders, the anterior shoulder rests beneath the symphysis pubis. The posterior shoulder is born, followed by the anterior shoulder and the rest of the body.

Assessment

When Labor Begins

History and Baseline Data

1. Introduce yourself; ask for name of woman's midwife or physician and if he or she has been notified that

Figure 25-2. Mechanism of delivery for a vertex presentation (Whitley N. *A Manual of Clinical Obstetrics.* Philadelphia, JB Lippincott, 1985)

the woman was coming to the hospital or birth center.
2. Establish baseline information.
    a. Gravidity, parity, expected date of delivery or confinement (EDC)
    b. When did contractions begin? How far apart are they? How long do they last?
    c. Have the membranes ruptured? color? consistency? amount of fluid?
    d. Is there any bloody show?

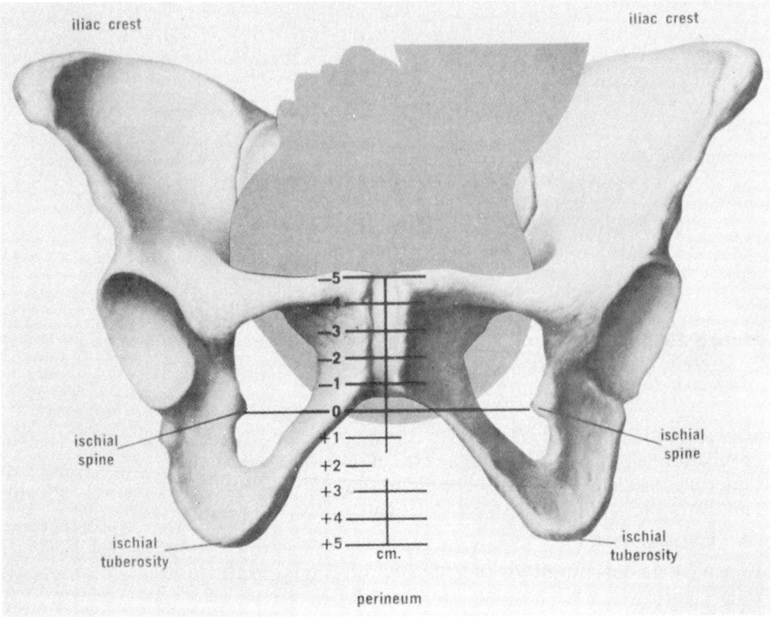

Figure 25-4. Stations of presenting part. The location of the presenting part in relation to the level of the ischial spines is designated *station*, and indicates the degree of advancement of the presenting part through the pelvis. Stations are expressed in centimeters above (*minus*) or below (*plus*) the level of the ischial spines (*zero*). (Courtesy of Ross Laboratories)

e. How much discomfort is the woman experiencing?
f. What, if any, problems has the woman had in this pregnancy? Problems in past pregnancies?
g. Blood type and Rh?

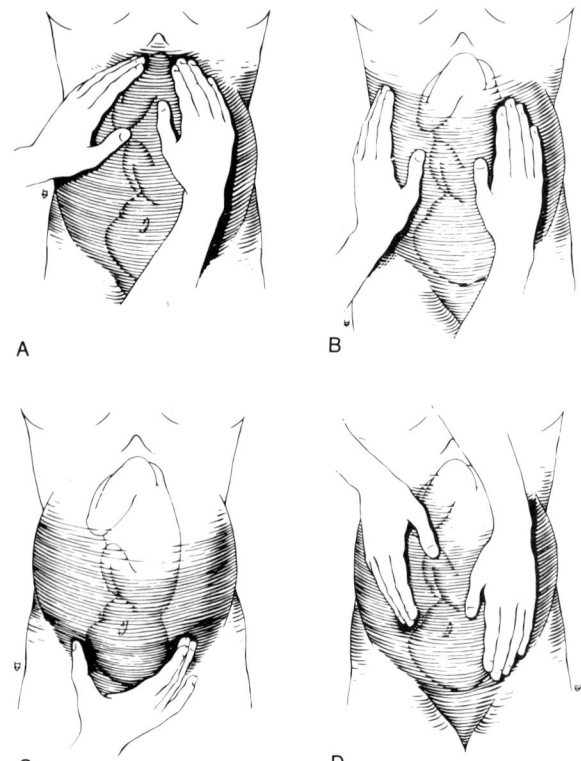

Figure 25-5. Leopold maneuvers.

3. Establish baseline vital signs.
   a. Temperature—elevation suggests infection.
   b. Blood pressure—measure between contractions.
   c. Pulse—some elevation of pulse, respiration, and blood pressure may be due to anxiety; blood pressure elevations of 140 mm. Hg systolic and 90 mm. Hg diastolic suggest hypertensive disorder of pregnancy.
   d. Respirations.

Methods for Determining Fetal Presentation

A. Vaginal Examination and Determination of Fetal Landmarks Presenting

B. Leopold Maneuvers

Determined by abdominal palpation (Leopold maneuvers; Fig. 25-5).

1. First maneuver (Fig. 25-5*A*)—to determine if fetal head or breech is in uterine fundus. Palpate sides of uterus and fundus. Head feels hard and round, freely movable and ballotable; breech feels large, nodular, softer.
2. Second maneuver (Fig. 25-5*B*)—to determine the position of the fetal extremities, the fetal back, and the anterior shoulder. Place hands on the sides of the abdomen to identify the location of the back and small parts. Palpate down sides of uterus applying gentle but deep pressure. On side of fetal back, a long continuous structure will be felt; side with fetal extremities will feel nodular, reflecting portions of fetal extremities.
3. Third maneuver (Fig. 25-5*C*)—to determine the portion of the fetus that is presenting and if engagement has occurred. Grasp the lower uterine segment between the thumb and fingers of one hand to feel the presenting part. If presenting part is movable, engagement has not occurred; if engagement has occurred, fetal part feels fixed in the pelvis. The head is at inlet or in pelvis in 90% of women.
4. Fourth maneuver (Fig. 25-5*D*)—to confirm the findings of the third maneuver and to determine the

flexion of the vertex. Turn and face the woman's feet. Gently move the fingers down the sides of the uterus. The cephalic prominence is felt on the side where there is greater resistance to the descent of the fingers into the pelvis.

C. Ultrasonography (see p. 972)

D. X-Ray—rarely used today; replaced by ultrasonography

Assessing Fetal Heart Tones

Heart tones are auscultated with DeLee–Hillis fetoscope (over the head) or Leffscope (stethoscope with a large weighted bell).

1. Note location, rate, and character.
2. Determine the position, presentation, and lie of the fetus by palpation. As internal rotation and descent occur, the location of the fetal heart tone (FHT) changes, swinging gradually from the right or left quadrant to the midline and dropping until immediately before delivery, when it is found above the pubic bone (Figs. 25-6 and 25-7).
3. Place the fetal stethoscope on the abdomen over the back or chest of the fetus, depending on which is closer to the uterine exit.
4. Listen and count the beat for 1 minute.
5. Check the rate before, during, and after a contraction to detect slowing or irregularities.
   Normal rate: 120–160 beats/minute.
6. Avoid friction noises caused by fingers on abdominal surface area.
7. Differentiate between FHT and other abdominal sounds.
   a. *Fetal heart tone*—a very rapid, somewhat muffled ticking sound.
   b. *Uterine bruit*—a soft murmur caused by the passage of blood through dilated uterine vessels; it is synchronous with the maternal pulse.
   c. *Funic souffle*—a hissing sound produced by passage of blood through the umbilical arteries; it is synchronous with the fetal heart rate (FHR).
8. Check FHT immediately following the rupture of the membranes; sudden release of fluid may cause prolapse of the umbilical cord.

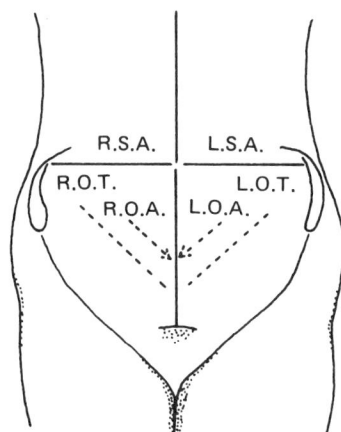

Figure 25-6. Fetal heart tone locations on the abdominal wall indicating possible corresponding fetal positions and the effects of the internal rotation of the fetus.

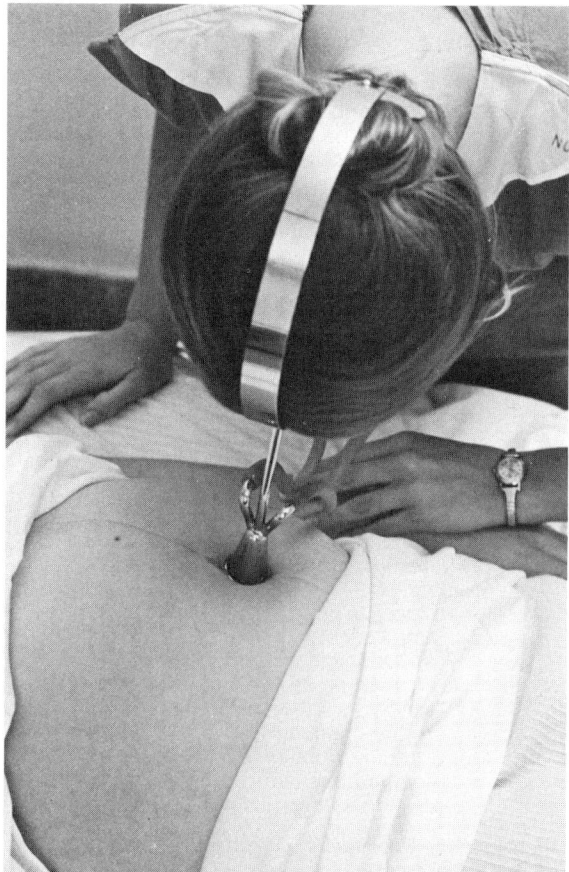

Figure 25-7. Auscultation of the fetal heartbeat using the fetoscope.

Assessing Uterine Contractions

Intensity. frequency. duration:

1. Place fingertips gently on the fundus.
2. As contraction begins, tension will be felt under the fingertips. Uterus will become harder, then slowly soften.
3. The intensity may be described as follows:
   a. Mild—the uterine muscle is somewhat tense.
   b. Moderate—the uterine muscle is moderately firm.
   c. Strong—the uterine muscle is so firm that it seems almost board-like.
4. The frequency is measured in minutes—represents the time from the beginning of one contraction until the beginning of the next.
5. Duration of a contraction is timed from the moment the uterus first begins to tighten until it relaxes again.
6. As labor progresses, the character of the contractions changes and they last longer.
7. When the cervix becomes completely dilated (the transition stage) the contractions become very strong, last for 60 seconds, and occur at 2- to 3-minute intervals.

▶ **NURSING ALERT:** If any contraction lasts longer than 70 seconds and is not followed by a period of uterine muscle relaxation, notify the attending physician immediately. Uterine rupture and fetal hypoxia may occur.

8. Take urine specimen—test for glucose and protein (if membranes are ruptured, protein will be positive).

Vaginal Examination (Fig. 25-8)

1. Place the woman in lithotomy position.
2. Conduct examination gently, under aseptic conditions.
3. Evaluate the following:
   a. Condition of cervix
      (1) Hard or soft (in labor cervix is soft)
      (2) Effaced and thin or thick and long (in labor cervix is thin and effaced)
      (3) Easily dilatable or resistant
      (4) Closed or open (dilated); degree of dilation
   b. Presentation
      (1) Breech, cephalic (head) or shoulder
      (2) Caput succedaneum (edema occurring in and under fetal scalp) present (small or large)
      (3) Station identified (see Fig. 25-4) engaged; floating
   c. Position
      (1) Cephalic presentation (identification of the sagittal suture and of its direction)
      (2) Location of posterior fontanelle
   d. Membranes
      (1) Intact
      (2) Ruptured
         (a) Drainage of fluid
         (b) Passage of meconium
      (3) Usually increases frequency and intensity of uterine contractions
      (4) Contraindicated in presence of vaginal bleeding, premature labor, or abnormal fetal presentation or position

Assessing Woman's/Couple's Expectations and Concerns

1. What are their concerns?
2. How anxious are they?
3. What has been their preparation for labor (type, by whom, and when)?
4. What is their understanding of the labor process?
5. What are their expectations of the labor and delivery process (prepared childbirth, anesthesia, analgesics, use of birthing room etc.)?
6. How well are they coping and how well are they communicating with each other?

Fetal Monitoring

The purposes of *continuous fetal monitoring* during labor are (1) to monitor the progress of a woman's contraction pattern and (2) to monitor the condition of the fetus in response to the stress of uterine contractions. Women's reactions to being monitored vary:

1. Some women are reassured by hearing the continuous fetal heart sounds.
2. Some women/couples use the printout of the contraction pattern to assist them in using breathing techniques since they can see when the contraction begins.
3. Some women experience discomfort because of the abdominal straps and their interference with effleurage, as well as difficulty assuming a comfortable position.

External Monitoring (indirect monitoring)

Separate transducers are secured to the woman's abdomen; a tokodynamometer translates abdominal tension, and an ultrasound transducer translates fetal heart sounds into electrical signals that are recorded on a strip chart (Fig. 25-9). The measurement by external monitoring of the intensity of uterine contractions is not accurate. External monitoring, however, does provide a pattern of the woman's contractions.

1. The ultrasonic transducer device should be applied over the area of the abdomen where the sharpest fetal heart sound is heard. Lubricate the face of the

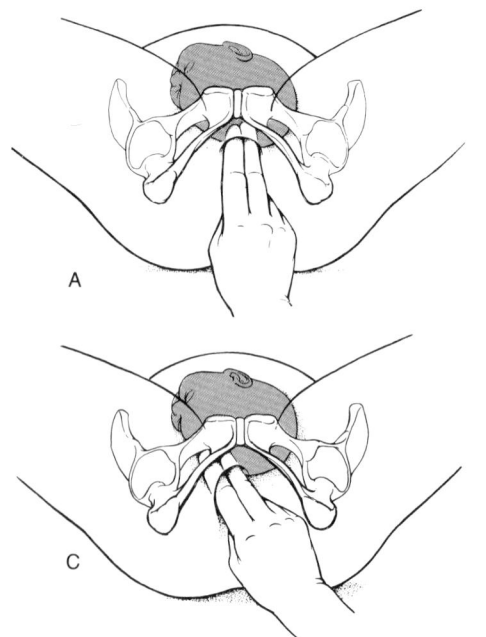

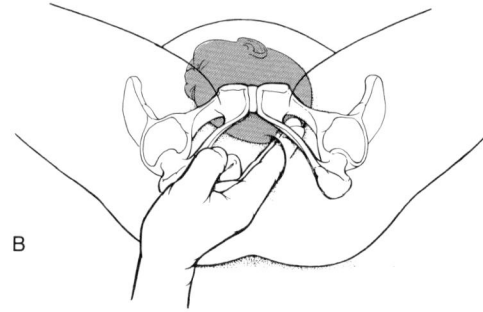

Figure 25-8. Vaginal examination. (A) Determining the station and palpating the sagittal suture. (B) Identifying the posterior fontanelle. (C) Identifying the anterior fontanelle.

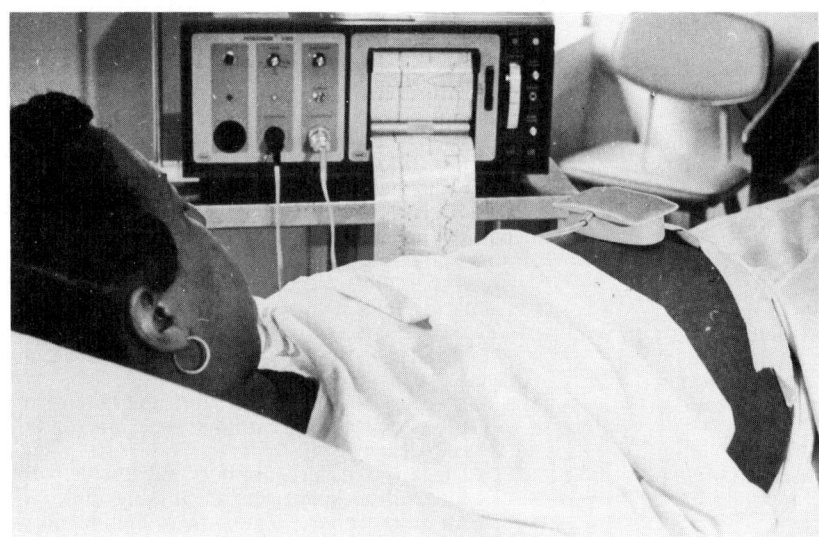

Figure 25-9. Patient with external fetal monitor applied. Note that the monitor function can be observed by the patient.

transducer with a thin layer of ultrasonic gel to aid in the transmission of sounds.

2. The transducer will need to be readjusted when the fetus changes positions.

3. The tokodynamometer recording uterine contractions will need to be reapplied over the fundus as the fetus and uterus descend during labor.

Internal Monitoring (direct monitoring)

A method of recording intrauterine pressure and the fetal heart rate (FHR) through internal measurements—more accurate than external monitoring (Fig. 25-10).

1. Fetal electrocardiograph—obtained by a small electrode clipped to the presenting part (membranes

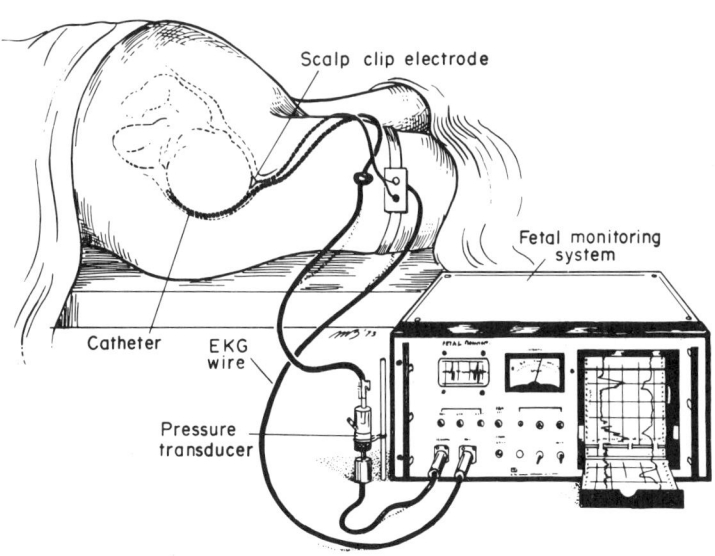

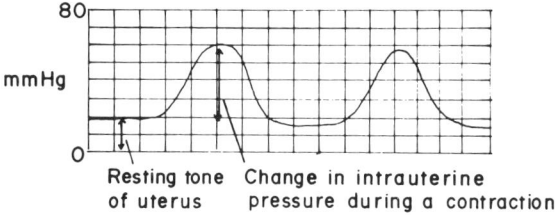

Figure 25-10. Fetal monitoring system for intrauterine determination of uterine pressure and fetal heart rate. (From Roux, Jacques F. Monitoring of labor in high-risk centers. In Aladjem S and Brown AK [eds]: Clinical Perinatology. St. Louis, CV Mosby

must be ruptured, the cervix must be dilated 3–4 cm., and the station must be at −2 or lower).
2. Uterine contractions are recorded by means of a catheter placed in the uterine cavity behind the presenting part.
   a. The catheter is filled with distilled water and is connected to an external transducer that converts pressure values into an electronic signal.
   b. Monitor strips record the quality of the uterine contractions and fetal heart patterns simultaneously.

Interpretation

1. Fetal heart rate (FHR) must be checked initially for *baseline rate* (FHR in the absence of or between contractions). A change from the baseline is termed a *fluctuation* and is either an *acceleration* or a *deceleration.*
2. Tachycardia—a sustained elevation of the FHR (often accompanies fetal hypoxia, fetal immaturity, or breech presentation).
   a. Moderate: 161–180 beats/minute.
   b. Severe: over 180 beats/minute
3. Bradycardia—persistent FHR levels below 120 beats/minute.
   a. Moderate: 120–90 beats/minute
     (1) Usually not associated with significant fetal acidosis.
     (2) Congenital heart disease may be related to persistently slow FHR.
   b. Marked: 89–70 beats/minute
   Associated with progressive fetal acidosis.
   c. Severe: less than 70 beats/minute
4. Short-term FHR fluctuations (variability) reflect the state of the nervous mechanisms controlling the fetal heart and are indicative of a healthy fetus. Normal variability ranges between 6 and 25 beats/minute from baseline; variability is considered by many clinicians to be the most reliable indicator of a normal fetus. A *lack* of this type of irregularity may indicate the following:
   a. A serious fetal compromise reflecting an acidotic fetal nervous system unable to make parasympathetic or sympathetic responses.
   b. Maternal use of central nervous system depressant drugs (narcotics, tranquilizers, anesthetic agents).
   c. Immature fetal nervous control mechanisms.
5. Periodic FHR changes
   a. Accelerations or decelerations of the FHR are due to:
     (1) Mechanical effects or uterine pressure applied directly to the fetal head and/or umbilical cord
     (2) Uterine pressure applied indirectly to the intervillous space, decreasing blood flow
   b. Acceleration of more than 60 beats/minute above baseline is considered severe and indicates fetal compromise.
   c. Deceleration
   Early deceleration (Fig. 25-11*A*)
     (1) Waveform approximates a mirror image of the pattern of intrauterine pressure.
     (2) Pattern is often uniform in appearance from one contraction to another.
     (3) Early deceleration begins near the onset of the contraction.
     (4) Lowest level of the FHR deceleration occurs at the peak of the uterine contraction.

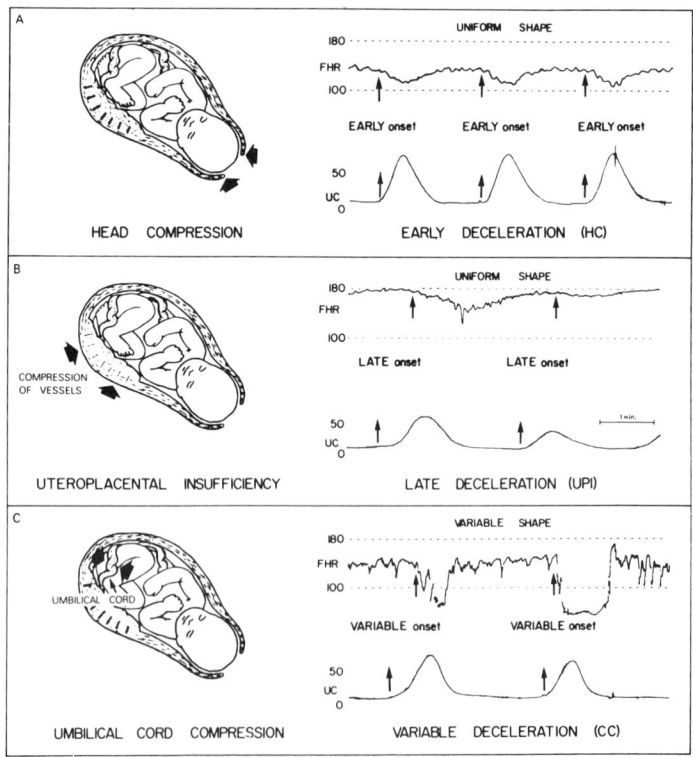

Figure 25-11. Three FHR deceleration patterns. (From Hon EH. An Atlas of Fetal Heart Rate Patterns. New Haven, Harty Press)

(5) FHR does not fall below 100 beats/minute, and duration is less than 90 seconds.
(6) Early deceleration does not usually cause a change in fetal acid–base status.
(7) This type of deceleration is considered benign, caused by fetal head compression. No intervention is required.

Late deceleration (Fig. 25-11*B*)
(1) Also manifests a smooth uniform heart rate pattern and reflects the pattern of uterine pressure.
(2) Begins later in contracting phase of uterus (as the contraction reaches its peak).
(3) Usually less than 90 seconds in duration.
(4) Markedly altered by maternal hypoxia.
(5) Frequently associated with fetal tachycardia.
(6) FHR irregularity and passage of meconium may occur.
(7) Associated with progressive fetal hypoxia and acidosis; if prolonged, hypoxia may have a direct effect on the fetal myocardium and possibly on the conduction system of the heart.
(8) Late deceleration pattern due to acute uteroplacental insufficiency as a result of a decreased intervillous space blood flow.

d. Deceleration of the FHR may be avoided in part by the following measures:
(1) Careful maintenance of the maternal blood pressure within normal limits
(2) Careful infusion of oxytocics
(3) Extremely careful administration of agents such as conduction anesthesia, which may produce maternal hypotension

e. Deceleration may be modified or corrected by measures that improve uteroplacental blood flow and oxygen transfer across the placenta.
(1) Discontinue oxytocin if it is being given.
(2) Change the woman's position to the left side to facilitate emptying of the vena cava into the heart and to correct hypotension caused by supine position. Elevation of the woman's legs may also be effective.
(3) Administer oxygen by face mask.
(4) Administer IV fluids and ephedrine.
(5) Obtain fetal blood sample to measure degree of fetal hypoxia; fetal compromise causes the following changes:
pH decrease (normal 7.30–7.40)
PCO_2 increase
PO_2 decrease
(6) If ominous FHR pattern persists, labor may be terminated by forceps delivery or cesarean birth.

f. *Variable deceleration* (Fig. 25-11*C*)—due to umbilical cord compression.
(1) Nonuniform periodic changes in FHR bear no consistent relationship to the uterine contractions.
(2) Often preceded and followed by acceleration.
(3) FHR usually falls below 100 beats per minute and may fall as low as 50–60 beats/minute.
(4) Duration of deceleration varies from a few seconds to minutes.
(5) Usually associated with baseline FHR in normal or near-normal range.

(6) Condition corrected by changing the woman's position to relieve pressure on the cord.
(7) When severe variable deceleration is present, prolapse of the cord should be suspected.

g. *Combined FHR deceleration patterns*—combination of 2 or 3 patterns may exist since a single uterine contraction may evoke all 3 types simultaneously; visual identification of the patterns thus becomes very difficult or impossible.

Nursing Interventions for Fetal Monitoring

1. Provide explanations to the woman and her family; ideally these should be given in the prenatal period during tours of the labor and delivery rooms or by means of films.
Information should include the following:
a. Why the monitor is being used and the benefits derived from its use.
b. What the monitor does and what causes the "bleeps."
c. How the monitor is applied.
d. What limitations of movement will be necessary, if any.
2. Provide comfort measures.
a. Give back rubs.
b. Assist the woman to change position; changes should be noted on graph since slight variations may occur.
c. Reposition external monitors.
d. Assist the woman with general hygiene; she may be concerned about disturbing the attachments.
3. Assist the woman to cope with anxieties and discomfort she may have.
Use relaxation techniques and comfort measures.

Patient Problems/Nursing Diagnoses

1. Anxiety related to uncertainties/misconceptions of the labor and birthing process, hospital environment, physical stressors, fear for self and baby
2. Pain and discomfort related to uterine contractions, passage of baby through birth canal, possible tearing of perineum
3. Potential for ineffective coping related to length and discomfort of labor process, fatigue, decreased energy
4. Potential for blood loss related to complications
5. Potential for infection related to ruptured membranes

Nursing Interventions

Reduce anxiety.
1. Monitor the woman's/couple's concerns.
2. Keep the woman/couple up to date on the woman's progress during labor.
3. Explain any procedures that need to be performed or any unexpected events that may occur.
4. If the woman is in true labor, the perineal area (vulva and perineal area) may be shaved. Rationale has been that it promotes cleanliness, reduces postpartum infection, and makes episiotomy repair easier. Research indicates there is no difference in infection rates, and thus perineal shaves are no longer done in many settings.
5. An enema (soapsuds) may be necessary if colon is very full.
a. Increases space available for passage of the fetus
b. Decreases fecal contamination of the field during delivery
Reduce pain and discomfort; promote effective coping throughout the state of labor as described in following section.

First Stage of Labor—Latent Phase (0–4 cm.)

1. Monitor progress of labor—take and record blood pressure, pulse, respirations, contractions (usually 5–10 minutes apart, lasting 20–40 seconds), fetal heart sounds every 1–2 hours; temperature every 4 hours unless elevated, in which case it may be taken every 2 hours.
2. Provide clear liquids if permitted (varies with midwife or physician).
3. Allow the woman to walk about, provided presenting part is engaged and membranes have not ruptured (may also vary with physician).
4. Encourage diversionary activity such as reading or watching television.
5. Evaluate and/or teach breathing techniques helpful in coping with active and transitional phases of first

Table 25-2 Obstetrical Analgesia and Anesthesia

Method	Comment	Precautions
Obstetrical Analgesia		
Prepared childbirth (Read, Lamaze methods)	Requires preparation and psychological support, controlled breathing, voluntary muscle relaxation	Requires commitment of woman and partner and support of obstetric staff
Hypnosis		Requires a willing woman, considerable prenatal training
Narcotics (such as meperidine and pentazocine)	Decrease fear and anxiety, promote physical relaxation and rest between contractions; may cause nausea and vomiting	
Tranquilizers (ataractics)	May be used in combination with narcotics; reduced dose of narcotic required; allay anxiety	
Barbiturates	Given in combination with analgesic; produce sedation and hypnosis	May depress infant for many hours after birth
Trichloroethylene (Trilene)—inhalation anesthetic agent	Usually is self-administered by cannister and face mask	For best results, the woman must be carefully instructed on how to use the equipment Prolonged use may cause confusion and overdose eliminating protective mechanism; if vomiting occurs, respiratory obstruction and asphyxia may result
General Anesthesia		
Nitrous oxide with oxygen	Administered in low concentrations to allow fetal oxygenation	
Halothane	Produces good uterine relaxation quickly; useful in tetanic contractions; useful for intrauterine manipulations such as removal of retained placenta. Because of its potent relaxant effect, postpartum hemorrhage may be a problem.	
Thiopental (Pentothal sodium)	For rapid induction of anesthesia for cesarean deliveries	
Cyclopropane	Rapid induction and recovery and can be used with high concentrations of oxygen; disadvantage is its flammability; if deep anesthesia is required, can cause fetal and maternal respiratory depression	
Ether	Inexpensive and easy to administer; wide margin of safety; high incidence of nausea and vomiting; irritates respiratory tract	

stage, and breathing and pushing techniques for second stage.
   a. Early first stage
      Relax, take 1 deep breath and exhale slowly and completely. Breathe deeply, slowly, rhythmically throughout contraction. Follow with another deep, complete breath.
   b. Late first stage
      Take 1 deep breath and exhale slowly and completely. Breathe regularly at more shallow level. When stronger contraction occurs, breathe more quickly with very light breaths. Then take deep breath and exhale slowly.
   c. Transition stage
      Concentrate on breathing in controlled manner. Take a deep breath and exhale slowly and completely. At beginning of contraction, take a fairly deep breath. Then engage in shallow breathing. If there is an urge to push, puff out every 3rd, 4th, or 5th breath. Take deep breath at end of contraction.
   d. Second stage
      When pushing (as directed), catch breath as needed. Relax pelvic floor and go limp between contractions. During contractions pant and push gently as directed.
6. Involve partner or support person in the woman's care.
   a. Coach during breathing.
   b. Help by timing contractions.
   c. Provide lower back massage.
7. Provide privacy for the couple between periods of giving care.
8. Encourage the woman to void approximately every 2 hours to keep bladder empty.

First Stage of Labor—Active Phase (4–7 cm.)

Contractions are usually 2–5 minutes apart lasting 30–50 seconds; one half to two thirds of labor has been completed near the beginning of the active phase.

1. Monitor progress of labor—take and record blood pressure, pulse, respirations, contractions, fetal heart sounds every 30 minutes (if continuous fetal monitoring is not being used).
2. Be aware that the woman may begin to feel unable to cope with discomfort and may begin to lose control.
3. Partner or nurse should help the woman to concentrate on breathing and relaxation techniques with each contraction.
4. Provide comfort measures.
   a. Side-lying position is usually more comfortable; removes pressure of gravid uterus on inferior vena cava and increases blood flow to the placenta.
   b. Provide sacral hand pressure and backrest.
   c. Change damp or soiled linen.
   d. Assist with mouth care.
   e. Sponge bathe face, neck, and back.
   f. Continue to provide encouragement and information.
   g. Administer prescribed analgesia as needed (Table 25-2)
   h. Assist with regional anesthesia if needed (Table 25-3)
5. Maintain hydration and glucose level of woman (low-

Table 25-3 **Regional Analgesia and Anesthesia**

Type	Method	Advantages	Disadvantages	Nursing Actions
1. Local infiltration	Regional anesthesia produced by local infiltration of the nerves of the perineum	Simple to administer Does not affect fetus Useful for perineal repair	No value for analgesia during labor Takes time for infiltration and for agent to take effect	
2. Pudendal block	Local anesthetic injected transvaginally or transperineally into pudendal nerves near the ischial spines	Does not interfere with uterine contractions Does not affect fetus Simple and safe method of securing perineal analgesia for normal deliveries	Difficult to administer No relief of pain of contractions Short duration; may be done in woman's room 30 minutes before delivery (may need to be repeated) May fail to produce adequate pain relief Woman must be cooperative	Help woman relax during administration Observe for signs of hematoma or rectal puncture
3. Paracervical block	Local anesthetic agent injected along base of broad ligament, in walls of lower uterine segment, and in vaginal fornix lateral to cervix	Does not interrupt woman's ability to push with contractions	Relieves pain in first stage but not perineal pain in 2nd and 3rd stage Fetal bradycardia associated with the block—avoided when uteroplacental insufficiency is suspected If woman's cervix is 8 cm. dilated or more, chance of anesthetic being injected accidently into fetal scalp	Monitor fetal heart rate frequently Monitor fetal heart rate and maternal vital signs continuously for 15 minutes following block
4. Subarachnoid blocks a. Spinal	Anesthesia introduced into cerebrospinal fluid in subarachnoid space between L4 and L5	Relative simplicity of procedure Is rapid, certain, and has lasting action Low failure rate Low incidence of side effects when properly performed	Used for pain of second stage; therefore does not provide continuous pain relief in first stage Postspinal headache may occur	Assist in positioning woman for procedure Monitor maternal vital signs for indications of hypotension Monitor fetal vital signs Woman will have trouble moving her legs—assist her when position changes are needed
b. Saddle	Anesthesia introduced into cerebrospinal fluid in subarachnoid space between L4 and L5	Same as spinal	Same as spinal	Same as spinal
5. Extradural blocks a. Caudal	Blocking of nerves in the peridural space at the sacral hiatus Can be given as single or continuous injection. If continuous, plastic catheter is passed into peridural space and taped to back. Anesthetic is injected periodically to maintain pain relief.	Provides analgesia in the 1st and 2nd stages of labor and anesthesia for delivery Woman is awake Has little effect on fetus Better than narcotics for women with metabolic diseases or lung or heart disease, and for some women with hypertensive disorders of pregnancy	Specially trained anesthesiologist is needed Produces hypotension (agents are vasodilators) May prolong labor in primigravida Higher incidence of forceps deliveries if unassisted with pushing May prolong labor if intensity of contractions is decreased Sacral hiatus may be difficult to locate Difficult to keep site clear	Explain procedure Have woman void Monitor maternal and fetal vital signs every 15 minutes and every 2 minutes for 20 minutes immediately following injection of anesthetic If maternal hypotension occurs, turn woman on left side, increase IV fluids, administer oxygen by mask Observe for inadvertent injection of anesthetic into a blood vessel—symptoms are light headedness, tingling, metallic taste in mouth (notify physician immediately) Keep woman's bladder empty Coach her in pushing when pushing is needed in stage 2
b. Lumbar epidural	Extradural analgesia produced by injection of a local anesthetic into the epidural space in the lumbar region Can be given in single or continuous injection. If continuous, plastic catheter is passed into peridural space and taped to back. Anesthetic is injected periodically to maintain pain relief. The passage of the catheter often elicits a neurologic response in the leg or hip if the tip of the catheter touches a nerve in the space. Amount of agent is determined by progress of labor and need for pain relief.	Provides analgesia in the 1st and 2nd stages and anesthesia for delivery Woman is awake and cooperative No effect on fetus unless hypotension occurs Useful when general anesthesia is contraindicated or when woman has diabetes, cardiovascular disease, or pulmonary, renal, or hepatic disease, or is in premature labor	Risk of dural puncture greater than in caudal May cause hypotension Requires expert administration by anesthesiologist Woman requires assistance in pushing Greater incidence of uterine atony following delivery May prolong labor if decreases intensity of contractions Higher incidence of forceps delivery if woman unable to push effectively	Same as for caudal

ered blood glucose levels decrease intensity of uterine contractions). Intravenous fluids may be necessary

First Stage of Labor—Transitional Phase
(7–10 cm.)

A. Characteristics

1. Contractions are usually 2–3 minutes apart, lasting 50–60 seconds.
2. This stage averages 10 contractions or 20 minutes for multigravidas and 20 contractions or 40 minutes for primigravidas.
3. Generally this is the most difficult of the phases of the first stage.
4. Bloody show increases as more capillary vessels in the cervix rupture.
5. Nausea and vomiting may occur because of reflex action as the cervix stretches and begins to retract over the fetal head.
6. Woman may experience feelings of rectal pressure.
7. Woman may have partial amnesia between contractions; she may be restless and may cry during contractions.

B. Nursing Interventions

1. Monitor progress of labor—take and record blood pressure, pulse, respirations, contractions, and fetal heart sounds every 15 minutes.
2. Assist with controlled breathing as contractions occur.
3. Discourage the woman from bearing down until cervical dilation is complete.
4. Encourage the woman to rest between contractions to conserve energy.
5. Since the woman may be irritable during this phase, provide concise and brief explanations.
6. Remind the woman that labor is nearing an end.
7. Prepare the woman for movement to the delivery room since she is usually taken to the delivery room toward the end of this phase (multigravida) or when approximately 2–4 cm. of the fetal head can be seen between contractions (primigravida).

Second Stage of Labor

A. Characteristics

1. Full cervical dilation occurs—infant is delivered.
2. Usually primigravidas have an average of 20 contractions and multigravidas an average of 10 contractions.

B. Nursing Interventions

1. Monitor fetal heart sounds, contractions, and blood pressure approximately every 5 minutes during this stage.
2. Assist the woman into lithotomy position (on delivery table or in birthing bed). Delivery chair may be used in some institutions, as may alternate birthing positions. Elevate both of the woman's legs simultaneously (to avoid backache, injury or ligament strain) and position in stirrups. Adjust stirrups to leg length and provide padding to prevent pressure on the popliteal nerves and veins.
3. Coach for most effective pushing—only with contraction; use of abdominal muscles.
4. If partner or support person is present, have him or her positioned to support woman and see birth if desired.
5. Adjust delivery mirror so the woman can see birth if desired.
6. Cleanse vulva and perineal area.
7. Move delivery table with instruments, drapes, etc. for easy access by midwife or physician.
8. Check equipment needed for infant resuscitation should it be necessary—gather equipment needed for normal newborn care.
9. Keep the woman/couple informed of progress of delivery.
10. The woman may need to be catheterized if bladder is full (avoids bladder trauma and allows presenting part to descend more easily).
11. When the head is encircled by the vulvovaginal ring, an episiotomy (perineal incision) may be performed by midwife or physician to prevent tearing of the perineum.
12. When head is delivered, mucus is wiped from face and aspirated (with bulb syringe) from the nose and mouth.
13. If loops of umbilical cord are around the infant's neck, they are loosened and slipped from around the neck; if unable to be loosened the cord is clamped with 2 clamps and cut between them
14. When the body is delivered, the infant is shown to the mother/couple, then given to the nurse or pediatrician for normal newborn care, and finally returned to the mother/couple (see following section).
15. Placenta usually separates and is delivered within 15–20 minutes following delivery (Fig. 25-12).

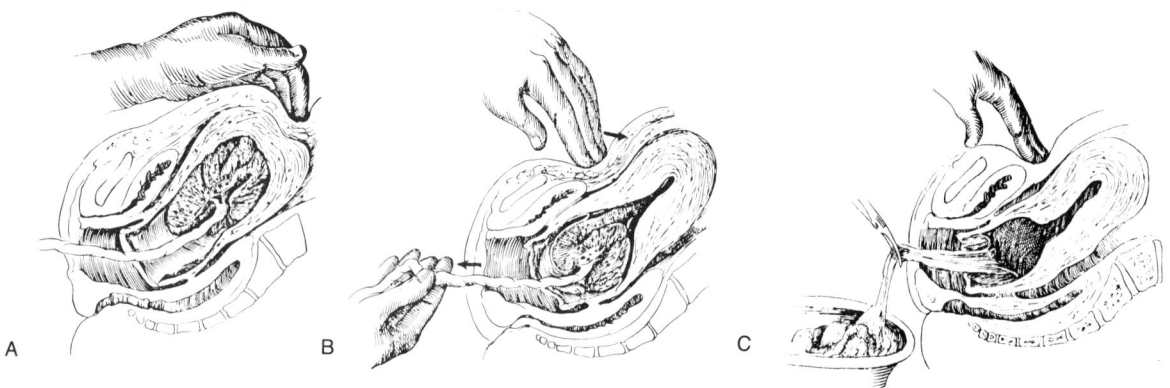

A   B   C

Figure 25-12. Delivery of the placenta. (From Willson JR. Atlas of Obstetric Technic, 2nd ed. St. Louis, CV Mosby)

16. Vaginal canal and cervix are inspected for lacerations or injury; if episiotomy has been performed, it is now sutured.
17. The woman's perineal area is cleansed and a sterile perineal pad applied.
18. The woman is assisted from delivery table to a bed or stretcher; she is moved with her newborn to the recovery room and accompanied by a support person.

Expected Outcomes

1. Manages anxiety; pulse rate and blood pressure at acceptable levels; expresses feelings and concerns

2. Copes with pain—uses breathing techniques; relaxes after contractions; dozes between contractions; uses diversionary techniques; effleurages abdominal area; focuses on one contraction at a time
3. Remains in control; interacts with significant other and health professionals; asks questions about the status of the labor process; listens when status of labor process is explained
4. Absence of untoward bleeding; vital signs within acceptable range
5. No evidence of infection

Immediate Care of the Newborn

The sequence of procedures may differ from one birth setting to another. In more traditional settings, the care is performed immediately after birth. In other settings, many aspects are performed after the parents have had an hour or more to become acquainted with their newborn.

Assessment and Interventions

1. Immediately after delivery, dry the infant—a wet small newborn loses up to 200 calories/kilogram/minute in the delivery room through evaporation, convection, and radiation. Drying the infant cuts this heat loss in half.
2. Aspirate mucus from the mouth and pharynx with suction catheter
3. Evaluate infant's condition by Apgar scoring system (Table 25-4) at 1 and 5 minutes after birth.
    a. Infants scoring 7–10 are free of immediate stress.
    b. Infants scoring 4–6 are moderately depressed.
    c. Infants scoring 0–3 are severely depressed.
4. *Cord care*—cord is tied off approximately 2.5 cm. (1 inch) from abdominal wall using a cotton cord tie, plastic clamp, or rubber band. Count the number of vessels in the cord; fewer than 3 vessels has been associated with renal and cardiac anomalies.
5. *Eye care*—prophylactic treatment against ophthalmia neonatorum (gonorrheal conjunctivitis) is mandatory in all states. Two drops of a 1% silver nitrate solution is placed in the conjunctival sac of the infant's eye. Some clinicians prefer to rinse the eye of mucus, etc., prior to instilling the silver nitrate. No rinse (sterile water) is needed following silver nitrate instillation. The infant of a mother with known gonococcal disease should receive penicillin intramuscularly.
6. *Vitamin K*—1 mg. of vitamin K may be administered

in the delivery room or nursery. The newborn has no intestinal flora to manufacture vitamin K which is important in preventing hemorrhagic disease in the newborn period.
7. *Identification*
    a. Apply ID band or bracelet to infant's arm; include mother's name, hospital number, infant's sex, and time and date of birth.
    b. Apply bracelet with same information on mother's wrist.
    c. After cleansing the soles of the infant's feet, take footprints of the infant and fingerprints of the mother.
8. Weigh and measure the infant.
9. Assess the infant for gestational age and general well-being.

Resuscitation of the Newborn

If after a minute the infant remains moderately depressed, appears limp and cyanotic, has shallow, irregular, or gasping respirations but has a heart rate above 100, he needs ventilatory assistance.
1. A laryngoscope is passed and the airway cleared of mucus or particles; artificial airway is inserted (Fig. 25-13).
2. Oxygen is administered via face mask attached to a hand-operated bag.
3. Newborn's chest should rise with each insufflation, and breath sounds should be heard in both lungs.
4. If color and respiration do not improve or heart rate drops below 100, endotracheal intubation is performed and the infant is given oxygen through a bag attached to the endotracheal tube.

Table 25-4 APGAR Scoring Chart

Sign	0	1	2
Heart rate	Absent	Slow (less than 100)	Over 100
Respiratory effort	Absent	Slow, irregular	Good, crying
Muscle tone	Flaccid	Some flexion of extremities	Active motion
Reflex irritability	No response	Cry	Vigorous cry
Color	Blue, pale	Body pink, extremities blue	Completely pink

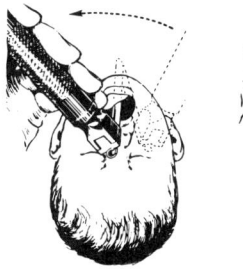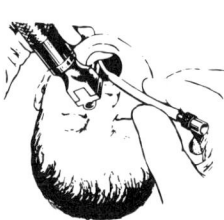

Figure 25-13. Laryngoscope is used to intubate a very depressed infant.

5. If heart rate remains depressed, external cardiac massage is started; compress heart 120 times per minute.
6. Prolonged hypoxia is accompanied by metabolic acidosis; this is treated with 7.5% solution of sodium

bicarbonate through the umbilical vein, provided cardiac activity is adequate
7. Keep the infant warm; IV glucose is usually given to maintain blood sugar.
8. Keep the parents informed of the infant's progress.

Childbirth Approaches

Prepared Childbirth

In the past, the term *natural childbirth* was used to describe one approach to giving birth. To some, natural childbirth meant delivery without analgesic or anesthesia, whereas to those who had developed the approach it simply meant being prepared for childbirth through prenatal education and training. This preparation gave the woman a method of coping with the discomforts of labor and delivery. To avoid the suggestion that analgesia or anesthesia are unavailable to the woman during labor and delivery should she need it, the term *"prepared childbirth"* is now used instead of natural childbirth.

Method of Grantly Dick-Read

1. This method is based on the idea that fear and anticipation of pain arouse natural protective tensions in the body, both psychic and muscular.
2. Fear stimulates the sympathetic nervous system and causes the circular muscle of the cervix to contract.
3. The longitudinal muscles of the uterus then have to act against increased cervical resistance, causing tension and pain.
4. Tension and pain aggravate fear, which produces a vicious cycle of tension, pain, and fear.
5. A minor degree of pain, magnified by fear, becomes unbearable.
6. According to Dick-Read, prenatal courses and training reduce fear, overcome ignorance, and build a woman's self-confidence. Included in this method are:
   a. Explanations of fetal development and childbirth
   b. Descriptions of methods available to relieve pain
   c. Exercises that strengthen certain muscles and relax others
   d. Breathing techniques that will enable the woman to relax in the first stage of labor and work effectively with muscles used during delivery
   e. Explanations of the value of improved physical health and emotional stability for childbirth
   f. The woman is not told that labor and delivery will be painless; analgesia and anesthesia are available if needed or desired
   g. The woman is given empathetic understanding and support during labor by her partner, the nurse, and the physician

Psychoprophylactic or Lamaze Method

1. Psychoprophylactic childbirth has a rationale based on Pavlov's concept of pain perception and his theory of conditioned reflexes (the substitution of favorable conditioned reflexes for unfavorable ones). The Lamaze method is an example of this technique.
2. The woman is taught to replace responses of restlessness, fear, and the loss of control with more useful activity. A high level of activity can excite the cerebral cortex efficiently to inhibit other stimuli, such as pain in labor.

3. The mother-to-be is taught exercises that strengthen the abdominal muscles and relax the perineum.
4. Breathing techniques to help the process of labor are practiced.
5. The woman is conditioned to respond with respiratory activity and disassociation or relaxation of the uninvolved muscles, while controlling her perception of the stimuli associated with labor.
6. One method of control consists of breathing normally while silently mouthing the words to a song and simultaneously tapping the rhythm with the fingers.
7. Similarity between the Dick-Read and Lamaze methods:
   a. Fear, which enhances the perception of pain, may diminish or disappear when the woman understands the physiology of labor.
   b. Since psychic tension enhances perception of pain, relaxation is achieved more easily in a calm, agreeable atmosphere with supportive persons nearby.
   c. Muscular relaxation and a specific type of breathing diminish or abolish the pains of labor.

The Leboyer Method of Delivery

1. The *Leboyer method* is based on the premise that the infant suffers psychological shock at the time of delivery. An effort is made to reduce the contrast between the intrauterine environment and the outside world.
2. Gentle, controlled delivery—prenatal education, support from family and personnel to decrease anxiety, fear, and tension.
3. Emphasis on providing protection to the craniosacral axis by gently supporting the newborn infant's head, neck, and sacrum. The craniosacral axis is completely relaxed, and lost body heat restored in a warm water bath.
4. Avoiding overstimulation of the newborn sensorium—the infant is allowed to breathe spontaneously; cutting the cord is delayed to permit placental blood transfusion for improved respiration.
5. Importance of maternal–infant bond—skin-to-skin contact with mother is provided, and infant is fondled and stroked.

Home Delivery

1. *Home delivery,* although controversial, has won increasing support in recent years.
2. Motivations for home delivery:
   a. Belief that home birth has significant advantages for the family and the newborn infant.
   b. Objection to the impersonal and authoritarian atmosphere of the hospital environment with enforced separation of woman and family.
   c. Desire to avoid such practices as routine cesarean delivery for breech presentation, episiotomy, for-

ceps delivery, oxytocin stimulation, routine monitoring of the FHT, and other practices associated with hospitals.

    d. Risk of in-hospital infections; belief that infant is immune to own-home bacteria.

    e. Rising costs of hospitalization.

3. Contraindications

    a. High-risk indications for infant or mother.

    b. Patient with history of premature or postdate delivery in previous pregnancy.

    c. Women with medical or emotional complications.

    d. Patients who cannot be quickly transported to a hospital.

4. Alternatives

    a. Alteration of hospital setting to a family-centered approach.

    b. Birthing centers for low-risk women with adequate facilities for emergency care.

    c. Properly educated and motivated support personnel.

Emergency Delivery

In delivery under emergency conditions, consider the woman and infant as a unit; work to prevent infection, injury, and hemorrhage in woman and infant and to establish respirations in the newborn.

Interventions

1. Have the woman assume a lithotomy position.

2. If time permits, the person attending the delivery should wash his/her hands and cleanse the mother's perineum.

3. Using a clean or sterile towel, exert gentle pressure against the head of the fetus to control its progress and prevent too rapid a delivery.

    a. Prevents undue stretching of the perineum

    b. Prevents sudden expulsion through the vulva with subsequent infant and maternal complications

4. Encourage the woman to pant at this time to prevent bearing down

5. If membranes have not ruptured by the time the head is delivered, they must be removed immediately by tearing them at the nape of the infant's neck

6. Wipe the infant's face with clean towel.

7. Holding the infant's head in both hands, gently exert downward pressure toward the floor, thereby slipping the anterior shoulder under the symphysis pubis (see Fig. 25-2).

8. If the cord is looped around the infant's neck, gently slip it over the head. If the cord is too tight to permit this, it must be clamped in 2 places and cut between the clamps before the rest of the body is delivered.

9. Support the infant's body and head as it is born.

10. Pick up the infant gently by feet, with head down to help drain mucus; wipe away excess mucus from mouth and nose; gentle rubbing of the back may stimulate breathing.

11. After the infant cries, place him gently on mother's abdomen where she can see him.

12. Avoid touching perineal area to prevent infection.

13. Avoid pulling on cord, which might break and cause hemorrhage.

14. Watch for signs of placental separation.

15. When placenta is delivered, do the following:

    a. Clamp cord with surgical clamp when cord stops pulsating. If clamp is not available, tie off cord with any suitable material several centimeters from the infant's abdomen

    b. Do not cut cord; the physician or midwife will cut it later under more sterile conditions

    c. Wrap the infant and placenta in a blanket; keep the infant warm and close to the mother.

16. Check fundal contractions; massage if indicated. Putting the baby to breast may help the uterus to contract.

17. Place identification of some kind on mother and infant.

18. Give the woman fluids.

19. If the woman is not in bed or a place where she can lie down, she should be assisted to move to a more suitable environment.

20. Do not leave the woman alone.

21. Teach the woman to massage her fundus; explain why the cord has not been cut.

22. Record the time and date of birth.

Bibliography

Books

Aladjem S. Obstetric Practice. St Louis, CV Mosby, 1980

Cibils LA. Electronic Fetal–Maternal monitoring. Boston, PSG Publishing, 1981

Danforth DN (ed). Obstetrics and Gynecology, 4th ed. Philadelphia, Harper & Row, 1982

Freeman RK and Garite TJ. Fetal Heart Rate Monitoring. Baltimore, Williams & Wilkins, 1981

Horsley JA and Crane J. Pain: Deliberative Nursing Intervention. New York, Grune & Stratton, 1982

Oxorn H. Human Birth and Delivery, 4th ed. New York, Appleton-Century-Crofts, 1980

Perez RH. Fetal monitoring. In Protocols for Perinatal Nursing Practice. St Louis, CV Mosby, 1981

Pritchard J, MacDonald PC, and Gant NF. Williams Obstetrics, 17th ed. New York, Appleton-Century-Crofts, 1985

Articles

Affonso DD and Stichler JF. Cesarean birth: Women's reactions. Am J Nurs 1980 Mar; 80:466–468

Anderson CJ. Enhancing reciprocity between mother and neonate. Nurs Res 1981 Mar/Apr; 30:89–93

Andrews C and Andrews E. Nursing, maternal postures and fetal position. Nurs Res 1983 Nov/Dec; 32(6):336–341

Bloom K. Assisting the unprepared woman during labor. JOGN Nurs 1984 Sept/Oct; 13(5):303–306

Boehm FH et al. The effect of electronic fetal monitoring on the incidence of cesarean section. Am J Obstet Gynecol 1981 Jun 1; 140:295–298

Brampton B et al. Initial mothering patterns of low-income black primiparas. JOGN Nurs 1981 May/Jun; 10(3):174–178

Britton GR. Early mother–infant contact and infant temperature stabilization. JOGN Nurs 1980 Mar/Apr; 9:84–86

Brown JL. Effects of suctioning newborn stomach contents during resuscitation. N Engl J Med 1982 Jun 3; 306(22): 1366

Bryant B. Unit dose erythromycin ophthalmic ointment for neonatal ocular prophyloxes. JOGN Nurs 1984 Mar/Apr; 13(2):83–87

Butani P et al. Mothers' perceptions of their labor experiences. Matern Child Nurs J 1980 Summer; 9:73–82

Campbell A and Worthington EL. Teaching expectant fathers how to be better childbirth coaches. MCN 1982 Jan/Feb; (7):28–32

Carmarck B and Corwin T. Nursing care of the schizophrenic maternity patient during labor. MCN 1980 Mar/Apr; 5: 107–113

Challis JR and Mitchell BF. Hormonal control of preterm and term parturition. Semin Perinatol 1981 Apr; 5:192

Chaney JA. Birthing in early America. J Nurse Midwife 1980 Mar/Apr; 25:5–13

Christo S. Infant resuscitation, a postpartum emergency for all concerned. Can Nurse (Suppl) 1983 May; 79(5):36–40

Clark RB. Conduction anesthesia. Clin Obstet Gynecol 1981 Jun; 24(2):601–617

Cranston CS. Obstetrical nurses' attitudes toward fetal monitoring. JOGN Nurs 1980 Nov/Dec; 9:344–347

Currie W. Physiology of uterine activity. Clin Obstet Gynecol 1980 Mar; 23(1): 33–49

Davis JA. The place of birth. Arch Dis Child 1982 June; 57:406–409

Dean PG et al. Making baby's acquaintance: A unique attachment strategy. MCN 1982 Jan/Feb; 7:37–41

Dilts PV. Narcotic analgesia. Clin Obstet Gynecol 1981 Jun; 24(2):597–600

Dunn DM and White DG. Interactions of mothers with their newborns in the first half-hour of life. J Adv Nurs 1981 Jul; (6):271–275

Fullerton JDT. Choice of in-hospital or alternative birth environment as related to the concept of control. J Nurse Midwife 1982 Mar/Apr; 27:17–22

Genest M. Preparation for childbirth—evidence for efficacy, a review. JOGN Nurs 1981 Mar/Apr; 10:82–85

Goodin RC et al. Determinants of maternal temperature during labor. Am J Obstet Gynecol 1982 May 1; 143:97–103

Griffith S. Childbearing and the concept of culture. JOGN Nurs 1982 May/Jun; 11(3):181–185

Heggenhougen HK. Father and childbirth: An anthropological perspective. J Nurse Midwife 1980 Nov/Dec; 25:21–26

Higgings PG and Wayland JR. Labour and delivery in North America. Nurs Times 1981 Sep 16; 77(midwifery suppl):44

Howley C. The older primipara: Implications for nurses. JOGN Nurs 1981 May/Jun; 10:182–185

Humenick SS. Mastery: The key to childbirth satisfaction? A review. Birth Fam J 1981 Summer; 8:79–83

Huszar G et al. Biochemistry and pharmacology of the myometrium and labor regulation at the cellular and molecular levels. Am J Obstet Gynecol 1982 Jan 15; 142:225–237

Klein RP et al. A study of father and nurse support during labor. Birth Fam J 1981 Fall; 8:161–164

Krebs HB et al. Intrapartum fetal heart rate monitoring. Am J Obstet Gynecol 1982 Feb 1; 142:297–305

Lavin JP et al. The effects of bupivacaine and chloroprocaine as local anesthetics for epidural anesthesia on fetal heart rate monitoring parameters. Am J Obstet Gynecol 1981 Nov 15; 141:717–722

Lederman RP et al. Relationship of psychological factors in pregnancy to progress in labor. Nurs Res 1979 Mar/Apr; 28:94–97

MacLaughlin SM and Taubenheim AM. Epidural anesthesia for obstetric patients. JOGN Nurs 1981 Jan/Feb; 10:9–15

May K and Di Tolla K. In-hospital alternative birth centers: Where do we go from here? MCN 1984 Jan/Feb; 9(1):48–51

McDonough M, Sheriff D and Zimmel P. Parents' responses to fetal monitoring. MCN 1981 Jan/Feb; 6:32–4

McKay S. Squatting: An alternate position for the second stage of labor. MCN 1984 May/Jun; 9:181–183

McKay SR. Second stage labor—has tradition replaced safety? Am J Nurs 1981 May; 81(5):1016–1019

Mercer RT. A theoretical framework for studying factors that impact on the maternal role. Nurs Res 1981 Mar/Apr; 30:73–77

Meissner JE. Predicting a patient's anxiety level during labor: A two part assessment tool. Nursing '80 1980 Jul; 10:50–51

Modanlou HD and Freeman RK. Sinusoidal fetal heart rate pattern: Its definition and clinical significance. Am J Obstet Gynecol 1982 Apr 15; 142: 1033–1038

Molfese V, Sunshine P and Bennett A. Reactions of women to intrapartum fetal monitoring. Obstet Gynecol 1982 Jun; 5(6):705–709

Morrison JC et al. Meperidine metabolism in the parturient. Obstet Gynecol 1982 Mar; 59(3):359–365

NAACOG Technical Bulletin. The nurses' role in electronic fetal monitoring. No. 7, 1980

Noble E. Controversies in maternal effort during labor and delivery. J Nurse Midwife 1981 Mar/Apr; 26:13–22

Okita JR et al. Initiation of human parturition. Am J Obstet Gynecol 1982 Feb 15; 142:432–435

Rayburn WF et al. Umbilical cord length and intrapartum complications. Obstet Gynecol 1981 Apr; 57(4):450–452

Richardson P. Significant relationships and their impact on childbearing a review. Matern Child Nurs J 1982; Spring; (11):17–40

Scott-Palmer J et al. Pain during childbirth and menstruation: A study of locus of control. J Psychosom Res 1981 May/Jun; 25(3):151–155

Smith C. Epidural anesthesia in labor: Various agents employed. JOGN Nurs 1984 Jan/Feb; 13(1):17–21

Stewart P. Spontaneous labor: When should the membranes be ruptured? Br J Obstet Gynecol 1982 Jan; 89:39–43

Worthington EL et al. Which prepared childbirth coping strategies are effective? JOGN Nurs 1982 Jan/Feb; (11):45–51

Care of the Mother and Newborn During the Postpartal Period

26

The Puerperium

Physiologic Changes of the Puerperium

The *puerperium* is the period beginning after delivery and ending when the woman's body has returned as closely as possible to its prepregnant state. The period lasts approximately 6 weeks.

1. Uterine changes
   a. The fundus is usually midline and about at the level of the woman's umbilicus after delivery and for the following day. After this, the level of the fundus descends about 1 finger breadth (or 1 cm.) each day until by the 10th day, it has descended into the pelvic cavity and can no longer be palpated.
   b. Postdelivery, *lochia* (a vaginal discharge), consisting of fatty epithelial cells, shreds of membrane, decidua, and blood, is red (*lochia rubra*) for about 2–3 days. It then progresses to a paler or more brownish color (*lochia serosa*), followed by a whitish or yellowish color (*lochia alba*) in the 7th to 10th day. Lochia usually ceases by three weeks and the placental site is completely healed by the 6th week.
2. The vaginal walls, uterine ligaments, and muscles of the pelvic floor and abdominal wall regain most of their tone during the puerperium.
3. Postpartum diuresis occurs between the 2nd and 5th postpartum days, as extracellular water accumulated during pregnancy begins to be excreted. A diuresis may also occur shortly after delivery if urinary output was obstructed because of the pressure of the presenting part or if intravenous fluids were given to the woman during labor.
4. Breasts
   a. With loss of the placenta, circulating levels of estrogen and progesterone decrease while levels of prolactin increase, thus initiating lactation in the postpartum woman.
   b. *Colostrum,* a yellowish fluid containing more minerals and protein but less sugar and fat than mature breast milk and having a laxative effect on the infant, is secreted for the first 2 days postpartum.
   c. Mature milk secretion is usually present by the 3rd postpartum day but may be present earlier if a woman breast-feeds immediately following delivery.
   d. Breast engorgement with milk, venous and lymphatic stasis, and swollen, tense, and tender breast tissue may occur between days 3 and 5 postpartum.

Emotional and Behavioral Status

1. Following delivery, the woman may progress through Rubin's stages of "taking in" and "taking hold."
   a. "Taking in"
      (1) May begin with a refreshing sleep following delivery
      (2) Woman exhibits passive, dependent behavior
      (3) Woman is concerned with sleep and the intake of food, both for herself and for the infant
   b. "Taking hold"
      (1) Woman begins to initiate action and to function more independently
      (2) Woman may require more explanation and reassurance that she is functioning well, especially caring for her infant
      (3) As the woman meets success in caring for the newborn, her concern extends to other family members and their activities
2. Some women may experience a euphoria in the first few days following delivery and set unrealistic goals for activities following discharge from the birthing place.
3. Many woman may experience temporary mood swings during this period because of the discomfort, fatigue, and exhaustion following labor and delivery and because of hormonal changes following delivery.
4. Some mothers may experience "postpartum blues" about the third postpartum day and exhibit irritability, poor appetite, insomnia, tearfulness, or crying. This is a temporary situation. Severe or prolonged depression is usually a sign of a more serious condition.
5. Nursing research findings indicate that new mothers identified the following postpartum needs: Coping with
   a. the physical changes and discomforts of the puerperium, including a need to regain their prepregnancy figure.
   b. changing family relationships and meeting the needs of family members including the infant.
   c. fatigue, emotional stress, feelings of isolation, and being "tied down."
   d. a lack of time for personal needs and interests.

Assessment

Immediate Postpartum Assessment

The first hour after delivery of the placenta ("4th stage of labor") is a critical period; postpartum hemorrhage is most likely to occur at this time.

1. Check fundus frequently and massage gently if fundus is not firm.
2. Inspect perineum frequently for visible signs of bleeding.
3. Evaluate vital signs at frequent intervals as determined by the woman's condition.
4. Avoid leaving the woman alone at this time since changes in condition can occur precipitously.

Subsequent Postpartum Assessment

A. For Postpartum Bleeding

1. Check firmness of the fundus at regular intervals.
2. Inspect the perineum regularly for frank bleeding.
   a. Note color, amount, and odor of the lochia (perineal discharge).
   b. Count the number of perineal pads that are saturated in each 8-hour period.
3. Assess vital signs at least once daily and more frequently if indicated.

Patient Problems/Nursing Diagnoses

1. Potential bleeding related to vaginal delivery, uterine atony, cesarean delivery, episiotomy, complications
2. Discomfort (backache, uterine cramping, breast engorgement, edema of episiotomy, hemorrhoids) related to process of labor and delivery
3. Urinary retention related to bladder trauma
4. Constipation related to decrease in muscle tone of intestines, lack of food and fluid during labor, perineal tenderness, episiotomy, hemorrhoids
5. Infection related to prolonged labor, vaginal delivery, lacerations, anemia
6. Knowledge deficit related to inadequate/lack of childbirth/parenting preparation, lack of self-confidence
7. Impaired maternal–child bonding related to age of mother, marital status, socioeconomic factors
8. Anxiety related to inability to integrate labor experience, adapting to new family member, chronic fatigue

Planning and Implementation

Nursing Interventions: Immediate Postoperative Care

A. First Hour After Delivery (4th Stage of Labor)

1. Provide a quiet environment for the woman to promote as much rest as possible
2. Evaluate the woman's vital signs every 15 minutes or less frequently, depending on her condition.
3. Evaluate fundal height and position when checking vital signs. Height should be at the umbilicus or below, and at the midline.
   a. If uterus is displaced to right or left, the woman's bladder may be full.
   b. If fundus is not firm, massage gently and express clots that may be collecting in the uterine cavity.
   c. Teach the woman to feel her fundus and explain the reasons for your actions as you proceed.
4. Inspect perineum for signs of bleeding including hematoma formation. An ice pack on the perineum will promote comfort and help to reduce swelling of the tissue.
5. Evaluate the amount of vaginal bleeding.

Nursing Interventions: Subsequent Postpartum Care

A. General Measures

1. Promote a quiet environment to allow frequent rest periods for the woman.
2. Assess height and firmness of the fundus and vital signs once daily or more frequently if indicated.
3. Inspect the woman's perineum daily for healing and signs of bleeding or infection.

B. Perineal Care

1. Teach the woman to carry out perineal care—warm water over the perineum after each voiding and/or bowel movement and routinely several times a day to promote comfort, cleanliness, and healing.
2. Sitz baths may be used for the same purpose.
3. Teach the woman to apply perineal pads by touching the outside only, thus keeping clean the portion that will touch her perineum.
4. Teach the woman to use witch hazel compresses or anesthetic sprays or ointments for relief of perineal discomfort.
5. Teach the woman to contract her buttocks before sitting to reduce perineal discomfort while sitting in a chair.

C. Voiding

1. Check the woman's voiding pattern. Most women void in sufficient amounts within 8 hours of delivery.
2. If the woman's meatus or bladder has been traumatized during delivery, she may need to be catheterized until the urinary tract swelling has subsided.
3. Teach the woman to void every several hours to keep her bladder empty. This may help reduce uterine cramping and promote comfort.

D. Breast Care

1. Assess the condition of the woman's breasts and nipples (a) Inspect nipples for reddening, erosions, or fissures. Reddened areas may be improved with A&D ointment, a lanolin cream, and air drying for 15 minutes several times a day.
2. Teach the woman to wash her breasts with warm water to avoid removing protective skin oils.
3. Teach the woman to wear a brassiere or breast binder that provides good support night and day.
4. Lactation suppressants such as estrogens and androgens, or bromocriptine mesylate may be given to bottle-feeding mothers to suppress milk production and breast engorgement.
5. Check the breasts for signs of engorgement (swollen, tender, tense, shiny breast tissue).
   a. If breasts are engorged and the woman is breast-feeding:
      (1) Allow warm to hot shower water to flow over the breasts to improve comfort.
      (2) Hot compresses on the breasts may improve comfort.
      (3) Express some milk manually or by breast pump to improve comfort and make nipple more available for infant feeding.
      (4) A mild analgesic may be used to improve comfort (see Guidelines on Breast-Feeding, p. 991).
   b. If breasts are engorged and the mother is bottle-feeding:
      (1) Teach the woman to wear a supportive breast binder night and day.

(2) Teach the woman to avoid handling her breasts since this stimulates more milk production.

(3) Suggest ice bags to the breasts to provide comfort.

(4) Moderately strong analgesics may be needed to provide comfort.

E. Diet and Elimination

1. Review the woman's dietary intake with her.
2. Emphasize foods high in iron, protein, and vitamins to aid the healing process. Foods such as fresh fruits and vegetables with high fiber will help reestablish normal bowel habits.
3. Remind the woman that not all of her weight gain during pregnancy was lost at delivery; approximately 5 pounds will be lost during the puerperium.
4. If the woman is breast-feeding, she should add between 500 and 900 additional calories daily for milk production. She also needs 20 gm. more protein than before she was pregnant, and additional calcium, phosphorus, vitamins D, A, C, E, B_1, and B_2, niacin, zinc, and iodine.

F. Exercise

1. Review postpartum exercises aimed at regaining muscle tone and body shape and promoting comfort (see Postpartum Exercises, p. 1001).

G. Rest and Ambulation

1. Most mothers ambulate within 8–12 hours after delivery or sooner.
2. When assisting the woman to ambulate for the first time, have her sit on the edge of the bed for 5 minutes, then ambulate only with assistance to avoid falling because of dizziness and fainting.
3. Counsel the woman to rest for at least 30 minutes after she arrives home from the hospital and to rest several times during the day for the first few weeks.
4. Counsel the woman to confine her activities to 1 floor if possible and avoid stair climbing as much as possible for the first several days at home.

H. Resumption of Sex

1. Intercourse may be resumed when perineal and uterine wounds have healed.
2. Healing occurs within 2–4 weeks; however, evaluation by the midwife or physician during the follow-up visit is necessary. Methods of contraception should be reviewed.
3. For women who are bottle-feeding, menstruation usually returns within 4–8 weeks.
4. For women who are breast-feeding, menstruation usually returns within 4 months, but may return between 2–18 months postpartum.

▶ **Patient Education** *Alert:* Nursing mothers may ovulate even if experiencing amenorrhea, and so a form of contraception should be used if pregnancy is to be avoided.

I. Personal Needs

1. Counsel the woman to provide quiet times for herself at home and help her establish realistic goals for resuming her own interests and activities.
2. Counsel the couple to provide times to reestablish their own relationship and to renew their social interests and relationships.

Evaluation
Expected Outcomes

1. Absence of untoward bleeding; uterus firm; decreasing color and amount of lochia; normal vital signs; normal hematocrit values; level of fundus at normal position; no clots/tissues passed vaginally
2. Reports decrease in discomfort; able to care for self and infant
3. Voids freely and without discomfort
4. Lack of constipation; eats high-fiber foods and uses stool softeners
5. Absence of infection; normal vital signs and laboratory values; no abnormal redness of perineum; no purulent discharge nor foul odor of lochia, no urinary complaints, no pain or swelling in legs
6. Demonstrates ability to perform infant care; shows confidence in caring for infant
7. Shows maternal–child bonding—maintains eye contact; calls infant by name; talks to infant; strokes infant and holds him close between feedings; shows she is moving into "taking hold" phase; participates in daily care of infant
8. Verbalizes diminishing anxiety; talks about labor and delivery experience; discusses infant's schedule; making plans for household help and for renewing some social activities

Guidelines: Breast-Feeding

Procedure

Action	Rationale/Amplification
1. Have the mother wash her hands before breast-feeding.	1. Protects the infant and mother's breasts from infection.
2. Have the mother breast-feed very soon after delivery.	2. Stimulates earlier milk production; gives the infant full benefit of colostrum; aids in contraction of the mother's uterus.
3. Have the mother assume a comfortable position—lying on her side, sitting upright, tailor sitting, etc.—with the infant facing the mother (Fig. 26-1).	3. Enhances milk letdown, more complete emptying of the breasts, lessens nipple trauma.
4. When beginning breast-feeding, have the mother "point up" the nipple by gently pressing the areola between two fingers.	4. Helps the infant get a firm grasp on the nipple and areola.
5. Make sure the infant has both the areola and nipple in his mouth.	5. Sucking on only the nipple causes nipple pain and trauma.

(continued)

Guidelines: Breast-Feeding (continued)

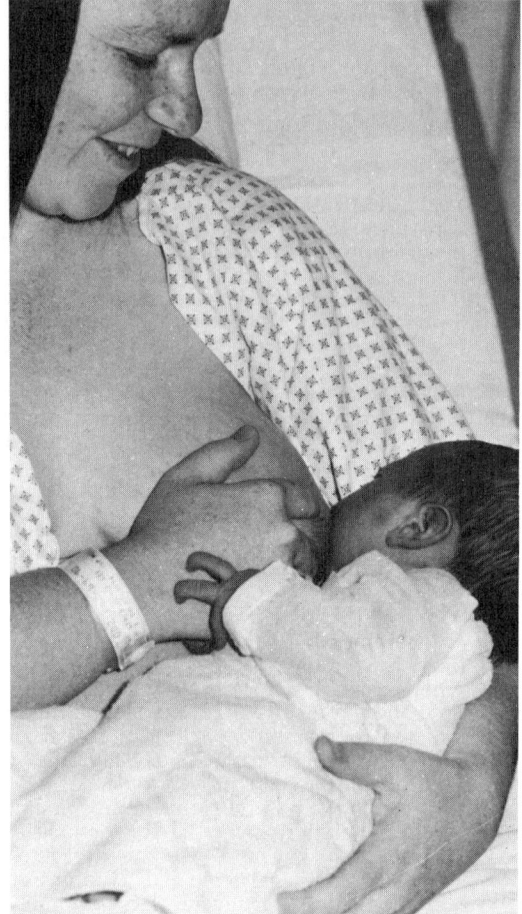

Figure 26-1. The mother may prefer to assume a sitting position when nursing her infant.

Procedure
(Cont.)

Action	Rationale / Amplification
6. Make sure the infant's nasal pathway is open. If the infant's nose is flat against the mother's breast, have her indent her breast near the infant's nose to ensure an open breathing space.	6. An obstructed nasal pathway will cause the infant to stop breast feeding
7. Have the mother alternate the breast she begins breast-feeding with at each feeding.	7. The infant's sucking is most rigorous at the beginning of breast-feeding. Alternating the breast used first at each feeding will reduce nipple pain and trauma.
8. Have the mother use each breast at each feeding. Begin with 5 minutes at each breast, then increase the time at each breast, allowing the infant to suck until he stops sucking actively. Pin a safety pin to the bra as a reminder of which breast to start with at the next feeding.	8. Empties each breast and maintains milk supply.
9. Have the mother breast-feed frequently and on a demand schedule (every 2–4 hours).	9. Frequent feedings maintain the milk supply, and prevent overly vigorous sucking on the nipple and nipple trauma.
10. Have the mother break the infant's suction by placing her finger in the corner of his mouth.	10. Prevents nipple trauma.
11. Have the mother air dry her nipples for 15–20 minutes after each feeding.	11. Prevents or reduces nipple trauma.
12. Have the mother bubble the infant at the end or midway through the feeding.	12. Releasing air in the infant's stomach will make him more satisfied and less fretful.

Procedure
(Cont.)

Action	Rationale/Amplification
13. Alert the mother that uterine cramping may occur, especially in multiparous women.	13. Nursing stimulates release of oxytocin causing uterine cramping which can be worse in women with lessened uterine tone.
14. Teach the mother to provide for adequate rest and to avoid tension, fatigue, and a stressful environment.	14. Maternal fatigue, stress, and tension inhibits the letdown reflex and makes breast milk less available to the infant at feeding.
15. Avoid taking medications and drugs.	15. Many substances pass into breast milk and can reduce milk production or have a deleterious effect on the infant.

Postpartum Exercises

Exercises for the Immediate Postpartum Period
(can be performed in bed)

Toe Stretch (tightens calf muscles)
While lying on your back, keep your legs straight and point your toes away from you, then pull your legs toward you and point your toes toward your chest. Repeat 10 times.

Pelvic Floor Exercise (tightens perineal muscles)
Contract your buttocks for a count of 5 and relax. Contract your buttocks and press thighs together for a count of 7 and relax. Contract buttocks, press thighs together, and draw in anus for a count of 10 and relax.

Exercises for Later Recovery Period (after first postpartum visit)
Bicycle (tightens thighs, stomach, waist)
Lie on your back on the floor, arms at sides, palms down. Begin rotating your legs as if you were riding a bicycle, bringing the knees all the way in toward the chest and stretching the legs out as long and straight as possible. Breathe deeply and evenly. Do the exercises at a moderate speed and do not tire yourself.
Buttocks Exercise (tightens buttocks)
Lie on your stomach and keep your legs straight. Raise your left leg in the air, then repeat with your right leg (feel the contraction in your buttocks). Keep your hips on the floor. Repeat 10 times.
Twist (tightens waist)
Stand with legs wide apart. Hold your arms at your sides, shoulder level, palms down. Twist your body from side to front and back again. Feel the twist in your waist.

Physiology of the Newborn

Transitional Stages
The first 24 hours of life constitute a highly vulnerable time during which the infant must make several adjustments to extrauterine life. During this period of transition, 6 overlapping stages have been identified:
Stage 1. Receives stimulation (during labor) from the pressure of the uterine contractions and from changes in pressure when the membranes rupture.
Stage 2. Encounters a variety of foreign stimuli—light, cold, gravity, and sound.
Stage 3. Initiates breathing.
Stage 4. Changes from fetal to neonatal circulation.
Stage 5. Undergoes alteration in metabolic processes with activation of liver, renal and gastrointestinal tracts for passage of meconium.
Stage 6. Achieves a steady level or equilibrium in metabolic processes (production of enzymes, increased blood oxygen saturation, decrease in acidosis associated with birth, and recovery of the neurologic tissues from the trauma of labor and delivery).

Respiratory Changes
A. Initiation of Respiration
A combination of physical, sensory, and chemical factors.
1. *Physical*—sudden change from intrauterine life produces stimulation needed to initiate respiration.
2. *Chemical*—changes in the blood as a result of transitory asphyxia include the following:
   a. Lowered oxygen level
   b. Increased carbon dioxide level
   c. Lowered pH—if asphyxia is prolonged, depression of the respiratory center (rather than stimulation) occurs, and resuscitation is necessary
3. *Sensory*—maximum effort is required to expand the lungs and fill the collapsed alveoli.
   a. Surface tension in the respiratory tract, resistance in the lung tissue, the thorax, the diaphragm, and the respiratory muscles must be overcome.
   b. First active inspiration comes from a strong contraction of the diaphragm, which creates a high negative intrathoracic pressure causing a marked retraction of the ribs and distention of the alveolar space. (Any remaining fluid is reabsorbed rapidly if the pulmonary capillary blood flow is adequate, since the fluid is hypotonic and passes easily into the capillaries.)

B. Character of Normal Respirations
1. The infant begins life with intense activity; diffuse, purposeless movements alternate with periods of relative immobility.
2. Respirations are rapid, as high as 80 breaths per minute, accompanied by tachycardia, 140–180 beats per minute.

3. Relaxation occurs and the infant usually sleeps; he then awakes to a second period of activity. Oral mucus may be a major problem during this period.
4. Respirations are reduced to 35–50 breaths per minute and become quiet and shallow; respiration is carried out by the diaphragm and abdominal muscles.
5. Period of dyspnea and cyanosis may occur suddenly in an infant who is breathing normally; this may indicate an anomaly or a pathologic condition.

Circulatory Changes

A. Anatomic Changes (see Chapter 24)

B. Blood Volume

85–100 ml./kg. at birth
Factors that influence blood volume:
1. Maternal blood volume (affected by maternal diseases and iron intake)
2. Placental function
3. Uterine contractions during labor
4. Amount of blood loss associated with delivery
5. Placental transfusion at birth—increase in blood volume of 60% if cord is clamped and cut after pulsation ceases

C. Peripheral Circulation

Residual cyanosis in hands and feet for 1–2 hours after birth because of sluggish circulation.

D. Pulse Rate

1. Generally follows pattern similar to that of respiration.
2. Apical pulse rate is more accurate.
3. Normal rate 120–150 beats per minute.
4. May rise to 180 when the infant is crying or drop to 70 during sleep.

E. Blood Pressure

70/45 at birth; 100/50 by 10th day

F. Blood Coagulation

Coagulability is temporarily diminished because of lack of bacteria in the intestinal tract that contribute to the synthesis of vitamin K.
1. Coagulation time, 3–4 minutes
2. Bleeding time, 2–4 minutes
3. Prothrombin, 50% decreasing to 20%–30%

G. Blood Elements

Values for blood components in the neonate
1. Hemoglobin, 16–22 gm.
2. Reticulocytes, 2.5%–6.5%
3. Leukocytes, 15,000–20,000 cu. mm.
(See Appendix III, p. 1534, for detailed pediatric hematology table.)

Temperature Regulation

1. Mechanism not fully developed; heat production low.
2. Infant responds readily to environmental heat and cold stimuli.
3. There may be heat loss of 2°–3°C. at birth by evaporation, convection, conduction, and radiation.
4. The infant develops mechanisms to counterbalance heat loss.
   a. Vasoconstriction—blood directed away from skin surfaces.
   b. Insulation—from subcutaneous adipose tissue.
   c. Heat production—by nonshivering thermogenesis elicited by the sympathetic nervous system's response to decreased temperatures; activated by adrenalin.

Basal Metabolism

1. Surface area of infant is large in comparison with weight.
2. Basal metabolism per kg. of body weight is higher than that of adult.
3. Calorie requirements are high—117 calories per kilogram of body weight per day.

Renal Function

Low arterial blood pressure and increased renal vascular resistance lead to the following effects:
1. Decreased ability to concentrate urine because of low tubular reabsorption rate and low levels of antidiuretic hormone.
2. Limited ability to maintain water balance by excretion of excess water or retention of needed water.
3. Decreased ability to maintain acid–base mechanism; slower excretion of electrolytes, especially sodium and the hydrogen ions, results in accumulation of these substances, which predisposes the infant to dehydration, acidosis, and hyperkalemia.
4. Excretion of large amount of uric acid during newborn period—appears as "brick dust" stain on diaper.

Hepatic Function

Function limited because of lack of gastrointestinal tract activity and limited blood supply; consequences include the following:
1. Decreased ability to conjugate bilirubin (rationale for physiologic jaundice).
2. Decreased ability to regulate blood sugar concentration (rationale for neonatal hypoglycemia).
3. Deficient production of prothrombin and other coagulation factors that depend on vitamin K for synthesis (rationale for neonate's predisposition to hemorrhage).

Endocrine Function

Endocrine glands are better organized than other systems; disturbances are most often related to maternally provided hormones, which can cause the following:
1. Vaginal discharge (and/or bleeding) in female infants.
2. Enlargement of mammary glands in both sexes—related to increased estrogen, luteal, and prolactin activity.
3. Disturbances related to maternal endocrine pathology (e.g., diabetic mother or mother with inadequate iodine intake).

Gastrointestinal Changes

The newborn's intestinal tract is proportionately longer than the adult's; however, elastic tissue and musculature are not fully developed, and neurologic control is variable and inadequate.
1. Most digestive enzymes are present, with the exception of pancreatic amylase and lipase. Protein and carbohydrates are easily absorbed, but fat absorption is poor.
2. Limitations relate primarily to anatomic structures and neutrality of the gastric contents.
3. Imperfect control of the cardiac and pyloric sphincters and immaturity of neurologic control cause mild regurgitation or slight vomiting.

4. Irregularities in peristaltic motility slow stomach emptying.
5. Peristalsis increases in the lower ileum, resulting in stool frequency—1–6 stools per day. Absence of stool within 48 hours after birth is indicative of intestinal obstruction.

Neurologic Changes

Neurologic mechanisms are immature; they are not fully developed anatomically or physiologically, and as a result, uncoordinated movements, labile temperature regulation, and poor control over musculature are characteristic of the infant. Reflexes are important indices of infant neural development. (See Chapter 29, pages 1066–1068, for a detailed discussion of the pediatric neurologic examination. See also Chapter 30, Pediatric Concepts, Growth and Development [pp. 1074–1087], which describes reflexes of the newborn and traces appearance and disappearance of the various reflexes.)

Pertinent History

1. Mother's age, socioeconomic status, ethnic or cultural group, educational level, marital status
2. Mother's/family's past medical history
3. Mother's past obstetrical history
4. Mother's prenatal history with this pregnancy
5. Labor and delivery

Physical Findings and Physiologic Functioning

A. Posture

1. Full-term newborn assumes symmetric posture; face turned to side, flexed extremities; hands tightly fisted with thumb covered by fingers.
2. Asymmetric posture may be caused by fractures of clavicle or humerus or by nerve injuries commonly of the brachial plexus.
3. Infants born in breech position may keep knees and legs straightened or in frog position depending on the type of breech birth.

B. Length

Average length of full-term newborn is 51 cm. (20 inches); range 46–56 cm. (18–22 inches).

C. Weight

Average weight of male infants is 3,400 gm. (7½ lbs.); female infants, 3,200 gm. (7 lbs.). Range of 80% of full-term newborns is 2,900 to 4,100 gm. (6 lbs., 5 oz.–9 lbs., 2 oz.).

D. Skin

Examine under natural light for:
1. Hair distribution—term infant will have some lanugo over back; most will have disappeared on extremities and other areas of the body.
2. Turgor—term infant should have good skin turgor.
3. Color
   a. Cyanosis—*acrocyanosis,* bluish color in hands and feet, is common due to immature peripheral circulation.
   b. Pallor—may indicate cold, stress, anemia, or cardiac failure.
   c. Plethora—reddish coloration may be due to excessive red blood cells from intrauterine intravascular transfusion (twins), cardiac disease, or diabetes in the mother.
   d. Jaundice—physiologic jaundice due to immaturity of liver is common beginning on day 2,

peaking at 1 week and disappearing by the 2nd week. First appears in skin over face or upper body then progresses over larger area; can also be seen in conjunctivae of eyes.
   e. Meconium staining—staining of skin, fingernails, and umbilical cord indicates compromise in utero unless infant was in breech position.
4. Dryness/peeling—marked scaliness and desquamation are a sign of postmaturity.
5. Vernix—in full-term infants, most vernix is found in skin folds under the arms and in the groin.
6. Nails—should reach end of fingertips and be well-developed in the full-term infant.
7. Edema—some edema may be present over buttocks, back, and occiput if the infant has been supine; pitting edema may be due to erythroblastosis, heart failure, electrolyte imbalance.
8. Ecchymoses—may appear over the presenting part in a difficult delivery; may also indicate infection or bleeding problem.
9. Petechiae—pinpoint hemorrhages on skin due to increased intravascular pressure, infection or thrombocytopenia; regresses within 24–48 hours.
10. Erythema toxicum—newborn rash appearing on trunk and diaper areas; regresses within 48 hours.
11. Hemangiomas—vascular lesions present at birth; some may fade, but others may be permanent.
12. Telangiectatic nevi (stork bites)—flat red or purple lesions most often found on back of neck, lower occiput, upper eyelid, and bridge of nose; regress by 2 years of age.
13. Milia—enlarged sebaceous glands found on nose, chin, cheeks, and forehead; regress in several days to a week or two.
14. Mongolian spots—blue pigmentation on lower back, sacrum and buttocks; common in Blacks, Asians, and infants of Southern European heritage; regress by 4 years of age.
15. Café-au-lait spots—brown macules, usually not significant; large numbers may indicate underlying neurofibromatosis.
16. Harlequin color change—when on side, dependent half turns red, upperhalf pale; due to gravity and vasomotor instability.

E. Head

1. Examine head and face for symmetry, paralysis, shape, swelling, movement.
   a. *Caput succedaneum*—swelling of soft tissues of the scalp because of pressure; swelling crosses suture lines.
   b. *Cephalohematoma*—subperiosteal hemorrhage with collection of blood between periosteum and bone; swelling does not cross suture lines.
   c. *Molding*—overlapping of skull bones caused by compression during labor and delivery (disappears in a few days).
   d. Examine symmetry of facial movements.
2. Measure biparietal circumference—33–35 cm. (13–14 inches); approximately 2 cm. (1 inch) larger than chest.
3. Fontanelles—area where more than 2 skull bones meet; covered with strong band of connective tissue; also called "soft spot."
   a. Enlarged or bulging—may indicate increased intracranial pressure.
   b. Sunken—often indicates dehydration.
   c. Size—posterior may be obliterated because of

molding—generally closes in 2–3 months; anterior is palpable—generally closes in 12–18 months.

4. Sutures—junctions of adjoining skull bones
   a. Overriding—due to molding during labor and delivery.
   b. Separation—extensive separation may be found in malnourished infants and with increased intracranial pressure.

F. Face

1. Eyes—examine the following:
   a. Color—sclerae in most full-term infants is white; eye color usually gray–blue in white infants, brown in dark-skinned infants; final eye color is evident by 6–12 months.
   b. Hemorrhagic areas—subconjunctival hemorrhages may appear as a red band from pressure during delivery; regresses within 2 weeks.
   c. Edema—of the eyelids may be due to pressure on the head and face during labor and delivery.
   d. Conjunctivitis or discharge—may be due to instillation of silver nitrate or infections from organisms such as staphylococcus or gonococcus.
   e. Jaundice—may be seen in sclera because of physiologic jaundice or, if severe, blood group incompatibility.
   f. Pupils—equal and should constrict in bright light.
   g. Infant can see and discriminate patterns; limited by imperfect oculomotor coordination and inability to accommodate for varying distances.
2. Nose—examine the following:
   a. Patency—necessary since infants breathe through the nose, not the mouth.
   b. Nasal flaring—may indicate respiratory distress.
   c. Discharge—due to congestion or possibly infection.
3. Ears—examine the following:
   a. Formation—large, flabby ears that slant forward may indicate abnormalities of kidney or other parts of urinary tract.
   b. Position in relation to eye—helix (top of ear) on same plane as eye; low-set ears may indicate chromosomal or renal abnormalities.
   c. Cartilage—full-term infant has sufficient cartilage to make ear feel firm.
   d. Hearing—auditory canals may be congested for a day or two following birth; the infant should hear well in a few days.
4. Mouth—examine the following:
   a. Size—small mouth found in trisomy 18 and 21; corners of mouth turn down ("fish mouth") in fetal alcohol syndrome.
   b. Palate—examine hard palate for closure.
   c. Size of tongue in relation to mouth—excessively large tongue seen in congenital anomalies such as cretinism and trisomy 21.
   d. Teeth—predeciduous teeth are found on rare occasion; if they interfere with feeding, they may be removed.
   e. Epstein's pearls—small white nodules found on sides of hard palate (often mistaken for teeth); regress in a few weeks.
   f. Frenulum linguae—thin ridge of tissue running from base of tongue along undersurface to tip of tongue; formerly believed to cause tongue tie; no treatment necessary.
   g. Sucking blisters—thickened areas on midline of upper lip; no treatment necessary.
   h. Infections—*thrush,* caused by *Candida albicans* may appear as white patches on tongue that do not wash away with fluids; treated with nystatin suspension.

G. Neck

Examine the following:
1. Mobility—infant can move head from side to side; palpate for lymph nodes; palpate clavicle for fractures, especially following a difficult delivery.
2. Torticollis—appears as a spasmodic, one-sided contraction of neck muscles; generally from hematoma of sternocleidomastoid muscle; usually no treatment required.
3. Excessive skin folds may be associated with congenital abnormalities such as trisomy 21.
4. Stiffness and hyperextension may be due to trauma or infection.

H. Chest

Examine the following:
1. Circumference and symmetry—average circumference is 30–33 cm. (12–13 inches), approximately 2 cm. smaller than head circumference.
2. Breast
   a. Engorgement—may occur at day 3 because of withdrawal of maternal hormones, especially estrogen; no treatment required—regresses in 2 weeks.
   b. Nipples and areolae—less formed and pronounced in preterm infants.

I. Respiratory System

1. Rate—normally between 40 and 60 breaths per minute; influenced by sleep–wake status, when last fed, drugs taken by mother.
2. Rhythm—respirations may be shallow with irregular rhythm.
   a. Respiratory movements are mainly diaphragmatic because of weak thoracic muscles.
   b. Periodic breathing—resumption of respiration after 5–15 second period without respiration; decreases over time; more common in preterm infant.
   c. Observe for abnormal respiratory signs.

J. Cardiovascular System

1. Rate—ranges between 100 and 160 beats per minute; influenced by behavioral state, environmental temperature, medication; take apical count for 1 full minute.
2. Rhythm—common to find periods of deceleration followed by periods of acceleration.
3. Heart sounds—2nd sound higher in pitch and sharper than 1st; 3rd and 4th sounds rarely heard; murmurs common—great majority are transitory.
4. Examine for presence of brachial, radial, pedal, and femoral pulses; lack of femoral pulses indicative of inadequate aortic blood flow.
5. Examine for cyanosis—acrocyanosis of distal extremities is common; record location of any cyanosis, color changes over time, and when crying.
6. Newborns over 3 kg. have systolic blood pressure between 60 and 80 mm. Hg; diastolic, between 35 and 55 mm. Hg.

K. Abdomen

1. Shape—cylindrical, protrudes slightly, moves synchronously with chest in respiration.
2. Distention may be due to bowel obstruction, organ enlargement, or infection.
3. Auscultate abdomen for masses; gap between rectus muscles is common; palpate liver and spleen.
   a. Liver has decreased ability to conjugate bilirubin (rationale for physiologic jaundice).
   b. Liver has decreased production of prothrombin and factors that depend on vitamin K for synthesis (rationale for neonate's predisposition to hemorrhage).
4. Palpate kidneys for size and shape:
   a. Infant has decreased ability of kidney to concentrate urine, excrete a solute load, maintain water and electrolyte balance.
   b. Urine may contain uric acid crystals which appear on diaper as reddish blotches; uric acid crystals may yield false-positive result when the infant's urine is tested for protein.
5. Examine umbilical cord:
   a. Normally contains 2 arteries, 1 vein; single artery associated with renal and other congenital abnormalities.
   b. Signs of infection around insertion into abdominal wall—redness, discharge.
   c. Meconium staining—associated with intrauterine compromise or postmaturity.
   d. By 24 hours, yellowish brown, dries and falls off in about 7–10 days.
   e. Umbilical hernia—defect in abdominal wall.
6. Genitalia
   a. Female
      (1) Labia majora cover labia minora in full-term female infants.
      (2) Hymenal tag (tissue) may protrude from vagina—regresses within several weeks.
      (3) Vaginal discharge—white or pink discharge may be present because of the drop in maternal hormones; no treatment necessary.
   b. Male
      (1) Full-term—testes in scrotal sac; scrotal sac markedly wrinkled.
      (2) Edema may be present in scrotal sac if the infant was born in breech presentation; a frank collection of fluid in the scrotal sac is a *hydrocele*—regresses in about a month.
      (3) Examine glans penis for urethral opening—normally central; opening ventral (*hypospadias*); opening dorsally (*epispadias*); abnormally adherent foreskin (*phimosis*).

L. Back

1. Examine spinal column for normal curvature and closure.
2. Examine anal area for anal opening, response of anal sphincter, fissures.

M. Musculoskeletal System

1. Examine extremities for fractures, paralysis, range of motion, irregular position.
2. Examine fingers and toes for number and separation; extra digits—*polydactyly;* fused digits—*syndactyly.*
3. Examine hips for dislocation—with the infant in supine position, flex knees and abduct hips to side and down to table surface; clicking sound indicates dislocation.

N. Neurologic System

1. Neurologic mechanisms are immature anatomically and physiologically; as a result, uncoordinated movements, labile temperature regulation, and lack of control over musculature are characteristic of the infant.
2. Examine muscle tone, head control, and reflexes.
3. Reflexes are important indices of infant neural development (see p. 1066).

Behavioral Assessment

1. Response to stimulation—newborns exhibit predictable, directed responses when in social interactions with nurturing adults or in response to attractive auditory or visual stimuli.
2. Newborn responses are influenced by states of consciousness such as:
   a. Quiet, deep sleep—no spontaneous activity, eyes closed, respirations regular
   b. Light, active sleep—random startles, eyes closed, rapid eye movements, frequent change of state with response to stimulation
   c. Drowsy awake—eyes open or closed, eyelids flutter, variable activity level, mild startles periodically, delayed response to stimulation
   d. Quiet alert—eyes open, little motor activity, focuses on source of stimulation
   e. Alert active—eyes open, much motor activity, increase in startles in response to stimulation
   f. Crying—intense crying that is difficult to interrupt with stimulation
3. Behavioral examinations have been developed that test neurologic adequacy and behavioral responses to environmental stimuli (see Behavioral Assessment, below). Understanding how an infant responds can help the parents respond to and care for him, and alter the environment to be most helpful to him.

Behavioral Assessment

1. Response decrement to repeated visual stimuli
2. Response decrement to repeated auditory stimuli
3. Response decrement to pinprick
4. Orienting responses to inanimate visual and auditory stimuli
5. Quality and duration of alert periods
6. General muscle tone
7. Motor maturity
8. Traction responses as infant is pulled to sitting position
9. Responses to being cuddled by the examiner
10. Defensive reactions to a cloth over the face
11. Consolability with intervention by examiner
12. Attempts to control self and to control state behavior
13. Rapidity of buildup to crying state
14. Peak of excitement and capacity for self control
15. Irritability during the examination
16. General assessment of kind and degree of activity
17. Tremulousness
18. Amount of startling
19. Lability of skin color
20. Lability of states during the examination
21. Hand-to-mouth activity

Brazelton TB. Clinical Obstetrics and Gynecology 1973; 16:59.

4. Sleeping pattern
   a. Length of sleep cycles (REM active and quiet sleep) changes normally with maturation of the central nervous system.
   b. Quiet sleep should increase over time in relation to REM sleep.
   c. Newborns usually sleep 20 hours per day.
5. Feeding pattern
   a. Most newborns eat 6–8 times per day with 2–8 hours between feedings; establish fairly regular feeding patterns in about 2 weeks.
   b. Calorie requirements are high—110–130 calories per kg. of body weight daily.
   c. Most digestive enzymes are present at birth.
   d. Imperfect control of cardiac and pyloric sphincters; immaturity results in regurgitation.
6. Pattern of elimination
   a. Stool
      (1) Meconium is usually passed in 24 hours.
      (2) Passage of meconium (tarry green–black stools) continues for 48 hours, followed by transitional stools (combination of meconium and yellow of milk stools). Milk stools (yellow) are passed by day 5.
      (3) Newborn has up to 6 stools per day in the first weeks after birth.

   b. Voiding
      (1) Newborn voids within first 24 hours.
      (2) After first few days, infant voids from 10–15 times a day
7. Temperature regulation
   a. Infant's body responds readily to changes in environmental temperature.
   b. Heat loss at birth may occur via evaporation, convection, conduction, and radiation.
   c. Physiologic mechanisms to avoid heat loss include:
      (1) Vasoconstriction
      (2) Nonshivering thermogenesis elicited by sympathetic nervous system in response to decreased temperature
      (3) Adipose tissue and brown fat—the latter contains many small blood vessels, fat vacuoles, and mitochondria, and is a site of heat production. Brown fat is found between scapulae, around neck and thorax, behind sternum, and around kidneys and adrenals.
      (4) Flexed position of full-term newborn

Nursing Care of the Newborn

See Guideline on page below.

Guidelines: Nursing Care of the Newborn

Purposes
1. To continue appraisal of the newborn by observing and recording vital signs, daily weight loss or gain, bowel and bladder function, activity or sleep.
2. To provide safeguards against infection.
3. To initiate feeding.
4. To provide health counseling to the parents.

Procedure

Nursing Action	Rationale/Amplification
General Considerations	
1. Carry out hospital policy for gowning and 3-minute scrub.	1. Utilizes basic principles of nursing care.
2. Never leave the infant alone.	2. Ensures safety factors.
3. Prevent undue exposure; provide warm environment (24°–27°C. [75°–80°F.]) and bath water (37°–38°C. [98°–100°F.]).	3. Prevents cold stress. Neonates have little adipose tissue to protect them.
Weight, Temperature, and Blood Pressure	
1. Weigh infant and record weight.	1. Infant may lose 5%–10% of birth weight because of minimal intake of nutrients and fluid and loss of excess fluid.
2. Take axillary temperature by placing thermometer in axilla and pressing infant's arm gently but firmly against it for 3 minutes.	2. Use of rectal thermometer predisposes to irritation of rectal mucosa.
3. Take blood pressure.	3. Hypotension may be present and require remedial action.
Bathing Technique	
1. Use cotton balls or soft, disposable wash cloths to wipe eyes, face, and outer ear. Eyes are wiped from inside corner outward.	1. Start from cleanest areas to most soiled.
2. Use a neutral soap—check pH. Clear water may be used if infant's skin is dry.	2. Prevents irritation of skin. The use of hexachlorophene to prevent staphylococcal infection is controversial. Hexachlorophene may cause brain damage if a sufficient quantity is absorbed through the skin.
3. Wash infant's head, using gentle circular motions.	3. Prevents cradle cap from forming, especially over the frontal areas.
4. Tilt head back to cleanse neck.	4. Exposes neck folds for more thorough cleansing.

Procedure
(Cont.)

Nursing Action	Rationale/Amplification

5. Bathe torso and extremities quickly.
6. Inspect umbilical cord. Check area for bleeding or foul odor. A drying agent such as 70% alcohol or merthiolate is applied several times daily. Dressings are not used.
7. Cleanse genital area of male infants.
   a. Retract foreskin gently for cleaning, and replace quickly.
   b. Circumcision care—keep area clean. Place sterile petrolatum gauze over area for first 24 hours; change after voiding. Observe hourly for bleeding. Position infant and diaper to avoid friction.
8. Cleanse genital area of female infants.
   a. Gently separate folds of the labia and remove secretions.
   b. Wipe vaginal area with cotton ball, using 1 stroke in a front-to-back direction.
9. Bathe buttocks, using a gentle, patting motion. Keep area clean and dry.
10. Prevent diaper rash. If rash does occur, protective ointment (zinc oxide or A & D) may be used.
    Exposure of buttocks to air or heat lamp is helpful.

5. Prevents unnecessary exposure and chilling.
6. Minimizes colonization by bacteria.

   a. Replacing foreskin quickly prevents edema.

   b. Prevents infection and promotes healing. Bleeding can be controlled by pressure or by application of adrenalin solution. Prevents discomfort.

   a. Vaginal discharge and smegma must be removed.

   b. Front-to-back cleansing prevents contamination of vagina.
9. Area is susceptible to skin breakdown because of acid reaction of urine and feces.

Stool Observation

1. Observe stool pattern—meconium during first 2–3 days.
2. Transitional stools—change from tarry black to greenish black, to greenish brown to brownish yellow to greenish yellow.
3. Number, color, and consistency are recorded daily.

1. Material composed of epithelial and epidermal cells, lanugo, and bile pigments.
2. Changes reflect intake of milk—stools are composed of both meconium and milk stools.
3. For early identification of abnormalities.
   a. No stool within 48 hours indicates an intestinal obstruction.
   b. Passage of meconium only (without other stool) suggests obstruction in the ileum.
   c. Thick, putty-like meconium may indicate cystic fibrosis.
   d. Diarrhea may be caused by overfeeding or by gastroenteritis.
   e. Blood in the stool is an indication of intestinal bleeding.

Nutritional Considerations

1. Provide for nutritional intake.
2. Promote feeding method of choice (see page 999 for Guidelines for breast-feeding).
3. Test urine glucose using reagent strip test and blood glucose using enzymatic strip test.
4. First feeding is sterile water. If retained, formula is given at next feeding.

5. Instruct the parent in technique of bottle-feeding.
   a. Hold baby in semi-upright position.
   b. Position bottle so that neck of bottle is filled.
   c. Insert nipple into baby's mouth so that baby's tongue is under nipple.
   d. Burp during feeding by holding infant upright.
6. Phenylketonuria (PKU) testing:
   Usually done on 3rd day before discharge from hospital.

1. Infants vary in their readiness to feed.

3. Infant may be hypoglycemic and require feeding sooner than usual 4- to 6-hour wait.
4. Glucose water, if aspirated, is dangerous to lung tissue. Most hospitals use prepared milk mixture in disposable containers. Various formulas are available.

   a. Gravity assists flow of milk into stomach.
   b. Prevents the baby from swallowing air.
   c. Sucking and swallowing reflexes are used in feeding.
   d. Allows air to escape from stomach, preventing distention or milk regurgitation.
6. Most states require by law routine testing of newborn infants for phenylketonuria (abnormal amino acid metabolism).
   For test to be accurate, infant must be receiving formula or breast milk in order to provide a supply of phenylalanine-containing protein.

Discharge Planning

1. Preparation for home care. Instruction is given concerning infant bathing and care, preparation of formula, and infant feeding. Written formula with instructions for preparation is provided to parents.
2. Provide ample opportunity for parent contact.

1. Instruction for infant care is a combined responsibility of the medical and nursing staffs.

2. Early attachment results in improved parent–child relationships.

Parent Teaching

A. Teach the parents infant feeding techniques.

1. Allow the infant to feed on demand.
2. Hold and talk to the infant while feeding.
3. For discussion of breast-feeding, see page 999.
4. Formula should be at room temperature for feeding.
5. Do not prop the bottle; leaking of milk into infant's ear can result in infection.
6. Bubble the infant (upright position) following feeding and during feeding if he appears to be getting air with the feeding.
7. Place the infant on right side or abdomen following feeding—safer positions should he regurgitate.

B. Teach the parents infant-bathing techniques.

1. Never leave the infant alone.
2. Prevent undue exposure—room temperature, 24°–31°C. (75°–88°F.); bath water, 36.6°–37.7°C. (98°–100°F.).
3. Use cotton balls or soft disposable wash cloths to wipe eyes, face, and outer ear. Eyes are wiped from inside corner outward.
4. Use a mild soap—clear water may be used if the infant's skin is dry.
5. Wash the infant's head using gentle circular motions; wash trunk and extremities quickly to avoid chilling the infant.
6. Inspect umbilical cord. Check area for bleeding or foul odor. A drying agent such as 70% alcohol is applied several times daily. Dressings are not usually used.
7. Cleanse genital area of male infants:
   a. Retract foreskin gently for cleansing.

b. Circumcision care—keep area clean. Place sterile petrolatum gauze over area for first 24 hours; change after voiding. Observe for bleeding. Position the infant and diaper to avoid friction.

8. Cleanse genital area of females:
   a. Use wet cotton ball.
   b. Separate labia.
   c. Wipe from front to back and discard cotton ball.

C. Discuss with the parents the infant's behavioral responses.

1. Sleeping pattern
2. Response to environmental stimuli
3. Response to soothing attempts
4. Ways in which environmental changes, tone of voice, and approaches to soothing may enhance the infant's responses

D. Teach the parents to take the infant's temperature.

Take axillary temperature by placing thermometer in axilla and pressing the infant's arm gently but firmly against it for 3 minutes.

E. Teach the parents to recognize reportable signs and symptoms.

1. Pallor or cyanosis
2. Anorexia, vomiting, diarrhea
3. Abnormal respirations
4. Irritability, lethargy, fever, or hypothermia

F. Have the parents identify location and time of first infant checkup following discharge.

Bibliography

Books

Postpartal Period

Barglow P. Postpartum mental illness: Detection and treatment. In Sciarra JJ (ed). Gynecology and Obstetrics, vol. 2, Philadelphia, Harper & Row, 1982

Bille DA. Practical Approaches to Patient Teaching. Boston, Little, Brown & Co, 1981

Clark AL. Culture and Childrearing. Philadelphia, FA Davis, 1981

Danforth DN. Obstetrics and Gynecology, 4th ed. Philadelphia, Harper & Row, 1982

Klaus MH and Kennell JH. Parent–Infant Bonding, 2nd ed. St Louis, CV Mosby, 1982

Lawrence RA. Breastfeeding: A Guide for the Medical Profession. St Louis, CV Mosby, 1980

Miller M and Brooten D. The Childbearing Family: A Nursing Perspective. Boston, Little, Brown & Co, 1983

The Newborn

Avery GB. Neonatology. Philadelphia, JB Lippincott, 1981

Benitz WE and Tatro DS. The Pediatric Drug Handbook. Chicago, Year Book Medical Publishers, 1981

Kempe CH et al. Current Pediatric Diagnosis and Treatment. Los Altos, CA, Lange Medical Publications, 1982

Klaus MH and Kennell JH. Parent–Infant Bonding, 2nd ed. St Louis, CV Mosby, 1982

Korones S. High-Risk Newborn Infants. St Louis, CV Mosby, 1981

Moore ML. Newborn Family and Nurse. Philadelphia, WB Saunders, 1981

Oehler JM. Family-Centered Neonatal Nursing Care. Philadelphia, JB Lippincott, 1981

Powell ML. Assessment and Management of Developmental Changes and Problems in Children, 2nd ed. St Louis, CV Mosby, 1982

Rong ML. Manual of Newborn Care Plans. Boston, Little, Brown & Co, 1981

Articles

Postpartal Period

Austin SEJ. Family-centered discharge planning classes . . . postpartum instruction. MCN 1980 Mar–Apr; 5(2): 96–97

Avant KC. Anxiety as a potential factor affecting maternal attachment. JOGN Nurs 1981 Nov–Dec; 10(6):416–419

Bowes WA. The effect of medications on the lactating mother and her infant. Clin Obstet Gynecol 1980 Dec; 23(4): 1073–80 (33 ref)

Brooten D et al. A comparison of four treatments to prevent and control breast pain and engorgement in non-nursing mothers. Nurs Res 1983 Jul–Aug; 32(4):225–229

Burd B. Encouragement counts in breast-feeding. Am J Nurs 1981 Aug; 81(8):1491

Carek DJ et al. Mothers' reactions to their newborn infants. J Am Acad Child Psychiatry 1981 Winter; 20(1): 16–31

Carr KC and Walton VE. Early postpartum discharge. JOGN Nurs 1982 Jan–Feb; 11(1):29–30

Clarke-Pearson DL and Creasman WT. Diagnosis of deep venous thrombosis in obstetrics and gynecology by impedance phlebography. Obstet Gynecol 1981 Jul; 58(1):52–57

Crowder DS. Maternity nurses' knowledge of factors promoting successful infant breastfeeding: A survey at two hospitals. JOGN Nurs 1981 Jan–Feb; 10(1):28–30

Ellis D and Hewat R. Mothers' postpartum perceptions of spousal relationships. JOGN Nurs 1985 Mar/Apr; 14(2):140–146

Horn BM. Cultural concepts and

postpartal care. Nurs Health Care 1981 Nov; 11(9):516–527

Inglis T. Postpartum sexuality. JOGN Nurs 1980 Sep–Oct; 9(5):298–300

Jarrett GE. Childbearing patterns of young mothers: Expectations, knowledge and practices. MCN 1982 Mar/Apr; 7(2):119–121

Jennings B and Edmundson M. The postpartum period: After confinement: The fourth trimester. Clin Obstet Gynecol 1980 Dec; 23(4):1093–1103

Kunst-Wilson W et al. Nursing care for the emerging family: Promoting paternal behavior. Res Nurs Health 1981 Mar; 4(1):201–211 (97 ref)

Leonard LG. Breastfeeding twins: Maternal–infant nutrition. JOGN Nurs 1982 May–Jun; 11(3):148–153

Mayfield et al. Temperature measurement in neonates. J Pediatr 1984 Feb; 104(2):271–275

Mercer RT. The nurse and maternal tasks of early postpartum. MCN 1981 Sept/Oct; 6(5):341–345

Moss JR. Concerns of multiparas on the third postpartum day. JOGN Nurs 1981 Nov–Dec; 10(6):421–424

Petrick, J. Postpartum depressions identification of high risk mothers. JOGN Nurs 1984 Jan–Feb; 13(1):37–40

Reiser SL. A tool to facilitate mother–infant attachment. JOGN Nurs 1981 Jul–Aug; 10(4):294–297

Riordan JM and Countryman BA. Basics of breastfeeding Part IV: Preparation for breastfeeding and early optimal functioning. JOGN Nurs 1980 Sep–Oct; 9(5):277–283

Riordan JM and Countryman BA. Basics of breastfeeding Part VI: Some breastfeeding problems and solutions. JOGN Nurs 1980 Nov–Dec; 9(6):361–366

Senie RT. Possible related risks to breastfeeding. JOGN Nurs 1982 Jan–Feb; 11(1):34–36

Sheehan F. Assessing postpartum adjustment: A pilot study. JOGN Nurs 1981 Jan–Feb; 10(1):19–22

Vanden Bergh RL. Postpartum depression. Clin Obstet Gynecol 1980 Dec; 23(4):1105–1111

Wainwright S. How to promote successful breastfeeding. Nurs Times 1981 Aug 5; 77(32):1397–1399

The Newborn

Beske E, Garvis M and Mullett S. Research-important factors in breastfeeding success. MCN 1982 May/Jun; 7(3):174–179

Borovies D. Assessing and managing pain in breastfeeding mothers. MCN 1984 Jul–Aug; 9(4):272–276

Brooten D et al. Breastmilk jaundice. JOGN Nurs 1985 May–June; 14(3):220–223

Crummette BD and Munton MT. Mothers' decisions about infant nutrition. Pediatr Nurs 1980 Nov–Dec; 6(6):16–19

Dallman PR. Inhibition of iron absorption by certain foods. Am J Dis Child 1980 May; 134(0):453–454

Davis V. The structure and function of brown adispose tissue in the neonate. JOGN Nurs 1980 Nov–Dec; 9(6):368–372

Driggers DA. Infant nutrition made simple. Am Fam Physician 1980 Oct; 22(4):113–116

Dunn DM and White DG. Interactions of mothers with their newborns in the first half hour of life. J Adv Nurs 1981 Jul; 6(4):271–275

Giefer M and Nelson C. A new method to help fathers develop parenting skills. JOGN Nurs 1981 Nov–Dec; 10(6):455–457

Gill N, White M and Anderson G. Transitional newborn infants in a hospital nursery: From first oral cue to first sustained cry. Nurs Res 1984 Jul–Aug; 33(4):213–217

Lauri S. The public health nurse as a guide in infant child care and education. J Adv Nurs 1981 Jul; 6(4):297–303

L'esperance C. and Frantz K. Time limitation for early breastfeeding. JOGN Nurs 1985 Mar–Apr; 14(2):114–118

Lubchenco LO. Routine neontal circumcision: A surgical anachronism. Clin Obstet Gynecol 1980 Dec; 23(4):1135–1140

Mansell K. Mother–baby units: The concept works. MCN 1984; 9:132

Osborne LM et al. Hygienic care in uncircumcised infants. Pediatrics 1981 Mar; 67(3):365–367

Palma PA and Adcock EW. Human milk and breastfeeding. Am Fam Physician 1981 Jul; 24(1):173–181

Peters D and Worthington-Roberts B. Infant feeding practices of middle-class feeding mothers. Birth 1982 Summer; 9(2):91–95

Picciano MF and Deering RH. The influence of feeding regimens on iron status during infancy. Am J Clin Nutr 1980 Apr; 33(4):746–753

Poland R, Schulty G and Garg G. High milk lipase activity associated with breast milk jaundice. Pediatr Res 1980 Dec; 14(12):1328–31

Reifsnider E and Taylor S. Employed mothers can breastfeed too! MCN 1985 Jul–Aug; 10(4):256–259

Rhodes P and Puchett CG. Staphylococcus aureus infections in the newborn Perinatol/Neonatol 1983 May; 69–77

Riordan J and Riordan M. Drugs in breastmilk. MCN 1984 Mar; 84(3):328–332

Schraeder B and Medoff-Cooper B. Development and temperament in very low birthweight infants—the second year. Nurs Res 1983 Nov–Dec; 32(6):331–335

Siegel E et al. Hospital and home support during infancy: Impact on maternal attachment, child abuse and neglect, and health care utilization. Pediatrics 1980 Aug; 66(2):183–190

Stefanski M et al. A scoring system for states of sleep and wakefulness in term and preterm infants. Pediatr Res 1984 Jan; 18(1):58–62

Van Poppel, Ray D and Estok P. Infant feeding choice and the adolescent mother. JOGN Nurs 1984 Mar/Apr 13(2):115–118

Verzemnieks I. Developmental stimulation for infants and toddlers. Am J Nurs 1984 Jun; 84(6):748–752

White PL et al. Comparative accuracy of recent abbreviated methods of gestational age determination. Clin Pediatr 1980 May; 19(5):319–321

Yoos L. Developmental issues and the choice of feeding method of adolescent mothers. JOGN Nurs 1985 Jan/Feb; 14(1):68–72

Complications of Pregnancy

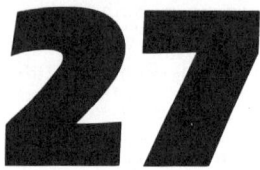

Ectopic Pregnancy

Ectopic pregnancy is any gestation located outside the uterine cavity. Although the majority of ectopic pregnancies are tubal implantations, other types include cervical, abdominal, or ovarian implantations. It is a major cause of maternal mortality because of rupture of the site and subsequent hemorrhage (Fig. 27-1).

Assessment

A. Contributing Causes (History)

1. Salpingitis
2. Pelvic inflammatory disease
3. Endometriosis
4. Congenital anatomic irregularity (often presence of diverticula of uterine tube)
5. Previous tubal surgery

B. Clinical Manifestations

1. Vary with the site of implantation and usually occur after tubal rupture
2. Tubal implants most common; most frequent are:
   a. Ampullary (implant grows and may extrude into abdominal cavity)
   b. Isthmus (tube ruptures after about 4–5 weeks' growth of embryo)
   c. Interstitial (cornua also hypertrophies; rupturing of this area may not occur until beginning of 2nd trimester—rupture similar to uterine rupture with massive, sudden hemorrhage)
3. Early signs and symptoms
   a. Menstrual irregularities
   b. Symptoms of early pregnancy
   c. Dull pain on affected side
4. Signs and symptoms of tubal rupture
   a. Pain—sudden, severe and unilateral; later, generalized and radiating to shoulder and neck because of diaphragmatic irritation
   b. Nausea, vomiting, faintness
   c. Shock manifested by pallor with slight cyanosis around the lips; yawning; weak, rapid pulse
   d. Normal or low temperature—fever important in distinguishing ruptured tubal pregnancy from acute salpingitis
   e. Tenderness over abdomen upon palpation
   f. Pelvic mass—posterior or lateral to uterus
   g. Cervical pain during vaginal examination and movement of the cervix
   h. Distention of the posterior fornix with blood in the cul-de-sac

C. Diagnostic Evaluation

1. *Culdocentesis*—aspiration of fluid from the cul-de-sac of Douglas. Presence of bloody fluid indicates intraperitoneal bleeding.
2. *Culdoscopy*—visualization of the pelvic organs through the punctured posterior fornix.

Patient Problems/Nursing Diagnoses

1. Shock related to effects of rupture (pain, blood loss)
2. Potential fluid volume deficit related to blood loss
3. Pain related to rupture and outpouring of blood into peritoneal cavity
4. Anxiety related to uncertainty about condition and potential loss of childbearing capacity.

Nursing Interventions

A. Preventing/Treating Shock

1. Monitor vital signs—assess for indications of impending shock.
2. Start IV fluids/blood as prescribed.
3. Provide constant monitoring, noting any changes in the woman's condition.
4. Inspect for vaginal bleeding.
5. Prepare the woman for surgery.

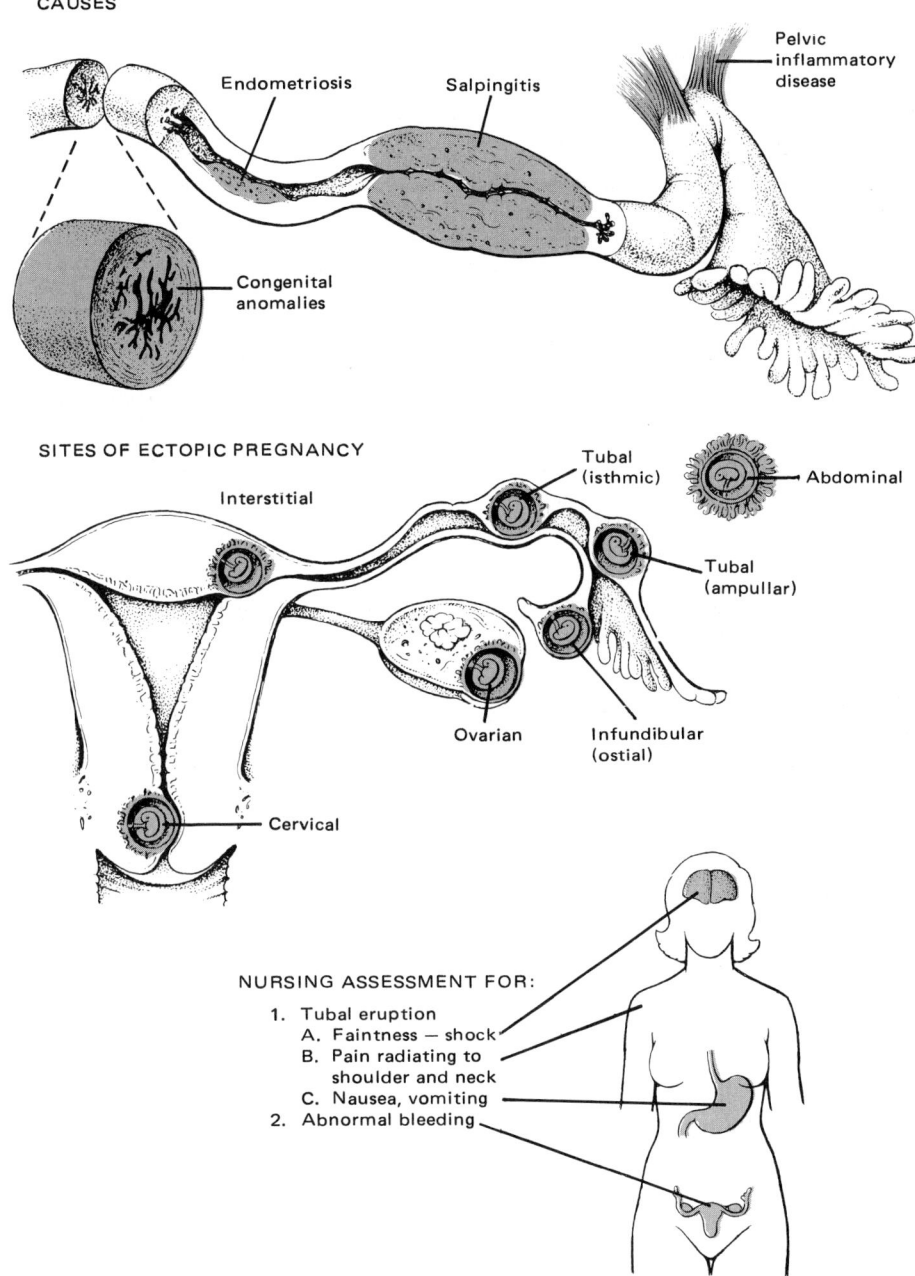

Figure 27-1. Ectopic pregnancy.

6. Postoperative care is the same as for the patient who has had an abdominal laparotomy.

B. Establishing Fluid Volume

1. Maintain ongoing record of IV intake and urinary output.
2. See above.

C. Reducing Pain

1. Remain with woman as much as possible and provide psychosocial support.

2. Administer analgesics as needed/prescribed.
3. Explain procedures that need to be performed to reduce anticipation of additional discomfort.

D. Coping with Anxiety

1. Listen empathetically to the woman's account of what has happened.
2. Reinforce physician's decisions/explanation of future childbearing potential.
3. Ask the woman to explain her understanding of future childbearing potential; correct misinformation and reinforce positive aspects.

Evaluation

1. Attains/maintains vital signs within physiologic limits
2. Achieves fluid volume equilibrium; absence of untoward bleeding

3. Verbalizes pain relief
4. Demonstrates lessening anxiety; talks freely about experience; asks questions; relates to hospital personnel in a positive manner; talks realistically about childbearing potential

Hydatidiform Mole

Hydatidiform mole is a developmental anomaly of the placenta resulting in the conversion of the chorionic villi into a mass of clear vesicles.
1. It is one of the most common lesions anteceding choriocarcinoma, a malignant tumor of the trophoblast with a tendency toward rapid and widespread metastasis.
2. There may be no fetus, or a degenerating fetus may be present.
3. It is believed to be derived from the paternal haploid, X-carrying set of chromosomes that reaches 46XX status by its own duplication.

Incidence

1. Occurs in about 1 of every 2,000 pregnancies.
2. Frequency in women over 45 is 10 times higher than in women aged 20–40.

Assessment

A. Clinical Manifestations

1. Enlargement of the uterus is out of proportion to what it normally is at a specific time in pregnancy.
2. Continuous or intermittent red or brownish bloody discharge about the 12th week of pregnancy; may also pass villi.
3. Signs and symptoms of preeclampsia, proteinuria, hypertension, or edema occurring earlier than 20 weeks' gestation
4. Hyperemesis gravidarum (pernicious vomiting) experienced by 30% of women with this condition
5. Human chorionic gonadotropin (HCG) titer is markedly increased beyond the 90th day of gestation, when normally expected to drop

6. No fetal heart tones by auscultation or amplification; no fetal skeleton found on ultrasound or X-ray.

Nursing Interventions

A. Preoperative and Postoperative Care

1. Replace blood as prescribed.
2. Prepare the woman for surgery—mole is removed by dilatation and curettage, suction curettage, or hysterotomy (if more than 14 weeks).
3. Administer antimetabolite drugs, if prescribed, before and following removal of mole.
4. Observe for complications—recurrent hemorrhage and uterine perforation.
5. Advise the woman that she should be followed routinely for 1 year for gonadotropin activity; HCG levels should be negative within 6 weeks of removal of mole. Chest x-rays are done at intervals to screen for metastasis.
6. Counsel the woman to avoid attempting pregnancy for 6 months–1 year to allow HCG levels to be monitored without pregnancy.

B. Promoting a Healthy Self-Concept

1. Encourage the woman to discuss her feelings regarding the abnormality.
2. Determine the woman's understanding of what causes the abnormal development; correct misinformation and reinforce correct information.
3. Help the woman to understand that the abnormal development was a "quirk of nature" and not caused by her or her partner's actions or genetic makeup.

Hyperemesis Gravidarum

Hyperemesis gravidarum is exaggerated nausea and vomiting during pregnancy, persisting past the 1st trimester.

Assessment

Predisposing Factors

1. Hormonal changes of pregnancy—chorionic gonadotropin levels are high.
2. Emotional factors—some clinicians believe that insecurity, anxiety, or a negative attitude toward the pregnancy are contributing factors.

Clinical Manifestations

1. Frequent vomiting, especially when stomach is empty
2. Tendency to become nauseated at mention, sight, or smell of food
3. Weight loss
4. Dehydration
5. Increased pulse rate

6. Signs of vitamin deficiency
7. Thirst
8. Heartburn
9. Constipation
10. Scanty, concentrated urine

Patient Problems/Nursing Diagnoses

1. Fluid volume and electrolyte deficit related to prolonged vomiting
2. Inadequate nutritional intake related to prolonged vomiting
3. Potential ineffective coping related to stress

Nursing Interventions

A. Maintaining Fluid and Electrolyte Balance

1. If vomiting is severe, the woman is hospitalized and oral intake is restricted for 24–48 hours; IV fluids are administered.

2. Oral liquid intake is resumed slowly; usually high in carbohydrates, of the type preferred by the woman.
3. Hot or cold beverages are usually tolerated better than warm ones.

B. Improving Nutritional Intake

1. Offer small meals, mainly carbohydrates of the type most preferred by the woman (usually 6 per day) when symptoms subside.
2. Avoid strong food odors.
3. Avoid greasy foods.
4. Give vitamin supplementation as directed.
5. Antiemetics may also be given.

C. Developing Coping Abilities

1. Have the woman discuss her perception of the problem and the difficulties it has created.
2. Discuss possible resolutions to problems identified.

3. Hospitalization often removes the woman from pressing duties and responsibilities.
4. Often, restriction of visitors, including most family members, removes further stress; restriction of visitors is eliminated as condition improves.

Expected Outcomes

1. Attains/maintains fluid and electrolyte balance in physiologic range; taking oral fluids; shows normal tissue turgor; urine appears less concentrated and has a normal specific gravity
2. Eats small meals; absence of vomiting; does not complain of nausea
3. Shows some coping ability; identifies her problems and discusses possible solutions; uses stress-reduction techniques (relaxation and breathing exercises)

Abortion

Abortion is the termination of pregnancy at any time before the fetus has attained viability (20 weeks' gestation or fetal weight of 500 gm. [1.1 lbs.]).

Types of Abortion

1. Spontaneous (Table 27-1)
   a. Threatened abortion
   b. Inevitable abortion
   c. Habitual abortion
   d. Incomplete abortion
   e. Missed abortion
2. Therapeutic

Spontaneous Abortion

A. Incidence

1. Frequent complication of pregnancy
2. One pregnancy in every 5–7 terminates in spontaneous abortion

B. Predisposing Factors

1. Faulty germ plasm—imperfect ova or sperm cells; abnormal development

2. Decrease in production of progesterone—insufficient progesterone leads to increased uterine sensitivity and contractions which cause expulsion of the embryo.
3. Incompetent cervix—mechanical defect in the cervix causes dilatation and effacement in early pregnancy (women with history of induced abortion have increased incidence of incompetent cervix).
4. Acute infections—cause fetal death by:
   a. Transmission of bacterial toxins from mother to fetus
   b. Passage of microorganisms from mother to fetus
   c. High temperature, which may stimulate uterine contractions
5. Environmental or workplace hazards
   a. Certain chemicals; heavy metal poisoning
   b. Radiation
   c. Anesthetic or illuminating gases
6. Systemic disease in parents
   a. Maternal thyroid dysfunction
   b. Severe maternal anemia

Table 27-1   Types of Spontaneous Abortions

Classification	Clinical Manifestations	Management
1. Threatened	Vaginal bleeding or spotting Mild cramps Tenderness over uterus, simulates mild labor or persistent low backache with feeling of pelvic pressure Cervix closed or slightly dilated Symptoms subside or develop into an inevitable abortion	Vaginal examination Bed rest (some clinicians citing the abnormal number of embryos that are aborted will not limit activity in belief that the embryo will be aborted anyway) Pad count
2. Inevitable	Bleeding more profuse Cervix dilated Membranes rupture Painful uterine contractions	Embryo delivered, followed by D&C
3. Habitual abortion	Spontaneous abortion occurs in successive pregnancies (3 or more)	D&C Treatment of possible causes: hormonal imbalance, tumors, thyroid dysfunction, abnormal uterus, incompetent cervix; with treatment, 70%–80% carry a pregnancy successfully Hysterogram to rule out uterine abnormalities, infections Surgical suturing of the cervix if incompetent cervix is a causative factor
4. Incomplete abortion	Fetus usually expelled Placenta and membranes retained	D&C
5. Missed abortion	Fetus dies in utero and is retained Maceration No symptoms of abortion, but symptoms of pregnancy regress (uterine size, breast changes)	Real time ultrasound, and if 2nd trimester, fetal monitoring to determine if fetus is dead If fetus is not passed after diagnosis, oxytocin induction may be used. Retained dead fetus may lead to development of disseminated intravascular coagulation (DIC) or infection Fibrinogen concentrations should be measured weekly

Therapeutic Abortion

Therapeutic abortion is the termination of pregnancy before the time of fetal viability for the purpose of safeguarding the health of the mother.

1. Legal aspects
   According to US Supreme Court ruling of January 22, 1973, pregnancy may be terminated as follows:
   a. In the 1st trimester of pregnancy, the abortion decision is to be left to the woman and her physician.
   b. During the 2nd trimester, the state may not prohibit abortion, but may regulate its practice in the interest of protecting the woman's health.
   c. During the final weeks of pregnancy, the state may choose to protect the potential life of the fetus by prohibiting abortion except when necessary to preserve the life or health of the woman.
   d. The religious beliefs of the patient are always respected.

2. Indications
   According to the therapeutic abortion policy established by the American College of Obstetricians and Gynecologists, therapeutic abortion may be performed for the following medical indications:
   a. When continuation of the pregnancy may threaten the life of the woman or seriously impair her health. In determining whether there is such a risk to health, account may be taken of the woman's total environment, actual or reasonably foreseeable.
   b. When pregnancy has resulted from rape or incest. In this case, the same medical criteria should be employed in the evaluation of the patient.
   c. When continuation of the pregnancy is likely to result in the birth of a child with grave physical deformities or mental retardation.

3. Counseling before elective abortion
   a. Reasons for the abortion should be identified and discussed
   b. Discussion of possible resolution of reasons for abortion
   c. Discussion of alternatives to abortion

Patient Problems/Nursing Diagnoses
(following abortion)

1. Potential for hemorrhage related to abortion
2. Infection related to cervical dilatation; abortion procedure
3. Pain related to uterine cramping
4. Grieving related to lost pregnancy

Nursing Interventions

A. Preventing Hemorrhage

1. Take and record vital signs.
2. Monitor blood loss (pad count); note character and amount of blood.
3. Save all tissue and clots passed for examination.

B. Preventing Infection

1. Be sure that examinations, etc. are done under aseptic conditions.
2. Give antimicrobial agent as directed.

C. Reducing Pain

1. Stay with hospitalized woman if she is in labor—reduces anxiety and pain.
2. Administer analgesics as needed.
3. If abortion is inevitable, explain to the woman that pain from contractions will cease when embryo and membranes are passed.
4. Teach controlled breathing and relaxation techniques.

D. Dealing with Grieving and Coping with Difficulties Associated with Pregnancy Loss

1. Determine if this was a planned pregnancy.
2. Assist the woman to discuss her feelings about the pregnancy and the meaning of its loss to her.
3. Allow the woman time and opportunity to grieve.
4. Do *not* tell the woman she "can get pregnant again"; each pregnancy has meaning, *this* pregnancy is a loss that cannot be replaced.
5. Contact clergy if the woman so desires.
6. Ensure that the physician talks with woman regarding her future childbearing potential and any treatment that may be necessary to carry a pregnancy to term.

Expected Outcomes

1. Absence of hemorrhage; vital signs within normal limits; hematocrit and hemoglobin levels are in acceptable range; decreasing amount of vaginal bleeding noted
2. Absence of infection; no evidence of fever; no foul discharge or abnormal urinary symptoms
3. Achieves relief of pain; uses controlled breathing and relaxation techniques
4. Goes through grieving process; talks about her experience and loss; has names of health care professionals if she feels more support is needed

Placenta Previa

Placenta previa is the development of the placenta in the lower uterine segment, partially or completely covering the internal cervical os (Fig. 27-2).

Assessment

A. Incidence

1. One of the major causes of bleeding during the last trimester
2. Occurs once in every 200 deliveries
3. As parity increases, placenta previa becomes more common

B. Contributing causes

1. Largely unknown, although multiparity and advancing age favor occurrence
2. Unfavorable decidua in upper uterine segment (fibroid tumors, poorly vascularized endometrium)

C. Clinical Manifestations

1. Painless vaginal bleeding in the latter half of pregnancy; occurs without warning in the absence of trauma.
2. Initial episode of bleeding is rarely fatal; in each subsequent episode, bleeding is heavier.

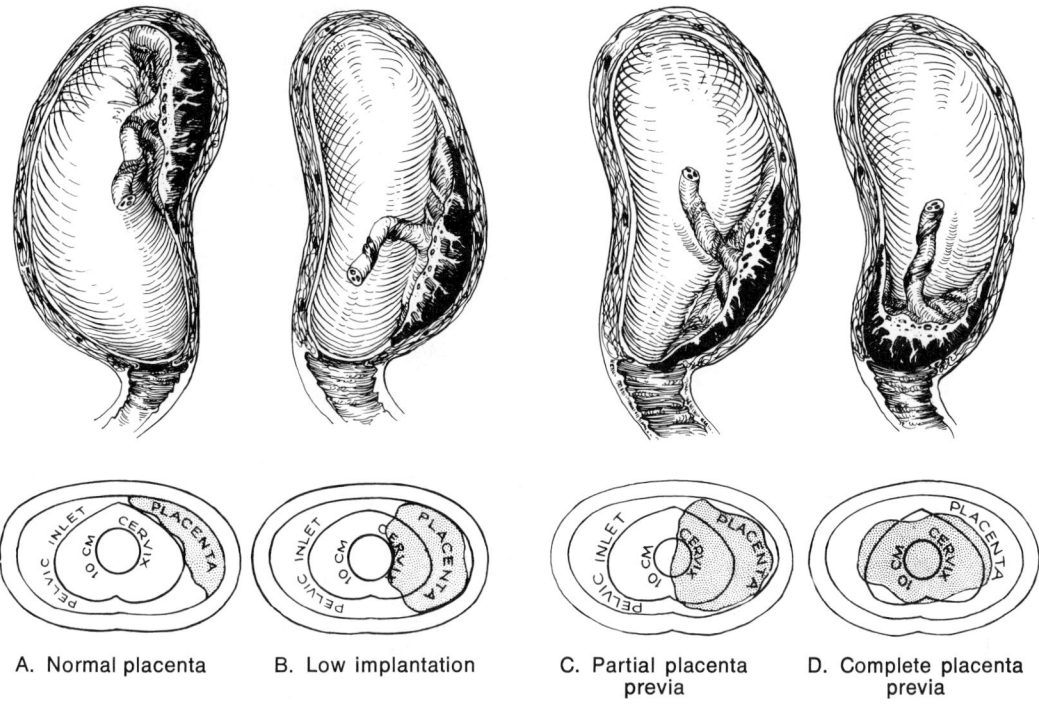

A. Normal placenta   B. Low implantation   C. Partial placenta previa   D. Complete placenta previa

Figure 27-2. Placenta previa. (From Benson RC. Handbook of Obstetrics and Gynecology. Los Altos, CA, Lange Medical Publications)

3. Placenta previa may not cause bleeding until labor begins or until complete dilation has occurred.
4. Bleeding occurs earlier and is more profuse with total placenta previa.

Nursing Interventions

A. Preventing Premature Delivery

1. Monitor hemoglobin, hematocrit, WBC, and differential counts.
2. Determine amount of bleeding, length of bleeding, any previous episodes.
3. Monitor vital signs, including fetal heart tones.
4. Evaluate contractions, if present.
5. Since the diagnosis is usually made by ultrasound, prepare the woman for the procedure.
6. See that the woman is maintained on bed rest; delivery delayed to increase fetal maturity.
   a. If bleeding is light, and the woman becomes stabilized and is able to remain at rest, she may be maintained on bed rest at home. (Referrals for homemaking service are often helpful.)
   b. If the woman is hospitalized, bed rest is enforced.
7. Continue to monitor vital signs (including fetal heart rate) and vaginal bleeding, Hb, and Hct.
8. Be ready to prepare the woman for delivery.
   a. If profuse hemorrhage occurs, cesarean delivery will be performed using the classic approach to avoid incision into placenta in lower uterine segment.
   b. In rare instances, vaginal delivery may be used; membranes are ruptured and pressure of fetal presenting part applies pressure to bleeding site.

Note: The incidence of postpartum hemorrhage is greater than normally expected since the lower uterine segment has less muscle fiber and cannot contract well, thus occluding vessels at the placental site.

Abruptio Placentae

Abruptio placentae is premature separation of the normally implanted placenta (Fig. 27-3).

Predisposing Factors

1. Hypertensive disease
2. Renal disease
3. Increased incidence in women over 30
4. Increased incidence in women with parity of 5 or more
5. Interference of flow of blood to intervillous space

Altered Physiology

Separation of the placenta is accompanied by hemorrhage, either concealed or external

1. Concealed hemorrhage—placental separation occurs centrally; large amount of accumulated blood is stored under placenta
2. External hemorrhage—blood flows outward from the edge of the placenta, under the membranes and through the cervix

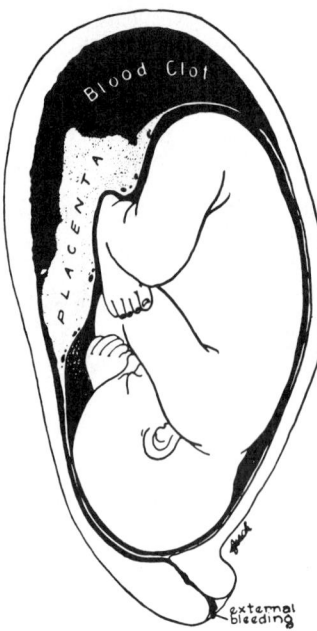

Figure 27-3. Abruptio placentae with large blood clot between placenta and uterine wall.

Clinical Manifestations

1. Vaginal bleeding
2. Sudden onset of severe, continuous abdominal pain and/or low back pain
3. Rigid, tender, irritable uterus
4. Amniotic fluid color may be dark red
5. If bleeding is severe, the myometrium may be infiltrated with blood and may fail to contract following delivery (Couvelaire uterus)
6. If bleeding is severe, hypofibrinogenemia may develop.
7. Fetal activity may be increased because of fetal hypoxia; with severe complete abruption, fetal heart tones may not be heard.
8. If bleeding is severe, the woman may go into shock.

Patient Problems/Nursing Diagnoses

1. Possible shock related to hemorrhage
2. Fluid volume deficit related to hemorrhage
3. Trauma to fetus related to hypoxia or anoxia
4. Anxiety regarding safety of fetus and self

Nursing Interventions

A. Fluid Replacement

1. Administer IV fluids and whole blood to replace blood loss, as prescribed.
2. Monitor fibrinogen levels.
3. Monitor blood pressure, pulse, respiration, and fetal heart tones—to detect impending shock and to assess fetal condition.
4. Monitor vaginal bleeding and height of fundus to detect increasing concealed hemorrhage.

B. Ensuring Blood Flow and Oxygen

1. Administer fluids or blood as prescribed.
2. Monitor fetal heart tones continuously to assess fetal well-being.
3. Provide oxygen therapy if prescribed.
4. Maintain the woman in side-lying position to keep uterus off vena cava, thereby improving blood flow to intervillous spaces.
5. Prepare the woman for immediate delivery—vaginally if the abruption is slight and the cervix dilated; cesarean delivery is used most frequently because it allows immediate delivery of infant.

C. Reducing Anxiety

1. Keep the woman/couple informed of what is happening and of the plan of care.
2. Reinforce positive aspects of the woman's condition without giving false reassurance; have the couple listen to fetal heart sounds.
3. Explain procedures that might be needed.
4. Do not leave the woman/couple alone.
5. Following delivery
   a. Provide nursing surveillance during the puerperium—for early detection of complications.
   b. Monitor vital signs and uterine muscle tone—traumatized myometrium may cause uterine atony.
   c. Be alert for indications of postpartum infections—blood loss and shock greatly reduce resistance to infections.

Characteristics of Abruptio Placentae and Placenta Previa

Characteristic	Abruptio Placentae	Placenta Previa
Onset	Third trimester	Third trimester (commonly in eighth month)
Bleeding	May be concealed, external dark hemorrhage, or bloody amniotic fluid	Mostly external, small to profuse in amount, bright red
Pain and uterine tenderness	Usually present; irritable uterus, progresses to board-like consistency	Usually absent; uterus soft
Fetal heart tone	May be irregular or absent	Usually normal
Presenting part	May or may not be engaged	Usually not engaged
Shock	Moderate to severe depending on extent of concealed and external hemorrhage	Usually not present unless bleeding is excessive
Delivery	Immediate delivery, usually by cesarean	Delivery may be delayed, depending on size of fetus and amount of bleeding

d. Observe urinary output for oliguria or hematuria.
e. Otherwise, give routine postpartum care for type of delivery.

Expected Outcomes

1. Absence of shock; demonstrates stable vital signs; absence of bleeding
2. Attains/maintains adequate fluid balance; urine output and laboratory values within acceptable range; absence of excessive thirst
3. Infant appears stable; color good
4. Demonstrates lessening of anxiety; asking questions; responds to infant in a positive manner

Pregnancy-Induced Hypertension

Hypertensive disorders induced by pregnancy or complicated by pregnancy rank among the leading causes of maternal mortality and make a significant contribution to perinatal mortality.

Types of Hypertensive Disorders

The American College of Obstetricians and Gynecologists has classified the hypertensive states of pregnancy as:

A. Gestational Edema

The occurrence of a general and excessive accumulation of fluid in the tissues of greater than 1+ pitting edema after 12 hours' rest in bed, or of a weight gain of 2½ kg. (5 lbs.) or more in 1 week caused by pregnancy.

B. Gestational Proteinuria

The presence of proteinuria during pregnancy, in the absence of hypertension, edema, renal infection, or known intrinsic renovascular cause.

C. Gestational Hypertension

The development of hypertension during pregnancy or within the first 24 hours postpartum in a previously normotensive woman.

D. Preeclampsia

1. The development of hypertension with proteinuria, edema, or both caused by pregnancy or a recent pregnancy.
2. It occurs after the 20th week of gestation but may develop before this time in the presence of trophoblastic disease.
3. Preeclampsia is predominantly a disease of primigravidas.

E. Eclampsia

The occurrence of one or more convulsions, not attributable to other cerebral disorders such as epilepsy or cerebral hemorrhage, in a patient with preeclampsia.

F. Superimposed Preeclampsia or Eclampsia

1. The development of preeclampsia or eclampsia in a patient with chronic hypertensive, vascular, or renal disease.
2. When the hypertension antedates the pregnancy, as established by previous blood pressure recordings, the following criteria are used to establish the diagnosis:
   a. A rise in the systolic pressure of 30 mm. Hg
   b. A rise in the diastolic pressure of 15 mm. Hg
   c. The development of proteinuria, edema, or both

G. Chronic Hypertensive Disease

The presence of persistent hypertension, of whatever cause, before pregnancy or prior to the 20th week of gestation, or persistent hypertension beyond the 42nd day of the postpartum period.

Preeclampsia (formerly termed toxemia)

1. Major hypertensive disorder of pregnancy
2. Characterized by development of hypertension, edema, and proteinuria (Table 27-2)
3. Usually relieved by termination of pregnancy
4. Edema usually first symptom to appear; observed as rapid weight gain; followed by rise in blood pressure and proteinuria
5. Preeclampsia appears in approximately 5% of all pregnancies; eclampsia (with convulsions) now rare because of improved treatment

Etiology

1. Unknown
2. Theories include:
   a. Uterine ischemia
   b. The woman is extremely sensitive to vasopressor agents (implicated—catecholamines, prolactin, vasopressin, prostaglandins)
   c. Autoimmune disease
   d. Deficiency of dietary protein
3. Contributing factors
   a. Age and parity—appears most frequently in young primigravidas
   b. Socioeconomic status—greater incidence in lower socioeconomic groups
   c. Greater incidence in women with diabetes, multiple pregnancies, polyhydramnios, molar pregnancies, obesity, and history of previous hypertension in pregnancy

Table 27-2 Symptoms and Signs of Preeclampsia

Symptoms & Signs	Definition
Mild preeclampsia	
Hypertension	Increase of 30 mm. Hg or more systolic, or systolic level of 140 mm. Hg or more; increase of 15 mm. Hg or more diastolic, or diastolic level of 90 mm. Hg or more
Proteinuria	+1 or +2 or 1 gm./liter in midstream or catheterized urine specimen (found in 2 specimens at least 6 hours apart)
Edema	Generalized, facial, hands, and fingers; reflected in a rapid weight gain of over 0.7 kg. (1.5 lbs.) per week
Severe preeclampsia	
Hypertension	160/110 mm. Hg or above
Proteinuria	5 gm. or more in 24-hour urine collection or +3 or +4 reading on turbidometric analysis
Edema	In addition to generalized edema, possibly pitting edema; weight gain may be 0.9 kg. (2 lbs.) or more over a period of 1 week or less
Headache	
Blurred vision	
Oliguria (less than 400 ml. in 24-hour urine collection)	
Epigastric pain	

Clinical Manifestations (see Table 27-2)

1. Weight gain—first indication, over 0.7 kg. (1.5 lbs.) per week, as early as the 20th week
2. Ankle edema, digital swelling, periorbital edema, then pretibial fluid collection
3. Optic fundi—reveal segmental or generalized arteriolar spasms
4. Hypertension—140/90 or increase of 30 mm. Hg systolic or 15 mm. Hg diastolic
5. Proteinuria
6. Cerebral and neurologic involvement—frontal headache, vertigo, tinnitus, visual disturbance, drowsiness, hyperreflexia, apprehension, excitability, nausea, and vomiting
7. *Positive rollover test*—a procedure carried out between the 28th and 32nd weeks in which the blood pressure is checked with the woman first on her side and then on her back. A test is positive when there is an increase of 20 mm. Hg in diastolic pressure. Eighty percent to ninety percent of women with a positive rollover test develop pregnancy-induced hypertension. Some clinicians report less success with the test as a screening device.

▶ **NURSING ALERT:** Epigastric pain may herald onset of convulsions or coma.

8. Possible complications
   a. Eclampsia
   b. Abruptio placentae
   c. Pulmonary edema
   d. Congestive heart failure
   e. Cerebral edema
   f. Detached retina
   g. Renal damage (monitor output carefully for oliguria)

Nursing Interventions

A. During Pregnancy

1. When symptoms appear, the woman is placed on bed rest in left lateral recumbent position; increases renal and uterine blood flow promoting diuresis and reducing blood pressure
2. Monitor blood pressure every 4 hours (if at home, family member or friend may do this); deep tendon reflexes are also monitored.
3. Take daily weight; and measure intake and urinary output.
4. Offer high-protein diet and normal fluid intake.
5. Sodium is not restricted unless edema is severe or cardiac complications occur.
6. Fetal condition is monitored via nonstress tests, urinary estriol determinations and ultrasound measurements of fetal growth.
7. If preeclampsia is severe, drugs may be used to control hypertension; magnesium sulfate is used most commonly (Table 27-3); magnesium sulfate (administered intramuscularly in 50% solution with 1% procaine; injection is painful and may cause abscess formation. Continuous IV infusion may be preferred; depresses myoneural junction, decreases hyperreflexia, and increases vasodilatation.

▶ **NURSING ALERT:** Repeat doses of magnesium sulfate only if (1) deep tendon reflexes are present, (2) respirations are above 12 per minute, and (3) urine output is at least 100 ml. per 6 hours. Calcium gluconate 10% IV must be available to counteract magnesium toxicity.

8. Sedatives may be used to promote rest.
9. Pregnancy is maintained until at least the 36th week.
10. In instances of severe eclampsia:
    a. Provide a quiet environment, avoiding stimuli that could provoke seizures.
    b. Evaluate vital signs through continuous monitoring.

Table 27-3   Medications Used in Treatment of Hypertensive Disorders of Pregnancy

Drug	Use	Dose	Adverse Reactions
Magnesium sulfate	Anticonvulsant; depresses CNS function, especially at neuromuscular junction; reduces muscle excitability; peripheral vasodilation; in large doses acts as osmotic diuretic	IM: 10 gm. initially as 50% solution followed by 5 gm. every hour until reflexes are reduced IV: loading dose of 4 gm. given over 10 minutes; followed by 1 gm./hour until therapeutic blood levels of 6–7 mEq./liter are reached	Respiratory depression, depression of deep tendon reflexes; IM injections may produce pain and swelling at injection site
Sodium amobarbital (Sodium Amytal)	Anticonvulsant; sedative used in eclampsia when convulsions persist	IV: up to 0.25 gm. injected over a 3-minute period	
Diazepam (Valium)	Anticonvulsant; used to control or reduce convulsions	IV: 5 mg. IM: 10 mg. Dose is administered every 2 hours until convulsions are controlled	Fetal tachycardia and loss of fetal heart rate variability, newborn lethargy, hypotonia, respiratory depression, failure to suck
Phenobarbital	Sedative; anticonvulsant (raises threshold for seizures)	Oral: 30–100 mg. BID or TID in preeclampsia IM or IV; large doses for eclampsia	Tolerance may develop; rashes; ataxia
Hydralazine (Apresoline)	Antihypertensive; dilation of vascular smooth muscle, especially arterioles	IV: when diastolic blood pressure is 110 mm. Hg, test dose 5 mg. followed by 10 mg., repeated until diastolic blood pressure is 90–100 mm. Hg (usual dose—5–20 mg.)	Chills, fever, depression, headache, palpitations, dizziness, vomiting, tachycardia, sweating
Hydrochlorothiazide	Diuretic; used in treating women with chronic hypertension; not used in prevention of preeclampsia (no documented advantage)	Oral: 50 mg. BID	Fatigue, weakness, anorexia, heartburn, nausea, vomiting, decreased fetal birth weight

c. Provide safety measures; be prepared for sudden seizures.
  (1) Have padded siderails in place.
  (2) Have tongue blade available.
  (3) Have emergency equipment (oxygen, suction, airway, tracheostomy tray) ready for immediate use.
  (4) Have emergency medications immediately available; IV sedation and inhalation anesthesia may be needed to control convulsions; IV fluids to be initiated.
  (5) Observe for indications of uterine contractions; convulsions may initiate labor.
  (6) Provide continuous observation and care.
  (7) Position the woman to promote drainage of respiratory passages; maintain clear airway; monitor for pulmonary edema.
  (8) Insert indwelling catheter to monitor output and renal status.

B. Restriction of Activity or Bed Rest

1. Discuss with the woman the importance of bed rest in promoting diuresis and controlling blood pressure.
2. Assist the woman/couple in planning how this might be accomplished at home if condition permits.

3. Assist the woman/couple in mobilizing family or community resources needed.
4. Assist the woman in developing passive exercise program which might be used while on bed rest.
5. Assist the woman in planning recreational, hobby, or work activities that can be done while on bed rest.
6. Assist the woman/couple in planning ways of maintaining family contacts during activity restriction, yet allowing woman adequate periods of rest and relaxation.

C. Treatment During Labor and Delivery

1. Management is based on assessment of the disease and viability of the fetus.
2. If fetus is thought to be viable and disease is not controlled, induction or cesarean delivery is usually recommended.

D. Management During Postpartum

1. Signs and symptoms usually decrease rapidly after delivery, however, danger of seizures does not pass until 48 hours following delivery.
2. Sedation may be continued.
3. Hypertension may recur with next pregnancy.
4. Follow-up care is essential.

Multiple Pregnancy

Multiple pregnancy results in twins in approximately 1 of 80 pregnancies, in triplets in 1 of 6,400 pregnancies, and in quadruplets in 1 of 512,000 pregnancies.

Types of Twinning

1. Monozygotic (identical) twinning occurs at random in about 1 of 200 pregnancies. May have:
  a. One chorion, 2 amnions (70%)
  b. Two chorions, 2 amnions (30%)
  c. Always same sex
2. Dizygotic (fraternal) twinning occurs more frequently in some families, has a higher incidence in Blacks, occurs in response to greater levels of follicle-stimulating hormone (FSH). Always have:
  a. Two chorions, 2 amnions
  b. May be different sexes

Clinical Manifestations

1. Uterus larger than expected for length of gestation
2. Two fetal heart tones can be counted simultaneously
3. Abdominal palpation yields many small parts by 6–7 months
4. Ultrasound usually used to confirm diagnosis
5. Premature labor is more common
6. Oversized uterus and increased abdominal pressure often lead to:
  a. Digestion difficulties
  b. Constipation
  c. Hemorrhoids and other varicosities

  d. Dyspnea
  e. Backache
7. One twin may be in breech position

Nursing Interventions

A. Preventing Premature Delivery

1. Encourage the woman to keep appointments for more frequent checkups.
2. Counsel the woman to rest frequently during the day in the 3rd trimester; assist family to mobilize support system for this purpose.
3. Teach the woman reportable signs and symptoms of premature labor.
4. Advocate a diet high in protein, iron, and calcium; 300–1,000 calories should be added to normal pregnancy diet according to needs of the individual woman.
5. Monitor for hypertensive disorders which occur more frequently in women with multiple pregnancies.
6. Following delivery, monitor the woman for postpartum hemorrhage due to overdistended uterus.

B. Health Teaching

1. Counsel the woman to rest frequently on her side to minimize the effects of increased abdominal pressure and decreased venous return from lower portion of the body
2. Encourage pelvic rocking exercises and sitting with legs elevated to help relieve backache.
3. Teach the woman that small, frequent meals will aid digestion.

Polyhydramnios

Polyhydramnios is an excessive amount of amniotic fluid.
Associated with:
1. Maternal disease such as diabetes, heart disease, kidney disease
2. Multiple gestation
3. Fetal abnormalities (atresias and neural tube defects)

Clinical Manifestations
1. Excessive uterine enlargement
2. Difficulty breathing
3. Difficulty ambulating, getting from chair to standing position
4. Difficulty finding a comfortable sleeping position
5. Varicosities
6. Pain in abdomen, back, and thighs due to increased pressure
7. Nausea and vomiting
8. Fetus may be difficult to palpate; fetal heart tones may be difficult to locate and hear

Management
1. Fluid may need to be removed by amniocentesis to reduce symptoms and enhance maternal comfort; carefully monitor the woman's vital signs during procedure.
2. Encourage the woman to rest on side in semirecumbent position to increase blood flow to uterus and fetus and to relieve symptoms.
3. Monitor carefully for signs of abruptio placentae, abnormal fetal presentation, and postpartal hemorrhage.

Oligohydramnios

Oligohydramnios is a small amount of amniotic fluid.
Associated with:
1. Fetal renal agenesis
2. Postmaturity

Clinical Manifestations
1. Small uterine size
2. Labor may be premature
3. Uterine contractions may be ineffectual and labor prolonged
4. Fetal hypoxia may occur because of cord compression

Management
1. Monitor fetal status carefully during pregnancy and labor
2. Monitor the woman for labor complications

Medical Disorders Complicating Pregnancy

Cardiac Disease

The woman with cardiac disease should be counseled prior to becoming pregnant about the restrictions that will be placed on her during pregnancy, the diet she will need, and the statistical chances of her delivering a live infant. Maternal mortality associated with heart disease ranges between 1% and 5%, the major cause of death being cardiac decompensation and heart failure. Most heart disease found in pregnant women is the result of congenital heart disease.

Physiologic Impact of Childbearing
1. Imposes a significant circulatory burden on the woman because of increased cardiac output, oxygen consumption, and blood volume
2. Burden begins in the 1st trimester, increases throughout the 2nd trimester, and persists to term
3. During labor, cardiac output increases 20%–30% during each uterine contraction; pulse rate, blood pressure, and left ventricular work also increase
4. Following delivery, fluid from interstitial spaces is shifted to general circulation, increasing blood volume; elevated plasma volume continues for approximately 2 weeks

Classification
The New York Heart Association's functional classification of patients with cardiac disease:
   Class 1. No limitation of physical activity; no symptoms of cardiac insufficiency or anginal pain
   Class 2. Slight limitation of physical activity; comfortable at rest; excessive fatigue, palpitations, dyspnea, or anginal pain with ordinary physical activity
   Class 3. Marked limitation of physical activity; comfortable at rest; excessive fatigue, palpitations, dyspnea, or anginal pain with less than ordinary physical activity
   Class 4. Inability to perform any physical activity without discomfort; symptoms of cardiac insufficiency or anginal syndrome possible at rest; discomfort increased with physical activity
1. Most women in classes 1 and 2 are able to handle the physiologic demands of pregnancy
2. The cardiac status of women in all classifications should be evaluated very early in pregnancy if not before; examination should include chest x-ray, electrocardiogram, and tests for vital capacity.
3. Cardiac status and functional capacity are monitored carefully throughout pregnancy.
4. Monitor for signs of cardiac decompensation: crackles at the bases of lungs, cough, hemoptysis, dyspnea on exertion, cyanosis, labored respirations, increased pulse, edema of face, ankles, and hands

Management
1. Rest is most important—10 hours sleep per night and rest throughout the day.
2. Physical exertion is to be avoided since it is an important cause of heart failure.
3. Stress, emotional as well as physical, is to be avoided.
4. Infection must be avoided and, if contracted, treated immediately.

5. A well-balanced diet, high in iron, protein, vitamins, and minerals is recommended to prevent anemia.
6. Hospitalization prior to delivery is usual for women with classes 1 or 2 cardiac disease to evaluate cardiac status before labor; women in class 3 are hospitalized somewhat earlier.
7. Any woman showing signs of cardiac failure during pregnancy is hospitalized and may remain hospitalized for the duration of the pregnancy.
8. During labor and delivery
   a. The woman labors upright, on side.
   b. The woman's vital signs and fetal heart tones are monitored continuously.
   c. The woman may receive oxygen during course of labor.
   d. Regional anesthesia may be used to reduce pain in labor and during delivery.
   e. To avoid having the mother push, the infant may be delivered by forceps.
   f. Cesarean birth is avoided because of:
      (1) Greater blood loss
      (2) Risk of infection
      (3) Risk of thromboembolism
9. During postpartum
   a. Monitor carefully for postpartum hemorrhage, infection, thromboembolism
   b. Restrict visitors; promote rest
   c. Ambulate to avoid thromboembolism
   d. Prophylactic antibiotics may be used to avoid infection

Nursing Interventions

1. Discuss plan of care and what the woman may expect during hospitalization, labor, delivery, and postpartum
2. Teach the woman reportable signs when at home and whom she should contact if these occur.
3. As pregnancy progresses, congratulate the woman on her progress to date and reinforce her current well-being and that of her fetus.
4. Discuss procedures as they need to be done and any changes in the care plan.
5. At each visit and during labor, have the woman/couple listen to fetal heart sounds.
6. Stay with the woman in labor to reduce anxiety.

The Pregnant Diabetic Woman

Pregnancy imposes an additional physiological stress on a diabetic woman. Successful delivery of a healthy infant requires much teaching, support, adherence to dietary control, and work of the entire health care team.

Physiologic Considerations

A. Prior to Pregnancy

1. The woman's diabetes must be in control (ketoacidosis is a major reason for early abortion in diabetics).
2. The woman's nutritional status should be good.
3. The woman should develop a plan to avoid stresses, including avoidance of infections.
4. Counseling is done to explain changes that occur during pregnancy and restrictions that may need to be carried out for pregnancy to be successful.

B. Physiology Altered by Pregnancy

1. Increased peripheral resistance to insulin
2. Placental insulinase increases the rate of destruction of insulin
3. Chorionic somatomammotropin (human placental lactogen [HPL]) spares carbohydrate (glucose) for fetal use, transferring it across the placenta while mobilizing lipids for maternal energy use. This action antagonizes the action of insulin.
4. Nausea and vomiting of pregnancy may further compound the problem of blood glucose regulation.

Assessment

1. Blood sugar levels are monitored closely to prevent episodes of hypoglycemia and ketoacidosis. Some diabetics experience episodes of hypoglycemia during the 1st trimester.
2. Assess the woman's ability to monitor blood sugar either through home glucose monitoring (see p. 702) or indirectly through urine testing for glucose. Insulin regulation throughout pregnancy is determined according to changes in blood sugar. Insulin requirements may increase during the 2nd trimester and will increase greatly during the 3rd trimester as amounts of HPL increase.
3. Assess the woman's understanding of diabetes, and changes that may occur during pregnancy.
4. Assess the woman's/family's understanding of hypoglycemia and acidosis and what to do if signs and symptoms of either become evident.
5. Assess the woman's support system since hospitalization may be necessary sometime during pregnancy.

Management

A. Maintenance of blood sugar within normal range; term delivery

1. The woman monitors her blood sugar several times a day either through home blood glucose monitoring or urine testing. In the latter months of pregnancy, some glucose may be lost normally in the urine as the glomerular filtration rate increases without a concomitant increase in tubular reabsorption.
2. Insulin requirements may remain the same in the first half of pregnancy or increase somewhat; insulin requirements increase greatly in 3rd trimester (may be as high as 70%–100% above prepregnancy needs). Mixtures of insulins (intermediate and short-acting in a 2:1 ratio) are most effective during pregnancy.
3. The woman whose diabetes is controlled through diet alone may require insulin during pregnancy.
4. Oral hypoglycemics are not effective during pregnancy and may be teratogenic.
5. Some women will exhibit signs and symptoms of diabetes only while pregnant (gestational diabetics; see Classification of Diabetes in Pregnancy, p. 1022); if these women receive insulin during the last trimester of pregnancy, their infants tend not to become macrosomic (large body size and high weight) as will infants of uncontrolled diabetic mothers.
6. The woman's diet during pregnancy is usually 30–35 K calories per kilogram of ideal body weight. The usual calorie range is 1,800–2,400 with 125 gm. of protein and carbohydrate distributed 30, 30, 30, and 10 for breakfast, lunch, dinner, and an evening snack.
7. Nonstress tests may be performed weekly after the 30th week; estriol levels and monthly ultrasound scans are all used to assess fetal well-being.
8. Periods of hypoglycemia on the woman's usual doses of insulin for that period may signal placental dysfunction. Decreased amounts of placental hormones reduce insulin antagonism and destruction, resulting in hypoglycemia due to higher functioning levels of insulin.
9. Monitor the woman for hypertensive disorder, poly-

hydramnios, infection, and after delivery, for post-partum infection
10. Delivery may be vaginal (induced) or if placental dysfunction occurs, by cesarean birth. Woman is usually hospitalized several days prior to delivery.
11. Infants of diabetic mothers tend to be larger, encounter more respiratory difficulties following birth, and have an increased incidence of congenital anomalies (major cause of death for these infants).

Classification of Diabetes in Pregnancy
(Duration of Disease More Important than Age at Onset)

Class A Gestational Diabetic (90% of all patients with diabetes seen by the obstetrician)
1. Normal fasting blood sugar
2. Abnormal glucose tolerance test
3. Usually controlled by diet
4. Infant may be large for gestational age (LGA)

Class B
1. Onset after age 20
2. Present less than 10 years
3. No vascular complications
4. May have been controlled by diet; now insulin-dependent
5. Infant may be LGA.

Class C
1. Onset between ages 10 and 19
2. Present 10–19 years
3. No vascular complications
4. Insulin-dependent before pregnancy; now insulin requirements increase
5. Infant may be LGA.

Class D
1. Onset before age 10
2. Present 20 years or more
3. Peripheral vascular disease
4. Retinal changes
5. Hypertension
6. Insulin-dependent
7. Infant may be small for gestational age (SGA)

Class F
1. Includes neuropathy with proteinuria and decreased creatinine clearance
2. Infant SGA

Class R
1. Proliferative retinopathy, which may intensify
2. Therapeutic abortion may be a consideration

Class G
1. When many failures have occurred in pregnancy; it is thus possible to have Class A-G

Class H
1. Includes patients with cardiopathy (may be symptomatic) Classes may change during pregnancy!

(Modified from White P. Diabetes mellitus in pregnancy. Clin Perinatol 1974; 1[2]:331)

12. Postpartum considerations
    a. Monitor the woman for postpartum hemorrhage.
    b. Monitor to see that insulin requirements begin to return to prepregnant levels.

Nursing Interventions
1. Develop plan of care with the woman/couple, reviewing and updating it at each visit.
2. Have the woman discuss her perceptions of how well she is progressing; reinforce positive feelings; provide reassurance and encouragement.
3. Have the woman/couple listen to fetal heart sounds at each visit; keep them updated on progress of fetus.
4. Have the woman meet nursing staff and tour hospital units on which she is likely to be.

Anemia

It is generally accepted that hemoglobin levels less than 1.0 gm. per dl. during pregnancy or the puerperium are considered an indication of anemia.

Types of anemia
1. Iron deficiency—major cause during pregnancy
2. Sickle cell
3. Anemia due to infection
4. Anemia due to folic acid deficiency

Clinical Manifestations
1. Fatigue
2. Pallor
3. Increased susceptibility to infection
4. In sickle cell anemia, crisis (precipitated by hypoxemia)
    a. Pain (abdominal and joint) as hemoglobin assumes a sickle shape, thus obstructing blood flow through small capillaries
    b. More frequent episodes of asymptomatic bacteriuria

Nursing Interventions
A. Improvement in Nutritional Status
1. Provide diet counseling emphasizing a well-balanced diet high in iron
2. Administer iron supplementation (ferrous sulfate, 300 mg. TID) if prescribed
3. If iron is supplemented, counsel the woman to increase fluids and fiber (avoids side effect of constipation) and to increase intake of foods high in vitamin C (enhances iron absorption).
4. Folic acid supplements (1 mg. folic acid a day) may be necessary with folic acid deficiency. Diets higher in animal protein and green leafy vegetables also are important.
5. In severe anemia, intramuscular iron or transfusions of packed red cells may be necessary.

B. Improvement in Fetal Nutrition and Oxygenation
1. Improved diet with vitamin and mineral supplementation will improve fetal nutrition.
2. Oxygenation to fetus can be improved or maintained by:
    a. Improving maternal hemoglobin levels (may require transfusions of packed red cells for woman with sickle cell anemia).
    b. Avoidance of maternal infections which can reduce Hb levels and increase metabolic rate and oxygen consumption.

Infections During Pregnancy

Although pregnant women, in general, are no more susceptible to acute infectious disease than are other women, infections may have serious consequences for the developing fetus (Table 27-4).

Urinary Infection

A. Incidence and Effect

1. Urinary tract infection is the most common renal problem encountered in pregnancy.
2. Chronic renal disease, especially if accompanied by hypertension, may cause fetal growth retardation and increase risk of perinatal mortality.

B. Predisposing Factors

1. Hormonal changes, mainly the effect of progesterone, cause dilatation of the ureters and increase the collecting space and decrease peristalsis of the ureters.
2. Mechanical pressure caused by the uterus pressing the ureters against the pelvic brim results in urinary stasis and increased risk of infection.

C. Clinical Manifestations

1. Chills and fever
2. Frequency of urination
3. Dysuria
4. Pain in the area of the kidney
5. Uterine irritability (may result in premature labor)

D. Management

1. Urine culture and antimicrobial sensitivity studies are carried out.
2. Appropriate antimicrobial is given for 2 weeks, then urine is recultured since recurrences are common.
3. Fluid intake is increased to approximately 3,000 ml. per day; IV fluids may be necessary.

▶ **NURSING ALERT:** The usual antibiotics and sulfonamides may be contraindicated since they may produce hemolysis, hyperbilirubinemia, or kernicterus in the fetus.

Drug Effects on the Fetus

During pregnancy and labor, the mother may be exposed to a variety of drugs for a number of reasons. The effects of these drugs on the fetus are indicated in Table 27-5.

Pseudocyesis

Pseudocyesis or false pregnancy is usually seen in women with a very strong desire to be pregnant.

Clinical Manifestations

1. Irregular or absent menses
2. Morning sickness
3. Increased abdominal size
4. May have breast enlargement with pigmentary changes
5. Intestinal gas or intestinal contractions may be interpreted as fetal movements
6. Uterus generally remains small

Management

1. Following physician's diagnosis and discussion with the woman, evaluate her understanding of the situation.
2. Reinforce the woman's correct understanding of the situation and facts; correct misunderstanding and, provide additional information as needed.
3. Help family members understand and accept situation.

Complications of Labor

Preterm Labor

Preterm labor is uterine contractions occurring after 20 weeks' gestation and before 37 completed weeks of gestation. Contractions are less than 10 minutes apart, resulting in progressive cervical changes or cervical dilation of 2 cm. or effacement of 75%.

Assessment

Risk factors for preterm labor:

A. Socioeconomic Risk Factors

1. Low socioeconomic status
2. More than 2 children at home with no household help
3. Maternal age less than 18 or more than 35 years
4. No prenatal care
5. Poor nutrition
6. Lack of childbirth experience or childbirth education

B. Medical/Obstetrical Risk Factors

1. Previous preterm labor and/or delivery
2. Spontaneous or induced abortion
3. Uterine anomalies; incompetent cervical os
4. Less than 1 year between last birth and present conception
5. Diethylstilbestrol (DES) exposure in utero

6. Pregnancy weight below 45.8 kg. (100 lbs.); maternal height less than 150 cm. (5 ft.)

C. Life-style Risk Factors

1. Smoking more than 10 cigarettes per day; alcohol or drug abuse
2. Factors that cause excessive fatigue
3. Event or series of events that precipitate unusual anxiety (death in family, separation or divorce, etc.)

D. Risk Factors in Current Pregnancy

1. Uterine overdistention
2. Bleeding
3. Weight gain < 10 pounds by 26 weeks' gestation
4. Fetal or placental malformations
5. Maternal illness or disease
6. Premature rupture of membranes

Management

A. Prevention of Premature Delivery

1. If woman is currently in preterm labor, she is admitted to a hospital and:
   a. Placed on bed rest lying on her side
   b. Uterine contractions and uterine irritability are evaluated and monitored every 1–2 hours

Table 27-4   Effects of Maternal Infection on Fetus and Neonate

Infection	Effect(s) on Fetus and Neonate	Associated Factors	Prognosis of Infant
Coxsackie virus	? Congenital malformations in 1st trimester Transplacental meningoencephalitis and/or myocarditis Acquired infections	Maternal infection mild	Depends on the extent of the disease
Cytomegalic inclusion body disease	Intrauterine death Premature delivery Severe generalized disease—jaundice, hemolytic anemia, thrombocytopenia, hepatosplenomegaly, central nervous system disease (including cerebral calcification and chorioretinitis), microcephaly, and undergrowth	Half the women in early childbearing years show no immunologic response to this virus; mothers are most often asymptomatic	Early death in majority of severely affected infants; severe mental and motor retardation in some survivors
Hepatitis B	Abortion Neonatal hepatitis	Newborn infection most common in symptomatic mother	
Herpes simplex	Mild infection with a few skin lesions; infant does not appear ill Viremia, severe generalized disease, CNS involvement ? Congenital malformations	Maternal herpetic vulvovaginitis usually present Transplacental infection of fetus may occur	Mild disease—recovery Severe disease—usually fatal
Influenza	Increased incidence of abortion and premature labor Occasional association of congenital malformations, especially anencephaly and meningomyelocele	Active immunization by an attenuated vaccine should not be given during pregnancy for fear of fetal damage	
Listeriosis	Infants infected either through direct invasion or from birth contamination Generalized disease, skin rash, meningitis, pneumonia, etc. Fetal involvement with scattered foci of necrosis (granulomatosis infantiseptica) Delayed infection of the newborn infant, usually listerial meningitis	4% of pregnant women harbor *Listeria monocytogenes* in the cervix or vagina	Mortality and morbidity high, especially from CNS complications; persistent fetal circulation
Malaria	Direct transmission of *P. falciparum* occurs rarely	Placental involvement 10 times more frequent than fetal involvement	
Mumps	Abortion, premature birth, or stillbirth uncommon ? Cause of endocardial fibroelastosis		
Poliomyelitis	Abortion Rare congenital or acquired poliomyelitis Growth retardation in chronic, severe, maternal, paralytic poliomyelitis	Widespread use of immunization procedures has all but eliminated this disease as a pregnancy problem Use of Sabin live virus vaccine during pregnancy is contraindicated May safely administer Salk vaccine	Fetal and neonatal loss: 33%
Rubella	Abortion Congenital malformations of heart, eye, ear, brain, dermatoglyphic abnormalities Systemic involvement with or without malformation, anemia, thrombocytopenia with purpura, jaundice, hepatosplenomegaly, bone changes, myocarditis, encephalitis, pneumonia, etc.	Maternal infection usually mild, occasionally arthritis and/or encephalitis Strict isolation for neonates with congenital rubella as long as virus is present in pharynx or urine for extended period of time	Residua and sequelae for the neonate depend on time during pregnancy when mother acquires the disease, virulence of the virus, and extent of the infectious process Incidence of malformation in the infant is 35% in 1st month, 25% in 2nd month, and 16% in 3rd month of gestation. After 4th month, abnormalities are uncommon
Rubeola	Interruption of pregnancy Congenital or neonatal measles, with or without bronchopneumonia (typical dermal lesions are in same stage as those in mother)	Measles vaccine should be given to all nonimmune women prior to but not during gestation	Maternal rubeola at any time during pregnancy is responsible for increased perinatal death rate Great majority of infants are normal
Smallpox and vaccinia	Increased fetal wastage in all stages of pregnancy Congenital malformations not more frequent, but congenital infections with skin lesions reported	Primary vaccination and revaccination against smallpox must be deferred until after delivery because vaccinia often causes fatal widespread fetal visceral and cutaneous lesions	
Syphilis	Major cause of mid-trimester abortion, fetal death in utero, or premature labor and delivery	If maternal infection occurs less than 1–2 years prior to gestation, fetus may be affected	40%–50% of infants affected in untreated mothers 40% of above show clinical signs at birth

Table 27-4   Effects of Maternal Infection on Fetus and Neonate (continued)

Infection	Effect(s) on Fetus and Neonate	Associated Factors	Prognosis of Infant
	Early congenital syphilis (septicemia, skin lesions, anemia, jaundice, periostitis) Late congenital syphilis	If exposed 3 months before pregnancy 1 year duration: Penicillin G 2.4 million units (half in each buttock) Procaine penicillin G, 600,000 units per day for 8 days If had disease more than 1 year: Penicillin G, 2.4 million units (IM) weekly for 3 weeks Erythromycin used for women allergic to penicillin Following treatment, serologic test may remain positive: a. Maternal—up to 8 months b. Newborn—up to 3 months	
Gonorrhea	If present at time of birth, ophthalmia neonatorum acquired during birth	Acute inflammation is found in urethra, vulvar glands, and vaginal and vulvar epithelium Treatment: Procaine penicillin G, 4.8 million units (IM) half in each buttock following 1 gm. of probenecid ingested before the injections	Silver nitrate 1% eyedrops at birth are preventive
Toxoplasmosis	High incidence of abortion Premature delivery Generalized disease—hepatosplenomegaly, jaundice, chorioretinitis, microphthalmia, convulsions Later manifestations—hydrocephalus or microcephaly, mental retardation, cerebral calcifications		Poor
Tuberculosis	Small infants born to mothers with active disease Congenital tuberculosis (rare) Acquired infection readily contracted	Severe maternal disease and malnutrition Essential to segregate mother with pulmonary tuberculosis from her infant to avoid neonatal infection Treatment: Isoniazid; ethambutol or rifampin Possibly streptomycin (auditory effects on fetus) Rest and diet high in protein, vitamins, and calories	Great majority of infants unaffected
Ureaplasma urealyticum (T mycoplasma	Chronic reproductive failure Low birth weight	Mycoplasma isolated from genital and lower urinary tracts of women and men	Abortion in early pregnancy
Varicella (chicken pox)	Premature delivery Congenital varicella	Low maternal immunity; most mothers have had the disease and developed immunity in childhood: therefore, congenital varicella is rare	Mortality high

(Klaus M and Fanaroff A. *Care of the High-risk Neonate.* Philadelphia; WB Saunders, 1979; Pritchard J and MacDonald P. *Williams Obstetrics.* New York; Appleton-Century-Crofts, 1980)

c. Cervical consistency (hard or soft), dilation, and effacement are evaluated

d. Symptoms are monitored to determine if they are increasing or decreasing

e. IV fluids are started if drug therapy is a possibility; see drugs used (Table 27-6, p. 1028)

f. Intake and output monitored

2. Once contractions have been stopped and the woman's condition has stabilized, she may be discharged and the following done to prevent subsequent occurrences:

a. Bed rest maintained

b. Nutritional status is improved; vitamins and iron are supplemented

c. Usual activity level is evaluated and restricted if necessary when the woman resumes activity

d. Chronic illness is monitored closely; acute illnesses are treated promptly

e. Life-style change is strongly recommended if life-style is associated with preterm labor and delivery

f. Oral medication (for premature labor) may be continued at home

g. The woman is instructed to call physician if symptoms of preterm labor recur

h. Prenatal visits are made weekly for remainder of pregnancy

B. Patient Teaching

1. Teach the symptoms of preterm labor:

a. Uterine contractions in regular pattern for more than 1 hour while at rest

b. Intermittent or constant uterine cramps or thigh pain

c. Low, dull backache

d. Intestinal cramping

Table 27-5 **Drugs Reported to Affect the Fetus**

	Effect		
Drug	Morphological	Functional	Delayed
Analgesics			
Narcotics		Withdrawal syndrome ↓ Hyperbilirubinemia	?
Salicylates	↑ Minor anomalies	Platelet dysfunction ↓ Factor XII	
Anesthetics			
General		Depression	
Local		Depression Bradycardia Acidosis Methemoglobinemia	
Antidiabetic Agents			
Tolbutamide	Anomalies	Thrombocytopenia	?
Chlorpropanide	Anomalies	Severe hypoglycemia	?
Cyclamates		?	?
Saccharin		?	?
Hormones			
Cortisone	Cleft palate ?	? Hemorrhages ? Hypoglycemia	
Prednisolone	Anencephaly ? Low birth weight ?	Normal adrenal activity ? Hemorrhages ? Hypoglycemia Normal adrenal activity	
Androgens	Masculinization female	Tomboyish behavior	Higher IQ
Progestins	Masculinization female	Tomboyish behavior	Higher IQ
Diethylstilbestrol	Clitoris hypertrophy		Adenocarcinoma vagina (adolescence)
Smoking			
	Low birth weight ↑ Stillborn		Smaller at 1 year of age
Alcohol			
Chronic intake	Intrauterine growth failure		
Acute administration		Withdrawal symptoms	?
Pollutants and Pesticides			
Mercury		Severe neurologic defects	Severe handicaps Mental retardation
Lead	Low birth weight	↑ Abortions Anemia Enzyme induction	
DDT and metabolites			
Parathion	? Teratogen		
Fungicides	?	?	
Herbicides	?	?	
Miscellaneous			
Atropine		Tachycardia	
Hexamethonium		Ileus	
Tubocurarine	? Arthrogryposis Multiplex congenita	Muscular paralysis	
LSD	? Minor limb deformities		
Chloroquine		Deafness	
Antimicrobials			
Sulfonamides		Kernicterus	
Nitrofurantoin		Hemolysis	
Tetracyclines	Teeth staining Enamel hypoplasia		
Streptomycin		8th nerve damage	Deafness
Isoniazid		Encephalopathy	

Table 27-5 Drugs Reported to Affect the Fetus (continued)

Drug	Effect		
	Morphological	Functional	Delayed
Anticonvulsants			
Phenytoin	Cleft-lip and palate	Coagulation defects	?
Phenobarbital		Coagulation defects	?
		Enzymes induction	?
Barbiturates		Addiction	
		Enzymes induction ↓ Sucking	
Anticoagulants			
Coumarin		↓ Prothrombin time	
		Hemorrhages	
Diuretics			
Thazides		Thrombocytopenia	?
		Hyponatremia	?
		? Electrolyte imbalance	
Antihypertensive Drugs			
Reserpine		Nasal stuffiness	
Cancer Chemotherapeutic Drugs			
Aminopterin	Bone defects		Retarded growth
	Intrauterine growth retardation		
Methotrexate	Malformation of head		
Chlorambucil	Unilateral absence of kidney and ureter		
Immunosuppressants			
Azathioprine	?	?	?
Psychopharmacologic Drugs			
Phenothiazine		?	?
			Behavioral changes
Chlorpromazine	? (Eyes)	Extrapyramidal dysfunction	
Imipramine	? Limb defects		
Lithium	?	Toxicity	
Diazepam		? Temperature	
Antithyroid			
Potassium iodide	Goiter		
Thiouracil	Goiter	↓ Thyroxine synthesis	?
I^{131}		Hypothyroidism	? Malignant changes

Avery GB. Neonatology, Pathophysiology and Management of the Newborn. Philadelphia: JB Lippincott)

    e. Change in vaginal discharge
    f. Rupture of membranes
2. Teach the woman the importance of avoiding stress and strenuous activity, and of getting adequate rest.
3. Assist the woman to plan a nutritious diet and understand its relationship to preterm labor.
4. Help the woman make life-style changes that are important in preventing preterm labor.
5. Teach the woman to recognize and be able to time uterine contractions.
6. Discuss with the woman the importance of limiting or stopping intercourse if uterine contractions occur following sexual activity.

C. **Reducing Anxiety About Delivering a Preterm Infant**

1. Discuss with the woman how changes in health practices (see previous section) have been found to prevent premature labor.
2. Discuss how these changes in health-care practices provide the woman with some control of eventual outcome of pregnancy.
3. Note that some instances of preterm labor occur despite the most careful health care practices; however, by having carried out the most favorable health-care practices the woman has done all she can to prevent preterm labor.
4. Provide support and encouragement for the woman at each prenatal visit.

Induction of Labor

Induction of labor is the deliberate initiation of uterine contractions prior to their spontaneous onset. Methods include:
1. *Amniotomy*—artificial rupture of the membranes; presenting part now puts greater pressure on cervix; contractions are stronger.
2. *Stripping the membranes*—separating the membranes

Table 27-6 Pharmacologic Agents Used for Preterm Labor

Agent	Dose and Method of Administration	Maternal Side Effects	Fetal Effects
Betamimetic Drugs			
Ritodrine hydrochloride (Yutopar)	Intravenously administered by calibrated infusion pump; initial dose 50–100 μg./minute, increased by 50 μg./minute every 10 minutes until contractions stop, unacceptable side effects develop, or the maximum dose of 350 μg./minute is reached	Increase in heart rate, decrease in blood pressure, widening pulse pressure, tremor, palpitations, nervousness, restlessness, ketoacidosis in patients with diabetes	Increase in heart rate, increase in blood pressure
	Oral therapy is started 30 minutes before the infusion is stopped with a dosage of 10 mg.; 10 mg. every 2 hours or 20 mg. every 2 hours for first 24 hours (maximum dose, 120 mg./day)		
Isoxsuprine hydrochloride (Vasodilan)	Initial intravenous infusion followed by oral or intramuscular doses; oral 10–20 mg. 3 or 4 times daily; intramuscular 5–10 mg. 2 or 3 times daily	Increase in heart rate, drop in diastolic blood pressure	Increase in heart rate, drop in diastolic blood pressure
Terbutaline sulfate (Bricanyl, Brethine)		Similar to those of isoxsuprine	Similar to those of isoxsuprine
Magnesium Sulfate	4 gm. as a loading dose intravenously, followed by a continuous infusion of 2 gm./hour in a 10% or 20% solution (not very effective)	Hypermagnesemia: flushing, sweating, extreme thirst, hypotension, sedation, confusion, depressed reflexes, muscle weakness	Hypermagnesemia
Ethanol	10% solution of ethanol in 5% aqueous dextrose is infused at the rate of 7.5 ml./hour for each kg. of body weight. After infusing this loading dose for 2 hour, the rate of infusion is reduced from 7.5 ml. to 1.5 ml./hour, which is then maintained for up to 12 hours	Nausea, vomiting, overt intoxication, hypoglycemia, lactic acidemia	Intoxication, metabolic derangements, respiratory distress if labor cannot be arrested

from the lower uterine segment without rupturing the membranes. Usually done during vaginal examination; membranes and amniotic fluid now act as a wedge to dilate cervix.

3. *Administration of oxytocin*—used to initiate and sustain uterine contractions; given IV; maternal and fetal vital signs and length, intensity, and frequency of contractions are monitored carefully.

Assessment

A. Indications

1. When the woman's life or well-being is in danger or if the fetus may be compromised by remaining in the uterus any longer
   a. Maternal hypertensive disease
   b. Diabetes of mother
   c. Premature rupture of membranes
   d. Maternal renal disease
   e. Fetal postmaturity
   f. Erythroblastosis
   g. Placental insufficiency
   h. History of rapid labors and living a long distance from birth center

B. Prerequisites for Successful Induction

1. The woman must be at or near term with a mature fetus
2. Cervix should be soft with moderate amount of effacement and dilation
3. No cephalopelvic disproportion
4. Fetal head fixed in inlet

Management and Nursing Interventions

A. Initiation of Labor

1. Rupture of membranes (amniotomy)
   a. Procedure is explained to the woman; fetal heart tones recorded (character and rate).
   b. Vulva is cleansed.
   c. Amniohook or Allis clamp is inserted through cervix to hook and rupture membranes.
   d. Note and record amount and quality of fluid (clear, color, bloody, meconium stained, etc.).
   e. Take and record fetal heart tones to assess how fetus tolerated procedure.
   f. Artificial rupture of the membranes is often done to augment labor already in progress. Since the membranes serve as a barrier against infection, delivery is usually accomplished soon after the membranes have been ruptured artificially.
2. Stripping of the membranes
   a. Often performed in conjunction with oxytocin administration to initiate labor.
   b. Performed by physician during sterile vaginal examination.
3. Oxytocin administration
   a. 10 IU of oxytocin added to 1 liter of 5% dextrose in water or to a balanced salt solution. This dilution provides 10 milliunits of oxytocin per each milliliter of solution.
   b. Initial dose using two-bottle system (one with oxytocin, one without medication) is 2 milliunits per minute via constant infusion pump.

c. Dose is increased every 15–20 minutes until dose is 20 milliunits per minute. Rarely necessary to exceed this dose; if satisfactory contractions have not been established with 30–40 milliunits per minute, it is unlikely that a greater dose will induce them.

d. Monitor the woman's blood pressure, pulse, respirations, contractions, and fetal heart tones every 15 minutes.

e. If fetal heart rate indicates distress or if contractions last 70 seconds or more, reduce or discontinue the IV oxytocin administration immediately. Increase IV solution without oxytocin, give the woman oxygen, turn her on her left side, and call the physician.

f. Satisfactory labor has usually been initiated when the woman has 3 contractions in 10 minutes, averaging 50 millimeters of mercury in intensity.

B. Reducing Anxiety

1. Explain proposed plan of labor initiation.
2. Explain all procedures as they are performed.
3. Keep the woman up to date on progress of labor.
4. If induction fails, have physician explain and discuss subsequent options.
5. Reassure the woman of fetal well-being.

Precipitate Labor

A *precipitate labor* is one that lasts less than 3 hours from the time of the first contraction to delivery of baby.

Assessment

A. Predisposing Factors

1. Multiparity
2. Large pelvis
3. Lax and unresistant soft tissue
4. Small baby in good position
5. Induction of labor by rupture of membranes and oxytocin infusion

B. Patient Problems/Nursing Diagnoses

1. Trauma to mother and fetus from strong, frequent uterine contractions
2. Maternal anxiety resulting from unexpected and unusual labor pattern

Management and Nursing Interventions

A. Prevention of Maternal and Fetal Trauma

1. Monitor fetal heart sounds every 15 minutes to detect distress resulting from fetal hypoxia (impaired intervillous blood flow due to strong and frequent contractions).
2. Anesthesia (e.g., pudendal block) is sometimes used to decrease strength of contractions or prevent involuntary pushing during delivery. Watch for signs of impending uterine rupture.
3. Following birth, evaluate infant carefully for signs of injury; inform nursery personnel of the tumultuous labor.
4. Examine the woman for cervical, vaginal, and perineal lacerations.

B. Reducing Anxiety

1. Explain precipitate labor and what is happening.
2. Assist the woman in retaining a sense of control over what is happening to her. Provide her with as many choices in her care as she desires or is able to handle.

3. Following the birth, have the woman hold her infant as soon as possible for reassurance that all is well. Provide time for the woman/couple (with their infant) to regain their composure and begin to incorporate recent labor events into reality.

Dystocia

Dystocia, or difficult labor, may be due to either mechanical or functional factors or to a combination of both.

Mechanical Dystocia

1. *Maternal causes*
   a. Contracted pelvis
   b. Obstructive tumors (ovarian or uterine fibromyoma
2. *Fetal causes*
   a. Failure of the vertex to rotate, as in occiput posterior or occiput transverse
   b. Malpresentations (shoulder, brow, face, or breech)
   c. Malformation of the fetus (as in hydrocephalus) or excessive size of the infant

Functional Dystocia (Uterine Dysfunction or Inertia)

Conditions in which uterine contractions deviate from the normal. Contractions may be extremely forceful with a rapid and traumatic labor and precipitate delivery. More commonly, the contractions are ineffectual.

A. Contributing Factors

1. Uterine anomalies
2. Overdistention such as hydramnios or multiple pregnancy
3. Chronic disease
4. Cervical scar tissue from previous surgery
5. Excessive analgesia or analgesia given too early in labor

Assessment

A. Mechanical Dystocia

1. Evaluate fetal presentation, position, and size.
2. Nonengagement of fetal head may indicate a contracted pelvis.
3. Note any known uterine or fetal anomalies.
4. X-ray pelvimetry is used for evaluation of cephalopelvic disproportion.
5. Monitor maternal vital signs, contraction pattern, and fetal heart rate every 15 minutes if the woman is to undergo a trial labor (6-hour labor to evaluate progress).

B. Functional Dystocia

1. Contractions may differ in quality and synchronization of activity. Contractions may be strong but localized to one portion of the uterus or may begin in lower segment and move upward rather than downward. The resultant decreased pressure on the cervix causes it to remain closed.
2. Contractions may also have inadequate intensity (hypotonic).
3. Evaluate contraction quality and pattern by manual evaluation of fingers on fundus and lower portion of uterine body; also evaluate via electronic monitoring (see p. 986).
4. Prolonged labor may be evident within 6–8 hours if labor has been plotted on a graph with normal labor curve for comparison.

5. Monitor and evaluate progress of cervical dilation and descent and rotation in birth canal.

Management and Nursing Interventions

A. Mechanical Dystocia

1. If occiput posterior position:
   a. Relieve back pain as much as possible by sacral pressure, back rubs, frequent change of position from side to side (may also assist fetal head to rotate).
   b. Observe the character and frequency of contractions and monitor fetal heart rate.
   c. IV fluids are used to prevent dehydration and provide glucose needed for effective contractions.
   d. When cervix is completely dilated, fetal head may be rotated by physician.
   e. Provide encouragement and reassurance to the woman throughout the labor.
2. If breech presentation:
   a. Labor may be longer, since in a breech delivery, the soft buttocks do not aid in cervical dilation as well as the head does in a vertex presentation.
   b. Analgesia may be limited in order not to interfere with the mother's ability to push effectively.
   c. Amniotomy is not done until breech is well engaged because there is greater danger of prolapse of the cord with footling presentation or breech that does not fill the pelvic cavity.
   d. Breech presentations may be delivered spontaneously with strong contractions, particularly in multiparae.
   e. More aid is indicated (application of Piper forceps to the aftercoming head) for the majority of women, especially primigravidas.
   f. Cesarean delivery is a better approach than difficult extraction.
3. Cesarean birth is performed when there is a shoulder presentation, when the size of the fetus is excessive for the maternal pelvis, or when there is a persistent occipital posterior presentation in which forcep rotation may be difficult.

B. Functional Dystocia

1. Hypertonic uterine dysfunction—muscle of the uterus is in a state of greater than normal tension, so that contractions are ineffective for accomplishing dilation. Contractions may be uncoordinated and involve only portions of the uterus.
   a. Provide rest with aid of sedatives (morphine, 16 mg., on prescription, usually stops contractions).
   b. Provide fluids to maintain hydration and electrolyte balance.
   c. Observe for normal contractions when woman awakens.
2. Hypotonic uterine dysfunction—contractions are inadequate (lack intensity); usually occurs in active phase of labor.
   a. Pelvis is reevaluated for size.
   b. IV fluids are provided to maintain hydration and electrolyte balance.
   c. Oxytocin administration is begun if pelvic size is adequate and fetal position, presentation, and station are normal.
      (1) Monitor fetal heart rate and contractions for character and frequency. If contractions last more than 60–70 seconds, decrease or stop infusion. (Tetanic contractions may cause premature separation of the placenta, rupture of the uterus, and fetal hypoxia.)
      (2) Observe IV drip; be certain infusion is running at prescribed rates.
      (3) Report any maternal or fetal distress immediately.
   d. Amniotomy may be performed to augment labor (see p. 1028).

C. Anxiety-Reducing Measures

1. Keep the woman/couple informed of the progress of labor and any changes in plan of care.
2. Promote rest and comfort.
   a. Keep room lights low and noise to a minimum, and limit the number of visits by nonessential personnel.
   b. Give frequent back rubs and massage sacral area.
   c. Assist the woman's labor coach if needed or coach the woman in breathing and relaxation techniques during contractions.
   d. Administer sedatives or analgesics as needed and prescribed.
   e. Encourage the woman's partner to take a break; provide assurance that you will be with her during his absence.
   f. Encourage the woman to sleep or rest with eyes closed between contractions.
   g. If the woman loses control, give her brief directions regarding assuming a comfortable position, breathing with you during contractions, resting between contractions, etc.; woman who has lost her own control during labor may panic and respond poorly to being given a choice of turning on her side, having back rubbed, etc.
3. Periodically tell the woman how well she is coping and how labor is progressing.
4. Following delivery, observe the woman and infant for physical injury resulting from prolonged labor; observe maternal–infant interaction for signs of difficulty resulting from prolonged labor.

Uterine Rupture

Uterine rupture is a spontaneous or traumatic rupture of the uterus.

Assessment

A. Causes

1. Rupture of the scar from a previous cesarean delivery or hysterotomy
2. Prolonged or obstructed labor
3. Forced delivery of fetus with abnormalities (e.g., hydrocephalus)
4. Ill-advised podalic version
5. Application of forceps and extraction before cervical os has completely dilated
6. Injudicious use of oxytocin
7. Excessive manual pressure applied to the fundus during delivery

B. Clinical Manifestations

1. Complete rupture
   a. Sudden sharp abdominal pain during contractions
   b. Abdominal tenderness

c. Cessation of contractions
d. Bleeding into the abdominal cavity and sometimes into the vagina
e. Fetus easily palpated; fetal heart tones cease
f. Signs of shock—rapid, weak pulse; cold, clammy skin; pale color; flaring of nostrils due to air hunger
2. Incomplete rupture—develops over a period of a few hours
a. Abdominal pain during contractions
b. Contractions continue, but cervix fails to dilate
c. Vaginal bleeding may be present
d. Rising pulse rate and skin pallor
e. Loss of fetal heart tones

Management and Nursing Interventions

A. Maintaining Maternal Fluid Balance and Fetal Gas Exchange

1. Administer IV fluids and blood as directed.
2. Administer oxygen to the woman.
3. Prepare the woman for emergency surgery.
4. Monitor maternal and fetal vital signs until surgery begins
5. Uterus may be repaired if rupture is not extensive; if extensive, hysterectomy is necessary.

B. Reducing Fear

1. While working swiftly and effectively, keep the woman informed about procedures being done; answer her questions as positively and as realistically as possible.
2. Fetal prognosis is very poor unless delivery can be accomplished immediately.
3. Maternal prognosis is guarded, especially in uterine rupture of traumatic origin (5%–10% mortality rate).

Amniotic Fluid Embolism

Amniotic fluid embolism is the escape of amniotic fluid containing debris such as meconium, lanugo, and vernix caseosa into the maternal circulation, usually resulting in deposition of fluid or debris in the pulmonary arterioles; may also cause disseminated intravascular coagulation (DIC). Amniotic fluid embolism is rare and usually fatal.

Assessment

A. Predisposing Conditions—myometrial vessels are exposed, usually at placental site, and contractions are especially forceful.

1. Marginal placental separation
2. Uterine rupture
3. Hysterectomy

B. Clinical Manifestations

1. Sudden dyspnea and chest pain
2. Cyanosis
3. Tachycardia
4. Pulmonary edema
5. Profound shock due to:
a. Anaphylaxis, which causes vascular collapse
b. Uterine bleeding with development of hypofibrinogenemia

Management and Nursing Interventions

A. Improving Tissue Perfusion and Cardiopulmonary Function

1. Administer oxygen as soon as situation is recognized.
2. Provide assisted ventilation.

B. Maintaining Fluid Volume and Correction of DIC

1. Administer fresh whole blood and fibrinogen.
2. Administer IV fluids and plasma.
3. Provide continuous monitoring of maternal and fetal signs.

C. Delivery of Fetus

1. Since fetus is in great danger, delivery is performed as soon as possible.
2. If cervix is dilated, forcep delivery is used to deliver fetus.

Prolapsed Umbilical Cord

Prolapsed umbilical cord—prolapses in front of or alongside the fetal presenting part.

Assessment

A. Causes

1. Rupture of membranes, when the presenting part is not engaged in the pelvis
2. More common in shoulder and foot presentations
3. Prematurity—small fetus allows more space around presenting part
4. Hydramnios—causes greater amount of fluid to be released with greater force when membranes rupture
5. Contracted pelvis
6. Placenta previa

B. Clinical Manifestations

1. Cord may be seen protruding from vagina.
2. Cord can be palpated in the vaginal canal or cervix.
3. Fetal distress may occur as the cord is compressed between the presenting part and the bony pelvis.
4. If cord is exposed to cold room air, there may be reflex constriction of umbilical blood vessels restricting oxygen flow to the fetus.
5. Fetal heart rate pattern may be irregular with periodic fetal bradycardia.

Management and Nursing Interventions

A. Maintaining Oxygen Supply to Fetus

1. Place the woman in deep Trendelenburg position.
2. Administer oxygen (5 liters) by mask.
3. Place sterile gloved hand in vagina and push the infant's head upward to relieve compression of the cord.
4. Prepare for immediate vaginal delivery if cervix is dilated.
5. Prepare for immediate cesarean delivery if cervix is incompletely dilated.
6. In home situation, cover protruding cord with clean, wet dressings, elevate the woman's hips and transport to hospital immediately.

B. Reducing Anxiety

1. Have the woman/couple hear fetal heart tones for reassurance.
2. Explain sequence of procedures and keep the woman informed of procedures being performed.
3. When infant is born and stabilized, have the woman/couple hold infant as soon as possible for reassurance.

Inverted Uterus

Inverted uterus—the uterus is inverted, or turned inside out, usually during the delivery of the placenta.

Assessment

A. Causes

1. Excessive traction on the cord when the placenta is firmly attached to the uterine wall
2. Markedly lax or thin uterine walls
3. Fundal pressure when the uterus is relaxed
4. May occur spontaneously

B. Clinical Manifestations

1. Shock with faintness, severe uterine pain, and hemorrhage

2. Mild symptoms observed with incomplete version in the later postpartum period

Management and Nursing Interventions

A. Replacement of Uterus

1. Uterus is replaced manually while the woman is under anesthesia.
2. IV oxytocin administration helps keep uterus well contracted and in position.
3. Indwelling urinary catheter helps keep uterus contracted and helps in calculating urinary output and renal status.

B. Maintaining Fluid Volume

1. Administer IV fluids and blood, depending on amount of blood lost.
2. Monitor intake and output carefully.

Operative Obstetrics

Operative obstetrics refers to a number of procedures (episiotomy, forceps delivery, cesarean delivery) that may be used to assist the mother in labor and delivery.

Episiotomy

An *episiotomy* is an incision of the perineum during delivery to:
1. Substitute a straight surgical incision for the laceration that may otherwise occur.
2. Facilitate repair of laceration and to promote healing.
3. Spare the infant's head from prolonged pressure and pushing against the rigid perineum, which may result in brain damage, especially in the premature infant
4. Shorten the 2nd stage of labor

Types of Episiotomies

1. Median
   a. Incision is made in the middle of the perineum and directed toward the rectum (Fig. 27-4).
   b. This method is believed to heal with few com-

plications, is more comfortable for the woman during healing, and is easy to repair.
   c. If a larger incision is needed during delivery, however, it may necessitate incision into anal sphincter.
2. Mediolateral
   a. Incision is made laterally in the perineum.
   b. This method avoids the anal sphincter if enlargement is needed.
   c. Women find it very uncomfortable during healing.

Management and Nursing Interventions

A. Patient Teaching

1. Explain reasons for episiotomy.
2. Discuss methods to reduce discomfort and promote healing.
3. Explain that with good hygienic measures, healing should be complete in several weeks.
4. Inspect area daily for signs of infection.

B. Reduction of Pain and Discomfort

1. Apply ice pack after procedure to reduce edema and promote comfort.
2. Encourage sitz baths to promote healing and comfort.
3. Use local analgesic sprays to promote comfort.

Forceps Delivery

The obstetric *forceps* consists of 2 pieces: a right blade, which is slipped into the right side of the mother's pelvis, and a left blade, which is slipped into the left side (Table 27-7). Forceps are designed for rotating or extracting the fetal head.

Conditions Requiring Forceps Delivery

A. Fetal Conditions

1. Fetal distress
2. Cord prolapse
3. Excess pressure on the fetal head from arrested descent
4. Abruptio placentae

B. Maternal Conditions

1. Eclampsia
2. Heart disease

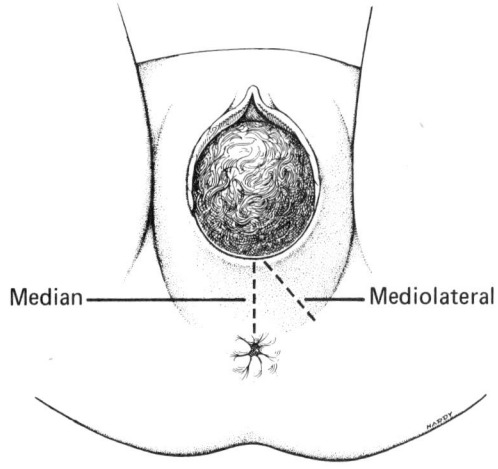

Median   Mediolateral

Figure 27-4. Types of episiotomies.

3. Maternal hemorrhage
4. Maternal exhaustion
5. Intrapartum infection
6. Failure of progress in the 2nd stage because of poor uterine contractions, rigid perineum

C. Prerequisites for Application of Forceps

1. Pelvis should be adequate, with no disproportion
2. Fetal head must be engaged—preferably deeply engaged
3. Cervix must be completely dilated
4. Accurate diagnosis of position and station must be made (see p. 975)
5. Membranes must be ruptured
6. Some form of anesthesia should be used
7. Rectum and bladder should be empty

Types of forceps deliveries

1. Low forceps operation
   Forceps are applied after the head has reached the perineal floor with the sagittal suture in the antero-posterior diameter of the outlet.
2. Midforceps delivery
   a. Forceps are applied before the criteria for low forceps are met but after engagement has taken place.
   b. Any forceps delivery requiring rotation, regardless of the station, is considered a midforcep delivery.
3. High forceps operation
   Forceps are applied before engagement has taken place (has been replaced by cesarean delivery).

Management and Nursing Interventions

A. Reducing Anxiety

1. Explain need for forceps delivery.
2. Keep the woman informed of procedure's progress.
3. Focus on positive outcome of the birth.

B. Reducing Potential for Trauma and Subsequent Complications

1. Assist the woman to relax between contractions, using abdominal muscles to push with a contraction when needed and to avoid pushing when not needed.
2. Have the woman empty her bladder.
3. Monitor the woman for signs and symptoms of complications following forceps delivery:
   a. Lacerations of vagina and cervix—excessive vaginal bleeding, decrease in blood pressure and increased pulse
   b. Rupture of uterus—signs and symptoms of massive hemorrhage
   c. Injury to bladder or rectum
4. Examine the infant for complications following forceps delivery:
   a. Facial paralysis
   b. Injury to eyes or skull
   c. Abrasions and bruises of the face

Vacuum Extraction

A *vacuum extractor* applies suction to the fetal head creating an artificial caput within the suction cup, thus allowing adequate traction for delivery of the infant's head.

Uses

1. Dysfunctional labor
2. Fetal distress

Table 27-7 Representative Types of Forceps*

Major Classifications	Use
1. Simpson—separated shanks (DeLee forcep is one example)	Extract fetus with elongated, molded head; commonly used with nulliparas who have long labors
2. Elliot—overlapping shanks (Tucker–McLean is one example)	Extract fetus with unmolded, rounder heads; commonly used with multiparas who have briefer labors
3. Specialized types	
a. Piper	Deliver aftercoming head in a breech presentation
b. Kielland	Rotate head from transverse or posterior position to an anterior position; used to deliver women with anthropoid pelves
c. Barton	Rotate head from transverse to an anterior position; designed for use in women with flat pelves

* There are more than 600 types of forceps.

3. Maternal cardiopulmonary disease
4. Hypertensive disorders of pregnancy
5. Abruptio placentae
6. Instances in which the thickness of forceps between the birth canal and presenting fetal head is to be avoided

Nursing Interventions

A. Explain procedure to the woman and why it is needed.

1. Help the woman relax during application of suction to fetal scalp.
2. Coach the mother to push with contraction when needed (time when traction is used with vacuum extractor to aid descent and delivery of fetal head).

B. Following delivery

1. Examine the infant for scalp lacerations, cephalhematoma, or intracranial hemorrhage.
2. Examine the woman for cervical or vaginal lacerations.
3. Explain to the woman that fetal caput will regress in a few days.

Cesarean Delivery

Cesarean delivery is removal of the infant from the uterus through an incision made in the abdominal wall and in the uterus. This type of delivery is used in the following situations:

1. Cephalopelvic disproportion
2. Uterine dysfunction, inertia, inability of cervix to dilate
3. Neoplasm obstructing birth canal or pelvis
4. Malposition and malpresentation
5. Previous uterine surgery (cesarean delivery, myomectomy, hysterotomy) or cervical surgery
6. Complete or partial placenta previa
7. Premature separation of the placenta
8. Prolapse of the umbilical cord
9. Fetal distress

Types of Cesarean Delivery

A. Low Segment (operation of choice)
Incision made transversely in lower segment of uterus

1. Incision is made in thinnest portion so that blood loss is minimal and uterus is easier to open.

2. Lower segment is area of least uterine activity.
3. Postoperative convalescence is more comfortable.
4. Possibility of later rupture is lessened.
5. Peritoneal flap is brought over uterine incision, preventing lochia from entering peritoneal cavity.
6. Incidence of postoperative adhesions and danger of intestinal obstruction are reduced.

B. Classic
Vertical incision is made directly into the wall of the body of the uterus.

1. Useful when bladder and lower segment are involved in extensive adhesions
2. Selected when anterior placenta previa exists
3. Useful when fetus is in a transverse lie

C. Extraperitoneal
The tissue around the bladder is dissected, providing access to lower uterine segment without entering into the peritoneal cavity.

1. Devised to prevent peritonitis
2. Availability of blood and antibiotics has reduced use of this method

D. Cesarean Delivery and Hysterectomy
(Porro's operation)
Cesarean delivery followed by removal of the uterus.
Indications:

1. Hemorrhage due to uterine atony, after conservative therapy fails
2. Uncontrollable hemorrhage from placenta previa and abruptio placentae
3. *Placenta accreta* (abnormal attachment of placenta to uterine endometrium)
4. Rupture of the uterus, not repairable
5. Gross multiple fibromyomas

Nursing Interventions

A. Promoting coping abilities

1. Have the woman discuss her perception of why the cesarean delivery is needed; correct misinformation, provide further information.
2. Have the woman/couple listen to fetal heart sounds to reassure them of the well-being of the fetus.
3. Research indicates that women react more positively to cesarean birth when they feel they have some control of and choice in aspects of the delivery.
4. Encourage woman/couple to view cesarean delivery as an alternate delivery method in which many of the woman's/couple's original expectations about delivery can be fulfilled

B. Reducing anxiety

1. Explain preoperative procedures as they are performed:
   a. Shave abdomen and perineum.
   b. Insert a retention urinary catheter.
   c. Monitor fetal heart tones.
   d. Monitor uterine contractions, if any.
   e. Examine results of routine laboratory studies: Hb, Hct, WBC, differential, urinalysis, type and cross match.
   f. Administer prescribed preoperative atropine; narcotics are avoided in order not to depress the fetus.
   g. Initiate IV infusion.
   h. Notify pediatrician and nursery staff; pediatrician may be present for the birth if a depressed infant is expected.
2. Explain postoperative care and procedures.
   a. Provide postoperative care similar to that following abdominal surgery.
   b. Observe for hemorrhage.
      (1) Inspect perineal pads and abdominal dressings.
      (2) Assess vital signs frequently.
   c. Administer oxytocics as prescribed.
   d. Check fundus for firmness.
   e. Continue IV fluids as prescribed.
   f. Check urinary output from indwelling catheter for amount and for evidence of bleeding.
   g. Provide medication for relief of pain.
   h. Encourage the woman to turn from side to side, to breathe deeply, and to cough.
   i. Assist the woman out of bed on 1st postoperative day.
   j. As soon as possible, have the woman hold and care for infant to reassure her of infant's well-being.

Postpartum Complications

Puerperal Infection

Puerperal infection is a postpartum infection of the genital tract, usually of the endometrium, that may remain localized or may extend to various parts of the body.

Causes
Bacterial organisms either are introduced from external sources or are normally present in the generative tract and are carried to the uterus.

Predisposing Factors

1. Prolonged labor
2. Postpartum hemorrhage
3. Premature rupture of membranes
4. Infections elsewhere in the body
5. Intrauterine manipulation
6. Anemia
7. Retention of placental fragments
8. Malnutrition

Clinical Manifestations
Diagnosis is made by sustained fever of 38°C. (100.4°F.) or higher occurring on any 2 of the first 10 days postpartum, excluding the first 24 hours. Symptoms depend on site and extension of infection.

A. Endometritis—postpartum infection involving the endometrium

1. Uterus usually larger than expected for postdelivery day.
2. Lochia may be profuse, bloody, and foul smelling.
3. Woman may have chills and fever if lochial discharge is obstructed by clots.

4. Infection may spread to myometrium, parametrium, uterine (fallopian) tubes, peritoneum, and blood.

B. **Parametritis** (pelvic cellulitis)—infection of the pelvic connective tissue

1. Chills, fever, tachycardia, severe unilateral or bilateral pain in lower abdomen, and tenderness on vaginal examination usually occur about the 4th postpartum day.
2. May result from infected wound in the cervix, vagina, perineum, or lower uterine segment.
3. Uterus may be larger than expected for postdelivery day and sensitive to touch.
4. Uterus may become fixed, the pelvic area warm, with one extremely sensitive spot due to an abscess underneath.
5. Incision and drainage is performed if an abscess forms.

C. **Thrombophlebitis** (inflammation of a venous wall with clot formation)—puerperal infection commonly spreads along the veins resulting in thrombophlebitis involving several sites

1. *Pelvic thrombophlebitis*—infection of veins supplying uterine wall and broad ligament
   a. Symptoms usually begin during 2nd week following delivery.
   b. The woman may have severe chills and intermittent high fever 40.6°C. (105°F.).
   c. Blood cultures are taken to isolate the organism.
2. *Femoral thrombophlebitis*—infection of the leg veins
   a. Pain, tenderness, and turgidity of the calf
   b. Redness, increased skin temperature, edema of the calf or thigh
   c. Positive Homan's sign

D. **Bacteremia** (presence of bacteria in the bloodstream)—result of infected thrombi breaking loose

1. Severe chill, fever, and rapid respirations
2. Pale skin; lips and fingers may become cyanotic
3. Lochial discharge may increase and have a foul odor

E. **Peritonitis** (inflammation of the peritoneum)

1. Clinical picture resembles surgical peritonitis; however, abdominal rigidity is minimal or absent.
2. Chills, high fever, rapid pulse, vomiting, severe abdominal pain

Diagnostic Evaluation

1. Clinical history and findings from physical examination
2. Culture and sensitivity tests of blood, lochia, or cervical discharge
3. Lung scan, chest roentgenogram, arterial blood gases, central venous pressure, and pulmonary angiography

Management and Nursing Interventions

1. Determine source of woman's anxiety and fear regarding complication and its implications.
2. Explain prescribed treatment regimen.
3. Correct misinformation regarding complication.
4. Monitor the woman's condition and implement plan of care.
   a. Continue monitoring (q 2–4 hours) temperature, pulse, and respiration.
   b. Isolate the woman with infection from other postpartal women.
   c. Maintain fluids and electrolytes.
   d. Blood may be necessary to combat severe anemia.

e. Antibiotic therapy.
f. Monitor site of infection—pain, rigidity, edema, redness, elevated skin temperature, and amount of lochial or wound drainage to evaluate progress of infection.
g. Provide diet with increased calories, protein, and vitamin C to promote healing.

5. Institute comfort measures.
   a. Good skin care
   b. Soothing sponge baths
   c. Frequent change of perineal pads
   d. Analgesics for pain
6. Determine needed resources if hospitalization will be prolonged.
7. Assist the woman/family in planning for child care or other contingencies required by prolonged hospitalization.

Postpartum Hemorrhage

Postpartum hemorrhage involves a loss of 500 ml. or more of blood; it occurs most frequently in the 1st hour following delivery.

Assessment

A. **Causes**

1. Uterine atony—relaxation of the uterus secondary to:
   a. Multiple pregnancy—causes overdistention of uterus and a larger placental site
   b. Polyhydramnios (excessive amniotic fluid)
   c. High parity
   d. Prolonged labor with maternal exhaustion
   e. Deep anesthesia
   f. Fibromyomata—prevents uterus from contracting
   g. Retained placental fragments
2. Retained placental fragments—results from:
   a. Manual removal of placenta
   b. Succenturiate (additional) lobe
   c. Abnormal adherent placenta (placenta acreta)
3. Laceration of the vagina, cervix or perineum secondary to:
   a. Forceps delivery, especially rotation forceps
   b. Large infant
   c. Multiple pregnancy

B. **Clinical Manifestations**

1. Uterine atony—uterus is soft or boggy, often difficult to palpate, and will not remain contracted; excessive vaginal bleeding.
2. Retained placental fragments—hemorrhage usually occurs about the 10th postpartum day.
3. Lacerations of the vagina, cervix, or perineum—bleeding is bright red; fundus is firm.
4. Marked fluctuations in blood pressure and pulse will not usually occur until a large amount of blood has been lost.
5. Excessive blood loss—pallor, restlessness, dyspnea, thready pulse, lowered blood pressure, chills, and air hunger.

Management and Nursing Interventions

1. Monitor changes in physiologic status.
   a. Monitor vital signs frequently.
   b. Describe number and saturation of perineal pads used per hour.
   c. Describe character and amount of vaginal bleeding.
   d. Evaluate uterine firmness, height, and position.

2. Restore fluid/blood volume.
   a. Administer IV fluids as prescribed to restore fluid volume.
   b. Administer blood as prescribed.
3. When cause has been determined, prepare the woman for further treatment.
   a. Lacerations—prepare for return to delivery room for inspection and repair.
   b. Retained placental fragments—prepare for curettage of uterus.
   c. Uterine atony—administer oxytocins as prescribed (usually ergonovine for sustained uterine contractions).
4. Help reduce anxiety.
   a. Determine major source of the woman's anxiety.
   b. Explain current status and prescribed treatment regimen.
   c. Correct misinformation regarding status or potential complications.
   d. Keep the woman/family informed of changes in physiologic status or treatment plan with emphasis on improvements in condition.

Mastitis

Mastitis is inflammation of breast tissue. It may involve:
1. Formation of a subareolar abscess in the underlying milk glands
2. The lacteriferous tubules (parenchymatous of glandular mastitis)
3. Connective tissue and fat around the lobes and lobules (intramammary mastitis)

Assessment

A. Cause

Usually due to *Staphylococcus aureus* derived from the nursing infant's nose and throat.

B. Clinical Manifestations

1. Symptoms may occur at the end of the 1st postpartum week but usually appear in 3rd to 4th week postpartum.
2. Marked breast engorgement
3. Chills
4. Elevated temperature (usually not above 39.4°C. [103°F.])
5. Increased pulse rate
6. Hardness and reddening of breasts
7. Pain in breasts

Nursing Interventions

1. Implement plan of care.
   a. Use comfort measures—breast support, tight binder or brassiere; analgesics for pain.
   b. Applications of heat to affected breast if suppuration is present.
   c. Antibiotics as prescribed.
   d. If breast milk is contaminated, breast-feeding on affected side may be discontinued; empty breast on affected side with breast pump and discard milk until infection is controlled.
   e. If abscess forms, incision and drainage may be necessary.
2. Describe complication and prescribed treatment regimen.
3. Correct misinformation regarding complication
4. Keep the woman/family informed of changes in physiologic status and treatment plan.

Postpartum Hematomas

Postpartum hematomas are localized collections of blood in loose connective tissue beneath the skin that covers the external genitalia, beneath the vaginal mucosa, or in the broad ligaments

Assessment

A. Causes

1. Trauma during spontaneous labor.
2. Trauma during forceps application or delivery.
3. Inadequate suturing of an episiotomy.

B. Clinical Manifestations

1. Vulvar hematoma—development of a sensitive swelling covered by discolored skin; pain.
2. Vaginal hematoma—feeling of vaginal pressure, inability to void; purple mass may be seen at introitus.

Nursing Interventions

1. Explain and implement plan of care.
   a. Application of ice may minimize hematoma initially, depending on amount and site of bleeding.
   b. Warm compresses may be applied to hematomas after 24 hours to promote comfort and healing.
   c. Incision, drainage, and ligation of bleeding point may be necessary.
   d. Comfort measures—cold or warm compresses, comfortable positioning, analgesics for pain.
2. Describe complication and prescribed treatment regimen.
3. Correct misinformation regarding complication.
4. Keep the woman/family informed of changes in physiologic status and treatment plan.

Subinvolution

Subinvolution is the slowing or halting of normal postpartum return of reproductive organs to their prepregnancy state

Assessment

A. Causes

1. Pelvic infection
2. Retention of placental fragments
3. Fibroid tumors
4. Any other factor that interferes with myometrial contractions

B. Clinical Manifestations

1. Uterus larger or softer than expected for postpartum date
2. Prolonged lochial discharge (after 1 month or more)
3. Irregular uterine bleeding
4. Backache or sensation of weight in pelvis

Nursing Interventions

1. Explain and implement plan of care.
   a. Administration of ergonovine maleate or methylergonovine maleate as prescribed to increase uterine contractility
   b. Prepare the woman for uterine curettage if placental fragments have been retained.
   c. Administer prescribed antibiotics for infection.
   d. Instruct the woman to report signs of infection, vaginal bleeding, or any tissue passed vaginally.
2. Describe complication and usual treatment regimen.
3. Correct misinformation the woman may have regarding complication.

Postpartum Urinary Tract Infection

Assessment

A. Causes

1. Bladder trauma during delivery
2. Urinary retention due to anesthesia, excessive intravenous fluids causing overdistention of the bladder
3. Frequent catheterization

B. Clinical Manifestations

1. Elevated temperature 37.8°C. (100°–101°F.)
2. Urinary frequency
3. Pain on urination
4. Flank pain
5. Chills

Nursing Interventions

1. Explain and implement plan of care.
   a. Monitor the woman's vital signs, degree, and site of pain.
   b. Instruct the woman to increase fluid intake
   c. Instruct woman to empty her bladder completely each time she urinates.
   d. Administer antibiotics and urinary tract antispasmodics as prescribed.
   e. Administer analgesics as needed.
   f. Encourage the woman to rest.
2. Describe complication and general treatment regimen.
3. Correct misinformation regarding complication.

Postpartum Psychosis

Psychosis occurring within 4–6 weeks after delivery.

Assessment

A. Causes—unknown, although approximately 33% of women probably had a mental illness prior to pregnancy; stresses of pregnancy, delivery, and new responsibilities of parenthood.

B. Clinical Manifestations

1. Clouding of consciousness
2. Depression, withdrawal
3. Hostility
4. Fear and suspiciousness
5. Feelings of inadequacy
6. Hallucinations

Nursing Interventions

A. Reducing anxiety and hostility

1. Have the woman state her perception of her current situation and reasons for her anxiety and hostility.
2. Have the woman describe how she might cope with current situation.
3. Explore potential resources the woman/family might use to reduce stresses.
4. Administer psychotropic drugs as prescribed.
5. Make referrals to appropriate health team members and/or agencies to increase resources available to the woman/family.

B. Patient Teaching

1. Teach the woman/family parenting skills—feeding, bathing, soothing of infant, dressing, normal characteristics, and activities of newborns when appropriate and possible.
2. Have the woman/family member return demonstration of parenting skills when able.

Bibliography

Books
Complications of Pregnancy

Borg S and Lasker J. When Pregnancy Fails. Boston, Beacon Press, 1981

Burrow GN and Ferris GF. Medical Complications During Pregnancy, 2nd ed. Philadelphia, WB Saunders, 1982

Danforth D (ed). Obstetrics and Gynecology, 4th ed. Philadelphia, Harper & Row, 1982

Gant NF and Worley RJ. Hypertension in Pregnancy: Concepts and Management. New York, Appleton-Century-Crofts, 1980

Guthrie DW and Guthrie RA. Nursing Management of Diabetes Mellitus, 2nd ed. St Louis, CV Mosby, 1982

Iffy L and Kaminetzky HA (eds). Principles and Practice of Obstetrics and Perinatology. New York, John Wiley & Sons, 1981

Pritchard JA, MacDonald PC and Gant NF. Williams Obstetrics, 17th ed. New York, Appleton-Century-Crofts, 1985

Complications of Labor and Delivery

Affonso DD. Impact of Cesarean Childbirth. Philadelphia, FA Davis, 1981

Babson S et al. Diagnosis and Management of the Fetus and Neonate at Risk. St Louis, CV Mosby, 1980

Burrow G and Ferris T. Medical Complications During Pregnancy. Philadelphia, WB Saunders, 1982

Carter FB and Wolber PG. Episiotomy. In Sciarra JJ (ed). Gynecology and Obstetrics, Vol. 2, Chap. 67. Hagerstown, Harper & Row, 1980

Danforth DN and Dignam WJ. Obstetrics and Gynecology, 4th ed. Philadelphia, Harper & Row, 1982

Johnson G. Oxytocics for the Induction of Labor. White Plains, NY, The March of Dimes Birth Defects Foundation, 1981

Miller M and Brooten D. The Childbearing Family: A Nursing Perspective. Boston, Little, Brown & Co, 1983

National Institute of Child Health and Human Development. Cesarean Childbirth. Bethesda, National Institutes of Health, 1982. NIH Publication No. 82-2067-G

Pritchard JA, MacDonald PC and Gant NF. Williams Obstetrics, 17th ed. New York, Appleton-Century-Crofts, 1985

Reeder S, Mastroianni L and Martin L.

Maternity Nursing. Philadelphia, JB Lippincott, 1983

Quilligan E and Kretchmer N. Fetal and Maternal Medicine. New York, John Wiley & Sons, 1980

Complications of the Postpartum

Aladjem S. Obstetric Practice. St Louis, CV Mosby, 1980

Bash D and Gold W. The Nurse and the Childbearing Family. New York, John Wiley & Son, 1981

Clark AL. Culture and Childrearing. Philadelphia, FA Davis, 1981

Danforth DN (ed). Obstetrics and Gynecology, 4th ed. Philadelphia, Harper & Row, 1982

Jensen M, Benson R and Bobak I. Maternity Care, 2nd ed. St Louis, CV Mosby, 1981

Jensen MD and Bobak IM. Maternity and Gynecologic Care: The Nurse and Family, 3rd ed. St. Louis, CV Mosby, 1985

Klaus MH and Kennell JH. Parent–Infant Bonding, 2nd ed. St Louis, CV Mosby, 1982

Miller M and Brooten D. The Childbearing Family: A Nursing

Perspective. Boston, Little, Brown & Co, 1983

Niswander K. Obstetrics. Boston, Little, Brown & Co, 1981

Olds S et al. Maternity–Newborn Nursing. Menlo Park, CA, Addison-Wesley, 1984

Pritchard J, MacDonald P and Gant NF. Williams Obstetrics, 17th ed. New York, Appleton-Century-Crofts, 1985

Reeder S, Mastroianni L and Martin L. Maternity Nursing. Philadelphia, JB Lippincott, 1983

Quilligan E and Kretchmer N. Fetal and Maternal Medicine. New York, John Wiley & Son, 1980

Articles

Complications of Pregnancy

Affonso DD and Harris TR. Postterm pregnancy: Implications for mother and infant, challenge for the nurse. JOGN Nurs 1980 May–Jun; 9(3):139–145

Auman G. Ritodrine Hydrochloride in the control of premature labor. Implications for use. JOGN Nurs 1982 Mar–Apr; 11(2):75–79

Bartlet D and Davis A. Recognizing fetal alcohol syndrome in the nursery. JOGN Nurs 1980 Jul–Aug; 9(4):223–225

Bills BJ. Nursing considerations: Administering labor-suppressing medications. MCN 1980 Jul/Aug; 5(4):252–256

Boehm FH et al. Management of genital herpes simplex virus infection occurring during pregnancy. Am J Obstet Gynecol 1981 Dec 1; 141(7):735–740

Brengman S. Ritodrine hydrochloride and preterm labor. Am J Nurs 1983 Apr; 83(3):537–539

Burns E. Diabetes Mellitus and Pregnancy. Nurs Clin North Am 1983 Dec; 18(4):673–685

Cahrache S et al. Management of sickle cell disease in pregnant patients. Obstet Gynecol 1980 Apr; 55(4):407–410

Caritis SN et al. Pharmacodynamics of ritodrine in pregnant women during preterm labor. Am J Obstet Gynecol 1983 Dec; 147(7):752–759

Caritis SN. Treatment of preterm labour. A review of therapeutic options. Drugs 1983 Sep; 26(3):243–261

Carr B. The endocrinology of pregnancy-induced hypertension. Clinics in Perinatology. 1983 Oct; 10(3):737–761

Castle B. The presence or absence of fetal breathing movements predicts the outcome of preterm labor. Lancet 1983 Aug 27; 2(8348):471–473

Chesley L. The control of hypertension in pregnancy. Obstet Gynecol Ann 1981; 10:69–106

Coustan D. The pregnant patient with overt diabetes: Practical guide to management. Perinatol Neonatol 1982 Jan/Feb; 29–34

Cunningham F. Pregnancy and sickle cell hemoglobinopathies: Results with and without prophylactic transfusions.

Obstet Gynecol 1983 Oct; 62(4):419–424

Dignan P. Teratogenic risk and counseling in diabetes. Clin Obstet Gynecol 1981 Mar; 24(1):149–159

Elliot J. Magnesium sulfate as a tocolytic agent. Am J Obstet Gynecol 1983 Oct 1; 147(3):277–284

Fawcett J and Burritt J. An exploratory study of antenatal preparation for cesarean birth. JOGN Nurs 1985 May–Jun; 14(3):224–230

Floyd CC. Pregnancy after reproductive failure. Am J Nurs 1981 Nov; 81(11):2050–2053

Fuchs F. Prevention of premature births. Clin Perinatol 1980 Mar; 7(1):3–15

Gabbe S. Diabetes mellitus in pregnancy: Have all problems been solved? Am J Med 1981 Mar; 70(3):613–618 (29 ref)

Gabbe S. General obstetric management of the diabetic pregnancy. Clin Obstet Gynecol 1981 Mar; 24(1):91–105

Grossman JH III et al. Management of genital herpes simplex virus infection during pregnancy. Obstet Gynecol 1981 Jul; 58(1):1–4

Hammer R, Bower E and Messina L. The prenatal use of Rh. (D) immune globulin. MCN 1984 Jan–Feb; 9(1):29–31

Hansen et al. Effects of maternal ritodrine on neonatal renal function. J Pediatr 1983 Nov; 103(5):774–780

Harger J et al. Etiology of recurrent pregnancy losses and outcome of subsequent pregnancies. J Obstet Gynecol 1983 Nov; 62(5):574–581

Harger J et al. Characteristics and management of pregnancy in women with genital herpes simplex virus infection. Am J Obstet Gynecol 1983 Apr 1; 145(7):784–791

Harman C et al. Severe Rh disease—Poor outcome is not inevitable. Am J Obstet Gynecol 1983 Apr; 145(7):823–829

Himell K. Genital herpes: The need for counseling. JOGN Nurs 1981 Nov–Dec; 10(6):446–450

Hollingsworth D. Alternations of maternal metabolism in normal and diabetics pregnancies: Differences in insulin-dependent, non-insulin dependent and gestational diabetes. Am J Obstet Gynecol 1983 Jun 15; 146(4):417–429

Huddleston F. Preterm Labor. Clin Obstet Gynecol 1982 Mar; 25(1):123–136

Hutchison CPT et al. Maternal and neonatal death due to pneumococcal infection Obstet Gynecol 1984 Jan; 63(1):130–131

Kelley M and Mongiello R. Hypertension in pregnancy: Labor, delivery and postpartum. Am J Nurs 1982 May; 85(5):813–822

Kucynski HJ. The pros and cons of douching: the nurse's role in counseling. JOGN Nurs 1980 Mar–Apr; 9(2):90–93

Kuntz W. Supine pressor (roll over) test: An evaluation. Am J Obstet Gynecol 1980 Aug; 137(7):764–768

Lake M. The role of a grief support team following stillbirth. Am J Obstet Gynecol 1983 Aug 15; 146(8):877–881

Leman R and Assey M. Heart disease and pregnancy. South Med J 1981 Aug; 74(8):944–946

Leveno K. Dilemmas in management of pregnancy complicated by diabetes. Med Clin North Am 1982 Nov; 66(6):1325–46

Lipson J. Repeat cesarean births: Social and psychological issues. JOGN Nurs 1984 May–Jun; 13(4):157–162

Luke B. Megavitamins and pregnancy: A dangerous combination. MCN 1985 Jan–Feb; 10(1):18–23

Mcanulty JH, Metcalfe J and Ueland K. General guidelines in the management of cardiac disease. Clin Obstet Gynecol 1981 Sep; 24(3):773–788

Moore D. Nursing care of the pregnant women with diabetes. JOGN Nurs 1981 May–Jun; 10(3):188–194

Nissen JC. Treatment of hypertensive emergencies of pregnancies. Clin Pharmacol 1982 Jul–Aug; 1(4):334–343

Peckham CS. Cytomegalovirus infection in pregnancy: Preliminary findings from a prospective study. Lancet 1983 Jun 18; 1(8338):1352–1355

Peckham C. Cytomegalovirus: Mastering a problem virus. Nurs Mirror 1982 Jan; 154(4):39–40

Perkins RP. Management of the hypertensive pregnant patient. Clin Perinatol 1980 Sep; 7(2):313–325

Quirk JG Jr and Bowes WA Jr. Intrapartum monitoring of the low birthweight fetus. Clin Perinatol 1982 Jun; 9(2):363–380

Rafferty TD and Berkowitz RL. Hemodynamics of patients with severe toxemia during labor and delivery. Am J Obstet Gynecol 1980 Oct 1; 138(3):263–270

Reedy N et al. Maternal–fetal transport: A nurse team. JOGN Nurs 1984 Mar–Apr; 13(2):91–100

Riblett B. Diabetes today. Insuring a safe pregnancy for your diabetic patient. RN 1983 Feb; 46(2):50–55

Rosenthal M. Intrapartum intensive care management of the cardiac patient. Clin Obstet Gynecol 1981 Sep; 24(3):789–807

Schutte MF et al. Threatened preterm labor: The influence of time factors on the incidence of RDS. Obstet Gynecol 1983 Sep; 62(3):287–293

Ship-Horowitz T. Nursing care of the sickel cell anemic patient in labor. JOGN Nurs 1983 Nov–Dec; 12(6):381–386

Souney PF et al. Pharmacotherapy of preterm labor. Clin Pharmacol 1983 Jan–Feb; 2(1):29–44

Srinwasan O et al. Congential syphilis: A diagnostic and therapeutic dilemma. Pediatr Infect Dis 1983; 2(6):436–441

Sullivan JM. The hypertensive diseases of pregnancy and their management. Adv Intern Med 1982; 27:407–433

Triolo P. Nonobstetric surgery during pregnancy. JOGN Nurs 1985 May–Jun; 14(3):179–183

Ueland K. Intrapartum management of the cardiac patient. Clin Perinatol 1981 Feb; 8(1):155–64

Well SG. The unspoken needs of families during high risk pregnancies. Am J Nurs 1981 Nov; 81(11):2047–2049

Welt SI et al. Effects of prophylactic management and therapeutics in hypertensive disease in pregnancy preliminary studies. Obstet Gynecol 1981 May; 57(5):557–565

Wheeler L and Jones ME. Pregnancy-induced hypertension. JOGN Nurs 1981 May–Jun; 10(3):212–232

Willis SE. Hypertension in pregnancy: pathophysiology. Am J Nurs 1982 May; 82(5):792–797

Willis SE and Sharp ES. Hypertension in pregnancy: Perinatal detection and management. Am J Nurs 1982 May; 82(5):798–808

Zlatnik FL and Burmeister LF. Dietary protein and preclampsia. Am J Obstet Gynecol 1983 Oct 1; 147(3):345–346

Complications of Labor and Delivery

Affonso D and Stichler J. Cesarean birth: Women's reactions. Am J Nurs 1980 Mar; 80(3):468–470

Amirikia H et al. Cesarean section: A 15 year review of changing incidence, indications, and risks. Am J Obstet Gynecol 1981 May 1; 140(1):81–90

Banta D and Thacker SB. The risks and benefits of epistomomy: A review. Birth. 1982 Spring; 9(1):25–30

Baxi LV et al. Induction of labor with low dose prostaglandin and oxytocin. Am J Obstet Gynecol 1980 Jan; 136(1):28–31

Bocchese J and Merker A. Seizure disorders in the neonate. Crit Care Nurse 1983 Nov/Dec; 3:42–51

Boyd S and Mahon P. The family centered cesarean delivery. MCN 1980 May–Jun; 5(3):176–180

Britton G. Early mother–infant contact and infant temperature stabilization. JOGN Nurs 1980 Mar–Apr; 9(2):84–86

Caritis SN et al. Fetal acid base state following spinal or epidural anesthesia for cesarean section. Obstet Gynecol 1980 Nov; 56(5):610–615

Coats PM et al. A comparison between midline and mediolateral episiotomies. Br J Obstet Gynecol 1980 May; 87(5):408–412

Cranston CS. Obstetrical nurses' attitudes toward fetal monitoring. JOGN Nurs 1980 Nov–Dec; 9(6):344–347

Crowell DH et al. Effects of induction of labor on the neurophysiologic functioning of newborn infants. Am J Obstet Gynecol 1980 Jan 1; 136(1):48–53

Chyun D. Pregnancy and cardiac valvular prostheses. JOGN Nurs 1985 Jan–Feb; 14(1):38–44

Fawcett J. Needs of cesarean birth parents JOGN Nurs 1981 Sep–Oct 10; (5):372–376

Flood B and Naeye R. Factors that predispose to premature rupture of the fetal membranes. JOGN Nurs 1984 Mar–Apr; 13(2):119–122

Frigoletto FD et al. Maternal mortality rate associated with cesarean section: An appraisal. Am J Obstet Gynecol 1980 Apr 1; 136(7):969–970

Frink B and Chally P. Managing pain responses to cesarean childbirth. MCN 1984 Jul–Aug; 9(4):270–272

Greis JB et al. Comparison of maternal and fetal effects of vacuum extraction with forceps or cesarean deliveries. Obstet Gynecol 1981 May; 57(5):571–577

Hart G. Maternal attitudes in prepared and unprepared cesarean deliveries. JOGN Nurs 1980 Jul–Aug; 9(4):243–245

Hawrylyshyn PA et al. Risk factors associated with infection following cesarean. Am J Obstet Gynecol 1981 Feb 1; 139(3):294–8

Hedahl K. Cesarean birth: A real family affair. Am J Nurs 1980 Mar; 80(3):471–472

Hodnett E. Patient control during labor: Effects of two types of fetal monitors. JOGN Nurs 1982 Mar–Apr; 11(2):94–99

Jagani N et al. Role of the cervix in the induction of labor. Obstet Gynecol 1982 Jan; 59(1):21–25

Kappy KA. Vacuum extractor. Clin Perinatol 1981 Feb; 8(1):79–86

Lavin JP et al. Vaginal delivery in patients with prior cesarean section. Obstet Gynecol 1982 Feb; 59(2):135–48

McDonough M, Sheriff D and Simmel P. Parents' response to fetal monitoring. MCN 1981 Jan/Feb; 6(1):32–34

McKay S and Roberts J. Second stage labor: What is normal? JOGN Nurs Mar–Apr; 14(2):101–106

McManus K and Angelini D. Meconium aspiration syndrome in the newborn. Crit Care Nurse 1983 Nov/Dec; 3:66–72

O'Driscoll K et al. Traumatic intracranial haemorrhage in first born infants and delivery with obstetric forceps. Br J Obstet Gynaecol 1981 Jun; 88(6):577–581

Pakzad KG. Risks occurring in birth induction without considering cervix maturity. J. Perinat Med 1980 8(1):27–37

Stewart P et al. A comparison of aestradiol and prostaglandin, E_2 for ripening the cervix. Br J Obstet Gynecol 1981 Mar; 88(3):236–239

Stichler JF and Affonso DD. Cesarean birth. Am J Nurs 1980 Mar; 80(3):468–470

Tradel-Korenchuk DM. Informed consent: Client participation in childbirth decisions. JOGN Nurs 1982 Nov–Dec; 11(6):379–481

Ulmsten U. Intracervical application of prostaglandin gel for induction of term labor. Obstet Gynecol 1982 Mar; 59(3):336–339

Vadurro J and Butts P. Reducing anxiety and pain of childbirth through hypnosis. Am J Nurs 1982 Apr; 82(4):620–623

VanDorsten JP et al. Randomized control trial of external cephalic version with tocolysis in late pregnancy. Am J Obstet Gynecol 1981 Oct 15; 141(4):417–424

Wall-Haas. Women's perception of first trimester spontaneous abortion. JOGN Nurs 1985 Jan–Feb; 14(1):50–53

Wise D and Engstrom. The predictive validity of fundal height curves in the identification of small and large for gestational age infants. JOGN Nurs 1985 Mar–Apr; 14(2):87–92

Young BK et al. Intravenous dexamethasome for prevention of neonatal respiratory distress—A prospective controlled study. Am J Obstet Gynecol 1980 Sep 15; 138(2):203–209

Complications of the Postpartum

Griffith S. Childbearing and the concept of culture. JOGN Nurs 1982 May–Jun; 11(3):181–184

Mince C. A program for helping grieving parents. MCN 1985 Mar–Apr; 10(2):118–122

Petrick J. Post-partum depression: Identification of high-risk mothers. JOGN Nursing 1984 Jan/Feb; 13(1):37–40

Renaud MT. Effect of discontinuing cover gowns on a postpartal ward upon cord colonization of the newborn. JOGN Nurs 1983 Nov–Dec; 12(6):399–401

Watson P. Postpartum hemorrhage and shock. Clin Obstet Gynecol 1980 Dec; 23(4):985–1001

Pediatric Nursing

Pediatric History Taking

28

General Principles

A. Information About a Child is Elicited for Several Reasons

1. To establish a relationship with the child and family
2. To assess what a family understands about their child's health
3. To formulate an individual plan of care
4. To correct any misinformation the family may have

B. Focus on Specific Topics in the History Depending on the Child's Age

1. Infant—stress pre- and postnatal history
2. Toddler—home environment, safety issues
3. School age—school, friends, reaction to previous hospitalizations
4. Adolescent—alcohol, drugs, friends, sexual history

Identifying Information

A. Type of Information Needed

1. Date and time
2. Hospital name and telephone number, if known
3. Patient's name, address, telephone number, birth date
4. Referring health care source (e.g., physician, nurse practitioner, health care agency, etc.)
5. Insurance data

B. Method of Collecting Data

1. Identify the "care person" in charge of the patient by name and relationship to the patient; obtain relative's or care person's address, home and work telephone numbers, if different from those of the patient.
2. To make the informant feel more at ease, the questions should begin in a friendly, nonthreatening manner. Questions addressed to the parent should be phrased appropriately.
3. Casual, friendly responses or remarks on the part of the interviewer may also help break the ice.
   a. "Whoever takes care of this baby certainly does a good job."
   b. "That's a lovely outfit the baby is wearing." (Remember that families will often put a new dress or suit on a baby for a visit to a health care agency.)
4. Sometimes repeat the information in order to verify data. This will give you a better judgment of the care person's cooperation and reliability.

Chief Complaint

A. Method of Recording

1. Write an exact description of the complaint.
2. Use quotation marks to clearly indicate that the informant's words are being used. It is helpful to explain:
   a. "I'll write it down so there will be no mistake."
   b. "Let me read this back to you to be sure it is correct."
3. Quotation of the care person's exact words may give an indication of how he/she feels about the symptoms; may reflect fear, guilt, defensiveness, etc.

B. Method of Collecting Information

1. Begin with a helpful open-ended question. That is the first overture made to this patient.
   a. "How may I help you?"
   b. "Please tell me the reason for your coming here today."
   c. "What do you think is wrong with the baby?"
2. Avoid confusing questions that may elicit funny-sounding or "smart" answers.
   a. "What brings you here?" (Answer: "The bus.")
   b. "Why are you here?" ("That's what I came to find out.")

C. Duration of Complaint

1. The information obtained may indicate the natural history of the disease, if one is present, and its gradual evolution. Pursue the information with a series of probing questions.
   a. "How long has the baby (child) had this problem?"
   b. If the informant cannot remember, try another route:
      "When did he last act well?"
      "Do you remember last Christmas? Did the baby have the trouble then?"
2. Write down the responses; try to assess, as more questions are asked, how accurate the informant's answers may be.

History of Present Illness

A. Type of Information Needed

When the patient is an infant or a preverbal child, information will consist mainly of what the informant has been able to observe. Having established what the chief complaint is, identify further problems, if any. Obtain the following information for each problem:

1. Body location—of pain, itching, weakness, etc.
2. Quality of complaint—both type (a burning pain) and severity (knife-like, comes and goes).
3. Degree of symptom—(e.g., pain, how severe; cough, day and night; eye drainage, how much).
4. Chronology—indicate time sequence and whether

problem is episodic (lasts for a while and then clears up completely).

5. Environment or setting—where and when the symptoms occur.
6. Aggravating and alleviating factors—what makes the pain worse or better?
7. Associated manifestations or symptoms—accompanied by vomiting, blurred vision, etc.

B. Importance of Detail

1. A carefully written description of a symptom will frequently be the source of a future diagnosis and will serve all who are involved in helping the patient.
2. Do not worry about large volume of notes at first.
3. You will be able to recheck this information when you do the review of systems.

Past History

A. Prenatal

1. Pregnancy—planned or not; source of care; date (approximately) of seeking care; birth order of this pregnancy, including miscarriages. This area of the history may be one of great sensitivity. Try to make the questions gentle and supportive.
   a. "Did you plan a baby around this time?"
   b. "When did you manage to get your first check-up for the pregnancy?"
   c. "Were there any unusual problems related to your pregnancy or delivery?"
2. Maternal health—includes illnesses and dates, abnormal symptoms (e.g., fever, rash, vaginal bleeding, edema, hypertension, urine abnormalities, sexually transmitted disease). Avoid technical words, if possible.
   a. "Did you have trouble with swollen feet?"
   b. "Were your rings tight?"
   c. "Do you know if your blood pressure went up?"
   d. "Did you have trouble with your urine?"
3. Weight gain—validate by trying to get a figure for nonpregnant weight and weight at delivery.
4. Medicines taken—(e.g., vitamins, iron, calcium, aspirin, cold preparations, tranquilizers (nerve medicine), antibiotics; use of ointments, hormones, injections during pregnancy, special or unusual diet, radiation exposure, sonography, amniocentesis.
5. Quality of the fetal movements; when felt, how brisk?

B. Natal

1. Expected date of delivery and approximate duration of pregnancy.
2. Place of delivery and who conducted the delivery.
3. Labor—spontaneous or induced; duration and intensity.
4. Analgesia or anesthesia.
5. Presentation—vaginal, breech, or vertex; cesarean delivery, forceps.
6. Episiotomy
7. Complications (e.g., need for blood transfusion, delay in delivery, etc.)

C. Neonatal

1. Condition of infant
2. Color (if seen) at delivery
3. Activity of infant
4. Crying heard
5. Breathing abnormality
6. Birth weight and length
7. Problems occurring immediately at birth

D. Postnatal

1. Duration of hospitalization of the mother and infant
2. Problems with baby's breathing or feeding
3. Need of supportive care (e.g., oxygen, incubator, special care nursery, isolation, medications)
4. Weight changes, weight at discharge if known
5. Color—cyanosis or jaundice
6. Bowel movements—when
7. Problems—seizures, deformities identified, consultation required
8. Mother's contact with the baby and her first impression
   a. "How did the baby look to you?"
   b. "What did the baby do when you were first together?"

E. Nutrition

1. Breast- or bottle-fed; what formula? how prepared?
2. Amounts offered and consumed
3. Frequency of feeding; weight gain
4. Addition of juice and/or solid foods
5. Food preferences or allergies
6. Feeding problems—variations in appetite
7. Age of weaning
8. Vitamins—type, amount, regularity
9. Pattern of weight gain
10. Current diet; frequency and content of meals

F. Growth and Development

1. Past weights and lengths if available
2. Milestones—sat alone unsupported; walked alone; used words, then sentences
3. Teeth—eruption, difficulty, cavities
4. Toilet training
5. Current motor, social, and language skills
6. Sexual development
   a. Infant—swollen breast tissue, vaginal discharge, hypertrophy of the labia
   b. Toddler or school child—early development of breasts or pubic hair
   c. Prepubertal or pubertal child—in females, time of development of breasts, pubic hair; onset of menstruation. In males, time of enlargement of testes, penis; development of pubic and facial hair; voice changes; acne

G. Health Maintenance

1. Immunizations—smallpox, rubella, rubeola, mumps, polio, diphtheria, pertussis, tetanus toxoid, BCG, influenza
   Indicate number and dates.
2. Screening procedures—hematocrit, tuberculin testing, visual and auditory acuity; rubella antibodies; syphilis testing; gonorrhea screen, Pap smear
3. Dental care—source and frequency of care, dental hygienist visits, fillings or extractions

H. Acute Infectious Diseases

Rubella, rubeola, mumps, chicken pox, scarlet fever, rheumatic fever, hepatitis, infectious mononucleosis, sexually transmitted disease, tuberculosis. Recent exposure to communicable disease.

I. Hospitalizations and Operations

1. Dates, hospital, physician
2. Indications, diagnosis, procedures

3. Complications
4. Reactions to previous hospitalizations

J. Injuries

1. Emergency department visits—frequency and diagnosis
2. Fractures—location and treatment
3. Trauma, burns, bruises
4. Ingestions

K. Medications

1. For general use such as vitamins, antihistamines, laxatives
2. Special or fad diets
3. Recent antibiotics
4. Routine use of aspirin
5. Oral contraceptives—types and dose, duration
6. Drugs, narcotics, marijuana, hallucinogens, mood elevators, tranquilizers, alcohol
7. Determine when last dose of medication was taken; is medication with patient? How does the child take the medication?

L. Radiation

1. Diagnosis requiring, number and occasion of exposures
2. Accidental exposure
3. Routine x-rays (chest, dental)
4. For injury, follow-up of fracture, etc.

Personal History

A. Type of Information Needed

1. Hygiene, exercise
2. Activities and hobbies, special talents
3. Friends
4. Sibling and parent relationships
5. Expression of emotions
   a. Blows up easily
   b. Rather quiet
6. Idiosyncratic behavior and habits (e.g., thumb sucking, nail biting, temper tantrums, head banging, pica, breath holding, rituals, tics, etc.)

B. Method of Collecting Data

1. Straightforward questions to a child (e.g., "What grade are you in?" "Who are your friends?")
2. Three wishes offered to the child:
   a. "If Christmas were here, what would you ask for?"
   b. "If you had your way, who would you like to be?"
   c. "What would be the best thing that could happen to you?"
3. "Who's your best friend?"
4. Adolescents—may want to interview without parents present

School History

A. Type of Information Needed

1. Present and past schooling, grade, and performance
2. Favored and least favored subjects
3. School-related behavior—anxious to go, anxious to stay home
4. General attitude towards school and any career plans

B. Method of Collecting Data

Emphasize the positive (e.g., "What's your best subject?" "Have you repeated a grade?" "Do you see your friends after school?")

Social History

A. Type of Information Needed

1. Environment—rural, urban
2. Housing—type, location, heating, sewage, water supply, family pets, other animal exposure
3. Parents' occupations (employment) and marital status
4. Number of individuals living in home, sleeping arrangements
5. Any religious affiliations
6. Utilization of social agencies previously
7. Health insurance and usual source of care

B. Method of Collecting Data

Parents are proud, so be careful with some of the questions. Ask permission.

1. "Can you tell me a little bit about your home?"
2. "I need to know more about how you live in order to help you with your child's problem."

Review of Systems

A. Type of Information Needed

1. General—activity, appetite, affect, sleep patterns, weight changes, edema, fever
2. Allergy—eczema, hay fever, asthma, hives, food or drug allergy, sinus disorders
3. Skin—rash or eruption, nodules, pigmentation or texture change, sweating or dryness, infection, hair growth, itching
4. Head—headache, head trauma, dizziness
5. Eyes—visual acuity, corrective lenses, strabismus, lacrimation, discharge, itching, redness, photophobia
6. Ears—auditory acuity, earaches (frequency), infection, drainage
7. Nose—colds and runny nose (frequency), infection, drainage
8. Teeth—hygiene practices, general condition
9. Throat—sore throat, tonsillitis, difficulty swallowing
10. Speech—peculiarity of or change in voice; hoarseness, clarity, enunciation, stammering
11. Respiratory—difficulty breathing, shortness of breath, chest pain, cough, wheezing, croup, pneumonia, tuberculosis or exposure
12. Cardiovascular—cyanosis, fainting, exercise intolerance, murmurs
13. Hematologic—pallor, anemia, tendency to bruise or bleed
14. Gastrointestinal—appetite (amount, frequency, cravings), nausea, vomiting, abdominal pain, abnormal size, bowel habits and nature of stools, parasites, encopresis (incontinence of feces), colic
15. Genitourinary—age of toilet training, frequency of urination, straining, dysuria, hematuria (or unusual color or odor of infant's soiled diaper), previous urinary tract infection, enuresis; urethral or vaginal discharge. Females: last menses, cramps, changes in interval and duration
16. Musculoskeletal—deformities, fractures, sprains, joint pains or swelling, limitation of motion, abnormality of nails
17. Neurologic—weakness or clumsiness, coordination, balance, gait, dominance, fatigability, tone, tremor. Seizures or paroxysmal behavior. Personality changes.

Bibliography

Books

Alexander M and Brown M. Pediatric History Taking and Physical Diagnosis for Nurses, 2nd ed. New York, McGraw-Hill, 1979

Athreya B. Clinical Methods in Pediatric Diagnosis. New York, Van Nostrand Reinhold, 1980

Bernstein L et al. Interviewing: A Guide for Health Professionals, 3rd ed. New York, Appleton-Century-Crofts, 1980

Christie-Seely J. Working With the Family in Primary Care—A Systems Approach to Health and Illness. New York, Praeger, 1984

Duldt BW et al. Interpersonal Communication in Nursing. Philadelphia, FA Davis, 1984

Frankenburg WK et al. Pediatric Developmental Diagnosis. New York, Thieme-Stratton, 1981

Green M. Pediatric Diagnosis— Interpretation of Symptoms and Signs in Different Age Periods, 3rd ed. Philadelphia, WB Saunders, 1980

Sherman JL and Fields SK. Guide to Patient Evaluation: History Taking, Physical Examination and the Problem-Oriented Method, 4th ed. Garden City, New York, Medical Examination Publishers, 1982

Waechter EH, Phillips J and Holaday B. Health assessment and health supervision. In Nursing Care of Children, 10th ed. Philadelphia, JB Lippincott, 1985

Whaley LF and Wong DL. Communication and the health interview. In Essentials of Pediatric Nursing. St Louis, CV Mosby, 1985 pp. 62–83

Articles

Mengel A. Getting the most from patient interviews. Nursing '82 1982 Nov; 12(11):46–49

Ross DM and Ross SA. The importance of type of question, psychological climate and subject set in interviewing children about pain. Pain 1984 May; 19(1):71–79

Talento B and Crockett-McKeever L. Improving interviewing techniques. Nurs Outlook 1982 Jul–Aug; 31(4): 234–235

Wasserman RC et al. Pediatric clinicians' support for parents makes a difference: An outcome-based analysis of clinician–parent interaction. Pediatrics 1984 Dec; 74(6):1047–1053

Pediatric Physical Examination

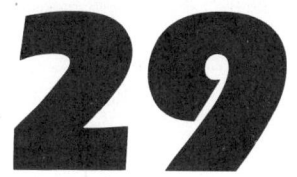

General Principles

1. Establish the order of all data collection according to the needs of the patients. For example:
   a. An exhausted parent with a screaming baby will not give a careful, comprehensive history.
   b. Alternative care may not be available for preschoolers when the newborn comes in for the first checkup.
2. If the parent has come in with more than 1 child, try to organize some supervision of the other children so that you can have a little time with the parent alone.
3. Remember that the safest place for any child is on the parent's knee. Privacy may not be possible because of the presence of other children.
4. Attempt to develop rapport with the young patient from the moment you first see or meet him or her.
5. Explain to the teenager what you are looking for as you proceed with the examination.

Approach to the Patient

1. Begin the examination with the patient on the parent's knee.
2. To evaluate the chest properly, you need to listen through 10 heartbeats when the child is not screaming; therefore, the chest is a good place to begin the examination.
3. The part to be examined should be completely exposed, but if an apprehensive child objects to having his clothes removed, slip your stethoscope under the shirt.
4. Forget the orderly and systematic approach, but remember to examine everything. Fortunately, children are small and one can check several systems very quickly over a small area.
5. As you examine each region, be aware that everything is confined to a small space.
6. Gradually remove the child's clothes, if you can; look for asymmetry very carefully in the bodies of all children.
7. Develop a pattern appropriate to the patient's age.
   a. Whistling is a great distraction.
   b. Keep a small music box or toy readily available.
8. Using a cold stethoscope may result in a frightened and screaming child, so warm the stethoscope before bringing it into contact with the child.
9. Some children are less frightened if able to hold the examining equipment first.
10. Show the child the procedure by demonstrating on the parent first.

Equipment

1. Have equipment ready and in working order before beginning.
2. Equipment is similar to that used in the adult physical examination:

Thermometer	Stethoscope
Oto-ophthalmoscope	Reflex hammer
Flashlight	Tuning fork

Tongue depressor   Disposable gloves
Cotton applicator stick   Lubricant

3. Additional equipment:
Sphygmomanometer cuffs in different sizes
Denver Developmental Test materials (see Appendix B, p. 1071)
Items for distraction—music box, toys

Vital Signs

Refer to Chapter 32, Pediatric Techniques—Measuring vital signs in children.

Technique	Findings

Standing Height, Head Circumference, and Chest Circumference

1. Use tape measure to obtain accurate head circumference. Measure widest part of head.

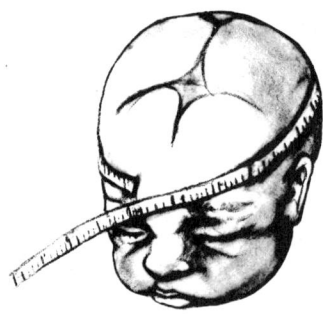

2. Record height and weight at each visit. Plot on growth chart.
3. Trends in growth are as important as the basic measurements.

Head and Chest Circumference

Age	Head Circumference		Chest Circumference	
Yr. Mo.	Inch	Cm.	Inch	Cm.
Birth	13.8	35.0	13.0	33.0
3	15.9	40.4	15.8	40.2
6	17.1	43.4	17.1	43.4
9	17.8	45.3	18.0	45.7
1–0	18.3	46.6	18.6	47.3
1–6	18.9	47.9	19.4	49.2
2–0	19.3	48.9	19.8	50.4
3–0	19.6	49.8	20.6	52.5
3–6	—	—	20.8	52.8
4–0	19.8	50.4	21.0	53.4
5–0	20.0	50.8	21.5	54.6

(From Studies at Harvard School of Public Health.)

General Appearance

1. Begin observations with the first contact with the patient, taking into account that there are at least 2 people to observe (child and parent).
2. The patient's interaction with the caretaker, whether it be the mother, a babysitter, an older sibling, or a friend of the family, is vital in the assessment of the child.

As you observe for race, sex, general physical development, nutritional state, mental alertness, evidence of pain, restlessness, body position, clothes, apparent age, hygiene, and grooming, remember that many of these things are part of the parent's caretaking.

1. If the child is easily distracted or sleepy, it may be naptime.
2. Careful observation of the general state of the child will provide many clues about the child's relationship to the family and their response to the child.

Skin

Examine as you move through each body region. (Include hair as well as skin.)

Inspection

Inspection of the skin is the same as for the adult (see p. 21).

1. Observe for skin color, pigmentation, lesions, jaundice, cyanosis, scars, superficial vascularity, moisture, edema, color of mucous membranes, hair distribution.
2. Describe any variation in color, particularly in children with increased pigmentation. Absence of pigment, or vitiligo, in darker children can be noted.
3. Birthmarks of any type are recorded. (May change as child grows older.)
4. Bruises or unusual marks of any kind, wounds or insect bites, scratch marks, scars, etc., may have particular significance.

1. In young babies, the skin is soft, smooth, and velvety in texture.

2. Pigmentations vary in children, depending on race, and will change as the child gets older.

3. A suntan, freckles, small, light-brown patches or café-au-lait spots may occur.

4. Bruises are particularly important because of the possibility of child abuse.

Technique	**Findings**

5. Draw a picture of anything unusual like a scar, and measure the dimensions of the lesion when recording the findings.

6. To ascertain suspected jaundice, take the child to the window to get a true picture of the color of the skin.
(A room with yellow walls and artificial lighting may create a wrong impression when jaundice is suspected.)

7. The skin of newborn infants will still be covered with vernix caseosa, the oily material that covers the fetus's body while in the utero.

8. Postmature infants may have scaliness that persists for several weeks after birth, particularly around the feet. The color of the skin may change as the child gets a little older.

9. Note the presence of striae.

Palpation

1. Use the tips of the fingers to palpate. (Fingertips are more sensitive.)

2. Feel the tension of the skin by pinching up a fold of skin.
Normal skin quickly falls back, but dehydrated skin remains in pinched position.

5. If you have difficulty in describing something, use ordinary words rather than inaccurate technical terms.

6. Carotenemia, which causes the nose and palms of the hands to have a yellowish tinge, may lead the parents to suspect jaundice; however, carotenemia is due to eating an excessive amount of yellow vegetables (carrots, sweet potatoes, squash, etc.). In carotenemia, the sclerae are clear; this is not so in jaundice.

7. Swollen sebaceous glands over the nose and chin are frequently seen right after birth and are called *milia.*

8. The blotchy, pink patches over the eyelid, bridge of the nose, and the back of the neck may persist until the child is nearly 2.

9. May indicate rapid weight gain.

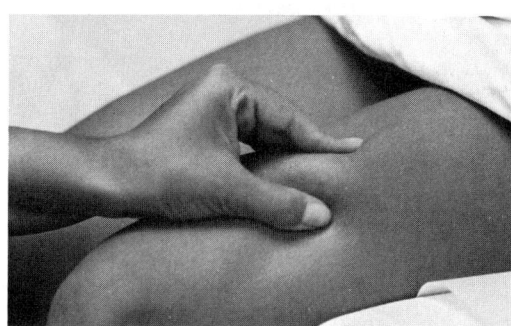

3. Feel the skin for texture, moisture, temperature, turgor, elasticity, masses, tenderness.

3. Skin that is rough and dry in texture may actually have a discrete rash that can be felt but not seen.

Nails

1. Observe for color, shape, irregularities in surface and general nail care—cleanliness, evidence of biting, etc.

2. Palpate the skin around the fingernails for firmness. Palpate any part that appears inflamed.

1. The nailbeds should be pink, the nails convex.

2. General care of the child is frequently reflected in good care of the nails.

Hair

1. Observe for color and distribution.
    a. Note according to the age of the child and race.
    b. Be aware that tufts of hair over the spine or sacral area may mark an underlying abnormality.

2. Note any change in pigmentation.

3. Palpate the hair for texture and thickness.

4. Examine to see if there are any patches where hair is missing on the head.

1. *Newborn:* Normally varies from no hair to a thick bush.
Infant: Consists of lanugo, a soft, downy covering frequently seen over the shoulders, back, arms, face, and sacral area, especially in dark-skinned children.
Race: Variations in hairiness.

2. Remember, children frequently experiment with mother's hair dye or rinse.

3. Texture may be thick or thin, coarse or fine, straight or curly.

4. May denote underlying skin infection; however, some children pull their hair out; sometimes the hair is braided so tightly that it falls out.

Technique	**Findings**
5. Separate thick hair on the head to get a good view of the scalp. Check for dandruff or scaliness in older children.	5. Look carefully for broken hairs, for scaliness on the scalp or cradle cap in infants.
6. Check scalp for any signs of lice infestation.	6. Nits (louse eggs) appear on the hair as little white dots. Lice may be seen on the scalp; they move quickly and may jump.
7. Inspect in the axillae and over the pubis as well as the extremities for the presence and quantity of hair, to gauge the development and level of puberty.	7. The child need not be totally undressed; a prepubertal child will usually be embarrassed if all of his or her clothes are removed.

Head and Neck

1. Unless specifically requested to do otherwise, examine the eyes and ears at the very last, especially in the younger child.
2. Also, examine the throat toward the last, unless the child exhibits concern about the "throat stick." It is then best to examine the throat right away in order to "get it over with."
3. To avoid frightening the child when palpating the head, make a game out of it—ask, "Where's your nose?" "Where are your eyes?"

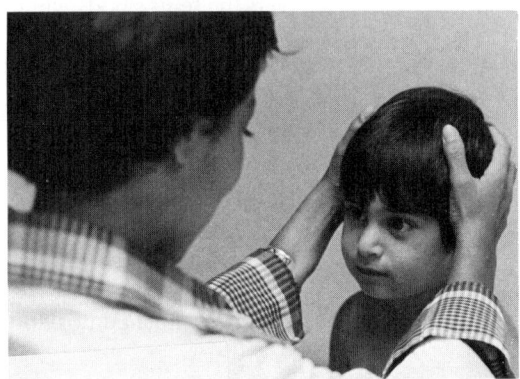

Inspection

1. Observe the face and skull for asymmetry, deformity, and abnormal or limited movements.

2. Closely observe facial expressions, blinking, etc., if the child is not crying. This may be one of your few moments to see the child when he is not crying.
   If you are examining a crying baby, watch particularly for asymmetry of the face.

3. Observe the movement of the head on the neck as the baby looks around. When turning an infant over, observe the head for control, position, and movement.

4. Since an infant's neck is often short and there are often several folds of skin under the chin, it is necessary to lift the chin a little to observe the skin completely—to see that it is clear and free of perspiration rash or irritation.

Findings

1. A baby's head may be asymmetrical because of pressure during pregnancy and delivery. The rounded head of the baby born by breech delivery contrasts with the long, pointed head of a baby who is a firstborn and whose head was moulded during a prolonged labor.

2. In a baby born by forceps delivery, there may be signs of weakness of the facial nerve caused by pressure of the forceps over the front of the ear where the facial nerve emerges. When the baby cries, the involved side will show weakness and downturning of the mouth.

3. There should be very little head lag beyond the age of 3 months.

4. In the back, the neck should be free of webbing or extra folds of skin extending from just beneath the ear toward the shoulder.

Palpation

1. Palpate the skull for the suture lines. Feel the face for any masses, noting size, consistency, surface, temperature, and tenderness.

2. Palpate the anterior and posterior fontanelles.

Findings

1. The suture lines of the skull may be felt to override as a result of the pressure applied when contractions occurred during labor. This is usually most marked between the frontal and the parietal bone where the coronal suture is located.

2. The fontanelles are soft and flat. Tense or bulging fontanelles may indicate hydrocephalus. Depressed fontanelles are often a sign of dehydration. The fontanelles usually close by 18 months.

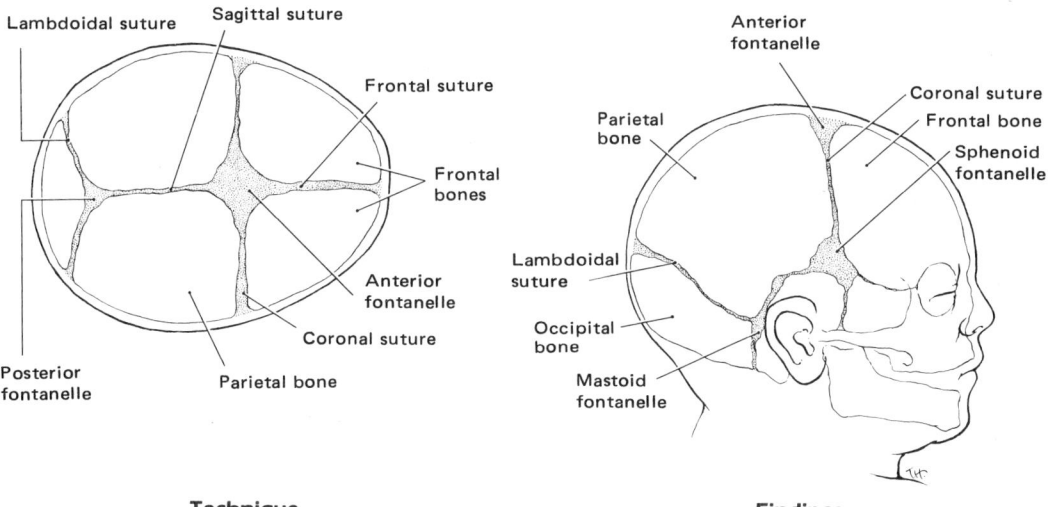

| **Technique** | **Findings** |

3. Palpate along the lambdoidal suture at the back of the head between the parietal bones and the occipital bone.

4. Palpate the neck for swollen lymph nodes, noting tenderness, mobility, location, and consistency.

4. Palpation of the lymph nodes may reveal slightly enlarged nodes in the anterior cervical chain secondary to sore throat.

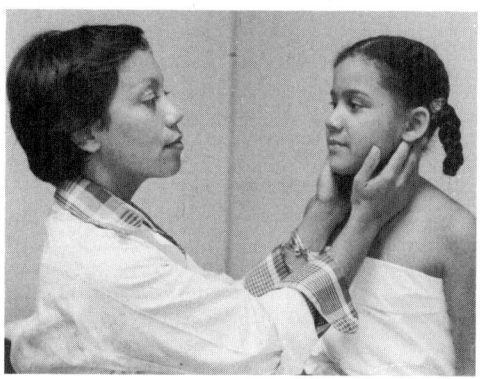

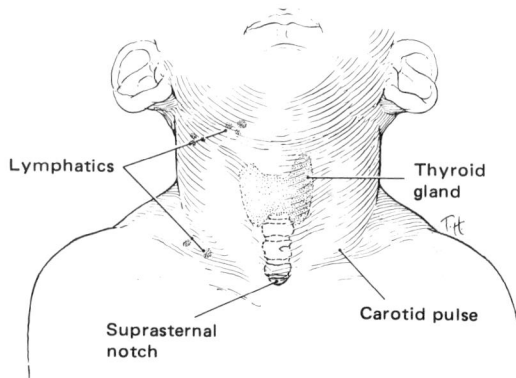

5. Note that there other nodes, which are normally not palpable.

5. These include the pre- and postauricular, the posterior cervical (behind the sternomastoid), the submental and submandibular (under the jaw), and the occipital nodes (along the prominence of the occiput).

6. Feel the pulses in the neck for location, strength, and equality.
7. Check the thyroid for enlargement, position, texture, and tenderness.
8. Locate the trachea in the suprasternal notch for position in the center of the neck.

Percussion

1. Percussion of the face may elicit tenderness over the sinuses.
2. Percuss over the head and neck directly with the fingertips, usually the middle finger of the right hand.
3. Percuss over the forehead for tenderness in the sinuses and across the zygoma, or cheekbone.

1. Tenderness may be due to a tooth cavity.

2. Gentle tapping over the skull elicits a typical noise when the sutures are open and a different sound when the sutures are closed.
3. This is to determine underlying tenderness in the maxillary sinus.

Technique	Findings

Auscultation

Auscultate the skull and carotid arteries in the neck.

To determine presence of bruits.

Eye and Vision

Equipment

Ophthalmoscope and pen light. Be sure batteries are new and lights are bright.

Inspection

(Similar to adult examination; p. 21)

1. Pay particular attention to the lacrimal duct.

1. Discharge from the eyes along the lower lid or from the lacrimal duct can occur as a result of infection or reaction to silver nitrate administered to the neonate.

2. Note the distance between the eyes and the distribution of the eyebrows.

2. Hypertelorism denotes a wider area between the eyes than normal. Excessively long and full eyebrows that meet in the midline and extra long eyelashes may signify a developmental abnormality.

3. Test the eyes for light perception.

3. It is difficult to prevent children from blinking their eyes or closing them when testing light response.

Palpation

If the child is old enough, have him squeeze his eyes tightly. (Not possible in younger children.)

Weakness of the muscles around the eyes is difficult to demonstrate in the young child. Muscle strength or weakness can be evaluated when the child cries.

Fundoscopic Examination

1. Check to see that the child's eyes move in conjugate fashion.
   Ask the mother if she has noticed any signs of squinting, especially when the child is tired.

1. Loss of vision can occur if the eyes are not working together properly. Squinting can indicate vision problems.

2. This is a difficult examination to conduct since children tend to watch the light and stare directly at you, which constricts their pupils. If the child cannot cooperate, it may be necessary to dilate the pupil to see the fundus.

2. A picture can be pinned to the wall opposite the child, who is then instructed to look at the picture during the examination. If the child is examined while lying down, a picture can be placed on the ceiling.

3. Start your examination at about ⅓ meter (1 foot) from the patient. Look for the red reflex, which should be readily observable.

4. Look for any opacities and then slowly approach the patient, turning the ophthalmoscopic dial to the smaller plus (+) numbers. Start originally at +8 to +10.
   (Wearing glasses or contact lenses may make a difference in the type of lens you use in the ophthalmoscope.)

4. The red reflex is diminished if there is something obstructing your view. A cataract or an opacity in the retina can cause this, as would a tumor filling the posterior chamber. If there is any paleness in the red reflex or difficulty in identifying it, a consultation should be sought immediately.

5. To help guide your gaze, put your hand on top of the child's head, with your thumb at the corner of the eye at the outer edge. If you lose the fundus, you can return to your thumb and get your bearings by directing your gaze medial to the tip of your thumbnail.

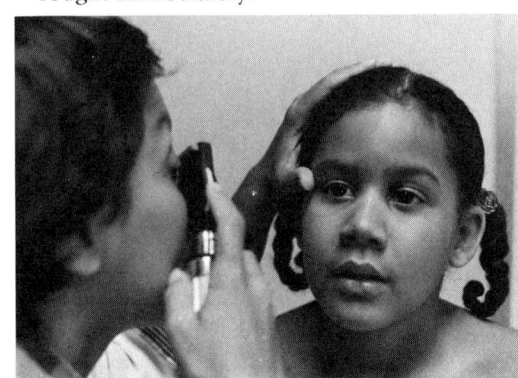

<table>
<tr><td align="center">**Technique**</td><td align="center">**Findings**</td></tr>
</table>

Ear and Hearing

Equipment

Tuning fork and otoscope
Small speculum for child's ear

Fresh batteries to ensure a bright light

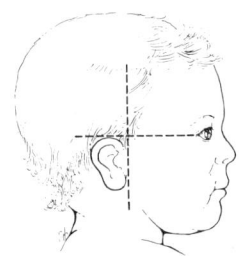

Inspection

1. When examining the external ear, the auricle, or the pinna, be sure to note the position of the ear.
   The top of the ear should cross an imaginary line drawn between the edge of the eye and the back of the occiput. If the ear is positioned more obliquely or is low-set, some underlying abnormality, particularly of the genitourinary system, may be present.

2. If you cannot get the child to cooperate by offering an explanation or by playing a game, the child will have to be restrained.

   a. The child can be seated on the parent's knee with the child's legs wedged between the parent's knees and the head held firmly with one hand while the baby's hands are controlled with the other hand.

   b. An older child may be held in a supine position, with the parent holding the child's arms above the head and controlling the head.

   c. If the child is very restless and apprehensive, examine the child from the top while the parent leans over the child's body, holds the arms down with her elbows, and at the same time grasps the child's head with her hands.

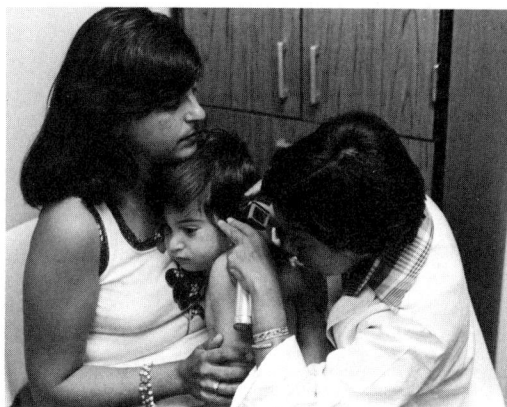

If the child is in a supine position, be sure to remove the shoes, because some children will kick when frightened.

Inspection with Otoscope

1. Hold the otoscope gently with the handle between the thumb and forefinger. This will enable you to control the head of the otoscope while keeping your hand steady on the child's head.

1. Small children will jerk about, so be careful not to push the speculum into the eardrum.

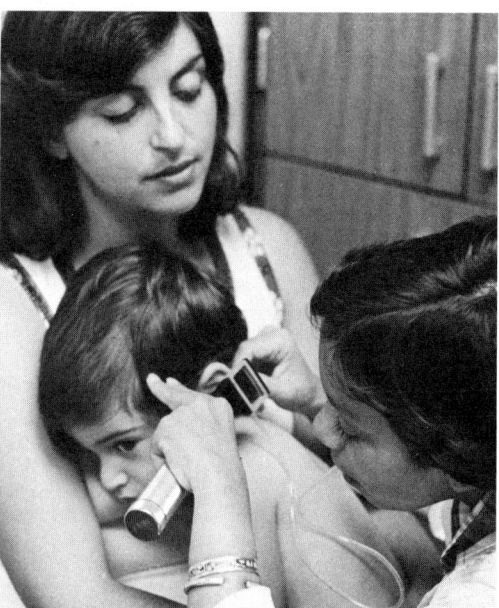

Technique	**Findings**
2. With your free hand, pull the pinna back and slightly upward to straighten the canal. Examine the canal.	2. Cerumen or wax may interfere with your view of the eardrum.
3. Inspect the eardrum and test for mobility by means of the pneumatoscope (the tube attachment of the otoscope).	3. The normal eardrum moves slightly when a soft breath is blown into the ear canal.

3. (continued)
   a. Attach one end of the tube to the otoscope and place the other end in your mouth.
   b. Blow gently through the tube.
      By blowing through plastic tubing it is possible to see the normal eardrum move back and forth. If the eardrum does not move, this may be indicative of infection behind the drum (serous otitis media).
   c. This method is preferred to the squeeze bulb because it allows for greater control of the force with which the air is introduced into the ear.

Palpation	
Palpate behind the ear over the mastoid process.	Tenderness behind the ear denotes infection. Sometimes a lymph node can be felt in this area.

Mechanical	
1. Most children will be able to respond to a test of gross hearing.	A small bell, such as the kind found in the Denver kit, can be used to determine hearing ability by noting if the child stops moving when the bell is rung and turns his head toward the sound.
2. More specific tests using an electric screening device are used prior to school age.	

Nose and Sinuses

Equipment

Nasoscope, small speculum

Inspection

1. Observe for general deformity.	
2. With nasoscope, examine nasal septum, mucous membranes and turbinates, and for discharge and nasal obstruction (see Adult Physical Examination, p. 25).	2. Dry mucous membranes may bleed and cause clots of blood to form in the nares. Scratches may also occur if child picks at nose or scratches when itching occurs.
3. Check for presence of any foreign body. Always remember that any child who has a "strange" odor may have a foreign body in the nose or ear. (In a female child, do not forget the vagina.)	3. A foreign body in the nose will cause a foul odor, purulent discharge, and may possibly cause bleeding.

Palpation

Palpate the sinuses, remembering the order of development.	Sinuses develop in a set order; the ethmoid and maxillary sinuses are present at birth; the frontal sinus develops at around 7, and the sphenoid after puberty.

Mouth and Throat

Equipment

Penlight, tongue depressor

1. Shining the light into the mouth or around the lips and teeth is not a threatening gesture.
2. However, the tongue blade, which is used to press against the inside of the cheek to allow for examination of the mucous membranes and which is also used to push the tongue out of the way, is a threatening instrument.
3. When the tongue depressor is placed on the tongue, it can have the unpleasant effect of making the child gag.

Technique	**Findings**

4. To avoid this unpleasant occurrence, encourage the child to stick out his tongue, breathe deeply, and say "ah." This may allow for easy visualization of the palate and uvula, without need for the "stick."

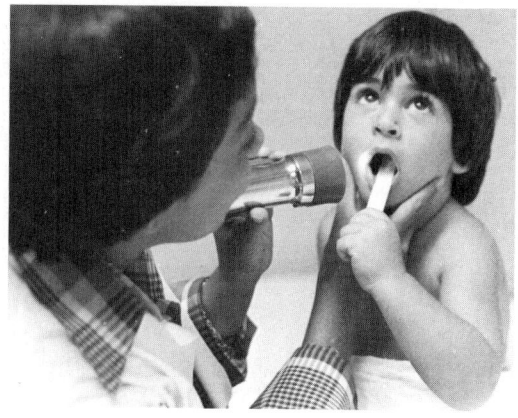

5. If these steps are not feasible, then the child may need to be restrained. If such is the case, examining the throat should be left to last, so as not to frighten the child.

A child may also be allowed to place the tongue blade directly on his own tongue while you guide him with your hand.

Inspection

1. Observe the lips, noting the color. (Remember that cyanosis is difficult to detect in a black child.)

1. *Infants:* There may be a protuberance on the upper lip, the so-called "sucking blister." *Children:* May have dry lips and redness around the lips due to an allergy or to some such activity as blowing bubble gum.

2. Count the teeth and note any extra or missing teeth, and any evidence of caries, staining, tartar, and malocclusion.

Time of eruption of deciduous teeth

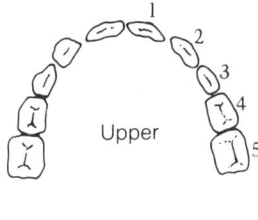

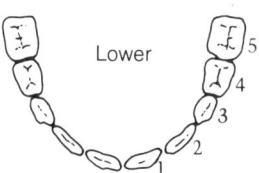

	(Upper)	(Lower)
1 Central incisor	8–12 mos.	5–9 mos.
2 Lateral incisor	8–12 mos.	12–18 mos.
3 Cuspid		18–24 mos.
4 First molar		12–18 mos.
5 Second molar		24–30 mos.

Time of eruption of permanent teeth

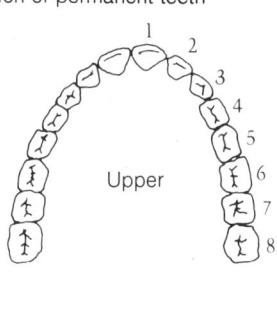

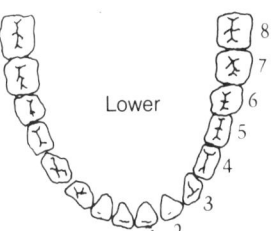

	(Upper)	(Lower)
1 Central incisor	6–7 yr.	7–8 yr.
2 Lateral incisor	7–8 yr.	8–9 yr.
3 Cuspid	9–10 yr.	11–12 yr.
4 First bicuspid	10–11 yr.	10–11 yr.
5 Second bicuspid	11–12 yr.	10–12 yr.
6 First molar	6–7 yr.	6–7 yr.
7 Second molar	11–13 yr.	12–13 yr.
8 Third molar	17 yr.	17–18 yr.

Technique	**Findings**
3. Check the gums for swelling and signs of easy bleeding. Also note mouth odor.	
4. Check the tongue for movement, color, and the presence of taste buds on the surface. Check to see that the frenulum under the tongue is of the proper length.	4. If the frenulum is too short, the child may be tongue-tied (meaning that the baby cannot advance the tip of the tongue beyond the lips), although this is not thought to interfere with sucking or speech.
5. As the gag reflex is elicited, note how the palate moves upward and the uvula springs into view.	5. It should be midline and single, although occasionally it will be divided or bifid.
6. Examine the roof of the mouth.	6. The roof of the mouth at the junction of the hard and soft palate will frequently reveal whitish lesions, or Epstein's pearls, which persist through infancy.
7. Inspect the height of the arch of the palate.	7. With experience, an unusually high arch is easily recognizable.
8. Note the tonsils on each side of the uvula and immediately posterior to it for position, surface, size, equality, and color.	8. Any coating with pus or ulcers or a pocket or cryptic appearance should be recorded.
9. As the baby cries, note the odor of the breath and any hoarseness of the voice; note difficulty on inspiration, as in croup, or wheezing on expiration.	9. These signs may indicate throat and chest disturbances.

Palpation

1. Palpate the lips and cheeks manually using a finger cot or glove.	1. By comparing one side with the other, differences due to abnormality can be detected.
2. Note any evidence of swelling.	

Breast and Thorax

1. Sometimes young children object to having their clothes removed.
2. The following approaches may overcome this problem:
   a. Distract the child by having him listen to a few heartbeats.
   b. Have the parent (while the child is on his or her knee) remove the underclothing while you stand by.
   c. For an older child entering puberty, provide an examining sheet, but stay in the room while the child puts on the gown, provided he or she is not embarrassed by your presence. During such preparation, you are able to make a superficial appraisal of the chest.

Breast

1. Check to see if there are any small extra nipples present.	1. These would appear along a line extending from the anterior axillary line through the normal nipple down toward the symphysis pubis.
2. In the newborn infant, the nipples appear a little darker than normal, and breast tissue underneath may form a small knot with occasional leakage of milk.	2. This leakage is a secondary effect of the hormone level in the mother; instruct the mother not to try to express the milk, because of the danger of infection.
3. In the older child, a lump found under the nipple in either male or female may cause some concern for cancer.	3. Such lumps are usually secondary to hormone stimulation and occur toward puberty.
4. Occasionally, the breasts begin to develop earlier than normal, at around 5 or 6 years.	4. This should be a reason for referral to a physician.

Thorax

Inspection

1. Observe the entire thorax as the child breathes; note symmetry and equal expansion of both sides as the lungs inflate.	1. In babies and young children (especially an infant lying on the parent's knee), diaphragm excursion is more marked than intercostal expansion. Thus the abdomen goes up and down more than the chest expands.
2. Confirm the respiratory rate as you observe the child with his shirt off.	

Technique	Findings

Percussion

Percussion of the child's chest is difficult. Because the underlying structures are crowded, not too much is elicited.

The heart edge is difficult to outline, and percussing the chest may be frightening to the child.

Very light percussion is necessary; a hyperresonant note may be elicited over air, particularly of a stomach bubble that projects up into the left side of the chest.

Palpation

1. Use warmed hands as you palpate the shape and angle of the sternum. Note if there is any sinking in of the sternum.

2. Palpate the costochondral junctions for tenderness and enlargement.

3. As you palpate, hoarse sounds (as in bronchitis) may be felt through your hands.

4. Vocal fremitus is difficult to elicit in the smaller child since it is difficult to have him make repetitive sounds on command.

1. The shape of the sternum may vary, although there may be a sinking in of the sternum (funnel sternum) which may cause subsequent trouble because of pressure on underlying structures. This should be referred to the pediatrician.

2. May suggest an underlying inflammatory response.

3. Normal inspiration and expiration do not give a sensation under the fingers, except for the expansion of the chest.

4. In the older child, it is worth trying, in order to obtain transmission of sound through the lung tissue.

Auscultation

The difficulty with examining a child is that everything sounds muddled and mixed. The examiner has to sort out breathing that is rapid from a heart rate that is also rapid, and must also differentiate between inspiration and expiration and the 1st and 2nd heart sounds.

1. Try to examine a baby before he begins crying.

2. Warm the stethoscope before using by rubbing it between your hands.

3. Be aware that breathing is louder in younger children with slightly increased length of inspiration, almost to the point of bronchovesicular breathing in the adult.

4. Crackles (discontinuous; interrupted, explosive sounds) may be heard more easily in children.

1. Note, however, that crying increases lung expansion.

2. A cold stethoscope will startle the child.

3. Bronchial breathing with equal inspiration and expiration is very loud and easy to hear if the patient has pneumonia.

4. Added coarse-quality sounds in the chest are commonly associated with mucus in the trachea or even in the back of the nose.

Heart

Inspection

In thin children, the apical beat or the point of maximal impulse (PMI) can easily be seen, particularly if you look obliquely across the chest wall.

As in all areas of the pediatric examination, measurement and documentation of the distance from the midline and the exact rib space are worth noting.

Palpation

The apical beat may be felt in the 6th intercostal space about 5 cm. (2 inches) from the midline in the school-age child. It is more difficult to feel in the baby, particularly a plump child, and would not be so far out towards the anterior axillary line.

The apical beat will be deviated to the left with cardiac enlargement or a collapsed lung on that side.

The apical pulse could be pushed toward the right by a tumor or a collapsed lung on the right. Pneumothorax under tension will push the heart away from the side of the increased pressure.

Auscultation

1. Identify the 1st heart sound (S_1). (Occurs during systole.)
    a. Locate the apical beat (closing of the mitral valve) by placing the stethoscope over the maximum impulse area, concentrating on the first heart sound. (As the ventricle on the left contracts, pushing the blood up into the aorta, the sound of the mitral valve closing is heard.)

1. Consists of the "lub" portion of the "lub-dub" heart sound.

Technique	**Findings**

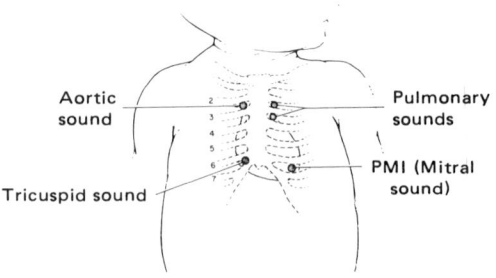

b. That sound can be identified by placing the thumb on the carotid pulse of the neck, which will coincide very closely with the heart sounds.

2. Identify the 2nd heart sound (S_2).
   a. Move the stethoscope up toward the sternum and to the left.
   b. At the base of the heart, both over the aortic and pulmonic areas, S_2 is louder than S_1.

2. Represents the "dub" portion of the "lub-dub" heart sound.

   b. In a child, S_2 can be heard as 2 heart sounds, since the 2 valves in the aorta and pulmonary vessels do not close at quite the same time. The "dub-dub" will disappear if you can get the child to cooperate and breathe deeply.

3. Move the stethoscope in small jumps from the apical area medially towards the sternum. Go up to the left side of the sternum, listening at each interspace next to the sternum.

3. This represents the area of maximum intensity of sound of the pulmonary vessels.

4. Move next to the patient's right second intercostal space—again next to the sternum.

4. It is at this area that you will hear the aortic sound best.

5. Descend down the right side of the sternum to the lower end where you will hear best the tricuspid valve from the right of the heart.

6. Listen to only 1 sound; concentrate on that to the exclusion of all others. Can you identify this sound? Is it clear? Compare it with your own heart sound or that of the parent.

6. The child will enjoy this comparison if he is allowed to listen.

7. If there is any question of a heart murmur or added sounds, refer to the physician.

8. As you listen to the heart sounds, you are also listening to the rhythm to confirm your findings on pulse.
   a. If he breathes in and out deeply, the sinus arrhythmia will be obvious.
   b. If a child holds his breath, the sinus arrhythmia will disappear.

8. The typical rhythm of a child is called *sinus arrhythmia*. As the heart speeds up, the child is breathing in; the heart slows down on expiration.

9. Be sure to count a rapid heart that is heard even when the child is quiet.

9. This may be indicative of a tachycardia that requires further investigation.

10. In the infant, heart sounds are just a series of taps; they occur so fast that it is impossible to make out which sound is the 1st heart sound.

10. In the infant, the 1st and 2nd heart sounds are equal in intensity.

Abdomen

1. For examination of the abdomen, the child should be lying down, relaxed, and not crying. Placing a small child, particularly around the age of 1–3 years, on a high table on cold paper, can be very frightening; as a result, the abdomen will not be relaxed.

2. Babies up to about 1 year do not seem to be perturbed and will often lie down and play very nicely as long as they can see the parent, who should be stationed at the head of the child while you examine the abdomen.

3. Having the child lie across the parent's knees with the legs dangling on one side and the head cradled in his or her arms, will enable you to feel the abdomen quite well.
   a. You may find that with the baby's head in the parent's left arm, you can use your left hand to examine the baby's abdomen on the right, feeling up under the right costal margin and into the right hypochondrium.

Technique	**Findings**

b. You may need to turn the baby around and use your right hand to examine the left side of the child's abdomen.

4. Do not discard the idea of using the floor.
   a. If the child is young, ask the parent if he or she minds putting the child on the floor on a sheet.
   b. The toddler will usually enjoy crawling around the floor and has probably been doing so while the history was being taken.

Inspection

1. Observe the abdomen for contour and any markings both while the child is standing and when he is lying down. As you inspect, you may see some abdominal movement with respiration. (Remember that the diaphragm, as it goes up and down, will move the contents of the abdomen.)	1. Sometimes superficial veins are seen on the abdomen, particularly in a very blond infant. Striae are often noticed on the flank following rapid loss or gain of weight.
2. Check for early signs of puberty as evidenced by pubic hair over the symphysis pubis.	2. Early pubic hair in younger children (8–10) may appear long and silky. This will ultimately become curly toward the onset of puberty.
3. Carefully inspect the umbilicus for cleanliness and the presence of any scar tissue.	3. A deep umbilicus may be difficult to keep clean. Immediately after the cord has dropped off, scar tissue or a granuloma may occur.

Auscultation

1. Since percussion and palpation will stimulate the small bowel and increase bowel sounds, auscultation should precede these 2 techniques.	1. Bowel sounds are heard as tinkling, irregular sounds that indicate that fluid is moving from one section of the bowel to the next.
2. To obtain the child's cooperation, you can conduct a running commentary as you listen, saying such things as, "I can hear the Cheerios in there."	2. In a quiet baby who has just eaten, not many bowel sounds will be heard. In a hungry child, noisy bowel sounds can be heard, even without a stethoscope.

Percussion

1. On the right side, percuss for the liver. Confirm on palpation.	1. Liver dullness can frequently be outlined.
2. Percuss over the left upper quadrant.	2. Percussion over a gas-filled bowel or stomach gives a high-pitched, hollow sound.
3. Percuss the lower abdomen, particularly above the symphysis pubis.	3. Above the symphysis pubis, a filled bladder can produce a confusing sound, as does a pregnant uterus. (A mass in the abdomen of a girl over 10 may be a fetus.)

Palpation

1. Divide the abdomen into 4 imaginary quadrants, palpating each with the fingertips.
2. In the right upper quadrant, palpate for the liver edge.
   a. Although the liver is easily palpable in most children, you may have to press quite firmly.
   b. The liver is frequently felt about 1 cm. (⅜ inch) below the right costal margin and in some instances as low as 2 cm. (¾ inch). This is a common finding in the newborn and through the early school-age years.

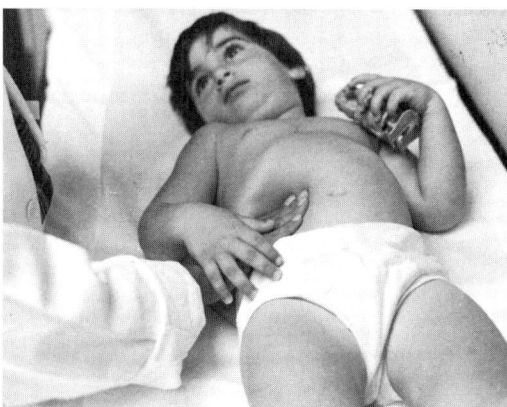

3. In the left upper quadrant, palpate for the spleen. Less resistance is encountered as you feel up under the left costal margin.	3. Only the tip of the spleen can be felt in the upper outer left quadrant, in the early months of life and in very thin children of preschool age.

Technique	Findings
4. In the upper quadrants also try to palpate for the kidneys. Deep palpation for both kidneys should routinely be a part of the examination to make sure there is no enlargement of the kidney. Normally, the kidney is not palpable.	4. Kidney palpation is difficult, but during the newborn period, the lower pole of the right kidney can frequently be felt and sometimes the left as well. (This applies to the period immediately following delivery, when the infant's abdomen is relaxed and the bowel is not distended.)
5. In the iliac fossa or the left lower quadrant, palpate for the descending bowel.	5. The descending colon can be felt, particularly if filled with firm stool. It may be slightly tender, but it should not cause severe pain on gentle palpation.
6. Palpate on the right lower quadrant (RLQ) where the appendix is located.	6. In the RLQ, usually the only sensation is that of gas-filled bowel. Tenderness in this area could be related to an inflamed appendix.
7. If the child has pain in any area or has pointed to the umbilicus when asked to show where the pain is, avoid the area demonstrated and leave it until last.	7. If the painful area is palpated first, the child may tense up when the other areas of the abdomen are examined.
8. Palpate around the umbilicus for any masses which may indicate a hernia, especially in black children. As you press over the protruding hernia you can feel the sensation of gurgling under your fingers as the bowel returns to the abdomen.	8. Most of these hernias heal naturally by the age of 6 years. A hernia above the umbilicus can be revealed by asking the child to lift his head from the table. (Widening of the muscles above the umbilicus is called *diastasis recti.*)

Rectum and Anus

1. Rectal examinations are rarely necessary in infants and young children.
2. If the child will be examined by a physician who will examine the rectum, it is not necessary to duplicate this part of the examination.
3. Rectal examinations are embarrassing and uncomfortable for most children. Explain the procedure before performing the examination.
4. Positioning for a rectal examination:
   a. Infants can be placed on their abdomens, sides, or backs with the legs raised to the chest.
   b. Young children and teenagers can be positioned on their sides.

Inspection

1. When examining a baby or toddler, place the child on a flat surface so that the weight is evenly distributed on the front of the pelvis. As the baby moves about on his abdomen, observe the entire back, the lower back, the upper thigh, and the tightening of the buttocks.	1. If one buttock is larger than the other, you will see that side projected above the other. Weakness of one side will be obvious as the baby moves around, although a child in the early stages of crawling will normally tend to use one knee as a predominant leader, dragging the other behind.
2. Notice particularly the lower part of the back for hairiness.	2. This may indicate an underlying abnormality of the vertebrae.
3. As the child moves away, part the buttocks and look at the cleft between them.	3. A pilonidal dimple or sinus may be seen over the lip of the coccyx at the superior end of the internatal cleft. This is a common finding, but parents should be told about it for cleaning purposes.
4. Pay careful attention to the outer appearance of the anus and the perineal body, the underside of the scrotum in the male, and the labia majora in the female. (Male genitalia, below and to pp. 1061–1062) (Female genitalia, pp. 1063–1064)	4. The anus is inspected for blood, fissures, or splitting in the external tissue, redness, swelling, or pads of extra flesh. On occasion, small white pinworms may be seen adhering to the anal skin.

Palpation

1. Take into consideration the child's age and feelings; ask the mother to assist if need be.	
2. Start by parting the buttocks with the left hand and introducing a well-lubricated finger (with finger cot) into the anus.	2. When an infant is being examined, the small finger should be used.

Technique	Findings
3. Gently apply pressure on the anal sphincter to allow the muscles to relax and the fingertip to slide into the rectum.	3. Apply pressure with pulp of the finger rather than jab at the anus with the fingertip.
4. Gently palpate the inner ring, feeling for areas of thickening and tenderness and simultaneously judging the sphincter tone.	4. As the perianal area is pressed upon from the inside, tenderness will be elicited if a deep fissure exists or if an infection has occurred around a fissure.
5. If the rectum is full of feces, it will be impossible to feel any other mass.	5. In the young child, particularly the infant, dilatation provided by the finger will result in a bowel movement. In the older child, a suppository or even an enema may be required.
6. Palpate the walls of the rectum.	6. Within the rectum, the mucosal walls should be smooth, and deep palpation should elicit mild tenderness and no acute pain.
7. As the finger reaches up from the rectum towards the right iliac fossa, place your other hand over the right iliac fossa, trying in effect to roll the appendix between your hands.	7. With an acutely inflamed appendix, this will elicit a great deal of pain and thus constitutes a significant finding.
8. In the male, gently turn your finger through 180 degrees and feel the posterior surface of the prostate. Note size, consistency, tenderness, and contour.	
9. In the female, perform a bimanual examination and palpate the cervix.	

Male Genitalia

1. This part of the examination requires a direct, matter-of-fact approach. Acknowledge that it is normal to feel embarrassed during an examination of the genitals. Explain what you are looking for as you proceed through the examination with a teenager.
2. Reassure the child after the examination that his genitals are normal. This decreases anxiety.

Scrotum and Testes

Inspection

1. Before touching the child, determine by observation of the testes whether they are in the scrotum.	1. Retraction of the testes into the abdomen occurs very frequently in young children; the development of the scrotum depends on the presence of the testes.
2. Observe the skin over the scrotum for color and surface appearance, noting the presence of wrinkles, or rugae.	2. The skin over the scrotum varies in color, being a darker brown to black in the more pigmented races and reddish in the fair-skinned. The wrinkles, or rugae, are more developed as the child grows older.

Palpation

1. Check the scrotum wall for swelling or sensitivity. Gently feel the testes, palpating across the upper pole and feeling for the epididymis. (Remember the scrotum is extremely sensitive to pressure.)	1. The epididymis is a ridge of soft, bumpy tissue extending from the superior pole and running down and behind the testis.
2. Estimate the size of the testes and identify the spermatic cord, tracing it from the testis up toward the groin.	2. The spermatic cord, with the vas deferens, feels firm and is accompanied by softer nerves, arteries, veins, and a few muscle fibers.
3. Make a special effort to locate the testis in a young child whose testes may be retracted into the abdomen via a hyperactive cremasteric reflex. a. If the testes cannot be felt in the scrotum, gently run the skin of the upper scrotum between your fingers, moving superiorly and approaching the external inguinal ring.	3. The presence of the testes in the scrotum is vital in the preschool or early school-age child. Nondescent of the testes requires that the child be referred to a physician. During this period the testis is about 1.5–2 cm. (½–¾ inch) in length. In the quiescent period prior to puberty, the male genitalia remain fairly infantile.

Technique	Findings

b. Try to milk the testis down towards the scrotum from above with your hand.

c. If this fails, have the child sit cross-legged to abolish the reflex of the cremaster muscle.

4. When examining a boy in the early stages of puberty, it is important to note the size of the testis as well as the greater number of rugae on the scrotum and the appearance of pubic hair around the penis.

4. In early puberty, the testes start to grow. Onset of puberty varies, occurring in some boys by age 10 and in others as late as 14. In most teenagers, the findings are similar to those in adults.

Penis

1. Evaluate the penis on all sides by lifting up the shaft.

1. The shaft of the penis contains the urethra on the under, or ventral surface and is easily palpable.

2. If the child is not circumcised, partially retract the foreskin to observe the glans and meatus.

2. The foreskin may adhere to the glans for the first few years of life. It is not necessary for the parent to "stretch" the foreskin by retraction.

Whitish discharge around the glans under the foreskin is normal and not a sign of infection. The foreskin should completely circle around the glans.

3. Observe the position of the meatus and evert the lips of the meatus to reveal an adequate orifice.

3. The meatus may be positioned off center. Refer the child to a physician if the meatus is located on the dorsal or ventral surface of the shaft.

4. In the older child, inspect the penis for ulcers, sores, or discharge from the meatus.

4. Consider sexually transmitted diseases in the older child and teenager.

Inguinal Area

1. Palpate for hernia over the external inguinal ring. Have the child cough to enhance your observation.

1. Having the child stand either with the parent holding him or placing him against his or her knee will help you in locating a hernia in the inguinal area.

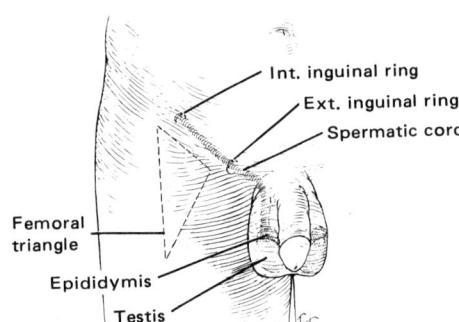

Int. inguinal ring
Ext. inguinal ring
Spermatic cord
Femoral triangle
Epididymis
Testis

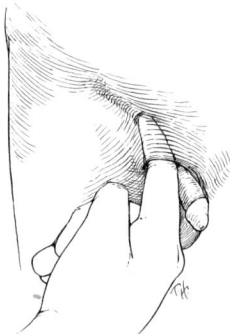

2. An increased cough reflex or swelling in the area should be checked by carefully placing the finger on the scrotal skin and invaginating the skin over your fingers toward the external ring. You are trying to follow the course of a hernia that would descend into the scrotum while you feel the external ring from below. A hernia in the inguinal region presents as a bulge which can be either seen or felt from below by placing the finger in the scrotum pointing up toward the external inguinal ring.

Technique	Findings
3. Also palpate for the inguinal lymph nodes.	3. The inguinal lymph nodes in an infant are palpable as small and "shotty." Anything more than this should alert you to possible infection, since the perianal area drains into the superficial inguinal lymph nodes. Thus, any signs of diaper rash will explain enlargement of the lymph nodes, which should be noted and reported.

Femoral Area

Palpate the femoral triangle carefully for a hernia and for lymph nodes.	In the femoral area, a swelling which can be reduced with a gurgling sound is an unusual finding.

Auscultation

If you are trying to reduce a mass, listen over the scrotum to see if there is a gurgling sound.	This will locate the bowel for you and confirm the presence of a hernia.

Transillumination

1. To locate the testis, darken the room and shine a bright light from behind the scrotum. In a normal child, the testis will stand out as the darker area.	1. Testes which are swollen by fluid (hydrocele) will transilluminate. Fluid around the testes or cord must be differentiated from a hernia.
2. Transilluminate any suspicious mass to help locate a hernia.	2. Any mass in this area must be reported to a physician immediately.

Female Genitalia

1. If the child will be examined by a physician who will examine the genitalia, it is not necessary to duplicate this part of the examination.
2. Place the infant or toddler on the table or on the parent's knee while he or she holds the knees in an abducted and flexed position.
3. A preschool child can be allowed to lean over her parent's knee. However, remember that the structures are being visualized upside down.
4. The older child or teenager should be draped as an adult would and should be placed in a lithotomy position with the aid of stirrups.

Equipment

Disposable gloves, speculum, light source

1. Carefully inspect the perineal area for cleanliness, inflammation, and abnormality.	1. This includes the mons pubis, clitoris, labia, urethra, and perineal body.
2. Fold back the labia majora and note the labia minora.	2. The labia minora are seen as 2 slender folds of tissue inside the labia majora.
3. Part the labia and note the clitoris and the meatus at the anterior end. (The clitoris is a hook-like structure that extends over the opening of the urethral meatus.) The meatus appears as a slit that is slightly darker in color against the pink of the mucosa about 2 cm. (¾ inch) posterior to the clitoris.	3. In some instances, adhesions of the labia minora occur because of the lack of natural hormones. The opening of the vagina is obscured by the two lateral flaps, which stick together, sometimes to the degree that urination is difficult because the urethral meatus is covered. This should be referred to a physician.
4. Having parted the labia, check for any signs of inflammation, discharge, tenderness, or infection. Include the urethral meatus, periurethral glands, the vagina, and the greater vestibular glands (Bartholin's). (Tenderness of these glands is unusual in young children, but may occur in adolescents.)	4. Inflammation and pus-like discharge from the urethra may be noted on palpation. The periurethral glands may be tender because of infection—possibly due to gonococci. If discharge is collected from the vagina, it should be cultured.

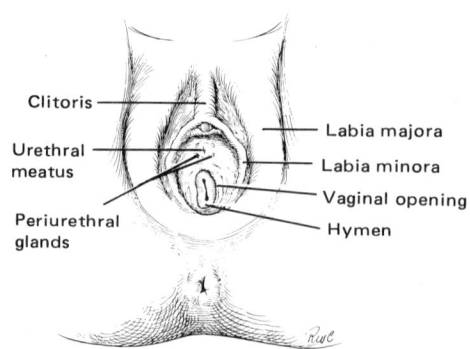

Technique

5. If the mother of a newborn infant has noted a bloody discharge from the infant's vagina during the first few days of life, reassure her that this is not an uncommon occurrence; the discharge will disappear, as will any swelling of the labia majora and clitoris and any enlargement of the infant's breasts.

6. Note the vaginal opening, which may vary in size because of the presence of a thin membrane, the hymen.
The hymen varies in appearance according to the age of the child.

7. In the young child, it is usually unnecessary to examine inside the vagina. Should you suspect the presence of a foreign body, insert a finger into the rectum and milk anteriorly to allow you to feel the lower part of the cervix and any firm foreign body within the vagina.

8. In an older child, the little finger can be inserted gently into the vagina and anterior pressure applied.

9. Turn the finger gradually, sweeping down the right side of the vagina, back over the rectum, and up on the left side of the vagina. Turn your finger, arm, and wrist so that undue pressure is not made on the child's tissues.

10. Once the genitalia are examined, lower the child's legs somewhat so that the femoral and inguinal areas can be palpated the same way as in the male.

Findings

5. Hormone stimulation from the mother's body accounts for this occurrence. The discharge usually stops once the hormones are excreted. The bloody appearance on the diaper may be confused with the presence of urates, which are also orange-red and which appear quite normally in the urine.

6. The lack of an opening into the vagina may result in the retention of menstrual fluid when the child reaches puberty. In the sexually active adolescent, vestigial remains of the hymen may appear as small particles (caruncles) at the fringe of the vagina.

7. A foreign body may be suspected if there is vaginal discharge (of any quantity) that is blood-tinged or has an odor. In the older child, vaginal discharge of this type may be due to gonorrhea.

8. Anterior pressure and milking downwards palpates the urethra towards the meatus. The periurethral glands are located on each side of the urethra.

10. Enlargement of the lymph nodes in the presence of a hernia in the femoral triangle may be found. Similarly, enlargement of the inguinal nodes may occur.

Musculoskeletal System

1. Evaluation of the musculoskeletal system can be done both in an informal manner while watching the child at rest and at play and in a formal manner as specific findings are methodically checked.

2. In the newborn, observe the position of the extremities during sleep and the quality of movement when the infant is awake.

3. Various aspects of size, shape, and movement are evaluated as the baby is observed pushing up on his arms and turning his head towards his mother.

4. The infant in the early stages of walking offers many opportunities for evaluation of muscle strength and movement.
At the same time, rapport with the mother can be reinforced by your admiring the baby's ability and by inquiring if she is concerned about the manner in which the baby is walking.

5. A more mobile child can be evaluated as you watch him play and explore the room.

6. Having the older child reach for crayons, run after a ball, or walk around the room enables you to evaluate the musculoskeletal system and the child's sense of balance.

Technique	Findings

Upper Extremities

1. In the infant, evaluate the status of the clavicles when examining the skull and neck.

2. Carefully examine the hands to note shape of the hand, shape and length of the fingers, changes in the nails, and the presence of creases on the palms.

1. During a difficult delivery, the clavicle that has been exposed to traction may snap. A lump can be felt on the bone at about 3 weeks of age.

2. Any variation in the hands or unusual length of the fingers should be noted. An incurved little finger or low-set thumb with the single Simian crease may reflect Down's syndrome, or mongolism.

Lower Extremities

1. Examine the appearance of the infant's foot, noting arch formation.

2. Inspect the angle of the foot and lower leg and then manipulate the ankle to evaluate the range of motion.

3. Place the knees together and see how far the ankles are separated.

4. Evaluate the baby's ability to walk, noting the appearance of the legs and foot placement. Remember to look at the child's shoes and see which side of the sole is worn down.

1. The foot of an infant is usually flat and appears broad since the arch on the inside of the foot is covered by a fat pad. Parents may need reassurance in this regard.

2. Full flexibility of the foot (plantar flexion) rules out underlying abnormality. The foot should return to the neutral position after manipulation. Frequently, the foot will turn in, or adduct. Such a finding should be recorded.

3. Normally there is only a small space between the ankles when the knees are held together. Marked bowing of the legs will be demonstrated by a wide distance between the ankles. This is particularly important following assumption of the upright position.

4. When babies first start to walk, their legs appear bowlegged. The feet are kept wide apart and turn slightly in, so that the ankles seem curved when viewed from behind.

Hip

1. When examining children under 1 year of age, check to see if there signs of hip dislocation. Refer to Chapter 44, Children With Orthopedic Conditions, Congenital Dislocation of the Hip, page 1449.

1. Any difficulties with hip examination call for immediate medical consultation because of possible congenital dislocation of the hip.
In the normal infant, the lateral aspect of each knee will touch the examining table without difficulty.

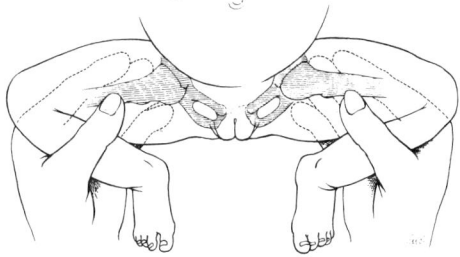

Spine

1. Check the spine for any signs of abnormal curvature.

2. Observe the child from the side and back in the standing position to see forward curving of the shoulders.

3. Have the child bend forward with the arms hanging down. A unilateral rib prominence will be seen in children with scoliosis.

1. The normal child has a curve inward at the lumbar region (lordosis), but this should not be exaggerated.
Abnormal curvatures include the following:
Kyphosis: Forward curvature of the shoulders.
Scoliosis: Side-to-side curvature of the spine.

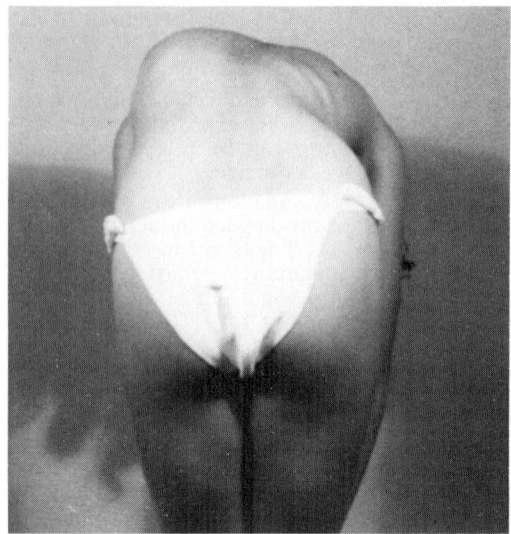

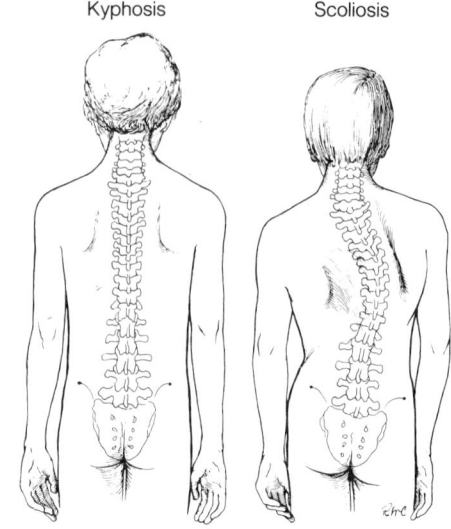

Kyphosis   Scoliosis

(O'Connor BJ. Scoliosis: Classification and diagnosis in pediatric orthopedics. ONAJ 3:84, Mar 1976)

Technique	**Findings**

Neurologic Examination

1. The neurologic system at birth is different from that of the baby of a few months. There is an even greater contrast between the baby on the one hand and children and adults on the other.
2. The central nervous system at birth is underdeveloped and the functions tested are below the level of the cortex.

Equipment

Flashlight, noisemaker, ophthalmoscope, tongue depressor, tuning fork

Procedure for the Newborn and Young Infant

(See Guidelines: Physical Appraisal of the Newborn, p. 1006.)

1. Observe the newborn for general appearance, positioning, activity, crying, and alertness. Take note of the posture—including head, neck, and extremities.

    1. Stiffness of the neck or marked attraction of the head will cause a position of opisthotonos.

2. Note the pitch, volume, and character of the cry.

    2. The high-pitched cry of the infant who has intracranial irritation is very distinctive.

3. Observe the infant's facial expression and the symmetry of the face when crying or sucking.

    3. Poor sucking, with dribbling, is abnormal. Transient weakness of the mouth due to 7th cranial nerve paralysis is frequently seen as a result of a forceps delivery in which the forceps is pressed on the facial nerve where it emerges from the ear.

4. Most of the cranial nerves are difficult to check at this early age.

Automatic Reflexes

1. *Blinking reflex due to loud noise*
   Clap your hands or produce a loud clicking noise, being careful not to clap near the baby so that a wave of air passes over his eyes and causes him to blink them anyway.

    1. Lack of a blink in response to a loud noise may indicate deafness.

2. *Blinking reflex due to bright light*
   Shine a bright light into the infant's eyes to elicit blinking reflex.

    2. Failure to blink may indicate blindness.

   a. Cranial nerve 10 can be checked by using a tongue depressor to gag the infant.

      a. Palate moves.

   b. Cranial nerve 12 (hypoglossal) can be tested by pinching the nose closed as the baby sucks.

      b. The infant opens the mouth and raises the tip of the tongue reflexly.

Technique	**Findings**
3. *Palmar grasp reflex* Place your fingers across the baby's palm from the ulnar side. The baby needs to be in a relaxed position with his head in a central position. Reinforcement may be offered by having the baby suck on the bottle at the same time.	3. Both hands will flex and can be compared for strength. Weakness on 1 side may be indicated by a failure to grasp when the palm is stimulated.
4. *Rooting reflex* Touch the edge of the baby's mouth.	4. The baby's mouth will open, and the head will turn toward the side stimulated. This reflex is marked during the early weeks of life. (Persistence time varies.)

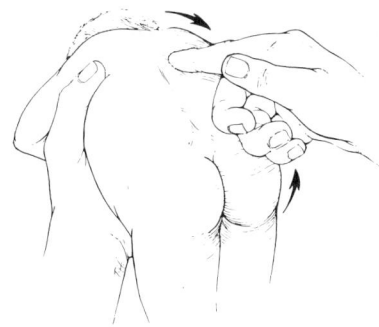

5. *Incurving of the trunk* Hold the baby horizontally and prone in one arm while using the other hand to stimulate 1 side of the infant's back from the shoulders to the buttocks. The trunk curves toward the stimulated side as the shoulders and pelvis move toward the stroking hand (persists until infant is about 2 months old).	
6. *Vertical suspension position* Place your hands under the baby's axillae with thumbs supporting the back of the head and hold the baby upright.	6. The legs flex at the hips and knees (persists for about 4 months).
7. *Stepping response* Hold the baby under its axillae with thumbs supporting the back of the head. Allow baby's foot to touch firm surface.	7. Normally the baby responds by lifting 1 knee and hip into a flexed position and moving the opposite leg forward—making a series of stepping movements (*A*). a. Difficulty with the stepping reflex and stiffness or spasticity connected with crossing of the feet and scissoring (*B*) is indicative of spastic paraplegia or diplegia. b. It should be noted that the stepping response may be affected by breech delivery. (It may also be affected by weakness.) c. The stepping response is evident toward the end of the 1st week and persists for a variable time.

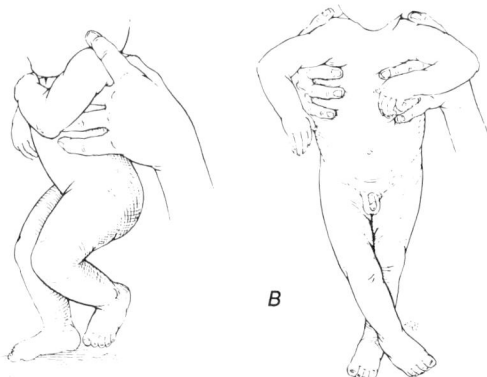

A   *B*

8. *Tonic neck reflex* Hold the baby in a supine position with the head turned to one side and the jaw held in place over the shoulder.	8. a. The arm and leg on the side to which the head is turned will extend, whereas those on the other side will flex (the so-called "bow and arrow position"). b. This reflex persists for about 6 months; it may be present at birth or delayed until the baby is 6 or 8 weeks old. c. Persistence beyond 6 months suggests major cerebral damage.

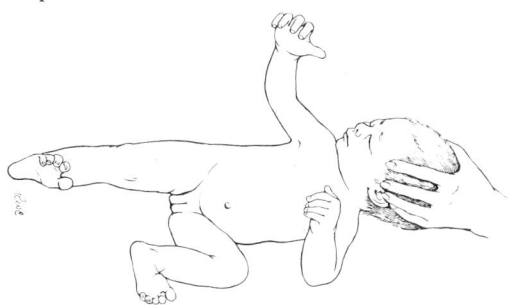

Technique	**Findings**

9. *Mass reflexes (Moro or startle reflex)*
Hold the baby along your arm with the other hand below the lower legs. Lower the feet and body in a sudden motion.

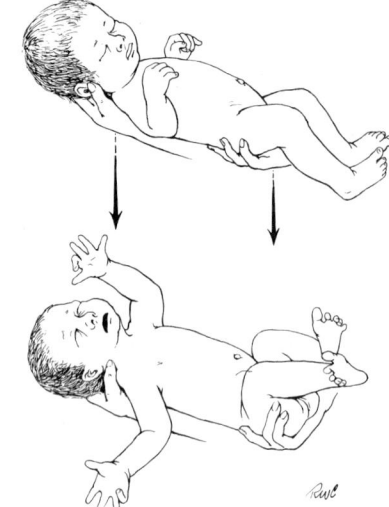

9. The arms will spring up and out, abducting and extending; the fingers are also extended. The arms then return forward over the body with a clasping motion. At the same time, the legs flex slightly and the hips abduct.
   a. The Moro reflex is present at birth and disappears at about the end of the 3rd month. Persistence beyond 6 months is significant.
   b. Asymmetric response may be due to paralysis of the arm following a difficult delivery, tension and injury to the brachial plexus, or a fracture of the clavicle or humerus. A dislocated hip would produce an asymmetrical response in the lower extremities.

10. *Perez reflex*
Hold the baby in a prone position along your arm; place the thumb of the other hand on the sacrum and move it firmly toward the head, along the entire length of the spine.

10. The head and spine will extend and the knees will flex upward.

Summary

1. Some of the jerking and shaking movements seen in infants are normal, but they should be rechecked frequently during the first few weeks of life.
2. Plantar stimulation will elicit a Babinski response (toes curl upward) in most children until the age of 2; this is a normal finding.
3. Variants in the findings due to the baby's sleepiness or hunger should be taken into account and reevaluations should be carried out under different conditions.
4. Severe neurologic damage may be completely asymptomatic and impossible to detect during the first few weeks of life.

Neurologic Examination of the Toddler and Early School-Age Child

1. The neurologic examination for the toddler and the early school-age child is very similar to that for the adult.
2. The Draw-A-Person Test* and the Denver Developmental Assessment† are both excellent methods for testing areas in the development of the child.
3. Beyond the newborn period, specific gross and fine motor coordination testing, accompanied by appropriate evaluation of the Denver test, will assist in assessing the child's level of development.
4. These tests also assess social and language development and are important screening devices.
5. Interview techniques‡ can also be useful in assessing development in the preschool child.

* See Appendix A, page 1070.
† See Appendix B, page 1071.
‡ See Appendix C, page 1073.

Bibliography

Books

Barness LA. Manual of Pediatric Physical Diagnosis, 5th ed. Chicago, Year Book Medical Publishers, 1981

Bates B. A Guide to Physical Examination, 3rd ed. Philadelphia, JB Lippincott, 1983

Brown MS and Murphy MA. Ambulatory Pediatrics, 2nd ed. New York, McGraw-Hill, 1981

Burns KR and Johnson PJ. Health Assessment in Clinical Practice. Englewood Cliffs, NJ, Prentice-Hall, 1980

DeGowin EL. Bedside Diagnostic Evaluation, 4th ed. New York, Macmillan, 1981

Ferholt JDL. Clinical Assessment of Children: A Comprehensive Approach to Primary Pediatric Care. Philadelphia, JB Lippincott, 1980

Goodenough FL. Measurement of Intelligence by Drawings. Chicago, World Book, 1926

Harris DB. Children's Drawing as a Measure of Intellectual Maturity. New York, Harcourt, Brace & Jovanovich, 1963

Malasanos L et al. Health Assessment, 2nd ed. St Louis, CV Mosby, 1981

Stangler S et al. Screening Growth and Development of Preschool Children: A Guide for Test Selection. New York, McGraw-Hill, 1980

Waechter EH, Phillips J and Holaday B. Principles of physical assessment. In Nursing Care of Children. Philadelphia, JB Lippincott, 1985, pp. 121–170

Whaley LF and Wong DL. Physical assessment of the child. In Essentials of Pediatric Nursing. St Louis, CV Mosby, 1985, pp. 84–131

Zelle RS and Coyner AB. Developmentally Disabled Infants and Toddlers: Assessment and Intervention. Philadelphia, FA Davis, 1983

Ziai M et al. Assessment of the Newborn—A Guide for the Practitioner. Boston, Little, Brown & Co, 1984

Ziai M. Bedside Pediatrics: Diagnostic Evaluation of the Child. Boston, Little, Brown & Co, 1983

Articles

Balk SJ et al. Examination of genitalia in children: The remaining taboo. Pediatrics 1982 Nov; 70(5):751–753

Cavanaugh RM. Genital self-examination in adolescent males. Am Fam Physician 1983 Sept; 28(3):199–201

Cavanaugh RM. Pelvic examination of adolescent girls. Am Fam Physician 1982 Oct; 26(4):105–108

Diaz C et al. Pediatric screening procedures. Adv Pediatr 1982; 29:409–469

Ellenberg JH and Nelson KB. Early recognition of infants at high risk for cerebral palsy: Examination at age four months. Dev Med Child Neurol 1981 Dec; 23(6):705–716

Kilmon C and Helpin M. Recognizing dental malocclusion in children. Ped Nurs 1983 May–June; 9(3):204–208

Moss JR. Predicting young children's cooperation with the physical exam. Pediatr Nurs 1983 May–June; 9(3): 188–190

O'Connor F. Ear, nose and throat examination in general practice. Practitioner 1981 Nov; 225(1361): 1546–1552

Phillips S et al. Teenagers preferences regarding the presence of family members, peers and chaperones during examination of the genitalia. Pediatrics 1981 Nov; 68(5):665–669

Reinecke RD. Ophthalmic examination of infants and children by the pediatrician. Pediatr Clin North Am 1983 Dec; 30(6):995–1002

Runyon DK. The pre-participation examination of the young athlete: Defining the essentials. Clin Pediatr 1983 Oct; 22(10):674–679

Welch NM et al. The value of the preschool examination in screening for health problems. J Pediatr 1982 Feb; 100(2):232–234

Williams JK. Evaluating the dysmorphic child. Pediatr Nurs 1983 Jul–Aug; 9(4):241–248

Appendix A: Goodenough–Harris Draw-a-Person Test

This test provides one of the methods of measuring the level of mental development of children between 3 and 10 years of age. It was originally described in 1926 and appears to be a sound one; there is a significant degree of correlation in the results of this test and IQ. Subsequently Harris brought the test up-to-date with specific scoring for drawings of a man or a woman.

1. *Procedure:* The child is supplied with a pencil (preferably a No. 2 with eraser) and a sheet of blank paper and instructed to "Draw a person," "Draw the best person you can." No additional directions are necessary. Encouragement may be supplied if necessary. Under no condition should the examiner suggest that the child's production needs to be supplemented or changed in any way—the only exception being the drawing of the stick figure. In this case the examiner is permitted to encourage the child to "draw a whole person."

2. *Scoring:* The child receives one point for each detail present according to the following scoring guides:

Drawing of a Woman

 1. Head present
 2. Neck present
 3. Neck, 2 dimensions
 4. Eyes present
 5. Eye detail: brow or lashes
 6. Eye detail: pupil
 7. Nose present (not round ball)
 8. Nose, 2 dimensions
 9. Bridge of nose (straight to eyes, narrower than base)
10. Nostrils shown
11. Mouth present
12. Lips, 2 dimensions
13. Both nose and lips in 2 dimensions
14. Both chin and forehead shown
15. Hair I (any scribble)
16. Hair II (more detail)
17. Necklace or earrings
18. Arms present
19. Fingers present
20. Correct number of fingers shown
21. Opposition of thumb shown (must include fingers)
22. Hands present
23. Legs present
24. Feet (any indication)
25. Shoe "feminine" (any attempt such as high heels, open toe, strap)
26. Attachment of arms and legs I (to trunk anywhere)
27. Attachment of arms and legs II (to trunk at correct point)
28. Clothing indicated (any)
29. Sleeve
30. Neckline (any indication)
31. Trunk present
32. Trunk in proportion, 2 dimensions (length greater than breadth)

Drawing of a Man

 1. Head present
 2. Neck present
 3. Neck, 2 dimensions
 4. Eyes present
 5. Eye detail: brow or lashes
 6. Eye detail: pupil
 7. Nose present
 8. Nose, 2 dimensions (not round ball)
 9. Mouth present
10. Lips, 2 dimensions
11. Both nose and lips in 2 dimensions
12. Both chin and forehead shown
13. Bridge of nose (straight to eyes; narrower than base)
14. Hair I (any scribble)
15. Hair II (more detail)
16. Ears present
17. Fingers present
18. Correct number of fingers shown
19. Opposition of thumb shown (must include fingers)
20. Hands present
21. Arms present
22. Arms at side or engaged in activity
23. Feet; any indication
24. Attachment of arms and legs I (to trunk anywhere)
25. Attachment of arms and legs II (at correct point of trunk)
26. Trunk present
27. Trunk in proportion, 2 dimensions (length greater than breadth)
28. Clothing I (anything)
29. Clothing II (2 articles of clothing)

3. *Norms:* Minimum score for child to be within one standard deviation of age-appropriate mean.

	Drawing of man		Drawing of woman	
Age	by boys	by girls	by boys	by girls
3	4	5	4	6
4	7	7	7	8
5	11	12	11	14
6	13	14	13	16
7	16	17	16	19
8	18	20	20	23

Appendix B: Denver Developmental Screening Test

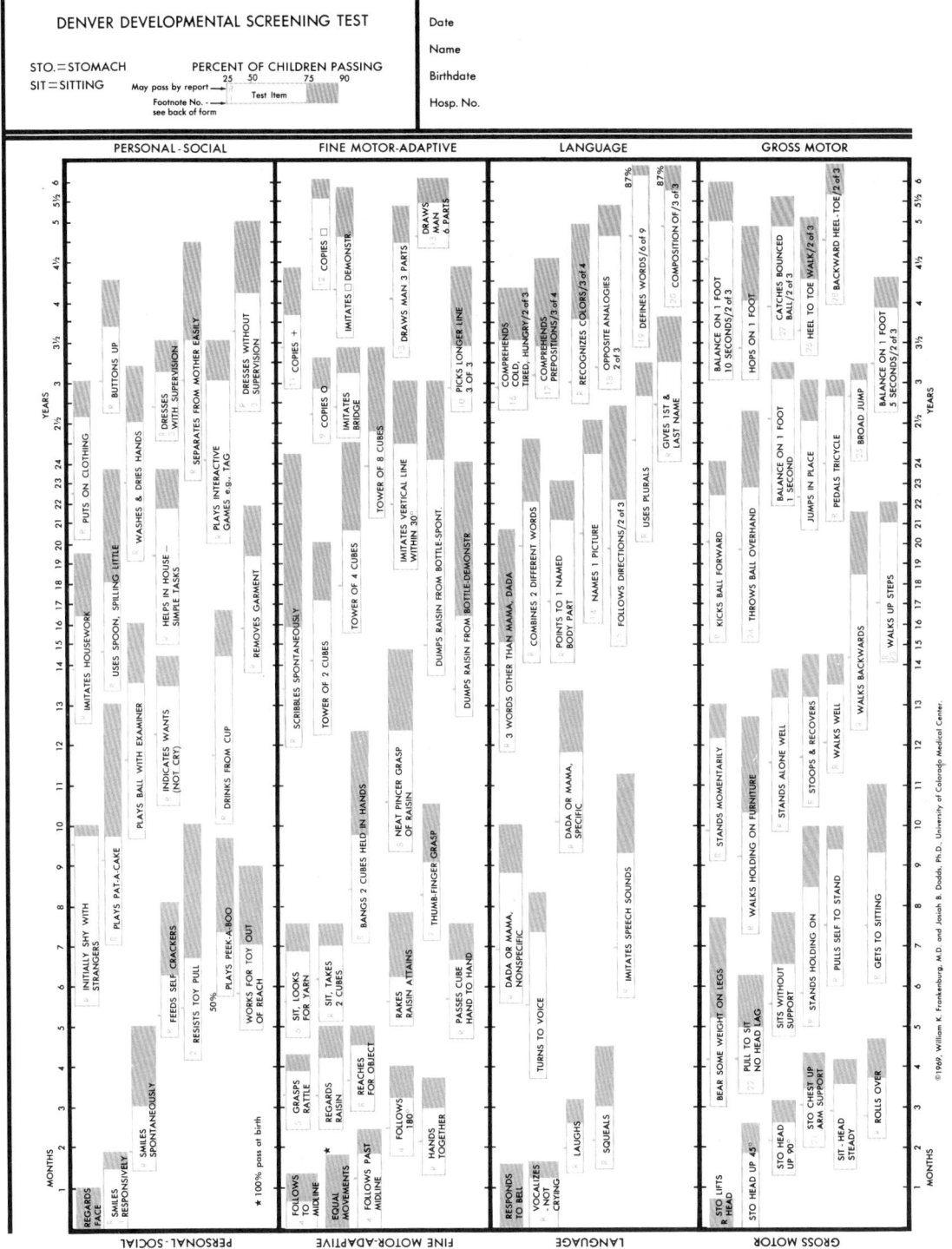

The Denver Developmental Assessment method developed by William K. Frankenburg, M.D., and his colleagues, is presented in a manual called Denver Developmental Screening Test. The test materials can be ordered from: Lodaco Project & Publishing Foundation, Inc., East 51st Avenue and Lincoln Street, Denver, Colorado 80216.

	DATE
DIRECTIONS	NAME
	BIRTHDATE
	HOSP. NO.

1. Try to get child to smile by smiling, talking or waving to him. Do not touch him.
2. When child is playing with toy, pull it away from him. Pass if he resists.
3. Child does not have to be able to tie shoes or button in the back.
4. Move yarn slowly in an arc from one side to the other, about 6″ above child's face. Pass if eyes follow 90° to midline. (Past midline; 180°)
5. Pass if child grasps rattle when it is touched to the backs or tips of fingers.
6. Pass if child continues to look where yarn disappeared or tries to see where it went. Yarn should be dropped quickly from sight from tester's hand without arm movement.
7. Pass if child picks up raisin with any part of thumb and a finger.
8. Pass if child picks up raisin with the ends of thumb and index finger using an over hand approach.

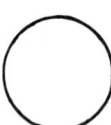 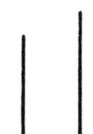 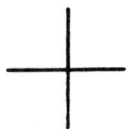 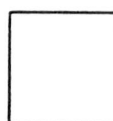

9. Pass any enclosed form. Fail continuous round motions.
10. Which line is longer? (Not bigger.) Turn paper upside down and repeat. (3/3 or 5/6)
11. Pass any crossing lines.
12. Have child copy first. If failed, demonstrate

When giving items 9, 11 and 12, do not name the forms. Do not demonstrate 9 and 11.

13. When scoring, each pair (2 arms, 2 legs, etc.) counts as one part.
14. Point to picture and have child name it. (No credit is given for sounds only.)

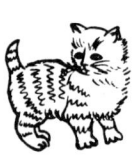 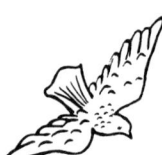 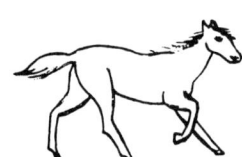 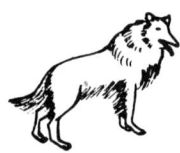 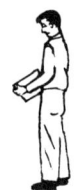

15. Tell child to: Give block to Mommie; put block on table; put block on floor. Pass 2 of 3. (Do not help child by pointing, moving head or eyes.)
16. Ask child: What do you do when you are cold? . .hungry? . .tired? Pass 2 of 3.
17. Tell child to: Put block <u>on</u> table; <u>under</u> table; <u>in front</u> of chair, <u>behind</u> chair. Pass 3 of 4. (Do not help child by pointing, moving head or eyes.)
18. As child: If fire is hot, ice is ?; Mother is a woman, Dad is a ?; a horse is big, a mouse is ?. Pass 2 of 3.
19. Ask child: What is a ball? . .lake? . .desk? . .house? . .banana? . .curtain? . .ceiling? . .hedge? . .pavement? Pass if defined in terms of use, shape, what it is made of or general category (such as banana is fruit, not just yellow). Pass 6 of 9.
20. Ask child: What is a spoon made of? . .a shoe made of? . .a door made of? (No other objects may be substituted.) Pass 3 of 3.
21. When placed on stomach, child lifts chest off table with support of forearms and/or hands.
22. When child is on back, grasp his hands and pull him to sitting. Pass if head does not hang back.
23. Child may use wall or rail only, not person. May not crawl.
24. Child must throw ball overhand 3 feet to within arm's reach of tester.
25. Child must perform standing broad jump over width of test sheet. (8½ inches)
26. Tell child to walk forward,   ⚭⚭⚭➤   heel within 1 inch of toe. Tester may demonstrate. Child must walk 4 consecutive steps, 2 out of 3 trials.
27. Bounce ball to child who should stand 3 feet away from tester. Child must catch ball with hands, not arms, 2 out of 3 trials.
28. Tell child to walk backward,   ◄⚭⚭⚭⚭   toe within 1 inch of heel. Tester may demonstrate. Child must walk 4 consecutive steps, 2 out of 3 trials.

<u>DATE AND BEHAVIORAL OBSERVATIONS</u> (how child feels at time of test, relation to tester, attention span, verbal behavior, self-confidence, etc,):

Appendix C: Developmental Assessment by Interview

A method has been developed of evaluation by utilizing an interview technique asking parents a list of questions regarding milestones in achievements which most will remember. Developed by Drs. Capute and Biehl, it has been very successful in its use at the John F. Kennedy Institute for the Habilitation of Handicapped Children at Johns Hopkins Hospital.

Age	Gross Motor	Fine Motor	Language	Social
3 mo.	A. Does he support himself on forearms when lying? B. Does he hold his head up steadily while on his stomach?	A. Are his hands usually open at rest? B. Does he pull at his clothing?	A. Does he laugh or make happy noises? B. Does he turn his head to sounds?	A. Does he smile at you? B. Does he reach for familiar people or objects?
6 mo.	A. Does he lift his head when lying on his back? B. Does he roll from back to front?	A. Does he transfer a toy from one hand to the other? B. Does he pick up small objects?	A. Does he "babble," repeat sounds together (i.e., mum-mum-mum)? B. Is he frightened by angry noise?	A. Does he stretch his arms out to be picked up? B. Does he show his likes and dislikes?
9 mo.	A. Does he sit for long periods without support? B. Does he pull up on furniture?	A. Does he pick up objects with his thumb and one finger? B. Does he finger-feed any foods?	A. Does he understand "no-no," "bye-bye"? B. Will he imitate any sounds or words if you make them first?	A. Does he hold his own bottle? B. Does he play any nursery games ("peek-a-boo," "bye-bye")?
12 mo.	A. Is he walking (alone or with hand held)? B. Does he pivot when sitting?	A. Does he throw toys (objects)? B. Does he give you toys (let go) easily?	A. Does he have at least one meaningful word other than "mama," "dada"? B. Does he shake his head for "no"?	A. Does he cooperate in dressing? B. Does he come when you call him?
18 mo.	A. Does he walk upstairs with help? B. Can he throw a toy while standing without falling?	A. Does he turn book pages (2 or 3 at a time)? B. Does he fill spoon and feed self?	A. Does he have at least 6 real words besides his "jargon"? B. Does he point at what he wants?	A. Does he copy you in routine tasks (sweeping, dusting, etc.)? B. Does he play in the company of other children?
2 yr.	A. Does he run well without falling? B. Does he walk up and down stairs alone?	A. Does he turn book pages one at a time? B. Does he remove his own shoes, pants?	A. Does he talk in short (2–3 word) sentences? B. Does he use pronouns ("me," "you," "mine")?	A. Does he ask to be taken to the toilet? B. Does he play in company of other children?
2½ yr.	A. Does he jump, getting both feet off the floor? B. Does he throw a ball overhand?	A. Does he unbutton any buttons? B. Does he hold a pencil or crayon adult fashion?	A. Does he use plurals or past tense? B. Does he use the word "I" correctly most of the time?	A. Does he tell his first and last name if asked? B. Does he get himself a drink without help?
3 yr.	A. Does he pedal a tricycle? B. Does he alternate feet (one stair per step) going upstairs?	A. Does he dry his hands (if reminded)? B. Does he dress and undress fully including front buttons?	A. Does he tell little stories about his experiences? B. Does he know his sex?	A. Does he share his toys? B. Does he play well with another child? Take turns?
4 yr.	A. Does he attempt to hop or skip? B. Does he alternate feet going downstairs?	A. Does he button clothes fully? B. Does he catch a ball?	A. Does he say a song or a poem from memory? B. Does he know all his colors?	A. Does he tell "tall tales" or "show off"? B. Does he play cooperatively with a small group of children?
5 yr.	A. Does he skip, alternating feet? B. Does he jump rope or jump over low obstacles?	A. Does he tie his own shoes? B. Does he spread with a knife?	A. Can he print his first name? B. Does he ever ask what a word means?	A. Is he a "mother's helper"—likes to do things for you? B. Does he play competitive games and abide by the rules?

Pediatric Health Maintenance

Growth and Development

Reflexes of the Newborn

1. *Pupillary reflexes*—ipsilateral (pertaining to the same side) constriction to light.
2. *Rooting*—when corner of mouth is touched and object is moved toward cheek, infant will turn head toward object and open mouth.
3. *Palmar grasp*—pressure on palm of hand will elicit grasp.
4. *Plantar grasp*—pressure on the sole of foot behind toes will cause flexion of toes.
5. *Tonic neck reflex*—sudden jolt will cause head to turn to one side with leg and arm on that side extended, while the extremities on the other side flex.
6. *Neck righting*—when head is turned to one side, the shoulder and trunk, followed by the pelvis, will turn to that side.
7. *Moro reflex*—response to sudden loud noise, causing body to stiffen and arms to go up and out, then forward and toward each other. Thumb and index finger will assume C-shape.
8. *Positive-supporting reflex*—when held in an erect position, baby will stiffen lower extremities and support his weight.
9. *Babinski's sign*—scratching sole of foot causes great toe to flex and toes to fan.
10. *Crossed extensor reflex*—when one leg is extended and the knee is held straight, while the sole of foot is stimulated, the opposite leg will flex.
11. *Landau's sign*—when baby is suspended horizontally with head depressed against trunk and neck flexed, legs will flex and be drawn up to trunk.
12. *Optical blink reflex*—when light is suddenly shone into open eyes, the eyes will close quickly with a quick dorsal flexion of head.
13. *Auditory blink reflex*—eyes quickly close if examiner loudly claps her hands about 30 cm. (11.5 inches) from infant's head.
14. *Recoil of arm*—when both arms are extended simultaneously by pulling outward grasping wrists, both arms will flex at elbows when released.
15. *Withdrawal reflex*—pricking sole of foot will result in the baby's leg being flexed at hip, knee, and ankle.
16. *Stepping reflex*—when infant is held upright with dorsum of foot gently touching edge of table, he will bend his hips and knees and put foot on table. This will elicit stepping response in the opposite foot. Series of alternating stepping actions will result when infant is moved forward so that 1 foot at a time touches the firm surface.
17. *Parachute reflex*—while the infant is held prone and lowered quickly toward a surface, he will extend arms and legs.
18. *Side-turning*—placing baby prone with head in midline will elicit the baby's turning his head to the side.
19. Other characteristics of the newborn:
    a. Cries
    b. Sucks
    c. Has extremely sensitive skin
    d. Makes discriminating sounds
    e. Sleeps for long intervals
    f. Has little head control (head lag)

Infant to Adolescent

See table on pages 1074–1087.

Childhood Diseases

See table on pages 1088–1094.

Nutrition of Pediatric Patients

See table on pages 1094–1100.

Infant to Adolescent: Growth and Development

Age and Physical Characteristics	Behavior Patterns	Nursing Implications/ Parental Guidance
Birth–4 weeks (1 month)	*Motor Development* Momentary visual fixation on objects and adult face. Eyes follow bright moving objects.	*Play Stimulation* Use human face—smile and talk. Dangle bright and moving object in field of vision (mobile).

Age and Physical Characteristics	Behavior Patterns	Nursing Implications/ Parental Guidance
	Lies awake on back with head averted. Immediately drops objects placed in hands. Responds to sounds of bell and other similar noises. Keeps hands fisted.	Hold, touch, caress, fondle, kiss. Rock, pat, change position. Play soft music or have infant listen to ticking clock, sing. Talk to infant, call him by name.
	Socialization and Vocalization Mews and makes throaty noises. Shows interest in human face. *Cognitive and Emotional Development* Reflexive. External stimuli are meaningless. Responses are generally limited to tension states or discomfort. Gains satisfaction from feeding and being held, rocked, fondled, and cuddled. Has an intense need for sucking pleasure. Quiets when picked up.	*Parental Guidance* Begin to expose infant to different household sounds. Change crib location in room. Use bright-colored clothing and linen. Keep infant nearby. Allow him to sleep. Play with him when he is awake. Hold him during feeding.
8 weeks (2 months) Crossed extensor reflex disappears.	*Motor Development* Reflexive behavior is slowly being replaced by voluntary movements. Turns from side to back. Begins to lift head momentarily from prone position. Shows eye coordination to light and objects. If bell is sounded near him, he will stop activity and listen. Eyes follow better, both vertically and horizontally. Focuses well.	*Play Stimulation* Arrange mobile over crib so infant's movement will set it in motion. Hang wind chimes near infant. Hang bright-colored pictures on wall (yellow and red-colored stripes, for example). Use cradle gym and infant seat. Use rattles. Hold infant and walk around room. Allow freedom of kicking with clothes off.
	Socialization and Vocalization Begins vocalization—coos, especially to a voice. Crying becomes differentiated. Visually looks for sounds. May squeal with delight when stimulated by touching, talking, or singing. Begins social smile. Eyes follow person or object more intently. *Cognitive and Emotional Development* Recognizes familiar face. Becomes more aware and interested in environment. Anticipates being fed when in feeding position. Enjoys sucking—puts hand in mouth.	*Parental Guidance* Talk to him and smile; get excited when he coos. Place infant seat near mother's activities but where he cannot fall off or tip over. Put in prone position in bed or on floor. Expose infant to different textures. Exercise infant's arms and legs. Sing to infant. Provide tactile experience during bathing, diapering, feeding. First DTP and TOPV immunization should be given.
12 weeks (3 months) Landau reflex appears at 3–4 months; stepping reflex disappears.	*Motor Development* When prone, he will rest on forearms and keep head in midline—makes crawling move-	*Play Stimulation* Encourage socialization, smiling, laughing. Place on mat on floor.

(continued)

Age and Physical Characteristics	Behavior Patterns	Nursing Implications/ Parental Guidance
	ments with legs, arches back, and holds head high, he may get chest off surface.	Continue to introduce new sounds.
Positive support reflex disappears. Posterior fontanelle closes.	Indicates preference for prone or supine position. Discovers hands—strikes at objects while watching hands. Holds objects in hands and brings to mouth. Has fairly good head control.	*Parental Guidance* Take on daily outing as weather permits. Bounce on bed. Play with infant during feeding. Rattles can be used effectively for visual following and for hand play.
	Socialization and Vocalization Smiles more readily. Babbles and coos. Stops crying when mother enters room or when he is caressed. Enjoys playing during feeding. Stays awake longer without crying. Turns head to follow familiar person.	
	Cognitive and Emotional Development Shows active interest in environment. Recognizes familiar faces and objects. Focuses and follows objects. Shows repetitiveness in play activity. Is aware of strange situations. Derives pleasure from sucking— purposefully gets hand to mouth. Begins to establish routine preceding sleep.	
16 weeks (4 months) Stepping reflex disappears. Rooting reflex disappears. By 4–5 months infant's weight approximately doubles birth weight. Birth to 6 months Average weekly weight gain, 140–200 gm. (4–7 ounces). Average monthly height gain, 2.5 cm. (1 inch). End of first year weighs three times birth weight. Pulse rate slows to 100–140 Respirations, 20–40/minute	*Motor Development* Eyes focus on small objects; he may pick a dangling ring. Holds head up (when being pulled to sitting position). Becomes more interested in environment. Hand comes to meet rattle. Listens—turns head to familiar sound. Sits with minimal support. Intentional rolling over, back to side. Reaches for offered objects. Grasps objects with both hands, and everything goes into mouth.	*Play Stimulation* Encourage mirror play. Provide soft squeeze toys in vivid colors of varying texture. Allow infant to splash in bath. Infant still enjoys holding and playing with rattles. Enjoys old-fashioned clothespins and playing pat-a-cake, peek-a-boo.
	Socialization and Vocalization Laughs and chuckles socially. Demands social attention by fussing. Recognizes mother. Begins to respond to "No, no." Enjoys being propped in sitting position.	*Parental Guidance* Be certain button eyes on toys and other small objects cannot be pulled off. Hold rattle for him and let him reach and grasp it. When baby is in highchair, strap in. Let him play with food; give finger foods. Move mobile out of reach—he may grab it and cause injury. Repeat child's sounds to him. Talk in varying degrees of loudness. Begin looking at and naming pictures in book. Begin roughhousing play by both parents.
	Cognitive and Emotional Development Actively interested in environment. Enjoys attention; becomes bored	

Age and Physical Characteristics	Behavior Patterns	Nursing Implications/ Parental Guidance
	when alone for long periods of time. Recognizes bottle. More interested in mother. Indicates increasing trust and security. Sleeps through night; has defined nap time.	Second DTP and TOPV immunization should be given. Give space in playpen or on sheet on floor to practice rolling over.
26 weeks (7 months) By 5–6 months, tonic neck reflex disappears. By 6–7 months, palmar grasp disappears. By 7–9 months, develops eye-to-eye contact while talking; engages in social games. 2 central lower incisors erupt.	*Motor Development* Shows momentary sitting, with hand support. Bounces and bears some weight when held in standing position. Transfers and mouths objects in one hand. Discovers feet. Bangs objects together. Rolls over well. May begin some form of mobility. *Socialization and Vocalization* Discriminates between strangers and familiar figures. Crows and squeals. Starts to say "Ma," "Da." Self-play is self-contained. Laughs out loud. Makes "talking" sounds in response to others' talking. Begins fear of strangers, 8½–10 months *Cognitive and Emotional Development* Secures objects by pulling on string. Searches for lost objects that are out of sight. Inspects objects; localizes sounds. Likes to sit in highchair. Drops and picks up objects. Displays exploratory behavior with food. Exhibits beginning fear of strangers. Becomes fretful when mother leaves. Shows much mouthing and biting.	*Play Stimulation* Enjoys social games, hide-and-seek with adult, toys, large blocks. Likes to bang objects. Plays in bounce chair, walker. Enjoys large nesting toys (round rather than square). Likes to drop and retrieve things. Likes metal cups, wooden spoons, and things to bang with. Loves crumpled paper. Enjoys squeeze toys in bath. Likes peek-a-boo, bye-bye, and pat-a-cake. *Parental Guidance* Will play as long as you can. Tie toys to chair with short string. Let play with extra spoon at feeding. Give soft finger foods. Since infant puts everything in mouth, *use safety precautions.* Keep small items away from him; he could choke on them. Show excitement at his achievements. Supply kitchen items for toys. Third DTP and TOPV immunization at 6 months.
40 weeks (10 months) 4 upper incisors erupt around 7–9 months. By 9–12 months, plantar reflex disappears. By 9–12 months, neck-righting reflex disappears. 6–12 months Average weekly weight gain, 85–140 gm. (3–5 ounces). Average monthly height gain, 1.25 cm. (½ inch).	*Motor Development* Sits without support. Recovers balance. Manipulates objects with hands. Unwraps objects. Creeps. Pulls self upright at crib rails. Uses index finger and thumb to hold objects. Rings a bell. Can feed himself a cracker and can hold bottle. Can control lips around cup. Does not like supine position. Can hold index finger and thumb in opposition.	*Play Stimulation* Encourage use of motion toys—rocking horse, stroller. Water play. Imitate animal sounds. Allow exploration outdoors. Provide for learning by imitation. Offer new objects (blocks). Child likes freedom of creeping and walking, but closeness of family is important. Good toys: milk carton; bean bag for tossing; fabric books; things to move around, fill up, empty out; pile-up and knock-down toys.

(continued)

Age and Physical Characteristics	Behavior Patterns	Nursing Implications/ Parental Guidance
	Socialization and Verbalization Claps hands on request. Responds to own name. Is very aware of social environment. Imitates gestures, facial expressions, and sounds. Smiles at image in mirror. Offers toy to adult, but does not release it. Begins to test parental reaction during feeding and at bedtime. Will entertain self for long periods of time. *Cognitive and Emotional Development* Begins to imitate. Shows more interest in picture books. Enjoys achievements. Has strong urge toward independence—locomotion, feeding, dressing.	*Parental Guidance* Do things with him. Protect him from dangerous objects—cover electrical outlets, block stairs, remove breakable objects from tables. Use plastic bottle. Have child with family at mealtime. Offer cup.
12 months (1 year) By 12–18 months, Babinski sign disappears. By 12–24 months, Landau reflex disappears. By 10–14 months, anterior fontanelle closes. Weight should approximately triple birth weight. 2 lower lateral incisors appear. 4 first molars appear by 14 months. *Child Development Theories* Freudian: Behavior Birth–1 year—Oral Stage Eriksonian: Emotion/Personality Birth–1 year—Sense of Trust vs. Mistrust Piagetian: Intellectual Activity (Thought Process) Birth–2 years—Sensorimotor Period	*Motor Development* Cruises around furniture. Beginning to stand alone and toddle. Turns pages in book. Tries tossing object. Shows hand dominance. Navigates stairs; climbs on chairs. Builds a tower of 2 blocks. Puts balls in box. May use spoon. Can release objects at will. Has regular bowel movements. *Socialization and Verbalization* Uses jargon. Points to indicate wants. Loves give-and-take game. Responds to music. Enjoys being center of attention and will repeat laughed-at activities. *Cognitive and Emotional Development* Shows fear, anger, affection, jealousy, anxiety, and sympathy. Experiments to reach new goals. Displays intense determination to remove barriers to action. Begins to develop concepts of space, time, and causality. Has increased attention span.	*Play Stimulation* Ball play Cloth doll Motion objects and toys Transporting objects Name and point to body parts. "Put-in" and "take-out" toys Sand box with spoons and other similar objects. Blocks Music *Parental Guidance* Allow self-directed play rather than adult-directed play. Continue to expose to foods of different textures, taste, smell, substance. Offer cup. Show affection and encourage child to return affection. Tuberculin test as well as measles, mumps, and rubella immunization should be given at 15 months.
18 months NOTE: Between 1 and 3 years the child is called a "toddler." Anterior fontanelle closed. Abdomen protrudes, arms and legs lengthen.	*Motor Development* Walks up stairs with help, creeps downstairs. Walks without support and with balance. Falls less frequently.	*Play Stimulation* Allow unrestricted motor activity (within safety limits). Offer push-pull toys. Child selects favorite toy. Child likes blocks, pyramid toys, teddy bears, dolls, pots and pans,

Age and Physical Characteristics	Behavior Patterns	Nursing Implications/ Parental Guidance
Big muscles become well developed. 4 cuspids appear by 18 months. Fine muscle coordination begins to develop. Toddler Average yearly weight gain, 2–3 kg. (4½–6½ lbs.). Average height gain during second year, 12 cm. (4¾ inches).	Throws ball. Stoops to pick up toys, look at bug. Turns pages of book. Holds and lifts cup. Builds 3-block tower. Picks up and places small beads in container. Begins to use spoon. *Cognitive and Emotional Development* Has vocabulary of 10 words that have meanings. Uses phrases, imitates words. Points to objects named by adult. Follows directions and requests. Imitates adult behavior. Retrieves toy from several hiding places. Is beginning to develop symbolic thought. *Psychosocial Development* Develops new awareness of strangers. Wants to explore everything in reach. Plays alone, but near others. Is dependent upon parents, but begins to reach out for autonomy. Finds security in a blanket, toy, or thumbsucking.	cloth picture books with colorful large pictures, telephone, musical top, nested blocks. *Parental Guidance* Begin to teach tooth brushing to establish good dental habits. Safety teaching: Child gets into everything within his reach. Place medications in safe, locked place. Create a safe environment for child. DTP and TOPV booster immunization. Limits need to be set that give toddler sense of security, yet encourage exploration. Identify behavior changes common in toddler.
2 years Protruding abdomen less noticeable. Landau reflex disappears. During first 2 years 35 cm. (14–15 inches) are added to height.	*Motor Development* Walks up and down stairs. Opens doors; turns knobs. Has steady gait. Holds drinking cup well with 1 hand. Uses spoon without spilling food (may prefer fingers). Kicks a ball in front of him without support. Builds a tower of 4–6 blocks. Scribbles. Rides tricycle or kiddie car (without pedals). *Cognitive Development* Has 200–300 words in vocabulary. Begins to use short sentences. Refers to self by pronoun. Obeys simple commands. Does not know right from wrong. Begins to learn about time sequences. *Psychosocial Development* Uses word "mine" constantly. Is possessive with toys. Displays negativism—uses "no" as assertion of self. Routine and rituals are important. Begins cooperation in toilet training.	*Play Stimulation* Shows parallel play, although he enjoys having other children around him. Has very short attention span. Enjoys same toys as child of 18 months. Likes doll play, ball. Imitates parents in domestic activities. Likes swing, hammering, paper, large crayons. *Parental Guidance* Has need for peer companionship, although he displays his immaturity by his inability to share and take turns. A decrease in appetite normally occurs at this stage. Toilet training should be started (each child follows his own pattern). Begin to have child eat his meals with family if he has not already done so. Begin to read to child; child likes storybooks with large pictures.

(continued)

Age and Physical Characteristics	Behavior Patterns	Nursing Implications/ Parental Guidance
	Resists restrictions on freedom. Has fear of parents' leaving. Shows parallel play. Dawdles. Resists bedtime—uses transitional objects (blanket, toy). Vacillates between dependence and independence.	
2–3 years Height approximates half his adult height. Legs are about 34% of body length. Begins 2+ kg (5 lbs.) weight gain per year until 5 years old. At 2½ years has full set (20) of baby teeth. 4 second molars appear by 2½ years. Height gain, 6–8 cm. (2⅜–3¼ inches). Lordosis and protuberant abdomen of toddler disappear.	*Motor Development* Throws objects overhead. Pedals tricycle. Walks backward. Washes and dries hands. Begins to use scissors. Can string large beads. Can undress himself. Feeds himself well. Tries to dance. Jumps in place. Builds tower of 8 blocks. Balances on one foot. Swings and climbs. Can eat an ice cream cone. Drinks from a straw. Chews gum without swallowing it. *Cognitive Development* Shows increased attention span. Gives first and last name. Begins to ask "why." Is egocentric in thought and behavior. Beginning ability to reflect on own behavior. Talks in short sentences. Uses plurals. May attempt to sing simple songs. Has vocabulary of 900 words. Begins fantasy. Begins to understand what it means to take turns. Can repeat 3 numbers. Shows interest in colors.	*Play Stimulation* Plays simple games with other children. Enjoys story-telling and dress-up play. Plays "house." Colors. Uses scissors and paper. Rides tricycle. Read simple books to him. Will assist in developing memory skills, visual discrimination skills, and language. *Parental Guidance* From 2–3 years, the child develops a seeming maturity; do not expect more of him than he is able to do. Arrange first visit to the dentist to have teeth checked. Be aware that negativistic and ritualistic behavior is normal. Be consistent in discipline. Control temper tantrums. Begin to teach traffic safety. Supervise outdoor play.
Child Development Theories Freudian: 1–3 years—Anal Stage Eriksonian: 1–3 years—Sense of Autonomy vs. Shame and Doubt Piagetian: 2–7 years—Preoperational Period; shows egocentrism and centering	*Psychosocial Development* Negativism grows out of child's sense of developing independence—says "no" to every command. Ritualism is important to toddler for his security (follows certain pattern, especially at bedtime). Temper tantrums may result from toddler's frustration in wanting to do everything himself. Shows parallel play as well as beginning interaction with others. Engages in associative play. Fears become pronounced. Continues to react to separation from parents but shows increasing ability to handle short periods of separation.	

Age and Physical Characteristics	Behavior Patterns	Nursing Implications/ Parental Guidance
	Has daytime bladder control and is beginning to develop nighttime bladder control. Becomes more independent. Begins to identify sex (gender) roles. Explores environment outside the home. Can create different ways of getting desired outcome.	
3–4 years NOTE: Between 3 and 5 years, the child is called a "pre-schooler."	*Motor Development* Drawings have form and meaning, not detail. Copies a circle and a cross. Buttons front and side of clothes. Laces shoes. Bathes self, but needs direction. Brushes teeth. Shows continuous movement going up and down stairs. Climbs and jumps well. Attempts to print letters. *Cognitive Developments* Awareness of body is more stable; child becomes more aware of own vulnerability. Is less negativistic. Learns some number concepts. Begins naming colors. Can identify longer of 2 lines. Has vocabulary of 1,500 words. Uses mild profanities and name-calling. Uses language aggressively. Asks many questions. Can be given simple explanation as to cause and effect. Thinks very concretely; demonstrates irreversibility of thought. Has beginning understanding of past and future. Is egocentric in thought. *Psychosocial Development* Is more active with peers and engages in cooperative play. Performs simple tasks. Frequently has imaginary companion. Dramatizes experiences. Is proud of accomplishments. Exaggerates, boasts, and tattles on others. Can tolerate separation from mother longer without feeling anxiety. Is keen observer. Has good sense of "mine" and "yours." Behavior still frequently ritualistic. Becomes curious about life and sex. Often indulges in masturbation.	*Plays Stimulation* Plays and interacts with other children. Shows creativity. Likes ring-around-the-rosy. "Helps" adults. Likes costumes and enjoys dramatic play. Toys and games: record player, nursery rhymes, housekeeping toys, transportation toys (tricycle, trucks, cars, wagon), blocks, hammer and peg bench, floor trains, blackboard and chalk, easel and brushes, clay, crayon and finger paints, outside toys (sandbox, swing, small slide), books (short stories, action stories), drum, scrapbook. *Parental Guidance* Base your expectations within child's limitations. Provide limited frustrations from environment to assist him in coping. Give small errands to do around the house (putting silverware on table, drying a dish). Expand child's world with trips to the zoo, to the supermarket, to restaurant, etc. Prevent accidents. Provide for brief, nonthreatening separation from parents and home. Reinforce correct use of language. Utilize opportunities for simple sexual education as child's needs arise. Accept masturbation as a normal phenomenon to be discouraged in public. Provide consistent discipline, motivated by love not anger. Prepare child for nursery school.

(continued)

Age and Physical Characteristics	Behavior Patterns	Nursing Implications/ Parental Guidance

4–5 years
By 2–5 years adds 25 cm. (9–10 inches) to height.
At age 4, legs comprise about 44% of body length.
 	
Child Development Theories
Freudian:
   3–6 years—Phallic Stage
Eriksonian:
   3–6 years—Sense of Initiative vs. Guilt
Piagetian:
   2–7 years—Preoperational Period; shows egocentrism and centering
	Motor Development
	Hops 2 or more times.
	Dresses without supervision.
	Has good motor control—climbs and jumps well.
	Walks up stairs without grasping handrail.
	Walks backwards.
	Washes self without wetting clothes.
	Prints first name and other words.
	Adds 3 or more details in drawings.
	Draws a square.
	
	Cognitive Development
	Has 2,100-word vocabulary.
	Talks constantly.
	Uses adult speech forms.
	Participates in conversations.
	Asks for definitions.
	Knows age and residence.
	Identifies heavier of two objects.
	Knows weeks as time units.
	Names days of week.
	Begins to understand kinship.
	Knows primary colors.
	Can count to 10.
	Can copy a triangle.
	Has high degree of imagination.
	Questioning is at a peak.
	Begins to develop power of reasoning.
	
	Psychosocial Developments
	May have an imaginary companion.
	Has a sense of order (likes to finish what he has started).
	Is obedient and reliable.
	Is protective toward younger children.
	Begins to develop an elementary conscience with some influence in governing his behavior.
	Has increased self-confidence.
	Accepts responsibility for acts.
	Is less rebellious.
	Has dreams and nightmares.
	Is cooperative and sympathetic.
	Shows generosity with toys.
	Begins to question parents' thinking.
	Identifies strongly with parent of same sex.
		Play Stimulation
		Demonstrates gross motor activity—likes to jump rope, skip, climb on jungle gyms, etc.
		Prefers group play and cooperates in projects.
		Plays simple letter, number, form, and picture games.
		Plays with cars and trucks.
		Still likes being read to.
		Continues to enjoy fantasy play.
		
		Parental Guidance
		Child no longer takes an afternoon nap.
		Prepare child for kindergarten.
		Tell him stories.
		Provide opportunities and reassurance for group play; have his friends visit for lunch and an afternoon of playing.
		Prevent accidents.
		Between 4 and 6 years DTP and TOPV booster immunizations are needed.
		Encourage child's participation in household activities.

Middle Childhood (5–9 years)
Growth rate is slow and steady.
Child gains an average of 3.18 kg. (7 lbs.) per year. Height increases approximately 6.25 cm. (2½ inches) per year.
Among children there is considerable variation in height and weight.
Child appears taller and slimmer.
	Motor Development
	6 years
	   Is active and impulsive.
	   Balance improves.
	   Uses hands as manipulative tools in cutting, pasting, hammering.
	   Can draw large letters or figures.
	7 years
	   Has lower activity level.
	   Capable of fine hand movements; can print sentences.
		Family atmosphere continues to have impact on child's emotional development and his future response within the family.
		The child needs ongoing guidance in an open, inviting atmosphere. Limits should be set with conviction. Deal with only one incident at a time. When punishment is

Age and Physical Characteristics	Behavior Patterns	Nursing Implications/ Parental Guidance

Early lordosis disappears.
Child begins to lose baby teeth; permanent teeth appear at a rate of about 4 teeth per year from 7–14 years.
Neuromuscular and skeletal development allows improved coordination.
Eyes become fully developed; vision approaches 20/20.
 	
Child Development Theories
Freudian:
    5–9 years—Beginning of Latency Period
Eriksonian:
    5–9 years—Industry vs. Inferiority
Piagetian:
    5–9 years—Enters stage of concrete operations
	Nervous habits such as nail biting are common.
	Muscular skills such as ball throwing have improved.
	8 years
	  Moves with less restlessness.
	  Has developed grace and balance, even in active sports.
	  Has developed coordination of fine muscles, allowing him to write in script.
	9 years
	  Uses both hands independently.
	  Has become skillful in manual activities because of improved eye–hand coordination.
	
	Cognitive Development
	6 years
	  Begins to learn to read. Defines objects in terms of use. Time sense is as much in past as present.
	  Is interested in relationship between home and neighborhood; knows some streets.
	  Uses sentences well; uses language to share others' experiences; may swear or use slang.
	  Distinguishes morning from afternoon.
	7 years
	  More reflective and has deeper understanding of meanings.
	  Interested in conclusions and logical endings. Begins to have scientific interests in cause and effect.
	  More responsible in relation to time, is more punctual. Sense of space is more realistic; child wants some space of own.
	  Knows value of coins.
	8 years
	  Thinking is less animistic. Is aware of impersonal forces of nature. Begins to understand logical reasoning, conclusions, implications.
	  Less self-centered in thinking. Personal space is expanding; goes places on own. Aware of time; plans events of day. Understands right from left.
	9 years
	  Intellectually energetic and curious. Realistic; reasonable in
		necessary, the child should not be humiliated. He should know that it was the *act* that the adult found undesirable, not the child.
		
		Needs assistance in adjusting to new experiences and demands of school. Should be able to share experiences with family. Parents need to have communication with the teacher in order to work together for the health of the child.
		Convey love and caring in communication. The child understands language directed at feelings better than at intellect. Get down to eye level with the child.
		Focus attention on child's abilities and accomplishments rather than his shortcomings and limitations.
		
		Child is sex-conscious. He should be able to discuss his questions at home rather than with his friends. Requires simple, honest answers to questions.
		Common problems include teasing, quarreling, nail-biting, enuresis, whining, poor manners, swearing. These are usually fleeting phases and should not be handled negatively. The causes for such behavior should be investigated and dealt with constructively.
		The child needs order and consistency in his life to help him cope with doubts, fears, unacceptable impulses, and unfamiliar experiences.
		Encourage peer activities as well as home responsibilities and give recognition to child's accomplishments and unique talents.
		Television may stimulate learning in several spheres, but should be monitored.
		Accidents are a major cause of disability and death. Safety practices should be continued. (Refer to section on safety, pp. 1104–1107.)
		Exercise is essential to promote motor and psychosocial development. The child should have a safe place to play and simple pieces of equipment.
		A school health program should be available and concerned with the child's physical, emotional, mental, and social health. This should

(continued)

Age and Physical Characteristics	Behavior Patterns	Nursing Implications/ Parental Guidance
	thinking. Able to plan in advance. Breaks complex activities into steps. Focuses on detail. Sense of space includes the entire earth. Participates in family discussions. Likes to have secrets.	be augmented by information and example at home. Medical supervision should continue with yearly examination to detect developmental delay, disease. Appropriate immunizations should be administered. Child frequently has "quiet days"— periods of shyness, which should be tolerated as part of growing up and deciding who he is. Child may be subject to nightmares, a situation which requires reassurance and understanding.
	Psychosocial Development (The following characteristics apply to the child in the 5–9-year group.) Still requires parental support, but pulls away from overt signs of affection. Peer groups provide companionship in widening circle of persons outside the home. Child learns more about self as he learns about others. "Chum" stage occurs at about 9–10 years of age. Child chooses a special friend of same sex and age in whom to confide. This is usually child's first love relationship outside of home, when someone becomes as important to him as himself. Play teaches the child new ideas and independence. He progressively utilizes tools of competition, compromise, cooperation, and beginning collaboration. Body image and self-concept are quite fluid because of rapid physical, emotional, social changes. Latency-stage sexual drive is controlled and repressed. Emphasis is on the development of skills and talent.	Parents, teachers, and health professionals should be available and able to provide information and answer questions about the physical changes which occur.
	Patterns of Play 6–7 years Child acts out ideas of family and occupational groups with which he has contact. Painting, pasting, reading, simple games, watching television, digging, running games, skating, riding bicycle, and swimming, are all enjoyed activities. 8 years Child enjoys collections; loosely formed, short-lived clubs; table games; card games; books; television; records.	

Age and Physical Characteristics	Behavior Patterns	Nursing Implications/ Parental Guidance
Late Childhood (9–12 years) Vital signs approach adult values. Loses childish appearance of face and takes on features that will characterize him as an adult. Growth spurt occurs, and some secondary sex characteristics appear: in females, at age 10–12 years; in males, at age 12–14 years. Physical changes of puberty: Increased height and weight, increased perspiration and activity of sebaceous glands; vasomotor instability; increased fat deposition. Physical changes in female: Pelvis increases in transverse diameter; hips broaden; tenderness in developing breast tissue; enlargement of areola diameter; appearance of pubic hair. Physical changes in male: Size of testes increases; scrotum color changes; breasts enlarge, temporarily; height and shoulder breadth increase. Appearance of lightly pigmented hair at base of penis. Increase in length and width of penis. *Child Development Theories* Freudian: 9–12 years—Latency period continues Eriksonian: 9–12 years—Industry vs. Inferiority continues Piagetian: 9–12 years—Stage of concrete operations continues	*Motor Development* Energetic, restless, active movements such as finger-drumming or foot-tapping appear. Has skillful manipulative movements nearly equal to those of adults. Works hard to perfect physical skills. *Cognitive Development* 10 years Likes to reason, enjoys learning. Thinking is concrete, matter of fact. Wants to measure up to challenge. Likes to memorize, identify facts. Attention span may be short. Space is rather specific (i.e., where things are). Can write for relatively long time with speed. 11 years Likes action in learning. Concentrates well when working competitively. Can understand relational terms such as weight and size. Perceives space as nothingness that goes on forever. Able to discuss problems. Can describe some abstract terms. 12 years Enjoys learning. Considers all aspects of a situation. Motivated more by inner drive than by competition. Able to classify, arrange, generalize. Likes to discuss and debate. Begins conceptual thinking. Verbal, formal reasoning now possible. Can recognize moral of a story. Defines time as duration; likes to plan ahead. Understands that space is abstract. Can be critical of own work. *Psychosocial Development* Gang becomes important, and gang code takes precedence over nearly everything. Often gang codes are characterized by collective action against the mores of the adult world. Here, children begin to work out own social patterns without adult interference. Early gangs may include both sexes; later gangs are separated by sex. May strive for unreasonable independence from adult control.	Continue appropriate nursing interventions related to early childhood. Continue sex education and preparation for adolescent body changes. Understanding is important. Encourage participation in organized clubs, youth groups. Democratic guidance is essential as child works through a conflict between dependence (on his parents) and independence. Child needs realistic limits set. Needs help channeling energy in proper direction—work and sports. Requires adequate explanation of body changes. Special understanding required for the child who lags in physical development. Continue consistent disciplinary style.

(continued)

Age and Physical Characteristics	Behavior Patterns	Nursing Implications/ Parental Guidance
	Often interested in religion, morality. Has increased interest in sexuality. May reach puberty; resurgence of sexual drives causes recapitulation of oedipal struggle. *Patterns of Play* Continues to enjoy reading, T.V., table games. More interested in active sports as a means to improve skills. Creative talents may appear; may enjoy drawing, modeling clay. By age 10, sex differences in play become profound. Occasional privacy is important. Begins to have vocational aspirations.	
Early Adolescence (females: 12–14 years; males: 14–18 years) Phase of development begins when reproductive organs become functionally operative; phase ends when physical growth is completed. Skeletal system grows faster than supporting muscles. Hands and feet grow proportionally faster than rest of body. Large muscles develop more quickly than small muscles. Females: Physical changes include appearance of menarche; growth of axillary and perineal hair; deepened voice; ovulation; further development of breasts. Male: Physical changes include growth of axillary, perineal, facial, chest hair; deepening of voice; production of spermatozoa; nocturnal emissions. *Child Development Theories* Freudian: 12–14 years—Begins stage of sexuality Eriksonian: 12–14 years—Identity vs. Role Diffusion Piagetian: 12–14 years—Begins stage of formal operations	*Motor Development* Often uncoordinated; has poor posture. Tires easily. *Cognitive Development* Mind has great ability to acquire and utilize knowledge. Categorizes thoughts into usable forms. May project thinking into the future. Is capable of highly imaginative thinking. *Psychosocial Development* Interest in opposite sex increases. Often revolts from adult authority to conform to peer-group standards. Continues to rework feelings for parent of opposite sex and unravel the ambivalence toward parent of same sex. Affection may turn temporarily to an adult outside of the family (for example, crush on family friend, neighbor, or teacher). Utilizes peer-group dialect—highly informal language or specially coined terminology. Peer groups are especially important and help adolescent to define own identity, to adapt to changing body image, to establish more mature relationships with others, and to deal with heightened sexual feelings. Cliques may develop. Dating generally progresses from groups of couples to double dates and finally single couples. Teenage "hangouts" become important centers of activity. Begins questioning existing moral values.	Stresses frequently result from conflicting value systems between generations. Parents may need help to see that the adolescent is a product of the times and that his actions reflect what is happening around him. Parents' limits and rules should be realistic and consistent. They should convey the love and concern of parents and should be a source of comfort and reassurance, protecting the child from activities for which he is not ready. The home should be an accepting, emotionally stable environment. Continue sex education, including discussion of ovulation, fertilization, menstruation, pregnancy, contraception, masturbation, nocturnal emissions, and hygiene. Adolescents have an increased need for rest and sleep, because they are expending large amounts of energy and are functioning with an inadequate oxygen supply. Recreational interests should be fostered. Favorite activities include sports, dating, reading, dancing, hobbies, and television. Talking on the telephone, listening to records are favorite pastimes. Adolescent health problems which require preventive education are accidents, obesity, acne, pregnancy, sexually transmitted disease, drug abuse. Allow adolescent to handle his own affairs as much as possible, but be aware of physical and psychosocial problems with which he will need help. Encourage independence but allow child to lean on

Age and Physical Characteristics	Behavior Patterns	Nursing Implications/ Parental Guidance
		parents for support when frightened or unable to attain his goals.
		Adolescents with special problems should have access to specialists such as adolescent clinics, and psychologists.
		Requires reassurance and help in accepting his changing body image. Parents should make the most of his positive qualities.
		Give gentle encouragement and guidance regarding dating. Avoid strong pressures in either direction.
		Understand his conflicts as he attempts to deal with social, moral, and intellectual issues.
		Provide opportunities for adolescents to earn their own money; allow some financial independence.
		Provide safety education—especially regarding driving.
		Provide assistance to develop good attitudes toward health—smoking, drinking, drugs, nutrition, etc.
Late Adolescence Begins when physical growth is completed and extends from age 15–18 years for females and from 18–20 for males. Wisdom teeth erupt. Males: Genitals and pubic hair are adult in appearance. Physique is that of mature male. Females: Breasts and pubic hair are adult in appearance. *Child Development Theories* Freudian: 15–18 years—Stage of adult sexuality Eriksonian: 15–18 years—May begin Intimacy vs. Isolation Piagetian: 15–18 years—Stage of formal operations	*Motor Development* Energy is increased as growth spurt ends. Muscular ability and coordination increase. *Cognitive Development* Spends large amount of time in abstract and analytical thinking. Begins to develop workable philosophy of life. May accept or reject the family religion. *Psychosocial Development* Tasks include achievement of ego identity, establishment of heterosexual relationships, planning for the future and for occupational and marital choices. Dating emphasis shifts to sharing and to intimate relationship. Sexual experimentation is common in various forms—masturbation, necking, petting, intercourse. May seek alternatives to marriage— "living together," communes, etc. Ability to love becomes a major concern. Values include fidelity, friendship, cooperation. Ability to work is the culmination of the developmental life that began with play. Achieves emotional independence from parents and other adults.	Continue appropriate nursing interventions related to early adolescence. Provide guidance in selection of and preparation for a vocation. Encourage discussion regarding mate selection and alternatives to marriage. Parents themselves may require assistance facing the loss of a child once dependent on them.

Childhood Diseases

Disease: *a*. Agent. *b*. Mode of transmission. *c*. Age when most common	Incubation (*I*) and Communicability (*C*) Periods	Symptoms
Rubella (German/3-day measles) a. Rubella virus, RNA togavirus b. Droplets or direct contact with infected persons or articles freshly contaminated with nasopharyngeal secretions, feces, urine c. School age, young adult; winter, spring *Diagnostic tests:* Tissue culture of throat, blood or urine; serologic studies (hemagglutination inhibition and complement fixation) *Passive immunity:* Birth to about 1 year of age if mother is immune prior to pregnancy	*I:* 14–21 days after exposure *C:* Virus can be passed from 7 days before to 5 days after rash appears.	a. Rash—enlarged lymph nodes in postauricular, suboccipital, and cervical areas b. In adolescents—headache, anorexia, low-grade fever, sore throat, coryza, conjunctivitis, generalized malaise 1–5 days before rash appears *Duration:* 3–5 days *Rash characteristics:* Pinpoint (or larger) red spots on soft palate (Forchheimer's spots) spread to face and downward toward the feet, covering entire body at end of first day; maculopapular eruption. Rash begins to subside on 2nd day in same order
Roseola infantum (exanthema subitum) a. Presumably caused by virus. May be syndrome due to many different viruses, not specifically roseola virus. b. Transmission not known c. 6 months–2 years; late fall–early spring	*I:* 5–15 days *C:* Not known—believed not to be highly contagious	a. Fever of 40°–40.5°C. (104°–105°F.), either intermittent or sustained 3–4 days; decrease in appetite; slightly irritable b. Fever suddenly drops and rash of red measles or maculopapules 2–3 mm. appears *Duration:* 1–2 days Rash fades on pressure. It appears first on trunk and spreads upward and downward.
Rubeola (hard, red, 7-day measles) a. Measles virus, RNA-containing paramyxovirus b. Direct contact with droplets from infected persons *Diagnostic tests:* Serologic procedures *Passive immunity:* Birth to about 1 year of age if mother is immune prior to pregnancy c. School-age; spring	*I:* 10–12 days *C:* 5th day of incubation to first 5–7 days of rash	a. Fever, lethargy, cough b. 48 hours—Koplik's spots on buccal mucosa (spots are reddened areas with grayish-blue center) c. 2 days later, rash appears at hairline and spreads to feet in one day, maculopapular eruption which begins to clear after 3–4 days d. Lymphadenopathy e. Anorexia f. Pruritus
Mumps a. Mumps virus, paramyxovirus b. Urine, blood, and saliva by direct contact or droplets *Diagnostic tests:* Complement fixation; cell culture from throat, urine, spinal fluid *Passive immunity:* Birth to 3–4 months of age if mother had antibodies against mumps prior to pregnancy c. School-age	*I:* 14–21 days *C:* 5 days before to 9 days after swelling appears; virus in saliva greatest just before and after parotitis onset	a. Headache, anorexia, generalized malaise; fever 1 day before glandular swelling; fever lasts 1–6 days. b. Glandular swelling, usually of parotid c. Enlargement and reddening of Wharton's duct and Stensen's duct

Treatment	Complications	Special Considerations
Symptomatic Isolation	In adolescent and adult: Arthritis; arthralgias Encephalitis Thrombocytopenic	Exposure of nonimmune pregnant women in first trimester results in high percentage of affected fetuses and infants born with various birth defects: cataracts, heart murmur, deafness
Symptomatic—antipyretic	Convulsions due to high fever Encephalitis (rare)	
Bed rest: isolation from onset of catarrh through 3rd day of rash *Treatment of itching:* Cornstarch bath, mitt hands, application of calamine lotion to lesions, keeping fingernails trimmed	Otitis media, pneumonia, laryngitis, mastoiditis, encephalitis	

Isolation until swelling has subsided
Symptomatic
  Analgesics
  Hydration
  Alimentation
  Antipyretics
  Rest
	Meningoencephalitis
	Auditory nerve involvement, resulting in deafness
	Orchitis (if disease occurs after puberty)
		Passive Immunization (immune globulin—human)—should be administered (0.25 mg./kg.) within 5 days; when susceptible child under 1 year has known exposure; especially important when child not immunized because of contraindications.
		0.5 ml./kg. of IG for immunocompromised child, not to exceed 15 ml. of IG

(continued)

Disease: *a*. Agent. *b*. Mode of transmission. *c*. Age when most common	Incubation (*I*) and Communicability (*C*) Periods	Symptoms
Chickenpox a. Varicella-zoster b. Highly communicable; acquired via direct contact, indirect contact, droplet spread, airborne transmission c. 2–8 years *Diagnostic tests:* Scrapings from vesicle; staining reveals multinucleated giant cells *Passive immunity:* Best accomplished by varicella-zoster immune globulin	*I:* 14–21 days after exposure *C:* Onset of fever (1 day prior to first lesion) until last vesicle is dried (5–7 days)	a. General malaise and fever for 24 hours b. Rash—macules to papules and vesicles to crusts within several hours c. Itching of lesions may be severe, and scratching may cause scarring *Rash characteristics:* Rash appears first on head and mucous membranes, then becomes concentrated on body and sparse on extremities, papulovesicular eruption

Diphtheria
a. *Corynebacterium diphtheriae*
b. Acquired through secretions of carrier or infected individual by direct contact with contaminated articles and environment
c. Incidence increased in autumn and winter
Diagnostic tests: Cultures of nose and throat
	I: 2–6 days
	C: 2–4 weeks untreated; 1–2 days with antibiotic treatment
		a. Pharyngeal and tonsillar diphtheria:
		  (1) General malaise, low-grade fever, anorexia
		  (2) 1–2 days later, whitish-gray membranous patch on tonsils, soft palate, and uvula
		  (3) Lymph node swelling, fever, rapid pulse
		b. Nasal diphtheria:
		  (1) Coryza with increasing viscosity, possibly epistaxis, low-grade fever
		  (2) Whitish-gray membrane may appear over nasal septum
		c. Laryngeal diphtheria:
		  (1) Usually spread from pharynx to larynx
		  (2) Fever, harsh voice, barking cough; respiratory difficulty with inspiratory retraction
		d. Nonrespiratory diphtheria: affects eye, ear, genitals, or, rarely, skin

Pertussis (whooping cough)
a. *Bordetella pertussis*
b. Direct contact, droplet spread; indirect contact with contaminated articles
c. Infants and young children; incidence higher in spring and summer
Diagnostic test—culture of nasopharyngeal mucus
	I: 5–21 days
	C: 7 days after exposure (greatest just before catarrhal stage) to 3 weeks after onset of paroxysms
		a. Stage I (catarrhal stage)
		  (1) Lasts 1–2 weeks
		  (2) Coryza, sneezing, tearing, tickling/dry cough, fever, loss of appetite
		b. State II (paroxysmal stage)
		  (1) Lasts 4–6 weeks
		  (2) Severe, violent coughing attacks occurring in clusters leading to vomiting, cyanosis, and exhaustion
		c. Stage III (convalescent stage)
		  (1) Lasts 4 months–2 years
		  (2) Coughing attacks decrease, but return with each respiratory infection
		Duration: 9 months–2 years

Tetanus (lockjaw) a. *Clostridium tetani*—prevalence in soil and animal feces; can be introduced into body through any break in skin or intestinal tract	*I:* 3 days–3 weeks; 8 days average *C:* None	a. Stiffening of striated muscles, usually the jaw b. 1–2 days later, stiffening leads to spastic rigidity and spreads down body to the extremities

Treatment	Complications	Special Considerations
Symptomatic: Short fingernails to prevent scratching Oral antihistamines to decrease pruritus Isolation until all lesions have crusted—about 5–6 days Treatment of itching: Mix baking soda (sodium bicarbonate) with warm water and pat on lesions drying lotion (i.e., calamine) *DO NOT GIVE* salicylates	Complications are rare in normal children Hemorrhagic varicella, encephalitis, pneumonia, and bacterial skin infection are not common, but they can occur Reye's syndrome	Severe in neonate and pregnant women Varicella-zoster immune globulin (VZIG) is available from Centers for Disease Control (Atlanta, GA) for high-risk susceptible children who have been exposed to varicella zoster. This should be given within 72 hours of exposure to varicella-zoster. If VZIG is unavailable, immune globulin at a dose of 0.6–1.2 ml./kg. body weight; promptly given, may modify varicella
Diphtheria antitoxin Antibiotic therapy (penicillin, erythromycin) Supportive treatment Respiratory support Isolation until 2–3 cultures are negative after antibiotic therapy is completed	Myocarditis Neuritis Paralysis	
Supportive: Bed rest Suctioning Antipyretics Antibiotics: erythromycin, ampicillin Increase fluids; nutrition and electrolyte balance Place in an environment with reduced stimuli to reduce coughing Sedation Isolation 4 weeks after coughing begins and continued for 7 days after onset of therapy with erythromycin	Respiratory: pneumonia, atelectasis, emphysema, bronchopneumonia Neurologic: brain damage	
Reduce muscular spasm with medication, quiet, dark room Antibiotics: penicillin or tetracycline*	Convulsion with laryngospasms leading to death Asphyxia from dysphagia and secretions	

* Not given to children under 9 years old

(continued)

Disease: *a.* Agent. *b.* Mode of transmission. *c.* Age when most common	Incubation (*I*) and Communicability (*C*) Periods	Symptoms
b. Direct or indirect contact with wound c. All ages *Diagnostic tests:* Wound culture anaerobically for *Clostridium tetani*		

Poliomyelitis (polio)
a. Virus serotypes 1, 2, and 3; incidence is higher in summer and fall
b. Virus is harbored in GI tract and is transmitted through saliva, vomitus, and feces
c. Predisposing factors that increase risk of disease: recent tonsillectomy, tooth extraction or DTP injections, pregnancy, physical exhaustion
Diagnostic tests: Isolation of polio virus from feces and throat
	I: 7–14 days, paralytic or nonparalytic; 3–5 days for prodromal or minor illness
	C: Increases around onset when virus is in throat and is excreted in feces; virus is present in throat 1 week after onset, in stool 4–6 weeks after
		a. Nonparalytic polio:
		  (1) Headache, lethargy, anorexia, vomiting, fever
		  (2) Muscle pain and stiffness
		b. Paralytic polio:
		  (1) Same as nonparalytic type, lasting about 1 week
		  (2) Then 1–2 days of CNS symptoms: loss of deep tendon reflexes, positive Kernig's and Brudzinski's signs, lethargy
		  (3) 1–2 days later, weakening of muscles and paralysis

Streptococcal pharyngitis ("strep throat") a. Beta hemolytic streptococcus—group A strain b. Direct or indirect contact with nasopharyngeal secretion of infected person or recently established carrier c. Not under 3 years of age, 5–16 years; incidence higher in winter and spring *Diagnostic tests:* nasopharyngeal (throat) culture	*I:* 2–5 days *C:* Greatest during acute phase of illness	a. Onset is generally acute: high fever, headache, vomiting, scarlatina rash b. After 12–24 hours—sore throat of varying degrees of severity, dryness of throat, cervical lymphadenopathy, white tongue coating that gives way to strawberry-red tongue
Impetigo a. Group A streptococcus (more common in older children) *Staphylococcus aureus* (more common in younger children) b. Usually direct contact often initiated by abrasions/insect bites; Streptococcal skin lesions often precede URI colonization *Diagnostic tests:* Lesions cleansed; culture on blood agar fluid from intact bleb or base of crusted lesion, no active or passive immunity	*I:* 2–5 days *C:* Until lesions healed	Lesions: Vesicular, become confluent and rapidly progress to pustular and crusting stage; do not appear in crops. Commonly involves nasolabial area and others easily scratched; typical lesion is a thick, adherent amber-colored crust Bullous impetigo usually caused by staphylococci Purulent crusting lesions caused by hemolytic streptococci or staphylococci
Rabies a. Rabies virus—a rhabdovirus b. Saliva via a bite of an infected animal (most common)	*I:* 9 days–several months; 20–60 days most common	a. During incubation—signs of inflammation and wound healing b. Prodrome—2–10 days nonspecific (i.e., malaise, anorexia, fatigue, fever, headache, apprehension, anxiety, agitation, irritability, depression, insomnia)
c. All ages *Diagnostic tests:* *Infected animal*—specific fluorescence in brain tissue		c. Acute neurologic (excitation stage)—2–7 days; objective signs of CNS involvement (i.e., hydrophobia, hyperactivity, aphasia,

Treatment	Complications	Special Considerations
Tetanus immune globulin Human—(TIG), preferred to equine tetanus antitoxoid (TAT) Debridement of wound Fluid and nutrition		
Nonparalytic: Supportive (i.e., relief of pain) Analgesics, heat Enteric isolation Bed rest With muscle weakness: Hospitalize Fluid and electrolytes Rest Relief of muscle pain and spasms Respiratory support	Respiratory paralysis Hypertension	
Isolation for 1 day while starting prescription Antibiotic therapy: penicillin G Symptomatic	Acute glomerulonephritis, 1–2 weeks after acute stage Rheumatic fever, 2–3 weeks after acute stage Peritonsillar abscess, cervical adenitis Pneumonia, otitis media, meningitis	Throat cultures are considered for entire household when: others are symptomatic concurrently or within past 3 weeks frequent or relapsing infections. Repeat throat cultures are recommended after treatment if child has clinical relapse or family members have rheumatic fever or glomerulonephritis.
Specific: Systemic antimicrobial therapy for extensive impetigo—oral Pen V or penicillin G for injection; others as indicated Symptomatic: Careful cleansing of lesions with soap and water; short fingernails to prevent scratching	Glomerulonephritis	Isolation necessary for hospitalized child; observe for skin lesions and treat promptly
Immediate and thorough cleansing of wound with 20% tincture of green soap with subsequent use of 70% alcohol Debridement as necessary Tetanus immunization Antibiotics	Coma Death due to vascular collapse and respiratory arrest Disease may be severe in children with prominent CNS disorders cardiac symptoms, splenomegaly	Passive immunity: Human rabies immune globulin (HRIG) 20 IU/kg.; ½ injected around wound and ½ given intermuscular Active immunity: Human diploid cell vaccine (HDCV) five 1-ml. injections over 28 days: 0-3-7-14-28 with booster at 90 days.
Immediate postexposure prophylaxis: Concurrent use of active and passive immunity (human products preferable)	Local reaction to antirabies treatment; systemic and allergic reactions	Duck embryo vaccine (DEV) use only if HDCV unavailable, check sensitivity to duck or chicken

(continued)

Disease: *a.* Agent. *b.* Mode of transmission. *c.* Age when most common	Incubation (*I*) and Communicability (*C*) Periods	Symptoms
Human—fluorescence of corneal smear		disorientation, hallucinations, seizures, bizarre behavior, nucal rigidity, increased deep tendon reflexes, progressive paralysis, (paralysis stage) coma and/or sudden death
Rocky Mountain Spotted Fever a. *Rickettsia rickettsii* b. Bite of infected wood tick, American dog tick or Lone Star tick c. All ages; spring and summer *Diagnostic tests:* 1. Immunofluorescent identified virus in skin lesion by punch biopsy 2. Indirect fluorescent antibody 3. Complement fixation to specific antibody formation	*I:* 1–10 days, usually 1 week	a. 3–7 days after exposure: headache, decreased appetite, sore throat, photophobia, nausea, abdominal pain, joint pain b. 3–4 days after illness begins: high spiking fever, nonpitting edema, rash *Rash characteristics:* Rash appears 1–5 days after fever, macular with light rosy hue, blanching with pressure—concentrated on distal extremities, especially wrist and ankles. Rash becomes papular, frequently petechial, dark red, or dusky and slowly moves to trunk and head.

Nutrition in Children*

Age and Developmental Influence on Nutritional Requirements and Feeding Patterns	Feeding Pattern/Diet	Nursing Implications/ Parental Guidance

Neonate
(birth–4 weeks)
Newborn's rapid growth makes him especially vulnerable to dietary inadequacies, dehydration, and iron deficiency anemia.
Feeding process is basis for infant's first human relationship, his formation of trust. Feeding reinforces mother's sense of "motherliness."
Because of limited nutritional stores, neonates require vitamin and mineral supplements.
Neonates require more fluid relative to their size than do adults.
Sucking ability is influenced by individual neuromuscular maturity.
	Breast milk or formula is generally given in 6–8 feedings per day, spaced 3–4 hours apart.
	Feeding schedules should be individualized according to infant's needs.
		Provide information to help parents make decision concerning breast- or bottle-feeding.
		Support parents in their decision.
		Breast-fed infant (see p. 999):
		1. Help mother assume comfortable and satisfying position for self and baby.
		2. Help mother to determine schedule, timing, and when infant is satisfied.
		3. Provide specific information about the following:
		   a. Feeding technique: position, "bubbling"
		   b. Care of breasts
		   c. Manual expression of milk from breast
		   d. Maternal diet

* For recommended daily dietary allowances, refer to Appendix II, page 1530.

Treatment	Complications	Special Considerations
There is no evidence that treatment of established illness with RIG is effective Isolation Supportive Airway Fluids Temperature control Staff protection—especially of respiratory secretions		protein, given subcutaneous in abdomen—1 ml./dose. Injection every day for 21 days if wound is below waist, or Injection two times a day for 7 days, then every day for 7 days if wound is above waist. Booster #1 in 10 days. Booster #2 in 20 days after completion of primary course
Early recognition (Fever, rash, edema) Antibiotics—chloramphenicol and tetracyclines (not used for child under 9 years old) Supportive Bed rest Adequate fluid High-protein diet Antipyretics Public education—prevention is best treatment	When treatment is delayed: Brain damage Heart impairments Thrombocytopenia Death	During tick season, care should be given to frequent inspection of body of child for ticks twice daily. Prompt removal is important. To remove tick, use tweezers or fingers covered with tissue to prevent contamination and disease transmission. Grasp tick close to site of its attachment to skin. Using firm, steady traction pull tick away. Wash site with soap and water and apply antiseptic or antibiotic ointment, H_2O_2 or alcohol

CDC, Atlanta, Georgia 30333; #(404) 329-3727 days; 329-3644 nights

Age and Developmental Influence on Nutritional Requirements and Feeding Patterns	Feeding Pattern/Diet	Nursing Implications/ Parental Guidance
		Bottle-fed infant: 1. Provide specific information concerning a. Type of formula b. Preparation of formula: measuring and sterilization c. Equipment—types of bottles, nipples, etc. d. Sterilization of equipment e. Technique of feeding: position, "bubbling" 2. Help mother to determine when infant is satisfied; develop schedule for feeding. Provide information concerning normal characteristics of stools, signs of dehydration, constipation, colic, milk allergy. Discuss need for vitamin supplements and how to administer.

(continued)

Age and Developmental Influence on Nutritional Requirements and Feeding Patterns	Feeding Pattern/Diet	Nursing Implications/ Parental Guidance
		Discuss need for additional fluids during periods of hot weather, and with fever, diarrhea, and vomiting.
		Observe for evidence of common problems and intervene accordingly:
		1. Overfeeding
		2. Underfeeding
		3. Difficulty digesting formula because of its particular composition.
		4. Improper feeding technique; holes in nipples too large or too small; formula too hot or too cold; uncomfortable feeding position; failure to "bubble"; improper sterilization.
		5. Emotional problems in family may cause irritability, colic, and other similar disturbances.
Infant (3 months–1 year)	Number of feedings per day decreases through the first year.	New foods should be offered one at a time and early in the feeding while the infant is still hungry.
Increased neuromuscular development allows infant to make transition from a totally liquid diet to a diet of milk and solid foods as well as to more active participation in the feeding process.	By a year of age, most infants are satisfied with 3 meals and additional fluids throughout the day.	The person feeding should be calm, gentle, relaxed and patient in approach.
3–6 months	By 4–6 months of age, the infant is generally ready to begin eating strained foods. The usual sequence of foods is cereal followed by fruits, vegetables, and meats. This sequence may vary according to individual preferences of pediatrician and family.	When the child is first offered puréed foods with a spoon, he expects and wants to suck. The protrusion of his tongue, which is needed in sucking, makes it appear that he is pushing the food out of his mouth. This response should not be interpreted as dislike for the food; it is a result of immature muscle coordination and surprise at the taste and feel of the new food.
Sucking reflex becomes voluntary and chewing action begins; infant can approximate lips to rim of cup and may begin drinking from cup at 6 months.		
6–12 months	Mashed table foods or junior foods generally are started at 6–8 months, when infant begins chewing action.	
Eyes and hands can work together; infant is able to sit without support and has developed grasp; able to feed self a biscuit; bangs objects on table; able to hold own bottle at 9–12 months; has "pincher" approach to food; able to be weaned as child becomes developmentally able to take sufficient fluids from the cup.	Infant begins to enjoy finger foods at 10–12 months.	The baby foods selected should be those which are high in nutrients without providing excessive calories. Personal and cultural preferences should be considered.
	The transition from iron fortified formula or breast milk to cow's milk is usually advised at about 12 months of age.	Infants should be observed for allergic reactions when new foods are added. Common allergies are to citrus juices and egg white.
Food provides the infant with a variety of learning experiences; motor control and coordination in self-feeding; recognition of shape, texture, color; stimulation of speech movement through use of mouth muscles.		Finger foods should be selected for their nutritional value. Good choices include teething biscuits, cooked vegetables, meat, cheese sticks, and enriched cereals. Avoid nuts, raisins and raw vegetables, which can cause choking.
Mealtime allows the infant to continue his development of trust in a consistent, loving atmosphere. The infant is forming his lifetime eating habits; it is therefore important to make mealtime a positive experience.		Parents can be taught to prepare their own strained or junior foods using a commercial baby food grinder or blender.
		Weaning is a gradual process.
		1. Assist parents to recognize indications of readiness.

Age and Developmental Influence on Nutritional Requirements and Feeding Patterns	Feeding Pattern/Diet	Nursing Implications/ Parental Guidance
		2. Do not expect the infant to completely drop his old pattern of behavior while learning a new one; allow overlap of old and new techniques.
		3. Evening feedings are usually the most difficult to eliminate, because the infant is tired and in need of sucking comfort.
		4. During illness or household disorganization, the infant may regress and return to sucking to relieve his discomfort and frustration.
		SPECIAL CONSIDERATIONS: Hospitalized infant
		Obtain a thorough nursing history that includes the following:
		Feeding pattern and schedule; types of foods that have been introduced; likes and dislikes; breast- or bottle-fed, type of bottle; temperature at which infant prefers foods and fluids.
Toddler (1–3 years) Growth slows at the end of the first year. The slower growth rate is reflected in a decreased appetite. The toddler has a total of 14–16 teeth, making him more able to chew foods. Increased self-awareness causes the toddler to want to do more for himself. Refusals of food or of assistance in feeding are common ways in which the toddler asserts himself. Since body tissues, especially muscles, continue to grow quite rapidly, protein needs are high.	Appetite is sporadic; specific foods may be favored exclusively or refused from time to time. Child may be ritualistic concerning food preferences, schedule, manner of eating, etc. Diet should include a full range of foods: milk, meat, fruits, vegetables, breads, and cereals. Older toddler can be expected to consume about one-half the amount of food that an adult consumes.	Provide foods with a variety of color, texture, and flavor. Toddlers need to experience the feel of foods. Offer small portions. It is fun for the child to ask for more. It is more effective to give small helpings than to insist that he eat a specified amount. Maintain a regular mealtime schedule. Provide appropriate mealtime equipment: 1. Silverware scaled to size. 2. Dishes—colorful, unbreakable; shallow, round bowls are preferable to flat plates. 3. Plastic bibs, placemats, and floor coverings permit a relaxed attitude toward child's self-feeding attempts. 4. Comfortable seating at good height and distance from table. Adults who help toddlers at mealtime should be calm and relaxed. Avoid bribes or force feeding because this reinforces negative behavior and may lead to a dislike for mealtime. Encourage independence, but provide assistance when necessary. Do not be concerned about table manners. Avoid the use of soda or "sweets" as rewards or between-meal snacks. Instead, substitute fruit, juice, or cereal. Toddlers who show little interest in

(continued)

Age and Developmental Influence on Nutritional Requirements and Feeding Patterns	Feeding Pattern/Diet	Nursing Implications/ Parental Guidance
		eggs, meat, or vegetables should not be permitted to appease their appetite with carbohydrates or milk because this may lead to iron-deficiency anemia (see page 1281). SPECIAL CONSIDERATIONS: Hospitalized toddler Nursing history should include the following: Feeding pattern and schedule; food likes and dislikes; food allergies; special eating equipment and utensils; whether or not child is weaned and whether he takes bottle to bed; what child is fed when ill.
Preschooler (3–5 years of age) Increased manual dexterity enables child to have complete independence at mealtime. Psychosocially, this is a period of increased imitation and sex identification. The preschooler identifies with parents at the table and will enjoy what parents enjoy. Additional nutritional habits are developed which become part of the child's lifetime practices. Slower growth rate and increased interest in exploring his environment may decrease the preschooler's interest in eating. Eating assumes increasing social significance. Mealtime promotes socialization and provides the preschooler with opportunities to learn appropriate mealtime behavior, language skills, and understanding of family rituals.	Appetite tends to be sporadic. Child requires the same basic 4 food groups as the adult, but in smaller quantities. Generally likes to eat one food from plate at a time. Likes vegetables that are crisp, raw, and cut into finger-sized pieces. Often dislikes strong-tasting foods.	Emphasis should be placed on the quality rather than the amount of food ingested. Foods should be attractively served, mildly flavored, plain, as well as being separated and distinctly identifiable in flavor and appearance. Nutritional foods (e.g., crackers and cheese, yogurt, fruit) should be offered as snacks. Desserts should be nutritious and a natural part of the meal, not used as a reward for finishing the meal or omitted as punishment. Unless they persist, periods of overeating or not wanting to eat certain foods should not cause concern. The overall eating pattern from month to month is more pertinent to assess. Frequent causes of insufficient eating: 1. Unhappy atmosphere at mealtime 2. Overeating between meals 3. Parental example 4. Attention-seeking 5. Excessive parental expectations 6. Inadequate variety or quantity of foods 7. Tooth decay 8. Physical illness 9. Fatigue 10. Emotional disturbance Measures to increase food intake: 1. Allow child to help with preparations, planning menu, setting table, and other simple chores. 2. Maintain calm environment with no distractions. 3. Avoid between-meal snacks. 4. Provide rest period before meal. 5. Avoid coaxing, bribing, threatening.

Age and Developmental Influence on Nutritional Requirements and Feeding Patterns	Feeding Pattern/Diet	Nursing Implications/ Parental Guidance
		SPECIAL CONSIDERATIONS: Hospitalized preschooler
		Consider cultural differences.
		Allow parents to bring in favorite foods or eating utensils from home.
		Encourage family members to be present at mealtime.
		Place children in small groups, preferably at tables during mealtime.
		Provide simple foods in small portions. Peanut butter and jelly sandwiches are often favorites.
		Allow and encourage children to feed themselves.
		Utilize nursing histories as described for toddlers (see p. 1097).
		Do not punish children who refuse to eat. Offer alternative foods.
School-Age Child Slowed rate of growth during middle childhood results in gradual decline in food requirements per unit of body weight. The preadolescent growth spurt occurs about age 10 in girls and about age 12 in boys. At this time, energy needs increase and approach those of the adult. Intake is particularly important, since reserves are laid down for the demands of adolescence. The child becomes dependent on peers for approval and makes food choices accordingly. The child experiences increased socialization and independence through opportunities to eat away from home—for example, at school and homes of peers.	By this time, food practices are generally well-established, a product of the eating experiences of the toddler and preschool period. Many children are too busy with other affairs to take time out to eat. Play readily takes priority unless a firm understanding is reached and mealtime is relaxed and enjoyable.	Nutrition education should help the child to select foods wisely and to begin to plan and prepare meals. Parental attitudes continue to be important as the child copies parental behavior (e.g., skipping breakfast, not eating certain foods). Most children require a nutritious breakfast to avoid lassitude in late morning. Mealtime should continue to be relaxed and enjoyable. Diversions such as television and other children should be avoided. Calcium and vitamin D intake warrant special consideration. They must be adequate to support the rapid enlargement of bones. Parents and health professionals should be alert to signs of developing obesity. Intake should be altered accordingly. Table manners should not be overemphasized. The young child often stuffs his mouth, spills foods, and chatters incessantly while eating. Time and experience will improve his habits. Provide some companionship and conversation at the child's level during meals. Peers should be invited occasionally for meals. SPECIAL CONSIDERATIONS: Hospitalized child

(continued)

Age and Developmental Influence on Nutritional Requirements and Feeding Patterns	Feeding Pattern/Diet	Nursing Implications/ Parental Guidance
		Nursing history should include the following: Food preferences; mealtime patterns and snacks; food allergies; food preferences when ill. Provide opportunities for children to eat in small groups at tables. Consider cultural differences. Allow parents to bring in favorite foods from home. Allow child to order his own meal.
Adolescent (approximately 11–17 years of age) Dietary requirements vary according to stage of sexual maturation, rate of physical growth, and extent of athletic and social activity. When rapid growth of puberty appears, there is a corresponding increase in energy requirements and appetite.	Previously learned dietary patterns are difficult to change. Food choices and eating habits may be quite unusual and are related to the adolescent's psychological and social milieu. Generally, a significant percentage of the daily caloric intake of the adolescent comes from snacking.	Continue nutrition education, with special emphasis on the following: 1. Selecting nutritious foods. 2. Nutritional needs related to growth. 3. Preparing favorite "adolescent foods." 4. Kinds of foods that may aggravate acne. 5. Foods and physical fitness. Informal sessions are generally more effective than lectures on nutrition. Special problems requiring intervention: Obesity Excessive dieting Extreme fads—eccentric and grossly restricted diets Anorexia Adolescent pregnancy Provide nutritious foods relevant to the adolescent's life style. Discourage cigarette smoking, which may contribute to poor nutritional status by decreasing appetite and increasing the body's metabolic rate. SPECIAL CONSIDERATIONS: Hospitalized adolescent Allow patient to choose own foods, especially if on a special diet. Provide a refrigerator in the recreation room for snacks, or utilize a snack cart. Serve foods that appeal to adolescents. Utilize a nursing history similar to that for the school-age child.

Preventive Pediatrics

Immunization

General Considerations

1. Immunizations may be started at any age. If an immunization program is not begun in infancy, a slightly different schedule may be followed, depending upon the child's age and the prevalence of specific infections at the time.
2. An interrupted primary series of immunizations need not be restarted; it need only be continued, regardless of the length of time that has elapsed.

3. The immunoresponse is limited in a significant proportion of young infants, and the recommended booster doses are designed to ensure and maintain immunity.
4. A time lapse of 8 weeks is recommended between the first 3 DTP injections for desirable maximum effects.
   a. The combination of depot antigens is preferred, because it is more immunogenic.
   b. Because of the increased risk of possible reactions to either diphtheria or pertussis antigen. Td (adult-type tetanus and diphtheria toxins) is recommended for children over 6 years of age.
   c. For contaminated wounds, a booster dose of tetanus should be given if more than 5 years have elapsed since the last dose. No booster is needed for clean, minor wounds if immunizations are up to date and no more than 10 years has elapsed since last dose.
5. *Pertussis*
   a. Protection of infants against pertussis should begin early.
   b. In newborn infants, the best protection against pertussis is avoidance of household contacts by adequate immunization of older siblings.
6. *Tuberculin test*
   a. It is recommended that the tuberculin test be given before or simultaneously with the measles vaccine.
      (1) The measles vaccine may invalidate the tuberculin test, giving a false negative, if given within 6 weeks after measles immunization.
      (2) Theoretically, measles vaccine could activate latent tuberculosis.
   b. Frequency of repeated tuberculin testing depends upon the following:
      (1) Risk of exposure of the child.

(2) Prevalence of tuberculosis in the population group.
(3) High-risk situations; intervals between routine testing should not exceed 6 months.
7. *Measles vaccine* is most effective when given at about 12–15 months of age. At this age, all maternal transplacental antibody has been catabolized.
   Measles vaccine may be administered at 6 months of age when child is at a high risk of contact with natural measles. A second dose should be given at 12–16 months of age if the original vaccine was given prior to 1 year of age, since rate of seroconversion before 1 year of age is variable.
8. Live trivalent oral polio virus vaccine is preferred to the inactivated form, because administration is easier and the immunologic effects are broader and longer.
9. *Mumps vaccine*—all preadolescent or older males who have not had mumps should be immunized.
10. *Rubella vaccine*
    a. Live vaccine is recommended for boys and girls between 1 year of age and puberty.
    b. Children in kindergarten should be given priority, because they are the major source of viral dissemination.
    c. A history of rubella illness is not reliable enough to exclude children from immunization.
11. Immunizations should be deferred if child has an acute febrile infection or illness. The common cold, without fever, is not a contraindication to immunization.
12. Contraindications to receiving measles, mumps, and rubella vaccines include the following: pregnancy; generalized malignancy; cell-mediated immunodeficiency disorders; current immunodepressive therapy; sensitivity to animal species used in vaccine preparation; transfusion of immune globulin, plasma, or blood.

Recommended Schedule for Active Immunization of Normal Infants and Children

Recommended Age	Vaccine(s)	Comments
2 mo	DTP,[1] OPV[2]	Can be initiated earlier in areas of high endemicity
4 mo	DTP, OPV	2-mo interval desired for OPV to avoid interference
6 mo	DTP (OPV)	OPV optional for areas where polio might be imported (e.g., some areas of Southwest United States)
12 mo	Tuberculin Test[3]	May be given simultaneously with MMR at 15 mo (see text)
15 mo	Measles, Mumps, Rubella (MMR)[4]	MMR preferred
18 mo	DTP, OPV	Consider as part of primary series—DTP essential
4–6 yr[5]	DTP, OPV	
14–16 yr	Td[6]	Repeat every 10 years for lifetime

[1] DTP—Diphtheria and tetanus toxoids with pertussis vaccine.
[2] OPV—Oral, attenuated poliovirus vaccine contains poliovirus types 1, 2, and 3.
[3] Tuberculin test—Mantoux (intradermal PPD) preferred. Frequency of tests depends on local epidemiology. The Committee recommends annual or biennial testing unless local circumstances dictate less frequent or no testing (see Tuberculosis for complete discusson).
[4] MMR—Live measles, mumps, and rubella viruses in a combined vaccine (see text for discussion of single vaccines versus combination).
[5] Up to the seventh birthday.
[6] Td—Adult tetanus toxoid (full dose) and diphtheria toxoid (reduced dose) in combination.
For all products used, consult manufacturer's brochure for instructions for storage, handling, and administration. Biologics prepared by different manufacturers may vary, and those of the same manufacturer may change from time to time. The package insert should be followed for a specific product.
(From Report of the Committee on Infectious Diseases, 19th Ed, American Academy of Pediatrics, Evanston, IL, 1982, p. 7)

Recommended Immunization Schedules for Infants and Children Not Initially Immunized at Usual Recommended Times in Early Infancy

Timing	Recommended Schedules				Comments
	Preferred Schedule	Alternatives			
		#1	#2	#3	
First visit	DTP #1, OPV #1, Tuberculin test (PPD)	MMR, PPD	DTP #1, OPV #1, PPD	DTP #1, OPV #1, MMR, PPD DTP #2	MMR should be given no younger than 15 mo old.
1 mo after first visit	MMR	DTP #1, OPV #1	MMR, DTP #2		
2 mo after first visit	DTP #2, OPV #2	—	DTP #3, OPV #2	DTP #3, OPV #2	—
3 mo after first visit	(DTP #3)	DTP #2, OPV #2	—	—	In preferred schedule, DTP #3 can be given if OPV #3 is not to be given until 10–16 mo.
4 mo after first visit	DTP #3 (OPV #3)	—	(OPV #3)	(OPV #3)	OPV #3 optional for areas for likely importation of polio (e.g., some southwestern states).
5 mo after first visit	—	DTP #3 (OPV #3)	—	—	
10–16 mo after last dose	DTP #4, OPV #3 or OPV #4	DTP #4, OPV #3 or OPV #4	DTP #4, OPV #3 or OPV #4	DTP #4, OPV #3 or OPV #4	—
Preschool	DTP #5, OPV #4 or OPV #5	DTP #5, OPV #4 or OPV #5	DTP #5, OPV #4 or OPV #5	DTP #5, OPV #4 or OPV #5	Preschool dose not necessary if DTP #4 or #5 given after fourth birthday.
14–16 yr old	Td	Td	Td	Td	Repeat every 10 yr.

Alternative #1 can be used in those more than 15 months old if measles is occurring in the community.
Alternative #2 allows for more rapid DTP immunization.
Alternative #3 should be reserved for those whose access to medical care is compromised by poor compliance.
DTP = Diphtheria and tetanus toxoids with pertussis vaccine.
OPV = Oral, attenuated poliovirus vaccine contains types 1, 2, and 3.
Tuberculin test = Mantoux (intradermal PPD) preferred. Frequency of tests depends on local epidemiology. The Committee recommends annual or biennial testing unless local circumstances dictate less frequent or no testing.
MMR = Live measles, mumps, and rubella viruses in a combined vaccine (see text for discussion of single vaccines).
Td = Adult tetanus toxoid (full dose) and diphtheria toxoid (reduced dose) in combination.
For all products used, consult manufacturer's brochure for instructions for storage, handling, and administration. Biologics prepared by different manufacturers may vary, and those of the same manufacturer may change from time to time. The package insert should be followed for a specific product.
(From Report of the Committee on Infectious Diseases, 19th Ed, American Academy of Pediatrics, Evanston, IL, 1982, pp. 18 and 19)

If any of these contraindications exist, immunizations may be temporarily deferred or an alternative vaccine preparation may be used.

13. *Smallpox vaccination*
   a. No longer recommended in US.
   b. Where indicated (i.e., while traveling), initial smallpox vaccine may be given at any time between 12 and 24 months of age (after age 12, it may be given every 3–10 years).
14. A good nursing history will include determining whether or not the child has been exposed to any communicable disease or has experienced such. Surveillance in this area will prevent unnecessary disease and allow for proper immunization for the child and his family.
15. Strict adherence to the manufacturer's storage recommendations is vital. Failure to observe these pre-cautions and recommendations may reduce the potency and effectiveness of the specific vaccine. Read manufacturer's package insert for volume of individual dose.

Dental Care

Primary Teeth

1. Eruption
   a. Two lower central incisors—appear by 6–7 months
   b. Four upper incisors—appear by 9 months
   c. Two lower lateral incisors—appear by 1 year
   d. Four first molars—appear by 14 months
   e. Four cuspids—appear by 18 months
   f. Four second molars—appear by 2–2½ years

2. Importance of primary teeth and dental care for primary teeth
Toothbrushing and oral cleansing should be started early. The infant's oral cavity can be cleansed by wiping area with a damp wash cloth daily to prevent plaque formation. In the very young child, parents should brush the teeth with plain water.
   a. At about 2 years of age, toothbrushing should be started. At this age, most of the primary teeth have erupted, and the child's muscle coordination has developed enough to allow some form of brushing. The primary goal is to clean teeth.
   b. By age 3, the child should be examined by a dentist when all primary teeth have erupted.
   c. When decayed primary teeth are neglected, they endanger the child's health and may cause abscesses, fever, and excessive pain. The infected teeth may damage the permanent tooth that is forming within the jaw. A child with advanced tooth decay finds it difficult to chew some foods that are essential to a well-balanced diet.
   d. Primary teeth act as a guide for the proper positioning of permanent teeth. Each primary tooth is holding the space for a permanent tooth that will replace it. If a primary tooth is lost prematurely, there will be a loss of space. This can result in crowding of permanent teeth, ultimately requiring orthodontic work when a child is older.
   e. Primary teeth serve as a stimulus for growth of the jaws, aid in the development of speech, and serve a cosmetic function.
      (1) A young person can become very self-conscious when he loses a tooth in the front of his mouth and realizes that he looks different.
      (2) Indirectly, a child's speech may be affected if self-consciousness about his loss of teeth prevents him from opening his mouth for proper talking.
      (3) Ability to use the teeth for pronunciation is acquired entirely with the aid of the primary teeth. Early loss of front teeth may lead to difficulty in pronouncing "s," "f," "l," "z," and "th."
      (4) Even after the permanent teeth erupt, difficulty in pronouncing "s," "z," and "th" may persist to the point that the child requires speech correction.

Permanent Teeth

1. Eruption
   a. Four "6-year molars" appear between the age of 6 and 7 years.
   b. From this point onward, until 12–13 years of age, the primary teeth loosen, one by one, and each is replaced by a permanent tooth.
   c. Four additional molars appear at 12–13 years of age.
   d. Four molars ("wisdom teeth") appear at 17–21 years.
2. Importance of early dental care
Care of teeth during infancy and childhood is necessary in order to:
   a. Promote proper development of the teeth.
   b. Prevent dental caries and periodontal disease.
   c. Establish good dental habits for optimal dental health.

Nursing Management

1. Take advantage of incidental opportunities to teach children and their parents information that will promote dental health.
   a. Emphasize that inflammatory periodontal disease and dental caries are the results of dental plaque. *Dental plaque* is a mass composed primarily of microorganisms that adhere to the tooth surface. As these microorganisms grow, they form products that are destructive to the underlying tissue. Removal of this plaque and prevention of its collection is a major part of dental care.
   b. Provide a well-balanced diet that is necessary for tooth development. Stress the importance of diet control in dental care. The microorganisms that form dental plaque need a sucrose substrate which comes from refined sugars for rapid growth. Therefore, decreasing the intake of such refined sugars is important.
   c. Start child on the correct procedure by having a good attitude toward brushing. Parents serve as role models as well as assist the young child to care for his teeth.
2. Provide supplemental fluoride if the local drinking water supply does not contain fluoride. Fluoride makes the tooth surface more resistant to disease.
   a. Topical application of fluoride should be done twice a year.
   b. Daily fluoride rinse after brushing is effective in decreasing dental caries in children.
   c. Daily use of a dentifrice-containing fluoride is another source of protection.
3. Maintain the child's general health.
4. Encourage parents to arrange a dental visit when child is 2½–3 years old.
5. Teach child and parents good brushing technique and dental habits.
   a. Use soft-bristle nylon brush with polished ends. Brushes for small children should be ¼–⅓ smaller than adult brushes with a flat brushing surface, firm, resilient bristles, and head sufficiently small to allow access to all surfaces of the teeth.
   b. Place bristles at the gingival margin at a 45-degree angle to the tooth. The brush rotates from gingival toward occlusal surface. Occlusal surfaces are brushed with scrubbing motion with small strokes in every direction.
   c. Stress that the length of time and thoroughness of brushing are important.
   d. Disclosing tablets can be used during teaching program to show the location of dental plaque before and after brushing.
   e. Daily flossing should be started at age 8–9 years.
6. The adolescent needs special encouragement and attention to maintain good dental habits.
   a. Stress importance of dietary control of refined sugars.
   b. Encourage proper brushing technique. The circular motion method: the brush is carried up, back, and forward, then up again without twisting hand.
   c. Encourage daily flossing in which floss is used correctly. (Improper use can cause traumatic injury to the gingiva.) Flossing is accomplished by passing the floss between the teeth with a back and forth motion. Place floss against tooth and move it up and down 6–7 times against the

tooth as far as the gingiva permits. Repeat process on side of adjacent tooth. Repeat until all sides of all teeth are cleansed.

7. Practice measures that will aid in avoiding cavities.
   a. Bottle-mouth syndrome—high incidence of dental caries in child 18 months–3 years is the result of taking bottle of milk or juice to bed. This syndrome can be prevented. Do not let child take a bottle to bed with him; if child does take a bottle, put plain water in it.
   b. Have the child brush teeth after every meal and at bedtime. If brushing is not possible after meals, rinse mouth with water.
   c. Reduce the amounts of sugar and sweets eaten by the child.
   d. Beware of foods that contain large amounts of sugar:
      Bubble and chewing gum
      Cola drinks
      Peanut butter and jelly on white bread
      Candies, cookies, cakes
      Jelly, jam, honey
      Malted and sweet chocolate drinks
      Synthetic orange juice (artificially sweetened)
      White bread and raisin bread
      Sugar-coated cereals

Safety

Incidence of Childhood Accidents

1. Accidents are the leading cause of death for children in the US.
2. Approximately 1 of every 3 children in the US is injured seriously enough each year to require medical treatment.

Role of the Nurse

1. Identify environmental hazards and take action to reduce or eliminate them.
2. Identify behavioral characteristics in individual children which may be related to accident liability and caution parents accordingly. Pay particular attention to children who show the following:
   a. Characteristics that increase exposure to hazards, such as excessive curiosity, inability to delay gratification, hyperactivity, and daring.
   b. Characteristics that reduce the child's ability to cope with hazards, such as aggressiveness, stubbornness, poor concentration, low frustration threshold, lack of self-control.
3. Provide anticipatory guidance about child development as it relates to accidents. Direct preventive teaching toward individuals or groups, toward children or adults.
4. Participate in policy-setting for accident prevention in institutions and communities.

Principles of Safety

1. The child's developmental stage influences the types of accidents that are likely to occur.
   Potential accident situations may be foreseen by parents who have knowledge of their own child's typical patterns of growth and development.
2. Children are naturally curious, impulsive, and impatient. The young child needs to touch, feel, and investigate.
   a. Patient adult supervision will enable the child

to learn what he wants to know within the limits of safety for his stage of growth and development.
   b. Young children should never be left alone at home.
3. Children copy the behavior of their parents and absorb parental attitudes.
   Parents and other adults should be certain that their ways of doing things are safe.
4. Children become less careful and less willing to listen to warnings and to observe routine safety precautions when they are tired or hungry.
5. An estimated 90% of all accidents are preventable.

General Areas of Adult Safety Responsibility

A. Motor Vehicle

1. All automobiles should be maintained in good mechanical condition.
2. Seat belts should be worn at all times.
3. Driver should look carefully in front of and in back of the car before accelerating.
4. All car doors should be locked when a child travels in the vehicle.
5. Young children should never be left alone in a car.
6. Heavy or sharp objects should not be placed on the same seat with a child.

B. Sports and Recreation

1. Keep equipment in good condition and proper working order.
2. Wear appropriate clothing for the activity.
3. Do not attempt activities beyond one's physical endurance.
4. Keep firearms and ammunition locked up.

C. Electrical and Mechanical Equipment

1. Only underwriter-approved devices should be installed; they should be inspected periodically.
2. Dry hands before touching appliances.
   Keep radios, fans, portable heaters, and hair dryers out of the bathroom.
3. Disconnect appliances after use and before attempting minor repairs.
4. Keep garden equipment and machinery in a restricted area.
   Teach proper use of the equipment as soon as the child is old enough.
5. Avoid overloading electrical circuits.
6. Discourage children from playing with or being in area where appliances or power tools (e.g., washing machine, clothes dryer, saw, lawn mower) are in operation.

D. Prevention of Falls

1. Keep stairs well-lighted and free from clutter.
2. Provide sturdy railings.
3. Anchor small rugs securely.
4. Use rubber mats in the bathtub and shower.
5. Use only sturdy ladders for climbing.

E. Poisonings and Ingestions

1. Do not mix bleaches with ammonia, vinegar, and other household cleaners.
2. See section on ingested poisons, page 944; poisoning (pediatric), page 1485.

F. Fire

1. Maintain an adequate fire escape plan and routinely conduct home fire drills.

Teach the child escape routes as soon as he is old enough.
2. Keep a pressure-type hand fire extinguisher on each floor.
   Instruct all family members who are old enough in its use.
3. Fit fireplaces with snug fireplace screens.
4. Store gasoline and other flammable fluids in tightly covered containers that are clearly labeled and away from heat and sparks.
5. Dispose of paint- and oil-soaked cloth quickly.
6. Utilize flame-retardant sleepwear.
7. Mark children's rooms so that they are obvious to firemen.
8. Teach children about the danger of smoke inhalation.

G. Swimming Pools

1. Completely enclose pool with a fence that complies with local regulations. The gate should be self-closing and have a lock.
2. Indicate water depth with numbers on the edge of the pool. Place a safety float line where the bottom slope begins to deepen.
3. Install at least 1 ladder at each end of the pool. Ladders should have handrails on both sides, and the diameter of the rails should be small enough for a child to grasp.
4. Use nonslip materials on ladders, deck, and diving boards.
5. Install underwater lighting as well as outdoor lights if the pool is used at night. A ground fault circuit interrupter should be installed on the pool circuit to cut off electrical power and thus prevent electrocutions should electrical fault occur.
6. Instruct children about safety rules such as not swimming alone, and not running around the pool or pushing others. Avoid using radios or other electrical appliances near the pool.
7. Keep essential rescue devices and first-aid equipment close to the pool.

H. Emergency Precautions

1. Record emergency telephone numbers in an obvious and easily accessible place.
2. Keep a well-stocked first-aid kit immediately available for emergencies.
3. Give instruction in principles of first aid to all family members who are old enough.
   a. Responsible adults should enroll in first-aid courses offered by the Red Cross, adult education programs, etc.
   b. Be aware of first-aid procedures for:
      Burns
      Electric shock
      Poisoning
      Bites and stings
      Cuts, scrapes, and punctures
      Drowning
      Fractures
      Cardiopulmonary arrest
4. Know the location of gas, water, and electrical switches and how to turn them off in an emergency.

I. Miscellaneous

1. Take advantage of preventive health care.
   a. Obtain recommended immunizations.
   b. Have regular physical examinations.

2. Seek immediate treatment of all diseases and health problems.
3. Balance periods of work, rest, and exercise in daily living.

Specific Safety Concerns Related to Child's Stage of Growth and Development

A. Infants

Newborn babies are helpless and need absolute protection. When they begin to move about they need close supervision.
1. Infants may wiggle, roll, and shift position.
   a. The crib should conform to the requirements of the Consumer Product Safety Commission.
   b. The sides of the crib should be kept up at all times.
   c. The crib should not be placed near a radiator or heating unit.
   d. The crib should be away from windows with blinds or draperies, to prevent the infant from becoming fatally entangled in a dangling cord.
   e. Babies should not be left unattended on anything from which they might fall.
      Infant seats should not be left on tables, beds, or other furniture.
   f. Infants should be strapped carefully in feeding chairs, infant seats, etc.
      A means should be provided to prevent the child from slipping down and being strangled by his waist strap.
   g. No strings should be placed around the infant's neck.
   h. Well-constructed infant carriers should be used for traveling.
      (1) *For all children under 4 years of age or weighing less than 40 pounds, the standard seat belt is not safe.* Special restraint devices should be used, beginning with the ride home from the nursery.
      (2) Infant car seats and car beds should meet the vehicle safety standards of the Department of Transportation for child-seating systems.
         (a) There should be a means of anchoring the device to the seat of the vehicle with the standard lap belt.
         (b) A harness should keep the child contained within the device.
         (c) The device should include a head support to minimize the danger of whiplash injury.
      (3) For older infants and toddlers, special devices are available which dispense with the harness and instead surround the child with a protective shield that distributes collision forces evenly.
      (4) Adults should be aware of state laws regarding infant restraint during travel.
   i. Diaper pins should always be kept closed, even when not in use.
2. Infants may start to suck on toys, crib slats, and other objects.
   a. Paints containing lead should not be used on toys, furniture, or any other objects that the child is likely to put into his mouth.
   b. Stuffed toys should be checked carefully to be

certain that button eyes and other small, attached parts cannot be pulled off and eaten by the child.

 c. Small objects should not be left within the reach of the infant.

 d. All plastic bags should be tied in knots and discarded to avoid danger of suffocation. Under no circumstances should mattresses be covered with thin plastic.

3. Children are helpless in water for the next several years.

 a. The temperature of the bath water should be checked carefully to avoid scalding.

 b. The child should never be left unattended in the bathtub for any reason.

4. Infants are frequently victims of rats in highly populated metropolitan areas.

 a. The rats should be exterminated before the baby is discharged from the hospital.

 b. Infant beds should be high above the floor.

5. Infants should be carried from one place to another.

 a. The adult who carries the infant should avoid walking on slippery floors or where toys or other small objects have been scattered.

 b. *Hospitalized infants* should always be transported in cribs or strollers and never carried from place to place in the arms of the nurse.

B. Toddlers

Toddlers are adventurous and are eager to explore everything around them. Although they sometimes seem very mature and independent, they still require close adult supervision.

1. Toddlers want to roam all over the house.

 a. Gates should be used at the head and foot of stairways to prevent falls.

 b. Fireplaces should be screened.

 c. Radiators should be enclosed or covered.

 d. Cords on blinds or draperies should be tied or cut so that children cannot get their heads through the loops.

2. Toddlers poke and probe with their index fingers.

 a. Sharp objects such as scissors, and nail files should be kept out of reach.

 b. Bureau drawers and cabinets with anything potentially dangerous in them should be locked.

 c. Unused light sockets should be taped or capped.

 d. Electric fans or heaters should be out of reach.

 e. Electrical cords should be kept in good repair.

3. Toddlers are curious about many things, especially those things higher than their eye level.

 a. They should be lifted occasionally to satisfy their curiosity.

 b. Furniture should be balanced to prevent the child from pulling it over on himself.

 c. Hot, scalding foods should be kept out of the reach of the children.

 d. All handles of pots and pans should be turned to the back of the stove.

 e. Tablecloths should not hang over the edge of the table.

 f. A small child should never be left alone in the kitchen. Appliances such as hot ovens, toasters, coffee pots, and irons pose a special threat to small children.

4. A toddler puts almost anything into his mouth.

 a. Medicines, lye, and household cleaning products should be locked up out of the reach of children.

 b. Pins, buttons, and needles should be put away.

 c. Unbreakable toys that have no small, removable parts should be used.

 d. The child should be closely supervised if he plays with a balloon. Aspiration of rubber from broken balloons can be fatal.

 e. Foods such as popcorn and peanuts should not be offered to toddlers because of the danger of aspiration.

 f. Poisonous plants should be removed from the home.

5. Toddlers climb onto things.

 a. Toddlers should be protected from falls.

  (1) Windows should have guards on them.

  (2) Screens should be firm and securely fastened.

 b. Car doors should be locked.

 c. Special equipment for climbing (e.g., small wooden grates) should be provided, and climbing should be done under adult supervision.

6. They like to play outside and in water.

 a. The toddler must have close supervision while playing outside.

 b. His play yard should be fenced.

 c. Ponds, pools, wells, and other similar outdoor structures should be fenced or covered. Wading pools should be emptied immediately after use.

 d. The child should never be left alone in a wading pool.

 e. Caution should be used in allowing the toddler to play with older children. He may easily be injured by bats, hard balls, bicycles, and rough play.

C. Preschool Children

Preschool children are very active and inquisitive. They begin to develop increased self-control, but still have an immature understanding of danger. They are at an ideal age to learn simple safety routines.

1. Preschoolers can reach doorknobs and are eager to explore the world beyond.

 a. Doors that open to potential danger should be locked.

 b. Bathroom doors should have locks that can be opened from the outside to prevent the child from locking himself in the room.

 c. Unused refrigerators, freezers, and trunks should have doors, handles and/or hinges removed to prevent small children from climbing into them and becoming trapped inside.

2. Preschoolers enjoy taking things apart, putting them together again, and experimenting with their use.

 a. Dangerous items such as knives and electrical equipment should be put away.

 b. Matches and lighters should be kept well out of the child's reach.

3. Preschoolers are nimble on their feet and usually in a hurry.

 a. The child should not be allowed to walk or run while eating a lollipop.

 b. Stairs should have strong railings. They should be clear of objects or defective coverings on which a child can trip.

 c. Stairs and floors should not be highly waxed.

 d. Area rugs should be fixed.

4. Preschoolers often enjoy cooperative play with others.

 a. Toy trucks or wagons should be strong enough

to bear their weight as well as that of their playmates.
  b. They should be taught to ride tricycles on the sidewalk and to watch for cars in driveways.
  c. They should be cautioned not to run after the ball if it rolls into the street or driveway.
  d. Clothes should allow the child freedom of action and shoes should be suitable for running and climbing.
  e. The play area should be checked for such hazards as old refrigerators, deep holes, construction, broken glass, and trash heaps.
  f. Swings and other equipment should be properly installed and maintained.
5. Preschoolers are proud to run simple errands. They should not be asked to do anything hazardous such as crossing the street or carrying a knife or glass container.
6. Preschoolers can take verbal directions, and their attention span is lengthening. They can be instructed in the following areas:
  a. Personal safety
    (1) To supply information such as their name, address, and telephone number.
    (2) To identify firemen, policemen, and other safety officials.
    (3) Not to accept gifts or rides from strangers.
  b. Home safety
    (1) The reasons for various safety measures such as keeping the floor clear of their toys.
    (2) The safe way to use tools.
    (3) Kitchen safety
    (4) The danger of matches, open flames, hot objects, and gas and electric equipment.
  c. Recreational safety
    Swimming instructions
  d. Motor vehicle and pedestrian safety
    (1) Safety rules and the dangers of traffic.
    (2) Obedience to the rules.
    (3) Appropriate use of automobile restraint systems.

D. School-Age Children

School-age children are usually fairly independent. They still need discipline and rules, but they also need to know *why* precautions are necessary and what the consequences are for failing to follow the rules.
1. School-age children are eager to make things and participate in household activities.
  a. They should be taught the proper use and storage of equipment such as those listed below:
    (1) Saws
    (2) Nails and hammer
    (3) Kitchen implements
    (4) Sewing machines
    (5) Gas and electric appliances
  b. They should be taught to wear protective devices over their eyes when doing anything potentially dangerous to their vision.
2. School-age children enjoy holding and attending parties, carnivals, and other similar gatherings. Party costumes and equipment should be checked to be certain that they are flameproof.
3. School-age children enjoy sports and outdoor play.
  a. Their whereabouts should be known at all times.
  b. The play areas should be inspected for broken glass, rusty nails, etc.

  c. They should be instructed regarding the dangers of playing in sand pits, old refrigerators, excavations, rickety shacks, and deserted buildings.
  d. They must learn the rules of the sports that they play. They should have the proper equipment and keep it in good working condition.
  e. Ice skating and other water sports should always be closely supervised.
  f. They should be taught how to climb a tree safely. Tree houses that are sturdily constructed under adult supervision may help prevent falls from trees.
4. Areas for teaching:
  a. The rules of cycling safety should be emphasized. A child with a bicycle must learn the rules of the road as well as respect for the traffic officers and their directions.
  b. Pedestrian safety rules should also be stressed because motor accidents are the most common cause of accidental injury in this age-group.
  c. Swimming instruction should be continued.
  d. The older child should be taught respect for fire, its uses, and its dangers.
  e. Safety with firearms should be discussed.
  f. Children should be taught to read labels and recognize symbols indicating poisons.

E. Adolescents

Adolescents are increasingly independent. They should be able to build on their past experiences and accept responsibility for their own safety. Limits must still be set, and direction given by adults because adolescents may lack emotional maturity.
1. Adolescents may obtain driving licenses.
  a. They should learn to maintain their automobiles in good mechanical condition.
  b. Seat belts should be worn at all times.
  c. They must be aware of traffic regulations and the penalty for not obeying them.
  d. They should be encouraged to participate in driver education and safety programs at school.
  e. Proper clothes should be worn while riding on motorcycles, motor scooters, or motorbikes. A safety helmet is essential.
2. Adolescents enjoy competing in competitive sports. Safeguards should be taken to prevent physical trauma when they want to do something beyond their physical endurance.
3. The values and habits of adolescents are greatly influenced by their peer groups and cliques.
  a. Parents should be aware of their child's activities.
  b. Constructive group activities should be encouraged.
  c. Formal instructions should be continued in the areas of sex education, drug and alcohol abuse, and smoking.
    Open discussions with responsible adults should be encouraged.
4. Older adolescents are capable of assuming some responsibility for family safety measures.
  a. They should be included in safety planning.
  b. Their opinions and suggestions should be considered.
  c. Specific areas of responsibility may be delegated to them.

Bibliography

Books

General

Bennett LC and Searl S. Communicable Disease Handbook. New York, John Wiley & Sons, 1982

Chinn P. Child Health Maintenance: Concepts in Family Centered Care, 2nd ed. St Louis, CV Mosby, 1979

Feigin RD and Cherry JD. Textbook of Pediatric Infectious Diseases, Vols. I and II. Philadelphia, WB Saunders, 1981

Furhold JDL. Clinical Assessment of Children: A Comprehensive Approach to Primary Care. Philadelphia, JB Lippincott, 1980

Greenspan S. The Clinical Interview of the Child. New York, McGraw-Hill, 1981

Heagarty M. Child Health: Basics for Primary Care. New York, Appleton-Century-Crofts, 1980

Horowitz J, Hughes C and Perdue B. Parenting Reassessed. A Nursing Perspective. Englewood Cliffs, NJ, Prentice-Hall, 1982

Howe J (ed). Nursing Care of Adolescents. New York, McGraw-Hill, 1980

Hymovich D and Barnard M (eds). Family Health Care, Vol 1, General Perspectives, and Vol 2, Developmental and Situational Crises. New York, McGraw-Hill, 1979

Johnson SH. High-Risk Parenting: Nursing Assessment and Strategies for the Family at Risk. Philadelphia, JB Lippincott, 1979

Krugman S and Katz SL. Infectious Diseases in Children, 7th ed. St Louis, CV Mosby, 1981

Lesner PA. Pediatric Nursing. Albany, Delmar, 1983

Levine MO et al. Developmental-Behavioral Pediatrics. Philadelphia, WB Saunders, 1983

Pillitteri A. Child Health Nursing. Boston, Little, Brown and Co, 1981

Powell ML. Assessment and Management of Developmental Changes and Problems in Children. St Louis, CV Mosby, 1981

Pringle SM and Ramsey BE. Promoting the Health of Children: A Guide for Caretakers and Health Care Professionals. St Louis, CV Mosby, 1982

Steele S. Child Health and Family. New York, Masson, 1981

Whaley LF and Wong DL. Nursing Care of Children, 2nd ed. St Louis, CV Mosby, 1983

Wieczorek RR and Natapoff JN. A Conceptual Approach to the Nursing Care of Children. Philadelphia, JB Lippincott, 1981

McCollum AT. The Chronically Ill Child. A Guide for Parents and Professionals. New Haven, Yale University Press, 1981

Kleinberg S. Educating the Chronically

Ill Child. Rockville, MD, Aspen Systems, 1982

Growth and Development

Anthony E and Chiland C (eds). The Child in His Family: Children and Their Parents in a Changing World. New York, John Wiley & Sons, 1978

Anthony E and Chiland C (eds). The Child in His Family: Children in Turmoil: Tomorrow's Parents. New York, John Wiley & Sons, 1982

Aten M and McAnarney E. A Behavioral Approach to the Care of Adolescents. St Louis, CV Mosby, 1981

Better Health For Our Children. The Report of the Select Panel for the Promotion of Child Health; Vol. 1 Major Findings and Recommendations. US Dept of HHS. Pub. #79-55071 Washington, DC, 1981

Boynton R, Dunn E and Stephens G. Manual of Ambulatory Pediatrics. Boston, Little, Brown and Co, 1984

Cave E et al. A Pediatrician's Guide to Child Behavior Problems. New York, Masson, 1979

Chilman C. Adolescent Sexuality in a Changing American Society: Social and Psychological Perspectives. Bethesda, US Dept. of HEW, Public Health Service, NIH, 1980

Chinn P and Leitch C. Child Health Maintenance: A Guide to Clinical Assessment. St Louis, CV Mosby, 1979

Clements IW and Roberts FB. Family Health—A Theoretical Approach to Nursing Care. New York, John Wiley & Sons, 1983

Evans J. Adolescent and Pre-Adolescent Psychiatry. New York, Academic Press, Grune & Stratton, 1982

Ginsburg H and Opper S. Piaget's Theory of Intellectual Development, 2nd ed. Englewood Cliffs, Prentice-Hall, 1979

Lipsitt LP and Field TM (ed). Infant Behavior and Development: Perinatal Risk and Newborn Behavior. Norwood, NJ, Ablex, 1982

Mercer RT. Perspectives on Adolescent Health Care. Philadelphia, JB Lippincott, 1979

Murray R and Zentner J. Nursing Assessment and Health Promotion Through the Life Span, 2nd ed. Englewood Cliffs, NJ, Prentice-Hall, 1980

Mussen P, Conger J and Kagen J. Child Development and Personality, 5th ed. New York, Harper & Row, 1979

Powell M. Assessment and Management of Developmental Changes in Children. St Louis, CV Mosby, 1981

Prugh D. Psychosocial Aspects of Pediatrics. Philadelphia, Lea & Febiger, 1983

Rutter M. Changing Youth in a Changing Society: Patterns of Adolescent Development and Disorder. Cambridge, Harvard University Press, 1980

Sahler OJ and McAnarney E. The Child from Three to Eighteen. St Louis, CV Mosby, 1981

Shafii M and Shafii SL. Pathways of Human Development. New York, Thieme-Stratton, 1982

Simon N. Don't Worry, You're Normal: A Teenager's Guide to Self Health. New York, Thomas Y Crowell, 1982

Skolnick A and Skolnick J. Family in Transition. Boston, Little Brown & Co, 1977

Stone LJ et al. Childhood and Adolescence: A Psychology of the Growing Person. New York, Random House, 1979

Sutterly D and Donnelly G. Perspectives in Human Development, 2nd ed. Philadelphia, JB Lippincott, 1980

Tudor M (ed). Child Development. New York, McGraw-Hill, 1981

Nutrition

Krieger I. Pediatric Disorders of Feeding, Nutrition and Metabolism. New York, John Wiley & Son, 1983

Lansky V. Feed Me, I'm Yours. New York, Bantam Books, 1979

Pipes P. Nutrition in Infancy and Childhood, 2nd ed. St Louis, CV Mosby, 1981

Suskind RM (ed). Textbook of Pediatric Nutrition. New York, Raven Press, 1981

Williams SR. Nutrition and Diet Therapy, ed 4. St Louis, CV Mosby, 1981

Preventive Pediatrics

McDonald RE and Avery DR. Dentistry for the Child and Adolescent. St Louis, CV Mosby, 1983

Stallard RE. A Textbook of Preventive Dentistry, 2nd ed. Philadelphia, WB Saunders, 1982

Stewart RE et al. Pediatric Dentistry. St Louis, CV Mosby, 1982

Stewart RE and Troutman KC. Pediatric dentistry in the hospital. In Hooley JR and Daun LG (eds). Hospital Dental Practice. St Louis, CV Mosby, 1980, pp. 291–310

Safety

Arena J and Bachar M. Child Safety is No Accident. Chapel Hill, Duke University Press, 1978

Illingsworth C. The Diagnosis and Primary Care of Accidents and Emergencies in Children. St Louis, CV Mosby, 1982

Articles

Growth and Development

Alder SP. In Maurer HM (ed). Infectious disease in Pediatrics. New York, Churchill Livingstone, 1983, pp. 327–372

Amonker RG. What do teens know about the facts of life? J Sch Health 1980 Nov; 50(9):527–530

Bax M. Developmental assessment.

Health Visitor 1980 Nov; 53(11):461–463

Bell RS. The Gesell developmental schedules: Arnold Gesell (1880–1961). J Abnorm Child Psychol 1977 Sept; 5(3):233–239

Betz CL. Faith development in children. Pediatr Nurs 1981 Mar/Apr; 7(2):22–25

Bruhn JG. The school as a setting for health education, health promotion and health care. Fam Community Health 1982 Feb; 4(2):57–69

Brunell PA. Rabies: Deciding when you should immunize. Consultant 1983 May; 23(5):258

Budassi SA. A case of tetanus. J Emerg Nurs 1981 Sept/Oct; 7(5):191–194

Brayton JB, Coleman WP and Johnson JE. Tracking down pet-associated diseases. Patient Care 1981 Mar 30; 15(6):18–20

Byrne KM, Lattanzi SM and Morrissey M. Don't let me fall. Am J Nurs 1982 Aug; 82(8):1242–1245

Castiglia PT and Aquilina S. Streptococcal pharyngitis: A persistent challenge. Pediatr Nurs 1982 Nov/Dec; 8(6):377–381

Cherry JD. The 'New' epidemiology of measles and rubella. Hosp Practice 1980 July; 15(7):49–57

Child AA et al. Depression in children: Reasons and risks. Pediatr Nurs 1980 July/Aug; 6(4):9–13

Clochesy JM and Habeck TJ. Nursing care of the patient with rabies. Heart Lung 1982 Nov/Dec; 11(6):541–544

Crosby R. Self concept development. J Sch Health 1982 Sept; 52(7):432–436

Dowie E. Rabies. Physician Assist Health Practit 1982 July; 6(7):28

Dowie E. Expanded guidelines for use of varicella-zoster immune globulin. Pediatrics 1983 Dec; 72(6):886–889

Ferguson CK and Roll LJ. Human rabies. Am J Nurs 1981 June; 81(6):1175–1179

Florey LG. Studies of play: Implications for growth, development, and for clinical practice. Am J Occup Ther 1981 Aug; 35(8):519–524

Ford K. School phobia: The school anxiety symptom. Pediatr Nurs 1980 Sept/Oct; 6(5):9–13

Fosson A and deQuan MM. Reassuring and talking with hospitalized children. Child Health Care 1984 Summer; 13(1):37–44

Fraiberg S (ed). Clinical studies in infant mental health: The first year of life. New York, Basic Books, 1983

Gardner H. The developmental psychology after Piaget: An approach in terms of symbolization. Hum Dev 1979; 22(1):73–78

Gibes RM. Clinical uses of the Brazelton Neonatal Behavioral Assessment Scale in nursing practice. Pediatr Nurs 1981 May/June; 7(3):23–26

Gohsman B. The hospitalized child and the need for mastery. Issues Comp Pediatr Nurs 1981 Mar/Apr; 5(2):67–76

Gratz RR and Zemke R. Piaget, preschoolers and pediatric practice.

Phys Occup Ther Pediatra 1980 Fall; 1(1):3–9

Hammer D et al. Child discipline: What we know and what we can recommend. Pediatr Nurs 1981 May/June; 7(3):31–35

Hart NAC et al. Adolescent suicide. Pediatr Nurs 1979 Nov/Dec; 5(6):22–28

Hayes JS. The McCarthy Scales of Children's Abilities: Their usefulness in developmental assessment. Pediatr Nurs 1981 July/Aug; 7(4):35–37

Heisler AB et al. Adolescence: Psychological and social development. J Sch Health 1980 Sept; 50(7):381–385

Hurff JM. A play skills inventory: A comprehensive monitoring tool for the 10 year old. Am J Occup Ther 1980 Oct; 34(10):651–656

Hurff JM. It's not fun to be sticked by a needle. Emerg Med 1982 Aug 15; 14(4):28–32

Jamison-Smith P and Hamm P. Infection control update! Rubella. Crit Care Update 1982 Dec; 9(12):34–36

Jellinek B et al. Adolescent consent: Questions, confusion, and conflicts. Pediatr Nurs 1981 Jan/Feb; 7(1):33–34

Judelsohn RG, Fleissner ML and O'Mara DJ. School-based measles outbreaks: Correlation of age at immunization with risk of disease. Am J Pediatr Health 1980 Nov; 70(11):1162–1165

Katz SL. The campaign against pertussis vaccination. Perinatol Neonatol 1984 Jan/Apr; 8(1):72–73

Knecht L. Consent and confidentiality: Legal issues in adolescent health care for the school nurse. J Sch Health 1981 Nov; 51(9):607–609

Kolbe LJ et al. Research in school health education: A needs assessment. Health Educ 1980 Jan/Feb; 11(1):3–8

Koster M. Self-care: Health behavior for the school-age child. Top Clin Nurs 1983 Apr; 5(1):29–40

Kuhnen K et al. Barry: A computer for teaching sex education. MCN 1983 Sept/Oct; 8(5):350–353

Ludington-Hoe SM. What can newborns really see? Am J Nurs 1983 Sept; 83(9):1286–1289

Nelms BC. What is a normal adolescent? MCN 1981 Nov/Dec; 6(6):402–406

Niparko N. The effect of prematurity on performance on the Denver Developmental Screening Test. Phys Occup Ther Pediatra 1982 Spring; 2(1):29–50

Nugent JK. The Brazelton Neonatal Behavioral Assessment Scale: Implications for intervention. Pediatr Nurs 1981 May/June; 7(3):18–21

Ode D. A viewpoint on school nursing. Am J Nurs 1981 Sept; 81(9):1677–1678

O'Pray M. Developmental screening tools: Using them effectively. MCN 1980 Mar/Apr; 5(2):126–130

Peach EH. Counseling sexually active very young adolescent girls. MCN 1980 May/June; 5(3):191–195

Pontious SL. Practical Piaget: Helping children understand: Piaget's theory of

cognitive development. AJN 1982 Jan; 82(1):114–117

Post CW et al. A "good beginning for families"—parent group education. Pediatr Nurs 1980 July/Aug; 6(4):32–36

Reres ME. Stressors in adolescence. Fam Community Health 1980 April; 2(4):31–41

Rice MA. Identifying the adolescent substance abuser. MCN 1983 Mar/Apr; 8(2):139–142

Robinson T. School nurse practitioners on the job. Am J Nurs 1981 Sept; 81(9):1674–1676

Roesel R. The nurse's role in primary prevention in sexual health. Imprint 1980 Dec; 27(5):27–28

Sapala S et al. Adolescent sexuality—Use of a questionnaire for health teaching and counseling. Pediatr Nurs 1981 Nov/Dec; 7(6):33–34

Seffrin JR. Making tobacco education relevant to the school-age child. Health Educ 1981 Mar/Apr; 12(2):11–15

Spadero DC. Assessing readability to patient information materials. Pediatr Nurs 1983 July/Aug; 9(4):274–278

Taussig WC. Sixth grade children's questions regarding sex. J Sch Health 1982 Sept; 52(7):412–416

Thornburg HD. Adolescent sources of information on sex. J Sch Health 1981 Apr; 51(4):274–277

Tishler CH et al. Assessment of suicidal potential in adolescents. J Emerg Nurs 1980 Mar/Apr; 6(2):24–26

Valenti SM. Stressors at school age. Fam Community Health 1980 April; 2(4):15–29

Valenti S. Suicide in school aged children: Theory and assessment. Pediatr Nurs 1983 Jan/Feb; 9(1):49–51

Vipperman JF. Childhood coping: How nurses can help. Pediatr Nurs 1980 Mar/Apr; 6(2):11–18

Webster-Stratton C. Recognizing and assessing conduct disorders in children. MCN 1983 Sept/Oct; 8(5):330–335

Yoos L. A developmental approach to physical assessment. MCN 1981 May/June; 6(3):168–170

Childhood Diseases

Baxley LM. Tetanus is still deadly. Occup Health Nurs 1981 Aug; 29(8):40–42

Brodoff AS. Think Rocky Mountain spotted fever! Patient Care 1982 July 15; 16(13):21–25

Massey K. Rocky mountain spotted fever: A national disease. MCN 1982 Mar/Apr; 7(2):104–109

Mortimer E et al. Tetanus prophylaxis in wound management. Patient Care 1981 May 30; 15(10):102–103

Mortimer E. New tactics in the war on tetanus. Emerg Med 1981 Mar 15; 13(5):73–75

Nichols AO. Taking the fear out of rabies treatment. Nursing 1983 June; 13(6):42–43

Preblud SR and Plotkin SA. Rubella:

Current diagnosis and prevention. Hosp Med 1983 Mar; 19(3):89–91

Preblud SR and Plotkin SA. Rabies vaccine too much of a bad thing. Emerg Med 1980 June 30; 12(12):53–56

Roderick MA. Tetanus. Nursing '82 1982 July; 12(7):63

Shahan MR. Mumps. Nursing '83 1983 Feb; 13(2):43

Shahan MR. The latest rules on rubella. Emerg Med 1981 April 30; 13(8):119

Sloane PD. Sore throats: They're common, but full of surprises. Consultant 1982 May; 22(5):110–113

White MJ. Rabies update. Nursing '80 1980 Aug; 10(8):53

Williams L. Childhood immunizations. Pediatr Nurs 1982 Jan/Feb; 8(1):18–21

Nutrition

American Academy of Pediatrics, Committee on Nutrition. Toward a prudent diet for children. Pediatrics 1983; 71(1):78–79

Coates JT et al. Heart healthy eating and exercise: Introducing and maintaining changes in health behaviors. Am J Public Health 1981 Jan; 71(1):15–23

Crummette BD et al. Mothers' decisions about infant nutrition. Pediatr Nurs 1980 Nov/Dec; 6(6):16–19

Fomon SJ. Recommendations for feeding normal infants. Pediatrics 1979 Jan; 63(1):52–59

Frankle RT. It's never too early for nutrition education. J Sch Health 1980 Sept; 50(7):387–391

Getchell E and Howard R. Nutrition in development. In Scipien G et al (eds). Comprehensive Pediatric Nursing, 2nd ed. New York, McGraw-Hill, 1979

Gross J. My child, the vegetarian. Fam Health 1981 Apr; 13(4):34–37

Hagenbuch VEG. Obesity and the school-age child. Nurs Clin North Am 1982 June; 17(2):207–216

Hennerman A et al. Preschool feeding problems: It's not nutritious unless they eat it. Issues Compr Pediatr Nurs 1980 Sept/Dec; 4(5–6):7–12

Langford RW. When your client has a weight problem. Teenagers and obesity. Am J Nurs 1981 Mar; 81(3):556–559

Mallick MJ. Health hazards of obesity and weight control in children: A review of the literature. Am J Public Health 1983 Jan; 73(1):78–82

Mandelbaum J. The food square: Helping people of different cultures understand balanced diets. Pediatr Nurs 1983 Jan/Feb; 9(1):21–24

Mangham DB et al. Introducing nutrition education. J Sch Health 1981 Feb; 51(2):110–112

Mowery BD. Family oriented approach to childhood obesity. Pediatr Nurs 1980 Mar/Apr; 6(2):40–44

Narins DM. Nutrition and the growing athlete. Pediatr Nurs 1983 May/June; 9(3):163–168

Nguyen TT et al. Food habits and preferences of Vietnamese children. J Sch Health 1983 Feb; 53(2):144–147

Rowe NR. Childhood obesity growth

charts vs. calipers. Pediatr Nurs 1980 Mar/Apr; 6(2):24–27

Smith MK et al. Curriculum guides for nutrition education. J Sch Health 1980 Sept; 50(7):371–376

Termini R. Good food habits for life: Developing a comprehensive nutrition education program. Health Educ 1982 Jul/Aug; 13(4):26–27

Williams CL. Teaching children self-care for chronic disease prevention: Obesity reduction and smoking prevention. Patient Counsel Health Educ 1980 2nd quarter; 2:92–98

Preventive Pediatrics

Abrams RG and Josell SD. Common oral and dental emergencies and problems. Pediatr Clin North Am 1982 June; 29(3):681–715

Adams C and Dering N. Preventing dental caries. J Nurs Care 1980 May; 13(5):18–20

Adams C and Dering N. A shortcut to diagnosing strep throat. Emerg Med 1980 June 30; 12(12):29

Adams C and Dering N. An update on DPT vaccine. Emerg Med 1981 Oct 15; 13(17):132–133

Barsky NH and Londereek. First Aid procedures for dental emergencies. J School Health 1982 Jan; 52(1):43–45

Beall S and Hurley RS. The humanistic approach: A model for dental health curriculums. J Sch Health 1982 Jan; 52(1):29–32

Boraz RA. Preventive dentistry for the pediatric patient. Issues Compr Pediatr Nurs 1981 Mar/Apr; 5(2):89–97

Brunell PA. Varicella vaccination: Where do we go from here? Hosp Practice 1980 Sept; 15(9):91–93

Casamassimo PS and Castaldi CR. Considerations in the dental management of the adolescent. Pediatr Clin North Am 1982 June; 29(3):631–651

Clarke SJ. Whooping cough vaccination: Some reasons for non-completion. J Adv Nurs 1980 May; 5(3):313–319

Claypool JM. Rubella protection for maternal child health care providers. MCN 1981 Jan/Feb; 6(1):53–56

Cooley RV and Sobel RS. Dental treatment considerations for the medically compromised child. Pediatr Clin North Am 1982 June; 29(3):613–629

Farrington FH. Teeth. In Maurer HM (ed). Pediatrics. New York, Churchill Livingstone, 1983, pp. 311–326

Fields WT. Dental myths: A baker's dozen. J Sch Health 1982 Jan; 52(1):33–35

Fulginiti VA. The problems of poliovirus immunization. Hosp Practice 1980 Aug; 15(8):61–67

Jaffe AC. Animal bites. Pediatr Clin North Am 1983 April; 30(2):405–413

Kamholtz JD and Wood B. Competing with Ronald McDonald, Cap'n Crunch and the Pepsi Generation. J Sch Health. 1982 Jan; 52(1):17–18

Kilmon C and Helpin ML. Update on dentistry for children. Pediatr Nurs 1981 Sept/Oct; 7(5):41–44

Levy RL, Lodish D, and Pawlak-Floyd C. Teaching children to take more responsibility for their own dental treatment. Social Work in Health Care. 1982 Spring; 7(3):69–76

Livingston JF and Muirden DM. Supervised toothbrush instruction for pre-school children. Australian Nurses J 1980 Mar; 9(8):44–46

Miller RE and Rosenstein DI. Children's dental health: Overview for the physician. Pediatr Clin North Am 1982 June; 29(3):429–438

Mortimer EA. Pertussis immunization: Problems, perspectives, prospects. Hosp Practice 1980 Oct; 15(10):103–107

Oda DS, Fine JI and Heilbron DC. School nursing and dental referrals. J Sch Health 1980 Sept; 50(7):393–396

Oda DS, Fine JI and Heilbron DC. Report of the Committee on Infectious Disease, 19th ed. Evanston, The American Academy of Pediatrics, 1982

Shelton PG and Ferretti GA. Maintaining oral health. Pediatr Clin North Am 1982 June; 29(3):653–668

Shelton PG and Ferretti GA. The choices in polio immunization. Emerg Med 1982 May 15; 14(9):97–98

Thompson S. Summertime and ticks. Am J Nurs 1983 May; 83(5):786–789

Watson ML. The relationship between dietary factors and dental caries. J Sch Health 1982 Jan; 52(1):39–41

Safety

Adams D. Children's response to a belt restraint program . . . seat belt use. Pediatr Nurs 1982 Jan/Feb; 8(1):28–30

Agran P and Dunkle D. Motor vehicle occupant injuries to children in crash and noncrash events. Pediatrics 1982 Dec; 70(6):993–996

Arena JM. The pediatrician's role in the poison control movement and poison prevention. Am J Dis Child 1983 Sept; 137(9):870–873

Betz C. Bicycle safety: Opportunities for family education. Pediatr Nurs 1983 Mar/Apr; 8(2):109–111

Eicholz J. What to do if your child is burned. Life Health 1981 Jan; 96(1):20–22

Ford AH. Use of automobile restraining devices for infants. Nurs Res 1980 Sept/Oct; 29(5):281–284

Gilles C et al. Management of pediatric poisoning. Pediatr Nurs 1980 Sept/Oct; 6(5):33–44

Hoadley MR et al. Child safety programs: Implications affecting use of child restraints. J Sch Health 1981 May; 51(5):352–355

Kavanaugh C and Banco B. The infant walker—A previously unrecognized health hazard. Am J Dis Child 1982 Mar; 136(3):205–206

Keim K. Preventing and treating plant poisonings in young children. Pediatr Nurs 1983 July/Aug; 8(4):287–289

Litt IF and Steinerman PR. Compliance with automotive safety devices among adolescents. J Pediatr 1981 Sept; 98(3):484–486

Luther SL et al. Burns and their

psychological effects on children. J Sch Health 1981 Aug; 51(6):419–422

Marcus D. Child car seats: A must for safety. Pediatr Nurs 1981 May/June; 7(3):13–18

Meier EM. The pediatric emergency patient. Emerg Med 1981 Aug 15; 13(14):28–37

Mofenson H and Wheatley G. Prevention of childhood injuries: Morbidity and mortality—An overview. Pediatr Ann 1983 Oct; 12(10):716–719

Morris NM. Pediatric health promotion through risk reduction. Fam Community Health 1980 May; 3(1): 63–76

Othersen H. Burns and scalds. Pediatr Ann 1983 Oct; 12(10):753–760

Ray G. Developmental risks . . . home accidents. Community Outlook 1982 Aug; 217–218

Reinhard SC. Nursing responsibility in infant car safety. MCN 1980 Jan/Feb; 5(1):26–27

Righi F and Krozy R. The child in the car: What every nurse should know about safety. Am J Nurs 1983 October; 83(10):1421–1424

Robertson LS. Crash involvement of teenaged drivers when driver education is eliminated from high school. Am J Public Health 1980 June; 70(6):599–603

Sovie MD et al. The burned person: Initial assessment and care. J Burn Care Rehab 1983 Mar/Apr; 4(2):119–125

Surveyor JA et al. Age-related burn injuries and their prevention. Pediatr Nurs 1981 Sept/Oct; 7(5):29–34

Suggested Additional Reading for Staff and Parents

Anderson JW. Dental care for the learning disabled child. Life Health 1980 Apr; 95(4):13–14

Becker W. Parents Are Teachers. Champaign, Research Press, 1971

Brazelton TB. Infants and Mothers. New York, Dell, 1969

Brazelton TB. Neonatal Behavioral Assessment Scale. Philadelphia, JB Lippincott, 1973

Brazelton TB. Toddlers and Parents. New York, Dell Publishing Co., 1974

Caplan F. The First Twelve Months of Life. New York, Grossett & Dunlap, 1973

Cecil B. Dear Nurse: You should know that . . . Life Health 1980 Feb; 95(2):4

Christophersen, ER. Little People. Lawrence, H&H Enterprises, 1977

Dodson F. How to Parent. New York, New American Library, 1971

Fraiberg S. The Magic Years. New York, Charles Scribner's Sons, 1959

Friedman DE, for Carnegie Corp of NY. Encouraging Employer Support to Working Parents: Community Strategies for Change. New York, Center for Public Advocacy Research, Inc, 1983

Giancarlo H. Dear Parent: I want you to know. . . . Life Health 1980 Feb; 95(2):5–6

Gordon I. Baby Learning Through Baby Play. New York, St Martin's Press, 1970

Holt J. How Children Learn. New York, Dell, 1967

Kamerman SB and Hayes CD (eds). Families that Work: Children in a Changing World. Washington, DC, National Academy Press, 1982

Kaye K. The Mental and Social Life of Babies: How Parents Create Persons. Chicago, University of Chicago Press, 1982

Kramer R. In Defense of the Family: Raising Children in America Today. New York, Basic Books, 1983

Painter G. Teach Your Baby. New York, Simon & Schuster, 1971

Parent–Child Bonding: The Development of Intimacy. Stanley Greenspan. Pamphlet from National Committee for the Prevention of Child Abuse

Sparking J and Lewis I. Learning Games for the First Three Years. New York, Berkley Books, 1978

National Center for Education in Maternal–Child Health, 3520 Prospect Street NW, Washington, DC 20007

Guidelines for Early Intervention Programs, 1980

Healthy Infants, 1980 Pub #HSA 80-5244

Healthy Mothers, Healthy Babies, 1981 Pub #PHS 81-50175 (collection of publications and films)

Healthy Mothers, Healthy Babies—Coalition Directory of Educational Materials, 1982

Healthy Preschoolers Through Community Action. National Committee for the Prevention of Child Abuse, 1982

Compendium of Resource Materials on Adolescent Health, 1981 #HSA 81-5246

Ross Laboratories. Series on Child Development. Ross Laboratories, Columbus, OH 43216

Nutrition

National Center for Education in Maternal–Child Health, 3520 Prospect Street NW, Washington, DC 20007

Building a Better Diet. USDA Food and Nutrition Service, 1979

Nutrition and Your Health #OM 81-2002

Nutrition Checkups for Children. #HSA 81-5113

Nutritional Screening for Children: A Manual for Screening and Follow-up. 1981, #HSA 81-5114

Safety

American Academy of Pediatrics, PO Box 1034, 1801 Hinman Avenue, Evanston, IL 60204

Highway Safety Institute, Watergate 600, Washington, DC 20037

National Fire Protection Association, Batterymarch Park, Quincy MA 02269

National Safety Council, 444 N. Michigan Avenue, Chicago, IL 60611

Project Burn Prevention, Education Development Center, 55 Chapel Street, Newton, MA 02160

US Consumer Product Safety Commission. Washington, DC 20207

The Hospitalized Child

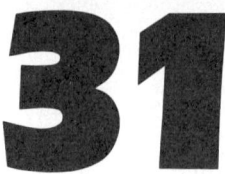

General Principles of Care

Emotional and Social Needs

1. The child has the same basic emotional and social needs during hospitalization as he does at home.
   a. He needs a chance to develop the following:
      (1) Motor skills
      (2) Social skills
      (3) Language skills
      (4) Psychological strengths
         (a) A sense of autonomy
         (b) Ego strength
         (c) A sense of identity
      (5) Patterns of behavior
   b. To help him accomplish these skills and strengths, he needs:
      (1) The continuing and reliable presence of someone who is important to him.
      (2) An appropriately stimulating environment.
      (3) Opportunities to explore and play.
      (4) Information and explanations concerning the hospital, illness and how sick people get better, treatments, procedures, routines, people, and expectations of him both before and during hospitalization. The child needs to know and to be able to predict how he will interact with his environment. Thus when he knows what to expect in an unfamiliar situation, he will be better able to cope and not feel so helpless.
2. The hospitalized child has special needs—to deal with the many new problems that confront him.
   a. Separation from home—implying loss of:
      (1) Consistent person who nurtures
      (2) Family associations
      (3) Familiar environment
      (4) Daily activities and routines
      (5) Peer associations
      (6) Independence
   b. Problems concerning the illness itself
   c. Hospital rules and regulations
   d. Surgery
   e. Death

Essential Elements

1. Parents must be closely involved with the child's hospitalization and the plan for his care. Parent participation is to be encouraged.
2. Nursing care should allow the child dependence, thereby helping him to develop confidence and trust in the situation and at the same time assisting him to develop independence (refer to Chap. 30).
3. Nursing histories should be taken when the child is admitted to the hospital. Specific questions should be asked to obtain information related to the following:
   a. Family home situation; parental anxieties
   b. Toilet habits and means of communicating
   c. Dietary habits
   d. Home routines and rituals
   e. Schooling
   f. Friends, peers
   g. Experience with illness
   h. Preparation for hospitalization
   i. Favorite toy, object, etc.
   j. How child handles frustration or stressful situations; his pattern for coping with strange situations and fears that arise
   k. Disciplinary practices at home
   l. Comforting practices at home
   m. Parental plans for visiting
4. Attempt to maintain home ties. Continuation of the ties within the existing family unit is a critical aspect of meeting the psychological needs of the child (refer to Family-Centered Care, p. 1117).
   a. Continue established rituals—rocking and story before bedtime.
   b. Have family photograph at the child's bedside.
   c. Use tape recorder to listen to tapes made of family conversations.
   d. Encourage use of the telephone, sending letters and pictures home, incoming cards.
   e. Talk about the people at home with the child.
   f. For the adolescent: assign roommate of same age, encourage use of telephone, encourage socialization with communal mealtimes and recreation periods.
5. Thorough explanations of the treatment plan and preparation for special tests, procedures, and surgery are essential. Unless the child is prepared for these experiences, he has minimal chance to mobilize his coping mechanisms to help him through his hospital experience.
   a. Listen to him repeat descriptions of his experience and continue to correct any misconceptions with factual information. Negative preparation of

the child results in chaos, panic, doubt or fear, or fantasy.
  b. Make sure preparation is appropriate to:
    (1) The child's age and personality
    (2) Level of comprehension and developmental norms
    (3) The child's attempt to cope with his frustrations and problems
  c. Be creative; avoid using terminology that may have unintended alternate meanings to the child, and that may cause him undue stress because of an inability to understand what is being said.
  d. Use metaphors appropriate for cognitive age.
  e. Include parents in the preparation process. Children through age 6 are dependent on their parents for identity and a sense of well-being, and will need their support. The parents know their child better than anyone and can serve as interpreters for child and health-care personnel.
6. Play is a natural part of nursing care. It is a means to help the child cope with an unpleasant experience; it allows him to project his fears to the outside world, and it helps him to attain a feeling of independence and control of the situation. It is important for the child's physical, emotional, and social development. Therapeutic play allows the child to explore real and simulated equipment that will be used during procedures. It will allow the child to learn to cope with his fears, concerns, and fantasies.
7. Nursing care should relate illness to the child's personality, individual reaction, and previous experiences. Recognition must be given to:
  a. What the child comes from
  b. What he is returning to
  c. What he is experiencing during his hospitalization
8. The ultimate goal in pediatric nursing is directed toward:
  a. Reduction of stress
  b. Increasing the child's feeling of well-being and a sense of mastery about the situation
9. Postprocedural sessions and support should be part of the total nursing care of the child. This allows the child to
  a. Acquire a less stressful and more realistic perspective of what has happened
  b. Develop appropriate coping behaviors
  c. Develop a sense of mastery over the situation
10. Nursing care is successful when its outcome is therapeutic and encompasses growth.

Parental Support

1. Parental presence and involvement with the hospitalized child will decrease anxieties of the child. Parents, however, need encouragement, support, and education to be of the greatest help possible to their hospitalized child. Parental reactions to hospitalization affect the child's reaction.

  a. Identify anxieties the parents may have regarding hospitalization of the child:
    (1) Relinquishing their child's care to others
    (2) Preparation for surgery or surgical outcome
    (3) Opinions they feel others have of their child
    (4) Guilt feelings regarding disciplining the sick and hospitalized child
    (5) Dealing with the child upon return to the home
  b. Establish at an early stage the degree to which parents are able and want to participate in the care of their child. Reassess this periodically, and provide opportunities for parents to give continuity of care, thus promoting continued close parent–child relationships (refer to Family-Centered Care, p. 1117).
    (1) Keep the family informed regarding the condition of the child.
    (2) Reassure parents that someone is available to help them.
    (3) Answer questions regarding hospital policy, procedures, or other concerns.
2. Begin early preparation and education of parents for possible posthospital behavior of their child.
  a. Frequently there are behavioral changes following hospitalization, especially in the child 18 months through 6 years of age. Behavioral changes may include increased demands for attention, withdrawal, violent reactions to temporary separation, changes in sleep patterns, shyness, increased clinging, bedwetting, temper tantrums, new fears, and changes in eating habits.
  b. Assist parents in anticipating these changes in their child's behavior. Help them to feel more adequate in coping with and responding to these temporary changes. Parents' reactions to post-hospital behavior can either help to reinforce, prolong, and perpetuate these behaviors or gradually diminish these behaviors. Aid parents in identifying their reactions and feelings towards any posthospital alterations in their child's behavior.
    Include parents in postprocedural sessions.
    (1) Establish a parent–teacher, anticipatory–guidance program for parents.
    (2) Provide staff support to parents during and following hospitalization.
3. Consider effects of child's illness and hospitalization on siblings. They, too, need a plan of care and support, both by hospital staff and parents.
  a. Periodic visitation to sick child
  b. Evaluate the response of well siblings to illness of the sister or brother. Identify siblings at risk or who are not coping well, determine their needs, and initiate a plan of action that will help them with their coping and adjustment.

Impact of Hospitalization on the Child's Stage of Development

Neonate
Birth–1 Month
A. Primary Concern
1. Bonding—hospitalization interrupts the early stages of the development of a healthy mother–child rela-

tionship, thus early stages of the development of trust are missing.
2. Sensory–motor deprivation—tactile, visual, auditory, kinesthetic
3. Sensory bombardment

B. Reactions

1. Impairment of maternal–child attachment.
2. Impairment of mother's ability to love and care for her baby.
3. Risking of infant's emotional and physical well-being.

C. Nursing Interventions

1. Provide for continual contact between baby and his parents (eye contact and touch).
2. Minimize isolation and strangeness by explaining and reexplaining equipment, procedures, etc., to parents.
3. Actively involve parents in caring for their baby—provide for rooming in.
4. Foster good neonate–sibling relationships as appropriate.
5. Identify areas of infant deprivation and/or overstimulation. Plan a schedule of appropriate stimulation (i.e., hold and rock every 3–4 hours, eye contact).
6. Provide sensory–motor stimulation as appropriate.
7. Allow individuality to begin to emerge.
8. Provide consistent caretaker.

Infant

1–4 Months

A. Primary Concern

1. Separation—mother is learning to identify and meet the needs of her infant. Infant is learning to make his needs known and to trust his mother to meet them.
2. Sensory–motor deprivation
3. Needs—security, motor activity, comforting measures

B. Reactions

Separation anxiety is different from that of older child, because for the infant, his mother seems to be a part of him. Development of trust is disturbed when infant is separated from mother.

C. Nursing Interventions

1. Encourage mother to stay and care for her baby, thus minimizing separation. When mother is absent, give infant attention and frequent handling from a limited number of personnel.
2. Provide opportunity for sensory stimulation, motor development, and social responsiveness.
3. Help parents to work through their anxieties. Remember, a mother's touch communicates her comfort or discomfort to her infant.

4–8 Months

A. Primary Concern

Separation from mother—infant now recognizes his mother as a separate person from himself. He rejects strangers.

B. Reactions

Separation anxiety—crying, terror, somatic upset, blank facial expression, extreme preoccupation.

C. Nursing Interventions

1. Encourage mother to stay and care for her baby.
2. Attempt to adjust schedule to home routines.
3. Become friends with the infant through the mother.
4. The infant is beginning to develop purposeful activities and to strive toward independence. Provide opportunities and encouragement for this development to continue and provide ways for him to use newly acquired skills.

8–12 Months

A. Primary Concern

Separation—infant becomes more possessive of mother and clings to her at the time of separation.

B. Reactions

Separation anxiety—tolerance is very limited. Fear of strangers, excessive crying, clinging, and overdependence on mother.

C. Nursing Interventions

1. Have the mother stay and care for her child.
2. Relieve some of his tensions and loneliness with "transference" object (i.e., blanket, toy).
3. Prepare the child for procedures—allow him to become familiar with simple equipment. Have the mother comfort child during procedures.
4. Provide for sensory stimulation and motor development appropriate for age. Provide opportunities for child to continue using skills he has acquired, such as feeding himself and drinking from cup.
   Child needs opportunity to foster increased independence, curiosity and exploration, locomotion and language skills. Use infant seats, swing; give him room to move around in crib, playpen or floor; use color, texture and sound; physical stroking, rocking, and talking.

Toddler (1–3 years)

A. Primary Concerns

1. Separation anxiety—relationship with mother is intense. Separation represents the loss of family and familiar surroundings, resulting in feelings of insecurity, grief, anxiety, and abandonment. The toddler's emotional needs are intensified by his mother's absence.
2. Changes in rituals and routines, all of which are important to his sense of security, become a source of concern.
3. Inability to communicate—beginning use and understanding of language affords him limited communication between himself and the world. Limited capacity to understand reality, passage of time.
4. Loss of autonomy and independence—his egocentric view of life helps him develop a sense of autonomy. He expresses himself as a separate being with some potential control of his body and environment.
5. Body integrity—incomplete and inaccurate understanding of the body results in fear, anxiety, frustration, and anger.
6. Decrease in mobility—restricting his mobility causes frustration. He wants to keep moving for the pleasure it gives him as well as for the feeling of independence, the opportunity to learn about his world, and the route it provides for coping with frustrations that cannot be verbally expressed. Physical interference with this freedom results in a sense of helplessness.

B. Reactions

1. Protest:
   a. Has urgent desire to find mother.
   b. Expects that she will answer his cries, "I want mommy."
   c. Frequently cries and shakes crib.
   d. Rejects attention of nurses.
   e. When with mother, child shows signs of distrust with anger and/or tears.

2. Despair:
   a. Feels increasingly hopeless about finding his mother.
   b. Becomes apathetic, anorectic, listless; looks sad.
   c. May cry continuously or intermittently.
   d. Uses comfort measures—thumbsucking, fingering lip, tightly clutching a toy.
3. Denial:
   a. Represses all feelings and images of his mother.
   b. Does not cry when she leaves.
   c. May seem more attached to nurses—will go to anyone.
   d. Finds little satisfaction in relationships with people.
   e. Accepts care without protest.
   f. Regresses to an earlier state of development.
4. Regression:
   Temporarily ceases use of newly acquired skills in an attempt to retain or regain control of a stressful situation.

C. Nursing Interventions

1. Rooming-in, unlimited visiting.
   Parental visits provide:
   a. Opportunity for child to express some of his feelings about his situation.
   b. Assurance that his parents are not abandoning him or punishing him.
   c. Periods of comfort and reassurance that allow for the reestablishment of family bonds.
2. Attempt to continue routines used at home, especially with regard to sleeping, eating, and bathing. Reestablish trust through body contact and comfort.
3. Set limits.
4. Obtain from parents key words in communicating with child. Find out about his nonverbal behavior as well.
5. Allow child to make choices when possible. Arrange physical setting to encourage independence. Allow child to explore the environment.
6. A Band-Aid may give the child security of wholeness after an injection.
7. Replace lost mobility with another form of motion: moving about in a wheelchair, cart, or bed. Exercise restrained extremity. Provide opportunity for the child to release energy suppressed by decreased mobility (i.e., by pounding, throwing). Provide opportunity to continue learning about world through sensory modalities such as water play and diversional play.
8. Discharge:
   If rooming-in has not occurred during hospitalization, parents must be prepared for the possible posthospital behavior of their toddler. They will need support in understanding and handling these behaviors. The child may do any of the following:
   a. Show lack of affection or resist close physical contact. Parents may interpret this as rejection.
   b. Regress to an earlier stage of development.
   c. Cling to mother, unable to tolerate any separation from her. Show excessive need for love and affection.
9. Appropriate parental response to the child's behavior is vital if relationships are to be reestablished.
   a. Extra love and understanding will help restore the child's trust.
   b. Hostility and withdrawal of love will cause the child further loss of trust, self-esteem, and independence.

Preschool Child (3–5 years)

A. Primary Concerns

1. Separation—although cognitive and coping capabilities have increased and the child responds less violently to separation from parents, separation and hospitalization represent stress beyond the coping mechanisms and adaptive capabilities of the preschool child. Loneliness and insecurities are experienced. Language is important; although the child may not verbally express what he is feeling, there is an attempt at this in the 4- or 5-year-old.
2. Unfamiliar environment—this requires coping with a change in daily routine and represents a loss of control and security.
3. Abandonment and punishment—fantasies and thought may contain vengeful wishes for other persons, for which the child expects retribution. Illness may be interpreted as punishment for thoughts. Enforced parental separation may be interpreted as loss of parental love and represents abandonment by them.
4. Body image and integrity—hospitalization and intrusive procedures provide a multitude of threats of both bodily mutilation and loss of identity, which are just beginning to develop along with the acquisition of autonomy.
5. Immobility—mobility is the child's dominant form of self-expression and adaptation to the environment. He has a great urge for locomotion and exercise of large muscles. It represents his main expression of emotion and release of tension.
6. Loss of control—this influences the preschooler's perception of and reaction to separation, pain, and illness.

B. Reactions

1. *Regression*—child temporarily stops using newly acquired skills in an attempt to retain or regain control of a stressful situation. Preschooler may return to behavior of the infant or toddler.
2. *Repression*—child may attempt to exclude the undesirable and unpleasant stresses from consciousness.
3. *Projection*—preschooler may transfer his own emotional state, motives, and desires to others in his environment.
4. *Displacement/sublimation*—emotions are permitted to be redirected and expressed in other situations such as art or play.
5. *Identification*—the child assumes characteristics of the aggressor in an attempt to reduce fear and anxiety and to feel that he is in control of the situation.
6. *Aggression*—hostility is direct and intentional; physical expression takes precedence over verbal expression.
7. *Denial and withdrawal*—the child is able to ignore interruptions and disavow any thought or feeling that would result in a painful experience.
8. *Fantasy*—a mental activity to help the child to bridge the gap between reality and fantasy through imagination. The child has difficulty separating reality from fantasy because of lack of experience.
9. The preschooler may simply show similar behaviors (protest, despair, denial) to those of the toddler, although the stage of protest is usually less aggressive and direct.

C. Nursing Interventions

1. Minimize stress of separation by providing for parental presence and participation in care. Strive to shorten

the hospital stay. Help parents understand what hospitalization means to the child.

2. Identify defense mechanisms apparent in the child and help him through the stressful situation by accepting him, showing him love and concern, and being alert to his readiness to relinquish them.
3. Set limits for the child. Let him know that someone is there. Help the child become master of something in the situation.
4. Provide opportunity and encouragement for child to verbalize.
5. Careful preparation for all procedures should be done on the child's level of development and comprehension.
6. Be sure the child has opportunities for play. Play is one important medium through which the child can overcome his fear and anxiety. A body outline, doll, and simple visual aids are appropriate teaching tools. Provide for self-expression; role reversal through puppets, dolls, drawings.
7. Encourage activities with other children.
8. Provide consistency in nursing personnel and approach to care.
9. Encourage the child to participate in his care and self-hygiene as appropriate.
10. Deal specifically with castration and mutilation fears. If the child is having surgery, describe exactly which body part will be repaired, and provide reassurance that nothing else will be removed or repaired.
11. Whenever appropriate, reassure the child that no one is to blame for his illness or hospitalization.

School-Age Child (5–12 years)

A. Concerns

1. Many fear loss of recently mastered skills.
2. Many worry about separation from school and peers. They may fear loss of former roles.
3. Mutilation fantasies are common.
4. Some may believe that they or their parents magically caused the illness merely by thinking that the event would occur.
5. Often they have increased concerns related to modesty, privacy.
6. The imposed passivity may be interpreted as punishment.
7. Children may feel their body no longer is their own, but rather is controlled by doctors and nurses.

B. Reactions

1. Regression
2. Separation anxiety—especially early school-age period
3. Negativism
4. Depression
5. Tendency to be phobic (normal)
   a. Fears include that of the dark, doctors, hospitals, medication, and death.
   b. Unrealistic fears are commonly attached to needles, x-ray procedures, and blood.
6. Conscious attempts at mature behavior
7. Suppression or denial of symptoms

C. Nursing Interventions

1. Help parents to prepare the child for elective hospitalizations.
2. Obtain a thorough nursing history, including information regarding health and physical development, hospitalizations, social–cultural background, and normal daily activities. Utilize this information to plan care.
3. Provide for continuity of nursing personnel.
4. Provide order and consistency in the environment whenever possible.
5. Establish and enforce reasonable policies to protect the child and to increase his sense of security in his environment.
6. Arrange the environment to allow for as much mobility as possible (i.e., make sure articles are appropriately placed; move the bed if the child is immobilized).
7. Respect the child's need for privacy and respect modesty during examinations, bathing, etc.
8. Utilize treatment rooms whenever possible when performing painful or intrusive procedures.
9. Help young children identify problems and questions (often through play). Then help them to find the answers.
10. Provide information about the illness and hospitalization based on assessment of what facts the child needs and wants and how this information can be made readily understandable to him.
11. View all nursing care activities as teaching situations. Explain the function of equipment and allow the child to handle it. Teach scientific terminology for body parts, procedures, etc.
12. When explaining a procedure, make sure that the child knows its purpose, what will be done, and what will be expected of him. Reassure the child during the procedure by continuing the explanations and support.
13. Reassure the child having surgery; explain where the organ to be removed or repaired is located, and that no other body part will be removed.
14. Carefully assess pain and provide appropriate relief.
15. Utilize play whenever appropriate to provide information about the hospital experience and to identify and decrease the child's fantasies and fears.
16. Reassure the child that he or his parents are not to blame for his illness.
17. Facilitate discharge of energy and aggression through appropriate play activities or through sharing aspects of ward management.
18. Encourage the child's participation in his care and self-hygiene.
19. Support intellectual potential through the use of games, books, puzzles, school work, and drawings.
20. Assist the child's family to understand his reactions to illness and hospitalization so that family members can facilitate positive coping patterns.
21. Let the child know that his normal status as a family member remains intact during his hospitalization. Encourage a consistent visiting pattern and allow sibling visits.
22. Help parents to deal with their own anxieties about hospitalization and assist them to help their child cope with the situation.
23. Encourage parental participation in the child's care when appropriate.
24. Encourage written communication with peers, and allow peer visiting when appropriate.
25. Begin discharge planning early, including plans for physical and emotional needs. Alert families to possible behavioral changes, including phobias, nightmares, regression, negativism, and disturbances in eating and learning.

Adolescent

A. Concerns

1. Physical illness, exposure, and lack of privacy may cause increased concern about body image and sexuality.
2. Separation from security of peers, family, and school may cause anxiety.
3. Interference with his struggle for independence and emancipation from his parents is a concern.
4. The adolescent may be very threatened by helplessness. He may see illness as a punishment for feelings not mastered or for breaking rules imposed by his parents or physician.

B. Reactions

1. Anxiety or embarrassment related to loss of control
2. Insecurity in strange environment
3. Intellectualization about disease details in order to avoid addressing actual concerns
4. Rejection of treatment measures, even if previously accepted
5. Anger, (may be directed toward parents or staff), because goals are being thwarted
6. Depression
7. Increased dependency on parents, staff
8. Denial or withdrawal
9. Demanding or uncooperative behavior (usually an attempt to assert control)
10. Capitalization on gains from illness or pain

C. Nursing Interventions

1. Help parents to prepare the adolescent for elective hospitalizations.
2. Assess the impact of illness on the adolescent by considering factors such as timing, nature of illness, new experiences imposed, changes in body image, and expectations for the future.
3. Introduce the adolescent to the hospital staff and to regular routines soon after admission.
4. Obtain a thorough nursing history that includes information about hobbies, school, family, illness, hospitalization, food habits, and recreation.
5. Encourage adolescents to wear their own clothes, and allow them to decorate their beds or rooms to express themselves.
6. Have drawers and closets available to store personal items.
7. Allow the adolescent access to a telephone.
8. Allow adolescents control over appropriate matters (i.e., timing of bath, selection of food, etc.).
9. Respect their need for periodic isolation and privacy.
10. Have a well-supervised recreational and activities program available that is planned by a professional child care worker.
11. Accept adolescent's level of performance. Allow regression with expectation of growth.
12. Involve the adolescent in planning his care so that he will be more accepting of restrictions and receptive to health teaching. He should be accepted as a vital member of the health-care team. His consent should be obtained for procedures and surgery.
13. Explain clearly all procedures, routines, expectations, and restrictions imposed by illness. If necessary, clarify the adolescent's interpretation of illness and hospitalization. Plan separate teaching sessions for parents.
14. Facilitate verbal rejection of treatment measures to protect the adolescent from harming himself physically by stopping treatment.
15. Assess the adolescent's intellectual skills and provide him with the necessary information to allow him to use problem-solving to deal with his illness and hospitalization.
16. Recognize positive and negative coping behaviors as attempts to adjust to a threatening situation. Attempt to deal with the feeling that caused the behavior as well as with the behavior itself.
17. Be a good listener. Maintain a sense of humor.
18. Provide opportunities such as writing, art work, and recreational activities to allow nonverbal adolescents to express themselves.
19. Foster interaction with other hospitalized adolescents and continuation of peer relationships with outside friends.
20. Establish regular group meetings to allow patients to meet with staff members and with each other to comment and to ask questions about their hospital experiences.
21. Set necessary limits to encourage self-control and ensure the rights of others.
22. Help adolescents work through sexual feelings. Avoid behavior which could be interpreted as provocative or flirtatious. Masturbation, unless excessive, may be considered a psychological healthy way to discharge sexual tension.
23. Interpret the needs and reactions of hospitalized adolescents to parents. Emphasize the adolescent's need to be respected as a unique individual, separate from his parents.
24. Assist parents to cope with the illness and hospitalization as well as to deal effectively with the adolescent's response to related stress.
25. Encourage continuation of education.
26. Stress the confidential nature of conversations between nurse and patient, and physician and patient.

Family-Centered Care

Family-centered care provides an opportunity for the family to care for the hospitalized child with nursing support.

The *goal* of family-centered care is to maintain or strengthen the roles and ties of the family with the hospitalized child in order to promote normality of the family unit.

Benefits for Parents and Child

1. Continued close family interactions during stress.
2. Absence of separation anxiety.
3. Reactions of protest, denial, and despair are decreased or nonexistent.
4. Greater sense of security for the child.

5. Opportunity for family to fulfill their needs to care for their child physically and emotionally.
6. Allows parents to feel useful and important rather than making them dependent and destroying their confidence.
7. Lessening of parental guilt feelings.
8. Opportunities for parents to increase their competence and confidence in caring for the sick child.
9. Comfort for the family provided by other families.
10. Greater absorption of staff teaching by the family.
11. Posthospitalization reactions are diminished.

Implementation Strategies

Implementation of family-centered care will depend on regulations of the particular health-care setting as well as the capabilities of the individual family unit. Examples of activities that can facilitate and strengthen family ties include:

1. Rooming-in for parents of young children
2. Parent participation in the child's physical care
3. Flexible visiting regulations for family members, including siblings
4. Having pictures of family members available at the hospital
5. Encouraging telephone contact
6. Use of family tape recordings

General Principles of Family-Centered Care

1. The nurse must be equipped with a broad knowledge base from the physical and behavioral sciences. Special emphasis is required in such areas as growth and development, family dynamics, socialization, and communication. Continuing education programs must be designed to support and improve family-centered care.
2. Staff must realize that parents are not time savers for nurses when they are participating in their child's care. The parents are not there to relieve the nurse of her routines and care.

   Additional nursing time is necessary to answer questions, to orient parents to the unit, to teach child care, and to comfort parents.
3. Family-centered care places a great deal of responsibility on the nurse and offers an opportunity to administer total patient care to the child and his family.
4. Family-centered care units should present a relaxed, comfortable atmosphere.
   a. Do not require parents to stay, but allow them to stay if they desire.
      (1) Some mothers may feel too anxious or guilty to participate.
      (2) Outside responsibilities may prohibit parents' staying.
   b. Provide physical comfort for participating parents.
      (1) Folding chair or bed in child's room
      (2) Comfortable lounge or waiting room
      (3) Eating facilities
      (4) Bathroom facilities, including showers
   c. Encourage parent(s) to take appropriate breaks from attending to the child.
      (1) Provides rest for the parent.
      (2) Helps child learn parent(s) will return and not abandon him.
5. When parents are active participants in their child's care, they too have certain needs, because they are concerned about their ill child.
   a. They want to care for their child as they would do at home.

b. They are interested in working with the staff and learning from the staff how they can help their child.
c. They like to have something to do for the child while visiting. This lessens their feeling of helplessness.
d. Supports should be available (e.g., parent advocates, child care for well siblings, parent surrogates for times when parents cannot stay).
6. If parents know what is expected of them and what they can expect of the staff, many problems can be avoided. It helps parents feel more comfortable.
   a. Nursing and medical observations and care will be continued with or without the parents (or mother) present.
   b. Parents should be encouraged to assume a nurturing, comforting role. They should also be allowed to participate in the child's physical care to the extent that they desire or that will be necessary after the child's discharge. This requires encouragement, support, and education from the nurse.
   c. Parents should allow child to become involved with peers on the unit.
   d. Parents should not ask for personal services.
7. Families of hospitalized children can offer a great deal of support to one another. Many times they have similar problems.
   a. Allow families to gather in groups—informal or formally planned group meetings.

Role of Parents

1. To serve as the child's primary resource of security and support so that he will be better able to tolerate unfamiliarity and discomfort and will be able to emerge from the experience with less likelihood of posthospitalization reactions.
2. To serve as the child's advocate in order to ensure that his basic human rights will be respected.
3. To teach nurses specific ways in which they can support the child.
4. To serve as role models and to support other families who may be dealing with similar problems.

Role of Nurse

1. To create an environment conducive to maintaining family integrity and unity. The nurse should:
   a. Help to maintain a healthy parent–child relationship. (Parents should not feel threatened by the nurse.)
   b. Facilitate a supportive marital relationship.
   c. Include siblings in planning and intervention as appropriate.
   d. Supplement the family in the common goal of the child's welfare.
2. To assist parents to make decisions about when to stay with their child.
   a. Parents' presence is especially important if the child is 5 years or younger, is especially anxious or upset, or is in medical crisis.
   b. The parents' decision is influenced by needs of other family members, as well as by job and home responsibilities.
   c. The nurse should try to alleviate guilty feelings of parents who are unable to stay with their child.
3. To develop trusting, goal-directed relationship with families.

a. Obtain a thorough nursing history that provides information to assess strengths, relationships, and concerns.
b. Plan with the family toward mutual, realistic goals.
c. Recognize good care that the child receives from parents.

4. To observe the parent–child relationship in order to do the following:
   a. Evaluate the degree of participation of the parents in physical and emotional care.
   b. Observe parents' attitudes, skills, and techniques and the child's behavior and response to them.
   c. Assess what teaching needs to be done.
   d. Detect problems in parent–child relationships.

5. To teach parents knowledge, understanding, and skills necessary to function effectively with the hospitalized child. The nurse should:
   a. Perform nursing techniques safely and efficiently.
   b. Interpret the behavior of the hospitalized child to parents so that they can understand it and intervene appropriately (refer to the section, Impact of Hospitalization on the Child's Stage of Development).
   c. Interpret and reinforce what physician has told parents. Answer questions thoroughly and honestly as knowledge permits.
   d. Interpret medical procedures and diagnostic tests.
   e. Provide health teaching.
   f. Offer anticipatory guidance.

6. To help parents adapt to the situation and to develop their own feeling of value by coping with the child's illness.
   a. Be aware of common parental reactions to the stress experienced by families of children who have severe or chronic illness.
   b. Be aware that defense mechanisms, if employed in moderation, are constructive and may facilitate optimal coping.
   c. Help parents recognize their own feelings.
   d. Identify parental support systems as well as adaptive and maladaptive coping.
   e. Be perceptive of parents' physical and emotional needs and limitations.
      (1) Do not allow parents to become fatigued.
      (2) Allow parents to leave, take a break.

7. To assist families as appropriate in dealing with normal family developmental tasks.
   a. Be aware that the child's hospitalization is often only one of many stresses a family experiences at a given time. Others frequently include:
      (1) Interpersonal problems
      (2) Debt, unemployment, job change
      (3) Recent changes in dwelling place and consequent disruption
      (4) Problems associated with child care and discipline
      (5) Concurrent illness of other family members

8. To ensure continuity of family-centered care between the hospital and home.

Pediatric Intensive Care Unit

Nursing Role and Responsibilities in a Pediatric Intensive Care Unit

1. To provide continuing, comprehensive physical care and supportive treatment required to maintain life and to aid recovery of acutely ill children.
2. To provide emotionally supportive care to acutely ill children.
3. To provide empathetic support to parents and families of children in the intensive care unit.
4. To act as an integral and essential member of the health care team by assessing patient needs as well as by planning care and evaluating its effectiveness.
5. To act as child advocate by ensuring that basic human rights are respected.
6. To serve as nursing care consultants when children who require some intensive care nursing skills are admitted to regular pediatric units.
7. To serve as members of appropriate hospital committees (e.g., committees that decide policy on emergency care, protocol for admission to the pediatric ICU, etc.).
8. To teach intensive care nursing principles and skills to appropriate groups (e.g., nursing students, resident physicians, persons in continuing education programs).
9. To function effectively and safely, the ICU nurse should demonstrate the following capabilities:
   a. Good physical and emotional health required to withstand the strain of continually nursing critically ill patients
   b. Understanding of pathophysiology underlying disease
   c. Knowledge and understanding of sophisticated monitoring equipment and special apparatus
   d. Ability to reason objectively and to judge and be aware of rapidly changing situations
   e. Ability to interpret data and to take rapid, decisive action
   f. Ability to perform complex technical skills correctly and in an organized manner
   g. Understanding of the impact of illness and hospitalization on the life of the child
   h. Understanding of parental responses and ways of coping with the stress of a critically ill child
   i. Ability to record data concisely, accurately, and thoroughly

Physical Care of the Child

1. Apply understanding of the pathogenesis of the disease in assessing patient needs and in planning care.
2. Perform complex technical skills to monitor and support the child (see text for specific procedures). These may include:
   a. Cardiac, respiratory, and blood pressure monitoring
   b. Basic interpretation of ECG tracing
   c. Endotracheal suctioning
   d. Oxygen administration and monitoring
   e. Tracheostomy care
   f. Ventilator management
   g. Monitoring central venous pressure
   h. Monitoring intracranial pressure
   i. Measuring arterial pressure
   j. Hyperalimentation

    k. Collection of specimens
    l. Chest drainage
3. Perform nursing activities related to life support of the child (see text for specific procedures). These activities include the following:
    a. Cardiopulmonary support
    b. Respiratory management
    c. Observation of neurologic signs
    d. Fluid and nutritional assessment and management
    e. Observations for complications and changing status
4. Apply general nursing measures for patient comfort and prevention of complications:
    a. Positioning—to prevent contractures, to drain secretions from the lungs, and to minimize pressure effects on skin
    b. Monitoring and regulation of body temperature
    c. Skin care—to prevent breakdown
    d. Eye care—to prevent conjunctivitis and injury to the cornea in unconscious children
    e. Fluid balance—record daily fluid intake by all routes and losses of urine, stool, vomit, blood, and other drainage; be sensitive to weight loss and gain
    f. Mouth care—to cleanse mouth of secretions, vomitus, especially in unconscious patient or patient with endotracheal tube
    g. Control of infection
5. Provide careful, continuous clinical observations of the child.

Emotional Support of Child

1. Refer to the section on the impact of hospitalization on the developmental stage of the child, page 1113.
2. If possible, familiarize the child with the unit before admission.
3. Provide immediate physical care that communicates strength and facilitates trust.
4. Be alert to behavioral changes that may indicate physical distress.
5. Facilitate parent–child interaction.
6. Question parents concerning the child's own way of responding to emotional stress. Utilize particular comforts that are most soothing to the child.
7. Support parents so that they will be best able to support their child.
8. Time activities; dim lights to allow for adequate sleep whenever possible.
9. Do everything possible to reduce the amount of pain that the child must endure.
10. Provide age-appropriate stimulation when indicated

by the child's condition (TV, games, books, toys, etc.).
11. Provide opportunities for the child to express his fears and concerns.
12. If possible, avoid exposing an alert child to the death or resuscitation of another child. If the child is exposed, provide adequate explanation. The child must also be helped to express and work through the experience.
13. Prepare the child for transfer from the intensive care unit by implementing a nursing care plan similar to that which the child will experience on a regular unit (e.g., decrease frequency of monitoring of vital signs, encourage independence). Give a thorough report to the receiving nurse during transfer.

Emotional Support to Family

1. Orient parents to the unit and its waiting areas. Clarify visiting policies and hospital expectations.
2. Encourage liberal visiting hours and unlimited phone calls from parents to the intensive care unit.
3. Assure parents that everything possible is being done for their child. Whenever possible, allow them to see child receiving treatment.
4. Make certain that parents are informed of important changes in the child's clinical status. Reinforce medical interpretations.
5. Explain special equipment and changes in nursing management.
6. Provide opportunities for parents to ask questions and have them answered.
7. Encourage parents to interact verbally and physically with their child. Support them in this endeavor.
8. Facilitate expressions of parental grief.
9. Provide opportunities for parents to talk to a person with whom they can share their concerns and fears. Be sure this person can see them as often as they require.
10. Provide opportunities for parents to meet together to share experiences and offer mutual support.
11. Be sensitive to parents' additional commitments to family and home as well as to their need to remain with their child. Whenever possible, allow visiting at a mutually convenient time.
12. Help parents provide anticipatory guidance for siblings and extended family members.
13. Refer parents to appropriate community resources for help with financial, environmental, or psychologic problems.
14. Offer follow-up contact to parents if appropriate.
15. Refer to section on Family-Centered Care.

Child Life Programs

Many hospitals have established programs with a specially trained staff whose job it is to concern themselves solely with the social and emotional welfare of every pediatric patient. Such programs are called by a variety of names, including "Child Life," "Children's Activities," "Recreational Therapy," "Play Therapy," and others.

Rationale for Child Life Programs

1. Hospitalization separates a child from his home, family, and all that is familiar, and places him in an institution where he may experience intrusive, em-

barrassing, painful, and mutilating invasion of his body.
2. The short-term and long-term effects of illness and hospitalization on the intellectual, social, and emotional development of children have been documented by observations and research.
3. A separate child life department to meet the social and emotional needs of patients is justified, because such work requires the following:
    a. Special expertise and training.
    b. Adequate time that is free of other responsibilities.

c. A special role definition of the staff member so that the child knows that this is a person who will not become involved in his medical care.

Staffing of Child Life Programs

1. Staffing of child life departments differs among institutions according to their needs and resources.
   In most settings, they are staffed entirely by professionals who work with aides and volunteers.
2. Most child life workers have bachelor's or master's degrees in child-related professions such as preschool, kindergarten, and elementary education; nursing; social work; child development; and recreational therapy.
   a. Various educational institutions offer courses and areas of concentration in "The Hospitalized Child."
   b. Most child life departments offer their own in-service training programs so that the staff may learn to work with the hospitalized child.

Goals of Child Life Programs

1. To prevent some of the emotional pain and fear associated with illness and hospitalization.
   a. Child life workers may assume primary responsibility or a supportive role in the preparation of patients for hospitalization, surgery, and/or particular procedures.
   b. In many hospitals, child life workers arrange preadmission tours, puppet shows, and similar activities to which all children who are planned pediatric admissions are invited.
2. To provide a comfortable, accepting, and nonthreatening environment where the child may play and interact with other children and with an adult who is not involved with his health care.
   a. Ideally, there is a separate child life playroom in every unit. However, there may be only an open area at the end of a corridor or in the middle of the ward.
   b. Generally, there is a specific regulation that no medical procedures (even relatively benign ones such as taking a child's temperature) are to be carried out in the play area.
   c. In many settings, children are encouraged to have their meals in the playroom. Generally, they not only enjoy the opportunity to eat with others but also seem to eat better.
3. To provide the child with an opportunity for choice.
   a. The child may choose whether or not he wishes to come to the playroom. Once there, he may choose what to do.
   b. A variety of craft and play materials, including real and miniature medical equipment, is available.
   c. Should the child choose to sit and watch or be held and rocked, these activities are seen as acceptable choices.
4. To provide a continuing educational program.
   a. In some settings, teachers are paid by the hospital and are an integral part of the child life program. In others, teachers are provided by the local public schools, and they work in close cooperation with the child life department.
   b. In most hospitals, the educational program includes special activities for preschoolers and toddlers as well as a program of infant stimulation.

Role and Responsibilities of the Child Life Worker

1. To serve as advocate for the child.
   a. The worker serves as spokesperson for the child in his interaction with the health care delivery system.
   b. Serves as an instrument of change when the delivery system does not seem to be in the best interests of a large group of children.
2. To alleviate distress.
   a. Supports and tries to help children who have already been traumatized by their illness, surgery, and hospitalization.
   b. Is available for immediate crisis intervention such as comforting children during painful or frightening procedures, consoling children when expected visits from parents do not occur, and in other similar situations.
3. To provide therapeutic and recreational activity programs.
   a. The worker provides programs on the unit— both for individuals (at bedside) and for groups of children able to come to the play area.
   b. Utilizes play to allow the child to do the following:
      (1) Master his fears about an anticipated procedure or one that he has already experienced.
      (2) Express his feelings.
      (3) Give life to his fantasies and clarify misconceptions.
      (4) Try other roles (particularly those of doctor and nurse).
      (5) Distract himself.
      (6) Relieve boredom and simply have fun.
   c. The nature of such programs, the facilities for them, and the time allowed will necessarily vary from one hospital to the next.
4. To serve as a diagnostic observer.
   a. As a trained observer of the development and behavior of children, the child life worker acts as a member of the diagnostic team.
   b. Records observations and shares them with other members of the health team.
5. To participate in patient planning.
   Acts as a member of the health team to ensure that consideration is given to the child's social and emotional needs during and after hospitalization.
6. To serve as a source of support for parents.
   a. Is available to parents as needed to help them deal with their own anxieties as well as those of their children.
   b. In most settings, parents are encouraged to join their children in the play area.
7. To serve as teacher to physicians, nurses, and other hospital personnel.
   Teaches others in the areas of child development and behavior and the reactions of children to illness and hospitalization.

Shared Goals and Responsibilities

1. A child life department can exist only as one part of a hospital's total commitment to the social and emotional welfare of all children who enter the hospital.
2. Child life staff and nursing staff must work closely together and must complement each other's efforts.

Intensive Care Nursery

Nurse's Role and Responsibilities in an Intensive Care Nursery

1. The nurse is an active, integral part of the essential nurse–physician team in caring for the sick newborn.
   a. The nurse has a major responsibility in caring for the sick newborn. Much credibility is given to her observations because of continual contact with and care of the infant and past experience in making similar observations.
   b. It is not enough to follow the written prescription of the physician. The nurse must use initiative (i.e., must employ independent nursing judgment) in evaluating the infant's condition and must make changes in therapy when there are signs of deterioration or be able to handle a medical emergency. Subtle changes in behavior or condition of the infant detected early by the nurse and related to the physician often result in treating the infant before he is critically ill or beyond the point where permanent damage may have occurred.
2. The nurse must have an understanding of pathogenesis of diseases of the newborn in order to program nursing activities in caring for the infant. The nurse must be informed about the following:
   a. Specific diseases of the newborn
   b. The treatment of their problems
   c. The uses of the equipment employed in caring for these infants
3. In addition, the nurse must possess the following qualities:
   a. Improved clinical awareness
   b. Increased diagnostic skills
   c. Ability to make nursing assessments
   d. Skills in performing special procedures
4. Working with the critically ill infant requires technical skills in several areas. Some of these include:
   a. Respiratory care
      (1) Endotracheal suctioning
      (2) Oxygen administration and monitoring
      (3) Ventilatory management
   b. Cardiac and vascular monitoring
      (1) Blood pressure assessment
      (2) Exchange transfusion and blood administration
      (3) Umbilical catheterization
      (4) Blood gas monitoring
   c. Other treatment and assessment modalities
      (1) Laboratory and roentgen studies
      (2) Phototherapy
      (3) Temperature control
   d. Equipment control
      Equipment working properly, etc.
5. The knowledge acquired in caring for the critically ill newborn will equip the nurse to compare signs such as respiration, fluctuating blood pressure, heart rate, subtle movement or lack of movement, and provide:
   a. Cardiopulmonary support
   b. Respiratory management
   c. Fluid and nutritional assessment and management
   d. Observation for complications and other illnesses
6. Infection control is within the realm of nursing responsibilities. Constant surveillance and strict adherence to procedures directed toward preventing infection must be practiced.
   a. Good handwashing technique:
      (1) 2- to 3-minute scrub with a brush and hexachlorophene or iodophor at the start of each tour of duty
      (2) 15-second scrub before and between infants
   b. Consider contact with Isolette or bassinet the same as contact with the infant himself.
   c. Nonhuman areas of contact and sources of possible contamination might be scales, examining table, and washing areas.
   d. Need for adequate and appropriate nurse–baby ratio.
   e. Surveillance of infant to recognize evidence of illness and source of infection to others.
   f. Removal from the area of individuals experiencing viral or bacterial illness.
   g. Effective cord care of the newborn—application of antiseptic dye (triple dye) or neomycin–polymyxin–bacitracin ointment.
   h. If staphylococcal or streptococcal infection develops in the area, the following procedures should be followed:
      (1) Periodic bathing of infants with a 0.1N dilution (0.3%) of hexachlorophene solution is effective in controlling infection by these organisms. Blood levels of hexachlorophene are lower if this solution is used rather than the 3% solution.

▶ **NURSING ALERT:** Hexachlorophene should be used cautiously and under strict and specific medical supervision in order to prevent neurotoxicity in the infant.

      (2) The Isolette and incubator serve as effective isolation when good handwashing is practiced.
   i. Invasive monitoring devices and procedures and ventilatory support, bypass local defenses and can allow for bacteria to colonize, resulting in infection.
7. The nurse must begin to help form a bond between infant and his mother as well as to build cohesiveness of the family immediately upon the infant's admission to the intensive care unit (see Caring for Parents of Infant in Intensive Care Nursery).
8. Research indicates that to enhance the quality of the life saved and to provide the best chance for the child to achieve his potential, early environmental, emotional, and psychosocial stimulation is essential. By virtue of involvement, the nurse has a tremendous responsibility and opportunity in this area (see p. 1123).
9. It is vitally important that the nurse practice meticulous recording and documentation for the protection of the infant as well as the nurse:
   a. Always record routine procedures (i.e., hourly ventilator care).
   b. Record physician visits to infant and any contact by nurse with physician.

c. Never erase. Errors should be crossed out with a single line, marked "error," and initialed.
d. Record events accurately (e.g., emergency treatment).

Classification of High-Risk Neonate Requiring Intensive Care

1. *Premature*—problems are related to general immaturity: feeding, respiratory distress and/or apneic spells, hyperbilirubinemia.
2. *Small for gestational age*—problems include hypoglycemia, poor temperature control, and high susceptibility to infection.
3. *Medical problems*—these include respiratory distress, hypoglycemia, hyperbilirubinemia, erythroblastosis, sepsis neonatorum, hypocalcemia, infant of diabetic mother (IDM), drug withdrawal, and neurologic conditions.
4. *Surgical problems*—these include tracheoesophageal fistula, myelomeningocele, cleft palate, imperforate anus, and distended abdomen.
5. *Congenital malformations*—these include cardiac problems, genetic defects.

Caring for Parents of Infant in Intensive Care Nursery

Research has documented that infant–mother bonding is significantly influenced by events before and immediately after delivery and may greatly influence later maternal behavior and the infant–mother relationship. Mother's attachment to her infant is critical for his optimal growth and development, since he depends entirely on his mother to satisfy his needs.

A. Barriers to healthy mother–infant bonding

1. Grief, guilt, anger, fear, and anxiety felt by the mother at the birth of a child she expected to be perfect. Mother may mourn over loss of this child.
2. Maternal background factors—socioeconomic status, educational training, own childhood experiences, emotional stability.
3. Expectations and attitudes of the mother toward her infant.
4. Separation of mother and her infant at a time when her sensitivity may be at a maximum for attachment to her infant.
5. Anticipatory grieving for possible loss of this infant and emotional withdrawal from infant.
6. Maternal attitude about herself—her lack of self-confidence in her ability to care for her infant; her negative feelings about her inability to carry her infant to term or to produce a normal child.
7. Disruption of care-eliciting behaviors by the infant; the infant serves as a stimulus for mother in helping her identify her offspring and promote her caretaking behaviors.
8. Stress elicited by physical presence of infant in intensive care nursery (i.e., realization of severity of illness of infant, emergency atmosphere, sensory deprivation)—all tend to diminish the mother's self-confidence—since she cannot give her own infant the special care he needs.
9. Maternal behaviors give clues to an altered relationship with her infant (i.e., lack of early claiming behavior and attachment, repulsion at infant's medical diagnosis or unrealistic view of infant's problems, infrequent visiting, anger towards staff, or inability to discuss problems).

B. Nursing intervention to help foster mother–infant bonding as well as eventual appropriate parenting behaviors

1. Allow mother to see and touch her infant immediately after delivery and again as soon and as often as possible. This minimizes any fantasies that may develop.
2. Describe in detail all the equipment surrounding the infant in the intensive care nursery, prior to the mother's seeing the infant and again when she is near him.
3. Talk with mother on a personal basis; call her by name; make personal comments. Encourage parents to name their baby and refer to him by that name.
4. Encourage mother to enter the intensive care nursery as soon as possible and allow unlimited visiting except during specialized procedures. If daily visits are not always possible, encourage phone contact with nursery staff. The nurse should also call the mother.
5. Carefully consider the mother's concerns and feelings. Being the parent of a critically ill infant is emotionally devastating. Communicate to her your caring concern.
6. Encourage mother to touch her infant.
   a. This will help her to see him as real and will decrease some of her fears.
   b. Touching is the first step in the mother's developing her own self-confidence.
   c. Show mother how she can gradually assume more of infant's care and how she is better at mothering than the nurse.
7. Open communication channels with parents early.
   a. Meet parents in hospital of origin.
   b. Reinforce information given.
   c. Share good news—first feeding, physical activity, less oxygen needed, etc.
   d. Support them when discouraging news (e.g., discontinued feedings, increased apneic spells) is given.
   e. Often there develops a closeness between the mother and nurse that allows her to participate knowledgeably and confidently with the nurse in evaluating the infant's progress.
8. Observe the intensive care nursery physical setting in terms of parental needs (i.e., need for rocking chairs, bright pictures on the walls, parents' visiting area inside the nursery, pictures of past ICN babies who are growing and thriving).
9. Encourage active participation by the mother in the care of her infant (as the infant's condition permits). For example, instruct the mother on how to enter the Isolette; allow her to visit during feeding and to do something in connection with feeding.
   a. Explain how her visits and contact will benefit the baby.
   b. Assist her in touching and talking to her infant as necessary.
   c. Show her that increasing her physical contact with the infant will increase her involvement and confidence in caring for the child. Foster a sense of mastery and coping and of accomplishment within the mother. As the infant improves, the parents should become increasingly involved

and ultimately competent and comfortable in caring for their infant.

    d. Continually assess the parents' (the mother's, in particular) ability to be involved; be sensitive to their tolerance for handling the infant and their degree of emotional tolerance.

10. There should be continuous focus on the family. Parents and infant must be treated as a unit.
    a. Priorities for this are:
      (1) Crisis intervention
      (2) Continual parent contact
      (3) Encouragement of parenting behaviors
    b. Goals are:
      (1) To develop mother's self-confidence and ability to rely on her own instincts and common sense in caring for her infant.
      (2) To assist the father in becoming involved emotionally and in developing competence in taking care of his family after discharge as well as in taking pleasure in his infant.

11. There is a necessity to decrease the social isolation that is often inherent in the birth of a critically ill baby.
    a. Initiate social service and community health nurse support early.
    b. Provide mother (parents) with an opportunity to talk with other mothers (or parents) of infants with similar conditions, thus affording them the opportunity to express their feelings and concerns and to realize that they are not alone in feelings of guilt, failure, and fear.
    c. Permit visits to infant and parents by others who will be a support to them.
    d. The stress on older siblings of the birth of a sick infant can be overwhelming, and this affects parents and their fantasies of the child. Sibling visits can often help reduce these fantasies, fears, and anxieties with the support of parents and staff.

12. Provide some mechanism by which information concerning parents can be evaluated and trouble areas can be recognized early. Document information such as the following:
    a. Parental involvement (phone calls, visits, handling and caring for infant).
    b. Specific or special procedures observed by, taught to, and performed by parents.
    c. Specific information discussed with parents—by whom and when.
    d. Discharge teaching and plans.

13. Some interventions that may help parents become attached to their sick infant include transporting mother to be near infant, rooming-in, parent groups, transporting healthier infant to mother's room or to a hospital closer to her residence.

Stimulation: The Infant in Intensive Care Nursery

Every infant has the emotional need and right to recognize his mother's face, touch, and voice. The sick infant or premature infant is forced to accept less. Research documents that problems can arise from early sensory deprivation. The intensive care nursery is devoid of much sensory and perceptual stimuli—a situation that is harmful to the infant, the mother, and the mother–infant interactions. To maximize the potential to which the infant can develop, an early stimulation program should be planned.

1. Each stimulation program should be individualized for the specific infant–parent unit, based on:
    a. Familiarization with the infant's physical condition and limitations.
    b. Assessment of the infant's behavioral skills, developmental status, areas of deprivation or over-stimulation.
    c. Assessment of the parents' abilities to be involved in stimulating their child.
    d. A program of infant stimulation adds specific sensory–motor activities and techniques to daily care activities for a specific area of development. It is not random activity meant to excite the infant.

2. Some general guidelines for establishing a psychosocial stimulation environment to be adapted for each infant include the following:
    a. Provide for the continuity of the same caretaker each day, tour of duty. This will benefit both infant and parents.
    b. Make the baby as attractive as possible—clean, colorful linen, lotion on skin, ribbon in hair. The general appearance of a "preemie" or sick infant makes it difficult for mother to relate to her infant.
    c. Help infant establish a day/night cycle. Dim lights or cover infant's eyes.
    d. Place an active mobile or colorful object in baby's line of vision, and adjust as his vision accommodation changes with age—about 23 cm. (9 inches) for newborn. This will increase visually directed reaching.
    e. Encourage personnel to talk to and touch infant when caring for him. Hold him at feedings as well as between feedings when infant's condition allows this. Have personnel attempt to have infant focus upon their face and follow their head movement with his eyes.
    f. Encourage personnel to follow specific procedure when feeding if infant is able to tolerate it.
      (1) Hold infant in nursing position to aid in establishing en face.
      (2) Rock, talk to, fondle, and pat infant before, during, and after feeding. Hold infant in upright position when burping to aid in this visual orientation.
    g. Encourage parent participation in this program.
      (1) Assist the infants so that they become emotionally involved with the baby.
      (2) Point out specific responses and behavior of the infant they can look for and what these responses mean. This will help them learn to pay attention to the baby's behavior and to respond to his needs. Talk about this behavior and the parents' feelings about it.
      (3) Encourage parents to visit during feeding time and to participate in the procedure. Even if gavage feedings are done, parents can hold infant, give him a pacifier, fondle him, and relate to him in many ways.
    h. Be aware of specific sensory stimulation for the infant.
      (1) Olfactory—mother's article of clothing near infant.
      (2) Visual—change position of infant; change location of Isolette; use of mobiles or bright objects; imitate infant's movements.

(3) Auditory—music box, tape of mother's voice; imitate infant's sounds.

Discharge Planning Begins Early

1. Maternal behaviors are learned. In order to provide the mother with an opportunity to build self-confidence and to develop to her potential, active participation with her infant during the infant's hospitalization is essential. Mother–infant bonding must be started and allowed to grow during this time for the well-being of both infant and mother.
2. Detailed preparation for home care is essential and must be given in advance.
   a. Specific or special procedures and medications.
   b. Information concerning routine baby care.
   c. Crying pattern of the newborn.
3. Initiate social service and/or community nurse referrals long before discharge.
   a. This provides parents with continual support by someone they know.
   b. Initiating these referrals also gives the nurse feedback about the home situation and possible areas where problems can be averted.
   c. Continual support by the community health nurse is important. Follow-up care can be directed also at assessing family interaction and parenting behaviors as well as development of the baby.
4. Evaluate the parents' willingness and ability to accept the child into their total care.
   Permit the mother a special nesting period when she can have close physical contact with her infant in privacy and can provide complete care for her infant. Nursing support and help are readily available for the mother to call on if needed.

a. Instructions, demonstrations, and practice of procedures should have occurred prior to this time.
b. It is possible that this period may enhance normal maternal attachment behaviors days or weeks after birth.
5. Encourage parents to continue psychosocial and intellectual stimulation of their infant at home.
   Provide a resource for parents so that they can assess child's readiness for the next step and promote it.

Realities of Nursing in the Intensive Care Nursery

Nursing in an intensive care nursery can be an emotionally draining experience; it can be difficult and depressing as well as hopeful and rewarding. Nurses frequently become surrogate mothers, grieving and rejoicing as the infant's condition changes. To minimize the personal agony frequently encountered, certain areas should be explored and opened to discussion.

1. Each nurse working in the intensive care nursery setting must be completely and totally educated to work in the area.
2. Discussions on grief and grieving should be open and frequent to allow each nurse to explore her own feelings.
3. Patient-centered discussions should be part of the routine to allow the nurse to express feelings about a particular patient.
4. Parent-centered discussions should focus on the parent's coping behaviors and stages of grief.
5. Each nurse must explore and acknowledge her feelings about the work in which she is involved.

The Child Undergoing Surgery

Preoperative Care

1. Provide emotional support, psychological preparation, and preoperative teaching appropriate for the age of the child. Such preparation and support will minimize stress and will help the child cope with his fears.
   a. Potential threats for the hospitalized child anticipating surgery are:
      (1) Physical harm—bodily injury, pain, mutilation, death
      (2) Separation from parents
      (3) The strange and unknown—possibility of surprise
      (4) Confusion and uncertainty about his limits and expected behavior
      (5) Relative loss of control of his world, his autonomy
      (6) Fear of anesthesia
      (7) Fear of the surgical procedure itself
   b. All preparation and support must be based on the child's age, developmental stage, and level; personality; past history and experience with health professionals and hospitals; background— including religion, socioeconomic group, culture, and family attitudes.
      (1) Know what information the child has already received.

(2) Determine from the child what he knows or expects.
(3) Additional guidelines in preparation include the following: Use illustration of a child's body, concrete examples and simple terms (not medical jargon); identify changes that may occur as a result of the procedure, both body and routine; give the explanation slowly and clearly, saving anxiety-producing aspects until the end.
   Make use of child's creative ability and logical thinking powers to aid in preparation for procedures.
   c. Orient patient and family to the unit, room, location of playroom, operating room, and recovery room and introduce them to other children, parents, and some of the personnel.*
   Make arrangements for the child to meet anesthesiologist as well as the operating room nurse and recovery room nurse.
   d. Allow and encourage questions. Give honest answers.*
      (1) Such questions will give the nurse a better

---

* Other aspects of preparation for procedures to be emphasized.

understanding of the child's fears and perceptions of what is happening to him.

(2) Infants and young children need to form a trusting relationship with those who care for them.

(3) The older child tends to be reassured by the information he receives.

e. Provide opportunity for child and parent to work out concerns and feelings (play, talk).

Such supportive care should result in less upset behavior and more cooperation.

f. Prepare child for what to expect postoperatively (i.e., equipment to be used or attached to child, different location, how he will feel, what he will be expected to do, diet, new health caretakers).*

2. Assist in physical preparation of patient for surgery.

a. Assist with necessary laboratory studies. Explain to child what is going to happen prior to procedure and how he can respond. Give continual support during procedure.

b. See that patient has nothing by mouth (NPO) (from Latin *nil per os*).

Explain to child and parents what NPO means.

c. Assist with fever reduction.

(1) Fever will result from some surgical diseases (i.e., intestinal obstruction).

(2) Fever increases risk of anesthesia and need for fluids and calories.

d. Administer appropriate medications as prescribed.

Sedatives and drugs to dry the secretions are often given on the unit.

e. Establish good hydration.

Parenteral therapy may be necessary to hydrate the child, especially if he is NPO, vomiting or febrile.

3. Support parents during this time of crisis. The attitudes of the parents towards hospitalization and surgery largely determine the attitudes of their child.

a. The experience may be emotionally distressing.

b. Parents may have feelings of fear or guilt.

c. The preparation and support should be integrated for parent and child.

d. Give individual attention to parents; explore and clarify their feelings and thoughts; provide accurate information and appropriate reassurance.

e. Stress parents' importance to the child. Help mother understand how she can care for her child.

4. Special considerations should be made for the mentally retarded child requiring surgery. (See section on the mentally retarded child.)

a. Remember that the parents know their child and his behaviors best and should be encouraged to share this knowledge with staff. Continue to work closely with parents throughout the hospitalization.

b. Encourage parent(s) to remain with child to help him maintain a sense of security and to decrease his fears.

c. Do not isolate the child. When placing him with others, explain his behavior to his peers in preparation for this social contact.

d. Design play activities for his behavioral age.

* Other aspects of preparation for procedures to be emphasized.

e. Communicate your knowledge of his behaviors, handicaps, etc. to others who will care for him.

Postoperative Care

A. Immediate

1. Maintain a patent airway and prevent aspiration.

a. Position the child on his side or abdomen to allow secretions to drain and prevent tongue from obstructing pharynx.

b. Suction any secretions present.

2. Make frequent observations of general condition and vital signs.

a. Take vital signs every 15 minutes until child is awake and his condition stable.

b. Note respiratory rate and quality, pulse rate and quality, blood pressure, skin color.

c. Watch for signs of shock.

(1) All children in shock have signs of pallor, coldness, increased pulse, and irregular respirations.

(2) Older children have decreased blood pressure and perspiration.

d. Change in vital signs may indicate airway obstruction, hemorrhage, or atelectasis.

e. Restlessness may indicate pain or hypoxia.

Medication for pain is not usually given until anesthesia has worn off.

f. Check dressings for drainage or constriction and pressure.

3. See that all drainage tubes are connected and functioning properly.

Gastric decompression relieves abdominal distention and decreases the possibility of respiratory embarrassment.

4. Monitor parenteral fluids as prescribed (see p. 1160).

5. Be physically near the child as he awakens to offer soothing words and a gentle touch. Reunite parents and child as soon as possible after the child recovers from anesthesia.

If a language barrier exists, the parents should be with the child as he recovers from anesthesia.

B. After Recovery from Anesthesia

After undergoing simple surgery and receiving a small amount of anesthesia, the child may be ready to play and eat in a few hours. More complicated and extensive surgery debilitates the child for a longer period of time.

1. Continue to make frequent and astute observations in regard to behavior, vital signs, dressings or operative site, and special apparatus (IV, chest tubes, oxygen).

a. Note signs of dehydration.

(1) Dry skin and membranes

(2) Sunken eyes

(3) Poor skin turgor

(4) Sunken fontanelle in infant

b. Record any passage of flatus or stool, bowel sounds.

Observe for intestinal ileus, since crying children swallow air and even a minimal of ileus may cause gastric distention.

c. Record voiding time, amount, characteristics.

2. Record intake and output accurately.

a. Parenteral fluids and oral intake.

b. Drainage from gastric tubes or chest tubes, colostomy, wound, and urinary output.

Dressing may need to be weighed for more accurate estimate of output.

c. Parenteral fluid is evaluated and prescribed by considering output and intake.

Parenteral fluid is usually maintained until the child is taking adequate oral fluids.

3. Advance diet as tolerated, according to the child's age and the physician's directions.

a. First feedings are usually clear fluids; if tolerated, advance slowly to full diet for age.

Note any vomiting or abdominal distention.

b. Since anorexia may occur, offer the child what he likes in small amounts and in an attractive manner.

4. Prevent infection.

a. Keep the child away from other children or personnel with respiratory or other infections.

b. Change the child's position every 2–3 hours— prop infants with a blanket roll.

c. Encourage the child to cough and breathe deeply—let the infant cry for short periods of time, unless contraindicated.

d. Keep operative site clean.

   (1) Change dressing as needed.
   (2) Keep diaper away from wound.

5. Provide good general hygiene.

a. Good skin care will increase circulation and prevent pressure sores.

b. Provide proper rest and sleep periods.

c. Allow child exercise and movement out of bed when he feels better.

Advance gradually.

d. Allow diversional activity at intervals appropriate for age.

6. Offer the child measures of comfort.

a. See that the child is warm and changes position as needed.

b. Provide mouth care.

c. Allow the child to have and hold favorite toy or object.

d. Anticipate his needs.

e. Holding and rocking the infant or young child may be comforting.

f. Relief of pain with narcotics should be balanced against the risk of respiratory depression.

7. Provide emotional support and psychological security.

a. Encourage the child to talk about his operation.

b. Allow the child to play out his feelings.

c. Return often to see and talk to the child.

d. Reassure him that things are going well. Talk about going home, if appropriate.

8. Continue to offer support to the parents.

a. Help to maintain healthy family relationships. (Encourage parents to care for their child.)

b. Encourage parents to talk about their concerns.

c. Begin early to prepare for discharge.

   (1) Teach any special procedures to be continued at home. Provide written instructions.
   (2) Arrange for community nurse referral.
   (3) Determine limits of activity for the child.
   (4) Make follow-up appointments.
   (5) Anticipate reactions of the child as a result of the hospitalization.

9. Do a follow-up evaluation of the hospitalization with telephone contact or letter–questionnaire.

Transcultural Nursing in Pediatrics
(Cross-Cultural Knowledge of Health–Illness Behavior)

General Principles

1. Comprehensive nursing should include being alert and responsive to the many cultural cues present in daily nursing situations. A conscious effort should be made to become knowledgeable about cultural diversity, and distinctiveness and similarities of the culture most likely to be served in nursing practice so that cues will be more meaningful and will be incorporated into patient assessment and care.

2. The nurse should be aware that cultural beliefs affect how a family perceives, experiences, and copes with health and illness. Culture influences how a family communicates about its health problems, the manner in which symptoms are presented, when and to whom members go for care, how long they remain in care, and how the care is evaluated.

3. It is possible that some health behaviors generated from cultural beliefs may be anxiety-producing and threatening to the nurse. Knowledge of and sensitivity to cultural diversity will decrease these anxieties, thus facilitating effective interactions and relationships with the child and his family.

4. The nurse should be aware of the beliefs of the popular (family, community) and folk (nonprofessional healers) domains of health care available to her client as well as the accepted views of the medical profession so that discrepancies can be discussed and resolved. This folk health system can work with the professional health system to provide meaningful and therapeutic health services.

5. Knowledge of the cultural beliefs of the patient will assist the nurse in understanding behaviors that may seem negative, confusing, illogical, or primitive, and help in producing a response that is more appropriate for the client's condition.

Because of cultural influences, the patient may experience fear, anxiety, and loneliness, and have lack of knowledge regarding routine and inability to communicate with the nurse.

Assessment

Cultural background determines issues nurses should be aware of when caring for a child and his family.

1. Areas to consider when involved in cultural assessment*:

a. Patterns or life-style of an individual or cultural group

b. Specific cultural values, norms, and experiences of the client regarding health and illness

c. Cultural taboos and myths

* Leininger M. Transcultural Nursing: Concepts, Theories and Practices, p. 88+. New York, John Wiley & Sons, 1978

d. The world view or ethnocentric tendencies
e. The extent of assimilation into the mainstream cultural group
f. Health and life-care rituals or rights of passage to maintain health and avoid illness
g. Folk and professional approaches to healing
h. Objectives and methods of caring for self and others
i. Indicators of cultural change or adaptive behavior

2. In an attempt to become knowledgeable about cultural beliefs relating to pediatric nursing, the nurse must determine the following by talking with the patient and family about health values, beliefs, and practices*:
   a. What is the meaning of children in the culture?
   b. Do cultural patterns determine infant or child care? What are these patterns?
   c. Do cultural patterns determine parental responses to behaviors and appearances of the infant or child?
   d. What meaning does language or nonverbal communication have in the culture?

3. The acceptance of health care by a family or subculture may depend on the nurse's knowledge of the cultural beliefs and behaviors and her attempt to understand their values while working within given guidelines. It is essential to know how the family unit is culturally defined, the family's functions, and the functions of the child in order to work effectively with that unit.

4. The following questions may be helpful in eliciting the family's perception of the illness and related cultural beliefs†:
   a. What do you think caused the problem?
   b. Why do you think it started when it did?
   c. What do you think your child's illness does to him?
   d. How severe is your child's illness? Will it have a short or long course?
   e. What kind of treatment do you think your child should receive?
   f. What results do you hope to receive from this treatment?
   g. What are the major problems your child's illness has caused you?
   h. What do you fear most about your child's illness?

5. In addition to health care, cultural patterns and bereavement behaviors must also be understood in order to provide effective psychological services and support for family.

Bibliography

Books

Impact of Hospitalization on the Child's Stage of Development

Anthony E and Koupecnic C (eds). The Child in His Family: The Impact of Disease and Death. New York, John Wiley & Sons, 1973

Aten M and McAnarney E. A Behavioral Approach to the Care of Adolescents. St Louis, CV Mosby, 1981

Avery G. Neonatology, 2nd ed. Philadelphia, JB Lippincott, 1981

Beuf A. Biting off the Bracelet, A Study of Children in Hospitals. Philadelphia, University of Pennsylvania Press, 1979

Copeland DR, Pfefferbaum B and Stovall AJ (eds). The Mind of the Child Who is Said to Be Sick. Springfield, IL, Charles C Thomas, 1983

Duvall E. Marriage and Family Development, 5th ed. Philadelphia, JB Lippincott, 1977

Friedman S and Hoekelman R. Behavioral Pediatrics—Psychosocial Aspects of Child Health Care. New York, McGraw-Hill, 1980

Gellert E. Psychosocial Aspects of Pediatric Care. New York, Grune & Stratton, 1978

Goodnow J. Children Drawing. Cambridge, Harvard University Press, 1977

Hall J and Weaver B (eds). Nursing of Families in Crisis. Philadelphia, JB Lippincott, 1979

Hardgrove C and Dawson RB. Parents and Children in the Hospital. Boston, Little, Brown & Co, 1972

Henning J (ed). The Rights of Children: Legal and Psychological Perspectives, 2nd ed. Springfield, IL, Charles C Thomas, 1982

Hofman A (ed). Adolescent Medicine. Menlo Park, CA, Addison-Wesley, 1983

Howe J. Nursing Care of Adolescents. New York, McGraw-Hill, 1980

Hymovich DP. Nursing of Children: A Family-Centered Guide for Study, 3rd ed. Philadelphia, WB Saunders, 1982

Hymovich DP and Barnard M. Family Health Care, vol 2. Developmental and Situational Crises. New York, McGraw-Hill, 1979

Hymovich DP and Chamberlin RW. Child and Family Development: Implications for Primary Health Care. New York, McGraw-Hill, 1980

Jolly J. The Other Side of Pediatrics—A Guide to the Everyday Care of Sick Children. Baltimore, University Park Press, 1981

Klaus MH and Fanaroff A. Care of the High-Risk Neonate. Philadelphia, WB Saunders, 1982

Klaus MH and Kennell JH. Maternal–Infant Bonding. St Louis, CV Mosby, 1983

Klepsch M and Logie L. Children Draw and Tell: An Introduction to the Projective Uses of Children's Human Figure Drawings. New York, Brunner/Mazel, 1982

Klinzing D and Klinzing D. The Hospitalized Child: Communication Techniques for Health Personnel. Englewood Cliffs, NJ, Prentice-Hall, 1977

Lesner PA. Pediatric Nursing. Albany, Delmar, 1983

Lindheim R et al. Changing Hospital Environments for Children. Cambridge, Harvard University Press, 1972

McCaffrey M. Nursing Management of the Patient With Pain, 2nd ed. Philadelphia, JB Lippincott, 1979

McCollum, A. The Chronically Ill Child. A Guide for Parents and Professionals. New Haven, Yale University Press, 1981

McCormick R and Gilson-Parkevich T. Patient and Family Education—Tools, Techniques and Theory. New York, John Wiley & Sons, 1979

Melton G. Child Advocacy: Psychological Issues and Interventions. New York, Plenum Press, 1983

Oremland E and Oremland J (eds). The Effects of Hospitalization on Children. Springfield, IL, Charles C Thomas, 1974

Petrillo M and Sanger M. Emotional Care of Hospitalized Children. Philadelphia, JB Lippincott, 1980

Robinson G and Clarke H. The Hospital Care of Children—A Review of Contemporary Issues. New York, Oxford University Press, 1980

---

* Leininger M. Transcultural Nursing: Concepts, Theories and Practices, p. 88+. New York, John Wiley & Sons, 1978

† Kleinman A, Eisenberg L, and Good B. Culture, illness and care. Ann Intern Med 1978 Feb; 88(1):251–258

Rubin J. Child Art Therapy: Understanding and Helping Children Grow Through Art. New York, Van Nostrand-Reinhold, 1978

Schaefer C and O'Connor K. Handbook of Play Therapy. New York, John Wiley & Sons, 1983

Schulman J. Coping with Tragedy: Successfully Facing the Problems of a Seriously Ill Child. Chicago, Follett, 1976

Scipien G et al. Comprehensive Pediatric Nursing. New York, McGraw-Hill, 1979

Smith M. Child and Family: Concepts of Nursing Practice. New York, McGraw-Hill, 1982

Smith M (ed). Chronic Disorders in Adolescence. Boston, Wright, 1983

Steele S. Health Promotion of the Child with Long-Term Illness, 3rd ed. Norwalk, CT, Appleton-Century-Crofts, 1983

Tackett J and Hunsberger M. Family Centered Care of Children and Adolescents. Philadelphia, WB Saunders, 1981

Whaley L and Wong D. Nursing Care of Infants and Children, 2nd ed. St Louis, CV Mosby, 1983

Wieczorek R and Natapoff J. A Conceptual Approach to the Nursing of Children. Philadephia, JB Lippincott, 1981

Family-Centered Care

Azarnoff P and Hardgrove C. The Family in Child Health Care. New York, John Wiley & Sons, 1981

Farkas S. Hospitalized Children: The Family's Role in Care and Treatment. Washington, DC, National Center for Family Studies, Catholic University, 1983

Miller J and Janosik E. Family Focused Care. New York, McGraw-Hill, 1980

Pediatric Intensive Care

American Association of Critical Care Nurses. Critical Care Nursing of Children and Adolescents. Philadelphia, WB Saunders, 1981

Hazinski M. Nursing Care of the Critically Ill Child. St Louis, CV Mosby, 1984

Levin D, Morriss F and Moore G. A Practical Guide to Pediatric Intensive Care, 2nd ed. St Louis, CV Mosby, 1984

Smith J. Pediatric Critical Care. New York, John Wiley & Sons, 1983

Vestal K (ed). Pediatric Critical Care Nursing. New York, John Wiley & Sons, 1981

Intensive Care Nursery

Klaus M and Fanaroff A. Care of the High-Risk Neonate. Philadelphia, WB Saunders, 1981

Krones SB. High-risk Newborn Infants, 3rd ed. St Louis, CV Mosby, 1981

Lancaster J. Impact of Intensive Care on the Parent–Infant Relationship. In Krones SB. High-Risk Newborn Infants, 3rd ed. St Louis, CV Mosby 1981, pp. 354–365

Levin D, Morriss F and Moore G. A

Practical Guide to Pediatric Intensive Care. St Louis, CV Mosby, 1983

Nelson JD. Control of infection acquired in the nursery. In Remington JS and Klein JO (eds). Infectious Diseases of the Fetus and Newborn Infant. Philadelphia, WB Saunders, 1983, pp. 1035–1052

Child Undergoing Surgery

Raffensperger JG. Swenson's Pediatric Surgery, 4th ed. New York, Appleton-Century-Crofts, 1980

Steele S. Child Health and the Family. New York, Masson, 1981

Transcultural Nursing in Pediatrics

Leininger M. Transcultural Nursing: Concepts, Theories and Practices. New York, John Wiley & Sons, 1978

Schmidt VE and McNeil E. Cultural Awareness. Washington, DC, The National Association for the Education of Young Children, 1978

Articles

Impact of Hospitalization on the Child's Stage of Development

Abu-Saad H. The assessment of pain in children. Issues Compr Pediatr Nurs 1981 Dec; 5(5–6):327–335

Abu-Saad H and Hozemer W. Measuring children's self-assessment of pain. Issues Compr Pediatr Nurs 1981 Dec; 5(5–6):337–349

Ack M. Psychosocial effects of illness, hospitalization and surgery. Child Health Care 1983 Spring; 11(4):132–136

Acord LT. One five year old boy's use of play. Matern Child Nurs J 1980 Spring; 9(1):29–35

Anderson L. Is this the liberry? JACCH 1981; Winter 9(3):77–79

Beal JA. Preparing children for hospital procedures. In Issue and Adv Pract in Pediatr Nurs, Reston, VA, Reston Publishing, 1983, pp. 3–23

Betz CL. After the operation—postprocedural sessions to allay anxiety. MCN 1982 July/Aug; 7(4):260–263

Bibace R and Walsh ME. Development of children's concepts of illness. Pediatrics 1980 June; 66(6):912–918

Birchfield ME. Nursing care for hospitalized children based on different stages of illness. MCN 1981 Jan/Feb; 6(1):46–52

Bjornsdittir S. Creative therapy for hospitalized children. Pediatrician 1980; 9(3–4):198–202

Blackburn S. Fostering behavioral development of high-risk infants. JOGN Nurs (supplement) 1983 May/Jun; 12(3):76s–86s

Carl DB. Helping the hospitalized child—A caring approach. NITA 1982 May/Jun; 5(3):195–196

Cartier TM. Anal compulsive behaviors of one four-and-a-half year old hospitalized boy. Matern Child Nurs J 1980 Summer; 9(2):117–126

Conlin JB. Role-playing with Paddy. Nursing '80 1980 May; 10(5):136

Craft M. Preferences of hospitalized

adolescents for information providers. Nurs Res 1981 Jul/Aug; 30(4):205–211

Daniel WA Jr (ed). Psychological effects of illness in adolescence. Anxiety, self-esteem and perception of control. Part 1 J Pediatrics 1980 July; 97(1):126–131; Impact of illness in adolescents—crucial issues and coping styles. Part 2 J Pediatrics 1980 July; 97(1):132–138

Facteau LM. Self-care concepts and the care of a hospitalized child. Nurs Clin North Am 1980 Mar; 15(1):145–155

Fletcher B. Psychological upset in posthospitalized children: A review of the literature. Matern Child Nurs J 1981 Fall; 10(3):185–195

Fletcher B and Johnson C. The myth of formal operations: Rethinking adolescent cognition in clinical contexts. Child Health Care 1982 Summer; 11(1):17–21

Frauman A and Sypert N. Sexuality in adolescents with chronic illness. MCN 1979 Nov/Dec; 4(6):371–375

Gohsman B. The hospitalized child and the need for mastery. Issues Compr Pediatr Nurs 1981 Mar/Apr; 5(2):67–76

Griffiths SS. Body image concerns of a four year old boy with meningitis. Matern Child Nurs J 1980 Summer; 9(2):127–136

Gross S and Gardner G. Child pain: Treatment and approaches. In Smith W, Mersky H and Gross S (eds). Pain: Meaning and Management. New York, Spectrum Books, 1980, pp. 127–142

Hansen BD and Evans ML. Preparing a child for procedures. MCN 1981 Nov/Dec; 6(6):392–397

Harvey S. The value of play therapy in hospital. Paediatrician 1980 9(3–4):191–197

Hodapp RM. Effects of hospitalization on young children: Implications of two theories. Child Health Care 1982 Winter; 10(3):83–89

Kieffer ML and Vaughn DK. Homelike surroundings lessen stress of care for pediatric patients. Hospitals 1981 Feb 16; 55(4):107–111

King J and Ziegler S. The effects of hospitalization on children's behavior: A review of the literature. Child Health Care 1981 Summer; 10(1):20–28

Klein CB and Satterthwaite M. Preparation and the hospitalized child. JACCH 1980 Winter; 8(3):60–63

Knafl KA. Parents' views of the response of siblings to a pediatric hospitalization. Res Nurs Health 1982 March; 5(1):13–20

Kornhauser P. Preschool and school programme in humanizing children's hospital stay. Paediatrician 1980 9(3–4):231–241

LaMontagne L. Three coping strategies used by school-aged children. Pediatr Nurs 1984 Jan/Feb; 10(1):25–28

Lamb J and Rodgers D. Assisting the hostile, hospitalized child. MCN 1983 Sep/Oct; 8(5):336–339

Lindquist I. Influencing attitudes toward children's emotional care. Child Health Care 1981 Winter; 9(3):73–76

Lindsey KE. The value of music for hospitalized infants. Child Health Care 1981 Spring; 9(4):104–107

Linenkugel N. Programs prepare children for hospital procedures. Hosp Prog 1982 Jan; 63(1):64

Lollar D, Smits S and Patterson D. Assessment of pediatric pain: An empirical perspective. J Pediatr Psychol 1982 Sep; 7(3):267–277

May B and Sparks M. School age children: Are their needs recognized and met in the hospital setting? Child Health Care 1983 Winter; 11(3):118–121

McCain GC. Parent created tape recordings for hospitalized children. Child Health Care 1982 Winter; 10(3):104–105

McCain G and Bies D. Television viewing and the hospitalized child. Pediatr Nurs 1983 Jan/Feb; 9(1):33–36

McGuire S and Dizard S. Managing pain in the young patient. Nursing '82 1982 August; 12(8):53–55

Medenwald NA. Children's liberation in a hospital! MCN 1980 July/Aug; 5(4):232

Meissner J. How you can improve care of the hospitalized child. Nursing '80 1980 Oct; 10(10):50–51

Meng A and Zastowny T. Preparation for hospitalization: A stress inoculation training program for parents and children. Matern Child Nurs J 1982 Summer; 11(2):87–94

Menke E. Schoolaged children's perception of stress in the hospital. Child Health Care 1981 Winter; 9(3):80–85

Nadler H. Art experience and hospitalized children. Child Health Care 1983 Spring; 11(4):160–164

Nelson M. Identifying the emotional needs of the hospitalized child. MCN 1981 May/Jun; 6(3):181–183

Newman L and Lind J. The child in hospital: Early stimulation and therapy through play. Paediatrician 1980; 9(3–4):147–150

Off to a good start: A Resource for Parents, Professionals and Volunteers. USDHHS Pub #81-30304, Apr 1981

O'Meara K et al. Preadmission programs: Development, implementation and evaluation. Child Health Care 1983 Spring; 11(4):137–141

Perrin E and Gerrity P. There's a demon in your belly: Children's understanding of illness. Pediatrics 1981 June 67(6):841–849

Perrin E and Perrin J. Clinician's assessment of children's understanding of illness. Am J Dis Child 1983 Sept; 137(9):874–878

Pidgon V. Functions of preschool children's questions in coping with hospitalization. Res Nurs Health 1981 June; 4(2):229–235

Piserchia EA, Boagg CF and Alvarez MM. Play and play areas for hospitalized children. Child Health Care 1982 Spring; 10(4):135–138

Poston LJ. Finding time to play. MCN 1982 Jan/Feb; 7(1):19–20

Puskar K. Structure for the hospitalized adolescent . . . structure in the environment as a therapeutic tool. J Psychiatr Nurse 1981 Jul; 19(7):13–16

Rae W. Hospitalized latency-age children: Implications for psychosocial care. JACCH 1981 Winter; 9(3):59–63

Rappazzo JA. Psychoesthetic environmental design for pediatric care facilities. JACCH 1980 Spring; 8(4):85–93

Ritchie JA, Caty S and Ellerton ML. Patterns of concern in hospitalized chronically-ill young children: A preliminary report. Nurs Papers 1982 Spring; 14(1):3–13

Riffee DM. Self-esteem changes in hospitalized school-age children. Nurs Res 1981 Mar/Apr; 30(2):94–97

Ritter FL and Klinzing KMB. FPO—For parents only. Child Health Care 1980 Fall; 9(2):31–34

Rothenberg MB. The unique role of the child life worker in children's health care settings. Child Health Care 1982 Spring; 10(4):121–124

Rumfelt JJM. How five year old children perceive the role of the nurse. Matern Child Nurs J 1980 Spring; 99(1):13–28

Savedra M et al. Description of the pain experience: A study of school-age children. Issues Compr Pediatr Nurs 1981 Dec; 5(5–6):373–380

Schreier A and Kaplan D. The effectiveness of a preoperative preparation program in reducing anxiety in children. Child Health Care 1983 Spring; 11(4):142–147

Shrewsbury J. Painting: A coping device for preschool children. Matern Child Nurs J 1982 Spring; 11(1):11–16

Shuler SN and Reich CA. Sibling visitation in pediatric hospitals: Policies, opinions and issues. Child Health Care 1982 Fall; 11(2):54–60

Taylor SC. Siblings need a plan of care too. Pediatr Nurs 1980 Nov/Dec; 6(6):9–13

Tesler M. Coping with hospitalization: A study of school-age children. Pediatric Nurs 1981 Mar/Apr; 7(3):35–38

Tesler M et al. Coping strategies of children in pain. Issues Compr Pediatr Nurs 1981 Dec; 5(5–6):351–359

Vipperman JF and Rager PM. Childhood coping: How nurses can help. Pediatric Nursing 1980 Mar/Apr; 6(2):11–18

Waechter-Shikora N. Pain theories and their relevance to the pediatric population. Issues Compr Pediatr Nurs 1981 Dec; 5(5–6):321–326

Wood S. School aged children's perception of the cause of illness. Pediatr Nurs 1983 Mar/Apr; 9(2):101–104

Family-Centered Care

Bingley L et al. Comprehensive management of children on a pediatric ward: A family approach. Arch Dis Child 1980 July; 55(7):555–561

Chan J and Leff P. Parenting the chronically ill child in the hospital: Issues and concerns. Child Health Care 1982 Summer; 11(1):9–16

Clark D. Parents' meeting in a pediatric unit: Helping parents cope with their child's hospitalization. JACCH 1979 Fall; 8(2):32–35

Coucouvanis J and Solomons H.

Handling complicated visitation problems of hospitalized children. MCN 1983 Mar/Apr; 8(2):131–134

Fore C and Holmes S. A care-by-parent unit revisited. MCN 1983 Nov/Dec; 8(6):408–410

Knafl K et al. How parents manage jobs and a child's hospitalization. MCN 1982 Mar/Apr; 7(2):125–127

Koss T and Teter M. Welcoming a family when a child is hospitalized. MCN 1980 Jan/Feb; 5(1):51–54

Marino B. When nurses compete with parents. JACCH 1980; Spring 8(4):94–98

Oberlander R. Parent Care units bring home to the hospital. Hospitals 1980 Nov 1; 54(21):81–85

Sciarillo W. Using Hymovich's framework in the family-oriented approach to nursing care. MCN 1980 Jul/Aug; 5(4):242–248

Shuler S and Reich C. Sibling visitation in pediatric hospitals: Policies, opinions, and issues. Child Health Care 1982 Fall; 11(2):54–60

Taylor S. The effects of chronic childhood illnesses upon well siblings. Matern Child Nurs J 1980 Summer; 9(2):109–116

Pediatric Intensive Care

Bellack JP et al. The young child in the critical care unit. Crit Care Update 1981 May; 8(5):26–31+

Betz C. Sensory disturbances among children in the ICU. DCCN 1982 May/Jun; 1(3):145–151

Carry R. Observed behaviors of preschoolers to intensive care. Pediatr Nurs 1980 Jul/Aug; 6(6):21–26

Green M. Parent care in the intensive care unit. Am J Dis Child 1979 Nov; 133(11):1119–1120

Hedenkamp E. Humanizing the intensive care unit for children. Crit Care Q 1980 Jun; 3(1):63–73

Lewandowski L. Stresses and coping styles of parents of children undergoing open-heart surgery. Crit Care Q 1980 June; 3(1):75–84

Miles M and Carter M. Assessing parental stress in intensive care units. MCN 1983 Sep/Oct; 8(5):354–359

Miles M and Carter M. Sources of parental stress in pediatric intensive care units. Child Health Care 1982 Fall; 11(2):65–69

Pearson JER et al. Pediatric intensive care unit patients: Effects of play intervention on behavior. Crit Care Med 1980 Feb; 8(2):64–67

Rothstein P. Psychological stress in families of children in a pediatric intensive care unit. Pediatr Clin North Am 1980 Aug; 27(3):613–620

Soupios M, Gallagher J and Orlowski J. Nursing aspects of pediatric intensive care in a general hospital. Pediatr Clin North Am 1980 Aug; 27(3):621–632

Stevens K. Humanistic nursing care for critically ill children. Nurs Clin North Am 1981 Dec; 16(4):611–622

Teyber E and Littlehales D. Coping with feelings: Seriously ill children, their families and hospital staff. JACCH 1981 Fall; 10(2):58–62

Vanek C. How school age children perceive the intensive care unit environment. J NY State Nurses Assoc 1979 Dec; 10(4):30–33

Vestal K and Richardson K. The nature of pediatric critical care nursing: Perspectives of patient, family and staff. Nurs Clin North Am 1981 Dec; 16(4):605–610

Intensive Care Nursery

Allen DA et al. The predictive validity of neonatal intensive care nurses' judgments of parent–child relationships: A nine-month follow-up. J Pediatr Psychol 1982 Jun; 7(2):125–134

Blackburn J. The neonatal ICN: A high-risk environment. Am J Nurs 1982 Nov; 82(11):1708–1712

Bromberger PI. Premature infants' nutritional needs 1. Preterm breast milk. Perinatol Neonatol 1982 Jul/Aug; 6(4):79–80+

Chaze BA and Ludington-Hoe SM. Sensory stimulation in the NICU. Am J Nurs 1984 Jan; 84(1):68–71

Davidson S and Leonard LG. Appearance, behavior and capabilities. Can Nurs 1981 Feb; 77(2):37–39

Gay J. A conceptual framework of bonding. JOGN Nurs 1981 Nov/Dec; 10(6):440–444

Goldson E. The family care center: Transitional care for the sick infant and his family. Child Today 1981 July/Aug; 10(4):15–20

Hansen FH. Nursing care in the neonatal intensive care unit. JOGN Nurs 1982 Jan/Feb; 11(1):17–20

Huzuka BT. Prevention of infection in the nursery. Nurs Clin North Am 1980 Dec; 15(4):825–831

Jenkins RL and Westhus NK. The nurse role in parent–infant bonding. JOGN Nurs 1981 Mar/Apr; 10(2):114–118

Kennedy J. Evacuation of a neonatal unit. Can Nurs 1983 May; 79(5):26–29

Klaus M and Kennell J. Interventions in the premature nursery: Impact on development. Pediatr Clin North Am 1982 Oct; 29(5):1263–1273

Kutnik ML. Assessing the family of the special-care infant. Perinatol Neonatol 1983 Aug; 7(8):33–34+

Leclair JM. Control of nosocomial neonatal viral infection. Crit Care Q 1980 Dec; 3(3):71–77

Levitt E. Neonatal I.V. therapy. NITA 1980 Sept/Oct; 3(5):169–174

Lund C and LeFrak L. Discharge planning for infants in the intensive care nursery. Perinatol Neonatol 1982 Mar/Apr; 6(2):49–50+

Miles MS and Carter MC. Assessing parental stress in intensive care units. MCN 1983 Sep/Oct; 8(5):354–359

Schwab F et al. Sibling visiting in a neonatal intensive care unit. Pediatrics 1983 May; 71(5):835–838

Trykowski LE, Kirkpatrick BV, Leonard EL. Enhancement of nutritive sucking in premature infants. Phys Occup Ther Pediatr 1981 Summer; 1(4):27–33

Varner B, Ossenkop D and Lyon J. Prematures, too, need rooming-in and care-by-parent programs. MCN 1980 Nov/Dec; 5(6):431–432

Wranesh BL. The effects of sibling visitation on bacterial colonization rate in neonates. JOGN Nurs 1982 July/Aug; 11(4):211–213

Child Undergoing Surgery

Abrams L. Resistance behaviors and teaching media for children in day surgery. AORN J 1982 Feb; 35(2):244+

Brown C. The pediatric patient undergoing surgical intervention. Point View 1982 Jan; 19(1):18–19

Chan JM. Preparation for procedures and surgery through play. Paediatrician 1980 9(3–4):210–219

Crocker E. Preparation for elective surgery: Does it make a difference? Child Health Care 1980 Summer; 9(1):3–11

Gatch G. Caring for children needing anesthesia. AORN J 1982 Feb; 35(2):219–226

Linenkugel N. Programs prepare children for hospital procedures. Hosp Pract 1982 Jan; 63(1):64

Meng AL. Parents' and childrens' reactions toward impending hospitalization for surgery. Matern Child Nurs J 1980 Summer; 9(2):83–98

McClintic J. Preoperative care of the pediatric patient. Today's OR Nurs 1980 Jul; 2(5):7–10

Nurse R and Deber R. Conquering fear of surgery. Dimens Health Serv 1982 Mar; 59(3):34–36

Schreier A and Kaplan D. The effectiveness of a preoperation preparation program in reducing anxiety in children. Child Health Care 1983 Spring; 11(4):142–147

Trouten F. Psychological preparation of children for surgery. Dimensions Health Serv 1981 Mar; 58(3):9–10+

Transcultural Nursing in Pediatrics

Anderson J and Chung J. Culture and illness: Parents' perceptions of their child's long term illness. Nurs Papers 1982 Winter; 14(4):40–52

Baker CM and Mayer GG. One approach to teaching cultural similarities and differences. JNE 1982 April; 21(4):17–22

Cohen FS. Transcultural nursing: Benefits for the nurse. Nurs Leadership 1982 Mar; 5(1):10–14

Davies M and Yoshida M. A model for cultural assessment of the new immigrant. Can Nurs 1981 Mar; 77(3):22–23

Diaz-Duque O. Overcoming the language barrier: Advice from an interpreter. Am J Nurs 1982 Sept; 82(9):1380–1382

Flaherty MJ. Cultural nursing: A point of view. Image 1982 Jun; 14(2):37–39

Germain CP. Cultural concepts in critical care. Crit Care Q 1982 Dec; 5(3):61–78

Grasska MA and McFarland T. Overcoming the language barrier: Problems and solutions. Am J Nurs 1982 Sep; 82(9):1376–1379

Griffith S. Childbearing and the concept of culture. JOGN Nurs 1982 May/Jun; 11(3):181–184

Grosso C et al. The Vietnamese American family . . . And grandma makes three. MCN 1981 May/Jun; 6(3):177–180

Henley A and Clayton J. Catering for all tastes. Health Soc Serv J 1982 July 22; 92:888–889

Johnston M. Cultural variations in professional and parenting patterns. JOGN Nurs 1980 Jan/Feb; 9(1):9–13

Kubricht DW and Clark JA. Foreign patients: A system for providing care. Nurs Outlook 1982 Jan; 30(1):55–57

Leininger MM. Transcultural nursing: Its progress and future. Nurs Health Care 1981 Sept; 11(7):365–371

Rackosky I. Nurses, nursing and culture. Superv Nurs 1980 July; 11(7):20–22

Rojas D. Effects of maternal expectations and child-rearing practice on the development of white and Puerto Rican children. Matern Child Nurs J 1980 Spring; 9(1):99–107

Ross HM. Societal/cultural views regarding death and dying. Top Clin Nurs 1981 Oct; 3(3):1–16

Ruiz MCJ. Open-closed mindedness, intolerance of ambiguity and nursing faculty attitude toward culturally different patients. Nurs Rev 1981 May/Jun; 30(3):177–181

Salzer JL and Nelson NA. Health care of Ethiopian refugees. Pediatr Nurs 1983 Nov/Dec; 96(6):449–452

Santopietro MCS and del Bueno DJ. How to get through to a refugee patient. RN 1981 Jan; 44(1):42–48

Shubin S. Nursing patients from different cultures. Nursing '80 1980 Jun; 80(6):78–81

Slevin KF. Motherhood, culture, and change. Pediatr Nurs 1982 Nov/Dec; 8(6):403–409

Spector RE. The role of the pediatric nurse clinician/practitioner: Cultural implications. In Beal JA (ed). Issues and Advanced Practice in Pediatric Nursing. Reston, VA, Reston Publishing Co, 1983, pp. 189–202

Additional Reading for Staff and Parents

Books

Grollman E. Talking About Death—A Dialogue Between Parent and Child. Boston, Beacon Press, 1976

Hardgrove C and Dawson R. Parents and Children in the Hospital. Boston, Little, Brown & Co, 1972

McCollum A. Coping with Prolonged Health Impairment in Your Child. Boston, Little, Brown & Co, 1975

Martinson I. Home Care for the Dying Child: Professional and Family Perspective. New York, Appleton-Century-Crofts, 1976

Resources for Staff and Parents

Brown CC. Childhood Learning Disabilities and Prenatal Risk. Pediatric Round-Table: No 9, 1982

Brown CC (ed). Infants at Risk: Assessment and Intervention, An Update for Health Care Professionals and Parents. Pediatric Round-Table Series No 5: 1981

Brown CC. The Many Facets of Touch. Pediatric Round-Table: No 10, 1984

Chance P. Learning Through Play. Pediatric Round-Table: No 3, 1979

Klaus MH, Legar T and Trause MA (ed).

Maternal Attachment and Mothering Disorders. Pediatric Round-Table: No 1, 1981, 2nd ed

Klaus MH and Robertson MO (ed). Birth, Interaction and Attachment. Pediatric Round-Table: No 6, 1982

Reilly AP (ed). The Communication Game. Pediatric Round-Table: No 4, 1980

Thomas EB and Trotter S (ed). Social Responsiveness of Infants. Pediatric Round-Table: No 2, 1978

The above are from:
Johnson & Johnson Baby Products Co, Grandview Road, Skillman, NJ 08558
Outside NJ: 1-(800)526-3967; NJ only: (800)942-7764

Learning about Hospitals and Health Care. School Kits: A fund and educational box for teachers and school nurses to help their students learn about hospitals and health care. Available from ACCH (see below for address)

Additional Information

Association for the Care of Children's Health, 3615 Wisconsin Avenue, Washington, DC 20016; for information and listings regarding films and books related to children's health issues

Zero to Three. Bulletin of the National Center for Clinical Infant Programs, 733 15th Street, NW, Suite 912, Washington, DC 20005

Transcultural Nursing Society, Dr. Madeline M. Leininger, University of Utah College of Nursing, 25 Medical Drive, Salt Lake City, UT 84112

National Center for Education in Maternal and Child Health, 3520 Prospect Street NW, Washington, DC 20007:

Altshuler A. Books That Help Children Deal With the Hospital Experience, HSA Pub. #78-5224, 1978

Readers Guide for Parents of Children with Mental, Physical, or Emotional Disabilities. HSA Pub. #79-5290, 1979

The Surgeon General's Workshop on Children with Handicaps and Their Families. PHS Pub. #83-50194, 1983

The Hospital Play Equipment Company, 1122 Judson Avenue, Evanston, IL 60202 (sells miniature hospital furniture and equipment, puppets, dolls, and books for children and parents about hospitalization)

For Children

Books

Ciliotta C and Livingston C. Why am I Going to the Hospital? Secaucus, NJ, Lyle Stuart, 1983

Clark B. Pop-up Going to the Hospital. Westminster, MD, Random House, 1971

Droske SC and Francis SA. Pediatric

Diagnostic Procedures with Guidelines for Preparing Children for Clinical Tests. New York, John Wiley & Sons, 1981

Howe J. The Hospital Book. New York, Crown Publishers, 1981

Marino BP. Eric Needs Stitches. Reading, MA, Addison-Wesley, 1979

Shay A. What Happens When You Go to the Hospital? Chicago, Henry Regnery, 1969

Sobol HL and Agre P. Jeff's Hospital Book. New York, Henry Z Walck, 1975

Steedman J. Emergency Room: An ABC Tour. McLean, VA, Windy Hill Press, 1974

Stein SB. A Hospital Story, New York, Walker & Co, 1974

Films

Care Through Parents
University of California Extension Media Center, Berkeley, CA, 94720; color; 14 minutes
Emphasizes the role of parents in caring for the young hospitalized child. Depicts a program in which parents are actively involved in the care of their children

Play in the Hospital
Campus Films Distribution Corporation, 14 Madison Avenue, Valhalla, NY 10595; color, 55 minutes
Portrays many ways in which hospitalized children are helped by a special play program. Filmed in a variety of settings. Gives a good picture of children's special concerns and needs and offers particular ways of dealing with these

To Prepare a Child
Media Center, Children's Hospital National Medical Center, Washington, DC 20010; color, 32 minutes (available in 16 mm. sound and videocassette)
This is an account of one hospital's approach to the preparation of children for hospitalization and surgery. Three children (one is an out-patient emergency case and the other two are surgical in-patients) are followed through their preparation for surgery and diagnostic procedures

A Hospital Visit with Clipper
Media Center, Children's Hospital National Medical Center, Washington, DC 20010; color, 15 minutes (available in 16 mm. sound and videocassette)
A professionally produced puppet show about a little girl coming into the hospital for a tonsillectomy. The script pays special attention to the most common concerns children have about hospitalization and surgery.

First Do No Harm
Media Center, Children's Hospital National Medical Center, Washington, DC 20010
This film illustrates how hospitals can and must adapt facilities, policies, staffing patterns, and routines to meet the psychosocial needs of children and their families. The film portrays

the real life hospital experiences of children in each major stage of child development

Hospital Adventure
Media Resources Librarian, Naval Health Sciences Education and Training Command, National Naval Medical Center, Bethesda, MD 20014; color, 15 minutes
This cartoon takes the child through a typical hospital and presents some of the most common experiences and procedures. It focuses on the misconceptions and concerns that children may have.

Let's Talk About
. . . *Going to the Hospital;*
. . . *Having an Operation;*
. . . *Wearing a Cast*
Mr. Rogers—Family Communications, Arthur Greenwald, Project Director, 4802 Fifth Avenue, Pittsburgh, PA 15213; videocassettes, 20 minutes each
. . . *Going to the Hospital:* A general introduction to the hospital and to the sights, sounds, and feelings children may experience there.
. . . *Having an Operation:* A more specific program for children scheduled for simple surgery. Helping them know what to expect and encouraging them to express their feelings in words and play.
. . . *Wearing a Cast:* A program about how casts are applied and removed, and how children can do many things for themselves while wearing a cast.

Preparing a Child for O.R., Anesthesia, Recovery Room and I.C.U.
Campus Film Distributors Corporation, 14 Madison Avenue, Valhalla, NY 10595; filmstrips, 8 minutes
Filmstrips for staff development when preparing children for procedures. Developed and written by Madeline Petrillo.

The Children's Medical Series—a series of eight videotapes (Asthma, Diabetes, Vocal Nodules, Hemophilia, Having a Sibling Go to the Hospital, Plastic Surgery, Accidents, Seizures) with Susan Linn and her puppets. Human Services Development, 1616 Soldiers Field Road, Boston, MA 02135; 8- to 12-minute videotape

Jasper Enters the Hospital; 16½ minutes. *The Day of Jasper's Operation;* 13½ minutes. Videocassettes—16 mm. Kids Corner, 2027 North Tejon Street, Colorado Springs, CO 80907
These two films take us through Jasper the Monster's hospital stay and shows that children experience many strange faces, sights, and sounds while in the hospital. Through questions and answers Jasper's fears and concerns are alleviated.

My Brother is Sick; 12½ minutes. Video/Film. Kids Corner (see above).
Portrays a grandmother helping a young girl understand why things are happening as they are because her brother is sick and in the hospital.

Pediatric Techniques

Measuring Vital Signs in Children

Normal Vital Sign Ranges in Children

Temperature
Oral 36.4°–37.4°C. (97.6°–99.3°F.)
Rectal 36.2°–37.8°C. (97°–100°F.)
Axillary 35.9°–36.7°C. (96.6°–98°F.)

Pulse and Respiratory Rates

Age	Pulse	Respirations
Newborn	70–170	30–50
11 months	80–160	26–40
2 years	80–130	20–30
4 years	80–120	20–30
6 years	75–115	20–26
8 years	70–110	18–24
10 years	70–110	18–24
Adolescence	60–110	12–20

General Considerations for Measuring Vital Signs

1. Vital sign values provide the nurse with only rough estimates of physiological activity. It is important to identify trends, sudden discrepancies, and wide deviations from normal.

2. Vital signs should be taken as often as the nurse thinks necessary. They should not be delayed until the next scheduled time if it is suspected that a trend is developing.

Temperature

1. Normal body temperature represents a balance between the body heat produced and body heat lost.
2. The mode for taking the temperature should be kept as constant as possible. (Refer to Table 32-1 for methods of measuring body temperature in infants and children.)
3. Never leave the child alone when taking his temperature.
4. For security, safety, and accuracy, keep one hand on the thermometer when it is in place.
5. Record the temperature value and method used.
6. Report an elevated or subnormal temperature and initiate whatever nursing measures are indicated by the child's condition.
7. If using an electronic thermometer, follow manufacturer's directions explicitly.
8. Question the accuracy of any temperature reading

Table 32-1 Methods of Measuring Body Temperature in Infants and Children

Method	Advantages	Disadvantages	Length of time required for accurate measurement with mercury-in-glass thermometer
Rectal	1. Safe for children who are unable to cooperate and who may bite the thermometer. 2. Not directly influenced by the ingestion of hot or cold fluids, smoking. 3. Method of choice if child has seizures or breathing difficulties; has had oral surgery.	1. Values may be altered by the presence of stool. 2. Emotional response may be negative. 3. Damage to rectal mucosa may occur. 4. Replication of the thermometer placement is difficult. 5. Contraindicated when child has diarrhea and following rectal surgery.	3–5 min.*
Oral	1. Easily accessible. 2. Replication of thermometer placement is easy. 3. Responds more quickly and regularly to changes in arterial temperature than does rectal method. 4. More aesthetically pleasing.	1. Value is readily influenced by ingestion of hot or cold fluids. 2. Requires child's cooperation to keep mouth closed and not to bite the thermometer. 3. Contraindicated if child has had oral injuries or surgery.	6–9 min.*
Axillary	1. Safe and easily accessible. 2. Avoids the danger of rectal or colon perforation. 3. Avoids initiating the defecation stimulus. 4. Often recommended for infants under 1 year.	1. Value is more readily influenced by environmental temperature and airflow. 2. Requires a relatively long period of time to obtain accurate reading.	9–11 min.*

* Time is generally decreased if an electronic thermometer is used.

that does not correlate with the child's signs and symptoms.

Pulse

1. Take apical rate on an infant.
   a. Place stethoscope between left nipple and sternum.
   b. Take heart rate for 1 full minute.
2. With an older child, the pulse rate may be obtained easily at the radial, temporal, or carotid locations. (The pulse may be taken for 30 seconds and multiplied by 2.)
3. Take pulse rate prior to taking temperature because child may cry when temperature is taken; this increases the pulse rate and makes it more difficult to hear the apical rate.
4. Record accurately the following:
   a. Rate
   b. Rhythm (regular or irregular)
   c. Strength of beat (full, bounding, weak, faint)
   d. Activity of child at time pulse is taken (sleeping, crying, etc.)
5. Report immediately any changes in pulse characteristics, and initiate whatever nursing measures are indicated by the child's condition.

Respirations

1. Count respirations on an infant for 1 full minute. Observe chest movement as well as abdominal movements.
2. Respirations may be counted for 30 seconds and multiplied by 2 in the older child.
3. Obtain respiratory rate prior to taking temperature and pulse since the child may cry during these procedures.
4. Note and record accurately the following:
   a. Respiratory rate
   b. Depth of respirations
      (1) Feel exhaled air to estimate adequacy of tidal volume.
      (2) Observe excursions of the chest and diaphragm.
   c. Quality of respirations
      (1) Determine if respirations are predominantly costal or abdominal. Dyspnea should be suspected in a school-age child who is breathing primarily with the abdomen.
      (2) Listen for unusual noises such as expiratory grunts, crowing noises, wheezing, or inspiratory stridor.
      (3) Observe for signs of dyspnea:
         (a) Restlessness
         (b) Retractions—sternal or intercostal
         (c) Nasal flaring
         (d) Cyanosis
   d. Activity of the child during the procedure.
5. Report immediately any change in respiratory status. Initiate whatever nursing measures are indicated by the child's condition.

Blood Pressure

Generally, the technique for taking the blood pressure of a child is the same as for the adult. The following principles are important to observe when dealing with the pediatric patient.

A. General Considerations

1. The cuff should cover no less than ½ and no more than ⅔ the length of the upper arm or leg. Even small variations in cuff size may produce significant differences in blood pressure reading.
   a. A cuff that is too narrow will produce an apparent increase in blood pressure.
   b. A cuff that is too wide will produce an apparent decrease in blood pressure.
   c. Using a flexible blood pressure cuff that can be folded to the correct size is frequently easier and more effective for the nurse than choosing among several assorted premeasured cuffs.
   d. The cuff should be of consistent width each time

that a child's blood pressure is measured during hospitalization.

2. If the child is excited or uncomfortable or if he distrusts the person taking the blood pressure, the systolic pressure may rise significantly.
   a. The blood pressure should be taken when the child is at rest and in a consistent position.
   b. The procedure should be explained to the child before it is done.
      (1) He should know that it will not hurt.
      (2) He should be allowed to handle the equipment, pump the cuff, etc.
      (3) It may be helpful for the child to use the equipment on his parents, the nurse, or a doll in order for him to overcome his fears and understand its use.

B. Methods Used in Obtaining Blood Pressure Measurements in Pediatrics

1. *Auscultatory method* (method of choice whenever possible)
   a. Center the bladder of the cuff over the artery.
   b. Apply the cuff evenly and snugly over the bare arm with the lower edge about 1.25 cm. (½ inch) above the antecubital space.
   c. Support the arm in a slightly flexed and abducted position at the level of the child's heart.
   d. Palpate the brachial artery and inflate the cuff until the palpated pulse is lost. Then pump for an additional 20–30 mm. Hg beyond that.
   e. Deflate the cuff slowly at a rate of about 5 mm. Hg/second.
   f. Deflate the cuff rapidly and completely when all sounds disappear.
   g. Record the reading and compare it with previous values.
      There continues to be a controversy as to what best indicates diastolic pressure. Therefore, it is good practice to record all 3 readings:
      (1) Systolic—point at which pulse becomes audible
      (2) Diastolic—point of muffling of sound
      (3) Point of disappearance of sounds
   h. The blood pressure may be obtained by the same method in the leg, using the popliteal artery.
2. *Palpatory method* (This method provides only an approximate mean pressure which lies between the systolic and diastolic pressures obtained by the auscultatory method.)
   a. Follow steps 1–3 of the auscultatory method.
   b. Inflate the cuff to about 200 mm. Hg.
   c. Take the reading when the pulse distal to the cuff becomes palpable in the course of deflation.

3. *Flush method* (This method is especially useful with infants, but also has the disadvantage of providing only an approximate mean pressure.)
   a. The infant should be quiet and in the supine position.
   b. Apply a blood pressure cuff to the upper or lower extremity, just above the wrist or ankle.
   c. Squeeze the extremity distal to the cuff with a hand or firm wrapping to force blood into the upper extremity. This will blanch the child's arm or leg below the cuff.
   d. Pump the manometer to 120–140 mm. Hg.
   e. Release the hand or the wrapping.
   f. Slowly deflate the cuff.
   g. Take the reading at the point at which blood reenters the hand or foot, causing a sudden flushing.
4. *Electronic and ultrasonic methods*
   a. Equipment utilizes electronic circuitry or reflected sound to detect blood flow or movement of an arterial wall under an occluding cuff.
   b. Sophisticated equipment is available which can inflate and deflate the cuff and either hold or automatically record the measurement.
   c. Advantages
      (1) Especially useful in infants when the Korotkoff sounds may be inaudible by ordinary methods.
      (2) The child is subjected to minimal handling despite frequent monitoring of the blood pressure.
      (3) Observer bias is minimized since pressures are analyzed electronically rather than by the human ear. Therefore, blood pressure readings are more consistent.
      (4) Ultrasonic measurements correlate closely with intra-arterial pressures.
   d. Nursing considerations
      (1) Read specific instructions before operating the device.
      (2) Note specifically what sounds are being measured, and whether the equipment measures muffling or silence, or both as the diastolic pressure.

C. Principles Related to Pediatric Blood Pressure Values
(See Figs. 32-1 and 32-2.)

1. The blood pressure varies with the age of the child and is closely related to his height and weight.
2. Variability of blood pressure among children of approximately the same age and body build is normal.
3. When the cuff technique is used, the pressure measurement in the legs may be slightly higher than that in the arms in children over 1 year of age.

Nursing Management of the Child with Fever

Fever is any abnormal elevation of body temperature. Prolonged elevation of temperature above 40°C. (104°F.) may produce dehydration and harmful effects on the central nervous system.

Causes
1. Infection
2. Inflammatory disease
3. Dehydration
4. Tumors
5. Disturbance of temperature regulating center
6. Extravasation of blood in the tissues
7. Drugs or toxins

Assessment
1. Consider basic principles related to temperature regulation in pediatric patients.
   a. Usually an infant's temperature does not stabilize before he is 1 week old. A newborn's temperature varies with the temperature of his environment.

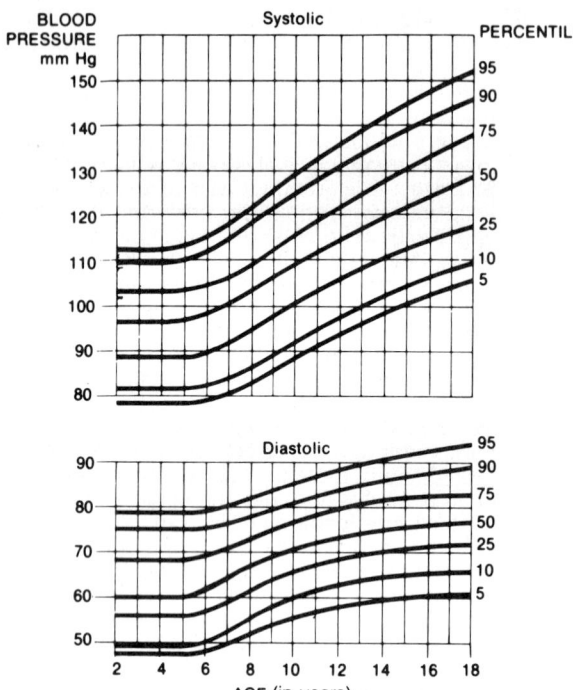

Figure 32-1. Percentiles of blood pressure measurements in boys (right arm, seated).

b. The degree of fever does not always reflect the severity of the disease. A child may have a very serious illness with a normal or subnormal temperature.

c. Fever, itself, may cause convulsions in some children when the temperature goes very high, very quickly.

d. The range for normal temperature varies widely in children. A common explanation for "fever" is misinterpretation of a normal temperature reading (refer to Measuring Vital Signs in Children, p. 1133).

e. The child's temperature is influenced by activity and by time of day; temperatures are highest in late afternoon.

2. Be certain that accurate technique is used for temperature measurement. The mode should be appropriate for the child's age and condition, and the thermometer should be left in place for the required period of time (refer to Measuring Vital Signs in Children, p. 1133).

3. Assist the physician in determining the cause of the illness.

  a. History

    Information should be elicited regarding:

      Age of the child

      Pattern of the fever

      Length of the illness

      Change in normal patterns of eating, elimination, recreation, etc.

      Other symptoms

      Exposure to any illnesses

      Recent immunizations or drugs

      Treatment of the fever and effectiveness of treatment

      Previous experiences with fever and its control

b. Physical examination

  Of special significance are:

    General appearance of the child

    Inspection of the skin for rashes, sores, flushed appearance

    Inspection of eyes, ears, nose, and throat for redness and/or drainage

    Auscultation of lungs for abnormal sounds

    Neurological observation for changes in state of consciousness, pupillary reaction, strength of grip, abnormal muscle movement or lack of movement

    Inspection of the external genitals for redness and/or drainage

    Presence of abdominal or flank pain

  (Refer to Pediatric Physical Assessment, p. 1047)

c. Laboratory tests

  Initial tests frequently include complete blood count, urinalysis, cultures of the throat, nasopharynx, urine, blood, and spinal fluid, and x-ray of the chest.

4. Attempt to identify the pattern of the fever. Take the child's temperature by the same method every hour until stable, then every 2 hours until normal, then every 4 hours for 24 hours.

Nursing Measures to Reduce Fever

Fever itself does not necessarily require treatment. The presence of fever should not be obscured by the indiscriminate use of antipyretic measures. However, if the child is uncomfortable or appears toxic because of fever, an attempt should be made to reduce it by any of the following nursing measures or by a combination of these measures (see p. 1137).

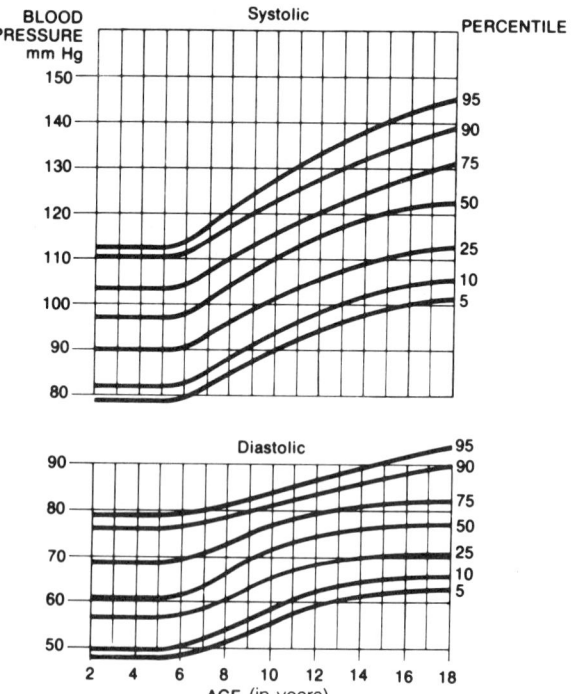

Figure 32-2. Percentiles of blood pressure measurement in girls (right arm, seated).

Nursing Action	Rationale/Amplification
1. Increase the child's fluid intake to prevent dehydration.	1. Fever increases the child's fluid requirements by increasing the metabolic rate.
2. Expose the skin to the air by leaving the child lightly dressed in an absorbent material. Avoid warm, binding clothing and blankets.	2. Loss of heat from the skin by radiation is the main temperature regulating mechanism available to the infant or small child.
3. Administer a tepid sponge bath (see Guidelines; Administering a Tepid Water Sponge, below.)	3. The temperature is lowered by evaporation of water from the surface of the skin.
4. Administer antipyretic drugs.	4. Although effective in reducing fever, antipyretic drugs may obscure the clinical picture and cause numerous side effects including diaphoresis, skin eruptions, nausea, vomiting, hematologic changes, and fever.
5. Utilize tub or a hypothermia blanket.	5. A tub bath is less frightening and is the preferred method for reducing fever if the child is able to cooperate.
6. Utilize ice bags for local comfort.	6. These should not be used for infants since they may produce chilling.

Guidelines: Administering a Tepid Water Sponge for Fever

A *tepid water sponge* is bathing of the body for a period of time to reduce fever.

Equipment

Basin of tepid water (21.1°–27°C. or 70°–80°F.)
Plastic sheet
2 bath blankets
Hot water bottle with cover
Towels
6 washcloths

▶ **NURSING ALERT:** Cold water or alcohol sponges should not be administered to pediatric patients. Cold water may produce vasoconstriction and shivering, which raise central body temperature. Alcohol sponges may reduce the temperature too rapidly, leading to convulsions in small children. In addition, the fumes may be toxic.

Procedure

Nursing Action	Rationale/Amplification
Preparatory Phase	
1. Secure the child's cooperation.	1. This helps to increase the effectiveness of the procedure. A tub bath in tepid water is less frightening and is the preferred method for reducing a fever if the child is able to cooperate. When using this technique, it is best to start with warm water and gradually add cool water to the tub. This prevents sudden chilling of the child.
a. Explain the procedure to the child in language he can understand.	
b. A small infant may be held during sponging.	
c. Allow the child or his parent to participate in the procedure.	
d. Discontinue sponging if the child is extremely upset and uncooperative.	
2. Take temperature, pulse, and respiration before starting the sponge.	2. This serves as a baseline for comparison to determine the effectiveness of treatment.
3. Give antipyretic medication as prescribed 15–20 minutes before starting the sponge.	3. There is a more rapid reduction of fever when sponging is combined with administration of antipyretic medication.
Performance Phase	
1. Place a plastic sheet covered with a bath blanket under the child.	
2. Place a bath blanket over the child, and remove top bedding.	
3. Place cold moist cloths in each axilla and groin and on the forehead.	3. This aids in lowering body temperature. The cloths should be changed as they become warm.
4. Expose the body area to be sponged. Place a towel under the area.	

(continued)

Guidelines: Administering a Tepid Water Sponge for Fever (continued)

Procedure
(Cont.)

Nursing Action	Rationale/Amplification
5. Slowly stroke the extremities with long, soothing strokes of the washcloth.	
a. Stroke each arm from the neck to the axilla and down to the palm of the hand.	
b. Stroke each leg from the groin to the foot.	
c. Bathe the back and buttocks.	
6. Use gentle friction to bring the blood to the surface.	6. This increases the effectiveness of the treatment and prevents chilling.
7. Change the water as often as necessary to maintain a water temperature of 21.1°–27°C. (70°–80°F.).	
8. Continue this procedure until temperature is adequately reduced, more drastic measures are prescribed, or the child's condition indicates that it should be discontinued.	8. Generally, the sponge should not last more than 30 minutes. Observe for shivering. If this occurs, cover the child and wait a few minutes before proceeding. Stop the sponge if cyanosis, mottling, or chilling do not stop when friction is applied to the skin. These symptoms indicate a change in vasomotor tone.
9. Pat dry with towel.	

Follow-up Phase

1. Remove bath blankets and plastic sheet. Place a dry gown on the child.	
2. Record vital signs 30 minutes after the sponge is finished.	2. Postsponge values indicate whether or not treatment has been effective.

Administering Medications to Children

Purpose

To safely administer medications to the child as prescribed by the physician.

Important Considerations

1. The nurse's manner of approach should indicate that she firmly expects the child to take the medication. This manner often convinces the child of the necessity of the procedure. Establishing a positive relationship with the child will allow him to express feelings, concerns, and fantasies regarding medications.
2. Explanation about the medication should appeal to the child's level of understanding (i.e., color, comparison to something familiar).
3. The nurse must mask her own feelings regarding the medication.
4. Always be truthful when the child asks, "Does it taste bad?" or "Will it hurt?" Respond by saying, "The medicine does not taste good, but I will give you some juice as soon as you swallow it," or "It will hurt for just a minute, like a mosquito bite."
5. It is often necessary to mix distasteful medications or crushed pills with a small amount of coke or cherry syrup, honey, or applesauce.
6. Never threaten a child with an injection if he refuses an oral medication.
7. Medications should not be mixed with large quantities of food or with any food that is taken regularly (e.g., milk).
8. Medications should not be given at mealtime unless specifically prescribed.
9. The nurse must know the following about each medication she is administering: common usages and dosages, contraindications, side effects, and toxic effects.
10. When preparing intramuscular injections, draw in 0.2 ml. of air after the correct amount of solution is in the syringe. This serves to clear all medication from the needle upon injection and prevents backflow and the depositing of medication in subcutaneous fat upon withdrawal of the needle.

Calculating the Pediatric Dosage

Although it is not the nurse's responsibility to determine the dosage of a drug, it *is* her responsibility to know the safe dosage range of any medication administered to children.

1. Know what factors determine the amount of drug prescribed.
   a. Action of the drug, absorption, detoxification, excretion are related to the maturity and metabolic rate of the child.
   b. The neonate and premature infants require a reduced dosage because of:
      (1) Deficient or absent detoxifying enzymes
      (2) Decreased effective renal function
      (3) Altered blood–brain barrier and protein-binding capacity
   c. Dosages recommended according to age-groups are not satisfactory since a child may be much smaller or larger than the average child in his age-group.
   d. Dosage calculations based on weight have limitations.

2. Be alert to a prescription that would be inappropriate for a child.
3. Consult drug literature for recommended dosage and other information.

Body Surface Area

The following formulas are used to estimate the pediatric dosage based on the child's body surface area. Body surface area (BSA) calculations are generally preferred because many physiologic processes in the child (i.e., blood volume, glomerular filtration) are related to BSA.

1. Surface area in sq. meters $\times$ Dose per sq. meter

$$= \text{Approximate child dose}$$

2. $\dfrac{\text{Surface area of child}}{\text{Surface area of adult}} \times \text{Dose of adult}$

$$= \text{Approximate child dose}$$

3. $\dfrac{\text{Surface area of child in sq. meters}}{1.75} \times \text{Adult dose}$

$$= \text{Child dose}$$

Clark's Rule

The following rule may be used as an estimate of the pediatric dosage based on the child's weight in respect to the adult dose of the drug.

$\dfrac{\text{Child's weight in pounds}}{150} \times \text{Adult dose}$

$$= \text{Approximate dose for child}$$

Identifying the Patient

Always check a child's identification bracelet with medication card before administering a medication. Ask the older child his name.

Oral Medications

A. Infants

1. Draw up medication in a plastic dropper or disposable syringe.
2. Elevate infant's head and shoulders; depress chin with thumb to open mouth.
3. Place dropper or syringe on the middle of the tongue and slowly drop the medication on the tongue.
4. Release thumb and allow child to swallow.
5. Once the correct amount of medication has been measured, it can be placed in a nipple and the infant can suck the medication through the nipple.
6. If the nurse feels comfortable managing the infant in her lap, it is acceptable to hold him for medication administration.

B. Toddlers

1. Draw up liquid medication in syringe or measure into medicine cup. Medications may be placed in medicine cup or spoon after being measured accurately in a syringe.
2. Elevate the child's head and shoulders.
3. Squeeze cup and put it to the child's lips; or place the syringe (without the needle) in the child's mouth, positioning the syringe tip in space between cheek mucosa and gum, and slowly expel the medicine. Child may prefer using the familiar teaspoon.

4. Allow the child time to swallow.
5. Allow the child to hold the medicine cup by himself, if he is able, and to drink it at his own pace. (This may be a more agreeable method.) Offer his favorite drink as a "chaser," if not contraindicated.
6. The small, safe, disposable medicine cups can be given to the child for play.

C. School-Age Children

1. When a child is old enough to take medicine in pill or capsule form, he should be taught to place the pill near the back of his tongue and immediately swallow fluid such as water or fruit juice. If the swallowing of the fluid is emphasized, the child will no longer think about the pill.
2. Always praise a child after he has taken his medication.
3. If the child finds it particularly difficult to take oral medications, the nurse must let him know that she understands some of his fear and displeasure and that she wants to help him.

Intramuscular Medications

A. General Considerations for IM Injections

1. After medication is drawn from vial, draw up an additional 0.2–0.3 ml. of air into syringe, thus clearing needle of medication and preventing medication seepage from injection site.
2. When injecting less than 1 ml. of medication, use a tuberculin syringe for accuracy.
3. Cleanse site thoroughly, using friction with an antiseptic solution; let site dry.
4. Establish anatomic landmarks (Fig. 32-3). Alternate injection site and keep record at bedside or on medication card.
5. After penetrating site, aspirate to check for blood vessel puncture. If this occurs, withdraw needle, discard medication, and start again.
6. Following injection, massage site (unless contraindicated). The complication of fibrosis and contracture of the muscle can be diminished by massage, warm soaks, and range-of-motion exercises to disrupt and stretch immature scar tissue when multiple injections are being administered.

B. Infants

1. Acceptable site selection:
   Vastus lateralis (middle third)
   Rectus femoris (mid-anterior thigh)
   Ventrogluteal—these areas are relatively free of major nerves and blood vessels.
   The gluteus maximus and deltoid muscles are underdeveloped in the infant and use of these sites can result in nerve damage.
2. Administration
   a. *Rectus femoris*
      (1) Place the child in a secure position to prevent movement of the extremity.
      (2) Do not use a needle longer than 2.5 cm. (1 inch).
      (3) Use upper outer quadrant of the thigh.
      (4) Insert needle at a 45-degree angle in a downward direction, toward the knee.
   b. *Vastus lateralis*
      (1) Place the child in prone or supine position.
      (2) Area is a narrow strip of muscle extending along a line from the greater trochanter to lateral femoral condyle below.
      (3) Insert needle perpendicular to skin 2–4 cm. deep—needle parallel to floor.

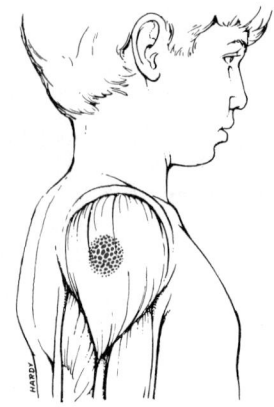

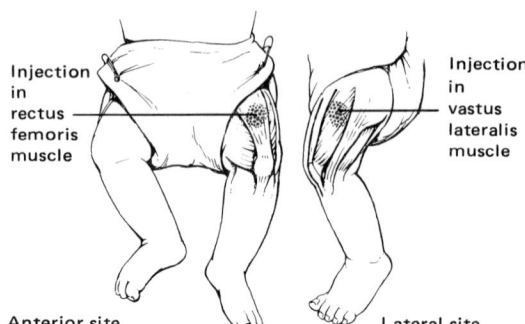

Anterior site   Lateral site

Arm for older child   Leg for small infant

Figure 32-3. Sites for IM injections in children.

c. *Ventrogluteal*—see below.

Following administration of medication, hold and cuddle infant. This site is also used on the older child who may be difficult to restrain.

C. Toddlers and School-Age Children

1. Site selection
   a. *Posterogluteal-upper outer quadrant*
      (1) Gluteal muscles do not develop until the child begins to walk; they should be used only when the child has been walking for 1 year or more.
          Complications include sciatic nerve injury or subcutaneous injury due to medication being injected and poor absorption.
      (2) Upper outer quadrant of the young child's buttock is smaller in diameter than that of an adult; thus accuracy in determining the area comprising the upper outer quadrant is essential.
      (3) Administration
          (a) Do not use a needle longer than 2.5 cm. (1 inch).
          (b) Position the child in a prone position.
          (c) Place thumb on the trochanter.
          (d) Place middle finger on the iliac crest.
          (e) Let index finger drop at a point midway between the thumb and middle finger to the upper outer quadrant of the buttock. This is the injection site.
          (f) Insert needle perpendicular to the surface on which the child is lying, not perpendicular to the skin.
   b. *Ventrogluteal*
      (1) This site provides a dense muscle mass that is relatively free of the danger of injuring the nervous and vascular systems.
      (2) The disadvantage is that the injection site is visible to the child.
      (3) Administration
          (a) Place the child on his back.
          (b) Place index finger on the anterosuperior spine.
          (c) With the middle finger moving dorsally, locate the iliac crest; drop finger below

the crest. The triangle formed by the iliac crest, index finger, and middle finger is the injection site.
          (d) Inject needle perpendicular to the surface on which the child is lying.
   c. *Deltoid*
      (1) May be used for older, larger children.
      (2) Determine injection site as with an adult.
      (3) Inject needle perpendicular to skin 2–3 cm. deep.
   d. *Lateral and anterior aspect of the thigh*
      (1) Do not use a needle longer than 2.5 cm. (1 inch).
      (2) Use the upper outer quadrant of the thigh.
      (3) Insert needle at a 45-degree angle in a downward direction, toward the knee.
2. Nursing support
   a. Explain to the child where you are going to give him the injection (site) and why he must receive the injection.
   b. Allow the child to express his fears.
   c. Carry out procedure quickly and gently. Have needle and syringe completely prepared and ready prior to contact with child.
   d. Numb site of injection by rubbing skin firmly with cleansing swab or with ice (older child may assist with this), and change needle after drawing medication through rubber stopper on medicine vial. Minimize pain of intramuscular injection by injecting needle into muscle with a quick, darting motion.
   e. Always secure the assistance of a second nurse to help immobilize the child and divert his attention as well as to offer him support and comfort.
   f. Praise the child for his behavior after the injection. Often, allowing him to assist with applying a Band-Aid will give him some feeling of comfort.
   g. Also encourage activity that will use the muscle site of injection—promotes dispersal of medication and decreases soreness. This can also be done by firmly massaging muscle following injection, unless contraindicated.
   h. Record accurately the injection site to ensure proper site rotation.

Intravenous Medications

(See intravenous infusions, p. 1160)

A. Intravenous Drip

1. Selecting the proper site for injecting medication into an intravenous line depends on the correct dilution for the drug, the rate of fluid administration, and the amount of intravenous fluid tolerated by the child.
   a. *Piggyback*—a second container holding the drug and a relatively small volume of fluid and an administration set are attached at the injection site of the primary administration set tubing, and allowed to flow over a period of time from 20 minutes–2 hours. This method maintains fluid schedule without fluid overload.
   b. *Bolus*—a rapid injection of a small volume of drug directly into the intravenous tubing or cannula by means of a syringe and needle.
   c. *Volume-control*—inject drug into gum-rubber injection port of volume control administration set. This allows for further dilution of drug with primary fluid or separate fluid reservoir. Then administer total fluid containing the drug in 30–60 minutes.
2. Prepare mixtures aseptically (laminar-flow hood) and use sterile technique when violating the line. (Sepsis is a constant threat when a child is receiving intravenous medications.)
3. Be aware that an exaggerated pharmacologic effect may exist with intravenous medications. As with any medication, know the use, side effects, and toxic effects of the drug, as well as the pharmacologic effect on the body.
4. Dilute intravenous medications and inject slowly—never less than 1 minute (this allows peripheral blood flow through the entire circulating system to dilute the medication and prevent high concentrations of the drug from reaching the brain and heart).
5. Be knowledgeable regarding compatibilities of drugs, electrolytes in IV solutions, and the fluid itself.
6. Observe IV site frequently. Restrain child, as needed, to prevent infiltration. Infiltration of fluids containing medications can cause rapid and severe tissue necrosis.

B. Heparin Lock (see adult, p. 109).

Venipuncture setup with 3½-inch tubing ending in a resealing rubber diaphragm creating a closed system.

1. The use of a heparin lock allows children who need repeated doses of chemotherapeutic agents to be fully mobile while reducing the trauma of repeated injections.
2. Heparin solution (0.25 heparin, 1000 USP/ml. to 10 ml. sterile water) is administered prior to and following instillation of medication, and regular heparin flushing is done every 8 hours to maintain patency.
3. The heparin lock can be connected to standard pediatric administration sets so that larger volumes of vehicle solutions can be used for dilution of medications.
4. The heparin lock should be securely taped in place to prevent dislodgement. Patency of vein must be determined prior to administration of fluids or medications.

Enema

An *enema* is the insertion of fluid into the rectum for the purpose of cleansing the lower bowel, or cooling to reduce temperature. An enema for an infant or a young child is based on the same principles as for an adult and is essentially the same, except that *less fluid and pressure are used than in an adult.*

Guidelines: Administering an Enema to a Child

Equipment

Solution measurements:

Soap suds enema—add 8 ml. (2 drams) soap jelly to 500 ml. (1 pint) of water

Saline enema—add 4 ml. (1 dram) salt to 500 ml. (1 pint) of water or 1 teaspoon salt to 500 ml H_2O

Procedure

Nursing Action	Rationale / Amplification
Preparatory Phase	
1. Explain procedure to the child according to his level of understanding.	1. Even though the child may not fully understand, an explanation will soothe him and build his trust in you.
2. Position	
a. *Older child:* Have him lie on his left side with his upper leg flexed.	a. This position places the descending colon at the lowest point.
b. *Infant:* Place infant in supine position, with a pillow under his head and back and a small bedpan under his buttocks. Gentle restraint may be needed—diaper placed under the bedpan, brought over thighs, and then pinned.	b. Infants and small children cannot retain enema fluid. Properly placed pillows promote body alignment.

(continued)

Guidelines: Administering an Enema to a Child (continued)

Procedure
(Cont.)

Nursing Action	Rationale/Amplification
Performance Phase	
1. Insert rectal tube 3.7–10 cm. (1½–4 inches) into the rectum just within the anal sphincter.	
2. Hang solution reservoir no higher than 25 cm. (10 inches) above the rectum.	2. This allows the solution to run slowly with minimal pressure.
3. Do not administer more than 300 ml. (10 oz.) of solution to infant unless otherwise prescribed.	3. Fluid volume may range from 30–300 ml. (1–10 oz.) depending on the size of the child. Suggested amounts: Birth to 3 months: 30–100 ml. Infant: 150–250 ml. Child: 200–500 ml. Older child: 500–1000 ml.
4. Once the rectal tube is removed, the abdomen can be gently massaged, if there are no contraindications.	4. This gentle massage will help relax the infant and assist in expelling the solution.
5. If young child is "potty trained," have a small potty chair available for his use.	5. The familiarity of a potty chair will provide great comfort for the child and eliminate the possible embarrassment of a soiled bed or pants.
6. When a retention enema is administered, the buttocks may be held or taped together to assist retention of fluid. Keep child as quiet as possible.	

Protective Measures to Limit Movement (Restraints)

Protective measures to limit movement are mechanisms for restraining children (Fig. 32-4).

Purposes

1. To maintain the child's safety and protect him from injury.
2. To facilitate examination and minimize the child's discomfort during special tests, procedures, and specimen collections.

Underlying Principles

1. Protective devices should be used only when necessary and never as a substitute for careful observation of the child.
2. The reason for using the protective device should be explained to the child and his parents to prevent misinterpretation and to ensure their cooperation with the procedure. Restraints are often interpreted as punishment by children.
3. Any protective device should be checked frequently to make sure that it is effective. It should be removed periodically to prevent skin irritation or circulation impairment.
4. Protective devices should always be applied in a manner that maintains proper body alignment and ensures the child's comfort.
5. Any protective device that requires attachment to the child's bed should be secured to the bed springs or frame, *never* the mattress or side rails. This allows the side rails to be adjusted without removing the restraint or injuring the child's extremity.
6. Any knots that are required should be tied in a manner that permits their quick release. This is a safety precaution.
7. When a child must be immobilized, an attempt should be made to replace the lost activity with another form of motion. For example, even though restrained, a child can be moved in a stroller, wheelchair, or in his bed. When arms are restrained, the child may be allowed to play kicking games. Water play, mirrors, body games, and blowing bubbles are helpful replacements.

Mummy Device

The *mummy device* involves securing a sheet or blanket around the child's body in such a way that his arms are held to his sides and his leg movements are restricted (see Fig. 32-4).

A. Purpose

To restrain infants and small children during treatments and examinations involving the head and neck.

B. Equipment

Small sheet or blanket
Several large safety pins

C. Nursing Action

1. Place the blanket or sheet flat on the bed.
2. Fold over 1 corner of the blanket.
3. Place the child on the blanket with his neck at the edge of the fold.
4. Pull the right side of the blanket firmly over the child's right shoulder.
5. Tuck the remainder of the right side of the blanket under the left side of the child's body.
6. Repeat the procedure with the left side of the blanket.
7. Separate the corners of the bottom portion of the sheet, and fold it up toward the child's neck.
8. Tuck both sides of the sheet under the infant's body.

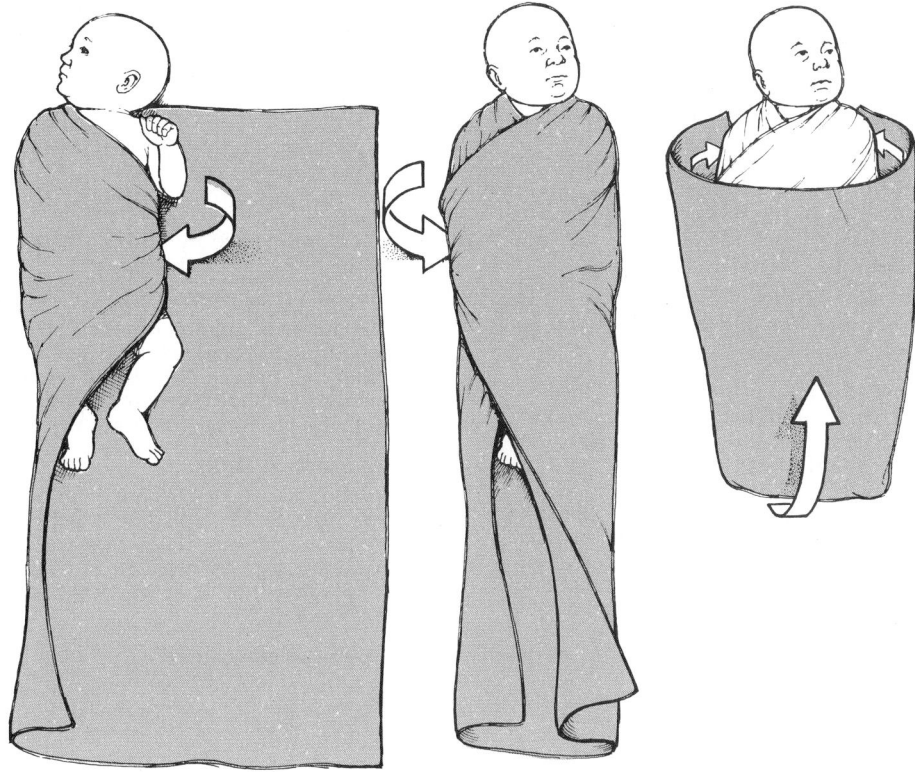

Mummy device

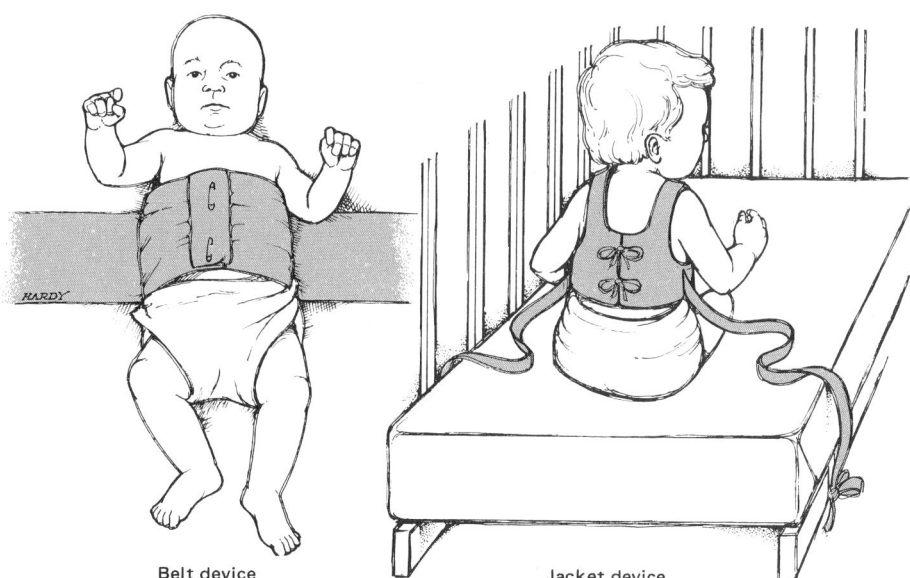

Belt device   Jacket device

Figure 32-4. Types of restraints.

9. Secure by crossing 1 side over the other in the back and tucking in the excess, or by pinning the blanket in place.

D. Special Precautions

Make certain that the child's extremities are in a comfortable position during this procedure.

Jacket Device

The *jacket device* is a piece of material that fits the child like a jacket or halter. Long tapes are attached to the sides of the jacket (see Fig. 32-4).

A. Purpose

To keep the child in his wheelchair, highchair, or crib.

B. Nursing Action

1. Put the jacket on the child so that the opening is in the back.
2. Tie the strings securely.
3. Position the child in his highchair, wheelchair, or crib.
4. Secure the long tapes appropriately:
   a. Under the arm supports of a chair.
   b. Around the back of the wheelchair or highchair.
   c. To the springs or frame of the crib.

C. Special Precautions

The child in a crib must be observed frequently to make certain that he does not entangle himself in the long tapes of the jacket device.

Belt Device

The *belt device* is exactly like the jacket method of restraining, except that the material fits the child like a wide belt and buckles in the back (see Fig. 32-4).

Elbow Device

The *elbow device* consists of a piece of material into which tongue depressors have been inserted at regular intervals. It is especially useful for infants receiving a scalp-vein infusion, those with eczema or cleft lip repair, and children having eye surgery.

A. Purpose

To prevent flexion of the elbow.

B. Equipment

    Elbow cuff
    Tongue depressors
    Safety pins, tapes, or string

C. Nursing Action

1. Insert tongue depressors into the appropriate places in the elbow cuff.
2. Place the child's arm in the center of the elbow cuff.
3. Wrap the cuff around the child's arm.
4. Secure the cuff with pins, tapes, or string.

D. Special Precautions

1. The tongue depressors should be cut to about 10 cm. (4 inches) in length if the elbow cuff is to be used for an infant—for greatest comfort.
2. Additional security may be provided by dressing the child in a long-sleeved shirt prior to the application of the elbow cuff. The ends of the shirt can then be turned back over the cuff and pinned securely.

Devices to Limit Movement of the Extremities

There are many different kinds of devices to limit motion of 1 or more extremities. One commercial variety consists of a piece of material with tapes on both ends to be secured to the frame of the crib. The material also has 2 small flaps sewn to it for securing the child's ankles or wrists. Similar devices are available which utilize sheepskin flaps. These should be used when the device will be necessary over a prolonged period, or for children with very sensitive skin.

A. Purpose

To restrain infants and young children for such procedures as intravenous therapy and urine collection.

B. Equipment

    Extremity restraint of appropriate size for the child (small, medium, or large)

    Several safety pins
    Cotton wadding covered with gauze

C. Nursing Action

1. Secure the device to the crib frame.
2. Pad the extremities to be restrained with cotton wadding covered with gauze or other suitable material.
3. Pin the small flaps securely around the child's ankles or wrists.
4. Adjust the device by pinning a tuck in the center of the material, if it is too large.

D. Special Precautions

1. The infant's fingers or toes should be observed frequently for coldness or discoloration and the skin under the device checked for signs of irritation.
2. The device should be removed periodically to provide skin care and range-of-motion exercises.

Abdominal Device

The *abdominal device* is used for restraining a small child in his crib. It operates exactly like the method described for limiting the movement of the extremities. However, the strip of material is wider and has only 1 wide flap sewn in the center for fastening around the child's abdomen.

Clove-Hitch Device

The *clove-hitch device* is a mechanism for restraining an extremity by tying gauze strips or a diaper in a special way.

A. Equipment

    Cotton wadding covered with gauze
    Gauze bandage cut in lengths of 1.37 meters (1½ yards)

B. Nursing Action

1. Pad the extremity to be restrained with cotton wadding that is covered with gauze or other suitable material.
2. Spread out the gauze strip on the bed.
3. Make a figure-8 loop in the center of the gauze strip.
4. Place the child's wrist or ankle in the loop of the device.
5. Pull the ends of the device to the desired tightness.
6. Tie the ends to the crib springs or frame.
7. Check the device to make certain that it does not tighten when both ends are pulled taut or slip over the child's hand or foot.

Mitts

Mitts are used to prevent a child from injuring himself with his hands. They are especially useful for children with dermatologic conditions, such as eczema or burns. Mitts can be purchased commercially or made by wrapping the child's hands in Kling gauze.

   Special Precaution
       Mitts should be removed at least twice during each tour of duty to permit skin care and to allow the child to exercise his fingers.

Crib Top Device

A *crib top device* is used to prevent an infant or small child from climbing over the crib sides. Several types of commercial devices are available, including nets, plastic tops, and domes. A crib top device should be applied to the crib of any infant capable of climbing over the crib sides.

Special Precaution

In all instances, it is essential to be certain that the crib sides are kept all of the way up and latched securely. There should be no space between the top of the crib sides and the bottom of the crib top device.

Feeding and Nutrition

Guidelines: Breast-Feeding the Ill or Hospitalized Infant*

Breast-feeding is suckling of an infant at the mother's breast to provide him with nourishment.

Purposes

1. To provide psychological and emotional satisfaction for the infant and the mother.
2. To feed the infant a natural and ideal food that will supply him with adequate nutrition, immunologic and anti-infection advantages.
3. To have milk always available at the right temperature.
4. To prevent chance of gastrointestinal disturbances and development of allergies.
5. To provide physical closeness of baby to mother during feeding.
6. To provide comfort after a frightening or painful procedure.

Points to Consider

1. The breast-fed infant up to 6 months of age may not have been started on solid foods.
2. The mother (at home) may give other liquids only by spoon or cup, not by bottle and nipple.
3. The infant may nurse frequently if mother is available.
4. Because breast milk is more easily and quickly digested, shorter periods of NPO both pre- and postoperatively may be used with the breast-fed infant.
5. Stress of hospitalization and illness experienced by the mother may decrease her milk supply and inhibit her "let down" reflex, as well as increase or decrease the infant's desire to suckle.
6. The infant in time of stress may cope with breast-feeding better than with bottle-feeding. Do not attempt to wean if avoidable.

Equipment

Clear water
Cotton balls

Procedure

Nursing Action	Rationale / Amplification
Preparatory Phase	
1. When an infant who is nursing is hospitalized, it is the nurse's responsibility to encourage the mother to continue breast-feeding if the infant's condition does not contraindicate it. Explain to the mother that: a. Supplemental artificial formula can be given to the infant if she is not available; or b. She can pump her breasts and bring in her milk to be given to the infant via bottle when she is not available.	1. Some mothers have very strong feelings about wanting to nurse their baby. It gives them an emotional satisfaction that is vitally important to the mother–child relationship since it is an integral part of the total mothering process. The nurse must help to foster this relationship as much as she can.
2. When nursing is to be done in the hospital pediatric setting, the physical surroundings may need to be altered somewhat. Provide the mother and infant with a relatively quiet area that is as private as possible and free from interruption.	2. This will provide the mother and infant with an opportunity to continue to develop their relationship during the crisis of illness and hospitalization.
3. Provide the mother with a comfortable armchair or pillow so that she can assume a comfortable position during the feeding. A footstool should also be available so that she can support her feet and the infant.	3. Proper and comfortable position of the mother will enable her to hold the baby correctly and support him while he is at the breast.
4. The infant should be awake and dry before the feeding is started.	4. If the infant is awake and comfortable, he will settle down and feed better.

* See page 999 for breast-feeding the newborn.

(continued)

Guidelines: Breast-Feeding the Ill or Hospitalized Infant (continued)

Procedure
(Cont.)

Nursing Action	Rationale/Amplification
5. Dress the infant appropriately so that he is not too warm or too cool during the feeding. The infant should also be hungry.	5. If he is too warm, he may fall asleep after the first few sucks of milk. A sleepy baby will not nurse well. If he is too cool, he may be fussy and restless.
6. Have mother wash her hands. Then she should wash her nipples with clear water and cotton balls.	6. Washing the nipples will remove any old milk that may have leaked and dried on them, providing a good medium for the growth of bacteria that can cause gastrointestinal disturbance in the infant.
7. Position the baby at breast. Put him in a semi-sitting position with his face close to the breast and supported by 1 arm and hand. A pillow may be used under the baby to support him. The breast may need to be supported by mother's other hand.	7. Proper positioning will provide the infant with comfort and security and make it easier for him to suck and swallow. This makes the nipple more easily accessible to the infant's mouth and prevents obstruction of nasal breathing.

Performance Phase

1. When the feeding is to start, let the breast touch the infant's cheek. Do not hold his cheek and try to help him find the nipple.	1. The rooting reflex will take over and the infant will turn his head toward the breast with his mouth open. If his cheek is touched with a hand, he will become confused, perhaps turning toward the hand.
2. The infant's lips should be out over the areola and not just around the nipple before he begins to suck.	2. Since the nipple is so small, suction cannot be achieved merely by grasping it. The areola must be in the infant's mouth in order to establish suction and make the suck effective.
3. Note the presence or absence of the "let-down" reflex during the nursing period.	3. Milk flowing from the other breast during nursing is quite normal. It is not usually present when the mother is worried.
4. The length of feeding time may vary from 5–30 minutes. Let the infant nurse until he is satisfied.	4. When the infant is satisfied and has nursed well, he is relaxed and usually falls asleep. He will stop sucking.
5. Instruct the mother to bubble the baby during and at the end of the feeding.	5. When the infant is sucking, he swallows some air. Bubbling will help prevent abdominal distention and discomfort as well as regurgitation.
6. One or both breasts may be used at each feeding. It makes no difference as long as (a) baby is satisfied at the end of the feeding and (b) 1 breast is completely emptied at the feeding.	6. Regular and complete emptying of the breast is the only stimulation for the production of milk.
7. Once the infant has stopped sucking, he likes to cling to the breast. To break this suction, instruct mother to put her finger to the corner of the baby's mouth and gently pull.	7. Gentle pulling will not hurt mother or infant.

Follow-up Phase

1. When the infant has finished feeding, change his diaper if it is wet or soiled.	1. To provide comfort for a restful sleep and to prevent diaper rash.
2. Position infant on his right side or on his abdomen in his bed.	2. This facilitates emptying of the stomach and decreases the possibility of regurgitation.
3. Note if baby appears satisfied or still seems to be hungry.	3. Mother may not have enough milk to satisfy the baby. Supplemental formula may be necessary.

4. Record descriptively and accurately:
  a. How baby fed
  b. How baby went to breast
  c. Satiety or hunger after feeding
  d. Breast or breasts used; which breast was emptied and which breast was nursed from thereafter.
	d. If both breasts were used, the second breast is not usually emptied and should be used first at the next feeding.

5. For the new mother–infant nursing team:
  a. Provide the mother with anticipatory guidance for possible problems (i.e., breast engorgement).
  b. Promote maternal confidence in handling and nursing her infant.
  c. Increase mother's knowledge about the mechanics of breast-feeding.
  d. Provide mother with literature and resources:
    (1) Resources for Nursing Mothers:
      Riordan J. A Practical Guide to Breast Feeding. St. Louis, CV Mosby, 1983
	5. To help establish and maintain successful breast-feeding that will be continued following discharge. Encourage mother to continue to get adequate rest and nutrition during and following infant's discharge.

Procedure
(Cont.)

Nursing Action	Rationale/Amplification

The Womanly Art of Breast Feeding, 2nd ed.
LaLeche League International, 9616 Minneapolis
Avenue, Franklin Park, IL 60131
(2) Agency:
LaLeche League International, 9616 Minneapolis
Avenue, Franklin Park, IL 60131

Guidelines: Artificial or Nipple Feeding

Artificial or *nipple feeding* is a method of supplying nutrition to the infant by oral feedings, using a bottle and nipple set-up.

Purposes
1. To provide the baby adequate fluid and calorie intake for appropriate growth.
2. To supplement breast-feeding with formula or water.
3. To provide additional fluid intake between feedings.

Equipment

Sterile nipple and bottle
Sterile formula or feeding fluid

Procedure

Nursing Action	Rationale/Amplification

Preparatory Phase

1. Baby should be awake and hungry. Change wet or soiled diaper.	1. A sleepy baby will not feed well. A dry diaper will provide comfort so that the baby will settle down and eat more easily.
2. Check formula for correct type and amount.	2. To prevent error.
3. Sit in a comfortable chair. Cradle baby with 1 hand and arm, while supporting baby against your body or lap.	3. Proper position will provide the baby with comfort and security and will make it easier for him to suck and swallow. Holding infant will enhance trust-building and provide sensory stimulation.

Performance Phase

1. Let the baby root for the nipple by touching the corner of his mouth with the nipple. When he opens his mouth, insert the nipple.	1. Place the nipple on top of the tongue and far enough in his mouth so suction can be created when he sucks.
2. Hold the bottle at an angle to completely fill the nipple with fluid.	2. This prevents the baby from sucking and swallowing excessive amounts of air.
3. NEVER prop the bottle or leave the baby unattended during feeding.	3. This is unsafe. Should vomiting occur, aspiration is more likely.
4. The bottle should be handled so as not to contaminate the nipple or fluid.	4. Contamination will increase the chances of gastrointestinal disturbances.
5. Baby's feeding time will vary from 10–25 minutes. Position baby so eye contact can be established (en face) during feeding. Soothing talk and fondling can provide additional comfort to the baby.	5. The length of time will depend on the age of the baby and how vigorously he sucks.
6. Bubble the baby at least once during the feeding and at the end of the feeding. a. Place the baby in sitting position in nurse's lap, tilt him slightly forward, and gently rub or pat his back or abdomen. Elevate head of mattress 30 degrees with young infant to prevent regurgitation and aspiration. b. Place the baby in prone position on nurse's shoulder and gently pat or rub his back. c. Place the baby in prone position on nurse's lap and gently rub or pat his back.	6. Most babies swallow some air during feeding. These positions aid in expelling air and thus prevent abdominal distention, discomfort, and regurgitation. Vigorous handling or patting may result in the infant spitting up or regurgitating feeding.
7. Take nipple out of mouth periodically.	7. To allow baby to rest and to let air into the bottle so that the nipple does not collapse.

(continued)

Guidelines: Artificial or Nipple Feeding (continued)

Procedure
(Cont.)

Nursing Action	Rationale / Amplification

Follow-up Phase

1. After final bubbling, change wet or soiled diaper and place baby in crib on his abdomen or right side.
2. Check baby in a few minutes. If he is restless, pick him up and bubble him. Note if any spitting-up has occurred.

3. Accurate and descriptive recording:
   a. What was fed and amount
   b. How feeding was tolerated
   c. Any regurgitation or emesis—amount and material
   d. Length of time of feeding
   e. How baby sucked and took the feeding; behavior before, during, and following feeding.

1. This position aids in emptying the stomach and prevents regurgitation.
2. Some babies relieve themselves of air when in the crib and also bring up small amounts of formula at the same time.

NOTE: When feeding a premature infant, the same principles apply. The premature infant, however, will tire more easily and fall asleep. Allow him frequent rest periods and use a soft nipple so that less energy is needed to suck. To stimulate this infant to suck, the nurse can brush the infant's cheek with her finger, place thumb or finger under the infant's chin or move the nipple slowly back and forth in his mouth. Feeding time should not exceed 30 minutes. Keep the infant warm during feeding.

Guidelines: Gavage Feeding

Gavage feeding is a means of providing food via a catheter passed through the nares or mouth, past the pharynx, down the esophagus, and into the stomach, slightly beyond the cardiac sphincter.

Purposes
1. To provide a method of feeding or administering medications that requires minimal patient effort, when the infant is unable to suck or swallow (i.e., infant under 32 weeks' gestation or under 1650 gm.).
2. To provide a route that allows adequate calorie or fluid intake.
3. To prevent fatigue or cyanosis which is apt to occur from nipple feeding.
4. To provide a safe method of feeding a limp and listless patient.

Equipment

Sterile rubber or plastic catheter, rounded-tip, size 5–10 (French Argyle feeding tube)
Clear, calibrated reservoir for feeding fluid
Syringe
Stethoscope
Water for lubrication
Tape—hypoallergenic
Feeding fluid, room temperature
Pacifier

Procedure

Nursing Action	Rationale / Amplification

Preparatory Phase

1. Position the infant on his side or back with a diaper roll placed under his shoulders. A mummy restraint may be necessary to help maintain this position.
2. Measure feeding catheter and mark with tape; measure distance from tip of nose to ear to xiphisternum.
3. Have suction apparatus readily available.

1. This position allows for easy passage of the catheter, facilitates observation, and helps avoid obstruction of the airway.
2. Premeasuring the catheter provides a guideline as to how far to insert catheter.
3. Suctioning clears the airway and prevents aspiration if vomiting occurs.

Performance Phase

1. Lubricate catheter with sterile water or saline.
2. Stabilize the patient's head with 1 hand; use the other hand to insert catheter.
   Push nose up to widen nostril.

1. Do not use oil because of danger of aspiration.

Procedure
(Cont.)

Nursing Action	Rationale/Amplification

a. *Insertion through nares:* slip the catheter into nostril and direct toward the occiput in a horizontal plane along floor of nasal cavity.

b. *Insertion through the mouth:* pass the catheter through the mouth toward the back of the throat. Depress anterior portion of tongue with forefinger, insert catheter along forefinger, and tilt head slightly forward.

a. This direction will follow the nares passageway into the pharynx. Do not direct the catheter upward. Positioning in nares may cause partial airway obstruction; therefore, observe for respiratory distress. Avoid this route if there is critical airway compromise.

3. If the patient swallows, passage of the catheter may be synchronized with the swallowing. Do not push against resistance.

3. Swallowing motions will cause esophageal peristalsis, which opens the cardiac sphincter and facilitates passage of the catheter. Perforation occurs with very little pressure.

4. If there is no swallowing, insert the catheter smoothly and quickly.

4. Because of cardiac sphincter spasm, resistance may be met at this point. Pause a few seconds, then proceed.

5. In the infant, especially, observe for vagal stimulation (i.e., bradycardia [slow heart rate] and apnea).

5. The vagus nerve pathway lies from the medulla through the neck and thorax to the abdomen. Above the stomach, the left and right branches unite to form the esophageal plexus. Stimulation of these nerve branches with the catheter will directly affect the cardiac and pulmonary plexus.

6. Once the catheter has been inserted to the premeasured length, tape the catheter to the patient's face (Fig. 32-5).

6. This prevents movement of catheter from the premeasured, preestablished correct position. Alternative method: loop narrow cloth tape around tube just below nostril, then secure it above lip or nose with tape. Some movement of tube may be seen with swallowing.

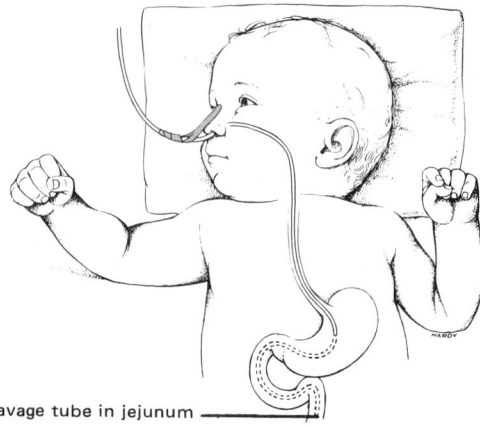

Gavage tube in jejunum

Figure 32-5. *Gavage feeding.*

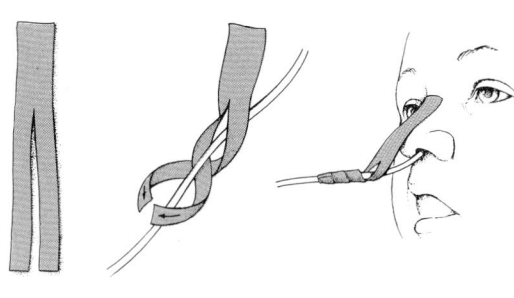

Steps in preparing adhesive tape to retain gavage tube

7. Test for correct position of the catheter in the stomach:
   a. Inject 0.5–5 ml. air into the catheter and stomach. At the same time listen to the typical growling stomach sound with a stethoscope placed over the epigastric region.
   b. Aspirate injected air from the stomach.
   c. Aspirate small amount of stomach content and test acidity by pH tape.

   d. Observe and gently palpate abdomen for tip of catheter. Avoid inserting catheter into the infant's trachea. (An infant's anatomy makes it relatively difficult to enter the trachea since esophagus is behind the trachea.)
8. The feeding position should be supine or right side-lying, with head and chest slightly elevated. Attach

a. Aids in ensuring proper location of catheter.

b. This prevents abdominal distention.
c. Failure to obtain aspirate does not indicate improper placement; there may not be any stomach content or the catheter may not be in contact with the fluid.
d. If improper placement occurs and the catheter enters the trachea, the patient may cough, fight, and become cyanotic. Remove the catheter immediately and allow the patient to rest before attempting intubation again.

8. This position allows the flow of fluid to be aided by gravity. The use of the pacifier will relax the infant,

(continued)

Guidelines: Gavage Feeding (continued)

Procedure
(Cont.)

Nursing Action	Rationale/Amplification
reservoir to catheter and fill with feeding fluid. Allow infant to suck on pacifier during feeding. Hold infant when possible.	allowing for easier flow of fluid as well as provide for normal sucking needs. Sucking will help develop muscles, and provide a positive association between sucking and relief of hunger.
9. Aspirate tube before feeding begins. a. If over ½ the previous feeding is obtained, withhold the feeding. b. If small residual of formula is obtained, return it to stomach and subtract that amount from the total amount of formula to be given.	9. This is done to monitor for appropriate fluid intake, digestion time, and overfeeding that can cause distention. Note an increase in gastric residual contents.
10. The flow of the feeding should be slow. Do not apply pressure. Elevate reservoir 15–20 cm. (6–8 inches) above the patient's head.	10. The rate of flow is controlled by the size of the feeding catheter; the smaller the size, the slower the flow. If the reservoir is too high, the pressure of the fluid itself increases the rate of flow.
11. Food taken too rapidly will interfere with peristalsis, causing abdominal distention and regurgitation.	11. The presence of food in the stomach stimulates peristalsis and causes the digestive process to begin. Also, when tube is in place, incompetence of the esophageal–cardiac sphincter may result in regurgitation.
12. Feeding time should last approximately as long as when a corresponding amount is given by nipple, 5 ml./5–10 minutes or 15–20 minutes total time.	
13. When the feeding is completed, the catheter may be irrigated with clear water. Before the fluid reaches the end of the catheter, clamp it off and withdraw it quickly.	13. Clamp the catheter before air enters the stomach and causes abdominal distention. Clamping also prevents fluid from dripping from the catheter into the pharynx, causing the patient to gag and aspirate.
14. Discard feeding tube and any leftover solution.	

NOTE: Intermittent gavage feeding is often preferred to indwelling gavage feeding. An indwelling catheter may coil and knot, perforate the stomach, and cause nasal airway obstruction, ulceration, irritation of the mucous membranes, incompetence of esophageal–cardiac sphincter, and epistaxis. However, if intermittent intubation is not well-tolerated and the indwelling method is used, the catheter should be clamped to prevent loss of feeding or entry of air and changed every 48–72 hours. (Use alternate sides of the nares.) Constant alertness to the above problems should be stressed. Indwelling method may be preferred with older infant or child.

Follow-up Phase

1. Burp or bubble the patient.	1. Adequate expulsion of air swallowed or ingested during feeding will decrease abdominal distention and allow for better tolerance of the feeding.
2. Place the patient on right side or on abdomen for at least 1 hour.	2. To facilitate gastric emptying and minimize regurgitation and aspiration.
3. Observe condition after feeding; bradycardia and apnea may still occur.	3. Because of vagal stimulation as mentioned above.
4. Note any vomiting or abdominal distention.	4. Due to overfeeding or too rapid feeding. Regurgitation of 1–2 ml. may occur in the premature infant as the musculature of the sphincter of the gastrointestinal tract is relaxed and allows for easy reflux.
5. Note infant's activity.	5. Fatigue or peaceful sleep.
6. Accurately describe and record procedure, including time of feeding, type of gavage feeding, type and amount of feeding fluid given, amount retained or vomited, how the patient tolerated feeding, and activity before, during, and following feeding.	6. Observe for readiness of the infant to feed by nipple—note sucking activity and sleep–wake cycle in relation to feeding.

Guidelines: Gastrostomy Feeding

Gastrostomy feeding is a means of providing nourishment and fluids via a tube that has been surgically inserted via a stab wound through the abdominal wall into the stomach.

Purposes
1. To provide a method of nutrition and fluids that requires minimal effort when the patient is unable to suck or swallow for long periods of time.
2. To allow for better decompression of stomach (because of large tube size) following a surgical procedure.

Purposes
(Cont.)

3. To provide a safe method of feeding a hypotonic patient or one who cannot tolerate alternative methods. Specific indications may include duodenal atresia, tracheal esophageal fistula, and omphalocele.
4. To provide a route that allows adequate calorie and/or fluid intake in a child with chronic lung disease or in one who does not have continuity of the gastrointestinal tract (i.e., esophageal atresia).

Equipment

Warm feeding fluid
Pacifier
Reservoir syringe or funnel
Syringe for aspirating

Procedure

Nursing Action	Rationale / Amplification
Preparatory Phase	
1. Gastrostomy tube may be in one of 3 positions between feedings: a. Lowered and open to start drainage. b. Open, connected to reservoir (funnel, syringe) that is elevated 10–12 cm. (4–4¾ inches). c. Clamped.	a. Constant decompression. b. To serve as safety valve outlet to prevent esophageal reflux and increased stomach pressure. c. Most ''normal'' physiologic setup, preparation for home care or tube removal.
2. The nurse may be directed to check residual stomach contents prior to any feeding. a. Attach syringe and aspirate stomach contents. b. Measure. c. Residual fluid may be returned to stomach or discarded, depending on amount.	2. This is done to monitor for appropriate fluid intake, digestion time, and overfeeding that can cause distention.
3. A Y-tube that is connected at the point where reservoir and gastrostomy tube join may be used during feeding.	3. To provide simultaneous decompression during feeding.
4. When feeding is about to begin, infant/child should be placed in comfortable position in bed—either flat or with head slightly elevated. If condition permits, the nurse should hold the infant. A pacifier can be given to him.	4. When the infant/child is comfortable and relaxed, feeding fluid will flow more easily into stomach. Pacifier will satisfy normal sucking activity, provide exercise for jaw muscles, and relax musculature as well as provide pleasure normally associated with feeding.
Performance Phase	
1. Attach reservoir syringe to tube (if not already open to continuous elevation) and fill reservoir with feeding fluid prior to unclamping tube.	1. Prevents air from entering tube (and then stomach), which may cause distention.
2. Elevate tube and reservoir to 10–12 cm. (4–4¾ inches) above abdominal wall. Do not apply any pressure to start flow.	2. This elevation level will allow for slow, gravity-induced flow. Pressure may cause a backflow of fluid into the esophagus.
3. Feed slowly, taking 20–45 minutes. Fill reservoir with remaining fluid before it is empty to avoid instillation of air.	3. Too rapid a feeding will interfere with normal peristalsis and will cause abdominal distention and backflow into reservoir or esophagus.
4. Continue to provide infant with pleasant feelings associated with feeding.	
5. When feeding is completed: a. Instill clear water (10–30 ml., or 0.3–1 oz.) if tube is to be clamped. Apply clamp before water level reaches end of reservoir. b. Leave tube unclamped and open to continuous elevation.	a. This rinses tubing and will prevent clogging. b. Feeding fluid is allowed to return to reservoir if infant cries or changes position, and thus decreases pressure on the stomach.
6. Often when oral feedings are started, they are given simultaneously with gastrostomy feedings.	6. This allows the infant to learn or reestablish the sucking-swallowing process as well as to build up tolerance to eating without compromising nutritional intake.
Follow-up Phase	
1. Check dressing and skin around point of tube entry for wetness. Clean skin and apply skin barrier (petrolatum, Maalox, aluminum paste, etc.). See that there is no pull on tube.	1. Skin breakdown is caused by continued exposure to stomach contents that may be leaking out around tube causing excoriation and infection. Constant pulling on tube can cause widening of skin opening and subsequent leakage.

(continued)

Guidelines: Gastrostomy Feeding (continued)

Procedure
(Cont.)

Nursing Action	Rationale/Amplification
2. Leave the infant dry and comfortable. If unable to hold him during feeding, this may be a good time to hold, fondle, and provide him with warmth and love. Place him on right side or in Fowler's position.	2. To promote relaxation and improved digestion of feeding.
3. Accurately describe and record procedure, including time of feeding, type and amount of feeding fluid given, amount and characteristics of residual (if any) and what was done with it, how the patient tolerated feeding, any abdominal distention, and activity following feeding.	

NOTE: Should infant pull gastrostomy tube out, cover ostomy site with sterile dressing and tape, notify physician and accurately record events.

Guidelines: Nasojejunal Feeding

Nasojejunal feeding is a means of providing full enteral feeding via a catheter passed through the nares, past the pharynx, down the esophagus, bypassing the stomach through the pylorus into the jejunum.

Purposes
1. To provide a method of feeding that requires minimal patient effort when the infant is unable to tolerate alternative feeding methods (i.e., low birth weight, persistent respiratory distress).
2. To provide a route that allows for adequate calorie or fluid intake (a full enteral feeding) via intermittent or continuous drip.
3. To provide a method of feeding a critically ill infant that minimizes regurgitation, aspiration, and gastric distention.
4. To provide a route for administration of oral medications (controversial).

Equipment

*Sterile radiopaque silicone or polyvinyl nasojejunal (N-J) tube, 1 meter (39 inches), No. 19, No. 21, or No. 23—may or may not have weighted tip
Tape
pH paper
Reservoir for feeding
Possibly an infusion pump
3-way stopcock
Syringe—0.5 ml. normal saline or sterile water
Equipment for N-G tube insertion; introducer catheter

Procedure

Nursing Action	Rationale/Amplification
Preparatory Phase	
1. Attach cardiac monitor to infant.	1. To allow for continuous monitoring of heart rate and rhythm. The vagus nerve pathway lies from the medulla through the neck and thorax to the abdomen. Above the stomach, the left and right branches unite to form the esophageal plexus. Stimulation of these nerve branches with the catheter will directly affect the cardiac and pulmonary plexus.
2. Tube is generally inserted by a physician. a. Measure from glabella (prominent point between eyebrows) to the heel for estimated length. b. Measure and mark the remaining length of tubing and record.	b. This serves as a double check to ensure that tube has not advanced farther than intended.
3. Place the infant on his right side with hips slightly elevated. Gentle restraint or soft mittens may have to be applied.	3. Facilitates passage of tube. Restraints prevent infant from pulling out tube before the tip passes the pylorus. Do not place on left side.
4. Tube is inserted by threading the N-J vinyl catheter into a No. 10 French feeding catheter and introducing both	4. Oral insertion may cause increased salivation, air swallowing, and regurgitation.

* See Gavage Feeding, page 1148.

Procedure
(Cont.)

Nursing Action	Rationale / Amplification
through the nostril into the stomach. The feeding tube is then withdrawn, and the N-J feeding tube is allowed to advance through the pylorus.	
5. Check intestinal aspirate for pH every 1–2 hours. Infant may be positioned on right side, back, or abdomen. Once the tube is past the pylorus, abdominal postero-anterior and lateral x-rays are taken to confirm that tip of catheter is at the ligament of Treitz.	5. When aspiration fluid reaches a pH of 5–7 or bile-colored fluid is obtained, the tip of the tube has passed the pylorus and duodenum into the jejunum.
6. A No. 5 French nasogastric feeding tube may be passed through the other nostril at this time and left indwelling. This is used to check stomach for residual fluid and regurgitation through the pylorus.	6. If gastric residual is significant, it will interfere with prescribed feeding. Notify physician. (4 ml/kg [0.12 oz/ 2.21 lbs] reflux in stomach is usually tolerated.) Do not remove N-G tube since it will adhere to N-J tube during withdrawal and pull out N-J tube also.
7. N-J feedings can generally be started following this progression:	
a. D$_5$W for 6–12 hours	
b. ½ strength formula with low osmolality for 6–12 hours.	b. Low solute formulas include SMA, Similac, Enfamil, (20 calories/30 ml., or 20 calories/1 oz.).
c. Full strength low osmolality formula.	c. Low osmolality formula is used to prevent loss of fluid into intestine and possible necrotizing enterocolitis.
d. The volume of feeding is increased 2 ml. (0.06 oz.) at a time until infant's daily calorie and fluid requirements are being administered.	d. 150 ml./kg. (4.5 oz./2.2 lbs.) fluid requirement is generally used (130–150 cal./kg.).
e. Medications may be given via the N-J tube if prescribed. A 3-way stopcock will have to be placed at the connection of the N-J tube and the line from the feeding fluid. Alternative method for administering oral medications is by passing an oral–gastric or nasogastric feeding tube; in this way the stomach and process of digestion and absorption are not by-passed.	e. Flush tubing with 0.5 ml. (.015 oz.) normal saline solution or sterile water after medication is administered to ensure that infant receives entire dosage prescribed and to prevent any sediment from remaining in tubing.

Performance Phase

Nursing Action	Rationale / Amplification
1. N-J feedings can be given as follows:	
a. Intermittently (i.e., every 1–3 hours)	
b. In a continuous slow drip.	b. Generally the preferred method to minimize the satiety–hunger cycle and large-volume instillation.
2. If intermittent feeding is the method used, the feeding techniques are the same as for nasogastric (gavage) feeding.	2. Feeding is given at room temperature. Avoid cold fluid, which may cause infant discomfort. If breast milk is used, gently rotate reservoir periodically to mix settled-out fat content.
3. If slow continuous drip method is used, the setup used is similar to the pediatric IV infusion using an infusion pump and small (100–250 ml., or 3.0–7.5 oz.) closed chamber for reservoir.	
a. Reservoir chamber and tubing should be changed every 8–24 hours.	a. To prevent growth of bacteria.
b. Record input every hour. Fill reservoir as needed, with no more than 3 hours worth of feeding fluid.	b. To ensure a constant flow and minimize overinfusion directly into the jejunum.

Follow-up Phase

Nursing Action	Rationale / Amplification
1. Be constantly alert for mechanical problems:	1. Tube clogging due to inadequate rinsing. Tube advancing too far into jejunum; check protruding tube measurement. Fluid overload, causing aspiration.
a. Check for abdominal distention due to the infant's inability to handle ingested amount of fluid:	
• palpate abdomen;	
• observe for ripple of intestines;	
• measure abdominal girth every 3–8 hours;	
• check residual formula in jejunum every 3–8 hours;	
• discard or refeed as prescribed.	
b. Check stools for occult blood, pH, and sugar every voiding or 4–8 hours to determine tolerance of feeding fluid.	
c. Check emesis for blood and report to physician immediately—may be a sign of necrotizing entero-colitis.	

(continued)

Guidelines: Nasojejunal Feeding (continued)

Procedure
(Cont.)

Nursing Action	Rationale / Amplification
2. Position infant in recumbent position.	2. Less likely for "dumping syndrome" to occur.

3. Observe infant closely to avoid potential dangers as tube passes the pylorus.
  a. Close attention to amount, type, concentration, and osmolality of feeding fluid is stressed.
  b. Check heart rate and BP.
	3. Diarrhea; as the tube passes through the pylorus, it (the tube) becomes stiff because of the change in pH. A stiff tube has been reported to cause intestinal perforation. If tube becomes clogged or dislodged, it must be removed.

4. Hold, fondle, and give positive stimulation to the infant if conditions permit (see Premature Infant, p. 1228).	4. This procedure limits the normal pleasures associated with feeding. Infant needs some attention to his psychological needs in order to thrive.
5. Accurately describe and record condition of infant and procedure, including type and amount of feeding given, amount of residual and characteristics, any signs of impending infant distress or problems.	

Specimen Collection

Guidelines: Assisting with Blood Collection

Blood collection from a venous puncture in the extremity of an infant or young child is the same as for an adult, with the following exceptions or additions.

Equipment

No. 23–19 gauge short needle or scalp-vein needle
Smaller volume or micro blood-collecting tubes
Smaller tourniquet (rubber band may be used with infant)

Procedure

Nursing Action	Rationale / Amplification
Preparatory Phase	
1. Immobilize the child by placing him in a mummy restraint if necessary (see p. 1142).	1. Infants and young children squirm. Immobilizing them allows easier access to the venipuncture site. It also helps keep the infant warm.

2. Position the patient.
  a. *Femoral venipuncture:* place the child on his back with legs in frog-like position. Nurse places her hands on child's knees (see position for bladder puncture, p. 1156).
  b. *External jugular venipuncture:* place the child in mummy restraint and lower his head over the side of the bed or table. Turn head to side and stabilize. Crying will make external jugular vein visible and causes blood to flow more readily.
  c. *Antecubital fossa venipuncture:* place the child in a supine position. The nurse stands on the side opposite the site to be used (across from the person drawing the specimen). The nurse positions her right arm across the upper part of the child's chest and grasps the shoulder at the axilla position. Her left arm is placed across the lower part of the child's chest and is used to extend the child's arm at the wrist.
	2. These positions allow for optimal visualization and stabilization of the patient. Cover perineum to protect site and operator, should infant void.
	
	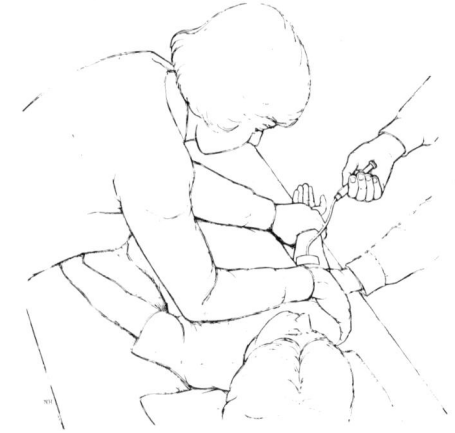

d. *Infant—heel, toe, or digital puncture:* warm area with warm compress for 5–10 minutes.	d. This dilates vessels allowing blood to flow more freely.

Procedure
(Cont.)

Nursing Action	Rationale/Amplification
Performance Phase	
1. After the specimen is collected and the needle is removed, apply pressure to the site with dry gauze for 3–5 minutes.	1. Both the femoral and jugular veins are large vessels. Since respiratory pressure is great, bleeding, oozing, and hematoma formation may result. External pressure prevents this from happening.
a. *Jugular venipuncture:* while applying pressure to the site, place the patient in an upright sitting position. Do not apply excessive pressure that may compromise circulation or respiration.	
b. *Capillary:* clean area with antiseptic and dry with dry sterile 2 × 2 gauze. Hold heel firmly and with free hand quickly puncture with microlancet or sterile No. 21 gauge needle on most medial or lateral part of plantar surface. Puncture deeply enough to get free-flowing blood—never deeper than 2.4 mm. Discard first drop of blood; rapidly collect specimen in proper capillary tube.	
2. When the bleeding has been stopped, soothe and comfort the child before leaving him.	2. Crying and thrashing about may initiate bleeding.
Follow-up Phase	
1. Check the patient frequently for an hour after the procedure for oozing, bleeding, or evidence of a hematoma.	1. Reapply pressure and report if oozing continues.
2. Record carefully and accurately:	
a. Site of venipuncture	
b. How the patient tolerated procedure	
c. Bleeding stopped or continued and for how long	
d. For what test was the specimen collected?	

Guidelines: Collecting a Urine Specimen from the Infant or Young Child

Urine collection is a safe method of obtaining urine for a specified purpose.

Purposes
1. To check urine for presence of sugar, acetone, bacteria, and other urinary products.
2. To aid in diagnosis.
3. To determine the condition of the patient.
4. To determine effectiveness of therapy.

Equipment

Collecting device—plastic, disposable urine bag or collector (Hollister, Inc. U-Bag, double chamber)
Cleansing agent
Wiping material—4 × 4's or cotton balls
Clean or sterile water
Containers for solutions
Specimen container

Procedure

Nursing Action	Rationale/Amplification
Preparatory Phase	
1. Offer the young child fluids he likes to drink 30–60 minutes prior to procedure, if no contraindications.	
2. Position the patient so that genitalia are exposed by placing him on his back with legs in frog-like position. Assistance may be needed to hold the legs of the young child in proper position.	2. Proper positioning will facilitate cleansing and allow for proper placement of collection device.
3. When small samples of urine are needed for pH, Clinitest, etc., to be done by the nurse, urine can be extracted from the diaper using a syringe or dropper.	

(continued)

Guidelines: Collecting a Urine Specimen from the Infant or Young Child (continued)

Procedure
(Cont.)

Nursing Action	Rationale/Amplification
Performance Phase	
1. Cleanse genital area.	1. This method of cleansing the female will prevent contamination of the genitalia from the anus, and will prevent contamination of the urine specimen obtained.
a. *Female:* using cotton balls, dip into cleansing agent, wipe labia majora from top to bottom (clitoris to anus) only once with each cotton ball. Repeat this once more. Wipe again with clear water. Then spread labia apart with one hand while wiping the labia minora in the same manner with other hand. Wipe area dry.	During the cleansing be gentle to avoid any injury or possible stimulation of urination.
b. *Male:* wipe tip of penis in circular motion down towards the scrotum. Be certain to retract foreskin if present. Wipe first with cleansing agent 2–3 times, then clear water. Dry the area.	
2. Apply collecting bag firmly so that the opening is exposed to receive urine.	2. If collecting bag is properly and securely placed, the procedure will not have to be repeated.
a. *Female:* stretch perineum taut during application. Attach bag to perineum first, then proceed up to symphysis.	a. This should ensure leak-proof contact.
Elevate head of bed or place the child in an infant seat, if appropriate.	To aid flow of urine by gravity.
b. *Male (small boys):* place penis inside bag.	
3. Apply diaper to patient and comfort him; possibly give him additional clear fluids.	
4. Check the patient frequently (30–45 minutes) to see if he has voided. When the patient has voided, remove bag gently. Cleanse area and reapply diaper to the child. If child has not voided within 45 minutes, procedure must be repeated.	4. The adhesive on the collecting bag may tend to be sticky. Careful removal of the bag will prevent skin injury on and around genitalia. Also avoid spilling urine out of the bag during removal. Reapplication of bag will decrease the possibility of unreliable test results.
Follow-up Phase	
1. Pour specimen into proper collecting container. Send specimen to the laboratory within 30 minutes or refrigerate.	1. Prompt delivery of specimen to the laboratory will prevent growth of organisms in an uncontrolled environment and distortion of the test results.
2. Accurately chart and describe the following in the nurse's notes:	2. Guideline for weighing diaper, excluding weight of dry diaper, 1 gm. = 1 ml. urine.
a. Time specimen collection was started and ended	
b. Amount of urine voided	
c. Color of urine (cloudy, clear, any sediment)	
d. Type of test to be done	
e. Condition of skin of perineal area	

    Note: If 24-hour urine collection is needed, use a collection bag that has a long tube attachment that drains into collecting receptacle. Adherence of bag to skin can be improved by applying a thin coating of tincture of benzoin to skin and allowing this to dry before attaching collection bag.

Guidelines: Assisting with a Percutaneous Suprapubic Bladder Aspiration

    Percutaneous bladder aspiration is an aseptic method of entering the bladder in the suprapubic location with a needle to obtain a urine specimen.

Purposes
1. To obtain urine in an aseptic manner for culture.
2. To aid in diagnostic workup.
3. To determine condition of the patient and aid in treatment.

Equipment

Antiseptic skin cleansing solution
Band-Aid
Sterile 4 × 4's
   Gloves
   Needle, No. 20–22 gauge, 3.7 cm. (1½ inches) long
   Syringe, 20 ml.
   Specimen container

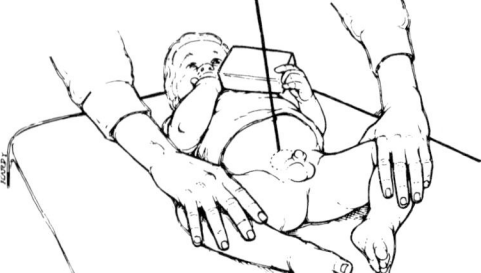

Outline of bladder

Procedure

Nursing Action	Rationale/Amplification
Preparatory Phase	
1. Check diaper for wetness. If the child has just voided, report this to the physician or report last voiding time. At least 1 hour should pass without voiding.	1. In order to perform a successful bladder aspiration, enough urine must be present to distend the bladder up above the pubic symphysis—so that bladder is accessible.
2. Position the child on his back on the examining table. His head should be toward nurse, his feet toward the physician. Spread his legs apart in a frog-like position. Place hands on his knees and thumbs along his sides at the hip level.	2. This position allows the nurse to stabilize the child. It also gives a full view of the child, making it easier to observe him, talk to him, and soothe him.
3. Ensure that the skin over the puncture site is cleansed in an antiseptic manner.	3. To prevent infection from being introduced into the bladder by inserting the needle through unclean skin which would contaminate the specimen.
Performance Phase	
1. While the procedure is being performed, note the condition of the patient and any signs of distress. Comfort him by talking to him and smiling at him.	1. Report any changes in color or respiration rate or other signs. Soothing the child will help him to relax so that he will not move about so much. Crying increases the muscle tone of the lower abdomen, making it more difficult to insert the needle.
2. To prevent urination during procedure, compress the infant's urethra: a. *Male:* pressure on penis. b. *Female:* digital pressure upward on urethra from rectum.	
3. When urine has been obtained or the procedure is discontinued and the needle is removed, apply pressure over the puncture site with a 4 × 4 and fingers.	3. This prevents any bleeding from occurring either internally or externally. Pressure should be maintained about 3 minutes or until oozing ceases and coagulation has taken place.
4. Apply a Band-Aid if necessary. Reapply diaper. Hold and comfort him for a few minutes.	4. Holding the child will help to restore and maintain a good nurse–patient relationship and will help the child to relax after a frightening and painful procedure.
Follow-up Phase	
1. Check the child periodically for 1 hour after procedure to see that bleeding or oozing has not occurred.	1. This is not likely if pressure was applied properly after procedure and the patient was left quiet.
2. Note time of first voiding after procedure. Note color of urine (it may be pink). Bloody urine should be reported to the physician.	2. It is important to note any changes in voiding pattern following the procedure since change might indicate injury. The first voided urine may be bloody because of a small amount of local capillary bleeding at the time of the procedure.
3. Accurately describe and chart the procedure, including: a. Time of procedure b. Whether or not a specimen was obtained c. How the patient tolerated the procedure d. Description and amount of urine obtained e. Patient's condition and activity following the procedure	

Guidelines: Collecting a Stool Specimen

Stool collection is a method of obtaining a stool specimen from the patient.

Purposes
1. To check stool for presence of specific material (i.e., blood, ova, and parasites or bacteria).
2. To aid in diagnosis.
3. To determine condition or status of the patient.
4. To determine effectiveness of therapy.

Equipment

Diaper
Cellophane or plastic liner (used when stool is loose or watery)
Tongue blade
Specimen container

NOTE: Collecting a stool specimen from an older child who is toilet-trained is the same as collecting such a specimen from an adult.

(continued)

Guidelines: Collecting a Stool Specimen (continued)

Procedure

Nursing Action	Rationale / Amplification
Preparatory Phase	
1. If a specimen is needed from a patient whose stools are loose or watery enough to be absorbed in the diaper, line the diaper with a piece of cellophane or plastic. Place this liner between the diaper and the skin. Then apply diaper to the child and position him so that his head is slightly elevated. If stools are soft or formed, apply diaper.	1. The liner and position will allow the loose stool specimen to collect in the liner and not be absorbed by the diaper.
Performance Phase	
1. Check the child frequently to see if stooling has occurred.	1. A fresh specimen should be obtained so that test results will not be distorted by time-lapse. This will also decrease the chance of contamination of the stool with urine and will prevent skin irritation from the stool.
2. Remove soiled diaper from child. Clean perineal area, apply clean diaper, and leave the child comfortable.	
3. Remove small amount of stool from diaper with the tongue blade and place it in the specimen container.	
4. Send labeled specimen to the laboratory promptly.	4. Prompt delivery to the lab will prevent changes from taking place in the specimen that could alter the test results.
Follow-up Phase	

1. Accurately describe and record the following:
   a. Time specimen was collected
   b. Color, amount, and consistency of stool (Note any foul smell.)
   c. Type of specimen collected
   d. Nature of test for which the specimen was collected
   e. Condition of the skin	

Guidelines: Assisting with a Spinal Tap—Lumbar Puncture

A *spinal tap* in an infant or young child is based on the same principles and is essentially the same as for an adult, with the following exceptions.

Equipment

No. 21–20 gauge, 3.5-cm. (1½-inch) long spinal needle

Procedure

Nursing Action	Rationale / Amplification
Preparatory Phase	

1. Position the patient.
   a. *Side position* (similar to the adult): wrap the lower extremities in a sheet; if an older child, place the patient on his side facing the nurse; flex knees and neck by placing one hand on his shoulders and head and the other hand on buttocks and upper thigh.
   b. *Sitting position:* this position is primarily used with small infants. Place infant in sitting position; extend legs and arms in front of the infant; flex his neck so chin is almost resting on chest; back is rounded by placing thumbs on his shoulders and hands along side of his hips.
	1. In either position the patient may squirm. Hold him securely to prevent him from moving and causing injury to himself or causing the spinal needle to be inserted too far, resulting in a traumatic tap.

▶ **NURSING ALERT:** Observe for signs of respiratory distress. Because the trachea in the infant is so soft, it can kink very easily when the neck is flexed. If this happens and the airway is obstructed, the infant will stop breathing. This is an emergency situation.

Follow-up Phase

1. It is not usually necessary to keep the infant or young child flat in bed following the procedure unless there are contraindications to his being up and physician has prescribed that he be kept in bed. It may be helpful to institute play activity and offer fluids to the child.

Fluid and Electrolyte Balance in Children

Basic Principles

1. Infants and small children have different proportions of body water and body fat than do adults (Table 32-2).
   a. The body water of a newborn infant approaches 80% of his body weight, compared to that of an average adult male, which approaches 60%.
   b. The normal infant demonstrates a rapid physiological decline in the ratio of body weight to body water during the immediate postpartum period.

Table 32-2 Body Fluids Expressed as Percent of Body Weight

Fluid	Adult		Infant
	Male	Female	
Total Body Fluids	60%	54%	75%
(1) Intracellular	40%	36%	40%
(2) Extracellular	20%	18%	35%

Table 32-3 Common Abnormalities of Fluid and Electrolyte Metabolism

Substance	Major Function	Abnormality	Cause	Clinical Manifestation	Laboratory Data
Water	Medium of body fluids, chemical changes, body temperature, lubricant	Volume deficit	1. Primary—inadequate water intake 2. Secondary—loss following vomiting, diarrhea, excessive gastrointestinal obstruction, etc.	Oliguria, weight loss, signs of dehydration including dry skin and mucous membranes, lassitude, sunken fontanelles, lack of tear formation, increased pulse rate, decreased blood pressure	Concentrated urine, azotemia, elevated hematocrit, hemoglobin and erythrocyte count
		Volume excess	1. Failure to excrete water in presence of normal intake such as in congestive heart failure, renal disease 2. Water intake in excess of output	Weight gain, peripheral edema, signs of pulmonary congestion	Variable urine volume, low specific gravity of urine, decreased hematocrit
Potassium	Intracellular fluid balance, regular heart rhythm, muscle and nerve irritability	Potassium deficit	1. Excessive loss of potassium due to vomiting, diarrhea, prolonged cortisone, ACTH or diuretic therapy, diabetic acidosis 2. Shift of potassium into the cells such as occurs with the healing phase of burns, recovery from diabetic acidosis	Signs and symptoms variable, including weakness, lethargy, irritability, abdominal distention, and eventually cardiac arrhythmias	Low plasma K^+ level (may be normal in some situations); hypochloremic alkalosis; ECG changes
		Potassium excess	Excessive administration of potassium-containing solutions, excessive release of potassium due to burns, severe kidney disease, adrenal insufficiency	Variable, including listlessness, confusion, heaviness of the legs, nausea, diarrhea, ECG changes, ultimately paralysis and cardiac arrest	Elevated potassium plasma level
Sodium	Osmotic pressure, muscle and nerve irritability	Sodium deficit	Water intake in excess of excretory capacity, replacement of fluid loss without sufficient sodium; excessive sodium losses	Headache, nausea, abdominal cramps, confusion alternating with stupor, diarrhea, lacrimation, salivation, later hypotension; early polyuria, later oliguria	Sodium plasma level may be high, low, or normal
		Sodium excess	Inadequate water intake especially in the presence of fever or sweating; increased intake without increased output; decreased output	Thirst, oliguria, weakness muscular pain, excitement, dry mucous membranes, hypotension, tachycardia, fever	Elevated Na^+ plasma level, high plasma volume
Bicarbonate	Acid–base balance	Primary bicarbonate deficit	Diarrhea (especially in infants), diabetes mellitus, starvation, infectious disease, shock or congestive heart failure producing tissue anoxia	Progressively increasing rate and depth of respiration—ultimately becoming Kussmaul respiration, flushed, warm skin, weakness, disorientation progressing to coma	Urine pH usually less than 6 Plasma bicarbonate less than 20 mEq./liter Plasma pH less than 7.35
		Primary bicarbonate excess	Loss of chloride through vomiting, gastric suction, or the use of excessive diuretics, excessive ingestion of alkali.	Depressed respiration, muscle hypertonicity, hyperactive reflexes, tetany and sometimes convulsions	Urine pH usually above 7.0, plasma bicarbonate above 25 mEq./liter (30 mEq./liter in adults), plasma pH above 7.45

c. Proportion of body water declines more slowly throughout infancy and reaches the characteristic value for adults by approximately 2 years of age.

2. Compared to adults, a greater percentage of the body water of infants and small children is contained in the extracellular compartment.
   a. Infants—approximately ½ of the body water is contained in the cell.
   b. Adults—approximately ⅔ of the body water is contained in the cell.

3. Compared with adults, the water turnover rate per unit of body weight is 3 or more times greater in infants and small children.
   a. The child's metabolic rate is about 3 times that of an adult.
   b. The child has more body surface in relation to weight.
   c. The immaturity of kidney function in infants may impair their ability to conserve water.

4. Electrolyte balance is dependent on fluid balance and cardiovascular, renal, adrenal, pituitary, parathyroid, and pulmonary regulatory mechanisms.

5. Infants and children are more vulnerable to disorders of hydration than are adults.
   a. The basic principles relating to fluid balance in children make the magnitude of fluid losses considerably greater in children than in adults.
   b. Children are prone to severe disturbances of the gastrointestinal tract that result in diarrhea and vomiting.
   c. Young children cannot independently respond to increased losses by increased intake. They depend on others to provide them with adequate fluid.

Common Fluid and Electrolyte Abnormalities

See Table 32-3, page 1159.

General Goals of Fluid and Electrolyte Therapy

1. Repair of preexisting deficits which may occur with prolonged or severe diarrhea or vomiting.
   a. Deficits are estimated and corrected as soon and as safely as possible.
      (1) Initial therapy is aimed at restoring blood and extracellular fluid volume in order to relieve or prevent shock and restore renal function.
      (2) Intracellular deficits are replaced slowly over 8- to 12-hour period after the circulatory status is improved.

2. Provision of maintenance requirements
   a. Maintenance requirements occur as a result of normal expenditures of water and electrolytes due to metabolism.
   b. Maintenance requirements bear a close relationship to metabolic rate and are ideally formulated in terms of caloric expenditure.

3. Correction of concurrent losses which may occur via the gastrointestinal tract by vomiting, diarrhea, or drainage of secretions.

   Replacement should be similar in type and amount to the fluid being lost.

   Replacement is usually formulated as ml. of fluid and mEq. of electrolytes replaced per ml. of fluid and mEq. of electrolytes lost.

Guidelines: Intravenous Fluid Therapy

Intravenous therapy refers to the infusion of fluids directly into the venous system. This may be accomplished through the use of a needle or by venous cutdown and insertion of a small catheter directly into the vein (Fig. 32-6).

Purpose   To restore and maintain the child's fluid and electrolyte balance and body homeostasis when his oral intake is inadequate to serve this purpose.

Equipment

A. Needle Method

IV solution
   The kind of solution is specified by the physician.
   For small children, 250-ml bottles should be used for purposes of safety.
IV pole
IV administration set
   The set should include a closed reservoir with a minidropper to ensure that the child will not receive an excessive amount of fluid in a brief period of time.
Micropore filter
Syringe, 5 or 10 ml.—approximately ½–⅔ filled with normal saline
Butterfly needle or catheter of appropriate gauge
   The size of the needle depends on the age and size of the child and the type of fluid to be administered.
Alcohol sponges, dry sponges
Betadine or other antibacterial cleansing solution
Normal saline
Small tourniquet or rubber band
Hypoallergenic tape, 1.2 cm. (½ inch), 2.5 cm. (1 inch), 5 cm. (2 inches)
Padded armboard
Gauze bandage for securing the extremity to the armboard
Restraining devices—bath blanket, extremity restraint, covered sandbags

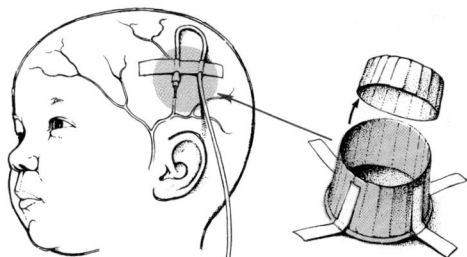

Venipuncture of scalp vein

Paper cup taped over ve-
nipuncture site for protection. A clear plastic cup
may also be used.

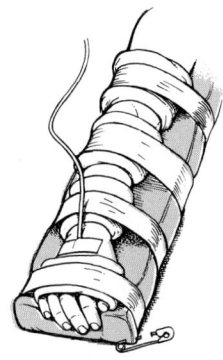

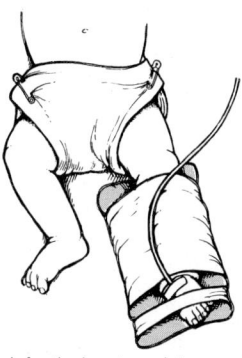

Restraint of arm when hand
is site of infusion

Infant's leg taped to sandbag for immobilization

Figure 32-6. IV fluid therapy.

Equipment
(Cont.)

The type of restraint depends on the child's age, his level of cooperation, and the kind of IV to be started.
Safety razor (if scalp vein is to be used)

B. Cutdown Method
IV solution, IV pole, IV administration set
Alcohol sponges
Hypoallergenic tape, 1.2 cm. (½ inch), 2.5 cm. (1 inch), 5 cm. (2 inches)
Padded armboard
Dry sponges
Gauze bandage
Sterile cutdown tray
  The tray should include the following equipment: medicine cups, treatment towels, wound towel, syringe, No. 1–25
  gauge 1.5-cm. (⅝-inch) needle, No. 1–20 gauge 2.5-cm. (1-inch) needle, knife handle and No. 15 blade, forceps,
  scissors, gauze sponges, 4–0 black silk suture, needle holder
Assorted sizes of sterile polyethylene tubing and Luer adapters
5–0 black silk suture with a straight eye needle
1%–2% procaine
Normal saline
Tourniquet
Sterile gloves
Restraining devices

Procedure

Nursing Action	Rationale/Amplification
Preparatory Phase	
1. Obtain the IV solution.	1. Although the type of solution and the rate of flow are prescribed by the physician, the nurse should be aware of the composition of common parenteral solutions and should know how to calculate maintenance therapy (Table 32-4).

(continued)

Guidelines: Intravenous Fluid Therapy (continued)

Table 32-4 Composition of Frequently Used Parenteral Fluids

Liquid	CHO	Prot.*	Cal/L	Na	K	Cl	HCO₃**	Ca	P†
	gm./100ml.				mEq./liter††			mg./dl.	
D₅W	5	—	170	—	—	—	—	—	—
D₁₀W	10	—	340	—	—	—	—	—	—
Normal saline (0.9% NaCl)	—	—	—	154	—	154	—	—	—
1/2 Normal saline (0.45% NaCl)	—	—	—	77	—	77	—	—	—
D5 (0.2% NaCl)	5	—	170	34	—	34	—	—	—
3% Saline.	—	—	—	513	—	513	—	—	—
8.4% Sodium Bicarbonate (1 mEq./ml.)	—	—	—	1000	—	—	1000	—	—
Ringer's	0–10	—	0–340	147	4	155.5	—	4.5	—
Ringer's lactate	0–10	—	0–340	130	4	109	28	3	—
Amino acid 8.5% (Travasol)	—	8.5	340	3	—	34	52	—	—
Plasmanate	—	5	200	110	2	50	29	—	—
Albumin 25% (salt poor)	—	25	1000	100–160	<1	<120	—	—	—
Intralipid (Cutter)§	2.25	—	1100	2.5	0.5	4.0	—	—	0.8

* Protein or amino acid equivalent
** Bicarbonate or equivalent (citrate, acetate, lactate)
† Approximate values: actual values may vary somewhat in various localities depending on electrolyte composition of water supply used to reconstitute solution
§ Values are approximate—may vary from lot to lot
(Cole H [ed]. Johns Hopkins Hospital: The Harriet Lane Handbook, 10th ed. Copyright 1984, Year Book Medical Publishers, Chicago, Used by permission.)

Procedure
(Cont.)

Nursing Action	Rationale/Amplification
2. Check the IV fluid for sediment or contaminant by holding the container up to the light.	2. Contaminant is most easily identified with the container in this position. If sediment is observed, the solution should be discarded.
3. Check the container for cracks.	3. If a flash of light can be seen through the bottle, it has a razor-thin crack and should be discarded.
4. Attach a micropore filter to the end of the infusion tubing which attaches to the needle. Use aseptic technique.	4. A 0.45-micron filter prevents entry into the vein of larger particles, air emboli, and most bacterial and fungal organisms except some pseudomonas organisms. A 0.22-micron filter prevents entry of any organisms but requires the use of an IV pump.
5. Remove the metal seal from the IV container without touching the rubber top.	5. Do not use the solution if the seal has been broken. It is not necessary to cleanse the sterile, rubber top with alcohol unless it has been accidentally contaminated.
6. Following product information, insert the end of the administration set into the container's opening. Fill the tubing with solution.	
7. Promote the cooperation of the child. a. *Infant:* provide with a pacifier. b. *Older child:* explain the procedure and its purpose.	7. The procedure will be least traumatic for the child if he is able to cooperate and is not frightened or resistant.
8. Position the child so that he is comfortable.	
9. Restrain the child as necessary. a. *Infant or young child:* restraints may include mummy wrappings, jacket or elbow restraints, or small sandbags. b. *Older child:* the extremity to be used should be comfortably restrained on the armboard. Free extremities may also require light restraints to remind the child not to move.	9. Protective devices may be necessary to prevent the child from dislodging the IV needle. The type and size of such devices should be appropriate for the child's age and the position of the IV. b. Toes and fingers should be visible to avoid compromising blood flow. The restraint board must be padded and the main pressure points (heel, palm), padded with gauze. Before strapping an extremity to the armboard, back the adhesive with tape or gauze wherever it touches the skin (see Fig. 32-6).

Performance Phase

1. Assist the physician as necessary.	1. The nurse may insert the IV.

Procedure
(Cont.)

Nursing Action

2. A simple method of applying a rubber band tourniquet is illustrated here.
   a. When applying the tourniquet, a second rubber band is placed crosswise under it.
   b. To remove the tourniquet, grasp the unstretched rubber band, pull up, and cut the tourniquet.

3. Check the restraints at intervals and adjust them as necessary.

4. Comfort and reassure the child.

5. Regulate the IV flow at the designated rate.
6. Record:
   Type of solution being used
   Reading on the container or reservoir
   Rate of flow
   Time that the infusion began
   Name of the physician or nurse who started the IV
   Site of administration
   Reaction of the child to the procedure
7. Return the child to his room.

Follow-up Phase
1. Check the child at least hourly.
   a. Note the location of the IV.
   b. Note the color of the skin at the needle point.
   c. Check for swelling of the skin at the needle point.
      (1) If in a hand or foot, compare with the opposite extremity.
      (2) If in the head, look at the face to determine asymmetry.
   d. Feel the area around the IV site for sponginess or leakage.
   e. Check for blood return into the tube when the flow of fluid is stopped.
   f. Make certain that the child is adequately restrained.

2. Observe closely for complications.
   a. *Local reactions:*
      (1) Compromised circulation
      (2) Pressure sores
      (3) Thrombophlebitis
   b. *Fluid and/or electrolyte disturbances:*
      (1) Maintain an accurate record of intake and output.
         (a) Total the intake and output every 8 hours.
         (b) Describe carefully the amount and consistency of all stools and vomitus.
         (c) Collect all urine and weigh diapers if more accurate measurement of the child's output is necessary.
      (2) Weigh the child at regular intervals, using the same scales each time.
      (3) Report:
         (a) Decreased skin turgor
         (b) Marked increase or decrease in urination
         (c) Fever

Rationale/Amplification

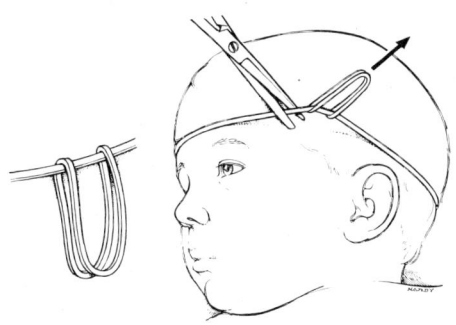

3. The restraints may become loose after a period of time and must be secured to ensure the child's safety. They may also become too tight and require loosening to maintain adequate circulation.

4. The procedure is usually disturbing for the child. This should be acknowledged. If crying and upset, the child should be reassured that his behavior is acceptable.

1. The child must be observed frequently to make certain that the IV is not infiltrating and is functioning properly. Report any swelling, discoloration, or leakage.

2. Complications associated with the administration of intravenous fluids to infants and children are very serious and may have fatal consequences. Any signs of complications must be reported immediately.

   b. Refer to Table 32-3, page 1159.

      (2) An increase or decrease of 5% within a relatively brief period of time is usually significant and should be reported.

(continued)

Guidelines: Intravenous Fluid Therapy (continued)

Procedure
(Cont.)

Nursing Action	Rationale/Amplification
(d) Sunken or bulging fontanelles in an infant	
(e) Sudden change in weight or vital signs	
(f) Diarrhea	
(g) Weakness, apathy, or lethargy	
c. Pyrogenic reactions	c. If severe, the IV should be discontinued. The solution should be saved for possible analysis.
3. Record essential information.	
a. Reading on the container or reservoir	
b. Amount of fluid absorbed in the hour	
c. Total amount of fluid absorbed (compare with the total amount of fluid intended to have been absorbed)	
d. Rate of flow	
e. Apparent condition of the child	
4. Regulate the rate of flow as necessary by any of the following methods:	
a. Raising the height of the container	
b. Adjusting the flow regulator	
c. Adjusting the position of the extremity	
d. Removing excess tubing or coiling it on the bed	d. If excess tubing falls below the level of the bed, the flow is slowed because the fluid must run uphill.
e. Adjusting the restraint	e. If an extremity is restrained too snugly, the restraint acts as a tourniquet, and the flow of solution will be slowed or stopped.
5. Irrigate the IV as necessary.	5. Irrigation may be required to dislodge small clots in the needle or to maintain the infusion rate of a sluggish IV.
a. Gather equipment:	
(1) Syringe with 1–3 ml. of normal saline solution	
(2) Several alcohol wipes	
b. Clamp off the IV solution.	
c. Disconnect the IV tubing at the needle insertion site. Keep it sterile.	
d. Remove the needle from the syringe.	
e. Connect the syringe to the tubing at the needle insertion site.	
f. Slowly inject the normal saline solution.	f. Great force of injector should be avoided because this may cause the vein to rupture or the needle to become dislodged from the vein.
g. Disconnect the syringe and reconnect the IV tubing to the needle insertion site.	
h. Unclamp the IV and regulate the flow of the solution.	
i. Check frequently to make certain that the IV is functioning properly.	
6. Change the IV container and tubing every 24 hours.	6. The IV set-up should be changed daily to maintain sterility and prevent contamination of the IV fluid during IV therapy.
7. If a catheter is used, check the dressing every tour of duty and change according to policy.	7. This reduces the incidence of infection and other local complications.
8. Disconnect the IV when prescribed or if it has obviously infiltrated	
a. Gather equipment	
(1) Scissors	
(2) 4 × 4 gauze square	
(3) Band-Aid	
b. Explain the procedure to the child, depending on his age.	
c. Clamp off the flow of the IV fluid.	
d. Determine the location of the needle.	
e. Loosen the tape around the needle, holding the needle firmly in position so that it does not slip out.	
f. Hold the 4 × 4 lightly over the insertion site and remove the needle quickly and carefully.	f. Inspect an Intracath or plastic needle to ensure that no portion has been left in the vein. If this is suspected, notify the physician. Alcohol sponges should not be used for removing IV needles because the stinging of alcohol on the puncture site causes unnecessary discomfort.
g. Apply pressure to the site immediately and hold until bleeding stops.	

Procedure
(Cont.)

Nursing Action	Rationale/Amplification
h. Apply Band-Aid.	h. The Band-Aid should not be applied until all bleeding has stopped to minimize the possibility of prolonged or unnoticed bleeding.

i. Remove the tape and armboard from the extremity.
j. Comfort the child as required.
k. Note the fluid level on the container or reservoir and complete recordings.
l. Record that the IV was discontinued.

For additional information relating to intravenous therapy, including criteria for selecting a suitable vein for venipuncture, guidelines for administering an infusion using the antecubital fossa, and complications of intravenous therapy, refer to The Patient Receiving Intravenous Therapy, pages 96–114.

Infusion Pumps

Infusion pumps are often used in pediatrics to provide a constant, slow rate of infusion. Several units are available and can be used with standard, commercial IV administration sets.

Types of Pumps

1. Peristaltic pumps—move fluid by compressing IV tubing.
2. Piston and cylinder pumps—move fluid by pushing it through a cylinder.

Indications for Use

1. When a constant rate of infusion is necessary, such as for administration of medication with a short half-life (e.g., insulin, lidocaine, catecholamines)
2. When a constant volume must be ensured per unit of time (e.g., prevention of volume overload in small infants, administration of parenteral hyperalimentation)
3. When patency of a vessel, usually an artery, must be preserved

Nursing Responsibilities

1. All nurses who operate a pump should be educated to do so correctly. Manufacturer's operating manuals and instruction sheets should be available.
2. Follow manufacturer's recommendations:
   a. In assembling equipment, initiating and maintaining infusion
   b. Before using an IV filter; some filters will blot out at infusion pump pressures, others can cause rate inaccuracies
   c. Before using a pump to infuse blood; some models can cause hemolysis
   d. In checking all parts of the pump frequently
3. Every hour, check:
   a. Delivery rate
   b. For infiltration, since many pumps will continue to infuse solution even if infiltration has occurred
4. Restart the pump promptly after it has been turned off to prevent the catheter from becoming clogged.
5. Turn off pump as soon as the infusion is completed. Failure to do so may damage some machines.
6. Be certain that the pump is tested for current leakage at least every 6 months to reduce electrical hazard.

Guidelines: Total Parenteral Nutrition (Hyperalimentation)

Hyperalimentation is a method of providing complete nutrition entirely by the intravenous route. It involves the infusion of hypertonic solutions of glucose, a nitrogen source, water, vitamins, minerals, and electrolytes at a constant rate.

Types of Hyperalimentation

1. *Central line total parenteral nutrition (TPN):* Infusion occurs through an indwelling catheter placed in a central vein, usually the superior vena cava. It is the method of choice for long-term therapy or if a high concentration of infused glucose (20–25 gm./100 ml.) is necessary.
2. *Peripheral line TPN:* Infusion occurs through a single needle set, catheter, or cutdown into a peripheral vein, usually in the scalp or extremities. It is the method of choice for intralipid infusion, but generally restricts infused glucose concentrations to 10 gm./100 ml.

Purpose   To sustain life and promote growth in patients when oral or gastrointestinal tube intake is either impossible, potentially hazardous, or insufficient for an extended period of time.

1. The procedure has been used successfully in children with gastrointestinal diseases such as chronic diarrhea, malabsorption syndrome, bowel fistulas, esophageal atresia or obstruction, and omphalocele.
2. It is also useful when a child's condition produces excessive nutritional needs, as in the case of burns, neurosurgical procedures, major trauma, large wound infections, and cancer.
3. Hyperalimentation has been successful in the treatment of premature infants of very low weights and infants with malnutrition or failure to thrive.

(continued)

Guidelines: Total Parenteral Nutrition (Hyperalimentation) (continued)

Equipment

Hyperalimentation solution:

The type, amount, and composition of the solution is prescribed by the physician.

The initial solution provides adequate daily fluid and minerals but less than optimal calories and nitrogen. The concentrations of caloric substances are increased daily over 3–5 days as the child tolerates higher glucose loads.

Micropore filter

IV extension tubing

Silastic catheter of appropriate size

Constant infusion pump

Alcohol wipes

Betadine

Benzoin

Antibacterial ointment

All of the equipment listed in the procedure for intravenous fluid therapy by cutdown method; see IV Fluid Therapy, cutdown method, page 1161.

Procedure—Central Line TPN

Nursing activities for all phases of the administration of hyperalimentation solution are the same as those specified in the procedure for intravenous fluid therapy, with the following additions:

Nursing Action	Rationale / Amplification
Preparatory Phase	
1. Prepare the child and family for the procedure.	
2. Administer preliminary medication, if prescribed.	
3. Assemble necessary equipment.	
Performance Phase	
1. Assist the physician with the insertion of the hyperalimentation catheter. This may involve obtaining equipment, positioning and restraining the child, etc.	
a. The hyperalimentation catheter should be inserted under sterile surgical conditions. It is often inserted in the operating room.	a. Violation of aseptic techniques at the time of insertion may result in overwhelming septicemia and death.
b. In infants and small children, the vena cava is usually approached through one of the common facial, internal jugular, or (usually) external jugular veins. The free end of the catheter is passed through a subcutaneous tunnel and is anchored in place at the parietal scalp (Fig. 32-7).	b. This prevents catheter displacement by the child's movements and allows asepsis to be maintained away from the child's oral and nasal secretions.
Follow-up Phase	
1. Until x-ray confirmation of the location of the catheter tip, infuse only isotonic solutions at a slow, "keep open" rate.	1. A chest x-ray confirms proper placement of the line and rules out complications such as pneumothorax or hemothorax which may be associated with catheter insertion. Infusing an isotonic solution minimizes the possibility of complications arising from the infusion of solution through a misplaced catheter.
2. Do not use the catheter for the administration of medications or for blood sampling.	2. This increases the risk of infections and the possibility of dislodging the catheter.
3. Before hanging the solution, check: a. Content label against the physician's request b. Expiration date and time c. Container for defects d. Solution for cloudiness or separation	3. Preparation of the solution should be done in the pharmacy using a closed system such as the laminar flow filtered air hood. Solutions should be prepared every 24 hours and refrigerated until used. Fat emulsions do not require refrigeration.
4. Check the infusion rate every ½–1 hour to make certain that the solution is infused continuously and at a constant rate. a. Use a constant-infusion pump. b. Reset the rate to that prescribed by the physician as necessary, but do not slow or increase the drip to make up for an excess or deficit without consulting the physician.	4. Continuous infusion is necessary to prevent such metabolic complications as osmotic diuresis, hypoglycemia, and pulmonary edema. b. Increasing the rate may cause hyperglycemia with osmotic diuresis. Slowing the rate may cause hypoglycemia.
5. Change the container, tubing, and filter at least once each day. a. Remove the tape that secures the filter to the dressing.	5. This is another attempt to prevent contamination and reduce the possibility that the child will develop infection.

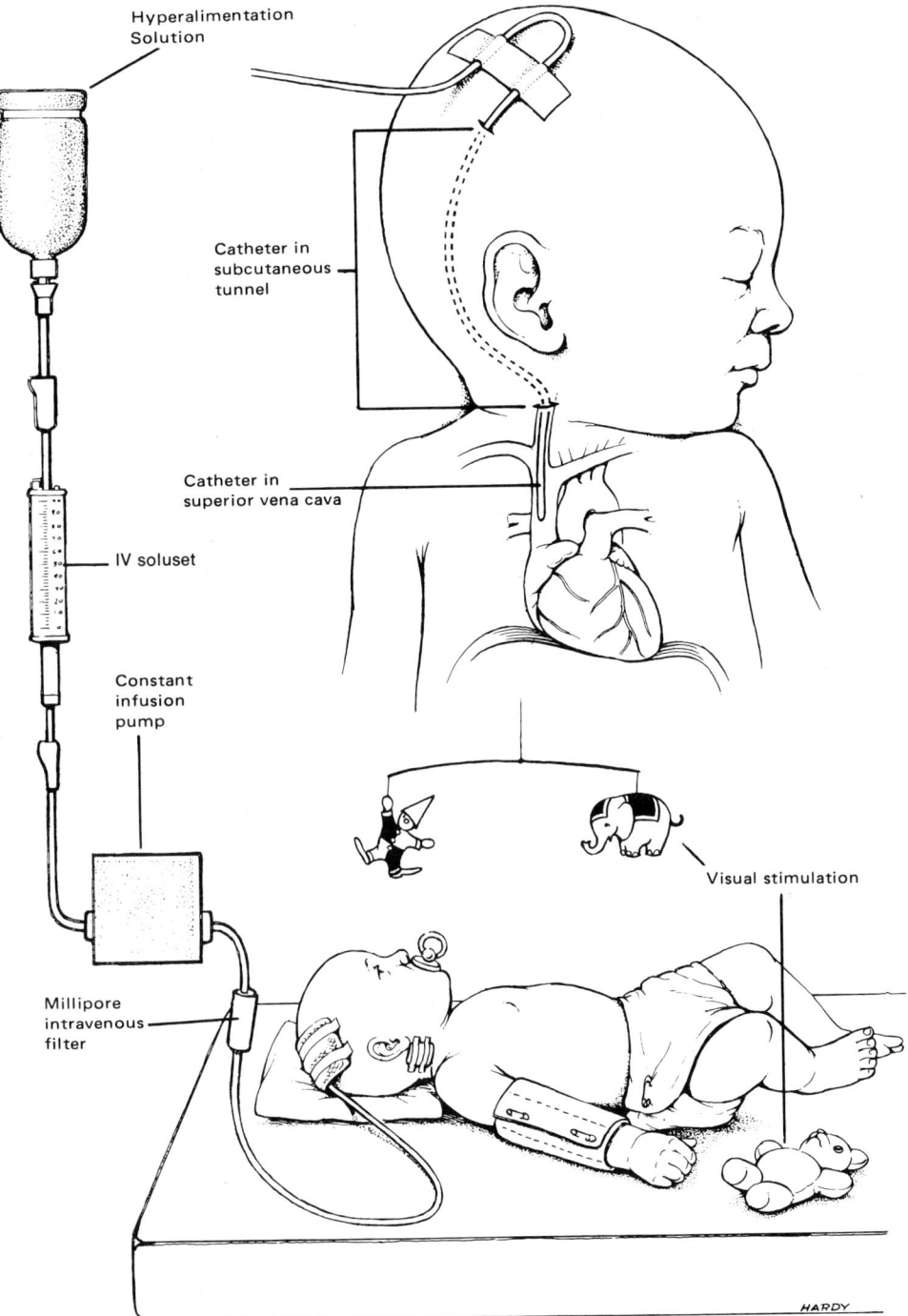

Figure 32-7. Hyperalimentation.

(continued)

Guidelines: Total Parenteral Nutrition (Hyperalimentation) (continued)

Procedure—Central Line TPN
(Cont.)

Nursing Action	Rationale/Amplification
b. Attach a new infusion set to the new container.	b. Cleanse each connecting point with Betadine.
c. Prime tubing and tap the end gently.	c. This dislodges any glucose droplets.
d. Connect the infusion set to the new filter housing carefully.	d. Avoid contamination of the filter.
e. Hang the new container on the pole.	
f. Remove the protective covering from the distal end of the filter and discard.	
g. Hold the filter parallel to the floor and run solution through the entire line.	g. This position allows for complete filling of the filter housing.
h. Gently tap the filter housing to dispel air and tap the end to free glucose droplets. Be careful not to contaminate the end of the filter.	h. Air bubbles will cause difficulty in maintaining constant flow.
i. Change the IV line at the catheter union rapidly, with the patient flat in bed or in low Fowler's position. Instruct the patient to perform Valsalva's maneuver. Use a sterile Kelly clamp to grasp the catheter hub for leverage during the tubing change.	i. This technique minimizes the danger of air embolism. Using a Kelly clamp helps reduce traction on the catheter and the chance of dislocation.
j. Anchor the filter to the dressing.	j. This prevents tension on the catheter.
k. Cleanse all connection sites with Betadine; allow to dry, and wrap with sterile 2 × 2 gauze pads.	
l. Secure all IV tubing joints with adhesive tape.	l. This prevents accidental separation of the tubing from the catheter and prevents air embolus.
m. Readjust flow rate.	
n. Write time and date on new tubing.	
o. Culture the filter each time it is changed.	o. It is possible, by culturing the filter, to detect microbial contamination prior to the development of clinical signs. Cultures should include fungal studies since a special danger of hyperalimentation is fungal septicemia.
6. Change the dressing around the catheter at least 3 times each week, using strict aseptic technique. Face masks should be worn by all persons at the head of the bed to prevent airborne contamination of the insertion site by nasopharyngeal organisms. If possible, the child should also wear a mask and turn his head away from the dressing.	6. This reduces the possibility of infection at the catheter site. The dressing should be changed immediately if it becomes soiled or wet. Most health care agencies have established policies for catheter care.
a. Remove the dressing carefully.	a. Extreme care is necessary to avoid dislodging the catheter.
b. Using an alcohol wipe, cleanse a large area surrounding the insertion site. Move in a circular motion from the center to the periphery.	b. This removes surface skin fats that might harbor organisms and removes remaining traces of adhesive tape that have adhered to the skin.
c. Paint the skin with Betadine solution and allow to dry.	
d. Apply a prescribed antibacterial ointment directly to the catheter insertion site and 2–3 cm. down the catheter.	
e. Apply a small dressing around the catheter. Using sterile scissors, cut a slit in the lower piece of a 3 × 3 gauze sponge. Slide it under the catheter to cover insertion site and hub only. Fold sponge over catheter.	e. Transparent dressings may be used in place of the gauze and tape dressing.
f. Apply benzoin to the area where tape will be applied. Allow to dry.	f. Even nonirritating tape may produce damage to the underlying skin with prolonged use.
g. Secure dressing with porous tape.	g. A waterproof dressing should be used if it is exposed to moisture such as tracheal secretions or humidified oxygen.
h. Tape looped tubing to the skin.	h. This prevents tension on the catheter.
i. Label dressing with date, time, and initials.	
j. Record the dressing change, how the child tolerated the procedure, and any relevant condition.	j. Consider condition of the skin, drainage, catheter placement, placement of needle guard, and presence of suture.

Procedure—Central Line TPN
(Cont.)

Nursing Action	Rationale / Amplification
7. In infants with a cutdown site on the neck, change the dressing as needed, using aseptic technique. Discontinue the dressing when the wound is healed.	7. Since this site is closest to the vascular bed, it should be observed closely for signs of infection. Wound sepsis can easily lead to bacteremia.
8. Monitor fractional urine specimens for glucose, acetone, pH, blood, protein, and specific gravity every 2–8 hours.	8. Some children require supplemental parenteral insulin to utilize the required amount of infused glucose. Children receiving certain drugs may show false-positive results. Positive urine sugars are confirmed by blood glucose levels.
9. Keep an accurate record of the child's total intake and output, including bowel movements, emesis, and gastric drainage. If the child is allowed oral intake, a calorie count should be kept.	9. This helps to provide a clear picture of the child's fluid and electrolyte balance.
10. Monitor the child's weight daily. Weigh at the same time each day, with the same amount of clothing, and on the same scales.	10. Weight gain is one of the most reliable indications of a positive response to therapy.
11. In infants, measure length and head circumference weekly.	11. Hyperalimentation promotes growth in these dimensions.

12. Observe for signs of complications resulting from therapy.
  a. Complications related to the catheter
    (1) Septicemia
    (2) Thrombosis of a major blood vessel
    (3) Plugging or dislodging of the catheter
    (4) Local skin infection
    (5) Cardiac arrhythmia
    (6) Leak around catheter or hole in catheter
    (7) Air embolism
  b. Metabolic complications
    (1) Hyperglycemia
    (2) Hypoglycemia
    (3) Dehydration
    (4) Metabolic acidosis
    (5) Electrolyte imbalances
    (6) Amino acid imbalance
    (7) Postinfusion hypoglycemia
	12.
	  a. Three fourths of the major complications of therapy are of this variety. Sepsis accounts for more than half of these problems.
	
	  b. Careful clinical and chemical monitoring, especially during the initial period of hyperalimentation, can greatly reduce the incidence of these types of complications.

13. Provide mouth care.
  a. If allowed, use a variety of mouthwashes to provide some change in taste.
  b. Apply lip balm flavored with fruit or mint.
  c. Offer crushed ice flavored with juice or syrup.
	13. In patients who are NPO, the tongue, throat, and mouth tend to become dry, inflamed and uncomfortable. The total absence of taste is unpleasant for older children.

14. Provide the infant with a pacifier.	14. It is especially important to meet the sucking needs of the infant since hyperalimentation therapy may be necessary for several weeks or months.

15. Discontinue the infusion when directed to do so by the physician. (In many hospitals this is the responsibility of the physician.)
  a. Turn the flow rate off.
  b. Remove the dressings.
  c. Cut and remove the stay suture.
  d. Pull the catheter out.
  e. Apply pressure with a sterile 4 × 4 gauze for 5–10 minutes.
  f. Cleanse the site with Betadine and apply a sterile dressing.
  g. Record time and date procedure was discontinued, by whom, cultures sent, and child's condition.
  h. Send the tip of the catheter, the filter, and the fluid in the tubing to the laboratory for culture.
	15. The child is gradually tapered off from hyperalimentation to allow for adjustment to decreased levels of glucose. Final cessation is often followed by isotonic glucose infusion for at least 12 hours to protect against rebound hypoglycemia from still high insulin levels. During the weaning process, the child's oral intake is gradually increased as the hyperalimentation solution is proportionally decreased.

Procedure—Peripheral Line TPN

Nursing activities are essentially the same as for central line TPN although dressing changes are not indicated. However, peripheral sites should be checked and cared for at regular intervals to avoid infiltration and vascular inflammation. For additional information, refer to the following procedure for the administration of intralipids.

Guidelines: Intralipids—Intravenous Fat Emulsion

(See adult, p. 430.)

Purpose Used in conjunction with partial parenteral (peripheral) nutrition (PPN) as an additional source of calories and essential fatty acids.

Equipment

*Intralipid 10% fat emulsion—isotonic emulsion composed of 10% soybean oil (a triglyceride), 1.2% egg yolk phospholipids, 2.2% glycerin and water for injection. Total caloric value is 1.1 calorie/ml. Intralipid 10%.

Antiseptic wipe	Complete infusion IV line	Tape
IV tubing and sterile needle	Constant infusion pump	

Procedure

Nursing activities for the administration of Intralipid 10% are the same as those specified in the procedure for intravenous fluid therapy and total parenteral nutrition, with the following exceptions.

Nursing Action	Rationale/Amplification
Preparatory Phase	
1. Prior to therapeutic administration of Intralipid 10%, a test dose of 0.1 ml./minute (10 mg.) is given in 10–15 minutes; afterwards, the rate is increased to permit 1 gm./kg. to run over 4 hours.	1. To identify any sensitivity the child may have to the emulsion.
a. Observe for immediate reactions of dyspnea, flushing, rash, sweating, sleepiness, headache, tachycardia, bradycardia, acidosis in infants.	▶ **NURSING ALERT:** Treatment of premature and low-birth-weight infants with IV fat emulsions must be based on careful evaluation of the potential benefits weighed against the potential risks of fat accumulation in the lungs.†
b. Should any of these signs appear, stop infusion and notify physician.	
2. Ensure that prescribed laboratory studies are done prior to commencement of test dose (i.e., cholesterol, triglycerides, platelets). Once testing has been accomplished, Intralipid 10% is administered as part of PPN, 1–4 gm./kg./24 hours based on age and size of the child.	2. To serve as baseline before test dose.
3. Ensure that nothing is added to emulsion (i.e., drugs, electrolytes, vitamins, or other nutrients).	3. May cause lipid to separate or cause a fat embolus.
4. Be aware of conditions that may contraindicate the use of Intralipid 10%—sepsis, hyperbilirubinemia, severe respiratory distress.	4. Prevents further compromise of the child: fat is taken up by the reticuloendothelial system; it displaces bilirubin from albumin and can plug small vessels in the lungs.
Performance Phase	
1. Once the IV lines have been purged with the emulsion, connect the line to the existing peripheral or central line via piggyback or Y-connector just proximal to the infusion site. Tape connection. Do not pass solution through a bacterial filter because this can clog filter and break down emulsion. Peripheral line administration can be used.	1. Infuse emulsion as a separate line that is added into the existing IV. The emulsion is administered in the self-contained solution container from manufacturer, syringe, and tubing or pediatric infusion set. The emulsion is not added to the TPN solution bottle to avoid disturbing the stability of the emulsion. It is administered with another fluid to decrease the high concentration of fat. (Intralipid is isotonic.)
2. Administer emulsion using separate continuous flow pump from that of PPN. (Pumps with electric eye may not be effective because of the opaque solution.)	2. Allows flow rate of each solution to be controlled independently.
3. Monitor hourly the amount of emulsion infused.	3. To control fluid intake. Emulsion can be infused continuously or in 4–5 separate doses over 2- to 6-hour time periods.
4. Change bottle and tubing:	4. To assist in preventing infection.
a. Intermittent administration—each administration	
b. Continuous administration—every 8 hours	
Follow-up Phase	
1. Once prescribed emulsion has been infused, discontinue. Flush line with normal saline solution. Check to be sure there is no leaking at point where connection was made.	1. To prevent infection and inaccurate account of fluid intake as a result of the line being violated. Prevents coagulation of Intralipid in IV line.
2. Record time procedure was discontinued, by whom, amount given, and the child's condition.	

* Cutter Laboratories
† Levene MI, Wigglesworth JS and Desai R. Pulmonary fat accumulation after intralipid infusion in preterm infant. Lancet 1980 Oct 18; 2(8199):815–818

Procedure (Cont.)	Nursing Action	Rationale/Amplification
	3. Ensure that prescribed laboratory studies are done at designated times—usually 2–6 hours after emulsion is discontinued or weekly (i.e., lipid and triglyceride levels).	3. To see if fat has been metabolized and utilized and to detect any early signs of complications.
	4. Continue to observe the child for any delayed adverse reactions: hepatomegaly, splenomegaly, thrombocytopenia, transient increase in liver function tests, system overload.	4. To detect any early signs of complications in addition to physical assessment of the child, serum studies may include liver function, bilirubin, alkaline phosphatase, CBC or platelet count.

Pediatric Home Hyperalimentation

Home hyperalimentation programs have been developed to provide an alternative to hospitalization for children who require long-term TPN.

Benefits of Home Hyperalimentation
1. The child is able to maintain a more normal lifestyle in his home environment.
2. Stress is reduced for the child and his family.
3. Cost is greatly reduced.

Resources Necessary for an Effective Program
1. A pharmacy to prepare the solution
2. A physician available to deal with problems
3. A reliable microchemistry laboratory
4. Someone to deal with equipment procurement, maintenance, and problems
5. An insurance agency willing to cooperate with such a program
6. Effective community health nursing support

Criteria for Determining Family Readiness and Ability to Cope with Home TPN
1. Does the family comfortably participate in the technical procedures in the hospital?
2. Do the parents state a desire to perform the TPN procedure in the home?
3. Do the parents respond to cues from the child and deal with them appropriately?
4. Do the parents interact effectively with the child by providing nurturing care and comfort measures, which they will have to continue at home?
5. Do parents have support from the nuclear and extended family in conducting home TPN?
6. Are community support systems available?

Health Education
1. Explain the principles and concepts of TPN.
2. Instruct the parents concerning the methods, procedures, and prevention of complications of TPN administration.
3. Demontrate TPN procedures to the parents.
4. Have parents demonstrate their ability to perform TPN procedures.
5. Encourage parents to carry out complete management of TPN until the child is discharged.
6. Provide means for continued education and problem solving during home TPN.
7. Evaluate treatment and follow-up.

Guidelines: Assisting with Exchange Transfusion

Exchange transfusion is replacement of circulating blood by withdrawing blood and injecting donor's blood in equal amounts.

Purposes
1. To prevent accumulation of bilirubin in the blood above a dangerous level.
2. To prevent kernicterus (brain damage—occurs when there is yellow staining of brain tissue from deposits of indirect bilirubin).
3. To prevent accumulation of other by-products of hemolysis from hemolytic disease (i.e., ABO incompatibility).
4. To raise a very low hemoglobin.
5. To replace red blood cells which have poor oxygen-releasing capacity and poor carbonic anhydrase activity (i.e., as in a premature infant).
6. To remove toxic metabolites.
7. To treat irreversible acidosis, overwhelming neonatal septicemia, DIC.

Equipment

Fresh donor blood—with hematocrit 50% ± 5%
Monitoring equipment
Sterile disposable exchange transfusion set containing:
    Stopcock with extension tubing
    Extra extension tubing
    Umbilical catheters sizes No. 5 and 8, French
    2 20-ml. syringes
    1 5-ml. syringe and No. 23 gauge needle

Gauze sponges
Transfusion record
Cleansing solution
Means of warming infant
Means of warming blood
Calcium gluconate in 5-ml. syringe
50% glucose solution in 10-ml. syringe
Sodium bicarbonate in 10-ml. syringe

(continued)

Guidelines: Assisting with Exchange Transfusion (continued)

Equipment
(Cont.)

Waste-blood container
Blood administration set

Sterile gown and gloves for physician
Resuscitative equipment

General Considerations

1. Volume of blood given is 160–180 ml./kg. infant weight (2-volume exchange, replacing approximately 85% of the infant's blood).
2. The infant's blood volume is 80–90 ml./kg. body weight
3. Blood type used:
   Rh sensitivity = Rh-negative blood used (typed and cross-matched to mother's serum).
   ABO disease—group O blood used.

Procedure

Nursing Action	Rationale/Amplification
Preparatory Phase	
1. Place the infant under heat lamps or radiant heating unit to keep his temperature within the thermoneutral zone. Environment temperature of 32°C. (86°F.) will usually maintain correct infant body temperature, depending on size of infant.	1. Chilling of the infant during the procedure can result in apnea and in increased caloric need and oxygen consumption, which can be exhausting to a baby with already limited amount of energy. Abnormal decrease in blood pH leading to acidosis can result from the stress of prolonged chilling. Hypothermia may also hinder albumin and bilirubin binding capacity. Hyperthermia may cause destruction of erythrocytes of donor blood.
2. If the infant has not been NPO for 3–4 hours, it may be necessary to empty stomach contents via stomach tube.	2. To prevent aspiration, should vomiting occur during the procedure.
3. Albumin (1 gm./kg.) may be given 1–2 hours prior to exchange transfusion.	3. The albumin may increase the effectiveness of the transfusion by yielding more bilirubin binding sites.
4. Attach electronic cardiac monitoring device to infant if available. Otherwise place stethoscope over apex of heart. Also attach temperature-monitoring device. Monitor continuously.	4. Apnea, bradycardia, and cardiac arrest are complications of an exchange transfusion. Close monitoring will allow for immediate observation of signs of trouble.
5. Place infant on his back. Restrain all 4 extremities.	5. This will prevent the infant from moving and inadvertently pulling out the exchange catheter.
6. Have resuscitative equipment ready for immediate use: oxygen supply, mask, intubation equipment, laryngoscope, breathing bag, suction, sodium bicarbonate, and 50% glucose solution.	6. Should the infant develop bradycardia, hypoglycemia, or cyanosis during procedure, these items will be necessary for immediate and supportive treatment.
7. Check donor blood for type, age, and other identifying data. Check blood pH. It should be corrected to pH 7.1 or as specified by physician.	7. Heparinized blood must be used within 24 hours of collection. Optimal age of ACD (heparin, acid–citrate–dextrose) or CPD (citrate–phosphate–dextrose) blood is less than 3 days old. CPD lasts longer—has better carbonic anhydrase level. Acidemia may result when fresh blood is not used because of the acid metabolites. Cardiac arrest may also occur from elevated potassium in donor blood.
8. Assist the physician in setting up blood and exchange equipment. Blood should be run through a coil of tubing through a water bath at 38°C., (100°F.). Ensure that lines and connections are securely closed.	8. Although hypothermia (i.e., rapid chilling of the infant) is a primary concern, increased blood viscosity and ventricular fibrillation can also result from administering cold blood.
Performance Phase	
1. The infant's skin is cleansed with soap and water followed by an antiseptic solution. Sterile drapes are applied by the physician who is gowned and gloved. Strict attention should be paid to maintaining aseptic technique.	1. To prevent infection or sepsis. A foreign body introduced into the blood vessel is always a potential for infection due to an infected cord stump or contaminated equipment. The umbilicus can be grossly contaminated and is impossible to sterilize.
2. Once the umbilical catheter is in place in the umbilical vein, the initial venous pressure is measured (although it is not usually accurate) and the exchange is begun. (Preferred site is the umbilical vein; jugular or femoral vessels may be used.)	2. Record the venous pressure. This will be maintained at about 10–12 cm. by equal volume exchanges. An increase in pressure during the procedure is an indication to stop and assess the infant.
3. Note and record the time the exchange started. Record each successive withdrawal and infusion of blood stating exact amount and time. Report to the physician when each 100 ml. of blood is exchanged (see Record Chart, p. 1173).	3. Blood is exchanged slowly in amounts of 5–20 ml., depending on the infant's size and condition. The total amount exchanged is about 170 ml. of blood/kilogram of body weight (80 ml./pound). About 75%–93% of the infant's total blood volume is exchanged.

EXCHANGE TRANSFUSION RECORD

HOSPITAL NO. _____

NAME OF BABY: *Johnson, Clarence David*

NAME OF MOTHER: *Marsha Johnson*

BIRTH WEIGHT: *3580 grams*

BLOOD GROUP: *O neg.*

TIME COMMENCING EXCHANGE: *3:45 pm*

TIME FINISHING EXCHANGE: *4:17 pm*

DATE OF DELIVERY: *8-29-86*

TIME: *4:10 am*

APGAR SCORE AT DELIVERY: *8 at 1 min* / *9 at 5 min*

INITIAL HEMOGLOBIN: *42*

BILIRUBIN: *16.3*

POST-EXCHANGE BILIRUBIN: *11.8*

AGE OF BABY IN HOURS: *30*

TIME	OUT Amount	OUT Total	IN Amount	IN Total	PULSE	RESPI-RATION	VENOUS PRESSURE	MEDI-CATION	COMMENTS
3:45	20	20	20	20			10 cm		
3:48	20	40	20	40					
3:51	20	60	20	60					
3:55	20	80	20	80					
3:58	20	100	20	100	150	48		Ca 1ml	
4:02	20	120	20	120			10 cm		
4:06	20	140	20	140					
4:10	20	160	20	160					
4:13	20	180	20	180					
4:17	20	200	20	200	160	56			

Procedure
(Cont.)

Nursing Action

This will prevent system overload from excessive infusion—resulting in cardiac failure and shock from too-rapid removal of infant's blood.

4. After each 100 ml. of blood is exchanged, 0.5–1.0 ml./kg. 10% calcium gluconate may be injected to prevent hypocalcemia. Blood-bank donor blood is calcium-defi-

Rationale/Amplification

The exchange should take about an hour. Rapid exchange can aggravate cardiovascular changes and prevent normal metabolism of infused acid and citrate.

4. Calcium decreases the irritability and irregularity of the heart. Too rapid an injection will cause bradycardia. Especially important when CPD donor blood is used.

(continued)

Guidelines: Assisting with Exchange Transfusion (continued)

Procedure
(Cont.)

Nursing Action	Rationale/Amplification
cient. Monitor cardiac rate very carefully during the injection.	
5. Constant monitoring of the cardiac rate is imperative. Also note respirations, skin color, and color of withdrawn blood. Keep transfusion lines tightly secured to prevent air embolus or exsanguination.	5. Observation and monitoring will allow immediate treatment if untoward signs appear. Bradycardia may occur at any time during the procedure due to a low pH of donor blood or old blood.
6. Protamine sulfate may be given after the transfusion is completed.	6. Because heparinized blood will affect the coagulation potential of the infant from 4–6 hours postexchange.

Follow-up Phase

Nursing Action	Rationale/Amplification

1. When transfusion is completed, umbilical catheter may be:
  a. Left in place with an IV plug or intravenous infusion or
  b. Removed
	1a. If catheter is left in place, it is usually done for future exchange transfusions, easy withdrawal of blood for blood studies, administration of intravenous fluids and medications. Keep infant restrained.
	1b. If catheter is removed, apply small pressure dressing and observe for any bleeding. Check the area every hour for 3 hours, then every 3 hours for 24 hours.

2. Record:
  a. Time transfusion was completed
  b. Total amount blood withdrawn and infused
  c. Any changes in vital signs
  d. Medications administered during exchange
  e. Infant's color and current vital signs
  f. Catheter removed or left indwelling
  g. How infant tolerated the procedure
  h. Any blood samples taken before or after exchange	

3. Monitor infant for any signs of post-exchange transfusion complications: a. Hypoglycemia—Dextrostix test every hour × 4	a. Hypoglycemia frequently occurs with erythroblastosis fetalis. Incidence is also increased because of fasting prior to and during procedure.
b. Hemolytic reaction	b. Reaction from donor blood.
c. Thrombocytopenia and hemorrhage—check for bleeding at catheter site and petechiae.	c. This results from overheparinized blood or when citrated blood is given without calcium replacement.
d. Intestinal perforation—observe for bloody stools, bile-stained vomitus, abdominal distention, respiratory distress, pallor.	d. Ischemia of bowel.
e. Metabolic acidosis—observe for deep, increased respirations; decreased consciousness; acid urine.	e. Resulting from old donor blood.
f. Hyperkalemia	f. From donor blood

The Child Undergoing Dialysis

Dialysis refers to the process of separating substances in solution by movement through a semipermeable membrane.

Purpose

To preserve life by acting as a substitute for kidney function during renal failure.
1. Aids in the removal of toxic substances and metabolic wastes.
2. Removes excessive body fluid.
3. Assists in regulating the body's fluid and electrolyte balance.

Types of Dialysis

A. Peritoneal Dialysis
1. Mechanism
  a. The peritoneal lining is used as the semipermeable membrane.
  b. A catheter is inserted through the anterior abdominal wall, and the dialysate is instilled into the abdominal cavity.
  c. After an equilibration time (about 30 minutes), the fluid is drained by gravity and fresh dialysate is instilled.
2. Major uses
  a. Acute, reversible uremic episodes such as those due to sudden illness, trauma, poisoning, or drug intoxication.
  b. In terminal illness, to keep the child comfortable for as long as possible.
  c. Prior to acceptance in a long-term hemodialysis and transplantation program.
  d. In selected cases of chronic renal failure.
    (1) The child may be dialyzed at night through a semi-permanently implanted abdominal cannula by an automatic, continually recycling machine.

(2) Continuous ambulatory peritoneal dialysis, (see p. 522) has been used successfully by many children.

3. Advantage

Relatively safe and readily available.

4. Disadvantages
   a. Long periods of time required to effectively remove waste products.
   b. May cause abdominal pain and discomfort.
   c. Sterile dialysate is required.
   d. Complications
      (1) Peritonitis
      (2) Bowel perforation during insertion of the catheter
      (3) Respiratory distress caused by upward displacement of the diaphragm by fluid in the peritoneal cavity
      (4) Shock due to excessive fluid loss
      (5) Protein loss because serum proteins pass through the peritoneal membrane during dialysis
      (6) Bleeding and leakage at the catheter insertion site
      (7) Inadequate fluid return
      (8) Nausea, vomiting, diarrhea

B. Hemodialysis

1. Mechanism
   a. The semipermeable membrane is located in a machine through which the child's blood is directed.
   b. Access to the circulation is provided via a Teflon–Silastic arteriovenous shunt or a subcutaneously implanted arteriovenous fistula.
   c. The child's blood is diverted through the machine adjacent to the semipermeable membrane to equilibrate with dialysate on the other side of the membrane.

d. Selection of the dialyzer depends on the size of the child. Considerations include:
   (1) Amount of blood the machine holds relative to the amount that the child can safely spare from the body at one time.
   (2) Efficiency of the machine relative to the child's weight.
   (3) Speed with which fluid can be removed by the machine.

Note: Dialysis can be dangerous if it is too rapid.

2. Major uses
   a. Long-term therapy for chronic renal failure.
   b. Holding procedure prior to kidney transplant.
3. Advantages
   a. Shorter period of time required to effectively remove waste products.
   b. Does not require sterile dialysate.
   c. Is less traumatic to initiate once access to the circulation is made.
   d. Home dialysis is available in selected situations.
4. Disadvantages
   a. It is costly.
   b. There are inherent moral, legal, logistical, and technical problems.
   c. Complications
      (1) Clotting, infection, accidental separation of shunt
      (2) Anemia—because a small amount of blood remains behind in the machine with each run
      (3) Malaise, headache, nausea, and vomiting during dialysis
      (4) Hepatitis due to transfusions necessitated by uremic anemia
      (5) Seizures—possibly related to large changes in sodium osmolarity.

Guidelines: Caring for the Child Undergoing Dialysis

Nursing Care

Nursing Action	Rationale/Amplification
1. Prepare the child for the procedure.	1. Dialysis is threatening to most children and may evoke fears of pain, mutilation, immobilization, helplessness, and dependency. Many children have fears of losing all of their blood in this process. A child who is well-prepared will be less frightened and better able to cooperate during the procedure.

a. Explain the procedure to the child in terms that he can understand.
     (1) Allow the child to handle equipment similar to that which will be used during dialysis.
     (2) Encourage the child to express his fears so that misinterpretations can be corrected.
     (3) Provide simple pictures and diagrams, if appropriate.
     (4) Allow the child to talk with peers who have undergone dialysis.
   b. Explain the procedure to the family and answer questions so that they will be in the best position to support their child.	

2. Protect the child from infection.
   a. Keep the dressings and area around the catheter or shunt clean and dry.
   b. Use aseptic technique throughout the dialysis procedure.
   c. Avoid exposure to children or adults with infection.
	2. These children are prone to infection because of their general debilitated state and because of protein loss and anemia.

(continued)

Guidelines: Caring for the Child Undergoing Dialysis (continued)

Nursing Care
(Cont.)

Nursing Action	Rationale/Amplification
d. Provide supplemental vitamins since a protein-restricted diet is poor in vitamins. e. Provide meticulous daily hygiene.	
3. Provide a high calorie diet which is low in sodium, potassium, and protein. Restrict fluids. Since the child often experiences anorexia, it may be helpful to allow him to choose foods from his allowances and offer small, frequent meals.	3. Fluids and sodium are restricted to prevent fluid overload. Potassium is limited to prevent complications related to hyperkalemia. Protein restriction reduces elevated BUN. The child may see dietary restrictions as punishment and must be helped to realize the purpose of the restrictions.
4. Maintain careful records of intake and output, vital signs, blood pressure, and daily weights.	4. These provide valuable information about the effectiveness of the therapy.

Procedure

Nursing Action	Rationale/Amplification

5. Support the child during the dialysis procedure.
  a. Provide symptomatic relief of nausea, vomiting, malaise, or headache.
    Notify the physician if these symptoms are severe.
  b. Be alert to clues from the child for helpful methods of offering support.
    (1) Young children often cling to stuffed toys or blankets or depend on parent's presence at the bedside.
    (2) Older children may benefit from radio, television, magazines, or contact with peers.	

6. Provide an environment that is as normal as possible.
  a. Encourage the family to bring in articles that will make the child's room appear more home-like (i.e., pictures, posters, etc.).
  b. Encourage the child to be as independent as possible in his daily care.
  c. Provide for age-appropriate recreation and/or diversion.
  d. Help the child to keep up with his school work by initiating a referral to a tutor, providing study times, etc.
	6. Although life is preserved, it is by no means normal during the time on dialysis or between dialyses. These measures may increase the child's feeling of self-esteem and diminish regression and social isolation. By serving as role models, health professionals may encourage parents to recognize and foster the normal, healthy aspects of the child's daily life.

7. Offer appropriate support to the family.
  a. Provide opportunity for family members to discuss their feelings, fears, and frustrations and to ask questions.
  b. Allow family members to become involved in the child's care to the extent that they wish and that is helpful for the child and family.
  c. Provide for continuity of personnel.
  d. Initiate appropriate referrals. These may include referrals to a social worker, psychiatrist, dietitian, community health agency, other families who are coping with dialysis.
	7. Families often need extensive support from many health professionals to cope with the physical, psychological, financial, and logistical aspects of renal failure and dialysis. Attention must be focused on siblings as well as parents since sibling relationships are often strained and difficult.

8. Teach the child and family about all of the important aspects of renal failure and dialysis, including:
  a. Signs and symptoms of uremia
  b. Shunt care and protection
  c. Protection from infection
  d. Dietary restrictions and recommendations; ways of incorporating the special diet into the family meal plan
  e. Dialysis schedule
  f. Medications
  g. Emergency procedures
	8. The family should be prepared to care for the child at home well before the day of discharge. Learning about the child's care also helps restore some sense of control in a frightening situation.

Peritoneal Dialysis: Specific Nursing Responsibilities

Refer to Guidelines: Assisting the Patient Undergoing Peritoneal Dialysis, page 519. In addition, the following principles should be considered by the nurse working with pediatric patients.

1. Because of the child's smaller size, the volume of dialysate required is less.

Peritoneal Dialysis: Specific Nursing Responsibilities
(Cont.)

2. Because the child may be unable to hold still, it may be necessary to apply protective measures to limit motion in order to avoid contamination of the sterile field or injury to the child (see p. 1142).
3. Because of the possibility of nausea and vomiting, oral intake should be limited to ice chips and small amounts of fluids during the first 12–24 hours of dialysis. Frequent mouth care should be provided.
4. Because the child may develop fears and fantasies about the equipment, it should be stored out of sight when not in use.

Hemodialysis: Specific Nursing Responsibilities

1. Care for the arteriovenous shunt (refer to Guidelines, below).
2. Assist in teaching the child and/or family proper care and protection of the shunt.
3. When possible, avoid giving subcutaneous or intramuscular injections because the child is anticoagulated with heparin at least twice weekly during dialysis, and extensive bleeding could occur as a result of such injections.
4. Care for the child during dialysis. (This aspect of nursing care is not presented since it is generally provided by specially trained personnel in a dialysis unit.)

Guidelines: Care of the Arteriovenous Shunt

Purpose   To preserve shunt function and prevent separation of the cannulas.

Equipment

2 shunt clips
Dressing tray with:
  2 sterile plastic basins
  Sterile 2 × 2-inch sponges
  Sterile 4 × 3-inch sponges
  Kling bandage
  Hydrogen peroxide
  Betadine
  Normal saline solution
  Sterile applicators
  Sterile scissors
  Mask
  Sterile gloves

Procedure

Nursing Action	Rationale/Amplification
1. Place shunt clips on the dressing and keep with the child at all times.	1. The clamps are used to close the shunt in case it separates at its connection.
2. Use another extremity for:	2. Disturbing the shunt in any way can encourage clotting and infection.
a. Taking blood pressure	a. Inflation of blood pressure cuff may precipitate clotting by slowing the flow of blood through the tubing.
b. Giving medications c. Giving infusions	b. c. Injections in the extremity increase the possibility of thrombosis of the vein.
d. Taking blood samples	d. A rubber puncture site may be added to the shunt. This can be punctured with a needle to obtain blood specimens.

NOTE: The silastic tubing should never be punctured since it will not seal.

3. Cleanse the area around the shunt and change the dressing with each dialysis treatment, or p.r.n.	
a. Remove old dressing.	a. Never use scissors to remove the dressing to avoid accidentally cutting the cannulas.
b. Observe the shunt for malalignment or kinks.	b. These factors increase the possibility of clot formation and must be corrected.
c. Observe the area around the cannula insertion sites for signs of inflammation (redness, swelling, drainage).	c. If noted, report signs of inflammation, and take culture before cleansing the area.
d. Using aseptic technique, clean the venous insertion site first with hydrogen peroxide and then with Betadine. Take new swabs and clean the arterial site in the same manner.	d. Do not use the same swabs to clean both sites as this may cause cross-infection. When cleaning, begin at the insertion site and move outward in a circular motion.

(continued)

Guidelines: Care of the Arteriovenous Shunt (continued)

Procedure
(Cont.)

Nursing Action	Rationale / Amplification
e. Allow to dry. Rinse well with normal saline solution and dry with a sterile 4 × 4 gauze pad.	e. Avoid leaving Betadine on the cannula because this could make connections slippery.
f. Apply dry, sterile dressing to the areas of cannula insertion.	f. A 2 × 2 gauze pad under the cannula at each insertion site will lessen tension at the site and increase comfort.
g. Wrap arm with compression bandage firmly, but not tightly, leaving a small section of the shunt in view.	g. Leave a section small enough that it cannot be pulled out by the child. If protective devices to limit movement are indicated, apply below the shunt.
h. Retape shunt clips to outer dressing in full view.	
4. Check frequently for shunt obstruction.	
a. Use stethoscope or place fingertips on area between cannula insertion points to detect bruit.	a. Presence of bruit indicates free flow of blood through shunt.
b. Observe child for signs of pain in the extremity.	
c. Observe color of blood in tubing.	c. Blood should appear smooth and should be of uniform color. Fibrin may appear as white specks along the cannula wall.
d. Report clotting immediately to the physician.	d. Clotting is indicated by separation of blood (i.e., presence of a darkened clot and clear serum). The shunt feels cool rather than warm to the touch. Delay in declotting may necessitate replacement of the entire shunt.
5. Be prepared for emergency action if the shunt should separate or the cannula should become dislodged.	5. These are emergency situations which may result in severe hemorrhage and possible exsanguination.
a. Identify source of bleeding by unwrapping bandage.	
b. Separation of shunt;	
(1) Clamp tubes with shunt clips and rejoin shunt— or	
(2) Pinch off tubes with fingers and rejoin shunt.	
c. Dislodgment of arterial or venous cannula:	
(1) Apply firm pressure over bleeding cannula site and clamp remaining cannula.	
(2) Notify physician.	
6. Teach the child and parents how to care for the shunt.	
a. Dressing changes and cleansing of area around shunt.	
b. Observation for signs of inflammation, infection, obstruction.	
c. Bathing	c. These activities are allowed at the discretion of the individual physician.
(1) Some children are permitted to bathe the shunted extremity, soaping the area at the beginning and at the end of the shower or bath.	
(2) Swimming may be permitted if the extremity is completely protected with a waterproof covering.	
d. Prevention of clotting	
(1) Avoid constricting clothing which may impair blood flow through the shunt.	
(2) Avoid keeping the extremity acutely flexed for long periods of time.	
(3) Avoid sleeping on the shunted arm.	
e. Emergency measures in case of accidental separation or dislodging of the cannula.	

Chest Physical Therapy and Respiratory Measures

Guidelines: Promoting Postural Drainage in the Pediatric Patient

Postural drainage is the positioning of the patient so that gravity will assist in the movement of secretions from the smaller bronchial airways to the main bronchus and trachea, from which the secretions can be removed by coughing or suctioning.

Procedure

Nursing Action	Rationale / Amplification

Preparatory Phase

1. Assess the child's respiratory status.
   a. Obtain a baseline respiratory rate.
   b. Observe for respiratory distress, retractions, nasal flaring, etc.
2. Identify the involved portion(s) of the lung by auscultation, percussion, and/or examination of the x-ray report.
3. Explain the procedure to the child and/or the parent.

4. Make the child comfortable.
   a. Remove constricting clothes.
   b. Flex the child's knees and hips.

   c. Have tissues and an emesis basin available.
   d. Have several pillows available.
5. Provide bronchodilator and/or nebulization therapy if indicated.

1. This is necessary in order to evaluate the effectiveness of the therapy.

2. The positions selected for drainage will depend on what portion of the lung is involved.
3. This allays anxiety and helps to secure the child's cooperation.

   b. To assist in relaxing and decreasing strain on the abdominal muscles during coughing.
   c. To collect mucus.
   d. To facilitate positioning.
5. It is easier to raise mucus mechanically after the bronchi are dilated and the secretions are thinned.

Performance Phase

1. Place the child in a series of appropriate positions.
   a. The area to be drained should be elevated and its respective bronchus placed in a vertical position. (Specific drainage positions are described in Table 32-5, below.)
   b. The spine should be as straight as possible to permit optimal expansion of the rib cage.

1. The positions are selected and modified according to the lung area involved, the child's age and general condition, and equipment such as IV, tracheostomies, monitors, ventilators, etc.

   b. Infants are positioned on the nurse's lap, in the isolette, or in the crib; older children may be treated on a tilt board or in bed.

Table 32-5 Postural Drainage Positions

Area of Lung to be Drained	Position	Area of Percussion
Upper lobes, left and right anterior apical segments	Child sitting, leaning slightly backward	Percuss over the top of shoulder and anterior thorax. Hand, in cupped position, should be over the clavicle.
Upper lobes, left and right posterior apical segments	Child sitting, leaning slightly forward	Percuss over the upper posterior thorax. Fingers should be contoured over the top of the child's shoulders.
Upper lobes, left posterior segment	Child sitting, slightly reclined and rotated to the right. (Infant may be positioned on stomach with left shoulder elevated on therapist's arm.)	Percuss over the left scapula.
Upper lobes, right posterior segment	Child lying flat and rotated onto the left side. (Infant may be positioned on stomach with right shoulder elevated on therapist's arm.)	Percuss over the right scapula.
Upper lobes, left and right anterior segments	Child lying flat on back	Percuss the anterior chest directly under the clavicles. Avoid direct pressure on the sternum.
Upper lobes, lingular segment	Child lying on right side, rotated back one-quarter turn and tilted 30 degrees	Percuss over the left breast.
Right middle lobe	Child rotated one-quarter turn from supine position onto the left side and tilted 30 degrees	Percuss over the right breast.
Lower lobes, left and right apical segments	Child lying flat in prone position	Percuss below the inferior angle of the scapula.
Lower lobes, left and right anterior basal segments	Child lying on back, tilted about 45 degrees	Percuss slightly above the lower ribs.
Lower lobe, left lateral basal segment	Child lying on right side, tilted about 45 degrees	Percuss the left lateral thorax at the level of the 8th rib.
Lower lobe, right lateral basal segment	Child lying on left side, tilted about 45 degrees	Percuss the right lateral thorax at the level of the 8th rib.
Lower lobes, left and right posterior basal segment	Child lying on stomach, tilted about 45 degrees	Percuss just above the 11th and 12th ribs.

(continued)

Guidelines: Promoting Postural Drainage in the Pediatric Patient (continued)

Procedure
(Cont.)

Nursing Action	Rationale/Amplification
2. Unless contraindicated, cup the chest wall for 1–2 minutes. (Description of cupping and vibration can be found below.)	2. More secretions can be raised in a shorter period of time when cupping and vibration are added to posturing.
3. Have the child inhale deeply; then, as he exhales, vibrate the chest wall during 3–5 exhalations.	
4. Encourage the child to cough.	4. Infants and young children may require suctioning.
5. Allow the child to rest for a minute, then repeat cupping, vibration, and coughing until no more mucus is produced or the child's condition indicates that the procedure should be stopped.	5. Total treatment time should generally not exceed 20–30 minutes.
	a. In acute conditions such as atelectasis, postural drainage may be done for 5 minutes out of every hour.
▶ **NURSING ALERT:** Postural drainage should not be done immediately after meals since it may induce vomiting.	b. In chronic conditions such as cystic fibrosis, postural drainage may be done 2–5 times per day for 15–30 minutes.
6. Provide for patient safety.	6. Stay with the child during the procedure, especially when he is in a head-down position.

Follow-up Phase

Nursing Action	Rationale/Amplification
1. Assist the child to slowly resume a normal position.	1. It may take a few minutes for the child to regain his equilibrium.
2. Provide oral hygiene.	2. This removes residual mucus from the child's mouth and promotes comfort.
3. Assess and record the effectiveness of the procedure and how well it was tolerated by the child.	

Cupping and Vibrating the Pediatric Patient

1. Cupping, or percussion, should be performed with a cupped hand, contoured to the thorax. For infants, it may be more effective to use cupped fingers or a small face mask from a self-inflating bag. (If this method is used, the rim should be filled with air so that it is firm.)
2. Light clothing or a single thickness diaper may be used between the therapist's hand and the child's chest to minimize discomfort during the procedure.
3. A hollow sound should be produced by the trapped air between the cupped hand and the patient. A slapping sound indicates that the hand is not cupped enough.
4. Cupping should not be performed directly over recent incisions, open wounds, or drainage tubes.
5. Cupping should be discontinued immediately if the percussion site is noted to be reddened.
6. To do vibration, the nurse must first observe the child for exhalation. With the upper arm stiffened, gently shake the child's chest; keep upper arm stiff and extend wrist. The older the child, the more force should be applied.
7. For infants who are breathing rapidly it is usually easier to vibrate with every second or third exhalation rather than with each exhalation. Hand electric vibrators may be easier to use with small infants.
8. For additional information, including the purpose, indications, contraindications, and procedure for administering cupping and vibration, refer to Guidelines: Percussion and Vibration, page 150.

Guidelines: Assisting the Patient to Cough

Coughing is the process of expelling air suddenly and noisily from the lungs through the glottis. Purpose: To clear secretions from the airways.

Procedure

Nursing Action	Rationale/Amplification
Preparatory Phase	
1. Position the child to help loosen and drain secretions.	1. a. Turn from side to side.
	b. Position for postural drainage as indicated (see p. 1179).

Procedure
(Cont.)

Nursing Action	Rationale/Amplification

2. Administer appropriate medications and allow time for them to take effect.

3. Explain the procedure to the child and/or parents.

4. Position the child for optimal chest expansion.

2. Medications may be utilized to loosen secretions or decrease pain awareness.

3. This helps to secure the child's cooperation.

4. The head should be elevated as high as possible.

Performance Phase

1. If the child has had surgery, splint the operative area with a pillow or by placing your hands on either side of the operative site.

2. Have the child take 3–4 deep breaths with emphasis on complete exhalation. Have him attempt to cough at the end of a series of deep breaths.

3. Repeat the procedure according to the child's tolerance until the airways are cleared.

4. Additional techniques for stimulating a cough in pediatric patients:
   a. Offer cold fluids or ice chips.
   b. Have the child swallow several times in sequence.
   c. Apply manual pressure by using an up-and-down movement of the finger with firm, steady pressure over the trachea above the manubrial arch.
   d. Pass a sterile suction catheter to produce endotracheal stimulation.

1. This decreases the pain associated with the procedure by decreasing movement in the area.

2. This helps to stimulate the cough reflex. Full exhalation causes secretions to be moved into the larger airways where mechanical cough receptors are present.

3. Suctioning may be indicated if the child is unable to produce an effective cough.

4. These techniques cause an irritating sensation in the trachea, triggering the cough reflex.

   d. The catheter is introduced through the child's nose and advances until coughing occurs (refer to the procedure for suctioning, p. 1182).

Follow-up Phase

1. Provide oral hygiene.

2. Assess and record the effectiveness of the cough, the amount and nature of the secretions, and successful techniques for stimulating the child to cough.

3. Auscultate the lungs.

1. This removes residual mucus from the child's mouth and promotes comfort.

3. This helps determine the extent of airway clearing.

Assisting the Pediatric Patient with Breathing Exercises

Nursing Considerations*

1. Breathing exercises must be performed routinely and diligently to be effective. Whenever possible, the same nurse should instruct and work with the child.
2. The respiratory tract should be free of secretions. If indicated, aerosol treatments, postural drainage, coughing, or suctioning should be done prior to deep breathing exercises.
3. The child should be relatively free of pain. If necessary, pain medication should be administered and time allowed for it to take effect before breathing exercises are initiated.
   Operative incisions should be splinted.
4. The nurse should be relaxed and unhurried. Her tone of voice, approach, and mannerisms affect the child's ability to relax.
5. The child should be positioned to eliminate excessive muscular activity.
   a. Flexion of the hips and knees reduces tension of the abdominal muscles, aiding inspiration.

   b. Supporting the upper extremities on pillows relieves the thorax of this additional weight during inspiration.
   c. The position for breathing exercises depends on the specific pulmonary problem and its severity as well as on the child's age and general condition.
6. Techniques to facilitate diaphragmatic breathing
   a. Have the child place a book on his abdomen.
   b. Instruct him to make the book fall off as he takes air in and makes his abdomen round.
   c. Have him watch his abdomen get flat as he blows all the air out.
   d. The chest should move as little as possible.
7. Techniques to facilitate pursed-lip breathing
   a. Blow cotton balls or Ping-Pong balls across a bedside table.
   b. Blow bubbles.
   c. Blow a harmonica or party favor.
   d. Blow a pinwheel.
   e. Suspend a Ping-Pong ball on a string from a doorframe. Have the patient see how long he can keep it propelled away before he needs to inhale. He should attempt to increase his time.
8. Techniques to facilitate deep breathing
   a. Rebreathing tube
   b. Incentive spirometry (see p. 208)
   c. Blowing up balloons or examining gloves
   d. Blowing bubbles

* For additional information, including the purpose of and instructions for diaphragmatic and pursed-lip breathing, refer to pages 151–153.

Guidelines: Suctioning

Suctioning is a method for removing excessive secretions from the airway. Suction may be applied to the oral, nasopharyngeal, or tracheal passages.

Procedure

To provide a patent airway by keeping it clear of excessive secretions.

Equipment

Suction source
Suction catheter with vent
Connecting tube
Sterile basin (for tracheal and tracheostomy suctioning)
Sterile distilled water
Tissues
Sterile towel
Sterile gloves (for tracheal and tracheostomy suctioning)
Collection bottle
Manometer to measure amount of vacuum applied
Padded tongue blades, p.r.n.

Procedure

Nursing Action	Rationale/Amplification

Oral Suctioning

Preparatory Phase

1. Gather equipment, including extra catheters of the appropriate size. Connect collection bottle and tubing to vacuum source.
2. Establish the need for suctioning by observing respirations and auscultating lungs.

3. Wash hands thoroughly.
4. Turn on suction to check system and regulate pressure if indicated and if equipment makes it possible.

5. Fill basin with sterile distilled water.
6. Position the child on his side, with his head slightly lowered. If necessary, seek an assistant to help maintain the child in this position.
7. Attach catheter to suction tubing; use a glove when handling catheter.
8. Place catheter tip in the basin and draw sterile distilled water through it.

1. Since suctioning is often done on an emergency basis, it is mandatory that the nurse keep the necessary equipment at the bedside.
2. The frequency of suctioning will vary with each patient. The need will be evidenced by noisy, moist respirations in a child who is unable to cough adequately.

4. Recommendations for *negative pressure*

Wall suction	
Infants	60–100 mm. Hg
Children	100–120 mm. Hg

6. This position aids in pooling and draining secretions.

7. Wear a glove to keep the catheter clean and to keep the nurse's hand clean.
8. This checks the patency of the system, lubricates catheter, and allows some water in the collection bottle which will prevent aspirated secretions from sticking to it.

Performance Phase

1. Use padded tongue blades to separate upper from lower teeth, if necessary.
2. Leave vent open to air and introduce catheter into the area to be suctioned.

3. Occlude vent with thumb and slowly withdraw catheter while rotating it between the thumb and finger. If catheter "grabs," remove thumb to stop suction.
4. Dip catheter in and out of the basin, drawing sterile distilled water through it to clean it.

5. Repeat steps 1–4 as necessary, suctioning no longer than 10 seconds at a time and allowing 1–3 minutes between suctioning periods (unless abundance of secretions makes this impossible).

1. This prevents the child from biting the catheter.

2. Area may include cheeks, beneath the tongue, and back of mouth. Avoid overstimulation of the gag reflex to prevent vomiting.
3. If catheter is allowed to remain in one place, the mucous membrane will be drawn against it. This will occlude the catheter and injure the tissues.
4. Use 50–100 ml. of water to adequately clean catheter. The bubbles created by the interrupted flow of water through the catheter increase the mechanical cleansing action.
5. Prolonged suctioning can produce laryngospasm, profound bradycardia and/or cardiac arrhythmias from vagal stimulation and loss of oxygen.

Procedure
(Cont.)

Nursing Action	Rationale/Amplification

Follow-up Phase

1. Turn off suction source, detach catheter from tubing, and wrap tubing in sterile towel. Discard disposable catheter.
2. Make the child comfortable and give mouth care.
3. Assess effectiveness by observing respirations and auscultating lungs.
4. Record the following:
   a. Amount, color, and consistency of secretions
   b. Coughing
   c. Dyspnea
   d. Cyanosis
   e. Frequency of suctioning
   f. Any bleeding
   g. Response of child to suctioning
5. Empty and rinse collection bottle before it fills completely and at the end of each tour of duty.

1. Preferably, a new catheter is used each time suctioning is required. The connecting tube should be changed at the end of each tour of duty, or more often if necessary.

3. Respirations should be quiet and occur with less effort.

Nasopharyngeal Suctioning

Preparatory Phase

This is the same as for oral suctioning.
In addition, the nurse should:
   Measure the distance between the tip of the child's nose and the tragus of the ear to determine how far to insert catheter.

The catheter tip will reach the nasopharynx.

Performance Phase

1. Leaving the vent in the catheter open, elevate the tip of the nose, and introduce the catheter along the floor of the nose (with the patient facing straight ahead).
2. If obstruction is encountered, do not force, but remove and insert at another angle or try the other nostril.
3. Follow steps 3–5 of the procedure for oral suctioning. Alternate nostrils when introducing the catheter.

1. This position will facilitate introduction of the catheter.

2. Some resistance should be expected when the catheter reaches the nasopharynx.
3. Alternating nostrils will ensure cleaning of both nasal passages and will minimize trauma to either side

Follow-up Phase

This is the same as for oral suctioning.

Tracheostomy Suctioning

1. Refer to Guidelines: Aspirating the Tracheostomy Tube, pp. 1184–1185.
2. Additional considerations for the pediatric patient include:
   a. Wall suction should be set at 50–95 mm. Hg for infants or at 90–115 mm. Hg for children.
   b. If sodium chloride solution is used to dilute secretions, the amount should be less (generally 1 ml. for infants and 1–5 ml. for children).
   c. The infant or young child should not be suctioned for more than 5 seconds at a time.
   d. The child's heart rate and color should be monitored throughout the procedure. In the event of irregularity, suctioning should be discontinued and oxygen or assisted ventilation administered.

Nasotracheal Suctioning

Preparatory Phase

1. Follow steps 1–4 of the Guidelines for oral suctioning.
2. Set wall suction at 50–95 mm. Hg for infants and 95–115 mm. Hg for children.
3. Make certain that an oxygen source is available.

4. Using aseptic technique, fill a sterile basin with sterile distilled water.
5. Position the child facing straight ahead with his head slightly tilted back. The infant should be placed in the "sniffing" position with chin up, head tipped slightly backward.

3. This procedure may produce hypoxia and necessitate oxygen therapy.
4. Tracheal suctioning should be done with sterile equipment to minimize the danger of infection.
5. This position facilitates introduction of the catheter.

(continued)

Guidelines: Suctioning (continued)

Procedure
(Cont.)

Nursing Action	Rationale/Amplification
6. Open the package containing the sterile catheter. Wear a sterile glove on the hand that will handle the catheter. Attach the catheter to the suction tubing.	6. From now until termination of the procedure, this hand should touch only the catheter.
7. Place catheter tip in the basin and draw sterile distilled water through it.	7. This checks the patency of the system, lubricates catheter, and allows some water in the collection bottle which will prevent aspirated secretions from sticking to it.

Performance Phase

Nursing Action	Rationale/Amplification
1. Leaving the vent in the catheter open, elevate the tip of the nose and introduce the catheter along the floor of the nose (with the patient facing straight ahead).	1. This position will facilitate introduction of the catheter.
2. If obstruction is encountered, do not force, but remove and insert at another angle or try the other nostril.	2. Some resistance should be expected when the catheter reaches the nasopharynx.

3. Move catheter forward slowly until it enters the trachea— when the following may happen:
  a. Child may cough.
  b. Air will be felt from vent in catheter on expiration.
  c. Voice or cry may change.
  d. Child may show marked anxiety.
	3. Attempt to enter the trachea carefully and on inspiration only. Tracheal tickle may be applied to stimulate coughing and ease the passage of the catheter into the trachea. Gentle pressure at the level of the vocal cords may also be helpful.

4. When catheter is in the trachea, occlude vent with the thumb of the ungloved hand and slowly withdraw catheter while rotating it between the thumb and finger.	4. If catheter grabs, remove thumb from vent to stop suction.
5. Remove thumb from vent for several seconds between inspirations.	5. Suctioning must be stopped at intervals to prevent hypoxia. During normal suction, 4 liters of air will be pulled out of the lungs in 15 seconds. Never suction for longer than 5 seconds.
6. Dip catheter in and out of the basin, drawing sterile distilled water through it to clean it.	6. Use 50–100 ml. of water to adequately clean catheter. The bubbles created by the interruped flow of water through the catheter increase the mechanical cleansing action.
7. Repeat steps 1–6 as required, suctioning no longer than 5 seconds at one time and allowing 1–3 minutes between suctioning periods (unless the secretions are too abundant).	7. If child is receiving oxygen, provide oxygen during these rest periods.
8. Monitor the child's heart rate and color throughout the procedure.	8. Discontinue suctioning and administer oxygen or assisted ventilation in the event of any irregularity.

▶ **NURSING ALERT:** Tracheal suction can result in laryngospasm. This may be recognized as obstructed respiration (rapid and labored with inspiratory stridor) and may rapidly progress to complete apnea. The nurse should call for assistance; she should straighten the airway by hyperextending the patient's neck and pulling his jaw forward and should administer oxygen.

Follow-up Phase
1. Follow the same procedure as for oral suctioning.
2. Administer oxygen if it is required by the patient's condition.

Guidelines: Care of a Child with a Tracheostomy

For information concerning purposes for tracheostomy, kinds of tracheostomy tubes, techniques for performing a tracheostomy, and nursing management, refer to the section on tracheostomy in adults, pages 211–223.

Kinds of Tracheostomy Tubes for Pediatric Patients

1. Plastic (polyvinyl chloride or Silastic) tubes, usually without an inner cannula (most common).
2. Silver tubes consisting of 3 parts: obturator, inner cannula, and outer cannula.
3. Cuffs are not generally used for infants and small children since the tracheostomy tube itself is big enough relative to the size of the trachea to act as its own sealer.

Common Reasons for Performing Tracheostomies in Pediatric Patients

1. Laryngotracheal bronchitis
2. Congenital abnormalities such as laryngeal stenosis, choanal atresia, and various anomalies of the heart and lung
3. Foreign bodies lodged in the hypopharynx or larynx
4. Severe chest trauma
5. Burns of the head and neck
6. Laryngeal edema from prolonged intubation
7. Management of secretions and provision of assisted ventilation postoperatively
8. Problems requiring ventilatory support

Nursing Management

Nursing Action	Rationale / Amplification
Physical Care of the Patient	
1. Provide adequate humidity, usually via a ventilator, humidifier, or tent.	1. The natural humidifying pathway of the oropharynx is no longer used. Mist will loosen mucus and secretions and reduce the chances of a mucous plug.
2. Aspirate secretions (using sterile technique) whenever indicated by noisy respiration, retractions, poor color, or change in vital signs (refer to procedure for aspirating a tracheostomy, pp. 220–223).	2. It takes a very small amount of secretions to obstruct a small tube.
3. Suction the child after he has had nebulization therapy, chest therapy, and postural drainage.	3. The secretions will be more liquid, more copious, and more easily removed following these procedures.
4. Observe closely for rising pulse rate and restlessness.	4. These are the first clinical signs of respiratory insufficiency and should be followed by careful tracheobronchial toilet.
5. Monitor respirations frequently and observe for unequal chest expansion.	5. This might indicate the development of a pneumothorax.
6. Keep the area around the tube clean and dry: a. Cleanse area with an applicator dipped in hydrogen peroxide. b. Observe the site for bleeding and irritation. c. Place an unfrayed sterile dressing around the tube and under the tapes that hold the tube in position.	6. To minimize irritation and the risk of infection.
7. Observe the child closely to prevent accidental removal of the tube. Arm restraints may be necessary. a. Have necessary equipment available at the bedside: Duplicate tracheostomy tubes with tapes attached. Tracheostomy set for emergency tracheostomy Materials for suctioning and cleansing tubes Materials for cleansing stomal site b. Never immerse the child in a full bath.	7. These are safety precautions. b. To prevent fluids from entering the airway.
8. Make certain that the tapes that hold the tube in place are tied securely with the proper amount of tension.	8. This prevents the tube from slipping out of place as the child becomes distressed or frightened or moves about.
9. Change ties as needed.	9. The knot should be at the side of the neck to prevent pressure while the child is lying on his back. Old ties should remain in place until the new ties are secured.
10. If an inner cannula is used it should be removed and cleaned of debris as needed, about every 4 hours.	
Special Considerations for the Infant	
1. Position the infant with his neck extended by placing a small roll under his shoulders.	1. An infant has a tendency to occlude the tube with his chin when his neck is flexed.
2. Support the infant's head when moving him.	2. Sudden movements of the head and neck can cause the tube to slip out.
3. When feeding, cover the tracheostomy with a moist piece of gauze. A bib may be used for older infants and young children.	3. This prevents food particles from dropping into the tube.
Psychosocial Care of Patients	
1. Explain, at the level of the child's understanding, the reasons for the tracheostomy and for all procedures and treatments.	1. The child's fantasies about what is happening and why may be more frightening than the truth. He may need reassurance that his voice will return once he is able to breathe normally again.
2. Allay fears and anxieties of parents by explanations and support.	2. Parental attitudes are conveyed to the child.
3. Provide some means of communication such as gestures, lip reading, magic slate, pad and pencil. An older child may enjoy alphabet letters or a word board.	3. The child is unable to communicate verbally.

(continued)

Guidelines: Care of a Child with a Tracheostomy (continued)

Nursing Management
(Cont.)

Nursing Action	Rationale/Amplification
4. Make sure that a call bell is within easy reach of the child, and answer it promptly.	4. The child is dependent on others to meet even his most basic needs. Prompt attention to his needs will help the child build trust in the nursing personnel.

Nursing Considerations if the Child is Discharged with a Tracheostomy Tube in Place

1. Involve the parents with the child's care as soon as possible. First, explain procedures and their rationale, and have them observe. Gradually turn more of the procedure over to them under nursing supervision.
2. Teach at the parent's level and pace of understanding.
3. Help parents to obtain necessary equipment. Make sure that they have a very specific list of the equipment (and the amounts needed).
4. Be alert to financial difficulties associated with securing equipment or nursing services. Refer to social worker if appropriate.
5. Make certain that parents know what to do and where to go in an emergency.
6. If possible, put parents in contact with other families who have managed children at home with tracheostomies.
7. If appropriate, initiate a community health nursing referral for nursing intervention after discharge.
8. Provide the parents with a written procedure to study and take home.
9. Assist parents to appreciate the normalcy of their child and to recognize his needs for an environment that will support developmental potentials.
10. Reference for parents:
    Tracheotomy Handbook for Parents. Chevalier Jackson Pediatric Tracheotomy Unit, St. Christopher's Hospital for Children. Philadelphia, PA 19133

Guidelines: Oxygen Therapy for Children

For additional information concerning the purpose, general considerations, and procedures for administering oxygen therapy, refer to Oxygen Therapy, pages 188–204.

General Nursing Responsibilities

Nursing Action	Rationale/Amplification
1. Explain the procedure to the child and allow him to feel the equipment and the oxygen flowing through the tube, mask, etc.	1. The child will be reassured if he understands the procedure and knows what to expect.
2. Maintain a clear airway by suctioning, if necessary.	2. The delivery of oxygen requires a clear airway.
3. Provide a source of humidification.	3. Oxygen is a dry gas and requires the addition of moisture to prevent drying of the tracheobronchial tree and thickening and consolidation of secretions.
4. Measure oxygen concentrations every 1–2 hours when a child is receiving oxygen via incubator hood, tent, or Croupette. a. Measure when the oxygen environment is closed. b. Measure the concentration close to the child's airway. c. Record oxygen concentrations and simultaneous measurements of the pulse and respirations.	4. It is desirable to keep the oxygen concentration as low as possible while still providing for physiologic requirements. This minimizes the danger of the child's developing retrolental fibroplasia or pulmonary oxygen toxicity. (Desired oxygen concentrations are determined by the arterial oxygen tension measurement.) The oxygen analyzer itself should be calibrated daily on both room air and 100% oxygen. The concentration of oxygen within the space is determined by the liter flow, the efficiency of the equipment, and the frequency with which it is opened to the external environment.
5. Observe the child's response to oxygen.	5. Desired response includes: a. Decreased restlessness b. Decreased respiratory distress c. Improved color d. Improved vital sign values
6. Organize nursing care so that interruption of therapy is minimal.	6. Interruption of therapy may result in the return of anoxia and defeat the goals of therapy.
7. Periodically check all equipment during each tour of duty.	7. For optimal functioning, the equipment should be clean, undamaged, and in good working order.
8. Clean equipment daily and change it at least once each week. (Tubing and nebulizer jars should be	8. Unclean equipment may be a source of contamination.

General Nursing Responsibilities
(Cont.)

Nursing Action	Rationale/Amplification
changed daily.) Take cultures of oxygen tubing, water, nebulizers, and the interior of incubators at least every 3 days.	
9. Keep combustible materials and potential sources of fire away from oxygen equipment. a. Avoid using oil or grease around oxygen connections. b. Do not use alcohol or oils on a child in an oxygen tent. c. Do not permit any electrical devices in or near an oxygen tent. d. Avoid the use of wool blankets and those made from some synthetic fibers because of the hazards resulting from static electricity. e. Prohibit smoking in areas where oxygen is being used. f. Have a fire extinguisher available.	9. Oxygen supports combustion.
10. Terminate oxygen therapy gradually. a. Slowly reduce liter flow. b. Open air vents in incubators. c. Open zippers or flip a section of the canopy over the top of the tent.	10. This allows the child to adjust to normal atmospheric oxygen concentrations.
11. Continually monitor the child's response during weaning. Observe for restlessness, increased pulse rate, respiratory distress, cyanosis.	11. These are indications that the child is unable to tolerate reduced oxygen concentration.

Specific Methods for Administering Oxygen to Pediatric Patients

Nursing Action	Rationale/Amplification
Oxygen by Nasal Cannula or Catheter 1. Refer to Guidelines: Administering oxygen by nasal cannula or catheter, pages 189–191.	
Oxygen by Mask 1. Choose an appropriate size mask that covers the mouth and nose but not the eyes.	1. Extra space under the mask and around the face is added dead space and decreases the effectiveness of the therapy.
2. Use a mask that is capable of delivering the desired oxygen concentration (refer to Table 32-6, below).	2. Venturi masks, available for use in pediatrics, deliver low to moderate concentrations of oxygen: 24%, 28%, 35%, or 40%.
3. Place the mask over the child's mouth and nose so that it fits securely. Secure the mask with an elastic head grip.	3. Make sure that the mask is adjusted properly over the mouth and nose. Do not allow the oxygen to blow in child's eyes. Small pieces of cotton may be placed above the ears to help relieve pressure and discomfort caused by the head strap.

Table 32-6 Oxygen Flow Required to Achieve Desired Oxygen Concentration in Mask Therapy*

Oxygen Flow Required liter/minute	Oxygen Concentration Desired†	
	Non-rebreathing Oxygen Mask	Pediatric Medium Concentration Oxygen Mask
6–8	40–50%	35–45%
8–10	50–60%	45–55%
10–12	60–95%	55–60%

* Tables from Lough MD and Doershuk CF. Oxygen therapy. In Lough MD, Doershuk C and Stern H. Pediatric Respiratory Therapy. Copyright © 1979 by Year Book Medical Publishers, Inc. Chicago. Used by permission.
† Indicates approximate figures.

(continued)

Guidelines: Oxygen Therapy for Children (continued)

Specific Methods for Administering Oxygen to Pediatric Patients
(Cont.)

Nursing Action	Rationale/Amplification
4. Remove the oxygen mask at hourly intervals; wash the face and dry.	4. Makes the patient feel more comfortable.
5. Do not use masks for comatose infants or children.	5. Such children are more likely to vomit. The risk of aspiration may be increased with mask therapy because of obstruction of the flow of vomitus.
6. For additional information, refer to Guidelines: Administering Oxygen by Venturi Mask (p. 191) and by Fask Mask (p. 193).	

Face Tent

1. Face tents are available in the adult size only. They can be used effectively in pediatric patients if inverted to create a smaller reservoir and better fit.	1. Face tents combine the positive qualities of aerosol masks and mist tents. The child is accessible and may continue to play without feeling confined.
2. A flow of 8–10 liters should be used to flush the system and provide a stable oxygen concentration.	2. Larger children will require higher flows.

T-Bars and Tracheostomy Masks

1. These devices are used to delivery oxygen to intubated patients.	
2. The flow rate must be set to meet the minute volume requirements of the child and to provide a 100% source of gas.	2. T-bars require a short, flexible tube on the distal end to act as a reservoir and prevent room-air entrapment.

Oxygen Tent

1. Select the smallest tent and canopy which will achieve the desired concentration of oxygen and maintain patient comfort.	1. This increases the efficiency of the unit.
2. Pad the metal frame which supports the canopy.	2. This protects the child from injury.
3. Maintain the tent temperature at 17.8°–21.1°C. (64°–70°F.).	3. This is done by placing ice in a trough on the back of the tent. It should be checked periodically and replaced as needed. Open-top tents do not require cooling.
4. Analyze and record the tent atmosphere every 1–2 hours. Concentrations of 30%–50% can be achieved in well-maintained tents.	4. The concentration varies with the efficiency of the tent, the rate of flow of oxygen, and the frequency with which the tent is opened to the outside environment.
5. Maintain a tight-fitting canopy. Whenever possible, provide nursing care through the sleeves or pockets of the tent.	5. This prevents oxygen leakage and disruption of the tent atmosphere. a. Fastening the canopy to the bedsprings with wooden clothespins may be helpful. b. If the child is extremely restless or uncooperative, it may be useful to permit a parent to hold the child's hand through a small opening in the zipper of the canopy.
6. Make certain that the cribsides are up.	6. The canopy, when tucked into the mattress, often gives the illusion of a safe, confined environment.
7. Select toys that retard absorption, are washable, and will not produce static electricity.	7. The child needs toys for stimulation and diversion. They should be safe and practical.

Croupette

1. This is an oxygen tent equipped with a high-humidification system (refer to procedure under oxygen tent).	1. If the child's condition requires high humidity but not oxygen, the unit can be operated with compressed air.
2. Change the child's clothing and bed linen when damp. Cover the child with a cotton blanket.	2. This prevents chilling in an environment of cooled, supersaturated, aerated mist.
3. Check the child frequently.	3. Condensation on the canopy may make it difficult to see the child.
4. If possible, remove the child from the mist periodically.	4. This prevents maceration of the skin. Mist may be delivered via nebulizer tubing or mask during these periods.
5. Promote postural drainage and suction the child as necessary.	5. Rapid mobilization of secretions may follow initiation of mist tent therapy.
6. Observe the small infant for signs of overhydration.	6. This occasionally results from intensive use of an ultrasonic nebulizer especially if a saline solution is nebulized.

Closed Incubators/Isolettes

1. The incubator is used to provide a controlled environment for the neonate.	1. The unit is able to provide precise environmental control of temperature, oxygen, humidity, and isolation.
2. Adjust the oxygen flow to achieve the desired oxygen concentration.	2. Refer to Table 32-7, p. 1189.

Table 32-7   Incubator Oxygen Therapy*

Red Flag in Horizontal Position		Red Flag in Vertical Position	
Flow of Oxygen liters/minute	Concentration of Oxygen	Flow of Oxygen liter/minute	Concentration of Oxygen
4	28%–31%	4	Flow not sufficient for high concentration
6	32%–36%	8	70%–75%
8	37%–40%	10	75%–80%
		12	80%–85%

* Tables from Lough MD and Doershuk CF. Oxygen therapy. In Lough MD, Doershuk CF and Stern RC. Pediatric Respiratory Therapy. Copyright © 1979 by Year Book Medical Publishers, Inc., Chicago. Used by permission.

Specific Methods for Administering Oxygen to Pediatric Patients
(Cont.)

Nursing Action	Rationale/Amplification
a. An oxygen limiter prevents the oxygen concentration inside the incubator from exceeding 40%.	a. This is desirable because it reduces the hazard of the child's developing retrolental fibroplasia.
b. Higher concentrations (up to 85%) may be obtained by placing the red reminder flag in the vertical position.	b. This operates by reducing the air intake.
3. Secure a nebulizer to the inside wall of the incubator if mist therapy is desired.	3. This should be cleaned and autoclaved daily. Sterile solutions are used to keep the bacteria count at a minimum.
4. Keep sleeves of incubator closed to prevent loss of oxygen	4. When incubator or sleeves are opened, supply supplemental oxygen with oxygen mask to face and nose.
5. Periodically analyze the incubator atmosphere.	5. To be certain that the child is receiving the desired concentration of oxygen.
Oxygen Hood	
1. Warmed, humidified oxygen is supplied via a plastic container that fits over the child's head (Fig. 32-8).	1. This is especially useful when high concentrations of oxygen are desired. The hood may be used in an incubator or with a warming unit. Oxygen should not be allowed to blow directly into the infant's face.
2. Continuously monitor the oxygen concentration, temperature, and humidity inside the hood.	2. Oxygen should be warmed to 31°–34°C. (87.8°–93.2°F.) to prevent a neonatal response to cold stress—including oxygen deprivation, metabolic acidosis, rapid depletion of glycogen stores, and reduction of blood glucose levels.

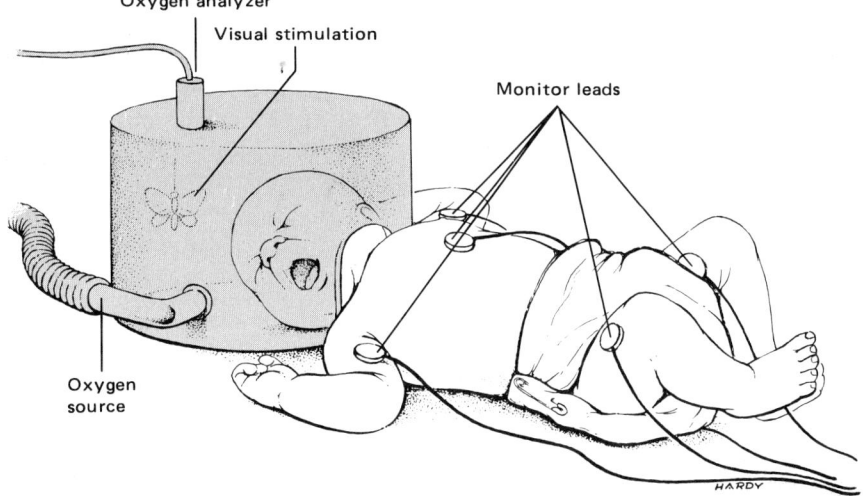

Figure 32-8. Oxygen hood.

(continued)

Specific Methods for Administering Oxygen to Pediatric Patients
(Cont.)

Nursing Action	Rationale/Amplification
3. Open the hood or remove the baby from it as infrequently as possible.	3. This prevents fluctuations of heat and oxygen which may further debilitate the young infant.
4. Several different designs are available for use. The manufacturer's directions should be carefully followed.	4. This is a safety consideration.

Nursing Care of the Child Requiring Mechanical Ventilation

Characteristics of the Ventilator

Available ventilators have a wide range of capabilities, versatility, and clinical application. Some are more suitable for use with infants, others with children. It is wise for the nurse to be well-acquainted with the characteristics of the machine that is being used and to be able to answer the following questions.

A. Rate Control

1. How is the rate controlled?
2. Can the patient initiate the cycle? (assisted ventilation)
3. What is the response time? (time elapsed between the initiation of respiration and response of the ventilator) This must be rapid in infants.
4. Is there a sensitivity control which allows the machine to be more or less sensitive to the patient's efforts to initiate respiration?
5. Is an IMV (intermittent mandatory ventilation) feature present? This allows the patient to breathe on his own and, at certain intervals, a mandatory inspiration is provided by the ventilator.

B. Volume Control

1. How is the volume controlled?
   a. Automatically preset (i.e., the Bennett MA-1, Ohio 560 and Bourn LS 104-150)
   b. Variable, with a preset pressure
2. What is the range of inspiratory flow rate capability? A very low flow rate is required by neonates; the rate will increase with the size of the child.

C. Cycling

1. What controls the cycle of the machine?
   a. Time cycle—inspiration is terminated at the end of a preset period that is controlled by a timing device. The volume delivered is usually a function of flow per unit of time.
   b. Volume cycle—the inspiratory phase is terminated after the predetermined volume of gas has been delivered. The pressure generated is dependent on the characteristics of the lung.
   c. Pressure cycle—the inspiratory phase ceases when a preset pressure is achieved. The volume of gas delivered and the time required to achieve the preset pressure are dependent on the characteristics of the lungs.
   d. Mixed cycle—many ventilators have 2 or more cycling modes.

D. Humidification

1. How is moisture added to the inspired air?
   a. Humidification
   b. Nebulization
2. Is there a means of controlling the temperature of the inspired air?
   Many models provide an adjustable thermostat on the humidifier controls.

E. Oxygen Control

1. What is the oxygen source?
2. How is the oxygen concentration controlled?

F. Pressure Control

1. How is the pressure controlled?
   a. Automatically preset (i.e., the Bennett Pr-2, Bird, Mark 7, 8, and 14, Baby-bird, and Bourns P200 infant ventilator)
   b. Variable, with a preset volume
2. What do the pressure gauges indicate and how are they read?
   a. Airway pressure indicator
   b. Machine pressure indicator
3. What is the peak effective pressure capability?

G. Ratio of Inspiration to Expiration (I/E ratio)

1. Is this variable?
2. How is it controlled?

H. PEEP (positive end-expiratory pressure)

Does the ventilator have this feature? How is it controlled?
1. PEEP refers to positive airway at end expiration.
2. This helps minimize alveolar volume loss during expiratory pauses and thus decreases the tendency toward atelectasis.

I. CPAP (continuous positive airway pressure)

Does the ventilator have this feature? How is it controlled? Refer to pages 1192–1194.

J. Sigh

Does the ventilator have this feature? How is it regulated?
1. Works by adding additional volume to the established tidal volume.
2. Has the effect of taking a deep breath and may expand alveoli, which tend to be collapsed at low volume ventilation.

K. Alarm Systems

What are the alarm systems to warn of possible problems?
1. Low pressure or disconnect alarm system.

2. High pressure alarm system to indicate rising pressures within the lung.
3. Electrical failure alarm system.
4. Volume and rate monitor
    a. Acceptable low and high rates and tidal volumes are set for the alarm.
    b. If either rate or tidal volume are outside acceptable parameters, an alarm sounds.

Nursing Management

Refer to Guidelines for managing the patient requiring mechanical ventilation, pages 225–232. In addition, the following considerations should be kept in mind by the nurse who is caring for a pediatric patient.

A. Setting Controls

In setting controls, inspiratory flow rate will be less, and the respiratory rate will be greater than in the adult patient. These depend on the patient's size and condition and are determined by the physician and/or respiratory therapist.

B. Humidification

1. Because of their small diameters, pediatric endotracheal tubes easily become obstructed by thickened secretions. Therefore, adequate humidification must be maintained to keep secretions loose.
2. During ventilation of an infant in an incubator, the amount of ventilator tubing outside the incubator should be kept to a minimum. The warm temperature inside the incubator helps decrease the amount of condensation in the tubing and thus provides higher water content in the inspired gas.

C. Oxygen Concentration

1. Inspired concentrations of oxygen should always be kept as low as possible (while still providing for physiologic requirements), to prevent the development of retrolental fibroplasia or pulmonary O_2 toxicity.
2. The oxygen concentration should be checked periodically with an analyzer.

D. Blood Gases

1. The arterialized capillary sample method is inaccurate for infants in respiratory distress because the constricted peripheral circulation may not reflect the arterial blood gases accurately.
2. An umbilical artery catheter is most frequently used to obtain arterial blood samples.

E. Sterile Precautions

The newborn has only those antibodies transferred across the placenta from the mother. Therefore, sterile precautions are essential.
1. Ventilator tubing should be changed every 24 hours.
2. Routine cultures should be taken after intubation; there should be daily gram-staining of secretions.
3. Suctioning requires aseptic technique.

F. Tubing Support

1. Special frames are available to support ventilator tubing; this helps to prevent accidental decannulation in infants and small children.
2. Infants may require folded diapers or padding on either side and at the top of their heads to decrease mobility and take up space between the head and the frame.

G. Monitoring the Ventilator

1. Pressure gauges should be checked at frequent intervals since this gives an indication of changing compliance or increased airway resistance.
2. Volume measurements are difficult to obtain in infants since most spirometers incorporated into ventilators and meters (such as the Wright respirometer) do not read accurately at low volumes and flows. However, they are helpful with older children.
3. Measure respiratory rates of the machine and the patient at least every hour.

Weaning the Pediatric Patient From the Ventilator

A. Method I—Permits the patient to breathe spontaneously for short periods of time:

1. Often used when ventilation has been solely for apnea.
2. The length of time without ventilator assistance is gradually increased, while observing that the infant does not become fatigued.
3. This method is often facilitated by applying continuous positive pressure to the airway when the infant is off the ventilator.
4. The CPAP (continuous positive airway pressure) can then be gradually decreased until the infant can breathe without assistance (see pp. 1192–1194).
5. A T-piece is generally attached to the child's artificial airway during this process to provide oxygen enrichment and humidification.

B. Method II—Switches from the "control" to the "assist" mode to permit the child to trigger respiration by his own effort.

1. This method is preferred for children with lung disease.
2. The ventilator is switched to the "assist" mode.
3. The trigger sensitivity is gradually decreased as the patient is encouraged to provide greater effort until he is able to ventilate adequately without the assistance of the machine.
4. The patient is then taken off the ventilator for progressively longer periods until use of the ventilator can be discontinued completely.
5. CPAP can be used with this method during the periods that the patient is off the ventilator.

C. Nursing Management

1. Weaning children from a ventilator is frequently a long and tedious process. The child and/or his parents may need a lot of support and encouragement.
2. Frequent blood gas determinations are necessary to determine if the child is maintaining adequate oxygenation.
3. The child should be observed closely for signs of respiratory difficulty including fatigue, nasal flaring, increased pulse rate, sweating, facial pallor and cyanosis, and rising blood pressure.
4. A calm atmosphere should be maintained.
5. Whenever possible, the ventilator should remain at the bedside until the child is satisfied that he can breathe without it.

Guidelines: CPAP (Continuous Positive Airway Pressure)

CPAP is a system of applying a constant distending or gas pressure which is greater than atmospheric pressure to the airway during spontaneous breathing. This system is also referred to as CPPB (continuous positive pressure breathing).

Purposes
1. To prevent alveolar collapse during expiration by keeping the alveoli open with pressure while avoiding overdistending already-expanded alveoli.
2. To prevent intrapulmonary right-to-left shunting.
3. To increase the oxygenation of the lungs, which in turn decreases potential for hypoxia, bradycardia, or apnea.
4. To decrease the work of breathing on the part of the infant.
5. To increase FRC (functional residual capacity).

Equipment (Fig. 32-9)

A source of gas—mixture of air and oxygen; warmth and humidity device for varying the pressure in the system.
Means of connecting the system to the infant's airway
    Endotracheal tube
    Nasal prongs (cannula)—insert to a depth of at least 1 cm.
    Face mask
    Head hood
    Negative pressure in NP respirator around chest
Extra equipment for administering mechanical ventilation
Equipment for immediate treatment of pneumothorax

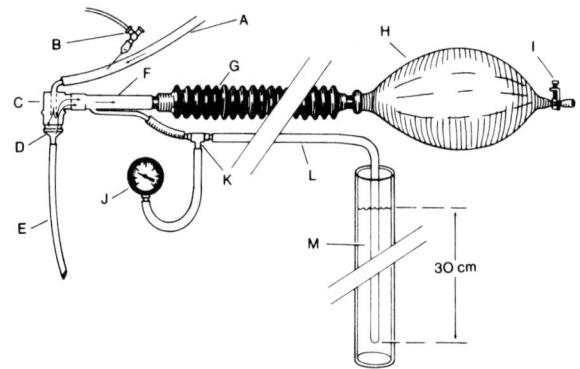

Figure 32-9. System for applying continuous positive airway pressure through an endotracheal tube. (*A*) Represents gas inflow, (*B*) oxygen sampling port, (*C*) Norman elbow (modified T piece), (*D*) endotracheal tube connector, (*E*) endotracheal tube, (*F*) Sommers T piece, (*G*) corrugated anesthesia hose, (*H*) reservoir bag (500 ml.) with open tail piece, (*I*) screw clamp, (*J*) aneroid pressure manometer, (*K*) plastic T connector, (*L*) plastic tubing (1-cm. internal diameter), and (*M*) underwater "pop-off." Arrows indicate direction of gas flow. (From Gregory et al. N Engl J Med 284(24):1333–1343, 1971) (Note: Although newer ventilator equipment can provide CPAP, the principles are the same.)

Procedure

Nursing Action	Rationale / Amplification
Preparatory Phase	
1. The CPAP system is generally set up by the physician and/or respiratory therapist. The accepted early criteria for initiating CPAP are: a. Infant breathing spontaneously b. PaO_2 (arterial O_2 tension) < 60 mm. Hg (breathing) in 60%–65% oxygen less than 24 hours of age c. F_1O_2 (inspired oxygen) > 80% at any time	1. The nurse must be in attendance to monitor the infant during application and must know and understand the workings of the CPAP system.
2. The connecting systems used may be nasal cannula or endotracheal tube.	
Nasal Cannula	
1. Lubricate cannula with a hydrocortisone cream before insertion.	1. Orogastric tube may be inserted and opened to straight drainage to allow for gastric decompression. Lubrication helps to prevent the inflammatory reaction.
2. Prepare headband and place around infant.	2. This keeps the nasal cannula in place.

Procedure
(Cont.)

Nursing Action	Rationale/Amplification

Endotracheal Tube

1. Lubricate endotracheal tube with hydrocortisone cream prior to insertion.
2. Set up sterile suction equipment.

Performance Phase

1. The infant's status can change quickly. Carefully observe the condition of infant:
   a. Skin color—cyanotic, dusky, or too pink.

   b. Respiratory pattern—rate, retractions, grunting, apnea, decreased breath sounds.

   c. Cardiac pattern—rate, especially bradycardia, blood pressure, femoral pulses.
   d. Activity—sudden increase or decrease in movement.

2. Observe closely for problems or malfunctions connected with CPAP system.
   a. Check inspired O_2 levels being delivered to the infant.

   b. Blood gases are checked frequently and always 20 minutes after any change is made in the system. O_2 changes are usually made in 5% increments unless the PaO_2 is >100 mg./dl.
   c. Pressure levels should be maintained as prescribed. Check all lines and connections.

   d. Maintain O_2 humidification and temperature.

1. CPAP can cause overdistention of lung alveoli leading to complications.
   a. Changes may be signs of pneumothorax, reduced cardiac output, low PaO_2, too much O_2 administration, infant too hot or cold.
   b. Change in respirations may indicate that the patient is not tolerating CPAP or that pneumothorax has occurred.
   c. Hypocalcemia, hypoglycemia, or opening of ductus arteriosus should be suspected when changes occur.
   d. Check for hypocalcemia, hypoglycemia, respiratory obstruction.

   a. O_2 needs are determined by the PaO_2 values and the infant's condition. Allowing elevated levels is detrimental to the infant.

   c. Any change in the pressure should be observed immediately and the cause determined. Increase in pressure indicates an obstruction in the baby or in the system tubing. Decrease in pressure indicates a leak in the system. Keep the patient's mouth closed when administering nasal CPAP. CPAP levels are usually increased or decreased by 1- to 2-cm. H_2O increments.
   d. The air O_2 mixture must be properly humidified for the following reasons:
      (1) To prevent drying of mucous membranes and thick secretions caused by too little moisture.
      (2) Possible aspiration or water intoxication can occur from a collection of droplets accumulating on walls of tubing and flowing to infant.
      Proper humidification is present when the tubing is evenly fogged with a fine mist.

▶ **NURSING ALERT:** Improper temperature of the air-oxygen mixture can lead to hypo- or hyperthermia and can increase oxygen consumption, resulting in acidosis and apnea. Proper temperature is just below body temperature and is not warm or cold when passing over one's skin.

3. Observe for signs of complications inherent with a premature infant (see p. 1216), respiratory distress syndrome (see p. 1268), and ventilation
   a. Spontaneous tension pneumothorax

   b. Metabolic acidosis

   c. Hyperbilirubinemia
   d. Infection, systemic

   e. Cardiac output reduction

   a. Presenting signs include decreased chest movements and breath sounds on affected side, tachypnea, cyanosis, bradycardia, inspiratory pressure elevated on manometer, decrease in systolic blood pressure.
   b. The blood pH is less than 7.3. This occurs because of tissue hypoxia and anaerobic metabolism.
   c. See page 1236.
   d. Temperature instability may be first indication of infection. Apnea, irritability, vomiting, diarrhea, change in status should be reported immediately.
   e. Results from CPAP set at too-high levels for improving compliance of lungs. CPAP is transmitted through the lungs to the large vessels of mediastinum. The increasing pressure may cause the vessels to partially collapse, affecting the return of blood to the heart; this causes a decrease in cardiac output.

(continued)

Guidelines: CPAP (Continuous Positive Airway Pressure) (continued)

Procedure
(Cont.)

Nursing Action	Rationale / Amplification
f. Hypocalcemia (blood calcium less than 8 mg./100 ml.) Hypoglycemia (blood sugar less than 20 mg./100 ml.)	f. Symptoms are nonspecific: jitteriness, sweating, tachypnea or apnea, lethargy, convulsions, cyanosis.
g. Hypovolemia (1) Accurate records should be kept of blood removed. (2) Monitor blood pressure.	g. This occurs from placenta previa or abruptio placentae, loss of blood into the placenta due to rapid clamping, or iatrogenically from too much sampling without replacement.
h. Abdominal distention—caused by inflation of air. (1) To decompress stomach use an NG (nasogastric) tube or aspirate air prior to NG (gavage) feedings. (2) Elevate the infant's head if possible during feeding and attempt to burp him. (3) NG (nasogastric) tube may be kept in place and connected to elevated open reservoir between feedings to serve as overflow safety valve.	h. Most common when using nasal, mask, or hood CPAP. Abdominal distention and increasing gastric residuals may be first sign of necrotizing enterocolitis.
4. Additional nursing care responsibilities to consider when caring for infant being treated with CPAP: a. Provide and maintain thermal stability of infant (p. 1222). b. Provide adequate fluid and caloric intake to meet the infant's needs via intravenous fluids and/or nasojejunal (N-J), gavage, or other methods. c. Administer proper and adequate physical therapy to infant to help reduce the potential for pneumonia.	c. Physical therapy includes percussion or vibrating, postural drainage, suctioning, and position change. This prevents airway obstruction as a result of the presence of mucus anywhere along the respiratory tract.
d. Mechanical ventilation with anesthesia bag may be administered at specific times. e. Assist in obtaining blood gases at appropriate times. (1) Observe the infant for signs that would indicate need for special blood gas studies. Also done after CPAP settings are changed and to monitor the infant's progress and condition. (2) When drawing blood, use a needle and syringe that have been rinsed with heparin. Avoid too much heparin since it will alter pH value. Store blood sample on ice while transporting to laboratory. Know normal blood gas values as well as the patient's "normal" values.	d. To help decrease PCO_2, assist a tiring infant, increase O_2 levels prior to any CPAP change or suctioning. e. Blood gases are always taken 20–30 minutes after CPAP settings are changed—this allows infant to stabilize with new settings. Arterial capillary blood is obtained from warmed heel blood. Arterial blood is drawn from umbilical artery indwelling catheter, radial or temporal artery puncture.
f. Avoid irritation and drying of mouth and nares. The mouth should be cleansed frequently with lemon–glycerin or normal saline swabs.	f. Prevents crust formation, which can lead to breakdown, by using an antibiotic ointment.
g. Keep skin clean and dry. Massage reddened areas gently. Change position every 1–2 hours. Avoid using large quantities of tape.	g. Give good skin care to prevent breakdown and eventual ulceration and infection.
h. Provide the infant with pleasant stimulation and love.	h. Colorful objects or pictures can be placed around the infant. Small musical toys and a pleasant, soothing voice combined with gentle touching can provide the necessary stimulation.

Follow-up Phase

1. When the infant can maintain adequate arterial oxygenation with CPAP at 1–2 cm. H_2O for 2–4 hours, he is ready to come off CPAP.

2. Once CPAP is discontinued, the infant is placed in an environment that provides 10%–20% more oxygen than he was breathing while on CPAP. Blood gases are checked as O_2 concentration is decreased as tolerated (see Respiratory Distress Syndrome [RDS], p. 1268, for further in-depth discussion).

Cardiac and Respiratory Monitoring

Cardiac and respiratory monitoring refers to electrical surveillance of heart and respiratory rates and patterns. It is indicated in all patients whose conditions are unstable or potentially unstable.

Nursing Management

1. Select a monitor that is appropriate for the child's needs. This will depend on the child's age, ability to cooperate, purpose for monitoring, information desired, and equipment available.
2. Stabilize the device to reduce the amount of mechanical noise and for safety considerations.
3. Reduce the child's anxiety:
   a. Provide age-appropriate explanations of the equipment.
   b. When possible, involve the child in his own care, including change of electrodes.
4. Select lead placement sites according to equipment specifications:
   a. Cardiac monitors frequently employ 3 leads located at:
      (1) Right upper lateral chest wall below clavicle
      (2) Left lower chest wall in the anterior axillary line
      (3) Upper left chest wall
   b. Respiratory monitors frequently employ 3 electrodes located:
      (1) On either side of the chest (anterior axillary line in fourth or fifth intercostal space)
      (2) At a reference electrode placed on the manubrium or other suitable distal point
5. Apply electrodes by:
   a. Cleaning the appropriate areas on the chest with alcohol
   b. Placing a small amount of conductive gel at each

area of contact unless pre-gelled, disposable electrodes are used
   c. Applying the electrode firmly to completely dry skin
6. Plug the leads into the lead cable at appropriate insertion points.
7. Be certain that the monitor alarms are in the "on" position. High and low alarm limits should be set according to the child's age and condition so that apnea, tachypnea, bradycardia, and tachycardia can be readily detected.
8. Avoid skin breakdown by changing lead placement sites as needed. Clean and dry old sites and expose them to the air.
9. Check integrity of the entire system at least once each tour of duty.
   a. Carefully inspect lead wires and cable for breaks and proper attachment.
   b. If malfunction is suspected, change equipment and notify the engineering department immediately.
10. Continue to count respiratory and apical rates at frequent intervals.
    a. Compare with monitor rates to verify accuracy of equipment.
    b. It must be remembered that monitors cannot substitute for close observation of the child.
11. Apnea mattresses or pads that employ sensing devices may be used for infants, eliminating the need for electrodes.
    a. Although less susceptible to cardiovascular artifact, these devices may record physical impact, vibrations, or body movements as breaths.
    b. In addition, older infants can easily roll or crawl off the pad.

Cardiopulmonary Resuscitation

Cardiopulmonary resuscitation involves measures instituted to provide effective ventilation and circulation when the patient's respiration and heart have ceased to function.

Underlying Considerations

A. Cardiac Arrest
1. Signs—absence of heartbeat and absence of carotid and femoral pulses.
2. Causes—asystole, ventricular fibrillation, or cardiovascular collapse related to arterial hypotension.

B. Respiratory Arrest
1. Signs—apnea and cyanosis.
2. Causes—obstructed airway, depression of the central nervous system, neuromuscular paralysis.

C. Emergency Preparation
1. Every hospital should have a well-defined and organized plan to be carried out in the event of cardiac or respiratory arrest.
2. Emergency carts should be placed in strategic locations in the hospital and checked daily to ensure that all equipment is available.

Equipment
Emergency cart—assembled and ready for use
   Positive pressure breathing bag with nonrebreathing valve and universal 15-mm. adapter
   Masks (premature infant, infant, child, adult sizes)
   Oropharyngeal airways, sizes No. 0 to No. 4
   Laryngoscope with blades of various sizes
   Extra batteries and light bulbs for laryngoscope
   Endotracheal tubes with connectors (complete sterile set, 2.5–8.0 mm. I.D.)
   Portable suction equipment and sterile catheters of various sizes
   Bulb syringe, DeLee trap
   Oxygen source—portable supply gauge and tubing, masks of various sizes
   Cardiac board (30 by 50 cm.)
   Emergency drugs

Sodium bicarbonate	Calcium chloride 10%
Epinephrine	
Isoproterenol	Dextrose 50%
Dextrose	Lidocaine (xylocaine)
Saline solution (for dilution)	Atropine

Diphenhydramine hydrochloride (Benadryl)
Diazepam (Valium)
Hydrocortisone sodium succinate
Digoxin
Naloxone (Narcan)
Calcium gluconate

Phenytoin sodium (Dilantin)
Insulin
Procainamide (Pronestyl)
Propranolol (Inderal)
Dopamine

Intracardiac needles, No. 20 and 22 gauge, 6–8 cm. (2⅜–3⅛ inches) long
IV equipment
  Fluids
  Infusion set
  Tourniquet
  Armboards
  Tape
  Scalp-vein needles of various sizes

  Longdwell catheters of various sizes
  3 way stopcock
  Cutdown set
  Pole
  Labels

Nasogastric tubes of various sizes
Other equipment
  Syringes of various sizes
  Needles of various sizes
  Alcohol wipes
  Tongue blades
  Sterile 4 × 4 gauze sponges
  Sterile hemostat
  Sterile scissors
  Blood specimen tubes
Electrocardiograph and monitor
Lubricating jelly
Defibrillator and paddles (pediatric and adult)

Artificial Ventilation

Technique for Artificial Ventilation

A. Mouth to Mouth

1. *Infants*
   a. Slightly extend neck by gently pulling chin up and forward and the head back. Place a rolled towel or diaper under the infant's shoulders, or use 1 hand to support the neck in an extended position. Do not hyperextend the neck since this narrows the airway.
   b. Check the mouth and throat and clear mucus or vomitus with finger or suction, if necessary.
   c. Take a breath.
   d. Make a tight seal with your mouth over the infant's mouth and nose.
   e. Gently blow air from the cheeks and observe for chest expansion.
   f. Remove your mouth from infant's mouth and nose and allow the infant to exhale.
   g. If spontaneous respirations do not return, continue breathing at a rate and volume appropriate for the size of the infant (usually 20 times per minute or 1 breath every 3 seconds).

2. *Older children and adolescents*
   a. Clear mouth of mucus or vomitus with finger or suction.
   b. Hyperextend neck with 1 hand or a rolled towel.
   c. Clamp the nostrils with the fingers of 1 hand which also continues to exert pressure on the forehead to maintain the neck extension.
   d. Take a deep breath.
   e. Make a tight seal with your mouth over the child's mouth.
   f. Force air into the lungs until chest expansion is observed.

g. Release your mouth from the child's mouth and release nostrils to allow the child to exhale passively.
h. Repeat approximately 12–15 times/minute or 1 breath every 4–5 seconds.

B. Hand-Operated Ventilation Devices

1. Remove secretions from mouth and throat and move mandible forward.
2. Appropriately extend the neck with one hand or place a diaper roll behind the neck.
3. Select an appropriate size mask to obtain an adequate seal, and connect mask to the bag.
4. Hold the mask snugly over the mouth and nose, holding the chin forward and the neck in extension.
5. Squeeze the bag, noting inflation of the lungs by chest expansion.
6. Release the bag, which will expand spontaneously. The child will exhale and the chest will fall.
7. Repeat 12–20 times per minute (depending on size of the child).
8. Since this technique is often difficult to master, it should be practiced in advance, under supervision.

Indications of Effective Technique

1. Victim's chest rises and falls.
2. Rescuer can feel in his own airway the resistance and compliance of the victim's lungs as they expand.
3. Rescuer can hear and feel the air escape during exhalation.
4. Victim's color improves.

Management of Complications

1. Gastric distention (occurs frequently if excessive pressures are used for inflation)
   a. Turn victim's head and shoulders to one side.
   b. Exert moderate pressure over the epigastrium between the umbilicus and the rib cage.
   c. A nasogastric tube may be used to decompress the stomach.
2. Vomiting
   a. Turn patient on side for drainage.
   b. Clear the airway with fingers or suction.
   c. Resume ventilations.

Artificial Circulation

General Principles Related to Artificial Circulation

(Technique of Artificial Circulation [Table 32-8, Fig. 32-10])

1. A backward tilt of the head lifts the back in infants and small children. A firm support beneath the back is therefore essential if external cardiac compression is to be effective.
2. A supine position on a firm surface is mandatory. Only in this position can chest compression squeeze the heart against the immobile spine enough to force blood into the systemic circulation.
3. External cardiac compression must always be accompanied by artificial ventilation for adequate oxygenation of the blood.
4. Compressions must be regular, smooth, and uninterrupted. Avoid sudden or jerking movements.
5. Relaxation must immediately follow compression; relaxation and compression must be of equal duration.
6. Between compressions, the fingers or heel of the hand must completely release their pressure but should remain in constant contact with the chest.

Table 32-8 Technique of Artificial Circulation

Size of Child	Preparatory Phase	Action Phase	Distance of Compression	Rate
Neonate, premature, or small infant	1. Place in supine position 2. Encircle the chest with the hands, with thumbs over the midsternum *or* Use method for a larger infant, at a rate of 100–120/min.	1. Compress midsternum with both thumbs, gently but firmly	2/3 distance to the spine or 1.3–1.8 cm. (½–¾ inch)	100–120/minute
Larger infant	1. Place on a firm, flat surface 2. Support the back with 1 hand or use a small blanket under the shoulders 3. Place the tips of the index and middle fingers of one hand over the midsternum	Compress the midsternum with the tips of the index and middle fingers	1.3–2.5 cm. (½–1 inch)	100 per minute
Small child	1. Place on a firm, flat surface 2. Support the back by slipping 1 hand beneath it, or use a small blanket under the shoulders 3. Place the heel of 1 hand over the midsternum, parallel with the long axis of the body	1. Apply a rapid downward thrust to the midsternum, keeping the elbow straight 2. Hold for approximately 0.4 second 3. Instantly and completely release the pressure so the chest wall can recoil 4. Do not remove the heel of the hand from the chest	2.5–3.8 cm. (1–1½ inches)	80–100/minute
Larger child, adolescent	1. Place on a flat, firm surface or place a board under the thorax 2. Place the heel of one hand on the lower half of the sternum, about 2.5–3.8 cm. (1–1½ inches) from the tip of the xiphoid process and parallel with the long axis of the body 3. Place the other hand on top of the first one (may interlock fingers) 4. Place shoulders directly over child's sternum, in order to use own weight in application of pressure	1. Exert pressure vertically downward to depress lower sternum, keeping elbows straight 2. Hold for approximately 0.4 second 3. Instantly and completely release the pressure so the chest wall can recoil 4. Do not remove the hands from the chest	3.8–5.0 cm. (1½–2 inches)	80 per minute

7. Fingers should not rest on the patient's ribs during compression. Pressure with fingers on the ribs or lateral pressure increases the possibility of fractured ribs and costochondral separation.
8. Never compress the xiphoid process at the tip of the sternum. Pressure on it may cause laceration of the liver.
9. Indications of effective technique include:
   a. A palpable femoral or carotid pulse
   b. Decrease in size of pupils
   c. Improvement in the patient's color

Nursing Management in Cardiopulmonary Resuscitation

1. Recognize cardiac and/or respiratory arrest.
2. Send for assistance and note time.
3. If alone:
   a. First ventilate the child's lungs rapidly 4 times, using appropriate technique (p. 1196), then palpate the carotid or brachial pulse. If a pulse is palpated, continue ventilatory support.
   b. If no pulse is felt, institute artificial circulation using appropriate technique (p. 1196).
   c. For an infant, interpose 1 breath after each series of 5 compressions. For a child or adolescent,

interpose 2 breaths after each series of 15 compressions.
   d. Continue repeating this cycle until help arrives.
4. When help arrives:
   a. One rescuer performs mouth-to-mouth resuscitation or institutes bag breathing.
   b. Another rescuer performs cardiac compressions.
   c. A ratio of 5 compressions to 1 breath is maintained for both infants and children.
   d. Cardiac compression should not be stopped for respiration. Breaths should be interposed on the upstroke of each fifth cardiac compression.
5. Anticipate and assist with emergency procedures and medications.
   a. Assist with intubation, monitoring, placement of cutdown, administration of intravenous fluids, defibrillation, and other definitive measures.
   b. Prepare and administer emergency medications as prescribed. Record dose and time.
6. After resuscitation:
   a. Care for the child as required.
   b. Determine if family members have been notified and are being cared for.
   c. Record all events.
   d. Restock emergency cart.

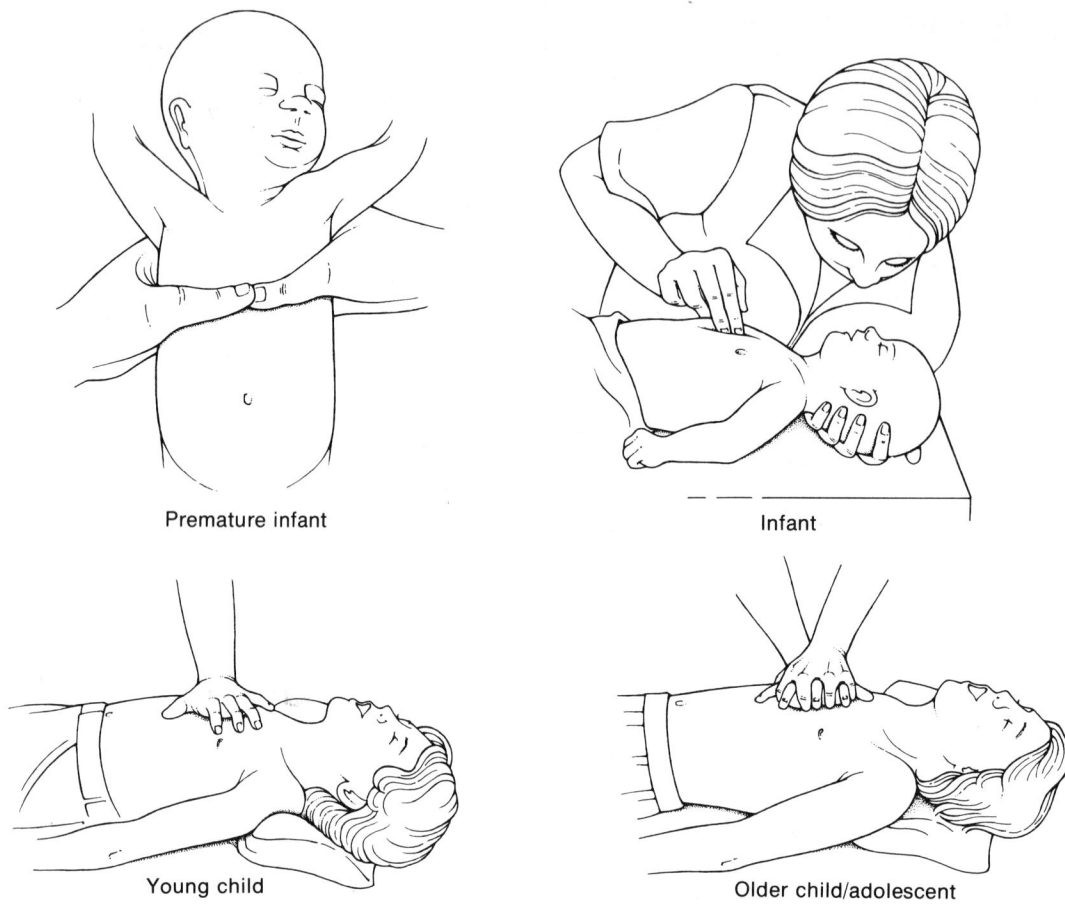

Premature infant

Infant

Young child

Older child/adolescent

Figure 32-10. Cardiopulmonary resuscitation in children. In the young child, the heel of the hand is placed over the lower sternum. In older children and adolescents, both hands are used.

Traction

Traction refers to the extension of an injured extremity in the direction and position which will promote healing and optimal functioning. It is accomplished by the use of weights which pull a part in the desired direction in the presence of countertraction.

Purposes

1. To foster and/or maintain the realignment of fractured segments of a bone.
2. To prevent deformities from resulting in the presence of injury or inflammation.
   a. Fractures
   b. Arthritis
   c. Trauma
3. To correct existing deformities.
   a. Congenital dislocation of the hip
   b. Flexion contractures of the knees
4. To lessen muscle spasm.

5. To immobilize a part.
6. To reduce dislocation.

Types of Traction

1. Skin traction
   a. Used for younger children when the condition of the skin is good and mild forces of traction are sufficient.
   b. Traction is applied to the skin of the affected body part:
      (1) Moleskin, adhesive, or foam rubber extensions are fastened firmly to the skin.
      (2) Elastic bandages are applied to hold them in place.
      (3) Weights are attached to the extensions by cords which pass over one or more pulleys.
2. Skeletal traction
   a. Used in children when greater traction force is required or if the skin is damaged.
   b. Force is exerted against the bone by means of a

metallic device such as a pin, wire, or Crutchfield tongs.

3. Traction may be continuous or intermittent, depending on its purpose.

a. Continuous traction cannot be interrupted for dressing or other activities.

b. Intermittent traction may be temporarily disconnected as specified by the physician.

Guidelines: Care of a Child in Traction

Equipment

Strips of moleskin
Adhesive tape
Elastic bandages
Square wooden blocks
Ropes, weights, pulleys
Traction bars
Slings

Procedure

Nursing Action	Rationale / Amplification
1. Explain the procedure to the child and his parents.	1. If the traction is to be effective, it is essential that the parents understand the procedure and cooperate while the child is in traction.
2. Maintain even, constant traction:	2. Traction must be kept constant in order to achieve the desired results. Any change in the amount of weights or countertraction affects the entire traction system.
a. Do not add or remove weights.	
b. Allow the weights to hang free at all times. Do not allow them to touch the floor or bed.	
c. Be certain that the ropes are in the wheel grooves of the pulleys.	
d. Keep the weights out of the child's reach.	
e. Wrap knotted areas of the ropes with adhesive tape to prevent slipping.	
f. Do not elevate the head or foot of the bed without consulting the physician.	
g. Supervise the child's position so that the purpose of the traction is accomplished.	

3. Check for disturbance of circulation by observing:
   a. Skin color—for redness, pallor, cyanosis
   b. Joint motion
   c. Skin temperature
   d. Tingling, numbness
   e. Swelling
	3. Compare the affected extremity with the unaffected one.

4. Provide skin care.	4. Immobilized children readily develop areas of pressure unless meticulous skin care is provided.
a. Pad bony prominences (ankles) with cotton padding before wrapping with elastic bandages.	a. Protects skin from injury.
b. Wash and dry all exposed areas thoroughly.	
c. Massage the child's back and sacral area at least 2–3 times daily. If indicated, apply cornstarch.	c. Cornstarch absorbs moisture and prevents maceration of the skin.
d. Inspect the heels, ankles, popliteal space, and top of the foot for signs of pressure from elastic bandages.	d. These are the areas most prone to breakdown.
e. Keep the linen clean, and free from wrinkles and crumbs.	e. When a large bed is used, 2 folded sheets are often more easily managed than 1 large sheet. One is used to cover the upper half of the bed, and 1 to cover the lower half. This facilitates changing the bed and makes the procedure less uncomfortable for the child.
f. Do not allow any traction cords to dig into the child's skin.	
g. Utilize a fracture bedpan.	g. This is less awkward and more comfortable for the child.
5. Plan for short periods of muscle exercise every day. a. Encourage the child to move and exercise his unaffected extremities.	5. Disuse of muscles can result in atrophy and deformities.

(continued)

Guidelines: Care of a Child in Traction (continued)

Procedure
(Cont.)

<table>
<tr><th>Nursing Action</th><th>Rationale/Amplification</th></tr>
<tr><td>

b. Provide diversional therapy that requires the use of these muscles.

c. Assist the child to exercise his toes.

6. Have the child breathe deeply at intervals. Provide him with soap bubbles, whistles, or party favors to make this more fun. An older child may use blow bottles.

7. Keep a record of the child's intake and output and do periodic urinalyses.

8. Provide a diet high in fiber and fluids (especially fruit juices) and low in calcium.

9. Provide daily diversion and encourage the child's family to visit frequently.

a. Attempt to replace the lost activity with another form of motion.

b. Suspend toys over the child's head so he can reach them. (Punching bag can help child relieve hostility.)

c. Provide continuing education for the school-age child.

d. Encourage projects that will allow child a feeling of accomplishment: painting, puzzles, knitting, ceramics.

e. Patients who are immobilized in traction or casts should be grouped together.

10. If not contraindicated, supply the child with an overhead trapeze.

11. Record:

a. Color, temperature, and appearance of the affected extremity

b. Skin condition

c. Evidence of local edema

d. Body alignment

e. Functioning of traction ropes, weights, and pulley

f. Response of the child to therapy

12. Make certain that countertraction is provided.

a. The foot of the child's bed may have to be raised or placed on shock blocks to counteract the traction weight and prevent the child from being pulled to the end of the bed.

13. Never disturb the traction device.

14. Avoid jarring the bed or swinging the weights.

15. Do not allow the weights to hang directly over the child's body.

</td><td>

6. Prolonged periods of immobilization may cause the child to develop hypostatic pneumonia.

7. Immobilization renders the child prone to developing urinary retention and renal calculi.

8. This helps to prevent constipation and the development of renal calculi.

9. Enforced bed rest makes time pass very slowly and can be very traumatic for a small child.

a. Water play, mirrors, body games are helpful replacements. Often the child can be moved in his bed into the playroom or hall.

10. This will facilitate movement and self-help.

12. Usually, the patient's body acts as the counterweight which keeps the extremity aligned and immobilized.

a. The child's weight is often insufficient to provide countertraction.

13. If it appears to need adjustment, notify the physician.

14. This may cause pain and is upsetting to the child.

15. This is a safety precaution.

</td></tr>
</table>

Skin Traction

<table>
<tr><td>

1. Shave the area if hair is present and paint the skin with tincture of benzoin.

</td><td>

1. This allows the adhesive to grasp the skin more firmly. Benzoin also disinfects the skin, allays itching, and prevents skin breakdown under the tape.

</td></tr>
</table>

Skeletal Traction

<table>
<tr><td>

1. Treat all entry sites, pins, wires, or tongs as surgical wounds.

a. Wipe the insertion site with Betadine and apply an antibiotic ointment at least daily. Cover with a sterile 4 × 4 gauze—or

b. Dress the insertion site with a 4 × 4 sterile gauze treated with an antiseptic prescribed by the physician.

c. Check the entry site regularly for any signs of infection and to be certain that the pin has not slipped through the bone.

2. Place corks or plastic guards over the exposed ends of the pins

</td><td>

a. This is an attempt to reduce the hazard of infection along the track of the pin. Some physicians prefer to let these areas crust over or cover them with plaster.

c. Notify the physician of either of these conditions.

2. This is a safety precaution to prevent injury to the nurse or patient.

</td></tr>
</table>

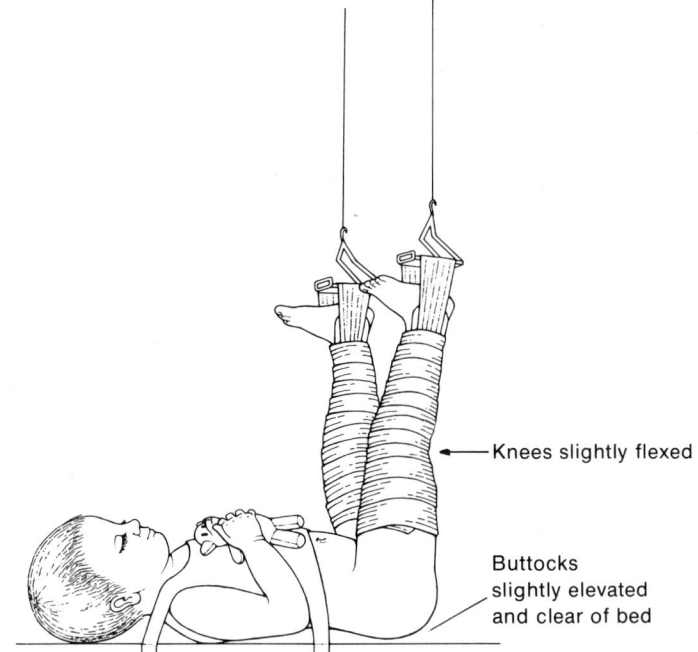

Knees slightly flexed

Buttocks
slightly elevated
and clear of bed

Figure 32-11. Bryant's traction

Procedure
(Cont.)

Nursing Action	Rationale/Amplification

Bryant's Traction (Fig. 32-11)

Purpose

Used to reduce fractured femurs in small children.

Mechanism of Action

Involves bilateral, vertical extension of the child's legs. The child's weight serves as countertraction to the vertical pull of the weights. Skin traction is applied to both legs in order to minimize potential trauma to the affected leg and maintain the stability of the position.

1. Maintain the child in the appropriate position.
   a. The legs are extended at right angles to the body.
   b. The hips are elevated slightly from the bed.
   c. The buttocks are elevated and clear of the bed.
   d. The heels and ankles are free from pressure.
   e. The child is flat in bed and unable to turn from side to side.
2. Check the position of the elastic bandages and rewrap if necessary and permitted by the physician.

1. This position is essential in order to achieve the desired results.

   e. A jacket or abdominal restraint is usually necessary.
2. The bandages should be wrapped snugly around the legs without compromising circulation. They should not slip and cause pressure on the dorsa of the feet. If rewrapping is necessary, traction must be maintained by a second person during the procedure.

Russell's Traction (Fig. 32-12)

Purpose

To reduce contractures of the knee or hip, reduce dislocated hips, immobilize the knee or hip postoperatively, or reduce fractures of the femoral shaft.

Mechanism of Action

Force is exerted on the long axis of the lower leg, and a knee sling is used under the distal thigh to provide flexion of the knee and hip.

1. Application of elastic bandages:
   a. Wrap bandages from the ankle to the thigh on patients under 18 months of age.

   a. The length of the leg from the knee to the foot is usually not long enough to maintain traction.

(continued)

Guidelines: Care of a Child in Traction (continued)

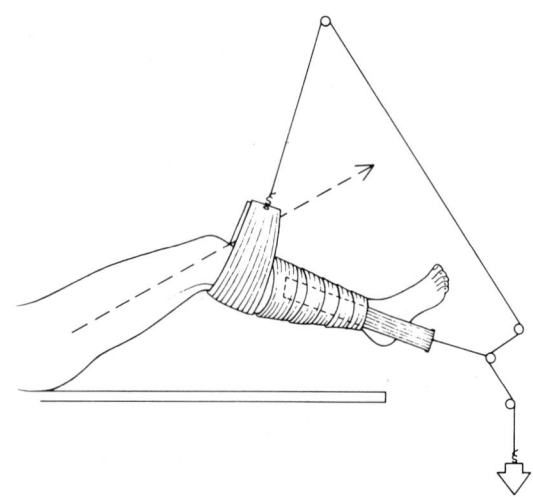

Figure 32-12. Russell's traction.

Procedure
(Cont.)

Nursing Action	Rationale/Amplification
b. Wrap bandages from the ankle to the knee on patients over 18 months of age.	b. This length in an older child is sufficient to maintain traction.
2. Place foot supports against the soles of both feet.	2. Prevents foot drop.
3. If necessary, place a small pillow under the thigh to maintain hip flexion at approximately 20 degrees.	3. Prevents hip contractures.
4. Keep the heel free of the bed.	4. Prevents pressure sore of the heel.
5. Carefully check the popliteal space for pressure sores. Make certain that the knee sling is positioned so that it does not exert pressure on the popliteal space.	5. Line the knee sling with a piece of felt or sheepskin for additional protection against pressure.
6. Make certain that the bandages do not exert pressure over the dorsalis pedis artery (inside of top of foot) or the Achilles tendon (back of heel).	6. Prevents discomfort, pressure sores, and circulatory complications.
7. Make certain that the footplate or spreader is wide enough to prevent irritation of the skin but not so wide that the tapes tend to pull from the skin	

90-Degree–90-Degree Traction (90–90 Traction) (Fig. 32-13)

Purpose
Used to reduce a fractured femur when skin traction is not adequate.

Mechanism of Action
Both the affected knee and hip are flexed at a 90-degree angle. Traction is applied by a skeletal pin drilled through the distal femur. A short leg cast or polyfoam boot is used to suspend the lower leg.

Buck's Extension

Purposes
Used to correct knee and hip contractures, to rest the leg, and for other short-term immobilization. For additional information, refer to Guidelines: Application of Buck's Extension Traction, page 835.

Balanced Traction with Thomas Splint and Pearson Attachment

Purposes
Used in older children and adolescents for fractured femurs, to rest the hip and knee, or to immobilize the hip and knee postoperatively.
Refer to Fracture of the Femur, page 823.

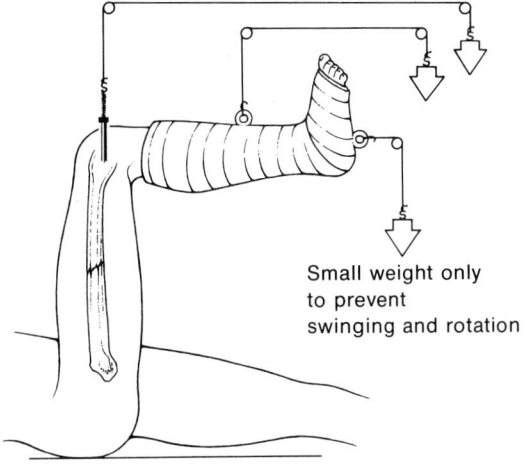

Small weight only
to prevent
swinging and rotation

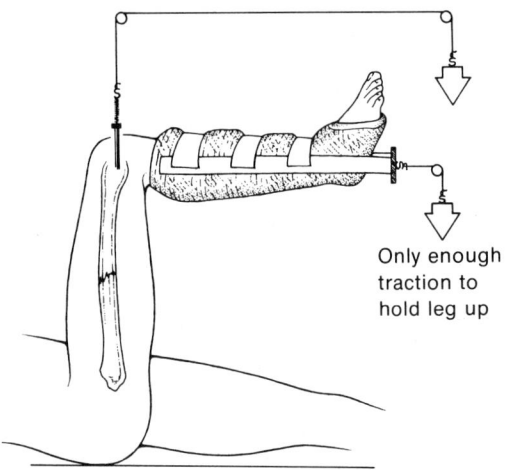

Only enough
traction to
hold leg up

Figure 32-13. 90–90 traction.

Procedure
(Cont.)

Nursing Action	Rationale / Amplification

Dunlop's Traction (Fig. 32-14)

Purpose
Used to treat fractures or injuries of the humerus, shoulder, or shoulder girdle.

Mechanism of Action
Longitudinal traction on the humerus is applied using a soft sling to pull against the forearm or using a pin drilled through the olecranon. A suspension apparatus is applied to the forearm with traction straps and an elastic bandage, using only enough weight to hold the forearm upright and the elbow just touching the bed. The elbow is kept flexed at slightly more than 90 degrees.

1. Be certain that the sling at the proximal forearm is well padded and that the margin does not create a ridge at the bend of the elbow.

2. Check the child's fingers frequently for signs of circulatory impairment. Immediately report any coldness, pallor, cyanosis, swelling, pain, or limited sensation.

1. This is a precaution to avoid pressure on the ulnar nerve.

2. Prolonged circulatory impairment may lead to ischemia and Volkmann's contraction (clawhand) and flexion at the wrist and elbow.

(continued)

Guidelines: Care of a Child in Traction (continued)

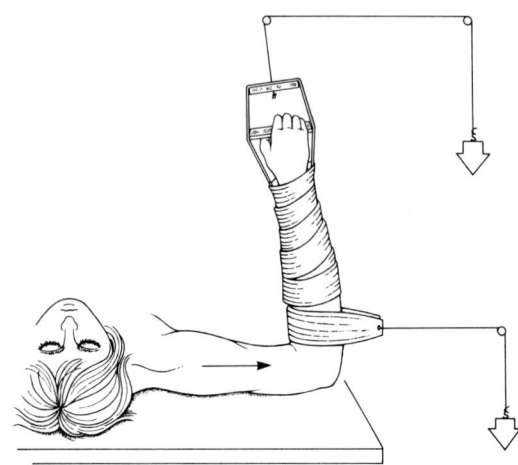

Figure 32-14. Dunlop's traction.

Procedure
(Cont.)

Nursing Action	Rationale/Amplification

Cervical Traction

Purposes
Used for children with spinal fractures, muscle spasms, or spinal injuries to provide immobilization in a neutral position that causes the least pressure on the spinal cord.

Mechanism of Action
Applied directly to the skull bone by a device such as the Crutchfield tong, or indirectly by using a head halter.

Cervical Skin (Head Halter) Traction (Fig. 32-15)

1. Check the position of the head halter frequently:
   a. The halter should not press on the ears.
   b. The rope should not rest against the skin.
   c. The chin piece should not press on the throat.
   d. Protect the chin halter when feeding the child.

2. Keep the position of the bed flat unless otherwise prescribed by the physician. Avoid lifting the child's head or flexing the neck.

3. Keep the child flat on his back.

4. Diversion
   a. Position an adjustable mirror at the head of the bed so that the child can see around the room.
   b. Encourage companionship:
      (1) Place the child in a room with other children his age.
      (2) Allow liberal visiting by parents, older siblings and friends.
   c. Place colorful objects, cards, pictures, etc. within sight of the child.
   d. Utilize audiovisual stimulation—records, radio, television, etc.
   e. Provide for continuing education for the child of school age.

Rationale:

1. It is important to prevent continuous pressure and rubbing on these areas in order to avoid skin breakdown.

2. Raising the head increases countertraction, which may be undesirable.

Cervical Skeletal Traction

1. If possible, place the child on a Stryker frame or CircOlectric bed.

2. Make certain that the neck is held in steady longitudinal traction.
   When the child is lying on his abdomen, support his arms on pillows at his sides and at the level of the bed.

Rationale:

1. Allows the child to be turned in one motion.

2. The neck should never be flexed since this may cause permanent spinal cord injury.
   The head should be in a neutral position in relation to the spine. The arms should not droop and the shoulders should not be hunched.

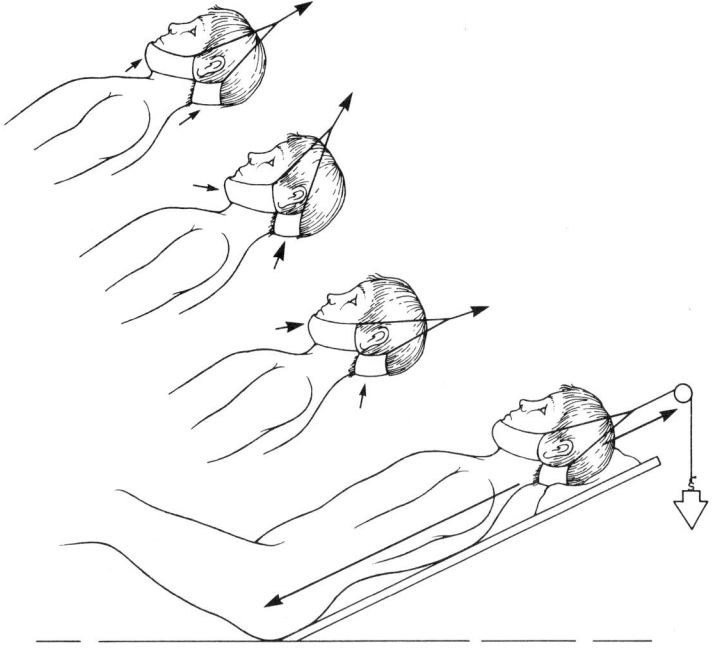

Figure 32-15. Cervical traction.

Procedure
(Cont.)

Nursing Action	Rationale/Amplification
3. Do not allow the patient to reach for objects.	3. Reaching can disrupt spinal alignment.
4. Provide the child with adjustable mirrors at the head of the bed, and with prism glasses.	4. These aids enable the child to look around the room, watch television, or read while on his back.
5. Brush the child's teeth and frequently rinse his mouth with an antiseptic mouthwash. 　a. Instruct the child to try not to breathe through his mouth since this may cause dryness of the mucosa. 　b. Apply lemon–glycerin or a lip balm to his lips to prevent dryness and cracking	5. This prevents mouth sores and is refreshing.

Cotrel's Traction

Purpose

To provide traction to the spine prior to surgery or to the application of a scoliotic brace.

Mechanism of Action

Traction is applied primarily to the occipital bone by means of a head harness which fits onto the chin and reaches around to the occiput. Pelvic straps maintain the pelvis in a fixed position.

1. Check the head halter for proper placement. 　a. The chin pad should not compress the child's throat. 　b. The hair should be free from entanglement. 　c. The halter should not pinch the ears.	1. This helps to ensure effectiveness of the treatment and prevents skin breakdown.
2. Check the facial skin, chin, occiput, and iliac crests for possible irritation and breakdown.	
3. Check the child frequently for maintenance of alignment.	3. It is relatively easy for the child to become malaligned in this type of traction.

Halo–Femoral Traction

Purposes

Utilized to correct severe and resistant spinal curvatures, and for treatment of vertebral fractures.

Mechanism of Action

An aluminum halo is fixed to the cranium with 4 threaded pins, and Steinman pins are placed in the distal ends of the femur. Upward traction is applied to the halo and downward traction to the femurs to pull the spine into alignment.

(continued)

Guidelines: Care of a Child in Traction (continued)

Procedure
(Cont.)

<table>
<tr><td align="center">Nursing Action</td><td align="center">Rationale/Amplification</td></tr>
</table>

Frequently, a suspension assembly is attached to the halo by threaded traction rods, the entire assembly being supported by a hoop attached to the pelvic pins. This apparatus allows control of position in all 3 planes plus progressive traction application. Femoral pins may be removed and countertraction applied by securing the halo device to a body jacket cast. This allows the child to be ambulatory.

Nursing Action	Rationale/Amplification
1. Prepare the child and the parents for the procedure.	1. The appearance of the apparatus may be overwhelming and frightening. Diagrams and visual aids will enhance comprehension and allay fear.
a. Explain the purpose, method of application, and approximate time required for the therapy. The child should know that the treatment is relatively pain-free and that the device does not penetrate the brain.	
b. If possible, introduce the child to other patients in the apparatus or those who have previously experienced it.	
c. Emphasize that this will provide optimal correction of the deformity and allow the child to appear more normal	c. These children are often very sensitive about their body image, and will develop a more positive attitude if they realize that the deformity is being improved.

2. Observe the child carefully while traction is being increased for:
  a. Neck pain
  b. Respiratory distress
  c. Nerve injury
	2. Alteration of neurologic or respiratory status is regarded as a warning sign and a release of several turns on the extension bars may be carried out by the physician as an emergency measure. Neck pain is a less serious sign. The amount of traction is usually not increased until the pain disappears.

3. *Symptoms of injury*
  a. Spinal cord
    (1) Weakness, numbness in legs
    (2) Loss of bladder function
    (3) Up- or downturning of toes
    (4) Clonus of ankles or knees
  b. Cranial nerves
    (1) Double vision
    (2) Difficulty in swallowing
    (3) Difficulty in coughing
    (4) Voice changes
    (5) Tongue weakness
  c. Upper extremities
    (1) Difficulty in moving hand, shoulder, or arm
    (2) Numbness or weakness in hand (check grip)	

4. Make certain that all of the fixtures on the apparatus are tightened.	4. Looseness and excessive movement of the apparatus may cause pain and infection. The physician should be notified.
5. Report complaints of pain or drainage at the pin sites.	5. Most children have mild pain and headache for the first few days. Thereafter, pain at the pin site usually means that the pin is loose or infected, and it may be necessary to change the pin.
6. Have an Allen wrench and torque wrench available.	6. The Allen wrench is used to release vest bolts quickly if CPR is necessary. The torque wrench is used to adjust the amount of traction on the bars.

Guidelines: Assisting the Child on a Bradford Frame

A *Bradford frame* is a piece of equipment that facilitates the nursing of young children who must be immobilized for extensive periods of time. It is frequently used for young infants with meningoceles, children in hip-spica casts, and children with extensive burns.

Purposes
1. To ensure correct positioning.
2. To facilitate the collection of urine and stools.
3. To protect the child from injury.

Equipment

Frame of appropriate size for the child
2 pieces of canvas of appropriate size to cover the head and foot of the frame

Equipment
(Cont.)

Plastic sheeting
2 crib sheets or draw sheets
Bedboard
Linen for the bed
Plastic drawsheet
Heavy blocks for supporting the frame
Material such as canvas strips for attaching the frame to the bed
Protective device to limit the child's movement

Procedure

Nursing Action	Rationale/Amplification
Preparatory Phase	
1. Select frame according to the size of the child.	1. Frame should be approximately 15 cm. (6 inches) longer and 5 cm. (2 inches) wider than the patient.

2. Cover the head and foot areas with canvas.
  a. Leave an open area between the head and foot sections for the drainage of urine and feces.
  b. Stretch the canvas tightly over the frame.
	
	  a. Make sure that the size of the opening is adequate for the size of the child.
	  b. If the canvas is not tight, it will stretch.

3. Cover the top and bottom sections of the canvas with heavy plastic sheeting.	3. This protects the canvas from becoming soiled.
4. Place a small sheet tightly over each section of the frame.	
Performance Phase	
1. Place a bedboard on the mattress.	1. A firm base is required for proper use of the frame.
2. Place 2 draw sheets on the bed, 1 at each end.	2. The entire bed will not require changing when only one part is soiled.
3. Place a plastic draw sheet under the center opening of the frame.	3. This is the area most likely to become soiled by urine or feces.
4. Place blocks on the bed. Place the frame on the blocks.	4. The position of the blocks and frame will be prescribed by the physician. The blocks should always be placed under the child's shoulders, never directly under his head if the head of the frame is to be elevated.
5. Secure the frame to the bed at the head and foot.	5. This is a safety precaution to prevent slipping.

6. Place the bedpan below the center opening.
  a. Plastic sheeting may be draped over the top and bottom edges of the opening of the frame.
  b. Place diapers over the plastic.
	
	  a. This permits urine and feces to drain into the bedpan if the child is incontinent.
	  b. This prevents irritation of the skin.

7. Place the child on the frame. a. Maintain his position by use of a jacket restraint. (See procedure for protective measures to limit movement.)	
8. Place pillows at the sides of the frame to support the child's arms.	8. It is important to maintain proper body alignment.
Follow-up Phase	

1. Check the following frequently:
  a. Position of the frame on the blocks.
  b. Security of all knots and materials which are used to fasten the frame to the bed.
  c. Position of the child on the frame.
	1. These are principles of safety (see procedure for protective devices to limit movement).

2. Provide meticulous general hygiene:
  a. Empty the bedpan frequently.
  b. Check the linen for soiling by urine or feces and change it if necessary.
  c. Cleanse the buttocks after each bowel movement and apply lotion or cornstarch.
  d. Bathe daily and provide skin care frequently.
	2. See procedure for traction and for care of a child in a spica cast.

3. Provide for the prevention of contractures, muscle wasting, and the development of hypostatic pneumonia.	3. See procedure for traction.
4. Provide diversion. Move the child's bed from room to room for a change of scenery or out into the hall so that he can watch unit activities.	4. See procedures for traction and care of a child in a spica cast.

(continued)

Guidelines: Assisting the Child on a Bradford Frame (continued)

Procedure
(Cont.)

Nursing Action	Rationale/Amplification

5. Reconstruct the child's frame as necessary.
  a. The child can usually be placed on a firm bed or stretcher while his frame is being changed.
  b. If a second frame is available, this can be prepared and placed on another bed. The child can then be easily transferred from one frame to another.
	a. Special care must be taken to ensure correct body alignment during this procedure.

Casts

Nursing Considerations

Nursing activities related to the application and care of casts are essentially the same for pediatric and adult patients. The following points of consideration are important.

1. The child is usually more troubled by immobilization than the adult. A special attempt should be made to ensure that his activities are as normal as possible and that full use is made of his unaffected joints and muscles.
2. The younger child may not be able to understand why the cast is necessary. He may attempt to remove it, put pieces of toys or food under it, etc.
   a. An attempt should be made to allow the child to work through his questions and feelings via play (e.g., give him a doll with a cast).
   b. Close supervision is necessary to prevent the child from destroying the cast or injuring himself.
3. There is danger of soiling a long-leg or hip-spica cast with feces or urine. (The area of the cast near the buttocks and genitalia should be protected with waterproof material.)
4. Children may be especially frightened by removal of the cast. They often think of the cast as part of their body and may be helped by analogies of having fingernails or hair cut. Age-appropriate explanations and demonstration should be provided (refer to adult section, p. 830).
5. Parents should be instructed in care following cast removal. Daily soaking of the area may be necessary to remove desquamated skin and secretions. Oil or lotion may provide comfort. Exercises should be done as prescribed to increase strength and function.
6. For additional information, including types of casts, methods of application, complications, etc., refer to pages 828–833.

Guidelines: Care of a Child in a Spica Cast

Procedure

Nursing Action	Rationale/Amplification
1. If possible, prepare the child for the application of the cast.	1. This can best be accomplished by allowing the child to put a cast on a doll. Older children should see a picture of the cast that is going to be applied and receive an explanation of the method of application.
2. Facilitate drying and accurate molding of the cast	2. About 24–48 hours are required for a cast to dry completely. A cast dries from the outside to the inside. It may feel dry to the touch but still be wet on the inside.
a. Place a bedboard under the mattress.	a. Prevents sagging of the bed from pressure of the cast.
b. Support the curves of the cast with small, plastic-covered pillows.	b. Prevents cracking while the cast is drying.
c. Avoid placing a pillow under the head and shoulders.	c. Causes pressure on the chest by thrusting it forward in the cast.
d. Keep the cast uncovered and turn the child every 1–2 hours.	d. Allows moisture to evaporate from the surface.
e. Handle moist cast with the palms of hands.	e. Fingers may cause indentation in the moist plaster.

3. Observe for complications resulting from pressure of the cast.
  a. Impaired circulation to the toes
    (1) Discoloration or cyanosis
    (2) Impaired movement
    (3) Loss of sensation
    (4) Edema
	3. Vascular insufficiency due to unrelieved swelling can cause necrosis and pressure sores. It may be necessary to bivalve the cast.

Procedure
(Cont.)

Nursing Action	Rationale/Amplification

(5) Temperature change
(6) Absent pedal pulses
  b. Complaints of pain or pressure in any area where the cast fits closely over the body.

4. Provide good skin care.
  a. Bathe accessible skin and massage with emollient lotion. Pay special attention to the buttocks and genital area.
  b. Massage the skin underneath the cast with alcohol.
  c. Inspect the skin for signs of irritation:
    (1) Around cast edge.
    (2) Under the cast—pull skin taut and inspect under the cast, using a flashlight for illumination.
  d. Investigate complaints of pain or burning or an offensive odor from the inside of the cast.

  e. Relieve itching by blowing cool air through the cast with an asepto syringe or hair dryer.

  f. Do not allow a small child to put objects inside his cast.
    (1) Keep small toys away from the child.
    (2) Pad the edges of the cast with cotton padding or cover cast with a towel to prevent food particles and foreign objects from being inserted by the child.

5. Prevent the skin around the edge of the cast from becoming excoriated.
  a. Smooth the edges of the cast and petal it with waterproof adhesive tape.

  b. Do not lift infants by their legs to change diapers.

6. Prevent urine and feces from soiling the cast.
  a. Offer the bedpan frequently.
    (1) Elevate the child's head slightly higher than his feet to prevent urine from running under the cast.
    (2) Place a sheet of plastic under the front and back edges of the cast opening for the buttocks and genitalia.
    (3) Slip the fracture pan beneath the buttocks.
    (4) Allow the ends of the plastic strips to hang into the pan.
  b. Place the child who is not toilet-trained on a Bradford frame.
    (1) See procedure for care of the child on a Bradford frame, page 1206.
    (2) Line the edges of the cast with waterproof material such as plastic or cellophane.
    (3) Tuck a folded diaper or perineal pad under the cast edges and change it frequently.
  c. Keep the perineum clean
    (1) Wash the skin under the edge of the cast whenever necessary and dry it thoroughly.
    (2) Change diapers immediately after they become soiled.
  d. Clean the cast by rubbing it with a small amount of scouring agent on a damp cloth, then dry it promptly.

7. Plan for short periods of muscle exercise every day.
  a. Encourage the child to move and exercise his unaffected extremities. Provide diversional therapy that requires the use of these muscles.
  b. Exercise the child's toes.

8. Have the child breathe deeply at intervals. Provide him with soap bubbles, whistles, or party favors to make this more fun. An older child may use blow bottles.

Rationale/Amplification

4. Prevents the development of pressure sores.

  d. These may indicate that a pressure sore is forming or has become infected. It may be necessary to create a "window" in the cast.
  e. Some physicians insert a strip of gauze through the cast which can be used to gently massage the skin. Do not use sharp objects such as coat hangers or knitting needles.
  f. A small hand vacuum cleaner may be used to remove crumbs from inside the cast.

  a. This prevents flakes of plaster from breaking off and slipping under the cast. It also facilitates cleansing of the cast.

6. A soiled cast will cause skin irritation, become odorous, and may mildew or partially disintegrate.

  d. A solution of zephiran chloride 1:750 may be used sparingly to eliminate odor-causing bacteria from cast.

7. Disuse of muscles can result in atrophy and deformities.

8. Prolonged periods of immobilization may cause the child to develop hypostatic pneumonia.

(continued)

Guidelines: Care of a Child in a Spica Cast (continued)

Procedure
(Cont.)

Nursing Action	Rationale/Amplification

9. Turn the child at least every 4 hours.
   a. Move the child to the side of the bed, using a steady, pulling motion.
   b. Place 1 hand under the head and back and 1 hand under the leg portion of the cast, and turn the child on his side.
   c. Second nurse accepts support of the child and cast as he is turned completely.
	9. Do not use the supporting bar between the legs as a lever when turning the child.

10. Assess the child's bowel and bladder function.
   a. Provide an adequate fluid intake, especially fruit juices.
   b. Check the urine for signs of infection.
	10. Immobilization may cause constipation and poor urinary drainage. Suppositories or mild laxatives may be necessary for the constipated child.

11. Maintain correct position of the cast. a. Support the contour of the cast with pillows. Allow the heel to extend beyond the pillow to avoid pressure sores.	11. This prevents cracking or flattening of the cast.

12. Provide as normal an environment as possible.
   a. Place the child on a cart or a stretcher so that he may leave his room. The child may be taken outdoors if the weather is suitable.
   b. Allow the child to be dressed. (Wide, flared pants are especially suitable.)
   c. Encourage contact with peers.
   d. Provide for play activities.
     (1) Provide the young child with large toys which he cannot put into his cast.
     (2) Television is a good method of diversion if used with discretion.
     (3) Older children often enjoy checkers, sewing, art work, building models, etc.
   e. Provide for education.
     (1) Refer the child to a visiting teacher service.
     (2) Provide for study time during each day.
	12. Enforced immobility is often traumatic for the child and may cause regression.

13. Evaluate the home situation for feasibility of home care.
   a. The child's place in the family and the number of siblings.
   b. Additional needs of the parents, such as pursuing their vocations.
   c. Physical setup of the home
   d. Financial situation
   e. Ability of the family to keep follow-up appointments	

14. Assist the family in caring for the child after discharge.
   a. Initiate the appropriate referrals.
     (1) Community health nurse
     (2) Social service agency
     (3) Home tutoring service
     (4) Physical therapy
   b. Begin teaching early.
     (1) Instruct the parent on all aspects of the child's care.
	(1) Teach only a few aspects of care each day. Have the parent(s) participate in the child's care until capable of providing total nursing care under supervision.

(2) Emphasize safety measures such as elevating the child's head during meals to prevent choking; preventing the small child from dropping objects into his cast; using good body mechanics when lifting and transporting the child, etc. (3) Provide with detailed, written instructions.	

15. Assist with cast removal.
   a. Prepare the child for the procedure.
     (1) Describe the sensations that the child will feel (warmth, vibration, etc.) as well as the procedure itself.
     (2) Allow the child to observe as the saw is lightly touched to the operator's palm.
	15. Children often believe that the saw will cut off an extremity, and are frightened by the loud noise.

Procedure
(Cont.)

Nursing Action	Rationale/Amplification
b. Immobilize the child as necessary so that the procedure can be carried out quickly and safely.	
16. Care for the child after cast removal.	
a. Support the part with pillows	a. Maintain the same position that existed in the cast.
b. Move the extremity gently.	b. It will be very weak and stiff.
c. Wash the skin gently with mild soap and apply oil or lanolin.	c. An accumulation of sebaceous material and dead skin causes the skin to appear brown and flaky. Vigorous rubbing will cause skin trauma.
d. Encourage the child to do prescribed exercises.	d. These will strengthen muscles and relieve joint stiffness.
e. Elevate the extremity when sitting.	e. Minimizes the development of edema.

Bibliography

Books

General

Avery GB (ed). Neonatology, 2nd ed. Philadelphia, JB Lippincott, 1981

Cole C. The Harriet Lane Handbook, 10th ed. Chicago, Year Book Medical Publishers, 1984

Droske S and Francis S. Pediatric Diagnostic Procedures. New York, John Wiley & Sons, 1981

Fletcher MA, McDonald MG and Avery GB (eds). Atlas of Procedures in Neonatology. Philadelphia, JB Lippincott, 1983

Gellis S and Kagan B (eds). Current Pediatric Therapy, vol 10. Philadelphia, WB Saunders, 1982

Hughes W and Buescher E. Pediatric Procedures. Philadelphia, WB Saunders, 1981

King E, Wieck L and Dyer M. Pediatric Nursing Procedures. Philadelphia, JB Lippincott, 1983

Leifer G. Principles and Techniques in Pediatric Nursing. Philadelphia, WB Saunders, 1982

Levin D, Morriss F and Moore G. A Practical Guide to Pediatric Intensive Care, 2nd ed. St Louis, CV Mosby, 1984

Nursing Pediatric Patients—Nursing Photobook. Nursing 82 Books, Intermed Communications, Inc. Springhouse, PA, 1982

Nussbaum E (ed). Pediatric Intensive Care. Mt Kisco, New York, Futura, 1983

Pikl B (ed). Massachusetts General Hospital Manual of Pediatric Nursing Practice. Boston, Little, Brown & Co, 1981

Schreiner RL. Care of the Newborn. New York, Rowen Press, 1981

Scipien G et al. Comprehensive Pediatric Nursing, 2nd ed. New York, McGraw-Hill, 1979

Sheldon RE, and Dominiak PS. The Expanding Role of the Nurse in Neonatal Intensive Care. New York, Grune & Stratton, 1980

Shirkey HC. Pediatric Therapy, 6th ed. St Louis, CV Mosby, 1980

Silver H, Kempe CH and Bruyn H. Handbook of Pediatrics, 14th ed. Los Altos, Lange Medical Publications, 1983

Smith J. Pediatric Critical Care. New York, John Wiley & Sons, 1983

Whaley LF and Wong DL. Nursing Care of Infants and Children. St Louis, CV Mosby, 1983

Whitson B and McFarlane J. The Pediatric Nursing Skills Manual. New York, John Wiley and Sons, 1980

Wong DL and Whaley LF. Clinical Handbook of Pediatric Nursing. St Louis, CV Mosby, 1981

Winters RW. Principles of Pediatric Fluid Therapy, 2nd ed. Boston, Little, Brown & Co, 1982

Vital Signs

Assessing Vital Signs Accurately (Nursing Skillbook Series). Horsham, Intermed Communications, 1978

Medications

Sager DP and Bomar SK. Intravenous Medications. Philadelphia, JB Lippincott, 1980

Feeding and Nutrition

Kitzinger S. The Experience of Breastfeeding. New York, Penguin Books, 1980

Lawrence RA. Breast-Feeding. A Guide for the Medical Profession, 2nd ed. St Louis, CV Mosby, 1985

Fluid and Electrolyte Balance

Burgess A. The Nurse's Guide to Fluid and Electrolyte Balance. New York, McGraw-Hill, 1979

Finberg L et al. Water and Electrolytes in Pediatrics: Physiology, Pathophysiology and Treatment. Philadelphia, WB Saunders, 1982

Gans SC. Surgical Pediatrics—Nonoperative Care. New York, Grune & Stratton, 1980

Kerner J (ed). Manual of Pediatric Parenteral Nutrition. New York, John Wiley and Sons, 1983

Metheny N and Snively W. Nurses'

Handbook of Fluid Balance, 4th ed. Philadelphia, JB Lippincott, 1983

Monitoring Fluids and Electrolytes Precisely (Nursing Skillbook Series). Horsham, Intermed Communications, 1978

Winters R. Principles of Pediatric Fluid Therapy, 2nd ed. Boston, Little Brown & Co, 1982

Dialysis

Gutch C and Stoner M. Review of Hemodialysis for Nurses and Dialysis Personnel, 4th ed. St Louis, CV Mosby, 1983

Chest Physical Therapy and Respiratory Measures

Lough M, Doershuk C and Stern R (eds). Pediatric Respiratory Therapy, 3rd ed. Chicago, Year Book Medical Publishers, 1985

Luce J, Tyler M and Pierson D. Intensive Respiratory Care. Philadelphia, WB Saunders, 1983

Mosher K and Spragg R. Respiratory Emergencies, 2nd ed. St Louis, CV Mosby, 1982

Providing Respiratory Care. (Nursing Photobook Series). Horsham, PA, Intermed Communications, 1979

Rattenborg C and Via-Reque E. Clinical Use of Mechanical Ventilation. Chicago, Year Book Medical Publishers, 1981

Using Monitors. (Nursing Photobook Series). Horsham, PA, Intermed Communications, 1981

Wade J. Respiratory Nursing Care: Physiology and Technique, 3rd ed. St Louis, CV Mosby, 1982

Cardiopulmonary Resuscitation

Dazé A and Scanlon J. Code Pink: A Practical System for Neonatal/Perinatal Resuscitation. Baltimore, University Park Press, 1981

Traction and Casts

Lewis R. Handbook of Traction, Casting and Splinting Techniques. Philadelphia, JB Lippincott, 1977

Rang M. Children's Fractures. Philadelphia, JB Lippincott, 1983

Williams P. Orthopedic Management in Childhood. St Louis, CV Mosby, 1982

Articles

Vital Signs

Adams F and Landaw E. What are healthy blood pressures for children? Pediatrics 1981 Aug; 68(2):268–270

Barrus D. A comparison of rectal and axillary temperatures by electronic thermometer measurement in preschool children. Pediatr Nurs 1983 Nov/Dec; 9(6):424–426

Britton C. Blood pressure measurement and hypertension in children. Pediatr Nurs 1981 July/Aug; 7(4):13–17

Eoff M and Joyce B. Temperature measurements in children. Am J Nurs 1981 May; 81(5):1010–1011

Haddock N. Blood pressure monitoring in neonates. MCN 1980 Mar/Apr; 5(2): 131–135

Hasler M and Cohen J. The effect of oxygen administration on oral temperature assessment. Nurs Res 1982 Sept/Oct; 31(5):265–268

Hill M. What can go wrong when you measure blood pressure. Am J Nurs 1980 May; 80(5):942–946

How to take your child's temperature. Patient Care 1980 Sep 30; 14(16):141–148

Kirkendall W, Feinleib M and Mark AL. American Heart Association recommendations for human blood pressure determination by sphygmomanometer. Circulation 1980 Nov; 62(5):1145A–1155A

Pituch D and Klein M. Axillary or rectal temperatures in children? Lancet 1981 Jul 4; 2(8236):43

Scharping E. Physiological measurements of the neonate—methods for accurately measuring vital signs are constantly being refined. MCN 1983 Jan/Feb; 8(1):70–73

Schiffman R. Temperature monitoring in the neonate: A comparison of axillary and rectal temperatures. Nurs Res 1982 Sept/Oct; 31(5):274–277

Shann F and Mackenzie A. Axillary or rectal temperatures in children? Lancet 1981 Aug 8; 2(8241):310

Fever

Levi M. On managing the febrile child. Emerg Med 1981 Dec 15; 13(21):114–115+

McCarthy PL et al. History and observation variables in assessing febrile children. Pediatrics 1980 June; 65(6):1090–1095

Schmitt B. Fever phobia: Misconceptions of parents about fevers. Am J Dis Child 1980 Feb; 134(2):176–181

Yaffe S. Management of fever in infants and children, pp. 225–233. In Lipton J (ed) Fever. New York, Raven Press, 1980

Medications

Bergeson PS, Singer SA and Kaplan AM. Intramuscular injections in children. Pediatrics 1982 Dec; 70(6):944–948

Drehobl P. Quadriceps contracture. Am J Nurs 1980 Sept; 80(9):1650–1651

Evans MC and Hansen BD.

Administering injections to different-aged children. MCN 1981 May/Jun; 6(3):194–199

Funk MJ, Mullins LL and Olson RA. Teaching children to swallow pills: A case study. Child Health Care 1984 Summer; 13(1):20–23

Lenz CL. Make your needle selection right to the point. Nurs 1983 Feb; 13(2):50–51

Rimar JM. Guidelines for the intravenous administration of medications used in pediatrics. MCN 1982 May/Jun; 7(3):184–187

Rimar JM. Sticking little muscles. Emerg Med 1983 May 15; 15(9):185–186+

Tureo SJ. Basic concepts in IV therapy. Am J IV Ther Clinic Nutr 1980 Jun; Spec issue:13–16+

Protective Devices to Limit Movement

Misik J. About using restraints—with restraint. Nursing '81 1981 Aug; 11(8): 50–55

Feeding and Nutrition

Albers RM. Emotional Support for the breast-feeding mother. Issues in Compr Pediatr Nurse. 1981 Mar/Apr; 5(2):109–124

Anderson GC et al. Development of sucking in term infants from birth to four hours postbirth. Res Nurs Health 1982 Mar; 5(1):21–27

Beer AE and Billingham RE. Immunology and the breast. Perinat/Neonatol 1981 Jan/Feb; 5(1):13–14+

Broome ME. Breastfeeding and the working mother. JOGN Nurs 1981 May/Jun; 10(2):201–202

Burd B. Encouragement counts in breast feeding. Am J Nurs 1981 Aug; 81(8): 1491

Field T et al. Nonnutritive sucking during tube feedings: Effects on preterm neonates in an intensive care unit. Pediatrics 1982 Sep; 70(3):381–384

Gartner C. Nourishment for the critically ill child. Emerg Med 1980 Apr 15; 12(7):133–135+

Gasson JE. Feeding stomas: Gastrostomy and jejunostomy. Part I: Surgical procedures and complications. Clin Gastroenterol 1982 May; 11(2):337–344

Grinde JG and Volden C. Gastrointestinal intubation. Crit Care Update 1982 Mar; 9(3):5–12

Lawrence RA. Practices and attitudes toward breast-feeding among medical professionals. Pediatrics 1982 Dec; 70(6):912–920

Leonard LG. Breastfeeding twins. JOGN Nurs 1982 May/Jun; 11(3):148–153

McDonald E et al. A Comparison of four holding devices for anchoring nasogastric tubes. J Neurosurg Nurs 1982 Feb; 14(1):90–93

Measel CP. A practical popular pacifier. Crit Care Nurs 1983 Mar/Apr; 3(2):47–48

Riordan J. The ill breastfeeding child. In Riordan J. A Practical Guide to Breastfeeding. St Louis, CV Mosby, 1983, pp. 157–170

Riordan J and Countryman BA. Basics of

breastfeeding Part II: The anatomy and psychophysiology of lactation. JOGN Nurs 1980 Jul/Aug; 9(4):210–213; Part III: The biological specificity of breast milk. JOGN Nurs 1980 Sept/Oct; 9(5):273–277; Part IV: Preparation for breastfeeding and early optimal functioning. Sep/Oct; 9(5):277–283; Part V: Self-care for continued breast feeding. 357–361; Part VI: Some breastfeeding problems and solutions. JOGN Nurs 1980 Nov/Dec; 9(6):361–366

Schlegel AM. Observations on breast-feeding technique: Fact and fallacies. MCN 1983 May/Jun; 8(3):204–208

Shepherd SC and Yarrow RE. Breastfeeding and the working mother. J Nurse–Midwife 1982 Nov/Dec; 27(6):16–20

Stevens PJ. Feeding stomas: Gastrostomy and jejunostomy. Part 2: Stoma care. Clin Gastroenterol 1982 May; 11(2): 345–350

Taylor LS. Newborn feeding behaviors and attaching. MCN 1981 May/Jun; 6(3):201–202

Specimen Collection

Hutton NM and Schreiner RL. Urine collection in the neonate. JOGN Nurs 1980 May/Jun; 9(3):165–169

Robinson GS. Techs, tots and fingersticks—without fear. Med Lab Observer 1983 Apr; 15(4):105–106

Shetler M. Collection and handling of specimens. Crit Care Update 1981 Dec 8; (12):26–34

Stevens DC, Schreiner RL and Gresham EL. Suprapubic bladder aspiration in the neonate. Perinatol Neonatol 1981 Jan/Feb; 5(1):47–50

Strohbach ME and Kratina SH. Diaper versus bag specimens: A comparison of urine specific gravity values. MCN 1982 May/Jun; 7(3):198–201

Fluid and Electrolyte Balance

Felver L. Understanding the electrolyte maze. Am J Nurs 1980 Sep; 80(9): 1591–1595

Glaeseman P. Pediatric fluid and electrolyte requirements. DCCN 1983 Sept/Oct; 2(5):280–284

Lander JD. Nursing care of children with fluid and electrolyte disorders. Issues Compr Pediatr Nurs 1980 Apr; 4(2): 41–52

McGrath B. Fluids, electrolytes and replacement therapy in pediatric nursing. MCN 1980 Jan/Feb; 5(1):58–62

Perkins R and Levin D. Common fluid and electrolyte problems in a pediatric intensive care unit. Pediatr Clin North Am 1980 Aug; 27(3):567–586

Wink D. Fluid induced hyponatremia in infancy: A preventable problem. Am J Nurs 1983 May; 83(5):765–767

Intravenous Infusion

Haessler R. Transparent I.V. dressings vs. traditional dressings. NITA 1983 May/Jun; 6(3):169–170

Huey F. Using the machines—setting up

and trouble shooting. Am J Nurs 1983 Jul; 83(7):1026–1028

Marshall J. Pediatric nursing considerations in intravenous therapy. NITA 1981 Nov/Dec; 4(6):404–405

Parent B. Are in-line IV filters really worthwhile? Nursing '81 1981 Aug; 81(8):58–60

Peterson PJ et al. Use of a transparent polyurethane dressing for peripheral intravenous catheter care. NITA 1982 Nov/Dec; 5(6):387–390

Piercy S. A care plan that really works for children on long-term I.V. therapy. Nursing '81 1981; 81(9):66–69

Poundstone W. Spotlight on neonatal infusion. Perinatol Neonatol 1982 Jul/Aug; 6(4):91+

Recommended standards of practices, policies, and procedures for intravenous therapy. National Coordinating Committee on Large Volume Parenterals. Am J of Hospital Pharmacy 1980 May; 37(5):660–663

Steel J. Too fast or too slow—The erratic I.V. Am J Nurs 1983 Jun; 83(6):898–910

Wittig P and Semmler-Bertanzi D. Pumps and controllers—A nurse's assessment guide. Am J Nurs 1983 July 83(7):1023–1025

Total Parenteral Nutrition

Bjeletick J and Kichman R. The Hickman indwelling catheter. Am J Nurs 1980 Jan; 80(1):62–65

Cannon R et al. Home parenteral nutrition in infants. J Pediatr 1980 June; 96(6):1098–1104

Fleming CR, Witzke DJ and Beart RW. Catheter-related complications in patients receiving home parenteral nutrition. Ann Surg 1980 Nov; 192(5):593–599

Heird W and Greene H. Panel report on nutritional support of pediatric patients. Am J Clin Nutr 1981 June 34(6—supplement):1223–1228

Hennessy K. HHNK Dehydration. Am J Nurs 1983 Oct; 83(10):1425–1426

Morrow A et al. Nursing care of the pediatric patient on parenteral nutrition, pp. 239–269. In Kerner J (ed). Manual of Pediatric Parenteral Nutrition. New York, John Wiley & Sons, 1983

Palidar P, Simonwitz D and Oreskovich M. Use of op-site as an occlusive dressing for total parenteral nutrition catheters. JPEN 1982 Mar/Apr; 6(2):150

Parfitt D and Thompson V. Pediatric home hyperalimentation. Educating the family. MCN 1980 May/Jun; 5(3):196–202

Sterk M. Understanding parenteral nutrition: A basis for neonatal nursing care. JOGN Nurs (Suppl) 1983 May/Jun; 12(3):455–503

Walsh E. Psychosocial aspects of pediatric parenteral nutrition, pp. 271–279. In Kerner J (ed). Manual of Pediatric Parenteral Nutrition. New York, John Wiley & Sons, 1983

Intralipids

Black CD and Popovich NG: A study of intravenous emulsion compatibility:

Effects of dextrose, amino acids, and selected electrolytes. Drug Intell Clin Pharm 1981 Mar; 15(3):184–193

Forlaw L. Parenteral nutrition in the critically ill child. Crit Care Q 1981 Mar; 3(4):1–20

Higbee KC and Lamy PP. The use of Intralipid in neonates and infants. Hosp Formul 1980 Feb; 15(2):117–119+

Hutchison MG. Administration of fat emulsions. Am J Nurs 1982 Feb; 82(2):275–277

Levene MI, Wigglesworth JS and Desai R. Pulmonary fat accumulation after intralipid infusion in preterm infant. Lancet 1980 Oct 18; 2(8199):815–818

Samson LF. Use of a premie needle. Crit Care Nurs 1982 Sept/Oct; 2(5):6

Tanner S. IV bolus leaves no room for error. RN 1981 Oct; 44(10):54–55

Exchange Transfusion

Carey B, Larson B and Goold G. A neonatal teaching tool: Working with unbilical catheters. MCN 1980 Nov/Dec; 5(6):393–397

For infant sepsis, a change for the better. Emerg Med 1981 Apr 15; 13(7):115

Vain NE et al. Role of exchange transfusion in the treatment of severe septicemia. Pediatrics 1980 Nov; 66(5):693–697

Dialysis

Binkley L. Keeping up with peritoneal dialysis. Am J Nurs 1984 Jun; 84(6):729–735

Davis V and Lavandero R. Caring for the catheter carefully . . . before, during and after peritoneal dialysis. Nursing '80 1980 Dec; 10(12):67–71

Ceccarelli C. Hemodialytic therapy for the patient with chronic renal failure. Nurs Clin North Am 1981 Sep; 16(3):531–550

Chambers J. Assessing the dialysis patient at home. Am J Nurs 1981 Apr; 81(4):750–754

Denniston D and Burns K. Home peritoneal dialysis. Am J Nurs 1980 Nov; 80(11):2022–2026

Fine R. Dialysis. In Gellis S and Kagan B (eds). Current Pediatric Therapy, vol 10. Philadelphia, WB Saunders, 1982, pp. 363–369

Gross S. Teaching young patients—and their families—about home peritoneal dialysis. Nursing '80 1980 Oct; 10(10):72–73

Grossman MB. Self-care for children and adolescents on dialysis. Am Assoc Nephrol Nurse Tech 1981 Aug; 8(4):36, 42

Sampson N. Peritoneal dialysis as a treatment modality. Nephrol Nurse 1980 Jan/Feb; 2(1):15–17

Sorrels P. Peritoneal dialysis: A rediscovery. Nurs Clin North Am 1981 Sep; 16(3):515–529

Chest Physical Therapy

Epstein MF. Neonatal and pediatric respiratory care: An update on research. Resp Care 1982 Mar; 27(3):295–297

Pryor JA et al. A comparison of

mechanical and manual percussion as adjuncts to postural drainage in the treatment of cystic fibrosis in adolescents and adults. Physiotherapy 1981 May; 67(5):140–141

Rivington-Law B. Review of literature in chest physical therapy: Dearth of well designed clinical trials. Physiother Can 1981 Sep/Oct; 33(5):269–275

Tecklin J. Positioning, percussing and vibrating patients for effective bronchial drainage. Nursing '79 1979 Mar; 9(3):64–71

Suctioning

McFadden R. Decreasing respiratory compromise during infant suctioning. Am J Nurs 1981 Dec; 81(12):2158–2161

Norris S et al. Nursing procedures and alterations in transcutaneous oxygen tension in premature infants. Nurs Res 1982 Nov/Dec; 31(6):330–336

Tracheostomy

Aradine C. Home care for young children with long term tracheostomies. MCN 1980 Mar/Apr; 5(2):121–125

Eigen H. Tracheostomy care, pp. 645–649. In Shirkey H (ed), Pediatric Therapy, 6th ed. St Louis, CV Mosby, 1980

Kennedy A, Johnson W and Sturdevant E. An educational program for families of children with tracheostomies. MCN 1982 Jan/Feb; 7(1):42–49

Rathlev M et al. Teaching families to give trach care at home . . . a child going home with tracheostomy. Nursing '82 1982 Jun; 12(6):70–71

Wills J. Concerns and needs of mothers providing home care for children with tracheostomies. Matern Child Nurs J 1983 Summer; 12(2):89–107

Oxygen Therapy

Administering oxygen safely: When, why, how. Nursing '80 1980 Oct; 10(10):54–56

Avery M and Stern L. Oxygen therapy, pp. 272–279. In Shirkey H (ed). Pediatric Therapy, 6th ed. St Louis, CV Mosby, 1980

Fuchs P. Getting the best out of oxygen delivery systems. Nursing '80 1980 Dec; 10(12):34–43

Glassanos MR. Infants who are oxygen dependent—Sending them home. MCN 1980 Jan/Feb; 5(1):42–45

Neilson L. Pulmonary oxygen toxicity and other hazards of oxygen therapy. Am J Nurs 1980 Dec; 80(12):2213–2215

Ventilatory Support and Monitoring

Dingle R et al. Continuous transcutaneous O_2 monitoring in the neonate. Am J Nurs 1980 May; 80(5):890–893

Finer N. Newer trends in continuous monitoring of critically ill infants and children. Pediatr Clin North Am 1980 Aug; 27(3):553–566

Finer N et al. Optimal ventilation for the neonate: Mechanical ventilation. Perinatol Neonatol 1983 Jan; 7(1):63–66, 68–70

Johnson B et al. Continuous positive airway pressure: Modes of action in relation to clinical applications. Pediatr Clin North Am 1980 Aug; 27(3):687–699

Kacmarek R. Technical aspects of positive end-expiratory pressure (PEEP): PEEP with spontaneous ventilation, part 3. Respir Care 1982 Dec; 27(12):1505–1518

Mason T. A hand ventilation technique for neonates. MCN 1982 Nov/Dec; 7(6):366–369

Murphy P and Schare B. Timely techniques in caring for the patient with an endotracheal tube, Part 1. Nursing '81 1981 Sept; 11(9):70–73

Nielson L. Mechanical ventilation: patient assessment and nursing care. Am J Nurs 1980 Dec; 80(12):2191–2217

Nielson L. Potential problems of mechanical ventilation. Am J Nurs 1980 Dec; 80(12):2206–2213

Nielson L. Ventilators and how they work. Am J Nurs 1980 Dec; 80(12):2201–2205

Neilson L. Weaning patients from mechanical ventilation. Am J Nurs 1980 Dec; 80(12):2214–2217

Pirie G et al. Options for ventilating the pediatric patient: Circuits and humidification systems, part 3. Respir Ther 1983 Sep/Oct; 13(5):73–74

Pirie G et al. Options for ventilating the pediatric patient: Mechanical

properties of three generations of ventilators, Part I. Respir Ther 1983 May/Jun; 13(3):65–71

Schroeder B. A creative approach to caring for the ventilator-dependent child. MCN 1979 May/June; 4(3):165–170

Thibeault D et al. Minimizing the risks of ventilator therapy in preterm infants. Respir Ther 1982 Jan/Feb; 12(1):67–70+

Cardiopulmonary Resuscitation

Hoops E. Cardiopulmonary resuscitation of children. Nurs Clin North Am 1981 Dec; 16(4):623–634

Matlock M et al. Pediatric resuscitation. J Emerg Nurs 1982 Jan/Feb; 8(1):55–56

Orlowski J. Cardiopulmonary resuscitation in children. Pediatr Clin North Am 1980 Aug; 27(3):495–512

Rehm R. Teaching cardiopulmonary resuscitation to parents. MCN 1983 Nov/Dec; 8(6):411–414

Taylor R and Gideon M. Cardiac arrest: A crisis for all people. Nursing '80 1980 Sep; 10(9):42–45

Thompson S. How to use the Heimlich maneuver on choking infants and children. Pediatr Nurs 1983 Jan/Feb; 9(1):13–16

Standards and Guidelines for Cardiopulmonary Resuscitation (CPR) and Emergency Cardiac Care (ECC). JAMA 1980 Aug 1; 244(5):453–509

Zenk K. Sharpen your knowledge of

drugs used in a pediatric code. Nursing '83 1983 Jul; 13(7):5–7

Zigelman D et al. Unique medication cart developed for pediatric emergencies helps avoid error . . . saves lives. Nephrol Nurse 1982 Jan/Feb; 4(1):35–36

Casts

Holland S. Up-to-date home care of a baby in a hip spica cast. Pediatr Nurs 1983 May/Apr; 9(2):114–115

Howard M and Corbo-Pelaia S. Psychological after effects of halo traction and a review of acute care. Am J Nurs 1982 Dec; 82(12):1839–1843

Lane P. New synthetic casts: What nurses need to know. Orthop Nurs 1982 Nov/Dec; 1(6):13–20

Laughlin R et al. Neurovascular examination of the injured extremity. Orthop Nurs 1982 Jan/Feb; 1(1):43–48

Moratz VA. Adapting shirts to fit over a halo vest. Am J Occup Ther 1979 Aug; 33(8):524–525

Rutecki B and Seligson D. Caring for the patient in a halo apparatus. Nursing '80 1980 Oct; 10(10):73–77

Swanson V. The school-age traction patient: Toward better behavior patterns. JACCH 1980 Summer; 9(1):12–14

Villalon D et al. At home with traction—Buck's traction at home. Pediatr Nurs 1982 Jan/Feb; 8(1):15–16

Problems of Infants

33

Management of the Premature Infant

The *premature infant* is a viable infant born before the completion of 37 weeks' gestation.

A *low-birth-weight (LBW)* infant is one whose birth weight is 1,501–2,500 gm. (3 lbs. 5 oz.–5 lbs. 8 oz.) without regard to gestational age.

A *very low birth weight (VLBW)* infant is one whose birth weight is below 1,500 gm. without regard to gestational age.

Etiology

1. Unknown
2. Maternal factors associated with prematurity:
   a. Chronic poor nutrition
   b. Diabetes
   c. Multiple births
   d. Drug abuse
   e. IUD in gravid uterus
   f. Chronic disease
      (1) Heart disease
      (2) Kidney disease
      (3) Infection
   g. Complications of pregnancy
      (1) Toxemia
      (2) Bleeding
      (3) Placenta previa or abruptio placentae
      (4) Incompetent cervix
      (5) Premature rupture of membranes
      (6) Polyhydramnios
   h. Multigravida under 18 years of age; primigravida over 35 years of age
3. Fetal factors associated with prematurity:
   a. Chromosomal abnormalities
   b. Anatomic abnormalities
      (1) Tracheoesophageal atresia or fistula
      (2) Intestinal obstruction
   c. Fetoplacental unit dysfunction

Altered Physiology

The premature infant has altered physiology due to immature and often poorly developed systems. The severity of any problem that occurs depends on the gestational age of the infant.

A. Respiratory System*

1. Alveoli begin to form at 26–28 weeks' gestation; therefore, lungs are poorly developed.

* Systems and situations that are most likely to cause problems in the premature.

2. Respiratory muscles are poorly developed.
3. Chest wall lacks stability.
4. Production of surfactant is reduced.
5. There is reduced compliance and low functional residual capacity of the lung.
6. Breathing may be labored and irregular with periods of apnea and cyanosis.
7. Infant is prone to atelectasis.
8. Gag and cough reflexes are poor; thus, aspiration may be a problem.

B. Digestive System*

1. The stomach is small, and vomiting is likely to occur because of poor muscle tone at the cardiac sphincter. It is difficult to provide caloric requirement in early days.
2. Tolerance is decreased related to decreased enzymes.
3. Lacks bile salts that aid digestion of fats and absorption of vitamin D and other fat-soluble vitamins.
4. Limited ability to convert glucose to glycogen and break down glycogen to glucose.
5. Limited and immature ability to release insulin in response to glucose.
6. Lacks coordinated sucking–swallowing reflex before 32–34 weeks' gestational age. Immature esophageal motility.

C. Poor Thermal Stability*

1. Has very little subcutaneous fat; thus, there is no heat storage or insulation. Poor glycogen and lipid stores.
2. Limited ability to shiver; has poor vasomotor control of blood flow to skin capillaries.
3. There is a relatively large surface area in comparison to body weight.
4. Sweat glands are decreased; infant cannot perspire under 32 weeks' gestation.
5. Has reduced muscle and fat deposits that restrict metabolic rate and heat production.
6. Usually is less active.
7. Posture flaccid—increasing surface area exposed.

D. Renal Function

1. Sodium excretion is probably increased, which may lead to hyponatremia; there is difficulty in excreting potassium.
2. Ability to concentrate urine decreases; thus, when vomiting or diarrhea occurs, dehydration is likely to follow. Decreased ability to conserve or excrete fluid.

1215

3. Ability to acidify urine decreases.
4. Glomerular tubular imbalance accounts for sugar, protein, amino acids, and sodium present in urine.

E. Nervous System

1. Response to stimulation is slow.
2. Suck, swallow, and gag reflexes are poor; feeding and possible aspiration therefore are problems.
3. Cough reflex is weak or absent.
4. Centers that control respirations, temperature, and other vital functions are poorly developed.

F. Infection* (see p. 1242, Sepsis Neonatorum)

1. Actively formed antibodies are lacking at birth (active immunity).
2. No IgM is present at birth.
3. Limited chemotaxis (reaction of cell to chemical stimuli).
4. Decreased opsonization (preparation of cells for phagocytosis).
5. Limited phagocytosis (digestion of bacteria by cells).
6. Hypofunctioning adrenal gland contributes to a decreased anti-inflammatory response.

G. Liver Function

1. Does not have good ability to handle and conjugate bilirubin.
2. Does not store or release sugar well; thus, there is a tendency toward hypoglycemia.
3. There is a steady decrease in hemoglobin after birth and in the production of blood; therefore, anemia may occur.
4. Does not make or store vitamin K; thus, infant is susceptible to hemorrhagic disease.

H. Eyes

1. Oxygen may cause retinal arteries to constrict, resulting in anoxic damage.
2. The retinae detach from the surface of posterior chambers, and a fibrous mass forms, resulting in an inability to receive visual stimulation. This is *retrolental fibroplasia* (RLF).
3. There are many stages of RLF.
4. The exact amount and level of oxygen needed to produce RLF is unknown. An infant under 1,000 gm. is at high risk for RLF. It is also related to sepsis, transfusions, chronic disease, hypoxia, etc.

I. Skin

1. Sensitive because of permeability and collagen instability.
2. Decreased cohesion between epidermis and dermis.
3. Decreased thickness of stratus corneum (outer layer of epidermis).
4. Delayed skin pH recovery to acidity following washing with alkaline-base soap, creams, and emollients.
5. Increased risk of toxicity from topical application and percutaneous absorption of drugs and substances.

Complications in Premature Infants

1. The severity of any problem that occurs in the premature infant depends on the gestational age of that infant.
   a. Hyaline membrane disease (respiratory distress syndrome)
   b. Aspiration
   c. Infection

*Systems and situations that are most likely to cause problems in the premature.

d. Hypoglycemia
e. Hypocalcemia
f. Patent ductus arteriosus
g. Apnea
h. Feeding intolerance
i. Intracranial hemorrhage
j. Hyperbilirubinemia

2. Major complications related to low-birth-weight infants include:
   a. Hypoxia, hyperoxia
   b. Hypoglycemia, hyperglycemia
   c. Difficulty feeding with malnutrition
   d. Dehydration
   e. Chronic lung disease—bronchopulmonary dysplasia
   f. Retrolental fibroplasia
   g. Hearing loss
   h. Psychological and behavioral problems
   i. Psychomotor retardation

Clinical Manifestations

1. Physical appearance
   Hair—lanugo, fluffy
   Poor ear cartilage
   Skin—very thin; capillaries are visible (may be red and wrinkled)
   Lack of subcutaneous fat
   Sole of foot is smooth
      (36 weeks' gestation—anterior ⅓ of foot is creased)
      (38 weeks' gestation—⅔ of foot is creased)
   Breast buds 5 mm.
      (36 weeks' gestation—none)
      (38 weeks' gestation—3 mm.)
   Testes—undescended
   Labia minora—undeveloped
   Rugae of scrotum—very fine
   Fingernails—soft
   Abdomen—relative large
   Thorax—relatively small
   Head—appears disproportionately large
   Facies resembles "an old man"
   Muscle tone poor—reflexes weak
2. Generally, maturation and growth rate increase after birth.

Assessment

A. Accurate body measurements (Fig. 33-1)— including:

1. Head circumference—frontal–occipital circumference (FOC) one finger above eyebrows, using parallel lines of tape around head.
2. Chest circumference—at nipple line.
3. Abdominal girth—one finger above umbilicus, mark location.
4. Heel–crown—used to calculate nasotracheal tube length.
5. Shoulder to umbilicus—used to calculate proper length of catheter for umbilical arterial catheter placement.
6. Weight

B. Assessment to determine gestational age (Table 33-1)

Ballard scoring system (recommended by Committee of Fetus and Newborn of American Academy of Pediatrics): Observation of physical and neurologic characteristics that change predictably with growth and maturation.

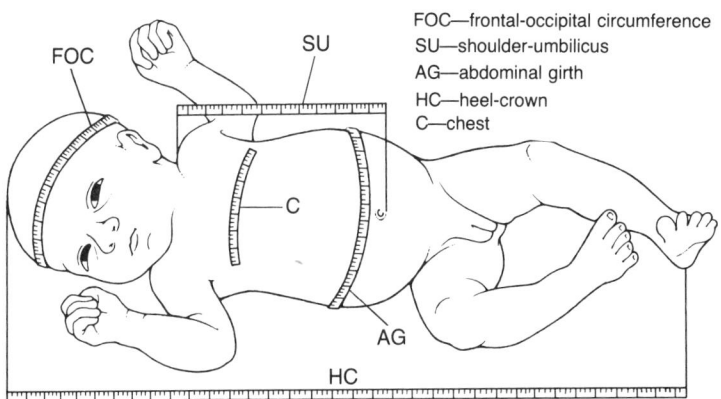

Figure 33-1. Infant measurements: FOC, frontal–occipital circumference; SU, shoulder–umbilicus; AG, abdominal girth; HC, heel–crown; C, chest. (Adapted from Levin DC, Morriss FC, and Moore GC. A Practical Guide to Pediatric Intensive Care. St Louis, CV Mosby, 1979, p. 8)

Ideally done at 1–2 hours after birth and repeated after 48 hours of life.

1. Physical assessment of maturity (i.e., sole creasing, presence of lanugo, skin transparency)
2. Neurologic assessment
   a. Maturation of the nervous system progresses at its own pace, and its rate is not increased by birth.
   b. The value of a neurologic evaluation increases after 48 hours of life.
   c. This examination is used primarily to estimate the infant's gestational age.
   d. The examination should be done when the infant is awake and quiet.
   e. Examination includes evaluation of muscle tone and evaluation of reflexes and reactions.
3. Assessment for appropriateness of size for gestational age—Colorado Intrauterine Growth Chart acknowledges that maturation is based on age, not size.
   a. Once weight, length, head circumference, and gestational age have been determined, these criteria are plotted on the intrauterine growth curve to determine if the infant is small, appropriate, or large for his gestational age.
   b. This knowledge will aid in anticipating potential problems that may occur in the infant.
   c. Brazelton Neonatal Assessment Scale—can assist in identifying interactive capabilities of the infant and in assessing the impact of these capabilities on the parents. Use of this information can enhance parent–infant interactions and relationships.
      Tool used from 3–30 days of age on full-term infant.
   d. Adjusted or corrected age:
      Once the infant reaches term (40 weeks after conception), his chronological age is adjusted for prematurity by taking gestational age minus 40 plus chronological age = developmental or corrected age; this is the age the infant would have been if he had been born at 40 weeks' gestation.
   e. Laboratory data as appropriate:
      (1) Blood gases
      (2) Blood sugar or Dextrostix
      (3) CBC or Hb and Hct
      (4) Lecithin/sphingomyelin ratio (L/S ratio) assessment of lung maturity
      (5) Electrolytes
      (6) Bilirubin
      (7) Calcium, potassium
      (8) Albumin

Potential Problems/Nursing Diagnoses

1. Potential complications related to immature development of systems; respiratory distress, apnea, thermal instability, aspiration, infection, hypoglycemia, intracranial hemorrhage, hyperbilirubinemia, poor nutrition and weight gain, fluid and electrolyte imbalance, alteration in skin integrity, altered cardiac status (PDA), hypocalcemia, and hyponatremia
2. Sensory deprivation related to hospitalization and altered nurturing activities
3. Potential for injury related to treatment (i.e., infiltrated intravenous infusions, altered skin integrity, etc.)
4. Alteration in parenting activities and parent–infant bonding related to illness, parental feelings, hospitalization and separation
5. Parental anxiety related to lack of understanding of infant's condition; infant's small size and physical appearance; presence of tubes, monitors, and other equipment

Nursing Interventions
Admission to the Nursery

A. Observe for any gross abnormalities as in the case of a full-term infant on admission, and pay special attention to respirations, heart rate, blood pressure, muscle tone, and activity.

1. Respirations above 40/minute over a period of time may be indicative of respiratory difficulty.
   a. Expiratory grunting, retractions, chest lag, or nasal flaring should be reported immediately (Retractions chart, Fig. 33-2).
   b. Cyanosis (other than acrocyanosis—coldness and cyanosis of hands and feet) should be watched for along with other signs of respiratory distress.
2. Increased (above 180/minute) or irregular heart rate may indicate cardiac or circulatory difficulties.
3. Muscle tone and activity should be evaluated.
4. Hypotension, indicated by blood-pressure measurement, may be due to hypovolemia.

B. Maintain a patent airway.

1. Have oxygen, suction, and resuscitation equipment readily available.
2. Suction mouth and pharynx if mucus is present—to prevent aspiration. Premature infants often have an excess amount of mucus as well as poor cough, swallow, and gag reflexes.

(Text continues on p. 1220)

Table 33-1 Clinical Estimation of Gestational Age

(Reproduced with permission from Kempe, C.H., Silver, H.K., and O'Brien, D. (eds.) Current Pediatric Diagnosis and Treatment, 4th ed. Lange Medical Publications, 1976.)

Examination First Hours — WEEKS GESTATION (20–48)

PHYSICAL FINDINGS		Progression across weeks of gestation
Vernix		Appears (21) → Covers body, thick layer (24–28) → On back, scalp, in creases (38–40) → Scant, in creases (40–41) → No vernix (43)
Breast tissue and areola		Areola and nipple barely visible, no palpable breast tissue (22–24) → Areola raised (34–35) → 1–2 mm nodule (36) → 3–5 mm (38) → 5–6 mm (39) → 7–10 mm (40) → ?12 mm (44)
Ear	Form	Flat, shapeless (22) → Beginning incurving superior (33–34) → Incurving upper 2/3 pinnae (37) → Well-defined incurving to lobe (39)
	Cartilage	Pinna soft, stays folded (22) → Cartilage scant, returns slowly from folding (32–33) → Thin cartilage, springs back from folding (38) → Pinna firm, remains erect from head (42)
Sole creases		Smooth soles without creases (22–26) → 1–2 anterior creases (32) → 2–3 anterior creases (35) → Creases anterior 2/3 sole (37) → Creases involving heel (40) → Deeper creases over entire sole (43)
Skin	Thickness & appearance	Thin, translucent skin, plethoric, venules over abdomen, edema (22–29) → Smooth, thicker, no edema (33–34) → Pink (37) → Few vessels (39) → Some desquamation, pale pink (40) → Thick, pale, desquamation over entire body (43)
	Nail plates	Appear (20–21) → Nails to finger tips (33) → Nails extend well beyond finger tips (44)
Hair		Appears on head (22) → Eye brows and lashes (24) → Fine, woolly, bunches out from head (30) → Silky, single strands, lays flat (38) → ?Receding hairline or loss of baby hair, short, fine underneath (43)
Lanugo		Appears (20) → Covers entire body (24) → Vanishes from face (33) → Present on shoulders (38) → No lanugo (43)
Genitalia	Testes	Testes palpable in inguinal canal (28) → In upper scrotum (37) → In lower scrotum (39)
	Scrotum	Few rugae (29) → Rugae, anterior portion (36) → Rugae cover (40) → Pendulous (43)
	Labia & clitoris	Prominent clitoris, labia majora small, widely separated (30–32) → Labia majora larger, nearly cover clitoris (36) → Labia minora and clitoris covered (44)
Skull firmness		Bones are soft (22) → Soft to 1" from anterior fontanelle (28–30) → Spongy at edges of fontanelle, center firm (36) → Bones hard, sutures easily displaced (38) → Bones hard, cannot be displaced (43)
Posture	Resting	Hypotonic, lateral decubitus (21–25) → Hypotonic (27) → Beginning flexion, thigh (30) → Stronger hip flexion (32) → Frog-like (34) → Flexion, all limbs (37) → Hypertonic (39) → Very hypertonic (42)
	Recoil - leg	No recoil (21) → Partial recoil (32) → Begin flexion, no recoil (34) → Prompt recoil (40)
	Arm	No recoil (21) → Begin flexion, no recoil (35) → Prompt recoil, may be inhibited (37–40) → Prompt recoil after 30" inhibition (41)

Confirmatory Neurologic Examination To Be Done After 24 Hours

Weeks Gestation: 20 21 22 23 24 25 26 27 28 29 30 31 32 33 34 35 36 37 38 39 40 41 42 43 44 45 46 47 48

Category	Physical Findings	Progression across weeks of gestation
Tone	Heel to ear	No resistance → Some resistance → Impossible
	Scarf sign	No resistance → Elbow passes midline → Elbow at midline → Elbow does not reach midline
	Neck flexors (head lag)	Absent → Head in plane of body → Holds head
	Neck extensors	Head begins to right itself from flexed position → Good righting cannot hold it → Holds head few seconds → Keeps head in line with trunk >40'' → Turns head from side to side
	Body extensors	Straightening of legs → Straightening of trunk → Straightening of head and trunk together
	Vertical positions	When held under arms, body slips through hands → Arms hold baby, legs extended? → Legs flexed, good support with arms
	Horizontal positions	Hypotonic, arms and legs straight → Arms and legs flexed → Head and back even, flexed extremities → Head above back
Flexion angles	Popliteal	No resistance; 150° → 110° → 100° → 90° → 80°
	Ankle	45° → 20° → 0 (A pre-term who has reached 40 weeks still has a 40° angle)
	Wrist (square window)	90° → 60° → 45° → 30° → 0
Reflexes	Sucking	Weak, not synchronized with swallowing → Stronger, synchronized → Perfect → Perfect, hand to mouth
	Rooting	Long latency period slow, imperfect → Hand to mouth → Brisk, complete, durable → Complete
	Grasp	Finger grasp is good, strength is poor → Stronger → Stronger → Can lift baby off bed, involves arms → Hands open
	Moro	Barely apparent → Weak, not elicited every time → Complete with arm extension, open fingers, cry → Arm adduction added → ?Begins to lose Moro
	Crossed extension	Flexion and extension in a random, purposeless pattern → Extension, no adduction → Still incomplete → Extension, adduction, fanning of toes → Complete
	Automatic walk	Minimal → Begins tiptoeing, good support on sole → Fast tiptoeing → Heel-toe progression, whole sole of foot → A pre-term who has reached 40 weeks walks on toes → ?Begins to lose automatic walk
	Pupillary reflex	Absent → Appears
	Glabellar tap	Absent → Appears
	Tonic neck reflex	Absent → Appears
	Neck-righting	Absent → Appears → Present after 37 weeks

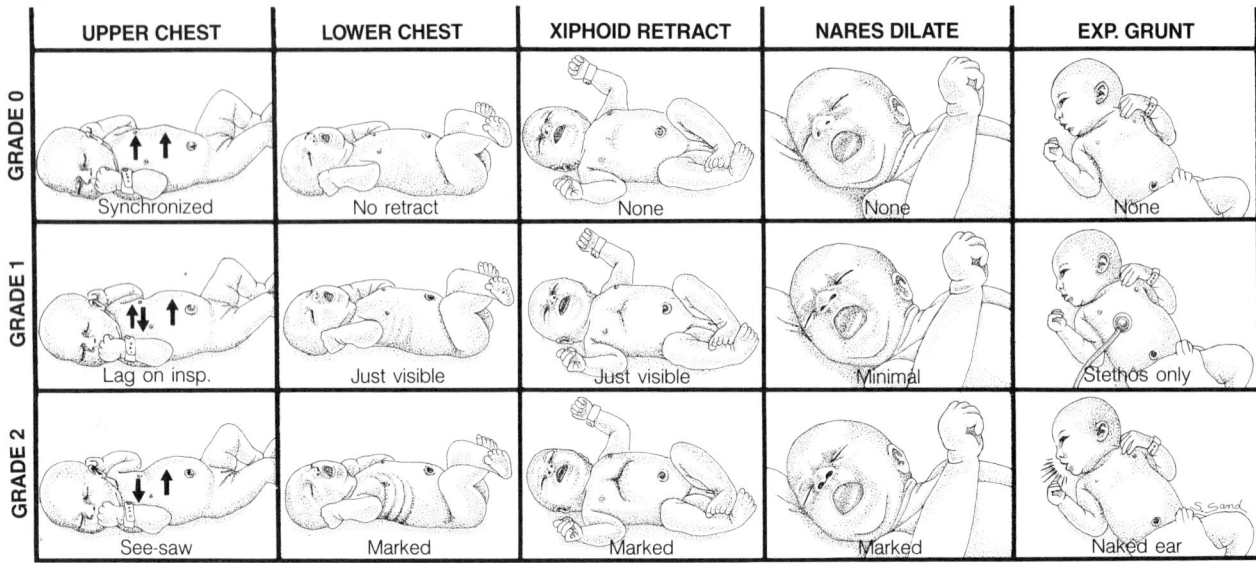

	UPPER CHEST	LOWER CHEST	XIPHOID RETRACT	NARES DILATE	EXP. GRUNT
GRADE 0	Synchronized	No retract	None	None	None
GRADE 1	Lag on insp.	Just visible	Just visible	Minimal	Stethos only
GRADE 2	See-saw	Marked	Marked	Marked	Naked ear

Figure 33-2. Observation of retractions. An index of respiratory distress is determined by grading each of five arbitrary criteria. Grade 0 indicates no difficulty; grade 1 indicates moderate difficulty; and grade 2 indicates maximum respiratory difficulty. The retraction score is the sum of these values; a total score of 0 indicates no dyspnea, whereas a total score of 10 denotes maximal respiratory distress.

3. Position infant in Isolette or radiant heater to allow for easy drainage of mucus from his mouth.
   a. Very small premature infants—place on side.
   b. Larger premature infants—place on abdomen.
   c. Head may be tilted down—this may be contraindicated because of increased intracranial pressure or increased respiratory distress due to liver pushing against diaphragm decreasing lung expansion, especially in the asphyxiated infant.
4. Obtain blood gas values.
5. Administer emergency oxygen to just barely relieve cyanosis.

C. Provide and maintain thermal neutrality of the premature infant.
1. Obtain weight and temperature; then attach cardiac monitor leads quickly and place infant in warm environment (Isolette, radiant heater). Omit bath until infant's temperature has stabilized.
2. The premature infant's ability to control his own body temperature is inhibited by many factors related to his immaturity (see p. 1215).

D. Ensure that prophylactic measures have been administered against ophthalmia neonatorum and that vitamin K_1 has been administered.
Since the premature infant is frequently taken from the delivery room as soon as possible after birth, prophylactic measures may have been omitted.

E. Be aware of early complications that may arise as a result of complications of the pregnancy, labor, or delivery.
1. Maternal medication
   a. Drugs pass quickly from mother's blood, across the placenta into the infant's blood.
   b. Infant may be drowsy and have slowed respirations.

   c. Because of poor development, respiratory difficulty may occur.
2. Blood incompatibility of mother and infant
   a. Premature infant is more susceptible to jaundice, even without incompatibilities.
   b. Observe closely for early signs of jaundice (see p. 1237, hyperbilirubinemia).
3. Maternal conditions that may predispose to infant problems.
   a. Infection or illness
   b. Diabetes
   c. Drugs
4. Neonatal asphyxia
   a. Apgar score of less than 5 at 1 minute and less than 7 at 5 minutes
   b. *Asphyxia* is lack of oxygen.
      Secondary problems:
      (1) Hypoxia (reduced oxygen available)
      (2) Anoxia (total lack of oxygen)
      (3) Hypercapnia (inability to eliminate CO_2)
      (4) Acidosis
   c. Causes of asphyxia or hypoxia can originate in the mother, the placenta, or the infant, or may be a result of the delivery.

The First 24–48 Hours of Life

This period after birth is the most critical time for the premature infant.

A. Be constantly aware of the infant's condition and make frequent observations.
1. This poorly developed, immature infant is prone to sudden and rapid changes in condition.
2. Early recognition of symptoms and reporting observations to physician are the most valuable contributions the nurse can make in caring for and saving the premature infant's life.

3. Note bleeding from the umbilical cord.
   a. Should bleeding occur, apply pressure.
   b. Estimate amount of bleeding and record.
   c. Notify the physician immediately—replacement transfusion may be necessary.
4. Note first voiding.
   a. This may occur up to 36 hours after birth, but it usually occurs within the first 24 hours. Report any 4- to 6-hour period when voiding does not occur.
   b. Note amount, color, and frequency of voidings; 2–3 ml./kg./hour; specific gravity 1.003–1.010.
   c. Lack of voiding may indicate renal system anomalies, shock, or poor circulation.
5. Note stools.
   a. Note when first stool occurred and its characteristics.
   b. Abdominal distention and lack of stool may indicate intestinal obstruction or other intestinal tract anomalies. Measure abdominal girth at regular intervals.
6. Note activity and behavior.
   a. Note amount of lethargy or activity or need for stimulation.
   b. Look for sucking movement, hand-to-mouth maneuver. This can help to determine oral feeding initiation.
   c. Note quality of cry.
7. Observe for a tense and bulging fontanelle; feel suture lines noting separation or overriding.
   a. Full fontanelle may indicate intracranial hemorrhage.
   b. Be alert to twitching and seizures.
8. Note color of skin.
   a. Cyanosis
      (1) Circulatory or cardiac difficulties may be present.
      (2) Respiratory effort may be ineffective.
   b. Jaundice may indicate:
      (1) Infection
      (2) Enclosed hemorrhage; bruising
9. Carefully monitor, record, and report vital signs.

B. Maintain respirations.

1. Immediate emergency support may be necessary, since respiratory system is poorly developed and ability to control respirations is often barely sufficient.
2. Have available resuscitative equipment, oxygen, and suction apparatus.
   a. Mucus may not be handled well, because of poor gag, cough, and swallowing reflexes.
      (1) Clearing the airway is of major importance.
      (2) A rubber ear bulb syringe is often all that is necessary for clearing the mouth.
      (3) Frequent suctioning of the pharynx may not be necessary.
3. Position infant to allow for easy ventilation.
   a. Supine position permits free expansion of the thoracic cage (infant's body weight is on the chest and abdomen when he is prone).
   b. Elevate head and trunk to decrease pressure on diaphragm from abdominal organs.
   c. Slight neck extension affords opening of trachea; place small roll under shoulders.
   d. Do not constrict abdominal area, since abdominal muscles are used to aid respiratory effort.
   e. Flex and abduct arms to enhance chest expansion.
   f. Change position from side to side. Perform postural drainage every 2 hours to aid in draining fluid accumulation in thoracic cavity.
4. Use only the percentage of oxygen necessary to maintain appropriate blood gas values.
   a. Oxygen is used with moisture to prevent mucous membranes from drying and becoming irritated.
   b. Monitor oxygen with analyzer every hour to ensure consistency in percentage used.
   c. Transcutaneous PO_2 monitor may be used (Tc PO_2)—values should correlate with blood gases.
      (1) Ensure that site of probe is changed every 2–6 hours; probe placement is on chest, abdomen, back (depending on size of infant).
      (2) Monitor is calibrated according to manufacturer's directions.
      (3) Complication of transcutaneous monitor probe is in a skin reaction: red marks at site of electrode placement; burn.
5. Note any changes in respiratory effort and report these to the physician.
   a. Note quality and rate particularly.
   b. Use retractions score for continual, consistent assessment of the respiratory status (see Fig. 33-2).
   c. Hyaline membrane disease or respiratory distress syndrome occurs during the first 24 hours of life. Observe for and report immediately any signs and symptoms of respiratory difficulty:
      (1) Increased respiratory rate (usually above 60/minute)
      (2) Thoracic retractions
      (3) Nasal flaring
      (4) Cyanosis
      (5) Expiratory grunting
      (6) Developing exhaustion
      (7) Periods of apnea
6. Hypoxemia is associated with birth asphyxia and recurrent apneic episodes. Serum PaO_2 less than 40 mm.Hg.
7. Hypoventilation—tendency to retain CO_2 because of irregular breathing, poor respiratory muscle activity, and flexible thoracic cage. PCO_2 greater than 50 mm.Hg.
8. Identify periodic breathing versus apneic episodes.
   a. *Periodic breathing*—cessation of breathing for short periods (5–10 seconds) followed by ventilation for 10–15 seconds at an increased rate.
   b. *Apneic episodes*—nonbreathing periods of more than 20 seconds' duration may be accompanied by bradycardia (heart rate below 100) and cyanosis, and is related to immature respiratory center. Infant is hypotonic and unresponsive.
      (1) Stimulation or resuscitation is required to restart breathing and increase heart rate.
      (2) Provocative conditions that increase apneic spells include:
      Hyperthermia, hypothermia
      Hypoglycemia
      Hypocalcemia
      Acidosis
      Hyperbilirubinemia
      CNS disease—intraventricular hemorrhage
      Pulmonary insufficiency
      Infection
      PDA (patent ductus arteriosus)
      Sodium disturbances
      Hypoxemia

Pneumonia/sepsis
RDS
Low hematocrit
Airway obstruction
    (3) Apnea may cause hypoxemia (decreased oxygen in blood) leading to hypoxia (decreased oxygen in tissues), which may result in complications (i.e., intracranial hemorrhage, PDA, atelectasis and hypoglycemia).
    (4) Theophylline or aminophylline may be given to reduce the frequency of apneic episodes. It is believed that the drug acts centrally by increasing the respiratory center activity and increasing the infant's sensitivity to CO_2.
        Observe for tachycardia (heart rate of 180–190/min); toxicity.
        Ensure that serum theophylline levels are checked frequently, since excretion of the drug is limited and toxic levels may be quickly reached.
        Toxic serum levels—20 mg./ml.; therapeutic levels—3–15 mg./ml.
    (5) Waterbed or tactile stimulation schedule every hour may help decrease frequency of apnea.
    (6) Keep infant's temperature close to the low range of the thermal neutral zone.

C. Conserve the infant's energy while providing necessary care.
1. Be organized in caring for the infant.
    Collect all equipment before starting care, do what needs to be done, and then let the infant rest. Infant's position will affect his ability to rest.
2. Premature infants tire very easily.
    a. Any activity increases oxygen need, thus increasing respiratory rate, taxing already limited energy.
        Holding the infant, suctioning, linen change, chest physical therapy, repositioning often cause significant lowering of PaO_2. Recovery to adequate PaO_2 depends upon the drop in PaO_2.
    b. Watch TcO_2 monitor—stop procedure if necessary or possible if TcO_2 levels fall.
    c. Adjust the infant's environment so that rest and sleep are not hindered. Decrease the risk of causing hypoxia.
    d. Interventions must be evaluated for their relative value versus the trauma they entail.

D. Provide and maintain thermal neutrality of the premature infant.
1. Maintain infant's temperature at the thermo-neutral zone (i.e., at the environmental temperature in which the resting infant maintains normal body temperature and still utilizes minimum energy–oxygen consumption and calories).
    a. Infant's core temperature (rectal temperature) should be maintained at 36.5–37.2°C. (98.6°F.). Axillary and abdominal skin temperature should be 36.0–36.8°C. (96.8–97.2°F.).
    b. Keep environmental (ambient) temperature ranges from 32°–35°C. (89.6–95.0°F.). Smaller premature infants may need higher temperature, 35°C. (95°F.); larger premature infants, around 32°C. (89.6°F.).
        Generally, ambient temperature is 1°–1.5°C. warmer than abdominal skin temperature; thus oxygen consumption is minimal.

2. Be aware that the infant loses heat by radiation, conduction, convection, and evaporation; thus, the nurse must be alert to conditions that influence heat loss or gain by the infant.
    a. Note location of warming unit in relation to air conditioners, direct sunlight, and drafts. Move the unit, if necessary.
    b. Minimize porthole entrance activities into Isolette; keep portholes tightly closed when they are not in use or tightly fitting around arm when entering Isolette.
    c. Infant should be undressed to allow direct body contact with warm air.
    d. To minimize heat loss by radiation, consider the possibility of partially lining the Isolette with foil, being careful not to obstruct view of infant. Covering infant from shoulders to feet with a plastic (kitchen plastic material) bubble may also aid in maintaining a stable temperature. Commercial products are also available.
3. Avoid constant or drastic changing of temperature-control dial (decreases risk of missing infection).
    a. If ambient temperature rises, skin and core temperature of the infant will rise resulting in increased metabolic rate and insensible water loss. The infant may exhibit weight loss, abdominal distention, regurgitation of feeding, and irritability.
    b. Decrease in ambient temperature will result in a decrease of the infant's skin temperature and an increase in metabolic rate in an attempt to increase heat production. Skin temperature reflects thermal stress first.
        (1) If the infant cannot compensate for the increased heat loss, his body temperature will drop.
        (2) Hypothermia results in tachycardia, hypoglycemia, metabolic acidosis, apnea, and inactivity.
4. Skin temperature probe should be placed on the trunk of the infant rather than extremities which are more susceptible to changes in peripheral circulation.
    a. Prevent the infant from lying on thermistor.
    b. Cover skin probe with a heat-reflecting material (foil) to decrease influence of ambient temperature on sensor.
5. Monitor both the infant's temperature and Isolette or radiant warmer temperature. Temperature-control centers are poorly developed in the premature infant, and his temperature is easily influenced by his environment. Hypermetabolic state and inadequate peripheral circulation predispose the premature infant to hyperthermia. When caring for the premature infant under the radiant warmer:
    a. Use white linen to increase efficiency of the unit.
    b. Monitor temperature every 30–60 minutes to determine specific temperature needed to keep the infant at correct temperature. Start unit setting at 37°–37.5°C. and adjust slowly. Increase temperature only 0.5°C. per hour (1.5°C. warmer than skin temperature) until the infant's temperature is stable. Then monitor every 1–4 hours.
    c. Keep alarm for overheating in operation.
    d. Be aware of the complications associated with the use of radiant warmer:
        (1) Overheating—increase in the infant's oxygen consumption
        (2) Flash burns—avoid oil on the infant's skin

(3) Cataracts—observe closure of eye lids

(4) Excess drying of skin and tissue breakdown

6. When assessing temperature regulation of the premature infant, consider the following:

   a. Note if the infant's body or extremities are cool to touch—possibly due to underheated incubator or heat loss from radiation.

   b. Note activity—restlessness or hyperactivity may indicate inappropriate temperature for comfort.

   c. Be aware of reasons for increased temperature of infant—overheated incubator, early sign of illness, incorrect placement of sensor.

   d. Be aware of causes for drop in temperature of infant—underheated incubator, infection, faulty sensor–skin contact from feces or bony prominence, vasoconstriction, iatrogenic (cold O_2).

7. When humidity is increased in the incubator, it will reduce infant heat loss and insensible water loss.

8. Avoid measuring rectal temperature.

   a. Stimulates defecation, resulting in fluid and caloric loss.

   b. Rectal perforation—at a depth of 3 cm., infant's colon changes from an anterior to posterior angle.

9. Insensible water loss is increased with use of radiant warmer by evaporation. Monitor fluid volume, urine output, and specific gravity.

10. Rocker bed and tactile and auditory stimulation may contribute to maintaining thermal neutrality in the infant.

E. Prevent infection in this very susceptible premature infant.

1. The premature infant is particularly susceptible to viral, fungal, and gram-negative and gram-positive bacterial infections. Septicemia, meningitis, and urinary tract infections are a constant hazard postnatally.

2. Specific techniques should be employed to ensure the control of infection (see p. 1122).

   a. Scrupulous handwashing must be practiced by all personnel handling the infant and entering the nursery.

   b. Use gown and mask technique as prescribed by the health agency. Short-sleeved gowns allow for proper handwashing up to the elbows.

   c. Minimize the infant's contact with unsterile equipment; equipment should be individualized.

   d. Minimize the number of persons who come in contact with the infant.

   e. Exclude from nursery any person who is febrile, has draining lesions, or has acute respiratory or gastrointestinal infections.

▶ **NURSING ALERT:** Routine use of hexachlorophene for infant bathing is to be avoided. Data indicate a marked association between its use and neuropathologic lesions.

3. Early symptoms of infection may include (see p. 1243):

   a. Hypothermia or hyperthermia

   b. Jaundice

   c. Lethargy

   d. Poor eating

   e. Apneic spells

4. Factors predisposing to infection

   a. Maternal infection

   b. Difficult and prolonged labor

   c. Prolonged rupture of membranes

   d. Manipulative measures—resuscitation, umbilical catheterization, surgery

F. Maintain fluid balance.

1. Monitor fluid intake and output and urine specific gravity.

2. Increased fluid may result in pulmonary edema, congestive heart failure, and 2nd-degree PDA, and may increase risk of BPD and possibly intraventricular hemorrhage.

3. Too little fluid may lead to dehydration, hypotension, acidosis, or electrolyte imbalance.

4. All infants under 1,500 gm. receive intravenous infusion of $D_{10}W$.

G. Provide appropriate skin care to protect skin integrity.

1. Skin provides important functions: protects internal organs; intact skin provides protection against foreign substances and organisms, helps regulate body temperature, stores fats, discharges electrolytes and water, and provides for tactile stimulation.

2. Specific techniques should be employed to ensure skin integrity.

   a. Avoid use of alkaline-base soaps which may cause alteration of skin pH. (Acid pH skin surface provides bacteriocidal quality).

   b. Increased permeability and large surface area put infant at risk of toxicity from topical application of drugs, lotions, etc.

   c. Lubrication of dry, flaky skin is not recommended. If cracking or fissures occur, a thin layer of nonperfumed emollient may be used.

   d. Avoid the use of adhesive—epidermis may be pulled off upon removal, increasing the risk of infection.

   e. Remove adhesive substances with cotton balls soaked in water or soapy solution while gently pulling edges back, or use commercial adhesive remover with care and rinse skin with clear water following use.

   f. Evaluate skin-care techniques used (i.e., tincture of Benzoin, Hollihesive, Op-site, Skin-gel).

   g. Zinc deficiencies may result in skin breakdown especially around the mouth, buttocks, fingers, toes, and creases.

H. Protect the infant's eyes from injury.

1. Protect eyes from too much light, especially when eyes are dilated.

   a. During procedures and from bright sunlight

   b. Intensive light may contribute to RLF or other retinal damage.

2. Corneas need protection when the infant's eyes remain open, (i.e., when the infant is receiving Pavulon).

I. Be aware of complications that occur in the premature infant and be alert for early signs indicating a change in condition.

1. *Hypoglycemia*

   a. Hypoglycemia—serum sugar levels are less than 40 mg./100 ml.; whole blood level, 20 mg./100 ml.

   b. Hypoglycemia is most likely to occur in first 12 hours after birth and as late as 48 hours after birth.

   c. Hypoglycemia is likely to occur in the premature infant because of the reduced glycogen storage he has at birth and his limited carbohydrate tolerance.

   d. Symptoms are nonspecific. Many infants with clinical hypoglycemia may be asymptomatic.

     (1) Jitteriness
     (2) Tachypnea or apnea
     (3) Lethargy, listlessness
     (4) Cyanosis
     (5) Convulsions
     (6) High-pitched or weak cry
     (7) Pallor
     (8) Temperature instability
     (9) Sweating
    (10) Tachycardia
    (11) Poor feeding

   e. Predisposing factors include:

     (1) Infant of diabetic mother—2–72 hours
     (2) Erythroblastosis fetalis—4–72 hours
     (3) Sepsis
     (4) Intrauterine malnutrition—2 hours–1 week
     (5) Development defects
     (6) Asphyxia
     (7) Respiratory distress
     (8) Hypothermia

   f. Blood sugar levels should be accurately monitored. Dextrostix screening can be done by the nurse.

     (1) When a blood specimen is collected, ideally a capillary tube should be used to prevent the reactive tip from coming in contact with the skin, which may give a false reading.
     (2) Specimen should remain on reactive tip for 60 seconds, then forcefully rinsed with clear running water.
       When Dextrostix* values are below 40 mg.%, a blood glucose should be done. Chemstrip bG† and Dextrometer should be used when available for more accurate values.
     (3) Check urine for excess levels of sugar.

   g. Treatment is to increase blood sugar intake by oral feeding or intravenously. If IV glucose is given too rapidly, hyperglycemia may occur because of poor insulin response. Maintain blood sugar at greater than 45 mg./100 ml.

   h. Hyperglycemia (blood sugar above 125 mg.%) not uncommon in the infant less than 1,000 gm. This infant often requires use of insulin to ensure adequate calories and has reduced ability to absorb adequate amounts.

2. *Hypocalcemia*

   a. Hypocalcemia—serum calcium levels are less than 7 mg./100 ml. (3.5 mEq./liter).

   b. Low blood calcium is reached the first day of life.

   c. Symptoms are nonspecific:

     (1) Twitching
     (2) Convulsions (late sign)
     (3) Hypotonia
     (4) Lethargy
     (5) High-pitched cry
     (6) Increased apneic spells
     (7) Abdominal distention with ileus

   d. Hypocalcemia occurs in the premature infant

---

because of reduced calcium storage at birth and reduced ability to absorb adequate amounts

   e. Predisposing factors:

     (1) Hypoglycemia
     (2) Previous maternal abortion
     (3) Low infant Apgar rating—asphyxia
     (4) Hyaline membrane disease
     (5) Lack of intake
     (6) Treatment of acidosis with bicarbonate
     (7) Decreased renal capacity for phosphorus excretion

   f. Try to maintain serum calcium above 8 mg./100 ml.

   g. Treatment is to give calcium intravenously or orally.
     Intravenous calcium given too rapidly will cause bradycardia.

3. *Hypoxia* or anoxia at birth

   a. The degree of asphyxia is judged immediately after delivery by Apgar scores and blood gas changes.

   b. Specific problems to be anticipated include:

     (1) Hyaline membrane disease
     (2) Profound acidosis
     (3) Hypoglycemia
     (4) Abnormal clotting function
     (5) Hyperbilirubinemia
     (6) Apneic episodes
     (7) Poor temperature control
     (8) Intracranial hemorrhage
     (9) Cardiac failure

4. Patent ductus arteriosus (PDA)

   a. PDA occurs frequently in premature infants with respiratory distress syndrome and in less mature infants (24–30 weeks' gestation) with associated congestive pulmonary failure.
     A majority of very low birth weight infants recovering from respiratory distress syndrome develop serious signs of this disease.
     The preterm infant is at risk for left-to-right shunting of blood through the patent ductus.

   b. Clinical signs include:

     (1) Bounding peripheral pulses
     (2) Chest retractions with mild cyanosis
     (3) Diminished breath sounds on auscultation
     (4) Moist crackles
     (5) Elevated PCO_2
     (6) Apneic periods
     (7) Systolic murmur—clicking sound
     (8) Tachypnea
     (9) Deterioration of general condition
    (10) Inability to wean from ventilator

   c. Treatment:

     (1) Medical—fluid restriction, maintenance of normal blood pH, oxygen as needed, maintenance of adequate hemoglobin levels, digitalization, when CHF is present, diuretics, indomethacin for closure.
       When indomethacin is used, the nurse should observe for diminished urine output, azotemia, and creatinemia. Contraindications: if the infant has bilirubin levels greater than 10 mg. (drug binds to albumin), bleeding tendencies (may alter platelet formation), renal problems, or necrotizing enterocolitis.
     (2) Surgical—ligation of ductus arteriosus

   d. Spontaneous closure of the PDA in the premature infant is likely to occur 2–6 weeks after birth.

---

* Dextrostix: Ames Laboratory, Elkhart, IN 46514

† Chemstrip: Bio-Dynamics, 9115 Hague Road, Indianapolis, IN 46250

5. *Sodium disturbances*
   a. Hypernatremia—serum sodium level above 150 mEq./liter; generally occurs because of inadequate hydration or overuse of $NaHCO_3$ for acidosis.
      Hypernatremia occurs frequently in the very low birth weight infant regardless of sodium intake.
   b. Hyponatremia—serum sodium level below 125–130 mEq./liter is generally secondary to loss of sodium in urine and inadequate intake.
6. *Intracranial hemorrhage* (most likely to occur in sick premature infants)
   a. Intracranial hemorrhage is a common cause of death in extremely premature infants.
   b. Factors predisposing infant to CNS bleeding
      (1) Immaturity
      (2) Respiratory distress syndrome
      (3) Hypoxia in fetus or neonate
      (4) Pneumothorax or any air leak
   c. Clinical signs
      Signs may be slow and subtle in appearance, or sudden, catastrophic neurologic deterioration may take place.
      (1) Labored respirations
      (2) Hypoventilation
      (3) Cyanosis
      (4) Apnea
      (5) High-pitched cry
      (6) Convulsions
      (7) Bulging fontanelle
      (8) Clinical deterioration; shock-like appearance
   d. Intracranial hemorrhage occurs more frequently in the preterm under 1,500 gm. and 35 weeks' gestation. Generally occurs 1–7 days after birth with a peak at 12–36 hours.
      Prevention of intraventricular hemorrhage is the best treatment, because once bleeding begins, it is difficult to control.
      (1) Keep the infant adequately oxygenated. Prevent asphyxia and hypercapnia.
         Stabilize PaO_2 early (low PaO_2 increases risks).
      (2) Maintain thermo-neutral environment.
      (3) Maintain normal acid–base balance.
      (4) Maintain normal blood volume.
7. *Hypertension*
   a. Hypertension may occur in infants with a history of indwelling artery catheter, patent ductus arteriosus, or perinatal hypoxia. These conditions put infant at risk for renal artery thrombosis and hypertension.
   b. Signs include:
      (1) Increasing blood pressure and considerable fluctuation in blood pressure
      (2) Tachypnea and cyanosis
      (3) Lethargy
      (4) Tremors
      (5) Apnea
   c. Treatment:
      Diuretics and/or antihypertensive medications
8. *Hypotension*—indicative of hypovolemia, sepsis, abdominal or intracranial hemorrhage, shock
9. *Hypothermia*—cold stress
   a. Temperature instability in the premature may result in hypothermia. Cold stress results when norepinephrine is released to activate brown fat metabolism (nonshivering thermogenesis).

   b. This hypermetabolic state requires increased oxygen and calories in the already compromised infant.
   c. By-products of brown fat metabolism are heat production and acidosis from ketones and lactic acid. Hypoglycemia also occurs because of rapid depletion of stored glucose.
   d. As this state continues, the infant is at risk for apnea, intracranial hemorrhage, acidosis, and hypoglycemia.
10. *Hyperthermia*
    This results when the infant attempts to dissipate heat.
    a. Skin vessels dilate, metabolic rate increases, oxygen and caloric consumption increases, and respiratory effort is increased.
    b. The infant is at risk for intracranial hemorrhage.
11. *Iatrogenic complications*
    Procedures performed on the preterm infant to assist him through the clinical course may result in additional problems related to noise, tape altering skin integrity, radiation exposure, burns, intravenous infiltration with tissue sloughing, sensory deprivation, etc.

J. Offer support to the parents of the premature infant during this crucial period.

1. Most parents, particularly mothers, are physically and emotionally unprepared for the early arrival of their baby.
2. Allow the parents to see their infant and touch him if this is feasible, and they are able to cope with doing so.
3. Listen to the parents talk and express their concerns. Encourage them, but do not give them false hope.
   a. Assess where they are in their grief, in coping, and in accepting their infant.
   b. Be alert to the father who may be overwhelmed with concern for the infant and mother (who also is hospitalized) and who may not know how to help or meet the needs of the mother at this time. Provide appropriate support.
   c. Refer to social worker as necessary.
4. If this pregnancy occurred outside of marriage, the premature birth may precipitate other feelings of guilt or punishment in the parents. The parents may need help in identifying and working through these feelings in order to progress towards a more healthy attitude.

The Growing or Older Premature Infant

After the first few days have passed without any complications, the premature infant is very busy growing. During this time, however, it must be remembered that other complications can occur. Be constantly alert to signs and symptoms of complications. The areas of concern mentioned above are still important, along with the following:
1. Aspiration
   a. The growing premature infant may still have poor gag and cough reflexes.
   b. The premature infant will show signs of respiratory distress.
      Suction mouth and pharynx immediately and get medical assistance.
2. Latent acidosis of prematurity (developing after 3 days of life). This is less common when new infant formulas are used.
   a. Metabolic acidosis occurring during first few

weeks (pH and bicarbonate or base excess drops) is associated with immaturity of the kidneys and is unrelated to major cardiovascular or respiratory problems.

    (1) Infant may hyperventilate to blow off excess CO_2.

    (2) Urine pH varies from 6.0–7.5; blood pH ranges from 7.25–7.30 with base deficit.

  b. Symptoms are subtle:

    (1) Infant begins to feed poorly and takes longer to eat. He is sleepy and needs stimulation to keep awake; he displays lethargy.

    (2) The infant shows increased frequency and severity of apneic spells.

    (3) The infant may remain vigorous and take adequate fluid and calories, yet fail to gain weight.

    (4) Inadequate weight gain or loss when there is large caloric intake.

    (5) Stools become watery.

    (6) Skin may take on a gray pallor.

  c. Treatment consists of replacing bicarbonate lost through excretion and adjusting the intake via formula to decrease in amount of protein load and total calories.

3. Fluid retention

  a. Abnormal fluid retention results from the infant's inability to excrete solutes or to excrete water.

  b. Symptoms include:

    (1) Excessive weight gain

    (2) Pitting edema of feet, then body

    (3) Chest retractions

    (4) Inspired air diminished on auscultation with possible crackles

    (5) Increase in oxygen need; increase in PCO_2

  c. Treatment consists of giving diuretic agent and possibly decreasing fluid intake.

  d. Predisposing factors that lead to fluid retention include:

    (1) Patent ductus arteriosus with borderline heart failure

    (2) Bronchopulmonary dysplasia

    (3) Low total serum proteins

4. Wilson–Mikity syndrome

  a. Chronic form of respiratory distress. Infant may or may not have had respiratory distress syndrome.

  b. Insidious symptoms include:

    (1) Gradual increase in chest retractions

    (2) Decrease in inspired air on auscultation

    (3) Slowly increasing need for oxygen to about 30%–40%

    (4) Characteristic streaky pattern of lungs, progressing to soap-bubble appearance on x-ray

5. Hyperbilirubinemia (see p. 1236)

  a. Bilirubin concentrations are generally higher in the premature infant because of the impaired ability to conjugate bile in the liver.

  b. If infant is bruised from delivery or is plethoric, the risk of hyperbilirubinemia is increased.

  c. Hypoproteinemia and acidemia increase risk of low bilirubin kernicterus.

6. Necrotizing enterocolitis (NEC)

  a. Iatrogenic disease of the intestine of uncertain etiology; the bowel has patches of necrotic mucosa, with intramural gas (pneumatosis intestinalis).

    (1) It is thought to result from hypoxia leading to bowel ischemia, ileus, and stasis.

    (2) This, in turn, allows for bacterial invasion, proliferation, and damage to intestinal wall.

  b. Predisposing factors:

    (1) Prematurity, especially less than 34 weeks' gestation

    (2) Low birth weight, especially below 2,500 gm.

    (3) Shock of any type

    (4) Perinatal or neonatal asphyxia, low Apgar score

    (5) Exchange transfusion

    (6) Association with postnatal infection

    (7) Mother having had prolonged ruptured membranes or fever at delivery

    (8) Nasojejunal tube feeding

    (9) Respiratory distress

    (10) Polycythemia

    (11) Patent ductus arteriosus

    (12) Umbilical artery catheterization

    (13) Early milk feeding

  c. Signs and symptoms—the onset of symptoms occurs suddenly between 1 and 14 days of life, most often between 4 and 7 days of life; the infant has generally been tolerating feedings.

    (1) Abdominal distention, delayed gastric emptying, vomiting, increased gastric residuals

    (2) Jaundice

    (3) Apnea

    (4) GI bleeding; bloody diarrhea

    (5) Toxic-looking, lethargic

    (6) Temperature instability

    (7) Acidosis

    (8) Decreased urine output; increased specific gravity

    (9) X-ray findings show distended, thickened bowel loops; they may show streaks of intramural gas in bowel wall and sometimes peritoneal air from perforation.

  d. Supportive treatment

    (1) Gastric decompression with nasogastric tube; NPO

    (2) Antibiotic therapy—intravenously and orally to treat sepsis

    (3) IV hyperalimentation, intralipids

    (4) Fluids and electrolyte balance

    (5) Proper thermal and environmental factors

    (6) Diagnostic workup

      (a) Electrolytes

      (b) Platelet count

      (c) Bleeding times

      (d) Blood gases

      (e) Bilirubin

      (f) Blood sugar

      (g) X-ray of abdomen

      (h) Cultures to determine causative agent, if any.

    (7) Surgery—resection of gangrenous bowel

  e. Prevention

    (1) Prevention is the best method of treatment. NEC can recur.

    (2) Suggested interventions to prevent NEC in the compromised premature infant include:

      (a) Caution with enteral feeding; NPO first week of life; introduce and advance feedings slowly.

      (b) Use iso-osmolar milk at start of feedings; MCT may be added for calories.

      (c) Feed via N-G or O-G tube to allow

amount of gastric residual to be monitored.

(d) Prevent gastric distention from high-volume feedings.

(e) Monitor abdominal girth.

(f) Check stool for reducing substance (sugar).

(g) Breast milk may be used, since it contains living macrophages that combat infection, has a high pH which inhibits growth of *E. coli, Shigella,* and yeasts, and contents limit growth of *E. coli* and *Salmonella,* and has a high content of IgA which may protect against intestinal infection.

(h) Enteral antibiotics to combat proliferation of intestinal bacteria resulting from feeding (controversial).

f. Nursing responsibilities

(1) Acute, constant observations—place the infant in an Isolette or a radiant warmer.

(2) Close monitoring of vital signs and general condition; report even minute changes in the infant.

  (a) Stop oral feeding.

  (b) Abdominal girth measurement; note distention or rigidity, redness or shininess, erythema, observable bowel loops.

  (c) Check bowel sounds with stethoscope with minimal abdominal palpation.

  (d) Check stools for occult blood and reducing substance; save specimen as appropriate for examination by physician.

(3) Prevent additional stress to infant by maintaining stability in environment, IV intake, and gastric decompression.

(4) Minimize handling and trauma to abdomen—x-rays may be taken frequently to evaluate status.
Place the infant in a supine position; undress to decrease pressure on abdomen.

(5) Do not take rectal temperatures.

(6) Provide meticulous skin care when diarrhea and vomiting are present.

(7) Prevent dehydration and electrolyte imbalance by monitoring fluids.

(8) Prevent acute respiratory distress with positioning, temperature control, etc.

7. Bronchopulmonary dysplasia (BPD)

a. Chronic lung disorder characterized by coarse cystic-appearing lungs with hyperinfiltration, obstructive bronchiolitis, and pulmonary fibrosis from respiratory distress syndrome with high concentrations of oxygen and positive-pressure ventilation.

b. Other factors associated with BPD include:

(1) Endotracheal tube

(2) Patent ductus arteriosus

(3) Pulmonary edema from increased fluid loads in first days of life

(4) Smaller premature infant with severe respiratory distress syndrome

c. Signs and symptoms include:

(1) Tachycardia

(2) Difficulty weaning from oxygen or ventilator

(3) Respiratory distress

(4) Cyanosis

(5) CO_2 retention

(6) Increased apnea

(7) Pulmonary hypertension; right heart failure

(8) Generalized edema associated with low serum protein

d. Treatment—supportive

(1) Respiratory support—O_2, ventilator

(2) Sodium-free albumin

(3) Diuretics and digitalization as indicated

(4) Maintain nutritional support and fluid and electrolyte balance.

(5) Vitamin E—may help protect retina and lungs from toxic effects of oxygen, although this has not been proved.

e. Nursing responsibilities include:

(1) Support respiratory effort with gentle airway suctioning, chest physical therapy, and positioning.

(2) Observe and record frequency of persistent apnea, cyanotic episodes, tachypnea, retractions, and crackles.

(3) Allow infant to rest during feeding regardless of method used (nipple or gavage). He will tire easily and respond with apnea.

(4) Exercise constant vigilance to avoid respiratory infection in the infant, which could lead to death.

(5) Help to maintain a meaningful parent–infant relationship through the long duration of treatment.

B. Provide and maintain adequate nutrition to allow for growth and development.

1. The growth rate of the premature infant should parallel the expected in utero growth rate: about 20 gm./24 hours after 30 weeks' gestation and 30 gm./24 hours as the infant approaches term.
From birth to 5–10 days of age there will be a 5%–10% weight loss; then the infant should begin to gain weight.
The smaller the infant, the greater the weight loss.

2. The premature infant has a small gastric capacity but a great need for calories.
110–140 Kcal./kg./24 hours (40%–45% of total calorie intake should be provided by carbohydrates)
Caloric intake is dependent on age and birthweight of the premature infant. RDS and metabolic stress may also require caloric manipulation
120–150 ml./kg./24 hours of fluid
70 ml./kg./24 hours at birth
100 ml./kg./24 hours at 1 week
140–150 ml./kg./24 hours at 2 weeks
This, however, depends on the size of the infant.
2–4 gm. protein/kg./24 hours
If more than 4 gm./kg./24 hours of protein is given, the premature infant may present with signs of acidosis, azotemia, and other problems leading to neurologic abnormalities.

a. Generally, the premature infant (except the very low birth weight infant) has adequate gastric capacity, intestinal motility, and absorption to tolerate small, frequent feedings.

b. The gastric capacity expands during the first few weeks of life; this enables the infant to tolerate larger feedings.

c. Overfeeding increases the risk of vomiting. Vomiting can lead to dehydration, loss of hydrochloric acid, alkalosis, and aspiration.

d. The premature infant regurgitates feedings easily because of poor muscle tone at the cardiac sphincter. Expect small amount after feeding, especially with burping.

e. Bubble the infant frequently during feeding.

f. Formula should be adequate in calories, fluid, electrolytes, iron, and vitamins to meet the needs of the infant.

3. Considerations for enteral feeding:

a. Breast milk of the preterm-delivered mother appears to have higher protein and mineral content than milk from the term-delivered mother; provides protein and fat that is more easily metabolized and provides immunologic and anti-infective factors. It is low in calcium and phosphorus; supplemental vitamins are always given.

b. Special premature formulas are available that provide appropriate concentrations of protein, CHO, sodium, and phosphorus with an osmolality of 300 mOsm./kg. water.

c. Diluted formula should be used for early feedings to decrease stress and test the infant's tolerance.

d. Vitamins E and D may be supplemented, as well as calcium for the low-birth-weight infant.

4. Inappropriate weight gain in relation to caloric intake can indicate problems.

a. Unusually large weight gain for caloric intake may indicate excessive fluid retention.

b. No weight gain or a loss with adequate caloric intake may indicate acidosis, sepsis, or malabsorption.

5. Allow the infant to rest prior to feeding. The premature infant tires easily from procedures and will eat better if rested.

6. Feed appropriately for the individual infant.

a. Gavage is indicated for very small premature infant who does not demonstrate good sucking or synchronized sucking and swallowing. Diarrhea may result from malabsorption if feeding is advanced too rapidly.

b. Dropper or nipple feeding is indicated for a vigorous premature infant with good suck, gag, and swallowing reflexes.

c. Consider demand feeding for the growing premature above 1,800 gm. and over 5 days of age. Use cues from the infant regarding his sleep–wake cycle.

d. Constant drip feeding may be best for the very low birth weight or chronically ill infant.

7. Anemia frequently occurs in the premature infant.

a. Premature infants develop anemia (hemoglobin less than 8–10 gm./100 ml.). Reasons for the development of anemia include the following:

(1) Total body iron content is less.

(2) There is a proportionately larger blood loss from sampling.

(3) Relative body growth is more rapid, and there is an expanding blood volume.

b. Supplemental iron is needed to supply new iron stores. The iron is generally started when the infant is 2 months of age.

Folic acid and vitamin B_{12} may also be supplemented.

c. Blood transfusions are indicated to replace sampling blood in the sick preterm infant. Keep accurate records of blood output.

d. Symptomatic O_2 deficiency with anemia may present as minimal weight gain, decreased activity, temperature instability, poor feeding, apnea, tachycardia, tachypnea, PDA, pallor, or poor perfusion.

C. Meet the psychological needs of the premature infant, who is an individual in his own right.

1. At first, even though handling is minimal, the nurse should talk to and caress the infant while performing procedures.

a. Stroking and gentle handling will provide necessary sensory stimulation, especially after feeding.

b. A soft musical sound may also be comforting.

2. Once the premature infant is able to leave the Isolette even for short periods of time, he should be held for feedings.

a. While holding him, stroke him and talk to him.

b. Keep him warmly wrapped; this will also give him a feeling of security.

3. If the infant is restless in his incubator, he may be calmed by propping him against a blanket or diaper roll.

The freedom of movement, restrained only by the mattress, cannot offer much security to the infant.

4. Remember that the infant's ability to hear, see, smell, and touch are intact. Give him the opportunities to develop these capabilities and encourage the development of his interaction potential by providing sensory input.

Use the infant's cues to initiate visual and auditory stimulation. Recognize signs of infant stress and respond appropriately.

a. Physical contact is important for a sense of security.

b. Arrange environment so eye-to-eye contact can be established between caretaker or mother and infant.

c. Allow the infant freedom of movement for self-stimulation.

d. Change the infant's position and location of Isolette to encourage him to see his environment. Avoid sudden position changes; be slow and gentle. Avoid bumping into the Isolette.

5. Include parents in this activity to help them get to know their infant and incorporate these activities into their behavior so they will continue this at home.

D. Provide the premature infant with an environment that helps him to emerge successfully into a state of well-being and to become a healthy growing baby.

1. Conserve his energy.

a. Promote rest and sleep by the following:

(1) Appropriate handling

(2) Organizing and controlling interruptions

(3) Proper positioning of infant

b. Support physiologic functions and provide assistance as necessary (i.e., monitor respiration, temperature, and nutrition).

2. Assess stress of infant caused by medical procedures, response to stimuli and environment.

3. Change position every 2 hours. This does the following:

a. Stimulates circulation

b. Facilitates respirations

c. Prevents stasis of accumulated secretions

d. Minimizes skin irritation

e. Provides infant with opportunity for different stimulation input

4. Provide for physical safety and comfort.

a. Bathing—gives nurse opportunity to observe infant thoroughly.

b. Protect infant from self-inflicted injury by own random movements.
c. Protect from injury by equipment.
d. Use protective devices as necessary but allow the infant some unrestricted self-stimulation.
e. Keep portholes of Isolette closed.
f. Keep the infant warm when out of the Isolette— wrap with blanket and cover head with bonnet.

E. Foster healthy family relationships with the premature baby.

1. Encourage the parents to make frequent visits to the nursery so they can become familiar with all aspects of care of their infant.
   a. When they visit, explain the equipment and procedures that may be foreign to them.
   b. Help them to feel comfortable and confident in handling their infant.
   c. Parents may lose interest in the infant if the hospitalization is long. If parents cannot visit daily, encourage them to call, or call them at predetermined times.
2. Help the mother to see her infant as an individual and to develop mothering behaviors based on the infant's behavior.
   a. The infant's size and physical characteristics are generally unexpected and are different from those of the expected full-term baby.
   b. The premature infant's reflexes and responses to his environment are immature. The mother's expectations of his responses are based on those of a full-term baby.
   c. Explain these discrepancies between expectations and reality. The mother may associate her infant's responses with her inadequacies rather than those of the baby.
   d. Be aware of reflexes and responses that may elicit reactions in the mother. For example:
      (1) Uncoordinated sucking and swallowing— the mother experiences disappointment in not being able to feed, especially if she wanted to breast-feed her infant.
      (2) Gag reflex—the mother fears choking of the infant.
      (3) Respiratory immaturity—periodic breathing frightens the mother.
      (4) Grasp reflex—the mother is disappointed if her infant does not grasp her finger.
      (5) Moro reflex—exaggerated Moro reflex may make the mother feel she has frightened her infant.
   e. Reassure the mother that as the infant matures, he will change his response and reflex behaviors.
3. The support and help given to parents during hospitalization will make home care easier.
   a. Observe and assess behaviors as an aid to assessing attachment or bonding relationships and ability to relate to the infant.
   b. Teach the mother how to care for her infant. Thorough and careful preparation of the mother in feeding and caring for her infant often results in earlier discharge.
   c. The small size of the infant often is the single factor that frightens parents the most.
4. Initiate community-nurse referral if the parents seem anxious about caring for their baby at home.
   a. If this premature infant is the first baby, the referral may be particularly helpful to the mother.
   b. Home follow-up will enable the nurse to assess family interactions, parenting behaviors, and infant developmental screening.
5. Encourage parents to talk about their feelings or fears concerning their infant and how they will care for him.
   a. By listening, the nurse can gain some insight as to what to talk about or to teach the parents.
   b. Parents' feelings can frequently interfere with appropriate home care.
   c. Parents often treat the "preemie" as if he were fragile and more prone to illness. Overconcern is potentially harmful.
   d. Parents worry about how to feed and protect the infant.
6. Help the family prepare for the time when their new baby will arrive home.
   a. Because of the early, unexpected arrival of the infant, things such as clothing, bed, and bottles may not be ready.
   b. If there are other children at home, they need to be prepared for the homecoming of the premature infant. This preparation should begin early—using, for example, pictures of the infant and conversations about him.
   c. The readiness for the premature infant to go home is evaluated and assessed in terms of the following:
      (1) The infant's weight and progress
      (2) Maternal attachment to the infant
      (3) Maternal competence in caring for the infant
7. Consider transfer to community hospital once the infant is stable and growing.

Health Education

1. Help the family to understand that caring for the premature infant at home should not be any different from caring for a full-term infant.
   a. Special treatment may lead to behavior problems later.
   b. At first a little extra caution should be practiced. Cyanotic spells and severe infection are major concerns for the premature infant during first few weeks at home.
      (1) Keep room temperature fairly constant.
      (2) Sponge-bathe the infant instead of bathing in tub and keep him warm during procedure.
      (3) Feed the infant the recommended amount of formula to be certain he receives the necessary calories for continual growth. Maintain iron therapy.
      (4) Keep the infant away from crowds and people who have colds.
2. Spend enough time with the mother teaching her how to feed and care for her infant.
   Show her how, then watch her and help her improve and gain confidence.
      (1) The infant needs gentle, firm handling.
      (2) The infant needs to be mothered and kept comfortable with minimal tension.
      (3) A soothing voice can be comforting.
      (4) Sucking provides a pleasant experience.
3. Stress the importance of medical follow-up for the baby after discharge from the hospital.
   Anemia and failure to thrive are common long-term side effects of prematurity.
4. Help mother understand the importance of good, early prenatal care for subsequent pregnancies.

Once a woman has had one premature infant, this classifies her as high-risk for another premature delivery with future pregnancies.

5. Discharge planning implemented long before discharge of the high-risk infant should include:
   a. Assessing and reassessing needs of the infant
   b. Assessing and reassessing needs of the caretaker
   c. Establishing and implementing a teaching plan
   d. Identifying and acquiring equipment needed at home
   e. Initiating a community-agency referral as necessary
   f. Verbalizing and demonstrating an understanding of teaching plan by caretaker

Expected Outcomes

1. Premature infant progresses to wellness with no or minimal complications; respirations within expected range; gaining weight; demonstrates thermal stability; absence of infection, jaundice, etc.
2. Responds to auditory, visual, and tactile input; stroking, cuddling, verbal stimulation, and eye contact
3. Absence of injury and complications from treatment protocols
4. Parents demonstrate appropriate parent–infant bonding; interact with the infant; maintain eye contact while feeding
5. Parents demonstrate diminishing anxiety, make frequent visits to the nursery to see the infant, participate in care, handle the infant gently and firmly

Small-for-Gestational-Age Infant

The *"small-for-gestational-age infant" (SGA)* is a newborn who shows a discrepancy between growth and gestational age or whose weight is 2 standard deviations below expected weight for duration of gestation, or is plotted below the 10th percentile on intrauterine growth chart.

Intrauterine growth retarded (IUGR) is used interchangeably with SGA.

Etiology

IUGR may be due to reduction of total number of cells in the body (hypoplastic), to a reduction in cell size (hypotrophic), or to both.

While the etiological factors are unknown in many cases, other cases may result from the following causes.

A. Maternal Factors

1. Undernutrition
2. Diminished uterine blood flow
   a. Preeclampsia
   b. Toxemia
   c. Chronic hypertensive vascular disease
   d. Diabetes mellitus
3. Small stature
4. Smoking
5. Inadequate prenatal care
6. Low socioeconomic class
7. Heart disease
8. Low maternal age
9. Primiparity
10. Grand multiparity
11. Low prepregnant weight
12. Narcotic usage
13. Hemoglobinopathy
14. Phenylketonuria

B. Environmental Factors

1. High altitude
2. Teratogens
3. Irradiation

C. Placental Lesions

1. Infarcts
2. Premature placental separation
3. Hemangiomas
4. Thrombosis of fetal vessels
5. Single umbilical artery
6. Avascular terminal villi

D. Fetal Causes

1. Genetic dwarfs
2. Anencephaly
3. Infections (rubella, cytomegalovirus, toxoplasmosis, herpes simplex)
4. Chromosomal aberrations
   a. Turner's syndrome
   b. Down's syndrome
   c. Trisomy syndromes
   d. Cri-du-chat syndrome
5. Congenital anomalies
   a. Osteogenesis imperfecta
   b. De Lange's syndrome
   c. Cystic fibrosis
   d. Galactosemia
   e. Pierre Robin syndrome
   f. GI tract malformations

Altered Physiology

Although, in general, the physiologic maturity of fetal organs develops according to gestational age, there are exceptions to organ maturation being consistent with gestational age that result in problems (conditions) associated with IUGR.

1. Poor glucose control
   a. Hyperglycemia related to severe IUGR—symptoms include weight loss, dehydration, fever, and glucosuria.
   b. Hypoglycemia is probably due to rapid depletion of hepatic glycogen stores and to ineffective functioning of hepatic enzyme system responsible for gluconeogenesis.
2. Limited temperature control
   a. The infant has relatively large surface area per unit of body weight.
   b. The infant lacks energy stores and subcutaneous fat insulation; decreased brown fat stores.
   c. The infant can assume position of flexion of extremities—reduces surface area exposed to environment and decreased heat loss by radiation and convection.
   d. Has vasomotor control over peripheral circulation to dilate or constrict capillaries as needed.
   e. Sweating mechanism is intact.
3. High hemoglobin, increased plasma volume, and enlarged extracellular fluid volume per kilogram of

body weight, putting the infant at risk for respiratory distress, cardiac and circulatory problems, and hyperbilirubinemia.
4. Minimal weight loss with rapid initial weight gain
   a. Weight gain is not maintained throughout first year.
   b. Rapid initial weight gain may suggest rehydration as well as tissue growth.
5. Late anemia
   Secondary to rapid weight gain and poor iron stores present at birth, especially in the premature infant.
6. Elevated immunoglobulin (IgM) in infants with intrauterine infection.
7. High nonprotein nitrogen levels, possibly due to:
   a. Increase in fetal catabolism—or
   b. Impaired placental excretion of fetal waste products
8. Prone to postasphyxial problems
   a. The asphyxial process of normal labor is associated with metabolic acidosis.
   b. Fetal malnutrition, in addition to the birth process, predisposes the infant to asphyxia neonatorum.
9. Limited fat and glycogen reserves due to intrauterine growth retardation
10. X-ray findings:
    a. Atrophy of thymus
    b. Thin ribs

Complications

1. Problems associated with asphyxia neonatorum and meconium aspiration syndrome
2. Hypoglycemia and hypocalcemia
3. Polycythemia
4. Pulmonary hemorrhage
5. Prematurity with intrauterine growth retardation
6. Infection associated with maternal conditions
7. Hypothermia
8. Late anemia
9. Future growth retardation (depends on cause of IUGR)
10. Delays in developmental and motor skills; difficult behavior styles (depends on cause of IUGR)

Assessment
Clinical Manifestations

Clinical manifestations of the SGA infant are related to the duration, intensity, and time of onset of the influence (factors) causing intrauterine growth retardation.
1. Chronic IUGR—growth of the fetus has been curtailed by insult for weeks or months prior to birth. Note the following characteristics (hypoplastic stage):
   a. Body proportions remain unaltered—weight, length, and possibly head circumference are below normal for gestational age.
   b. Creases on soles of feet
   c. Coarse, straight, silky hair
   d. Well-developed ear cartilage
   e. Firm skull bones
2. Subacute IUGR—growth of fetus has been curtailed by insult only a few days or weeks prior to birth (hypotrophic stage).
   a. Weight is diminished; length of body and head circumference may be normal.
   b. Wasted look with loose, thin skin
   c. Long, thin appearance
   d. Face has look of "worried little old man"
   e. Scaphoid abdomen

f. Skin dry, cracked, and peeling
g. Thin umbilical cord that dries and hardens rapidly
h. Widened skull sutures

Diagnostic Evaluation

1. Evaluate general appearance of the infant.
2. Determine gestational age using physical characteristics and neurologic examination (see Table 33-1, pp. 1218–1219).
3. The infant can be SGA and preterm, SGA and term, or SGA and postterm.
4. Measure weight, length, and head circumference; plot on Colorado intrauterine growth chart and compare relative percentiles.
5. Determine blood sugar.
6. Obtain hematocrit (HCT) and hemoglobin to determine polycythemia and hyperviscosity (venous HCT over 65%).

Potential Problems/Nursing Diagnoses

The small-for-gestational-age infant is prone to complications and should be considered at-risk.
1. Complications related to SGA: pulmonary hemorrhage and infection
2. Problems associated with asphyxia neonatorum or meconium aspiration related to fetal distress
3. Hypoglycemia related to rapid depletion of glycogen stores
4. Hypothermia related to lack of energy stores and subcutaneous fat
5. Problems related to polycythemia (i.e., jaundice, tachypnea, tachycardia, respiratory distress)
6. Malnutrition and feeding problems related to low birth weight
7. Other problems related to hospitalized premature infant (see Preterm, p. 1217)

Planning and Implementation
Nursing Interventions

The nursing management of the SGA infant in many aspects is similar to that for the premature infant (see p. 1217). The following are major interventions of the nurse caring for the SGA neonate:

A. Observe for any gross and less obvious congenital anomalies as in the case of any infant upon admission to the nursery.

1. Congenital anomalies are often associated with intrauterine growth retardation.
   Genitourinary, cardiovascular and skeletal complications and syndromes are common problems.
2. Certain types of intrauterine infection account for intrauterine growth retardation and may present signs of skin rash, petechiae and ecchymoses, hepatomegaly, splenomegaly, early-onset of obstructive jaundice, chorioretinitis, lethargy, and irritability.
3. Report any suspicious findings and observations to the physician immediately.

B. Observe for problems associated with asphyxia neonatorum.

The SGA neonate has an increased incidence of asphyxia neonatorum. His lessened metabolic stores of carbohydrates lower his ability to handle the stresses of delivery. Acidosis may develop quickly.
1. Be aware of the Apgar scores which will help in determining degree of asphyxia (Apgar less than 5 at 1 minute or less than 7 at 5 minutes).

2. See that blood gas studies are done to confirm adequate oxygenation and acidosis. Frequent monitoring should be continued.
3. Observe for signs of respiratory distress.
   a. Adequate oxygenation is imperative for improving prognosis.
   b. Suction and oxygen equipment should be available and ready for immediate use.
   c. Aspiration pneumonia and pulmonary hemorrhage are postasphyxiation problems.
4. Check vital signs frequently and note behavior (i.e., reflex responses, irritability; cardiac function can be affected and CNS damage can occur with severe asphyxia.
5. Check and record intake and output. Renal damage is a common sequel of severe asphyxia.
6. Observe for abnormal clotting function and hyperbilirubinemia.
7. Postasphyxial hypocalcemia may occur.
8. Record and report all observations appropriately.

C. Screen for hypoglycemia, beginning soon after birth.

1. The SGA infant has reduced carbohydrate stores at birth. Glycogen reserves are depleted almost immediately after birth. Gluconeogenesis is inadequate because of reduced stores of muscle protein and fat tissue, as well as reduced hyperglycemic response to norepinephrine and glucagon, which activate the gluconeogenesis process.
2. Hypoglycemia is most likely to occur from 12–48 hours after birth.
   Severely hypoxic, hypothermic SGA infants can become hypoglycemic as early as 6 hours after birth.
3. Blood sugars should be monitored frequently (every 30–60 minutes) by Dextrostix during the first few hours after birth and during IV glucose therapy.
   a. If Dextrostix evaluation is below 40 mg./100 ml., report this to physician immediately because measurement of serum glucose should be done.
   b. Keep Dextrostix bottle tightly covered and out of direct sunlight to avoid false reading on Dextrostix.
4. When IV infusion of glucose is used to prevent or treat hypoglycemia, particular care must be given to prevent infiltration and subsequent slough and necrosis of tissue.
5. With the infant at risk for hypoglycemia, oral feeding should be started as early as 2 hours after birth (if there are no contraindications).
6. Signs of hypoglycemia include:
   a. Jitteriness
   b. Sweating
   c. Tachypnea or apnea
   d. Cyanosis
   e. Convulsions
   f. Respiratory distress
7. Report all observations to the physician and record accurately.

D. Prevent hypothermia and maintain thermal stability of the SGA neonate (see p. 1220–1222).

1. Ensure that adequate environmental heat is provided to maintain the infant's abdominal skin temperature at 36.0°–36.5°C. (96.8°F.), thus decreasing calories needed for heat production, which would slow growth rate.
2. Prevent the infant from lying on the thermistor.

E. Take measures to deal with polycythemia.

Polycythemia, which is increased red blood cell volume, is frequently seen in SGA infants when growth retardation is due to placental insufficiency.

1. Polycythemia is identified by a high hematocrit or hemoglobin level (i.e., venous blood HCT over 65%); Hb of 20–22 gm./100 ml.). Hyperviscosity can result from this condition.
2. Signs and symptoms of viscosity include:
   a. Plethora
   b. Jaundice
   c. Tachypnea
   d. Tachycardia
   e. Peripheral cyanosis
   f. Grunting
   g. Nasal flaring, intercostal retractions
   h. Scrotal edema
   i. Priapism (persistent, abnormal erection of penis)
   j. Tremors, irritability, possibly seizures
3. Ensure that the HCT or Hb is monitored during the first 6–12 hours after birth in the high-risk infant.
4. Treatment for HCT above 70% usually consists of partial exchange transfusion. The nurse must be prepared to assist with this by using fresh frozen plasma or whole blood.

F. Provide adequate nutrition for growth.

1. Parenteral nutrition may be considered if the infant cannot tolerate enteral feedings by 3rd day of life.
2. Synchronized suck–swallow reflex does not become effective until 32–34 weeks' gestational age.
   Alternate gavage and nipple feeding are used when weight is above 1,800 gm. and the infant is of 34 weeks' gestation or more.

G. Prevent spread of infection to personnel and other neonates if infant IUGR is due to congenital infection.

1. Initiate isolation precautions according to health agency policy.

H. Accurately measure and record daily weights and monitor length and head circumference.

Rapid weight gain is expected the first few days and weeks.

I. Support the parents of the infant (see Premature Infant, p. 1225).

1. The long-term outcome of the SGA infant often represents an increase in long-range sequelae frequently manifested in lowered intellectual achievement resulting from malnutrition during peak intrauterine brain growth (depends on cause of IUGR).
2. Long-term prognosis depends on adequate treatment of problems encountered immediately after birth, etiology of problems, and subsequent home environment.
3. Teach parents about their infant: temperament, behavior styles, what comforts or irritates the infant, corrected gestational age as a criterion for developmental expectations.
4. Establish parent–infant bonding.
5. Emphasize importance of follow-up medical care.

Evaluation
Expected Outcomes

1. Absence of complications; no evidence of pulmonary hemorrhage; normal breathing pattern for gestational age; no temperature elevation

2. Maintains normal respiratory status and adequate oxygenation; absence of respiratory distress; appropriate PaO_2.
3. Shows no signs of hypoglycemia; normal serum glucose

4. Maintains temperature stability; avoids fever and infections
5. Shows no signs of polycythemia; normal hematocrit and hemoglobin values
6. Receives adequate nutrition; gaining weight

Postmature Infant

The *postmature infant* is one whose gestation is 42 weeks or longer and who may show signs of weight loss with placental insufficiency.

Etiology

1. Not known in many cases.
2. Maternal factors associated with postmaturity:
   a. Primigravida and high-parity mother at any given age.
   b. Prolonged gestation in preceding pregnancies.

Altered Physiology

1. The postmature infant appears to have suffered from intrauterine malnutrition and hypoxia.
   Before the termination of the pregnancy, but at the point when the birth should have occurred, the placental function begins to diminish, resulting in impaired oxygen exchange and inadequate nutrient transfer to the fetus.
2. There are stages of postmaturity—severity of associated problems is determined by length of gestation (i.e., the longer the gestation, the more severe the problems).

Assessment

Clinical Manifestations

Physical appearance—the following characteristics are most often seen in infant of 44 weeks' gestation or more:
1. Reduced subcutaneous tissue—loose skin, especially of buttocks and thighs
2. Long, curved fingernails and toenails
3. Reduced amount of vernix caseosa
4. Abundant scalp hair
5. Wrinkled, macerated skin; possibly pale, cracked, parchment-like skin.
6. Having the alert appearance of a 2- to 3-week old infant following delivery
7. Greenish-yellow staining of skin, indicating fetal distress

Diagnostic Evaluation

1. Evaluate general appearance.
2. Determine gestational age—give neurologic examination.
3. Measure weight, length, and head circumference, and plot on Colorado intrauterine growth chart. Compare percentiles.
4. Determine blood sugar. In hypoglycemia, the serum sugar level is below 40 mg./100 ml.
5. Assessment of asphyxia neonatorum.
   a. Apgar score
   b. Blood gas analysis

Potential Problems/Nursing Diagnoses

1. Respiratory distress related to meconium aspiration, asphyxia neonatorum, pulmonary hemorrhage, pneumonia or pneumothorax, polycythemia
2. Hypoglycemia related to decreased glycogen stores and malnutrition due to placental dysfunction

3. Birth injury related to large size
4. Other complications related to sick infant and hospitalization (see Premature Infant, p. 1223)

Complications

1. Meconium aspiration
2. Hypoglycemia and hypocalcemia
3. Polycythemia
4. Pulmonary hemorrhage
5. Problems associated with asphyxia neonatorum
6. Pneumonia
7. Pneumothorax

Planning and Implementation
Nursing Interventions

Problems and nursing care encountered in the postmature infant may include the metabolic disturbances of the SGA infant and complications of asphyxia neonatorum as well as polycythemia (see SGA, p. 1232). Massive meconium aspiration causes specific problems for the postmature infant (refer to nursing objectives for the premature infant, p. 1231 and SGA, p. 1217).

A. Be alert for respiratory distress that may indicate meconium aspiration.

1. The stage is set for meconium aspiration when placental function diminishes and oxygen transport to the fetus decreases, leading to cerebral hypoxia.
   a. The anal sphincter relaxes and meconium passes into the surrounding amniotic fluid.
   b. The asphyxiated fetus gasps and aspiration occurs.
2. Signs and symptoms of meconium aspiration—severity depends on amount and thickness of meconium aspirated, as well as the location of the aspirate in the respiratory tract.
   a. Tachypnea, increasing signs of cyanosis; difficulty breathing, with need for ventilation
   b. Tachycardia
   c. Inspiratory nasal flaring and retraction of chest
   d. Expiratory grunting
   e. Increased anteroposterior diameter of the chest
   f. Palpable liver
   g. Crackles and rhonchi on chest auscultation
   h. Concomitant cerebral irritation—jitteriness, hypotonia, seizures
   i. X-ray—classic coarse, patchy, irregular pulmonary infiltrates ranging in severity
   j. Additional signs: metabolic acidosis, hypotension, hypoglycemia, hypocalcemia
3. Mainly supportive treatment
   a. Warmth—maintain thermally neutral environment so the infant uses fewer calories and less oxygen
   b. Adequate oxygenation and humidification to maintain PaO_2 at 50–70 mm. Hg.
   c. Respiratory support with ventilator
      (1) Be aware that metabolic disturbances often accompany respiratory problems.

(2) Ensure that monitoring of blood gases and pH is done.

(3) Carefully record blood sampling.

d. Adequate administration of calories and fluid Accurately record intake and output—assess possible alteration in kidney function due to hypoxia.

e. Antibiotics

(1) Prophylactically—meconium may lead to a chemical pneumonia and the growth of gram-negative bacteria. Therefore, antibiotics specifically for gram-negative bacteria may be used.

(2) Treatment—antibiotics used only when clinical evidence indicates infection.

f. Pulmonary physical therapy—every 30–60 minutes first few hours

(1) Postural drainage (p. 1178)

(2) Pulmonary lavage—using nonirritating solution and immediate suctioning of mouth, pharynx, and trachea; bag ventilate using high concentrations of oxygen between lavage procedures

(3) Change position from side to side frequently and elevate head by adjusting the mattress to a 20-degree angle

(4) Complications of meconium aspiration

(a) Pneumothorax and/or pneumomediastinum

(b) Secondary pneumonia

(c) Pulmonary hypertension with persistent fetal circulation

(d) Respiratory failure

(e) Death

(5) Prevention

Most cases of meconium aspiration can be prevented if meconium is removed from the mouth and trachea by proper suctioning, prior to the infant's taking his first breath.

Note: If ventilator management is indicated, treatment is similar to that of the infant with hyaline membrane disease (p. 1270).

B. Be aware that the postmature infant is particularly prone to hypoglycemia within hours after birth (see SGA, p. 1232).

1. Oral feeding or IV glucose is usually initiated soon after birth. If oral feedings are not contraindicated, they can begin 1–2 hours after birth.

2. Close and careful monitoring of blood sugar should be done with Dextrostix every hour until condition stabilizes.

3. Persistent hypoglycemia may contribute to CNS problems.

4. Be alert to signs and symptoms of hypoglycemia and report to physician.

C. Support the parents of the infant (see Premature Infant, p. 1225, and ICN, p. 1225).

The long-term sequelae common in the postmature infant are associated with central nervous system (neurologic) problems.

Evaluation

Expected Outcomes

1. Maintains adequate oxygen–carbon dioxide exchange; no evidence of respiratory distress

2. Shows no signs of hypoglycemia; taking oral feedings; maintaining appropriate serum glucose levels

3. Demonstrates no signs of birth injuries

4. No signs of complications related to hospitalization (see premature infant, p. 1230)

Infant of Diabetic Mother

The *infant of a diabetic mother (IDM)* is the infant born to a mother with diabetes. The mother may be an overt diabetic or gestational diabetic. The severity of infant problems depends on the severity of the maternal diabetes (Table 33-2).

Altered Physiology

Hyperinsulinemia in utero secondary to decreased epinephrine and glucose response result in the following in the infant:

1. Increased amount of body fat, not edema.

a. Total body water is somewhat reduced at birth.

b. High urinary output during first 2 days of life, probably from freeing of intracellular water.

2. Hypoglycemia

a. Occurs within first 2–12 hours of life; may occur within minutes after birth.

b. The infant's response to glucose is excessive (i.e., insulin blood level will have a slight elevation, will drop and then peak within 1 hour). This is probably due to maternal hyperglycemia.

c. The infant's cord insulin levels may not be higher than in a normal infant unless a large amount of glucose is given.

d. IDM may be symptomatic or asymptomatic with blood sugars below 20 mg./100 ml.

3. Hypocalcemia

a. Associated with prematurity, difficult labor and delivery, and/or asphyxia at birth.

b. Generally occurs during first 24–48 hours of life.

Table 33-2 White's Classification of Diabetes in Pregnancy

Class A	Highest probability of fetal survival No insulin, little dietary regulation Includes gestational diabetes and prediabetes
Class B	Onset at age 20 or older Duration less than 10 years before pregnancy No vascular disease
Class C	Onset between 10 and 19 years of age Duration between 10 and 19 years Minimal vascular disease (retinal arteriosclerosis, calcification of vessels in the legs only)
Class D	Onset before age 10 years Duration 20 years or more Moderately advanced vascular disease (diabetic retinopathy, transient albuminuria, and hypertension)
Class E	Characteristics of class D plus calcification of pelvic vessels
Class F	Characteristics of class D plus nephritis
Class R	Active retinitis

(Krones SB. High-Risk Newborn Infant: The Basis for Intensive Nursing Care, 3rd ed. St Louis, CV Mosby, 1981, p. 307)

4. Hyperbilirubinemia
   a. Most likely to occur within 48–72 hours after birth.
   b. Immature liver results in inability to conjugate bilirubin.
   c. HCT is higher on the 3rd day after birth and extracellular volume is decreased.
   d. Because of large size, birth trauma may increase risk of enclosed hemorrhage.
5. Prematurity
   a. May be premature or small for gestational age when associated with placental insufficiency in classes D–F mothers (Table 33-1).
   b. Respiratory function is similar to that of other premature infants—thus the infant is prone to hyaline membrane disease.
6. Polycythemia
   a. Venous hematocrit greater than 65% or venous hemoglobin 22 gm./100 ml.
   b. Polycythemia increases the risks of occurrence of renal vein thrombosis, respiratory distress, hypoglycemia, and hypocalcemia.
7. Congenital anomalies
   a. Increased incidence of congenital anomalies may be due to:
      (1) Divergent gene pattern
      (2) Glucose homeostasis in utero
   b. Most common anomalies are skeletal and cardiac.
8. Infection
   a. Prematurity and lowered passive immunity
   b. Possible maternal urinary tract infection and bacteria crossing the placenta

Assessment
Diagnostic Evaluation

1. Maternal history of diabetes
2. Physical assessment of infant and determination of gestational age
3. Blood studies
   a. Glucose
   b. Calcium, phosphorus
   c. HCT and Hb
   d. Blood gas analysis
   e. Magnesium (if indicated)
   f. Electrolytes
   g. Bilirubin

Clinical Manifestations

1. Macrosomia
2. Cardiomegaly
3. Hepatomegaly
4. Large umbilical cord and placenta
5. Plethora
6. Full-face
7. Tendency to be large for gestational age; some may be normal weight or SGA; IUGR when mother has had long-standing insulin dependency
8. Abundant fat, hair, and vernix caseosa

Complications

1. Hypoglycemia
2. Hypocalcemia
3. Hyaline membrane disease
4. Polycythemia and renal vein thrombosis
5. Infection
6. Hyperbilirubinemia
7. Hypermagnesemia or hypomagnesemia
8. Congenital anomalies

9. Birth injuries—cephalohematomas, facial nerve paralysis, fractured clavicles, brachial nerve plexus
10. Prematurity
11. Congestive heart failure secondary to congenital heart disease, subaortic stenosis, asymmetrical ventricular septal hypertrophy
12. Asphyxia neonatorum
13. Organomegaly
14. Neurologic instability

Potential Problems/Nursing Diagnoses

1. Respiratory distress and infection related to prematurity
2. Hypoglycemia and hypocalcemia related to prematurity
3. Birth injuries related to large size
4. Potential for other problems related to hospitalization of premature infant (see preterm infant, p. 1217)

Planning and Implementation
Nursing Interventions

Except for specific considerations discussed below, the nursing care of the infant of a diabetic mother (IDM) is the same as for the premature infant (p. 1217).

A. Observe closely for hypoglycemia.

Report any irregularities immediately to physician.
1. Monitor serum glucose levels every 30–60 minutes beginning immediately after birth for 24 hours or every 4–8 hours until stabilized. Glucose levels are lowest 1–2 hours after birth; at 2–6 hours, glucose levels even off and gradually increase. Warm the extremity prior to capillary sampling to prevent false-low value resulting from stasis.
2. The infant with hypoglycemia (premature infant: below 20 mg./100 ml.; term infant: below 30 mg./100 ml.) may be symptomatic or asymptomatic. Signs include:
   a. Jitteriness
   b. Tremors
   c. Convulsions
   d. Sweating
   e. Cyanosis
   f. Weak or high-pitched cry
   g. Refusal to eat
   h. Hypotonia (reduced muscle tone)
   i. Apnea
   j. Temperature instability
   k. Rotating eye movements
3. Hypoglycemia may be prevented or treated by early feedings of 10%–20% glucose or formula by nipple or gavage.
   a. IV glucose, 10%–15%, may be given for very low serum glucose levels or when infant's condition prevents oral feeding.
   b. Glucose levels should be maintained in the low-normal range.
   c. Overfeeding or excessive IV infusion of glucose may result in a rebound effect causing insulin levels to increase and hypoglycemia to reappear.
   d. IV glucose must not be discontinued abruptly in order to prevent rebound hypoglycemia.

B. Monitor infant closely for changes in acid–base status, respiratory distress, temperature, hypocalcemia, and sepsis.

C. Observe for hyperbilirubinemia.

1. Infants of diabetic mothers have a higher incidence of hyperbilirubinemia.

Levels will be elevated 48–72 hours after birth.
Other predisposing factors include prematurity and polycythemia, which increases the load of bilirubin from the natural process of RBC breakdown to be cleared, decreased extracellular fluid, and birth trauma related to increased birth weight.

2. The infant may need an exchange transfusion at relatively lower bilirubin levels (as in the premature infant) to prevent kernicterus. Phototherapy may need to be initiated early.

3. The blood sugar must be monitored during and following exchange transfusion.
CPD (citrate phosphate dextrose) contains large amounts of dextrose which may subsequently cause rebound hypoglycemia.

D. Assist in the prevention of dehydration and maintenance of fluid and electrolyte balance.

1. Because of the increase in fatty tissue and decrease in total amount of body water, the freeing of intracellular water after birth will increase urinary output. This, along with inability to concentrate urine, increases the risk of dehydration. Dehydration increases risk of polycythemia.

2. Accurately record intake and output; administer prescribed fluids and evaluate laboratory studies to determine current status.

E. Be aware of the infant who is predisposed to hypomagnesemia or hypermagnesemia and observe for signs and symptoms of each.

1. Hypermagnesemia may occur when the preeclamptic mother was treated with magnesium sulfate.
   a. Signs and symptoms may include:
      (1) Hypotonia
      (2) Weak or absent cry
      (3) Severe respiratory distress with apnea or cyanosis
   b. Treatment is an exchange transfusion.

2. Hypomagnesemia may accompany hypocalcemia or follow an exchange transfusion.
   a. Severe neuromuscular excitability may be the presenting symptom.
   b. IM magnesium sulfate is the treatment.

F. Be alert for development of renal vein thrombosis in the infant during the first few days of life.

1. Polycythemia, transient dehydration, and decreased extracellular fluid may be causes.
2. Observe for hematuria and proteinuria.
3. Flank masses may be palpable.

G. Observe the infant for possible cardiac anomalies (see p. 1292).

Monitor cardiac and respiratory rates.

H. Support the mother who may have feelings of severe guilt or inadequacy, since she is directly related to the problems her infant may be having.

1. Encourage and allow the mother to talk about these feelings.
2. Encourage her, when appropriate, to have close obstetrical care for subsequent pregnancies.
3. Stress importance of a periodic evaluation for diabetes in her child.

Evaluation
Expected Outcomes

1. Reveals no signs of respiratory distress; normal vital signs; laboratory values within acceptable ranges
2. Achieves physiologic balance soon after birth; normal serum glucose values; absence of tremors, convulsions, etc.
3. Has no evidence of birth injury
4. Shows no evidence of other complications related to prematurity (see preterm infant, p. 1230)

Jaundice in the Newborn (Hyperbilirubinemia)

Hyperbilirubinemia (jaundice) in the newborn is an accumulation of serum bilirubin above normal levels.

Etiology

1. Increased bilirubin load
   a. Hemolytic disease—Rh and ABO incompatibility
   b. Morphologic abnormalities of red blood cells
   c. Red blood cell enzyme defects
   d. Physiologic jaundice (see later discussion of "physiologic jaundice")
2. Extravascular blood
   a. Cephalohematoma
   b. Pulmonary or cerebral hemorrhage
   c. Any enclosed occult blood
3. Decrease or inhibition of bilirubin conjugation
   a. Inherited bilirubin conjugation defect: Crigler–Najjar syndrome (deficiency of glucuronyl transferase).
   b. Acquired bilirubin conjugation defect: breast-milk jaundice, Lucey–Driscoll syndrome, infant of diabetic mother, asphyxiated infant with respiratory distress
4. Increased extrahepatic circulation
Intestinal obstruction

5. Polycythemia
   a. Twin–twin transfusion
   b. Maternofetal transfusion
   c. Infant of diabetic mother
   d. Small-for-gestational-age infant
6. Mixed jaundice—increased bilirubin load and decreased clearance resulting in elevated indirect and direct bilirubin levels
   a. Sepsis
   b. Severe hemolytic disease
   c. Intrauterine transfusion
   d. Galactosemia
   e. Biliary atresia—absence of extrahepatic ducts or presence of cordlike structures without a lumen
7. Hypothyroidism
8. Familial, transient—associated with inhibiting factor in plasma
9. Unknown

Altered Physiology

A. Bilirubin Production

1. 75% of the bilirubin present in the newborn is from RBC breakdown.

a. The red blood cell is broken down into protein and globin combined with heme, which is an iron–porphyrin complex.
b. In the presence of the enzyme called heme oxygenase:
   (1) Globin is reduced to amino acids.
   (2) Iron is broken off and stored.
   (3) Porphyrin moiety is broken into biliverdin, which is reduced to bilirubin.
c. This bilirubin is unconjugated or indirect and is fat-soluble.
d. Indirect bilirubin, bound to albumin, is present in circulating blood and tissues.
e. The liver selectively removes this albumin-bound bilirubin from the blood.
f. Once the unconjugated bilirubin is in the liver, it is converted to direct or conjugated water-soluble bilirubin with the aid of enzymes, one of which is glucuronyl transferase.
g. From the liver, conjugated bilirubin is excreted via the bile into the intestine and is excreted in the stool or is hydrolyzed to unconjugated bilirubin in the intestine and reabsorbed across the intestinal mucosa into the circulation (entero-hepatic circulation).

2. 25% of the bilirubin present in the newborn is from non–erythrocyte-containing heme proteins.

B. Physiologic Jaundice

1. Increased load of bilirubin on liver cells.
   a. Increased bilirubin production—more rapid hemolysis because of higher level of circulating RBCs per kg. (2.2 lbs.) of body weight and a shorter RBC life span.
   b. Enterohepatic circulation—reabsorption of unconjugated bilirubin.
2. Decreased clearance of bilirubin from plasma.
   a. Predominant bilirubin-binding protein in liver cells may be deficient the first days of life.
   b. Glucuronyl transferase enzyme activity may be decreased, resulting in impaired conjugation of bilirubin.
   c. Liver may show decreased ability to excrete large amounts of conjugated bilirubin.
   d. Poor portal blood supply may decrease the liver's capacity to act effectively.
   e. Open ductus venosus may allow blood to bypass liver.

C. Erythrocyte Destruction

1. Erythroblastosis fetalis (isoimmunization due to Rh factor or ABO incompatibility)
   a. Immune hemolysis or Rh/ABO blood group incompatibility; the mother's and fetus' blood are different.
      Rh factor; different ABO blood groups (see Coomb's test, next column).
   b. Mother produces antibodies against the antigen of the fetus' blood. Fetal cells frequently cross the placenta.
   c. Antibodies of the mother's blood are present in the infant's blood at birth, causing the following conditions:
      (1) There is hemolysis of the infant's red blood cells.
      (2) Hemolysis leads to a rising level of indirect bilirubin.
2. Glucose-6-phosphate dehydrogenase deficiency (G-6-PD)—nonimmune hemolytic disease (erythrocyte biochemical factor)
   a. Deficiency results in reduced stability to oxidative destruction from substances that act as oxidizing agents (i.e., vitamin K, naphthalene, salicylates).
   b. X-linked recessive disease that affects primarily Black and Mediterranean–Oriental groups.
   c. Screen maternal blood for carrier state and screen neonate blood in high-risk groups.
3. Other conditions associated with increased erythrocyte destruction:
   a. Infection—bacterial, viral, and/or protozoan
   b. Structural abnormal erythrocyte
   c. Sequestered blood (i.e., cephalohematoma, ecchymoses)

D. Other Considerations

1. Each gram of hemoglobin breakdown forms 35 mg. of bilirubin.
2. An unmeasurable amount of bilirubin does not bind to albumin. Free indirect bilirubin is very toxic to the cells of the CNS.
3. The enzyme system responsible for conjugation of bilirubin is oxygen-dependent and altered by infant's pH, temperature, etc. Thus infants who are acidotic, hypoxic, or hypothermic tend to present with higher levels of bilirubin.

Clinical Manifestations

1. Onset of clinical jaundice seen when serum bilirubin levels are less than 5–7 mg./100 dl.
   a. Physiologic jaundice—occurs 3–5 days after birth.
      (1) Increase in unconjugated bilirubin levels; levels must not exceed 5 mg./100 dl. per day.
      (2) Peak bilirubin levels not to exceed 12 mg./100 dl. in full-term infant and 15 mg./100 dl. in premature infant.
      (3) Full-term peak levels (6 mg./100 dl.) are reached by 48–72 hours after birth; clinical jaundice declines in 1 week, and normal bilirubin levels are reached in 2 weeks.
      (4) Premature peak levels (10–15 gm./100 dl.) are reached by 4–6 days of age; clinical jaundice declines in 2 weeks and normal bilirubin levels are reached in 3–4 weeks.
   b. Erythroblastosis—may occur within 24 hours after birth.
2. Signs and symptoms may include:
   a. Sclerae appearing yellow before skin appears yellow
   b. Skin appearing light to bright yellow
   c. Lethargy
   d. Dark amber, concentrated urine
   e. Poor feeding
   f. Dark stools

Diagnostic Evaluation

1. All infants who have clinical signs of hyperbilirubinemia should be given the following work-up:
   a. Serum bilirubin levels—total and direct
   b. Peripheral smear—for evidence of red blood cell morphology and reticulocyte count
   c. Reticulocyte count—to determine rate of hemolysis
   d. Coombs' test—to check for Rh and ABO or other group incompatibility between the mother and infant—direct Coombs' test on infant serum

e. Blood typing of mother and infant
f. Total serum protein—to measure binding capacity
g. Hematocrit or hemoglobin
h. Acid–base status
i. Albumin-binding test—to measure reserve binding sites (if available)
2. There are 3 current approaches to measuring risk of bilirubin toxicity:
   a. Sephadex G—25 level
   b. HBABA dye-binding
   c. Salicylate saturation index
3. Measuring the bilirubin–albumin binding capacity of the plasma can also be valuable in determining the risk of kernicterus (see below) and the need for an exchange transfusion. This test defines the upper limits to which serum bilirubin is allowed to rise when an exchange transfusion is done.
   a. $\dfrac{\text{Total bilirubin}}{\text{Total serum protein}} =$

      (1) If less than 3.7—no danger of kernicterus
      (2) If greater than 3.7—treatment by exchange transfusion is indicated.
   b. Total serum protein × 3.7 = level of bilirubin at which to do exchange transfusion.
4. The level of bilirubin at which the infant is at risk for brain damage depends on the degree of prematurity, presence of acidosis, hypoxia, or drugs which bind albumin indirect bilirubin (20 mg. of bilirubin/100 ml. of blood in term infant is not necessarily the upper limit of bilirubin as formerly thought).
5. Appropriate cultures when infection is suspected.
6. Serum glucose levels.

Complications—Kernicterus

Kernicterus is a yellow discoloration of specific areas of brain tissue by unconjugated bilirubin; can be confirmed only by death and autopsy.
   Bilirubin encephalopathy best describes the occurrence of the syndrome and the accompanying neurologic sequelae in neonates.
1. Early signs of kernicterus
   a. Poor feeding
   b. Vomiting
   c. Lethargy
   d. High-pitched cry
   e. Hypotonia
   f. Decrease of normal reflexes, Moro reflex
2. Later signs
   a. Opisthotonus; spasticity
   b. Apnea
   c. Irritability
   d. Seizures
   e. Deafness to high-pitched sounds
3. Occurrence of kernicterus at low levels of bilirubin may be seen in infants with
   a. Previous asphyxia (acidosis)
   b. Respiratory distress
   c. Sepsis
   d. Hypothermia
   e. Prematurity; especially low birth weight
   f. Hypoglycemia
4. Bilirubin is nephrotoxic and especially compromises renal concentrating capacity.
5. Bilirubin increases affinity of RBC for oxygen.
6. Controversy exists as to the actual mechanics and causes involved with the development of kernicterus

and the serum bilirubin levels at which exchange transfusions are done.

Treatment

1. Exchange transfusion—to mechanically remove bilirubin.
2. Phototherapy—to allow for utilization of alternate pathways for bilirubin excretion.
3. Enzyme induction agent—to reduce bilirubin levels by inducing hepatic enzyme system involved in bilirubin clearance (i.e., phenobarbital, ethanol).

Potential Problems/Nursing Diagnoses

1. Alteration in fluid and electrolyte balance related to decreased oral fluid intake and hyperthermia
2. Potential behavioral changes in the infant (i.e., poor sucking, irritability) related to increased serum bilirubin
3. Trauma and discomfort to the infant related to procedures (i.e., blood drawing, phototherapy, exchange transfusion)
4. Alteration in skin integrity related to increased pigmentation, diarrhea
5. Psychosocial and sensory deprivation related to phototherapy treatment
6. Altered parenting behaviors related to hospitalization and separation from infant
7. Parental anxiety related to uncertainty about outcome

Nursing Interventions

A. Observe the infant's skin for appearance of or increase in jaundice.

1. Make observations in daylight, sunlight, or white fluorescent light.
2. Blanch the skin during the observation to clear away capillary coloration: forehead, cheeks and clavicle sites allow for clear view. Record findings at least twice daily.
3. Be aware of any blood incompatibility between the infant's and mother's blood.
4. Be alert to the infant's age in connection with the appearance of jaundice.

B. Note any changes in urine pigmentation and frequency of urination.

Careful notation of frequency, amount, and color of urine should be made so changes will be noticed immediately. Test for presence of bilirubin (urobilinogen).

C. Maintain adequate fluid intake.

1. Be aware of feeding history and amount of fluid taken.
2. If the infant is a slow eater, feed small amounts frequently.
3. The amount of fluid intake determines the amount of hydration and in turn determines the excretion of bilirubin. Early feeding is a good preventive prescription for hyperbilirubinemia.
4. If the infant is receiving intravenous fluid, keep an accurate hourly record of fluid intake. Do not allow intake to fall behind prescribed rate. Observe IV site for infiltration so IV can be discontinued and restarted immediately.

D. Be alert for any behavior changes and report them to the physician.

Note particularly increasing lethargy, change in sucking activity or quality, or vomiting.

E. Be alert to signs of kernicterus (bilirubin encephalopathy) **and report them to the physician.**

Observe for signs of decreased muscle tone, no sucking, no hand grasp, or regurgitation of feedings not previously observed. In time, the infant becomes opisthotonic and irritable.

F. Administer the treatment of phototherapy safely and properly, should it be prescribed.

1. The shining of daylight fluorescent bulbs or blue light directly on the exposed skin of the infant reduces tissue bilirubin, which in turn reduces serum bilirubin by:
    a. Photo-oxidizing tissue bilirubin to biliverdin, to secondary yellow pigments, to colorless, nontoxic compounds excreted in bile and urine.
    b. Causing tissue–serum bilirubin equilibrium, or as the bilirubin decreases in tissue, pulling bilirubin from the serum into the tissue to maintain this equilibrium. The *flux,* which is the unit of measurement of energy output of lamps, at 425–475 nm. is important in bilirubin degradation.
        (1) The distance of the infant from the light should be 45–60 cm.
        (2) Check light intensity for therapeutic range daily. Use commercial Bililight.
        (3) Effectiveness of phototherapy depends on: intensity of illumination; area of skin exposed; initial phototherapy effect on bilirubin in skin appears to have greater influence.
2. The physician will determine the length of time the infant is to be under the lights based on serum bilirubin levels and clinical condition of the infant.

Nursing Care Related to Photophobia

A. General Measures

1. Have the infant completely undressed so entire skin surface is exposed to light.
2. Keep the infant's eyes covered to protect them from the constant exposure to high-intensity light which may cause retinal injury. Do not apply pressure when the eyes are covered because this may cause corneal ulceration. Be certain both eyes are occluded with protective cover and that eyelids are closed. Change protective covers routinely and check for conjunctivitis. Make sure nose is not occluded. Cover scrotum.
3. Develop a systematic schedule of turning infant so all surfaces are exposed (i.e., every 2 hours).
4. Maintain thermo-neutrality—measure incubator or Isolette temperature as well as that of the infant. Light affects the ambient temperature.
    a. Do not expose the thermistor probe to the lights without the probe's being covered with an opaque tape.
    b. Avoid hyperthermia. Monitor temperature every 2–4 hours.
5. Adequate fluid intake should be provided either orally or intravenously. Vasodilatation increases insensible water loss, and there is excess stool loss from occasional diarrhea. Keep urine specific gravity below 1.015.
6. The infant should be shielded (by Plexiglas) from direct exposure of the lights to filter out and protect him from the ultraviolet radiation of daylight and cool white fluorescent lights. This shield will also protect the infant from injury should the lights break.
7. Ensure that serum bilirubin levels are obtained as prescribed. The diminishing icterus (i.e., the lowering of unconjugated bilirubin from cutaneous tissue) does not reflect the serum bilirubin concentration.
    a. Lights should be turned off when blood is being collected to eliminate false-low bilirubin levels.
    b. When phototherapy has been discontinued, check serum bilirubin levels within 4 hours to determine rebound.
8. If possible, remove the infant from under the lights, remove eye covers, and hold the infant for feedings. This will allow for some human contact and pleasure during feeding and a chance to open his eyes and look around, and perhaps will encourage parental involvement in the infant's care.
9. Note sleeping and eating patterns. The feeding schedule may need to be adjusted to the infant's pattern for better feeding. Obtain daily weight. Increased metabolic rate may increase caloric needs.
10. Develop a schedule for changing light bulbs. The effectiveness of light of this wavelength decreases after 800 hours of use; thus, the bulbs should be changed at that time. A record of hours of use will be helpful. Measure effective light life with light meter.

B. Side Effects of Phototherapy

1. Lethargy
2. Loose, green stools
3. Dark urine
4. Temperature elevation
5. Skin changes—rash due to capillary dilatation; Black infant skin may darken
6. Priapism—turn the infant on his abdomen for short periods of time, and this will cease.
7. Dehydration from increased insensible water loss
8. Possible damage to photo receptors of retinae when eyes not shielded
9. Airway obstruction from slippage of eye shield
10. Possible decreased ability of albumin binding to bilirubin.
11. Possible effect on biological rhythm
12. Obscures diagnosis of other problems
13. Increased platelet turnover

Other Measures

A. Be aware of drugs that may compete with bilirubin for binding to albumin free fatty acids (sulfonamides, chloramphenicol, salicylates, caffeine, novobiocin).

Their administration will result in increasing serum level of "free" unconjugated bilirubin.

B. Observe for hypoglycemia in the infant with erythroblastosis resulting from islet cell hyperplasia, and increased insulin secretion.

Hypoglycemia may occur shortly after birth or exchange transfusion.

C. Assist in the treatment of exchange transfusion (see p. 1171).

1. Used to stop hemolytic process (erythroblastosis fetalis), correct anemia, and treat potential/actual bilirubinemia.
2. Complications: hypoglycemia, necrotizing enterocolitis.

D. Foster a healthy family–child relationship.

1. Encourage parents to visit infant as much as possible during hospitalization.

2. Allow the parents to fondle, care for, hold, and feed the infant as much as possible or as his condition permits.
3. Initiate a community-nursing referral if the parents are particularly anxious about caring for their infant at home after discharge.
4. If breast-feeding is temporarily discontinued, encourage the mother to pump her breasts; be supportive.

Health Education

1. Help the family to understand what is wrong with their baby. Explain in simple terms what the doctor has already told them. Allow them to ask questions about the baby and treatment.
2. If the baby has erythroblastosis fetalis, help the parents understand the importance of prenatal care and monitoring should another pregnancy occur.
3. Stress the importance of close follow-up of the baby after hospital discharge. Anemia is a common long-term side effect of red blood cell hemolysis and exchange transfusion. The baby's hemoglobin level should be monitored for some time after illness so appropriate treatment can be initiated if necessary.

4. Unsensitized Rh-negative mother, after delivery of an Rh-positive infant, should receive Rho immune globulin (RhoGAM)* to prevent isoimmunization with subsequent pregnancies.

Expected Outcomes

1. Achieves and maintains fluid and electrolyte balance; adequate urine output and specific gravity; gaining weight; shows adequate serum electrolyte values
2. Demonstrates minimal behavioral changes; achieves normalization of serum bilirubin levels
3. Experiences minimal trauma and discomfort; normal vital signs; no abnormal crying; comforted when held and cuddled
4. Maintains skin integrity; no signs of skin breakdown
5. Demonstrates normal developmental behavior; no evidence of sensory or psychological deprivation while in nursery
6. Parent–infant bonding observed; parents show willingness to visit child, hold him, and participate in his care
7. Parents show lessening of anxiety; ask appropriate questions; verbalize that they understand treatment protocols

Failure to Thrive

"Failure to thrive" syndrome is a term used to identify infants characterized by growth and developmental failure along with psychosocial disruption.

Etiology

1. Unknown
2. Organic
   a. Central nervous system
   b. Cardiovascular
   c. Renal
   d. Gastrointestinal
   e. Respiratory
   f. Endocrine
   g. Metabolic
3. Nonorganic
   a. Inadequate caloric intake; disturbed feeding patterns
   b. Maternal deprivation or faulty mother–child relationship
   c. Family problems (socioeconomic problems)
   d. Environmental deprivation

Clinical Manifestations

1. Weight measurement falls below 2 standard deviations from mean for age (weight and length fall below that expected for gestational and postnatal age).
2. Infant fails to gain weight or loses subcutaneous fat and muscle mass.
3. Possible presenting manifestations that are associated with maternal deprivation:
   a. Developmental retardation
   b. Disturbed psychosocial development
      (1) Inappropriate response for age to strangers
      (2) Avoidance of eye contact with another person
      (3) Exaggerated self-comfort measures
      (4) Withdrawn—no interest in environment
4. Somatic manifestations
   a. Gastrointestinal
      (1) Anorexia
      (2) Vomiting
      (3) Diarrhea
      (4) Rumination
      (5) Dehydration
   b. Respiratory—coughing
5. Most frequently seen at age 6–16 months

Diagnostic Evaluation

1. Detailed history—including dietary and family (social)
2. Physical examination—accurate measurements of length, weight, and head circumference—general condition
3. Laboratory data—preliminary tests should be minimal, unless history or examination indicates a specific line of inquiry. Include the following tests:
   a. Complete blood count
   b. Urinalysis and culture
   c. Stool for fat, occult blood, ovum and parasites, and pH, trypsin
   d. Levels of serum sodium, potassium, CO_2, chlorides, creatinine, calcium
   e. Tine test
4. Observe systematic behavioral distortions.

Treatment

(When no organic reasons have been found)
1. Adequate caloric intake for weight gain (120–150 cal./kg./day based on appropriate weight for gestational and postnatal age). Significant weight gain will usually occur within 7–10 days.
2. Appropriate "mothering"—nurturing activities and environmental stimulation. Investigation has suggested that weight gain will occur when adequate nutrition is taken independent of nurturing activities; however, one is also dealing with a hospitalized

* Ortho Diagnostic Systems, Raritan, NJ 08869

child who is subjected to parental separation or deprivation.

3. If, after a trial of adequate caloric ingestion, the infant does not gain weight, intensive investigation is done. Trial period may have to be 7–10 days in some instances.

4. Provide a nurturing environment that will enhance positive patterns of behavior toward interaction of the family unit.

Prognosis

1. Prognosis generally depends on the etiology, severity, and duration of the condition, as well as on the home situation to which the child returns.

2. Long-term—continued impaired growth rate and failure to thrive, lowered intelligence, and emotional disorders.

Potential Problems/Nursing Diagnoses

1. Alteration in nutritional status related to decreased oral intake

2. Alteration in developmental level related to inappropriate nutrition

3. Alteration in behavior and coping mechanisms related to inappropriate maternal–child relationship and/or stimulation

4. Parental anxiety related to lack of knowledge, guilt, or concern for child

5. Altered mother–infant bonding/relationship related to lack of understanding, frustration, and anxiety

Nursing Interventions

A. Make an assessment of the infant's general condition, level of development, coping mechanisms, and behavior.

1. Carefully note what behaviors need attention and/or modifying.

2. Accurately record findings in nursing notes.

3. Obtain and record accurate height, weight, and head circumference.

B. Develop a detailed nursing care plan that is workable based on:

1. The infant's physical condition and limitations

2. Medical management

3. Nursing history

4. Input from other multidiscipline team members

C. Understand that the reason for this child's condition may not totally be the mother's fault.

1. Lack of food availability may be a result of socioeconomic situation.

2. Disturbed feeding patterns may have continued despite attempts by mother to correct them.

3. Disturbed mother–infant relationship resulting from separation at neonatal period.

D. Provide and maintain nutritional intake that will allow for weight gain.

1. Determine if a feeding problem does exist. Document feeding behaviors (i.e., sleep/wake cycle related to eating, clues of hunger, response to offered food).

2. Infant may need to be taught to eat appropriately for his age (i.e., cup, solids, spoon, finger food).

3. If the child vomits, then smaller, more frequent feedings may be necessary; prop him up in sitting position for feeding.

   a. Assess what effect environment, position, and

other factors have on vomiting and feeding behavior.

   b. Prevent ruminating or self-induced vomiting.

   c. Daily weights and accurate input and output are necessary to evaluate progress.

E. Gently and warmly provide nurturing to this infant.

1. Assess what the infant can tolerate and base activities on this, slowly increasing TLC and physical contact as infant can accept it.

2. Encourage the development of a trusting relationship between 1 or 2 persons and the infant.

3. Use each opportunity presented by daily care to develop the relationship, help the infant become interested in and enjoy his environment and eventually reach out to explore himself and people and things around him.

4. Part of nurturing activities include the therapeutic use of tactile, visual, and auditory stimulation through play. Do not force this on child if he is unable to tolerate it. Have items within reach, occasionally showing infant how they operate.

5. Talk to the infant, use his name; slowly help him to tolerate eye-to-eye contact.

6. Document the infant's reactions and responses to handling, playing, etc.

F. Establish a relationship with the mother (parents) **that will allow for open communication and cooperative efforts.**

1. Accept the mother as a person, one who may have problems with which she cannot cope. She may be young and inexperienced or have doubts about her ability to be a mother, as well as socioeconomic problems.

2. A trusting relationship between the nurse and mother will enhance identifying infant-care problems the mother may be experiencing as well as make her more receptive to any teaching or information the nurse may offer.

3. The mother (parents) must be allowed to express her (their) feelings.

G. Work as a contributing integral part of the multidiscipline team caring for this infant and family.

1. The physician—responsible for medical diagnosis and management of the family with regard to the child's illness.

2. The social worker—helps the parents handle the stress that prevents them from assuming their parenting roles.

3. The nurse—coordinates infant care and participates in teaching infant care to the mother.

4. The parents—must be included in the team because the plan of approach must be acceptable and understood in order to be used by them.

5. Other members of the team may include a psychiatrist, child-life worker, physical therapist, occupational therapist.

H. Help the mother and infant establish a healthy relationship that will continue to grow when the infant is discharged (see also ICN, p. 1123).

1. Encourage the mother to be active in the plan of treatment. Identify areas of involvement in the nursing care plan.

2. Praise the mother's positive efforts; gradually redirect negative aspects.
3. Identify and interpret the infant's behavior pattern for the mother.
   a. Help her to understand the discrepancies between her expectations and reality.
   b. Teach her expected growth and development.
4. Help the mother to understand her importance to the infant and that the relationship is based on reciprocal needs and responses between the mother and infant.
5. Observe and document mother–infant interactions.
   a. Mother—holding, interest in infant, comforting activities
   b. Infant—response to mother (i.e., looking at the mother, squirming, cuddling, crying, cooing).
6. The mother may actually need to be taught "mother craft"—how to cuddle, feed, play, and react to her child.

I. Initiate community-nurse referral before discharge and/or communicate with community nurse already involved.

1. Provides the parents with continual support by someone they know.

2. Gives feedback as to the home situation and possible areas where problems can be avoided.

J. Help the mother (parents) **understand and accept the need for continual follow-up care of her** (their) **infant.**

1. Be certain the mother knows where and when to obtain this care.
2. Encourage the mother to seek support from appropriate resources as necessary.

Expected Outcomes

1. Demonstrates improved nutritional status; eating; gaining weight
2. Shows advances in developmental level; shows appropriate behavior for age; reaching out; accepts physical contact
3. Responds to nurturing; tolerates eye-to-eye contact; shows evidence of establishing trusting relationship; accepts comforting
4. Parents demonstrate an understanding of the causes of the child's illness; express their feelings and concerns
5. Mother begins to establish infant–mother bonding; holds and comforts the infant; is reading materials on growth and development

Septicemia Neonatorum

Septicemia neonatorum (sepsis) is a generalized infection which may occur in the neonate and is characterized by the proliferation of bacteria in the bloodstream and frequently involves the meninges (as distinguished from simple bacteremia, congenital infection, septicemia following major diseases or surgery, or major congenital anomalies).

Etiology

1. The distribution of etiologic agents varies from year to year and from institution to institution.
2. Gram-negative organisms:
   E. coli
   Klebsiella (enterobacteriaceae)
   Pseudomonas
   Proteus
   Salmonella
   H. influenzae
3. Gram-positive organisms:
   Group B beta-hemolytic *Streptococcus*
   Listeria monocytogenes
   Staphylococcus aureus—coagulase-negative and coagulase-positive
   Staphylococcus epidermidis
   Streptococcus pneumoniae
   Streptococcus faecalis
4. Predisposing factors
   a. Sex—male predominance
   b. Perinatal factors
      (1) Maternal complications
          Prolonged rupture of membranes
          Prolonged and difficult labor; precipitous delivery
          Chorioamnionitis
          Endometritis
          Urinary tract infection
          Toxemia
          Abruptio placentae
          Maternal illness
          Cardiovascular disease
          Colonization of organisms in genital tract
      (2) Infant complications
          Prematurity or low birth weight
          Congenital heart disease
          Intracranial bleeding
          Respiratory distress syndrome
          Skin infections
          Difficult/traumatic labor or delivery
   c. Iatrogenic or environmental factors
      (1) Related to type of equipment used in caring for infant
          Catheters
          Oxygen and humidity
          Resuscitative
      (2) Defective or unclean equipment
      (3) Obstetric and nursery practices
      (4) Surgical procedures
5. Mode of entry
   a. Infection may gain access into the amniotic sac either prior to or after rupture of the membranes; the fetus may aspirate some of this infected fluid.
   b. Bacteria may enter the fetal circulation following invasion of the decidua from the amniotic cavity.
   c. After birth, bacteria may enter the infant's circulation by a variety of routes. Infection may originate in the skin, umbilical stump, or mucous membranes of the eyes, nose, pharynx, and ear as well as the respiratory, gastrointestinal, and genitourinary tracts.
   d. Iatrogenic—equipment, resuscitation.

Altered Physiology

1. Temporary breakdown or depression of the infant's defense mechanisms for unknown reason
   a. Possibly due to stress of labor and delivery
   b. Predisposing factors (see under Etiology)
2. The defense systems of the newborn, especially the low-birth-weight infant, are ineffective with regard to:
   a. Active immunity
      (1) Significant formation of IgG (immunoglobulin G) begins at 1–3 months of age
      (2) Significant formation of IgM (immunoglobulin M) begins at birth to 7 days
   b. Passive immunity
      Born without IgM antibodies and bactericidal protection against gram-negative organisms
   c. Phagocytosis and minimal inflammatory response
      Neutrophils are less active in response to chemotactic stimuli and migrate more slowly to areas of inflammation
   d. Unknown factors

Complications

1. Meningitis—very common complication
2. Shock
3. Adrenal hemorrhage
4. Disseminated intravascular coagulation
5. Metabolic derangements
6. Pneumonia
7. Urinary tract infection
8. Congestive heart failure
9. High mortality rate

Assessment and Clinical Manifestations

1. The early signs of sepsis are usually vague and subtle. The infant is often described as not doing well. The signs often include:
   a. Poor feeding; gastric retention
   b. Lethargy, limpness
   c. Temperature alteration—generally hypothermia, but infant may have hyperthermia
2. Later signs and symptoms may include any of the following:
   a. Pallor, cyanosis or apneic episodes, respiratory distress
   b. Jaundice
   c. Abdominal distention
   d. Vomiting and/or diarrhea
   e. Paronychia
   f. Petechiae or purpura
   g. Vesicles or pustules
   h. Hepatosplenomegaly
   i. Irritability, convulsion
   j. Bulging fontanelles
   k. Hypotonia

Diagnostic Evaluation

1. History of predisposing factors
2. Physical findings
3. Laboratory—recovery of organism from blood cultures must be obtained for a diagnosis of sepsis neonatorum
   a. Cultures to detect specific organism
      (1) Blood
      (2) Urine
      (3) Spinal fluid—delay in unstable infant
      (4) Umbilical stump
      (5) Skin lesions
      (6) Nose, throat, rectal
      (7) External auditory canal
      (8) Gastric fluid
   b. WBC and differential—nonspecific test; may be difficult to interpret
   c. Hemoglobin, hematocrit—red blood cell counts may hemolyze with some bacteria
   d. Blood chemistries—sugar, calcium, pH, electrolytes
   e. C-reactive protein and erythrocyte sedimentation rate
   f. Acid–base studies
   g. Bilirubin
   h. TORCH (toxoplasmosis–rubella–cytomegalic inclusion virus—herpes—other)—detect antibodies against common intrauterine-infective agents or specific IgMs and cultures for CMV
4. Chest x-ray—may demonstrate pulmonary infection
5. Urinalysis

Treatment

A. **Antibacterial Therapy**—based on the identified organism

1. Before the specific organism is identified, and after cultures have been obtained, the antibacterial therapy is based on the more common causative agents and their anticipated susceptibilities.
   a. Knowledge of particular nursery offenders and their antibiotic susceptibilities is needed for proper drug selection for both gram-negative and gram-positive organisms.
   b. Therapy duration is generally 5–10 days after clinical improvement, but may be as long as 3–4 weeks with complicated infections.
   c. Serum levels

B. **Supportive Therapy**

1. Observation
2. Isolation, if indicated
3. Fluid and caloric maintenance
4. Oxygen therapy
5. Regulation of thermal environment
6. Blood transfusion to correct anemia, shock
7. Others, as indicated
8. Exchange transfusion (controversial)
9. Protect from further infection

Potential Problems/Nursing Diagnoses

1. Complications related to infection and its systemic effects: meningitis, shock, disseminated intravascular coagulation, congestive heart failure, apnea, jaundice
2. Hypothermia related to unstable central temperature control and stress of infection
3. Alteration of nutritional status related to infection
4. Other complications related to hospitalized infant (see premature infant, p. 1216)

Nursing Interventions

(See also ICN, p. 1122)

A. **Review maternal history. Identify infants at risk for infection.**

B. **Practice measures which will prevent the transmission of infection in the nursery.**

1. Practice careful handwashing technique and serve as a model of good technique.
2. Personnel with infection should avoid contact with infants.

a. Seek health care for infection. (Cultures should be done.)
b. Remain out of the nursery.
c. Wear a mask when it is necessary to enter the nursery.
3. Teach parents and other persons entering the nursery proper handwashing and gown techniques.
4. Maintain sterile technique when procedures demanding this technique are performed.
5. Promote general cleanliness of the nursery environment.
Infected equipment and stagnant water provide excellent conditions for bacterial growth.

C. Observe infants for the vague symptoms that appear early in the course of sepsis.

1. Observe for the following:
   a. Lethargy, decreased activity, and loss of muscle tone
   b. Poor feeding or refusal to feed
   c. Temperature alterations, especially hypothermia
   d. Alteration in vital signs
   e. Skin color and condition
   f. Intake and output
   g. Examine each body system
2. Be consistent in planning for the care of infants to provide a means whereby these early symptoms may be detected.
   a. Accurate charting of the infant's previous behavior
   b. Assigning the same nurse to care for an infant on successive days
3. Report to the physician the symptoms observed.
4. When neonatal sepsis is caused by B group streptococci, the disease may take one of two courses:
   a. Early onset—within 12–24 hours after birth and within 3 days of age.
      (1) Acute septicemia with fulminant clinical course; high mortality and severe neurologic sequelae in survivors.
      (2) There is generally a history of obstetric complications, and the serotypes of streptococci from the mother's birth canal and the infant are the same.
      (3) Signs and symptoms include respiratory symptoms—in particular, acute respiratory distress, hypoxia, leading to shock.
   b. Delayed onset—occurs 10 days to 6–12 weeks after birth
      (1) Illness is severe and associated with meningitis.
      (2) Normal obstetric history; probably acquired infection from environment.
      (3) Disease is characterized by meningeal symptoms, including bulging fontanelle and seizures.
5. Observe for signs of complications—meningitis, urinary tract infection, pneumonia.

D. Observe for episodes of apnea and initiate measures to stimulate respiration.

1. Observe the infant closely for apnea or place the infant on a respiratory monitor.
2. Stimulate the infant when apnea does occur.
3. Report frequent periods of apnea to physician.
4. Report length of apneic episode and response to stimulation.

E. Observe the infant for convulsions which may occur with sepsis.

1. Immediately report to the physician any twitching or convulsive activity.

a. Remain with the infant.
b. Suction mouth and nose if the infant has secretions or vomitus in his mouth.
c. Turn head to side.
d. Protect the infant from banging against side of Isolette or incubator or falling from radiant warmer.
e. Provide oxygen if cyanosis or respiratory distress occurs.
f. Administer any medication prescribed to control the convulsions.
2. Record the length of and the type of convulsion, the parts of the body involved, the infant's general appearance before and following the convulsion, and response to any therapy given.

F. Ensure that evaluation and diagnostic tests be initiated promptly and correctly to avoid altered results from contamination.

1. Tests should be completed prior to starting antibiotics.
2. Since the infective organism must be recovered in blood cultures, strict antiseptic technique in obtaining cultures is vital.
   a. Peripheral venipuncture is the site of choice (the umbilical vessels are already contaminated, and the femoral vein offers possible contamination from perineum).
   b. Cleanse skin with an antiseptic solution (e.g., iodine solution). For maximal aseptic effect, allow the solution to dry.

G. Provide for the nutritional needs of the infant in order to provide for his caloric needs.

1. During the acute phase of the illness, the infant may not be able to take or tolerate oral feedings.
   a. Monitor the administration of intravenous fluids. Nasogastric tube may be in place to aid in preventing abdominal distention.
   b. Provide for the sucking needs of the infant by giving him a pacifier.
   c. Gavage feedings may be given to the infant.
2. Initiate oral feedings of formula as soon as the infant's condition improves.
   a. Begin by offering small feedings and observe following responses:
      Vomiting
      Abdominal distention
      The infant's interest in feeding and ability to suck
      Whether the infant tires with feeding
   b. Nipple feedings may be supplemented with gavage feedings.
   c. Gradually increase amount of feeding.
      Do not force feedings—vomiting associated with diarrhea may result, leading to dehydration.
   d. Resume regular feeding schedule based on the infant's ability to tolerate feeding.
3. Hold the infant for feedings as soon as his condition warrants it.

H. Provide measures to maintain the infant's temperature within normal range.

1. Take the infant's temperature at hourly intervals.
2. Adjust the Isolette temperature to maintain the infant's temperature between 36° and 37°C. (96.8° and 98.6°F.).
3. When the infant is placed in an open crib, maintain temperature and cover the infant appropriately.
4. Report hypothermia or hyperthermia to the physician.

I. Administer the prescribed antibiotic therapy to control the infection.

1. Administer the prescribed medications.
   a. Be aware of the action and side effects of the specific medications.
   b. Be aware of the route of excretion.
   c. Be aware of drug incompatibilities.
2. Observe the infant's apparent response to therapy.
   a. Note the child's activity, feeding behavior, and weight.
   b. Observe for the development of new symptoms.

J. Be prepared to assist with blood transfusions used to correct anemia and shock (see Exchange Transfusions, p. 1171).

Adult whole blood also provides specific factors that enhance the phagocytic abilities of neonate leukocytes.

K. Observe for the occurrence of septic shock and report immediately.

Early phase—associated with peripheral vasodilatation and hypotension with metabolic acidosis.

Later phase—peripheral vasoconstriction occurs with deterioration of heart and lung function. Decrease in cardiac output and arterial blood pressure is associated with increased central venous pressure.

1. Monitor blood pressure.
2. Check peripheral resistance in pulses in all extremities; note color and temperature.
3. Monitor hourly urine output for evaluation of renal function.

L. Provide for the emotional needs of the infant.

1. Place bright, colorful objects in the crib or Isolette.
2. Talk gently and quietly while caring for the infant.
3. Touch and gently stroke the infant.
4. Encourage the parents to visit and allow them to hold the infant as soon as possible.

M. Involve the parents in the infant's care in the hospital and prepare them for the infant's discharge.

1. Encourage the parents to visit the infant.
   a. Allow them to hold and feed the baby.
   b. Answer questions they may have regarding the infant's progress and care.
   c. Provide them with an opportunity to explain their concerns.
2. Discuss symptoms of complications that may occur and should be watched for following discharge.
3. Give specific instruction regarding medications to be given at home.

Expected Outcomes

1. No complication as evidenced by stable function of body systems.
2. The infant maintains stable temperature.
3. The infant achieves and maintains appropriate nutrition as evidenced by weight gain.
4. The parents and infant experience no other complications related to their hospitalization experience (see preterm infant, p. 1230).

Infant of Addicted Mother

An *infant of an addicted mother* is one who is born to a mother who is narcotic- or methadone-dependent and who takes the drug or drugs in varying dosages for varying periods during her pregnancy.

Etiology

A. Maternal use of narcotics or methadone or both drugs during pregnancy

1. The drugs cross the placental barrier and enter the fetal circulation.
2. The supply to the infant is abruptly terminated at delivery.
3. Other agents (i.e., phenobarbital, alcohol, propoxyphene) are capable of causing withdrawal symptoms.

B. Fetal alcohol syndrome—etiology

1. Direct ethanol toxicity to developing fetus
2. Maternal malnutrition—vitamin deficiency
3. Hypoglycemia, maternal
4. Concurrent drug abuse
5. Smoking
6. Alcohol-induced illness (i.e., gastric hemorrhage, cirrhosis of liver)
7. Alcohol freely crosses placenta and is found in amniotic fluid and cord blood.
8. Maturity of infant's metabolic and excretory mechanism is important.

Prognosis

A. For Drug Addiction

1. The long-term biologic effects on the infant of a drug-dependent mother are not fully known. These children may have:
   a. Abnormal psychomotor development associated with intrauterine growth retardation
   b. Behavioral disturbances such as hyperactivity, brief attention spans, temper tantrums
2. The unstable environment that the drug-addicted mother (or parents) may provide is a major threat to the child's health and development.

B. For Fetal Alcohol Syndrome

1. Intellectual impairment
2. Poor fine motor control
3. Difficulty feeding
4. Hyperactive
5. Developmental delay of gross motor skills
6. Minimal brain dysfunction
7. Slow postnatal catching up

Complications

A. For Drug Addiction

1. Prematurity
2. Intrauterine growth retarded infant (IUGR); small-for-gestational-age infant (SGA)
3. Fetal anoxia with meconium aspiration
4. Infection-associated maternal sexually transmitted disease or hepatitis
5. Hypoglycemia
6. Hypocalcemia
7. RDS related to prematurity
8. Septicemia
9. Hyperbilirubinemia

B. For Fetal Alcohol Syndrome

1. Metabolic imbalance
2. Hypoglycemia

3. Respiratory distress
4. Neurologic pathology
5. Craniofacial anomalies
6. Congenital heart disease

Clinical Manifestations (of neonatal withdrawal)

A. Drug Addiction

1. The degree of withdrawal symptoms the infant manifests may be related to the duration of the mother's drug habit, the type and dosage requirements of her addiction, and her drug level immediately prior to her delivery.
   a. The closer to delivery the mother received her last dose, the longer her addiction and the higher her dose need, the longer the delay of withdrawal symptoms, and the more severe the symptoms will be in the infant.
   b. Although heroin and methadone produce similar withdrawal symptoms in the infant, those same symptoms are generally more severe with methadone withdrawal—probably because of the high level of the mother's dose, the pharmacologic characteristics of the drug itself, and the use by the mother of other drugs simultaneously.
2. Onset of symptoms
   a. Heroin—several hours after birth to 3–4 days of life
   b. Methadone—7–10 days after birth to several weeks of life
3. Cardinal signs of neonatal narcotic withdrawal
   a. Coarse, flapping tremors
   b. Irritability; hyperactivity; hypertonicity
   c. Prolonged, persistent, high-pitched cry
   d. Restlessness; sleepiness
4. Other signs and symptoms of acute withdrawal:
   a. Vigorous, ineffective sucking; poor feeding
   b. Excessive tearing; excessive sweating
   c. Increased salivation
   d. Sneezing, nasal stuffiness
   e. Vomiting and/or diarrhea
   f. Muscle rigidity
   g. Yawning
   h. Convulsions—with methadone withdrawal
   i. Tachypnea with associated respiratory alkalosis
   j. Exaggerated reflexes
   k. Hyperpyrexia
   l. Hiccoughs
5. Prematurity
   High incidence of infants born to addicted mothers are premature and/or small for gestational age.

B. Fetal Alcohol Syndrome

(Develop within first 24 hours of life)
1. Difficulty establishing respirations
2. Metabolic problems
3. Irritability
4. Increased muscle tone, tremulousness
5. Lethargy
6. Opisthotonus
7. Poor sucking reflex
8. Abdominal distention
9. Seizure activity

Diagnosis

1. Thorough maternal history, including drug habits
2. Physical assessment; Kahn's* criteria of tremulousness and irritability:

* Kahn EJ et al. The course of heroin withdrawal syndrome in newborn infants treated with phenobarbital or chlorpromazine. J Pediatr 75:495

   a. Grade I—signs recognizable but mild
   b. Grade II—signs marked but only when the infant is disturbed
   c. Grade III—signs marked and occurring at frequent intervals, even when the infant is undisturbed
3. Laboratory studies
   a. Urine for toxicologic studies
   b. Blood glucose
   c. Serum calcium, pH, and total protein
   d. Acid–base status studies, respiratory alkalosis
   e. Serologic studies for syphilis
   f. Appropriate cultures if systemic bacterial infection is suspected
4. Many of the clinical signs of neonatal narcotic withdrawal are nonspecific and may indicate other problems: hypoglycemia, hypocalcemia, CNS disorders or hemorrhage, infection, other, nonnarcotic drug withdrawal

Treatment

A. Drug Addiction

1. Narcotic antagonist for narcotic-induced respiratory depression at birth (morphine addiction)
2. Drug therapy for alleviation of signs of narcotic withdrawal. Duration of therapy using decreasing dosages may be from 4–40 days
   a. Paregoric (camphorated tincture of opium) orally
   b. Phenobarbital, orally
   c. Chlorpromazine (Thorazine) orally
   d. Diazepam (Valium) intramuscularly
3. Supportive therapy as appropriate

B. Fetal Alcohol Syndrome

1. Quiet environment with minimized auditory and sensory stimulation
2. Drug therapy to control seizures
3. Intravenous therapy for dehydration which accompanies alcohol withdrawal
4. Supportive therapy as appropriate

Potential Problems/Nursing Diagnoses

1. Alteration in metabolic status—(hypoglycemia) related to prematurity or SGA
2. Altered nutritional status related to poor intake
3. Withdrawal symptoms (complications) related to maternal substance abuse
4. Respiratory distress related to prematurity, SGA, meconium aspiration
5. Infection related to maternal disease
6. Alteration in maternal–infant bonding related to maternal addiction and status

Nursing Interventions

A. Be familiar with withdrawal symptoms in order to facilitate early diagnosis, which in turn will decrease incidence of morbidity and mortality of high-risk infants.

1. Recognize cardinal as well as other symptoms.
2. Identify infants likely to have symptoms.
3. Report to physician any suspicious behavior.

B. Ensure that prophylactic measures have been administered against ophthalmia neonatorum.

There is a high incidence of gonococcal infection in drug-addicted pregnant women.

C. Ensure that diagnostic measures are carried out.

Collect urine for toxicologic studies within 24 hours after birth, since narcotic metabolites disappear rapidly.

D. Administer nursing care appropriate for the symptoms of withdrawal the infant is experiencing.

1. Irritability and restlessness, high-pitched crying
   a. Swaddle (be aware that this may increase the infant's temperature).
   b. Minimize handling—holding may aggravate irritability; some infants respond well to close contact and body movement.
   c. Decrease environmental stimuli (i.e., light, noise).
   d. Organize care to allow for periods of uninterrupted sleep.
   e. Prone positioning may help the infant organize his motor movements.
   f. Give medications with meals unless there is vomiting; then 30 minutes before.
2. Floppy tremors
   a. Protect skin from irritation and abrasions:
      (1) Use sheep skin.
      (2) Change position frequently.
      (3) Give good frequent skin care—keep the infant clean and dry.
3. Frantic sucking
   a. Give pacifier between feedings.
   b. Protect the infant's hands from excoriation.
4. Poor feeding—similar to the premature infant's inability to take an adequate amount at feedings
   a. Give small, frequent feedings.
   b. Maintain caloric and fluid intake requirement for the infant's desired weight.
5. Vomiting/diarrhea
   a. Position the infant to prevent aspiration.
   b. Provide good skin care to areas exposed to vomitus or stool.
6. Muscle rigidity—hypertonicity
   a. Change position frequently to minimize development of pressure areas.
   b. Use sheep skin.
   c. Skin care.
7. Increased salivation and/or nasal stuffiness
   a. Aspirate nasopharynx; suction tracheal mucus.
   b. Provide frequent nose and mouth care.
   c. Note respiration rate and characteristics and the infant's color.
8. Tachypnea
   a. Note onset and severity of accompanying signs of respiratory distress; place the infant on respiratory monitor.
   b. Position the infant for easier ventilation—semi-Fowler's position; tilt head back slightly.
   c. Minimize handling.
   d. Have resuscitative equipment available.

E. Record accurately and in detail all symptoms, including the following:

1. Time of onset
2. Duration and frequency
3. Severity
4. Treatment initiated and the infant's response
   Example: extent of irritability, changes in feeding behavior, tolerance of handling, characteristics and frequency of stool
5. Vital signs

F. Maintain caloric and fluid requirements and balance.

1. Keep accurate intake and output records to prevent dehydration.

2. Maintain IV fluids as appropriate when the infant experiences vomiting or diarrhea.
3. The infant may feed better on a demand schedule.
4. The infant may need increased calories because of increased activity.

G. Support drug therapy when used to control symptoms of withdrawal.

1. When diazepam (Valium) is used, be alert for the appearance of jaundice.
   Sodium benzoate is used as a preservative in preparation and interferes with binding of albumin with unconjugated bilirubin.
2. Methadone withdrawal symptoms are frequently more difficult to control than those of heroin withdrawal.
3. Note appearance of side effects of depression from oversedation:
   a. Respiratory distress
   b. Lethargy
   c. Decreased sucking activity
   d. Hypotonia

H. Protect the infant from pathophysiologic processes to which he is predisposed because of prematurity or being small for gestational age.

1. Hypoglycemia
2. Hypocalcemia
3. Hypothermia
4. Hypoxia
5. Sepsis

I. Encourage multidisciplinary conferences in an attempt to treat the whole family.

1. Initiate early referrals as needed to social services, child welfare agency, and/or community nurse to provide for continuity of care after discharge.
   a. The unstable environment into which the infant may be discharged offers a threat to the child's future well-being and development.
   b. Discharge to a foster home may be considered.
2. Evaluate the mother's attitude toward her infant.
   a. She may be able to accept the responsibility of her child and to accept help offered her.
   b. She may become nonfunctioning as a result of the birth of her infant; she may feel inadequate, angry, guilty or see the infant as an added economic burden.

J. Encourage parental involvement in the care of this infant.

Frequently the infant may not be discharged with the mother. Promote early mother–infant attachment and foster their relationship.
1. Encourage frequent mother–infant contact.
2. Have the mother feed the infant.
3. Pace the growth of the relationship between the infant and mother based on the infant's progress and the mother's positive reactions.
4. Keep in mind that methadone and heroin can be detected in breast milk and may lead to permanent addiction of the infant should the mother breastfeed.

Health Education

1. Carefully planned follow-up care for the infant is essential.
   a. Explain to the mother the need for consistent follow-up care of her infant.
   b. Infants of drug-dependent mothers are at risk; they may show failure to thrive, experience bat-

tering, succumb to sudden infant death syndrome, and may be at risk for AIDS.
c. Involve the community health nurse in the planning early in hospitalization. This early involvement may offer mother some security.
d. Social work involvement may be indicated to determine ability of the parents to care for the child at home.
e. It is often difficult to maintain contact for follow-up.
2. The mother may be accepting of rehabilitation during the postpartum period. Contact appropriate people or provide appropriate information for her; incorporate her into total care of the infant prior to discharge
3. Help the mother understand what she should expect in the infant's behavior upon discharge.
a. Many infants are irritable and restless for several months after birth.

b. Discuss with the mother the feelings she may have as a result of a strained mother–child relationship.

Expected Outcomes

1. The infant maintains normal metabolic status: normal serum glucose levels.
2. Achieves adequate intake as evidenced by weight gain.
3. The infant proceeds through withdrawal with minimal complications as evidenced by calm behavior, weight gain, and stable vital signs.
4. The infant maintains adequate oxygenation and does not experience respiratory distress.
4. The infant is free of infection as demonstrated by normal vital signs and laboratory values.
5. Maternal–infant bonding is established and demonstrated during hospitalization.

Neonatal or Prolonged Sleep Apnea of Infancy (Near-miss SIDS)

1. *Apnea of infancy* is the cessation of breathing for more than 20 seconds, or a shorter episode associated with bradycardia, cyanosis, or pallor; frequently identified as an infant, usually between 2 weeks and 6 months of age, who is brought to medical attention because of an unexplained frightening respiratory or cardiac event, usually occurring while the infant is asleep.
2. Sudden infant death syndrome (SIDS)
"The sudden death of any infant or young child, which is unexplained by history, and in which a thorough postmortem examination fails to demonstrate an adequate cause of death."*

Etiology

1. Unknown—may result from many different pathologic processes.
2. Apnea related to organic disorders:
a. Seizure disorders
b. Gastroesophageal reflux
c. Significant anemia
d. Sepsis, severe infection
e. Hypoglycemia
f. Impaired regulation of breathing
3. Current theories relating to the cause of SIDS:
a. Prolonged sleep apnea
b. Chronic oxygen deficiency
c. Enzyme abnormalities
Although many feel that some infants with prolonged sleep apnea are at risk for SIDS, a definitive causal relation between the two has not been scientifically established.
4. Characteristics that may identify infants at risk for SIDS include:
a. Prematurity
b. Neonatal conditions with apnea
c. History of apnea
d. History of SIDS in family
5. Characteristics of SIDS pattern include:
a. Prematurity
b. Preceding cold or URI

* Second International SIDS Conference, 1965

c. Peak age, 2–4 months
d. Occurs in males in a ratio of 3:2

Management

1. Cardiopulmonary monitoring—is critical
2. Specific treatment of any underlying cause
3. Consultation with infant apnea team
4. Theophylline—may be used to decrease apneic spells
5. Long-term follow-up for physiologic and neurologic behavioral functions

Prognosis

1. Infants who have experienced infant apnea may be at risk for recurrent apnea, hypoxia, and sudden death.
2. Because of hypoxemia that may have occurred, child should be assessed for learning difficulties (hearing, eyesight), discrete neurologic impairments, personality disorders, etc.

Clinical Manifestations

1. The infant is usually found by parents or caretaker to be:
a. Limp
b. Cyanotic
c. Pale
d. No respiration
e. Cool to touch
f. Normal muscle tone
2. Some form of resuscitation may be required—mouth-to-mouth respiration or cardiopulmonary assistance.
3. The infant usually exhibits symptoms when asleep, although the syndrome may occur during waking hours.
4. Types of sleep apnea include:
a. Central or diaphragmatic—chest movement ceases, absence of airflow
b. Obstructive—chest and diaphragm move but there is no air-exchange.
c. Mixed—cessation of airflow and chest movement, followed by respiratory effort without airflow.

Diagnostic Evaluation

It must be established that a primary life-threatening failure in physiologic homeostasis has occurred, ruling out other medical problems that could result in respiratory failure as a secondary cause. To accomplish this the following procedures are generally included:

1. Detailed history of the event including information concerning what happened, appearance of infant, type of intervention, how the infant responded, conditions prior to the event, special past medical history, special family history
2. Medical evaluation of the infant (physical examination)
3. Laboratory data—generally minimal unless history or examination indicates a specific line of inquiry
   a. Complete blood count with differential
   b. Serum glucose
   c. Electrolytes
   d. Calcium and phosphate
   e. Magnesium
   f. Blood gases, as indicated
4. Chest x-ray
5. Electrocardiogram
6. Electroencephalogram (may not be routine) and neurologic examination
7. Respiratory studies—a pneumogram 12- to 24-hour tape recording of small changes in electrical resistance with each breath or respiratory pattern; multichannel sleep test with continuous print-out
8. Continuous cardiac and apnea monitoring for recurrence of event, prolonged apnea, or bradycardia
9. Barium swallow for gastroesophageal reflux

Potential Problems/Nursing Diagnoses

1. Recurrent hypoxemia related to alteration/cessation of respirations
2. Parental knowledge deficit as to cause and explanation of what is happening
3. Parental anxiety related to frightening episode of infant apnea
4. Potential for alteration in parenting related to parental anxieties and fears

Nursing Interventions

A. Be prepared for the infant's admission.

Have all equipment, including apnea monitor, ready for use.

1. Select a room that is clearly visible from the nursing station; the room should be quiet in order to reduce sensory stimulation, which may reduce the likelihood of a recurring episode.
2. The family has just experienced the extreme stress of feeling that their infant has almost died. Professional efficiency and empathy at the time of admission is reassuring and builds parental confidence in nursing care.

B. Obtain a nursing history with special attention to:

1. The parents' description of the events that preceded hospitalization, and their understanding of prolonged apnea.
   a. This information may provide clues for factors to observe during hospitalization and provides data for the development of a teaching plan.
   b. It also allows for the correction of misinformation and misconceptions.
2. Have the parents describe sleep patterns, feeding habits, prior health problems, immunizations, and medications; this information may provide data regarding possible influencing factors or causes of the condition.
3. Have the parents describe a typical day in the life of the infant and the family unit. This provides important data on how home-monitoring may affect family life, and contributes to the effective development of home management and family teaching plans; it also provides a basis for continuity of care for the infant.

C. Orient the parents to the unit and the equipment used in the infant's care.

Explain the visiting policy and encourage the parents to visit as much as possible.

1. The parents must be willing and available for comprehensive instruction in their infant's condition and necessary interventions so that they feel competent in the infant's care prior to discharge.
2. Assignment of consistent nursing (primary nurse) is helpful so that families can develop a trusting relationship that will help them deal with the emotional aspects of the diagnosis and the complexities of the treatment plan.
3. Preparing the parents for all diagnostic tests that will be performed helps reduce the fear surrounding these procedures.

D. Monitor constantly, and document any apneic event the infant may experience.

1. Condition of the infant
   a. Awake/asleep
   b. Respirations—none, normal, shallow; color of infant
   c. Monitor reading—apnea, bradycardia and rate
   d. Position of infant—limp, vomited, etc.
2. Intervention
   a. Nothing—infant all right or self-corrected
   b. Gentle stimulation
   c. Vigorously shaken
   d. Resuscitation

E. Serve as a role model for the family in the following areas of infant care.

1. Use of the infant monitor (i.e., electrode placement, operation of controls, care of lead wires to prevent damage, etc.). Discussion of home-monitoring should not take place until it has been determined that this procedure will be used.
2. Methods of responding to alarms. Respond to all alarms immediately according to established procedures (i.e., observation and assessment of infant, stimulation, resuscitation, etc.).
3. Recording procedure—complete documentation of any apneic episode; record each time alarm sounds.
4. Administration of theophylline, if prescribed.
   a. Observe for signs of toxicity: apical rate above 200, vomiting, and agitation.
   b. Although the mechanism by which theophylline reduces or prevents apnea in some infants is not understood, research indicates it may act by:
      (1) Inducing rapid shallow breathing
      (2) Increasing metabolic rate with an increase in alveolar ventilation in proportion to increased CO_2 production.
5. Continue the infant's normal activities whenever possible (i.e., holding him for feedings, playing with him, disconnecting him from monitor for bathing); allow for continuation of usual eating or sleeping patterns. Simulating the home environment as much as possible will encourage deep-sleep patterns, which

may stimulate apnea in some infants (valuable diagnostic information).

F. Effectively prepare parents for eventual discharge of infant.

Since the parents have experienced at least one apneic episode prior to hospitalization, the fear of their infant's sudden death has been heightened. When discharged, the parents have direct and full responsibility for appropriate action should the infant's breathing cease.

1. Assess what parents know and understand about apnea. Correct any misconceptions and provide accurate information.
2. Make sure parents know about feeding precautions—frequent burping, no bottle in bed, upright position after feeding, elevation of the head of the bed, position on abdomen for sleep.
3. Have parents contact local emergency service to discuss prolonged apnea of infancy and CPR, and to be certain they have infant resuscitation equipment. It may be possible to arrange for the power company to notify the parents if power supply is to go off.
4. Instruct the parents in the administration of any medications (i.e., theophylline).
5. Teach CPR to the parents as well as to another responsible person, relative, or friend, to provide some relief for the parents from infant care.

G. Teach and prepare the parents for home-monitoring, if necessary.

1. Show the parents how to operate and maintain the monitor. Reinforce teaching by equipment supplier. Be sure they know how to contact a monitor technician.
2. Describe apnea recording procedure to be used (see D).
3. Teach methods of responding to alarms—what to observe (i.e., color, presence or absence of breathing) and how to respond (gentle and vigorous stimulation, CPR).
4. Discuss adjustments in daily living that will be necessary. Start by identifying a typical family day, then discuss anticipated changes.
   a. Emphasize that this responsibility must be shared by both parents.
   b. Discuss the possible impact on siblings.
   c. Caution the parents to eliminate noises that would interfere with their ability to hear the alarm (i.e., showering, vacuum cleaning) when only one parent is present. Someone must always be available to hear and respond to the alarm.
   d. Avoid traveling long distances alone with infant.
   e. Encourage the parents to maintain their relationship with one another by using another person trained in CPR to assume infant care occasionally.
5. Use anticipatory guidance in preparing parents for complication of home monitoring:
   a. Increased anxiety and tension
   b. Constant worry about the alarm—even when it does not go off
   c. Fatigue
   d. The financial and emotional burdens encountered by the entire family
   e. Loss of "normal, healthy child"—parents then grieve when given the diagnosis
6. Emphasize the healthy aspects of the infant. Encourage the parents to continue as many usual routines as possible. Provide specific things parents can do to encourage normal development and a healthy parent–child relationship.

7. Encourage the parents to provide total care for their infant for 24 hours prior to discharge.

H. Continue to observe family dynamics.

1. Assess for family conflicts or problems that can be alleviated.
2. Families who are overly stressed or demonstrate a maladaptive response may require social service or psychiatric consultation.
3. Modification of the management plan may be indicated.

I. Document patient/family progress in order to facilitate comprehensive care and discharge planning.

Daily notes should include:
1. Frequency and type of monitor alarms; intervention required
2. Teaching
3. Family dynamics
   a. Who visited and for how long
   b. Description of parent–child interaction
   c. Description of parent interaction
   d. Amount of care done by parents
   e. Assessment of parental competence in providing care

J. Ensure adequate follow-up support.

Most families are frightened by the responsibility of home-monitoring and will require support after discharge.
1. Some may need a community health nurse—homemaker/home health aide.
2. Instruct the parents regarding when and how to obtain assistance for medical, technical, and psychosocial problems.
3. Facilitate contact with other parents of infants with prolonged apnea.
4. Assist the parents with arrangements for competent babysitting help.

K. Be aware that successful outcome for every baby with prolonged apnea cannot be certain, despite continuous surveillance with or without monitors and appropriate intervention.

L. Participate in community education regarding prolonged apnea and SIDS.

Expected Outcomes

1. Infant regains normal breathing pattern; does not experience recurring apnea; vital signs stable
2. Parents verbalize some understanding of the apnea event
3. Parents recall what to observe in infant; demonstrate appropriate interventions (CPR; use of apnea monitoring equipment) when apnea occurs
4. Parents appear to reestablish and maintain normal parenting relationship with the infant

Available Resources

National Sudden Infant Death Syndrome Foundation (NSIDF), Dept. NB3, 2 Metro Plaza, Suite 205, 8240 Professional Plaza, Landover, MD 20785.

The International Guild for Infant Survival, Inc., 1515 Reistertown Road, Suite 300, Baltimore, MD 21208, (301) 484-0111.

National Foundation for Sudden Infant Death, 1501 Broadway, New York, NY 10036.

Bibliography

Books

Avery GB. Neonatology, 2nd ed. Philadelphia, JB Lippincott, 1981

Avery ME and Taeusch WH. Diseases of the Newborn. Philadelphia, WB Saunders, 1984

Butnarescu FG, Tillotson DM and Villarreal PP. Perinatal Nursing, Vol. 2: Reproductive Risk. New York, John Wiley & Sons, 1980

Cloherty JP and Stark AR (eds). Manual of Neonatal Care. Boston, Little, Brown & Co, 1980

Fanaroff AA and Martin RJ (eds). Behrman's Neonatal–Perinatal Medicine. St Louis, CV Mosby, 1983

Henig RM and Fletcher AB. Your Premature Baby. New York, Rawson Associates, 1983

Hodson WA and Truog WE. Critical Care of the Newborn. Philadelphia, WB Saunders, 1983

Hyperbilirubinemia in the Newborn. Report of the Eighty-fifth Conference in Ross Pediatric Research. Columbus, OH, Ross Laboratories, 1983

Johnson SH. High-Risk Parenting: Nursing Assessment and Strategies for the Family at Risk, 2nd ed. Philadelphia, JB Lippincott, 1986

Klaus MH and Kennell JH. Maternal–Infant Bonding. St Louis, CV Mosby, 1983

Klaus MH and Fanaroff AA. Care of the High-Risk Neonate. Philadelphia, WB Saunders, 1982

Krones SB. High-Risk Newborn Infant: The Basis for Intensive Nursing Care, 3rd ed. St Louis, CV Mosby, 1981

Milunsky H, Friedman EA and Gluck L (eds). Advances in Perinatal Medicine, Vol. 1. New York, Plenum, 1981

Perez RH. Protocols for Perinatal Nursing Practice. St Louis, CV Mosby, 1981

Schreiner RL (ed). Care of the Newborn. New York, Raven Press, 1981

Stahler-Miller K (ed). Neonatal and Pediatric Critical Care Nursing. New York, Churchill Livingstone, 1983

Stern L. Hyaline Membrane Disease: Pathogenesis and Pathophysiology. New York, Grune & Stratton, 1984

Tilden JT, Roeder LM and Steinschneider A (eds). Sudden Infant Death Syndrome. New York, Academic Press, 1983

Warshaw JB and Hobbins JC (eds). Principles and Practice of Perinatal Medicine. Reading, MA, Addison-Wesley, 1983

Whaley LF and Wong DL. Nursing Care of Infants and Children, 2nd ed. St Louis, CV Mosby, 1983

Articles

Anderson JV, Martin RJ and Fanaroff AA. Neonatal respiratory control and apnea of prematurity. Perinatol/Neonatol 1983 Jul; 7(7):65–68+

Ariagno RL. Evaluation and management of infantile apnea. Pediatr Ann 1984 Mar; 3(3):210–213+

Ariagno RL et al. "Near-miss" for sudden infant death syndrome infants: A clinical picture. Pediatrics 1983 May; 71(5):726–730

A screen for neonatal sepsis. Emerg Med 1982 May 30; 14(10):71

Bakke K and Dougherty J. Sudden infant death syndrome and infant apnea: Current questions, clinical management, and research directions. Issues Compr Pediatr Nurs 1981 Mar/Apr; 5(2):77–88

Bejar R, Coen RW and Gluck L. Hypoxic–ischemic and hemorrhagic brain injury in the newborn. Perinatal/Neonatol 1982 July/Aug; 6(4):69–70+

Bejar R et al. Neonatal intraventricular hemorrhage. Perinatol/Neonatal 1982 Sep/Oct; 6(5):107–109

Bhat R et al. Patent ductus arteriosus: Recent advances in diagnosis and management. Pediatr Clin North Am 1982 Oct; 29(5):1117–1136

Blackburn S. Fostering behavioral development of high-risk infants. JOGN Nurs (Supplement) 1983 May/Jun; 12(3):76s–86s

Blackburn S. The neonatal ICU: A high-risk environment. Am J Nurs 1982 Nov; 82(11):1708–1712

Boggs KR and Rau PK. Breastfeeding the premature infant. Am J Nurs 1983 Oct; 83(10):1436–1439

Bomberger PI. Premature infants' nutritional needs—Part 1: Preterm breast milk. Perinatol/Neonatol 1982 Jul/Aug; 6(4):79–80+

Bragdon DB. A basis for the nursing management of feeding the premature infant. JOGN Nurs (Supplement) 1983 May/Jun; 12(3):51s–57s

Braune KW and Lacey L. Common hematologic problems of the immediate newborn period. JOGN Nurs (Supplement) 1983 May/Jun; 12(3):19s–30s

Brooks JG. Apnea of infancy and sudden infant death syndrome. Am J Dis Child 1982 Nov; 136:1012–1023

Brown EG and Sweet AY. Neonatal necrotizing enterocolitis. Pediatr Clin North Am 1982 Oct; 29(5):1149–1170

Brown JV et al. Nursery-based intervention with prematurely born babies and their mothers: Are there effects. J Pediatr 1980 Sep; 97(3):487–491

Brown MS. The anemia of prematurity. Perinatol/Neonatol 1983 Sep; 7(9):32–4+

Brooten D. Issues for research on alternative patterns of care for low birthweight infants. Image 1983 Summer; 15(3):80–83

Cain LP, Kelly DM and Shannon DC. Parents' perceptions of the psychological and social impact of home monitoring. Pediatrics 1980 July; 66(1):37–41

Camfield P et al. Infant apnea syndrome. Clin Pediatr 1982 Nov; 21(10):684–687

Capobianco JA. Keeping the newborn warm: How to safeguard the infant against life-threatening heat loss. Nursing '80 1980 May; 10(5):64–67

Carey B, Larson B and Goold G. A neonatal teaching tool: Working with umbilical catheters. MCN 1980 Nov/Dec; 5(6):393–397

Carey BE. Intraventricular hemorrhage in the preterm infant. JOGN Nurs (Supplement) 1983 May/Jun; 12(3):60s–68s

Cashore WJ and Stern L. Neonatal hyperbilirubinemia. Pediatr Clin North Am 1982 Oct; 29(5):1191–1203

Chang JHT. Necrotizing enterocolitis. Perinatol/Neonatol 1980 May/Jun; 4(3):51–53

Collinge JM et al. Demand vs. scheduled feedings for premature infants. JOGN Nurs 1982 Nov/Dec; 11(6):362–367

Cowett RM and Schwartz R. The infant of the diabetic mother. Pediatr Clin North Am 1982 Oct; 29(5):1213–1231

Cranley MS. Perinatal risk. JOGN Nurs (Supplement) 1983 May/Jun; 12(3):13s–18s

Davis N and Bakke K. Evaluation of a home apnea monitoring program. Perinatol/Neonatol 1983 Aug; 7(8):15–16+

Davis V. The structure and function of brown adipose tissue in the neonate. JOGN Nurs 1980 Nov/Dec; 9(6):368–372

Deal AW and Bordeaux BR. The phenomenon of SIDS. Pediatr Nurs 1980 Jan/Feb; 6(1):48–50

Devore NE, Jackson VM and Piening SL. TORCH infections. Am J Nurs 1983 Dec; 82(12):1660–1665

DeMaggio GT and Sheetz AH. The concerns of mothers caring for an infant on an apnea monitor. MCN 1983 July/Aug; 8(4):294–297

Dingle RE, et al. Continuous transcutaneous O_2 monitoring in the neonate. Am J Nurs 1980 May; 80(5):890+

Duncan JA and Webb LZ. Teaching families home apnea monitoring. Pediatr Nurs 1983 May/Jun; 9(3):171–175

Eager M and Exoo R. Parents visiting parents for unequalled support. MCN 1980 Jan/Feb; 5(1):35–36

Fantazia D. Physiologic basis of host susceptibility. JOGN Nurs (Supplement) 1983 May/Jun; 12(3):27s–30s

Finnegan LP. Substance abuse: Implications for the newborn. Perinatol/Neonatol 1982 Jul/Aug; 6(4):17–23

Gennaro S. Listerial infection: Nursing care of mother and infant. MCN 1980 Nov/Dec; 5(6):390–392

Gennaro S. Necrotizing enterocolitis: Detecting it and treating it. Nursing '80 1980 Jan; 10(1):52–55

Gibes RM. Clinical use of the Brazelton Neonatal Behavioral Assessment Scale in nursing practice. Pediatr Nurs 1981 May/Jun; 7(3):23–26

Graber HP and Balas-Stevens S. A discharge tool for teaching parents to monitor infant apnea at home. MCN 1984 May/Jun; 9(3):178–180

Griffith RA, Falterman CG and Richardson CJ. Care of low-birth-weight infant. Perinatol/Neonatol 1981 Jan/Feb; 5(1):19–27

Griffith RA, Falterman CG and Richardson CJ. Care of the low-birth-weight infant, part 2. Perinatol/Neonatol 1981 Mar/Apr; 5(2):13+

Gunn S. Critical care concepts related to maturation problems. Crit Care Q 1981 Jun; 4(1):1–7

Haddock N. Blood pressure monitoring in neonates. MCN 1980 Mar/Apr; 5(2):131–135

Harmon RJ, Glicken AD and Good WV. A new look at maternal–infant bonding. Perinatol/Neonatol 1982 Sep/Oct; 6(5):27–31

Harris MC and Polin RA. Neonatal septicemia. Pediatr Clin North Am 1983 Apr; 30(2):243–258

Hathaway WE. Neonatal hyperviscosity. Pediatrics 1983 Oct; 72(4):567–569

Hawkins-Walsh E. Diminishing anxiety in parents of sick newborns. MCN 1980 Jan/Feb; 5(1):30–34

Hayes JS. Premature infant development: The relationship of neonatal stimulation, birth condition and home environment. Pediatr Nurs 1980 Nov/Dec; 6(6):33–36

Hinkes P. Persistent apnea and bradycardia of prematurity. Perinatol/Neonatol 1984 Jan/Feb; 8(1):17+

Hodgman JE. Sepsis in the neonate. Perinatol/Neonatol 1981 Nov/Dec; 5(6):45–46+

Jay SS. The effects of gentle human touch on mechanically ventilated very-short-gestation infants. Matern Child Nurs J 1982 Winter; 11(4):199–259

Kanto WP and Wilson R. Epidemiology of necrotizing enterocolitis, with etiologic implications. Perinatol/Neonatol 1983 Oct; 7(1):63–68

Kelly DM and Shannon DC. Sudden infant death syndrome and near sudden infant death syndrome: A review of the literature, 1964–1982. Pediatr Clin North Am 1982 Oct; 29(5):1241–1261

Klijanowicz A. Protocol for the nursing care of hospitalized infants with prolonged apnea. Infant Apnea Center Handbook. Rochester, University of Rochester School of Medicine and Dentistry and School of Nursing, 1980

Korner AF, Ruppel EM and Rho JM. Effects of waterbeds on the sleep and motility of theophylline-treated preterm infants. Pediatrics 1982 Dec; 70(6):864–869

Kotsubo CZ. Helping families survive S.I.D.S. Nursing '83 1983 May; 13(5):94–96

Kuller JM, Lund C and Tobin C. Improved skin care for premature infants. MCN 1983 May/Jun; 8(3):200–203

LaRossa MM and Brown JV. Foster grandmothers in the premature

nursery. Am J Nurs 1982 Dec; 82(12):1834–1835

Lemons JA. Neonatal glucose metabolism and the infant of the diabetic mother. Crit Care Q 1981 Jun; 4(1):59–69

Lemons JA et al. Considerations in feeding the very-low-birth-weight infant. Perinatol/Neonatol 1982 May/Jun; 6(3):75–84

Lemons PM. Prenatal addiction: A duel tragedy. Crit Care Q 1981 Jun; 4(1):79–88

Levitt E. Neonatal IV therapy. NITA 1980 Sep/Oct; 3(5):169–174

Longo A. Teaching parents CPR. Pediatr Nurs 1983 Nov/Dec; 9(6):445–449

Lund C and Lefrak L. Discharge planning for infants in the intensive care nursery. Perinatol/Neonatol 1982 Mar/Apr; 6(2):49–50+

Lundeen KW. When baby makes three . . . challenges. Nursing '82 1982 May; 12(3):74–75

Mahan CK. Care of the family of the critically ill neonate. Crit Care Q 1981 Jun; 4(1):89–103

Mandell F, McAnulty EH and Carlson A. Unexpected death of an infant sibling. Pediatrics 1983 Nov; 72(5):652–657

Mayer CL, Mahan CK and Schreiner RL. Transfer of newborns to community hospitals. Perinatol/Neonatol 1982 Mar/Apr; 6(2):75–78

McCarthy PA. Fetal alcohol syndrome and other alcohol-related birth defects. Nurs Pract 1983 Jan; 8(1):33–34+

Measel CP. A practical popular pacifier. Crit Care Nurs 1983 Mar/Apr; 8(3):47–48

Medoff-Cooper B and Schraeder BA. Development trends and behavioral styles of very low birth weight infants. Nurs Res 1982 Mar/Apr; 31(2):68–72

Merritt TA and Valdes-Dapena M. SIDS research update. Pediatr Ann 1984 Mar; 3(3):193–195+

Mohan Rao HK and Elhassani SB. Primum non nocere: Iatrogenic complications of procedures performed on the newborn, part 3. Perinatol/Neonatol 1981 Mar/Apr; 5(2):23–26+

Murant I. The efficacy of caffeine in the treatment of recurrent idiopathic apnea in premature infants. J Pediatr 1983 Dec; 99(6):984–989

Neonatal Drug withdrawal. Pediatrics 1983 Dec; 72(6):895–902

Newborn and near death. Emerg Med 1983 Mar 15; 15(5):114–118+

Norris S, Campbell LA and Brenkert S. Nursing procedures and alterations in transcutaneous oxygen tension in premature infant. Nurs Res 1982 Nov/Dec; 31(6):330–336

Nugent J. Intra-arterial blood pressure monitoring in the neonate. JOGN Nurs 1982 Sep/Oct; 11(5):281–287

Nugent JK. The Brazelton Neonatal Behavioral Assessment Scale: Implications for intervention. Pediatr Nurs 1981 May/Jun; 7(3):18–21+

Ogata ES. Metabolic problems of the premature infant. Perinatol/Neonatol 1983 May; 7(5):49–50+

Ogata ES. Diabetes-related problems of the newborn. Perinatol/Neonatol 1984 Jan/Feb; 8(1):48–53

Paukert S. Maternal–infant attachment in a traditional hospital setting. JOGN Nurs 1982 Jan/Feb; 11(1):23–26

Peterson DR, Chinn NM and Fisher LD. The sudden infant death syndrome: Repetitions in families. J Pediatr 1980 Aug; 97(2):265–267

Phelps DL. Neonatal oxygen toxicity—Is it preventable? Pediatr Clin North Am 1982 Oct; 29(5):1233–1240

Philip AGS. Noninvasive diagnostic techniques in newborn infants. Pediatr Clin North Am 1983 Oct; 29(5):1275–1298

Rausch PB. Effects of tactile and kinesthetic stimulation on premature infants. JOGN Nurs 1981 Jan/Feb; 10(1):34–37

Rehm R. Teaching cardiopulmonary resuscitation to parents. MCN Nov/Dec; 8(6):411–416

Reid TJ. Newborn cyanosis. Am J Nurs 1982 Aug; 82(8):1230–1234

Rigatto H. Apnea. Pediatr Clin North Am 1982 Oct; 29(5):1105–1116

Rosenn DW, Loeb LS and Jura MB. Differentiation of organic from nonorganic failure to thrive syndrome in infancy. Pediatrics 1980 Nov; 66(5):698–704

Sahu S. Birthweight, gestational age, and neonatal risks. Perinatol/Neonatol 1984 Jan/Feb; 8(1):28–30+

Sasso SC. Prostaglandin E, for infants with congenital heart disease. MCN 1983 Jan/Feb; 8(1):29

Scanlon KB et al. Placement of umbilical artery catheters. High vs. low. JOGN Nurs 1982 Nov/Dec; 11(6):355–357

Scott CB et al. Diaphragm strength in near-miss Sudden Infant Death Syndrome. Pediatrics 1982 Jun; 69(6):782–784

Schanler RJ. Human milk for the very low-birthweight infant. Perinatol/Neonatol 1983 Nov/Dec; 7(11):17–20a+

Scharping EM. Physiological measurements of the neonate. MCN 1983 Jan/Feb; 8(1):70–73

Schiffman RF. Temperature monitoring in the neonate: A comparison of axillary and rectal temperatures. Nurs Res 1982 Sep/Oct; 31(5):274–277

Seaman CK. Monitoring the critically ill neonate. Crit Care Q 1981 Jun; 4(1):9–17

Sinatra FR and Merritt RJ. Nutritional needs of the premature infant. Perinatol/Neonatol 1983 May; 7(5):61–66

Silvio KT. SIDS and apnea monitoring: A parent's view. Pediatr Ann 1984 Mar; 3(3):229–230+

Smith JC. Psychosocial aspect of infantile apnea and home monitoring. Pediatr Ann 1984 Mar; 3(3):219–220+

Southall DP et al. Undetected episodes of prolonged apnea and severe bradycardia in preterm infants. Pediatrics 1983 Oct; 72(4):541

Steinschneider A, Weinstein SL and Diamond E. The sudden death syndrome and apnea/obstruction during neonatal sleep and feeding. Pediatrics 1982 Dec; 70(6):858–863

Stephens CJ. The fetal alcohol syndrome: Cause for concern. MCN 1981 Jul/Aug; 6(4):251–256

Sterk MB. Understanding parenteral nutrition. JOGN Nurs (Supplement) 1983 May/Jun; 12(3):45s–50s

Stevens DC, Kleiman MB and Schreiner RL. Early-onset pseudomonas sepsis of the neonate. Perinatol/Neonatol 1982 Sep/Oct; 6(5):75–77

Strodtbeck F. Critical care concepts related to neonatal septicemia and septic shock. Crit Care Q 1981 Jun; 4(1):71–77

Tarby JT and Volpe JJ. Intraventricular hemorrhage in the premature infant. Pediatr Clin North Am 1982 Oct; 29(5):1077–1104

Thibeault DW and Callenbach JC. Drug therapy in neonatal lung disease. Perinatol/Neonatol 1983 Apr; 7(4):39–40+

Trotter CW, Chang P and Thompson T. Perinatal factors and the developmental outcome of preterm infants. JOGN Nurs 1982 Mar/Apr; 11(2):83–90

Trykowski LE, Kirkpatrick BV and Leonard EL. Enhancement of nutritive sucking in premature infants. Phys Occup Ther Pediatr 1981 Summer; 1(4):27–33

Varner B, Ossenkop D and Lyon J. Prematures, too, need rooming-in and care-by-parent programs. MCN 1980 Nov/Dec; 5(6):431–432

Webb LZ. Developmental care in the neonatal ICU. DCCN 1980 Jul/Aug; 1(4):221–231

Webb LZ and Duncan JA. Selecting the right home apnea monitor. Pediatr Nurs 1983 May/Jun; 9(3):179–182

Weinstein SL and Steinschneider A. Prolonged infantile apnea: Diagnostic and therapeutic dilemma. J Respir Dis 1980 Jul/Aug; 1(8):76–77+

Wright LL et al. The effect of early feeding on plasma glucose levels in SGA infants. Clin Pediatr 1983 Aug; 22(8):539–541

Wu PYK. Phototherapy. Perinatol/Neonatol 1982 Mar/Apr; 6(2):21–24+

Wu PYK. Phototherapy update: Factors affecting efficiency of phototherapy. Perinatol/Neonatol 1981 Sep/Oct; 5(5):45–46+

Yoos L. Taking another look at failure to thrive. MCN 1984 Jan/Feb; 9(1):32–36

Zebal BH and Friedman SB. Sudden infant death syndrome and infantile apnea. Pediatr Ann 1984 Mar; 3(3):188–190

Zebal BH and Woolsey SF. SIDS and the family: The pediatrician's role. Pediatr Ann 1984 Mar; 3(3):237–238+

Zukowsky K and Dulczak S. Maintaining the infant's skin integrity. Crit Care Nurs 1982 Jul/Aug; 2(4):53

Additional Pertinent References

Cagan J and Meier PA. A discharge planning tool for use with families of high-risk infants. JOGN Nurs 1979 May/Jun; 8(3):146–148

Caring for your Hospitalized Baby. Washington, DC, Association for the Care of Children's Health, 1984

Metcalf SC. Getting to Know Your Premature Baby. Louisville, The National Foundation March of Dimes

Schraeder BD. Attachment and parenting despite lengthy intensive care. MCN 1980 Jan/Feb; 5(1):37–41

Whaley PA, Gosling CG and Schreiner RL. Relieving parental anxiety—A booklet for parents of an infant in NICU. JOGN Nurs 1979 Jan/Feb; 8(1):49–55

Audio-Visual Materials

Brazelton Film No. 1: An Introduction
Education Development Center
39 Chapel Street
Newton, MA 02160
In this 16-mm., 20 minute film, Dr. T. Berry Brazelton briefly describes the Neonatal Behavioral Assessment Scale while he examines a normal 2-day-old infant. He assesses the infant's initial state of rest and then tests his habituation to various stimuli and responses to different experiences.

Inservice education modules: Series I— First Six Hours of Life, Neonatal Thermoregulation, Hypoglycemia, Early Parent–Infant Relationships, Assessment of Risk in the Newborn.
March of Dimes–Birth Defect Foundation
1275 Mamaroneck Avenue
White Plains, NY 10605

Children With Conditions of the Respiratory Tract

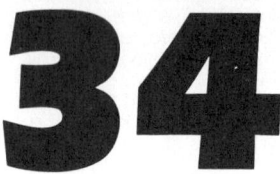

Overview of Childhood Respiratory Disorders

Common Types of Respiratory Disorders

Examples of common childhood respiratory disorders can be found in Table 34-1. The following disorders are included:
1. Bacterial pneumonia
2. Viral pneumonia
3. Pneumocystis carinii pneumonia
4. Mycoplasma pneumonia
5. Bronchiolitis
6. Croup

Assessment

Physical Assessment

Determine the severity of the respiratory distress that the child is experiencing. Make an initial nursing assessment.
1. Observe the respiratory rate and pattern.
   a. Count the respirations for 1 full minute.
   b. Observe the child for retractions, and note severity and location.
   c. Listen to the chest with a stethoscope to determine if crackles are present and to evaluate the breath sounds.
2. Observe the child's color, and note any presence of cyanosis.
3. Observe for nasal flaring.
4. Evaluate the child's degree of restlessness, apprehension, and motor tone.
5. Note any wheezing, stridor, or hoarseness.

Potential Problems/Nursing Diagnoses

1. Hypoxemia related to impaired oxygen–carbon dioxide exchange
2. Alteration in comfort related to respiratory distress, infectious process, and treatments
3. Alteration in fluid and electrolyte balance related to increased respiratory effort, nausea and vomiting, and decreased appetite
4. Potential for infection related to underlying disease condition
5. Anxiety related to respiratory distress and hospitalization
6. Parental anxiety related to uncertainty about the child's well-being

Planning and Implementation

Nursing Interventions

A. Provide a humidified environment enriched with oxygen in order to combat anoxia and to liquefy secretions.

1. Place the child in a Croupette with cool mist or use ultrasonic mist in tent (see Oxygen Therapy, p. 1186).

▶ **NURSING ALERT:** At no time should the mist be allowed to become so dense that it obscures clear visualization of the patient's respiratory pattern.

2. Observe the child's response to this environment.
3. Place the child in a comfortable position to promote easier ventilation.
4. Frequent changing of clothing and bed linen will prevent chilling and will provide comfort.

B. Provide the child with adequate hydration.

1. Maintain the administration of intravenous fluids at the prescribed rate.
2. When the child is in severe respiratory distress, he is given nothing by mouth because of the danger of aspiration.
3. Offer the child small sips of clear fluid when the respiratory status improves.
   a. Note any vomiting or abdominal distention after the oral fluid is given.
   b. As the child begins to take more fluid by mouth, notify the physician so that intravenous fluid rate may be adjusted in order to prevent fluid overload.
   c. Do not force the child to take fluids orally that he does not want, since this may cause increased distress and possibly vomiting. Anorexia often accompanies acute febrile infection. Generally, do not awaken a sleeping child just to give frequent fluids.
4. Record the child's intake and output.
   a. Measure urinary output and record.
   b. Check specific gravity of urine.

C. Provide the child with both physical and psychological rest.

1. Disturb the child as little as possible by organizing nursing care, and protect him from unnecessary interruptions.
2. Be aware of the age of the child and be familiar with his level of growth and development as it applies to hospitalization.
3. The presence of the child's parents will alleviate some of his apprehension.
4. Provide opportunities for quiet play as the child's condition improves.
5. Explain procedures and hospital routine to the child as appropriate for his age.
6. Reduce anxiety and apprehension to aid in decreasing psychological distress, which will help the child relax and ease respiratory effort.

D. Provide good skin care to prevent skin excoriation from secretions, accompanying diarrhea, and skin breakdown from confinement to bed.

E. Provide measures to improve ventilation of affected portion of the lung.

1. Change position frequently.
2. Provide postural drainage if prescribed.
3. Relieve nasal obstruction that contributes to breathing difficulty.
   Instill saline solution or prescribed nose drops and apply nasal suctioning.
4. Crying can be an effective method for ventilating the lungs.
5. Coughing is a normal tracheobronchial cleansing procedure. Constant coughing can be relieved temporarily by allowing the child to sip water; use extreme caution to prevent aspiration.
6. Abdominal distention frequently accompanies respiratory infection and can be painful and a hindrance to respiration.
   a. Place in semi-Fowler's position.
   b. Rectal tube, small enema, or suppository may give relief.
   c. Nasogastric tube may be prescribed to relieve distention.

(Text continues on p. 1260)

Parental Education
When Your Child has a Croup Attack*

If your child develops hoarseness and croupy cough with a cold, or if he wakes up in the middle of the night with a croup attack, here is the way to handle it:

1. **Take your child's temperature, then call your doctor.** He or she will want to know whether the child has a fever or has been sick and may want to listen to the child breathe or cry over the phone. If the doctor suggests going to the emergency room, do so without delay.
2. Humidification is the most effective treatment for croup since it loosens secretions and eases breathing. While waiting for the doctor to get back to you or after talking with him (unless he recommends that you go to the emergency room), take the child into the bathroom, close the door, and turn the hot water on in the shower. Do the same in the bathtub if there is no shower. Keep the child in the steamy bathroom—not in the tub or shower stall, where he might get burned—until breathing becomes easier and the cough is less dry. Call back the doctor if you see no improvement in breathing comfort within 10–15 minutes.
3. After breathing has improved, humidify the child's room with a cool-mist humidifier, located in a safe place but still close to the child. If the night air is cool and moist, open the bedroom window or take the child outside for a while.
4. Give your child liquids that you know he likes (avoid milk) every hour he's awake. Drinking plenty of fluids helps liquefy secretions and is very important in helping him get over croup.
5. If the child has a fever, you may give acetaminophen (30–40 milligrams per kilogram [1 kilogram = 2.2 pounds] of the child's weight over a 24-hour period) every 4 hours. If necessary, your doctor can help you determine the appropriate dose.
6. Stay in the child's room for the rest of the night or check on him or her periodically. Worsening symptoms may not waken the child. Allow child to choose the position in which he is most comfortable.
7. **Call the doctor immediately if any of the following happens:**
   - The child's condition worsens (noisier and more difficult breathing, high fever).
   - The child becomes more restless (repeatedly sitting up, then lying down or rapidly moving about trying to find a comfortable position).
   - You notice a sinking in of the soft skin area below the top of the shoulder (above the collar bone), beneath the Adam's apple, or between and below the ribs and in the pit of the child's stomach.
   - The lips or fingernails appear very pale or bluish in color.
   - The child clearly is quite sick regardless of the exact degree of breathing difficulty.
8. Some things are not helpful in treating a croup attack. **Avoid** giving the child cough syrup or preparations for relieving a cold; these may worsen breathing distress by inhibiting the natural tendency to clear the throat by coughing or by drying and thickening secretions.
9. Call the doctor's office the next day and ask whether the child needs to be seen, even if symptoms are gone.

* Adapted from Patient Care, Nov 30, 1982, Copyright 1982 Miller and Fink Corp., 16 Thorndale Circle, Darien, CT 06820. All rights reserved.

Table 34-1 **Respiratory Disorders**

Condition and Causative Agent	Age and Incidence	Clinical Manifestations
I. Bacterial Pneumonia		

A. Streptococcus pneumonia
Streptococcus pneumoniae (gram-positive)
This type of bacterial pneumonia is most frequent in children.
	Birth–4 years
	Winter and spring
	(especially in patients with sickle cell disease and patients without spleens)
		Mild upper respiratory infection (URI) with sudden symptoms
		Infants
		  Refusal to eat
		  Vomiting, diarrhea
		  Hypo- or hyperthermia
		May be
		  Tachypnea
		  Grunting
		  Retractions
		  Nasal flaring
		Older child
		  Prodromal upper respiratory infection
		  Headache
		  Anorexia
		  Malaise
		  Dry cough
		  Fever
		  Restlessness
		  Pleuritic pain
		  Grunting with shallow, rapid respirations
		  Possibly abdominal pain

B. Streptococcal pneumonia Beta-hemolytic streptococcus Group A (gram-positive)	3–5 years	Commonly superimposed on febrile respiratory infection in a child already ill with a viral exanthem Shows sudden increased fever, worsening cough, chills, pleuritic pain, respiratory distress
C. Staphylococcal pneumonia Coagulase-positive *Staphylococcus aureus* (gram-positive)	Birth–2 years	History of predisposing factors. Gradual onset with respiratory symptoms or sudden onset with systemic involvement (very toxic child) Presence of coarse, bubbly crepitations
D. *Haemophilus influenzae,* Type B (less common in healthy child)	6 months–3 years	Similar to other lobar pneumonias and bronchopneumonia with spasmodic cough, "toxic" appearance
II. Viral Pneumonia Respiratory syncytial virus (RSV) (most common) Parainfluenza virus, types 1-2-3 Adenoviruses Influenza viruses	Birth–2 years; higher incidence in females than in males Winter and early spring	Gradual onset following an upper respiratory infection RSV turns into extension of bronchiolitis Parainfluenza virus causes coryza, pharyngitis, cough may succeed pneumonia Adenovirus causes pharyngitis and cervical adenitis, may succeed pneumonia

Diagnostic Evaluation	Treatment and Nursing Management	Complications

X-ray—patchy area around bronchi
Positive cultures
   Sputum
   Nasopharyngeal secretions
   Blood
	Penicillin G
	Symptomatic
	   Rest, with gradually increasing exercise
	   Fluids—I & O
	   Antipyretics
	   O_2 mist
	   Position change
	Bronchodilators
		Rare with antibiotic prescription
		May see
		   Otitis media
		   Sinusitis
		   Empyema
		   Bacteremia

X-ray—usually patchy, but may show
   disseminated infiltrate
WBC increased—polymorphic leukocytosis
Erythrocyte sedimentation rate (ESR) increased
Positive culture from:
   Respiratory secretions
   Empyema fluid
	Penicillin G
	Symptomatic
		Empyema
		Pneumatocele to pneumothorax
		Permanent pulmonary fibrosis and pleural
		   thickening (fibrothorax)

X-ray—patchy consolidation of one or more lobes;
   pneumatocele abscesses
Culture, sputum, or gastric aspirate, pulmonary
   fluid or lung aspirate
WBC—elevated in older child
	Methicillin or penicillin G
	   Rapid treatment is important
	   Symptomatic special attention to fluid balance,
	     treatment of pleural complications, treatment
	     of anemia; O_2 mist
	Be alert to signs of tension pneumothorax; abrupt
	   onset of pain, cyanosis, dyspnea, diminished
	   chest movement on one side
	Ampicillin—if organism is not resistant
	Other: penicillin G, chloramphenicol
		Empyema
		Pneumothorax
		Lung abscess
		Osteomyelitis
		Staphylococcal pericarditis
		Bronchiectasis

Culture: blood, nasal secretions: WBC shows an
   increase—lymphocytosis
X-ray—lobar consolidation (may also have pleural
   effusion)
	Symptomatic cough suppression	Empyema

X-ray—infiltration of one or more lobes is more
   extensive than clinical picture would suggest
Culture: nasopharyngeal
Increase titer of specific antibody
	Broad-spectrum antibiotic therapy (until
	   confirmation of organism is established)
	Symptomatic and supportive	

(continued)

Table 34-1   Respiratory Disorders (continued)

Condition and Causative Agent	Age and Incidence	Clinical Manifestations

III. *Pneumocystis carinii* Pneumonia
Pneumocystis carinii—parasite of uncertain systemic status; presumed to be a sporozoan
	Predisposing factors:
	   Prematurity, immature debilitated infant, infectious disease, especially cytomegalic inclusion disease; serious compromising disease (e.g., cystic fibrosis)
	Children receiving immunosuppressive medication for malignant diseases
	Immunodeficiency disease especially in children under 1 year of age
		Onset is generally slow, taking 3–6 weeks to peak, with increasing tachypnea, extreme grayish cyanosis and dyspnea at rest, cough, O_2 desaturation
		   Presence of predisposing factors

IV. Mycoplasma Pneumonia *Mycoplasma pneumoniae* (pleuropneumonia-like organism) Microorganisms with properties between bacteria and viruses	5–15 years Late fall and winter	Onset is insidious Malaise, headache, low-grade fever, sore throat irritating cough, vomiting, possible crepitation
V. Bronchiolitis Respiratory syncytial virus (RSV) Adenovirus Parainfluenza virus, types 1 and 3 Influenza virus *Mycoplasma pneumoniae*	Most common in infants and children under 6 months; may occur in child up to 2 years of age Greater incidence in males than in females Winter–spring	Onset is often gradual and associated with exposure to respiratory infection Coryza of 1–3 days, tachypnea Intercostal and suprasternal retraction Expiratory rhonchi Dry cough; paroxysmal cough; may have wheezing Fever Cyanosis Possible dehydration Tachypnea

VI. Croup and Epiglottitis
   A. Croup (see box, p. 1255)
      Acute laryngotracheobronchitis (LTB); laryngotracheitis
      Parainfluenza virus 1-2-3 (most common virus)
      Respiratory syncytial virus
      Influenza virus during epidemics
      Rhinovirus
	3 months–3 years
	Winter
		Generally onset is gradual and progresses slowly, following 1 to several days after an upper respiratory infection
		Coryza
		Croupy cough, barking cough
		Inspiratory stridor
		Hoarseness
		Low-grade fever
		Increasing respiration and pulse rate
		Apprehension, restlessness, anxiety

B. Epiglottitis–supraglottitis (Fig. 34-1)
      Bacterial
      Hemophilus influenzae type B (most common)
      Pneumococci
      Staphylococcus aureus
      Beta-hemolytic streptococcus
	3–10 years
	Seasonal variations
		Onset and progression are rapid—may follow short duration of coryza
		Severe inspiratory stridor with marked supraclavicular and intercostal retractions
		Sore throat—refusal to eat, dysphagia
		High fever 39°–40°C. (102°–104°F.)
		Drooling, respirations may be shallow, hoarseness; paleness and exhausted appearance, may insist on sitting up—condition worsens when lying down; cherry-red epiglottis; apprehension; restlessness; anxiety; cannot swallow; mouth open and chin thrust forward with tongue out

Diagnostic Evaluation	Treatment and Nursing Management	Complications

X-ray shows bilateral diffuse alveolar densities, especially perihilar
Observe cysts in special stained smear in material obtained from lung biopsy (not reliable)
Lung aspiration by needle
Endotracheal brush catheter technique
	Trimethroprim-sulfamethoxazole
	Supportive: maintain oxygen and respirations; administer immunoglobulins, possibly withhold immunosuppressive chemotherapy, maintain fluid, electrolyte, and acid–base balance, maintain nutrition
	Be alert to early signs and predisposing factors that will aid in early diagnosis
	Carefully observe for adverse effects of drug therapy: abscess formation and necrosis of injection site, if pentamide isethionate used
	   Hypoglycemia
	   Nephrotoxicity
	   Hypotension
	   Tachycardia
	   Hypocalcemia
	   Nausea and vomiting
	   Skin rash
	   Anemia
	   Hyperkalemia
	   Thrombocytopenia
	   Isolation
		Pneumothorax from diagnostic tests, concomitant bacterial pneumonia or sepsis
		Death

X-ray shows peribronchial infiltrate in lower lobes Increase in complement fixation test Positive sputum culture Cold agglutinins	Erythromycin Supportive antipyretic cough suppression Secretion precautions	
X-ray demonstrates overinfiltration of lungs Virologic or serologic studies to isolate virus on throat swab PaO_2 decreases, $PaCO_2$ increases (late finding)	Antibiotic therapy given to severely ill child until laboratory confirmation is established Humidified O_2 to relieve arterial hypoxemia Monitoring blood gases and correction of acidosis Possible ventilatory assistance Maintain fluid–electrolyte–acid/base and nutritional balance Keep nasal airway open and clear of mucus to decrease respiratory difficulty, because infant is an obligatory nose breather Position baby in infant seat inside Croupette; it may provide some respiratory assistance Be alert to signs of impending respiratory acidosis and dehydration, and cardiac involvement Epinephrine theophylline or racemic epinephrine via IPPB may relieve bronchospasm	Exhaustion and anoxia Secondary bacterial infection Pneumothorax and pneumomediastinum (occasional) Apneic spells Circulatory collapse Increase—predisposed to asthma
History and clinical evaluation—Laboratory findings PCO_2 increased (late finding), PO_2 decreased Normal—mild leukocytosis X-ray of neck—subglottic edema (below vocal cords) Normal supraglottic structures	Supportive: high humidification with oxygen, as necessary; hydration; nebulized racemic epinephrine with or without IPPB, minimal handling; allow undisturbed sleep; monitor vital signs Teach parents home management of croup (see below) Syrup of ipecac may be beneficial in reducing coughing in spasmodic croup	Airway obstruction Anorexia
History and clinical evaluation— Laboratory findings PCO_2 increased (late finding); PO_2 decreased Leukocytosis X-ray of neck—epiglottic edema (above vocal cords); normal trachea and larynx	Medical emergency: endotracheal/nasotracheal intubation or tracheostomy; "cool humidified oxygen" Antibiotic therapy Chloramphenicol Fluids Rest Observe carefully for signs and symptoms of increasing respiratory distress; have in readiness equipment for intubation or tracheostomy (see p. 1184) Teach parents home care of tracheostomy Community health nurse referral	Airway obstruction Death Other: bacteremia, pneumothorax, mediastinal emphysema, interstitial bronchopneumonia

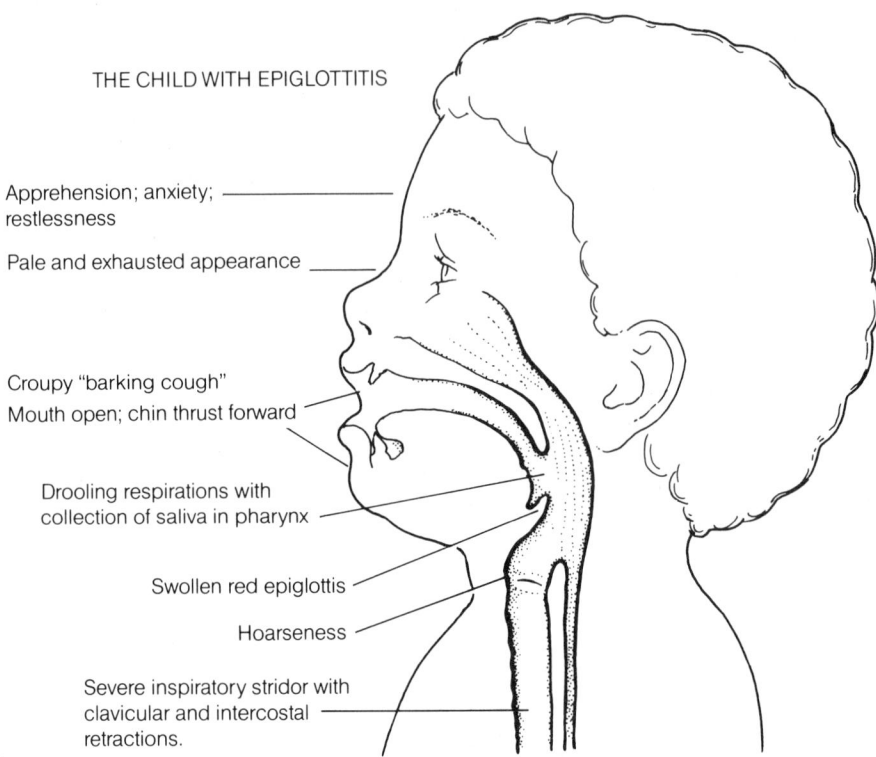

THE CHILD WITH EPIGLOTTITIS

Apprehension; anxiety; restlessness

Pale and exhausted appearance

Croupy "barking cough"
Mouth open; chin thrust forward

Drooling respirations with collection of saliva in pharynx

Swollen red epiglottis

Hoarseness

Severe inspiratory stridor with clavicular and intercostal retractions.

Figure 34-1. Epiglottitis.

F. Assist in the control of fever.

1. Give antipyretics as prescribed.
2. Increase evaporation from skin with cool sponges.

G. Provide for adequate nutrition to meet the growth and development needs of the child.

1. Determine the child's food preferences.
2. Offer the child small meals.

H. Administer appropriate antibiotic therapy.

1. Observe for drug sensitivity.
2. Observe the child's response to therapy.

I. Be alert for the appearance of specific complications that may accompany respiratory infection and notify physician immediately (see Table 34-1).

J. Include parents in the planning of care and in caring for the child.

Recognize the parents' anxieties. The mother may be exhausted from caring for her sick child prior to his hospitalization.

▶ **NURSING ALERT:**
To minimize spasm and sudden blockage of airway:
Avoid:
 Making the child lie flat
 Forcing the child to drink
 Looking down the child's throat

Evaluation
Expected Outcomes

1. Shows no signs of complications of respiratory distress; stable vital signs; normal blood gas values
2. Experiences minimal respiratory distress as evidenced by stable vital signs, by statements that discomfort has subsided and appropriate age-related behaviors
3. Attains/maintains fluid and electrolyte balance; normal laboratory values; appropriate intake and output
4. Absence of infection; temperature normal; lessening of colored sputum; thinning of secretions
5. Experiences lessening of anxiety as evidenced by appropriate coping behaviors; appears relaxed and at ease
6. Parents verbalize understanding of illness; making appointment for follow-up care

Tonsillectomy and Adenoidectomy

Tonsillectomy and *adenoidectomy* are the surgical removal of the adenoidal and tonsillar structures, part of the lymphoid tissue that encircles the pharynx.

Function of Tonsils and Adenoids

1. Serve as a first line of defense against respiratory infections

2. Because the growth of the tonsils and adenoids in the first 10 years of life exceed general somatic growth, these structures appear especially large in the child.

Clinical Manifestations

1. Acute or chronic infection of tonsils and adenoids
2. Hypertrophy produces obstruction to:
   a. Breathing
   b. Swallowing
   c. Auditory (eustachian) tube

Diagnostic Evaluation

Since bleeding is a likely complication of surgery in this highly vascular area, preoperative blood studies must be completed.

1. Clotting time
2. Smear for platelets
3. Prothrombin time
4. Partial prothrombin time
5. Others specific for general anesthesia

Complications

1. Hemorrhage—although unusual, it can occur
2. Emotional/psychological sequelae
3. Reactions to anesthesia
4. Otitis media; bacteremia
5. Lung abscess; pneumonia; septicemia—all very rare

Treatment

Tonsillectomy and adenoidectomy are separate procedures with separate indications. Controversy exists among experts as to indications, necessity, and benefits of surgery.

A. Indications for Tonsillectomy

1. Conservative:
   a. Recurrent or persistent tonsillitis with documented streptococcal infection 4 times in 1 year
   b. Marked hypertrophy of tonsils, which distorts speech, causes swallowing difficulties, and causes subsequent weight loss
   c. Tonsillar malignancy
   d. Diphtheria carrier
   e. Cor pulmonale due to obstruction
2. Controversial:
   a. Peritonsillar abscess or retrotonsillar abscess
   b. Suppurative cervical adenitis with tonsillar focus
   c. Persistent hyperemia of anterior pillars
   d. Enlarged cervical nodes

B. Indications for Adenoidectomy

1. Conservative:
   a. Adenoid hypertrophy resulting in obstruction of airway leading to hypoxia, pulmonary hypertension, and cor pulmonale
   b. Hypertrophy with nasal obstruction accompanied by breathing difficulty and severe speech distortion
   c. Hypertrophy associated with chronic suppurative or serous otitis media and sensorineural or conductive hearing loss, chronic mastoiditis, or cholesteatoma
   d. Mouth-breathing due to hypertrophied adenoids
2. Controversial:
   Enlarged adenoids, chronic otitis media, and no evidence of complications

Contraindications to Surgery

1. Bleeding or coagulation disorders
2. Uncontrolled systemic disorders (i.e., diabetes, rheumatic fever, cardiac, renal disease)
3. Child under the age of 5–6 years—unless life-threatening situation
4. Presence of upper respiratory infection in child or immediate family
5. Specific for adenoidectomy—certain palate abnormalities (i.e., cleft palate or submucus cleft palate)

Potential Problems/Nursing Diagnoses

1. Anxiety and fear of child and parents related to surgery
2. Potential postoperative hemorrhage related to surgery in the highly vascular area of tonsils and/or adenoids.
3. Discomfort related to surgery.
4. Parental anxiety related to surgical procedure

Preoperative Nursing Interventions

A. Assess upon admission the psychological preparation of the child for hospitalization and surgery.

1. The child should know why he has been admitted to the hospital and what will happen to him.
2. When the parents have not told the child about hospitalization, it may be because they cannot.
   a. They do not know what will happen.
   b. They do not know how to tell the child because of their own anxieties.
   c. They do not understand the importance of telling the child the truth in order to perpetuate the child's trust in the parents.
3. Help the parents in preparing the child by talking at first in general terms about hospitalization.
4. The child may have preconceived ideas from parents and peers about what to expect. (These may pose a threat to the child.)
   a. Introduce the child to other children on the unit, especially those who have had and are recovering from surgery.
   b. Talk about and show the child the new things he will see.
   c. Correct any misunderstandings the child may have.
5. The preschool child is very vulnerable to psychological trauma as a result of this experience.
   a. Tell the child the truth.
   b. Include parents when helping the child.

B. Take nursing history from parents at the time of admission to obtain any pertinent information that would contraindicate surgery.

1. Infection
   a. When was the most recent infection?
      It is desirable for the patient to be free of respiratory infection for at least 2–3 weeks.
   b. Has child been exposed to any communicable diseases?
2. Safety
   a. Does the child have any loose teeth?
   b. Are there any bleeding tendencies in child or family?

C. Maintain adequate hydration prior to surgery, since blood loss may be extensive during surgery.

1. Encourage the child to drink fluids the night before surgery.
2. The child usually is NPO a few hours prior to surgery.

D. Prepare the child specifically (appropriate for age) **for what to expect postoperatively.**

1. Where he will wake up.
2. Sore throat, emesis of blood, position, foul taste and smell in mouth
3. Ice collar, medications
4. Fluid regimen

E. Encourage the mother to stay with her young child the day and night of surgery or at least before surgery and when the child returns to his room and is waking up.

Prepare the mother as to what to expect when she sees the child postoperatively.
   1. Vomiting
   2. Skin color
   3. Crying, angry, or frightened

F. Know if the child has a history of chronic infection or rheumatic fever so antibiotics may be given pre- and postoperatively.

G. Ensure that preoperative bleeding and clotting time blood studies have been done.

Postoperative Nursing Interventions

A. Administer good postoperative care based on general principles and observe for usual postoperative complications (see p. 1126).

B. Assist the child in maintaining a patent airway, by draining secretions and preventing aspiration of vomitus.

1. Place the child prone or semiprone before he becomes alert with head turned to side.
2. Allow the child to assume position of comfort when he is alert. (Mother may hold the child.)
3. The child may vomit old blood initially.
   If suctioning is necessary, avoid trauma to oropharynx.
4. Remind the child not to cough or clear throat unless necessary.

C. Observe the child constantly until he is awake, and then frequently thereafter; monitor vital signs and be alert to signs of hemorrhage.

1. Indications of hemorrhage (the most frequent complication)
   a. Increasing rapid pulse
   b. Frequent swallowing
   c. Pallor
   d. Restlessness
   e. Clearing of throat and vomiting of blood
   f. Continuous slight oozing of blood over a number of hours postoperatively
   g. Check vomitus for any fresh bleeding
   h. Inspect throat for signs of oozing
2. Have emergency equipment readily available.
   a. Suction equipment
   b. Packing material

D. Offer measures of comfort to the child.

1. Cool liquids offer some relief from sore throat, as well as prevent dehydration and temperature elevation.

   a. Give ice chips 1–2 hours after awakening.
   b. When vomiting has ceased, advance to clear liquids cautiously.
   c. Offer cool, synthetic fruit juices and milk at first since they are best tolerated; then offer Popsicles, cool water for first 12–24 hours.
2. Ice collar to neck may provide some comfort. (Remove ice collar if child becomes restless.)
3. Give analgesic, especially to older child.
4. Rinse mouth with cool water or alkaline solution.
5. Keep child and environment free from blood-tinged drainage to help decrease anxiety.
6. There is some controversy regarding intake of milk and ice cream the evening of surgery: it can be soothing and reduce swelling but it does coat the mouth and throat, causing child to clear throat more often and this may initiate bleeding.

E. Provide opportunity for the child to have as much rest as possible.

1. Encourage the mother to be with the child when he awakens since he is usually frightened. (The mother's presence can be very comforting.)
2. When mother must leave, reassure the child that she will return.
3. Keep the child in bed in a quiet room.

Health Education

1. Explain and write instructions as to the care of the child at home after discharge (usually the day after surgery).
   a. Diet should still consist of large amounts of fluids as well as soft, cool, nonirritating foods. (Supply list of suggestions.)
   b. Eating helps promote healing since it increases the blood supply to tissues.
   c. Bed rest should be maintained for a couple of days, then daily rest periods for about a week. Resume normal activities about 2 weeks following surgery.
   d. Avoid contact with persons with infections.
   e. Discourage the child from frequent coughing and clearing of throat.
   f. Avoid gargling. Mouth odor may be present for a few days after surgery; only mouth rinsing is acceptable.
   g. If signs and symptoms of impending trouble occur, the physician should be called immediately.
      (1) Earache accompanied by fever
      (2) Any bleeding, often indicated only by frequent swallowing; most common about 5th–10th day when membrane sloughs from surgical site.
   h. How to give any medications the physician may prescribe.
   i. The telephone number of the physician or emergency department if trouble occurs.
2. Discuss with the mother (parents) what results they can expect from the surgery.
   a. Decreased number of sore throats
   b. Lessened evidence of obstructive symptoms
   c. Decreased incidence of cervical lymphadenitis
   d. Improvement in nutritional status
   e. Will not improve nasal allergies
   f. Will not improve secretory otitis media
3. Guide parents in helping the child think of the

hospital experience as a positive one once he has returned home.
a. Talk about what happened.
b. Let the child play out his feelings.

Expected Outcomes

1. Experiences minimal anxiety and fear evidenced by appropriate coping behaviors

2. Achieves stabilized postoperative condition; vital signs normal; no unusual bleeding

3. Experiences minimal discomfort as evidenced by normal vital signs, ability to swallow, and relaxed behavior

4. Parents verbalize postoperative plan of care at home (i.e., diet, activities, follow-up)

Asthma

Asthma is a recurrent, reversible condition of the lungs in which there is airway obstruction due to spasm of the bronchial smooth muscle, edema of the mucosa, and increased mucous secretions in the bronchi and bronchioles that have been brought on by various stimuli.

Classification of Asthma

1. *Spasmodic*—sporadic in nature, with varying intervals of freedom from difficulty and with precipitating factors often readily defined.
2. *Continuous*—no outward signs or symptoms of asthma, but there is some shortness of breath on occasion, transitory wheezing on strenuous exercise, and wheezy crackles heard during deep inspiration.
3. *Intractable asthma*—persistent wheezing requiring regular, daily medication, for either the control of symptoms or the ability to function.
4. *Status asthmaticus*—severe attack in which the patient deteriorates in spite of adequate treatment with sympathomimetic drugs.

Etiology

The stimuli responsible for triggering attacks of asthma are as follows:
1. Extrinsic—antigen–antibody reaction, a positive reaction to certain allergens. IgE or IgA antibodies are activated by allergens resulting in bronchospasm, edema, and increased secretions of mucus (allergy to pollen, animal dander, feathers, foods, house dust, and mites).
2. Intrinsic—symptoms caused by other nonallergic factors—little evidence of IgE antibodies.
   a. Infection—respiratory syncytial virus, parainfluenza virus (types I and II), mycoplasmal pneumonia
   b. Physical factors
      (1) Cold
      (2) Meteorologic factors (i.e., humidity, sudden changes in temperature and barometric pressure)
   c. Inheritable tendencies
   d. Irritants
      (1) Chemicals
      (2) Air pollutants (e.g., sulfur dioxide, carbon monoxide, particulate matter)
   e. Psychic or emotional factors (i.e., tension, fear, anxiety)
   f. Physical stress—fatigue, excessive exercise

Incidence

1. The incidence of asthma in infancy exists but increases in children 3 years and older.
   a. In younger children, the incidence is greater in males.
   b. Incidence is equal in males and females during adolescence.
2. Childhood asthma may decrease at puberty.
3. Approximately 3% of school-age children have symptoms of asthma.

Altered Physiology

1. The turbinates warm and moisten all air that passes into the lung.
2. Inspired air contains particulate matter which is removed by the blanket of mucus present in the tracheobronchial tree. This mucus is kept moistened by inspired moist air.
3. The blanket of mucus is moved constantly upward by the propelling action of the cilia, and if mucus becomes thickened or inspissated it cannot be moved.
4. An increased local deposition and concentration of allergens occur.
5. This produces intrabronchial accumulation and stagnation of mucus which is the primary cause of the respiratory embarrassment.
6. Chemical mediators in asthma:
   a. Primarily involved are histamine and SRS-A (slow-reacting substance of anaphylaxis). SRS-A appears after histamine release, and persists for a longer period. It is not inhibited by the action of the antihistamines.
   b. These materials are primarily responsible for changes in the blood vessels and mucous membrane in the bronchi and bronchioles, as well as for the initiation of bronchospasm.
7. During an asthma attack, abnormal constriction of muscles surrounding the bronchioles (spasm) results in narrowed bronchiolar lumen and decreased oxygen supply in alveoli.
   a. In addition, edema, inflammation, and increased mucus production further compromise respirations.
   b. Hyperresonance and decreased breath sounds may be observed (ominous sign).
8. There are bronchial smooth muscle hypertrophy, bronchial spasms, mucus gland hypertrophy, and edema of respiratory mucosa, and mucus plugging.

Complications

1. Infections—bronchiectasis, pneumonia, bronchiolitis
2. Status asthmaticus
3. Atelectasis
4. Pneumothorax
5. Emphysema
6. Cor pulmonale
7. Misuse of medications
8. Emotional and behavioral problems
9. Dehydration

10. Hypotension, hypertension
11. Cardiac arrhythmias
12. Infants (up to 2 years)—serious respiratory failure due to the stage of development of their anatomic structures and physiologic mechanisms that are unable to cope with the insult and compensatory demands of the disease.

Clinical Manifestations

1. The onset of an asthmatic attack may be gradual, with nasal congestion, sneezing and a watery nasal discharge present before the attack.
2. Attacks may occur suddenly, often at night, when the child awakens with the following symptoms.
   a. Wheezing which occurs primarily with expiration
   b. Anxiety and apprehension
   c. Diaphoresis
   d. Uncontrollable cough
   e. Dyspnea, with increased effort during expiration
3. With treatment, the attack may be controlled. The asthmatic attack may progress, however, and the child will develop the following symptoms.
   a. Increasing dyspnea
   b. Thick, tenacious mucus
   c. Coarse and fine musical crackles
   d. Flaring of the alae nasi
   e. Use of accessory muscles for respiration
   f. Cyanosis
   g. Hypoxemia
   h. Respiratory alkalosis leading to respiratory acidosis
   i. Hypercapnia
   j. Increased heart and respiratory rates
   k. Abdominal pain from severe coughing
   l. Vomiting
   m. Extreme anxiety and apprehension
4. Chronic cough relieved by bronchodilators
5. Nonspecific episodic dyspnea unrelated to exercise
6. Hypersecretions and recurrent lung infiltration and atelectasis
7. Frequent hospital admissions for acute symptoms.
8. Physical characteristics
   a. May be smaller in size
   b. Anterior–posterior chest diameter may be increased
   c. Excessive nasal secretions
   d. Mouth gaping
   e. Inspiratory and expiratory wheeze

Diagnostic Evaluation

1. Eosinophilia in peripheral blood, nasal secretions, and sputum
2. Polymorphonuclear leukocytosis in the presence of infection
3. Pulmonary function studies—diminished maximal breathing capacity, tidal volume and timed vital capacity; spirometric picture of obstruction
4. Determination of blood gases and pH—respiratory acidosis and later metabolic acidosis
5. Gross and microscopic examination of sputum—bronchial casts and eosinophilia
6. Serum CBC
7. Chest x-ray—to exclude presence of other diseases; child may show hyperventilation during asthma attack; air trapping, atelectasis, pulmonary hypertension, edema
8. Routine skin testing may help determine allergic causes

Treatment

A. Acute or Emergency Care

Relieve symptoms and increase ventilatory capacity.
1. Bronchodilators—intravenous aminophylline; subcutaneous epinephrine; inhalation sympathomimetics
2. Continual assessment of respiratory status, blood gas studies
3. Maintain patent airway and oxygenation; suction viscous secretion; ensure humidity and oxygenation; position correctly
4. Reestablish and maintain fluid and electrolyte balance
5. Cardiac monitoring—monitor for hypertension and right-sided heart failure and arrhythmias
6. Maintain rest and physical comfort
7. Give patient and parental reassurance
8. Anti-inflammatory agents; expectorants as indicated
9. Intubation and ventilation if necessary

B. Long-Term Care

Prevention of acute asthmatic episodes and school absences; maximum control of symptoms with minimal medications and treatments, participation in normal activities, normalization of pulmonary function tests, and normal growth and development.
1. Removal of suspected stimulus—allergen, irritant, exercise, emotional factors
2. Desensitization in order to build up the child's resistance to his allergens
3. Drug therapy to control symptoms
4. Chest physical therapy—bronchial drainage, breathing exercises
5. Supportive:
   a. Adequate hydration
   b. Adequate oxygenation
   c. Appropriate treatment of any existing infection
   d. Correct acid–base imbalance
   e. Relieve fatigue

Assessment

History and Physical Examination

A. Become informed regarding the child's symptomatology and the medical plan of care.

1. Make a base-line nursing assessment of the child's condition in order to determine the severity of the attack and the degree of respiratory distress.
   a. Observe the child's breathing pattern:
      (1) Determine whether the expiratory phase of respiration is increased.
      (2) Determine whether the child is wheezing. (In severe attacks, wheezing is audible at a distance from the child.) Assess for inspiratory as well as expiratory wheeze.
      (3) Determine whether the child is using accessory muscles for breathing.
   b. Listen to the child's chest with a stethoscope to determine whether crackles and wheezing are present, and to determine whether all areas of the lung fields are being aerated.
   c. Assess the child's level of anxiety and apprehension.
   d. Observe for flaring of the alae nasi.
   e. Observe the child for the development of cyanosis, utilizing adequate light.
2. Determine the heart and respiratory rates; record and report to the physician any significant change.

3. Identify what medications were administered at home and when.
4. Discuss with the physician the plan of medical care.

Potential Problems/Nursing Diagnoses

1. Alteration in respiratory function (respiratory alkalosis or acidosis and hypoxemia) related to impaired gas exchange
2. Alteration in hydration related to hyperventilation and decreased oral intake
3. Alteration in electrolyte balance related to respiratory acidosis and dehydration
4. Alteration in comfort related to respiratory distress
5. Anxiety related to difficult breathing and hospitalization
6. Potential for cardiac malfunction related to overhydration or medications
7. Potential for atelectasis or pneumothorax related to hyperinfiltration of lungs

Planning and Implementation
Nursing Interventions

A. Provide measures to relieve the respiratory distress the child is experiencing.

1. Position the child in high Fowler's position to allow maximum lung expansion.
   a. Raise the head of the bed to achieve high Fowler's position.
   b. Place an overbed table padded with a pillow in front of the child and have him extend his arms over the table—this provides a comfortable position and allows maximum utilization of accessory muscles for breathing.
2. Administer oxygen when signs of air hunger are present.
   a. Do not wait for the appearance of cyanosis before administering oxygen.
   b. Oxygen must be administered with caution since the child with severe respiratory distress may be dependent upon his low PO_2 to stimulate spontaneous respiration. In the face of a rising PCO_2 and a potential CO_2 narcosis, the administration of oxygen may remove the last stimulus to spontaneous respirations.
      Mild asthma attacks cause respiratory alkalosis, but as air flow obstruction worsens, the $PaCO_2$ rises causing respiratory acidosis. When there is bronchospasm, hypoxemia, and a normal $PaCO_2$, this a sign that the child is tiring. Blood gases should be monitored.
3. Humidity may be used with or without oxygen to help liquefy secretions and reduce mucosal inflammation and edema.
4. Explain to the child the purpose of the oxygen equipment before oxygen is administered and allow the child to feel and touch the equipment.
5. Use aerosolized bronchodilators, or inhaler with bronchodilators.

B. Relieve the anxiety and apprehension that results from the respiratory embarrassment.

1. Place the child in a quiet, clean room, where he can be closely observed.
2. Provide the child with maximum reassurance.
   a. Allow the parents to remain with the child.
      (1) Keep the parents informed of the child's progress—what is being done and why—in order to relieve their apprehension. Parental anxiety is readily transmitted to the child.
      (2) Talk calmly and quietly to the child.
      (3) Assure the child that you will not leave him alone.
      (4) Allow the child to have his favorite security object.
3. Organize care so as to avoid disturbing the child any more than necessary.
4. Evaluate the need for sedation.
5. When the child falls asleep, allow him to continue to sleep and do not disturb him unless absolutely necessary.

C. Provide adequate hydration in order to liquefy and mobilize bronchial secretions and maintain electrolyte balance.

Dehydration occurs secondary to decreased fluid intake, excessive perspiration, vomiting, increased respiration and infection; some bronchodilators may cause dehydration.

1. Observe for signs of dehydration.
   a. Lack of skin turgor
   b. Lack of tears
   c. Dry, parched lips
   d. Depressed fontanelle
   e. Decreased urinary output—high specific gravity; concentrated appearance.
2. Maintain parenteral fluid administration.
3. Encourage oral fluid intake.
   a. Determine the child's fluid preferences.
   b. Offer small sips of fluid frequently, when respiratory effort improves.
   c. Avoid iced fluids which may provoke bronchospasm.
   d. Avoid carbonated beverages when wheezing.
4. Allow the child to return to a regular diet as soon as possible.
5. Observe for signs of overhydration and pulmonary edema, related to high negative pleural pressure generated during bronchospasm.

D. Be aware of the action and side effects of drugs used in the treatment of asthma.

1. *Aminophylline*—bronchodilator
   a. Toxic reaction may occur, but it is more likely to happen with prolonged overdose or when given in conjunction with epinephrine or ephedrine without reducing aminophylline dosage.
      (1) Serum drug levels should be done.
      (2) Toxic reactions include:
         Fever, restlessness, nausea and vomiting, hypotension, abdominal distention.
   b. Side effects—irritability, excitability, continued dehydration, vomiting, diuresis and tachycardia, hematemesis, proteinuria, stupor, convulsions, coma, death. Hypotension occurs with IV use. Avoid ingestion of stimulants.
   c. Occasionally cyanosis and syncope may appear after only a small amount of the prescribed dose. This is considered an idiosyncracy, and the drug should be discontinued.
   d. Use caution when other medications are also given in order to determine drug interaction.
2. *Epinephrine*—relaxes bronchial smooth muscle and constricts bronchial mucosal vessels, thereby reducing congestion and edema; acts as a bronchodilator.
   a. The smallest dose affording relief should be used.

b. Side effects—insomnia, headache, nervousness, palpitations, precordial pain, hypertension, hypoxemia, tachycardia, nausea, sweating, urinary retention. (It may potentiate aminophylline toxicity.)

3. *Ephedrine*—relaxes bronchial smooth muscle and constricts bronchial mucosal vessels, thereby reducing congestion and edema. Acts as a bronchodilator.
   a. Has the advantage of prolonged action and oral administration.
   b. Side effects—same as for epinephrine.
   c. Do not allow child to drink cola, tea, or coffee, since they may increase nervousness.

4. *Pseudoephedrine*
   a. Has prolonged action and can be administered orally.
   b. Side effects—relatively free

5. *Isoproterenol (Isuprel)*—bronchodilator
   a. Toxic reaction—headache, flushing, dizziness, tremors, nausea and vomiting.
   b. Side effects—nervousness, palpitations, pink saliva or sputum if administered orally.
   c. Do not use concurrently with epinephrine.

6. *Expectorants*—given as an adjunct to hydration; thins secretions and helps the child to cough productively (i.e., saturated solution of potassium iodide, Robitussin).

7. *Aerosolized bronchodilator*—Bronkosol

8. *Inhaled sympathomimetics*—(beta-adrenergic agonists): metaproterenol, isoetharine, isoproterenol.
   a. Can use aerosol compressor/nebulizer system for the child under 6 or metered-dosed inhalers for the older child.
   b. Side effects may be shakiness and cardiac stimulation.

9. *Corticosteroids*—anti-inflammatory agents; diminish the inflammatory component of asthma, thus reducing airway obstruction.
   a. Produce beneficial effects only after several hours.
   b. Used when other drugs fail to bring relief from an asthmatic attack.
   c. Side effects—persistent use for mild attacks may lead to suppression of adrenal activity. Prolonged use may lead to growth retardation and steroid dependency.
   d. Corticosteroids via inhaler (Vanceril/Beclovent)

10. *Cromolyn sodium prophylaxis*—adjunct to existing treatment, especially for steroid-dependent child. It inhibits the release of histamine and the slow-reacting substance of anaphylaxis (SRS-A). It has prophylactic action; it should not be used in acute attack. This medication is used only as an inhalant.

11. During the transition from intravenous to oral bronchodilators, respirations should be monitored carefully and frequently.

E. Encourage the child and his parents to practice measures that will help to maintain optimal health, to prevent acute attacks, to ameliorate chronic symptoms, and to prevent onset of progression of respiratory disabilities.

1. General health measures
   a. Provide a well-balanced diet and increased fluid intake.
   b. Ensure sleep, rest, and reasonable exercise; avoid fatigue and chilling.
   c. Avoid known irritants.

2. Psychologic measures
   a. Attempt to keep the child emotionally calm and at ease.
   b. Maintain optimistic attitude.

3. Regular medical follow-up
   a. Ensure strict adherence to medication regimen.
   b. Give prompt attention when infection is present and new or progressive respiratory symptoms appear.

F. Teach the child and involve the parents in the teaching of proper breathing habits.

The exercises strengthen the diaphragm so that breathing will become much better and the total lung capacity will be increased. Breathing exercises used with postural drainage may lessen the need for continuous medication and contribute to increased expectoration of mucus that causes respiratory difficulty.

1. Instruct the child to clear his nasal passages before beginning exercises.

2. Each exercise should start with a short, gentle inspiration through the nose, followed by a prolonged expiration through the mouth.

3. During inspiration, the upper portion of the thorax should be kept immobilized.

4. During expiration, abdominal muscles should be pulled in.

5. On no account should the child take a deep inspiration during the exercise, but instead he should see how long he can continue the expiration.
   a. *Exercise I—Abdominal Breathing*
      (1) Lie on back with knees drawn up, body relaxed, and hands resting on upper abdomen.
      (2) Exhale slowly (through mouth), gently sink the chest and then upper abdomen until retracted at end of expiration.
      (3) Relax upper abdomen (bulges forward) while taking brief inspiration through nose (chest is not raised).
         Repeat 8–16 times; rest 1 minute; repeat.
   b. *Exercise II—Side Expansion Breathing*
      (1) Sit relaxed in a chair and place palms of hands on each side of lower ribs.
      (2) Exhale slowly through mouth, contracting upper part of thorax, then lower ribs, then compress palms against ribs. (This expels air from base of lungs.)
      (3) Inhale, expanding lower ribs against slight pressure from hands.
         Repeat 8–16 times; rest 1 minute; repeat.
   c. *Exercise III—Forward Bending*
      (1) Sit with feet apart, arms relaxed at sides.
      (2) Exhale slowly, drop head forward and downward to knees, while retracting abdominal muscles.
      (3) Raise trunk slowly while inhaling and expand upper abdomen.
      (4) Exhale quickly, sinking chest and abdomen, but remain erect.
      (5) Inhale, expanding upper abdomen.
   d. *Exercise IV—Elbow Arching*
      (This exercise is performed between breathing exercises.)
      (1) Sit leaning slightly forward, back straight, and fingers on shoulders.
      (2) Move elbows in circles forward, upward, backward, and downward.
         Repeat 4–8 times; rest; repeat.

e. *General Instructions*
Perform exercises:
(1) In the morning before breakfast when the child is feeling fresh
(2) At night, before getting into bed to clear the lungs before sleep, and
(3) At the first sign of an impending attack to prevent asthma from developing.

6. Less complicated exercises using same principles can be blowing of a cotton ball or ping pong ball across a table top—keeping score of the distance achieved (make a game of activity), and blowing large soap bubbles.

7. Regular exercise not only improves the lung capacity but also the general physical and emotional well-being of the child.

8. Special exercise programs and camps have been developed throughout the United States to help children with asthma.

Note: Many patients can abort their attacks entirely by doing simple exercises gently. Should the child become short of breath or wheeze slightly, take single dose of whatever medication relieved him before beginning the exercises. Exercise may occasionally produce wheezing or coughing at the end of exercise. It may distress the child, but with perseverance the mucus in the bronchial tubes becomes loosened, and the patient may be able to cough it up with consequent relief of attack.

Health Education

A. Assist the parents to develop a realistic attitude toward the child's illness.

1. Try to treat the child as a completely normal child who needs only a few additional restrictions imposed because of his illness.
   a. Accept him as a unique individual with unique contributions to make.
   b. Let him know he is capable, loved, and respected.
   c. Set consistent behavior limits. Do not accept child triggering attack to gain secondary rewards.

2. Allow the child the same duties and rights as other children in the family.

3. Try to explain why he must watch for certain things and why he is restricted in some ways.

4. Teach the child the symptoms of an asthma attack and how to relax.
   a. Give explanations instead of orders and show him confidence and respect.
   b. Be honest with him and express empathy.
   c. Help him to express his feelings rather than use his illness as an excuse for physically aggressive hostility or manipulative behavior.

5. Avoid overprotection and unnecessary surveillance.

6. Teach the child to gradually manage for himself rather than to be dependent on parents.
   a. Allow him to actively explore his limitations and capabilities.
   b. Teach him all the symptoms of asthma—will aid in early treatment.
   c. Encourage him to keep a daily diary of symptoms, activity, environment, etc., noting any changes.
   d. Explain to him what medications he is taking and why and when they are taken.
   e. Show him the importance of a regular exercise program.
   f. Teach him to recognize signs of respiratory infection and to seek medical attention when appropriate.

g. Encourage him to become involved in hyposensitization (if used). Perhaps he can even administer his own medications.
   h. Teach him the importance of increasing fluid intake, especially during an asthma attack when fluid is needed to compensate for fluid loss resulting from dyspnea and diaphoresis.
   i. Teach him to keep records of activities, symptoms, weather, etc.
   j. Teach him when to seek medical help—when usual medication fails to provide relief, when asthma suddenly worsens, with onset of fever or other signs of infection.
   k. Teach proper use of airflow meter and inhaler as appropriate.

7. If the child is too much engrossed with his illness, he can be diverted with kindly scolding, friendly minimizing of his ailments, or by encouraging other interests, so that he forgets his troubles as much as possible.
   a. Encourage him to build on his interests; help him to find activities that will not hurt him.
   b. The child's ability to control his breathing problems, in addition to learning that he can participate in some way with his peers, will increase his self-confidence and self-value, and result in beneficial physical and attitudinal changes.
   c. Involvement in physical activity should be encouraged, as should rest at signs of fatigue.

8. Do not talk about the child's illness any more than necessary—do not allow secrecy or whispering. Recognize the child's feelings about his illness and allow him to talk about them with parents and family.

9. Inform friends and relatives of problems so that the necessary consideration is given him.
   a. Plan a team conference involving parent(s), school nurse, and teacher.
   b. The school nurse should be provided with information relating to: child's activity, what to do during an attack, medications to be taken during school hours, especially inhaler, who to call for information or if problems arise that cannot be handled at school.

10. Create an atmosphere at home that is not provoking or upsetting—but is still not artificially calm.

11. Prepare the child for approaching events (if bursts of emotions have an effect on his illness).

12. Teach the child special skills.
    a. Let him develop special hobbies and interests that can be combined with his illness.
    b. Remember that accomplishments that develop respect and admiration in peers are particularly desirable and aid in building self-confidence and a feeling of security.

13. Both parents and child feel greater assurance if they are aware of how the child should be treated at certain stages of the disease.
    Have special instructions and medications on hand.

14. If the child takes medications for his allergy or specific symptoms, administer them in a matter-of-fact manner without making any fuss. Encourage taking medication when stomach is empty, drinking adequate amount of fluid.

15. Child needs security, self-confidence, and love. (Do not force these on the child.) Exaggeration is never beneficial.

16. Provide information and literature for the family. Encourage contact with the local chapter of the

American Lung Association or Asthma and Allergy Foundation of America for information on existing programs in which other children with asthma and their parents come together.

B. Teach the child and his parents protective measures that will encourage environmental control and help to avoid the offending allergen, as well as practice measures that will help control asthma attacks.

1. Keep the child's bedroom as free from dust as possible.
    a. Keep in bedroom only the furniture that is absolutely necessary.
    b. Remove upholstered furniture, draperies, carpets, pictures, books, toys, and unnecessary dust-collecting objects.
    c. Use washable curtains and cotton or synthetic rugs.
    d. Use cotton or synthetic blankets and washable bedspreads (not chenille or tufted types).
    e. Do not use insect or other sprays in the bedroom.
    f. Do not store outer clothing or household articles in bedroom closets.
    g. Enclose mattresses, box-springs, and pillows in dustproof covers (unless they are synthetic).
    h. Blankets and clothing that have been stored should be thoroughly aired before use.
2. Avoid irritating odors such as paint, tobacco smoke, insect powders, pine oils, and jellies, and irritating cooking odors.
3. If possible, use an exhaust fan in the kitchen to remove cooking odors.
4. Remove all overstuffed furniture and rugs.
5. Avoid sitting and playing on overstuffed furniture and down pillows.
6. Avoid carbonated drinks, such as ginger ale and colas (especially when wheezing).
7. Avoid any physical exertion that causes wheezing or excessive shortness of breath.
8. Avoid using irritating salves on chest or in nose.
9. Avoid dusty and musty places (basements, storerooms, etc.).
10. Avoid felt rug pads because of animal hair content.
11. Purchase foam furniture and foam rubber pads if possible when refurnishing the home.
12. If home is heated by a circulating hot-air system, shut it off in the bedroom (use electric heater if necessary). A central air filter in the furnace is desirable; clean or replace it frequently.
13. Take only drugs prescribed by the physician.
14. Report for treatment as directed by physician.

C. Help foster a healthy mother–child relationship by understanding the feelings of anxiety, guilt, or frustration the mother may have.

1. Remember that the mother's life-style may have changed with the diagnosis of asthma in her child, resulting in loss of sleep, constant care, etc.
2. Listen to her and provide appropriate support.
3. Initiate social service referral as indicated.

Evaluation

Expected Outcomes

1. Demonstrates improved respiratory function; rapid abatement of symptoms; normal blood gas values
2. Demonstrates adequate hydration; urine specific gravity and vital sign measurements within normal ranges; normal tissue turgor
3. Attains/maintains normal electrolyte balance and blood gas values
4. Experiences increasing comfort; improved respiratory status; normal vital signs and behavior.
5. Shows minimal anxiety; has relaxed behavior and improved respiratory status
6. Reveals normal cardiac function; normal vital signs; ECG, heart auscultation, and chest x-ray results normal
7. Exhibits normal respiratory function; no atelectasis or pneumothorax; normal vital signs
8. Patient/parents demonstrate understanding of disease and care; demonstrate breathing exercises; verbalize information concerning medications, activities needed to remove trigger mechanisms, follow-up visits, etc.

Respiratory Distress Syndrome (Hyaline Membrane Disease)

Respiratory distress syndrome (RDS) is a syndrome of immature infants that is characterized by a progressive and frequently fatal respiratory disorder resulting from atelectasis and immaturity of the lungs.

Etiology

The exact etiology of respiratory distress syndrome is not clearly defined.
1. Adequate pulmonary function at birth depends on the following:
    a. Adequate amount of surfactant (a lipoprotein mixture) lining the alveolar cells, which allows for alveolar stability and prevents alveolar collapse at the end of expiration.
    b. Adequate surface area in air spaces to allow for gas exchange (i.e., sufficient pulmonary capillary bed in contact with this alveolar surface area).
2. Respiratory distress syndrome is the result of decreased pulmonary surfactant.

3. Contributing factors—any factor that decreases surfactant, such as
    a. Prematurity and immature alveolar lining cells
    b. Acidosis
    c. Hypothermia
    d. Hypoxia
    e. Hypovolemia
    f. Diabetes
    g. Unknown
    It should be noted that some situations result in the acceleration of surfactant (steroid therapy; heroin-addicted mother).

Incidence

Respiratory distress syndrome occurs most frequently in:
1. Premature infants (primarily weighing between 1,000–1,500 gm. [2.2–3.3 lbs.]) and between 28–37 weeks' gestation; incidence increases with increased degree of prematurity.

2. Infants of mothers who have diabetes
3. Infants delivered by cesarean section—probably related to underlying indication for surgery
4. Infants of mothers who have experienced intrauterine vaginal bleeding

Altered Physiology

1. Immature lung—underdeveloped and uninflated alveoli, immature pulmonary capillary bed.
2. Surfactant lowers surface tension at alveolar surface, giving alveoli stability; at end of expiration, some of the air remains in the lung (called the functional residual capacity or FRC), thus requiring less negative pressure and exertion to take next breath. When surfactant is deficient, surface tension is higher and alveoli are unstable and collapse at end of expiration. There is decreased FRC; thus, the next breath requires almost as much effort as the first breath after birth.
3. Sequence of events resulting in hyaline membrane disease:
   a. Deficient surfactant
      (Although some surfactant may be present at birth, it may not be regenerated at a rate commensurate with disappearance.)
      (1) Alveoli inflate unequally on inspiration and collapse on expiration.
      (2) More oxygen and energy are required by the infant to expand the alveoli with each breath that he inhales, causing him to tire.
      (3) The number of alveoli that expand progressively decreases.
   b. Alveolar instability and atelectasis.
      (1) Pulmonary vascular resistance increases—hypoperfusion of lung.
      (2) Fetal circulation right-to-left shunt results, leading to hypoxemia and hypercapnia, which lead to respiratory and metabolic acidosis.
   c. Hypoxemia and pulmonary vascular pressure causes ischemia in the alveoli.
      (1) Effusion of plasma through capillary walls (transudate) into aveoli.
      (2) Necrotic cells and fibrin form a membranous layer in alveoli.
      (3) Gas exchange becomes inhibited.
      (4) Lungs become stiff (decreased compliance), requiring more pressure to expand them.
   d. Airway obstruction leads to increased asphyxia and vasoconstriction, and the cycle continues.
4. RDS is usually a self-limited disease and symptoms peak in about 3–4 days, at which time surfactant synthesis begins to accelerate and pulmonary function and clinical appearance begin to improve.
   a. Moderately ill infants or those who do not require assisted ventilation show the following:
      (1) Slow improvement by about 48 hours.
      (2) Rapid recovery over next 3–4 days; few complications.
   b. Severely ill and very immature infants who require some ventilatory assistance:
      (1) Demonstrate rapid deterioration (see Clinical Manifestations).
      (2) Ventilatory assistance may be required for several days; chronic lung disease is a frequent complication.
      (3) Iatrogenic harm more likely (i.e., infection, necrotizing enterocolitis, etc.).

Complications

1. Complications related to respiratory therapy:
   a. Air leak: pneumothorax—pneumomediastinum, pneumopericardium, and pneumoperitoneum
   b. Pneumonia—especially gram-negative organisms
   c. Pulmonary interstitial emphysema
2. Patent ductus arteriosus
3. Intraventricular hemorrhage—epecially in infant less than 1,500 gm. (3.3 lbs.)
4. Disseminated intravascular coagulation
5. Chronic problems associated with long-term use of oxygen:
   a. Bronchopulmonary dysplasia—lungs cystic-appearing with hyperinfiltration, obstructive bronchiolitis, dysplastic changes, and pulmonary fibrosis
   b. Chronic respiratory infections
6. Necrotizing enterocolitis
7. Tracheal stenosis
8. Retinopathy of prematurity (retrolental fibroplasia)
9. Other complications related to prematurity

Clinical Manifestations

Symptoms are usually observed soon after birth and may include

A. Primary Signs and Symptoms

1. Expiratory grunting or whining (when infant is not crying)
2. Sternal, suprasternal, substernal, and intercostal retractions progressing to paradoxical seesaw respirations (see Observation of retractions, Fig. 33-2, p. 1220)
3. Inspiratory nasal flaring
4. Tachypnea
5. Hypothermia
6. Cyanosis when child is in room air (infants with severe disease may be cyanotic even when given oxygen), increasing need for oxygen
7. Decreased breath sounds and dry "sandpaper" breath sounds—on auscultation of chest
8. As the disease progresses:
   a. Seesaw retractions become marked with marked abdominal protrusion on expiration.
   b. Peripheral edema increases.
   c. Muscle tone decreases.
   d. Cyanosis increases.
      (1) Body temperature drops.
      (2) Short periods of apnea occur.
      (3) Bradycardia may occur.
   e. Asphyxia becomes more severe
      (1) Apneic episodes develop.
      (2) Changes in distribution of blood throughout body result in pale gray skin color.

B. Secondary Signs and Symptoms

1. Hypotension
2. Edema of hands and feet
3. Bowel sounds absent early in the illness
4. Urine output decreased

Diagnostic Evaluation

1. Laboratory tests
   a. PCO_2—elevated
   b. PO_2—low
   c. Blood pH—low due to metabolic acidosis
   d. Calcium—low
2. Chest x-ray—demonstrates a diffuse, fine granularity; air bronchograms show "ground glass" appearance

representing atelectasis of some alveoli, surrounded by hyperdistended bronchioles.
3. Pulmonary function studies—demonstrate stiff lung with a reduced effective pulmonary blood flow.

Treatment

1. Early recognition is imperative so that treatment may be instituted immediately.
2. Transportation to a facility providing specialized care is desirable when possible.
3. The objectives of treatment include supportive measures:
    a. Maintenance of oxygenation—PaO_2 at 60–80 mm. Hg—to prevent hypoxia
    b. Maintenance of respiration with ventilatory support if necessary
    c. Maintenance of thermoneutral state—to prevent hypothermia
    d. Maintenance of fluid, electrolyte, and acid–base balance
    e. Maintenance of nutrition
    f. Antibiotic is indicated only when hyaline membrane disease cannot be differentiated from early onset of sepsis
    g. Constant observation for complications
    h. Care appropriate for small premature infant

Assessment
History and Physical Examination

A. Check the birth history for pertinent information to assist in determining the intensity of observation and care that the infant may require.

1. The Apgar score 1 minute after birth and 5 minutes after birth (see p. 993)
2. The type of resuscitation required
3. Any treatment or medication administered
4. Any medication or anesthesia the mother received during labor
5. Estimated gestational age

B. Make a generalized nursing assessment of the infant's condition immediately upon admission.

Early diagnosis is critical to increasing survival rate.
1. Record and report any findings to physician immediately.
2. Determine the degree of respiratory distress.
    a. Observe the type of retraction.
        (1) Determine the type of retraction (see Fig. 33-2, p. 1220)
        (2) Determine the degree and severity of retractions.
    b. Count the respiratory rate for 1 full minute.
        (1) Observe and determine if respirations are regular or irregular.
        (2) Observe to determine if the infant experiences any periods of apnea.
            (a) Note the length of apnea.
            (b) Note what type of stimulation initiates breathing.
        (3) Note the infant's activity at the time respirations are recorded (e.g., crying, sleeping).
    c. Listen for expiratory grunting or whining sounds from the infant when he is not crying. This partial Valsalva maneuver is expiration against a partially closed glottis in an attempt to maintain a positive end-expiratory pressure and FRC

(functional residual capacity) to prevent alveoli from collapsing.
    d. Observe for nasal flaring.
    e. Observe for cyanosis.
        (1) Note location of cyanosis.
        (2) Note if cyanosis improves with oxygen administration.
    f. Listen to the chest with a stethoscope.
        (1) Note diminished breath sounds and location.
        (2) Note the presence of crackles.
3. Determine the infant's cardiac rate and rhythm.
    a. Count the apical pulse for 1 full minute.
    b. Note any irregularity in the heart rate; bounding pulses.
4. Observe the infant's general activity.
    a. Determine if the infant is lethargic or listless.
    b. Determine if the infant is active and responds to stimuli.
    c. Determine if the infant cries.
5. Observe the infant's skin color; note:
    a. Cyanosis as to degree and location.
    b. Evidence of jaundice.
    c. Skin mottling.
    d. Paleness or grayness.
6. Observe the general appearance of the infant's body.
    a. Note edema and location (face, hands, feet, etc.).
    b. Note any other abnormal appearance of body.
7. Check the infant's body temperature.
8. Listen to abdomen with a stethoscope to determine if bowel sounds are present. Note any stool passed and observe and record type of stool.
9. Note any urinary output—assess fluid balance.
    a. Apply urine collector to obtain sample of urine.
    b. Observe color of urine.
    c. Check specific gravity of urine and frequency.
    d. Record amount of urine and frequency.

Potential Problems/Nursing Diagnoses

(Refer to the Premature Infant, p. 1217 for potential problems related to prematurity)
1. Hypoxia, acidosis, atelectasis, and insufficient oxygen–carbon dioxide exchange related to decreases in surfactant and immaturity of lungs
2. Compromised respiratory status and respiratory distress related to pneumothorax, patent ductus arteriosus, and later chronic lung disease
3. Cerebral hemorrhage related to hypoxia
4. Potential for necrotizing enterocolitis related to hypoxia
5. Alteration in nutritional status related to prematurity and respiratory status
6. Alteration in maternal–infant bonding related to separation as a result of life-support equipment attached to infant

Planning and Implementation
Nursing Interventions

The reader is referred to specific areas throughout this text for in-depth discussion of specific conditions.

A. Provide measures to relieve respiratory distress.

1. Have emergency equipment readily available for use in the event of cardiac or respiratory arrest.
2. Provide measures for monitoring ECG and respiratory rate.
3. Place the infant in an oxygen-rich environment.

a. Incubator with oxygen at prescribed concentration.
b. Plastic hood with oxygen at prescribed concentration.
c. Plastic hood with oxygen at prescribed concentration when using radiant warmer.
d. Measure oxygen concentration every hour and record.
e. Monitor blood gases as appropriate
4. Observe the infant's response to oxygen.
   a. Observe for improvement in color, respiratory rate and pattern, and nasal flaring (see retraction score, p. 1220)
   b. Note response by improvement in pH, PO_2, PCO_2 (arterial), or capillary blood gas.
5. Observe closely for apnea.
   a. Stimulate infant if apnea occurs.
   b. If unable to produce spontaneous respiration with stimulation within 15–30 seconds:
      (1) Call for help.
      (2) Clear airway.
      (3) Tilt head back.
      (4) Apply hand resuscitator attached to an oxygen supply, or apply mouth-to-mouth resuscitation (see pp. 1196–1198).
      (5) Intubation may be necessary:
         (a) Obtain heart rate during intubation by physician.
         (b) Initiate cardiac massage if severe bradycardia or asystole occurs.
         (c) Listen to breath sounds after intubation; make sure that they are equal bilaterally and that x-ray for tube position is taken and checked.
         (d) Attach infant to appropriate ventilator. Secure endotracheal tube. Suction tube to maintain patency.
         (e) Continue to monitor vital signs.
   c. Record events.
6. Position the infant to allow for maximal lung expansion.
   a. Prone position provides for a larger lung volume because of the position of the diaphragm but may be contraindicated when umbilical-artery catheter is in place.
   b. Change position frequently.
7. Suction as needed—because the gag reflex is weak and cough is ineffective.

B. Be familiar with the methods of providing assisted or controlled ventilation and the nursing implications for each.

The objective of ventilation therapy is to ventilate the infant effectively, using the lowest possible FIO_2 pressures and cycling frequency to eliminate oxygen toxicity and to minimize mechanical trauma, thus reducing complications of treatment.
1. Positive end-expiratory pressure (PEEP)
2. Continuous positive airway pressure (CPAP)
3. Positive or negative pressure respirator
4. Face mask and bag

C. Continue the administration of intravenous fluids necessary to meet the metabolic demands of the infant.

Hypovolemia can affect pulmonary perfusion by associated metabolic acidosis resulting in pulmonary vasoconstriction.
1. Monitor flow.
2. Observe site for infiltration or infection.

3. If umbilical-artery catheter is in place, observe for bleeding.
4. Record the amount of blood drawn for laboratory analysis (small infants can become anemic from having large amounts of blood removed for samples).
5. Prepare and administer prescribed medications.

D. Provide adequate caloric intake (80–120 kcal./kg./24 hours) **as indicated.**

1. Nasojejunal
2. Nasogastric
3. Parenteral nutrition
4. Monitor for hypoglycemia—especially common during stress

E. Maintain the infant's abdominal skin temperature between 36.0° and 36.5°C. (97° and 98°F.), **thus minimizing oxygen consumption rate.**

Hypothermia may result in vasoconstriction and acidosis increasing complications in the already compromised infant.
1. Adjust Isolette or radiant warmer accordingly.
   a. For the infant under 1,250 gm., the radiant warmer should be used with caution because of increase of water loss and potential for hyperglycemia.
2. Prevent frequent opening of Isolette.
3. Ensure that O_2 is warmed to 32°–34°C (87.6°–93.2°F.) with 60%–80% humidity.

F. Constantly and carefully observe for any complications that may occur from ventilatory assistance, prematurity, or the disease itself.

Record and report observations to physician immediately.

G. Assist the physician in other supportive measures used to treat the infant.

1. Ventilatory assistance, oxygen therapy
2. Endotracheal tube, suctioning, physical therapy
3. Monitoring blood values
4. Monitoring vital signs, including blood pressure, and general condition
5. Monitoring machines

H. Provide an environment that allows infant rest and minimal disturbance balanced with necessary procedures and treatment based on the infant's condition.

Infants undergoing multiple procedures lasting 45 minutes to 1 hour have shown a moderate decrease in PO_2 on continuous PO_2 measurement.

I. Provide for the psychological needs of the infant with respiratory distress syndrome.

Do not neglect his need for tactile, visual, and auditory stimulation.

J. Support the parents of this critically ill infant.

1. Help them work through their grief.
2. Assist them with psychological, emotional, and physical attachment to the infant as appropriate.

Health Education

A. Prepare the family for long-term follow-up as appropriate.

Infants with BPD (bronchopulmonary dysplasia, chronic lung disease) may eventually go home on oxygen therapy.

Note: The premature infant with respiratory difficulty

should continue to be observed very closely and his therapy should be adjusted as his condition changes. When his condition stabilizes, resume care as for a premature infant (see p. 1217).

Evaluation

Expected Outcomes

1. The infant achieves adequate oxygenation as indicated by blood gas studies and stable respiratory status

2. The infant shows stable condition (no evidence of cerebral hemorrhage; stable vital signs and normal neurologic status)
3. No signs of necrotizing enterocolitis: stable abdominal girth measurement, normal elimination pattern, tolerance of enteral feeding
4. Attains and maintains normal nutritional status as evidenced by weight gain
5. Begins appropriate infant–maternal bonding as demonstrated by parental behaviors and verbalization and response of infant

Cystic Fibrosis

Cystic fibrosis is a generalized multisystem disorder affecting the exocrine glands so that the substances they secrete are abnormally viscous, affecting primarily pulmonary and gastrointestinal function.

Etiology and Incidence

1. Condition is inherited as an autosomal mendelian recessive trait.
2. Underlying cause of the abnormal secretions is unknown.
3. Incidence is estimated to be 1:1,800–1:2,000 in predominantly white population. About 4%–5% of Caucasian population are carriers.

Altered Physiology

1. The secretions of the exocrine glands are thick and sticky rather than thin and slippery.
2. Pulmonary involvement
   a. Decreased ciliary action
   b. Metaplasia and hyperplasia of squamous cells of mucus-secreting cells leading to increased production of thick secretions (increased risk of infection).
   c. Bronchi and bronchioles become plugged, resulting in bronchiectasis and bronchiolitis.
   d. Atelectasis and hyperinfiltration of lungs results.
   e. Irreversible fibrotic changes occur in lungs.
3. Gastrointestinal and pancreatic involvement
   a. Acini and ducts of pancreas become filled with thick mucus and are obstructed.
   b. Trypsin, chymotrypsin, lipase, and amylase do not reach the small intestine.
   c. Digestion is impaired; especially protein, carbohydrates, and fat
   d. There is abnormality of stools, loss of foodstuff in feces (fat and nitrogen [protein])—malabsorption syndrome.
   e. Meconium ileus in infant—bowel obstructed by thick intestinal secretions.
   f. Biliary cirrhosis—intrahepatic biliary tract obstructed by thick secretions.
4. Involvement of sweat glands
   Secretions contain excessive amount of sodium and chloride, leading to excessive loss of these substances—especially in hot weather, when child experiences fever or becomes overheated with activity. Saliva also contains an excess of sodium and chloride.

Complications

1. Pulmonary infections
   a. Most frequently caused by *Pseudomonas aeruginosa, Staphylococcus,* and *Haemophilus influenzae*
   b. Also bronchiectasis and bronchiolitis
2. Other lung complications
   a. Emphysema
   b. Atelectasis
   c. Pneumothorax
3. Biliary cirrhosis—portal hypertension, esophageal varices, splenomegaly
4. Pancreatic fibrosis; islets of Langerhans may be fibrotic, resulting in glucose intolerance; diabetes
5. Cor pulmonale
6. Enlarged and plugged mucus-secreting glands; chronic sinusitis
7. Rectal polyps (3 months–3 years)
8. Intussusception (under 2 years of age)
9. Pancreatitis
10. Nasal polyps
11. Heat prostration
12. Fibrosis of epididymis and vas deferens in male; aspermia
13. Hemoptysis
14. Growth retardation

Clinical Manifestations

1. Diagnosis is frequently made prior to 6 months of age—can be made at any age.
2. Meconium ileus is found in newborn.
3. Other presenting signs:
   a. Salty taste when skin is kissed
   b. Cough (dry and hacking to loose and productive); wheezing
   c. Failure to gain weight or grow in the presence of a good appetite
   d. Frequent, bulky, and foul-smelling stools; excessive flatus
   e. Protuberant abdomen—pot belly
   f. Wasted buttocks
   g. Vomiting following coughing
   h. Recurrent pulmonary infections
   i. Clubbing of fingers—in older child
   j. Increased anteroposterior chest diameter
   k. Decreased exertional endurance

l. Maldigestion; steatorrhea (loss of lipid-soluble fat and vitamins in stool)

m. Hyperglycemia, glucosuria with polyuria and weight loss

Diagnostic Evaluation

1. Check for family history of cystic fibrosis, failure to thrive, and unexplained infant death; check the child's history and physical condition. Carefully listen for subtle information that may be suggestive of cystic fibrosis.

2. Measurement of sodium and cloride level in sweat—chloride level of more than 60 mEq./liter is virtually diagnostic.
   a. 40–60 mEq./liter is borderline and repeated.
   b. Sodium levels greater than 70 mEq./liter are diagnostic.

3. Measurement of trypsin concentration in duodenal secretions—absence of normal concentration is virtually diagnostic.

4. Analysis of digestive enzymes (trypsin and chymotrypsin) in stool
   Level is lower—used for initial screening for cystic fibrosis.

5. Chest x-ray
   a. May be normal initially.
   b. Later shows increased areas of infection, overinflation, bronchial thickening and plugging, atelectasis, and fibrosis.

6. Analysis of stool for steatorrhea.

7. BMC (Boehringer–Mannheim Corp.)—meconium strip test includes lactose and protein content, both present in babies with cystic fibrosis, used for screening.

8. Pulmonary function studies (after 4 years old)
   a. Decreased vital capacity and flow rates
   b. Increased residual volume and/or increased total lung capacity

9. Diagnosis is made when a positive sweat test is seen in conjunction with one or more of the following:
   a. Positive family history for cystic fibrosis
   b. Typical chronic obstructive lung disease
   c. Documented exocrine pancreatic insufficiency

Treatment

1. Prevent and control pulmonary infection.
   a. Antimicrobial therapy as indicated for pulmonary infection.
   b. Bronchodilators and vasoconstrictors—for relief of bronchospasm.
   c. Aerosol, expectorants, and mucolytic agents—decrease viscosity of secretions.
   d. Antihistamines (controversial)—for hayfever-like symptoms.
   e. Physical therapy—bronchial drainage
      (1) Postural drainage
      (2) Breathing exercises
   f. Bronchopulmonary lavage—treatment of atelectasis and mucoid impaction, using large volumes of saline (used in some institutions in country).
   g. Lobectomy—resection of symptomatic lobar bronchiectasis to retard progression of lesion to total pulmonary involvement.

2. Establish and maintain good nutrition.
   a. Pancreatic enzyme supplement with each feeding.

   b. Increased caloric (carbohydrates) and protein intake.
   c. Decrease in fat intake.
   d. Daily intake of water-soluble vitamins.
   e. Supplementary fat-soluble vitamins.
   f. Adequate fluid and salt intake.

3. Promote normal growth and development.
   a. Treat the child as a normal person.
   b. Encourage normal relationships with peers and family.
   c. Promote positive self-image.

Physical Assessment

A. Assist in the diagnosis and assessment of the child being evaluated for cystic fibrosis by careful observation, recording, and reporting.

1. Characteristics of stool
2. Respiratory status
3. General behavior and activity
4. Compliance to test being done
5. The child's response to any treatments done

Potential Problems/Nursing Diagnoses

1. Decreased oxygen–carbon dioxide gas exchange related to thick pulmonary secretions
2. Alteration in comfort related to illness and treatments
3. Alteration in nutritional status related to decreased appetite and/or inadequate absorption
4. Potential for infection related to thick pulmonary secretion
5. Anxiety related to hospitalization and disease process
6. Alteration in parent–child relationships related to hospitalization, disease, and inappropriate coping behaviors
7. Knowledge deficit of appropriate home care

Nursing Interventions

A. Establish and maintain adequate nutrition to allow for growth and development.

1. Diet composed of food that is high in calories, high in protein, and low to moderate in fat is usually recommended. (Absorption of food is incomplete.) Infant may receive medium-chain triglyceride supplement in formula. Fat tolerance may be adequate and decreased fat may not be part of diet regimen.

2. Fat-soluble vitamins in water-miscible solution are given in quantities that are 2–3 times the normal dose. (The child shows difficulty in absorption.)
   a. Vitamins A, D, and E are given daily.
   b. Vitamin K may be given when the child has infection and is being treated with antibiotics.

3. Absent pancreatic enzymes are replaced with extracts of animal pancreas to obtain normal stools, nutrition, and growth.
   a. Give with each meal and snacks.
   b. Mix capsule, granules, or powder with small portion of food for infant or small child (e.g., mashed banana, applesauce). Never mix in formula.
   c. Offer the older child capsules or tablets.
   d. May not be given if the child is taking only a clear liquid diet (e.g., postoperative vomiting).

4. Salt intake will need to be increased during hot weather or during excessive exercise when sweating increases, to prevent salt depletion and heat prostration and cardiovascular collapse. During periods of

profuse sweating, infant may become hyponatremic and alkalotic.
5. Use patience when feeding the child.
   a. The child may be irritable and fussy.
   b. Breathing may be difficult; coughing and vomiting may be common.
6. Supplemental diet that is readily absorbed and requires a minimum of digestive enzymes may be prescribed.

B. Assist in preventing or treating lung infections and support respirations by thinning secretions and clearing them from the respiratory tract.

1. Intermittent aerosol therapy
   a. Usually done prior to postural drainage. (Treatment may also be done following drainage, or both.)
   b. Provides small amount of medication or water in droplet form to penetrate respiratory tract.
   c. Treatment is 3–4 times daily.
2. Mist tent (controversial)
   a. Frequently used only with patients that have already used mist; not started on newly diagnosed patients.
   b. High humidity loosens secretions.
   c. Used primarily at night or nap time.
   d. Check temperature often and maintain below 26.6°C. (80°F.).
   e. Mist inhalation therapy may be used when secretions are particularly thick or copious.

▶ **NURSING ALERT:** Mist therapy may cause airway resistance to increase in some patients.

3. Chest physical therapy (see Chest Physical Therapy, p. 1178, and Fig. 34-2)
   a. Usually follows aerosol therapy 3–4 times per day for 20–30 minutes.
      (1) May need to be increased if infection is present.
   b. Treatment ideally done 1 hour after eating to prevent vomiting or discomfort.
   c. Place child in position that gives greatest access to affected lobes of lung and facilitates gravity drainage of mucus from specific lung area (Fig. 34-2). The following positions are useful:
      (1) Leaning over side of bed
      (2) Infant held in lap
      (3) Using pillow
   d. Clapping with cupped hands and vibrating for 1–2 minutes in each area loosens plugs of mucus. Clapping is usually done 20–30 minutes, 3–4 times a day; may need to be increased when infection is present.
   e. A relaxed patient will cough more easily; coughing should be encouraged after postural drainage. Suctioning of an infant or young child may be necessary when the child will not cough.
4. Breathing exercises
   Have the child exhale slowly with pursed lips to increase the duration of exhalation.

C. Understand what medications are given in treatment and why they are given.

1. Antibiotics
   a. Frequently given when a child is not doing well generally
   b. Broad-spectrum antibiotics to treat specific organism causing infection

c. Specific antibiotics to treat specific organism causing infection—often given intravenously
2. Expectorants are used to thin bronchial mucous secretions.
3. Bronchodilators are used to increase width of bronchial tubes, allowing free passage of air into lungs.

D. Give meticulous attention and care in hygiene to the patient and prevent infection.

1. Provide good skin care and position changes to prevent skin breakdown of malnourished child.
2. See that diaper area is clean to reduce offensive odor from stool and to prevent diaper rash.
3. Because child may perspire freely, change clothing as often as necessary to keep him dry.
4. Mouth care is important, since mucus is present so frequently.
5. Shampooing and bathing will provide comfort by removing sticky residue from mist and aerosol therapy.
6. Restrict contact with person with respiratory infection.

E. Support the child's emotional, psychological, and intellectual needs and development.

1. Explain each procedure (new or routine), medications, etc. to the child in a manner that is appropriate for his age.
2. Allow the child to show his frustrations, fears, and feelings by talking, complaining, or crying.
   a. Support him during these times.
   b. Comfort him by talking to him and holding him.
3. Provide diversional activities appropriate for age, during or between treatments.
4. The older child may begin to take responsibility for treatments with minimal supervision.
   a. Teach him about his disease (i.e., food, medications, treatments, equipment).
   b. Help him identify his strengths and limitations, and to feel good about himself as a person.
   c. Foster independence.
5. Frequently the child will manifest his anger, fear, and other emotions by resistance to chest-physical therapy. Allowing child to engage in normal activities (e.g., swimming) within his physical tolerance can help to redirect these feelings as well as to improve respiratory function.

F. Make and record observations of the child and his condition and behavior which will give information concerning his condition.

1. Characteristics of stools: color, size, consistency, frequency
2. Eating habits
   a. Foods taken or refused
   b. Appetite—good or poor
3. Coughing and description of secretions produced
4. Daily weight to determine weight gain or loss
5. General behavior
   a. Irritability
   b. Cooperativeness
6. Conservation of energy—periods of rest, nonstrenuous activity

G. Encourage parental participation in learning to care for and handle the child and foster acceptance of the child and his illness by his parents and family.

1. Provide opportunities for the parents to learn all aspects of care of their child.

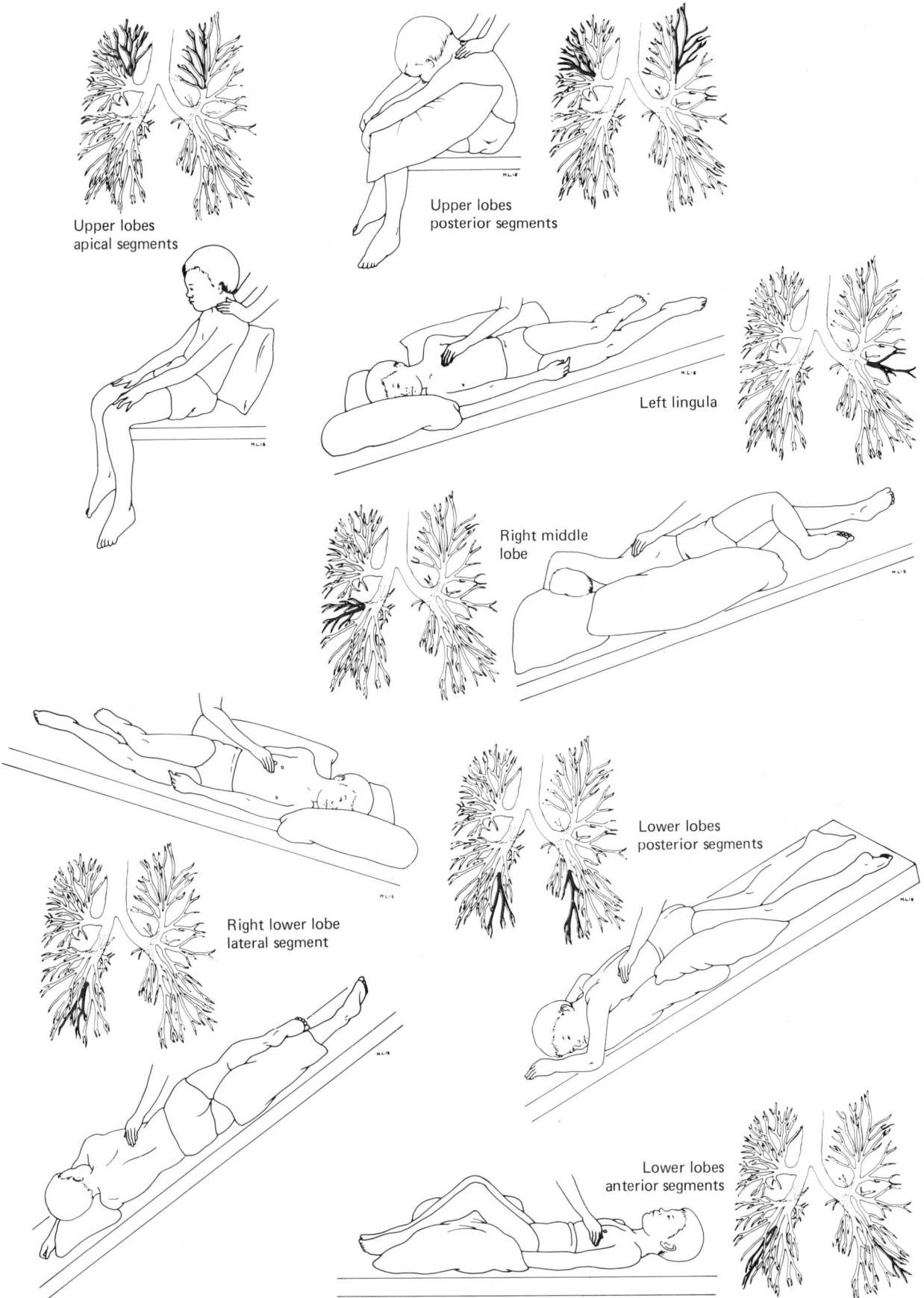

Figure 34-2. Postural drainage. Position for draining upper lobes, anterior segments, is the same as the position for draining lower lobes, anterior segments.

2. Note that all the support and help given the parents during hospitalization will make home care easier.
3. Initiate community nurse referral, which provides the following:
   a. Facilitates preparing the home for the child's entry, both emotionally and physically.
   b. Can assist the family in properly carrying out treatments.
4. Initiate social work referral. The social worker can help the parents to better understand their family situation and their feelings about their child and cystic fibrosis; she can arrange for financial assistance if appropriate. The worker can be an emotional support to the mother who may be physically and emotionally exhausted from caring for the child with cystic fibrosis.
5. Inform friends and relatives of the child's illness so that necessary consideration is given him. Plan a team conference including the parent(s), school nurse, teacher, and physical education teacher, as appropriate.
6. Assist with interpretation of the disease to family and patient. Help them to talk about their feelings and fears. Be honest with the parents and child; help them understand there may be gradual lung involvement.
7. Initiate a teaching program for the child and his family early. Offer them available literature and help them to become familiar with the Cystic Fibrosis Foundation* and the nearest chapter.
   a. Multidiscipline team approach and cooperation is vital.
   b. Incorporate teaching program into nursing care plan. Be consistent with information and methods.

Health Education

Education of the parents is important in preparing them to continue the child's care at home.
1. The parents must have a thorough understanding of the dietary regimen. Help them to know what types of foods the child is allowed to have and which foods are restricted. Talk about ways to make each meal or certain foods attractive. Discuss need for salt replacement—free access to salt; increase salt intake on hot summer days or when vomiting and diarrhea occur.
2. Help the parents to become thoroughly familiar with the pulmonary therapy regimen. Do not rush your explanation; take time to demonstrate and explain procedures. Then allow the parents to demonstrate all the treatments to be done at home.
3. Help the family to plan the most normal family

---

* Cystic Fibrosis Foundation
6000 Executive Blvd, Suite 309
Rockville, MD 20852
Publications from CF Foundation:

What everyone should know about Cystic Fibrosis

Cystic Fibrosis: A summary of symptoms, diagnosis and treatment

Your Child and Cystic Fibrosis

Living with Cystic Fibrosis—A Guide for the Young Adult.
A Teacher's Guide to Cystic Fibrosis.
Listing of Publications and Educational Materials for Physicians and Scientists

---

pattern of living in relation to treatment of their child.
   a. Consider the marriage needs of the parents and the needs of other members of the family.
   b. Encourage family activities, vacations, etc. during the child's remission of symptoms.
4. Help the parents to understand and to provide emotional support of their child. Explain that he will experience the usual problems of growing up as well as the problems of cystic fibrosis and hospitalizations. The child needs love, understanding, and security—not overprotection. He needs growing independence, peer relationships, and personal achievements.
5. Help the parents understand the rebellious and uncooperative behavior of their adolescent. It is a normal part of this age; however, it may be directed toward the illness and treatment. Be firm with the child—optimistic, yet realistic, understanding, and loving.
6. Help the parents understand the value of genetic counseling and support the information given to them through counseling.
   a. Diagnosis may cause family discord and anger.
   b. A period of grief and mourning is normal following diagnosis.
7. Impress upon the parents the importance of regular medical follow-up care:
   a. Routine immunizations—measles vaccine and influenza given early in infancy.
   b. Continuing evaluation and supervision in home management.
   c. New developments through research that may change therapy.
   d. Detection or prevention of complications.
8. Inform parents of the future of their child in society.
   a. With the medical advancements that have occurred, there is every reason to believe that, depending upon pulmonary involvement and complications, the child with cystic fibrosis may grow to adulthood. When the child grows up, he may be smaller and shorter than expected.
   b. Play and school participation depends upon severity of illness.
   c. Have the parents discuss the child's problem with the school nurse, teacher, and other responsible adults who have close contact with the child.
   d. Encourage the parents to allow the child to participate in as well as take additional responsibility for his own care and treatment as he gets older.
   e. Support agency, see footnote, first column

Expected Outcomes

1. Child demonstrates improved oxygen–carbon dioxide gas exchange; improved general respiratory status; normal blood gas values
2. Experiences minimal discomfort; shows relaxed behavior; engages in play activities appropriate for age
3. Demonstrates improved nutritional status evidenced by weight gain
4. Experiences lessening anxiety; appropriate behavior for age; interacting with other children and personnel
5. Parent–child relationship appropriate as evidenced by verbalization and behavior
6. Parents show understanding of disease and can explain home care requirements

Bibliography

Books

Avery GB. Neonatology, 2nd ed. Philadelphia, JB Lippincott, 1981

Avery ME and Taeusch HW. Schaffer's Diseases of the Newborn, 5th ed. Philadelphia, WB Saunders, 1984

Behrman RE and Vaughan VC. Nelson Textbook of Pediatrics. Philadelphia, WB Saunders, 1983

Eigan H and Scott PH. Asthma and allergic rhinitis. In Ambulatory Pediatrics. Green M and Haggerty RJ (eds). Philadelphia, WB Saunders, 1984, pp. 378–391

Falliers CJ. Asthma, eczema, and related allergies. In Levine MD (ed). Developmental—Behavioral Pediatrics. Philadelphia, WB Saunders, 1983, pp. 474–482

Fanaroff AA and Martin RJ. Behrman's Neonatol–Perinatol Medicine, 3rd ed. St Louis, CV Mosby, 1982

Feigin RD and Cherry JD. Textbook of Pediatric Infectious Diseases, Vol 1. Philadelphia, WB Saunders, 1981

Fleisher G and Ludwig S. Textbook of Pediatric Emergency Medicine. Baltimore, Williams & Wilkins, 1983

Hoeprich PD. Infectious Diseases, 3rd ed. Philadelphia, Harper & Row, 1983

Krugman S and Katz SL. Infectious Diseases of Children. St Louis, CV Mosby, 1981

Plant TF. Children with Asthma: A Manual for Parents. Amherst, MA, PediPress, 1983

Schreiner RL and Kisling JA. Practical Neonatal Respiratory Care. New York, Raven Press, 1982

Whaley LF and Wong DL. Nursing Care of Infants and Children. St Louis, CV Mosby, 1983

Wieczorek RR and Natapoff JN. A Conceptual Approach to the Nursing of Children. Philadelphia, JB Lippincott, 1981

Articles

General

Amin NM. Managing the growing threat of *Pneumocystis carinii* infections. Consultant 1983 Jan; 23(1):71–73+

Davis HW et al. Acute upper airway obstruction: Croup and epiglottitis. Pediatr Clin North Am 1981 Nov; 28(5):859–880

Hannallah RF. Management of croup and epiglottitis in children. Curr Rev Respir Ther 1983 12(5):95–100

Holbrook PR. On opening the airway. Emerg Med 1982 Jan 15; 14(1):137+

Huang HN and Palmer J. Management of patients with cystic fibrosis. Respir Ther 1981 1. Clinical Manifestations 1981 Jan/Feb; 11(1):49–53 2. Principles of Treatment Mar/Apr; 11(2):65+ 3. Treatment of pulmonary infections May/Jun; 11(3):81+

Johnson MP. Self-instruction for the family of a child with cystic fibrosis. MCN 1980 Sept/Oct; 5(5):345–348

Katz AE. Tonsillectomy and adenoidectomy: Recommendations that make sense. Consultant 1982 Jan; 22(1):207–209+

Levinson M, Tabachnik E, Newth CJL. Wheezing in infancy, croup and epiglottitis. Curr Prob Pediatr 1982 Jan; 12(3):2–65

Long SS. Treatment of acute pneumonia in infants and children. Pediatr Clin North Am 1983 Apr; 30(2):297–322

McBride MM and Sack WH. Emotional management of children with acute respiratory failure in the ICU. Heart Lung 1980 Jan/Feb; 9(1):98–106

Mendelsohn J. Pediatric respiratory emergencies. In Pierog JE and Pierog LJ (eds). Pediatric Critical Illness and Injury. Rockville, MD, Aspen Publications, 1984, pp. 37–46

Munoz AI. Haemophilus influenzae infections. Clin Pediatr 1980 Feb; 19(2):86–90

Neonatal screening for cystic fibrosis: Position paper Ad Hoc Committee Task Force in Neonatal Screening, CF Foundation. Pediatrics 1983 Nov; 72(6):741–745

Page HS. Croup and epiglottitis: Sudden trouble for young children. Am Lung Assoc Bull 1981 Mar; 67(2):9–11

Pierog JE. Acute supraglottitis (epiglottitis) in children. In Pierog JE and Pierog LJ (eds). Pediatric Critical Illness and Injury. Rockville, MD, Aspen Publications, 1984, pp. 47–60

T & A: Overdone, yet underdone. Emerg Med 1981 June 15; 13(11):136–137+

Treating peritonsillar abscess without tonsillectomy. Emerg Med 1983 Jul 15; 15(13):130+

Walsh S. Parents of asthmatic kids (PAK): A successful parent support group. Pediatr Nurs 1981 May/Jun; 7(3):28–29

When a child's symptoms suggest croup (based on interviews with Gershon AA, etc.). Patient Care 1982 Nov 30; 16(20):15–18+

Wolf SI. Exercise, the asthmatic child and PL 94-142. Pediatr Nurs 1980 Nov/Dec; 6(6):21–23

Respiratory Distress Syndrome

Budd RA. The "Logan Bar" method for securing endotracheal tube in neonates. Crit Care Nurse 1982 May/Jun; 2(3):27–28

Cohen S, Perez RC and Strodtbeck F. Newborn respiratory paralysis for severe respiratory distress: A nursing protocol. DCCN 1982 Nov/Dec; 1(6):340–349

Emami CL and Delbianco LM. An improved technique for securing nasoendotracheal tubes. MCN 1981 Sept/Oct; 6(5):337–340

Fick RB and Reynolds HY. Respiratory infections and lung defenses. Respir Ther 1982 Jan/Feb; 12(1):31–32+

Finer NN and Kelly MA. Optimal ventilation for the neonate: Part I: Continuous positive airway pressure. Respir Ther 1983 Jan/Feb; 13(1):43–44+

Glassanose MR. Infants who are oxygen dependent—sending them home. MCN 1980 Jan/Feb; 5(1):42–45

Hallman M and Gluck L. Respiratory distress syndrome—update 1982. Pediatr Clin North Am 1982 Oct; 29(5):1057–1075

McFadden R. Decreasing respiratory compromise during infant suctioning. Am J Nurs 1981 Dec; 81(12):2158–2161

Nugent TJ. Acute respiratory care of the newborn. JOGN Nurs (Suppl) 1983 May/Jun; 12(3):31s–44s

Price GE and Cain DC. Options for ventilating the pediatric patient. Part 2: Choosing the right techniques. Respir Ther 1983 Jul/Aug; 13(4):60–62+

Schreiner RL and Kisling JA. Treatment of the newborn in respiratory distress. Crit Care Q 1981 Jun; 4(1):19–31

Tabor LH. Ribavirin aerosol treatment of bronchiolitis associated with respiratory syncytial virus infection in infants. Pediatrics 1983 Nov; 72(5):613–618

Tanswell AK. Continuous distending pressure in the respiratory distress syndrome of the newborn: Who, when and why? Respir Care 1982 Mar; 27(3):257–266

Thibeault DW and Callenbach TC. Drug therapy in neonatal lung disease. Perinatol/Neonatol 1983 Apr; 7(4):39–47

Asthma

Acetaminophen and the asthmatic child. Emerg Med 1983 May 30; 15(10):96

Brodoff AS. Asthma roundtable Part V: When your patient's asthma's mild, 115–117+; Part VI: When asthma causes "moderate" trouble. Patient Care 1981 Nov 15; 15(19):143–145+

Burns KL. Behavioral health care in asthma. Public Health Review 1982 Jul/Dec; 10(3/4):339–381

Freydenburg N et al. The impact of bronchial asthma on school attendance and performance. J Sch Health 1980 Nov; 50(9):522–526

Gortmaker SL et al. Parental smoking and the risk of childhood asthma. Am J Pub Health 1982 Jun; 72(6):574–579

Holbreich M and Strunk RC. Precipitating factors in childhood asthma. Respir Ther 1981 Jan/Feb; 11(1):74–77

Inhalation for acute asthma. Emerg Med 1983 Mar 15; 15(5):172+

Janson-Bjerklie S. The role of emotions and suggestion in triggering asthma. Respir Ther 1983 May/Jun; 13(3):17–21+

Jennings C. Controlling the home environment of the allergic child. MCN 1982 Nov/Dec; 7(6):376–381

Kandel G and Aberman A. Asthma: Diagnostic and therapeutic strategies that work. Consultant 1983 Jun; 23(6): 143–145+

Kiblawi SSO and Jay SJ. Management of status asthmaticus. Respir Ther 1981 Mar/Apr; 11(2):48–49+

Kinilloff LM and Tibbals SC. Drugs for asthma. Am J Nurs 1983 Jan; 83(1): 55–61

Kinsman RA, Dirks JF, Schraa JC. Psychomaintenance in asthma. Respir Ther 1981 Mar/Apr; 11(2):39–41+

Lee HS. Proper aerosol inhalation technique for delivery of asthma medications. Clin Pediatr 1983 Jun; 22(6):440–443

Lee H and Evans HE. Aerosol bag for administration of bronchodilators to young asthmatic children. Pediatrics 1984 Feb; 73(2):230–232

McCaully ME. Breathing exercises as play for asthmatic children. MCN 1980 Sep/Oct; 5(5):340–344

McGrath DM. Nursing management of the child in status epilepticus. Issues Compr Pediatr Nurs 1981 Sep–Dec; 5(5–6):273–277

McLaughlin FJ and Dozor AJ. Cold air inhalation challenge in the diagnosis of asthma in children. Pediatrics 1983 Oct; 72(4):503–509

Orton R. The asthmatic child and exercise. Part I. Respir Ther 1981 Jan/Feb; 11(1):37+

The asthmatic child and exercise. Part II. Respir Ther 1981 Mar/Apr; 11(2): 33–35

Pituch M and Bruggeman J. Lungs unlimited: A self-care program for asthmatic children and their families. Child Today 1982 Jul/Aug; 11(3):7–10

Richards W and Church JA. Self-help for asthmatic children. Respir Ther 1982 Nov/Dec; 12(6):45–48+

Rifas ME. Teaching patients to manage acute asthma. Nursing '83 1983 April; 13(4):77–80

SanJoaquin VH, Reyes S, Marks MI. Influenza vaccination in asthmatic children on maintenance theophylline therapy. Clin Pediatr 1982 Dec; 21(2): 724–726

Shaman D. Tots play games to beat asthma. Am Lung Assoc Bull 1982 May; 68(4):5–9

Silver RB and Ginsburg CM. Early prediction of the need for hospitalization in children with acute asthma. Clin Pediatr 1984 Feb; 23(2): 81–84

Yeh TF et al. Improved lung compliance following indomethacin therapy in premature infant with patent ductus arteriosus. Chest 1981 Dec; 80(6): 698–700

Additional Suggested Reading for Staff and Parents

Asthma and You. New York, Winthrop Laboratories, Jan 1973

Asthma: Facts About Your Lungs. Am Lung Assoc Pub Apr 1978

Barron H.: The Strange Case of the White Rabbit. Am Lung Assoc Pub, Jun 1976

Kendig EL and Chernick V. Disorders of the Respiratory Tract in Children. Philadelphia, WB Saunders, 1983

Leffert F. Your Child and Asthma. Denver, Nat Jewish Hosp and Research Center, Jan 1975

Lloyd-Still JD (ed). Textbook of Cystic Fibrosis. Boston, John Wright, 1983

Oseid S and Edwards AM. The Asthmatic Child in Play and Sports. London, Pitman, 1983

Parcel GS et al. Teaching Myself About Asthma. St Louis, CV Mosby, 1979 Teaching Myself about Asthma is a patient education teaching aid designed for 7- to 12-year-old children with asthma.

Silverstein A and Silverstein V. Itch, sniffle and sneeze: All About Asthma, Hay Fever & Other Allergies. New York, Four Winds, 1978 (grades 3–8)

Blood Disorders in Children

35

Anemia

Anemia refers to a deficit of red blood cells or hemoglobin in the blood. It is the most frequent hematologic disorder encountered in children.

Etiology

1. Blood loss
2. Impairment of red blood cell production
   a. Nutritional deficiency
      (1) Iron deficiency
      (2) Folic acid deficiency
      (3) Vitamin B_{12} deficiency
      (4) Vitamin B_6 deficiency
   b. Decreased erythrocyte production
      (1) Pure red cell anemia
      (2) Secondary hemolytic anemias associated with infection, renal disease, chronic disorders
      (3) Aplastic anemias
      (4) Invasion of bone marrow
         (a) Leukemia
         (b) Tumors
3. Increased erythrocyte destruction
   a. Drugs and chemicals
   b. Infections
   c. Antibody reactions
   d. Burns
   e. Poisons, including lead poisoning
   f. Abnormalities of the red cell membrane
   g. Enzymatic defects—G6PD (glucose-6-phosphate dehydrogenase) deficiency
   h. Hemolytic disease of the newborn
   i. Abnormal hemoglobin synthesis
      (1) Abnormal hemoglobins—sickle cell disease
      (2) Thalassemic syndromes

Altered Physiology

A. General Considerations

1. Red cells and hemoglobin are normally formed at the same rate at which they are destroyed.
2. Whenever formation of red cells or hemoglobin is decreased or their destruction is increased, anemia results.
3. The ability of red blood cells to carry hemoglobin is decreased.
4. The ability of hemoglobin to oxygenate the tissues and remove carbon dioxide for excretion by the lungs is also decreased.
5. Less hemoglobin is available to act as a buffer in regulating the pH of the blood.

B. Specific Anemias

1. Iron deficiency anemia (hypochromic anemia)
   a. Iron deficiency occurs most commonly between the age of 6 months and 2 years, but it also occurs frequently during adolescence.
   b. Initially the neonate's iron requirements are usually met by reserves acquired during fetal life, but after 3–4 months of age, additional iron must be derived from the diet.
   c. A positive iron balance is necessary for optimal formation of red blood cells.
   d. Results of iron deficiency:
      (1) Decreased hemoglobin formation
      (2) Red cells with less color and smaller in size
      (3) Low plasma iron
      (4) Low body stores
      (5) Low levels of transferrin, which binds and transports iron
   e. Causes of iron deficiency
      (1) Insufficient supply
         (a) Dietary insufficiency (most common)
         (b) Inadequate stores at birth (in premature infants, twins)
      (2) Excessive demands
         (a) Growth requirements
         (b) Chronic illness
      (3) Blood loss
         (a) Hemorrhage
         (b) Parasitic infection
      (4) Impaired absorption (rare)
         (a) Diarrhea
         (b) Malabsorption syndrome
2. Megaloblastic anemias
   a. Folic acid and vitamin B_{12} are necessary for the synthesis of nucleoproteins which are essential for the maturation of red blood cells.
   b. Deficiencies of folic acid or vitamin B_{12} or disturbances in their normal metabolism interfere with the synthesis of nucleoproteins.
   c. Red blood cells are immature and larger than normal at every stage of their development.
   d. The number of circulating red blood cells is decreased.
   e. Each red blood cell may carry a normal amount of hemoglobin.
3. Hypoplastic anemias
   The bone marrow is unable to manufacture new red blood cells and hemoglobin at a rate necessary to

maintain a normal concentration of these substances in the circulating blood.

4. Aplastic anemia
   a. Formation of red blood cells stops altogether.
   b. There is usually an associated defective synthesis of other elements in the blood such as platelets and white blood cells.
5. Anemia of infection
   a. Life span of the red blood cell is moderately decreased.
   b. The ability of the bone marrow to produce red blood cells is significantly decreased. (This is the principal factor in determining the degree of anemia.)
6. Hemolytic anemias
   a. The red blood cells are destroyed at abnormally high rates.
   b. The activity of the bone marrow increases to compensate for the shortened survival time of the red blood cells.
   c. Products of red cell breakdown increase with hemolysis.
   d. Jaundice results when the liver is unable to clear the blood of the pigment resulting from the breakdown of hemoglobin from destroyed red cells.
   e. Bone marrow hypertrophies and occupies a larger than normal share of the inner structure of bones.
7. Sickle cell anemia (see p. 1282)

Assessment
Clinical Manifestations

1. Condition may be acute or chronic
2. Early symptoms
   a. Listlessness
   b. Fatigability
   c. Anorexia
3. Late symptoms
   a. Pallor
   b. Weakness
   c. Tachycardia
   d. Palpitations
4. Eventual symptoms
   a. Mental and physical sluggishness
   b. Cardiac enlargement and symptoms of congestive heart failure
   c. Inability to carry out the usual childhood activities
5. Prognosis
   a. Varies with the type of anemia
   b. Death may result because of cardiac failure

Potential Problems/Nursing Diagnoses

1. Fatigue related to decreased ability of blood to transport oxygen to the tissues
2. Activity intolerance related to fatigue
3. Anxiety related to hospitalization and painful diagnostic procedures (venipunctures, finger sticks)
4. Inadequate nutritional intake related to general sense of malaise
5. Danger of infection related to generally debilitated state
6. Parental knowledge deficit regarding recommended dietary allowances and iron supplementation

Planning and Implementation
Nursing Interventions

A. Make a baseline assessment of the child's condition.

1. Examine skin and mucous membranes for evidence of pallor.

2. Estimate the child's current functional level, including exercise tolerance and level of frustration.
3. Question the parents regarding the child's normal level of activity, any symptoms that they have observed (pallor, decreased appetite, excessive fatigue, etc.), ways that their child indicates frustration, fatigue.
4. Obtain a history related to possible causative factors:
   a. Dietary habits
   b. Persistent infection, chronic disease
   c. Access to drugs, poisons, etc.

B. Prevent infection and assess for signs of infection.

1. See that the child maintains good general body hygiene.
2. Provide a diet high in vitamins, calories, and iron.
   a. Be aware of the child's food preferences and plan his diet accordingly.
   b. Offer small amounts of food at frequent intervals.
   c. Reward the child for positive attempts to eat.
   d. Allow the child to participate in selection of foods and in preparation of his meal tray.
   e. Avoid tiring activities and unpleasant procedures at mealtime.
   f. Make mealtime as pleasurable as possible (refer to section on Nutrition, p. 1094).
   g. Provide food supplements and vitamins when necessary.
3. Ensure adequate rest.
   a. Plan nursing care to allow for lengthy periods when the child is not disturbed by hospital routines, procedures, treatments, etc.
   b. Observe for early signs of fatigue such as irritability, hyperactivity, etc.
   c. Encourage sedentary rather than active projects.
4. Avoid exposure to other children with colds, infections, etc.
5. Always be sure to wash hands thoroughly and advise visitors to do the same.
6. Report any temperature elevation to the physician.

C. Administer blood and maintain the transfusion.

1. The procedure is similar to the administration of IV fluids (see p. 1160).
   The blood administration set contains a filter in the drip chamber. The blood level should cover the filter.
2. Packed cells are frequently administered to enable the child to receive a high concentration of erythrocytes in a small quantity of fluid.
   The bag should be squeezed every 20–30 minutes during the transfusion to prevent settling of the red cells.
3. Take special precautions.
   a. The patient's name, physician's name, hospital number, and blood type must correspond with the information on the blood container from the blood bank.
   b. Identifying information such as donor type and number, patient's name on the blood label, kind of blood, and expiration date should always be checked by 2 people.
   c. The blood should be checked for abnormal cloudiness or color and for gas bubbles.
   d. The child's temperature should be taken as a baseline measurement before the transfusion is begun.
   e. Normal saline should be hung so that the tubing can be flushed before and after blood is administered and when medications must be given (a separate infusion line for IV medications is preferable).

▶ **NURSING ALERT:** Medications should not be given in the infusing blood. Blood should never be given with a dextrose and water solution because hemolysis and clotting in the IV tubing can occur.

    f. Blood should be run through new IV tubing, and after blood administration, the tubing should be changed before IV fluids are resumed.

    g. The rate of flow should be carefully regulated to prevent circulatory overload, especially in those children receiving multiple transfusions. Blood is administered slowly at first as a precautionary measure in case of transfusion reaction, and to allow the blood to reach room temperature.

    h. The same blood should not be left running over a long period of time (usually not over 4 hours).

    i. Recommendations of the blood bank for storage and administration of blood should be followed explicitly.

4. Observe the child for signs of transfusion reaction.

    a. Reaction usually occurs within 15–20 minutes from the start of the transfusion. Stay with the patient during this time.

    b. Signs and symptoms:
      (1) Restlessness
      (2) Irritability
      (3) Chills
      (4) Elevation of temperature
      (5) Sudden changes in pulse and respiration
      (6) Rash or change in the color of the skin
      (7) Changes in the appearance or quantity of urine output
      (8) Hemorrhagic phenomena
      (9) Pain, sensation of tightness in the chest

    c. Notify the physician immediately if a transfusion reaction is suspected. Discontinue the transfusion, but keep the intravenous line open with saline solution.

5. For additional information, refer to Transfusion Therapy and Guidelines: Administering Blood Transfusions (Adult), pp. 263 and 273.

D. Minimize the child's anxieties and ensure his cooperation during hospitalization.

1. Allow the child to handle equipment used for tests and procedures (tourniquets, syringes, etc.).
2. Explain all procedures and the treatment plan to the child in a way that he can understand.
3. Allow the older child to look through a microscope at a blood smear.
4. Permit the child to cleanse the area for a venipuncture or finger stick.

Nursing Management of Specific Anemias

A. Iron Deficiency Anemia

1. Administer iron as prescribed by the physician.

    a. Oral iron preparations
      (1) Administer shortly after meals to minimize gastric distress.
      (2) Administer with a dropper or straw, or dilute with water or fruit juice to prevent staining of teeth.
      Dental stains can be removed by brushing the teeth with sodium bicarbonate or hydrogen peroxide and then rinsing with water.
      (3) Observe for side effects.
        (a) Gastric distress
        (b) Colic pain
        (c) Diarrhea or constipation
      (4) Caution the mother that iron medication causes the child's stools to be dark green or black.
      (5) Stress to the parents the importance of continuing the iron therapy according to the physician's directions even though the child may not appear ill.
      (6) Warn the parents that medications containing iron are a leading cause of poisoning in children. The medication should always be stored well out of reach.

▶ **NURSING ALERT:** There is a great deal of variation in the elemental iron content of the commercially available liquid preparations containing iron. To avoid confusion, the dosage should be expressed in terms of elemental iron and then converted to the proper amount of the therapeutic agent selected.

    b. Intramuscular iron preparations
      (1) Dosage
        (a) Calculated by the physician
        (b) Depends on the child's weight and hemoglobin level
      (2) Special precautions
        (a) Should be injected into a large muscle, preferably the gluteus maximus (buttock).
        (b) Injection sites should be recorded and rotated.
        (c) The injection site should not be massaged. Any pressure on the site may force the medication out of the muscle into the subcutaneous tissue. Walking will help absorption.
        (d) Parenteral iron should be administered with discretion and only to those children whose anemia is not amenable to oral iron therapy.
        (e) Parenteral iron is contraindicated in children sensitive to the preparation or in anemias other than iron deficiency anemia.
      (3) Technique of administration
        (a) Use a separate needle to withdraw the medication from the ampule and for injection.
        (b) Use a needle which is 5 cm. (2 inches) long. Medication must be injected deeply into the muscle to avoid staining the tissue.
        (c) Allow 0.5 ml. of air in the syringe before injecting.
        (d) Retract the skin over the muscle laterally before inserting the needle.
        (e) Insert the needle and withdraw the plunger to check against entry into a blood vessel.
        (f) Inject the medication and the 0.5 ml. of air following the injection—to clear the needle and prevent leakage of the medication along the injection track when needle is withdrawn.
        (g) Wait 10 seconds after injection before removing the needle.
      (4) Observe for side effects
        (a) Local
        Pain at the injection site
        Skin discoloration
        Local inflammation with lymphadenopathy

(b) Systemic toxicity (occurs within 10 minutes of injection)
Headache
Muscle and joint pain
Nausea and vomiting
Dizziness
Tachycardia
Bronchospasm with dyspnea
Circulatory collapse (rare)

▶ **NURSING ALERT:** Because of the possibility of anaphylaxis, a test dose should be given before initiating parenteral iron therapy.

2. Initiate and reinforce good dietary habits.
   a. Determine from the parents the type and amount of foods customarily eaten, the feeding methods, and the child's reaction to eating.
   b. Introduce foods rich in iron such as certain meats, fortified cereals, vegetables, and fruits.
   c. Do not allow the child to drink excessive quantities of milk to the exclusion of other foods that contain more iron. Limit milk intake to 1 liter (1 quart) per day.
   d. Provide vitamin supplements if necessary. Vitamin C appears to enhance the absorption of iron.
   e. Explain the reasons for diet change to parents in language they can understand. Visual aids and pictures may be helpful.
   f. Assist the parents to select iron-rich foods that are acceptable to the child, within the family's food budget, and culturally acceptable.
   g. Make mealtime a pleasurable experience (refer to section on nutrition, p. 1094).
3. Investigate social and economic problems that may contribute to the child's disease.
   Complete a referral to a community health nurse if it appears that the mother will need support in dealing with the child's chronic disease.

B. Anemia of Infection

1. Provide supportive care relative to the underlying disease.
2. Administer antibiotics as directed by the physician.

C. Megaloblastic Anemias

Administer folic acid or vitamin B_{12} as directed by the physician.

1. Folic acid (pteroylmonoglutamic acid)
   a. Dosage—must be determined by trial for each patient.
   b. Route
      (1) Oral route is preferred.
      (2) May be administered intramuscularly if malabsorption is suspected.
   c. Toxic effects—none
2. Vitamin B_{12} (cyanocobalamin)
   a. Dosage—regulated by individual trial for each patient
   b. Route
      (1) Intramuscular injection is preferred.
      (2) Oral administration is also possible. (This method is more expensive and less reliable.)
   c. Side effects—none
   d. Points of emphasis
      Regular administration of the medication is essential. Patients may be tempted to miss injections because they are not in distress before the injection or do not feel significantly better after it.

Health Education

1. Discuss general hygiene measures, including adequate rest, diet, sunshine, fresh air.
2. Encourage regular medical and dental evaluations.
3. Explain that infection may be prevented by dressing the child according to the weather and keeping him away from persons with colds, sore throats, and other infections.
4. Teach the parents how to administer medication.
5. Alert the parents to signs of disease progress.

Evaluation

Expected Outcomes

1. The child experiences less fatigue evidenced by increasing activity, improved appetite
2. Indicates basic understanding of diagnostic tests either verbally or through play
3. Remains free of infection; normal temperature
4. Parents indicate understanding of anemia and its treatment through compliance with management recommendations; the child does not have a recurrence of anemia

Sickle Cell Disease (Sickle Cell Anemia)

Sickle cell disease is a severe, chronic, hemolytic anemia occurring in persons who are homozygous for the sickle gene. The clinical course is characterized by episodes of pain due to the occlusion of small blood vessels by sickled red cells. Persons heterozygous for the sickling gene are said to possess sickle cell trait which is associated with a benign clinical course.

Etiology

1. Genetically determined, inherited disease
2. Each person inherits 1 gene from each parent which governs the synthesis of hemoglobin (Table 35-1).

Incidence

1. Found almost entirely in American Blacks and persons of Spanish–American ancestry.

2. Approximately 8% of Black Americans have sickle cell trait.
3. Approximately 1 of every 600 Black infants born in the US has sickle cell anemia.

Altered Physiology

1. Each hemoglobin molecule consists of 4 molecules of heme folded into 1 molecule of globin.
2. Each globin molecule consists of 2 alpha chains and 2 beta chains.
3. The amino acid sequence on the beta chain is altered in sickle cell hemoglobin.
   Valine is substituted for glutamic acid in the 6th position.
4. Sickle cell hemoglobin aggregates into elongated crystals under conditions of low oxygen concentration.

5. This distorts the membrane of the red blood cell causing it to assume a crescent or sickle shape. The cells easily become entangled and enmeshed leading to increased blood viscosity.
6. Sickled red cells are fragile and are rapidly destroyed in the circulation.
7. Anemia results when the rate of destruction of red cells is greater than the rate of production.

Prognosis

1. Variable; improving with new forms of treatment.
2. Greatest risk of death is in children under 5 years of age.
3. Crises usually become less frequent and severe as a child becomes older.

Preventive Measures

1. Every Black child admitted to the hospital should be tested for sickle cell anemia.
2. Parents at risk should be counseled regarding the genetic aspects of sickle cell anemia.
3. All siblings of any child who is admitted to the hospital with sickle cell anemia should be tested for the disease.

Assessment

Clinical Manifestations

A. Symptoms

1. Children are rarely symptomatic until late in the first year of life.
2. Clinical manifestations are sporadic.
   a. The child may be asymptomatic for several months.
   b. Periods of crisis occur at variable intervals.
   c. Precipitating factors of crisis include:
      (1) Dehydration
      (2) Infection
      (3) Trauma
      (4) Strenuous physical exertion
      (5) Extreme fatigue
      (6) Cold exposure
      (7) Hypoxia
3. Signs of crisis
   a. Loss of appetite
   b. Paleness
   c. Weakness
   d. Fever
   e. Pain in abdomen, back, joints, and/or extremities
   f. Swelling of joints, hands, or feet ("hand–foot syndrome")
   g. Irritability
   h. Jaundice

B. Thrombocytic Crisis

(Most common form of crisis)
1. Small blood vessels are occluded by the sickle-shaped cells, causing distal ischemia and infarction.
2. Extremities
   a. Bony destruction
   b. Periosteal reaction
   c. Ulcers
3. Spleen
      Abdominal pain
4. Cerebral occlusion
   a. Strokes
   b. Hemiplegia
   c. Blindness
5. Pulmonary infarction, thromboses

Table 35-1 Transmission of Sickle Cell Disease

Genotype of Parents	Probability of Abnormal Hemoglobin in Offspring		
	Normal	Trait	Disease
1 parent with trait	50%	50%	0
Both parents with trait	25%	50%	25%
1 parent with trait; 1 parent with disease	0	50%	50%
Both parents with disease	0	0	100%

6. Cardiac decompensation
7. Impaired liver function
8. Convulsions, cerebral infarction
9. Retinal damage, blindness

C. Sequestrian Crisis

1. Large amounts of blood become pooled in the liver and spleen.
2. Spleen becomes massively enlarged.
3. Signs of circulatory collapse develop rapidly.
4. Frequent cause of death in infant with sickle cell disease.

D. Aplastic Crisis

Bone marrow ceases production of red blood cells.

E. Chronic Symptoms

1. Jaundice
2. Gallstones
3. Progressive impairment of kidney function
4. Fibrotic spleen
5. High susceptibility to salmonella, osteomyelitis, and pneumococcal septicemia
6. Growth failure
7. Delayed puberty
8. Decreased life span

Diagnostic Evaluation

1. Stained blood smear
   a. Done by finger stick.
   b. Sickle cells are viewed under the microscope on a stained smear of blood.
   c. Cells are seen only in persons with sickle cell anemia (not sickle cell trait).
2. Sickle cell prep
   a. Done by finger stick.
   b. Oxygen is removed from a drop of blood.
   c. The blood is observed under the microscope for the presence of sickle-shaped cells.
   d. Does not distinguish between persons with sickle cell trait and disease.
3. Sickledex
   a. Done by finger stick.
   b. A small amount of blood is placed in a solution containing a chemical reducing agent.
   c. The presence of sickle hemoglobin is indicated if the solution turns cloudy.
   d. Also does not distinguish between persons with sickle cell trait and disease.
4. Hemoglobin electrophoresis
   a. Requires venipuncture.
   b. Hemoglobin is subjected to an electric current which separates the various types and determines the amounts present.
   c. A person is diagnosed as having sickle cell trait

if 2 types of hemoglobin are demonstrated in approximately equal amounts.

A person is diagnosed as having sickle cell anemia if the majority of his hemoglobin is sickle hemoglobin.

5. Antenatal diagnosis is available to the high-risk group through amniocentesis and gene mapping.

Potential Problems/Nursing Diagnoses

1. Pain related to agglutination of sickled cells within the small blood vessels
2. Hypoxia related to increased blood viscosity and increased destruction of red blood cells
3. Increased danger of infection related to fibrotic changes in the spleen
4. Potential for injury related to IV therapy
5. Parental guilt related to hereditary nature of the disease
6. Knowledge deficit regarding sickle cell anemia and its management

Planning and Implementation
Nursing Interventions

A. Dilute the blood and reverse the agglutination of sickled cells within the small blood vessels.

1. Maintain intravenous therapy if indicated (see procedure for the administration of intravenous fluids, p. 1160).
2. Increase the amount and frequency of liquid intake.
   a. Offer fruit juice, water, milk, etc.
   b. Offer the child a choice in selection of fluids and method of drinking (straw, etc.).
3. Record the child's intake and output accurately.
4. Assist with a partial exchange transfusion if required. This technique is designed to remove some of the sickled cells and replace them with normal ones.

B. Reduce the child's fever which may aggravate dehydration.

1. Make frequent assessments of the child's temperature.
2. Administer antipyretic drugs as prescribed by the physician.
3. Refer to the section on fever, p. 1135.

C. Alleviate the child's pain during a crisis.

1. Identify effective measures to alleviate pain by questioning parents and by personal trial and error. Consider any of the following measures:
   a. Carefully position and support painful areas.
   b. Hold or rock the infant.
   c. Distract the child by singing to him, reading stories, providing play activities.
   d. Provide familiar objects; encourage visits by familiar persons.
   e. Bathe the child in warm water, applying local heat or massage.
   f. Give suitable medications.
   g. Maintain bed rest.
2. Share effective methods of reducing pain with other nursing staff and family.

D. Treat associated or precipitating infections.

1. Treatment will depend on the specific nature of the infection.
2. Administer antibiotics as prescribed by the physician.

E. Administer blood in cases of severe anemia.

1. Refer to information on blood transfusion, p. 1280.
2. Be especially alert for signs of transfusion reaction, which is a very serious problem.

F. Decrease surgical risk.

1. Administer preoperative blood transfusion(s) as prescribed.
   Preoperative blood is usually prescribed to suppress the formation of new sickle cells and to reduce the threat of anoxia.
2. Prepare the child emotionally for surgery.
3. Maintain adequate hydration before and after surgery.
4. Avoid sedatives and analgesics which depress the respiratory center.
5. Observe the child closely for evidence of infection, especially of the respiratory tract.

G. Provide emotional support to the child and his parents.

1. Encourage parents to talk about their child, his disease, and how they feel about it.
   a. Expect such feelings as guilt, shock, frustration, depression, and resentment.
   b. Accept negative feelings.
   c. Counsel the parents concerning ways to recognize and alleviate their child's apprehension.
   d. Provide factual information so that parents are prepared to answer their child's questions.
      (1) The recessive nature of the inheritance should be explained.
      (2) Make certain that the parents understand the difference between sickle cell trait and sickle cell anemia.
2. Alleviate the child's anxieties concerning his illness.
   a. Role playing and play activities are useful in identifying his fears.
   b. Explain what is happening to him in a way that he can understand.
      Numerous teaching tools such as coloring books are available for this purpose.
   c. Adolescents should be assured that although sexual development is delayed, they will eventually catch up with their peers.
3. Stress the positive aspects of his disease.
   a. Sickle cell disease does not affect intelligence.
   b. Between periods of crisis the child can usually participate in peer group activities with the exception of some strenuous sports.
   c. Discuss the positive achievements of recent research and correct misconceptions.
4. Encourage quiet activities in which the child can excel—art, painting, leather work, metal and woodworking, chess, etc.
5. Plan for the child to continue his education.
   a. Encourage the parents to bring school work to the child during a lengthy hospitalization.
   b. Refer the child to a home teacher if necessary.
   c. Be certain that the child receives vocational guidance if appropriate.
6. Inform parents of community resources, such as the school nurse or groups for parents and/or children.

H. Make certain that the child receives coordinated and continuous care.

Send a nursing care summary to the community health nurse or school nurse who will work with the child after he is discharged from the hospital.

Health Education

1. Provide factual information about the disease and its cause. Encourage questions.
2. Discuss the genetic implications of sickle cell disease and offer genetic counseling to the family.

3. Instruct the parents in ways that they can help their child to avoid sickling episodes.
   a. Do not allow the child to become chilled or to wear tight clothing that might impede circulation.
   b. Maintain adequate hydration. Give the parents written instructions regarding the minimum amount of fluid required by their child each day. Discuss implications of abnormal fluid loss (i.e., vomiting, excessive sweating). Instruct parents how to recognize signs of dehydration.
   c. Instruct the child to avoid strenuous physical activity.
   d. Provide prompt treatment of cuts, sores, mosquito bites, etc. Notify the physician if the child is exposed to a communicable disease.
   e. Maintain good dental hygiene and be certain that the child receives frequent dental checkups.
   f. Be certain that the child receives regular medical supervision, including all the normal childhood immunizations and a PPD (purified protein derivative) test for tuberculosis every 2–3 years. In addition, children over 2 years of age should be immunized against pneumococcal infection, and children over 5 years of age should receive meningococcal vaccine.
   g. Teach the child to avoid undue emotional stress.
   h. Instruct the child to avoid areas of low oxygen concentration (i.e., high mountains and unpressurized airplanes).
4. Teach the parents that the child has the same needs as a normal, healthy child for a balanced diet, good fluid intake, adequate rest, and daily exercise. The child will learn his own activity limitations and will rest when he becomes fatigued. He should not be pampered, but should receive the same love, discipline, privileges, and responsibilities of a normal child his age.
5. Sexually active adolescents should receive contraceptive information and should be helped to make informed choices.
6. Teach parents how to recognize the signs of mild crisis:
   a. Fever
   b. Decreased appetite
   c. Irritability
   d. Pain or swelling in abdomen, extremities, back
7. Instruct the parents regarding home management of mild crisis.
   a. Encourage adequate hydration. Teach techniques for increasing fluid intake.
   b. Administer antipyretic medications.
   c. Encourage rest.
   d. Keep the child warm.
   e. Hospitalize child if pain becomes severe or if IV hydration is required.
8. Teach the parents the signs of severe crises:
   a. Pallor
   b. Lethargy and listlessness
   c. Difficulty in awakening
   d. Irritability
   e. Severe pain
   f. High fever or a moderate fever that persists for 2 days
9. Instruct the parents to have emergency information available to those involved in the child's care (school nurse, teacher, babysitter, family members, etc.).
   a. Name and phone number of physician and alternate physician
   b. Closest emergency facility and ambulance number
   c. Child's blood type, allergies, medications, and hospital chart number
   d. Name of informed neighbor or relative to be notified in an emergency
   e. Discuss the genetic implications of sickle cell disease with the child early, so that when he is old enough, he can avail himself of counseling concerning marriage and family planning.
10. Stress the benefit of wearing a Medic-Alert tag.

Teaching Aids

The following may be useful in providing information to the parents and child:
1. National Sickle Cell Disease Program, National Institutes of Health, Bethesda, MD 20892
2. National Association for Sickle Cell Disease, Inc., 3460 Wilshire Blvd, Suite 1012, Los Angeles, CA 90010
3. National Center for Education in Maternal and Child Health, 3520 Prospect Street, NW, Washington, DC 20007

Evaluation

Expected Outcomes

1. The child experiences relief of pain: appears more comfortable and does not cry or complain of pain
2. Does not become hypoxic, as demonstrated by normal laboratory evaluation
3. The child remains free of infection; temperature normal
4. The parents discuss their feelings and work out any sense of guilt
5. The parents accurately describe sickle cell anemia and discuss the major management principles; the parents manage mild crises successfully at home

Hemophilia

Hemophilia is an inherited, congenital blood dyscrasia which is characterized by a disturbance of blood clotting factors. It appears in males but is transmitted by females.

Etiology

1. Hereditary (about 80% of patients)
   a. Sex-linked, recessive trait
      (1) Caused by a gene carried on the X chromosome, one of the sex chromosomes.
      (2) Transmitted by asymptomatic females who carry the hemophilic gene on 1 of their X chromosomes.
      (3) Appears in males who have the hemophilic gene on their only X chromosome.
      (4) Affected males may carry a latent form of the disease to female offspring
      (5) May appear in females if a female carrier mates with a male hemophiliac.

Table 35-2 Transmission of Hemophilia

| | Probability of Abnormality in Offspring | | | | |
| | Female | | | Male | |
Genotype of Parents	Normal	Carrier	Hemophiliac	Normal	Hemophiliac
Female carrier/normal male	50%	50%	0	50%	50%
Noncarrier female/hemophiliac male	0	100%	0	100%	0
Female carrier/hemophiliac male	0	50%	50%	50%	50%

2. Spontaneous mutations may cause the condition when the family history is negative for the disease (about 20% of patients).

Transmission of Hemophilia

See Table 35-2.

Altered Physiology

1. Hemophilia results from the absence or malfunction of any one of the blood clotting factors from the plasma.
2. These blood clotting factors are necessary for the formation of prothrombin activator, which acts as a catalyst in the conversion of prothrombin to thrombin.
   a. The rate of formation of thrombin from prothrombin is almost directly proportional to the amount of prothrombin activator available.
   b. The rapidity of the clotting process is proportional to the amount of thrombin formed.
3. The most common types of hemophilia and the clotting factors involved are shown in the chart below.

Assessment

Clinical Manifestations

A. General Considerations

1. Seldom diagnosed in infancy unless excessive bleeding is observed from the umbilical cord or after circumcision.
2. Usually diagnosed after the child becomes active.
3. Varies in severity depending on the plasma level of the coagulation factor involved.
   a. Children with factor levels of less than 1% of normal are considered severe hemophiliacs and often demonstrate severe clinical bleeding.
   b. Children with factor levels of above 5% but less than 25% of normal are considered moderately afflicted. These children may be free of spontaneous bleeding, and may not manifest the potentially severe bleeding disorder until after trauma.
   c. Children with factor levels of 25%–50% of normal are considered mildly afflicted. They usually lead normal lives and bleed only with severe injury or surgery.

d. Degree of severity tends to be constant within a given family.

B. Clinical Signs and Symptoms

1. Easily bruised
2. Prolonged bleeding from the mucous membranes of the nose and mouth or from lacerations
3. Spontaneous soft-tissue hematomas
4. Hemorrhages into the joints—especially elbows, knees, and ankles (hemarthrosis)
   a. Causes pain, swelling, limitation of movement
   b. Repeated hemorrhages may produce degenerative changes with osteoporosis and muscle atrophy
5. Spontaneous hematuria
6. Gastrointestinal bleeding

C. Complications

1. Airway obstruction due to hemorrhage into the neck and pharynx
2. Intestinal obstruction due to bleeding into intestinal walls or peritoneum
3. Compression of nerves with paralysis due to hemorrhaging into deep tissues
4. Intracranial bleeding
5. Secondary complications associated with therapy—liver disease, immunologic problems, thrombotic complications

D. Prognosis

1. Uncertain—a normal life span is possible for many hemophiliacs because of advances in therapy.
2. Cycles may occur with periods of little bleeding followed by periods of severe bleeding.
3. Death may result from intracranial hemorrhage or from exsanguination following any serious hemorrhage.

Diagnostic Evaluation

1. Routine bleeding and clotting tests—often normal
2. Partial thromboplastin time (PTT)—prolonged
3. Prothrombin consumption—decreased
4. Thromboplastin generation—increased
5. Specific assays for clotting factors—abnormal

Most Common Types of Hemophilia

Type of Hemophilia	Clotting Factor
Hemophilia A (classic hemophilia)	Factor VIII (antihemophilic globulin)
Hemophilia B (Christmas disease)	Factor IX (plasma thromboplastin component)
Hemophilia C	Factor XI (plasma thromboplastin antecedent)

Potential Problems/Nursing Diagnoses

1. Danger of shock or exsanguination related to inability of blood to clot
2. Potential for injury from blood replacement therapy
3. Pain related to bleeding into joints
4. Anxiety and coping difficulty related to the need for frequent transfusions
5. Activity intolerance related to painful joints
6. Maternal guilt related to hereditary nature of the disease
7. Parental overprotection related to fear of injury
8. Knowledge deficit regarding hemophilia and its management

Planning and Implementation
Nursing Interventions

A. Provide emergency care for bleeding wounds.

1. Cleanse wound thoroughly.
2. Immobilize the affected part and elevate above the level of the heart.
3. Administer cryoprecipitate or plasma concentrate containing the necessary factor (see procedure for the administration of intravenous fluid, p. 1160, and for blood transfusion, p. 1280).
   a. Avoid rapid administration to minimize the possibility of transfusion reaction.
   b. Stop the transfusion if hives, headaches, tingling, chills, flushing, or fever occur.
4. Apply local measures for control of bleeding.
   a. Apply pressure on the area for 10–15 minutes to allow clot formation.
   b. Place fibrin foam or absorbable gelatin foam in the wound.
5. Keep the child quiet during treatment.
   a. Remain calm.
   b. Sedate the child if necessary.
6. Take special precautions.
   Suturing and cauterization should be avoided.

B. Provide supportive care for the child with hemarthroses.

1. Control bleeding.
   a. Immobilize the joint in a position of slight flexion.
   b. Elevate the affected part.
   c. Apply ice packs.
   d. Administer plasma or therapeutic concentrate as directed by the physician.
2. Alleviate pain.
   a. Administer sedatives or narcotics as prescribed by the physician.
   b. Avoid excessive manipulation of the child.
   c. Use a bed cradle to keep the weight of the bedcovers off the affected part.
3. Prevent further bleeding.
   a. Continue immobilization of the joint. (A bivalve plaster cast may be necessary.)
   b. Maintain the child on bed rest. (Careful handling of the child is essential.)
4. Prevent permanent deformities and crippling.
   a. Begin gentle, passive exercise after the acute phase. Progress to active exercises.
   b. Refer the child for physical therapy on an outpatient basis if this is indicated by:
      (1) Presence of persistent deformity.
      (2) Need to use orthopedic devices such as crutches, braces, splints, etc.
      (3) Need for specialized programs such as whirlpool baths, electrical stimulation, increased physical exercises.
   c. Reconstructive orthopedic surgery may be required.
5. Assess the child for evidence of disease progress:
   a. Increased pain
   b. Further swelling of joints
   c. Limitation of movement
   d. Flexion contractures

C. Prevent hemorrhage during nursing procedures.

1. Temperature measurement
   Insert the thermometer very gently.
2. Injections
   a. Administer medications orally whenever possible.
   b. Choose injection sites carefully and rotate them. The subcutaneous route is preferred.
   c. Inject the medication slowly.
   d. Apply pressure to the area for 5 minutes.

▶ **NURSING ALERT:** Children with hemophilia should not receive aspirin or compounds containing aspirin because this medication affects platelet function and prolongs bleeding time.

D. Maintain a safe environment during hospitalization.

1. Pad crib rails.
2. Inspect toys for sharp or rough edges.
3. Offer foods and fluids in plastic or paper containers.
4. Supervise small children when they are ambulatory.
5. Utilize protective devices which the child brings from home. (Many children wear helmets, knee pads).
6. Continually assess environment for potential hazards.

E. Provide emotional support to the child and his family.

1. Permit the child to participate in as many normal activities as possible within the realm of safety.
2. Allow the child to handle equipment used in his care.
   Use play to help the young child adjust to his illness by "transfusing" his teddy bear, etc.
3. Encourage the child's continuing education.
   a. Have parents bring assignments from the child's teacher.
   b. Refer to a home teacher if indicated.
   c. Investigate the possibility of a school-to-home telephone service.
4. Encourage parental participation in the child's care.
   a. Refer to section on family-centered care, page 1117.
   b. Assess the parents' attitudes and understanding about the disease. Clarify information if necessary.
   c. Teach the parents aspects of their child's care which must be continued after discharge. Have them practice appropriate techniques with nursing supervision until they achieve competence and are comfortable in the situation (see Health Education, p. 1288).
5. Counsel the parents concerning:
   a. Financial problems caused by repeated hospitalizations and transfusions.
   b. Feelings of guilt at having given birth to the child or resentment at having to care for him.

c. Refer the parents to a social worker or psychiatrist if indicated.

6. Introduce the child and his family to other hemophiliac families.
   a. Information concerning the location of parent groups may be obtained from the National Hemophilia Foundation, 19 West 34th Street, Room 1204, New York, NY, 10001.
   b. Numerous specialized hemophilia centers have been established in the United States.

7. Initiate a community health nursing referral if appropriate.

Health Education

1. Protecting the child from trauma
   a. Select toys that are soft and without rough edges.
   b. Pad the sides of cribs, playpens, etc.
   c. Offer food and liquids in plastic containers to avoid laceration.
   d. Guard against child's falling when he is learning how to stand and walk.
      (1) Remove potential sources of injury from furniture.
      (2) Pad the child's knees and buttocks.
      (3) Use a helmet for the child's head.
   e. Supervise play closely.
   f. Inform the child's teacher and playmates, the school nurse, and other adults of his condition so that they can be supportive of the child's needs and know what to do in an emergency.
   g. Have the child wear a Medic-Alert bracelet.
   h. Do not administer aspirin to the child.

2. Emergency treatment for hemorrhage
   a. Immobilize the part.
      This may be done with splints or an elastic compression bandage. (These materials should be immediately available in the home.)
   b. Apply ice packs.
      Parents should keep 2 or 3 plastic bags of ice immediately available in the freezer.
   c. Consult the child's physician and initiate additional recommended therapy.

3. Regular medical and dental supervision
   Preventive dental care is important. Soft-bristled or sponge-tipped toothbrushes should be used to prevent bleeding. Hospitalization may be necessary for extensive dental work and extractions.

4. Diet
   Diet is important to avoid overweight which places additional strain on the child's weight-bearing joints and predisposes him to hemarthrosis.

5. Information concerning the disease itself
   The child should be helped to understand the exact nature of his illness as early as possible. Special attention should be given to the signs of hemorrhage, and the child should be told of the need to report even the slightest bleeding to an adult immediately.

6. Avoidance of overprotection—this can be more disabling than the disease itself.
   a. Promote a sense of independence and self-care within the patient's limitations.
   b. Encourage healthful activity and reasonably aggressive pursuits. Reinforce self-judgment of child or teenager in selection of safe physical activities.
   c. Help parents understand the importance of vocational guidance for their child—emphasis given to occupations using intellect or skills rather than physical effort.

7. Genetic counseling and family planning services

These should be offered to the family and to the adolescent patient.

8. Home care program
   a. Home care programs teach the parents and children to administer infusion therapy at home when a hemorrhage episode begins.
   b. Advantages of home treatment:
      (1) Can be initiated immediately
      (2) Earlier recovery of joint functions
      (3) Greater self-sufficiency for patient and family
      (4) Fewer absences from school or work
      (5) Less anxiety related to traveling
      (6) Decrease in the cost of treatment
   c. General criteria for acceptance into program:
      (1) Adequate knowledge of the disease
      (2) Willingness to learn venipuncture technique
      (3) Demonstrated ability to follow directions
      (4) Acceptance of the necessity for follow-up care
      (5) Emotional stability sufficient to accept the responsibility
   d. Teaching is usually done by the nurse in the specialty clinic and includes instruction and practice in the following:
      (1) Storage and preparation of replacement factors
      (2) Venipuncture technique
      (3) Transfusion management
      (4) Record keeping
      (5) Awareness of signs of transfusion reaction
      (6) Recognition of indications of need for subsequent transfusions
   e. Hospital nursing responsibilities:
      (1) Screen patients and families who may be eligible for home care programs.
      (2) Facilitate appropriate self-management by children and families enrolled in home care programs if hospitalization becomes necessary. Establish communication with the clinic nurse.

9. Reference:
   Understanding Hemophilia—A Guide for Parents (1979), Hemophilia Foundation of Illinois, 327 South LaSalle Street, Chicago, IL 60604

10. Agencies
    National Hemophilia Foundation, 19 West 34th Street, Room 1204, New York, NY 10001

    National Center for Education in Maternal and Child Health, 3520 Prospect Street NW, Washington, DC 20007

Evaluation

Expected Outcomes

1. The child or parents achieve prompt control of bleeding episodes by administration of adequate treatment

2. Appears more comfortable as joint pain is relieved, achieves improved range of motion and does not demonstrate permanent joint deformities

3. Is not unduly anxious about transfusions, evidenced by his verbal and nonverbal communication

4. Demonstrates an age-appropriate level of independence

5. The parents are able to talk about their concerns/guilt

6. The family gains an understanding of hemophilia and its treatment

Thalassemia Major (Cooley's Anemia)

Beta-thalassemia (β-thalassemia) refers to an inherited group of blood disorders characterized by a reduction or absence of the beta globulin chain in hemoglobin synthesis. Homozygous β-thalassemia is the most severe of the β-thalassemia syndromes and is also know as thalassemia major or Cooley's anemia.

Etiology

1. Genetically determined, inherited disease.
2. Autosomal-recessive pattern of inheritance.
   Two types of β-thalassemia genes produce different severities of the disease.

Incidence

1. Most prevalent in the Mediterranean basin, Middle East, India, Pakistan, Southeast Asia, and Africa.
2. In the United States, it is most common in children of Italian, Greek, or Chinese ancestry.

Altered Physiology

1. Insufficient beta globulin synthesis allows large amounts of unstable alpha chains to accumulate.
2. The precipitates of alpha chains that form cause red blood cells to be rigid and easily destroyed, leading to severe anemia and resultant chronic hypoxia.
3. Erythroid activity is markedly increased in an attempt to overcome the increased rate of destruction, resulting in enormous expansion of bone marrow.
4. Rapid destruction of defective red blood cells, decreased production of hemoglobin, and increased absorption of dietary iron due to the body's response to anemia result in an excess supply of available iron.
5. In response to the low level of adult hemoglobin, large concentrations of fetal hemoglobin, which does not contain beta chains, are produced.

Prognosis

1. No known cure
2. Unable to predict which severely afflicted children will follow a more favorable course
3. Often fatal in late childhood or early adolescence

Preventive Measures

1. Parents of a child with thalassemia should be tested for the trait, and referred for genetic counseling (refer to p. 1481).
2. Prenatal diagnosis is possible through fetal blood sampling early enough to allow the opportunity to terminate the pregnancy.

Management

1. Frequent and regular blood transfusions to maintain hemoglobin levels above 9–10 gm./dl
   a. Washed, packed red cells are usually used to minimize the possibility of transfusion reactions.
   b. The frequency and amount of transfusions depend on the size of the child, with older children often reaching a peak requirement of 500 ml. of packed cells every 2–3 weeks.
2. Iron chelation therapy to reduce the toxic side effects of excess iron
3. Supportive management of complications

Assessment

Clinical Manifestations

1. Onset is usually insidious, with symptoms noted toward the end of the first year of life.
2. Symptoms are primarily related to the progressive anemia, expansion of the marrow cavities of the bone and the development of hemosiderosis (excess iron storage in various body tissues).
3. Early symptoms often include progressive pallor, poor feeding, and protuberant abdomen due to hepatosplenomegaly.
4. Further signs of progressive anemia include headache, bone pain, exercise intolerance, and listlessness.

Complications

A. Splenomegaly

1. Uniformly present because of extramedullary hemopoiesis and rapid destruction of defective red blood cells
2. Causes abdominal discomfort, pressure on other organs, and increased transfusion requirements
3. Usually requires splenectomy for improved well-being and to decrease the need for transfusions

B. Growth and Endocrine Complications

1. Growth retardation in 2nd decade.
2. Delayed development of secondary sex characteristics.
   a. The majority of males fail to undergo puberty.
   b. Most females experience alteration in menstruation.
3. Diabetes mellitus is often seen in older patients.
4. Adrenal and pituitary dysfunction, hypoparathyroidism, hypothyroidism, and pancreatic exocrine deficiency have been reported.

C. Skeletal Complications

1. Becoming less common because of early transfusion therapy.
2. Excessive expansion of the erythroid marrow may cause:
   a. Frontal bossing
   b. Maxillary hypertrophy
   c. Broad ribs
   d. Premature fusion of epiphyses of long bones
   e. Generalized skeletal osteoporosis
3. Pathologic fractures of the long bones and vertebrae collapse may occur.

D. Cardiac Complications

1. Arrhythmias
2. Pericarditis
3. Congestive heart failure
   This is the usual cause of death in thalassemic patients.

E. Liver Enlargement

1. This is initially due to extramedullary hemopoiesis.
2. Later, the liver becomes the main storage area for excess iron resulting in fibrosis and eventually cirrhosis.
3. May lead to coagulation abnormalities.

F. Gallbladder Disease

1. Gallstones are common by late adolescence.
2. May require cholecystectomy.

G. Megaloblastic Anemia

1. Folic acid deficiency may be sporadically present.
2. Prevented by daily, oral supplementation.

H. Skin

May have brown pigmentation because of iron deposits in the dermis and jaundice.

I. Leg Ulcers

Uncommon in well transfused patients.

Diagnostic Evaluation

1. Hemoglobin level—decreased.
2. Red cell indices—microcytosis and hypochromia.
3. Peripheral blood smear—many anisopoikilocytes, nucleated red cells, and basophilic stippling.
4. Reticulocyte count—low, usually less than 10%.
5. Hemoglobin electrophoresis—elevated levels of HbF and HbA$_2$.

Patient Problems/Nursing Diagnoses

1. Bone pain and headache related to progression of disease
2. Activity intolerance related to bone pain
3. Inadequate nutritional intake related to poor feeding behavior
4. Knowledge deficit regarding thalassemia and its management
5. Altered body image related to endocrine and skeletal complications
6. Increased susceptibility to infection related to progressive anemia
7. Anxiety related to the need for frequent transfusions
8. Parental guilt related to the hereditary nature of the disease
9. Coping difficulties related to presence of a potentially fatal diagnosis
10. Financial concerns related to the costs of treatment

Planning and Implementation

Nursing Interventions

A. Increase circulating hemoglobin and prevent tissue hypoxia.

1. Administer blood transfusions (refer to Care of the Child with Anemia, p. 1279).
   a. Because the chance of usual complications (sensitization, febrile reactions, hives, and hepatitis) is increased with the frequency of transfusions, it is essential to observe the child closely for signs indicative of a reaction.

B. Prevent infection and assess for signs of infection (refer to Care of the Child with Anemia, p. 1279).

▶ **NURSING ALERT:**
Because of the excess iron deposition in children with thalassemia, dietary iron should be decreased as much as possible.

1. Splenectomy is often required, and it results in further increased susceptibility to infection.
   a. These children should be maintained on oral penicillin prophylaxis.
   b. Vaccination against Haemophilus flu and pneumococcal infections should be considered.
   c. Prompt medical attention is essential for fever or signs of infection.

C. Eliminate the toxic side effects of excess iron.

1. Deferoxamine (Desferal) is used as a chelating agent to increase iron excretion through the urine and feces.
   a. Parents are usually taught to administer the drug subcutaneously during an overnight infusion.
   b. Daily, oral administration of vitamin C may be used as an adjunct to chelation therapy. Its usefulness should be assessed on an individual basis as vitamin C may also contribute to cardiac toxicity.
2. Dietary iron should be decreased as much as possible.

D. Prevent megaloblastic anemia.

1. Administer daily, oral folic acid supplementation.

E. Provide supportive care for the child in congestive heart failure (refer to Care of the Child with Congestive Heart Failure, p. 1303).

F. Assist the child to cope with thalassemia and its management.

1. Alleviate the child's anxieties about his illness.
   a. Role playing and play activities are useful in identifying concerns.
   b. Explain what is happening in a way that the child can understand.
   c. Explore the child's feelings about being different from other children.
   d. Adolescents may require counseling to deal with their feelings about delayed or absent sexual maturity.
   e. Discuss the positive achievements of recent research and correct misconceptions.
2. Plan treatment so that it interferes minimally with the child's regular activities and social interactions.
3. Encourage less strenuous activities in which the child can excel.
4. Encourage interaction with peers.
5. Plan for the child to continue his education.
6. Assist the child with vocational planning.
7. Include child in a support group of other children with thalassemia.
8. Provide supportive care to the dying child (refer to p. 1495).

G. Provide emotional support to the parents.

1. Encourage the parents to express their thoughts about their child's disease.
   a. Feelings of guilt, shock, frustration, depression, and resentment are common.
2. Counsel parents regarding ways to recognize and alleviate their child's apprehension.
3. Provide factual information about thalassemia and its management.
4. Inform parents of community resources which may provide financial, social, or other types of support.
5. Include parents in a support group if one is available.
6. Help the parents deal with the potentially fatal nature of the disease (refer to Care of the Dying Child, p. 1495).

Parental Education

1. Provide factual information about thalassemia, including its etiology, usual course, and treatment.
2. Discuss the genetic implications of thalassemia and offer genetic counseling to the family (refer to p. 1481).
3. Explain that the child has the same developmental needs as any healthy child. He should be encouraged

to participate in the usual activities of childhood to the extent that he is safely able to do so. The child should not be pampered, but should receive the same love, discipline, privileges, and responsibilities as a healthy child of his age.

4. Provide detailed instruction regarding:
   a. Prevention and prompt treatment of infections.
   b. Medications
   c. Home chelation therapy
   d. Dietary modifications
   e. Activity restrictions including avoidance of activities that increase the risk of fractures.
   f. Signs of complications
5. Encourage parents to provide information about the child's condition to significant adults who are involved with the child (teacher, school nurse, babysitter, scout leader, etc.).

Evaluation

Expected Outcomes

1. The child becomes more comfortable: does not cry in a distressed manner or complain of pain; engages in more activity; appears relaxed
2. Engages in age-related activity
3. Continues to develop in accordance with age
4. Increases nutritional intake and demonstrates willingness to eat
5. Copes well with body-image problems
6. Avoids infection (temperature normal; improved blood counts)
7. The parents are able to express their feelings and concerns about their child's illness
8. The parents gain an understanding of their child's illness and the necessary treatment

Bibliography

Books

Biggs R (ed). The Treatment of Haemophilia A and B and von Willebrand's Disease. London, Blackwell Scientific Publications, 1978

Hilgartner M. Hemophilia in The Child and Adult. New York, Masson, 1982

Johnson SH. High Risk Parenting. Philadelphia, JB Lippincott, 1986

Lanzkowsky P. Pediatric Hematology-Oncology. New York, McGraw-Hill, 1980

Lichtman MA. Hematology for Practitioners. Boston, Little, Brown & Co, 1978

Nathan D and Oski F. Hematology of Infancy and Childhood, 2nd ed. Philadelphia, WB Saunders, 1981

Sherwood W and Cohen A (eds). Transfusion Therapy: The Fetus, Infant and Child. New York, Masson, 1980

Varni J. Clinical Behavioral Pediatrics. Elmsford, NY, Pergamon Press, 1983

Whaley L and Wong D. Nursing Care of Infants and Children. St Louis, CV Mosby, 1983

Williams WJ (ed). Hematology, 3rd ed. New York, McGraw-Hill, 1983

Wintrobe M. Clinical Hematology. Philadelphia, Lea & Febiger, 1981

Articles

Buchanan GR. Hemophilia. Pediatr Clin North Am 1980 May; 27(2):309–326

Cohen A, Markenson A and Schwartz E. Transfusion requirements and splenectomy in the thalassemia major. J Pediatr 1980 Jul; 97(1):100–102

Conyard S et al. Psychosocial aspects of sickle cell anemia in adolescents. Health Soc Work 1980 Feb; 5(1):20–26

Dallman P, Siimes M and Stekel A. Iron deficiency in infancy and childhood. Am J Clin Nutr 1980 Jan; 33(1):86–118

Damiano ML et al. Hemophilia: The role of the school nurse. J Sch Health 1980 Oct; 50(10):451–454

Dressler D. Understanding and treating hemophilia. Nursing '80 1980 Aug; 10(8):72–73

Flanagan C. Home management of sickle cell anemia. Pediatr Nurs 1980 Mar/Apr; 6(2):B–D

Gever L. Parenteral iron supplements. Nursing '80 1980 Aug; 10(8):60

Inman M et al. Hemophilia: Information for school personnel. J Sch Health 1980 Mar; 50(3):137–140

Jones J et al. Antenatal diagnosis of sickle cell disease: Amniotic fluid cell DNA analysis. Obstet Gynecol 1982 Apr; 59(4):484–489

Karpatkin M. Screening tests in hemostasis. Pediatr Clin North Am 1980 Nov; 27(4):831–841

Klein H. Transfusion with young erythrocytes (neocytes) in sickle cell anemia. Am J Pediatr Hematol Oncol 1982 Summer; 4(2):162–165

Landesman S, Rao S and Ahonkhai V. Infections in children with sickle cell anemia. Am J Pediatr Hematol Oncol 1982 Winter; 4(4):407–415

McIntosh S et al. Fever in young children with sickle cell disease. J Pediatr 1980 Feb; 96(2):199–204

Mentzer W and Wang W. Sickle-cell disease: Pathophysiology and diagnosis. Pediatr Ann 1980 Aug; 9(8): 287–296

Nash K. Overview of humanistic progress in sickle cell anemia during the past 10 years. Am J Pediatr Hematol Oncol 1983 Winter; 5(4): 352–359

Ohene-Frempong K and Schwartz E. Clinical features of thalassemia. Pediatr Clin North Am 1980 May; 27(2):403–420

Oski F and McMillan J. Iron in infant nutrition, pp. 153–162. In Suskind R (ed). Textbook of Pediatric Nutrition. New York, Raven Press, 1981

Oski F and Stockman J. Anemia due to inadequate iron sources or poor iron utilization. Pediatr Clin North Am 1980 May; 27(2):237–253

Reindorf C. Sickle cell anemia: Current concepts. Pediatr Nurs 1980 Mar/Apr; 6(2):E–G

Reis E et al. Using a standard form to collect psychosocial data about hemophilia patients. Health Soc Work 1982 Aug; 7(8):206–214

Sarnaik S and Lusher J. Neurological complications of sickle cell anemia. Am J Pediatr Hematol Oncol 1982 Winter; 4(4):387–394

Scott R. Sickle cell diseases: Challenges of the eighties. Am J Pediatr Hematol Oncol 1982 Summer, 4(2):161

Sergis-Davenport E and Varni J. Behavioral techniques in teaching hemophilia factor replacement procedures to families. Pediatr Nurs 1982 Nov/Dec; 8(6):416–419

Shepherd MJ and Swearington P. Z-Track injection. Am J Nurs 1984 Jun; 84(6):746–747

Smith J. Management of sickle cell disease: Progress during the past 10 years. Am J Pediatr Hematol Oncol 1983 Winter; 5(4):360–365

Weeks H. Iron supplements. MCN 1980 Sep/Oct; 5(5):345

Children with Cardiovascular Disorders

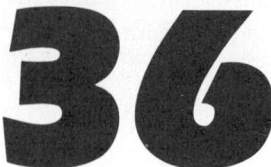

Congenital Heart Disease

Congenital heart disease is a structural malformation of the heart or great vessels, present at birth.

Etiology

1. Exact cause is unknown
2. Results from abnormal embryonic development or the persistence of fetal structure beyond the time of normal involution
3. Possible causes
   a. Fetal and maternal infection occurring during first trimester (primarily rubella)
   b. Teratogenic effects of drugs
   c. Maternal dietary deficiencies
   d. Genetic factors
4. Frequently associated with other congenital defects

Incidence

1. Approximately 25,000 infants are born each year with congenital heart disease.
2. As a category, congenital heart disease is the most common congenital malformation.

Common Congenital Heart Malformations
(Table 36-1)

A. Acyanotic

1. Obstructive lesions
   a. Aortic valvular stenosis
   b. Pulmonic stenosis
   c. Coarctation of the aorta
2. Left-to-right shunts
   a. Patent ductus arteriosus
   b. Atrial septal defect
   c. Ventricular septal defect

B. Cyanotic

Right-to-left shunts
1. Tetralogy of Fallot
2. Tricuspid atresia
3. Transposition of great arteries

Aortic Valvular Stenosis

Aortic valvular stenosis occurs when there is obstruction to the left ventricular outflow at the level of the valve. This is the most common form of aortic stenosis, others being hypertrophic subaortic stenosis and supravalvular stenosis.

Pathophysiology

1. Blood flows from the left ventricle through the obstructed aortic valve into the aorta.
2. Left ventricular pressure increases to overcome the resistance of the obstructed valve.
3. Myocardial ischemia may occur as a result of an imbalance between the increased oxygen requirements of the hypertrophied left ventricle and the amount of oxygen that can be supplied to the myocardium.

Clinical Manifestations

1. Rarely symptomatic during infancy; in severe cases, infants may demonstrate evidence of decreased cardiac output, such as faint peripheral pulses or exercise intolerance.
2. Older children may experience chest pain, dyspnea, and fatigue with exertion.
3. Narrow pulse pressure.
4. Weak peripheral pulses.

Diagnostic Evaluation

1. Auscultation:
   a. Harsh, low-pitched systolic ejection murmur, maximal at the second right intercostal space, radiates to apex, back, neck.
   b. Ejection click at fourth interspace to the left of the sternum (mild or moderately severe cases).
   c. Single or narrowly split second heart sound.
2. Chest x-ray—dilated ascending aorta and varying degrees of left ventricular enlargement.

3. Electrocardiogram—normal or left ventricular hypertrophy. Strain pattern (T-wave inversion) is evidence of severe stenosis. S–T segment depression indicates myocardial ischemia.
4. Cardiac catheterization
5. Angiography

Complications

1. Congestive heart failure
2. Myocardial infarction
3. Bacterial endocarditis
4. Sudden death

Treatment

Aortic valvulotomy or prosthetic valve replacement (indicated for children who are symptomatic or have evidence of left ventricular strain on electrocardiogram).

Pulmonic Stenosis

Pulmonic stenosis refers to any lesion that obstructs the flow of blood from the right ventricle.

Pathophysiology

1. Blood flows from the right ventricle through the obstructed pulmonary valve into the pulmonary artery.
2. Right ventricular pressure increases to maintain normal cardiac output.
3. Right ventricular hypertrophy develops.
4. Right-sided heart failure occurs in severe cases.

Clinical Manifestations

1. Generally asymptomatic; the child may have decreased exercise tolerance.
2. With severe obstruction, the child may have dyspnea, generalized cyanosis.
3. May complain of precordial pain.

Diagnostic Evaluation

1. Auscultation
   a. Systolic ejection murmur over pulmonic area
   b. Often will hear an ejection click and a widely split second sound
2. Chest x-ray—right ventricular enlargement, main pulmonary artery enlargement, normal pulmonary vascularity, and normal left side. In severe stenosis, right atrial hypertrophy is also observed.
3. Electrocardiogram—moderate or severe cases demonstrate right ventricular hypertrophy.
4. Cardiac catheterization
5. Angiocardiography

Complications

1. Anoxic spells in infants with severe lesions
2. Bacterial endocarditis
3. Sudden death at any age

Treatment

1. Surgery (valvulotomy) is generally indicated for all patients with severe stenosis and for symptomatic patients with moderate stenosis.
2. Asymptomatic children with moderate pulmonic stenosis should be evaluated at regular intervals for progression of the lesion.

Coarctation of the Aorta

Coarctation of the aorta is a narrowing or constriction of the vessel at any point. Most commonly, the constriction is located just distal to the origin of the left subclavian artery in the vicinity of the ductus arteriosus.

Altered Physiology

1. The narrowing of the aorta obstructs blood flow through the constricted segment of the aorta, thus increasing left ventricular pressure and work load.
2. Collateral vessels develop, arising chiefly from the branches of the subclavian and intercostal arteries, bypassing the coarcted segment of the aorta and supplying circulation to the lower extremities.

Clinical Manifestations

1. Usually asymptomatic in childhood—growth and development are normal.
2. May demonstrate:
   a. Occasional fatigue
   b. Headache
   c. Nose bleeds
   d. Leg cramps
3. Absent or greatly reduced femoral pulsations.
4. Hypertension in upper extremities and diminished blood pressure in lower extremities.
5. Symptoms secondary to hypertension (rare in children).
6. Severe anomalies cause symptoms in infants, including growth failure, tachypnea, dyspnea, peripheral edema, and severe congestive heart failure.

Diagnostic Evaluation

1. Auscultation—nonspecific systolic murmur heard along the left sternal border
2. Chest x-ray:
   a. Prominent aorta.
   b. Rib notching is a common finding in children over 10 years of age.
   c. Seriously ill infants demonstrate significant cardiomegaly with increased pulmonary vascularity.
3. Electrocardiogram—normal or varying degrees of left ventricular hypertrophy
4. Cardiac catheterization
5. Angiography

Complications

1. Cerebral hemorrhage
2. Rupture of the aorta
3. Infective endocarditis
4. Congestive heart failure

Treatment

1. Infants—vigorous management of congestive heart failure and surgical correction is indicated for infants who present in the first 6 months of life with heart failure.
2. Asymptomatic older child—surgical resection is recommended for children between the ages of 2–4 years with significant coarctation.
3. Surgery—resection of the coarcted segment and end-to-end anastomosis or graft.

(Text continues on p. 1296)

Table 36-1 Congenital Heart Abnormalities*

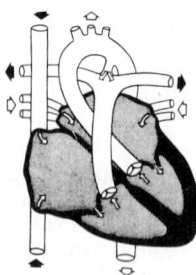

Patent Ductus Arteriosus

The patent ductus arteriosus is a vascular connection that, during fetal life, short circuits the pulmonary vascular bed and directs blood from the pulmonary artery to the aorta. Functional closure of the ductus normally occurs soon after birth. If the ductus remains patent after birth, the direction of blood flow in the ductus is reversed by the higher pressure in the aorta.

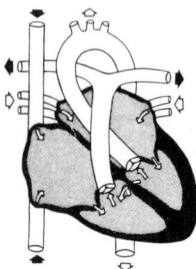

Ventricular Septal Defects

A ventricular septal defect is an abnormal opening between the right and left ventricle. Ventricular septal defects vary in size and may occur in either the membranous or muscular portion of the ventricular septum. Due to higher pressure in the left ventricle, a shunting of blood from the left to right ventricle occurs during systole. If pulmonary vascular resistance produces pulmonary hypertension, the shunt of blood is then reversed from the right to the left ventricle, with cyanosis resulting.

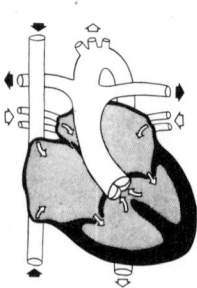

Truncus Arteriosus

Truncus arteriosus is a retention of the embryologic bulbar trunk. It results from the failure of normal septation and division of this trunk into an aorta and pulmonary artery. This single arterial trunk overrides the ventricles and receives blood from them through a ventricular septal defect. The entire pulmonary and systemic circulation is supplied from this common arterial trunk.

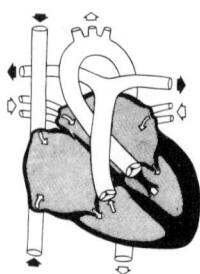

Subaortic Stenosis

In many instances, the stenosis is valvular with thickening and fusion of the cusps. Subaortic stenosis is caused by a fibrous ring below the aortic valve in the outflow tract of the left ventricle. At times, both valvular and subaortic stenosis exist in combination. The obstruction presents an increased work load for the normal output of the left ventricular blood and results in left ventricular enlargement.

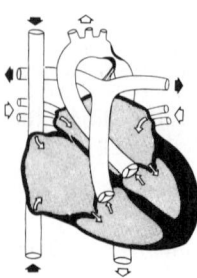

Coarctation of the Aorta

Coarctation of the aorta is characterized by a narrowed aortic lumen. It exists as a preductal or postductal obstruction, depending on the position of the obstruction in relation to the ductus arteriosus. Coarctations exist with great variation in anatomical features. The lesion produces an obstruction to the flow of blood through the aorta causing an increased left ventricular pressure and work load.

* Courtesy, Ross Laboratories.

Table 36-1   Congenital Heart Abnormalities (continued)

Tetralogy of Fallot

Tetralogy of Fallot is characterized by the combination of 4 defects: (1) pulmonary stenosis, (2) ventricular septal defect, (3) overriding aorta, (4) hypertrophy of right ventricle. It is the most common defect causing cyanosis in patients surviving beyond 2 years of age. The severity of symptoms depends on the degree of pulmonary stenosis, the size of the ventricular septal defect and the degree to which the aorta overrides the septal defect.

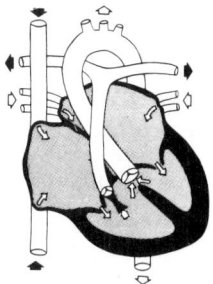

Complete Transposition of Great Vessels

This anomaly is an embryologic defect caused by a straight division of the bulbar trunk without normal spiraling. As a result, the aorta originates from the right ventricle, and the pulmonary artery from the left ventricle. An abnormal communication between the 2 circulations must be present to sustain life.

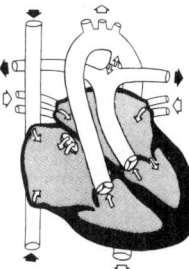

Atrial Septal Defects

An atrial septal defect is an abnormal opening between the right and left atria. Basically, 3 types of abnormalities result from incorrect development of the atrial septum. An incompetent foramen ovale is the most common defect. The high ostium secundum defect results from abnormal development of the septum secundum. Improper development of the septum primum produces a basal opening known as an ostium primum defect, frequently involving the atrioventricular valves. In general, left to right shunting of blood occurs in all atrial septal defects.

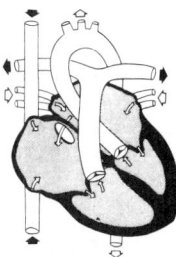

Tricuspid Atresia

Tricuspid valvular atresia is characterized by a small right ventricle, large left ventricle and usually a diminished pulmonary circulation. Blood from the right atrium passes through an atrial septal defect into the left atrium, mixes with oxygenated blood returning from the lungs, flows into the left ventricle and is propelled into the systemic circulation. The lungs may receive blood through 1 of 3 routes: (1) a small ventricular septal defect, (2) patent ductus arteriosus, (3) bronchial vessels.

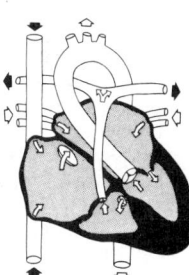

Anomalous Venous Return

Oxygenated blood returning from the lungs is carried abnormally to the right heart by one or more pulmonary veins emptying directly, or indirectly through venous channels, into the right atrium. Partial anomalous return of the pulmonary veins to the right atrium functions the same as an atrial septal defect. In complete anomalous return of the pulmonary veins, an interatrial communication is necessary for survival.

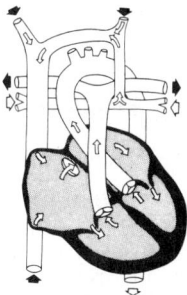

Patent Ductus Arteriosus

Patent ductus arteriosus is the persistence of a fetal connection (ductus arteriosus) between the pulmonary artery and the aorta.

Altered Physiology

1. During fetal life, the ductus arteriosus allows most of the right ventricular blood to bypass the nonfunctioning lungs by directing blood from the pulmonary artery to the aorta.
2. After birth, with the initiation of respiration, the ductus arteriosus is no longer necessary. It should functionally close within several hours after birth and anatomically close within several weeks after birth.
    a. The smooth muscle in the wall of the ductus arteriosus contracts to obliterate the lumen.
    b. Within several weeks after birth, degenerative changes occur in the ductus arteriosus and it becomes a cord of fibrous connective tissue (ligamentum arteriosum).
3. When the ductus arteriosus remains patent, oxygenated blood from the higher pressure systemic circuit (aorta) flows to the lower pressure pulmonary circuit (pulmonary artery) through the patent ductus arteriosus.
4. The volume of blood that the heart must pump in order to meet the demands of the peripheral tissues is increased. A greater volume burden is placed on the lungs and eventually on the left heart.

Clinical Manifestations

1. Small patent ductus arteriosus—usually asymptomatic
2. Large patent ductus arteriosus—may develop symptoms in very early infancy
    a. Slow weight gain
    b. Feeding difficulties
    c. Frequent respiratory infections
    d. Congestive heart failure

Diagnostic Evaluation

1. Auscultation—continuous machinery-like murmur at the left intraclavicular area is heard in most older children. Neonates with patent ductus have a variety of murmurs.
2. May have a wide pulse pressure and/or bounding posterior tibial and dorsalis pedis pulses.
3. Chest x-ray:
    a. Symptomatic infants usually demonstrate gross cardiomegaly and increased pulmonary vasculature.
    b. Older children show normal or slightly increased pulmonary arterial markings and prominent main pulmonary artery.
4. Electrocardiogram—may be normal; may demonstrate left ventricular hypertrophy.
5. Echocardiogram
6. Cardiac catheterization—may not be necessary.
7. Angiocardiography

Complications

1. Congestive heart failure
2. Infective endocarditis

Treatment

Surgical division of the patent ductus arteriosus:
1. In early infancy if congestive heart failure develops and cannot be controlled
2. Electively by 1–2 years

Note: Indomethacin appears to trigger the natural closing of the ductus. It is the treatment of choice for many preterm infants.

Atrial Septal Defect

Atrial septal defect is an abnormal opening in the septum between the left atrium and the right atrium.
1. *Ostium secundum type*—located in the center of the atrial septum (most common).
2. *Ostium primum type*—large gap at the base of the atrial septum frequently associated with deformities of the mitral and tricuspid valves and/or a small, high ventricular septal defect (endocardial cushion defects).

Altered Physiology

1. The pressure in the left atrium is greater than the pressure in the right atrium and promotes the flow of oxygenated blood from the left atrium to the right atrium.
2. The oxygenated blood that flows through the defect enters the right atrium and mixes with the systemic venous blood returning to the lung. The blood flow through the shunt recirculates through the lung, thus increasing the total blood flow through the lung.
3. The major hemodynamic abnormality is volume overload of the right ventricle.
4. If the pulmonary resistance is great, this may increase right atrial pressure, thus causing a reversal of the shunt, with unoxygenated blood flowing from the right atrium to the left atrium. (This situation will produce cyanosis.)

Clinical Manifestations

1. Ostium secundum type—generally asymptomatic even when this defect is large.
2. Ostium primum type—generally asymptomatic, although the following may occur:
    a. Slow weight gain
    b. Fatigability
    c. Dyspnea with exertion
    d. Frequent respiratory infections
    e. Congestive heart failure

Diagnostic Evaluation

1. Auscultation
    a. Systolic, medium-pitched ejection murmur heard best at the second left interspace.
    b. Fixed widely split second sound.
    c. May have mid-diastolic filling sound at the lower left sternal border.
    d. A holosystolic murmur of mitral insufficiency is often heard at the apex in patients with primum defects.
2. Chest x-ray—prominent main pulmonary artery, right atrial and right ventricular enlargement, increase in vascular markings of the lungs. Radiologic findings are influenced by associated lesions in primum defects.
3. Electrocardiogram may demonstrate right ventricular hypertrophy and right axis deviation (ostium secundum defect); left axis deviation, P-wave changes indicating atrial enlargement, and prolonged P–R interval are common in ostium primum defects.
4. Echocardiogram
5. Cardiac catheterization
6. Angiocardiography

Complications

(Rare in children)
1. Infective endocarditis
2. Cardiac failure
3. Pulmonary hypertension
4. Coronary artery disease
5. Atrial fibrillation

Treatment

Surgical closure with cardiopulmonary bypass by suture or patch

Ventricular Septal Defect

Ventricular septal defect is an abnormal opening in the septum between the right and left ventricles. It may vary in size from very small defects (Roger's defect) to very large defects, and may occur in either the membranous or muscular portion of the ventricular septum.

Altered Physiology

1. The pressure in the left ventricle is greater than the pressure in the right ventricle and promotes the flow of oxygenated blood from the left ventricle to the right ventricle.
2. The oxygenated blood that flows through the defect mixes with the blood returning from the right atrium. The blood flow through the shunt recirculates through the lungs, thus increasing the total blood flow through the lungs.
3. The major hemodynamic abnormalities are:
   a. Increased right ventricular and pulmonary arterial pressure
   b. Increased blood flow to the right ventricle, pulmonary arteries, left atrium, and left ventricle
4. If the pulmonary resistance is great, this may increase right ventricular pressure, thus causing a reversal of the shunt with unoxygenated blood flowing from the right ventricle to the left ventricle (this situation, termed *Eisenmenger's complex,* will produce cyanosis).

Clinical Manifestations

1. Small ventricular septal defects—usually asymptomatic (many close spontaneously)
2. Large ventricular septal defects—may develop symptoms as early as 1–2 months of age
   a. Slow weight gain
   b. Feeding difficulties
   c. Pale, delicate-looking, scrawny appearance
   d. Frequent respiratory infections
   e. Tachypnea
   f. Excessive sweating
   g. Congestive heart failure

Diagnostic Evaluation

1. Auscultation—harsh holosystolic murmur, heard best at the fourth interspace to the left of the sternum. Elevated pulmonary resistance is manifested by a loud, banging, pulmonic component of the second sound.
2. Chest x-ray—ranges from normal (small defect) to varying degrees of biventricular hypertrophy, left atrial enlargement, pulmonary artery enlargement, and increased pulmonary vascular markings.
3. Electrocardiogram—normal or biventricular hypertrophy, left atrial enlargement
4. Echocardiogram

5. Cardiac catheterization
6. Angiocardiography

Complications

1. Infective endocarditis
2. Congestive heart failure

Treatment

1. Medical management of congestive heart failure if this occurs in infancy.
2. If congestive heart failure is intractable to medical management, surgical closure is indicated.
3. Patients with pulmonary arterial hypertension require early surgery (before 2 years of age) to avoid irreversible pulmonary bed changes.
4. Surgery is contraindicated in patients with Eisenmenger's complex.

Tetralogy of Fallot

Tetralogy of Fallot consists of 4 abnormalities: (1) right ventricular-outflow stenosis or atresia, (2) ventricular septal defect, (3) overriding of the aorta, and (4) right ventricular hypertrophy.

Altered Physiology

1. Obstruction of the blood flow from the right ventricle to the pulmonary circulation is caused by obstruction at the pulmonary valve level or the infundibular area of the right ventricle below the pulmonary valve.
2. Unoxygenated blood is shunted from the right ventricle through the ventricular septal defect directly into the aorta.
3. The right ventricle is hypertrophied because of high right ventricular pressure.

Clinical Manifestations

1. The clinical manifestations are variable and depend on the size of the ventricular septal defect and the degree of right ventricular outflow obstruction.
2. Cyanosis
   a. Initially, the shunt through the ventricular septal defect may be from left to right. Many infants with this defect are not cyanotic at birth, but they develop cyanosis as they grow and as the stenosis becomes relatively more severe.
   b. Cyanosis may at first be observed only with exertion and crying, but during the first few years of life, the child may become cyanotic even at rest.
   c. Infundibular stenosis may be minimal so that cyanosis never develops ("pink tetralogy").
3. Clubbing of the fingers and toes
4. Squatting (a posture characteristically assumed by children with this defect once they have reached the walking stage)
5. Slow weight gain
6. Dyspnea on exertion
7. Hypoxic spells, transient cerebral ischemia

Diagnostic Evaluation

1. Auscultation
   a. Single second sound (aortic component)
   b. Systolic ejection murmur at the second and third interspaces to the left of the sternum
   c. Prominent ejection click heard immediately after the first heart sound
2. Chest x-ray

a. Heart size normal
b. Pulmonary segment small and concave ("boot-shaped heart")
c. Diminished pulmonary vascular markings
3. Electrocardiogram—right axis deviation; right ventricular hypertrophy
4. Cardiac catheterization
5. Angiocardiography
6. Laboratory data
   a. Polycythemia
   b. Increased hematocrit

Complications

1. Congestive heart failure—may occur in newborn but is uncommon beyond infancy
2. Infective endocarditis
3. Cerebral vascular accident (due to thrombosis or severe hypoxia)
4. Brain abscess
5. Iron deficiency anemia

Treatment

Goal:
Improve oxygenation of arterial blood.

1. Palliative
   a. Blalock–Taussig shunt—anastomosis between the right or left subclavian artery and the right pulmonary artery (preferred method).
   b. Waterston shunt—anastomosis between the posterior lateral aspect of the ascending aorta and the right pulmonary artery.
2. Total correction
   a. Removal of shunt if previously performed.
   b. With cardiopulmonary bypass, ventricular septal defect is repaired and right ventricular-outflow obstruction is relieved.
   c. Total correction is increasingly being advocated for all infants in whom pulmonary arteries are of sufficient size.

Transposition of the Great Arteries

Transposition of the great arteries occurs when the pulmonary artery originates posteriorly from the left ventricle and the aorta originates anteriorly from the right ventricle.

Altered Physiology

1. This defect results in 2 separate circulations; the right heart manages the systemic circulation, and the left heart manages the pulmonary circulation.
2. In order for life to be sustained, there must be an accompanying defect that provides for the mixing of oxygenated and unoxygenated blood between the 2 circulations.
3. The mixing of oxygenated and unoxygenated blood occurs through one or more of the following shunts:
   a. Atrial septal defect
   b. Ventricular septal defect
   c. Patent ductus arteriosus
   d. Patent foramen ovale

Clinical Manifestations

Influenced predominantly by the extent of intercirculatory mixing:

1. Cyanosis, usually developing shortly after birth (degree depends on the type of associated malformations)

2. Congestive heart failure manifested by tachypnea, cardiomegaly, hepatomegaly
3. Fatigability
4. Slow weight gain
5. Clubbing of the fingers and toes

Diagnostic Evaluation

1. Auscultation—murmurs may be absent in infancy; may be a murmur of an associated defect.
2. Chest x-ray—cardiomegaly, narrow mediastinum, egg-shaped cardiac silhouette, increased vascular markings (decreased vascular markings in children with associated pulmonary stenosis). Neonatal x-ray is often normal.
3. Electrocardiogram—right axis deviation, right or biventricular hypertrophy. Variable findings depending on age and anatomic factors.
4. Echocardiogram
5. Laboratory tests
   a. Polycythemia
   b. Thrombocytopenia
6. Cardiac catheterization
7. Angiocardiography

Complications

1. Congestive heart failure
2. Infective endocarditis
3. Brain abscess
4. Cerebral vascular accident (due to thrombosis or severe hypoxia)

Treatment

1. Vigorous medical management of congestive heart failure
2. Palliative procedures
   a. *Rashkind procedure*—the creation of an atrial septal defect with a balloon catheter during cardiac catheterization
   b. *Blalock-Hanlon procedure*—surgical creation of an atrial septal defect
   c. Pulmonary artery banding (indicated for infants with ventricular septal defects with large pulmonary blood flow)
   d. Systemic–pulmonary anastomosis (indicated for some infants with severe pulmonary stenosis).
3. Complete correction
   a. *Mustard procedure*—with cardiopulmonary bypass, the atrial septum is removed and a baffle of Dacron velour and/or pericardium is sutured in place in such a way that the pulmonary venous blood is directed toward the right ventricle and the systemic venous blood is directed toward the left ventricle
   b. *Senning procedure*—with cardiopulmonary bypass, the systemic and pulmonary returns are rerouted by arranging flaps of the interatrial septum and right atrial free wall to form the new venous channels.
   c. *Rastelli procedure*
      (1) Surgery of choice for transposition with ventricular septal defect and left ventricular outflow-tract obstruction.
      (2) With cardiopulmonary bypass, the ventricular septal defect is closed in such a way that the left ventricle communicates with the aorta. The pulmonary artery is ligated, and the right ventricle is connected to the distal

portion of the pulmonary artery by means of a valve bearing tubular graft.

d. Recent procedures have been developed for anatomic correction of transposition of the great arteries by direct contraposition of the transposed vessels. This may become the preferred treatment in the future.

e. As with other types of congenital cardiac surgery, the question of optimum timing for surgery is controversial. Increasingly, total correction is recommended when feasible.

Tricuspid Atresia

Tricuspid atresia is a condition in which there is (1) atresia of the tricuspid valve so that there is no communication between the right atrium and right ventricle, (2) interatrial septal defect, and (3) a hypoplastic right ventricle.

Pathophysiology

1. Blood from the systemic circulation is shunted from the right atrium through an interatrial communication to the left atrium and then to the left ventricle.
2. Pulmonary blood flow is established either through a patent ductus arteriosus, bronchial circulation, or a ventricular septal defect.

Clinical Manifestations

1. Severe cyanosis in the neonatal period
2. Respiratory distress
3. Clubbing
4. Hypoxic spells
5. Delayed weight gain
6. Right heart failure (may occur)

Diagnostic Evaluation

1. Auscultation
    a. First sound single and accentuated
    b. Commonly no murmur or murmur of associated defect

2. Chest x-ray—patients with diminished pulmonary blood flow have a normal to mildly increased cardiac silhouette, concavity in the region of the main pulmonary artery, and diminished pulmonary vascular markings; those with increased pulmonary flow have cardiac enlargement and plethoric pulmonary vasculature (less common)
3. Electrocardiogram—right atrial, left atrial, left ventricular hypertrophy, left axis deviation
4. Echocardiogram—demonstrates diminutive right ventricular chamber and no tricuspid valve
5. Cardiac catheterization
6. Angiocardiography

Complications

1. Cerebral vascular accident
2. Brain abscess
3. Bacterial endocarditis

Treatment

1. Palliative procedures to increase pulmonary blood flow:
    a. *Waterston shunt*—anastomosis between the ascending aorta and right pulmonary artery
    b. *Glenn procedure*—side-to-end anastomosis of the superior vena cava to the right pulmonary artery
    c. *Blalock-Taussig shunt*—subclavian to pulmonary artery anastomosis
2. Complete correction:
    a. *Fontan procedure*—involves placement of a tubular conduit with a valve between the right atrium and main pulmonary artery. The atrial defect is closed and the main pulmonary artery is ligated just above the pulmonary valve.
    b. Has been done successfully in a limited number of older, symptomatic patients with diminished blood flow.

Treatment and Nursing Management of the Child With a Congenital Heart Defect

Nursing Process Overview

Assessment

History and Physical Examination

A. **Become informed about the child's symptomatology and the plan of medical care.**

1. Obtain a thorough nursing history to become familiar with the child and his family in order to recognize normal and abnormal patterns (color, respirations, murmur, feeding, exercise tolerance, etc.).
2. Discuss with the physician the plan for medical care.
3. Make a baseline nursing assessment of the child's condition.
    a. Observe and record information relevant to the child's growth and development (motor coordination, muscular development, emotional maturity).

(1) Compare data with that for siblings, other family members.
(2) Plot appropriate information on growth chart.
    b. Observe and record the child's level of exercise tolerance.
(1) Observe the child at play:
    Is play interrupted to rest?
    How does he play as compared with his peers?
    Does he squat during play? (Squatting is a characteristic position a cyanotic child assumes when resting after exertion.)
(2) Observe infants while feeding.
    Does the infant stop feeding to rest, or does he fall asleep during feeding?
    c. Observe the child's skin and mucous membranes for color changes.

(1) Skin
Color changes vary from pink, dusky, mottled, to cyanotic.
Earlobes are good indicators of the degree of oxygen saturation.
Circumoral cyanosis occurs with oxygen deprivation.
Nailbeds are good indicators of color change.
(2) Mucous membranes
Lips and tongue indicate color change because they are very vascular areas and contain superficial blood vessels; *mucous membranes are the best places to observe for cyanosis.*
(3) Record where cyanosis was observed (localized or generalized), when it was observed and the duration (continuous or intermittent, whether variable with exercise).
d. Observe for clubbing (rounding) of the fingers, especially the thumbnails, with thickening and shininess of the terminal phalanges—may occur in cyanotic children by 2–3 months of age.
e. Observe for chest deformities.
(1) Visible pulsations
(2) Left- or right-sided prominence
f. Observe respiratory pattern.
(1) Remove any clothing or covers which obscure visualization of the chest.
(2) Count respirations for at least 30 seconds.
(3) Count respirations while a child is at rest; if unable to soothe the child, document that he is crying, irritable, etc.
(4) Observe for increased respiratory rate, grunting, retractions, nasal flaring, irregularity of respirations.
(5) Record all signs of respiratory distress including change from usual pattern, when it occurred, duration, etc.
g. Palpate the child's pulses.
(1) Radial or dorsalis pedis is difficult to feel in the newborn.
(2) Femoral pulsations are easily felt in the inguinal region and can be compared with brachial pulsations.
(3) Record the strength of the pulse (full, bounding, weak, or faint).
(4) When a pulse is difficult to locate, mark its location with a pen to facilitate locating it the next time.
h. Auscultate the child's heart to:
(1) Count apical pulse rate.
(2) Determine cardiac rhythm or change in rhythm.
(3) Become familiar with a known murmur.
(4) Determine the presence of new murmurs.
i. Record vital signs (apical pulse, blood pressure, respirations)
(1) Have child quiet for base-line vital signs.
(2) Record which extremity is used for blood pressure measurement.
(3) Refer to vital sign procedure (see p. 1133).

Patient Problems/Nursing Diagnoses

1. Respiratory distress related to altered pulmonary blood flow or oxygen deprivation
2. Altered cardiac output related to the specific anatomical defect

3. Inadequate nutrition related to the excessive energy demands required by increased cardiac workload
4. Increased potential for infection related to hematologic abnormalities and poor nutritional status
5. Anxiety related to diagnostic procedures and hospitalization
6. Developmental delay related to inadequate nutrition, physical limitations, and social isolation
7. Alteration in parenting, (overprotection, lack of discipline) related to parental perception of the child as vulnerable

Planning and Implementation
Nursing Interventions

A. Provide adequate nutritional and fluid intake to maintain the growth and developmental needs of the child.

1. Feed slowly in a semierect position; burp infants after each ounce.
2. Utilize soft nipples with large holes which make it easier for the infant to suck.
3. Provide small, frequent feedings.
4. Feeding should generally be completed within 45 minutes or sooner if the infant tires.
5. Provide foods that have high nutritional value.
6. Determine the child's likes and dislikes and plan meals with the dietitian, taking into consideration the child's preferences.
7. Observe the child at mealtime; does a poor appetite represent a lack of interest in food, or does the child become fatigued while eating?
8. Report vomiting and specify the amount, type, and relationship to feeding or to medications.
9. Report diarrhea and specify type and amount.
10. Maintain adequate hydration in the cyanotic child when he is vomiting, has diarrhea or fever, or is exposed to high environmental temperatures since polycythemia predisposes him to thrombosis.

B. Prevent infection.

1. Prevent exposure to communicable disease, including exposure to children with upper respiratory infections, diarrhea, wound infections, etc.
2. Check with the parents to be certain the child's immunizations are up to date.
3. Practice careful handwashing technique and teach this to the child.
4. Report temperature elevation, diarrhea, vomiting, and upper respiratory symptoms promptly.
5. Be certain that the child receives prophylactic medication for infective endocarditis before genitourinary instrumentation or dental work (refer to American Heart Association recommendations).

C. Prepare the child for diagnostic and treatment procedures.

1. Explain to the child what is going to be done in simple terms (refer to section on hospitalized child, p. 1112).
2. Encourage the child to express his fears and fantasies verbally or through play.
3. Diagnostic procedures may include:
   a. Electrocardiogram
   b. Vectorcardiogram
   c. Phonocardiogram
   d. Echocardiogram
   e. Chest x-ray
   f. Barium swallow

g. Cardiac catheterization and angiocardiography
h. Complete blood count
i. Platelet count
j. Blood gases

D. Explain the cardiac problem to child and parents.

1. Discuss with the parents the importance of being truthful with the child about his heart condition.
2. The time to tell the child is generally when the child begins asking questions as to why he visits the doctor so frequently and why the doctor listens to his heart so closely.
3. The child's questions should be answered truthfully in a simple way.

E. Relieve the respiratory distress associated with increased pulmonary blood flow or oxygen deprivation.

1. Determine the degree of respiratory distress.
   a. Infants—respirations greater than 60 per minute are indicative of respiratory difficulty.
   b. Young children—respirations greater than 40 per minute are indicative of respiratory difficulty.
   c. Observe the regularity of the respiratory pattern.
   d. Observe for retractions (drawing in of soft tissue in the rib interspaces or below the costal margin with each inspiration; may be barely visible, mild or severe).
   e. Observe for nasal flaring; listen for grunting.
2. Include specific information in nursing record.
   a. Number of respirations per minute
   b. Regularity of respirations
   c. Type and severity of retractions
   d. Presence of nasal flaring, grunting
   e. Response to oxygen therapy
   f. Response to positioning
   g. Color changes
   h. Irritability or anxiety observed
3. Position the child at a 45-degree angle to decrease pressure of the viscera on the diaphragm and increase lung volume.
   a. Infant—place in an infant seat.
   b. Children—elevate head of the bed and support the arms with pillows.
4. Pin diapers loosely; provide loose-fitting pajamas for older children.
5. Feed slowly, allowing frequent rest periods.
   a. Rapid respirations and frequent coughing predispose the child to aspiration.
   b. May require gavage feeding.
   c. Observe for abdominal distention which may increase respiratory difficulty.
6. Tilt the infant's or child's head back slightly.
7. Suction the nose and throat if the child is unable to adequately cough up secretions.
8. Provide oxygen therapy as indicated.

F. Relieve the hypoxic spells associated with cyanotic types of congenital heart disease (primarily tetralogy of Fallot).

1. Observe for hypoxic spells (attacks of acute oxygen deprivation), characterized by:
   a. Increased rate and depth of respiration
   b. Increasing cyanosis
   c. Murmur that becomes less intense, may disappear
   d. Bradycardia
   e. Progressive limpness and syncope
   f. The possibility of convulsions

2. Be aware that these attacks frequently occur in the morning after awakening from sleep, during or after crying, during or after defecation, or during or immediately following feeding.
3. Once an attack is recognized, call for assistance and immediately:
   a. Place child in knee–chest position.
   b. Administer oxygen via mask.
   c. Be prepared to administer medications as prescribed.
      Morphine sulfate
      NaHCO₃ to correct acidosis
      Propranolol
   d. Assume a calm, reassuring attitude.
4. Observe the child closely following recovery from an attack. Encourage fluid intake.
5. Record observations in the following areas:
   a. Condition and activity before the attack
   b. Response to positioning and medication
   c. Vital signs during and after attack

G. Improve oxygenation so that body functions may be maintained.

1. Provide a safe, effective oxygen environment (refer to procedure on oxygen therapy, p. 1186).
2. Explain to the child how oxygen will help; orient him to equipment before it is used on him (e.g., tent, mask).
3. Observe the child's response to oxygen therapy.
   a. Improvement of color
   b. Change in rate and character of respiration
   c. Change in anxiety level
4. Observe the child's response while he is being weaned from oxygen.
   Reduce liter flow gradually and observe response after each reduction.
5. Measures that are directed to relieve respiratory distress will aid in improving oxygenation.

H. Reduce the work load of the heart since decreased activity and expenditure of energy will decrease oxygen requirements.

1. Organize nursing care to provide periods of uninterrupted rest.
2. Avoid unnecessary activities such as frequent, complete baths and clothing changes.
3. Prevent excessive crying.
   a. Use pacifier.
   b. Hold the infant.
   c. Feed when hungry.
   d. Keep the infant comfortable.
4. Explain to the child the need for rest.
5. Provide diversional activities that require limited expenditures of energy.
6. Avoid discussing the child's condition or the condition of other children in the presence of the patient in order to prevent unnecessary anxiety.
7. Support the child during diagnostic and therapeutic procedures.

I. Observe the child for symptoms of congestive heart failure which occur frequently as a complication of congenital heart disease. (For nursing management, refer to section on congestive heart failure, p. 1303.)

1. Respiratory distress (tachypnea; retractions, nasal flaring, grunting, voice changes)
2. Tachycardia, gallop heart rhythm
3. Fatigue (as evidenced by poor feeding in infants)

4. Edema
   Periorbital edema is often observed in infants; older children develop swelling of the hands and feet.
5. Weight gain
6. Irritability
7. Sweating
8. Liver enlargement
9. Splenomegaly
10. Orthopnea
11. Neck vein distention (rarely seen in infants)
12. Murmurs (may appear, or the characteristics of previously heard murmur may change)
13. Cyanosis (may occur)
14. Pulmonary crackles (may occur)

J. Observe for the development of symptoms of infective endocarditis which may occur as a complication of congenital heart disease.

1. Be aware of the symptoms of infective endocarditis.
   a. Spiking fever
   b. Petechiae
   c. Anorexia
   d. Pallor
   e. Fatigue
2. Be aware of the need for infective endocarditis prophylaxis for selected children undergoing surgery, dental work, and laceration repair.
3. For nursing management, refer to section on infective endocarditis, p. 1312.

K. Observe for the development of thrombosis which may occur as a complication of cyanotic heart disease.

1. Be aware of the signs and symptoms of thrombosis:
   a. Irritability and restlessness
   b. Convulsion, coma, neurologic signs
   c. Paralysis
   d. Rapid onset of edema
   e. Anuria, oliguria, hematuria
2. Be aware that thrombosis is more likely to occur during phases of acute dehydration, fever, and vomiting.

L. Refer the family to appropriate resources concerned with the financial and/or emotional aspects of caring for a child with congenital heart disease.

1. Social worker
2. Crippled children's program
3. Parents and organized parent groups
4. American Heart Association

Health Education

1. Instruct the family in necessary measures to maintain the child's health:
   a. Complete immunization
   b. Adequate diet and rest
   c. Prevention and control of infections
   d. Regular medical and dental checkup
      The child should be protected against infective endocarditis when undergoing certain dental procedures (refer to American Heart Association Protocol).
   e. Regular cardiac checkups
2. Teach the family about the defect and its treatment.
   a. Pathophysiology and natural history
   b. Signs and symptoms of disease progress
   c. Signs and symptoms of complications
   d. Signs of infection, dehydration
   e. Medications and side effects
   f. Special diets
   g. Emergency precautions related to hypoxic attacks, pulmonary edema, cardiac arrest (if appropriate)
3. Encourage the parents and other persons (teachers, peers, etc.) to treat the child in as normal a manner as possible.
   a. Avoid overprotection and overindulgence.
   b. Avoid rejection.
   c. Facilitate performance of the usual developmental tasks within the limits of the child's physiological state.
      With most congenital cardiac defects it is not necessary to restrict the child's activity; the child will rest when he becomes tired and then will resume his play.
   d. Prevent adults from projecting their fears and anxieties onto the child.
4. Initiate a community health nursing referral if indicated.

Evaluation
Expected Outcome

1. The child breathes with little or no difficulty as evidenced by decreased respiratory rate, increased regularity of breathing, and decreased retractions and grunting
2. Maintains adequate or improved oxygenation as evidenced by normal color, decreased cyanosis, and improved blood gases.
3. Demonstrates adequate weight gain according to his normal curve
4. Remains free of infections (normal temperature) or receives prompt treatment if fever occurs
5. Effectively expresses his thoughts and fears about his illness and hospitalizations either verbally or through play
6. Achieves age-appropriate developmental milestones
7. The parents encourage and promote the child's normal development
8. The parents accurately explain the child's diagnosis and treatment, administer prescribed therapies, and recognize and report changes in the child's condition, signs of complications, and side effects of medications

Congestive Heart Failure

Congestive heart failure occurs when the cardiac output is inadequate to meet the metabolic demands of the body and results in accumulation of excessive blood volume in the pulmonary and/or systemic venous system.

Etiology

1. Congenital heart disease (primary cause in the first 3 years of life)
2. Acquired heart disease—rheumatic heart disease, endocarditis, myocarditis
3. Noncardiovascular causes—acidosis, pulmonary disease, various metabolic diseases

Altered Physiology

1. For any number of reasons, cardiac output is inadequate to meet the oxygenation and nutritional requirements of vital organs.
2. Various compensatory mechanisms occur.
   a. Stroke volume increases and cardiomegaly develops.
   b. Tachycardia occurs in an effort to maintain adequate stroke volume.
   c. Catecholamines are released by the sympathetic venous system that increase systemic vascular resistance and venous tone and decrease cutaneous, splanchnic, and renal blood flow.
   d. Glomerular filtration decreases, and tubular reabsorption increases, causing diminished urinary output and sodium retention.
   e. Diaphoresis occurs.
3. Cardiac output decreases further as compensatory mechanisms fail.
4. The pulmonary vascular bed is not emptied efficiently, causing engorgement of the pulmonic system with subsequent pulmonary hypertension and edema.
5. There is diminished blood return to the heart, with venous congestion and a rise in venous pressure.

Complications

1. Respiratory infections
2. Pulmonary edema
3. Intractable congestive heart failure
4. Myocardial failure

Assessment

Clinical Manifestations

1. Dyspnea and tachypnea
2. Tachycardia
3. Orthopnea
4. Peripheral edema—often scrotal or periorbital
5. Feeding difficulties, anorexia
6. Restlessness
7. Easy fatigability
8. Pallor
9. Weight gain
10. Diaphoresis
11. Growth failure
12. Nonproductive, irritative cough
13. Neck vein distention
14. Hepatomegaly

Diagnostic Evaluation

1. Palpation
   a. May have weak peripheral pulses.
   b. Hepatomegaly (feature of right heart failure).
   c. Abnormal precordial activity may occur.
2. Auscultation
   a. Gallop rhythm (frequent).
   b. Cardiac murmurs may or may not be present.
   c. Crackles (infrequent in infants).
3. Chest x-rays—cardiomegaly; pulmonary congestion
4. Laboratory data:
   a. Dilutional hyponatremia
   b. Hypochloremia
   c. Hyperkalemia

Patient Problems/Nursing Diagnoses

1. Decreased cardiac output related to the specific anatomic defect
2. Fluid volume excess related to the inability of the heart to pump blood from the ventricle(s), and decreased blood flow to the kidney
3. Impaired gas exchange related to pulmonary engorgement
4. Activity intolerance related to fatigue
5. Growth failure related to general weakened state
6. Inadequate nutritional intake related to poor feeding
7. Anxiety of child or parent related to their perception(s) of the child's condition and potential for death
8. Knowledge deficit about congestive heart failure and its treatment

Planning and Implementation

Nursing Interventions

A. Improve myocardial efficiency.

1. Administer digoxin as prescribed by the physician.
   a. Carefully calculate dosage; digoxin is given to infants and children in very small amounts.
   b. Count apical pulse for 1 full minute before administering.
      Be aware of the heart rate at which the physician wants the medication withheld.
   c. Report vomiting, which may occur following administration of digoxin, to determine if physician desires dose to be repeated.
   d. Observe for the development of premature ventricular contractions when digoxin is initially started; report this to physician.
   e. Be aware of signs of digitalis intoxication.
      (1) Altered emotional status, "digitalis blues"
      (2) Decreased appetite
      (3) Bradycardia
      (4) Arrhythmias
      (5) Gastrointestinal symptoms

B. Reduce energy requirements.

1. Organize nursing care to provide periods of uninterrupted rest.
2. Avoid unnecessary activities such as frequent complete baths and clothing changes.
3. Prevent excessive crying.
   a. Use pacifier.
   b. Hold baby.
   c. Eliminate sources of distress (e.g., hunger, wet diapers).
4. Explain to the child the need for rest.
5. Provide diversional activities that require limited expenditure of energy.

C. Remove accumulated sodium and fluid.

1. Administer diuretics as prescribed by the physician.
   a. Be aware of the side effects of the prescribed medication.
   b. Weigh the child at least daily to observe response.
   c. Maintain an accurate record of intake and output. Record urine specific gravity.
   d. Encourage foods such as bananas and orange juice that have a high potassium content to prevent potassium depletion associated with many diuretics.
      (1) Hypokalemia may cause weakened myocardial contractions and may precipitate digoxin toxicity.
      (2) Oral potassium supplements may be indicated when a child is on diuretics for an extended period of time.
2. Restrict sodium intake
   a. The child may be placed on a low-sodium diet.
   b. Be aware of the prescribed diet and the amount of sodium in foods and fluids offered to the child.
   c. Question the child about his likes and dislikes so that the diet can be made as appealing as possible.
   d. Interpret the diet and its purpose to the child and his parents.
   e. Infants may require low-sodium formulas.

D. Relieve the respiratory distress associated with pulmonary engorgement.

Refer to section on Congenital Heart Disease, pp. 1292–1302.

E. Improve tissue oxygenation.

1. Administer oxygen therapy—refer to procedure, pp. 1186–1190.
2. Maintain the infant in a neutral thermal environment.

F. Provide adequate nutrition to meet the caloric requirements of the child.

1. Provide foods that the child enjoys in small amounts, because he may have a poor appetite due to liver enlargement.
2. Infant feeding:
   a. Feed frequently in small amounts.
   b. Feed slowly in a sitting position, allowing frequent rest periods.
   c. Supplement oral feedings with gavage feeding if the infant is unable to take an adequate amount of formula by mouth.
   d. Record the amount of formula taken.
   e. Place the child in an infant seat following feeding to prevent pressure of the viscera on the diaphragm.
   f. Observe for distention and vomiting following feeding.

G. Decrease the danger of infection.

1. Practice careful handwashing technique.
2. Avoid exposure to other children with upper respiratory infections, diarrhea, etc.
3. Report changes such as temperature elevation, diarrhea, vomiting, and upper respiratory symptoms promptly.

H. Observe for signs of disease progress or response to treatment.

1. Record and report in detail presence or disappearance of signs and symptoms.
2. Monitor vital signs frequently and report any significant changes.

I. Explain the condition and treatment to the child and family.

1. Utilize terminology that the child and/or parents can understand.
2. Correct misinterpretations—parents and children frequently interpret congestive heart failure to be synonymous with myocardial infarction, or they may fear that the heart is about to stop beating.

Health Education

1. Describe symptoms to be aware of and to be reported.
2. Teach them how to administer medications and about the side effects.
3. Explain dietary and/or activity restrictions.
4. Explain methods to prevent infection.
5. Initiate a community health nursing referral if indicated.

Evaluation
Expected Outcomes

1. The child achieves improved cardiac output, evidenced by his clinical condition and laboratory measurements
2. Achieves and maintains fluid and electrolyte balance, evidenced by decreased edema and laboratory measurements
3. Maintains or improves oxygenation, evidenced by normal color, decreased cyanosis, and improved blood gas values
4. Conserves energy and rest in accordance with needs
5. Achieves normal growth pattern as evidenced by weight, height, and developmental tasks
6. Maintains adequate nutritional intake
7. The parents discuss their concerns about the child's condition with one another
8. The parents accurately describe congestive heart failure and its treatment, correctly administer digoxin and diuretics, and recognize signs and symptoms of complications

Nursing Care of the Child Undergoing Cardiac Catheterization

Cardiac catheterization involves introducing a radiopaque catheter into a vein or artery in the groin or in the arm, either percutaneously or by means of a cutdown. The catheter is advanced into the cardiac chambers and vessels, where pressures are measured and samples for oxygen concentration are obtained. The procedure is usually done in conjunction with angiography, the injection of radiopaque material into various chambers of the heart.

Purposes

1. To establish the diagnosis of cardiovascular defect.
2. To identify the severity of the defect.

3. To evaluate the effects of the defect on cardiovascular function.

Preoperative Nursing Interventions

A. Prepare the child and parents for the procedure.

1. Reinforce explanations of the procedure to the child and parents.
   a. Provide specific information about:
      (1) Time of the test
      (2) Preparation for the procedure (NPO, sedation, etc.)
      (3) Site of the venipuncture (if known)
      (4) What the child will see (atmosphere of the catheterization room)
      (5) What will be expected of the child during the procedure
      (6) Routines after the procedure
   b. Detail, length, and timing of explanations should be appropriate to the child's age and level of cognitive development.
      (1) Photographs or a miniature replica of the cardiac laboratory and equipment may facilitate understanding of explanations.
      (2) Older children and parents may benefit from an opportunity to see the room where the procedure will be done.
      (3) It is helpful for some children to handle the mask and other equipment that will be used.
   c. Parents should be provided with an opportunity for private discussion of the anticipated procedure.
2. Maintain adequate hydration (especially important for children with cyanotic heart disease).
   Offer fluids just prior to NPO period.
3. Cleanse proposed catheterization site thoroughly. Clean fingernails and/or toenails.
4. Obtain baseline set of vital signs—including blood pressure—just prior to the time of catheterization.
5. Administer sedation if prescribed.
   a. Raise and secure side rails after the child has been medicated.
   b. Observe the child closely for depressed respirations.

Postoperative Nursing Interventions

A. Observe for and prevent postoperative complications.

1. Monitor vital signs frequently and report:
   a. Sudden drop in blood pressure
   b. Changes in pulse rate or rhythm
   c. Increased or depressed respirations
   d. Faintness, weakness
   e. Elevated temperature
2. Observe for complications resulting from damage to the vessels through which the catheter was passed.
   a. Check the dressing or puncture site for bleeding.
   b. Observe site for redness, swelling, pain, or induration.
   c. Observe for numbness, pallor, decreased temperature, decreased motion, cyanosis, or mottling of affected extremity.
   d. Palpate pulses in affected extremity and compare with pulses in the opposite extremity.
3. Keep the child warm to avoid the risk of hypothermia.
   This is especially important for small infants and children who may already be hypoxic because of their cardiac condition.
4. Maintain the child in a reclining position for several hours after catheterization to avoid:
   a. Possibility of sudden drop in blood pressure that may accompany an abrupt assumption of an upright position.
   b. Bleeding at the site of catheter entry.
5. Offer fluids as soon as the child is able to take them to avoid dehydration.
   This is especially important for cyanotic children who are polycythemic and prone to thrombus formation.

B. Prepare the child and parents for discharge.

1. Reinforce discharge information. Parents should be informed about:
   a. Care of the incision, puncture site
   b. Dressing change (if any)
   c. Activity limitations (if any)
   d. Observation for and reporting of late complications (especially infection)
   e. Follow-up medical care
2. If the child is a candidate for surgery, utilize appropriate opportunities to prepare him and his family for the experience.
   a. Encourage contact with children who are convalescing from surgery.
   b. Answer immediate questions of the parents.

Reference for Teaching

Dee Dee's Heart Test, Children's Hospital of Philadelphia, 34th and Civic Center Blvd, Philadelphia, PA 19104.

Cardiac Surgery

Generally, nursing care of children who require cardiac surgery is the same as that of adults (refer to pp. 328–334). In addition, the following considerations should be kept in mind by the nurse who works with pediatric patients.

Preoperative Nursing Interventions

A. Prepare the child and parents for surgery.

1. Prepare the parents for the experience prior to the day of admission for surgery.
   a. Parents frequently ask questions about:
      (1) What to tell the child
      (2) When to begin preparation
      (3) What to bring to the hospital
      (4) Anticipated sequence of events
      (5) Separation—rooming-in, whether or not to leave at night, etc.
   b. Utilize opportunities for teaching—physician's office, catheterization episode, puppet shows, telephone calls, contact with other patients.

2. Prepare the child for what he will experience during hospitalization.
   a. Consult with the parents prior to beginning explanation. Their desires regarding how much information to give the child should be respected, and they should be active participants in preparation of the child.
   b. Most children need information about:
      (1) Preparation for surgery:
         (a) Diagnostic tests
         (b) Antibacterial skin preparation or baths
         (c) NPO period
         (d) Injections—antimicrobials and/or sedatives
         (e) Time of the surgery
         (f) Transportation to the operating room
      (2) Postoperative expectations:
         (a) Incision (location)
         (b) Chest tube
         (c) Dressings
         (d) Nasogastric tube
         (e) IVs
         (f) Monitors
         (g) Endotracheal tube, ventilator
         (h) Suctioning
         (i) Oxygen equipment
         (j) Pain (ability to relieve)
         (k) Restraints
         (l) Bed scale (may fantasize that it is a stretcher to return child to the OR)
         (m) Appearance of intensive care unit; visiting regulations for parents
   c. Have the child practice coughing and deep-breathing exercises (see procedure, p. 1180).
   d. Detail, length, and time of explanations should be appropriate to the child's age and level of cognitive development.
      (1) Photographs or a miniature replica of the intensive care unit may facilitate understanding of explanations.
      (2) Older children and parents often benefit from an opportunity to see the intensive care unit.
      (3) It is helpful for some children to have an opportunity to manipulate some of the equipment that will be used.
   e. Test the child's comprehension of teaching by asking him simple questions, having him place equipment on a doll, demonstrating coughing and deep breathing, and other similar activities.
   f. Allow opportunity for the child to express his concerns, either verbally or in play situations.
3. Provide opportunity for private discussions with the parents about the anticipated surgery.
   a. Parents need the same type of information as their child. They also need information about the following:
      (1) Scheduled time of surgery
      (2) Whether or not they can accompany their child to the operating room
      (3) Waiting area
      (4) Usual length of surgery
      (5) Intensive care unit expectations and policies
   b. Provide emotional support to the parents and answer their questions so that they are in the best position to support their child.
      (1) The parents may need help dealing with guilt feelings that they had a role in causing the disease, that they did not seek medical advice soon enough, etc.
      (2) Parents frequently have fears that the child will suffer excessive pain or die.
      (3) Parents may ask technical questions relating to such matters as the heart–lung machine, and the type of material used for patching defects.

B. Make baseline assessments which are essential in planning postoperative care:

1. Height and weight
2. Vital signs
3. Sleep/wake patterns
4. Elimination patterns
5. Fluid intake

C. Observe for any indications that surgery may need to be cancelled.

1. Signs of infection or inflammation (upper respiratory infection, hoarseness, elevated temperature, vomiting, diarrhea, skin lesions, etc.).
2. Congestive heart failure (see p. 1302)
3. Anemia (see p. 1279)

D. Perform appropriate nursing activities associated with congenital heart disease (see p. 1299).

Immediate Postoperative Nursing Interventions

A. Ensure continuity of care.

1. Send the nursing history and care plan to the intensive care unit and relay information about the child and family to appropriate personnel.

B. Provide safe physical care to the child.

1. Refer to:
   Postoperative Nursing Management (adults), pp. 85–96
   Cardiac Arrhythmias, pp. 339–351
   Respiratory Procedures, pp. 1178–1195
   Cardiopulmonary Resuscitation, pp. 1195–1196
   Managing the Patient Undergoing Water-seal Chest Drainage, p. 183
   Direct Current Countershock Procedures for Ventricular Fibrillation, p. 292
   Measuring Central Venous Pressure, p. 286
   Assisting with Obtaining Blood for Blood Gas Analysis, p. 143
   Intensive Care, p. 1119

C. Observe the child for complications.

1. Be aware of specific complications which may occur following surgery for congenital heart disease.
   a. Patent ductus arteriosus (rare)
      Recurrent laryngeal nerve injury
   b. Coarctation of the aorta
      Paradoxical hypertension
      Abdominal pain, distention
   c. Atrial septal defect
      (1) Atrial arrhythmias
      (2) Transient or permanent heart block
   d. Ventricular septal defect (VSD)
      (1) Complete heart block
      (2) Recurrent VSD
   e. Tetralogy of Fallot
      (1) Low cardiac output
      (2) Pulmonary insufficiency

(3) Complete heart block
(4) Recurrent VSD
(5) Residual pulmonary outflow tract obstruction
f. Transposition of great arteries (Mustard procedure)
   (1) Superior vena cava obstruction
   (2) Pulmonary venous obstruction, pulmonary edema
   (3) Complete heart block
   (4) Residual atrial shunts
   (5) Arrhythmias
g. Aortic stenosis
   Aortic insufficiency

D. Provide emotional support to the parents.

1. Support the parents during the time that the child is in the intensive care unit.
   a. Accompany the parents when they first visit their child following surgery. Since this may be traumatic, do not force them to maintain lengthy contact with the child.
   b. Address parental concerns and answer questions such as:
      (1) How they should react to their child
      (2) Amount of parental participation that is beneficial
      (3) Fears and fantasies during lengthy periods when they are unable to visit child
      (4) Concern for other children and families
      (5) Technical questions
   c. Provide the parents with the telephone number of the intensive care unit if they elect to leave.
   d. Make certain that parents have a comfortable place to sleep if they elect to stay at the hospital.
   e. Reassure the parents that it is normal for children to regress following such extensive surgery.

Convalescent Nursing Interventions

A. Observe for late complications.

1. Respiratory (atelectasis, pneumothorax, pulmonary edema)
   a. Continue coughing and deep-breathing exercises.
   b. Ambulate child as tolerated.
   c. Note changes in the character of respirations, dyspnea, chest pain, tachycardia, and cyanosis.
2. Infection
   a. Monitor temperature at regular intervals.
   b. Observe incision(s) for redness, swelling, drainage.
3. Congestive heart failure
   See Nursing Management, pp. 1303–1304.
4. Postpericardiotomy syndrome
   Symptoms include fever, pericardial friction rub, and pericardial and pleural effusion.
5. Postperfusion syndrome

Symptoms include fever, hepatosplenomegaly, leukocytosis, malaise, and maculopapular rash.
6. Infective endocarditis, (see p. 1312)

B. Provide emotional support to the child and parents:

1. Explain procedures, medications, special diet to the child and parents.
2. Encourage the child to attend to his personal needs as he is able.
3. Allow the child to make some decisions in order to give him a feeling of control.
4. Provide the child with appropriate diversion and play materials.
5. Encourage parental participation in the child's care.
   a. Teach the parents those aspects of the child's care that they can assume (e.g., coughing and breathing exercises).
   b. Discuss usual convalescent expectations of patient with parents (e.g., fatigue, itching at incision, emotional reactions).

C. Prepare the child and parents for discharge.

1. Active parental participation in the child's care facilitates discharge teaching.
2. Provide the family with oral and written discharge recommendations including:
   a. Activity restrictions
   b. Care of incision
   c. Medications—exact amounts and times of administration
   d. Special diet (low sodium is often indicated)
   e. Emotional reactions—child may demonstrate:
      (1) Regression in toilet habits, feeding and other learned skills
      (2) Nightmares
      (3) Increased dependency
      (4) Decreased appetite
      (5) Demanding behavior—need to set limits
   c. Observation for complications:
      (1) Fever
      (2) Increased heart rate
      (3) Chest pain
      (4) Shortness of breath
      (5) Problems with the incision
      (6) Vomiting or diarrhea
      (7) Rash
3. Provide the parents with the names and telephone numbers of persons to call for questions and emergencies.

Reference for Teaching

Margaret's Heart Operation, Children's Hospital of Philadelphia, 34th and Civic Center Blvd, Philadelphia, PA 19104.

Acute Rheumatic Fever

Acute rheumatic fever is a systemic disease characterized by inflammatory lesions of connective tissue and endothelial tissue.

Etiology

1. The exact pathogenesis is unknown, but it is thought to be an autoimmune response to group A beta hemolytic streptococcus.

2. Most first attacks of rheumatic fever are preceded by streptococcal infection of the throat or upper respiratory tract at an interval of several days to several weeks.

Altered Physiology

1. The unique pathologic lesion of rheumatic fever is the Aschoff body.

2. The basic changes consist of exudative and proliferative inflammatory reactions in the mesenchymal supporting tissue of the heart, joints, blood vessels, and subcutaneous tissues.
3. The inflammatory process involves all layers of the heart.
4. The inflammation may involve the leaflets and/or chordae tendinae of the heart valves, most frequently the mitral and/or aortic valves.

Assessment
Clinical Manifestations and Diagnostic Evaluation

No single clinical or laboratory finding is characteristic of rheumatic fever. The diagnosis is based on a combination of manifestations characteristic of this disease and in the absence of other diseases that may mimic it.

1. For this reason, the Jones Criteria, as established by a committee of the American Heart Association, are utilized.
2. The presence of 2 major criteria, or 1 major and 2 minor criteria, plus evidence of a preceding streptococcal infection are required to establish a diagnosis.

A. Major Manifestations

1. Carditis—manifested by significant murmurs, signs of pericarditis, cardiac enlargement, or congestive heart failure.
2. Polyarthritis—almost always migratory and manifested by swelling, heat, redness and tenderness, or by pain and limitation of motion of 2 or more joints.
3. Chorea—purposeless, involuntary, rapid movements often associated with muscle weakness.
4. Erythema marginatum—an evanescent, pink rash.
   a. The erythematous areas have pale centers and round or wavy margins.
   b. They vary greatly in size and occur mainly on the trunk and extremities.
   c. The erythema is transient, migrates from place to place, and may be brought out by the application of heat.
5. Subcutaneous nodules—firm, painless nodules seen or felt over the extensor surface of certain joints, particularly elbows, knees, and wrists, in the occipital region, or over the spinous processes of the thoracic and lumbar vertebrae; the skin overlying them moves freely and is not inflamed.

B. Minor Manifestations

1. *Clinical*
   a. History of previous rheumatic fever or evidence of preexisting rheumatic heart disease
   b. Arthralgia—pain in one or more joints without evidence of inflammation, tenderness to touch, or limitation of motion
   c. Fever—temperature in excess of 38°C. (100.4°F.)
2. *Laboratory*
   a. Erythrocyte sedimentation rate—elevated
   b. C-reactive protein—positive
   c. Electrocardiographic changes—mainly P–R interval prolongation
   d. Leukocytosis

C. Supporting Evidence of Streptococcal Infection

1. Increased titer of streptococcal antibodies (antistreptolysin O, or ASO titer)
2. Positive throat culture for group A streptococci
3. Recent scarlet fever

Patient Problems/Nursing Diagnoses

1. Pain related to polyarthritis
2. Inadequate cardiac output related to heart damage
3. Altered body-image related to chorea and/or steroid therapy
4. Potential for injury related to chorea
5. Activity intolerance related to muscle weakness
6. Potential for infection related to steroid therapy
7. Knowledge deficit about rheumatic fever and its treatment
8. Potential for disease recurrence

Planning and Implementation
Nursing Interventions

A. Become informed about the child's symptomatology and the medical plan of care.

1. Discuss with the physician the plan for medical treatment.
2. Make a baseline nursing assessment of the child's condition.
   a. Listen to the child's chest with a stethoscope to become familiar with the murmur or to determine the presence of a murmur not previously heard; listen for a friction rub.
   b. Determine from the child whether he is experiencing any pain or discomfort (also observe the child's facial expression as he moves since children may deny pain, thinking they will be able to go home).
   c. Describe the pain as to location, when it occurs, whether there is any heat, swelling, redness or tenderness.
   d. Examine the knees, elbows, wrists, occipital region and spine for nodules; describe location.
   e. Determine whether the child has any muscle weakness or rapid, purposeless movements.

B. Initiate specific preventive teaching in order to prevent a recurrence or an additional case of rheumatic fever within the family.

1. Have all family members screened for streptococcus by referring them for throat cultures.
2. All persons with positive cultures should be treated.
3. Teach the specific symptoms of streptococcal infections.

C. Treat the precipitating streptococcal infection.

Administer antibiotics as prescribed by the physician (generally intramuscular penicillin G).

▶ **NURSING ALERT:** Before administering penicillin, elicit a history for possible drug allergy.

D. Evaluate the child for evidence of response to treatment or progression of disease.

1. Observe for the development or disappearance of any major or minor manifestations of the disease.
2. Monitor carditis by careful documentation of the child's pulse, respirations, and blood pressure.
   a. The pulse should be counted for 1 full minute.
   b. The sleeping pulse is a good indicator of the extent of carditis.

E. Provide symptomatic management of the child's fever.

1. Refer to section on fever, p. 1135.
2. Antipyretic drugs are usually withheld during the diagnostic period.

F. Suppress the rheumatic inflammatory process by administering appropriate medications.

1. Salicylates (generally prescribed for patients without carditis)
   a. Observe for gastrointestinal upsets, ringing in the ears, headaches, bleeding, and disturbances in the mental state.
   b. Administer milk or antacids with salicylates.
   c. Report side effects promptly.
   d. Aspirin therapy should be monitored by salicylate levels in the blood.
2. Steroids (generally prescribed for patients with carditis; as steroids are tapered, administration of salicylates is begun)
   a. Prepare the child and his family for the expected side effects of steroid therapy.
      (1) Body appearance may change through rounding facial contour
      (2) Localized fat deposits
      (3) Appearance of acne or excessive hair
      (4) Weight gain with linear markings appearing in the stretched skin
   b. Mental and emotional disturbances may necessitate discontinuance of the medication.
   c. Hypertension and the tendency to retain water and sodium may result from steroid therapy.
      (1) Provide a low-sodium diet.
      (2) Weigh the child daily—report sudden weight increases.
   d. Steroids diminish the child's resistance to infection and may mask symptoms of infection.

▶ **NURSING ALERT:** Do not place a child with an infectious disease in the room with the child with rheumatic fever.
   Restrict visitors and personnel with infectious diseases from contact with the child on steroid therapy.

   e. A combination of steroid therapy and stress may lead to the development of gastric ulcers.
3. Administer medications punctually and at regular intervals to achieve constant therapeutic blood levels.
4. Report signs of increased rheumatic activity as salicylates or steroids are being tapered.

G. Alleviate the child's anxiety about the functioning of his heart, because anxiety utilizes energy and produces fatigue.

1. Give the child information about rheumatic fever in terms that he can understand, e.g., "Rheumatic fever is a hard thing to understand because you can't see it. When you scratch yourself, you can see the mark, and you can see the scratch heal. Rheumatic fever is something like that—only you can't see the healing because it happens to the tissue underneath the skin. (And sometimes it happens to the valves in the heart)"
2. Assure the child that physicians know how to treat rheumatic fever.
3. Communicate information about the child's reactions to all staff members in order to provide consistent information.

H. Decrease the cardiac workload until the acute inflammatory reaction has subsided.

1. Explain to the child the need for rest (usually prescribed for 4–12 weeks, depending on the severity of the disease and physician's preference).

2. Assure the child that bed rest will be imposed no longer than necessary.
3. Organize nursing care to provide periods of uninterrupted rest.
4. Assure the child that his needs will be met.
   a. Give the child a bell to call the nurse.
   b. Answer his calls promptly.
5. Assist the child to resume activity very gradually once he is asymptomatic at rest and indicators of acute inflammation have become normal.
   a. Allow the child to participate in decisions about such matters as timing his periods of activity.
   b. Monitor the pulse rate carefully after periods of activity in order to assess the degree of cardiac compensation.

I. Provide frequent and comfortable changes in position to aid in relaxation and to prevent tissue breakdown.

1. Elevate the back of the bed and support the arms with pillows when child is dyspneic.
2. Position the legs in good body alignment—use a footboard.
3. When the joints are painful, move the child gently, supporting the extremity.
4. Provide meticulous skin care.

J. Provide nursing care for the child with congestive heart failure.

Refer to section on congestive heart failure, pp. 1302–1304.

K. Provide safe, supportive care for the child with chorea.

1. Place the child in a bed with padded side rails, especially if uncontrolled body movements are severe.
2. Feed the child slowly and carefully because of incoordinate movements of the head, mouth, and swallowing muscles. Avoid the use of sharp eating utensils.
3. Provide frequent feedings that are high in calories, protein, vitamins, and iron, because constant movements cause the child to burn calories at a rapid rate.
4. Spend time talking with the child even though his speech may be defective. If severe, utilize other methods of communication.
5. Administer sedation, if prescribed.
6. Reassure the child about the cause of his instability and tell him that his symptoms will subside.
7. Encourage positive parent–child relationships which may have been strained if the onset of symptoms was insidious (lack of concentration at school, mood swings, irritability, etc.).
8. Help the child regain his former skills once symptoms begin to subside.
   a. Support the child during periods of ambulation.
   b. Provide activities that require the use of large muscles and progress to materials that require fine coordination.

L. Assist the child to develop a realistic attitude toward his illness and encourage him to discuss his concerns.

1. Help the child to realize the restrictions he must face and the fact that progress is slow.
2. Attempt to avoid negative connotations related to activity restrictions. Emphasize what the child is allowed to do—that is, say, "You may be up in the

chair for 2 hours every day," rather than "You have to stay in bed all day, except for 2 hours."

3. Alleviate the child's anxieties about keeping up with his class and school activities.
    a. Initiate a referral for a hospital-based school teacher to see him on a regular basis.
    b. When this service is not available, encourage the parents to contact his teacher, who will prepare lesson plans and short assignments for him—encourage the parents to maintain this contact with the teacher.
    c. Plan time each day on a regular basis for the child to complete his assignments.

M. Provide for diversional activity that will help the child feel a sense of achievement and satisfaction.

1. Initiate some long-term projects.
2. Refer to section on the hospitalized child, p. 1112.

N. Assist the family to deal with the emotional and financial stresses caused by the illness and hospitalization.

1. Assess the family's needs in this area and initiate a referral to a social worker if indicated.
2. Refer to section on family-centered care, p. 1117.

O. Prevent a recurrent attack of rheumatic fever by reinforcing the need for prophylactic antimicrobial therapy.

1. Penicillin is the drug of choice—either intramuscular benzathine G every 28 days or oral penicillin V or G twice daily.
2. Continuous prophylaxis is recommended throughout the childhood years and well into adult life, often indefinitely.
3. Utilize creativity in recommending methods to remind families about administering the medication.
    a. The child should be taught to assume responsibility for his own medication at an early age so that it becomes habitual.
    b. Some children profit from the use of a calendar or special chart. Others find it useful to associate their medication schedule with other routine tasks, such as brushing their teeth.
4. Be certain that the child receives his prophylactic medication on schedule during his hospitalization

and during subsequent hospitalizations (including hospitalization for treatment of other illnesses).

5. When indicated, additional prophylaxis should be utilized for prevention of infective endocarditis. The American Heart Association's recommendations for the prevention of endocarditis should be observed for children undergoing certain dental procedures as well as for surgery or instrumentation of the upper respiratory tract, genitourinary tract, or lower gastrointestinal tract.

P. Begin to prepare for discharge early enough with the parents in order that sufficient adjustments and preparation may be made.

1. The child should have a bed of his own and, preferably, a room of his own.
2. A responsible adult must be in the home to care for him.
3. Provide information about:
    a. Activity restrictions
    b. Medications—dosage, schedule, side effects
    c. Dietary instruction
    d. Symptoms to report—pain, malaise, anorexia, tachycardia, tachypnea, weight gain
    e. Telephone number of physician
    f. Follow-up appointment
4. Initiate a community nursing referral—this may be done prior to discharge if a home evaluation is desired.

For nursing care of the adult patient with rheumatic heart disease, refer to page 317.

Evaluation
Expected Outcomes

1. The child experiences relief of pain evidenced by facial expressions
2. Copes effectively with altered body-image evidenced by relaxed behavior
3. Conserves energy by resting and limiting activity
4. Engages in quiet activity that promotes cognitive development
5. Avoids injury during choreic movements
6. Avoids infection during treatment for rheumatic fever; or infections are recognized and treated promptly
7. Family accurately describes rheumatic fever and its treatment
8. The child does not have a recurrent attack of rheumatic fever

Myocarditis

Myocarditis is an inflammatory disease of the heart. The inflammation is rarely confined to the myocardium (isolated myocarditis), but is usually part of a pancarditis such as acute rheumatic carditis.

Etiology

1. Often unknown
2. Coxsackie B virus (most common pediatric cause)
3. Rheumatic fever
4. Other infectious agents—viruses, bacteria, fungi, spirochetes, rickettsiae, and parasites

5. Toxic causes—diphtheria, endotoxin, chemotherapeutic agents
6. Various multisystem diseases

Pathophysiology

1. The inflammatory process interferes with the effectiveness of myocardial contractility.
2. Cardiac enlargement occurs, and congestive heart failure frequently results.
3. Residual myocardial fibrosis may occur, causing sub-

sequent myocardial insufficiency and cardiac enlargement.
4. Prognosis is related to age at onset, extent of inflammation, response to therapy, and presence or absence of recurrences

Assessment

Clinical Manifestations

1. Variable, depending on age of child, extent of inflammation, and capacity of myocardium to recover; varies from total absence of clinical manifestations to sudden, unexpected death.
2. Neonate—often presents with sudden onset of congestive heart failure. Signs include respiratory distress, tachycardia, pale skin which is cool and clammy, peripheral cyanosis, diaphoresis, edema, and enlarged liver.
3. Older child:
   a. Onset may often be insidious, with complaints of fatigue, low-grade fever, respiratory illness, malaise, and gradual development of cardiac findings.
   b. Onset may be rapid with sudden temperature elevation, dyspnea, and rapid pulse.

Diagnostic Evaluation

1. Auscultation
   a. Heart sounds often indistinct, muffled, or dull.
   b. Systolic murmurs frequently present.
   c. Gallop rhythm common.
   d. Pulmonary crackles may be heard.
2. Palpation
   a. Peripheral pulses often rapid, weak, thready.
   b. May demonstrate pulsus alternans—a pulse in which there is regular alternation of weak and strong beats.
   c. May have hepatomegaly.
3. Chest x-ray—shows generalized cardiomegaly involving all four chambers of the heart. Pulmonary venous congestion is often visualized, and pneumonitis may be present.
4. Electrocardiogram is variable. It may reveal arrhythmias, conduction disturbances, and S–T segment changes.
5. Laboratory tests—cultures of blood, stool, nose, and throat; serial antibody testing.

Patient Problems/Nursing Diagnoses

1. Potential for sudden death related to cardiac arrhythmia and/or congestive heart failure
2. Respiratory distress related to decreased oxygen intake
3. Problems related to congestive heart failure (see p. 1303)
4. Fatigue related to reduced cardiac output
5. Potential for side effects of steroid therapy, including hypertension, altered body-image, gastrointestinal bleeding, decreased resistance to infection

Planning and Implementation

Nursing Interventions

A. Control the underlying disease causing myocarditis.

1. Administer specific therapy for treatable conditions such as rheumatic fever, toxoplasmosis, and trichinosis.

2. Administer steroid therapy as prescribed by the physician.
   a. Be aware that steroids are generally not recommended except for the treatment of rheumatic myocarditis with cardiac failure—to suppress the inflammatory process associated with connective tissue disorders, or in situations that are considered life-threatening.
   b. Prepare the child and his family for any expected side effects of steroid therapy:
      (1) Body appearance may change—for example, rounding of facial contours
      (2) Localized fat deposits
      (3) Appearance of acne or excessive hair
      (4) Weight gain with linear markings appearing in the stretched skin
   c. Be aware of serious side effects of steroid therapy and report promptly:
      (1) Gastrointestinal bleeding, ulcer
      (2) Hypertension and the tendency to accumulate water and sodium within tissues
         (a) Provide a low sodium diet.
         (b) Weigh the child daily—report sudden weight gain.
      (3) Diminished resistance to infection; may mask symptoms of infection.

▶ **NURSING ALERT:** Do not place a child with an infectious disease in the room with a child receiving steroid therapy. Restrict visitors and personnel with infectious diseases from contact with the child.

3. Maintain bed rest during the acute phase of the illness, usually 10–14 days.

B. Treat congestive heart failure.

1. Refer to section on congestive heart failure, page 1302.
2. Be aware that children with myocarditis frequently show increased sensitivity to digitalis and may require a lower dose. Assess for the toxic symptoms.

C. Observe for the development of cardiac arrhythmias.

1. Be aware that children with myocarditis are prone to develop arrhythmias.
2. Initiate continuous cardiac monitoring, especially if the child demonstrates dysrhythmias, anginal pain, or congestive heart failure. If appropriate, transfer the child to the intensive care unit.
3. Have equipment for resuscitation, cardiac defibrillation, and cardiac pacing available in the event of life-threatening arrhythmia.

D. Provide supportive nursing care to the severely ill or dying child.

Refer to section on the dying child, page 1495.

E. Evaluate the child for evidence of response to treatment or progression of disease.

1. Observe for the development or disappearance of signs of congestive heart failure.
2. Monitor and record the child's pulse, respirations, and blood pressure at frequent intervals.
   a. Count pulse for 1 full minute. Record rate and rhythm.
   b. Monitor the pulse when the child is asleep.

For additional nursing considerations, refer to the section

on Nursing Management of the Patient with Rheumatic Endocarditis, page 316.

Evaluation

Expected Outcomes

1. Absence of arrhythmias; shows no evidence of signs and symptoms of congestive heart failure

2. Regains normal breathing patterns and oxygen exchange as evidenced by normal vital signs and laboratory values
3. Remains on bed rest or reduces activity to conserve energy
4. Does not demonstrate side effects of steroid therapy
5. Copes effectively with the illness and treatment as evidenced by his verbal and nonverbal communication

Infective Endocarditis

Infective endocarditis refers to infection of the endocardial surface of the heart or the intimal surface of certain arterial vessels. It is a rare condition that is usually associated with preexisting cardiovascular disease (congenital or rheumatic) but may develop in a normal heart during a course of septicemia.

For etiology, clinical manifestations, pathophysiology, treatment and nursing management, refer to discussion on adult, page 314. In addition, the following points of management should be considered by the pediatric nurse.

Nursing Management

1. Although any child with heart disease is at risk for developing endocarditis, those most at risk are older (over 10 years of age) children with:
   a. Prosthetic valves
   b. Congenital aortic stenosis (repaired)
   c. Valvular deformities
   d. Systemic artery to pulmonary artery anastomosis
   e. Ventriculoatrial shunts
   f. Intravascular lines for medications or monitoring
   g. Transvenous pacemakers
2. Long-term (usually at least 4–6 weeks) intravenous administration of antimicrobials is indicated in all cases.
   a. Careful management of intravenous therapy is essential.
      (1) Refer to Intravenous Therapy Procedure, page 1160.
      (2) Drugs must be administered according to schedule to maintain constant therapeutic levels.
      (3) Notify appropriate personnel immediately if the IV infiltrates, so that it can be restarted.
      (4) Heparin locks may be utilized to allow the child freedom of movement between intervals of medication.

   b. Appropriate measures should be initiated to help the child maintain his level of development during the lengthy hospitalization.
      (1) Refer to The Hospitalized Child, page 1112.
      (2) Arrange for continuation of school work.
      (3) Facilitate interaction with family, including siblings.
      (4) Provide diversional activities that will help the child feel a sense of achievement and satisfaction.
      (5) Facilitate contact with peers through written correspondence, telephone, or selected visiting.
3. Prevention is an important nursing responsibility.
   a. Procedures which increase the risk of bacteria gaining access to the bloodstream include:
      (1) Tooth extraction, oral surgery, and periodontal procedures.
      (2) Tonsillectomy and adenoidectomy
      (3) Bronchoscopy
      (4) Instrumentation of the genitourinary tract
      (5) Surgery or instrumentation of the lower gastrointestinal tract
      (6) Childbirth
   b. Almost all children with congenital or rheumatic heart disease should receive prophylactic antibiotics in conjunction with these procedures to reduce bacteremia and prevent bacterial implantation. The current recommendations of the American Heart Association for chemoprophylaxis should be observed.
   c. The child and family should be instructed regarding the importance of good dental hygiene.
   d. Families of children with heart disease should be instructed about prevention of endocarditis, as well as about signs and symptoms of the disease.

Atherosclerosis

Atherosclerosis is a condition characterized by fatty deposits on the walls of arteries. It may lead to narrowing and obstruction of major vessels such as the coronary arteries, the arteries of the neck and brain, and those of the lower extremities. It is a cause of coronary heart disease and cerebrovascular disease.

Although the major clinical manifestations of atherosclerosis occur in middle-age and older adults, the pre-

cursors of atherosclerosis may become established in childhood. Thus, the pediatric nurse should be aware of the following factors:

1. Although much is known about the pathology of atherosclerosis and its evolution in adults, there is still much to be learned about its earlier stages.
2. The atherosclerotic process is probably influenced by a variety of inheritance factors, including vascular

structure and metabolism as well as environmental factors such as diet.

3. Data indicate that irreversible atherosclerotic changes may occur by 20 years of age. Therefore, the pediatric patient must be identified as being at risk in order for medical treatment to be instituted early enough to alter the course of the disease meaningfully.

Identified Risk Factors

1. Serum lipid disorders—may be genetically determined (e.g., inherited hypercholesterolemia) or acquired—probably resulting from an excess intake of saturated fat and cholesterol
2. Hypertension—probably caused by a hereditary predisposition, interacting with environmental factors such as obesity, increased sodium intake, and endogenous and exogenous vasoconstrictors
3. Impaired glucose tolerance
4. Obesity
5. Sedentary living habits, lack of regular exercise
6. Smoking

Nursing Interventions

A. Screen all children at risk for lipid abnormalities and correct these by diet or other procedures as indicated.

1. Infants of families with any history of familial hypercholesterolemia or premature cardiovascular disease should be studied for lipid abnormality. If negative, these children should receive periodic reevaluation.
2. All siblings of hyperlipoproteinemic children should be tested.

B. Screen children for hypertension at periodic intervals, and initiate appropriate treatment.

1. Refer to Procedure for Taking Blood Pressure, page 1134 and Normal Vital Sign Values, page 1133.

C. Initiate diet counseling.

1. Discourage the common habit of adding salt to childhood diets because the habit of adding salt to practically all foods is developed early in life.
2. Teach parents to read labels to learn the sodium content of commercial food products, including baby foods.
3. Counsel parents to provide meals that are low in cholesterol and saturated fats. Emphasize skimmed milk and dairy products derived from skimmed milk, legumes, fruits, whole grains, lean meats, poultry, and fish. Substitute margarine for butter. Deemphasize egg yolks, animal fat, and organ meats.
4. Discourage overeating and overfeeding.
5. Refer to section on Pediatric Nutrition, page 1094.

D. Encourage physical activity.

1. Discuss the benefits of physical activity with parents and encourage them to set an example for their children.
2. Encourage participation in physically active games and sports; this helps to establish a pattern for a physically active way of life in adulthood.

E. Discourage cigarette smoking.

1. Discuss the dangers of smoking with parents and encourage them to set a positive example for their children.
2. Make children aware of the dangers of smoking at an early age so that they will be less inclined to develop the habit during adolescence or adult life.

Bibliography

Books

Adams F and Emmanouilides G (eds). Heart Disease in Infants, Children, and Adolescents, 3rd ed. Baltimore, Williams & Wilkins, 1983

Anthony C and Arnon R. Textbook of Pediatric Cardiology. New Hyde Park, Medical Examination Publishing Co, 1983

Berenson G. Cardiovascular Risk Factors in Children. The Early Natural History of Atherosclerosis and Essential Hypertension. New York, Oxford University Press, 1980

Berwick D. Cholesterol, Children and Heart Disease. New York, Oxford University Press, 1980

Borman J and Gotsman M. Rheumatic Valvular Disease in Children. New York, Springer-Verlag, 1980

Eldredge W, Goldberg H and Lemole G. Current Problems in Congenital Heart Disease. New York, Spectrum Publications, 1979

Ingelfinger J. Pediatric Hypertension. Vol XXIV in the Series Major Problems in Clinical Pediatrics. Philadelphia, WB Saunders, 1982

Krovetz L, Gessner I and Schieber G. (eds). Handbook of Pediatric Cardiology, 2nd ed. Baltimore, University Park Press, 1979

Lauer R and Shekelle R. Childhood Prevention of Atherosclerosis. New York, Raven Press, 1980

Levin D, Morriss F and Moore G (eds). A Practical Guide to Pediatric Intensive Care, 2nd ed. St Louis, CV Mosby, 1984

Michaelson C (ed). Congestive Heart Failure. St Louis, CV Mosby, 1983

Moller J. Essentials of Pediatric Cardiology, 2nd ed. Philadelphia, FA Davis, 1978

Mustard W et al (eds). Pediatric Surgery, 3rd ed, Vol I. Chicago, Year Book Medical Publishers, 1979

Petrillo M and Sanger S. Emotional Care of Hospitalized Children, 2nd ed. Philadelphia, JB Lippincott, 1980

Rao PS (ed). Tricuspid Atresia. Mt. Kisco, NY, Futura Publishing Co, 1982

Rowe R and Freedom R. The Neonate with Congenital Heart Disease, 2nd ed, Vol V. In the Series: Major Problems in Clinical Pediatrics. Philadelphia, WB Saunders, 1981

Smith J. Pediatric Critical Care. New York, John Wiley & Sons, 1983

Whaley L and Wong D. Nursing Care of Infants and Children. St Louis, CV Mosby, 1983

Articles

Arciniegas E et al. Surgical closure of ventricular septal defect during the first twelve months of life. J Thorac Cardiovasc Surg 1980 Dec; 80(6):921–928

Bender H et al. Comparative operative results of the Senning and Mustard procedures for transposition of the great arteries. Circulation 1980 Suppl. I; 62(I):197–203

Berenson G et al. Cardiovascular risk factors in children: Should they concern the pediatrician? Am J Dis Child 1982 Sep; 136(9):855–863

Britton C. Blood pressure measurement and hypertension in children. Pediatr Nurs 1981 Jul/Aug; 7(4):13–17

Cleary T and Kohl S. Anti-infective therapy of infectious endocarditis. Pediatr Clin North Am 1983 Apr; 30(2):349–364

Cloutier J and Measel C. Home care for

the infant with congenital heart disease. Am J Nurs 1982 Jan; 82(1): 100–103

Cohen P, Maguire J and Weinstein L. Infective endocarditis caused by gram-negative bacteria: A review of the literature, 1945–1977. Prog Cardiovasc Dis 1980 Jan/Feb; 22(4):205–242

Cohen S. New concepts in understanding congestive heart failure. Part I. How the clinical features arise. Am J Nurs 1981 Jan; 81(1):119–142

Cohen S. New concepts in understanding congestive heart failure. Part II. How the therapeutic approaches work. Am J Nurs 1981 Feb; 81(2):357–380

Committee on Nutrition, American Academy of Pediatrics. Toward a prudent diet for children. Pediatrics 1983 Jan; 71(1):78–80

Committee on Rheumatic Fever and Infective Endocarditis of the Council on Cardiovascular Disease in the Young. Circulation 1984 Dec; 70(6): 1123A–1127A

Crow T et al. Assessing potential predisposition of elementary school children to heart disease. Prevention of bacterial endocarditis. J Sch Health 1982 Dec; 52(10):601–604

Diehl A. Clinical aspects of rheumatic fever: An update. Issues Compr Pediatr Nurs 1980 Apr; 4(2):69–76

DiSciascio G and Taranta A. Rheumatic fever in children. Am Heart J 1980 May; 99(5):635–658

Engle M. Heart sounds and murmurs in diagnosis of heart disease. Pediatr Ann 1981 Mar; 10(3):18–31

Engle M. Management of the child after cardiac surgery. Pediatr Ann 1981 Apr; 10(4):53–60

Furgal C. Pediatric cardiology: stressors, reactions and interventions. Issues Compr Pediatr Nurs 1981 Jan/Feb; 5(1):21–32.

Fyler D. Report of the New England Regional Infant Cardiac Program. Pediatrics 1980 Feb; 65(2, Suppl):377–461

Gale A et al. Fontan procedure for tricuspid atresia. Circulation 1980 Jul; 62(1):91–96

Gay W. Cardiac surgery in infancy. Pediatr Ann 1981 Apr; 10(4):145–148

Gersony W and Bierman F. Cardiac catheterization in the pediatric patient. Pediatrics 1981 May; 67(5):738–740

Hazinski M. Critical care of the pediatric cardiovascular patient. Nurs Clin North Am 1981 Dec; 16(4):671–697

Heyman S. Correcting transposition of the great arteries. AORN J 1982 Jul; 36(1):35–44

Jatene A et al. Anatomic correction of transposition of the great arteries. J Thorac Cardiovasc Surg 1982 Jan; 83(1):20–26

Jones Criteria (revised) for guidance in the diagnosis of rheumatic fever. Circulation 1984 Jan; 69(1):204A–208A

Lewandowski L. Stresses and coping styles of parents of children undergoing open-heart surgery. Crit Care Q 1980 Jun; 3(1):75–84

Lewis A et al. Side effects of therapy with prostaglandin E. in infants with critical congenital heart disease. Circulation 1981 Nov; 64(5):893–898

Marsh B, Dubes M and Boosinger J. Adolescent hypertension and significant variables: Weight, height and skinfold thickness. Pediatr Nurs 1983 Jul/Aug; 9(4):287–289

Miller W et al. Pediatric cardiology—minimizing the risks of adult heart disease . . . The young cardiac patient: management considerations. Pediatr Nurs 1980 Jan/Feb; 5(1):29–38

Neal W et al. Care of the critically ill neonate with heart disease. Crit Care Q 1981 Jun; 4(1):47–58

Nora J. Identifying the child at risk for coronary disease as an adult. A strategy for prevention. J Pediatr 1980 Nov; 97(5):706–714

Slota M. Pediatric cardiac catheterization: Complications and interventions. Crit Care Nurse 1982 May/Jun; 2(3):22+

Strattford M, Griffiths S and Gersony W. Coarctation of the aorta: A study in delayed detection. Pediatrics 1982 Feb; 69(2):159–163

Turley K, Tucker W and Ebert P. The changing role of palliative procedures in the treatment of infants with congenital heart disease. J Thorac Cardiovasc Surg 1980 Feb; 79(2):194–201

Yeh T et al. Intravenous indomethacin therapy in premature infants with patent ductus arteriosus. Am J Dis Child 1982 Sep; 136(9):803–807

Agencies

American Heart Association
7320 Greenville Avenue
Dallas, TX 75231

National Heart, Lung and Blood Institute
National High Blood Pressure Education
Program
National Institutes of Health
Bethesda, MD 20892

Digestive Disorders, Pediatric Considerations

37

Dental Caries

Dental caries involves loss of tooth structure or the formation of a cavity as a result of bacterial attack—first on the enamel, which is the hard surface of the tooth, and then progressing inward toward the pulp.

Etiology and Altered Physiology

A. Bacteria

1. Acidogenic organisms—decalcify the hard tissue by producing acids on the tooth surface.
2. Proteolytic organisms—digest the product of tooth surface (decalcification thus produces odor and discoloration).
3. Leptotrichae organisms—form structures on the smooth tooth surface which houses acidogenic organisms.

B. Contributing Factors

1. Age—most susceptible age-groups are children, 4–8 years (primary teeth), and adolescents, 12–18 years (permanent teeth).
2. Diet—large intake of simple sugars between meals, milk-bottle caries in infants and toddlers.
3. Familial tendency to tooth decay.
4. Lack of proper oral hygiene.
5. Poor state of health (illness alters the normal bacteriostatic quality of saliva), chronic disease.

Complications

As a result of missing teeth or multiple caries, the child may experience many problems:
1. Poor nutrition
   a. Refusal to eat foods that need chewing
   b. Teeth drift and cause malocclusion
2. Faulty speech habits and articulation
   a. Weak jaw muscles
   b. Abnormal alveolar bone development
3. Psychological problems
   Embarrassment caused by appearance of teeth and oral odor
4. Oral foci of infection
   Subacute bacterial endocarditis may result in child with congenital heart disease.

Prevention

1. Regular frequent dental observation by dental professional

2. Decreased eating between meals
3. Fluoridation of water supply
4. Biannual topical application of fluoride to teeth
5. Decreased eating of sucrose-containing snacks
6. Removal of plaque and debris from tooth surface with brushing

Clinical Manifestations

1. Decay is acute and rapidly penetrates the tooth in children.
2. Caries occur where food debris collects.
   a. Pits and fissures
   b. Between teeth
   c. At neck of tooth
3. Discoloration of teeth.
4. Decay odor.
5. Pain, abscess, or infection.

Treatment

1. Removal of decay and restoration of tooth surfaces involved.
2. Removal of diseased tooth or teeth that are decayed beyond restoration.

Patient Problems/Nursing Diagnoses

1. Anxiety related to hospitalization and surgery
2. Potential for alteration in nutrition related to long-standing caries or missing teeth and malocclusion
3. Potential for faulty speech habits and articulation related to weak jaw muscles, abnormal alveolar bone development, and missing teeth
4. Potential for infection related to poor oral hygiene
5. Knowledge deficit of adequate nutrition and oral hygiene practices

Nursing Interventions

Hospitalization of a child for treatment of dental caries is likely only when special behavior difficulties are anticipated in treatment, when medical problems complicate dental treatment or when extensive repair is necessary. (See Preventive Pediatrics, Dental Care, p. 1102.)

A. Prevent dental caries in all patients.

The nurse should be an active member on the dental health care team in preventive education by motivating the child and family toward good dental hygiene and nutritional practices.

B. Know that there is a direct relationship between incidence of dental caries in children and dental health education or knowledge of parents.

1. Assess parental knowledge and use opportunities to teach parents preventive care.
2. Encourage parental participation with the young child during teeth-brushing exercise.

C. Know the principles of good oral hygiene and practice them when caring for each pediatric patient.

1. Encourage mouth rinsing or teeth brushing after eating.
Brush before bedtime to decrease bacteriogenic activity in the warm, undisturbed mouth during sleep.
2. Encourage proper brushing of teeth.
   a. Brush crosswise with a soft-bristled brush.
   b. Electric tooth brush cleans teeth and stimulates the gingivae.
3. Supervise brushing in young children. (Dentrifice is not necessary.)

D. Know the value of good nutrition and its effect in preventing dental caries.

1. No between-meal snacking with refined-sugar foods. No gum chewing, except of sugarless gum.
   a. Improves appetite at meals.
   b. Substitute fresh fruit for refined sugars. (No lollipops between meals; give after meal before brushing.)
2. Discourage a bottle, other than water, at bedtime or before sleep.
Residue is left on teeth during long periods of sleep and results in rampant decay.

E. Know the value of periodic dental examination and preventive measures used to decrease decay.

1. Encourage patient and parent to participate in regular dentist visits.
   a. Regular visits for cleaning and checking for decay; repair if necessary.
   First visit is to familiarize the young child with the dentist and equipment.

(1) Usually age 18–30 months—or when all primary teeth have erupted
(2) Should not be when the child has a toothache
   b. During childhood and adolescence, visits are every 3–6 months.
   New decay appears suddenly in multiple areas and advances rapidly.
2. If fluoridation is not supplied in community water, topical application is advisable.
   a. Most effective when applied on newly erupted teeth.
   b. Fluoride makes enamel more resistant to decay as it strengthens calcification of the developing dental tissue.

F. Keep the adolescent aware of his diet and its effect on dental decay.

1. Keep in mind diet fads and peer-group pressure.
2. Have the patient keep a dietary record for 1 week. Then evaluate it against an example of a good, nutritious diet. Encourage the patient to make his own evaluation.

Health Education

1. After assessment of parental knowledge has been made, embark on a teaching program.
Main areas of concern:
   a. Proper technique of dental hygiene
   b. Value of good nutrition
   c. Value of fluoridation
   d. Importance of regular visits to the dentist every 3–6 months.
2. American Dental Association, 211 East Chicago Avenue, Chicago, IL 60611

Expected Outcomes

1. Experiences minimal anxiety; relaxed behavior; restful sleep; willingness to engage in play activities
2. Achieves improved nutritional status; alert appearance; weight gain
3. Demonstrates improved speech habits and articulation
4. Is free of infection as evidenced by normal vital signs and laboratory values
5. Patient/parent verbalize understanding of nutritional practices and demonstrate care of the child's teeth

Cleft Lip and Palate

Cleft lip and palate facial malformation results when fusion involving the first brachial arch fails to take place during embryonic development.

Etiology

1. Failure of embryonic development—cause not known
2. Hereditary factor
3. May be related to mutant genes, chromosomal abnormalities, teratogens

Incidence

1. Cleft lip—approximately 1:1,000 births; more frequent in males (with or without cleft palate).
2. Cleft palate—approximately 1:2,500 births; more frequent in females.
3. Combination of cleft lip and palate account for about 50%, cleft lip about 25%, and cleft palate about 25%.

Altered Physiology

1. The lip and palate develop independently; thus, any combination of defects can occur.
   a. Cleft lip—prealveolar cleft
      (1) Varies from a notch in the lip to complete separation of the lip into the nose.
      (2) May be unilateral or bilateral.
      (3) Failure of maxillary process to fuse with nasal elevations on frontal prominence—normally occurs during 5th–6th week of gestation.
      (4) Merging of upper lip at midline is complete between 7th and 8th week of gestation.
   b. Isolated cleft palate—postalveolar cleft
      (1) Cleft of uvula
      (2) Cleft of soft palate

(3) Cleft of both soft and hard palate through roof of mouth
(4) Unilateral or bilateral
(5) Failure of mesodermal masses of lateral palatine process to meet and fuse—normally occurs between 7th and 12th week of gestation.
c. Cleft lip and palate combined
Any degree of involvement
d. Submucous cleft
(1) Muscles of soft palate are not joined.
(2) Not recognized until child talks; cannot be seen at birth.
2. Associated problems
a. Eating
(1) Suction cannot be created for effective sucking
(2) Food returns through the nose
b. Nasal speech
c. Lack of normal dental function and appearance
d. Repeated bouts of otitis media with subsequent hearing loss

Complications

1. Associated problems:
a. Pierre Robin syndrome
b. Intellectual deficits
2. Long-term problems:
a. Speech impairment
b. Improper tooth placement
c. Recurring otitis media
d. Hearing impairment
e. Faulty social adjustment related to poor self-concept and abnormal speech

Clinical Manifestations

Physical appearance of cleft lip or palate
1. Incompletely formed lip
2. Opening in roof of mouth felt with examiner's finger on palate

Treatment

1. General management is focused on closure of the cleft(s), prevention of complications, habilitation, and facilitation of normal growth and development of the child.
2. The cleft lip is generally repaired before the palate defect.
a. Immediate repair, or
b. Repair done when infant is 6–12 weeks of age, hemoglobin 10 g./dl., steady weight gain seen.
3. Cleft palate repair may be done anytime between 6 months and 5 years—based on degree of deformity, width of oropharynx, neuromuscular function of palate and pharynx, and surgeon preference.

Patient Problems/Nursing Diagnoses

1. Alteration in facial and/or oral integrity related to failure of embryonic development
2. Alteration in nutritional intake and status related to facial/oral deformity
3. Infection and aspiration related to cleft palate
4. Speech and hearing problems related to oral malformation
5. Altered parent–child relationship related to the child's appearance
6. Faulty social adjustment related to self-image and abnormal speech

7. Patient anxiety related to hospitalization and treatments

Planning and Implementation
Nursing Intervention
Newborn

A. Show acceptance of the baby.

1. The nurse must maintain her composure and not show shock when handling the infant. The manner in which the nurse handles the baby can make a lasting impression on the parents.
a. The baby with a cleft lip can be unattractive and can cause shock when first seen.
b. When showing a newborn baby to parents for the first time, support them by accepting both the baby and the parents' feelings. Parents may be grieving about the perfect infant they did not have and may harbor ambivalent feelings about this baby.
c. The sequence of normal parental responses may include shock and disbelief, sadness, anxiety and anger, and then proceed to a state of equilibrium and reorganization.
d. Be supportive of the parents by reassuring them that reparative surgery can be done with much success.
(1) The time when reparative surgery is done depends on the surgeon, the condition of the baby, and the degree to which the parents have accepted the baby.
(2) Lip surgery may be done several hours after birth or when the infant is 2–3 months of age or has gained 4.54 kg. (10 lbs), and hemoglobin is 10 g./dl.
2. Reparative surgery of the palate is usually done between 12 and 24 months of age.
At this age, speech patterns have not been set, yet growth of involved structures allows for improved surgical repair.
b. If repair is delayed to age 4 or 5 years, a special denture palate is used to help occlude the cleft and aid in establishing speech patterns.

B. Establish and maintain adequate nutrition for growth and development.

1. Babies with just a cleft lip may feed well if a soft nipple with enlarged holes is used.
2. With certain types and combinations of cleft lips and palates, the baby is unable to create a vacuum and is thus unable to suck.
a. Several types of nipples and feeding devices are available to make feedings easier.
b. A soft base or disposable bottle can be helpful by applying gentle, constant pressure to maintain flow.
c. Feeding devices include regular nipple with enlarged holes: Lamb's nipple, Duckey nipple, Brecht feeder, Beniflex disposable nurser,* and Premi nipple.
d. Rubber-tipped asepto syringe or dropper. (Rubber extension should be long enough to extend back into the mouth to prevent regurgitation through the nose.)
3. Feed baby in an upright, sitting position to decrease

---

* Mead Johnson & Company.

possibility of fluid being aspirated or returned through the nose, or back to the auditory canal.

   a. Feed slowly; place the nipple in the infant's mouth so it can be compressed between the existing palate and tongue.
   b. Bubble frequently during feeding, because these babies swallow a great deal of air.
   c. Avoid repeated removal of nipple from the infant's mouth because of fear of choking because this only frustrates the infant, causing him to cry and increasing chances of aspiration.
   d. Smaller but more frequent feedings may be necessary if the infant tires or requires an extended period of time to eat.
4. Advance diet as appropriate for age and needs of the baby.
   Eating often improves when solids are introduced, since they are easier for the baby to manipulate.
5. Encourage the mother to begin feeding the infant herself as soon as possible. Use feeding time to help mother and infant develop their relationship.

C. Prevent infection in the child so that surgery will not have to be delayed.

1. Avoid patient contact with anyone who has an infection.
2. Change the baby's position frequently.
3. Clean the cleft after each feeding with clear water and a cotton-tipped applicator.

D. Support the respiratory efforts and the feeding and nutritional needs of the infant with Pierre Robin syndrome. (Features of Pierre Robin syndrome are cleft palate, glossoptosis [tongue falls back on pharynx], and micrognathia [underdeveloped mandible].)

1. Prevent respiratory obstruction, especially on inspiration and when the infant is quiet.
   a. Place the infant in prone position so that tongue and jaw fall forward.
   b. Tilt head back as best tolerated by the infant and slightly elevate upper trunk.
   c. Stockinette cap securely attached to the infant's head and suspended from an overhead support may be of some benefit in assisting the infant to maintain a position for easy ventilation.
   d. Suction nasopharynx as needed.
   e. The tongue may be sutured to pull it forward; if this is done, observe for slipping, cut tongue, and infection.
2. When this infant is fed, consideration must be given to his respiratory effort, flaccid tongue and cleft palate. Generally, feeding can be done with a nursing bottle (feeding techniques similar to those used for cleft palate).
   a. Use orthopneic position—vertical and slightly forward; this allows infant to push jaw forward to suck and also allows the feeder a clear view of the infant.
   b. Gentle finger pressure by feeder at mandibular attachment can aid in bringing jaw forward.
   c. Feed slowly.
3. By 3–4 months of age, the mandible has grown enough to accommodate the tongue, and respiratory difficulty is greatly diminished.
4. Additional complications associated with Pierre Robin syndrome are slow weight gain and ear infections.

E. Assist parents in preparing to take the newborn home from the nursery before lip and palate surgery have been done.

Health Education

1. Prepare the mother for home feedings. She should have several days to practice feeding in order to become familiar with the baby's feeding pattern.
   a. Home equipment should be used in the hospital.
   b. The mother should be aware of difficulties with feeding and how to manage them.
      (1) Formula returning through the nose
      (2) Respiratory distress
      (3) Longer time necessary for feeding
   c. Suggest that about a week or so prior to scheduled admission for surgery, the mother begin using feeding technique preferred by surgeon for postoperative feeding.
      (1) Side of spoon
      (2) Rubber-tipped dropper
      (3) Toddler cup
2. Encourage the parents to prepare siblings at home for the arrival of this baby. (Pictures of the new baby might be suggested.)
3. Initiate a community nurse referral to continue emotional support and teaching program at home.
4. Offer parents available literature about children with cleft lip and palate.*
5. Parents should know what plans have been started for surgical treatment.
6. Social work referral may be indicated.
   a. To listen to the mother express her concerns regarding management at home with a handicapped child.
   b. To arrange financial assistance.

F. Be aware of the complexity of long-range care and the importance of the many disciplines involved in the eventual outcome. The nurse should know all the ramifications and potential problems for this child and his family.

1. The organization of trained professional people from the many disciplines that become involved include pediatrician, plastic surgeon, otologist, general dentist, orthodontist, prosthodontist, medical-social worker, nurse, speech therapist, and psychologist.
2. Long-term follow-up and reparative surgery:
   a. Chronic otitis media and hearing loss (The auditory canal is abnormally located.)
   b. Lip, palate, and orthodontic repair
   c. Speech therapy
   d. Psychological insult to the child
3. Financial burden on the family
   State programs for crippled children can offer relief.
4. Psychological trauma to the family

* Snyder GB et al. *Your Cleft Lip and Palate Child: A Guide for Parents.* Florida CP Association, Mead Johnson & Company Laboratory, (ND)
   The Child with a Cleft Palate, US Department of Health and Human Services, Social and Rehabilitation Service.
Booklets sponsored by Mead Johnson & Company Laboratories, Evansville, IN 47721:
   Road to Normalcy for the Cleft Lip and Palate Child
   Steps in Habilitation for the Cleft Lip and Palate Child

G. **Emphasize the importance of the mother's role in caring for the child during outpatient treatment and the many hospitalizations required.**

The mother can offer a great deal of security to the child when he is subjected to the trauma and frightening experiences of treatment.

Preoperative Care of the Child with a Cleft Lip

A. **Prepare the infant for postoperative care so that it will be familiar to him, less frightening, and easier for him to accept after surgery.**

1. Practice the feeding method to be used as preferred by the surgeon
   a. Rubber-tipped syringe or asepto syringe
   b. Side of spoon
2. Elbow restraints may be used for short periods of time.
   a. Let the child play with them if he is old enough.
   b. Allow the mother to become involved in their use.
   c. Jacket restraint may be necessary in the older child to prevent him from rolling over, and rubbing against the sheets
3. Help the infant get used to being on his back or propped on his side for long periods of time.

B. **Prepare the mother** (parents) **as to what to expect when she sees the child postoperatively.**

1. Explain the use of the Logan bow (a curved metal wire that prevents stress on the suture line) and restraints.
2. Encourage the mother to be with the infant, especially when he wakes up from anesthesia, to offer him security and comfort.

Postoperative Care of the Child with a Cleft Lip

A. **Administer good postoperative care based on general principles and observe for usual postoperative complications.**

B. **Prevent injury to the suture line of the lip.**

1. Elbow restraints are the most effective way to prevent busy hands from reaching the lip, yet still allow some freedom of movement.
   a. Pad restraint and place it from the axilla to inner aspect of the wrist.
   b. Remove restraints occasionally, one at a time, to exercise the arms.
   c. Restraints or cuff of shirt may need to be pinned to the bed to decrease chances of the infant rubbing his lip with his upper arm.
2. Logan bow, butterfly-type adhesive, or Band-Aid placed cheek-to-cheek across top of lip prevents lateral tension.
   Prevent wetting tape, or it will loosen.
3. Prevent the infant from crying, because crying also increases tension on the suture line.
   a. Encourage the mother to hold and cuddle the infant.
   b. Keep the infant dry, fed, and comfortable.
4. Position the infant on his back or propped on his side to keep him from rubbing his lip on the sheets. An infant seat may be useful for variation of position, comfort, and entertainment. Provide for appropriate diversional activity, hanging toys, mobiles, etc.

C. **Maintain adequate nutrition and fluid intake for weight gain, growth, and prevention of dehydration.**

1. For several days postoperatively, feeding will have to be accomplished without tension on the suture line.
   a. Dropper or syringe with a rubber tip, inserted from the side to avoid suture line or to avoid stimulating sucking.
   b. Side of spoon (Never put spoon into the mouth.)
   c. Nasogastric gavage—usually last treatment of choice
2. Advance slowly to nipple feeding as indicated by physician preference.
   The infant should be able to suck more efficiently with the lip repaired.
3. Encourage the mother to participate as much as possible in the care of the infant. It is good for both infant and mother to continue their relationship.

D. **Keep the suture line clean to decrease infection and eliminate crust formation which enlarges the resulting scar.**
   The sutures are removed from 3–14 days after surgery.

1. Clean suture line after every feeding.
   a. The cleansing solution used is usually the physician's choice.
      (1) Water
      (2) Hydrogen peroxide
      (3) Saline solution
   b. Gently and frequently wipe with a wet cotton-tipped applicator.
   c. Gently dry by patting.
      (1) May use antibiotic ointment or petrolatum after drying.
      (2) May be left open to the air.
   d. Water should be given after feeding to cleanse the mouth.

Preoperative Care of the Child with a Cleft Palate
(Repair may require several operations.)

A. **Be familiar with growth and development as well as the emotional and psychological needs of the toddler, 12–18 months old.** (This is the age most common for palate repair.)

1. Primary objectives for palate repair are to improve speech and to minimize maxillary growth retardation and dental alveolar deformity.
2. This toddler age is selected because the anatomical structures involved are still growing.
3. The toddler finds the hospital strange and frightening (see p. 1114).
   a. Encourage the mother to stay with the child if possible.
   b. Encourage play.

B. **Prepare the child for postoperative care; if he is familiar with the procedures and routines, he will be less frightened and more likely to cooperate.**

1. Use elbow restraints frequently for short periods of time.
2. Do not allow the child to suck from a bottle. Ideally, he has been taught to drink from a cup. Feed him in the manner in which he will be fed postoperatively.

3. Practice frequent mouth irrigations using the same solution and equipment to be used postoperatively. Allow the child to handle and become familiar with equipment.

C. Prevent infection by keeping the child away from anyone with infection.

D. Prepare the parents as to what to expect when they see the child postoperatively.

Include the parents in the preparation of the child. Then, with the parents alone discuss in more depth what to expect.

Postoperative Care of the Child with a Cleft Palate

A. Administer good postoperative care and observe for possible postoperative complications.

1. Breathing with a closed palate is different from the child's customary way of breathing; the child must also contend with increased mucous production.
2. Note respiratory effort.
3. Croup tent with mist decreases occurrence of respiratory problems and provides moisture to mucous membranes which may become dry because of mouth breathing.
4. Infant may lie on abdomen.

B. Prevent injury to the suture line in the mouth.

1. Use elbow restraints.
2. Do not put anything into the mouth. Do not allow the use of straws, eating utensils, fingers.
3. Prevent the child from crying. Blowing, sucking, talking, and laughing put strain on the suture line.

C. Keep the suture line and mouth clean to prevent infection.

1. Irrigate the mouth with normal saline solution or water.
   a. Direct a gentle stream over the suture line using an ear bulb syringe.
   b. Have the child in sitting position with his head forward.
2. Keep the mouth moist to promote healing and provide comfort.
3. Rinse the mouth after each feeding.

D. Maintain adequate nutrition for growth and to promote healing.

1. Diet progresses from clear liquids to full liquids to soft foods.
   Soft foods are usually continued for about 1 month after surgery at which time a regular diet is started, excluding hard food.
2. Check weight periodically to see if adequate nutrition is being maintained.
3. Feed the child in the manner used preoperatively (cup, side of spoon, or rubber-tipped syringe). Never use straw, nipple, or plain syringe.

E. Administer antibiotics as prescribed.

The mouth and suture line are constantly contaminated.

F. Provide opportunities for social relationships and play as soon as possible.

1. While the child must be restrained, he especially needs to have some stimulation and diversional activity.
2. A satisfactory relationship with the mother or the nurse can minimize frustration and discomfort from surgery and restraints.

G. Continue support of parents who have already encountered many frustrations in caring for the child, and foster continual parental acceptance of the child and his handicap.

1. Solicit assistance of social worker if appropriate; the mother may talk about problems she is having rearing a handicapped child.
2. Sincerely compliment the parents for the good work they have already done with this child.
3. Help the parents understand that this child can live a normal life in the community.

H. Begin discharge planning and health teaching soon after admission so the parents can learn how to care for the child at home.

1. Continued protection of the mouth.
   a. May need to use elbow restraints.
   b. A child this age will put everything into his mouth—restrict this.
   c. No sucking or blowing.
2. Diet of soft foods will need to be continued. Do not give this child lollipops.
3. Infection must be prevented.
   Continue to cleanse his mouth after eating.

Health Education

1. There are 3 specific times when parental teaching is vitally important for continual, effective management of the child:
   a. Management of the child with cleft lip and palate not yet repaired
   b. Preparing for lip or palate surgery
   c. Preparing for the patient's discharge following surgery
2. In each case specific instructions need to be given in the following areas:
   a. Good nutrition and feeding techniques
   b. Proper oral hygiene
   c. Prevention of injury to operative site
   d. Prevention of infection
   e. Function of therapy; purpose of any appliances plus proper use and care
   f. Plan for follow-up, especially after surgery
   g. Psychological and social development of the child—including speech therapy, hearing tests, and understanding of the normal sounds at specific stages of growth and development
3. Other members of the family must be considered.
   a. The child with a cleft lip or palate should not be thought of as sick, but as a child who has special needs. It is important to promote his individual growth and development, but he does not require attention all the time.
   b. The family should be included in his care, but they also must have a life of their own.
   c. The parents need time to themselves.
4. Help the parents realize that even though rehabilitation of the child is long, drawn-out, and expensive, the child can live a normal life.
   a. Have the parents discuss the child's problem with the school nurse, the teacher and other responsible adults who will have close contact with the child.
   b. Long-range planning should include detailed communication between the family and various disciplines.

(1) Collaborative effort between disciplines promotes the effectiveness of each discipline.
(2) Parents may need help in understanding the value of each discipline for the future well-being of their child.
Speech therapy is often one area where the value is not completely understood. This needs to be emphasized.

Support Agencies

Special Child Health Services, 2023 W. Ogden Avenue, Chicago, IL 60612
National Institute of Dental Research, Westwood Bldg, 5333 Westbard Avenue, Bethesda, MD 20205

Expected Outcomes

1. Demonstrates appropriate nutritional intake and status as evidenced by weight gain and eating habits
2. Is free of infection and aspiration as evidenced by normal vital signs and laboratory values
3. Parents show appropriate bonding and ability to care for child as evidenced by their actions, verbalization and demonstration of feeding and handling, etc., of child.
4. Develops a positive self-image and socialization as evidenced by play activity, interest in surroundings and outgoing behavior
5. Experiences minimal anxiety as evidenced by appropriate coping behaviors

Esophageal Atresia with Tracheoesophageal Fistula

Esophageal atresia is failure of the esophagus to form a continuous passage from the pharynx to the stomach during embryonic development. *Tracheoesophageal fistula* is the abnormal connection between the trachea and esophagus.

Etiology

1. Failure of embryonic development
2. Cause unknown in most cases

Altered Physiology

1. Failure of proper separation of the embryonic channel into the esophagus and trachea occurring during the 4th and 5th weeks of gestation.
2. Classification of esophageal atresia of most common types (see Fig. 37-1)
Type I—Proximal and distal segments of esophagus are blind; there is no connection to trachea—10%–15% of cases.
Type II—Proximal segment of esophagus opens into trachea by a fistula; distal segment is blind—very rare.
Type III—Proximal segment of esophagus has blind end: distal segment of esophagus connects into trachea by a fistula (most common; discussion is limited to this type—80%–90% of cases).
Type IV—Esophageal atresia with fistula between both proximal and distal ends of trachea and esophagus—very rare.
Type V—Both proximal and distal segments of esophagus open into trachea by a fistula; no esophageal atresia (H-type)—not usually diagnosed at birth.
3. Type III—Tracheoesophageal Fistula (TEF)
   a. Child is unable to swallow effectively.
   b. Saliva or formula accumulates in upper esophageal pouch and is aspirated into airway from spillover.
   c. Regurgitation of gastric acid through distal fistula.
      (1) Abdominal distention occurs as a result of air entering the lower esophagus via the fistula and passing into the stomach, especially when the child is crying.
      (2) Gastric distention may be severe enough to cause respiratory distress by elevation of the diaphragm.

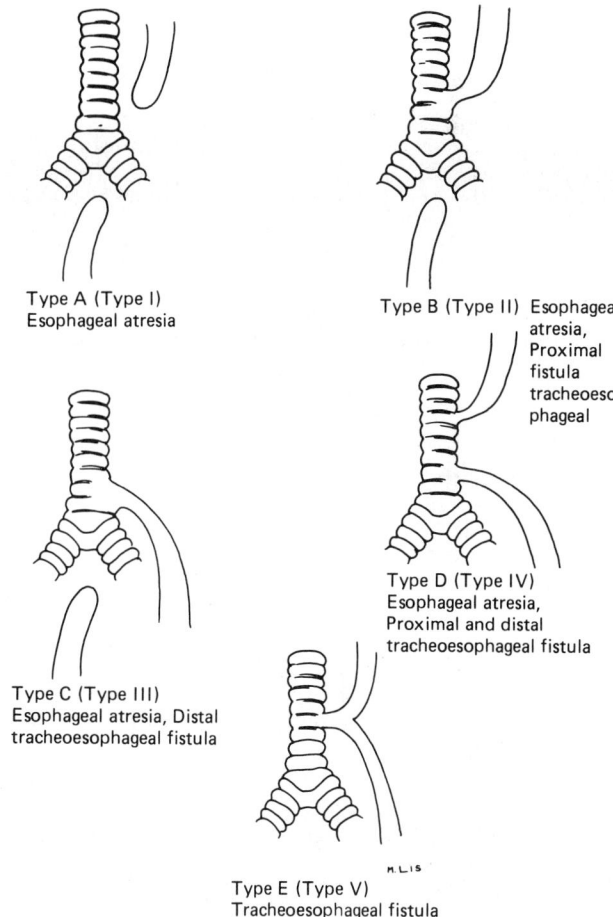

Type A (Type I)
Esophageal atresia

Type B (Type II) Esophageal atresia, Proximal fistula tracheoesophageal

Type C (Type III)
Esophageal atresia, Distal tracheoesophageal fistula

Type D (Type IV)
Esophageal atresia, Proximal and distal tracheoesophageal fistula

Type E (Type V)
Tracheoesophageal fistula (H-type)

Figure 37-1. Types of esophageal atresia: esophageal atresia and tracheoesophageal fistula (TE fistula). (Wieczorek RR and Natapoff JN. A Conceptual Approach to the Nursing of Children. Philadelphia, JB Lippincott, 1981, p. 370)

Complications Associated with TEF

1. Pneumonitis—secondary to
   a. Salivary aspiration
   b. Gastric acid reflux
2. Concomitant lesions
   a. Congenital heart disease
   b. Gastrointestinal anomalies, particularly imperforate anus
   c. Skeletal and muscular deformities
3. Prematurity

Postoperative Complications

1. Leak at anastomosis site
2. Recurrent fistulas
3. Esophageal strictures
4. Abnormal function of distal esophagus sphincter (gastroesophageal reflux) and esophagitis
5. Tracheomalacia
6. Feeding problems with the older child

Clinical Manifestations

Appear soon after birth
1. Excessive amount of secretions
   a. Constant drooling
   b. Large amount of secretions from nose
2. Intermittent cyanosis—unexplained; laryngospasm caused by aspiration of accumulated saliva in blind pouch
3. Abdominal distention
   Inspired air from trachea passes through fistula into stomach.
4. If fed, the infant will respond violently after first or second swallow.
   a. The infant coughs and chokes.
   b. Fluid returns through nose and mouth.
   c. Cyanosis occurs.
   d. The infant struggles.
5. Inability to pass catheter through nose or mouth into stomach—tip of catheter will stop at blind pouch, or atresia.

Note: Be aware of coiling of catheter; coiling may make catheter *appear* to be descending into stomach.

Diagnostic Evaluation

1. Recognize infants at risk for TEF. Two major groups are at risk:
   a. Infants with polyhydramnios
   b. Premature infants
2. Observations of specific symptoms manifested by infant.
3. Inability to pass a stiff, radiopaque 10–14 Fr. catheter into stomach through nose or mouth.
4. X-ray, flat plate of abdomen and chest—reveals presence of gas in stomach and tip of catheter in blind pouch

Treatment

1. Immediate treatment
   a. Propping infant at 30-degree angle to prevent reflux of gastric content
   b. Suctioning of upper esophageal pouch with Replogle tube or sump drain
   c. Gastrostomy to decompress stomach and prevent aspiration; later used for feedings
2. Appropriate treatment of any existing pathologic processes—either acquired complications, such as pneumonitis, or complications from concomitant lesions, such as congestive heart failure.

3. Supportive therapy—meeting nutritional requirements, IV fluids, antibiotics, respiratory support, maintaining thermally neutral environment
4. Surgery
   a. Prompt primary repair—division of fistula followed by esophageal anastomosis of proximal and distal segments (infant is greater than 2,000 gm and is without pneumonia).
   b. Short-term delay—subsequent primary repair—used to stabilize infant and to prevent deterioration when the patient's condition contraindicates immediate surgery.
   c. Staging—initial fistula division and gastrostomy with later secondary esophageal anastomosis. Approach may be used with a very small premature infant or a very sick neonate, or when severe congenital anomalies exist.
   d. Circular esophagomyotomy—on proximal pouch to gain length and allow for primary anastomosis at initial surgery.
   e. Cervical esophagostomy—when ends of esophagus are too widely separated; esophageal replacement with segment of intestine is done at 18–24 months of age.

Patient Problems/Nursing Diagnoses

1. Respiratory distress and altered oxygen–carbon dioxide exchange related to excessive nasopharyngeal secretions and gastric secretions refluxing into the tracheobronchial tree
2. Alteration in nutritional intake related to tracheal–esophageal reflux
3. Potential for alteration in electrolyte and fluid balance related to lack of oral nutrition and gastric fluid loss
4. Potential for complications (i.e., temperature instability) related to prematurity
5. Parental anxiety related to the child's illness and insecurity in caring for the child

Preoperative Nursing Intervention

A. Position the infant with head and chest elevated 20–30 degrees to prevent or decrease reflux of gastric juices into the tracheobronchial tree.

1. This position may also ease respiratory effort by dropping the distended intestines away from the diaphragm.
2. Prone position will allow gastric juices to pool anteriorly away from the esophagus. Turn frequently to prevent atelectasis and pneumonia.

B. Assist in removing nasopharyngeal secretions from esophageal blind pouch and support the infant's respiration.

1. Intermittent nasopharyngeal suctioning or indwelling Replogle tube (double lumen tube) or sump tube with constant suction is used.
   a. Tip of tube is placed in the blind pouch.
   b. Replogle or sump tube allows air to be drawn in via a second lumen and prevents tube obstruction by mucous membrane of pouch.
   c. Maintain indwelling tube patency by irrigating with 1 ml. normal saline solution frequently.
   d. Change indwelling tube as needed and at least once every 12–24 hours (by the physician); alternate nostrils. Take care to prevent necrosis of nostrils from pressure by catheter.

2. Place the infant in an Isolette or under a radiant warmer with high humidity to aid in liquefying secretions and thick mucus. Give mouth care.
3. Administer oxygen as needed.
4. Suction mouth to keep clear of secretions and prevent aspiration.
5. Be alert for indications of respiratory distress:
   a. Retractions
   b. Circumoral cyanosis
   c. Restlessness
   d. Nasal flaring
   e. Increased respiration and heart rate
6. The infant is to receive nothing by mouth.

C. Administer antibiotics and other medications prescribed.

Give to prevent or treat associated pneumonitis.

D. Monitor parenteral fluids as prescribed in order to prevent dehydration and electrolyte imbalance (see p. 1159).

1. Supplies water and caloric and mineral requirements.
2. The infant does not receive oral feedings.

E. Observe infant carefully for any change in condition; report changes immediately.

1. Check vital signs, color, amount of secretions, abdominal distention, and respiratory distress.
2. Also be alert for complications that can occur in any neonate or premature infant.

F. Prevent infection by using the principles of isolation.

Isolette may be used for environmental isolation.

G. Be available and recognize need for emergency care or resuscitation.

Accompany the infant to the x-ray department or the operating room in Isolette with portable oxygen and suction equipment.

H. Administer supportive nursing care that will prevent any deterioration of infant's condition and will assist in preparation for surgery.

1. Careful observations, recording and reporting of any signs or symptoms that may indicate additional congenital anomalies or complications.
2. Maintain the infant's temperature in thermoneutral zone.
3. Gastrostomy tube may be placed prior to definitive surgery to aid in gastric decompression and prevention of reflux. The gastrostomy tube is generally attached to straight gravity drainage, and irrigation is not done before surgery.

I. Ensure that bougie dilatation (should it be done) **remains undisturbed.**

Postoperative Nursing Interventions

There are 2 types of surgery considered for esophageal atresia with tracheoesophageal fistula: (1) fistula division and esophageal anastomosis (called *primary repair*) and (2) palliative surgery temporarily using a gastrostomy and cervical esophagostomy until the infant gains weight so that a bowel transplant or anastomosis can be done. Generally the nursing care is essentially the same for either procedure.

A. Administer good postoperative care and observe for signs of possible complications.

B. Maintain a patent airway to prevent oxygen starvation, apnea, and aspiration of secretions.

1. Request that the physician mark a suction catheter, indicating how far the catheter can be safely inserted without disturbing the anastomosis.
   a. Suction frequently—every 5–10 minutes may be necessary; at least every 1–2 hours.
   b. Observe for signs of obstructed airway.
2. Administer chest physiotherapy as prescribed by physician.
   a. Change the infant's position by turning; stimulate him to cry so that he fully expands his lungs.
   b. Head and shoulders elevated 20–30 degrees.
   c. Mechanical vibrator (to minimize trauma to anastomosis) may be used 2–3 days postoperatively, followed by more vigorous physical therapy after the 3rd day. Care should be taken not to hyperextend the neck, causing stress to the operative site.
3. Continue use of Isolette or radiant warmer with humidity. Either device does the following:
   a. Provides an environment in which infant can maintain his temperature in thermoneutral zone.
   b. Provides humidity to liquefy secretions.
   c. Allows for observation of and easy access to infant.
4. Be prepared to function in an emergency.
   Have emergency equipment available:
   (1) Suction machine, catheter
   (2) Oxygen
   (3) Laryngoscope, endotracheal tubes in varying sizes

C. Be aware of type of chest drainage present, which may be determined by surgical approach, and provide appropriate care.

1. Retropleural—small tube in posterior mediastinum; may be left open for drainage.
2. Transthoracic—chest tube placed in pleural space and connected to suction.
   a. Keep tubing free from clots; keep it unkinked and without tension.
   b. If a break occurs in the closed drainage system, immediately clamp tubing close to the infant to prevent pneumothorax.

D. Assist in maintaining adequate nutrition to promote healing, growth, and development.

Feedings may be given by mouth, by gastrostomy, or—rarely—by a feeding tube into the esophagus, depending on the type of operation performed and the infant's condition. The gastrostomy is generally attached to gravity drainage for 3 days postoperatively, then elevated and left open to allow for air escape and passage of gastric secretions into the duodenum for a period of time before feedings are begun.

1. Gastrostomy feeding
   a. Gastrostomy feeding can be started prior to esophageal healing—adequate nutrition is an important factor in healing. Give the infant a pacifier to suck during feedings, unless contraindicated.
   b. Gastrostomy feedings may be continued until the infant can tolerate full feedings orally.
   c. Care should be taken not to allow air to enter the stomach, thereby causing gastric distention and possible reflux.
   d. Check with the surgeon before allowing the

infant to suck on a pacifier during gastrostomy feeding.
2. Oral feedings may begin 10–14 days postoperatively following anastomosis.
   a. Feed slowly to allow the infant time to swallow.
   b. Use upright sitting position.
   c. Burp frequently.
   d. Demand feeding may be more successful and pleasant for the infant than strictly scheduled feeding.
   e. Do not allow the infant to become overtired at feeding time. Note cardiac rate.
   f. Try to make each feeding a pleasant experience for the infant. Use a consistent approach and patience. Encourage parental involvement.

E. Care appropriately for cervical esophagostomy (artificial opening in neck which allows for drainage of the upper esophagus).

1. Keep the area clean of saliva.
   a. Wash with clear water.
   b. Place an absorbent pad over the area.
2. As soon as possible, allow the infant to suck a few milliliters of milk at the same time gastrostomy feeding is being done. Advance the infant to solid foods as appropriate if esophagostomy is maintained for a few months.
   a. Encourage sucking and swallowing.
   b. Familiarize the infant with food, so that when he is able to eat orally, he will be used to it.

F. Be aware of impending complications of esophageal repair.

1. Leak at the anastomosis (development of mediastinitis, pneumothorax, and saliva in chest tube).
   a. Hypothermia or hyperthermia
   b. Pneumothorax
      (1) Severe respiratory distress
      (2) Cyanosis
      (3) Restlessness
      (4) Weak pulses
2. Stricture at the anastomosis
   a. Difficulty in swallowing
   b. Vomiting or spitting up of ingested fluid
   c. Refusing to eat
   d. Fever—secondary to aspiration and pneumonia
3. Recurrent fistula
   a. Coughing, choking, and cyanosis associated with feeding
   b. Excessive salivation
   c. Difficulty in swallowing associated with abnormal distention
   d. Repeated episodes of pneumonitis
   e. General poor physical condition—no weight gain
4. Atelectasis or pneumonitis
   a. Aspiration
   b. Respiratory distress

G. Provide for the infant's emotional and social needs.

The extent of hospitalization and long-term care puts a strain on the normal opportunities in these areas (see ICN, p. 1122).
1. Hold and cuddle the infant for feedings and/or after feedings.

2. Encourage mother (parents) to cuddle and love the infant.
3. Provide for visual, auditory, and tactile stimulation as appropriate for the infant's physical condition and age.

H. Encourage parental participation in learning to care for and handle the infant and to foster acceptance of the child by his parents and family.

1. Provide opportunities for the parents to learn all aspects of care of their infant.
2. Initiate a teaching program for the parents early. Offer them available literature and help them become familiar with community resources.
3. Initiate a community nurse referral for continuity of care in the home.
4. Encourage the parents to talk about their feelings, fears, and concerns.
5. Help to develop a healthy parent–child relationship.
   a. Frequent visiting
   b. Phone calls
   c. Physical contact of child and parents

Health Education

1. Teach carefully and thoroughly all procedures to be done at home. Show the parents how; then watch return demonstration of the following procedures:
   a. Gastrostomy feedings and care
   b. Esophagostomy care with feeding technique
   c. Suctioning
   d. Identifying signs of respiratory distress
2. Help the parents understand the psychological needs of the infant for sucking, warmth, comfort, stimulation, and love. Suggest that activity be appropriate for age.
3. Encourage the parents to continue close medical follow-up and help them learn to recognize possible problems.
   a. Dilatation of esophagus to treat stricture at the site of the anastomosis
   b. Raspy cough for 6–24 months
   c. Eating problems, especially when solids are introduced
   d. Repeated respiratory tract infection
   e. Occurrence of stricture at site of anastomosis weeks to months later—recognized by difficulty in swallowing; spitting of ingested fluid; fever
4. Help the parents understand the need for good nutrition and the need to follow the diet regimen suggested by the physician.

Expected Outcomes

1. Shows no signs of respiratory distress; maintains adequate oxygen–carbon dioxide exchange; normal blood gas values; stable vital signs
2. Receives adequate nutritional intake; demonstrates willingness to eat; shows weight gain
3. Maintains normal fluid and electrolyte balance; has adequate intake and output; normal laboratory values
4. Experiences minimal complications of prematurity (i.e., thermal stability); laboratory values within normal range; stable vital signs; improved appearance
5. The parents verbalize an understanding of illness and follow-up care; becoming involved in child care and the bonding process

Gastroesophageal Reflux

Gastroesophageal reflux (GER) is a malfunction of the distal end of the esophagus permitting return of stomach content into the esophagus.

Etiology

1. The cause is undetermined in most patients.
2. Possible causes:
   a. Neuromuscular imbalance; delayed development
   b. Cerebral defects
   c. Obstruction at or just below the pylorus
   d. Physiologic immaturity

Altered Physiology

1. The lower esophageal sphincter is a physiologic rather than an anatomic segment that forms an anti-reflux barrier
   a. The segment is 2–5 cm. in length.
   b. The segment is characterized by a pressure greater than that found proximally in the esophagus or distally in the stomach.
   c. Constitutes an effective barrier to protect the esophageal mucosa from damage by gastric contents (acid, pepsin, bile salts).
2. GER—consequence of incompetence or malfunctioning of this lower esophageal sphincter.
   a. Filling of the esophagus from the stomach upon inspiration, leading to vomiting
   b. Increased intra-abdominal pressure

Complications

Resulting from frequent and sustained reflux of gastric contents into lower esophagus:
1. Recurrent pulmonary disease; aspiration pneumonia
2. Chronic esophagitis
3. Failure to thrive
4. Anemia
5. Cyanotic episodes
6. Esophageal stricture from scarring; esophagitis
7. Asthma
8. Hiatal hernia frequently associated with chalasia

Clinical Manifestations

A. Infant

1. Vomiting (unexplained)
   a. Immediately after feeding, especially when the infant is placed in a prone position
   b. Usually regurgitation rather than projectile vomiting
2. Onset usually soon after birth
3. Weight loss or failure to gain weight; rumination
4. Dehydration
5. Recurrent pulmonary symptoms

B. Older Child:

1. Substernal burning
2. Upper abdominal discomfort; pressure or "squeezing" feeling
3. Persistent pulmonary problems
4. Dysphagia as evidenced by irritability during eating
5. Anemia

Diagnostic Evaluation

1. Upper GI barium x-ray with fluoroscope
   Barium enters stomach but then is regurgitated back into the esophagus.
2. Monitor pH in esophagus
3. Serum studies
   a. Calcium level—may be lowered
   b. Alkalosis—pH greater than 7.45
   c. Hemoglobin and Hematocrit

Treatment

1. Propping in an upright position
   a. Infant—60-degree angle, supine; 30-degree angle, prone; 60 minutes postfeeding to constant 24 hours
   b. Older child—raise head of bed with 8-inch blocks
2. Antacid between feedings if esophagitis is present (forms a floating barrier)
3. Infant—thickened feedings; small, frequent feedings. Older Child—nothing to eat 2 hours before bedtime; possible avoidance of certain foods
4. Medication to stimulate lower esophageal sphincter pressure (tone) and increase peristaltic wave amplitude and clearance rate (bethanechol or metoclopramide)
5. Surgical reconstruction of esophagogastric junction—if conservative management does not improve condition

Patient Problems/Nursing Diagnoses

1. Alteration in oxygen–carbon dioxide exchange and respiratory distress related to frequent and sustained reflux of gastric contents into tracheobronchial tree
2. Alteration in nutritional status related to decreased oral intake
3. Alteration in fluid and electrolyte balance related to frequent vomiting
4. Alteration in comfort related to inadequate nutrition and vomiting
5. Potential for infection related to malnourishment
6. Parental anxiety and concern related to the child's illness

Nursing Interventions

A. Assist in treatment of dehydration.

1. Monitor intravenous therapy (see p. 1160).
2. Observe and record accurately urinary output.
   a. Amount, frequency, color, and concentration
   b. Specific gravity
3. Promote good skin care to prevent lesions of dry and delicate tissues.
   a. Change position frequently.
   b. Change soiled diapers often.
   c. Apply lotion and gently massage any reddened areas.

B. Maintain adequate nutrition and to prevent vomiting.

1. Thicken formula for each feeding.
   a. May use cereal.
   b. Enlarge nipple hole so that formula can be more easily extracted.

2. Prop the infant in upright position.
   a. 60-degree, supine; 30-degree, prone—constantly
   b. Suggested methods: elevate mattress, Anti-Reflux saddle,* infant seat
3. Handle the infant gently, with minimal movement during and after feeding.
4. Bubble frequently during and at completion of feeding.
5. Record accurately activity of infant.
   a. Amount of feeding taken; whether retained
   b. Emesis, estimated amount, type, occurrence in relation to feeding
   c. Any change in behavior as a result of feeding technique

C. Support the family, especially the mother, and encourage them to participate in care and feeding of the infant.

1. The mother may be overly concerned about the infant and blame herself and feeding technique for the infant's condition.
   a. Help the mother understand it is not her fault; she is not a "bad mother."
   b. Let her talk about her concerns.
2. Encourage the mother to take an active part in caring for the infant—provides a good opportunity to guide the mother in correct or preferred methods of handling baby with this condition.

Health Education

1. Plan a program of intensive parental teaching on how to handle and care for the infant. Be certain the parents understand why this is being done. Ensure they have proper equipment for propping the infant.
   Help the parents understand that it is not necessary to keep infant in infant seat or propped at all times.
   (1) Bathe or play with the infant *prior to feeding.*
   (2) Change position about 1 hour after feeding.
   (3) During the night after feeding, the infant can sleep in an upright position.
   (4) Expect occasional small amounts of vomiting.
2. Help parents to understand that chalasia is self-limited—symptoms usually disappear within 12 months.
3. If a temporary gastrostomy is done, ensure that the parents know how to use the tube, clear it, and replace it.
4. Help the parents understand the importance of follow-up of weight gain and development.

Expected Outcomes

1. Breathes more easily and shows minimal respiratory distress; normal blood gas values and vital signs; lungs clear on auscultation
2. Ingests adequate amount of food; shows willingness to eat; gaining weight
3. Maintains balanced fluid and electrolyte values
4. Experiences minimal discomfort; stable vital signs; shows calm behavior; engages in play activities
5. Absence of infection; stable vital signs; normal laboratory values
6. The parents have overcome their anxiety; appear more relaxed; express sense of relief; becoming involved in the child's care

Hypertrophic Pyloric Stenosis

Hypertrophic pyloric stenosis is congenital, progressive hypertrophy of the muscle of the pylorus, causing partial or total obstruction of the stomach outlet (pyloric sphincter).

Etiology

1. Unknown
2. Possibly, immature pyloric ganglion cells

Incidence

1. 1:500
2. 4:1 ratio, with males predominantly

Altered Physiology

1. Increase in size of the circular musculature of the pylorus with thickening (size and shape of an olive). The pylorus muscle becomes elongated and thickened and is enlarged—about twice the usual size.
2. Hypertrophy of the pylorus musculature occurs with narrowing of the pyloric lumen.
3. Constriction of the lumen of the pyloric canal (at the distal end of the stomach) causes the stomach to become dilated.
4. Gastric emptying is delayed; vomiting after feeding and obstruction also occur.

* Continuity of Care Committee, Children's Hospital Medical Center, Cincinnati, OH (1979).

Clinical Manifestations

Onset is within the first 2 months after birth.
1. Vomiting—onset may be gradual and intermittent or sudden and forceful. The following characteristics may be noted:
   a. Occasional, nonprojectile vomiting at first, gradually increasing in frequency and intensity
   b. Projectile vomiting, not bile-stained
2. Constipation—decreased quantity of stools
3. Loss of weight or failure to gain weight
4. Visible gastric peristaltic waves, left to right
5. Excessive hunger—willingness to eat immediately after vomiting
6. Dehydration—electrolyte disturbance with alkalosis
7. Decreased urinary output
8. Palpable pyloric mass in upper right quadrant of abdomen, to the right of the umbilicus and best felt during feeding or immediately after vomiting

Diagnostic Evaluation

1. Palpation of pyloric mass ("olive") in conjunction with persistent, projectile vomiting with associated alkalosis
2. Tests for metabolic alkalosis—due to loss of hydrochloric acid and potassium from vomiting
   a. Serum sodium—decreases
   b. Serum chloride—decreases
   c. Serum potassium—decreases

d. Serum pH—increases above 7
e. Serum CO_2—increases
3. Urinalysis—urine becomes alkaline and concentrated
4. Blood hematocrit and hemoglobin—elevated due to hemoconcentration
5. Flat film of abdomen—dilated, air-filled stomach; nondilated pyloric canal
6. X-ray examination with barium
   a. Narrowing of pyloric canal
   b. Delayed gastric emptying time
   c. Enlarged stomach
   d. Increased peristaltic waves
   e. Gas distal to stomach

Treatment

1. Initial treatment:
   a. Rehydrate and correct electrolytes
   b. Correct alkalosis
2. Surgical—pyloromyotomy

Patient Problems/Nursing Diagnoses

1. Alteration in fluid and electrolyte balance related to frequent vomiting
2. Alteration in nutritional status (failure to thrive) related to vomiting
3. Alteration in comfort related to frequent hunger and/or surgical procedure
4. Parental anxiety related to the child's illness and insecurity in caring for child

Preoperative Nursing Intervention

A. Assist in restoring hydration and electrolyte balance.

1. Intravenous therapy is usually initiated (see p. 1160). Corrects dehydration, metabolic alkalosis, and electrolyte deficiency.
2. Careful observation of output, amount, and characteristics.
   a. Urine (Check specific gravity.)
   b. Vomiting
   c. Stools
3. Accurate daily weight—serves as a guide for calculating need for parenteral fluid.

B. Prevent or decrease the likelihood of vomiting.

1. Patient may be NPO with indwelling nasogastric tube to remove any residual barium and retained formula. Ensure proper functioning of tube and note drainage.
2. Oral feedings may be continued.
   a. Feed small, frequent feedings, given slowly.
   b. Bubble frequently, before, during, and after feeding.
   c. Thickened formula may be prescribed.
3. Proper positioning (see Fig. 37-2).
   Prop the patient in upright position.
   (1) Elevate head of bed, mattress, or infant seat at a 75- to 80-degree angle.
   (2) Place slightly on right side—to aid in gastric emptying.
   (3) Handle gently and minimally after feeding.

C. Make frequent, accurate observations of the infant's condition.

1. Dehydration
2. Vomiting
3. Stools and urine output
4. Vital signs
5. Electrolyte imbalance

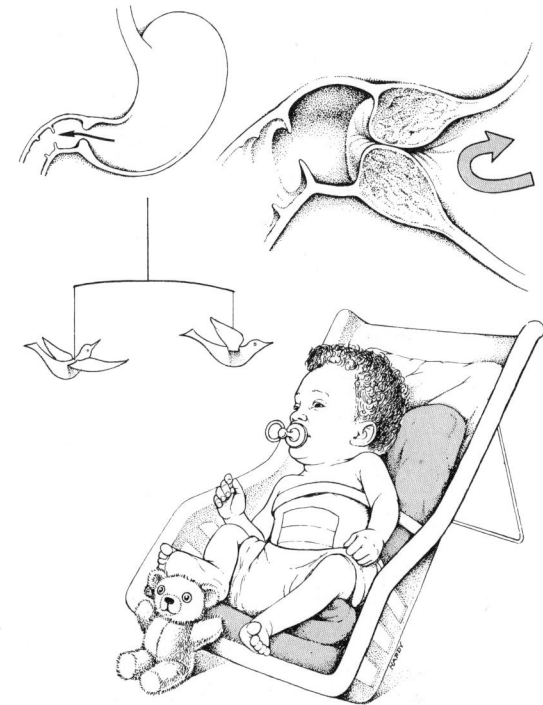

Figure 37-2. Pyloric stenosis. (*A*) Normal passage through pyloric sphincter. (*B*) Stoppage of flow due to stenotic sphincter. (*C*) Postoperative treatment: child propped on right side after feeding to aid gastric emptying.

▶ **NURSING ALERT:** Respiratory rate may be irregular with apnea when the patient is in severe alkalosis.

D. Provide comfort for the infant.

1. Mouth care—wet lips
   Let the infant suck on a pacifier.
2. Physical contact or nearness of the nurse or mother
3. Audio or visual stimulation may be soothing
4. Minimal palpation of pyloric "olive"—will decrease risk of postoperative wound infection from bruising abdominal wall and excoriation of tissue in operative site

E. Prevent infection.
   The infant is at increased risk for infection because of his decreased nutritional status.

F. Support the parents, who are usually very concerned and worried.

1. The mother may feel guilty (i.e., she may feel she has a poor feeding technique)
   Help her understand that she did not do anything to cause this deformity.
2. Prepare the parents for the surgery of their child.
   a. Be honest with them.
   b. Inform them of the expected postoperative appearance of the infant.
   c. Show them where the operating room and recovery room are located and where to wait during surgery.
3. Encourage the parents to maintain a good relationship with the infant. Allow them to hold the infant.

4. Encourage them to get some rest.
   The mother may be tired and frustrated because of the extensive care she has had to give to the child prior to hospitalization.

Postoperative Nursing Interventions

A. Give good postoperative care and observe for the usual postoperative complications
(see p. 1126).

B. Monitor parenteral fluids in order to maintain hydration.

Intravenous therapy may be continued until adequate oral intake is obtained.

C. Assist in resuming oral feedings.

1. Feeding is usually resumed 2–8 hours after surgery.
   a. Feedings usually start with small, frequent feedings of glucose water and slowly advance to full-strength formula and regular diet.
   b. Report any vomiting—the amount and characteristics. Feeding schedule may be withheld 4 hours and then restarted.
   c. Feed slowly and bubble frequently.
   d. Note how feeding is taken and if it is retained.
   e. The amount of feeding is increased as the time interval between feedings is lengthened.
2. Continue to elevate the infant's head and shoulders after feeding for 45–60 minutes for several feedings after surgery. Place on right side to aid gastric emptying.
3. Regurgitation may continue for a short period after surgery.

D. Encourage the parents to resume care—especially feeding—of their infant.

1. This will help to restore their confidence in caring for their baby.
2. This activity provides an opportunity for the nurse to teach.
3. If the mother was breast-feeding, she should resume this as soon as possible.

Health Education

1. Help the parents to understand that surgery has corrected the pyloric stenosis.
   a. Discharge of baby may be from 2–5 days after surgery.
   b. Proper care of the operative site can be done by the mother.
   c. A modified method of feeding technique will be continued at home for only a short period of time.
2. Since this may be a new mother, and the infant may be under 6 weeks of age, the mother may need help with routine infant care.

Expected Outcomes

1. Attains/maintains fluid and electrolyte balance; appears well hydrated; experiences fewer vomiting episodes; normal skin turgor
2. Shows improved nutritional status; retains feedings; shows more alert appearance; has weight gain
3. Appears more comfortable; rests for longer periods; appears satisfied after feeding; no signs of excessive peristalsis or abdominal distention
4. The parents participate in their child's care and express understanding of follow-up care of wound site and feeding

Celiac Disease

Celiac disease, also called gluten-sensitive enteropathy, is a disease of the small intestines characterized by a permanent inability to tolerate dietary gluten.

Etiology

1. Unknown. Although the relationship of gluten to mucosal abnormalities is established, the way in which these mucosal changes occur is not clear.
2. Genetics
   a. Familial incidence
   b. Mode of inheritance is not clear, probably autosomal recessive with incomplete penetrance
3. Environmental inference likely—role of other "allergens" unclear
4. Current theories being investigated include the following:
   a. Immunological (autoimmune vs. specific immune abnormality, aberrant immunologic response to gluten)
   b. Search to identify deficient enzymes that digest gluten, or possible lack of intestinal enzymes that detoxifies gluten
   c. Altered epithelial cell surfaces—allow gluten or gluten-fragment-binding with resultant cellular toxicity.

Altered Physiology

1. Characteristics of celiac disease include
   a. Impaired intestinal absorption
   b. Histologic abnormalities of the small intestine
   c. Clinical and histological improvement with wheat- and rye-free (possibly also barley- and oat-free) diet
   d. Recurrence of clinical manifestations and histological changes after reintroduction of dietary gluten
2. Histologic changes in mucosa of small bowel, especially duodenum and jejunum resulting from dietary gluten include
   a. Irregularity of epithelial cells
   b. Loss of normal villous pattern
   c. Obliteration of intervillous spaces which are infiltrated with plasma cells and eosinophils
   d. Loss of epithelial cell brush border
3. This mucosal damage results in
   a. Disaccharidase deficiency
   b. Depression of peptidase activity
4. Subsequent malabsorption probably results from
   a. Decreased area of absorption in small bowel
   b. Impaired enzyme activity

5. Inability to absorb fats, fat-soluble vitamins (A, D, K, and E), minerals, and some protein and carbohydrates. The severity of symptoms of the disease depends on the extent of intestine with histologic changes.
   a. The extent of affected intestine is variable.
   b. Generally, proximal small intestine mucosal damage is most severe and condition decreases in severity distally.

Complications
1. Recurrence of symptoms if diet is not followed
2. Possible predisposition to malignant lymphoma of small intestine at later age, if dietary restrictions are terminated
3. Refractory sprue
4. Associated disorders
   a. Dermatitis herpetiformis
   b. Insulin-dependent diabetes mellitus
   c. Cystic fibrosis

Clinical Manifestations
The age and mode of presenting signs and symptoms are extremely variable. Diagnosis is most commonly made by 6–24 months of age; however, it can be made in the adult.
1. 3–9 months of age
   a. Acutely ill
   b. Severe diarrhea and vomiting
   c. Possibly failure to thrive
2. 9–18 months of age (age when "typical" celiac appearance is seen)
   a. Impaired growth
      (1) Normal growth during early months of life
      (2) Slackening of weight and weight loss follow
   b. Abnormal stools
      (1) Pale
      (2) Soft
      (3) Bulky
      (4) Having offensive odor
      (5) Greasy—steatorrhea
      (6) May increase in number
   c. Abdominal distention
   d. Anorexia
   e. Muscle wasting—most obvious in buttocks and proximal parts of extremities
   f. Hypotonia
   g. Mood changes—ill humor, irritability, temper tantrums, shyness
   h. Mild clubbing of fingers
   i. Vomiting—often occurring in evening
3. Older child
   a. Signs and symptoms often related to nutritional or secondary deficiencies resulting from disease
   b. May have abnormal stools and growth impairment
   c. May have colicky abdominal pain with constipation and large, pale stools
4. Manifestations secondary to malabsorption
   a. Anemia, vitamin deficiency
   b. Hypoproteinemia with edema
   c. Hypocalcemia
   d. Hypoprothrombinemia—resulting from impaired vitamin K absorption
   e. Disaccharide intolerance—with acid-sugar-containing stools (secondary to the altered small bowel mucosa)
5. Celiac crisis—most often seen in very young child and toddler (although rare)
   a. Profound anorexia
   b. Severe vomiting and diarrhea
   c. Weight loss
   d. Marked dehydration and acidosis (secondary to intractable diarrhea and vomiting)
   e. Immobility
   f. Grossly distended abdomen
      (1) Fluid rattle is present.
      (2) Abdomen flattens with passage of large liquid stool.
      (3) The patient appears shock-like.
   g. Looks profoundly depressed

Diagnostic
1. Thorough evaluation of history and general status of child
2. Small bowel biopsy—demonstrates abnormal mucosa Diagnostic criteria:
   a. Severely damaged or flat, villous lesions
   b. Clinical response to gluten elimination
   c. Histologic recovery following gluten elimination
   d. Histologic recurrence of villous injury within 2 years of gluten reintroduction
3. D-Xylose absorption—less 20–25 mg./dl. at 60 minutes
4. Red blood count smear—hypochromia
5. Serum iron and folate—folic acid reduced
6. Immunoglobulin determination—IgA may be increased in acute stage of disease
7. Determination of fat absorption—fecal fat excretion—24-hour collection 3 times
8. Measurement of hemoglobin levels—may be reduced
9. Prothrombin time—before intestinal biopsy
10. Radiologic studies—skeletal x-rays commonly show
    a. Demineralization
    b. Retarded bone age
11. Sweat test and pancreatic function studies to rule out cystic fibrosis

Treatment
1. *Lifelong* gluten-free diet
   a. Avoid *all* foods containing wheat or rye gluten. The exclusion of barley and oats is controversial; however, it is often wise to err on the safe side or to offer specific challenges and to test with biopsy.
   b. The small intestine mucosa will always respond abnormally to dietary gluten, even though clinical signs may not be immediately evident.
   c. Biopsy reverts to normal with appropriate diet.
   d. Clinical signs of improvement should be seen 1–4 weeks after proper diet is initiated.
2. Adequate caloric intake
3. Supplemental vitamins and minerals
   a. Folic acid for 1–2 months
   b. Vitamin D
   c. Iron for 1–2 months
4. Reduction of fat intake (rare)
5. Possible elimination of lactose from diet for 6–8 weeks—based on reduced disaccharidase activity
6. Treatment of celiac crisis
   a. IV restoration of electrolyte balance and fluids for replacement of blood volume
   b. Steroids
   c. Parenteral hyperalimentation with amino acids, medium chain triglycerides, and glucose—for short periods of time may be necessary

d. Initial oral feedings may need to be disaccharide- or completely sugar-free

Patient Problems/Nursing Diagnoses

1. Alteration in nutritional status related to malabsorption of nutrients, diarrhea, and vomiting
2. Infection related to malnourishment and anemia
3. Alteration in behavior related to dietary restrictions
4. Potential for celiac crises related to vomiting and diarrhea
5. Anxiety and fear related to illness, hospitalization, treatments, and separation from parents
6. Parental anxiety related to the child's illness and lack of understanding of condition

Nursing Interventions

A. Assist with diagnostic evaluation.

1. Prepare the child for diagnostic tests appropriate for age. Assist him during the procedure to aid in compliance and reduce fear and anxiety.
2. Collect stool specimens for 3 days for fat analysis.
3. Ensure that the child is appropriately prepared for special blood studies (i.e., glucose tolerance test).

B. Follow explicitly the dietary regimen that has been calculated by the physician and dietitian to include enough calories for weight gain yet to exclude wheat, rye, barley, and oat glutens that produce enteropathy.

1. Initial diet is high in protein, relatively low in fat, and starch-free.
   a. Milk protein or skim milk is sweetened with sucrose or banana powder.
   b. Infants and young children may have a problem in intestinal fat absorption; therefore, fat intake may be reduced.
2. Proteins and sugars should be added gradually.
   a. Individual foods are added one at a time at several-day intervals. Foods included and added are lean meat, cottage cheese, egg white, and raw ground apple.
   b. Starchy foods are added to diet last.
   c. Wheat and rye are never added to diet.
3. The child is given nothing by mouth during the initial treatment of celiac crisis or during diagnostic testing.
4. If the child is ambulatory, take special precautions to ensure that he does not eat restricted foods.
5. The child may have anorexia; feeding him can be difficult.
   a. Make mealtime pleasant.
   b. Serve small, attractive portions.
   c. Do not force him to eat.
6. Note carefully the child's reaction to food. Close observation of the child's responses to food may reveal other intolerances. Note and record:
   a. Intake, foods refused
   b. Appetite
   c. Change in behavior after eating
   d. Characteristics and frequency of stools
   e. General disposition—behavior improvement often seen within 2–3 days after diet control is initiated
7. New foods may be temporarily eliminated if symptoms increase.

C. Prevent infection in this child who is malnourished, anemic, and very susceptible to respiratory infection, which in turn will increase indigestion.

1. Avoid exposing the child to anyone with an infection of any kind.
2. The child usually perspires freely and has a subnormal temperature with cold extremities.
   a. Keep him dry.
   b. Cover the child lightly when the room is cool.
3. If the child remains quiet in bed, change his position frequently because he is prone to upper respiratory infections.
4. Promote good hygiene.

D. Be aware of the child's behavior or change in behavior and care for him accordingly.

1. Diet and eating have a direct effect on behavior. A hungry child may be irritable.
2. Behavior is indicative of how the child is feeling.
3. The child is prone to mood swings—from having temper tantrums to being very timid, nervous, or unstable.
   a. Allow the child to express his feelings freely. Provide different types of media for child to express himself.
      (1) An older child talks or complains.
      (2) A baby cries and whines.
   b. The nurse must exhibit patience.
   c. Socialize routine procedures.
4. Record changes in behavior, especially in relation to eating and diet.
5. Avoid conflicts or emotionally upsetting situations; these may precipitate diarrhea, vomiting, and celiac crisis.
6. Teach the older child how to adjust his diet. He can eat buckwheat, millet, corn (maize), and rice.

E. Meet the child's emotional and psychological needs and provide diversional activities appropriate for his age and severity of disease.

1. This child may be withdrawn and indulge in self-play.
   Provide opportunity for play with other children, especially when the child begins to feel better.
2. Frequently, play is more passive than active.
   Activity may be very exhausting. Provide appropriate material for constructive activities.
3. The toddler may cling to infantile habits for security. Allow this behavior; it may disappear as his physical condition improves and he feels better.
4. The nurse must show the child she understands his mood swings and irritability by being patient with him. He needs a great deal of emotional satisfaction and support.
5. Offer the child other sensory stimulation to compensate for lack of eating pleasure.

F. Support the parents and foster continuing parental acceptance of the child, his disease, and his behavior.

Help the parents maintain a healthy relationship with their child. The most important aspect in working with parents and child is stressing health and family counseling.

1. Encourage the parents to visit and care for the child as much as possible. Comforting and holding the

child can be very helpful. The child needs much love and understanding, especially from his parents.
2. Start teaching the parents early about the disease and how they should care for the child at home.
   a. Acquaint them with available literature, parent groups, and community resources.
   b. Initiate community-nurse referral to provide for continued support and teaching at home.
3. Listen to parental concerns and questions.
   a. Give simple, honest answers.
   b. Reinforce what the physician has told them.
4. Allow the parents to continue to maintain what other responsibilities they may have outside the hospital. Do not insist they stay at the hospital and attend only to this child.
5. Help the parents to understand that after initial rapid weight gain further improvement may be slow.

G. Be aware of the signs and symptoms of celiac crisis and attend to the child's care according to medical plans.

Initial treatment:
1. Replace fluids and electrolytes by parenteral therapy.
2. Give nothing by mouth, especially if child is vomiting. Nasogastric tube may be prescribed.
3. Observe the child carefully.

H. Be familiar with the medications used in the treatment of celiac disease and their implications.

1. Vitamins A and D—not absorbed well
2. Vitamin B complex and vitamin C—given if the child is receiving antibiotics
3. Iron—given if the child is anemic
4. Vitamin K—for hypothrombinemia and bleeding
5. Calcium lactate—given if milk is restricted from diet
6. Water-miscible vitamins and minerals should be used
7. When nutrients and drugs are essential, intravenous infusion may be used since absorption is poor

I. Assist with gluten-challenge diet, if used, to evaluate histologic and clinical response.

1. After an extended period of time on dietary regimen, the child may dislike gluten-containing foods.
2. The child and parents may be extremely apprehensive about the possible effects of gluten.
3. The child may have mild gastrointestinal symptoms (i.e., loose stools, vague abdominal pain, etc.). These may be related to anxiety.
4. Support the family and provide reassurance. The gluten-challenge diet may last 3–4 months before bowel biopsy is repeated.

Health Education

1. Help the parents to understand what celiac disease is and how it is controlled by diet.
   a. Provide a specific list of restricted foods as well as foods the child is allowed to eat.
   b. Teach the mother (parents) how to read labels on foods to identify those containing wheat and rye glutens, thus avoiding them.
   c. Grains—corn, rice, soybean flour and gluten-free starch are used as substitutes for wheat, rye, barley, and oats.

d. Help the mother become comfortable and proficient in situation problem-solving (e.g., What can be done when her child is invited to a birthday party where cake will be served? Bake gluten-free cupcakes and take to party).
   e. Provide opportunity for mother, dietitian, and nurse to come together and talk about diet. At the same time, foster a positive feeling toward dietary controls.
   f. Be certain the parents understand the importance of the vitamin regimen.
   g. Help the parents understand the importance of continued adherence to diet, even though the child is feeling well, eating well, and has normal stools. Advancing diet too rapidly may result in a setback.
2. Impress upon the parents the importance of regular medical follow-up.
   a. Encourage the parents to seek prompt medical attention if the child has an upper respiratory infection which might trigger celiac crisis if untreated.
   b. Ensure that the parents understand measures to prevent celiac crisis—dietary control, dangers of prolonged fasting, inform unfamiliar physician of celiac disorder, and use of anticholinergic drugs.
3. Encourage the parents to practice good hygiene to prevent infection.
   This child is especially prone to infection because of malnutrition and anemia.
4. Help the parents to understand that the emotional climate in the home and around the child is vitally important in maintaining the child's medical and physical stability.
   a. The parents must exhibit patience with the child.
   b. Have the parents set defined limits of behavior for the child; everyone in the family should know what these limits are.
   c. Avoid conflicts or any emotional upsets in the child's presence.
   d. A social worker may need to become involved if there is domestic disharmony.
   e. Other children and their needs must also be considered in the total family picture.
5. Help the parents to understand that the child's physical condition and behavior problems are related to the disease.
   a. The parents may feel guilty or ambivalent toward the child.
   b. Show them how they may avoid becoming overprotective of the child.
6. Help the parents to understand that the disorder is lifelong; however, changes in the mucosal lining of the intestine and in general the clinical condition of their child are reversible when dietary gluten is avoided.
7. Offer parents available literature about the American Celiac Society; help them to become familiar with the society and the chapter nearest them.*

* American Celiac Society, 45 Gifford Avenue, Jersey City, NJ 07304.

Expected Outcomes

1. Attains and maintains adequate nutritional status; appropriate weight gain; normal range of laboratory values
2. Is free of infection; normal vital signs and laboratory values
3. Demonstrates normalization of behavior; absence of temper tantrums; becoming more social; adheres to diet
4. Absence of celiac crises
5. Experiences minimal anxiety and lessening of fear; normalization of behavior; engaging in play activities
6. Reduction in parental anxiety; verbalize understanding of illness, treatment and follow-up care

Diarrhea

Diarrhea is an excessive loss of water and electrolytes that occurs with passage of one or more unformed stools. It is a symptom of many conditions and may be caused by many diseases (Table 37-1).

Etiology

Often the cause is difficult to determine; occasionally it is unknown. The numerous causes of diarrhea in infants and young children include:

1. Acute and infectious factors
   a. Bacterial
      (1) Enteropathogenic *Escherichia coli*
      (2) *Salmonella*
      (3) *Shigella*
      (4) *Yersinia enterocolitica*
      (5) *Campylobacter fetus*
   b. Viral
      (1) Enteroviruses—ECHO viruses
      (2) Adenoviruses
      (3) Human reovirus-like agent (HRVL)
      (4) *Rotovirus*
   c. Normal intestinal tract inhabitants act as pathogens in certain circumstances (i.e., after ingestion of antibiotics)
   d. Fungal—*Candida* enteritis

Table 37-1 Some Malabsorption Syndromes—Based on Types of Stool*

Disease	Diagnostic Studies	Etiology
A. Watery Stools		

1. Disaccharide intolerance
 a. Lactose
  (lactose → glucose, galactose)
    ↑
   enzyme lactase
	1. Stool pH
	2. Stool reducing substances
	3. Lactose intolerance test
	4. Enzyme assay
		Primary—congenital absence of enzyme lactase
		Secondary—any disease that damages epithelium of small intestine (e.g., gastroenteritis, cow's milk sensitivity, celiac sprue)

b. Sucrose
  (sucrose → glucose, fructose)
    ↑
   enzyme sucrase
	1. Stool pH
	2. Stool reducing substances
	3. Sucrose tolerance
	4. Enzyme assay
		Primary—congenital absence of enzyme sucrase
		Secondary—any disease that damages epithelium of small intestine

2. Monosaccharide intolerance (glucose–galactose)	1. Stool pH 2. Stool-reducing substances 3. Glucose–galactose tolerance tests 4. Trial carbohydrate elimination, using fructose	Primary—congenital defect in glucose transport Secondary—damage to and decrease of epithelium of intestine from acute gastroenteritis or persistent diarrhea, showing intolerance to fructose, glucose, and galactose
3. Cow's milk protein sensitivity	1. Lactose tolerance test 2. Elimination of cow's milk from diet 3. Rechallenge with cow's milk will produce same symptoms	Unknown Sensitivity to cow's milk
B. Parasites		
Strongyloidiasis (roundworm)	Examination of intestinal content for rhabtidiform larvae	*Strongyloides*
Giardia lamblia (protozoan)	Stool examination for *Giardia* cysts; duodenal aspirate for trophozoites	Protozoan *Giardia lamblia*
C. Fatty Stool		
Cystic fibrosis, celiac sprue (see above discussion) Pancreatic insufficiency and bone marrow failure (Schwachman syndrome) Short-bowel syndrome Biliary tract obstruction	Pancreatic enzymes abnormal; sweat test normal; neutropenia	Familial pancreatic enzymes are probably reduced Inadequate absorptive surfaces Extensive bowel resection, increase in gastric acidity and production rate (hypersecretion), which in turn may inactivate pancreatic enzymes Biliary atresia Choledochal cyst Obstructive neonatal hepatitis
D. Normal Stools		
Juvenile pernicious anemia (vitamin B_{12} malabsorption)		Absence of intrinsic factor activity—cannot absorb vitamin B_{12}

* Adapted from Ament, ME. J. Pediatr. 81:685, 1976
Nursing care plans can be adapted from discussions on diarrhea, celiac disease, and cystic fibrosis.

e. Parasitic—*Giardia lamblia*
f. Protozoal
2. Noninfectious factors
  a. Allergy to certain foods—milk, wheat protein
  b. Metabolic disorders
    (1) Celiac disease
    (2) Cystic fibrosis of pancreas
  c. Disaccharidase deficiencies
  d. Infant exposed to overfeeding; displaying emotional excitement and fatigue
  e. Direct irritation of gastrointestinal tract by foods
  f. Inappropriate use of laxatives and purgatives
3. Mechanical disorders
  a. Malrotation
  b. Incomplete small bowel obstruction
  c. Intermittent volvulus
4. Congenital anomalies—Hirschsprung's disease

Altered Physiology

1. The particular etiology of diarrhea does not influence the potentially dangerous cycle of events as much as does the virulence of the organism and the general condition of the child.
2. The effects of diarrhea present more of a threat to infants and young children than to the older child and adult.
  a. Extracellular fluid volume is proportionately larger in the infant and young child
  b. Nutritional reserves are relatively smaller in the young child
3. Major alterations in physiology
  a. Dehydration—extracellular fluid loss—results from the following:
    (1) Large loss of fluid and electrolytes in watery stools
    (2) Losses with repeated vomiting
    (3) Decreased fluid intake
    (4) Increased insensible fluid losses from skin and lungs resulting from fever and rapid respirations
    (5) Continued urine excretion
  b. Electrolyte imbalance
    (1) Potassium—varies
    (2) Chloride; sodium; hypotonic, isotonic, or hypertonic dehydration may occur
  c. Acid–base imbalance—metabolic acidosis may result from
    (1) Large losses of potassium, sodium, and bicarbonate in stools
    (2) Impairment of renal function

Complications

1. Direct disturbances caused by diarrhea itself
  a. Dehydration
  b. Acidosis
  c. Hypernatremia
  d. Alterations in potassium levels
  e. Monosaccharide intolerance
2. Infection
  a. Local (i.e., site of cutdown, injection site)
  b. Respiratory tract
  c. Middle ear (otitis media)
3. Nervous system, hemorrhage
4. Iatrogenic
  a. Potassium depletion—"washing out"
  b. Hypernatremia—sodium chloride overload
  c. Edema—excessive amount of parenteral fluids

Clinical Manifestations

A. Classification of Diarrhea

1. Mild diarrhea—hospitalization may not be indicated.
2. Severe diarrhea with gradual onset.
3. Severe diarrhea with sudden onset—incidence of death is high in infant.

B. Symptoms

All classifications have symptoms, the severity of which depends on the intensity of diarrhea and type of onset.
1. Fever—low-grade to 41.1°C. (100°F.)
2. Anorexia
3. Mild and intermittent to severe vomiting
4. Stools
  a. Appearance of diarrhea varies from a few hours to 3 days
  b. Loose and fluid in consistency
  c. Greenish or yellow–green color
  d. May contain mucus, pus, or blood
  e. Frequency varies from 2–20/day
  f. Expelled with force; may be preceded by pain
5. Behavior change
  a. Irritability and restlessness
  b. Weakness/pallor
  c. Extreme prostration
  d. Stupor and convulsions
  e. Flaccidity
6. Respirations
  a. Rapid
  b. Hyperpneic
7. Dehydration
  a. Little to extreme loss of subcutaneous fat
  b. Up to 50% total body weight loss
  c. Urinary output decreases or stops
  d. Poor skin turgor and dry skin
  e. Fontanelles and eyes sunken
  f. Collapse imminent, low blood pressure, high pulse

Diagnostic Evaluation

1. Thorough history of onset of diarrhea and cause
2. Evaluation of general physical appearance and condition of child, including weight
3. Studies to establish nature of the child's condition
  a. Electrolyte status and kidney function
    (1) Serum sodium
    (2) Serum chloride
    (3) Serum potassium
    (4) BUN (blood urea nitrogen)
  b. Acid–base imbalance
    (1) Serum pH (acidosis)
    (2) Serum CO_2 content or combining power
  c. Plasma volume by hematocrit and hemoglobin; also complete blood count, sedimentation rate, and culture
  d. Urinalysis
  e. Stool pH, reducing substances
4. Studies to determine cause of diarrhea
  a. Bacteriologic cultures of stool
  b. Bacteriologic cultures of rectal swab
  c. Serologic studies for viral pathogens or direct visualization under electron microscope (i.e., HRVL)

Treatment

1. Prevent spread of disease—suspect disease to be communicable until proven otherwise. Isolation; use enteric isolation precautions.

2. Supportive care—maintain hydration and electrolyte balance; record IV fluids, weights, fluid loss from diarrhea, urine, and vomiting.
3. Specific antimicrobial therapy
   Complications:
   (1) Dehydration
   (2) Protracted diarrheal state
   (3) Transient lactase deficiency—lactose intolerance

Patient Problems/Nursing Diagnoses

1. Alteration in fluid and electrolyte balance related to diarrhea and extracellular fluid loss
2. Potential for additional infection related to debilitated state and altered nutritional status
3. Alteration in nutritional status related to malabsorption
4. Alteration in comfort related to effects of disease and treatments
5. Anxiety and fear related to hospitalization and illness
6. Parental anxiety related to the child's illness, hospitalization, and lack of understanding of the child's condition

Nursing Interventions

A. Monitor intravenous fluid therapy (both amount and rate), which has been appropriately calculated by the physician.

1. Fluid prescribed as maintenance or replacement, depending on degree of patient's dehydration, must be checked.
2. Fluid is calculated carefully so as not to overload circulatory system.
   a. Check flow rate and amount absorbed hourly and totally.
   b. Check IV site for infiltration or improper flow so site can be changed as necessary.
3. Use appropriate protective devices to prevent the patient from moving and injuring himself or causing IV to malfunction.
4. When preparing solution for therapy, use sterile solution and equipment.
5. Weigh the patient daily to serve as a guide for specific fluid needs and current patient status.
6. When oral feedings are given in conjunction with IV fluid, careful adherence to prescribed volume is vital to prevent circulatory overload.

B. Provide physical comfort for the patient.

1. If protective devices are used, passive range of motion may help to keep the patient's joints from stiffening.
2. While the patient is given nothing by mouth, special mouth care should be administered.
   An infant may find comfort in sucking a pacifier. Bubble him frequently to help expel air he has swallowed during sucking.
3. Change position and give good skin care to prevent lesions that may occur because of dehydration.
   Change soiled diapers quickly, because diarrheal stool will cause excoriation. Clean perineum thoroughly after each stool; application of ointment to skin may help protect it from contact with stool. Ointment must be completely removed after each stool. Leave diaper area exposed to air.

C. Make frequent observations and be constantly alert to the patient's condition.

Record and report any changes immediately. Careful observations can give clues to improvement or deterioration in the patient's condition and can serve as a guide to medical care.

1. Note any changes in vital signs.
2. Note stool characteristics and number.
   a. Abnormal constituents
   b. Foul odor
   c. Test stool for pH, reducing substances (Clinitest tablets), and occult blood.
3. Note activity, level of consciousness, and neurologic signs.
4. Note vomiting—frequency and characteristics.
5. Record urinary output—amount, frequency, and characteristics.
6. Check for presence of edema, and skin characteristics.
7. Assess the child's behavior to determine how he feels.
   a. Eating and restful sleep indicates he feels fairly good.
   b. Crying or legs drawn up to abdomen usually indicates pain.

D. Prevent spread of infection by using good handwashing and gown techniques as indicated by hospital policy.

1. Many hospitals use isolation technique for children admitted with diarrhea until the cause has been determined. (Infectious pathogens can spread rapidly and easily among infants and young children.)
2. Follow hospital policy as to care of diapers.

E. Meet the emotional and psychological needs of the patient.

1. Hospitalization is frightening—especially when it is sudden, as with diarrhea.
2. Many treatments and procedures are painful—give reassurance to the child before, during, and after treatment.
   a. Talk to the child.
   b. Hold him and comfort him after the procedure.
   c. Explain to him in language appropriate for his age what is to be done.
3. Provide some means of pleasant stimulation, entertainment, or diversion—especially while he must remain in bed.
   a. Infant—mobile, musical toy
   b. Young child—read to him, something appropriate for age
4. A hungry child is not easily comforted. Physical closeness may be helpful.
   a. Petting, stroking
   b. Holding and rocking

F. Provide and assist in resuming adequate caloric and volume of oral intake.

1. If diarrhea is mild, oral electrolyte solution may be given. (Do not advance too quickly—base administration of solution on number of stools.)
2. Fluid is usually advanced slowly from clear liquids, such as gelatin-flavored water, to half-strength formula, to regular diet. Older child may advance more rapidly.
3. As diet is advanced, note any vomiting or increase in stools and report it immediately. Oral feedings should not be resumed too early or advanced too rapidly, because diarrhea may recur.

G. Provide support for the family, especially the mother.

1. Reassure the mother that she is not the cause of her child's illness.

2. Explain procedures and need for treatment in easy-to-understand language. Be sure family understands the following:
   a. Why the infant's hair was shaved off his head for an IV
   b. Reason for not giving the child anything to eat or drink
   c. Need for protective devices
3. Allow mother (parents) to care for and comfort the child as much as possible.
4. Allow her to leave the hospital and attend to other family members and matters. Invite the parents to call the hospital when they cannot be there.
5. Initiate a community-nurse referral, especially if other children at home are ill or if home conditions have precipitated the diarrhea.

Health Education

1. After the cause of the diarrhea is determined, it may be necessary to teach proper formula or food preparation, handling, and storage.
   It is especially important to be certain that the mother knows proper formula and bottle sterilization procedures.
2. Parents may need help in understanding the symptoms of a sick child.
3. Help the parents understand the importance of medical care and general good hygiene.

Expected Outcomes

1. Shows proper hydration; maintains acid–base and fluid and electrolyte balance; has normal laboratory values; demonstrates weight gain
2. Is free of secondary infection; normal vital signs and laboratory values
3. Reestablishes a more normal bowel elimination pattern; gains weight; eating more solid foods
4. Shows minimal discomfort; lessening of abdominal cramps; resting; fewer complaints; stable vital signs
5. Shows lessening of anxiety; more relaxed; willing to play; takes interest in surroundings
6. The parents gain an understanding of the child's treatment; verbalize the dietary protocol and measures to prevent recurrences

Hirschsprung's Disease

Hirschsprung's disease (congenital aganglionic megacolon) is a congenital absence of the parasympathetic ganglion nerve cells from within the muscle wall of the intestinal tract, usually at the distal end of the colon.

Etiology

1. An arrest in embryologic development affecting the migration of parasympathetic nerves (innervation) of the intestine, occurring prior to the 12th week of gestation
2. The cause is unknown—may be familial

Incidence

1. 1:5,000 births; accounts for about 25% of all intestinal obstructions in the newborn
2. 4:1 male ratio

Altered Physiology

1. Absence or reduced number of the parasympathetic ganglion cells in Auerbach's plexus within the intestinal tract muscle wall, usually the distal end of the colon and the rectum. Most commonly affected site is the rectosigmoid colon.
2. No peristalsis occurs in the affected portion of intestine (i.e., spastic and contracted).
   a. This section is usually narrow; therefore, no fecal material passes through it.
   b. The intestine above the affected section has an accumulation of fecal material.
3. Proximal to the narrow affected section, the colon is dilated.
   a. Filled with fecal material and gas.
   b. Hypertrophy of muscular coating.
   c. In newborn, may see ulceration of mucosa.
4. The internal rectal sphincter fails to relax and evacuation of fecal material and gas is prevented. Abdominal distention and constipation result.

Complications

1. Prior to primary surgery
   a. Enterocolitis—a major cause of death
   b. Hydroureter or hydronephrosis
   c. Water intoxication from tap water enemas
   d. Cecal perforation
2. Postoperative
   a. Enterocolitis
   b. Leaking of anastomosis and pelvic abscess
   c. Temporary sudden inability to evacuate colon
3. Postoperative—colostomy
   a. Abdominal distention
   b. Respiratory distress
   c. Infection
   d. Hemorrhage, shock

Clinical Manifestations

Vary depending on degree of involved bowel
1. Appearing at birth or within first weeks of life.
   a. No meconium passed
   b. Vomiting—bile-stained or fecal
   c. Abdominal distention
   d. Constipation
   e. Overflow-type diarrhea
   f. Anorexia
   g. Temporary relief of symptoms with enema
2. Older child—symptoms not prominent at birth
   a. History may reveal obstipation at birth
   b. Distention of abdomen—progressive enlarging
   c. Thin abdominal wall—superficial veins are visible
   d. Peristaltic activity observable
   e. Constipation
      (1) Never has fecal soiling
      (2) Relieved temporarily with enema
   f. Stool appears ribbon-like, fluid-like or in pellet form

g. Failure to grow
   (1) Loss of subcutaneous fat
   (2) Appears malnourished; perhaps has stunted growth

Diagnostic Evaluation

1. Rectal examination—exhibits absence of fecal material
2. Roentgen examination with barium enema
   a. Narrow segment of intestine proximal to anus
   b. Dilated intestine proximal to narrow segment
3. Rectal biopsy—absence or reduced number of ganglion nerve cells
4. Anorectal manometry—records the reflex response of sphincter

Treatment

Definitive treatment is removal of the aganglionic, non-functioning, dilated segment of the bowel, followed by anastomosis, and improved functioning of internal rectal sphincter.
1. Initially a colostomy or ileostomy is performed to decompress intestine, divert fecal stream, and rest the normal bowel
2. Definitive surgery (abdominoperineal pullthrough) may be delayed until age 9–12 months or until child is 6.8–9.0 kg. (15–20 lb.).
3. In older child when symptoms are chronic but not severe, treatment may consist of isotonic enemas, stool softeners and low residue diet.

Patient Problems/Nursing Diagnoses

1. Respiratory distress in infant related to abdominal distention
2. Alteration in nutritional status related to poor intake
3. Discomfort and pain related to abdominal distention
4. Acid–base imbalance and dehydration related to vomiting
5. Alteration in elimination related to decreased peristalsis in affected bowel
6. Potential skin breakdown around colostomy stoma related to drainage and excoriation
7. Anxiety and fear, especially in older child, related to illness, hospitalization, and treatments
8. Potential for altered parent–child relationship related to illness of child, hospitalization, and temporary colostomy

Preoperative Nursing Interventions

A. Assist in emptying the bowel and in preparing for surgery.

1. Give repeated enemas and colonic irrigations.
   a. Procedure for enema in an infant is similar to that in an adult, except that less fluid and pressure are used.
   b. Chemotherapeutic agents are used to reduce the bacterial flora.
   c. Physiologic saline solution (warmed) should be used for irrigations.
      Tap water may result in large quantities of water being absorbed and in water intoxication.
   d. Carefully note return from irrigation and degree of abdominal distention.
      Measure returned fluids; retained fluid may be absorbed and result in water intoxication and cerebral edema.
   e. If enema is not expelled, siphoning may be indicated.

f. Continuous use of a rectal tube may be prescribed; ensure that it is properly located and remains in place.
2. Note and record frequency and characteristics of stools. (Obstipation is likely to occur.)
3. Prevent injury to mucosa by taking axillary temperature.

B. Observe for abdominal distention and its effect on the patient's condition.

1. Note any change in degree of distention before and after irrigation. Record if location of distention changes (i.e., upper or lower abdomen).
2. Respiratory embarrassment may result from abdominal distention.
   Elevate head and chest of infant by tilting mattress.
3. Note degree of abdominal tenderness.
   a. Legs of infant drawn up
   b. Chest breathing
4. Note color of abdomen and presence of gastric waves; take sequential measurements of abdominal girth.

C. Assist in establishing and maintaining hydration and adequate nutrition so that growth and weight gain may take place.

1. Monitor parenteral fluids appropriately. Measure all output.
2. Feeding may cause additional discomfort because of distention and nausea.
3. Offer small, frequent feedings. (Low-residue diet will aid in keeping stools soft.)
   a. Appetite is poor.
   b. The child must be fed slowly.
   c. Provide as comfortable a position as possible for child during feedings.

D. Obtain a dietary history regarding food and eating habits.

1. This will contribute to planning dietary alterations.
2. Eating problems are common with Hirschsprung's disease.

E. Properly care for the patient when a nasogastric tube is used to aid in decreasing abdominal distention.

1. Note drainage from nasogastric tube and chart characteristics.
2. Check for patency.
   a. Saline irrigations may be requested.
   b. Carefully record input and output.
   c. Note increasing distention; measure abdominal girth.
3. Give adequate mouth care.
4. Alternate nares when changing nasogastric tube every 24 hours. (Use minimal amount of tape to prevent skin irritation.)

F. Provide emotional and psychological support needed by the child.

1. Encourage the mother to visit, even for short periods.
2. Irritable child may be calmed with holding and rocking.
3. Provide suitable diversion appropriate for age.

Postoperative Nursing Interventions

One of 2 surgical procedures may be done in treatment of Hirschsprung's disease: (1) primary resection of aganglionic segment or (2) temporary colostomy above the narrowed section; when condition of child is stabilized or weight is obtained, resection is done and colostomy closed (most common).

A. Give good postoperative care and observe for possible postoperative complications (see p. 1126).

B. Prevent infection.

1. At the site of the surgical wound.
   a. Dressing change, using sterile technique.
   b. Prevent contamination from diaper.
      (1) Apply diaper below dressing.
      (2) Change frequently.
      (3) Prevent perianal and anal excoriation by frequent changing, thorough cleansing, and use of ointments.
   c. Use careful handwashing technique.
   d. Report any redness, swelling or drainage, evisceration, or dehiscence immediately.
2. Of the tracheobronchial tree and lungs.
   a. Suction secretions frequently.
   b. Encourage frequent coughing and deep breathing.
      Allow the infant to cry for short periods.
   c. Change position frequently to increase circulation and allow for aeration of all lung areas.

C. Properly care for colostomy and understand its purpose.

1. Proper functioning of colostomy.
   a. Note drainage from colostomy—characteristics, frequency, fecal material, or liquid drainage.
   b. Note abdominal distention.
   c. Measure fluid loss from colostomy as the amount will affect fluid replacement.
2. Signs of obstruction from peritonitis, paralytic ileus, handling bowel, or swelling.
   a. No output from colostomy
   b. Increased tenderness
   c. Irritability
   d. Vomiting
   e. Increased temperature
3. Good skin care to prevent breakdown around colostomy.
   a. Change soiled dressing or diaper frequently.
   b. Wash skin with clear water.
   c. Use karaya gum, aluminum paste, Maalox, or other means to protect skin from contact with secretions.
   d. Keep area open to air occasionally.

D. Prevent abdominal distention.

1. Nasogastric tube may be used immediately postoperatively.
   a. Check patency.
   b. Watch for increasing abdominal distention; measure abdominal girth.
   c. Measure fluid loss because amount will affect fluid replacement.
2. Once oral feeding is begun, the nasogastric tube will be removed.
   a. Avoid overfeeding.
   b. Bubble frequently during feeding.
   c. Proper positioning after feeding.

E. Continue taking axillary temperatures.

1. Avoids injury
2. Allows for more accurate reading

F. Continue to provide emotional support to the patient (see p. 1334, diarrhea).

1. Recognize the effects of immobility, less handling, and less activity than is generally given the healthy infant.
2. Allow the infant to derive some satisfaction from using a pacifier. Hold him often during this time if condition permits.
3. Prepare the parents for what they will see postoperatively (i.e., equipment, dressings, stoma).

G. Help the parents understand and accept the child and the disease, as well as all that has happened.

1. Even a temporary colostomy can be a difficult procedure to accept and to learn to care for.
   a. Support the parents when teaching them to care for the colostomy. Include them, soon after surgery, in dressing changes.
   b. Try to help them treat the baby or child as normally as possible.
2. Encourage the parents to talk about their fears and anxieties.
   Anticipating future surgery for resection may be confusing and frightening.
3. Initiate community-nurse referral to help the parents care for the child at home away from the comfortable situation of the hospital, and obtain necessary equipment.

Ostomy Care

Colostomy and ileostomy care in the infant and young child is based on the same principles and is essentially the same as that for an adult (see pp. 447–459), with the following exceptions:

1. Colostomy irrigation is not part of management in small children. Irrigation is primarily for the purpose of regulating the colostomy to empty at regular intervals. Since children have bowel movements at more frequent intervals, this type of control is not feasible. Irrigation should only be done in preparation for tests or surgery and occasionally for the treatment of constipation.
2. Dehydration occurs quickly in the infant or small child; therefore, it is particularly important to observe drainage for amount and characteristics. It should be measured to provide an accurate basis for computation of fluid replacement.
3. Prevention and treatment of skin excoriation around the stoma is of primary concern and is a nursing challenge. With the advent of better skin shields and equipment that is designed especially for the pediatric patient, keeping an ostomy appliance in place is much less of a problem than it has been in the past. Through careful application and by trying different types of pouches until a proper fit is obtained, most children can be kept clean and dry for at least 24 hours between changes. This is a very significant factor in preventing skin breakdown and subsequent infections in the peristomal area. It is helpful to remember, however, that in the infant, dressings must be checked frequently:
   a. Dressings and collection bags may not adhere well or stay in place.
   b. Skin breakdown is more frequent.
   c. Infant elimination is more frequent than in the older child.

4. Helping agency for parents:
United Ostomy Association, 2001 W. Beverly Boulevard, Los Angeles, CA 90057
5. Some companies manufacturing pediatric size ostomy equipment:
United Surgical (Division of Howmedia, Inc.), Largo, FL 33540
Coloplast, C.R. Bard Inc., 713 Central Avenue, Murray Hill, NJ 07974
Hollister, Inc., 211 E. Chicago Avenue, Chicago, IL 60611
6. Suggested reading:
Jeter K. These Special Children. Palo Alto, CA, Bull Publishing Co, 1982; written specifically for parents of children with colostomies, ileostomies, and urostomies

Health Education

1. Begin early to teach thoroughly and carefully what the colostomy is for, how it works, and how to care for it and the child.
   a. Involve the whole family in teaching colostomy care to enhance acceptance of body change of the child.
   b. An older child should become totally responsible for his colostomy care.
   c. Procedures needed to be thoroughly understood and practiced include preparation of skin, application of collecting appliance, care of appliance, and control of odor.
   d. Signs of stomal complications: ribbon-like stool, diarrhea, failure of evacuation of stool or flatus, bleeding.
   e. Dilatation of stoma with finger may need to be taught and practiced.
   f. Increased fluid intake is needed because colon absorption is decreased; low-residue food is needed to decrease bulk of stool.

g. Prepare parents and older child for colostomy closure as appropriate.
2. The parents may also need to know gastrostomy feeding techniques as well as procedures for care and dilation of anus.
3. Allow the parents to learn and practice these procedures long before the infant is to be discharged.
4. Emphasize the importance of treating the child as normally as possible to prevent behavior problems later.
5. Good nutrition and diet need to be understood by parents prior to discharge. Involve the dietitian as necessary.
6. Encourage close medical follow-up and general good health and hygiene.
   a. Nutrition
   b. General growth and development
   c. Immunizations

Expected Outcomes

1. Regains normal breathing pattern; shows relief of abdominal distention; stabilization of vital signs; blood gas values returning to normal
2. Takes small frequent feedings or receives parenteral feedings; shows weight gain
3. Achieves normal acid–base balance; has good skin turgor and moist mucous membranes; normal laboratory values
4. Demonstrates appropriate elimination pattern following surgery
5. Maintains skin integrity around colostomy site
6. Becomes less irritable when held and rocked
7. Parents express fears and anxieties about child's condition; engage in appropriate parent–child relationships
8. Parents demonstrate colostomy care; verbalize need for follow-up care

Intussusception

Intussusception is the invagination or telescoping of a portion of the intestine into an adjacent, more distal section of the intestine.

Etiology

1. Not usually known
   May be due to increased mobility of intestine and hyperperistalsis present in young children.
2. Possible contributing causes in older child
   a. Meckel's diverticulum
   b. Polyps, cysts in the bowel
   c. Malrotation of intestines
   d. Acute enteritis
   e. Abdominal injury
   f. Abdominal surgery; intestinal intubation
   g. Cystic fibrosis
   h. Celiac disease

Altered Physiology

1. Mesentery is pulled into intestine when invagination occurs.
2. Progression to obstruction
   a. Intestine becomes curved, sausage-like—blood supply is cut off.

b. Bowel begins to swell—hemorrhage may occur.
   c. Complete intestinal obstruction results—necrosis of involved segment.
3. Classification of location.
   a. *Ileocecal* (most common)—ileum invaginates into ascending colon
   b. *Ileocolic*—ileum invaginates into colon
   c. *Colocolic*—colon invaginates into colon
   d. *Ileo-ileo*—(enteroenteric) small bowel invaginates into small bowel

Clinical Manifestations

1. Incidence is rare in first month of life.
   a. 4–10 months is most common age of onset (50%–70%).
   b. 1–2 years of age—frequency of occurrence is high.
2. Onset is sudden.
   a. Paroxysmal abdominal pain
   b. Currant jelly-like stools
      (1) Blood and mucus present in stool
      (2) One or more stools with this characteristic
      (3) Presence of bloody mucus on finger following rectal examination

c. Vomiting
d. Increasing absence of stools
e. Increasing abdominal distention and tenderness
f. Sausage-like mass palpable in abdomen
g. Dehydration and fever
h. Shock-like state
   (1) Rapid pulse
   (2) Pale skin
   (3) Marked sweating

Diagnostic Evaluation

1. General condition and appearance of child; history
2. X-ray examination
   a. Flat plate of abdomen—reveals staircase pattern (invagination appears like stair steps on x-ray)
   b. Barium enema under fluoroscopy—coil-like appearance of bowel

Treatment

1. Hydrostatic reduction of telescoped bowel with barium enema used during first 48 hours after onset.
2. Surgical reduction of intussusception; resection if bowel is gangrenous.

Patient Problems/Nursing Diagnoses

1. Alteration in comfort related to paroxysmal abdominal pain, fever, and treatments
2. Alteration in fluid and electrolyte balance related to vomiting
3. Alteration in elimination related to intestinal obstruction
4. Respiratory distress related to abdominal distention
5. Anxiety related to pain, hospitalization and treatments
6. Parental anxiety related to suddenness of child's illness and lack of understanding of disease and its consequences

Preoperative Nursing Interventions

A. Assist in maintaining or restoring hydration and electrolyte balance.

Monitor parenteral fluids (see IV Therapy, p. 1160)

B. Prevent vomiting and aspiration.

1. Stomach may be deflated by insertion of nasogastric tube.
2. Maintain patency of nasogastric tube if one is inserted.
   a. Irrigate at frequent intervals.
   b. Note drainage and return from irrigation.
3. Patient is likely to be NPO.
   a. Wet lips and give mouth care.
   b. Give infant pacifier to suck.

C. Be aware of the patient's condition by frequent observations, thereby contributing to the total care of the patient.

1. Respirations are affected because of abdominal distention.
   a. Grunting
   b. Shallow and rapid if patient is in shock-like state
2. Abdominal distention and unusual appearance of anus—intussusception may look like rectal prolapse.

▶ **NURSING ALERT:** When anus has an unusual appearance, take axillary temperatures to prevent injury.

3. Behavior
   a. Irritable—very sensitive to handling (Be gentle!)
   b. Lethargic or unresponsive

   c. Behavior indicative of presence or absence of pain

D. Prepare the patient for surgery when he is shock-like or febrile.

1. Blood or plasma is given to restore circulating blood volume—observe for transfusion reactions.
2. Observe pulse rate carefully—safe range is below 140/minute.
3. Reduce temperature—fever increases metabolism and makes oxygenation during anesthesia more complicated.

E. Offer support to the parents during this time of crisis and fear.

1. Encourage the parents to verbalize their concerns.
2. Reinforce what the physician has told them.
3. Encourage them to be with the child whenever possible.
4. Help them understand the basic defect and the reason for surgery.

Postoperative Nursing Interventions

A. Give good postoperative care and observe for possible postoperative complications (see p. 1126).

B. Be constantly alert for complications arising from surgery for intussusception.

1. Fever is usually present.
   a. As a result of absorption of foreign protein
   b. From absorption of bacteria through the damaged intestinal wall
2. Diarrhea—from exposure to others who are infected
3. Shock
4. Dehydration
5. Toxicity
6. Peritonitis

C. Assist in maintaining stomach decompression until first stool is passed.

1. See that indwelling nasogastric tube is functioning properly.
   a. Tube is usually connected to constant intermittent suction.
   b. Note returns from drainage and irrigation.
2. The patient is usually given nothing by mouth. Give mouth care.
3. Note passing of flatus or stool and report—indicates peristalsis has returned to normal activity.
   Oral feedings may start.

D. Gradually resume full caloric intake and volume of oral intake appropriate for age and weight.

Progression will vary with physician and will depend on whether bowel reduction or resection was the surgical procedure.

1. Oral fluid is usually begun after the first stool is passed—about 4–5 days after surgery. When only a reduction was performed, oral fluid may be resumed when abdominal peristaltic activity is audible.
2. Give frequent, small feedings.
   a. Start with glucose water or water.
   b. Note and report any abdominal distention or vomiting.

E. Provide emotional support and meet the psychological needs of the child.

(See Diarrhea, p. 1334)

F. Support the parents and help them to maintain a good relationship with their child.
1. Encourage them to visit and call. Allow the parents to become involved in caring for their child.
2. Help the parents to understand that recurrence is rare, but that certain short-term limits must be placed on the child's activity after discharge.

Expected Outcomes
1. Experiences increasing comfort; shows more normal breathing pattern; more restful behavior; decrease in distressed crying; has relaxed body posture

2. Attains/maintains fluid and electrolyte balance; normal laboratory values and skin turgor
3. Passes stool within 4–5 days following surgery; has audible abdominal peristaltic activity; ingests prescribed feedings without signs of abdominal distention or vomiting
4. Exhibits decrease in abdominal girth; absence of respiratory distress
5. Responds to comfort measures with more relaxed behavior
6. Parents participate in child's care; show an understanding of the treatment protocol

Imperforate Anus

The term *imperforate anus* is used to describe all congenital abnormalities of the anorectal canal or in the location of the anus within the perineum.

Etiology and Incidence
1. An arrest in embryologic development of the anus, lower rectum, and urogenital tract at the 8th week of embryonic life
2. Cause unknown
3. 1:4,000–1:5,000 incidence
4. Closely associated with other congenital deviations, including:
   a. Congenital heart disease
   b. Esophageal atresia
   c. Spinal malformations
   d. Hydronephrosis
   e. Low birth weight

Types
1. Low imperforate anus (transelevator)—implies that the rectum has descended below the pubococcygeal line (puborectalis muscle) and is in normal anatomical relationship to levator sling and puborectus muscle (Fig. 37-3).
   a. Female
      (1) 90% of females with this condition present with low imperforate anus.
      (2) Fistula is present; rectum ends in fistula which presents in any location from low in vagina to normal position of anus.
   b. Male
      (1) 50% of males with imperforate anus present with this type.
      (2) Perineal fistula is present and is located from

anterior or normal position of anus to ventral surface of penis. (supraelevator)
2. High imperforate anus (supraelevator)—term implies that the rectal pouch is at or above the pubococcygeal line or the levator musculature (75%).
   a. Male
      (1) 50% of males with imperforate anus present with this type.
      (2) If fistula is present, it will usually communicate with the posterior urethra.
   b. Female
      (1) 10% of females with imperforate anus present with this type.
      (2) Fistula will end high in vagina.

Complications
1. Rectal stenosis or prolapse, usually confined to mucosa
2. Separation of anastomosis
3. Urethral injury or stricture
4. Urinary retention and infection
5. Recurrent urinary fistulas
6. Fecal impaction or incontinence
7. Small bowel obstruction

Clinical Manifestations
Condition is usually discovered immediately after birth or within several hours.
1. No anal opening
2. Thermometer or small finger cannot be inserted into rectum
3. Absence of meconium stool
4. Green-tinged urine—if fistula is present (high, male)
5. Progressive abdominal distention

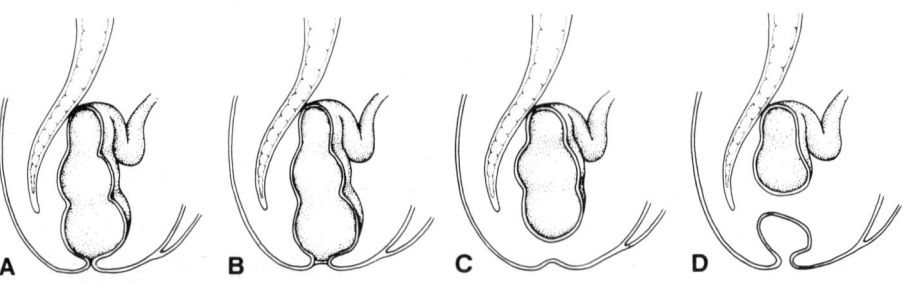

Figure 37-3. Anorectal malformations.

A Anal stenosis

B Imperforate anal membrane

C Anal agenesis

D Rectal agenesis

6. Fistula is likely to be present
    a. Female—occurs between rectum and vagina or perineum.
    b. Male—occurs between rectum and urinary tract, scrotum or perineum.

Diagnostic Evaluation

1. Visual examination
    a. Presence of perineal fistula
    b. Meconium coming from vagina or presence of meconium-stained urine
2. General examination and/or presence of other associated manifestations
3. Urine examination for presence of meconium and epithelial debris—indicates presence of fistula.
4. Voiding cystourethrogram
5. Wangensteen–Rice x-ray (upside-down position)
    a. Limited accuracy in locating rectal pouch
    b. Useful only after infant is 24 hours of age
6. Sonography
7. Neurologic examination

Treatment

1. Low—female
    a. Decompression of bowel with catheter irrigations
    b. Dilatation of fistula for 8–12 months thereafter
    c. Definitive repair
2. Low—male
    a. Rectal cutback anoplasty or Y–V plasty
    b. Local dilatation of fistula
3. High—male
    a. Colostomy for decompression
    b. Definitive pull-through surgery—deferred until about 1 year of age or when child attains 6.75–9 kg. (15–20 lbs.)
4. High—female
    a. Colostomy
    b. Definitive repair done when infant is 1 year of age or 6.75–9 kg. (15–20 lbs.)

Preoperative Nursing Interventions

A. Assist in maintaining stability in the patient's general condition prior to emergency surgery.

1. Feedings are usually withheld. Note any vomiting, color and amount.
2. Nasogastric tube may be passed to decompress the stomach. Measure abdominal girth.
3. Observe the patient carefully for any signs of distress and report these to physician. Check vital signs frequently. Maintain temperature stability.

B. Observe the infant carefully for any other anomalies or changes in condition.

1. Use an Isolette or radiant warmer.
2. Observe for stool coming from a fistula.
3. Note that urine may be green-tinged.
4. Keep area clean.

Postoperative Nursing Interventions

Depending on the location of the rectum (see types of imperforate anus), and sex of child, 1 of 3 surgical approaches may be used: (1) anoplasty, (2) temporary colostomy with definitive pull-through at a later time when the child is older and larger, or (3) abdominal or sacroperineal pull-through.

A. Give good postoperative care and to observe for possible postoperative complications.

(See p. 1126.)
Especially note any vomiting or stooling.

B. Provide appropriate care for perineal anoplasty, prevent infection of suture line, and promote healing.

1. Do not put anything in rectum.
2. Expose perineum to air.
3. Position the infant for easy access to perineum for cleansing and minimal irritation to site (i.e., place the infant on abdomen, possibly with hips elevated, to prevent pressure on perineal surfaces; turn side-to-side).

C. Provide good colostomy care and prevent skin breakdown.

(See Hirschsprung's disease, p. 1337)

D. Provide appropriate care for definitive pull-through surgery.

1. Carry out perineal care as stated above.
2. Provide proper care of gastrostomy or nasogastric tube used to decompress the gastrointestinal tract until peristalsis returns.
3. Provide proper care of bladder catheter, if used, and measure urinary output accurately.
4. Observe carefully for abdominal distention, bleeding from perineum, and respiratory embarrassment.

E. Maintain adequate nutrition as well as caloric and fluid intake to prevent dehydration and electrolyte imbalance.

1. Oral feedings are usually started within hours after an anoplasty.
2. Oral feedings are usually withheld until peristalsis returns. When primary repair is done, nasogastric suction may be maintained until feedings are started.
3. Monitor parenteral fluids (see p. 1160).

F. Foster acceptance of the child and his diagnosis by his parents.

1. Assure the parents that colostomy is temporary.
2. Encourage the parents to become involved in care of the child and to give him the emotional security he needs.
3. Support teaching program of surgeon for special care needed at home.
    a. Colostomy care
    b. Anal dilatation to prevent a stricture at site of anastomosis from scar tissue after instructions by physician
4. Initiate referral to community nurse, especially if the parents are particularly anxious about caring for the child at home.
5. Encourage the parents to talk about their concerns.

Health Education

1. Provide careful, thorough teaching of special care and procedures to be continued at home—colostomy care, anal dilatation. Develop a plan for return demonstration by mother.
2. Help the parents to understand situations that may be encountered as a result of imperforate anus as the baby gets older:
    a. Fecal impaction due to lack of sensation to defecate
    b. Future surgery—if primary repair was not done
    c. Toilet training
    d. Inability to control fecal seepage from rectum

Bibliography

Books

Cooper HK et al (eds). Cleft Palate and Cleft Lip: A Team Approach to Clinical Management and Rehabilitation of the Patient. Philadelphia, WB Saunders, 1979

Gryboski J and Walker WA. Gastrointestinal Problems in the Infant, 2nd ed. Philadelphia, WB Saunders, 1983

Lebenthal E (ed). Textbook of Gastroenterology and Nutrition in Infancy, Vol. 2: Gastrointestinal Disease and Nutritional Inadequacies. New York, Raven Press, 1981

Raffensperger JG. Swenson's Pediatric Surgery, 4th ed. New York, Appleton-Century-Crofts, 1980

Silverberg M. Pediatric Gastroenterology. Garden City, NY, Medical Examination Publishing Co, 1983

Silverberg A and Roy CC. Pediatric Clinical Gastroenterology, 3rd ed. St Louis, CV Mosby, 1983

Whaley LF and Wong DL. Nursing Care of Infants and Children. St Louis, CV Mosby, 1983

Wieczorek RR and Natapoff JN. A Conceptual Approach to the Nursing of Children. Philadelphia, JB Lippincott, 1981

Articles

Alvear DT and Solenberger MD. Constipation in infants and children: Personal observations and management. J Enterostom Ther 1983 Jan/Feb; 10(1):14–18

Barsky NH and Londeree K. First aid procedures for dental emergencies. J Sch Health 1982 Jan; 52(1):43–45

Boyd CW. Postural therapy at home for infants with gastroesophageal reflux. Pediatr Nurs 1982 Nov/Dec; 8(6):395–398

Carreto V. Maternal responses to an infant with cleft lip and palate: A review of literature. Matern Child Nurs J 1981 Fall; 10(3):197–205

Chapparo CJ, et al. Incidence of sensory integrative dysfunction among children with orofacial cleft. AJOT 1981 Feb; 35(2):96–100

Diagnosis and management of acute diarrhea. Report of the Thirteenth Ross Roundtable on Clinical Approaches to Common Pediatric Problems in collaboration with the Ambulatory Pediatric Association. Ross Lab, Columbus OH, 1982

Elhassani SB. Surgically treatable neonatal respiratory distress: Part 2. Perinatol/Neonatol 1983 Jan; 7(1):47–48+

Euler AR. Gastroesophageal reflux among pediatric-age patients. Hosp Formulary 1981 Mar; 16(3):258–263

Falchuk ZM. Gluten-sensitive enteropathy. Clin Gastroenterol 1983 May; 12(2):475–494

Haase GM and Lilly JR. Advances in newborn surgery. Perinatol/Neonatol 1982 Jun; 6(3):21–24+

Hartwig MS. Sticking to a gluten free diet. Am J Nurs 1983 Sep; 83(9):1308–1310

Hatten CL. The importance of good nutrition in dental health. Point View 1983 July; 20(3):19

Hayward JR. Cleft lip and cleft palate. In Kruger GO (ed). Textbook of Oral and Maxillofacial Surgery, 6th ed. St Louis, CV Mosby 1984, pp. 456–483

Jeter KF. Pediatric problems associated with stomas, Part 2: Special needs of paediatric patients. Clin Gastroenterol 1982 May; 11(2):360–372

Kilmon C and Helpin ML. Recognizing dental malocclusion in children. Pediatr Nurs 1983 May/Jun; 9(3):204–208

Kurfiss-Daniels D. Positioning as treatment for infant gastroesophageal reflux. Am J Nurs 1982 Oct; 82(10):1535–1537

Labenthal E and Branski D. Childhood celiac disease—a new appraisal. J Pediatr 1981 May; 98(95):681–690

Labenthal E, Wynn R and Labenthal H. Digestive disorders in neonates, Part 2: Congenital and acquired disease. Perinatol/Neonatol 1983 Apr; 7(4):53–56+

Luce M and Sande D. Oral health in children: Prevention of dental caries. Nurs Pract 1983 Mar; 8(3):43, 47+

Martin K, Grosfeld J and Perez RC. Care of the neonate with surgical problems. Crit Care Q 1981 Jun; 4(1):33–46

Meyers WF and Herbst JJ. Effectiveness of positioning therapy for gastroesophageal reflux. Pediatrics 1982 Jun; 69(6):768–772

Nixon HH. Pediatric problems associated with stomas, Part 1: Intestinal surgical problems. Clin Gastroenterol 1982 May; 11(2):351–359

Ochoa JB. Diagnosis and management of gastroesophageal reflux in children. In Nyhus LM (ed). Surgery Annual. New York, Appleton-Century-Crofts, 1981 13:123–137

Page-Goertz SS and Stewart DR. Is the baby just spitting? Consideration of the gastroesophageal reflux. Issues Compr Pediatr Nurs 1980 Apr; 4(2):53–66

Peacock JL and Starr P. An outreach program for families of infants with a cleft lip and/or palate. Child Today 1980 Sep/Oct; 9(5):23–24

Pickering LK. Antimicrobial therapy of gastrointestinal infections. Pediatr Clin North Am 1983 Apr; 30(2):373–388

Puri P et al. Delayed primary anastomosis following spontaneous growth of esophageal segments in esophageal atresia. J Pediatr Surg 1981 Apr; 16(2):180–183

Ramenofsky ML and Leape LL. Continuous upper esophageal pH monitoring in infants and children with gastroesophageal reflux, pneumonia, and apneic spells. J Pediatr Surg 1981 Jun; 16(3):374–378

Sasso SC. Metoclopramide and chalasia. MCN 1983 Sep/Oct; 8(5):361

Schneider PL. Care of the cleft lip and cleft palate patient. Physician Assist 1982 Feb; 6(2):19–21+

Styler GW and Freeh K. Feeding infants with cleft lip and/or palate. JOGN Nurs 1981 Sep/Oct; 10(5):329–332

Sugar EC. Hirschsprung's Disease. Am J Nurs 1981 Nov; 81(11):2065–2067

Taitz L. Managing toddler diarrhea. Health Visit 1983 Jan; 56(1):9–10

Walker RM. Surgery for the child ostomate. JET 1982 Jul/Aug; 9(4):18–20

White JE and Owsley VB. Helping families cope with milk, wheat, and soy allergies. MCN 1983 Nov/Dec; 8(6):423–428

Children with Conditions of the Kidneys, Urinary Tract, and Reproductive System

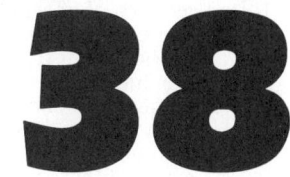

Acute Glomerulonephritis

Glomerulonephritis refers to inflammation of the kidneys caused by an antigen–antibody reaction following an infection in some part of the body. Acute glomerulonephritis is predominantly a disease of childhood and is the most common type of nephritis in children.

Etiology

1. Presumed cause—antigen–antibody reaction secondary to an infection elsewhere in the body
2. Initial infection
   a. Usually either an upper respiratory infection or a skin infection
   b. Most frequent causative agent—nephritogenic strains of group A beta hemolytic streptococcus

Incidence

1. Unknown—milder cases are not recognized
2. More common in males than females
3. Most common in preschool and early school-age groups
4. Rare in children under 2 years of age
5. Varies with the prevalence of nephritogenic strains of streptococci and the likelihood of cross infection

Altered Physiology

1. The organisms responsible for nephritis contain antigens similar to those of the basement membrane of the renal glomeruli.
2. Antibodies produced to fight the invading organism also react against the glomerular tissue, forming immune complexes.
3. The immune complexes become trapped in the glomerular loop and cause an inflammatory reaction in the affected glomeruli.
4. Changes in the glomerular capillaries reduce the amount of the glomerular filtrate, allow passage of blood cells and protein into the filtrate, and reduce the amount of sodium and water that is passed to the tubules for reabsorption.
5. General vascular disturbances, including loss of capillary integrity and spasm of arterioles, are secondary to kidney changes and are responsible for much of the symptomatology of the disease.

Assessment

Clinical Manifestations

A. Onset

1. Usually 1–3 weeks after the onset of the initiating infection
2. May be abrupt and severe, or mild and detected only by laboratory measures

B. Signs and Symptoms

1. Urinary symptoms
   a. Decreased urine output
   b. Bloody or brown-colored urine
2. Edema
   a. Present in most patients
   b. Usually mild
   c. Often manifested by periorbital edema in the morning
   d. May appear only as rapid weight gain
   e. May be generalized and influenced by posture
3. Hypertension
   a. Present in over 50% of patients
   b. Usually mild
   c. Rise in blood pressure may be sudden
   d. Usually appears during the first 4–5 days of the illness
4. Malaise
5. Mild headache
6. Gastrointestinal disturbances, especially anorexia and vomiting

Diagnostic Evaluation

1. Urinalysis
   a. Decreased output—may approach anuria
   b. Microscopic or gross hematuria
   c. Specific gravity—moderately elevated
   d. Proteinuria (3+ to 4+)
   e. Microscopic—red blood cells, leukocytes, epithelial cells and casts
2. Serum complement level—usually reduced
3. BUN and creatinine—often mildly to moderately elevated
4. ASO or antistreptokinase titer—elevated

5. Sedimentation rate—elevated
6. Chest x-ray—may show pulmonary congestion, cardiac enlargement
7. Renal function studies—normal in 50% of the patients

Prognosis

1. At least 95% of affected children recover completely.
   a. Acute symptoms usually disappear in 1–3 weeks.
   b. Blood chemistry is usually normal by the end of the 2nd week.
   c. Urine sediment may be abnormal for months or even years following the acute episode.
   d. Sedimentation rate may remain elevated for several months.
2. Death during the acute phase is very uncommon, but may occur due to the effects of hypertensive encephalopathy or heart failure.
3. A small percentage of children develop chronic nephritis.

Complications

(Occur infrequently)

A. Hypertensive Encephalopathy

1. Manifestations
   a. Restlessness
   b. Stupor
   c. Convulsions
   d. Vomiting
   e. Severe headache
   f. Visual disturbances
2. Cause—probably ischemia secondary to vasospasm
3. No correlation with the degree of renal impairment or fluid retention
4. Duration
   a. Usually 1–2 days
   b. Ends spontaneously with decreased blood pressure

B. Congestive Heart Failure

1. Cardiac failure may occur due to persistent hypertension, hypervolemia, and peripheral vasoconstriction.
2. Manifestations
   a. Dyspnea
   b. Tachycardia
   c. Gallop rhythm
   d. Liver engorgement
3. Duration
   a. Variable
   b. Usually subsides rapidly with the onset of diuresis and the fall in blood pressure

C. Uremia (rare)

Manifestations
1. Evidence of acidosis
2. Drowsiness
3. Coma
4. Stupor
5. Muscular twitching
6. Convulsions

D. Anemia

Usually caused by hypervolemia rather than a loss of red blood cells in the urine

Patient Problems/Nursing Diagnoses

1. Development of life-threatening complications, including hypertensive encephalopathy, congestive heart failure, and acute renal failure

2. Reduced urine output related to glomerular dysfunction
3. Fluid volume excess related to kidney failure
4. Headache and discomfort related to toxic buildup in blood
5. Reduced nutritional intake related to anorexia
6. Anxiety related to uncertain course of disease and hospitalization
7. Activity intolerance related to fatigue caused by underlying disease
8. Knowledge deficit regarding acute glomerulonephritis and its management
9. Nonadherence to dietary and fluid restrictions

Planning and Implementation
Nursing Interventions

A. Promote healing and prevent disease complications.

1. No specific measures have been demonstrated to modify the inflammatory process.
2. General measures
   a. Maintain bed rest during the acute phase of the illness, at least until gross hematuria has disappeared and child is no longer hypertensive.
      (1) Organize nursing activities to allow the child to have periods of uninterrupted rest.
      (2) Explain to the child why it is necessary for him to stay in bed. (Bed rest is often interpreted by the child as punishment.)
      (3) Administer sedation if required to keep the child quiet and at rest.
      (4) Provide diversion appropriate for the child's age.
      (5) Place the child's bed in a position where he can watch the activities of the unit and other children.
      (6) Provide alternative means of rest for children who are too young to understand the necessity of remaining in bed. (Such children can be held by the mother or nurse in a chair.)
      (7) Observe the child closely for fatigue once ambulation is begun.
   b. Protect the child from infection.
      (1) Avoid placing the child in a room with patients who have fevers, upper respiratory infections, or any other contagious disease.
      (2) Administer therapeutic doses of antibiotics as prescribed by the physician to eradicate existing infection.
         (a) A 10-day course of intramuscular penicillin is often prescribed.
         (b) Points of emphasis.
            Inject the medication into a large muscle.
            Rotate the site of injection.
            Observe the child closely for adverse reactions such as skin rash, urticaria, serum sickness, and anaphylaxis.
      (3) Protect the child from chilling or overheating.
      (4) Provide scrupulous daily hygiene, including mouth care. Keep the skin clean and dry.
   c. Provide a diet in conformity with the child's age and the recommendation of his physician.
      (1) A regular diet without added salt is usually prescribed during the acute phase in noncomplicated cases.

(2) A diet restricted in protein and potassium is necessary for children who demonstrate some degree of renal failure.

(3) Fluids must be restricted in children with hypertension, edema, congestive failure, or renal failure.

(4) Explain all dietary restrictions to the child and his parents.

(5) Obtain a careful history of dietary preferences and patterns so that the child's meals can be as acceptable as possible.

(6) Place a sign indicating dietary restrictions on the child's bed so that anyone approaching him will be aware of his special needs.

(7) If the child is to be given a restricted amount of fluids, offer small amounts of fluids spaced at regular intervals throughout the day and evening.
Use a cup of appropriate size for the amount of fluid being offered.

(8) Refer to section on nutrition, p. 1094.

B. Observe and record disease progress.

1. Maintain a complete record of the child's intake and output.
   a. Measure fluids accurately in graduated containers. Do not estimate fluid intake or output.
   b. Place a sign on the child's bed to ensure that no urine is accidentally discarded and that all intake is recorded.
   c. Total the intake and output every 8 hours.
      (1) Notify the physician if output does not appear adequate.
      (2) In children who are not toilet trained, a fairly accurate record of output can be obtained by weighing diapers before and after voiding.
   d. Record other causes of fluid loss such as the number of stools per day, perspiration, etc.
2. Weigh the child daily.
   a. An increase in weight may indicate fluid retention.
   b. Weigh the child on the same scale and at the same time each day.
      (1) It is usually advantageous to weigh the child before breakfast.
      (2) The child should be weighed in a consistent manner, with minimal clothing.
3. Record the blood pressure at frequent intervals.
   a. Refer to the method for determining blood pressure, page 1134.
   b. A diastolic pressure of 100 mm. Hg is an indication of concern and should be reported to the physician immediately.
   Place the child into bed and observe him closely for cerebral changes.
4. Observe for signs of complications.
   a. Increased blood pressure
   b. Fluid retention or edema
   c. Changes in vital signs, especially more rapid pulse or respirations
   d. Changes in activity status, especially lethargy, restlessness, stupor, or coma
   e. Vomiting
   f. Visual disturbances
   g. Severe headache
   h. Convulsions

5. Record appearance of urine.
Note the persistence of hematuria or whether the urine appears to be clearing.

C. Reduce hypertension.

1. Limit the fluid intake according to the physician's recommendation.
2. Maintain bed rest.
3. Administer antihypertensive drugs as prescribed by the physician.
   a. Reserpine is the drug most frequently used.
      (1) Route of administration—intramuscular or intravenous
      (2) Side effects—nasal stuffiness, dryness of mouth, diarrhea
   b. Hydralazine (Apresoline) is often combined with reserpine in refractory cases.
      (1) Route of administration
         (a) Intramuscular
         (b) This drug may be given orally once initial control of hypertension is established.
      (2) Side effects
         (a) Nausea, vomiting, diarrhea, anorexia
         (b) Headache
         (c) Tachycardia

D. Provide appropriate nursing care to the child with disease complications.

1. Encephalopathy (see the section on care of the child with seizures, p. 1429)
2. Congestive heart failure
3. Anemia
4. Renal failure

E. Provide emotional support to the child and his family during hospitalization.

1. Explain all aspects of the diagnostic tests and treatment in terms that the family can understand.
2. Formulate a nursing care plan that facilitates a consistent approach to the child's care.
3. Allow the child to make some decisions and to participate in his care. He may decide when he wants his bath and should be allowed to make some dietary choices, etc.
4. Maintain discipline. Establish and enforce appropriate limits for the child's behavior.
5. Provide diversion appropriate for the child's age.
6. Arrange for the continued education of the school-age child.

F. Prepare the child and his parents for discharge.

1. Encourage as much family participation as possible during the child's hospitalization (see the section on family-centered care, p. 1117).
2. Help the family plan for adaptation of the child's nursing care to the home environment.
   a. Review the medication schedule.
   b. Suggest means of implementing a sodium-restricted diet.
      (1) Provide the family with a list of commercial foods and fluids that are normally high in sodium content, so that they can avoid these.
      (2) Help the parents to plan sample menus.
      (3) Provide suggestions for low-sodium cooking and baking.
   c. Discuss activity and fluid restrictions if appropriate.

3. Make certain that the family has an appointment for continued medical supervision.
4. Initiate appropriate referrals.
   a. Community health nurse
   b. Home tutor

Health Education

1. Medical explanation of the disease process should be reinforced.
   a. The need for medical evaluation and culture of all sore throats should be emphasized.
   b. The family should be made aware of signs and symptoms of disease recurrence.
2. Tonsillectomy or other oral surgery is not recommended for several months after the acute phase of glomerulonephritis.
   If this type of surgery is necessary later, penicillin may be recommended before and after the procedure to prevent bacterial infection.

Evaluation

Expected Outcomes

1. Absence of life-threatening complications
2. Demonstrates increasing urinary output
3. Adheres to prescribed fluid restriction; maintains weight within acceptable level for condition
4. Copes with discomfort; engages in diversional activities in accordance with age
5. Eats prescribed diet
6. Adheres to treatment protocol; parents gaining an understanding of child's illness as evidenced by their questions, conversation and participation in child's care

Nephrotic Syndrome

Nephrotic syndrome refers to a symptom complex characterized by edema, marked proteinuria, hypoalbuminemia, and hypercholesterolemia. Although there are many types of the disease, minimal change nephrotic syndrome is the most common in children.

Etiology

1. The symptom complex results from large losses of protein in the urine, too great for the body to replenish by albumin synthesis.
2. The syndrome may be classified as primary (associated with a primary glomerular disease) or secondary (resulting from a wide variety of disease states or nephrotoxic agents).

Incidence

1. Annually afflicts about 2–3 children per 100,000 under the age of 8 years in the US
2. More common in males than in females
3. Most common age of onset—between 1½ and 3 years

Altered Physiology

1. For unknown reasons, the glomerular membrane, usually impermeable to large proteins, becomes permeable.
2. Protein, especially albumin, leaks through the membrane and is lost in the urine.
3. Plasma proteins decrease as proteinuria increases.
4. The colloidal osmotic pressure that holds water in the vascular compartments is reduced because of the decrease in amount of serum albumin. This allows fluid to flow from the capillaries into the extracellular space, producing edema.
5. Accumulation of fluid in the interstitial spaces and peritoneal cavity is also increased by an overproduction of aldosterone, which causes retention of sodium.
6. There is increased susceptibility to infection because of decreased gamma globulin.
7. Generalized edema is responsible for most of the physical characteristics of the disease, including respiratory distress, gastrointestinal symptoms, umbilical and inguinal hernias, rectal prolapse, decreased ambulation, loss of body tissue, and malnutrition.

Clinical Course and Prognosis

1. The severity and duration of the clinical course is variable and affects the prognosis.
2. Most children experience remission following the initial course of treatment.
   a. Of these responders, most will relapse once or not at all during the subsequent 6 months.
   b. About ⅓ of the responders experience multiple relapses following the initial remission.
3. The majority of affected children eventually have a complete recovery.
4. Death may occur from profound sepsis, progressive renal insufficiency, or congestive heart failure.

Assessment

Clinical Manifestations

A. Onset

1. Insidious
2. Edema is often the presenting symptom.
   a. Initially, usually slight and inconstant
   b. Usually first apparent around the eyes

B. Signs and symptoms

1. Irritability and depression
2. Gastrointestinal disturbances, including vomiting and diarrhea
3. Anorexia—malnutrition may become severe
4. Recurrent infections
5. Edema—may be minimal or massive
   a. Ascites may be severe
   b. Intense scrotal edema is common
   c. Peripheral edema is dependent and shifts with the child's position
   d. Striae may appear on the skin from overstretching
6. Profound weight gain; the child may actually double his normal weight
7. Decreased urine output during the edematous phase
8. Wasting of skeletal muscles may occur because of the continuous drain of plasma protein nitrogen into the urine
9. Nephrotic crisis
   a. Abdominal pain
   b. Fever

c. Erysipeloid skin eruption possible
d. Symptoms subside within a few days
e. Often followed by spontaneous diuresis

Diagnostic Evaluation

1. Urinalysis
   a. Proteinuria—marked
   b. Casts—numerous
   c. Hematuria—absent or transient
2. Renal function tests—variable, often normal
3. Blood
   a. Total serum protein—reduced
   b. Serum albumin—reduced
   c. Total serum globulin—normal or increased
      Gamma fraction—reduced
   d. Cholesterol and lipoproteins—increased
   e. Serum calcium—reduced
4. Blood pressure—usually normal although mild hypertension may be present

Patient Problems/Nursing Diagnoses

1. Fluid volume excess related to glomerular dysfunction
2. Impaired skin integrity related to edema
3. Altered urinary pattern related to glomerular dysfunction
4. Increased susceptibility to infection related to disease process and steroid therapy
5. Pain and discomfort
6. Altered body image (round face; hirsutism) related to side effects of medications
7. Inadequate nutritional intake related to anorexia
8. Anxiety and frustration related to the up-and-down course of the disease
9. Knowledge deficit about nephrotic syndrome

Planning and Implementation
Nursing Interventions

A. Relieve edema and other manifestations of the nephrotic state.

1. Administer steroids as recommended by the physician.
   a. Steroid therapy is the preferred approach to treatment because steroids appear to affect the basic disease process in addition to controlling edema.
   b. Prednisone is usually the drug of choice because it is less likely to induce salt retention and potassium loss.
      There is no standard program of therapy, but most children receive 2–3 mg./kg. until complete remission occurs; this is followed by low-dose maintenance therapy or an intermittent schedule for several months.
   c. Children with nephrotic syndrome may respond to steroid therapy in several ways:
      (1) Steroid-sensitive—children respond to a single short course of steroids without evidence of relapse after cessation of therapy.
      (2) Steroid-dependent—children respond incompletely or tend to relapse on lowered dosages of steroids and require additional supportive treatment.
      (3) Steroid-resistant—children become resistant to steroid therapy or cannot be maintained in remission without developing serious side effects of treatment.
   d. Observe for evidence of side effects and complications of therapy.

(1) Cushing's syndrome
   (a) Manifestations include increased body hair (hirsutism), rounding of the face ("moon face"), abdominal distention, striae, increased appetite with weight gain, and aggravation of adolescent acne.
   (b) The child should have access to a mirror so that he can observe gradual physical changes in his body.
   (c) The child and his parents should be provided with opportunities to discuss their feelings about the child's altered body image. Play therapy may be helpful for the young child.
   (d) It should be stressed that these physical changes are not harmful nor permanent, and will disappear after the steroid treatment is stopped.
(2) Serious side effects and uncommon complications
   (a) Masking of infections
      The child should be observed very closely for signs of inflammation or infection.
   (b) Peptic ulceration
      Give medication with milk or an antacid. Test all stools with Hematest.
   (c) Growth suppression
   (d) Precipitation of diabetes mellitus
   (e) Increased intracranial pressure manifested by headache, anorexia, vomiting, diplopia, and seizures
   (f) Osteoporosis
   (g) Cataracts
   (h) Thromboembolism
   (i) Adrenal suppression and insufficiency

▶ **NURSING ALERT:** No vaccinations or immunizations should be given during active episodes of nephrosis or while the child is receiving immunosuppressive therapy.

2. Administer immunosuppressive drugs as prescribed by the physician.
   a. Cyclophosphamide is the drug of choice.
   b. This therapy is generally reserved for children with steroid-dependent or steroid-resistant nephrosis because of severe side effects. It should be administered only with informed consent of the patient or parent.
   c. Observe for complications of therapy.
      (1) Decreased white blood count renders the child very susceptible to infection.
      (2) Hair loss—the child should be prepared for this complication and should be helped to deal with the change in body image. Head scarves or wigs may minimize the child's distress.
      (3) Cystitis—the drug should be given in the morning and large volumes of fluid given orally to prevent concentration of the drug in the urine.
      (4) Sterility may result in both sexes from long-term use.
3. Administer diuretics as recommended by the physician.
   a. Be aware of those diuretics which may cause potassium depletion.

(1) Offer foods high in potassium, such as orange juice or bananas.

(2) Supplemental potassium chloride may be administered orally if the urine output is adequate.

4. Maintain the child on bed rest during periods of severe edema.

See the section on acute glomerulonephritis, page 1344.

5. Administer a diet low in sodium and high in potassium.

a. Moderate sodium restriction is usually indicated. Excessively salty foods are excluded, and extra salt is eliminated.

b. Potassium may be provided in juices, fruits (especially oranges, grapes, and bananas), and milk.

6. Restrict fluids as requested by the physician.

a. Fluid restriction is usually imposed only during the extreme edematous phases.

b. Restriction is carefully calculated at frequent intervals, based on the urine output of the previous day plus estimated insensible losses.

c. Offer small amounts of fluids spaced at regular intervals throughout the day and evening.

Use a cup of appropriate size for the amount of fluid being offered.

d. Measure fluids accurately in graduated containers. Do not estimate fluid intake or output.

e. Place a sign on the child's bed to ensure that no urine is accidentally discarded and that all intake is recorded.

f. Determine total intake and output every 8 hours. In children who are not toilet trained, a fairly accurate record of output can be obtained by weighing diapers before and after voiding.

g. Record other causes of fluid loss such as the number of stools per day, perspiration, etc.

7. Assist with abdominal paracentesis when this is required because of marked ascites (see Guidelines, p. 1349).

B. Protect the child from infection.

1. Apply measures stated in the section on acute glomerulonephritis, page 1344.

2. Closely observe the child who is on steroids for signs of infection since this medication masks such symptoms.

3. Provide meticulous skin care to the edematous areas of the body.

a. Bathe the child frequently and apply powder. Areas of special concern are the moist parts of the body and edematous male genitalia.

Support the scrotum with a cotton pad held in place by a T-binder, if necessary, for the child's comfort.

b. Position the child so that edematous skin surfaces are not in contact.

Place a pillow between the child's legs when he is lying on his side, etc.

c. Irrigate swollen eyes and cleanse the surrounding area several times daily to remove exudate.

Elevate the child's head to reduce edema.

4. If possible, avoid femoral venipunctures and intramuscular injections in the buttocks.

In addition to the risk of infection, the child may be predisposed to thromboembolism because of hypovolemia, stasis, and increased plasma concentration of clotting factors.

C. Restore lost plasma and tissue proteins.

1. Offer a high-protein, high-calorie diet.

a. Salt restriction is usually not necessary, except during periods of edema and hypertension.

2. Obtain a complete history of dietary preferences and patterns so that the child's meals can be as acceptable as possible.

3. Place a sign on the child's bed indicating any dietary restrictions, so that anyone approaching him will be aware of his special needs.

4. Permit additional amounts of food at the child's discretion.

5. See the section on nutrition, page 1094.

D. Observe for disease progress.

1. Apply nursing measures outlined in objective B in the section on acute glomerulonephritis, page 1345.

2. Observe the child's entire body at frequent intervals for edema.

a. Record areas of transient edema.

b. Measure abdominal girth.

3. Measure all urine and test for protein, blood, and specific gravity.

Record findings. Report:

a. Decreased urine output

b. Increased amount of protein

c. Cloudiness

d. Hematuria

4. Observe for side effects of all medications.

5. Observe for indications of thrombosis and report these to the physician immediately.

E. Provide emotional support to the child and his family.

1. Encourage frequent visiting.

a. Allow as much parental participation in the child's care as possible.

b. See the section on family-centered care, page 1117.

2. Allow the child as much activity as he can tolerate.

a. Bed rest should be enforced during periods of hypertension.

b. Balance periods of rest, recreation, and quiet activities during the convalescent phase.

c. Allow the child to eat his meals with other children.

3. Encourage the child to verbalize his fears.

a. Young children frequently fear abandonment by their parents or loss of body integrity. (The boy who is unable to visualize his penis because of extensive edema may think that he has been castrated and needs reassurance that his body is intact.)

b. See the section on the hospitalized child, page 1112.

4. Assist the parents to verbalize their fears, frustrations, and questions.

a. Parents often express frustration regarding the uncertainties associated with the cause of the disease, the clinical course, and prognosis.

b. Parents may question the difference between nephritis and nephrosis.

F. Prepare for the child's discharge.

1. Begin discharge planning early.

a. Have the dietitian discuss special diets with the parents. Encourage them to plan sample menus.

b. Encourage the parents to administer the child's medication prior to discharge.

c. Instruct the parents about urine testing.
d. Provide suggestions regarding activity restriction at home.
2. Provide written discharge instructions concerning:
   a. Diet
   b. Prevention of infection
   c. Skin care
   d. Administration of medications
   e. Activity restrictions, if any
   f. Urine testing
   g. Symptoms of relapse
   h. Appointment for continued medical supervision.
3. Initiate a community health nursing referral if necessary for reinforcement of teaching.

Health Education

1. Reinforce medical interpretation of the child's disease. Stress the importance of attention to the details of the child's care and continued medical supervision.
2. Discuss the problem of discipline with the parents. Encourage them to set consistent limits on and expectations of their child's behavior.
3. Emphasize the necessity of taking medication according to the prescribed schedule and for an extended period of time. Discuss complications encountered with steroid therapy.

Evaluation

Expected Outcomes

1. Shows reduction in edema and ascites; cooperates with prescribed reduced fluid intake; abdominal girth decreasing
2. No signs of skin breakdown
3. Demonstrates urine output within acceptable range; laboratory values indicate trend toward recovery; no signs of hematuria
4. Absence of infection; no elevation of temperature
5. Appears more comfortable; engaging in play activities
6. Adheres to prescribed drug therapy; verbalizes that side effects are result of medications
7. Consumes prescribed diet
8. Demonstrates improved coping ability through play, interaction with other children, and normalization of behavior
9. Parents able to describe nephrotic syndrome and treatment program; discuss feelings and frustration with personnel

Guidelines: Assisting with Pediatric Abdominal Paracentesis

Purpose   To withdraw fluid from the peritoneal cavity in order to relieve pressure symptoms and respiratory distresss

Equipment

Sterile equipment
   Hypodermic syringe
   Hypodermic and aspiration needles
   Novocain
   Scalpel
   Cannula
   Trocar
   Rubber tubing
   Needle holder
Nonsterile equipment
   Preparation tray
   Test tubes
   Pail for the collection of fluid

Suture needles and sutures
Forceps
Gloves
Towels
Graduated receptacle
Cotton balls
Gauze squares
Abdominal dressing
Abdominal binder
Safety pins

Procedure

Nursing Action	Rationale/Amplification
Preparatory Phase	
1. Explain the procedure to the child in terms he can understand. Stress that he will feel better after the procedure.	1. To allay his fears and ensure his cooperation.
2. Have the child void just prior to the procedure.	2. To avoid puncturing the bladder during the procedure.
3. Secure the help of a second person.	3. To observe the child and assist the physician during the procedure.
4. Position the child correctly: a. Place him close to the edge of the examining table b. Support his back with your body c. Hold his hands	
Performance Phase	
1. Maintain the child's position.	1. To avoid injury.
2. Talk to the child frequently and hold his hands. Praise him for his cooperation.	2. To offer emotional support.
3. Observe the child's color and respirations.	3. Symptoms of shock develop if too much fluid is removed.

(continued)

Guidelines: Assisting with Pediatric Abdominal Paracentesis (continued)

Procedure
(Cont.)

Nursing Action	Rationale/Amplification

Follow-up Phase

1. Apply abdominal binder snugly.
2. Place the child in bed.
3. Record the amount and character of the drainage and the child's condition.
4. Observe frequently for signs of shock and note the drainage on the bandages.

Urinary Tract Infection

Urinary tract infection refers to an infection within the urinary system. Either the lower urinary tract (urethra, bladder, or the lower portion of the ureters) or the upper urinary tract (upper portion of the ureters or kidney) or both may be involved.

Etiology

1. Causative organisms—*E. coli* (most common)
2. Route of entry
   a. Ascent from the urethra (most common)
   b. Circulating blood
3. Contributing causes
   a. Obstruction, usually congenital
   b. Vesicoureteral reflux
   c. Infections elsewhere in the body
      (1) Upper respiratory
      (2) Gastrointestinal: diarrhea
   d. Poor perineal hygiene
   e. Short female urethra
   f. Catheterization and instrumentation
   g. Entrance of an irritant into the bladder
   h. Inherent defect in the ability of the bladder mucosa to protect it from microbial invasion

Incidence

1. Most common renal disease in children.
2. Almost 10 times more common in females than in males, except in the neonatal period.

Altered Physiology

1. Inflammatory changes occur in the affected portions of the urinary tract.
2. Clumps of bacteria may be present.
3. Inflammation results in urinary retention and stasis of urine in the bladder. There may be backflow of urine into the kidneys through the ureters.
4. There are inflammatory changes in the renal pelvis and throughout the kidney when this organ is involved.
5. Scarring of the kidney parenchyma occurs in chronic infection and interferes with kidney function, particularly with the ability to concentrate urine.
6. Eventually, the kidney becomes small, tissue is destroyed, and renal function fails.

Prognosis

1. Generally good in uncomplicated cases.
2. There is a tendency for recurrent infection.
3. Children with obstructive lesions of the urinary tract

and those with severe vesicoureteral reflux are at highest risk for kidney damage.

Assessment
Clinical Manifestations

A. Onset

1. May be abrupt or gradual
2. May be asymptomatic

B. Signs and Symptoms

1. Fever
   a. May be moderate or severe
   b. May fluctuate rapidly
   c. May be accompanied by chills or convulsions
2. Anorexia and general malaise
3. Urinary frequency, urgency, dysuria, dribbling
4. Daytime or nocturnal enuresis
5. Foul odor or change in the appearance of urine
6. Abdominal or suprapubic pain
7. Tenderness over one or both kidneys
8. Irritability
9. Vomiting
10. Failure to thrive in infancy

Diagnostic Evaluation

1. Urine culture
   a. Documentation of pathogenic organisms in the urine is the only means of definitive diagnosis.
   b. A urine culture demonstrating more than 100,000 bacteria per milliliter indicates significant bacteriuria.
2. Urinalysis
   a. Pus is present in abnormal amounts.
   b. Casts, especially white cell casts, may be present and are indicative of intrarenal infection.
   c. Hematuria—occurs occasionally.
3. Renal concentrating ability—decreased
4. Urologic and radiologic studies:
   A voiding cystourethrogram and IVP should be done after the initial infection subsides to identify abnormalities, which might contribute to the development of infection, and to identify existing kidney changes due to recurrent infection.

Patient Problems/Nursing Diagnoses

1. Alteration in urination (frequency, burning, pain, dribbling, and/or enuresis) related to infection
2. Pain related to inflammatory changes in urinary tract

3. Potential development of toxic effects of antimicrobial therapy
4. Body image concerns related to exposure and manipulation of the genitourinary tract
5. Knowledge deficit about urinary tract infections and prevention

Planning and Implementation
Nursing Interventions

A. Obtain a clean urine specimen for examination or culture.

1. A freshly voided early morning specimen is most accurate. (This urine is usually acid and concentrated, which tends to preserve the formed·elements.)
2. See the procedure for the collection of urine specimens, page 1155.
3. Obtain a midstream specimen whenever possible.
4. Catheterization may be necessary to obtain a sterile specimen in older girls.
   Defer this procedure whenever possible in order to avoid emotional trauma and the accidental introduction of additional bacteria.
5. The urine should be sent to the laboratory immediately or refrigerated to avoid a falsely high bacterial count.

B. Eradicate infective organisms.

1. Administer antibiotics as prescribed by the physician (Table 38-1).
2. Antibiotic therapy is generally determined by the results of urine cultures and sensitivities, and by the child's response to therapy.

C. Provide for symptomatic relief of the child's discomfort during the febrile period.

1. Maintain bed rest.
2. Administer analgesic and antipyretic drugs as recommended by the physician.
3. Encourage fluids to reduce the fever and dilute the concentration of the urine.
   a. Obtain a complete nursing history regarding the child's fluid preferences and method of taking them.
   b. Administer intravenous fluids if necessary (see Guidelines, p. 1160).

4. Refer to the section on care of the child with fever, page 1135.

D. Observe for progress of disease.

Nursing notes should include:
1. Frequent recording of the child's temperature
2. Accurate measurement of intake and output
3. Description of the color and odor of the urine, especially if it is abnormal
4. Presence of any of the following symptoms
   a. Frequency of urination
   b. Burning or pain with voiding
   c. Enuresis
   d. Urinary retention
5. General behavior and activity status of the child
6. Signs of untoward or toxic effects of drugs
7. Pain, especially in the kidney area

E. Provide emotional support to the child and his parents.

1. Reinforce medical explanations of the disease and its therapy.
2. Explain all diagnostic tests and procedures to the child before they are carried out.
3. Encourage the verbal child to talk about his experience and how he feels about it. Correct any misconceptions he may have, and particularly address concerns that the functioning of the urinary tract is separate from any sexual functions. The child should be reassured that the tests and treatment are for a problem that he did not cause.
4. Provide an environment that is as close to normal as possible during hospitalization. Include opportunities for the child to play.

F. Prepare the child and his family for discharge.

1. Discuss any treatment that will be required at home. Provide written discharge instructions regarding:
   a. Rest
   b. Fluid intake
   c. Administration of medications
   d. Appointment for continued medical supervision
2. Communicate or have the parents communicate with the school nurse if it is necessary for the child to receive medications at school.

Table 38-1 Antimicrobial Agents Commonly Used in the Management of Childhood Urinary Tract Infection

Drug	Toxic Effects	Nursing Considerations
Amoxicillin	Occasional nausea, vomiting, diarrhea Hypersensitivity reactions of skin	Readily absorbed. May be taken with food.
Ampicillin	Diarrhea, urticaria Anaphylactic reaction	Contraindicated in penicillin-sensitive children. Package insert should be consulted regarding reconstitution, administration, and storage of intramuscular and intravenous preparations. Absorption of oral preparations may be decreased with food. Dose must be repeated every 6 hours to ensure therapeutic blood levels.
Cephalexin	Diarrhea, nausea, vomiting	May be taken with food. Dose should be reduced if renal function is impaired.
Gentamicin	Renal and auditory toxicity; respiratory paralysis	Toxic effects can be minimized by slow intravenous infusion (over 1 hour).
Kanamycin	Renal and auditory toxicity	Keep the child well hydrated to minimize renal irritation. Warm soaks may relieve pain at injection sites.
Nitrofurantoin	Fever, nausea, vomiting, peripheral neuropathy	Recommended for prolonged use. Give with food or milk to decrease GI side effects. May cause urine to be amber or brown in color. Contraindicated in renal failure and in infants under 3 months of age.
Sulfonamides	Nausea, vomiting, drug fever, rashes, photosensitivity	Keep the child well hydrated to avoid crystallization of the drug in the urine. Contraindicated if known drug sensitivity and in infants under 2 months of age.
Trimethoprim–sulfamethoxazole	Same as with other sulfonamides	Commonly used if bacterial resistance is anticipated or the child fails to respond to initial therapy.

3. Complete a community nursing referral if reinforcement of discharge teaching appears necessary.

Health Education

1. Long-term therapy is often prescribed to prevent recurrence of urinary tract infections.
   Schedules for prolonged therapy vary from several months to continuous prophylaxis.
2. The child should be kept under continued medical surveillance because of the possibility of disease recurrence.
   a. Emphasis should be placed on the fact that even though this disease may have few symptoms, it can lead to very serious, permanent disability.
   b. Periodic urine cultures are indicated for 2 years following the acute infection.
3. Measures of prevention:
   a. Spread of bacteria from the anal and vaginal areas to the urethra can be minimized in female children by cleansing the perianal area from the urethra back toward the anus.

b. Bubble baths should not be used because of the bladder-irritant effect of these solutions.
c. Encourage adequate fluid intake, especially water.
d. Acidify urine with juices (e.g., cranberry).
e. Encourage the child to void frequently and to empty the bladder completely with each voiding.

Evaluation
Expected Outcomes

1. Is asymptomatic within 24–48 hours after initiation of treatment; decrease/cessation of urinary frequency, urgency, dysuria, burning on urination, and fever
2. Absence of complaints of pain during/after voiding; adheres to program of bed rest
3. Takes food and fluid with antimicrobial medication to avoid nausea, gastrointestinal side effects, etc.
4. Shows less anxiety about hospitalization; appears more relaxed about appearance, body image, tests, etc.
5. Parents discuss home care needs: rest, fluid intake, medications, possibility of recurrence, prevention of infection; follow-up care

---

Abnormalities of the Genitourinary Tract That Require Surgery

Exstrophy of the Bladder

In *exstrophy of the bladder,* the anterior surface of the bladder lies open on the lower part of the abdomen, allowing constant passage of urine to the outside. There are usually associated defects including separation of the pubic rami and epispadias in both sexes: cleft scrotum, undescended testes, and a shortened penis in males; cleft clitoris, separated labia, or shortened vaginal orifice in females.

Etiology

Results from failure of the abdominal wall and its underlying structures to fuse in utero.

Clinical Manifestations

1. Constant dribbling of urine excoriates the skin.
2. Infection and ulceration of the bladder mucosa may occur.
3. Genitalia may be ambiguous.
4. Affected children walk with a waddling or unsteady gait.

Management

1. Complete correction by means of reconstructive and orthopedic surgery is the preferred treatment.
2. Urinary diversion may be necessary.

Patient Problems/Nursing Diagnoses

1. Altered patterns of urination related to the nature of the defect
2. Body image concerns related to the appearance of the abdomen and genitalia
3. Increased danger of urinary tract infection or trauma to the exposed bladder

Nursing Interventions
A. Preoperative Care

1. Protect the bladder area from trauma and irritation.
   a. Position the infant on his back or side.
   b. Cleanse the area frequently with mild soap and water. Pat the area dry.

c. Expose the area to warm, dry air, sunlight, or artificial light at least once or twice each day.
d. Cover the defect with sterile gauze to which a bland ointment, such as petrolatum, has been applied, or with a layer of Saran wrap placed directly over the bladder.
e. Change the gauze covering and the infant's diaper frequently.
2. Observe the infant closely for signs of infection.
3. Collect urine specimens by holding the infant over an emesis basin in a position that allows urine to drip into the container.
4. Assist the parents to deal with their emotional reactions regarding the child's defect.
5. Teach the parents how to care for the child at home. Initiate a community nursing referral if reinforcement of teaching or maternal support appears necessary.
6. Prepare the child and his parents for the proposed surgery (see p. 1125).

B. Postoperative Care

1. Provide care for the ureteral and urethral catheters. Observe and record the amount of urinary drainage, catheter positions, and occurrence of bladder spasms.
2. The child is often placed in a body cast for several weeks (see Guidelines: Care of a Child in a Spica Cast, p. 1208).
3. An ileal conduit may be necessary (see p. 1355).
4. Observe for complications:
   a. Urinary or incisional infections
   b. Fistulae in the suprapubic or penile incisions
5. Long-term support will be necessary for many children and families to help them deal with such fears as appearance of genitalia, potential inability to procreate, and rejection by peers. Ongoing discussion groups for parents and children may be helpful.

C. Resource for Parents

Parents of Children with Exstrophy, Children's Health Center, 2525 Chicago Avenue, South, Minneapolis, MN 55403

Evaluation

Expected Outcomes

1. Demonstrates adequate absorption (by diaper) of continually draining urine; free of odor
2. Parents/child show acceptance of altered body image evidenced by their verbal and nonverbal communication
3. Absence of urinary tract infection; absence of trauma to bladder; parents verbalize signs and symptoms of complications

Patent Urachus

Patent urachus is persistence of the embryonic connection between the umbilicus and the bladder. In many patients only a cyst persists, located at the upper end of the tract, under the umbilicus.

Clinical Manifestations

1. Urine dribbles from the umbilicus when entire urachus is present.
2. Midline swelling is present in cases of a cyst.
3. Infection of urachal cysts is common.

Treatment

1. Eradication of infection
2. Removal of cysts
3. Surgical obliteration of the patent urachus

Obstructive Lesions of the Lower Urinary Tract

Types of Obstruction

1. Urethral valves
   a. Filamentous valves that obstruct urine flow
   b. Most commonly found in males
2. Congenital narrowing of the urethra
3. Bladder neck obstruction
   Most common site of lower urinary tract obstruction
4. Meatal stricture
5. Neuromuscular dysfunction (see the section on spina bifida, p. 1421)
6. Severe phimosis (rare)

Clinical Manifestations

Abnormal urination
1. Dysuria
2. Frequency
3. Enuresis
4. Dribbling
5. Reduced force of urine stream
6. Difficulty starting urine stream
7. Straining during urination
8. Abrupt cessation during urination

Altered Physiology

1. Urinary tract becomes distended proximal to the point of obstruction.
2. The bladder dilates and hypertrophies.
3. Stasis of urine occurs.
4. The ureters become elongated, dilated, and tortuous.
5. Hydronephrosis and destruction of kidney tissue inevitably result.

Treatment

1. Prevention or eradication of infection (see the section on urinary tract infection, p. 1351)
2. Dilation of urethral stenosis or stricture
3. Surgical relief of the obstruction

Obstructive Lesions of the Upper Urinary Tract

Types of Obstruction

1. Stricture of a ureter
2. Congenital absence of 1 ureter
3. Duplication of the ureter of 1 kidney
4. Compression of a ureter by an aberrant blood vessel

Clinical Manifestations

1. Often asymptomatic. (There is seldom any problem with voiding.)
2. Vague symptoms such as failure to thrive may be present.
3. Urinary tract infections may be frequent.
4. Hypertension may occur.

Treatment

Same as for obstructions of lower urinary tract.

Hypospadias

Hypospadias is malposition of the urethral opening.

Altered Physiology

A. **Males**
1. The urethra opens on the lower surface of the penis, proximal to its usual site.
2. In severe cases, the urethra may open on the shaft of the penis, at its base, or on the perineum.
3. Frequently associated with congenital chordee in males—cord-like defect that extends from the scrotum up the penis and deflects the penis downward.

B. **Females**
The urethra opens into the vagina (rare).

Clinical Manifestations

1. Inability to void with the penis in the normal elevated position.
2. Severe forms interfere with the ability to procreate.

Treatment

Plastic surgery

Cryptorchidism (Undescended Testis)

Cryptorchidism is the absence of one or both testes from the scrotum. The tests may be located in the abdominal cavity or inguinal canal.

Etiology

Caused by delayed descent, prevention of descent by some mechanical lesion, or endocrine disorders (rare).

Clinical Manifestations and Altered Physiology

1. Normal development of secondary sex characteristics.
2. Degeneration of the sperm-forming cells occurs after puberty because of the higher temperature of the abdomen compared with the normal location in the scrotum. Sterility results.
3. Emotional disturbances often occur when the child discovers that he is different from his peers.
4. Associated hernias are found in more than 50% of the patients.

Treatment

1. Orchiopexy (placement of the testes in the scrotum) Surgery should be performed by the time the child is 5 years of age to prevent damage to the tissues and to lessen emotional concerns related to body image.
2. Plastic surgery in patients with an absent testis.
3. Administration of chorionic gonadotropin—has produced descent of the testes in some children. (Testes would probably have descended spontaneously in these cases.)

Nursing Management

A. Preoperative Care

1. Encourage the child and his parents to express their feelings about the condition.
   Expect anxieties regarding sterility and homosexuality and perceptions of the child as defective or inadequate.
2. Discuss the condition and surgery frankly, in terms the child can understand.
   a. Maintain a matter-of-fact attitude.
   b. Clarify any misconceptions the child may have.
3. Provide privacy for medical examinations.

B. Postoperative Care

1. Maintain traction.
   a. A suture is placed in the lower portion of the scrotum and is attached to a rubber band that is fastened to the upper aspect of the inner thigh by a piece of adhesive.
   b. This traction anchors the testis to the scrotum and is removed in approximately 5–7 days.
2. Prevent contamination of the suture line.
3. Administer antibiotics as prescribed to prevent infection.

Ambiguous Genitalia

Female Pseudohermaphroditism

1. Most common problem of sexual differentiation.
2. A deficiency of hydrocortisone results in adrenocortical hyperplasia and an overproduction of androgens.
3. *Manifestations*—masculinization of the external genitalia in the female infant.
4. *Treatment:*
   a. Close observation for adrenal crisis
   b. Administration of hydrocortisone in children with adrenal hyperplasia
   c. Corrective plastic surgery, if needed
   This should be undertaken as early as possible, before social adjustment becomes a severe problem.

Male Pseudohermaphroditism

True Hermaphroditism

1. May be either genetic males or females.
2. Have both ovarian and testicular tissue.
3. Genitalia are usually ambiguous.
4. Gender choice is based on the infant's anatomy.

Diagnostic Evaluation

1. Buccal smear to determine the presence or absence of sex chromatin
2. Endoscopy and x-ray studies to reveal presence, absence, and nature of internal genital structures
3. Chromosomal analysis to identify genetic sex
4. Biochemical tests of urinary steroid excretion patterns
5. Laparotomy or gonad biopsy

Nursing Management

1. Recognize the situation as a social emergency.
   Support the parents while they wait for gender assignment for the infant. This should be done as soon as possible, but may require several days or weeks for results of studies.
2. Reinforce medical explanations of the anatomic problems and treatment. Approach the situation in a matter-of-fact manner.
3. Initiate appropriate referrals for family support and counseling. These may include:
   a. Social work
   b. Psychiatry
   c. Community health nursing
   d. Child guidance clinic
   e. Genetic counseling

Care of the Child Requiring Urologic Surgery

Patient Problems/Nursing Diagnoses

1. Potential alterations in urination related to the nature of disease, especially if ileal conduit is required
2. Body image concerns related to appearance of genitalia or presence of stones
3. Potential for infection related to catheterization and aftereffects of surgery
4. Anxiety related to proposed surgery
5. Knowledge deficit about surgery
6. Increased danger of fluid and electrolye imbalance related to surgery

Preoperative Care

1. Determine the child's fantasies regarding his illness and hospitalization. Correct any misconceptions that he reveals.

Type	Treatment
1. Normal female genitalia with testes internally	1. a. Surgical removal of testes b. Administration of estrogens at puberty c. Child reared as female
2. Predominantly male genitalia with testes internally	2. a. Surgical removal of all nonmale structures b. Child reared as male
3. Ambiguous genitalia	3. a. Plastic reconstruction b. Gender assignment based on internal and external anatomy

2. Provide an explanation of the anatomy and physiology of the urinary system in terms that the child can understand.
   a. Use a body outline appropriate for the age of the child.
   b. Explain how the child differs from the normal. Relate his defect to his symptoms whenever possible.
3. Explain all diagnostic tests prior to their occurrence. These may include urinalysis, 24-hour urine collections, intravenous and retrograde pyelography, angiography, and cystoscopy.
   a. Descriptions should include such information as:
      (1) Preparation required—fasting, enemas, etc.
      (2) Location of the test—operating room, radiology department, etc.
      (3) Appearance and attire of personnel
      (4) Positioning
      (5) Anesthesia
      (6) Pain or discomfort
      (7) Expectations following the procedure—diet, rest, urine collections, etc.
   b. Determine the child's understanding of the procedure.
      (1) Ask him simple, direct questions.
      (2) Allow him to perform the procedure on a doll or demonstrate it on a diagram.
4. Explain the surgical procedure.
   a. Explanations should include:
      (1) Preparation required—fasting, enemas, etc.
      (2) Description of the operating room including the appearance of the personnel
      (3) Anesthesia
      (4) Postoperative appearance
         (a) Urinary drainage tubing and collection devices
         (b) Appearance of urine
         (c) Sutures
         (d) Bandages
         (e) Intravenous infusion
   b. Determine the child's understanding of his surgery and reinforce teaching when necessary.
5. Points of emphasis during the preparation:
   a. The child is in no way to blame for his illness.
   b. No other part of the body will be operated on.

Postoperative Care

1. Care for all catheters and urinary tubes according to hospital procedure. Maintain appropriate position of tubes.
2. Observe and record:
   a. Amount and appearance of urinary drainage
   b. Occurrence of bladder spasms
   c. Symptoms of urinary or incisional infection

Care of the Child Who Has an Ileal Conduit
(Ileoloop)

A. Definition of the Procedure

One or both ureters are anastomosed to a segment of ileum, which then serves to carry urine to the external body surface of the abdomen.

Preoperative Care

1. Refer to the preceding section on the emotional preparation of the child and his family for urologic surgery.

2. Allow the child to try on the ileal conduit apparatus in order to become familiar with it.
   Observe for discomfort and skin reactions to the adhesive or cement.
3. Administer antimicrobials as prescribed by the physician.
   Be aware of the action, side effects, and contraindications of the prescribed therapy.
4. Provide the child and his parents with opportunities to express their fears and ask questions about the procedure.
   Expect concerns related to sterility, location and appearance of the stoma, activity restrictions, clothing, and management.
5. Reassure the child and his parents that they will be taught to manage the conduit before leaving the hospital.
6. If appropriate, introduce the family to a rehabilitated individual who has had the same surgery.
   Trained volunteers from the United Ostomy Association may be able to provide valuable psychological support.

Postoperative Care

1. Maintain the urinary collection apparatus. (A temporary collection bag is usually worn in the immediate postoperative period and may be replaced by a permanent appliance once edema of the stoma subsides.)
   a. Cleanse the area around the stoma with mild soap and water and dry it well.
   b. Keep the skin around the stoma completely dry during application of the appliance to ensure that it will remain attached.
   c. Place the adhesive plate of the appliance securely around the stoma.
      The opening in the adhesive plate should be of a size that fits snugly over the stoma but does not compromise circulation.
   d. Empty the appliance every 2 hours or whenever it contains approximately 100 ml. of fluid. (During the night, the appliance may be attached via tubing to a collection bottle.)
   e. Nursing observations related to the appliance:
      (1) Leaking around the appliance
      (2) Skin irritation
      (3) Improper fit of the appliance
   f. Points of emphasis:
      (1) A properly applied apparatus should remain in place 3–5 days. It needs to be changed only when it begins to leak or becomes uncomfortable.
      (2) It is normal for the urine to contain some mucus; it may be blood tinged.
2. Offer generous amounts of fluids to maintain hydration and keep the urine dilute and clear.
   Cranberry juice should be included in the diet because it helps to keep the urine acid.
3. Carefully monitor intake and output.
   Decreased urine output may indicate dehydration, obstruction of ureters, urine drainage into the peritoneal cavity, or compromised kidney function.
4. Observe for complications.
   a. Wound infection
   b. Leaking at the site of anastomosis
   c. Peritonitis
   d. Paralytic ileus
   e. Intestinal obstruction

f. Stenosis of the stoma

g. Fluid and electrolyte disturbances

5. Assist the child and his family with problems related to altered body image.

   a. Assume a calm, understanding, and matter-of-fact attitude.

   b. Keep equipment used in the management of the conduit out of sight to avoid embarrassment when visitors appear.

   c. Encourage the child to wear his own clothes so he is reassured that the appliance is invisible under clothing.

   d. Take precautions to prevent or eliminate odors (e.g., immediate cleansing of used collection bags, etc.).

   e. Help the child and family to achieve control by teaching them to manage the care as soon as possible.

   f. Encourage early resumption of as many normal activities as possible.

6. Prepare the family for discharge.

   a. Provide written information regarding the equipment that the child is using and where to obtain it.

   b. Provide at least a 2-week supply of equipment for the family to take home.
   Advise the parents to order new supplies before the old ones are depleted.

   c. Initiate appropriate referrals.

      (1) Community nursing agency

      (2) Local "ostomy" clubs

Health Education

1. Involve the child and his family in his self-care as soon as possible.
   Teaching should include how to assemble, apply, empty, change, and cleanse the appliance.

2. Explain that appliances can be adapted to meet the individual patient's needs.
   Some experimentation will probably be necessary before the most suitable equipment can be identified.

3. Adequate fluid intake (approximately 125 ml./kg. [1.7 oz./lb.]) is essential for maintaining good urine flow.

4. Two appliances should be available, one in use and the other as a spare.

5. The appliance should be cleaned and aired regularly to avoid odor or crusting.

   a. A few drops of Lysol to a quart of water whitens and deodorizes the bags.

   b. Crusting can be removed by a solution of white vinegar and water (approximately 1 cup of white vinegar to a quarter of water).

   c. A mild soap and warm water should be used to clean the appliance.

6. New appliances should be purchased approximately every 6 months or whenever old ones begin to feel thin or worn.

7. Activity limitations are usually not necessary unless the child has associated physical problems.

8. Clothing may have to be altered slightly to fit over the pouch of the appliance.

9. References for Parents
   Norris C. All About Jimmy. Los Angeles, United Ostomy Association, 1973
   United Ostomy Association, 2001 West Beverly Blvd, Los Angeles, CA 90057

Expected Outcomes

1. The child/parents attain ability to care for stoma, ostomy appliance, equipment, etc.

2. Shows a positive self-image evidenced by verbal and nonverbal communication

3. Absence of infection; vital signs normal; urine clear

4. Attains/maintains fluid and electrolyte balance; taking fluids well; laboratory values within acceptable range

5. Shows reduction of anxiety; no distressful crying; playing with toys; interacts with personnel; makes his needs known

6. Child/parent demonstrates application of appliance; monitoring of urinary output, care of collecting pouch

Acute Renal Failure

Nursing care of the children with acute renal failure is generally the same as that of adults (see pp. 516–517). The following considerations are important for pediatric patients.

Causes of Acute Renal Failure in Children

1. Prerenal causes (resulting from decreased perfusion to a normal kidney and collecting system)

   a. Dehydration (the most common cause of acute and renal failure in children)

   b. Surgical shock

   c. Trauma

   d. Burns

2. Postrenal causes

   a. Uncommon, except for obstructive uropathies in the first year of life

   b. Renal function is restored with relief of the obstruction

3. Renal causes (the largest group to require extended medical management)

   a. Disease of the kidney

   b. Tubular destruction secondary to nephrotoxins, transfusion reactions

Clinical Course

1. The length of the oliguric phase is highly variable.

   a. Shorter in infants, children, and milder cases (3–5 days)

   b. Longer in older children and adolescents (10–14 days)

2. The diuretic phase is also highly variable from mild and lasting only a few days, to profound.

3. 75% of children with acute renal failure attain complete recovery.

Management

1. Fluids are restricted to an amount needed to maintain zero water balance, calculated on the basis of endogenous water formation and sensible and insensible losses.

2. The child is weighed at least once each day, and is

expected to lose 10–20 gm. per kg. of original body weight per day.
3. A major nursing goal is to support parents who may feel anxious and/or guilty about the child's condition.

4. Refer to the following sections:
   a. Pediatric Intensive Care, page 1119
   b. Dialysis, page 1174
   c. The Dying Child, page 1495

Chronic Renal Failure

Nursing care of children with chronic renal failure is similar to that of adults (see pp. 517–519). The following considerations are important for pediatric patients.

Etiology of Chronic Renal Failure in Children

1. Congenital renal and urinary tract abnormalities (most common cause under 5 years of age)
2. Glomerular disease ⎫
3. Hereditary renal disease ⎬ Most common causes from 5–15 years
4. Renal vascular disorders ⎭

Clinical Manifestations (usually emerge only late in the course of the disease, similar to adults)

1. Decreased interest in usual activities such as school and play
2. Bedwetting
3. Bone or joint pain
4. Delayed or absent sexual maturation
5. Secondary amenorrhea in girls past puberty
6. Growth retardation
7. Dryness and itching of skin

Management

1. Rapid correction of acidosis may precipitate tetany in the hypocalcemic child. Therefore, correction of acidosis is most safely attempted after calcium levels are elevated.
2. When serum phosphate levels are in the normal range, vitamin D in increasing doses or dihydrotachysterol is administered to increase the absorption of calcium via the gastrointestinal tract.
3. Growth retardation may be reduced by the administration of the anabolic steroid, oxandrolone.
4. Intercurrent infections are common and must be treated immediately. The dosage of antimicrobials excreted through the kidneys is usually reduced and the interval between doses extended to avoid toxic effects.

Clinical Course and Prognosis

1. Once symptoms of uremia appear, the disease progresses rapidly and terminates in death unless end-stage renal care is initiated.
2. Children are regarded as having end-stage renal disease when the glomerular filtration rate falls below 10 ml./min./1.73 m.^{2}.
3. End-stage renal disease is treated by dialysis or transplantation.

Nursing Interventions

1. Numerous psychosocial issues may interfere with the child's psychological and social development and education. A major nursing goal, is to help the child and family to cope with:
   a. Uncertainty regarding the course of the disease and ultimate prognosis
   b. Stress of repeated hospitalizations and recurring need for painful medical procedures
   c. Abnormal life-style necessitated by dialysis
   d. Burden of dialysis and continuous administration of medications
   e. Problems of adjustment related to growth failure
   f. Fear of death, present in most children and adolescents
   g. Need for urinary diversion and manipulation of the genital area in cases of urologic abnormalities
   h. Transplantation involving major surgery, prolonged hospitalization followed by altered body image due to high doses of steroids and potential for rejection which may threaten survival
2. Refer to:
   a. The Child Undergoing Dialysis, page 1174
   b. Pediatric Renal Transplantation, see below
   c. The Dying Child, page 1495

Pediatric Renal Transplantation

Kidney transplantation is the treatment of choice for end-stage renal failure in the pediatric age-group. With transplantation, there is a greater likelihood of complete rehabilitation and better growth than with dialysis, although post-transplantation growth is variable and related to caloric intake, corticosteroid dosage, bone age at transplantation, and rejection episodes. Nursing care of children experiencing kidney transplantation is similar to that of adults (see p. 526). The following special considerations apply to pediatric patients.

Donor Selection (in order of priority)

1. Identical twin sibling
2. Sibling
   It is important to note that siblings cannot be used

as donors until they are of legal age to give consent for removal of a kidney.
3. Parent
4. Aunt or uncle
5. Unrelated live donor (seldom used) or cadaver donor

Operative Procedure

Small children may require placement within the abdomen with vessel anastomosis to the aorta and inferior vena cava.

Potential Emotional Concerns of Children with Transplants

1. The concept of a foreign body, especially a cadaver kidney inside his own body may be disturbing.

2. Fear that the kidney may wear out sooner if it is from an older person.
3. Altered body image due to growth failure and the effects of steroid therapy.
4. Guilt feeling if a live-donor transplant fails.

Nursing Care

Refer to sections on:
1. Chronic Renal Failure, page 1357
2. Care of the Child Requiring Urologic Surgery, page 1354

Bibliography

Books

Belman AB and Kaplan G. Genitourinary Problems in Pediatrics. Major Problems in Clinical Pediatrics, Vol. 23. Philadelphia, WB Saunders, 1981

Brundage B. Nursing Management of Renal Problems, 2nd ed. St Louis, CV Mosby, 1980

Chisholm TC and McParland FA. Exstrophy of the urinary bladder. In Ravitch MM (ed). Pediatric Surgery, 3rd ed. Chicago, Year Book Medical Publishers, 1979, pp. 1239–1254

Gauthier B, Edelmann C and Barnett H. Nephrology and Urology for the Pediatrician. Boston, Little, Brown & Co, 1982

Hallerstein S. Urinary Tract Infections in Children. Chicago, Year Book Medical Publishers, 1982

Hollerman C. Pediatric Nephrology. Garden City, Medical Examination Publishing Co, 1979

Josso N (ed). The Intersex Child. New York, S Karger, 1981

Kunin CM. Detection, Prevention and Management of Urinary Tract Infections, 3rd ed. Philadelphia, Lea & Febiger, 1979

Lancaster L (ed). The Patient with End Stage Renal Disease, 2nd ed. New York, John Wiley & Sons, 1984

Petrillo M and Sanger S. Emotional Care of Hospitalized Children, 2nd ed. Philadelphia, JB Lippincott, 1980

Whaley L and Wong D. Nursing Care of Infants and Children. St Louis, CV Mosby, 1983

Articles

Burgess M. Protective support for children following renal transplant. Physiotherapy 1982 Nov; 68(11):368

Burnett J. Congenital adrenocortical hyperplasia. Am J Nurs 1980 Jul; 80(7):1304–1308

Fine R. Treatment of end-stage renal disease in children. Pediatric Ann 1981 Jan; 10(1):65–73

Frauman AC. Health care for the child with a renal transplant. AANNT J 1982 Feb; 9(1):33–34+

Ginsburg C and McCraken G. Urinary tract infections in young infants. Pediatrics 1982 Apr; 69(4):409–412

Grossman H, Kirks D and Merten D. Imaging of the pediatric urinary tract. Pediatr Ann 1981 Jan; 10(1):25–40

Higgerson J. A descriptive study concerning the psychosocial dimensions of living related kidney donation. AANNT J 1982 Dec; 9(6): 27–31

Hooper S. Primary transplantation: An alternative. AANNT J 1981 Feb; 8(1): 27–29

Ingelfinger J et al. Growth acceleration following renal transplantation in children less than 7 years of age. Pediatrics 1981 Aug; 68(2):255–259

Irvin B. Teaching the transplant recipient. AANNT J 1981 Feb; 8(1): 30–34

Krensky A, Inglefinger J and Grupe W. Peritonitis in childhood nephrotic syndrome, 1970–1980. Am J Dis Child 1982 Aug; 136(8):732–736

Lansing L and McLaughlin P. Establishing a teaching plan for adolescents awaiting a cadaver or living related donor transplant. AANNT J 1981 Feb; 8(1):35–41

Levi M. The psychological dilemmas confronting the adolescent transplant patient . . . a social worker's response . . . a nurse's response. Nephrol Nurse 1982 Nov/Dec; 4(6):42–45

Mazur T. Ambiguous genitalia: detection and counseling. Pediatr Nurs 1983 Nov/Dec; 9(6):417–422

McCoy J. Preliminary diagnosis of urinary tract infection in symptomatic children. Nurse Pract 1982 Jan; 7(1): 28–29

McCraken G et al. Evaluation of short-term antibiotic therapy in children with uncomplicated urinary tract infections. Pediatrics 1981 June; 67(6):796–801

Moncrief J. Continuous ambulatory peritoneal dialysis: Impact on management of patients with end-stage renal disease. Nephron 1981; 27(4–5):226–228

Report of the International Reflux Study Committee. Medical versus surgical treatment of primary vesicoureteral reflux. Pediatrics 1981 Mar; 67(3):392–400

Report of International Study of Kidney Disease in Children. Minimal change nephrotic syndrome in children: Deaths during the first 5 to 15 years' observation. Pediatrics 1984 Apr; 73(4):497–501

Report of International Study of Kidney Disease in Children. The primary nephrotic syndrome in children. Identification of patients with minimal change nephrotic syndrome from initial response to prednisone. J Pediatr 1981 Apr; 98(4):561–564

Rizzoni G et al. Renal transplantation in children less than 5 years of age. Arch Dis Child 1980 Jul; 55(7):532–536

Rodriquez D. Teaching the preschooler with two ostomies. J Enterostom Ther 1982 Jan/Feb; 9(1):18–19

Roy S. Disorders of genitourinary system. In Shirkey H (ed). Pediatric Therapy. St Louis, CV Mosby, 1980

Seldon R et al. Managing urinary tract infections in children. Pediatr Ann 1981 Jan; 10(1):12–24

Sidor T and Resnick M. Urinary tract infection in children. Pediatr Clin North Am 1983 Apr; 30(2):323–333

Siegel S et al. Urinary infections in infants and preschool children. Am J Dis Child 1980 Apr; 134(4):371–372

Southby JR et al. Nursing diagnosis for a child with end-stage renal disease. AANNT J 1983 Jun; 10(4):23–27

Stevens M and Reinitz M. Nursing a child through exstrophic bladder reconstruction surgery. MCN 1980 Jul/Aug; 5(4):265–270

Thomas C. Childhood urinary tract infection. Pediatr Nurs 1982 Mar/Apr; 8(2):114–119

Toper M. Renal transplantation in children. AANNT J 1981 Feb; 8(1):14–18

Vehaskari M and Robson A. The nephrotic syndrome in children. Pediatr Ann 1981 Jan; 10(1):42–62

Walker R. Surgery for the child ostomate. J Enterostom Ther 1982 Jul/Aug; 9(4):18–20

Resources for Children and Parents

National Kidney Foundation
Two Park Avenue
New York, NY 10016

Pamplin H, Light J and Hyman L. Sidney Kidney—A Book for Children and Parents About Renal Disease, Hemodialysis and Transplantation. Washington, DC, Walter Reed Army Medical Center 20012. Sale by Superintendent of Documents, US Government Printing Office, Washington, DC 20402

Skin Problems in Children

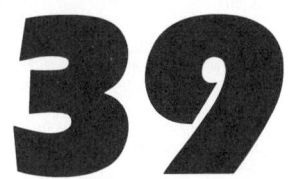

Burns in Children

Burns are a frequent form of childhood injury. The following types are considered very serious:
1. Second-degree burn of 10% or more of the body surface; 5% or more full-thickness
2. Burns of face, hands, feet, or perineum in a child younger than 1 year
3. Electrical burns of the mouth
4. Presence of other injuries
5. When home situation is not adequate for optimal care

The effects of burns are not limited to the burn area.

Incidence and Etiology

1. Burns are the second most important cause of accidental deaths in childhood, with the highest incidence of burns occurring in children under 5 years of age.
2. Causes of burns in children
   a. Burns from hot water
      (1) Child (left unsupervised in tub) turns on the hot water tap
      (2) Child placed in tub of hot water that has not been tested
      (3) Spilling of hot coffee, tea on child; spilling occurs especially when pot handles stick out on top of stove; hot liquids and foods removed from microwave oven
      (4) Most common in children under 3 years
   b. Burns from open flames
      (1) House fires
      (2) Child climbing up to stove—clothing catches fire
      (3) Child playing with matches
      (4) Playing/working with gasoline
      (5) Gas tank explosion during automobile accident
      (6) Most common in children under 3 years
   c. Electrical burns
      (1) Child playing with electrical outlets or appliances
      (2) Child playing with extension cords
      (3) Child playing on railroad tracks; climbing trees and touching high tension wires, lightning
      (4) Most common in toddlers and adolescents
   d. Caustic acid or alkali burns of mouth and esophagus—child ingesting strong household cleaning products
   e. Chemical burns of the skin—child playing with gasoline that comes in contact with skin (often the gasoline ignites)
   f. Burns inflicted upon the child as a result of neglect or child abuse—20%–30% of all burns
   g. Smoke inhalation and inhalation from plastic combustion
   h. Radiation burns—resulting from the sun and radiation secondary to cancer therapy

Altered Physiology

See section on burns in adults, page 630.

Complications

Depend upon severity of burn injury and are usually the rule rather than the exception, especially with severe burn injury.

A. Acute
1. Infection
   a. Burn wound sepsis
   b. Pneumonia
   c. Urinary tract infection
   d. Phlebitis
2. Curling's ulcer, GI hemorrhage—most likely to occur in burns >20% body surface area
3. Acute gastric dilation, paralytic ileus—especially in child under 2 years of age with greater than 20% injury
4. Renal failure
5. Respiratory failure
6. Postburn seizures
7. Hypertension
8. CNS dysfunction
9. Vascular ischemia
10. Anema and malnutrition
11. Fecal impaction
12. Depression—secondary to hospitalization and changing body image
13. Malnutrition may resolve once burned area is covered

B. Long-term
1. Malnutrition
2. Scarring
3. Contractures
4. Psychological trauma

Assessment

Clinical Manifestations
1. The characteristics of burn wounds are classified as follows (Table 39-1):

Table 39-1 **Classification of Depth of Burns**

Degree (Depth)	Appearance of Burn	Sensitivity to Pain	Tissue Involvement	Healing Time and Prognosis
First-degree (superficial)	Erythema; no blister formation; slight edema (gradual onset)	Intense pain–hyperesthesia; sensitivity to pinprick	Outer layer of epidermis (stratum corneum)	7–10 days; no scarring
Second-degree (partial-thickness but superficial)	Blister formation with oozing; subcutaneous edema	Pain–hyperesthesia; sensitivity to pinprick	All of epidermis, parts of stratum germinativum intact	5–21 days; as scabs fall off, skin remains red for several weeks. Ability to regenerate epithelium is intact; can scar
Second-degree (partial-thickness but deep)	Blister formation moist; subcutaneous edema; mottled red or pink	Pain variable; may be insensitive to pinprick due to depth in dermal layer of skin	Deep dermis; cutaneous nerve endings may be damaged	21–35 days; firm eschar formation; regeneration takes place from epithelial lining of hair follicles and sweat glands. Pigmentation rarely returns to normal. *Please note:* Deep dermal burns are hard to distinguish from third-degree burns. In case of infection, injury may progress to third-degree.
Third-degree (full-thickness)	Blistering is not usual. Blanched, reddish, black; hard and leathery to touch; rapid edema; mottled	No pain because of destruction of nerve endings and anesthesia	Dermis and corium; deep third-degree burns extend into subcutaneous fat, muscles, and bones	Prolonged hospitalization; scarring; requires grafting since no regeneration of skin layers

(Wieczorek RR and Natapoff JN. A Conceptual Approach to the Nursing of Children. Philadelphia, JB Lippincott, 1981, p. 562)

a. First-degree burns (partial-thickness—epidermal) involve superficial epidermis; the skin is pink or red in appearance and is painful to touch.
b. Second-degree burns (partial-thickness—superficial or deep dermal) involve the entire epidermis; the skin is red, blistered, moist with exudate, and painful to pinprick or touch. Deep dermal injury penetrates into corium and may be anesthetic for 1–2 days after burn injury.
c. Third-degree burns (full-thickness—subdermal) involve the dermis or underlying fat, muscle, or bone; the skin appears white, dry, or charred and has little pain. Often it is difficult to tell the degree of burn, especially in the young child.
d. Electrical burn—(especially of mouth when child is under 2 years of age chews or sucks on live wire) Takes several days before injury becomes demarcated.

2. Symptoms of shock appear soon after the burn:
a. Rapid pulse
b. Subnormal temperature
c. Pallor
d. Prostration
e. Low blood pressure

3. Symptoms of toxemia may develop within 1–2 days after the initial burn:
a. Prostration
b. Fever
c. Rapid pulse
d. Glucosuria
e. Vomiting
f. Edema

Note: These symptoms may progress to coma or death.

4. Burns of the respiratory tract result in symptoms of upper airway obstruction from acute edema and inflammation of the glottis, vocal cords, and upper trachea.

a. Rapid breathing
b. Dyspnea
c. Stridor, hoarseness, substernal retraction, and intercostal breathing
d. Nasal flaring
e. Restlessness

5. Smoke inhalation may cause no initial symptoms other than mild bronchial obstruction during the initial phase following the burn. Within 6–48 hours the child may develop sudden onset of the following conditions:
a. Bronchiolitis
b. Pulmonary edema
c. Severe airway obstruction
d. Damage from smoke inhalation—can present up to 7 days after the burn injury

Treatment

See the adult section on burns, page 634.

Goals:
Replace fluid loss from burn surface.
Maintain circulation.
Prevent renal failure.
Prevent or treat infection.
Aim toward early repair of the burn wound.
Restore the child to the best possible state of physical and psychological functioning.
Maintain airway secondary to inhalation injury or edema.

1. Calculation of the burn area
a. Evans' "rule of nine" (used in assessment of extent of burns in adults) has proved quite inexact when applied to young children. May be acceptable to use in child over 10 years of age.
(1) During infancy and early childhood, the relative surface area of different parts of the body varies with age.
(2) The younger the child, the greater the proportion of the surface area constituted by

BURN SHEET

Name _____ Age _____ Number _____

Date of Observation _____

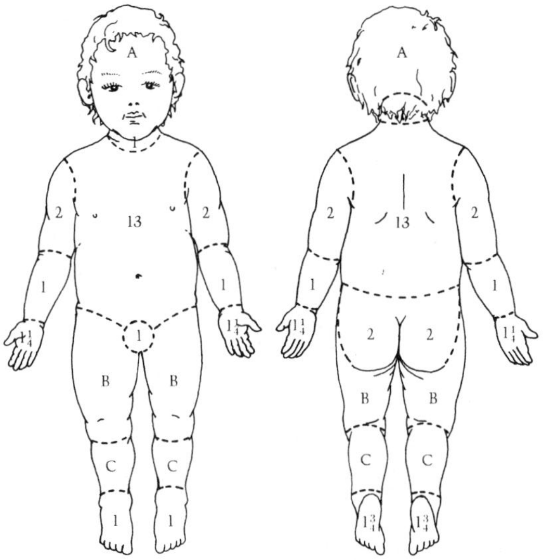

Relative Percentages of Areas Affected by Growth			
Area	Age 0	1	5
A = $\frac{1}{2}$ of head	$9\frac{1}{2}$	$8\frac{1}{2}$	$6\frac{1}{2}$
B = $\frac{1}{2}$ of one thigh	$2\frac{3}{4}$	$3\frac{1}{4}$	4
C = $\frac{1}{2}$ of one leg	$2\frac{1}{2}$	$2\frac{1}{2}$	$2\frac{3}{4}$

	% Burn by Areas			
Probable 3rd burn	Head _____ Neck _____ Body _____ Upper arm _____			
	Forearm _____ Hands _____ Genitals _____ Legs _____			
	Buttocks _____ Thighs _____ Feet _____			
Total burn	Head _____ Neck _____ Body _____ Upper arm _____			
	Forearm _____ Hands _____ Genitals _____ Legs _____			
	Buttocks _____ Thighs _____ Feet _____			
Sum of all areas _____	Probable 3rd _____		Total burn _____	

Figure 39-1. Calculation of burn surface area. (Redrawn from Pascoe DJ and Grossman M. Quick Reference to Pediatric Emergencies. Philadelphia, JB Lippincott; appears in Waechter EH, and Blake FG. Nursing Care of Children, 9th ed. Philadelphia, JB Lippincott)

the head and the lesser the proportion of the surface area constituted by the legs.

b. Calculation of percentage of burn surface area is based on Lund and Browder's design (Fig. 39-1). This design compensates for the changes in percentage of body surface resulting from growth.

c. A rough estimate can be obtained by using child's hand that is equal to 1%.

2. Categorization of seriousness of burn is based on
   a. Total area injured
   b. Depth of injury
   c. Location of injury
   d. Age of child
   e. Condition of patient (i.e., level of consciousness)
   f. Previous medical history (i.e., chronic disease)
   g. Additional injuries

3. Schematic classification of burn severity*:
   a. Minor burn:
      (1) 10% Total body surface area, first- and second-degree burn
   b. Moderate burn:
      (1) 10%–20% Total body surface area, second-degree burn
      (2) 2%–10% Total body surface area, third-degree burn not involving eyes, ears, face, or genitals
   c. Major burn:
      (1) 20% Total body surface area, second-degree burn
      (2) All third-degree burns greater than 10%; depending on age of child, 5% is sometimes used
      (3) All burns involving hands, face, eyes, ears, feet, and/or genitals
      (4) All electrical burns

* Adapted from Helm PA. Burn injury: Rehabilitation management: 1982. J Burn Care Rehabil 1983 Nov/Dec; 4(6):411

   (5) Complicated burn injuries involving fracture or other major trauma
   (6) All poor-risk patients (i.e., head injury, cancer, lung disease, diabetes)

Patient Problems/Nursing Diagnoses

(See burns in adults, p. 639)

1. Shock related to fluid loss, hypermetabolic state, and loss of skin integrity
2. Infection related to injury, altered skin integrity, decreased circulation, etc.
3. Alteration in respiratory status related to inhalation injury or edema
4. Alteration in gastrointestinal status, (Curling's ulcer, paralytic ileus) related to stress
5. Alteration in nutritional status related to hypermetabolic state and poor appetite
6. Alteration in mobility related to dressings, pain, and contractures
7. Alteration in comfort related to dressing changes, physical therapy, itching, and treatments/procedures
8. Alteration in self-image and self-esteem related to pain, scarring, and disfigurement
9. Anxiety related to pain, treatments, procedures, and hospitalization
10. Altered parent–child relationship related to crisis situation, prolonged hospitalization, and disfigurement
11. Parental anxiety related to fear, guilt, and lack of understanding of the treatment protocols

Planning and Implementation
Nursing Intervention

A. Recognize the symptoms of shock and use support measures to restore and maintain circulation.

1. Be alert to the symptoms of shock that occur very shortly after a severe burn.

a. Tachycardia
b. Hypothermia
c. Hypotension
d. Pallor
e. Prostration
f. Shallow respirations
g. Anuria

2. Monitor the administration of intravenous fluid, since major burns are followed by a reduction in blood volume due to outflow of plasma into the tissues.
   a. Maintain the administration of intravenous fluid—usually lactated Ringer's solution is used during first 24 hours after injury because of its similarity to plasma.
   b. Obtain weight—this measurement is critical for accurate intravenous fluid volumes to be determined.
   Infants and small children: 4 ml./kg./% burn
   Older child: 2–3 ml./kg./% burn
   c. Fluid loss from transcapillary leakage is greatest during the first 12 hours postinjury and diminishes to almost zero 12–24 hours postinjury. Fluid loss after 48 hours is due to vaporization of water from wound.
   d. Maintain the administration of other intravenous fluids as directed.

3. Maintain an accurate record of intake and output.
   a. Record time and amount of all fluids given.
   b. Measure accurate urinary output every ½ hour to 1 hour.
      (1) With severe burn injuries, an indwelling catheter may be used the first 3 days.
      (2) Urine flow is a most helpful clinical guide to fluid replacement and kidney function.
      (3) Estimate urine output: 1 ml./kg./hour or
      10–20 ml./hour under 2 years of age
      20–30 ml./hour 3–5 years of age
      30–50 ml./hour over 5 years of age
      (4) Check specific gravity.
      (5) Report diminishing urinary output.

4. Provide a rich oxygen environment in order to combat hypoxia, as necessary.

5. Provide sedation to relieve pain.
   a. Sedatives are given to children in very small amounts in order to prevent their depressant effect.
   b. In severe burn injury, sedation should be given intravenously because of lack of absorption of intramuscular medication during emergency phase and the possibility of the child receiving a large bolus once capillary integrity is restored. Morphine or meperidine are generally drugs of choice; however, their use is kept to a minimum in order to assess accurately brain perfusion by observation of sensorium. Serum titrate levels are closely monitored.

6. Provide a source of heat over the child's bed, since additional heat may be necessary to maintain body temperature.

7. Request laboratory results and record on special flow sheet.
   a. Hematocrit or RBC count serves as a rough guide to the adequacy of initial treatment, since the loss of plasma results in concentration of red blood cells.
   b. Electrolytes serve as a guide to fluid replacement.

8. Maintain close observation of vital signs in order to evaluate continuously the state of peripheral circulation; check for clear sensorium. Report immediately any significant changes.

9. Observe for additional complaints or circumstances that might suggest associated injury.
   a. GI hemorrhage
   b. Acute gastric dilatation may occur, especially if the child has greater than 20% injury, associated injury, or tachypnea. Nasogastric tube may be inserted to prevent vomiting, aspiration, and paralytic ileus.
   c. Ileus—associated with circulatory problems in small children; may be alleviated with insertion of nasogastric tube.

10. Determine need for tetanus inoculation.

B. Observe for symptoms of respiratory distress and initiate measures to alleviate distress.

Most common form of airway obstruction in young child is from edema of the head and neck, and the glottic and subglottic areas.

1. Be alert for symptoms of respiratory distress:
   a. Dyspnea
   b. Stridor
   c. Rapid respirations
   d. Restlessness
   e. Cyanosis

2. Report these symptoms.

3. Provide an oxygen source in order to combat anoxia.

4. Monitor blood gases—serum dioxide (indicated only initially)

5. Intubation or tracheostomy may be performed.

C. Obtain medical history of the child: childhood diseases, immunizations, current medications, and recent infections.

D. Provide scrupulous skin care in order to prevent infection and promote healing.

1. Burn treatment:
   a. Exposure—after cleansing, wound remains exposed to air: maintains a dry surface, produces early formation of a protective eschar, and predisposes patient to less infection; usually combined with the use of antibacterial creams and daily soaking in Hubbard tank to remove cream and dead tissue; can allow for increased movement.
   b. Occlusive dressing—burns are kept covered with dressings that have been soaked in a solution, or topical medication is applied followed by dressing. Dressings are changed every 8–24 hours. Burned areas are soaked daily in Hubbard tank. Children appear to be more mobile when burn injury is covered since they are in less pain.
   c. Primary excision of burn—necrotic eschar is immediately removed, allowing site to be grafted. Grafting may be postponed 24–48 hours with temporary cover of porcine xenograft or comparable biosynthetic material (i.e., Biobrane)
   d. Escharotomy—incision through eschar to relieve severe constriction and compromised circulation, when burn eschar is circumferential. It is done within first 12–24 hours after injury.
   e. Physicians have their own preferences as to which method is used. The goals remain the same—to prevent infection, to remove dead tissue, and to provide for early closure of wound.
   f. Maintain sterility in working with the burn area

regardless of whether the open or closed method is used.

2. Cleansing the wound and changing the dressing is critical for preventing infection, preserving tissue, promoting early closure of the wound, and maintaining function.
   a. Hubbard tank is treatment of choice for cleansing.
   b. Use clean technique—gown, cap, mask, gloves, and plastic apron.
   c. Limit tubbing to 20 minutes to prevent hypothermia, hyponatremia, and hemodilution.
   d. Isotonic solution may be needed for large wounds and small children.
   e. Gaining popularity is the use of a shower to facilitate the loosening and removal of sloughing tissue, eschar, exudate, and topical medications. The child is suspended over a tub in a fine-mesh nylon sling. The shower, water about 32°C. (90°F.) flows over the child; then debridement is done. The wound is air-dried before dressings are applied.

3. The Bradford frame may be used to facilitate skin care.
   a. Provides a method for the collection of urine and feces and maintains cleanliness of the burn areas and dressings.
   b. Contractures may be prevented by maintaining functional position of extremities and good body alignment.
   c. Two Bradford frames may be used to change position of the child from back to stomach and vice versa without having to handle the severely burned child.

4. Alternating water bed or sand bed may also be used.
5. Position the child and turn him frequently.
6. Apply protective devices to prevent the child from scratching the burn area, or give prescribed antipruritic drug when necessary.
7. Administer antibiotics as prescribed.
   Specific antibiotic therapy may be necessary for complicating infection.
8. Ensure that serial wound biopsy and quantitative cultures are done if prescribed.
9. Topical antibacterial therapy may include:
   a. 1% silver sulfadiazine cream (Silvadene)—treatment of choice as present; especially for partial-thickness burn.
      (1) Easy to apply—applied 1–2 times daily
      (2) Does not hurt the child upon application, but the child may complain of cold
      (3) Allergic reactions occur very rarely
      (4) Nontoxic
      (5) Bactericidal for up to 48 hours
      (6) Effective against gram-negative and gram-positive bacteria and *Candida albicans*
   b. Povidone-iodine (Betadine ointment)
      (1) Allergic reaction fairly common
      (2) Apparently nontoxic
      (3) Effective against broad spectrum of organisms
      (4) Associated with pain
      (5) Eschar becomes stained and stiff
      (6) Elevation of protein-bound iodine
   c. 10% mafenide acetate (Sulfamylon) cream
      (1) Allergic reaction (rash)—common
      (2) Painful immediately after application where there is partial-thickness burn

      (3) Metabolically active in kidney as carbonic anhydrase inhibitor resulting in metabolic acidosis and hyperventilation
      (4) Most effective for extensive burns with thick eschar
      (5) Easily applied
      (6) Effective against many gram-positive and gram-negative organisms (i.e., *Pseudomonas* and *Clostridium*)
   d. ½% silver nitrate soaks
      (1) Solution is hypo-osmolar, leading to electrolyte deficiencies
      (2) Soaks are continuous, messy, and turn everything they touch black
      (3) Hypoallergenic
      (4) Effective in controlling *Pseudomonas* and *Staphylococcus*

10. Heterograft or homografts (Table 39-2) are used to:
    a. Restore water vapor barrier and decrease protein loss
    b. Decrease pain
    c. Decrease bacterial count at the wound as graft adheres to the site

E. Monitor parenteral fluids to prevent electrolyte imbalance and dehydration.

1. Injury-induced fluid loss is greatest up to 48 hours postburn, at which time reabsorption of these fluids results in diuresis if renal function is intact; accurate urinary output measurement is critical during this time.
2. Decreasing water loss by evaporation can be accomplished by keeping ambient air warm and moist, thus reducing high energy requirements and the chance of metabolic derangements. This, however, sets up an excellent environment for bacterial growth, especially of *Pseudomonas*.
3. When parenteral hyperalimentation is used, there is increased risk of infection in the burned patient. Be alert to early signs and symptoms of infection.

F. Provide a high-protein, high-calorie diet in order to provide nutrition necessary for healing and for the growth and developmental needs of the child.

1. Hypernutrition is important, because of the extreme hypermetabolism related to large burn injuries.
   a. High-caloric—to support hypermetabolic state; protein synthesis; calories should come from carbohydrates.
   b. High-protein—to replace protein lost by exudation; support synthesis of immunoglobulins and structural protein; prevent negative nitrogen balance
   c. Vitamin and mineral supplement—particularly vitamins B and C, and iron and zinc
2. Anorexia is common in the burned child.
   a. Tell the child why eating is important.
   b. Offer small amounts of food, perhaps 4–5 feedings rather than 3 per day.
   c. Give him a choice of foods; determine his favorite foods.
   d. Offer high-protein, high-calorie dietary supplements.
   e. Make meals a pleasant time, unassociated with treatments or unpleasant interruptions.
   f. Nasogastric tube feedings may be necessary to supply high nutritive needs.

Table 39-2 **Wound Closure**

Types of Coverage	Source
Permanent grafts	
Autograft	Tissue obtained from uninjured area on the child's own body.
Isograft	Histocompatible tissue obtained from genetically identical individual (i.e., child's identical twin).
Temporary grafts	
Homograft (allograft)	Tissue obtained from genetically different individual of same species—living or dead. Can be fresh or frozen.
Heterograft (xenograft)	Tissue obtained from other species—pigskin.
Human amnion	Material obtained by stripping the amniotic membrane from the placenta.
Biobrane (Woodroof Laboratories, Inc., Santa Ana, CA 92704)	Semisynthetic material consisting of knitted elastic, flexible, nylon fabric, which is bonded to silastic membrane.

Types of Grafts	Methods of Covering Application
Full-cover graft	Sheet of skin from donor site is applied as one piece on recipient site.
Postage-stamp graft	Donor site sheet of skin, cut into postage-stamp size and applied on recipient site with spaces between grafts, which allows for drainage.
Mesh, lace, or split graft	Donor site sheet of skin that has mechanically had splits made in it, which stretches to cover area about three times its size.

G. Maintain a planned physical therapy program in order to achieve the greatest functional capacity for the child.

1. Carry out physical therapy procedures to minimize joint and skin complications:
   a. Position—position joint in opposite direction of expected contracture.
   b. Splints—aid joint positioning and decrease skin contractures and hypertrophy.
   c. Exercise—gain and maintain optimal range of motion.
   d. Pressure garment—aid circulation, protect newly healed skin, and prevent and treat hypertrophic scar formation by promoting dermal collagen fiber growth in parallel direction. It may be necessary to wear pressure garments 12–18 months after injury at which time healed skin has matured and becomes supple.
2. Plan the time each day for the therapy to be carried out. Movement, a normal activity for a child, is now painful because of crusts, dressings, and pain from the burn area.
3. Utilize play opportunities to help the child accept the program (e.g., tricycle riding may be used as form of exercise).
4. Allow the child to be ambulatory as soon as he is able.

H. Prepare the child for the many painful surgical and other procedures that he must undergo.

1. Explain to the child what will happen before each procedure.
2. Explain to the child what will happen before he goes to the operating room, where he will wake up, and who will be there when he wakes up.
3. Explain and demonstrate what equipment will be used following surgery or other procedures.
4. Puppet or doll play, water play, clay or Play-Doh and drawings can all be helpful in letting the child work through his feelings about all that is happening to him.

I. Provide emotional support for the child who has been very frightened and traumatized by this painful experience.

1. The child may be suffering from all-encompassing physical pain for which he has no previous experience to prepare him; he becomes confused and frightened, and he may regress.
   a. Coupled with physical pain is psychological pain resulting from isolation, separation from parents, reliving the experience of being burned, fear of rejection, fear of death, immobilization, chronic pain, and repeated surgery.
   b. Prepare the child for dressing changes and debridement. Provide comfort after procedure.
2. Encourage the child to talk about the way he feels.
   a. The child may feel guilty and think that the burn is punishment for some wrong deed.
   b. Allow the child opportunities at play where he may be able to begin to work out his feelings.
3. The child will be concerned about his appearance.
   a. Continually inform the child that you love him even though he has a bad burn.
   b. Encourage early contact with other children.
   c. Adjustment to disfigurement can be long and painful.
4. Psychiatric consultation is very frequently necessary in order to assist the child to work out his feelings. Signs may include:
   a. Persistent refusal to eat
   b. Resisting all nursing procedures
   c. Resisting socialization
5. Contact with the child's parents, siblings, and nurse will help him with his feelings of fear, isolation, and rejection.
6. Arrange for services of a schoolteacher for the school-age child as soon as his condition permits.

J. Support the parents during this very difficult time. They are under extreme stress, because a burned child creates a crisis.

1. Use knowledge about the family's psychosocial status in planning care.
   a. A medical social worker may offer beneficial psychosocial support to the family.
   b. Be aware of siblings at home and that they may have needs that are being neglected as a result of this crisis.
2. Encourage the parents to visit their child often.
   a. Attempt to have them become actively involved in the child's care when they are ready to do so.

b. If the parents are unable to visit, telephone calls and family photographs are helpful.
3. Give the parents the opportunity to discuss their feelings.
   Parents frequently feel very guilty because they feel they did not give the child the appropriate supervision he should have had when the accident occurred.
4. Keep the parents informed of the child's progress.
   a. Begin initial teaching at admission with supportive words and limited technical information.
   b. Education and orientation to the facility and the burn injury will decrease some anxiety and begin to build rapport on which future support can be based.
   c. Parents' meetings can help the parents cope with trauma.
5. Psychiatric consultation is frequently required in order to assist the parents in coping with their feelings.
K. Prepare the child and family for discharge with the understanding that rehabilitation is long-term.*
1. Separation from the hospital environment, caretakers, and other patients can produce excessive anxiety. Short-time home passes (overnight, weekend) are helpful prior to final discharge.
2. If the child is school age, prepare for school reentry—visit classroom and tell peers what to expect; at the same time teach how to prevent burn injuries.
3. Social re-entry can be painful for the child who may have to respond to questions and stares from strangers and rejection by friends.
4. Hospitalization and future scar revisions may be necessary.
5. Special skin care is necessary following burn injury. Give written specific instructions to parents.
   a. Avoid exposure to sunlight.
   b. Use pressure garments to prevent hypertrophic scar and keloid formation.
   c. Use lotions and creams to prevent drying, cracking and itching.
   d. Burn area has decreased sensation to touch, heat, and pressure, thus precautions need to be practiced to prevent injury to area.
6. Psychological support of the child is necessary because of the trauma resulting from the burn injury, the actual event, and hospitalization.
7. Physical therapy must be continued.
L. Provide educational activities in the community to prevent burn injuries.
Health Education
1. Teach parents and children the prevention of burn injury. Parents can be taught commonsense safety

measures as well as being aware of other fire hazards (i.e., turn pot handles toward stove rather than letting them extend over stove edge, avoid electrical cords hanging over table or counter edge, cover electrical outlets, do not leave small children alone in bathroom or kitchen, etc.).
2. Children can be taught the hazards of flame and other devices that can cause injury.
3. Parents can be taught first-aid emergency care for burn injury (i.e., cool burned area with cool water; remove clothing; parents should know when to seek medical assistance.
4. Children can be taught what to do in case of fire or if their clothes catch on fire (i.e., stop, drop and roll, crawl to safety, etc.).
5. Community groups, media, clinics, and public areas can all be used for public education in prevention of burn injury.

Evaluation

Expected Outcomes

(See adult, p. 645)

1. Absence of shock; stabilization of vital signs; normal serum and electrolyte values
2. Absence of infection as demonstrated by normal laboratory values, clean wound, and normal vital signs
3. Is free of respiratory distress as demonstrated by stable vital signs, respiratory status, and blood gases
4. Shows no signs of gastrointestinal complications as evidenced by normal bowel sounds, normal elimination, stable vital signs
5. Maintains adequate nutritional status as demonstrated by weight gain and wound healing
6. Demonstrates improved mobility as evidenced by involvement in play and other activities
7. Experiences minimal discomfort as evidenced by stable vital signs, verbalization, involvement in play, and other activities
8. Develops a more positive self-image as evidenced by verbalization, socialization, and other behaviors
9. Experiences minimal anxiety as evidenced by appropriate coping behavior
10. Demonstrates appropriate parent/child relationships as evidenced by verbalization and other behaviors
11. Parents reveal lessening of anxiety and demonstrate behaviors of appropriate parent–child relationships, and understanding of illness, treatments, and follow-up care

---

Atopic Eczema (Infantile and Childhood Eczema)

Atopic eczema is a term that describes any inflammatory dermatosis that is characterized by erythema, papulovesiculation, oozing, crusting, and scaling in various phases of resolution.

* Cunningham G with Sand GX. Never Quit. Lincoln, VA, Chosen Books, 1981. *Never Quit* would be a valuable resource for adolescents facing a long illness or handicap resulting from burn injury.

Etiology and Incidence

1. Infantile eczema usually manifests itself between the 2nd and 6th month of age, up to 2 years.
2. This type of dermatitis is the most common, earliest manifestation of allergy.
3. Atopic eczema is not a disease but, rather, a reaction state of the skin.
4. The exact etiology is not known. Many infants with

eczema have a positive family history of allergy and later develop asthma or hay fever.
5. The following may be triggering factors affecting the day-to-day appearance of the lesions:
   a. Bacterial, viral, or fungal infections
   b. Particulate matter and contact irritants
   c. Environmental factors
      (1) Temperature and humidity
      (2) Inhalants
   d. Foods
   e. Emotional or physical stress
   f. Drugs

Altered Physiology

1. The dermatitis involves the epidermis and the vascular layer of the cutis.
2. The dermatitis goes through a cycle involving areas of erythema, papules, vesicles, wheal reactions, and, ultimately, scaling eruption. There is no distinct primary cutaneous lesion. Pruritus followed by scratching and trauma leads to excoriation.
3. With superimposed infection, there is exudation, pustulation, and crust formation.
4. Various stages of the dermatoses can be present on different parts of the child's body.
5. The patient is subject to remissions and exacerbations.
6. Secondary infections may occur from scratching.

Complications

1. Acute infection—pyogenic infection may develop.
2. Long-term—eczema may progress to allergic rhinitis or asthma.

Assessment
Clinical Manifestations

1. Infants—lesions
   a. Erythematous, papular, and weeping lesions develop.
   b. Oozing and crusting of the lesions occur, along with excoriation.
   c. Cheeks, forehead, neck, behind ears, and the crawling surfaces of arms and legs are the areas most frequently involved.
   d. Lesions are more concentrated on the head and body than on the extremities; however, they may progress to cover the body.
2. Older children—lesions
   a. Erythematous, papular, and weeping lesions develop.
   b. Oozing and crusting of the lesions occur.
   c. The flexor surfaces of the upper and lower extremities, antecubital and popliteal fossae, in addition to the face and neck are areas frequently involved.
   d. As the disease becomes chronic, lichenification (leatheriness and hardening of skin) and hyperpigmentation develop.
3. Pruritus—may be mild or severe.
4. Excessive itching may cause restlessness, sleeplessness, and irritability.
5. Excessive scratching may result in an inflammatory reaction and excoriation, bleeding, and subsequent infection.
6. The color of lesions is red (possibly intense red).

Diagnosis

1. Family history of allergies
2. Positive dermal reaction

3. Presence of circulating Prausnitz–Küstner antibodies
4. Tendency to develop blood eosinophilia
5. Clearing of skin with removal of specific allergen and reappearance of dermal reaction upon reexposure

Treatment

1. Symptomatic and supportive
   a. Trial period of hypoallergenic diet to eliminate any responsible food
   b. Avoidance by patient of any other known allergen; wool clothing, blankets, etc.
   c. Control of any complicating skin infection
   d. Relief of itching and irritability; sedation may be necessary
   e. Measures to improve condition of involved skin:
      (1) Prevent scratching
      (2) Cleansing
      (3) Topical steroid
      (4) Tar preparations
      (5) Lubricants
   f. Medications to relieve itching (chloral hydrate, diphenhydramine hydrochloride, Periactin)
   g. Antibiotics/antibacterials—as necessary to control infection
2. Preventive—teach the mother how to keep condition under control

Patient Problems/Nursing Diagnoses

1. Infection related to altered skin integrity and scratching
2. Alteration in comfort related to itching and crusted lesions
3. Anxiety related to discomfort and hospitalization
4. Decreased mobility related to discomfort upon movement of crusted flexor surfaces of extremities

Planning and Implementation
Nursing Interventions

A. Institute measures that prevent the child from scratching himself when he experiences severe itching in order to prevent further irritation and possible infection of the skin.

1. Apply protective devices to prevent the child from scratching himself.
   a. Any one or combination of the following protective devices may be used (elbow cuff, ankle and wrist restraint, face mask, jacket restraint).
   b. Apply these protective devices only when absolutely necessary—when scratching cannot be controlled by other methods.
   c. Apply protective devices securely enough to prevent scratching, yet not so tight as to impair circulation. Check circulation frequently when protective devices are used.
   d. When protective devices are used, the device should be removed at frequent intervals.
      (1) Allow for free movement and active range of motion.
      (2) Allow the child to sit on the nurse's or mother's lap.
      (3) Attempt to divert the child's attention by playing with him and reading to him.
      (4) Allow the child to eat his meals free from protective devices; this requires direct supervision.
   e. When the child experiences severe itching and uncontrollable scratching, remove only one protective device at a time so that scratching can be controlled.

f. Anger and frustration are frequently displayed in violent scratching.
  (1) Keep the child comfortable and anticipate his needs.
  (2) Provide as much personal contact and supervision as possible.
  (3) Allow play activities that afford the child the opportunity to act out his anger and frustrations.
  (4) Provide infants with a cradle gym and a pacifier.
2. Cotton hand mitts and booties may be applied to prevent the child from scratching himself.
3. Trim fingernails and toenails and keep them clean.
4. Provide safe toys that will not be used by the child to scratch himself. (Use soft playthings made of hypoallergenic material.)
5. Administer prescribed medications.
  a. Sedatives
  b. Antihistamines
  c. The use of local anesthetics to relieve itching is contraindicated because of their potential for skin sensitization.
  d. Antipruritics
  e. Topical steroids

B. Provide measures that will improve the condition of the involved skin.

1. Bathe the child by the prescribed method.
  a. Water and soap are often irritating.
  b. Starch baths may be used; oil baths may be soothing.
  c. Oil may be used if the skin is dry and crusted. (Apply oil with a soft cloth.)
  d. While giving the child a bath, keep him from scratching himself. (It may be necessary to maintain protective devices at this time.)
2. Local care of the skin is aimed at removing the debris and allaying the inflammatory reaction and pruritus.
  a. Wet soaks of Burow's solution may be applied to the affected areas.
    (1) These soaks are continuous and must be kept wet. Solution should be at room temperature.
    (2) These bulky, wet dressings may serve to immobilize the child sufficiently so that he does not require other protective devices.
  b. Lassar's paste or another hydrophilic preparation may be applied to the affected areas.
    (1) Local medications must be kept on the skin constantly.
    (2) Caution must be exercised to keep ointment out of the child's eyes.
      (a) Remove all old ointment before applying new ointment.
      (b) Starch bath may be used to remove ointment.
    (3) Routine urine examination should be done because of possible toxic effect of medications on kidneys.
    (4) Coal tar preparations should be used with caution during the summer when exposure to the sun is more likely, because they have a photosensitizing effect.
3. Prevent skin irritation from bedding. Padding may be used.
4. Change diapers frequently to prevent skin excoriation.
5. Avoid extreme ambient temperatures.

C. Promote measures that will prevent contact with dietary and environmental allergens.

1. Review the child's chart and question the parents about known allergies.
  a. Note the known allergens on the Kardex and place a tag on the head of the bed to indicate that the child has an allergy.
  b. Inform the dietitian of the child's food allergies.
2. Avoid substances that have a high potential for sensitization.
  a. Foods such as milk, eggs, chocolate, wheat cereal, and orange juice are to be avoided.
  b. Wool and dust are to be avoided.
3. Observe the child's reactions when an elimination diet is prescribed.
  a. A minimal diet is prescribed. Trial diet may be composed of:
    (1) Milk substitute
    (2) Rice cereal
    (3) 2 fruits
    (4) 2 vegetables
    (5) Beef
    (6) Aqueous multivitamins
    (7) No egg products
  b. A new food is added to the diet every 3–5 days, during which time the response to that food is observed.
  c. An allergic response occurring during this 3- to 5-day period indicates sensitivity to that food; that particular food is then eliminated from the diet.
  d. If no response is apparent, that food is added to the child's diet.
  e. Another food substance is then added, and the child is observed for the following 3 to 5-day period. This method is followed until the food allergen is determined.
4. Provide a substitute for cow's milk when the child is allergic to it.
  a. Goat's milk may be used.
  b. Commercial formulas made from meat or vegetable protein substances are available.

D. Protect the child from sources of infection.

1. Protect the child from exposure to sources of infection known to cause exacerbations and severe infections.
  a. Contact with other children, visitors, and personnel who have the herpes simplex virus is to be avoided.
  b. Use single-patient rooms.

▶ **NURSING ALERT:** If the child needs to be vaccinated against smallpox, it should not be done until his skin has been free from eczema for several months. Use caution with routine immunizations. Skin testing may be advisable.

  c. The child should not be exposed to individuals who have a fresh vaccine lesion.
2. When the child is immobilized, his position should be changed frequently to prevent respiratory complications.

E. Provide the emotional support needed by any child his age who is hospitalized; provide love and attention, and give the child freedom to express his feelings.

(*Text continues on p. 1374*)

Common Skin Problems

Disorder/Organism	Clinical Manifestations	Treatment/Prevention	Specific Nursing Goals and Interventions*	Comments

Impetigo
Bacterial infectious disease affecting the superficial layers of the skin and characterized by the formation of vesicles, crusts, or bullae.
 	
Etiology and Incidence
1. Bullous impetigo in neonate and infant—lesions are large, flaccid bullae containing pus and supernatant clear serum that rupture and leave raw edges. Lesions are more prominent in axillae and groin.
2. Impetigo contagiosa in the older child—lesions appear with thick, yellow crusts.
3. Impetigo is caused by staphylococci (bullous) or streptococci (crusted).
4. Occurs most frequently when personal hygiene is poor.
5. Occurs most frequently in children under 10 years of age.
6. Spread by contact—easily conveyed from person to person (using same handkerchief, towels, napkins, pencils, toys, etc.); plastic wading pools in summer—when spilled water is replaced and no antiseptic or disinfectant is used. Very contagious.
7. Any abrasion of skin may serve as portal of entry.
 	
Diagnosis
1. Aspiration and culture of bullae.
2. Culture after removal of crust.
	(Impetigo contagiosa)
	1. Incubation period of 1–5 days.
	2. Lesion first appears as pink-red macules that quickly change to vesicles which, in turn, enlarge, become pustular, develop crusts, and leave temporary superficial erythematous areas.
	  a. Bullous (newborn and older child)—broken blisters form thin, light brown, liquor-like crust.
	  b. Crusted (preschool-age—seen more often in summer on exposed body parts)—skin around crusts is red and weeping with satellite lesions.
	3. Face, scalp, and hands are commonly involved, but other areas may be affected.
	4. Regional lymphadenopathy—common with secondary infection of insect bites, eczema, poison ivy, scabies.
		Based on etiology and type of infection.
		1. Removal of undermined skin, crusts and debris: 1:20 Burow's solution compresses to affected area. Remove crusts when softened.
		2. Topical application of bactericidal medication (Bacitracin, Neomycin, Neosporin, or Garamycin, Betadine).
		3. Systemic antibiotic—when severe or recurrent (penicillin)
		4. Prevention—avoid contact with child and his siblings.
			Be aware of the appearance of the characteristic lesion of impetigo.
			1. Observe the condition of the child's skin upon admission to the hospital.
			2. Report any suspicious-appearing lesions.
			3. Record the appearance and location of the lesion.
			4. Initiate appropriate measures to prevent the spread of the infection.
			  a. Place the child in a single room.
			  b. Maintain medical aseptic technique.
			5. Watch for the development of new lesions.
			
			Provide measures to prevent secondary infections.
			1. Provide mittens or protective devices to prevent the child from scratching the lesions.
			2. Trim the child's fingernails and toenails.
			3. Maintain the cleanliness of fingernails and toenails.
			
			Provide measures to ensure the child's comfort until healing has occurred and the child is free from infection.
			1. Hold the child frequently and release from any necessary protective device.
			2. Provide diversional therapy.
			3. Administer medication and treatment to relieve itching—local medications or packs which relieve itching and promote healing may be used.
				Practice good general health measures and provide teaching for the child and his parents that will be helpful in preventing spread and further infection.
				1. General measures to improve personal cleanliness should be encouraged.
				2. Minor wounds should be adequately cleansed and treated.
				3. The child should be isolated if at home.
				4. The child should be kept out of school until the lesions have healed.

* See Eczema for Patient Problems/Nursing Diagnoses, general goals and interventions, and Evaluation.

Disorder/Organism	Clinical Manifestations	Treatment/Prevention	Specific Nursing Goals and Interventions*	Comments
	5. Pruritus may occur.		4. Provide the child with a diet adequate to meet his growth and development needs.	
Ringworm of the scalp (*tinea capitis*)	1. The lesions usually develop in the occipital, temporal, and parietal areas of the scalp.	1. Griseofulvin—an antifungal antibiotic that is administered orally, 5 mg./kg./dose b.i.d. × 6–8 weeks; 20 mg./kg./day for 7–14 days.	Recognize the characteristic lesions of ringworm of the scalp.	Teach the child and his family methods to prevent further episodes.
A fungal infection of the scalp and hair follicles.	2. Pruritus usually occurs in the area.	2. Topical agents—applied b.i.d.	1. Observe the condition of the hair and scalp as a part of the routine assessment of the child on admission to the hospital and at daily bath.	1. Teach general hygiene measures—regular shampooing and bathing.
Etiology and Incidence	3. The involved areas of the scalp appear as patches, rounded or oval in outline, covered by scales and lusterless, irregularly broken hairs.	Antifungal—clotrimazole, haloprogin, or miconazole nitrate, Whitfield's ointment	2. Report suspicious-appearing lesions.	2. Advise them to avoid the sharing of hats, combs, brushes, etc.
1. Ringworm of the scalp is caused by different species of the *Microsporum canis*, *Tricbopbyton tonsurans* (most common).		For *T. tonsurans*—selenium sulfide lotion, 2.5% (Selsun Brown, Exsel)	3. Record the appearance and location of the lesions.	3. Stress the importance of wearing a cap continuously until the infection has been eliminated.
2. Ringworm of the scalp is seen primarily in children before puberty.	4. Single patches or multiple patches may occur; alopecia.	3. Cut hair short, keep head clean, and avoid scratching. Wear cap to prevent broken hair pieces from falling.	4. Initiate the appropriate isolation techniques (as per hospital policy).	4. All lesions must be dry before child can return to school.
3. Most commonly seen in ages 3–10 years.	5. Systemic manifestations are absent.		Be aware of the side effects of the medications used in the treatment of ringworm of the scalp.	
Altered Physiology	6. Evaluation		1. Griseofulvin may produce headache, heartburn, nausea, epigastric discomfort, diarrhea, and urticaria.	
1. The fungal infection produces an inflammation of the scalp that causes alopecia and broken hairs.	a. Wood's lamp—a filtered ultraviolet radiation causes microsporon infections to fluoresce with a brilliant, greenish light.		2. Record and report to the physician any side effects observed.	
2. The lesions of the scalp may have papulovesicular erythematous borders or may appear only as scaling with a few broken hairs.	b. Microscopic evaluation of infected hair follicles and fungal culture to identify *Tricbopbyton* which fluoresces poorly under Wood's lamp—spores coat hair in a visible way.		3. A diet high in fat may be prescribed to enhance intestinal absorption.	
3. *Kerion*, an acute inflammation that produces edema, pustules, and granulomatous swelling, may occur.			Be aware of the case-finding measures to prevent additional cases and to identify the earliest evidence of infection.	
4. The infection may be spread through child-to-child contact, as well as through the common use of towels, combs, brushes, hats. Kittens and puppies may be the source of the infection.			1. All family contacts should be screened.	
			2. The school should be notified so that appropriate case-finding techniques may be initiated.	
			Be aware of the psychological trauma associated with loss of hair, especially in a girl, and provide support as appropriate.	

(continued)

Disorder/Organism	Clinical Manifestations	Treatment/Prevention	Specific Nursing Goals and Interventions*	Comments
Pediculosis The infestation of human beings by lice *Etiology* 1. Three types of lice affect human beings: a. *Pediculosis capitis*—head louse b. *Pediculosis corporis*—body louse (rare in US) c. *Phthirus pubis*—pubic louse/crab louse (seldom found in children) can attach only to curly hair—pubes, axillae, eyebrows 2. Each type of louse generally remains in the area designated by its name, but it may occasionally be seen in other areas of the body. Lice are transmitted by personal contact with people harboring them or through contact with articles that temporarily harbor them. *Altered Physiology* 1. The eggs of lice (nits) are attached to the hair or clothing by a sticky substance that hardens. The eggs hatch within 1 week—the lice reach maturity within 1 month and are then capable of reproducing. 2. The lice on the skin produce itching; the longer the infestation persists, the more severe the skin reaction becomes and the more severe the lesions appear. 3. The lice live on clothing and go to the body for feeding; thus, they produce visible scratch marks and points of puncture.	1. Severe itching in the area affected is the primary symptom of pediculosis; scratch marks will be evident in these areas. 2. In children, pubic lice are found most frequently in the eyelashes and eyebrows. 3. Infested scalp areas may become secondarily infected from scratching. 4. Crusts, pediculi, nits, and dirt may combine to cause a foul odor and matted hair. 5. Body lice may produce minute red lesions.	Eliminate and remove nits and pediculi (lice) and treat the irritated skin. 1. *Pediculosis capitis* may be treated with lindane 1% (Kwell), benzyl benzoate emulsion, or crotamiton (see package inserts). Eggs are not killed by 5-minute wash; must repeat in 1 week when they hatch. Over-the-counter products (RID) appear to be safe and effective 2. *Pediculosis corporis* may be treated with the above plus chlorophenothane powder.	Maintain technique that will prevent the spread of the infection. Institute measures to carry out medical asepsis. Perform the treatments prescribed to destroy and eliminate the parasite. Observe and record the response to treatment. 1. Note the change in the degree of discomfort caused by itching. 2. Observe infected areas for changes in the characteristics of the lesions. 3. Observe for systemic manifestations of infection. Provide measures to prevent the child from scratching himself. 1. Provide mittens or protective devices to prevent the child from scratching. 2. Trim fingernails and toenails and keep them clean. 3. Provide the child with diversional therapy to distract him from itching. 4. Hold the child frequently and release him from the protective devices.	Use of wigs or scarves may provide some relief of embarrassment. Hair loss is usually temporary. Provide appropriate teaching for the family to prevent recurrences. 1. Wash linens in water temperature above 52°C. (120°F.) for 10 minutes or store in a closed bag for 10 days. 2. Caution against using same hairbrush and comb. Do not wear one another's hats. 3. Screen the whole family for parasitic infection. Nurses caring for affected child should wear gloves and protective cap during examination and treatment.

Disorder/Organism	Clinical Manifestations	Treatment/Prevention	Specific Nursing Goals and Interventions*	Comments

Scabies
 	
A disease of the skin produced by the burrowing action of a parasite mite resulting in irritation and the formation of vesicles or pustules.
 	
Etiology
1. Scabies is caused by the itch mite, *Sarcoptes scabiei*.
2. Scabies occurs most frequently in individuals living in areas of poverty, where cleanliness is lacking.
3. Scabies occurs as a result of direct contact with infected persons or by indirect contact through soiled bed linen, clothing, etc.
 	
Altered Physiology
1. Both the male and female parasite live on the skin.
2. The female parasite burrows into the superficial skin to deposit her eggs.
3. The burrow is seen most commonly between the fingers but may occur in any natural fold of the skin or in pressure areas (e.g., heel of palm, axillary and buttock folds, male genitalia, female breasts).
4. The burrows may occur in any part of the body in infants and small children and are easily identifiable.
5. Pruritus occurs, and the scratching of the skin may produce secondary infection. Scattered follicular eruptions contain immature mites.
6. Inflammation may produce pustules and crusts.
7. Eggs hatch in 4 days. Larvae undergo a series of molts before becoming adult. The life cycle is complete in 1–2 weeks.
	1. Itching, particularly at night, is the primary symptom. The itching is usually very severe.
	2. Scratching frequently produces secondary skin infection.
	3. Systemic manifestations are absent, unless they result from the secondary infection (i.e., fever, leukocytosis).
		Destroy the parasite, to relieve itching, and to reduce skin irritation.
		
		1. Scrubbing, soaking, use of soap and water bath to remove scaling and crusting debris.
		2. Application of a scabicide:
		  a. Lindane 1% (Kwell)—cream or lotion. Apply topically from the neck down and remove with bath after 8–12 hours.
		  b. Crotamiton (Eurax) cream or lotion—recommended for use in infants, because Kwell may produce neurotoxic symptoms. Massage into skin nightly 2 times; 24 hours after second application, wash off thoroughly.
		  c. 6%–10% precipitate of sulfur in petrolatum.
		3. Contagion unlikely 24 hours after treatment.
		4. Launder all clothing and bedding
			Same as for pediculosis (see above).	Nurses caring for affected children should wear gloves. All infected members of the family should be treated at the same time.

(continued)

Disorder/Organism	Clinical Manifestations	Treatment/Prevention	Specific Nursing Goals and Interventions'	Comments
		with sufficient heat to kill mites. 5. Itching may continue 2–3 weeks after destruction of mites. This can be controlled by using a topical antipruritic.		
Diagnosis Presence on skin of female mite, ova, and feces. Skin scrapings.				
Oral Candidiasis (Thrush)/ **Candidal Diaper Dermatitis** *Oral candidiasis* is a mycotic stomatitis characterized by the appearance of white plaques on the oral mucous membrane, the gums, and the tongue. *Candidal diaper dermatitis* is a rash characterized by red, scaly, sharply circumscribed but moist patches with pustular satellite lesions. *Etiology* 1. Caused by *Candida albicans.* 2. Most frequently seen in newborns, but may be seen in older infants, usually as a complication of antibiotic therapy or underlying disease (malignant neoplasm, immune deficiency disorders). 3. Maternal vulvovaginal candidiasis is the primary source of neonatal thrush. 4. The growth of the organisms is favored by: a. Lack of cleanliness	*Thrush* 1. The infant develops small plaques on the oral mucous membrane, tongue, or gums; these plaques appear like curds of milk but cannot be wiped out of the mouth. 2. Thrush often appears to cause the infant no pain or discomfort, unless the case is severe and there is erosion and ulceration of the mucosa. 3. The mouth may be dry. 4. Occasionally, the infant may appear	*Thrush* 1. Oral administration of nystatin in suspension 3–4 times daily (treatment of choice). Apply over affected surfaces of oral cavity after feeding, allowing the child to swallow any medication to treat any lesions along the gastrointestinal tract. 2. Amphotericin B, clotrimazole, or miconazole is used for candidiasis resistant to nystatin. *Diaper dermatitis* 1. Keep dry and clean.	Recognize the appearance of thrush and be aware of the infant who is particularly susceptible to the development of the condition. 1. Newborns and infants who have particular susceptibility include: a. Sick, debilitated infants b. Infants who are on antibiotic therapy c. Infants with cleft lip and palate, hyperparathyroidism, and neoplasms 2. Inspect mouth *before* every feeding for presence of thrush. 3. Report the appearance of thrush to the physician and record this information on the nursing record. Practice measures that prevent the development and spread of thrush. 1. Practice careful handwashing techniques.	

Disorder/Organism	Clinical Manifestations	Treatment/Prevention	Specific Nursing Goals and Interventions	Comments
b. Malnutrition c. Diabetes d. Antibiotic treatment (destroys normal flora) e. Neoplasms f. Hyperparathyroidism 5. The infection may be acquired from: a. Contaminated hands b. Contaminated feeding equipment c. Contaminated bedding d. Another patient 6. Thrush frequently occurs in children with cleft lip and palate. *Altered Physiology* *Thrush:* 1. Spores lodge between epithelial cells and gradually separate the layers. 2. The infection then spreads to the surface of the mucous membrane. 3. Growth usually begins in several discrete areas of the oral mucous membrane with gradual spreading to the point where a continuous membrane may be formed.	to have some difficulty in swallowing, or eat less vigorously. 5. Enteric infection is frequently associated with oral thrush. *Diaper dermatitis* 1. Buttock rash consisting of erythematous maculopapular eruption with perianal distribution. 2. Generally causes discomfort, especially with wetting and cleansing.	2. Topical application of nystatin or miconazole nitrate cream or ointment. 3. Nystatin may be given orally if rash is persistent.	2. Practice techniques that ensure that nipples, bottles, or any other object that comes into direct or indirect contact with the infant's mouth is clean. Recognize the appearance of candidal diaper dermatitis and report to physician immediately. Teach parents the general principles of preventing diaper dermatitis. 1. Change diaper as soon as possible after wetting or soiling. Check diaper every hour in newborn. 2. Wash entire diaper area thoroughly and dry area before applying clean diaper. 3. Allow the infant to go without a diaper for short periods. 4. Use clean diapers that are soft to the touch and absorbent. 5. Use terminal aseptic rinse when washing diapers to neutralize ammonia produced when infant urinates; use vinegar, Borax, or Diaparene. 6. Avoid powder and oil which tend to clog pores and cake on skin, retaining bacteria. 7. Avoid occlusive plastic coverings, tightly pinned or double diapers, all of which tend to increase production and retention of body heat and moisture.	

Health Education

A. Assist the parents in providing for the child's care following hospitalization.

1. Explain to parents the usual causes of the problem. Help them to understand that eczema is chronic—that there is no cure—but that a therapeutic regimen can be followed that will control it. Home care is preferred, and a home care program is essential.
2. Demonstrate the application of topical medications and the application of dressings. Explain timing of application of medicine. Stress the importance of several thin applications rather than one thick layer.
   a. Weeping and moist areas—apply cream or lotion
   b. Drier areas—paste applied thickly or ointment
3. Give specific information about diet. Emphasize the foods that are allowed rather than foods to be avoided.
4. Demonstrate the application of protective devices and the precautions in using them.
5. Additional information in home management may include the following:
   a. Launder clothes with a neutral pH soap and double rinse.
   b. Control environment.
   c. Use apron to cover clothing when holding child.
   d. Avoid exposure of child to extreme heat or cold or to rapid changes in ambient temperature; have him avoid strenuous activity (can swim), soap, perfume, detergents, and stress.
   e. Keep the child's fingernails clean and cut short.
   f. Do not leave the child alone to entertain himself when itching is severe; prevent play with toys that can be injurious if used to scratch the skin.
   g. Baths may be effective in relieving itching—Alpha-Keri, Domol, Lubath; give bath using 2 cups cornstarch in tub of tepid water. Lubricate dry skin after bath.
6. Encourage the parents to hold and cuddle the child as much as possible to encourage the body contact that is frequently impossible because of protective devices and ointments.
7. Encourage the parents to discuss their feelings and concerns about the child's illness.
   a. The appearance of the child may be very disturbing to them.
   b. They need to feel adequate in caring for the child at home.
8. A community health nurse referral may be indicated to provide support to the family, especially during initial phases of adjustment.

Evaluation

Expected Outcomes

1. Absence of infection as evidenced by stable vital signs, normal laboratory values, and clean wound surfaces
2. Reveals minimal discomfort as evidenced by stable vital signs, behavior, and verbalization
3. Shows minimal anxiety demonstrated by appropriate behavior
4. Remains mobile and participates in activities of daily living

Bibliography

Books

Coleman WP and McBurney EI. Pediatric Dermatology: New Directions in Therapy. Garden City, NY, Medical Examination Publishing Co, 1981

Green M and Haggerty RJ. Ambulatory Pediatrics, 3rd ed. Philadelphia, WB Saunders, 1984

Hills SW and Birmingham JJ. Burn Care. The Fleschner Series in Critical Care. Bethany, CT, Fleschner Publishing Co, 1981

Maddin S (ed). Current Dermatologic Therapy. Philadelphia, WB Saunders, 1982

Orkin M, Juranek DD and Maibach HI. Treatment of Household and Sexual Contacts of Patients with Scabies. In Epstein E (ed). Controversies in Dermatology. Philadelphia, WB Saunders, 1984, pp. 433–435

Sauer GC. Manual of Skin Diseases. Philadelphia, JB Lippincott, 1980

Whaley LF and Wong DL. Nursing Care of Infants and Children. St Louis, CV Mosby, 1983

Wieczorek RR and Natapoff JN. A Conceptual Approach to the Nursing of Children. Philadelphia, JB Lippincott, 1981

Articles

Allen HB et al. Selenium sulfide: Adjunctive therapy for tinea capitis. Pediatrics 1982 Jan; 69(1):81–83

Burn Therapy: "Here's my idea of best burn care." Patient Care 1981 Oct 15; 15(17):13–16+

Charnock EL and Meehan JJ. Postburn respiratory injuries in children. Pediatr Clin North Am 1980 Aug; 27(3):661–676

Clare ER. Lice: Ancient pest with new resistance. Pediatr Nurs 1983 Sep/Oct; 9(5):347–350

Cook T and Zeanah G. Burn prevention as a component of health care in a pediatric hospital. J Burn Care Rehabil 1982 Sep/Oct; 3(5):289–290+

Dittemore IL. Behavioral response in the early recovery of a severely burned 4-year-old child. Matern Child Nurs J 1983 Spring; 12(1):21–34

Fleming JW. Common dermatologic conditions in children. MCN 1981 Sep/Oct; 6(5):346–354

Foutes JA, et al. Policy decisions in scabies control. J Sch Health 1981 Dec; 51(10):673–675

Frank DH, et al. Comparison of Biobrane, porcubine, and human allograft as biologic dressings for burn wounds. J Burn Care Rehabil 1983 May/Jun; 4(3):186–190

Goldstein N. Scabies and pediculosis: Persistent, pruritic and puzzling conditions. Consultant 1980 Sep; 20(9):36–37+

Guzzetta PC and Randolph J. Burns in children: 1982. Pediatr Rev 1983 Mar; 4(9):271–278

Helm PA et al. Burn injury: Rehabilitation management in 1982. J Burn Care Rehabil 1982 Nov/Dec; 4(6):411–422

Kavanaugh C. A new approach to dressing change in the severely burned child and its effect on burn-related psychopathology. Heart Lung 1983 Nov; 12(6):612–619

Krowchuk DP, et al. Current status of

the identification and management of tinea capitis. Pediatrics 1983 Nov; 72(5):625–631

Lushbaugh MA. Critical care of the child with burns. Nurs Clin North Am 1981 Dec; 16(4):635–646

McGrath PJ and Vair C. Psychological aspects of pain management of the burned child. Child Health 1984 Summer; 13(1):15–19

McLaury P. Head lice: Pediatric social disease. Am J Nurs 1983 Sep; 83(9): 1300–1303

O'Neill JA. Burns. Top Emerg Med 1982 Oct; 4(3):28–35

Puczynski M, Rademaker D and Gaston RL. Burn injury related to the microwave oven. Pediatrics 1983 Sep; 72(5):714–715

Quay NB and Alexander LL. Preparation of burned children and their families for discharge. J Burn Care Rehabil 1983 Jul/ Aug; 4(4):288–290

Roche J and Jackson D. Developing a patient/family burn unit information booklet. J Burn Care Rehabil 1983 Nov/Dec; 4(6):451–452

Rose MP and Deitch EA. The effective use of a tubular compression bandage, Tubigrip, for burn scar therapy in the growing child. J Burn Care Rehabil 1983 May/Jun; 4(3):197–201

Schanberger JE. Inflicted burns in children. Top Emerg Med 1981 Oct; 3(3):85–92

Stap L, Brock R and Zissermann L. The tactile functions of burned children. J Burn Care Rehabil 1983 Jul/Aug; 4(4): 291–302

Wooldridge-King M. Nursing considerations of the burned patient during the emergent period. Heart Lung 1982 Jul/Aug; 11(4):353–361

Metabolic Disturbances in Children

40

Major Endocrine Disorders of Childhood

Gland	Disorder	Etiology
Anterior pituitary	Growth retardation, dwarfism	Growth hormone deficiency
	Tall stature (Pituitary gigantism)	Growth hormone excess
Posterior pituitary	Diabetes insipidus (see p. 1381)	Vasopressin (antidiuretic hormone) deficiency
Thyroid	Hypothyroidism	Thyroxine (T_4) and Triiodothyronine (T_3) deficiency*
	Cretinism (see p. 673)	
	Thyrotoxicosis (see p. 1384)	Thyroxine and triiodothyronine excess*
Parathyroid	Hypoparathyroidism (hypocalcemia, tetany, increased serum phosphorus)	Parathyroid hormone (PTH) deficiency
	Hyperparathyroidism (hypercalcemia, hypophosphatemia) [rare in children]	Parathyroid hormone excess
Islands of Langerhans of pancreas	Diabetes mellitus (see below)	Insulin deficiency
Adrenal cortex	Adrenal insufficiency	Deficiency of adrenal hormones*
	Addison's disease (weakness, fatigue, weight loss, pigmentation of skin)	
	Cushing's syndrome (obesity of the face, trunk and abdomen)	Cortisol excess*
	Adrenogenital syndrome	Androgen excess*
	Ambiguous genitalia (see p. 1354)	
Ovaries	Lack of or repressed female sexual development	Estrogen deficiency*
	Precocious puberty of female	Estrogen excess*
Testes	Delayed male sexual development	Testosterone deficiency*
	Eunuchoidism	
	Precocious puberty of male	Testosterone excess*

 * May also result from deficiency or excess of appropriate stimulating hormones from the anterior pituitary (that is, thyrotropin (TSH), adrenocorticotropic hormone (ACTH), gonadotropins, (follicle-stimulating hormone [FSH], luteinizing hormone [LH]).

Diabetes Mellitus

Diabetes mellitus is a disorder of carbohydrate metabolism resulting in high serum levels of glucose and the spilling of glucose in the urine. The disease is also associated with abnormal metabolism of fat and protein. With few exceptions, diabetes in children is of the type I insulin-dependent variety.

Etiology
1. Believed to be related to inheritance of certain HLA antigens which predispose an individual to autoimmune destruction of pancreatic islets.
2. Factors, in addition to genetic ones, are also involved in provoking the clinical manifestations of the disease.

3. Viral infection has been suggested as a triggering factor in individuals with a genetic predisposition for diabetes.

Incidence

1. Diabetes mellitus is the most common endocrine disorder of children.
2. Affects approximately 1.9 per 1,000 school-age children.
3. Age-related peaks of presentation occur among 5–7 year olds and at puberty.

Altered Physiology

1. The pancreas produces an insufficient amount of insulin.
2. The body is unable to oxidize glucose properly.
3. Hyperglycemia results from the deficient oxidation of glucose and the inability of tissues to use glucose as fuel.
4. Glucosuria results when the serum level of glucose exceeds the renal threshold.
5. Diuresis is initiated and may progress to dehydration and impaired renal function.
6. Protein and fat are oxidized at abnormal rates.
7. Ketones accumulate in the blood when fat is oxidized at abnormal rates.
8. Ketones are excreted in the urine.
9. Acidosis occurs when ketosis is severe enough to lower the CO_2-combining power of the blood. Diabetic coma may result.

Assessment

Clinical Manifestations

1. Rapid onset (usually over a period of a few weeks)
2. Major symptoms
   a. Increased thirst
   b. Increased urination, eneuresis
   c. Increased food ingestion
   d. Weight loss
   e. Fatigue
3. Minor symptoms
   a. Skin infections
   b. Dry skin
   c. Monilial vaginitis in adolescent girls
4. Diabetic acidosis
   a. Precomatose state
      Drowsiness
      Dryness of skin
      Cherry red lips
      Increased respirations
      Nausea
      Vomiting
      Abdominal pain
   b. Comatose state
      Extreme hyperpnea (Kussmaul breathing)
      Soft, sunken eyeballs
      Rigid abdomen
      Rapid, weak pulse
      Decreased temperature
      Decreased blood pressure
   c. Circulatory collapse and renal failure may follow, resulting from the combination of lowered pH, electrolyte deficiency, and dehydration.
5. Side effects
   a. Stunting of growth

Complications

(Appear to be related to the degree of control of diabetes)
1. Retinopathy and cataracts
2. Neuropathy
3. Renal disease
4. Increased incidence of gangrene, myocardial infarction, and stroke

Patient Problems/Nursing Diagnoses

1. Potential for developing diabetic ketoacidosis and hypoglycemic reactions related to imbalances between insulin requirements and supply
2. Potential disruption in skin integrity related to daily administration of insulin
3. Potential nutritional imbalance related to problems in following a regulated diet plan
4. Body image concerns related to limits imposed by treatment, stunting of growth, and delayed puberty
5. Prolonged dependence on parents related to treatment regimen
6. Knowledge deficit of parents and child regarding diabetes and its management

Planning and Implementation

Nursing Interventions

A. **Recognize signs of diabetic acidosis** (see Clinical Manifestations) **and provide supportive care to the child should this develop.**

1. Be aware of common causes of diabetic acidosis
   a. Untreated diabetes
   b. Inadequate insulin coverage
   c. Failure to adhere to the prescribed diet
   d. Chronic or repeated infections
   e. Stress
   f. Vomiting
2. Apply the principles of nursing care of the comatose child (see Nursing the Unconscious Patient, p. 760).
3. Maintain intravenous therapy (see IV Procedure, p. 1160).
   a. Be prepared to administer intravenous sodium bicarbonate if pH <7.2 (use somewhat controversial).
   b. Have intravenous glucose available should the child suddenly become hypoglycemic.
      Care is taken to avoid reducing the blood glucose to hypoglycemic levels.
   c. Parenteral fluids may need to be changed frequently because of continued polyuria and results of electrolyte determinations.
4. Be prepared to administer relatively large quantities of regular insulin.
   a. A variety of acceptable formulas are available for insulin therapy.
   b. A recent technique involves:
      (1) IV push injection of 0.1 unit of insulin per kg. body weight.
      (2) This is followed by a constant infusion of 0.1 unit of insulin per kg. body weight per hour until blood glucose reaches 300 mg./dl.
      (3) Insulin infusion is then discontinued, IV is changed to $D_5\frac{1}{2}NS$, and sliding-scale insulin therapy is begun.
5. Insert a nasogastric tube to relieve abdominal distention and prevent vomiting.

6. Monitor urine output exactly.
   Test each specimen for ketones.
7. Provide emotional support to the child and his family.
   a. Respond immediately to the child's needs for physical comfort.
   b. Discuss the child's treatment plan and expected response with his parents to alleviate their anxiety.
8. Reinstitute oral feedings when the child is sufficiently responsive and can tolerate them.
   a. This is usually after 12–16 hours of parenteral therapy.
   b. Begin with a low-fat, liquid diet.
   Observe closely for signs of insulin shock or recurrent acidosis once oral feedings are reinstituted.
9. Begin a teaching program with the child as soon as possible to allay his worries concerning his physical status, prognosis, and treatment.

B. **Provide a diet adequate for the child's normal growth and development and sufficient to satisfy his appetite.**

1. Nutritional requirements are determined by the child's symptomatology, family and cultural characteristics, and physician preference.
   a. Most prescribed diets are of the unmeasured type.
   The diet plan eliminates concentrated sweets, follows recommended allowances from all of the 4 basic food groups, but otherwise does not require measuring or rigidity.
   b. Occasionally a more rigid, strictly controlled diet is necessary.
   c. The diet should be composed of approximately 55% carbohydrate, 30% fat, and 15% protein.
   (1) Most diets are restricted in carbohydrates, saturated fats, and cholesterol, and may be based on the exchange method as recommended by the American Diabetes Association.
   (2) Approximately 70% of the carbohydrate content should be derived from complex carbohydrates such as starch.
   (3) Foods with high fiber content should be encouraged.
   (4) All diets must supply sufficient caloric intake for activity and growth, sufficient protein for growth, and the required vitamins and minerals.
   d. Foods are distributed throughout the day to accommodate varying peak action of insulin.
   Distribution may be adjusted for increased or decreased amounts of exercise.
2. Determine the child's usual dietary habits so that adherence to his controlled diet will be easier.

3. Include the child and his parents in his meal planning as soon as possible.
4. Allow the child normal activity while hospitalized so that the observed result of his dietary control will be valid.
5. Allow the child to eat with other children.
6. Make certain that the child adheres to his prescribed diet and understands the rationale for this.

C. **Administer insulin in an amount adequate to maintain the child's approximate glycemic equilibrium.**

1. The dosage and kinds of insulin are determined from the results of blood glucose monitoring.
   a. Generally, a combination of about ⅓ short-acting insulin and ⅔ intermediate-acting insulin are prescribed, to be administered either once or twice daily.
2. Insulin should be given ½ hour before breakfast. If split-dose insulin is prescribed, it should be given ½ hour before breakfast and ½ hour before the evening meal.
3. Be aware of the major types of insulin and their effect (Table 40-1).
4. Develop a systematic plan for injections that emphasizes rotation of sites. In this way, it will be several weeks before it is necessary to return to the same site.
   a. The upper arms and thighs are the most acceptable sites for injection in children, but the outer areas of the abdomen or hips may also be used.
   b. A diagram showing injection sites should be used to maintain the rotation (Fig. 40-1).
   The sites can be checked off each day until the routine is familiar.
   c. Injections are begun at an upper corner of the area to be used.
   d. Subsequent injections are given about 2.5 cm. (1 inch) apart, working in rows.
   e. When all rows in one area are completed, injections are begun in the next area.
   f. Guidelines for site location:
   (1) *Arms*—Begin below the deltoid muscle and end one hand breadth above the elbow. Begin at the midline and progress outward laterally using the external surface only.
   (2) *Thighs*—Begin 1 hand breadth below the hip and end 1 hand breadth above the knee. Begin at the midline and progress outward laterally using only the outer, anterior surface.
   (3) *Abdomen*—Avoid the beltline and 1 inch around the umbilicus.
   (4) *Buttocks*—Use the upper outer quadrant of the buttocks.
5. Be certain that the measuring scale of the syringe matches the unit strength on the bottle of insulin.
   a. Insulin is available in strengths of 40, 80, and 100 units per ml.
   b. U-100 insulin is preferred since it allows the smallest possible amount to be given.
   c. New purified forms of insulin are available but should not be used unless recommended by the physician because use may require a decrease in insulin dose.
6. Use insulin that is at room temperature.
   a. The bottle in use may be kept at room temperature without losing appreciable strength.
   b. Extra bottles should be stored in the refrigerator.

Table 40-1   Types of Insulin and Their Effects

Type of Insulin	Onset (hours)	Maximal Activity (hours)	Duration (hours)
Regular	½–1	2–4	6–8
Semi-Lente	½–1	2–4	10–12
NPH	2	4–12	24
Lente	2	8–10	24
Ultralente	4–8	14–20	36

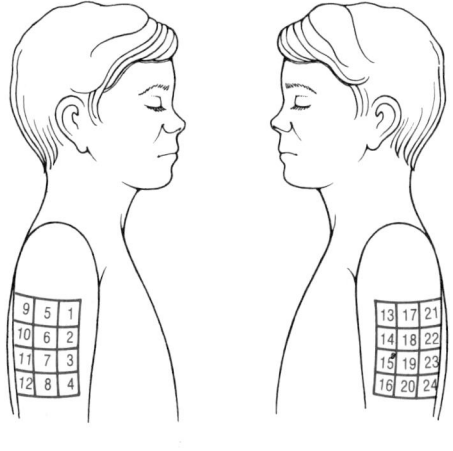

Figure 40-1. Rotating injection sites for insulin in the pediatric patient.

7. Mix the solution by rotating the vial between the hands. Do not shake vigorously.

8. Administer insulin subcutaneously and not too near the skin to prevent local skin reactions and to promote absorption.

9. Following injection, exert firm pressure with an alcohol sponge to prevent bleeding.

10. Observe the skin closely for signs of irritation. Avoid the injection site for several weeks if signs of local irritation are observed.

11. Observe the skin for a rash indicating an allergic reaction to the insulin.

12. Be aware of factors that vary the need for and utilization of insulin, particularly exercise and infection.
    a. Exercise
       (1) Tends to lower the blood sugar level.
       (2) Encourage normal activity, regulated in amount and time.
    b. Infection
       (1) Increases the child's insulin requirement
       (2) Be alert for signs of infection.

13. Encourage the child to express his feelings about the injections.
    The child may be helped to master his fear of injections by gaining control of the situation through play and active participation in the procedure.

14. Insulin can also be administered by constant, subcutaneous infusion using a pump.
    a. The pump delivers fixed small amounts of insulin continuously.
    b. Before meals, the child (or parent) uses the pump to deliver a bolus dose of insulin.
    c. The amount of insulin is adjusted by the child (or parent) based on self-monitoring of blood glucose.
    d. Because of the expense and commitment required, pump therapy is most suited to older children and adolescents who have experienced control problems with conventional insulin therapy.

D. Be aware of the symptoms and treatment of hypoglycemic reactions.

1. Common causes
   a. Overdose of insulin
   b. Reduction in diet or increased exercise without sufficient caloric coverage

2. Symptoms

Trembling	Drowsiness
Shaking	Odd behavior
Sweating	Mental confusion
Apprehension	Seizures
Tachycardia	Coma
Hunger	

3. Be prepared to give orange juice or other food containing readily available simple sugars.

4. Have glucose available for intravenous injection or glucagon available for intramuscular or subcutaneous injection.

E. Monitor the child's blood glucose level to evaluate diabetic control, and adjust insulin dosage and nutritional needs.

1. This method of monitoring control is being used increasingly for children of all ages.

2. The procedure requires a drop of blood, obtained by finger stick, a reagent strip, and a reflectance meter.

3. Specific instructions for performing the procedure vary with the equipment being utilized and must be followed explicitly.

4. Blood glucose measurements are usually made 4 times per day, before meals and at bedtime.

5. Additional blood tests are helpful during episodes of hypoglycemic symptoms or other problem situations.

6. Urine tests for ketones should be continued if the child is ill or if blood glucose is greater than 240 mg./100 ml.

7. Record the results of blood glucose testing accurately.
   a. Use a standard form for recording so that the information will be clear and readily available.
   b. Help the child to understand how his disease is controlled by teaching him to test his own blood,

record results and report information to health care personnel or parents.

F. Prevent infection.

1. Bathe daily.
2. Maintain meticulous skin care through such activities as frequent ambulation of the child and application of body lotion.
3. Keep fingernails and toenails clean and well trimmed.
4. Provide prompt treatment for any violations of the skin (bruises, abrasions, lacerations, etc.).

G. Foster acceptance on the part of the child that he is a normal, healthy person and able to compete with his peers.

1. Include the child and his parents in the treatment plan in its earliest stages.
2. Emphasize that daily management of his disease can become as routine as matters of personal hygiene.
3. Permit and encourage the development of the child's natural talents. Do not allow him to use his disease as a crutch.
4. Allow the child independence in his care as soon as possible, but provide the necessary direction.
5. Initiate a teaching program for the child and his parents early. Offer them available literature.
6. If appropriate, group diabetic children together on the unit. Initiate group discussions for diabetic adolescents.
7. Invite the parents to join a group of parents of diabetic children if such a group is available in the area.
8. Initiate a community nursing referral if the parents or the child appears apprehensive or seems to lack confidence.

Health Education

Patient or parental education is one of the most important aspects in the nursing care of the diabetic child. Thorough instruction is essential in the following areas:

1. Influence of exercise, emotional stress, and other illnesses on both insulin and diet needs
2. Recognition of the symptoms of insulin shock and diabetic acidosis and knowledge of related emergency management
3. Prevention of infection
   a. Attend to regular body hygiene with special attention to foot care.
   b. Report any breaks in the skin. Treat them promptly.
   c. Use only properly fitted shoes; do not wear vinyl or plastic which do not permit ventilation. Avoid calluses and blisters.
   d. Dress the child appropriately for the weather.
   e. See that the child receives regular dental check-ups and maintenance.
   f. Follow routine immunizations according to the recommended schedule.
4. Blood testing
   a. Demonstrate the procedure.
   b. Have the child and his parent demonstrate to the nurse.
   c. Allow the child to do the procedure under supervision until his accuracy is certain.
   d. Encourage the child to assume responsibility for his own blood testing.
   e. Help the child to develop an easy method of recording blood glucose results.
      A record should be used that includes blood test

results, kind and amount of insulin given, and additional remarks, such as child's activity, insulin reactions, etc.
   f. Be certain the parents understand what results are desirable for the child and the appropriate action to take when test results are other than those desired.
5. Administration of insulin
   a. Both the child and his parents should be taught how to do this procedure and what effects the various forms of insulin have.
   b. Give parents an opportunity to express their feelings about the injection.
   c. Explain the procedure simply and demonstrate it.
   d. Discuss the procedure for rotation of sites and the rationale for this method.
   e. Allow the parent and child to practice by injecting normal saline into the nurse.
   f. Have the parent inject his child under supervision.
   g. Have the child inject himself.
      (1) Most children over the age of 8 can be taught to give insulin to themselves.
      (2) Generally, the earlier this responsibility is given to the child, the easier it is for him.
   h. Carefully check the dosage measured by the child and his parent until you are certain of their accuracy.
   i. Complete a community nursing referral for assistance with this procedure at home if indicated.
6. Diet
   a. Review the prescribed diet with the family.
   b. Discuss acceptable modifications of exchanges.
   c. Allow the child to manage his own diet as early as possible.
   d. Emphasize that the diet is based on normal household foods. The purchase of special, expensive dietetic foods is usually not necessary.
   e. Stress that food labels must be scrutinized. A label of "dietetic" or "low-calorie" does not necessarily mean that the food is acceptable for the child.
   f. Inform the parents and children of the exchange lists available from many of the national fast-food restaurants.
7. Precautionary measures
   a. Have the child carry with him an identifying card that states that he has diabetes and includes his name, address, telephone number, and his physician's name and telephone number.
   b. See that the child has orange juice, a lump of sugar, or a bar of candy available in case of an insulin reaction.
   c. Have the family discuss the child's disease with the school nurse and with other responsible adults who are in close contact with the child (teachers, scout leaders, etc.).
   d. Advise the parents that vials of insulin should be kept on one's person when traveling, because baggage may be subjected to extreme temperatures and pressures incompatible with the stability of insulin. If necessary, a thermos can be used to keep the insulin at the appropriate temperature.
8. Teaching materials and Resources for Children and Parents:
   Faro B et al. Diabetic Teaching Manual for Children

and Parents. Unpublished manuscript. University of Rochester, School of Nursing, Rochester, NY 14642

Kipnis L and Adler S. You Can't Catch Diabetes From A Friend. Gainesville, Triad Scientific Publishers, 1979

Travis LB. An Instructional Aid on Juvenile Diabetes Mellitus, 6th ed. Galveston, TX, Department of Pediatrics, University of Texas, Medical Branch, 1980

9. Agency:
   American Diabetes Association
   2 Park Avenue
   New York, NY 10020

Evaluation

Expected Outcomes

1. Blood glucose levels stay within normal range (no signs of ketoacidosis or hypoglycemia); carries identification stating diabetic condition; carries candy bar to offset potential insulin reaction
2. Child's skin remains intact without signs of irritation or infection
3. Child adheres to treatment regimen, demonstrates the proper method of insulin administration; adheres to diet restriction
4. Maintains healthy self-concept; participates in self-care, engages in normal activities for age; works toward independence
5. Assumes age-appropriate responsibility for his own care (A reasonable expectation is for total independence by the age of 12–13 years.)
6. The parents and child demonstrate understanding of the essentials of diabetes care; insulin administration; diet; infection control; signs of hypoglycemia; blood and urine testing; precautionary measures to avoid insulin reaction

Diabetes Insipidus

Diabetes insipidus is a disorder of water metabolism caused by a deficiency of vasopressin, the antidiuretic hormone (ADH) secreted by the posterior pituitary.

Etiology

1. Deficient secretion of vasopressin (antidiuretic hormone)
   a. Primary
      (1) Genetic transmission (autosomal dominant or X-linked inheritance)
      (2) Idiopathic
   b. Secondary
      (1) Brain tumors, especially those in the hypothalamic area (most frequent cause)
      (2) CNS malformation or degenerative disease
      (3) Head trauma or neurosurgery
      (4) Infections of the central nervous system
      (5) Vascular disease—aneurysm, thrombosis
2. Failure of the renal tubules to respond to vasopressin (nephrogenic diabetes insipidus)
   a. Hereditary (X-linked) disease
   b. Found almost exclusively in males

Altered Physiology

1. Vasopressin normally acts on the distal tubules and collecting ducts of the kidney to facilitate reabsorption of water.
2. Pathology of the pituitary or hypothalamus results in a deficiency of vasopressin.
3. The kidney is unable to produce a concentrated urine without sufficient vasopressin.
4. Nephrogenic diabetes insipidus
   a. Vasopressin secretion is normal.
   b. The renal tubules do not respond to vasopressin.
   c. The kidney is unable to produce a concentrated urine.

Clinical Manifestations

1. Onset—usually sudden
2. Symptoms
   a. Depend on the age of the child, the extent of vasopressin deficiency, and the primary lesion
   b. Universal symptoms
      (1) Polydipsia (excessive thirst)
      (2) Polyuria (excessive urine output)
      (3) Inability to concentrate urine
   c. Symptoms in infants
      (1) Excessive crying (quieted with water rather than additional milk)
      (2) Hyperthermia
      (3) Vomiting
      (4) Constipation
      (5) Rapid weight loss
      (6) Dehydration
      (7) Growth failure
   d. Symptoms in older children
      (1) Excessive thirst which may interfere with play and sleep
      (2) Enuresis, and/or nocturia
      (3) Anorexia
      (4) Pale and dry skin
      (5) Reduced sweating
      (6) Viscid saliva

Diagnostic Evaluation

A. Water Deprivation Test

1. After a 24-hour period of adequate hydration and stable weight, fluids are restricted for 6 hours.
2. Urine volumes and osmolality and the child's weights are recorded hourly.
3. Serum sodium and osmolality are measured at the beginning and end of the test.
4. Persistent excretion of dilute urine, a rise in serum sodium (>145 mEq./liter) and serum osmolality (>290 mOsm./kg.), and a weight loss of 3%–5% are suggestive of diabetes insipidus.

▶ **NURSING ALERT:** The test should be terminated if weight loss approaches 5%, indicating moderate dehydration.

B. Vasopressin Sensitivity Test

1. A reduction of urine flow and an increase in urine concentration are observed following the administration of antidiuretic hormone.

2. This test should be used after it has been demonstrated that the child is unable to concentrate urine during the water deprivation test.

Nursing Interventions

A. Participate in the diagnostic evaluation of diabetes insipidus.

1. Explain the purpose of appropriate laboratory tests and the protocol that the child and family will be asked to follow.
2. Supervise the child closely to avoid surreptitious fluid intake during fasting periods.
3. Observe the child closely for evidence of fluid and electrolyte disturbances while the test is in progress.
   a. Dehydration and shock may occur in severely affected children during the water deprivation test.
   b. Overhydration may occur in patients with primary psychogenic polydipsia during the vasopressin sensitivity test.
4. Collect urine specimens as requested by the physician.

B. Prevent dehydration and restore electrolyte balance.

1. Nursing actions when the disorder is caused by a deficiency of vasopressin.
   a. DDAVP (a synthetic analog of vasopressin), is the drug of choice for replacement therapy.
      (1) Dosage-regulated by trial for each child; goal is to eliminate polyuria except for brief periods prior to the next dose
      (2) Route of administration—nasal spray
      (3) Duration—8–24 hours, depending on the child's state of hydration
      (4) Special precautions
         (a) If the child is treated with a single, daily dose, it should be given in the evening so that polyuria will not interfere with sleep or school.
         (b) Excess mucus such as occurs with upper respiratory infections or allergic rhinitis may interfere with hormone absorption.
   b. Pitressin tannate in oil may also be used as replacement therapy. It has the advantage of being much less expensive.
      (1) Dosage—regulated by trial for each child
      (2) Route of administration—intramuscular injection
      (3) Duration—approximately 48 hours
      (4) Special precautions
         (a) Careful attention must be given to adequate suspension of the pitressin tannate in oil.
         (b) Hold the ampule under hot water to reduce the viscosity of the suspending medium. (Immersion of the ampule in boiling water destroys the hormone.)
         (c) Shake the ampule vigorously until the active ingredient is smoothly dispersed.
         (d) Inject the medication with a 2.5-cm. (1-inch) No. 20–22 gauge needle.

         (e) Inject the medication deeply into the muscle.
         (f) Establish a pattern of systematic rotation of injection sites.

▶ **NURSING ALERT:** Water intoxication is a dangerous complication if Pitressin is given too frequently.

   c. Aqueous vasopressin is available as a nasal spray, but the duration of action is so brief that administration is required every 3–4 hours.
2. Nursing actions when the disorder is caused by failure of the kidney to respond to vasopressin.
   a. Administration of Pitressin is ineffective.
      These children already produce a sufficient quantity of vasopressin.
   b. Administer water at frequent intervals and in sufficient volume to prevent dehydration.
   c. Administer a low-sodium, low-solute residue diet to reduce the osmolar load on the kidney.
   d. Administer thiazide therapy as prescribed by the physician.
      This causes sodium diuresis, which acts to promote proximal tubular sodium reabsorption.

C. Observe and record the child's response to therapy.

1. Intake and output
   a. Total the intake and output record every 8 hours.
   b. Record the urine specific gravity of each voiding.
2. Temperature—be alert for the development of fever.
3. Skin turgor—decreased skin turgor is sign of dehydration.
4. Color
5. Appetite—record the child's intake accurately with each meal.

D. Provide emotional support to the family.

Prognosis depends on the underlying condition.
1. Hereditary and idiopathic types—favorable with adequate treatment.
2. Trauma—spontaneous recovery often occurs.
3. Tumor
   a. Varies with the site of the lesion and type of tumor.
   b. Needs of the family accentuated by many problems including surgery and facing the death of the child.

Health Education

1. Explain the condition with specific clarification that diabetes insipidus and diabetes mellitus are very different disorders.
2. Teach the parents the correct procedure for preparation and administration of vasopressin.
3. Encourage the child to assume full responsibility for his care when he is old enough.
4. The child should wear a Medic-Alert tag, which identifies his condition.
5. The older child should carry nasal spray for temporary relief of symptoms if necessary.
6. School personnel and other significant adults should be made aware of the child's problem.

Hypothyroidism

Hypothyroidism is an endocrine disease resulting from deficient production of thyroid hormone. It may be either congenital (cretinism) or acquired.

Etiology

A. Congenital

1. Embryonic defect with partial or complete absence of the thyroid gland
2. Defect in the synthesis of thyroid hormone
3. Destruction of fetal thyroid as a result of antigen–antibody reaction
4. Iodide deficiency (endemic cretinism)
5. Toxic substances encountered during pregnancy causing maldevelopment or atrophy of the fetal thyroid gland. These may rarely include some medications administered during pregnancy.

B. Acquired

1. Chronic lymphocytic thyroiditis
2. Subacute thyroiditis
3. Medications
   a. Iodides
   b. Thiouracil
4. Thyroidectomy
5. Hypothalamic or pituitary disease
6. Peripheral resistance to thyroid hormones
7. Congenital thyroid disorders that do not decompensate until later childhood, appearing acquired

Altered Physiology

Same as in the adult.

Clinical Manifestations

1. Depend on age at onset, the specific defect, the extent of thyroid deficiency, and its duration
2. Congenital hypothyroidism
   a. Clinical manifestations usually nonspecific and subtle
   b. Prolonged jaundice
   c. Lethargy
   d. Constipation
   e. Feeding problems
   f. Cool to touch
   g. Poor muscle tone—umbilical hernia
   h. Hoarse cry
   i. Hypotonia, slow reflexes
   j. Dry skin
3. Acquired hypothyroidism
   a. Decreased growth rate
   b. Goiter
   c. Increase in upper to lower body segment ratio
   d. Delayed dentition
   e. Mild obesity
   f. Delayed puberty
   g. Developmental delay
   h. Decreased school performance
4. Classic signs and symptoms of untreated hypothyroidism
   a. Generalized puffiness
   b. Skin—dry, thick, scaly, coarse, cool, and pale
   c. Facial characteristics

(1) Bridge of nose—flat, broad, and undeveloped
(2) Eyes—widely spaced with swollen eyelids
(3) Anterior fontanelle widely open
(4) Tongue—thick and protruding
   d. Hair—frequently dry, coarse, brittle, slow-growing
   e. Short stature
   f. Slow pulse and decreased blood pressure
   g. Protuberant abdomen and buttocks
   h. Delayed reflexes
   i. Dull, placid expression
   j. Poor appetite
   k. Constipation
   l. Lethargy
   m. Delayed motor and mental development
5. Clinical manifestations may be delayed in breast-fed infants until the child is weaned because of the thyroid hormone contained in breast milk.

Diagnostic Evaluation

1. X-ray shows retarded bone age.
2. Thyroid function test results are abnormal.
3. Thyroid scan reveals decreased uptake.
4. Neonatal screening is possible and is mandatory in most states.

Prognosis

1. Depends on the child's age at onset and the effectiveness of his therapy.
2. Congenital hypothyroidism is one of the most common preventable causes of mental retardation.
   a. If untreated, mentally deficient dwarf results.
   b. When treated:
      (1) Normal physical growth and development can occur.
      (2) Mental development can be normal.
         (a) The best results are obtained by giving continuous, full therapy as early as possible (within the first 3–6 weeks of life).
         (b) The best outlook is for children who have active thyroid tissue during the fetal life, have adequate treatment, and show a high family intelligence quotient.
3. Acquired hypothyroidism
   a. Risk of permanent intellectual impairment is small if hypothyroidism develops beyond age 2 or 3 years.
   b. All changes should be reversible.

Nursing Interventions

A. Administer replacement therapy for the deficient hormone.

1. Sodium-1-thyroxine is the most reliable replacement therapy.
2. Dosage
   a. Individualized for each child.
   b. Adjusted according to clinical response and results of thyroid function tests.
   c. Goal is to achieve normal growth and development.

3. Route of administration
    a. Always administer thyroid replacement orally.
    b. The tablet may be crushed and mixed with fruit for infants.
4. Special precautions
    a. The total daily requirement is given as a single dose.
    b. Administer the medication at the same time each day.
5. Observe for toxic effects.
    a. Excitability
    b. Nervousness
    c. Tachycardia
    d. Tremors
    e. Cramps

B. Provide a complete, well-balanced diet.

1. Special problems related to nutrition
    a. Increased skeletal development
        (1) Increases the need for additional vitamin D.
        (2) Encourage the child to drink 3–4 glasses of milk daily.
    b. Constipation
        Provide foods that are high in fiber such as raw fruits and vegetables.
2. Determine the child's dietary preferences and use this information to plan his menus.
    a. Include the child in menu planning when this is possible.
    b. See the section on nutrition, page 1094.

C. Provide emotional support to the child and his family.

1. Assess the child's capabilities and establish realistic expectations and limits.

2. Assist the parents to adjust to alterations in their child's behavior as he responds to treatment.
    The child may develop new enthusiasm for the naturally disturbing antics of childhood.
3. Allow the parents to discuss their feelings about the child's condition. Parents often feel guilty that they misinterpreted the child's symptoms, resulting in delayed treatment.

D. Provide support to the parents of a mentally retarded child.

(See the section on mental retardation, p. 1473)

Health Education

A. Medication

1. Give the medication conscientiously at the same time every day.
2. Adjust the dosage (by the physician) to the needs of each individual child.
    a. Regular medical follow-up and frequent reevaluation are essential.
    b. Dose may have to be increased during puberty and the reproductive period.
3. Observe for signs of drug toxicity, especially rapid pulse, irritability, insomnia, fever, sweating and weight loss. Teach parents how to measure the pulse and to consult the physician if the rate is above a certain value.
4. The medication must be continued throughout life.
5. Allow the parents to administer the medication during the child's hospitalization so that they will gain confidence in their ability to carry out the procedure.
6. Encourage parents to help the child accept increasing responsibility for his medications as he grows older.

Thyrotoxicosis (Grave's Disease)

Thyrotoxicosis is an endocrine disease resulting from an excessive secretion of thyroid hormone. It is frequently characterized by an enlarged thyroid gland (goiter) and prominent eyeballs (exophthalmos).

Etiology

1. Autoimmune process—most common
    a. Probable genetic basis
    b. Occasionally precipitated by stress
2. Tumors
3. Inappropriate secretion of thyroid stimulating hormone (TSH)

Altered Physiology

Same as in the adult.

Clinical Manifestations

1. Rare and less severe in children as compared with adults.
2. More common in females than males.
3. Onset is usually between 10 and 15 years of age (usually gradual onset).
4. Signs and symptoms
    a. Enlarged thyroid gland (goiter)
    b. Exophthalmos
    c. Nervousness and motor hyperactivity
        (1) Inability to sit still
        (2) Decreased attention span
        (3) Mood shifts
            Irritable

            Excitable
            Cries easily
        (4) Tremors
    d. Increased appetite and food intake
    e. Weight loss or no weight gain
    f. Heat intolerance
    g. Skin
        (1) Warm
        (2) Moist
        (3) Flushed
    h. Muscular weakness and fatigue
    i. Tachycardia, palpitation, and dyspnea
    j. Increased systolic blood pressure; increased pulse pressure
    k. Accelerated growth rate
    l. Delayed sexual maturation
    m. Possible amenorrhea in females
    n. Thyroid "crisis" or "storm" (very rare in children)

Diagnostic Evaluation

1. High serum levels of T_4 and T_3
2. Radioactive iodine uptake—rapid
3. Thyroid antibody titers—increased

Treatment

1. Antithyroid drugs (recommended initial treatment)
2. Destruction of thyroid by radioiodine (not advocated until the child has reached maturity)
3. Subtotal thyroidectomy

Prognosis

1. Permanent remission using medical therapy is achieved in 36%–61% of children.
2. Predictors of recurrence
   a. Noncompliance with medical therapy
   b. Long history of illness
   c. Large goiter
   d. Severe toxicity
   e. Strongly positive microsomal titer
3. Recurrences are generally treated surgically

Nursing Interventions

Nursing care of the child with hyperthyroidism is similar to that of the adult (see section on hyperthyroidism). The following objectives are of special importance in pediatrics:

A. Avoid excitement.

1. Provide a quiet environment.
   a. Avoid assigning the child to a large room with several other patients.
   b. Limit the number of playmates that the child has at any one time.
   c. Maintain a fairly constant schedule of daily activities
   d. Sedate the child if necessary.
      (1) Barbiturates or tranquilizers are the drugs of choice.
      (2) Sedation may be especially beneficial at bedtime.
2. Encourage quiet rather than strenuous activities. Interest the child in diversionary activities which do not require lengthy mental concentration.
3. Maintain constant but gentle discipline.

B. Provide a diet high in protein, calories, and vitamins.

1. Offer between-meal snacks such as milk shakes.
2. Vitamin supplements may be necessary.
3. Offer foods that can be easily swallowed if the child is experiencing dysphagia.

C. Administer antithyroid drugs.

1. Propylthiouracil (PTU) is the drug of choice
   a. Dosage
      (1) Must be individually regulated for each child.
      (2) It is essential to space the dose at regular intervals (every 6–8 hours) throughout a 24-hour period.
      Each dose is fully effective for only a few hours.
   b. Observe for
      (1) Clinical response
         (a) It is usually apparent in 2–3 weeks.
         (b) Exophthalmos may not reverse, but it should not advance.
         (c) Record disappearance of symptoms, including decreased enlargement of the thyroid gland.
2. Side effects
   a. Pruritus
   b. Skin rash

c. Arthralgia
d. Nausea and vomiting
3. Severe reaction—agranulocytosis
   a. Sudden onset of fever
   b. Skin rash
   c. Sore throat
4. Signs of overdose
   a. Lethargy
   b. Somnolence
5. Signs of relapse when the drug is discontinued
   a. Usually discontinued after 2–3 years of administration if the child is euthyroid.
   b. Relapse usually occurs within 6 months of discontinuing the drug.

D. Demonstrate understanding of the child's physical and emotional problems.

1. The disease frequently has its onset during adolescence when the child is very concerned with his body image.
2. Encourage the child to talk about his disease and how he feels about it.
   Correct misinformation and misinterpretations as necessary.
3. Assist the adolescent girl to apply make-up which can significantly reduce the obviousness of her exophthalmos.
4. Discuss the child's disease and treatment with his parents and teachers so that their demands and expectations will be realistic.

E. Care for the child who requires thyroidectomy.

(Refer to adult text, p. 679)
1. Indications for surgery in juvenile hyperthyroid patients include:
   a. Toxicity to antithyroid drugs
   b. Failure to cure after an adequate course of medical therapy
   c. Lack of parent or patient compliance
2. Psychological preparation for surgery is essential. The child may associate death with the thought of having his throat cut at the incisional site.

Health Education

A. Medication

1. Allow the parent to administer the child's medication under supervision during his hospitalization to ensure accuracy after discharge.
2. Points of emphasis
   a. The medication must be administered in the exact amount that was prescribed.
   b. Daily administration of the drug at regular intervals is essential.
   c. The child must be observed for signs and symptoms of drug toxicity.

B. Medical Supervision

Close medical follow-up is necessary in order to evaluate the child's progress and regulate his drug dosage.

Bibliography

Books

Bacon G et al. A Practical Approach to Pediatric Endocrinology, 2nd ed. Chicago, Year Book Medical Publishers, 1982

Brook C (ed). Clinical Pediatric Endocrinology. Oxford, Blackwell Scientific Publications, 1981

Collu R, Ducharme J and Guyda H

(eds). Pediatric Endocrinology. New York, Raven Press, 1981

Frasier S. Pediatric Endocrinology. New York, Grune & Stratton, 1980

Guthrie D and Guthrie R (eds). Nursing Management of Diabetes Mellitus, 2nd ed. St Louis, CV Mosby, 1982

Kaplan S (ed). Clinical Pediatric and Adolescent Endocrinology. Philadelphia, WB Saunders, 1982

Laron Z and Galatzer A (eds). Pediatric and Adolescent Endocrinology, Vol. 10, Psychological Aspects of Diabetes in Children and Adolescents. Basel, Switzerland, S Karger, 1982

Laron Z and Galatzer A (eds). Pediatric and Adolescent Endocrinology, Vol. 11, Recent Progress in Medico-Social Problems in Juvenile Diabetes. Basel, Switzerland, S Karger, 1983

Muthe N. Endocrinology, A Nursing Approach. Boston, Little, Brown, & Co, 1981

Traisman H. Management of Juvenile Diabetes Mellitus. St Louis, CV Mosby, 1980

Articles

Arky R. Nutrition therapy for the child and adolescent with type I diabetes mellitus. Pediatr Clin North Am 1984 Jun; 31(3):711–720

Baumer J et al. Impact of home blood glucose monitoring on childhood diabetes. Arch Dis Child 1982 Mar; 58(3):195–199

Brouhard B. Control and monitoring for the child with insulin-dependent diabetes. Am J Dis Child 1983 Aug; 137(8):787–794

Brown A et al. Racial differences in the incidence of congenital hypothyroidism. J Pediatr 1981 Dec; 99(6):934–936

Cerreto M and Travis L. Implications of psychological and family factors in the treatment of diabetes. Pediatr Clin North Am 1984 Jun; 31(3):689–710

Coody D. Congenital hypothyroidism. Pediatr Nurs 1984 Sep/Oct; 10(5): 342–346

Daneman D, Becker D and Drash A. Factors affecting glycosylated hemoglobin values in children with insulin-dependent diabetes. J Pediatr 1981 Dec; 99(6):847–853

Dexter D. The new insulins. Am J Nurs 1981 Jan; 81(1):146–148

Evanier D. When the child has hypothyroidism. Patient Care 1983 Mar 15; 17(5):53–56, 59–61

Faro B. Maintaining good control in children with diabetes. Pediatr Nurs 1983 Sep/Oct; 9(5):368–373

Fendya D and Flynn K. Nursing care for children with hypoglycemia due to hyperinsulinism. MCN 1981 Mar/ Apr; 6(2):100–105

Fort P, Waters S and Lifshitz F. Low-dose insulin infusion in the treatment of diabetic ketoacidosis: Bolus versus no bolus. J Pediatr 1980 Jan; 96(1):36–40

Fow S. Home blood glucose monitoring in children with insulin-dependent diabetes. Pediatr Nurs 1983 Nov/Dec; 439–442

Fredholm N, Vignati L and Brown S. Insulin pumps, the patients' verdict. Am J Nurs 1984 Jan; 84(1):36–38

Fredholm N. The insulin pump: New method of insulin delivery. Am J Nurs 1981 Nov; 81(11):2024–2026

Geffner M, Kaplan S and Lippe B. Home blood glucose monitoring (HBGM) is effective and well-accepted in the management of children with diabetes. Diabetes 1982 May; 31(Suppl):35A

Giordano B et al. Home blood glucose monitoring in children. Diabetes 1982 May; 31(Suppl):80A

Grey M, Genel M and Tamborlane W. Psychosocial adjustment of latency aged diabetics: Determinants and relationship to control. Pediatrics 1980 Jan; 65(1):69–72

Hurwitz LS. Symposium on endocrine disorders. Nursing implications of selected pediatric endocrine problems. Nurs Clin North Am 1980 Sep; 15(3):524–534

Jackson R. Education of the parents of a child with diabetes. Nutr Today 1980 May/Jun; 15(3):30–34

Jackson R. Growth and maturation of children with insulin-dependent diabetes mellitus. Pediatr Clin North Am 1984 Jun; 31(3):545–568

Jackson R. Management and treatment of the child with diabetes. Nutr Today 1980 Mar/Apr; 15(2):6–12, 27–29

Kaye R. Juvenile diabetes. In Shirkey HC (ed). Pediatric Therapy, 6th ed. St Louis, CV Mosby, 1980

Kiser D. The Somogyi effect. Am J Nurs 1980 Feb; 80(2):236–238

Kohler E et al. A developmentally staged curriculum for teaching self-care to the child with insulin-dependent diabetes mellitus. Diabetes Care 1982 May/Jun; 5(3):300–304

Koivisto V and Felig P. Alterations in insulin absorption and in blood glucose control associated with varying insulin injection sites in diabetic patients. Ann Intern Med 1980 Jan; 92(1):59–61

Kosub S and Kosub C. Assessing perceptions of stress in diabetic children. Children's Health Care 1982 Summer; 11(1):4–8

Langdon D, Frederick D and Sperling M. Comparison of single and split-dose insulin regimens with 24-hour monitoring. J Pediatr 1981 Dec; 99(6): 854–861

Lebovitz H. Etiology and pathogenesis of diabetes mellitus. Pediatr Clin North Am 1984 Jun; 31(3):521–530

Lessick M. Genetic counseling of families with endocrine disorders. Issues Compr Pediatr Nurs 1980 Apr; 4(2):27–40

Lillo R and Masteller D. Outpatient management of children in diabetic ketoacidosis. Pediatr Nurs 1982 Nov/Dec; 8(6):383–385

Lobo M. Nursing implications in camps for children with diabetes. In Chinn P and Leonard K (eds). Current Practice in Pediatric Nursing, Vol 3. St Louis, CV Mosby, 1980

Miller B and White N. Diabetes assessment guide. Am J Nurs 1980 Jul; 80(7):1314–1316

New England Congenital Hypothyroidism Collaborative. Characteristics of infantile hypothyroidism discovered on neonatal screening. J Pediatr 1984 Apr; 104(4):539–544

Novogoder M. Neonatal screening for congenital hypothyroidism. Pediatr Clin North Am 1980 Nov; 27(4):881–890

Ory M and Dronenfeld J. Living with juvenile diabetes mellitus. Pediatr Nurs 1980 Sep/Oct; 6(5):47–50

Plasse N. Monitoring blood glucose at home. A comparison of three products. Am J Nurs 1981 Nov; 81(11):2028–2029

Reiter E et al. Childhood thyromegaly: Recent developments. J Pediatr 1981 Oct; 99(4):507–518

Rosenbloom A, Kohrman A and Sperling M. Classification and diagnosis of diabetes in children and adolescents. J Pediatr 1981 Aug; 99(2):320–323

Saucier C. Self concept and self-care management in school-age children with diabetes. Pediatr Nurs 1984 Mar/Apr; 10(2):135–138

Schechter K and Carney R. Increasing compliance to the treatment regimen in insulin dependent diabetic children. Diabetes 1982 May 31(Suppl):110A

Schneider A. Starting insulin therapy in children with newly diagnosed diabetes, an outpatient approach. Am J Dis Child 1983 Aug; 137(8):782–786

Sharkey P and Myer S. Hyperthyroidism. Crit Care Update 1981 May; 8(5):12–24

Sharkey PL et al. Hypothyroidism . . . cretinism. Crit Care Update 1981 Jun; 8(6):5–8+

Slama G et al. Multiple use of disposable insulin syringe–needle units. JAMA 1980 Jul 18; 244(3):266–267

Smith J. Nursing management of diabetes insipidus. J Neurosurg Nurs 1981 Dec; 13(6):313–317

Sperling M. Diabetic ketoacidosis. Pediatr Clin North Am 1984 Jun; 31(3):591–610

Stevens A. Monitoring blood glucose at home. Who should do it? Am J Nurs 1981 Nov; 81(11):2026–2027

Tamborlane W. Insulin infusion pump treatment of type I diabetes. Pediatr Clin North Am 1984 Jun; 31(3):721–734

Tamborlane W et al. Outpatient treatment of juvenile onset diabetes with a pre-programmed portable subcutaneous insulin infusion system. Am J Med 1980 Feb; 68(2):190–196

Wong D. The significance of dead space in syringes. Am J Nurs 1982 Aug; 82(8):1237

Children with Eye and Ear Conditions

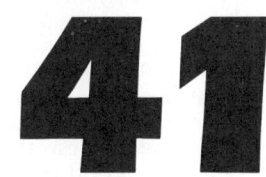

1: Conditions of the Eye

The Blind Child

Impaired vision (blindness) refers to insufficient or inadequate vision in varying degrees.

Etiology
1. Familial factors
      Genetic determination
2. Prenatal or intrauterine factors
      a. Rubella
      b. Toxoplasmosis
      c. Syphilis
3. Perinatal factors
      a. Prematurity
      b. Oxygen toxicity—retrolental fibroplasia
      c. Infections
4. Postnatal factors
      a. Injury or trauma
      b. Infections
      c. Inflammatory disease

Altered Physiology
1. Defective visual fields
2. Impaired color vision
3. Decreased visual acuity
4. No vision—or a small percentage of vision (may have light perception)

Complications
Developmental delays in motor, communication, ego, and behavior

Assessment
Clinical Manifestations

A. Infant
1. No eye-to-eye contact, especially with the mother
2. Abnormal eye movements
3. Does not follow objects at 2 months of age
4. Failure to locate distant objects at 6–12 months of age
5. Mother senses "something is wrong"

B. Older Child
1. Squinting, frequent blinking
2. Bumping into things
3. Frequent rubbing of eyes

Diagnostic Evaluation
1. Legal definition—visual acuity 20/200 or less with correction
2. Tunnel vision—peripheral field of vision has an angular distance not greater than 20 degrees

Treatment
1. Surgical repair of defect
2. Glasses
3. Special training
      a. Language development and acquisition
      b. Mobility–perceptual motor training
      c. Early stimulation therapy

Patient Problems/Nursing Diagnoses
1. Anxiety and feelings of isolation related to stranger anxiety; fear of unknown
2. Sensory deprivation related to inability to see items in surroundings
3. Alteration in parent–child relationship related to lack of eye contact and inadequate communication
4. Potential for injury related to falls and tendency to bump into things
5. Self-care deficit related to limitations imposed by visual impairment
6. Developmental delays related to altered visual stimulation and possible overprotective behavior of parents

Planning and Implementation
Nursing Intervention
The nurse may become involved with the blind child in the hospital in 3 critical situations: (1) before diagnosis has been made when she may detect a visual loss, usually in an infant, (2) at time of diagnosis, and (3) after diagnosis has been made and she is giving nursing care to the hospitalized child who is blind.

Detection; Early Care of the Blind Child After Diagnosis
A. Be familiar with the normal pattern of visual development and recognize deviations as well as manifestations of visual impairment.
1. Knowing the stages of growth and development can be helpful in recognizing or suspecting visual impairment in the individual child.

2. The appreciation of vision by the infant begins at about 3 months of age.
3. Be alert to and assess the child's response to visual stimulation.
   a. Does the infant follow the human face or bright object with his eyes according to his stage of development?
   b. Does the infant reach for objects?
   c. Does the 9- to 12-month-old child move around?

B. Be familiar with the causes of visual impairment and blindness in order to recognize from the history whether or not the child is in a high-risk category.

1. Neonatal and perinatal factors
   a. Prematurity
   b. Oxygen therapy
   c. Infections
2. Past infections—inflammatory disease
3. Trauma

C. Record observations and report any suspicious behavior by the infant or child indicating visual impairment.

1. Early diagnosis is the key to successful habilitation and optimal development of the child's capabilities.
2. The complication of complete withdrawal of the child can be avoided by early diagnosis and proper stimulation and emotional support.

D. Help the family of a newly diagnosed visually impaired child.

1. Parents must be allowed time to understand and accept what has happened.
2. They will experience guilt, anger, and depression. How they accept the child will depend on how they feel about having a handicapped child.
3. Their life-style will have to change; they will need to find new ways to adjust socially and personally.

E. Work with physician and parents in helping the child master certain developmental tasks, thus aiding the child in achieving his fullest potential.

Parents need help in recognizing the clues the child presents indicating his need and readiness for new learning experiences. The child must also learn in his own natural way.

1. Continued communication must be fostered between parents, mother, and child.
   a. The mother must learn techniques of touching, handling, and talking to her child.
   b. Mother should make a special effort to help her baby associate her voice and body with receiving pleasure.
   c. Encourage touching by both mother and baby during feeding times, as well as other times. Touch is a good nonverbal form of communication.
2. *The child and parents must be helped to develop a discriminating relationship;* specific consistent clues of handling the child can be built into behavior.
   a. Each parent shares some special, individualized activity with the child.
   b. Voice and touch bring parents and child together.
3. The child must be allowed and encouraged to use his hands for exploring his world. Child must also learn appropriate use of hands.
   a. Give the child objects of different shapes, sizes,

and textures. Use toys that make noise and that are within reach and stay there.
   b. Give finger food to child during meals—when the child is about 8 months of age or when he sits up.
   c. Extra tactile opportunities provided for child will compensate to some extent for loss of visual input.
4. The child needs to learn to become mobile.
   a. The mother's voice can encourage child to move toward her.
   b. A favorite toy placed in front of child can encourage him to move toward it.
5. The child needs much help in learning to talk.
   a. Expose the child to sounds that have a specific function—cleaning equipment, dishes.
   b. Mother should talk a great deal to the child. The child cannot benefit from gestures and facial expression used in language.
6. The child needs social exposure to his peers. Nursery school can be very helpful.

F. Foster continuous acceptance of the child by his parents and provide support for them.

1. Evaluate the parents' emotional status and offer them reassurance and explanations.
   a. Parental acceptance and a healthy home atmosphere are vitally important in helping the visually impaired or blind child to accept and adjust to his limitations.
   b. The child can sense his parents' approval or disapproval and the degree to which they love and accept him.
2. Help the parents to understand and accept their responsibilities in the care of their child. Parents who have received appropriate information and guidance in handling their child can enrich the time spent with the child and prevent further handicapping and management problems. Indicate that they should do the following:
   a. Provide proper stimulation for the child to learn that which is ordinarily learned through vision. Frustration often occurs when the child gives little feedback. Efforts may decrease as a consequence.
   b. The voice is often used to protect the child.
   c. Reinforce that this child has the same needs for growth and development as any child.
3. Help parents understand how they can develop the child's skills in interpreting information through the senses of hearing, touch, smell, and taste. They can learn to understand their blind child.
   a. Hearing
      (1) Help the child to determine distance by ringing a bell.
      (2) Familiarize him with appliances, birds, voices.
      (3) Use voice—tone, expression, etc. because nonverbal cues go unnoticed.
      (4) A tape recorder can be helpful in teaching the child to recognize different sounds.
   b. Touch
      Allow the child to handle different textured materials.
   c. Smell
      Acquaint the child with flowers, perfume, kitchen odors.

d. Taste
Help the child distinguish different kitchen substances.
e. Memory
Have the child practice retelling stories, his telephone number, address, etc.
4. Initiate referral to the community nurse who can make home visits to reinforce and interpret what the mother has heard from the physician and to encourage the mother in her efforts.
5. Encourage the parents to discuss their feelings about caring for a handicapped child at home.
Initiate a social worker referral. (The social worker can help parents deal with their feelings.)
6. Help the parents understand the problems the child faces and will face as he gets older.
a. The child with probably be delayed in development. There can be a delay of up to 5 months in creeping and 7 months in walking, even though posture and balance for such activities are similar to those of sighted child.
b. The child is likely to develop ''blindisms''— habits or mannerisms of blind children; these are a manifestation of inadequate impulse control. The child may also show self-stimulatory behavior.
c. Vision is the primary elicitor of the smile, thus, the infant will be late in development of the social smile. Subtle expressions used in communication will be missed by the infant, and skills will not be developed by imitation.

G. Be familiar with the community resources and the professional team to be involved in habilitation of the visually impaired child.

Several types of school programs are available to the child, depending on his confidence and coping abilities.
1. Residential schools.
a. Used when nothing is available in the local community.
b. Preferred when the home care of the child would be detrimental to his progress.
2. Day schools for the blind. (The child attends school during day but lives at home.)
3. Public school where the blind child is integrated with sighted child. (The child receives special training in braille.)
4. Vocational habilitation programs (training for some occupation).
5. Public law 94-142 provides for public education of all handicapped children.

H. Evaluate how well the child who was once able to see accepts visual impairment—in terms of his physical abilities and psychologic dependence. (Vision helps to maintain contact with reality.)

1. A serious impairment in relationships with people can result when the child is unable to express his innermost sentiments.
2. Allow the child to express his feelings, especially those of fear and anger. Talk, play, and certain activities help the child express these feelings.

Hospital Care of the Visually Impaired or Blind Child

Many of the important areas discussed above must be considered when caring for the child in the hospital situation. In addition, emphasis must be placed on the following goals:

A. Interview the parents at the time of admission to learn as much as possible about the child and his care and activities at home.

1. Be aware of the child's schedule and activities during the day. Know what activities he can or cannot do, and what he likes to do.
2. Become familiar with how he is oriented to his new surroundings.
a. How much does he ambulate?
b. What precautions are necessary?
3. Be aware of how the parents comfort and discipline the child.
How does he comfort himself or seek security?
4. What special care or treatment must be continued while the child is hospitalized?
5. Share this information with nursing staff in a nursing care plan so that continuity of care from home to hospital can minimize fear and frustration in the child.

B. Attend to the child's needs according to the medical problem that required his hospitalization.

C. Plan and provide for the appropriate type of play, activities program, and stimulation for the child.

1. Assess the child's level of growth and development and use the information obtained from parents.
2. Allow the child as much independence as possible in his care, but provide guidance as necessary.
Orient the ambulatory child thoroughly to his room and surroundings.
3. Encourage the development of the child's abilities. Avoid overprotecting him.
4. Provide activities that will increase his learning and give him pleasure (e.g., talking records).
5. Provide emotional preparation for procedures and surgery, as appropriate.

D. Meet the psychological and emotional needs of the visually impaired or blind child for protection and security against harm.

1. The nurse should always speak to the child prior to touching him so as not to frighten or startle him.
2. Always use a warm and gentle touch.
3. Explain strange sounds that may be frightening.
Tape recording of sounds he may hear help put them into proper perspective.
4. Plan frequent nurse–patient interactions to increase the child's sense of security.
5. Place items he needs and uses within his reach.
a. Familiar items that give the child security should also be close to him.
b. Tell him if they are moved.
6. During any procedure, talk to the child the entire time. Explain what is going on around him.

E. Avoid overemphasizing the child's handicap and be unobtrusive about meeting his needs.

Allow the child to explore and learn about his new environment and the hospital.

Health Education

A. Provide continual parental support.

1. Encourage the parents to become involved in the care of their child to help maintain or develop a healthy parent–child relationship.

Separation from the parents can be extremely traumatic and has severe implications for the blind child.
2. Encourage the parents to talk about their fears and feelings concerning this child. Help them relax.
The parents can be invaluable in increasing the security and decreasing the fear the child may have as a result of being in a strange place.
3. Discuss realistically long-term and short-term planning for the child (i.e., educational opportunities).
    a. Encourage the parents to tell teachers and adults responsible for his care about his special needs.
    b. Avoid overemphasis on educational achievements.
4. Help the parents understand that discipline, order and consistency are necessary in the child's environment to give him security.
5. Emphasize that the parents' role is to give this child love and physical care as well as to stimulate and influence him so he may have satisfactory mental, social, and emotional growth.
6. Help the parents see that other members of the family must also be considered.
    a. Their handicapped child does need special attention, but he does not need all the attention all the time.
    b. Other members of the family should be included in his care, but they also have a life of their own and need as much attention from parents as they would have if the handicapped child were not present in the family.

c. Parents need time to themselves. They should be encouraged to go out alone together and to give time to their marriage.
7. Help the parents realize that even though habilitation of their blind child is long, drawn out, and expensive, the child may be able to live a normal life in the community.
    a. Are the parents aware of and do they accept the short- and long-term goals?
    b. Many blind people are successful as technicians and professionals.

Evaluation
Expected Outcomes

1. Demonstrates lessening of anxiety; interacts with others in environment
2. Shows awareness of sensory stimulation; has access to auditory stimulation (records; radio; verbal communication); tactile stimulation, etc.
3. The parents demonstrate appropriate parenting behaviors; talking with child, touching, encouraging independence, establishing normal discipline, and order; exploring educational opportunities
4. Avoids injury through use of protective measures; accepts normal limits on behavior; adheres to social rules
5. Attempts to fulfill developmental tasks through age-related activities (within limits of visual impairment; tries to do things for himself)

Eye Defects Requiring Surgery

Eye defects requiring surgery are (1) structural manifestations of the eye present at birth or (2) acquired conditions of the eye. They can be extraocular or intraocular conditions.

Etiology

1. Congenital
    a. Hereditary tendencies
    b. Birth injury
    c. Innervational factors
    d. Intrauterine influences
2. Disease
    a. Metabolic
    b. Infection
3. Trauma to the eye

Strabismus

Strabismus is the inability to balance the extraocular muscles; thus the eyes cannot function together at the same time.

Altered Physiology

1. The visual axis of only 1 eye goes to the object being observed. The person appears to be looking in 2 directions at once.
2. Specific deviations
    a. Paralytic strabismus—muscles of 1 eye are underactive.
    b. Concomitant strabismus—both eyes move, but the deviation between the eyes is always the same.

c. Hypertropia—eye deviation is upward.
d. Hypotropia—eye deviation is downward.
e. Vertical—vertical separation of visual axes.
f. Esotropia—1 eye deviates toward other eye; convergent—"cross-eye."
g. Exotropia—1 eye deviates away from the other eye; divergent—"wall-eye."

Complications

1. Amblyopia—poor vision in eye not used.
2. Emotional problems resulting from cosmetic aspect of deformity.
3. Repeated surgery may be necessary.

Clinical Manifestations

1. Deviations of the eye (constant or intermittent)
2. Squinting
3. Closing one eye to see
4. Tilting head
5. Stumbling or clumsy behavior
6. Inaccuracy in picking up objects
7. Double vision

Treatment

1. Corrective glasses (lenses)
2. Patching nondiverging eye
3. Surgery
    a. Lengthening or shortening of extraocular structures
See page 1391 for nursing management.

Cataract

Cataract is an opacification or milk-white appearance of the eye lens.

Altered Physiology

Inability of light to pass through the clouded lens in adequate amounts—loss of vision as lens becomes more opaque; loss of transparency.

Clinical Manifestations

1. Gradual diminution of visual acuity
2. Strabismus
3. Nystagmus
4. Gray opacities of lens

Diagnostic Evaluation

Ophthalmoscopic examination reveals opacification of the lens.

Treatment

1. Medication—dilation of pupil with mydriatic eye drops
2. Surgery
   a. Optical iridectomy
   b. Lens fragmentation, irrigation, and aspiration, or cutting and aspiration
   c. Intraocular lens implantation

Complications

A. Untreated Cataract

1. Bilateral cataract
   a. Nystagmus
   b. Stimulus-deprivation amblyopia
2. Unilateral cataract
   a. Strabismus
   b. Stimulus-deprivation amblyopia

B. Following Surgery for Congenital Cataract

1. Retinal detachment several years later
2. Average vision only 20/70
3. Need for glasses or contact lenses to replace refracting power of lens
   See below for nursing management.

Trauma

Trauma is injury to the globe, adnexa, and surrounding tissue of the eye as a result of blunt objects (baseball, rock) striking the eye area, or sharp items (scissors, knife) penetrating the eye area.

Altered Physiology

A. Blunt Injury

1. Subconjunctival hemorrhage and suffusion of blood into eyelid
2. Secondary hemorrhage occurring days after injury
   a. Accumulation of blood in anterior chamber and blocking of overflow channels
   b. Rapid rise of intraocular pressure (glaucoma)
3. Retinal edema, hemorrhages, and detachment

B. Penetrating Injury

1. Loss of aqueous fluid, development of cataract
2. Bleeding into anterior chamber and vitreous
3. Retinal detachment

C. Corneal Abrasions (i.e., from fingernail)

1. Common in young children
2. Treated for 24 hours with patching and antibiotic ointment

Complications

Sympathetic ophthalmia—inflammation of the uninjured eye probably due to an allergic reaction to pigment released from injured eye. This condition can lead to significant visual loss.

Nursing Management of the Child Undergoing Eye Surgery

Nursing Interventions

Preoperative Care

A. Help the child and his parents know and understand what the surgery entails.
(Explanations should be appropriate for the age of the child.)

1. Take a trip to the operating and recovery rooms if the child is not on bed rest due to trauma.
2. Practice applying eye patches for short frequent periods.
   a. Allow the child to handle the equipment.
   b. Explain that the patches will only be temporary.
3. Help the child become familiar with the protective devices if they are to be used postoperatively.
4. Discuss and practice postoperative exercises if feasible.
5. Relieve the child's fears by telling him that there will be a little pain—as if something is in the eye.

B. Assess the child and his needs according to age and specifically to his eye problem.

1. Can the child read or watch television?
2. Does the child wear glasses? When? Help him to learn to protect his glasses when not in use.

C. Provide as much comfort and reassurance to the child as possible to diminish his fears especially concerning hospitalization and impending surgery.

1. Room assignment can be significant.
   a. A quiet room with subdued lighting can be more comfortable for trauma patients.
   b. Placement in a room with other children (without infection) may be comforting for elective surgery patients.
2. Allow the child to have familiar tactile and auditory stimulating objects around him.

Postoperative Care

A. Administer effective postoperative care and observe for possible postoperative complications (see p. 1126).

Be alert to the care and considerations for specific eye defect.
1. Strabismus
   a. Frequently the child is discharged on the day of surgery, following recovery from anesthesia.
   b. Surgery is extraocular; no postoperative ocular rupture hazards exist.
   c. Activity is not restricted.
   d. Eye bandages may or may not be used.
   e. Eyes will probably be blood-tinged and will

drain. Eyes may feel uncomfortable. Black eye is normal, as is postoperative swelling.
  f. Eyes may be difficult to open the morning after surgery. Gently separate lids from above and below. Do not force lids open. Tears will soften secretions.
  g. Child may have photosensitivity.
2. Cataract or intraocular surgery
  a. The child is generally positioned on his back; thus, prevention of aspiration is a concern.
  b. Avoid sudden head movement, crying, and vomiting, because these increase intraocular pressure; they cause strain on sutures and subsequent bleeding.
  c. Avoid surprising the patient and making him jump. Avoid loud noises. Speak gently before touching the child.

B. Prevent the child from pulling off the dressing and causing injury or contamination.

1. Sedation may be warranted until the child becomes accustomed to having his eye continually bandaged.
2. Protective devices may be used only if necessary. Rest is necessary during the immediate postoperative period, and a child struggling because of restraints can defeat their intended purpose.
3. Diet should be increased slowly to prevent vomiting; this could cause possible injury to the eye because of increased pressure.

C. Provide emotional and psychological reassurance and support to the child who is anxious because his eyes are bandaged preventing him from seeing.

1. Encourage the parents to be with their child, especially when he is waking up from anesthesia. Someone should be with the child if the parents are unable to be present.
  a. Sit with child, stroke him, and speak gently and softly to him.
  b. Let him hold a familiar object.
  c. Hold him if there are no contraindications to his being lifted and held.
2. Always speak to child before touching him so as not to startle him.
   Explain what is going to be done to him before doing it.
3. Tell the child what foods are on his tray.
   Allow him to finger feed himself.
4. Explain sounds. (Sounds in the world without sight can be very frightening.)
5. Reassure the child that patches will be removed soon, and he will be able to see again (if he is going to see).
6. Provide appropriate diversional activities for the child.
  a. Read him stories
  b. Provide radio or phonograph
  c. Talk with him

D. Administer appropriate eye medications and change dressing as prescribed.

1. First dressing change is usually done by the physician.
  a. Strabismus—dressing removed day after surgery.
  b. Cataract—dressing may be used for 5–10 days after surgery.
2. Be familiar with types of eye medications used.
  a. Mydriatic—used to dilate pupil.
  b. Miotic—constricts pupil and decreases increased intraocular pressure in early glaucoma.
  c. Anti-inflammatory drugs
  d. Antibiotics
3. Be familiar with the principles of instilling eye medications (drops, ointments, and irrigations).
  a. Have the room darkened—light may be uncomfortable.
  b. Try to gain the confidence and cooperation of the child and reassure him by talking to him during the procedure.
  c. Assistance may be necessary to stabilize the child's head and prevent injury. Have the child close his eye; drop medication onto the inner canthus; open the eye and the drop will roll in.
  d. Irrigate from the inner canthus outward.
  e. To instill drops, pull the lower lid down and drop the medication onto the conjunctiva from a dropper parallel to the lid. If drops are instilled on the conjunctiva and not on the cornea, the patient tolerates the medication better.
  f. Do not force the lid open.
  g. Blot away excess fluid with a paper tissue or cotton ball; do not rub the eye.
  h. Avoid contaminating the dressing.
  i. Always wash hands before and after contact with the eye for any procedure.

E. Involve the parents and child in preparation for discharge.

1. Teach the parents how to instill eye medications (see above).
2. Postoperative patches or glasses may be necessary. Help the parents and child understand the value and importance of the patching or glasses.
3. Encourage the parents to contact the school nurse and other adults responsible for child's care to explain special exercises or specific care for the child.
4. Encourage follow-up as advised by the physician.

Health Education

1. Help the parents understand what was wrong with the child, what was done to help correct the problem and what the parental responsibilities are in continuing any recommended therapy with the child.
   Be certain the parents understand what special care is to be given and how it is to be accomplished.
2. Prevention is the best treatment for eye injury; eye-protective devices should be used during sports. Street glasses are not a protection in contact sports; and special protectors (with built-in prescription) are advised.

2: Conditions of the Ear

The Child with Impaired Hearing

Impaired hearing occurs when there is a hearing loss in speech frequencies of over 20 decibels, and the child does not learn to talk in the normal way. Speech essentially may have no meaning.

Etiology

1. Unknown
2. Familial factors—genetically transmitted; family history of hearing impairment*
3. Prenatal or intrauterine factors
   a. Rubella*
   b. Preeclampsia or eclampsia
   c. Drugs
   d. Congenital syphilis
4. Perinatal factors
   a. Prematurity*—especially <1,500 gm.
   b. Anoxia at birth—asphyxia with acidosis
   c. Hyperbilirubinemia*
   d. Erythroblastosis fetalis
   e. Neonatal sepsis,* meningitis
5. Postnatal factors
   a. Ototoxic drugs
   b. Acquired disorders of the central nervous system
   c. Acute infections, otitis media
   d. Injury
   e. Structural defects*
6. Chromosomal anomalies
   a. Trisomy 13-14-15
   b. Trisomy 18

Altered Physiology

A. Conductive Hearing Loss

1. Impairment in the mechanism of conducting sound waves to the cochlea; sound not transmitted well, distorted
   a. Blockage of sound waves from outer ear, external canal, or middle ear (lack of loudness)
   b. Tympanic membrane damage and scarring
   c. Dislocation or disturbance of tiny ossicular bones in the middle ear
2. Often recognized in the school-age child

B. Sensorineural Hearing Loss

1. Malfunction of inner ear apparatus or 8th cranial nerve—medically irreversible
   a. Lack of loudness
   b. Distorted sounds because of defect of cochlea or neural pathways to temporal lobe of the brain
   c. Problems with discrimination of sound

C. Mixed Hearing Loss

Both sensorineural and conductive hearing loss in some children

D. Central Hearing Loss

1. Middle ear transformer mechanics; the cochlea and nerves are probably functioning normally.
2. There is abnormal or inability to process auditory signals within the brain.

Complications

1. In childhood when there is a hearing disorder, there is a delay of speech and language development; thus, there is a loss of contact between the individual, his peers, and his environment.
2. Biological, behavioral, and social complications may result when there is a breakdown of the normal communicative process.
3. The seriousness of the total problem depends on the nature and extent of auditory involvement and on the age of onset and length of time before the hearing problem is detected.

* Criteria for high risk of impaired hearing.

Clinical Manifestations

A. Infant

1. Little or no interest in sounds of his environment
   a. Does not blink at loud noise
   b. Does not turn eyes toward sound of musical toy or mother's voice at 3 months of age
   c. Does not turn toward whispered voice within 1 meter (3 feet) at 8–12 months of age
   d. Hyperactivity or gesturing may increase
2. Lack of or minimal vocalization
   a. Does not coo or gurgle
   b. May not smile
   c. Babbling decreases after 6–8 months of age
3. Lack of neonatal startle reflex to noise 1–2 meters (3–6 feet) away

B. Toddlers

1. Little or no vocalization
   a. Sounds produced poorly
   b. Will not repeat a word with single stimulus
   c. Uses gestures to express needs
2. Little interest in environmental sounds—does not respond to name, doorbell, or telephone

C. Preschool and School-age Child

1. Behavioral disturbances
   a. Intense, contant activity
   b. Temper tantrums
   c. Inattentiveness
   d. Slow learner
2. May show abrupt change in social or communicative behavior.

D. Sensorineural vs. Conductive Hearing Loss

1. Sensorineural
   a. The child may talk more loudly than necessary.
   b. The child may not respond to average loudness but responds to loud sounds.
   c. When intensity of sound is increased above the threshold of sensitivity, the child shows some type of response.
2. Conductive
   a. The child has a tendency to talk in a relatively soft voice.
   b. The child hears better in a noisy environment.
   c. The child can hear loud speech and sounds.

Diagnostic Evaluation

1. Otolaryngologic examination (inspection of external ear and tympanic membrane)—to rule out involvement of conductive apparatus
2. Audiologic examination—to establish the extent of hearing loss and to determine type of hearing aid needed
   a. Observation of the child's response to sounds calibrated for intensity and frequency
   b. Objective measuring techniques of hearing loss, (i.e., cortical audiometry)
3. Hearing loss classification (see also Table 17-2, p. 743)
   Pure tone audiometry hearing threshold level:
   > 0–20 db—Normal hearing
   > 21–40 db—Mild hearing impairment
   > 41–55 db—Moderate hearing loss
   > 56–70 db—Moderately severe hearing loss
   > 71–90 db—Severe hearing loss
   > 91+ db—Profound hearing loss
4. Limited high-risk register (to identify infants at high risk for hearing loss)

a. Family history of child with hearing impairment
b. Rubella or other nonbacterial infection
c. Defects of ear, nose or throat, low set or absent pinnae, cleft lip/palate
d. Birth weight less than 1,500 gm.
e. Hyperbilirubinemia (greater than 20 mg./100 ml.)

Treatment

1. Conductive hearing loss
   a. Surgical correction of defect
   b. Hearing aid
2. Sensorineural hearing loss
   a. Hearing aid
   b. Special training
      (1) Language acquisition
      (2) Auditory training
      (3) Speech therapy
      (4) Perceptual motor training

Potential Problems/Nursing Diagnoses

1. Impaired communication related to inability to hear or express self through understandable speech pattern
2. Social isolation related to inability to interact verbally
3. Delayed developmental growth related to lack of auditory stimulation
4. Potential for injury related to failure to detect warning sounds
5. Alteration in parent–child relationships related to inappropriate communication
6. Anxiety and coping difficulties related to reduced social interaction
7. Parental anxiety related to having a child with impaired hearing

Nursing Interventions

The nurse may become involved with the child with impaired hearing in the hospital in 3 situations: (1) before diagnosis has been made when she may detect a hearing loss, (2) at the time of diagnosis, and (3) after diagnosis has been made when giving nursing care to the hospitalized child.

Detection; Early Care After Diagnosis

A. Be familiar with the normal pattern of language and learning development and the manifestations of hearing loss in the infant and child.

1. Knowing the stages of growth and development can be helpful in recognizing and suspecting hearing impairment in the individual child.
2. Be alert to and assess the child's response to auditory stimulation.
   a. Does the infant stop activity and listen to vocal sounds?
   b. Does the child respond to his name?
   c. Does the child have unusual visual alertness at age 1 year?
3. The critical period of learning or language development is from birth to 16 months.

B. Be familiar with the causes of hearing impairment and recognize from the history if the child may be in a high-risk category.

1. Ensure that follow-up hearing evaluation is planned.
2. Criteria for high risk of impaired hearing (see limited high-risk register, p. 1393)

C. Record observations and report to physician any suspicious behavior by the infant or child that indicates possible hearing loss.

1. Early diagnosis is the key to successful habilitation and optimal development of the capabilities of the child. Early intervention is aimed toward the child's acquisition of heard and spoken language.
   a. After 16 months of age, habilitation is more difficult.
   b. If hearing loss occurs after the time of critical language development, rehabilitation is less difficult, as the groundwork for verbal communication has been established.
2. The impulse for learning spontaneous speech and acquiring most of the basic verbal skills as well as the structure on which mature use of language and speech is built is reached during the first 3–4 years of life.
3. A current screening device is the Crib-O-Gram*—an automated method of recording responses of the infant's motor activity before and after test sound.

D. Be familiar with community resources and the professional team involved in habilitation.

1. Each child must be treated as an individual.
2. Knowing general philosophies and training techniques of the involved resource can be helpful. Help the child to capitalize on assets and minimize limitations.

E. Be familiar with the guidelines and techniques of educating a child with impaired hearing.

1. The main mode of communication for the child with impaired hearing is visual, supplemented by auditory clues.
   a. Educational task is to develop the child's understanding and expression of language.
   b. Speech can be learned through a multisensory approach, using visual, tactile, kinesthetic, and auditory stimulation.
2. The child with a less severe hearing loss uses auditory stimulation, supplemented by visual clues, as his main mode of communication. The educational task is to develop adequate speech and language and the best use of residual hearing.
3. The 3 basic methods currently used in educating deaf children include:
   a. *Oral Approach*—emphasizes verbal communication, speech reading, and auditory training. Most useful when child has some hearing.
   b. *Manual Communication*—sign language.
   c. *Total Communication Approach*—combines sign language with auditory training and speech reading. Language modes—child-devised gestures, sign, speech, speech reading, finger spelling, reading, and writing.
4. Cued speech, which visually pinpoints a single sound being spoken by using a manual supplement to lip reading of hand shapes used near the mouth to make language sounds look different on the lips or hand. The tool is made up of 12 hand shapes and positions.
5. Whatever method of education and communication is used, it is *critical for parents* to enter the educational process so that they can establish communication with their child.

* Telesensory System, Inc., Palo Alto, CA

F. **Be familiar with hearing devices that are available and may be used by the child.**

1. Hearing aids
   a. In the ear
   b. Behind the ear
   c. On the body or in the pocket
   d. Eyeglass model
2. Technical aids—telecommunication device for the hearing impaired

G. **Help the family cope with and accept a newly diagnosed hearing impairment in their child.**

1. Encourage the physician to have both parents present when he tells them the diagnosis. This allows the parents to support each other.
2. Do not focus all your attention on the child. Show your concern for and interest in the parents.
3. Be aware that parents must be given time to adjust to this usually drastic and unexpected change in their lives before they can deal constructively with meeting the needs of the child.
4. At this time, parents need general information—good literature that is specific to their child's problem. Contact with other parents who have made successful adjustments to living with their hearing-impaired children can be helpful to parents. Acquaint them with organizations dealing with deafness (see below).

H. **Be aware of the problems facing the parents (and family) of a hearing-impaired child.**

Offer them specific guidance in handling and caring for the child.

1. Problems encountered
   a. Lack of knowledge of principles of parenting methods that govern the child's development.
   b. Unaware of cues from their child that are familiar to most parents.
   c. Limited feedback from their child in speech (vocalization), emotional response, or achievement—all of which increase spontaneous parenting. Communication limitations tend to restrict early parent–child relationships.
      Child is not equipped to show his attachment to his parents.
   d. The parent must be in close contact with the child to control and regulate his behavior.
   e. The child is lacking in impulse control and is unable to understand and order his world.
   f. The parents may show embarrassment because of their child's behavior.
   g. There is a possible tendency to neglect or deny common childhood conflicts and/or problems.
   h. Frustration—they do not know how to help their child.
2. Specific guidance to offer parents:
   a. Allow and encourage the parents to communicate with the child through mime, gestures, and body language. There is an increased need for stimulation and physical contact.
   b. Optimize the auditory environment.
   c. Teach the parents how to talk to their child—to use verbal and nonverbal reinforcement of behavior.
   d. Help the baby develop "watching behavior" by rewarding him with pleasure and praise.
   e. Encourage the parents to look directly into the child's eyes when they talk to him and to use appropriate facial expressions.
   f. Help them to understand that their child is probably unable to express his anxieties; frustration leads to anger and sudden rage or temper tantrums. Help them to gain confidence in their own resourcefulness and care by anticipating the child's random behavior through their knowledge of its coincidence with certain situations.
   g. Teach them the stages of language development.

Care of the Hospitalized Child with a Hearing Loss

A. **Interview the parents at the time of admission to learn as much as possible about the child and his activities at home.**

1. What is the child's way of communicating his needs? How do the parents communicate with the child?
2. Be aware of the child's schedule and activities at home.
   Know what activities he can or cannot do and what he likes to do.
3. Be aware of how the parents discipline the child and how they comfort him.
4. Does the child wear a hearing aid? When? Any special exercises or training that needs to be continued?
5. Share this information with nursing staff in the nursing care plan to ensure continuity of care from home to hospital and to minimize fear and frustration in the child.

B. **Attend to the child's needs according to the medical or surgical problem that required his hospitalization.**
   Properly prepare the child for procedures, etc., using increased sense of touch and visual sense.

C. **Plan and provide for the appropriate type of play program and stimulation for the child.**

1. Assess the child's level of development and growth and use information provided by parents.
2. Allow the child as much independence as possible in his care, but provide guidance as necessary—prevent boredom.
3. Encourage the development of the child's abilities.

D. **Meet the emotional needs of the child with impaired hearing for closeness and belonging.**

1. Place the child in a room with a friendly, outgoing child.
2. Plan frequent nurse–patient interactions.
   a. Gentle touch
   b. Games or activities he enjoys
3. Encourage the parents, especially the mother, to take an active part in his care, thus decreasing fear of desertion.
4. Be aware of coping behaviors seen in the child, including visual information gathering, avoidance, and comfort-seeking measures.
5. Adolescents may need special consideration since at this developmental stage they normally may be experiencing a time of confusion.

Health Education

A. **Foster continuous parental acceptance of the child and provide support for the family.**

1. Invite the parents to become involved in the care of their hospitalized child as much as possible.
2. Help the parents to understand the problems the child faces and will face as he gets older.

a. Although hearing impairment does alter life experiences for the child, it does not limit intelligence or capacity for emotional response and normal growth and development.

b. The child may not be able to participate in activities in which sounds and verbal commands are used.

c. Often the referral agency will become very involved in supporting the family.

3. Help the parents become aware of their importance in the success of the habilitation of the child.

a. Parents have the most important educational influence on their child.

b. Opportunities to use effective ways of stimulating the child's awareness and understanding of speech occur daily in the home.

c. The child needs the warmth and security of a family setting.

4. Help the parents to understand what can be accomplished in their child's education to enable him to be a contributing member of society.

5. Stress the importance of close follow-up by the specialists caring for the child.

6. Help the parents to understand the use and importance of the hearing aid their child is using.

a. Most children with a hearing loss have enough residual hearing to respond to and/or recognize sounds with use of an aid.

b. Use of the aid does not approximate normal hearing; the child receives sound differently.

c. Parents must be convinced of the value of the aid but not pay too much attention to it.

d. Young child does not have much difficulty in adjusting to the hearing aid if the ear mold is comfortable and the sound amplification is not too unpleasant. Place the aid on the child and have him wear it during waking hours.

e. For the older child who has become used to the aid as a youngster, it is part of his body image and he is dependent on the sound.

f. Parents should be sensitive to their child's reactions to the aid.

g. Follow-up care is vital; a malfunctioning aid can cause the child to lose interest in its use.

7. Help shape healthy parental attitudes about their child and guide them through this difficult time.

a. Prevent denial.

b. Parents need sympathetic understanding during the time of diagnosis and immediately following when they are bewildered and grieving.

c. Parental attitudes may be the primary factor in determining the success or failure of the child's progress.

8. Help the parents to maintain continued awareness of normal growth and development of their child and the normal stresses and needs during each stage.

9. Encourage the parents to write for literature from appropriate agencies.*

B. Offer continuing parental support.

1. Help the parents to think of their child as a child first, then as a child with special needs.

2. Emphasize their importance in the habilitation of their child. Point out the value of the home environment in his development.

a. Talk about the daily routines.

b. Talk about mother's role in stimulating the child's interest in sounds and speech.

c. Encourage the use of hearing aids and the learning program set up by specialists in hearing problems in children, as appropriate.

d. Expose the child to other children his own age who have hearing impairment.

e. An adult who is deaf (if parents are not) may also help the child.

f. With the passage of Public Law 94-142, public education is provided for all handicapped children.

g. Residential placement may be considered when local facilities are nonexistent or when the home environment would be detrimental to the child's progress.

3. Encourage the parents to talk about their fears, frustrations, and feelings in caring for the child at home. Initiate a social worker referral, if a social worker is not already involved from the special training center.

Expected Outcomes

1. Communicates through sign language, touch, eye contact, and visual clues

2. Interacts with people in the environment; uses assistive measures to communicate; undergoing auditory and speech training

3. Engages in play activities suitable for age; becoming less dependent

4. Practices safety measures; wears hearing aid

5. Interacts with parents; parents verbalize understanding of the child's stage of growth and development

6. Reveals lessening of anxiety; assumes a more confident manner; plays with other children; learning techniques to augment communication.

7. The parents are reinforcing tactile and visual methods of communication with the child; working out their own grief, anxiety and guilt feelings; exploring community resources; displaying an accepting, loving attitude toward child

---

* Organizations for parents concerned with hearing problems include the following:

1. Alexander Graham Bell Association for the Deaf, 3417 Volta Place, NW, Washington, DC 20007

2. The John Tracy Clinic, 806 West Adams Blvd, Los Angeles, CA 90007. This clinic offers a free home correspondence course (in English and Spanish) for parents that provides them with information, guidance, and encouragement in training their child.

3. National Association of the Deaf, 814 Thayer Avenue, Silver Spring, MD 20910

4. National Easter Seal Society for Crippled Children and Adults, Inc., 2023 W. Ogden Avenue, Chicago, IL 60612

5. Bill Wilkerson Hearing and Speech Center, 1114 19th Avenue, South, Nashville, TN 37212

6. National Association for Hearing and Speech Action, 10801 Rockville Pike, Rockville, MD 20852

7. Gallaudet College, 800 Florida Avenue NE, Washington, DC 20002

Otitis Media

Otitis media is an infection of the middle ear. It may or may not be infectious or be accompanied by effusion.

Classification

1. *Acute otitis media*—suppurative or purulent
2. *Chronic otitis media* with effusion (also called secretory, serous, nonsuppurative otitis media, and "glue ear." Chronic effusion may be serous, mucoid, or purulent)—Inflammatory process of the middle ear with effusion collection as a result of auditory canal blockage. Can occur with or without infection. Bacterial or viral agents cause purulent exudate to collect in the space of the middle ear behind the eardrum (tympanic membrane).

Etiology

1. Suppurative otitis media
   a. Bacteriologic
      (1) *Haemophilus influenzae*
      (2) Beta hemolytic streptococci
      (3) Pneumococci
   b. Secondary
      (1) Cold
      (2) Measles
      (3) Scarlet fever
2. Nonsuppurative otitis media
   a. Allergy
   b. Auditory canal dysfunction
      (1) Obstruction
      (2) Abnormal patency
   c. Often unknown—nonsuppurative
3. Predisposing factors
   a. Auditory canal in children is shorter, wider, and more horizontal, thus making the middle ear more accessible to invasion of organisms.
   b. Anatomic immaturity of tubal muscles and cartilage in children under 2 years of age.
   c. Certain craniofacial congenital defects (i.e., cleft palate, Down's syndrome).

Incidence

1. Suppurative—children under 5 years of age, with highest incidence under 2 years of age
2. Nonsuppurative—school-age children
3. Increased incidence during winter and early spring

Altered Physiology

All related to alteration in function of auditory canal
1. Obstruction of the auditory canal by swelling of the mucous membranes.
   a. Air exchange does not take place between the pharynx and middle ear.
   b. Obstruction impedes drainage of secretions to the nasopharynx.
2. Secretions and bacteria becomes trapped in the middle ear (suppurative).
   a. Bacteria multiply rapidly in that environment, spread to mastoid bone or inner ear, and cause permanent damage.
   b. Examination reveals hyperemic, opaque, and bulging tympanic membrane with hypomobility, with or without effusion.

3. Fluid and exudate replace air in the middle ear. Fluid changes from watery secretions to viscous gluelike substance (nonsuppurative).
   a. Examination reveals tympanic membrane that is opaque, but if translucent, an air fluid level or air bubbles may be seen. Amber or bluish fluid may be seen in the middle ear; hypomobility and tympanic membrane may be retracted or convex.
   b. Tympanic membrane may rupture.

Complications

From untreated or ineffective treatment of acute otitis media
1. Chronic otitis media
2. Mastoiditis
3. Septicemia
4. Meningitis and brain damage
5. Chronic otitis media with mastoiditis and perforated eardrum may lead to impaired hearing or deafness
6. Transient or permanent hearing loss
7. Nonsuppurative otitis media (and tympanosclerosis; adhesive otitis media)
8. Cholesteatoma tympani

Clinical Manifestations

1. History of cold for several days
2. Fever
3. Older child
   a. Pain in affected ear; fullness
   b. Indistinct hearing
   c. Headache
   d. Vomiting
4. Infant
   a. May rub ear; (pain)
   b. Anorexia
   c. Turns head from side to side
   d. Diarrhea
5. Decrease in hearing

Diagnostic Evaluation

1. Examination will reveal bulging, red eardrum, partial or complete obstruction of bony landmarks, and lack of normal luster; ruptured drum may be obscured by secretions. Absence of light reflex, impaired mobility of eardrum when using pneumatic otoscope. Eardrum usually will be retracted.
2. Culture and sensitivity determination of drainage from ruptured drum or through myringotomy in order to select appropriate antibiotic therapy.
3. *Tympanometry*—the use of an electroacoustic impedance bridge with which a tympanogram can be obtained. The tympanograms produced show the dynamics of the tympanic membrane, middle ear, auditory canal system.
4. Acoustic emittance measurements—test for conductive hearing loss.

Treatment

A. Medical

Identify etiology
1. Antibiotics—appropriate for organism; usually ampicillin or penicillin

2. Acetaminophen or aspirin—for fever
3. Analgesic
4. Ear drops for relief of pain; may not be given as this may obscure view of tympanic membrane
5. Antihistamines and decongestant—to clear nasal pharyngitis and inflammation of auditory canals (controversial)
6. Follow-up hearing tests

B. Surgical

1. *Myringotomy*—surgical incision of the tympanic membrane to allow drainage and relieve pressure; done when fluid remains in middle ear despite medical treatment, or performed for diagnostic reasons.
   Heat probe may also be used.
2. *Tympanostomy ventilating tube*—Small plastic tube is inserted into the middle ear through a myringotomy incision, creating an artificial auditory canal to equalize pressure on both sides of the eardrum.
   a. The tube projects through the drum into the external auditory canal.
   b. This tube is a substitute for the eustachian tube, allowing the following to occur:
      (1) Continuous ventilation of the middle ear
      (2) Drainage of fluid into the external auditory canal
      (3) Promotion of healing of lining membranes
      (4) Prevention of premature closing of incision
   c. The tube may be left in place several weeks to several months. The perforation closes in about a week after the tubes are removed.
   d. Hearing will improve in children with middle ear fluid
   e. Most common age for treatment is between 2 and 7 years.
   f. Complications of tympanostomy tube include:
      (1) Recurring otitis media or suppurative otitis media
      (2) Plugging of tube with blood, cerumen, or exudate
      (3) Early spontaneous extrusion of tube
      (4) Permanent perforations
      (5) Tympanosclerosis
      (6) Local or diffuse atrophy of tympanic membrane
   g. Specific postoperative considerations
      Do not allow water to get into ears (during swimming or bathing) because of the infection potential. Emphasize the advantage—improvement of hearing.
3. *Tympanocentesis*—aspiration of middle ear fluids
4. Follow-up hearing tests

Patient Problems/Nursing Diagnoses

1. Potential for brain injury related to spread of infection
2. Pain and discomfort related to alteration in eustachian tube function
3. Skin encrustation related to drainage from ear
4. Anxiety related to procedures and treatment
5. Sensory deprivation (loss of hearing) related to effusion/disease process
6. Potential for delay in developmental growth related to inability to react/relate to sounds in environment
7. Potential for knowledge deficit of parents

Nursing Interventions

A. Administer medications and treatments as prescribed.

1. Give appropriate antibiotics according to sensitivity of organisms. Usual course of treatment is 10–14 days.
2. Instill nose drops and decongestant (controversial). May help to shrink mucous membranes and allow drainage from obstructed auditory canal.
3. Give ear irrigations and instill glycerin or oil for relief of pain.
   a. The child may need to be held, or "mummy" restraint used.
   b. For the child under 3 years old—pull auricle down and back.
   c. For the child over 3 years old—pull auricle up and back.
   d. Position the child so the affected ear is up—allows fluid to run onto the eardrum.

B. Prevent mixed infection and reduce the chances of complications arising from present infection.

1. Always wash hands prior to any treatment or contact with the ear.
2. Change position of the child as appropriate.
   a. Position affected ear up to instill medications or to irrigate ear.
   b. Position affected ear down to facilitate drainage when the child is resting.
3. Clean any exudate present from myringotomy or perforated drum.
   Prevents excoriation from drainage.

C. Provide physical comfort for the child while continuing therapy.

1. Local heat
   a. Use hot water bottle containing water not over 38.9°C. (102°F.).
      Heating pad may be used with an older child (set on low).
   b. Place the child on his side, with affected ear on top of bottle to facilitate drainage.
   c. Ice pack may provide comfort by decreasing edema and pressure.
2. A mild analgesic may be necessary if the child is restless and indicates pain.
3. Myringotomy may be done in cases where there is severe pain.
   Small incision of the tympanic membrane to relieve pressure and prevent a jagged opening from a spontaneous rupture. Prepare the child for procedure. Use model of ear anatomy for teaching. Show him and let him handle ventilating tubes.
4. If there is drainage, keep the external ear clean to prevent excoriation by using cotton pledgets soaked in hydrogen peroxide.
5. Encourage fluid intake to help maintain hydration since the child may have a fever.
6. Give a soft diet; chewing may cause increased pain.

D. Observe for signs of complications and report them.

1. Mastoiditis
   a. Pain behind the affected ear
   b. Increasing irritability

c. Onset or increase of fever
d. Tenderness, redness, and swelling over mastoid area
2. Meningitis
   a. Sudden onset of high fever
   b. Stiffness of neck
   c. Irritability
   d. Headache
   e. Lethargy
3. Chronic otitis media with perforation of tympanic membrane
   Usually not observed until follow-up care by physician
4. Cholesteatoma—results from squamous epithelium of the external canal growing into the middle ear, to the mastoid antrum, and eroding the bone. It is seen as a shiny white mass. It is a complication of chronic suppurative otitis media and should be reported to the physician immediately.

E. Provide emotional and psychological support appropriate for child's age and degree of illness.

1. Encourage the child to participate in diversional activities.
2. Reassure the child.
   a. Talk to him gently.
   b. Allow the child to express his feelings, fears, and frustrations by talking, playing and drawing.
   c. Hold and rock the younger child.
3. Encourage parental visits and involvement in the child's care.
   a. Ensure that the parents understand the diagnosis, pathology involved, and treatment.
   b. Help them to understand the necessity for follow-up and return visit following the episode, and the possible complications.

F. Assess for signs of hearing loss and social and language retardation.

Health Education

A. Help the parents understand that prevention of recurring otitis media is vitally important for the future well-being of the child.

1. Explain the value of preventing and treating the common cold and preventing otitis media.
   a. Feed the child in a sitting or upright position.
   b. Teach the child to use gentle nose blowing during a cold.
   c. Replace air in the middle ear—bubble blowing, chewing sugarless gum, blowing up balloon, Valsalva's maneuver by forcing air into a closed mouth while holding nose.
2. Removal of hypertrophied and infected adenoid tissue

may be necessary at a later date upon the recommendation of the physician.
3. Explain that the child may have decreased hearing for several weeks following this episode of illness.
4. Help the parents learn what signs indicate recurrent otitis media and the need for immediate medical intervention.
   a. Prompt treatment can prevent permanent hearing loss.
   b. Identify the relationship between hearing and language development.
   c. Teach the parents signs of hearing loss and to monitor speech and language as well as social development.
5. Help the parents understand the necessity of continuing administration of antibiotics for the prescribed time even though the child may no longer appear sick.
6. Assess the need for community agency referral.

B. Help the parents and child understand treatment and expectations related to ventilating tubes.

1. Following surgery, antibiotic ear drops may be prescribed to aid in keeping tubes patent.
2. Hearing may not improve for 1–3 weeks postoperatively.
3. Tubes will remain in place from 2–10 months, and are designed to extrude into the external ear canal.
4. When tubes extrude, slight pain and a small amount of bloody drainage may occur. Physician should be notified that the tubes are out.
5. Water should be prevented from entering the external ear canal—use custom made ear plugs, cottonballs coated with petroleum, etc.
6. Prepare the parents and child for possible occurrence of otorrhea.
7. Stress the importance of regular medical follow-up to evaluate proper functioning of tubes.

Expected Outcomes

1. Shows recovery from infection; temperature returning to normal; taking prescribed antimicrobial medication
2. Experiences minimal discomfort; does not rub ear or have distressful cry; sleeping in a restful manner; no complaints of pain
3. Avoids skin breakdown in area of ear drainage
4. Shows reduced level of anxiety; complies with treatment; interacts with personnel; demonstrates appropriate age-related behaviors
5. Demonstrates improved hearing; responding to auditory stimulation
6. Parents demonstrate understanding by explaining illness, complications, and treatment

Bibliography

Books

Bluestone CD and Stool SE (eds). Pediatric Otolaryngology. Vol 1, Philadelphia, WB Saunders, 1982

Gallender D. Symbol Communication for the Severely Handicapped.

Springfield, IL, Charles C Thomas, 1980

Harley RD (ed). Pediatric Ophthalmology, 2nd ed. Vol 1 & Vol 2. Philadelphia, WB Saunders, 1983

Whaley LF and Wong DL. Nursing Care of Infants and Children. St Louis, CV Mosby, 1983

Wieczorek RR and Natapoff JN. A Conceptual Approach to the Nursing of Children: Health Care from Birth through Adolescence. Philadelphia, JB Lippincott, 1981

Wybar K and Taylor D. Pediatric Ophthalmology—Current Concepts. New York, Marcel Dekker, 1983

Eye

Articles

Greenwald MJ. Visual development in infancy and childhood. Pediatr Clin North Am 1983 Dec; 30(6):977–994

Holt JE. Prevention and management of sport-related injuries. Consultant 1983 Jul; 23(17):117–121+

Lovelace BM. The blind child in the hospital. AORN J 1980 Feb; 31(2): 256+

Moller MA. The visually handicapped child. Pediatr Clin North Am 1983 Dec; 30(6):1185–1194

Nelson LB. Diagnosis and management of strabismus and amblyopia. Pediatr Clin North Am 1983 Dec; 30(6):1003–1014

Rogow SM. Rhythms and rhymes: Developing communication in very young blind and multihandicapped children. Child Care Health Dev 1982 Sep/Oct; 8(5):249–260

Smigielski PA and Steinmann MJ. Teaching sex-education to multiple handicapped adolescents. J Sch Health 1981 Apr; 51(4):238–241

Stengel TJ. Developmental and nondevelopmental obstacles to blind-infant–sighted mother attachment. Phys Occup Ther Pediatr 1981 Summer; 1(4):1–19

Sykanda AM and Levitt S. The physiotherapist in the developmental management of the visually impaired child. Child Care Health Dev 1982 Sep/Oct; 8(5):261–270

Villeneuve ME, Mevey E and Steinberg F. Self-care for the totally blind diabetic: It is possible. RN 1983 Jun; 46(6):38–40

Wassenberg C. Common visual disorders in children. Nurs Clin North Am 1981 Sep; 16(3):479–485

Wright KW. Pediatric ophthalmology: An update on amblyopia and strabismus. Consultant 1982 Nov; 22(11):97–99+

Ear

Articles

Adams JL, Evans GA and Roberts JE. Diagnosis and treating otitis media with effusion. MCN 1984 Jan/Feb; 9(1):22–28

Aranosian RD. Dealing with the deaf. Emerg Med 1983 Mar 30; 15(6):28–32, 37–39

Bluestone CD. Otitis media in children: To treat or not to treat? N Engl J Med 1982 Jun 10; 306(33):1399–1404

Bluestone CD. Recent advantages in the pathogenesis, diagnosis and management of otitis media. Pediatr

Clin North Am 1981 Nov; 28(4):727–756

Bluestone CD and Klein JO. Otitis media with effusion, atelectasis and eustachian tube dysfunction. In Bluestone CD and Stool SE (eds). Pediatric Otolaryngology. Philadelphia, WB Saunders, 1982, pp. 356–512

Boffman JH and Boffman RT. Early detection of hearing impairment. Issues Comp Pediatr Nurs 1981 Jan/Feb; 5(1):11–20

Calhoun JH. Cataracts in children. Pediatr Clin North Am 1983 Dec; 30(6):1061–1070

Cantekin EI et al. Lack of efficacy of a decongestant-antihistamine combination for otitis media with effusion ("secretory" otitis media) in children. N Engl J Med 1983 Feb 10; 308(6):297–301

Castiglia PT, Aquilina SS and Kemsley M. Focus: Nonsuppurative otitis media. Pediatr Nurs 1983 Nov/Dec; 9(6):427–431

Chambers LW et al. Serving the needs of hearing impaired preschool children in rural areas. Can J Pub Health 1981 May/Jun; 72(3):173–180

Craig WN. Education of the deaf. In Bluestone CD and Stool SE (eds). Pediatric Otolaryngology. Philadelphia, WB Saunders, 1982, pp. 1569–1580

Effgen SK. Effect of an exercise program on the static balance of deaf children. Phys Ther 1981 Jun; 61(6):873–877

Fria TJ. Assessment of hearing. Pediatr Clin North Am 1981 Nov; 28(4):757–776

Fria TJ. The assessment of hearing and middle ear function in children. In Bluestone CD and Stool SE (eds). Pediatric Otolaryngology. Philadelphia, WB Saunders, 1982, pp. 152–185

Grundfast KM. Hearing loss. In Bluestone CD and Stool SE (eds). Pediatric Otolaryngology, Vol 1. Philadelphia, WB Saunders 1982, pp. 229–260

Liden CB. Audiologic aspects of learning and behavior. Pediatr Clin North Am 1981 Nov; 28(4):981–990

Magian VC and Eadie JA. The risk register for infant deafness as implemented in Manitoba. Can J Pub Health 1981 May/Jun; 72(3):181–185

Merchant CD and Shurin PA. Therapy in otitis media. Pediatr Clin North Am 1983 Apr; 30(2):281–296

McDermott JC. Immittance screening for aural problems in school children. J Sch Health 1982 Oct; 52(8):462–468

Morgan RH. Breaking through the sound barrier. Nurs 1983 Feb; 13(2):112–114

Paradise JL. Tonsillectomy and adenoidectomy. Pediatr Clin North Am 1981 Nov; 28(4):881–892

Paradise JL. Otitis media during early life: How hazardous to development? A critical review of the evidence. Pediatrics 1981 Dec; 68(6):869–873

Paradise JL. Otitis media in infants and children. Pediatrics 1980 May; 65(5): 917–943

Sasso SC. Erythromycin/sulfisoxazole treatment for otitis media. MCN 1983 May/Jun; 8(3):193

Sataloff RT, Colton CM. Otitis media: A common childhood infection. Am J Nurs 1981 Aug; 81(8):1480–1483

Schwartz DM and Konkle DF. Hearing aids for children. In Bluestone CD and Stool SE (eds). Pediatric Otolaryngology. Philadelphia, WB Saunders, 1983, pp. 1543–1568

Teele DW et al. Middle ear disease and the practice of pediatrics. JAMA 1983 Feb 25; 249(8):1026–1029

Thomson LR. Understanding tympanometry. Pediatr Nurs 1982 May/Jun; 8(3):193–197

Wagner JA and Kloepper C. Children and parents and otitis media. JEN 1982 Nov/Dec; 8(6):306–307

Books for Parents/Patient Education

Eyerly J. The Seeing Summer. New York, JB Lippincott, 1981. A story of friendship between two 10-year-old girls who are alike, even though one cannot see.

Freeman RD, Carbin CF and Boese RJ. Can't your child hear? A guide for those who care about deaf children. Baltimore, University Park Press, 1981

Kastein, Spaulding and Scharf: Raising the Young Blind Child. Human Sciences Press, Inc. 72 Fifth Avenue, New York, NY 10011

Lipke L and Allen P. Your changing body: A Guide for Self-exploration. Grand Rapids, MI, Institute for Development of Creative Child Care, 1974

Preschool Learning Activities for the Visually Impaired Child: A Guide for Parents. ERIC Document Reproduction Service, Computer Microfilm International, PO Box 190, Arlington, VA 22210

Raynor S and Drouillard R. Get a Wiggle On. AAHPER Publications–Sales, 1201 61st Street, NW, Washington, DC 20036

Raynor S and Drouillard R: Move It! AAHPER Publications–Sales, 1201 61st Street, NW, Washington, DC 20036

Scott EP, Jan JE and Roger DF. Can't your child see? Baltimore, University Park Press, 1977

Ulrich S and Wolf AWM. Elizabeth. Ann Arbor, The University of Michigan Press, 1972

Agencies

American Printing House for the Blind, Inc.
1839 Frankfort Avenue
Louisville, KY 40206

Library of Congress
Division for the Blind and Physically Handicapped
1291 Taylor Street, NW
Washington, DC 20542

National Association for Visually
 Handicapped
305 E 24th Street
New York, NY 10010

Helen Keller National Center for Deaf–
 Blind Youths and Adults
111 Middle Deck Road
Sands Point, NY 11050

National Society to Prevent Blindness,
 Inc.
70 Madison Avenue
New York, NY 10016

Telesensory Systems, Inc.
3408 Hillview Avenue
PO Box 10099
Palo Alto, CA 94304

Association for Retarded Citizens
PO Box 6109
Arlington, TX 76011

National Association of the Deaf, Inc.
814 Thayer Avenue
Silver Spring, MD 20910

National Braille Association
422 South Clinton Avenue
Rochester, NY 14620

Office of Education, Bureau of Education
 for the Handicapped
7th and D Streets, SW
Washington, DC 20202
(202) 245-7134

American Foundation for the Blind
15 W Sixteenth Street
New York, NY 10011
(212) 620-2000

Connective Tissue Disease in Children

42

Juvenile Rheumatoid Arthritis

Juvenile rheumatoid arthritis (JRA) is a chronic inflammatory, generalized, systemic disease that involves a wide spectrum of manifestations, including joint, connective tissue, and visceral lesions throughout the body.

Etiology and Incidence

1. The cause of juvenile rheumatoid arthritis is unknown.
2. Current hypotheses
   a. Infection from an unidentified organism
   b. Autoimmune process or hypersensitivity to unknown stimuli
3. Peak stages of onset .
   a. 18 months–5 years of age
   b. 8½–12 years of age

Altered Physiology

1. In the early stages, one or many joints show signs of inflammation.
2. The inflammation is initially localized in a joint capsule, primarily in the synovium. The tissue becomes thickened from congestion and edema.
3. A characteristic inflammatory response develops in the form of a synovial proliferation which invades the interior of the joint.
4. The inflammatory tissue extends into the interior of the joint along the surface of the articular cartilage to which it may be adherent, so that it deprives the cartilage of nutrition.
5. By starvation and invasion, this inflammatory tissue slowly destroys the articular cartilage.
6. Synovial tissue eventually frees the joint space leading to narrowing, fibrous ankylosis and bony fusion.
7. Growth centers next to inflamed joints may undergo either premature epiphyseal closure or accelerated epiphyseal growth.
8. Tendons and tendon sheaths may develop inflammatory changes similar to the synovial tissues.
9. Inflammation of muscle may occur.
10. Rheumatoid nodules are uncommon in children.

Complications

1. Bony deformities—crippling from progressive polyarthritis
2. Psychological and social reactions to this chronic illness
3. Iridocyclitis—leading to cataracts, glaucoma, or blindness
4. Pericarditis

Modes of Onset and Clinical Manifestations

A. Acute Febrile–Systemic Onset (Still's Disease)

1. Highest incidence of onset is in children under 7 years of age
2. Distribution about equal between males and females
3. Represents 20% of cases
4. Initially joint involvement is variable—from no joint pain to generalized florid arthritis
5. Systemic characteristics:
   a. Irritability, anorexia, and malaise
   b. Intermittent fever—1 or 2 spikes a day over 38.9°C. (102°F.); occurrence of subnormal temperature between elevations; possible seizures
   c. Rash consisting of small, discrete, pink macules with pale centers occurring on trunk and extremities; rash may be transient.
   d. Hepatosplenomegaly
   e. Generalized lymphadenopathy
   f. Anemia
   g. Periorbital edema
   h. Carditis—tachycardia (disproportionate to fever), tachypnea, pericarditis, myocarditis
   i. Pleuritis or pneumonitis independent of carditis
6. WBC count and sedimentation rate may be elevated
7. More than half those with systemic onset will progress to polyarthritic disease

B. Polyarticular Onset

1. Highest incidence of onset is in children 6–12 years of age
2. Higher incidence in females than males
3. Represents about 30% of cases
4. Characterized by arthritis of more than 4 joints
   a. Acute onset is manifested by painful swelling of joints.
   b. Insidious onset—minimal or no joint pain; however, the child may wince on movement or may limp on walking.
   c. Large joints most often involved are knees, wrists, ankles, and elbows.
   d. Other areas are often involved.
      (1) Rheumatoid foot—metatarsophalangeal joints swollen and tender; pain in heel
      (2) Cervical spine and hip—tenderness and restricted movement
5. Systemic manifestations occur less frequently than in acute febrile onset; may see low-grade fever and general lymphadenopathy

6. May have positive rheumatoid factor and antinuclear antibody (ANA) test
7. Incidence of disabling arthritic disease is high when rheumatoid factor is present

C. Pauciarticular Onset
1. Incidence
   a. Type I—onset in early childhood, under age 3 years; predominantly female
   b. Type II—onset in late childhood, over age 9 years; predominantly male
   c. Represents about 50% of presenting cases
2. Characterized by arthritis of 1 or up to 4 joints, primarily of lower extremities
   a. Child under 5 years may be listless and irritable, have low-grade fever, and fail to grow at normal rate.
   b. Older child does not appear ill.
3. Systemic manifestations are few.
   a. May see rash, low-grade fever, lymphadenopathy, and splenomegaly.
   b. There is increased incidence of iridocyclitis.
      (1) Type I—chronic iridocyclitis
      (2) Type II—acute iridocyclitis
4. ANA test positive in about half cases
   HLA–B27—positive (human lymphocyte antigen)

Generalized Clinical Manifestations

A. Joints (changes may occur with or without systemic symptoms)
1. Symptoms may develop gradually with progressive stiffness, swelling and impaired motion of a joint or joints.
2. Symptoms may develop rapidly with sudden appearance of symptomatic arthritis in one or more joints.
3. Knees, ankles, feet, wrists, or fingers are usually involved initially.
4. Joints are swollen and warm.
5. Pain and stiffness of joint may appear before objective changes develop.
6. Limitation of motion of inflamed joints occurs.
7. Characteristic posture is one of guarding joints from movement; an anxious pained expression (with polyarthritis) is common.
8. Morning stiffness of joints occurs following periods of inactivity.
9. Atrophy and weakness of muscles near the affected joints may develop.
10. Skin over inflamed joints may be pigmented.
11. Chronically affected joints may become dislocated, deformed, or fused.
12. Subcutaneous nodules may appear over pressure points (knees, elbows, etc.).
13. Condition may ultimately affect any joint in the body (knees, ankles, wrists, feet, fingers, toes, shoulders, elbows, neck, jaw, hips and sacroiliac joints are frequently involved).
14. Small, deformed feet result from foot involvement in early childhood.
15. Micrognathia (unusually small lower jaw), as a result of temporomandibular arthritis, is one hallmark of juvenile rheumatoid arthritis.
16. Spindling or fusiform changes of the fingers may occur.

B. Inflammation of the Eye (unilateral or bilateral uveitis; iridocyclitis)

Child may have no early symptoms. If symptoms occur late, child may develop irreversible eye damage, including scarring and adhesions of the iris and cataracts.

1. Redness
2. Pain
3. Photophobia
4. Decreased visual acuity
5. Nonreactive pupil

C. Generalized growth retardation
1. During periods of remission, growth spurts may occur.
2. Treatment with long-term steroid therapy as well as the disease process may contribute to growth failure.

Diagnostic Evaluation

(of limited value)
1. Elevated sedimentation rate (usually)
2. Leukocytosis
3. High total serum proteins
4. Positive creatine protein
5. High frequency of serum antinuclear antibodies with pauciarticular onset
6. Possible alteration in serum proteins (increased alpha and gamma; decreased albumin)
7. Changes in bone, demonstrated by x-rays—initially nonspecific

Treatment

Goals:
Relieve joint inflammation and pain.
Maintain and increase joint range of motion, muscle strength, and tone, and prevent physical deformities.
Preserve total growth and development potential.
Support emotional outlook of patient and his family.

1. Although this is a painful disease of long duration, the outlook for remission is good.
2. There is no specific cure; treatment is supportive:
   a. Drug therapy to reduce inflammation; analgesia
   b. Exercise program to promote joint movement
3. Surgery
   a. Synovectomy—(to maintain function) when extensive synovitis develops, especially around wrists
   b. Joint replacement—with severe destructive arthritis (ankylosing spondylitis)

Patient Problems/Nursing Diagnoses

1. Alteration in mobility related to decreased joint range and muscle strength from the disease
2. Alteration in comfort related to joint inflammation
3. Potential or actual nonadherence to treatment program related to psychological reactions to illness and/or lack of understanding
4. Anxiety related to hospitalization, pain, and treatments
5. Altered self-image and self-esteem related to decreased mobility and deformities
6. Potential for gastric upset or aspirin toxicity related to treatment doses

Nursing Interventions

A. Offer the patient and his parents realistic encouragement.

1. Although the response to medication is slow, the recovery is slow, and episodes of acute illness recur, the long-term outlook is generally good.
2. The child may be hospitalized during an acute attack and systemic illness, or to receive intensive physical therapy.

B. Discuss with the parents and the child what they know about the disease and what they expect from treatment.

1. Determine what information has been given to them by the physician.
2. The child and his family must understand the disease and treatment. This is a chronic disease and has an unpredictable course; however, compliance with prescribed treatment will minimize crippling from progressive polyarthritis and allow the child to grow and develop to his potential.

C. Be an effective member of the special team caring for this patient and his family.

The team often includes pediatrician, rheumatologist, social worker, physical therapist, occupational therapist, psychologist/psychiatrist, ophthalmologist, hospital nurse, and community health nurse.

D. Assist in the program of physical therapy in order to maintain or increase joint range of motion and muscle strength and tone (Figs. 42-1, 42-2, and 42-3).

1. The parents and child are instructed in the exercises. Encourage development of program (with parental involvement) while patient remains in the hospital.

2. Night splints for the wrists, knees, hip, and ankle may be prescribed to do the following:
   a. Give rest and relief of pain.
   b. Prevent or correct deformity.
   c. Maintain damaged joint in a functional position.
3. Know proper application of splint and help the patient to adjust to it.
4. A hot tub bath prior to the exercises and following long rest periods may make the exercises less painful. Whirlpool treatment will aid in decreasing stiffness.
5. Full range of motion exercises should be performed every day. Inactivity results in stiffness.
   a. Encourage the child to do his own exercises as soon as possible.
   b. Isometric exercise may be done when active free exercise may be too much strain for an arthritic joint, or when they are impractical because of physical location (riding in car, sitting at desk in school).
6. Orthopedic surgery may be required to correct some deformities.

E. Provide the child with the freedom to engage in as much activity as he is able to tolerate.

1. Children will limit their own activity.
   Play is an effective therapeutic modality.

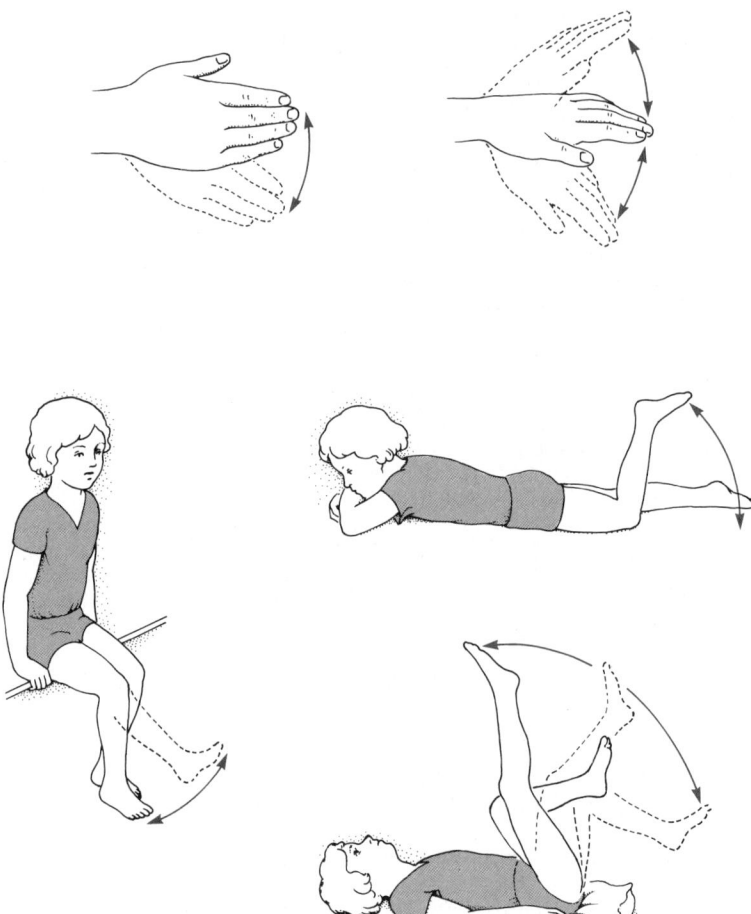

Figure 42-1. Therapeutic exercise: active range of motion for wrists, knees, and hips.

2. Those activities that produce overtiring or cause joint pain should be avoided.
3. Diversional activities should encourage movement based on the child's tolerance.
4. Encourage the child to be as self-sufficient as possible.
5. Allow the child to make some decisions himself (e.g., when he prefers to do his exercises).
6. Limit the use of wheelchairs. Tricycles and pedal cars provide good modes of mobility and exercise.

F. Use the principles of proper body mechanics and posture whether the child is at rest or is active.

1. Provide firm mattress to prevent sagging joints.
2. Use thin pillow (nor more than 5 cm. [2 inches] thick) to prevent dowager hump. Do not place pillows under joints.
3. The child may attempt to protect joints by assuming a position of flexion to ease discomfort.

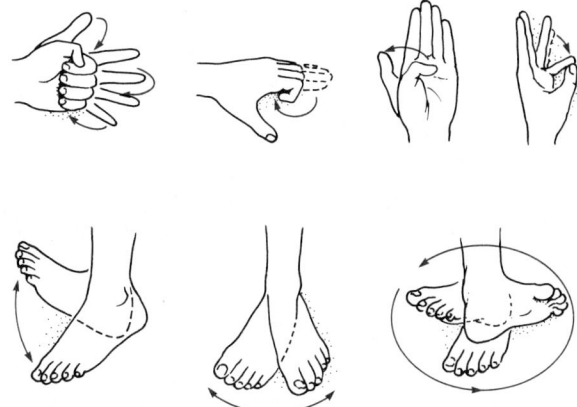

Figure 42-3. Therapeutic exercise: active range of motion for fingers and ankles.

G. Administer medications used to treat JRA. Know usage, side effects, and screening tests to be done during therapy.

Drug classes include:
1. *Nonsteroid anti-inflammatory drugs*
   a. Aspirin is the drug of choice.
      (1) Therapeutic serum levels are 20–30 mg./dl.
      (2) Enteric-coated aspirin reduces incidence of gastrointestinal symptoms.
      (3) Salicylates
         (a) Anti-inflammatory, analgesic, antipyretic
         (b) See Salicylates and Steroids, under Rheumatic Fever, page 1309, for side effects.
   b. Tolmetin
      (1) Used when aspirin is not effective or tolerated
      (2) Causes less gastric upset
      (3) May increase risk of anemia
      (4) Excreted quickly; therefore, must be given 3–4 times daily

▶ **NURSING ALERT:** Because of the increased association of aspirin and Reye's syndrome, discontinue use of aspirin when the child has a viral illness.

2. *Analgesics*
   a. Aspirin
   b. Acetaminophen
3. *Corticosteroids*
   a. Used in addition to salicylates when salicylates alone are not effective. Their use does not prevent complications of severe arthritis or influence ultimate prognosis.
   b. See the reference to salicylates and steroids, under Rheumatic Fever.
   c. Tuberculin test should be done prior to starting steroid therapy.
   d. Monitor for glucosuria.
4. *Long-acting, disease-modifying agents*
   a. Water-soluble gold salts (sodium aurothiomalate)
      (1) Used in conjunction with salicylates when improvement is not apparent or progression is not halted after several months. Injection given weekly for several months.

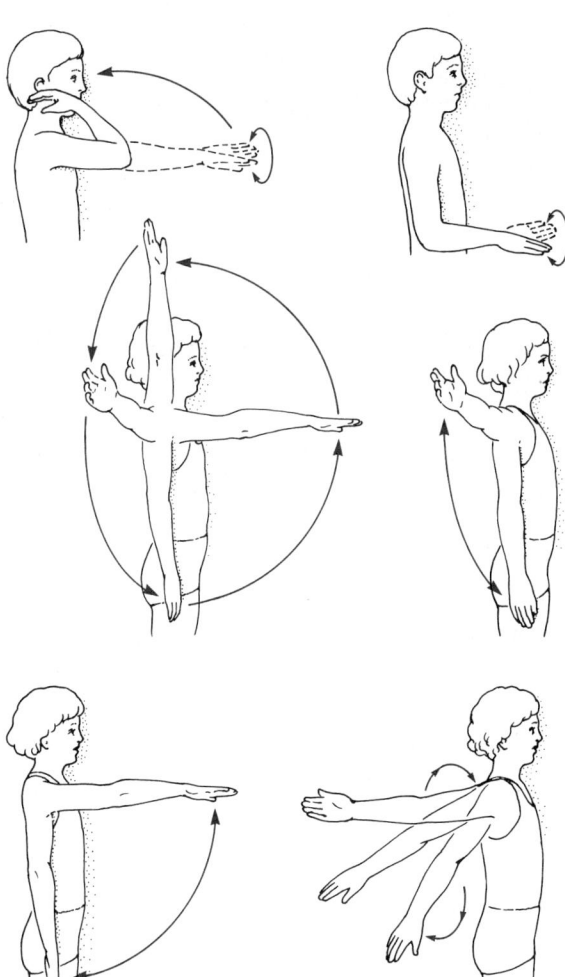

Figure 42-2. Therapeutic exercise: active range of motion for wrists, elbows, and shoulders.

(2) Side effects include skin rash, nephritis with hematuria or proteinuria, thrombocytopenia, and neurotoxicity, gastric upset, leukopenia, anemia, and mucosal ulcers

(3) Monitor urine for protein.

b. *Antimalarial with anti-inflammatory activity* (hydroxychloroquine or chloroquine)

(1) May cause gastric upset

(2) Blindness—due to deposition of the compound in pigmented tissue, especially eyes; eye examination every 3–6 months is advocated

(3) Used primarily with polyarticular disease

D. Promote general good health.

1. Well-balanced diet
2. Regular exercise and play appropriate for age
3. Avoid exposure to infections; seek medical treatment for infections
4. Ensure adequate rest
5. Schedule regular medical and ophthalmologic examinations

Health Education

A. Educate and motivate parents and child in continuing program of treatment at home.

Help parents to understand the needs of the child.

1. Extra rest—but not bed rest, which will contribute to contractures and muscle atrophy.
2. Program of daily exercise—this can be adjusted to fit in with the mother's or family's routine.
3. The child should attend school regularly and participate in regular school activities.
   a. This participation will allow the child to obtain social and scholastic achievement.
   b. Teachers should be informed of the child's condition and needs.
      (1) Child should get out of his seat and walk around room every hour.
      (2) Desk and chair should properly fit the child (i.e., when child is sitting with his back in the chair, his feet should be on the floor at right angles to legs; the seat should be deep enough to support thighs without pressure on popliteal arteries).
   c. Recreation is important—swimming is a beneficial sport activity.

4. Compensate for activities of daily living—help the child understand he must do as much for himself as possible.
Adapt items he uses to make their use easier (e.g., lift toilet seat several inches).

5. Provide nutritionally balanced diet to eliminate obesity that puts additional weight on joints.

6. Do not force unnecessary restrictions on the child that can produce acute behavioral upsets and interfere with his social development.

7. This disease affects the whole family. Remind parents to devote time to other members of the family and to their marriage. Various agencies can provide pertinent literature and can direct the family to helpful local resources.*

8. The child needs continual follow-up after hospitalization.
   a. Community health nurse can assist in home management of exercise program.
   b. Social worker can assist in helping parents work out their emotions and seek financial assistance.
   c. Ophthalmologist—must examine patient every 3–6 months for occurrence of iridocyclitis. Encourage the parents to report any eye symptoms that the child may develop.
   d. The physician must be consulted when any new symptoms occur, in an acute attack, or when progression is apparent, as well as for routine care.

Expected Outcomes

1. Demonstrates improved joint range of motion and muscle strength as evidenced by increased mobility, involvement in diversional activities, increased self-sufficiency, limited use of wheelchair or other assistive devices

2. Experiences minimal discomfort as evidenced by stable vital signs, increased mobility, play activity, interest in becoming involved with friends, use of proper body mechanics

4. Is free of complications related to aspirin use: absence of gastrointestinal upset and anemia

5. The patient/parents understand and can describe home-care measures to ensure rest, daily exercise, regular school attendance, maximum independence as able, proper diet

Systemic Lupus Erythematosus

Systemic lupus erythematosus (SLE) is a disease of the connective tissue with vascular and perivascular fibrinoid changes that may involve any organ or system.
Discoid lupus affects only the skin.

Incidence and Etiology

1. Incidence higher in females than in males; most common during the childbearing period (15–44 years of age). However, it can affect children 5–15 years of age.
2. Cause is unknown.
3. General theory of etiology is autoimmunity—believed to be an abnormal response of the body against its own connective tissue. Possible causes of this include the following:

   a. Genetic predisposition
   b. Viral—nonspecific antibody rise as part of general immunologic hyperactivity

4. Possible factors that trigger or unmask initial symptoms:
   a. Exposure to sunlight; snow on bright day
   b. Injury
   c. Stress
   d. Radiation therapy
   e. Vaccination
   f. Antitoxins
   g. Other drugs (e.g., anticonvulsants, antibiotics)

* Contact the Arthritis Foundation, 1314 Spring Street, NW, Atlanta, GA 30309

Altered Physiology

1. Connective tissue in different organs develops non-specific aberrations such as fibrinoid change in collagen and cellular infiltration, either in the walls of small blood vessels or elsewhere.
2. Alteration of collagen and subendothelial thickening of small blood vessels obstruct the flow of blood. These changes may be widespread or limited in distribution.

Complications

1. Sepsis—primarily resulting from steroid and immunosuppressive therapy
2. Renal involvement; chronic nephritis; renal failure
3. Cardiac complications
4. Neurologic involvement
5. Allergic reactions to drugs
6. Chronic fatigue
7. Pulmonary lupus and myocardial infarction
8. Growth retardation related to steroids and immunosuppressive therapy

Clinical Manifestations

1. General characteristic signs and symptoms may include:
   a. Malar erythema which usually spreads over bridge of nose. (Butterfly rash may consist only of an erythematous blush or scaly erythematous papules; rash may be photosensitive.)
      Rash spreads from face and scalp to neck, chest, and extremities.
   b. Acute polyarthritis, arthralgia
   c. Fever
   d. Fatigue, malaise
   e. Anorexia, weight loss
   f. Cardiac involvement—pleurisy or pericarditis most diagnostic
   g. Nephritis—at onset or during course of disease
      (1) Hematuria
      (2) Proteinuria
   h. CNS involvement—during course of disease
      (1) Behavior disturbances
      (2) Convulsions
      (3) Coma
   i. Splenomegaly
   j. Hepatomegaly
   k. Lymphadenopathy
   l. Anemia, thrombocytopenia
   m. Hypoglobulinemia
   n. Raynaud's phenomenon
2. Onset may be gradual, with no specific signs and symptoms
   a. Aching joints
   b. Morning stiffness
   c. Butterfly rash
3. Onset may be abrupt, with the development of any of the following:
   a. High fever
   b. Dyspnea, chest pain
   c. Arthritis without severe deformities
   d. Abdominal pain

Diagnostic Evaluation

1. Thorough physical examination; patient and family history
2. Primary laboratory studies
   a. Fluorescent antinuclear antibody test (FANA) to detect antibodies that react with nucleus of cells
   b. Lupus erythematosus (LE) cell test if FANA is positive—most diagnostic
   c. Serum sedimentation rate—elevated
   d. Serum complement studies—lowered
   e. CBC—leukopenia and mild to moderate anemia; can be hemolytic anemia
   f. Serum thrombotic accelerator (STA) (serology)—false-positive
   g. Blood chemistry—evaluate:
      (1) BUN—elevated
      (2) Blood sugar
      (3) Plasma protein—abnormal electrolytes
3. Kidney function studies
   a. Urine sediment—shows RBCs and granular casts, increased protein, leukocyturia
   b. Serum creatinine—elevated
   c. Urine protein—elevated
   d. Creatinine clearance
4. Presence of 4 or more of criteria for SLE proposed by American Rheumatism Association*
   a. Facial erythema
   b. Discoid lupus erythema (uncommon in children)
   c. Photosensitivity
   d. Oral or nasopharyngeal ulceration
   e. Raynaud's phenomenon
   f. Alopecia—focal or diffuse
   g. Arthritis—without severe deformity
   h. LE cells
   i. Chronic false-positive serology—syphilis
   j. Profuse proteinuria
   k. Cellular casts in urine
   l. Pleurisy or pericarditis
   m. Psychosis or convulsions
   n. Hemolytic anemia, leukopenia, or thrombocytopenia

Treatment

1. Control of symptoms with medication
   a. Salicylates—relieve joint symptoms, fever, fatigue
   b. Antimalarials such as hydroxychloroquine sulfate (Plaquenil) to relieve joint symptoms and skin rash
   c. Steroids such as prednisone—used when there is renal or neurologic involvement or hemolytic anemia; TB test should be done prior to starting steroid therapy
   d. Immunosuppressive agents such as azathioprine and cyclophosphamide—used in severe disease, especially with nephritis or steroid-resistant patients
   e. Topical steroid preparations—may help suppress cutaneous lesions
2. Careful and controlled monitoring of drug therapy and reassessment of clinical and laboratory picture
3. Supportive
   a. Rest
   b. Adequate nutrition
   c. Treatment of existing complications
   d. Early identification and treatment of opportunistic infection

Patient Problems/Nursing Diagnoses

1. Altered activity and mobility related to muscle weakness and joint pain

* Cohen AS et al. Preliminary criteria for the classification of systemic lupus erythematosus. Bull Rheum Dis 1976 May; 21: 643–648

2. Alteration in nutritional status related to anemia and possible medication effects
3. Potential for neurologic complications (excitability, headaches, seizures) related to neurologic involvement
4. Potential altered respiratory status related to inflamed serous lining of lungs, pleurisy, or pericarditis
5. Potential renal complications related to glomerular inflammation
6. Alteration in body image related to body changes from the disease and/or drugs
7. Nonadherence to treatment program related to lack of understanding

Nursing Interventions

A. Provide opportunities for the patient and the parents to discuss the disease—their understanding of it and their expectations.

Assist the child and his family to adjust to the limitations and treatments of the disease.

1. Determine what information has been given to them by the physician.
2. Provide supportive care to help them work out feelings of fear, anxiety, and uncertainty.
3. Support them in accepting this condition as a long-term illness, with exacerbations and remissions.
   a. They will need continuing support. Initiate early referral to community health nurse and social worker.
   b. Provide available literature and encourage contact with the nearest chapter of the Lupus Erythematosus Foundation.*

B. Assist the child in developing a realistic attitude about his illness and to assist him in expressing his feelings about his illness.

1. Provide the child with the opportunity to openly discuss his feelings about illness when he is able to verbalize these feelings.
2. Provide the child with the opportunity to express his feelings; utilize play as a method.
3. Arrange for a visiting teacher so that the child may have the opportunity to continue his education.
4. Encourage the child to continue contact with his peers (i.e., via telephone, letter writing, etc.).
5. Allow the child to make some decisions and become involved in planning his own care.

C. Be aware of the action and side effects of medications used in the treatment of systemic lupus erythematosus.

Steroids and salicylates (see section on juvenile rheumatoid arthritis, p. 1405).

D. Observe closely for the development of symptoms that may indicate development of complications.

1. Observe for the development of renal symptoms. There is usually some degree of renal involvement.
   a. Record intake and output.
   b. Record specific gravity of urine.
   c. Observe the color and characteristics of urine, especially proteinuria.
   d. Observe for the development of edema.

---

* Lupus Foundation of America, 11921 Olive Blvd, St. Louis, MO 63141
National Lupus Erythematosus Foundation, 5430 Van Nuys Avenue, Van Nuys, CA 91401

2. Observe for the development of sepsis.
3. Report to the physician any abnormal findings.

E. Assist the child and family in understanding ways to prevent exacerbations and complications of the disease.

1. Important "do's":
   a. Get enough rest.
   b. Avoid anxiety and tension.
   c. Follow treatment plan and medication schedule.
   d. Avoid contact with persons with infectious diseases.
   e. Follow prescribed diet, especially when receiving steroids.
   f. Seek medical attention at times of illness or stress.
   g. Recognize warning signs of exacerbation.
   h. Become knowledgeable about SLE.
2. Important "don'ts":
   a. Do not overexert.
   b. Do not alter prescribed medications.
   c. Do not use over-the-counter drugs.
   d. Do not ignore treatment plan.
   e. Do not expose self to sun and reflected sun through clouds, on snow, water, or white concrete, or fluorescent lighting.

F. Be aware of the special situation when a neonate is born to a known SLE mother.

1. Positive ANA and LE factor transmitted transplacentally
   a. Infant may have clinical and/or nonclinical evidence of lupus erythematosus. Discoid lesions may be present.
   b. Other infants may have no clinical symptoms.
2. Symptoms usually resolve in 3–4 months; however, the child may develop SLE later in life.

Health Education

A. Inform the parents about requirements for caring for the child at home.

1. Prevent direct exposure to the sun; if exposure to the sun cannot be avoided, a sunscreen lotion with PABA should be used.
   a. The child can go outside in early morning or late afternoon.
   b. The child should avoid snow on bright days, cement, and white buildings because of photosensitivity.
2. Discuss with the parents and be certain they are aware of and understand each of the following:
   a. Side effects of any medications being administered at home and what to do about these reactions
   b. Signs of worsening of the disease
   c. Factors that precipitate flare-up or early warning signs of flare-up: chills, fever, anorexia, and fatigue
   d. Problems that may be associated with the adolescent—i.e., body image, relationship with peers
3. Provide measures that will be helpful in preventing infection:
   a. Avoid exposure to individuals with infections.
   b. Practice general measures of personal hygiene.
   c. Provide a well-balanced diet.
4. Continual medical follow-up
   a. Disease progress needs reevaluation.
   b. Drug therapy must be strictly controlled, and it

    is based on the condition of the child as well as laboratory studies.

    c. Renal function specifically needs to constantly be evaluated.

Expected Outcomes

1. Demonstrates increased mobility and activity
2. Shows improved nutritional status as evidenced by appropriate intake and weight gain and laboratory values
3. Is free of neurologic complication such as headache or seizures
4. Maintains normal respiratory function and cardiac output as reflected by vital signs, behavior, and laboratory studies
5. Shows normal kidney function; normal urine output, specific gravity, color, and protein content
6. Avoids exposure to sunlight or sun glare
7. Demonstrates a self-confident attitude and improved self-image as reflected in play activity, willingness to interact with others, regular attendance at school, and eagerness to make decisions and to be independent
8. Adheres to the treatment regimen: gets rest, takes medication, follows diet
9. Parents understand and can explain home-care protocols for avoiding sunlight, side effects of medications, signs of exacerbation, the need for relaxed attitude, measures for maintaining social interactive skills

---

Schönlein–Henoch Purpura (Anaphylactoid Purpura)

Schönlein–Henoch purpura is a diffuse disease resulting from inflammatory reaction around capillaries and arterioles involving the skin, intestines, joints, and kidneys.

Incidence and Etiology

1. Slightly higher incidence in males than in females. Increased incidence of onset is between ages 2 and 8 years.
2. Possible cause is an allergic reaction to a variety of antigenic stimuli such as infection (e.g., beta streptococci), allergens, insect bites, food, and drugs.
3. Cause is unknown.
4. Disease is usually self-limiting.

Altered Physiology

1. Acute vasculitis
   a. Swelling and edema of capillaries, small venules, and arterioles
   b. Fibrin is deposited in the glomeruli of the kidney
2. Vasculitis results in skin manifestations (purpura), arthritis, and gastrointestinal symptoms.

Complications

1. Acute nephritis or nephrosis that may lead to chronic nephritis (urinalysis should be done 6 and 12 months after episode).
2. Colicky abdominal pain, related to vasculitis and edema of the bowel; steroids may be used.
3. Intussusception

Clinical Manifestations

1. Rash—sudden onset may precede or follow other manifestations.
   a. Typical rash begins with itching, urticarial wheals and then proceeds to maculopapular erythematous lesions.
   b. These lesions become less raised and more petechial or purpuric in character and do not fade with pressure. They blanch initially, then progress to ecchymotic areas until they fade.
   c. Several stages of the rash may be present at one time.
   d. Rash appears primarily on buttocks, lower back, extensor aspects of arms and legs, and face.
2. Arthritis of knee and ankle joints develops; the condition is moderately severe, with painful swelling due to periarticular edema. Movement is limited.
3. Local edema—especially of scrotum.
4. Colicky abdominal pain—from submucosal hemorrhage.
5. Nausea and vomiting
6. Proteinuria
7. Microscopic hematuria
8. Symptoms may appear acutely or gradually.

Diagnostic Evaluation

1. Appearance of rash
2. Blood studies—not diagnostic
   a. Platelet count—normal
   b. Erythrocyte sedimentation rate (ESR)—elevated
   c. Anemia possible
   d. Azotemia (with severe kidney involvement)
   e. pH and prothromboplastin tests
3. Urine studies
   a. Proteinuria
   b. Microscopic hematuria
   c. Casts
4. Stool—shows occult or gross blood

Treatment

Treatment is primarily symptomatic and supportive.
1. Encourage bed rest until the child is able to ambulate and can do so without increasing edema of feet.
2. Remove allergen if it is known.
3. Give antibiotic therapy if acute episode was preceded by infection, especially streptococcal.
4. Manage complicating abdominal or renal involvement:
   a. Steroids (prednisone) may relieve abdominal symptoms and prevent intussusception.
   b. Immunosuppressive therapy (azathioprine or cyclophosphamide) may be given to stabilize persistent renal involvement.

Patient Problems/Nursing Diagnoses

1. Alteration in comfort related to arthritis, nausea, vomiting, and abdominal pain, and itching
2. Alteration in mobility related to arthritis and edema
3. Potential for complications of intussusception and nephritis related to vasculitis and edema of gastrointestinal tract and glomeruli
4. Potential skin breakdown related to erythematous lesions and itching
5. Anxiety and fear related to discomfort and hospitalization

6. Parental anxiety related to sudden onset of disease and lack of understanding

Nursing Intervention

A. Offer the patient and his parents realistic encouragement.

The long-term outlook is good when renal involvement is minimal.

B. Assist the child in expressing his feelings about illness and hospitalization.

1. Provide the child with an opportunity to openly discuss his feelings about illness and his situation when he is able to verbalize these feelings.
2. Provide the child with the opportunity to express his feelings; utilize play as a method.
3. Allow the child to make some decisions (appropriate for his age), and to become involved in planning his own care.
4. Consider his age and then allow and encourage parental participation.

C. Provide physical comfort for the child's painful and swollen joints.

Salicylates are found not to be particularly effective (see Juvenile Rheumatoid Arthritis, p. 1405).

D. Observe for developing signs and symptoms of complications.

1. Renal
   a. Record intake and output.
   b. Record specific gravity of urine.
   c. Observe color and characteristics of urine.
   d. Observe development of or increase in edema.
2. Intussusception—sudden onset
   a. Paroxysmal abdominal pain
   b. Currant jelly-like stools
   c. Vomiting
   d. Increasing absence of stools
   e. Increasing abdominal distention and tenderness

E. Observe and record the child's general condition and the current status of the rash.

F. Be aware of the action and side effects of medications used in the treatment of anaphylactoid purpura.

See Juvenile Rheumatoid Arthritis, page 1405.

Health Education

1. Reassure the parents that symptoms are self-limiting.
2. Ensure that parents understand treatment and signs and symptoms of complications.
3. Make community health nurse referral as needed.
4. Encourage the parents to return the child for follow-up urinalysis 6 and 12 months following acute episode.

Expected Outcomes

1. Shows relief of pain evidenced by verbalization and/or behavior
2. Increases mobility as arthritis and edema decrease
3. Maintains normal gastrointestinal function; shows no signs of intussusception: abdominal pain, vomiting, distention, failure to pass stool
4. Maintains normal urinary function: normal output, specific gravity; no edema
5. Demonstrates lessening anxiety; expresses feelings; engages in play activities; and has a more relaxed behavior
6. The parents gain an understanding of the child's illness, are supportive of the child, become involved in care and follow through with home care in relation to medications and avoidance of complications

Kawasaki Disease (Mucocutaneous Lymph Node Syndrome)

Kawasaki disease is a multisystem vasculitis identified by a febrile illness with several distinguishing features that attack vital body systems.

Etiology and Prevalence

1. Cause is unknown.
2. Peak age of occurrence is about 3 years; 1:5 male ratio.
3. There seems to be no familial, seasonal, socioeconomic, or communicability prevalence associated with the disease.

Altered Physiology

1. Although vasculitis is a multisystem disease, the cardiovascular system seems to be primarily involved.
2. Initially: stage I
   a. Perivasculitis of arterioles, venules, and capillaries
   b. Coronary arteries are included—pancarditis
3. As disease progresses: stage II and III
   a. Panvasculitis and perivasculitis of coronary arteries
   b. Aneurysm formation, pericarditis, myocarditis, endocarditis, and phlebitis may result.
4. Stage IV
   a. Coronary arterial scarring, stenosis, calcification
   b. Myocardial fibrosis and endocardial fibroelastosis
   c. Healing begins

Complications

1. Cardiac involvement during illness
2. Aspirin toxicity
3. Posthospital (postillness) cardiac involvement

Clinical Manifestations

A. Acute Febrile Phase—Stage I: The child appears severely ill and irritable (days 1–14).

*1. High, spiking fever, 5 or more days
*2. Bilateral congestion of ocular conjunctivae
*3. Oropharyngeal erythema, "strawberry" tongue, red and dry lips
*4. Indurative edema of hands and feet or erythema of palms and soles
*5. Erythematous rash of trunk
*6. Cervical lymphadenopathy
7. Carditis—pericarditis, myocarditis, cardiomegaly, congestive heart failure, coronary thrombosis

B. Subacute Phase—Stage II: Acute symptoms of Stage I subside as temperature returns to normal. The child remains irritable and anorexic (days 10–25).

* Six major criteria—CDC requires that fever and four of the remaining symptoms be present for diagnosis. (Adapted from Emergency Medicine, Jan 30 1982)

1. Dry, cracked lips with fissures (part of third criterion)
2. Desquamation of toes and fingers (part of fourth criterion)
3. Arthralgia, arthritis
4. Coronary thrombosis, aneurysms

C. **Convalescent Phase—Stage III:** The child appears well (days 25–60).

1. Transverse grooves of fingers and toenails (Beau's lines)
2. Coronary thrombosis; aneurysms (may occur)

Diagnostic Evaluation

A. **Demonstration of criteria seen above**

B. **ECG and echocardiographic abnormalities**

C. **Although there are no specific laboratory tests, the following may help support diagnosis or rule out other diseases:**

1. White blood cell count—leukocytosis during acute stage
2. ESR—elevated during acute stage
3. Erythrocytes and hemoglobin—slight decrease
4. C-reactive protein—positive
5. Platelet count—increased during 2nd and 3rd week of illness
6. IgM, IgA, IgG, and IgF—transiently elevated
7. Urine—proteinuria and leukocytes present

Treatment (controversial among authorities)

1. Treatment goal is to prevent coronary thrombosis leading to coronary aneurysm and death.
2. Aspirin
   a. High dose during acute phase as antipyretic and anti-inflammatory.
   b. Lower doses used as platelet aggregation inhibitor in subacute phase and continued until sedimentation rate is normal.
3. Supportive
   a. Maintain fluid and electrolyte balance; nutritional support.
   b. Provide comfort.
   c. Employ careful monitoring of cardiac status.

Patient Problems/Nursing Diagnoses

1. Parental anxiety and stress related to uncertainty about disease
2. Alteration in comfort related to fever, conjunctival inflammation, edematous and peeling skin, oral lesions, and immobility
3. Alteration in skin integrity related to edema, dehydration
4. Cardiac complications related to vasculitis
5. Potential for aspirin toxicity related to high-dose treatment
6. Dehydration related to hyperthermia and decreased fluid intake
7. Sensory deprivation related to presence of eye patches in treating conjunctivitis
8. Mobility intolerance related to joint pain and enforced bed rest
9. Patient anxiety and fear related to hospitalization, pain, and body changes that occur with the disease

Nursing Interventions

A. **Promote comfort and rest of the febrile child, and prevent dehydration.**

1. Although aspirin is given in high doses in an attempt to control the quickly spiking temperature, it is often ineffective.

2. Give tepid sponge baths for temperature over 38.3°C. (101°F.), or a cooling blanket should be employed (see Child with Fever, p. 1137).
3. Monitor vital signs every 1–2 hours.
4. Offer clear liquids every hour when the child is awake (Popsicles are often accepted and may be soothing to sore oral mucous membranes).
5. Monitor urinary output and specific gravity.
6. Monitor intravenous infusion hourly.
7. Weigh daily in the morning.
8. Assess skin turgor, tears, etc. to aid in assessment of hydration status.
9. Pad side rails and have airway and suction available; seizures may occur because of rapid temperature rise.

B. **Carry out continual cardiac monitoring and assessment for complications.**

1. Take vital signs and blood pressure every 2 hours; report abnormalities.
2. Ensure proper functioning of cardiac monitor; observe for and report any arrhythmias.
3. Assess the child for signs of myocarditis: tachycardia, gallop rhythm, chest pain.
4. Monitor the child for congestive heart failure: dyspnea, nasal flaring, grunting, retractions, cyanosis, orthopnea, crackles, moist respirations, distended neck veins, and edema.

C. **Monitor the child for signs of aspirin toxicity when high-dose aspirin is prescribed** (see Rheumatic Fever, p. 1309).

(Serial aspirin serum levels are monitored.)

D. **Provide measures of comfort for the child with altered skin integrity and conjunctival inflammation.**

1. Comfort measures related to skin
   a. Cool, moist compresses to skin. Avoid use of soap because it tends to dry skin and make it more likely to break down.
   b. Elevate edematous extremities.
   c. Use sheepskin, egg crate mattress, and smooth sheets.
   d. If clothes are used, they should be of soft flannel or terry cloth.
2. Comfort measures related to eyes—conjunctivitis can cause photosensitivity
   a. Darken room; cover eyes with cool cloth or sunglasses.
   b. Instruct the child to avoid rubbing eyes.
   c. Consider using artificial tear drops to increase comfort.
3. Comfort measures related to altered oral mucous membranes
   a. Offer cool liquids—(ice chips and popsicles)
      (1) Progress to soft, bland foods.
      (2) Encourage the child to eat meats and snacks to prevent nutrition deficit.
      (3) Encourage the parents to participate in selecting food and feeding activities.
   b. Give mouth care every 1–4 hours—special mouth swabs; soft tooth brush only after healing has occurred.
   c. Apply petrolatum to dried, cracked lips.
   d. Observe the mouth frequently for signs of infection.
4. Comfort measures related to joint pain and tender lymph nodes
   a. Employ passive range of motion exercises every

4 hours while the child is awake because movement may be restricted.

b. Allow and encourage the child to move about freely under supervision.

c. Provide soft toys and quiet play and encourage use of hands and fingers.

E. Provide for emotional support and diversional activities appropriate for age.

1. The child is generally irritable, uncomfortable, and lethargic because of his illness and hospitalization.
2. Play therapy—both active and passive—can help the child express his feelings.
3. Explain procedures to the child.
4. Encourage the parents to be involved in care and help them offer support to their child.
5. Allow the child periods of uninterrupted rest—should decrease irritability.

F. Provide emotional support for the parents who are distressed and concerned about their child.

1. Help the parents understand what is happening; they need to be told what changes they will see (i.e., fever spikes, eye changes, desquamation of hands and feet, irritable behavior, decreased appetite).
2. Encourage them appropriately; usually the disease is self-limiting, but there is potential for cardiac involvement.
3. Involve the parents in comforting and care of the child to help relieve some of their anxieties and feelings of helplessness.
4. Encourage the parents to verbalize their concerns, fears, and questions.

Health Education

1. Long-term care following discharge is critical because complications can occur during period of convalescence or months following acute illness. Medical observation, ECGs and echocardiograms should be done every 3 months during the 1st year.
2. The parents should be given instructions (verbal and written) and demonstrate that they understand the specific information and instructions related to cardiac problems (i.e., color change, shortness of breath, chest pain, and lethargy).

3. The parents need to understand what medications are prescribed; dose, action, frequency of administration, and signs of toxic effects.
4. Anticipatory guidance is needed in terms of behavioral context.
   a. Do not overprotect the child.
   b. Allow him to be as active as he wants.
   c. Discuss regression that might occur as a result of hospitalization and how to deal with these changes.
5. Initiate community health nurse and/or social work referral as indicated.

Expected Outcome

1. Child experiences increasing comfort as evidenced by appropriate behavior (i.e., less irritable, increased fluid intake, interest in diversional activities, ability to rest easily)
2. Maintains normal cardiac function as evidenced by normal echocardiogram, ECG, and vital signs; does not complain of chest pain
3. Shows no signs of aspirin toxicity as evidenced by normal gastric function and appropriate serum aspirin levels
4. Remains well hydrated as evidenced by adequate intake and output, normal urine specific gravity and skin turgor
5. Engages in range of motion exercises and other activities to improve mobility
6. Skin remains intact; good turgor; no evidence of pressure
7. The parents comfort the child and participate in care when possible
8. The parents verbalize understanding of their home-care responsibilities in relation to detecting possible complications; administering medications, watching for side effects and continuing with follow-up medical observation every 3 months for the 1st year

Bibliography

Books

Behrman RE and Vaughan VC. Nelson Textbook of Pediatrics. Philadelphia, WB Saunders, 1983

Brewer EJ, Giannini EH and Person DA. Juvenile Rheumatoid Arthritis, 2nd ed (Vol VI in series, Major Problems in Clinical Pediatrics). Philadelphia, WB Saunders, 1982

Coleman WP and McBurney EI. Pediatric Dermatology: New Directions in Therapy. Garden City, NY, Medical Examination Publishing Co, 1981

*Horgan B. Arthritis in Children: A Practical Guide. Melbourne, Australia, Dominion Press, Fontana/Collins, 1982

Hoeprich PD (ed). Infectious Diseases,

3rd ed. Philadelphia, Harper & Row, 1983

Whaley LF and Wong DL. Nursing Care of Infants and Children. St Louis, CV Mosby, 1983

Wieczorek RR and Natapoff JN. A Conceptual Approach to the Nursing of Children. Philadelphia, JB Lippincott, 1981

*Williams GF. Children with Chronic Arthritis. Littleton, MA, PSG Publishing Co, 1981

Articles

Anderson DJ and Thibault J. Nursing management of the pediatric patient with Kawasaki's disease. Issues Compr Pediatr Nurs 1981 Jan/Feb; 5(1):1–11

Ascheim JH. The adolescent and systemic lupus erythematosus: A developmental and educational approach. Issues Compr Pediatr Nurs 1981 Sep–Dec; 5(5–6):293–307

Baum J. Treatment of juvenile arthritis. Hosp Pract 1983 Sep; 18(9):121–124+

Calabro JJ. Kawasaki disease: Inscrutable and unmistakable. Emerg Med 1982 Jan 30; 14(2):24–29+

Dix PE and Ridder ME. The adolescent with a stroke. J Neurosurg Nurs 1983 Apr; 15(2):80–86

Englund JA and Lucas RV. Cardiac complications in children with systemic lupus erythematosus. Pediatrics 1983 Nov; 72(5):724–729

Kadlowec N, Price JH and Forouzesh M. Systemic lupus erythematosus. J Nurs Care 1981 Aug; 14(8):6–9

Kawasaki T et al. A new infantile acute febrile mucocutaneous lymph node syndrome (MLNS) prevailing in Japan. Pediatrics 1974 Sep; 54(3):271–276

Kinash RG. Systemic lupus erythematosus: The psychological dimension. Can Mental Health 1983 Jun; 3(2):19–22

* Suggested Parent Reading

Litt IF, Cuskey WR and Rosenberg A. Role of self-esteem and autonomy in determining medication compliance among adolescents with juvenile rheumatoid arthritis. Pediatrics 1982 Jan; 69(1):15–17

L'Orange C and Werner-McCullough M. Kawasaki disease: A new threat to children. Am J Nurs 1983 Apr; 83(4): 558–562

Lynch MH and Gray JL. Kawasaki disease. Pediatr Nurs 1982 Mar/Apr; 8(2):96–101

Melish ME, Hicks RV and Reddy V. Kawasaki syndrome: An update. Hosp Pract 1982 Mar; 17(3):99–106

Morens DM, Anderson LJ and Hurwitz ES. National surveillance of Kawasaki disease. Pediatrics 1980 Jan; 65(1):21–25

Sealy S. Kawasaki disease: A worldwide problem. MCN 1980 Sep/Oct; 5(5): 331–334

Shapiro SR et al. Cardiac evaluation of children with mucocutaneous lymph node syndrome. Clin Proc Childrens Hospital National Medical Center 1982 Jan/Feb; 38(1):6–9

Useful laboratory findings in systemic lupus erythematosus. Hosp Med 1983 Feb; 19(2):99–100

Waring NP and DeShazo RD. JRA diagnosis: Why it can be confusing, even for the experts. Consultant 1983 May; 23(5):93–97+

Patient, Family and Teacher Education Materials

Arthritis Foundation
1314 Spring Street, NW
Atlanta, GA 30309

Action for Childhood Arthritis Guide, 1985
Contains a reference list of materials about childhood arthritis

American Juvenile Arthritis Organization
1314 Spring Street, NW
Atlanta, GA 30309

Arthritis Information Clearinghouse
PO Box 9782
Arlington, VA 22209
Provides bibliographies and listings of educational materials concerned with arthritis and related diseases

National Lupus Erythematosus Foundation
5430 Van Nuys Avenue
Van Nuys, CA 91401

Children with Neurologic and Neurosurgical Problems

Cerebral Palsy

Cerebral palsy is a comprehensive diagnostic term used to designate a group of nonprogressive disorders resulting from malfunction of the motor centers and pathways of the brain. Although there are varying degrees and clinical manifestations of cerebral palsy, it is generally characterized by paralysis, weakness, incoordination, and/or ataxia. Cerebral palsy is a major cause of disability among children in the US.

Etiology

A. Prenatal Factors

1. Infection, rubella, toxoplasmosis, herpes simplex, cytomegalic inclusions and other viral or infectious agents
2. Maternal anoxia, anemia, placental infarcts, abruptio placentae
3. Prenatal cerebral hemorrhage, maternal bleeding, maternal toxemia, Rh or ABO incompatibility
4. Prenatal anoxia, twisting or kinking of the cord
5. Genetic factors
6. Miscellaneous—toxins, drugs

B. Perinatal Factors

1. Anoxia from any cause
    a. Anesthetic and analgesic drugs administered to the mother may cause anoxia in the infant's brain
    b. Prolonged labor
    c. Placenta previa or abruptio placentae
    d. Respiratory obstruction
2. Cerebral trauma during delivery
3. Complications of birth
    a. "Small for date" babies, prematurity, immaturity, postmaturity
    b. Hyperbilirubinemia
    c. Hemolytic disorders
    d. Respiratory distress
    e. Infections
    f. Electrolyte disturbances (hypoglycemia, hypocalcemia)

C. Postnatal Factors

1. Head trauma
2. Infections
    a. Meningitis
    b. Encephalitis
    c. Brain abscess
3. Vascular accidents
4. Anoxia
5. Neoplastic and late neurodevelopmental defects

Altered Physiology

A. Spastic Type

1. Defect in the cortical motor area or pyramidal tract causes abnormally strong tonus of certain muscle groups.
2. Attempt to move a joint causes muscles to contract and block the motion. Permanent contractures develop without muscle training.

B. Athetotic Type

Lesions of the extrapyramidal tract and basal ganglia cause involuntary, uncoordinated, uncontrollable movements of muscle groups.

C. Ataxia

Disturbances of balance result from cerebellar involvement.

Clinical Manifestations

A. Early Signs—may include one or more of the following:

1. Asymmetry in motion or contour
2. Listlessness or irritability
3. Difficulty in feeding, sucking, or swallowing
4. Excessive or feeble cry
5. Long, thin infants who are slow to gain weight

B. Late Signs—may include one or more of the following:

1. Failure to follow normal pattern of motor development
   Delayed gross motor development is a universal manifestation of cerebral palsy.
2. Persistence of infantile reflexes
3. Weakness
4. Apparent preference for one hand before the infant is 12–15 months old
5. Abnormal postures
6. Delayed or defective speech
7. Evidence of mental retardation

C. Common Associated Findings

1. Seizures
2. Hearing deficiency
3. Visual defect
4. Perceptual disorders
5. Mental retardation
6. Language disorders

Diagnostic Evaluation

1. History, including prenatal and perinatal factors
2. Neurologic examination
3. Laboratory data—pneumoencephalogram or tomography may be helpful in some instances
4. Psychological testing to determine cognitive functioning
5. Psychosocial assessment, including family adaptation

Classification of Cerebral Palsy

A. Clinical Type

1. Spasticity—in 50%-60% of patients
   a. Generally appears before 6 months of age.
   b. Characterized by hypertonicity, uneven tone distribution, persistent primitive reflexes, lack or delay of normal postural control, and spastic paresis.
   c. Motor activity is impaired because of disharmony of muscle movements.
      (1) Arms
         (a) The child often holds his arm pressed against his body with the forearm bent at right angles to the upper arm and the hand bent against the forearm. The fist may be clenched tightly.
         (b) The child with mild involvement may demonstrate an overextended appearance of the fingers and rotation of the wrists when he reaches for things.
      (2) Legs—may be more (usually) or less involved than arms.
         (a) Mild case may be evident only when the child walks, demonstrating wide-based gait (with arms outstretched). The fingers may be alternately clenched and extended.
         (b) The child with moderate involvement may demonstrate slow and labored movements. Walking is jerky and unrhythmic. Balance is poor.
         (c) The child with severe involvement may be unable to sit or walk unsupported.
         (d) When both legs are involved, bilateral contractures may cause "scissoring." (The child crosses his legs and points his toes.)
2. Dyskinesia—in 20%-25% of patients
   a. Characterized by involuntary, extraneous motor activity; accentuated by emotional stress.
   b. Athetosis is the most common manifestation of this group.
      (1) Characterized by uncontrollable, jerky, irregular, twisting movements of the extremities, especially the fingers and wrists, except when at rest or asleep.
      (2) Any or all extremities may be involved.
      (3) If legs are involved, the child may walk in a writhing, lurching, stumbling manner with noticeable incoordination of the arms. When calm and well-rested, he may walk well.
3. Ataxia—in 1%-10% of patients
   a. Characterized by inability to achieve balance or awkwardness in maintaining it, with associated gross and/or fine motor incoordination.
   b. Gait is often high-stepping, stumbling, or lurching.
   c. Nystagmus is common.

d. Manifested in varying degrees depending on the pathology.
4. Mixed types—in 15%-40% of patients
   Consists of various combinations of the above types—most frequently, athetosis combined with spasticity.

B. Topographical Classification

1. *Hemiplegia*—findings are limited to 1 side of the body (35%-40% of patients); arm usually involved more than leg.
2. *Diplegia*—similar parts on both sides of the body involved (10%-20%), legs usually involved more than the arms.
3. *Paraplegia*—the legs only are involved (10%-20%).
4. *Quadriplegia*—all 4 extremities are involved (15%-20%); upper and lower extremities equally affected.
5. *Monoplegia*—only 1 extremity is involved (rare).
6. *Triplegia*—3 extremities are involved (rare).

C. Degree of Severity

1. Mild—impairment only of fine precision movement.
2. Moderate—gross and fine movements and speech are impaired, but the child is able to perform usual activities of living.
3. Severe—inability to perform adequately the usual activities of daily living (i.e., walking, using hands, communicating verbally).

Treatment

A. Goal—Normalization. The aim is to help each child reach optimal functional ability in adulthood. Broad aims of therapy include:

1. To gain optimal appearance and integration of motor function.
2. To establish locomotion, communication, and self-help skills.
3. To correct associated defects.
4. To provide opportunities for education appropriate for the individual child's needs and capabilities.

B. Management

1. Requires comprehensive evaluation and intervention, including:
   a. General health care
   b. Correction or alleviation of specific neuromotor deficits and/or associated disabilities
   c. Developmental enrichment experiences
   d. Development of prevocational, vocational, and socialization skills
   e. Emotional, behavioral, and social adjustments
2. Requires coordination and integration of the contributions of numerous health care professionals as well as societal institutions.
3. The ability of the family to carry out both supportive and participant roles in rehabilitation is a key determinant of the success of any comprehensive management program.

Prognosis

Factors influencing the prognosis
1. Extent of the manifestations
2. Existence of associated defects, especially mental retardation
3. Ability of the family to cope and to see what is right and normal about their child
4. Type and availability of community resources

Patient Problems/Nursing Diagnoses

1. Ineffective family coping: parental feelings of guilt, disappointment, grief, and/or anxiety at learning of the child's diagnosis
2. Developmental delay related to the nature and extent of the disorder
3. Self-care deficits related to the nature and extent of the disorder
4. Social isolation and coping difficulties related to the nature of the defect, the demands of daily management and resultant changes in family life
5. Knowledge deficit of care requirements
6. Potential for injury related to deficit in motor activity

Nursing Interventions

Like other children, the child with cerebral palsy receives the bulk of his care at home and within his community. The nursing role is no longer confined to care within the hospital setting. Within the expanded role, nurses are involved in working with the family on household routines, integrating the child into the family unit, and helping to "mainstream" the child into regular schools, recreational activities, dating situations, etc.

However, the child with cerebral palsy may experience several hospitalizations for diagnostic evaluation, orthopedic management, and/or medical care. The nurse should consider the following guidelines when caring for the hospitalized child with cerebral palsy:

A. Assist the parents with initial coping and with long-range adaptation to the child's disability.

1. Encourage the parents to express their feelings about the child and his diagnosis and help them to deal with these feelings.
2. Assist the parents to appraise the child's assets so that they may capitalize on these positive features.
   a. Early recognition of the extent of the child's handicap and realistic direction for obtainable goals are essential.
   b. Help the parents to recognize immediate needs and identify short-term goals which can be integrated into the long-range plan.
3. Encourage the parents to care for the child during his hospitalization so that they will feel secure about meeting his daily physical needs (feeding, exercise, braces, etc.).
   See Family-Centered Care, page 1117.
4. Introduce the parents to members of the health team who will be involved with the child's care and management.
5. Begin parental teaching about the disability.
   a. Provide the parents with appropriate reading material. Encourage their questions and provide them with the information they need.
   b. See Health Education, page 1417.
6. Assist the parents in interpreting the child's diagnosis and needs to other family members, teachers, and friends.
7. Initiate appropriate referrals.
   a. Community agencies for disabled children
   b. Community health nurse
   c. Day-care centers
   d. Clinics
   e. Local branch of the United Cerebral Palsy Association
   f. Parent groups

B. Promote the attainment of developmental milestones as much as possible.

1. Evaluate the child's developmental level and then assist him to build one skill upon another. (Refer to sections on Growth and Development and the Hospitalized Child, pp. 1074 and 1112.)
2. Provide for continuity of care from home to hospital.
   a. Obtain a thorough history from the mother regarding the child's usual home routines, and use this in planning the child's care during hospitalization.
      (1) Feeding
      (2) Sleeping
      (3) Physical therapy
      (4) Stage of growth and development
      (5) Play
      (6) Special interests, security objects, etc.
   b. Ask the parents to bring to the hospital any special devices or equipment the child uses in his daily activities.
   c. Encourage the child's parents to participate in the child's care if they so desire and if it is medically feasible (See Family-Centered Care, p. 1117).
3. Be alert for associated defects which could be corrected.
   a. Hearing
   b. Speech
   c. Vision
      (1) Squinting
      (2) Failure to follow objects
      (3) Bringing objects very close to the face

C. Provide emotional support to the parents.

1. Acknowledge the numerous challenges of daily management and the changes in family life associated with caring for a child with cerebral palsy.
2. Allow the parent(s) to express frustrations they may feel because of the many demands placed on them, with few rewards.
3. Acknowledge the parents' feelings of frustration and anger as legitimate and understandable.
4. Provide positive feedback for effective parenting skills and positive approaches to caring for the child.
5. Assist the parents to deal with siblings' responses to the disabled child.
6. Assist the parents to secure respite from the day-to-day care of the child, as appropriate.

D. Provide for the child's physical care needs.

1. Safety
   a. Evaluate the child's need for specific safety measures (suction machine, helmet, seizure precautions, etc.), and modify the environment as appropriate to ensure the child's safety.
   b. Select toys that are safe.
2. Nutrition
   a. Maintain a pleasant environment, free from distractions.
      (1) Provide a comfortable chair.
      (2) Serve the child alone, initially. After he begins to master the task of eating, he may enjoy eating with other children.
      (3) Do not attempt feedings if the child is very fatigued.
   b. Encourage independence, but do not force the child.

(1) Find the eating position in which the child can do the most for himself.

(2) Allow the child to hold the spoon even if he has to be fed with another one.

(3) Stand behind the child and reach over his shoulder to guide the spoon from the plate to his mouth.

(4) Serve foods that stick to the spoon, like thick applesauce, mashed potato, etc.

(5) Encourage finger foods that the child can handle alone.

(6) Provide appropriate special equipment for the child to use in feeding himself.

    (a) Spoon and fork with special handles

    (b) Plate and glass holders, etc.

    (c) Feeding chair

(7) Disregard "messy" eating.

    (a) Place newspapers around the feeding chair.

    (b) Use a large plastic bib or towel to protect the child's clothes.

  c. If the child must be fed, do so slowly and carefully. The child may have difficulty sucking and swallowing because he cannot control the muscles of his throat.

(1) Offer foods that the child likes.

(2) Cut solid foods into small pieces.

(3) Place the food back on the tongue for ease in swallowing.

3. Exercise

  a. Carry out appropriate exercises under the direction of the physical therapist.

  b. Use appropriate appliances to facilitate muscle control and improve body functioning.

(1) Splints

(2) Casts

(3) Braces

  c. Encourage active motions that are functionally useful.

  d. Use play (games, peg boards, puzzles, etc.) as techniques to improve coordination.

  e. Maintain good body alignment to prevent contractures.

4. Rest

  a. Avoid exciting events before rest or bedtime.

  b. Administer tranquilizing agents or anticonvulsants, etc., as prescribed by the physician.

  c. Avoid stress and frustration during the child's program of physical therapy.

E. Ensure continuity of care.

1. Communicate with representatives of all of the disciplines involved with the child's management.

2. Communicate with community agencies already involved with the child and his family (school, cerebral palsy center, community health nursing agency, etc.).

3. Formulate a consistent nursing care plan which is well coordinated with the plans and goals of related disciplines and meets the needs of the *entire* child and his family.

4. On discharge, send a report of the child's hospitalization, including a summary of nursing problems, to the appropriate community agencies.

Health Education

1. Instruct the parent in all areas of the child's physical care.

2. Reinforce teaching done by physical therapists. Assist the parents to integrate therapy into play activities.

3. Assist the parents to modify equipment and activities to facilitate home care.

4. Provide practical suggestions for feeding, holding, bathing, infant stimulation, etc.

5. The child needs regular medical and dental evaluations.

  a. It is important for the child to receive his childhood immunizations.

  b. He should be taken to the dentist every 6 months starting at the age of 2 years.

  c. He may require some adaptations of his toothbrush in order to use it effectively.

(1) The handle can be built up with a sponge or a more sophisticated enlarging device.

(2) Brushes with specially bent handles are available.

6. The child needs discipline in order to feel secure and relaxed.

  a. He should have realistic limits set, within which he can function successfully.

  b. The parents should be firm but not rejecting.

7. References for Parents:

Brightman A. Hollis. New York, Scholastic Book Services, 1978

Napear P. Brain Child, A Mother's Diary. New York, Harper & Row, 1974

Trevarton J. Amy Maura. Syracuse, Human Policy Press, 1975

United Cerebral Palsy Association, 66 E 34th Street, New York, NY 10016

Expected Outcomes

1. The parents discuss feelings with each other and with appropriate health care personnel

2. The child achieves sequential developmental milestones consistent with his condition

3. Achieves independence in feeding, dressing and personal hygiene to the extent that is possible; develops realistic goals

4. The child/family participates in activities (school, church, etc.); seeks respite care on occasion

5. The parents take an active part in learning about child's condition; make plans for future; join a support group

6. Absence of injury; child wears helmet; plays with safe toys

Hydrocephalus

Hydrocephalus is a condition of imbalance between the production of cerebrospinal fluid and its absorption over the surface of the brain into the circulatory system. It is characterized by an abnormal increase in cerebrospinal fluid volume within the intracranial cavity and by enlargement of the head in infancy.

Etiology and Incidence

1. Obstruction in the system between the source of cerebrospinal fluid production and the area of its reabsorption (the obstruction may be partial, intermittent or complete)
   a. The majority of cases are of this type
   b. Causes:
      (1) Congenital—etiology largely unknown
      (2) Acquired
         (a) Infections
         (b) Trauma
         (c) Spontaneous intracranial bleeding
         (d) Neoplasms
2. Failure in the absorption system—cause unknown
3. Excessive production of cerebrospinal fluid—tumor or unknown causes (rare)
4. Approximately 3–4 cases per 1,000 births, including those associated with spina bifida

Types of Hydrocephalus

A. Noncommunicating Hydrocephalus

An obstruction is located within or at the outlets of the ventricular system, preventing any or all of the cerebrospinal fluid from leaving the ventricles and entering the subarachnoid space.

B. Communicating Hydrocephalus

1. There is free communication between the ventricles and the subarachnoid space.
2. Abnormal reabsorption of the cerebrospinal fluid in the subarachnoid space occurs.

Altered Physiology

1. The ventricular system is greatly distended.
2. The increased ventricular pressure results in thinning of the cerebral cortex and cranial bones, especially in the frontal, parietal, and temporal areas.
3. The floor of the third ventricle commonly bulges downward, compresses the optic nerves, dilates the sella turcica, and often compresses the hypophysis cerebri.
4. The basal ganglia, brain stem, and cerebellum remain relatively normal but compressed.
5. The choroid plexus is usually atrophied to some degree.

Clinical Manifestations

1. May be rapid, slow and steadily advancing, or remittent.
2. Clinical signs depend on the age of the child, whether or not the anterior fontanelle has closed, whether the cranial sutures have fused, and the type and duration of hydrocephalus.
   a. Infants
      (1) Excessive head growth (may be seen up to 3 years of age)
      (2) Delayed closure of the anterior fontanelle Fontanelle may become tense and elevated above the surface of the skull.
      (3) Signs of increased intracranial pressure include:
         (a) Vomiting
         (b) Restlessness and irritability
         (c) High-pitched, shrill cry
         (d) Alteration in vital signs
            Increased systolic blood pressure
            Decreased pulse
            Decreased and irregular respirations
         (e) Pupillary changes
         (f) Seizures (possible)
         (g) Lethargy
         (h) Stupor
         (i) Coma
      (4) Alteration of muscle tone of the extremities
      (5) Later physical signs
         (a) Forehead becomes prominent.
         (b) Scalp appears shiny with prominent scalp veins.
         (c) Eyebrows and eyelids may be drawn upward, exposing the sclera above the iris.
         (d) Infant cannot gaze upward, causing "sunset eyes."
         (e) Strabismus, nystagmus, and optic atrophy may occur.
         (f) Infant has difficulty in holding head up.
         (g) Child may experience physical and/or mental developmental lag.
   b. Older children who have closed sutures
      (1) Signs of increased intracranial pressure include:
         (a) Headache
         (b) Vomiting
         (c) Lethargy, fatigue, apathy
         (d) Personality changes
         (e) Separation of cranial sutures (may be seen in children up to 10 years of age)
         (f) Double vision, constricted peripheral vision, sudden appearance of internal strabismus, pupillary changes
         (g) Alteration in vital signs similar to those seen in infants
         (h) Difficulty with gait
         (i) Stupor
         (j) Coma

Diagnostic Evaluation

1. Transillumination of the infant's head may show varying degrees of localized glowing indicative of abnormal fluid collection.
2. Percussion of the infant's skull may produce a typical "cracked pot" sound (Macewen's sign).
3. Ophthalmoscopy may reveal papilledema.
4. CAT scan (computed tomography) provides a noninvasive means of diagnosing some types of hydrocephalus by computer analysis of x-ray transmission data. It is the diagnostic tool of choice.
5. Ventriculography (rarely used)—abnormalities are visualized in the ventricular system or the subarachnoid space.
6. Pneumoencephalography (rarely used)
   a. Dilated ventricles
   b. Extent of the brain damage and the location of the obstruction
7. Radiologic findings show the following:
   a. Widening of the fontanelle and sutures
   b. Erosion of intracranial bone

Surgical Treatment

A. General Techniques

1. Direct operation on the lesion causing the obstruction (rarely feasible).
2. Intracranial shunts—useful in selected cases of noncommunicating hydrocephalus to divert fluid from the obstructed segment of the ventricular system to the subarachnoid space beyond the block.

3. Extracranial shunts—divert fluid from the ventricular system to an extracranial compartment, frequently the peritoneum or right atrium. Preferred method for treating most cases of communicating hydrocephalus and cases of noncommunicating hydrocephalus not amenable to direct surgery or intracranial shunts.

B. **Common Extracranial Shunt Procedures**

1. Ventriculoperitoneal shunt (V–P shunt)
   a. Diverts cerebrospinal fluid from a lateral ventricle or the spinal subarachnoid space to the peritoneal cavity.
   b. A tube is passed from the lateral ventricle through an occipital burr hole subcutaneously through the posterior aspect of neck and paraspinal region to the peritoneal cavity through a small incision in the right lower quadrant.
2. Ventriculoatrial shunt (V–A shunt)
   a. A tube is passed from the dilated lateral ventricle through a burr hole in the parietal region of the skull.
   b. It is then passed under the skin behind the ear and into a vein down to a point where it discharges into the right atrium or superior vena cava.
   c. The tube passes at one point through a one-way pressure sensitive system.
   d. The valve or valves close to prevent reflux of blood into the ventricle and open as ventricular pressure rises, allowing fluid to pass from the ventricle into the bloodstream.
3. *Complications*
   a. Need for shunt revision frequently occurs because of occlusion, infection, or malfunction.
   b. Shunt revision may be necessary because of growth of the child. Newer models, however, include coiled tubing to allow the shunt to grow with the child.
   c. Shunt dependency frequently occurs. The child rapidly manifests symptoms of increased intracranial pressure if the shunt does not function properly.
   d. Children with ventriculoatrial shunts may experience endocardial contusions and clotting leading to bacterial endocarditis, bacteremia and ventriculitis, or thromboembolism and cor pulmonale.
   e. Late complications occur with discouraging frequency the longer an operative series is followed.

Prognosis

1. Prognosis is dependent on early diagnosis and prompt therapy.
2. The outcome of treatment depends on the time it is begun, the success of the surgical procedure, good follow-up care, and the child's innate motor and intellectual capabilities.
   a. With improved diagnostic and management techniques, the prognosis is becoming considerably better. Many children experience normal motor and intellectual development.
   b. The severity of neurologic deficits is directly proportional to the interval between onset and the time of diagnosis.
3. Spontaneous arrest sometimes occurs as a result of natural compensatory mechanisms or rupture of the ventricle into the subarachnoid space.
4. A child with postmeningitic hydrocephalus might also undergo spontaneous remission following gradual disappearance of adhesions.
5. Approximately two thirds of patients will die at an early age if they are not given surgical treatment.

Patient Problems/Nursing Diagnoses

1. Potential for neurologic complications related to increased intracranial pressure and shunt failure
2. Infection related to bacterial infiltration of the shunt
3. Potential for skin breakdown and contractures related to immobility
4. Alteration in nutrition/electrolyte balance related to reduced oral intake and vomiting
5. Parental anxiety related to the diagnosis and surgery
6. Knowledge deficit about hydrocephalus and its treatment

Preoperative Nursing Interventions

A. **Observe for and record disease progress.**

1. Measure head.
   a. Measure at the occipitofrontal circumference (OFC)—point of largest measurement.
   b. Measure the head at approximately the same time each day.
   c. Use a centimeter measure for greatest accuracy.
2. Observe for evidence of increased intracranial pressure. Note especially:
   a. Vomiting
   b. Changes in vital signs
      (1) Increased systolic blood pressure
      (2) Decreased pulse rate
      (3) Decreased or irregular respirations
   c. Pupillary changes
   d. Change in level of consciousness
3. Note especially these changes in appearance:
   a. Increased head size, prominent forehead (noticeable over days or weeks)
   b. "Sunset" eyes
   c. Opisthotonic positioning—occurs with brain stem herniation

B. **Provide adequate nutrition.**

1. Feeding is often a problem because the child may be listless, anorectic, and prone to vomiting.
2. Complete nursing care and treatments before feeding so that the child will not be disturbed after feeding.
3. Hold the infant in a semi-sitting position with head well supported during feeding. Allow ample time for bubbling.
4. Offer small, frequent feedings.
5. Place the child on his side with his head elevated after feeding to prevent aspiration.

C. **Assist with diagnostic procedures.**

1. Be familiar with the procedure that is being performed (see diagnostic tests).
2. Explain the procedure to the child and his parents at their levels of comprehension.
   a. Make certain that they understand what will happen before and after as well as during the procedure.
   b. Play is frequently helpful for explaining the procedure to a young child.
3. Administer prescribed sedatives.
   a. Give the sedative exactly at the prescribed time to ensure its effectiveness.
   b. Organize activities so that the child is permitted to rest after administration of the medications.

▶ **NURSING ALERT:** Sedatives are contraindicated in many cases because of increased intracranial pressure. If they are administered, the child should be observed very closely for evidence of respiratory depression.

4. Apply protective measures to limit motion as necessary (see section on pediatric procedures: restraints, p. 1142, and positioning for a lumbar puncture, p. 1158).
5. Observe the child closely following the procedure for:
   a. Leaking of cerebrospinal fluid from the sites of subdural or ventricular taps
      These tap holes should be covered with a small piece of gauze or cotton saturated with collodion.
   b. Reactions to the sedative, especially respiratory depression
   c. Changes in vital signs indicative of shock
   d. Signs of increased intracranial pressure which may occur if air has been injected into the ventricles.

D. **Provide supportive nursing care as indicated by the child's condition.** (Without treatment, the child becomes more helpless as head size increases.)

1. Prevent pressure sores and the development of contractures.
   a. Place the child on a sponge rubber or lamb's wool pad or an alternating-pressure mattress to keep his weight evenly distributed.
   b. Keep the scalp clean and dry.
   c. Turn the child's head frequently; change his position every 2 hours.
      (1) When turning the child, rotate his head and body together to prevent strain on the neck.
      (2) A firm pillow may be placed under the head and shoulders for further support when lifting the child.
   d. Provide meticulous skin care to all parts of the body.
      (1) Observe the skin for evidence of pressure sores.
      (2) Pressure sores on the head are a frequent problem.
   e. Give passive range-of-motion exercises to the extremities, especially the legs.
2. Keep the eyes moistened if the child is unable to close his eyelids normally. This prevents corneal ulcerations and infections.
3. Provide for the child's emotional need for love and affection.
   a. Hold and cuddle the infant as much as possible.
   b. Play with the child according to his mental development.

E. **Provide emotional support to the parents.**

1. Encourage the parents to visit and to participate in the child's care as much as possible.
2. Encourage the parents to talk about the child's problem and how they feel about it. Parents are generally fearful of any procedure involving the brain, and may have fears about mental retardation or brain damage.
3. Provide the parents with appropriate information concerning the defect. Answer their questions directly and honestly. Correct any misconceptions that they may have such as fear that the child's head may burst.

Postoperative Nursing Interventions

A. **Provide immediate supportive nursing care.**

1. Monitor the child's temperature, pulse, respiration, blood pressure, and pupillary size and reaction every 15 minutes until fully reactive; then monitor every 1–2 hours.
2. Avoid hypothermia or hyperthermia.
   a. Provide appropriate blankets or covers as indicated by body temperature.
   b. An Isolette or warming cradle may be used for an infant.
   c. An older child may profit from use of the hypothermia blanket.
   d. Administer a tepid sponge bath or antipyretic medication for temperature elevation (see section on fever, p. 1137).
3. Aspirate mucus from the nose and throat as necessary to prevent respiratory difficulty.
4. Turn the child every 2 hours.
5. Use a nasogastric tube if necessary for abdominal distention.
   a. This is most frequently used when a ventriculoperitoneal shunt has been performed.
   b. Measure the drainage and record the amount and color.
6. Give frequent mouth care to prevent dryness of the mucous membranes.
7. Observe for pallor or mottled condition of the skin, coldness, or clamminess of the body and decreased level of consciousness.
8. Administer prescribed prophylactic antibiotics.

B. **Allow for optimal draining of cerebrospinal fluid through the shunt.**

1. Pump the shunt and position the child as directed by the physician.
   a. If pumping is prescribed, carefully compress the valve the specified number of times at regularly scheduled intervals.
   b. Report any difficulties in pumping the shunt to the physician.

C. **Prevent the development of pressure sores on the skin overlying the shunt reservoir.**

1. Place cotton behind and over the ears under the head dressing.
2. Avoid positioning the child on the area of the valve or the incision until the wound is well healed.

D. **Maintain fluid and electrolyte balance.**

1. Accurately measure and record total fluid intake and output.
2. Administer intravenous fluids as prescribed (see procedure, p. 1160).
3. Begin oral feedings once the child is fully recovered from the anesthetic and displays interest.
   a. Begin with small amounts of 5% dextrose and water.
   b. Gradually introduce formula.
   c. Introduce solid foods suitable to the child's age and tolerance (see section on nutrition, p. 1145).
   d. Encourage a high protein diet.

E. Observe for signs of complications.

1. Increased intracranial pressure indicates shunt malfunction (see listing of symptoms under clinical manifestations).
   a. Older children should also be observed for changes in customary behavior, sleep patterns, and developmental capabilities.
2. Dehydration may be manifested in the following ways:
   a. Sunken fontanelle (Without additional signs of dehydration, this may indicate only a successful shunt.)
   b. Decreased urine output, increased specific gravity
   c. Diminished skin turgor and dryness of mucous membranes
   d. Lethargy
3. Infection may be manifested by:
   a. Fever (Temperature normally fluctuates during the first 24 hours after surgery.)
   b. Purulent drainage from the incision
   c. Swelling, redness, and tenderness along the shunt tract
4. Excessive drainage of fluid from the cranial cavity, manifested by
   a. Sunken fontanelle, agitation, restlessness (infant)
   b. Decreased level of consciousness (older child)

F. Provide continued emotional support to the parents.

1. Begin discharge planning early (see Health Education).
2. Accompany all instructions with reassurance necessary to prevent the parents from becoming anxious or fearful about assuming the care of the child.
   Describe the success that other mothers have had in dealing with similar infants.
3. Encourage the parents to treat the child as normally as possible, providing him with appropriate toys and love.
4. Help the parents with problems of assisting siblings and grandparents to deal with the child's needs.
5. Initiate appropriate referrals.
   a. Social worker
   b. Community health nurse
   c. Parent groups
   d. Community agencies
   e. Specialty clinics and schools

Health Education

1. Parents should be given complete explanations of the disease, the surgery, the changes that the surgery

may produce, and the follow-up care that will be required.
2. Physical nursing care
   a. Special attention should be directed toward specific techniques of supportive nursing care, for example:
      (1) Turning
      (2) Skin care
      (3) Play
      (4) Exercises to strengthen the child's muscles
   b. Feeding techniques and patterns
   c. Pumping of shunt
3. Symptoms of increased intracranial pressure, shunt malfunction, infection, and dehydration must be treated. Parents should be taught not only to recognize these complications (see prior listing of signs of complications) but also to report them immediately to the physician.
4. Illnesses that cause vomiting and diarrhea or that prevent an adequate fluid intake are a great threat to the child who has had a shunt procedure. The parents should be instructed regarding:
   a. Prevention of such illnesses
   b. Early recognition of warning symptoms
   c. Necessity of seeking immediate medical care so that the child can receive intravenous therapy to replace fluid and electrolyte loss
5. The child's emotional needs should be stressed. Parents should be encouraged to treat the child as normally as possible. Generally, few restrictions need to be placed on his daily activities.
6. If appropriate, refer to the section on mental retardation for additional areas of parent teaching (see p. 1475).

Expected Outcomes

1. Avoids neurologic complications; no changes in vital signs or head size; parents recognize early signs of increased intracranial pressure
2. Shows no signs of developing infection; shunt site appears clean; vital signs stable
3. Maintains skin integrity and musculoskeletal function
4. Maintains adequate nutritional status; normal tissue turgor; normal serum electrolyte values; absence of vomiting
5. The parents discuss their feelings about hydrocephalus and surgery with one another and with appropriate health professionals
6. Parents verbalize an understanding of the cause and consequence of hydrocephalus and its treatment

Spina Bifida

Spina bifida refers to a malformation of the spine in which the posterior portion of the laminae of the vertebrae fails to close. Several types of spina bifida are recognized, of which the following 3 are most common (Fig. 43-1):

1. *Spina bifida occulta*, in which the defect is only in the vertebrae. The spinal cord and meninges are normal.
2. *Meningocele*, in which the meninges protrude

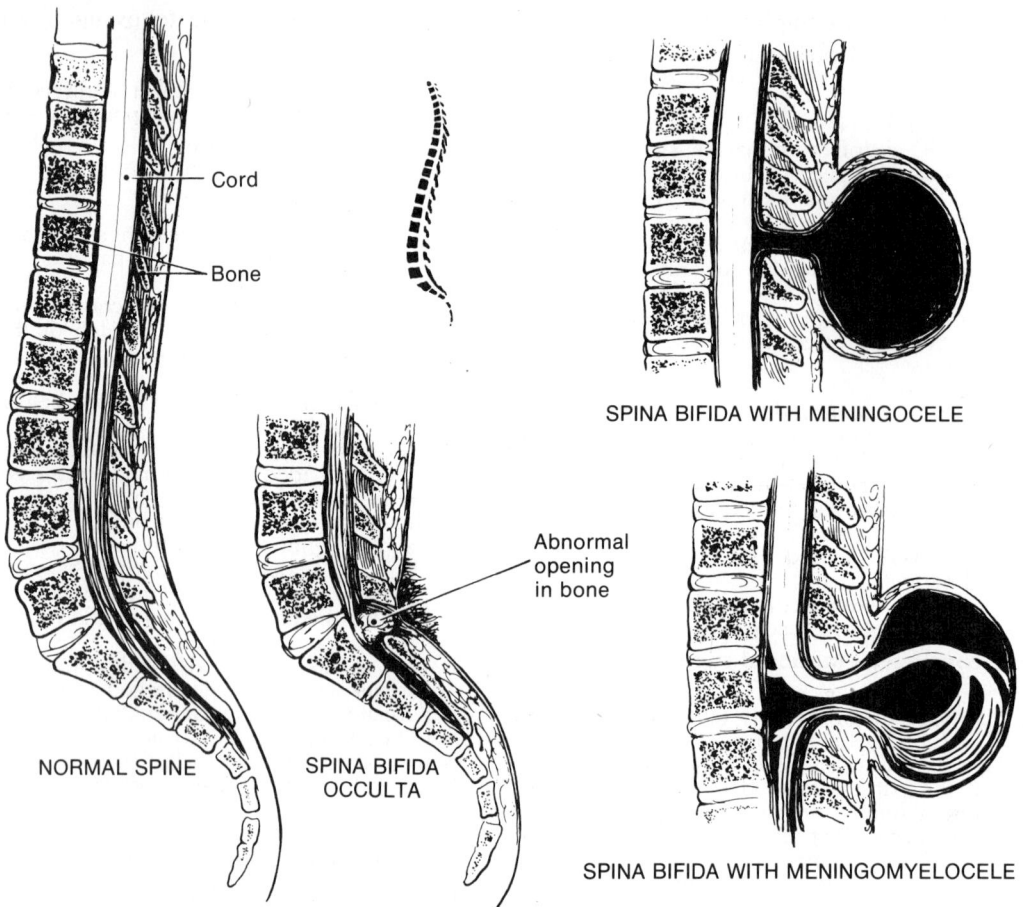

Figure 43-1. Spina bifida. (From Spina Bifida: Hope Through Research, PHS Pub. No. 1023, Health Information Series No. 103, 1970)

through the opening in the spinal canal, forming a cyst filled with cerebrospinal fluid and covered with skin.
3. *Meningomyelocele* (or myelomeningocele), in which both the spinal cord and cord membranes protrude through the defect in the laminae of the spinal canal. Meningomyeloceles are covered by a thin membrane.

Etiology

1. Unknown but generally thought to result from genetic predisposition triggered by something in the environment.
2. Involves an arrest in the orderly formation of the vertebral arches and spinal cord that occurs between the 4th and 6th week of embryogenesis.
   Theories of causation:
   (1) There is incomplete closure of the neural tube during the 4th week of embryonic life.
   (2) The neural tube forms adequately but then ruptures.

Incidence

1. Geographical distribution and incidence vary widely.
2. Condition occurs in approximately 1 per 1,000 live births in the US.

3. Most common developmental defect of the central nervous system.
4. More common in Caucasians than in nonwhite population.
5. Condition may have other congenital anomalies associated with it.
6. Women who have spina bifida and parents who have one affected child have an increased risk of producing children with neural tube defects.

Altered Physiology and Clinical Manifestations

A. Spina Bifida Occulta

1. Most common type; may occur in as many as 25% of otherwise normal children.
2. The bony defect may range from a very thin slit separating one lamina from the spinous process to a complete absence of the spines and laminae.
3. A thin, fibrous membrane sometimes covers the defect.
4. The spinal cord and its meninges may be connected with a fistulous tract extending to and opening onto the surface of the skin.
5. Most patients have no symptoms.

a. They may have a dimple in the skin or a growth of hair over the malformed vertebra.

b. There is no externally visible sac.

c. With growth, the child may develop foot weakness or bowel and bladder sphincter disturbances.

B. Meningocele

1. An external cystic defect can be seen in the spinal cord, usually in the center line.
   a. The sac is composed only of meninges and is filled with cerebrospinal fluid.
   b. The cord and nerve roots are usually normal.
2. The defect may occur anywhere on the cord. Higher defects (from thorax and up) are usually meningoceles.
3. There is seldom evidence of weakness of the legs or lack of sphincter control.
4. Surgical correction is necessary to prevent rupture of the sac and subsequent infection.
5. Hydrocephalus may be an associated finding and may be aggravated after surgery for a meningocele.
   a. Occurs in about 9% of patients.
   b. Usually not associated with the Arnold–Chiari malformation.
6. Prognosis is good with surgical correction.

C. Meningomyelocele (Myelomeningocele)

1. Most common type of open spinal defect—occurs 4–5 times more frequently than meningocele.
2. A round, raised, and poorly epithelialized area may be noted at any level of the spinal column. However, the highest incidence of the lesion occurs in the lumbosacral area.
3. The lesion contains both the spinal cord and cord membranes. A bluish area may be evident on the top because of exposed neural tissue.
4. The sac may leak in utero or may rupture after birth, allowing free drainage of cerebrospinal fluid. This renders the child highly susceptible to meningitis.
5. Prognosis
   a. Influenced by the site of the lesion and the presence and degree of associated hydrocephalus. Generally, the higher the defect, the greater the extent of neurologic deficit and the greater the likelihood of hydrocephalus.
   b. In the absence of treatment, most infants with meningomyelocele die early in infancy.
   c. Surgical intervention is most effective if it is done early in the neonatal period, preferably within the first few hours of life.
   d. Even with surgical intervention, infants can be expected to manifest associated neurosurgical, orthopedic, and/or urologic problems.
   e. New techniques of treatment, intensive research, and improved services have increased life expectancy and have greatly enhanced the quality of life for most children who receive treatment for the defect.

Clinical Problems Commonly Associated with Meningomyelocele

A. Neurologic Problems

1. Arnold–Chiari malformation
   a. Associated malformation involving the brain stem and cerebellum.
   b. Causes a block in the flow of cerebrospinal fluid through the ventricles and leads to failure in the reabsorption mechanism of cerebrospinal fluid.
   c. Produces significant hydrocephalus in approximately two-thirds of children with meningomyelocele.
2. Loss of motor control and sensation below the level of the lesion.
   These conditions are highly variable and depend on the size of the lesion and its position on the cord. For example:
   a. A low thoracic lesion may cause total flaccid paralysis below the waist.
   b. A small sacral lesion may cause only patchy spots of decreased sensation in the feet.

B. Mobility and Orthopedic Problems

1. Contractures may occur in the ankles, knees, and/or hips. Hips may be pulled out of the sockets.
   a. Nature and degree of involvement depends on size and location of lesion.
   b. Occurs because some threads of innervation do get through. One side of a hip, knee, or ankle may be innervated while the opposing side may not be. The unopposed side then becomes pulled out of position.
2. Clubfeet are a common accompanying anomaly.
   This anomaly is thought to be related to the position of paraplegic feet in the uterus.
3. Scoliosis is common in later years.
   a. Occurs in approximately 50% of patients.
   b. Caused by the congenital lesion in the spinal column.
4. Ambulation and ability to be upright are possible through various types of bracing and equipment.
   Extent of bracing will depend on extent of sensory and motor loss. Children with low sacral lesions can ambulate with small, short leg braces. Older children with significant loss may choose to use a wheelchair.

C. Urologic Problems

1. Almost all lesions affect the sacral nerves that innervate the bladder. The bladder fails to respond to normal messages that it is time to void, and simply fills and overflows. Usually, the bladder does not empty completely, causing two sets of problems:
   a. Susceptibility to urinary tract infections because of constant stasis
   b. Incontinence, because the bladder is never completely empty and fails to receive signals to void
2. Management
   a. Children must be followed routinely with IVP, voiding cystoureterogram, urine culture and sensitivity. BUN and creatinine levels must be measured to assess renal status.
   b. Continence management
      (1) Usually achieved with clean, intermittent self-catheterization.
         (a) Children can generally be taught to catheterize themselves by the age of 6–7 years.
         (b) Parents can catheterize younger children.
      (2) Surgically implanted mechanical urinary sphincters and bladder pacemakers are being used with increasing frequency.
      (3) Indwelling catheters or external collecting devices are used by some children.
      (4) Urinary diversion may be necessary in some cases.

c. Medications
(1) Antibiotics are used periodically or prophylactically to prevent urinary tract infections.
(2) Medications such as imipramine hydrochloride (Tofranil) and ephedrine sulfate are used to help children retain their urine until it can be voided at one time (rather than to dribble continuously). When self-catheterization is used in conjunction with medication, many children can stay dry for 3–4 hours at a time.
d. Dietary recommendations
(1) Adequate fluid intake is essential to maintain good urinary flow.
(2) Foods such as cranberry juice or medications such as vitamin C are often prescribed to acidify the urine thus preventing stone formation.
e. The ability to stay dry for reasonable time intervals is one of the greatest factors in enhancing self-esteem and positive body image.

D. Bowel Problems

1. Fecal incontinence and constipation are promoted by poor innervation of the anal sphincter and bowel musculature.
2. To compensate for decreased sensation, children are placed on a toileting schedule and are taught to push. Medications such as stool softeners, suppositories, or enemas may be utilized to help determine scheduling.
3. Remaining unconstipated is essential to any type of fecal control. High-bulk, high-fiber, and/or high-fluid diets as well as medications may be used to increase bulk or soften stool.

E. Skin Problems

1. Areas of decreased sensation have a tendency to break down. Braces and shoes should be checked frequently for rubbing.
2. During hospitalization, the nurse should be particularly watchful for areas of skin breakdown. The use of air mattresses, lamb's wool, and other similar materials may help to prevent skin breakdown in bedridden children.

F. Dietary Problems

1. Many children become overweight because of activity limitations.
2. Dietary control is necessary to prevent obesity.

G. Developmental Problems

1. Most children have average intellectual ability despite hydrocephalus.
a. Most children are able to learn in a "mainstreamed" normal school, provided they are able to overcome other barriers (architectural and attitudinal).
2. The most significant problems are secondarily handicapping conditions that develop when a child has a disability of this degree.
3. Disabled children need exposure to all activities and to rules and regulations for the nondisabled.

Prevention and Treatment of Meningomyelocele

A. Prenatal Detection

Prenatal detection is now possible through amniocentesis and measurement of alphafetoprotein. This testing should be offered to all women at risk (women who are affected themselves or have had other affected children).

B. Surgical Intervention

1. Procedure
Laminectomy and closure of the open lesion and/or removal of the sac usually can be done soon after birth.
2. Purpose
a. To prevent further deterioration of neural function
b. To minimize the danger of rupture and infection, especially meningitis
c. To improve cosmetic effect
d. To facilitate handling of the infant by parents and nurses

C. Multidisciplinary Follow-up for Associated Problems

1. A coordinated team approach will help maximize the physical and mental potential of each affected child.
a. A group of health care personnel (including a neurologist, neurosurgeon, orthopedic surgeon, urologist, pediatrician, nurse, social worker, and physical therapist) should be available to the child and family.
b. A continuing, stable relationship with one person on the health care team who is coordinating efforts for the child is of great benefit.
2. Numerous neurosurgical, orthopedic, and urologic procedures and operations may be necessary to help the child achieve his maximum potential.

Patient Problems/Nursing Diagnoses

1. Parental difficulties in bonding related to the birth of a defective child
2. Potential for infection related to contamination of the meningomyelocele site or urinary stasis
3. Fecal incontinence/constipation related to impaired innervation of anal sphincter and bowel musculature
4. Potential for skin breakdown related to immobility and reduced sensation
5. Excessive weight related to inactivity
6. Potential developmental problems related to neurologic deficits or locomotion restrictions
7. Body-image concerns related to the child's appearance, difficulties with locomotion, and lack of control over excretory functions
8. Prolonged dependence related to need for help in physical care and transportation
9. Family stress related to long-term demands of caring for a disabled child

Preoperative Nursing Interventions for Initial Surgery in the Neonatal Period

A. Prevent leakage of cerebrospinal fluid or rupture of the sac or lesion.

1. Position the infant on his abdomen.
a. Avoid placing the infant on his back, because this would cause pressure on the sac.
b. A Bradford frame may be used to facilitate positioning (see procedure for the use of the Bradford frame, p. 1206).
c. Check the position of the child at least once every hour.
2. Do not place a diaper or other covering directly over the sac.
3. A doughnut-shaped sterile padding may be placed around the sac.

4. Observe the sac frequently for evidence of irritation or leakage of cerebrospinal fluid.

B. Prevent infection.

1. Infection of the sac
   a. This is most commonly caused by contamination by urine and feces.
   b. Keep the buttocks and genitalia scrupulously clean.
      (1) Do not diaper the infant if the defect is in the lower portion of the spine.
      (2) Utilize a divided Bradford frame to allow urine and feces to drain away from the body (see technique, p. 1206).
      (3) A small plastic drape taped between the defect and the anus may help to prevent contamination.
   c. A sterile gauze pad or towel or a sterile, moistened dressing may be applied according to the physician's preference.
      (1) When the sterile covering is used, it should be changed frequently to keep the area free of exudate and to maintain sterility.
      (2) Care must be taken to prevent the covering from adhering to and damaging the sac.
2. Infection of the bladder and urinary tract
   a. Infection is frequently caused by stasis of urine.
   b. Use the Credé method for emptying the bladder if recommended by the physician.
      (1) Apply firm, gentle pressure to the abdomen, beginning in the umbilical area and progressing toward the symphysis pubis.
      (2) Continue the procedure as long as urine can be manually expressed.
      (3) This technique is often contraindicated for infants with vesicoureteral reflux.
   c. Encourage fluid intake to dilute the urine.
   d. Administer prescribed prophylactic antibiotics.

C. Prevent deformities and ulcerations of lower extremities.

1. Maintain the infant in the prone position with hips only slightly flexed to decrease tension on the sac.
2. Place a foam rubber pad covered with a soft cloth between the infant's legs to maintain the hips in abduction and to prevent or counteract subluxation. A diaper roll or small pillow may be used in place of the foam rubber pad.
3. Allow the baby's feet to hang freely over the pads or mattress edge to prevent aggravation of foot deformities.
4. Change the infant's position when permissible to relieve pressure.
5. Provide meticulous skin care to all areas of the body—especially ankles, knees, tip of nose, cheeks, and chin.
6. Provide passive range-of-motion exercises for those muscles and joints that the infant does not use spontaneously. Hip exercises should not be done unless recommended by the physician.
7. Use a foam or fleece pad to reduce pressure of the mattress against the infant's skin.

D. Provide adequate nutrition and hydration.

1. Hold the infant for feedings if permissible. This provides the needed position change and affection and facilitates feeding.
   Position the infant in such a way that pressure on the back is eliminated. This may be accomplished by holding the infant in a normal feeding position with elbow rotated to avoid touching the sac. Alternatives include feeding the infant on his side or while he is prone on the nurse's lap.
2. The child who must be fed in the prone position should have his head turned to one side and tilted upward.
3. Stop the feeding frequently so that the baby can rest and air can be expelled.
   a. These infants cannot be bubbled in the same way as normal babies.
   b. Small, frequent feedings may be necessary.
4. Monitor the infant's weight pattern to ensure adequate gain.

E. Provide normal infant stimulation.

1. Establish eye contact with the infant by sitting at the crib with your face at the level of his.
2. Provide appropriate toys, such as bright mobiles or musical toys.
3. Refer to section on growth and development, page 1074.

F. Monitor neurologic status and observe for signs of complications.

1. Hydrocephalus
   a. Irritability
   b. Feeding difficulty, vomiting, decreased appetite
   c. Increased head circumference
   d. Tense fontanelle
   e. Temperature fluctuations
   f. Decreased alertness
2. Infection
   a. Oozing of fluid or pus from the sac
   b. Fever
   c. Irritability or listlessness
   d. Convulsions
   e. Concentrated or foul-smelling urine
3. Record the following:
   a. Frequent vital signs
   b. Behavior of the infant
   c. Movement of the legs
   d. Degree of continence
   e. Evidence of urine retention or fecal impaction
   f. Daily measurement of head circumference
   g. Evidence of complications

G. Provide initial emotional support to the family.

1. Encourage the parents to talk about their child and how they feel about the defect.
2. Provide them with basic information about the condition.
3. Encourage them to become involved with the child's care from the beginning.
   a. Demonstrate techniques for holding and feeding the child and for providing routine care.
   b. Emphasize what is *normal* and *well* about their infant.
4. Initiate communication with appropriate members of the multidisciplinary team that manages infants with these problems.

For nursing management of the infant with hydrocephalus or clubfoot, refer to Hydrocephalus, page 1419, and Clubfoot, page 1450, in the pediatric section.

Postoperative Nursing Interventions

A. Prevent postoperative complications.

1. Shock
   a. Keep the infant warm by placing him in an Isolette or infant warmer.

2. Respiratory problems
   a. Periodically change the infant's position if permitted by his condition and by the extent of surgery.
   b. Have oxygen available if necessary.
   c. Report abdominal distention which may interfere with breathing and feeding.
3. Nutritional problems
   a. The infant may be fed intravenously for several days or may be fed via gavage if he is unable to take oral feedings (see procedures for intravenous therapy, p. 1160, and gavage feeding, p. 1148).
   b. Apply previously stated principles when bottle-feeding the infant.
4. Infection
   a. Keep the surgical dressing clean and dry.
   b. Observe the dressing frequently for drainage.
   c. Apply previously stated principles to prevent infection.
   d. Administer prescribed antibiotics.
5. Nursing observations—record the following:
   a. Frequent measurements of temperature, pulse, and respiration
   b. Color
   c. Neurologic status
   d. Evidence of abdominal distention
   e. Condition of dressing
   f. Evidence of infection
   g. Degree of continence
   h. Behavior of the infant
   i. Evidence of hydrocephalus

B. Continue appropriate preoperative nursing activities.

1. Once the infant's back is well healed, he may be placed in a supine position for brief periods, which are gradually increased as the skin tolerates it.
2. The infant may also be positioned on his side at no more than a 45-degree angle for brief periods. This position, however, has the disadvantage of placing the hips in flexion and reduces the desirable use of the arms.
3. Special positioning may be requested by the orthopedic surgeon or the physical therapist.
4. Bikini diapers may be used once the back is well healed.

C. Provide continued emotional support to the family.

1. Encourage continued participation by parents in the infant's care.
2. Facilitate communication and interaction with appropriate members of the multidisciplinary clinic for birth defects.
   It is essential that open lines of communication exist between clinic members and the staff that provides daily care for the infant. This ensures that families receive consistent information and facilitates continuity of care.
3. If a multidisciplinary team is not available, initiate appropriate individual referrals—to social worker, clergyman, community health nurse, physical therapist, etc.
4. Foster the goal of helping the child to become as independent as possible.
   a. Emphasize habilitation which makes use of the normal parts of the body and minimizes the disabilities.

b. Focus on immediate planning in areas such as ambulating and bowel and bladder management.
5. Begin discharge teaching early (see below).
6. Provide support for dealing with the usual problems of a newborn baby. Answer questions related to formula, bath, problems of growth and development, and discipline.

Health Education

1. Prepare the parents to feed, hold, and stimulate their infant as normally as possible.
   Include information related to the management of the usual neonatal problems such as bathing, feeding, formula preparation, and sleeping (see section on growth and development, p. 1074).
2. Teach the parents any special techniques that may be required for the infant's physical care. Examples:
   a. Methods of holding and positioning the infant
   b. Techniques of feeding
   c. Care of the incision
   d. Provision for adequate elimination:
      (1) Procedure for bladder Credé method
      (2) Administration of prescribed prophylactic antibiotics
      (3) Signs of constipation and alleviation of the problem through diet regulation
   e. Physical therapy exercises if prescribed
3. Infant stimulation
   Teach the parents ways to help the infant to accomplish developmental tasks of his age level within the limits imposed by his disabilities.
4. Safety
   The child with decreased sensation in the extremities should be protected from prolonged pressure, from burns or trauma due to bath water that is too warm, and from contact with hot or sharp objects.
5. Familiarize the parents with signs of associated problems, especially signs of increased intracranial pressure or shunt malfunction and signs of infection.
   Instruct the parents to notify the physician if a problem does occur.
6. Be certain that a mechanism is developed for the family to receive continued support and teaching following discharge.
   a. This is best provided through a birth defects center.
   b. A community health nursing referral is helpful for many families.
7. References for Parents:
   Allum N. Spina Bifida: The Treatment and Care of Spina Bifida Children. London, George Allen and Unwin, 1975
   Pieper E. The Teacher and the Child With Spina Bifida. Chicago, Spina Bifida Association of America, 1977
   Reid R. My Children, My Children. New York, Harcourt Brace Jovanovich, 1977
   White P. Janet At School. New York, Thomas Y Crowell, 1978
   Swinyard C. The Child With Spina Bifida. Chicago, Spina Bifida Association of America, 1977
8. Agencies:
   March of Dimes Birth Defects Foundation, 1375 Mamaroneck Avenue, White Plains, NY 10605
   Spina Bifida Association of America, 343 S Dearborn Avenue, Chicago, IL 60604

Expected Outcomes

1. The parents demonstrate bonding in their interaction with the infant
2. Avoids infection; signs of infection are recognized promptly and treatment is initiated
3. Adjusts to toileting schedule; eating diet high in fiber; maintains adequate fluid intake
4. Maintains skin integrity; avoids prolonged pressure; checks potential pressure areas from braces or prolonged sitting
5. Attains/maintains normal weight; adheres to dietary regimen
6. Accomplishes appropriate developmental tasks within limits imposed by disability
7. Attains/maintains a positive body image evidenced by verbal and nonverbal communication
8. Achieves maximum independence within limits imposed by his disability
9. The family discusses feelings associated with caring for disabled child; seeks help when necessary

Bacterial Meningitis

Bacterial meningitis is an inflammation of the meninges that follows the invasion of the spinal fluid by a bacterial agent.

Etiology

1. The proportion of cases due to a specific organism varies from year to year; there is also considerable geographic difference.
2. The organisms most commonly causing bacterial meningitis in different age-groups are:
   a. Birth–2 months
      Escherichia coli
      Streptococcus, group B
   b. 2 months–3 years
      Haemophilus influenzae
      Streptococcus pneumoniae
      Neisseria meningitidis
   c. 3–16 years
      Streptococcus pneumoniae
      Neisseria meningitidis

Altered Physiology

1. Bacterial meningitis is almost always preceded by an upper respiratory infection, which is complicated by bacteremia.
2. Bacteria in the circulating blood then invade the spinal fluid.
3. Bacterial meningitis may occur as an extension of a local bacterial infection such as otitis media, mastoiditis, or sinusitis (less common).
4. Bacteria may also gain direct entry through a penetrating wound, spinal tap, surgery, or anatomic abnormalities.
5. The infective process results in inflammation, exudation, and varying degrees of tissue damage in the brain.

Clinical Manifestations

1. Signs and symptoms are variable, depending on the patient's age, the etiologic agent, and the duration of the illness when diagnosed.
   a. Infants less than 1 month of age display the following symptoms:
      (1) Irritability
      (2) Lethargy
      (3) Vomiting
      (4) Lack of appetite
      (5) Seizures
      (6) High-pitched cry
   b. Infants up to 2 years of age manifest symptoms similar to those of the young infant and in addition may have:
      (1) Fever
      (2) Tenseness of the fontanelle
      (3) Neck rigidity
      (4) Positive Kernig's and/or Brudzinski's signs
         (a) *Kernig's sign*
            With the child in the supine position and knees flexed, the leg is flexed at the hip so that the thigh is brought to a position perpendicular to the trunk. An attempt is then made to extend the knee. If meningeal irritation is present, this cannot be done and attempts to extend the knee result in pain.
         (b) *Brudzinski's sign*
            Spontaneous flexion of the lower limbs following passive flexion of the neck.
   c. Children over 2 years of age:
      (1) Common initial symptoms
         (a) Vomiting
         (b) Headache
         (c) Mental confusion
         (d) Lethargy
      (2) Later symptoms
         (a) Neck rigidity within 12–24 hours after onset
         (b) Positive Kernig's and/or Brudzinski's sign
         (c) Seizures
         (d) Progressive decline in responsiveness
2. Onset may be insidious or fulminant.
3. Petechiae or purpura may develop.
   a. Characteristic skin lesions are most often observed in cases of meningococcal or *Pseudomonas* infection.
   b. Hemorrhagic rashes may occur in any child with overwhelming bacterial sepsis because of disseminated intravascular coagulation.
4. Septic arthritis suggests either meningococcal or *Haemophilus influenzae* infection.

Diagnostic Evaluation

1. Diagnosis is usually established by performance of a lumbar puncture and examination of the cerebrospinal fluid.
   a. Cloudy or turbid appearance
   b. Elevated cerebrospinal fluid pressure

    c. High cell count with mostly polymorphonuclear cells

    d. Low glucose level

    e. Elevated protein level (may also be normal)

    f. Gram stain and cultures positive—to identify the causative organism

2. Additional laboratory studies

    a. Complete blood count (Total white blood cell count is often increased, with a preponderance of young neutrophils in the differential blood count.)

    b. Platelet count

    c. Urinalysis

    d. Blood, urine, and nasopharyngeal cultures

    e. Serum electrolytes—often demonstrate hyponatremia and hypochloremia

    f. Serum glucose

    g. Blood urea nitrogen (BUN) and creatinine

    h. Tuberculin skin test

    i. Skull and chest x-rays

Treatment

1. Intravenous administration of the appropriate antimicrobial agents to promote rapid destruction of the bacteria and to suppress the emergence of resistant strains

2. Recognition and treatment of hyponatremia

3. Supportive management of the comatose child or the child with seizures

4. Appropriate prophylactic treatment provided for contacts when indicated

Complications

1. Seizures

2. Cerebral edema

3. Subdural effusion

4. Hydrocephalus

5. Cerebral infarction or abscess

6. Diffuse residual effects, including slowed development

Patient Problems/Nursing Diagnoses

1. Potential for serious complications including, shock, peripheral circulatory collapse, disseminated intravascular coagulation, syndrome of inappropriate antidiuretic hormone secretion, seizures, and respiratory compromise

2. Pain related to neurologic effects from the disease process

3. Inadequate nutritional intake related to inability to eat

4. Parental anxiety related to the life-threatening nature of the child's illness

5. Potential for permanent sequelae including impairment of learning or vision, paralysis, and behavioral defects

Nursing Interventions

A. Practice measures that will prevent the transmission of infection.

1. Place the child in isolation until at least 24 hours after initiation of antibiotic therapy.

2. Practice careful handwashing technique.

3. Personnel with infection should avoid contact with infants.

    a. Seek medical care for infection. (Cultures should be taken.)

    b. Remain out of the nursery.

    c. Wear a mask when it is necessary to enter the nursery.

4. Teach parents and other visitors proper handwashing and gown technique.

5. Maintain sterile technique when procedures demanding this technique are performed.

6. Identify close contacts or high-risk children who might benefit from meningococci vaccination.

B. Assess the child for evidence of disease progression or response to therapy.

1. Determine baseline data at admission. Include the following information:

    a. Weight

    b. Head circumference

    c. Vital signs

    d. Blood pressure

    e. Neurologic status

    f. History related to present illness

    g. Usual behavior and feeding patterns

2. Monitor vital signs, blood pressure, and neurologic status at frequent intervals.

3. Monitor intake and output continuously.

4. Monitor weight and head circumference at least daily.

5. Observe for and report the appearance or disappearance of any of the previously listed clinical manifestations.

    a. Be especially alert for vague symptoms that appear early in the course of meningeal irritation in infants:

        (1) Lethargy

        (2) Irritability

        (3) Poor feeding or refusal to feed

        (4) Weight loss

        (5) Temperature changes

    b. Be consistent in planning for the care of infants to provide a means by which these early symptoms may be detected.

        (1) Accurate charting of the infant's previous behavior

        (2) Assigning the same nurse to care for an infant on successive days

C. Administer the prescribed antibiotic therapy to control the infection.

1. Administer medications at the specified time to achieve optimal serum levels.

2. Since medications are generally administered intravenously for 2–3 weeks, restrain the child in a functional position which safeguards the integrity of the IV. Refer to sections on intravenous therapy, page 1160, and protective devices to limit movement, page 1142.

3. Observe medication sites for evidence of infiltration or development of tissue irritation.

4. Be aware of the actions, proper dilution, and side effects of specific medications.

5. Be aware of drug interactions and incompatibilities.

D. Observe for evidence of complications of the disease.

Report the following:

1. Decreased respirations, decreased pulse rate, increased systolic blood pressure, visual disturbances, pupillary changes, or decreased responsiveness, which may indicate increased intracranial pressure.

2. Decreased urine volume and increased body weight,

which may indicate inappropriate secretion of anti-diuretic hormone.

3. Sudden appearance of a skin rash and bleeding from other sites, which may indicate disseminated intravascular coagulation.

4. Persistent or recurring fever, bulging fontanelle, signs of increased intracranial pressure, focal neurologic signs, seizures, or increased head circumference which may indicate subdural effusion.

5. Hearing disturbances and apparent deafness.

E. Reduce fever

1. Possible adverse effects of the increased cerebral metabolic rate associated with fever in the child with cerebral swelling and cerebral vascular compromise

2. Increased potential for seizures in the febrile child

3. Refer to section on management of fever, page 1135

F. Provide for the nutritional needs of the patient.

1. During the acute phase of the illness, the patient may be unable to take or tolerate oral feedings.
   a. Carefully monitor the administration of intravenous fluids.
   b. Provide nasogastric feedings if necessary (see section on feeding methods, p. 1152).
   c. Provide for the sucking needs of the infant by offering a pacifier.

2. Initiate oral feedings as soon as the patient's condition improves.
   a. Infants
      (1) Begin by offering small feedings and observe for the following responses:
         (a) Vomiting
         (b) Abdominal distention
         (c) The infant's interest in feeding and ability to suck
         (d) The infant tires with feeding
      (2) Supplement oral feedings with gavage feedings if necessary.
      (3) Gradually increase amount of feeding.
      (4) Resume regular feeding schedule based on the infant's ability to tolerate it.
      (5) Hold the infant for feedings as soon as his condition warrants it.
   b. Older children—refer to section on nutrition, page 1094.

3. Carefully monitor the child's weight to ensure that caloric needs are being met.

G. Provide a supportive environment during the stage of irritability.

1. Reduce the general noise level around the child and shield child from sudden loud noises.

2. Organize nursing care to provide for periods of uninterrupted rest. Disturb only when necessary.

3. Keep general handling of the child at a minimum. When necessary, approach the child slowly and gently.

4. Maintain subdued lighting as much as possible.

5. Speak in a low, well-modulated tone of voice to reduce anxiety.

H. Provide therapeutic care for the child who experiences seizures.

(See section on seizures, below.)

I. Observe for episodes of apnea and initiate measures to stimulate respiration.

1. Observe the infant closely for apnea or have the infant placed on a respiratory monitor.

2. Stimulate the infant when apnea does occur.
   a. Pinch feet and provide more vigorous stimulation if necessary.
   b. When spontaneous respiration does not occur within 15–20 seconds, apply hand resuscitator or perform mouth-to-mouth resuscitation.

3. Report frequent periods of apnea to physician.

4. Record length of apnea episode and response to stimulation on nursing record.

J. Provide supportive care for the child during the convalescent phase of illness.

1. Record disappearance of symptoms and indications that the child is returning to his normal state.

2. Provide for the emotional needs of the child (see the section on the hospitalized child, p. 1112).

3. Encourage parental visiting and family-centered care.

4. Note any evidence that the child is developing sequelae of the illness, such as deafness, brain abnormality, or hydrocephalus.

Health Education

1. Encourage the parents to visit their child.
   a. Encourage their participation in the child's care.
   b. Provide them with an opportunity to express their concerns.
   c. Answer questions they may have regarding the infant's progress and care.

2. Discuss symptoms the parents should watch for as signs of possible complications.

3. Give specific instruction regarding medications to be administered at home.

Expected Outcomes

1. Absence of serious complications; maintains normal respiratory, circulatory, and neurologic functions

2. Achieves pain relief; does not appear distressed

3. Receives adequate nutritional support; taking feedings; absence of vomiting and abdominal distention

4. The parents discuss their feelings about the child's illness with each other and with appropriate health care professionals

5. Recovers with no evidence of permanent sequelae of meningitis; no signs of visual or hearing impairment; no paralysis or developmental retardation noted

Convulsive Disorders *(Seizure Disorders, Epilepsy)*

Convulsive disorder is a term used to encompass a number of varieties of episodic disturbances of brain function. Convulsions should not be regarded as one specific disease, but as a symptom of an underlying disorder. They are relatively common in children, being more prevalent during the first 2 years than at any other time in life.

Etiology

1. Idiopathic
2. Prenatal factors
   a. Genetic predisposition
   b. Congenital structural anomalies
   c. Fetal infections
   d. Maternal diseases
3. Perinatal factors
   a. Trauma
   b. Hypoxia
   c. Jaundice
   d. Infection
   e. Prematurity
   f. Drug withdrawal
4. Postnatal factors
   a. Primary infection of the central nervous system
   b. Infectious diseases of childhood with encephalopathy
   c. Head trauma
   d. Circulatory diseases
   e. Toxic encephalopathy
   f. Allergic encephalopathy
   g. Metabolic encephalopathy
   h. Degenerative diseases
   i. Cerebral neoplasms
   j. Renal disease
   k. Anoxia

Altered Physiology

1. The basic mechanism for all seizures appears to be prolonged depolarization causing brain cells to become overactive and to discharge in a sudden, violent, disorderly manner.
2. This paroxysmal burst of electrical energy spreads to adjacent areas or may jump to distant areas of the central nervous system. A seizure results.
3. The biochemical basis of seizures is incompletely understood.
4. Some seizures appear to occur under the influence of a triggering factor.
   a. Hormonal factors, such as those related to the menstrual period, menarche, and menopause
   b. Nonsensory factors, such as hyperthermia, hyperventilation, metabolic disorders, sleep deprivation, emotional disturbances, and physical stress
   c. Sensory factors, such as those related to vision, hearing, touch, the startle reaction, and those that are self-induced
5. For international classification of epileptic seizures refer to a neurology textbook.

Types of Seizures

A. Grand Mal Epilepsy (Generalized Seizures)

1. Onset
   a. Onset is abrupt.
   b. May occur at night.
   c. An aura (peculiar sensation, often dizziness) occurs in about ⅓ of epileptic children prior to a grand mal seizure.
2. Tonic spasm
   a. The child's entire body becomes stiff.
   b. He loses consciousness.
   c. The face may become pale and distorted.
   d. His eyes are frequently fixed in one position.
   e. His back may be arched with his head held backward or to one side.
   f. His arms are usually flexed and his hands clenched.
   g. If standing, the child falls to the ground.
   h. He may utter a peculiar, piercing cry.
   i. He is often unable to swallow his saliva.
   j. Breathing is ineffective and cyanosis results if spasm includes the muscles of respiration.
   k. The pulse may become weak and irregular.
3. Clonic phase
   a. Characterized by rhythmic, jerking movements which follow the tonic state.
   b. Usually start in one place and become generalized, including the muscles of the face.
   c. The child may be incontinent and may bite his tongue or cheek. (This occurs because of sudden forceful contraction of his jaw and abdominal muscles.)
4. Duration
   a. Varies, from a few seconds to 30 minutes or longer.
   b. Usually, convulsions cease after a few minutes.
5. Postconvulsive (postictal) state of child
   a. Usually is sleepy or exhausted.
   b. May complain of headache.
   c. May appear to be in a dazed state.
   d. Often performs relatively automatic tasks without being able to recall the episode.
6. Secondary symptomatology
   a. Represents the patient's response over a long period of time to the injurious attitudes of other people toward the child and the diagnosis.
   b. The child develops a self-image consistent with his perception of how others view him.
7. Electroencephalogram (EEG)
   a. Definite abnormalities can usually be demonstrated in the interval between seizures.
      (1) Random spike discharges
      (2) Diffuse high-voltage slow waves
      (3) Pattern abnormal for child's chronologic age
   b. Multiple high-voltage spike discharges are demonstrated during the seizure.
   c. Asymmetries between the 2 hemispheres and diffuse slowing may be observed after the seizure.

B. Status Epilepticus

1. Refers to grand mal seizures which occur in series without the patient's regaining consciousness between attacks.
2. Transient postictal (i.e., period following seizures) signs and symptoms include ataxia, aphasia, and mental sluggishness.
3. Irreversible brain damage may occur secondary to prolonged cerebral hypoxia.
4. This condition should be treated as a medical emergency.

C. Petit Mal Epilepsy

1. Onset—rarely appears before 5 years of age.
2. Clinical signs
   a. Loss of contact with the environment for a few brief seconds:
      (1) The child may appear to be staring or daydreaming.
      (2) If reading or writing, the child will suddenly discontinue the activity and may resume it when the seizure has ended.

b. Minor manifestations include rolling of the eyes, nodding of the head, slight hand movements, and smacking of the lips.
3. Duration—usually 5–10 seconds.
4. Frequency—varies from 1 or 2 per month to several hundred each day.
5. Precipitating factors may include hyperventilation, fatigue, hypoglycemia, and stress.
6. Postconvulsive state
   a. Child appears normal.
   b. Is not aware of having had a convulsion.
7. Electroencephalogram (EEG)
   Has characteristic 3-per-second spike and wave pattern during the seizure.

D. Focal Seizures

1. Psychomotor
   a. Occur most frequently in children from 3 years of age through adolescence.
   b. Seizure discharge usually originates in the temporal lobe and may be referred to as "temporal lobe seizures."
   c. Clinical signs:
      (1) Frequently experiences a sense of fullness rising from the abdomen to the thorax.
      (2) Aura, if present, often includes bad odor or taste.
      (3) May experience complex auditory or visual hallucinations, déjà vu feeling, or strong sense of fear and anxiety.
      (4) Perceptual alterations may occur.
      (5) Dysphagia or aphasia may be present.
      (6) Most common motor symptom is drawing or jerking of the mouth and face.
      (7) May perform coordinated but inappropriate movements repeatedly in a stereotyped manner (e.g., clutching, kicking, picking at clothes, walking in circles, chewing, licking, spitting).
      (8) Consciousness may be impaired but is rarely completely lost.
   d. Duration—brief, usually from 30 seconds to 5–10 minutes.
   e. Postconvulsive state—the child is usually drowsy or sleeps after an attack. Confusion and amnesia are common.
2. Focal motor
   a. Clinical signs
      (1) Sudden jerking movements occur in a particular area of the body, such as the face, thumb, or toe.
      (2) Consciousness may or may not be disturbed.
      (3) Clonic movements occasionally begin in 1 area of the body and spread to adjacent areas on the same side in a fixed progression (Jacksonian seizures).
   b. Prognosis—seizures may become more extensive as the child matures, leading to grand mal seizures.
3. Focal sensory (rare in children)—sensations occur, such as numbness, tingling, and coldness in the part of the body controlled by the area of the brain cell overactivity.

E. Infantile Myoclonic Seizures (Massive Myoclonic Spasms)

1. These seizures are peculiar to infants; they are second in incidence only to grand mal seizures in this age-group.

2. Peak incidence is in children between 3 and 6 months; onset after 2 years of age is rare.
3. Clinical signs
   a. Sudden, forceful, myoclonic contractions involving the musculature of the trunk, neck, and extremities.
      (1) Flexor type—the infant adducts and flexes his extremities, drops his head, and doubles upon himself.
      (2) Extensor type—the infant extends neck, spreads arms out, and bends body backward in a position described as "spread eagle."
   b. A cry or grunt may accompany severe attacks.
   c. The infant may grimace, laugh, or appear fearful during or after the attack.
4. Duration—momentary (usually under 1 minute).
5. Frequency—varies from a few attacks per day to hundreds per day.
6. EEG—random, high-voltage slow waves and spikes suggestive of a diffuse disorganized state.
7. Prognosis
   a. Almost always associated with cerebral abnormalities.
   b. Usually this type of seizure disappears spontaneously by the time the child reaches 4 years of age.
   c. Subsequent grand mal or other types of seizures often develop.
   d. Mental retardation usually accompanies this disorder.

Chemotherapy

A. General Principles Related to the Administration of Medications

1. Selection of the most effective drug(s) depends on correct identification of the clinical seizure type.
2. A desirable drug level is one that will prevent attacks without producing undesirable side effects.
3. Dosages are adjusted according to blood level and clinical signs.
4. Accurate timing is essential to prevent seizures.
   This is especially true when there is a tendency for the child to have convulsions at a certain period each day.
5. Enteric coated tablets which have a delayed effect should be used for children who are prone to attacks during sleep.
6. Most anticonvulsants are available in liquid form as well as in capsules or tablets.
   Tablets can be crushed and given to infants and small children in coke syrup or applesauce.
7. It may take several months to find the best combination of medications and the best dosages of each to control the child's seizures.
8. One hundred percent control of symptoms may not be achieved in every patient.
9. Dosage adjustment may be required from time to time because of the child's growth.
10. Blood counts, urinalyses, and liver-function studies are done at regular intervals in children receiving certain anticonvulsants.
11. Medication is often not discontinued until 2–3 years after the last attack
12. Weaning from medication should always be gradual, with stepwise reduction of dosage and withdrawal of 1 drug at a time.

B. Drugs Commonly Used for the Control of Seizures in Children

1. Phenobarbital
   a. Dosage
      (1) An initial loading dose is usually given intramuscularly or intravenously for an acute, ongoing seizure, because it takes from days to weeks to achieve therapeutic blood levels by the oral route alone.
      (2) The dosage is reduced for maintenance therapy and is generally administered orally.
   b. Indications and advantages
      (1) Drug of choice for initial trial, except for petit mal seizures
      (2) One of the safest anticonvulsant drugs
      (3) Relatively inexpensive
   c. Untoward effects
      (1) Excitement, hyperactivity
      (2) Rash
      (3) Gastrointestinal symptoms
      (4) Dizziness, ataxia
      (5) Aggravated psychomotor seizures
      (6) Drowsiness
      (7) Irritability
      (8) Depression
   d. Toxic effects (rare, except in overdose, accidental ingestion)—respiratory, circulatory, or renal depression
   e. Contraindications
      (1) Severe hepatic or renal dysfunction
      (2) Hypersensitivity
2. Phenytoin (Dilantin)
   a. Route—oral
   b. Indications and advantages
      (1) Does not produce excessive drowsiness
      (2) Safest drug for the management of psychomotor epilepsy
      (3) Often used with phenobarbital
   c. Untoward effects
      (1) May accentuate petit mal seizures
      (2) Hypertrophy of the gums—daily gum massage is an important aspect of nursing care for a patient taking phenytoin
      (3) Hirsutism
      (4) Rickets
      (5) Nystagmus
      (6) Ataxia
      (7) Rash
      (8) Nausea and vomiting
      (9) Decreased alertness
      (10) Agitation
   d. Toxic effects—(rare, except in overdose, accidental ingestion)
      (1) Blood dyscrasia
      (2) Liver damage
3. Ethosuximide (Zarontin)
   a. Route—oral
   b. Indications and advantages
      (1) Used for petit mal seizures
      (2) Occurrence of blood dyscrasia is less common following administration of ethosuximide than with trimethadione (Tridione)—the other medication frequently used to control petit mal seizures.
   c. Untoward effects
      (1) Drowsiness
      (2) May increase grand mal seizures

      (3) Gastrointestinal symptoms—administer with food
      (4) Lethargy
      (5) Euphoria
   d. Toxic effects
      (1) Blood dyscrasias
      (2) Psychiatric symptoms
   e. Contraindications—hepatic or renal disease
4. Primidone (Mysoline)
   a. Route—oral
   b. Indications and advantages
      (1) Used alone or with other anticonvulsants to control mixed-type seizure patterns.
      (2) May control grand mal seizures not responsive to treatment by other anticonvulsant therapy.
   c. Untoward effects
      (1) More common
         (a) Ataxia
         (b) Vertigo
      (2) Occasional
         (a) GI symptoms
         (b) Fatigue
         (c) Diplopia
         (d) Nystagmus
         (e) Skin eruption
   d. Toxic effects
      (1) Megaloblastic anemia may occur as a rare idiosyncratic response to the drug.
      (2) Drowsiness in nursing newborns of primidone-treated mothers indicates that breast-feeding should be discontinued.
   e. Contraindications
      (1) Patients who are hypersensitive to phenobarbital
      (2) Patients with porphyria
5. Diazepam
   a. Route—oral, intravenous, or intramuscular
   b. Indications and advantages
      (1) Intravenous or intramuscular diazepam is indicated in the treatment of status epilepticus and severe recurrent convulsive seizures.
      (2) Oral diazepam may be used adjunctively in maintenance therapy for convulsive disorders.
   c. Special precautions
      (1) If administered intravenously, give slowly over 3 minutes. Avoid intra-arterial administration or extravasation.
      (2) Administer intravenously with caution to children with limited pulmonary reserve, because of the possibility that apnea and/or cardiac arrest may occur.
      (3) Tonic status epilepticus has been precipitated in patients treated with intravenous diazepam for petit mal seizures.
      (4) Concomitant use of barbiturates, alcohol, or other central nervous system depressants may potentiate the action of diazepam with increased risk of apnea.
      (5) Administer with caution to children with compromised renal function.
   d. Untoward effects
      (1) More common
         (a) Ataxia
         (b) Drowsiness

           (c) Fatigue
           (d) Venous thrombosis and phlebitis at in-
               jection site
       (2) Less common
           (a) GI symptoms
           (b) Confusion, depression
           (c) Headache
           (d) Tremor
           (e) Vertigo
           (f) Incontinence or urinary retention
           (g) Visual disturbances
           (h) Skin rash
           (i) Anxiety
           (j) Sleep disturbance
           (k) Neutropenia
           (l) Jaundice
    e. Toxic effects
       (1) Somnolence
       (2) Confusion
       (3) Diminished reflexes
       (4) Hypotension
       (5) Coma
       (6) Apnea
       (7) Cardiac arrest
6. Carbamazepine (Tegretol)
    a. Route—oral
    b. Indications and advantages—especially useful in
       treatment of major motor and psychomotor sei-
       zures.
    c. Special precautions—administration with phe-
       nytoin (Dilantin) reduces the half-life of phe-
       nytoin. The phenytoin dose may need to be
       increased when carbamazepine is added.
    d. Untoward effects (most likely to occur during
       the initial phases of therapy)
       (1) Dizziness
       (2) Drowsiness
       (3) Nausea and vomiting
    e. Toxic effects
       (1) Bone marrow depression (aplastic anemia,
           thrombocytopenia, agranulocytosis, and leu-
           kopenia)
       (2) Early toxic signs and symptoms
           (a) Fever
           (b) Sore throat
           (c) Ulcers in mouth
           (d) Easy bruising
           (e) Petechial or purpuric hemorrhage
    f. Contraindications
       (1) History of previous bone marrow depression
       (2) Known hypersensitivity to the drug
       (3) Used with caution in patients with cardiac,
           hepatic, or renal problems

Prognosis

1. General prognosis depends on type and severity of
   seizure disorder, coexisting mental retardation, organic disorders, and the type of medical management.
    a. Medically treated seizures—spontaneous cessa-
       tion of seizures may occur. Drugs may be grad-
       ually discontinued when the child has been free
       from attacks for an extensive period and his EEG
       pattern has reverted to normal.
    b. Nontreated epilepsy—seizures tend to become
       more numerous.

2. Mental development
    a. Convulsive episodes do not in themselves usually
       cause irreversible brain damage.
    b. Hypoxia during seizures can cause mental retar-
       dation.
    c. Epileptic children with normal mentality can be
       expected to remain normal with proper control
       of seizures.

Patient Problems/Nursing Diagnoses

1. Potential for injury during a convulsive seizure
2. Potential ineffective breathing/cyanosis related to
   spasms of respiratory musculature
3. Disorientation following seizure related to disruption
   of cerebral function
4. Possible nonadherence to treatment regimen (anticonvulsant medications)
5. Potential for undesirable/toxic effects of anticonvulsant medications
6. Anxiety related to hospitalization and the diagnostic
   procedures
7. Knowledge deficit about convulsive disorders and
   their management
8. Social isolation related to the child's feelings about
   his illness and/or public fears and misconceptions

Nursing Interventions

A. Control the seizures.

Administer medications as prescribed.

B. Protect the child from injury during a convulsive episode.

1. Preventive measures
    a. Remove hard toys from the bed. Keep a padded
       tongue blade or rubber bite block immediately
       available to put between the child's teeth to
       prevent him from biting his tongue.
    b. Pad the sides of the crib.
    c. Have a suction machine available to remove
       secretions during a seizure.
    d. Have an emergency oxygen source in the room
       in case of sudden respiratory difficulty.
2. Emergency actions
    a. Clear the area around the child if he is not in
       bed.
    b. Do not restrain him.
    c. Loosen the clothing around his neck.
    d. If the child is standing, ease him to his bed or
       the floor.
    e. Turn the child on his side so that saliva can flow
       out of his mouth.
    f. Place a small, folded blanket under the head to
       prevent trauma if the seizure occurs when the
       child is on the floor.
    g. Place a padded tongue blade or airway between
       the teeth to prevent damage to the tongue and
       cheeks and to facilitate respiration if this can be
       done without difficulty (procedure is controver-
       sial). If the teeth have clamped shut, do not
       attempt to force them open.
    h. Suction the child and administer oxygen as nec-
       essary.
    i. Do not give anything by mouth.
    j. After the seizure, place the child on his side in
       bed, if he is not already there.

C. Accurately record the seizures—include the following:

1. Significant preseizure events, such as noise, excitement, lethargy
2. Behavior before the seizure, aura
3. Types of movements observed
4. Time seizure began and ended
5. Site where twitching or contraction began
6. Areas of the body involved
7. Movements of the eyes and changes in pupil size
8. Incontinence
9. Amount of perspiration
10. Respiratory changes
11. Color change—pallor, cyanosis, flushing
12. Mouth—teeth clenched, movement, tongue bitten, foaming at the mouth
13. Apparent degree of consciousness during the seizure
14. Behavior after the seizure
    a. Degree of memory for recent events
    b. Types of speech
    c. Coordination
    d. Paralysis or weakness
    e. Sleeping after the attack
    f. Pupil reaction
    g. Vital signs
    h. Unusual sensations

D. Observe the child for recurrent seizures.

1. Place the child where he can be watched closely.
2. Monitor vital signs and assess neurologic status frequently.
3. Check the child frequently. Report:
    a. Behavior changes
    b. Irritability
    c. Restlessness
    d. Listlessness

E. Provide emotional support to the child's parents.

1. Describe completely any examinations, evaluations, treatments that the child is receiving.
    a. EEG
    b. Pneumoencephalogram
    c. Blood studies
    d. Medications
2. Provide information regarding the disease itself.
    a. Epilepsy is *not* contagious, is seldom dangerous, and does *not* indicate insanity or mental retardation.
    b. Most children with epilepsy have infrequent seizures and with medications can completely control their convulsions.
    c. The child may have normal intelligence and can live a useful and productive life.
    d. The child's medication is not addicting when used as prescribed. It should in no way influence his mental ability or personality or cause him to become a drug addict.
    e. It is impossible to predict accurately the possibility of the convulsive disorder appearing in siblings or offspring of the affected child.
3. Observe the parent–child reaction for evidence of rejection or overprotection.
   Offer reassurance and praise for achievements in dealing with the child's problem.
4. Prepare the parents for the fact that it may take several months of regulating drug dosages before adequate control is obtained.

5. Provide the parents with appropriate literature.
6. Refer the family to appropriate community resources and services.
    a. Social worker
    b. Community health nurse
    c. School nurse
    d. Psychiatrist
    e. Parent groups
    f. Voluntary agencies

F. Minimize anxiety during the child's hospitalization.

1. Rationale—the therapeutic value of anticonvulsant drugs is decreased if the child has more anxiety than he can handle
2. Explain the diagnostic and treatment plan to the child in a manner that he can understand.
3. Allow the child as much normal activity as possible. Allow him to be dressed if desired.
4. If the child does have a seizure, stay with him and remain calm.
    a. Stay with the child after a convulsion and reassure him and his parents that he is all right.
    b. Help the child to adjust to reality if he has difficulty remembering the episode.
    c. Older children may require intervention to deal with guilt and embarrassment secondary to incontinence and the loss of body control.
    d. Maintain a quiet environment if the child has had a long convulsive period.
5. Provide diversion appropriate for the child's age. Play equipment should be such that it will not cause injury during a seizure.
6. Avoid unnecessary stimulation.

Health Education

1. The child should be in an environment that is as normal as possible.
    a. Attendance at a regular school with healthy children should be encouraged.
        (1) Contact should be made with the school nurse who can help the child's teacher understand his disease, emergency treatment of seizures, etc.
        (2) The child should be allowed to participate in organizations and outside activities with limited restrictions.
            (a) Each child must be treated individually; the kind of activity depends on the degree of control.
            (b) Generally, children with seizure disorders should not be allowed to climb in high places or to swim alone.
            (c) Responsible adults should be made aware of the child's disease.
        (3) The child should not be made to feel that he can never be left alone.
        (4) He needs to be disciplined as a normal child.
            He should not gain attention directly or indirectly by having seizures.
2. The child should be given appropriate information regarding his diagnosis and treatment. He is less confident of his body and his control over it and therefore less confident of himself.
    a. He should be included in conferences with the physician.

b. He needs an opportunity to ask questions which should be answered honestly.

c. He should be aware of his restrictions and helped to deal with them.

d. He should gradually be given responsibility for taking his own medications faithfully.

e. He should be encouraged to wear a Medic-Alert bracelet.

3. The older child or adolescent should be helped to achieve independence.

a. He should be given the opportunity for privacy to discuss his diagnosis with his physician.

b. He should be allowed to use his own judgment in his daily activities.

c. He should be helped to develop realistic educational and career goals.

(1) The assistance of a social worker or psychiatrist may be invaluable during this period.

(2) Genetic counseling may be indicated in some cases.

(a) People with epilepsy can marry and have children.

(b) There is no proof that epilepsy is hereditary although there may be a tendency to transmit a low convulsive threshold.

(3) Counseling regarding matters such as securing a driver's license and obtaining life, health, and automobile insurance should be available.

d. Fantasies that "there is nothing wrong with me" or the refusal to take medications requires prompt intervention.

4. Factors that may precipitate a convulsive episode should be avoided.

a. The seizures should be treated matter of factly. A calm, reassuring attitude is essential during and after a seizure. The attitude of adults when the child has a seizure influences the attitude of other children toward him.

b. The child should be kept in optimal physical condition with special attention to the status of his teeth and eyes and to the prevention of infection.

c. Excessive fatigue, overhydration, and hyperventilation should be avoided.

d. Irregular, fluctuating schedules are detrimental. A routine of daily living should be encouraged.

5. Medical care and supervision to control convulsions are essential. Instructions regarding medical and nursing care should be stressed.

(1) Administration of medications and side effects of prescribed drugs

(2) Emergency care during a seizure

(3) Observations

(a) Signs of impending seizure

(b) Behavior during and after the seizure

(4) Diet—ketogenic diets are no longer widely used, except in difficult cases

6. Parents should be referred to appropriate support groups for help in dealing with their feelings, concerns, and problems related to their child.

7. References for parents:

Lagos J. Seizures, Epilepsy and Your Child. New York, Harper & Row, 1974

Sands H and Minters F. The Epilepsy Fact Book. Philadelphia, FA Davis, 1977

Svoboda W. Learning About Epilepsy. Baltimore, University Park Press, 1979

Volle F and Heron P. Epilepsy and You. Springfield, IL, Charles C Thomas, 1978

Ziegler R and Erba G. Does Your Child Have Epilepsy? Baltimore, University Park Press, 1983

8. Agency:

Epilepsy Foundation of America, 4351 Garden City Drive, Landover, MD 20785

Expected Outcomes

1. Avoids injury during a convulsive episode; takes protective measures; wears helmet

2. Regains normal breathing pattern following a seizure

3. Becomes oriented to time, place, and person after a seizure episode

4. Takes medications as prescribed

5. Does not experience untoward effects of his anticonvulsant medication; no dizziness, nausea, vomiting, mouth ulcers, fever

6. The child shows decreasing anxiety; asks appropriate questions; expresses his feelings through verbal and nonverbal communication and with play

7. The child and parents describe his disease; verbalize the importance of medication and follow-up

8. Participates in age-appropriate social activities

Febrile Convulsions

Febrile convulsions refer to seizures that occur in the context of a febrile illness in a previously normal child. The seizures are brief and generalized. They should be distinguished from focal or prolonged seizures which occur in a child with an underlying seizure disorder that is exacerbated by fever.

Etiology

1. Accompany intercurrent infections—especially viral illness, tonsillitis, pharyngitis, and otitis.

2. Appear to occur in a familial pattern, although exact pattern of inheritance is incompletely understood.

Incidence

1. Febrile convulsions occur in approximately 3%–5% of all children.

2. The vast majority of first febrile seizures occur in children between the ages of 6 months and 3 years of age.

3. Febrile seizures are unusual after 5 years of age.

Clinical Manifestations

1. Most febrile convulsions consist of generalized tonic–clonic seizures.

2. Seizures generally last less than 15 minutes.
3. Fever is usually high—over 38.8°C. (101.8°F.) rectally.
4. Seizures usually occur near the onset of fever rather than after prolonged fever.

Diagnostic Evaluation

Measures are directed toward delineating the cause of any seizure as precisely as possible so that its implications and prognosis may be discussed with the parents. Diagnostic methods include:

1. Physical examination with special attention to neurologic status
2. Cerebrospinal fluid examination
3. Complete blood count and urinalysis
4. Cultures of nasopharynx, blood, or urine as appropriate to determine cause of fever
5. Blood sugar, calcium, and electrolyte levels
6. EEG
   a. Demonstrates mild, post ictal slowing soon after the attack
   b. Pattern is generally normal after a few days

Prognosis

1. The likelihood of febrile seizure recurrence is about 40%–50% for a second febrile seizure.
2. Factors influencing recurrence rate
   a. The younger the child is at the time of the first seizure, the greater the risk for additional febrile seizures.
   b. Children with a positive family history of febrile convulsions have a greater risk of recurrent febrile convulsions.
3. The risk for development of nonfebrile convulsions is relatively low (about 3%). At risk are those children who demonstrate the following characteristics:
   a. Multiple febrile seizures during 1 day
   b. Prolonged febrile seizures
   c. Persistent electroencephalographic abnormalities
   d. Central nervous system infections

Nursing Interventions

A. Assess and reduce fever.

Refer to section on fever, page 1135.

B. Intervene appropriately during and after the seizure episode(s).

See Nursing Interventions A–D in previous section, pages 1433–1434.

Health Education

1. Remain calm and efficient if the child has a seizure in the presence of his parents.
2. Reinforce realistic, reassuring information such as:
   a. A convulsion does not necessarily imply that the underlying disease is a serious one.
   b. Children rarely die in seizures.
   c. The prognosis depends on the cause of the convulsion.
      (1) A single febrile seizure is not indicative of later chronic epilepsy.
      (2) Children who have a tendency to develop febrile convulsions usually lose it as they grow older.
      (3) Occasional, brief convulsions have no adverse effects on the child's ultimate development.
3. Discuss and demonstrate emergency management of seizures.
4. Stress that medical evaluation is indicated as soon as the child develops a fever.
   a. Review technique of temperature measurement.
   b. Prompt administration of antipyretic measures is necessary when the child is febrile.
5. Reinforce medical instructions regarding anticonvulsant therapy.
   a. The advisability of long-term anticonvulsant medications in normal children with simple febrile convulsions is currently controversial. Recommendations vary among physicians from no medication to maintenance therapy with phenobarbital.
   b. Intermittent therapy with phenobarbital during febrile episodes is apparently of no value because of the length of time required to achieve therapeutic serum levels of the drug.

Subdural Hematoma

Subdural hematoma refers to an accumulation of fluid, blood, and its degradation products within the potential space between the dura and arachnoid (subdural space). Subdural hematomas are classified as acute, subacute, or chronic, depending on the time period between injury and the onset of symptoms.

Etiology

1. Direct or indirect trauma to the head.
   a. Birth trauma
   b. Accidental causes
   c. Purposeful violence, as in the battered child syndrome (see p. 1490)
2. Meningitis

Classification*

A. Acute

Syndrome presents as an acute problem, closely related to the time of presumed injury.

B. Chronic

1. Signs and symptoms are nonlocalizing and subacute.
2. Most common type of subdural hematoma in children.

* Classification does not imply any basic differences in the disease process but refers only to the duration of the lesion before it becomes manifest. The classification varies slightly among several sources.

3. It is often difficult to delineate the exact time and type of injury, since the precipitating episode may appear relatively insignificant.

Altered Physiology

1. Trauma to the head causes tearing of the delicate subdural veins, resulting in small hemorrhages into the subdural space. (Bleeding may be of arterial origin in cases of acute subdural hematoma.)
2. As the blood breaks down, there is an increased capillary permeability and effusion of blood cells and protein into the subdural space.
3. The breakdown products of blood stimulate the growth of connective tissue and capillaries largely from the dura.
4. A membrane is formed that usually extends frontally and laterally over the hemispheres, surrounding the clot.
5. Fluid accumulates within the membrane and increases the width of the subdural space.
6. Further hemorrhages occur.
7. The lesion enlarges, expanding the skull, and, if unrelieved, ultimately causes cerebral atrophy or death from compression and herniation.
8. The lesion may arrest spontaneously at any point.
9. Further bleeding may occur into an already existing sac and may increase symptoms.
10. In long-standing subdural hematoma, the fluid may disappear, leaving a constricting membrane which prevents normal brain growth.

Clinical Manifestations

A. Acute

1. Often present with continuous unconsciousness from the time of injury, but child may present with a lucid interval.
2. Ensuing manifestations include deterioration of level of consciousness, evidence of progressive hemiplegia, focal seizures, and signs of brain stem herniation (pupillary enlargement, changes in vital signs, development of decerebrate state, and respiratory failure).

B. Chronic

1. Insidious onset
2. Symptoms are variable and are related to the age of the child.
   a. Infants
      (1) Early signs
         (a) Anorexia
         (b) Difficulty feeding
         (c) Vomiting
         (d) Irritability
         (e) Low grade fever
         (f) Retinal hemorrhages
         (g) Failure to gain weight
      (2) Later signs
         (a) Enlargement of the head
         (b) Bulging and pulsation of the anterior fontanelle
         (c) Tight, glossy scalp with dilated scalp veins
         (d) Strabismus, pupillary inequality, ocular palsies (rare)
         (e) Hyperactive reflexes
         (f) Seizures
         (g) Retarded motor development

   b. Older children
      (1) Early signs
         (a) Lethargy
         (b) Anorexia
         (c) Symptoms of increased intracranial pressure
            (1) Vomiting
            (2) Irritability
            (3) Increased blood pressure
            (4) Decreased pulse
            (5) Decreased or irregular respirations
            (6) Headache
      (2) Later signs (may occur immediately if bleeding takes place rapidly)
         (a) Convulsions
         (b) Coma

Diagnostic Evaluation

1. CAT scan is the procedure of choice for diagnosing subdural hematomas.
2. Bilateral subdural taps may provide the diagnosis as well as immediate relief of increased intracranial pressure.
3. Angiography may be used if CAT scan is unavailable.

Complications

1. Mental retardation
2. Ocular abnormalities
3. Seizures
4. Spasticity
5. Paralysis

Treatment

1. Acute subdural hematoma—requires evacuation of the clot through a burr hole or craniotomy.
2. Chronic subdural hematoma
   a. Repeated subdural taps are done to remove the abnormal fluid.
      (1) In infants, the needle can be inserted through the fontanelle or suture line.
      (2) In older children, burr holes into the skull are necessary before the needle can be inserted.
      (3) The subdural taps may be the only treatment required if the fluid disappears entirely and symptoms do not recur.
      (4) Concurrently, treatment is instituted to correct anemia, electrolyte imbalance, and malnutrition.
   b. Shunting procedure may be indicated if repeated taps fail to reduce significantly the volume or protein content of the subdural collections. Shunting is generally to the peritoneal cavity.

Prognosis

1. Treatment is usually successful when the diagnosis is made early—before cerebral atrophy and a fixed neurologic deficit have occurred. In such cases, subsequent development is normal.
2. Prognosis depends on the effect of the initial trauma on the brain as well as the effect of continued fluid collection.
3. Mortality in massive, acute subdural bleeding is very high, even if promptly diagnosed.

Nursing Interventions

A. Assess the child's neurologic status in order to help evaluate the effectiveness of treatment or to identify disease progress.

Observe for and document the following:

1. General behavior—especially irritability, lethargy, and evidence of personality changes.

   It is important to obtain a thorough history from the child's parents regarding his normal behavior and level of functioning so that abnormalities can be more easily recognized.
2. Appetite and feeding difficulties, including vomiting.
3. Signs of increased intracranial pressure.
   a. Vital signs, including pulse, respiration, and blood pressure should be monitored frequently.
   b. Be alert for:
      (1) Increased systolic blood pressure
      (2) Increased pulse pressure
      (3) Decreased pulse or irregularities
      (4) Changes in respiratory rate or difficulty breathing
4. Level of consciousness—describe findings explicitly. The following "levels" may be useful as guidelines:
   a. Alert and responds immediately and appropriately to visual, auditory, and tactile stimuli.
   b. Lethargic, drowsy, and inactive but can be aroused to an alert state.
   c. Lethargic and dull; responds with vigorous stimulation, but quickly returns to lethargic state.
   d. Can be aroused only to a very low level of response with vigorous stimulation.
   e. Moderate coma with rudimentary physiologic or psychomotor responses.
   f. Totally nonresponsive, even to deep pain stimuli.
5. Pupillary changes—especially dilated pupil, double vision, lack of response to light, alterations in visual acuity, and decreased integrity of eye movements.
6. Seizures
7. Motor function, including ability to move all extremities. The ability to grasp should be checked and compared bilaterally.
8. Drainage of cerebrospinal fluid from the nose or ears.

B. Observe for signs of complications.

1. Infection
   a. Record temperature frequently.
   b. Report purulent drainage from the site of the subdural tap.
2. Recurrent bleeding—note rapid changes in vital signs indicating shock or increased intracranial pressure.
3. Paralysis

C. Avoid additional increase in intracranial pressure.

1. Maintain a quiet environment.
2. Avoid sudden changes in position.
3. Organize nursing activities to allow for long periods of uninterrupted rest.
4. Administer laxatives or suppositories to prevent straining during a bowel movement.

D. Assist with subdural taps.

1. Wrap the infant or young child in a mummy restraint (see procedure on protective devices to limit motion, p. 1142).
2. Hold the child securely to avoid injury caused by sudden movement.

3. Apply firm pressure over the puncture site(s) for a few minutes after the tap has been completed to prevent fluid leakage along the needle tract.
4. Observe the child frequently after the procedure for:
   a. Shock
   b. Drainage from the site of the tap
      (1) Note whether this is serous drainage or frank blood.
      (2) Reinforce the dressing, if present, to prevent contamination of the wound.

E. Provide adequate nutrition.

Apply principles stated in the section on hydrocephalus, page 1419.

F. Provide supportive care to the child in coma.

1. Keep the child's eyes well lubricated to prevent corneal damage.
2. Suction the child as necessary to remove secretions in the mouth and nasopharynx.
3. Provide frequent mouth care.
4. Maintain adequate nutrition and hydration through nasogastric feedings (see procedure, p. 1152).
5. Carefully regulate fluid administration to avoid danger of rapidly increasing intracranial pressure.
6. Measure urine output and record specific gravity.
7. Administer suppositories or enemas as necessary to prevent constipation and impaction.
8. Change the child's position frequently and provide meticulous skin care to prevent hypostatic pneumonia and pressure sores.
9. Prevent contractures.
   a. Apply passive range of motion exercises to all extremities.
   b. Place pillows appropriately to support the child's body in good alignment.
   c. Use a footboard for the older child.
10. Have emergency equipment available for cardiopulmonary resuscitation, respiratory assistance, blood transfusion, subdural tap, etc.
11. Avoid discussing the child's condition near the bedside. Even though comatose, the child may be able to hear.
12. Observe for the development of the following complications:
    a. Respiratory problems (infection, aspiration, obstruction, atelectasis)
    b. Fluid and electrolyte imbalance
    c. Infection (urinary or central nervous system)
    d. Bladder and gastrointestinal distention

G. Care for the child with a craniotomy.

See section on the postoperative care of the child with a brain tumor, page 1464.

H. Provide for the child's emotional needs.

1. Hold and cuddle the infant as much as possible according to his condition.
2. Provide diversion according to the child's age.
   a. Infants—mobiles or musical toys
   b. Older children—quiet games, reading, etc.

I. Provide emotional support to the parents.

1. Encourage as much parental participation in the child's care as possible.
2. Reassure the parents that the prognosis is favorable with adequate treatment.
3. Avoid blaming the parents for the child's injury
   a. Attempt to alleviate their guilt feelings if present.

b. Refer the parents to a social worker or psychiatrist if this problem is severe.

Health Education

Reinforce explanations in the following areas:
1. The condition
2. The causes of the child's specific symptoms
3. The need and rationale for treatment
4. Postoperative and recovery expectations
5. Signs of recurrent bleeding
6. Safety measures to prevent accidents in the future

Reye's Syndrome

Reye's syndrome in children has been clinically characterized as a complex of signs and symptoms including encephalopathy and fatty degeneration of the viscera, mainly affecting the liver, brain, and kidneys.

Etiology and Incidence

1. Unknown
2. Most consistent single factor is an antecedent viral infection
   a. Influenza B—clustered geographically, occurring in older children (mean age is 11 years)
   b. Varicella—sporadic occurrence in younger children (mean age is 6 years)
   c. Gastroenteritis
   d. Upper respiratory tract infection
3. Other related viruses include adenovirus, coxsackie, ECHO, herpes simplex and zoster, reovirus, and polio type I.
4. Other controversial possibilities (contributors)
   a. Genetic make-up of individual child that increases his susceptibility triggered by virus, toxins, drugs, or endogenous factors.
   b. Environmental factors—chemical toxins (i.e., pesticides or fertilizers).
   c. Clinical—salicylates and phenothiazines, acetaminophen.
5. Occurs more commonly in Caucasian children living in rural or suburban areas under the age of 16 years. Occurs more frequently in Black infants from lower socioeconomic urban areas than white infants.
6. Peak seasonal occurrences are in winter and spring.

Altered Physiology

1. Mitochondrial injury or change is primary in all tissues.
   Dysfunctioning mitochondri result in decreased enzymes for proper functioning of specific metabolic pathways.
2. Liver—enlarged and bright yellow; fatty infiltration in the form of small lipid droplets; mitochondria are large and swollen with some decrease of enzymatic activity, particularly for ammonia detoxification, thus hyperammoniemia.
   a. Liver function studies are elevated—SGOT, SGPT.
   b. Clotting disturbances result in decreased clotting factor and prolonged prothrombin time and partial prothrombin time.
   c. Dysfunction of gluconeogenetic enzymatic pathway and depleted supply of glycogen stores. Hypoglycemia leads to the increased production of ammonia and fatty acidemia. Hypoglycemia seen in younger children is related to less liver reserve of glycogen and a higher metabolic rate.
3. Brain—cerebral edema with small ventricles, possible neuronal necrosis, findings consistent with hypoxia, inflammatory reaction absent, grossly enlarged mitochondria; and pervasive watery blebs.
   a. Hypoxia and/or hypoglycemia are evidenced by neuronal degeneration.
   b. Cerebral spinal fluid is usually normal, except in later stages of disease when pressure is elevated.
4. Kidney—fatty degeneration of loop of Henle and proximal convoluted tubules with a few lipid droplets in distal tubular cells.
   Renal vasculature and glomeruli are normal.
   Renal insufficiency occurs. Edema, decreased urinary output, increased BUN and creatinine, and loss of autoregulation lead to decrease in cerebral blood flow, tissue hypoxia, and neuronal death.
5. Heart—fatty accumulation in fibers; bundle of His, and bundle branches.

Prognosis and Complications

1. Complete recovery
2. Recovery with brain damage—developmental delays, motor impairment, or mental retardation
3. Posthospital anxiety and apprehension

Clinical Manifestations

▶ **NURSING ALERT:** Early diagnosis is critical because of the rapidly fatal course of the disease.

1. Prodromal illness (see etiology) that may be improving
2. Sudden pernicious vomiting—fever usually not present
3. Irrational behavior
4. Altered sensorium—from mild lethargy to progressive stupor and coma
5. Hyperventilation, tachypnea
6. Hepatomegaly
7. Stages—children with Reye's syndrome advance through definite stages of progression. After diagnosis is made, the child should be categorized as fitting within one of the stages, with any progression noted. Generally, the more rapid the progression through these stages, the poorer the prognosis.
   Lovejoy's Stages of Progression* follow:
   Stage I: Vomiting, lethargy, difficult to arouse, liver dysfunction, type I EEG†
   Stage II: Disorientation, delirium, combativeness, hyperventilation, hyperactive reflexes, liver dysfunction, type II EEG
   Stage III: Decorticate positioning, obtundent, coma,

---

* From Lovejoy FH et al. Clinical staging in Reye's syndrome. Am J Dis Child 1974 July; 128(1):36–41
† See bibliography for EEG typing references.

hyperventilation, liver dysfunction, presence of pupillary light reaction, type II EEG

Stage IV: Deepening coma, decerebrate rigidity, costal–caudal progression of brain stem dysfunction, loss of oculocephalic reflexes, fixed and dilated pupils, improvement of liver dysfunction, type III EEG

Stage V: Seizures, loss of reflexes, flaccidity, respiratory arrest, correction of liver dysfunction, isoelectric EEG

Diagnostic Evaluation

1. General condition and appearance of child: History of prodromal illness—mild upper respiratory infection or other infection with sudden development of pernicious vomiting, presence of other symptoms.
2. Differential diagnosis—acute toxic encephalopathy, hepatic coma, hepatitis, meningitis, or encephalitis. History to rule out ingestion of medications or toxic materials.
3. Laboratory data
   * a. Serum ammonia—elevated 48 μg./100 ml.
   * b. Liver enzymes (SGOT, SGPT)—elevated
   * c. Clotting factors (PT and PTT)—prolonged
   * d. Serum glucose—hypoglycemia
   e. Creatinine—elevated
   f. BUN—elevated
   g. Amino acid, free fatty acids—elevated
   h. Acid–base status—acidemia
   i. CBC
   * j. Serum bilirubin—mild, transient elevations to normal less than 3%
   k. Electrolytes
   l. Serum osmolality
   m. Serum levels of salicylates, acetaminophen, and phenothiazines
   n. Urine: analysis, electrolytes, and osmolality
4. Lumbar puncture—done if cerebrospinal fluid is needed to rule out other diagnoses. If symptoms of increased intracranial pressure exist, the performance of a lumbar puncture is to be avoided to prevent rapid decompression and herniation of the brain.
5. Liver biopsy—usually done, however the biopsy may not be done unless evidence is insufficient to make a definite diagnosis (shows microvesicular fatty degeneration of liver).

Medical and Nursing Management

A. General Considerations

1. Because this is a multisystem disease, it must be emphasized that:
   a. Intracerebral integrity is of utmost priority, and if the brain can be supported through the course of the illness, the chances of the other organs running their course uneventfully are very high and are of less concern.
   b. The multidisciplinary team must have a leader who initiates, coordinates, and supervises *all* activities and medical planning. It may be the physician, neurosurgeon, endocrinologist, or the attending pediatrician. However, it should be the person with the knowledge and capability of monitoring and directing care 24 hours a day.
2. Treatment is supportive by maintaining adequate levels of circulating glucose and cerebral perfusion

* Essential for diagnosis

while preventing or controlling IICP (increased intracranial pressure).

Treatment is aimed toward normalizing organ function and protection of the brain from irreversible damage.

B. Supportive Interventions*

1. Admission to an intensive care unit. Multisystem invasive monitoring: complex coordination of care (medical and nursing) of all systems is essential in order to control and reduce IICP.
   a. It takes many hours to several days after control of the disease process is achieved to begin to withdraw therapy or liberalize intervention without having recurring IICP symptoms.
   b. The nurse is the most constant and consistent person at the bedside in most institutions and must be alert to all aspects of this very complex critical-care problem.
   c. The nursing input may have a very significant impact on the morbidity of the patient; a knowledgeable nurse can make very important judgments concerning the timing of interventions and can anticipate problems and needs.
   d. Nursing responsibilities include assessment, reassessment, anticipation, and documentation of physical status, environmental impacts, and therapeutic interventions.
2. General supportive care includes:
   a. Correction of hypoglycemia
   b. Correction of fluid and electrolyte imbalance
   c. Correction of acidosis
   d. Prevention or correction of hypoxia
   e. Prevention of or treatment of increased intracranial pressure
   f. Correction of metabolic abnormalities
   g. Continuous monitoring of cardiopulmonary and neurologic status
   h. Evaluation of laboratory data
   i. Monitoring vital signs for signs of shock
3. Supportive care of the child in stage I or II (noncomatose):
   a. Hourly neurologic checks—see Glasgow Coma Scale (Table 43-1)
   b. Nothing by mouth
   c. Strict intake and output record
   d. Maintain serum glucose; 150–200 mg./dl. intravenous hypertonic glucose solution given
   e. Monitor body weight
   f. Administer phytonadione—to combat coagulation defects
   g. Sedation—to decrease anxiety and potential for IICP
4. Management of the child in stage III or IV (comatose):
   a. Insert intraventricular pressure catheter or subarachnoid bolt with pressure monitoring and control of IICP.† Goal is to maintain intracranial pressure within normal range of 10–15 torr.

* Miller J and Arsenault L. Reye's syndrome. J Neurosurg Nurs 1983 Jun; 15(3):154–164

† Hausman KA. Critical care of the child with increased intracranial pressure. Nurs Clin North Am 1981 Dec; 16(4):647–656

Shaywitz BA, Rothstein P and Venes JL. Monitoring and management of increased intracranial pressure in Reye's syndrome: Results in 29 children. Pediatrics 1980 Aug; 66(2):198–202

Table 43-1   Glasgow Coma Scale

Eyes open	Spontaneously	4
	To speech	3
	To pain	2
	No response	1
Best Verbal Response	Oriented	5
	Confused	4
	Inappropriate words	3
	Incomprehensible sounds	2
	None	1
Best Motor Response	Obeys commands	5
	Localizes pain	4
	Flexion to pain	3
	Extension to pain	2
	None	1

A deterioration in sensorium is indicated by decreasing score (Trauner DA. Treatment of Reye's syndrome. J Nat Reye's Syn Foundation 1980; 1(2):85–89)

b. Intubate (endo- or nasotracheal) and ventilate— to provide optimal cerebral blood flow. (Auto regulation − ↓ PCO_2 = ↓ size blood vessels = ↓ vol = ↓ ICP.)
Maintain $PaCO_2$ about 25 mm. torr and PaO_2 at 100–150 torr. Muscle relaxants and short-acting barbiturates are also used.

c. Establish arterial line for pressure monitoring and blood sampling.

d. Insert indwelling urethral catheter.
   (1) Accurately record intake and output every 1–4 hours.
   (2) Measure urine specific gravity.

e. Insert nasogastric tube and measure drainage. Give an antacid every 2–4 hours to maintain gastric pH above 4. Neomycin may be given via nasogastric tube to aid in reduction of ammonia accumulation.

f. Limit fluid intake—peripheral IV fluids given at a rate of ⅔ maintenance because of potential cerebral edema and IICP. Calculate administered medications as part of fluid intake.

g. Monitor blood glucose—give IV glucose to prevent any neurologic deterioration (hypertonic solution up to 15%–20% IV drip through a central line). Keep serum glucose 200–300 mg./dl, serum osmolality 300–310 mOsm./liter.

5. Additional measures directed at controlling intracranial pressure:

a. Maintain core body temperature at 36.5°–37°C. (97.7°–98.6°F.). Moderate hypothermia (controversial) may be employed using a cooling blanket.

b. Position supine with head of bed elevated 30 degrees; keep head still—aids in intracranial venous drainage.

c. Provide chest physical therapy—to prevent infection and atelectasis, increased intrathoracic pressure, thus increasing intracranial pressure. The risk of increasing intracranial pressure must be weighed against the benefit of the procedure.

d. Observe for complications—cardiac arrhythmias, heme concentration, decreased urinary output, decreased mean arterial pressure, fluid overload (↑ CVP 6–8 cm. H_2O, urine output ↑ 2 ml./kg./hour, clinical edema), hypovolemia (mean arterial pressure ↓ 65 mm. Hg).

e. Monitor EEG continuously.

f. Monitor nursing activities that may cause an increase in intracranial pressure: suctioning, turning,* chest physical therapy, painful (intrusive) procedures, conversation at bedside about diagnosis.

g. Prevent and control IICP with drugs.
   (1) Muscle relaxation (pancuronium bromide) while on ventilator
   (2) Sedation (diazepam, chloral hydrate)
   (3) Osmotic diuretic (mannitol or glycerol)
   (4) Barbiturate therapy (thiopental, phenobarbital)†

h. Provide secondary infection coverage—especially staphylococcus (neurologic and lung).

6. When all intensive medical and nursing support has been exhausted and ICP is still uncontrollable or cardiovascular status is unstable, consideration for bilateral decompression craniectomies must be made by the medical team.

Patient Problems/Nursing Diagnoses

1. Inadequate respiratory function related to apnea, pulmonary congestion and obstruction, and coma
2. Alterations in cardiac function related to hypovolemia, dehydration/or fluid overload, altered electrolytes, cardiac instability, and impaired autoregulatory mechanism
3. Increased intracranial pressure related to cerebral edema
4. Hypoglycemia related to altered liver function
5. Potential for complications (i.e., skin breakdown, corneal injury, etc., related to comatose state)
6. Anxiety and altered coping behaviors of family related to lack of knowledge, fear, and/or guilt.
7. Anxiety related to acuteness of illness, procedures, hospitalization and on recollection of events that occurred during critical phase of illness.

Nursing Interventions

A. Provide acute and intensive nursing care.

1. During the acute phase of the disease, the child should be cared for in an intensive care unit.
2. Refer to:
   Respiratory procedures, page 1178
   Cardiopulmonary resuscitation, page 1195
   Assisting with obtaining blood for gas analysis, page 143
   Intensive care, page 1119
   Intravenous therapy, page 1160
   Increased intracranial pressure, page 1418
   Care of the comatose patient, page 760
   NG tube procedures, page 1152
   Catheter procedure, page 505

B. Be aware of the medical plan of treatment and be alert to the rapidity of the course of the disease.‡ Particularly important factors:

1. Note and report immediately any changes in the child's status or stage of progression (see clinical manifestations).

---

* Suggested reading: Lipe HP and Mitchell PH. Positioning the patient with intracranial hypertension: How turning and head rotation affect the internal jugular vein. Heart Lung 1980 Nov/Dec; 9(6):1031–1037

† Suggested reading: Marshall LF, Shapiro HM, Rauscher A and Kaufman NM. Phenobarbital therapy for intracranial hypertension in metabolic coma. Crit Care Med 1978 Jan/Feb; 6(1):1–5

‡ Suggested reading: Nikas DC and Konkoly R. Nursing responsibilities in arterial and intracranial pressure monitoring. J Neurosurg Nurs 1975 Dec; 7(2):116–122

2. Therapy is directed at maintaining normal intracranial pressure and adequate cerebral perfusion.
3. Protect the child from complications that may result from the comatose condition or life-saving medical intervention.
4. Maintain fluid and electrolyte balance.
5. Before any procedure is done for the child, consider the effects on his intracranial pressure.

C. **Support parents during the time that the child may be in the intensive care unit.**

1. Prior to the first visit, explain in detail what the child will look like. Accompany the parents when they first visit their child. Since this may be traumatic, do not force them to maintain lengthy contact with the child.
2. Address parental concerns and answer questions regarding:
   a. How they should react to their child
   b. Amount of parental participation that is beneficial
   c. Fears and fantasies during lengthy periods when they are unable to visit child
   d. Concerns for other children and other family members, and their reactions to the illness
   e. Technical questions
3. Provide the parents with the telephone number of the intensive care unit.
4. Make sure the parents have a comfortable place to sleep if they elect to stay at the hospital.
5. Help the parents who request consultation—social service for ICU, chaplain, Reye's Syndrome Foundation parent group (if appropriate and available).
6. Help the family express their feelings about what has happened and how it is affecting them.
   a. Assess how they are coping; their family support systems.
   b. Initiate referrals to appropriate social agencies as needed.
   c. The lack of knowledge of the disease and rapid course from a mild to a critical illness may be difficult for parents to understand. They may have extreme feelings of guilt, and blame themselves or others for not recognizing the seriousness of the illness sooner. They may have other children at home with similar prodromal viral infection who may be experiencing guilty feelings about the ill sibling.

D. **Provide psychological and emotional support to the child.**

1. Although the child may be heavily sedated, comatose, or paralyzed from muscle relaxants, he perceives in varying degrees what is happening to him and to his environment.
2. Explain procedures to the child while they are being done.
3. Conversations about the child, his condition, or other children should take place away from the sick child.
4. Encourage parents to bring in a favorite toy or security object.
5. Show a constant awareness of any activity, noise, etc. that increases or changes intracranial pressure.
6. When a sedated or comatose child awakens, he may be disoriented and have no memory of previous events. Provide explanations and reassurance as appropriate.
7. Parental separation may increase anxiety; support as necessary.

E. **Provide continued support of the child and his family when the child is transferred from the critical care unit to the pediatric nursing unit.**

1. Once the child is alert, his condition stable, and he is recovering, he should be transferred to the regular pediatric unit.
2. The child recovering from Reye's syndrome without any neurologic sequelae should recover fairly rapidly. Provide support as needed.
3. When the child has experienced sequelae or complications, attention to his physical manifestations will be needed according to the child's specific deficit (i.e., physical therapy). A multidisciplinary team approach to treatment will continue to provide for optimal functioning.
4. The child and his family will continue to need emotional support during this period.
5. A critical role of the nurse is to educate herself, other members of the staff, and the community about Reye's syndrome.*
   a. Learn to recognize the symptoms that may lead to a diagnosis of the illness.
   b. Be prepared for the course of the illness, from a mild disease to one that is life-threatening.
   c. Support parent groups and other community groups to educate parents about Reye's syndrome, and to seek medical consultation when symptoms may indicate the disease.

Health Education

1. Encourage the family to maintain a close physical and emotional relationship with the child during his illness
   a. Helps the child feel less disoriented
   b. Helps the family work through feelings of guilt and helplessness
2. Ensure that the parents understand the importance of medical follow-up, especially related to any complications associated with the illness
3. Become involved in community education to help caretakers recognize early signs and symptoms suggestive of Reye's syndrome

Expected Outcomes

1. Demonstrates adequate respiratory function as evidenced by appropriate respiratory status, normal vital signs, and normal arterial blood gases
2. Achieves adequate circulatory function and cerebral perfusion as evidenced by normal CVP values, normal urinary output, and normal sinus rhythm
3. Maintains integrity of cerebral blood flow and oxygenation and is free of neurologic deterioration as evidenced by intracranial pressures ↓ <15 torr, absence of clinical signs of deterioration and absence of hyperthermia
4. Shows no signs of hypoglycemia as evidenced by appropriate serum glucose levels
5. Avoids complications of immobility and comatose state as evidenced by intact skin, absence of secondary infections, etc.
6. Reveals minimal anxiety and disorientation as evidenced by behaviors
7. The parents demonstrate and verbalize understanding of disease and events

* National Reye's Syndrome Foundation, 436 N. Lewis, Bryan, OH 43506
Reye's Syndrome Society, PO Box RS, 7045 Traverse Avenue, Benzonia, MI 49616

Bibliography

Books

Bell W and McCormick W. Neurologic Infections in Children, 2nd ed. Volume XII in the Series, Major Problems in Clinical Pediatrics. Philadelphia, WB Saunders, 1981

Behrman RE and Vaughan VC. Nelson Textbook of Pediatrics. Philadelphia, WB Saunders, 1983

Chess S and Fernandez P. The Handicapped Child in School: Behavior and Management. New York, Brunner/Mazel, 1981

Conway-Rutkowski B. Carini and Owen's Neurological and Neurosurgical Nursing, 8th ed. St Louis, CV Mosby, 1982

Danilova L. Methods of Improving the Cognitive and Verbal Development of Children with Cerebral Palsy. New York, World Rehabilitation Fund, 1983

Darling R and Darling J. Children Who Are Different: Meeting the Challenges of Birth Defects in Society. St Louis, CV Mosby, 1981

Dobbing J (ed). Prevention of Spina Bifida and other Neural Tube Defects. New York, Academic Press, 1982

Downey J and Low N (eds). The Child with Disabling Illness: Principles of Rehabilitation, 2nd ed. New York, Raven Press, 1982

Farmer T (ed). Pediatric Neurology, 3rd ed. Philadelphia, Harper & Row, 1983

Fraser B and Hensinger R. Managing Physical Handicaps: A Practical Guide for Parents, Care Providers and Educators. Baltimore, Paul H Brookes, 1983

Hickey J. The Clinical Practice of Neurological and Neurosurgical Nursing. Philadelphia, JB Lippincott, 1981

Hicks DA. Cerebral edema. In Pierog JE and Pierog LJ (eds). Pediatric Critical Illness and Injury. Rockville, MD, Aspen Publication, 1984

Hoeprich PD (ed). Infectious Diseases, 3rd ed. Philadelphia, Harper & Row, 1983

Hopkins A. Epilepsy: The Facts. New York, Oxford University Press, 1981

Kaktis JV. An introduction to monitoring intracranial pressure in critically ill children. In Pierog JE and Pierog LJ (eds). Pediatric Critical Illness and Injury. Rockville, MD, Aspen Publication, 1984

Krugman S and Katz S. Infectious Diseases of Children, 7th ed. St Louis, CV Mosby, 1981

Levin D, Morriss F and Moore G (eds). A Practical Guide to Pediatric Intensive Care, 2nd ed. St Louis, CV Mosby, 1984

Levitt S. Treatment of Cerebral Palsy and Motor Delay, 2nd ed. London, Blackwell Scientific Publications, 1982

Oakes A (ed). Critical Care Nursing of Children and Adolescents. Philadelphia, WB Saunders, 1981

Pellock J and Myer E (eds). Neurologic Emergencies in Infancy and Childhood. Philadelphia, Harper & Row, 1984

Powell M. Assessment and Management of Developmental Changes and Problems in Children, 2nd ed. St Louis, CV Mosby, 1981

Roessler R and Bolton B. Psychosocial Adjustment to Disability. Baltimore, University Park Press, 1978

Rudy E. Advanced Neurological and Neurosurgical Nursing. St Louis, CV Mosby, 1984

Schafer M and Dias L. Myelomeningocele: Orthopedic Treatment. Baltimore, Williams & Wilkins, 1983

Scheiner A and Abrams I. The Practical Management of the Developmentally Disabled Child. St Louis, CV Mosby, 1980

Scherzer A and Tscharnuter I. Early Diagnosis and Therapy In Cerebral Palsy. New York, Marcel Dekker, 1982

Section of Pediatric Neurosurgery of the American Association of Neurological Surgeons (eds). Pediatric Neurosurgery: Surgery of the Developing Nervous System. New York, Grune & Stratton, 1982

Smith J (ed). Pediatric Critical Care. New York, John Wiley & Sons, 1983

Snyder M. A Guide to Neurological and Neurosurgical Nursing. New York, John Wiley & Sons, 1983

Swaiman K and Wright F. The Practice of Pediatric Neurology. St Louis, CV Mosby, 1982

Thompson G, Rubin I and Bilenker R. Comprehensive Management of Cerebral Palsy. New York, Grune & Stratton, 1982

Varni J. Clinical Behavioral Pediatrics. New York, Pergamon Press, 1983

Vestal K (ed). Pediatric Critical Care Nursing. New York, John Wiley & Sons, 1981

Wedgwood RJ, et al. Infections in Children. Philadelphia, Harper & Row, 1982

Whaley L and Wong D. Nursing Care of Infants and Children, 2nd ed. St Louis, CV Mosby, 1983

Worcester CC. Reye's Syndrome. In Pierog JE and Pierog LJ (eds). Pediatric Critical Illness and Injury. Rockville, MD, Aspen Publication, 1984

Woodbury D, Penry J and Pippenger C. Antiepileptic Drugs, 2nd ed. New York, Raven Press, 1982

Zucman E. Childhood Disability in the Family. New York, World Rehabilitation Fund, 1982

Articles

Arcinue EL. Reye's syndrome: Contending with a mysterious and increasingly common disease. Consultant 1982 Nov; 22(11):165–167+

. . Aspirin and Reye's Syndrome. Am J Dis Child 1982 Nov; 136(11):971–972

Benjamin R and McKay R. Working with a brain-injured child. J Assoc Care Child Health 1980 Spring; 8(4):99–104

Berkowitz C and Jones C. The PNP's role in evaluation and management of febrile seizures. Pediatr Nurs 1983 Nov/Dec; 9(6):432–434

Boutros AR, et al. Reye syndrome: A predictable curable disease. Pediatr Clin North Am 1980 Aug; 27(3):539–552

Brink J, Imbus C and Woo-Sam J. Physical recovery after severe closed head trauma in children and adolescents. J Pediatr 1980 Nov; 97(5):721–727

Bruce D. The child's injured head: Trauma in the young. Emerg Med 1983 Aug 15; 15(14):45, 49–50, 55–56

Budd RA and Hobdell EF. Reye's syndrome. Crit Care Nurse 1983 Mar/Apr; 3(2):94–97

Budd RA and Rothwell R. Spotting Reye's syndrome while there's still time. RN 1983 Dec; 46(12):38–42+

Camfield P et al. The first febrile seizure—antipyretic instruction plus either phenobarbital or placebo to prevent recurrence. J Pediatr 1980 Jul; 97(1):16–21

Cecconi C et al. Model instructional program for mainstreaming handicapped children . . . designed to teach normal children about cerebral palsy. Phys Ther 1980 Aug; 60(8):1022–1025

Clarke K et al. Reye's syndrome nursing protocol. J Nat Reye's Syn Found 1980 1(2):82–84

Chee D. Seizure disorders. Nurs Clin North Am 1980 Mar; 15(1):71–82

Clarkson J. Self-catheterization training of a child with myelomeningocele. AJOT 1982 Feb; 36(2):95–98

Coffey R. Pediatric neurological emergencies. Top Emerg Med 1982 Jul; 4(2):67–78

Colgan M. The child with spina bifida. Am J Dis Child 1981 Sep; 135(9):854–858

Consensus Development Panel. Febrile seizures: Long term management of children with fever-associated seizures. Pediatr Rev 1981 Jan; 2(1):209–212

Coulter D. The psychosocial impact of epilepsy in childhood. Child Health Care 1982 Fall; 11(2):48–53

Dalgas P. Reye's syndrome update. MCN 1983 Sep/Oct; 8(5):345–349

Dunne RS and Perez RC. Reye's syndrome: A challenge not limited to critical care nurses. Issues Compr Pediatr Nurs 1981 Jul/Aug; 5(4):253–263

Edwards M and Baker C. Complications and sequelae of meningococcal infections in children. J Pediatr 1981 Oct; 99(4):540–545

Ferry P. Computed cranial tomography in children. J Pediatr 1980 Jun; 96(6):961–967

Gaddy D. Meningitis in the pediatric population. Nurs Clin North Am 1980 March; 15(1):83–97

Graziani L et al. Ultrasound studies in preterm infants with hydrocephalus. J Pediatr 1980 Oct; 97(4):624–631

Griffiths S. Body image concerns of a four year old boy with meningitis. Matern Child Nurs J 1980 Summer; 9(2):127–136

Grow DH. Reye's syndrome. Nursing '81 1981 Nov; 11(11):156+

Gururaj V. Febrile seizures: Current concepts. Clin Pediatr 1980 Nov; 19(11):731–738

Hahn JF. Cerebral edema and neurointensive care. Pediatr Clin North Am 1980 Aug; 27(3):587–592

Haller J. Intracranial pressure monitoring in Reye's syndrome. Hosp Pract 1980 Feb; 15(2):101–108

Hausman KA. Critical care of the child with increased intracranial pressure. Nurs Clin North Am 1981 Dec; 16(4):647–656

Icenogle D and Kaplan A. A review of congenital neurologic malformations. Clin Pediatr 1981 Sep; 20(9):565–576

Jackson P. Increased intracranial pressure in infants and young children. Crit Care Q 1981 Mar; 3(4):47–59

Jackson P. Peritoneal shunting for hydrocephalus. Crit Care Update 1983 Apr; 10(4):33–39

Jackson P. Ventriculo–peritoneal shunts. Am J Nurs 1980 Jun; 80(6):1104–1109

Jamison-Smith P and Hamm P. Reye's syndrome. Crit Care Update 1983 Jul; 10(7):54–55

Jeffries J, Killam P and Varni J. Behavioral management of fecal incontinence in a child with myelomeningocele. Pediatr Nurs 1982 Jul/Aug; 8(4):267–270

Johnson LK. If your patient has increased intracranial pressure, your goal should be: No surprises. Nursing '83 1983 Jun; 13(6):58–63

Johnson M and Freeman J. Pharmacologic advances in seizure control. Pediatr Clin North Am 1981 Feb; 28(1):179–194

Kaplan S and Feigin. Treatment of meningitis in children. Pediatr Clin North Am 1983 Apr; 30(2):259–270

Killam P et al. Behavioral pediatric weight rehabilitation for children with myelomeningocele. MCN 1983 Jul/Aug; 8(4):280–286

Kolata GB. Reye's syndrome: A medical mystery. Science 1980 Mar 28; 207(4438):1453–1454

Kunkel J. Nursing management of the head injured patient. Crit Care Update 1981 Mar; 8(3):22–24+

Lovejoy FC et al. Clinical staging in Reye's syndrome. Am J Dis Child 1974 Jul, 128:36–41

Manella K and Varni J. Behavior therapy in a gait-training program for a child with myelomeningocele. Phys Ther 1981 Sep; 61(9):1284–1287

Martelli ME. Teaching parents about Reye's syndrome. Am J Nurs 1982 Feb; 82(2):260–263

McElroy D. Hydrocephalus in children. Nurs Clin North Am 1980 Mar; 15(1):23–34

McGrath D. Video recording seizure activity in children. MCN 1983 May/Jun; 8(3):218–220

Meir E. Evaluating head trauma in infants and children. MCN 1983 Jan/Feb; 8(1):54–57

Miller J and Arsenault L. Reye's syndrome. J Neurosurg Nurs 1983 Jun; 15(3):154–164

Mills G. Preparing children and parents for cerebral computerized tomography. MCN 1980 Nov/Dec; 5(6):403–407

Mitchell PH, Ozuna J and Lipe HP. Moving the patient in bed: Effects on intracranial pressure. Nurs Res 1981 Jul/Aug; 30(4):212–218

Norman S. The pupil check. Am J Nurs 1982 Apr; 82(4):588–591

Norman S and Browne T. Seizure disorders. Am J Nurs 1981 May; 81(5):985–994

Orlowski J, Rothner D and Lueders H. Submersion accidents in children with epilepsy. Am J Dis Child 1982 Sep; 136(9):777–780

Parrish MA. A comparison of behavioral side effects related to commonly used anticonvulsants. Pediatr Nurs 1984 Mar/Apr; 10(2):149–152

Passo S. Malformations of the neural tube. Nurs Clin North Am 1980 Mar; 15(1):5–21

Pinyerd B. Siblings of children with myelomeningocele: Examining their perceptions. Matern Child Nurs J 1983 Spring; 12(1):61–70

Pleasants D. Managing hydrocephalus with a ventricular shunt. AORN J 1982 Apr; 35(5):885–892

Pressman S. Myelomeningocele: A multidisciplinary problem. J Neurosurg Nurs 1981 Dec; 13(6):333–336

Raphaely R et al. Management of severe pediatric head trauma. Pediatr Clin North Am 1980 Aug; 27(3):715–727

Reye RD, Morgan G and Barae J. Encephalopathy and fatty degeneration of the viscera—a disease entity in children. Lancet 1963 Oct 12; 2(7310):749–752

. . . . Reye Syndrome and aspirin use: The role of prodromal illness severity in the assessment of relative risk. Pediatrics 1982 Jun; 69(6):812–822

Rothner A and Erenberg G. Status epilepticus. Pediatr Clin North Am 1980 Aug; 27(3):593–602

Ruben F et al. Epidemiologic factors of Reye syndrome seen in southwestern Pennsylvania 1970–1980. AJPH 1983 Sep; 73(9):1063–1065

Santilli N and Tonelson S. Screening for seizures. Pediatr Nurs 1981 Mar/Apr; 7(2):11–15

Sasso S. Phenytoin for seizure disorders. MCN 1984 Jul/Aug; 9(4):279

Scarff T et al. Myelomeningocele: A review and update. Rehabil Nurs 1981 Nov/Dec; 6(6):26–29

Shaw L. A teaching plan for cerebroventricular shunting for hydrocephalus. AORN J 1982 Apr; 35(5):893–898

Shurtleff D. Myelodysplasia: Management and treatment. Curr Probl Pediatr 1980 Jan; 10(3):1–56

Smith EE. Reye's syndrome: Deadly threat to children. Am Lung Assoc Bull 1982 May; 68(4):11–12

. . . . Take two aspirin and call me in the morning: Salicylate use and Reye's syndrome. Am J Dis Child 1982 Nov; 136(11):973–974

Thurston J et al. Prognosis in childhood epilepsy: Additional follow-up of 148 children 15 to 23 years after withdrawal of anticonvulsant therapy. N Engl J Med 1982 Apr; 306(14):831–836

Trauner DA. Reye's syndrome. Current Probl Pediatr 1982 May; 12(7):2–31

Tucker C. Complex partial seizures. Am J Nurs 1981 May; 81(5):996–1000

Vigliarolo D. Managing bowel incontinence in children with meningomyelocele. Am J Nurs 1980 Jan; 80(1):105–107

Waldman RJ et al. Aspirin as a risk factor in Reye's syndrome. JAMA 1982 Jun; 247(22):3089–3094

Wallack C. Head trauma in children. Nurs Clin North Am 1980 Mar; 15(1):115–117

Walson P et al. Once daily doses of phenobarbital in children. J Pediatr 1980 Aug; 97(2):303–305

Wink D. Bacterial meningitis in children. Am J Nurs 1984 Apr; 84(4):456–460

Ziff S. The sexual concerns of the adolescent woman with cerebral palsy. Issues Health Care Women 1981 Jan/Feb; 3(1):55–63

Children with Orthopedic Conditions

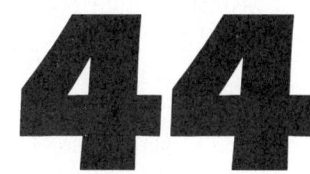

Fractures

Generally, nursing care of the child with a fracture is similar to that of an adult. The child is usually hospitalized only for application of a cast (see procedure for cast care, p. 1208) or to be placed in traction (see procedure for traction, p. 1199). The nurse should be aware of the following principles concerning fractures in pediatrics.

General Considerations

1. Children's bones are softer and more pliable than adult's bones. They can tolerate a greater degree of deformity before breaking.
2. Greenstick fractures in normal bones are unique to children.
   a. The bone breaks at one cortex and bends at the other.
   b. There is no complete loss of bony continuity.
   c. The younger the child, the more likely he is to sustain a greenstick fracture.
   d. The radius, ulna, clavicle, or long bone in the hand are most likely to sustain a greenstick fracture.
3. Comminuted fractures are less common in pediatric patients.
4. Injuries of the epiphyseal plate are unique to children.
   a. The epiphyseal plate is weaker than normal tendons, ligaments, or the joint capsule.
   b. Injury resulting in a torn ligament or dislocation in the adult is more likely to produce a separation of the epiphysis in a child.
   c. The lower radial epiphysis is more frequently separated than any other.
   d. This type of injury may cause growth disturbance.
5. Fractures in pediatric patients heal more readily than those in adults.
   a. The younger the child, the more rapidly the fracture unites.
   b. The thick periosteum and abundant blood supply make nonunion rare.
6. End-to-end apposition of fracture surfaces is not essential in pediatric patients.
   a. The long bones may be allowed to unite with side-to-side apposition in children up to 11–12 years of age.
   b. Subsequent molding will produce a normal bone by the end of growth.
7. Following injury, the extremities in children are likely to swell much more rapidly and the swelling to disappear more quickly than in an adult.
8. Function is usually restored rapidly and sometimes spontaneously following injury in children.

Common Fractures in Children

Fracture of the Clavicle

A. Cause
1. Compression of the shoulders during delivery of a baby
2. Transmitted force caused by falling on an outstretched hand, elbow, or side of the shoulder
3. Direct force (rare)

B. Treatment
1. Immobilization in a figure 8 bandage or clavicle strap.
2. Closed reduction and use of a plaster figure 8 cast, or bed rest and side arm traction may be necessary in older children with displaced fractures.

C. Healing Time
1. Younger children: 3–4 weeks
2. Older children: 5–6 weeks

Fracture of the Neck of the Humerus

A. Cause
1. Indirect force from a fall on an outstretched hand
2. Direct force by blow or fall on the lateral aspect of the shoulder

B. Treatment
1. Minimal displacement—immobilization of the shoulder and upper extremity with stockinette collar and sling
2. Considerable displacement
   a. Reduction under anesthesia may be done.
   b. Immobilization of the shoulder and upper extremity in a collar and cuff sling or a shoulder spica.
   c. Dunlop traction followed by use of a shoulder spica cast may be required in severe cases.

C. Healing Time
1. Minimal displacement: 3–4 weeks
2. Considerable displacement: 4–6 weeks

Fractures of the Shaft of the Humerus

A. Cause
1. Birth injury—most common long bone to be fractured at that time

2. Direct force, such as a fall on the side of the arm
3. Indirect force, such as the child throwing a ball, or a caretaker grabbing the child's arm to prevent a fall or pulling an arm in or out of a sleeve roughly

B. Treatment

1. Reduction of the fracture
2. Immobilization
   a. Infants and young children
      (1) A U-slab of plaster is used to keep the arm against the chest with the elbow at a 90- to 45-degree angle.
      (2) Skin traction may be necessary for 2–3 weeks if the fracture is unstable or oblique with much overriding of the fragments.
         The arm is then immobilized as described above until healing is complete.
   b. Older children or adolescents
      (1) A shoulder spica cast is used for an unstable fracture.
      (2) Skeletal traction and suspension of the forearm and hand are indicated if the local skin and soft tissue conditions do not permit skin traction.
      (3) A hanging cast may be used for an older adolescent.
         (a) This type of cast permits the child to be ambulatory and active.
         (b) Erect position should be maintained as much as possible during the day.
         (c) The child should sleep in a semirecumbent position.
         (d) There should be no support at the elbow.
         (e) Pressure from clothing or anything that might compress the arm against the body must be avoided as it interferes with traction.

C. Healing Time

4–6 weeks

Supracondylar Fracture of the Humerus

A. Cause

Fall on an outstretched hand with hyperextension of the elbow (most common type of elbow fracture in children and adolescents)

B. Treatment

1. Should be managed as an acute emergency because of the danger of neurovascular complications.
2. Minimally displaced fractures—immobilization in a collar and cuff sling.
3. Moderately displaced fractures
   a. Closed reduction under anesthesia.
   b. Immobilization in a long arm cast or collar and cuff sling.
   c. Need for Dunlop skin traction for a period of 5–7 days until swelling subsides and a long-arm cast can be applied. Circulation and neural function should be carefully assessed.
4. Severely displaced fractures
   a. Closed reduction under anesthesia.
   b. Skeletal traction with the shoulder abducted 60 degrees and the arm elevated 20 degrees above the horizontal until the fracture is stable. Circulation and neural function should be carefully assessed.

c. Continued immobilization in a long-arm cast or collar and cuff sling.

C. Healing Time

1. 6–8 weeks
2. Several months may be required for complete restoration of function.

D. Complications

1. Malunion and changes in carrying angle.
2. Vascular complications—the extremity should be observed for pallor, pain, absent pulse, paresthesia, and paralysis.

Fractures of the Distal Third of the Radius and Ulna

A. Cause

1. Fracture may result from indirect force, such as falling on an outstretched hand.
2. Bones may break at different levels, and each fracture may be complete or greenstick.

B. Treatment

1. Greenstick fracture
   a. Closed reduction if the degree of angulation exceeds 30 degrees in infants or 15 degrees in children
   b. Immobilization in a long-arm cast
2. Complete fracture
   a. Reduction under anesthesia
   b. Immobilization in an above-elbow cast

C. Healing Time

4–6 weeks

Fractures Involving the Distal Radial Physis

A. Cause

1. Indirect force by falling on an outstretched hand
2. Most common physical injury

B. Treatment

1. Closed reduction
2. Immobilization in a long-arm cast

C. Healing Time

3–4 weeks

Fractures of the Phalanges

A. Cause

Direct force to the finger

B. Treatment

1. Distal phalanx
   a. Aluminum finger splint
   b. Splinting of adjoining finger
2. Middle phalanx
   a. Manual traction and flexion of the distal fragment
   b. Immobilization in a below-elbow plaster cast with a padded aluminum splint
   c. Unstable fractures—need for skeletal traction with a pin through the distal phalanx

C. Healing Time

2–5 weeks

Femoral Shaft Fracture

A. Cause

Major force, either direct or indirect, such as that sustained in automobile accidents or falls from a height

B. Treatment

1. Requires treatment as serious injury because of the blood loss and potential shock which may accompany the primary trauma
2. Infants and children under 2 years of age
   a. Bryant's traction for 2–3 weeks until the fracture is stable
   b. Immobilization in a 1½ hip spica cast until solid union occurs
3. Older children and adolescents
   a. Undisplaced fracture—immobilization in a hip spica cast
   b. Displaced fracture
      (1) Reduction and traction until fracture is stable. Traction type depends on location and manner of displacement—usually Russell, split Russell, or balanced traction with Thomas splint and Pearson attachment.
      (2) Immobilization in a spica cast until bony union is firm.

C. Healing Time

3–12 weeks, depending on the child's age and the type of fracture

D. Complications

1. Discrepancy in extremity length
2. Angular deformities of the femoral shaft

Fracture of the Tibia or Fibula

A. Cause

1. Direct force
2. Indirect rotational twisting force

B. Treatment

1. Closed reduction
2. Immobilization in a long leg cast—during the final weeks of healing, partial weight-bearing in a walking cast may be permitted.
3. Careful evaluation of neurologic and vascular function is imperative.

C. Healing Time

3–6 weeks, depending on the age of the child and the type of fracture

Osteomyelitis

Osteomyelitis is an infection that may involve all parts of a bone.

Etiology

1. Pathogenic bacteria commonly associated with osteomyelitis
   a. *Staphylococcus aureus*—responsible for the majority of cases (up to 90%)
   b. Streptococcal organisms
   c. *Salmonella*
   d. *H. influenzae*
2. Exogenous osteomyelitis—acquired by direct invasion of the bone by extension from the outside, as from a penetrating wound, fracture, etc.
3. Hematogenous osteomyelitis (more common)—caused by hematogenous spread of organisms from another focus
   Identifiable primary infections:
   a. Skin abscesses
   b. Otitis media
   c. Urinary tract infections
   d. Pneumonia
   e. Abscessed teeth
4. Preconditions favoring development of osteomyelitis in children
   a. Bone regions that have suffered trauma
   b. Bone that suffers from low oxygen tension of sickle cell anemia

Incidence

1. Most frequent occurrence between 5 and 14 years of age
2. More frequent in males than in females

Altered Physiology

1. Infection starts in the soft, medullary tissues.
2. This causes hyperemia, changes in the capillary permeability, and edema of the tissue.

3. Granulocytic leukocytes infiltrate the area and are destroyed by bacteria, liberating a proteolytic enzyme which causes tissue necrosis.
4. The inflammatory reaction causes thrombosis of vessels, producing irregular areas of bone ischemia.
5. Pus forms and spreads toward the diaphysis and extends through the cortex of the bone.
6. A subperiosteal abscess is formed with elevation of the periosteum.
7. There is further interference of blood supply to the bone shaft.
   a. Vascular supply may remain sufficient to maintain life of bone tissue:
      (1) New bone is created.
      (2) Bone healing occurs.
   b. Vascular supply may be diminished below that necessary to maintain life of bone tissue:
      (1) Bone dies and becomes inert.
         Small pieces of dead bone may be completely destroyed by granulation tissue from contiguous living tissue.
      (2) Large pieces of dead bone cannot be completely destroyed.
         (a) Central residual remains as a sequestrum composed of cancellous or cortical bone or a combination.
         (b) New bone is laid down beneath the elevated periosteum and tends to form an encasement (involucrum) around the sequestrum.
         (c) The involucrum is punctured by numerous channels through which pus may escape from the inside.
         (d) Pockets of infection are walled off in which organisms can lie dormant for long periods of time.
         (e) Chronic sinuses may form which eventually reach the surface and drain.

(f) Drainage continues until infection quiets once more.

Channels become plugged with granulations and remain closed until the pressure of the pus builds up and causes the sinuses to reopen or reach the surface via new channels (chronic osteomyelitis).

(g) Complete healing takes place only when all of the dead bone has been destroyed, discharged, or excised.

Clinical Manifestations

A. Onset

1. Usually abrupt
2. May be altered when osteomyelitis follows an infection which has been treated by antimicrobials.

B. Initial Symptoms

1. Pain in the involved area
2. Fever
3. Malaise

C. Later Symptoms

1. Swelling, redness, and warmth over the affected bone
2. Weakness
3. Irritability
4. Generalized signs of sepsis

D. Common Sites of Infection in Children

1. Large, cylindrical bones of the extremities
   a. Femur
   b. Tibia
   c. Humerus
   d. Radius

Diagnostic Evaluation

1. Leukocytosis
2. Blood culture—usually positive
3. Sedimentation rate usually elevated
4. Positive needle aspiration of the bone
5. X-ray data
   a. Progressive findings
      (1) Periosteal reaction
      (2) Areas of radiolucency secondary to bone destruction
      (3) Evidence of the formation of involucrum (reactive, living bone)
   b. Progress of the disease not seen on x-ray for at least 5 days in small children; as long as 8–10 days in older children
6. Bone scans—helpful in documenting the progress of the disease, but may be normal in the early period

Treatment

1. Intravenous administration of antimicrobial therapy
2. Immobilization of the affected extremity
3. Surgical decompression of the infected bony area may be necessary with insertion of drains

Prognosis

1. Mortality rate markedly improved with the advent of modern antimicrobial agents
2. Depends on early institution of appropriate therapy and adequate continuation

Patient Problems/Nursing Diagnoses

1. Pain related to the infectious process and required intravenous therapy
2. Immobility related to pain and possible traction as part of treatment
3. Potential for adverse reaction to long-term antimicrobial therapy
4. Anxiety related to hospitalization and painful procedures
5. Social isolation related to possible isolation technique and long-term hospitalization
6. Parental knowledge deficit about osteomyelitis and its treatment
7. Parental coping difficulties related to feelings of guilt

Nursing Interventions

A. Treat the infection with antimicrobial therapy.

1. Administer intravenous antimicrobials as prescribed by the physician.
   a. Administer medication exactly on schedule in order to maintain consistent blood levels.
   b. Monitor intravenous infusion carefully.
      (1) Notify the appropriate person if infiltration is suspected, so that the IV can be restarted.
      (2) A venous cutdown is often necessary, especially for a small child.
      (3) A constant infusion pump may be helpful if the infusion rate is slow.
      (4) A heparin lock may be useful because it allows the child to be more active between medication doses.
2. Perform irrigations of the infected area with antimicrobial solutions as prescribed by the physician.
3. Be alert for evidence of drug reactions.
4. Consider drug stability and compatability with other intravenous antibiotics when planning schedule for administration.

B. Increase the child's comfort.

1. Administer analgesics as prescribed by the physician.
2. Rest the affected extremity.
   a. Traction or splints may be used to reduce pain and prevent contractures in the soft tissues.
   b. Avoid excessive handling of the infected extremity, because this is very painful and may spread infection.
      (1) Bed linens should be changed only when necessary.
      (2) When it is necessary to move the extremity, support the joints above and below the affected part as well as the area itself.
      (3) Move the extremity in a smooth, unhurried, and gentle manner.

C. Protect other patients and personnel from the infectious organism.

1. Isolate children with draining wounds.
2. Utilize careful handwashing procedure.
3. Utilize strict aseptic technique when performing irrigations, changing dressings, and handling drainage.

D. Facilitate wound healing.

Maintain adequate nutrition and hydration.
1. Offer abundant fluids according to the child's preference.
2. Provide a diet rich in protein and vitamin C.
3. Allow the child to participate in selection of foods and preparation of his meal tray.
4. Refer to section on nutrition, p. 1094.

E. Observe for evidence of response to treatment or progress of disease.

1. Monitor the child's temperature at frequent intervals and record the pattern. Notify the physician of a sudden increase in temperature.
2. Monitor and record the extent of swelling, redness,

pain, and limitation of movement in the affected extremity.

3. Monitor and record the amount and nature of drainage if the infection has been drained.

F. Provide emotional support to the parents.

1. Parents often feel guilty if they did not recognize early signs of the disease.
2. Assist the parents to express and deal with their feelings. Initiate a social service referral if appropriate.
3. See section on family-centered care, p. 1117.

G. Assist the child to maintain many of his normal activities during the lengthy hospitalization.

1. Allow the child to be dressed during the convalescent period.
2. Encourage the child to attend playroom activities, even if he must be moved in his bed.
3. Initiate plans for the child's continuing education, and provide time each day for his school work.
4. Encourage liberal visiting by family and friends.

H. Provide for continuity of care following the child's discharge from the hospital.

1. Encourage parents to participate in all aspects of the child's care during hospitalization.
   a. Parents should be instructed and should have an

opportunity to practice (under nursing supervision) all procedures which will be required at home. (Procedures often include changes of dressing, application of a splint, or use of appliances such as crutches.)
   b. The child should not be discharged until both the parents and the nurse are satisfied with the parents' level of competency.
2. Instruct the parents to observe for evidence of complications, such as deformity, stiffness of joints, fracture, and disease recurrence.
3. Initiate a community health nursing referral if appropriate.

Expected Outcomes

1. Takes analgesics, rests extremity to relieve pain
2. Regains mobility function gradually
3. Adheres to drug therapy with no signs of adverse reaction to the drugs
4. Behaves in a less anxious manner
5. Participates in age-appropriate diversional and educational activities
6. Parents express an understanding of osteomyelitis and its treatment
7. Parents work out their guilt over the child's condition by talking about their feelings and realizing that they did not cause the problem

Congenital Dislocation of the Hip

Congenital dislocation of the hip refers to a malposition of the head of the femur in the acetabulum. The head of the femur is usually dislocated posterosuperiorly. Dislocation may be either partial or complete and may be either unilateral or bilateral.

Etiology

1. Unknown
2. Possible causes
   a. Abnormal development of the joint caused by:
      (1) Fetal position
      (2) Genetic factors
   b. Abnormal relaxation of the capsule and ligaments of the joint caused by hormonal factors
   c. Environmental factors such as breech delivery

Incidence

1. More common in female infants than in males.
2. Recurrence risk among siblings is greater when one child in the family has been affected.

Altered Physiology

1. Acetabulum tends to be shallow and extremely oblique.
2. Head of the femur tends to be smaller than normal.
3. Ossification centers are delayed in appearance.

Clinical Manifestations

(May not be observed until 1–2 months of age)

1. Asymmetry of the gluteal folds with deeper creases apparent on the affected side.
2. Limited ability to abduct the hip when the infant is lying on his back with his knees and hips flexed to 90 degrees. Normally, the hips will abduct at least 65 degrees.
3. Trendelenburg's sign—pelvis drops on the normal side if the child stands on his abnormal leg.

4. Leg length inequality with unilateral complete dislocation.
5. Delayed walking
6. Limp
   a. Trunk dips when the child puts weight on his involved leg.
   b. Waddling gait is observed in children with bilateral dislocation.

Diagnostic Evaluation

1. *Barlow's maneuver*
   a. With the infant on a firm surface, the examiner grasps the symphysis pubis in front and the sacrum in back with one hand. The second hand grasps the thigh on the side of the hip being tested.
   b. Slight outward pressure is applied over the proximal thigh by the thumb while longitudinal pressure is applied in an effort to dislocate the hip out of its socket.
   c. Sensation of abnormal movement indicates a dislocation.
2. *Ortolani's maneuver*
   a. The examiner positions his hands in the same manner as for Barlow's maneuver.
   b. The thigh is brought away from the midline of the body into a position of abduction.
   c. A sensation or sound of a clicking or jerking into place may be detected with reduction of the head into the socket.
3. X-ray data (helpful only after the age of 4–5 months, when the hip bones are sufficiently developed).
   a. Acetabular angle greater than 40 degrees
   b. Upward and outward displacement of the femoral head.

Treatment

1. Varies with age and extent of the defect
2. Early stages
   a. Reduction by gentle manipulation
   b. Splinting the hip in abduction by means of double or triple diapers, an abduction splint, or a cloth harness
3. Later stages
   a. Preliminary traction
   b. Closed reduction
   c. Immobilization in a hip spica cast or splint
4. Older child
   a. Preliminary traction
   b. Possible need for open reduction or osteotomy
   c. Immobilization in a hip spica cast

Prognosis

1. Depends on the age of the child when the condition is diagnosed.

2. Delay in diagnosis prolongs treatment and may preclude formation of a normal hip.

Nursing Interventions

Generally, nursing care of the child with congenital dislocation of the hip is provided at home. Nursing activities during hospitalization are those related to the child's care when he is in traction or after application of a hip spica cast (see p. 1208).

Health Education

1. If the child is to be treated with an abduction splint, explain its purpose and demonstrate its application to the parents.
   a. Allow the parents to practice application of the splint with nursing supervision.
   b. Clarify with parents the times that the splint is to be worn and if it can be removed for bathing, dressing, diaper changes, etc.
   c. Demonstrate handling of the child in such a way that the hips are kept abducted.

Congenital Clubfoot (Talipes Equinovarus)

Congenital clubfoot refers to a deformity in which the affected foot and leg have a club-like appearance. Talipes equinovarus is one of the most common congenital deformities of the foot, occurring in approximately one in 1,000 live births.

Etiology

1. Exact cause unknown.
2. Evidence indicates a mixed genetic and environmental causation.
3. Tends to recur in families already having 1 affected child.
4. Males are affected twice as often as females.

Altered Physiology

1. Pathologic anatomy
   a. Inversion and adduction of the forepart of the foot
   b. Inversion of the heel
2. Soft tissue changes are adaptive in nature, conforming to the skeletal deformity. The soft tissues on the medial and posterior aspect of the foot and ankle are shortened.

Clinical Manifestations

1. Varies in severity from a mild deformity to one in which the toes touch the medial side of the lower leg.
   a. Rigid type
      (1) Very severe deformity
      (2) Corrected only minimally by passive manipulation
      (3) Usually accompanied by moderate atrophy of the leg
   b. Flexible type—the condition can be readily corrected to neutral position by passive manipulation
2. Deformity increases progressively, and contractures become more rigid if the deformity is untreated.
   a. Child bears weight on the lateral border of the foot.
   b. Ambulation is difficult and gait is awkward.

c. Callosities and bursae may develop over the lateral side of the foot.

Diagnostic Evaluation

1. Diagnosis is determined by clinical manifestations.
2. X-ray valuable for the following:
   a. Determination of the degree of varus and equinus deformity
   b. Demonstration of the deranged mechanics of the hindfoot
   c. Accurate assessment of the amount of correction obtained with treatment

Treatment

1. Manipulation of the foot into normal position, with or without serial casting.
2. Maintenance of correction until normal muscle balance is regained.
3. Surgical procedures may be necessary for some children.

Nursing Interventions

A. Manipulate the foot into normal position.

1. Passive stretching exercises
   a. Technique of manipulation should be demonstrated to the nurse and parents by the physician, because there are many variations in the manner of performing the manipulation.
   b. Manipulation should be done before feedings, because it may cause some discomfort for the baby.
2. Manipulation and casting
   a. A plaster of paris cast is applied from the toes to the groin with the knee flexed.
      Casts are changed frequently; with each cast change, the foot is manipulated to obtain further correction.
   b. Once the deformity is fully corrected, the foot is held in an overcorrected position in a solid cast for 3–6 weeks.

(1) The parents should be instructed in cast care (see p. 1208).

(2) The parents should be alerted that if the foot portion of the cast becomes thin or worn, the cast should be reapplied.

(3) The parents can be taught to soak off old casts prior to clinic visits by immersing the cast in a solution of 1 part vinegar to 4 parts water and then unwrapping the plaster.

3. Denis Browne splint

a. The splint is composed of a flexible horizontal bar attached to a pair of footplates.

(1) The infant's feet are attached to the footplates by means of special shoes or adhesive tape.

(2) The desired position of the foot is controlled by positioning the abduction bar and the footplates.

(3) The infant provides his own corrective manipulation by his normal activity.

b. Parents should be instructed in the following details of care:

(1) Application and removal of the splint

(2) Times the splint is to be worn

(3) Protection of the feet by socks

(4) Skin care

(5) Use of splint key to tighten the shoes against the bar if they become loose

4. Continued treatment

a. Treatment is continued until the child is able to walk normally and until the wear on several pairs of shoes demonstrates that there has been no recurrence of deformity.

b. Foot is held in an overcorrected position at night by means of bivalved casts or a Denis Browne splint.

c. A prewalker clubfoot shoe with valgus strap may be prescribed for the infant's use during the day.

d. An older child may require special shoes that promote walking in the overcorrected position.

e. Passive stretching exercises are continued.

5. Indications for surgical measures

a. Failure of conservative methods to correct the deformity

b. In older children, severe and rigid deformities that obviously will not respond to nonsurgical measures

Legg-Calvé-Perthes Disease (Coxa Plana)

Legg-Calvé-Perthes disease is an aseptic necrosis of the capital femoral epiphysis secondary to ischemia.

Etiology

Unknown

Incidence

1. Males between the ages of 4 and 10 years of age are most frequently affected.

2. Condition tends to recur in families.

3. White children are affected 10 times more frequently than black children.

Altered Physiology

A. Stage I (Avascularity)

1. Spontaneous interruption of the blood supply to the upper femoral epiphysis occurs.

2. Bone-forming cells in the epiphysis die and bone ceases to grow.

3. Slight widening of the joint space occurs.

4. Swelling of the soft tissues around the hip occurs.

B. Stage II (Revascularization)

1. Growth of new vessels supplies the area of necrosis; both bone resorption and deposition take place.

2. The new bone is not strong, and pathologic fractures may occur.

3. Abnormal forces on the weakened epiphysis may produce progressive deformity.

C. Stage III (Reossification)

1. The head of the femur gradually reforms.

2. Nucleus of the epiphysis breaks up into a number of fragments with cyst-like spaces between them.

3. New bone starts to develop at the medial and lateral edges of the epiphysis which becomes widened.

4. Dead bone is removed and is replaced with new bone which gradually spreads to heal the lesion.

D. Stage IV (Postrecovery Period)

1. Without treatment

a. Head of the femur flattens and becomes mushroom shaped.

b. Incongruity between the head of the femur and the acetabulum persists.

c. Degenerative changes develop later in life.

2. Complete recovery

a. Head of the femur remains spherical.

b. Acetabulum appears normal.

c. Width of the neck of the femur is normal.

Clinical Manifestations

(May be intermittent initially)

1. Synovitis causing limp and pain in the hip.

2. Referred pain to the knee, inner thigh, and groin

3. Limited abduction and internal rotation of the hip

4. Mild to moderate muscle spasm

Diagnostic Evaluation

1. X-ray findings are related to the stage of the disease, and may be normal early after its onset.

2. Bone scans—helpful in identifying those patients with extensive epiphyseal infarction early in the course of the disease.

Treatment

(Depends on type of involvement)

1. First goal—to restore full range of motion of the hip joint by alleviating synovitis and muscle spasm. Bed rest with or without traction.

2. Second goal—to locate the femoral head deep in the acetabulum, thereby protecting it while revascularization and growth occur.

a. Non–weight-bearing abduction cast or brace.

b. Weight-bearing abduction casts or braces may be used once full range of motion has been restored except in older children with major femoral head involvement.

    c. Femoral osteotomy—indicated in cases of severe involvement of the femoral head.

3. Final goal—return to unassisted weight-bearing.

    a. Unassisted weight-bearing can be resumed once the increased density in the femoral head disappears, usually 6–15 months.

    b. The child's time out of the brace is gradually increased, and his hip motion is evaluated frequently. Loss of motion is an indication that a longer period of bracing is necessary.

Prognosis

1. Appears to be directly related to the initial extent of femoral head involvement.
2. Influenced by the stage at which the disease was diagnosed and treatment was instituted.
3. Limitation of motion and incongruity of joint surfaces may result if treatment is ineffective; condition may lead to degenerative joint disease in later life.

Nursing Interventions

A. Care for the child requiring traction or a spica cast.

See procedures, pages 1199 and 1208.

B. Evaluate the home and provide guidance to the family regarding the child's home care.

1. This guidance is important, because treatment may be continued in the home for an extended period.
2. Encourage family participation in the child's care so that members can become familiar with the details of his management (see section on family-centered care, p. 1117).
3. Appropriate referrals may include the following:
    a. Community health nurse
    b. Social service
    c. Home teacher
    d. Physical therapy
    e. Occupational therapy

C. Enable the child to participate in as many normal activities of life as possible.

1. Plans must be made for continuing education.
2. Diversion is an extremely important consideration.
3. Play should include exercise for uninvolved extremities.
4. Special activities with peers should be arranged.

D. Provide emotional support to the child and his family because of the long-term nature of the illness.

1. Provide the family with frequent opportunities to express their feelings and concerns. Techniques of therapeutic play should be used with the child.
2. Point out even small indications of the recovery process.
3. Introduce the family to other families with similarly affected children, if possible.

Health Education

1. General techniques of home nursing
    a. Bathing and skin care
    b. Maintenance of good muscle tone, proper body alignment, and prevention of contractures
    c. Provision for elimination
    d. Nutritional considerations
    e. Bedmaking
    f. Special equipment (e.g., traction, casts)
2. Pathology of the disease and rationale of treatment
    a. Reinforce medical explanations and clarify interpretations as necessary.
    b. Allow the child to view his own x-rays with his parents, to increase his knowledge of the disease.
    c. Emphasize that complete recovery can occur only with strict adherence to the treatment regimen.
3. Necessity of regular medical follow-up for evaluation of the child's progress.

Structural Scoliosis

Structural scoliosis is a lateral curvature of the spine characterized by a defect in the bones and surrounding tissues of the spine.

Etiology

1. Idiopathic
    a. Accounts for 80% of cases
    b. Possible familial incidence
2. Congenital
    a. Failure of vertebral formation
    b. Failure of segmentation
3. Neuropathic—results from conditions such as poliomyelitis, cerebral palsy, paralysis, and neurofibromatosis
4. Myopathic—associated with conditions such as muscular dystrophy and myopathies
5. Osteopathic—results from conditions such as fractures, bone disease, arthritis, and infection
6. Trauma such as fractures, burns, thoracoplasty
7. Irritative phenomena such as spinal cord tumor or nerve root irritation

8. Miscellaneous—Marfan's syndrome, postirradiation, metabolic, nutritional, or endocrinic factors

Classification

1. According to the spinal segment involved
    a. Thoracic
    b. Lumbar
    c. Thoracolumbar
2. According to age-group
    a. Infantile—birth–3 years
    b. Juvenile—4–9 years
    c. Adolescent—10 years to cessation of growth (usually found in females, with a right thoracic curve most common)

Altered Physiology

1. Lateral flexion of a scoliotic spine causes the trunk to shift away from the midline, altering the center of gravity and causing shortening of the spine.
2. Simultaneously, the spine rotates on its longitudinal

axis, contributing to many of the clinical manifestations.
3. The vertebrae become permanently wedge-shaped.
4. The scoliosis is increased by additional factors:
    a. The weight of the trunk itself.
    b. The muscles on the concave side, being contracted, have a mechanical advantage over the lengthened muscles on the convex side.
    c. Disturbed forces on active growing vertebral elements bring about structural changes in the bone.
5. Changes occur in the shape of the rib cage.
    a. The thoracic cavity narrows.
    b. The ribs do not move in a plane that allows normal expansion of the lungs.
6. Untreated scoliosis may cause back pain, degenerative arthritis, and disturbances in cardiopulmonary function in later life.

Clinical Manifestations

1. Presenting complaints (see Pediatric Physical Examination, p. 1047)
    a. Poor posture
    b. One shoulder higher than the other
    c. Hemline hanging unevenly
    d. One hip that seems more prominent
    e. Crooked neck
    f. Lump on back
    g. Waistline uneven
    h. One breast appearing larger
2. Visualization of deformity
3. Back pain

Diagnostic Evaluation

1. Detailed history from patient, parent, and other family members
2. Thorough examination of the back with patient first in the forward bent position and then standing erect
3. Assessment of the neurologic status of the lower extremities
4. Inclusion of clinical photographs in the record for future reference
5. X-rays of the spine to identify and measure primary and compensating curves
6. Pulmonary function studies for children who require surgery to predict risk of postoperative respiratory complications
7. Intravenous pyelography for children with congenital scoliosis because of a high evidence of associated renal anomalies

Treatment

A. Brace Management

1. Most effective for thoracic, thoracolumbar, and lumbar curves of less than 30–40 degrees which are not associated with extreme deformity.
2. Goal is to prevent progression of the curve.
3. Brace programs usually last 4–6 years and require faithful compliance.

B. Surgery

1. Indications:
    a. Curve is too severe to be braced
    b. Progression occurs despite bracing
    c. Brace management is not feasible
2. Preoperative casting or traction may be employed to increase curve flexibility prior to surgery
3. Types of surgery

a. Harrington instrumentation and posterior spinal fusion
b. Dwyer instrumentation and anterior spinal fusion
4. A protective cast is ordinarily required for 6 months–1 year following spinal fusion

Prognosis

Best when curve is mild at the time of initial diagnosis and effective treatment is initiated early.

Patient Problems/Nursing Diagnoses

1. Body-image concerns related to the appearance of the deformity and/or immobilization in unattractive devices
2. Pain related to the extent of the defect and/or surgery
3. Impaired skin integrity related to pressure from braces, traction, or casts
4. Potential for serious postoperative complications (neurologic impairment, shock, infection, urinary retention, paralytic ileus) related to surgery
5. Anxiety related to hospitalization and surgery
6. Decreased independence related to immobilization
7. Social isolation and coping difficulties related to hospitalization and immobilization
8. Knowledge deficit regarding scoliosis and its management

Nursing Interventions

A. Care for the child who is using a brace.

1. Educate the child and parents concerning the brace and supplemental exercise program.
    a. Clarify goals of therapy with the family.
    b. Offer incentives for compliance with the recommended treatment program.
2. Prevent break in tissue integrity.
    a. Provide meticulous skin care to areas in contact with the brace.
    b. Use a smooth-fitting undershirt or stockinette under the brace to protect the skin.
    c. Examine skin surfaces for evidence of pressure areas.
    d. Have brace adjusted if skin breakdown occurs because of improper fit.
3. Assist the child and family to modify normal activities such as bathing and dressing to accommodate the brace.
    a. Clothing must be loose or must be purchased in larger sizes to fit over the outside of the appliance.
    b. Underpants should be worn over the brace to facilitate toileting.

B. Prepare the child for surgical correction (spinal fusion).

1. Explain to the child and his parents the nature of the care immediately before surgery, the anesthesia, postoperative care, and appearance.
2. Introduce the child and his parents to a nurse from the intensive care unit if the child will be transferred there postoperatively.
3. Have the child practice aspects of the anticipated therapy, such as deep-breathing and other respiratory routines, leg exercises, logrolling, use of the Stryker frame or CircOlectric bed, and use of the fracture bedpan.

C. Provide postoperative care to the child following spinal fusion.

1. Observe for signs of hypotension.
    a. Monitor fluid balance.

b. Maintain blood pressure at desired level; report changes.
2. Observe wound for bleeding, hematoma, or infection.
   a. Maintain aseptic technique when caring for the wound.
   b. Report any redness, swelling, drainage, or heat in the incisional area.
3. Relieve pain.
   a. Identify causes of pain through discussion with the child and through observation.
   b. Administer analgesic therapy as prescribed by the physician.
4. Maintain tissue integrity.
   a. Turn the child as prescribed (usually by logrolling at 2-hour intervals).
   b. Provide skin care with each turning maneuver.
   c. Use sheepskin under pressure areas.
5. Prevent respiratory complications—utilize breathing exercises, blow bottles, and/or intermittent positive pressure to increase respiratory exchange.
6. Observe for neurologic deficits.
   Assess neurologic status each tour of duty, including dorsiflexion, mobility of legs, perineal sensation, and bladder function.
7. Observe for evidence of urinary retention which may develop as an effect of anesthesia, neurologic trauma, hypovolemia, or drugs.
   a. Maintain careful record of intake and output.
   b. Notify the physician if the child does not void within 8 hours following surgery.
   c. Care for the urethral catheter if present (see procedure, pp. 502–512).
8. Observe for signs of paralytic ileus.
   Note hypoactive and hyperactive bowel sounds, nausea, vomiting, or abdominal pain as diet is gradually increased.
9. Prevent development of thrombophlebitis.
   a. Have the patient do leg exercises.
   b. Apply elastic stockings.
   c. Observe for leg swelling, redness, or pain upon dorsiflexion; also note chest symptoms such as dyspnea, chest pain, or hemoptysis.
10. Prevent displacement of the rod or hook.
    a. Do not lift the child under the axillae.
    b. Use a turning sheet.
    c. Instruct the child not to lift hands over head.
11. Maintain adequate nutrition and hydration.
    a. Be aware of normal requirements for size and age.
    b. Evaluate nutritional value of diet and provide appropriate supplements.
12. Provide a safe environment for the patient.
    a. Place the bed so that it is not easily jolted.
    b. Be certain that all equipment is in good working order and that personnel are instructed in its use.

D. Care for the child following application of a jacket cast.

1. Stay with the child during the casting procedure to provide emotional support because of the unfamiliar, frightening, and embarrassing nature of the experience.
2. Observe for evidence of compromised circulation. Report changes in color, sensation, temperature of extremities, respiratory compromise, or abdominal distress.

3. Prevent potential trauma.
   a. Help the child to accept the realities of activity limitation by providing safe alternatives.
   b. Facilitate the child's getting in and out of bed by use of a hospital bed.
   c. Teach the child safe methods of becoming mobile.
4. Instruct the child/parents about how to arrange for cast changes as required either by growth of the child or by soiling of the cast.
5. For additional information related to cast care, see the section on casts, page 1208.

E. Provide emotional support for the child.

1. Allow the child to continue as many of his normal activities as possible.
   a. Continue schooling.
   b. Encourage peer visiting or telephone contact.
2. Provide diversional activities.
   a. Assess the child's interests and provide things that he can do within the limits of his position.
   b. Use prism glasses, mirrors, bedboards, and easels.
   c. Bring others into the child's room and transport the child in his bed to the recreation room as soon as his condition allows.
   d. Establish schedules and make each day meaningful.
3. Be sensitive to the child's concerns about body image and intervene appropriately.
   a. Many adolescent girls express concerns that the cast will prevent growth or change the shape of their breasts, or that menstruation will temporarily cease while they are in the cast.
   b. Children may feel vulnerable because of the restrictions imposed by casts or traction.
4. Provide as much privacy as possible especially during bathing, toileting, and cast changing.
5. Refer to section on the hospitalized adolescent, page 1117.

Health Education

1. Have the child and family practice cast care during hospitalization.
2. Demonstrate techniques of personal hygiene, including matters such as special skin care and hair shampooing.
3. Assist the child to develop an exercise program within his limitations but adequate to maintain tonicity.
4. Provide dietary instructions, including basic nutritional needs for age and modifications necessary because of immobilization.
5. Provide assistive devices to facilitate physical care needs.
6. Arrange for home equipment with available services.
7. Provide continuity by referral to appropriate community agencies.
8. Arrange for transportation and/or social service assistance if needed.
9. Act as a liaison between the child and his school to encourage the school nurse to supervise patient compliance after the return to school and provide support for the child with adjustment problems.
10. References for patients and parents:
    Brower E. Children Should Be Seen . . . A Handbook for Teachers. University Youth Spine Center, 2074 Abington Road, Cleveland, OH 44106

Scoliosis—A Handbook for Patients. Scoliosis Research Society, 444 N Michigan, Suite 1500, Chicago, IL 60611

Schatzinger L. What if You Need An Operation for Scoliosis and Brace Yourself—Scoliosis and the Milwaukee Brace. University Youth Spine Center, 2074 Abington Road, Cleveland, OH 44106

Expected Outcomes

1. Maintains a positive body image, evidenced by verbal and nonverbal communication
2. Experiences relief of pain
3. Maintains skin integrity; wears undershirt under brace; adjusts brace when necessary
4. Recovers from surgery with no complications; vital signs within normal limits; moves extremities; incision healing
5. Appears less anxious about condition; discusses concerns about outcome
6. Engages in diversional activities and interacts with family and friends
7. Adjusts to immobilization; learns to use trapeze to turn, etc.; exercises within limits of enforced bed rest
8. The parents learn about cast care, special hygienic measures for skin care and washing hair, exercise, diet, assistive home equipment, and transportation needs

Bibliography

Books

Edmondson A and Crenshaw A. Campbell's Operative Orthopedics, 6th ed. St Louis, CV Mosby, 1980

Farrell J. Illustrated Guide to Orthopedic Nursing, 2nd ed. Philadelphia, JB Lippincott, 1982

Ferguson A. Orthopedic Surgery in Infancy and Childhood, 5th ed. Baltimore, Williams & Wilkins, 1981

Gershwin ME and Robbins D (eds). Musculoskeletal Diseases of Children. New York, Grune & Stratton, 1983

Hensinger R and Jones E. Neonatal Orthopedics. New York, Grune & Stratton, 1981

Hilt N and Cogburn S. Manual of Orthopedics. St Louis, CV Mosby, 1980

Keim H. The Adolescent Spine, 2nd ed. New York, Grune & Stratton, 1982

Rang M. Children's Fractures, 2nd ed. Philadelphia, JB Lippincott, 1983

Rothman R and Simeone F. The Spine, 2nd ed. Philadelphia, WB Saunders, 1982

Salter R. Textbook of Disorders and Injuries of the Musculoskeletal System, 2nd ed. Baltimore, Williams & Wilkins, 1983

Scoles P. Pediatric Orthopedics in Clinical Practice. Chicago, Year Book Medical Publishers, 1982

Sharrard W. Paediatric Orthopaedics and Fractures, Vols 1 and 2. London, Blackwell Scientific Publications, 1979

Whaley L and Wong D. Nursing Care of Infants and Children, 2nd ed. St Louis, CV Mosby Co, 1983

Winter R. Congenital Deformities of the Spine. New York, Thieme–Stratton, 1983

Articles

Brown C. Nursing care of the child having anterior spinal surgery. Orthop Nurs 1982 Mar/Apr; 1(2):33–35

Buckwalter K et al. Musculo-skeletal conditions and sexuality. Sex Disabl 1982 Fall; 5(3):131–142

Chaston M. School nurses' learning experiences related to providing services for mainstreamed orthopedically impaired children. J Sch Health 1983 Dec; 53(10):621–623

Davis S and Lewis S. Managing scoliosis: Fashions for the body and mind. MCN 1984 May/Jun; 9(3):186–187

Dunwoody C et al. Scoliosis. Nursing '83 1983 Sep; 13(9):24–25

Eckerson L. Lateral electrical surface stimulation as an alternative to bracing in the treatment of idiopathic scoliosis: Treatment protocol and patient acceptance. Phys Ther 1984 Apr; 64(4):483–490

Farady J. Current principles in the non-operative management of structural adolescent idiopathic scoliosis. Phys Ther 1983 Apr; 63(4):512–523

Gore D et al. Scoliosis screening: Results of a community project. Pediatrics 1981 Feb; 67(2):196–200

Griffin P. The child's broken bones: Trauma in the young. Emerg Med 1983 Aug 15; 15(14):38–39

Gurnham R. Adolescent compliance with spinal brace wear. Orthop Nurs 1983 Nov/Dec; 2(6):18–19

Holland S. Up-to-date home care of a baby in a hip spica cast. Pediatr Nurs 1983 Mar/Apr; 9(2):114–115

Howard M and Corbo-Pelaia S. Psychological aftereffects of halo traction. Am J Nurs 1982 Dec; 82(12):1839–1843

Ibrahim K. An overview of childhood fractures. Pediatr Nurs 1984 Jan/Feb; 10(1):57–65

Kryschyshen P and Fischer D. External fixation for complicated fractures. Am J Nurs 1980 Jan; 80(1):156–159

Kylberg H. Descriptions of growth disturbances in children with osteomyelitis at different ages. Orthop Nurs 1983 Nov/Dec; 2(6):28–32

Lonstein J et al. Voluntary school screening for scoliosis in Minnesota. J Bone Joint Surg 1982 Apr; 64A(4):481–488

Love-Mignogna S. Taping and splinting. Seven common problems . . . and how to solve them. Nursing '80 1980 Apr; 10(4):88–92

Mubarak S et al. Pitfalls in the use of the Paulik harness for treatment of congenital dysplasia, subluxation and dislocation of the hip. J Bone Joint Surg 1981 Oct; 63-A:1239–1248

Mulley D. Harnessing babies' dysplastic hips. Am J Nurs 1984 Aug; 84(8):1006–1008

Nelson J. Suppurative arthritis and osteomyelitis. In Shirkey HC (ed). Pediatric Therapy, 6th ed, St Louis, CV Mosby, 1980, pp. 468–473

Rutechi B and Seligson D. Caring for the patient in a halo apparatus. Nursing '80 1980 Oct; 10(10):73–77

Sherk H, Pasquariello P and Watters W III. Congenital dislocation of the hip: A review. Clin Pediatr 1981 Aug; 20(8):513–523

Staheli L and Griffin L. Corrective shoes for children: Survey of current practice. Pediatrics 1980 Jan; 65(1):13–17

Swanson A. Congenital limb deformities: Classification and treatment. Clin Symp 1981; 33(3):3–32

Swanson V. The school-age traction patient: Toward better behavior patterns. J Assoc Care Child Health 1980 Summer; 9(1):12–14

Thomas P. Nursing care of patients undergoing posterior spinal fusion with segmental (Luque) spinal instrumentation. Orthop Nurse 1983 May/Jun; 2(3):13–20

Tibbits C. Adolescent idiopathic scoliosis. Nurse Pract 1980 Mar/Apr; 5(2):11–13+

Villalon D and Smith M. At home with traction. Pediatr Nurs 1982 Jan/Feb; 8(1):15–16

Wenger D. The limping child. Orthop Nurs 1982 Jul/Aug; 1(4):29–35

Pediatric Oncology

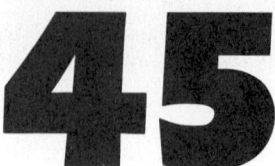

General Considerations

Incidence

1. Cancer is the leading cause of death from disease in children from 1–14 years of age.
2. Cancer affects approximately 10 per 100,000 children annually in the US.
3. The incidence of specific cancers is related to sex, age, and ethnic backgrounds.

Types

A. Common Types of Cancer in Children (in order of frequency)

1. Leukemia
2. Cancer of the central nervous system
3. Lymphoma
4. Neuroblastoma
5. Rhabdomyosarcoma
6. Wilms' tumor
7. Bone tumor
8. Retinoblastoma

Warning Signals of Cancer in Children

1. Marked change in bowel or bladder habits; nausea and vomiting for no apparent cause
2. Bloody discharge of any kind; failure to stop bleeding in the usual time
3. Presence of swelling, lump, or mass anywhere in the body
4. Any change in the size or appearance of moles or birthmarks
5. Unexplained stumbling in the child
6. Generally run-down condition
7. Unexplained pain or persistent crying of an infant or child

Treatment Modalities*

A. Surgery

B. Radiation Therapy

Nursing considerations:
1. Prepare the child and his family for the procedure.
2. Do not wash off any marks placed by the radiologist to indicate the area to be treated.

---

* For additional information, see Chapter 22, Nursing the Person with Cancer (Adult), page 903.

3. Initiate comfort and support measures when the child demonstrates any side effects of treatment.
   a. General malaise and headache
   b. Nausea and vomiting
   c. Diarrhea
   d. Anorexia
   e. Skin irritation and breakdown
   f. Lethargy
4. See the adult text, section on radiation in diagnosis and therapy, page 912.

C. Chemotherapy

Nursing considerations:
1. Be aware of the chemotherapeutic agents most frequently used to treat childhood cancer, their side effects, and precautions for administration. See Table 45-1, page 1458.
2. Care for the child who develops side effects of chemotherapy.
   a. Prepare the child and his family for the possible side effects of the chemotherapeutic agents he is receiving. Explain to the child that the medicine is to help him feel better but that when he first begins to take the medicine he may feel sicker. If this is explained prior to the development of symptoms, the child will be more trusting and less frightened.
   b. Nausea and vomiting
      (1) Administer antiemetics as prescribed.
      (2) Plan activities and meals according to the medical schedule. Many children prefer to receive chemotherapeutic agents that cause nausea and vomiting during the evening so that they can sleep through the hours of greatest nausea.
      (3) Carefully observe the sleeping child who is prone to vomiting. Position him in a manner that prevents aspiration.
      (4) Offer foods and fluids that are most appealing to the child (e.g., warm tea, carbonated beverages, soups).
      (5) Record the nature of the nausea and vomiting.
      (6) Report any prolonged or delayed nausea or vomiting which may be an indication that the medication should be withheld or that the dosage should be reduced.

c. Anorexia
  (1) Create a pleasant eating environment that is free of sights, sounds, and odors that cause nausea or that discourage or distract the child.
  (2) Encourage the child to eat in the playroom with other children.
  (3) Give good mouth care prior to eating.
  (4) Provide frequent, small meals.
d. Extreme fluctuations in appetite—be aware that this is temporary and that eventually normal eating patterns will be established. Reassure the parents of this fact.
e. Gastrointestinal mucosal cell damage causing stomatitis, gastrointestinal ulceration, rectal ulceration, diarrhea, or bleeding
  (1) Provide meticulous oral hygiene. Local anesthetics may be prescribed for painful mouth ulcers.
  (2) If diarrhea or rectal ulcers occur, keep the skin clean and dry to prevent maceration and secondary infection.
  (3) These signs of toxicity are generally indications for temporary discontinuation of therapy or a reduction of dosage.

f. Alopecia
  (1) Assist the family in obtaining wigs or caps in preparation for hair loss.
  (2) Reassure the child and family that the hair will grow back, although it might be of a different color and texture.
g. For side effects and nursing interventions associated with specific drugs, see Table 45-1, Drugs Commonly Used in the Treatment of Childhood Cancer.

Prevention

1. Children and adults should be educated about the hazards of known carcinogens, especially cigarette smoking, and excessive exposure to sunlight or radiation.
2. Female adolescents should be instructed concerning the method of breast self-examination. Males should be taught to do testicular self-examination. Periodic examinations should be encouraged for cancer screening.
3. Parents should be taught the warning signals of childhood cancer.

Acute Lymphocytic Leukemia

Acute lymphocytic leukemia (ALL) is a primary disorder of the bone marrow in which the normal marrow elements are replaced by immature or undifferentiated blast cells. When the quantity of normal marrow is depleted below the level necessary to maintain peripheral blood elements within normal ranges, anemia, neutropenia, and thrombocytopenia occur.

Etiology

1. The exact cause of acute leukemia is unknown.
2. Environmental causes, infectious agents (especially viruses), genetic factors, and chromosomal abnormalities are suspected in some cases.

Incidence and Classification

1. Acute leukemia is the most common malignancy in children, occurring in nearly 4 per 100,000 children under 15 years of age.
2. Acute leukemia is classified according to the cell type involved.
3. The incidence of ALL is more common among Caucasian children.

Altered Physiology

1. Acute lymphocytic leukemia results from the growth of an abnormal type of nongranular, fragile leukocyte in the blood-forming tissues, particularly in the bone marrow, spleen, and lymph nodes.
2. The abnormal cell has little cytoplasm and a round, homogeneous nucleus which resembles that of a lymphoblast.
3. Normal bone marrow elements may be displaced or replaced in this type of leukemia.
4. The changes in the blood and bone marrow result from the accumulation of leukemic cells and from the deficiency of normal cells.

a. Red cell precursors and megakaryocytes from which platelets are formed are decreased, causing anemia, prolonged and unusual bleeding, and tendency to bruise easily.
b. Normal white cells are markedly decreased, predisposing the child to infection.
c. The bone marrow is hyperplastic with a uniform appearance due to the presence of leukemic cells.
5. Leukemic cells may infiltrate into lymph nodes, spleen, and liver, causing diffuse adenopathy and hepatosplenomegaly.
6. Expansion of marrow or infiltration of leukemic cells into bone results in bone or joint pain.
7. Invasion of the central nervous system by leukemic cells may cause headache, vomiting, cranial nerve palsies, convulsions, and coma.
8. Weight loss, muscle wasting, and fatigue may occur when the body cells are deprived of nutrients because of the immense metabolic needs of the proliferating leukemic cells.

Assessment
Clinical Manifestations

1. Manifestations depend on the degree to which the bone marrow has been compromised and the location and extent of extramedullary infiltration.
2. Presenting symptoms
   a. Fatigability
   b. General malaise, listlessness
   c. Persistent fever of unknown cause
   d. Recurrent infection
   e. Prolonged bleeding following simple surgical procedures (e.g., dental extractions and tonsillectomy)

Table 45-1 Drugs Commonly Used in the Treatment of Childhood Cancer

Drug Category	Administration	Side Effects/Toxicity	Specific Nursing Implications
Adriamycin (doxorubicin): antibiotic	IV	Nausea and vomiting, alopecia, stomatitis, myelosuppression, cardiotoxicity, red urine Causes chemical irritation on extravasation	1. Use the same precautions when administering this medication as with vincristine. 2. Use only sterile water as a diluent. 3. Observe for changes in heart rate or rhythm.
Bleomycin (Blenoxane): antibiotic	IV, IM, subcutaneous	Allergic reaction, anaphylaxis, nausea and vomiting, stomatitis, cumulative effects involving the skin and lung (pneumonitis, pulmonary fibrosis)	1. Administer test dose before giving a therapeutic dose. 2. Be prepared for allergic reaction, especially with first few doses.
Carmustine: (BiCNU)	IV	Facial burning and flushing on infusion, burning pain along IV infusion, nausea and vomiting, bone marrow depression	1. Avoid extravasation.
Chlorambucil (Leukeran): alkylating agent	PO	Nausea and vomiting, diarrhea, myelosuppression	1. Side effects usually related to high doses.
Cisplatin (Platinol)	IV	Severe renal toxicity, 8th nerve damage, severe nausea and vomiting, myelosuppression, neurotoxicity, anaphylactic reactions	1. Assess renal function before administration. 2. Maintain hydration before and during therapy. 3. Administer antiemetic. 4. Be prepared for allergic reaction. 5. Instruct the parents to report signs of hearing loss or neurotoxicity.
Cyclophosphamide (Cytoxan): alkylating agent	Oral or IV	Alopecia, nausea and vomiting, myelosuppression, hemorrhagic cystitis, mucous membrane ulceration, immunosuppression, infertility, hyperpigmentation	1. To prevent exposure of the bladder to chemical irritants, maintain liberal hydration for 48 hours after weekly dose and continuously when given daily. Have the child empty his bladder frequently after the drug is administered, including at least once during the night. 2. Protect child from infection.
Cytarabine hydrochloride (Cytosar-U): antimetabolite; pyrimidine antagonist	IV, IM, subcutaneous, or intrathecal (IT)	Nausea and vomiting, myelosuppression, mucous membrane ulcerations, hepatotoxicity, immunosuppression	1. Anticipate severe nausea and vomiting during or soon after administration. 2. May require premedication with antiemetics. 3. Protect the child from infection. 4. Do not enter vial twice for IT use.
Dacarbazine	IV	Nausea and vomiting (especially after the first dose), flu-like syndrome, bone marrow depression	1. Used with caution in children with renal dysfunction.
Daunorubicin: antibiotic	IV	Cardiotoxicity, myelosuppression, nausea and vomiting, abdominal pain, fever, skin rash, red urine Causes chemical irritation on extravasation	1. Use the same precautions when administering this medication as those followed with vincristine.
L-Asparaginase: enzyme	IV	Hypersensitivity reaction, nausea and vomiting, lethargy, somnolence, fever, hepatotoxicity, coagulopathy Hyperglycemia Renal failure	1. Observe for hypersensitivity reaction. Have epinephrine and resuscitation equipment available. 2. Observe for confusion, irritability, convulsions, and other neurologic signs. 3. Do not shake vial. 4. Use clear solution only.
Lomustine: CCNU	PO	Nausea and vomiting, bone marrow depression	1. Administer 4 hours after meals on an empty stomach.
Mechlorethamine (nitrogen mustard): alkylating agent	IV, IT	Nausea and vomiting, myelosuppression, alopecia, local phlebitis	1. Use caution when mixing drug—wear eyeglasses or goggles. Rinse skin immediately if solution comes in contact with skin. 2. Use immediately after mixing. 3. Check patency of IV line before infusing and inject drug cautiously.
6-Mercaptopurine: antimetabolite—purine antagonist	Oral	Nausea and vomiting, myelosuppression, anorexia, dermatitis, mucous membrane ulceration, hepatotoxicity, abdominal pain	1. Dosage should be reduced to one-third of the usual dosage if a child is also receiving allopurinol, since this drug inhibits the degradation of 6-mercaptopurine.
Methotrexate: antimetabolite—folic acid antagonist	Oral, IV, IM, or IT	Nausea and vomiting, GI mucosal ulceration, myelosuppression, pneumonitis, osteoporosis, hepatotoxicity, hyperpigmentation Sensitivity to sun	1. Avoid side effects of meningeal irritation during IT injection by diluting the drug in a preservative-free vehicle, bringing it to room temperature and filtering it through a 0.22-millimicron Millipore filter. 2. Do not enter vial twice for IT use.

Table 45-1   Drugs Commonly Used in the Treatment of Childhood Cancer (continued)

Drug Category	Administration	Side Effects/Toxicity	Specific Nursing Implications
			3. Method of IT injection: a. A lumbar puncture is performed. b. A volume of spinal fluid equal to the volume of drug to be injected is removed. c. Without aspiration, the medication is injected in a continuous infusion (15–30 seconds/10 ml. of solution. d. The stylet is reinserted, and the needle is removed. e. The child may be required to remain in the Trendelenburg position for 30 minutes after the injection to ensure optimal circulation of the medication throughout the central nervous system. f. Use of an Ommaya reservoir may eliminate the need for repeated lumbar punctures. 4. Avoid use of salicylates and sulfonamides which increase toxicity of methotrexate.
Prednisone: adrenocorticosteroid	Oral	Increased appetite, weight gain, fluid retention, hypertension, Cushing's syndrome, immunosuppression, psychosis, GI tract ulceration	1. Avoid excessive sodium intake. 2. Observe for evidence of GI bleeding. 3. Protect from infection.
Procarbazine	PO	Severe nausea and vomiting, lethargy, dermatitis, arthralgia, bone marrow depression, stomatitis	1. Central nervous system depressants (phenothiazines and barbiturates) enhance CNS symptoms. 2. Acts as an MAO inhibitor—sympathomimetic drugs and natural foods such as yogurt, aged cheese, and bananas should be avoided.
Vincristine (Oncovin): periwinkle alkaloid	IV	Alopecia, constipation, peripheral neuropathy, mild myelosuppression Causes chemical irritation on extravasation	1. Use different needles to withdraw and inject. Check patency of IV line with saline flush before injecting. Inject cautiously, observing for signs of infiltration. Follow injection with saline flush. 2. Observe for constipation; report condition promptly. Keep well hydrated. Administer laxatives or stool softeners as prescribed. 3. Alter activities appropriately if weakness of hands, feet, or legs occurs or if the child becomes easily fatigued. 4. Prepare children and parents for the possibility of numbness and tingling of fingers and toes.
Vinblastine (Velban): plant alkaloid	IV	Nausea and vomiting, alopecia, myelosuppression, neurotoxicity	1. Same as for vincristine.

f. Tendency to bruise easily
g. Pallor
h. Enlarged lymph nodes
i. Abdominal pain due to organomegaly
j. Bone and joint pain
k. Headache and vomiting (with CNS involvement)
3. Presenting symptoms may be isolated or in any combination or sequence.

Diagnostic Evaluation

A. Physical Findings

1. Pallor, especially of the mucous membranes
2. Scattered petechiae and ecchymoses
3. Generalized lymphadenopathy
4. Enlarged liver and spleen
5. Unexplained bruising
6. Continued bone and joint pain
7. Fever

B. Laboratory Evaluation

1. May have altered peripheral blood counts. Blood studies may show the following:
   a. Low hemoglobin, red blood cell count, hematocrit, and platelet count
   b. Decreased, elevated, or normal white blood cell count
2. Stained peripheral smear and bone marrow examination show large numbers of lymphoblasts and lymphocytes.
3. Lumbar puncture—to determine if there is central nervous system involvement.
4. Renal and liver function studies—to determine any contraindications or precautions for chemotherapy.

Treatment

A. Supportive Therapy—to control disease complications such as hyperuricemia, infection, anemia, and bleeding.

B. **Specific Therapy**—to eradicate malignant cells and to restore normal marrow function.

1. Chemotherapy is utilized to achieve complete remission with restoration of normal peripheral blood and physical findings.
2. There is no universally accepted standard therapy for the treatment of children with acute leukemia, but most centers have similar protocols which utilize a combination of drugs (see Table 45-1).
3. Components of therapy
   a. Induction—course of therapy designed to achieve a complete remission.
   b. Central nervous system prophylaxis—treatment begun early in the course of the illness to destroy leukemic cells that have infiltrated the central nervous system. It generally consists of intrathecal administration of methotrexate with or without cranial irradiation.
   c. Maintenance or continuation therapy—to prevent reappearance of the disease (usually continued for about 3 years).
   d. Reinduction therapy to reinduce remission if relapse occurs.
   e. Extramedullary disease therapy.
4. Research is continuing to determine the optimal method of inducing and maintaining remission with the least risk to the patient.
5. Bone marrow transplantation has been used successfully for treating children who fail to respond to conventional treatment.

Complications

1. Infection—most frequently occurs in the lungs, gastrointestinal tract, or skin
2. Hemorrhage—usually due to thrombocytopenia
3. Central nervous system involvement
4. Bony involvement
5. Testicular involvement
6. Urate nephropathy

Prognosis

1. At least 90% of children with ALL can be expected to achieve an initial remission if treated in a specialized center.
2. At least 50% of children with ALL will survive more than 5 years.
3. Children with good prognostic features may have a 60%–70% chance of long-term survival.
4. The prognosis becomes poorer with each relapse the child experiences.
5. The term "cure" is difficult to define because later relapses still occur after long remissions.
6. Prognosis appears to be related to the child's age and white blood cell count on diagnosis, and the exact cell type of the leukemia.

Patient Problems/Nursing Diagnoses

1. Parental feelings of anxiety/grief at learning of the diagnosis
2. Danger of infection related to decreased numbers of normal white blood cells
3. Danger of hemorrhage related to decreased numbers of platelets
4. Alterations in nutrition, (less than body requirements) related to anemia and anorexia, nausea, and vomiting and mucosal ulceration secondary to chemotherapy and/or irradiation

5. Pain related to the progress of the disease and to diagnostic and treatment procedures
6. Activity intolerance related to fatigue resulting from disease and treatment
7. Anxiety of the child related to hospitalization and to diagnostic and treatment procedures
8. Alteration in body image related to alopecia associated with chemotherapy
9. Knowledge deficit about leukemia and its treatment
10. Concerns about death and dying (see p. 1495)

Planning and Implementation
Nursing Interventions

A. **Provide emotional support to the parents when the diagnosis of leukemia is made known to them.**

1. Be available to the parents when they feel that they want to discuss their feelings.
2. Kindness, concern, consideration, and sincerity toward the child and his parents help to serve as a source of consolation.
3. Contact the family's clergyman or the hospital chaplain if the parents desire this.
4. Utilize the services of a social worker as appropriate to help the family work out their feelings.
5. Avoid discussing life expectancy in terms of the time element—offer the hope that therapy will be effective and will prolong life.
6. Allow the parents to participate in the child's care so that they will feel that they are actually doing something for the child. This also helps the family feel more secure (see the section on family-centered care, p. 1117).
7. Assess family dynamics and coping mechanisms and plan intervention accordingly.

B. **Give skillful, supportive care in the early stages of treatment and sustain life until antileukemic agents have had a chance to become effective.**

1. Initiate nursing activities associated with anemia (see p. 1280).
2. Provide adequate hydration.
   a. Maintain parenteral fluid administration.
   b. Offer small amounts of oral fluids if tolerated.
   c. Record and report vomiting if this occurs.
3. Observe renal function carefully.
   a. Measure and record urinary output.
   b. Check specific gravity.
   c. Observe the urine for any evidence of gross bleeding.
4. Provide a highly nutritious diet if the child can tolerate it.
   a. Determine the child's likes and dislikes.
   b. Offer frequent, small meals.
   c. Offer supplemental feedings high in calories and protein.
   d. Encourage the parents to assist at mealtime.
   e. Allow the child to eat with a group at a table if his condition allows this.
5. Protect the child from sources of infection.
   a. Family, friends, personnel, and other patients who have infections should not visit or care for the child.
   b. Do not place a child with an infection in the room with a child with leukemia.
   c. Reverse isolation procedure may be utilized (a protective technique that provides the child with

protection from those people with whom he has contact)—gowns and masks.

Explain to both the child and his parents the purpose of this protective technique.

d. Observe the child closely and be alert to signs of impending infection.
   (1) Observe any area of broken skin or mucous membrane for signs of infection.
   (2) Report any febrile incidents.
e. Teach preventive measures at discharge (i.e., handwashing, isolation from children with communicable disease).

C. Be alert for the symptoms of hemorrhage that may occur when the platelet count is diminished or may appear as side effects of antileukemic therapy.

1. Record vital signs and report any changes that may indicate hemorrhage.
   a. Tachycardia
   b. Lowered blood pressure
   c. Pallor
   d. Diaphoresis
   e. Increasing anxiety and restlessness
2. Give careful oral hygiene since the gums and mucous membranes of the mouth bleed easily.
   a. Use a soft toothbrush.
   b. If the child's mouth is bleeding or painful, clean the teeth and mouth with a moistened cotton swab.
   c. Use a nonirritating rinse for the mouth (e.g., hydrogen peroxide).
   d. Apply petrolatum to cracked, dry lips.
3. Observe for gastrointestinal bleeding.
   a. Hematemesis
   b. Tarry or bloodstained stools
4. Move and turn the child gently since hemarthrosis may occur and cause movement to be very painful.
   a. Handle the child in a gentle manner.
   b. Turn frequently to prevent pressure sores.
   c. Place the child in proper body alignment, in a position comfortable for him.
   d. Allow the child to be out of bed in a chair if this position is more comfortable for him.
5. Avoid intramuscular injections if possible.
6. Handle catheters as well as drainage and suction tubes carefully to prevent mucosal bleeding.
7. Protect the child from injury by monitoring his activities and environmental hazards.
8. Be aware of emergency procedures for control of bleeding:
   a. Careful application of local pressure so as not to interfere with clot formation.
   b. Administration of blood and blood components (see the section on anemia, p. 1279).

D. Prepare the child for diagnostic and treatment procedures.

1. Utilize knowledge of growth and development to prepare the child for procedures such as bone marrow aspirations, blood transfusions, and chemotherapy (see the section on the hospitalized child, p. 1112).
2. Provide a means for talking about the experience. Play, storytelling, or role-playing may be helpful.
3. Convey to the child an acceptance of his fears and anger.

E. Control hyperuricemia which may occur because of rapid cell turnover and tumor lysis.

1. Administer allopurinal as prescribed to neutralize the effects of uric acid on the kidney.
2. Provide liberal oral and/or IV hydration.
3. Administer sodium bicarbonate or acetazolamide (Diamox) as prescribed to alkalize the urine.
4. Collect urine specimens to monitor urinary excretion of uric acid.

F. Be aware of chemotherapeutic agents and the side effects of these agents that are capable of inducing remissions in children with acute leukemia.

1. Induction—usually includes a combination of vincristine and prednisone. A third drug, such as 6-mercaptopurine, L-asparaginase, daunorubicin, adriamycin, or cytosine arabinoside, may be added.
2. Maintenance—usually includes daily oral administration of 6-mercaptopurine and weekly oral administration of methotrexate with intermittent administration of other drugs such as vincristine, prednisone, cyclophosphamide, cytosine arabinoside, or daunorubicin.
3. Reinduction—remissions can often be reinduced using the same initial drugs or with other agents.
4. See Table 45-1, Drugs Commonly Used in the Treatment of Childhood Cancer.

G. Provide symptomatic care for the child who develops the side effects of chemotherapy.

See the section on chemotherapy, page 1456.

H. Observe for the possibility of CNS involvement.

Report changes in behavior or personality: persistent nausea and vomiting, headache, lethargy, irritability, dizziness, ataxia, convulsions, or alteration in state of consciousness.

I. Provide supportive nursing care to the child receiving cranial irradiation.

Refer to section on radiation therapy, page 1456.

J. Provide pain relief.

1. Position the child so that he is most comfortable. Water beds and beanbag chairs are often helpful.
2. Administer medications on a preventive schedule before pain becomes severe. Individualize medication schedule for each patient.
3. Manipulate the environment as necessary to increase the child's comfort and minimize unnecessary exertion.

K. Provide emotional support to the child.

1. Provide for continuity of care.
2. Encourage family-centered care (see p. 1117).
3. Prepare the child for potential changes in his body image (alopecia, weight loss, wasting, etc.) and help him cope with related feelings.
4. Facilitate play activities for the child and utilize opportunities to communicate with him through play.
5. Maintain some discipline, placing calm limitations on unacceptable behavior.
6. Provide appropriate diversional activities.
7. Encourage independence and provide opportunities which allow the child to control his environment.
8. Avoid exposing the child to activities that he will be unable to accomplish.

L. Provide continued emotional support to the parents throughout the course of hospitalization.

1. Assist the parents to feel comfortable on the unit.
2. Provide guidelines concerning how parents and the treatment team can work together most profitably.
3. Encourage parental participation in care—to the extent that they feel comfortable.
4. Suggest tasks that the parents may do to reduce their feelings of helplessness and anxiety.
5. Provide for continuity of care so that the parents are able to establish trusting relationships with a few nurses.
6. Assist the parents to deal with anticipatory grief.
7. Assist the parents to deal with other family members, especially siblings and grandparents, and friends.
8. Encourage the parents to discuss concerns about limiting their child's activities, protecting him from infection, disciplining him, and having anxieties about the illness.
9. Answer parental questions related to such matters as home management, the purpose of periodic tests, treatments and clinic visits, side effects of medications, and indications for medical intervention.
10. Facilitate communication with the clinic nurse and/or clinical specialist who may interact with the child during the entire course of illness.
11. Initiate appropriate referrals (e.g., to social worker, parent group, clergy, and community health nurse).

M. Provide supportive care to the terminally ill or dying child.

See the section on care of the dying child, page 1495.

N. References for children and parents

Baker LS. You and Leukemia—A Day At A Time. Philadelphia, WB Saunders, 1978

Sherman M. The Leukemic Child, DHEW Pub No (NIH) 78-863 National Cancer Program, National Cancer Institute, Bethesda, MD 20892

Leukemia Society of America, 733 Third Avenue, New York, NY 10017

See the Bibliography, page 1472.

Evaluation
Expected Outcomes

1. The parents discuss their feelings about the child's diagnosis
2. The child avoids infection
3. The child shows no signs of excessive bleeding—vital signs normal; no hematemesis or tarry stools
4. Eats at mealtime; takes between meal feedings
5. Experiences relief from pain (no crying or expression of pain)
6. Demonstrates lessened anxiety (talks about his feelings or shows them in play; participates in other age-appropriate activities
7. Maintains a positive body image; does not become overly self-conscious or shy about appearance
8. The parents indicate that they understand what leukemia is and how it is treated

Brain Tumors in Children

Brain tumors are expanding lesions within the skull. About 20% of the malignant tumors that occur in children are brain tumors.

Etiology

The etiology of brain tumors is unknown.

Clinical Manifestations

(Signs and symptoms are directly related to the location and size of the tumor.)

1. Headache
   a. May occur at any time, but usually is more severe in the early morning hours.
   b. May be intermittent and disappear for days or weeks—may be due to yielding of the sutures.
2. Nausea or vomiting
   a. May occur at any time, but frequently occurs in the early morning hours.
   b. Vomiting may be projectile.
3. Visual disturbances
   a. Nystagmus
   b. Diplopia
   c. Blurred vision
   d. Loss of peripheral vision
   e. Significant loss of visual acuity
4. Muscular problems
   a. Lack of balance
   b. Incoordination
   c. Deficits in muscle functioning—eyes, face, extremities
   d. Paralysis
   e. Spasticity
5. Behavioral changes
   a. Arrest or regression in development
   b. Irritability or lassitude
   c. Lack of attentiveness
   d. Deterioration in school performance
   e. Personality changes
   f. Loss of sphincter control
   g. Disturbances in sleep and eating patterns
6. Slow cerebration
   a. The child answers questions after a considerable delay.
   b. The child appears to talk slowly.
   c. The child responds to any stimulus in a slow manner.
7. Seizures—usually focal, psychomotor, or generalized

Diagnostic Evaluation

Determined by the type of tumor that is suspected; usually includes many or all of the following procedures:

1. Thorough neurologic examination
   a. Fundoscopic examination
   b. Tests for cerebral function (level of consciousness, orientation, intellectual performance, mood, behavior, etc.)
   c. Assessment of cranial nerves
   d. Tests for cerebellar function (e.g., balance and coordination)
   e. Evaluation of the motor system—especially muscle size, tone, strength, and abnormal muscle movements
   f. Evaluation of the sensory system
   g. Assessment of reflexes

2. Electroencephalogram—of limited value, but possibly useful when seizures are manifested
3. Skull x-ray
4. Computed tomography
   a. Safe, noninvasive procedure using a combination of sophisticated electronic and computer technology.
   b. Scanning of head by a slit x-ray beam passing through at a multitude of angles.
   c. Absorption values, varying with the density of tissues and fluids, are calculated and analyzed. This allows for differentiation of normal and abnormal brain tissue and ventricular sizes and configurations.
5. Isotopic brain scanning
6. Angiography
7. Air-contrast studies

Treatment

1. Surgery is performed to determine the type of the tumor, the extent of invasiveness, and to excise as much of the lesion as possible.
2. Radiation therapy is usually initiated as soon as the diagnosis is established and the surgical wound healed.
3. Chemotherapy is used to induce remissions in recurrent brain tumors, especially astrocytomas and medulloblastomas. The role of chemotherapy for treatment of primary tumors is currently being investigated. Commonly used drugs include nitrosoureas, vincristine, methotrexate, procarbazine, and steroids.

Prognosis

1. Prognosis is improved in cases involving early diagnosis and adequate therapy.
2. Prognosis is related to completeness of surgical removal, extent of invasion, and rate of tumor growth.
3. Five-year survivors are increasing, especially in children with low-grade astrocytomas or ependymomas.

Cerebellar Astrocytoma

Cerebellar astrocytoma is a slow-growing, often cystic type of tumor of the cerebellum which accounts for about 20% of all pediatric brain tumors.

Clinical Manifestations

Insidious onset and slow course
1. Evidence of increased intracranial pressure—especially headache, visual disturbances, papilledema, and personality changes
2. Cerebellar signs—ataxia, dysmetria, (inability to control the range of muscular movement), nystagmus
3. Behavioral changes

Pathophysiology

1. The tumor produces slowly increasing intracranial pressure.
2. Condition classified according to its malignancy—from grade I (least malignant) to grade IV (most malignant).

Treatment

Surgical removal—the tumor can often be removed with few sequelae.

Medulloblastoma

Medulloblastoma is a highly malignant, rapidly growing tumor usually found in the cerebellum.

Incidence

1. Medulloblastoma is the single most common tumor of the central nervous system in children.
2. About 75% of medulloblastomas occur in males.

Clinical Manifestations

1. Similar to manifestations of cerebellar astrocytoma, but condition develops more rapidly.
2. The child may present with unsteady gait, anorexia, vomiting, and early morning headache and later develop ataxia, nystagmus, papilledema, and drowsiness.

Pathophysiology

1. The tumor grows rapidly and produces evidence of increased intracranial pressure progressing over a period of weeks.
2. As the tumor grows, it seeds along cerebrospinal fluid (CSF) pathways.

Treatment

1. Partial excision or decompression of the posterior fossa (complete removal is rarely possible)
2. Radiation of site and spinal canal
3. Chemotherapy
4. Shunt to relieve CSF obstruction

Brain Stem Glioma

Brain stem glioma is a tumor of the brain stem. It accounts for approximately 15% of brain tumors in children.

Clinical Manifestations

1. Cranial nerve palsies
   a. Strabismus
   b. Weakness, atrophy, and fasciculations of the tongue
   c. Swallowing difficulties
2. Hemiparesis
3. Cerebellar ataxia
4. Signs of increased intracranial pressure (rare)

Altered Physiology

Through its growth, this type of tumor interferes early with the function of cranial nerve nuclei, pyramidal tracts, and cerebellar pathways.

Treatment

1. Surgical removal is not possible
2. Radiation of site

Ependymoma of the Fourth Ventricle

Ependymoma is a tumor derived from the ependyma, or lining, of the central canal of the spinal cord and cerebral ventricles. It frequently arises on the floor of the fourth ventricle, causing obstruction of the flow of cerebrospinal fluid. Ependymomas represent about 9% of all intracranial neoplasms.

Clinical Manifestations

1. Nausea or vomiting
2. Headache
3. Unsteady gait
4. Signs of increased intracranial pressure

Altered Physiology
1. Tumors grow with varying speed.
2. Because of location, tumors can invade the cardio-respiratory center, cerebellum, and spinal cord.
3. Graded according to degree of differentiation, as are the astrocytomas.

Management
1. Partial surgical removal
2. Radiation therapy, including the entire craniospinal axis

Nursing Process Overview of Care of the Child Undergoing Surgery for Brain Tumor

Assessment
History and Physical Assessment
Assess the child's neurologic status in order to help locate the site of the tumor and the extent of involvement; identify signs of disease progress.
1. Obtain a thorough nursing history from the child and his parents—particularly data related to normal behavioral patterns and presenting symptoms.
2. Perform portions of the neurologic examination as appropriate. Assess muscle strength, coordination, gait, and posture.
3. Observe for the appearance or disappearance of any of the clinical manifestations previously described. Report these to the physician and record each of the following in detail:
   a. Headache—duration, location, severity
   b. Vomiting—time occurring, whether or not projectile
   c. Convulsions—activity prior to seizure; type of seizure; areas of body involved; behavior during and after seizure
4. Monitor vital signs frequently, including blood pressure and pupillary reaction.
5. Monitor ocular signs. Check pupils for size, equality, reaction to light, and accommodation.
6. Observe for signs of brain stem herniation—should be considered a neurosurgical emergency.
   a. Attacks of opisthotonos
   b. Tilting of the head; neck stiffness
   c. Poorly reactive pupils
   d. Increased blood pressure; widened pulse pressure
   e. Change in respiratory rate and nature of respirations
   f. Irregularity of pulse or lowered pulse rate
   g. Alterations of body temperature

Patient Problems/Nursing Diagnoses
1. Parental anxiety related to the nature of the diagnosis and usual need for surgery
2. Pain related to increased intracranial pressure and surgery
3. Alteration in nutrition (less than body requirements) related to nausea and vomiting associated with increased intracranial pressure and to irradiation
4. Potential for serious postoperative complications (shock, increased intracranial pressure, respiratory arrest) related to surgery
5. Fatigue related to radiation therapy
6. Anxiety of the child related to hospitalization and to diagnostic and treatment procedures

7. Alteration in body image related to appearance of the incision, shaved head, and/or changes due to irradiation
8. Knowledge deficit regarding brain tumors and their treatment
9. Concerns about death and dying (see p. 1495)

Planning and Implementation
Nursing Interventions
A. Provide the parents and child with emotional support during the very stressful preoperative period.
1. Assess the family unit and its coping mechanisms.
2. Allow parents to ask questions and encourage them to discuss their fears and concerns. Many parents feel guilty for not seeking help earlier because they either did not recognize or dismissed symptoms.
3. Deliver nursing care to the child in a manner that provides support.
   a. Assume a gentle, concerned attitude toward both parents and child.
   b. Make the child as comfortable as possible.

B. Provide appropriate nursing care for the child undergoing diagnostic tests.
1. Prepare the child and parents for each procedure.
2. If prescribed, administer preliminary sedative on time. (If the child is not adequately sedated, completion of the test may be impossible.)
3. Refer to adult section, page 755, for nursing care related to specific procedures.

C. Prepare the child and parents for surgery.
1. Refer to section on preparation for surgery, page 1125.
2. Determine physician's plans regarding shaving the head, bandages, and other procedures, and prepare the child accordingly.
   a. Encourage the child to express his feelings regarding the threat to his body image.
   b. Reassure the child that he will be able to wear a wig or hat after recovery.
   c. If the area is to be shaved, allow the child and parents the option of saving the hair.
3. Prepare the parents for the postoperative appearance of their child and for the fact that he might be comatose immediately following surgery.
4. If appropriate, introduce the child and his family to intensive care nursing personnel and arrange a tour of the unit.
5. Prepare the child for postoperative expectations (i.e., he may feel sleepy or have a headache and will need to remain quiet).

D. Provide an adequate diet for the child preoperatively.
1. Refeed the child when he vomits. (Vomiting is not usually associated with nausea.)
2. Allow the child to participate in the selection of foods and the preparation of his tray.
3. Maintain IV hydration if indicated.

E. Provide care for the child during the immediate postoperative period. (This is usually provided in an intensive care unit.)
1. Position the child according to physician's request—usually on his unaffected side with his head level.
   a. Raising the foot of the bed may increase intracranial pressure and bleeding.
   b. Post a sign above the bed noting the exact position of the head.

2. Check the dressing for bleeding and for drainage of cerebrospinal fluid.
3. Monitor the child's temperature closely.
   a. A marked rise in temperature may be due to trauma, to disturbance of the heat-regulating center, or to intracranial edema.
   b. If hyperthermia occurs, utilize appropriate measures to reduce it (see the section on fever, p. 1137).
      Temperature should not be reduced too rapidly.
4. Observe child closely for signs of shock, increased intracranial pressure, and alterations in level of consciousness.
5. Assess the child for edema of the head, face, and neck.
   a. Edema may inhibit respirations and impair circulation of lacrimal secretions.
   b. Apply cold compresses to the affected areas, being careful not to dampen the dressing.
   c. Instill prescribed ophthalmologic drops in the eyes to prevent corneal damage.
6. Carefully regulate fluid administration in order to prevent increased cerebral edema.
7. Change the child's position frequently and provide meticulous skin care to prevent hypostatic pneumonia and pressure sores.
   a. Move the child carefully and slowly, being certain to move the head in line with the body.
   b. Support paralyzed or spastic extremities with pillows, rolls, or other means.
8. Avoid discussing the child's condition in his presence, even if he appears to be unconscious.
9. Have equipment readily available for cardiopulmonary resuscitation, respiratory assistance, oxygen-inhalation, blood transfusion, ventricular tap, and other potential emergency situations.
10. Continue to support parents who may be very frightened and upset by the appearance of their child and necessary emergency procedures.

F. Provide care for the child during the convalescent phase.

1. Maintain adequate nutrition and hydration.
   a. Encourage the child to eat increasingly larger meals.
   b. Provide tube feedings if the child is unable to eat.
2. Allow and encourage the child to regain his independence as his condition improves.
3. Facilitate the return of normal parent–child relationships.
   a. The parents may tend to be overprotective.
   b. Help the parents to see the child's increasing capabilities and encourage them to foster independence.
4. Make provisions for play activities.
   a. Allow the child to meet and play with other children.
   b. Provide the child with quiet play activities when it is necessary to encourage rest.

c. Be careful that the child does not hit his head or fall until he is completely healed.
   A head dressing, football helmet, or wig may be used to prevent trauma should the child fall.
5. Assist the child to adjust to his altered body image.
   a. Utilize stocking caps, surgical caps, head scarves, hats, or wigs as appropriate.
   b. If the child's hair has not been totally shaved, it may be combed so that the area of baldness is not evident.
   c. Reassure the child that his hair will grow back.
6. For care of children with residual effects from surgery, refer to adult text, section on rehabilitation concepts, page 51.

G. Care for the child receiving radiation therapy.

See the section on radiation therapy, page 1456.

H. Care for the child receiving chemotherapy.

Refer to section on chemotherapy, page 1456.

I. Prepare the child and his family for discharge.

1. Provide parents with written information regarding the child's needs—medications, activity, care of incision, follow-up appointments, etc.
2. Initiate a referral to a community health nurse to reinforce teaching and to maintain therapeutic support for the family.
3. Encourage the parents to contact the child's teacher and the school nurse before the child returns to school so that they can prepare his classmates for his return and help them to deal with their feelings.
4. Provide the parents with the phone number of the nursing unit so that they may call if questions occur to them after discharge.
5. See the Bibliography, page 1472, for additional resources.

J. Provide supportive care to the terminally ill child.

See the section on the dying child, page 1495.

Evaluation

Expected Outcomes

1. The parents discuss their feelings about the child's diagnosis and surgery
2. The child experiences relief from pain
3. Nutritional intake is adequate to meet body requirements
4. Does not develop life-threatening postoperative complications (shock, increased intracranial pressure, respiratory problems, edema)
5. Participates in age-appropriate activities within limitations imposed by fatigue
6. Demonstrates lessened anxiety through verbalization, play, or other age-appropriate activities
7. Maintains a positive body image, evidenced by his verbal and nonverbal communication
8. Parents accurately describe the brain tumor and its treatment

Neuroblastoma

Neuroblastoma refers to a malignant tumor arising from the sympathetic nervous system.

Etiology
Unknown

Incidence

1. Most common extracranial solid tumor of childhood
2. Occurs in approximately 1 per 10,000 live births
3. Primarily affects infants and young children

Altered Physiology

1. Tumors arise from embryonic neural crest cells anywhere along the craniospinal axis.
2. Histologic picture varies greatly from tumor to tumor and even within the same tumor.
3. Tumors are staged primarily on the basis of the extent of disease, from stage I (tumor is confined to the organ or structure of origin) to stage IV (there is remote disease involving the skeleton, parenchymal organs, soft tissue, or distant lymph glands). Stage IV-S refers to cases with remote disease confined to only 1 or more sites, either the liver, skin, or bone marrow without x-ray evidence of skeletal metastasis.
4. Neuroblastoma is one of the few tumors that may demonstrate spontaneous remission.

Clinical Manifestations

1. Symptoms depend on the location of the tumor and the stage of the disease.
2. Most tumors are located within the abdomen and present as firm, nontender, irregular masses that cross the midline.
3. Other common signs:
   a. Bowel or bladder dysfunction resulting from compression by a pelvic tumor
   b. Neurologic symptoms because of compression by the tumor on nerve roots or because of tumor extension
   c. Supraorbital ecchymosis, periorbital edema, and exophthalmos resulting from metastases to the skull bones and retrobulbar soft tissue
   d. Lymphadenopathy, especially in the cervical area
   e. Bone pain with skeletal involvement
   f. Swelling of the neck or face, and cough with thoracic masses
   g. General symptoms of pallor, anorexia, weight loss, and weakness with widespread metastasis

Diagnostic Evaluation

To document the extent of the disease:
1. X-rays of the chest, skull, abdomen, and long bones
2. Intravenous pyelogram
3. Bone marrow aspiration
4. Complete blood count with platelet count
5. 24-hour urine collection—elevated excretion of homovanillic acid (HVA) and vanillylmandelic acid (VMA)
6. Bone scan
7. Histologic confirmation
8. Additional studies
   a. CT scan
   b. Ultrasound examination
   c. Liver/spleen scan
   d. Inferior vena cavography
   e. Arteriography

Medical/Surgical Management

1. Management is controversial and depends on the stage of the child's disease at the time of diagnosis.

2. When complete surgical resection of a stage I tumor is possible, this may be the only treatment required.
3. Children with other than stage I disease generally receive a combination of surgery, radiation therapy, and chemotherapy.
   Drugs of choice include vincristine, dacarbazine, and cyclophosphamide.

Prognosis

1. Overall survival rate is about 30%–35%, with almost all recurrences or deaths occurring within the first 2 years after diagnosis.
2. Influencing factors:
   a. Stage of disease—the earlier the stage, the better the prognosis.
   b. Age—infants under 1 year of age demonstrate the best survival.
   c. Pattern of metastasis—children with metastases to the bone marrow, liver, and skin have better prognoses than those with radiographic bone involvement.
   d. Site of primary tumor—children with tumors of the thorax, pelvis, or neck appear to do better than children with abdominal tumors.
3. Neuroblastoma is one of few childhood tumors that has not responded dramatically to modern antitumor therapy.
4. The use of newer chemotherapeutic drugs and other techniques, such as immunotherapy, may improve survival rates for these children.

Nursing Management

Nursing care for children with neuroblastoma is similar to that of children with other types of cancer.
Points of emphasis:
1. The child must be prepared for diagnostic tests and treatments in ways that are appropriate for his age and level of development.
2. General principles of preoperative and postoperative care should be applied for children who require abdominal, thoracic, or cranial surgery. See the sections on Wilms' tumor, cardiovascular surgery, page 1467, or brain tumor, page 1464.
3. For nursing care of the child receiving chemotherapy, see page 1456.
4. For nursing care of the child receiving radiation therapy, see page 1456.
5. Parents should be encouraged to express their feelings about the child's disease, and should be supported in their efforts to cope with the child's illness.
   Many parents feel guilty for not recognizing or reporting early signs of the illness. They may express anger toward health professionals or place blame on one another.
6. For nursing care of the terminally ill child, see page 1495.

Rhabdomyosarcoma

Rhabdomyosarcoma is a highly malignant soft tissue tumor which arises from the embryonic mesenchymal cells that form striated muscle.

Etiology

1. Unknown.
2. Genetic and environmental factors have been implicated.

Incidence

1. Most common soft tissue tumor in childhood.
2. Accounts for 4%–8% of all malignant disease in children under 15 years of age.
3. Peak incidence is between 2 and 5 years of age.

Altered Physiology

1. Classified in 4 pathologic categories based on histologic characteristics.
2. Tumor spreads either by local extension or by metastasis via the venous and lymphatic system.
3. Frequent sites of metastasis include the regional lymph nodes, lungs, bone marrow, bones, and brain.
4. Tumor staging is on the basis of the extent of the disease:
   a. Stage I: localized tumor, completely resected
   b. Stage II: regional disease, resected
   c. Stage III: localized disease, not completely resected
   d. Stage IV: metastatic disease at diagnosis

Clinical Manifestations

1. Often presents as an asymptomatic lump noted by the patient or parent.
2. Signs and symptoms variable and reflect the location of the tumor and metastases.
   a. Orbit—proptosis, chemosis, ocular paralysis
   b. Nasopharynx—epistaxis, pain, dysphagia, nasal voice, airway obstruction
   c. Sinuses—swelling, pain, discharge, sinusitis
   d. Middle ear—pain, chronic otitis, facial nerve palsy
   e. Neck—hoarseness, dysphagia
   f. Truncal, extremities, testicular areas—enlarging soft tissue masses
   g. Prostate, bladder—urinary tract symptoms
   h. Retroperitoneal tumors—gastrointestinal and urinary tract obstruction

Diagnostic Evaluation

To document the extent of the disease and provide objective criteria for measuring response to therapy

1. Complete blood count
2. Urinalysis
3. Chest x-ray
4. Bone scan and/or skeletal survey
5. Bone marrow aspiration
6. Liver scan
7. CAT scan of the chest and primary lesion
8. Skull x-ray, tomogram, CAT scan and lumbar puncture—for children with cranial lesions
9. Lymph angiography and/or CAT scan for patients with lower extremity and genitourinary lesions
10. Open biopsy of the primary tumor—definitive diagnostic procedure

Treatment

1. Surgery—to biopsy the lesion, determine the stage of the disease, and completely remove or reduce the primary tumor—increasingly, chemotherapy/radiation therapy is used prior to surgery to avoid the disability associated with radical surgery for selected anatomic sites, (head, neck, and pelvis).
2. Radiation—high-dose radiation is generally recommended for the primary tumor and metastasis.
3. Chemotherapy
   a. Used for all patients, usually in combination with irradiation.
   b. Commonly used drugs include actinomycin D, vincristine, cyclophosphamide, and doxorubicin.

Prognosis

1. Survival rates have improved considerably in recent years.
2. Overall survival rate is approximately 70%.
3. Prognosis is related to the stage of the disease at diagnosis and the location of the primary tumor.

Nursing Management

Nursing care is similar to that for a child with neuroblastoma (see p. 1466).

Wilms' Tumor

Wilms' tumor is a malignant renal tumor.

Etiology

1. The etiology of Wilms' tumor is not known.
2. Genetic inheritance has been documented in a small percentage of cases.

Incidence

1. Wilms' tumor is the most common neoplasm involving the retroperitoneal space in children.
2. It constitutes approximately 30% of all pediatric renal masses and 7% of all childhood tumors.
3. 75% of cases occur before the child is 5 years of age.

Altered Physiology

1. Wilms' tumor has a capacity for very rapid growth and usually grows to a large size before it is diagnosed.
2. The effect of the tumor on the kidney depends on the site of the tumor.
3. In most cases, the tumor expands the renal parenchyma, and the kidney becomes stretched over the surface of the tumor.
4. The covering of the tumor may be very thin and easily torn.
5. The tumor is often exceedingly vascular, soft, mushy, or gelatinous in character.
6. Wilms' tumors present various histologic patterns from patient to patient.
7. The neoplasms metastasize early, either by direct extension or by way of the bloodstream. They may invade perirenal tissues, lymph nodes, the liver, the diaphragm, abdominal muscles, and the lungs. Invasions of bone and brain are less common.
8. Staging of Wilms' tumor is done on the basis of clinical and anatomical findings. It ranges from group I (tumor is limited to the kidney and is completely resected) to group IV (metastases are present in the liver, lung, bone, or brain). Group V includes those cases in which there is bilateral involvement either initially or subsequently.

Clinical Manifestations

1. A firm, nontender upper quadrant abdominal mass is usually the presenting sign; it may be on either side. (It is frequently observed by the parents.)
2. Abdominal pain, which is related to rapid growth of the tumor, may occur. As the tumor enlarges, pressure may cause constipation, vomiting, abdominal distress, anorexia, weight loss, and dyspnea.
3. Less common are hypertension, fever, hematuria, and anemia.
4. Associated anomalies:
   a. Hemihypertrophy
   b. Aniridia (absence of the iris)
   c. Genitourinary anomalies

Diagnostic Evaluation

1. IVP—to demonstrate the tumor and to assess the status of the opposite kidney
2. X-ray of chest and skeletal survey to identify metastases
3. CBC and peripheral smear
4. Urinalysis
5. Blood chemistries, especially serum electrolytes, uric acid, renal function tests (BUN and creatinine), and liver function tests (bilirubin, SGOT, SGPT, LDH, total protein, albumin, and alkaline phosphatase)
6. Coagulation studies—PT, PTT, and fibrinogen
7. Urinary VMA
8. Echograms to search for tumor extension
9. Ultrasonography to distinguish between a variety of renal masses
10. Radioisotope scans and tomography to rule out metastasis (often postponed until after surgery)

Treatment

1. Determined by the stage of the tumor
2. Includes a combination of surgery, radiation therapy, and chemotherapy

Prognosis

1. Overall survival rates for Wilms' tumor are the highest among all childhood cancers.
2. High cure rate associated with early diagnosis and optimal treatment.
3. Prognosis best in children whose tumor is classified as group I or II and who receive multimodal therapy.
4. About 12% of children with Wilms' tumor have histologic features that are associated with a poor prognosis.

Nursing Interventions

A. Support the family and the child at the time the diagnosis is made.

1. Discuss with the physician what specific information has been given to the parents.
2. Provide the parents with the opportunity to express their concerns.
3. Provide the parents with a place where they may have some privacy when they wish to be alone.
4. Convey a compassionate attitude to the parents in talking with them, and assure them that their child's needs will be met.
5. See the section on family-centered care, page 1117.

B. Exercise caution in the manipulation of the child in order to avoid inadvertently increasing the danger of metastasis.

1. Bathe the child carefully, avoiding manipulation of the abdomen.

2. Hold the child carefully to prevent abdominal pressure.
3. Communicate the need for this caution to all staff members.
4. Place a sign on the child's bed to reduce indiscriminate palpation.

C. Explain to the child and his parents the elements of preoperative and postoperative care.

1. Utilize knowledge of growth and development to plan a teaching program for the child that will include diagnostic tests, preoperative care, and postoperative care (see the section on the hospitalized child, p. 1112).
2. Involve the parents in the teaching plan and encourage them to support the child at this time.
3. See the Bibliography, page 1472, for additional references.

D. Provide preoperative and postoperative care for the child.

1. See the section on the child undergoing surgery, page 1125.
2. Many children require gastric suction postoperatively to prevent distention or vomiting.
   a. See Guidelines: Nasogastric Intubation, page 412.
   b. Monitor gastric output accurately and replace it with appropriate IV fluids as prescribed by the physician.
   c. When oral feedings are resumed, begin with small amounts of clear fluids.
3. Continue to avoid abdominal manipulation, because cells may have escaped locally from the excised tumor.

E. Care for the child receiving radiation therapy.

1. Radiation therapy is given to the tumor bed postoperatively to render nonviable all cells that have escaped locally from the excised tumor. It is usually indicated for all children with Wilms' tumor except those under 18 months of age with stage I disease.
2. Alterations in the growth and development of bones, joints, and musculature may occur as a result of radiation therapy.
3. Be aware that acute skin reactions occasionally occur when dactinomycin is given concomitantly with or following administration of radiation therapy.
4. See the section on radiation therapy, page 1456.

F. Care for the child receiving chemotherapy.

1. Chemotherapy is initiated postoperatively to achieve maximal killing of tumor cells.
2. The usual chemotherapeutic agents employed are actinomycin D, vincristine, and doxorubicin.
3. Prepare the child and his family for chemotherapy.
4. See the section on chemotherapy, page 1456.

G. Provide diversional therapy for the child.

Provide the child with the opportunity for play as his condition permits.

H. Provide supportive care appropriate for the dying child when the tumor metastasizes and the child's condition deteriorates.

See the section on the dying child, page 1495.

Osteogenic Sarcoma

Osteogenic sarcoma is a malignant tumor of the bone.

Etiology

Unknown

Incidence

1. Most frequent malignant bone cancer in children.
2. Peak incidence between 10 and 25 years of age.
   a. Most common at the peak of the adolescent growth spurt.
   b. Males are affected more often than females, with a ratio of 1.5:1.
3. Common sites of occurrence—distal femur, proximal tibia, proximal humerus, pelvis, phalanges, and jaw.

Altered Physiology

1. Presumably arises from bone-forming mesenchyme tissue.
2. Produces malignant spindle-cell stroma, which gives rise to malignant osteoid tissue.
3. Most osteogenic sarcomas are fully malignant but may appear in relatively nonmalignant forms.
4. Most commonly metastasize to lungs and other bones.

Clinical Manifestations

1. Pain in the affected site, frequently causing limp or limitation of motion
2. Palpable, tender, fixed bony mass
3. Additional symptoms related to site of metastasis, if present

Diagnostic Evaluation

1. X-ray examination—to visualize the tumor
2. Serum alkaline phosphatase—often elevated
3. Bone scan—helpful in detecting initial extent of malignancy, planning therapy, and evaluating effects of treatment
4. Biopsy of lesion—to confirm the diagnosis and provide histologic data for the selection of a treatment plan
5. Chest x-ray, tomography, or CAT scan—to identify lung metastasis
6. Renal and liver function tests—to screen for problems prior to initiating chemotherapy

Medical/Surgical Management

1. Radical amputation of the affected extremity, and often the joint proximal to the involved area, is required in most cases.
2. Newer techniques include transmedullary amputation and limb-salvaging surgery, such as total femur replacement.
3. Chemotherapy is advocated for 1–3 years following surgery. It is also used preoperatively for patients undergoing resectional surgery and for metastatic disease.
   a. High-dose methotrexate with citrovorum factor rescue is the drug of choice.
   b. Other drugs administered in combination with methotrexate include doxorubicin, vincristine, cyclophosphamide, cisplatin, derivatives of nitrogen mustard, bleomycin, and dactinomycin.

Prognosis

1. Survival has greatly improved with the aggressive use of multimodal therapy.
2. Approximately 50%–60% of patients who undergo surgery followed by chemotherapy can expect to be disease-free after 3 years.
3. Limb-saving surgery has improved the quality of life for many survivors.

Nursing Management

Nursing care of the child with osteogenic sarcoma is essentially the same as care of the adult. See page 853.
Points of emphasis:
1. The child must be prepared for diagnostic tests, surgery, and chemotherapy in ways that are appropriate for his age and level of development.
2. Radical body alterations caused by surgery and chemotherapy are especially upsetting for adolescents.
   a. They need time and support to accept the diagnosis and surgery, and to grieve for their lost body part.
   b. They can be helped to select clothing that camouflages the prosthesis yet is sexually appealing.
   c. Wigs, scarves, or hats are useful for children experiencing hair loss.
3. Discharge planning should be done to promote normalcy and resumption of appropriate presurgical activities.
   a. Accessibility of home and school should be assessed and environmental handicaps alleviated.
   b. The school nurse should be contacted to facilitate reentry into school.
   c. Visits by peers should be encouraged, and the child should be helped to deal with questions and reactions from peers.
   d. A tutor should be arranged for students who must remain out of school for lengthy periods.
   e. A community health nursing referral should be initiated if appropriate.
   f. See the Bibliography, page 1472, for additional references.
4. For nursing care of the hospitalized adolescent, see page 1117.
5. For nursing care of the child receiving chemotherapy, see page 1456.

Retinoblastoma

Retinoblastoma is a malignant, congenital tumor arising in the retina of one or both eyes.

Etiology

1. Nonhereditary somatic mutations:

a. Account for approximately 60% of all retinoblastomas.

b. Always demonstrate unilateral involvement.

2. Hereditary germinal mutations:
   a. Account for approximately 40% of all retinoblastomas.
   b. May be bilateral or unilateral.
   c. Mode of inheritance is autosomal-dominant.
3. Can be associated with chromosomal aberrations.

Incidence

1. Relatively rare tumor, usually diagnosed in patients before 2 years of age.
2. Occurs in 1 in 18,000 live births, or approximately 200 children in the US each year.
3. Incidence is increasing because of prolonged survival of affected children with transmission of the tumor to their offspring and increased exposure to mutagenic agents.

Altered Physiology

1. Retinoblastomas probably arise in the photoreceptor cells in the retina.
2. Usually arise in multiple foci rather than a single tumor.
3. Most tumors (endophytic type) arise in the internal nuclear layers of the retina and grow forward into the vitreous cavity.
4. Some tumors (exophytic type) arise in the external nuclear layer and grow into the subretinal space, with detachment of the retina.
5. Extension of the tumor may occur into the choroid, the sclera, and optic nerve.
6. Hematogenous spread of the tumor may occur to the bone marrow, skeleton, lymph nodes, and liver.
7. Tumor staging reflects the extent of the disease and the probability of preserving useful vision in the affected eye, from Group I = very favorable to Group V = very unfavorable.

Clinical Manifestations

1. "Cat's eye" reflex—whitish appearance of the pupil, represents visualization of the tumor through the lens as light falls on the tumor mass
2. Strabismus
3. Red and painful eye—usually indicates extensive disease
4. Limited vision or blindness—late sign
5. Symptoms of distant metastasis

Diagnostic Evaluation

1. Careful history regarding visual changes and tumor occurrence in relatives
2. Bilateral indirect ophthalmoscopy under general anesthesia
3. Skull x-ray
4. CAT scan
5. Determinations of lactic acid dehydrogenase (LDH) isoenzymes in the aqueous humor
6. Bone marrow aspiration, lumbar puncture, and skeletal and liver surveys—done if metastasis is suspected

Treatment

1. Depends on the stage of the disease at the time of diagnosis.
2. Unilateral tumors in stages I, II, or III are usually treated with external beam irradiation.
   a. Goal of treatment is to eradicate the tumor(s) and preserve useful vision.

b. Radiation is usually administered over a period of 3–4 weeks.

3. Surgery (enucleation) is the treatment of choice for advanced tumor growth, especially with optic nerve involvement.
4. Bilateral disease often requires enucleation of the severely diseased eye and irradiation of the least affected eye.
   a. Every attempt is made to salvage whatever vision there may be.
   b. Bilateral enucleation is indicated with extensive bilateral retinoblastoma where there is no hope of vision.
5. Radioactive applicators, light coagulation, and cryotherapy are sometimes used to treat small, localized tumors.
6. Chemotherapy is used for cases of extensive involvement to prevent or treat distant metastasis.
   Drugs commonly used include cyclophosphamide, vincristine, actinomycin D, and doxorubicin.

Prognosis

1. Overall survival rate is high (86%–88%), even in severe cases.
2. Heritable retinoblastoma is associated with a high incidence of spontaneous and radiation-related new tumors, particularly sarcomas.

Patient Problems/Nursing Diagnoses

1. Parental feelings of guilt related to the genetic implications of the diagnosis
2. Parental anxiety related to the nature of the diagnosis and treatment
3. Potential for side effects (skin changes, loss of lashes, fat atrophy, impaired bone growth, dry eye) related to irradiation
4. Alteration in body image and coping difficulties related to enucleation and need for an eye prosthesis
5. Anxiety of the child related to hospitalization and to diagnostic and treatment procedures
6. Parental knowledge deficit regarding retinoblastoma and its treatment

Nursing Interventions

A. **Provide emotional support to the parents at the time the diagnosis is made.**

1. The parents often feel guilty about transmitting the disease to the child or because they did not notice the symptoms earlier.
2. The parents may exhibit anger toward one another or the physicians for ignoring parental remarks or postponing a thorough examination.

B. **Care for the child receiving radiation therapy.**

1. Sedate the child as requested by the physician.
   a. Administer the medication in a timely manner so that sedation is adequate for current positioning of the child.
   b. Observe for possible side effects of irradiation and prepare the parents for their occurrence.
      (1) Skin changes at the temples
         (a) Use soap sparingly in these areas.
         (b) Avoid exposure to the sun.
         (c) Apply a nonirritating lubricant.
      (2) Loss of lashes
      (3) Fat atrophy with ptosis
      (4) Delayed wound healing
      (5) Dry eye
      (6) Permanent radiation dermatitis
      (7) Impaired bone growth

C. Provide preoperative care for the child.

1. Encourage the parents to "room-in" and participate in the child's care to minimize separation anxiety.
2. Prepare the child and parents for all diagnostic procedures.
3. Describe the surgery and anticipated postoperative appearance of the child.
   a. The parents should be reassured that the operation is not extremely bloody or mutilating.
   b. All adnexal structures of the eye are left intact.
   c. A surgically implanted sphere maintains the shape of the eyeball.
   d. The child's face may be edematous and ecchymotic.
   e. A small dressing is used to cover the site.
4. Offer the family the opportunity to talk with another parent who has gone through the experience or to see pictures of another child with an artificial eye.
5. See nursing management of the child undergoing eye surgery, page 1391.

D. Provide postoperative care for the child.

1. Change the dressing and cleanse the operative site as requested by the physician.
2. Encourage the parents to see the socket and participate in dressing changes soon after the surgery, since they will need to do this after discharge.
3. See nursing management of the child undergoing eye surgery, page 1391.

E. Care for the child receiving chemotherapy.

See the section on chemotherapy, page 1456.

F. Encourage the parents to seek genetic counseling.

1. Discuss the benefit of consultation about the probability of having another affected child.
   a. Risk ranges from approximately 1%–10%, depending on family history and whether the affected child had unilateral or bilateral disease.
   b. The reportedly high lifelong cancer burden among retinoblastoma patients may also be important to parents in making informed decisions.
   c. Support parental decisions regarding future pregnancies.

2. Encourage the parents to seek genetic counseling for the affected child when he reaches puberty.
   a. The risk to his offspring is from 1%–50%, depending on family history and whether he had unilateral or bilateral disease.
   b. Among his affected offspring, there is a high probability (>50%) of bilateral disease.

Health Education

The parents should receive instruction concerning:

1. Care of the socket
2. Care of the prosthesis—initial instructions are provided by the ocularist and should be reinforced by the nurse.
3. Protection of the remaining eye from accidental injury.
4. Coping with limited vision, loss of peripheral vision, or blindness (see the section on childhood blindness, p. 1387)
5. Need to have subsequent children carefully evaluated for retinoblastoma.
   a. An ophthalmologic examination under anesthesia is usually recommended at about 2 months of age.
   b. The child should receive frequent examinations thereafter until he is judged safe from developing retinoblastoma, usually about age 3 years.

Expected Outcomes

1. The parents participate in genetic counseling
2. The parents have an opportunity to discuss their feelings about retinoblastoma and its treatment and to express any sense of guilt they might have
3. The child deals with side effects of radiation therapy—skin changes, possible ptosis, loss of lashes
4. Develops and maintains a positive body image—accepts the presence of the prosthesis and is not inhibited in his behavior
5. The child demonstrates lessened anxiety by his ability to participate in age-appropriate activities
6. The parents gain an understanding of retinoblastoma and its treatment as reflected in their conversation and participation in the child's care

Bibliography

Books

Abeloff M (ed). Complications of Cancer: Diagnosis and Management. Baltimore, Johns Hopkins University Press, 1980

Backer B, Hannon N and Russell N. Death and Dying. New York, John Wiley & Sons, 1982

Blume K and Petze L (eds). Clinical Bone Marrow Transplantation. New York, Churchill Livingstone, 1983

Fochtman D and Foley G (eds). Nursing Care of the Child with Cancer. Boston, Little, Brown & Co, 1984

Kellerman J. Psychological Aspects of Childhood Cancer. Springfield, IL, Charles C Thomas, 1980

Koocher G and O'Malley J. The Damocles Syndrome: Psychosocial Consequences of Surviving Childhood Cancer. New York, McGraw-Hill, 1981

Levine A (ed). Cancer in the Young. New York, Masson Publishers, 1982

McIntire S and Cioppa A. Cancer Nursing: A Developmental Approach. New York, John Wiley & Sons, 1984

Petrillo M and Sanger S. Emotional Care of Hospitalized Children. Philadelphia, JB Lippincott, 1979

Pochedly C (ed). Pediatric Cancer Therapy. Baltimore, University Park Press, 1979

Schulman J and Kupst M. The Child with Cancer: Clinical Approaches to Psychosocial Care: Research in Psychosocial Aspects. Springfield, IL, Charles C Thomas, 1980

Spinetta J, Deasy-Spinetta P and Brandt S (eds). Living with Childhood Cancer. St Louis, CV Mosby, 1981

Sutow W, Ferbach D and Vietti T. Clinical Pediatric Oncology, 3rd ed. St Louis, CV Mosby, 1984

Van Eys J (ed). The Normally Sick Child. Baltimore, University Park Press, 1979

Whaley L and Wong D. Nursing Care of Infants and Children, 2nd ed. St Louis, CV Mosby, 1983

Williams C. All About Cancer. New York, John Wiley & Sons, 1983

Articles

Baskin C et al. Helping teachers help children with cancer: A workshop for school personnel. Child Health Care 1983 Fall; 12(2):78–83

Belasco J and D'Angio G. Wilms' tumor. CA 1981 Sep/Oct; 31(5):258–270

Bersani G and Carl W. Oral care for cancer patients. Am J Nurs 1983 Apr; 83(4):533–536

Blumberg B et al. Developing materials to meet the educational needs of adolescents with cancer. Oncol Nurs Forum 1983 Winter; 10(1):35–39

Cameron C and Wallace N. Having a bone marrow test: A child's perspective. Child Health Care 1983 Summer; 12(1):41–42

Cleaveland M. Nursing care in childhood cancer: Brain tumor. Am J Nurs 1982 Mar; 82(3):422–425

Collins M. The leukemic child. Issues Compr Pediatr Nurs 1980 Feb; 4(1): 49–59

Croft M et al. Nursing care in childhood cancer: Coping. Am J Nurs 1982 Mar; 82(3):440–442

Daeffler R. Oral hygiene measures for patients with cancer, II. Cancer Nurs 1980 Dec; 3(6):427–432

Dasson M. A chance to be normal again Cancer Nurs 1982 Dec; 5(6):453–459

Dax J and Greenwood R. A very special camp. Am J Nurs 1982 Aug; 82(8): 1218–1219

DeMoss C. Giving intravenous chemotherapy at home. Am J Nurs 1980 Dec; 80(12):2188–2189

D'Angio G et al. Wilms' tumor: An update. Cancer 1980 Suppl; 45(7): 1791–1798

Dodd M and Mood D. Chemotherapy: Helping patients to know the drugs they are receiving and their possible side effects. Cancer Nurs 1981 Aug; 4(4):311–318

Ertel I. Brain tumors in children. CA 1980 Nov/Dec; 30(6):306–321

Evans A. Staging and treatment of neuroblastoma. Cancer 1980 Suppl; 45(7):1799–1802

Fife B. Childhood cancer is a family crisis. J Psych Nurs 1980 Oct; 18(10): 29–34

Gaddy D. Nursing care in childhood cancer: Update. Am J Nurs 1982 Mar; 82(3):416–421

Greene P and Fergusson J. Nursing care in childhood cancer: Late effects of therapy. Am J Nurs 1982 Mar; 82(3): 443–446

Griffiths S. Changes in body image caused by neoplastic drugs. Issues Compr Pediatr Nurs 1980 Feb; 4(1): 17–27

Hayes V. The adolescent unit: A holistic approach to cancer management. Oncol Nurs Forum 1980 Summer; 7(3):9–12

Healy G. Malignant tumors of the head and neck in children: Diagnosis and treatment. Otolaryngol Clin North Am 1980 Aug; 13(3):483–488

Hutchinson M and Itoh K. Nursing care of the patient undergoing bone marrow transplantation for acute leukemia. Nurs Clin North Am 1982 Dec; 17(4):697–711

Jenkin D and Sonley M. Soft-tissue sarcomas in the young. Cancer 1980 Aug 1; 46(3):621–629

King D and Clatworthy W Jr. The pediatric patient with sarcoma. Semin Oncol 1981 Jun; 8(2):215–221

Koocher G et al. Psychological adjustment among pediatric cancer survivors. J Child Psychol Psychiatry 1980 Apr; 21(2):163–173

Krakoff I. Cancer chemotherapeutic agents. CA 1981 May/Jun; 31(3):130–140

Kramer R et al. Childhood cancer: meeting the special needs of healthy siblings. Cancer Nurs 1983 Jun; 6(3): 213–217

Krulik T. Helping parents of children with cancer during the mid-stage of illness. Cancer Nurs 1982 Dec; 5(6): 441–445

LaFortune S and Gloriant F. Nursing diagnosis in cancer chemotherapy in theory and in practice. Am J Nurs 1981 Nov; 81(11):2013–2022

Levenson P et al. Sources of information about cancer as perceived by adolescent patients, parents and physicians. Patient Couns Health Educ 1981 2nd quarter; 3(2):71–76

Lipman A. Drug therapy in cancer pain. Cancer Nurs 1980 Feb; 3(1):39–46

Mackey C and Hopefl A. Keeping infections down when risks go up. Nursing '80 1980 Jun; 10(6):69–73

Manchester P. The adolescent with cancer: Concerns for care. Topics Clin Nurs 1981 Jan; 2(4):31–37

Mattia M and Blake S. Hospital hazards: Cancer drugs. Am J Nurs 1983 May; 83(5):759–762

Maul S. Childhood brain tumors: A special nursing challenge. MCN 1984 Apr; 9(2):123–129

Miller D. Acute lymphoblastic leukemia. Pediatr Clin North Am 1980 May; 27(2):269–291

Mills G. Preparing children and parents for cerebral computerized tomography. MCN 1980 Dec; 5(6): 403–407

Newberger P and Sallan S. Chronic pain: Principles of management. J Pediatr 1981 Feb; 98(2):180–189

Nilsen J. Nursing care in childhood cancer: Adolescence. Am J Nurs 1982 Mar; 82(3):436–439

Nuscher R et al. Bone marrow transplantation. Am J Nurs 1984 Jun; 84(6):764–772

Olness K. Imagery (self-hypnosis) as adjunct therapy in childhood cancer. Am J Pediatr Hematol/Oncol 1981 Fall; 3(3):313–321

Ritchie J. Nursing the child undergoing limb amputation. MCN 1980 Mar/Apr; 5(2):114–120

Ross J et al. Facilitating the pediatric cancer patient's return to school. Soc Work 1982 May; 27(3):256–261

Sachs M. Helping the child with cancer go back to school. J Sch Health 1980 Aug; 50(6):328–331

Sallan S, Weinstein H and Nathan D. The childhood leukemias. J Pediatr 1981 Nov; 99(5):676–688

Schaffner A. Safety precautions in home chemotherapy. Am J Nurs 1984 May; 84(5):346–347

Shields J and Augsburger J. Current approaches to the diagnosis and management of retinoblastoma. Surv Ophthalmol 1981 May/Jun; 25(6): 347–372

Smithson W, Gilchrist M and Burgert E. Childhood acute lymphocytic leukemia. CA 1980 May/Jun; 30(3): 159–177

Stream P, Harrington E and Clark M. Bone marrow transplantation: An option for children with acute leukemia. Cancer Nurs 1980 Jun; 3(3): 195–199

Taylor M et al. Use of therapeutic play in the ambulatory pediatric hematology clinic. Cancer Nurs 1980 Dec; 3(6):433–437

Teitell B. Complications of pediatric cancer chemotherapy. NITA 1982 Nov/Dec; 5(6):361–366

Toal D. Tumor cell kinetics and cancer chemotherapy. Am J Nurs 1980 Oct; 80(10):1802–1804

Walter J. Care of the patient receiving antineoplastic drugs. Nurs Clin North Am 1982 Dec; 17(4):607–629

Walters J. Coping with leg amputation. Am J Nurs 1981 Jul; 81(7):1349–1352

Wegmann J and Ogrinc M. Oncology nursing conflict: A case presentation of holistic care and the family in crisis. Cancer Nurs 1981 Feb; 4(1):43–48

Welch D and Lewis K. Chemotherapy and alopecia. Am J Nurs 1980 May; 80(5):903–905

Wiley F et al. Allogenic bone marrow transplantation for children with acute leukemia. Oncol Nurs Forum 1983 Summer; 10(3):49–53

Wolf W and Bancroft B. Early detection of childhood malignancies. Pediatr Nurs 1980 Jan/Feb; 5(1):43–46

Wong D and Dornan L. Nursing care in childhood cancer: Retinoblastoma. Am J Nurs 1982 Mar; 82(3):425–430

Additional References/Agencies

American Cancer Society
90 Park Avenue
New York, NY 10016

Candlelighters Foundation
2025 Eye Street, NW
Suite 1011
Washington, DC 20006

Center for Attitudinal Healing
19 Main Street
Tiburon, CA 94920

Copeland D, Copeland K and Pfferbaum B. The Andy Anderson Coloring Book. University of Texas System Cancer Center. M. D. Anderson Hospital and Tumor Institute, Parent Education Program. 6723 Bertner Avenue, Houston, TX 77030 (available in Spanish)

US Department of Health and Human Services
Public Health Service
National Institutes of Health
Office of Cancer Communications
National Cancer Institute
Bethesda, MD 20892

The Child at Risk—Special Pediatric Problems

46

Mental Retardation

Mental retardation refers to significantly subaverage general intellectual functioning existing concurrently with deficits in adaptive behavior and manifested during the developmental period.*

Etiology

A. General

1. Congenital lack of brain cells
2. Later destruction of cells originally present

B. Prenatal Factors

1. Heredity
2. Fetal irradiation
3. Infection—maternal or fetal
4. Kernicterus due to Rh or ABO incompatibility
5. Anoxia
6. Cranial anomalies
    a. Hydrocephalus
    b. Craniosynostosis
7. Chromosomal abnormalities
8. Disorders of metabolism

C. Natal Factors

1. Anoxia
    a. Maternal
    b. Placental
    c. Respiratory obstruction
2. Breech delivery with delay in delivery of the head
3. Cerebral injury
    a. Trauma
    b. Cephalopelvic disproportion
    c. Precipitate delivery
    d. Prematurity
4. Infection
5. Intracranial hemorrhage

D. Postnatal Factors

1. Central nervous system infection
2. Brain injury, hemorrhage, or tumor
3. Cerebral degenerative disease
4. Anoxia
5. Poisoning

---

* Definition of the American Association on Mental Deficiency. In Heber R (ed). A Manual on Terminology and Classification in Mental Retardation. (Monograph Supplement). Am J Ment Defic 1958; 64:3

6. Vascular disorders
7. Social and cultural factors

E. Unknown

1. No identifiable organic or biologic cause for 65%–75% of retardation in children.
2. Suspected causes include sociocultural or environmental deprivation or poverty.
3. Generally, these children are more mildly retarded than children with associated organic and physical defects.

Incidence

1. It is estimated that approximately 125,000 infants born each year in the US will at some time in their lives be classified as mentally retarded.
2. A decrease in infant deaths, a longer life span, and improved case finding have caused a rise in the total number of persons classified as mentally retarded.

Classification*

1. Mental retardation is most often classified according to the child's educational potential, based on the IQ score:
    a. Mild (educable)—IQ of 50–55 to approximately 70
    b. Moderate (trainable)—IQ of 30–40 to 50–55
    c. Severe—IQ of 20–25 to 35–40
    d. Profound (custodial)—IQ of below 20 or 25
2. Although the IQ score may be helpful in assessing and planning for retarded children, low IQ in itself is not sufficient to make a diagnosis of mental retardation.
3. Both intellectual level and adaptive behavior level (the effectiveness or degree with which the individual meets the standards of personal independence and social responsibility expected of his age and cultural group) should be considered when one makes the classification.
4. Scales have been developed for measuring and classifying adaptive behavior based on the following expectations:
    a. *Infancy and early childhood*
        (1) Sensory–motor skills development

---

* Grossman H (ed). Classification in Mental Retardation. Washington, DC, American Association on Mental Deficiency, 1983, pp. 11–26

(2) Communication skills (including speech and language)
(3) Self-help skills
(4) Socialization
  b. *Childhood and early adolescence*
    (1) Application of basic academic skills in daily life activities
    (2) Application of appropriate reasoning and judgment in mastery of environment
    (3) Social skills, group activities
  c. *Late adolescence and adult life*
    Vocational and social responsibilities and performances
5. Only those children who demonstrate deficits in both intellectual level and adaptive behavior should be classified as mentally retarded.

Prognosis

1. Factors that influence the prognosis
   a. Degree of retardation
   b. Existence of additional, physical defects
   c. Family and community resources available to help the child to use his mental resources
2. Factors that favor improvement in intelligence
   a. Modification of the environment to eliminate stress and deprivation

b. Improvement in learning opportunities
c. Increased social acceptance
d. Early intervention
3. The prognosis is best for the mildly retarded child without a coexistent physical defect.

Clinical Manifestations

1. Developmental delay—failure to meet normal motor, mental, and/or social milestones for age
2. Physical
   a. Approximately 75% of retarded individuals have no obvious physical stigma.
   b. Mentally retarded children have a greater percentage of sensory defects, language disorders, neuromuscular impairment, seizures, and physical anomalies than the general population.

Diagnostic Evaluation

1. Diagnosis is difficult and is most reliable when the determination is made by a comprehensive team that offers medical, psychological, social, and educational examinations.
2. Care must be taken to ensure that no child is mislabeled as mentally retarded.

Down's Syndrome (A Specific Cause of Mental Retardation)

Down's syndrome is a chromosomal abnormality involving an extra chromosome (number 21), characterized by a typical physical appearance and mental retardation.

Etiology

A. Trisomy 21

1. The abnormality is an error in cell division.
   a. Both number 21 chromosomes in the pair instead of just one of the pair migrate to one daughter cell during meiosis.
   b. 47 chromosomes are present in the new individual rather than the normal 46.
   c. There are 3 number 21 chromosomes, thus extra genetic material.
2. Occurrence is associated with advanced maternal age.
   a. Risk is increased after maternal age of 35.
   b. Occurrence in the same set of parents is rare, but dependent on maternal age.
3. This form of Down's syndrome is not inherited.

B. Translocation

1. Chromosome number 21 attaches to another chromosome, usually the 13–15 group.
2. This abnormal attachment occurs in the parent.
   a. The parent passes on to the offspring an extra dose of chromosome 21, plus a normal chromosome 21.
   b. The child with this type of Down's syndrome has 46 chromosomes.
3. This form of Down's syndrome is inherited.
   In most cases, it is a fresh occurrence, and for chromosomally normal parents there is small risk of a future child with Down's syndrome. In one third of the cases, one parent is a balanced translocation carrier; thus, there is risk of recurrence.

Incidence

About 1 in 660/700 live births each year will be diagnosed as having Down's syndrome.

Altered Physiology

1. The normal person, without Down's syndrome, has 46 chromosomes (23 pairs).
   a. One pair of chromosomes is sex-determining.
   b. 22 pairs of chromosomes are non–sex-determining and are called *autosomes.*
2. The individual with Down's syndrome has an extra chromosome—number 21. He carries extra genetic material.
3. Abnormalities that are present at birth occurred during fetal growth.
   a. There has been interference with normal fetal growth.
   b. This interference affects mainly the heart, brain, eyes, hands, and general growth.
4. Specific physical characteristics are apparent as a result of the extra chromosome.

Complications

1. Recurrent infections of upper respiratory tract
2. Skin infections
3. Complications secondary to physical anomalies present at birth:
   a. Eye problems—strabismus; error in refractions
   b. Elevated leukocyte enzymes
      (1) Small percentage of affected children born with fatal leukemia
      (2) Leukemia—acute type developing in first 2–3 years
4. Serious behavioral problems

Assessment

Clinical Manifestations

1. Physical stigmata recognized at birth:
   a. Marked hypotonia and floppiness
   b. Joint hyperextension or hyperflexibility
   c. Tendency to keep mouth open with tongue protruding; high, arched palate; furrowed tongue
   d. Brachycephaly with relatively flat occiput
   e. Eyes slant upward and outward with internal epicanthal folds
   f. Excess skin on back of neck
   g. Flattened nasal bridge and flat facial profile
   h. Small ears, often incompletely developed
   i. Spade-like hands; there is inward curving of distal phalanx of fifth finger; simian crease
   j. Short, broad feet; there is a wide separation between first and second toe (plantar furrow)
   k. Small male genitalia
   l. Absence of Moro reflex (Response to sudden loud noise, causing body to stiffen and arms to go up and out, then forward and toward each other. Thumb and index finger will assume "C" shape.)
2. Complications most likely to be present at birth:
   a. Congenital cardiac defects, especially atrial septal defect
   b. Duodenal stenosis and other intestinal obstruction
3. Later findings in the child (up to 1 year of age):
   a. Slow intellectual development (IQ of 20–75; mean, 50)
   b. Slow motor development

Diagnostic Evaluation

1. Chromosomal analysis (karyotyping) will show how the third chromosome, number 21, is attached to another autosome in translocation or nondisjunction.
2. Pelvic x-ray will show inner edge of ilium flattened, iliac wings are widened resulting in reduced acetabular and iliac angles.

The following sections pertain to mental retardation with special emphasis on Down's syndrome.

Nursing Interventions

The Infant

A. Support the parents during the initial period of diagnosis.

1. Provide time for the parents to comprehend the extent of their problem and to mobilize their resources to work on its solution.
   a. When the parents appear ready, offer counseling and verbal support at a slow pace, one step at a time.
   b. Be sensitive to clues concerning the type of support that is most helpful to each family.
2. Encourage both parents to talk about the diagnosis and how they feel about it.
   a. The parents' reaction will be individually determined by factors such as the nature of the diagnosis, the manner in which the family is told of the diagnosis, the perceived attitude of health professionals, the parents' previous life experiences, their attitudes toward retardation, their marital relationship, and their personal aspirations.
   b. Expect attitudes of guilt, shame, and self-pity;

feelings of grief, hostility, and ambivalence; expressions of denial; thoughts that they might be unable to care for the child.
   c. Provide privacy for discussions.
   d. Express sympathetic understanding of the family's problems and show acceptance of their attitudes. Reassure them that many parents react to the diagnosis with grief and sorrow.
3. Assure the family that their child has had the benefit of the best diagnostic procedures and has been given every treatment that is indicated.
4. If appropriate, initiate a referral to a social worker, a psychiatrist, or any other professional who may assist the family to deal with their immediate reactions and may plan for the child's long-term care.
   Many parents benefit from the continuous or intermittent support of a variety of health professionals.
5. Communicate a genuine concern for the parents as individuals and an understanding of the responsibilities that they have outside the hospital (i.e., care of other children, work, etc.).

B. Encourage parental participation in caring for and handling the infant and to foster acceptance of the child by his parents and family.

1. Provide opportunities for the parents to learn all aspects of caring for their baby. The basic needs of the baby with Down's syndrome are the same as those of other infants.
   Emphasize the need for parents to appreciate the child for his unique attributes; he can be lovable and can be enjoyed as a person, but he requires special attention.
2. All the support and help given the parents during hospitalization will make home care easier. Early intervention and support should strengthen and support the parental role.
   a. Encourage the physician to have both parents present, possibly with the infant, when he tells them of the child's diagnosis. In this way, they can turn to one another for support.
   b. Make special efforts to involve the father. Respond to his needs—he may require special attention, support, and guidance.
   c. Adaptation by both parents is critical for the continual improvement of the child's functioning and to foster optimal growth and development.
   d. Help the parents to be honest in their thoughts and emotions concerning the baby.
   e. Help the parents to accept the fact that their child has Down's syndrome and to accept the child for himself.
3. Assist the parents in learning what Down's syndrome is and how it alters a child's mental and physical development.
   a. Provide appropriate literature (see the Bibliography, p. 1501, for some suggestions).
   b. Inform them of local or national organizations.
   c. Alert the parents to some common physical deviations that occur with Down's syndrome and the consequent effect of these deviations on behavior. If possible, provide an adjusted time table of development that takes into account the child's retardation.
4. Invite the parents to join a group of parents who have children with Down's syndrome. Counseling

can also alleviate the parents' loss of self-concept and feeling of self-worth.

5. Be aware of problems that new parents of a Down's syndrome baby may encounter.
   a. Grief for the loss of the expected normal child.
   b. Poor communication with the baby's physician.
   c. Difficulty in telling family and friends.

6. Emphasize the infant's need for love, affection, consideration, and individual attention.

C. Foster acceptance of the child by his parents and family and increase feelings of self-worth and self-confidence in the parents.

1. Serve as a role model by interacting with the child in a manner that conveys acceptance, respect, and love.

2. Help the parents to develop a fundamental understanding of what has happened to their child and what this means in terms of his future development.
   a. Clarify and support medical speculations regarding the cause of the retardation.
      (1) Genetic counseling as indicated, especially in familial types of retardation.
      (2) Answer parental questions sensitively but directly.
      (3) Provide explanations in terms they can understand.
      (4) Avoid vague generalities, such as "the child is slow," and demoralizing words, such as "moron" or "imbecile."
   b. Provide as much specific information as possible. Parents have the right to know what diagnostic tests have been done, what positive or negative conclusions have been made, what uncertainties remain, and what general prognosis can be made.

3. Involve both parents in the child's care so that they may gain a realistic concept of his ability.
   a. Point out the child's areas of strengths and weaknesses and show how these can be considered in his management.
   b. Emphasize the *well* part of the child and that he has the same needs as a normal child for love and security.

4. Include the family as soon as possible with other members of the health team in planning for the child's future care.
   a. The plan should be based on the degree of the child's retardation, the reaction of the family to the diagnosis, and the availability of community resources.
   b. The family should be supported in the decisions they make.
   c. The family should be guided to make decisions for the child's care which will allow for maximum utilization of his capabilities.

5. Discuss with the parents their plans for dealing with the siblings of the retarded child.
   a. Adequate explanations and information should be given to siblings early to avoid any misconceptions later.
   b. Siblings often need help in explaining the retarded child's abnormality to their friends.
   c. Caution the parents to guard against intense sibling rivalry; the other children often feel neglected because of the amount of time devoted to the retarded child.

6. If appropriate, initiate a community health nursing referral for assistance with planning and implementing home care.

D. Observe carefully for any signs of physical complications that may occur with Down's syndrome. Record and report them immediately.

1. Intestinal obstruction (duodenal stenosis)
   a. Observe for abdominal distention and its association with feeding.
   b. Note vomiting—what is vomited and when.
      (1) Bile-stained emesis indicates lower tract obstruction.
      (2) Partially digested milk indicates upper tract obstruction.
   c. Note absence of stools.

2. Congenital cardiac defect
   a. When taking vital signs, note any irregularity of the heart rate. Murmurs may not be evident to the untrained ear. Note any respiratory distress or labored respirations.
   b. Note any cyanosis and when it occurs—with crying, feeding, or all the time.
   c. Be particularly alert to the infant tiring easily during feeding.

E. Provide a safe environment for the infant.

1. Infant is usually very floppy because of poor muscle tone. When handling the infant, support him well with a firm grasp.

2. Position the infant so that if vomiting should occur he will not aspirate.
   a. If he is on his abdomen, be certain that he can turn his head to the side.
   b. Prop him with a diaper roll so that position will be maintained.
   c. This infant is not usually very active; thus, his position will need to be changed frequently.

F. Establish and maintain adequate nutrition to allow for growth and development.

1. The diet is calculated according to the infant's needs.

2. Because of poor muscle tone and a protruding tongue, the infant may be a poor eater with a weak and ineffective suck.
   a. Provide the appropriate nipple so that minimal sucking effort is needed to feed.
   b. Allow adequate time for feeding. Do not allow the infant to become overly tired.
   c. Note and report poor eating and insufficient sucking.

G. Provide proper stimulation according to the child's age.

1. Be aware that this infant needs stimulation from the very start to begin to help him develop to his potential. Develop a plan of stimulation so that your activity and actions lead toward this goal.
   a. Infants with Down's syndrome who are quiet and undemanding tend to be understimulated, so they do not reach their full potential.
   b. Begin a program of mental stimulation early—one that can be continued at home.
      (1) Program should include exercises built around existing reflexes; these can reduce hypotonia.
      (2) Encourage exercises to develop eye–hand coordination and later finger–thumb grasp.

2. Offer positive and effective sensory stimulation. Hold and fondle the infant, especially during feeding.

3. When the infant is awake, the adult face in his visual

field is good stimulation and should interest him for a few seconds.

4. The gentle sound of talking or music can provide a pleasant auditory experience. The infant should stop activity and listen.

The Older Child

The older child with Down's syndrome is usually admitted to the hospital because of some medical complication, such as an acute respiratory infection.

A. Be aware of nursing activities associated with hospitalization of a child previously diagnosed as mentally retarded.

1. Apply all of the previously outlined principles.
2. Obtain a thorough nursing history from the parent and/or child regarding the child's usual home routines.
   a. Feeding
   b. Sleeping
   c. Toilet habits
   d. Learning activities
   e. Play
   f. Vocabulary
   g. Discipline
3. Utilize the information obtained to develop a nursing care plan that provides for continuity of care from home to hospital in order to maintain the child's sense of security and minimize his regression.
   a. Counsel the mother that some regression can be anticipated even in normal children who require hospitalization.
   b. Know what activities the child can or cannot do and what he likes to do.
   c. Plan the child's day according to what he is used to as much as possible.
4. Encourage parental participation to the extent that it is therapeutic for both the child and the parent(s).
5. Provide a safe environment appropriate to the child's needs.
   a. This environment is best determined by observing the child and from information obtained during the admission interview.
   b. If possible, use the type of bed with which the child is familiar.
   c. Remove any objects that are potentially injurious to the child.
6. Whenever possible, assign the same nursing personnel to care for the child.
7. Explain procedures to the child using communication methods appropriate for his level of cognitive development.
   Share this information with nursing staff to ensure continuity of care from home to hospital to minimize fear and frustration in the child.

B. Attend to the child's needs according to the medical problem that required his hospitalization.

The child may need to be watched and assessed more frequently for pain, frustration, and distress.

C. Plan and provide for the appropriate type of play program and stimulation for the child.

1. Assess the child's level of growth and development and consider this in the plan.
2. Do not try to teach the child new or different things because he may react adversely to the newness.
3. Allow the child as much independence as possible in his care, but provide guidance as necessary.

4. Permit the development of the child's abilities. Minimize frustrating situations.

D. Teach the child basic skills with the long-range goal of developing independent behavior at the highest level possible according to the child's potential.

1. Determine the child's care plan according to his individual areas of strengths and weaknesses and coordinate it with the plans of the related health professionals.
2. Because a retarded child has a limited attention span, present a smaller amount of material to him at a slower rate and over a longer period of time than to a normal child.
3. Provide organized, consistent, and repetitive experiences.
4. Employ techniques of positive reinforcement.
   a. Give rewards for positive responses so that the probability of recurrence of that response will be strengthened.
      Rewards should be given consistently and immediately after the approved response.
   b. Do not reward unacceptable behaviors.
5. Break complex behaviors down into small steps which the child can easily achieve.
   a. This is very important in the areas of feeding, dressing, and toilet training.
   b. Do not expect the child to transfer learning from one situation to another.
6. Base expectations for the child on his mental ability, *not* on his chronological age.
7. Maintain a relaxed learning environment.

E. Reduce destructive behavior and encourage that which is socially acceptable.

1. Establish a routine of daily living so that the child knows precisely what is expected of him.
2. Employ consistent discipline.
   a. Use language that the child understands so that he can comprehend his misdeed.
   b. When punishment is necessary, it should follow the misdeed immediately.
3. Provide immediate reinforcement for positive behaviors and ignore undesirable behaviors.

F. Prepare the mentally retarded individual so that he may cope successfully (within his potentiality) with the problems and adjustments of adult life.

1. Help the parents identify areas of home responsibilities that may be delegated to the retarded child.
2. In the child's early learning activities, provide habits that are essential to his later vocational life.
   a. Getting to places on time
   b. Cooperating
   c. Focusing and holding attention on the task at hand
   d. Establishing acceptable interpersonal relationships
3. Help the child to develop a set of attitudes and behaviors that will motivate him to work.
4. Identify attainable occupational goals early in the child's educational experience.
   Early education should tie into later social and vocational programs.

G. Foster continuing parental acceptance of the child and provide support for them.

1. Invite the parents to care for their child as much as they can. Rooming-in may be advisable.

2. Help the parents to understand why the child behaves as he does.
3. Encourage the parents to talk about their feelings or problems they have with the child. Reemphasize the need for parents to appreciate their child for his unique attributes and special characteristics, such as sociability and sensitivity to the feelings of others.
4. Initiate a teaching program for the child and his parents early. Continued educational experiences are vital. Offer the family available literature and help them to become familiar with community resources.
   a. Parents can provide positive and effective sensory training.
   b. Help the child to socialize with other children and provide an environment that will stimulate him mentally.
5. Allow the parents to continue to maintain what other responsibilities they may have outside the hospital (i.e., other children, work).
   Do not insist that they stay at the hospital and attend only to this child.

H. Help modify existing social attitudes toward retardation.

1. Assess and work through your own feelings about the retarded, including personal attitudes and defenses which are used to avoid personal involvement in the care of retarded children and their families.
2. Utilize opportunities to influence the attitudes of other hospitalized children and their families.
   a. Serve as a role model in your own interactions with retarded children.
   b. Encourage hospitalized children to socialize with the retarded child during play programs or other activities, and help them to understand and accept the child.
   c. Provide opportunities for other parents to discuss their feelings about retardation and to ask questions. Correct any misconceptions they may have.
3. Initiate and/or support community educational and service programs.
4. Support federal legislation relating to funding for research and services for the mentally retarded.

Health Education

Parental education is one very important aspect in the nursing care of a child with Down's syndrome, especially in the following areas:

1. The environment has an influence on the rate of the child's progress in performance, behavior, growth, and development.
   a. The role of the parents is critical. A nurturing and loving environment gives the child the best chance to develop to his full potential.
   b. Encourage the entire family to be included in the child's care.
   c. The child will usually be lovable and quiet, affectionate, and socially responsive if he is loved and if individual attention is given to his specific needs.
   d. Patience and understanding must be developed by parents and family.
2. The mentally retarded child may require more medical supervision than the normal child. Regular dental care is also essential.
   a. The child is often more susceptible to infections.
   b. He may eat poorly.
   c. He may be underweight or overweight.

d. He may have poor motor coordination.
   e. He often has speech and language problems.
3. Secondary handicaps such as visual or hearing problems should be treated.
4. The child's environment has a greater influence on his behavior, growth, and development. It should provide experiences that contribute to a positive self-concept of a person who is loved, wanted, valued, and respected.
5. Parents need to be helped to recognize their child's method of communicating so that they can respond to his needs.
6. Parents should be assisted to identify learning readiness in their child in order to help him achieve his maximum level of development without subjecting him to unnecessary experiences of failure and frustration.
7. Practical, tangible suggestions relative to everyday living should be offered to the parents.
   a. Selection of toys
   b. Techniques of feeding
   c. Patterns for toilet training
   d. Methods of discipline
   e. Sex education for the adolescent
8. Special precautions may be necessary to provide a safe environment for the child.
   His delayed motor, intellectual, and social development make him more vulnerable to the usual childhood accidents.
9. The child should have the opportunity of participating in social, religious, and recreational activities.
   a. Organizations should be selected in which the probability of success is the highest.
   b. The parent should discuss the situation with the group leader and the leader should have an opportunity to meet the child so that both child and leader can assess each other.
   c. Help the parents to understand that in spite of signs of slow mental growth, the child can make steady progress. In early life, the child with Down's syndrome should not be stereotyped in behavior. His behavior is similar to the norm when mental age is considered. Help parents not to lower their expectations.
      (1) The child needs a great deal of repetition in all areas of learning.
      (2) He usually has a good memory, can acquire a fairly large vocabulary and can learn to spell. Arithmetic may be more difficult for him.
      (3) Speech may lag behind walking by 1–2 years. He may encounter trouble in pronouncing certain words. Stammering may occur if the child is under pressure.
      (4) Parents need help in learning to recognize the child's readiness to learn these skills.
      (5) A general decrease of IQ score occurs with increasing age and should be an expected occurrence because of the increasing verbal and abstract content of test materials at the higher mental age.
10. The child's motor development is slow. The degree of hypotonia probably greatly influences the early motor development; genetic potential and environmental stimulation of the child also influence motor development.
    a. Encourage motor coordination. It will take time for the child to learn to sit. At age 5 or 6 years,

he may still walk like a 2-year-old child. Toilet training usually can be accomplished.
   b. He may always have trouble with fine motor skills.
   c. Encourage the child to do as much for himself as he can.
11. Parents need to know that they are important as people. They each should be encouraged to lead a normal life. They should be helped to feel that they are not their child's only resource, but that others care and are willing to help.
   Other members of the family must be considered.
   a. The child should not be thought of as a sick child, but as a child who needs special handling to promote his individual growth and development. But he does not need all the attention all the time.
   b. The family should be included in his care, but they also must have a life of their own and as much parental attention as they would receive if the child were not present in the family.
   c. Parents need time to themselves. They should be encouraged to go out alone together and to give time to their marriage.
   d. Encourage parents to be open with the family and to discuss concerns. Children are sensitive to parental distress. Lack of communication can create and increase parental isolation and can cause unrealistic concerns.
   e. Sibling reactions generally reflect the parents' reactions toward the child with Down's syndrome.
   f. Assist parents to assess their family situation to promote healthy family relationships. Do the following situations exist?
      (1) Are older siblings frequent caretakers of the child with Down's syndrome?
      (2) Is there excessive parental attention to the afflicted child at expense of other siblings?
      (3) Do the parents show hostility toward the child?
      (4) Are there excessive expectations of other children?
      (5) Is the family dominated by the destructiveness or overactivity of child with Down's syndrome?
12. Available literature should be offered to parents; they should also be made aware of community resources (see the Bibliography, pp. 1500–1501).
   a. Community nursing agencies or special preschool programs
   b. Day-care centers
   c. Foster grandparent programs, foster home
   d. Nursery groups
   e. Special schools
   f. Parent groups
   g. Volunteer organizations
   h. Specialized diagnostic facilities
   i. Recreational programs
   j. Vocational training
   k. Residential settings
   l. National associations
   m. Sheltered workshop
13. Parents should be assisted in making decisions regarding residential placement.
   a. Alternatives to home care and reasons for placement should be discussed as appropriate.
   b. Parents should be helped to select the best alternative to home care and establish ways to maintain contact with the child.
14. Future in society
   a. The child with Down's syndrome should go to school. He learns by copying. Have the parents discuss the child's problem with the school nurse, the teacher, and other adults who have close contact with the child.
   b. Education enables the child with Down's syndrome to be productive to some extent in society, to have a fuller life, and to take pride in his accomplishments. Such children can learn routine housework, gardening, or farming. They can run errands, learn to obey traffic rules, and ride buses.
15. References for parents:
   American Association on Mental Deficiency, 1719 Kalorama Road, NW, Washington, DC 20009
   Association for Retarded Citizens, Inc., PO Box 6109, Arlington, TX 76011
   National Information Center for Handicapped Children and Youth, PO Box 1492, Washington, DC 20013
   National Down Syndrome Congress, 1640 W Roosevelt Road, Chicago, IL 60608 (publishes *Down's Syndrome News,* booklets, bibliographies for articles, etc.)
   National Down Syndrome Society, 70 W 40th Street, New York, NY 10018
   Parents of Down's Syndrome Children, % Montgomery County Association for Retarded Citizens, 11600 Nebel Street, Rockville, MD 20852

Minimal Brain Dysfunction

Minimal brain dysfunction (*MBD*) is a general term used to refer to a legion of disorders involving children of normal intelligence who have learning or behavioral disabilities associated with deviations of function of the central nervous system. MBD has been used synonymously with terms such as hyperkinesis, attention deficit disorder, learning disabilities, and dyslexia.

Etiology

1. Unknown
2. Probably represents a result of highly complex interactions between individual neuropsychologic endowments and environmental factors.
3. Contributing factors
   a. Genetic variations
   b. Some insult, usually mild, during the early developmental months
   c. Biochemical irregularities
   d. Dietary sensitivity to specific foods or food additives
   e. Psychosocial factors

Incidence

1. Estimated to occur in as many as 15% of children.
2. Males are affected more frequently than females.
3. Most important cause of school underachievement.

Management

A multi-faceted approach involving some or all of the following aspects is necessary:
1. Family education and counseling concerning MBD
2. Medication—central nervous system stimulants such as Benzedrine, Dexedrine, and Ritalin used alone or in combination are effective in reducing many of the symptoms of some children with MBD.
3. Environmental manipulation to decrease external stimuli and encourage desirable behavior patterns
4. Remedial education focused on the specific area(s) of deficit
5. Psychiatric or psychologic therapies

Clinical Manifestations

The child usually demonstrates a constellation of the following features:
1. Behavioral characteristics
   a. Hyperactivity—stimulus-bound behavior which lacks consistent direction and frequently shifts focus. Usually manifested in mild to moderate degrees.
   b. Short attention span—inability to focus on the task at hand because of low threshold to distracting stimuli.
   c. Impulsivity—inability to delay gratification. Difficulty restraining impulses to move or speak.
   d. Labile emotions—poorly modulated emotional response. Results in extreme reactions of pleasure and displeasure triggered by relatively minor stimuli.
   e. Perseveration—inability to shift attention appropriately from one activity to another.
   f. Impaired interpersonal relations and antisocial behavior.
   g. Hypoactivity—much less common than hyperactivity.
2. Learning disability—specific deficit of learning, such as listening, thinking, reading, writing, or arithmetic.
3. Neurologic features
   a. Poor motor integration or coordination.
   b. Perceptual deficits—difficulty with perception of time, space, form, sound, and sequence resulting in confusion of right to left, before and after, etc.

Diagnostic Evaluation

1. Detailed medical, developmental, and behavioral history
2. Neurologic examination to detect abnormalities
3. Psychologic testing to determine the exact nature of cognitive or perceptual dysfunctions that may be present
4. Additional testing depends on the child's symptomatology and frequently includes EEG and hearing evaluation

Nursing Interventions

A. Identify minimal brain dysfunction.

1. Be aware of the clinical features of MBD.
2. Observe the child's behavior for evidence of abnormality.

3. Include developmental and behavioral components in the nursing history.
4. Make appropriate referrals for diagnosis in suspected cases of MBD.

B. Provide emotional support to the family.

1. Provide parents with opportunities to express their feelings and concerns about the diagnosis.
2. Expect such reactions as guilt, disbelief, relief, anger, and frustration. Reassure the parents that these feelings are normal and acceptable.
3. Provide factual information about the disorder and treatment plan.
4. Assist the parents to deal with identified problems, and provide them with positive feedback when appropriate.
5. Help the parents anticipate and deal with the reactions and needs of siblings.
6. Assist the family to find appropriate programs to meet the child's special needs.
7. Serve as coordinator of services between family, school, physician, and other agencies.
8. Refer to a parent support group if one is available.

C. Reduce symptoms.

1. Administer prescribed medications.
   a. The child is usually started on a small dose, which is gradually increased until the desired response is achieved.
   b. Evaluate the child's response to medication by direct observation and consultation with others, such as parents and teachers.
   c. Observe for side-effects, including appetite suppression, sleep disturbance, stomach upset, and blurred vision.
      These usually disappear after a few weeks of therapy or with alteration of dosage.
2. Provide controlled diet if prescribed.

D. Provide a therapeutic physical environment.

1. Assist the parents to manipulate the home environment to reduce stimulation and stress.
   a. Maintain regular sleeping, eating, working, and playing routines.
   b. Provide a minimum of external stimuli and alternatives.
   c. Divide tasks and expectations into small, manageable parts. Give only one or two instructions at a time.
   d. Set firm but reasonable limits on behavior and carry through with consistent discipline.
   e. Avoid situations that cause excessive excitement, stimulation or fatigue.
2. Evaluate the environment for safety hazards and eliminate them.
3. Provide for energy release.
   a. Plan for periods of physical activity, vocal outlet, and outdoor play.
   b. Channel need for movement into safe, appropriate activities.

E. Care for the hospitalized child previously diagnosed with MBD.

1. Elicit a detailed history emphasizing management techniques currently used by the family.
2. Continue home management techniques during the hospitalization as much as possible.
3. Manipulate the hospital environment to reduce unnecessary stimulation and stress.

4. Eliminate any safety hazards.
5. Observe the child for response to hospitalization and his therapeutic regimen.
6. Provide continued support to parents.
7. Teach the child about his health problem.
   a. The teaching plan should be divided into short, concrete steps.
   b. Select a learning environment with minimal distraction. Limit interruptions.
   c. Use learning materials that are clear and specific. Avoid presenting too much equipment at one time.
   d. Select reading materials carefully, according to the reading ability of the child. Do not assume that the child understands the material simply because he can read it.
   e. Encourage eye-to-eye contact when talking with the child.

F. Participate in community programs.

1. Take advantage of opportunities to teach about MBD.
2. Assist with related screening programs.

Health Education

1. Provide factual information about the disorder, clearly differentiating MBD from mental retardation, autism, and other disabilities.

2. Teach parents regarding all aspects of the management program.
   a. Medication
      (1) Parents should be instructed concerning the dosage and schedule, desired effects and side effects of medication.
      (2) They should be helped to think of the use of medication for MBD as a necessity, much as insulin is used for the diabetic, rather than as a tranquilizer.
      (3) They can be assured that there is no evidence that the drugs produce any euphoric effect or addiction in children.
   b. Diet—parents may need help in locating sources for the proper foods.
   c. Environmental manipulation to reduce stimulation and stress
   d. Consistent and appropriate disciplinary techniques
   e. Remedial education—assist parents to understand, select, and demand the best alternatives for their child's education.
3. Caution the parents about unproven approaches that profess a single solution to the problem of MBD.
4. Resources for parents:
   Association for Children With Learning Disabilities, 4156 Library Road, Pittsburgh, PA 15234

Genetic Counseling

Genetic counseling is the process of providing families with information about hereditary and congenital disorders. It involves determining the risk of occurrence or recurrence, interpreting the findings, and assisting the family in making a reasonable decision.

Inheritance of Disease

Disease may be inherited by:
1. Chromosomal rearrangement
   a. Nonhereditary—risk increases with maternal age
   b. Chromosome translocation
2. Single gene inheritance
   a. Dominant—1 abnormal gene
   b. Recessive—2 abnormal genes
   c. X-linked—from female carrier to male offspring
   d. A schematic outline is shown in Table 46-1.
3. Polygenic inheritance—inheritance of many genes
   a. Related to the total number of genes received from each parent; genetic component gives predisposition to congenital malformation
   b. May include meningocele, congenital dislocated hip

Indications for Prenatal Diagnosis of Genetic Disorders

1. Increased risk of chromosomal disorders
   a. Advanced maternal age—woman 35 years of age or older
   b. Parent known to be a carrier of chromosomal disorder
   c. Previous pregnancy resulting in child with chromosomal disorder
   d. Previous multiple congenital anomalies—when no cytogenetic analysis was done
   e. History of spontaneous abortions
2. Known risk for significant metabolic disorders
3. Known risk for significant sex-linked genetic disorders
4. Willingness to consider termination of the pregnancy if an abnormal fetus is detected

Parental Barriers to Counseling

1. Lack of knowledge or misinformation
2. Social and/or psychological implications
3. Cultural–religious beliefs
4. Financial

Table 46-1   Single Gene Inheritance

Inheritance Pattern	Number of Abnormal Genes	Risk with Each Pregnancy	Example
Autosomal-dominant	1	50%—if parent affected	Congenital cataracts
Autosomal-recessive	2	25% from 2 normal parents	Cystic fibrosis
X-linked recessive	1 on sex chromosome	50% for male—if mother is carrier	Duchenne's muscular dystrophy

Prenatal Diagnosis of Genetic Disorders

Genetic screening provides information for discovering cases of treatable diseases before irreversible damage has taken place, provides reproductive options, and facilitates research.

A. Amniocentesis (see Obstetrics, p. 973)

1. Method of obtaining amniotic fluid of a pregnant woman by inserting a needle transabdominally through the uterus.
2. Examination is made of amniotic fluid, amniotic fluid cells, and cultured amniotic fluid cells.
3. Procedure done at 12–16 weeks' gestation.
4. Useful in diagnosing some inborn errors of metabolism.

B. Roentgenography

1. Useful in diagnosing anencephaly, hydrocephaly, achondroplasia, osteogenesis imperfecta congenita, myelomeningocele, and bilateral cleft palate.
2. Many diagnoses are established only in the last trimester.
3. Risk of radiation exposure to fetus is high if done prior to third trimester.

C. Amniography–Fetography

1. A technique of intra-amniotic injection of a contrast material, which opacifies the fluid and displaces the fetal soft tissue parts; is swallowed by fetus.
2. Useful in diagnosing soft tissue and gastrointestinal malformations (gastrointestinal obstruction, diaphragmatic hernia, meningocele), intrauterine growth retardation, and multiple gestation.
3. This test is usually done when the AFP (alpha-fetoprotein) is abnormally increased in the amniotic fluid.

D. Ultrasonography

1. Sound frequencies, when applied to the body, reflect back when they meet boundaries and between tissues of different densities, thus outlining anatomic structures.
2. Used in conjunction with other clinical, laboratory, and sometimes radiologic studies in diagnosing malformations of the central nervous system.
3. Used to determine the size of the fetus and the fetal head, to locate the placenta and fetus prior to amniocentesis, to identify multiple gestation, neural tube defects (anencephaly, meningocele, hydrocephalus), sternal agenesis, enlarged cystic kidneys, and some skeletal abnormalities, and to determine accurately gestational age.

E. Fetoscope

1. Visualization of fetus in utero by endoscopic instruments (investigational)
2. Provides tissue sampling
   a. Fetal blood for thalassemia, hemophilia, chronic granulomatous diseases, and muscular dystrophy.
   b. Fetal skin biopsy for ichthyosiform erythroderma and epidermolysis bullosa.

Goals of Genetic Counseling

1. To provide clients with information about the genetic defect in question. Identifies risks and provides information regarding severity of condition.
2. To communicate to clients the risk of transmitting the defect to subsequently conceived children.
3. To enable individuals and couples to make informed decisions regarding marriage and/or parenthood (e.g., having children, adopting children, continuing or terminating an existing pregnancy).
4. To provide psychological support to assist clients with their decision-making process and the necessary reordering of their lives.
5. To reduce the number of individuals affected by genetic disease.
6. To alert other health professionals involved with the family of the possibility of genetic disease in the family background.
7. In order to provide effective counseling one must have:
   a. Correct and accurate diagnosis
   b. Detailed and accurate family history
   c. Current information about the diagnosis or problem

Major Genetic Disorders

See Table 46-2.

Diagnostic Studies Performed from Amniocentesis

A. Amniotic Fluid

1. Steroid levels
2. Enzyme studies
3. Mucopolysaccharide determinations
4. Alpha-fetoprotein (AFP) levels

B. Amniotic Cells

1. Enzyme studies
2. Sex chromatin and Y-body fluorescence

C. Amniotic Fluid Cells, Cultured

1. Cytogenetic studies (karyotype)
2. Enzyme studies
3. Autoradiographic studies
4. Histochemistry

Nursing Interventions

A. Identify families who need genetic counseling and to whom the service should be offered.

1. Be alert to information in the family history that would indicate referral for genetic counseling.
2. Be aware of evidence of deviation from normal growth and development and of other abnormalities (e.g., a single umbilical artery, low-set ears, or defects of the genitalia) that may indicate genetic problems.
3. Offer the opportunity for counseling to any family that has a child with a known genetic problem.

B. Assist families to acquire sufficient and correct information about the genetic problem in question.

1. Be aware of local and regional centers for genetic counseling and other available resources.
2. Be knowledgeable about the types of genetic disorders and their probability of occurrence (see Table 46-2).

C. Serve as a liaison between the genetic counselor and the family.

Note: In some situations, the nurse acts as the counselor.

1. Prepare parents for the experience of counseling. Help them know what to anticipate to lower their anxiety level and to make the counseling sessions a better experience.

2. If possible, attend the counseling session. This facilitates reinforcement of information and makes it easier to answer questions adequately.
3. Assess the family's need for additional counseling sessions, and initiate these if the need is recognized.

D. Help families handle the information received and guide them in coping with this crisis in their lives.

1. Utilize interviewing skills to facilitate discussion regarding parental feelings.
   Consider factors such as timing and privacy.
2. Alleviate parental feelings of guilt and shame.
   a. If a recessive trait is involved, both parents may blame themselves. A parent who is a carrier of a dominant anomaly may blame himself, and the other parent may blame him as well even if she (or he) does not outwardly express these feelings.
   b. Emphasize that a person has no choice or responsibility in acquiring the genes that cause the problem.
   c. Reassure the parents that information gathered is important for determining an accurate diagnosis and the nature of inheritance; assure them that it will be kept confidential.
   d. It may be helpful to inform the parents that many other people have hidden, recessive genes.
3. Anticipate parental questions and areas of difficulty and conflict.
   a. Many parents are afraid to ask questions. They may fear they will sound stupid; they may not know what to ask—much less how to ask questions.
   b. Listen carefully for parental areas of unanswered or unasked questions.
   c. Help parents formulate questions. Utilize statements such as, "Many parents have questions about _____."
   d. Be available to parents when they have something to ask.
   e. Listen carefully to parents' questions and answer them whenever possible.
4. Remain objective.
   a. Be aware of personal feelings about specific genetic disorders.
   b. Come to terms with your own emotional difficulty related to genetic disorders and issues such as abortion.
   c. Avoid letting personal reactions affect your attitude toward counseling and behavior toward the family.
      (1) If the nurse avoids the situation, parents are tacitly given professional sanction to do the same thing.
      (2) A nurse who conveys the impression that he/she cannot cope with the fact of genetic disease is unlikely to convey assurance that a family should be able to cope with the consequences of the disease.
5. Reinforce information about the genetic disorder, probability, possible interventions to correct the defect or minimize the disability, self-care goals, and limitations requiring adaptation.
   a. Frequently parents do not understand the meaning of the risk ratio quoted to them, or they may attach too much or too little importance to it.

b. Be certain that parents understand specifically what the predictions imply.
6. Clarify understanding of all family members.
   Have both parents present for discussions as frequently as possible to prevent misinterpretations and distortions from being passed from one to the other. Include grandparents and siblings as appropriate.
7. Assist the parents to evaluate the total situation and to see the ramifications of any decision they may make.
   Facilitate realistic assessment of the expected burden to the parents, the child, and society; have them evaluate their capacity for dealing with the situation and expected problems.
8. Provide psychological support to allow parents to make and carry out decisions.
   a. Parents who decide against having children should be given information about contraception and/or sterilization.
   b. Parents who elect pregnancy should be informed about appropriate techniques of prenatal diagnosis of genetic disorders.
   c. Parents who elect adoption should be given the opportunity for additional advice when the adoption is being undertaken.

E. Ensure continued and comprehensive nursing care for the affected child and the family.

1. Continue to educate parents about the defect the child may have. Even though they may have received genetic counseling, if they have a child with the defect they may not fully understand what it is and what it means.
2. In order to be more effective in supporting parents after the birth of an affected baby, it is important to understand the phases of adjustment they go through.
   a. Shock and disorganization—denial of the infant's defect while dealing with their own emotions
   b. Adjustment—partial acceptance along with anger
   c. Reintegration—resumption of effective and realistic functioning
3. Complete necessary referrals to appropriate professionals and to community resources. These may include infant stimulation programs, preschool programs, parent groups, social service agencies, and other similar resources.

Health Education

1. Provide information regarding known genetic risk factors to the general public.*
   a. Support the concept of premarital counseling.
   b. Support prenatal counseling to increase awareness of potential hazards of infections such as rubella, to the impact of drugs on the fetus, and to pollution of water and foodstuffs by pesticides and fertilizers.

---

* Professional Education Department, March of Dimes Birth Defects Foundation, 1275 Mamaroneck Avenue, White Plains, NY 10605 (for information on location of genetic services)

National Clearinghouse for Maternal and Child Health, 3520 Prospect Street, NW, Suite 1, Washington, DC 20057 (centralized source of materials and information in the area of human genetics and child health)

Table 46-2   Common Genetic Disorders

Types	Incidence	Characteristics	Risk	Discussion
Chromosomal Disorders				
1. Autosomal abnormalities Down's syndrome (trisomy 21) (see p. 1474)	1 in 600–800 live births; varies with maternal age; meiotic nondisjunction Young mother: 1 in 1,000 live births Mother over 35: 1 in 300 live births	Brachycephalic skull; oblique palpebral fissures; epicanthal folds; Brushfield's spots; multiple eye defects; flat nasal bridge; protruding, fissured tongue; growth retardation; short extremities; dry, scaly skin; clinodactyly and simian line; mental retardation; congenital heart disease	Insufficient data Spontaneous abortion rates are high (10%–60%)	Chromosomal disorders result from: 1. Failure of a chromosome to separate at cell division (nondisjunction), causing loss or gain of genetic material. 2. Cell division error causing a chromosomal imbalance or rearrangement of genetic material. Error is associated with major structural changes. Most of the variations and abnormalities are directly transmitted to offspring from parent.
2. Monosomy (autosomal)	Product of conception rarely survives			
3. Sex chromosome abnormalities Klinefelter's syndrome (XXY abnormality)	1 in 500–750 male live births	Diagnosis is rare before puberty; mentally retarded; body may be tall, slim, and underweight; small testes; pubertal development delayed; azoospermia and infertility; psychosocial, learning, or school adjustment problems		
Turner's syndrome (X abnormality; also monosomy sex chromosome, applies to phenotype female with genotype 45; XO)	1 in 1,500–3,000 female live births	Face is heart-shaped; premature aging of face; multiple eye defects; micrognathia; short stature; webbed neck; infantile external genitalia; underdeveloped breasts; lymphedema of hands and feet during infancy; mentally retarded		
Mendelian Disorders—Single Gene				
1. Autosomal dominant Achondroplasia, classic	1 in 10,000 live births	Brachycephaly; frontal bossing; depressed nasal bridge; dwarfism; short extremities; lumbar lordosis; bowed legs; pelvic tilt	Usually sporadic occurrence. Affected parent has a 50% chance of having affected offspring with each pregnancy.	Mendelian inheritance: A single deleterious gene can cause multiple anomalies or isolated malformations.
Skeletal disorders (e.g., syndactyly)				
2. Autosomal recessive Sickle cell anemia* Cystic fibrosis*	1 in 400 live births of Blacks 1 in 1,800 live births (predominantly white)		Risk of affected parent having affected offspring is 25% per pregnancy; 50% carrier state	
Tay–Sachs disease Inherited metabolic disorders (e.g., galactosemia)	50 live births per year (occurs mainly in Jewish children)	Lack of CNS maturation; impaired motor development; cherry-red spot on eyes; early death		Carrier can be identified.
3. Sex-linked recessive Glucose 6-phosphate dehydrogenase (G6PD) Hemophilia, classic*	10%–14% of male live births in Blacks 24% of female live births in Blacks 1 in 10,000 male live births		If affected male reproduces, offspring will be as follows: Males are normal; females are carriers. Unaffected female carrier offspring: 50% male affected 50% male normal 50% female carrier 50% female normal	Sex-linked disorders occur mainly in males, although the female is the carrier. Most sex-linked disorders are recessive.
Duchenne's muscular dystrophy	1 in 7,000 live births	Onset in early childhood; muscles seem well-developed but weak; slow to walk and climb—no gross motor milestones; Gower's sign (when in sitting position will climb up legs to stand; mental retardation		
4. Sex-linked dominant (rare) Vitamin D-resistant rickets		Lateral bowing deformity of legs; frontal bossing; costochondral beading; en-	Transmitted from affected male to all female offspring. Male offspring	

* See text under the specific subject.

Table 46-2   Common Genetic Disorders (continued)

Types	Incidence	Characteristics	Risk	Discussion
		larged wrists; dental defects; hyphosphatemia; short stature	are normal. Affected female—50% of all offspring will be affected.	
Multifactorial–Polygenic Disorders				
Neural tube defects* (myelomeningocele)	0.2–4.2 in 1,000 live births		Risk varies with racial background. Recurrence risk is usually 2%–7% but is related to outcome of previous pregnancies.	Polygenic disorders are probably the result of several deleterious genes combined with environmental factors.
Cleft lip and cleft palate*	1 in 1,000 live births			These disorders are difficult to prove, because they are mainly the result of slight variations at multiple gene loci.
Pyloric stenosis*	1 in 200–300 male live births 1 in 1,000 female live births			

* See text under the specific subject.

2. Follow-up support of the family is needed to ensure that they understand the information they received and to help them integrate it into their lives.
3. Parents need a resource readily available to help them in time of crisis
   a. Supply community resources, providing telephone numbers and office hours.
   b. Written material should provide information regarding the clinical course of the genetic disorder, recurrent risk factors, etc.

Poisoning

Ingested Poisons

Poisoning by ingestion refers to the oral intake of a harmful substance which, even in a small amount, can damage tissues, disturb bodily functions, and cause possible death. In the pediatric population, poisoning is often caused by the ingestion of medications as well as toxic household substances such as furniture polish, charcoal lighter, kerosene, paint remover, cleansers, and lye.

Etiology
1. Improper or dangerous storage
2. Poor lighting—causes errors in reading
3. Human factors
   a. Failure to read label properly
   b. Failure to return poison to its proper place
   c. Failure to recognize the material as poisonous

Clinical Manifestations
1. Gastrointestinal symptoms (common in metallic, acid, alkali, and bacterial poisonings)
   a. Anorexia
   b. Abdominal pain
   c. Nausea
   d. Vomiting
   e. Diarrhea and/or intestinal cramping
2. Central nervous system symptoms
   a. Convulsions—common in poisoning due to ingestion of central nervous system stimulants such as camphor and strychnine.
   b. Coma—common in poisoning due to ingestion of central nervous system depressants such as alcohol, atropine, chloral hydrate, and barbiturates.
   c. Dilated pupils—common in poisoning due to atropine, nicotine, cocaine, and ephedrine.
   d. Pinpoint pupils—common in poisoning due to opiates.
3. Skin symptoms
   a. Rashes
   b. Burns
   c. Eye inflammation
   d. Skin irritation
   e. Stains around the mouth or lesions of the mucous membranes
   f. Cyanosis—cyanide and strychnine poisoning
4. Cardiopulmonary symptoms
   a. Dyspnea
   b. Cardiopulmonary depression or arrest

Diagnostic Evaluation
Analysis reveals presence of toxic substances in:
1. Blood
2. Urine
3. Gastric washings
4. Vomitus
5. Stool

Nursing Interventions
A. Assist the family by telephone management.
1. Calmly obtain and record the following information:
   a. Name, address, and telephone number of caller
   b. Age and condition of the child
   c. Name of the ingested product, approximate amount ingested, and time of ingestion.
2. Instruct the caller regarding appropriate emergency actions (see the section on patient and parental education).
3. Direct the patient to the nearest emergency department. Dispatch an ambulance if necessary.
4. Instruct the parents to save vomitus, unswallowed

liquid or pills, and the container, and to bring them to the hospital as aids in identifying the poison.

B. Identify the poison.

1. Determine the nature of the ingested substance from the child's history or by reading the label on the container.
2. If necessary, call the nearest poison control center or toxicology section of the medical examiner's office to identify the toxic ingredient and obtain recommendations for emergency treatment.
3. Save vomitus, stool, and urine for analysis once the child reaches the hospital.

C. Remove the poison from the body.

1. Dilute with water if advised.
2. Induce vomiting unless contraindicated.

▶ **NURSING ALERT: Do *not* induce vomiting if:**
1. The child is convulsing, semiconscious, or comatose.
2. Poison is known to be a strong acid or alkali, strychnine, or a hydrocarbon (e.g., lighter fluid, gasoline, kerosene, paint remover, or fingernail polish remover). Strong acids or alkalis may damage the esophagus for a second time during emesis, and hydrocarbons can cause severe pneumonia if aspirated.

    a. For children over 1 year of age, administer syrup of ipecac according to the directions on the label. (The usual dose is 15 ml. [about 1 tablespoon] mixed in a glass of warm water.)

▶ **NURSING ALERT: Do not use tincture of ipecac; it is much stronger than the syrup and is itself a poison.**

    b. Stimulate the posterior pharynx with a finger.
    c. Position the child with his head down or on his side to prevent aspiration of vomitus.
3. Administer gastric lavage. (This is indicated when vomiting is impossible because of the child's condition or age, or when induction of vomiting has been unsuccessful.) See Guidelines, page 945.
    a. A cuffed endotracheal tube may be inserted prior to lavage to protect the child from aspiration.
    b. Use the largest size tube that can be passed orally—preferably one with a double lumen.
    c. Place the child on his left side with his head lower than his stomach.
    d. Aspirate the stomach.
    e. Lavage with small, repeated introductions and withdrawals of normal saline, ½ normal saline, or special lavage solution.
    f. Do not leave a large amount of water in the child's stomach.
    g. Follow lavage with a cathartic to hasten removal of the poison from the gastrointestinal tract.
    h. Be aware of the dangers associated with lavage:
        (1) Esophageal perforation—may occur in corrosive poisoning
        (2) Gastric hemorrhage
        (3) Impaired pulmonary function resulting from aspiration
        (4) Cardiac arrest
        (5) Convulsions—may result from stimulation in strychnine ingestion

D. Reduce the effect of the poison by administering an antidote.

1. An antidote may either react with the poison to prevent its absorption or counteract the effects of the poison after its absorption.

2. Not all poisons have specific antidotes.
3. Information regarding appropriate antidotes for specific poisons is available through all poison control centers and in many pediatric textbooks. Antidotes for the most common poisons should be listed in the emergency department of the hospital.
4. Effectiveness of the antidote usually depends on the amount of time that elapses between ingestion of the poison and administration of the antidote.
5. Activated charcoal absorbs all poisons except cyanide. Administer orally, after vomiting has occurred, in a dose of 5–10 grams per gram of ingested poison in 177–237 ml. (6–8 oz.) of water.

E. Eliminate the absorbed poison.

1. Force diuresis.
    a. Administer large quantities of fluid either orally or intravenously.
    b. Carefully monitor intake and output.
2. Assist with kidney dialysis which may be necessary if the child's own kidneys are not functioning effectively.
3. Assist with exchange transfusion if this method is indicated for removing the poison.

F. Observe the child for progression of symptoms and provide supportive care should these develop.

1. Central nervous system involvement
    a. Observe for restlessness, confusion, delirium, convulsions, lethargy, stupor, or coma.
    b. Administer sedation with caution—in order to avoid depression and masking of symptoms.
    c. Avoid excessive manipulation of the child.
    d. See nursing care of the child with seizures, page 1433.
    e. See nursing care of the unconscious patient, page 760.
2. Respiratory involvement
    a. Observe for respiratory depression, obstruction, pulmonary edema, pneumonia, or tachypnea.
    b. Have an artificial airway available.
    c. Be prepared to administer oxygen and provide artificial respiration.
    d. Other nursing concerns:
        (1) Nursing care of the child on a ventilator, page 1190.
        (2) Procedures for administration of oxygen, page 1186.
        (3) Procedure for cardiopulmonary resuscitation, page 1195.
3. Cardiovascular involvement
    a. Observe for peripheral circulatory collapse, disturbances of heart rate and rhythm, or cardiac failure.
    b. Maintain intravenous therapy as directed: See procedure for the administration of intravenous fluids, page 1160.
    c. Be prepared for cardiac arrest (see procedure for cardiopulmonary resuscitation, p. 1195).
4. Gastrointestinal involvement
    a. Observe for nausea, pain, abdominal distention, and difficulty in swallowing.
    b. Maintain intravenous therapy to replace water and electrolyte losses (see procedure for intravenous therapy, p. 1160).
    c. Offer a diet that is easily swallowed and digested.
        (1) Begin with clear liquids.
        (2) Progress to full liquids, soft foods and then a regular diet as the child's condition improves.

5. Kidney involvement
   a. Observe the child for decreased urine output. Record urine output exactly.
   b. Observe for hypertension.
   c. Insert indwelling catheter if necessary for urinary retention.
   d. Administer appropriate amounts of fluids and electrolytes.
   e. See nursing care of the child with renal failure, page 1356.
6. General considerations
   a. Maintain adequate caloric, fluid and vitamin intake. Oral fluids are preferable if they can be retained.
   b. Avoid hypo- or hyperthermia.
      (1) Control of body temperature is impaired in many types of poisoning.
      (2) Monitor the child's temperature frequently.
   c. Observe closely for infection.
      (1) This is especially important in ingestion of kerosene or other hydrocarbons, which cause chemical pneumonitis.
      (2) Isolate the patient from other children, especially those with respiratory infections.
      (3) Administer antibiotics as prescribed by the physician.

G. Provide emotional support for the child and his family.

1. Remain calm and efficient while working rapidly.
2. Discourage anxious parents from handling, caressing, and overstimulating their child.
3. Counsel parents who often feel guilty about the accident.
   a. Encourage parents to talk about the poisoning.
   b. Emphasize how their quick action in getting treatment for the child has helped.
   c. Discuss ways that they can be supportive to their child during his hospitalization.
   d. Do not allow prolonged periods of self-incrimination to continue. Refer the parents to a social worker or psychiatrist for assistance in resolving these feelings if necessary.
4. Involve the young child in therapeutic play to determine how he views the situation.
   a. The child often sees nursing measures as punishments for his misdeed involving the poisoning.
   b. Explain the child's treatment and correct his misinterpretations in a manner appropriate for his age.

H. Prevent further poisoning episodes.

1. Initiate patient and parental teaching once the acute episode is over.
2. Initiate a community health nursing referral.
   A home assessment should be made so that underlying problems are recognized and appropriate help is provided.

Health Education

A. Prevention

1. Information concerning poison prevention should be available on every hospital pediatric unit.
   a. Many free booklets and home safety checklists are available from sources such as insurance companies and drug companies.
   b. Teaching may be done with any parent regardless of the reason for the child's hospitalization.
2. General precautions
   a. Keep medicines and poisons out of the reach of children.
   b. Provide locked storage for highly toxic substances.
   c. Do not store poisons in the same area as foods.
   d. Be certain all containers are properly marked and labeled. Keep medicines, drugs, and household chemicals in their original containers.
   e. Do not discard poisonous substances in receptacles where children can reach them.
   f. Teach children not to taste or eat unfamiliar substances.
   g. Medications
      (1) Clean out medicine cabinets periodically.
         (a) Dispose of old medications in containers out of the reach of children.
         (b) Prescription medications should be discarded when the illness for which they were prescribed has run its course.
         (c) Keep medications in "child-proof" containers that are securely closed.
      (2) Read all labels carefully before each use.
         (a) Follow exact directions on the label.
         (b) Never take a drug from an unlabeled bottle.
      (3) Do not give medicines prescribed for one child to another child.
      (4) Never refer to drugs as candy or bribe children with such inducements.
      (5) Never give or take medications in the dark.
   h. Never puncture or burn aerosol containers.
   i. Store lawn and garden pesticides in a separate place under lock and key outside of the house.
   j. Keep a 30-ml. (1-ounce) bottle of ipecac syrup and a can of activated charcoal available in the home.
   k. Keep a list of emergency telephone numbers including the poison control center, physician's number, nearest hospital, and ambulance service.
   l. Be prepared to act in cases of poisoning. Keep a list of emergency actions readily available.

B. Emergency Actions

1. Suspect poisoning with the occurrence of sudden, bizarre symptoms or peculiar behavior in toddlers and preschoolers.
2. Read the label on the ingested product or call the physician, hospital, or poison control center for instructions regarding treatment for the poisoning. Give all relevant information about the child, his condition, and the substance he took.
3. Maintain an adequate airway in a child who is convulsing or who is not fully conscious.
4. Dilute the poison with water if advised.

▶ **NURSING ALERT:** Be careful not to administer such large quantities of fluid that the poison is forced through the pylorus.

5. Make the child vomit if so directed. Do not induce vomiting if any of the following occurs:
   a. The child is unconscious or convulsing.
   b. Ingested poison was a strong corrosive such as lye or drain cleaner.
   c. Ingested poison contains gasoline, kerosene, or other petroleum distillates.
6. Directions for making the child vomit:
   a. Administer 1 tablespoon of ipecac syrup with at least 250 ml. (about 1 cup) of warm water.
   b. If vomiting does not occur in 20 minutes, this dose may be repeated once only.

c. Vomiting may also be induced by touching the back of the throat with a finger to stimulate the gag reflex.
7. Transport the child promptly to the nearest medical facility.
    a. Wrap the child in a blanket to prevent chilling.
    b. Bring the container and any vomitus or urine to the hospital with the child.
8. If transportation to a medical facility is impossible, do the following:

a. Continue to induce vomiting until vomitus is a clear liquid.
b. Administer activated charcoal between vomiting episodes.
9. Avoid excessive manipulation of the child.
10. Act promptly but calmly.
11. Do not assume the child is safe simply because the emesis shows no trace of the poison or because the child appears well. The poison may produce a delayed reaction or may have reached the small intestine, where it is still being absorbed.

Lead Poisoning

Lead poisoning (plumbism) results from the consumption of lead in some form.
1. Each year, approximately 4% of children aged 6 months to 5 years in the US have evidence of excessive serum lead levels.
2. A small number of these victims die, and many are left with chronic neurologic handicaps, mental deficiency, and/or behavioral problems.

Etiology

1. Ingestion of substances containing lead
    a. Toys, furniture, windowsills, household fixtures, and plaster painted with lead-containing paint. (New legislation stipulates that toys, children's furniture, and the interior of homes be painted with lead-free paint; however, the problem may continue if the deeper layers of paint and plaster are contaminated with lead.)
    b. Lead toys
    c. Cigarette butts and ashes
    d. Acidic juices or foods served in pottery made with lead glazes
    e. Colored paints used in newspapers, magazines, children's books, matches, playing cards, and food wrappers
    f. Water from lead pipes
    g. Fruit covered with insecticides
    h. Dirt containing lead fallout from automobile exhaust
    i. Antique pewter, particularly when used to serve acidic juices or foods
    j. Lead weights (curtain weights, fishing sinkers)
2. Inhalation of fumes containing lead (less common cause in children)
    a. Motor fuel
    b. Burning storage batteries
    c. Dust-containing lead salts
    d. Dust in the air at shooting galleries and in enclosed firing ranges with poor ventilation
    e. Cigarette smoke

Altered Physiology

1. Lead salts are absorbed by the blood from the respiratory tract or the intestines.
2. Normally, lead is deposited in the bone, where it is stored in an inert form.
3. Excess lead is deposited in the soft tissues, causing damage primarily to the nervous system, blood, and kidneys.
    a. Nervous system
        (1) Brain—edema, vascular damage; destruction of brain cells, causing convulsive disorders; neurologic deficits; learning difficulties
        (2) Peripheral nerve palsies
    b. Blood
        (1) Increases in the concentration of hemoglobin precursors in body fluids
        (2) Inhibition of a number of steps in the biosynthesis of heme, thus reducing the number of red blood cells, increasing fragility, and reducing half-life
    c. Kidneys—injury to the cells of the proximal tubules, causing abnormal excretion of amino acids, protein, glucose, and phosphate
4. Lead is slowly transferred from soft tissues to bone.
    a. It is deposited in insoluble form with calcium.
    b. The deposition causes increased thickness and density of long bones.
    c. Decalcification is associated with the release of lead from bone.

Epidemiologic Factors

1. Slums and old neighborhoods are high-risk areas because of old, deteriorating housing.
2. Pica (a habit of eating nonfood items such as paint chips, often involving a craving type of behavior) is a common precondition.
    a. Poisoning associated with pica is a chronic process.
    b. Clinical manifestations appear after 3–6 months of fairly steady lead ingestion.

Incidence

1. Highest in children between 1 and 6 years of age, especially those between 1 and 3 years
2. High in Blacks and Spanish-speaking individuals living in old homes or slum areas
3. No significant difference in sex
4. High among siblings
5. Symptomatic lead poisoning usually occurs in the summer months
6. Recurrence rate is high

Clinical Manifestations

1. Gastrointestinal symptoms
    a. Vomiting
    b. Vague abdominal pain
    c. Colic
    d. Constipation
    e. Loss of appetite
    f. Weight loss

2. Central nervous system symptoms (common in children)
   a. Falling, clumsiness, loss of coordination
   b. Irritability
   c. Dispositional changes
   d. Convulsions with or without local paralysis
   e. Drowsiness, coma
   f. Peripheral nerve palsies
3. Hematologic symptoms
   a. Anemia
   b. Pallor
4. Cardiovascular symptoms
   a. Hypertension
   b. Bradycardia
5. Symptoms depend on the amount of lead in the soft tissues and blood:
   a. Onset is insidious.
   b. Usually progresses from mild to severe manifestations as the lead slowly accumulates.
   c. Infants and toddlers may present severe manifestations initially.
   d. Symptoms may be intermittent for several months.

Diagnostic Evaluation

1. Detailed history with emphasis on the presence or absence of clinical symptoms, evidence of pica, family history of lead poisoning, possible source of exposure to lead, recent change in behavior, developmental delay, or behavior problems.
2. Erythrocyte protoporphyrin (EP) level—often used as the initial screening test. Children with values ≥50 μg./100 ml. should have a blood level determination done.
3. Blood lead level—values above 50-60 μg./100 ml. often indicate need for treatment, depending on the results of a more complete medical and laboratory examination of the individual child.
4. Hematologic evaluation for anemia.
5. Flat plate of abdomen—may reveal radiopaque material if lead has been ingested during the preceding 24–36 hours.
6. X-ray of long bones—may show increased density at the epiphyseal lines.
7. Calcium disodium EDTA mobilization test—demonstrates increasing levels of lead in the urine over a 24-hour period following injection of calcium disodium EDTA.
8. Urinary coproporphyrin (UCP) level—elevated with high blood lead levels.
9. Urinary delta-aminolevulinic acid (ALA) level—20 μg./100 ml. is considered abnormal.

Prognosis

1. Improving, with increased emphasis on prevention and screening.
2. Children with central nervous system involvement have a poor prognosis for normal development. Residual effects on the nervous system are permanent and progressive.
   Late symptoms of mental retardation may appear 3–9 years after treatment. Specific intellectual defect may interfere with the child's progress at school.

Nursing Interventions

A. Collect a urine specimen as a diagnostic tool.

A 24-hour specimen is more accurate than a single voided specimen (see the section on specimen collection).

B. Prevent absorption of lead.

1. Administer cleansing enemas if radiopaque lead particles are observed on abdominal x-rays.
2. Make certain that all sources of lead are removed from the child's environment, including the hospital environment.

C. Increase excretion of lead from the body.

Administer appropriate chelating agents (editate calcium disodium; dimercaprol).
1. Action—react with lead to form nontoxic compounds which are excreted by the body.
2. Dosage—depends on individual drug, the child's weight, severity of poisoning, prior history, and whether or not other chelating agents are being used simultaneously.
3. Appropriate play activities should be planned to prepare the child for the injections, and as an outlet for the pain and anger he feels.

D. Provide supportive care to the child with encephalopathy.

1. Observe for:
   a. Rising blood pressure
   b. Papilledema
   c. Slow pulse
   d. Convulsions
   e. Unconsciousness
2. See the section on pediatric neurologic problems, page 1414.
3. Maintain seizure precautions and have respiratory arrest equipment at the bedside.

E. Observe for factors associated with lead poisoning.

1. Pica
   a. Observe and record the child's eating habits and food preferences.
   b. Report any attempted eating of nonfood substances.
   c. Provide regular meals and make mealtime a pleasurable time for the child.
   d. Discourage oral activity and substitute activity that contributes to play, social skills, and ego development.
   e. Refer the family for additional social or psychiatric casework if indicated to reduce the psychological or cultural factors that result in pica in the child.
2. Altered parent–child relationships—record when family members visit as well as the nature of their interaction with the child.

F. Provide the child with social and motor stimulation.

1. Assess the child's level of development. The DDST (Denver Developmental Screening Test) may be useful for this purpose (see pp. 1071–1072).
2. Provide and encourage activities that will help the child to learn and progress from his present developmental state (see the section on growth and development, p. 1074).
3. Initiate appropriate referrals in cases of obvious developmental delays. Such referrals may be to such professionals as psychologists, psychiatrists, and specialists in early child education.
4. Share the results of developmental testing with the parent(s) and discuss ways to provide stimulation for the child at home.

G. Provide emotional support to the parent(s) and/or caretakers.

1. Utilize sensitivity in interviewing and teaching to avoid causing or increasing guilt feelings about the poisoning and to establish a positive, trusting relationship between the family and the health care facility.
2. Explain the treatment and its purpose, since parents are frequently faced with putting an asymptomatic child through painful treatments.

H. Prevent reexposure of the child to lead.

1. Instruct the parents regarding the seriousness of repeated exposure to lead.
2. Initiate a referral to a community health nurse to determine if exposure to lead is continuing and to provide continuing support to the family.
3. Advise the parents to require their landlord to remove lead paint from the walls; assist them with this process.
   a. Refer the parents to the housing authority.
   b. Do not allow the child in the home while lead paint is being removed. Place the child temporarily in a convalescent home or foster home if necessary.
4. When it is impossible to eliminate lead hazards from the home:
   a. Scrape loose or chipped paint and plaster from the window sills, woodwork, moldings, etc., and tape the areas with masking tape or contact paper.
   b. Remove all crumbling plaster and replaster or cover the area with wallboard or contact paper.
5. Suggest periodic, focused household cleaning to remove the lead dust.
6. Encourage handwashing before meals and at bedtime to eliminate lead consumption from normal hand-to-mouth activity.
7. Make certain that the family is able to provide close supervision of the child or assist them to make arrangements to ensure that the child is adequately supervised at home.

I. Participate in the prevention of lead poisoning.

1. Initiate and support educational campaigns through schools, day-care centers, and news media to alert parents and children to hazards and symptoms of lead poisoning.
2. Provide in clinics, waiting rooms, and other appropriate settings literature stressing the hazards of lead, sources of lead, and signs of lead intoxication.
3. Inquire about the presence of pica in all children under 6 years of age.
4. Screen siblings of known cases immediately.
5. Screen all children from high-risk areas.
6. Provide follow-up to all children suffering from lead poisoning as well as to those in the early stage of undue lead absorption to prevent their becoming poisoned.
7. Support legislation to study the nature and extent of the lead poisoning problem, to detect and treat such poisoning, and to eliminate the causes of lead poisoning.

Health Education

Parental education is an extremely important part of the nursing care of a child with lead poisoning. It should include the following points of emphasis:
1. Long-term medical follow-up is essential.
   a. Residual lead is liberated gradually after treatment.
      (1) May result in the renewal of symptoms.
      (2) May increase serum lead to a dangerous level.
      (3) Additional damage to the central nervous system may become apparent for several months (after discharge from the hospital).
   b. Acute infections must be recognized and treated promptly. (These may reactivate the disease.)
   c. Some children are placed on D-penicillamine for long-term chelation. If this drug is used, it should be given on an empty stomach, 2 hours before breakfast.
   d. Many children require supplemental iron therapy. Parents should be instructed regarding its administration and side effects.
2. Reexposure to lead must be prevented.
3. Siblings and playmates should be screened for lead poisoning.
4. Literature stressing the causes and prevention of lead poisoning should be provided.*
5. Nutritional teaching may be indicated (see the section on nutrition, p. 1094).

The Abused Child (Child Abuse and Neglect)

Child abuse and neglect refers to "a child under the age of 18 who is suffering from physical injury (inflicted upon him by other than accidental means), or sexual abuse, or malnutrition, or suffering physical or emotional harm or substantial risk thereof by reason of neglect. Reporting of neglect shall take into account the accepted child-rearing practices of the culture of which he or she is part."*
Child abuse and neglect includes the following conditions:
1. Battering—physical injury
2. Nutritional neglect—deliberate omission of adequate nutrition. "Failure to thrive" results when the child's weight is below the 3rd percentile for age and sex and the child has no predisposing physical abnormality.
3. Drug abuse—intentional administration of harmful drugs
4. Medical neglect—intentional omission of basic preventive-medicine practices or specific treatment for medical problems

* Clinical Proceedings. Washington, DC Children's Hospital National Medical Center, Vol. 30, No. 2, Feb 1974, p. 38

* Literature is available from the Lead Industries Association, 292 Madison Avenue, New York, NY 10017 and from the US Dept. of Health and Human Services, Superintendent of Documents, US Government Printing Office, Washington, DC 20402.

5. Sexual abuse
   a. Sexual assault or molestation (nonfamily offender)
   b. Incest (family offender)
6. Safety neglect—intentional omission of safety precautions appropriate for age of child
7. Emotional abuse—scapegoating, belittling, humiliating, lack of mothering
8. Child neglect—lack of providing the child with basic needs of survival: shelter, clothing, stimulation, development of trust, etc.

Etiology

Child abuse is not a uniform phenomenon with one set of causal factors, but a multidimensional phenomenon. The phenomenon may be related to the combined presence of 3 factors: special kind of child, special kind of parent, special circumstances of crisis.
1. Psychopathology of the abuser
2. Cultural, social, and economic factors
3. Specific child characteristics (i.e., premature, debilitated, child needing special care)

Contributing Factors (Not Unicausal)

1. Incidents of child abuse may develop as a result of disciplinary action taken by the abuser who responds in uncontrolled anger to real or perceived misconduct of the child. The parents may confuse punishment with discipline. "Good parenting" may be equated with physical contact to eradicate undesirable child behavior.
2. Incidents of child abuse may develop from a general attitude of resentment or rejection on the part of the abuser toward the child.
3. Atypical child behavior (e.g., hyperactivity) may provoke the abuser. This may be child-initiated or child-provoked abuse.
   Some children contribute to their own abuse by inappropriate use of learned behaviors.
4. Incidents of child abuse may develop out of a quarrel between the caretakers. The child may come to the aid of one parent, may find himself in the midst of the quarrel, or may object to the quarrel.
5. The abuser may be a stern, authoritarian disciplinarian.
6. The abuser may be under a great deal of stress because of life circumstances (debt, poverty, illness) and may thus resort to child abuse. Crisis and stress may be ongoing. The abuser may have a low frustration tolerance level and may not have a well-developed means of coping with stress in general.
7. The abuser may be intoxicated with alcohol or drugs at the time of the abuse.
8. Child abuse frequently occurs while the mother is out of home and the child is left in the care of a babysitter or boyfriend.
9. Lack of early mothering, inappropriate mother–child bonding, and punitive treatment as a child may contribute to child neglect.
10. Specific characteristics evident in many abusing parents include:
    a. Low self-esteem—a sense of incompetence in role; unworthiness; unimportance
    b. Unrealistic attitudes and expectations of child; little regard for the child's own needs and age-appropriate abilities
    c. Fear of rejection—a deep need to feel wanted and loved, but a feeling of rejection when love is not obvious; a crying infant may elicit a feeling of rejection
    d. Inability to accept help—isolation from the community; loneliness
    e. Unhappiness due to unsatisfactory relationships; may look to child for satisfaction of own emotional needs
11. The abused or neglected child may be seen by the parent as "special." The premature infant or one having a serious illness may have resulted in failure of emotional-bonding. The parents perhaps could not provide special care to the child because of their own psychological variables or situation.
12. A breakdown of parent–child interaction.

Clinical Manifestations

A. **Physical characteristics utilized as an index of suspicion.**

1. Child usually under 3 years of age. School-age child is also subject to abuse, however.
2. General health of the child indicates neglect (diaper rash, poor hygiene, malnutrition).
3. Characteristic distribution of fractures (scattered over many different parts of body).
4. Disproportionate amount of soft tissue injury.
5. Evidence that injuries occurred at different times (healed and new fractures, resolving and fresh bruises).
6. Cause of recent trauma in question.
7. History of similar episodes in past.
8. No new lesions occurring during the child's hospitalization.
9. The child may develop behaviors through interaction with parents and peers that place him at risk for abuse.

B. **Injuries or types of abuse that may occur:**

1. Bruises, welts (linear or loop-like)
2. Abrasions, contusions, lacerations (most common)
3. Wounds, cuts, punctures
4. Burns (cigarette, radiator, etc.), scalding—stocking, glove distribution
5. Bone fractures (including skull)
6. Sprains, dislocations
7. Subdural hemorrhage or hematoma
8. Brain damage
9. Internal injuries
10. Drug intoxication
11. Malnutrition (deliberately inflicted)
12. Freezing, exposure
13. Whiplash-type injury
14. Eye injuries
15. Periorbital injuries; ear bruises
16. Dirty, infected wounds or rashes
17. Unexplained coma in infant

C. **Possible characteristics of the child suspected of being abused or neglected:**

1. May show a wide range of reactions—may be either very withdrawn or overactive. The child may be anxious, tense, or nervous.
2. Avoids physical contact with parents; does not look to parents for comfort; shows distinct preference for one parent, while fearfully withdrawing from the other.
3. Is fearful, constantly alert for danger; seeks information as to what is going to happen next; is mistrustful of environment.

4. May show unusual affection for strangers or may be overly fearful of adults and avoid any physical contact with them.

D. Identifying behavior common in abusing or neglecting parent(s):

(Be aware that not all abusing parents exhibit these behaviors.)

1. Anxiously volunteers information or withholds information.
2. Gives an explanation of the injury that does not fit the condition or gets story confused concerning the injury.
3. Shows inappropriate reaction to severity of injury.
4. Becomes irritable about questions being asked.
5. Seldom touches or speaks to the child; does not respond to him. May be critical of the child or indicate unreal expectations of him.
6. Delays seeking medical help; refuses to sign permit for diagnostic studies. Frequently changes hospitals or physicians.
7. Shows no involvement in care of the hospitalized child; does not inquire about the child.
8. The problem of abuse is a total family problem—family dysfunction.

Treatment

1. Prevention is the most critical aspect of treatment.
   a. Early recognition for potential abuse—identify family or child at risk: alcohol/drug abuser, adolescent parent, low-income single-parent family, multiple births, or unwanted child; sickly and more demanding child or premature with long separation from mother at birth.
   b. Use community resources and special programs (i.e., "hot lines," crisis nurseries, self-help groups) to aid the parent in preventive support.
2. Once abuse or neglect is suspected:
   a. Public Law 94-247 (Child Abuse and Neglect Act—1973) requires that professionals report suspected abuse. Notify the appropriate officials.
   b. Since other children in the family may be involved, they should be examined by a physician as soon as possible.
   c. Establish and maintain a therapeutic relationship with the parents. Generally a team approach is recommended to assess family needs and determine the most effective use of community resources to protect the child and help the family. The parents are the focus of treatment. They are helped to develop a sense of self-esteem and confidence and to relinquish their abusive behavior.
   d. Specific counseling and/or psychiatric intervention for the abused child focusing on the emotional impact of the event(s).

Nursing Interventions

A. Inspect every child's body upon admission to the hospital for evidence of abuse.

1. Describe on nursing record all bruises, lacerations, etc., as to location and state of healing. Look carefully at areas generally covered with clothing (i.e., buttocks, underarms, behind knees, bottom of feet). Be alert for abuse of the school-age child. Most often the child's injury is not severe enough to require medical attention, but the child may be hospitalized for some other medical problem.

2. Discuss with the physician the case of any child suspected of being abused.
   a. Every state (as well as the District of Columbia) has mandatory reporting laws. All states provide statutory immunity for those who report real or suspected child abuse. There is no immunity from civil or criminal liability for failure to report such.
   b. Every nurse is morally and legally responsible to report and provide protective services for the abused child.
   c. Become familiar with laws, procedures, and protective services in your community and state.

B. Be prepared to effectively care for the child who is the victim of sexual assault or incest.

1. Sexual abuse should be suspected when the young, prepubital child presents with:
   a. Trauma not readily explained
   b. Gonorrhea, syphilis, or other sexually transmitted organisms
   c. Blood in urine or stool
   d. Painful urination or defecation
   e. Penile or vaginal infection or itch
   f. Penile or vaginal discharge
   g. Report of increased, excessive masturbation
   h. Report of increased, unusual fears
2. Establish a relationship with the child based on mutual respect, empathy, and sensitivity.
   a. The child may be extremely calm or hysterical. She/he may verbally express a desire to talk about the incident. Take into consideration the different ways emotions are expressed by children at different developmental stages.
   b. Consideration of the child's emotions in conjunction with a good relationship may encourage the child to express his or her feelings either verbally or through drawings or play.
   c. Prepare the child both physically and psychologically for the necessary physical and pelvic examination.
   d. Talk with the child without the presence of the parents, especially when incest is possible.
3. Know the state laws regarding the reporting of suspected child abuse, as well as the legal definition of sexual deviation. In 1974, Public Law 93-237 established a National Center on Child Abuse and Neglect* to provide financial assistance for prevention, identification, and treatment of child abuse and neglect.
   a. Document any physical findings—bruises, abrasions, telltale secretions in mouth or pharynx, on hair or skin, in and around buttocks, clothes.
   b. Collect any necessary specimens for identification of organisms, sperm, or semen.
   c. Take colored photographs.
4. Participate in the therapeutic approach.
   a. Talk with the child and parents alone. Be honest with the mother.
   b. Prevent sexually transmitted disease, pregnancy, and tetanus. Prophylactic treatment should be given for penile penetration of any orifice.
   c. Support the parents who may have feelings of guilt, anger, and helplessness. Explain to them the extent of trauma and educate them regarding

---

* National Center on Child Abuse and Neglect, US Dept. of Health and Human Services, 400 Sixth Street, SW, Washington, DC 20013

pediatric gynecology; allow them to ventilate their feelings. Support their parental role in handling the child (i.e., allow the child to talk about or play out the incident, but do not force it).

    d. Encourage compliance with the treatment selected for the child, parents, and family (i.e., group counseling, psychiatry).

C. Observe and record pertinent information regarding the parent–child relationship.

1. Do the parents visit the child? Do parents become involved in caring for child?
2. How do(es) the parent(s) respond to the child? Does the parent talk to the child, touch him, hold him, and play with him?
3. How does the child react to the parent? Is he excited when the parent arrives? Does he appear frightened and withdrawn? Does he cry when the parent leaves?
4. What does the parent expect of the child? Are his expectations appropriate for the child? Is there role-reversal between parent and child?

D. Obtain a thorough nursing history in order to establish a nursing care plan that is individualized to meet specific needs of the child.

1. Information should be obtained relating to the child's sleeping habits, toilet habits, favorite foods and eating habits, favorite toy or security objects, play habits and favorite playmate, names and ages of siblings, nickname, previous hospital experience, developmental assessment, and persons who will visit the child.
2. Care and good judgment must be used in obtaining this information from parents, because they undoubtedly have already been asked many questions by many people. Use chart information already obtained to eliminate repetition.
3. Obtaining a nursing history in a nonthreatening, nonjudgmental manner can convey to parents that you have a genuine interest in caring for their child, and that you respect the knowledge they have as parents of their child. Getting the history will also allow you to assess the parents' knowledge and expectations of their child and will set a positive atmosphere for a continued relationship.

E. Provide for the child a milieu to reduce trauma similar to that of any hospitalized child placed in the strange and frightening environment of the hospital by implementing the principles of emotional support (see p. 1112).

The child must be treated as an individual. He may need extra help in the following areas:

1. Having ambivalent feelings toward his parent or parents
2. Overcoming his low self-image and the fear that something is wrong with him
3. Fearing future abuse upon his return home
4. Satisfying his strong need for attention, affection, and having a trusting relationship with an adult
5. Learning alternate ways of expressing his needs and feelings

F. Foster a trusting relationship with the child who may be fearful of adults.

1. Assign one nurse to care for the child over a period of time. Select the right nurse for the right patient.

2. Make no threatening moves toward the child. The child will indicate his readiness and awareness of the environment by his verbal or facial expressions.
3. Touch the child gently.
4. Provide nonthreatening physical contact (hold the child frequently and cuddle him). Pick him up and carry him around; encourage any exploration of your face, hair, etc.
5. Enlist the cooperation of volunteers to provide additional mothering.
6. Provide appropriate opportunities for play.
7. Set limits for him.

G. Come to terms with your own feelings of anger, disgust, and contempt for the parents.

A critical part of working in this area is learning to recognize, examine, and work with these feelings. It may help to do the following:

1. Realize that most abusing parents do love their child and want the best for him in spite of their ambivalent feelings for him.
2. Understand the dynamics of child abuse and neglect. This crisis is due to the stress with which the parents are unable to cope and to the deprivations they have themselves suffered in their past.
3. Focus on the needs of the parents rather than on the injuries of the child. Treatment is aimed at helping the parents reach their maximum potential as parents.
4. Expect repeated rejection from the parents who lack self-esteem and trust.
5. Understand that these parents are often difficult to like under ordinary conditions. They are experiencing terror, guilt, and remorse; they are fearful and yet expect criticism and condemnation.

H. Foster a relationship with the parents that will encourage them to accept guidance and will help in dealing with the problem.

1. Assume a nonjudgmental attitude that is neither punitive nor threatening. The desire to help must be conveyed.
2. Refrain from questioning them about the incident of abuse. (The suspected abuser will be interviewed by the physician, the social worker, and the authority who investigates the case.)
3. Include the parents in the hospital experience (i.e., orient them to the unit and to any procedure to be done for the child). Serve as role model in the management of the child's behavior as well as their own. Try to give the parents as much information as possible about the care of their child. Listen to what they are saying.
4. Refrain from challenging all the information they may give.
5. Express appropriate concern and kindness. Remain objective yet empathetic. This will help foster the parents' self-respect and improve their self-image and dignity.
6. Discuss the reporting to the authorities with them because of the widespread nature of the problem and the need for public attention and education.

I. Foster a healthy mother–child relationship.

1. Build a relationship by working with the mother's strengths rather than her weaknesses. Use compliments as positive reinforcement.
2. Serve as a role model of appropriate methods of child care in areas such as feeding, bathing, and play.

3. Provide the mother with psychological support and reinforcement for appropriate mothering behaviors she does exhibit.
4. Work with the mother in planning for the child's future care.
5. Determine in what areas the mother needs help: Does the baby cry a lot? How does this make her feel? How does she comfort him? When she is alone, is there someone she can call for help? Does she feel the child understands what she expects of him?
6. By forming a helping relationship with the mother, the nurse will strengthen the protective ability of the mother and bind her to her child.

J. Be aware of the entire scope of nursing responsibilities in dealing with the abused and neglected child.

1. Case finding—identify the potential (or suspected) abused and neglected child. Be a participating and contributing member of the multidisciplinary team in treating the abused child and his family.
2. Nurse–parent relationship—develop therapeutic, trusting relationships that will help parents develop to their full potential.
3. Support community assistance programs to help parents overcome isolation—crisis nurseries, parent aids, Parents Anonymous, foster care facilities, and day-care centers.
4. Support public reeducation to enhance the parenting capabilities of every man and woman: Education for Parenting, Home Start, and adolescent parenthood programs.

K. Be aware that the goal of treatment of the parents is to ensure the physical and emotional safety of the child.

1. It is estimated that 90% of abusing parents can be rehabilitated.
2. The ideal approach is to return the child to his biological parents.
3. Treatment is offered to help the parents to do the following:
   a. Understand and redirect their anger.
   b. Develop an adequate parent–child relationship.
   c. See their child as an individual with his own needs and differences.
   d. Enjoy their child.
   e. Develop realistic expectations of their child.
   f. Decrease their use of criticism.
   g. Increase their own sense of self-esteem and confidence.
   h. Establish supportive relationships with others.
   i. Improve economic situation (if appropriate).
   j. Show progress toward physical, emotional, and intellectual development.
4. Inform the parents of organizations designed to help them:
   a. Parents Anonymous, 2230 Hawthorne Blvd, Suite 208, Torrance, CA 90505. This is a private organization of self-help groups for parents who have abused or fear they might have abused their children. *Frontiers* is their publication.
   b. C. Henry Kempe National Center for the Prevention and Treatment of Child Abuse and Neglect, 1205 Oneida Street, Denver, CO 80220

L. Be aware of the child who has the potential for being abused and provide anticipatory guidance for prevention of abuse.

1. The premature infant, the hyperactive child, the chronically ill child, the retarded child, the child who requires a great deal of care and confines the mother to the home, the child involved in a disturbed mother–infant bond all have the potential for being abused.
2. Encourage early participation of mother (parents) in the care of the child during hospitalization.
3. Prepare the mother for the fact that the child does require a great deal of care, but encourage her to find outlets for her frustrations.
4. Provide her with the name and telephone number of someone at the hospital to whom she can look for help (e.g., social worker).
5. Initiate a community nursing referral.

Health Education

A. Teach the parents about normal growth and development.

(See the section on growth and development, p. 1074.)
1. Give specific information about and examples of the types of behavior to expect at the various stages of development. Point out in a nonthreatening way normal behavior exhibited by their child.
2. Give specific information on dealing with this behavior.
3. Serve as a role model and teacher; minimize intensity when the parents become threatened.

B. Teach the parents how to use discipline without resorting to physical force.

1. Discipline must be consistent. Offer suggestions for alternative ways of handling undesirable behavior.
2. Rewards may be used for acceptable behavior (e.g., a trip to the zoo, staying up later than usual for a special television show, a special treat).
3. Rewards are withheld for unacceptable behavior.

C. Support the parent and the child when a decision is made to have the child removed from the home.

1. The decision is made for the safety and protection of the child.
2. The parents are afforded the opportunity to have counseling to help them learn to deal with their problem.
3. The child must be prepared for his removal from the home and placement plans. He must be allowed time to work through his feelings.

D. Support the parents and child in preparation for discharge to home.

1. Both parents and child (if age is appropriate) need to know and understand any specific instructions relative to injury and follow-up care.
2. The parents need to be made aware of the most common posthospitalization behavior children may have (see p. 1113).
3. Make known to parents your continued concern and your availability as a source of help. Stress the need for follow-up care. Help them to use community resources available (i.e., homemaker, community health nurse, therapy for parents, etc.).

Agencies and organizations dealing with abuse:
International Institute of Children's Nature and Their Rights, 1615 Myrtle Street, NW, Washington, DC 20012; (202) 726-3341; publishes journal
National Center on Child Abuse and Neglect, 400 Sixth Street, SW, Washington, DC 20013
National Committee for Prevention of Child Abuse,

322 S Michigan Avenue, Suite 1250, Chicago, IL 60604; (312) 565-1100; publishes *Caring* (quarterly) and monographs

Society's League Against Molestation (SLAM), 524 S First Avenue, Arcadia, CA 91106; publishes *Guardian* (bimonthly) and a brochure; works to prevent sex abuse and molestation and to educate public through media

The Dying Child

Nursing Interventions

A. Analyze one's own feelings about death and develop a philosophy that enables the nurse to support the dying child and his family.

1. Become familiar with literature about death and dying and use it as a resource in planning nursing care.
2. Recognize that the goal is to assist the child and family to cope with the experience in such a way that it will promote growth rather than destroy family integrity and emotional well-being.
3. Share personal feelings about death and dying with colleagues. It is not unusual for the nurse to experience personal feelings of anger, frustration, helplessness, and guilt.

B. Recognize the stages of dying as identified by E. Kübler-Ross and utilize this knowledge in planning and implementing care (see Stages of Dying as Identified by Dr. Elizabeth Kübler-Ross, see below).

1. Be aware that dying children, their families, and the staff will all progress through these stages, not necessarily at the same time.
2. Children experience the stages with much variation. They tend to pass more quickly through the stages and may merge some of these stages.

3. The nursing goal is to be aware of one's own stage of reaction and to accept the child and family wherever they are, not to push them through the stages.

C. Understand the meaning of illness and death to the child at the various stages of growth and development and utilize this information in planning and implementing care.

1. See Stages in the Development of a Child's Concept of Death, page 1496.
2. Be aware of other factors that influence a child's personal concept of death. Of particular importance are:
   a. The amount and type of direct exposure a child has had to death.
   b. Cultural values, beliefs, and patterns of bereavement.
   c. Religious beliefs about death and an afterlife.

D. Utilize the knowledge about children's interpretation of the meaning of death at the various stages of growth and development in talking to the child about his illness and in answering questions concerning death.

1. Research indicates that children generally can cope with more than adults will allow, and that children appreciate the opportunity to know and understand what is happening to them.

Stages of Dying as Identified by Dr. Elizabeth Kübler-Ross

Stage	Nursing Implications
I. Denial. Shock. Disbelief.	Accept denial, but function within a reality sphere. Do not tear down the child's (or family's) defenses. Be aware that denial usually breaks down in the early morning when it may be dark and lonely. Be certain that it is the child or family who is using denial, not the staff.
II. Anger. Rage. Hostility.	Accept anger and help the child express it through positive channels. Be aware that anger may be expressed toward other family members, nursing staff, physicians, and other persons involved. Help families to recognize that it is normal for children to express anger for what they are losing.
III. Bargaining (from "No, not me." to "Yes, me, but . . .")	Recognize this period as a time for the child and family to regain strength. Encourage the family to finish any unfinished business with the child. This is the time to do things such as take the promised trip or buy the promised toy.
IV. Depression. (The child and/or family experiences silent grief and mourns past and future losses.)	Recognize this as a normal reaction and expression of strength. Help families to accept the child who does not want to talk and excludes help. This is a usual pattern of behavior. Reassure the child that you can understand his feelings.
V. Acceptance.	Assist families to provide significant loving human contact with their child.

Stages in the Development of a Child's Concept of Death

Age of Child	Stage of Development
Child up to 3 years	At this stage, the child cannot comprehend the relationship of life to death, since he has not developed the concept of infinite time. The child fears separation from protecting and comforting adults. The child perceives death as a reversible fact.
Preschool-age child	At this age the child has no real understanding of the meaning of death; he feels safe and secure with his parents. The child may view death as something that happens to others. The child may interpret his illness as a type of punishment for real or imagined wrongdoing. The child may interpret the separation that occurs with hospitalization as punishment; the painful tests and procedures that he is subjected to support this idea. The child may become depressed because he is not able to correct these wrongdoings and regain the grace of adults. The concept may be connected with magical thoughts and mystery.

School-age child	The child at this age sees death as the cessation of life; he understands that he is alive and that he can become "not alive"; he fears dying.
	The child differentiates death from sleep. Unlike sleep, the horror of death is in pain, progressive mutilation, and mystery.
	The child is vulnerable to guilt feelings related to death because of difficulty in differentiating between death wishes and the actual event.
	The child learns the meaning of death from his own personal experiences.
	    Pets
	    Death of family members, political figures, etc.
	Television and movies have contributed to his concepts of death and understanding of the meaning of illness.
	    Develops more knowledge in the meaning of diagnosis
	    Death may occur violently

Adolescent	The adolescent comprehends the permanence of death much as the adult does, although he may not comprehend death as an event occurring to persons close to himself. He wants to live—he sees death as thwarting pursuit of his goals: independence, success, achievement, physical improvement, and self-image. He fears death before fulfillment. The adolescent may become depressed and resentful because of bodily changes that may occur, dependency, and the loss of his social environment. The adolescent may feel isolated and rejected, since his own adolescent friends may withdraw when faced with his impending death. The adolescent may express rage, bitterness, and resentment. He especially resents the fact that he is fated to die.

2. It is important that the child's questions be answered simply, but truthfully, and that they be based on his particular level of understanding.
3. The following responses have been suggested by Eassom in *The Dying Child* and may be useful as a guide:
   a. Preschool-age child
      (1) When the child at this age is comfortable enough to ask questions about his illness, his questions should be answered. When death is anticipated at some future time and the child asks, "Am I going to die?" a response might be, "We will all die someday, but you are not going to die today or tomorrow."
      (2) When death is imminent and the child asks, "Am I going to die?" the response might be, "Yes, you are going to die, but we will take care of you and stay with you."
      (3) The parents should be allowed to stay with the child to provide him with protection and support.
      (4) When the child asks, "Will it hurt?" the response should be truthful and factual. Death may be described as a form of sleep— a sleep where he will be secure in the love of those around him. (Some children may fear sleep as the result of this type of explanation.)
      (5) Parents can express to the child the fact that they do not want him to go and that they will miss him very much; they feel sad, too, that they are going to be separated.
   b. School-age child
      (1) Responses to the school-age child's questions about death should be answered truthfully. The child looks for support from those he trusts.
      (2) The school-age child should be given a simple explanation of his diagnosis and its meaning; he should also receive an explanation of all treatments and procedures.
      (3) The child should be given no specific time in terms of days or months, since each individual and each illness is different.
      (4) When the school-age child asks, "Am I going

to die?'' and death is inevitable, he should be told the truth. The school-age child does have the emotional ability to look to his parents and those he trusts for comfort and support.

    (5) The school-age child believes in his parents. He should be allowed to die in the comfort and security of his family.

    (6) The school-age child knows death means final separation, and he knows what he will miss. He must be allowed to mourn this loss as he dies. He may be sad and bitter and demonstrate aggressive behavior. He must be allowed the opportunity to verbalize this if he is able to do so.

  c. Adolescent

    (1) The adolescent should be given an explanation of his illness and all necessary treatment procedures.

    (2) The adolescent feels deprived and reasonably resentful regarding his illness because he wants to live and reach fulfillment.

    (3) As death approaches, the adolescent becomes emotionally closer to his family.

    (4) The adolescent should be allowed to maintain his emotional defenses—he may deny absolutely. The adolescent will indicate by his questions what kind of answer he wants.

    (5) If the adolescent states, "I am not going to die," he is pleading for support. Be truthful and state, "No, you are not going to die right now."

    (6) The adolescent may ask, "How long do I have to live?" He is able to face reality more directly and can tolerate more direct answers. No absolute time should be given since that blocks all hope. If an adolescent has what is felt to be a prognosis of approximately 3 months, the response might be, "People with an illness like yours may die in 3 to 6 months, but some may live much longer."

    (7) The bitterness and resentment of the fact that he is fated to die may interrupt necessary procedures and treatments. This behavior must be appropriately handled.

E. Confer with the parents regarding their feelings about discussing the illness with the child and give them information that will be helpful in allowing them to play a more supportive role.

1. Determine what information they have given the child about his illness, and how the child reacted to this information.
2. Determine what specific questions the child has asked about his illness and how the parents have responded.
3. Share with parents your assessment of what the child knows about his illness and what he wants to know.
4. Discuss with the parents how children of various age levels interpret the meaning of death and offer suggestions as to how children's questions regarding death may be answered.
5. Provide the parents with helpful literature about explaining death to children (see references for parents, p. 1505).
6. Assist the parents to explain the child's illness to siblings and to answer their questions. If appropriate, help the parents to identify ways that siblings can share in the child's care.

F. Assist the parents in dealing with their adaptation to their child's illness and anticipated death.

1. Develop a plan of care that includes the following approach:
  a. The primary responsibility for communicating with the parents should be designated to one nurse.
  b. Information regarding the parents' concerns should be communicated to all staff members.
2. Accept parental feelings about the child's anticipated death and help parents deal with these feelings.
  a. It is not unusual for parents to reach the point of wishing the child dead and to experience guilt and self-blame because of this thought.
  b. The parents may withdraw emotional attachments to the child if the process of dying is lengthy. This occurs because the parents complete most of the mourning process before the child reaches biological death. They may relate to the child as if he were already dead.
3. Provide anticipatory guidance regarding the child's actual death and immediate postdeath decisions and responsibilities.
  a. Describe what the death will probably be like and how to know when it is imminent. This is necessary to dispel the horrifying fantasies that many parents have.
  b. Clarify the parents' wishes about being present at the child's death and respect their desires.
  c. If appropriate, allow the parents to discuss their feelings about issues such as autopsy and transplant in order that they may make appropriate decisions.
  d. If necessary, assist the parents to think about funeral arrangements.
4. Be aware of factors that affect the family's capacity to cope with fatal illness, especially social and cultural features of the family system, previous experiences with death, present stage of family development, and resources available to them.

G. Perform the nursing measures that provide the child with both physical and emotional care during illness.

1. Provide physical care that makes the child as comfortable as possible. Deliver care in a calm, assured, gentle manner.
2. Talk to the child and answer his questions truthfully.
3. Provide an atmosphere that offers the child the greatest security (e.g., room with another child, room near the nurses' station, etc.).
4. Provide opportunities for play therapy as the child's condition permits.
5. Plan for consistency of assignment so that the child can experience continuity of contact with a few nurses who inspire confidence and trust.
6. Encourage active involvement in living to the extent that the child is able (e.g., participation in activities of daily living, play, schooling, socialization).
7. Observe children carefully during play for clues to their symbolic language. Watch carefully what they do and listen to what they say. Drawings and self portraits may also help the child to express his feelings.
8. Communicate caring through touch. The child is comforted by being held, especially by his parents.
9. Allow the child opportunity to direct activities and to let his wishes be known.

10. Set realistic limits for the child when necessary, and enforce them consistently.

H. Encourage the parents to spend as much time as possible with the child and participate in the child's care (see the section on Family-Centered Care, p. 1117).

1. Allow the parents to bathe the child and to do procedures within their ability and desire. This allows the parents the feeling that they are doing something for their child.
2. Teach the parents those aspects of the child's care with which they are not familiar.
3. Provide the parents with a place to stay and be comfortable. They should be told where they can find privacy when they want to be alone.
4. Assure the parents that their child will be well cared for in their absence.

I. Utilize appropriate services and resources in planning the care of the child and family.

1. Team members often include:
   a. Physician
   b. Nurse
   c. Child
   d. Family
   e. Social worker
   f. Psychiatrist
   g. Clergyman
   h. Community health nurse
   i. School nurse
   j. Parent groups

2. Teamwork is essential because:
   a. Terminally ill children and their families may require different kinds of assistance at different points in time.
   b. They face many problems that are nonmedical in nature.
   c. The child's need for assistance may be very different from that required by his family.
   d. Team members may support one another.
3. To be effective team members, nurses must:
   a. Communicate, collaborate, and cooperate with other members of the team.
   b. Accept responsibility for their contribution to the plan of care and be accountable for the outcome.

J. Provide emotional support to the parents following the death of the child.

1. Allow families who wish it the opportunity to spend some time alone with the child after death.
2. Provide privacy for parents to express their grief in whatever manner they choose.
3. If appropriate, compliment the parents on the excellent care they gave their child.
4. Be aware that your compassionate silence may be more helpful to families than small talk.
5. Assist families to contact other relatives and funeral home as appropriate.
6. Make certain that families have a safe and comfortable means to get home.
7. Invite the parents to call if they have lingering questions or concerns that they wish to discuss.
8. See the bibliography for additional resources.

Trauma—Prehospital Management of the Injured Child

Trauma is a wound or injury that compromises the functioning of major organ systems (i.e., burns, drowning, ingestion, blunt or penetrating injury).

Etiology

External forces—mechanical, chemical, electrical, or radiation in nature.

Incidence

See Table 46-3.

Immediate Intervention—Primary Survey

Perform the primary survey (initial assessment) in a systematic fashion to recognize and manage life-threatening injuries to the respiratory (airway and ventilation), circulatory (shock), and neurologic systems. Intervention also includes child and family crisis management.

As first responder, the nurse:
1. Notifies the emergency medical services via bystander, or self if feasible.
2. Does *not* move the child until the airway is patent and cervical spine immobilization is secured.
3. Airway management with cervical spine immobilization
   a. Clear the airway of any debris: blood, vomitus, or broken teeth.
   b. Relieve potential obstruction from the tongue falling into the posterior pharynx with a chin lift

or jaw thrust maneuver. The chin lift maneuver is performed by placing the thumb into the mouth and the index finger on the chin and pulling outward to pull the tongue out of the posterior pharynx.

The jaw thrust maneuver is performed by placing the finger at the temporal–mandibular joint and

Table 46-3 Leading Causes of Death in Children Age 1–14 Years*

	Age 1–4		Age 1–14	
	Deaths	Death Rate†	Deaths	Death Rate†
All causes	8,108	64.2	11,146	31.5
Accidents	3,349	26.5	5,689	16.1
Motor-vehicle	1,239	9.8	2,952	8.3
Fires, burns	693	5.5	552	1.6
Drowning	690	5.5	908	2.6
Ingestion food/object	155	1.2		
Firearms			315	0.9
Falls	104	0.8	121	0.3
Congenital anomalies	1,021	8.1	578	1.6
Cancer	578	4.6	1,552	4.4

* Accident Facts, National Safety Council, Chicago, IL, 1983
† Deaths per 100,000 population in each age group.

sliding the mandible forward to pull the tongue out of the posterior pharynx (Fig. 46-1*A*).

  c. In traumatic injury, always anticipate the possibility of a fractured cervical vertebra.

  d. Manually keep the head in midline by providing inline traction on the cervical spine. Inline traction is performed by placing the two middle fingers on the mastoid process of the occipital skull and pulling toward the rescuer who is at the child's head (Fig. 46-1*B*).

4. Respiratory
  a. Look, listen, and feel for spontaneous breathing if the airway is open.
  b. If the child is not breathing, initiate cardiopulmonary resuscitation (see CPR, p. 1195).
  c. If a chest wound is present, apply an airtight dressing to avoid spontaneous pneumothorax.

5. Circulation
  a. Apply direct pressure to the area of external bleeding.
  b. Apply direct pressure to the supplying artery to control the hemorrhage. (Children can bleed significantly from small wounds or lacerations.)
  c. Elevate the injured extremity.
  d. Place the child in Trendelenburg position if no head injury or respiratory difficulty is present.
  e. Apply a tourniquet as a last resort.

6. Neurologic
  a. Level of consciousness
    (1) Alert
    (2) Verbal response
    (3) Pain response
    (4) Unresponsive—comatose
  b. Pupil size
  c. Pupil reaction to light
  d. Symmetry of pupils
  e. Thermoregulation
    (1) Children have a larger surface area to body mass ratio. Their body temperature drops

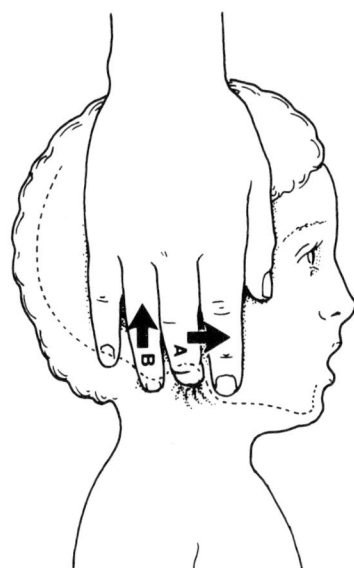

Figure 46-1. (*A*) Jaw thrust maneuver. (*B*) In-line manual traction.

more rapidly than that of adults. If body temperature falls below 36° to 37°C. (98°–98.6°F.) resuscitative efforts are more difficult.
    (2) Prevent heat loss by applying any covering such as a blanket, jacket, or other clothing article.
  f. Head injury—elevate the patient to a semi-recumbent position. *Caution:* Do not bend head at neck; assume the existence of a cervical spine fracture.

Continued Intervention—Secondary Survey

Once life-threatening injuries are recognized and stabilized, the secondary survey is performed.

1. The secondary survey consists of a rapid head-to-toe evaluation for additional injuries.
  a. Head
    (1) Skull depression or deformities
    (2) Scalp, mouth, and facial lacerations
  b. Eyes
    (1) Foreign body or hemorrhage
    (2) Periorbital bruising around the eyes may indicate skull fracture (raccoon's sign)
  c. Ears
    (1) Ecchymotic area over the mastoid process may indicate a skull fracture (Battle's sign)
    (2) Clear fluid discharge may indicate a skull fracture
  d. Nose—clear fluid drainage may indicate a skull fracture
  e. Abdomen
    (1) Distention
    (2) Ecchymosis
    (3) Tenderness
  f. Extremities
    (1) Swelling
    (2) Deformity
    (3) Pain or tenderness
    (4) Loss of motion
    (5) Loss of sensation
    (6) Presence or absence of pulse
    (7) Color: pale or cyanotic

Complications

Permanent neurologic compromise (disability) or death

Clinical Manifestations

1. Airway—obstructed, semi-obstructed, stridor
2. Respirations—tachypnea, dyspnea, cyanosis, nasal flaring, subclavicular, or suprasternal retractions, paradoxical movement of the chest during inspiration and expiration
3. Circulation
  a. Signs and symptoms of shock occur after 20%–25% of the total blood volume has been depleted.
  b. Observe for tachycardia, pallor, cold, clammy skin surface, altered sensorium, delayed capillary refill.
    (1) Capillary refill is determined by depressing the thumb nailbed and observing the return blood flow.
    (2) Normal capillary refill returns within 2 seconds or the amount of time it takes to mentally say, "capillary refill." Anything greater than 2 seconds indicates that the child is in shock.

4. Neurologic
   a. Eye opening
      (1) Spontaneous
      (2) To voice
      (3) To pain
      (4) None
   b. Verbal response
      (1) Oriented
      (2) Confused
      (3) Inappropriate words
      (4) Incomprehensible words
      (5) None
   c. Motor response
      (1) Obeys commands
      (2) Localizes pain
      (3) Withdraw (pain)
      (4) Flexion (pain)
      (5) Extension (pain)
      (6) None
   d. Check pupil size for equality and observe for any deviation of the eye(s) from normal center.
5. Extremity injury—immobilize injured or fractured extremity with minimal movement to prevent additional damage.
6. Child's and family's reactions—range from hysteria, indifference, shock, anger, controlled, or cooperative.
7. Child and family crisis intervention
   a. Remain calm.
   b. Use a reassuring voice.
   c. Empathize with the child's pain and fear.
   d. Solicit the parents to aid and comfort the child if they are able.
   e. Reassure the child and family that everything possible is being done before and during transport to an emergency facility.
8. Transfer the child to the emergency medical services for rapid transport to a hospital emergency facility.

Diagnostic Evaluation

The nurse will not have access to diagnostic tools at the scene of the injury. She should use observational skills and understanding of the altered physiology caused by traumatic injury to help prevent death and disability at the scene by following the primary and secondary survey approach.

Nursing Interventions

A. Prevent death.

Recognize life-threatening injuries and provide initial resuscitative efforts by:

1. Providing a patent airway
2. Covering open chest wounds
3. Control of obvious bleeding

B. Ensure that the child avoids permanent disability.

1. Maintain adequate airway and ventilation for oxygen perfusion to the brain.
2. Prevent paralysis by providing cervical spine immobilization.
3. Keep the child calm through reassurance in an effort to avoid unnecessary movement.
4. Keep movement of possible extremity fractures to a minimum to avoid blood vessel, nerve, and tissue damage.

C. Assist the child to achieve psychological homeostasis with minimal emotional disruption.

1. Encourage the child to ventilate his feelings to avoid short- and long-term psychological maladjustment to the traumatic incident.
2. Permit the child to cry and verbalize discomfort at the scene.
3. Keep the parents at the child's side to give support at the scene of injury.

D. Ensure that the child is transported rapidly to a hospital emergency facility.

1. Notify the emergency medical services by telephoning 911 or its equivalent.
2. Enlist the family and bystanders to render assistance under the direction of the nurse while the child awaits emergency transport.

Health Education

1. Know the principles of safety for each developmental age-group of children.
2. Be aware of potentially dangerous toys and products for children.
3. Keep matches, chemicals, medication, etc. out of the reach of children.
4. Teach children to respect traffic laws and look each way before crossing the street.
5. Be aware of infant and child automobile restraint laws.
6. Encourage children to play in designated areas.
7. Teach bicycle safety.
8. Encourage the use of protective sporting gear.
9. Teach the appropriate telephone number to access the emergency medical services of the community.

Bibliography

Books

Mental Retardation and Down's Syndrome

Accardo P and Capute A. The Pediatrician and the Developmentally Delayed Child. Baltimore, University Park Press, 1979

Berg J (ed). Perspectives and Progress in Mental Retardation. Report of Sixth Congress of the International Association for the Scientific Study of Mental Deficiency, Vol. 1—Social, Psychological and Educational Aspects; Vol. 2—Biomedical Aspects. Baltimore, University Park Press, 1984

Camino FJ and Reeve RE. General issues in working with parents of handicapped children. In Abidin RR (ed). Parent Education and Intervention Handbook. Springfield, IL, Charles C Thomas, 1980, pp. 82–106

Edgerton R. Mental Retardation. Cambridge, MA, Harvard University Press, 1979

Gollin E. Malformations of Development: Biological and Psychological Sources and Consequences. New York, Academic Press, 1984

Grossman H (ed). Classification in Mental Retardation. Washington DC, American Association on Mental Deficiency, 1983

Hutt M and Gibby R. The Mentally Retarded Child: Development, Training and Education, 4th ed. Boston, Allyn and Bacon, 1979

Jakab J (ed). Mental Retardation. New York, Karger, 1982

Kearsley R and Sigel I. Infants at Risk: Assessment of Cognitive Functioning. New York, Lawrence Erlbaum Associates, 1979

Matson J and Andrasik F. Treatment Issues and Innovations in Mental Retardation. New York, Plenum Press, 1983

Matson J and Breuning S. Assessing the Mentally Retarded. New York, Grune & Stratton, 1983

Matson J and McCartney J (ed). Handbook of Behavior Modification with the Mentally Retarded. New York, Plenum Press, 1981

Plog S and Santamour M (ed). The Year 2000 and Mental Retardation. New York, Plenum Press, 1980

*Pueschel SM (ed). Down Syndrome: Growing and Learning. Kansas City, Sheed Andrews & McMeel, 1978

Pueschel SM. The Young Child with Down Syndrome. New York, Human Science Press, 1983

Pueschel SM and Rynders JE. Down Syndrome: Advances in Biomedical and the Behavioral Sciences. Cambridge, Mass, The Ware Press, 1982

*Ross BM. Our Special Child. New York, Walker & Co, 1981

Wacht MA. The Mentally Disabled Child. In Johnson SH (ed). High-Risk Parenting. Philadelphia, JB Lippincott, 1979, pp. 132–143

Warkany J, Lemire M and Cohen M. Mental Retardation and Congenital Malformations of the Central Nervous System. Chicago, Year Book Medical Publishers, 1981

Minimal Brain Dysfunction

Guralnick M and Richardson H (eds). Pediatric Education and the Needs of Exceptional Children. Baltimore, University Park Press, 1980

Levine M et al. A Pediatric Approach to Learning Disabilities. New York, John Wiley & Sons, 1980

Rie HE and Rie ED (eds). Handbook of Minimal Brain Dysfunction. New York, John Wiley & Sons, 1980

Small L. The Minimal Brain Dysfunctions: Diagnosis and Treatment. New York, Free Press, 1982

Genetic Counseling

Behrman RE and Vaughan VC. Nelson Textbook of Pediatrics. Philadelphia, WB Saunders, 1983

Finley SC, Finley WH and Flowers CE (ed). Birth Defects: Clinical and Ethical Consideration. New York, Alan R Liss, 1983, March of Dimes Birth Defects Foundation. Birth Defects: Original Article Series Vol. 19, No. 5, 1983

Fuhrmann W and Vogel F. Genetic Counseling, 3rd ed. New York, Springer-Verlag, 1983

Muir BL. Essentials of Genetics for Nurses. New York, John Wiley & Sons, 1983

Leavitt MB. Families at Risk: Primary

Prevention in Nursing Practice. Boston, Little, Brown & Co, 1982

Levine MD et al. Developmental–Behavioral Pediatrics. Philadelphia, WB Saunders, 1983

Tschudin V. Counselling Skills for Nurses. London, Bailliere Tindall, 1982

Willey AM et al. Clinical Genetics: Problems in Diagnosis and Counseling. New York, Academic Press, 1982

Poisoning

Goldfrank L. Toxicologic Emergencies: A Comprehensive Handbook in Problem Solving, 2nd ed. New York, Appleton Century Crofts, 1982

Hanenson I. Quick Reference to Clinical Toxicology. Philadelphia, JB Lippincott, 1980

Matthew H and Lawson A. Treatment of Common Acute Poisonings. 4th ed. New York, Churchill Livingstone, 1979

Pascoe DJ and Grossman M. Quick Reference to Pediatric Emergencies, 3rd ed. Philadelphia, JB Lippincott, 1984

Reece RM and Chamberlain JW. Manual of Emergency Pediatrics, 3rd ed. Philadelphia, WB Saunders, 1984

Abuse

Garbarino J and Garbarino AC. Emotional Maltreatment of Children. Chicago, Nat'l Comm for Prevention of Child Abuse, 1982

Kempe CH and Helfer RE. The Battered Child, 3rd ed. Chicago, University of Chicago Press, 1982

Michalek JB. Nursing and child protection. In Newberger EH (ed). Child Abuse. Boston, Little, Brown & Co, 1982, pp. 217–234

Newberger EH (ed). Child Abuse. Boston, Little, Brown & Co, 1982

Vines DW. Sexual abuse in children. In Beal JA (ed). Issues and Advanced Practice in Pediatric Nursing. Reston, VA, Reston Publishing Co, 1983, pp. 49–68

The Dying Child

Arnold J and Gemma P. A Child Dies: A Portrait of Family Grief. Rockville, Aspen Systems Corp, 1983

Buckingham R. A Special Kind of Love, Care of the Dying Child. New York, Continuum Publishing Co, 1983

Easson W. The Dying Child: The Management of the Child or Adolescent Who is Dying. Springfield, IL, Charles C Thomas, 1981

Franz T and Hansen J. Death and Grief in the Family. Rockville, MD, Aspen Systems Corp, 1984

Garfield C (ed). Stress and Survival: The Emotional Realities of Life-Threatening Illness. St Louis, CV Mosby, 1979

Grollman E. Explaining Death to Children. Boston, Beacon Press, 1967

Kastenbaum RJ. Death, Society and Human Experience, 2nd ed. St Louis, CV Mosby, 1981

Kübler-Ross E. Living with Death and Dying. New York, Macmillan, 1981

Kübler-Ross E. On Children and Death. New York, Macmillan, 1983

Kübler-Ross E. On Death and Dying. New York, Macmillan, 1970

Martinson I. Home Care for the Dying Child: Professional and Family Perspectives. New York, Appleton-Century-Crofts, 1976

Osterweis M, Solomon F and Green M (eds). Bereavement: Reactions, Consequences, and Care. Washington, DC, National Academy Press, 1984

Sahler OJ. The Child and Death. St Louis, CV Mosby, 1978

Schneider J. Stress, Loss, and Grief. Baltimore, University Park Press, 1984

Weinstein S. (ed). Mental Health Issues in Grief Counseling: Summary of Proceedings, National Conference on Mental Health Issues Related to Sudden Infant Death Syndrome. Rockville, MD, US Dept of HEW, Public Health Service, 1979

Trauma—The Prehospital Management of the Injured Child

American Academy of Orthopaedic Surgeons. Emergency Care and Transportation of the Sick and Injured. Syracuse, American Academy of Orthopaedic Surgeons, 1981

Caroline NL. Emergency Medical Treatment. A Textbook for EMT-A's and EMT Intermediates. Boston, Little, Brown, & Co, 1982

Committee on Trauma, American College of Surgeons. Advanced Trauma Life Support Course, Instructor Manual. Chicago, American College of Surgeons, 1981

Eichelberger MR. Pediatric trauma. In Edlich RF and Spyker DA (eds). Current Emergency Therapy '84. Norwalk, CT, Appleton-Century-Crofts, 1984, pp. 307–318

Johnson TR, More WM and Jefferies JE. Children are Different: Development Physiology. Columbus, OH, Ross Laboratories, 1978

Ravenscroft K. Psychological considerations for the child with acute trauma. In Randolph J et al (eds), The Injured Child: Surgical Management. Chicago, Year Book Medical Publishers, 1979, pp. 31–42

Reece RM. Manual of Emergency Pediatrics. Philadelphia, WB Saunders, 1984

Smith RM. Anesthesia for Infants and Children. St Louis, CV Mosby, 1980

Articles

Mental Retardation and Down's Syndrome

Bromley D. What parents want . . . holiday relief for parents with a mentally handicapped child. Health Soc Serv J 1981 Feb; 90(2):191–193

Browder JA. The pediatrician's orientation to infant stimulation programs. Pediatrics 1981 Jan; 67(1): 42–44

Buzinski P. Groups for brothers and sisters of developmentally disabled children: One component of a family-centered approach. Issues Compr

Pediatr Nurs 1980 Sep/Dec; 4(5-6): 45-50

Caparulo F et al. Sexual health needs of the mentally retarded adolescent female. Issues Health Care Women 1981 Jan/Feb; 3(1):35-46

Crowe TK. Father involvement in care, intervention programs. Phys Occup Ther Pediatr 1981 Spring; 1(3):35-46

Deaton J. Down's Syndrome: Reappraising treatment of children and adults. Consultant 1981 Apr; 21(4):249-251+

DeLa Cruz FF and Muller JZ. Facts about Down syndrome. Child Today 1983 Nov/Dec; 12(6):2-7

Denhoff E. Current status of infant stimulation or enrichment programs for children with developmental disabilities. Pediatrics 1981 Jan; 67(1): 33-36

Erickson MP. Responding to the needs of sick children with mental retardation. Child Today 1980 Jan/Feb; 9(1):24-25

Ferry PC. On growing new neurons: Are early intervention programs effective? Pediatrics 1981 Jan; 67(1):38-41

*Gerver JM. A grandparent's view. Child Today 1983 Nov/Dec; 12(6):12-13

Harris SR. Relationship of mental and motor development in Down syndrome infants. Phys Occup Ther Pediatr 1981 Spring; 1(3):13-18

Harris SR. Transdisciplinary therapy model for the infant with Down's syndrome. Phys Ther 1980 Apr; 60(4): 420-423

Huether CA. Projection of Down's syndrome births in the United States 1979-2000, and the potential effects on prenatal diagnosis. Am J Pub Health 1983 Oct; 73(10):1186-1189

Hunt PJ. Oral motor dysfunction in Down's syndrome: Contributing factors and interventions. Phys Occup Ther Pediatr 1981 Summer; 1(4):69-78

*Kihlstnom A. A very special boy. Child Today 1983 Nov/Dec; 12(6):8-11

Lydic JS. Motor development in children with Down syndrome. Phys Occup Ther Pediatr 1982 Winter; 2(4):53-74

Maxwell B. The special olympics. Nurse Pract 1983 Nov/Dec; 8(10):65, 68

Mivla ES. A "rightful" life: A nurse's reflections. Perinat Press 1983; 7(8): 117-118

Montgomery P. Assessment and treatment of the child with mental retardation: Guidelines for a public school therapist. Phys Ther 1981 Sep; 61(9):1265-1272

Plawecki JA and Plawecki HM. An unpopular patient—The mentally retarded child. Child Health Care 1981 Spring; 9(4):114-117

Ramey C et al. Children at risk: Identification and intervention . . . The mildly retarded are associated more with socio-cultural factors. Child Today 1980 Nov/Dec; 9(6):12-16

Roberts MJ and Canfield M. Behavior

modification with a mentally retarded child. Am J Nurs 1980 Apr; 80(4):679

Schild S. Beyond diagnosis: Issues in recurrent counseling of parents of the mentally retarded. Soc Work Health Care 1982 Fall; 8(1):81-93

Smigielski P et al. Teaching sex education to a multiply handicapped adolescents. J Sch Health 1981 Apr; 51(4):238-241

Sparling J. Use of taxonomies to sequence clinical objectives . . . feeding intervention with the delayed child. AJOT 1982 Jun; 36(6):388-395

Stephens C. The fetal alcohol syndrome: Cause for concern. MCN 1981 Jul/Aug; 6(4):251-256

Temple MJ. Chromosomal syndrome. Hosp Pract 1983 Feb; 18(2):124A+

Wasch S. Hospitalization of profoundly and severely mentally retarded children. Child Health Care 1981 Spring; 9(4):126-131

Williams JK. Reproductive decisions: Adolescents with Down's syndrome. Pediatr Nurs 1983 Jan/Feb; 9(1):43-44+

Wilson B. Toilet training the mentally handicapped child. Dev Med Child Neurol 1980 Apr; 22(2):225-229

Minimal Brain Dysfunction

Bassett L, Gudas L and McAnulty E. The learning disabled child: Recognition, evaluation and management. Pediatr Nurs 1982 Sep/Oct; 8(5):325-330

Brown R and Wynne M. Sustained attention in boys with attention deficit disorder and the effect of methylphenidate. Pediatr Nurs 1984 Jan/Feb; 10(1):35-41

Carey WB and McDevitt S. Minimal brain dysfunction and hyperkinesis. Am J Dis Child 1980 Oct; 134(10): 926-927

Deuel RK. Minimal brain dysfunction, hyperkinesis, learning disabilities, attention deficit disorder. J Pediatr 1981 Jun; 98(6):912-915

Erb L and Anderson BD. Hyperactivity: A possible consequence of maternal alcohol consumption. Pediatr Nurs 1981 Jul/Aug; 7(4):30-33

Forness S et al. Identifying children with school learning and behavior problems served by interdisciplinary clinics and hospitals. Child Psychiatry Hum Dev 1980 Winter; 11(2):67-78

Hansen C and Cohen D. Multimodality approaches in the treatment of attention deficit disorders. Pediatr Clin North Am 1984 Apr; 31(2):499-514

Huber CJ et al. Symposium on central nervous system disorders in children. Minimal brain dysfunction syndrome. Nurs Clin N Am 1980 Mar; 15(1):51-69

Levine MD and Obeikaid F. Hyperactivity. Am J Dis Child 1980 Apr; 134(4):409-414

Palfrey J et al. An analysis of observed attention and activity patterns in preschool children. J Pediatr 1981 Jun; 98(6):1006-1011

Robinson LA. Food allergies, food additives and the Feingold diet.

Pediatr Nurs 1980 Nov/Dec; 6(6):38-39

Ryan B. We played a game with Jill . . . and Jill won . . . a hyperactive teenager with minimal brain damage. Nursing '80 1980 Dec; 10(12):44-46

Shaywitz S and Shaywitz B. Diagnosis and management of attention deficit disorders. Pediatr Clin North Am 1984 Apr; 31(2):429-458

Sleator EK et al. Can the physician diagnose hyperactivity in the office? Pediatrics 1981 Jan 67(1):13-17

Whalen C and Henker B. Hyperactivity and the attention deficit disorders: Expanding frontiers. Pediatr Clin North Am 1984 Apr; 31(2):397-428

White J. Special nursing needs of hospitalized children with learning disabilities. MCN 1983 May/Jun; 8(3): 209-212

Genetic Counseling

Alper JC. Genetic counseling: Extending your help beyond treatment. Consultant 1982 May; 22(5):159-160+

Anderson CE. Diabetes mellitus: Explaining the genetic risk for siblings and offspring. Consultant 1982 Oct; 22(10):285-287, 290-292+

Black RB. Risk taking behavior: Decision making in the face of genetic uncertainty. Soc Work Health Care 1982 Fall; 7(1):11-25

Childs B. Genetic decision making and pastoral care: The dimensions of the problem. Hosp Pract 1982 Dec; 17(12):96E+

Ente G et al. Ultrasound as a tool for prenatal diagnosis of chondrodystrophia calcificans congenita. Perinatol/Neonatol 1981 Sep/Oct; 5(5):27-29

Golbus MS. The current scope of antenatal diagnosis. Hosp Pract 1982 Apr; 17(4):179-186.

Jones OW. Genetic counseling: General concepts and principles. Perinatol/Neonatol 1981 May/Jun; 5(3):32-33

LaRue L. Fetal genes: Easy access, early treatment. Lab World 1981 Jan; 32(1): 15-18

Nevin NC. Genetic disorders. Clin Obstet Gynecol 1982 Apr; 9(1):3-28

Rozovsky LE and Rozovsky FA. Genetic screening: Public health and the law. Can J Pub Health 1981 Jan/Feb; 72(1):15-16

Temple MJ. Genetic decision making and pastoral care: Chromosomal syndromes. Hosp Pract 1983 Feb; 18(2):124A+

Tishler CL. The psychological aspect of genetic counseling. Am J Nurs 1981 Apr; 81(4):732-734

Weitz R. The public, the primary physician and genetic counselling. Patient Couns Health Educ 1981 First Quarter; 3(1):13-16

Poisoning

Benirschke K. Time bomb of lye ingestion. Am J Dis Child 1981 Jan; 135(1):17-18

Chisolm J. Poisoning from heavy metals (mercury, lead, and cadmium). Pediatr Ann 1980 Dec; 9(12):28-42

---

* Suggested parent reading.

Ford P. Management of pediatric poisoning, update on first aid management. Pediatr Nurs 1980 Sep/Oct; 6(5):35–36

Foster D. In case of emergency: ipecac syrup. MCN 1982 Jul/Aug; 7(4):277

Gillies C. Management of pediatric poisoning, role of the nurse practitioner. Pediatr Nurs 1980 Sep/Oct; 6(5):33–35

Greensher J and Mofenson H. Emergency room care of the poisoned child. Issues Compr Pediatr Nurs 1980 Jun; 4(3):1–21

Keim K. Preventing and treating plant poisonings in young children. MCN 1983 Jul/Aug; 8(4):287–289

Krenzelok E and Garber R. Teaching poison prevention to preschool children, their parents, and professional educators through child care centers. Am J Pub Health 1981 Jul; 71(7):750–752

Lovejoy F. Management of pediatric poisoning. Part I. Pediatr Nurs 1980 Sep/Oct; 6(5):37–39

Marcum L et al. Prehospital management of the poisoned patient. Crit Care Q 1982 Mar; 4(4):25–31

Moutinho M et al. Acute mercury vapor poisoning. Am J Dis Child 1981 Jan; 135(1):42–44

Oderda G et al. General management of the poisoned patient. Crit Care Q 1982 Mar; 4(4):1–16

Saracino M, Flowers J and Lovejoy F. The epidemiology of poisoning from drug products. Am J Dis Child 1980 Aug; 134(8):763–765

Syrup of ipecac still number one choice. Am Pharm 1981 Feb; NS21(2):46

Temple A. Management of pediatric poisoning, Part II. Pediatr Nurs 1980 Sep/Oct; 6(5):40–43

Wasserman G. Hydrocarbon poisoning. Crit Care Q 1982 Mar; 4(4):33–41

Poisoning—Additional Resources

American Association of Poison Control Centers
% Dr. Gary Oderda
Maryland Poison Center
20 N Pine
Baltimore, MD 21201

Food and Drug Administration
Department of Health and Human Services
5401 Westbard Avenue
Bethesda, MD 20016

National Planning Council for National Poison Prevention Week
PO Box 1543
Washington, DC 20013

National Safety Council
444 N Michigan Avenue
Chicago, IL 60611

US Consumer Product Safety Commission
Washington, DC 20207

Lead Poisoning

Charney E, Sayre J and Coulter M. Increased lead absorption in inner city children: Where does the lead come from? Pediatrics 1980 Feb; 65(2):226–231

Chisholm J. Poisoning from heavy metals (mercury, lead, and cadmium). Pediatr Ann 1980 Dec; 9(12):28–42

Cohen A, Trotzky M and Pincus D. Reassessment of the microcytic anemia of lead poisoning. Pediatrics 1981 Jun; 67(6):904–906

Dolcourt J et al. Hazard of lead exposure in the home from recycled automobile storage batteries. Pediatrics 1981 Aug; 68(2):225–230

Drummond A. Lead poisoning in children. J Sch Health 1981 Jan; 51(1):43–47

Ehrnman K. Community involvement in the prevention of childhood lead poisoning. Health Educ 1982 Jul/Aug; 13(4):38–41

Ernhart C et al. Subclinical levels of lead and developmental deficit: A multivariate follow-up reassessment. Pediatrics 1981 Jun; 67(6):911–919

Langner B, Modrcin-McCarthy M. Lead poisoning: An ongoing pediatric nursing concern. Issues Compr Pediatr Nurs 1980 Jun; 4(3):23–36

Lipnickey S. Lead poisoning: A need for education. Health Educ 1981 Mar/Apr; 12(2):7–10

Miller S. Nursing care of the lead-burdened child: A problem oriented approach. Pediatr Nurs 1981 Sep/Oct; 7(5):47–52

Lead Poisoning—Additional Resource

National Clearinghouse for Education in Maternal and Child Health
3520 Prospect Street, NW
Washington, DC 20007

Abuse

Adler R and Kane-Nussen B. Erythema multiforme: Confusion with child battering syndrome. Pediatrics 1983 Nov; 72(5):718–720

Besharov DJ. The third international congress on child abuse and neglect: Conference highlights. Child Today 1981 Sep/Oct; 10(5):12–15+

Braen GR. Rape and sexual assault of the adolescent and adult female. Top Emerg Med 1982 Jun; 3(4):55–62

Bross DC. Professional and agency liability for negligence in child protection. Law, Medicine, Health Care 1983 Apr; 11(2):71–75

Bruckman P and Ferguson L. Two steps forward and one back. Can Nurs 1981 May; 77(5):29–34

Burgess AW, McCausland MP and Wolbert WA. Children's drawings as indicators of sexual trauma. Perspect Psych Care 1981 Mar/Apr; 19(2):50–58

Christensen ML, Schommer BL and Velasquez J. Child Abuse. Part 1: An interdisciplinary approach to preventing child abuse. MCN 1984 Mar/Apr; 9(2):108–112; Part 2: Intensive services help prevent child abuse. MCN 1984 Mar/Apr; 9(2):113–117

Critchley DL. Therapeutic group work with abused pre-school children. Perspect Psych Care 1982 Jun; 20(2):79–85

Dietrich KN, Starr RH and Weisfeld GE. Infant maltreatment: Caretaker-infant interaction and developmental consequences at different levels of parenting failure. Pediatrics 1983 Oct; 72(4):532–540

Engel NS and Law AD. Nursing care for adolescent urban nomad. MCN 1983 Jan/Feb; 8(1):74–77

Erlen JA. Reporting suspected child abuse: Is the decision clear-cut? Point View 1983 Jul 1; 20(3):10–11

Feldman KW and Brewer DK. Child abuse, cardiopulmonary resuscitation, and rib fractures. Pediatrics 1984 Mar; 73(3):339–342

Grindley JF. Child abuse: The nurse and prevention. Nurs Clin North Am 1981 Mar; 16(1):167–177

Harrison TG and Gatch G. When the abused child comes to surgery. AORN J 1981 Oct; 34(4):643–649

Hayes P. The long-term treatment of victims of child abuse. Nurs Clin North Am 1981 Mar; 16(1):139–147

Heindl MC. Dealing with feelings: Who is the victim? Nurs Clin North Am 1981 Mar; 16(1):117–125

Helberg JL. Documentation in child abuse. Am J Nurs 1983 Feb; 83(2):236–239

Hodge D et al. The bacteriologically battered baby: Another case of Munchausen by proxy. Ann Emerg Med 1982 Apr; 11(4):205–207

Jason J et al. Epidemiologic differences between sexual and physical child abuse. JAMA 1982 Jun; 247(24):3344–3348

Jaudes PK. Comparison of radiography and radionuclide bone scanning in the detection of child abuse. Pediatrics 1984 Feb; 73(2):166–168

Josten L. Prenatal assessment guide for illuminating possible problems with parenting. MCN 1981 Mar/Apr; 6(2):113–117

Khan M and Sexton M. Sexual abuse of young children. Clin Pediatr 1983 May; 22(5):369–372

Kreitzer M. Legal aspects of child abuse: Guidelines for the nurse. Nurs Clin North Am 1981 Mar; 16(1):149–160

Lieske AM. Incest: An overview. Perspect Psych Care 1981 Mar/Apr; 19(2):59–63

Ludwig S. A multidisciplinary approach to child abuse. Nurs Clin North Am 1981 Mar; 16(1):161–165

Marder JH. Child abuse: Fallout in adulthood. AORN J 1981 Oct; 34(4):651–658+

McCown DE. Father/daughter incest: A family problem. Pediatr Nurs 1981 Jul/Aug; 7(4):25–28

McIvor DL and Adolf EE. Working with incest victims: The children. Can J Psychiatr Nurs 1983 Jan/Feb/Mar; 24(1):8–10

McKittrick CA. Child abuse: Recognition and reporting by health professionals. Nurs Clin North Am 1981 Mar; 16(1):103–115

Millor GK. A theoretical framework for nursing research in child abuse and neglect. Nurs Res 1981 Mar/Apr; 30(2):78–83

Murphy JF et al. Objective birth data and the prediction of child abuse. Arch Dis Child 1981 Apr; 56(4):295–297

Nalepka C, O'Toole R and Turbett JP. Nurses' and physicians' recognition and reporting of child abuse. Issue Compr Pediatr Nurs 1981 Jan/Feb; 5(1):33–44

Nix H. Why parents anonymous? J Psychiatr Nurs 1980 Oct; 18(10):23–28

Prince J. Father–daughter incest: An attempt to maintain the family and to meet human needs. Fam Community Health 1981 Aug; 4(2):35–44

Queen PS and Queen JA. In-service workshop on child abuse. J Sch Health 1980 Oct; 50(8):441–446

Raimer BJ, Raimer SS and Hebeler JR. Cutaneous signs of abuse. Am Acad Dermatol 1981 Aug; 5(2):203–212

Riggs RS. Incest: The school's role. J Sch Health 1982 Aug; 52(6):365–370

Rimsza ME and Niggemann EH. Medical evaluation of sexually abused children: A review of 311 cases. Pediatrics 1982 Jan; 69(1):8–14

Robarge JP, Reynolds ZB and Groothuis JR. Increased child abuse in families with twins. Res Nurs Health 1982 Dec; 5(4):199–203

Rodriguez-Trias H. Abused or neglected children in the emergency department. Top Emerg Med 1983 Jan; 4(4):51–56

Rosenberg N and Bottenfield G. Fractures in infants: A sign of child abuse. Ann Emerg Med 1982 Apr; 11(4):176–180

Rosenberg NM, Meyers S and Shackleton N. Prediction of child abuse in an ambulatory setting. Pediatrics 1982 Dec; 70(6):879–882

Schanberger JE. Inflicted burns in children. Top Emerg Med 1981 Oct; 3(3):85–92

Schultz LG and Jones P. Sexual abuse of children: Issues for social service and health professionals. Child Welfare 1983 Mar/Apr; 62(2):99–107

Shah CP, Holloway CP and Valkil DV. Sexual abuse of children. Ann Emerg Med 1982 Jan; 11(1):18–23

Shaw A. Child abuse. Top Emerg Med 1982 Oct; 4(3):75–79

Smith JB. Care of the hospitalized abused child and family. Nurs Clin North Am 1981 Mar; 16(1):127–137

Stark E. The unspeakable family secret. Psychol Today 1984 May; 18(5):38–39+

Thomas JN and Rogers CM. Sexual abuse of children: Case finding and clinical assessment. Nurs Clin North Am 1981 Mar; 16(1):179–188

Tokarski PA. Management of child abuse. Top Emerg Med 1982 Jan; 3(4):23–30

Tokarski PA. Sexual abuse of the child. Top Emerg Med 1982 Jan; 3(4):15–21

Triplett JL and Arbeson SW. Working with children of alcoholics. Pediatr Nurs 1983 Sep/Oct; 9(5):317–320

Tush BAR. Bruising in healthy 3-year-old children. Matern Child Nurs J 1982 Fall; 11(3):165–179

Weaver BM and McCarthy P. Sexual misuse of children: An emergency department nursing perspective. J Emerg Nurs 1981 Mar/Apr; 7(2):59–62

Weaver BM and Vines DW. Case recognition and assessment of father–daughter incest. Issues Compr Pediatr Nurs 1980 Sep/Dec; 4(5–6):67–76

Wegmann MP and Lancaster J. Child neglect and abuse. Fam Community Health 1981 Aug; 4(2):11–17

Young L. Physical child neglect. Child Today 1981 Sep/Oct; 10(5):12+

Young L. Radiological assessment in suspected child abuse. Top Emerg Med 1982 Jan; 3(4):33–53

Suggested Readings Related to Child Abuse Programs

Birch TL. The children's trust fund. Child Today 1983 Jul/Aug; 12(4):25, 41

Coolsen P. Community involvement in the prevention of child abuse and neglect. Child Today 1980 Sep/Oct; 9(5):5–8

Davidson HA. The guardian ad litem: An important approach to the protection of children. Child Today 1981 Mar/Apr; 10(1):20–23

Depanfilis D. Clients who refer themselves to child protection services. Child Today 1982 Mar/Apr; 11(1):21–25

Foster PH et al. Medical foster care: An alterative nursing practice. MCN 1982 Jul/Aug; 7(4):245–248

Gordon M. Families under stress—Children at Risk. Melbourne, Australia, Melbourne City Council, 1982

Hall M, DeLa Cruz A and Russell P. Working with neglecting families. Child Today 1982 Mar/Apr; 11(1):6–9+

Harling PR and Haines JK. Specialized foster homes for severely maltreated children. Child Today 1980 Jul/Aug; 9(4):16–18

Abuse—Additional Suggested Reading for Staff

deYoung M. The Sexual Victimization of Children. Jefferson, NC, McFarland & Co, 1982

Ebeling NB and Hill DA ed. Child Abuse and Neglect. Boston, John Wright, 1983

Giarretto H. Integrated Treatment of Child Sexual Abuse: A Treatment and Training Manual. Palo Alto, CA, Science and Behavior Books, 1982

Henning JS ed. The Rights of Children: Legal and Psychological Perspectives. Springfield, IL, Charles C Thomas, 1982

Kelly JA. Treating Child-Abusive Families. New York, Plenum Press, 1983

Lynch MA and Roberts J. Consequences of Child Abuse. New York, Academic Press, 1982

O'Doherty N. The Battered Child: Recognition in Primary Care. London, Bailliere Tindall, 1982

Sgroi SM. Handbook of Clinical Intervention in Child Sexual Abuse. Lexington, MA, Lexington Books, DC Heath & Co, 1982

Teenage Prostitution and Child Pornography. Hearings before the Subcommittee on Select Education of the Committee on Education and Labor—House of Representatives, 1982; US Government Printing Office, Washington, DC

What Everyone Should Know about Child Abuse. (DHEW Pub #1645E-6-78) Washington, DC, US Government Printing Office, 1979

Warner CG and Braen GR (eds). Management of the Physically and Emotionally Abused: Emergency Assessment, Intervention and Counseling. Norwalk, CT, Appleton-Century-Crofts, 1982

Publications from the National Committee for Prevention of Child Abuse, 323 S Michigan Avenue, Suite 1250, Chicago, IL 60604

Cohn AH. An Approach to Preventing Child Abuse

Young L. Physical Child Neglect

Elmer E. Growth and Development through Parenting

Green SI. Parent–Child Bonding. The Development of Intimacy

Readings for Staff and Parents:

Herman JL. Father–Daughter Incest. Cambridge, MA, Harvard Press, 1981

Schmitt B et al. Guidelines for the Hospital and Clinic Management of Child Abuse and Neglect. Public #80-30167, USDHEW, Office of Human Develop Services, 1979

Selected Readings on Adolescent Maltreatment:

DDHS, OHDS, ACYF, CB, National Center on Child Abuse and Neglect. Publication No. (OHDS)81-30301, 1981. Single copies free from LSDS, Dept 76-B1, Washington, DC 20402

Sometimes It's OK to Tattle and Some Secrets Should be Told. The Mass Society for the Prevention of Cruelty to Children. Family Information Systems, 1982

A program for elementary school children about sexual abuse. Obtain from Family Information Systems, 69 Clinton Rd, Brookline, MA 02146; (617) 232-3737

What Everyone Should Know About the Sexual Abuse of Children. South Deerfield, MA, Channing L Bete, 1981

The Dying Child

Carnevale F. Child death in the hospital: The survivor's perspective. Focus AACN 1982 Aug/Sep; 9(5):7–9

Chee CM. A child's right to die. MCN 1982 Mar/Apr; 7(2):81+

Cordell AS et al. Family support in infant death. JOGN Nurs 1981 Jul/Aug; 10(4):281–285

Delisle RG et al. Children's perceptions of death: A look at the appropriateness of selected picture books. Death Educ 1981 Spring; 5(1):1–13

Farrell R et al. Living until death: Adolescents with cancer. Health Soc Work 1980 Nov; 5(4):35–38

Greenham D. Children facing death:

Recurring patterns of adaptation. Health Soc Work 1982 May; 7(2):89–94

Goodell A. Responses of nurses to the stresses of caring for pediatric oncology patients. Issues Compr Pediatr Nurs 1980 Jan/Feb; 4(1):1–6

Hutton LM. Annie is alone: The bereaved child. MCN 1981 Jul/Aug; 6(4):274–277

Johnson-Soderburg S. The development of a child's concept of death. Oncol Nurs Forum 1981 Winter; 8(1):23–26

Lang D. Death education: An integral part of school health education. Health Educ 1981 Mar/Apr; 12(2):38–39

Lauer M and Camitta B. Home care for dying children: A nursing model. J Pediatr 1980 Dec; 97(6):1032–1035

Moldow D and Martinson I. From research to reality—Home care for the dying child. MCN 1980 May/Jun; 5(3):159–166

Salladay SA and Royal ME. Children and death: Guidelines for grief work. Child Psychiatry Hum Dev 1981 Summer; 11(4):203–212

Smith M et al. When a child dies at home. Nursing '82 1982 Aug; 12(8):66–67

Williams H, Frederick P and Rothenburg M. The child is dying: Who helps the family? MCN 1981 Jul/Aug; 6(4):261–265

Wong D. Bereavement: The empty-mother syndrome. MCN 1980 Nov/Dec; 5(6):385–389

Wooten B. Death of an infant. MCN 1981 Jul/Aug; 6(4):261–265

Zelauskas B. Siblings: The forgotten grievers. Issues Compr Pediatr Nurs 1981 Jan/Feb; 5(1):45–52

The Dying Child—Additional Resources

Conley B. Children and Death. Elburn, IL, Thum Printing, 1981

DeFrain J, Taylor J and Ernst L. Coping with Sudden Infant Death. Lexington, MA, Lexington Books, 1982

Donnelly K. Recovering from the Loss of a Child. New York, Macmillan, 1982

Hickman M. I Will Not Leave You Desolate: Some Thoughts for Grieving Parents. Nashville, The Upper Room, 1982

Jewett C. Helping Children Cope with Separation and Loss. Harvard, Harvard Common Press, 1982

Johnson W and Olson R. Each Day a Gift. New York, William Morrow and Co, 1982

LaTour K. For Those Who Live: Helping Children Cope with the Death of a Brother or Sister. Kathy LaTour, PO Box 141182, Dallas, TX 75214, 1983

Louern P et al. Our Child Died—An Attempt to Help You Endure By Some Who Have. Lynchburg, VA, Virginia Baptist Hospital, 1981

Schiff H. The Bereaved Parent. New York, Crown Publishers, 1977

The Dying Child—Agencies

Pediatric Projects, Inc
PO Box 2175
Santa Monica, CA 90406

The Compassionate Friends
PO Box 1347
Oak Brook, IL 60521

Children's Hospice International
501 Slaters Lane #207
Alexandria, VA 22314

Appendixes and Index

Appendix I:
Diagnostic Studies and Their Meaning

Table of Abbreviations

kg. = kilogram	L. = liter	mm. = millimeter
gm. = gram	dl. = 100 milliliters	μ. = micron or micrometer
mg. = milligram	ml. = milliliter	mm. Hg = millimeters of mercury
μg. = microgram	cu. mm. = cubic millimeter	mU = milliunit
$\mu\mu$g. = micromicrogram	nM. = nanomolar	μU = microunit
ng. = nanogram		mEq. = milliequivalent
pg. = picogram		IU = International Unit
		mIU = milliInternational Unit

Determination	Normal Range	Clinical Significance
A$_2$ hemoglobin	1.5%–3.5% of total hemoglobin	Increased in certain types of thalassemia
Bleeding time	2–8 min.	Prolonged in thrombocytopenia, defective platelet function, and aspirin therapy
Factor V assay	60%–140%	Pro-accelerin factor
Factor VIII assay (antihemophiliac factor	50%–200%	Deficient in classical hemophilia
Factor IX assay (plasma thrombo)	75%–125%	Deficient in Christmas disease (pseudohemophilia)
Factor X (Stuart factor)	60%–140%	Stuart clotting defect
Fibrinogen	200–400/dl.	Increased in pregnancy, infections accompanied by leukocytosis and nephrosis
		Decreased in severe liver disease, abruptio placentae
Fibrin split products	less than 10 mg./L.	Increased in disseminated intravascular coagulation
Fibrinolysins (whole blood clot lysis time)	No lysis in 24 hr.	Increased activity associated with massive hemorrhage, extensive surgery, and transfusion reactions
Partial thromboplastin time (activated)	20–45 sec.	Prolonged in deficiency of fibrinogen and of factors II, V, VIII, IX, X, XI, and XII and in heparin therapy
Prothrombin consumption	Over 20 sec.	Impaired in deficiency of factors VIII, IX, and X
Prothrombin time	9.5–12 sec.	Prolonged by deficiency of factors I, II, V, VII, and X, fat malabsorption, severe liver disease, and coumarin–anticoagulant therapy
Erythrocyte count	Males: 4,600,00–6,200,000 per cu. mm. Females: 4,200,000–5,400,000 per cu. mm.	Increased in severe diarrhea and dehydration, polycythemia, acute poisoning, and pulmonary fibrosis Decreased in all anemias, in leukemia, and after hemorrhage, when blood volume has been restored
Erythrocyte indices Mean corpuscular volume (MCV)	80–94 (cu. μ.)	Increased in macrocytic anemias, decreased in microcytic anemia
Mean corpuscular hemoglobin (MCH)	27–32 $\mu\mu$g. per cell	Increased in macrocytic anemias, decreased in microcytic anemia
Mean corpuscular hemoglobin concentration (MCHC)	33%–38%	Decreased in severe hypochromic anemia
Reticulocytes	0.5%–1.5% of red cells	Increased with any condition stimulating increase in bone marrow activity (i.e., infection, blood loss [acute and chronic]); following iron therapy in iron deficiency anemia, polycythemia rubra vera Decreased with any condition depressing bone marrow activity, acute leukemia, late stage of severe anemias
Erythrocyte sedimentation rate (ESR) (Westergren)	Males under 50 yr.: <15 mm./hr. Males over 50 yr.: <20 mm./hr. Females under 50 yr.: <20 mm./hr. Females over 50 yr.: <30 mm./hr.	Increased in tissue destruction, whether inflammatory or degenerative, and during menstruation, pregnancy, and in acute febrile diseases

(continued)

* Laboratory values vary according to the techniques used in different laboratories.

Normal Ranges—Hematology* (continued)

Determination	Normal Range	Clinical Significance
Erythrocyte sedimentation ratio (Zeta centrifuge)	41%–54% in both sexes	Significance similar to ESR
Hematocrit	Males: 42%–50% Females: 40%–48%	Decreased in severe anemias, anemia of pregnancy, acute massive blood loss Increased in erythrocytosis of any cause, and in dehydration or hemoconcentration associated with shock
Hemoglobin	Males: 13–18 gm./dl. Females: 12–16 gm./dl.	Decreased in various anemias, pregnancy, severe or prolonged hemorrhage, and with excessive fluid intake Increased in polycythemia, chronic obstructive pulmonary diseases, failure of oxygenation because of congestive heart failure, and normally, in people living at high altitudes
Hemoglobin F	Less than 2% of total hemoglobin	Increased in infants and children, in thalassemia and many anemias
Leukocyte alkaline phosphatase	Score of 40–100	Increased in polycythemia vera, myelofibrosis and infections Decreased in chronic granulocytic leukemia, paroxysmal nocturnal hemoglobinuria, hypoplastic marrow, viral infections, and, particularly, infectious mononucleosis
Leukocyte count Neutrophils Eosinophils Basophils Lymphocytes Monocytes	Total: 5,000–10,000 cu. mm. 60%–70% 1%–4% 0%–0.5% 20%–30% 2%–6%	Elevated in acute infectious diseases—predominantly in the neutrophilic fraction with bacterial diseases, and in the lymphocytic and monocytic fractions in viral diseases. Eosinophils elevated in collagen diseases, allergy, intestinal parasitosis. Elevated in acute leukemia, following menstruation, and following surgery or trauma. Depressed in aplastic anemia, agranulocytosis, and by toxic agents, such as chemotherapeutic agents used in treating malignancy
Osmotic fragility of red cells	Increased if hemolysis occurs in over 0.5% NaCl Decrease if hemolysis is incomplete in 0.3% NaCl	Increased in congenital spherocytosis, idiopathic acquired hemolytic anemia, isoimmune hemolytic disease, ABO hemolytic disease of newborn Decreased in sickle cell anemia, thalassemia
Platelet count	100,000–400,000 per cu. mm.	Increased in malignancy, myeloproliferative disease, postoperatively, rheumatoid arthritis; about 50% of patients with unexpected increase of platelet count will be found to have a malignancy Decreased in thrombocytopenic purpura, acute leukemic aplastic anemia, and during cancer chemotherapy, infections, and drug reactions

Normal Ranges—Serum, Plasma, Whole Blood Chemistries

Determination	Normal Adult	Clinical Significance	
		(Increased)	(Decreased)
Acetoacetate and acetone	0.3–2.0 mg./dl.	Diabetic acidosis Fasting Toxemia of pregnancy Carbohydrate-free diet High-fat diet	
Adrenocorticotropic hormone (ACTH) (plasma), RIA*	Less than 50 pg./ml.	Pituitary-dependent Cushing's syndrome Ectopic ACTH syndrome Primary adrenal atrophy	Adrenocortical tumor Adrenal insufficiency secondary to hypopituitarism
Aldolase	3–8 Sibley–Lehninger U/dl. at 37°C.	Hepatic necrosis Granulocytic leukemia Myocardial infarction Skeletal muscle disease	
Aldosterone (plasma), RIA	Supine: 3–10 ng./dl. Upright: 5–30 ng./dl. Adrenal vein: 200–800 ng./dl.	Primary (Conn's syndrome) Secondary aldosteronism	Addison's disease
Alpha-1-antitrypsin	200–400 mg./dl.		Certain forms of chronic lung and liver disease in young adults

* By radioimmunoassay

Normal Ranges—Serum, Plasma, Whole Blood Chemistries (continued)

Determination	Normal Adult	Clinical Significance	
		(Increased)	(Decreased)

Alpha-1-fetoprotein	None detected	Hepatocarcinoma
		Metastatic carcinoma of liver
		Germinal cell carcinoma of the testis
		    or ovary
		Prenatal fetal neural tube defects—
		    elevation in maternal serum	

Alpha-hydroxybutyric dehydrogenase	Up to 140 mU/ml.	Myocardial infarction Granulocytic leukemia Hemolytic anemias Muscular dystrophy	
Ammonia (plasma)	40–80 μg./dl. (enzymatic method) varies considerably with method	Severe liver disease Hepatic decompensation	

Amylase	60–160 Somogyi U/dl.	Acute pancreatitis
		Mumps
		Duodenal ulcer
		Carcinoma of head of pancreas
		Prolonged elevation with pseudocyst
		    of pancreas
		Increased by drugs that constrict
		    pancreatic duct sphincters:
		    morphine, codeine, cholinergics
			Chronic pancreatitis
			Pancreatic fibrosis and atrophy
			Cirrhosis of liver
			Pregnancy (2nd and 3rd trimesters)

Arsenic	6–20 μg./dl.; if >50μg./dl., suspect toxicity	Accidental or intentional poisoning Excessive occupational exposure	

Ascorbic acid (vitamin C)	0.4–1.5 mg./dl.	Large doses of ascorbic acid as a
		    prophylactic against the
		    common cold	

Bilirubin	Total: 0.1–1.2 mg.dl. Direct: 0.1–0.2 mg./dl. Indirect: 0.1–1.0 mg./dl.	Hemolytic anemia (indirect) Biliary obstruction and disease Hepatocellular damage (hepatitis) Pernicious anemia Hemolytic disease of newborn	
Calcitonin	Basal: Nondetectable (<400 pg./ml.)	Medullary carcinoma of the thyroid Some nonthyroid tumors Zollinger–Ellison syndrome	
Calcium	8.5–10.5 mg./dl.	Tumor or hyperplasia of parathyroid Hypervitaminosis D Multiple myeloma Nephritis with uremia Malignant tumors Sarcoidosis Hyperthyroidism Skeletal immobilization Excess calcium intake—milk–alkali syndrome	Hypoparathyroidism Diarrhea Celiac disease Vitamin D deficiency Acute pancreatitis Nephrosis After parathyroidectomy
CO_2 content	Adults: 24–32 mEq./L. Infants: 18–24 mEq./L. (Venous)	Tetany Respiratory disease Intestinal obstruction Vomiting	Acidosis Nephritis Eclampsia Diarrhea Anesthesia

Carcinoembryonic antigen (CEA), RIA	0–2.5 ng./ml.	The repeatedly high incidence of this
		    antigen in cancers of the colon,
		    rectum, pancreas, and stomach
		    suggest that CEA levels may be
		    a useful adjunct in the diagnosis
		    of these conditions and
		    therapeutic monitoring	

Catecholamines, plasma, RIA	Recumbent: 200–600 ng./L. Upright: 300–1000 ng./L.	Pheochromocytoma	
Ceruloplasmin	Males: 29–80 mg./dl.		Wilson's disease (hepatolenticular degeneration)
Chloride	95–105 mEq./L.	Nephrosis Nephritis Urinary obstruction Cardiac decompensation Anemia	Diabetes Diarrhea Vomiting Pneumonia Heavy metal poisoning Cushing's syndrome Burns Intestinal obstruction Febrile conditions
Cholesterol	150–250 mg./dl.	Lipemia Obstructive jaundice	Pernicious anemia Hemolytic anemia

(continued)

Normal Ranges—Serum, Plasma, Whole Blood Chemistries (continued)

		Clinical Significance	
Determination	Normal Adult	(Increased)	(Decreased)
		Diabetes Hypothyroidism	Hyperthyroidism Severe infection Terminal states of debilitating disease
Cholesterol esters	60%–70% of total		The esterified fraction decreases in liver disease
Cholinesterase	Serum: 0.61–1.60 delta pH Red cells: 0.60–1.00 delta pH	Nephrosis Exercise	Nerve gas intoxication (greater effect on red cell activity) Insecticides, organic phosphates (greater effect on plasma activity)
Chorionic gonadotrophin, beta subunit, RIA	0–5 IU/L.	Pregnancy Hydatidiform mole Choriocarcinoma	
Complement, human C_3	Males: 88–252 mg./dl. Females: 88–206 mg./dl.	Some inflammatory diseases	Acute glomerulonephritis Disseminated lupus erythematosus with renal involvement
Complement, C_4	14–51 mg./dl.	Some inflammatory diseases	Often decreased in immunologic disease, especially with active SLE Hereditary angioneurotic edema
Complement, total (hemolytic)	90%–94% complement	Some inflammatory diseases	Acute glomerulonephritis Epidemic meningitis Subacute bacterial endocarditis
Copper	70–165 μg./dl.	Cirrhosis of liver Pregnancy	Wilson's disease
Cortisol, RIA	8 AM: 7–25 μg./dl. 4 PM: 2–9 μg./dl.	Stress: infectious disease, surgery, burns, etc. Pregnancy Cushing's syndrome Pancreatitis Eclampsia	Addison's disease Anterior pituitary hypofunction
C-peptide reactivity	1.5–10 ng./ml.	Insulinoma	Diabetes
Creatine	0.2–0.8 mg./dl.	Pregnancy Skeletal muscle necrosis or atrophy Starvation Hyperthyroidism	
Creatine phosphokinase (CPK)	Males: 50–325 mU/ml. Females: 50–250 mU/ml.	Myocardial infarction Skeletal muscle diseases Intramuscular injections Crush syndrome Hypothyroidism Delirium tremens Alcoholic myopathy Cerebrovascular disease	
Creatine phosphokinase isoenzymes	MM band present (skeletal muscle): MB band absent (heart muscle)	MB band increased in myocardial infarction, ischemia	
Creatinine	0.7–1.4 mg./dl.	Nephritis Chronic renal disease	Kidney diseases
Creatinine clearance	100–150 ml. of blood cleared of creatinine/min.		
Cryoglobulins, qualitative	Negative	Multiple myeloma Chronic lymphocytic leukemia Lymphosarcoma Systemic lupus erythematosus Rheumatoid arthritis Subacute bacterial endocarditis Some malignancies Scleroderma	
11-Desoxycortisol	0–2 μg./dl.	Hypertensive form of virilizing adrenal hyperplasia due to an 11-beta hydroxylase defect.	
Dibucaine number	Normal: 70%–85% inhibition Heterozygote: 50%–65% inhibition Homozygote 16%–25% inhibition		Important in detecting carriers of abnormal cholinesterase activity who are susceptible to succinyldicholine anesthetic shock
Dihydrotestosterone	Males: 50–210 ng./dl. Females: None detectable		Testicular feminization syndrome
Estradiol, RIA	Females: Menstruation: 1.5–7.6 ng./dl.	Pregnancy	Depressed or failure to peak— ovarian failure

Normal Ranges—Serum, Plasma, Whole Blood Chemistries (continued)

Determination	Normal Adult	Clinical Significance	
		(Increased)	(Decreased)
	Follicular phase: 2.0–20 ng./dl. Midcycle: 12–40 ng./dl. Luteal phase: 10–30 ng./dl. Postmenopausal: 1.0–5.0 ng./dl. Males: 0.5–5.0 ng./dl.		

Estriol, RIA	Nonpregnant females: <0.5 ng./ml.
	Pregnant females:
	  1st trimester—up to 1.0 ng./ml.
	  2nd trimester—0.8—7.0 ng./ml.
	  3rd trimester—5.0—25.0 ng./ml.
		Pregnancy	Depressed or failure to peak—
			  ovarian failure

Estrogens, total, RIA	Females:
	  Menstrual flow: 43–67 ng./dl.
	  Follicular phase: 40–103 ng./dl.
	  Ovulation peak: 75–139 ng./dl.
	  Luteal phase: 47–113 ng./dl.
	Males: 47–74 ng./dl.
		Pregnancy
		Measured on a daily basis can be
		  used to evaluate response of
		  hypogonadotrophic,
		  hypoestrogenic women to
		  human menopausal or pituitary
		  gonadotropin
			Fetal distress
			Ovarian failure

Estrone, RIA	Females:
	  Day 1–10: 4.3–18.0 ng./dl.
	  Day 11–20: 7.5–19.6 ng./dl.
	  Day 21–30: 13.0–20.0 ng./dl.
	Males: 2.5–7.5 ng./dl.
		Pregnancy	Depressed or failure to peak—
			  ovarian failure

Ferritin, RIA	Males: 10–270 ng./ml. Females: 5–100 ng./ml.	Nephritis Hemochromatosis Certain neoplastic diseases Acute myelogenous leukemia Multiple myeloma	Iron deficiency
Folic acid, RIA	4–16 ng./ml.		Megaloblastic anemias of infancy and pregnancy Inadequate diets Liver disease Malabsorption syndrome Severe hemolytic anemia

Follicle stimulating hormone (FSH),
  RIA
	Normal females:
	  Follicular phase: 5–20 mlU/ml.
	  Peak of middle cycle:
	    12–30 mlU/ml.
	  Luteinic phase: 5–15 mlU/ml.
	Menopausal females:
	  40–200 mlU/ml.
	Normal males: 5–25 mlU/ml.
		Menopause and primary ovarian
		  failure
			Pituitary failure

Galactose-1-phosphate uridyl
  transferase
	Above 18 units of activity per gram
	  of hemoglobin
	0.05–1.5: Possibly galactosemic
	0–0.05: Galactosemic
			Galactosemia

Gamma glutamyl transpeptidase	Males: <45 IU/L. Females: <30 IU/L.	Hepatobiliary disease Anicteric alcoholics Drug therapy damage Myocardial infarction Renal infarction	

Gastrin, RIA	Fasting: 50–155 pg./ml.
	Postprandial: 80–170 pg./ml.
	Zollinger-Ellison syndrome: 200–over
	  2000 pg./ml.
	Pernicious anemia: 130–2,260 (mean
	  912) pg./ml.
		Zollinger–Ellison syndrome
		Peptic ulceration of the duodenum
		Pernicious anemia	

Glucose	Fasting: 60–110 mg./dl. Postprandial (2 hr.): 65–140 mg./dl.	Diabetes Nephritis Hyperthyroidism Early hyperpituitarism Cerebral lesions Infections Pregnancy Uremia	Hyperinsulinism Hypothyroidism Late hyperpituitarism Pernicious vomiting Addison's disease Extensive hepatic damage

Glucose tolerance (oral)	Features of a normal response:
	  1. Normal fasting between 60–125
	    mg./dl.
	  2. No sugar in urine
	  3. The upper limits of normal are:
	    fasting—125
	    1 hour—190
	    2 hours—140
	    3 hours—125
		(Flat or inverted curve)
		Hyperinsulinism
		Adrenal cortical insufficiency
		  (Addison's disease)
		Anterior pituitary hypofunction
		Hypothyroidism
		Sprue and celiac disease
			(High or prolonged curve)
			Diabetes
			Hyperthyroidism
			Primary adrenal cortical tumor or
			  hyperplasia
			Severe anemia
			Certain central nervous system
			  disorders

(continued)

Normal Ranges—Serum, Plasma, Whole Blood Chemistries (continued)

Determination	Normal Adult	Clinical Significance	
		(Increased)	(Decreased)
Glucose-6-phosphate dehydrogenase (red cells)	Screening: Decolorization in 20–100 min Quantitative: 1.86–2.50 IU/ml. RBC		Drug-induced hemolytic anemia Hemolytic disease of newborn
Glycoprotein (alpha-1-acid)	40–110 mg./dl.	Neoplasm Tuberculosis Diabetes complicated by degenerative vascular disease Pregnancy Rheumatoid arthritis Rheumatic fever Infectious liver disease Lupus erythematosus	
Growth hormone, RIA	<10 ng./ml.	Acromegaly	Failure to stimulate with arginine or insulin—hypopituitarism
Haptoglobin	50–250 mg./dl.	Pregnancy Estrogen therapy Chronic infections Various inflammatory conditions	Hemolytic anemia Hemolytic blood transfusion reaction
Hemoglobin (plasma)	0.5–5.0 mg./dl.	Transfusion reactions Paroxysmal nocturnal hemoglobinuria Intravascular hemolysis	
Hexosaminidase, total	Controls: 333–375 nM./ml./hr. Heterozygotes: 288–644 nM./ml./hr. Tay–Sachs disease: 284–1232 nM./ml./hr. Diabetics: 567–3560 nM./ml./hr.	Diabetes Tay–Sachs disease	
Hexosaminidase A	Controls: 49%–68% of total Heterozygotes: 26%–45% of total Tay-Sachs disease: 0–4% of total Diabetics: 39%–59% of total		Tay–Sachs disease and heterozygotes
High-density lipoprotein cholesterol (HDL cholesterol)	Age (yr) / Males (mg./dl.) / Females (mg./dl.): 0–19: 30–65 / 30–70; 20–29: 35–70 / 35–75; 30–39: 30–65 / 35–80; 40–49: 30–65 / 40–85; 50–59: 30–65 / 35–85; 60–69: 30–65 / 35–85		It has been claimed that HDL cholesterol is lower in patients with increased risk for coronary heart disease. This however, has not been universally accepted.
17-Hydroxyprogesterone, RIA	Males: 0.4–4.0 ng./ml. Females: 0.1–3.3 ng./ml. Children: 0.1–0.5 ng./ml.	Congenital adrenal hyperplasia Pregnancy Some cases of adrenal or ovarian adenomas	
Immunoglobulin A	Adult: 50–300 mg./dl. (In children the normals are lower and vary with age.)	Gamma A myeloma Wiskott–Aldrich syndrome Autoimmune disease Hepatic cirrhosis	Ataxia telangiectasis Agammaglobulinemia Hypogammaglobulinemia, transient Dysgammaglobulinemia Protein-losing enteropathies
Immunoglobulin D	0–30 mg./dl.	IgD multiple myeloma Some patients with chronic infectious diseases	
Immunoglobulin E	20–740 ng./ml.	Allergic patients and those with parasitic infestations	
Immunoglobulin G	Adults: 635–1400 mg./dl.	IgG myeloma Following hyperimmunization Autoimmune disease states Chronic infections	Congenital and acquired hypogammaglobulinemia IgA myelomas, Waldenstrom's (IgM) macroglobulinemia Some malabsorption syndromes Extensive protein loss
Immunoglobulin M	Adult: 40–280 mg./dl.	Waldenstrom's macroglobulinemia Parasitic infections Hepatitis	Agammaglobulinemias Some IgG and IgA myelomas Chronic lymphatic leukemia
Insulin, RIA	5–25 μU/ml.	Insulinoma Acromegaly	Diabetes mellitus
Iodine, butanol extractable	3.5–6.5 mg./dl.	Hyperthyroidism	Hypothyroidism
Iodine, protein-bound	4.0–8.0 μg./dl.	Hyperthyroidism	Hypothyroidism
Iron	65–170 μg./dl.	Pernicious anemia Aplastic anemia Hemolytic anemia Hepatitis Hemochromatosis	Iron deficiency anemia
Iron-binding capacity	IBC: 150–235 μg./dl. TIBC: 250–420 μg./dl. % Saturation: 20–50	Iron deficiency anemia Acute and chronic blood loss Hepatitis	Chronic infectious diseases Cirrhosis

Normal Ranges—Serum, Plasma, Whole Blood Chemistries (continued)

Determination	Normal Adult	Clinical Significance	
		(Increased)	(Decreased)
Isocitric dehydrogenase	50–180 U	Hepatitis: cirrhosis Obstructive jaundice Metastatic carcinoma of the liver Megaloblastic anemia	
Lactic acid (whole blood)	Venous: 5–20 mg./dl. Arterial: 3–7 mg./dl.	Increased muscular activity Congestive heart failure Hemorrhage Shock Some varieties of metabolic acidosis Some febrile infections May be increased in severe liver disease	
Lactic dehydrogenase (LDH)	100–225 mU/ml.	Untreated pernicious anemia Myocardial infarction Pulmonary infarction Liver disease	

Lactic dehydrogenase isoenzymes
  Total lactic dehydrogenase
  LDH-1
  LDH-2
  LDH-3
  LDH-4
  LDH-5
	100–225 mU/ml.
	20–35%
	25–40%
	20–30%
	0–20%
	0–25%
	up to 40 µg./dl.
		LDH-1 and LDH-2 are increased in
		  myocardial infarction,
		  megaloblastic anemia, and
		  hemolytic anemia
		LDH-4 and LDH-5 are increased in
		  pulmonary infarction, congestive
		  heart failure, and liver disease	

Lead (whole blood)		Lead poisoning	
Leucine aminopeptidase	80–200 µ./ml.	Liver or biliary tract diseases Pancreatic disease Metastatic carcinoma of liver and pancreas Biliary obstruction	
Lipase	0.2–1.5 U/ml.	Acute and chronic pancreatitis Biliary obstruction Cirrhosis Hepatitis Peptic ulcer	
Lipids, total	400–1000 mg./dl.	Hypothyroidism Diabetes Nephrosis Glomerulonephritis Hyperlipoproteinemias	Hyperthyroidism

Lipoprotein phenotype

Summary of Findings in the Primary Hyperlipoproteinemias

Type	Frequency	Appearance	Triglyceride	Cholesterol	Lipoprotein Staining				Secondary Causes
					Beta	Pre-Beta	Alpha	Chylomicrons	
Normal		Clear	Normal	Normal	Moderate	Zero to moderate	Moderate	Weak	
I	Very rare	Creamy	Markedly increased	Normal to moderately increased	Weak	Weak	Weak	Markedly increased	Dysglobulinemia
II	Common	Clear	Normal to slightly increased	Slightly to markedly increased	Strong	Zero to strong	Moderate	Weak	Hypothyroidism, myeloma, hepatic disease, nephrotic syndrome, macroglobulinemia, and high dietary cholesterol
III	Uncommon	Clear, cloudy or milky	Increased	Increased	Broad intense band	Extends into beta	Moderate	Weak	
IV	Very common	Clear, cloudy or milky	Slightly to markedly increased	Normal to slightly increased	Weak to moderate	Moderate to strong	Weak to moderate	Weak	Hypothyroidism, diabetes mellitus, pancreatitis, glycogen storage diseases, nephrotic syndrome, myeloma, pregnancy, and oral contraceptives
V	Rare	Cloudy to creamy	Markedly increased	Increased	Weak	Moderate	Weak	Strong	Diabetes mellitus, pancreatitis, and alcoholism

Types I and II are fat induced; III and IV are carbohydrate induced; type V is fat and carbohydrate induced.

(continued)

Normal Ranges—Serum, Plasma, Whole Blood Chemistries (continued)

Determination	Normal Adult	Clinical Significance (Increased)	(Decreased)
Lithium	Usual maintenance level: 0.5–1.0 mEq./L.		
Low-density lipoprotein cholesterol (LDL cholesterol)	Age (yr.) mg./dl. 0–19 50–170 20–29 60–170 30–39 70–190 40–49 80–190 50–59 80–210	LDL cholesterol is claimed to be higher in patients with increased risk for coronary heart disease. This claim, however, is not universally accepted.	

Luteinizing hormone, RIA	Males: 6–30 mIU/ml.
	Females:
	  Follicular phase: 2–30 mIU/ml.
	  Ovulatory peak: 40–200 mIU/ml.
	Luteal phase: 0–20 mIU/ml.
	Postmenopausal: 35–120 mIU/ml.
		Pituitary tumor
		Ovarian failure
			Depressed or failure to peak—pituitary failure

Lysozyme (muramidase)	2.8–8.0 μg./ml.	Certain types of leukemia (acute monocytic leukemia) Inflammatory states and infections	Acute lymphocytic leukemia
Magnesium	1.3–2.4 mEq./L.	Excess ingestion of magnesium-containing antacids	Chronic alcoholism Severe renal disease, diarrhea Defective growth
Manganese	0.08–0.26 μg./dl.		
Mercury	up to 10 μg./dl.	Mercury poisoning	
Myoglobin, RIA	up to 85 ng./ml.	Myocardial infarction Muscle necrosis	
Nonprotein nitrogen	20–35 mg./dl.	Acute nephritis Polycystic kidneys Obstructive uropathy Peritonitis Congestive heart failure Pregnancy	
5′ Nucleotidase	3.2–11.6 IU/L.	Hepatobiliary disease	
Osmolality	280–300 milliosmoles/kg.	Useful in the study of electrolyte and water balance	Inappropriate secretion of antidiuretic hormone

Oxygen, arterial (Whole blood):
  Partial pressure pO$_2$
  Saturation
	95–100 mm. Hg
	94%–100%
		Polycythemia
		Anhydremia
			Anemia
			Cardiac decompensation
			Chronic obstructive pulmonary disease

pCO$_2$ (whole blood) arterial	35–45 mm. Hg	Respiratory acidosis Metabolic alkalosis	Respiratory alkalosis Metabolic acidosis
pH (whole blood) arterial	7.35–7.45	Vomiting Hyperpnea Fever Intestinal obstruction	Uremia Diabetic acidosis Hemorrhage Nephritis
Parathyroid hormone	163–347 pg./ml.	Hyperparathyroidism	Conditions which decrease gastric acidity
Pepsinogen	200–425 U/ml.		Pernicious anemia Achlorhydria
Phenylalanine	1.2–3.5 mg./dl. first week 0.7–3.5 mg./dl. thereafter	Phenylketonuria	
Phosphatase, acid, total	0–11 IU/L.	Carcinoma of prostate Advanced Paget's disease Hyperparathyroidism Gaucher's disease	
Phosphatase, acid, prostatic, RIA	0–10 ng./ml. Borderline: 2.5–3.3 IU/L.	Carcinoma of prostate	
Phosphatase, alkaline	Adults: 30–115 mU/ml.	Conditions reflecting increased osteoblastic activity of bone Rickets Hyperparathyroidism Liver disease	
Phosphatase, alkaline, thermostable fraction	Thermostable fraction greater than 35%: hepatic disease and combined disease with predominant hepatic component Thermostable fraction between 25% and 35%: combined hepatic and skeletal disease	Hepatic disease	

Normal Ranges—Serum, Plasma, Whole Blood Chemistries (continued)

Determination	Normal Adult	Clinical Significance	
		(Increased)	(Decreased)
	Thermostable fraction <25%: skeletal disease with increased osteoblastic activity		
Phosphohexose isomerase	20–90 IU/L.	Malignancy Diseases of heart, liver, and skeletal muscles	
Phospholipids	125–300 mg./dl.	Diabetes Nephritis	
Phosphorus, inorganic	2.5–4.5 mg./dl.	Chronic nephritis Hypoparathyroidism	Hyperparathyroidism Vitamin D deficiency
Potassium	3.8–5.0 mEq./L.	Addison's disease Oliguria Anuria Tissue breakdown or hemolysis	Diabetic acidosis Diarrhea Vomiting
Progesterone, RIA	Follicular phase: up to 0.8 ng./ml. Luteal phase: 10–20 ng./ml. End of cycle: <1 ng./ml. Pregnant: up to 50 ng./ml. in 20th week	Useful in evaluation of menstrual disorders and infertility and the evaluation of placental function during pregnancies complicated by toxemia, diabetes mellitus, or threatened miscarriage	
Prolactin, RIA	6–24 ng./ml.	Pregnancy Functional or structural disorders of the hypothalamus Pituitary stalk section Pituitary tumors	
Protein, total Albumin Globulin	6.0–8.0 gm./dl. 3.5–5.0 gm./dl. 1.5–3.0 gm./dl.	Hemoconcentration Shock Multiple myeloma (globulin fraction) Chronic infections (globulin fraction) Liver disease (globulin)	Malnutrition Hemorrhage Loss of plasma from burns Proteinuria
Electrophoresis (Cellulose acetate) Albumin Alpha$_1$ globulin Alpha$_2$ globulin Beta globulin Gamma globulin	3.3–5.0 gm./dl. 0.2–0.4 gm./dl. 0.6–1.0 gm./dl. 0.6–1.2 gm./dl. 0.7–1.5 gm./dl.		
Protoporphyrin, erythrocyte (whole blood)	15–100 μg./dl.	Lead toxicity Erythropoietic porphyria	
Pyridoxine	3.6–18 ng./ml.		A wide spectrum of clinical conditions such as mental depression, peripheral neuropathy, anemia, neonatal seizures, and reactions to certain drug therapies
Pyruvic acid (whole blood)	0.3–0.7 mg./dl.	Diabetes Severe thiamine deficiency Acute phase of some infections, possibly secondary to increased glycogenolysis and glycolysis	
Renin (plasma), RIA	*Normal diet:* Supine: 0.3–1.9 ng./ml./hr. Upright: 0.6–3.6 ng./ml./hr. *Low-salt diet:* Supine: 0.9–4.5 ng./ml./hr. Upright: 4.1–9.1 ng./ml./hr.	Renovascular hypertension Malignant hypertension Untreated Addison's disease Primary salt-losing nephropathy Low-salt diet Diuretic therapy Hemorrhage	Frank primary aldosteronism Increased salt intake Salt-retaining steroid therapy Antidiuretic hormone therapy Blood transfusion
Riboflavin (whole blood)	0.9–1.31 (activity coefficient)		Riboflavin deficiency
Sodium	135–145 mEq./L.	Hemoconcentration Nephritis Pyloric obstruction	Alkali deficit Addison's disease Myxedema
Sulfate	0.5–1.5 mg./dl.	Nephritis Nitrogen retention	
Testosterone, RIA	Females: 25–100 ng./dl. Males: 300–800 ng./dl.	Females: Polycystic ovary Virilizing tumors	Males: Orchidectomy for neoplastic disease of the prostate or breast Estrogen therapy Klinefelter's syndrome Hypopituitarism Hypogonadism Hepatic cirrhosis

(continued)

Normal Ranges—Serum, Plasma, Whole Blood Chemistries (continued)

Determination	Normal Adult	Clinical Significance (Increased)	Clinical Significance (Decreased)
T_3 uptake	25%–35%	Hyperthyroidism TBG deficiency Androgens and anabolic steroids	Hypothyroidism Pregnancy TBG excess Estrogens and antiovulatory drugs
T_3, triiodothyronine (total circulating), RIA	75–200 ng./dl.	Pregnancy Hyperthyroidism	Hypothyroidism
T_4, thyroxine, RIA	4.5–11.5 µg./dl.	Hyperthyroidism Thyroiditis Elevated thyroxine-binding proteins caused by oral contraceptives Pregnancy	Primary and pituitary hypothyroidism Idiopathic involvement Cases of diminished thyroxine-binding proteins caused by androgenic and anabolic steroids Hypoproteinemia Nephrotic syndrome
T_4, thyroxine, free	1.0–2.2 ng./dl.	Euthyroid patients with normal free thyroxine levels may have abnormal T_3 and T_4 levels caused by drug preparations	
Thyroid stimulating hormone (TSH), RIA	0–10 µIU/ml.	Primary hypothyroidism	
Thyroid-binding globulin	10–26 µg./dl.	Hypothyroidism Pregnancy Estrogen therapy Oral contraceptives Genetic and idiopathic	Androgens and anabolic steroids Nephrotic syndromes Marked hypoproteinemia Hepatic disease
Transaminase (SGOT) (aspartate aminotransferase)	7–40 mU/ml.	Myocardial infarction Skeletal muscle disease Liver disease	
Transaminase (SGPT) (Alanine aminotransferase)	10–40 mU/ml.	Same conditions as SGOT, but increase is more marked in liver disease than SGOT	
Transferrin	230–320 mg./dl.	Pregnancy Iron-deficiency anemia due to hemorrhaging Acute hepatitis Polycythemia Oral contraceptives	Pernicious anemia in relapse Thalassemic and sickle cell anemia Chromatosis Neoplastic and hepatic diseases
Triglycerides	10–150 mg./dl.	See lipoprotein phenotype	
Tryptophan	1.4–3.0 mg./dl.		Tryptophan-specific malabsorption syndrome
Tyrosine	0.5–4.0 mg./dl.	Tyrosinosis	
Urea nitrogen (BUN)	10–20 mg./dl.	Acute glomerulonephritis Obstructive uropathy Mercury poisoning Nephrotic syndrome	Severe hepatic failure Pregnancy
Uric acid	2.5–8.0 mg./dl.	Gouty arthritis Acute leukemia Lymphomas treated by chemotherapy Toxemia of pregnancy	Xanthinuria Defective tubular reabsorption
Viscosity	1.4–1.8 relative to water at 37°C. (98.6°F.)	Patients with marked increases of the gamma globulins	
Vitamin A	50–220 µg./dl.	Hypervitaminosis A	Vitamin A deficiency Celiac disease Sprue Obstructive jaundice Cystic fibrosis Giardiasis Parenchymal hepatic disease
Vitamin B_1 (thiamine)	1.6–4.0 µg./dl.		Anorexia Beriberi Polyneuropathy Cardiomyopathies
Vitamin B_6 (pyridoxal phosphate)	3.6–18.0 ng./ml.		Chronic alcoholism Malnutrition Uremia Neonatal seizures Malabsorption, such as celiac syndrome
Vitamin B_{12}, RIA	130–785 pg./ml.	Hepatic cell damage and in association with the	Strict vegetarianism Alcoholism

Normal Ranges—Serum, Plasma, Whole Blood Chemistries (continued)

		Clinical Significance	
Determination	Normal Adult	(Increased)	(Decreased)
		myeloproliferative disorders (the highest levels are encountered in myeloid leukemia)	Pernicious anemia Total or partial gastrectomy Ileal resection Sprue and celiac disease Fish tapeworm infestation
Vitamin E	0.5–2.0 mg./dl.		Vitamin E deficiency
Xylose absorption test	2 hr. 30–50 mg./dl.		Malabsorption syndrome
Zinc	55–150 µg./dl.	Zinc is essential for the growth and propagation of cell cultures and the functioning of several enzymes	

Normal Ranges—Urine Chemistry

		Clinical Significance	
Determination	Normal Range	Increased	Decreased
Acetone and acetoacetate	Zero	Uncontrolled diabetes Starvation	
Acid mucopolysaccharides	Negative	Hurler's syndrome Marfan's syndrome Morquio–Ulrich disease	

Aldosterone	*Normal salt:*
	Normal: 4–20 µg./24 hr.
	Renovascular: 10–40 µg./24 hr.
	Tumor: 20–100 µg./24 hr.
	Low salt:
	Normal: 10–40 µg./24 hr.
	Renovascular: 20–100 µg./24 hr.
	Tumor: 20–100 µg./24 hr.
		Primary aldosteronism (adrenocortical tumor)
		Secondary aldosteronism
		  Salt depletion
		  Potassium loading
		  ACTH in large doses
		  Cardiac failure
		  Cirrhosis with ascites formation
		  Nephrosis
		  Pregnancy	

Alpha amino nitrogen	64–199 mg./24 hr.	Leukemia Diabetes Phenylketonuria Other metabolic diseases	
Amylase	35–260 units excreted/hr.	Acute pancreatitis	
Arylsulfatase A	Greater than 2.4 units/ml.		Metachromatic leukodystrophy
Bence–Jones protein	None detected	Myeloma	
Calcium	Less than 150 mg./24 hr.	Hyperparathyroidism Vitamin D intoxication Fanconi syndrome	Hypoparathyroidism Vitamin D deficiency
Catecholamines	Total: 0–275 µg./24 hr. Epinephrine: 10%–40% Norepinephrine: 60%–90%	Pheochromocytoma Neuroblastoma	
Chorionic gonadotrophin, qualitative (pregnancy test)	Negative	Pregnancy Chorionepithelioma Hydatidiform mole	
Copper	20–70 µg./24 hr.	Wilson's disease Cirrhosis Nephrosis	
Coproporphyrin	50–300 µg./24 hr.	Poliomyelitis Lead poisoning Porphyria hepatica Porphyria erythropoietica Porphyria cutanea tarda	
Cortisol, free	20–90 µg./24 hr.	Cushing's syndrome	
Creatine	0–200 mg./24 hr.	Muscular dystrophy Fever Carcinoma of liver Pregnancy	

(continued)

Normal Ranges—Urine Chemistry (continued)

Determination	Normal Range	Clinical Significance	
		Increased	Decreased
Creatinine	0.8–2.0 gm./24 hr.	Hyperthyroidism Myositis Typhoid fever Salmonella infections Tetanus	Muscular atrophy Anemia Advanced degeneration of kidneys Leukemia
Creatinine clearance	100–150 ml. of blood cleared of creatinine/min.		Measures glomerular filtration rate Renal diseases
Cystine and cysteine	10–100 mg./24 hr.	Cystinuria	
Delta amino-levulinic acid	0.00–0.54 mg./dl.	Lead poisoning Porphyria hepatica Hepatitis Hepatic carcinoma	
11-Desoxycortisol	20–100 µg./24 hr.	Hypertensive form of virilizing adrenal hyperplasia due to an 11-beta hydroxylase defect	
Estriol (placental)	Weeks of pregnancy — mg./24 hr. 12 — less than 1 16 — 2–7 20 — 4–9 24 — 6–13 28 — 8–22 32 — 12–43 36 — 14–45 40 — 19–46		Decreased values occur with fetal distress of many conditions, including preeclampsia, placental insufficiency, and poorly controlled diabetes mellitus
Estrogens, total (fluorimetric)	Females: Onset of menstruation: 4–25 µg./24 hr. Ovulation peak: 28 µg./24 hr. Luteal peak: 22–105 µg./24 hr. Menopausal: 1.4–19.6 µg./24 hr. Males: 5–18 µg./24 hr.	Hyperestrogenism due to gonadal or adrenal neoplasm	Primary or secondary amenorrhea
Etiocholanolone	Males: 1.9–6.0 mg./24 hr. Females: 0.5–4.0 mg./24 hr.	Adrenogenital syndrome Idiopathic hirsutism	
Follicle stimulating hormone, RIA	Females: Follicular: 5–20 IU/24 hr. Luteal: 5–15 IU/24 hr. Midcycle: 15–60 IU/24 hr. Menopausal: 50–100 IU/24 hr. Males: 5–25 IU/24 hr.	Menopause and primary ovarian failure	Pituitary failure
Glucose	Negative	Diabetes mellitus Pituitary disorders Intracranial pressure Lesion in floor of 4th ventricle	
Hemoglobin and myoglobin	Negative	Extensive burns Transfusion of incompatible blood Myoglobin increased in severe crushing injuries to muscle	
Homogentisic acid, qualitative	Negative	Alkaptonuria Ochronosis	
Homovanillic acid	Up to 15 mg./24 hr.	Neuroblastoma	
17-hydroxycorticosteroids	2–10 mg./24 hr.	Cushing's syndrome	Addison's disease Anterior pituitary hypofunction
5-hydroxyindoleacetic acid, qualitative	Negative	Malignant carcinoid tumors	
Hydroxyproline	25–77 mg./24 hr.	Paget's disease Fibrous dysplasia Osteomalacia Neoplastic bone disease Hyperparathyroidism	
17-ketosteroids, total	Males: 10–22 mg./24 hr. Females: 6–16 mg./24 hr.	Interstitial cell tumor of testes Simple hirsutism, occasionally Adrenal hyperplasia Cushing's syndrome Adrenal cancer, virilism Arrhenoblastoma	Thyrotoxicosis Female hypogonadism Diabetes mellitus Hypertension Debilitating disease of mild to moderate severity Eunuchoidism Addison's disease Panhypopituitarism Myxedema Nephrosis

Normal Ranges—Urine Chemistry (continued)

Determination	Normal Range	Clinical Significance	
		Increased	Decreased
Kynurenic and xanthurenic acids	Kynurenic acid: up to 18.0 mg./24 hr. Xanthurenic acid: up to 4.0 mg./24 hr.	Vitamin B_6 deficiency Acute typhoid fever Sandfly fever Tularemia	
Lead	up to 150 μg./24 hr.	Lead poisoning	

Luteinizing hormone	Males: 5–18 IU/24 hr.
	Females:
	  Follicular phase: 2–25 IU/24 hr.
	  Ovulatory peak: 30–95 IU/24 hr.
	  Luteal phase: 2–20 IU/24 hr.
	  Postmenopausal: 40–110 IU/24 hr.
		Pituitary tumor
		Ovarian failure
			Depressed or failure to peak—pituitary failure

Metanephrines, total	Less than 1.3 mg./24 hr.	Pheochromocytoma, a few patients with pheochromocytoma may have elevated urinary metanephrines but normal catecholamines and VMA	

Osmolality	Males:
	  390–1090 millimoles/kg.
	Females:
	  300–1090 millimoles/kg.
		Useful in the study of electrolyte and water balance	

Oxalate	up to 40 mg./24 hr.	Primary hyperoxaluria	
Phenylpyruvic acid, qualitative	Negative	Phenylketonuria	
Phosphorus, inorganic	0.8–1.3 gm./24 hr.	Hyperparathyroidism Vitamin D intoxication Paget's disease Metastatic neoplasm to bone	Hypoparathyroidism Vitamin D deficiency
Porphobilinogen, qualitative	Negative	Chronic lead poisoning Acute porphyria Liver disease	
Porphobilinogen, quantitative	0–1.0 mg./24 hr.	Acute porphyria Liver disease	
Porphyrins, qualitative	Negative	See porphyrins, quantitative	
Porphyrins, quantitative (coproporphyrin and uroporphyrin)	Coproporphyrin: 50–160 μg./24 hr. Uroporphyrin: up to 50 μg./24 hr.	Porphyria hepatica Porphyria erythropoietica Porphyria cutanea tarda Lead poisoning (only coproporphyrin increased)	
Potassium	40–65 mEq./24 hr.	Hemolysis	

Pregnanediol	Females:
	  Proliferative phase: 0.5–1.5 mg./24 hr.
	  Luteal phase: 2–7 mg./24 hr.
	  Menopause: 0.2–1.0 mg./24 hr.
	  Pregnancy:
	  (Weeks of gestation) mg./24 hr.
	  10–12 5–15
	  12–18 5–25
	  18–24 15–33
	  24–28 20–42
	  28–32 27–47
	Males: 0.1–2.0
		Corpus luteum cysts
		When placental tissue remains in the uterus following parturition
		Some cases of adrenocortical tumors
		Pregnancy
			Placental dysfunction
			Threatened abortion
			Intrauterine death

Pregnanetriol	0.4–2.4 mg./24 hr.	Congenital adrenal androgenic hyperplasia	
Protein	up to 100 mg./24 hr.	Nephritis Cardiac failure Mercury poisoning Bence–Jones protein in multiple myeloma Febrile states Hematuria	
Sodium	130–200 mEq./24 hr.	Useful in detecting gross changes in water and salt balance	
Titratable acidity	20–40 mEq./24 hr.	Metabolic acidosis	Metabolic alkalosis
Urea nitrogen	9–16 gm./24 hr.	Excessive protein catabolism	Impaired kidney function
Uric acid	250–750 mg./24 hr.	Gout	Nephritis

(continued)

Normal Ranges—Urine Chemistry (continued)

		Clinical Significance	
Determination	Normal Range	Increased	Decreased
Urobilinogen	Random urine: <0.25 mg./dl. 24-hr. urine: up to 4 mg./24 hr.	Liver and biliary tract disease Hemolytic anemias	Complete or nearly complete biliary obstruction Diarrhea Renal insufficiency
Uroporphyrins	up to 50 μg./24 hr.	Porphyria	
Vanillylmandelic acid (VMA)	0.7–6.8 mg./24 hr.	Pheochromocytoma Neuroblastoma Coffee, tea, aspirin, bananas, and several different drugs	
Xylose absorption test (5 hour)	16%–33% of ingested xylose		Malabsorption syndromes
Zinc	0.15–1.2 mg./24 hr.	Zinc is an essential nutritional element	

Normal Values—Cerebrospinal Fluid

		Clinical Significance	
Determination	Normal Value	Increased	Decreased
Albumin	15.5–32.0 mg./dl.	Certain neurologic disorders Lesion in the choroid plexus or blockage of the flow of CSF Damage to the blood–CNS barrier	
Cell count	0–5 mononuclear cells/cu. mm.	Bacterial meningitis Neurosyphilis Anterior poliomyelitis Encephalitis lethargica	
Chloride	100–130 mEq./L.	Uremia	Acute generalized meningitis Tuberculous meningitis
Glucose	50–75 mg./dl.	Diabetes mellitus Diabetic coma Epidemic encephalitis Uremia	Acute meningitides Tuberculous meningitis Insulin shock
Glutamine	6–15 mg./dl.	Hepatic encephalopathies, including Reye's syndrome Hepatic coma Cirrhosis	
IgG	0–6.6 mg./dl.	Damage to the blood–CNS barrier Multiple sclerosis Neurosyphilis Subacute sclerosing panencephalitis Chronic phases of CNS infections	
Lactic acid	Less than 24 mg./dl.	Bacterial meningitis Hypocapnia Hydrocephalus Brain abscesses Cerebral ischemia	
Lactic dehydrogenase	One-tenth that of serum	CNS disease	
Protein Lumbar Cisternal Ventricular	15–45 mg./dl. 15–25 mg./dl. 5–15 mg./dl.	Acute meningitides Tubercular meningitis Neurosyphilis Poliomyelitis Guillain–Barré syndrome	
Protein electrophoresis (cellulose acetate) Prealbumin Albumin Alpha₁ globulin Alpha₂ globulin Beta globulin Gamma globulin	% of total: 3.0–7.0 56.0–74.0 2.0–6.5 3.0–12.0 8.0–18.5 4.0–14.0	An increase in the level of albumin alone can be the result of a lesion in the choroid plexus or a blockage of the flow of CSF. An elevated gamma globulin value with a normal albumin level has been reported in multiple sclerosis, neurosyphilis, subacute sclerosing panencephalitis, and the chronic phase of CNS infections. If the blood–CNS barrier has been severely damaged during the course of these diseases, the CSF albumin level may also be elevated.	

Miscellaneous Values

Determinations	Normal Value	Clinical Significance
Acetaminophen	Zero	Therapeutic level = 10–20 μg./ml.
Aminophylline (theophylline)	Zero	Therapeutic level = 10–20 μg./ml.
Bromide	Zero	Therapeutic level = 5–50 mg./dl.
Carbon monoxide	0–2%	Symptoms with over 20% saturation
Chlordiazepoxide	Zero	Therapeutic level = 1–3 μg./ml.
Diazepam	Zero	Therapeutic level: 0.5–2.5 μg./dl.
Digitoxin	Zero	Therapeutic level = 5–30 ng./ml.
Digoxin	Zero	Therapeutic level = 0.5–2.0 ng./ml.
Ethanol	0–0.01%	Legal intoxication level = 0.10% or above 0.3–0.4% = marked intoxication 0.4–0.5% = alcoholic stupor
Gentamicin	Zero	Therapeutic level = 4–10 μg./ml.
Methanol	Zero	May be fatal in concentrations as low as 10 mg./dl.
Phenobarbital	Zero	Therapeutic level = 15–40 μg./ml.
Phenytoin	Zero	Therapeutic level = 10–20 μg./ml.
Primidone	Zero	Therapeutic level = 5–12 μg./ml.
Quinidine	Zero	Therapeutic level = 0.2–0.5 mg./dl.
Salicylate	Zero	Therapeutic level = 2–25 mg./dl. Toxic level = over 30 mg./dl.
Sulfonamide	Zero	Therapeutic levels: Sulfadiazine 8–15 mg./dl. Sulfaguanidine 3–5 mg./dl. Sulfamerazine 10–15 mg./dl. Sulfanilamide 10–15 mg./dl.

Gastric Analysis		Increased	Decreased
pH	<2.0		Pernicious anemia
Basal acid output	0–6 mEq./hr.	Peptic ulcer	Gastric carcinoma
Maximum acid	5–40 mEq./hr.	Zollinger–Ellison syndrome	Chronic atrophic gastritis Decreased normally with age

Appendix II:
Conversion Tables

Metric Units and Symbols

Quantity	Unit	Symbol	Equivalent
Length	millimeter	mm.	1000 mm. = 1 m.
	centimeter	cm.	100 cm. = 1 m.
	decimeter	dm.	10 dm. = 1 m.
	meter	m.	1000 m. = 1 km.
Volume	cubic centimeter	cc. or cm.^{3}	$1000 \frac{cc \text{ or } dm.^3}{ml.} = 1 \text{ cm.}^3 \text{ or liter}$
	milliliter	ml.	
	cu. decimeter	dm.^{3}	$1000 \frac{dm.^3}{1} = 1 \text{ m.}^3$
	liter	L.	
Mass	microgram	μg.	1000 μg. = 1 mg.
	milligram	mg.	1000 mg. = 1 g.
	gram	g.	1000 g. = 1 kg.
	kilogram	kg.	1000 kg. = 1 metric ton (t)

Table of Metric and Apothecaries' Systems*

(Approved *approximate* dose equivalents are enclosed in parentheses. Use exact equivalents in calculations.)

Conversion Factors

Metric	Apothecaries	Metric	Apothecaries
1 milligram (mg.)	$1/_{64}$ grain	3.888 cubic centimeters or grams	1 dram (4 cc. or grams)
64.79 milligrams	1 grain (65 mg.)	31.103 cubic centimeters or grams	1 ounce (30 cc. or grams)
1 gram	15.43 grains (15 grains)	473.167 cubic centimeters	1 pint (500 cc.)
1 cubic centimeter (cc.)	16 minims		

Weights

Metric	Apothecaries	Metric		Apothecaries
0.0001 gram—0.1 mg.—$1/_{640}$ grain ($1/_{600}$ grain)		0.057 gram —57	mg.—$7/_8$	grain
0.0002 gram—0.2 mg.—$1/_{320}$ grain ($1/_{300}$ grain)		0.06 gram —60	mg.—$9/_{10}$	grain (1 grain)
0.0003 gram—0.3 mg.—$1/_{210}$ grain ($1/_{200}$ grain)		0.065 gram —65	mg.—1	grain (60 mg.)
0.0004 gram—0.4 mg.—$1/_{150}$ grain		0.07 gram —70	mg.—$1\frac{1}{20}$	grains
0.0005 gram—0.5 mg.—$1/_{120}$ grain		0.08 gram —80	mg.—$1\frac{1}{5}$	grains
0.0006 gram—0.6 mg.—$1/_{100}$ grain		0.09 gram —90	mg.—1⅓	grains
0.0007 gram—0.7 mg.—$1/_{90}$ grain		0.097 gram —97	mg.—1½	grains (0.1 gram)
0.0008 gram—0.8 mg.—$1/_{80}$ grain		0.12 gram —120	mg.—2	grains
0.0009 gram—0.9 mg.—$1/_{75}$ grain		0.2 gram —200	mg.—3	grains
0.001 gram—1 mg.—$1/_{64}$ grain ($1/_{60}$ grain)		0.24 gram —240	mg.—4	grains (0.25 gram)
0.0011 gram—1.1 mg.—$1/_{60}$ grain		0.3 gram —300	mg.—4½	grains
0.0013 gram—1.3 mg.—$1/_{50}$ grain (1.2 mg.)		0.33 gram —330	mg.—5	grains (0.3 gram)
0.0014 gram—1.4 mg.—$1/_{48}$ grain		0.4 gram —400	mg.—6	grains
0.0016 gram—1.6 mg.—$1/_{40}$ grain (1.5 mg.)		0.45 gram —450	mg.—7	grains
0.0018 gram—1.8 mg.—$1/_{36}$ grain		0.5 gram —500	mg.—7½	grains
0.0020 gram—2 mg.—$1/_{32}$ grain ($1/_{30}$ grain)		0.53 gram —530	mg.—8	grains
0.0022 gram—2.2 mg.—$1/_{30}$ grain		0.6 gram —600	mg.—9	grains
0.0026 gram—2.6 mg.—$1/_{25}$ grain		0.65 gram —650	mg.—10	grains (0.6 gram)
0.003 gram—3 mg.—$1/_{20}$ grain		0.73 gram —730	mg.—11	grains
0.004 gram—4 mg.—$1/_{16}$ grain ($1/_{15}$ grain)		0.80 gram —800	mg.—12	grains (0.75 gram)
0.005 gram—5 mg.—$1/_{12}$ grain		0.86 gram —860	mg.—13	grains
0.006 gram—6 mg.—$1/_{10}$ grain		0.93 gram —930	mg.—14	grains
0.007 gram—7 mg.—$1/_9$ grain		1.0 gram —1000	mg.—15	grains
0.008 gram—8 mg.—$1/_8$ grain		1.06 grams—1060	mg.—16	grains
0.009 gram—9 mg.—$1/_7$ grain		1.13 grams—1130	mg.—17	grains
0.01 gram—10 mg.—$1/_6$ grain		1.18 grams—1180	mg.—18	grains
0.013 gram—13 mg.—$1/_5$ grain (12 mg.)		1.26 grams—1260	mg.—19	grains
0.016 gram—16 mg.—¼ grain (15 mg.)		1.30 grams—1300	mg.—20	grains
0.02 gram—20 mg.—⅓ grain		1.50 grams—1500	mg.—22	grains
0.025 gram—25 mg.—⅜ grain		2 grams—2000	mg.—30	grains (½ dram)
0.03 gram—30 mg.—$2/_5$ grain (½ grain)		4 grams	—1	dram (60 grains)
0.032 gram—32 mg.—½ grain (30 mg.)		5 grams	—75	grains
0.04 gram—40 mg.—$3/_5$ grain (⅔ grain)		8 grams	—2	drams (7.5 grams)
0.043 gram—43 mg.—⅔ grain (40 mg.)		10 grams	—2½	drams
0.05 gram—50 mg.—¾ grain		15 grams	—4	drams
		30 grams	—1	ounce

Liquid Measures†

Metric	Apothecaries	Metric	Apothecaries
0.03 cubic centimeter —½ minim		8 cubic centimeters—2	fluid drams
0.05 cubic centimeter —¾ minim		10 cubic centimeters—2½	fluid drams
0.06 cubic centimeter —1 minim		15 cubic centimeters—4	fluid drams
0.1 cubic centimeter —1½ minims		20 cubic centimeters—5½	fluid drams
0.2 cubic centimeter —3 minims		25 cubic centimeters—$5/_6$	fluid ounce
0.25 cubic centimeter —4 minims		30 cubic centimeters—1	fluid ounce
0.3 cubic centimeter —5 minims		50 cubic centimeters—1¾	fluid ounces
0.5 cubic centimeter —8 minims		60 cubic centimeters—2	fluid ounces
0.6 cubic centimeter —10 minims		100 cubic centimeters—3½	fluid ounces
0.75 cubic centimeter —12 minims		120 cubic centimeters—4	fluid ounces
1 cubic centimeter —15 minims		200 cubic centimeters—7	fluid ounces
2 cubic centimeters—30 minims		250 cubic centimeters—8	fluid ounces
3 cubic centimeters—45 minims		360 cubic centimeters—12	fluid ounces
4 cubic centimeters—1 fluid dram		500 cubic centimeters—1	pint
5 cubic centimeters—1¼ fluid drams		1000 cubic centimeters—1	quart

* (From Culver VM. Modern Bedside Nursing. Philadelphia, WB Saunders, 1969)

† Note: A cubic centimeter (cc.) is the approximate equivalent of a milliliter (ml.). The terms are used interchangeably in general medicine.

24-Hour Clock

From midnight to noon—12-hour time ⎱ identical
24-hour time ⎰ identical

From noon to midnight—Add 12 to P.M. time = 24-hour time

12-hour Time	24-hour Time
12:00 midnight	24:00
12:01 A.M.	00:01
12:59 A.M.	00:59
1:00 A.M.	01:00
12:00 noon	12:00
12:01 P.M.	12:01
1:00 P.M.	13:00
5:30 P.M.	17:30
10:08 P.M.	22:08
12:00 midnight	24:00

A useful clock for avoiding confusion about A.M. and P.M. designations

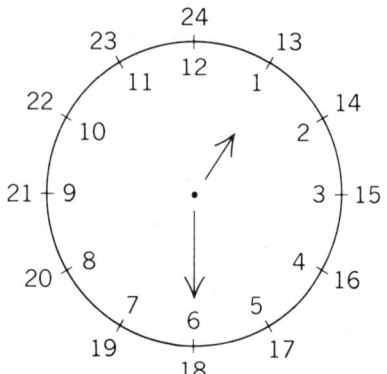

Celsius (Centigrade) and Fahrenheit Temperatures

Celsius (Centigrade) 0	Fahrenheit 32
36.0	96.8
36.5	97.7
37.0	98.6
37.5	99.5
38.0	100.4
38.5	101.3
39.0	102.2
39.5	103.1
40.0	104.0
40.5	104.9
41.0	105.8
41.5	106.7
42.0	107.6

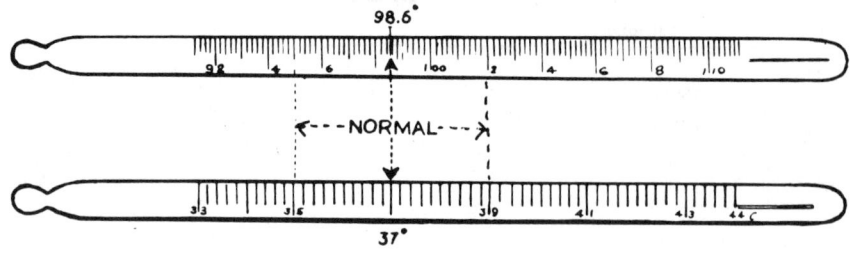

To convert degrees F. to degrees C.
Subtract 32, then multiply by 5/9
To convert degrees C. to degrees F.
Multiply by 9/5, then add 32

Nomogram for Estimating Surface Area of Infants and Young Children

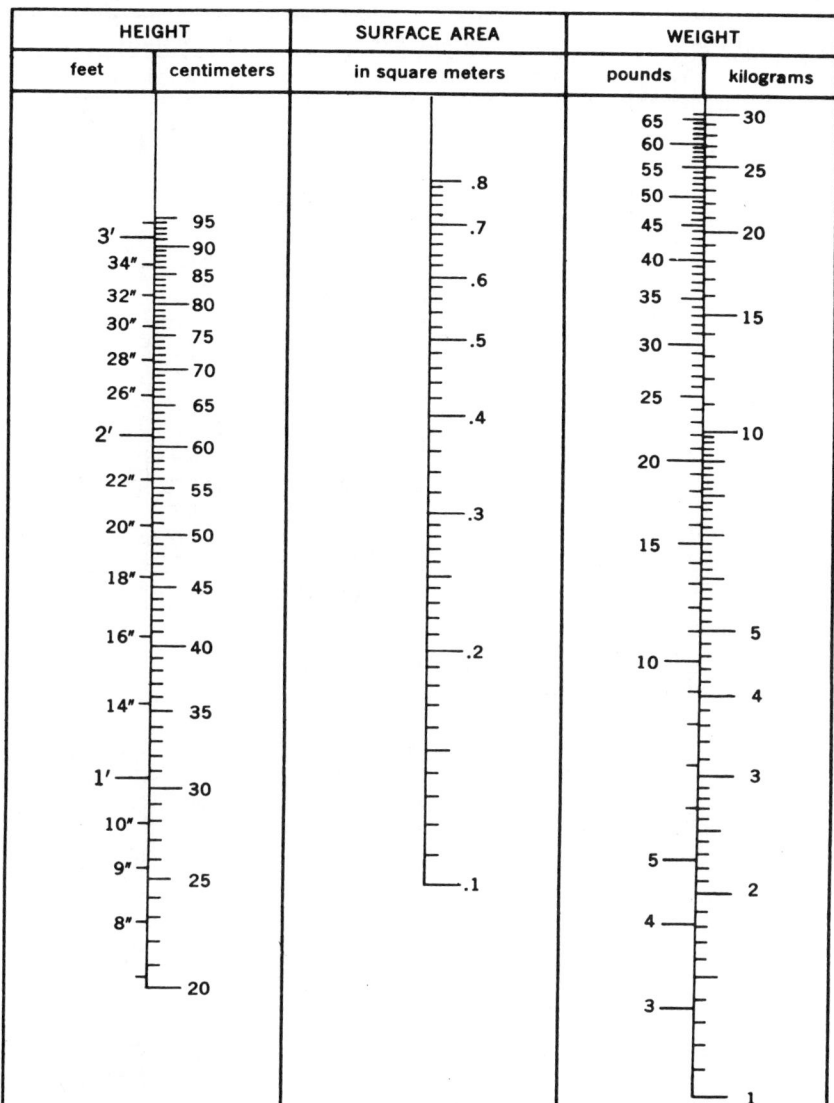

HEIGHT		SURFACE AREA	WEIGHT	
feet	centimeters	in square meters	pounds	kilograms

To determine the surface area of the patient, draw a straight line between the point representing his height on the left vertical scale to the point representing his weight on the right vertical scale. The point at which this line intersects the middle vertical scale represents the patient's surface area in square meters. (Courtesy of Abbott Laboratories)

Nomogram for Estimating Surface Area of Older Children and Adults

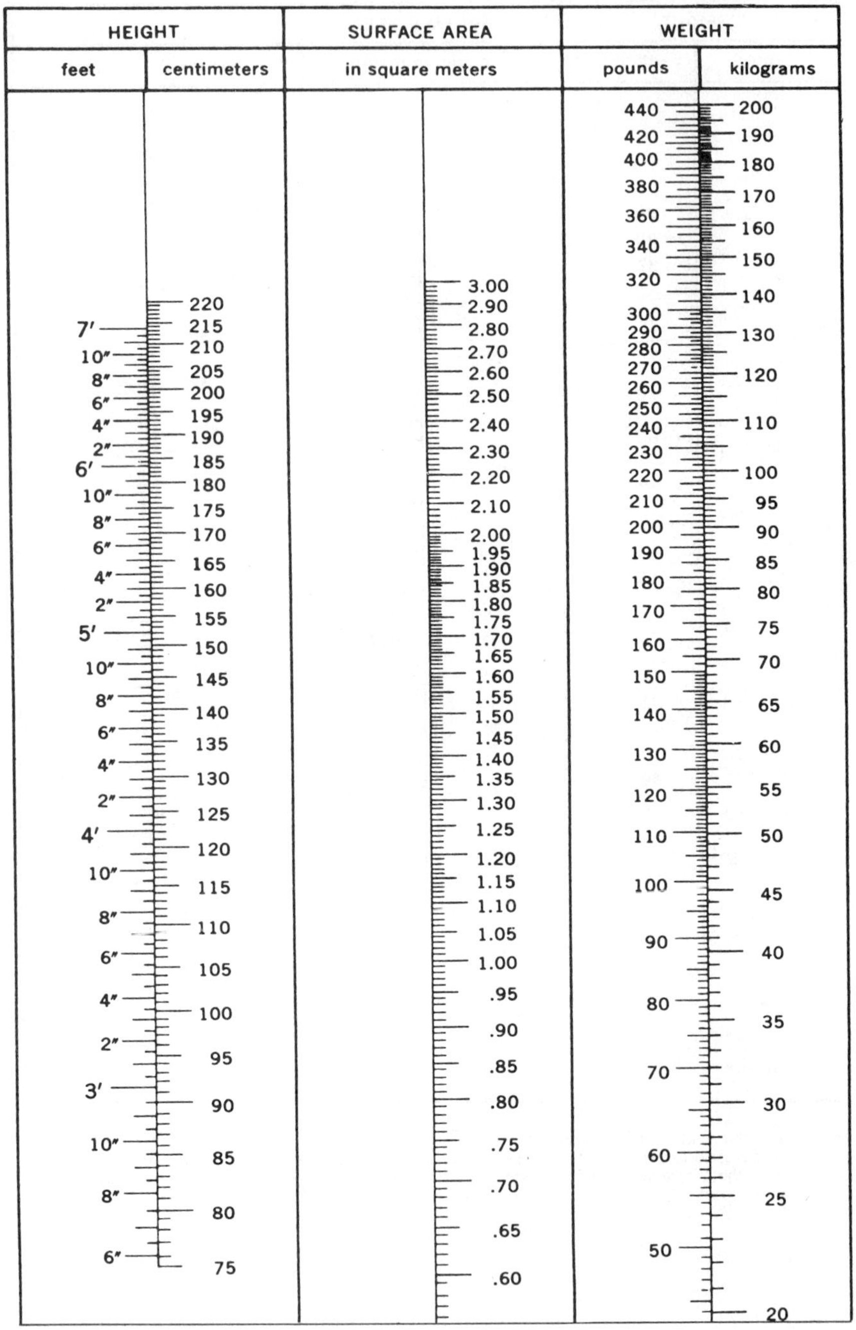
HEIGHT
SURFACE AREA
WEIGHT
feet
centimeters
in square meters
pounds
kilograms
7′ 10″ 8″ 6″ 4″ 2″ 6′ 10″ 8″ 6″ 4″ 2″ 5′ 10″ 8″ 6″ 4″ 2″ 4′ 10″ 8″ 6″ 4″ 2″ 3′ 10″ 8″ 6″
220 215 210 205 200 195 190 185 180 175 170 165 160 155 150 145 140 135 130 125 120 115 110 105 100 95 90 85 80 75
3.00 2.90 2.80 2.70 2.60 2.50 2.40 2.30 2.20 2.10 2.00 1.95 1.90 1.85 1.80 1.75 1.70 1.65 1.60 1.55 1.50 1.45 1.40 1.35 1.30 1.25 1.20 1.15 1.10 1.05 1.00 .95 .90 .85 .80 .75 .70 .65 .60
440 420 400 380 360 340 320 300 290 280 270 260 250 240 230 220 210 200 190 180 170 160 150 140 130 120 110 100 90 80 70 60 50
200 190 180 170 160 150 140 130 120 110 100 95 90 85 80 75 70 65 60 55 50 45 40 35 30 25 20

(Courtesy, Abbott Laboratories.)

Comparative Scales of Measures, Weights, and Temperatures*

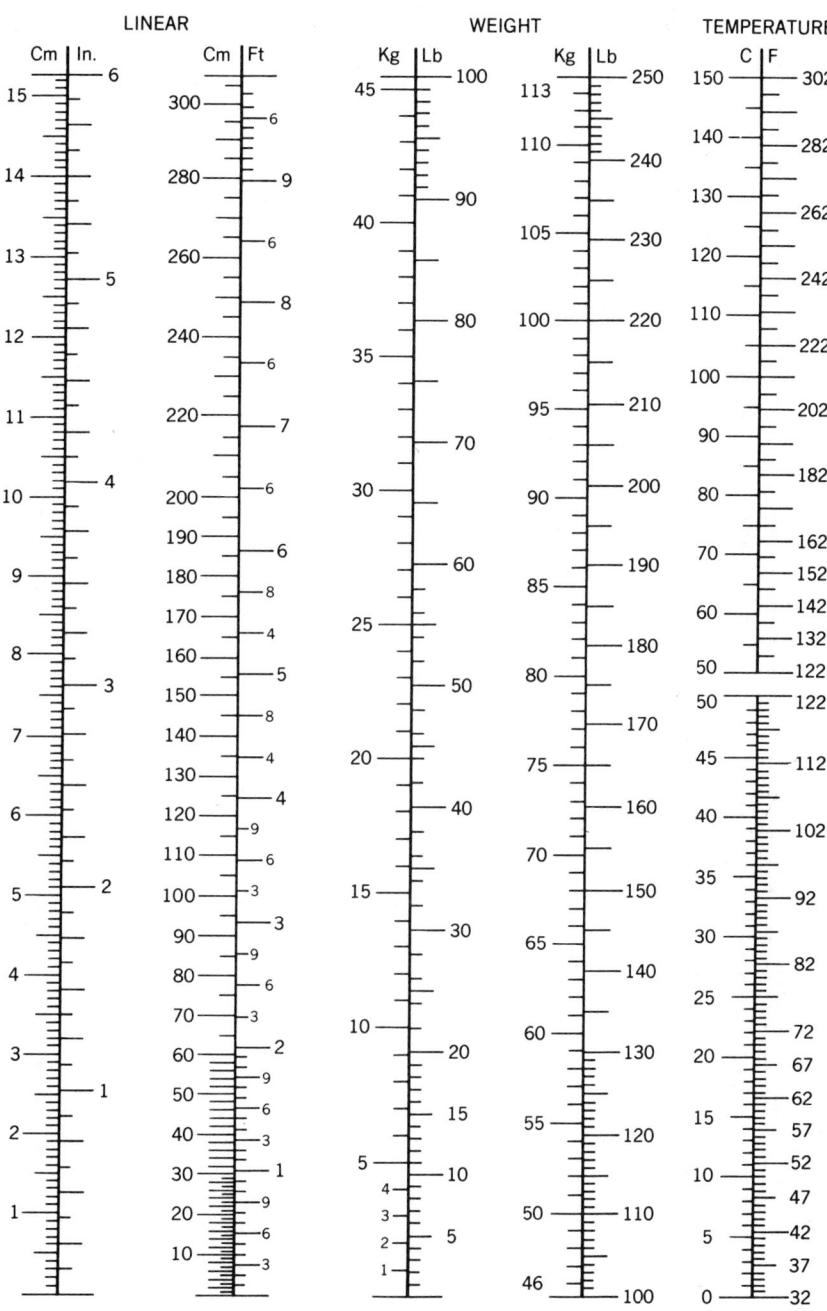

LINEAR	WEIGHT	TEMPERATURE

* 2.5 cm. = 1 inch   1 kg. = 2.2 lb.

Recommended Daily Dietary Allowances

Food and Nutrition Board, National Academy of Sciences—National Research Council
Recommended Daily Dietary Allowances,[a] Revised 1980

Designed for the maintenance of good nutrition of practically all healthy people in the USA

	Age (years)	Weight (kg.)	Weight (lb.)	Height (cm.)	Height (in.)	Protein (gm.)	Vitamin A (µg RE)[b]	Vitamin D (µg)[c]	Vitamin E (mg α-TE)[d]	Vitamin C (mg.)	Thiamin (mg.)	Riboflavin (mg.)	Niacin (mg NE)[e]	Vitamin B-6 (mg.)	Folacin[f] (µg.)	Vitamin B-12 (µg.)	Calcium (mg.)	Phosphorus (mg.)	Magnesium (mg.)	Iron (mg.)	Zinc (mg.)	Iodine (µg.)
Infants	0.0–0.5	6	13	60	24	kg. × 2.2	420	10	3	35	0.3	0.4	6	0.3	30	0.5[g]	360	240	50	10	3	40
	0.5–1.0	9	20	71	28	kg. × 2.0	400	10	4	35	0.5	0.6	8	0.6	45	1.5	540	360	70	15	5	50
Children	1–3	13	29	90	35	23	400	10	5	45	0.7	0.8	9	0.9	100	2.0	800	800	150	15	10	70
	4–6	20	44	112	44	30	500	10	6	45	0.9	1.0	11	1.3	200	2.5	800	800	200	10	10	90
	7–1	28	62	132	52	34	700	10	7	45	1.2	1.4	16	1.6	300	3.0	800	800	250	10	10	120
Males	11–14	45	99	157	62	45	1000	10	8	50	1.4	1.6	18	1.8	400	3.0	1200	1200	350	18	15	150
	15–18	66	145	176	69	56	1000	10	10	60	1.4	1.7	18	2.0	400	3.0	1200	1200	400	18	15	150
	19–22	70	154	177	70	56	1000	7.5	10	60	1.5	1.7	19	2.2	400	3.0	800	800	350	10	15	150
	23–50	70	154	178	70	56	1000	5	10	60	1.4	1.6	18	2.2	400	3.0	800	800	350	10	15	150
	51+	70	154	178	70	56	1000	5	10	60	1.2	1.4	16	2.2	400	3.0	800	800	350	10	15	150
Females	11–14	46	101	157	62	46	800	10	8	50	1.1	1.3	15	1.8	400	3.0	1200	1200	300	18	15	150
	15–18	55	120	163	64	46	800	10	8	60	1.1	1.3	14	2.0	400	3.0	1200	1200	300	18	15	150
	19–22	55	120	163	64	44	800	7.5	8	60	1.1	1.3	14	2.0	400	3.0	800	800	300	18	15	150
	23–50	55	120	163	64	44	800	5	8	60	1.0	1.2	13	2.0	400	3.0	800	800	300	18	15	150
	51+	55	120	163	64	44	800	5	8	60	1.0	1.2	13	2.0	400	3.0	800	800	300	10	15	150
Pregnant						+30	+200	+5	+2	+20	+0.4	+0.3	+2	+0.6	+400	+1.0	+400	+400	+150	h	+5	+25
Lactating						+20	+400	+5	+3	+40	+0.5	+0.5	+5	+0.5	+100	+1.0	+400	+400	+150	h	+10	+50

[a] The allowances are intended to provide for individual variations among most normal persons as they live in the United States under usual environmental stresses. Diets should be based on a variety of common foods in order to provide other nutrients for which human requirements have been less well defined.

[b] Retinol equivalents. 1 retinol equivalent = 1 µg retinol or 6 µg β carotene.

[c] As cholecalciferol. 10 µg. cholecalciferol = 400 IU of vitamin D.

[d] α-tocopherol equivalents. 1 mg. d-α tocopherol = 1 α-TE.

[e] 1 NE (niacin equivalent) is equal to 1 mg. of niacin or 60 mg. of dietary tryptophan.

[f] The folacin allowances refer to dietary sources as determined by Lactobacillus casei assay after treatment with enzymes (conjugases) to make polyglutamyl forms of the vitamin available to the test organism.

[g] The recommended dietary allowance for vitamin B-12 in infants is based on average concentration of the vitamin in human milk. The allowances after weaning are based on energy intake (as recommended by the American Academy of Pediatrics) and consideration of other factors, such as intestinal absorption.

[h] The increased requirement during pregnancy cannot be met by the iron content of habitual American diets nor by the existing iron stores of many women; therefore, the use of 30–60 mg. of supplemental iron is recommended. Iron needs during lactation are not substantially different from those of nonpregnant women, but continued supplementation of the mother for 2–3 months after parturition is advisable in order to replenish stores depleted by pregnancy.

Recommended Dietary Allowances, 9th ed. Washington DC, The National Research Council National Academy of Sciences. 1980

* Refer to Recommended Dietary Allowances, 9th ed. Washington, DC. The National Research Council National Academy of Sciences, 1980

Appendix III:
Pediatric Laboratory Values

(It should be noted that laboratory determinations vary from hospital to hospital depending on the techniques used by individual laboratories.)

Blood Chemistries

These values are compiled from the published literature, *Pediatric Clinical Chemistry* and the Johns Hopkins Hospital Department of Laboratory Medicine. They are the most widely accepted normal values. Normal values, however, vary with the analytic method used. If any doubt exists, consult your laboratory for its analytical method and normal range of values. (*Ref.*: Meites S. (ed). Pediatric Clinical Chemistry. Columbus, OH, Ross Laboratories, 1975; courtesy of Ross Laboratories, Columbus, OH).

Acid phosphatase:

Newborns	7.4–19.4 IU/ml.
2–13 years	6.4–15.2 IU/ml.
Adults	0.2–11.0 IU/ml.

Aldolase:

Adults	<11 IU/L.
Children	2×–4× adult values

Alkaline phosphatase:

Newborn	20–266 IU/L.
1 month–1 year	50–260 IU/L.
1–2 years	146–477 IU/L.
2–6 years	70–160 IU/L.
7–10 years	45–273 IU/L.
Puberty	56–253 IU/L. (average = 117)
Adults	13–40 IU/L.

Alpha-1-antitrypsin:

PI type M (normal)	2.1–5.0 gm./L.
PI type MZ	>75% normal pool
PI type SZ	55%–75% normal pool
PI type Z or null	30%–50% normal pool
	<40% normal pool

Alpha fetoprotein: <10 mg/dl

Ammonia nitrogen (venous sample):

Newborns	90–150 µg./dl.
0–2 weeks	70–129 µg./dl.
>1 month	20–79 µg./dl.
Infants–children	29–80 µg./dl.
Adults	13–48 µg./dl.

Amylase: 60–160 Somogyi U/dl.

Bicarbonate: 22–30 mEq./L.

Newborn:	
Premature	18–26 mEq./L.
Full-term	20–26 mEq./L.

Bilirubin (total):

Cord	<1.8 mg./dl.
24 hours	Premature: 1–6 mg./dl.
	Full-term: 2–6 mg./dl.
48 hours	Premature: 6–8 mg./dl.
	Full-term: 6–7 mg./dl.
3–5 days	Premature: 10–15 mg./dl.
	Full-term: 4–12 mg./dl.
1 month–adults	1 mg./dl.
Conjugated	<0.4 mg./dl.

Calcium (total):

Premature <1 week	6–10 mg./dl.
Full-term <1 week	7.0–12.0 mg./dl.
Children	8–11.0 mg./dl.
Adults	8.5–11.0 mg./dl.

Calcium (ionized): 4.4–5.4 mg./dl.

Carotenoids (carotenes):

Birth	70 µg./dl.
<1 year	70–340 µg./dl.
>3 years	100–150 µg./dl.

Ceruloplasmin: 20–40 mg./dl. (280–570 U)

Chloride: 94–106 mEq./L.

Cholesterol (total):

Full-term	50–120 mg./dl.
1–2 years	70–190 mg./dl.
2–16 years	135–250 mg./dl.
Adults	130–270 mg./dl.

Copper:

0–6 months	70 µg./dl.
6 months–5 years	27–153 µg./dl.
5–17 years	94–234 µg./dl.
Adults	70–155 µg./dl.

Creatine kinase (creatine phosphokinase):

Newborns	30–100 U/L.
Children	15–50 U/L.
Adults	5–10 U/L.

Creatinine (serum):

1–18 months	0.2–0.5 mg./dl.
2–12 years	0.3–0.8 mg./dl.
13–20 years	0.5–1.2 mg./dl.
Adults	0.8–1.5 mg./dl.

Ferritin:

Children	10–150 ng./ml.
Females (adult)	10–60 ng./ml.
Males (adult)	30–100 ng./ml.

(continued)

Blood Chemistries (continued)

Fibrinogen:	200–400 mg./dl.
Folic acid (folate):	5–21 ng./L. (microbiological assay)
Gastrin:	<300 pg./ml.

Glucose (serum):

Children	60–110 mg./L.
Premature	>30 mg./dl.
Full-term	>40 mg./dl.

Haptoglobin:

Newborn	Detectable in only 10%–20%
>1 year	400–1,800 mg. of Hb bound/L.

Iron (iron-binding capacity):

	Iron (μg./dl.)	Iron-Binding Capacity (μg./dl.)	Approximate Percent Saturation (μg./dl.)
Newborn	110–270	59–175	65%
4–10 months	30–70	250–400	25%
3–10 years	53–119	250–400	30%
Adults	87–279	250–400	35%

Ketones:

Qualitative:	negative
Quantitative:	up to 3 mg./dl.

Lactate:

Venous	0.5–1.6 mEq./L.
Arterial	0.3–1.0 mEq./L.

Lactate dehydrogenase:

Birth	290–501 U/L.
1 day–1 month	185–404 U/L.
1 month–2 years	110–244 U/L.
<4 years	60–170 U/L.
3–17 years	85–165 U/L.
Adults	30–90 U/L.

Lactate dehydrogenase isoenzymes (% total):

LD_1 heart	24%–34%
LD_2 heart, erythrocytes	35%–45%
LD_3 muscle	15%–25%
LD_4 liver, trace muscle	4%–10%
LD_5 liver, muscle	1%–9%

Lead:	<40 μg./dl.
Lipids (total):	450–1000 mg./dl.

Lipoproteins:

	Child–Adult	Newborn
Alpha	286–450 mg./dl.	71–176 mg./dl.
Pre-Beta	22–72 mg./dl.	—
Beta	276–438 mg./dl.	51–158 mg./dl.

Magnesium:

Newborns	1.52–2.33 mEq./L. (2.1–2.2 mg./100 ml.)
Children	1.4–1.9 mEq./L.
Adults	1.3–2.5 mEq./L. (1.8–3 mg/100 ml)

Mercury (urine):	<50 μg./24 hours

Metanephrine (urine):

Children	0.02–0.16 μg./mg. creatinine

Methemoglobin:	<0.3 gm./dl. or <3% of total Hb

Normetanephrine (urine):

Children	0.05–0.6 μg./mg. creatinine

5' Nucleotidase:	<1.6 U/L.
Osmolality:	285–295 mOsm./kg. (270–285 mOsm./L. plasma)
Phenylalanine:	<3 mg./dl.

Phospolipids:

Cord blood	0.48–1.6 gm./L.
2–13 years	1.66–2.47 gm./L.
3–20 years	1.93–3.38 gm./L.

Phosphorus (inorganic):

Newborn	4.0–10.5 mg./dl.
1 year	4.0–6.8 mg./dl.
5 years	3.6–6.5 mg./dl.
Adult	3.0–4.5 mg./dl.

Porcelain:	8–20 mEq./L.
Porphyrins:	<7.0 μg./dl.

Potassium:

<10 days of age	3.5–7.0 mEq./L.
>10 days of age	3.5–5.5 mEq./L.

Proteins: Average (range) in gm./dl.

Age	Total	Albumin	Globulin	Gamma Globulin
Premature	5.5 (4.0–7.0)	3.7 (2.5–4.5)	1.8 (1.2–2.0)	0.7 (0.5–0.9)
FT newborn	6.4 (5.0–7.1)	3.4 (2.5–5.0)	3.1 (1.2–4.0)	0.8 (0.7–0.9)
1–3 months	6.6 (4.7–7.4)	3.8 (3.0–4.2)	2.5 (1.0–3.3)	0.3 (0.1–0.5)
3–12 months	6.8 (5.0–7.5)	3.9 (2.7–5.0)	2.6 (2.0–3.8)	0.6 (0.4–1.2)
1–15 years	7.4 (6.5–8.6)	4.0 (3.2–5.0)	3.1 (2.0–4.0)	0.9 (0.6–1.2)

Pyruvate:	0.05–0.14 mEq./L.

Serotonin:

Children	127–187 ng./dl.
Adults	119–171 ng./dl.

Sodium:

Prematures	130–140 mEq./L.
Older	135–145 mEq./L.

Transaminase (SGOT):

1–3 days	16–74 U/L.
<6 months	20–43 U/L.
6 months–1 year	16–35 U/L.
1 year–5 years	6–30 U/L.
5 years–adults	19–28 U/L.
Adults	Male: 8–16 U/L. Female: 7–34 U/L.

Transaminase (SGPT):

Infants	<54 U/L.
Children	1–30 U/L.
Adults	0–19 U/L.

Triglycerides:	29–154 mg./dl.
Urea nitrogen:	6–23 mg./dl.
Uric acid:	2.5–8.0 mg./dl.

Blood Chemistries (continued)

Vitamin A retinol:

<6 months	20–90 µg./dl.
1–5 years	30–100 µg./dl.
5–16 years	60–100 µg./dl.
Adults	20–80 µg./dl.

Vitamin B$_{12}$: 330–1025 µg./dl.

Vitamin C: 0.4–1.5 mg./dl.

Vitamin E:

Newborns	>0.3 µg./dl.
Children–Adults	0.5–1.2 µg./dl.

Zinc:

0–1 year	Range: 74–146 µg./dl.
2–10 years	72–128 µg./dl.
11–18 years	65–125 µg./dl.
Adults	60–120 µg./dl.

* (Reproduced with permission from Johns Hopkins Hospital: The Harriet Lane Handbook, 9th edition, Jeffrey A. Biller and Andrew M. Yeager (eds). Copyright © 1981 by Year Book Medical Publishers, Inc., Chicago)

Term Infants—Normal Blood Chemistry Values

Determination	Sample Source	Cord	1–12 hr.	12–24 hr.	24–48 hr.	48–72 hr.
Sodium, mmol./L.*	Capillary	147 (126–166)	143 (124–156)	145 (132–159)	148 (134–160)	149 (139–162)
Potassium, mmol./L.		7.8 (5.6–12)	6.4 (5.3–7.3)	6.3 (5.3–8.9)	6.0 (5.2–7.3)	59 (5.0–7.7)
Chloride, mmol./L.		103 (98–110)	100.7 (90–111)	103 (87–114)	102 (92–114)	103 (93–112)
Calcium, mg./dl.		9.3 (8.2–11.1)	8.4 (7.3–9.2)	7.8 (6.9–9.4)	8.0 (6.1–9.9)	7.9 (5.9–9.7)
Phosphorus, mg./dl.		5.6 (3.7–8.1)	6.1 (3.5–8.6)	5.7 (2.9–8.1)	5.9 (3.0–8.7)	5.8 (2.8–7.6)
Blood urea, mg./dl.		29 (21–40)	27 (8–34)	33 (9–63)	32 (13–77)	31 (13–68)
Total protein, gm./dl.		6.1 (4.8–7.3)	6.6 (5.6–8.5)	6.6 (5.8–8.2)	6.9 (5.9–8.2)	7.2 (6.0–8.5)
Glucose, mg./dl.		73 (45–96)	63 (40–97)	63 (42–104)	56 (30–91)	59 (40–90)
Lactic acid, mg./dl.		19.5 (11–30)	14.6 (11–24)	14.0 (10–23)	14.3 (9–22)	13.5 (7–21)
Lactate, mmol./L.†		2.0–3.0	2.0			

(From Avery GB. Neonatology. Philadelphia, JB Lippincott, 1981. Original data from: *Acharya PT and Payne WW. Arch Dis Child 40:430, 1965; †Daniel SS, Adamsons K Jr and James LS. Pediatrics 37:942, 1966)

Low Birth Weight Infants—Normal Blood Chemistry Values
(Capillary Blood, First Day)

Determination	<1,000	1,001–1,500	1,501–2,000	2,001–2,500
Sodium, mmol./L.	138	133	135	134
Potassium, mrnol./L.	6.4	6.0	5.4	5.6
Chloride, mmol./L.	100	101	105	104
Total CO$_2$, mmol./L.	19	20	20	20
Urea, mg./dl.	22	21	16	16
Total protein, gm./dl.	4.8	4.8	5.2	5.3

(From Avery GB. Neonatology. Philadelphia, JB Lippincott, 1981. Original data from Pincus JB et al. Pediatrics 18:39, 1956)

Acid–Base Status

Determination	Vaginal Delivery	Birth	1st Hr.	3rd Hr.	24 Hr.	2 Days	3 Days
Vigorous Term Infants							
pH	Umbilical artery	7.26					
	Umbilical vein	7.29					
pCO_2 torr	Arterial	54.5	38.8	38.3	33.6	34	35
	Venous	42.8					
O_2 sat.	Arterial	19.8	93.8	94.7			
	Venous	47.6			93.2		
pH	Left atrial		7.30	7.34	7.41	7.39 (temp. artery)	7.38 (temp. artery)
CO_2 content, mmol./L.			20.6	21.9	21.4		
Premature Infants							
	Capillary						
pH	<1,250 g				7.36	7.35	7.35
pCO_2 torr					38	44	37
pH	>1,250 g				7.39	7.39	7.38
pCO_2 torr					38	39	38

(From Avery GB. Neonatology. Philadelphia, JB Lippincott, 1981. Data of Weisbort LM et al. J Pediatr 52:395, 1958; and Bucci E et al. Biol Neonate, 8:81, 1965)

Normal Values—Hematology

Age	Hgb (gm. %)	Hct (%)	MCV (fl.)	MCHC (gm./dl. RBC)	Retic (%)	WBC per mm^3 × 100 range (avg.)	% Neutrophils
28 week's gestation	14.5	45	120	31	—	—	
32 week's gestation	15.0	47	118	32	—	—	
Full-term							
1 day +	16.8–21.2	57–68	110–128	29.7–33.5	1.8–4.6	7–35 (18)	45–85
1 week +	15.0–19.6	46–62	107–129	30.4–33.6	0.1–0.9	4–20 (10)	30–50
1 month +	11.1–14.3	31–41	93–109	33.3–36.5	0.1–1.7	6–18 (10)	30–50
3–5 months	10.4–12.2	33	80–96	31.8–36.2	0.4–1.0	6–17 (10)	30–50
6–11 months	11.8	35	77	33	0.7–2.3	6–16 (10)	30–50
1 year	11.2	35	78	32	0.6–1.7	6–15 (10)	30–50
2–10 years	12.8	37	80	34	0.5–1.0	7–13 (9)	35–60
11–15 years	13.4	39	82	34	0.5–1.0	5–12 (8.5)	40–60
Adults							
Males	16.0 ± 2.0	47 ± 7			0.8–2.5		
			91 (82–101)	34 (31.5–36)		4.3–10 (7)	25–62
Females	14.0 ± 2.0	42 ± 5			0.3–4.1		

+Under 1 month of age, capillary Hgb exceeds venous: 1 hour—3.6-gm. difference
5 days—2.2-gm. difference
3 weeks—1.1-gm difference

Absolute eosinophil count: avg. 250/mm^3 (100–600/mm^3)

(*Ref.:* Am J Dis Child 93: 486, 1957; Acta Paed [Stockholm] 60:317, 1971; Wintrobe. Clinical Hematology, 7th ed. Philadelphia, Lea & Febiger, 1974; Mauer. Pediatric Hematology, New York, McGraw-Hill, 1969; Oski and Naiman. Hematologic Problems in the Newborn Infant, Philadelphia, WB Saunders, 1972)

(Reproduced with permission from Johns Hopkins Hospital: The Harriet Lane Handbook, 9th edition. Jeffrey A. Biller and Andrew M. Yeager (eds). Copyright © 1981 by Year Book Medical Publishers, Inc, Chicago)

Urinalysis—Ranges from Newborn/Infant to Adult

Determination		Age/Sex	Normal Range		
Addis count	Leukocytes		<10		
	Erythrocytes		< 5		
	Casts		occasional hyaline		
Colony count, colonies/ml. urine (fresh specimen)			*Clean Catch, Midstream**	*Catheterization*	*Suprapubic Bladder Puncture*
		Infant/Child	< 1,000	100	0
		Thereafter	<10,000	100	0
Microscopic	Leukocytes		0–4 per high-power field		
	Erythrocytes		rare per high-power field		
	Casts		rare per high-power field		
Osmolarity		Premature/Newborn	50–600 mOsm./L.		
		Thereafter	50–1400		
		Thereafter	>850 (after fluid restriction)		
pH		Newborn/Neonate	5.0–7.0		
		Thereafter	4.8–7.8		
Protein	qualitative		Negative		
	quantitative		10–100 mg/d (higher after strenuous exercise)		
Specific gravity, random		Newborn/Infant	1.001–1.020		
		Thereafter	1.001–1.030		
		Thereafter	>1.025 (after fluid restriction)		
Sugar, qualitative (including glucose)			Negative		
Volume		Newborn/Neonate	50–300 ml./d.		
		Infant	350–550		
		Child	500–1000		
		Adolescent	700–1400		
		Thereafter: M	800–2000		
		F	800–1600		

* Pure cultures with colony counts >100,000 are considered diagnostic in adults, whereas colony counts of >10,000 are usually considered diagnostic in children. Intermediate counts must be interpreted relative to the clinical situation. For females, the physician must be aware of the cleanliness and care used in collecting the specimen. Urine obtained by means of a plastic collection device or by voiding into a container without prior preparation of the patient is usually contaminated, and has limited usefulness in evaluating the possibility of urinary tract infections.

(From Vaughan, V.C., McKay, R.J., and Behrman, R.E.: Nelson's Textbook of Pediatrics. Philadelphia, W.B. Saunders, 1979.)

Normal Serologic Reference Values

Anti-streptolysin O titer	
Preschool	<1:85
School ages and adults	<1:170
Older adults	<1:85
Anti-hyaluronidase	<1:256
Anti-nuclear antibody	<1:40
C-reactive protein	Negative
C_3'	70–176 mg./dl.
C_4'	16–45 mg./dl.
Chorioembryonic antigen (CEA)	<2.5 nanograms/ml.
Febrile agglutinins	<1:80 or <fourfold rise in titer
Mononucleosis screen	Negative
Proteus OX-19 agglutinins	<1:80 or <fourfold rise in titer
Rheumatoid latex titer	1:80–1:160—doubtful
	1:40—negative
Rheumatoid screen	Negative
Tularemia agglutinins	<1:80 or <fourfold rise in titer
W. rose titer	1:10 Negative
	1:20–1:40—doubtful
	>1:80 Positive

Complement fixation tests should be negative or <1:8
  Brucellosis
  Cytomegalic inclusion disease
  Eastern and Western equine encephalitis
  Epidemic typhus
  Influenza type A (F.M.I. and P.R. 8)
  Influenza type B (Lee)
  Lymphocytic choriomeningitis
  Lymphogranuloma venereum
  Mumps
  Psittacosis
  Q fever (American)
  Rickettsial pox
  Rocky Mountain spotted fever
  St. Louis encephalitis
  Toxoplasmosis
  Tularemia

(Reproduced with permission from Johns Hopkins Hospital: The Harriet Lane Handbook, 8th edition, Kenneth C. Schulberth and Basil J. Zitelli (editors). Copyright © 1978 by Year Book Medical Publishers, Inc., Chicago.)

Cerebrospinal Fluid

Cell Count

Preterm mean: 9.0	(0–25.4 WBC/mm.^{3})
Term mean: 8.2	(0–22.4 WBC/mm.^{3})
>1 month	0–7

% PMNs

57%
61%
0

Glucose

Preterm	24–63 mg./dl.	(mean: 50)
Term	34–119 mg./dl.	(mean: 52)
Children	40–80 mg./dl.	

CSF Glucose/Blood Glucose (%)

Preterm	55–105
Term	44–128
Children	~50%

Lactic Acid Dehydrogenase

Mean: 20 U/ml. (range: 5–30 U/ml.)

Pandy

Negative, may be + in newborn

Pressure: Initial L.P.

Newborn	80–110 < 110 mm. H$_2$O
Infant/Child	<200 Lateral recumbent positions
Respiratory movements	5–10 mm./H$_2$O

Protein

Preterm	(mean 115)	65–150 mg./dl.
Term	(mean 90)	20–170 mg./dl.
Children	Ventricular	5–15 mg./dl.
	Cisternal	5–25 mg./dl.
	Lumbar	5–40 mg./dl.

(*Ref.:* Sarff LD et al. J. Pediatr 88:473–477, 1976)

(Reproduced with permission from Johns Hopkins Hospital: The Harriet Lane Handbook 9th edition, Jeffrey A. Biller and Andrew M. Yeager (eds). Copyright © 1981 by Year Book Medical Publishers, Inc, Chicago)

Conversion of Pounds and Ounces to Grams

POUNDS	OUNCES															
	0	1	2	3	4	5	6	7	8	9	10	11	12	13	14	15
0	—	28	57	85	113	142	170	198	227	255	283	312	340	369	397	425
1	454	482	510	539	567	595	624	652	680	709	737	765	794	822	850	879
2	907	936	964	992	1021	1049	1077	1106	1134	1162	1191	1219	1247	1276	1304	1332
3	1361	1389	1417	1446	1474	1503	1531	1559	1588	1616	1644	1673	1701	1729	1758	1786
4	1814	1843	1871	1899	1928	1956	1984	2013	2041	2070	2098	2126	2155	2183	2211	2240
5	2268	2296	2325	2353	2381	2410	2438	2466	2495	2523	2551	2580	2608	2637	2665	2693
6	2722	2750	2778	2807	2835	2863	2892	2920	2948	2977	3005	3033	3062	3090	3118	3147
7	3175	3203	3232	3260	3289	3317	3345	3374	3402	3430	3459	3487	3515	3544	3572	3600
8	3629	3657	3685	3714	3742	3770	3799	3827	3856	3884	3912	3941	3969	3997	4026	4054
9	4082	4111	4139	4167	4196	4224	4252	4281	4309	4337	4366	4394	4423	4451	4479	4508
10	4536	4564	4593	4621	4649	4678	4706	4734	4763	4791	4819	4848	4876	4904	4933	4961
11	4990	5018	5046	5075	5103	5131	5160	5188	5216	5245	5273	5301	5330	5358	5386	5415
12	5443	5471	5500	5528	5557	5585	5613	5642	5670	5698	5727	5755	5783	5812	5840	5868
13	5897	5925	5953	5982	6010	6038	6067	6095	6123	6152	6180	6209	6237	6265	6294	6322
14	6350	6379	6407	6435	6464	6492	6520	6549	6577	6605	6634	6662	6690	6719	6747	6776
15	6804	6832	6860	6889	6917	6945	6973	7002	7030	7059	7087	7115	7144	7172	7201	7228
16	7257	7286	7313	7342	7371	7399	7427	7456	7484	7512	7541	7569	7597	7626	7654	7682
17	7711	7739	7768	7796	7824	7853	7881	7909	7938	7966	7994	8023	8051	8079	8108	8136
18	8165	8192	8221	8249	8278	8306	8335	8363	8391	8420	8448	8476	8504	8533	8561	8590
19	8618	8646	8675	8703	8731	8760	8788	8816	8845	8873	8902	8930	8958	8987	9015	9043
20	9072	9100	9128	9157	9185	9213	9242	9270	9298	9327	9355	9383	9412	9440	9469	9497
21	9525	9554	9582	9610	9639	9667	9695	9724	9752	9780	9809	9837	9865	9894	9922	9950
22	9979	10007	10036	10064	10092	10120	10149	10177	10206	10234	10262	10291	10319	10347	10376	10404

(From Avery GB. Neonatology, 2nd ed. Philadelphia, JB Lippincott, 1981)

Index

The letter *f* after a page number indicates a figure; *t* following a page number indicates tabular material.

Joyce E Anderson

ISBN 0-397-54499-5

90000

9 780397 544998